Nursing 2021

DRUG

HANDBOOK®

D0004220

Photoguide to tablets and capsules

This photoguide includes 450 tablets and capsules, representing the most commonly prescribed generic and trade name drugs. These drugs, organized alphabetically by generic name, are shown in actual size and color with cross-references to drug information. Each product is labeled with its trade name and its strength.

ALENDRONATE SODIUM

Fosamax
(Page 93)

70 mg

ALFUZOSIN HYDROCHLORIDE

Uroxatral
(Page 1799)

10 mg

ALPRAZOLAM

Xanax
(Page 102)

0.25 mg

0.5 mg

1 mg

2 mg

AMLODIPINE BESYLATE

Norvasc
(Page 119)

2.5 mg

5 mg

ANASTROZOLE

Arimidex
(Page 134)

1 mg

APIXABAN

Eliquis
(Page 138)

2.5 mg

5 mg

ARIPIPRAZOLE

Abilify
(Page 146)

10 mg

15 mg

30 mg

ATAZANAVIR SULFATE

Reyataz
(Page 159)

200 mg

ATENOLOL

Tenormin
(Page 164)

25 mg   50 mg   100 mg

ATOMOXETINE HYDROCHLORIDE

Strattera
(Page 170)

10 mg   18 mg   25 mg

40 mg   60 mg

ATORVASTATIN CALCIUM

Lipitor
(Page 171)

10 mg   20 mg   40 mg

80 mg

AZITHROMYCIN

Zithromax
(Page 188)

250 mg   500 mg   600 mg

BENAZEPRIL HYDROCHLORIDE

Lotensin
(Page 203)

20 mg   40 mg

BUMETANIDE

Bumex
(Page 245)

0.5 mg   1 mg   2 mg

BUPROPION HYDROCHLORIDE

Wellbutrin SR
(Page 254)

100 mg   150 mg   200 mg

Zyban
(Page 254)

150 mg

CANDESARTAN CILEXETIL

Atacand
(Page 272)

4 mg   8 mg   16 mg

32 mg

CARISOPRODOL

Soma
(Page 289)

350 mg

CELECOXIB

CeleBREX
(Page 323)

100 mg   200 mg

CEPHALEXIN

Keflex
(Page 325)

250 mg   500 mg   750 mg

CIPROFLOXACIN

Cipro
(Page 345)

250 mg   500 mg   750 mg

CITALOPRAM HYDROBROMIDE

CeleXA
(Page 354)

20 mg   40 mg

CLONAZEPAM

KlonoPIN
(Page 368)

0.5 mg   1 mg   2 mg

CLOPIDOGREL BISULFATE

Plavix
(Page 373)

75 mg

CLOZAPINE

Clozaril
(Page 376)

25 mg   100 mg

CODEINE PHOSPHATE—ACETAMINOPHEN

Tylenol with Codeine #3
(Page 380)

30 mg/300 mg

COLCHICINE

Colcrys
(Page 388)

0.6 mg

COLESEVELAM HYDROCHLORIDE

Welchol
(Page 390)

625 mg

DABIGATRAN ETEXILATE MESYLATE

Pradaxa
(Page 404)

75 mg   150 mg

DARIFENACIN HYDROBROMIDE

Enablex
(Page 423)

7.5 mg   15 mg

DESLORATADINE

Clarinex
(Page 436)

5 mg

DESVENLAFAXINE SUCCINATE

Pristiq
(Page 442)

50 mg   100 mg

DEXLANSOPRAZOLE

Dexilant
(Page 448)

30 mg   60 mg

DEXMETHYLPHENIDATE HYDROCHLORIDE

Focalin XR
(Page 450)

5mg   10 mg   15 mg

20 mg   30 mg   40 mg

DIAZEPAM

Valium
(Page 457)

2 mg   5 mg   10 mg

DILTIAZEM HYDROCHLORIDE

Cardizem
(Page 474)

30 mg   90 mg

Cardizem CD
(Page 474)

120 mg   180 mg   240 mg

300 mg   360 mg

DILTIAZEM HYDROCHLORIDE

Cardizem LA
(Page 474)

180 mg

240 mg

360 mg

DIVALPROEX SODIUM

Depakote
(Page 1609)

125 mg

250 mg

500 mg

Depakote Sprinkle
(Page 1609)

125 mg

DONEPEZIL HYDROCHLORIDE

Aricept
(Page 489)

5 mg

10 mg

DOXAZOSIN MESYLATE

Cardura
(Page 492)

1 mg

2 mg

4 mg

8 mg

DULOXETINE HYDROCHLORIDE

Cymbalta
(Page 518)

20 mg

30 mg

60 mg

DUTASTERIDE

Avodart
(Page 521)

0.5 mg

ELETRIPTAN HYDROBROMIDE

Relpax
(Page 532)

20 mg   40 mg

ENALAPRIL MALEATE

Vasotec
(Page 551)

2.5 mg   5 mg   10 mg

20 mg

ERYTHROMYCIN BASE

Eryc
(Page 589)

250 mg

Ery-Tab
(Page 589)

333 mg

ESCITALOPRAM OXALATE

Lexapro
(Page 592)

10 mg   20 mg

ESOMEPRAZOLE MAGNESIUM

Nexium
(Page 599)

20 mg   40 mg

ESTROGENS (CONJUGATED)

Premarin
(Page 616)

0.3 mg   0.45 mg   0.625 mg

0.9 mg   1.25 mg

ESZOPICLONE

Lunesta
(Page 622)

1 mg   2 mg   3 mg

EZETIMIBE

Zetia
(Page 649)

10 mg

EZETIMIBE—SIMVASTATIN

Vytorin
(Page 1748)

10 mg/10 mg   10 mg/20 mg   10 mg/40 mg

10 mg/80 mg

FAMOTIDINE

Pepcid
(Page 652)

20 mg

40 mg

FENOFIBRATE

TriCor
(Page 656)

48 mg

145 mg

FINASTERIDE

Proscar
(Page 671)

5 mg

FLUCONAZOLE

Diflucan
(Page 677)

50 mg

100 mg

150 mg

200 mg

FLUOXETINE HYDROCHLORIDE

Prozac
(Page 691)

10 mg

20 mg

40 mg

FROVATRIPTAN SUCCINATE

Frova
(Page 723)

2.5 mg

FUROSEMIDE

Lasix
(Page 726)

20 mg   40 mg   80 mg

GABAPENTIN

Neurontin
(Page 728)

100 mg   300 mg   400 mg

GEMFIBROZIL

Lopid
(Page 738)

600 mg

GLIMEPIRIDE

Amaryl
(Page 747)

1 mg   2 mg   4 mg

GLIPIZIDE

Glucotrol
(Page 749)

5 mg   10 mg

Glucotrol XL
(Page 749)

2.5 mg   5 mg   10 mg

IBANDRONATE SODIUM

Boniva
(Page 793)

150 mg

INDINAVIR SULFATE

Crixivan
(Page 824)

200 mg   400 mg

IRBESARTAN

Avapro
(Page 872)

75 mg   150 mg   300 mg

LAMIVUDINE—ZIDOVUDINE

Combivir
(Page 1748)

150 mg/300 mg

LANSOPRAZOLE

Prevacid
(Page 916)

15 mg   30 mg

LEVODOPA—CARBIDOPA

Sinemet
(Page 936)

100 mg/10 mg   250 mg/25 mg

Sinemet CR
(Page 936)

100 mg/25 mg

LEVODOPA—CARBIDOPA—ENTACAPONE

Stalevo
(Page 939)

50 mg/12.5 mg/   100 mg/25 mg/   150 mg/37.5 mg/
200 mg   200 mg   200 mg

LEVOFLOXACIN

Levaquin
(Page 941)

250 mg   500 mg

LEVOTHYROXINE SODIUM

Levoxyl
(Page 947)

 25 mcg

 50 mcg

 75 mcg

 88 mcg

 100 mcg

 112 mcg

 125 mcg

 137 mcg

 150 mcg

 175 mcg

 200 mcg

Synthroid
(Page 947)

 25 mcg

  50 mcg

 75 mcg

 88 mcg

   100 mcg

  112 mcg

  125 mcg

 150 mcg

 175 mcg

 200 mcg

 300 mcg

LISDEXAMFETAMINE DIMESYLATE

Vyvanse
(Page 959)

 20 mg

 30 mg

 40 mg

 50 mg

 60 mg

 70 mg

LISINOPRIL

Prinivil
(Page 961)

 5 mg

 10 mg

 20 mg

 40 mg

Zestril
(Page 961)

 2.5 mg

5 mg

10 mg

 20 mg

 40 mg

LOPINAVIR—RITONAVIR

Kaletra
(Page 975)

 200 mg/50 mg

LORAZEPAM

Ativan
(Page 980)

 0.5 mg

 1 mg

 2 mg

LOSARTAN POTASSIUM

Cozaar
(Page 984)

25 mg   50 mg

LUBIPROSTONE

Amitiza
(Page 1770)

24 mcg

LURASIDONE HYDROCHLORIDE

Latuda
(Page 988)

20 mg   40 mg   80 mg

MEDROXYPROGESTERONE ACETATE

Provera
(Page 996)

2.5 mg   5 mg   10 mg

MEMANTINE HYDROCHLORIDE

Namenda
(Page 1005)

5 mg   10 mg

MEPERIDINE HYDROCHLORIDE

Demerol
(Page 1007)

50 mg   100 mg

METFORMIN HYDROCHLORIDE

Glucophage
(Page 1017)

500 mg   850 mg   1,000 mg

Glucophage XR
(Page 1017)

500 mg

METHADONE HYDROCHLORIDE
(Page 1020)

5 mg

10 mg

METHYLPHENIDATE HYDROCHLORIDE
Concerta
(Page 1034)

18 mg

36 mg

54 mg

Ritalin
(Page 1034)

5 mg

10 mg

20 mg

Ritalin-SR
(Page 1034)

20 mg

METHYLPREDNISOLONE
Medrol
(Page 1038)

4 mg

16 mg

METOPROLOL SUCCINATE
Toprol-XL
(Page 1047)

50 mg

100 mg

200 mg

METOPROLOL TARTRATE
Lopressor
(Page 1047)

50 mg

100 mg

MILNACIPRAN HYDROCHLORIDE
Savella
(Page 1061)

12.5 mg

25 mg

50 mg

MODAFINIL

Provigil
(Page 1077)

100 mg   200 mg

MONTELUKAST SODIUM

Singulair
(Page 1082)

4 mg   5 mg   10 mg

MOXIFLOXACIN HYDROCHLORIDE

Avelox
(Page 1093)

400 mg

NAPROXEN

Naprosyn
(Page 1113)

500 mg

NEBIVOLOL HYDROCHLORIDE

Bystolic
(Page 1121)

2.5 mg   5 mg   10 mg

20 mg

NIFEDIPINE

Procardia XL
(Page 1140)

30 mg   60 mg   90 mg

NITROFURANTOIN MACROCRYSTALS

Macrodantin
(Page 1144)

25 mg 50 mg 100 mg

NITROGLYCERIN

Nitrostat
(Page 1146)

0.4 mg

NORTRIPTYLINE HYDROCHLORIDE

Pamelor
(Page 1160)

10 mg 25 mg 50 mg

75 mg

OLANZAPINE

Zyprexa
(Page 1176)

2.5 mg 5 mg 7.5 mg

10 mg 15 mg 20 mg

OLMESARTAN MEDOXOMIL

Benicar
(Page 1180)

20 mg 40 mg

OLMESARTAN MEDOXOMIL—HYDROCHLOROTHIAZIDE

Benicar HCT
(Page 1745)

20 mg/12.5 mg   40 mg/12.5 mg   40 mg/25 mg

OMEGA-3–FATTY ACIDS

Lovaza
(Page 1190)

1 g

OSELTAMIVIR PHOSPHATE

Tamiflu
(Page 1203)

30 mg   45 mg   75 mg

OXYCODONE HYDROCHLORIDE

OxyCONTIN
(Page 1219)

10 mg   20 mg   40 mg

80 mg

PANTOPRAZOLE SODIUM

Protonix
(Page 1250)

20 mg   40 mg

PIOGLITAZONE HYDROCHLORIDE

Actos
(Page 1301)

15 mg   30 mg   45 mg

PRASUGREL HYDROCHLORIDE

Effient
(Page 1318)

5 mg   10 mg

PRAVASTATIN SODIUM

Pravachol
(Page 1320)

20 mg   40 mg

PREGABALIN

Lyrica
(Page 1330)

25 mg   50 mg   75 mg

100 mg   150 mg   200 mg

225 mg   300 mg

PROPRANOLOL HYDROCHLORIDE

Inderal LA
(Page 1348)

60 mg   80 mg   120 mg

160 mg

QUETIAPINE FUMARATE

Seroquel
(Page 1352)

25 mg

50 mg

100 mg

200 mg

300 mg

400 mg

QUINAPRIL HYDROCHLORIDE

Accupril
(Page 1356)

5 mg

10 mg

20 mg

40 mg

RABEPRAZOLE SODIUM

Aciphex
(Page 1361)

20 mg

RALOXIFENE HYDROCHLORIDE

Evista
(Page 1363)

60 mg

RANITIDINE HYDROCHLORIDE

Zantac
(Page 1375)

150 mg

300 mg

RANOLAZINE

Ranexa
(Page 1377)

500 mg

RASAGILINE MESYLATE

Azilect
(Page 1378)

0.5 mg   1 mg

RISEDRONATE SODIUM

Actonel
(Page 1397)

5 mg   35 mg

RISPERIDONE

Risperdal
(Page 1399)

0.25 mg   0.5 mg   1 mg

2 mg   3 mg   4 mg

RIVAROXABAN

Xarelto
(Page 1410)

15 mg   20 mg

RIVASTIGMINE TARTRATE

(Page 1413)

1.5 mg   3 mg   4.5 mg

6 mg

ROSIGLITAZONE MALEATE

Avandia
(Page 1421)

2 mg   4 mg   8 mg

ROSUVASTATIN CALCIUM

Crestor
(Page 1423)

5 mg   10 mg   20 mg

40 mg

SAXAGLIPTIN

Onglyza
(Page 1441)

2.5 mg   5 mg

SERTRALINE HYDROCHLORIDE

Zoloft
(Page 1449)

50 mg   100 mg

SILDENAFIL CITRATE

Viagra
(Page 1453)

25 mg   50 mg   100 mg

SIMVASTATIN

Zocor
(Page 1457)

5 mg

10 mg

20 mg

40 mg

SITAGLIPTIN PHOSPHATE

Januvia
(Page 1463)

100 mg

SOLIFENACIN SUCCINATE

VESIcare
(Page 1474)

5 mg

10 mg

SPIRONOLACTONE

Aldactone
(Page 1482)

25 mg

50 mg

100 mg

SUCRALFATE

Carafate
(Page 1488)

1 g

SULFAMETHOXAZOLE—TRIMETHOPRIM

Bactrim DS
(Page 1493)

800 mg/160 mg

SUMATRIPTAN SUCCINATE

Imitrex
(Page 1497)

25 mg   50 mg

SUNITINIB MALATE

Sutent
(Page 1500)

12.5 mg   25 mg   50 mg

TADALAFIL

Cialis
(Page 1506)

2.5 mg   5 mg   10 mg

20 mg

TAMSULOSIN HYDROCHLORIDE

Flomax
(Page 1510)

0.4 mg

TAPENTADOL HYDROCHLORIDE

Nucynta
(Page 1844)

50 mg   100 mg

Nucynta ER
(Page 1844)

100 mg

TELMISARTAN

Micardis
(Page 1514)

20 mg

40 mg   80 mg

TEMAZEPAM

Restoril
(Page 1516)

7.5 mg   15 mg   30 mg

TENOFOVIR DISOPROXIL FUMARATE

Viread
(Page 1519)

300 mg

TOLTERODINE TARTRATE

Detrol
(Page 1567)

1 mg   2 mg

TOPIRAMATE

Topamax
(Page 1571)

15 mg   25 mg   25 mg

50 mg   100 mg   200 mg

TORSEMIDE

Demadex
(Page 1578)

5 mg   10 mg   20 mg

100 mg

TRAMADOL HYDROCHLORIDE—ACETAMINOPHEN

Ultracet
(Page 1738)

37.5 mg/325 mg

VALACYCLOVIR HYDROCHLORIDE

Valtrex
(Page 1607)

500 mg   1,000 mg

VALSARTAN

Diovan
(Page 1613)

40 mg   80 mg   160 mg

320 mg

VALSARTAN—HYDROCHLOROTHIAZIDE

Diovan HCT
(Page 1746)

80 mg/12.5 mg   160 mg/12.5 mg   160 mg/25 mg

320 mg/12.5 mg   320 mg/25 mg

VARDENAFIL HYDROCHLORIDE

Levitra
(Page 1616)

5 mg	10 mg	20 mg

VARENICLINE TARTRATE

Chantix
(Page 1618)

0.5 mg	1 mg

VENLAFAXINE HYDROCHLORIDE

Effexor XR
(Page 1624)

75 mg	150 mg

VERAPAMIL HYDROCHLORIDE

Calan
(Page 1627)

80 mg	120 mg

Verelan
(Page 1627)

120 mg	180 mg	240 mg

VILAZODONE HYDROCHLORIDE

Viibryd
(Page 1632)

10 mg	20 mg	40 mg

WARFARIN SODIUM

Coumadin
(Page 1650)

1 mg

2 mg

2.5 mg

3 mg

4 mg

5 mg

6 mg

7.5 mg

10 mg

ZAFIRLUKAST

Accolate
(Page 1652)

10 mg

20 mg

ZIDOVUDINE

Retrovir
(Page 1656)

100 mg

ZIPRASIDONE HYDROCHLORIDE

Geodon
(Page 1658)

20 mg

40 mg

60 mg

80 mg

ZOLPIDEM TARTRATE

Ambien
(Page 1664)

5 mg

10 mg

Contents

Contributors and consultants

Janine Barnaby, BS Pharm, RPh, BCOP
Manager, Outpatient Hospital Pharmacy
Lehigh Valley Hospital
Allentown, PA

David Bruch, BS, PharmD
Associate Lecturer
University of Wyoming School of
  Pharmacy
Laramie

Lawrence Carey, PharmD, RPh, BS
Clinical Professor of Pharmacy Practice
Director of Experiential Education
Associate Chair Pharmacy Practice
Temple University School of Pharmacy
Philadelphia, PA

Jason Cooper, PharmD
Clinical Pharmacist
Medical University of South Carolina
Charleston

Lana Gettman, PharmD
Associate Professor, Department of
  Pharmacy Practice
Harding University College of Pharmacy
Searcy, AR

Toshal S. Hallowell, PharmD
Pharmacist
Edward M. Kennedy Community Health
  Center
Worcester, MA

AnhThu Hoang, PharmD
Instructor, Faculty of Applied Health and
  Community Studies
Sheridan College
Brampton, Ontario, Canada

Rebecca Hoover, PharmD, MBA, BCPS
Assistant Professor
Idaho State University
Pocatello

Lenka Janecka, BSPharm, RPh, CRE
Clinical Consultant
New York, NY

Jill Krabak, PharmD, BSPharm
Pharmacist
Rite Aid
Scranton, PA

Chung-Shien Lee, PharmD, BCPS, BCOP
Assistant Professor
St. John's University
Queens, NY

Hannah Livengood, PharmD
Formulary/Clinical Pharmacist
Health Partners Plans
Philadelphia, PA

Celia Lu, PharmD, BCACP
Assistant Professor
St. John's University
Queens, NY

Kristy H. Lucas, PharmD, FCCP, CTTS
Professor, Pharmacy Practice Department
University of Charleston School of Pharmacy
Charleston, WV

Kimberly E. Ng, PharmD, BCPS
Assistant Professor
St. John's University
Queens, NY

Michele Pisano, PharmD, BCGP, CDE
Associate Professor
St. John's University, College of Pharmacy
  and Health Sciences
Queens, NY

Christine Price, PharmD
Clinical Coordinator, PGY1 Pharmacy
  Residency Director
Morton Plant Hospital
Clearwater, FL

Janet Rader, BSN, RN
Clinical Consultant
New Tripoli, PA

Melissa Rinaldi, PharmD
Clinical Pharmacist
Independence Blue Cross
Philadelphia, PA

Kerry Rinato, PharmD, BCPS
Clinical Pharmacist
Sunrise Hospital
Las Vegas, NV

Maha Saad, PharmD, BCGP, BCPS
Associate Clinical Professor
Co-Director, Drug Information Services
St. John's University, College of Pharmacy
  and Health Sciences
Queens, NY

Michele F. Shepherd, PharmD, MS, BCPS
Clinical Specialist
Abbott Northwestern General Medicine
  Associates
Edina, MN

Michelle Smith, PharmD, BCPS, CPE
Consultant
Havre, MT

How to use *Nursing2021 Drug Handbook*®

The best-selling nursing drug guide for 41 years, *Nursing Drug Handbook* is meticulously reviewed and updated annually by pharmacists and nurses to include the most current, relevant information that practicing nurses and students need to know to administer medications safely in any health care setting. As in previous editions, *Nursing2021 Drug Handbook* emphasizes nursing and safety aspects of drug administration without attempting to replace detailed pharmacology texts. Only the most essential information is included, and helpful graphic symbols, logos, and highlighting draw special attention to critical details that can't be overlooked.

New and outstanding features

The 41st edition provides a wealth of the latest drug information right at your fingertips:
• Tabbed "New Drugs" section—ensures quick access to all 25 complete drug monographs introduced in this edition
• Thoroughly updated text featuring thousands of generic, brand, and combination drugs; 645 comprehensive drug monographs; and 63 generic drugs newly approved by the FDA
• Pregnancy-Lactation-Reproduction header in each monograph—captures all relevant information in one convenient place
• Drug safety always at the forefront—includes a special chapter with updated information on the safe administration of opioid analgesics; in addition, you'll find numerous appendices covering drug safety guidelines, dosage alerts, best practices to avoid medication errors, pediatric drugs commonly involved in drug errors, and elder care medication tips
• Addition of ISMP-recommended Tall Man letters to look-alike drug names
• Appendices on Prescription drug abuse: Identifying and treating toxicity; Understanding biosimilar drugs; and Safe disposal of unused drugs: What patients need to know
• Appendices covering Canadian drugs and safety concerns—Do Not Use list (ISMP Canada), decision tree, and the official Canadian National Drug Schedules
• Easy-to-spot icons and logos—Canadian drugs (maple leaf) and Do Not Crush logo—as well as Black Box Warnings and other special alerts

• Genetic icon throughout to highlight the key genetic considerations used to select and guide drug therapy
• Biosimilar drug banner highlighting FDA-approved biosimilar drug monographs
• Dialyzable drug logo under Contraindications & Cautions—indicates if drug levels can be reduced by hemodialysis and, if so, the percentage reduced
• Photoguide of 450 full-color, actual-sized tablets and capsules.

Introductory chapters

Chapter 1, "Drug actions, interactions, and reactions," explains how drugs work in the body. It provides a general overview of drug properties (absorption, distribution, metabolism, and excretion) and other significant factors affecting drug action (including protein binding, patient's age, underlying disease, dosage form, and route and timing of administration). Also discussed are drug interactions, adverse reactions, and toxic reactions. Chapter 2, "Drug therapy across the lifespan," discusses the danger associated with indiscriminate use of drugs during pregnancy and breastfeeding and the special precautions women should take when medications are necessary. This chapter also covers the unique challenges of giving drugs to children and elderly patients and offers practical suggestions on how to minimize problems with these special populations. Chapter 3, "Safe drug administration," explores the ongoing involvement of governmental and nongovernmental organizations weighing in on drug safety issues and the necessary measures nurses must take to prevent medication errors from occurring.

Chapter 4, "Selected therapeutic drug classifications," summarizes the indications, actions, and contraindications and cautions of more than 60 drug classes represented in *Nursing2021 Drug Handbook*. Generic drugs within each class are also listed, allowing nurses to quickly identify and compare similar drugs when patients can't tolerate or don't respond to a particular drug.

Drug monographs

Each generic drug monograph in *Nursing2021 Drug Handbook* includes the most pertinent clinical information nurses must know to administer medications safely, monitor for potential interactions and adverse effects, implement necessary care measures, and provide appropriate patient teaching. Entries are arranged alphabetically, with the generic drug name prominently displayed—along with its "tall man" lettering (if applicable), pronunciation, corresponding brand (or trade) names, therapeutic class, and pharmacologic class—on a shaded background for quick and easy identification. Banners or symbols to identify drugs that warrant a special safety alert, designate biosimilar drugs, or indicate drugs that appear in the color photoguide are also included in this highlighted area.

Specific information for each drug is then systematically organized under the headings below. Special icons and logos may be used throughout, as warranted, to point out the drug's safety concerns. For example, a clinical alert logo (🕲) provides important advice about life-threatening effects associated with the drug or its administration; a black box warning (**Black Box Warning**) represents a specific warning issued by the FDA. A special icon (📵) indicates oral drug forms that shouldn't be crushed or chewed. (See *Anatomy of a monograph,* on the inside book cover, for a visual guide to the various symbols that may appear within a drug entry.)

Available forms

This section lists the preparations available for each drug (for example, tablets, capsules, solutions for injection) and specifies available dosage forms and strengths. Dosage strengths specifically available in Canada are designated with a maple leaf (🍁). Preparations that may be obtained over the counter, without a prescription, are marked with an open diamond (◊). Liquid formulations that contain alcohol are indicated with an asterisk (*).

Indications & dosages

General dosage information for adults and children is found in this section. Dosage instructions reflect current trends in therapeutics and can't be considered absolute or universal. For individual patients, dosage instructions must be considered in light of the patient's condition.

Indications and dosages that aren't approved by the FDA are followed by a closed diamond (◆). It should be noted that only highly evidence-based off-label uses are included in

this edition. An *Adjust-a-dose* logo appearing within this section indicates the need for a special dosage adjustment for certain patients, such as elderly patients or those with renal or hepatic impairment. In some cases, a dosage adjustment may apply to all patient populations for all of the indications listed; this is marked accordingly.

Administration

Here, readers will find guidelines for safely administering drugs by all applicable routes, including PO, IV, IM, subcut, ophthalmic, inhalational, topical, rectal, vaginal, transdermal, and buccal. A special screened background highlights IV administration guidelines (including specific instructions on how to reconstitute, mix, and store IV medications) and the major potential IV incompatibilities.

Action

This section succinctly describes the mechanism of action—that is, how the drug provides its therapeutic effect. For example, although all antihypertensives lower BP, they don't all do so by the same process. Also included, in table form, are the onset, peak (described in terms of effect or peak blood level), and duration of drug action for each route of administration, if data are available or applicable. Values listed are for patients with normal renal function unless otherwise specified. The drug's half-life is also provided when known.

Adverse reactions

In this section, adverse reactions that are known to occur at a frequency of 1% or greater are listed according to body system. Life-threatening reactions appear in ***bold italic*** type.

Interactions

Within this section, readers can find each drug's confirmed, clinically significant interactions (additive effects, potentiated effects, and antagonistic effects) with other drugs, herbs, foods, beverages, and lifestyle behaviors (such as alcohol use, sun exposure, or smoking). Interactions with a rapid onset are highlighted in color; interactions with a delayed onset are in **bold** type.

Drug interactions are listed under the drug that's adversely affected. For example, because magnesium trisilicate, an antacid ingredient, interacts with tetracycline to decrease tetracycline's absorption, this interaction is listed under tetracycline. To check on the possible effects of using two or more drugs simultaneously, refer to the interaction section for each drug.

Effects on lab test results
This section lists increased and decreased levels, counts, and other values in lab test results that may be caused by the drug's systemic effects. It also indicates false-positive, false-negative, and otherwise altered results of lab tests a drug may cause.

Contraindications & cautions
This section outlines any conditions or special circumstances, such as diseases or conditions, in which use of the drug is undesirable or for which the drug should be given with caution. When applicable, specific signs and symptoms of drug overdose are listed as the last bulleted item under this heading and highlighted by a special logo (**⚠ *Overdose S&S:***) for easy identification.

Pregnancy–lactation–reproduction
This section provides nurses with targeted, easy-to-understand safety information about each drug's use during pregnancy and breastfeeding. It also provides information about fertility effects, contraception recommendations, and enrollment information for registries that monitor drug safety during pregnancy.

Nursing considerations
Within this section, readers can find practical information on patient-monitoring techniques and suggestions for the prevention and treatment of adverse reactions as well as helpful tips on promoting patient comfort.

Patient teaching
Concise guidelines for explaining the drug's purpose, encouraging compliance, ensuring proper use and storage, and preventing or minimizing adverse reactions are included in this section.

Appendices and other helpful aids
Nursing2021 Drug Handbook includes 28 appendices that provide nurses and students with hands-on access to a wealth of supportive data and clinical information.

Appendix 28, "Additional new drugs: Indications and dosages," introduces 38 brand-new FDA-approved drugs that couldn't be included as full monographs in time for publication of this edition.

A handy visual "Quick guide to special symbols, logos, and highlighted terms" and "Guide to abbreviations" immediately follow this "How to use" piece.

Photoguide to tablets and capsules
To enhance patient safety and help make drug identification easier, *Nursing2021 Drug Handbook* offers a 32-page full-color photoguide to the most commonly prescribed tablets and capsules. Shown in actual size, the drugs are arranged alphabetically by generic name for quick reference followed by the brand names and their most common dosage strengths. Below the name of each drug is a cross-reference to where information on the drug can be found in the book. Brand names of drugs that appear in the photoguide are shown in text with a special capsule symbol (**✔**). Page references to the drug photos appear in boldface type in the index (for example, **C12**).

Photos for certain brands were provided by the following companies for use in this book: Novartis Pharmaceuticals (Enablex); Sepracor, Inc. (Lunesta); Teva Pharmaceuticals (Azilect); and Pfizer (Sutent). Additional photos were provided by Jeff Sigler of SFI Medical Publishing.

Online Toolkit
A Toolkit containing a wide array of drug-related materials that practicing nurses and students can use on the job and for study—covering safety issues (such as an equianalgesic dosing chart), pharmacology, drug therapy guidelines, patient populations, and a host of other drug-specialty areas—can be found online at **NDHnow.com**. Included are a dosage calculator, pharmacology animations, English-Spanish translator, audio drug pronunciation guide, 325-question NCLEX®-style test, and access to free and discounted CE tests. Monthly FDA drug updates, drug warnings, and newsworthy drug information can also be accessed through this site.

Quick guide to special symbols, logos, and highlighted terms

The following symbols or highlighted features appear throughout drug monographs and select appendices in this edition.

Special symbols and logos	Usage or meaning
SAFETY ALERT!	Drug that presents a heightened avoidable danger
BIOSIMILAR DRUG	FDA-approved biosimilar drug
buPROPion	"Tall man" lettering for FDA-designated generic drug names prone to mix-ups
➤	Indication for drug
✳ *NEW INDICATION:*	New indication for drug
Adjust-a-dose:	Dosage adjustment needed for certain populations
Adjust-a-dose (for all indications):	Dosage adjustment needed for all indications
▓	Genetic considerations used to select and guide drug therapy
✪ *Alert:*	Clinical alert
✤	Available in Canada
◇	Over-the-counter (OTC)
◆	Off-label use
✎	Appears in Photoguide
*	Liquid contains alcohol
⬤	Drugs that shouldn't be crushed or chewed
Look alike–sound alike:	Drugs with easily confused names
Black Box Warning	FDA black box warning
⚠ *Overdose S&S:*	Overdose signs & symptoms
Highlighted reactions and interactions	
life-threatening	Life-threatening reaction
rapid onset	Causes interaction with rapid onset
delayed onset	Causes interaction with delayed onset

Guide to abbreviations

ACE	angiotensin-converting enzyme	CVAD	central venous access device
ACS	acute coronary syndrome	D_5W	dextrose 5% in water
ADH	antidiuretic hormone	DEHP	di(2-ethylhexyl) phthalate
ADHD	attention deficit hyperactivity disorder	DIC	disseminated intravascular coagulation
ADLs	activities of daily living	dL	deciliter
ADP	adenosine 5′ diphosphate	DMARD	disease-modifying antirheumatic drug
AEDs	antiepileptic drugs	DNA	deoxyribonucleic acid
AIDS	acquired immunodeficiency syndrome	DPP-4	dipeptidyl peptidase-4
ALS	amyotrophic lateral sclerosis	DRESS	drug reaction with eosinophilia and systemic symptoms
ALT	alanine transaminase		
ANA	antinuclear antibody	DVT	deep vein thrombosis
ANC	absolute neutrophil count	ECG	electrocardiogram
aPTT	activated partial thromboplastin time	EEG	electroencephalogram
		EENT	eyes, ears, nose, throat
ARB	angiotensin receptor blocker	eGFR	estimated glomerular filtration rate
ARDS	acute respiratory distress syndrome		
		ESRD	end-stage renal disease
AST	aspartate transaminase	ET	endotracheal
AV	atrioventricular	FDA	Food and Drug Administration
b.i.d.	twice daily		
BMI	body mass index	FSH	follicle-stimulating hormone
BP	blood pressure	5-FU	fluorouracil
BPH	benign prostatic hypertrophy	G	gauge
BSA	body surface area	g	gram
BUN	blood urea nitrogen	G6PD	glucose-6-phosphate dehydrogenase
CABG	coronary artery bypass graft		
CAD	coronary artery disease	GABA	gamma-aminobutyric acid
cAMP	cyclic 3′, 5′ adenosine monophosphate	G-CSF	granulocyte colony-stimulating factor
CBC	complete blood count	GERD	gastroesophageal reflux disease
CDAD	*Clostridium difficile*–associated diarrhea		
		GFR	glomerular filtration rate
CDC	Centers for Disease Control and Prevention	GGT	gamma-glutamyltransferase
		GI	gastrointestinal
CHF	congestive heart failure	gtt	drops
CK	creatine kinase	GU	genitourinary
CMV	cytomegalovirus	GVHD	graft-versus-host disease
CNS	central nervous system	H_1	histamine$_1$
COPD	chronic obstructive pulmonary disease	H_2	histamine$_2$
		Hb	hemoglobin
CrCl	creatinine clearance	HBsAg	hepatitis B virus surface antigen
CSF	cerebrospinal fluid	HBV	hepatitis B virus
CT	computed tomography	HCV	hepatitis C virus
CTCAE	Common Terminology Criteria for Adverse Events	HDL	high-density lipoprotein
		HER2	human epidermal growth factor receptor 2
CV	cardiovascular		

HF	heart failure	NNRTI	non-nucleoside reverse transcriptase inhibitor
HIV	human immunodeficiency virus	NRTI	nucleoside reverse transcriptase inhibitor
HMG-CoA	3-hydroxy-3-methyl-glutaryl coenzyme A	NSAID	nonsteroidal anti-inflammatory drug
HPA	hypothalamic-pituitary-adrenal	NSCLC	non-small-cell lung cancer
HR	heart rate	NSS	normal (0.9%) saline solution
HTN	hypertension	NYHA	New York Heart Association
IBS	irritable bowel syndrome	OCD	obsessive-compulsive disorder
ICP	intracranial pressure	ODT	orally disintegrating tablet
ICU	intensive care unit	OTC	over-the-counter
ID	intradermal	oz	ounce
Ig	immunoglobulin	PABA	para-aminobenzoic acid
ILD	interstitial lung disease	PAH	pulmonary arterial hypertension
IM	intramuscular		
INR	International Normalized Ratio	PCA	patient-controlled analgesia
		PCI	percutaneous coronary intervention
IOP	intraocular pressure	PDE5	phosphodiesterase type 5
IPPB	intermittent positive-pressure breathing	PE	pulmonary embolus
		P-gp	P-glycoprotein
ITP	idiopathic thrombocytopenic purpura	PO	by mouth
		PPI	proton pump inhibitor
IV	intravenous	PR	by rectum
kg	kilogram	p.r.n.	as needed
L	liter	PSA	prostate-specific antigen
lb	pound	PT	prothrombin time
LDH	lactate dehydrogenase	PTCA	percutaneous transluminal coronary angioplasty
LDL	low-density lipoprotein		
LFTs	liver function tests	PTT	partial thromboplastin time
LVEF	left ventricular ejection fraction	PVC	premature ventricular contraction
M	molar	PVD	peripheral vascular disease
m^2	square meter	q.i.d.	four times daily
MAO	monoamine oxidase	RA	rheumatoid arthritis
mcg	microgram	RAAS	renin-angiotensin-aldosterone system
mEq	milliequivalent		
mg	milligram	RBC	red blood cell
MI	myocardial infarction	RDA	recommended daily allowance
min	minute	REM	rapid eye movement
mL	milliliter	REMS	risk evaluation and mitigation strategy
mm^3	cubic millimeter		
mo	month	RNA	ribonucleic acid
MRI	magnetic resonance imaging	RSV	respiratory syncytial virus
MRSA	methicillin-resistant *Staphylococcus aureus*	SA	sinoatrial
		sec	second
MS	multiple sclerosis	SIADH	syndrome of inappropriate antidiuretic hormone
msec	millisecond		
MUGA	multigated acquisition scan	SJS	Stevens-Johnson syndrome
NG	nasogastric	SL	sublingual
NMS	neuroleptic malignant syndrome	SLE	systemic lupus erythematosus

SSNRI	selective serotonin and norepinephrine reuptake inhibitor		TLS	tumor lysis syndrome
			TNF	tumor necrosis factor
			TSH	thyroid-stimulating hormone
SSRI	selective serotonin reuptake inhibitor		tsp	teaspoon
			ULN	upper limit of normal
subcut	subcutaneous		URI	upper respiratory infection
T_3	triiodothyronine		USP	United States Pharmacopeia
T_4	thyroxine		UTI	urinary tract infection
TB	tuberculosis		VLDL	very low density lipoprotein
TCA	tricyclic antidepressant		WBC	white blood cell
TIA	transient ischemic attack		WHO	World Health Organization
t.i.d.	three times daily		wk	week

1

Drug actions, interactions, and reactions

Any drug a patient takes causes a series of physical and chemical events in the body. The first event, when a drug combines with cellular drug receptors, is the *drug action*. What happens next is the *drug effect*. Depending on the type of cellular drug receptors affected by a given drug, an effect can be local, systemic, or both. A systemic drug effect can follow a local effect. For example, when you apply a drug to the skin, it causes a local effect. But transdermal absorption of that drug can also produce a systemic effect. A local effect can also follow systemic absorption. For example, the peptic ulcer drug ranitidine produces a local effect after it's swallowed by blocking histamine receptors in the stomach's parietal cells. Diphenhydramine, on the other hand, causes a systemic effect by blocking histamine receptors throughout the body.

Drug properties

Drug absorption, distribution, metabolism, and excretion make up a drug's pharmacokinetics. These processes determine a drug's onset of action, peak concentration, duration of action, and bioavailability.

Absorption

Before a drug can act in the body, it must be absorbed into the bloodstream—usually after oral administration, the most common route. Before an oral drug can be absorbed, it must disintegrate into particles small enough to dissolve in GI secretions. Only after dissolving can the drug be absorbed. Most absorption of orally given drugs occurs in the small intestine because the mucosal villi provide extensive surface area. Once absorbed and circulated in the bloodstream, the drug is *bioavailable*, or ready to exert its action and produce a drug effect. The speed of absorption and whether absorption is complete or partial depend on the drug's effects, dosage form, administration route, interactions with other substances in the GI tract, and various patient characteristics. Oral solutions and syrups bypass the need for disintegration and dissolution and are usually absorbed faster than solid dosage forms. Some tablets have enteric coatings to prevent disintegration in the acidic environment of the stomach; others have coatings of varying thicknesses that simply delay release of the drug.

Drugs given IM must first be absorbed through the muscle into the bloodstream. Rectal suppositories must dissolve to be absorbed through the rectal mucosa. Drugs given IV are injected directly into the bloodstream and are bioavailable completely and immediately.

Distribution

After absorption, a drug moves from the bloodstream into the fluids and tissues in the body, a movement known as *distribution*. The volume into which a drug is distributed throughout the body is known as the *volume of distribution*. Individual patient variations can change the amount of drug distributed throughout the body. For example, in an edematous patient, a given dose is distributed into a larger volume than in a nonedematous patient. Occasionally, a dose is increased to account for this difference. In this case, the dose should be decreased after the edema is corrected. Conversely, a dose given to a dehydrated patient may need to be decreased to allow for its distribution into a much smaller volume. Patients who are very obese may present another problem when considering drug distribution. Some drugs—such as digoxin, gentamicin, and tobramycin—aren't well-distributed into fatty tissue. Sometimes, doses based on actual body weight may lead to overdose and serious toxicity. In these cases, doses must be based on lean body weight, or adjusted body weight, which may be estimated from mathematical formulas or actuarial tables that give an average weight range for height.

Metabolism

Most drugs are metabolized in the liver. Hepatic diseases may affect the liver's metabolic functions and may increase or decrease a drug's usual metabolism. Closely monitor all patients with hepatic disease for drug effect and toxicity.

The rate at which a drug is metabolized varies from person to person. Some patients metabolize drugs so quickly that the drug levels in their blood and tissues prove therapeutically inadequate. In other patients, the rate of metabolism is so slow that ordinary doses can produce toxicity or prolonged duration of action. Specific genetic tests can be performed to determine whether a patient is a slow or fast metabolizer.

Excretion

The body eliminates drugs by metabolism (usually hepatic) and excretion (usually renal). *Drug excretion* is the movement of a drug or its metabolites from the tissues back into circulation and from the circulation into the organs of excretion, where they're removed from the body. Most drugs are excreted by the kidneys, but some can be eliminated through the lungs, exocrine (sweat, salivary, or mammary) glands, liver, skin, or intestinal tract. Drugs also may be removed artificially by direct mechanical intervention, such as peritoneal dialysis or hemodialysis.

Other modifying factors

One important factor influencing a drug's action and effect is its tendency to bind to plasma proteins, especially albumin, and other tissue components. Because only a free, unbound drug molecule can act in the body, protein binding greatly influences the degree and duration of a drug's effect. Malnutrition, renal failure, and the presence of other protein-bound drugs can influence protein binding. When protein-binding behavior changes, the drug dosage may need to be adjusted accordingly.

The patient's age is another important factor. Elderly patients usually have decreased hepatic function, less muscle mass, diminished renal function, and lower albumin levels. These patients may need lower doses and sometimes longer dosage intervals to avoid toxicity. Neonates have underdeveloped metabolic enzyme systems and inadequate renal function, so they need highly individualized dosages and careful monitoring.

Underlying disease also may affect drug action and effect. For example, acidosis may cause insulin resistance. Genetic diseases, such as G6PD deficiency and hepatic porphyria, may turn drugs into toxins, with serious consequences. Patients with G6PD deficiency may develop hemolytic anemia when given certain drugs, such as sulfonamides. A genetically susceptible patient can develop acute porphyria if given a barbiturate. A patient with a highly active hepatic enzyme system, such as a rapid acetylator, can develop hepatitis when treated with isoniazid because of the quick intrahepatic buildup of a toxic metabolite.

Drug administration issues

The dosage form of a drug is important because it can also influence the drug's action in the body. Some tablets and capsules are too large to be easily swallowed by sick patients. An oral solution may be substituted, but it may produce higher drug levels than a tablet because the liquid is more easily and completely absorbed. When a potentially toxic drug (such as digoxin) is given in the liquid form, its increased absorption can cause toxicity. Sometimes a change in dosage form also requires a change in dosage.

Routes of administration aren't always interchangeable. For example, diazepam is readily absorbed PO but is slowly and erratically absorbed IM. On the other hand, gentamicin must be given parenterally because oral administration results in drug levels too low to effectively treat systemic infections.

Improper storage can alter a drug's potency. Most drugs must be stored in tight containers protected from direct sunlight and extremes in temperature and humidity that can cause them to deteriorate. Some drugs require special storage conditions, such as refrigeration. Patients should be cautioned not to store drugs in a bathroom because of the constantly changing environment.

The timing of drug administration can be important. Sometimes, giving an oral drug during, shortly before, or after a meal changes the amount of drug absorbed. Sometimes, the presence of food in the GI tract may be desirable, such as with aspirin or other irritating drugs. But penicillins and tetracyclines shouldn't be taken at mealtimes because certain foods can inactivate them. If in doubt about the effect of food on a certain drug, the nurse should check with a pharmacist.

The nurse should always document the patient's age, height, and weight (in kg). The prescriber will need this information when calculating the dosage for many drugs. It's especially important to record daily weights of intensive-care patients, neonates, and infants because their weights can change frequently. Children should always be weighed because most medications given to children are weight-based. The patient's medical record should also include all current laboratory data, especially results of renal and liver function studies, so the prescriber can adjust the dosage as needed.

The nurse should also watch for metabolic and physiologic changes (such as depressed respiratory function, acidosis, or alkalosis) that might alter drug effect.

The nurse should obtain a comprehensive family history from the patient or family, asking about past reactions to drugs, possible genetic traits that might affect drug response, and current use of other prescription and OTC drugs, illicit drugs, herbal supplements, and vitamin supplements. Multiple drug therapies can cause serious and fatal drug interactions and can dramatically change many drugs' effects.

Drug interactions

A *drug interaction* occurs when a drug given concomitantly with another drug alters the effect of either or both drugs. Usually the effect of one drug is increased or decreased. For instance, one drug may inhibit or stimulate the metabolism or excretion of the other or free it for further action by displacing the drug from protein-binding sites.

Combination therapy is based on drug interactions. One drug may be given to complement, enhance, or protect the effects of another. For example, imipenem and cilastatin are given together because cilastatin inhibits a renal enzyme that would degrade imipenem. In many cases, two drugs with similar actions are given together precisely because of the additive effect. For instance, acetaminophen and codeine are commonly given in combination because together they provide greater pain relief than if either is given alone.

Drug interactions are sometimes used to prevent or antagonize certain adverse reactions. The diuretics hydrochlorothiazide and spironolactone are often given together because the former is potassium-depleting and the latter potassium-sparing.

Not all drug interactions are beneficial. Many drugs interact to decrease efficacy or increase toxicity. An example of decreased efficacy occurs when a tetracycline is given with drugs or foods that contain calcium or magnesium (such as antacids or milk). These bind with tetracycline in the GI tract and cause inadequate drug absorption. An example of increased toxicity can be seen in a patient taking an NSAID and an anticoagulant such as warfarin. This combination of drugs increases the risk of GI bleeding. Avoid drug combinations that produce these effects, if possible.

Sometimes drug interactions occur after a drug that inhibits or increases the metabolism of another drug has been discontinued. After the drug is discontinued, the other drug's levels may increase or decrease, so the dosage may need adjustment.

Adverse reactions

Drugs cause adverse *effects;* patients have adverse *reactions.* An adverse reaction may be tolerated to obtain a therapeutic effect, or it may be hazardous and unacceptable. Some adverse reactions subside with continued use. For example, the drowsiness caused by paroxetine and the orthostatic hypotension caused by prazosin usually subside after several days, when the patient develops tolerance. But many adverse reactions are dose related and lessen or disappear only if the dosage is reduced. Most adverse reactions aren't therapeutically desirable, but a few can be put to clinical use. An example of this is the drowsiness caused by diphenhydramine, which makes it useful as a mild sedative.

Common Terminology Criteria for Adverse Events are standardized definitions that describe adverse events that may occur in the course of cancer therapy. An *adverse event* is considered any event that's unfavorable or has an unfavorable outcome to a patient due to a medication and not to the underlying condition of the patient. (See *Common Terminology Criteria for Adverse Events*, page 4.)

Drug hypersensitivity, or drug allergy, is the result of an antigen–antibody immune reaction that occurs in the body when a drug is given to a susceptible patient. Signs and symptoms of a drug allergy may include rash, itching, angioedema, or shortness of breath. One of the most dangerous of all drug hypersensitivities is penicillin allergy. In its most severe form, penicillin anaphylaxis can rapidly become fatal.

Rarely, idiosyncratic reactions occur. These reactions are highly unpredictable and unusual. One of the best known idiosyncratic adverse reactions is aspirin-induced asthma, which may be life-threatening. A more common idiosyncratic reaction is extreme sensitivity to very low doses of a drug or insensitivity to higher-than-normal doses.

To manage adverse reactions correctly, you need to be aware of changes in the patient's clinical condition, even subtle ones. Such changes may be an early warning of impending toxicity. Listen to the patient's complaints about reactions to a drug, and consider each objectively. You may be able to reduce adverse reactions in several ways. Dosage reduction can help. But,

Common Terminology Criteria for Adverse Events

The National Cancer Institute developed a classification system to grade and describe the severity of certain toxicities related to cancer treatment. This grading scale is used to manage the dosage and administration of the patient's chemotherapy and, in clinical trials, to provide standardized definitions of toxicities for scientific analysis. The CTCAE classification is applied to blood, cardiac, fatigue, GI, hepatobiliary, infusion reaction and extravasation, kidney and urinary tract, lung, metabolic, neurologic, pain, psychiatric, and skin-related adverse events.

The CTCAE classification consists of five different grades that define the severity of the adverse events and describe them. Each grade has specific parameters related to the physiologic or anatomic system involved.
Grade 1: Mild; asymptomatic or mild symptoms with no intervention needed
Grade 2: Moderate; minimal local or noninvasive; intervention indicated
Grade 3: Severe or medically significant but not immediately life-threatening; hospitalization or prolonged hospitalization stay indicated; disabling
Grade 4: Life-threatening; urgent intervention indicated
Grade 5: Death related to adverse event.

in many cases, so does a simple rescheduling of the dose. For example, the CNS stimulation that pseudoephedrine may produce may be managed if it's given early in the day rather than at bedtime. Similarly, drowsiness from antihistamines or tranquilizers can be less important if these drugs are given at bedtime. Most importantly, your patient needs to be told which adverse reactions to expect so that the patient won't become worried or even decide to stop taking the drug. Always advise the patient to report all adverse reactions to the prescriber, and teach the patient which adverse reactions must be reported immediately.

Your ability to recognize signs and symptoms of drug allergies or serious idiosyncratic reactions may save your patient's life. Ask each patient about the drugs currently being taken or those taken in the past and whether any unusual reactions occurred while taking them. If a patient claims to be allergic to a drug, ask for specific examples of what the patient experienced after taking the drug. The patient may be calling a harmless adverse reaction such as upset stomach an allergic reaction or may have a true history of anaphylaxis. In either case, you and

the prescriber need to be aware of the reaction. Record and report clinical changes throughout the patient's course of treatment. If you suspect a severe adverse reaction, withhold the drug until you can check with a pharmacist and the prescriber.

Toxic reactions

Chronic drug toxicities are usually caused by the cumulative effect and resulting buildup of the drug in the body. These effects may be undesired extensions of the desired therapeutic effect. For example, standard doses of glyburide normalize the blood glucose level, but higher doses can produce hypoglycemia.

Drug toxicities may also occur when a drug level rises as a result of impaired metabolism or excretion. For example, hepatic dysfunction impairs the metabolism of amiodarone, raising its concentration in the blood. Similarly, renal dysfunction may cause digoxin toxicity because this drug is eliminated by the kidneys. Excessive dosage can also cause toxic levels. For instance, tinnitus is usually a sign that the safe dose of aspirin has been exceeded.

Many drug toxicities are predictable, dosage-related, and reversible upon dosage adjustment or discontinuation. Monitor patients carefully for physiologic changes that might alter drug effect. Watch especially for hepatic and renal impairment. Warn the patient about signs of impending toxicity and tell the patient what to do if a toxic reaction occurs. Also, make sure to emphasize the importance of taking a drug exactly as prescribed. Warn the patient that serious problems could arise if the patient changes the dose or schedule or stops taking the drug without the prescriber's knowledge.

Pharmacogenetics

Prescribers typically follow a standardized approach to prescribing drugs. Although decisions are made based on evidence-based approaches and with the best of intentions, some result in the development of adverse drug reactions. It would be helpful to be able to accurately predict which patients will (and which will not) respond and to what degree when prescribed a certain drug. Pharmacogenetics—the study of how varied responses to a drug can be caused by genetic differences between individuals—attempts to do just this.

The first pharmacogenetic detection occurred when Pythagoras recognized the dangers of ingesting fava beans in 510 B.C., which eventually led to the discovery of G6PD in 1956. Shortly after, the term *pharmacogenetics* was coined and later defined as the study of variability in drug response due to heredity. The goals of pharmacogenetics include identification of innovative drug targets, consideration of DNA sequence variation on drug effects, development of new agents, and optimization of drug efficacy while minimizing drug toxicity.

Pharmacogenetics considers the existence of *polymorphisms*, which are genetic variations that occur in 1% or more of the population. If clinicians are able to predict which patients express polymorphisms, they can provide targeted therapy. Researchers have learned that many polymorphisms involve cytochrome P450 (CYP450) isoenzymes.

Polymorphisms play a significant role in determining whether a drug will be predictably metabolized. Patients fall into one of four classes of metabolizers: extensive, ultrarapid, intermediate, and poor. Patients considered extensive metabolizers possess an overwhelming capacity to metabolize certain drugs and may exhibit therapeutic failure, whereas patients who are poor metabolizers, such as those with G6PD deficiency, exhibit toxicities due to their inability to metabolize certain drugs. Ethnicity may also play a role in determining how patients are classified in regard to metabolism.

It's vital to recognize the importance of the CYP450 system. Approximately 60 CYP enzymes are found in humans, and many genes that encode for these enzymes are polymorphic. Polymorphism associated with CYP enzymes may be expressed via amino acid substitution (thereby reducing enzymatic activity) or by amplification or duplication of activity (thereby increasing enzymatic activity). It's thought that approximately one-third of all medications prescribed today are metabolized by CYP450, including TCAs, antiarrhythmics, beta-receptor antagonists, codeine, warfarin, phenytoin, and nicotine.

In addition, enzymes that metabolize cancer chemotherapy drugs, such as thiopurine S-methyltransferase, dihydropyrimidine dehydrogenase, and UDP-glucuronosyl transferase, can have therapeutic implications; for example, polymorphisms affecting these enzymes can result in serious adverse reactions, such as anemia and neurotoxicity. Finally, miscellaneous polymorphisms affecting drug transport proteins such as P-gp may affect drug response. P-gp acts as a safety mechanism to remove toxins from cells and has a role in the distribution of cancer chemotherapy drugs, digoxin, cyclosporine, and protease inhibitors.

As a nurse, you need to be aware of the clinical ramifications of pharmacogenetics—having an effective knowledge of which drugs, diseases, or ethnic groups are affected by these variations can help you anticipate issues that may arise with patients under your care. For example, some Asian patients have a significant reduction in enzyme activity secondary to amino acid substitution and, therefore, exhibit slower metabolism of certain drugs compared to patients from other ethnic groups. The effect of this on clinical practice is seen in the dosing of rosuvastatin; patients of Asian descent are typically started at 5 mg/day PO, whereas non-Asian patients are started at 10 mg/day. Giving a lower dose helps limit the development of serious adverse reactions in Asian patients.

Another example of how drug metabolism is affected by genetic polymorphism involves the drug warfarin. Studies have shown that CYP2C9, which is the primary enzyme responsible for warfarin metabolism, has two genetic variants. These variants are associated with up to an 80% decrease in enzymatic activity that can affect approximately 7% to 11% of patients. Patients with these variant genotypes have 2.4 times an increase in the risk of serious or life-threatening bleeding after usual doses of warfarin. Consequently, patients with these variants retain warfarin longer and need significantly lower maintenance dosages.

Fortunately, genetic testing for polymorphisms is available when issues such as these arise. Although testing isn't done for every patient, it can be helpful for those who seem to be refractory or overly sensitive to the effects of certain drugs or who meet other criteria.

2

Drug therapy across the lifespan

Drug therapy is a fact of life for millions of people of all ages, and certain aspects of a patient's life, such as age, growth, and development, can affect drug therapy.

Drugs and pregnancy

Drug administration during pregnancy has been a source of serious medical concern and controversy since the thalidomide tragedy of the late 1950s, when thousands of malformed infants were born after their mothers were given this mild sedative-hypnotic while pregnant. To identify drugs that may cause such teratogenic effects, preclinical drug studies include tests on pregnant laboratory animals. These studies may reveal gross teratogenicity but don't establish absolute safety. This is because different animal species react to drugs in different ways. Consequently, animal studies can't reveal all possible teratogenic effects in humans. For example, the preliminary animal studies on thalidomide gave no warning of its teratogenic effects, and it was subsequently released for general use in Europe.

What about the placental barrier? Once thought to protect the fetus from drug effects, the placenta isn't much of a barrier at all. Almost every drug a pregnant woman takes crosses the placenta and enters fetal circulation, except for drugs with exceptionally large molecular structures, such as heparin, an injectable anticoagulant. By this standard, heparin could be used in a pregnant woman without fear of harming the fetus, but even heparin carries a warning for cautious use during pregnancy. Conversely, just because a drug crosses the placenta doesn't necessarily mean it's harmful to the fetus.

One factor—stage of fetal development—seems clearly related to greater risk during pregnancy. During the first and third trimesters of pregnancy, the fetus is especially vulnerable to damage from maternal use of drugs. During these times, give *all* drugs with extreme caution.

Organogenesis—when fetal organs differentiate—occurs in the first trimester. This is the most sensitive period for drug-induced fetal malformation. Strongly advise your patient not to take medications, including OTC drugs and supplements, without first discussing them with her health care provider.

Fetal sensitivity to drugs is also of special concern during the third trimester. At birth, after maternal separation, the neonate must rely on its own metabolism to eliminate any remaining drug. Because the neonate's detoxifying systems aren't fully developed, any residual drug may take a long time to be metabolized and thus may induce prolonged toxic reactions. For this reason, discourage pregnant patients from taking drugs except when absolutely necessary and advised by their prescribers during the last 3 months of pregnancy.

In many circumstances, pregnant women must continue to take certain drugs. For example, a woman with a seizure disorder that is well controlled with an anticonvulsant may need to keep taking the drug during pregnancy. Similarly, a pregnant woman with a bacterial infection must receive antibiotics. In such cases, the potential risk to the fetus is outweighed by the mother's medical needs, and drugs with lower teratogenic potential are used whenever possible.

Complying with the following general guidelines can prevent indiscriminate and harmful use of drugs in pregnancy:
- Before a drug is prescribed for a woman of childbearing potential, ask the date of her last menstrual period and whether she may be pregnant. If a drug is a known teratogen (for example, isotretinoin), some manufacturers may recommend special precautions to ensure that the drug isn't given to a woman of childbearing potential until pregnancy is ruled out and may require that contraceptives be used throughout the course of therapy.
- Caution a pregnant woman to avoid all drugs (including OTC drugs and herbs and supplements) except those essential to maintain her pregnancy and health—especially during the first and third trimesters.
- Topical drugs may be subject to the same warning against use during pregnancy. Many topically applied drugs can be absorbed in amounts large enough to be harmful to the fetus.
- When a pregnant woman needs to be prescribed a medication, use the safest drug in the lowest dose possible to minimize harm to the fetus.

- Instruct a pregnant woman to check with her prescriber before taking any drug.
- Encourage a pregnant woman to enroll in the pregnancy exposure registry for drugs that have one. Registries compile data on pregnancy outcomes to further define the risks of drug exposure in human pregnancies.
- Advise a pregnant woman to give her prescriber a list of all drugs, herbs, and supplements she's currently taking.

Drugs and breastfeeding

Many drugs a breastfeeding mother takes appear in human milk. Drug levels in human milk tend to be high when drug levels in maternal blood are high, especially after each dose. Many manufacturers' instructions advise the mother to breastfeed *before* taking each drug dose, not *after*. Also, in general, drugs with short half-lives are preferred because they peak quickly and are then eliminated and are less likely to be excreted in human milk.

A mother who wants to breastfeed usually may continue to do so with her prescriber's advice. However, breastfeeding should be temporarily interrupted and replaced with bottle-feeding when the mother must take certain drugs, such as a tetracycline, a sulfonamide (during the first 2 weeks postpartum), some oral anticoagulants, a drug that contains iodine, or an antineoplastic.

Caution the breastfeeding patient to protect her infant by not taking drugs indiscriminately. Instruct the mother to first check with her prescriber to be sure she's taking the safest drug at the lowest dose. Also instruct her to give her prescriber a list of all drugs, herbs, and supplements she's currently taking.

Drug therapy in children

Providing drug therapy to infants, children, and adolescents is challenging. Physiologic differences between children and adults, including those involving vital organ maturity and body composition, significantly influence a drug's effectiveness.

Physiologic changes affecting drug action

As a child develops, the processes of absorption, distribution (including drug binding to plasma proteins), metabolism, and excretion undergo profound changes that affect drug dosage. To ensure optimal drug effect and minimal toxicity, consider these factors when giving drugs to a child.

Absorption

Drug absorption in children depends on the form of the drug, its physical properties, simultaneous ingestion of other drugs or food, physiologic changes, and concurrent disease.

The pH of neonatal gastric fluid is neutral or slightly acidic; it becomes more acidic as the infant matures, which affects drug absorption. For example, ampicillin is better absorbed in an infant than in an adult because of the infant's low gastric acidity.

Various infant formulas or milk products may increase gastric pH and impede absorption of acidic drugs. If possible and so advised, give a child oral drugs on an empty stomach.

Gastric emptying time and transit time through the small intestine—which takes longer in children than in adults—can affect absorption. Also, intestinal hypermotility (as occurs in patients with diarrhea) can diminish a drug's absorption.

A child's comparatively thin epidermis allows increased absorption of topical drugs, increasing the risk of adverse systemic reactions.

Distribution

As with absorption, changes in body weight and physiology during childhood can significantly influence a drug's distribution and effects. In a premature infant, body fluid makes up about 85% of total body weight; in a full-term infant, it makes up 55% to 70%; in an adult, 50% to 55%. Extracellular fluid (mostly blood) constitutes 40% of a neonate's body weight, compared with 20% in an adult. Intracellular fluid remains fairly constant throughout life and has little effect on drug dosage.

Extracellular fluid volume influences a water-soluble drug's concentration and effect because most drugs travel through extracellular fluid to reach their receptors. Compared with adults, distribution volume in children is proportionately greater because their fluid-to-solid body weight proportion is larger.

Because the proportion of fat to lean body mass increases with age, the distribution of fat-soluble drugs is more limited in children than in adults. As a result, a drug's fat or water solubility affects the dosage for a child.

Plasma protein binding

A decrease in albumin level or intermolecular attraction between drug and plasma protein causes many drugs to be less bound to plasma proteins in infants than in adults.

Highly protein-bound drugs may displace endogenous compounds, such as bilirubin or free fatty acids. Displacement of bound bilirubin can increase unbound (free) bilirubin, which can lead to increased risk of kernicterus at normal bilirubin levels. Conversely, an endogenous compound may displace a low protein-bound drug.

Because only an unbound drug molecule has a pharmacologic effect, a change in the ratio of a protein-bound to an unbound active drug can greatly influence the drug's effect.

Several diseases and disorders, such as nephrotic syndrome and malnutrition, can decrease plasma protein levels and increase the level of an unbound drug, which can either intensify the drug's effect or produce toxicity.

Metabolism

A neonate's ability to metabolize a drug depends on the integrity of the hepatic enzyme system, intrauterine exposure to the drug, and the properties of the drug itself.

Certain metabolic mechanisms are underdeveloped in neonates. Glucuronidation is a metabolic process occurring in the liver that renders most drugs more water soluble, facilitating renal excretion. This process isn't developed enough to permit larger doses of most drugs until the infant is 1 month old. The use of chloramphenicol sodium succinate in a neonate may cause gray baby syndrome because the infant's immature liver can't metabolize the drug; as a result, toxic levels accumulate in the blood. Reducing the dosage in a neonate and periodically monitoring drug levels are good ways to avoid toxicity. Conversely, intrauterine exposure to drugs may induce precocious development of hepatic enzyme mechanisms, thereby increasing the infant's capacity to metabolize potentially harmful substances.

Older children can metabolize some drugs (theophylline, for example) more rapidly than adults. This ability may arise from their increased hepatic metabolic activity. Doses larger than those recommended for adults may be required.

Also, more than one drug given simultaneously to a child may change hepatic metabolism and initiate production of hepatic enzymes. Phenobarbital, for example, induces hepatic enzyme production and accelerates the metabolism of some drugs taken concomitantly.

Excretion

Renal excretion of a drug is the net result of glomerular filtration, active tubular secretion, and passive tubular reabsorption. Many drugs are excreted in the urine. The degree of renal development or presence of renal disease can greatly affect a child's dosage requirements because if a child can't excrete a drug renally, the drug may accumulate to toxic levels.

Physiologically, an infant's kidneys differ from an adult's in that infants have a high resistance to blood flow and their kidneys receive a smaller proportion of cardiac output. Infants have incomplete glomerular and tubular development and short, incomplete loops of Henle. (A child's GFR reaches an adult value between ages 2½ and 5 months; the child's tubular secretion rate may reach an adult value between ages 7 and 12 months.) Infants also are less able to concentrate urine or reabsorb certain filtered compounds. The proximal tubules in infants also are less able to secrete organic acids.

Children and adults have diurnal variations in urine pH that correlate with sleep patterns. Changes in urine pH can affect the amount of drug excreted into the urine.

Special administration considerations

Biochemically, a drug displays the same mechanisms of action in all people. But the response to a drug can be affected by a child's age and size, as well as by the maturity of the target organ. To ensure optimal drug effect and minimal toxicity, consider the following factors when giving drugs to children.

Adjusting dosages for children

When calculating children's dosages, don't use formulas that modify adult dosages. A child isn't a scaled-down version of an adult. Base pediatric dosages on either body weight (mg/kg) or body surface area (mg/m^2).

Reevaluate dosages at regular intervals to ensure needed adjustments as the child develops. Although BSA provides a useful standard for adults and older children, use the body weight method in premature or full-term infants. Don't exceed the maximum adult dosage when calculating amounts per kilogram of body weight (except with certain drugs, such as theophylline, if indicated).

Obtain an accurate maternal drug history, including prescription and OTC drugs, vitamins, herbs, or supplements taken during pregnancy. Drugs passed into human milk can have adverse effects on the breastfeeding infant. Before giving a drug to a breastfeeding mother, investigate its potential effects on the infant.

For example, a sulfonamide given to a breastfeeding mother for a UTI appears in human milk and may cause kernicterus in an infant with low levels of unconjugated bilirubin. Also, high levels of isoniazid appear in the human milk of a mother taking this drug for TB. Because isoniazid is metabolized by the liver, the infant's immature hepatic enzyme mechanisms can't metabolize the drug, and the infant may develop CNS toxicity.

Giving oral drugs

Remember the following when giving oral drugs to a child:

If the patient is an infant, give drugs in liquid form, if possible. For accuracy, measure and give the preparation by oral syringe, never a parenteral syringe. It's very important to remove the syringe cap to keep the infant from swallowing or aspirating it. Be sure to instruct parents to do the same. Never use a vial or cup. Lift the patient's head to prevent aspiration of the drug, and press down on the chin to prevent choking. You may also place the drug in a nipple and allow the infant to suck the contents.

If the patient is a toddler, explain how you're going to give the drug. If possible, have the parents enlist the child's cooperation. Never call it "candy," even if it has a pleasant taste. Let the child take the liquid drug from a calibrated medication cup rather than a spoon. It's easier and more accurate. If the preparation is available only in tablet form, crush and mix it with an appropriate vehicle, such as jelly or applesauce. (First, verify with a pharmacist that the tablet can be crushed and mixed without compromising its effectiveness. For example, most long-acting or extended-release products shouldn't be crushed.)

If the patient is an older child who can swallow a tablet or capsule, have the child place the drug on the back of the tongue and swallow it with water or nonacidic fruit juice, because milk and milk products may interfere with drug absorption.

Giving IV infusions

For IV infusions in infants, use a peripheral vein or a scalp vein in the temporal region. The scalp vein is safe because the needle isn't likely to dislodge. However, the hair must be clipped around the site, and the needle and infiltrated fluids may cause temporary disfigurement. For these reasons, scalp veins aren't used as commonly today as they were in the past.

The arms and legs are the most accessible insertion sites, but because children tend to move about, take these precautions:

• Protect the insertion site to keep the catheter or needle from being dislodged. Use a padded arm board to reduce the risk of dislodgment. Remove the arm board during range-of-motion exercises.

• Place the IV tubing clamp out of the child's reach. If extension tubing is used to allow the child greater mobility, securely tape the connection.

• Explain in simple terms to the child why restraints must be used while the child is asleep, to alleviate anxiety and maintain trust.

During an infusion, monitor flow rates and check the child's condition and the insertion site at least every hour. Titrate the flow rate only while the patient is composed; crying and emotional upset can constrict blood vessels. Flow rate may vary if a pump isn't used. Flow should be adequate because some drugs (calcium, for example) can be irritating at low flow rates. Infants, small children, and children with compromised cardiopulmonary status are especially vulnerable to fluid overload with IV drug administration. To prevent this problem and help ensure that a limited amount of fluid is infused in a controlled manner, use a volume-control device in the IV tubing and an infusion pump or a syringe. Don't place more than 2 hours of IV fluid in the volume-control set at a time.

Giving IM injections

IM injections are preferred when a drug can't be given by other parenteral routes and rapid absorption is needed.

The vastus lateralis muscle is the preferred injection site in children age 2 and younger. For children ages 3 to 18, the deltoid muscle is the preferred site. Though rarely used in children, the ventrogluteal site can be used in certain circumstances, such as when the child's condition prevents administration in other sites. To select the correct needle size, consider the patient's age, muscle mass, nutritional status, and drug viscosity.

Record and rotate injection sites. Explain to the patient that the injection will hurt but that the drug will help the patient feel better. Swaddle an infant or use an assistant during the injection, if needed, and comfort the infant afterward.

Giving topical drugs and inhalants

When giving a child a topical drug or inhalant, consider the following:

Use eardrops warmed to room temperature. Cold drops can cause pain and vertigo. To give drops, turn the patient on the side, with the affected ear up. If the patient is younger than age 3, pull the pinna down and back; if age 3 or older, pull the pinna up and back.

Avoid using inhalants in young children because it's difficult to get them to cooperate. Before you try to give a drug to an older child through a metered-dose inhaler, explain how to use the inhaler. Then have the child hold the inhaler and close the lips around the mouthpiece. Have the child exhale and pinch the nostrils shut. When the child starts to inhale, release one dose of the drug into the child's mouth. Tell the patient to continue inhaling until the lungs feel full; then the child can breathe normally and unpinch the nostrils. Most inhaled drugs aren't useful if the drug remains in the mouth or throat—if you doubt the patient's ability to use the inhaler correctly, don't use it. Devices, such as spacers or assist devices, may help. Check with a pharmacist, the prescriber, or a respiratory therapist for suggestions.

Use topical corticosteroids cautiously because prolonged use in children may delay growth. When you apply topical corticosteroids to the diaper area of infants, don't cover the area with plastic or rubber pants, which act as an occlusive dressing and may enhance systemic absorption.

Giving parenteral nutrition

Give IV nutrition to patients who can't or won't take adequate food orally and to patients with hypermetabolic conditions who need supplementation. The latter group includes premature infants, children, and adolescents with burns or other major trauma, intractable diarrhea, malabsorption syndromes, GI abnormalities, emotional disorders (such as anorexia nervosa), and congenital abnormalities.

Before giving fat emulsions to infants and children, weigh the potential benefits against any possible risks. Fats—supplied as 10% or 20% lipid emulsions—are given both peripherally and centrally. Their use is limited by the child's ability to metabolize them. For example,

an infant or child with a diseased liver can't efficiently metabolize fats.

Some fats, however, must be supplied both to prevent essential fatty acid deficiency and to permit normal growth and development. A minimum of calories (2% to 4%) must be supplied as linoleic acid—an essential fatty acid found in lipids. Nevertheless, fat solutions may decrease oxygen perfusion and may adversely affect children with pulmonary disease. This risk can be minimized by supplying only the minimum fat needed for essential fatty acid requirements and not the usual intake of 40% to 50% of the child's total calories.

Fatty acids can also displace bilirubin bound to albumin, causing a rise in free, unconjugated bilirubin and an increased risk of kernicterus. Fat solutions may interfere with some bilirubin assays and cause falsely elevated bilirubin levels. To avoid this complication, draw a blood sample 4 hours after infusion of the lipid emulsion or, if the emulsion is infused over 24 hours, be sure the laboratory is aware so that the blood samples can be centrifuged before the assay is performed.

It isn't usually recommended to give other IV solutions or medications in the same line as parenteral nutrition because of the potential for precipitates to form. Refer to your facility's nutrition/pharmacy policy or contact a pharmacist for further information.

Drug therapy in elderly patients

If you're giving drugs to elderly patients, you'll need to understand the physiologic and pharmacokinetic changes in this population that may affect drug dosage, cause common adverse reactions, or create compliance problems.

Physiologic changes affecting drug action

As a person ages, gradual physiologic changes occur. Some of these age-related changes may alter the therapeutic and toxic effects of drugs.

Body composition

Proportions of fat, lean tissue, and water in the body change with age. Total body mass and lean body mass tend to decrease, but the proportion of body fat tends to increase.

Body composition varies from person to person, and these changes in body composition affect the relationship between a drug's concentration and distribution in the body.

For example, a water-soluble drug such as gentamicin isn't distributed to fat. Because there's relatively more fat tissue and less lean tissue in an elderly person, more drug remains in the blood. Fat-soluble drugs tend to accumulate in older patients, resulting in prolonged half-lives and more pronounced effects.

Gastrointestinal function
In elderly patients, decreases in gastric acid secretion and GI motility slow the emptying of stomach contents and movement through the entire intestinal tract. Research suggests that elderly patients may not absorb drugs as easily as younger patients. This is an especially significant problem with drugs that have a narrow therapeutic range, such as digoxin, in which any change in absorption can be crucial.

Hepatic function
The liver's ability to metabolize certain drugs decreases with age. This decrease is caused by diminished blood flow to the liver, which results from an age-related decrease in cardiac output, and from the lessened activity of certain liver enzymes. When an elderly patient takes a sleep medication such as flurazepam, for example, the liver's reduced ability to metabolize the drug as well as the lipophilic property of the drug can produce residual effects the next morning.

Decreased hepatic function may result in more intense drug effects caused by higher levels, longer-lasting drug effects because of prolonged levels, and a greater risk of drug toxicity.

Renal function
An elderly person's renal function is usually sufficient to eliminate excess body fluid and waste, but the ability to eliminate some drugs may be reduced by 50% or more.

Many drugs commonly used by elderly patients, such as digoxin, are excreted primarily through the kidneys. If the kidneys' ability to excrete the drug is decreased, high blood levels may result. Digoxin toxicity can occur in elderly patients who don't receive a reduced digoxin dosage to accommodate decreased renal function.

Drug dosages can be modified to compensate for age-related decreases in renal function. Aided by results of laboratory tests, such as BUN and creatinine levels, adjust drug dosages so the patient receives therapeutic benefits without the risk of toxicity. It's important to remember that serum creatinine is a function of muscle mass and that most elderly people lose muscle mass as they age. An elderly patient can have significant renal impairment even with a serum creatinine level in the normal range. Observe the patient for signs and symptoms of toxicity.

Special administration considerations
Aging is usually accompanied by a decline in organ function that can affect drug distribution and clearance. This physiologic decline is likely to be worsened by a disease or a chronic disorder. Together, these factors can significantly increase the risk of adverse reactions and drug toxicity, as well as noncompliance.

Adverse reactions
Compared with younger people, elderly patients experience twice as many adverse drug reactions, mostly from greater drug use, poor compliance, and physiologic changes.

Signs and symptoms of adverse drug reactions—including confusion, weakness, agitation, and lethargy—are often mistakenly attributed to senility or disease. If the adverse reaction isn't identified, the patient may continue to receive the drug and receive other, unnecessary drugs to treat the complications caused by the original drug. This prescribing cascade can sometimes result in a pattern of inappropriate and excessive drug use, causing polypharmacy.

Any drug can cause adverse reactions, but most of the serious reactions in the elderly are caused by relatively few drugs. Be particularly alert for toxicities resulting from diuretics, antihypertensives, digoxin, corticosteroids, anticoagulants, sleeping aids, and OTC drugs.

Diuretic toxicity
Because total body water content decreases with age, a normal dosage of a potassium-wasting diuretic, such as furosemide or hydrochlorothiazide, may result in fluid loss and even dehydration in an elderly patient.

These diuretics may deplete a patient's potassium level, making the patient feel weak, and they may raise blood uric acid and glucose levels, complicating gout and diabetes mellitus.

Antihypertensive toxicity
Many elderly patients experience lightheadedness or fainting when taking antihypertensives, partly in response to atherosclerosis and decreased elasticity of the blood vessels. Antihypertensives can lower BP too rapidly, resulting in insufficient blood flow to the brain, which can cause dizziness, fainting, or even a stroke.

Consequently, dosages of antihypertensives must be carefully individualized. In elderly patients, aggressive treatment of high BP may be harmful. Treatment goals should be reasonable. Elevated BP needs to be reduced slowly in elderly patients. Tell the patient to change positions slowly and maintain adequate fluid intake to avoid orthostatic hypotension.

Digoxin toxicity
As the body's renal function and rate of excretion decline, the digoxin level in the blood of an elderly patient may increase to the point of causing nausea, vomiting, diarrhea and, most seriously, cardiac arrhythmias. Monitor the patient's digoxin level and observe for early signs and symptoms of toxicity, such as appetite loss, confusion, or depression.

Corticosteroid toxicity
Elderly patients taking a corticosteroid may experience short-term effects, including fluid retention and psychological effects ranging from mild euphoria to acute psychotic reactions. Long-term toxic effects, such as osteoporosis, can be especially severe in elderly patients who have been taking prednisone or related steroidal compounds for months or even years. To prevent serious toxicity, carefully monitor patients on long-term regimens. Observe them for subtle changes in appearance, mood, and mobility and for impaired healing and fluid and electrolyte disturbances.

Anticoagulant effects
Elderly patients taking an anticoagulant have an increased risk of bleeding, especially when they take NSAIDs or aspirin at the same time. Be sure to evaluate all drugs the patient is taking for increased risk of bleeding. Because elderly patients are more likely to fall, they're also at increased risk for bleeding as a result of a fall. Monitor the patient's INR carefully, if applicable, and monitor for bruising and other signs and symptoms of bleeding.

Sleeping aid toxicity
Sedatives and sleeping aids, such as zolpidem and diphenhydramine, may cause excessive sedation or drowsiness. Keep in mind that consumption of alcohol may increase CNS depressant effects, even if the sleeping aid was taken the previous evening. Use these drugs sparingly in elderly patients.

Over-the-counter drug toxicity
Prolonged ingestion of aspirin, aspirin-containing analgesics, and other OTC NSAIDs (such as ibuprofen, ketoprofen, and naproxen) may cause GI irritation—even ulcers—and gradual blood loss resulting in severe anemia. Prescription NSAIDs may cause similar problems. Both OTC and prescription NSAIDs can cause renal toxicity in older adults. Anemia from prolonged aspirin consumption can affect all age groups, but elderly patients may be less able to compensate because of their already reduced iron stores. These drugs should be used very carefully and at the lowest effective doses.

Acetaminophen is found in a variety of prescription and OTC products. Liver injury may occur from inadvertently taking excess acetaminophen from multiple sources.

Laxatives may cause diarrhea in elderly patients, who are extremely sensitive to drugs such as bisacodyl. Long-term oral use of mineral oil as a lubricating laxative may result in lipid pneumonia from aspiration of small residual oil droplets in the patient's mouth.

Antihistamines such as diphenhydramine have anticholinergic effects and can cause confusion and mental status changes; they are also more likely to cause dizziness, sedation, and hypotension in elderly patients. OTC decongestants, including phenylephrine, can have systemic effects, such as hypertension, anxiety, insomnia, and agitation.

Noncompliance
Poor compliance can be a problem with patients of any age. Many hospitalizations result from noncompliance with a medical regimen. In elderly patients, factors linked to aging, such as diminished visual acuity, hearing loss, forgetfulness, the need for multiple drug therapy, and socioeconomic factors, can combine to make compliance a special problem. About one-third of elderly patients fail to comply with their prescribed drug therapy. They may fail to take prescribed doses or to follow the correct schedule. They may take drugs prescribed for previous disorders, stop drugs prematurely, or indiscriminately use drugs that are to be taken as needed. Elderly patients may also have multiple prescriptions for the same drug and inadvertently take an overdose.

Review the patient's drug regimen with the patient. Make sure the patient understands the dose amount, the time and frequency of doses, and why the drug has been prescribed. Also, explain in detail if a drug is to be taken with food, with water, or separate from other drugs. To verify the patient's understanding, ask the patient to repeat the instructions back to you.

Help the patient avoid drug therapy problems by suggesting the use of drug calendars, pill sorters, or other aids to help with compliance. Refer the patient to the prescriber, a pharmacist, or social services if further information or assistance with drug therapy is needed.

3

Safe drug administration

Medication therapy is a primary intervention for many illnesses. It greatly benefits many patients and yet is involved in many instances of unintended harm to patients and health care workers from either unintended consequences of therapy (adverse drug reactions or exposure to hazardous drugs) or medication-related errors (preventable adverse drug events). (See *Preventing and treating IV vesicant extravasation injury*, page 15.) Medication errors are a significant cause of patient morbidity and mortality in the United States. In 1999, the Institute of Medicine (IOM) published its first Quality Chasm report, "To Err is Human: Building a Safer Health System," which reported that errors related to medications accounted for approximately 1 out of 131 outpatient deaths, 1 out of 854 inpatient deaths, and more than 7,000 deaths annually. Recent research indicates that the number of medication errors may actually be much higher. Of all sentinel events reviewed between 2005 and 2017 (10,750) by The Joint Commission (a nonprofit organization that seeks to improve public health care through the voluntary accreditation of health care institutions), approximately 508 events were attributed to medication errors, and an additional 247 events were medication equipment–related.

Many governmental and nongovernmental organizations are dedicated to improving the safety of drug administration. One mission of the FDA, for example, is to protect the public health by assuring the safety, effectiveness, and security of human drugs, vaccines, and medical devices. In 2007, the Food and Drug Administration Amendments Act expanded the FDA's authority regarding assessing and communicating risks associated with drugs. One of the new provisions of the law granted the FDA authority to require drug manufacturers to submit Risk Evaluation and Mitigation Strategies. (See *Risk Evaluation and Mitigation Strategies*, page 16.) The U.S. Pharmacopeia (USP), a nonprofit, nongovernmental public health organization, sets official public standards for drugs and other health care products manufactured or sold in the United States. It also sets standards for the quality, purity, and strength of food ingredients and dietary supplements.

In 2005, The Patient Safety and Quality Improvement Act authorized the creation of patient safety organizations (PSOs) to improve the quality and safety of U.S. health care delivery. One of these PSOs, the Institute for Safe Medication Practices (ISMP), is a nonprofit organization entirely dedicated to preventing medication errors and using medications safely. In addition, The Joint Commission has established National Patient Safety Goals and standards to improve the safe use of medications in its accredited facilities.

The CDC has a number of campaigns and initiatives to promote medication safety by developing evidence-based policies and using collaborative interventions.

One important initiative of the CDC, FDA, and other organizations is to address the use and misuse of opioids in treating chronic pain (pain not related to cancer or palliative care that lasts longer than 3 months or past the time of normal tissue healing). According to the CDC, in 2016 more than 11.5 million individuals in the United States reported misusing prescription opioids in the past year, and from 1999 to 2017, almost 218,000 people died from prescription opioid-related overdose. The death rate continues to increase. (See *Safe opioid administration*, page 17.)

The CDC has developed an evidence-based guideline, "CDC Guideline for Prescribing Opioids for Chronic Pain–United States, 2016" (www.cdc.gov/mmwr/volumes/65/rr/rr6501e1.htm?s_cid=rr6501e1_w), which addresses "1) when to initiate or continue opioids for chronic pain; 2) opioid selection, dosage, duration, follow-up, and discontinuation; and 3) assessing risk and addressing harms of opioid use." The CDC has also developed the "Checklist for Prescribing Opioids for Chronic Pain" (https://stacks.cdc.gov/view/cdc/38025), which provides guidance for primary care providers treating adults with chronic pain.

The FDA has developed a comprehensive action plan that focuses on policies to reduce the impact of the opioid abuse epidemic on families and communities while providing patients access to safe and effective pain relief. The FDA opioid medication action plan includes consulting expert advisory committees

Preventing and treating IV vesicant extravasation injury

Extravasation injuries occur when vesicant IV solutions or drugs—those with the potential to cause significant tissue injury (such as certain chemotherapy drugs, antibiotics, electrolyte solutions, vasopressors, and antiemetics)—escape from blood vessels into surrounding tissue (extravasate) during administration. Drugs or solutions that produce inflammation rather than serious or lasting tissue injury from extravasation are considered irritants. Extravasation injuries may occur when vesicants are given centrally or peripherally. Such injury can cause significant harm, including necrotic ulcers that may require surgical intervention, infection, loss of a limb or limb function, or complex regional pain syndrome.

Signs and symptoms of peripheral extravasation include:

- changes in IV site appearance (blanching, bruising) or temperature (coolness, erythema)
- pain, tightness, or itching at or surrounding the insertion site
- IV site fluid leakage
- numbness or tingling, diminished capillary refill, or decreased motor function in the extremity.

Signs and symptoms of CVAD extravasation include:

- discomfort at the insertion site or along the CVAD path
- fluid leakage from the insertion site
- increased resistance to solution injection
- shoulder, neck, or chest edema.

Preventing extravasation

Use the following measures to prevent extravasation injuries:

- Know facility policy for administering vesicant drugs and solutions. Make sure you've been properly trained in prevention measures and extravasation recognition and management.
- When administering vesicants, know the specific antidote for the drug being given, and make sure that the antidote and equipment needed to manage extravasation are on hand. Some antidotes for vesicants and solutions include sodium thiosulfate for alkylating agents, hyaluronidase for electrolytes and antibiotics (nafcillin, vancomycin [Vancocin]), and phentolamine for vasopressors (dopamine, norepinephrine).

- Ensure that the IV access site or CVAD is patent before giving the drug. Make sure the insertion site is visible, and use an appropriate catheter stabilization device.
- Make sure the drug is given by the proper route according to facility policy. Most vesicants administered by continuous infusion should be given utilizing a CVAD. Know when an IV infusion pump device should and shouldn't be used.
- Frequently monitor the patient for extravasation signs and symptoms, and teach the patient to immediately report them.

Treating extravasation

- Follow facility policy for treatment of extravasation injury. Stop the drug, and aspirate any residual drug and blood from the IV catheter or CVAD.
- Estimate the amount of solution extravasated and notify the practitioner.
- If an antidote exists, prepare for administration through the existing IV catheter or CVAD. After antidote administration, remove the peripheral IV catheter, but avoid pressure to the site.
- For extravasation from a CVAD, prepare the patient for a CT scan to assess catheter placement and fluid collection, if appropriate.
- For peripheral extravasation, prepare for subcut injections of drug-specific antidote, if appropriate.
- Elevate the affected limb.
- Apply hot (for vasoconstrictors) or cold (for alkylating drugs) compresses, if ordered.
- Use a skin marker or photo for serial documentation of extravasation according to facility policy.
- Monitor the site for pain, erythema progression, induration, tissue necrosis, and possible compartment syndrome. Note that symptom development may be delayed for 48 hours.
- Document the date and time of the infusion, time when signs and symptoms were first noted, extravasation signs and symptoms, type and size of venous access device, estimated extravasation solution amount, treatment instituted, practitioner notification, and the patient's response to treatment. Patients with significant tissue damage may need surgery.

before new drug approvals for opioids without abuse-deterrent properties and for new labeling of appropriate opioid use in children, developing additional changes and warnings to immediate-release opioid labeling information to provide risk and safe prescribing guidance for physicians, strengthening the requirements for drug companies to generate postmarket data

on the long-term impact of using opioids to improve treatment of both addiction and pain, updating REMS requirements for opioids to increase pain management and safe prescribing training of prescribers and to decrease inappropriate opioid prescribing, supporting the development of and expanding the use of abuse-deterrent opioids, improving access to naloxone

Risk Evaluation and Mitigation Strategies

REMS is a risk management program that goes beyond the drug's package insert and is used when necessary to make certain that a drug's benefits outweigh its risks. The FDA can require a REMS at any stage of a drug's lifecycle (as part of a drug's New Drug Application or after approval as new safety information becomes available), and manufacturers who fail to comply with REMS requirements can face substantial monetary penalties.

When evaluating the necessity of REMS, the FDA takes into consideration such factors as:

- the number of patients most likely to use the drug
- the seriousness of the patient's disease
- the drug's benefit
- the projected duration of treatment
- the severity of known or potential adverse events
- whether the drug is a new molecular entity.

The FDA has issued an outline of specific components that manufacturers should use to develop a REMS proposal. These include the development of specific REMS goals and elements to ensure a drug's safe and appropriate use. The

REMS must also describe how the manufacturer plans to evaluate whether the REMS goal is being met and the timetable for periodic assessments and reassessments. The results of the evaluations must be reported to the FDA, and the FDA may require that the REMS be modified and will determine if additional actions must be taken.

REMS may contain one or all of the following components:

- **Medication guide:** Written safety information for patients that must be distributed by the pharmacist to each patient receiving the drug
- **Communication plan:** Plan that includes the tools to teach health care professionals how to use the drug safely and appropriately
- **Elements to Assure Safe Use (EASU):** Specific requirements and elements to ensure safe use of the drug, including requirements that each patient be enrolled in a registry, that essential laboratory monitoring be performed, that the drug may only be prescribed by a prescriber with a specific certification, and that the drug may only be distributed by a specialty pharmacy
- **Implementation plan:** Plan that describes how the EASUs will be put into action.

and other drug treatment options for opioid use disorders, and reexamining the risks and benefits of opioids and their effects on public health.

Causes of medication errors

The National Coordinating Council for Medication Error Reporting and Prevention (www.nccmerp.org) defines a *medication error* as "any preventable event that may cause or lead to inappropriate medication use or patient harm while the medication is in the control of the health care professional, patient, or consumer. Such events may be related to professional practice, health care products, procedures, and systems, including prescribing; order communication; product labeling, packaging, and nomenclature; compounding; dispensing; distribution; administration; education; monitoring; and use."

Medication errors were once thought to be caused by lapses in an individual's practice. Traditionally, teaching nurses to administer drugs safely focused on the individual nurse's practice and the application of the "rights" of safe medication administration. (See *The eight "rights" of medication administration*, page 18.)

Although individual nursing practice is still an extremely important part of safe drug administration, the focus of prevention efforts has widened. After medication errors had been systematically studied by numerous organizations who shared data, it became apparent that these errors are complex events with multiple factors and are most often caused by failures within systems. As a result of these findings, research has shifted to preventing medication errors by identifying their root causes and then developing and validating evidence-based prevention strategies. Organizational processes, management decisions, inadequate medication administration protocols, staffing shortages, environmental conditions, poor communication, inadequate drug knowledge and resources, and individual mistakes or protocol violations may all contribute to medication errors.

The medication administration process

Medication errors can occur from medication administration process problems or within any one or more than one of the five stages of medication administration. Because up to 40% of a nurse's time may be spent in medication administration and nursing practice intersects multiple stages, nurses may often be involved in

Safe opioid administration

Opioid analgesics are associated with adverse effects, most notably respiratory depression followed by sedation. Additional adverse effects include aspiration pneumonia, constipation, delirium, dizziness, falls, hallucinations, hypotension, and nausea and vomiting. Opioid analgesics are also linked with adverse drug events due to:

- lack of knowledge regarding differing potencies among opioids
- incorrect administration of multiple opioids, including their respective routes of administration
- inadequate monitoring of patients who take opioids.
  Nurses can help avoid opioid misuse use by:
- identifying conditions that put patients at a higher risk for oversedation and respiratory depression (sleep disorders, morbid obesity, older age, habitual opioid use, major organ dysfunction or failure, respiratory disorders, smoking, polypharmacy)
- screening patients for respiratory depression risk factors using screening tools, such as the Pasero Opioid-induced Sedation Scale (POSS), Richmond Agitation-Sedation Scale (RASS), Screener and Opioid Assessment for Patients with Pain (SOAPP and SOAPP-R), the Opioid Risk Tool (ORT), and the Screening Instrument for Substance Abuse Potential (SISAP)
- assessing the patient's opioid history, including possible abuse, adverse effects, and intolerance
- assessing the patient's skin for an existing opioid patch, implanted drug delivery system, or infusion pump
- starting opioid-naive patients with a nonnarcotic pain regimen before moving on to opioids
- starting opioid-naive patients with the lowest dosage of opioid possible and titrating upwards
- consulting a pharmacist when changing opioid medications or their administration routes
- dosing opioids based on the individual patient's condition and needs
- being mindful of when opioids are administered; for instance, not administering opioids before a patient transfer to avoid possible injury to the patient if drug levels peak during the time of transfer
- using patient-controlled analgesia (PCA) devices
- educating patients and their caregivers about opioid misuse and the steps to take to prevent this occurrence.

Tips for safe opioid administration include the following:

- Double-check the medication order, appropriateness of the medication, the dose, line placement for infusions, and pump settings.
- Ensure standing orders are available for reversal agents.
- Label all IV and epidural lines to avoid confusion.
- Monitor the patient closely if identified as being at high risk for adverse outcomes related to opioid treatment. Frequently assess respiration quality and rate, and observe for signs and symptoms of oversedation.
- Use capnography and pulse oximetry readings to help detect opioid toxicity.
- Keep oxygen and naloxone in the area where opioids are administered.
- Utilize established pain guidelines and standardized formats that are consistent with the patient's age, condition, and ability to understand to monitor and document the patient's pain.
- In collaboration with the multidisciplinary team, involve the patient in the pain management planning process. Develop realistic expectations and measurable goals that the patient understands for the degree, duration, and reduction of pain. Discuss objectives used to evaluate treatment progress (for example, relief of pain and improved physical and psychosocial function).
- Educate patients and their caregivers about PCA use before surgical procedures and warn against dosing by proxy.
- Regularly observe and monitor patients who are using PCA.
- Provide education on pain management, treatment options, and safe use of the opioid.
- Teach the patient and family about pain management strategies during discharge planning. Include information about the patient's pain management plan and adverse effects of pain management treatment.
- Teach the patient and family about safe use, storage, and disposal of opioids. Instruct patients who use fentanyl patches to store them in a secure manner to prevent access by children, pets, and drug-seekers. Educate patients about how to properly apply patches and to protect them from heat.

medication errors. Here are some of the types of errors that have been reported in each stage.

Stage 1: Ordering and prescribing
- Prescriber orders are incomplete or illegible.
- Contraindicated drugs (such as drugs to which the patient is allergic) are prescribed.

- The prescriber specifies the wrong drug, dose, route, frequency, or duration, or fails to specify the indication.
- Drugs are prescribed using inappropriate or inadequate verbal orders.

Stage 2: Transcribing and verifying
• An incorrect drug, dose, route, time, or frequency is transcribed into the medication administration record (MAR) by the pharmacist or nurse.
• Drug verification and documentation in the MAR by the pharmacist or nurse are inadequate.

Stage 3: Dispensing and delivery
• The prescribed drug is filled incorrectly.
• Failure to deliver the right drug to the right place for the right patient occurs.

Stage 4: Administering
• The wrong drug is given to the wrong patient by the nurse or other licensed professional.
• The wrong dose is calculated and given or infused by the nurse or other licensed professional.
• The right drug is incorrectly prepared (such as crushing a drug that shouldn't be crushed)

and is given by the nurse or other licensed professional.
• The correct drug is administered by the wrong route (such as an oral drug that is injected IV) by the nurse or other licensed professional.
• The correct drug is given at the wrong time or frequency by the nurse or other licensed professional.

Stage 5: Monitoring and reporting
• Monitoring of the patient by the nurse before and after medication administration is inadequate.
• Documentation and reporting of the patient's condition by the nurse before and after medication administration are inadequate.
• Hand-off communication between licensed professionals is inadequate.
• Reporting of medication errors is inadequate.

Elements contributing to safer drug administration

Ensuring the safe delivery of medication involves a system-wide, interdisciplinary approach, and research has shown that improvements in communication, education, and prevention of hazardous drug exposure can facilitate the safe delivery of medication.

Communication improvements

Communication issues have been implicated in approximately 60% of reported medication errors. Communication can be improved in many ways throughout the medication administration process. The traditional nursing process "rights" of safe drug administration are still important components of safe drug administration, but even when protocols are followed exactly, some medication errors still occur. For example, a nurse who's exactly following the eight "rights" might administer a drug to which a patient is allergic if the allergy information is incomplete or undocumented or hasn't been communicated effectively. Appropriate communication among all members of the health care team, including nurses, is vitally important.

Many health care facilities have instituted measures to help standardize and organize appropriate communication. One tool commonly used is SBAR (Situation, Background, Assessment, and Recommendation); its purpose is to logically organize information to optimize proper communication among health care providers.

Each institution must have tools and policies in place for the documentation of medication administration. Each prescribed medication order must be clearly written or entered into an electronic medical chart system, and verbal orders must be used and documented according to facility policy. Each verbal order should be read back and verified with the prescriber before the drug is administered. The patient's condition must be monitored after each medication is given, and the patient's response and any nursing interventions must be documented appropriately. Clear communication through documentation is essential to safe practice.

The Joint Commission has developed goals and standards regarding medication reconciliation—the process of comparing a patient's medication regimen at every transition in care (for example, on admission, upon discharge, and between care settings and levels). Medication reconciliation helps ensure that essential information about the patient's medication regimen is communicated to the health care team. Medication reconciliation helps prevent the inadvertent omission of needed medications, prevents medication duplication, and helps identify medications with potentially harmful interactions.

Education improvements

Lack of knowledge has been implicated in many medication errors; therefore, education about medications is essential to their safe administration. All health care team members involved in the process of medication administration, including the prescriber, pharmacist, and nurse, must have access to accurate information about each drug's indications, appropriate dosing regimen, appropriate route, appropriate frequency, possible drug interactions, appropriate monitoring, any cautions, and possible adverse effects. Each facility should have processes in place to educate staff and communicate important drug information.

Governmental and nongovernmental agencies are doing their part toward educating facilities, prescribers, and nurses. The FDA established the black box warning system to alert prescribers to drugs with increased risks to patients. These boxed warnings are the strongest labeling requirements for drugs that can have serious reactions. The Joint Commission requires accredited health care facilities to develop a list of abbreviations to avoid in all medication communications. The ISMP maintains a list of high-alert medications that may cause significant patient harm when given incorrectly. (Each facility should have protocols in place for administering high-alert medications with safeguards built into the process.) The FDA and ISMP have developed a list of drugs with similar names—sound-alike, look-alike (SALA) medications—that can be easily confused with each other. Dissimilarities in each drug's name are highlighted with uppercase letters (so each name has mixed-case letters, called tall-man lettering), making such mix-ups less likely to occur for each drug.

Patient education

Patients and their families should be active participants in the patient's care and should understand the patient's plan of care, including the purpose of newly prescribed medications. The patient and family need to be taught what to watch for, how the patient's condition will be monitored, what signs and symptoms to report, and to report anything that doesn't seem right, including unfamiliar medications. Before administering a medication, the nurse needs to verify with the patient medication allergies or unusual past reactions to medications.

The following general teaching guidelines will help ensure that the patient receives the maximum therapeutic benefit from the medication regimen and will help the patient avoid adverse reactions, accidental overdose, and harmful changes in effectiveness.

• Instruct the patient to learn the brand names, generic name, and dosages of all drugs and supplements (such as herbs and vitamins) being taken.

• Tell the patient to notify the pharmacist and prescriber about all medications the patient is taking, including prescription drugs, OTC drugs, and herbal or other supplements, and about any drug allergies or reactions.

• Advise the patient to always read the label before taking a drug, to take it exactly as prescribed, and to never share prescription drugs with others.

• Warn the patient not to change brands of a drug without consulting the prescriber, to avoid harmful changes in effectiveness.

• Tell the patient to check the expiration date before taking a drug.

• Teach the patient how to safely discard drugs that are outdated or no longer needed.

• Caution the patient to keep all drugs safely out of the reach of children and pets.

- Advise the patient to store drugs in their original containers, at the proper temperature, and in areas where they won't be exposed to sunlight or excessive heat or humidity. Sunlight, heat, and humidity can cause drug deterioration and reduce a drug's effectiveness.
- Encourage the patient to report all suspected adverse or unusual reactions to the prescriber, and teach proper techniques for self-monitoring the condition (for example, how to obtain a resting HR before taking digoxin).
- Suggest that the patient have all prescriptions filled at the same pharmacy or pharmacy system so that pharmacists can warn against potentially harmful drug interactions.
- Tell the patient to report the complete medication history to all health care providers involved in the patient's care, including the dentist.
- Instruct the patient to call the prescriber, poison control center, or pharmacist immediately and to seek immediate medical attention if the patient or someone else has taken an overdose. The National Poison Control Center emergency phone number is 1-800-222-1222. Tell the patient to keep this and other emergency numbers handy at all times.
- Advise the patient to make sure a sufficient supply of drugs is on hand when traveling. The patient should personally carry the drugs in their original containers and not pack them in luggage. Also, recommend that the patient carry a letter from the prescriber authorizing the use of a drug, especially if the drug is a controlled substance.
- Encourage the patient to keep a wallet card or cell phone app that lists all medications the patient is taking, including dose, route, frequency, and indication.

Improvements in preventing hazardous drug exposure

The CDC estimates that 8 million U.S. health care workers are potentially exposed to hazardous drugs in the workplace. Hazardous drugs, as defined by the American Society of Health-System Pharmacists and the National Institute for Occupational Safety and Health (NIOSH), have one or more of the following characteristics:

- carcinogenicity (cause cancer)
- teratogenicity (cause defects in the developing fetus) or cause other developmental toxicities
- reproductive toxicity
- organ toxicity at low doses
- genotoxicity (cause damage to DNA)

- a structure and toxicity profile that mimics that of existing hazardous drugs.

The NIOSH list of antineoplastics and other hazardous drugs can be found at https://www.cdc.gov/niosh/docs/2016-161. Health care workers can be exposed to hazardous drugs through inhalation, ingestion, skin contact/absorption, or injection; exposure is most likely from skin contact/absorption or inhalation. Potential exposure can occur in many ways, such as:

- preparing drugs for administration (reconstituting powdered drugs, crushing tablets for oral liquids, compounding powders, or counting out oral doses from multidose bottles)
- administering hazardous drugs IM, IV, intrathecally, or subcut
- directly contacting drugs on the contaminated exteriors of drug vials, on drug-contaminated work surfaces, and on IV tubing and syringes
- handling body fluids that contain drugs or drug-contaminated dressings, linens, or waste
- transporting hazardous drugs
- removing and disposing of personal protective equipment (PPE)
- cleaning contaminated work spaces and spills.

Protecting workers and minimizing exposure

Protecting health care workers and minimizing their exposure to hazardous drugs can be achieved through engineering and administrative controls and use of appropriate PPE.

Engineering controls include:
- class II or III biological safety cabinets (also known as *vertical flow hoods* or *ventilated cabinets*) for hazardous drug preparation
- closed-system drug transfer devices
- needleless systems.

Administrative controls include:
- implementing training, retraining, and testing programs to educate and monitor staff about best practices to prevent hazardous drug exposure
- developing and implementing management policies and protocols to reduce staff risk
- using monitoring programs to identify hazardous drugs and staff exposure or development of early disease.

Appropriate use of PPE includes:
- making sure PPE fits and is used and disposed of properly, following facility policies and protocols

- selecting PPE based on assessment of the potential for hazardous drug exposure:
  - Gloves: Select gloves appropriate for the potential exposure. Double gloving may be necessary depending on the potential exposure. Polyvinyl chloride exam gloves offer little hazardous drug protection. Look for test information provided by the glove manufacturer showing resistance to specific hazardous drugs. If gloves are made with latex, make sure your patient doesn't have a latex allergy.
  - Gowns: These should be long-sleeved, with tight-fitting cuffs. Disposable gowns coated with laminate materials provide better protection than noncoated gowns. Refer to the manufacturer for permeation information. Don't reuse gowns; change gowns immediately after a spill or splash.
  - Respirators: A properly fit-tested certified N-95 respirator or surgical N-95 respirator provides protection from most airborne particles. Other types of respirators may be necessary to protect from airborne gases. Surgical masks don't provide adequate respiratory protection from drug exposure.
  - Face shields: Using face shields with goggles protects against splashes to the face and eyes. Full-face respirators also provide protection. Face shields or eye glasses with side shields don't provide full eye and face protection.
  - Sleeve, hair, and shoe covers: These covers help provide additional protection. They may be required in certain environments such as drug-compounding areas.

Strategies for reducing error rates

In addition to improvements in communication and education, other strategies that have helped reduce medication administration error rates include:

- providing adequate nurse-to-patient staffing ratios
- designing drug preparation areas as safety zones that promote making correct choices during the medication administration process according to drug importance, frequency of use, and sequence of use
- improving the medication administration environment (reduce noise to 50 dB, improve lighting to at least 100 foot-candles, obtain nonglare computer screens)
- developing and using protocols that reduce distractions for nursing staff directly involved in administering medications

- dispensing medications in unit-dose or unit-of-use packaging
- restricting high-alert drugs and administration routes (limiting their number, variety, and concentration in patient care areas). For example, remove all neuromuscular blockers from units where patients aren't normally intubated. Remove highly concentrated electrolytes from unit stock in patient care units. Remove concentrated oral opioids from unit stock and dispensing cabinets. Apply additional strong warnings to drug labels. Make sure emergency equipment is always available.
- switching from IV to oral or subcut forms as soon as possible
- dispensing IV and epidural infusions only from the pharmacy
- labeling all medications both on and off the sterile field
- posting drug information in patient care units and having drug information available for all health care providers at the point of care; using infusion rate and dosing charts in patient care areas
- avoiding unapproved abbreviations
- using leading zeros; for example, use "0.5 mg" rather than ".5 mg"
- avoiding trailing zeros; for example, use "5 mg" rather than "5.0 mg"
- requiring that medication orders be prescribed by metric weight, not by volume (for example, in mg/kg not mL). Never rely on a patient's stated or historical weight. Weigh patients as soon as possible, and measure and document actual weights only in metric units in all electronic and written formats.
- establishing protocols and checklists to double-check and document unusual drugs, dosages, or regimens
- always recalculating doses before giving drugs to children or neonates. Make sure that the dose formula is included for calculating the dose. Have a second clinician (preferably a pharmacist) double-check the calculations.
- making sure each patient is monitored appropriately before and after drug administration. Have appropriate monitoring equipment (cardiac monitors, capnography, pulse oximeters) available as needed.

Using technology to promote safety

Technology is becoming an increasingly important part of providing safer drug administration. The goal of medication administration technology is to enhance individual practice and help build safeguards into the medication administration process. Information about ISMP and safe medication practices can be found at http://ismp.org/.

Computerized provider order entry

In computerized provider order entry (CPOE), the prescriber enters the medication orders into a computerized record, thus eliminating errors due to illegible handwriting. Such safeguards as immediate order checking for errors (such as incorrect dosing or routes of administration) and drug interactions, allergy checks, and administration protocols can be built into the system. Orders can be immediately transmitted to the appropriate department and can also be linked to drug information databases. CPOE can be used to monitor how drugs are utilized and can provide data for quality improvement.

Bar codes

Bar-code technology is widely used and was initially developed to help control and track inventory for industry. The use of this technology for safer drug administration, dispensing, inventory control, and drug storage and preparation has been endorsed by the IOM, The Joint Commission, Agency for Healthcare Research and Quality, and ISMP. With this technology, the patient wears a bar-code identifier on a wristband; the medication also has a bar code that uses the medication's own unique National Drug Code to identify the name, dose, manufacturer, and type of packaging. The nurse scans the bar code using an optical scanner, verifying the patient's identity and medication. The system supports but does not replace the traditional "rights" of safe medication.

Bar-code systems have been shown to reduce medication errors, but they aren't without disadvantages. For example, they don't save time in the medication administration process. Problems with the technology can cause delays in treatment. Wristbands can become unreadable due to wear, and scanners can malfunction. These problems may tempt nurses to develop dangerous shortcuts, such as attaching patients' wristbands to clipboards or giving the patient the medication first and then scanning the wristband.

Automated dispensing cabinets

Automated dispensing cabinets (ADCs) are computer-controlled medication distribution systems in the patient care unit or ancillary department that are used to store, track, and dispense medications. ADCs can provide nurses with near-total access to medications needed in their patient care area and promote the control and security of medications. They electronically track the use of drugs such as controlled substances. They may have bar-code capabilities for restocking and correct medication selection, and can be programmed to provide safeguards such as drug safety alerts. ADCs can be linked with external databases and billing systems to increase the efficiency of drug dispensing and billing.

"Smart" pumps

From 2005 through 2009, the FDA received 56,000 reports of adverse events and 500 deaths linked to infusion pumps. Currently, there are initiatives to improve infusion systems and technology. "Smart" IV pumps can have such features as programmable drug libraries and dosage limits, can perform automatic calculations, have dose-error reduction software, and can be programmed to signal dosage alerts. ISMP recommends administering high-alert IV medications using programmable infusion pumps with dose error-reduction software. They can be integrated with bar-code and CPOE technologies and can be wireless. Smart pumps can help alert nurses when incorrect dosages have been selected or to dosages that may exceed recommended levels.

Smart pumps can't detect all problems with IV drug infusions, however. For example, an incorrect drug can be selected from the library database and, with some pumps, it's possible to override safety alerts. Other infusion pump problems include software defects and failure of built-in safety alarms. Some pumps have ambiguous on-screen directions that can lead to dosing errors. The FDA recommends reporting all infusion-related adverse events, planning ahead in case a pump fails, labeling the channels and tubing to prevent errors, checking all settings, and monitoring patients for signs and symptoms of infusion problems. Nurses should perform independent calculation of all doses and infusion rates and not rely solely on the pump. It's essential to double-check each dose calculation. Nurses shouldn't bypass pump alarms and must verify that the pump is functioning properly before beginning an infusion.

Other technologies

Using oral syringes that don't have luer-locks to administer oral or enteral medications helps prevent oral or enteral medications from being administered via the wrong route. (The ISMP has reported cases in which oral medications were drawn into parenteral syringes and inadvertently injected into IV lines, resulting in patient deaths.) Utilizing special tubing that doesn't have side ports for epidural medication administration prevents inadvertent injection of an incorrect drug into the epidural catheter. Certain drugs such as vincristine should always be dispensed in a minibag (25 to 50 mL) of solution and never in a syringe, to avoid accidental intrathecal instead of IV administration. Oral liquid dosing devices, such as syringes, cups, and droppers, should display the metric scale only.

Reporting medication errors

Clearly, medication errors are a major threat to patient safety. Only by sharing and analyzing data and performing more research can evidence-based quality improvements be developed and validated. Several agencies and organizations provide voluntary reporting systems to study the causes and prevalence of medication errors. The FDA has its Adverse Event Reporting System, which is part of the MedWatch program. The USP maintains MEDMARX (a national database utilized to lower the incidence of hospital medication errors) and the Medication Errors Reporting Program (MERP). In addition, the USP works with the ISMP to compile voluntary reports of medication errors. The reports are analyzed by these watchdog agencies, and information is published about their findings. Nurses should be encouraged to report medication errors and "near misses" and to help identify problems within systems.

4
Selected therapeutic drug classifications

Alkylating drugs
bendamustine hydrochloride, busulfan, CARBOplatin, carmustine, chlorambucil, CISplatin, cyclophosphamide, dacarbazine, ifosfamide, lomustine, melphalan, oxaliplatin, temozolomide, thiotepa

INDICATIONS
➤ **Various tumors, especially those with large volume and slow cell-turnover rate**

ACTION
Alkylating drugs appear to act independently of a specific cell-cycle phase. Highly reactive, they primarily target nucleic acids and form links with the nuclei of different molecules. This allows the drugs to cross-link double-stranded DNA and to prevent strands from separating for replication, which may contribute to these drugs' ability to destroy cells. These polyfunctional compounds can be divided chemically into five groups: nitrogen mustards, ethyleneamines, alkyl sulfonates, triazines, and nitrosoureas.

ADVERSE REACTIONS
The most common adverse reactions are bone marrow depression, chills, diarrhea, fever, flank pain, hair loss, leukopenia, nausea, redness or pain at the injection site, sore throat, swelling of the feet or lower legs, thrombocytopenia, secondary leukemia, infertility, and vomiting.

CONTRAINDICATIONS & CAUTIONS
Black Box Warning Refer to individual drug monographs for black box warnings. ∎
• Contraindicated in patients hypersensitive to these drugs.
• Use cautiously in patients receiving other cell-destroying drugs or radiation.
• May cause fetal harm if administered during pregnancy. Females and males with female partners of childbearing potential should use effective contraception during therapy. Consult individual drug monographs for contraception recommendations after final dose of drug. Breastfeeding women should stop breastfeeding during therapy because drugs appear in human milk. Safety and effectiveness of many alkylating drugs haven't been established in children. Elderly patients are at increased risk for adverse reactions; monitor closely.

Alpha blockers (peripherally acting)
alfuzosin hydrochloride, doxazosin mesylate, phentolamine mesylate, prazosin hydrochloride, silodosin, tamsulosin hydrochloride, terazosin hydrochloride

INDICATIONS
➤ **HTN, or mild to moderate urinary obstruction in men with BPH**

ACTION
Selective alpha blockers decrease vascular resistance and increase vein capacity, thereby lowering BP and causing nasal and scleroconjunctival congestion, ptosis, orthostatic and exercise hypotension, mild to moderate miosis, interference with ejaculation, and pink, warm skin. They also relax nonvascular smooth muscle, especially in the prostate capsule, which reduces urinary problems in men with BPH. Because alpha$_1$ blockers don't block alpha$_2$ receptors, they don't cause transmitter overflow.

Nonselective alpha blockers antagonize both alpha$_1$ and alpha$_2$ receptors. Generally, alpha blockade results in tachycardia, palpitations, and increased renin secretion because of abnormally large amounts of norepinephrine (from transmitter overflow) released from adrenergic nerve endings as a result of the blockade of alpha$_1$ and alpha$_2$ receptors. Norepinephrine's effects are counterproductive to the major uses of nonselective alpha blockers.

ADVERSE REACTIONS
Alpha blockers may cause severe orthostatic hypotension and syncope, especially with the first few doses, an effect commonly called the *first-dose effect.* The most common adverse effects of alpha$_1$ blockade are dizziness, headache, drowsiness, somnolence, and malaise. These drugs also may cause tachycardia, palpitations, fluid retention (from excess renin secretion),

nasal and ocular congestion, weakness, and aggravation of respiratory tract infection.

CONTRAINDICATIONS & CAUTIONS

• Contraindicated in patients hypersensitive to these drugs or their components. Also contraindicated in combination therapy with PDE5 inhibitors (sildenafil, tadalafil, vardenafil) due to increased risk of hypotension. Discontinue if symptoms of angina or coronary insufficiency occur. May cause hypotension and increased risk of syncope. Use cautiously. Alfuzosin is contraindicated in patients with moderate or severe hepatic insufficiency and when given with potent CYP3A4 inhibitors.

• In pregnant or breastfeeding women, use cautiously. In children, safety and effectiveness of many alpha blockers haven't been established; use cautiously. In elderly patients, hypotensive effects may be more pronounced.

Alzheimer disease drugs

donepezil hydrochloride, galantamine hydrobromide, memantine hydrochloride, rivastigmine tartrate

INDICATIONS

➤ Treatment of mild to moderate dementia of the Alzheimer type

ACTION

Current theories attribute signs and symptoms of Alzheimer disease to a deficiency of cholinergic neurotransmission. It's suggested that these drugs improve cholinergic function by increasing acetylcholine levels through reversible inhibition of its hydrolysis by cholinesterase. Memantine is an N-methyl-D-aspartate (NMDA) receptor antagonist. Persistent activation of the NMDA receptors is thought to contribute to the symptoms of Alzheimer disease. No evidence indicates that these drugs alter the course of the underlying disease process.

ADVERSE REACTIONS

Weight loss, diarrhea, anorexia, nausea, vomiting, dizziness, headache, bradyarrhythmias; HTN and constipation (memantine).

CONTRAINDICATIONS & CAUTIONS

• Contraindicated in patients hypersensitive to these drugs or their components.

• May exaggerate neuromuscular blocking effects of succinylcholine-type and similar neuromuscular blockers used during anesthesia.

• Use cautiously with concomitant drugs that slow HR because of increased risk of heart block.

• Use cautiously with NSAIDs because the drugs increase gastric acid secretion. There is increased risk of developing ulcers and active or occult GI bleeding.

• Use cautiously in patients with moderate hepatic or renal impairment. Some drugs aren't recommended in severe hepatic impairment or severe renal impairment. Refer to manufacturer's instructions for use and dosage adjustments for patients with renal impairment.

• Use cautiously in patients with a history of asthma or COPD.

Aminoglycosides

amikacin sulfate, gentamicin sulfate, neomycin sulfate, tobramycin sulfate

INDICATIONS

➤ Septicemia; postoperative, pulmonary, intra-abdominal, and urinary tract infections; skin, soft-tissue, bone, and joint infections; aerobic gram-negative bacillary meningitis not susceptible to other antibiotics; serious staphylococcal, *Pseudomonas aeruginosa*, and *Klebsiella* infections; enterococcal infections; nosocomial pneumonia; TB; initial empirical therapy in febrile, leukopenic patients

ACTION

Aminoglycosides are bactericidal. They bind directly and irreversibly to 30S ribosomal subunits, inhibiting bacterial protein synthesis. They're active against many aerobic gram-negative and some aerobic gram-positive organisms and can be used with other antibiotics for short courses of therapy.

ADVERSE REACTIONS

Ototoxicity and nephrotoxicity are the most serious complications. Neuromuscular blockade also may occur. Oral forms (neomycin) most commonly cause diarrhea, nausea, and vomiting. Parenteral drugs may cause vein irritation, phlebitis, and sterile abscess.

DRUG CLASSES

CONTRAINDICATIONS & CAUTIONS

Black Box Warning Refer to individual drug monographs for black box warnings. ∎
• Contraindicated in patients hypersensitive to these drugs.

Black Box Warning Aminoglycosides are associated with significant nephrotoxicity and ototoxicity. Toxicity may develop even with conventional doses, particularly in patients with prerenal azotemia or impaired renal function. Evidence of renal function impairment or ototoxicity requires drug discontinuation or appropriate dosage adjustments. When possible, monitor serum drug concentrations. Avoid use with other ototoxic, neurotoxic, or nephrotoxic drugs. Aminoglycosides can cause fetal harm when given to pregnant women. ∎
• Use cautiously in patients with neuromuscular disorders and in those taking neuromuscular blockers.
• Use at lower dosages in patients with renal impairment.
• In pregnant women, use cautiously. Safety hasn't been established in breastfeeding women. In neonates and premature infants, the half-life of aminoglycosides is prolonged because of immature renal systems. In infants and children, dosage adjustment may be needed. Elderly patients have an increased risk of nephrotoxicity and commonly need a lower dose and longer dosage intervals; they're also susceptible to ototoxicity and superinfection.

Angiotensin-converting enzyme inhibitors

benazepril hydrochloride, captopril, enalaprilat, enalapril maleate, fosinopril sodium, lisinopril, moexipril hydrochloride, perindopril erbumine, quinapril hydrochloride, ramipril, trandolapril

INDICATIONS
➤ HTN, HF, left ventricular dysfunction (LVD), MI, and diabetic nephropathy

ACTION
ACE inhibitors prevent conversion of angiotensin I to angiotensin II, a potent vasoconstrictor. Besides decreasing vasoconstriction and thus reducing peripheral arterial resistance, inhibiting angiotensin II decreases adrenocortical secretion of aldosterone. This reduces sodium and water retention and extracellular fluid volume. ACE inhibition also causes increased levels of bradykinin, which results in vasodilation. This decreases HR and systemic vascular resistance.

ADVERSE REACTIONS
The most common adverse effects of therapeutic doses are angioedema of the face and limbs, dry cough, dysgeusia, fatigue, headache, hyperkalemia, hypotension, proteinuria, rash, and tachycardia. Severe hypotension may occur at toxic drug levels.

CONTRAINDICATIONS & CAUTIONS
• Contraindicated in patients hypersensitive to these drugs.

Black Box Warning When pregnancy is detected, discontinue drug as soon as possible. Drugs that act directly on the RAAS can cause fetal injury and death. ∎
• Use cautiously in patients with impaired renal function or serious autoimmune disease and in those taking other drugs known to decrease WBC count or immune response.
• Women of childbearing potential taking ACE inhibitors should report suspected pregnancy immediately to the prescriber. High risks of fetal morbidity and mortality are linked to ACE inhibitors, especially in the second and third trimesters. Some ACE inhibitors appear in human milk; instruct patient to stop breastfeeding during therapy. Safety in children hasn't been established for all products; for use in children, refer to manufacturer's instructions for individual products. Elderly patients may need lower doses because of impaired drug clearance.

Antacids

aluminum hydroxide, calcium carbonate, magnesium hydroxide, magnesium oxide, sodium bicarbonate

INDICATIONS
➤ Gastric hyperacidity; hyperphosphatemia (aluminum hydroxide); hypomagnesemia (magnesium oxide); postmenopausal hypocalcemia (calcium carbonate)

ACTION
Antacids reduce the total acid load in the GI tract and elevate gastric pH to reduce pepsin activity. They also strengthen the gastric mucosal barrier and increase esophageal sphincter

DRUG CLASSES

tone. Aluminum-containing antacids bind with phosphate ions in the intestine to form insoluble aluminum phosphate, which is excreted in feces. Calcium helps to prevent or treat negative calcium balance and bone loss in osteoporosis.

ADVERSE REACTIONS
Antacids containing aluminum may cause aluminum intoxication, constipation, hypophosphatemia, intestinal obstruction, and osteomalacia. Antacids containing magnesium may cause diarrhea or hypermagnesemia (in renal failure). Calcium carbonate, magnesium oxide, and sodium bicarbonate may cause constipation, milk-alkali syndrome, and rebound hyperacidity.

CONTRAINDICATIONS & CAUTIONS
• Calcium carbonate and magnesium oxide are contraindicated in patients with severe renal disease. Sodium bicarbonate is contraindicated in patients with HTN, renal disease, or edema; in those who are vomiting; in those receiving diuretics or continuous GI suction; and in those on sodium-restricted diets.
• Use magnesium oxide cautiously in patients with mild renal impairment.
• Give aluminum preparations and calcium carbonate cautiously in elderly patients; in those receiving antidiarrheals, antispasmodics, or anticholinergics; and in those with dehydration, fluid restriction, chronic renal disease, or suspected intestinal absorption problems.
• Pregnant and breastfeeding women should consult their prescriber before using antacids. Serious adverse effects from changes in fluid and electrolyte balance are more likely in infants; monitor them closely. Elderly patients have an increased risk of adverse reactions; monitor them closely.

Antianginals
ranolazine

Beta blockers
atenolol, bisoprolol fumarate, metoprolol, nadolol, propranolol hydrochloride

Calcium channel blockers
amLODIPine besylate, dilTIAZem hydrochloride, niCARdipine hydrochloride, NIFEdipine, verapamil hydrochloride

Nitrates
isosorbide (dinitrate; mononitrate), nitroglycerin

INDICATIONS
➤ **Moderate to severe angina (beta blockers); classic, effort-induced angina and Prinzmetal angina (calcium channel blockers); recurrent angina (long-acting nitrates and topical, transdermal, transmucosal, and oral extended-release nitroglycerin); acute angina (SL nitroglycerin and SL or chewable isosorbide dinitrate); unstable angina (IV nitroglycerin); chronic angina (ranolazine)**

ACTION
The mechanism of action of ranolazine's antianginal effects hasn't been determined. Beta blockers decrease catecholamine-induced increases in HR, BP, and myocardial contraction. Calcium channel blockers inhibit the flow of calcium through muscle cells, which dilates coronary arteries and decreases systemic vascular resistance, known as *afterload*. Nitrates decrease afterload and left ventricular end-diastolic pressure, or *preload*, and increase blood flow through collateral coronary vessels.

ADVERSE REACTIONS
Ranolazine may cause QT-interval prolongation, dizziness, constipation, and nausea. Beta blockers may cause bradycardia, cough, diarrhea, disturbing dreams, dizziness, dyspnea, fatigue, fever, HF, hypotension, lethargy, nausea, peripheral edema, and wheezing. Calcium channel blockers may cause bradycardia, heart block, confusion, constipation, depression, diarrhea, dizziness, dyspepsia, edema, elevated liver enzyme levels (transient), fatigue, flushing, headache, hypotension, insomnia, nervousness, and rash. Nitrates may cause flushing, headache, orthostatic hypotension, reflex tachycardia, rash, syncope, and vomiting.

CONTRAINDICATIONS & CAUTIONS
• Contraindicated in patients hypersensitive to these drugs.
Black Box Warning Abrupt discontinuation of beta blocker therapy has been associated with angina exacerbation and, in some cases, MI and ventricular arrhythmias. When discontinuation of beta blockers is planned, gradually reduce dosage over at least a few weeks. ■

DRUG CLASSES

• Ranolazine is contraindicated in patients taking strong inhibitors of CYP3A or inducers of CYP3A and in those with clinically significant hepatic impairment. Beta blockers are contraindicated in patients with cardiogenic shock, sinus bradycardia, heart block greater than first degree, or bronchial asthma. Calcium channel blockers are contraindicated in patients with severe hypotension or heart block greater than first degree (except with functioning pacemaker). Nitrates are contraindicated in patients with severe anemia, cerebral hemorrhage, head trauma, or glaucoma, and in patients using PDE5 inhibitors (sildenafil, tadalafil, vardenafil).

• Use beta blockers cautiously in patients with nonallergic bronchospastic disorders, diabetes mellitus, or impaired hepatic or renal function. Use calcium channel blockers cautiously in those with hepatic or renal impairment, bradycardia, HF, or cardiogenic shock. Use nitrates cautiously in those with hypotension or recent MI.

• Use beta blockers cautiously in pregnant women. Recommendations for breastfeeding vary by drug; use beta blockers and calcium channel blockers cautiously. Safety and effectiveness haven't been established in children. Check with the prescriber before giving these drugs to children. Elderly patients have an increased risk of adverse reactions; use cautiously.

Antiarrhythmics
adenosine

Class IA
disopyramide phosphate, procainamide hydrochloride, quiNIDine (gluconate; sulfate)

Class IB
lidocaine hydrochloride, mexiletine hydrochloride

Class IC
flecainide acetate, propafenone hydrochloride

Class II (beta blockers)
esmolol hydrochloride, propranolol hydrochloride, sotalol hydrochloride

Class III
amiodarone hydrochloride, dofetilide, dronedarone, ibutilide fumarate, sotalol hydrochloride

Class IV (calcium channel blockers)
dilTIAZem hydrochloride, verapamil hydrochloride

INDICATIONS
➤ Atrial and ventricular arrhythmias

ACTION
Class I drugs reduce the inward current carried by sodium ions, which stabilizes neuronal cardiac membranes. Class IA drugs depress phase 0, prolong the action potential, and stabilize cardiac membranes. Class IB drugs depress phase 0, shorten the action potential, and stabilize cardiac membranes. Class IC drugs block the transport of sodium ions, which decreases conduction velocity but not repolarization rate. Class II drugs decrease HR, myocardial contractility, BP, and AV node conduction. Class III drugs prolong the repolarization phase. Class IV drugs decrease myocardial contractility and oxygen demand by inhibiting calcium ion influx; they also dilate coronary arteries and arterioles.

ADVERSE REACTIONS
Most antiarrhythmics can aggravate existing arrhythmias or cause new ones. They also may produce CNS disturbances, such as dizziness or fatigue; GI problems, such as nausea, vomiting, or altered bowel elimination; hypersensitivity reactions; and hypotension. Some antiarrhythmics may worsen HF. Class II drugs may cause bronchoconstriction.

CONTRAINDICATIONS & CAUTIONS
Black Box Warning Refer to individual drug monographs for black box warnings. ∎
• Contraindicated in patients hypersensitive to these drugs.
• Many antiarrhythmics are contraindicated or require cautious use in patients with cardiogenic shock, digitalis toxicity, and second- or third-degree heart block (unless patient has a pacemaker or implantable cardioverter defibrillator).
• In pregnant women, use only if potential benefits to the mother outweigh fetal risks. Use cautiously in breastfeeding women; many antiarrhythmics appear in human milk. Monitor children closely because they have an increased

risk of adverse reactions. Use cautiously in elderly patients, who may exhibit physiologic alterations in CV system.

Antibiotic antineoplastics

bleomycin sulfate, DAUNOrubicin hydrochloride, DAUNOrubicin citrate (liposomal), DOXOrubicin hydrochloride, epiRUBicin hydrochloride, IDArubicin hydrochloride, mitoMYcin

INDICATIONS
➤ Various solid tumors, leukemia

ACTION
Although classified as antibiotics, these drugs destroy cells, thus ruling out their use as antimicrobials alone. They interfere with proliferation of malignant cells in several ways. Their action may be specific to cell-cycle phase, not specific to cell-cycle phase, or both. Some of these drugs act like alkylating drugs or antimetabolites. By binding to or creating complexes with DNA, antibiotic antineoplastics directly or indirectly inhibit DNA, RNA, and protein synthesis.

ADVERSE REACTIONS
The most common adverse reactions include anxiety, bone marrow depression, chills, confusion, diarrhea, ECG changes, extravasation, fever, flank or joint pain, hair loss, nausea, redness or pain at the injection site, sore throat, swelling of the feet or lower legs, vomiting, and cardiomyopathy.

CONTRAINDICATIONS & CAUTIONS
Black Box Warning Refer to individual drug monographs for black box warnings. ∎
• Contraindicated in patients hypersensitive to these drugs.
• In pregnant women, avoid antineoplastics. Breastfeeding during therapy isn't recommended. Safety and effectiveness of some drugs haven't been established in children; use cautiously. Use cautiously in elderly patients because of their increased risk of adverse reactions.

Anticholinergics

atropine sulfate, benztropine mesylate, dicyclomine hydrochloride, scopolamine

INDICATIONS
➤ Prevention of motion sickness, preoperative reduction of secretions and blockage of cardiac reflexes, adjunctive treatment of peptic ulcers and other GI disorders, blockage of cholinomimetic effects of cholinesterase inhibitors or other drugs, and (for benztropine) various spastic conditions, including acute dystonic reactions, muscle rigidity, parkinsonism, and extrapyramidal disorders

ACTION
Anticholinergics competitively antagonize the actions of acetylcholine and other cholinergic agonists at muscarinic receptors.

ADVERSE REACTIONS
Therapeutic doses commonly cause blurred vision, constipation, cycloplegia, decreased sweating or anhidrosis, dry mouth, headache, mydriasis, palpitations, tachycardia, urinary hesitancy, and urine retention. These reactions usually disappear when therapy stops. Toxicity can cause signs and symptoms resembling psychosis (disorientation, confusion, hallucinations, delusions, anxiety, agitation, and restlessness); dilated, nonreactive pupils; blurred vision; hot, dry, flushed skin; dry mucous membranes; dysphagia; decreased or absent bowel sounds; urine retention; hyperthermia; tachycardia; HTN; and increased respirations.

CONTRAINDICATIONS & CAUTIONS
• Contraindicated in patients hypersensitive to these drugs and in those with angle-closure glaucoma, renal or GI obstructive disease, reflux esophagitis, or myasthenia gravis.
• Use cautiously in patients with heart disease, GI infection, open-angle glaucoma, prostatic hypertrophy, HTN, hyperthyroidism, ulcerative colitis, autonomic neuropathy, or hiatal hernia with reflux esophagitis.
• Safety hasn't been established in pregnant women. In breastfeeding women, avoid anticholinergics because they may decrease milk production; some may appear in human milk and cause infant toxicity. Safety and effectiveness in children haven't been established. Patients older than age 40 may be more sensitive to these drugs. In elderly patients, use cautiously and reduce dosage, as indicated.

DRUG CLASSES

Anticoagulants

Heparin derivative
heparin sodium

Low-molecular-weight heparins
dalteparin sodium, enoxaparin sodium

Selective factor Xa inhibitors
apixaban, betrixaban, edoxaban,
fondaparinux sodium, rivaroxaban

Thrombin inhibitors
argatroban, bivalirudin, dabigatran
etexilate mesylate

Vitamin K inhibitor
warfarin sodium

INDICATIONS
➤ **PE, DVT, thrombus, DIC, unstable
angina, MI, atrial fibrillation, heparin-
induced thrombocytopenia, heparin-
induced thrombosis–thrombocytopenia
syndrome**

ACTION
Heparin derivatives accelerate formation of an
antithrombin–thrombin complex. They inactivate thrombin and prevent conversion of fibrinogen to fibrin. Thrombin inhibitors directly
bind to thrombin and inhibit its action. Selective
factor Xa inhibitors directly bind to factor Xa.
Warfarin inhibits vitamin K–dependent activation of clotting factors II, VII, IX, and X, which
are formed in the liver.

ADVERSE REACTIONS
Anticoagulants commonly cause bleeding and
may cause hypersensitivity reactions. Heparin derivatives may cause thrombocytopenia
and may increase liver enzyme levels. Non-
hemorrhagic adverse reactions associated with
thrombin inhibitors may include back pain,
bradycardia, and hypotension. Warfarin may
cause agranulocytosis, alopecia (long-term use),
anorexia, dermatitis, fever, nausea, tissue necrosis or gangrene, urticaria, and vomiting.

CONTRAINDICATIONS & CAUTIONS
Black Box Warning Refer to individual drug
monographs for black box warnings. ■
• Contraindicated in patients hypersensitive
to these drugs or their components; in patients with aneurysm, active bleeding, CV

hemorrhage, hemorrhagic blood dyscrasias,
hemophilia, severe HTN, pericardial effusions,
or pericarditis; and in patients undergoing major surgery, neurosurgery, neuraxial anesthesia,
spinal puncture, or ophthalmic surgery.
• Heparin formulations are contraindicated in
patients with history of heparin-induced thrombocytopenia or heparin-induced thrombosis–
thrombocytopenia syndrome.
• Use cautiously in patients with severe diabetes, renal impairment, severe trauma, ulcerations, or vasculitis.
• Most anticoagulants (except warfarin) may
be used in pregnancy only if potential benefit
to the mother outweighs potential risk to the fetus. In pregnant women and those who have just
had a threatened or complete spontaneous abortion, warfarin is contraindicated. Women should
avoid breastfeeding during therapy. Infants, especially neonates, may be more susceptible to
anticoagulants because of vitamin K deficiency.
Elderly patients are at greater risk for hemorrhage because of altered hemostatic mechanisms and age-related deterioration of hepatic
and renal functions.

Anticonvulsants

brivaracetam, carBAMazepine, cloBAZam,
clonazePAM, diazePAM, eslicarbazepine
acetate, felbamate, fosphenytoin
sodium, gabapentin, lacosamide,
lamoTRIgine, levETIRAcetam, magnesium
sulfate, OXcarbazepine, phenytoin
sodium, primidone, rufinamide,
tiaGABine hydrochloride, topiramate,
valproate sodium, valproic acid,
vigabatrin, zonisamide

INDICATIONS
➤ **Seizure disorders; acute, isolated
seizures not caused by seizure disorders;
status epilepticus; prevention of seizures
after trauma or craniotomy; neuropathic
pain**

ACTION
Anticonvulsants include six classes of drugs:
selected hydantoin derivatives, barbiturates,
benzodiazepines, succinimides, iminostilbene derivatives (carbamazepine), and val-
proic/carboxylic acid derivatives. Magnesium
sulfate is a miscellaneous anticonvulsant. Some
hydantoin derivatives and carbamazepine inhibit the spread of seizure activity in the motor

cortex. Some barbiturates and succinimides limit seizure activity by increasing the threshold for motor cortex stimuli. Selected benzodiazepines and valproic/carboxylic acid derivatives may increase inhibition of GABA in brain neurons. Magnesium sulfate interferes with the release of acetylcholine at the myoneural junction.

ADVERSE REACTIONS

Anticonvulsants can cause adverse CNS effects, such as ataxia, confusion, somnolence, and tremor. Many anticonvulsants also cause CV disorders, such as arrhythmias and hypotension; GI effects, such as vomiting; and hematologic disorders, such as agranulocytosis, bone marrow depression, leukopenia, and thrombocytopenia. SJS, other severe rashes, and abnormal LFT results may also occur.

CONTRAINDICATIONS & CAUTIONS

Black Box Warning Refer to individual drug monographs for black box warnings. ■
• Contraindicated in patients hypersensitive to these drugs.
• Carbamazepine is contraindicated within 14 days of MAO inhibitor use.
• Use cautiously in patients with blood dyscrasias. Also, use barbiturates cautiously in patients with suicidal ideation.
• In pregnant women, therapy may continue despite the fetal risks caused by some anticonvulsants. Refer to manufacturer's instructions for each product for use during pregnancy and breastfeeding. Children, especially young ones, are sensitive to the CNS depression of some anticonvulsants; use cautiously. Elderly patients are sensitive to CNS effects and may need lower doses. Also, some anticonvulsants may take longer to be eliminated because of decreased renal function, and parenteral use is more likely to cause apnea, hypotension, bradycardia, and cardiac arrest.

Antidepressants, tricyclic

amitriptyline hydrochloride, amoxapine, clomiPRAMINE hydrochloride, desipramine hydrochloride, doxepin hydrochloride, imipramine (hydrochloride; pamoate), nortriptyline hydrochloride, protriptyline hydrochloride, trimipramine

INDICATIONS

➤ **Depression, anxiety (doxepin), OCD (clomipramine), enuresis in children older than age 6 (imipramine), neuropathic pain**

ACTION

TCAs may inhibit reuptake of norepinephrine and serotonin in CNS nerve terminals (presynaptic neurons), thus enhancing the concentration and activity of neurotransmitters in the synaptic cleft. TCAs also exert antihistaminic, sedative, anticholinergic, vasodilatory, and quinidine-like effects.

ADVERSE REACTIONS

Adverse reactions include anticholinergic effects, orthostatic hypotension, and sedation. The tertiary amines (amitriptyline, doxepin, imipramine, and trimipramine) exert the strongest sedative effects; tolerance usually develops in a few weeks. TCAs may cause CV effects such as T-wave abnormalities, conduction disturbances, and arrhythmias.

CONTRAINDICATIONS & CAUTIONS

Black Box Warning Antidepressants can increase the risk of suicidal thinking and behavior. Appropriately monitor patients of all ages who are started on antidepressant therapy, and observe closely for clinical worsening, suicidality, or unusual changes in behavior. Advise families and caregivers of the need for close observation and communication with the prescriber. ■
• Contraindicated in patients hypersensitive to these drugs and in patients with urine retention or angle-closure glaucoma.
• TCAs are contraindicated within 2 weeks of MAO inhibitor therapy.
• Use cautiously in patients with suicidal tendencies, schizophrenia, paranoia, seizure disorders, CV disease, or impaired hepatic function.
• In pregnant and breastfeeding women, safety hasn't been established; use cautiously. In children younger than age 12, TCAs aren't recommended except for imipramine, which is used for enuresis in children age 6 and older. Elderly patients are more sensitive to therapeutic and adverse effects and need lower dosages.

DRUG CLASSES

Antidiabetics (type 2 diabetes)

acarbose, albiglutide, alogliptin benzoate, bromocriptine mesylate, canagliflozin, dapagliflozin propanediol, empagliflozin, exenatide, glimepiride, glipiZIDE, glyBURIDE, linagliptin, liraglutide, lixisenatide, metFORMIN hydrochloride, miglitol, nateglinide, pioglitazone hydrochloride, pramlintide acetate, repaglinide, rosiglitazone maleate, sAXagliptin hydrochloride, semaglutide, SITagliptin phosphate

INDICATIONS

➤ **Mild to moderately severe, stable, non-ketotic, type 2 diabetes mellitus that can't be controlled by diet alone**

ACTION

Antidiabetics come in several types. Sulfonylureas are sulfonamide derivatives that aren't antibacterial. They lower glucose levels by stimulating insulin release from the pancreas. These drugs work only in the presence of functioning beta cells in the islet tissue of the pancreas. After prolonged administration, they produce hypoglycemia by acting outside of the pancreas, resulting in effects that include reduced glucose production by the liver and enhanced peripheral sensitivity to insulin. The latter may result from an increased number of insulin receptors or from changes after insulin binding.

Meglitinides, such as nateglinide and repaglinide, are nonsulfonylurea antidiabetics that stimulate the release of insulin from the pancreas.

Metformin decreases hepatic glucose production, reduces intestinal glucose absorption, and improves insulin sensitivity by increasing peripheral glucose uptake and utilization. With metformin therapy, insulin secretion remains unchanged, and fasting insulin levels and all-day insulin response may decrease.

Alpha-glucosidase inhibitors, such as acarbose and miglitol, delay digestion of carbohydrates, resulting in a smaller rise in glucose levels. Pramlintide, a human amylin analogue, slows the rate at which food leaves the stomach, decreasing postprandial increase in glucose level, and reduces appetite.

Rosiglitazone and pioglitazone are thiazolidinediones, which lower glucose levels by improving insulin sensitivity. They are potent and highly selective agonists for receptors found in insulin-sensitive tissues, such as adipose tissue, skeletal muscle, and liver.

DPP-4 inhibitors, such as linagliptin and sitagliptin, increase insulin release by inhibiting the enzyme DPP-4. Sodium–glucose cotransporter 2 inhibitors, such as dapagliflozin and empagliflozin, reduce reabsorption of filtered glucose and lower plasma glucose concentration by increasing urinary excretion of glucose.

Glucagonlike peptide 1 receptor agonists (albiglutide, dulaglutide, and others) increase insulin secretion from pancreatic beta cells, suppress glucagon secretion, and slow gastric emptying.

ADVERSE REACTIONS

🕕 **Alert:** All antidiabetics have the potential to cause severe hypoglycemia.

Sulfonylureas cause dose-related reactions that usually respond to decreased dosage: anorexia, headache, heartburn, nausea, paresthesia, vomiting, and weakness.

The most serious adverse reaction linked to metformin is lactic acidosis. It's a rare effect and is most likely to occur in patients with renal dysfunction. Other reactions to metformin include dermatitis, GI upset, megaloblastic anemia, rash, and unpleasant or metallic taste.

Thiazolidinediones may cause fluid retention leading to or exacerbating HF. Alpha-glucosidase inhibitors can cause abdominal pain, diarrhea, and flatulence.

Sodium–glucose cotransporter 2 inhibitors may cause hypotension and abnormal renal function and may increase risk of UTIs.

DPP-4 inhibitors may cause GI reactions and antibody formation.

CONTRAINDICATIONS & CAUTIONS

Black Box Warning Refer to individual drug monographs for black box warnings. ∎

• Contraindicated in patients hypersensitive to these drugs, in patients with history of allergic reaction to sulfonamide derivatives (glimepiride), and in patients with diabetic ketoacidosis with or without coma. Metformin is also contraindicated in patients with renal disease or metabolic acidosis and generally should be avoided in patients with hepatic disease.

• Use sulfonylureas cautiously in patients with renal or hepatic disease or history of sulfonamide antibiotic hypersensitivity. Use metformin cautiously in patients with adrenal or

pituitary insufficiency and in debilitated and malnourished patients. Alpha-glucosidase inhibitors should be used cautiously in patients with mild to moderate renal insufficiency. Thiazolidinediones aren't recommended in patients with edema, HF, or liver disease.
• DPP-4 inhibitors may increase the risk of pancreatitis and are contraindicated in patients with a personal or family history of medullary thyroid cancer and in patients with multiple endocrine neoplasia syndrome type 2.
• Use is contraindicated in pregnant or breast-feeding women. Oral antidiabetics appear in small amounts in human milk and may cause hypoglycemia in the infant. Elderly patients may be more sensitive to these drugs, usually need lower dosages, and are more likely to develop neurologic symptoms of hypoglycemia; monitor these patients closely.

Antidiarrheals
bismuth subsalicylate, diphenoxylate hydrochloride–atropine sulfate, loperamide, octreotide acetate

INDICATIONS
➤ Mild, acute, or chronic diarrhea; certain cancers that cause diarrhea (octreotide acetate)

ACTION
Bismuth preparations may have a mild water-binding capacity, may absorb toxins, and provide a protective coating for the intestinal mucosa. Diphenoxylate and loperamide slow GI motility and excessive GI propulsion. Addition of atropine sulfate to diphenoxylate discourages abuse. Octreotide inhibits secretion of GI neurotransmitters and hormones to control diarrhea.

ADVERSE REACTIONS
Bismuth preparations may cause salicylism (with high doses), temporary darkening of tongue and stools, constipation, and abdominal cramps.

CONTRAINDICATIONS & CAUTIONS
• Contraindicated in patients hypersensitive to these drugs.
• Some antidiarrheals may appear in human milk; check individual drugs for specific recommendations. For children or teenagers recovering from flu or chickenpox, consult prescriber before giving bismuth subsalicylate. For elderly

patients, use caution when giving antidiarrheal drugs.

Antiemetics
aprepitant, dimenhyDRINATE, dolasetron mesylate, dronabinol, fosaprepitant dimeglumine, granisetron hydrochloride, meclizine hydrochloride, metoclopramide hydrochloride, ondansetron hydrochloride, palonosetron hydrochloride, prochlorperazine, prochlorperazine maleate, promethazine hydrochloride, rolapitant hydrochloride, scopolamine, trimethobenzamide hydrochloride

INDICATIONS
➤ Nausea, vomiting, motion sickness, and vertigo

ACTION
For antihistamines (dimenhydrinate, meclizine hydrochloride, trimethobenzamide), the mechanism of action is unclear. Phenothiazines (prochlorperazine, promethazine hydrochloride) work by blocking the dopaminergic receptors in the chemoreceptor trigger zone of the brain. Serotonin receptor antagonists (dolasetron, granisetron, ondansetron) block serotonin stimulation centrally in the chemoreceptor trigger zone and peripherally in vagal nerve terminals. Substance P/neurokinin 1 receptor (NK_1) antagonists (aprepitant, fosaprepitant, rolapitant) inhibit the NK_1 receptor.

ADVERSE REACTIONS
Antiemetics may cause asthenia, fatigue, dizziness, headache, insomnia, abdominal pain, anorexia, constipation, diarrhea, epigastric discomfort, gastritis, heartburn, nausea, vomiting, neutropenia, hiccups, tinnitus, dehydration, and fever. Metoclopramide and prochlorperazine may cause tardive dyskinesia. Rolapitant may cause neutropenia and anemia. Serotonin receptor antagonists may cause headache and increased QT interval.

CONTRAINDICATIONS & CAUTIONS
Black Box Warning Refer to individual drug monographs for black box warnings. ■
• Contraindicated in patients hypersensitive to these drugs or to any of their components.
• Contraindicated in severe vomiting until etiology of vomiting is established.

• Rolapitant is contraindicated in patients receiving CYP2D6 substrates with a narrow therapeutic index, such as thioridazine and pimozide, because of risk of QT-interval prolongation and torsades de pointes due to increased plasma levels of the substrates.

• Use cautiously in patients with tartrazine and sulfite sensitivities. Antiemetics may cause allergic-type reactions, including hives, itching, wheezing, asthma, and anaphylaxis.

Antifungals

amphotericin B (lipid complex; liposomal), anidulafungin, caspofungin acetate, clotrimazole, econazole nitrate, efinaconazole, fluconazole, flucytosine, griseofulvin, isavuconazonium sulfate, itraconazole, ketoconazole, luliconazole, micafungin sodium, miconazole nitrate, nystatin, posaconazole, sertaconazole nitrate, tavaborole, terbinafine hydrochloride, voriconazole

INDICATIONS
➤ **Various fungal infections**

ACTION
The amphotericin products bind to sterols in the fungal cell membrane, altering permeability and allowing intracellular components to leak out. These drugs usually inhibit fungal growth and multiplication, but if the level is high enough, the drugs can destroy fungi. Azole antifungals, nystatin, and terbinafine interfere with sterol synthesis in fungal cells, damaging cell membranes and increasing permeability. Caspofungin inhibits the synthesis of an integral component of fungal cell walls. Tavaborole inhibits fungal protein synthesis. Flucytosine penetrates into fungal cells and is converted to 5-FU, and then converted to several active metabolites, which inhibit protein synthesis. Griseofulvin inhibits cell mitosis at metaphase.

ADVERSE REACTIONS
Fluconazole may cause transient elevations of liver enzymes, alkaline phosphatase, and bilirubin levels, as well as dizziness, nausea, vomiting, abdominal pain, diarrhea, rash, headache, and hypokalemia. Adverse reactions to itraconazole include headache and nausea. The most common adverse reactions to ketoconazole are nausea and vomiting. Efinaconazole, lulicona-

zole, and tavaborole can cause local skin irritation. Adverse reactions to voriconazole are uncommon. However, the drug may alter renal function and cause vision changes. Common adverse reactions to caspofungin include paresthesia, tachycardia, anorexia, anemia, pain, myalgia, tachypnea, chills, and sweating. Reactions to nystatin seldom occur, but may include diarrhea, nausea, vomiting, and abdominal pain. Terbinafine may cause abdominal pain, jaundice, diarrhea, flatulence, nausea, anaphylaxis, headache, rash, and vision disturbances. Flucytosine may cause headache, diarrhea, abdominal pain, and bone marrow depression. Griseofulvin may cause confusion, rash, diarrhea, nausea, vomiting, and decreased granulocyte count.

CONTRAINDICATIONS & CAUTIONS
Black Box Warning Refer to individual drug monographs for black box warnings. ∎
• Contraindicated in patients hypersensitive to these drugs or to any of their components.
• Administer IV amphotericin under close clinical observation. Acute infusion reactions can occur, including fever, shaking chills, hypotension, anorexia, nausea, vomiting, and tachypnea.
• Use caution with concomitant use of caspofungin and cyclosporine because of the possibility of elevated liver enzymes.
• Amphotericin formulations aren't interchangeable and are each prescribed differently.

Antihistamines

cetirizine hydrochloride, chlorpheniramine maleate, desloratadine, diphenhydrAMINE hydrochloride, fexofenadine hydrochloride, levocetirizine dihydrochloride, loratadine, promethazine hydrochloride

INDICATIONS
➤ **Allergic rhinitis, urticaria, pruritus, vertigo, motion sickness, nausea and vomiting, sedation, dyskinesia, parkinsonism**

ACTION
Antihistamines are structurally related chemicals that compete with histamine for H_1-receptor sites on smooth muscle of bronchi, GI tract, and large blood vessels, binding to cellular receptors and preventing access to and subsequent activity of histamine. They don't directly alter histamine or prevent its release.

ADVERSE REACTIONS

First-generation antihistamines cause drowsiness and impaired motor function early in therapy. They also can cause blurred vision, constipation, and dry mouth and throat. Some antihistamines, such as promethazine, may cause cholestatic jaundice, which may be a hypersensitivity reaction, and may predispose patients to photosensitivity. Promethazine may also cause extrapyramidal reactions with high doses.

CONTRAINDICATIONS & CAUTIONS

Black Box Warning Refer to individual drug monographs for black box warnings. ∎
• Contraindicated in patients hypersensitive to these drugs and in those with angle-closure glaucoma, stenosing peptic ulcer, pyloroduodenal obstruction, or bladder neck obstruction. Promethazine is contraindicated in those taking MAO inhibitors.
• In pregnant women, safe use hasn't been established. During breastfeeding, antihistamines shouldn't be used because many of these drugs appear in human milk and may cause unusual excitability in the infant. Neonates, especially premature infants, may experience seizures. Children, especially those younger than age 6, may experience paradoxical hyperexcitability with restlessness, insomnia, nervousness, euphoria, tremors, and seizures; give cautiously. Elderly patients usually are more sensitive to the adverse effects of antihistamines, especially dizziness, sedation, hypotension, and urine retention; use cautiously and monitor these patients closely.

Antihypertensives

ACE inhibitors
benazepril hydrochloride, captopril, enalaprilat, enalapril maleate, fosinopril sodium, lisinopril, moexipril hydrochloride, perindopril erbumine, quinapril hydrochloride, ramipril, trandolapril

Angiotensin II receptor blockers
azilsartan kamedoxomil, candesartan cilexetil, eprosartan mesylate, irbesartan, losartan potassium, olmesartan medoxomil, telmisartan, valsartan

Beta blockers
atenolol, bisoprolol fumarate, carvedilol, labetalol hydrochloride, metoprolol (succinate; tartrate), nadolol, propranolol hydrochloride

Calcium channel blockers
amLODIPine besylate, dilTIAZem hydrochloride, felodipine, niCARdipine hydrochloride, NIFEdipine, nisoldipine, verapamil hydrochloride

Centrally acting alpha blockers (sympatholytics)
cloNIDine hydrochloride, guanFACINE hydrochloride, methyldopa

Direct renin inhibitor
aliskiren hemifumarate

Peripherally acting alpha blockers
doxazosin mesylate, prazosin hydrochloride, terazosin hydrochloride

Vasodilators
hydrALAZINE hydrochloride, nitroglycerin, nitroprusside sodium

INDICATIONS
➤ Essential and secondary HTN

ACTION
For information on the action of ACE inhibitors, alpha blockers, ARBs, beta blockers, calcium channel blockers, and diuretics, see their individual drug class entries. Centrally acting sympatholytics stimulate central alpha-adrenergic receptors, reducing cerebral sympathetic outflow, thereby decreasing peripheral vascular resistance and BP. Vasodilators act directly on smooth muscle to reduce BP.

ADVERSE REACTIONS
Antihypertensives commonly cause orthostatic changes in HR, headache, hypotension, nausea, and vomiting. Other reactions vary greatly among different drug types. Centrally acting sympatholytics may cause constipation, depression, dizziness, drowsiness, dry mouth, headache, palpitations, severe rebound HTN, and sexual dysfunction; methyldopa also may cause aplastic anemia and thrombocytopenia. Vasodilators may cause ECG changes, diarrhea, dizziness, HF, palpitations, pruritus, and rash.

DRUG CLASSES

CONTRAINDICATIONS & CAUTIONS

Black Box Warning When pregnancy is detected in patients receiving ACE inhibitors, ARBs, or direct renin inhibitors, discontinue therapy as soon as possible. Drugs that act directly on the RAAS can cause fetal injury and death. ■

Black Box Warning Abrupt discontinuation of beta blocker therapy has been associated with angina exacerbation and, in some cases, MI and ventricular arrhythmias. When discontinuation of beta blockers is planned, gradually reduce dosage over at least a few weeks. ■

Black Box Warning Refer to individual drug monographs for additional black box warnings. ■

• Contraindicated in patients hypersensitive to these drugs and in those with hypotension.

• Use cautiously in patients with hepatic or renal dysfunction.

• Refer to each manufacturer's instructions for use in pregnancy. In breastfeeding women, refer to manufacturer's instructions for use because some antihypertensives appear in human milk. Safety and effectiveness of many antihypertensives haven't been established in children; refer to individual manufacturer's instructions. Elderly patients are more susceptible to adverse reactions and may need lower maintenance doses; monitor these patients closely.

Antilipemics

alirocumab, atorvastatin calcium, cholestyramine, colesevelam hydrochloride, colestipol, evolocumab, ezetimibe, fenofibrate, fluvastatin sodium, gemfibrozil, lomitapide mesylate, lovastatin, mipomersen sodium, niacin, pitavastatin, pravastatin sodium, rosuvastatin calcium, simvastatin

INDICATIONS
➤ **Hyperlipidemia, hypercholesterolemia**

ACTION

Antilipemics lower elevated lipid levels. Bile-sequestering drugs (cholestyramine, colesevelam) lower LDL level by forming insoluble complexes with bile salts, triggering cholesterol to leave the bloodstream and other storage areas to make new bile acids. Fibric acid derivatives (gemfibrozil) reduce cholesterol formation, increase sterol excretion, and decrease lipoprotein and triglyceride synthesis. HMG-CoA reductase inhibitors (atorvastatin, fluvastatin, lovastatin, pitavastatin, pravastatin, rosuvastatin, simvastatin) interfere with the activity of enzymes that generate cholesterol in the liver. Selective cholesterol absorption inhibitors (ezetimibe, evolocumab) inhibit cholesterol absorption by the small intestine, reducing hepatic cholesterol stores and increasing cholesterol clearance from the blood.

ADVERSE REACTIONS

Antilipemics commonly cause GI upset. Bile-sequestering drugs may cause bloating, cholelithiasis, constipation, and steatorrhea. Fibric acid derivatives may cause cholelithiasis and have other GI or CNS effects. Use of gemfibrozil with HMG-CoA reductase inhibitors may affect liver function or cause rash, pruritus, increased CK levels, rhabdomyolysis, and myopathy. Alirocumab may cause hypersensitivity reactions.

CONTRAINDICATIONS & CAUTIONS

• Contraindicated in patients hypersensitive to these drugs. Also, bile-sequestering drugs are contraindicated in patients with complete biliary obstruction. Fibric acid derivatives are contraindicated in patients with primary biliary cirrhosis or significant hepatic or renal dysfunction. HMG-CoA reductase inhibitors and cholesterol absorption inhibitors are contraindicated in patients with active liver disease or persistently elevated transaminase levels.

• Use bile-sequestering drugs cautiously in constipated patients. Use fibric acid derivatives cautiously in patients with peptic ulcer. Use HMG-CoA inhibitors cautiously in patients who consume large amounts of alcohol or who have a history of liver or renal disease.

• In pregnant women, use bile-sequestering drugs and fibric acid derivatives cautiously and avoid using HMG-CoA inhibitors. In breastfeeding women, avoid using fibric acid derivatives and HMG-CoA inhibitors; give bile-sequestering drugs cautiously. In children ages 10 to 17, certain antilipemics have been approved to treat heterozygous familial hypercholesterolemia. Elderly patients have an increased risk of severe constipation; use bile-sequestering drugs cautiously and monitor patients closely.

Antimetabolite antineoplastics

azaCITIDine, capecitabine, cytarabine, decitabine, fludarabine phosphate, fluorouracil, gemcitabine hydrochloride, mercaptopurine, methotrexate, PEMEtrexed, PRALAtrexate, trifluridine–tipiracil hydrochloride

INDICATIONS
➤ Various tumors and hematologic conditions

ACTION
Antimetabolites are structurally similar to naturally occurring metabolites and can be divided into three subcategories: purine, pyrimidine, and folinic acid analogues. Most of these drugs interrupt cell reproduction at a specific phase of the cell cycle. Purine analogues are incorporated into DNA and RNA, interfering with nucleic acid synthesis (by miscoding) and replication. They also may inhibit synthesis of purine bases through pseudofeedback mechanisms. Pyrimidine analogues inhibit enzymes in metabolic pathways that interfere with biosynthesis of uridine and thymine. Folic acid antagonists prevent conversion of folic acid to tetrahydrofolate by inhibiting the enzyme dihydrofolic acid reductase.

ADVERSE REACTIONS
The most common adverse effects include anxiety, bone marrow depression (anemia, leukopenia, thrombocytopenia), chills, diarrhea, fever, flank or joint pain, hair loss, nausea, redness or pain at the injection site, stomatitis, swelling of the feet or lower legs, and vomiting.

CONTRAINDICATIONS & CAUTIONS
Black Box Warning Refer to individual drug monographs for black box warnings. ∎
• Contraindicated in patients hypersensitive to these drugs.
• Most drugs can cause fetal harm; women exposed to them during pregnancy should be informed of risk to the fetus. Breastfeeding isn't recommended for women taking these drugs. Safety and effectiveness of some drugs in children haven't been established. Elderly patients have an increased risk of adverse reactions; monitor them closely.

Antimigraine drugs

almotriptan malate, eletriptan hydrobromide, frovatriptan succinate, naratriptan hydrochloride, rizatriptan benzoate, SUMAtriptan succinate, ZOLMitriptan

INDICATIONS
➤ Migraines with or without aura

ACTION
The antimigraine drugs are serotonin 5-HT$_1$ agonists. These drugs constrict cranial vessels, inhibit neuropeptide release, and reduce transmission in the trigeminal nerve pathway.

ADVERSE REACTIONS
These drugs have a wide range of adverse reactions. These include weakness, drowsiness, tingling, warmth or hot sensations, flushing, nasal discomfort, visual disturbances, paresthesia, dizziness, fatigue, somnolence, chest pain, weakness, dry mouth, dyspepsia, nausea, sweating, injection-site reactions, and neck, throat, or jaw pain. Intranasal sumatriptan can cause nasal or throat discomfort and taste disturbances.

CONTRAINDICATIONS & CAUTIONS
• Contraindicated in patients hypersensitive to these drugs or to any of their components.
• Contraindicated in patients with ischemic heart disease, angina, previous MI, uncontrolled HTN or other significant underlying CV conditions, cerebrovascular disease, PVD, and ischemic bowel disease.
• Serotonin syndrome can occur, especially when used with other serotonergic drugs.
• Information regarding use during pregnancy is limited; however, other drugs exist that are preferred for migraine therapy in pregnant women. Sumatriptan and eletriptan appear in human milk; use cautiously in breastfeeding women. Refer to manufacturer's instructions for each drug.

DRUG CLASSES

Antiparkinsonian drugs

amantadine hydrochloride, apomorphine hydrochloride, benztropine mesylate, bromocriptine mesylate, diphenhydrAMINE hydrochloride, entacapone, levodopa–carbidopa, levodopa–carbidopa–entacapone, pramipexole dihydrochloride, rasagiline mesylate, rOPINIRole hydrochloride, selegiline hydrochloride, tolcapone

INDICATIONS
➤ **Signs and symptoms of Parkinson disease and drug-induced extrapyramidal reactions**

ACTION
Antiparkinsonians include synthetic anticholinergics, dopaminergics, and the antiviral amantadine. Anticholinergics probably prolong the action of dopamine by blocking its reuptake into presynaptic neurons and by suppressing central cholinergic activity. Dopaminergics act in the brain by increasing dopamine availability, thus improving motor function. Entacapone and tolcapone are reversible inhibitors of peripheral catechol-*O*-methyltransferase (commonly known as COMT), which is responsible for elimination of various catecholamines, including dopamine. Blocking this pathway when giving levodopa–carbidopa should result in higher levels of levodopa, thereby allowing greater dopaminergic stimulation in the CNS and leading to a greater effect in treating parkinsonian symptoms. Amantadine is thought to increase dopamine release in the substantia nigra.

ADVERSE REACTIONS
Anticholinergics may cause blurred vision, cycloplegia, constipation, decreased sweating or anhidrosis, dry mouth, headache, mydriasis, palpitations, tachycardia, urinary hesitancy, and urine retention. Dopaminergics may cause arrhythmias, confusion, disturbing dreams, dystonias, hallucinations, headache, muscle cramps, nausea, orthostatic hypotension, and vomiting. Amantadine also causes irritability, insomnia, and livedo reticularis (with prolonged use).

CONTRAINDICATIONS & CAUTIONS
Black Box Warning Refer to individual drug monographs for black box warnings. ∎

• Contraindicated in patients hypersensitive to these drugs.
• Use cautiously in patients with prostatic hyperplasia or tardive dyskinesia and in debilitated patients.
• NMS-like syndrome involving muscle rigidity, increased body temperature, and mental status changes may occur with abrupt withdrawal of antiparkinsonian agents.
• Safe use hasn't been established in pregnant women. Antiparkinsonians may appear in human milk; the patient should stop the drug or stop breastfeeding, taking into account the importance of the drug to the mother. Safety and effectiveness haven't been established in children. Elderly patients have an increased risk of adverse reactions; monitor closely.

Antiplatelet drugs

abciximab, aspirin, cangrelor tetrasodium, cilostazol, clopidogrel bisulfate, dipyridamole, eptifibatide, prasugrel, ticagrelor, ticlopidine hydrochloride, tirofiban hydrochloride, vorapaxar sulfate

INDICATIONS
➤ **Reduction of thrombotic events by reducing platelet aggregation; adjunct to PCI, prevention of cardiac ischemic complications, or treatment of unstable angina not responding to conventional therapy when PCI is planned within 24 hours (abciximab); ACS and PCI (eptifibatide); ACS (tirofiban); non-ST-segment elevation ACS and ST-segment elevation MI, recent MI, recent stroke or PVD (clopidogrel, ticlopidine, and vorapaxar)**

ACTION
The IV drugs abciximab, eptifibatide, and tirofiban antagonize the glycoprotein (GP)IIb/IIIa receptors located on platelets, which are involved in platelet aggregation. Clopidogrel, cangrelor, prasugrel, and ticagrelor are inhibitors of platelet aggregation that inhibit the binding of ADP to its platelet receptor and the subsequent ADP-mediated activation of the GPIIb/IIIa complex. Ticlopidine inhibits the binding of fibrinogen to platelets. Vorapaxar inhibits thrombin-induced and thrombin receptor agonist peptide-induced platelet aggregation.

ADVERSE REACTIONS
The IV drugs can cause serious bleeding, thrombocytopenia, and anaphylaxis. The most common adverse reactions to the oral agents include anaphylaxis, rash, stomach pain, nausea, and headache. Ticlopidine may cause neutropenia and elevated alkaline phosphatase and serum transaminase levels. Prasugrel and ticagrelor can cause atrial fibrillation, dyspnea, cough, and hypotension.

CONTRAINDICATIONS & CAUTIONS
Black Box Warning Refer to individual drug monographs for black box warnings. ■
• Contraindicated in patients hypersensitive to these drugs or their components.
• Contraindicated in active bleeding, bleeding disorders, intracranial neoplasm, AV malformation or aneurysm, cerebrovascular accident (within 2 years), recent major surgery or trauma, severe uncontrolled HTN, or thrombocytopenia.
• Avoid use of ticagrelor in patients with severe hepatic impairment.
• Because of its very long half-life, vorapaxar is effectively irreversible.
• Safe use in pregnant women hasn't been established. Refer to manufacturer's instructions. Drugs may appear in human milk. The patient should stop the drug or stop breastfeeding.

Antipsychotics
First generation (typical)
chlorproMAZINE hydrochloride, fluPHENAZine (decanoate; hydrochloride), haloperidol (decanoate; lactate), loxapine (hydrochloride; succinate), molindone hydrochloride, perphenazine, pimozide, prochlorperazine (edisylate; maleate), thioridazine hydrochloride, thiothixene hydrochloride, trifluoperazine hydrochloride

Second generation (atypical)
ARIPiprazole, ARIPiprazole lauroxil, asenapine maleate, brexpiprazole, cariprazine hydrochloride, cloZAPine, iloperidone, lurasidone hydrochloride, OLANZapine (pamoate), paliperidone (palmitate), QUEtiapine fumarate, risperiDONE, ziprasidone (hydrochloride; mesylate)

INDICATIONS
➤ Schizophrenia (all but pimozide); schizoaffective disorder (paliperidone); psychosis, acute agitation, depression, or mania in bipolar I disorder; depression, hiccups (chlorpromazine); autism irritability (aripiprazole, risperidone); child hyperactivity and severe behavioral problems (chlorpromazine, haloperidol); acute intermittent porphyria (chlorpromazine); nausea, vomiting (chlorpromazine, prochlorperazine); anxiety, tetanus (chlorpromazine); hiccups (chlorpromazine); Tourette syndrome (haloperidol, pimozide)

ACTION
Antipsychotics block several neurotransmitters, particularly dopamine. The exact mechanism of action and ideal combination of targeted neurotransmitters remain unknown.

ADVERSE REACTIONS
First-generation antipsychotics may cause cardiac arrhythmias, cardiac arrest, hypotension, tachycardia, agitation, akathisia, seizures, dizziness, sedation, dystonia, headache, insomnia, NMS, extrapyramidal symptoms, tardive dyskinesia, photosensitivity, pruritus, anorexia, constipation, dry mouth, nausea, weight gain, amenorrhea, galactorrhea, gynecomastia, impotence, urine retention, blurred vision, and hyperthermia/hyperpyrexia.

Second-generation antipsychotics may cause akathisia, dizziness, drowsiness, extrapyramidal symptoms, headache, constipation, nausea, QT-interval prolongation, weight gain, hyperprolactinemia, dyslipidemia, hyperglycemia, and hyperthermia/hyperpyrexia.

CONTRAINDICATIONS & CAUTIONS
Black Box Warning Elderly patients with dementia-related psychosis treated with antipsychotics are at increased risk for death. Antipsychotics aren't approved for treatment of patients with dementia-related psychosis. ■
Black Box Warning Refer to individual drug monographs for additional black box warnings. ■
• Contraindicated in patients hypersensitive to these drugs.
• Use cautiously and observe for tardive dyskinesia, which may be irreversible.
• Use cautiously and watch for signs and symptoms of NMS (muscle rigidity, fever, delirium),

DRUG CLASSES

especially with first-generation injectable antipsychotics.

• Use cautiously in depressed or agitated patients.

• Use cautiously with lithium because of risk of encephalopathic syndrome (weakness, lethargy, fever, confusion).

• Use cautiously in patients with MI, ischemic heart disease, HF, conduction abnormalities, or cerebrovascular disease, and in those at risk for hypotension.

• Use cautiously in patients with dyslipidemia or diabetes mellitus, particularly with second-generation antipsychotics.

• Use cautiously in patients with respiratory infections or chronic disorders because of increased pneumonia risk.

• Use cautiously in patients with blood dyscrasias.

• Use cautiously in patients with history of seizures.

• Use cautiously in patients with Parkinson disease or dementia with Lewy bodies.

• Use cautiously in patients with renal impairment; lower dosage or discontinue drug if BUN level is abnormal.

• Risk in pregnancy is unknown; refer to manufacturer's instructions for use in pregnancy and breastfeeding. When used during the third trimester, there is an increased risk of extrapyramidal symptoms or withdrawal symptoms in the newborn that can be severe and require hospitalization.

• Patients taking antipsychotics should use caution when driving or performing hazardous work due to drowsiness.

Antirheumatics (disease-modifying)

abatacept, adalimumab, certolizumab pegol, etanercept, golimumab, inFLIXimab, inFLIXimab-abda, inFLIXimab-dyyb, inFLIXimab-qbtx, leflunomide, tocilizumab, tofacitinib citrate

INDICATIONS

➤ **RA, ankylosing spondylitis, Crohn disease, psoriatic arthritis, plaque psoriasis (infliximab), ulcerative colitis (infliximab), giant cell arteritis, polyarticular juvenile idiopathic arthritis, systemic juvenile idiopathic arthritis, cytokine release syndrome**

ACTION

Activated T lymphocytes are found in the synovium of patients with RA. Some drugs bind to TNF so it can't bind to a receptor and exert an effect. TNF plays an important role in pathologic inflammation and joint destruction. Some drugs are antagonists of interleukin-6 receptor, which leads to reduction of cytokine production.

ADVERSE REACTIONS

The most serious adverse reactions include serious infections and malignancies in patients treated with abatacept, adalimumab, infliximab, leflunomide, and tocilizumab. The most common adverse reactions include rash, pruritus, hair loss, urticaria, nausea, vomiting, anorexia, flatulence, dyspepsia, anemia, leukopenia, thrombocytopenia, elevated liver enzymes, stomatitis, HTN, headache, and hematuria.

CONTRAINDICATIONS & CAUTIONS

Black Box Warning Refer to individual drug monographs for black box warnings. ■

• Contraindicated in patients hypersensitive to these drugs or their components.

• Use cautiously in patients receiving two antirheumatics with similar mechanisms of action.

• Use cautiously in patients with a history of recurrent infections, COPD, CNS disorders, demyelinating disorders, HF, and immunosuppression.

• Safety in pregnant women hasn't been established. Drugs may appear in human milk. Refer to manufacturer's instructions for use during pregnancy and breastfeeding.

Antituberculotics

bedaquiline fumarate, cycloSERINE, ethambutol hydrochloride, isoniazid, pyrazinamide, rifabutin, rifAMPin, rifapentine

INDICATIONS

➤ **Acute pulmonary and extrapulmonary TB, acute UTIs**

ACTION

Cycloserine and isoniazid inhibit cell-wall synthesis in susceptible strains of gram-positive and gram-negative bacteria, including *Mycobacterium tuberculosis*. Rifampin, rifapentine, and rifabutin inhibit DNA-dependent RNA polymerase activity in susceptible *M. tuberculosis* organisms. Ethambutol causes impaired cell metabolism. Bedaquiline inhibits an enzyme essential to generate energy in *M. tuberculosis* organisms. The mechanism of action for pyrazinamide is unknown.

ADVERSE REACTIONS

Adverse reactions primarily affect the GI tract, peripheral nervous system, and hepatic system. Use cautiously in patients with hepatic impairment. Isoniazid may precipitate seizures in patients with a seizure disorder and may produce optic or peripheral neuritis. Optic neuritis, blood dyscrasias, anaphylaxis, and hepatotoxicity may occur with ethambutol. Rifampin may cause epigastric pain, nausea, vomiting, flatulence, abdominal cramps, anorexia, and diarrhea. Cycloserine can cause seizures, confusion, dizziness, headache, and somnolence.

CONTRAINDICATIONS & CAUTIONS

• Contraindicated in patients hypersensitive to these drugs or their components.
• Multidrug regimens should be used.
• Discontinue drugs or reduce dosage if patients develop signs of CNS toxicity, including seizures, psychosis, somnolence, depression, confusion, hyperreflexia, headache, tremor, vertigo, paresis, or dysarthria.
• The use of medications for TB in pregnant women may outweigh risks to the fetus. Refer to manufacturer's instructions for use during pregnancy and breastfeeding.

Benzodiazepines

ALPRAZolam, chlordiazePOXIDE hydrochloride, cloBAZam, clonazePAM, diazePAM, flurazepam, LORazepam, midazolam hydrochloride, oxazepam, temazepam, triazolam

INDICATIONS

➤ **Seizure disorders (clobazam, clonazepam, diazepam, midazolam, parenteral lorazepam); anxiety, tension, and insomnia (chlordiazepoxide, clonazepam, diazepam, lorazepam, oxazepam, temazepam, triazolam); procedural/surgical sedation or amnesia (diazepam, lorazepam, midazolam); skeletal muscle spasm and tremor (oral forms of chlordiazepoxide and diazepam); delirium**

ACTION

Benzodiazepines act selectively on polysynaptic neuronal pathways throughout the CNS. Precise sites and mechanisms of action aren't fully known. However, benzodiazepines enhance or facilitate the action of GABA, an inhibitory neurotransmitter in the CNS. These drugs appear to act at the limbic, thalamic, and hypothalamic levels of the CNS to produce anxiolytic, sedative, hypnotic, skeletal muscle relaxant, and anticonvulsant effects.

ADVERSE REACTIONS

Therapeutic doses may cause drowsiness, impaired motor function, constipation, diarrhea, vomiting, altered appetite, urinary changes, visual disturbances, and CV irregularities. Toxic doses may cause continuing problems with short-term memory, confusion, severe depression, shakiness, vertigo, slurred speech, staggering, bradycardia, respiratory depression, respiratory arrest, or severe weakness. Prolonged or frequent use can cause physical dependency and withdrawal syndrome when drug is stopped.

CONTRAINDICATIONS & CAUTIONS

Black Box Warning Refer to individual drug monographs for black box warnings. ∎
• Contraindicated in patients hypersensitive to these drugs, in those with acute angle-closure glaucoma, and in those with depressive neuroses or psychotic reactions in which anxiety isn't prominent.
• Avoid use in patients with suicidal tendencies and in patients with a history of drug abuse. If drug is necessary, monitor patient carefully.
• Abrupt discontinuation can trigger withdrawal symptoms; withdraw drug gradually.
• Use cautiously in patients with chronic pulmonary insufficiency or sleep apnea and in those with hepatic or renal insufficiency.
• In pregnant patients, benzodiazepines increase the risk of congenital malformation if taken in the first trimester. Use during labor may cause neonatal flaccidity. A neonate whose mother took a benzodiazepine during pregnancy may have withdrawal symptoms. Benzodiazepines appear in human milk; women shouldn't breastfeed during therapy. In elderly patients, benzodiazepine elimination may be prolonged; consider a lower dosage.

DRUG CLASSES

Beta blockers

Beta₁-selective blockers
acebutolol hydrochloride, atenolol, betaxolol hydrochloride, bisoprolol fumarate, esmolol hydrochloride, metoprolol (succinate; tartrate), nebivolol hydrochloride

Beta₁ and beta₂ (nonselective) blockers
carvedilol phosphate (beta blocker and alpha₁ blocker), labetalol hydrochloride (beta blocker and alpha₁ blocker), nadolol, propranolol hydrochloride, sotalol hydrochloride, timolol maleate

INDICATIONS
➤ **HTN (most drugs), angina pectoris (atenolol, metoprolol, nadolol, propranolol), arrhythmias (acebutolol, esmolol, propranolol, sotalol), glaucoma (betaxolol, timolol), prevention of MI (atenolol, metoprolol, propranolol), prevention of recurrent migraine and other vascular headaches (propranolol), pheochromocytomas or essential tremors (selected drugs), HF (atenolol, carvedilol, metoprolol)**

ACTION
Beta blockers compete with beta agonists for available beta receptors; individual drugs differ in their ability to affect beta receptors. Some drugs are nonselective: they block beta₁ receptors in cardiac muscle and beta₂ receptors in bronchial and vascular smooth muscle. Several drugs are cardioselective and, in lower doses, inhibit mainly beta₁ receptors. Some beta blockers have intrinsic sympathomimetic activity and stimulate and block beta receptors, and thereby have less effect on slowing HR. Others stabilize cardiac membranes, which affects cardiac action potential.

ADVERSE REACTIONS
Therapeutic dose may cause bradycardia, dizziness, fatigue, and erectile dysfunction; some may cause other CNS disturbances, such as depression, hallucinations, memory loss, and nightmares. Toxic dose can produce severe hypotension, bradycardia, HF, or bronchospasm.

CONTRAINDICATIONS & CAUTIONS
Black Box Warning Abrupt discontinuation of beta blockers has been associated with angina exacerbation and, in some cases, MI and ventricular arrhythmias. When discontinuation of beta blockers is planned, gradually reduce dosage over at least a few weeks. ■

Black Box Warning Refer to individual drug monographs for additional black box warnings. ■

• Contraindicated in patients hypersensitive to these drugs and in those with cardiogenic shock, sinus bradycardia, heart block greater than first degree, or bronchial asthma.

• Beta blockers may mask signs and symptoms of hypoglycemia (palpitations, tachycardia, tremor).

• Use cautiously in patients with nonallergic bronchospastic disorders, diabetes mellitus, impaired hepatic or renal function, and HF.

• Use cautiously in pregnant women. Drugs appear in human milk. Safety and effectiveness haven't been established in children; use only if the benefits outweigh the risks. Use cautiously in elderly patients; patients may need reduced maintenance doses because of increased bioavailability, delayed metabolism, and increased adverse effects.

Calcium channel blockers
amLODIPine besylate, clevidipine butyrate, dilTIAZem hydrochloride, felodipine, isradipine, niCARdipine hydrochloride, NIFEdipine, niMODipine, nisoldipine, verapamil hydrochloride

INDICATIONS
➤ **Prinzmetal variant angina; chronic stable angina; unstable angina; HTN; arrhythmias; subarachnoid hemorrhage (nimodipine)**

ACTION
The main physiologic action of calcium channel blockers is to inhibit calcium influx across the slow channels of myocardial and vascular smooth muscle cells. By inhibiting calcium flow into these cells, calcium channel blockers reduce intracellular calcium levels. This, in turn, dilates coronary arteries, peripheral arteries, and arterioles and slows cardiac conduction.

When used to treat Prinzmetal variant angina, calcium channel blockers inhibit coronary spasm, which then increases oxygen delivery to the heart. Peripheral artery dilation reduces afterload, which decreases myocardial oxygen use. Inhibiting calcium flow into specialized cardiac conduction cells in the SA and

AV nodes slows conduction through the heart. Verapamil and diltiazem have the greatest effect on the AV node, which slows the ventricular rate in atrial fibrillation or flutter and converts supraventricular tachycardia to a normal sinus rhythm.

ADVERSE REACTIONS

Symptomatic hypotension can occur. Verapamil may cause bradycardia, hypotension, various degrees of heart block, and worsening of HF after rapid IV delivery. Nifedipine may cause flushing, headache, heartburn, hypotension, light-headedness, and peripheral edema. The most common adverse reactions to diltiazem are headache and dizziness; it also may induce dyspepsia, bradycardia, HF, edema, and various degrees of heart block.

CONTRAINDICATIONS & CAUTIONS

Black Box Warning Refer to individual drug monographs for black box warnings. ■
• Contraindicated in patients hypersensitive to these drugs and in those with MI (nifedipine), second- or third-degree heart block (except those with a pacemaker), and cardiogenic shock. Use diltiazem and verapamil cautiously in patients with HF.
• In pregnant and breastfeeding women, use cautiously and refer to individual manufacturer's instructions for use. Calcium channel blockers may appear in human milk; some drugs may need to be stopped during breastfeeding. In elderly patients, the half-life of calcium channel blockers may be increased as a result of decreased clearance.

Cephalosporins

First generation
cefadroxil, ceFAZolin sodium, cephalexin

Second generation
cefaclor, cefOXitin sodium, cefprozil, cefuroxime (axetil; sodium)

Third generation
cefdinir, cefditoren pivoxil, cefotaxime sodium, cefpodoxime proxetil, cefTAZidime, cefTRIAXone sodium

Fourth generation
cefepime hydrochloride

Fifth generation
ceftaroline fosamil

INDICATIONS

➤ **Infections of the lungs, skin, soft tissue, bones, joints, urinary and respiratory tracts, blood, abdomen, and heart; CNS infections caused by susceptible strains of *Neisseria meningitidis, Haemophilus influenzae*, and *Streptococcus pneumoniae*; meningitis caused by *Escherichia coli* or *Klebsiella;* infections that develop after surgical procedures classified as contaminated or potentially contaminated; penicillinase-producing *Neisseria gonorrhoeae;* otitis media and ampicillin-resistant middle ear infections caused by *H. influenzae***

ACTION

Cephalosporins are chemically and pharmacologically similar to penicillin; they act by inhibiting bacterial cell-wall synthesis, causing rapid cell destruction. Their sites of action are enzymes known as *penicillin-binding proteins.* The affinity of certain cephalosporins for these proteins in various microorganisms helps explain the differing actions of these drugs. They are bactericidal: They act against many aerobic gram-positive and gram-negative bacteria and some anaerobic bacteria but don't kill fungi or viruses.

First-generation cephalosporins act against many gram-positive cocci, including penicillinase-producing *Staphylococcus aureus* and *S. epidermidis, S. pneumoniae*, group B streptococci, and group A beta-hemolytic streptococci. Susceptible gram-negative organisms include *Klebsiella pneumoniae, E. coli, Proteus mirabilis*, and *Shigella.*

Second-generation cephalosporins are effective against all organisms susceptible to first-generation drugs and have additional activity against *Moraxella catarrhalis, H. influenzae, Enterobacter, Citrobacter, Providencia, Acinetobacter, Serratia*, and *Neisseria. Bacteroides fragilis* are susceptible to cefoxitin.

Third-generation cephalosporins are less active than first- and second-generation drugs against gram-positive bacteria but are more active against gram-negative organisms, including those resistant to first- and second-generation drugs. They have the greatest stability against beta-lactamases produced by gram-negative bacteria. Susceptible gram-negative organisms include *E. coli, Klebsiella, Enterobacter, Providencia, Acinetobacter, Serratia, Proteus, Morganella*, and *Neisseria.* Some third-generation drugs are active against *B. fragilis* and *Pseudomonas*.

Cefepime shows activity against a wide range of gram-positive and gram-negative bacteria. Cefepime exhibits resistance to beta-lactamases. Susceptible gram-negative bacteria include *Enterobacter, E. coli, K. pneumoniae, P. mirabilis*, and *Pseudomonas aeruginosa*. Susceptible gram-positive bacteria include *S. aureus, S. pneumoniae*, and *Streptococcus pyogenes*.

Ceftaroline has antimicrobial activity against gram-negative bacteria similar to third-generation cephalosporins. It is also active against gram-positive bacteria such as MRSA and methicillin-resistant *S. pneumoniae*.

ADVERSE REACTIONS
Many cephalosporins have similar adverse effects. Hypersensitivity reactions range from mild rashes, fever, and eosinophilia to fatal anaphylaxis and are more common in patients with penicillin allergy. Adverse GI reactions include abdominal pain, diarrhea, dyspepsia, glossitis, nausea, tenesmus, and vomiting. CDAD ranging in severity from mild to fatal colitis can occur during treatment or after treatment ends. Hematologic reactions include positive direct and indirect antiglobulin on Coombs test, thrombocytopenia or thrombocythemia, transient neutropenia, and reversible leukopenia. Minimal elevation of LFT results occurs occasionally. Adverse renal effects may occur with any cephalosporin; they are most common in older patients, those with decreased renal function, and those taking other nephrotoxic drugs. Some products increase risk of arrhythmia, chest pain, hypotension, and HTN.

Local reactions may occur after IV or IM administration; these reactions occur more often with higher doses and long-term therapy. Bacterial and fungal superinfections may result from suppression of normal flora.

CONTRAINDICATIONS & CAUTIONS
● Contraindicated in patients hypersensitive to cephalosporins and related antibiotics.
● Use cautiously in patients with renal or hepatic impairment, history of GI disease, or allergy to penicillins.
● In pregnant women, use only when potential benefits outweigh potential fetal hazards; safety hasn't been definitively established. In breastfeeding women, use cautiously because drugs appear in human milk. In neonates and infants, half-life is prolonged; use cautiously. Elderly patients are susceptible to superinfection and coagulopathies, commonly have renal impairment, and may need a lower dosage; use cautiously.

CNS stimulants
armodafinil, dexmethylphenidate hydrochloride, dextroamphetamine sulfate, doxapram hydrochloride, lisdexamfetamine dimesylate, methylphenidate hydrochloride, modafinil, phentermine hydrochloride

INDICATIONS
➤ **Stimulation of respiration in patients with drug-induced postanesthesia respiratory depression or CNS depression caused by overdose and as temporary measure in acute respiratory insufficiency (doxapram); obstructive sleep apnea (armodafinil, modafinil); narcolepsy (armodafinil, dextroamphetamine, methylphenidate, modafinil); shift-work sleep disorder (armodafinil, modafinil); obesity (phentermine); binge eating disorder (lisdexamfetamine); ADHD (dextroamphetamine, lisdexamfetamine, dexmethylphenidate, methylphenidate)**

ACTION
Doxapram produces respiratory stimulation through the peripheral carotid chemoreceptors. The exact mechanism of action of armodafinil and modafinil isn't known. Phentermine is a sympathomimetic amine. The exact mechanism of action in treating obesity isn't established. Dextroamphetamine, dexmethylphenidate, lisdexamfetamine, and methylphenidate promote nerve impulse transmission.

ADVERSE REACTIONS
The adverse effects of CNS stimulants are related to the stimulatory effect of these drugs and include HTN, palpitations, tachyarrhythmias, urticaria, constipation, decreased appetite, diarrhea, dizziness, excitement, insomnia, tremor, and restlessness. Armodafinil and modafinil may cause severe rash, including SJS.

CONTRAINDICATIONS & CAUTIONS
Black Box Warning Refer to individual drug monographs for black box warnings. ∎

• Contraindicated in patients hypersensitive to these drugs or their components.

• Use drugs cautiously in patients with psychiatric illness.

• Drugs have the potential for abuse and misuse.

• Doxapram is contraindicated in epilepsy, seizure disorders, mechanical disorders of ventilation such as muscle paresis, flail chest, pneumothorax, asthma, pulmonary fibrosis, head injury, stroke, cerebral edema, uncompensated HF, severe coronary disease, and severe HTN.

• Delay administration of doxapram in patients who have received general anesthesia utilizing a volatile agent until the volatile agent has been excreted. This will lessen the chance for arrhythmias, including ventricular tachycardia or ventricular fibrillation.

• Administer doxapram cautiously in patients taking MAO inhibitors or sympathomimetics because an added pressor effect may occur.

• Phentermine is contraindicated in agitated states, CV disease, history of drug abuse, severe HTN, hyperthyroidism, and glaucoma.

• Dextroamphetamine, phentermine, lisdexamfetamine, dexmethylphenidate, and methylphenidate are contraindicated during or within 14 days after use of MAO inhibitors.

• Drugs can cause arrhythmias, HTN, nervousness, and insomnia.

• Use lisdexamfetamine, dextroamphetamine, methylphenidate, dexmethylphenidate, and modafinil cautiously in patients with seizure disorder.

• Safety in pregnant women hasn't been established. Some amphetamines appear in human milk; breastfeeding isn't recommended.

Corticosteroids

beclomethasone dipropionate, betamethasone (dipropionate; valerate), budesonide, ciclesonide, cortisone acetate, deflazacort, dexamethasone (sodium phosphate), fludrocortisone acetate, flunisolide, fluticasone propionate, hydrocortisone (acetate; butyrate; cypionate; probutate; sodium succinate; valerate), methylPREDNISolone (acetate; sodium succinate), mometasone furoate, prednisoLONE (acetate; sodium phosphate), predniSONE, triamcinolone (acetonide; hexacetonide)

INDICATIONS

➤ **Duchenne muscular dystrophy; hypersensitivity; inflammation, particularly of eye, nose, and respiratory tract; to initiate immunosuppression; replacement therapy in adrenocortical insufficiency, dermatologic diseases, respiratory disorders, and rheumatic disorders**

ACTION

Corticosteroids suppress cell-mediated and humoral immunity by reducing levels of leukocytes, monocytes, and eosinophils; by decreasing Ig binding to cell-surface receptors; and by inhibiting interleukin synthesis. They reduce inflammation by preventing hydrolytic enzyme release into the cells, preventing plasma exudation, suppressing polymorphonuclear leukocyte migration, and disrupting other inflammatory processes.

ADVERSE REACTIONS

Systemic corticosteroid therapy may suppress the HPA axis. Excessive use may cause cushingoid symptoms and various systemic disorders, such as diabetes and osteoporosis. Other effects may include dermatologic disorders, edema, mood changes, fluid and electrolyte imbalances, gastritis or GI irritation, HTN, ocular changes, immunosuppression, increased appetite, insomnia, psychosis, and weight gain.

CONTRAINDICATIONS & CAUTIONS

• Contraindicated in patients hypersensitive to these drugs or their components and in those with systemic fungal infection.

• Use cautiously in patients with GI ulceration, renal disease, HTN, osteoporosis, varicella, vaccinia, exanthem, diabetes mellitus, hypothyroidism, thromboembolic disorder, seizures, myasthenia gravis, HF, TB, ocular herpes simplex, hypoalbuminemia, emotional instability, or psychosis.

• Avoid use in pregnant women, if possible, because of risk to the fetus. If use during pregnancy is necessary, use the lowest effective dose for the shortest duration. Inhaled drugs are preferred for treating asthma during pregnancy. Women should stop breastfeeding because these drugs appear in human milk and could cause serious adverse effects in infants. In children, long-term use should be avoided whenever possible because stunted growth may result. Elderly patients may have an increased risk of adverse reactions; monitor closely.

Diuretics, loop
bumetanide, ethacrynate sodium, ethacrynic acid, furosemide, torsemide

INDICATIONS
➤ Edema from HF, hepatic cirrhosis, or nephrotic syndrome; mild-to-moderate HTN; adjunctive treatment in acute pulmonary edema or hypertensive crisis

ACTION
Loop diuretics inhibit sodium and chloride reabsorption in the ascending loop of Henle, thus increasing excretion of sodium, chloride, and water. Like thiazide diuretics, loop diuretics increase excretion of potassium. Loop diuretics produce more diuresis and electrolyte loss than thiazide diuretics.

ADVERSE REACTIONS
Therapeutic doses commonly cause metabolic and electrolyte disturbances, particularly potassium depletion, and also may cause hyperglycemia, hyperuricemia, hypochloremic alkalosis, and hypomagnesemia. Rapid parenteral administration may cause hearing loss (including deafness) and tinnitus. High doses can produce profound diuresis, leading to hypovolemia and CV collapse. Photosensitivity also may occur.

CONTRAINDICATIONS & CAUTIONS
Black Box Warning Refer to individual drug monographs for black box warnings. ▮
• Use cautiously in patients with a sulfa allergy because of the potential for a cross-reaction.
• Contraindicated in patients hypersensitive to these drugs and in patients with anuria, hepatic coma, or severe electrolyte depletion.
• Use cautiously in patients with severe renal disease. Also use cautiously in patients with severe hypersensitivity to sulfonamides because allergic reaction may occur.
• Use cautiously in pregnant women. Don't use in breastfeeding women. Use cautiously in neonates; the usual pediatric dose can be used, but dosage intervals should be extended. If needed in elderly patients, use a lower dose and monitor patient closely; these patients are more susceptible to drug-induced diuresis.

Diuretics, potassium-sparing
aMILoride hydrochloride, eplerenone, spironolactone, triamterene

INDICATIONS
➤ Edema from hepatic cirrhosis, nephrotic syndrome, and HF; mild or moderate HTN; diagnosis of primary hyperaldosteronism; aid in treatment of hypokalemia; prophylaxis of hypokalemia in patients taking cardiac glycosides

ACTION
Amiloride and triamterene act directly on the distal renal tubule of the nephron to inhibit sodium reabsorption and potassium and hydrogen excretion. Spironolactone and eplerenone competitively inhibit aldosterone at the distal renal tubules, also promoting sodium excretion and potassium retention.

ADVERSE REACTIONS
Hyperkalemia is the most serious adverse reaction; it could lead to arrhythmias. Other adverse reactions include nausea, vomiting, headache, weakness, fatigue, bowel disturbances, cough, and dyspnea.

CONTRAINDICATIONS & CAUTIONS
Black Box Warning Refer to individual drug monographs for black box warnings. ▮
• Contraindicated in patients hypersensitive to spironolactone, in those taking other potassium-sparing diuretics or potassium supplements, and in those with anuria, acute or chronic renal insufficiency, severe hyperkalemia, or diabetic nephropathy.
• Use cautiously in patients with severe hepatic insufficiency because electrolyte imbalance may lead to hepatic encephalopathy and in patients with diabetes, who are at increased risk for hyperkalemia.
• No controlled studies of use in pregnant women exist. Refer to manufacturer's instructions for use during pregnancy and breastfeeding. Use cautiously in children, who are more susceptible to hyperkalemia. In elderly and debilitated patients, observe closely and reduce dosage, if needed; these patients are more susceptible to drug-induced diuresis and hyperkalemia.

Diuretics, thiazide and thiazide-like

Thiazide
hydroCHLOROthiazide

Thiazide-like
Indapamide, metOLazone

INDICATIONS
➤ **Edema from right-sided HF, mild to moderate left-sided HF, or nephrotic syndrome; edema and ascites caused by hepatic cirrhosis; HTN; diabetes insipidus, particularly nephrogenic diabetes insipidus**

ACTION
Thiazide and thiazide-like diuretics interfere with sodium transport across the tubules of the cortical diluting segment in the nephron, thereby increasing renal excretion of sodium, chloride, water, and potassium and decreasing calcium excretion.

Thiazide diuretics also exert an antihypertensive effect. Although the exact mechanism is unknown, direct arteriolar dilation may be partially responsible. In diabetes insipidus, thiazides cause a paradoxical decrease in urine volume and an increase in renal concentration of urine, possibly because of sodium depletion and decreased plasma volume. This increases water and sodium reabsorption in the kidneys.

ADVERSE REACTIONS
Therapeutic doses cause electrolyte and metabolic disturbances, most commonly potassium depletion. Other abnormalities include elevated cholesterol levels, hypercalcemia, hyperglycemia, hyperuricemia, hypochloremic alkalosis, hypomagnesemia, hyponatremia, and photosensitivity.

CONTRAINDICATIONS & CAUTIONS
Black Box Warning Refer to individual drug monographs for black box warnings. ∎
• Contraindicated in patients hypersensitive to these drugs and in those with anuria.
• Use cautiously in patients with severe renal disease, impaired hepatic function, or progressive liver disease.
• Use cautiously in pregnant women. Drugs appear in human milk; patient should either discontinue breastfeeding or discontinue drug. Safety and effectiveness haven't been established in children. If needed in elderly patients, reduce dosage and monitor patient closely; these patients are more susceptible to drug-induced diuresis.

Estrogens

esterified estrogens, estradiol (cypionate; hemihydrate; valerate), estrogens (conjugated), estropipate

INDICATIONS
➤ **Prevention of moderate to severe vasomotor symptoms linked to menopause, such as hot flushes and dizziness; stimulation of vaginal tissue development, cornification, and secretory activity; inhibition of hormone-sensitive cancer growth; female hypogonadism; female castration; primary ovulation failure; ovulation control; prevention of conception**

ACTION
Estrogens promote the development and maintenance of the female reproductive system and secondary sexual characteristics. They inhibit the release of pituitary gonadotropins and have various metabolic effects, including retention of fluid and electrolytes, retention and deposition in bone of calcium and phosphorus, and mild anabolic activity.

Estrogens and estrogenic substances given as drugs have effects related to endogenous estrogen's mechanism of action. They can mimic the action of endogenous estrogen when used as replacement therapy and can inhibit ovulation or the growth of certain hormone-sensitive cancers.

ADVERSE REACTIONS
Acute adverse reactions include abdominal cramps; bloating caused by fluid and electrolyte retention; breast swelling and tenderness; changes in menstrual bleeding patterns, such as spotting and prolongation or absence of bleeding; headache; loss of appetite; loss of libido; nausea; photosensitivity; swollen feet or ankles; and weight gain.

Long-term effects include benign hepatomas, cholestatic jaundice, elevated BP (sometimes into the hypertensive range), endometrial carcinoma (rare), and thromboembolic disease (risk increases greatly with cigarette smoking, especially in women older than age 35).

DRUG CLASSES

CONTRAINDICATIONS & CAUTIONS

Black Box Warning Refer to individual drug monographs for black box warnings. ∎

• Contraindicated in women with thrombophlebitis or thromboembolic disorders, unexplained abnormal genital bleeding, or estrogen-dependent neoplasia.

• Use cautiously in patients with HTN; metabolic bone disease; migraines; seizures; asthma; cardiac, renal, or hepatic impairment; blood dyscrasia; diabetes; family history of breast cancer; or fibrocystic disease.

• Contraindicated in pregnant or breastfeeding women. In adolescents whose bone growth isn't complete, use cautiously because of effects on epiphyseal closure. Postmenopausal women with a history of long-term estrogen use are at increased risk for endometrial cancer and stroke. Postmenopausal women also have increased risk of breast cancer, MI, stroke, and blood clots with long-term use of estrogen plus progestin.

Fluoroquinolones

ciprofloxacin, delafloxacin meglumine, gatifloxacin, gemifloxacin mesylate, levoFLOXacin, moxifloxacin hydrochloride, ofloxacin

INDICATIONS

➤ **Bone and joint infection, bacterial bronchitis, endocervical and urethral chlamydial infection, bacterial gastroenteritis, endocervical and urethral gonorrhea, intra-abdominal infection, empirical therapy for febrile neutropenia, pelvic inflammatory disease, bacterial pneumonia, bacterial prostatitis, acute sinusitis, skin and soft-tissue infection, typhoid fever, bacterial UTI (prevention and treatment), chancroid, meningococcal carriers, and bacterial septicemia caused by susceptible organisms; bacterial conjunctivitis (gatifloxacin)**

ACTION

Fluoroquinolones produce a bactericidal effect by inhibiting intracellular DNA gyrase and topoisomerase IV. These enzymes are essential catalysts in the duplication, transcription, and repair of bacterial DNA.

Fluoroquinolones are broad-spectrum, systemic antibacterial drugs active against a wide range of aerobic gram-positive and gram-negative organisms. Gram-positive aerobic bacteria include *Staphylococcus aureus, S. epidermidis, S. hemolyticus, S. saprophyticus;* penicillinase- and non–penicillinase-producing staphylococci and some methicillin-resistant strains; *Streptococcus pneumoniae;* group A (beta) hemolytic streptococci *(S. pyogenes);* group B streptococci *(S. agalactiae);* viridans streptococci; groups C, F, and G streptococci and nonenterococcal group D streptococci; and *Enterococcus faecalis.* Fluoroquinolones are also effective against gram-negative aerobic bacteria, including, but not limited to, *Escherichia coli, Neisseria meningitidis*, and most strains of penicillinase- and non–penicillinase-producing *Haemophilus ducreyi, H. influenzae, H. parainfluenzae, Moraxella catarrhalis, N. gonorrhoeae*, most clinically important *Enterobacteriaceae*, and *Vibrio parahaemolyticus.* Certain fluoroquinolones are active against *Chlamydia trachomatis, Legionella pneumophila, Mycobacterium avium-intracellulare, Mycoplasma hominis, M. pneumoniae,* and *Pseudomonas aeruginosa.*

ADVERSE REACTIONS

Adverse reactions that are rare but need medical attention include CNS stimulation (acute psychosis, agitation, hallucinations, tremors), hepatotoxicity, hypoglycemia or hyperglycemia, hypersensitivity reactions, interstitial nephritis, phlebitis, pseudomembranous colitis, and tendinitis or tendon rupture. Adverse reactions that need no medical attention unless they persist or become intolerable include CNS effects (dizziness, headache, nervousness, drowsiness, insomnia), GI reactions, and photosensitivity.

CONTRAINDICATIONS & CAUTIONS

Black Box Warning Fluoroquinolones are associated with increased risk of tendinitis and tendon rupture in all age-groups. The risk further increases in older patients (usually older than age 60), in patients taking corticosteroids, and in patients who have received kidney, heart, or lung transplants. For patients with sinusitis, bronchitis, and uncomplicated UTIs, use only if there are no alternative treatment options. ∎

Black Box Warning Fluoroquinolones may exacerbate muscle weakness in persons with myasthenia gravis. Avoid use in patients with known history of myasthenia gravis. ∎

• Contraindicated in patients hypersensitive to fluoroquinolones because serious, possibly fatal, reactions can occur.

- Most systemic fluoroquinolones can cause QT-interval prolongations. Avoid in patients with a history of QTc-interval prolongation or uncorrected electrolyte disorders (hypokalemia, hypomagnesemia) and in patients taking class IA or class III antiarrhythmics and other drugs that prolong the QT interval.
- Hypoglycemia or hyperglycemia may occur in patients with or without diabetes.
- Use cautiously in patients with known or suspected CNS disorders that predispose them to seizures or lower the seizure threshold, cerebral ischemia, severe hepatic dysfunction, or renal insufficiency.
- CDAD ranging in severity from mild to fatal colitis can occur during treatment or even more than 2 months after therapy ends.
- If phototoxicity occurs, discontinue drug.
- Refer to manufacturer's instructions for use during pregnancy and breastfeeding. In children, fluoroquinolones aren't recommended because they can cause joint problems. If needed in elderly patients, reduce dosage; these patients are more likely to have reduced renal function.

Hematopoietic agents
darbepoetin alfa, epoetin alfa, epoetin alfa-epbx

INDICATIONS
➤ **Anemia associated with chronic renal failure, zidovudine therapy in patients with HIV, and cancer chemotherapy; to reduce the need for allogeneic blood transfusions in surgical patients (epoetin alfa-epbx)**

ACTION
Epoetin alfa, epoetin alfa-epbx, and darbepoetin alfa stimulate RBC production in the bone marrow.

ADVERSE REACTIONS
Hematopoietics may cause fatigue, headache, chest pain, HTN, nausea, vomiting, diarrhea, mucositis, stomatitis, myalgias, fever, dyspnea, cough, sore throat, alopecia, rash, urticaria, seizures, and stinging at injection site.

CONTRAINDICATIONS & CAUTIONS
Black Box Warning Refer to individual drug monographs for black box warnings. ∎
- Contraindicated in patients hypersensitive to these drugs, their components, or human albumin.

- Contraindicated in uncontrolled HTN.
- Don't use darbepoetin alfa, epoetin alfa, or epoetin alfa-epbx in patients with breast, non-small-cell lung, head and neck, lymphoid, and cervical cancers, or for the treatment of cancers with curative potential.
- Use cautiously in patients with cardiac disease, seizures, and porphyria.
- In pregnant women, consider the benefits and risks for the mother and possible risks to the fetus before starting therapy. It isn't known if drugs appear in human milk. Consider the benefits and risk of breastfeeding and potential adverse effects on infant; use cautiously in breastfeeding women.

Histamine$_2$-receptor antagonists
cimetidine, famotidine, nizatidine, raNITIdine hydrochloride

INDICATIONS
➤ **Duodenal or gastric ulcer, Zollinger-Ellison syndrome, GERD**

ACTION
H_2-receptor antagonists inhibit the action of H_2 receptors in gastric parietal cells, reducing gastric acid output and concentration, regardless of stimulants, such as histamine, food, insulin, and caffeine, or basal conditions.

ADVERSE REACTIONS
H_2-receptor antagonists rarely cause adverse reactions. Cardiac arrhythmias, dizziness, fatigue, gynecomastia, headache, mild and transient diarrhea, and thrombocytopenia are possible.

CONTRAINDICATIONS & CAUTIONS
- Contraindicated in patients hypersensitive to these drugs.
- Use cautiously in patients with impaired renal or hepatic function.
- Use cautiously in pregnant women. Refer to manufacturer's instructions for use during breastfeeding as some drugs shouldn't be used. Elderly patients have increased risk of adverse reactions, particularly those affecting the CNS; use cautiously.

DRUG CLASSES

Immunosuppressants

anakinra, azaTHIOprine, basiliximab, belimumab, cycloSPORINE, etanercept, fingolimod, inFLIXimab, inFLIXimab-abda, inFLIXimab-dyyb, inFLIXimab-qbtx, lymphocyte immune globulin, mycophenolate mofetil, sirolimus, tacrolimus

INDICATIONS
➤ **Prevention of rejection in organ transplants; management of severe RA, MS, psoriasis, SLE, Crohn disease, ulcerative colitis**

ACTION
The exact mechanism of action is not fully known. Immunosuppressants act by suppressing cell-mediated hypersensitivity reactions and produce various alterations in antibody production, blocking the activity of interleukin, inhibiting helper T cells and suppressor T cells, and antagonizing the metabolism of purine, therefore inhibiting RNA and DNA structure and synthesis.

ADVERSE REACTIONS
Immunosuppressants may cause albuminuria, hematuria, proteinuria, renal failure, hepatotoxicity, oral *Candida* infections, gingival hyperplasia, tremors, and headache. The most serious reactions include leukopenia, thrombocytopenia, and risk of secondary infection.

CONTRAINDICATIONS & CAUTIONS
Black Box Warning Refer to individual drug monographs for black box warnings. ∎
• Contraindicated in patients hypersensitive to these drugs or their components.
• Use cautiously in patients with severe renal disease or severe hepatic disease.
• Refer to manufacturer's instructions for use in pregnancy and breastfeeding.

Inotropes

digoxin, DOBUTamine hydrochloride, DOPamine hydrochloride, milrinone lactate

INDICATIONS
➤ **HF and supraventricular arrhythmias, including supraventricular tachycardia, atrial fibrillation, and atrial flutter (digoxin); short-term HF and patients awaiting heart transplantation (milrinone); low cardiac output (dopamine)**

ACTION
Inotropics help move calcium into the cells, which increases cardiac output by strengthening contractility. Digoxin also acts on the CNS to slow HR. Dobutamine increases cardiac stroke volume and cardiac output without marked increases in HR. Milrinone relaxes vascular smooth muscle, decreasing peripheral vascular resistance (afterload) and the amount of blood returning to the heart (preload). Dopamine produces positive chronotropic and inotropic effects on the myocardium, resulting in increased HR and cardiac contractility.

ADVERSE REACTIONS
Inotropics may cause arrhythmias, nausea, vomiting, diarrhea, headache, fever, mental disturbances, visual changes, and chest pain. Milrinone may cause thrombocytopenia, hypotension, hypokalemia, and elevated liver enzymes.

CONTRAINDICATIONS & CAUTIONS
• Contraindicated in patients hypersensitive to these drugs or their components.
• Digoxin is contraindicated in ventricular fibrillation.
• Use cautiously in patients with renal insufficiency because of the potential for toxicity.
• Use digoxin cautiously in patients with sinus node disease or AV block because of the potential for advanced heart block.
• Refer to manufacturer's instructions for use during pregnancy and breastfeeding.

Laxatives
Bulk-forming
calcium polycarbophil, psyllium

Emollient
mineral oil

Hyperosmolar
glycerin, lactulose, lubiprostone, polyethylene glycol

Saline
magnesium (citrate; hydroxide; sulfate), sodium phosphates

Stimulant
bisacodyl

Stool softener, stool surfactant
docusate (calcium; sodium)

INDICATIONS
➤ **Constipation, IBS, diverticulosis**

ACTION
Laxatives promote movement of intestinal contents through the colon and rectum in several ways: bulk-forming, emollient, hyperosmolar, and stimulant.

ADVERSE REACTIONS
All laxatives may cause flatulence, diarrhea, and abdominal disturbances. Bulk-forming laxatives may cause intestinal obstruction, impaction, or (rarely) esophageal obstruction. Emollient laxatives may irritate the throat. Hyperosmolar and saline laxatives may cause fluid and electrolyte imbalances. Stimulant laxatives may cause urine discoloration, malabsorption, and weight loss.

CONTRAINDICATIONS & CAUTIONS
• Contraindicated in patients with GI obstruction or perforation, toxic colitis, megacolon, nausea and vomiting, or acute surgical abdomen.
• Use cautiously in patients with rectal or anal conditions, such as rectal bleeding or large hemorrhoids.
• Refer to manufacturer's instructions for use in pregnant and breastfeeding women. Infants and children have an increased risk of fluid and electrolyte disturbances; use cautiously. In elderly patients, dependence is more likely to develop because of age-related changes in GI function. Monitor closely.

Macrolide anti-infectives
azithromycin, clarithromycin, erythromycin (ethylsuccinate; lactobionate; stearate), fidaxomicin

INDICATIONS
➤ **Various common infections**

ACTION
Inhibit RNA-dependent protein synthesis by acting on a small portion of the 50S ribosomal unit. They're active against

Staphylococcus aureus, Streptococcus pneumoniae, Streptococcus pyogenes, Streptococcus agalactiae, Moraxella catarrhalis, Chlamydia trachomatis, Mycoplasma pneumoniae, Haemophilus influenzae, and *Neisseria gonorrhoeae.* Fidaxomicin is active against CDAD.

ADVERSE REACTIONS
These drugs may cause cardiac effects (prolonged QT interval, arrhythmias, torsades de pointes), nausea, vomiting, diarrhea, abdominal pain, palpitations, chest pain, vaginal candidiasis, nephritis, dizziness, headache, vertigo, somnolence, rash, and photosensitivity.

CONTRAINDICATIONS & CAUTIONS
• Contraindicated in patients hypersensitive to these drugs and their components.
• CDAD ranging in severity from mild to fatal colitis can occur during treatment or even more than 2 months after therapy ends (except fidaxomicin).
• Refer to manufacturer's instructions for use during pregnancy and breastfeeding.

Neuromuscular blockers
atracurium besylate, cisatracurium besylate, pancuronium bromide, rocuronium bromide, succinylcholine chloride, vecuronium bromide

INDICATIONS
➤ **To relax skeletal muscle during surgery, reduce intensity of muscle spasms in drug-induced or electrically induced seizures, and manage patients who are fighting mechanical ventilation**

ACTION
Nondepolarizing blockers (atracurium, cisatracurium, pancuronium, rocuronium, vecuronium) compete with acetylcholine at cholinergic receptor sites on the skeletal muscle membrane. This action blocks acetylcholine's neurotransmitter actions, preventing muscle contraction. Succinylcholine is a depolarizing blocker. This drug isn't inactivated by cholinesterase, thereby preventing repolarization of the motor endplate and causing muscle paralysis.

DRUG CLASSES

ADVERSE REACTIONS

Neuromuscular blockers may cause apnea, hypotension, HTN, arrhythmias, tachycardia, bronchospasm, excessive bronchial or salivary secretions, and skin reactions.

CONTRAINDICATIONS & CAUTIONS

Black Box Warning Refer to individual drug monographs for black box warnings. ■

• Contraindicated in patients hypersensitive to these drugs or their components.

• The drugs should be used only by personnel skilled in airway management and respiratory support.

• Refer to manufacturer's instructions for use during pregnancy and breastfeeding.

Nonsteroidal anti-inflammatory drugs

aspirin, celecoxib, diclofenac, diflunisal, etodolac, fenoprofen, ibuprofen, indomethacin, ketoprofen, ketorolac tromethamine, meloxicam, nabumetone, naproxen, piroxicam, sulindac

INDICATIONS

➤ **Mild to moderate pain, inflammation, stiffness, swelling, or tenderness caused by headache, arthralgia, myalgia, neuralgia, dysmenorrhea, RA, juvenile arthritis, osteoarthritis, dental or surgical procedures, or patent ductus arteriosus**

ACTION

The analgesic effect of NSAIDs may result from interference with the prostaglandins involved in pain. Prostaglandins appear to sensitize pain receptors to mechanical stimulation or to other chemical mediators. NSAIDs inhibit synthesis of prostaglandins peripherally and possibly centrally.

NSAIDs exert an anti-inflammatory effect that may result in part from inhibition of cyclooxygenase-1 and -2 enzymes and prostaglandin synthesis and release during inflammation. The exact mechanism isn't clear.

ADVERSE REACTIONS

Adverse reactions chiefly involve the GI tract, particularly erosion of the gastric mucosa. The most common symptoms are abdominal pain, dyspepsia, epigastric distress, heartburn, and nausea. CNS and skin reactions also may occur.

Flank pain with other evidence of nephrotoxicity occurs occasionally. Fluid retention may aggravate HTN or HF.

CONTRAINDICATIONS & CAUTIONS

Black Box Warning Refer to individual drug monographs for additional black box warnings. ■

Black Box Warning NSAIDs may increase risk of serious CV thrombotic events, MI, and stroke, which can be fatal, and are contraindicated after CABG surgery. ■

Black Box Warning NSAIDs increase risk of serious GI reactions, including inflammation, ulceration, and perforation of the stomach or intestines, which can be fatal. Elderly patients are at increased risk. ■

• Contraindicated in patients hypersensitive to these drugs.

❸ *Alert:* MI or stroke can occur as early as the first week of using an NSAID (except aspirin). The risk appears higher with higher doses. Use the lowest effective dose for the shortest duration possible.

❸ *Alert:* NSAIDs increase the risk of HF.

• Use cautiously in patients with HF, HTN, risk of MI (except low-dose aspirin), fluid retention, renal insufficiency, or coagulation defects.

• Safety in pregnant women hasn't been established. Use during the third trimester increases risk of premature closure of the ductus arteriosus. Patients older than age 60 may be more susceptible to toxic effects of NSAIDs because of decreased renal function.

Nucleoside reverse transcriptase inhibitors

abacavir sulfate, didanosine, emtricitabine, lamiVUDine, stavudine, zidovudine

INDICATIONS

➤ **HIV infection, AIDS, prevention of maternal-fetal HIV transmission, prevention of HIV infection after occupational exposure (such as needle stick or mucous membrane or nonintact skin contact) or nonoccupational exposure to blood, genital secretions, or other potentially infectious body fluids of an HIV-infected person when there's substantial risk of transmission**

ACTION

NRTIs inhibit DNA viral replication by chain termination, competitive inhibition of reverse transcriptase, or both.

ADVERSE REACTIONS

Because of the complexity of HIV infection, it's often difficult to distinguish between disease-related symptoms and adverse drug reactions. The most frequently reported adverse effects of NRTIs are anemia, leukopenia, and neutropenia. Thrombocytopenia is less common. Rare adverse effects of NRTIs are hepatotoxicity, myopathy, and neurotoxicity. Any of these adverse effects requires prompt medical attention.

Adverse effects that don't need medical attention unless they persist or are bothersome include headache, insomnia, myalgias, nausea, and hyperpigmentation of nails.

CONTRAINDICATIONS & CAUTIONS

Black Box Warning Refer to individual drug monographs for black box warnings. ∎
• Contraindicated in patients hypersensitive to these drugs and patients with moderate to severe hepatic impairment (abacavir) or pancreatitis (didanosine).
• Use cautiously in patients with mild hepatic impairment or risk factors for liver impairment, risk for pancreatitis (didanosine), or compromised bone marrow function (zidovudine).
• In pregnant women, use drug only if benefits outweigh risks. To reduce the risk of transmitting the virus, HIV-infected mothers shouldn't breastfeed. The pharmacokinetic and safety profiles of NRTIs are similar in children and adults. NRTIs may be used in children age 3 months and older, but the half-life may be prolonged in neonates. In elderly patients, elimination half-life may be prolonged.

Opioid analgesics

codeine, fentaNYL citrate, HYDROmorphone hydrochloride, meperidine hydrochloride, methadone hydrochloride, morphine sulfate, nalbuphine hydrochloride, oxyCODONE hydrochloride, oxyMORphone hydrochloride, pentazocine lactate

INDICATIONS

➤ **Moderate to severe pain from acute and some chronic disorders; management of pain severe enough to require** daily, around-the-clock, long-term opioid treatment; dry, nonproductive cough (codeine); management of opioid dependence (methadone); anesthesia support; sedation

ACTION

Opioids act as agonists at specific opioid-receptor binding sites in the CNS and other tissues, altering perception of pain.

ADVERSE REACTIONS

Respiratory and circulatory depression (including orthostatic hypotension) are the major hazards of opioids. Other adverse CNS effects include agitation, coma, depression, dizziness, dysphoria, euphoria, faintness, mental clouding, nervousness, restlessness, sedation, seizures, visual disturbances, and weakness. Adverse GI effects include biliary colic, constipation, nausea, and vomiting. Urine retention or hypersensitivity also may occur. Drug tolerance and psychological or physical dependence may follow prolonged use.

CONTRAINDICATIONS & CAUTIONS

Black Box Warning Refer to individual drug monographs for black box warnings. ∎
Black Box Warning Opioids should only be prescribed with benzodiazepines or other CNS depressants to patients for whom alternative treatment options are inadequate. ∎
• Contraindicated in patients hypersensitive to these drugs and in those who have recently taken an MAO inhibitor. Also contraindicated in those with acute or severe bronchial asthma or respiratory depression.
♦ *Alert:* When used concomitantly with serotonergic drugs, risk of serotonin syndrome increases.
♦ *Alert:* Use may lead to rare but serious decrease in adrenal gland cortisol production and, with long-term use, to decreased sex hormone levels.
• Use cautiously in patients with head injury, increased ICP or increased IOP, hepatic or renal dysfunction, mental illness, emotional disturbances, or drug-seeking behaviors.
• Use cautiously in pregnant or breastfeeding women. Prolonged maternal use of opioids during pregnancy can cause neonatal withdrawal syndrome in the newborn, which may be life-threatening if not recognized and treated according to protocols developed by neonatology experts. Breastfed infants of women taking

opioids may develop physical dependence. Safety and effectiveness of some opioids in children haven't been established. Elderly patients may be more sensitive to opioids, and lower doses are usually given.

Penicillins

Natural penicillins
penicillin G (benzathine; potassium; procaine; sodium), penicillin V potassium

Aminopenicillins
amoxicillin, amoxicillin–clavulanate potassium, ampicillin (trihydrate), ampicillin sodium–sulbactam sodium

Extended-spectrum penicillins
piperacillin sodium–tazobactam sodium

Penicillinase-resistant penicillins
dicloxacillin sodium, nafcillin sodium, oxacillin sodium

INDICATIONS
➤ Streptococcal pneumonia; enterococcal and nonenterococcal group D endocarditis; diphtheria; anthrax; meningitis; tetanus; botulism; actinomycosis; syphilis; relapsing fever; Lyme disease; pneumococcal infections; rheumatic fever; bacterial endocarditis; neonatal group B streptococcal disease; septicemia; gynecologic infections; infections of urinary, respiratory, and GI tracts; infections of skin, soft tissue, bones, and joints

ACTION
Generally bactericidal, penicillins inhibit synthesis of the bacterial cell wall, causing rapid cell destruction. They're most effective against fast-growing susceptible bacteria. Their sites of action are enzymes known as *penicillin-binding proteins* (PBPs). The affinity of certain penicillins for PBPs in various microorganisms helps explain the different activities of these drugs.

Susceptible aerobic gram-positive cocci include *Staphylococcus aureus;* nonenterococcal group D streptococci; groups A, B, D, G, H, K, L, and M streptococci; *Streptococcus viridans;* and *Enterococcus* (usually with an aminoglycoside). Susceptible aerobic gram-negative cocci include *Neisseria meningitidis* and non–penicillinase-producing *N. gonorrhoeae.*

Susceptible aerobic gram-positive bacilli include *Corynebacterium, Listeria,* and *Bacillus anthracis.* Susceptible anaerobes include *Peptococcus, Peptostreptococcus, Actinomyces, Clostridium, Fusobacterium, Veillonella,* and non–beta-lactamase–producing strains of *Streptococcus pneumoniae.* Susceptible spirochetes include *Treponema pallidum, T. pertenue, Leptospira, Borrelia recurrentis* and, possibly, *B. burgdorferi.*

Aminopenicillins have uses against more organisms, including many gram-negative organisms. Like natural penicillins, aminopenicillins are vulnerable to inactivation by penicillinase. Susceptible organisms include *Escherichia coli, Proteus mirabilis, Shigella, Salmonella, S. pneumoniae, N. gonorrhoeae, Haemophilus influenzae, S. aureus, S. epidermidis* (non–penicillinase-producing *Staphylococcus*), and *Listeria monocytogenes.*

Extended-spectrum penicillins offer a wider range of bactericidal action than the other three classes and usually are given in combination with aminoglycosides. Susceptible strains include *Enterobacter, Klebsiella, Citrobacter, Serratia, Bacteroides fragilis, Pseudomonas aeruginosa, Proteus vulgaris, Providencia rettgeri,* and *Morganella morganii.* These penicillins are also vulnerable to beta-lactamase and penicillinases.

Penicillinase-resistant penicillins are semisynthetic penicillins designed to remain stable against hydrolysis by most staphylococcal penicillinases and thus are the drugs of choice against susceptible penicillinase-producing staphylococci. They also act against most organisms susceptible to natural penicillins.

ADVERSE REACTIONS
With all penicillins, hypersensitivity reactions range from mild rash, fever, and eosinophilia to fatal anaphylaxis. Hematologic reactions include hemolytic anemia, leukopenia, thrombocytopenia, and transient neutropenia. Certain adverse reactions are more common with specific classes. For example, bleeding episodes are usually seen with high doses of extended-spectrum penicillins, whereas GI adverse effects are most common with ampicillin. In patients with renal disease, high doses (especially of penicillin G) irritate the CNS, causing confusion, twitching, lethargy, dysphagia, seizures, and coma. Hepatotoxicity may

occur with penicillinase-resistant penicillins, and hypokalemia and hypernatremia have been reported with extended-spectrum penicillins. Local irritation from parenteral therapy may be severe enough to warrant administration by subclavian or centrally placed catheter or may warrant stopping therapy.

CONTRAINDICATIONS & CAUTIONS

Black Box Warning Refer to individual drug monographs for black box warnings. ▪
- Contraindicated in patients hypersensitive to these drugs.
- Use cautiously in patients with history of asthma or drug allergy, mononucleosis, renal impairment, CV diseases, hemorrhagic condition, or electrolyte imbalance.
- May cause CDAD, requiring drug discontinuation and treatment with other drugs.
- Use cautiously in pregnant women. For breastfeeding women, recommendations vary depending on the drug. For children, dosage recommendations have been established for most penicillins. Elderly patients are susceptible to superinfection and renal impairment, which decreases excretion of penicillins; use cautiously and at a lower dosage.

Phenothiazines

chlorproMAZINE hydrochloride, fluPHENAZine decanoate, perphenazine, prochlorperazine maleate, promethazine hydrochloride, thioridazine hydrochloride, thiothixene, trifluoperazine hydrochloride

INDICATIONS

➤ **Agitated psychotic states, schizophrenia, hallucinations, manic-depressive illness, excessive motor and autonomic activity, nausea and vomiting, moderate anxiety, behavioral problems caused by chronic organic mental syndrome, tetanus, acute intermittent porphyria, intractable hiccups, itching; allergies (promethazine)**

ACTION

Phenothiazines are believed to function as dopamine antagonists by blocking postsynaptic dopamine receptors in various parts of the CNS. Their antiemetic effects result from blockage of the chemoreceptor trigger zone. They also produce varying degrees of anticholinergic effects and alpha-adrenergic receptor blocking.

ADVERSE REACTIONS

Phenothiazines may produce extrapyramidal symptoms, such as dystonic movements, torticollis, oculogyric crises, and parkinsonian symptoms ranging from akathisia during early treatment to tardive dyskinesia after long-term use. An NMS resembling severe parkinsonism may occur, most often in young men taking fluphenazine.

Other adverse reactions include abdominal pain, agitation, anorexia, arrhythmias, confusion, constipation, dizziness, dry mouth, endocrine effects, fainting, hallucinations, hematologic disorders, local gastric irritation, nausea, orthostatic hypotension with reflex tachycardia, photosensitivity, seizures, skin eruptions, urine retention, visual disturbances, and vomiting. Promethazine injection can cause severe chemical irritation and tissue damage with such reactions as burning, pain, thrombophlebitis, tissue necrosis, and gangrene. Preferred route is IM.

CONTRAINDICATIONS & CAUTIONS

Black Box Warning Refer to individual drug monographs for black box warnings. ▪
- Contraindicated in patients with CNS depression, bone marrow suppression, HF, circulatory collapse, coronary artery or cerebrovascular disorders, subcortical damage, or coma. Also contraindicated in patients receiving spinal and epidural anesthetics and adrenergic blockers.
- Use cautiously in debilitated patients and in those with hepatic, renal, or CV disease; respiratory disorders; hypocalcemia; seizure disorders; suspected brain tumor or intestinal obstruction; glaucoma; and prostatic hyperplasia.
- In pregnant women, use only if clearly needed; safety hasn't been established. Women shouldn't breastfeed during therapy because most phenothiazines appear in human milk and directly affect prolactin levels. Phenothiazines aren't recommended for children younger than age 12 unless otherwise specified; use cautiously for nausea and vomiting. Acutely ill children, such as those with chickenpox, measles, CNS infections, or dehydration, have a greatly increased risk of dystonic reactions. Elderly patients are more sensitive to therapeutic and adverse effects, especially cardiotoxicity, tardive dyskinesia, and other extrapyramidal effects; use cautiously and reduce doses, adjusting dosage to patient response.

DRUG CLASSES

Progestins

HYDROXYprogesterone caproate, medroxyPROGESTERone acetate, norethindrone (acetate), ulipristal acetate

INDICATIONS

➤ **Amenorrhea, endometrial hyperplasia, abnormal uterine bleeding, endometriosis, contraception**

ACTION

Progestins transform proliferative endometrium into secretory endometrium.

ADVERSE REACTIONS

Progestins may cause amenorrhea, breakthrough bleeding, spotting, changes in menstrual flow, breast enlargement and tenderness, alterations in weight, and mood changes.

CONTRAINDICATIONS & CAUTIONS

Black Box Warning Refer to individual drug monographs for black box warnings. ■
• Contraindicated in patients with impaired liver function or liver disease; known or suspected breast cancer; active DVT, PE, or history of these conditions; active or recent arterial thromboembolic disease; and undiagnosed vaginal bleeding. Also contraindicated in patients hypersensitive to these drugs and their components.
• Use cautiously in patients with depression, epilepsy, migraine headaches, asthma, cardiac dysfunction, or renal dysfunction.
• Use is contraindicated in pregnant women. Use cautiously in breastfeeding women because detectable amounts of progestins have been identified in human milk. Progestins aren't indicated in children.

Protease inhibitors

atazanavir sulfate, darunavir ethanolate, fosamprenavir calcium, indinavir sulfate, lopinavir, nelfinavir mesylate, ritonavir, saquinavir mesylate, tipranavir

INDICATIONS

➤ **HIV infection and AIDS, postexposure prophylaxis**

ACTION

Protease inhibitors bind to the protease active site and inhibit HIV protease activity. This enzyme is required for the proteolysis of viral polyprotein precursors into the individual functional proteins found in infectious HIV. The net effect is formation of noninfectious, immature virus particles.

ADVERSE REACTIONS

The most common adverse effects that require immediate medical attention include kidney stones, pancreatitis, diabetes or hyperglycemia, ketoacidosis, and paresthesia.

Common adverse effects that don't need medical attention unless they persist or are bothersome include generalized weakness, GI disturbances, headache, insomnia, and taste disturbance. Less common adverse effects include dizziness and somnolence.

CONTRAINDICATIONS & CAUTIONS

Black Box Warning Refer to individual drug monographs for black box warnings. ■
• Contraindicated in patients hypersensitive to these drugs or their components and in patients taking a drug highly dependent on CYP3A4 for metabolism.
• Use cautiously in patients with impaired hepatic or renal function and those with diabetes mellitus or hemophilia.
• In pregnant women, use drug only if benefits outweigh risks. To reduce the risk of transmitting HIV to the infant, HIV-infected mothers shouldn't breastfeed.

Proton pump inhibitors

dexlansoprazole, esomeprazole (magnesium; sodium), lansoprazole, omeprazole (magnesium), pantoprazole sodium, RABEprazole

INDICATIONS

➤ **Duodenal ulcers, gastric ulcers, erosive esophagitis, and GERD; hypersecretory conditions (Zollinger-Ellison syndrome)**

ACTION

The drugs reduce stomach acid production by combining with hydrogen, potassium, and adenosine triphosphate in parietal cells of the stomach to block the last step in gastric acid secretion.

ADVERSE REACTIONS
PPIs may cause abdominal pain, diarrhea, constipation, flatulence, nausea, dry mouth, headache, asthenia, URI, abnormal LFT results, and hyperglycemia.

CONTRAINDICATIONS & CAUTIONS
• Contraindicated in patients hypersensitive to these drugs or their components.
• May increase risk of osteoporosis-related bone fractures and CDAD. Use lowest effective dose for the shortest duration.
• May increase risk of GI infections, hypomagnesemia and, with prolonged use, vitamin B_{12} deficiency.
• Studies are limited in pregnant women; consider the benefits and risks before starting therapy. Some drugs may appear in human milk. Refer to manufacturer's instructions for use during breastfeeding.

Selective serotonin reuptake inhibitors
citalopram hydrobromide, escitalopram oxalate, FLUoxetine hydrochloride, fluvoxaMINE maleate, PARoxetine hydrochloride, sertraline hydrochloride, vilazodone hydrochloride

INDICATIONS
➤ **Major depression, OCD, bulimia nervosa (fluoxetine), premenstrual dysphoric disorders, panic disorders, posttraumatic stress disorder (sertraline)**

ACTION
SSRIs selectively inhibit the reuptake of serotonin with little or no effects on other neurotransmitters in the CNS, such as norepinephrine and dopamine.

ADVERSE REACTIONS
Common adverse effects include headache, tremor, dizziness, sleep disturbances, GI disturbances, and sexual dysfunction. Less common adverse effects include bleeding (ecchymoses, epistaxis), akathisia, breast tenderness or enlargement, extrapyramidal effects, dystonia, fever, hyponatremia, mania or hypomania, palpitations, serotonin syndrome, weight gain or loss, rash, urticaria, and pruritus.

CONTRAINDICATIONS & CAUTIONS
Black Box Warning Antidepressants can increase risk of suicidal thinking and behavior, particularly in children, adolescents, and young adults. Appropriately monitor patients of all ages who are started on antidepressant therapy; observe closely for clinical worsening, suicidality, or unusual behavior changes. Advise families and caregivers of the need for close observation and communication with the prescriber. ∎
• Contraindicated in patients hypersensitive to these drugs or their components, within 14 days of MAO inhibitor therapy, and with concurrent use of linezolid or methylene blue.
• Use cautiously in patients with hepatic, renal, or cardiac disease.
• In pregnant women, use drug only if benefits outweigh risks; use of certain SSRIs in the first trimester may cause birth defects. Neonates born to women who took an SSRI during the third trimester may develop complications that require prolonged hospitalization, respiratory support, and tube feeding. Some SSRIs appear in human milk. Refer to manufacturer's instructions for use during breastfeeding. Elderly patients may be more sensitive to the insomniac effects of SSRIs.

Skeletal muscle relaxants
baclofen, carisoprodol, cyclobenzaprine hydrochloride, dantrolene sodium, methocarbamol, orphenadrine citrate, tiZANidine hydrochloride

INDICATIONS
➤ **Painful musculoskeletal disorders, muscle spasticity**

ACTION
Baclofen may reduce impulse transmission from the spinal cord to skeletal muscle. Carisoprodol, cyclobenzaprine, methocarbamol, orphenadrine, and tizanidine's mechanisms of action are unclear. Dantrolene acts directly on skeletal muscle to decrease excitation and reduce muscle strength by interfering with intracellular calcium movement.

ADVERSE REACTIONS
Skeletal muscle relaxants may cause ataxia, confusion, depressed mood, dizziness, drowsiness, dry mouth, hallucinations, headache, hypotension, nervousness, tachycardia, tremor,

DRUG CLASSES

and vertigo. Baclofen also may cause seizures with abrupt withdrawal.

CONTRAINDICATIONS & CAUTIONS
Black Box Warning Refer to individual drug monographs for black box warnings. ∎
• Contraindicated in patients hypersensitive to these drugs.
• Use cautiously in patients with impaired renal or hepatic function.
• Refer to manufacturer's instructions for use in pregnant and breastfeeding patients. In children, recommendations vary. Elderly patients have an increased risk of adverse reactions; monitor carefully.

Sulfonamides
sulfADIAZINE, sulfamethoxazole–trimethoprim

INDICATIONS
➤ **Bacterial infections, nocardiosis, toxoplasmosis, chloroquine-resistant** *Plasmodium falciparum* **malaria**

ACTION
Sulfonamides are bacteriostatic. They inhibit biosynthesis of tetrahydrofolic acid, which is needed for bacterial cell growth. They're active against some strains of staphylococci, streptococci, *Nocardia asteroides* and *N. brasiliensis, Clostridium tetani* and *C. perfringens, Bacillus anthracis, Escherichia coli,* and *Neisseria gonorrhoeae* and *N. meningitidis.* Sulfonamides are also active against organisms that cause UTIs, such as *E. coli, Proteus mirabilis* and *P. vulgaris, Klebsiella, Enterobacter,* and *Staphylococcus aureus,* and genital lesions caused by *Haemophilus ducreyi* (chancroid).

ADVERSE REACTIONS
Many adverse reactions stem from hypersensitivity, including bronchospasm, conjunctivitis, erythema multiforme, erythema nodosum, exfoliative dermatitis, fever, joint pain, pruritus, leukopenia, Lyell syndrome, photosensitivity, rash, SJS, and toxic epidermal necrolysis. GI reactions include anorexia, diarrhea, folic acid malabsorption, nausea, pancreatitis, stomatitis, and vomiting. Hematologic reactions include agranulocytosis, granulocytopenia, hypoprothrombinemia, thrombocytopenia and, in G6PD deficiency, hemolytic anemia. Renal effects usu-

ally result from crystalluria caused by precipitation of sulfonamide in the renal system.

CONTRAINDICATIONS & CAUTIONS
• Contraindicated in patients hypersensitive to these drugs.
• Use cautiously in patients with renal or hepatic impairment, bronchial asthma, severe allergy, or G6PD deficiency.
• Use is contraindicated in pregnant women at term and in breastfeeding women; sulfonamides appear in human milk. Elderly patients are susceptible to bacterial and fungal superinfection and have an increased risk of folate deficiency anemia and adverse renal and hematologic effects.

Tetracyclines
doxycycline (hyclate; monohydrate), minocycline hydrochloride, tetracycline hydrochloride

INDICATIONS
➤ **Bacterial, protozoal, and rickettsial infections**

ACTION
Tetracyclines are bacteriostatic but may be bactericidal against certain organisms. They bind reversibly to 30S and 50S ribosomal subunits, which inhibits bacterial protein synthesis.

Susceptible gram-positive organisms include *Bacillus anthracis, Actinomyces israelii, Clostridium perfringens* and *C. tetani, Listeria monocytogenes,* and *Nocardia.*

Susceptible gram-negative organisms include *Neisseria meningitidis, Pasteurella multocida, Legionella pneumophila, Brucella* species, *Vibrio cholerae, Yersinia enterocolitica, Yersinia pestis, Bordetella pertussis, Haemophilus influenzae, Haemophilus ducreyi, Campylobacter fetus, Shigella* species, and many other common pathogens.

Other susceptible organisms include *Rickettsia akari, Rickettsia typhi, Rickettsia prowazekii,* and *Rickettsia tsutsugamushi; Coxiella burnetii; Chlamydia trachomatis* and *Chlamydia psittaci; Mycoplasma pneumoniae* and *Mycoplasma hominis; Leptospira* species; *Treponema pallidum* and *Treponema pertenue;* and *Borrelia recurrentis.*

ADVERSE REACTIONS

The most common adverse effects involve the GI tract and may be dose related; they include abdominal discomfort; anorexia; bulky, loose stools; colitis; epigastric burning; flatulence; nausea; and vomiting. Superinfections and CDAD can occur.

Photosensitivity reactions may be severe. Permanent discoloration of teeth occurs if drug is given during tooth formation in children younger than age 8.

CONTRAINDICATIONS & CAUTIONS

- Contraindicated in patients hypersensitive to these drugs.
- Use cautiously in patients with renal or hepatic impairment.
- Tetracyclines can cause fetal harm and shouldn't be used in pregnant women. Tetracyclines appear in human milk; the decision to continue or discontinue breastfeeding should take into account benefits to the mother and risks to the infant. Children younger than age 8 shouldn't take tetracyclines; these drugs can cause permanent tooth discoloration, enamel hypoplasia, and a reversible decrease in bone calcification. Elderly patients may have decreased esophageal motility; use these drugs cautiously, and monitor patients for local irritation from slow passage of oral forms.

Thrombolytics

alteplase, defibrotide sodium, reteplase, tenecteplase

INDICATIONS

➤ To lyse thrombi, often in acute or emergency situations
➤ Acute MI, acute ischemic stroke, PE, peripheral vascular occlusion; to restore patency to thrombosed grafts and IV access devices (alteplase); hepatic sinusoidal obstruction syndrome after hematopoietic stem cell transplant (defibrotide)

ACTION

Thrombolytics convert plasminogen to plasmin, which lyses thrombi, and degrades fibrin, fibrinogen, and other plasma proteins.

ADVERSE REACTIONS

The most common adverse reactions are bleeding and allergic responses. Other common adverse reactions include nausea, vomiting, fever, and hypotension.

CONTRAINDICATIONS & CAUTIONS

- Contraindicated in patients hypersensitive to drugs and their components and in combination with other fibrinolytics.
- Contraindicated in active bleeding, history of stroke, recent intracranial or intraspinal surgery or trauma, intracranial neoplasm, arteriovenous malformation or aneurysm, bleeding diathesis, or severe uncontrolled HTN.
- Pregnancy is considered to be a relative contraindication, but drugs shouldn't be withheld in life-threatening situations. It isn't known if drugs appear in human milk; use cautiously in breastfeeding women.

Vasopressors

DOBUTamine hydrochloride, DOPamine hydrochloride, ePHEDrine sulfate, EPINEPHrine hydrochloride, norepinephrine

INDICATIONS

➤ Correction of hemodynamic imbalances present in shock, trauma, septicemia, cardiac surgical procedures, spinal anesthesia, drug reactions, renal failure, and HF

ACTION

Dobutamine is a direct-acting inotrope whose primary activity results from stimulation of the beta receptors of the heart while producing mild chronotropic, hypertensive, arrhythmogenic, and vasodilatory effects. Dobutamine increases cardiac output by decreasing peripheral vascular resistance, reducing ventricular filling pressure, and increasing AV node conduction. Dopamine is a natural catecholamine, a precursor to norepinephrine in noradrenergic nerves, and a neurotransmitter in certain areas of the CNS. It produces positive chronotropic and inotropic effects on the myocardium, resulting in increased HR and cardiac contractility, by directly exerting agonist action on beta-adrenergic receptors. Epinephrine and related medications (ephedrine, norepinephrine) act on receptors in the heart to produce a positive chronotropic effect as well as constrict arteries in the skin, mucous membranes, and organs via action on alpha-adrenergic receptors.

DRUG CLASSES

ADVERSE REACTIONS

Adverse reactions to vasopressors may include ventricular arrhythmias, tachycardia, angina, palpitations, cardiac conduction abnormalities, widened QRS complex, bradycardia, hypotension, HTN, vasoconstriction, headache, anxiety, azotemia, dyspnea, phlebitis, peripheral cyanosis, and gangrene of the extremities. Difficult or painful urination can be seen with ephedrine. Less common are hypotension, thrombocytopenia, hypokalemia, and nausea.

CONTRAINDICATIONS & CAUTIONS

Black Box Warning Refer to individual drug monographs for black box warnings. ■

• Contraindicated in patients hypersensitive to these drugs or their components.

• Contraindicated in patients with pheochromocytoma, uncorrected tachyarrhythmias, or ventricular fibrillation.

• Dobutamine is contraindicated in patients with idiopathic hypertrophic subaortic stenosis.

• Before treatment, correct hypovolemia.

• Some vasopressors must be used cautiously in patients with a sulfite allergy, particularly asthmatic patients. Allergic-type reactions, including anaphylactic symptoms and severe asthmatic episodes, can occur.

• Administer infusion into a large vein to prevent extravasation into surrounding tissue, which can cause tissue necrosis.

• Use with extreme caution in patients taking MAO inhibitors or who have been treated with MAO inhibitors 2 to 3 weeks before infusion. Patients taking dopamine will require substantially reduced dosages.

• Dopamine, ephedrine, and norepinephrine shouldn't be used during cyclopropane and halothane anesthesia because of the risk of ventricular tachycardia or fibrillation.

• Use cautiously in patients with hyperthyroidism, bradycardia, partial heart block, myocardial disease, or severe arteriosclerosis.

• Give to pregnant women only if clearly indicated. Use cautiously in breastfeeding women. Safety and effectiveness in children haven't been established.

abacavir sulfate ⌘
ah-BAK-ah-veer

Ziagen

Therapeutic class: Antiretrovirals
Pharmacologic class: Nucleoside reverse transcriptase inhibitors

AVAILABLE FORMS
Oral solution: 20 mg/mL
Tablets: 300 mg

INDICATIONS & DOSAGES
➤ **HIV-1 infection**
Adults: 300 mg PO b.i.d. or 600 mg PO daily with other antiretrovirals.
Children ages 3 months and older: 8 mg/kg PO b.i.d. or 16 mg/kg PO once daily up to maximum of 600 mg PO daily, with other antiretrovirals.
Adjust-a-dose: In patients with mild hepatic impairment (Child-Pugh class A), give 200 mg (oral solution) PO b.i.d. Don't use in patients with moderate to severe (Child-Pugh class B or C) hepatic impairment.

ADMINISTRATION
PO
⌘ **Black Box Warning** Screen for the HLA-B*5701 allele before start of therapy and before reinitiating therapy in patients with unknown status who previously tolerated drug. ∎
• Drug is considered hazardous; use safe handling and disposal precautions according to facility policy.
• Always give drug with other antiretrovirals, never alone.
• Patient may take drug with or without food.

ACTION
Converted intracellularly to the active metabolite carbovir triphosphate, which inhibits activity of HIV-1 reverse transcriptase, terminating viral DNA growth.

Route	Onset	Peak	Duration
PO	Unknown	0.7–1.7 hr	Unknown

Half-life: 1 to 2 hours.

ADVERSE REACTIONS
CNS: fever or chills, headache, insomnia and sleep disorders, anxiety, depressive disorders, malaise, fatigue, dizziness. **EENT:** ear, nose, and throat infections. **GI:** diarrhea, nausea, vomiting. **Hepatic:** *lactic acidosis, hepatomegaly with steatosis.* **Skin:** rash. **Other:** *hypersensitivity reaction.*

INTERACTIONS
Drug-drug. *Methadone:* May slightly increase methadone elimination. Monitor effectiveness; increase methadone dosage if needed.
Drug-lifestyle. *Alcohol use:* May decrease elimination of drug, increasing overall exposure. Monitor alcohol consumption. Discourage use together.

EFFECTS ON LAB TEST RESULTS
• May increase ALT, AST, amylase, CK, and triglyceride levels.
• May decrease platelet and neutrophil counts.

CONTRAINDICATIONS & CAUTIONS
⌘ **Black Box Warning** Contraindicated in patients who carry the HLA-B*5701 allele because they are at high risk for hypersensitivity reactions; screen patients before start of therapy and before reinitiating therapy in those with unknown status who previously tolerated drug. ∎
Black Box Warning Serious and sometimes fatal hypersensitivity reactions have occurred. Contraindicated in patients with a prior hypersensitivity reaction to abacavir. ∎
• Contraindicated in patients with moderate to severe hepatic impairment.
۞ Alert: Due to increased risk of hepatotoxicity, use cautiously when giving drug to patients at risk for liver disease. Lactic acidosis and severe hepatomegaly with steatosis, including fatal cases, have been reported with the use of nucleoside analogues alone or in combination, including abacavir and other antiretrovirals. Stop treatment with drug and don't restart if events occur.
Dialyzable drug: Unknown.

PREGNANCY-LACTATION-REPRODUCTION
• Use cautiously in pregnant women because the effects are unknown. Use during

---

✤Canada   ◇OTC   ◆Off-label use   ✔Photoguide   ⊜Do not crush   *Liquid contains alcohol   ⌘Genetic pregnancy only if potential benefits outweigh risk. Register pregnant women with the Antiretroviral Pregnancy Registry at 1-800-258-4263.

• Drug is present in human milk. To avoid risk of postnatal transmission of HIV-1 infection, development of viral resistance in HIV-positive infants, and possible adverse reactions, instruct patients not to breastfeed.

NURSING CONSIDERATIONS

• Women are more likely than men to experience lactic acidosis and severe hepatomegaly with steatosis. Obesity and prolonged nucleoside exposure may be risk factors.

Black Box Warning Drug can cause fatal hypersensitivity reactions with multiple organ involvement; if patient develops signs or symptoms of hypersensitivity (such as fever, rash, fatigue, achiness, generalized malaise, nausea, vomiting, diarrhea, abdominal pain, cough, dyspnea, or pharyngitis), stop drug and notify prescriber immediately. ■

Black Box Warning Don't restart drug or any abacavir-containing product after a hypersensitivity reaction, regardless of HLA-B*5701 status, because severe signs and symptoms will recur within hours and may include life-threatening hypotension and death. ■

• Because of a high rate of early virologic resistance, triple antiretroviral therapy with abacavir, lamivudine, and tenofovir shouldn't be used as a new treatment regimen for treatment-naive or pretreated patients. Monitor patients currently controlled with this combination and those who use this combination in addition to other antiretrovirals, and consider modification of therapy.

• Monitor patient for immune reconstitution syndrome. Inflammatory response to indolent or residual opportunistic infection (*Mycobacterium avium* infection, CMV, *Pneumocystis jiroveci* pneumonia, or TB) may occur during initial treatment; autoimmune disorders (Graves disease, polymyositis, and Guillain-Barré syndrome) may occur at any time after start of therapy.

• Assess for CAD risk factors with antiretroviral use, and address modifiable risk factors (such as HTN, hyperlipidemia, diabetes mellitus, and smoking).

• Drug may mildly elevate glucose level, especially in children.

PATIENT TEACHING

• Inform patient that drug can cause a life-threatening hypersensitivity reaction. Warn patient who develops signs or symptoms of hypersensitivity (such as fever, rash, severe tiredness, achiness, a generally ill feeling, nausea, vomiting, diarrhea, stomach pain, cough, shortness of breath, or sore throat) to stop taking drug and notify prescriber immediately.

• Encourage patient to review information leaflet about drug with each new prescription and refill and to carry a warning card summarizing the signs and symptoms of hypersensitivity.

• Inform patient that drug doesn't cure HIV infection. Tell patient that drug doesn't reduce the risk of transmission of HIV to others through sexual contact or blood contamination and that its long-term effects are unknown.

• Caution patient not to stop anti-HIV medicines, even for a short time, because the virus count may increase and the virus may become harder to treat.

• Warn patient not to restart abacavir or other abacavir-containing drugs without being under medical care because of the risk of serious hypersensitivity reaction.

• Tell patient to take drug exactly as prescribed with or without food.

abatacept
ab-a-TA-sept

Orencia

Therapeutic class: Antirheumatics
Pharmacologic class: Selective costimulation modulators

AVAILABLE FORMS

Lyophilized powder for injection: 250 mg single-use vial (25 mg/mL when reconstituted)
Solution for subcut administration: 50 mg/0.4 mL, 87.5 mg/0.7 mL, 125 mg/mL single-dose prefilled syringe; 125 mg/mL prefilled autoinjector

---

Reactions in bold italics are *life-threatening*. Interactions may have a *rapid onset* or a *delayed onset*.

INDICATIONS & DOSAGES

➤ **To reduce signs and symptoms, induce major clinical response, inhibit disease progression and structural damage, and improve physical function in patients with moderate to severe RA. Used alone or with other DMARDs (except TNF antagonists and anakinra)**

Adults weighing more than 100 kg: 1 g IV over 30 minutes. Repeat 2 and 4 weeks after initial infusion and then every 4 weeks thereafter.

Adults weighing 60 to 100 kg: 750 mg IV over 30 minutes. Repeat 2 and 4 weeks after initial infusion and then every 4 weeks thereafter.

Adults weighing less than 60 kg: 500 mg IV over 30 minutes. Repeat 2 and 4 weeks after initial infusion and then every 4 weeks thereafter.

Adults (subcut): 125 mg subcut once weekly with or without IV loading dose. For patients receiving loading dose, give single IV dose based on weight. Then give 125 mg subcut within a day, followed by 125 mg subcut once weekly. Patients transferring from IV to subcut form should receive the first subcut dose instead of the next scheduled IV dose.

➤ **As monotherapy or with methotrexate to reduce signs and symptoms of moderately to severely active polyarticular juvenile idiopathic arthritis**

Children ages 6 and older weighing 75 kg or more: Use adult dosing regimen, not to exceed a maximum dose of 1,000 mg.

Children ages 6 and older weighing less than 75 kg: 10 mg/kg IV over 30 minutes. Repeat 2 and 4 weeks after initial infusion and then every 4 weeks thereafter. Maximum dose is 1,000 mg. Calculate dosing based on body weight before each dose is administered.

Children ages 2 and older weighing 50 kg or more: 125 mg subcut once weekly without an IV loading dose.

Children ages 2 and older weighing 25 to less than 50 kg: 87.5 mg subcut once weekly without an IV loading dose.

Children ages 2 and older weighing 10 to less than 25 kg: 50 mg subcut once weekly without an IV loading dose.

➤ **Adult psoriatic arthritis**

Adults weighing more than 100 kg: 1 g IV over 30 minutes. Repeat 2 and 4 weeks after initial infusion, then every 4 weeks thereafter.

Adults weighing 60 to 100 kg: 750 mg IV over 30 minutes. Repeat 2 and 4 weeks after initial infusion, then every 4 weeks thereafter.

Adults weighing less than 60 kg: 500 mg IV over 30 minutes. Repeat 2 and 4 weeks after initial infusion, then every 4 weeks thereafter.

Adults (subcut): 125 mg subcut once weekly without IV loading dose. Patients transferring from IV to subcut form should receive first subcut dose instead of the next scheduled IV dose.

ADMINISTRATION

IV

▼ Reconstitute vial with 10 mL of sterile water for injection, using only the silicone-free disposable syringe provided, to yield 25 mg/mL. Use an 18G to 21G needle for preparation.

▼ Gently swirl contents until completely dissolved. Avoid vigorous shaking.

▼ Vent the vial with a needle to clear away foam.

▼ Solution should be clear and colorless to pale yellow. Don't use if opaque particles, discoloration, or other foreign particles are present.

▼ Further dilute solution to 100 mL total volume with NSS. Infuse over 30 minutes using an infusion set and a sterile, nonpyrogenic, low–protein-binding filter (pore size 0.2 to 1.2 micron).

▼ Store diluted solution at room temperature or refrigerate at 36° to 46° F (2° to 8° C). Complete infusion within 24 hours of reconstituting.

▼ **Incompatibilities:** Don't infuse in the same line with other IV drugs.

Subcutaneous

• Prefilled syringes and autoinjectors aren't intended for IV administration.

• Remove prefilled syringe or autoinjector from refrigerator 30 to 60 minutes before administration so that it reaches room temperature.

- Abatacept should be clear and colorless to pale yellow; don't use if particulate matter or discoloration is present.
- Rotate injection sites.
- Never inject into tender, bruised, red, or hard areas.
- Safety and effectiveness of autoinjector for subcut injection haven't been studied in patients younger than age 18.

ACTION
Inhibits T-cell activation, decreases T-cell proliferation, and inhibits production of TNF-alpha, interferon-gamma, and interleukin-2.

Route	Onset	Peak	Duration
IV, subcut	Unknown	Unknown	Unknown

Half-life: IV, 13 days; subcut, 14.3 days.

ADVERSE REACTIONS
CNS: headache, dizziness, pyrexia. **CV:** HTN. **EENT:** nasopharyngitis, rhinitis, sinusitis. **GI:** nausea, diverticulitis, dyspepsia, diarrhea, abdominal pain. **GU:** acute pyelonephritis, UTI. **Musculoskeletal:** back pain, limb pain. **Respiratory:** URI, bronchitis, cough, pneumonia, rhonchi, dyspnea. **Skin:** cellulitis, rash. **Other:** infections, *malignancies,* herpes simplex, influenza, infusion reactions, injection-site reaction.

INTERACTIONS
Drug-drug. *Anakinra, TNF antagonists:* May increase risk of infection. Don't use together.
Live-virus vaccines: May decrease effectiveness of vaccine. Avoid giving vaccines during or for 3 months after abatacept therapy.
Drug-herb. *Echinacea:* May diminish the therapeutic effect of immunosuppressants. Avoid concurrent use.

EFFECTS ON LAB TEST RESULTS
- GDH-PQQ (glucose dehydrogenase pyrroloquinoline quinone)–based glucose monitoring systems may react with maltose present in abatacept, causing falsely elevated blood glucose readings on the day of infusion (IV form only).

CONTRAINDICATIONS & CAUTIONS
- Contraindicated in patients hypersensitive to drug or its components.
- Rare cases of severe hypersensitivity reactions have been reported. Reactions may occur with the first dose or within 24 hours of infusion. Discontinue drug and treat emergently if hypersensitivity occurs.
- Use cautiously in patients with active infection, history of chronic infections, or underlying conditions that may predispose patient to infection; scheduled elective surgery; or COPD.
- Patients should be screened for viral hepatitis before starting therapy. Antirheumatic treatment may cause reactivation of HBV.
- Patients who test positive for TB should be treated before receiving drug.
Dialyzable drug: Unknown.

PREGNANCY-LACTATION-REPRODUCTION
- Use cautiously in pregnant women and only if benefit to the mother justifies potential risk to the fetus.
- Register pregnant women with the pregnancy registry (1-877-311-8972).
- It isn't known if drug appears in human milk. Patient should discontinue breastfeeding or discontinue drug, taking into account the importance of drug to the mother.

NURSING CONSIDERATIONS
- Make sure patient has been screened for TB and viral hepatitis before giving drug.
- Monitor patient, especially an older adult, carefully for infections and malignancies.
- If patient develops a severe infection, notify prescriber; therapy may need to be stopped.
- **❸ Alert:** If patient has COPD, watch for worsening respiratory status.
- Ensure the availability of appropriate supportive measures to treat possible hypersensitivity reactions.
- Ensure that patients with juvenile idiopathic arthritis are up to date with all immunizations before start of therapy.
- **Look alike–sound alike:** Don't confuse Orencia with Oracea.

PATIENT TEACHING
- Instruct patient that TB and viral hepatitis screening is necessary before therapy.

Reactions in bold italics are *life-threatening*. Interactions may have a *rapid onset* or a **delayed onset**.

- Tell patient to continue taking prescribed arthritis drugs. Caution against taking anakinra or TNF antagonists, such as etanercept, infliximab, or adalimumab.
- Tell patient to avoid exposure to infections.
- Tell patient to immediately report signs and symptoms of infection, swollen face or tongue, and difficulty breathing.
- Tell patient with COPD to report worsening signs and symptoms.
- Advise patient to avoid live-virus vaccines during and for 3 months after therapy.
- Advise female patient to consult prescriber if she becomes pregnant or plans to breastfeed.
- Encourage pregnant patient to enroll in pregnancy registry at 1-877-311-8972.
- Advise patient to contact prescriber before taking any other drugs or herbal supplements.
- Remind patient to contact prescriber before scheduling surgery.

SAFETY ALERT!

abemaciclib ⚱
a-bem-a-SYE-klib

Verzenio

Therapeutic class: Antineoplastics
Pharmacologic class: Kinase inhibitors

AVAILABLE FORMS
Tablets ⓞ: 50 mg, 100 mg, 150 mg, 200 mg

INDICATIONS & DOSAGES
Adjust-a-dose (for all indications): For severe hepatic impairment (Child-Pugh class C), reduce abemaciclib dosing frequency to once daily. Refer to manufacturer's instructions for toxicity-related dosage adjustments. For concomitant use of strong CYP3A inhibitors, if recommended starting dose of abemaciclib is 150 or 200 mg b.i.d., reduce abemaciclib dose to 100 mg b.i.d. If a strong CYP3A inhibitor is begun and abemaciclib dose has been decreased to 100 mg b.i.d. due to adverse reactions, further reduce abemaciclib dose to 50 mg b.i.d. When a strong CYP3A inhibitor has been discontinued, increase abemaciclib dose

(after three to five half-lives of the inhibitor) to the dose that was used before the strong CYP3A inhibitor was begun.
➤ **Initial endocrine-based treatment of hormone receptor (HR)–positive, HER2–negative advanced or metastatic breast cancer, in combination with an aromatase inhibitor**
Postmenopausal women: 150 mg PO b.i.d. Coadminister fulvestrant 500 mg IM on days 1, 15, and 29, and monthly thereafter. Treat premenopausal and perimenopausal women with a gonadotropin-releasing hormone agonist per clinical practice standards. Continue treatment until disease progression or unacceptable toxicity occurs.
➤ **HR-positive, HER2-negative advanced or metastatic breast cancer with disease progression after endocrine therapy, in combination with fulvestrant** ⚱
Women: 150 mg PO b.i.d. Coadminister fulvestrant 500 mg IM on days 1, 15, and 29, and monthly thereafter. Treat premenopausal and perimenopausal women with a gonadotropin-releasing hormone agonist per clinical practice standards. Continue treatment until disease progression or unacceptable toxicity occurs.
➤ **Monotherapy for the treatment of HR-positive, HER2-negative advanced or metastatic breast cancer with disease progression after endocrine therapy and prior chemotherapy in the metastatic setting** ⚱
Adults: 200 mg PO b.i.d. Continue treatment until disease progression or unacceptable toxicity occurs.

ADMINISTRATION
PO
- Give drug at approximately the same time every day.
- Patient must swallow tablets whole and not chew, crush, or split them. Only administer intact tablets.
- May give without regard for food.
- If patient vomits or misses a dose, give the next dose at its scheduled time.
- Store at 68° to 77° F (20° to 25° C).

ACTION
An inhibitor of cyclin-dependent kinases 4 and 6 (CDK4 and CDK6). In estrogen

receptor–positive breast cancer cells, cyclin D1 and CDK4 and CDK6 promote cell-cycle progression and cell proliferation. Drug blocks progression from G1 into S phase of the cell cycle, resulting in cell aging and death.

Route	Onset	Peak	Duration
PO	Unknown	8 hr	Unknown

Half-life: 18 hours.

ADVERSE REACTIONS

CNS: fatigue, pyrexia, headache, dizziness. **CV:** peripheral edema, *venous thromboembolism, PE*. **GI:** diarrhea, nausea, abdominal pain, vomiting, stomatitis, constipation, dry mouth, dysgeusia, decreased appetite. **GU:** UTI, vaginal infection. **Hematologic:** *neutropenia*, anemia, *leukopenia, thrombocytopenia*. **Hepatic:** *hepatotoxicity*. **Metabolic:** weight loss, dehydration. **Musculoskeletal:** arthralgia. **Respiratory:** cough. **Skin:** alopecia, pruritus, rash. **Other:** infections, *sepsis*.

INTERACTIONS

Drug-drug. *Ketoconazole:* May significantly increase abemaciclib level. Avoid concomitant use.
Strong CYP3A inducers (rifampin): May decrease abemaciclib plasma level and lead to reduced activity. Avoid concomitant use; consider alternative agents.
Strong CYP3A inhibitors (clarithromycin, diltiazem, itraconazole, verapamil): May increase abemaciclib level and increase risk of toxicity. Decrease abemaciclib dosage.
Drug-food. *Grapefruit products:* May increase abemaciclib level. Avoid concomitant use.

EFFECTS ON LAB TEST RESULTS

• May increase ALT, AST, and creatinine levels.
• May decrease Hb level and hematocrit and WBC, RBC, neutrophil, and platelet counts.

CONTRAINDICATIONS & CAUTIONS

• Drug may cause GI toxicity (including diarrhea associated with dehydration and infection), bone marrow suppression, and hepatotoxicity.

• Venous thromboembolism has been reported in patients treated with abemaciclib with fulvestrant or with an aromatase inhibitor.
• Use in patients with severe renal impairment and ESRD hasn't been studied.
• Use cautiously in patients with severe hepatic impairment (Child-Pugh class C).
• Safety and effectiveness in children haven't been established.
Dialyzable drug: Unknown.

PREGNANCY-LACTATION-REPRODUCTION

• Drug may cause fetal harm. Advise women of the risk to a fetus.
• Pregnancy testing is recommended for women of childbearing potential before treatment.
• Women of childbearing potential should use effective contraception during treatment and for at least 3 weeks after final dose.
• There is potential for serious adverse reactions in breastfed infants. Women shouldn't breastfeed during treatment and for at least 3 weeks after final dose.
• Based on animal studies, drug may impair fertility in males of reproductive potential.

NURSING CONSIDERATIONS

• Monitor patients for loose stools and associated dehydration and infection. Initiate antidiarrheal therapy and increase oral fluids at first sign of diarrhea.
• Monitor CBC before therapy begins, every 2 weeks during therapy for the first 2 months, monthly for the next 2 months, then as clinically indicated.
• Monitor patients for signs and symptoms of hepatotoxicity (fatigue, right upper quadrant abdominal pain, loss of appetite) and bone marrow suppression (fatigue, unusual bleeding or bruising, fever, infection).
• Obtain LFTs before therapy begins, every 2 weeks during therapy for the first 2 months, monthly for the next 2 months, then as clinically indicated.
• Monitor patients for signs and symptoms of thrombosis (pain and swelling of the extremities) and PE (chest pain, dyspnea, tachycardia), and treat appropriately.

PATIENT TEACHING
• Teach patient to take drug at the same time each day, to take only whole tablets, and not to take damaged tablets.
• Tell patient to report all adverse reactions and to immediately report signs and symptoms of hepatotoxicity or venous thromboembolism.
• Advise patient to immediately report fever, particularly in association with other signs and symptoms of infection (malaise, pain, cough, shortness of breath, drainage, changes in urine).
• Instruct patient to begin antidiarrheal therapy (such as loperamide) at first sign of loose stools, to increase fluid intake, and to notify prescriber for further instructions and follow-up.
• Warn female patient of childbearing potential of the possible risk to a fetus. Advise her that a pregnancy test will be done before therapy begins, to use effective contraception during therapy and for at least 3 weeks after final dose, and to report known or suspected pregnancy.
• Remind female patient not to breastfeed during treatment and for at least 3 weeks after final dose.

SAFETY ALERT!

abiraterone acetate
a-bir-A-ter-one

Yonsa, Zytiga

Therapeutic class: Antineoplastics
Pharmacologic class: Androgen biosynthesis inhibitors

AVAILABLE FORMS
Tablets ⊕: 250 mg
Tablets (micronized) ⊕: 125 mg

INDICATIONS & DOSAGES
Adjust-a-dose (for all indications): For patients with baseline moderate hepatic impairment (Child-Pugh class B), reduce starting dosage of Zytiga to 250 mg PO once daily or Yonsa starting dosage to 125 mg once daily. If hepatotoxicity develops during treatment, refer to manufacturer's instructions for dosage adjustments.

➤ **Metastatic, castration-resistant prostate cancer**
Adult men: 1,000 mg Zytiga PO once daily, in combination with 5 mg prednisone PO b.i.d. Or, 500 mg Yonsa PO once daily in combination with 4 mg methylprednisolone PO b.i.d.
➤ **Metastatic, high-risk castration-sensitive prostate cancer (Zytiga only)**
Adult men: 1,000 mg PO once daily in combination with 5 mg prednisone PO daily.

ADMINISTRATION
PO
• Patients receiving abiraterone should also receive a gonadotropin-releasing hormone analogue concurrently (or have had a bilateral orchiectomy).
• Drug is hazardous: use safe handling and disposal precautions according to facility policy. Women who are pregnant or may become pregnant should wear gloves when handling tablets.
• Zytiga and Yonsa tablets aren't interchangeable; don't substitute between formulations.
• Give Zytiga tablets on an empty stomach; patient shouldn't eat for 2 hours before or 1 hour after receiving drug. Give Yonsa tablets without regard to food.
• Patient should swallow tablets whole with water and not crush or chew them.
• Store tablets at room temperature.

ACTION
Inhibits biosynthesis of androgen production and increases mineralocorticoid production by the adrenal glands.

Route	Onset	Peak	Duration
PO	Rapid	2 hr	Unknown

Half-life: 7 to 17 hours.

ADVERSE REACTIONS
CNS: fatigue, pyrexia, insomnia. **CV:** edema, hot flushes, HTN, *arrhythmias,* chest pain, *cardiac failure.* **EENT:** nasopharyngitis. **GI:** diarrhea, dyspepsia, constipation, vomiting. **GU:** UTI, hematuria, urinary frequency, nocturia. **Hematologic:** anemia, bruising, lymphopenia. **Hepatic:** *hepatotoxicity.* **Metabolic:** *hypokalemia, hypophosphatemia,*

hyperglycemia, hyperlipidemia, hypernatremia. **Musculoskeletal:** joint swelling, joint discomfort, muscle discomfort, fractures, groin pain. **Respiratory:** URI, cough, dyspnea. **Skin:** rash. **Other:** falls.

INTERACTIONS
Drug-drug. *Dextromethorphan, thioridazine, other CYP2D6 substrates:* May inhibit metabolism of these drugs, causing higher levels. Avoid using together. If drugs must be used together, consider reducing dosage of CYP2D6 substrate drug.
Strong CYP3A4 inducers (such as carbamazepine, phenobarbital, phenytoin, rifabutin, rifampin, rifapentine): May decrease abiraterone level. If drugs must be used together, increase Zytiga dosage to 1,000 mg b.i.d. or Yonsa dosage to 500 mg b.i.d. during concomitant use; decrease back to the previous dose and frequency if the CYP3A4 inducer is discontinued.
Drug-food. *Any food:* May significantly increase drug absorption of Zytiga. Patient must take Zytiga on an empty stomach; Yonsa may be taken without regard to food.

EFFECTS ON LAB TEST RESULTS
• May increase ALT, AST, bilirubin, alkaline phosphatase, glucose, sodium, cholesterol, and triglyceride levels.
• May decrease potassium, phosphate, and Hb levels.
• May decrease lymphocyte count.

CONTRAINDICATIONS & CAUTIONS
• Contraindicated in patients hypersensitive to drug or its components and in those with baseline severe hepatic impairment (Child-Pugh class C).
• Use cautiously in patients with a history of CV disease (HF, recent MI, ventricular arrhythmias) or liver disease.
• Safety in patients with LVEF of less than 50% or NYHA Class III or IV HF hasn't been established.
Dialyzable drug: Unknown.

PREGNANCY-LACTATION-REPRODUCTION
• Drug isn't indicated for use in women and is contraindicated in women who are pregnant, may become pregnant, or are breastfeeding.

• Because drug may harm a developing fetus, women who are pregnant or may become pregnant shouldn't handle drug without protection (gloves).
• Based on animal studies, male patients with female partners of childbearing potential should use effective contraception during treatment and for at least 3 weeks after final dose.

NURSING CONSIDERATIONS
• Monitor ALT, AST, and bilirubin levels in all patients at baseline, every 2 weeks for first 3 months, then monthly thereafter. For patients with moderate hepatic impairment, measure at baseline, every week during first month of treatment, every 2 weeks for next 2 months, and monthly thereafter.
• Monitor LFTs frequently for elevated results and signs and symptoms of hepatotoxicity (malaise, jaundice, abdominal pain, nausea, and vomiting). If AST or ALT level rises above 5 × ULN, or bilirubin level rises above 3 × ULN, interrupt treatment and closely monitor liver function.
• Monitor patient with a history of CV disease at least monthly for HTN, hypokalemia, and fluid retention. Monitor serum potassium level before treatment and at least monthly. Control HTN and correct hypokalemia before and during treatment.
• Monitor patient for signs and symptoms of adrenocortical insufficiency (chronic fatigue, loss of appetite, muscle weakness, weight loss, nausea, and vomiting). Patient may need an increased corticosteroid dosage before, during, and after stressful situations.

PATIENT TEACHING
• Teach patient to take Zytiga on an empty stomach and not to eat for at least 2 hours before or 1 hour after taking drug. Yonsa may be taken without regard to food. Advise patient to swallow tablets whole with water.
• Instruct patient that abiraterone and either prednisone or methylprednisolone must be used together.
• Warn patient not to stop abiraterone, prednisone, methylprednisolone, or other chemotherapy drugs without consulting prescriber.
• Advise patient that if a single dose of abiraterone, methylprednisolone, or prednisone

---

Reactions in bold italics are *life-threatening*. Interactions may have a *rapid onset* or a *delayed onset*.

is missed, to take the regular dose the next day. If more than one dose is missed, advise patient to inform prescriber.
• Teach patient that periodic blood tests will be needed to monitor tolerance to therapy.
• Warn patient, female caregivers, and female sexual partners about risk of fetal harm from abiraterone therapy. Teach women who are pregnant or may become pregnant to wear gloves while handling drug.
• Teach male patient and female sexual partners the importance of using condoms. If patient's partner is pregnant or of childbearing potential, patient should use a condom and another effective birth control method during treatment and for at least 3 weeks after final dose.

SAFETY ALERT!

acalabrutinib
a-KAL-a-BROO-ti-nib

Calquence

Therapeutic class: Antineoplastics
Pharmacologic class: Kinase inhibitors

AVAILABLE FORMS
Capsules ⬛: 100 mg

INDICATIONS & DOSAGES
➤ **Treatment of mantle cell lymphoma in patients who have received at least one prior therapy**
Adults: 100 mg PO approximately every 12 hours until disease progression or unacceptable toxicity occurs.
Adjust-a-dose: Refer to manufacturer's instructions for toxicity-related dosage adjustments. Avoid concomitant use with CYP3A inhibitors but if a CYP3A inhibitor is necessary and will be used short term (up to 7 days), interrupt acalabrutinib therapy. If patient is taking acalabrutinib with a moderate CYP3A inhibitor, reduce acalabrutinib dosage to 100 mg once daily. Avoid concomitant use with strong CYP3A inducers but if use together can't be avoided, increase acalabrutinib dosage to 200 mg b.i.d.

ADMINISTRATION
PO
• Make sure patient swallows capsule whole with water; don't open, break, or allow patient to chew capsules.
• May give drug with or without food.
• If a dose is missed by more than 3 hours, skip the dose and give next dose at its regularly scheduled time. Don't give an extra dose to make up for a missed dose.
• Store at 68° to 77° F (20° to 25° C).

ACTION
A selective and irreversible second-generation Bruton tyrosine kinase inhibitor that causes decreased malignant B-cell proliferation and survival.

Route	Onset	Peak	Duration
PO	Unknown	45 min	Unknown

Half-life: Acalabrutinib, 0.9 hour; active metabolite, 6.9 hours.

ADVERSE REACTIONS
CNS: headache, fatigue. **CV:** atrial fibrillation, atrial flutter, hematoma, *hemorrhage.* **EENT:** epistaxis. **GI:** diarrhea, nausea, abdominal pain, constipation, vomiting. **Hematologic:** *cytopenias,* anemia, *thrombocytopenia, neutropenia.* **Musculoskeletal:** myalgia. **Skin:** bruising, rash. **Other:** infection, *second primary malignancies.*

INTERACTIONS
Drug-drug. *Antacids (calcium carbonate):* May decrease acalabrutinib level. Separate antacid dosing from acalabrutinib by at least 2 hours.
Anticoagulants, antiplatelet agents: May increase risk of bleeding. Use cautiously together and monitor for hemorrhage.
H₂-receptor antagonists (famotidine, ranitidine): May decrease acalabrutinib level. Give drug 2 hours before H₂-receptor antagonist.
Moderate CYP3A inhibitors (diltiazem, erythromycin, fosamprenavir, verapamil): May increase acalabrutinib level. Reduce acalabrutinib dosage to 100 mg once daily.
PPIs (omeprazole): May decrease acalabrutinib level. Avoid concurrent use.

Strong CYP3A inducers (rifampin): May decrease acalabrutinib level. Avoid coadministration but if a strong CYP3A inducer can't be avoided, increase acalabrutinib dosage to 200 mg b.i.d.

Strong CYP3A inhibitors (itraconazole): May increase acalabrutinib level. Avoid coadministration but if inhibitor will be used short term (less than 7 days), interrupt acalabrutinib therapy.

Drug-lifestyle. *Sun exposure:* May increase risk of skin cancer. Protect skin from sun exposure.

EFFECTS ON LAB TEST RESULTS
• May increase creatinine level.
• May decrease Hb level and platelet and neutrophil counts.

CONTRAINDICATIONS & CAUTIONS
• Serious hemorrhagic events, including fatal events, have occurred in patients with hematologic malignancies. Consider benefits and risks of withholding drug for 3 to 7 days before and after surgery, depending on the type of surgery and the risk of bleeding.
• Serious infections (bacterial, viral, or fungal), including fatal events and opportunistic infections, have occurred. Patients at increased risk for infection may need prophylaxis.
• Second primary malignancies, including nonskin carcinomas and skin cancer, can occur.
• Safety and effectiveness in children haven't been established.
Dialyzable drug: Unlikely.

PREGNANCY-LACTATION-REPRODUCTION
• There are no available data in pregnant women concerning drug-associated risk. Based on animal studies, drug may cause fetal harm. Advise pregnant women of the potential risk to the fetus.
• Women shouldn't breastfeed during therapy and for at least 2 weeks after final dose.

NURSING CONSIDERATIONS
• Monitor patient for development of malignancies, including skin cancers.
• Monitor patient for atrial fibrillation and atrial flutter, and treat appropriately.

• Monitor patient for infection and treat as clinically indicated. Prophylactic therapy may be needed.
• Obtain CBC at least monthly to monitor for cytopenias.
• Monitor patient closely for hemorrhage, especially in patients on antiplatelet or anticoagulant therapy.
• Monitor and manage drug-related toxicities using treatment interruption, dosage reduction, or discontinuation according to manufacturer's instructions.

PATIENT TEACHING
• Teach patient to report all adverse reactions.
• Teach patient to swallow capsules whole with water.
• Instruct patient to immediately report signs or symptoms of severe bleeding (blood in stools, black stools, pink or brown urine, unexpected or uncontrolled bleeding, blood in vomit or sputum, dizziness, weakness, confusion, changes in speech, persistent headache).
• Caution patient that drug may need to be interrupted for major surgeries.
• Advise patient to immediately report signs or symptoms of infection (fever, chills, flu-like symptoms).
• Inform patient that blood tests will be needed to check blood counts at least once a month during therapy.
• Warn patient that other malignancies, including skin cancer, have been reported in patients who have been treated with this drug; advise patient to use sun protection.
• Counsel patient to seek medical attention for palpitations, light-headedness, dizziness, fainting, shortness of breath, and chest discomfort.
• Inform female patient of childbearing potential that drug may cause fetal harm.
• Caution patient not to breastfeed during treatment and for at least 2 weeks after final dose.

acamprosate calcium
a-kam-PRO-sate

Therapeutic class: Alcohol deterrents
Pharmacologic class: Synthetic amino acid neurotransmitter analogues

AVAILABLE FORMS
Tablets (delayed-release) ⊕: 333 mg

INDICATIONS & DOSAGES
➤ **Adjunct to management of alcohol abstinence**
Adults: 666 mg PO t.i.d.
Adjust-a-dose: In patients with CrCl of 30 to 50 mL/minute, give 333 mg t.i.d. Do not use in patients with severe renal impairment (CrCl 30 mL/minute or less).

ADMINISTRATION
PO
• Don't crush or break tablets.
• Give drug without regard for food.

ACTION
Restores the balance of neuronal excitation and inhibition, probably by interacting with glutamate and GABA neurotransmitter systems, thus reducing alcohol dependence.

Route	Onset	Peak	Duration
PO	Unknown	3–8 hr	Unknown

Half-life: 20 to 33 hours.

ADVERSE REACTIONS
CNS: abnormal thinking, amnesia, anxiety, asthenia, depression, dizziness, headache, insomnia, migraine, paresthesia, somnolence, *suicidal thoughts,* syncope, tremor, pain. **CV:** chest pain, HTN, palpitations, peripheral edema, vasodilation. **EENT:** abnormal vision, pharyngitis, rhinitis. **GI:** abdominal pain, anorexia, constipation, diarrhea, dry mouth, dyspepsia, flatulence, increased appetite, nausea, taste disturbance, vomiting. **GU:** erectile dysfunction. **Metabolic:** weight gain. **Musculoskeletal:** arthralgia, back pain, myalgia. **Respiratory:** bronchitis, dyspnea, increased cough. **Skin:** increased sweating, pruritus, rash. **Other:** accidental injury, chills, decreased libido, flulike symptoms, infection.

INTERACTIONS
None significant.

EFFECTS ON LAB TEST RESULTS
• May increase ALT, AST, bilirubin, blood glucose, and uric acid levels.

CONTRAINDICATIONS & CAUTIONS
• Contraindicated in patients hypersensitive to drug or its components and in those with CrCl of 30 mL/minute or less.
• Use cautiously in elderly patients, patients with moderate renal impairment, and patients with a history of depression and suicidal thoughts or attempts.
Dialyzable drug: Unknown.
⚠ *Overdose S&S:* Diarrhea, hypercalcemia in chronic overdose.

PREGNANCY-LACTATION-REPRODUCTION
• Use cautiously in pregnant women and only if potential benefit justifies potential risk to the fetus.
• It isn't known if drug appears in human milk. Use cautiously in breastfeeding women.

NURSING CONSIDERATIONS
• Use only after patient successfully becomes abstinent from drinking.
• Drug doesn't eliminate or reduce withdrawal symptoms.
⚙ *Alert:* Monitor patient for development of depression or suicidal thoughts.
• Drug doesn't cause alcohol aversion or a disulfiram-like reaction if used with alcohol.

PATIENT TEACHING
• Tell patient to continue the alcohol abstinence program, including counseling and support.
⚙ *Alert:* Advise patient to notify prescriber if depression, anxiety, thoughts of suicide, or severe diarrhea develops.
• Caution patient's family or caregiver to watch for signs of depression or suicidal ideation.
• Tell patient that drug may be taken without regard to meals, but that taking it with meals may help to remember it.
• Tell patient not to crush, break, or chew the tablets but to swallow them whole.

• Advise female patient to use effective contraception during therapy. Tell patient to contact prescriber if she becomes or plans to become pregnant.

• Explain that drug may impair judgment, thinking, or motor skills. Urge patient to use caution when driving or performing hazardous activities until drug's effects are known.

• Tell patient to continue taking acamprosate and to contact prescriber if patient resumes drinking alcohol.

acetaminophen (APAP, paracetamol)
a-seet-a-MIN-a-fen

ACET✢ ◇, Arthritis Pain Relief ◇, Atasol Forte✢ ◇, Fortolin✢, Ofirmev, Pediatrix✢ ◇, Rapid Action✢ ◇, Taminol✢, Triaminic Fever Reducer ◇, Tylenol ◇

Therapeutic class: Analgesics
Pharmacologic class: Para-aminophenol derivatives

AVAILABLE FORMS
Caplets: 500 mg ◇
Caplets (extended-release) ⓞⓣⓒ: 650 mg ◇
Capsules: 325 mg ◇, 500 mg ◇
Drops: 80 mg/mL✢ ◇
Elixir: 160 mg/5 mL✢ ◇*
Gelcaps: 500 mg ◇
Injection: 10 mg/mL
Oral liquid: 160 mg/5 mL✢ ◇, 500 mg/15 mL ◇
Oral solution: 80 mg/mL✢ ◇, 160 mg/5 mL✢ ◇, 167 mg/5 mL ◇
Oral suspension: 80 mg/0.8 mL ◇, 160 mg/5 mL✢ ◇
Oral syrup: 160 mg/5 mL ◇
Suppositories: 80 mg ◇, 120 mg ◇, 160 mg ◇, 325 mg ◇, 650 mg ◇
Tablets: 325 mg ◇, 500 mg ◇, 650 mg ◇
Tablets (chewable): 80 mg ◇, 160 mg ◇
Tablets (dispersible): 80 mg ◇, 160 mg ◇
Tablets (extended-release) ⓞⓣⓒ: 650 mg ◇

INDICATIONS & DOSAGES
Black Box Warning Maximum daily dose includes all routes of administration and all acetaminophen-containing products, including combination products. ∎

➤ **Mild pain or fever**
PO
Adults: 325 to 650 mg PO every 4 to 6 hours. Or, two extended-release caplets PO every 8 hours. Maximum, 3,250 mg daily unless under health care provider supervision, when 4 g daily (immediate-release) may be used. For long-term therapy, don't exceed 2.6 g daily unless prescribed and monitored closely by health care provider.
Children older than age 12: 325 to 650 mg PO every 4 to 6 hours or 1,300 mg PO every 8 hours (extended-release) p.r.n. Maximum dose for immediate-release is 3,250 mg/24 hours unless under health care provider supervision, when up to 4 g/24 hours may be used. Maximum dose for extended-release is 3,900 mg/24 hours.
Children ages 6 to 11 (immediate-release): 325 mg PO every 4 to 6 hours. Maximum daily dose is 1,625 mg/day PO. Don't use for more than 5 days unless directed by health care provider.
Children age 11 weighing 32.7 to 43.2 kg: 480 mg PO (oral suspension or chewable tablets) every 4 hours p.r.n. Maximum, five doses/day.
Children ages 9 to 10 weighing 27.3 to 32.6 kg: 400 mg PO (oral suspension or chewable tablets) every 4 hours p.r.n. Maximum, five doses/day.
Children ages 6 to 8 weighing 21.8 to 27.2 kg: 320 mg PO (oral suspension or chewable tablets) every 4 hours p.r.n. Maximum, five doses/day.
Children ages 4 to 5 weighing 16.4 to 21.7 kg: 240 mg PO (oral suspension or chewable tablets) every 4 hours p.r.n. Maximum, five doses/day.
Children ages 2 to 3 weighing 10.9 to 16.3 kg: 160 mg PO (oral suspension or chewable tablets) every 4 hours p.r.n. Maximum, five doses/day.
Children ages 1 to 2 weighing 8.2 to 10.8 kg: 120 mg PO (oral suspension or chewable tablets) every 4 hours p.r.n. Maximum, five doses/day.
Children ages 4 to 11 months weighing 5.4 to 8.1 kg: 80 mg PO (oral suspension, drops, or liquid) every 4 hours p.r.n. Maximum, five doses/day.

Reactions in bold italics are *life-threatening*. Interactions may have a *rapid onset* or a *delayed onset*.

Children ages 0 to 3 months weighing 2.7 to 5.3 kg: 40 mg PO (oral drops) every 4 hours p.r.n. Maximum, five doses/day.

Adjust-a-dose: For adults with GFR of 10 to 50 mL/minute/1.73 m^2, give every 6 hours; if GFR is less than 10 mL/minute/1.73 m^2, give every 8 hours. For patients receiving continuous renal replacement therapy, give every 6 hours. For infants, children, and adolescents with GFR less than 10 mL/minute/1.73 m^2, give every 8 hours. For infants, children, and adolescents receiving hemodialysis or peritoneal dialysis, give every 8 hours.

Rectal
Adults and children age 12 and older: 650 mg PR every 4 to 6 hours p.r.n. Maximum, 3.9 g daily. For long-term therapy, don't exceed 2.6 g daily unless prescribed and monitored closely by health care provider.
Children ages 6 to 11: 325 mg PR every 4 to 6 hours p.r.n. Maximum, 1,625 mg in 24 hours.
Children ages 3 to 6: 120 mg PR every 4 to 6 hours p.r.n. Maximum, 600 mg in 24 hours.
Children ages 1 to 3: 80 mg PR every 4 to 6 hours p.r.n. Maximum, 400 mg in 24 hours.
Children ages 6 to 11 months: 80 mg PR every 6 hours p.r.n. Maximum, 320 mg in 24 hours.

➤ **Mild to moderate pain; mild to moderate pain with adjunctive opioid analgesics; fever**
Adults and children age 13 and older weighing 50 kg or more: 1,000 mg IV every 6 hours or 650 mg IV every 4 hours. Maximum dose is 1,000 mg as a single dose and 4,000 mg/day.
Adults and children age 13 and older weighing less than 50 kg: 15 mg/kg IV every 6 hours or 12.5 mg/kg IV every 4 hours. Maximum dose is 15 mg/kg (up to 750 mg) as a single dose and 75 mg/kg (up to 3,750 mg)/day.
Children ages 2 to 12: 15 mg/kg IV every 6 hours or 12.5 mg/kg IV every 4 hours. Maximum dose is 15 mg/kg as a single dose and 75 mg/kg (up to 3,750 mg)/day.
Infants age 29 days to 2 years for fever: 15 mg/kg IV every 6 hours. Maximum dose

is 60 mg/kg/day, with minimum dosing interval of 6 hours.
Neonates (32 weeks' gestational age and greater) to age 28 days for fever: 12.5 mg/kg IV every 6 hours. Maximum dose is 50 mg/kg/day, with minimum dosing interval of 6 hours.
Adjust-a-dose: Longer dosing intervals and a reduced total daily dose may be warranted in patients with CrCl of 30 mL/minute or less.

ADMINISTRATION
PO
• Use liquid form for children and patients who have difficulty swallowing.
• Give drug without regard for food.
• Dispersible tablet should be allowed to dissolve in the mouth.
• Shake liquid formulations well before using.
• Give extended-release forms whole; don't crush, dissolve, or allow patient to chew extended-release forms.

IV
▼ Examine vial; don't use if particulate matter or discoloration is observed.
▼ For 1,000-mg dose, give by inserting a vented IV set through the septum of a 100-mL vial.
▼ For doses less than 1,000 mg, withdraw appropriate dose and place into a separate container before administration.
▼ Place small-volume pediatric doses of up to 60 mL in a syringe and use a syringe-pump.
▼ May administer without further dilution.
▼ Don't add other medications to IV solution.
▼ Give over 15 minutes.
▼ Entire 100-mL vial isn't for use in patients weighing less than 50 kg.
▼ Monitor end of infusion to prevent possibility of air embolism.
▼ Use within 6 hours of penetrating vial seal.
▼ Vial is for single use only. Discard unused portion.
▼ **Incompatibilities:** Diazepam, chlorpromazine hydrochloride. Don't admix with other drugs.

Rectal
• If suppository is too soft, refrigerate for 15 minutes or run under cold water in wrapper.

ACTION
Thought to produce analgesia by inhibiting prostaglandin and other substances that sensitize pain receptors. Drug may relieve fever through central action in the hypothalamic heat-regulating center.

Route	Onset	Peak	Duration
PO	<1 hr	30–60 min	4–6 hr
IV	5–30 min	15 min	4–6 hr
PR	Unknown	1½–5 hr	Unknown

Half-life: PO, 2 to 3 hours; IV, 2.4 to 7 hours; PR, 2 to 3 hours.

ADVERSE REACTIONS
CNS: agitation (IV), anxiety, fatigue, headache, insomnia, pyrexia. **CV:** HTN, hypotension, peripheral edema, periorbital edema, tachycardia (IV). **GI:** nausea, vomiting, abdominal pain, diarrhea, constipation (IV). **GU:** oliguria (IV). **Hematologic:** hemolytic anemia, *leukopenia, neutropenia, pancytopenia, anemia.* **Hepatic:** jaundice. **Metabolic:** hypoalbuminemia (IV), *hypoglycemia, hypokalemia,* hypervolemia, *hypomagnesemia,* hypophosphatemia (IV). **Musculoskeletal:** muscle spasms, extremity pain (IV). **Respiratory:** abnormal breath sounds, dyspnea, *hypoxia,* atelectasis, pleural effusion, *pulmonary edema, stridor,* wheezing (IV). **Skin:** rash, urticaria; infusion-site pain (IV), pruritus.

INTERACTIONS
Drug-drug. *Barbiturates, carbamazepine, hydantoins, rifampin:* High doses or long-term use of these drugs may reduce therapeutic effects and enhance hepatotoxic effects of acetaminophen. Avoid using together.
Busulfan: May increase busulfan level. Monitor patient closely.
Cholestyramine resin: May decrease acetaminophen absorption. Give at least 1 hour after acetaminophen or consider therapy change.
Dasatinib: May enhance hepatotoxic effects of dasatinib and increase acetaminophen level. Avoid use together.
Imatinib, mipomersen: May increase hepatotoxic effects of these drugs. Monitor patient closely.

Isoniazid: May increase risk of acetaminophen adverse effects. Monitor patient closely.
Lamotrigine: Prolonged acetaminophen use may decrease lamotrigine level. Monitor patient for therapeutic effects; adjust lamotrigine dosage as needed.
Lomitapide: May increase lomitapide level. Limit maximum adult dose of acetaminophen to 4 g or less daily for 3 or fewer days per week or consider therapy change.
Metyrapone, probenecid: May increase acetaminophen level and risk of hepatotoxicity. Avoid use together.
Warfarin: May increase hypoprothrombinemic effects with long-term use with high doses of acetaminophen. Monitor INR closely.
Drug-lifestyle. *Alcohol use:* May increase risk of hepatic damage. Discourage use together.

EFFECTS ON LAB TEST RESULTS
• May increase AST level. May decrease glucose, potassium, phosphorus, magnesium, albumin, and Hb level and hematocrit.
• May decrease neutrophil, WBC, RBC, and platelet counts.
• May cause false-positive test result for urinary 5-hydroxyindoleacetic acid. May falsely decrease glucose level in home monitoring systems.

CONTRAINDICATIONS & CAUTIONS
Black Box Warning Drug can cause acute liver failure, which may require a liver transplant or cause death. Most cases of liver injury are associated with drug doses exceeding 4,000 mg/day and often involve more than one acetaminophen-containing product. ▮
❸ *Alert:* May cause serious, potentially fatal skin reactions, including SJS, toxic epidermal necrolysis, and acute generalized exanthematous pustulosis. Reaction may occur with first or subsequent use when acetaminophen is used as monotherapy or when it is one component of combination drug therapy. Monitor for reddening of the skin, rash, blisters, and detachment of the

upper surface of the skin. Stop drug immediately if skin reaction is suspected.
• Contraindicated in patients hypersensitive to drug. IV form is contraindicated in patients with severe hepatic impairment or severe active liver disease.
• Use cautiously in patients with any type of liver disease, G6PD deficiency, chronic malnutrition, severe hypovolemia (dehydration, blood loss), or severe renal impairment (CrCl of 30 mL/minute or less).
• Use cautiously in patients with long-term alcohol use because therapeutic doses cause hepatotoxicity in these patients. Chronic alcoholics shouldn't take more than 2 g of acetaminophen every 24 hours.
Dialyzable drug: Unknown.
⚠ **Overdose S&S:** Stage 1 (up to 24 hours)—abdominal pain, diaphoresis, nausea, vomiting, malaise, pallor; stage 2 (24 to 36 hours)—right upper quadrant pain, elevated LFT results, prolonged PT; stage 3 (72 to 96 hours)—hepatic failure, encephalopathy, coma.

PREGNANCY-LACTATION-REPRODUCTION
• Use cautiously in pregnant and breastfeeding women. Embryo-fetal risk is very low.
• There are no studies of IV acetaminophen use in pregnant women. Use during pregnancy only if clearly needed.

NURSING CONSIDERATIONS
Black Box Warning Many OTC and prescription products contain acetaminophen; be aware of this when calculating total daily dose. ∎
Black Box Warning Use caution when prescribing, preparing, and administering IV acetaminophen to avoid dosing errors leading to accidental overdose and death. Be careful not to confuse dose in milliGRAMS and dose in milliLITERS. Be sure to base dose on weight for patients weighing less than 50 kg, to properly program infusion pump, and to ensure that total daily dose of acetaminophen from all sources doesn't exceed maximum daily limit. ∎
• Consider reducing total daily dose and increasing dosing intervals in patients with hepatic or renal impairment.

PATIENT TEACHING
• Tell parents to consult prescriber before giving drug to children younger than age 2.
• Advise parents that drug is only for short-term use; urge them to consult prescriber if giving to infants for longer than 3 days, children for longer than 5 days, or adults for longer than 10 days.
Black Box Warning Advise patient or caregiver that many OTC products contain acetaminophen and should be counted when calculating total daily dose. ∎
• Tell patient to consult prescriber for fever lasting longer than 3 days or recurrent fever.
❸ *Alert:* Warn patient that high doses or unsupervised long-term use can cause liver damage. Excessive alcohol use may increase the risk of liver damage. Caution long-term alcoholics to limit drug to 2 g/day or less.
• Caution patient to contact health care provider if signs and symptoms of liver damage (illogical thinking, severe dyspepsia, jaundice, inability to eat, weakness) occur.
• Tell breastfeeding patient that drug appears in human milk in low levels. Drug may be used safely if therapy is short-term and doesn't exceed recommended doses.
❸ *Alert:* Warn patient to stop drug and seek medical attention immediately if rash or other reactions occurs while using acetaminophen.

acetylcysteine
a-se-teel-SIS-tay-een

Acetadote, Cetylev

Therapeutic class: Mucolytics
Pharmacologic class: L-cysteine derivatives

AVAILABLE FORMS
Inhalation solution: 10%, 20%
IV injection: 200 mg/mL
Tablets (effervescent for oral solution): 500 mg, 2.5 g

INDICATIONS & DOSAGES
➤ **Adjunctive therapy for abnormal viscid or thickened mucous secretions in patients with pneumonia, bronchitis, bronchiectasis, primary amyloidosis of the lung, TB, cystic fibrosis, emphysema,**

atelectasis, pulmonary complications of thoracic surgery, or CV surgery
Adults and children: 1 to 2 mL 10% or 20% solution by direct instillation into trachea as often as every hour. Or, 1 to 10 mL of 20% solution or 2 to 20 mL of 10% solution by nebulization every 2 to 6 hours, p.r.n.

➤ **Diagnostic bronchial studies**
Adults and children: Two or three administrations of 1 to 2 mL of 20% solution or 2 to 4 mL of 10% solution by nebulization or intratracheal instillation before procedure.

➤ **Routine tracheostomy care**
Adults and children: 1 to 2 mL of 10% or 20% solution by direct instillation into tracheostomy every 1 to 4 hours.

➤ **Acetaminophen toxicity**
PO
Adults and children: Initially, 140 mg/kg PO; then 70 mg/kg PO 4 hours after initial dose, then every 4 hours for 17 doses (total).
IV
Adults and children weighing 41 to 100 kg or more: 150 mg/kg in 200 mL of diluent IV over 1 hour. Then, 50 mg/kg in 500 mL of diluent IV over 4 hours. Then, 100 mg/kg in 1,000 mL of diluent IV over 16 hours.
Adults and children weighing 21 to 40 kg: 150 mg/kg in 100 mL of diluent IV over 1 hour. Then, 50 mg/kg in 250 mL of diluent IV over 4 hours. Then, 100 mg/kg in 500 mL diluent IV over 16 hours.
Adults and children weighing 5 to 20 kg: 150 mg/kg in 3 mL/kg diluent IV over 1 hour. Then, 50 mg/kg in 7 mL/kg diluent IV over 4 hours. Then, 100 mg/kg in 14 mL/kg diluent IV over 16 hours.
Adjust-a-dose: Refer to manufacturer's instruction for dosing in patients weighing less than 40 kg and requiring fluid restriction.

ADMINISTRATION
PO
(inhalation formulation)
• Administer via the oral route. Dilute oral dose (used for acetaminophen overdose) with diet cola or other diet soft drinks or water. Dilute 20% solution to 5% (add 3 mL of diluent to each milliliter of drug). If patient vomits within 1 hour of receiving loading or maintenance dose, repeat dose. Use diluted solution within 1 hour.

• Drug smells strongly of sulfur. Mixing oral form with juice or cola improves its taste.
• Drug delivered through NG tube may be diluted with water.
• Store opened, undiluted oral solution in the refrigerator for up to 96 hours.
PO
(effervescent tablet formulation)
• Dissolve appropriate number of 2.5-g or 0.5-g tablets in volume of water specified in manufacturer's instructions, based on patient weight, and administer the solution immediately.
• Prepare fresh solution for each dose; use within 2 hours.
• If patient vomits within 1 hour of receiving loading or maintenance dose, repeat dose. May administer by nasoduodenal tube if necessary.
IV
▼ Drug may turn from a colorless liquid to a slight pink or purple color once the stopper is punctured. This color change doesn't affect the drug.
▼ Drug is hyperosmolar and is compatible with D_5W, half-NSS, and sterile water for injection.
▼ Adjust total volume given for patients who weigh less than 40 kg or who are fluid restricted.
▼ For patients who weigh 41 kg or more, dilute loading dose in 200 mL of D_5W, second dose in 500 mL, and third dose in 1,000 mL. Refer to manufacturer's instructions for dosage and dilution for patients weighing 40 kg or less.
▼ Reconstituted solution is stable for 24 hours at room temperature.
▼ Vials contain no preservatives; discard after opening.
▼ **Incompatibilities:** None listed by manufacturer. Consult a drug incompatibility reference for more information.
Inhalational
• Use plastic, glass, stainless steel, or another nonreactive metal when giving by nebulization. Hand-bulb nebulizers aren't recommended because output is too small and particle size too large.
• If only a portion of the solution in a vial is used for inhalation, store remainder in refrigerator and use within 96 hours.

Reactions in bold italics are *life-threatening*. Interactions may have a *rapid onset* or a *delayed onset*.

• **Incompatibilities:** Physically or chemically incompatible with inhaled tetracyclines, erythromycin lactobionate, amphotericin B, and ampicillin sodium. If given by aerosol inhalation, nebulize these drugs separately. Iodized oil, trypsin, and hydrogen peroxide are physically incompatible with acetylcysteine; don't add to nebulizer.

ACTION
Reduces the viscosity of pulmonary secretions by splitting disulfide linkages between mucoprotein molecular complexes. Also, restores liver stores of glutathione to treat acetaminophen toxicity.

Route	Onset	Peak	Duration
PO	Unknown	1–3½ hr	Unknown
Inhalation	5–10 min	1–2 hr	1 hr
IV	Unknown	½–1 hr	Unknown

Half-life: PO, 18.1 hours; inhalation, unknown; IV, 5.6 hours.

ADVERSE REACTIONS
CNS: fever, drowsiness. **CV:** chest tightness, flushing, tachycardia, edema. **EENT:** rhinorrhea, pharyngitis, throat tightness. **GI:** nausea, stomatitis, vomiting. **Respiratory:** *bronchospasm,* cough, dyspnea, rhonchi. **Skin:** clamminess, pruritus, rash, urticaria. **Other:** *anaphylactoid reaction,* chills, hypersensitivity reaction.

INTERACTIONS
Drug-drug. *Activated charcoal:* May limit acetylcysteine's effectiveness. Avoid using activated charcoal before or with oral acetylcysteine.

EFFECTS ON LAB TEST RESULTS
None reported.

CONTRAINDICATIONS & CAUTIONS
• Contraindicated in patients hypersensitive to drug.
🔴 **Alert:** Serious anaphylactoid reactions, including rash, hypotension, dyspnea, and wheezing, have been reported. Reactions usually occur 30 to 60 minutes after start of infusion and may require treatment and drug discontinuation.
• Use cautiously in elderly or debilitated patients with severe respiratory insufficiency.

Use IV form cautiously in patients with asthma or a history of bronchospasm, in those weighing less than 40 kg, and in patients requiring fluid restriction.
Dialyzable drug: Yes.

PREGNANCY-LACTATION-REPRODUCTION
• There are no adequate and well-controlled studies in pregnant women. Use cautiously in pregnant women and only if clearly indicated.
• It's unknown if drug appears in human milk. Use cautiously in breastfeeding women.

NURSING CONSIDERATIONS
• Monitor cough type and frequency.
🔴 **Alert:** Monitor patient for bronchospasm, especially if patient has asthma.
• Ingestion of more than 150 mg/kg of acetaminophen may cause hepatotoxicity. Measure acetaminophen level 4 hours after ingestion to determine risk of hepatotoxicity. See manufacturer's information for nomogram for estimating potential for hepatotoxicity from acute acetaminophen ingestion and need for acetylcysteine therapy.
🔴 **Alert:** Drug is used for acetaminophen overdose within 24 hours of ingestion. Start drug immediately; don't wait for results of acetaminophen level. Give within 10 hours of acetaminophen ingestion to minimize hepatic injury.
• For suspected acetaminophen overdose, obtain baseline INR and AST, ALT, bilirubin, BUN, creatinine, glucose, and electrolyte levels.
• Check acetaminophen, ALT, and AST levels and INR after the last maintenance dose. If acetaminophen level is still detectable, or if the ALT/AST level is still increasing or the INR remains elevated, the maintenance doses should be continued and the prescriber should contact a regional poison control center (1-800-222-1222) or a special health professional assistance line (1-800-525-6115) for assistance with dosing recommendations.
• Half-life elimination increases by 80% in patients with severe liver damage.
🔴 **Alert:** Monitor patient receiving IV form for anaphylactoid reactions. Reactions involving more than simple skin flushing or erythema should be treated as anaphylactoid

reactions. If anaphylactoid reaction occurs, stop infusion and treat reaction with antihistamines and epinephrine if needed. Once anaphylaxis treatment starts, carefully restart infusion. If anaphylactoid symptoms return, stop drug.

• Flushing and skin erythema may occur within 30 to 60 minutes of start of IV infusion and usually resolve without stopping infusion.

• When acetaminophen level is below toxic level according to nomogram, stop therapy.

• The vial stopper doesn't contain natural rubber latex, dry natural rubber, or blends of natural rubber.

• *Look alike–sound alike:* Don't confuse acetylcysteine with acetylcholine.

PATIENT TEACHING

• Warn patient that drug may have a foul taste or smell that may be distressing.

• For maximum effect, instruct patient to cough to clear airway before aerosol administration.

acyclovir
ay-SYE-kloe-ver

Sitavig, Zovirax

acyclovir sodium
Zovirax

Therapeutic class: Antivirals
Pharmacologic class: Nucleosides and nucleotides

AVAILABLE FORMS
Capsules: 200 mg
Cream: 5%
Injection: 500 mg/vial, 1 g/vial
Ointment: 5%
Solution (IV): 50 mg/mL
Suspension: 200 mg/5 mL
Tablets: 400 mg, 800 mg
Tablets (buccal) ⓄⓉⒸ: 50 mg

INDICATIONS & DOSAGES
Adjust-a-dose (for all indications): For patients receiving the IV form, if CrCl is 25 to 50 mL/minute/1.73 m^2, give 100% of dose every 12 hours; if CrCl is 10 to 25 mL/minute/1.73 m^2, give 100% of dose every 24 hours; if CrCl is less than 10 mL/minute/1.73 m^2, give 50% of dose every 24 hours.

For patients receiving the PO form, if normal dose is 200 mg every 4 hours five times daily and CrCl is less than 10 mL/minute/1.73 m^2, give 200 mg PO every 12 hours. If normal dose is 400 mg every 12 hours and CrCl is less than 10 mL/minute/1.73 m^2, give 200 mg every 12 hours. If normal dose is 800 mg every 4 hours five times daily and CrCl is 10 to 25 mL/minute/1.73 m^2, give 800 mg every 8 hours; if CrCl is less than 10 mL/minute/1.73 m^2, give 800 mg every 12 hours.

For patients who require hemodialysis, give additional dose after each dialysis.

➤ **First and recurrent episodes of mucocutaneous HSV (HSV-1 and HSV-2) infections in immunocompromised patients; severe first episodes of genital herpes in patients who aren't immunocompromised**
Adults and children age 12 and older: 5 mg/kg IV over 1 hour every 8 hours for 7 days. Give for 5 days for severe first episode of genital herpes.
Children younger than age 12: 10 mg/kg IV over 1 hour every 8 hours for 7 days.

➤ **First genital herpes episode**
Adults: 200 mg PO every 4 hours while awake, five times daily. Continue for 10 days.

➤ **Initial genital herpes; limited, non-life-threatening mucocutaneous HSV infections in immunocompromised patients**
Adults and children age 12 and older: Adequately cover all lesions every 3 hours six times daily for 7 days. Although dosage varies depending on total lesion area, use about ½-inch (1.3-cm) ribbon of ointment on each 4-inch (10-cm) square of surface area.

➤ **Intermittent therapy for recurrent genital herpes**
Adults: 200 mg PO every 4 hours while awake, five times daily. Continue for 5 days. Begin therapy at first sign of recurrence.

➤ **Long-term suppressive therapy for recurrent genital herpes**
Adults: 400 mg PO b.i.d. for up to 12 months. Or, 200 mg PO t.i.d. to five times daily for up to 12 months.

➤ **Varicella zoster infections in immuno-compromised patients**
Adults and children age 12 and older:
10 mg/kg IV over 1 hour every 8 hours for 7 days. Dosage for obese patients is 10 mg/kg based on ideal body weight every 8 hours for 7 days. Don't exceed maximum dosage equivalent of 20 mg/kg every 8 hours.
Children younger than age 12: 20 mg/kg IV over 1 hour every 8 hours for 7 days.

➤ **Varicella (chickenpox) infection in immunocompetent patients**
Adults and children weighing more than 40 kg: 800 mg PO q.i.d. for 5 days.
Children age 2 and older weighing less than 40 kg: 20 mg/kg (maximum, 80 mg/kg/day) PO q.i.d. for 5 days. Start therapy as soon as symptoms appear.

➤ **Acute herpes zoster infection in immunocompetent patients**
Adults and children age 12 and older:
800 mg PO every 4 hours five times daily for 7 to 10 days.

➤ **Herpes simplex encephalitis**
Adults and children age 12 and older:
10 mg/kg IV over 1 hour every 8 hours for 10 days.
Children ages 3 months to 12 years:
20 mg/kg IV over 1 hour every 8 hours for 10 days.

➤ **Neonatal HSV infections**
Children from birth to age 3 months:
10 mg/kg IV over 1 hour every 8 hours for 10 days. Although doses of 15 or 20 mg/kg (infused at a constant rate over 1 hour every 8 hours) have been used, the safety and efficacy of these doses aren't known.

➤ **Recurrent herpes labialis**
Adults and children age 12 and older: Apply cream five times daily for 4 days. Start therapy as early as possible after signs and symptoms occur. Or, apply ointment every 3 hours, six times daily for 7 days.

➤ **Recurrent herpes labialis in immuno-competent patients**
Adults: 50-mg buccal tablet as a single dose to upper gum region, on the same side as the symptoms, within 1 hour after onset of prodromal symptoms and before appearance of signs of cold sore.

ADMINISTRATION
PO
• Give drug without regard for meals, but give with food if stomach irritation occurs.
• Patient should take drug as prescribed, even after feeling better.
Buccal
• Patients shouldn't chew, suck, crush, or swallow tablets.
• Apply with dry finger immediately after taking tablet out of blister pack.
• Place tablet just above incisor tooth on upper gum on the same side of the mouth as prodromal symptoms appeared.
• Hold tablet in place with slight pressure over upper lip for 30 seconds to ensure adhesion. Place rounded side to gum for comfort, but either side can be applied.
• Tablet will stay in place and dissolve gradually.
• Food and drink can be taken normally with tablet in place.
• Patients should avoid chewing gum, touching or pressing tablet, wearing upper denture, brushing teeth, or other activity that may interfere with adhesion.
• Patients should drink plenty of liquids in case of dry mouth.
• If buccal tablet doesn't adhere or falls off within first 6 hours, reposition same tablet immediately. If tablet doesn't adhere, place a new tablet.
• If patient swallows buccal tablet within first 6 hours, have patient drink a glass of water; then apply a new tablet.
• If buccal tablet falls out or patient swallows it after first 6 hours, don't reapply.

IV
▼ Solutions concentrated at 7 mg/mL or more may cause a higher risk of phlebitis.
▼ Encourage fluid intake because patient must be adequately hydrated during infusion.
▼ Bolus injection, dehydration (decreased urine output), renal disease, and use with other nephrotoxic drugs increase the risk of renal toxicity. Don't give by bolus injection.
▼ Give IV infusion over at least 1 hour to prevent renal tubular damage.
▼ Monitor intake and output, especially during the first 2 hours after administration.
⚠ *Alert:* Don't give IM or subcut.

▼ **Incompatibilities:** None listed by manufacturer. Consult a drug incompatibility reference for more information.

Topical
• Apply with finger cot or rubber glove to prevent autoinoculation of other body sites and transmission of infection to others.
• Thoroughly cover all lesions.
• Topical form is for cutaneous use only; don't apply to eyes.

ACTION
Interferes with DNA synthesis and inhibits viral multiplication.

Route	Onset	Peak	Duration
PO	Unknown	2½ hr	Unknown
Buccal	Unknown	8 hr (in saliva)	Unknown
IV	Immediate	Immediate	Unknown
Topical	Unknown	Unknown	Unknown

Half-life: 2 to 3½ hours with normal renal function; up to 19 hours with renal impairment.

ADVERSE REACTIONS
CNS: headache, malaise, *encephalopathic changes (including lethargy, obtundation, tremor, confusion, hallucinations, agitation, seizures, coma).* **EENT:** gum pain, canker sores (buccal tablets). **GI:** nausea, vomiting, diarrhea. **GU:** *acute renal failure,* hematuria. **Hematologic:** *leukopenia, thrombocytopenia,* thrombocytosis. **Skin:** inflammation or phlebitis at injection site, rash, urticaria, eczema, dryness, pruritus, contact dermatitis, application-site reaction; mild pain, burning, or stinging (topical or buccal form); *SJS,* toxic epidermal necrolysis. **Other:** *angioedema, anaphylaxis.*

INTERACTIONS
Drug-drug. *Foscarnet:* May enhance nephrotoxicity. Don't use together.
Hydantoins, valproic acid: May decrease levels of these drugs. Monitor patient closely.
Probenecid: May increase acyclovir level. Monitor patient for possible toxicity.
Varicella vaccine: May diminish therapeutic effect of vaccine. Avoid use of acyclovir within 24 hours before vaccine administration and for 14 days after.
Zidovudine: May cause drowsiness or lethargy. Use together cautiously.

EFFECTS ON LAB TEST RESULTS
• May increase BUN and creatinine levels.
• May decrease WBC count. May increase or decrease platelet count.

CONTRAINDICATIONS & CAUTIONS
• Contraindicated in patients hypersensitive to drug.
• Use cautiously in patients with neurologic problems, renal disease, or dehydration, and in those receiving other nephrotoxic drugs.
• Drug increases risk of thrombotic thrombocytopenic purpura and hemolytic-uremic syndrome in immunocompromised patients, which can be fatal.
Dialyzable drug: Yes.
⚠ *Overdose S&S:* Agitation, coma, seizures, lethargy, elevated BUN and creatinine levels, renal failure.

PREGNANCY-LACTATION-REPRODUCTION
• Use cautiously in pregnant women and only if potential benefit outweighs potential risk to the fetus.
• Drug appears in human milk. Women with active herpetic lesions near or on the breasts should avoid breastfeeding.

NURSING CONSIDERATIONS
• Start therapy as early as possible after signs or symptoms occur.
• Drug isn't a cure for herpes, but it helps improve signs and symptoms.
🕑 *Alert:* Long-term acyclovir use may result in nephrotoxicity. In patients with renal disease or dehydration and in those taking other nephrotoxic drugs, monitor renal function.
🕑 *Alert:* If signs and symptoms of extravasation occur, stop IV infusion immediately and notify prescriber. Hyaluronidase may need to be injected subcut at extravasation site as an antidote.
• Encephalopathic changes are more likely to occur in patients with neurologic disorders and in those who have had neurologic reactions to cytotoxic drugs.
• *Look alike–sound alike:* Don't confuse acyclovir sodium (Zovirax) with acetazolamide sodium (Diamox) vials, which may look alike. Don't confuse Zovirax with Zyvox.

PATIENT TEACHING
• Tell patient to take drug as prescribed, even after feeling better.
• Tell patient drug is effective in managing herpes infection but doesn't eliminate or cure it. Warn patient that drug won't prevent spread of infection to others.
• Tell patient to avoid sexual contact while visible lesions are present. Virus transmission can occur during treatment.
• Teach patient about early signs and symptoms of herpes infection (such as tingling, itching, or pain) and to notify prescriber and get a prescription for drug before the infection fully develops. Early treatment is most effective.

BIOSIMILAR DRUG

adalimumab
ay-da-LIM-yoo-mab

Humira

Therapeutic class: Antiarthritics
Pharmacologic class: TNF blockers

AVAILABLE FORMS
Injection: 10 mg/0.1 mL, 10 mg/0.2 mL, 20 mg/0.2 mL, 20 mg/0.4 mL, 40 mg/0.4 mL, 40 mg/0.8 mL, 80 mg/0.8 mL pre-filled syringes or pens; 40 mg/0.8 mL single-use vial (institutional use only)

INDICATIONS & DOSAGES
➤ **RA; psoriatic arthritis; ankylosing spondylitis**
Adults: 40 mg subcut every other week. Patient may continue to take methotrexate, steroids, NSAIDs, salicylates, analgesics, or other DMARDs during therapy. Patients with RA who aren't also taking methotrexate may have the dose increased to 40 mg weekly, if needed.
➤ **Moderate to severe adult Crohn disease when response to conventional therapy is inadequate or when response to infliximab is lost or patient can't tolerate the drug; moderate to severe active ulcerative colitis when response to immunosuppressants (such as corticosteroids, azathioprine, or 6-mercaptopurine) is inadequate**

Adults: Initially, 160 mg subcut on day 1 given in 1 day or split over 2 consecutive days; then 80 mg 2 weeks later (day 15), followed by a maintenance dose of 40 mg every other week starting at week 4 (day 29). For ulcerative colitis, only continue in patients who have shown evidence of clinical remission by 8 weeks (day 57) of therapy.
➤ **Pediatric Crohn disease**
Children age 6 and older weighing 40 kg or more: Initially, 160 mg subcut on day 1 given in 1 day or split over 2 consecutive days; then 80 mg 2 weeks later (day 15), followed by a maintenance dose of 40 mg every other week starting at week 4 (day 29).
Children age 6 and older weighing from 17 to less than 40 kg: 80 mg subcut on day 1, followed by 40 mg 2 weeks later (day 15), followed by a maintenance dose of 20 mg every other week starting at week 4 (day 29).
➤ **To reduce the signs and symptoms of moderately to severely active polyarticular juvenile idiopathic arthritis**
Children age 2 and older weighing from 10 to less than 15 kg: 10 mg subcut every other week.
Children age 2 and older weighing between 15 and 30 kg: 20 mg subcut every other week.
Children age 2 and older weighing 30 kg or more: 40 mg subcut every other week. Patients may continue to take methotrexate, steroids, NSAIDs, and analgesics during therapy.
➤ **Moderate to severe chronic plaque psoriasis**
Adults: 80 mg subcut, followed by 40 mg subcut every other week starting 1 week after the initial dose. Treatment beyond 1 year has not been studied.
✳ *NEW INDICATION:* **Noninfectious intermediate uveitis, posterior uveitis, and panuveitis**
Adults: 80 mg subcut, followed by 40 mg subcut every other week starting 1 week after initial dose.
Children age 2 and older weighing 30 kg or more: 40 mg subcut every other week.
Children age 2 and older weighing 15 to less than 30 kg: 20 mg subcut every other week.
Children age 2 and older weighing 10 to less than 15 kg: 10 mg subcut every other week.

➤ **Moderate to severe hidradenitis suppurativa**

Adults and adolescents age 12 and older weighing 60 kg or more: Initially, 160 mg subcut given in 1 day or split over 2 consecutive days; then 80 mg subcut on day 15. Thereafter, starting on day 29, give 40 mg subcut weekly.

Adolescents age 12 and older weighing 30 to less than 60 kg: Initially, 80 mg subcut on day 1; then 40 mg subcut on day 8. Thereafter, give 40 mg subcut every other week.

ADMINISTRATION
Subcutaneous
• Inject subcut into abdomen or thigh at separate sites.
• Rotate injection sites.
• Don't give in an area that is bruised, tender, red, or hard.
• May leave drug (don't remove cap or cover) at room temperature for about 15 to 30 minutes before injecting.
• Don't use if particulates or discoloration is noted in autoinjector, pen, prefilled syringe, or single-use institutional-use vial.
• May store at room temperature (maximum, 77° F [25° C]) for up to 14 days. Discard after 14 days. Protect from light.
⚠ *Alert:* Needle caps of the Humira pen and prefilled syringe may contain latex. Check product packaging to confirm.

ACTION
A recombinant human IgG$_1$ monoclonal antibody that blocks human TNF-alpha. TNF-alpha participates in normal inflammatory and immune responses and in the inflammation and joint destruction of RA.

Route	Onset	Peak	Duration
Subcut	Variable	75–187 hr	Unknown

Half-life: 10 to 20 days.

ADVERSE REACTIONS
CNS: headache, syncope, hypertensive encephalopathy, confusion, paresthesia, subdural hematoma, tremor, myasthenia, fever.
CV: *hemorrhage,* HTN, arrhythmia, atrial fibrillation, chest pain, CAD, cardiac arrest, cardiac failure, MI, palpitations, pericardial effusion, pericarditis, tachycardia, edema, thrombosis. **EENT:** sinusitis,

cataract. **GI:** abdominal pain, nausea, cholecystitis, cholelithiasis, esophagitis, gastroenteritis, GI hemorrhage, vomiting, diverticulitis. **GU:** hematuria, UTI, cystitis, kidney stones, menstrual disorder. **Hematologic:** *leukopenia, pancytopenia, thrombocytopenia,* polycythemia, *agranulocytosis.* **Hepatic:** hepatic necrosis. **Metabolic:** hypercholesterolemia, hyperlipidemia, dehydration, ketosis. **Musculoskeletal:** back pain, bone disorder, bone necrosis, joint disorder, muscle cramps, synovitis, tendon disorder, pyogenic arthritis. **Respiratory:** URI, bronchitis, dyspnea, decreased lung function, pleural effusion, asthma, *bronchospasm,* pneumonia. **Skin:** rash, injection-site reactions (erythema, itching, pain, swelling), alopecia, cellulitis, erysipelas, *SJS.* **Other:** accidental injury, *anaphylaxis, malignancy,* allergic reactions, flulike syndrome, parathyroid disorder.

INTERACTIONS
Drug-drug. *Abatacept, anakinra, tocilizumab:* May increase risk of serious infections and neutropenia in patients with RA. Don't use together.
CYP450 substrates with narrow therapeutic index (cyclosporine, theophylline, warfarin): May affect CYP450 substrate level. Monitor levels closely when initiating or discontinuing adalimumab; adjust CYP450 substrate dosage as needed.
Live-virus vaccines: No data are available on secondary transmission of infection from live-virus vaccines. Avoid using together.

EFFECTS ON LAB TEST RESULTS
• May increase CK, alkaline phosphatase, and cholesterol levels.
• May decrease platelet and WBC counts.
• May cause positive ANA titer and development of antibodies.

CONTRAINDICATIONS & CAUTIONS
• Contraindicated in immunosuppressed patients and in those with an active chronic or localized infection.
⚠ *Alert:* Anaphylaxis and angioneurotic edema have been reported. If serious reaction occurs, discontinue drug immediately and treat appropriately.

Reactions in bold italics are *life-threatening*. Interactions may have a *rapid onset* or a *delayed onset.*

Black Box Warning Patients taking TNF-alpha blockers are at increased risk for developing serious infections that can lead to hospitalization or death. Most patients were taking concomitant immunosuppressants, such as methotrexate or corticosteroids. Reported infections include *Legionella* and *Listeria* infections, active TB, and invasive fungal infections. Consider empirical antifungal therapy for patients at risk for invasive fungal infections who develop systemic illness. Carefully consider risk and benefits of therapy before starting drug in patients with chronic or recurrent infections. ∎

Black Box Warning Lymphoma and other malignancies, some fatal, have been reported in children and adolescents treated with TNF blockers, including adalimumab. ∎

Black Box Warning Hepatosplenic T-cell lymphoma, a rare type of T-cell lymphoma, has occurred in adolescents and young adults with inflammatory bowel disease treated with TNF blockers, including adalimumab. ∎

• Use cautiously in patients with demyelinating disorders, a history of recurrent infection, those with underlying conditions that predispose them to infections, those who have lived in areas where TB and histoplasmosis are endemic, patients with HF, and elderly patients.

Dialyzable drug: Unknown.

PREGNANCY-LACTATION-REPRODUCTION
• Use during pregnancy only if clearly needed.
• Drug appears in human milk. Use cautiously in breastfeeding women.

NURSING CONSIDERATIONS
• Give first dose under supervision of prescriber.

Black Box Warning Patient should be evaluated and treated, if necessary, for latent TB before start of adalimumab therapy. Closely monitor patient for possible development of TB even if patient has tested negative before start of therapy. ∎

Black Box Warning Serious infections and sepsis, including TB and invasive fungal infections, may occur. If patient develops new infection during treatment, monitor closely; if infection becomes serious, stop drug. ∎

❸ *Alert:* Drug may increase the risk of malignancy. Patients with highly active RA may be at an increased risk for lymphoma.

❸ *Alert:* If patient develops anaphylaxis, a severe infection, other serious allergic reaction, or evidence of a lupuslike syndrome, stop drug.

• Drug may cause reactivation of HBV in chronic carriers.

❸ *Alert:* The needle covers may contain latex and shouldn't be handled by those with latex sensitivity.

• *Look alike–sound alike:* Don't confuse Humira with Humulin or Humalog.

PATIENT TEACHING
• Tell patient to report all adverse reactions and any evidence of TB or other infection.
• Teach patient or caregiver how to give drug.

❸ *Alert:* Warn patient to seek immediate medical attention for symptoms of blood dyscrasias or infection, including fever, bruising, bleeding, and pallor.

• Tell patient to rotate injection sites and to avoid tender, bruised, red, or hard skin.
• Teach patient to dispose of used needles and syringes properly and not in the household trash or recyclables.
• Tell patient to refrigerate drug in its original container before use. If necessary, drug may be stored at room temperature up to maximum of 77° F (25° C) for up to 14 days, protected from light.

adefovir dipivoxil
ah-DEF-oh-veer

Hepsera

Therapeutic class: Antivirals
Pharmacologic class: Nucleosides and nucleotides

AVAILABLE FORMS
Tablets: 10 mg

INDICATIONS & DOSAGES
➤ **Chronic HBV infection**
Adults and children age 12 and older: 10 mg PO once daily.

Adjust-a-dose: In adult patients with CrCl of 30 to 49 mL/minute, give 10 mg PO every 48 hours. In patients with CrCl of 10 to 29 mL/minute, give 10 mg PO every 72 hours. In patients receiving hemodialysis, give 10 mg PO every 7 days, after dialysis session. There are no dose recommendations for adolescents with renal impairment.

ADMINISTRATION
PO
• Give drug without regard for meals.

ACTION
An acyclic nucleotide analogue that inhibits HBV reverse transcription via viral DNA chain termination.

Route	Onset	Peak	Duration
PO	Unknown	½–4 hr	Unknown

Half-life: 7½ hours.

ADVERSE REACTIONS
CNS: asthenia, headache. **GI:** abdominal pain, diarrhea, dyspepsia, flatulence, nausea, vomiting. **GU:** *renal failure, renal insufficiency.* **Hepatic:** *hepatic failure,* hepatomegaly with steatosis, *severe acute exacerbation of hepatitis.* **Metabolic:** *lactic acidosis.* **Skin:** pruritus, rash.

INTERACTIONS
Drug-drug. *Ibuprofen:* May increase adefovir bioavailability. Monitor patient for adverse effects.
Nephrotoxic drugs (aminoglycosides, cyclosporine, NSAIDs, tacrolimus, vancomycin): May increase risk of nephrotoxicity. Use together cautiously.
Tenofovir disoproxil fumarate–containing products (Atripla, Cimduo, Complera, Delstrigo, Stribild, Symfi, Temixys, Truvada, Viread): Use together increases risk for lactic acidosis and hepatotoxicity. Contraindicated for use together.

EFFECTS ON LAB TEST RESULTS
• May increase ALT, amylase, AST, CK, creatinine, and lactate levels. May decrease phosphorus level.

CONTRAINDICATIONS & CAUTIONS
• Contraindicated in patients hypersensitive to components of drug.
• Use cautiously in patients with renal dysfunction, in those receiving nephrotoxic drugs, and in those with known risk factors for hepatic disease.
• Use cautiously in elderly patients because they're more likely to have decreased renal and cardiac function.
• Safety and effectiveness in children younger than age 12 haven't been established.
Dialyzable drug: 35%.
⚠ *Overdose S&S:* GI adverse reactions.

PREGNANCY-LACTATION-REPRODUCTION
• Use cautiously in pregnant women and only if potential benefit to the mother justifies potential risk to the fetus.
• To monitor fetal outcomes of pregnant women exposed to drug, health care providers should register patients in the antiretroviral pregnancy registry (1-800-258-4263).
• It isn't known if drug appears in human milk. Patient should discontinue breastfeeding or discontinue drug.

NURSING CONSIDERATIONS
Black Box Warning Due to increased risk of nephrotoxicity, monitor renal function, and adjust dosage if needed, especially in patients with renal dysfunction or those taking nephrotoxic drugs. ∎
Black Box Warning Patients may develop lactic acidosis and severe hepatomegaly with steatosis during treatment. Women, obese patients, and those taking antiretrovirals are at higher risk. Monitor hepatic function. Stop drug, if needed. ∎
Black Box Warning Stopping adefovir may cause severe worsening of hepatitis. Monitor hepatic function closely for at least several months in patients who stop anti-HBV therapy. ∎
• The ideal length of treatment hasn't been established.
Black Box Warning Offer patients HIV antibody testing; drug may promote resistance to antiretrovirals in patients with chronic HBV infection who also have unrecognized or untreated HIV infection. ∎

Reactions in bold italics are *life-threatening*. Interactions may have a *rapid onset* or a *delayed onset*.

PATIENT TEACHING
• Inform patient that drug may be taken without regard to meals.
• Tell patient to immediately report weakness, muscle pain, trouble breathing, stomach pain with nausea and vomiting, dizziness, light-headedness, fast or irregular heartbeat, and feeling cold, especially in arms and legs.
• Warn patient not to stop taking this drug unless directed because it could cause hepatitis to become worse.
• Instruct female patient to tell prescriber if she becomes pregnant or is breastfeeding.

SAFETY ALERT!

adenosine
a-DEN-oh-seen

Therapeutic class: Antiarrhythmics
Pharmacologic class: Nucleosides

AVAILABLE FORMS
Injection: 3 mg/mL

INDICATIONS & DOSAGES
➤ **To convert paroxysmal supraventricular tachycardia (PSVT) to sinus rhythm**
Adults and children weighing 50 kg or more: 6 mg IV by rapid bolus injection over 1 to 2 seconds, followed by a saline flush. If PSVT isn't eliminated in 1 to 2 minutes, give 12 mg by rapid IV push and repeat, if needed.
Children weighing less than 50 kg: Initially, 0.05 to 0.1 mg/kg IV by rapid bolus injection followed by a saline flush. If PSVT isn't eliminated in 1 to 2 minutes, give additional bolus injections, increasing the amount given in 0.05- to 0.1-mg/kg increments, followed by a saline flush. Continue, as needed, until conversion of the PSVT or a maximum single dose of 0.3 mg/kg (up to 12 mg) is given.
➤ **Stress-testing diagnostic aid**
Adults: 140 mcg/kg/minute infused over 6 minutes (total dose of 0.84 mg/kg).

ADMINISTRATION
IV
▼ Don't give single doses exceeding 12 mg.

▼ Crystals may form if solution is cold; gently warm solution to room temperature. Don't use solutions that aren't clear.
▼ In adults, avoid giving drug through a central line because central administration hasn't been studied.
▼ Give by rapid IV injection to ensure drug action.
▼ Give directly into a vein, if possible. When giving through an IV line, use the port closest to patient.
▼ Flush immediately and rapidly with NSS to ensure that drug quickly reaches the systemic circulation.
▼ Drug lacks preservatives. Discard unused portion. Don't refrigerate.
▼ **Incompatibilities:** Consult a drug incompatibility reference for information.

ACTION
Naturally occurring nucleoside that acts on the AV node to slow conduction and inhibit reentry pathways. Drug is also useful in treating PSVTs, including those with accessory bypass tracts (Wolff-Parkinson-White syndrome).

Route	Onset	Peak	Duration
IV	Immediate	Immediate	Unknown

Half-life: Less than 10 seconds.

ADVERSE REACTIONS
CNS: dizziness, light-headedness, numbness, tingling in arms, headache, nervousness. **CV:** chest pressure, facial flushing, hypotension, arrhythmias, first- or second-degree AV block. **EENT:** throat, neck, or jaw discomfort. **GI:** nausea. **Respiratory:** dyspnea.

INTERACTIONS
Drug-drug. *Carbamazepine:* May cause high-level heart block. Use together cautiously and consider using a lower initial adenosine dose.
Digoxin, verapamil: May cause ventricular fibrillation. Monitor ECG closely.
Dipyridamole: May increase adenosine's effects. Adenosine dose may need to be reduced. Use together cautiously.
Methylxanthines (caffeine, theophylline): May decrease adenosine's effects. Adenosine dose may need to be increased, or

patients may not respond to adenosine therapy.

EFFECTS ON LAB TEST RESULTS
None reported.

CONTRAINDICATIONS & CAUTIONS
• Contraindicated in patients hypersensitive to drug.
• Contraindicated in those with second- or third-degree heart block or sinus node disease (sick sinus syndrome and symptomatic bradycardia), except those with a pacemaker.
• Use cautiously in patients with obstructive lung disease not associated with bronchoconstriction (emphysema or bronchitis); avoid use in those with bronchoconstriction or bronchospasm (asthma).
• Drug may increase risk of seizures.
• Avoid use in patients with signs and symptoms of acute MI (unstable angina, CV instability). Drug may increase risk of serious CV reaction (fatal or nonfatal cardiac arrest, supraventricular tachycardia, MI). Make sure appropriate emergency equipment is readily available.
• Use cautiously in patients with autonomic dysfunction, stenotic valvular heart disease, pericarditis or pericardial effusions, stenotic carotid artery disease with cerebrovascular insufficiency, or uncorrected hypovolemia. Drug may increase risk of hypotensive complications.
Dialyzable drug: Unknown.

PREGNANCY-LACTATION-REPRODUCTION
• No studies have been performed in pregnant women. Use in pregnant women only if clearly indicated.
• There are no well-controlled studies in breastfeeding women. Patient should discontinue breastfeeding or discontinue drug, taking into account importance of drug to the mother.

NURSING CONSIDERATIONS
🜂 *Alert:* By decreasing conduction through the AV node, drug may produce first-, second-, or third-degree heart block. Patients who develop high-level heart block after a single dose shouldn't receive additional doses.

🜂 *Alert:* New arrhythmias, including heart block and transient asystole, may develop; monitor cardiac rhythm and treat as indicated.
• Monitor BP closely. Discontinue drug in patients who develop persistent or symptomatic hypotension.
• Monitor patient for seizures during therapy.
🜂 *Alert:* Don't confuse adenosine with adenosine phosphate.

PATIENT TEACHING
• Instruct patient to report adverse reactions promptly.
• Tell patient to report discomfort at IV site.
• Inform patient that flushing or chest pain lasting 1 to 2 minutes may occur.

SAFETY ALERT!

ado-trastuzumab emtansine ⚗
ADD-oh tras-TOOZ-oo-mab em-TAN-seen

Kadcyla

Therapeutic class: Antineoplastics
Pharmacologic class: Antibody drug conjugates

AVAILABLE FORMS
Injection (lyophilized powder for solution): 100 mg, 160 mg in single-use vials

INDICATIONS & DOSAGES
➤ **HER2-positive, metastatic breast cancer in patients who previously received trastuzumab and a taxane, separately or in combination. Patients should have either received previous treatment for metastatic disease or developed recurrence during or within 6 months of completing adjuvant treatment**
Adults: 3.6 mg/kg IV every 21 days until disease progression or unacceptable toxicity occurs. Maximum dose is 3.6 mg/kg.
Adjust-a-dose: Refer to manufacturer's instructions for toxicity-related dosage adjustments.

ADMINISTRATION

IV

Black Box Warning Don't confuse or substitute this drug with trastuzumab (Herceptin). These drugs aren't interchangeable. ■

❖ *Alert:* The manufacturer recommends that the trade name be used and clearly recorded (with the batch number) in patient record to avoid confusion.

▼ Drug is considered hazardous; use safe handling and disposal precautions according to facility policy.

▼ To reconstitute, slowly inject 5 mL sterile water for injection into 100-mg vial or 8 mL sterile water for injection into 160-mg vial to yield concentration of 20 mg/mL.

▼ Swirl gently until dissolved. Don't shake. Solution should be colorless to pale brown.

▼ Add reconstituted dose to 250 mL of NSS in infusion bag and administer immediately through IV line containing 0.2- or 0.22-micron in-line nonprotein adsorptive polyethersulfone filter.

▼ Administer initial infusion over 90 minutes. Don't administer as IV push or bolus. Monitor patient for infusion-related reactions during administration and for 90 minutes after completion. Slow or interrupt infusion for infusion-related events. Discontinue drug if life-threatening infusion-related reactions occur.

▼ May administer subsequent infusions over 30 minutes if initial infusion was uneventful. Monitor patient during infusion and for 30 minutes after completion.

▼ Observe for subcut infiltration during infusion.

▼ Give at dosage and rate patient tolerated at most recent infusion.

▼ If dose is delayed or missed, give as soon as possible; don't wait for next planned cycle. Adjust schedule to maintain a 3-week interval between doses.

▼ Reconstituted vials can be stored in refrigerator for 24 hours at 36° to 46° F (2° to 8° C). Don't freeze.

▼ **Incompatibilities:** Dextrose solution, other drugs.

ACTION

Drug contains both trastuzumab and DM1 (a microtubule inhibitor), linked by a covalent bond, and targets the HER2 receptor by combined mechanisms of trastuzumab and DM1. The recombinant monoclonal antibody, trastuzumab, binds to the HER2 receptor and intracellular lysosomal degradation releases the cytotoxic component, DM1, resulting in microtubule disruption and cell death.

Route	Onset	Peak	Duration
IV	Unknown	End of infusion	Unknown

Half-life: 4 days.

ADVERSE REACTIONS

CNS: chills, fatigue, headache, fever, asthenia, dizziness, peripheral neuropathy, insomnia. **CV:** *left ventricular dysfunction,* edema, HTN. **EENT:** dry eye syndrome, blurred vision, conjunctivitis, increased lacrimation, epistaxis. **GI:** nausea, constipation, stomatitis, abdominal pain, vomiting, diarrhea, dyspepsia, dry mouth, taste perversion. **GU:** UTI. **Hematologic:** *thrombocytopenia, neutropenia,* anemia, hemorrhage. **Hepatic:** elevated transaminase levels, increased alkaline phosphatase level, increased bilirubin level. **Metabolic:** *hypokalemia.* **Musculoskeletal:** musculoskeletal pain, arthralgia, myalgia, weakness. **Respiratory:** pneumonitis, dyspnea, cough. **Skin:** pruritus, rash. **Other:** chills, hypersensitivity reactions, infusion reaction.

INTERACTIONS

Drug-drug. *Anthracyclines:* May enhance cardiotoxic effects of anthracyclines. When possible, avoid anthracycline-based therapy for up to 7 months after stopping ado-trastuzumab emtansine. Monitor patients who must receive this combination closely for cardiac dysfunction.

Strong CYP3A4 inhibitors (atazanavir, clarithromycin, indinavir, itraconazole, ketoconazole, nefazodone, nelfinavir, ritonavir, saquinavir, telithromycin, voriconazole): May increase ado-trastuzumab level and potential toxicity. Avoid use together. If use together is necessary, stop CYP3A4 inhibitor and delay treatment until inhibitor clears from patient's circulation, or monitor patient carefully for adverse effects.

EFFECTS ON LAB TEST RESULTS
• May increase bilirubin, AST, and ALT levels. May decrease potassium level.
• May decrease Hb level and platelet and neutrophil counts.

CONTRAINDICATIONS & CAUTIONS
• Contraindicated in patients hypersensitive to drug or its components.
• Use cautiously in patients with liver failure, risk of hepatotoxicity, symptomatic HF, serious cardiac arrhythmia, history of MI, or unstable angina.
• Avoid use in patients with history of trastuzumab hypersensitivity or infusion-related events.
• Discontinue drug in patients diagnosed with ILD or pneumonitis.
• Patients with shortness of breath at rest due to advanced malignancy and comorbidities may be at increased risk for pulmonary toxicity.
• Use cautiously in patients taking anticoagulants and in those with preexisting thrombocytopenia.
▧ Patients of Asian ancestry may be at higher risk for thrombocytopenia.
Dialyzable drug: Unknown.
⚠ *Overdose S&S:* Thrombocytopenia, death.

PREGNANCY-LACTATION-REPRODUCTION
Black Box Warning Exposure to drug can result in embryo-fetal death or birth defects. ▮
• Verify pregnancy status before start of therapy.
Black Box Warning Women of childbearing potential should use effective contraception during treatment and for 7 months after last dose. Male patients with female partners of childbearing potential should use effective contraception during treatment and for 4 months after last dose. ▮
• May impair fertility in females and males of childbearing potential. It isn't known if the effects are reversible.
◑ *Alert:* Advise patient to immediately inform physician if she suspects or confirms pregnancy during therapy or within 7 months after last dose. Report drug exposure to manufacturer (1-888-835-2555) and encourage patient to participate in MotHER Pregnancy Registry (1-800-690-6720).

• It isn't known if drug appears in human milk. Advise women not to breastfeed during treatment and for 7 months after last dose.

NURSING CONSIDERATIONS
▧ Confirm HER2 testing with FDA-approved test by established laboratory. Only patients with HER2 protein overexpression should receive drug because those are the only patients studied for whom benefit has been shown.
• Infusion-related reactions, including hypersensitivity reactions, may occur. Closely monitor patient during and for 90 minutes after infusion for fever, chills, flushing, dyspnea, hypotension, wheezing, bronchospasm, or tachycardia. Slow or interrupt infusion as necessary. In most patients, these reactions resolve over the course of several hours to a day after the infusion is terminated.
• Monitor patient for extravasation, which may cause redness, tenderness, skin irritation, pain, or swelling at infusion site.
Black Box Warning Severe liver injury (including fatal liver damage, liver failure, and death) has been reported. Monitor serum transaminase and bilirubin levels before starting drug and before each dose. Dosage modifications or discontinuation of therapy may be necessary. ▮
Black Box Warning Drug may significantly reduce LVEF. Assess LVEF before starting drug and every 3 months during treatment. Withhold or discontinue drug as clinically indicated. ▮
◑ *Alert:* Permanently discontinue drug in patients diagnosed with ILD or pneumonitis.
• Monitor platelet count before treatment and before each dose.
• Discontinue drug in patients diagnosed with nodular regenerative hyperplasia of the liver.
▧ ◑ *Alert:* Asian patients may have increased incidence and severity of thrombocytopenia.

PATIENT TEACHING
• Inform patient that drug may cause severe liver damage that may be life-threatening.
• Tell patient to report unexplained nausea, vomiting, abdominal pain, jaundice, dark urine, generalized itchiness, or anorexia.

Reactions in bold italics are *life-threatening*. Interactions may have a *rapid onset* or a *delayed onset*.

- Caution patient that drug may cause heart problems, with or without symptoms. Instruct patient to report new-onset or worsening of shortness of breath, cough, swelling of the ankles or legs, palpitations, weight gain of more than 5 lb in 24 hours, fatigue, dizziness, or loss of consciousness.
- Advise patient that drug may cause lung problems. Tell patient to report trouble breathing, cough, or tiredness.
- Alert patient that drug may cause low platelet count. Instruct patient to contact prescriber if excessive bleeding occurs.
- Warn patient that drug may cause nerve damage. Instruct patient to report numbness or tingling, burning or sharp pain, sensitivity to touch, lack of coordination, or muscle weakness or loss of muscle function.

Black Box Warning Inform patient that drug may cause birth defects and fetal death. Advise female patient of childbearing potential to use effective contraception during treatment and for 7 months after last dose. Advise male patient with female partner of childbearing potential to use effective contraception during treatment and for 4 months after last dose. ■

🌢 *Alert:* Advise patient to immediately inform physician if she suspects or confirms pregnancy during therapy. Encourage her participation in MotHER Pregnancy Registry (1-800-690-6720) and advise her to report drug exposure to manufacturer (1-888-835-2555).

- Advise female patient not to breastfeed during treatment and for 7 months after last dose.

albuterol sulfate
al-BYOO-ter-ole

Airomir✣, ProAir HFA, ProAir RespiClick, Proventil HFA, Ventolin HFA

Therapeutic class: Bronchodilators
Pharmacologic class: Adrenergics

AVAILABLE FORMS
Inhalation aerosol: 100 mcg/actuation✣, 108 mcg/actuation
Inhalation powder: 108 mcg/actuation

Solution for inhalation: 0.021% (0.63 mg/3 mL), 0.042% (1.25 mg/3 mL), 0.083% (2.5 mg/3 mL), 0.5 mg/mL✣, 1 mg/mL✣, 2 mg/mL✣, 0.5% (5 mg/mL)
Syrup: 2 mg/5 mL
Tablets: 2 mg, 4 mg
Tablets (extended-release) 🚫: 4 mg, 8 mg

INDICATIONS & DOSAGES
➤ **To prevent or treat bronchospasm in patients with reversible obstructive airway disease**
Tablets (extended-release)
Adults and children older than age 12: 4 to 8 mg PO every 12 hours. Maximum, 32 mg daily.
Children ages 6 to 12: 4 mg PO every 12 hours. Maximum, 24 mg daily.
Tablets
Adults and children older than age 12: 2 to 4 mg PO t.i.d. or q.i.d. Maximum, 32 mg daily.
Children ages 6 to 12: 2 mg PO t.i.d. or q.i.d. Maximum, 24 mg daily.
Solution for inhalation
Adults and children age 12 and older: 2.5 mg by nebulizer, given over 5 to 15 minutes, t.i.d. or q.i.d. To prepare solution, use 0.5 mL of 0.5% solution diluted with 2.5 mL of NSS. Or, use 3 mL of 0.083% solution.
Children ages 2 to 12 weighing more than 15 kg: 2.5 mg by nebulizer given over 5 to 15 minutes t.i.d. or q.i.d., with subsequent doses adjusted to response. Don't exceed 2.5 mg t.i.d. or q.i.d.
Children ages 2 to 12 weighing 15 kg or less: 0.63 mg or 1.25 mg by nebulizer given over 5 to 15 minutes t.i.d. or q.i.d. with subsequent doses adjusted to response. Don't exceed 2.5 mg t.i.d. or q.i.d.
Syrup
Adults and children older than age 14: 2 to 4 mg PO t.i.d. or q.i.d. Maximum, 32 mg daily.
Children ages 6 to 14: 2 mg PO t.i.d. or q.i.d. Maximum, 24 mg daily.
Children ages 2 to 5: Initially, 0.1 mg/kg PO t.i.d. Starting dose shouldn't exceed 2 mg t.i.d. Maximum, 12 mg daily.
Inhalation aerosol
Adults and children age 4 and older: 1 to 2 inhalations every 4 to 6 hours as needed.

Regular use for maintenance therapy to control asthma symptoms isn't recommended.
Adjust-a-dose: For elderly patients and those sensitive to sympathomimetic amines, 2 mg PO t.i.d. or q.i.d. as oral tablets or syrup. Maximum, 32 mg daily.

Inhalational powder
Adults and children age 4 and older: 2 inhalations every 4 to 6 hours. In some patients, 1 inhalation every 4 hours may be sufficient.

➤ **To prevent exercise-induced bronchospasm**
Adults and children age 4 and older: 2 inhalations 15 to 30 minutes before exercise.

➤ **Adjuvant therapy for acute treatment of moderate to severe hyperkalemia ♦**
Adults: 10 to 20 mg via nebulization over 10 minutes, given in combination with other recommended therapy.

ADMINISTRATION
PO
• When switching patient from regular to extended-release tablets, remember that a regular 2-mg tablet every 6 hours is equivalent to an extended-release 4-mg tablet every 12 hours.
• Give extended-release tablets whole; don't break or crush tablets or mix them with food.

Inhalational
• If more than 1 inhalation is ordered, wait at least 2 minutes between inhalations.
• Inhalation powder inhaler device doesn't require priming. Use spacer device to improve drug delivery, if appropriate. Don't use ProAir RespiClick with a spacer or volume holding chamber.
• Discard ProAir RespiClick 13 months after opening foil pouch, when dose counter displays "0," or after expiration date on product, whichever comes first.
• Shake the aerosol inhaler well before use and prime inhaler according to manufacturer's instructions before first use, when it has been dropped, or when it hasn't been used for more than 2 weeks.
• Keep cap on inhaler closed during storage.

ACTION
Relaxes bronchial, uterine, and vascular smooth muscle by stimulating beta$_2$ receptors.

Route	Onset	Peak	Duration
PO	15–30 min	2–3 hr	4–8 hr
PO (extended)	Unknown	6 hr	12 hr
Inhalation (aerosol)	5–15 min	30–120 min	3–4 hr
Inhalation (powder)	Rapid	30 min	3–4 hr

Half-life: Oral, 5 to 6 hours; inhalation aerosol, 6 hours; inhalation powder, 5 hours.

ADVERSE REACTIONS
CNS: tremor, nervousness, headache, hyperactivity, insomnia, dizziness, weakness, CNS stimulation, malaise. **CV:** tachycardia, palpitations, HTN, chest pain, lymphadenopathy, edema. **EENT:** conjunctivitis, otitis media, dry and irritated nose and throat (with inhaled form), nasal congestion, epistaxis, hoarseness, pharyngitis, rhinitis. **GI:** nausea, vomiting, heartburn, anorexia, altered taste, increased appetite. **GU:** UTI. **Metabolic:** hypokalemia. **Musculoskeletal:** muscle cramps, back pain. **Respiratory:** *bronchospasm,* cough, wheezing, dyspnea, bronchitis, increased sputum. **Other:** hypersensitivity reactions, flulike syndrome, cold symptoms.

INTERACTIONS
Drug-drug. *Antiarrhythmics (amiodarone, bretylium, disopyramide, dofetilide, procainamide, quinidine, sotalol), arsenic trioxide, chlorpromazine, dolasetron, droperidol, mefloquine, mesoridazine, moxifloxacin, pentamidine, pimozide, tacrolimus, thioridazine, ziprasidone:* May prolong QT interval and increase risk of life-threatening arrhythmias, including torsades de pointes. Monitor QT interval and patient.
CNS stimulants: May increase CNS stimulation. Avoid using together.
Digoxin: May decrease digoxin level. Monitor digoxin level closely.
Diuretics (furosemide, thiazides): May cause ECG changes and hypokalemia. Monitor potassium level. Use caution when administered with non-potassium-sparing diuretics.
Linezolid, MAO inhibitors, TCAs: May increase adverse CV effects. Consider alternative therapy. Monitor patient closely if used together.

Reactions in bold italics are *life-threatening*. Interactions may have a *rapid onset* or a *delayed onset*.

Propranolol and other beta blockers: May cause mutual antagonism. Monitor patient carefully.

EFFECTS ON LAB TEST RESULTS
• May decrease potassium level.

CONTRAINDICATIONS & CAUTIONS
• Contraindicated in patients hypersensitive to drug or its ingredients.
• Use cautiously in patients with CV disorders (including coronary insufficiency and HTN), hyperthyroidism, or diabetes mellitus and in those who are unusually responsive to adrenergics.
• Use extended-release tablets cautiously in patients with GI narrowing.
Dialyzable drug: Unknown.
⚠ *Overdose S&S:* Exaggeration of adverse reactions, seizures, angina, hypotension, HTN, tachycardia, arrhythmias, nervousness, headache, tremor, dry mouth, palpitations, nausea, dizziness, fatigue, malaise, sleeplessness, hypokalemia, cardiac arrest.

PREGNANCY-LACTATION-REPRODUCTION
• There are no adequate and well-controlled studies in pregnant women. Use during pregnancy only if potential benefit justifies potential risk to the fetus.
• It isn't known if drug appears in human milk. Use cautiously in breastfeeding women.

NURSING CONSIDERATIONS
• Drug may decrease sensitivity of spirometry used for diagnosis of asthma.
• Syrup contains no alcohol or sugar and may be taken by children as young as age 2.
• In children, syrup may rarely cause erythema multiforme or SJS.
• Monitor patient for effectiveness. Using drug alone may not be adequate to control asthma in some patients. Long-term control medications may be needed.
⚙ *Alert:* Drug may cause paradoxical bronchospasm. Monitor patient closely; discontinue drug immediately and use alternative therapy if paradoxical bronchospasm occurs. Bronchospasm with inhaled formulations frequently occurs with first use of new canister or vial.

⚙ *Alert:* Patient may use tablets and aerosol together. Monitor these patients closely for signs and symptoms of toxicity.
• *Look alike–sound alike:* Don't confuse albuterol with atenolol or Albuten.

PATIENT TEACHING
• Warn patient about risk of paradoxical bronchospasm and advise patient to stop drug immediately if it occurs.
• Teach patient to perform oral inhalation correctly.
• If prescriber orders more than 1 inhalation, tell patient to wait at least 2 minutes before repeating procedure.
• Tell patient that use of a spacer device with appropriate inhaler may improve drug delivery to lungs.
• If patient is also using a corticosteroid inhaler, instruct patient to use the bronchodilator first and then to wait about 5 minutes before using the corticosteroid.
• Tell patient to remove canister and wash aerosol inhaler with warm, soapy water at least once a week.
• Warn patient not to wash or place any part of powder inhaler in water. If mouthpiece needs cleaning, advise patient to gently wipe it with dry cloth or tissue.
• Advise patient not to use more than prescribed and not to increase dose or frequency without consulting physician. Fatalities have been reported from excessive use.
• Instruct patient to report worsening symptoms.
• Advise patient not to chew or crush extended-release tablets or mix them with food.

SAFETY ALERT!

alectinib hydrochloride ⬥
al-EK-ti-nib

Alecensa

Therapeutic class: Antineoplastics
Pharmacologic class: Tyrosine kinase inhibitors

AVAILABLE FORMS
Capsules ⬤: 150 mg

INDICATIONS & DOSAGES
➤ **To treat anaplastic lymphoma kinase (ALK)-positive, metastatic NSCLC** ▨
Adults: 600 mg PO b.i.d. until disease progression or unacceptable toxicity.
Adjust-a-dose: Recommended dosage in patients with severe hepatic impairment (Child-Pugh class C) is 450 mg PO b.i.d. Refer to manufacturer's instructions for toxicity-related dosage adjustments.

ADMINISTRATION
PO
- Hazardous drug; use safe handling and disposal precautions according to facility policy.
- Give with food.
- Don't open or dissolve contents of capsule.
- If a dose is missed or vomiting occurs after taking a dose, give next dose at the scheduled time.
- Don't store above 86° F (30° C). Store in the original container to protect from light and moisture.

ACTION
A tyrosine kinase inhibitor that targets *ALK* and *RET* gene abnormalities that alter signaling and expression and result in increased cellular proliferation and survival in tumors that express these fusion proteins. Inhibiting ALK signaling decreases tumor cell viability.

Route	Onset	Peak	Duration
PO	Unknown	4 hr	Unknown

Half-life: 33 hours (parent drug).

ADVERSE REACTIONS
CNS: fatigue, headache. **CV:** *bradycardia,* edema. **EENT:** vision disorder. **GI:** vomiting, constipation, nausea, diarrhea. **Hematologic:** anemia, *lymphopenia,* neutropenia. **Hepatic:** hyperbilirubinemia, elevated alkaline phosphatase, AST, and ALT levels. **Metabolic:** increased weight, hypoalbuminemia, hypocalcemia, hyperglycemia, *hypokalemia, hyperkalemia,* hyponatremia, hypophosphatemia. **Musculoskeletal:** myalgia, back pain. **Respiratory:** dyspnea, cough. **Skin:** rash, photosensitivity.

INTERACTIONS
Drug-drug. *Bradycardia-causing drugs:* May increase risk of bradycardia. Monitor patient closely.
Drug-lifestyle. *Sun exposure:* May increase risk of photosensitivity. Discourage sun exposure and recommend use of broad-spectrum sunscreen and lip balm.

EFFECTS ON LAB TEST RESULTS
- May increase AST, ALT, alkaline phosphatase, CK, bilirubin, glucose, GGT, and creatinine levels. May decrease calcium, phosphorus, albumin, and sodium levels.
- May increase or decrease potassium level.
- May decrease WBC and RBC counts.

CONTRAINDICATIONS & CAUTIONS
▨ Drug is only approved for use in patients with metastatic NSCLC who test positive for the abnormal *ALK* gene.
- Drug may increase risk of hepatotoxicity, pulmonary toxicity (ILD or pneumonitis), intestinal perforation, endocarditis, and hemorrhage.
- Safety and effectiveness in children haven't been determined.
Dialyzable drug: Unlikely.

PREGNANCY-LACTATION-REPRODUCTION
- Drug may cause fetal harm. Women of childbearing potential should use effective contraception during treatment and for 1 week after therapy ends.
- Males with female partners of childbearing potential should use effective contraception during treatment and for 3 months after final dose.
- It's unknown if drug appears in human milk. Due to the potential for serious adverse reactions in breastfed infants, breastfeeding isn't recommended during treatment and for 1 week after therapy ends.

NURSING CONSIDERATIONS
- Monitor LFTs (ALT, AST, and total bilirubin levels) every 2 weeks during first 3 months of treatment, then once a month and as clinically indicated during treatment. Monitor patients for signs and symptoms of hepatotoxicity (dark urine, abdominal pain, nausea, vomiting, malaise) and intestinal

perforation (severe abdominal pain, fever, nausea, vomiting).
• Monitor patients for signs and symptoms of ILD or pneumonitis (worsening of respiratory symptoms, cough, dyspnea, fever). Withhold drug if patients are diagnosed with ILD or pneumonitis and permanently discontinue drug if it's the causative factor.
• Monitor patients for myalgia or musculoskeletal pain and assess CK level every 2 weeks for first month of treatment and as clinically indicated. Drug may need to be withheld or dosage reduced.
• Monitor patients for chest pain and monitor HR and BP regularly. Dosage modification isn't required in cases of asymptomatic bradycardia. Adjust dosage for non-life-threatening, symptomatic bradycardia and assess for concomitant bradycardia-contributing drugs. Treat life-threatening bradycardia appropriately.
• Monitor patients for abnormal bleeding.
• Monitor patients for signs and symptoms of photosensitivity.

PATIENT TEACHING
• Advise patient to report all drugs and supplements being taken before beginning therapy.
• Teach patient to report signs and symptoms of liver injury or intestinal perforation (tiredness, anorexia, jaundice, dark urine, pruritus, nausea, vomiting, right-sided stomach pain, sharp abdominal pain, fever, easy bleeding or bruising); explain the need for blood tests throughout treatment.
• Inform patient of the risks of severe ILD or pneumonitis. Advise patient to contact prescriber immediately for new or worsening respiratory symptoms.
• Educate patient about the possibility of muscle pain, tenderness, and weakness and to immediately report new, worsening, or persistent signs and symptoms of muscle pain or weakness.
• Counsel patient that drug may cause dizziness, light-headedness, syncope and, rarely, chest pain and to immediately report these symptoms to prescriber.
• Advise patient to report abnormal bleeding.
• Advise patient to avoid prolonged sun exposure while taking drug and for at least

7 days after last dose. Advise patient to use broad-spectrum sunscreen and lip balm (SPF 50 or higher) to protect from potential sunburn.
• Advise patient that if a dose is missed or if vomiting occurs after taking a dose, not to take an extra dose, but to take the next dose at the regular time.
• Caution female patient of childbearing potential of possible fetal harm if drug is taken during pregnancy. Advise her to use effective contraception during treatment and for 1 week after last dose and to inform prescriber immediately if she is or may be pregnant.
• Explain to male patient with female partners of childbearing potential the need to use effective contraception during and for 3 months after treatment ends.
• Warn female patient not to breastfeed during treatment and for 1 week after treatment ends.

alendronate sodium
ah-LEN-dro-nate

Binosto, Fosamax&

Therapeutic class: Antiosteoporotics
Pharmacologic class: Bisphosphonates

AVAILABLE FORMS
Oral solution: 70 mg/75 mL
Tablets: 5 mg, 10 mg, 35 mg, 40 mg, 70 mg
Tablets (effervescent): 70 mg

INDICATIONS & DOSAGES
➤ **Osteoporosis in postmenopausal women; to increase bone mass in men with osteoporosis**
Adults: 10 mg PO daily or 70-mg tablet or solution PO once weekly.
➤ **Paget disease of bone (osteitis deformans) (excluding Binosto and oral solution)**
Adults: 40 mg PO daily for 6 months.
➤ **To prevent osteoporosis in postmenopausal women (excluding Binosto and oral solution)**
Adults: 5 mg PO daily or 35-mg tablet PO once weekly.

➤ **Glucocorticoid-induced osteoporosis in patients receiving glucocorticoids in a daily dose equivalent to 7.5 mg or more of prednisone and who have low bone mineral density (excluding Binosto and oral solution)**
Adults: 5 mg PO daily. For postmenopausal women not receiving estrogen, recommended dose is 10 mg PO daily.

ADMINISTRATION
PO
• Give drug with 180 to 240 mL of plain water at least 30 minutes before patient's first food or drink of the day to facilitate delivery to the stomach and reduce esophageal irritation risk.
• Dissolve effervescent tablet in 120 mL of plain room-temperature water.
• Give at least 60 mL of water after oral solution.
• Don't allow patient to lie down for 30 minutes after taking drug and until after first food of the day.

ACTION
Suppresses osteoclast activity on newly formed resorption surfaces, which reduces bone turnover. Bone formation exceeds resorption at remodeling sites, leading to progressive gains in bone mass.

Route	Onset	Peak	Duration
PO	Unknown	Unknown	Unknown

Half-life: More than 10 years.

ADVERSE REACTIONS
CNS: headache. **GI:** abdominal pain, nausea, dyspepsia, constipation, diarrhea, flatulence, acid regurgitation, esophageal ulcer, vomiting, dysphagia, abdominal distention, gastritis, taste perversion, melena. **Musculoskeletal:** pain.

INTERACTIONS
Drug-drug. *Antacids, calcium supplements, multivitamins and minerals, many oral drugs:* May interfere with absorption of alendronate. Instruct patient to wait at least 30 minutes after taking alendronate before taking other drug orally.

Aspirin, NSAIDs: May increase risk of upper GI adverse reactions. Monitor patient closely.
PPIs: May diminish therapeutic effects of alendronate. Monitor therapy.
Ranitidine (IV form): May increase availability of alendronate. Reduce dosage as needed.
Drug-food. *Any food:* May decrease absorption of drug. Advise patient to take with full glass of plain water at least 30 minutes before food, beverages, or ingestion of other drugs.

EFFECTS ON LAB TEST RESULTS
• May decrease calcium and phosphate levels.

CONTRAINDICATIONS & CAUTIONS
• Contraindicated in patients hypersensitive to drug and in those with hypocalcemia or abnormalities of the esophagus that delay esophageal emptying.
• Oral solution contraindicated in patients at increased risk for aspiration.
• Drug isn't recommended for patients with CrCl of less than 35 mL/minute.
⊘ *Alert:* There may be an increased risk of atypical fractures of the thigh in patients treated with bisphosphonates.
• Contraindicated in patients unable to stand or sit upright for at least 30 minutes.
• Use cautiously in patients with active upper GI problems (dysphagia, symptomatic esophageal diseases, gastritis, duodenitis, ulcers) or mild to moderate renal insufficiency.
• Use cautiously in patients with known risk factors for osteonecrosis of the jaw (diagnosis of cancer; concomitant treatment with chemotherapy, radiotherapy, corticosteroids), poor oral hygiene, and comorbid disorders, such as preexisting dental disease, anemia, coagulopathy, or infection.
Dialyzable drug: No.
⚠ *Overdose S&S:* Hypocalcemia, hypophosphatemia, upset stomach, heartburn, esophagitis, gastritis, ulcer.

PREGNANCY-LACTATION-REPRODUCTION
• No data exist on fetal risk in humans, but there is a theoretical risk of fetal harm. Use during pregnancy only if potential benefit justifies potential risk to the fetus.

Reactions in bold italics are *life-threatening*. Interactions may have a *rapid onset* or a *delayed onset*.

- It isn't known if drug appears in human milk. Use cautiously in breastfeeding women.

NURSING CONSIDERATIONS

- Correct hypocalcemia and other disturbances of mineral metabolism (such as vitamin D deficiency) before therapy begins.
- When used to treat osteoporosis, disease may be confirmed by findings of low bone mass on diagnostic studies or by history of osteoporotic fracture.
- Patients at risk for vitamin D deficiency, such as those who are chronically ill, who are nursing home bound, who have a GI malabsorption syndrome, or who are older than age 70, may require vitamin D supplementation.
- In Paget disease, drug is indicated for patients with alkaline phosphatase level at least 2 × ULN, for those who are symptomatic, and for those at risk for future complications from the disease.
- Monitor patient's calcium and phosphate levels throughout therapy.
- Severe musculoskeletal pain has been associated with bisphosphonate use and may occur within days, months, or years of start of therapy. When drug is stopped, symptoms may resolve partially or completely.
- Patients who develop osteonecrosis of the jaw should receive care by an oral surgeon.
- Optimal length of treatment hasn't been determined. Reevaluate need for continued therapy periodically. Patients at low risk for fracture should be considered for discontinuation after 3 to 5 years of treatment.
- *Look alike–sound alike:* Don't confuse Fosamax with Flomax.

PATIENT TEACHING

- Stress importance of taking tablet only with 180 to 240 mL of plain water at least 30 minutes before ingesting anything else, including food, beverages, and other drugs. Tell patient that waiting longer than 30 minutes improves absorption.
- Warn patient not to lie down for at least 30 minutes after taking drug to facilitate delivery to stomach and to reduce risk of esophageal irritation.
- Tell patient who misses a once-weekly dose to take one dose on the morning after

remembering and then return to weekly dosing on the chosen day as originally scheduled.
- Advise patient to report adverse reactions immediately, especially chest pain or difficulty swallowing.
- Advise patient to take supplemental calcium and vitamin D if dietary intake is inadequate.
- Advise patient to discuss usage and timing of OTC medications with prescriber.
- Tell patient about benefits of weight-bearing exercises in increasing bone mass. If applicable, explain importance of reducing or eliminating cigarette smoking and alcohol use.

aliskiren hemifumarate
a-lis-KYE-ren

Rasilez✦ , Tekturna

Therapeutic class: Antihypertensives
Pharmacologic class: Renin inhibitors

AVAILABLE FORMS
Tablets: 150 mg, 300 mg

INDICATIONS & DOSAGES
➤ **HTN, alone or with other antihypertensives**
Adults: 150 mg PO daily; may increase to 300 mg PO daily.
Children age 6 and older weighing more than 50 kg: Dosing same as adult.
Children age 6 and older weighing 20 to less than 50 kg: Starting dose, 75 mg PO once daily, with a maximum dose of 150 mg.

ADMINISTRATION
PO
- Don't give drug with high-fat meal; may decrease drug's effectiveness.
- Give consistently at same time each day with or without meals. However, consistent administration with regard to meals is recommended.

ACTION
Decreases renin activity and inhibits conversion of angiotensin to angiotensin I, decreasing vasoconstriction and lowering BP.

Route	Onset	Peak	Duration
PO	Unknown	1–3 hr	Unknown

Half-life: 24 hours.

ADVERSE REACTIONS

CNS: headache, dizziness, fatigue, *seizures.* **CV:** hypotension. **GI:** abdominal pain, diarrhea, dyspepsia, gastroesophageal reflux. **Metabolic:** hyperuricemia, *hyperkalemia.* **Respiratory:** cough, URI. **Skin:** rash. **Other:** *angioedema.*

INTERACTIONS

Drug-drug. ⚠ *Alert: ACE inhibitors (benazepril, captopril, lisinopril, moexipril, perindopril, quinapril, ramipril, trandolapril), ARBs (azilsartan, candesartan, eprosartan, irbesartan, losartan, olmesartan, telmisartan, valsartan), other drugs that antagonize RAAS:* May increase risk of renal impairment, hypotension, and hyperkalemia. Concomitant use is contraindicated in diabetic patients. Avoid concomitant use in patients with moderate to severe renal impairment (GFR < 60 mL/minute).
Atorvastatin: May increase aliskiren levels. Use cautiously together.
CYP3A4/P-gp inhibitors (cyclosporine, itraconazole, ketoconazole, verapamil): May increase aliskiren concentration and risk of adverse reactions. Use with caution. Avoid concurrent use with cyclosporine or itraconazole.
Furosemide: May reduce furosemide peak levels. Monitor patient for effectiveness.
NSAIDs: May increase risk of renal toxicity. Monitor renal function periodically.
Potassium-sparing diuretics, potassium supplements: May increase risk of hyperkalemia. Use cautiously together.
Rifampin: May decrease aliskiren plasma concentration. Larger aliskiren doses may be needed.
Drug-food. *Fruit juices (apple, grapefruit, orange):* May decrease aliskiren plasma level. Advise patient to avoid products containing fruit juice.
High-fat meals: May substantially decrease plasma levels of drug. Monitor patient for effectiveness.

EFFECTS ON LAB TEST RESULTS

• May increase potassium, CK, BUN, uric acid, and serum creatinine levels.

CONTRAINDICATIONS & CAUTIONS

• Contraindicated in patients hypersensitive to drug or its components and in those with diabetes who are receiving ARBs or ACE inhibitors.
• Contraindicated in patients taking cyclosporine or itraconazole.
• Use cautiously in patients with history of angioedema, severe renal dysfunction (GFR of less than 30 mL/minute), history of dialysis, nephrotic syndrome, or renovascular HTN.
Dialyzable drug: No.
⚠ *Overdose S&S:* Hypotension.

PREGNANCY-LACTATION-REPRODUCTION

Black Box Warning Drug can cause fetal harm. Drugs that act on the RAAS can cause injury and death to the developing fetus. Discontinue drug as soon as possible once pregnancy is detected. ▮
• Women of childbearing potential should avoid becoming pregnant while taking drug.
• It isn't known if drug appears in human milk. Patient should discontinue breastfeeding or discontinue drug.

NURSING CONSIDERATIONS

• Monitor BP for hypotension, especially if used in combination with other antihypertensives.
• Monitor potassium levels, especially in patients also taking ACE inhibitors.
⚠ *Alert:* Rarely, angioedema may occur at any time during treatment. Discontinue drug for angioedema or anaphylaxis and don't readminister. Early emergency treatment is critical and may include intubation, antihistamines, steroids, and epinephrine.
• Monitor renal function. It's unknown how patients with significant renal disorders will respond to the use of this drug.
• Correct volume or salt depletion before giving drug or start therapy under close monitoring.
• Effect of any dose is usually seen within 2 weeks.
• Monitor patient for serious skin reactions (SJS, toxic epidermal necrolysis).

Reactions in bold italics are *life-threatening*. Interactions may have a *rapid onset* or a *delayed onset*.

PATIENT TEACHING
• Instruct patient not to take drug with a high-fat meal because this may decrease drug's effectiveness.
• Instruct patient to monitor BP daily, if possible, and to report low readings, dizziness, and headaches to prescriber.
• Tell patient to immediately report swelling of the face or neck or difficulty breathing.
• Advise patient of need for regular laboratory tests to monitor for adverse effects.

allopurinol ⚕
al-oh-PURE-i-nole

Zyloprim

allopurinol sodium ⚕
Aloprim

Therapeutic class: Antigout drugs
Pharmacologic class: Xanthine oxidase inhibitors

AVAILABLE FORMS
allopurinol
Tablets (scored): 100 mg, 200 mg✤, 300 mg
allopurinol sodium
Injection: 500 mg/30 mL vial

INDICATIONS & DOSAGES
Adjust-a-dose (for all indications): If CrCl is 10 to 20 mL/minute, give 200 mg PO or IV daily; if CrCl is 3 to 10 mL/minute, give 100 mg PO or IV daily; if CrCl is less than 3 mL/minute, give a maximum of 100 mg PO or IV at extended intervals.
➤ **Gout or hyperuricemia**
Adults: Initially, 100 mg PO daily; then titrate in 100-mg increments weekly until serum urate concentration falls to 6 mg/dL or less. Maximum, 800 mg daily. Dosage varies with severity of disease; can be given as single dose or divided, but doses greater than 300 mg should be divided.
➤ **Hyperuricemia caused by malignancies**
Adults and children older than age 10: 200 to 400 mg/m^2 daily IV as a single infusion or in equally divided doses every 6, 8, or 12 hours beginning 24 to 48 hours before initiation of chemotherapy. Maximum, 600 mg daily.

Children age 10 and younger: Initially, 200 mg/m^2 daily IV as single infusion or in equally divided doses every 6, 8, or 12 hours beginning 24 to 48 hours before initiation of chemotherapy. Then titrate according to uric acid levels. For children ages 6 to 10, give 300 mg PO daily or in three divided doses; for children younger than age 6, give 150 mg PO daily.
➤ **To prevent uric acid nephropathy during cancer chemotherapy**
Adults: 600 to 800 mg PO daily for 2 to 3 days, with high fluid intake.
➤ **Recurrent calcium oxalate calculi**
Adults: 200 to 300 mg PO daily in single or divided doses.

ADMINISTRATION
PO
• Give drug with or immediately after meals to minimize GI upset.
IV
▼ When possible, initiate therapy 24 to 48 hours before the start of chemotherapy known to cause tumor lysis.
▼ Dissolve contents of each 30-mL vial in 25 mL of sterile water for injection.
▼ Dilute solution to desired concentration (no greater than 6 mg/mL) with NSS for injection or D$_5$W. Can give as a single daily infusion or in equally divided infusions at 6-, 8-, or 12-hour intervals. Rate of infusion depends on volume of infusate.
▼ Store solution at 68° to 77° F (20° to 25° C) and use within 10 hours. Don't use solution if it contains particulates or is discolored.
▼ **Incompatibilities:** Amikacin, amphotericin B, carmustine, cefotaxime, chlorpromazine, cimetidine, clindamycin, cytarabine, dacarbazine, daunorubicin, diphenhydramine, doxorubicin, doxycycline, droperidol, floxuridine, gentamicin, haloperidol, hydroxyzine, idarubicin, imipenem–cilastatin, mechlorethamine, meperidine, methylprednisolone, metoclopramide, minocycline, nalbuphine, ondansetron, prochlorperazine, promethazine, sodium bicarbonate (or solutions containing sodium bicarbonate), streptozocin, tobramycin, vinorelbine.

ACTION
Reduces uric acid production by inhibiting xanthine oxidase.

Route	Onset	Peak	Duration
PO	Unknown	1½ hr (allopurinol); 4½ hr (oxypurinol)	1–2 wk
IV	Unknown	30 min	Unknown

Half-life: Allopurinol, 1 to 2 hours; oxypurinol, 19 to 28 hours.

ADVERSE REACTIONS
GI: nausea, vomiting, abdominal pain, diarrhea. **GU:** *renal failure.* **Musculoskeletal:** acute gout attack. **Skin:** rash, maculopapular rash.

INTERACTIONS
Drug-drug. *Amoxicillin, ampicillin:* May increase possibility of rash. Avoid using together.
Anticoagulants: May increase anticoagulant effect. Dosage may need to be adjusted.
Antineoplastics: May increase potential for bone marrow suppression. Monitor patient carefully.
Azathioprine, mercaptopurine: May increase levels of these drugs. Concomitant administration of 300 to 600 mg of oral allopurinol per day requires dosage reduction to ⅓ to ¼ of usual dose of azathioprine or mercaptopurine. Make subsequent dosage adjustments based on therapeutic response and appearance of toxic effects.
Chlorpropamide: May increase hypoglycemic effect. Avoid using together.
Cyclosporine: May increase cyclosporine level. Monitor cyclosporine level and adjust dosage as necessary.
Ethacrynic acid, thiazide diuretics: May increase risk of allopurinol toxicity. Reduce allopurinol dosage, and monitor renal function closely.
Theophylline: May increase theophylline level. Adjust theophylline dosage as needed.
Uricosurics: May have additive effect. May be used to therapeutic advantage.

EFFECTS ON LAB TEST RESULTS
• May increase alkaline phosphatase, ALT, and AST levels.

• May increase eosinophil count. May decrease Hb level, hematocrit, and granulocyte and platelet counts.
• May increase or decrease WBC count.

CONTRAINDICATIONS & CAUTIONS
• Contraindicated in patients hypersensitive to drug.
▓ ❸ *Alert:* To avoid risk of severe cutaneous adverse reactions (SCAR), avoid use of allopurinol in HLA-B*5801-positive patients. The American College of Rheumatology recommends HLA-B*5801 screening in patients at elevated risk for SCAR, including patients of Korean descent who have chronic kidney disease stage 3 or greater as well as patients of Han Chinese or Thai descent regardless of kidney function. Some experts suggest screening in all patients of Korean ethnicity regardless of renal function.
Dialyzable drug: Yes.

PREGNANCY-LACTATION-REPRODUCTION
• Use in pregnancy only if clearly needed.
• Drug appears in human milk. Use cautiously in breastfeeding women.

NURSING CONSIDERATIONS
❸ *Alert:* Rash can be followed by more severe hypersensitivity reactions (SJS, vasculitis, irreversible hepatotoxicity), which can be fatal. Discontinue drug at first sign of rash.
• Monitor uric acid level to evaluate drug's effectiveness.
• Monitor fluid intake and output; daily urine output of at least 2 L and maintenance of neutral or slightly alkaline urine are desirable.
• Periodically monitor CBC and hepatic and renal function, especially at start of therapy.
• Optimal benefits may need 2 to 6 weeks of therapy. Because acute gout attacks may occur during this time, concurrent use of colchicine may be prescribed prophylactically.
• Don't restart drug in patients who have a severe reaction.
• *Look alike–sound alike:* Don't confuse Zyloprim with ZORprin or zolpidem.

Reactions in bold italics are *life-threatening*. Interactions may have a *rapid onset* or a *delayed onset*.

PATIENT TEACHING
- To minimize GI adverse reactions, tell patient to take drug with or immediately after meals.
- ▧ ❸ *Alert:* Advise patient who is known to be HLA-B*5801-positive to avoid allopurinol.
- Encourage patient to drink plenty of fluids while taking drug unless otherwise contraindicated.
- Drug may cause drowsiness; tell patient not to drive or perform hazardous tasks requiring mental alertness until CNS effects of drug are known.
- If patient is taking drug for recurrent calcium oxalate stones, advise patient also to reduce dietary intake of animal protein, sodium, refined sugars, oxalate-rich foods, and calcium.
- Tell patient to stop drug at first sign of rash, which may precede severe hypersensitivity or other adverse reactions. Rash is more common in patients taking diuretics and in those with renal disorders. Tell patient to report all adverse reactions.
- Advise patient to avoid alcohol during therapy.
- Teach patient importance of continuing drug even if asymptomatic.

almotriptan malate
al-moh-TRIP-tan

Axert

Therapeutic class: Antimigraine drugs
Pharmacologic class: Serotonin 5-HT$_1$ receptor agonists

AVAILABLE FORMS
Tablets: 6.25 mg, 12.5 mg

INDICATIONS & DOSAGES
➤ **Acute migraine with or without aura**
Adults and adolescents ages 12 to 17:
6.25 mg or 12.5 mg PO, with one additional dose after 2 hours if headache is unresolved or recurs. The 12.5-mg dose tends to be more effective in adults. Maximum, two doses (total of 25 mg) within 24 hours.

Adjust-a-dose: For patients with hepatic or renal impairment, initially 6.25 mg, with maximum daily dose of 12.5 mg.

ADMINISTRATION
PO
- Give drug without regard for food.
- Give only one repeat dose within 24 hours, no sooner than 2 hours after first dose.

ACTION
May act as an agonist at serotonin receptors on extracerebral intracranial blood vessels, which constricts the affected vessels, inhibits neuropeptide release, and reduces pain transmission in the trigeminal pathways.

Route	Onset	Peak	Duration
PO	1–3 hr	1–3 hr	Unknown

Half-life: 3 to 4 hours.

ADVERSE REACTIONS
CNS: paresthesia, headache, dizziness, somnolence. **GI:** nausea, vomiting, dry mouth.

INTERACTIONS
Drug-drug. *Antiemetics (5-HT$_3$ antagonists), antipsychotics, metolazone, methylene blue, metoclopramide, opioid analgesics, tramadol:* May increase serotonergic effects and serotonin syndrome. Monitor therapy.
CYP3A4 inhibitors (such as ketoconazole): May increase almotriptan level. Monitor patient for potential adverse reaction. May need to reduce dosage. Avoid concomitant use in patients with renal or hepatic impairment.
Ergot-containing drugs, serotonin 5-HT$_{1B/1D}$ agonists: May cause additive effects. Don't use within 24 hours of almotriptan.
MAO inhibitors, verapamil: May increase almotriptan level. No dose adjustment is necessary.
SSNRIs, SSRIs: May cause additive serotonin effects, resulting in weakness, hyperreflexia, or incoordination. Monitor patient closely if given together.

EFFECTS ON LAB TEST RESULTS
None reported.

♣Canada   ◇OTC   ◆Off-label use   ✔Photoguide   ⊛Do not crush   *Liquid contains alcohol   ▧Genetic

CONTRAINDICATIONS & CAUTIONS
• Contraindicated in patients hypersensitive to drug.
• Contraindicated in patients with angina pectoris, history of MI, silent ischemia, coronary artery vasospasm, Prinzmetal variant angina, or other CV disease; uncontrolled HTN; PVD, including ischemic bowel disease; cerebrovascular disease (history of stroke or TIA); and hemiplegic or basilar migraine.
• Don't give within 24 hours after treatment with other 5-HT$_{1B/1D}$ agonists or ergot derivatives.
• Use cautiously in patients with renal or hepatic impairment and in those with cataracts because of the potential for corneal opacities.
• Use cautiously in patients with risk factors for CAD, such as obesity, diabetes, and family history of CAD.
• Use cautiously in patients with known hypersensitivity to sulfonamides.
• Drug isn't intended for migraine prophylaxis or treatment of cluster headaches.
Dialyzable drug: Unknown.
⚠ Overdose S&S: HTN, more serious CV symptoms.

PREGNANCY-LACTATION-REPRODUCTION
• Use during pregnancy only if potential benefit justifies potential risk to the fetus.
• It isn't known if drug appears in human milk. Use cautiously in breastfeeding women.

NURSING CONSIDERATIONS
• Patients with renal or hepatic impairment should receive a reduced dosage.
• Repeat dose after 2 hours, if needed, and don't give more than two doses (or 25 mg) in 24 hours.
• Overuse of acute migraine drugs for 10 or more days per month may lead to migraine-like daily headaches or a marked increase in frequency of migraine attacks (medication overuse headache). Withdrawal of the overused drugs may be necessary.
• Consider obtaining ECG with first dose of drug in patients with positive CAD risk factors.
• Assess patients with signs and symptoms of angina after almotriptan dose for CAD

and Prinzmetal or variant angina, including ECG monitoring.
❸ Alert: Combining triptans with SSRIs or SSNRIs may cause serotonin syndrome. Signs and symptoms include restlessness, hallucinations, loss of coordination, rapid heartbeat, rapid changes in BP, increased body temperature, overactive reflexes, nausea, vomiting, and diarrhea. Serotonin syndrome occurs more often when starting or increasing the dose of a triptan, SSRI, or SSNRI.
• **Look alike–sound alike:** Don't confuse Axert with Antivert.

PATIENT TEACHING
• Tell patient that drug can be taken with or without food.
• Advise patient to take drug only when having a migraine; explain that drug isn't taken on a regular schedule.
• Advise patient to use only one repeat dose within 24 hours, no sooner than 2 hours after first dose.
• Advise patient that other commonly prescribed migraine drugs can interact with almotriptan.
• Advise patient to report chest or throat tightness, pain, or heaviness.
• Teach patient to avoid possible migraine triggers, such as cheese, chocolate, citrus fruits, caffeine, and alcohol.

SAFETY ALERT!

alogliptin benzoate
AL-oh-GLIP-tin

Nesina

Therapeutic class: Antidiabetics
Pharmacologic class: DPP-4 inhibitors

AVAILABLE FORMS
Tablets: 6.25 mg, 12.5 mg, 25 mg

INDICATIONS & DOSAGES
➤ **Adjunct to diet and exercise to improve glycemic control in adults with type 2 diabetes**
Adults: 25 mg PO daily.
Adjust-a-dose: For patients with moderate renal impairment (CrCl of 30 to less than

60 mL/minute), give 12.5 mg PO daily.
For patients with severe renal impairment
(CrCl of 15 to less than 30 mL/minute) and
for those with ESRD (CrCl of less than
15 mL/minute) or requiring hemodialysis,
give 6.25 mg PO daily.

ADMINISTRATION
PO
• Give without regard for food.
• Store at room temperature.

ACTION
Slows inactivation of incretin, which increases blood concentrations of incretin and
reduces fasting or postprandial glucose in
patients with type 2 diabetes.

Route	Onset	Peak	Duration
PO	Unknown	1–2 hr	Unknown

Half-life: 21 hours.

ADVERSE REACTIONS
CNS: headache. **CV:** *HF.* **EENT:** nasopharyngitis. **GU:** decreased CrCl, decreased GFR. **Metabolic:** *hypoglycemia.*
Respiratory: URI.

INTERACTIONS
Drug-drug. *ACE inhibitors:* May enhance
the adverse effects of ACE inhibitor, especially angioedema. Monitor therapy.
Androgens (except danazol), pegvisomant:
May enhance hypoglycemic effect. Monitor
therapy.
*Danazol, fluoroquinolones, thiazide diuret-
ics:* May diminish hypoglycemic effect.
Monitor therapy.
Insulin, sulfonylureas: May enhance hypoglycemic activity. Adjust dosage of insulin
or sulfonylurea.
MAO inhibitors, salicylates, SSRIs: May
cause hypoglycemia. Monitor therapy.

EFFECTS ON LAB TEST RESULTS
• May increase ALT level.
• May decrease GFR and CrCl.

CONTRAINDICATIONS & CAUTIONS
• Contraindicated in patients hypersensitive
to drug or its components and in those with
type 1 diabetes mellitus or ketoacidosis.

• Use cautiously in patients with liver disease or injury, history of pancreatitis, gallstones, history of alcoholism, renal disease,
or history of angioedema with another
DPP-4 inhibitor.
● *Alert:* Use cautiously in patients with a
history of HF or renal disease. Drug may
increase risk of HF in these patients.
Dialyzable drug: No.

PREGNANCY-LACTATION-REPRODUCTION
• Use cautiously in pregnant women and
only if clearly needed.
• It isn't known if drug appears in human milk. Use cautiously in breastfeeding
women.

NURSING CONSIDERATIONS
● *Alert:* Monitor patient for signs and symptoms of HF (shortness of breath, orthopnea,
tiredness, weakness, fatigue, weight gain,
peripheral or abdominal edema). Drug may
need to be discontinued and other antidiabetics may be needed.
• Assess renal function at baseline and periodically during treatment.
• Monitor patient for hypersensitivity reactions, including SJS (rare). Stop drug immediately if hypersensitivity is suspected.
• Monitor patient for signs and symptoms
(rare) of acute pancreatitis (severe abdominal pain that may radiate to the back, with or
without vomiting).
• Assess LFTs before treatment. If liver injury (rare) is suspected during treatment
(fatigue, anorexia, abdominal discomfort,
dark urine, jaundice), obtain LFTs. If elevated LFT values are present, persist, or
worsen, withhold drug and determine probable cause. Restart drug only if cause isn't
alogliptin-related.
• Monitor blood glucose level if patient is
receiving concurrent antidiabetic medications; adjust dosages of these medications if
needed.
• Monitor patients for development of blisters or skin erosions; consider dermatologist referral for diagnosis and treatment if
present.
● *Alert:* May cause joint pain that can be severe and disabling. Report severe and persistent joint pain to prescriber; drug may need
to be discontinued.

PATIENT TEACHING
⊕ **Alert:** Instruct patient to immediately report signs and symptoms of HF. Patient shouldn't stop drug without first discussing with prescriber.
• Instruct patient to monitor blood glucose level carefully.
• Advise patient to report respiratory symptoms to prescriber.
• Caution patient to seek medical attention for signs and symptoms of pancreatitis (severe abdominal pain that may radiate to the back, with or without vomiting) or liver injury (fatigue, anorexia, abdominal discomfort, dark urine, or jaundice).

SAFETY ALERT!

ALPRAZolam
al-PRAH-zoe-lam

Apo-Alpraz✷, Apo-Alpraz TS✷, Xanax✐, Xanax XR

Therapeutic class: Anxiolytics
Pharmacologic class: Benzodiazepines
Controlled substance schedule: IV

AVAILABLE FORMS
Oral solution: 1 mg/mL (concentrate)
Tablets: 0.25 mg, 0.5 mg, 1 mg, 2 mg
Tablets (extended-release) ⒪ⓉⒸ: 0.5 mg, 1 mg, 2 mg, 3 mg
Tablets (ODTs): 0.25 mg, 0.5 mg, 1 mg, 2 mg

INDICATIONS & DOSAGES
Adjust-a-dose (for all indications): For debilitated patients or those with advanced hepatic disease, usual first dose is 0.25 mg PO b.i.d. or t.i.d. For extended-release tablets, 0.5 mg PO once daily.
➤ **Anxiety**
Adults: Usual first dose, 0.25 to 0.5 mg (immediate-release) PO t.i.d. Maximum, 4 mg daily in divided doses.
Elderly patients: Usual first dose, 0.25 mg PO b.i.d. or t.i.d. Maximum, 4 mg daily in divided doses. For extended-release tablets, 0.5 mg PO once daily. May increase gradually as needed and tolerated.

➤ **Panic disorders**
Adults: 0.5 mg PO t.i.d., increased at intervals of 3 to 4 days in increments of no more than 1 mg/day. Maximum, 10 mg daily in divided doses. For extended-release tablets, start with 0.5 to 1 mg PO once daily. Increase by no more than 1 mg/day every 3 to 4 days. Maximum daily dose, 10 mg.
Elderly patients: Usual first dose, 0.25 mg (immediate-release) PO b.i.d. or t.i.d. Maximum, 4 mg daily in divided doses.

ADMINISTRATION
PO
• Don't break or crush extended-release tablets.
• Mix oral solution with liquids or semisolid food, such as water, juices, carbonated beverages, applesauce, and puddings. Use only calibrated dropper provided with this product. Give drug immediately after mixing.
• Use dry hands to remove ODTs from bottle. Discard cotton from inside bottle.
• Discard unused portion if breaking scored ODT.
• Patients treated with divided doses of immediate-release tablets can be switched to extended-release tablets at same total daily dose. Patients should take extended-release tablets in the morning.

ACTION
Unknown. Probably potentiates the effects of GABA, depresses the CNS, and suppresses the spread of seizure activity.

Route	Onset	Peak	Duration
PO	Unknown	1–2 hr	Unknown
PO (extended-release)	Unknown	Unknown	Unknown

Half-life: Immediate-release, 6.3 to 26.9 hours; extended-release, 10.7 to 15.8 hours.

ADVERSE REACTIONS
CNS: insomnia, irritability, dizziness, headache, anxiety, confusion, drowsiness, light-headedness, sedation, somnolence, difficulty speaking, impaired coordination, memory impairment, fatigue, depression, *suicide,* mental impairment, ataxia, paresthesia, dyskinesia, hypoesthesia, lethargy, vertigo, malaise, tremor, nervousness, restlessness, agitation, nightmare, syncope,

---

Reactions in bold italics are *life-threatening*. Interactions may have a *rapid onset* or a *delayed onset*.

akathisia, mania. **CV:** palpitations, chest pain, hypotension. **EENT:** blurred vision, tinnitus, allergic rhinitis, nasal congestion. **GI:** diarrhea, dry mouth, constipation, nausea, increased or decreased appetite, anorexia, vomiting, dyspepsia, abdominal pain, increased or decreased salivation. **GU:** dysmenorrhea, sexual dysfunction, premenstrual syndrome, difficulty urinating. **Metabolic:** increased or decreased weight. **Musculoskeletal:** arthralgia, myalgia, arm or leg pain, back pain, muscle rigidity, muscle cramps, muscle twitch. **Respiratory:** URI, dyspnea, hyperventilation. **Skin:** pruritus, increased sweating, dermatitis. **Other:** influenza, injury, emergence of anxiety between doses, dependence, feeling warm, increased or decreased libido.

INTERACTIONS

Drug-drug. *Anticonvulsants, antidepressants, antihistamines, barbiturates, benzodiazepines, general anesthetics, narcotics, phenothiazines, protease inhibitors:* May increase CNS depressant effects. Avoid using together.

Carbamazepine: May induce alprazolam metabolism and may reduce therapeutic effects. May need to increase dose.

Cimetidine, fluoxetine, fluvoxamine, hormonal contraceptives: May increase alprazolam level. Use cautiously together, and consider alprazolam dosage reduction.

CYP3A strong inhibitors (atazanavir, clarithromycin, fluconazole, indinavir, itraconazole, ketoconazole, miconazole, nelfinavir, ritonavir, saquinavir, telithromycin, voriconazole), delavirdine: May increase and prolong alprazolam level, CNS depression, and psychomotor impairment. Use together is contraindicated.

Hydantoins (phenytoin): May decrease effects of alprazolam and increase hydantoin levels. Monitor patient closely.

Methadone: May significantly increase risk of respiratory depression. Use together cautiously.

Black Box Warning *Opioids:* May cause slow or difficult breathing, sedation, and death. Avoid use together. If use together is necessary, limit dosage and duration of each drug to the minimum necessary for desired effect. ∎

Rifamycins (rifampin): May decrease effects of alprazolam. Alprazolam dosage increase may be needed.

TCAs (amitriptyline, doxepin, imipramine, nortriptyline): May increase levels of these drugs. Monitor patient closely.

Drug-herb. *Kava, valerian root:* May increase sedation. Discourage use together.

St. John's wort: May decrease drug level. Discourage use together.

Drug-food. *Grapefruit juice:* May increase drug level. Discourage use together.

Drug-lifestyle. *Alcohol use:* May cause additive CNS effects. Discourage use together.

Smoking: May decrease effectiveness of drug. Monitor patient closely.

EFFECTS ON LAB TEST RESULTS
• May increase ALT and AST levels.

CONTRAINDICATIONS & CAUTIONS
• Contraindicated in patients hypersensitive to drug or other benzodiazepines and in those with acute angle-closure glaucoma.

Black Box Warning Opioids should only be prescribed with benzodiazepines or other CNS depressants to patients for whom alternative treatment options are inadequate. ∎

• Use cautiously in patients with hepatic, renal, or pulmonary disease or history of substance abuse.

• Use cautiously in elderly patients.

Dialyzable drug: No.

⚠ Overdose S&S: Somnolence, confusion, impaired coordination, diminished reflexes, coma.

PREGNANCY-LACTATION-REPRODUCTION
• Drug may cause fetal harm. Use isn't recommended during pregnancy.

• Drug appears in human milk. Use isn't recommended in breastfeeding women.

NURSING CONSIDERATIONS
Black Box Warning Monitor patient also taking an opioid for signs and symptoms of respiratory depression and sedation. ∎

• The optimum duration of therapy is unknown.

• Give smallest effective dose to prevent ataxia or oversedation, especially in elderly or debilitated patients.

◑ *Alert:* Don't withdraw drug abruptly; withdrawal symptoms, including seizures, may occur. Gradually reduce dosage. Abuse or addiction is possible.

• Monitor hepatic, renal, and hematopoietic function periodically in patients receiving repeated or prolonged therapy.

• Closely monitor addiction-prone patients.

◑ *Alert:* Panic disorder is associated with major depressive disorders and increased reports of suicide among untreated patients. Monitor patients with depression for suicidal ideation or plans for suicide.

• Consider giving same total daily dose of immediate-release formulation in divided doses more frequently in patients being treated for panic disorder who experience early-morning anxiety or anxiety symptoms between doses.

• *Look alike–sound alike:* Don't confuse alprazolam with alprostadil or lorazepam. Don't confuse Xanax with Fanapt, Zantac, Xopenex, or Tenex.

PATIENT TEACHING

Black Box Warning Caution patient or caregiver of patient taking an opioid with a benzodiazepine, CNS depressant, or alcohol to seek immediate medical attention if patient experiences dizziness, lightheadedness, extreme sleepiness, slowed or difficult breathing, or unresponsiveness. ∎

• Warn patient to avoid hazardous activities that require alertness and good coordination until effects of drug are known.

• Tell patient to avoid use of alcohol while taking drug.

• Advise patient that smoking may decrease drug's effectiveness.

• Warn patient not to stop drug abruptly because withdrawal symptoms or seizures may occur.

• Tell patient to swallow extended-release tablets whole.

• Tell patient using ODT to remove it from bottle using dry hands and to immediately place it on the tongue, where it will dissolve and can be swallowed with saliva.

• Tell patient taking half a scored ODT to discard the unused half.

• Advise patient to discard the cotton from the bottle of ODTs and keep it tightly sealed to prevent moisture from dissolving the tablets.

• Warn female patient not to use drug if she is pregnant or breastfeeding and to report pregnancy to prescriber.

alteplase
al-ti-PLAZE

Activase, Cathflo Activase

Therapeutic class: Thrombolytics
Pharmacologic class: Enzymes

AVAILABLE FORMS
Cathflo Activase injection: 2-mg single-patient vials
Injection: 50-mg, 100-mg vials

INDICATIONS & DOSAGES
➤ **Lysis of thrombi obstructing coronary arteries in acute MI (Activase)**
3-hour infusion
Adults weighing 65 kg or more: 100 mg by IV infusion over 3 hours, as follows: 60 mg in first hour, 6 to 10 mg of which is given as a bolus over first 1 to 2 minutes. Then 20 mg/hour infused for 2 hours.
Adults weighing less than 65 kg: 1.25 mg/kg in a similar fashion: 0.075 mg/kg bolus over 1 to 2 minutes, followed by 0.675 mg/kg in rest of first hour. Then 0.25 mg/kg/hour infused for 2 hours. Don't exceed total dose of 100 mg.
Accelerated infusion
Adults weighing more than 67 kg: 100 mg maximum total dose. Give 15 mg IV bolus over 1 to 2 minutes, followed by 50 mg infused over the next 30 minutes; then 35 mg infused over the next hour. Don't exceed total dose of 100 mg.
Adults weighing 67 kg or less: 15 mg IV bolus over 1 to 2 minutes, followed by 0.75 mg/kg (not to exceed 50 mg) infused over the next 30 minutes; then 0.5 mg/kg (not to exceed 35 mg) infused over the next hour. Don't exceed total dose of 100 mg.
➤ **To manage acute massive PE (Activase)**
Adults: 100 mg by IV infusion over 2 hours. Begin parenteral anticoagulation at end of infusion when PTT or thrombin time returns to twice normal or less. Don't exceed

100-mg dose. Higher doses may increase risk of intracranial bleeding.

➤ **Acute ischemic stroke (Activase)**
Adults: 0.9 mg/kg by IV infusion over 1 hour with 10% of total dose given as an initial IV bolus over 1 minute. Maximum total dose is 90 mg.

➤ **To restore function to CVADs (Cathflo Activase)**
Adults and children older than age 2: For patients weighing more than 30 kg, instill 2 mg in 2 mL sterile water into catheter. For patients weighing between 10 and 30 kg, instill 110% of the internal lumen volume of the catheter, not to exceed 2 mg in 2 mL sterile water. After 30 minutes of dwell time, assess catheter function by aspirating blood. If function is restored, aspirate 4 to 5 mL of blood in patients weighing 10 kg or more or 3 mL in patients weighing less than 10 kg to remove drug and residual clot, and gently irrigate the catheter with NSS. If catheter function isn't restored after 120 minutes, instill a second dose.

➤ **Acute ischemic stroke presenting 3 to 4½ hours after symptom onset (Activase)** ◆
Adults: 0.9 mg/kg by IV infusion over 1 hour with 10% of total dose given as an initial IV bolus over 1 minute. Maximum total dose is 90 mg.

ADMINISTRATION

IV
▼ Immediately before use, reconstitute solution with unpreserved sterile water for injection. Check manufacturer's labeling for specific information.
▼ Don't use 50-mg vial if vacuum isn't present; 100-mg vials don't have a vacuum.
▼ Using an 18G needle, direct stream of sterile water at lyophilized cake. Don't shake.
▼ Slight foaming is common. Let it settle before giving drug. Solution should be colorless or pale yellow.
▼ Drug may be given reconstituted (at 1 mg/mL) or diluted with an equal volume of NSS or D₅W to yield 0.5 mg/mL.
▼ Give drug using a controlled infusion device.
▼ Discard any unused drug after 8 hours.

Cathflo Activase
▼ Assess the cause of catheter dysfunction before using drug. Possible causes of occlusion include catheter malposition, mechanical failure, constriction by a suture, and lipid deposits or drug precipitates in the catheter lumen. Don't try to suction the catheter because you risk damaging the vessel wall or collapsing a soft-walled catheter.
▼ Reconstitute Cathflo Activase with 2.2 mL sterile water to yield 1 mg/mL. Dissolve completely to produce a colorless to pale yellow solution. Don't shake.
▼ Don't use excessive pressure while instilling drug into catheter; doing so could rupture the catheter or expel a clot into circulation.
▼ Solution is stable for up to 8 hours at room temperature.
▼ **Incompatibilities:** Bivalirudin, dobutamine, dopamine, heparin, morphine, nitroglycerin. Consult detailed reference for other specific incompatibilities.

ACTION

Converts plasminogen to plasmin by directly cleaving peptide bonds at two sites, causing fibrinolysis.

Route	Onset	Peak	Duration
IV	Unknown	Unknown	Unknown

Half-life: Less than 5 minutes.

ADVERSE REACTIONS

CNS: *cerebral hemorrhage,* fever. **CV:** *arrhythmias,* hypotension, edema, *cholesterol embolization, venous thrombosis.* **GI:** *bleeding,* nausea, vomiting. **GU:** *bleeding.* **Hematologic:** *spontaneous bleeding.* **Skin:** ecchymosis. **Other:** *anaphylaxis, sepsis (Cathflo Activase),* bleeding at puncture sites, hypersensitivity reactions.

INTERACTIONS

Drug-drug. *Aspirin, clopidogrel, dipyridamole, drugs affecting platelet activity (abciximab), heparin, warfarin, anticoagulants:* May increase risk of bleeding. Monitor patient carefully.
Nitroglycerin: May decrease alteplase serum concentration. Monitor therapy.

EFFECTS ON LAB TEST RESULTS
• May alter coagulation and fibrinolytic test results.

CONTRAINDICATIONS & CAUTIONS
• Contraindicated in patients hypersensitive to drug or its components.
• Activase therapy for acute MI or PE is contraindicated in patients with active internal bleeding; history of stroke; recent intracranial or intraspinal surgery or trauma; intracranial neoplasm, AV malformation, or aneurysm; known bleeding diathesis; or severe uncontrolled HTN.
• Activase therapy for acute ischemic stroke is contraindicated in patients with evidence of intracranial hemorrhage; suspected subarachnoid hemorrhage; recent (within 3 months) intracranial or intraspinal surgery; serious head trauma or previous stroke; history of intracranial hemorrhage; uncontrolled HTN (BP greater than 185 mm Hg systolic or 110 mm Hg diastolic) at time of treatment; seizure at onset of stroke; active internal bleeding; intracranial neoplasm, AV malformation, or aneurysm; bleeding diathesis (which may include current use of oral anticoagulants, INR greater than 1.7, PT longer than 15 seconds, platelet count less than $100,000/mm^3$, current use of direct thrombin inhibitors or direct factor Xa inhibitors with elevated sensitive laboratory tests, or patients who have received heparin within the previous 48 hours and who at presentation have a prolonged aPTT).
• In patients with acute ischemic stroke, Activase may be initiated before available coagulation study results. The infusion should be discontinued if either a pretreatment INR is greater than 1.7 or a prolonged aPTT is identified.
• Patients with severe neurologic deficits (National Institutes of Health Stroke Scale greater than 22) or who have major early infarct signs on a CT scan may have increased risk of bleeding.
• Use cautiously in patients who have had a recent major surgery or procedure or who have other conditions in which bleeding constitutes a significant hazard or would be difficult to control because of its location.
• Use cautiously in patients with previous puncture of a noncompressible vessel; concomitant oral anticoagulant therapy; organ biopsy; trauma (including cardiopulmonary resuscitation); GI or GU bleeding; cerebrovascular disease; systolic pressure of 175 mm Hg or higher or diastolic pressure of 110 mm Hg or higher; mitral stenosis, atrial fibrillation, or other conditions that may lead to left heart thrombus; acute pericarditis or subacute bacterial endocarditis; hemostatic defects caused by hepatic or renal impairment; septic thrombophlebitis; or diabetic hemorrhagic retinopathy.
• Use cautiously in patients receiving anticoagulants and in patients age 75 and older.
Dialyzable drug: Unknown.

PREGNANCY-LACTATION-REPRODUCTION
• Information related to use in pregnant women is limited; most guidelines consider pregnancy to be a relative contraindication. Drug shouldn't be withheld from pregnant women in life-threatening situations but should be avoided if safer alternatives are available.
• It isn't known if drug appears in human milk. Use cautiously in breastfeeding women.

NURSING CONSIDERATIONS
◑ *Alert:* When used for acute ischemic stroke, give drug within 3 hours after symptoms occur and only when intracranial bleeding has been ruled out.
• Drug may be given to menstruating women.
• To recannulize occluded coronary arteries and improve heart function, begin treatment as soon as possible after symptoms start.
• Anticoagulant and antiplatelet therapy is commonly started during or after treatment, to decrease risk of another thrombosis.
• Monitor vital signs and neurologic status carefully. Keep patient on strict bed rest.
• Coronary thrombolysis is linked with arrhythmias caused by reperfusion of ischemic myocardium. Such arrhythmias don't differ from those commonly linked with MI. Have antiarrhythmics readily available, and carefully monitor ECG.
• Avoid invasive procedures, IM injections, and nonessential handling of patient during thrombolytic therapy. Perform essential venipunctures carefully. Closely monitor

---

patient for signs of internal bleeding, and frequently check all puncture sites. Bleeding is the most common adverse effect and may occur internally and at external puncture sites.

• If an arterial puncture is necessary during Activase infusion, use an arm vessel that can be manually compressed. Apply pressure for at least 30 minutes followed by a pressure dressing. Check the site regularly for bleeding.

• If uncontrollable bleeding occurs, stop infusion (and parenteral anticoagulant) and notify prescriber.

• *Look alike–sound alike:* Don't confuse alteplase with Altace. Don't confuse Activase with Cathflo Activase or TNKase.

PATIENT TEACHING

• Explain use and administration of drug to patient and family.

• Tell patient to report adverse reactions promptly and to immediately report signs and symptoms of bleeding, urinary problems, abdominal pain, nausea, vomiting, confusion, severe headache, one-sided weakness, trouble speaking or thinking, visual disturbances, dizziness, passing out, chest pain, or catheter-site pain.

---

amantadine hydrochloride
a-MAN-ta-deen

Gocovri, Osmolex ER

Therapeutic class: Antivirals
Pharmacologic class: Synthetic cyclic primary amines

AVAILABLE FORMS
Capsules: 100 mg
Capsules (extended-release) ⓓⓝⓒ: 68.5 mg, 137 mg
Oral solution: 50 mg/5 mL
Tablets: 100 mg
Tablets (extended-release) ⓓⓝⓒ: 129 mg, 193 mg, 258 mg

INDICATIONS & DOSAGES
Adjust-a-dose (for all indications): Lower dosages are recommended for patients with renal impairment. Refer to the manufac-

turer's product information for specific dosage adjustments.
➤ **Parkinson disease**
Adults: Initially, if used as monotherapy, 100 mg PO b.i.d. In patients with serious illness or in those already receiving high doses of other antiparkinsonians, begin dose at 100 mg PO once daily. Increase to 100 mg b.i.d. if needed after at least 1 week. Some patients may benefit from 400 mg daily in divided doses. For extended-release tablet (Osmolex ER), 129 mg PO once daily; increase weekly to maximum daily dose of 322 mg. For extended-release capsule (Gocovri), 137 mg PO once daily; increase in 1 week to maximum daily dose of 274 mg.
➤ **To prevent or treat symptoms of influenza type A virus and respiratory tract illnesses**
Children age 13 and older and adults up to age 65: 200 mg PO daily as a single dose or 100 mg PO b.i.d.
Children ages 9 to 12: 100 mg PO b.i.d.
Children ages 1 to 8: 4.4 to 8.8 mg/kg PO as a total daily dose given once daily or in two equally divided doses. Maximum daily dose is 150 mg.
Elderly patients: 100 mg PO once daily in patients older than age 65 with normal renal function.

Begin treatment within 24 to 48 hours after symptoms appear and continue for 24 to 48 hours after symptoms disappear (usually 2 to 7 days). Start prophylaxis as soon as possible after exposure and continue for at least 10 days after exposure. May continue prophylactic treatment for the duration of known influenza A in the community because of repeated and unknown exposures if influenza vaccine is unavailable. If used with influenza vaccine, continue dose for 2 to 4 weeks until antibody response to vaccine has developed.
➤ **Drug-induced extrapyramidal reactions**
Adults: 100 mg PO b.i.d. May increase to 300 mg daily in divided doses. Extended-release (Osmolex ER), 129 mg PO once daily. Maximum daily dose, 322 mg.

ADMINISTRATION
PO
• Give without regard for food.

• Give extended-release tablets in the morning; extended-release capsules at bedtime.
• Don't crush or break extended-release forms. May sprinkle entire contents of capsule on a small amount (tsp) of soft food such as applesauce and administer immediately. Patient shouldn't chew extended-release forms.

ACTION

May exert its antiparkinsonian effect by causing the release of dopamine in the substantia nigra. As an antiviral, may prevent release of viral nucleic acid into the host cell, reducing duration of fever and other systemic symptoms.

Route	Onset	Peak	Duration
PO	Unknown	1½–8 hr	Unknown

Half-life: About 10 to 25 hours; with renal dysfunction, as long as 10 days.

ADVERSE REACTIONS

CNS: dizziness, insomnia, irritability, lightheadedness, depression, fatigue, confusion, hallucinations, anxiety, ataxia, headache, nervousness, dream abnormalities, agitation, somnolence, dystonia. **CV:** *HF,* peripheral edema, orthostatic hypotension. **EENT:** blurred vision, cataract, dry eye. **GI:** nausea, anorexia, constipation, vomiting, dry mouth, diarrhea. **GU:** UTI, BPH. **Musculoskeletal:** joint swelling, muscle spasms. **Respiratory:** cough. **Skin:** livedo reticularis, contusion. **Other:** falls.

INTERACTIONS

Drug-drug. *Anticholinergics:* May increase anticholinergic effects. Use together cautiously; reduce dosage of anticholinergic before starting amantadine.
CNS stimulants: May increase CNS stimulation. Use together cautiously.
Quinidine, sulfamethoxazole–trimethoprim, thiazide diuretics, triamterene: May increase amantadine level, increasing the risk of toxicity. Use together cautiously.
Thioridazine: May worsen Parkinson disease tremor. Monitor patient closely.
Drug-lifestyle. *Alcohol use:* May increase CNS effects, including dizziness, confusion, and orthostatic hypotension. Discourage use together.

EFFECTS ON LAB TEST RESULTS

• May increase CK, BUN, creatinine, alkaline phosphatase, LDH, bilirubin, GGT, AST, and ALT levels.

CONTRAINDICATIONS & CAUTIONS

• Contraindicated in patients hypersensitive to drug.
• Use cautiously in elderly patients and in patients with seizure disorders, psychosis, impulse control disorders, HF, peripheral edema, hepatic disease, mental illness, eczematoid rash, renal impairment, orthostatic hypotension, and CV disease.
• Avoid use in patients with untreated angle-closure glaucoma.
Dialyzable drug: No.
⚠ *Overdose S&S:* Arrhythmia, HTN, tachycardia, pulmonary edema, respiratory distress, increased BUN level, decreased CrCl, renal insufficiency, insomnia, anxiety, aggressive behavior, hypertonia, hyperkinesia, tremor, confusion, disorientation, depersonalization, fear, delirium, hallucinations, psychotic reactions, lethargy, somnolence, coma, seizures, hyperthermia.

PREGNANCY-LACTATION-REPRODUCTION

• Drug may cause fetal harm. Use during pregnancy only if potential benefit justifies potential risk to the fetus.
• Drug appears in human milk. Use isn't recommended in breastfeeding women.

NURSING CONSIDERATIONS

• Patients with Parkinson disease who don't respond to anticholinergics may respond to this drug.
🔵 *Alert:* Elderly patients are more susceptible to adverse neurologic effects. Monitor patient for mental status changes.
🔵 *Alert:* Suicidal ideation and attempts may occur in any patient, regardless of psychiatric history.
🔵 *Alert:* Sporadic cases of NMS have been reported with dosage reduction or drug withdrawal. Observe patient carefully when dosage is abruptly reduced or drug is discontinued.
• Drug can worsen mental problems in patients with a history of psychiatric disorders or substance abuse.
• Monitor renal function tests and LFTs.

Reactions in bold italics are *life-threatening*. Interactions may have a *rapid onset* or a *delayed onset*.

- Drug must be discontinued gradually. Abrupt discontinuation may cause an increase in signs and symptoms of Parkinson disease or cause delirium, agitation, delusions, hallucinations, paranoid reaction, stupor, anxiety, depression, or slurred speech.
- *Look alike–sound alike:* Don't confuse amantadine with amiodarone, rimantadine, or ranitidine.

PATIENT TEACHING
🛈 *Alert:* Tell patient to take drug exactly as prescribed because not doing so may result in serious adverse reactions or death.
- Advise patient that drug must be stopped gradually and not to stop taking drug or change the dose before consulting prescriber.
- Caution patient to report increases in Parkinson disease signs or symptoms or adverse effects.
- Stress importance of taking extended-release capsules at bedtime.
- If insomnia occurs, tell patient to take drug several hours before bedtime.
- Tell patient that if dizziness occurs when standing up, not to stand or change positions too quickly.
- Instruct patient to notify prescriber of adverse reactions, especially dizziness, depression, anxiety, nausea, and urine retention.
- Caution patient to avoid activities that require mental alertness until effects of drug are known.
- Encourage patient with Parkinson disease to gradually increase physical activity as symptoms improve.
- Advise patient to avoid alcohol while taking drug.

SAFETY ALERT!

ambrisentan
am-bree-SEN-tan

Letairis, Volibris✤

Therapeutic class: Antihypertensives
Pharmacologic class: Endothelin-receptor antagonists

AVAILABLE FORMS
Tablets ⊕: 5 mg, 10 mg

INDICATIONS & DOSAGES
➤ **PAH (WHO Group 1) to improve exercise tolerance and decrease rate of clinical worsening; in combination with tadalafil to reduce risks of disease progression and hospitalization for worsening PAH, and to improve exercise ability**
Adults: 5 mg PO once daily with or without tadalafil 20 mg once daily; at 4-week intervals, may increase ambrisentan to 10 mg PO once daily or tadalafil to 40 mg once daily if tolerated.

ADMINISTRATION
PO
- Drug is considered hazardous: use safe handling and disposal precautions according to facility policy.
- Give without regard for food.
- Give whole; don't crush or split tablets.

ACTION
Blocks endothelin-1 receptors on vascular endothelin and smooth muscle. Stimulation of these receptors in smooth muscle cells is associated with vasoconstriction and PAH.

Route	Onset	Peak	Duration
PO	Rapid	2 hr	Unknown

Half-life: 9 hours.

ADVERSE REACTIONS
CNS: asthenia, dizziness, fatigue, headache. **CV:** peripheral edema, flushing, *HF.* **EENT:** nasal congestion, sinusitis. **GI:** nausea, vomiting, dyspepsia. **Hematologic:** anemia. **Hepatic:** hepatic impairment. **Respiratory:** cough, bronchitis, *PAH.* **Other:** hypersensitivity reaction (*angioedema*, rash).

INTERACTIONS
Drug-drug. *Cyclosporine:* May increase ambrisentan level. Use together cautiously. Limit ambrisentan dosage to 5 mg daily.

EFFECTS ON LAB TEST RESULTS
- May increase AST, ALT, and bilirubin levels.
- May decrease Hb level and hematocrit.

CONTRAINDICATIONS & CAUTIONS
- Contraindicated in patients hypersensitive to drug or its components and in those with

idiopathic pulmonary fibrosis, including patients with pulmonary HTN.
• Use cautiously in patients with mild hepatic impairment. Not recommended in patients with moderate or severe hepatic impairment.
• Use cautiously in those with renal impairment; drug hasn't been studied in those with severe renal impairment.
⚠ *Alert:* Patients who develop acute pulmonary edema during initial treatment may have pulmonary veno-occlusive disease. Discontinue drug if pulmonary veno-occlusive disease is confirmed.
Dialyzable drug: Unknown.
⚠ *Overdose S&S:* Headache, flushing, dizziness, nausea, nasal congestion, hypotension.

PREGNANCY-LACTATION-REPRODUCTION
Black Box Warning May cause birth defects. Contraindicated in pregnant women. ∎
Black Box Warning Pregnancy must be excluded before therapy is begun. Obtain monthly pregnancy tests during treatment and 1 month after discontinuation. ∎
Black Box Warning Women of childbearing potential must use one highly effective form of contraception (intrauterine device [IUD], contraceptive implant, or tubal sterilization) or a combination of methods (hormonal method with a barrier method or two barrier methods) during treatment and for 1 month after treatment ends. If a partner's vasectomy is the chosen method of contraception, a hormonal or barrier method must also be used. ∎
Black Box Warning Because of risk of birth defects, ambrisentan is available to females only through the Letairis REMS Program. Only registered prescribers and pharmacies may prescribe and dispense ambrisentan and only to female patients enrolled in and meeting all the conditions of REMS at www.ambrisenatanrems.com or 1-866-664-5327. ∎
• It isn't known if drug appears in human milk. Patient should discontinue breastfeeding or discontinue drug.
• Drug may adversely affect spermatogenesis.

NURSING CONSIDERATIONS
• Treat women of childbearing potential only after negative pregnancy tests.

• Assess Hb level at initiation, at 1 month, and periodically thereafter. Use isn't recommended in patients with significant anemia.

PATIENT TEACHING
Black Box Warning Inform female patient that she'll need to have a pregnancy test done monthly and to report suspected pregnancy to prescriber immediately. ∎
⚠ *Alert:* Teach female patient of childbearing potential to use one highly effective form of contraception (IUD, contraceptive implant, or tubal sterilization) or a combination of methods (hormonal method with a barrier method or two barrier methods) during treatment and for 1 month after treatment ends. If her partner's vasectomy is the chosen method of contraception, patient must also use a hormonal or barrier method.
• Tell patient that monthly blood tests will be done to monitor for adverse effects.
• Advise patient to take the tablet whole and not to split, crush, or chew it.
⚠ *Alert:* Teach patient to notify prescriber immediately of signs or symptoms of liver injury, including anorexia, nausea, vomiting, fever, malaise, fatigue, right upper quadrant abdominal discomfort, itching, and jaundice.
• Tell patient to report edema and weight gain.
• Inform male patient of potential for decreased sperm count.

amikacin sulfate
am-i-KAY-sin

Therapeutic class: Antibiotics
Pharmacologic class: Aminoglycosides

AVAILABLE FORMS
Injection: 250 mg/mL vial

INDICATIONS & DOSAGES
Adjust-a-dose (for all indications): For adults with impaired renal function, initially, 7.5 mg/kg IM or IV. Subsequent doses and frequency determined by amikacin levels and renal function studies. For adults receiving hemodialysis, give supplemental doses of 50% of initial loading dose at end of each dialysis session. Monitor drug levels and adjust dosage accordingly.

➤ **Serious infections caused by sensitive strains of *Pseudomonas aeruginosa, Escherichia coli, Proteus, Klebsiella, Staphylococcus, Providencia, Enterobacter, Serratia,* or *Acinetobacter***
Adults and children: Maximum dosage is 15 mg/kg/day IM or IV infusion, in divided doses every 8 to 12 hours, for 7 to 10 days.
Neonates: Initially, loading dose of 10 mg/kg IV; then 7.5 mg/kg every 12 hours for 7 to 10 days. Don't exceed 1.5 g/day.
➤ **Uncomplicated UTI caused by organisms not susceptible to less toxic drugs**
Adults: 250 mg IM or IV b.i.d.

ADMINISTRATION

IV
▼ Obtain specimen for culture and sensitivity tests before giving first dose. Begin therapy while awaiting results.
▼ For adults, dilute IV drug in 100 to 200 mL of D_5W or NSS. For children, the amount of fluid will depend on the ordered dose.
▼ In adults and children, infuse over 30 to 60 minutes. In infants, infuse over 1 to 2 hours.
▼ Don't premix with other drugs.
▼ After infusion, flush line with NSS or D_5W.
▼ **Incompatibilities:** None listed by manufacturer. Consult a drug incompatibility reference for more information.

IM
• Obtain specimen for culture and sensitivity tests before giving first dose. Begin therapy while awaiting results.
• Obtain blood for peak level 1 hour after IM injection and 30 minutes to 1 hour after IV infusion ends; for trough levels, draw blood just before next dose. Don't collect blood in a heparinized tube; heparin is incompatible with aminoglycosides.

ACTION

Inhibits protein synthesis by binding directly to the 30S ribosomal subunit; bactericidal.

Route	Onset	Peak	Duration
IV	Immediate	30 min	8–12 hr
IM	Unknown	1 hr	8–12 hr

Half-life: Adults, 2 hours; patients with severe renal damage, 17 to 150 hours.

ADVERSE REACTIONS

CNS: *neuromuscular blockade.* **EENT:** ototoxicity. **GU:** azotemia, *nephrotoxicity,* increase in urinary excretion of casts. **Respiratory:** *apnea.*

INTERACTIONS

Drug-drug. **Black Box Warning** *Acyclovir, amphotericin B, bacitracin, cisplatin, colistin, paromomycin, polymyxin B, vancomycin, other aminoglycosides:* May increase nephrotoxicity. Avoid use together and monitor renal function test results. ∎
Cephalosporins, penicillins: May inactivate each other in vitro. Don't mix.
Dimenhydrinate: May mask ototoxicity symptoms. Monitor patient's hearing.
Black Box Warning *General anesthetics:* May increase neuromuscular blockade. Monitor patient for increased effects. ∎
Indomethacin: May increase trough and peak amikacin levels in premature infants. Avoid administering together. Monitor amikacin level.
Black Box Warning *IV loop diuretics (ethacrynic acid, furosemide):* May increase ototoxicity. Avoid use together and monitor patient's hearing. ∎
Black Box Warning *Neuromuscular blockers:* May increase effects of nondepolarizing muscle relaxants, including prolonged respiratory depression. Use together only when necessary, and expect to reduce dosage of nondepolarizing muscle relaxant. ∎
NSAIDs: May increase amikacin level in premature infants. Avoid administering together.

EFFECTS ON LAB TEST RESULTS

• May increase BUN, creatinine, nonprotein nitrogen, and urine urea levels.

CONTRAINDICATIONS & CAUTIONS

• Contraindicated in patients hypersensitive to drug or other aminoglycosides.
• Use cautiously in patients with sulfite sensitivity.
• Use cautiously in patients with impaired renal function, hypocalcemia, neuromuscular disorders (myasthenia gravis, parkinsonism), or hearing impairment; neonates and infants; and elderly patients.

• Drug can cause superinfection such as CDAD, which can be severe and can occur more than 2 months after therapy ends.
Dialyzable drug: Yes.
⚠ *Overdose S&S:* Nephrotoxicity, ototoxicity, neurotoxicity.

PREGNANCY-LACTATION-REPRODUCTION
• There are no well-controlled studies in pregnant women. Other aminoglycosides can cause fetal harm. Not recommended in pregnant women. If drug is used during pregnancy, or if patient becomes pregnant while taking drug, patient should be apprised of potential hazard to the fetus.
• It isn't known if drug appears in human milk. Patient should discontinue breastfeeding or discontinue drug.

NURSING CONSIDERATIONS
Black Box Warning Due to increased risk of ototoxicity, evaluate patient's hearing before and during therapy if patient will be receiving the drug for longer than 2 weeks. Notify prescriber if patient has tinnitus, vertigo, or hearing loss. ∎
Black Box Warning Weigh patient and review renal function studies before and periodically during therapy. ∎
• Correct dehydration before therapy because of increased risk of toxicity.
Black Box Warning Monitor serum amikacin peak and trough concentrations periodically during therapy. Peak drug levels greater than 35 mcg/mL and trough levels greater than 10 mcg/mL may be linked to a higher risk of toxicity. ∎
Black Box Warning Due to increased risk of nephrotoxicity, monitor renal function: urine output, specific gravity, urinalysis, BUN and creatinine levels, and CrCl. Report evidence of declining renal function to prescriber. Safe use for longer than 14 days hasn't been established. ∎
• Watch for signs and symptoms of superinfection (especially of upper respiratory tract), such as continued fever, chills, and increased pulse rate.
Black Box Warning Neuromuscular blockade and respiratory paralysis have been reported after aminoglycoside administration, especially in patients receiving anesthetics, neuromuscular blockers, or massive transfusions of citrate-anticoagulated blood. If blockade occurs, calcium salts may reverse these phenomena, but mechanical ventilation may be necessary. Monitor patient closely. ∎
• Therapy usually continues for 7 to 10 days. If no response occurs after 3 to 5 days, stop therapy and obtain new specimens for culture and sensitivity testing.
• *Look alike–sound alike:* Don't confuse amikacin with anakinra.

PATIENT TEACHING
• Instruct patient to promptly report all adverse reactions, especially changes in urine, weight gain, edema, hearing impairment, fever, diarrhea, and abdominal pain.
• Warn patient about risks to fetus if drug is taken during pregnancy and to report possible pregnancy to prescriber immediately.
• Encourage patient to maintain adequate fluid intake.

aMILoride hydrochloride
a-MILL-oh-ride

Midamor✤

Therapeutic class: Diuretics
Pharmacologic class: Potassium-sparing diuretics

AVAILABLE FORMS
Tablets: 5 mg

INDICATIONS & DOSAGES
➤ **HTN; hypokalemia; edema of HF, usually in patients also taking thiazide or other potassium-wasting diuretics**
Adults: 5 mg PO daily, increased to 10 mg daily if needed. If hypokalemia persists with 10 mg, dosage can be increased to 15 mg, then 20 mg with careful monitoring of electrolyte levels.

ADMINISTRATION
PO
• Give with food to minimize GI upset.

ACTION
Inhibits sodium reabsorption and potassium excretion in the distal tubules.

Route	Onset	Peak	Duration
PO	2 hr	3–4 hr	24 hr

Half-life: 6 to 9 hours.

ADVERSE REACTIONS

CNS: dizziness, fatigue, headache, weakness, *encephalopathy*. **GI:** abdominal pain, anorexia, appetite changes, constipation, diarrhea, nausea, vomiting, flatulence. **GU:** erectile dysfunction. **Metabolic:** hyperkalemia. **Musculoskeletal:** muscle cramps. **Respiratory:** cough, dyspnea.

INTERACTIONS

Drug-drug. *ACE inhibitors, ARBs, canagliflozin, cyclosporine, indomethacin, other potassium-sparing diuretics, potassium supplements, tacrolimus:* May cause severe hyperkalemia. Avoid use together if possible. Monitor potassium level closely if using together.
Digoxin: May affect digoxin clearance and decrease inotropic effects. Monitor digoxin level.
Lithium: May decrease lithium clearance, increasing risk of lithium toxicity. Monitor lithium level.
NSAIDs: May decrease diuretic effectiveness and cause severe hyperkalemia. Avoid use together.
Drug-food. *Foods high in potassium (such as bananas, oranges), salt substitutes containing potassium:* May cause hyperkalemia. Advise patient to choose diet carefully and to use low-potassium salt substitutes.

EFFECTS ON LAB TEST RESULTS

• May increase BUN and potassium levels. May decrease pH, Hb, and liver enzyme and sodium levels.
• May decrease neutrophil count.

CONTRAINDICATIONS & CAUTIONS

• Contraindicated in patients hypersensitive to drug, in those with potassium level greater than 5.5 mEq/L, and in those with anuria, acute or chronic renal insufficiency, or diabetic nephropathy.
• Contraindicated in patients receiving potassium supplementation or other potassium-sparing diuretics, such as spironolactone and triamterene.

• Use cautiously in patients with diabetes mellitus, cardiopulmonary disease, or severe hepatic insufficiency.
• Use cautiously in elderly or debilitated patients.
• Safety and effectiveness in children haven't been established.
Dialyzable drug: Unknown.
⚠ *Overdose S&S:* Dehydration, electrolyte imbalance.

PREGNANCY-LACTATION-REPRODUCTION

• Use during pregnancy only if clearly needed.
• It isn't known if drug appears in human milk. Patient should discontinue breastfeeding or discontinue drug.

NURSING CONSIDERATIONS

• To prevent nausea, give with meals.
Black Box Warning Carefully monitor potassium level because of the risk of hyperkalemia, especially in patients with renal impairment or diabetes and in elderly patients. Monitor potassium level when drug is initiated, when diuretic dosages are adjusted, and during an illness that could affect renal function. Alert prescriber immediately if potassium level exceeds 5.5 mEq/L; expect to stop drug. ∎
• Drug may cause severe hyperkalemia after glucose tolerance testing in patients with diabetes; stop drug at least 3 days before testing.
• *Look alike–sound alike:* Don't confuse amiloride with amiodarone or amlodipine.

PATIENT TEACHING

• Instruct patient to take drug with food to minimize GI upset.
• Advise patient to avoid sudden posture changes and to rise slowly to avoid dizziness.
• Caution patient not to perform hazardous activities if adverse CNS reactions occur.
• To prevent serious hyperkalemia, warn patient to avoid eating potassium-rich foods, potassium-containing salt substitutes, and potassium supplements.
• Advise patient to report signs of hyperkalemia, such as tingling, muscle weakness, muscle cramps, fatigue, and limb paralysis.

• Instruct patient to check with prescriber before taking new prescriptions or OTC drugs.

SAFETY ALERT!

amiodarone hydrochloride
am-ee-OH-dah-rohn

Nexterone, Pacerone

Therapeutic class: Antiarrhythmics
Pharmacologic class: Benzofuran derivatives

AVAILABLE FORMS
Injection: 50 mg/mL, 150 mg/100 mL, 360 mg/200 mL, 450 mg/9 mL, 450 mg/200 mL, 750 mg/500 mL, 900 mg/18 mL, 900 mg/500 mL, 1,000 mg/500 mL
Tablets: 100 mg, 200 mg, 400 mg

INDICATIONS & DOSAGES
Black Box Warning Amiodarone is intended for use only in patients with life-threatening recurrent ventricular fibrillation or recurrent hemodynamically unstable ventricular tachycardia unresponsive to adequate doses of other antiarrhythmics or when alternative drugs can't be tolerated. ■
➤ **Prevention of recurrent life-threatening ventricular arrhythmias, such as ventricular fibrillation or hemodynamically unstable ventricular tachycardia**
Adults: Give loading dose of 800 to 1,600 mg PO daily or divided into two equal doses daily for 1 to 3 weeks until first therapeutic response occurs; then 600 to 800 mg PO daily for 1 month, followed by maintenance dose of 400 mg PO daily or, for patients with severe GI intolerance, 200 mg PO b.i.d. Determine long-term maintenance dose according to antiarrhythmic effect.

Or, give loading dose of 150 mg IV over 10 minutes (15 mg/minute); then 360 mg IV over next 6 hours (1 mg/minute), followed by 540 mg IV over next 18 hours (0.5 mg/minute). After first 24 hours, continue with maintenance IV infusion of 720 mg/24 hours (0.5 mg/minute).

Maintenance infusion can continue cautiously for 2 to 3 weeks. To convert to oral form from IV (based on a 720-mg/day infusion): If IV infusion has been for less than 1 week, initial dose is 800 to 1,600 mg PO daily; if IV infusion has been from 1 to 3 weeks, initial dose is 600 to 800 mg PO daily; if IV infusion has been more than 3 weeks, initial dose is 400 mg PO daily.

If breakthrough episodes of ventricular fibrillation or hemodynamically unstable ventricular tachycardia occur, may give supplemental infusions of 150 mg IV over 10 minutes.

ADMINISTRATION
PO
• Divide oral loading dose into two or three equal doses and give with meals to decrease GI intolerance. Give maintenance dose once daily or divide into two doses with meals to decrease GI intolerance.
IV
▼ Give drug IV only if continuous ECG and electrophysiologic monitoring are available.
▼ Mix first dose of 150 mg in 100 mL of D_5W solution.
▼ If infusion will last 2 hours or longer, mix solution in glass or polyolefin bottles.
▼ If concentration is 2 mg/mL or more, give drug through a central line. If possible, use a dedicated line.
▼ Drug may be a vesicant; ensure proper needle or catheter placement before and during IV infusion and avoid extravasation.
▼ Use an in-line filter.
▼ Continuously monitor patient's cardiac status. If hypotension occurs, reduce infusion rate.
▼ IV amiodarone leaches out plasticizers from IV tubing and adsorbs to polyvinyl chloride (PVC) tubing, which can adversely affect male reproductive tract development in fetuses, infants, and toddlers when used at concentrations or flow rates outside of recommendations.
▼ **Incompatibilities:** Aminophylline, ampicillin sodium–sulbactam sodium, bivalirudin, cefazolin sodium, ceftazidime, digoxin, furosemide, heparin sodium, imipenem–cilastatin sodium, magnesium sulfate, micafungin, nitroprusside sodium, NSS, piperacillin sodium, piperacillin–tazobactam sodium, quinidine gluconate, sodium bicarbonate, sodium phosphates, potassium phosphates.

Reactions in bold italics are *life-threatening*. Interactions may have a *rapid onset* or a *delayed onset*.

ACTION

Inhibits adrenergic stimulation and blocks sodium and potassium channels, leading to a prolongation of action potential duration.

Route	Onset	Peak	Duration
PO	Variable	3–7 hr	Variable
IV	Unknown	Unknown	Variable

Half-life: Oral, 15 to 142 days; IV single dose mean range, 9 to 36 days.

ADVERSE REACTIONS

CNS: fatigue, malaise, tremor, peripheral neuropathy, ataxia, paresthesia, insomnia, sleep disturbances, headache, dizziness. **CV:** hypotension, *asystole,* atrial fibrillation, *bradycardia, arrhythmias, HF, heart block, sinus arrest,* edema, flushing. **EENT:** asymptomatic corneal microdeposits, visual disturbances, optic neuropathy or neuritis resulting in visual impairment, abnormal smell. **GI:** nausea, vomiting, abnormal taste, anorexia, constipation, abdominal pain, diarrhea. **Hematologic:** *coagulation abnormalities.* **Hepatic:** *hepatic failure,* hepatic dysfunction. **Metabolic:** hypothyroidism, hyperthyroidism. **Respiratory:** *ARDS, severe pulmonary toxicity, pulmonary edema, eosinophilic pneumonitis.* **Skin:** photosensitivity, solar dermatitis, blue-gray skin. **Other:** decreased libido.

INTERACTIONS

Drug-drug. *Antiarrhythmics:* May reduce hepatic or renal clearance of certain antiarrhythmics, especially flecainide, procainamide, and quinidine. Use of amiodarone with other antiarrhythmics, especially mexiletine, propafenone, disopyramide, and procainamide, may induce torsades de pointes. Avoid using together.
Azole antifungals, disopyramide, pimozide: May increase the risk of arrhythmias, including torsades de pointes. Avoid using together.
Beta blockers, calcium channel blockers: May potentiate bradycardia, sinus arrest, and AV block; may increase hypotensive effect. Use together cautiously.
Cimetidine: May increase amiodarone level. Use together cautiously.
Cyclosporine: May increase cyclosporine level, resulting in an increase in serum

creatinine level and renal toxicity. Monitor cyclosporine levels and renal function tests.
Dabigatran: May increase bleeding risk. Monitor patient closely.
Digoxin: May increase digoxin level 70% to 100%. Monitor digoxin level closely, and reduce digoxin dosage by half or stop drug completely when starting amiodarone therapy.
Fentanyl: May cause hypotension, bradycardia, and decreased cardiac output. Monitor patient closely.
Fluoroquinolones: May increase risk of arrhythmias, including torsades de pointes. Avoid using together.
HMG-CoA reductase inhibitors (lovastatin, simvastatin): May cause myopathy or rhabdomyolysis. Lovastatin dosage shouldn't exceed 40 mg daily. Simvastatin dosage shouldn't exceed 20 mg daily. Lower the dosages of other drugs in this class. Monitor patient carefully.
Loratadine, trazodone: May cause prolonged QT interval and torsades de pointes. Monitor closely.
Macrolide antibiotics (azithromycin, clarithromycin, erythromycin): May cause additive prolongation of the QT interval. Use with caution.
Phenytoin: May decrease phenytoin metabolism and increase phenytoin level. May decrease amiodarone level. Monitor phenytoin level and adjust dosages of drugs if needed.
Protease inhibitors (amprenavir, atazanavir, indinavir, lopinavir–ritonavir, nelfinavir, ritonavir, saquinavir): May increase the risk of amiodarone toxicity. Use of ritonavir or nelfinavir with amiodarone is contraindicated. Use other protease inhibitors cautiously.
Quinidine: May increase quinidine level, causing life-threatening cardiac arrhythmias. Avoid using together, or monitor patient closely if use together can't be avoided. Adjust quinidine dosage as needed.
Rifamycins: May decrease amiodarone level. Monitor patient closely.
Theophylline: May increase theophylline level and cause toxicity. Monitor theophylline level.
Warfarin: May increase anticoagulant response, with the potential for serious or fatal bleeding. Decrease warfarin dosage 33% to

50% when starting amiodarone. Monitor patient closely.

St. John's wort: May decrease amiodarone levels. Discourage use together.

Drug-food. *Grapefruit juice:* May inhibit CYP3A4 metabolism of drug in the intestinal mucosa, causing increased levels and risk of toxicity. Discourage use together.

Drug-lifestyle. *Sun exposure:* May cause photosensitivity reaction. Advise patient to take precautions.

EFFECTS ON LAB TEST RESULTS
• May increase alkaline phosphatase, ALT, AST, GGT, reverse T_3, and T_4 levels. May decrease T_3 level.
• May prolong PT and increase INR.

CONTRAINDICATIONS & CAUTIONS
• Contraindicated in patients hypersensitive to drug or to iodine.
• Contraindicated in those with cardiogenic shock, second- or third-degree AV block, severe SA node disease resulting in bradycardia unless an artificial pacemaker is present, and in those for whom bradycardia has caused syncope.
• Use cautiously in patients receiving other antiarrhythmics. Upon starting amiodarone, attempt to gradually discontinue prior antiarrhythmics.
• Use cautiously in patients with pulmonary, hepatic, or thyroid disease.
• **Alert:** Avoid use in patients with Wolff-Parkinson-White syndrome and preexcited atrial fibrillation or flutter.
Dialyzable drug: No.
⚠ Overdose S&S: AV block, bradycardia, hypotension, cardiogenic shock, hepatotoxicity.

PREGNANCY-LACTATION-REPRODUCTION
• Drug may cause fetal harm. Use during pregnancy only to treat life-threatening or refractory arrhythmias.
• Drug appears in human milk. Contraindicated in breastfeeding women.

NURSING CONSIDERATIONS
• Be aware of the high risk of adverse reactions.

• Obtain baseline pulmonary, liver, and thyroid function test results and baseline chest X-ray.
• **Alert:** Drug may cause hyperthyroidism or hypothyroidism. Hyperthyroidism can result in fatal thyrotoxicosis or arrhythmia. If hyperthyroidism or hypothyroidism occurs, reduce dosage or discontinue drug. Thyroid nodules and thyroid cancer have been reported. Use cautiously in patients with thyroid disease. Monitor thyroid function during treatment, particularly in elderly patients and those with underlying thyroid dysfunction.
Black Box Warning Give loading doses in a hospital setting and with continuous ECG monitoring because of the slow onset of antiarrhythmic effect and the risk of life-threatening arrhythmias. ∎
Black Box Warning Drug may pose life-threatening management problems in patients at risk for sudden death. Use only in patients with life-threatening, recurrent ventricular arrhythmias unresponsive to or intolerant of other antiarrhythmics or alternative drugs. ∎
Black Box Warning Drug is highly toxic. Watch carefully for pulmonary toxicity. Risk increases in patients receiving doses over 400 mg/day. Liver injury is also common and is usually mild but has been fatal in a few cases. ∎
• Watch for evidence of pneumonitis, exertional dyspnea, nonproductive cough, and pleuritic chest pain. Monitor pulmonary function tests and chest X-ray.
• Correct electrolyte imbalances before start of therapy and throughout treatment.
• Monitor LFTs and thyroid function test results and electrolyte levels, particularly potassium and magnesium.
• Monitor PT and INR if patient takes warfarin and digoxin level if patient takes digoxin.
• Instill methylcellulose ophthalmic solution during amiodarone therapy to minimize corneal microdeposits. About 1 to 4 months after starting amiodarone, most patients develop corneal microdeposits, although 10% or less have vision disturbances. Regular ophthalmic examinations are advised.
• Reevaluate amiodarone therapy and promptly refer patient for ophthalmic

---

Reactions in bold italics are ***life-threatening***. Interactions may have a *rapid onset* or a ***delayed onset***.

examination if diagnosis of optic neuropathy or optic neuritis is confirmed.
• Monitor BP and HR and rhythm frequently. Perform continuous ECG monitoring when starting or changing dosage. Notify prescriber of significant change in assessment results.
�835 *Alert:* Patients may continue to be at risk for drug-related adverse reactions or drug interactions after discontinuation of amiodarone.
�835 *Alert:* May cause life-threatening or fatal reactions, including SJS and toxic epidermal necrolysis. Discontinue drug immediately if such signs or symptoms as progressive rash with blisters or mucosal lesions occur.
• Safety and effectiveness in children haven't been established. Life-threatening gasping syndrome may occur in neonates given IV solutions containing benzyl alcohol.
• During or after treatment with IV form, patient may be transferred to oral therapy.
• *Look alike–sound alike:* Don't confuse amiodarone with amiloride.

PATIENT TEACHING
• Advise patient to wear sunscreen or protective clothing to prevent sensitivity reaction to the sun. Monitor patient for skin burning or tingling, followed by redness and blistering. Exposed skin may turn blue-gray.
• Advise patient to keep follow-up appointments, including eye exams and blood tests.
• Tell patient to report vision changes, weakness, "pins and needles" or numbness, poor coordination, weight change, heat or cold intolerance, neck swelling, progressive rash, or mucosal lesions.
• Tell patient to take oral drug with food if GI reactions occur.
• Inform patient that adverse effects of drug are more common at high doses and become more frequent with treatment lasting longer than 6 months, but are generally reversible when drug is stopped. Resolution of adverse reactions may take up to 4 months.
• Tell patient not to stop taking this medication without consulting with prescriber.

amitriptyline hydrochloride
a-mih-TRIP-ti-leen

Elavil ✦

Therapeutic class: Antidepressants
Pharmacologic class: TCAs

AVAILABLE FORMS
Tablets: 10 mg, 25 mg, 50 mg, 75 mg, 100 mg, 150 mg

INDICATIONS & DOSAGES
➤ **Depression (outpatients)**
Adults: 75 mg PO daily in divided doses. Or, 50 to 100 mg PO daily as single dose at bedtime or in divided doses. May increase by 25 to 50 mg, as needed, to a total of 150 mg/day. Make increases preferably in late afternoon or at bedtime. Continue for at least 3 months. Maintenance, 40 to 100 mg daily.
Elderly patients and adolescents: 10 mg PO t.i.d. plus 20 mg at bedtime daily.
➤ **Depression (hospitalized patients)**
Adults: Initially, 100 mg PO daily. If necessary, gradually increase to 200 to 300 mg daily. Maintenance dose is 40 to 100 mg daily. Continue for at least 3 months.

ADMINISTRATION
PO
• Give drug without regard for food.
• Give higher doses in late afternoon or at bedtime to minimize daytime sedation.

ACTION
Unknown. A TCA that increases the amount of norepinephrine, serotonin, or both in the CNS by blocking their reuptake by the presynaptic neurons.

Route	Onset	Peak	Duration
PO	Unknown	2–5 hr	Unknown

Half-life: 13 to 36 hours.

ADVERSE REACTIONS
CNS: *stroke, seizures, coma,* ataxia, tremor, peripheral neuropathy, anxiety, insomnia, restlessness, drowsiness, dizziness, weakness, fatigue, headache, extrapyramidal

reactions, hallucinations, delusions, disorientation. **CV:** orthostatic hypotension, tachycardia, *heart block, arrhythmias, MI,* ECG changes, HTN, edema, palpitations, syncope. **EENT:** blurred vision, mydriasis, increased IOP, tinnitus. **GI:** dry mouth, nausea, vomiting, anorexia, epigastric pain, diarrhea, constipation, paralytic ileus. **GU:** urine retention, altered libido, erectile dysfunction. **Hematologic:** *agranulocytosis, thrombocytopenia, leukopenia,* eosinophilia. **Metabolic:** *hypoglycemia,* hyperglycemia. **Skin:** rash, urticaria, photosensitivity reactions, diaphoresis. **Other:** hypersensitivity reactions.

INTERACTIONS
Drug-drug. *Barbiturates:* May increase amitriptyline metabolism. Consider therapy modification.
Cimetidine: May decrease TCA metabolism. Monitor therapy.
CNS depressants: May enhance CNS depression. Avoid using together.
Disulfiram: May increase pharmacologic effects of amitriptyline. May cause acute organic brain syndrome. Monitor patient. Stop amitriptyline or decrease amitriptyline dosage if an interaction is suspected.
Epinephrine, norepinephrine: May increase hypertensive effect. Use together cautiously.
Fluoxetine, fluvoxamine, hormonal contraceptives, paroxetine, sertraline: May increase TCA level. Consider therapy modification.
Linezolid, methylene blue: May cause serotonin syndrome. Avoid combination.
MAO inhibitors: May cause severe excitation, hyperpyrexia, or seizures, usually with high doses. Avoid using within 14 days of MAO inhibitor therapy.
Quinolones: May increase the risk of life-threatening arrhythmias. Monitor therapy.
Drug-herb. *SAM-e, St. John's wort, yohimbe:* May cause serotonin syndrome and decrease amitriptyline level. Discourage use together.
Drug-lifestyle. *Alcohol use:* May enhance CNS depression. Discourage use together.
Smoking: May lower drug level. Watch for lack of effect.

Sun exposure: May increase risk of photosensitivity reactions. Advise patient to take precautions.

EFFECTS ON LAB TEST RESULTS
• May increase or decrease glucose level.
• May increase eosinophil count and LFT values.
• May decrease granulocyte, platelet, and WBC counts.

CONTRAINDICATIONS & CAUTIONS
• Contraindicated in patients hypersensitive to drug, in those who have received an MAO inhibitor within the past 14 days, and in the acute MI recovery phase.
❸ **Alert:** Concomitant use with linezolid or methylene blue can cause serotonin syndrome (fever, mental status changes, muscle twitching, excessive sweating, shivering or shaking, diarrhea, loss of coordination). Use drug with linezolid or methylene blue only for life-threatening or urgent conditions when the potential benefits outweigh the risks of toxicity.
Black Box Warning Drug isn't approved for use in children younger than age 12. ▮
• Use cautiously in patients with history of seizures, urine retention, angle-closure glaucoma, or increased IOP; in those with hyperthyroidism, CV disease, diabetes, or impaired liver function; and in those receiving thyroid drugs.
• Use cautiously in elderly patients and in patients with suicidal ideation.
• Use cautiously in those receiving electroconvulsive therapy.
Dialyzable drug: No.
▲ **Overdose S&S:** Cardiac arrhythmias, severe hypotension, seizures, CNS depression, coma, impaired myocardial contractility, confusion, disturbed concentration, transient visual hallucinations, dilated pupils, disorders of ocular motility, agitation, hyperactive reflexes, polyradiculoneuropathy, stupor, drowsiness, muscle rigidity, vomiting, hypothermia, hyperpyrexia.

PREGNANCY-LACTATION-REPRODUCTION
• There are no adequate and well-controlled studies in pregnant women. Use during pregnancy only if potential benefit outweighs potential risk to the fetus.

• Drug appears in human milk. Patient should discontinue breastfeeding or discontinue drug.

NURSING CONSIDERATIONS

Black Box Warning Drug may increase the risk of suicidal thinking and behavior in children, adolescents, and young adults with major depressive disorder or other psychiatric disorder. Don't use in children younger than age 12. ∎

◑ Alert: If linezolid or methylene blue must be given, amitriptyline must be stopped and patient should be monitored for serotonin toxicity for 2 weeks, or until 24 hours after the last dose of methylene blue or linezolid, whichever comes first. Treatment with amitriptyline may be resumed 24 hours after last dose of methylene blue or linezolid.

• Amitriptyline has strong anticholinergic effects and is one of the most sedating TCAs. Anticholinergic effects have rapid onset even though therapeutic effect is delayed for weeks.

• Elderly patients may have an increased sensitivity to anticholinergic effects of drug; sedating effects of drug may increase the risk of falls in this population.

• If signs or symptoms of psychosis occur or increase, expect prescriber to reduce dosage. Record mood changes. Monitor patient for suicidal tendencies and allow only minimum supply of drug.

• Because patients using TCAs may suffer hypertensive episodes and arrhythmias during surgery, stop drug gradually several days before surgery.

• Monitor glucose level.

• Watch for nausea, headache, and malaise after abrupt withdrawal of long-term therapy; these symptoms don't indicate addiction.

• Don't withdraw drug abruptly.

• **Look alike–sound alike:** Don't confuse amitriptyline with nortriptyline or aminophylline. Don't confuse Elavil with Eldepryl or enalapril.

PATIENT TEACHING

Black Box Warning Advise family and caregivers to closely observe patient for increased suicidal thinking and behavior. ∎

◑ Alert: Teach patient to recognize and immediately report symptoms of serotonin toxicity (fever, mental status changes, muscle twitching, excessive sweating, shivering or shaking, diarrhea, loss of coordination).

• Advise patient to take full dose at bedtime when possible; however, caution patient that morning orthostatic hypotension may occur.

• Tell patient to avoid alcohol during drug therapy.

• Advise patient to consult prescriber before taking other drugs.

• Warn patient to avoid activities that require alertness and psychomotor coordination until CNS effects of drug are known. Drowsiness and dizziness usually subside after a few weeks.

• Inform patient that dry mouth may be relieved with sugarless hard candy or gum. Saliva substitutes may be useful.

• Advise patient to use a sunblock, wear protective clothing, and avoid prolonged exposure to strong sunlight.

• Warn patient not to stop drug abruptly.

• Advise patient that it may take as long as 30 days to achieve full therapeutic effect.

amLODIPine besylate
am-LOE-di-peen

Norvasc℘

Therapeutic class: Antihypertensives
Pharmacologic class: Calcium channel blockers

AVAILABLE FORMS
Tablets: 2.5 mg, 5 mg, 10 mg

INDICATIONS & DOSAGES
➤ **Chronic stable angina, vasospastic angina (Prinzmetal or variant angina); to reduce risk of hospitalization because of angina; to reduce risk of coronary revascularization procedure in patients with recently documented CAD by angiography and without HF or with LVEF less than 40%**
Adults: Initially, 5 to 10 mg PO daily. Most patients need 10 mg daily.
Elderly patients: Initially, 5 mg PO daily.

Adjust-a-dose: For patients who are small or frail or have hepatic insufficiency, initially, 5 mg PO daily.

➤ **HTN**

Adults: Initially, 5 mg PO daily. Dosage adjusted according to patient response and tolerance. Titration should occur over 7 to 14 days. Maximum daily dose is 10 mg.

Children ages 6 to 17: 2.5 to 5 mg PO once daily. Maximum dosage is 5 mg daily.

Elderly patients: Initially, 2.5 mg PO daily.

Adjust-a-dose: For patients who are small or frail, are taking other antihypertensives, or have hepatic insufficiency, initially, 2.5 mg PO daily.

ADMINISTRATION
PO
• Give without regard for food.

ACTION
Inhibits calcium ion influx across cardiac and smooth-muscle cells, dilates coronary arteries and arterioles, and decreases BP and myocardial oxygen demand.

Route	Onset	Peak	Duration
PO	Unknown	6–12 hr	24 hr

Half-life: 30 to 50 hours.

ADVERSE REACTIONS
CNS: headache, somnolence, fatigue, dizziness. **CV:** edema, flushing, palpitations. **GI:** nausea, abdominal pain. **Respiratory:** *pulmonary edema,* dyspnea. **Skin:** pruritus, rash.

INTERACTIONS
Drug-drug. *Conivaptan, moderate and strong CYP3A4 inhibitors (clarithromycin, itraconazole, ketoconazole, ritonavir):* May increase amlodipine plasma concentration. Monitor patient for hypotension and edema.
Cyclosporine (systemic), tacrolimus: May increase levels of both drugs. Monitor levels and patient.
Sildenafil: May increase risk of hypotension. Monitor BP closely.
Simvastatin: May increase risk of myopathy, including rhabdomyolysis. Simvastatin dosage shouldn't exceed 20 mg daily.

EFFECTS ON LAB TEST RESULTS
None reported.

CONTRAINDICATIONS & CAUTIONS
• Contraindicated in patients hypersensitive to drug.
• Use cautiously in patients receiving other peripheral vasodilators, especially those with severe aortic stenosis or hypertrophic cardiomyopathy with outflow tract obstruction, and in patients with HF with reduced LVEF. Because drug is metabolized by the liver, use cautiously and in reduced dosage in patients with severe hepatic disease.
Dialyzable drug: No.
⚠ *Overdose S&S:* Marked peripheral vasodilation with hypotension and possibly reflex tachycardia.

PREGNANCY-LACTATION-REPRODUCTION
• Use in pregnancy only if potential benefit justifies the risk to the fetus. Other antihypertensives are preferred during pregnancy.
• Drug appears in human milk. Patient should discontinue breastfeeding or discontinue drug.

NURSING CONSIDERATIONS
🛈 *Alert:* Monitor patient carefully. Some patients, especially those with severe obstructive CAD, have developed increased frequency, duration, or severity of angina or acute MI after initiation of calcium channel blocker therapy or at time of dosage increase.
• Monitor BP frequently during initiation of therapy. Because drug-induced vasodilation has a gradual onset, acute hypotension is rare.
• Notify prescriber if signs of HF occur, such as swelling of hands and feet or shortness of breath.
🛈 *Alert:* Abrupt withdrawal of drug may increase frequency and duration of chest pain. Taper dose gradually under medical supervision.
• *Look alike–sound alike:* Don't confuse amlodipine with amiloride.

PATIENT TEACHING
• Caution patient to report all adverse reactions and to continue taking drug, even when feeling better.

Reactions in bold italics are *life-threatening.* Interactions may have a *rapid onset* or a *delayed onset.*

• Tell patient SL nitroglycerin may be taken as needed when angina symptoms are acute. If patient continues nitrate therapy during adjustment of amlodipine dosage, urge continued compliance.

amoxicillin
a-moks-i-SIL-in

Amoxil, Apo-Amoxi✤, Novamoxin✤

Therapeutic class: Antibiotics
Pharmacologic class: Aminopenicillins

AVAILABLE FORMS
Capsules: 250 mg, 500 mg
Oral suspension: 50 mg/mL (pediatric drops), 125 mg/5 mL, 200 mg/5 mL, 250 mg/5 mL, 400 mg/5 mL (after reconstitution)
Tablets: 500 mg, 875 mg
Tablets (chewable): 125 mg, 250 mg

INDICATIONS & DOSAGES
Adjust-a-dose (for all indications): Adults with GFR of less than 30 mL/minute shouldn't receive the 875-mg tablet. Adults with GFR of 10 to 30 mL/minute should receive 250 or 500 mg every 12 hours depending on the infection. Adults with GFR of less than 10 mL/minute should receive 250 or 500 mg every 24 hours depending on the severity of infection. Adults on hemodialysis should receive 250 or 500 mg every 24 hours with an extra dose both during and at the end of dialysis.
➤ **Mild to moderate infections of the ear, nose, and throat; skin and skin structure; or GU tract**
Adults and children weighing 40 kg or more: 500 mg PO every 12 hours or 250 mg PO every 8 hours.
Children older than age 3 months weighing less than 40 kg: 25 mg/kg/day PO divided every 12 hours or 20 mg/kg/day PO divided every 8 hours.
Neonates and infants up to age 3 months: Up to 30 mg/kg/day PO divided every 12 hours.
➤ **Mild to severe infections of the lower respiratory tract and severe infections of the ear, nose, and throat; skin and skin structure; or GU tract**

Adults and children weighing 40 kg or more: 875 mg PO every 12 hours or 500 mg PO every 8 hours.
Children older than age 3 months weighing less than 40 kg: 45 mg/kg/day PO divided every 12 hours or 40 mg/kg/day PO divided every 8 hours.
Neonates and infants up to age 3 months: Up to 30 mg/kg/day PO divided every 12 hours.
➤ **Pharyngitis, tonsillitis, or both secondary to *Streptococcus pyogenes* infection**
Adults and children weighing 40 kg or more: 875 mg every 12 hours or 500 mg every 8 hours for at least 10 days.
Children older than age 3 months weighing less than 40 kg: 45 mg/kg/day PO divided every 12 hours or 40 mg/kg/day PO divided every 8 hours for at least 10 days.
Neonates and infants up to age 3 months: Up to 30 mg/kg/day PO divided every 12 hours for at least 10 days.
➤ ***Helicobacter pylori* eradication to reduce risk of duodenal ulcer recurrence**
Adults: Amoxicillin 1 g with lansoprazole 30 mg PO every 8 hours for 14 days (dual therapy). Or, amoxicillin 1 g, clarithromycin 500 mg, and lansoprazole 30 mg, all given PO every 12 hours for 14 days (triple therapy). Consult latest guidelines for recommendations due to increasing macrolide resistance.
➤ **Acute otitis media ◆**
Children age 6 and older with mild to moderate infection: 80 to 90 mg/kg PO daily in two divided doses for 5 to 7 days.
Children younger than age 2 and those with severe infection: 80 to 90 mg/kg PO daily in two divided doses for 10 days.

ADMINISTRATION
PO
• Before giving, ask patient about allergic reactions to penicillin. A negative history of penicillin allergy is no guarantee against allergic reaction.
• Obtain specimen for culture and sensitivity tests before giving first dose. Begin therapy while awaiting results.
• Give drug with or without food.
• For a child, place drops directly on child's tongue for swallowing or add to formula, milk, fruit juice, water, ginger ale, or other

---

cold drink for immediate and complete consumption.
• Store reconstituted oral suspension in refrigerator, if possible. Be sure to check individual product labels for storage information.

ACTION

Inhibits cell-wall synthesis during bacterial multiplication.

Route	Onset	Peak	Duration
PO	Unknown	1–2 hr	6–8 hr

Half-life: 1 to 1½ hours (7½ hours in severe renal impairment).

ADVERSE REACTIONS

CNS: *seizures,* anxiety, confusion, agitation, dizziness, reversible hyperactivity, anxiety, insomnia, behavioral changes. **GI:** diarrhea, nausea, *pseudomembranous colitis,* vomiting. **GU:** interstitial nephritis, nephropathy. **Hematologic:** *agranulocytosis, leukopenia, thrombocytopenia, thrombocytopenic purpura,* anemia, eosinophilia, hemolytic anemia. **Other:** *anaphylaxis,* hypersensitivity reactions, overgrowth of nonsusceptible organisms.

INTERACTIONS

Drug-drug. *Hormonal contraceptives:* May decrease contraceptive effectiveness. Advise use of additional form of contraception during penicillin therapy.
Live-virus vaccines: May decrease effectiveness of live-virus vaccines. Concurrent use isn't recommended.
Methotrexate: May increase methotrexate serum concentration. Monitor patient closely for toxicity.
Probenecid: May increase levels of amoxicillin and other penicillins. Probenecid may be used for this purpose.
Tetracyclines: May reduce therapeutic action of penicillins. Avoid administering together.
Warfarin: May enhance anticoagulant effect. Use together cautiously.
Drug-herb. *Khat:* May decrease antimicrobial effect. Discourage khat chewing, or tell patient to take drug 2 hours after khat chewing.

EFFECTS ON LAB TEST RESULTS

• May increase AST and ALT levels.
• May decrease Hb level.
• May increase eosinophil count. May decrease granulocyte, platelet, and WBC counts.
• May decrease aminoglycoside level. May alter results of urine glucose tests that use cupric sulfate, such as Benedict reagent and Clinitest.
• May cause transient decrease in total conjugated estriol, estriol glucuronide, conjugated estrone, and estradiol in pregnant women.

CONTRAINDICATIONS & CAUTIONS

• Contraindicated in patients hypersensitive to drug or other penicillins.
• Use cautiously in patients with other drug allergies (especially to cephalosporins) because of possible cross-sensitivity.
• Use cautiously in those with mononucleosis because of high risk of maculopapular rash.
Dialyzable drug: Yes.
⚠ *Overdose S&S:* Oliguric renal failure.

PREGNANCY-LACTATION-REPRODUCTION

• Use during pregnancy only if clearly needed.
• Drug appears in human milk. Use cautiously in breastfeeding women.

NURSING CONSIDERATIONS

• If large doses are given or if therapy is prolonged, bacterial or fungal superinfection may occur, especially in elderly, debilitated, or immunosuppressed patients.
• CDAD, ranging from mild diarrhea to fatal colitis, has been reported with nearly all antibacterial agents, including amoxicillin. Evaluate patient if diarrhea occurs.
• Amoxicillin usually causes fewer cases of diarrhea than ampicillin.
• *Look alike–sound alike:* Don't confuse amoxicillin with amoxapine.

PATIENT TEACHING

• Tell patient to take entire quantity of drug exactly as prescribed, even after feeling better.
• Instruct patient to take drug with or without food.

Reactions in bold italics are *life-threatening*. Interactions may have a *rapid onset* or a *delayed onset*.

- Tell patient to notify prescriber if rash, fever, or chills develop. A rash is the most common allergic reaction, especially if allopurinol is also being taken.
- Tell parent to place drops directly on child's tongue for swallowing or add to formula, milk, fruit juice, water, ginger ale, or other cold drink for immediate and complete consumption.

amoxicillin–clavulanate potassium
a-mox-i-SILL-in/KLAV-yu-lah-nate

Augmentin, Augmentin ES-600, Augmentin XR, Clavulin ✤

Therapeutic class: Antibiotics
Pharmacologic class: Aminopenicillins–beta-lactamase inhibitors

AVAILABLE FORMS
Oral suspension: 125 mg amoxicillin trihydrate, 31.25 mg clavulanic acid/5 mL (after reconstitution); 200 mg amoxicillin trihydrate, 28.5 mg clavulanic acid/5 mL (after reconstitution); 250 mg amoxicillin trihydrate, 62.5 mg clavulanic acid/5 mL (after reconstitution); 400 mg amoxicillin trihydrate, 57 mg clavulanic acid/5 mL (after reconstitution); 600 mg amoxicillin trihydrate, 42.9 mg clavulanic acid/5 mL (after reconstitution)
Tablets: 875 mg amoxicillin trihydrate, 125 mg clavulanic acid
Tablets (chewable): 200 mg amoxicillin trihydrate, 28.5 mg clavulanic acid; 250 mg amoxicillin trihydrate, 62.5 mg clavulanic acid; 400 mg amoxicillin trihydrate, 57 mg clavulanic acid
Tablets (extended-release) ⓓ: 1,000 mg amoxicillin trihydrate, 62.5 mg clavulanic acid
Tablets (film-coated): 250 mg amoxicillin trihydrate, 125 mg clavulanic acid; 500 mg amoxicillin trihydrate, 125 mg clavulanic acid

INDICATIONS & DOSAGES
➤ **Lower respiratory tract infections, otitis media, sinusitis, skin and skin-structure infections, and UTIs caused by susceptible strains of gram-positive and gram-negative organisms**
Adults and children weighing 40 kg or more: 250 mg PO, based on amoxicillin component, every 8 hours; or 500 mg every 12 hours. For more severe infections, 500 mg every 8 hours or 875 mg every 12 hours.
Children age 3 months and older weighing less than 40 kg: 20 to 45 mg/kg/day PO, based on amoxicillin component and severity of infection, daily in divided doses every 8 to 12 hours.
Children younger than age 3 months: 30 mg/kg/day PO, based on amoxicillin component of the 125 mg/5 mL oral suspension, in divided doses every 12 hours.
Adjust-a-dose: Don't give the 875-mg tablet to patients with CrCl of less than 30 mL/minute. If CrCl is 10 to 30 mL/minute, give 250 to 500 mg PO every 12 hours. If CrCl is less than 10 mL/minute, give 250 to 500 mg PO every 24 hours. Give hemodialysis patients 250 to 500 mg PO every 24 hours with an additional dose both during and after dialysis.
➤ **Community-acquired pneumonia or acute bacterial sinusitis caused by *H. influenzae, M. catarrhalis, H. parainfluenzae, Klebsiella pneumoniae,* methicillin-susceptible *Staphylococcus aureus,* or *S. pneumoniae* with reduced susceptibility to penicillin**
Adults and children weighing 40 kg or more: 2,000 mg/125 mg Augmentin XR tablets every 12 hours for 7 to 10 days for pneumonia; 10 days for sinusitis.
Adjust-a-dose: In patients with CrCl less than 30 mL/minute and patients receiving hemodialysis, don't use Augmentin XR.

ADMINISTRATION
PO
- Before giving drug, ask patient about allergic reactions to penicillin. A negative history of penicillin allergy is no guarantee against an allergic reaction.
- Obtain specimen for culture and sensitivity tests before giving first dose. Begin therapy while awaiting results.
- Give drug at the start of a meal to enhance absorption.

• Give drug at least 1 hour before a bacterio-static antibiotic.
• Avoid use of 250-mg tablet in children weighing less than 40 kg. Use chewable form instead.
• After reconstitution, refrigerate the oral suspension; discard after 10 days.

ACTION

Amoxicillin prevents bacterial cell-wall synthesis during replication. Clavulanic acid increases amoxicillin's effectiveness by inactivating beta-lactamases, which destroy amoxicillin.

Route	Onset	Peak	Duration
PO	Unknown	1–2½ hr	6–8 hr
PO (Aug-mentin XR)	Unknown	1–6 hr	Unknown

Half-life: 1 to 1½ hours. For patients with severe renal impairment, 7½ hours for amoxicillin and 4½ hours for clavulanate.

ADVERSE REACTIONS

CNS: agitation, anxiety, behavioral changes, confusion, dizziness, insomnia, headache, *seizures.* **GI:** nausea, vomiting, diarrhea, indigestion, gastritis, stomatitis, glossitis, black hairy tongue, enterocolitis, *pseudomembranous colitis,* mucocutaneous candidiasis, abdominal pain. **GU:** vaginal candidiasis, vaginitis. **Hematologic:** anemia, *thrombocytopenia, thrombocytopenic purpura,* eosinophilia, *leukopenia, agranulocytosis.* **Other:** hypersensitivity reactions, *anaphylaxis,* pruritus, rash, urticaria, *angioedema,* overgrowth of nonsusceptible organisms, serum sickness–like reaction.

INTERACTIONS

Drug-drug. *Allopurinol:* May increase risk of rash. Monitor patient for rash.
Hormonal contraceptives: May decrease hormonal contraceptive effectiveness. Advise use of additional form of contraception during penicillin therapy.
Live-virus vaccines: May decrease effectiveness of live-virus vaccines. Concurrent use isn't recommended.
Methotrexate: May increase risk of methotrexate toxicity. Monitor methotrexate levels.

Oral anticoagulants (warfarin): May prolong PT. Monitor PT closely during coadministration.
Probenecid: May increase levels of amoxicillin and other penicillins. Use together isn't recommended.
Tetracyclines: May reduce therapeutic action of penicillins. Avoid administering together.
Warfarin: May enhance anticoagulant effect. Use together cautiously.
Drug-herb. *Khat:* May decrease antimicrobial effect of certain penicillins. Discourage khat chewing, or tell patient to take amoxicillin 2 hours after khat chewing.

EFFECTS ON LAB TEST RESULTS

• May decrease platelet, leukocyte, and granulocyte counts. May increase or decrease eosinophil count.
• May decrease aminoglycoside level.
• May alter results of urine glucose tests that use cupric sulfate, such as Benedict reagent and Clinitest.

CONTRAINDICATIONS & CAUTIONS

• Contraindicated in patients hypersensitive to drug or other penicillins and in those with a history of amoxicillin-related cholestatic jaundice or hepatic dysfunction.
• Use cautiously in patients with other drug allergies (especially to cephalosporins) because of possible cross-sensitivity.
• Augmentin XR is contraindicated in patients receiving hemodialysis and those with CrCl of less than 30 mL/minute.
• Use cautiously in patients with hepatic dysfunction.
• Drug may increase risk of hepatic dysfunction (hepatitis, cholestatic jaundice), especially in elderly patients, males, and patients on prolonged treatment.
• Don't give ampicillin-class antibiotics to patients with mononucleosis due to high incidence of erythematous rash.
Dialyzable drug: Yes.
⚠ *Overdose S&S:* Crystalluria, oliguric renal failure, GI symptoms, rash, hyperactivity or drowsiness.

PREGNANCY-LACTATION-REPRODUCTION

• Use during pregnancy only if clearly needed.

Reactions in bold italics are *life-threatening*. Interactions may have a *rapid onset* or a *delayed onset*.

• Drug appears in human milk. Use cautiously in breastfeeding women.

NURSING CONSIDERATIONS

🚫 *Alert:* Ratios of amoxicillin and clavulanic acid aren't consistent from product to product. Therefore, formulations aren't equivalent. For example, don't substitute two 250-mg tablets for one 500-mg tablet or substitute one 250-mg film-coated tablet for one 250-mg chewable tablet.

• Each Augmentin XR tablet contains 29.3 mg (1.27 mEq) of sodium and 13 mg of potassium (0.33 mEq).

• Augmentin XR isn't indicated for treating infections caused by *S. pneumoniae* with penicillin minimum inhibitory concentration, or MIC, of 4 mcg/mL or greater.

• If large doses are given or therapy is prolonged, bacterial or fungal superinfection may occur, especially in elderly, debilitated, or immunosuppressed patients.

• CDAD, ranging from mild diarrhea to fatal colitis, has been reported with nearly all antibacterial agents, including amoxicillin–clavulanate. Evaluate patient if diarrhea occurs.

• Chewable tablets and powder for oral solution contain phenylalanine.

• Monitor LFTs periodically in patients with hepatic impairment. Discontinue drug if signs of hepatitis occur.

🚫 *Alert:* Don't interchange the oral suspensions because of varying clavulanic acid contents.

• 600 mg amoxicillin/42.9 mg clavulanic acid/5 mL is intended only for children ages 3 months to 12 years with persistent or recurrent acute otitis media.

🚫 *Alert:* Both 250- and 500-mg film-coated tablets contain the same amount of clavulanic acid (125 mg). Therefore, two 250-mg tablets aren't equivalent to one 500-mg tablet. Regular tablets aren't equivalent to Augmentin XR.

• This drug combination is particularly useful in clinical settings with a high prevalence of amoxicillin-resistant organisms.

• *Look alike–sound alike:* Don't confuse amoxicillin with amoxapine or Azulfidine.

PATIENT TEACHING

• Tell patient to take entire quantity of drug exactly as prescribed, even after feeling better.

• Instruct patient to take drug with food to prevent GI upset. Advise patient taking the oral suspension to keep drug refrigerated, to shake it well before taking it, and to discard remaining drug after 10 days.

• Tell patient to report all adverse reactions and to call prescriber if a rash occurs because rash may indicate an allergic reaction.

SAFETY ALERT!

amphotericin B lipid complex
am-foe-TER-i-sin

Abelcet

Therapeutic class: Antifungals
Pharmacologic class: Polyene antibiotics

AVAILABLE FORMS
Suspension for injection: 100 mg/20-mL vial

INDICATIONS & DOSAGES
➤ **Invasive fungal infections, including *Aspergillus* and *Candida* species, in patients refractory to or intolerant of conventional amphotericin B therapy**
Adults and children: 5 mg/kg daily IV as a single infusion given at rate of 2.5 mg/kg/hour.
Adjust-a-dose: Determine dosage based on overall clinical condition of individual patient.

ADMINISTRATION
IV

▼ To prepare, shake vial gently until there's no yellow sediment. Using aseptic technique, withdraw calculated dose into one or more 20-mL syringes using an 18G needle. More than one vial will be needed.

▼ Attach a 5-micron filter needle to syringe and inject dose into IV bag of D_5W. Volume of D_5W should be sufficient to yield 1 mg/mL (2 mg/mL for pediatric patients and those with CV disorders). One filter needle can be used for up to four vials of amphotericin B lipid complex.

▼ Don't use an in-line filter.

▼ If infusing through an existing IV line, flush first with D₅W.

▼ Use an infusion pump, and give by continuous infusion at 2.5 mg/kg/hour.

▼ If infusion time exceeds 2 hours, mix contents by shaking infusion bag every 2 hours.

▼ Monitor vital signs closely. Fever, shaking chills, and hypotension may appear within 2 hours of starting infusion. Slowing infusion rate may decrease risk of infusion-related reactions.

▼ If severe respiratory distress occurs, stop infusion, provide supportive therapy for anaphylaxis, and notify prescriber. Don't restart drug.

▼ Reconstituted drug is stable up to 48 hours if refrigerated (36° to 46° F [2° to 8° C]) and up to 6 hours at room temperature.

▼ Discard any unused drug because it contains no preservative.

▼ **Incompatibilities:** Electrolytes, other IV drugs, saline solutions.

ACTION

Binds to sterols of fungal cell membranes, altering cell permeability and causing cell death.

Route	Onset	Peak	Duration
IV	Unknown	Unknown	Unknown

Half-life: About 1 week.

ADVERSE REACTIONS

CNS: fever, headache, pain. **CV:** *cardiac arrest,* chest pain, HTN, hypotension. **GI:** *GI hemorrhage,* abdominal pain, diarrhea, nausea, vomiting. **GU:** *renal failure.* **Hematologic:** *leukopenia, thrombocytopenia,* anemia. **Hepatic:** hyperbilirubinemia. **Metabolic:** hypokalemia. **Respiratory:** *respiratory failure,* dyspnea, respiratory disorder. **Skin:** rash. **Other:** *multiple organ failure,* chills, *sepsis,* infection.

INTERACTIONS

Drug-drug. *Antineoplastics:* May increase risk of renal toxicity, bronchospasm, and hypotension. Use together cautiously.
Cardiac glycosides: May increase risk of digitalis toxicity from amphotericin

B–induced hypokalemia. Monitor potassium level closely.
Clotrimazole, fluconazole, itraconazole, ketoconazole, miconazole: May counteract effects of amphotericin B by inducing fungal resistance. Monitor patient closely.
Corticosteroids, corticotropin: May enhance hypokalemia, which could lead to cardiac toxicity. Monitor electrolyte levels and cardiac function.
Cyclosporine: May increase renal toxicity. Monitor renal function test results closely.
Flucytosine: May increase risk of flucytosine toxicity from increased cellular uptake or impaired renal excretion. Use together cautiously.
Leukocyte transfusions: May increase risk of pulmonary reactions, such as acute dyspnea, tachypnea, hypoxemia, hemoptysis, and interstitial infiltrates. Don't coadminister.
Nephrotoxic drugs (such as aminoglycosides, pentamidine): May increase risk of renal toxicity. Use together cautiously and monitor renal function closely.
Skeletal muscle relaxants: May enhance skeletal muscle relaxant effects of amphotericin B–induced hypokalemia. Monitor potassium level closely.
Zidovudine: May increase myelotoxicity and nephrotoxicity. Monitor renal and hematologic function.

EFFECTS ON LAB TEST RESULTS

• May increase alkaline phosphatase, ALT, AST, bilirubin, BUN, creatinine, GGT, and LDH levels. May decrease Hb and magnesium and potassium levels.
• May decrease platelet and WBC counts.

CONTRAINDICATIONS & CAUTIONS

• Contraindicated in patients hypersensitive to amphotericin B or its components.
• Anaphylaxis can occur. If patient develops severe respiratory distress, discontinue infusion, treat appropriately, and don't restart drug.
• Use cautiously in patients with renal impairment. Adjust dosage based on patient's overall condition. Renal toxicity is more common at higher dosages.
Dialyzable drug: No.
⚠ *Overdose S&S:* Cardiorespiratory arrest.

Reactions in bold italics are *life-threatening*. Interactions may have a *rapid onset* or a *delayed onset*.

PREGNANCY-LACTATION-REPRODUCTION
- Use cautiously during pregnancy, taking into account importance of drug to the mother.
- It isn't known if drug appears in human milk. Patient should discontinue breastfeeding or discontinue drug.

NURSING CONSIDERATIONS
🜂 **Alert:** Different amphotericin B preparations aren't interchangeable, so dosages will vary. Confusing the preparations may cause permanent damage or death.
- Hydrate before infusion to reduce risk of nephrotoxicity.
- Frequently monitor creatinine and electrolyte levels (especially magnesium and potassium), LFT values, and CBC during therapy.
- Acute infusion reactions, including fever and chills, may occur 1 to 2 hours after start of infusion and are more common with first few doses. Infusion has rarely been associated with arrhythmias, hypotension, and shock.
🜂 **Alert:** Immediately stop infusion if severe respiratory distress occurs. Patient shouldn't receive further infusions.
- **Look alike–sound alike:** Don't confuse Abelcet with AmBisome.

PATIENT TEACHING
- Inform patient that fever, chills, nausea, and vomiting may develop during infusion, but that these symptoms usually subside with subsequent doses.
- Instruct patient to report any redness or pain at infusion site.
- Teach patient to recognize and report to prescriber signs and symptoms of acute hypersensitivity, such as respiratory distress.
- Warn patient that therapy may take several months.
- Tell patient to expect frequent laboratory testing to monitor kidney and liver function.

amphotericin B liposomal
am-foe-TER-i-sin

AmBisome

Therapeutic class: Antifungals
Pharmacologic class: Polyene antibiotics

AVAILABLE FORMS
Powder for injection: 50-mg vial

INDICATIONS & DOSAGES
➤ **Empirical therapy for presumed fungal infection in febrile, neutropenic patients**
Adults and children: 3 mg/kg IV infusion over 2 hours daily.
➤ **Systemic fungal infections caused by *Aspergillus* species, *Candida* species, or *Cryptococcus* species refractory to conventional amphotericin B therapy; patients for whom renal impairment or unacceptable toxicity precludes use of conventional amphotericin B therapy**
Adults and children: 3 to 5 mg/kg IV infusion over 2 hours daily.
➤ **Visceral leishmaniasis in immunocompetent patients**
Adults and children: 3 mg/kg IV infusion over 2 hours daily on days 1 to 5, day 14, and day 21. A repeat course of therapy may be beneficial if initial treatment fails to clear parasites.
➤ **Visceral leishmaniasis in immunocompromised patients**
Adults and children: 4 mg/kg IV infusion over 2 hours daily on days 1 to 5, day 10, day 17, day 24, day 31, and day 38.
➤ **Cryptococcal meningitis in patients with HIV infection**
Adults and children: 6 mg/kg/day IV infusion over 2 hours.
➤ **Candidiasis (invasive) in HIV-exposed/infected patients ◆**
Infants and children: 5 mg/kg/dose IV once daily.
➤ **Coccidioidomycosis in HIV-exposed/infected patients with severe non-meningeal infection (diffuse pulmonary or extrathoracic, disseminated disease) ◆**

Adolescents: 3 to 5 mg/kg/dose IV once daily until clinical improvement; then initiate triazole therapy.

Infants and children: 5 mg/kg/dose IV once daily until clinical improvement; then initiate triazole therapy. May increase dosage to 10 mg/kg/dose IV once daily for life-threatening infection.

➤ **Histoplasmosis in HIV-exposed/ infected patients with moderately severe to severe infection ♦**

Adolescents: 3 mg/kg/dose IV once daily.

Infants and children: 3 to 5 mg/kg/dose IV once daily.

ADMINISTRATION

IV

▼ Don't reconstitute with bacteriostatic water for injection, and don't allow bacteriostatic product in solution.

▼ Don't reconstitute with saline solutions, add saline solutions to reconstituted concentration, or mix with other drugs.

▼ Reconstitute each 50-mg vial with 12 mL of sterile water for injection to yield 4 mg/mL. A yellow, translucent suspension will form.

▼ After reconstitution, shake vial vigorously for 30 seconds or until particulate matter disperses.

▼ Dilute to 1 to 2 mg/mL by withdrawing calculated amount of reconstituted solution into a sterile syringe and injecting it through a 5-micron filter into an appropriate amount of D_5W. Use only one filter needle per vial. Concentrations of 0.2 to 0.5 mg/mL may provide sufficient volume of infusion for children.

▼ Flush existing IV line with D_5W before infusing drug. If this isn't possible, give drug through a separate line.

▼ Use a controlled infusion device and an in-line filter with a mean pore diameter of 1 micron or larger.

▼ Initially, infuse drug over at least 2 hours. If drug is tolerated well, reduce infusion time to 1 hour. If discomfort occurs, increase infusion time.

▼ Store unopened vial at 36° to 46° F (2° to 8° C). Store reconstituted drug for up to 24 hours at 36° to 46° F. Use within 6 hours of dilution with D_5W. Don't freeze.

▼ **Incompatibilities:** Other IV drugs, saline solutions.

ACTION

Binds to sterols of fungal cell membranes, altering cell permeability and causing cell death.

Route	Onset	Peak	Duration
IV	Unknown	Unknown	Unknown

Half-life: About 4 to 6 days.

ADVERSE REACTIONS

CNS: fever, anxiety, confusion, headache, insomnia, asthenia, pain. **CV:** chest pain, hypotension, tachycardia, HTN, edema, flushing. **EENT:** epistaxis, rhinitis. **GI:** anorexia, constipation, nausea, vomiting, abdominal pain, diarrhea, *GI hemorrhage.* **GU:** hematuria, *renal failure.* **Hematologic:** anemia, thrombocytopenia, leukopenia. **Hepatic:** hyperbilirubinemia, *hepatotoxicity.* **Metabolic:** hyperglycemia, hypernatremia, hyponatremia, hypocalcemia, hypokalemia, *hypomagnesemia.* **Musculoskeletal:** back pain, weakness. **Respiratory:** increased cough, dyspnea, hypoxia, pleural effusion, lung disorder, hyperventilation. **Skin:** pruritus, rash, sweating. **Other:** chills, infection, *anaphylaxis, sepsis,* blood product infusion reaction.

INTERACTIONS

Drug-drug. *Antineoplastics:* May enhance potential for renal toxicity, bronchospasm, and hypotension. Use together cautiously.

Cardiac glycosides: May increase risk of digitalis toxicity caused by amphotericin B–induced hypokalemia. Monitor potassium level closely.

Clotrimazole, fluconazole, ketoconazole, miconazole: May induce fungal resistance to amphotericin B. Use together cautiously.

Corticosteroids, corticotropin: May increase potassium depletion, which could cause cardiac dysfunction. Monitor electrolyte levels and cardiac function.

Cyclosporine: May increase renal toxicity. Monitor renal function test results closely.

Flucytosine: May increase flucytosine toxicity by increasing cellular reuptake or impairing renal excretion of flucytosine. Use together cautiously.

Reactions in bold italics are *life-threatening*. Interactions may have a *rapid onset* or a *delayed onset*.

Leukocyte transfusions: Increases risk of pulmonary toxicity. Don't use together.
Other nephrotoxic drugs, such as antibiotics and antineoplastics: May cause additive nephrotoxicity. Use together cautiously; monitor renal function closely.
Skeletal muscle relaxants (tubocurarine): May enhance effects of skeletal muscle relaxants resulting from amphotericin B–induced hypokalemia. Monitor potassium level.

EFFECTS ON LAB TEST RESULTS
• May increase alkaline phosphatase, ALT, AST, bilirubin, BUN, creatinine, GGT, glucose, LDH, and sodium levels. May decrease calcium, magnesium, and potassium levels.
• May decrease Hb level and platelet count.

CONTRAINDICATIONS & CAUTIONS
• Contraindicated in patients hypersensitive to drug or its components.
• Use cautiously in patients with impaired renal function, in elderly patients, and in pregnant women.
Dialyzable drug: No.
⚠ *Overdose S&S:* Cardiorespiratory arrest.

PREGNANCY-LACTATION-REPRODUCTION
• Use during pregnancy only if potential benefits outweigh potential risks to the fetus.
• It isn't known if drug appears in human milk. Patient should discontinue breastfeeding or discontinue drug.

NURSING CONSIDERATIONS
• Patients also receiving chemotherapy or bone marrow transplantation and those with HIV disease are at greater risk for additional adverse reactions, such as cardiac arrest, hallucinations, seizures, arrhythmias, and thrombocytopenia. Refer to manufacturer's instructions for a complete list of reactions.
✪ *Alert:* Different amphotericin B preparations aren't interchangeable, so dosages will vary. Confusing the preparations may cause permanent damage or death.
• Premedicate patient with antipyretics, antihistamines, antiemetics and corticosteroids.
• Hydrate before infusion to reduce the risk of nephrotoxicity.

• Monitor BUN, creatinine, and electrolyte levels (particularly magnesium and potassium), LFT, and CBC.
• Watch for signs and symptoms of hypokalemia (ECG changes, muscle weakness, cramping, drowsiness).
• Patients treated with this drug have a lower risk of chills, elevated BUN level, hypokalemia, HTN, and vomiting than patients treated with conventional amphotericin B.
• Therapy may take several weeks or months.
• Observe patient closely for adverse reactions during infusion. If anaphylaxis occurs, stop infusion immediately, provide supportive therapy, and notify prescriber.
• *Look alike–sound alike:* Don't confuse amphotericin B liposomal with AmBisome.

PATIENT TEACHING
• Teach patient signs and symptoms of hypersensitivity, and stress importance of reporting them immediately.
• Warn patient that therapy may take several months; teach personal hygiene and other measures to prevent spread and recurrence of lesions.
• Instruct patient to report any adverse reactions that occur while receiving drug.
• Tell patient to watch for and report signs and symptoms of low blood potassium levels (muscle weakness, cramping, drowsiness).
• Advise patient that frequent laboratory testing will be needed.

ampicillin
am-pi-SIL-in

ampicillin sodium

Therapeutic class: Antibiotics
Pharmacologic class: Aminopenicillins

AVAILABLE FORMS
Capsules: 250 mg, 500 mg
Injection: 125 mg, 250 mg, 500 mg, 1 g, 2 g
Oral suspension (reconstituted): 125 mg/5 mL, 250 mg/5 mL

INDICATIONS & DOSAGES
➤ **Respiratory tract infections**
Adults and children weighing more than 20 kg: 250 mg PO every 6 hours.

Children weighing 20 kg or less: 50 mg/kg/day PO in equally divided doses every 6 to 8 hours. Maximum dose is 250 mg q.i.d.

➤ **GI infections or GU infections (excluding gonorrhea)**

Adults and children weighing 20 kg or more: 500 mg PO every 6 hours. For severe infections, larger doses may be needed.

Children weighing less than 20 kg: 100 mg/kg/day PO in equally divided doses every 6 hours. Maximum dose is 500 mg q.i.d.

➤ **Uncomplicated gonorrhea**

Adults and children weighing more than 20 kg: 3.5 g PO with 1 g probenecid given as a single dose.

➤ **Bacterial meningitis or septicemia**

Adults: 150 to 200 mg/kg/day IV in divided doses every 3 to 4 hours. May be given IM after 3 days of IV therapy. Maximum recommended daily dose is 14 g.

Children: 150 to 200 mg/kg IV daily in divided doses every 3 to 4 hours. Give IV for 3 days; then give IM.

➤ **GI infections and GU tract infections (including gonorrhea in females)**

Adults and children weighing 40 kg or more: 500 mg IV or IM every 6 hours.

Adults and children weighing less than 40 kg: 50 mg/kg/day IV or IM in equally divided doses every 6 to 8 hours.

➤ **Respiratory tract and soft-tissue infections**

Adults and children weighing 40 kg or more: 250 to 500 mg IV or IM every 6 hours.

Adults and children weighing less than 40 kg: 25 to 50 mg/kg/day IV or IM in equally divided doses every 6 to 8 hours.

➤ **Urethritis in males due to gonorrhea**

Adult men: Two doses of 500 mg each IV or IM at 8- to 12-hour intervals. May repeat or extend treatment if necessary.

ADMINISTRATION
PO

• Before giving drug, ask patient about allergic reactions to penicillin. A negative history of penicillin allergy is no guarantee against a future allergic reaction.

• Obtain specimen for culture and sensitivity tests before giving. Begin therapy while awaiting results.

• When given orally, drug may cause GI disturbances. Food may interfere with

absorption. Give drug with 8 oz of water ½ hour before or 2 hours after meals.

• Give drug IM or IV if infection is severe or if patient can't take oral dose.

IV

▼ Before giving drug, ask patient about allergic reactions to penicillin. A negative history of penicillin allergy is no guarantee against a future allergic reaction.

▼ Obtain specimen for culture and sensitivity tests before giving. Begin therapy while awaiting results.

▼ Give drug IM or IV only if infection is severe or if patient can't take oral dose.

▼ Give drug intermittently to prevent vein irritation. Change site every 48 hours.

▼ For direct injection, reconstitute with bacteriostatic water for injection. Use 5 mL for 250-mg or 500-mg vials, 7.4 mL for 1-g vials, and 14.8 mL for 2-g vials. Give drug over 10 to 15 minutes to avoid seizures. Don't exceed 100 mg/minute.

▼ For intermittent infusion, dilute in 50 to 100 mL of NSS for injection. Give drug over 15 to 30 minutes.

▼ Use first dilution within 1 hour. Follow manufacturer's directions for stability data when drug is further diluted for IV infusion.

▼ **Incompatibilities:** None listed by manufacturer. Consult a drug incompatibility reference for more information.

IM

• Before giving drug, ask patient about allergic reactions to penicillin. A negative history of penicillin allergy is no guarantee against a future allergic reaction.

• Obtain specimen for culture and sensitivity tests before giving. Begin therapy while awaiting results.

• Give drug IM or IV only if infection is severe or patient can't take oral dose.

ACTION

Inhibits cell-wall synthesis during bacterial multiplication.

Route	Onset	Peak	Duration
PO	Unknown	2 hr	6–8 hr
IV	Immediate	Immediate	Unknown
IM	Unknown	1 hr	Unknown

Half-life: 1 to 1.8 hours (10 to 24 hours in severe renal impairment).

Reactions in bold italics are *life-threatening*. Interactions may have a *rapid onset* or a *delayed onset*.

ADVERSE REACTIONS

GI: diarrhea, nausea, *pseudomembranous colitis,* abdominal pain, black hairy tongue, enterocolitis, gastritis, glossitis, stomatitis, vomiting. **Hematologic:** *leukopenia, thrombocytopenia, thrombocytopenic purpura,* anemia, eosinophilia, hemolytic anemia, *agranulocytosis.* **Other:** hypersensitivity reactions, overgrowth of nonsusceptible organisms.

INTERACTIONS

Drug-drug. *Allopurinol:* May increase risk of rash. Monitor patient for rash.
H₂ antagonists, PPIs: May decrease ampicillin absorption and level. Separate administration times. Monitor patient for continued antibiotic effectiveness.
Hormonal contraceptives: May decrease hormonal contraceptive effectiveness. Advise use of another form of contraception during therapy.
Live-virus vaccines: May decrease effectiveness of live-virus vaccines. Concurrent use isn't recommended.
Methotrexate: May increase methotrexate level, increasing risk of toxicity. Monitor methotrexate level.
Oral anticoagulants: May increase risk of bleeding. Monitor PT and INR.
Probenecid: May increase levels of ampicillin and other penicillins. Probenecid may be used for this purpose.
Drug-herb. *Khat:* May decrease antimicrobial effect of certain penicillins. Discourage khat chewing, or tell patient to take drug 2 hours after khat chewing.

EFFECTS ON LAB TEST RESULTS

• May decrease Hb level.
• May increase eosinophil count. May decrease granulocyte, platelet, and WBC counts.
• May decrease aminoglycoside level.
• May alter results of urine glucose tests that use cupric sulfate, such as Benedict reagent and Clinitest.

CONTRAINDICATIONS & CAUTIONS

• Contraindicated in patients hypersensitive to drug or other penicillins and in those with infections caused by penicillinase-producing organisms.

• Use cautiously in patients with other drug allergies (especially to cephalosporins) because of possible cross-sensitivity, and in those with mononucleosis because of high risk of maculopapular rash.
• Use cautiously in patients with renal impairment.
Dialyzable drug: Yes.

PREGNANCY-LACTATION-REPRODUCTION

• There are no adequate and well-controlled studies in pregnant women. Use during pregnancy only if clearly needed.
• Drug appears in human milk. Use cautiously in breastfeeding women.

NURSING CONSIDERATIONS

• Monitor sodium level because each gram of ampicillin sodium injection contains 2.9 mEq of sodium.
• If large doses are given or if therapy is prolonged, bacterial or fungal superinfection may occur, especially in elderly, debilitated, or immunosuppressed patients.
• Watch for signs and symptoms of hypersensitivity, such as erythematous maculopapular rash, urticaria, and anaphylaxis.
• Use lowest dosage compatible with effective treatment in neonates and infants because of incompletely developed renal function in these patients.
• Monitor patients for CDAD, which can be fatal and can occur even more than 2 months after therapy ends. Antibiotic may need to be stopped and other treatment begun.

PATIENT TEACHING

• Tell patient to take entire quantity of drug exactly as prescribed, even after feeling better.
• Instruct patient to take oral form with 8 oz of water on an empty stomach (½ hour before or 2 hours after meals).
• Inform patient to report all adverse reactions and to notify prescriber if rash, fever, or chills develop. A rash is the most common allergic reaction, especially if allopurinol is also being taken.
• Instruct patient to report diarrhea.

ampicillin sodium–sulbactam sodium

am-pi-SIL-in/sul-BAK-tam

Unasyn

Therapeutic class: Antibiotics
Pharmacologic class: Aminopenicillins–beta-lactamase inhibitors

AVAILABLE FORMS
Injection: Vials and piggyback vials containing 1.5 g (1 g ampicillin sodium and 0.5 g sulbactam sodium), 3 g (2 g ampicillin sodium and 1 g sulbactam sodium)

INDICATIONS & DOSAGES
Adjust-a-dose (for all indications): If CrCl in adults is 15 to 29 mL/minute/1.73 m^2, give 1.5 to 3 g every 12 hours; if CrCl is 5 to 14 mL/minute/1.73 m^2, give 1.5 to 3 g every 24 hours. Give dose after hemodialysis.
➤ **Intra-abdominal, gynecologic, and skin-structure infections caused by susceptible strains**
Adults: 1.5 to 3 g IM or IV every 6 hours. Don't exceed 4 g/day of sulbactam.
Children age 1 or older weighing 40 kg or more (skin and skin-structure infections only): 1.5 to 3 g IV or IM every 6 hours for no longer than 14 days. Don't exceed 4 g/day sulbactam.
Children age 1 or older weighing less than 40 kg (skin and skin-structure infections only): 300 mg/kg/day IV in divided doses every 6 hours for no longer than 14 days. Continue therapy with an appropriate oral anti-infective agent if necessary.

ADMINISTRATION
IV
▼ Before giving drug, ask patient about allergic reactions to penicillin. A negative history of penicillin allergy is no guarantee against future allergic reaction.
▼ Obtain specimen for culture and sensitivity tests. Begin therapy while awaiting results.
▼ Reconstitute powder with one of these diluents: NSS, sterile water for injection, D$_5$W, lactated Ringer injection, M/6 sodium lactate, dextrose 5% in half-NSS for injection, or 10% invert sugar.
▼ After reconstitution, let vials stand for a few minutes so foam can dissipate. Inspect solution for particles.
▼ Give drug at least 1 hour before giving a bacteriostatic antibiotic.
▼ For infusion, can give dose by slow IV injection over at least 10 to 15 minutes or can dilute in 50 to 100 mL of compatible diluent and infuse over 15 to 30 minutes.
▼ Stability varies with diluent, temperature, and concentration of solution.
▼ **Incompatibilities:** Acyclovir, aminoglycosides, amiodarone, amphotericin B cholesteryl, amphotericin B lipid complex, amphotericin B liposomal, caspofungin, chlorpromazine, ciprofloxacin, daunorubicin, dobutamine, ganciclovir, ondansetron, phenytoin, prochlorperazine, verapamil.
IM
● Before giving drug, ask patient about allergic reactions to penicillin. A negative history of penicillin allergy is no guarantee against future allergic reaction.
● Obtain specimen for culture and sensitivity tests. Begin therapy while awaiting results.
● For IM injection, reconstitute with sterile water for injection or 0.5% or 2% lidocaine hydrochloride injection. Add 3.2 mL to a 1.5-g vial (or 6.4 mL to a 3-g vial) to yield 375 mg/mL. Give deep into muscle within 1 hour after preparation.
● IM injection may cause pain at injection site.
● In children, don't use IM route.

ACTION
Inhibits cell-wall synthesis during bacterial multiplication.

Route	Onset	Peak	Duration
IV	Immediate	15 min	Unknown
IM	Unknown	30–52 min	Unknown

Half-life: 1 to 1½ hours (10 to 24 hours in severe renal impairment).

ADVERSE REACTIONS
CV: thrombophlebitis. **GI:** diarrhea. **Hematologic:** *agranulocytosis, leukopenia, thrombocytopenia, thrombocytopenic*

Reactions in bold italics are *life-threatening*. Interactions may have a *rapid onset* or a ***delayed onset***.

purpura. **Skin:** pain at injection site, thrombophlebitis, rash, urticaria. **Other:** hypersensitivity reactions.

INTERACTIONS
Drug-drug. *Allopurinol:* May increase risk of rash. Monitor patient for rash.
Hormonal contraceptives: May decrease hormonal contraceptive effectiveness. Strongly advise use of another contraceptive during therapy.
Live-virus vaccines: May decrease effectiveness of live-virus vaccines. Use together isn't recommended.
Methotrexate: May increase methotrexate level, increasing risk of toxicity. Monitor methotrexate level.
Oral anticoagulants: May increase risk of bleeding. Monitor PT and INR.
Probenecid: May increase ampicillin level. Probenecid may be used for this purpose.
Tetracycline: May decrease effectiveness of ampicillin–sulbactam. Avoid coadministration if possible.
Drug-herb. *Khat:* May decrease antimicrobial effect of certain penicillins. Discourage khat chewing, or tell patient to take drug 2 hours after khat chewing.

EFFECTS ON LAB TEST RESULTS
• May increase alkaline phosphatase, ALT, AST, bilirubin, BUN, CK, creatinine, GGT, and LDH levels. May decrease Hb level.
• May transiently decrease conjugated estriol, conjugated estrone, estradiol, and estriol glucuronide levels in pregnant women.
• May increase eosinophil count. May decrease granulocyte, platelet, and WBC counts.
• May alter results of urine glucose tests that use cupric sulfate, such as Benedict reagent and Clinitest.

CONTRAINDICATIONS & CAUTIONS
• Contraindicated in patients hypersensitive to drug or other penicillins, in those with sensitivity to multiple allergens, and in those with mononucleosis because of high risk of maculopapular rash.
• Contraindicated in patients with a history of cholestatic jaundice or hepatic dysfunc-

tion associated with ampicillin–sulbactam injection.
• Use cautiously in patients with other drug allergies (especially to cephalosporins) because of possible cross-sensitivity and in those with renal impairment.
Dialyzable drug: Yes.
⚠ *Overdose S&S:* Neuromuscular hyperexcitability, seizures.

PREGNANCY-LACTATION-REPRODUCTION
• There are no adequate and well-controlled studies in pregnant women. Use cautiously during pregnancy and only if clearly needed.
• Drug appears in human milk. Use cautiously in breastfeeding women.

NURSING CONSIDERATIONS
• Dosage is expressed as total drug. Each 1.5-g vial contains 1 g ampicillin sodium and 0.5 g sulbactam sodium.
• In patients with impaired renal function, decrease frequency of administration.
• Monitor LFT results during therapy, especially in patients with impaired liver function.
• If large doses are given or if therapy is prolonged, bacterial or fungal superinfection may occur, especially in elderly, debilitated, or immunosuppressed patients.
• Watch for signs and symptoms of hypersensitivity, such as erythematous maculopapular rash, urticaria, and anaphylaxis.
• Monitor for CDAD, which can be fatal. Antibiotic may need to be stopped and other treatment begun.

PATIENT TEACHING
• Tell patient to report all adverse reactions, including rash, fever, or chills. A rash is the most common allergic reaction.
• Warn patient that IM injection may cause pain at injection site.

anastrozole
an-AS-troh-zol

Arimidex◆

Therapeutic class: Antineoplastics
Pharmacologic class: Aromatase inhibitors

AVAILABLE FORMS
Tablets: 1 mg

INDICATIONS & DOSAGES
➤ First-line treatment of postmenopausal women with hormone receptor–positive or hormone receptor–unknown locally advanced or metastatic breast cancer; advanced breast cancer in postmenopausal women with disease progression after tamoxifen therapy; adjunctive treatment of postmenopausal women with hormone receptor–positive early breast cancer
Adults: 1 mg PO daily.
➤ Risk reduction for breast cancer in postmenopausal women ◆
Adults: 1 mg PO daily for 5 years.

ADMINISTRATION
PO
- Drug is a potential teratogen. Follow safe handling procedures when preparing, administering, or dispensing.
- Give drug without regard for meals.

ACTION
A selective nonsteroidal aromatase inhibitor that significantly lowers estradiol levels, which inhibits breast cancer cell growth in postmenopausal women.

Route	Onset	Peak	Duration
PO	<24 hr	2–5 hr	<7 days

Half-life: 50 hours.

ADVERSE REACTIONS
CNS: headache, asthenia, pain, dizziness, depression, paresthesia, anxiety, insomnia, stroke. **CV:** hot flashes, ***thromboembolic disease,*** chest pain, peripheral edema, HTN, vasodilation, cardiac ischemia. **EENT:** cataracts, pharyngitis, sinusitis. **GI:** nausea, vomiting, diarrhea, constipation, abdominal pain, anorexia, dry mouth, dyspepsia. **GU:** vaginal dryness, pelvic pain, UTI. **Metabolic:** weight gain, increased appetite. **Musculoskeletal:** bone pain, back pain, arthritis, arthralgia, osteoporosis, fractures. **Respiratory:** dyspnea, bronchitis, cough. **Skin:** rash, sweating. **Other:** lymphedema, flulike symptoms.

INTERACTIONS
Drug-drug. *Estrogen:* May decrease pharmacologic action of anastrozole. Use together isn't recommended.
Tamoxifen: May reduce anastrozole plasma level. Don't use together.

EFFECTS ON LAB TEST RESULTS
- May increase liver enzyme and cholesterol levels.

CONTRAINDICATIONS & CAUTIONS
- Contraindicated in patients hypersensitive to drug or its components.
- Use cautiously in patients with preexisting ischemic heart disease.
Dialyzable drug: Unknown.

PREGNANCY-LACTATION-REPRODUCTION
- Drug can cause fetal harm. Contraindicated in women who are or may become pregnant.
- Women of childbearing potential should use effective contraception during therapy and for at least 3 weeks after final dose.
- It isn't known if drug appears in human milk. Patient shouldn't breastfeed during therapy and for 2 weeks after final dose.

NURSING CONSIDERATIONS
- Give drug under supervision of a prescriber experienced in use of antineoplastics.
- Patients with hormone receptor–negative disease and patients who didn't respond to previous tamoxifen therapy rarely respond to anastrozole.
- For patients with advanced breast cancer, continue anastrozole until tumor progresses.
- Monitor bone mineral density because drug can decrease bone mineral density.
- Use drug only in postmenopausal women.
- Rule out pregnancy before starting drug.

PATIENT TEACHING

- Instruct patient to report adverse reactions, especially difficulty breathing, chest pain, or skin lesions or blisters.
- Tell patient to take medication at the same time each day.
- Stress need for follow-up care.
- Counsel female patient about risks of pregnancy during therapy and advise her to use effective contraception during therapy and for at least 3 weeks after final dose.
- Advise patient not to breastfeed during treatment and for 2 weeks after final dose.
- Tell patient that drug lowers estrogen level, which may lead to decreased bone strength and increased risk of fractures.

anidulafungin
ah-nid-doo-la-FUN-jin

Eraxis

Therapeutic class: Antifungals
Pharmacologic class: Echinocandins

AVAILABLE FORMS
Powder for injection: 50 mg/vial, 100 mg/vial

INDICATIONS & DOSAGES
➤ **Candidemia and other *Candida* infections (intra-abdominal abscess, peritonitis)**
Adults: A single 200-mg loading dose by IV infusion at no more than 1.1 mg/minute on day 1; then 100 mg daily for at least 14 days after last positive culture result.
➤ **Esophageal candidiasis**
Adults: A single 100-mg loading dose by IV infusion at no more than 1.1 mg/minute on day 1; then 50 mg daily for at least 14 days and for at least 7 days after symptoms resolve.

ADMINISTRATION
IV
▼ Obtain specimens for culture and sensitivity tests and baseline laboratory tests before starting therapy.
▼ Reconstitute each 50-mg vial with 15 mL of sterile water for injection. Reconstitute

each 100-mg vial with 30 mL of sterile water for injection.
▼ Reconstituted solution can be stored for up to 24 hours at room temperature before dilution into the infusion solution. Don't freeze.
▼ Further dilute with D_5W or NSS only.
▼ Add 50-mg dose (in 15 mL) to 50 mL of D_5W or NSS. Add 100-mg dose (in 30 mL) to 100 mL of D_5W or NSS. Add 200-mg dose (in 60 mL) to 200 mL of D_5W or NSS.
▼ Store infusion solution for up to 48 hours at room temperature or store frozen for at least 72 hours before administration.
▼ Don't infuse faster than 1.1 mg/minute. Minimum duration of infusion is 45 minutes for 50 mg, 90 minutes for 100 mg, and 180 minutes for 200 mg.
▼ **Incompatibilities:** Compatibility with other IV substances, additives, or drugs hasn't been established.

ACTION
Inhibits glucan synthase, which in turn inhibits formation of 1,3-β-D-glucan, an essential component of fungal cell walls.

Route	Onset	Peak	Duration
IV	<24 hr	Unknown	Unknown

Half-life: 40 to 50 hours.

ADVERSE REACTIONS
CNS: headache, fever, confusion, depression, insomnia. **CV:** *DVT,* hypotension, HTN, edema, chest pain. **EENT:** oral candidiasis. **GI:** nausea, vomiting, diarrhea, constipation, abdominal pain, dyspepsia. **GU:** UTI. **Hematologic:** *leukocytosis, anemia, thrombocytopenia.* **Metabolic:** hypokalemia, *hyperkalemia,* hyperglycemia, *hypoglycemia,* hypomagnesemia, dehydration. **Musculoskeletal:** back pain. **Respiratory:** dyspnea, pleural effusion, cough, respiratory distress, pneumonia. **Skin:** rash. **Other:** histamine-mediated symptoms (bronchospasm, dyspnea, flushing, hypotension, pruritus, rash, urticaria), infection, *sepsis.*

INTERACTIONS
None reported.

EFFECTS ON LAB TEST RESULTS
• May increase AST, ALT, alkaline phosphatase, GGT, amylase, lipase, bilirubin, CK, creatinine, urea, calcium, glucose, and sodium levels.
• May decrease glucose and magnesium levels. May increase or decrease potassium level.
• May prolong PT and decrease platelet count or increase WBC count.

CONTRAINDICATIONS & CAUTIONS
• Contraindicated in patients hypersensitive to drug, other echinocandins, or any component of the drug.
• Anaphylaxis has been reported. If reaction occurs, discontinue drug and give appropriate treatment.
• Use cautiously in patients with hepatic impairment and in elderly patients.
• Safety and effectiveness in children age 16 and younger haven't been established.
Dialyzable drug: No.

PREGNANCY-LACTATION-REPRODUCTION
• Use during pregnancy only if clearly needed.
• It isn't known if drug appears in human milk. Use cautiously in breastfeeding women.

NURSING CONSIDERATIONS
• Use only sterile water for injection to reconstitute powder and D_5W or NSS to infuse.
• To avoid histamine-mediated symptoms, such as rash, urticaria, flushing, itching, dyspnea, and hypotension, don't infuse faster than 1.1 mg/minute.
• Monitor patient closely for changes in liver function and blood cell counts during therapy.
• Notify prescriber about signs or symptoms of liver toxicity, such as dark urine, jaundice, abdominal pain, and fatigue.
• Patients with esophageal candidiasis who are HIV positive may need suppressive antifungal therapy after drug to prevent relapse.

PATIENT TEACHING
• Tell patient to immediately report rash, itching, trouble breathing, or other adverse reactions during infusion.

• Explain that blood tests will be needed to monitor the drug's effects.

SAFETY ALERT!

apalutamide
a-pa-LOO-ta-mide

Erleada

Therapeutic class: Antineoplastics
Pharmacologic class: Androgen receptor inhibitors

AVAILABLE FORMS
Tablets ⓞⓡⓖ: 60 mg

INDICATIONS & DOSAGES
➤ **Nonmetastatic, castration-resistant prostate cancer**
Adult males: 240 mg (four 60-mg tablets) PO once daily.
Adjust-a-dose: If grade 3 or greater toxicity occurs, withhold drug until symptoms improve to grade 1 or less or to original grade; then resume at same dosage or a reduced dosage (180 mg or 120 mg), if warranted.

ADMINISTRATION
PO
• Make sure patient swallows tablets whole. Don't break, crush, or allow patient to chew tablets.
• May give with or without food.
• Give a missed dose as soon as possible on the same day; then return to the normal schedule on the following day. Don't give extra tablets to make up for a missed dose.
• Store in original container; don't discard desiccant. Protect from light and moisture.

ACTION
Binds to androgen receptors to decrease tumor cell proliferation and increase apoptosis, leading to decreased tumor volume.

Route	Onset	Peak	Duration
PO	Unknown	2 hr	Unknown

Half-life: 3 days.

ADVERSE REACTIONS
CNS: fatigue, asthenia. **CV:** peripheral edema, HTN, hot flushes, *ischemic heart*

Reactions in bold italics are *life-threatening*. Interactions may have a *rapid onset* or a *delayed onset*.

disease, HF. **EENT:** conjunctivitis. **GI:** decreased appetite, diarrhea, nausea, stomatitis. **GU:** hematuria. **Hematologic:** anemia, leukopenia, lymphopenia. **Metabolic:** weight loss, hypothyroidism, hypercholesterolemia, hyperglycemia, hypertriglyceridemia, *hyperkalemia.* **Musculoskeletal:** arthralgia, fracture. **Skin:** rash, urticaria, pruritus. **Other:** fall.

INTERACTIONS
Drug-drug. *Strong CYP3A4/CYP2C8 inducers (rifampin):* May decrease apalutamide level. Monitor patient for loss of apalutamide activity.
Strong CYP3A4 (itraconazole, ketoconazole) or CYP2C8 (gemfibrozil) inhibitors: May increase apalutamide level. Monitor patient and reduce apalutamide dosage if necessary.
Substrates of CYP2C9 (warfarin), CYP2C19 (omeprazole), CYP3A4 (midazolam), and uridine diphosphate glycosyltransferase: May reduce levels of these drugs. Use other drugs as substitutes for these drugs if possible, or if use with apalutamide is necessary, monitor patient for loss of activity of these drugs.
Substrates of P-gp (fexofenadine), breast cancer resistance protein, and organic anion transporting polypeptide 1B1 (rosuvastatin): May reduce levels of these drugs. Use cautiously together if necessary. If use with apalutamide is necessary, monitor patient for loss of activity of these drugs.

EFFECTS ON LAB TEST RESULTS
• May increase TSH, potassium, cholesterol, glucose, and triglyceride levels.
• May decrease RBC, WBC, and lymphocyte counts.

CONTRAINDICATIONS & CAUTIONS
• Drug isn't indicated for use in females.
• Use cautiously in patients with a risk of falls and fractures.
• Drug may increase risk of seizures. Avoid use in patients with a history of seizures or with predisposing factors for seizures and in those receiving drugs known to decrease seizure threshold or to induce seizures.
• Drug may increase risk of hypothyroidism and CV disease.

• Safety and effectiveness in children haven't been established.
Dialyzable drug: Unknown.

PREGNANCY-LACTATION-REPRODUCTION
❸ *Alert:* Contraindicated for use in pregnant women. May cause fetal harm and loss of pregnancy.
• Patients with female partners of childbearing potential should use effective contraception during treatment and for 3 months after final dose. Patients with female partners who are pregnant should use a condom. Drug may impair fertility in males of reproductive potential.

NURSING CONSIDERATIONS
• Administer a gonadotropin-releasing hormone analogue concurrently unless patient has had a bilateral orchiectomy.
• Evaluate patient for risk of falls and fractures. Consider use of bone-targeted agents, if appropriate.
• Monitor patient for seizures. If seizure occurs, permanently discontinue drug.
• *Look alike–sound alike:* Don't confuse apalutamide with bicalutamide, flutamide, or nilutamide.

PATIENT TEACHING
• Instruct patient to take drug at the same time each day and to swallow tablets whole. Tell patient not to take extra tablets to make up for a missed dose.
• Inform patient receiving a gonadotropin-releasing hormone analogue that he will need to continue this drug while taking apalutamide.
• Warn patient that drug isn't indicated for use in females.
• Tell patient that drug may increase risk of falls and fractures.
• Caution patient that drug may increase the risk of seizures and to use care when involved in activities in which loss of consciousness could cause harm to himself or others.
• Tell patient to report all adverse reactions and to immediately report seizure, falls, or rash.
❸ *Alert:* Advise patient of reproductive potential to use effective contraception during treatment and for 3 months after final dose.

• Caution patient to use condoms while having sex with a pregnant woman. Drug may cause fetal harm.
• Educate patient of reproductive potential about the risk of impaired fertility. Advise patient not to donate sperm during treatment and for 3 months after final dose.

SAFETY ALERT!

apixaban
a-PIX-a-ban

Eliquis⬥

Therapeutic class: Anticoagulants
Pharmacologic class: Factor Xa inhibitors

AVAILABLE FORMS
Tablets: 2.5 mg, 5 mg

INDICATIONS & DOSAGES
➤ **Reduction of risk of stroke and systemic embolism in patients with nonvalvular atrial fibrillation**
Adults: 5 mg PO b.i.d.
Adjust-a-dose: Reduce dosage to 2.5 mg b.i.d. in patients with any two of the following characteristics: age 80 or older, body weight 60 kg or less, or serum creatinine 1.5 mg/dL or greater.
➤ **DVT prophylaxis after hip or knee replacement surgery**
Adults: 2.5 mg PO b.i.d. beginning 12 to 24 hours after surgery. Continue for 35 days after hip replacement surgery or for 12 days after knee replacement surgery.
➤ **DVT and PE**
Adults: 10 mg PO b.i.d. for 7 days followed by 5 mg PO b.i.d.; then, to reduce risk of recurrence after at least 6 months of treatment, 2.5 mg PO b.i.d.

ADMINISTRATION
PO
• May give without regard for food.
• Patient who doesn't take dose at the scheduled time should take the dose as soon as possible on the same day, then resume twice-daily administration. Patient shouldn't double the dose to make up for a missed dose.
• If patient can't swallow tablets, crush and suspend in water, D_5W, or apple juice or

mix with applesauce and give promptly PO, or crush and suspend in 60 mL of water or D_5W and give promptly through NG tube. Crushed tablets are stable in water, D_5W, apple juice, or applesauce for up to 4 hours.
• Store at room temperature.

ACTION
Selectively inhibits factor Xa, decreasing thrombin generation and thrombus development.

Route	Onset	Peak	Duration
PO	Unknown	3–4 hr	Unknown

Half-life: 12 hours.

ADVERSE REACTIONS
EENT: epistaxis. **GI:** nausea, rectal hemorrhage, bleeding gums. **GU:** hematuria, menorrhagia. **Hematologic:** *major bleeding,* anemia, bruising. **Respiratory:** hemoptysis.

INTERACTIONS
Drug-drug. *Aspirin and other antiplatelet agents/anticoagulants, heparin, NSAIDs, SSNRIs, SSRIs, thrombolytics:* May increase bleeding risk. Avoid use together.
Strong dual inducers of CYP3A4 and P-gp (carbamazepine, phenytoin, rifampin): May decrease apixaban concentration. Avoid use together.
Strong dual inhibitors of CYP3A4 and P-gp (clarithromycin, itraconazole, ketoconazole, ritonavir): May increase apixaban concentration. Decrease dosage by 50% in patients taking 5 or 10 mg b.i.d.; avoid use together in patients already taking 2.5 mg b.i.d.
Vorapaxar: May increase bleeding risk. Avoid use together.
Drug-herb. *Alfalfa, anise, bilberry:* May increase bleeding risk. Consider therapy modification.
St. John's wort: May decrease apixaban concentration. Avoid use together.
Drug-food. *Grapefruit juice:* May increase drug level and risk of bleeding. Use cautiously and monitor patient for bleeding.

EFFECTS ON LAB TEST RESULTS
• May increase LFT values.
• May prolong PT, INR, and aPTT.

Reactions in bold italics are *life-threatening*. Interactions may have a *rapid onset* or a *delayed onset*.

CONTRAINDICATIONS & CAUTIONS

• Contraindicated in patients hypersensitive to drug or its components and in those with active pathological bleeding.

• Use cautiously in patients at risk for severe bleeding (especially those concomitantly taking drugs that affect hemostasis).

Black Box Warning Discontinuing drug increases risk of thrombotic events. If anticoagulation with apixaban must be discontinued for a reason other than pathological bleeding, strongly consider coverage with another anticoagulant. ▪

Black Box Warning Consider potential risk of epidural or spinal hematoma versus benefit in patients scheduled for spinal procedures, such as spinal or epidural anesthesia or spinal puncture. Hematomas may result in long-term or permanent paralysis. Risk may increase with use of indwelling epidural catheters, concomitant use of drugs that affect hemostasis (NSAIDs, platelet inhibitors, anticoagulants), history of traumatic or repeated epidural or spinal punctures, or history of spinal deformity or surgery. ▪

🕄 **Alert:** Discontinue apixaban at least 48 hours before elective surgery or invasive procedures with a moderate or high risk of unacceptable or clinically significant bleeding.

🕄 **Alert:** Discontinue apixaban at least 24 hours before elective surgery or invasive procedures with a low risk of bleeding or when the bleeding would be noncritical in location and easily controlled.

• Bridging anticoagulation before the intervention isn't generally required. Restart apixaban as soon as adequate hemostasis has returned.

• Drug isn't recommended for patients with severe hepatic impairment or prosthetic heart valves.

• Bleeding risk is increased in patients with severe renal impairment.

Dialyzable drug: 14%.

⚠ *Overdose S&S:* Increased risk of bleeding.

PREGNANCY-LACTATION-REPRODUCTION

• Not recommended in pregnant women.

• It isn't known if drug appears in human milk. Not recommended for breastfeeding women.

NURSING CONSIDERATIONS

• Monitor patient for bleeding. Discontinue drug if acute pathologic bleeding occurs.

🕄 **Alert:** Promptly evaluate signs and symptom of blood loss. Drug can cause serious, potentially fatal bleeding.

Black Box Warning Monitor patients receiving neuraxial anesthesia or undergoing spinal puncture for neurologic impairment (midline back pain, sensory or motor deficits, such as numbness or weakness in lower limbs, bowel or bladder dysfunction). Treat impairment urgently. ▪

🕄 **Alert:** Removal of indwelling epidural or intrathecal catheters should be delayed for at least 24 hours after last dose of apixaban. Next dose of apixaban should be given no earlier than 5 hours after catheter removal. Don't give drug for at least 48 hours after traumatic or repeated epidural or spinal punctures.

• Administration of activated charcoal may be useful in the management of apixaban overdose or accidental ingestion. An agent to reverse the anti-factor Xa activity of apixaban is available.

• When switching from warfarin to apixaban, discontinue warfarin and start apixaban when INR is below 2.0.

• If switching from apixaban to warfarin, discontinue apixaban and begin both a parenteral anticoagulant and warfarin at the time the next dose of apixaban would have been taken. Discontinue the parenteral anticoagulant when INR reaches an acceptable range. Initial INR measurements during the transition to warfarin may not be useful because apixaban affects the INR.

• If switching between apixaban and anticoagulants other than warfarin, discontinue drug being taken and begin other drug at next scheduled dose.

PATIENT TEACHING

• Warn patient not to discontinue drug without first talking to prescriber, because of risk of clot formation and stroke.

• Tell patient to report all adverse reactions; caution patient that bruising or bleeding may occur more easily.

• Advise patient to report unusual bleeding.

• Instruct patient to inform all health care providers (including dentists) about taking this drug as well as other products known to affect bleeding (including nonprescription products, such as aspirin or NSAIDs) before scheduling surgery or medical or dental procedure and before taking any new drug.

• Tell female patient to inform practitioner if she is pregnant, plans to become pregnant, is breastfeeding, or intends to breastfeed during treatment.

apremilast
a-PRE-mi-last

Otezla

Therapeutic class: Antiarthritics
Pharmacologic class: Phosphodiesterase-4 inhibitors

AVAILABLE FORMS
Tablets ⓞⓣⓒ: 10 mg, 20 mg, 30 mg

INDICATIONS & DOSAGES
Adjust-a-dose (for all indications): In patients with severe renal impairment (CrCl less than 30 mL/minute), give doses according to a.m. schedule only (omit p.m. doses) from days 1 through 5. For day 6 and onward, give 30 mg once daily.

➤ **Active psoriatic arthritis; moderate to severe plaque psoriasis in patients who are candidates for phototherapy or systemic therapy**
Adults: Initially, 10 mg PO in a.m. on day 1; 10 mg PO b.i.d. (a.m. and p.m.) on day 2; 10 mg PO in a.m. and 20 mg PO in p.m. on day 3; 20 mg PO b.i.d. (a.m. and p.m.) on day 4; 20 mg PO in a.m. and 30 mg PO in p.m. on day 5; then 30 mg PO b.i.d. (a.m. and p.m.) on day 6 and thereafter.

ADMINISTRATION
PO
• Give without regard to meals.
• Don't crush, split, or allow patient to chew tablets.
• Store tablets below 86° F (30° C).

ACTION
Increases intracellular cAMP level. Its action in the treatment of psoriatic arthritis and psoriasis isn't well defined.

Route	Onset	Peak	Duration
PO	Unknown	2½ hr	Unknown

Half-life: 6 to 9 hours.

ADVERSE REACTIONS
CNS: headache, depression, fatigue, insomnia, migraine. **EENT:** nasopharyngitis. **GI:** anorexia, diarrhea, nausea, vomiting, upper abdominal pain, decreased appetite, dyspepsia, tooth abscess, GERD. **Metabolic:** weight loss. **Musculoskeletal:** back pain. **Respiratory:** URI, bronchitis. **Skin:** folliculitis.

INTERACTIONS
Drug-drug. *Strong CYP450 inducers (carbamazepine, phenobarbital, phenytoin, rifampin):* May decrease apremilast level, causing loss of effectiveness. Use together isn't recommended.
Drug-herb. *St. John's wort:* May decrease apremilast level. Consider therapy modification.

EFFECTS ON LAB TEST RESULTS
None reported.

CONTRAINDICATIONS & CAUTIONS
• Contraindicated in patients hypersensitive to drug or its components.
❸ *Alert:* Use cautiously in patients with history of depression or suicidal thoughts. Weigh risks and benefits of using drug in these patients.
• Use cautiously in patients with severe renal impairment.
• Safety and effectiveness in children haven't been established.
Dialyzable drug: Unknown.

PREGNANCY-LACTATION-REPRODUCTION
• Use cautiously in pregnant women and only if benefits outweigh risks to the fetus. Enroll pregnant patients in pregnancy exposure registry (1-877-311-8972) to monitor pregnancy outcomes.
• It isn't known if drug appears in human milk. Use cautiously in breastfeeding women.

Reactions in bold italics are *life-threatening*. Interactions may have a *rapid onset* or a *delayed onset*.

NURSING CONSIDERATIONS
• Titration to maintenance dose is intended to reduce GI symptoms with initial therapy.
• Monitor patient for depression or suicidal thoughts.
• Monitor patient regularly for unexplained or significant weight loss. Evaluate cause and consider discontinuing drug.

PATIENT TEACHING
• Explain to patient that drug may cause weight loss.
⚠ *Alert:* Warn patient and caregivers to immediately report signs and symptoms of depression or suicidal thoughts.
• Instruct patient to titrate drug as directed to reduce GI symptoms.
• Advise patient that drug may be taken without regard to food and not to crush, chew, or split tablets.
• Educate patient on possible adverse effects of this drug, such as headache, diarrhea, nausea, vomiting, upper abdominal pain, weight loss, or infections in the nose, throat, or lungs.

---

aprepitant
ah-PRE-pit-ant

Cinvanti, Emend

fosaprepitant dimeglumine
Emend

Therapeutic class: Antiemetics
Pharmacologic class: Substance P and neurokinin-1 receptor antagonists

---

AVAILABLE FORMS
aprepitant
Capsules: 40 mg, 80 mg, 125 mg
Injection (emulsion): 130 mg/18 mL single-dose vial
Powder for oral suspension (kit): 125 mg
fosaprepitant dimeglumine
Injection: 150-mg single-dose vial

INDICATIONS & DOSAGES
➤ **To prevent nausea and vomiting after highly emetogenic chemotherapy (HEC) (including cisplatin) and moderately emetogenic chemotherapy (MEC), with a 5-HT$_3$ antagonist and a corticosteroid**

Adults and children age 12 and older (capsules): On day 1 of chemotherapy, 125 mg PO 1 hour before treatment; on days 2 and 3, give 80 mg PO 1 hour before chemotherapy or if no chemotherapy is scheduled, give in the morning.
Adults and children age 12 and older (fosaprepitant): Single-day regimen: On day 1, 150 mg IV over 20 to 30 minutes given 30 minutes before chemotherapy. For 3-day dosage regimen in children ages 12 to 17: On day 1, 115 mg IV over 30 minutes given 30 minutes before chemotherapy; on days 2 and 3, give 80 mg PO 1 hour before treatment or, if no chemotherapy is scheduled, give in the morning.
Children ages 6 months to younger than age 12 years weighing at least 6 kg (fosaprepitant): Single-day regimen for children ages 2 to younger than 12: 4 mg/kg (maximum dose, 150 mg) IV over 60 minutes given 30 minutes before chemotherapy; for children ages 6 months to younger than 2 years: 5 mg/kg (maximum dose, 150 mg) IV over 60 minutes given 30 minutes before chemotherapy. For 3-day regimen in children ages 6 months to younger than 12 years: On day 1, 3 mg/kg (maximum dose, 115 mg) IV over 60 minutes given 30 minutes before chemotherapy; on days 2 and 3, give 2 mg/kg (maximum dose, 80 mg) PO 1 hour before chemotherapy or, if no chemotherapy is scheduled, give in the morning.
Adults unable to swallow capsules and children age 6 months to younger than 12 years weighing 6 kg or more (oral suspension): On day 1 of chemotherapy, 3 mg/kg PO 1 hour before treatment; maximum dose, 125 mg. On days 2 and 3, 2 mg/kg PO 1 hour before chemotherapy or, if no chemotherapy is scheduled, give in the morning; maximum dose, 80 mg.
Adults (aprepitant [Cinvanti]): Single dose regimen for HEC: On day 1, 130 mg IV over 30 minutes given 30 minutes before chemotherapy. Three-day regimen for MEC: On day 1, 100 mg IV over 30 minutes given 30 minutes before chemotherapy; on days 2 and 3, 80 mg PO 1 hour before chemotherapy or, if no chemotherapy is scheduled, give in the morning.

➤ **To prevent postoperative nausea and vomiting**
Adults: 40 mg PO within 3 hours before induction of anesthesia.

ADMINISTRATION
PO
• Give drug without regard for food.
• Drug may be given with other antiemetics.
• Oral suspension should be prepared by a health care provider, but once prepared may be administered by a health care provider, patient, or caregiver.
• Refer to manufacturer's instructions for preparing oral suspension.
• Refrigerate prepared oral suspension until administered. May store at room temperature for up to 3 hours before use. Discard any dose remaining after 72 hours.
IV
⬥ *Alert:* In children, administer drug through a CVAD.
Fosaprepitant (Emend)
▼ Reconstitute with 5 mL of NSS. Add the NSS along the vial wall to prevent foaming. Swirl gently and avoid shaking.
▼ Add entire reconstituted volume to infusion bag containing 145 mL of NSS. Total volume will be 150 mL and concentration will be 1 mg/mL.
▼ Gently invert the bag two to three times.
▼ For children age 12 and older, the volume to administer in mL is equal to the recommended dose in mg.
▼ In children age 6 months to younger than age 12, the volume to be administered is calculated as follows: Volume to administer (mL) = recommended dose (mg/kg) × weight (kg).
Aprepitant (Cinvanti)
▼ For 130-mg dose, aseptically prepare an infusion bag filled with 130 mL NSS or D_5W; then withdraw 18 mL from the vial and transfer it into infusion bag to yield a total volume of 148 mL.
▼ For 100-mg dose, aseptically prepare an infusion bag filled with 100 mL NSS or D_5W; then withdraw 14 mL from the vial and transfer it into infusion bag to yield a total volume of 114 mL.
▼ Gently invert the prepared bag four to five times. Avoid shaking.

▼ Before administering either drug, inspect bag for particulate matter and discoloration. Discard if particulates or discoloration is observed.
▼ Final fosaprepitant (Emend) solution is stable for 24 hours at ambient room temperature; Cinvanti is stable for 6 hours in NSS or 12 hours in D_5W.
▼ **Incompatibilities:** Any solutions containing divalent cations (e.g., Ca^{2+}, Mg^{2+}), including lactated Ringer solution and Hartmann solution.

ACTION
Inhibits emesis by selectively antagonizing substance P and neurokinin-1 receptors in the brain; appears to be synergistic with $5\text{-}HT_3$ antagonists and corticosteroids.

Route	Onset	Peak	Duration
PO	Unknown	3–4 hr	Unknown
IV	Unknown	<30 min	Unknown

Half-life: 9 to 13 hours.

ADVERSE REACTIONS
CNS: asthenia, fatigue, dizziness, fever, headache. **CV:** *bradycardia*, HTN, hypotension, dehydration. **EENT:** dry mouth, mucous membrane disorder, tinnitus. **GI:** anorexia, constipation, diarrhea, nausea, abdominal pain, flatulence, gastritis, heartburn, vomiting. **GU:** UTI. **Hematologic:** *neutropenia*, anemia. **Respiratory:** hiccups. **Skin:** pruritus, infusion-site pain, infusion-site induration. **Other:** dehydration, alopecia.

INTERACTIONS
Drug-drug. *Alprazolam, midazolam, triazolam:* May increase levels of these drugs. Watch for CNS effects, such as increased sedation. Decrease benzodiazepine dose by 50%.
Atazanavir, clarithromycin, diltiazem, erythromycin, itraconazole, ketoconazole, nefazodone, nelfinavir, ritonavir, troleandomycin, other CYP3A4 inhibitors: May increase aprepitant level and risk of toxicity. Use together cautiously.
Carbamazepine, phenytoin, rifampin, other CYP3A4 inducers: May decrease aprepitant level. Watch for decreased antiemetic effect.

Reactions in bold italics are *life-threatening*. Interactions may have a *rapid onset* or a *delayed onset*.

Dexamethasone, methylprednisolone: May increase levels of these drugs and risk of toxicity. Decrease PO corticosteroid dose by 50%; decrease IV methylprednisolone dose by 25%.

Diltiazem: May increase diltiazem level. Monitor HR and BP. Avoid using together.

Docetaxel, etoposide, ifosfamide, imatinib, irinotecan, paclitaxel, vinorelbine, vinblastine, vincristine: May increase levels and risk of toxicity of these drugs. Use together cautiously.

Hormonal contraceptives: May decrease contraceptive effectiveness. Female patients should use additional birth control method during therapy and for 1 month after last dose.

Paroxetine: May decrease paroxetine and aprepitant effects. Monitor patient for effectiveness.

Phenytoin: May decrease effectiveness of aprepitant. Avoid use together.

Pimozide: May increase pimozide level. Use together is contraindicated.

Warfarin: May decrease warfarin effectiveness. Monitor INR carefully for 2 weeks after each aprepitant treatment.

Drug-herb. *St. John's wort:* May decrease antiemetic effects by inducing CYP3A4. Discourage use together.

Drug-food. *Grapefruit juice:* May increase drug level and risk of toxicity. Discourage use together.

EFFECTS ON LAB TEST RESULTS
• May increase alkaline phosphatase, AST, ALT, BUN, creatinine, glucose, and urine protein levels. May decrease sodium level.
• May decrease WBC and neutrophil counts.

CONTRAINDICATIONS & CAUTIONS
• Contraindicated in patients hypersensitive to fosaprepitant, aprepitant, or their components. Hypersensitivity reactions have been reported. Also contraindicated in patients taking pimozide.
• Use cautiously in patients receiving chemotherapy drugs metabolized mainly via CYP3A4 and in those with severe hepatic disease.
• Drug isn't approved for prevention of postoperative nausea and vomiting in children.

Dialyzable drug: No.
⚠ *Overdose S&S:* Drowsiness, headache.

PREGNANCY-LACTATION-REPRODUCTION
• Use during pregnancy only if clearly needed.
• Cinvanti contains alcohol and shouldn't be used in pregnant women.
• Women taking hormonal contraceptives should use an additional form of contraception during therapy and for 1 month after final dose.
• It isn't known if drug appears in human milk. Patient should discontinue breastfeeding or discontinue drug.

NURSING CONSIDERATIONS
• Avoid giving drug for more than 3 days per chemotherapy cycle.
⚠ *Alert:* IV form is only given on day 1 of a 3-day antiemetic regimen.
⚠ *Alert:* Before giving drug, screen patient carefully for possible drug and herb interactions.
• Don't give drug for existing nausea or vomiting.
• Expect to give drug with other antiemetics to treat breakthrough emesis.
• Monitor CBC, LFT results, and creatinine level periodically during therapy.
• *Look alike–sound alike:* Don't confuse aprepitant (oral and IV form) with fosaprepitant (IV form). Don't confuse Emend with Vfend.

PATIENT TEACHING
• Advise patient to report all adverse reactions to prescriber.
• If nausea or vomiting occurs, instruct patient to take breakthrough antiemetics rather than more aprepitant.
• Urge patient to report use of any other drugs or herbs.
• Caution patient against taking drug with grapefruit juice.
• Advise female patient who takes a hormonal contraceptive to use an additional form of birth control during therapy and for 1 month after last dose.
• Tell patient who takes warfarin that PT and INR will be monitored closely for 2 weeks after therapy starts.

- Teach patient to take drug 1 hour before chemotherapy, then daily in the morning or as directed.

SAFETY ALERT!

argatroban
ahr-GAH-troh-ban

Therapeutic class: Anticoagulants
Pharmacologic class: Direct thrombin inhibitors

AVAILABLE FORMS
Injection: 1 mg/mL in 50-mL, 125-mL, and 250-mL vials; 100 mg/mL in 2.5-mL vial

INDICATIONS & DOSAGES
➤ **To prevent or treat thrombosis in patients with heparin-induced thrombocytopenia**
Adults without hepatic impairment: 2 mcg/kg/minute, given as a continuous IV infusion; adjust dose until the steady-state aPTT is 1½ to 3 times the initial baseline value, not to exceed 100 seconds; maximum dose, 10 mcg/kg/minute. See current manufacturer's label for recommended doses and infusion rates.
Adjust-a-dose: For adults with moderate or severe hepatic impairment, reduce first dose to 0.5 mcg/kg/minute, given as a continuous infusion. Monitor aPTT closely and adjust dosage as needed.
➤ **Anticoagulation in patients with or at risk for heparin-induced thrombocytopenia during PCI**
Adults: Start a continuous IV infusion at 25 mcg/kg/minute and give a 350 mcg/kg IV bolus over 3 to 5 minutes. Check activated clotting time (ACT) 5 to 10 minutes after bolus dose is completed. Proceed with procedure if ACT is more than 300 seconds.
Adjust-a-dose: Use the following table to adjust dosage.

Activated clotting time (ACT)	Additional IV bolus	Continuous IV infusion
<300 sec	150 mcg/kg	30 mcg/kg/min*
>450 sec	None needed	15 mcg/kg/min*

*Check ACT again after 5 to 10 minutes.

Once a therapeutic ACT (300 to 450 sec) has been achieved, continue this dose for the duration of the procedure. In case of dissection, impending abrupt closure, thrombus formation during the procedure, or inability to achieve or maintain an ACT exceeding 300 seconds, give an additional bolus of 150 mcg/kg and increase infusion rate to 40 mcg/kg/minute. Check ACT again after 5 to 10 minutes.

ADMINISTRATION
IV
▼ Before starting therapy, obtain a complete list of patient's prescription and OTC drugs and supplements, including herbs.
▼ Stop all parenteral anticoagulants before giving drug. Giving with antiplatelets, thrombolytics, and other anticoagulants may increase risk of bleeding.
▼ Before starting drug, get results of baseline coagulation tests, platelet count, Hb level, and hematocrit, and report any abnormalities to prescriber.
▼ Dilute each 2.5-mL vial 100-fold by mixing it with 250 mL of NSS, D_5W, or lactated Ringer injection to a final concentration of 1 mg/mL. Dilution isn't required for the 50-mL vial.
▼ Mix the solution by repeated inversion of the diluent bag for 1 minute.
▼ Don't expose solution to direct sunlight.
▼ See manufacturer's instructions for storage.
▼ **Incompatibilities:** Other IV drugs.

ACTION
Reversibly binds to the thrombin-active site and inhibits thrombin-catalyzed or -induced reactions: fibrin formation; coagulation factor V, VIII, and XIII activation; protein C activation; and platelet aggregation. Inhibits the action of free and clot-associated thrombin.

Route	Onset	Peak	Duration
IV	Rapid	1–3 hr	Duration of infusion

Half-life: 39 to 51 minutes.

ADVERSE REACTIONS
CNS: *cerebrovascular disorder, hemorrhage,* fever, pain, headache. **CV:** *atrial fibrillation, cardiac arrest,* hypotension, *ventricular tachycardia,* chest pain, angina,

---

Reactions in bold italics are *life-threatening*. Interactions may have a *rapid onset* or a *delayed onset*.

bradycardia, MI, groin or brachial bleeding. **GI:** abdominal pain, diarrhea, *GI bleeding,* nausea, vomiting. **GU:** abnormal renal function, hematuria, UTI. **Hematologic:** anemia, *bleeding.* **Respiratory:** cough, dyspnea, pneumonia, hemoptysis. **Other:** allergic reactions, infection, *sepsis.*

INTERACTIONS

Drug-drug. *Glycoprotein IIb/IIIa inhibitors (abciximab, eptifibatide, tirofiban), thrombolytics:* May increase risk of bleeding, including intracranial bleeding. Avoid using together. Safety and effectiveness of concurrent use haven't been established.
Heparin: May increase risk of bleeding. Allow sufficient time for heparin's effect on aPTT to decrease before starting argatroban.
Warfarin: May prolong PT and INR and may increase risk of bleeding. Monitor patient closely.
Drug-herb. *Herbs with anticoagulant or antiplatelet properties (alfalfa, anise, bilberry, others):* May increase risk of bleeding. Discourage use together.

EFFECTS ON LAB TEST RESULTS
• May decrease Hb level and hematocrit.

CONTRAINDICATIONS & CAUTIONS
• Contraindicated in patients who have overt major bleeding or who are hypersensitive to drug or any of its components.
• Use cautiously in patients with hepatic disease or conditions that increase the risk of hemorrhage, such as severe HTN.
• Use cautiously in patients who have just had lumbar puncture, spinal anesthesia, or major surgery, especially of the brain, spinal cord, or eye; patients with hematologic conditions causing increased bleeding tendencies, such as congenital or acquired bleeding disorders; and patients with GI ulcers or other lesions.
• Use cautiously in critically ill patients; reduced dosages may be needed.
Dialyzable drug: 20% during 4-hour hemodialysis session.
⚠ *Overdose S&S:* Excessive anticoagulation, with or without bleeding.

PREGNANCY-LACTATION-REPRODUCTION
• There are no adequate well-controlled studies in pregnant women. Use during pregnancy only if clearly needed.
• It isn't known if drug appears in human milk. Patient should discontinue breastfeeding or discontinue drug.

NURSING CONSIDERATIONS
• Check aPTT 2 hours after giving drug; dose adjustments may be required to get a targeted aPTT of 1.5 to 3 times the baseline, no longer than 100 seconds. Steady state is achieved 1 to 3 hours after starting drug.
• Draw blood for ACT every 20 to 30 minutes during prolonged PCI.
⚙ **Alert:** Patients can hemorrhage from any site in body. Unexplained decreases in hematocrit or BP or other unexplained symptoms may signify a hemorrhagic event.
• To convert to warfarin therapy, give expected daily dose of warfarin PO with argatroban at up to 2 mcg/kg/minute until INR exceeds 4 on combined therapy. If argatroban infusion rate is greater than 2 mcg/kg/minute, decrease rate to 2 mcg/kg/minute before administering warfarin. After argatroban is stopped, repeat INR in 4 to 6 hours. If the repeat INR is less than desired therapeutic range, resume IV argatroban infusion. Repeat procedure daily until desired therapeutic range on warfarin alone is reached.
• *Look alike–sound alike:* Don't confuse argatroban with Aggrastat or Aggrenox.

PATIENT TEACHING
• Tell patient that drug can cause bleeding and to report unusual bruising or bleeding (nosebleeds, bleeding gums) or tarry stools to prescriber immediately.
• Advise patient to avoid activities that carry a risk of injury and to use a soft bristle toothbrush and an electric razor during therapy.
• Advise patient to report use of any herbal therapy; many herbs have anticoagulant, antiplatelet, and fibrinolytic properties.
• Instruct patient to report wheezing, trouble breathing, or rash.
• Instruct female patient who is pregnant, has recently delivered, or is breastfeeding to notify prescriber.

• Tell patient to report GI ulcers or liver disease, recent surgery, radiation treatment, falling episodes, or injury to prescriber.

ARIPiprazole ⚇
air-eh-PIP-rah-zole

Abilify⬦, Abilify Maintena, Abilify MyCite

ARIPiprazole lauroxil ⚇
Aristada, Aristada Initio

Therapeutic class: Antipsychotics
Pharmacologic class: Quinolinone derivatives

AVAILABLE FORMS
Oral solution: 1 mg/mL
Suspension for IM use (extended-release): 300 mg, 400 mg (Abilify Maintena); 441 mg/1.6 mL, 662 mg/2.4 mL, 882 mg/ 3.2 mL, 1,064 mg/3.9 mL in prefilled syringes (Aristada); 675 mg/2.4 mL in prefilled syringe (Aristada Initio)
Tablets: 2 mg, 5 mg, 10 mg, 15 mg, 20 mg, 30 mg
Tablets (ODTs): 10 mg, 15 mg
Tablets (with sensor [Abilify MyCite]) ⓞⓝⓒ: 2 mg, 5 mg, 10 mg, 15 mg, 20 mg, 30 mg

INDICATIONS & DOSAGES
Adjust-a-dose (for all indications except adjunctive treatment of major depressive disorder): Refer to manufacturer's instructions for drug-interaction and missed dose dosage adjustments.
➤ Schizophrenia (oral, IM [Abilify Maintena])
Adults: Initially, 10 to 15 mg PO daily; increase to maximum daily dose of 30 mg, if needed, after at least 2 weeks. Continue responding patients on the lowest dosage needed to maintain remission. Periodically reassess patients to determine the need for maintenance treatment.
Or, 400 mg IM monthly. For patients who have never taken aripiprazole, establish tolerability with aripiprazole PO before initiating treatment with Abilify Maintena. It may take up to 2 weeks to fully assess tolerability. After the first IM injection, administer 10 to

20 mg aripiprazole PO for 14 days. For patients already stable on another oral antipsychotic and known to tolerate aripiprazole, after the first IM injection, continue treatment with the other antipsychotic for 14 days.
Maintenance dosage is 400 mg IM monthly, no sooner than 26 days after previous injection. If adverse reactions occur, consider reducing dosage to 300 mg IM monthly. Refer to manufacturer's instructions for dosage adjustments for missed doses.
Adolescents ages 13 to 17: Initially, 2 mg PO daily; increase to 5 mg after 2 days, then to recommended dose of 10 mg in 2 more days. May titrate to maximum daily dose of 30 mg in 5-mg increments. Responding patients should be continued on the lowest dosage needed to maintain remission. Patients should be periodically reassessed to determine the need for maintenance treatment.
➤ Schizophrenia (Aristada, Aristada Initio)
Adults: Establish tolerability with oral aripiprazole before initiating treatment with aripiprazole lauroxil, which may take up to 2 weeks. Base initial monthly dose of Aristada on current oral daily aripiprazole dose. If current oral aripiprazole dose is 10 mg/day, give 441 mg IM in the deltoid or gluteal muscle once per month. If current oral aripiprazole dose is 15 mg/day, give 662 mg once per month, 882 mg once every 6 weeks, or 1,064 mg once every 2 months IM in the gluteal muscle. If current oral aripiprazole dose is 20 mg/day or more, give 882 mg IM in the gluteal muscle once every month. Continue oral aripiprazole for 21 consecutive days after initiation of the first monthly dose or give a single injection of 675 mg Aristada Initio in the deltoid or gluteal muscle and one dose of oral aripiprazole 30 mg. Avoid injecting both preparations into the same deltoid or gluteal muscle.
The first Aristada injection may be administered on the same day as Aristada Initio or up to 10 days after.
Adjust-a-dose: Adjust dosage as needed; if a dose is required earlier than the recommended interval, don't administer earlier than 14 days after the previous injection.

Reactions in bold italics are *life-threatening*. Interactions may have a *rapid onset* or a *delayed onset*.

➤ Bipolar mania, including manic and mixed episodes, with or without psychotic features; adjunctive therapy with either lithium or valproate for treatment of manic and mixed episodes associated with bipolar I disorder with or without psychotic features

Adults: Initially, 15 mg PO once daily as monotherapy or 10 to 15 mg PO once daily as adjunctive therapy with lithium or valproate. Target dose is 15 mg/day as monotherapy or adjunctive therapy. May increase dose to maximum of 30 mg/day based on clinical response. For maintenance, continue responding patients on monotherapy on the lowest dosage needed to maintain remission. Periodically reassess patients to determine the long-term usefulness of maintenance treatment.

Children ages 10 to 17: Initially, 2 mg PO daily; increase to 5 mg PO daily after 2 days, then to recommended dose of 10 mg after 2 additional days. May titrate to maximum daily dose of 30 mg in 5-mg increments every 5 days. Give as monotherapy or as adjunct to lithium or valproate. For maintenance, continue responding patients on monotherapy on the lowest dosage needed to maintain remission. Periodically reassess patients to determine the need for maintenance treatment.

➤ Bipolar I disorder maintenance monotherapy

Adults: For patients who have never taken aripiprazole, establish tolerability with oral aripiprazole before initiating treatment with extended-release IM suspension. Once tolerability is established, give 400 mg (extended-release suspension) IM monthly. After first injection, continue oral aripiprazole for 14 consecutive days to achieve therapeutic aripiprazole concentrations during initiation of therapy. Maintenance dosage is 400 mg IM monthly, given no sooner than 26 days after previous injection.

▧ *Adjust-a-dose:* If adverse reactions occur with 400-mg dose or if patient is a poor metabolizer of CYP2D6, consider reducing dosage to 300 mg IM monthly. Refer to manufacturer's instructions for toxicity-related dosage adjustments.

➤ Adjunctive treatment of major depressive disorder

Adults: Initially, 2 to 5 mg PO daily. Dose range is 2 to 15 mg/day. Dosage adjustments of up to 5 mg/day should occur gradually, at intervals of no less than 1 week.

➤ Irritability associated with autistic disorder

Children ages 6 to 17: Initially, 2 mg PO daily for 7 days. Increase dosage to 5 mg/day, with subsequent increases to 10 or 15 mg/day if needed. Dosage adjustments of up to 5 mg/day should occur gradually, at intervals of no less than 1 week.

➤ Tourette disorder

Children ages 6 to 18 weighing 50 kg or more: Initially, 2 mg/day PO for 2 days; then increase to 5 mg/day with a target dose of 10 mg/day on day 8. If optimal control of tics isn't achieved, increase by 5 mg/day at intervals of no less than 1 week to maximum of 20 mg/day.

Children ages 6 to 18 weighing less than 50 kg: Initially, 2 mg/day PO, increasing to target dose of 5 mg/day after 2 days. If optimal control of tics isn't achieved, increase to 10 mg/day. Adjust dosage at intervals of no less than 1 week.

ADMINISTRATION
PO
• Give drug without regard for food.
• Substitute the oral solution on a milligram-by-milligram basis up to 25 mg. Give patients taking 30-mg tablets 25 mg of solution.
• Keep ODTs in blister package until ready to use. Don't split tablet.
• Abilify MyCite drug-device combination system consists of tablets with an embedded ingestible event marker (IEM) to track drug ingestion, a wearable patch containing a sensor that detects the signal from the IEM after ingestion and transmits data to a smartphone, a smartphone application (app) to display patient information, and a Web-based portal for health care professionals and caregivers. Refer to manufacturer's detailed instructions for use.
• Apply the MyCite patch when instructed by the app to the left side of the body just above the lower edge of the rib cage. Don't place patch over skin that is irritated, inflamed, or not intact, or is overlapping the area where the last patch was located.

- Patient must swallow tablets with sensor whole; don't divide, crush, or allow patient to chew these tablets.
- Don't repeat dose if tablet with sensor isn't detected after ingestion.
- Store oral solution at room temperature; it can be used up to 6 months after opening.

IM
- Inject slowly into the deltoid or gluteal muscle according to manufacturer's instructions; rotate injection sites.

⊙ *Alert:* Don't confuse IM dosage forms (Abilify Maintena, Aristada, Aristada Initio).

ACTION
Thought to exert partial agonist activity at dopamine 2 and 5-HT_{1A} receptors and antagonist activity at 5-HT_{2A} receptors.

Route	Onset	Peak	Duration
PO	Unknown	3–5 hr	Unknown
IM	Unknown	1–3 hr	Unknown
		4–7 days (Abilify Maintena)	

Half-life: About 75 hours in patients with normal metabolism. Abilify Maintena, 30 to 45 days; Aristada, 54 to 57 days; Aristada Initio, 15 to 18 days.

ADVERSE REACTIONS
CNS: headache, anxiety, insomnia, lightheadedness, somnolence, sedation, akathisia, *NMS, seizures,* extrapyramidal disorder (children), tremor, asthenia, depression, fatigue, dizziness, nervousness, hostility, manic behavior, confusion, abnormal gait, cogwheel rigidity, fever, tardive dyskinesia, restlessness, agitation, thinking abnormalities, impaired concentration, incoordination. **CV:** peripheral edema, chest pain, HTN, tachycardia, orthostatic hypotension, *bradycardia.* **EENT:** blurred vision, conjunctivitis, photophobia, ear pain, epistaxis, rhinitis, toothache, increased salivation, nasopharyngitis, pharyngolaryngeal pain. **GI:** nausea, vomiting, constipation, anorexia, dry mouth, dyspepsia, diarrhea, abdominal pain, esophageal dysmotility, increased appetite, toothache, GERD.
GU: urinary incontinence, decreased libido, erectile dysfunction, dysmenorrhea. **Hematologic:** ecchymosis, anemia, *neutropenia.*

Metabolic: weight gain, weight loss, hyperglycemia, hypercholesterolemia. **Musculoskeletal:** neck pain, neck stiffness, muscle cramps, myalgia, extremity pain.
Respiratory: dyspnea, pneumonia, cough, URI. **Skin:** rash, dry skin, pruritus, sweating, ulcer. **Other:** flulike syndrome, *suicidal ideation and behaviors.*

INTERACTIONS
Drug-drug. *Antihypertensives:* May enhance antihypertensive effects. Monitor BP.
Benzodiazepines: May cause excessive sedation and orthostatic hypotension. Monitor patient closely.
Carbamazepine and other CYP3A4 inducers: May decrease aripiprazole level and effectiveness. See manufacturer's instructions for dosage adjustments. Monitor patient closely.
CNS depressants: May lead to enhanced CNS depression. Use together with caution.
Ketoconazole and other CYP3A4 inhibitors: May increase risk of serious toxic effects. Start treatment with reduced dose of aripiprazole, and monitor patient closely.
Metoclopramide: May increase risk of extrapyramidal reactions. Use together is contraindicated.
Black Box Warning *Opioid class warning:* May cause slow or difficult breathing, sedation, and death. Avoid use together. If use together is necessary, limit dosage and duration of each drug to the minimum necessary for desired effect. ∎
Potential CYP2D6 inhibitors (fluoxetine, paroxetine, quinidine): May increase aripiprazole level and toxicity. See manufacturer's instructions for dosage adjustments.
Drug-food. *Grapefruit juice:* May increase drug level. Tell patient not to take drug with grapefruit juice.
Drug-lifestyle. *Alcohol use:* May increase CNS effects. Discourage use together.

EFFECTS ON LAB TEST RESULTS
- May increase CK and glucose levels.
- May decrease WBC count and ANC.

CONTRAINDICATIONS & CAUTIONS
- Contraindicated in patients hypersensitive to drug.

Black Box Warning *Opioid class warning:*
Opioids should only be prescribed with CNS
depressants such as aripiprazole and benzodiazepines to patients for whom alternative
treatment options are inadequate. ■

• Drug isn't approved for use in children
with depression.

Black Box Warning Elderly patients with
dementia-related psychosis treated with
atypical antipsychotics are at an increased
risk for death. Drug isn't approved for treatment of patients with dementia-related
psychosis. ■

• Use cautiously in patients with CV disease, cerebrovascular disease, or conditions
that could predispose patient to hypotension,
such as dehydration or hypovolemia.

• Life-threatening arrhythmias have occurred with therapeutic doses of antipsychotics.

• Use cautiously in patients with history of
seizures or with conditions that lower the
seizure threshold.

• Use cautiously in patients who engage in
strenuous exercise, are exposed to extreme
heat, take anticholinergics, or are susceptible
to dehydration.

• Use cautiously in patients with Lewy body
dementia or Parkinson disease; drug may
aggravate motor disturbances.

• Use cautiously in patients at risk for aspiration pneumonia, such as those with
Alzheimer disease.

• Use cautiously in patients at risk for falls,
including those who have diseases or conditions or are taking medications that may
cause somnolence, orthostatic hypotension,
or motor or sensory instability.

• Discontinue drug at first sign of blood
dyscrasia or if ANC is less than 1,000/mm³.

• Abilify MyCite drug-device product is
only approved for use in adults.

Dializable drug: Unlikely.

⚠ Overdose S&S: Somnolence, tremor, vomiting, acidosis, aggression, atrial fibrillation,
bradycardia, coma, confusion, seizures, depressed level of consciousness, HTN, hypokalemia, hypotension, increased AST and
blood CK levels, lethargy, loss of consciousness, aspiration pneumonia, prolonged QRS
complex, prolonged QT interval, respiratory
arrest, status epilepticus, tachycardia.

PREGNANCY-LACTATION-REPRODUCTION

• Safety of atypical antipsychotic use in
pregnant women hasn't been well studied;
routine use isn't recommended. Use during
pregnancy only if potential benefit justifies
potential risk to the fetus.

⊙ Alert: Neonates exposed to antipsychotics
during the third trimester are at risk for developing extrapyramidal signs and symptoms (repetitive muscle movements of the
face and body) and withdrawal signs and
symptoms (agitation, abnormally increased
or decreased muscle tone, tremors, sleepiness, severe difficulty breathing, difficulty
feeding) after delivery.

• Enroll pregnant women exposed to aripi-
razole in the National Pregnancy Registry
for Atypical Antipsychotics (1-866-961-
2388).

• Drug appears in human milk. Use in
breastfeeding women isn't recommended.

NURSING CONSIDERATIONS

⊙ Alert: NMS may occur. Monitor patient
for hyperpyrexia, muscle rigidity, altered
mental status, irregular pulse or BP, tachycardia, diaphoresis, and cardiac arrhythmias.

• If signs and symptoms of NMS occur, immediately stop drug and notify prescriber.

• Monitor patient for signs and symptoms
of tardive dyskinesia. Elderly patients, especially women, are at highest risk of developing this adverse effect.

⊙ Alert: Fatal cerebrovascular adverse events
(stroke, TIA) may occur in elderly patients
with dementia. Drug isn't safe or effective in
these patients.

Black Box Warning Drug may increase the
risk of suicidal thinking and behavior in children, adolescents, and young adults ages 18
to 24 during the first 2 months of treatment,
especially in those with major depressive
or other psychiatric disorder. Monitor patients for worsening or emergence of suicidal thoughts and behaviors. ■

⊙ Alert: Hyperglycemia may occur. Monitor patient with diabetes regularly. Patient
with risk factors for diabetes should undergo
fasting blood glucose testing at baseline
and periodically. Monitor all patients for
symptoms of hyperglycemia, including increased hunger, thirst, frequent urination,

and weakness. Hyperglycemia may resolve when patient stops taking drug.

⦿ *Alert:* Monitor patient for symptoms of metabolic syndrome (significant weight gain and increased BMI, HTN, hyperglycemia, hypercholesterolemia, and hypertriglyceridemia).

⦿ *Alert:* Monitor patient for new or increasing compulsive or uncontrollable urges to gamble, binge eat, shop, and have sex. Dosage may need to be reduced or drug discontinued if urges occur.

• Monitor patients with clinically significant neutropenia for fever or other signs and symptoms of infection; treat promptly if they occur. Discontinue drug if ANC is less than 1,000/mm^3 and monitor WBC count until recovery.

• Assess fall risk at start of treatment then periodically for patients who have diseases or conditions or are taking drugs that may cause somnolence, orthostatic hypotension, or motor or sensory instability.

• Monitor patient for abnormal body temperature regulation, especially if patient exercises, is exposed to extreme heat, takes anticholinergics, or is dehydrated.

▧ Dosage adjustments may be indicated in patients who are known CYP2D6 poor metabolizers.

• Treat patient with the smallest dose for the shortest time, and periodically reevaluate for need to continue.

• Give prescriptions only for small quantities of drug, to reduce risk of overdose.

• Change Abilify MyCite patch weekly or sooner, as needed. Patient should keep patch on while showering, swimming, or exercising.

• Remove Abilify MyCite patch before an MRI or if patch causes skin irritation.

• Detection of tablet by the sensor takes 30 minutes to 2 hours and may not occur in some cases.

• Tracking drug ingestion in "real time" or during an emergency isn't recommended because detection of sensor may be delayed or not occur, causing a false-negative reading.

• *Look alike–sound alike:* Don't confuse aripiprazole with rabeprazole, omeprazole, or pantoprazole. Don't confuse IM dosage forms (Abilify Maintena, Aristada, Aristada Initio).

PATIENT TEACHING

Black Box Warning Advise families and caregivers to closely observe patient for clinical worsening, suicidality, or unusual changes in behavior. ∎

Black Box Warning Caution patient or caregiver of patient taking an opioid with a benzodiazepine, CNS depressant, or alcohol to seek immediate medical attention if patient experiences dizziness, lightheadedness, extreme sleepiness, slowed or difficult breathing, or unresponsiveness. ∎

⦿ *Alert:* Advise patient and caregiver to notify prescriber if compulsive or uncontrollable urges occur.

⦿ *Alert:* Caution patient not to stop drug without first discussing with prescriber.

• Tell patient to use caution while driving or operating hazardous machinery because psychoactive drugs may impair judgment, thinking, or motor skills.

• Tell patient that drug may be taken without regard to meals.

• Advise patient that grapefruit juice may interact with aripiprazole and to avoid its use.

• Advise patient that gradual improvement in symptoms should occur over several weeks rather than immediately.

⦿ *Alert:* Warn patient with phenylketonuria that ODTs contain phenylalanine.

• Advise patient that each milliliter of oral solution contains 400 mg of sucrose and 200 mg of fructose.

• Tell patient to avoid alcohol use while taking drug.

• Advise patient to limit strenuous activity while taking drug to avoid dehydration.

• Tell patient to keep ODT in blister package until ready to use. Using dry hands, patient should carefully peel open the foil backing and place tablet on tongue. Advise patient not to split tablet.

• Tell patient to store oral solution at room temperature, and that the solution can be used for up to 6 months after opening.

• Teach patient that the Abilify MyCite drug-device combination product is used to track drug ingestion. Ensure that patient is capable and willing to use a smartphone and app, and that the app is compatible with the specific phone. Assist patient to download

---

app and encourage patient to follow instructions for use.
• Instruct patient to verify that app is paired with the sensor patch before use.
• Teach patient that app will direct patient to apply and remove the patch correctly. Tell patient to change the patch weekly and to keep it on while showering, swimming, or exercising.
• Tell patient that the Abilify MyCite patch will need to be removed before an MRI and then reapplied afterwards.
• Instruct patient to remove the patch if skin irritation occurs and to report this to prescriber.
• Instruct patient to take Abilify MyCite tablets whole.
• Teach patient that the Abilify MyCite tablets are usually detected within 30 minutes but there may be a delay of more than 2 hours for the smartphone app/Web portal to detect it. Inform patient that sometimes the tablet may not be detected at all. If tablet isn't detected, instruct patient not to repeat dose.
• Advise female patient not to breastfeed without first discussing with prescriber.

armodafinil
ar-moe-DAF-i-nil

Nuvigil

Therapeutic class: Stimulants
Pharmacologic class: CNS stimulants
Controlled substance schedule: IV

AVAILABLE FORMS
Tablets: 50 mg, 150 mg, 200 mg, 250 mg

INDICATIONS & DOSAGES
➤ **To improve wakefulness in patients with excessive sleepiness caused by narcolepsy, obstructive sleep apnea (OSA), or shift-work sleep disorder**
Adults: 150 to 250 mg PO daily in morning. For OSA, doses exceeding 150 mg daily may not be more effective. For shift-work sleep disorder, 150 mg PO daily, 1 hour before start of shift.
Adjust-a-dose: Reduce dosage in patients with severe hepatic impairment, with or

without cirrhosis. Consider lower doses in elderly patients.

ADMINISTRATION
PO
• Give drug consistently with or without food at same time each day. Food may delay effect of drug.

ACTION
Unknown. May be similar to sympathomimetics, such as amphetamine and methylphenidate. Also may inhibit dopamine reuptake.

Route	Onset	Peak	Duration
PO	Unknown	2–6 hr	Unknown

Half-life: 15 hours.

ADVERSE REACTIONS
CNS: agitation, anxiety, depression, dizziness, fatigue, headache, insomnia, migraine, nervousness, pain, paresthesia, pyrexia, tremor, disturbance in attention.
CV: increased BP, increased pulse rate, palpitations. **GI:** abdominal pain, anorexia, constipation, diarrhea, dry mouth, dyspepsia, loose stools, nausea, vomiting, decreased appetite. **GU:** polyuria. **Respiratory:** dyspnea, seasonal allergy. **Skin:** contact dermatitis, hyperhidrosis, rash. **Other:** allergic reactions, flulike illness, thirst.

INTERACTIONS
Drug-drug. *Drugs metabolized by CYP2C19 (clomipramine, diazepam, omeprazole, phenytoin, propranolol):* May increase levels of these drugs. Monitor patient and reduce doses as needed.
Drugs metabolized by CYP3A (cyclosporine, midazolam, triazolam): May decrease levels of these drugs. Adjust doses as needed.
Drugs that induce CYP3A (carbamazepine, phenobarbital, rifampin): May decrease armodafinil level. Adjust dosage as needed.
Drugs that inhibit CYP3A (erythromycin, ketoconazole): May increase armodafinil level. Monitor patient carefully and decrease dose as needed.
Hormonal contraceptives (ethinyl estradiol): May decrease effectiveness of these drugs. Alternative or concomitant contraceptive

methods are recommended during and for 1 month after armodafinil therapy.

Drug-food. *Any food:* May delay onset of action by several hours. Monitor effect and give drug consistently with or without food, at the same time daily.

Drug-lifestyle. *Alcohol use:* May counteract armodafinil's effect. Discourage use together.

EFFECTS ON LAB TEST RESULTS
• May increase GGT and alkaline phosphatase levels.

CONTRAINDICATIONS & CAUTIONS
• Contraindicated in patients hypersensitive to modafinil, armodafinil, or their inactive ingredients.
• Avoid use in patients with left ventricular hypertrophy and in those who have experienced mitral valve prolapse when previously given other CNS stimulants.
• Use cautiously in patients with a history of drug abuse or dependence.
• **Alert:** Use cautiously in patients with psychosis, depression, or mania; drug may increase the risk of mania, delusion, hallucinations, and suicidal ideation.
• Use cautiously in patients with cardiac disease, multiorgan hypersensitivity, severe hepatic impairment, or rash.
• Rare cases of serious or life-threatening rash, including SJS and toxic epidermal necrolysis, have been reported in adults and children.
• DRESS syndrome has been reported, which may be life-threatening. Discontinue drug if suspected.
• Use cautiously in elderly patients.
• Safety and effectiveness in patients younger than age 17 haven't been established.
Dialyzable drug: Unknown.
⚠ **Overdose S&S:** Excitation or agitation, insomnia, slight or moderate elevations in hemodynamic parameters, restlessness, disorientation, confusion, hallucinations, nausea, diarrhea, tachycardia, bradycardia, HTN, chest pain.

PREGNANCY-LACTATION-REPRODUCTION
• Use in pregnancy only when benefit to mother outweighs risk to fetus.

• Drug may reduce effectiveness of hormonal contraceptives when used together. Women using hormonal contraception should use an additional barrier method or nonhormonal method of contraception during treatment and for 1 month after final dose.
• Register women exposed to drug in the Nuvigil Pregnancy Registry (1-866-404-4106).
• It isn't known if drug appears in human milk. Use cautiously in breastfeeding women.

NURSING CONSIDERATIONS
• Obtain a thorough medication history to avoid potentially dangerous drug interactions.
• Obtain a complete cardiac history. Monitor patient for increased BP and pulse rate, ECG changes, chest pain, and arrhythmias.
• Monitor patient carefully for evidence of allergic reaction. If rash or other symptoms appear, stop drug immediately, notify prescriber, and monitor carefully.
• Monitor patient for signs or symptoms of angioedema or anaphylaxis, such as swelling of face, eyes, lips, tongue, or larynx; difficulty in swallowing or breathing; and hoarseness.
• Monitor patient for signs and symptoms of DRESS syndrome, including fever, rash, lymphadenopathy, and facial swelling, in association with other organ system involvement, such as hepatitis, nephritis, hematologic abnormalities, myocarditis, or myositis, sometimes resembling an acute viral infection.
• Stop drug and notify prescriber immediately at first sign of rash, skin or mouth sores, or blistering or ulceration, unless rash is clearly not drug-related.
• Monitor patient for signs of mania, delusions, hallucinations, suicidal ideation, and aggression, especially if there's a prior psychiatric history.
• Monitor patient for signs and symptoms of misuse or abuse, especially those with a history of drug or stimulant abuse.
• Assess patient for abnormal level of sleepiness. Don't allow patient to engage in dangerous activities, such as driving, until effect of medication is known.

• Patients receiving continuous positive airway pressure therapy for OSA should continue its use regardless of armodafinil therapy.

PATIENT TEACHING
🜄 *Alert:* Instruct patient to stop taking drug and notify prescriber if rash, hives, mouth sores, blister, peeling skin, trouble swallowing or breathing, facial swelling (eye, lips, tongue, larynx), lymphadenopathy, fever, or other symptoms of a reaction occur.
• Tell patient and family to immediately report signs of mania, delusions, hallucinations, suicidal ideation, and aggression.
• Tell patient not to perform hazardous tasks such as driving until drug's effects (including excessive sleepiness) are known.
• Tell patient to notify prescriber about all drugs being taken to avoid potentially dangerous drug interactions.
• Tell patient to take drug at the same time, consistently with or without food, every day.
• Advise patient that taking drug with food may delay its effects.
• Caution female patient of childbearing potential taking hormonal contraceptives to use alternative or additional methods of contraception during and for 1 month after armodafinil therapy is discontinued.
• Urge female patient to notify prescriber right away if she becomes pregnant or plans to breastfeed.

---

asenapine
a-SEN-a-peen

Saphris

Therapeutic class: Antipsychotics
Pharmacologic class: Dopamine–serotonin antagonists

AVAILABLE FORMS
Tablets (SL) 💊: 2.5 mg, 5 mg, 10 mg

INDICATIONS & DOSAGES
➤ **Schizophrenia (acute and maintenance therapy)**
Adults: 5 mg SL b.i.d. May increase up to 10 mg b.i.d. after 1 week based on tolerability. For maintenance therapy, give 5 to 10 mg SL b.i.d.

➤ **Acute manic or mixed episodes associated with bipolar I disorder as monotherapy or as adjunctive therapy with either lithium or valproate**
Adults: For monotherapy, 5 to 10 mg SL b.i.d. For adjunctive therapy, 5 mg SL b.i.d. Dosage may be increased to a maximum of 10 mg SL b.i.d.
Adjust-a-dose: If adverse effects occur, reduce dosage to 5 mg SL b.i.d.
➤ **Maintenance treatment of bipolar I disorder as monotherapy**
Adults: Continue dosage that patient received during stabilization (5 or 10 mg SL b.i.d.). Based on clinical response and tolerability, can decrease a dose of 10 mg SL b.i.d. to 5 mg SL b.i.d.
➤ **Acute manic or mixed episodes associated with bipolar I disorder as monotherapy**
Children ages 10 to 17: Initially, 2.5 mg SL b.i.d. May increase after 3 days to 5 mg SL b.i.d., then to 10 mg SL b.i.d. after 3 additional days based on tolerability.

ADMINISTRATION
Sublingual
• Obtain BP before starting drug, and monitor pressure regularly. Watch for orthostatic hypotension.
• Make sure patient doesn't split, crush, chew, or swallow tablet.
• Peel back colored tab on tablet pack, gently remove tablet, place under patient's tongue, and allow to dissolve completely.
• Advise patient not to eat or drink for 10 minutes after taking drug.

ACTION
Unknown. May block dopamine and 5-HT receptors.

Route	Onset	Peak	Duration
SL	Immediate	½–1½ hr	Unknown

Half-life: 24 hours.

ADVERSE REACTIONS
CNS: akathisia, anxiety, depression, dizziness, extrapyramidal symptoms, fatigue, headache, insomnia, irritability, somnolence, manic symptoms. **CV:** HTN, peripheral edema, tachycardia, temporary bundle-branch block. **EENT:** diplopia, blurred

vision, dry mouth, oral hypoesthesia, salivary hypersecretion, toothache, nasopharyngitis. **GI:** constipation, dyspepsia, increased appetite, stomach discomfort, taste perversion, nausea, vomiting, glossitis. **Hematologic:** anemia. **Metabolic:** weight gain, hyperinsulinemia. **Musculoskeletal:** arthralgia, extremity pain. **Respiratory:** URI. **Skin:** rash, photosensitivity. **Other:** suicidal ideation.

INTERACTIONS

Drug-drug. *Alpha₁ blockers (doxazosin, terazosin):* May increase risk of hypotension. Use together cautiously.

Antiarrhythmics, class IA (procainamide, quinidine) and class III (amiodarone, sotalol); antibiotics (gatifloxacin, moxifloxacin); antipsychotics (chlorpromazine, thioridazine, ziprasidone); citalopram: May prolong QTc interval, leading to lethal arrhythmias such as torsades de pointes. Avoid use together.

Antidepressants (fluvoxamine, imipramine, paroxetine): May increase asenapine level. Use together cautiously. Reduce paroxetine dosage by half if using with asenapine.

CNS agents: May enhance CNS depression. Use with caution.

Dextromethorphan: May increase dextromethorphan level. Use together cautiously.

Metoclopramide: May increase risk of extrapyramidal reactions. Avoid administering together.

Black Box Warning *Opioid class warning:* May cause slow or difficult breathing, sedation, and death. Avoid use together. If use together is necessary, limit dosage and duration of each drug to the minimum necessary for desired effect. ■

Drug-lifestyle. *Alcohol use:* May increase CNS effects. Discourage use together.

EFFECTS ON LAB TEST RESULTS
• May increase glucose, cholesterol, ALT, AST, and prolactin levels.
• May decrease WBC and neutrophil counts.

CONTRAINDICATIONS & CAUTIONS
Black Box Warning Elderly patients with dementia-related psychosis treated with atypical or conventional antipsychotics

are at increased risk for death. Antipsychotics aren't approved for the treatment of dementia-related psychosis. ■

Black Box Warning *Opioid class warning:* Opioids should only be prescribed with benzodiazepines or other CNS depressants to patients for whom alternative treatment options are inadequate. ■

◑ *Alert:* Contraindicated in patients with a known hypersensitivity and in patients with severe hepatic failure (Child-Pugh class C). Hypersensitivity reactions may occur as early as the first dose.

◑ *Alert:* Avoid use in patients with conditions that may increase risk of torsades de pointes and in those taking other drugs that prolong QTc interval.

• Use cautiously in patients with or at risk for diabetes; in those with known CV or cerebrovascular disease, preexisting low WBC count, difficulty swallowing, history of leukopenia or neutropenia, Parkinson disease, or history of seizures or conditions that lower the seizure threshold; and in antipsychotic-naive patients.

• Don't use in patients at risk for aspiration pneumonia.

• Use cautiously in patients at risk for falls, including those who have diseases or conditions or are taking medications that may cause somnolence, orthostatic hypotension, or motor or sensory instability.

• Safe and effective use for bipolar I disorder in children younger than age 10 or for schizophrenia in children younger than age 12 hasn't been established.

Dialyzable drug: Unknown.

⚠ **Overdose S&S:** Agitation, confusion, hypotension, circulatory collapse.

PREGNANCY-LACTATION-REPRODUCTION
• Drug may cause fetal harm. Safety of atypical antipsychotic use during pregnancy hasn't been well studied; routine use isn't recommended. Use during pregnancy only if potential benefit justifies potential risk to the fetus.

◑ *Alert:* Neonates exposed to antipsychotics during the third trimester are at risk for developing extrapyramidal signs and symptoms (repetitive muscle movements of the face and body) and withdrawal signs and symptoms (agitation, abnormally increased

---

Reactions in bold italics are *life-threatening*. Interactions may have a *rapid onset* or a ***delayed onset***.

or decreased muscle tone, tremors, sleepiness, severe difficulty breathing, difficulty feeding) after delivery.
• Pregnant women exposed to asenapine should be enrolled in National Pregnancy Registry for Atypical Antipsychotics (1-866-961-2388) or should visit https://womensmentalhealth.org/research/pregnancyregistry/
• It isn't known if drug appears in human milk. A decision should be made to discontinue breastfeeding or discontinue drug, taking into account risk to infant and importance of drug to mother.

NURSING CONSIDERATIONS
• Monitor ECG before and regularly during treatment for prolongation of QTc interval.
• Obtain BP before starting drug, and monitor BP regularly. Watch for orthostatic hypotension.
• Monitor patient for tardive dyskinesia, which may occur after prolonged use. It may disappear spontaneously or persist for life, despite stopping drug.
⊗ **Alert:** Watch for signs and symptoms of NMS (extrapyramidal effects, hyperthermia, autonomic disturbance), which are rare but can be fatal. Discontinue drug immediately if they occur, and monitor patient closely.
• Monitor patient for serious allergic reactions (anaphylaxis, angioedema, hypotension, difficulty breathing, wheezing, swollen tongue, rash).
• Drug may alter glucose control in diabetics. Monitor glucose levels closely.
• Monitor CBC frequently during first few months of therapy in those with history of leukopenia or neutropenia. If WBC count decreases, monitor patient for signs and symptoms of infection; if infection occurs, discontinue drug in the absence of another cause.
• Monitor patient for dysphagia, which can lead to aspiration and aspiration pneumonia.
• Dispense lowest appropriate quantity of drug, to reduce risk of overdose.
• Monitor patient for abnormal body temperature regulation, especially if patient exercises, is exposed to extreme heat, takes anticholinergics, or is dehydrated.
• Complete fall risk assessments at start of treatment then periodically for patients on

long-term therapy who have diseases or conditions or are taking medications that may cause somnolence, orthostatic hypotension, or motor or sensory instability.

PATIENT TEACHING
Black Box Warning *Opioid class warning:* Caution patient or caregiver of patient taking an opioid with a benzodiazepine, CNS depressant, or alcohol to seek immediate medical attention if patient experiences dizziness, light-headedness, extreme sleepiness, slowed or difficult breathing, or unresponsiveness. ■
• Instruct patient to peel back colored tab on tablet pack, gently remove tablet, place under the tongue, and allow to dissolve completely. Advise patient not to swallow tablet and not to eat or drink for 10 minutes after taking drug.
• Warn patient to avoid activities that require mental alertness, such as operating hazardous machinery or operating a motor vehicle, until drug's effects are known.
• Advise patient to contact prescriber if palpitations or rapid heartbeat occurs.
• Advise patient not to stand up quickly but to get up slowly from a sitting position to avoid dizziness.
• Inform patient that weight gain may occur.
• Warn patient against exposure to extreme heat because drug may impair body's ability to reduce temperature.
• Advise patient to avoid alcohol.

aspirin (acetylsalicylic acid, ASA)
AS-pir-in

Asaphen❁ ◇, Asatab❁ ◇, Bayer Aspirin ◇, Durlaza, Ecotrin ◇, Entrophen❁ ◇, Novasen❁ ◇, Rivasa❁ ◇

Therapeutic class: NSAIDs
Pharmacologic class: Salicylates

AVAILABLE FORMS
Capsules: 325 mg ◇
Capsules (extended release) ⊕: 162.5 mg

Suppositories: 60 mg ◇, 120 mg ◇,
150 mg✸ ◇, 160 mg✸ ◇, 200 mg ◇,
300 mg ◇, 600 mg ◇, 650 mg✸ ◇
Tablets: 325 mg ◇, 500 mg ◇
Tablets (chewable): 80 mg✸ ◇, 81 mg ◇
Tablets (delayed-release): 81 mg, 325 mg,
500 mg
Tablets (enteric-coated) ⓞⓝⓒ*:* 80 mg✸ ◇,
81 mg ◇, 162 mg✸ ◇, 325 mg ◇,
500 mg ◇, 650 mg✸ ◇, 975 mg✸ ◇

INDICATIONS & DOSAGES
➤ **RA, osteoarthritis, or other poly-
arthritic or inflammatory conditions**
Adults: Initially, 3 g PO daily in divided
doses. Increase as needed, with target plasma
salicylate levels of 150 to 300 mcg/mL.
➤ **Juvenile RA**
Children: 90 to 130 mg/kg/day PO in divided doses. Increase as needed, with
target plasma salicylate levels of 150 to
300 mcg/mL.
➤ **Mild pain or fever; spondyloarthrop-
athies**
*Adults: and children age 12 and older
weighing 50 kg or more:* 325 to 650 mg PO
or PR every 4 hours p.r.n. Or, for delayed-
release products, 1,300 mg PO followed by
650 to 1,300 mg PO every 8 hours. Maximum dose is 4,000 mg in 24 hours.
*Children ages 2 to 11 weighing less than
50 kg:* 10 to 15 mg/kg/dose PO or PR every
4 hours up to 90 mg/kg daily.
➤ **Suspected acute MI**
Adults: Initial dose of 160 to 325 mg PO
(non-enteric-coated) chewed or crushed as
soon as MI is suspected. Continue maintenance dose of 160 to 325 mg PO daily for
30 days after infarction. After 30 days, consider further therapy for prevention of MI.
➤ **To reduce risk of MI in patients with
previous MI, unstable angina, and chronic
stable angina pectoris**
Adults: 75 to 325 mg PO daily. Or, 162.5 mg
extended-release capsule PO daily.
➤ **To reduce risk of recurrent TIAs and
stroke or death in patients at risk**
Adults: 50 to 325 mg PO daily. Or, 162.5 mg
extended-release capsule PO daily.
➤ **Acute ischemic stroke**
Adults: 50 to 325 mg PO daily, started
within 48 hours of stroke onset; continue
indefinitely.

➤ **CABG**
Adults: 325 mg PO daily starting 6 hours
postprocedure.
➤ **PTCA ◆**
Adults: Initial dose of 81 to 325 mg PO at
least 2 hours before surgery, then 160 to
325 mg PO daily.
➤ **Carotid endarterectomy ◆**
Adults: 75 to 100 mg PO daily.
➤ **Primary/secondary prevention of colorectal adenomas in patients previously
diagnosed with colorectal cancer ◆**
Adults: 75 to 325 mg immediate-release PO
once daily.
➤ **Prevention of colorectal cancer in
patients who are carriers of hereditary nonpolyposis colon cancer (Lynch
syndrome) ◆**
Adults: 600 mg PO once daily for at least
2 years.
➤ **Venous thromboembolism extended
therapy to prevent recurrence (in patients who have completed anticoagulation treatment and have decided to stop
oral anticoagulation) ◆**
Adults: 100 mg PO once daily.

ADMINISTRATION
PO
• For patient with swallowing difficulties,
crush non–enteric-coated aspirin and dissolve in soft food or liquid. Give liquid immediately after mixing because drug will
break down rapidly.
• Give drug with food, milk, antacid, or
large glass of water to reduce GI effects.
• Give enteric-coated or extended-release
forms whole; don't crush or break these
tablets.
• For acute MI, have patient chew non-
enteric-coated tablet.
Rectal
• Refrigerate suppositories.

ACTION
Thought to produce analgesia and exert
its anti-inflammatory effect by inhibiting
prostaglandin and other substances that sensitize pain receptors. Drug may relieve fever
through central action in the hypothalamic
heat-regulating center. In low doses, drug
also appears to interfere with clotting by

keeping a platelet-aggregating substance from forming.

Route	Onset	Peak	Duration
PO (buffered)	5–30 min	1–2 hr	1–4 hr
PO (enteric-coated)	5–30 min	Variable	1–4 hr
PO (tablet)	5–30 min	25–40 min	1–4 hr
PO (extended-release)	Unknown	2 hr	4–8 hr
PR	Unknown	3–4 hr	Unknown

Half-life: 15 minutes to 6 hours (dose dependent).

ADVERSE REACTIONS
CNS: agitation, *cerebral edema, coma,* confusion, dizziness, headache, lethargy, *seizures, subdural or intracranial hemorrhage.* **CV:** *arrhythmias,* hypotension, tachycardia. **EENT:** tinnitus, hearing loss. **GI:** nausea, *GI bleeding,* dyspepsia, GI distress, occult bleeding, *pancreatitis,* vomiting. **GU:** *antepartum and postpartum bleeding,* interstitial nephritis, papillary necrosis, prolonged pregnancy and labor, proteinuria, renal insufficiency, renal failure. **Hematologic:** prolonged bleeding time, *leukopenia, thrombocytopenia,* coagulopathy, *DIC.* **Hepatic:** *hepatitis.* **Metabolic:** dehydration, *hyperkalemia,* hyperglycemia; *hypoglycemia* (children), *metabolic acidosis,* respiratory alkalosis. **Skin:** rash, bruising, urticaria, hives. **Other:** *angioedema, Reye syndrome,* hypersensitivity reactions, low birth weight (infants), stillbirth.

INTERACTIONS
Drug-drug. *ACE inhibitors:* May decrease antihypertensive effects. Monitor BP closely.
Acetazolamide: May cause accumulation and toxicity of acetazolamide, resulting in CNS depression, metabolic acidosis, anorexia, and death. Administer together with caution and monitor patient for toxicity.
Ammonium chloride and other urine acidifiers: May increase levels of aspirin products. Watch for aspirin toxicity.
Antacids in high doses and other urine alkalinizers: May decrease levels of aspirin products. Watch for decreased aspirin effect.

Anticoagulants, antiplatelet agents: May increase risk of bleeding. Use with extreme caution if these drugs must be used together.
Beta blockers: May decrease antihypertensive effect. Avoid long-term aspirin use if patient is taking antihypertensives.
Corticosteroids: May enhance salicylate elimination and decrease drug level. Watch for decreased aspirin effect. May increase risk of GI ulceration and bleeding. Monitor therapy.
Diuretics: May decrease effectiveness of diuretics in patients with underlying renal or CV disease. Monitor patient for effectiveness.
Heparin: May increase risk of bleeding. Monitor coagulation studies and patient closely if used together.
Ibuprofen, other NSAIDs: May negate the antiplatelet effect of low-dose aspirin therapy. Patients using immediate-release aspirin (not enteric-coated) should take ibuprofen at least 30 minutes after or more than 8 hours before aspirin. Patients using extended-release aspirin should take ibuprofen at least 2 to 4 hours after or more than 8 hours before aspirin. Occasional use of ibuprofen is unlikely to have a negative effect.
Influenza virus vaccine, live: Increased risk of Reye syndrome. Use together is contraindicated in children and adolescents.
Methotrexate: May increase risk of methotrexate toxicity. Avoid using together.
Oral antidiabetics: May increase hypoglycemic effect. Monitor patient closely.
Probenecid: May decrease uricosuric effect. Avoid using together.
Valproic acid: May increase valproic acid level. Avoid using together.
Drug-herb. *White willow:* Contains salicylates and may increase risk of adverse effects. Discourage use together.
Drug-food. *Caffeine:* May increase drug absorption. Watch for increased effects.
Drug-lifestyle. *Alcohol use:* May increase risk of GI bleeding. Discourage use together.

EFFECTS ON LAB TEST RESULTS
• May increase LFT values, BUN, creatinine, and potassium levels.
• May decrease platelet and WBC counts.

• May falsely decrease protein-bound iodine level.

• May interfere with urine glucose analysis with Diastix, Chemstrip uG, Clinitest, and Benedict solution; with urinary 5-hydroxyindoleacetic acid and vanillylmandelic acid tests; and with Gerhardt test for urine acetoacetic acid.

CONTRAINDICATIONS & CAUTIONS
• Contraindicated in patients hypersensitive to drug and in those with NSAID-induced sensitivity reactions, G6PD deficiency, or bleeding disorders, such as hemophilia, von Willebrand disease, telangiectasia, bleeding ulcers, and hemorrhagic states.

• Use cautiously in patients with GI lesions, impaired renal function, hypoprothrombinemia, vitamin K deficiency, thrombocytopenia, or thrombotic thrombocytopenic purpura.

• Avoid use in patients with severe hepatic impairment or history of active peptic ulcer disease.

◑ *Alert:* Oral and rectal OTC products containing aspirin and nonaspirin salicylates shouldn't be given to children or teenagers who have or are recovering from chickenpox or flulike symptoms with or without fever because of the risk of Reye syndrome.

• Safe use of extended-release capsules in children hasn't been established.

Dialyzable drug: Yes.

⚠ *Overdose S&S:* Severe acid-base and electrolyte disturbance, hyperthermia, dehydration, tinnitus, vertigo, headache, confusion, drowsiness, diaphoresis, hyperventilation, vomiting, diarrhea.

PREGNANCY-LACTATION-REPRODUCTION
• Use in pregnancy only if clearly needed and specifically directed to do so by a physician. Avoid use during third trimester.

• Drug appears in human milk. Breastfeeding women should avoid aspirin if possible.

NURSING CONSIDERATIONS
• For inflammatory conditions, rheumatic fever, and thrombosis, give aspirin on a schedule rather than as needed.

• Because enteric-coated tablets are slowly absorbed, they aren't suitable for rapid relief of acute pain, fever, or inflammation.

They cause less GI bleeding and may be better suited for long-term therapy, such as for arthritis.

• For patients who can't tolerate oral drugs, ask prescriber about using aspirin rectal suppositories. Watch for rectal mucosal irritation or bleeding.

• Febrile, dehydrated children can develop toxicity rapidly.

• Monitor elderly patients closely because they may be more susceptible to aspirin's toxic effects.

• Monitor salicylate level. Therapeutic salicylate level for arthritis is 150 to 300 mcg/mL. Tinnitus may occur at levels above 200 mcg/mL, but this isn't a reliable indicator of toxicity, especially in very young patients and those older than age 60. With long-term therapy, severe toxic effects may occur with levels exceeding 400 mcg/mL.

• During prolonged therapy, assess hematocrit, Hb level, PT, INR, and renal function periodically.

• Drug irreversibly inhibits platelet aggregation. Stop drug 5 to 7 days before elective surgery to allow time for production and release of new platelets.

• Monitor patient for hypersensitivity reactions, such as anaphylaxis and asthma.

• *Look alike–sound alike:* Don't confuse aspirin with Asendin or Afrin.

PATIENT TEACHING
• Tell patient who's allergic to tartrazine to avoid aspirin.

• Advise patient on a low-salt diet that 1 tablet of buffered aspirin contains 553 mg of sodium.

• Advise patient to take drug with food, milk, antacid, or large glass of water to reduce GI reactions.

• Tell patient not to crush or chew enteric-coated or extended-release forms but to swallow them whole.

• Advise patient to take extended-release capsules at same time each day.

• Warn patient not to drink alcohol 2 hours before or 1 hour after taking extended-release capsule and not to take extra capsule to make up for a missed dose.

• Remind patient taking drug for a chronic condition not to stop drug without first discussing with prescriber.

Reactions in bold italics are *life-threatening*. Interactions may have a *rapid onset* or a *delayed onset*.

- Instruct patient to discard aspirin tablets that have a strong vinegar-like odor.
- Tell patient to consult prescriber if giving drug to children for longer than 5 days or adults for longer than 10 days.
- Advise patient receiving prolonged treatment with large doses of aspirin to watch for small, round, red pinprick spots; bleeding gums; and signs of GI bleeding; advise patient to drink plenty of fluids. Encourage use of a soft-bristled toothbrush.
- Because of the many drug interactions with aspirin, warn patient taking prescription drugs to check with prescriber or pharmacist before taking aspirin or OTC products containing aspirin.
- Ibuprofen can interfere with the antiplatelet effect of low-dose aspirin therapy, negating its effect. Teach patient how to safely use ibuprofen in relation to aspirin therapy.
- Urge pregnant patient to avoid aspirin during last trimester of pregnancy unless specifically directed by prescriber.
- Drug is a leading cause of poisoning in children. Caution parents to keep drug out of reach of children. Encourage use of child-resistant containers.

atazanavir sulfate
A-ta-ZAN-a-veer

Reyataz⚯

Therapeutic class: Antiretrovirals
Pharmacologic class: Protease inhibitors

AVAILABLE FORMS
Capsules: 150 mg, 200 mg, 300 mg
Oral powder: 50 mg

INDICATIONS & DOSAGES
Adjust-a-dose (for all indications): In patients with Child-Pugh class B hepatic insufficiency who haven't experienced prior virologic failure, reduce dosage to 300 mg PO once daily. Treatment-naive patients with ESRD who are on hemodialysis should receive atazanavir 300 mg with ritonavir 100 mg. Don't give to treatment-experienced patients on hemodialysis.

➤ **HIV-1 infection, with other antiretrovirals in treatment-experienced patients**
Adults: Give 300 mg once daily, plus 100 mg ritonavir once daily with food. In patients also taking an H_2-receptor antagonist (H2RA) and tenofovir, give 400 mg PO once daily, plus 100 mg ritonavir.
Children and adolescents ages 6 to younger than 18 who are treatment-experienced and receiving ritonavir: For patients weighing 35 kg or more, give 300 mg with ritonavir 100 mg PO once daily. For patients weighing 15 to 34 kg, give 200 mg with ritonavir 100 mg PO once daily. For patients weighing 5 to 15 kg, capsules aren't recommended. Use oral powder.
Children at least age 3 months and weighing at least 5 kg and less than 25 kg: For patients weighing 15 to less than 25 kg, give 250 mg PO immediately followed by 80 mg ritonavir daily. For patients weighing 5 to less than 15 kg, give 200 mg PO immediately followed by 80 mg ritonavir daily.
➤ **HIV-1 infection, with other antiretrovirals, in treatment-naive patients**
Adults: Recommended regimen is 300 mg PO once daily with ritonavir 100 mg. When drug is given with efavirenz, give atazanavir 400 mg and ritonavir 100 mg as a single daily dose with food and efavirenz on an empty stomach, preferably at bedtime. For adults unable to tolerate ritonavir, give 400 mg PO once daily.
Adolescents at least age 13 and weighing at least 40 kg who can't tolerate ritonavir: 400 mg PO once daily with food.
Children and adolescents ages 6 to younger than 18: For patients weighing 35 kg or more, give 300 mg with ritonavir 100 mg PO once daily. For patients weighing 15 to less than 34 kg, give 200 mg with ritonavir 100 mg PO once daily. For patients weighing 5 to 15 kg, capsules aren't recommended. Use oral powder.
Children at least age 3 months and weighing at least 5 kg and less than 25 kg: For patients weighing 15 to less than 25 kg, give 250 mg PO immediately followed by 80 mg ritonavir daily. For patients weighing 5 to less than 15 kg, give 200 mg PO immediately followed by 80 mg ritonavir daily.

Adjust-a-dose: Administration with ritonavir in patients with any degree of hepatic impairment isn't recommended. In adults with mild hepatic impairment (Child-Pugh class A), give 400 mg PO daily; for moderate hepatic impairment (Child-Pugh class B), give 300 mg daily; for severe hepatic impairment (Child-Pugh class C), atazanavir isn't recommended.

➤ **HIV-1 infection, with other antiretrovirals, in pregnant patients**

Women: Give 300 mg PO daily with 100 mg ritonavir. For treatment-experienced patients during second or third trimester when given with either H2RA or tenofovir, give 400 mg PO daily with 100 mg ritonavir.

ADMINISTRATION
PO
• Give drug with food.
• Give to pregnant women only if potential benefit justifies risk to the fetus.
• Don't open capsules.
• Mix oral powder with food (such as applesauce or yogurt) or beverage (such as milk, infant formula, or water).
• When mixing with food, mix powder with a minimum of 1 tablespoon of food in small container and feed to child. Add additional tablespoon of food to container, mix, and feed residual mixture to child.
• When mixing with beverage, mix powder with minimum of 30 mL of beverage and give to child to drink. Add additional 15 mL of beverage to the drinking cup, mix, and give to child to drink residual mixture. If water is used, also give food at same time.
• For young infants who can't eat solid food or drink from a cup, mix powder with 10 mL of infant formula in a medicine cup and draw up into oral syringe. Give to infant into either inner cheek. Pour additional 10 mL of formula into medicine cup and mix. Give residual mixture to infant in the same manner. Don't give in an infant bottle.
• Give entire dose of powder after mixing within 1 hour of preparation. Additional food may be given after dose is given.

ACTION
Inhibits viral maturation in HIV-1–infected cells, resulting in the formation of immature noninfectious viral particles.

Route	Onset	Peak	Duration
PO	Unknown	2–3 hr	Unknown

Half-life: Unboosted, 7 to 8 hours; boosted with ritonavir, 9 to 18 hours.

ADVERSE REACTIONS
CNS: headache, depression, dizziness, fatigue, fever, insomnia, pain, peripheral neuropathy. **CV:** prolonged PR interval, first- and second-degree heart block, peripheral edema. **EENT:** nasal congestion, rhinorrhea, oropharyngeal pain. **GI:** abdominal pain, diarrhea, nausea, vomiting. **Hematologic:** *neutropenia.* **Hepatic:** hyperbilirubinemia, jaundice/scleral icterus. **Metabolic:** lipodystrophy, *hypoglycemia.* **Musculoskeletal:** arthralgia, myalgia. **Respiratory:** increased cough, wheezing. **Skin:** rash.

INTERACTIONS
Drug-drug. *Alfuzosin:* May increase alfuzosin plasma concentration, increasing risk of hypotension. Use together is contraindicated.
Antacids, buffered medications (didanosine buffered preparation): May reduce atazanavir plasma concentration. Administer atazanavir 2 hours before or 1 hour after these medications.
Antiarrhythmics (amiodarone, bepridil, systemic lidocaine, quinidine): May produce serious or life-threatening adverse reactions. Use cautiously. Monitor antiarrhythmic therapeutic concentration.
Anticoagulants (apixaban, warfarin): May cause serious or life-threatening bleeding. Monitor INR.
Antifungals (itraconazole, ketoconazole, posaconazole, voriconazole): May increase risk of toxicity of both antifungal and atazanavir. Use cautiously when high doses of ketoconazole or itraconazole are administered with atazanavir and ritonavir. Administration of voriconazole with atazanavir and ritonavir isn't recommended.
Aprepitant: May increase aprepitant serum concentration. Avoid combination.
Aripiprazole: May increase aripiprazole plasma concentration. Monitor patient and adjust aripiprazole dosage as needed when atazanavir is started or stopped.

Benzodiazepines (midazolam, triazolam): May increase plasma concentrations of these drugs. Oral midazolam and triazolam are contraindicated because of the potential for serious or life-threatening events, such as prolonged or increased sedation or respiratory depression. Use IV midazolam with caution and close monitoring. Consider reducing the IV midazolam dosage.

Bosentan: May decrease atazanavir plasma concentration when administered without ritonavir; coadministration of atazanavir and bosentan without ritonavir isn't recommended. May increase bosentan plasma concentration. Adjust bosentan dose when used with atazanavir/ritonavir. Consider therapy modification.

Brentuximab: May increase brentuximab plasma concentration. Close monitoring is warranted. Adjust brentuximab dosage as needed.

Cabazitaxel: May increase cabazitaxel plasma concentration. Avoid administering together.

Calcium channel blockers (amlodipine, diltiazem, felodipine, nicardipine, nifedipine, verapamil): May prolong PR interval in some patients; use caution. Consider reducing diltiazem dosage by 50% and titrating dosages of other calcium channel blockers. Monitor ECG.

Carbamazepine: May increase carbamazepine level. May decrease atazanavir level, resulting in antiretroviral treatment failure. If coadministration can't be avoided, monitor patient closely. Consider alternative therapy for carbamazepine.

Cilostazol: May increase cilostazol plasma concentration. Consider reducing cilostazol dosage.

Clarithromycin: May prolong QTc interval; reduce clarithromycin dosage by 50%. Significantly reduces concentration of active metabolite (14-OH clarithromycin); consider alternative therapy for indications other than *Mycobacterium avium* complex.

Colchicine: May increase plasma concentrations of colchicine. Don't give colchicine and atazanavir together to patients with hepatic or renal impairment. In those with normal renal and hepatic function, reduce colchicine dose. Consider therapy modification.

Corticosteroids (fluticasone, prednisone): May increase corticosteroid plasma concentration. Monitor patient for signs and symptoms of adrenal insufficiency. Consider alternatives to fluticasone for long-term use.

Crizotinib, docetaxel, dronedarone, ixabepilone, ticagrelor, toremifene: May increase plasma concentration of these drugs. Avoid administering together.

Delavirdine: May increase atazanavir plasma concentration and decrease delavirdine plasma concentration. Closely monitor patient and adjust therapy as needed.

Didanosine (buffered): May decrease atazanavir concentration. Give atazanavir 2 hours before or 1 hour after buffered formulation of didanosine. Coadministration of enteric-coated didanosine capsules and atazanavir decreases didanosine exposure. Separate atazanavir and didanosine administration times.

Digoxin: May prolong PR interval. Use with caution.

Eletriptan: May increase eletriptan plasma concentration. Avoid use together.

Eplerenone: May increase eplerenone plasma concentration. Avoid combination.

Ergot derivatives (dihydroergotamine, ergonovine, ergotamine, methylergonovine): May cause serious or life-threatening events such as acute ergot toxicity (peripheral vasospasm, ischemia of the extremities). Use together is contraindicated.

Erlotinib: May increase erlotinib plasma concentration. Monitor clinical response and watch for adverse reactions. Adjust erlotinib dosage as needed.

Eszopiclone: May increase eszopiclone plasma concentration. Monitor patient closely. Consider reducing eszopiclone dosage when administered with atazanavir.

Fluoxetine: May increase plasma concentrations of both drugs. Closely monitor patient for adverse reactions, including serotonin syndrome. Fluoxetine or atazanavir dosage reduction may be needed.

HMG-CoA reductase inhibitors (atorvastatin, lovastatin, rosuvastatin, simvastatin): May increase serum concentrations of these drugs, possibly increasing their toxicity, including rhabdomyolysis. Administration with simvastatin or lovastatin is contraindicated. If using atorvastatin or rosuvastatin,

---

✤Canada ◇OTC ◆Off-label use ✐Photoguide ⓓDo not crush *Liquid contains alcohol ✖Genetic start with lowest possible dosage with careful monitoring. Consider pravastatin or fluvastatin in combination with atazanavir.

Hormonal contraceptives (ethinyl estradiol, norethindrone, norgestimate): See manufacturer's instructions. Alternative methods of nonhormonal contraception are recommended.

H2RAs (famotidine): May decrease atazanavir plasma concentration, possibly causing development of resistance. See manufacturer's instructions for H2RA administration recommendations.

Iloperidone: May increase iloperidone plasma concentration. Reduce iloperidone dosage by half when administering with atazanavir. If atazanavir is discontinued, increase iloperidone dosage to original dosage.

Immunosuppressants (cyclosporine, sirolimus, tacrolimus): May increase levels of these drugs. Monitor immunosuppressant concentrations.

Irinotecan: May interfere with irinotecan metabolism, resulting in increased toxicity. Use together is contraindicated.

Lurasidone: May increase lurasidone plasma concentration. Use together is contraindicated if administered with ritonavir.

Maraviroc: May increase maraviroc plasma concentration. Monitor patient response and adjust maraviroc dosage as needed.

mTOR inhibitors (everolimus, temsirolimus): May increase plasma concentrations of these drugs. If coadministration can't be avoided, monitor clinical response and adjust mTOR inhibitor dosage as needed.

NNRTIs (efavirenz, nevirapine): May decrease atazanavir plasma level. In treatment-naive patients, administer atazanavir 400 mg with food and ritonavir 100 mg with efavirenz 600 mg on an empty stomach. Don't administer atazanavir with efavirenz in treatment-experienced patients. Nevirapine may decrease atazanavir exposure; administering them together may increase nevirapine exposure. Use together is contraindicated.

Opioid analgesics (buprenorphine, fentanyl, oxycodone, sufentanil): May increase plasma concentration and half-life of opioid; reduced opioid dosage may be needed. Closely monitor respiratory function during opioid administration and for a longer period than usual after stopping opioid. Atazanavir without ritonavir shouldn't be administered with buprenorphine.

PDE5 inhibitors (sildenafil, tadalafil, vardenafil): Coadministration of atazanavir and sildenafil for PAH is contraindicated. When used for erectile dysfunction, see manufacturer's instructions for dosage adjustments. Monitor patient closely.

Pimozide: May cause serious or life-threatening reactions (cardiac arrhythmias). Use is contraindicated.

Protease inhibitors (amprenavir, darunavir, fosamprenavir, indinavir, nelfinavir, ritonavir, saquinavir, tipranavir): Drug may increase concentration of other protease inhibitors. Atazanavir and indinavir are contraindicated together. Atazanavir/ritonavir isn't recommended with other protease inhibitors. Other combinations may require dosage changes. Consider therapy modification.

PPIs (omeprazole): Substantially decrease atazanavir plasma concentration, possibly causing development of resistance. In treatment-naive patients, administer PPI 12 hours before atazanavir dose. PPI shouldn't exceed dose equivalent to omeprazole 20 mg. Don't use PPIs in treatment-experienced patients receiving atazanavir.

Quetiapine: May increase quetiapine plasma concentration. Administer cautiously; closely monitor clinical response. Adjust quetiapine dosage to one-sixth of current dose.

Ranolazine: Increases risk of dose-related QTc-interval prolongation, torsades de pointes–type arrhythmias, and sudden death. Avoid use together.

Rifabutin: May increase rifabutin blood level. Rifabutin dosage reduction of up to 75% (150 mg every other day or three times/week) is recommended.

Rifampin: May decrease atazanavir plasma concentration, possibly causing development of resistance. Use together is contraindicated.

Risperidone: May increase risperidone plasma concentration. Closely monitor clinical response. Adjust risperidone dosage as needed.

Reactions in bold italics are *life-threatening*. Interactions may have a *rapid onset* or a *delayed onset*.

Romidepsin: May increase romidepsin plasma concentration, increasing risk of adverse reactions, including QT-interval prolongation. If use together can't be avoided, closely monitor clinical, laboratory, and ECG results. Adjust romidepsin dosage as needed.

Salmeterol: May increase salmeterol concentration, increasing risk of CV events, including QT-interval prolongation, palpitations, and sinus tachycardia. Use together isn't recommended.

Saxagliptin: May increase saxagliptin plasma concentration. Limit saxagliptin dosage to 2.5 mg daily.

TCAs (amitriptyline): May cause serious or life-threatening adverse reactions. Monitor TCA concentration.

Tenofovir: May decrease atazanavir area under the curve and minimum (trough) concentration. Don't administer atazanavir with tenofovir unless also administering ritonavir; administer as atazanavir 300 mg, ritonavir 100 mg, and tenofovir 300 mg. Atazanavir increases tenofovir concentration; watch for tenofovir-associated adverse reactions.

Tetracyclines (minocycline): May reduce atazanavir plasma concentration. Closely monitor atazanavir concentration and clinical response. Adjust atazanavir dosage as needed.

Trazodone: May increase trazodone plasma concentration. Use cautiously and reduce trazodone dosage.

Tyrosine kinase inhibitors (dasatinib, lapatinib, pazopanib, sorafenib, sunitinib): May increase tyrosine kinase inhibitor plasma concentrations. If use together can't be avoided, closely monitor clinical response and adjust tyrosine kinase inhibitor dosage as needed.

Vasopressin receptor antagonists (conivaptan, tolvaptan): May increase plasma concentration of these drugs. Avoid coadministration.

Vemurafenib: May increase vemurafenib plasma concentration. Avoid combination.

Vilazodone: May increase vilazodone plasma concentration. Reduce vilazodone dosage to 20 mg in patients receiving atazanavir.

Vinca alkaloids (vinblastine, vincristine): May increase pharmacologic effects of these drugs and risk of toxicity (characterized by profound neutropenia or severe neuropathy). Consider temporarily suspending atazanavir in patients experiencing hematologic or GI toxicity during administration of atazanavir and vinca alkaloids. Or, reducing vinca alkaloid dosage may decrease toxicity.

Drug-herb. *St. John's wort:* May decrease drug level, reducing therapeutic effect and causing drug resistance. Use together is contraindicated.

Drug-food. *Any food:* May increase bioavailability of drug. Tell patient to take drug with food.

EFFECTS ON LAB TEST RESULTS

• May increase ALT, AST, amylase, bilirubin, lipase, CK, glucose, triglyceride, and total cholesterol levels. May decrease glucose and Hb level.

• May decrease neutrophil and platelet counts.

CONTRAINDICATIONS & CAUTIONS

• Contraindicated in patients hypersensitive to drug or its ingredients.

• Contraindicated in patients taking drugs cleared mainly by CYP3A4 or drugs that can cause serious or life-threatening reactions at high levels (alfuzosin, dihydroergotamine, elbasvir/grazoprevir, ergonovine, ergotamine, indinavir, irinotecan, lovastatin, methylergonovine, midazolam [PO], nevirapine, pimozide, rifampin, sildenafil [Revatio], St. John's wort, simvastatin, triazolam).

• Don't use in patients with Child-Pugh class C hepatic insufficiency.

• Use cautiously in patients with cardiac conduction system disease, hepatic impairment, diabetes, or hemophilia types A and B.

• Use cautiously in elderly patients because of the increased likelihood of other disease, additional drug therapy, and decreased hepatic, renal, or cardiac function.

Dialyzable drug: No.

⚠ *Overdose S&S:* Asymptomatic bifascicular block, PR-interval prolongation, jaundice.

PREGNANCY-LACTATION-REPRODUCTION

• Use during pregnancy only if potential benefit justifies potential risk to the fetus.

The U.S. Department of Health and Human Services Perinatal HIV Guidelines recommend atazanavir as a preferred protease inhibitor in antiretroviral-naive pregnant women when combined with low-dose ritonavir boosting. Enroll pregnant women in the Antiretroviral Pregnancy Registry (1-800-258-4263).

• Drug appears in human milk. Breastfeeding is contraindicated in HIV-infected mothers because of risk of postnatal transmission of HIV.

NURSING CONSIDERATIONS

🛈 *Alert:* Drug may prolong the PR interval. Monitor ECG, especially in patients with preexisting conduction system disease.

• Monitor patient for hyperglycemia and new-onset diabetes or worsened diabetes. Insulin and oral antidiabetic dosages may need adjustment.

• Monitor patient with HBV or HCV infection for elevated liver enzyme levels or hepatic decompensation.

• Monitor patient for immune reconstitution syndrome. Evaluate and treat indolent or residual opportunistic infections, such as *Mycobacterium avium*, CMV, *Pneumocystis jiroveci* pneumonia, or TB. Some autoimmune disorders, such as Graves disease, polymyositis, and Guillain-Barré syndrome, have also occurred, even after many months of treatment.

• Watch for life-threatening lactic acidosis syndrome and symptomatic hyperlactatemia, especially in women and obese patients.

• If patient has hemophilia, watch for bleeding.

• Drug may cause nephrolithiasis or cholelithiasis. Evaluate patient for signs or symptoms of nephrolithiasis (flank pain) or cholelithiasis (abdominal pain, nausea, vomiting, jaundice); interrupt or discontinue drug as clinically indicated should signs or symptoms occur.

• Monitor patient for rash. Discontinue drug if rash occurs.

• Most patients have an asymptomatic increase in indirect bilirubin, possibly with yellowed skin or sclerae. This hyperbilirubinemia will resolve when therapy stops.

• Monitor liver enzyme levels before and periodically during treatment.

• Although cross-resistance occurs among protease inhibitors, resistance to drug doesn't preclude use of other protease inhibitors.

🛈 *Alert:* For patients with phenylketonuria, be aware that oral powder contains 35 mg of phenylalanine; capsules don't.

PATIENT TEACHING

• Urge patient to take drug with food every day and to take other antiretrovirals as prescribed.

• Explain that drug doesn't cure HIV infection and that patient may develop opportunistic infections and other complications of HIV disease.

• Caution patient that drug doesn't reduce the risk of transmitting HIV to others.

• Tell patient that drug may cause altered or increased body fat, central obesity, buffalo hump, peripheral wasting, facial wasting, breast enlargement, and a cushingoid appearance.

• Tell patient to report yellowed skin or eyes, dizziness, or light-headedness.

• Caution patient not to take other prescriptions or OTC or herbal medicines without first consulting prescriber.

SAFETY ALERT!

atenolol
a-TEN-o-loll

Tenormin◆

Therapeutic class: Antihypertensives
Pharmacologic class: Beta blockers

AVAILABLE FORMS
Tablets: 25 mg, 50 mg, 100 mg

INDICATIONS & DOSAGES
Adjust-a-dose (for all indications): If CrCl is 15 to 35 mL/minute/1.73 m^2, maximum dose is 50 mg daily; if CrCl is below 15 mL/minute/1.73 m^2, maximum dose is 25 mg daily. Hemodialysis patients need 25 to 50 mg after each dialysis session. For elderly patients, consider starting initial dose at 25 mg PO daily.

Reactions in bold italics are *life-threatening*. Interactions may have a *rapid onset* or a *delayed onset*.

➤ **HTN**
Adults: Initially, 50 mg PO daily alone or in combination with a diuretic as a single dose, increased to 100 mg once daily after 7 to 14 days. Dosages of more than 100 mg daily are unlikely to produce further benefit.

➤ **Angina pectoris**
Adults: 50 mg PO once daily, increased as needed to 100 mg daily after 7 days for optimal effect. Maximum, 200 mg daily.

➤ **Acute MI**
Adults: 100 mg PO daily or 50 mg b.i.d. for at least 7 days; may continue for 1 to 3 years if no contraindications.

ADMINISTRATION
PO
• Check apical pulse before giving drug.
• Give drug exactly as prescribed, at the same time each day.

ACTION
Selectively blocks beta$_1$-adrenergic receptors, decreases cardiac output and cardiac oxygen consumption, and depresses renin secretion.

Route	Onset	Peak	Duration
PO	1 hr	2–4 hr	24 hr

Half-life: 6 to 7 hours.

ADVERSE REACTIONS
CNS: depression, dizziness, fatigue, lethargy, vertigo, drowsiness, fever, lightheadedness. **CV:** orthostatic hypotension, *bradycardia, HF, heart block,* intermittent claudication, atrial fibrillation, *supraventricular tachycardia, cardiac arrest, ventricular tachycardia.* **GI:** nausea, diarrhea. **Musculoskeletal:** leg pain. **Respiratory:** *bronchospasm,* dyspnea, *PE,* wheezing. **Skin:** rash.

INTERACTIONS
Drug-drug. *Aluminum salts:* May reduce bioavailability of atenolol. Separate doses by at least 2 hours.
Amiodarone: May increase risk of bradycardia, AV block, and myocardial depression. Monitor ECG and vital signs.
Antihypertensives: May increase hypotensive effect. Use together cautiously.

Calcium carbonate, calcium citrate: May decrease atenolol level. Separate doses by at least 2 hours. Monitor patient and adjust atenolol dosage as needed.
Calcium channel blockers, hydralazine, methyldopa: May cause additive hypotension and bradycardia. Adjust dosage as needed.
Cardiac glycosides, diltiazem, verapamil: May cause excessive bradycardia and increased depressant effect on myocardium. Use together cautiously.
Catecholamine-depleting drugs (reserpine): May increase risk of hypotension and bradycardia. Use together cautiously.
Clonidine: May exacerbate rebound HTN if clonidine is withdrawn. Atenolol should be withdrawn before clonidine by several days or added several days after clonidine is stopped.
Dolasetron: May decrease clearance of dolasetron and increase risk of toxicity. Monitor patient for toxicity.
Insulin, oral antidiabetics: May alter dosage requirements in previously stabilized diabetic patient. Observe patient carefully.
IV lidocaine: May reduce hepatic metabolism of lidocaine, increasing risk of toxicity. Give bolus doses of lidocaine at a slower rate and monitor therapy.
NSAIDs: May decrease antihypertensive effects. Monitor BP.
Penicillins: May reduce bioavailability of atenolol. Monitor BP closely.
Prazosin: May increase the risk of orthostatic hypotension in the early phases of use together.
Rivastigmine: May enhance bradycardic effect of atenolol. Avoid combination.
Rifamycins: May reduce effects of atenolol. Monitor BP.
Salicylates: May reduce effects of atenolol. Consider lowering salicylate dosage or changing to a nonsalicylate antiplatelet.

EFFECTS ON LAB TEST RESULTS
• May increase alkaline phosphatase, BUN, creatinine, glucose, LDH, potassium, AST, ALT, and uric acid levels. May decrease glucose level.
• May increase platelet count.

CONTRAINDICATIONS & CAUTIONS

• Contraindicated in patients hypersensitive to drug or its components.
• Contraindicated in patients with sinus bradycardia, heart block greater than first degree, overt cardiac failure, untreated pheochromocytoma, and cardiogenic shock.
• Contraindicated in patients with acute MI and HF who don't promptly respond to IV furosemide or equivalent therapy.
• Use cautiously in patients at risk for HF and in those with diabetes, hyperthyroidism, and impaired renal or hepatic function.
• Beta blockers shouldn't be routinely used in patients with bronchospastic disease. Atenolol may be used cautiously in patients who don't respond to or can't tolerate other antihypertensive treatment. Use lowest possible dosage and have bronchodilator available. Consider divided doses if atenolol dosage must be increased.
• Safe use in children hasn't been established.

Dialyzable drug: Yes.

⚠ *Overdose S&S:* Lethargy, decreased respiratory drive, wheezing, sinus pause, bradycardia.

PREGNANCY-LACTATION-REPRODUCTION

• Drug can cause fetal harm. Use cautiously in pregnant women and inform women of the potential fetal hazard.
• Drug appears in human milk. Use cautiously in breastfeeding women.
• Neonates born to mothers receiving atenolol at parturition and breastfed infants of mothers receiving atenolol may be at risk for hypoglycemia and significant bradycardia.

NURSING CONSIDERATIONS

• Monitor BP, preferably just before next dose, to evaluate effectiveness.
• Monitor hemodialysis patients closely because of hypotension risk.
• Beta blockers may mask tachycardia caused by hyperthyroidism. In patients with suspected thyrotoxicosis, withdraw beta blocker gradually to avoid thyroid storm.
• Drug may mask signs and symptoms of hypoglycemia in diabetic patients.
• Drug may cause changes in exercise tolerance and ECG.

• Monitor patient for cardiac failure. Discontinue drug in patients who develop cardiac failure that doesn't respond to standard treatment.

Black Box Warning Avoid abrupt discontinuation of therapy. Withdraw drug gradually to avoid serious adverse reactions, such as severe exacerbations of angina, MI, and ventricular arrhythmias even in patients treated only for HTN. ■

• *Look alike–sound alike:* Don't confuse atenolol with timolol or albuterol.

PATIENT TEACHING

• Instruct patient to take drug exactly as prescribed, at the same time every day.

Black Box Warning Caution patient not to stop drug suddenly. ■

• Advise patient to report all adverse reactions to prescriber.
• Teach patient how to take pulse, when to withhold drug, and when to report HR according to prescriber's instructions.
• Tell female patient of childbearing potential to notify prescriber about planned, suspected, or known pregnancy.
• Advise breastfeeding patient to contact prescriber; drug may cause hypoglycemia or significant bradycardia in the infant.

SAFETY ALERT!

atezolizumab ⚕
a-te-zoe-LIZ-ue-mab

Tecentriq

Therapeutic class: Antineoplastics
Pharmacologic class: Monoclonal antibodies

AVAILABLE FORMS
Injection: 1,200 mg/20 mL single-dose vial

INDICATIONS & DOSAGES
Adjust-a-dose (for all indications): Dosage reductions aren't recommended for toxicities; drug is either withheld or permanently discontinued. Refer to manufacturer's instructions for toxicity-related treatment.

➤ **Locally advanced or metastatic urothelial carcinoma in patients who are not eligible for cisplatin-containing chemotherapy and whose tumors express PD-L1**

(PD-L1 stained tumor-infiltrating immune cells [IC] covering 5% or more of the tumor area), as determined by an FDA-approved test, or aren't eligible for platinum-containing chemotherapy regardless of PD-L1 status, or have disease progression during or after platinum-containing chemotherapy or disease progression within 12 months of neoadjuvant or adjuvant treatment; patients with metastatic NSCLC with disease progression during or after platinum-containing chemotherapy. (Patients with NSCLC and *EGFR* or *ALK* genomic tumor aberrations should have disease progression on FDA-approved therapy for these aberrations before starting drug. ⨳)

Adults: 1,200 mg IV over 60 minutes every 3 weeks until disease progression or unacceptable toxicity.

✴ NEW INDICATION: First-line treatment of patients with metastatic nonsquamous NSCLC with no *EGFR* or *ALK* genomic tumor aberrations

Adults: 1,200 mg IV over 60 minutes, followed by bevacizumab, paclitaxel, and carboplatin on the same day, every 3 weeks for a maximum of four to six cycles. After completion of chemotherapy, give atezolizumab 1,200 mg IV, followed by bevacizumab on day 1 of each 21-day cycle.

➤ Small-cell lung cancer (extensive-stage), first-line treatment ♦

Adults: 1,200 mg IV over 60 minutes on day 1 every 3 weeks in combination with carboplatin and etoposide for four cycles (induction), followed by maintenance therapy of single-agent atezolizumab 1,200 mg IV once every 3 weeks.

✴ NEW INDICATION: Treatment of unresectable locally advanced or metastatic triple-negative breast cancer (TNBC) tumors that express *PD-L1* as determined by an FDA approved test, in combination with paclitaxel protein-bound ⨳

Adults: 840 mg IV infusion over 60 minutes on days 1 and 15 of a 28-day cycle. Give paclitaxel protein-bound 100 mg/m² on days 1, 8, and 15 of the 28-day cycle following atezolizumab. If the first infusion of atezolizumab is tolerated, all subsequent infusions may be administered over 30 minutes.

For all new indications, continue treatment until disease progression or unacceptable toxicity occurs.

ADMINISTRATION

IV

▼ Visually inspect vial for particulate matter and discoloration. Discard vial if solution is cloudy or discolored or if particles are present. Don't shake vial.

▼ Withdraw 20 mL of atezolizumab and dilute in 250 mL polyvinyl chloride, polyethylene, or polyolefin infusion bag containing NSS.

▼ Mix diluted solution by gentle inversion; don't shake.

▼ Administer immediately once prepared and discard unused solution in vial.

▼ May give through IV tubing with or without a sterile, nonpyrogenic, low-protein-binding in-line filter (pore size 0.2 to 0.22 micron).

▼ Don't give as IV push or bolus. Administer as IV infusion over 60 minutes. If first infusion is tolerated, may give subsequent infusions over 30 minutes.

▼ If necessary, prepared solution can be stored up to 6 hours at room temperature, including administration time, or up to 24 hours in refrigerator at 36° to 46° F (2° to 8° C). Don't freeze.

▼ Store in original carton and protect from light.

▼ **Incompatibilities:** Don't dilute in any solution other than NSS or administer other drugs in same IV line.

ACTION

A monoclonal antibody that binds to PD-1, allowing activation of the antitumor immune response without inducing antibody-dependent cellular cytotoxicity.

Route	Onset	Peak	Duration
IV	Unknown	Unknown	Unknown

Half-life: 27 days.

ADVERSE REACTIONS

CNS: fatigue, fever, confusion. **CV:** peripheral edema, dehydration, *venous thromboembolism.* **GI:** nausea, constipation, abdominal pain, vomiting, decreased appetite, intestinal obstruction, immune-mediated colitis, diarrhea. **GU:** UTI, hematuria, urinary obstruction, acute kidney injury. **Hematologic:** anemia, *lymphopenia.* **Hepatic:** *immune-mediated hepatitis,* increased liver enzyme levels. **Musculoskeletal:** back pain, neck pain, arthralgia. **Respiratory:** dyspnea, cough, pneumonia, *immune-mediated pneumonitis, ILD.* **Skin:** rash, pruritus. **Other:** severe infection (*sepsis,* herpes encephalitis, mycobacterial infection), infusion-related reaction, hypothyroidism, hyperthyroidism.

INTERACTIONS

Drug-drug. *Belimumab:* May enhance adverse/toxic effect of belimumab. Avoid combination.

EFFECTS ON LAB TEST RESULTS

• May increase glucose, AST, ALT, alkaline phosphatase, potassium, magnesium, bilirubin, and creatinine levels.
• May decrease phosphorus, sodium, and albumin levels.
• May decrease hematocrit and lymphocyte count.

CONTRAINDICATIONS & CAUTIONS

• Drug increases risk of immune-mediated reactions, including myocarditis, nephritis, pneumonitis, hepatitis, colitis, endocrinopathy (thyroid disorders, pituitary gland inflammation, adrenal insufficiency), meningitis, and encephalitis.
• The FDA recommends providers select patients for the treatment of locally advanced or metastatic urothelial cancer using the criteria described in Section 14 of the Tecentriq product labeling as there has been an association with decreased survival in certain patient populations.
• Initiating drug in patients with moderate or severe hepatic impairment hasn't been studied.
• Safety and effectiveness in children haven't been established.
Dialyzable drug: Unknown.

PREGNANCY-LACTATION-REPRODUCTION

• Based on its mechanism of action, drug can cause fetal harm. If drug is used during pregnancy, or patient becomes pregnant during treatment, advise her of potential risk to the fetus.
• Women should use effective contraception during treatment and for at least 5 months after last dose.
• Drug may impair fertility in women of childbearing potential who are receiving treatment.
• It isn't known if drug appears in human milk. Patients shouldn't breastfeed during treatment and for at least 5 months after last dose.

NURSING CONSIDERATIONS

• Monitor patient for infusion reactions (rash, pruritus, chills, flushing, dyspnea, wheezing, dizziness, pain, facial swelling); if a mild or moderate reaction occurs, interrupt or slow infusion rate. Permanently discontinue drug in patients with grade 3 or 4 reactions.
• Monitor patient for signs and symptoms of immune-related pneumonitis (new or worsening cough, chest pain, dyspnea) and assess with radiographic imaging. For grade 2 or greater toxicities, drug may need to be withheld or discontinued and treatment with prednisone or equivalent begun.
• Monitor patient for immune-mediated hepatitis (jaundice, severe nausea, vomiting, right quadrant abdominal pain, lethargy, easy bruising, bleeding). For grade 2 or greater transaminase elevations, drug may need to be withheld or discontinued and treatment with prednisone or equivalent begun.
• Monitor patient for immune-related colitis or diarrhea (frequent or bloody stools, abdominal pain). Withhold drug for grade 2 symptoms. If symptoms persist for more than 5 days or recur, give 1 to 2 mg/kg/day of prednisone or equivalent. For grade 3 symptoms, withhold drug and treat with 1 to 2 mg/kg/day of IV methylprednisolone, then convert to oral steroids once patient improves. For grade 2 or 3 diarrhea or colitis, when symptoms improve to grade 1, taper steroids over 1 month or more. Resume drug if symptoms improve to grade 0 or 1 within 12 weeks and steroids have been tapered to 10 mg or less of oral prednisone per day. Permanently discontinue drug for grade 4 diarrhea or colitis.

Reactions in bold italics are *life-threatening*. Interactions may have a *rapid onset* or a *delayed onset*.

• Monitor patient for immune-related hypophysitis (pituitary gland inflammation). Treat with corticosteroids and hormone replacement as clinically indicated. Withhold drug for grade 2 or 3 hypophysitis; permanently discontinue for grade 4.

• Assess baseline thyroid levels and monitor thyroid function periodically during treatment. For symptomatic hypothyroidism (tiredness, feeling cold, dizziness, mood changes), give replacement therapy. Manage isolated hypothyroidism with replacement therapy without corticosteroids. For symptomatic hyperthyroidism (poor concentration, heat intolerance, tremors, palpitations), withhold drug and start antithyroid drugs as needed. Resume drug when symptoms are controlled and thyroid function improves.

• Monitor patient for adrenal insufficiency (fatigue, arthralgia, myalgia, nausea, vomiting, weakness, low BP, dizziness). For symptomatic adrenal insufficiency, withhold drug and give IV methylprednisolone 1 to 2 mg/kg/day followed by oral prednisone 1 to 2 mg/kg/day or equivalent once symptoms improve. Begin steroid taper when symptoms improve to grade 1 or less and taper over at least 1 month. May restart drug if symptoms improve to grade 1 or less within 12 weeks, corticosteroids have been reduced to 10 mg of oral prednisone per day or less, and patient is stable on replacement therapy.

• Monitor patient for signs and symptoms of new-onset diabetes with ketoacidosis (decreased alertness, dry skin, flushing, frequent urination or thirst, headache, fruity-smelling breath, nausea, vomiting). Initiate treatment with insulin. For grade 3 or more hyperglycemia, withhold drug. Resume drug when glucose metabolic control is achieved on insulin replacement therapy.

• Monitor patient for immune-related meningitis or encephalitis and permanently discontinue drug if these conditions occur. Treat with IV steroids and convert to oral steroids once patient has improved.

• Monitor patient for myasthenic syndrome, myasthenia gravis, Guillain-Barré syndrome, and signs and symptoms of sensory and motor neuropathy (severe muscle weakness, numbness or tingling of the hands or feet, confusion, mood changes, neck stiffness, photosensitivity). Permanently

discontinue drug if these occur. Treat as appropriate, and consider systemic prednisone 1 to 2 mg/kg/day.

• Monitor patient for acute pancreatitis (severe epigastric pain, nausea, vomiting, diarrhea, chills, tachycardia). Withhold drug for grade 3 or higher amylase or lipase levels (greater than $2 \times$ ULN) or grade 2 or 3 pancreatitis. Give IV methylprednisolone or equivalent per day and follow with oral prednisone or equivalent when symptoms improve. May resume drug if serum amylase and lipase levels improve to grade 1 or better within 12 weeks, symptoms have resolved, and corticosteroids have been reduced to 10 mg of oral prednisone or less. Permanently discontinue drug for grade 4 pancreatitis or any grade recurrent pancreatitis.

• Monitor patient for signs and symptoms of infection (fever, cough, pain while urinating, flulike symptoms), including sepsis, herpes encephalitis, and mycobacterial infections. UTI and pneumonia are the most common serious infections. Treat as clinically indicated for suspected or confirmed infection. Withhold drug for grade 3 or greater infection.

• Monitor patient for development of myocarditis or nephritis; withhold drug if signs or symptoms occur.

PATIENT TEACHING

• Teach patient signs and symptoms of immune-mediated reactions and that they may require corticosteroid treatment and interruption or discontinuation of therapy.

• Advise patient to immediately report infusion-related and hypersensitivity reactions.

• Caution patient to immediately report all adverse effects.

• Instruct patient to immediately report signs and symptoms of infection.

• Instruct patient that laboratory testing will be needed to monitor for adverse reactions related to treatment.

atomoxetine hydrochloride 🔒
AT-oh-mox-e-teen

Strattera✦

Therapeutic class: ADHD drugs
Pharmacologic class: Selective norepinephrine reuptake inhibitors

AVAILABLE FORMS
Capsules 🔵: 10 mg, 18 mg, 25 mg, 40 mg,
60 mg, 80 mg, 100 mg

INDICATIONS & DOSAGES
➤ **ADHD**
*Adults and children older than age 6 and
adolescents weighing more than 70 kg:*
Initially, 40 mg PO daily; increase after at
least 3 days to a total of 80 mg/day PO, as a
single dose in the morning or two evenly divided doses in the morning and late afternoon or early evening. After 2 to 4 weeks,
increase total dose to a maximum of 100 mg,
if needed.
*Children age 6 and older and adolescents
weighing 70 kg or less:* Initially, 0.5 mg/kg
PO daily; increase after a minimum of 3
days to a target total daily dose of 1.2 mg/kg
PO as a single dose in the morning or two
evenly divided doses in the morning and late
afternoon or early evening. Don't exceed
1.4 mg/kg or 100 mg daily, whichever is less.
🔒 *Adjust-a-dose:* In patients with moderate
hepatic impairment (Child-Pugh class B),
reduce to 50% of the normal dose; in those
with severe hepatic impairment (Child-Pugh
class C), reduce to 25% of the normal dose.
Poor metabolizers of CYP2D6 or those also
receiving strong CYP2D6 inhibitors may
require a reduced dose.
 In children and adults weighing more
than 70 kg who are also receiving strong
CYP2D6 inhibitors (fluoxetine, paroxetine,
quinidine) or are known CYP2D6 poor metabolizers, start at 40 mg daily and increase
to 80 mg daily only if symptoms don't improve after 4 weeks and if first dose is tolerated.
 In children weighing less than 70 kg
who are also receiving strong CYP2D6 inhibitors or are known CYP2D6 poor metabolizers, adjust dosage to 0.5 mg/kg daily and

increase to 1.2 mg/kg daily only if symptoms don't improve after 4 weeks and if first
dose is tolerated.

ADMINISTRATION
PO
• Give drug without regard for meals.
• Capsules should be swallowed whole and
not opened.

ACTION
May be related to selective inhibition of the
presynaptic norepinephrine transporter.

Route	Onset	Peak	Duration
PO	Rapid	1–2 hr	Unknown

Half-life: 5 hours; 24 hours in poor metabolizers.

ADVERSE REACTIONS
CNS: headache, insomnia, dizziness, somnolence, irritability, mood swings, fatigue,
sedation, depression, tremor, early-morning
awakening, paresthesia, abnormal dreams,
sleep disorder, syncope, anxiety. **CV:** orthostatic hypotension, tachycardia, HTN, palpitations, hot flashes. **EENT:** mydriasis, conjunctivitis, oropharyngeal pain, pharyngolaryngeal pain, sinus headache. **GI:** abdominal
pain, constipation, dyspepsia, nausea, vomiting, decreased appetite, dry mouth. **GU:**
urine retention, urinary hesitation, ejaculatory problems, difficulty in micturition,
dysmenorrhea, erectile disturbance, erectile
dysfunction, menstrual disorder, prostatitis.
Metabolic: weight loss. **Skin:** pruritus, increased sweating, rash. **Other:** decreased
libido, chills.

INTERACTIONS
Drug-drug. *Albuterol:* May increase CV
effects. Use together cautiously.
MAO inhibitors: May cause hyperthermia,
rigidity, myoclonus, autonomic instability with possible rapid fluctuations of vital
signs, and mental status changes. Avoid use
within 2 weeks of MAO inhibitor.
Pressor agents: May increase BP. Use together cautiously.
*Strong CYP2D6 inhibitors (fluoxetine,
paroxetine, quinidine):* May increase atomoxetine level. Start atomoxetine at usual
initial daily dose. Increase to the usual target
dose of 80 mg only if signs and symptoms

---

fail to improve after 4 weeks and the initial dose is well tolerated.

EFFECTS ON LAB TEST RESULTS
None reported.

CONTRAINDICATIONS & CAUTIONS
• Contraindicated in patients hypersensitive to drug or its components; in those with serious heart problems, current or history of pheochromocytoma, or angle-closure glaucoma; in those who are intolerant of increased BP or HR; and in those who have taken an MAO inhibitor within the past 2 weeks.
• Use cautiously in patients with HTN, tachycardia, hypotension, urine retention, or cerebrovascular disease.
• Safety and effectiveness in children younger than age 6 haven't been established.
Dialyzable drug: No.
⚠ *Overdose S&S:* Somnolence, agitation, hyperactivity, abnormal behavior, GI symptoms, mydriasis, tachycardia, dry mouth, prolonged QT interval, disorientation, hallucinations, seizures.

PREGNANCY-LACTATION-REPRODUCTION
• Don't use in pregnant women unless potential benefit justifies potential risk to the fetus. Women of childbearing potential should be advised to use effective contraception.
• It isn't known if drug appears in human milk. Use cautiously in breastfeeding women.

NURSING CONSIDERATIONS
• Use drug as part of a total treatment program for ADHD, including psychological, educational, and social intervention. Drug may be discontinued without tapering.
Black Box Warning Monitor children and adolescents closely for worsening of condition, agitation, irritability, suicidal thinking or behaviors, and unusual changes in behavior, especially the first few months of therapy or when dosage is increased or decreased. ∎
• Periodically monitor patients for changes in HR or BP.
• Assess patients carefully for cardiac disease, including family history of sudden death or ventricular arrhythmia. Evaluate

patients with new cardiac symptoms promptly.
• Patients taking drug for extended periods must be reevaluated periodically to determine drug's usefulness.
• Monitor growth during treatment. If growth or weight gain is unsatisfactory, consider interrupting therapy.
🜲 *Alert:* Severe liver injury may occur and progress to liver failure. Notify prescriber of any sign of liver injury: yellowing of the skin or the sclera of the eyes, pruritus, dark urine, upper right-sided tenderness, or unexplained flulike syndrome.
• Monitor BP and pulse rate at baseline, after each dosage increase, and periodically during treatment.
• Monitor patient for urinary hesitancy, urine retention, or sexual dysfunction. Drug may increase risk of priapism.

PATIENT TEACHING
Black Box Warning Advise patients to call prescriber immediately about unusual behavior or suicidal thoughts. ∎
• Instruct patient to immediately report chest pain, shortness of breath, or fainting.
• Tell patient to use caution when operating a vehicle or machinery until the effects of drug are known.
• Warn male patient to seek prompt medical attention for an erection that lasts more than 4 hours.
• Inform patient that therapy may be interrupted periodically to check ADHD symptoms.
• Tell female patient who is pregnant, planning to become pregnant, or breastfeeding to consult prescriber before taking atomoxetine.

---

atorvastatin calcium 🜲
ah-TOR-va-stah-tin

Lipitor✐

Therapeutic class: Antilipemics
Pharmacologic class: HMG-CoA reductase inhibitors

AVAILABLE FORMS
Tablets 🄰: 10 mg, 20 mg, 40 mg, 80 mg

INDICATIONS & DOSAGES

➤ **In patients with clinically evident CAD, to reduce risk of nonfatal MI, fatal and nonfatal strokes, angina, HF, and revascularization procedures**
Adults: Initially, 10 to 20 mg PO daily. May increase based on patient response and tolerance; usual dosage, 10 to 80 mg PO daily.

➤ **To reduce risk of MI, stroke, angina, or revascularization procedures in patients with multiple risk factors for CAD but who don't yet have the disease**
Adults: 10 to 80 mg PO daily.

➤ **To reduce risk of MI or stroke in patients with type 2 diabetes and multiple risk factors for CAD but who don't yet have the disease**
Adults: 10 to 80 mg PO daily.

➤ **Adjunct to diet to reduce LDL, total cholesterol, apolipoprotein B, and triglyceride levels and to increase HDL levels in patients with primary hypercholesterolemia (heterozygous familial and nonfamilial) and mixed dyslipidemia (Fredrickson types IIa and IIb); adjunct to diet to reduce triglyceride level (Fredrickson type IV); primary dysbetalipoproteinemia (Fredrickson type III) in patients who don't respond adequately to diet** 🔲
Adults: Initially, 10 or 20 mg PO once daily. Patient who requires a reduction of more than 45% in LDL level may be started at 40 mg once daily. Increase dose, as needed, to maximum of 80 mg daily as single dose. Dosage based on lipid levels drawn within 2 to 4 weeks of starting therapy and after dosage adjustment.

➤ **Alone or as an adjunct to lipid-lowering treatments, such as LDL apheresis, to reduce total and LDL cholesterol in patients with homozygous familial hypercholesterolemia** 🔲
Adults: 10 to 80 mg PO once daily.

➤ **Heterozygous familial hypercholesterolemia in pediatric patients who don't respond adequately to dietary treatment** 🔲
Children ages 10 to 17 (girls should be 1 year postmenarche): Initially, 10 mg PO once daily. Adjustment intervals should be at least 4 weeks. Maximum daily dose is 20 mg.

➤ **Intensive lipid-lowering after an ACS event regardless of baseline LDL; noncardioembolic stroke/TIA (secondary prevention)** ◆
Adults: Initially, 80 mg PO once daily. Adjust dosage based on tolerability.

ADMINISTRATION

PO
• Give drug without regard for meals.

ACTION

Inhibits HMG-CoA reductase, an early (and rate-limiting) step in cholesterol biosynthesis.

Route	Onset	Peak	Duration
PO	Unknown	1–2 hr	Unknown

Half-life: 14 hours.

ADVERSE REACTIONS

CNS: insomnia. **EENT:** nasopharyngitis, pharyngolaryngeal pain. **GI:** abdominal pain, diarrhea, dyspepsia, flatulence, nausea. **GU:** UTI. **Musculoskeletal:** *rhabdomyolysis,* arthralgia, myalgia, extremity pain, muscle spasms, musculoskeletal pain. **Skin:** rash.

INTERACTIONS

Drug-drug. *Amiodarone:* May increase risk of severe myopathy or rhabdomyolysis. Avoid use together or decrease atorvastatin dose.
Antacids, cholestyramine, colestipol: May decrease atorvastatin level. Separate administration times.
Boceprevir: May increase atorvastatin level and risk of myopathy and rhabdomyolysis. Atorvastatin dosage shouldn't exceed 40 mg daily.
Colchicine, **diltiazem,** *fibric acid derivatives,* **nefazodone,** *niacin, protease inhibitors,* **verapamil:** May decrease metabolism of HMG-CoA reductase inhibitors, increasing toxicity. Monitor patient for adverse effects and report unexplained muscle pain.
Cyclosporine, *tacrolimus, telaprevir, tipranavir plus ritonavir:* May increase statin level and risk of myopathy and rhabdomyolysis. Avoid use together.
Darunavir and ritonavir, fosamprenavir, fosamprenavir and ritonavir, saquinavir and

ritonavir: May increase atorvastatin level and risk of myopathy and rhabdomyolysis. Atorvastatin dosage shouldn't exceed 20 mg daily.

Digoxin: May increase digoxin level. Monitor digoxin level and patient for evidence of toxicity.

Fluconazole, itraconazole, ketoconazole, voriconazole: May increase atorvastatin level and adverse effects. Avoid using together or, if unavoidable, atorvastatin dosage shouldn't exceed 20 mg daily.

Gemfibrozil: May increase risk of myopathy/rhabdomyolysis. Avoid combination.

Hormonal contraceptives: May increase norethindrone and ethinyl estradiol levels. Consider increased drug levels when selecting an oral contraceptive.

Lopinavir and ritonavir: May increase statin level and risk of myopathy and rhabdomyolysis. Use together cautiously and at lowest atorvastatin dosage necessary.

Macrolides (azithromycin, clarithromycin, erythromycin, telithromycin): May increase atorvastatin level and risk of myopathy and rhabdomyolysis. Atorvastatin dosage shouldn't exceed 20 mg daily.

Nelfinavir: May increase statin level and risk of myopathy and rhabdomyolysis. Atorvastatin dosage shouldn't exceed 40 mg daily.

Drug-herb. *Jin bu huan, kava:* May increase risk of hepatotoxicity. Discourage use together.

Drug-food. *Grapefruit juice:* May increase drug levels when consumed in large quantities, increasing risk of adverse reactions. Discourage use together.

EFFECTS ON LAB TEST RESULTS
• May increase ALT, AST, and CK levels.

CONTRAINDICATIONS & CAUTIONS
• Contraindicated in patients hypersensitive to drug and in those with active liver disease or unexplained persistent elevations of transaminase levels.
• Some dosage forms contain polysorbate 80, which can cause delayed hypersensitivity reactions.
• Use cautiously in patients with hepatic impairment or heavy alcohol use, in patients with inadequately treated hypothyroidism,

with other drugs associated with myopathy, and in elderly patients.
• Withhold or stop drug in patients at risk for renal failure caused by rhabdomyolysis resulting from trauma; in serious, acute conditions that suggest myopathy; and in major surgery, severe acute infection, hypotension, uncontrolled seizures, or severe metabolic, endocrine, or electrolyte disorders.
🎗 Limit use in children to those older than age 10 with homozygous familial hypercholesterolemia.
Dialyzable drug: No.

PREGNANCY-LACTATION-REPRODUCTION
• Drug may cause fetal harm. Contraindicated in women who are pregnant or may become pregnant. Women of childbearing potential should use effective contraception during treatment and be apprised of potential hazards to the fetus.
• It isn't known if drug appears in human milk. Use is contraindicated in breastfeeding women.

NURSING CONSIDERATIONS
• Patient should follow a standard cholesterol-lowering diet before and during therapy.
• Before treatment, assess patient for underlying causes for hypercholesterolemia and obtain a baseline lipid profile. Obtain periodic LFT results and lipid levels before starting treatment and at 4 and 12 weeks after initiation, or after an increase in dosage and periodically thereafter.
• Watch for signs of myositis and myopathy (unexplained muscle pain, tenderness, weakness, malaise, dark urine, fever). Drug may need to be discontinued.
• *Look alike–sound alike:* Don't confuse atorvastatin with atomoxetine. Don't confuse Lipitor with Loniten, Levatol, or Zyrtec.

PATIENT TEACHING
• Teach patient about proper dietary management, weight control, and exercise. Explain their importance in controlling high fat levels.
• Warn patient to avoid alcohol.
• Tell patient to inform prescriber of all adverse reactions, such as muscle pain, malaise, and fever.

- Advise patient that drug can be taken at any time of day, without regard for meals.
- **⊕ Alert:** Tell female patient to stop drug and notify prescriber immediately if she is or may be pregnant or if she's breastfeeding.

atovaquone
a-TOE-va-kwon

Mepron

Therapeutic class: Antiprotozoals
Pharmacologic class: Ubiquinone analogues

AVAILABLE FORMS
Suspension: 750 mg/5 mL

INDICATIONS & DOSAGES
➤ **Acute, mild to moderate *Pneumocystis jiroveci* pneumonia in patients who can't tolerate sulfamethoxazole–trimethoprim**
Adults and adolescents age 13 and older: 750 mg (5 mL) PO b.i.d. for 21 days.
➤ **To prevent *P. jiroveci* pneumonia in patients who are unable to tolerate sulfamethoxazole–trimethoprim**
Adults and adolescents age 13 and older: 1,500 mg (10 mL) PO daily.

ADMINISTRATION
PO
- Give with food; taking with meals enhances absorption.
- Shake bottle gently before using.
- Give entire contents of foil pouch, which can be poured into a dosing spoon or cup or be taken directly into the mouth.

ACTION
May interfere with electron transport in protozoal mitochondria, inhibiting enzymes needed to synthesize nucleic acids and adenosine triphosphate.

Route	Onset	Peak	Duration
PO	Unknown	Unknown	Unknown

Half-life: 2 to 4 days.

ADVERSE REACTIONS
CNS: headache, insomnia, fever, pain, asthenia, anxiety, dizziness, depression.
CV: hypotension. **EENT:** sinusitis, rhinitis. **GI:** abdominal pain, nausea, diarrhea, oral candidiasis, vomiting, constipation, anorexia, dyspepsia, taste perversion. **Hematologic:** *neutropenia,* anemia. **Metabolic:** *hypoglycemia,* hyponatremia. **Musculoskeletal:** myalgia. **Respiratory:** cough, dyspnea. **Skin:** rash, diaphoresis, pruritus. **Other:** flulike syndrome.

INTERACTIONS
Drug-drug. *Indinavir:* May decrease indinavir trough level. Monitor patient closely for potential loss of effectiveness.
Metoclopramide: May decrease atovaquone bioavailability. Use another antiemetic.
Rifabutin, rifampin: May decrease atovaquone's steady-state level. Avoid using together.
Tetracycline: May decrease atovaquone level. Monitor patient for continued or reactivated infection.
Zidovudine: May elevate zidovudine level and lead to toxicity. Monitor closely.

EFFECTS ON LAB TEST RESULTS
- May increase glucose, amylase, alkaline phosphatase, ALT, and AST levels. May decrease Hb and sodium levels.
- May decrease neutrophil count.

CONTRAINDICATIONS & CAUTIONS
- Contraindicated in patients hypersensitive to drug.
- Serious hypersensitivity reactions have been reported.
- Use cautiously in patients with severe hepatic impairment.
- Use cautiously with other highly protein-bound drugs; if used together, assess patient for toxicity.
⊕ Alert: Patients with GI disorders may not absorb drug well and may not achieve adequate plasma levels. Consider parenteral therapy with alternative drugs.
Dialyzable drug: Unknown.
⚠ Overdose S&S: Methemoglobinemia, rash.

PREGNANCY-LACTATION-REPRODUCTION
- Use cautiously in pregnant women and only if potential benefit justifies potential risk to the fetus.

Reactions in bold italics are *life-threatening*. Interactions may have a *rapid onset* or a *delayed onset*.

- It isn't known if drug appears in human milk. Use cautiously in breastfeeding women.

NURSING CONSIDERATIONS
🔴 **Alert:** Monitor patient closely during therapy because of risk of pulmonary infection.
- Monitor patients with hepatic impairment closely.
- Monitor patient for GI disorders (nausea, vomiting, diarrhea) that might affect patient's ability to absorb drug.

PATIENT TEACHING
- Instruct patient to take drug with meals; food significantly enhances absorption.
- Stress importance of taking atovaquone as prescribed.
- Advise patient to report all adverse reactions and to immediately report nausea, vomiting, diarrhea, white mouth patches, flulike symptoms, dark urine, tiredness, lack of appetite, yellow skin, and light stools.

---

atovaquone–proguanil hydrochloride
a-TOE-va-kwon/pro-GWA-nil

Malarone, Malarone Pediatric

Therapeutic class: Antimalarials
Pharmacologic class: Hydroxynaphtho-quinone and biguanide derivatives

AVAILABLE FORMS
Tablets (adult-strength): 250 mg atovaquone and 100 mg proguanil hydrochloride
Tablets (pediatric-strength): 62.5 mg atovaquone and 25 mg proguanil hydrochloride

INDICATIONS & DOSAGES
➤ **To prevent *Plasmodium falciparum* malaria, including in areas where chloroquine resistance has been reported**
Adults and children weighing more than 40 kg: 1 adult-strength tablet PO once daily with food or milk, beginning 1 or 2 days before entering a malaria-endemic area. Continue prophylactic treatment during stay and for 7 days after return.
Children weighing 31 to 40 kg: 3 pediatric-strength tablets PO once daily beginning 1 or 2 days before entering endemic area.

Continue prophylactic treatment during stay and for 7 days after return.
Children weighing 21 to 30 kg: 2 pediatric-strength tablets PO once daily beginning 1 or 2 days before entering endemic area. Continue prophylactic treatment during stay and for 7 days after return.
Children weighing 11 to 20 kg: 1 pediatric-strength tablet PO daily beginning 1 or 2 days before entering endemic area. Continue prophylactic treatment during stay and for 7 days after return.
Adjust-a-dose: Don't use for malaria prophylaxis in patients with severe renal impairment (CrCl less than 30 mL/minute).
➤ **Acute, uncomplicated *P. falciparum* malaria**
Adults and children weighing more than 40 kg: 4 adult-strength tablets PO once daily for 3 consecutive days.
Children weighing 31 to 40 kg: 3 adult-strength tablets PO once daily for 3 consecutive days.
Children weighing 21 to 30 kg: 2 adult-strength tablets PO once daily for 3 consecutive days.
Children weighing 11 to 20 kg: 1 adult-strength tablet PO once daily for 3 consecutive days.
Children weighing 9 to 10 kg: 3 pediatric-strength tablets PO once daily for 3 consecutive days.
Children weighing 5 to 8 kg: 2 pediatric-strength tablets PO once daily for 3 consecutive days.

ADMINISTRATION
PO
- Give dose at same time each day, with food or milk.
- If patient has difficulty swallowing tablets, crush tablets and mix in condensed milk.
- If vomiting occurs within 1 hour of drug administration, repeat dose.
- Store tablets at controlled room temperature of 59° to 86° F (15° to 30° C).

ACTION
Thought to interfere with nucleic acid replication in the malarial parasite. Atovaquone selectively inhibits mitochondrial electron transport in the parasite. Cycloguanil, an active metabolite of proguanil hydrochloride,

inhibits dihydrofolate reductase. Atovaquone and cycloguanil are active against the erythrocytic and exoerythrocytic stages of *Plasmodium* species.

Route	Onset	Peak	Duration
PO	Unknown	Unknown	Unknown

Half-life: Atovaquone: 2 to 3 days in adults, 1 to 2 days in children; proguanil: 12 to 21 hours in adults and children.

ADVERSE REACTIONS
CNS: headache, asthenia, dizziness, dreams, insomnia. **GI:** abdominal pain, nausea, vomiting, diarrhea, anorexia, dyspepsia, gastritis, oral ulcers. **Respiratory:** cough. **Skin:** pruritus.

INTERACTIONS
Drug-drug. *Indinavir:* May decrease indinavir trough level. Monitor patient closely for potential loss of effectiveness.
Metoclopramide: May decrease atovaquone bioavailability. Use another antiemetic.
Rifabutin, rifampin: May decrease atovaquone level by about 50%. Avoid using together.
Tetracycline: May decrease atovaquone level by about 40%. Monitor patient closely for continued or reactivated infection.
Warfarin: May increase anticoagulation effect. Monitor INR.

EFFECTS ON LAB TEST RESULTS
• May increase alkaline phosphatase, ALT, and AST levels. May decrease Hb level and hematocrit.
• May decrease WBC count.

CONTRAINDICATIONS & CAUTIONS
• Contraindicated in patients hypersensitive to atovaquone, proguanil hydrochloride, or components of drug and in those with severe renal impairment or severe or complicated malaria.
• Use cautiously in patients who are vomiting.
• Use cautiously in elderly patients because they have a greater frequency of decreased renal, hepatic, and cardiac function.
• Safety and effectiveness haven't been established for prevention in children who weigh less than 11 kg or for treatment in children who weigh less than 5 kg.

Dialyzable drug: Unknown.
⚠ *Overdose S&S:* Rash, methemoglobinemia (atovaquone); epigastric discomfort, vomiting, reversible hair loss, scaling of the skin on the palms or soles, reversible aphthous ulceration, hematologic adverse effects (proguanil).

PREGNANCY-LACTATION-REPRODUCTION
• Use during pregnancy only if potential benefit justifies potential risk to the fetus.
• It isn't known if atovaquone appears in human milk, but proguanil does appear in small amounts. Use cautiously in breastfeeding women.

NURSING CONSIDERATIONS
• Persistent diarrhea or vomiting may decrease drug absorption. Patients with these symptoms may need a different antimalarial.
• Monitor patients on prophylactic therapy for elevated liver enzyme levels, hepatitis, and hepatic failure.

PATIENT TEACHING
• Tell patient to take dose at same time each day with food or milk.
• Tell patient or caregiver to crush tablets and mix in condensed milk if patient has difficulty swallowing tablets.
• Tell patient to repeat dose if vomiting occurs within 1 hour after dose.
• Advise patient to notify prescriber if patient can't complete the course of therapy as prescribed.
• Instruct patient to supplement preventive antimalarial with use of protective clothing, bed nets, and insect repellents.

SAFETY ALERT!

atropine sulfate
AT-troe-peen

AtroPen

Therapeutic class: Antiarrhythmics
Pharmacologic class: Anticholinergics–belladonna alkaloids

AVAILABLE FORMS
Injection: 0.05 mg/mL, 0.1 mg/mL, 0.4 mg/mL, 0.8 mg/mL, 1 mg/mL

Reactions in bold italics are *life-threatening*. Interactions may have a *rapid onset* or a *delayed onset*.

Prefilled autoinjectors: 0.25 mg, 0.5 mg, 1 mg, 2 mg
Prefilled syringe: 0.05 mg/mL in 5-mL syringe (pediatric), 0.1 mg/mL in 5- and 10-mL syringe

INDICATIONS & DOSAGES
➤ **Bradyasystolic cardiac arrest**
Adults: 1 mg IV (preferred) every 3 to 5 minutes; maximum total dose is 3 mg.
➤ **Organophosphorus or muscarinic mushroom poisoning**
Adults: 2 to 3 mg IV (preferred), IM, or subcut; may repeat every 20 to 30 minutes.
➤ **Initial treatment of muscarinic symptoms of insecticide (organophosphorus or carbamate) poisoning or organophosphorus nerve agent poisoning**
Adults and children weighing more than 41 kg: For severe symptoms, immediately give three AtroPen 2 mg IM injections in rapid succession. For mild symptoms, give one AtroPen 2 mg IM injection. If patient then develops severe symptoms, give two additional 2 mg IM injections in rapid succession 10 minutes after first injection.
Children weighing 18 to 41 kg: For severe symptoms, immediately give three AtroPen 1 mg IM injections in rapid succession. For mild symptoms, give one AtroPen 1 mg IM injection. If patient then develops severe symptoms, give two additional 1 mg IM injections in rapid succession 10 minutes after first injection.
Children weighing 7 to 18 kg: For severe symptoms, immediately give three AtroPen 0.5 mg IM injections in rapid succession. For mild symptoms, give one AtroPen 0.5 mg IM injection. If patient then develops severe symptoms, give two additional 0.5 mg IM injections in rapid succession 10 minutes after first injection.
Infants weighing less than 7 kg: For severe symptoms, immediately give three AtroPen 0.25 mg IM injections in rapid succession. For mild symptoms, give one AtroPen 0.25 mg IM injection. If patient then develops severe symptoms, give two additional 0.25 mg IM injections in rapid succession 10 minutes after first injection.
➤ **Preoperatively to diminish secretions and block cardiac vagal reflexes**

Adults: 0.5 to 1 mg IV (preferred), IM, or subcut 30 to 60 minutes before anesthesia. May repeat in 1 to 2 hours.
➤ **Stress echocardiography (adjunct chronotropic agent)** ◆
Adults: 0.25 to 0.5 mg IV up to a total dose of 1 to 2 mg until 85% of target HR is achieved.
➤ **Symptomatic bradycardia**
Adults: 0.5 mg IV push, repeated every 3 to 5 minutes, not to exceed a total of 3 mg or 0.04 mg/kg.
Children and adolescents: 0.02 mg/kg IV. May repeat once in 3 to 5 minutes; maximum dose is 1 mg.

ADMINISTRATION
IV
▼ Give into a large vein or into IV tubing over at least 1 minute.
▼ Slow delivery may cause slowing of the HR.
▼ **Incompatibilities:** None listed by manufacturer. Consult a drug incompatibility reference for more information.
Subcutaneous
• Document administration site.
IM
• Auto-injection may be given through clothing.
• Firmly jab tip into midlateral thigh at 90-degree angle.
• Hold auto-injector in place for at least 10 seconds to allow time for complete administration.
• Make sure needle is visible after removing auto-injector. If needle didn't engage, repeat injection, jabbing more firmly.
• Massage injection site for several seconds after removing auto-injector.
• In very thin or young patients, pinch the skin on the thigh together before injection.

ACTION
Inhibits muscarinic actions of acetylcholine at parasympathetic neuroeffector junction, blocking vagal effects on SA and AV nodes, enhancing conduction through AV node and increasing HR.

Route	Onset	Peak	Duration
IV	Immediate	Unknown	Unknown
IM	Rapid	3 min	4 hr
Subcut	Unknown	Unknown	Unknown

Half-life: IM: adults, 2 to 4 hours; children older than age 2, 1½ to 3½ hours; children younger than age 2, 4 to 10 hours.

ADVERSE REACTIONS

Severity and frequency of adverse reactions are dose-related. **CNS:** headache, restlessness, insomnia, dizziness, ataxia, disorientation, hallucinations, delirium, excitement, agitation, confusion, fever. **CV:** *bradycardia,* palpitations, tachycardia, *atrial and ventricular arrhythmias.* **EENT:** blurred vision, mydriasis, photophobia, cycloplegia, increased IOP. **GI:** dry mouth, constipation, thirst, nausea, vomiting. **GU:** urine retention, erectile dysfunction. **Hematologic:** leukocytosis. **Metabolic:** hyperglycemia, *hypoglycemia,* hyponatremia, *hypokalemia.* **Skin:** rash. **Other:** *anaphylaxis.*

INTERACTIONS

Drug-drug. *Anticholinergics, drugs with anticholinergic effects (amantadine, antiarrhythmics, antiparkinsonians, meperidine, phenothiazines, TCAs):* May increase anticholinergic effects. Use together cautiously. *Potassium chloride wax-matrix extended-release tablets:* May increase risk of mucosal lesions. Avoid combination.

EFFECTS ON LAB TEST RESULTS

• May increase BUN level.
• May decrease sodium and potassium levels.
• May increase or decrease glucose level.
• May increase or decrease Hb level. May increase RBC and WBC counts.

CONTRAINDICATIONS & CAUTIONS

• Contraindicated in patients hypersensitive to drug and in patients with hyperthermia.
• Drug may increase risk of acute angle-closure glaucoma, obstructive uropathy, obstructive disease of GI tract, and paralytic ileus, toxic megacolon, and intestinal atony.
• Use cautiously in patients with hyperthyroidism, CAD, HTN, HF, tachycardia, hiatal hernia with reflux esophagitis, prostatic

hypertrophy, myasthenia gravis, or renal or hepatic impairment, and in elderly patients.
• Use cautiously in patients with Down syndrome because they may be more sensitive to drug.
• Drug will be ineffective treatment of bradycardia in heart transplant patients due to lack of vagal nerve innervation.
Dialyzable drug: No.
⚠ *Overdose S&S:* Delirium, seizures, coma, tachycardia, fever, mydriasis, decreased salivation and sweating, urine retention, HTN, vasodilation, hyperthermia.

PREGNANCY-LACTATION-REPRODUCTION

• Use in pregnant women only if clearly needed.
• Safe use in breastfeeding women hasn't been established. Use cautiously in breastfeeding women.

NURSING CONSIDERATIONS

• Doses less than 0.5 mg in adults and less than 0.1 mg in children may increase risk of paradoxical bradycardia.
⊙ *Alert:* Watch for tachycardia in cardiac patients because it may lead to ventricular fibrillation.
• Monitor fluid intake and urine output. Drug causes urine retention and urinary hesitancy.

PATIENT TEACHING

• Instruct patient to report all adverse reactions and to immediately report urine retention, abnormal heartbeat, dizziness, passing out, difficulty breathing, weakness, tremors, and abdominal edema.
• Tell patient to protect the AtroPen from light and not to freeze it.

SAFETY ALERT!

axitinib
ax-I-ti-nib

Inlyta

Therapeutic class: Antineoplastics
Pharmacologic class: Kinase inhibitors

AVAILABLE FORMS
Tablets: 1 mg, 5 mg

Reactions in bold italics are *life-threatening*. Interactions may have a *rapid onset* or a *delayed onset*.

INDICATIONS & DOSAGES
➤ **Advanced renal cell carcinoma after failure of one prior systemic therapy**
Adults: 5 mg PO b.i.d. approximately 12 hours apart. If patient tolerates drug for at least 2 consecutive weeks with adverse reactions no greater than grade 2 CTCAE guidelines, is normotensive, and isn't receiving antihypertensives, may increase dosage to 7 mg b.i.d., then 10 mg b.i.d.
Adjust-a-dose: Base dosage adjustment on individual safety and tolerability. Management of adverse reactions may require temporary interruption or permanent discontinuation. If dosage reduction from 5 mg b.i.d. is needed, recommended dosage is 2 or 3 mg b.i.d. If a strong CYP3A4/5 inhibitor must be coadministered, decrease axitinib dosage by approximately half; may increase or decrease subsequent doses based on individual safety and tolerability. If strong CYP3A4/5 inhibitor is discontinued, return axitinib dosage to that used before initiation after inhibitor is out of system (3 to 5 half-life periods of the strong inhibitor). Reduce axitinib starting dose by approximately half in patients with baseline moderate hepatic impairment (Child-Pugh class B); may increase or decrease subsequent doses based on individual safety and tolerability.

ADMINISTRATION
PO
• Drug is considered hazardous: use safe handling and disposal precautions according to facility policy.
• May give without regard for food.
• Have patient swallow tablets whole with a glass of water.
• If a dose is missed or patient vomits, don't give an additional dose; give next prescribed dose at usual time.
• Store at 68° to 77° F (20° to 25° C); excursions permitted to 59° to 86° F (15° to 30° C).

ACTION
Inhibits receptor tyrosine kinase, which decreases cell proliferation, tumor growth, angiogenesis, and cancer progression.

Route	Onset	Peak	Duration
PO	Unknown	2½–4 hr	Unknown

Half-life: 2.5 to 6.1 hours.

ADVERSE REACTIONS
CNS: asthenia, fatigue, headache, dizziness, TIA. **CV:** cardiac failure, *hemorrhage,* HTN, *DVT.* **EENT:** dysphonia, mucosal inflammation, stomatitis, dysgeusia, epistaxis, tinnitus, retinal-vein occlusion thrombosis, glossodynia. **GI:** diarrhea, nausea, vomiting, constipation, abdominal pain, upper abdominal pain, dyspepsia, hemorrhoids, *GI perforation,* fistula formation, *rectal hemorrhage, hemoptysis.* **GU:** hematuria, proteinuria. **Hematologic:** anemia, *polycythemia.* **Metabolic:** decreased appetite, decreased weight, hypothyroidism, dehydration. **Musculoskeletal:** arthralgia, extremity pain, myalgia. **Respiratory:** cough, dyspnea, *PE.* **Skin:** alopecia, hand-foot syndrome, rash, dry skin, pruritus, erythema.

INTERACTIONS
Drug-drug. *Moderate CYP3A4/5 inducers (bosentan, efavirenz, etravirine, modafinil, nafcillin), strong CYP3A4/5 inducers (carbamazepine, dexamethasone, phenobarbital, phenytoin, rifabutin, rifampin, rifapentine):* May reduce axitinib level. Avoid concurrent use.
Strong CYP3A4/5 inhibitors (atazanavir, clarithromycin, indinavir, itraconazole, ketoconazole, nefazodone, nelfinavir, ritonavir, saquinavir, telithromycin, voriconazole): May increase axitinib level. Avoid concurrent use; if strong CYP3A4/5 inhibitor is absolutely necessary, reduce axitinib dosage.
Drug-herb. *St. John's wort:* May decrease axitinib plasma concentration. Discourage concurrent use.
Drug-food. *Grapefruit, grapefruit juice:* May increase axitinib plasma concentration. Discourage concurrent use.

EFFECTS ON LAB TEST RESULTS
• May increase potassium, amylase, lipase, alkaline phosphatase, ALT, AST, bilirubin, and creatinine levels.
• May decrease bicarbonate, calcium, albumin, phosphate, and thyroid hormone levels.

- May increase or decrease glucose, sodium, and TSH levels.
- May decrease Hb level and lymphocyte, neutrophil, and platelet counts.

CONTRAINDICATIONS & CAUTIONS

- Use isn't recommended in patients with recent GI bleeding or untreated brain metastases.
- Drug may be associated with impaired wound healing.
- Use cautiously in patients with HTN; in those at risk for GI perforation, HF, fistula formation, thyroid dysfunction, or arterial or venous thromboembolic events; and in patients with moderate hepatic impairment (Child-Pugh class B) or ESRD (CrCl less than 15 mL/minute). Drug hasn't been studied in patients with Child-Pugh class C hepatic impairment.
- Drug is associated with proteinuria.
- Cases of reversible posterior leukoencephalopathy syndrome (RPLS) have been reported.

Dialyzable drug: Unknown.

⚠ *Overdose S&S:* Dizziness, HTN, seizures, possible fatal hemoptysis.

PREGNANCY-LACTATION-REPRODUCTION

- Drug can cause fetal harm. Women of childbearing potential should be advised of potential hazard to the fetus and to avoid becoming pregnant during therapy.
- Women of childbearing potential should have a pregnancy test before starting drug.
- Women of childbearing potential and men with female partners of childbearing potential should use effective contraception during therapy and for 1 week after final dose.
- It isn't known if drug appears in human milk. Patient should discontinue breastfeeding or discontinue drug.

NURSING CONSIDERATIONS

- HTN should be well controlled before start of therapy. Monitor patient for increased BP; treat as indicated. If HTN persists despite antihypertensive use, decrease axitinib dosage, as ordered.
- Watch for hypotension if drug is withheld for any reason and patient continues antihypertensive use.

- Monitor patient for signs and symptoms of hematologic or neurologic disease, thromboembolic events, and GI disorders.
- Monitor patient for bleeding or hemorrhagic event. Temporarily interrupt treatment if bleeding occurs.
- Monitor use of all prescription drugs, OTC medications, grapefruit or grapefruit juice, and supplements.
- Obtain LFTs and renal and thyroid function tests before and periodically during therapy.
- Stop drug at least 24 hours before surgery; resume based on clinical judgment of wound healing. Monitor wound healing carefully.
- Monitor patient for signs and symptoms of RPLS (headache, seizures, lethargy, confusion, blindness, and other visual disturbances) and other neurologic signs and symptoms. Discontinue drug if these occur.
- Monitor patient for proteinuria before and during therapy. For moderate or severe proteinuria, reduce dosage or withhold drug.

PATIENT TEACHING

- Advise female patient and male patient with female partner of childbearing potential to use effective birth control during treatment and for 1 week after final dose.
- Instruct patient that drug may be taken without regard to meals and that patient should swallow capsules whole with a glass of water.
- Tell patient to avoid grapefruit and grapefruit juice while taking this drug.
- Caution patient that if a dose is missed, to wait until the next scheduled dose and never to take two doses at the same time to make up for a missed dose.
- Advise patient to report all adverse reactions, including stomach pain, bruising, bleeding, delayed wound healing, fatigue, high BP, or neurologic signs and symptoms (headache, seizures, lethargy, confusion, blindness, other visual changes).
- Teach patient to consult prescriber before starting new drugs or supplements.
- Instruct patient to keep laboratory test appointments as requested by prescriber to monitor drug's safety and effectiveness.

azaCITIDine
ay-za-SYE-ti deen

Vidaza

Therapeutic class: Antineoplastics
Pharmacologic class: Pyrimidine nucleoside analogues

AVAILABLE FORMS
Powder for injection: 100-mg vials

INDICATIONS & DOSAGES
➤ **Myelodysplastic syndrome, including refractory anemia, refractory anemia with ringed sideroblasts (if patient has neutropenia or thrombocytopenia, or needs transfusions), refractory anemia with excess blasts, refractory anemia with excess blasts in transformation, or chronic myelomonocytic leukemia**
Adults: Initially, 75 mg/m^2 subcut or IV daily for 7 days; repeat cycle every 4 weeks. May increase to 100 mg/m^2 if no response after two treatment cycles and nausea and vomiting are the only toxic reactions. Minimum of four treatment cycles are recommended. Continue treatment as long as patient continues to benefit.
Adjust-a-dose: Refer to manufacturer's instructions for toxicity-related dosage adjustments.
➤ **Acute myeloid leukemia ♦**
Adults: 75 mg/m^2/day subcut or IV for 7 days every 4 weeks for at least six cycles. May continue treatment as long as patient continues to benefit or until disease progression or unacceptable toxicity.

ADMINISTRATION
• Hazardous drug; use safe handling and disposal precautions.
• Discard unused portions of each vial properly. Don't save for future use.
IV
▼ Reconstitute drug with 10 mL of sterile water for injection.
▼ Vigorously shake or roll the vial until powder is dissolved. The resulting solution will be 10 mg/mL.
▼ Use only clear solution.

▼ Withdraw proper dose and mix in a total volume of 50 to 100 mL of NSS or lactated Ringer solution.
▼ Give the infusion over 10 to 40 minutes. Infusion must be completed within 1 hour of reconstitution.
▼ **Incompatibilities:** Dextrose 5%, hespan, bicarbonate solutions.
Subcutaneous
• Dilute using aseptic and hazardous substances techniques.
• Reconstitute with 4 mL sterile water for injection. Don't filter after reconstitution. Vigorously shake or roll the vial until a uniform suspension forms. The resulting cloudy suspension will be 25 mg/mL.
• Draw up suspension into syringes for injection (no more than 4 mL per syringe).
• Just before giving drug, resuspend drug by vigorously rolling the syringe between the palms for 30 seconds. Divide doses greater than 4 mL into two syringes and inject into two separate sites.
• Give new injections at least 1 inch (2.5 cm) from previous site, and never into tender, bruised, red, or hardened skin. Rotate sites (thigh, abdomen, upper arm).
• Reconstituted drug is stable for 1 hour at room temperature. Or, if refrigerated immediately after reconstitution at 36° to 46° F (2° to 8° C): When reconstituted using water for injection that hasn't been refrigerated, reconstituted drug may be stored for up to 8 hours refrigerated; when reconstituted using refrigerated water for injection, reconstituted drug may be stored for up to 22 hours refrigerated.
• After refrigeration, suspension may be allowed to warm for up to 30 minutes at room temperature.

ACTION
Causes hypomethylation of DNA and is toxic to abnormal hematopoietic cells in bone marrow. Hypomethylation may restore normal function to genes needed for proliferation and differentiation. Drug has little effect on nonproliferating cells.

Route	Onset	Peak	Duration
IV	Unknown	Unknown	Unknown
Subcut	Unknown	30 min	Unknown

Half-life: About 4 hours.

ADVERSE REACTIONS

CNS: anxiety, dizziness, fatigue, headache, insomnia, malaise, pain, weakness, lethargy, pyrexia. **CV:** chest pain, edema, hypotension, HTN, peripheral swelling. **EENT:** nasopharyngitis, pharyngitis, rhinitis, nasal congestion. **GI:** abdominal pain and tenderness, anorexia, constipation, diarrhea, nausea, vomiting, abdominal distention, dyspepsia, gingival bleeding, loose stools, stomatitis. **GU:** UTI. **Hematologic:** anemia, *febrile neutropenia, leukopenia, neutropenia, thrombocytopenia,* hematoma, postprocedural hemorrhage. **Metabolic:** decreased weight, *hypokalemia.* **Musculoskeletal:** arthralgia, bone pain, limb pain, myalgia, chest wall pain. **Respiratory:** dyspnea, pneumonia, URI. **Skin:** ecchymosis, erythema (including erythema at injection site), pallor, petechiae, pitting edema, rash, cellulitis, dry skin, granuloma, pigmentation, pruritus at injection site, skin nodules, swelling at injection site, urticaria. **Other:** rigors.

INTERACTIONS

Drug-drug. *Clozapine, deferiprone, tacrolimus:* May increase risk of neutropenia and toxicities. Avoid concurrent use.

EFFECTS ON LAB TEST RESULTS

• May increase BUN and creatinine levels. May decrease bicarbonate and potassium levels.
• May decrease neutrophil, platelet, and WBC counts.

CONTRAINDICATIONS & CAUTIONS

• Contraindicated in patients hypersensitive to azacitidine or mannitol and in patients with advanced malignant hepatic tumors.
• Use cautiously in patients with hepatic and renal disease and in elderly patients.
• Drug may cause fatal or serious TLS despite concomitant use of allopurinol.
Dialyzable drug: Unknown.
⚠ *Overdose S&S:* Diarrhea, nausea, vomiting.

PREGNANCY-LACTATION-REPRODUCTION

• Drug may cause fetal harm. Women of childbearing potential should be advised to avoid pregnancy during treatment.

• Men should be advised not to father a child during therapy.
• It isn't known if drug appears in human milk. Patient should discontinue breastfeeding or discontinue drug.

NURSING CONSIDERATIONS

• Check LFT and electrolyte results and creatinine level before therapy starts and before each cycle. If unexplained reductions in serum bicarbonate level less than 20 mEq/L or elevations of BUN or serum creatinine level occur, reduce dosage by 50% or withhold dose.
• Obtain CBC before each cycle or more often. Bone marrow suppression is common.
• Premedicate patient for nausea and vomiting.
• Monitor renal function at baseline, before each cycle, and more frequently if indicated. Monitor renal function closely in elderly patients and in renally impaired patients receiving drug because renal impairment may increase toxicity.
• Assess baseline risk of TLS; monitor patient and treat as appropriate.
• Verify pregnancy status of female patients of childbearing potential before therapy starts.
• *Look alike–sound alike:* Don't confuse azacitidine with azathioprine.

PATIENT TEACHING

• Advise patient to report all adverse reactions and to immediately report signs and symptoms of infection (fever, cough, malaise), liver problems (dark urine, abdominal pain, yellowing of skin or eyes), or renal problems (urine retention, change in amount of urine, edema); abnormal bleeding; chest pain; dizziness; or severe GI signs and symptoms.
• Inform patient that blood counts may decrease with febrile neutropenia, thrombocytopenia, and anemia.
• Advise male and female patient to use birth control during therapy.

Reactions in bold italics are *life-threatening*. Interactions may have a *rapid onset* or a *delayed onset*.

azaTHIOprine ⌧
ay-za-THYE-oh-preen

Azasan, Imuran

azaTHIOprine sodium ⌧
Imuran ✦

Therapeutic class: Immunosuppressants
Pharmacologic class: Purine antagonists

AVAILABLE FORMS
Powder for injection: 50-mg vial ✦,
100-mg vial
Tablets: 50 mg, 75 mg, 100 mg

INDICATIONS & DOSAGES
➤ **Immunosuppression in kidney transplantation**
Adults: Initially, 3 to 5 mg/kg PO or IV daily,
usually beginning on day of transplantation.
Maintained at 1 to 3 mg/kg daily based on
patient response and tolerance.
Adjust-a-dose: Give drug in lower doses to
patients with oliguria in the posttransplant
period and in those with impaired renal
function. In patients receiving allopurinol,
decrease azathioprine dose to ⅓ to ¼ of the
usual dose.
➤ **RA**
Adults: Initially, 1 mg/kg PO as single dose
or divided into two doses. Usual dose is 50
to 100 mg. If patient response isn't satisfactory after 6 to 8 weeks, dosage may be increased by 0.5 mg/kg daily to maximum of
2.5 mg/kg daily at 4-week intervals. Maintenance therapy should be at lowest effective dose. Attempt gradual dose reduction
once patient is stable. Reduce dosage by
0.5 mg/kg (about 25 mg daily) every
4 weeks.

ADMINISTRATION
PO
• Give drug after meals to minimize adverse
GI effects.
• Drug is a potential teratogen and mutagen.
Use safe-handling procedures.
IV
▼ Drug is a potential teratogen and muta-
gen. Use safe handling procedures.

▼ Use only in patients who can't tolerate
oral drugs.
▼ Reconstitute drug in 50-mg vial with
5 mL of sterile water for injection. Give by
direct IV injection, or further dilute in NSS
for injection or D₅W solution.
▼ Reconstitute drug in 100-mg vial with
10 mL of sterile water for injection. Dilute
further in NSS for injection or D₅W solution.
▼ When drug is diluted further, the final
volume depends on desired infusion time,
usually 30 to 60 minutes, but may be as
short as 5 minutes and as long as 8 hours
for the daily dose.
▼ Inspect for particles before use.
▼ **Incompatibilities:** None listed by manufacturer. Consult a drug incompatibility
reference for more information.

ACTION
May alter antibody production and suppress
T-cell effects.

Route	Onset	Peak	Duration
PO, IV	Unknown	1–2 hr	Unknown

Half-life: About 5 hours.

ADVERSE REACTIONS
CNS: fever. **GI:** nausea, vomiting, anorexia,
pancreatitis, abdominal pain. **Hematologic:** *leukopenia, myelosuppression,
pancytopenia, thrombocytopenia, immunosuppression.* **Hepatic:** *hepatotoxicity.*
Musculoskeletal: myalgia. **Other:** infections, *increased risk of neoplasia.*

INTERACTIONS
Drug-drug. *ACE inhibitors:* May cause se-
vere leukopenia and increase risk of anemia.
Monitor patient closely.
*Aminosalicylate derivatives (mesalazine,
olsalazine, sulfasalazine):* Inhibit thiopurine
S-methyltransferase (TPMT). Use together
cautiously.
⌧ *Allopurinol:* May impair inactivation of
azathioprine. Avoid using if possible; de-
crease azathioprine to ⅓ to ¼ usual dose.
Consider further dosage reduction or alter-
native therapy for patients with low or absent
TPMT activity.
Cyclosporine: May decrease cyclosporine
level. Monitor cyclosporine level closely.

Febuxostat: May increase risk of toxicity. Concomitant use is contraindicated.

DMARDs (abatacept, adalimumab, etanercept, hydroxychloroquine, leflunomide, methotrexate, minocycline, sulfasalazine, tocilizumab): Concomitant use hasn't been studied. Use together isn't recommended.

Live-virus vaccines: May reduce effectiveness of live-virus vaccines. Immunocompromised patients may be at increased risk for vaccine-induced infection. Defer live-virus vaccines until immune function improves.

Mercaptopurine: May increase risk of myelosuppression, including pancytopenia. Avoid concomitant use.

Ribavirin: May increase risk of severe pancytopenia and azathioprine-related myelotoxicity. Monitor CBC, including platelet count.

Sulfamethoxazole–trimethoprim and other drugs that interfere with myelopoiesis: May cause severe leukopenia, especially in renal transplant patients. Use together cautiously.

Tacrolimus (topical): May increase risk of adverse effects of immunosuppressants. Avoid use together.

Warfarin: May inhibit warfarin's anticoagulant effect. Monitor patient. Adjust warfarin dosage as needed.

Drug-herb. *Cat's claw, echinacea:* May increase immune function and reduce drug's therapeutic effects. Avoid using together.

EFFECTS ON LAB TEST RESULTS

• May increase alkaline phosphatase, ALT, AST, and bilirubin levels. May decrease uric acid level.

• May decrease Hb level and platelet, RBC, and WBC counts.

CONTRAINDICATIONS & CAUTIONS

• Contraindicated in patients hypersensitive to drug or its components.

Black Box Warning Long-term immunosuppression with this drug increases risk of neoplasia, including posttransplant lymphoma and hepatosplenic T-cell lymphoma in patients with inflammatory bowel disease. Prescribers using this drug should be very familiar with its risks, the mutagenic potential to both men and women, and possible hematologic toxicities. ∎

⧆ Patients with intermediate TPMT activity may be at increased risk for myelotoxicity if receiving conventional doses of drug. Patients with low or absent TPMT activity are at increased risk for developing severe, life-threatening myelotoxicity if receiving conventional doses of azathioprine. TPMT genotyping or phenotyping can help identify patients who are at increased risk for developing azathioprine toxicity.

• Use cautiously in patients with hepatic or renal dysfunction.

• Benefits must be weighed against risk when giving to patient with systemic viral infection, such as chickenpox or herpes zoster.

• Rare but life-threatening hepatic veno-occlusive disease has been reported in transplant patients. If this is suspected, permanently discontinue drug.

• Patients with RA previously treated with alkylating drugs, such as cyclophosphamide, chlorambucil, or melphalan, may be at increased risk for tumor development if treated with this drug. Use together is contraindicated.

Dialyzable drug: 45% in an 8-hour dialysis session.

⚠ **Overdose S&S:** Nausea, vomiting, diarrhea, abnormal liver function, leukopenia.

PREGNANCY-LACTATION-REPRODUCTION

• There are no adequate and well-controlled studies in pregnant women. Drug can cause fetal harm. Avoid use in pregnant women when possible. Don't use to treat RA in pregnant women. Women of childbearing potential should be advised to avoid becoming pregnant.

• Drug appears in human milk. Not recommended in breastfeeding women.

NURSING CONSIDERATIONS

⧆ Consider genotype or phenotype testing for TPMT. Patients with low or absent levels are at greater risk for the hematologic effects of and severe bone marrow toxicity from azathioprine therapy.

• To prevent bleeding, avoid all IM injections when platelet count is below 100,000/mm^3.

• Monitor CBC and platelet counts weekly for 1 month, twice monthly for 2 months,

then monthly unless more frequent monitoring is clinically indicated. Also monitor counts at dosage changes. Notify prescriber if counts drop suddenly or become dangerously low. Drug may need to be temporarily withheld.
• Watch for early signs and symptoms of hepatotoxicity (such as clay-colored stools, dark urine, pruritus, and yellow skin and sclera) and monitor patient periodically for increased alkaline phosphatase, bilirubin, AST, and ALT levels.
• Monitor patient for bacterial, viral, fungal, protozoal, and opportunistic infections, including reactivation of latent infections such as TB.
• Watch for new-onset neurologic symptoms. Patients on immunosuppressive therapy may be at increased risk for JC virus–associated infection resulting in multifocal leukoencephalopathy.
• Aspirin, NSAIDs, and low-dose glucocorticoids may be continued during azathioprine therapy.
• Therapeutic response usually occurs within 8 weeks. Patients not improved after 12 weeks can be considered refractory to treatment.
• *Look alike–sound alike:* Don't confuse azathioprine with Azulfidine. Don't confuse Imuran with Inderal.

PATIENT TEACHING
Black Box Warning Warn patient of the risk of malignancy. ▋
• Warn patient to report even mild infections (colds, fever, sore throat, malaise), because drug is a potent immunosuppressant.
• Warn patient that some hair thinning is possible.
• Tell patient taking drug for refractory RA that it may take up to 12 weeks to be effective.
• Advise patient to report unusual bleeding or bruising.
• Tell patient that drug may be taken with food to decrease nausea.
• Advise patient to use soft toothbrush and perform oral care cautiously.

azelastine hydrochloride
a-ZEL-as-teen

Astelin, Astepro

Therapeutic class: Antihistamines
Pharmacologic class: H$_1$-receptor antagonists

AVAILABLE FORMS
Intranasal: 0.1%, 0.15%
Ophthalmic solution: 0.05%

INDICATIONS & DOSAGES
➤ **Pruritus from allergic conjunctivitis**
Adults and children age 3 and older: Instill 1 drop into affected eye b.i.d.
➤ **Perennial allergic rhinitis (Astepro only)**
Adults and children age 12 and older: Instill 2 sprays (0.15%) per nostril b.i.d.
Children ages 6 to 11: Instill 1 spray (0.1% or 0.15%) per nostril b.i.d.
Children age 6 months to 5 years: Instill 1 spray (0.1%) per nostril b.i.d.
➤ **Seasonal allergic rhinitis**
Adults and children age 12 and older: Instill 1 to 2 sprays (0.1% or 0.15%) per nostril b.i.d. or 2 sprays (0.15%) per nostril once daily.
Children ages 6 to 11 (Astepro): Instill 1 spray (0.1% or 0.15%) per nostril b.i.d.
Children ages 5 to 11 (Astelin): Instill 1 spray (0.1%) per nostril b.i.d.
Children ages 2 to 5 (Astepro only): Instill 1 spray (0.1%) per nostril b.i.d.
➤ **Vasomotor rhinitis (Astelin only)**
Adults and adolescents age 12 and older: Instill 2 sprays (0.1%) per nostril b.i.d.

ADMINISTRATION
Ophthalmic
• Keep bottle tightly closed when not in use.
• Don't touch tip of dropper to any surface.
Intranasal
• Before initial use of nasal spray, prime the delivery system with 4 sprays (0.1%) or 6 sprays (0.15%), or until a fine mist appears.

✦Canada ◇OTC ◆Off-label use ✐Photoguide ⓓDo not crush *Liquid contains alcohol ▓Genetic

- If 3 or more days have elapsed since last use, reprime the delivery system with 2 sprays or until a fine mist appears.
- After each use, wipe spray tip with a clean tissue or cloth.

◑ Alert: Be aware of different concentrations of nasal spray as some aren't indicated for use in all indications or certain age-groups.

ACTION

Inhibits the release of histamine and other mediators from cells involved in the allergic response.

Route	Onset	Peak	Duration
Ophthalmic	3 min	Unknown	8 hr
Intranasal	Unknown	2–4 hr	Unknown

Half-life: 22 to 25 hours.

ADVERSE REACTIONS

CNS: anxiety, depression, dizziness, drowsiness, headache, fatigue, malaise, nervousness, sleep disorder, vertigo. **CV:** flushing, HTN, tachycardia. **EENT:** transient eye burning or stinging, conjunctivitis, eye pain, temporary blurring, pharyngitis, rhinitis, nasal discomfort, nasal congestion, sinusitis, postnasal drip, sneezing, epistaxis, bitter taste. **GI:** abdominal pain, constipation, diarrhea, nausea, vomiting, gastroenteritis, increased appetite. **GU:** hematuria, increased urinary frequency. **Respiratory:** *asthma, bronchospasm,* dyspnea, cough, URI. **Skin:** pruritus. **Other:** flulike syndrome, weight gain.

INTERACTIONS

Drug-drug. *Cimetidine:* May interfere with plasma concentrations of azelastine. Avoid use together.
CNS depressants: May enhance CNS depressant effect of azelastine. Avoid combination.
Drug-lifestyle. *Alcohol use:* May increase CNS depressant effect of azelastine. Avoid use together.

EFFECTS ON LAB TEST RESULTS

None reported.

CONTRAINDICATIONS & CAUTIONS

- Contraindicated in patients hypersensitive to drug or its components.

Dialyzable drug: Unknown.

PREGNANCY-LACTATION-REPRODUCTION

- Use cautiously in pregnant women and only if potential benefit justifies potential risk to the fetus.
- It isn't known if drug appears in human milk. Use cautiously in breastfeeding women.

NURSING CONSIDERATIONS

- Drug is for ophthalmic or intranasal use only. Don't inject or give orally.
- Don't use ophthalmic form for irritation caused by contact lenses.

PATIENT TEACHING

- Instruct patient not to touch any surface, eyelid, or surrounding areas with tip of eye dropper.
- Tell patient to keep bottle tightly closed when not in use.
- Advise patient not to wear contact lens if eye is red.
- Warn patient that soft contact lenses may absorb the preservative benzalkonium.
- Instruct patient who wears soft contact lenses and whose eyes aren't red to wait at least 10 minutes after instilling drug before inserting contact lenses.
- Tell patient to report all adverse reactions and to immediately report shortness of breath or severe nose irritation if taking intranasal form.
- Because drug may cause CNS depression, advise patient using intranasal form to avoid hazardous activities requiring complete mental alertness, such as driving or operating machinery.
- Advise patient and caregivers that different concentrations of nasal spray exist and may not be indicated for use in certain conditions or age-groups.

Reactions in bold italics are *life-threatening*. Interactions may have a *rapid onset* or a *delayed onset*.

azelastine hydrochloride-fluticasone propionate
a-ZEL-as-teen/floo-TIK-a-sone

Dymista

Therapeutic class: Antihistamines–corticosteroids
Pharmacologic class: H₁-receptor antagonists–corticosteroids

AVAILABLE FORMS
Nasal spray: 137 mcg azelastine hydrochloride and 50 mcg fluticasone propionate/spray

INDICATIONS & DOSAGES
➤ **Symptoms of seasonal allergic rhinitis**
Adults and children age 6 and older:
1 spray/nostril b.i.d.

ADMINISTRATION
Intranasal
• Shake gently before each use.
• Prime the spray before initial use; spray six times or until a fine mist appears. If the spray hasn't been used within the past 14 days, prime the spray again with 1 spray or until a fine mist appears.
• Store upright at room temperature with dust cap in place. Don't freeze or refrigerate.
• Protect from light.

ACTION
Azelastine inhibits release of histamine and other mediators from cells involved in the allergic response. Fluticasone may decrease inflammation by inhibiting mast cells, macrophages, and mediators such as leukotrienes.

Route	Onset	Peak	Duration
Intranasal	Rapid	½ hr (azelastine), 1 hr (fluticasone)	Unknown

Half-life: Azelastine, 25 hours; fluticasone, 7.8 hours.

ADVERSE REACTIONS
CNS: headache, fever, pain. **EENT:** epistaxis, nasal congestion, rhinitis, pharyngitis, oropharyngeal pain, otitis media, otitis externa. **GI:** diarrhea, dysgeusia, nausea, vomiting, upper abdominal pain. **Respiratory:** cough, URI. **Skin:** urticaria. **Other:** viral infection.

INTERACTIONS
Drug-drug. *CNS depressants:* May increase risk of drowsiness. Use together cautiously.
CYP3A4 inhibitors (fluconazole, ketoconazole): May increase fluticasone plasma level. Use together cautiously.
Desmopressin: Fluticasone may enhance hyponatremic effect of desmopressin. Avoid concurrent use.
Ritonavir: May increase fluticasone plasma level and risk of systemic corticosteroid effects, including Cushing syndrome and adrenal suppression. Avoid use together.
Drug-lifestyle. *Alcohol use:* May increase risk of somnolence and CNS impairment. Discourage use together.

EFFECTS ON LAB TEST RESULTS
None reported.

CONTRAINDICATIONS & CAUTIONS
• Contraindicated in patients hypersensitive to either drug or its components.
• Avoid use in patients with current nasal ulcers, nasal trauma, or nasal surgery until healing occurs.
• Use cautiously in patients with glaucoma, cataracts, ongoing infection, or history of adrenal suppression.
Dialyzable drug: Unknown.

PREGNANCY-LACTATION-REPRODUCTION
• Use cautiously in pregnant and breastfeeding women and only if benefits outweigh risks to the fetus or infant.

NURSING CONSIDERATIONS
• Monitor patient for fungal, bacterial, or viral infections.
• Monitor patient for localized nasopharyngeal *Candida albicans* infection with prolonged use.
• Ensure that patient receives regular eye exams to screen for cataracts and glaucoma with long-term use.
• Monitor growth rate in children using the spray long-term.

• Monitor patient for adrenal insufficiency (tiredness, weakness, nausea, vomiting, hypotension).

PATIENT TEACHING
• Instruct patient to shake bottle gently before each use and to prime the bottle by releasing six sprays or until a fine mist appears before initial use or if the spray hasn't been used in the past 14 days. Advise patient to follow full package directions for use.
• Caution patient to avoid spraying into eyes and, if exposure occurs, to flush eyes with water for 10 minutes.
• Warn patient to watch for changes in vision, which can indicate serious eye problems, such as glaucoma or cataracts. Advise patient to have regular eye exams while taking drug.
• Tell patient to watch for nasal problems, such as nosebleeds and nasal septal perforation.
• Advise patient that drug can decrease the body's ability to heal or fight infection. Tell patient to report fever, aches or pains, chills, fatigue, or exposure to chickenpox or measles. Caution patient to avoid exposure to communicable diseases.
• Warn patient that drug can cause drowsiness. Instruct patient to avoid alcohol and other drugs that cause drowsiness while taking this medication.
• Advise patient to avoid driving or tasks that require alertness until drug's effects are known.
• Instruct female patient to notify prescriber if she is pregnant, planning to become pregnant, or is breastfeeding.

azithromycin
ay-zi-thro-MY-sin

AzaSite, Zithromax✲

Therapeutic class: Antibiotics
Pharmacologic class: Macrolides

AVAILABLE FORMS
Injection: 500 mg
Ophthalmic solution: 1%
Powder for oral suspension: 100 mg/5 mL, 200 mg/5 mL; 1,000 mg/single-dose packet
Tablets: 250 mg, 500 mg, 600 mg

INDICATIONS & DOSAGES
➤ **Acute bacterial worsening of COPD caused by *Haemophilus influenzae, Moraxella catarrhalis,* or *Streptococcus pneumoniae;* uncomplicated skin and skin-structure infections caused by *Staphylococcus aureus, Streptococcus pyogenes,* or *Streptococcus agalactiae;* second-line therapy for pharyngitis or tonsillitis caused by *S. pyogenes***
Adults and adolescents age 16 and older: Initially, 500 mg PO as a single dose on day 1, followed by 250 mg daily on days 2 through 5. Total cumulative dose is 1.5 g. Or, for worsening COPD, 500 mg PO daily for 3 days.
➤ **Community-acquired pneumonia caused by *Chlamydophila pneumoniae, H. influenzae, Mycoplasma pneumoniae, S. pneumoniae, Legionella pneumophila, M. catarrhalis,* or *S. aureus***
Adults and adolescents age 16 and older: For mild infections, give 500 mg PO as a single dose on day 1; then 250 mg PO daily on days 2 through 5. Total dose is 1.5 g. For more severe infections or those caused by *S. aureus,* give 500 mg IV as a single daily dose for 2 days; then 500 mg PO as a single daily dose to complete a 7- to 10-day course of therapy. Switch from IV to oral therapy based on patient response.
➤ **Community-acquired pneumonia caused by *C. pneumoniae, H. influenzae, M. pneumoniae,* or *S. pneumoniae***
Children age 6 months and older: 10 mg/kg oral suspension PO (maximum of 500 mg) as a single dose on day 1, followed by 5 mg/kg (maximum of 250 mg) daily on days 2 through 5.
➤ **Acute bacterial sinusitis caused by *H. influenzae, M. catarrhalis,* or *S. pneumoniae***
Adults: 500 mg PO daily for 3 days.
Children age 6 months and older: 10 mg/kg oral suspension PO once daily for 3 days.
➤ **Chancroid**
Adults: 1 g PO as a single dose.
➤ **Nongonococcal urethritis or cervicitis caused by *Chlamydia trachomatis***
Adults and adolescents age 16 and older: 1 g PO as a single dose.

➤ **To prevent disseminated *Mycobacterium avium* complex in patients with advanced HIV infection**
Adults and adolescents: 1.2 g PO once weekly.

➤ ***M. avium* complex in patients with advanced HIV infection**
Adults: 600 mg PO daily with ethambutol 15 mg/kg daily.

➤ **Urethritis and cervicitis caused by *Neisseria gonorrhoeae***
Adults: 2 g PO as a single dose.

➤ **Pelvic inflammatory disease caused by *C. trachomatis, N. gonorrhoeae,* or *Mycoplasma hominis* in patients who need initial IV therapy**
Adults and adolescents age 16 and older: 500 mg IV as a single daily dose for 1 to 2 days; then 250 mg PO daily to complete a 7-day course of therapy. Switch from IV to oral therapy based on patient response.

➤ **Otitis media**
Children older than age 6 months: 30 mg/kg oral suspension PO as a single dose; or 10 mg/kg PO once daily for 3 days; or 10 mg/kg PO on day 1 and then 5 mg/kg once daily on days 2 to 5.

➤ **Pharyngitis, tonsillitis**
Children age 2 and older: 12 mg/kg oral suspension (maximum, 500 mg) PO daily for 5 days.

➤ **Bacterial conjunctivitis caused by coryneform group G, *H. influenzae, Staphylococcus aureus, Streptococcus mitis* group, and *S. pneumoniae***
Adults and children age 1 and older: Instill 1 drop in affected eye(s) b.i.d., 8 to 12 hours apart for first 2 days; then instill 1 drop in affected eye(s) once daily for next 5 days.

➤ **Cat scratch disease (*Bartonella henselae* infection) ◆**
Adults and children weighing 45.5 kg or more: 500 mg PO on day 1, then 250 mg PO daily on days 2 to 5.
Children weighing less than 45.5 kg: 10 mg/kg on day 1, then 5 mg/kg PO daily on days 2 to 5.

➤ **Severe cholera ◆**
Adults: 1 g PO as a single dose.

➤ **COPD, prevention of exacerbations ◆**
Adults: 250 to 500 mg PO three times/week or 250 mg PO once daily.

➤ **Cystic fibrosis to improve lung function and reduce exacerbations ◆**
Adults: 500 mg PO for patients weighing 40 kg or more or 250 mg PO for patients weighing less than 40 kg three times/week or 250 mg PO once daily. Screen patients before treatment; don't give to those who test positive for nontuberculous mycobacterial infection.

ADMINISTRATION
PO
• Obtain specimen for culture and sensitivity tests before giving first dose. Begin therapy while awaiting results.
• Reconstitute suspension packet with 2 oz (60 mL) of water. After patient has taken dose, rinse glass with additional 2 oz of water and have patient drink it to ensure entire dose has been taken. Packets aren't for children.

IV
▼ Reconstitute drug in 500-mg vial with 4.8 mL of sterile water for injection to yield 100 mg/mL.
▼ Shake well until all drug is dissolved.
▼ Further dilute in 250- or 500-mL NSS solution, half-NSS, D_5W, or lactated Ringer solution to yield a final concentration of 1 or 2 mg/mL, respectively.
▼ Infuse a 500-mg dose of azithromycin IV over 1 hour or longer. Never give it as a bolus or IM injection.
▼ Reconstituted solution and diluted solution are stable for 24 hours when stored below 86° F (30° C). Diluted solution is stable for 7 days when refrigerated at 41° F (5° C).
▼ **Incompatibilities:** Amikacin sulfate, aztreonam, cefotaxime, ceftazidime, ceftriaxone sodium, cefuroxime, ciprofloxacin, clindamycin phosphate, famotidine, fentanyl citrate, furosemide, gentamicin sulfate, imipenem–cilastatin sodium, ketorolac tromethamine, levofloxacin, morphine sulfate, piperacillin–tazobactam sodium, potassium chloride, tobramycin sulfate.

Ophthalmic
• Avoid contaminating applicator tip. Don't allow it to touch eye, fingers, or other surfaces.
• Invert closed bottle and shake once before each use. Remove cap with bottle still in the

inverted position. Tilt head back, and with bottle inverted, gently squeeze bottle to instill 1 drop into affected eye(s).

• Store unopened bottle under refrigeration at 36° to 46° F (2° to 8° C). Once bottle has been opened, store at 36° to 77° F (2° to 25° C) for up to 14 days. Discard after 14 days.

ACTION
Binds to the 50S subunit of bacterial ribosomes, blocking protein synthesis; bacteriostatic or bactericidal, depending on concentration.

Route	Onset	Peak	Duration
PO	Unknown	2–5 hr	Unknown
IV, ophthalmic	Unknown	Unknown	Unknown

Half-life: About 3 days.

ADVERSE REACTIONS
CNS: fatigue, headache, somnolence, dizziness. **CV:** chest pain, palpitations. **EENT:** eye irritation (ophthalmic). **GI:** abdominal pain, anorexia, diarrhea, nausea, vomiting, *pseudomembranous colitis,* dyspepsia, flatulence, melena. **GU:** candidiasis, nephritis, vaginitis. **Hepatic:** cholestatic jaundice. **Skin:** photosensitivity reactions, rash, pain at injection site, pruritus. **Other:** *angioedema.*

INTERACTIONS
Drug-drug. *Antacids containing aluminum and magnesium:* May lower peak azithromycin level (immediate-release form). Separate doses by at least 2 hours.
Antiarrhythmics (amiodarone, quinidine): May increase risk of life-threatening arrhythmias, including torsades de pointes. Monitor ECG rhythm carefully.
Carbamazepine, phenytoin: May increase levels of these drugs. Monitor drug levels.
Cyclosporine: May elevate cyclosporine concentrations, with increased risk of nephrotoxicity and neurotoxicity. Monitor cyclosporine levels and renal function.
Digoxin: May increase digoxin level. Monitor digoxin level.
Drugs that prolong QT interval (fluoroquinolones, lithium, methadone, paliperidone, perflutren): May prolong QT interval.

Use together with caution and monitor patient.
Ergotamine: May cause acute ergotamine toxicity. Monitor patient closely.
HMG-CoA reductase inhibitors (atorvastatin, lovastatin): May increase HMG-CoA reductase inhibitor levels, resulting in severe myopathy or rhabdomyolysis. Consider alternative therapy.
Nelfinavir: May increase azithromycin level. Monitor for liver enzyme abnormalities and hearing impairment.
Pimozide: May prolong QT interval and cause ventricular tachycardia. Concurrent use is contraindicated.
Theophylline: May increase theophylline level. Monitor theophylline level carefully.
Triazolam: May decrease triazolam clearance. Monitor patient closely.
Warfarin: May increase INR. Monitor INR carefully.
Drug-lifestyle. *Sun exposure:* May cause photosensitivity reactions. Advise patient to avoid excessive sunlight exposure.

EFFECTS ON LAB TEST RESULTS
• May increase ALT, AST, creatinine, LDH, and bilirubin levels.

CONTRAINDICATIONS & CAUTIONS
• Contraindicated in patients hypersensitive to azithromycin, erythromycin, or other macrolide or ketolide antibiotics and in those with history of cholestatic jaundice or hepatic dysfunction from prior use of azithromycin.
• Serious cases of allergic reactions, including angioedema, anaphylaxis, SJS, toxic epidermal necrolysis, and DRESS syndrome have been reported, some with fatalities. Prolonged observation and symptomatic treatment may be necessary.
• Infantile hypertrophic pyloric stenosis has been reported after the use of azithromycin in neonates (treatment up to 42 days of life).
• Don't use oral drug in patients with pneumonia or in those with moderate to severe illness or risk factors (such as cystic fibrosis, nosocomially acquired infections, known or suspected bacteremia; hospitalized, elderly, or debilitated patients; or patients with immunodeficiency or functional asplenia).

• Use cautiously in patients with impaired hepatic function or myasthenia gravis.
❸ *Alert:* Drug is not indicated for prophylaxis of bronchiolitis obliterans syndrome in patients undergoing hematopoietic stem cell transplantation (HSCT). Long-term exposure may increase the risk of hematologic malignancy relapse and death.
❸ *Alert:* Use cautiously in patients at increased risk for torsades de pointes and fatal arrhythmias, including those with known prolonged QT interval, history of torsades de pointes, congenital long QT syndrome, bradyarrhythmias, uncompensated HF, uncorrected hypokalemia or hypomagnesemia, clinically significant bradycardia, or concomitant use of drugs known to prolong the QT interval or class IA (procainamide, quinidine) or class III (amiodarone, dofetilide, sotalol) antiarrhythmics.
❸ *Alert:* Elderly patients may be at increased risk for drug-associated QT-interval effects.
• Drug may cause CDAD ranging in severity from mild diarrhea to fatal colitis, which may occur over 2 months after administration. If CDAD is suspected or confirmed, drug may need to be discontinued and appropriate treatment begun.
• Prolonged use of ophthalmic solution may result in overgrowth of nonsusceptible organisms, including fungi. If superinfection occurs, discontinue drug and institute alternative therapy.
Dialyzable drug: Unknown.

PREGNANCY-LACTATION-REPRODUCTION
• There are no adequate and well-controlled studies in pregnant women. Use during pregnancy only if clearly needed.
• Drug appears in human milk. Use cautiously in breastfeeding women.

NURSING CONSIDERATIONS
• Monitor patient for superinfection. Drug may cause overgrowth of nonsusceptible bacteria or fungi.
❸ *Alert:* Monitor patient for CDAD, which may range in severity from mild diarrhea to fatal colitis.
❸ *Alert:* Consider full risk profile when choosing appropriate antibiotic therapy. Alternative macrolide or fluoroquinolone class drugs also have the potential to cause QT-

interval prolongation and other significant adverse effects.
• Monitor patient for allergic and skin reactions. Discontinue drug if reactions occur. Be aware that allergic symptoms may recur when symptomatic therapy is discontinued; patient may require prolonged monitoring and treatment.
• Monitor patient for jaundice, hepatotoxicity, and hepatitis. Discontinue drug immediately if signs and symptoms (yellowing of skin or sclera, abdominal pain, nausea, vomiting, dark urine) occur.
❸ *Alert:* Exacerbation and new onset of myasthenia gravis have occurred with azithromycin use.

PATIENT TEACHING
• Tell patient to take drug as prescribed, even after feeling better.
• Advise patient to avoid excessive sunlight and to wear protective clothing and use sunscreen when outside.
• Tell patient to report adverse reactions promptly.
• Instruct parents and caregivers to contact prescriber if vomiting or irritability with feeding occurs during or after azithromycin use in neonates (treatment up to 42 days of life).
❸ *Alert:* Warn patient to seek immediate medical care for irregular heartbeat, shortness of breath, dizziness, or fainting.
• Advise patient not to stop taking drug without first contacting health care provider.
• Tell patient that tablets and suspension can be taken with or without food. Food may reduce GI upset.
• Instruct patient to thoroughly wash hands before instilling ophthalmic solution.
• Tell patient to avoid contaminating ophthalmic applicator tip and not to let tip touch eye, fingers, or other surfaces.
• Instruct patient how to instill ophthalmic solution.
• Advise patient to avoid contact lenses when diagnosed with bacterial conjunctivitis.

aztreonam
AZ-tree-oh-nam

Azactam, Cayston

Therapeutic class: Antibiotics
Pharmacologic class: Monobactams

AVAILABLE FORMS
Inhalation (Cayston): 75-mg ampule
Injection: 1-g vials, 2-g vials
Injection in premixed container: 1 g/50 mL,
2 g/50 mL

INDICATIONS & DOSAGES
➤ **UTI; septicemia; infections of lower respiratory tract, skin, and skin structures; intra-abdominal infections, surgical infections, and gynecologic infections caused by susceptible** *Escherichia coli, Klebsiella pneumoniae, Proteus mirabilis, Pseudomonas aeruginosa, Enterobacter cloacae, Klebsiella oxytoca, Citrobacter* **species, and** *Serratia marcescens;* **respiratory infections caused by** *Haemophilus influenzae*
Adults: 500 mg, 1 g, or 2 g IV or IM every 8 to 12 hours. For severe systemic or life-threatening infections, 2 g every 6 to 8 hours. Maximum dose is 8 g daily.
Children ages 9 months and older: 30 mg/kg IV every 6 to 8 hours. Maximum dose is 120 mg/kg/day.
Adjust-a-dose: For adults with CrCl of 10 to 30 mL/minute/1.73 m², give 1 to 2 g; then give 50% of the usual dose at usual interval. If CrCl is less than 10 mL/minute/ 1.73 m², give 500 mg to 2 g; then give 25% of the usual dose at usual interval. For serious infections, add ⅛ of the initial dose to maintenance doses after each hemodialysis session.
➤ **To improve respiratory symptoms in cystic fibrosis patients with** *P. aeruginosa* **infection (Cayston)**
Adults and children age 7 and older: 75 mg inhalation t.i.d. at least 4 hours apart for 28 days, followed by 28 days off.

ADMINISTRATION
Inhalational
• Patient should use bronchodilator before Cayston administration.
• Give short-acting bronchodilators 15 minutes to 4 hours before each dose of aztreonam or long-acting bronchodilators 30 minutes to 12 hours before each dose.
• Space doses at least 4 hours apart.
• Treatment order for patients on multiple therapies is bronchodilator, mucolytics, then aztreonam.
• Don't reconstitute until ready to give dose.
• Add one ampule of diluent to one amber glass vial of aztreonam. Replace rubber stopper on vial and gently swirl until contents have completely dissolved. Administer immediately.
• Don't use diluent or reconstituted drug if it's cloudy or if there are particles in the solution.
• Use only Altera Nebulizer System to administer drug.
• Never mix with other drugs in nebulizer.
• Administration usually takes 2 to 3 minutes.
IV
▼ Obtain specimen for culture and sensitivity tests before giving first dose. Begin therapy while awaiting results.
▼ For direct injection, reconstitute with 6 to 10 mL of sterile water for injection and immediately shake vial vigorously. Constituted solutions aren't for multiple-dose use. Discard unused solution.
▼ To give a bolus, inject drug over 3 to 5 minutes, directly into IV tubing.
▼ For infusion, reconstitute with a compatible IV solution to yield 20 mg/mL or less.
▼ Give infusions over 20 minutes to 1 hour.
▼ Give thawed solutions only by IV infusion.
▼ **Incompatibilities:** Acyclovir, amphotericin B, ampicillin sodium, azithromycin, chlorpromazine, daunorubicin hydrochloride, ganciclovir, lorazepam, metronidazole, mitomycin, mitoxantrone, nafcillin, prochlorperazine, streptozocin, vancomycin.
IM
• To prepare IM injection, add at least 3 mL of one of the following solutions per gram of aztreonam: sterile water for injection,

bacteriostatic water for injection, NSS, or bacteriostatic NSS.
• Give IM injections deep into a large muscle, such as the upper outer quadrant of the gluteus maximus or the side of the thigh.
• Give doses larger than 1 g by IV route.
❸ **Alert:** Don't give IM injection to children.
• Pain and swelling may occur at injection site.

ACTION
Inhibits bacterial cell-wall synthesis, ultimately causing cell-wall destruction; bactericidal.

Route	Onset	Peak	Duration
IV	Unknown	Immediate	Unknown
IM	Unknown	<1 hr	Unknown
Inhalation	Unknown	1 hr	Unknown

Half-life: 1½ to 2 hours.

ADVERSE REACTIONS
CNS: *seizures,* confusion, headache, insomnia, pyrexia. **CV:** hypotension, thrombophlebitis, chest discomfort. **EENT:** nasal congestion, sore throat. **GI:** *pseudomembranous colitis,* diarrhea, abdominal pain, nausea, vomiting. **Hematologic:** *neutropenia, pancytopenia, thrombocytopenia,* anemia, leukocytosis, thrombocytosis. **Respiratory:** bronchospasm, cough. **Skin:** discomfort and swelling at IM injection site, rash, erythema multiforme. **Other:** hypersensitivity reactions.

INTERACTIONS
Drug-drug. *Aminoglycosides:* May have synergistic nephrotoxic effects. Monitor renal function.
Cefoxitin, imipenem: May have antagonistic effect. Avoid using together.

EFFECTS ON LAB TEST RESULTS
• May increase ALT, AST, BUN, creatinine, and LDH levels. May decrease Hb level.
• May prolong PT and PTT, and increase INR.
• May decrease neutrophil and RBC counts. May increase or decrease platelet and WBC counts.
• May cause false-positive Coombs test result. May alter urine glucose determinations

using cupric sulfate (Clinitest or Benedict reagent).

CONTRAINDICATIONS & CAUTIONS
• Contraindicated in patients hypersensitive to drug or its components and in those taking other beta-lactam antibiotics.
• Use cautiously in elderly patients and in those with impaired renal or hepatic function. Dosage adjustment may be needed. Monitor renal function test results.
• Drug may cause CDAD ranging in severity from mild diarrhea to fatal colitis occurring up to 2 months after administration. If CDAD is suspected or confirmed, drug may need to be discontinued and appropriate treatment begun.
• Rare cases of toxic epidermal necrolysis have been reported in patients undergoing bone marrow transplant with multiple risk factors, including sepsis, radiation therapy, and concomitantly administered drugs associated with toxic epidermal necrolysis.
Dialyzable drug: Yes.

PREGNANCY-LACTATION-REPRODUCTION
• There are no adequate and well-controlled studies in pregnant women. Use during pregnancy only if clearly needed.
• Drug appears in human milk. Breastfeeding women should temporarily discontinue breastfeeding.

NURSING CONSIDERATIONS
• Observe patient for signs and symptoms of superinfection.
❸ **Alert:** Because drug is ineffective against gram-positive and anaerobic organisms, combine it with other antibiotics for immediate treatment of life-threatening illnesses.
❸ **Alert:** Patients allergic to penicillins or cephalosporins may not be allergic to this drug. Monitor closely those who have had an immediate hypersensitivity reaction to these antibiotics, especially to ceftazidime.
• Antibiotics may promote overgrowth of nonsusceptible organisms. Monitor patient for signs of superinfection.

PATIENT TEACHING
• Warn patient receiving IM drug that pain and swelling may occur at injection site.

❈Canada   ◇OTC   ◆Off-label use   ✐Photoguide   ⊕Do not crush   *Liquid contains alcohol   ⚍Genetic

- Tell patient to report discomfort at IV insertion site.
- Instruct patient to report adverse reactions and signs and symptoms of superinfection promptly.
- Instruct patient or caregiver in proper administration of drug by nebulizer.
- Teach patient or caregiver to use bronchodilator before using Cayston.

baclofen
BAK-loe-fen

Gablofen, Lioresal Intrathecal

Therapeutic class: Skeletal muscle relaxants
Pharmacologic class: Gamma-aminobutyric acid derivatives

AVAILABLE FORMS
Intrathecal injection: 50 mcg/mL, 500 mcg/mL, 1,000 mcg/mL, 2,000 mcg/mL
Tablets: 5 mg, 10 mg, 20 mg

INDICATIONS & DOSAGES
Adjust-a-dose (for all indications): For patients with impaired renal function, decrease oral and intrathecal doses.
➤ **Spasticity in MS; spinal cord injury**
Adults and children age 12 and older: Initially, 5 mg PO t.i.d. for 3 days; then 10 mg t.i.d. for 3 days, 15 mg t.i.d. for 3 days, 20 mg t.i.d. for 3 days. Increase daily dosage, based on response, to maximum of 80 mg (given as 20 mg q.i.d.).
Adjust-a-dose: For patients with psychiatric or brain disorders and for elderly patients, increase dose gradually.
➤ **To manage severe spasticity in patients who don't respond to or can't tolerate oral baclofen therapy**
Adults: For screening phase, after test dose to check responsiveness, give drug via implantable infusion pump. Give test dose of 1 mL of 50 mcg/mL dilution into intrathecal space by barbotage over 1 minute or longer. Significantly decreased severity or frequency of muscle spasm or reduced muscle tone should appear within 4 to 8 hours. If response is inadequate, give second test dose of 75 mcg/1.5 mL 24 hours after the first. If response is still inadequate, give final

test dose of 100 mcg/2 mL after 24 hours. Patients unresponsive to the 100-mcg dose shouldn't be considered candidates for implantable pump.
Children age 4 and older: Initial test dose is the same as that for adults (50 mcg); for very small children, initial dose is 25 mcg.
For maintenance therapy: Adjust first dose based on screening dose that elicited an adequate response. Double this effective dose and give over 24 hours. However, if screening dose effectiveness was maintained for 8 hours or longer, don't double dose. After first 24 hours, increase dose slowly as needed and tolerated by 10% to 30% increments at 24-hour intervals in spasticity of spinal cord origin. In children with spasticity of spinal cord origin and adults and children with spasticity of cerebral origin, increase by 5% to 15% increments at 24-hour intervals. During prolonged maintenance therapy, increase daily dose by 10% to 40% in spasticity of spinal cord origin, or increase daily dose by 5% to 20% in spasticity of cerebral origin, if needed; if patient experiences adverse effects, decrease dose by 10% to 20%. Maintenance dosages range from 12 to 2,003 mcg daily based on diagnosis, but experience with dosages of more than 1,000 mcg daily is limited. Most patients need 300 to 800 mcg daily for spasticity of spinal cord origin and 90 to 703 mcg daily for spasticity of cerebral origin.

ADMINISTRATION
PO
- Give drug with meals or milk to prevent GI distress.
Intrathecal
Black Box Warning Don't discontinue abruptly. This can result in high fever, altered mental status, exaggerated rebound spasticity, and muscle rigidity, which in rare cases, has led to rhabdomyolysis, multiple organ-system failure, and death. ∎
- Don't give intrathecal injection by IV, IM, subcut, or epidural route.
- Maintenance infusions that require dilution must be diluted with sterile preservative-free sodium chloride for injection.
- If patient suddenly requires a large intrathecal dose increase, check for a catheter

complication, such as kinking or dislodgment.

• With long-term intrathecal use, about 5% of patients may develop tolerance to drug. In some cases, this may be treated by hospitalizing patient and slowly withdrawing drug over a 2- to 4-week period. After the "drug holiday," drug may be restarted at the initial continuous infusion dose.

ACTION

Hyperpolarizes fibers to reduce impulse transmission. Appears to reduce transmission of impulses from the spinal cord to skeletal muscle, thus decreasing the frequency and amplitude of muscle spasms in patients with spinal cord lesions.

Route	Onset	Peak	Duration
PO	Unknown	30 min–4 hr	Unknown
Intrathecal	30 min–1 hr	4 hr	4–8 hr

Half-life: Oral, children with cerebral palsy, 4½ hours; adults, 2¾ to 4¾ hours. Intrathecal, 1½ hours over first 4 hours.

ADVERSE REACTIONS

CNS: agitation, drowsiness, dizziness, headache, weakness, fatigue, hypotonia, confusion, insomnia, *seizures with intrathecal use,* paresthesia, asthenia, pain, speech disorder, depression. **CV:** hypotension, peripheral edema. **EENT:** nasal congestion. **GI:** nausea, constipation, dry mouth, vomiting. **GU:** urinary frequency, urine retention, erectile dysfunction, incontinence. **Metabolic:** hyperglycemia, weight gain. **Musculoskeletal:** muscle rigidity or spasticity, muscle weakness. **Respiratory:** dyspnea, pneumonia. **Skin:** rash, pruritus, urticaria, excessive sweating. **Other:** chills, accidental injury.

INTERACTIONS

Drug-drug. *CNS depressants:* May increase CNS depression. Avoid using together.
Black Box Warning *Opioid class warning:* May cause slow or difficult breathing, sedation, and death. Avoid use together. If use together is necessary, limit dosage and duration of each drug to minimum necessary for desired effect. ∎
Drug-lifestyle. *Alcohol use:* May increase CNS depression. Discourage use together.

EFFECTS ON LAB TEST RESULTS

• May increase alkaline phosphatase, AST, CK, and glucose levels.
• May increase leukocyte count.

CONTRAINDICATIONS & CAUTIONS

• Contraindicated in patients hypersensitive to drug.
• Use cautiously in patients with impaired renal function, respiratory disease, or seizure disorder or when spasticity is used to maintain motor function.
• Use cautiously in patients with psychotic disorders, schizophrenia, or confusional states. Exacerbations of these conditions have occurred.
Black Box Warning Opioids should only be prescribed with benzodiazepines or other CNS depressants to patients for whom alternative treatment options are inadequate. ∎
• Safety and effectiveness in children younger than age 4 (intrathecal use) and age 12 (oral use) haven't been established.
Dialyzable drug: Yes.
⚠ *Overdose S&S:* Coma, dizziness, lightheadedness, diminished reflexes, vomiting, hypotonia, increased salivation, drowsiness, vision changes, respiratory depression, seizures.

PREGNANCY-LACTATION-REPRODUCTION

• Use in pregnant women only when potential benefits justify possible risks to the fetus.
• Oral drug appears in human milk. It isn't known if drug appears in human milk after intrathecal administration. Patient should avoid breastfeeding during therapy unless the potential benefit justifies the potential risks to the infant.

NURSING CONSIDERATIONS

❸ *Alert:* Don't use oral drug to treat muscle spasm caused by rheumatic disorders, cerebral palsy, Parkinson disease, or stroke because drug's effectiveness for these indications hasn't been established.
❸ *Alert:* Life-threatening CNS depression, CV collapse, and respiratory failure may occur with intrathecal use. Have trained staff and resuscitation equipment available during screening, dosage titration, and pump refill.
• Avoid contamination of sterile surfaces through contact with the nonsterile exterior

of the Gablofen prefilled syringe while refilling implantable intrathecal pumps. Use of the prefilled syringe in an aseptic setting (e.g., operating room) to fill sterile intrathecal pumps before implantation in patients isn't recommended unless external surface of syringe is treated to ensure sterility.

• Reservoir refilling must be performed by fully trained and qualified personnel following directions provided by the pump manufacturer.

◑ *Alert:* Use extreme caution when filling an FDA-approved implantable pump equipped with an injection port that allows direct access to the intrathecal catheter. Direct injection into the catheter through the catheter access port may cause a life-threatening overdose.

• Watch for sensitivity reactions, such as fever, skin eruptions, and respiratory distress.

• Expect an increased risk of seizures in patients with seizure disorder.

• The amount of relief determines whether dosage (and drowsiness) can be reduced.

• Some degree of muscle tone and spasticity may be necessary to sustain upright posture and balance with movement or to obtain optimal function, help support circulatory function, and prevent formation of DVT.

• When switching to intrathecal baclofen, attempt to discontinue concomitant oral antispasmodics to avoid overdose or increased adverse effects. Reduce oral antispasmodic dosage slowly while monitoring patient closely.

Black Box Warning Don't withdraw intrathecal drug abruptly after long-term use unless severe adverse reactions demand it; doing so may precipitate seizures, high fever, hallucinations, or rebound spasticity. ∎

• *Look alike–sound alike:* Don't confuse baclofen with Bactroban.

PATIENT TEACHING

Black Box Warning Advise patient and caregivers, especially patients with spinal cord injuries at T6 or above, communication difficulties, or history of withdrawal symptoms from oral or intrathecal baclofen, of risks associated with abrupt discontinuation of intrathecal form. Tell them to keep scheduled refill visits and teach them

the signs and symptoms of baclofen withdrawal. ∎

• Instruct patient to take oral form with meals or milk to reduce GI upset.

Black Box Warning *Opioid class warning:* Caution patient or caregiver of patient taking an opioid with a benzodiazepine, CNS depressant, or alcohol to seek immediate medical attention for dizziness, lightheadedness, extreme sleepiness, slowed or difficult breathing, or unresponsiveness. ∎

• Tell patient to avoid activities that require alertness until CNS effects of drug are known. Drowsiness usually is transient.

• Tell patient to avoid alcohol and OTC antihistamines while taking drug.

• Advise patient to follow prescriber's orders regarding rest and physical therapy.

• Teach patient and caregivers about the signs and symptoms of overdose and what to do if an overdose occurs.

• Teach patient and caregivers proper home care of pump and insertion site.

beclomethasone dipropionate (inhalation)
be-kloe-METH-a-sone

QVAR RediHaler

Therapeutic class: Antiasthmatics
Pharmacologic class: Corticosteroids

AVAILABLE FORMS
Oral inhalation aerosol: 40 mcg/metered spray, 80 mcg/metered spray

INDICATIONS & DOSAGES
➤ **Chronic asthma**
Adults and children age 12 and older: Starting dose, 40 to 80 mcg b.i.d. when patient previously used bronchodilators alone, or 40 to 320 mcg b.i.d. when patient previously used inhaled corticosteroids. If patient doesn't respond adequately to initial dosage after 2 weeks, increasing dosage may provide additional asthma control. Maximum, 320 mcg b.i.d.
Children ages 4 to 11: 40 mcg b.i.d. May increase to 80 mcg b.i.d. after 2 weeks if needed. Maximum, 80 mcg b.i.d.

Reactions in bold italics are *life-threatening*. Interactions may have a *rapid onset* or a *delayed onset*.

ADMINISTRATION
Inhalational
• No need to prime or shake RediHaler.
• Close the white cap to prepare the inhaler with medicine before each inhalation.
• Have patient rinse mouth and spit after use.
• Space doses 12 hours apart.
• Don't shake inhaler with cap open to avoid possible actuation.
• Don't wash or put any part of the inhaler in water; gently wipe mouthpiece with a dry cloth or tissue as needed.
• Don't use with a spacer or volume holding chamber.

ACTION
May decrease inflammation by decreasing the number and activity of inflammatory cells, inhibiting bronchoconstrictor mechanisms, producing direct smooth-muscle relaxation, and decreasing airway hyperresponsiveness.

Route	Onset	Peak	Duration
Inhalation	1–4 wk	½ hr	Unknown

Half-life: 2.8 hours.

ADVERSE REACTIONS
CNS: headache. **EENT:** hoarseness, throat irritation, fungal infection of throat, pharyngitis, rhinitis, sinusitis. **GI:** fungal infection of mouth, dry mouth. **Musculoskeletal:** back pain. **Respiratory:** cough, URI, exacerbation of asthma, wheezing. **Other:** *angioedema,* facial edema, hypersensitivity reactions, *adrenal insufficiency,* suppression of HPA function.

INTERACTIONS
None reported by manufacturer.

EFFECTS ON LAB TEST RESULTS
None reported.

CONTRAINDICATIONS & CAUTIONS
• Contraindicated in patients hypersensitive to drug or its ingredients and in those with status asthmaticus, nonasthmatic bronchial diseases, or asthma controlled by bronchodilators or other noncorticosteroids alone.
• Use cautiously, if at all, in patients with TB, ocular HSV, or untreated systemic fungal, bacterial, parasitic, or viral infections.
• Use cautiously in patients receiving systemic corticosteroid therapy.
Dialyzable drug: No.

PREGNANCY-LACTATION-REPRODUCTION
• Use during pregnancy only when potential benefits justify possible risks to the fetus. After delivery, evaluate neonates for adrenal suppression if mother received substantial doses during pregnancy.
• Serious adverse reactions may occur in breastfeeding infants. A decision should be made to discontinue breastfeeding or discontinue drug, taking into account importance of drug to the mother.

NURSING CONSIDERATIONS
• Check mucous membranes frequently for signs and symptoms of fungal infection.
• During times of stress (trauma, surgery, or infection), systemic corticosteroids may be needed to prevent adrenal insufficiency in previously corticosteroid-dependent patients.
• Periodic measurement of growth and development may be needed during high-dose or prolonged therapy in children.
• Cataracts and decreases in bone mineral density can occur. Closely monitor patients for vision changes and for decreased bone mineral content, especially patients with major risk factors.
❸ *Alert:* Taper oral corticosteroid therapy slowly. Acute adrenal insufficiency and death may occur in patients with asthma who change abruptly from oral corticosteroids to beclomethasone.
❸ *Alert:* Bronchospasm may occur after dosing; discontinue drug and treat immediately with a short-acting inhaled bronchodilator.

PATIENT TEACHING
• Tell patient inhaler doesn't need to be primed or shaken.
• Tell patient to close the white cap to prepare the inhaler with medicine before each inhalation.
• Inform patient that drug doesn't relieve acute asthma attacks.

• Tell patient who needs a bronchodilator to use it several minutes before beclomethasone.

• Instruct patient who hasn't had chickenpox or measles or been properly immunized to use particular care to avoid exposure.

• Instruct patient to carry or wear medical identification indicating patient's need for supplemental systemic corticosteroids during stress.

• Advise patient to hold breath for 5 to 10 seconds to enhance drug action.

• Tell patient it may take up to 4 weeks to feel the full benefit of the drug.

• Tell patient to keep inhaler clean by wiping it as needed with a dry tissue or cloth. Caution patient not to get it wet.

• Advise patient to prevent oral fungal infections by gargling or rinsing mouth with water after each use. Caution patient not to swallow the water.

• Tell patient to report evidence of corticosteroid withdrawal, including fatigue, weakness, arthralgia, orthostatic hypotension, and dyspnea.

• Instruct patient to store drug between 59° and 86° F (15° and 30° C).

---

beclomethasone dipropionate (intranasal)
be-kloe-METH-a-sone

Beconase AQ, Qnasl, Rivanase AQ✤

Therapeutic class: Corticosteroids
Pharmacologic class: Corticosteroids

AVAILABLE FORMS
Nasal aerosol solution: 40 mcg/actuation, 80 mcg/actuation
Nasal spray: 42 mcg/metered spray, 50 mcg/metered spray✤

INDICATIONS & DOSAGES
➤ **To relieve symptoms of seasonal or perennial allergic and nonallergic (vasomotor) rhinitis; to prevent nasal polyp recurrence after surgical removal (Beconase AQ)**
Adults and children age 12 and older: 1 or 2 sprays (42 to 84 mcg Beconase AQ) in each nostril b.i.d.

Children ages 6 to 12: Initially, 1 spray (42 mcg) in each nostril b.i.d. May increase to 2 sprays in each nostril b.i.d. Once adequate control is achieved, decrease to 1 spray in each nostril b.i.d. Maximum, 336 mcg daily.
➤ **To relieve symptoms of seasonal or perennial allergic rhinitis (Qnasl)**
Adults and children age 12 and older: 2 sprays (160 mcg total) in each nostril once daily. Maximum, 320 mcg/day.
Children ages 4 to 11: 1 spray (40 mcg) in each nostril once daily. Maximum, 80 mcg/day.

ADMINISTRATION
Intranasal
• Pump nasal spray six times or until a fine mist is produced before first use; repeat priming if nasal spray hasn't been used for 7 days (Beconase AQ). Qnasl doesn't need to be primed.
• Shake Beconase AQ well before use.

ACTION
May reduce nasal inflammation by inhibiting mediators of inflammation.

Route	Onset	Peak	Duration
Intranasal	5–7 days	3 wk	Unknown

Half-life: About 4½ hours (major active metabolite).

ADVERSE REACTIONS
CNS: headache, light-headedness, fever. **EENT:** mild, transient nasal burning and stinging; dryness, epistaxis, nasal congestion, nasopharyngeal fungal infections, rhinorrhea, sneezing, watery eyes. **GI:** nausea. **Metabolic:** growth velocity reduction in children and adolescents. **Skin:** rash, urticaria.

INTERACTIONS
None reported by manufacturer.

EFFECTS ON LAB TEST RESULTS
None reported.

CONTRAINDICATIONS & CAUTIONS
• Contraindicated in patients hypersensitive to drug.
• Not recommended for children younger than age 6 (Beconase AQ) or age 4 (Qnasl).

• Use cautiously, if at all, in patients with active or quiescent respiratory tract tuberculous infections, untreated local or systemic fungal or bacterial infections, systemic viral or parasitic infections, or ocular HSV infections.
• Avoid use in patients who have recently had nasal septal ulcers, nasal surgery, or trauma until wound healing occurs.
• Use cautiously in patients receiving systemic corticosteroid therapy.
Dialyzable drug: No.
⚠ *Overdose S&S:* Hypercorticism, adrenal suppression.

PREGNANCY-LACTATION-REPRODUCTION
• Use during pregnancy only when potential benefits justify possible risks to the fetus. After delivery, evaluate neonates for adrenal suppression if mother received substantial doses during pregnancy.
• It isn't known if drug appears in human milk. Use cautiously in breastfeeding women.

NURSING CONSIDERATIONS
• Observe patient for fungal infections.
• Drug isn't effective for acute exacerbations of rhinitis. Decongestants or antihistamines may be needed.
• Stop drug if no significant symptom improvement occurs after 3 weeks.
• Monitor growth routinely in pediatric patients; reduction in growth rate may occur.
• Glaucoma and cataracts can occur. Closely monitor patients for vision changes and increased IOP.
• Watch for hypercorticism and adrenal suppression with very high doses, or with standard doses in susceptible patients. If signs and symptoms occur, taper and discontinue drug.

PATIENT TEACHING
• Advise patient or parent to read package insert for instructions on drug use and canister and applicator care.
• Advise patient to pump Beconase AQ nasal spray four to six times until a fine mist is produced before first use. If nasal spray pump hasn't been used for 7 or more days in a row, it should be reprimed.

• To instill, instruct patient to blow nose to clear nasal passages, shake container, tilt head slightly forward, and insert nozzle into nostril, pointing away from septum. Tell patient to hold other nostril closed and inhale gently while spraying, hold breath for a few seconds, and exhale through the mouth. Next, have patient shake container and repeat in other nostril.
• Tell patient not to blow nose for 15 minutes after using Qnasl.
• Advise patient to use drug as prescribed, because its effectiveness depends on regular use.
• Explain that unlike decongestants, drug doesn't work right away. Most patients notice improvement within a few days, but some may need 2 to 3 weeks.
• Warn patient not to exceed recommended dosage because of risk of HPA axis suppression.
• Instruct patient who hasn't had chickenpox or measles or been properly immunized to use particular care to avoid exposure.
• Tell patient to notify prescriber if signs and symptoms don't improve within 3 weeks or if nasal irritation persists.
• Teach patient good nasal and oral hygiene.

---

belimumab ✂
beh-LIH-moo-mab

Benlysta

Therapeutic class: Immunosuppressants
Pharmacologic class: Human monoclonal antibodies

AVAILABLE FORMS
IV injection: 120 mg, 400 mg in single-use vials
Subcut injection: 200 mg/mL single-dose prefilled autoinjector or prefilled syringe

INDICATIONS & DOSAGES
➤ **Active, autoantibody-positive SLE**
Adults: 10 mg/kg IV infusion every 2 weeks for first three doses, then every 4 weeks thereafter. Or, 200 mg subcut once weekly.

ADMINISTRATION

IV

▼ Consider premedicating with an antihistamine and antipyretic for prophylaxis against infusion or hypersensitivity reactions.

▼ Store unopened vials in refrigerator.

▼ Once vial has been at room temperature for 10 to 15 minutes, reconstitute with sterile water: 1.5 mL for 120-mg vial and 4.8 mL for 400-mg vial.

▼ Direct stream of sterile water toward side of vial to minimize foaming. Gently swirl for 60 seconds every 5 minutes until dissolved. Don't shake. Protect solution from light while dissolving. Usual reconstitution time is 10 to 15 minutes but may take up to 30 minutes.

▼ Solution should be opalescent and colorless to pale yellow. Small air bubbles are expected and acceptable.

▼ Dilute only in NSS, half-NSS, or lactated Ringer solution to a volume of 250 mL.

▼ To dilute, withdraw a volume of fluid equal to amount of medication to be added from a 250-mL infusion bag, so total volume will remain at 250 mL when the medication is added. Add the medication to the 250-mL infusion bag and gently invert to mix the solution. Discard any unused drug solution.

▼ Protect unused reconstituted solution from light and store in refrigerator. Solutions in NSS, half-NSS, or lactated Ringer solution may be stored in refrigerator or at room temperature.

▼ Administer as an IV infusion over 1 hour. Don't give as an IV push or bolus.

▼ Complete infusion within 8 hours of reconstitution.

▼ **Incompatibilities:** Dextrose solution, other IV drugs.

Subcutaneous

• If changing from IV therapy to subcut administration, give first subcut dose 1 to 4 weeks after last IV dose.

• Administer by subcut injection in abdomen or thigh.

• Rotate injection sites weekly; never inject into areas where skin is tender, bruised, red, or hard.

• Remove from refrigerator and allow to sit at room temperature for 30 minutes before use.

• Inspect visually for particulate matter and discoloration before administration; use only if solution appears clear to opalescent and colorless to pale yellow.

• Administer once a week, preferably on the same day each week.

• If a dose is missed, administer injection as soon as possible; then resume schedule or start a new weekly schedule from the day that the missed dose was administered. Don't administer two doses on the same day.

ACTION

B-lymphocyte stimulator-specific inhibitor that inhibits survival of B cells, including autoreactive B cells, and reduces their differentiation into Ig-producing plasma cells.

Route	Onset	Peak	Duration
IV, subcut	Unknown	Unknown	Unknown

Half-life: IV, 19.4 days; subcut, 18.3 days.

ADVERSE REACTIONS

CNS: anxiety, headache, insomnia, migraine, depression, fever. **EENT:** nasopharyngitis, pharyngitis. **GI:** nausea, diarrhea, viral gastroenteritis. **GU:** cystitis, UTI. **Hematologic:** *leukopenia.* **Musculoskeletal:** extremity pain. **Respiratory:** bronchitis, URI. **Other:** infection, antibody detection, hypersensitivity reactions, infusion reactions.

INTERACTIONS

Drug-drug. *IV cyclophosphamide, other biological agents:* Use together hasn't been studied. Don't use together.

Live-virus vaccines: May impair response to vaccines. Don't give live-virus vaccines for 30 days before or concurrently with belimumab.

Drug-herb. *Echinacea:* May decrease drug's therapeutic effects. Consider therapy modification.

EFFECTS ON LAB TEST RESULTS

• May decrease leukocyte count.

Reactions in bold italics are *life-threatening*. Interactions may have a *rapid onset* or a *delayed onset*.

CONTRAINDICATIONS & CAUTIONS
• Contraindicated in patients with a history of anaphylaxis to belimumab.
• Use cautiously in patients with a history of chronic infection, hypersensitivity reactions, infusion reactions, depression, or malignancies.
▩ Use cautiously in black patients because response rate may be lower.
• More deaths occurred with belimumab than with placebo during the controlled period of the main clinical trials. No single cause of death predominated, but possible causes included infection, CV disease, and suicide.
• Use isn't recommended for patients with severe active lupus nephritis or severe active CNS lupus.
• Safety and effectiveness in children haven't been established.
Dialyzable drug: Unknown.

PREGNANCY-LACTATION-REPRODUCTION
• There are no adequate well-controlled studies in pregnant women. Use cautiously during pregnancy and only if potential benefit outweighs risk to the fetus. Pregnant women should enroll in a pregnancy registry that monitors maternal-fetal outcomes of exposure to belimumab by calling 1-877-681-6296.
• Women of childbearing potential should use adequate contraception during treatment and for at least 4 months after final dose.
• Monitor infant of a treated mother for B-cell reduction and other immune dysfunction; consider risks and benefits before giving live or live-attenuated vaccines to the infant.
• It isn't known if drug appears in human milk. A decision should be made to discontinue breastfeeding or discontinue drug, taking into account importance of drug to the mother.

NURSING CONSIDERATIONS
• Patient shouldn't receive live-virus vaccines for 30 days before or concurrently with drug.
• IV drug should be administered only by a health care professional prepared to manage anaphylaxis.

• Patient or caregiver may administer subcut after proper training and if prescriber determines it's appropriate.
• Watch for hypersensitivity reactions, even in patients who previously tolerated infusions.
• Monitor patient for infection. Serious and sometimes fatal infections have occurred in patients receiving immunosuppressants.
• Monitor patient for depression, suicidal ideation, malignancies, allergic reactions, and infusion reactions.
• Assess patients with new-onset or deteriorating neurologic signs and symptoms for JC virus–associated progressive multifocal leukoencephalopathy (PML). If PML is confirmed, therapy may have to be discontinued.

PATIENT TEACHING
• Warn patient not to skip appointments to ensure that drug is given on schedule to improve effectiveness of treatment.
• Tell patient to immediately report signs and symptoms of an allergic reaction (itching, hives, shortness of breath, swelling of the face, and throat closure) and new or worsening depression, suicidal thoughts, or other mood changes.
• Teach patient infection-prevention measures.
• Instruct patient to immediately report signs and symptoms of infection (fever, body aches, cough, and sore throat).
• Tell patient to report history of cancer to health care provider.
• Instruct patient not to receive live-virus vaccines while taking drug.
• If patient or caregiver will be administering subcut at home, provide training and instruct patient or caregiver to follow directions for administration provided in the "Instructions for Use."
• Advise patient to use a different injection site each week.
• Counsel female patient of childbearing potential to use adequate contraception during treatment and for at least 4 months after final dose.
• Advise female patient to tell prescriber if she is pregnant or breastfeeding.

SAFETY ALERT!

belinostat ⚖
be-LIN-oh-stat

Beleodaq

Therapeutic class: Antineoplastics
Pharmacologic class: Histone deacetylase inhibitors

AVAILABLE FORMS
Injection: 500-mg single-use vial

INDICATIONS & DOSAGES
➤ **Relapsed or refractory peripheral T-cell lymphoma**
Adults: 1,000 mg/m^2 IV infusion once daily on days 1 through 5 of a 21-day cycle over 30 minutes. Repeat cycles until disease progression or unacceptable toxicity occurs.
Adjust-a-dose: ⚖ For patients homozygous for the UGT1A1*28 allele, reduce starting dose to 750 mg/m^2 because drug clearance may be decreased. (This may affect 20% of the black population, 10% of the white population, and 2% of the Asian population.)

For obese patients, use patient's actual body weight for calculating BSA or weight-based dosing.

Refer to manufacturer's instructions for toxicity-related dosage adjustments.

ADMINISTRATION
IV
▼ Store vial at room temperature. Retain in original package until use.
▼ Follow safe handling and disposal procedures for cytotoxic drugs.
▼ Reconstitute each vial with 9 mL sterile water for injection to yield a concentration of 50 mg/mL. Swirl vial until there are no visible particles.
▼ May store reconstituted vial for up to 12 hours at ambient temperature (59° to 77° F [15° to 25° C]).
▼ Withdraw volume needed for required dose and transfer to infusion bag containing 250 mL NSS injection. The infusion bag with drug solution may be stored at ambient room temperature for up to 36 hours, including infusion time.

▼ Inspect solution for particulate matter. Don't use if solution is cloudy or contains particulates.
▼ Infuse drug over 30 minutes using 0.22-micron in-line filter. Infusion time may be extended to 45 minutes if infusion-site pain or other symptoms associated with the infusion occur.
▼ **Incompatibilities:** None listed by manufacturer. Consult a drug incompatibility reference for more information.

ACTION
Induces cell-cycle arrest or apoptosis of some transformed cells. Shows preferential cytotoxicity toward tumor cells compared to normal cells.

Route	Onset	Peak	Duration
IV	Rapid	Unknown	Unknown

Half-life: 1.1 hours.

ADVERSE REACTIONS
CNS: fatigue, pyrexia, chills, headache, dizziness. **CV:** peripheral edema, *prolonged QT interval,* hypotension, phlebitis. **GI:** nausea, vomiting, constipation, diarrhea, decreased appetite, abdominal pain. **GU:** increased creatinine level. **Hematologic:** anemia, *thrombocytopenia, leukopenia.* **Hepatic:** *hepatic impairment,* increased blood LDH level. **Metabolic:** *hypokalemia.* **Respiratory:** dyspnea, cough, *pneumonia.* **Skin:** rash, pruritus, injection-site pain. **Other:** infection, *sepsis, multiorgan failure.*

INTERACTIONS
Drug-drug. *Drugs that prolong QT interval:* May increase risk of prolonged QT interval. Monitor patient closely.
⚖ *Strong inhibitors of UGT1A1 allele (atazanavir, indinavir):* May increase belinostat blood level. Monitor patient closely. Avoid use together if possible.

EFFECTS ON LAB TEST RESULTS
• May increase creatinine and blood LDH levels. May decrease potassium level.
• May decrease RBC, platelet, neutrophil, and lymphocyte counts.

Reactions in bold italics are *life-threatening.* Interactions may have a *rapid onset* or a *delayed onset.*

CONTRAINDICATIONS & CAUTIONS
• Contraindicated in patients hypersensitive to drug or its components.
• Serious, sometimes fatal infections, including pneumonia and sepsis, can occur. Avoid giving to patients with an active infection. Those with history of extensive or intensive chemotherapy may be at increased risk for life-threatening infection.
• May cause hepatotoxicity, which may be fatal. Not recommended in patients with moderate to severe hepatic impairment; drug hasn't been studied in these populations.
• May cause TLS, especially in patients with advanced disease or high tumor burden. Monitor patient closely; if TLS occurs, begin appropriate treatment.
• Use cautiously in patients with renal insufficiency.
• Safety and effectiveness in children haven't been established.
Dialyzable drug: Unknown.

PREGNANCY-LACTATION-REPRODUCTION
• Avoid use in pregnant women because of potential for teratogenicity or embryo-fetal death.
• May impair male fertility.
• It isn't known if drug appears in human milk. Patient should discontinue breastfeeding or discontinue drug.

NURSING CONSIDERATIONS
• Monitor CBC at baseline and weekly, and adjust dosage as necessary.
• Monitor patients for infection.
• Before first dose of each cycle, obtain serum chemistry tests, including renal and hepatic function. Adjust dosage or interrupt or discontinue therapy as necessary.
• Monitor patients for signs and symptoms of TLS (lethargy, arrhythmia, edema, renal failure, metabolic acidosis, hyperkalemia, hyperuricemia, hypocalcemia). Report signs or symptoms immediately.
• Monitor patient for nausea, diarrhea, and vomiting. Treat symptomatically.
• *Look alike–sound alike:* Don't confuse belinostat with beractant.

PATIENT TEACHING
• Advise patient to immediately report GI signs or symptoms, such as diarrhea, vomiting, or nausea.
• Explain importance of obtaining laboratory studies as instructed.
• Tell patient to report signs and symptoms of hepatic injury (yellowing of skin or eyes, dark urine, itching, pain in right upper quadrant of abdomen).
• Caution patient to report signs and symptoms of infection (fever, flulike symptoms, cough, shortness of breath, burning on urination, muscle aches, worsening of skin problems).
• Instruct patient to report unusual bleeding or bruising, weakness, tiredness, pallor, dyspnea, or infection.
• Teach patient to immediately report signs and symptoms of TLS (lethargy, confusion, fatigue, rapid irregular heartbeat, rapid breathing, edema, low urine output, dark urine, nausea, tingling of arms or legs, aching joints, muscle weakness).
• Warn patient to avoid becoming pregnant and not to use drug while breastfeeding. Inform patient of potential hazard to fetus.
• Warn male patient taking belinostat that drug may impair fertility.

benazepril hydrochloride ✂
ben-A-za-pril

Lotensin✐

Therapeutic class: Antihypertensives
Pharmacologic class: ACE inhibitors

AVAILABLE FORMS
Tablets: 5 mg, 10 mg, 20 mg, 40 mg

INDICATIONS & DOSAGES
Adjust-a-dose (for all indications): If CrCl is below 30 mL/minute/1.73 m^2 or serum creatinine level is greater than 3 mg/dL, give 5 mg PO daily. Daily dose may be adjusted up to 40 mg.
➤ **HTN**
Adults: For patients not receiving a diuretic, 10 mg PO daily initially. Adjust dosage as needed and tolerated; usually 20 to 40 mg daily in one or two divided doses. For

patients receiving a diuretic, 5 mg PO daily initially.

Children age 6 and older: 0.2 mg/kg (between 0.1 and 0.6 mg/kg) PO daily. Adjust as needed up to 0.6 mg/kg (maximum 40 mg) PO daily.

ADMINISTRATION
PO
• Protect tablets from moisture.

ACTION
Inhibits ACE, preventing conversion of angiotensin I to angiotensin II, a potent vasoconstrictor. Less angiotensin II decreases peripheral arterial resistance, decreasing aldosterone secretion, which reduces sodium and water retention and lowers BP. Drug also acts as antihypertensive in patients with low-renin HTN.

Route	Onset	Peak	Duration
PO	1 hr	1–2 hr	24 hr

Half-life: 10 to 11 hours.

ADVERSE REACTIONS
CNS: headache, dizziness, somnolence. **CV:** symptomatic hypotension. **Respiratory:** cough.

INTERACTIONS
Drug-drug. *Aliskiren:* May increase risk of renal impairment, hypotension, and hyperkalemia in diabetic patients and those with moderate to severe renal impairment (GFR less than 60 mL/minute). Concomitant use is contraindicated in diabetic patients. Avoid concomitant use in those with moderate to severe renal impairment.

Angiotensin II receptor antagonists (telmisartan): May increase risk of renal dysfunction. Avoid concurrent use.

Antidiabetics, insulin: May increase risk of hypoglycemia. Monitor patient carefully.

Azathioprine: May increase risk of anemia or leukopenia. Monitor hematologic study results if used together.

Diuretics, other antihypertensives: May cause excessive hypotension. Stop diuretic or lower dosage of benazepril, as needed.

Everolimus, sirolimus: May increase risk of angioedema. Discontinue one or both agents if an interaction is suspected.

Gold salts: May increase risk of nitritoid reaction. Carefully monitor patients.

Iron salts (parenteral): May increase risk of adverse reactions to iron salts. Monitor patient closely.

Lithium: May increase lithium level and toxicity. Use together cautiously; monitor lithium level.

Nesiritide: May increase risk of hypotension. Monitor BP.

NSAIDs: May decrease antihypertensive effects. Monitor BP. May also increase risk of renal dysfunction. Monitor renal function periodically.

Pergolide, phenothiazines (chlorpromazine): May cause profound hypotension. Use with caution and monitor BP.

Potassium-sparing diuretics, potassium supplements: May cause hyperkalemia. Monitor potassium level and renal function.

Salicylates: May decrease hypotensive effects of benazepril. Consider increasing benazepril dosage or decreasing or stopping salicylate.

Thiazide diuretics: May attenuate potassium loss. Also may increase risk of renal failure. Monitor serum potassium level and renal function.

Trimethoprim: May increase risk of hyperkalemia. Monitor serum potassium level and clinical response.

Drug-herb. *Ma huang, yohimbe:* May decrease antihypertensive effects. Discourage use together.

Drug-food. *Salt substitutes containing potassium:* May cause hyperkalemia. Monitor potassium level and renal function.

EFFECTS ON LAB TEST RESULTS
• May increase BUN, creatinine, and potassium levels.
• May lead to false-negative aldosterone/renin ratio.

CONTRAINDICATIONS & CAUTIONS
• Contraindicated in patients hypersensitive to ACE inhibitors and in those with a history of angioedema regardless of prior ACE inhibitor use.
• Use cautiously in patients with impaired hepatic or renal function. If jaundice develops or liver enzyme levels are markedly elevated, discontinue drug.

Reactions in bold italics are *life-threatening*. Interactions may have a *rapid onset* or a *delayed onset*.

Dialyzable drug: Slightly.
⚠ *Overdose S&S:* Hypotension.

PREGNANCY-LACTATION-REPRODUCTION
Black Box Warning Drugs that act on the RAAS can cause injury and death to a developing fetus. Discontinue drug as soon as possible once pregnancy is detected. ∎
• Small amounts of drug appear in human milk. Patient should either discontinue drug or discontinue breastfeeding.

NURSING CONSIDERATIONS
• Monitor patient for hypotension. Excessive hypotension can occur when drug is given with diuretics. If possible, diuretic therapy should be stopped 2 to 3 days before starting benazepril to decrease potential for excessive hypotensive response. If drug doesn't adequately control BP, diuretic may be cautiously reinstituted.
🧬 Although ACE inhibitors reduce BP in patients of all races, they reduce it less in black patients taking ACE inhibitors alone. Black patients should take drug with a thiazide diuretic for a more favorable response.
🧬 Drug may increase risk of angioedema in black patients.
• Measure BP when drug level is at peak (2 to 6 hours after administration) and at trough (just before a dose) to verify adequate BP control.
• Assess renal and hepatic function before and periodically during therapy. Monitor potassium level.
• Monitor patient for excessive cough. Therapy may need to be changed if cough is intolerable.
• *Look alike–sound alike:* Don't confuse benazepril with Benadryl. Don't confuse Lotensin with lovastatin.

PATIENT TEACHING
• Instruct patient to avoid salt substitutes because they may contain potassium, which can cause high potassium level in patients taking drug.
• Inform patient that light-headedness can occur, especially during first few days of therapy. Tell patient to rise slowly to minimize this effect, to report dizziness to prescriber and, if fainting occurs, to stop drug and call prescriber immediately.

• Warn patient to use caution in hot weather and during exercise. Inadequate fluid intake, vomiting, diarrhea, and excessive perspiration can lead to light-headedness and fainting.
• Advise patient to report signs and symptoms of infection (such as fever and sore throat), easy bruising or bleeding; swelling of tongue, lips, face, eyes, mucous membranes, or extremities; difficulty swallowing or breathing; or hoarseness.
�› *Alert:* Tell female patient of childbearing potential to notify prescriber if she becomes pregnant. Drug will need to be stopped.
• Tell patient to contact physician if intolerable cough develops.

---

benztropine mesylate
BENZ-troe-peen

Cogentin

Therapeutic class: Antiparkinsonian drugs
Pharmacologic class: Anticholinergics

AVAILABLE FORMS
Injection: 1 mg/mL in 2-mL ampules
Tablets: 0.5 mg, 1 mg, 2 mg

INDICATIONS & DOSAGES
➤ **Drug-induced extrapyramidal disorders (except tardive dyskinesia)**
Adults: 1 to 4 mg PO, IV, or IM once daily or b.i.d.
➤ **Transient extrapyramidal disorders**
Adults: 1 to 2 mg PO, IV, or IM b.i.d. or t.i.d. After 1 or 2 weeks, withdraw drug to determine continued need.
➤ **Acute dystonic reaction**
Adults: 1 to 2 mg PO, IV, or IM; then 1 to 2 mg PO once daily or b.i.d. to prevent recurrence. IV or IM route is preferred for severe acute reactions.
➤ **Parkinsonism**
Adults: 0.5 to 6 mg PO, IV, or IM daily in a single dose at bedtime or divided in two to four doses. First dose is 0.5 to 1 mg, increased by 0.5 mg every 5 to 6 days. Adjust dosage to meet individual requirements. Maximum, 6 mg daily.

➤ **Postencephalitic parkinsonism**
Adults: 2 mg PO, IV, or IM daily in one or
more doses. In highly sensitive patients,
therapy may be initiated with 0.5 mg PO
or IM at bedtime, and increased as needed.
Maximum, 6 mg daily.

ADMINISTRATION
PO
• May give before or after meals, depending
on patient reaction. If patient is prone to excessive salivation, give drug after meals. If
patient's mouth dries excessively, give drug
before meals unless it causes nausea.

IV
▼ Reserve IV delivery for emergencies,
such as acute dystonic reactions.
▼ The IV form is seldom used because no
significant difference in onset exists between it and the IM form.
▼ Use filtered needle to draw up solution
from ampule.
▼ **Incompatibilities:** Haloperidol lactate.

IM
• Use filtered needle to draw up solution
from ampule.

ACTION
Unknown. May block central cholinergic receptors, helping to balance cholinergic activity in the basal ganglia.

Route	Onset	Peak	Duration
PO	1 hr	7 hr	24 hr
IV, IM	15 min	Unknown	24 hr

Half-life: Unknown.

ADVERSE REACTIONS
CNS: confusion, memory impairment, nervousness, depression, disorientation, hallucinations, toxic psychosis, fever. **CV:** tachycardia. **EENT:** dilated pupils, blurred vision.
GI: dry mouth, constipation, nausea, vomiting, paralytic ileus. **GU:** urine retention,
dysuria. **Musculoskeletal:** muscle weakness. **Skin:** decreased sweating. **Other:** heat
stroke.

INTERACTIONS
Drug-drug. *Amantadine, phenothiazines,
TCAs:* May cause additive anticholiner-
gic adverse reactions, such as confusion,

hallucinations, GI effects, fever, or heat intolerance. Reduce dosage before giving.
*Cholinergics (donepezil, galantamine, riv-
astigmine, tacrine):* May antagonize the
therapeutic effects of these drugs. If used together, monitor patient for therapeutic effect.

EFFECTS ON LAB TEST RESULTS
None reported.

CONTRAINDICATIONS & CAUTIONS
• Contraindicated in patients hypersensitive to drug or its components, in those with
angle-closure glaucoma, and in children
younger than age 3.
• Drug isn't recommended for use in
patients with tardive dyskinesia.
• Drug may produce anhidrosis. Use cautiously in hot weather, in patients with
mental disorders, in elderly patients, and in
children age 3 and older.
• Use cautiously in patients with prostatic
hyperplasia, arrhythmias, or seizure disorders.
Dialyzable drug: Unknown.
⚠ *Overdose S&S:* CNS depression preceded
or followed by stimulation; confusion, nervousness, listlessness, intensification of
mental symptoms or toxic psychosis (in patients with mental illness being treated with
neuroleptic drugs), hallucinations, dizziness,
muscle weakness, ataxia, dry mouth, mydriasis, blurred vision, palpitations, tachycardia, HTN, nausea, vomiting, dysuria, numbness of fingers, dysphagia, allergic reactions,
headache, delirium, coma, shock, seizures,
respiratory arrest, anhidrosis, hyperthermia,
glaucoma, constipation; hot, dry, flushed
skin.

PREGNANCY-LACTATION-REPRODUCTION
• Safe use during pregnancy hasn't been established.
• It isn't known if drug appears in human
milk. Anticholinergic agents may suppress
lactation.

NURSING CONSIDERATIONS
• Monitor vital signs carefully. Watch
closely for adverse reactions, especially
in elderly or debilitated patients. Call prescriber promptly if adverse reactions occur.

Reactions in bold italics are *life-threatening*. Interactions may have a *rapid onset* or a *delayed onset*.

• At certain doses, drug produces atropine-like toxicity, which may aggravate tardive dyskinesia.
• Watch for intermittent constipation and abdominal distention and pain, which may indicate onset of paralytic ileus.
• Monitor elderly patients closely as they are more prone to severe adverse effects.
◑ *Alert:* Never stop drug abruptly. Reduce dosage gradually.
• *Look alike–sound alike:* Don't confuse benztropine with bromocriptine.

PATIENT TEACHING
• Warn patient to avoid activities that require alertness until CNS effects of drug are known.
• Advise patient who takes a single daily dose to do so at bedtime.
• Advise patient to report signs and symptoms of urinary hesitancy or urine retention.
• Tell patient to relieve dry mouth with cool drinks, ice chips, sugarless gum, or hard candy.
• Advise patient to limit hot weather activities because drug-induced lack of sweating may cause overheating.

betamethasone dipropionate
bay-ta-METH-a-sone

Diprolene, Diprolene AF, Sernivo

betamethasone valerate
Luxiq

Therapeutic class: Corticosteroids
Pharmacologic class: Corticosteroids

AVAILABLE FORMS
betamethasone dipropionate
Cream: 0.05%
Gel: 0.05%
Lotion: 0.05%
Ointment: 0.05%
Spray: 0.05%
betamethasone valerate
Cream: 0.1%
Foam: 0.12%
Lotion: 0.1%
Ointment: 0.1%

INDICATIONS & DOSAGES
➤ **Inflammation and pruritus from corticosteroid-responsive dermatoses**
Adults and children older than age 12: Clean area; apply cream, ointment, lotion, or gel sparingly. Give dipropionate products once daily to b.i.d.; give valerate 0.1% lotion b.i.d., or valerate 0.1% cream or ointment once daily to t.i.d. Maximum dosage of augmented betamethasone dipropionate 0.05% ointment, cream, gel, or lotion is 45 g, 45 g, 50 g, or 50 mL per week, respectively. Therapy with augmented formulations shouldn't exceed 2 weeks.
➤ **Inflammation and pruritus from corticosteroid-responsive dermatoses of scalp (valerate only)**
Adults: Gently massage small amounts of foam into affected scalp areas b.i.d., morning and evening, until control is achieved. If no improvement is seen in 2 weeks, reassess diagnosis.
➤ **Mild to moderate plaque psoriasis**
Adults: Apply spray to affected skin areas b.i.d. for up to 4 weeks; rub in gently.

ADMINISTRATION
Topical
• Apply sparingly to affected areas. To prevent skin damage, rub in gently, leaving a thin coat.
• Decrease dosing frequency to once daily if clinical improvement is seen.
• Avoid applying near eyes or mucous membranes or in ear canal, groin area, or armpit.
• Don't dispense foam directly into warm hands because foam will begin to melt on contact.
• For patients with eczematous dermatitis whose skin may be irritated by adhesive material, hold dressing in place with gauze, elastic bandages, stockings, or stockinette.
• Shake spray well before use. Avoid use on face, scalp, axilla, groin, or other intertriginous areas.
◑ *Alert:* Foam product is flammable. Avoid fire, flame, or smoking during use. Don't expose to heat.
◑ *Alert:* Don't use occlusive dressings.
• Continue drug for a few days after lesions clear.

ACTION
Unclear. Is diffused across cell membranes to form complexes with receptors. Has anti-inflammatory, antipruritic, vasoconstrictive, and antiproliferative activity. Considered a medium-potency to very-high-potency drug (depending on product), according to vaso-constrictive properties.

Route	Onset	Peak	Duration
Topical	Unknown	Unknown	Unknown

Half-life: Unknown.

ADVERSE REACTIONS
GU: glycosuria (with dipropionate).
Metabolic: hyperglycemia. **Skin:** burn-ing, pruritus, irritation, dryness, erythema, folliculitis, striae, acneiform eruptions, pe-rioral dermatitis, hypopigmentation, hyper-trichosis, allergic contact dermatitis, sec-ondary infection, maceration, atrophy, mil-iaria with occlusive dressings, application-site pain. **Other:** *HPA axis suppression,* Cushing syndrome.

INTERACTIONS
None significant.

EFFECTS ON LAB TEST RESULTS
• May increase glucose level.
• May suppress the wheal and flare reactions to skin test antigens.

CONTRAINDICATIONS & CAUTIONS
• Contraindicated in patients hypersensitive to corticosteroids.
• Don't use as monotherapy in primary bacterial infections (impetigo, paronychia, erysipelas, cellulitis, angular cheilitis), rosacea, perioral dermatitis, or acne.
• Don't use augmented betamethasone dipropionate 0.05% ointment; betametha-sone dipropionate 0.05% gel, cream, and ointment; betamethasone 0.05% spray; or betamethasone valerate 0.1% ointment on the face, groin, or axilla.
Dialyzable drug: No.
⚠ *Overdose S&S:* Systemic effects.

PREGNANCY-LACTATION-REPRODUCTION
• There are no adequate and well-controlled studies in pregnant women. Use during pregnancy only if potential benefit justifies potential risk to the fetus.
• Use cautiously in breastfeeding women.

NURSING CONSIDERATIONS
• Drug isn't for ophthalmic use.
• Because of alcohol content of vehicle, gel products may cause mild, transient stinging, especially when used on or near excoriated skin.
• If antifungal or antibiotic combined with corticosteroid fails to provide prompt im-provement, stop corticosteroid until infec-tion is controlled.
• Systemic absorption is likely with pro-longed or extensive body surface treatment. Watch for symptoms of HPA axis suppres-sion, manifestations of Cushing syndrome, hyperglycemia, and glycosuria. If HPA axis suppression occurs, attempt to withdraw drug or substitute a less potent steroid. Withdraw gradually.
• Evaluate patient for HPA axis suppression by using the urinary free cortisol and corti-cotropin stimulation tests.
• Drug may increase risk of posterior sub-capsular cataracts and glaucoma. Consider referral to an ophthalmologist for evaluation if symptoms develop.
◑ **Alert:** Children may demonstrate greater susceptibility to HPA axis suppression and Cushing syndrome.
• Avoid using plastic pants or tight-fitting diapers on treated areas in young children. Children may absorb larger amounts of drug and be more susceptible to systemic toxicity.
◑ **Alert:** Diprolene and Diprolene AF may not be replaced with generics because other products have different potencies.

PATIENT TEACHING
• Teach patient how to apply drug.
• Emphasize that drug is for external use only.
• Tell patient to wash hands after application.
• Tell patient to stop drug and report signs of systemic absorption, skin irritation or ul-ceration, hypersensitivity, visual changes, or infection.
• Instruct patient not to use occlusive dressings.

• Discuss personal hygiene measures to reduce chance of infection.

bethanechol chloride
be-THAN-e-kole

Duvoid, Urecholine

Therapeutic class: Urinary stimulants
Pharmacologic class: Cholinergic agonists

AVAILABLE FORMS
Tablets: 5 mg, 10 mg, 25 mg, 50 mg

INDICATIONS & DOSAGES
➤ **Acute postoperative and postpartum nonobstructive (functional) urine retention, neurogenic atony of urinary bladder with urine retention**
Adults: 10 to 50 mg PO t.i.d. to q.i.d. Determine minimum effective dose by giving 5 or 10 mg and repeating same amount at hourly intervals until satisfactory response or maximum of 50 mg has been given.

ADMINISTRATION
PO
• Give drug 1 hour before or 2 hours after meals because drug may cause nausea and vomiting if taken soon after eating.

ACTION
Directly stimulates muscarinic cholinergic receptors, mimicking acetylcholine action, increasing GI tract tone and peristalsis and contraction of the detrusor muscle of the urinary bladder.

Route	Onset	Peak	Duration
PO	30 min	60–90 min	Up to 6 hr

Half-life: Unknown.

ADVERSE REACTIONS
CNS: headache, malaise, *seizures.* **CV:** *bradycardia,* profound hypotension with reflexive tachycardia, flushing. **EENT:** lacrimation, miosis. **GI:** abdominal cramps, diarrhea, excessive salivation, nausea, belching, borborygmus. **GU:** urinary urgency. **Respiratory:** *bronchoconstriction, asthma attack.* **Skin:** diaphoresis.

INTERACTIONS
Drug-drug. *Anticholinergics, atropine, belladonna alkaloids, procainamide, quinidine:* May reverse cholinergic effects. Observe patient for lack of drug effect.
Cholinesterase inhibitors (donepezil), cholinergic agonists: May cause additive effects or increase toxicity. Avoid using together.
Ganglionic blockers: May cause critical drop in BP, usually preceded by severe abdominal pain. Avoid using together.

EFFECTS ON LAB TEST RESULTS
• May increase amylase, lipase, and liver enzyme levels.

CONTRAINDICATIONS & CAUTIONS
• Contraindicated in patients hypersensitive to drug or its components and in those with uncertain strength or integrity of bladder wall, mechanical obstruction of GI or urinary tract, hyperthyroidism, peptic ulceration, latent or active bronchial asthma, obstructive pulmonary disease, pronounced bradycardia or hypotension, vasomotor instability, cardiac disease or CAD, AV conduction defects, HTN, seizure disorder, Parkinson disease, spastic GI disturbances, acute inflammatory lesions of the GI tract, peritonitis, or marked vagotonia.
• Safe use in children hasn't been established.
Dialyzable drug: Unknown.
⚠ *Overdose S&S:* Abdominal discomfort, excessive salivation, flushing, hot feeling, sweating, nausea, vomiting.

PREGNANCY-LACTATION-REPRODUCTION
• It isn't known if drug affects reproduction. Use during pregnancy only if clearly needed.
• It isn't known if drug appears in human milk. Patient should discontinue breastfeeding or discontinue drug.

NURSING CONSIDERATIONS
• Adverse effects are rare with oral use.
• Monitor vital signs frequently, especially respirations. Always have atropine injection available, and be prepared to give 0.6 mg subcut or by slow IV push. Provide respiratory support, if needed.

- Monitor patient for orthostatic hypotension.
- Watch closely for adverse reactions that may indicate drug toxicity.

PATIENT TEACHING
- Tell patient to take drug on an empty stomach and at regular intervals.
- Inform patient that drug is usually effective 30 to 90 minutes after use.

SAFETY ALERT!

betrixaban
be-TRIX-a-ban

Bevyxxa

Therapeutic class: Anticoagulants
Pharmacologic class: Factor Xa inhibitors

AVAILABLE FORMS
Capsules: 40 mg, 80 mg

INDICATIONS & DOSAGES
➤ **Prophylaxis of venous thromboembolism in patients hospitalized for an acute medical illness and who are at risk for thromboembolic complications**
Adults: 160 mg PO as a single dose on day 1 followed by 80 mg PO daily for 35 to 42 days.
Adjust-a-dose: If CrCl is 15 to less than 30 mL/minute (calculated using actual body weight in the Cockcroft-Gault equation) or patient is also taking a P-gp inhibitor, decrease initial dose to 80 mg PO followed by 40 mg PO daily for 35 to 42 days.

ADMINISTRATION
PO
- Give at the same time each day with food.
- Give a missed dose as soon as possible on the same day. Don't double the dose to make up for a missed dose.
- Store at room temperature (68° to 77° F [20° to 25° C]).

ACTION
A selective factor Xa inhibitor that blocks factor Xa and decreases thrombin formation.

Route	Onset	Peak	Duration
PO	Unknown	3–4 hr	>72 hr

Half-life: 19 to 27 hours.

ADVERSE REACTIONS
CNS: headache, *intracranial hemorrhage.*
CV: hypertension, *hemorrhage.* **EENT:** intraocular bleeding, epistaxis. **GI:** *GI bleeding,* constipation, diarrhea, nausea. **GU:** UTI, hematuria. **Metabolic:** *hypokalemia.*

INTERACTIONS
Drug-drug. *Anticoagulants, antiplatelet agents, NSAIDs, SSNRIs, SSRIs, thrombolytic agents:* May increase risk of bleeding. Use together cautiously.
P-gp inhibitors (amiodarone, azithromycin, clarithromycin, ketoconazole, verapamil): May increase betrixaban blood level and bleeding risk. Reduce betrixaban dosage in patients receiving or starting P-gp inhibitors.

EFFECTS ON LAB TEST RESULTS
- May decrease potassium level.

CONTRAINDICATIONS & CAUTIONS
- Contraindicated in patients with active bleeding or severe hypersensitivity to drug.
Black Box Warning Consider potential risk of epidural or spinal hematoma versus benefit in patients scheduled for spinal procedures, such as spinal or epidural anesthesia or spinal puncture. Hematomas may result in long-term or permanent paralysis. Risk may increase with use of indwelling epidural catheters, concomitant use of drugs that affect hemostasis (NSAIDs, platelet inhibitors, anticoagulants), history of traumatic or repeated epidural or spinal punctures, or history of spinal deformity or surgery. ■
- There is no specific antidote to reverse betrixaban.
- Use cautiously in patients with severe renal impairment (CrCl of 15 to less than 30 mL/minute). Drug may increase risk of bleeding. Avoid use in patients with severe renal impairment who are taking concomitant P-gp inhibitors.
- Use in patients with hepatic impairment isn't recommended as they may have intrinsic coagulation abnormalities.
- Drug may increase QTc interval.

• Safety and effectiveness in patients with prosthetic heart valves haven't been studied.
• Safety and effectiveness in children haven't been established.
Dialyzable drug: Unknown.

PREGNANCY-LACTATION-REPRODUCTION
• Use in pregnancy hasn't been studied; however, drug is likely to increase risk of hemorrhage during pregnancy and delivery. Use in pregnant women only if potential benefits outweigh risks to mother and fetus.
• It isn't known if drug appears in human milk. Use in breastfeeding patients only if potential benefits outweigh risk to infant.

NURSING CONSIDERATIONS
• Monitor patients for signs and symptoms of bleeding, especially those with impaired renal function, and promptly evaluate if bleeding occurs. Administer blood replacement as clinically indicated.
 Black Box Warning Frequently monitor patients who have had neuraxial anesthesia or spinal or epidural puncture for signs and symptoms of neurologic impairment (leg numbness or weakness, bowel or bladder dysfunction). Immediately notify prescriber if adverse reactions occur. ■
• Wait at least 72 hours after last dose of betrixaban before removing an epidural catheter. Wait 5 hours or more before giving next betrixaban dose.
• Wait at least 72 hours after a traumatic spinal or epidural puncture before giving betrixaban.
• *Look alike–sound alike:* Don't confuse betrixaban with apixaban. Don't confuse Bevyxxa with Byetta.

PATIENT TEACHING
• Tell patient to report all adverse reactions.
• Warn patient that it may take longer than usual for bleeding to stop and that bleeding or bruising may occur more easily than usual. Tell patient to notify prescriber of unusual bleeding.
 Black Box Warning Advise patient to immediately report signs and symptoms of spinal or epidural hematoma (numbness or weakness of the legs and feet, bowel or bladder dysfunction, back pain) after neuraxial

anesthesia or spinal puncture and to seek immediate medical attention if they occur. ■
• Instruct patient to inform all health care providers about taking betrixaban and any other products known to affect bleeding before surgical, medical, or dental procedures and before initiation of new drugs.
• Teach patient signs and symptoms of bleeding (unexpected bleeding; heavier than normal menstrual bleeding; red, pink, or brown urine; red or black stools; blood or blood clots in sputum or vomit; unexpected pain or swelling; joint pain; headache; dizziness; or weakness). Tell patient to immediately report such signs and symptoms to prescriber and to seek emergency medical care.
• Tell female patient to inform prescriber if she is or plans to become pregnant or plans to breastfeed during therapy.

SAFETY ALERT!
BIOSIMILAR DRUG

bevacizumab
beh-vah-SIZZ-yoo-mab

Avastin

bevacizumab-awwb

Therapeutic class: Antineoplastics
Pharmacologic class: Monoclonal antibodies

AVAILABLE FORMS
Solution: 25 mg/mL in 4-mL, 16-mL vials

INDICATIONS & DOSAGES
Adjust-a-dose (for all indications): Although there are no recommended dosage reductions, temporarily suspend or stop drug in patients with severe infusion reactions, severe HTN that isn't controlled with medical management, or moderate to severe proteinuria.
➤ **Platinum-resistant recurrent epithelial ovarian, fallopian tube, or primary peritoneal cancer (Avastin only)**
Adults: 10 mg/kg IV every 2 weeks in combination with paclitaxel, pegylated liposomal doxorubicin, or weekly topotecan; or 15 mg/kg IV every 3 weeks in combination with topotecan.

➤ **Platinum-sensitive recurrent epithelial ovarian, fallopian tube, or primary peritoneal cancer (Avastin only)**
Adults: Initially, 15 mg/kg IV every 3 weeks in combination with carboplatin and paclitaxel for six cycles up to eight cycles, followed by continued use of bevacizumab 15 mg/kg IV every 3 weeks as a single agent until disease progression. Or, give 15 mg/kg IV every 3 weeks in combination with carboplatin and gemcitabine for six cycles up to 10 cycles, followed by continued use of bevacizumab 15 mg/kg IV every 3 weeks as a single agent until disease progression.

✴ *NEW INDICATION:* **Stage III or IV epithelial ovarian, fallopian tube, or primary peritoneal cancer after initial surgical resection (Avastin only)**
Adults: 15 mg/kg every 3 weeks with carboplatin and paclitaxel for up to six cycles, followed by 15 mg/kg every 3 weeks as a single agent, for a total of up to 22 cycles.

➤ **Metastatic colorectal cancer with fluoropyrimidine-irinotecan–based or fluoropyrimidine-oxaliplatin–based chemotherapy for second-line treatment after progression on a first-line bevacizumab-containing regimen**
Adults: 5 mg/kg IV every 2 weeks or 7.5 mg/kg IV every 3 weeks.

➤ **Persistent, recurrent, or metastatic cervical cancer with paclitaxel and cisplatin or paclitaxel and topotecan**
Adults: 15 mg/kg IV infusion once every 3 weeks.

➤ **First- or second-line treatment, with 5-FU–based chemotherapy, for metastatic colon or rectal cancer**
Adults: If used with bolus irinotecan, 5-FU, and leucovorin (IFL) regimen, give 5 mg/kg IV every 14 days. If used with oxaliplatin, 5-FU, and leucovorin (FOLFOX 4) regimen, give 10 mg/kg IV every 14 days. Infusion rate varies by patient tolerance and number of infusions.

➤ **With carboplatin and paclitaxel as first-line treatment of unresectable, locally advanced, recurrent, or metastatic nonsquamous NSCLC**
Adults: 15 mg/kg IV infusion once every 3 weeks.

➤ **With interferon alfa for metastatic renal cell carcinoma; as single agent for progressive glioblastoma following prior therapy**
Adults: 10 mg/kg IV every 14 days.

➤ **Metastatic breast cancer ◆**
Adults: 10 mg/kg IV once every 2 weeks in combination with paclitaxel.

➤ **Unresectable malignant pleural mesothelioma ◆**
Adults: 15 mg/kg IV every 3 weeks in combination with pemetrexed and cisplatin for up to six cycles, followed by bevacizumab maintenance therapy at 15 mg/kg once every 3 weeks until disease progression or unacceptable toxicity.

➤ **Age-related macular degeneration ◆**
Adults: Intravitreal bevacizumab 1.25 mg (0.05 mL) monthly for 3 months; then may give scheduled (monthly) or as needed based on monthly ophthalmologic assessment.

➤ **Diabetic macular edema ◆**
Adults: Initially, intravitreal bevacizumab 1.25 mg (0.05 mL); repeat every 4 weeks depending on ophthalmologic response.

ADMINISTRATION

IV
▼ Don't freeze or shake vials.
▼ Dilute drug using aseptic technique. Withdraw proper dose and mix in a total volume of 100 mL NSS in an IV bag.
▼ Don't give by IV push or bolus.
▼ Give first infusion over 90 minutes and, if tolerated, second infusion over 60 minutes. Later infusions can be given over 30 minutes if previous infusions were tolerated.
▼ Discard unused portion; drug is preservative-free.
▼ Diluted drug is stable 8 hours if refrigerated at 36° to 46° F (2° to 8° C).
▼ Protect from light.
▼ **Incompatibilities:** Dextrose solutions.

ACTION

A recombinant humanized vascular endothelial growth factor inhibitor.

Route	Onset	Peak	Duration
IV	Unknown	Unknown	Unknown

Half-life: About 20 days.

ADVERSE REACTIONS

CNS: asthenia, dizziness, headache, abnormal gait, confusion, pain, syncope, fatigue, insomnia. **CV:** *intra-abdominal thrombosis,* HTN, *thromboembolism, DVT,* HF, hypotension, chest pain. **EENT:** excess lacrimation, epistaxis, rhinitis, sinusitis, gum bleeding, taste disorder, voice alteration. **GI:** anorexia, constipation, diarrhea, dyspepsia, flatulence, stomatitis, vomiting, *GI hemorrhage,* abdominal pain, colitis, dry mouth, nausea. **GU:** *vaginal hemorrhage,* proteinuria. **Hematologic:** *leukopenia, neutropenia, thrombocytopenia.* **Hepatic:** bilirubinemia. **Metabolic:** *hypokalemia, hyperkalemia,* weight loss, hyperglycemia, *hypomagnesemia,* hyponatremia, hypoalbuminemia, *hypocalcemia.* **Musculoskeletal:** back pain, myalgia, arthralgia, muscle weakness. **Respiratory:** *hemoptysis,* dyspnea, URI, cough. **Skin:** alopecia, dry skin, exfoliative dermatitis, nail disorder, palmar-plantar erythrodysesthesia, skin ulcer. **Other:** decreased wound healing, hypersensitivity.

INTERACTIONS
Drug-drug. *Antineoplastics (anthracyclines, systemic):* May increase cardiotoxic effects of antineoplastics. Monitor therapy.
Bisphosphonate derivatives: May increase risk of osteonecrosis of the jaw. Monitor therapy.
Live-virus vaccines: May reduce immune response. Avoid use together.
Sunitinib: May increase bevacizumab toxicities, including microangiopathic hemolytic anemia and HTN. Avoid combination.

EFFECTS ON LAB TEST RESULTS
• May increase bilirubin, glucose, and urine protein levels.
• May decrease magnesium, calcium, and sodium levels.
• May increase or decrease potassium level.
• May decrease neutrophil, platelet, and WBC counts.

CONTRAINDICATIONS & CAUTIONS
• Use cautiously in patients hypersensitive to drug or its components, in those who need surgery, are taking anticoagulants, or have significant CV disease.
Dialyzable drug: Unknown.
⚠ **Overdose S&S:** Headache.

PREGNANCY-LACTATION-REPRODUCTION
• Drug has shown teratogenic effects in animal studies. Avoid use in pregnant women.
• Because of bevacizumab's long half-life, patients should use adequate contraception during therapy and for 6 months after final dose.
⚠ **Alert:** May increase risk of ovarian failure and may impair fertility. Long-term effects on fertility are unknown.
• It isn't known if drug appears in human milk. Women shouldn't breastfeed during therapy and for 6 months after final dose.

NURSING CONSIDERATIONS
⚠ **Alert:** Posterior reversible encephalopathy syndrome (PRES)–associated symptoms (HTN, headache, visual disturbances, altered mental function, seizures) may occur 16 hours to 1 year after starting drug. PRES can be confirmed only by MRI. Monitor patient closely. If syndrome occurs, stop drug and provide supportive care.
⚠ **Alert:** Monitor patient for arterial thromboembolic events and venous thromboembolic events (VTEs). Patients treated for cervical cancer may be at increased risk for VTEs. Permanently discontinue drug for grade 4 VTE, including PE.
⚠ **Alert:** Drug may increase risk of developing fistula, including non-GI fistulae (tracheoesophageal, bronchopleural, biliary, vaginal, renal, or bladder), which can be fatal.
• Permanently stop drug if patient develops any fistula of an internal organ.
• Hypersensitivity reactions can occur during infusion. Monitor patient closely.
• If patient develops severe HTN, hypertensive crisis, serious hemorrhage, or GI perforation that needs intervention, stop drug.
⚠ **Alert:** Drug may increase risk of serious arterial thromboembolic events, including MI, TIAs, stroke, HF, and angina. Patients at highest risk are age 65 or older, have a history of arterial thromboembolism, and have taken drug before. If patient has an arterial thrombotic event, permanently stop drug.
Black Box Warning Drug may cause fatal GI perforation. Monitor patient closely. ∎
Black Box Warning Bevacizumab can result in life-threatening wound dehiscence. Permanently discontinue bevacizumab

therapy in patients who experience wound dehiscence that requires medical intervention. Discontinue drug at least 28 days before elective surgery and don't restart drug for at least 28 days after surgery and until the surgical wound is fully healed. ■

Black Box Warning Drug increases risk of severe or fatal hemorrhage, hemoptysis, GI bleeding, CNS hemorrhage, and vaginal bleeding. Don't give to patients with serious hemorrhage or recent hemoptysis. ■

• Monitor urinalysis for worsening proteinuria. Patients with 2+ or greater urine dipstick test should undergo 24-hour urine collection. Discontinue use in patients with nephrotic syndrome.
• Monitor patient's BP every 2 to 3 weeks.
• Adverse reactions occur more often in older patients.

PATIENT TEACHING
• Inform patient about potential adverse reactions.
• Tell patient to report adverse reactions immediately, especially abdominal pain, constipation, and vomiting.
• Advise patient that BP and urinalysis will be monitored during treatment.
• Caution female patient of childbearing potential to avoid pregnancy during treatment and for 6 months after final dose.
❸ *Alert:* Inform female patient of the potential for ovarian failure and impaired fertility before starting treatment.
• Urge patient to alert other health care providers about bevacizumab therapy and to avoid elective surgery during treatment.

---

bictegravir–emtricitabine–tenofovir alafenamide
bik-TEG-ra-veer/em-try-SYE-tah-been/ten-OF-oh-veer AL-a-FEN-a-mide

Biktarvy

Therapeutic class: Antivirals
Pharmacologic class: HIV-1 integrase strand transfer inhibitors–HIV-1 nucleoside analogue reverse transcriptase inhibitors

AVAILABLE FORMS
Tablets: 50 mg bictegravir, 200 mg emtricitabine, 25 mg tenofovir alafenamide

INDICATIONS & DOSAGES
➤ **To treat HIV-1 infection in adults who have no antiretroviral treatment history or to replace current antiretroviral regimen in patients who are virologically suppressed (HIV-1 RNA less than 50 copies/mL) on a stable antiretroviral regimen for at least 3 months with no history of treatment failure and no known substitutions associated with resistance to the individual components**
Adults: 1 tablet PO daily.

ADMINISTRATION
PO
• May give with or without food.
• Store below 86° F (38° C) in original container.

ACTION
Combination of three anti-HIV-1 drugs that work through different mechanisms to block HIV-1 replication.

Route	Onset	Peak	Duration
PO (bictegravir)	Unknown	2–4 hr	Unknown
PO (emtricitabine)	Unknown	1½–2 hr	Unknown
PO (tenofovir alafenamide)	Unknown	½–2 hr	Unknown

Half-life: Bictegravir, 17.3 hours; emtricitabine, 10.4 hours; tenofovir alafenamide, 0.5 hour; tenofovir diphosphate (active metabolite), 150 to 180 hours.

ADVERSE REACTIONS
CNS: headache, fatigue, abnormal dreams, dizziness, insomnia, depression. **GI:** diarrhea, nausea, vomiting, flatulence, dyspepsia, abdominal pain. **GU:** renal impairment. **Hematologic:** *immune reconstitution syndrome.* **Hepatic:** exacerbation of HBV infection, *hepatomegaly,* steatosis. **Metabolic:** *lactic acidosis.* **Skin:** rash. **Other:** autoimmune disorders.

INTERACTIONS
Drug-drug. *Antacids or laxatives containing aluminum, calcium, or magnesium; buffered medications; sucralfate:* May decrease bictegravir level. Give antiviral on an empty stomach 2 hours before these

---

Reactions in bold italics are *life-threatening*. Interactions may have a *rapid onset* or a *delayed onset*.

products. Administration of these products with or 2 hours after the antiviral isn't recommended.

Anticonvulsants (carbamazepine, oxcarbazepine, phenobarbital, phenytoin): May decrease bictegravir and tenofovir alafenamide levels. Consider use of noninteracting anticonvulsants.

Antimycobacterials (rifabutin, rifampin, rifapentine): May decrease bictegravir and tenofovir alafenamide levels. Coadministration with rifampin is contraindicated. Coadministration with rifabutin or rifapentine isn't recommended.

Calcium or iron supplements: May decrease bictegravir level. Don't give supplement with drug on an empty stomach or give drug within 2 hours after supplement. May give drug and supplement together with food.

Dofetilide: May increase dofetilide level and risk of serious or life-threatening events. Use together is contraindicated.

Metformin: May increase metformin level. Refer to metformin prescribing information to assess risk and benefit of coadministration.

Other antiretrovirals: Coadministration isn't recommended because drug is a complete anti-HIV-1 regimen.

Renally eliminated drugs (acyclovir, aminoglycosides, cidofovir, ganciclovir, NSAIDs, valacyclovir, valganciclovir): May increase emtricitabine and tenofovir alafenamide levels and increase risk of renal dysfunction. Discontinue drug if renal function decreases significantly or Fanconi syndrome develops.

Drug-herb. *St. John's wort:* May decrease bictegravir and tenofovir alafenamide levels. Don't use together.

EFFECTS ON LAB TEST RESULTS

• May increase amylase, ALT, AST, bilirubin, LDL cholesterol, CK, and serum creatinine levels.
• May decrease neutrophil count.

CONTRAINDICATIONS & CAUTIONS

Black Box Warning Severe acute exacerbations of HBV infection have been reported in patients who are coinfected with HIV-1 and HBV and have discontinued products containing emtricitabine or tenofovir disoproxil fumarate. Closely monitor hepatic function

for at least several months in patients who are coinfected with HIV-1 and HBV and discontinue Biktarvy. If appropriate, administer anti-HBV therapy. ∎
• Drug isn't recommended for use in patients with severe renal impairment (CrCl less than 30 mL/minute) or with severe hepatic impairment (Child-Pugh class C).
• Use cautiously in patients with impaired renal function and in those taking nephrotoxic agents, including NSAIDs. Drug may increase risk of renal-related adverse reactions.

❸ Alert: Drug may increase risk of suicidal ideation, suicidal attempt, and suicidal depression, especially in patients with a history of depression, prior suicide attempt, or psychiatric illness.
• Drug may increase risk of immune reconstitution syndrome. Initially, an inflammatory response to indolent or residual opportunistic infections, including *Mycobacterium avium* infection, CMV, *Pneumocystis jiroveci* pneumonia, or TB, may occur and should be evaluated and treated as clinically indicated. Autoimmune disorders (Graves disease, polymyositis, Guillain-Barré syndrome) may occur many months after initiation of therapy.
• Safety and effectiveness in children haven't been established.

Dialyzable drug: 30% emtricitabine, 54% tenofovir alafenamide.

PREGNANCY-LACTATION-REPRODUCTION

• Data on the use of drug during pregnancy are insufficient to determine drug-associated risk of birth defects and miscarriage.
• Enroll pregnant patients exposed to drug in the Antiretroviral Pregnancy Registry (1-800-258-4263).
• Emtricitabine has been shown to appear in human milk. Because of the potential for HIV transmission to HIV-negative infants, development of viral resistance in HIV-positive infants, and adverse reactions similar to those seen in adults, women shouldn't breastfeed during therapy.

NURSING CONSIDERATIONS

• Test patients for HBV infection before therapy begins.

Black Box Warning Monitor patients coinfected with HBV for exacerbations of HBV infection for at least several months after treatment. Consider anti-HBV therapy, especially in patients with advanced liver disease or cirrhosis. ■

• Obtain serum creatinine, estimated CrCl, urine glucose, and urine protein levels before and during therapy as clinically indicated.

• Monitor patients for signs and symptoms of inflammation and development of immune reconstitution syndrome, which occurs soon after drug initiation.

• Monitor patients for autoimmune disorders, including Graves disease, polymyositis, and Guillain-Barré syndrome, during and after therapy.

• Monitor patients for signs and symptoms and laboratory findings that suggest development of lactic acidosis or hepatotoxicity (hepatomegaly and steatosis with or without LFT elevations). Discontinue drug if they develop.

• Monitor serum phosphorus level in patients with chronic kidney disease or who develop clinically significant decreases in renal function or evidence of Fanconi syndrome.

PATIENT TEACHING

• Emphasize the importance of not missing doses, to avoid developing resistance.

• Caution patient not to discontinue drug without first discussing with prescriber.

☉ Alert: Instruct patient to immediately seek medical attention for signs or symptoms of lactic acidosis (weakness, fatigue, unusual muscle pain, shortness of breath, abdominal pain with nausea and vomiting, cold or blue extremities, dizziness or light-headedness, or a fast or abnormal heartbeat).

• Instruct patient to seek immediate medical attention for signs or symptoms of liver failure (jaundice, dark or tea-colored urine, light-colored stools, loss of appetite, nausea, or abdominal pain).

• Warn patient that immune reconstitution syndrome can develop soon after therapy begins in patient with dormant infections. Treatment for infections may be needed.

• Advise patient that blood and urine tests will be needed before therapy begins and during treatment.

• Warn patient that renal impairment can occur.

• Encourage pregnant patient to enroll in the Antiretroviral Pregnancy Registry (1-800-258-4263).

• Warn female patient not to breastfeed during therapy.

bisoprolol fumarate
BIS-oh-PROE-lol

Therapeutic class: Antihypertensives
Pharmacologic class: Selective beta blockers

AVAILABLE FORMS
Tablets: 5 mg, 10 mg

INDICATIONS & DOSAGES
Adjust-a-dose (for all indications): In patients with bronchospastic disease or hepatic or renal insufficiency (CrCl less than 40 mL/minute), initially give 2.5 mg; then titrate with caution.

➤ HTN
Adults: Initially, 2.5 to 5 mg PO daily alone or with other antihypertensives. May increase to 10 mg daily, then to 20 mg once daily if needed.

➤ HF with reduced ejection fraction ♦
Adults: 1.25 mg PO once daily. Titrate gradually to maximum tolerated dose while monitoring patient for signs and symptoms of HF. Maximum dose, 10 mg PO daily.

ADMINISTRATION
PO
• May give without regard to meals.
• Store at room temperature. Protect from moisture.

ACTION
Selectively blocks cardiac adrenoceptors, reducing resting and exercise HR, decreasing cardiac output, depressing renin secretion, and decreasing tonic sympathetic outflow from the vasomotor centers in the brain.

Reactions in bold italics are *life-threatening*. Interactions may have a *rapid onset* or a *delayed onset*.

Route	Onset	Peak	Duration
PO	1–2 hr	2–4 hr	Unknown

Half-life: 9 to 12 hours.

ADVERSE REACTIONS
CNS: headache, dizziness, hypoesthesia, insomnia, asthenia, fatigue. **CV:** chest pain, peripheral edema, bradycardia. **EENT:** dry mouth, pharyngitis, rhinitis, sinusitis. **GI:** diarrhea, nausea, vomiting. **Musculoskeletal:** arthralgia. **Respiratory:** cough, dyspnea, URI. **Skin:** sweating.

INTERACTIONS
Drug-drug. *Antiarrhythmics (disopyramide), calcium channel blockers (diltiazem, verapamil):* May increase myocardial depression or conduction delay. Use cautiously together.
Beta blockers: May increase beta blocker effects to unsafe level. Use together is contraindicated.
Catecholamine-depleting drugs (guanethidine, reserpine): May cause hypotension or bradycardia. Monitor patient closely.
Clonidine: May cause rebound HTN if clonidine is discontinued. Stop bisoprolol for several days before discontinuing clonidine.
Digoxin: May increase risk of slow AV conduction and bradycardia. Use together cautiously.
Insulin, oral antidiabetics: May mask signs and symptoms of hypoglycemia, particularly tachycardia. Use together cautiously.
Rifampin: May increase bisoprolol metabolism. Monitor patient for decreased bisoprolol effects.

EFFECTS ON LAB TEST RESULTS
• May increase serum triglyceride, AST, ALT, uric acid, creatinine, BUN, potassium, glucose, and phosphorus levels.
• May decrease WBC and platelet counts.
• May cause ANA conversion.

CONTRAINDICATIONS & CAUTIONS
• Contraindicated in patients hypersensitive to drug and in those with cardiogenic shock, overt cardiac failure, second- or third-degree AV block, or marked sinus bradycardia.

• Use cautiously in patients with hepatic or renal insufficiency, hyperthyroidism, HF, arterial insufficiency, PVD, or diabetes.
• Use cautiously in patients with a history of severe anaphylactic reaction to a variety of allergens. Patients may be more sensitive if allergen is reintroduced; usual epinephrine doses may not be effective.
• Use cautiously in patients with bronchospastic disease who don't tolerate or respond to other antihypertensive treatment. Patients should have a bronchodilator on hand in the event of an episode.
Dialyzable drug: No.

PREGNANCY-LACTATION-REPRODUCTION
• There are no adequate and well-controlled studies in pregnant women. Use during pregnancy only if potential benefit justifies potential risk to the fetus.
• It isn't known if drug appears in human milk. Use cautiously in breastfeeding women.

NURSING CONSIDERATIONS
• Monitor BP closely.
• Avoid use in patients with acute HF because of worsening of disease. If bisoprolol administration is necessary, monitor patient closely.
• Use cautiously in patients with known compensated HF. In patients without a history of HF, drug may precipitate signs and symptoms of new HF. Consider stopping drug at first indication of new HF. Drug may be continued while HF is being treated with other drugs.
• Drug interruption or abrupt discontinuation may exacerbate angina pectoris, MI, or ventricular arrhythmia and may exacerbate the signs and symptoms of hyperthyroidism, possibly leading to thyroid storm. If drug is to be discontinued, taper over approximately 1 week while monitoring patient. If withdrawal signs and symptoms occur, restart drug at least temporarily.
• A long-term bisoprolol regimen shouldn't be discontinued before major surgery. However, the impaired ability of the heart to respond to reflex adrenergic stimuli may increase risks of general anesthesia and surgical procedures.

• Drug may mask tachycardia caused by hyperthyroidism. In patients with suspected thyrotoxicosis, withdraw drug gradually to avoid thyroid storm.

• Drug may mask signs and symptoms of hypoglycemia in diabetic patients.

• Drug may cause or aggravate signs and symptoms of arterial insufficiency in patients with PVD.

PATIENT TEACHING

• Tell patient to report slowed heartbeat, difficulty breathing, or other signs of HF.

• Caution patient not to discontinue bisoprolol without first consulting health care provider.

• Warn diabetic patient that bisoprolol may mask signs and symptoms of hypoglycemia (such as tachycardia, dizziness, and weakness).

• Urge patient to use caution when operating automobiles and machinery or performing activities requiring alertness.

SAFETY ALERT!

bivalirudin
bye-VAL-ih-roo-din

Angiomax

Therapeutic class: Anticoagulants
Pharmacologic class: Direct thrombin inhibitors

AVAILABLE FORMS
Injection: 250-mg vial

INDICATIONS & DOSAGES

Adjust-a-dose (for all indications): For patients with CrCl of 30 mL/minute or less, decrease infusion rate to 1 mg/kg/hour. For patients on hemodialysis, reduce infusion rate to 0.25 mg/kg/hour. No reduction of bolus dose is needed.

➤ **Anticoagulation in patients with unstable angina undergoing PTCA; anticoagulation in patients with unstable angina undergoing PCI, with provisional use of a platelet glycoprotein (GP)IIb/IIIa inhibitor**
Adults: 0.75 mg/kg IV bolus followed by a continuous infusion of 1.75 mg/kg/hour

during the procedure. Check activated clotting time 5 minutes after bolus dose is given. May give additional 0.3 mg/kg bolus dose if needed. Infusion may continue for up to 4 hours after procedure. After 4-hour infusion, may give an additional infusion of 0.2 mg/kg/hour for up to 20 hours, if needed. Use with 300 to 325 mg aspirin.

➤ **Patients undergoing PCI who have or are at risk for heparin-induced thrombocytopenia (HIT) or heparin-induced thrombocytopenia–thrombosis syndrome (HITTS)**
Adults: 0.75 mg/kg IV bolus, followed by a continuous infusion of 1.75 mg/kg/hour throughout the procedure. Infusion up to 4 hours after procedure is optional. After 4 hours, may give an additional infusion of 0.2 mg/kg/hour for up to 20 hours. Use with 300 to 325 mg aspirin.

➤ **ST-elevation MI in patients undergoing primary PCI ◆**
Adults: 0.75 mg/kg IV bolus, followed by 1.75 mg/kg/hour IV infusion for duration of procedure. May give additional 0.3 mg/kg bolus dose if needed. Consider continuing infusion at 1.75 mg/kg/hour for up to 4 hours after procedure to mitigate risk of stent thrombosis. If infusion is continued and an additional infusion is clinically necessary, may continue infusion at a reduced dose of 0.2 mg/kg/hour for up to 20 hours.

➤ **Non-ST-elevation ACS (moderate to high risk) in patients undergoing an early invasive strategy ◆**
Adults: If initiating during PCI, give 0.75 mg/kg IV bolus, followed by 1.75 mg/kg/hour IV infusion for duration of procedure. May give additional 0.3 mg/kg bolus dose if needed. Consider continuing infusion at 1.75 mg/kg/hour for up to 4 hours after procedure to mitigate risk of stent thrombosis. If infusion is continued and an additional infusion is clinically necessary, may continue infusion at a reduced dose of 0.2 mg/kg/hour for up to 20 hours. *Note:* If patient received unfractionated heparin before procedure, wait 30 minutes before initiating bivalirudin.

If initiating before PCI or diagnostic angiography, give 0.1 mg/kg IV bolus, followed by 0.25 mg/kg/hour IV infusion. Continue until diagnostic angiography or

---

Reactions in bold italics are *life-threatening*. Interactions may have a *rapid onset* or a *delayed onset*.

PCI. Once PCI is necessary, give additional 0.5 mg/kg via IV bolus and increase infusion rate to 1.75 mg/kg/hour during PCI.

ADMINISTRATION

IV

▼ Reconstitute each 250-mg vial with 5 mL of sterile water for injection. Gently swirl until all material is dissolved.

▼ Reconstituted material will be a clear to slightly opalescent, colorless to slightly yellow solution.

▼ Withdraw and discard 5 mL from a 50-mL infusion bag containing D₅W or NSS. Then add contents of reconstituted vial to infusion bag to yield a final concentration of 5 mg/mL.

▼ To prepare low-rate infusion, withdraw and discard 5 mL from a 500-mL D₅W or NSS infusion bag. Then add contents of reconstituted vial to infusion bag to yield a final concentration of 0.5 mg/mL.

▼ Solutions with concentrations of 0.5 to 5 mg/mL are stable at room temperature for 24 hours. Discard remaining unused portion of reconstituted solution.

▼ **Incompatibilities:** Alteplase, amiodarone, amphotericin B, chlorpromazine, diazepam, dobutamine, prochlorperazine, reteplase, streptokinase, vancomycin. *Note:* Compatible with dobutamine at concentrations up to 4 mg/mL, but incompatible at concentration of 12.5 mg/mL.

ACTION

Binds specifically and rapidly to thrombin, inhibiting its effects, thereby producing an anticoagulant effect.

Route	Onset	Peak	Duration
IV	Rapid	Immediate	1–2 hr

Half-life: 25 minutes in patients with normal renal function.

ADVERSE REACTIONS

CNS: anxiety, headache, insomnia, nervousness, fever, pain. **CV:** *bradycardia*, HTN, hypotension. **GI:** abdominal pain, dyspepsia, nausea, vomiting. **GU:** urine retention. **Hematologic:** *severe, spontaneous bleeding (cerebral, retroperitoneal, GU, GI).* **Musculoskeletal:** back pain, pelvic pain. **Skin:** pain at injection site.

INTERACTIONS

Drug-drug. *GPIIa/IIIb inhibitors (abciximab, eptifibatide, tirofiban), heparin, thrombolytics, warfarin:* May increase risk of hemorrhage. Use together cautiously.
Drug-herb. *Herbs with anticoagulant or antiplatelet properties (alfalfa, anise, bilberry, ginseng):* May increase risk of bleeding. Discourage use together.

EFFECTS ON LAB TEST RESULTS

● May decrease Hb level and hematocrit.
● May decrease platelet count.
● INR measurements may not be useful for determining the appropriate warfarin dose.

CONTRAINDICATIONS & CAUTIONS

● Contraindicated in patients hypersensitive to drug or its components; in those with history of thrombocytopenia after tirofiban administration, major surgical procedure, or severe physical trauma within previous month; and in those with active major bleeding. Avoid using in patients with unstable angina who aren't undergoing PTCA or PCI or in patients with other acute coronary syndromes.
● Use cautiously in patients undergoing brachytherapy, in those with HIT or HITTS, in those with diseases linked to increased risk of bleeding, and in elderly patients.
Dialyzable drug: 25%.

PREGNANCY-LACTATION-REPRODUCTION

● Use cautiously in pregnant women and only if clearly indicated.
● It's unknown if drug appears in human milk. Use cautiously in breastfeeding women.

NURSING CONSIDERATIONS

● There is no antidote for drug.
● Monitor coagulation test results, Hb level, and hematocrit before starting therapy and periodically thereafter.
● Circumstances for provisional use of a GP inhibitor during PCI include decreased Thrombolysis in Myocardial Infarction (TIMI) flow (0–2) or slow reflow, dissection with decreased flow, new or suspected thrombus, persistent residual stenosis, distal embolization, an unplanned stent, suboptimal stenting, side-branch closure, abrupt

closure, clinical instability, and prolonged ischemia.

• Obtain a complete list of patient's prescription and OTC drugs and supplements, including herbs.

🕃 *Alert:* Hemorrhage can occur at any site in the body. If patient has unexplained decrease in hematocrit, decrease in BP, or other unexplained symptoms, suspect hemorrhage.

• Monitor venipuncture sites for bleeding, hematoma, or inflammation.

• Puncture-site hemorrhage and catheterization-site hematoma may occur in patients age 65 and older more often than in younger patients.

• Don't give drug IM.

PATIENT TEACHING

• Advise patient that drug can cause bleeding and to immediately report unusual bruising or bleeding (nosebleeds, bleeding gums) or tarry stools.

• Counsel patient that drug is given with aspirin. Caution patient to avoid other aspirin-containing drugs or NSAIDs while receiving this drug.

• Advise patient to consult with prescriber before initiating any herbal therapy; many herbs have anticoagulant, antiplatelet, and fibrinolytic properties.

• Advise patient to avoid activities that carry a risk of injury and to use a soft toothbrush and electric razor while taking drug.

SAFETY ALERT!

bleomycin sulfate
blee-oh-MYE-sin

Therapeutic class: Antineoplastics
Pharmacologic class: Cytotoxic glycopeptide antibiotics

AVAILABLE FORMS
Injection: 15-unit vials, 30-unit vials

INDICATIONS & DOSAGES
Adjust-a-dose (for all indications): For patients with CrCl of 40 to 50 mL/minute, give 70% of dose; for CrCl of 30 to 39 mL/minute, give 60% of dose; for CrCl of 20 to 29 mL/minute, give 55% of dose; for CrCl of 10 to

19 mL/minute, give 45% of dose; and for CrCl of 5 to 9 mL/minute, give 40% of dose.

➤ **Squamous cell carcinoma (head, neck, skin, penis, cervix, and vulva), non-Hodgkin lymphoma, testicular carcinoma**
Adults: Because an anaphylactoid reaction is possible, treat lymphoma patients with 2 units or less for first two doses. If no acute reaction occurs, then may follow regular dosage schedule: 0.25 to 0.5 units/kg (10 to 20 units/m^2) IV, IM, or subcut once or twice weekly to total of 400 units.

➤ **Hodgkin lymphoma**
Adults: Because an anaphylactoid reaction is possible, treat lymphoma patients with 2 units or less for first two doses. If no acute reaction occurs, then may follow regular dosage schedule: 0.25 to 0.5 units/kg (10 to 20 units/m^2) IV, IM, or subcut one or two times weekly. After 50% response, maintenance dose is 1 unit IV or IM daily or 5 units IV or IM weekly. Total cumulative dose is 400 units.

➤ **Malignant pleural effusion**
Adults: 60 units given as single-dose bolus intrapleural injection.

➤ **Hodgkin lymphoma (pediatric)** ◆
Children: Because an anaphylactoid reaction is possible, treat lymphoma patients with 2 units or less for first two doses. If no acute reaction occurs, then may follow regular dosage schedule: 5 to 10 units/m^2 based on treatment cycle and combination therapy (e.g., doxorubicin, vincristine, etoposide). Consult oncologist for specific dose for cycle/regimen.

ADMINISTRATION
IV

▼ Preparing and giving parenteral form of drug may be mutagenic, teratogenic, and carcinogenic. Use safe handling and disposal precautions according to facility policy.

▼ Drug may adsorb to plastic IV bags. For prolonged infusions, use glass containers.

▼ Reconstitute 15-unit or 30-unit vial with 5 or 10 mL, respectively, of NSS for injection to equal 3 units/mL solution.

▼ Administer slowly over 10 minutes.

▼ Use reconstituted solution within 24 hours.

Reactions in bold italics are *life-threatening*. Interactions may have a *rapid onset* or a *delayed onset*.

▼ Refrigerate unopened vials containing dry powder.

▼ Drug is an irritant and may cause phlebitis. It isn't known to cause tissue damage with extravasation. If signs or symptoms of extravasation occur, stop infusion immediately and institute appropriate care according to facility policy.

▼ **Incompatibilities:** Amino acids; aminophylline; amphotericin B conventional/lipid complex/liposome; ascorbic acid injection; cefazolin; dantrolene; diazepam; drugs containing sulfhydryl groups; fluids containing dextrose; furosemide; hydrocortisone; methotrexate; mitomycin; nafcillin; penicillin G; phenytoin; riboflavin; solutions containing divalent and trivalent cations, especially calcium salts and copper; terbutaline sulfate.

IM

• Dilute 15-unit vial in 1 to 5 mL or 30-unit vial in 2 to 10 mL of sterile water for injection, bacteriostatic water for injection, or NSS for injection.

• Monitor injection site for irritation.

Subcutaneous

• Dilute 15-unit vial in 1 to 5 mL or 30-unit vial in 2 to 10 mL of sterile water for injection, bacteriostatic water for injection, or NSS for injection.

• Monitor injection site for irritation.

Intrapleural

• For intrapleural use, dilute 60 units of drug in 50 to 100 mL NSS for injection; give drug through a thoracotomy tube.

• If patient's condition requires sclerosis, instill drug when chest tube drainage is 100 to 300 mL/24 hours; ideally, drainage should be less than 100 mL/24 hours. After instillation, clamp thoracotomy tube and move patient from the back to the left then right side several times for the next 4 hours. Remove clamp and reestablish suction. Length of time chest tube is left in place after sclerosis depends on patient's condition.

ACTION

May inhibit DNA synthesis and cause scission of single- and double-stranded DNA; also inhibits RNA and protein synthesis.

Route	Onset	Peak	Duration
IV, IM, subcut	Unknown	30–60 min	Unknown

Half-life: 2 hours.

ADVERSE REACTIONS

CNS: fever. **GI:** stomatitis, anorexia, nausea, vomiting, diarrhea. **Metabolic:** weight loss, hyperuricemia. **Respiratory:** *pneumonitis, pulmonary fibrosis.* **Skin:** erythema, hyperpigmentation, acne, rash, striae, skin tenderness, pruritus, reversible alopecia, hyperkeratosis, nail changes. **Other:** chills, *anaphylactoid reactions.*

INTERACTIONS

Drug-drug. *Anesthesia:* May increase oxygen requirements. Monitor patient closely.
Brentuximab: May increase risk of pulmonary toxicity. Use together is contraindicated.
Cisplatin: May decrease bleomycin elimination. Monitor renal function and adjust bleomycin dosage as needed.
Fosphenytoin, phenytoin: May decrease phenytoin and fosphenytoin levels. Monitor drug levels closely.
Live-virus vaccines: May increase risk of vaccine-induced adverse reactions. Avoid concomitant use.
Oxygen: May increase risk of pulmonary toxicity during surgery due to increased sensitization of lung tissue from bleomycin. Use together cautiously.

EFFECTS ON LAB TEST RESULTS

• May increase uric acid level.

CONTRAINDICATIONS & CAUTIONS

• Contraindicated in patients hypersensitive to drug.

• Severe idiosyncratic reactions can occur (hypotension, mental confusion, fever, chills, wheezing), usually after first or second dose. Monitor patient carefully.

• Use cautiously in patients with renal or pulmonary impairment.

Dialyzable drug: Unknown.

PREGNANCY-LACTATION-REPRODUCTION

• Drug can cause fetal harm when administered to pregnant women. If used during pregnancy, or if patient becomes pregnant

while receiving drug, apprise patient of the potential hazard to the fetus.
• Women of childbearing potential should avoid becoming pregnant during therapy.
• It isn't known if drug appears in human milk. Patient should discontinue breastfeeding during therapy.

NURSING CONSIDERATIONS

Black Box Warning Drug should be administered under the supervision of a physician experienced in the use of cancer chemotherapeutic agents. ∎
• Pulmonary toxicities are common. Obtain pulmonary function tests before start of treatment and at regular intervals during treatment. If tests show a marked decline, stop drug.

Black Box Warning Fatal pulmonary fibrosis may occur, especially when cumulative dose exceeds 400 units. ∎

Black Box Warning Monitor lymphoma patient for idiosyncratic reaction (hypotension, confusion, fever, chills, wheezing) after receiving drug. ∎

⊕ Alert: Adverse pulmonary reactions are more common in patients older than age 70. Also, in patients receiving radiation therapy, patients with lung disease, and patients who need oxygen therapy, pulmonary toxic adverse effects may be increased.
• Monitor chest X-ray every 1 to 2 weeks and listen to lungs regularly.
• Watch for fever, which may be treated with antipyretics. Fever usually occurs within 3 to 6 hours of administration.
• Hodgkin disease and testicular tumor improvement is prompt and noted within 2 weeks. If no improvement is seen by this time, improvement is unlikely. Squamous cell cancers sometimes require as long as 3 weeks before improvement is noted.
⊕ Alert: Watch for hypersensitivity reactions, which may be delayed for several hours, especially in patients with lymphoma. (Give test dose of 1 to 2 units before first two doses in patients with lymphoma. If no reaction occurs, follow regular dosage schedule.)

PATIENT TEACHING
• Warn patient that hair loss may occur but is usually reversible.

• Tell patient to report adverse reactions promptly and to take infection-control and bleeding precautions.
• Advise patient who is to receive anesthesia to inform anesthesiologist about taking this drug. High oxygen levels inhaled during surgery may enhance pulmonary toxicity of drug.

SAFETY ALERT!

bortezomib
bore-TEZ-uh-mib

Velcade

Therapeutic class: Antineoplastics
Pharmacologic class: Proteasome inhibitors

AVAILABLE FORMS
Powder for injection: 3.5 mg

INDICATIONS & DOSAGES
Adjust-a-dose (for all indications): Refer to manufacturer's instructions for toxicity-related dosage adjustments in patients with hepatic impairment or peripheral neuropathy and in those on combination therapies.
➤ **Previously untreated multiple myeloma**
Adults: 1.3 mg/m^2 IV bolus over 3 to 5 seconds or subcut in combination with oral melphalan and oral prednisone for nine 6-week treatment cycles. In cycles 1 to 4, bortezomib is given twice weekly (days 1, 4, 8, 11, 22, 25, 29, and 32). In cycles 5 to 9, bortezomib is given once weekly (days 1, 8, 22, and 29). Separate consecutive doses of drug by at least 72 hours. Prior to initiating any cycle, platelet count should be 70 × 10^9/L or greater, ANC should be 1 × 10^9/L or greater, and nonhematologic toxicities should have resolved to grade 1 or baseline.
➤ **Previously untreated mantle cell lymphoma**
Adults: 1.3 mg/m^2 IV bolus over 3 to 5 seconds in combination with IV rituximab, cyclophosphamide, doxorubicin, and oral prednisone for six 3-week treatment cycles. Bortezomib is administered first followed by rituximab. Bortezomib is given twice weekly for 2 weeks (days 1, 4, 8, and 11) followed by 10-day rest period on days 12 to 21. Patients who respond at cycle 6 should

---

receive two additional cycles for a total of 8 cycles. Separate consecutive doses of drug by at least 72 hours. Before initiating any cycle other than cycle 1, platelet count should be 100×10^9/L or greater, ANC should be 1.5×10^9/L or greater, Hb level should be at least 8 g/dL or greater, and nonhematologic toxicities should have resolved to grade 1 or baseline.

➤ **Multiple myeloma or mantle cell lymphoma that still progresses after at least one therapy**

Adults: 1.3 mg/m^2 by IV bolus over 3 to 5 seconds or subcut twice weekly for 2 weeks (days 1, 4, 8, and 11), followed by a 10-day rest period (days 12 through 21). This 3-week period is a treatment cycle. For therapy longer than eight cycles, may adjust dosage schedule to once weekly for 4 weeks (days 1, 8, 15, and 22) followed by a 13-day rest period (days 23 through 35). Separate consecutive doses of drug by at least 72 hours.

ADMINISTRATION

IV

▼ Drug is hazardous. Use appropriate precautions for handling and disposal.

▼ Use caution and aseptic technique when preparing and handling drug. Wear gloves and protective clothing to prevent skin contact.

▼ Reconstitute with 3.5 mL of NSS to a final concentration of 1 mg/mL and give by IV bolus over 3 to 5 seconds within 8 hours of preparation.

▼ Inspect solution before administration. Don't give if discolored or if particles are seen.

▼ Reconstituted drug may be stored in original vial or a syringe at 77° F (25° C); total storage time must not exceed 8 hours.

▼ Store unopened vial at a controlled room temperature, in original packaging, protected from light.

▼ **Incompatibilities:** None listed by manufacturer. Consult a drug incompatibility reference for more information.

Subcutaneous

• Reconstitute with 1.4 mL of NSS to a final concentration of 2.5 mg/mL and give within 8 hours of preparation.

• Inspect solution before administration. Don't give if solution is discolored or contains particles.

• Reconstituted drug may be stored in original vial or a syringe at 77° F (25° C); total storage time must not exceed 8 hours.

• Rotate injection sites. New injections should be given at least 1 inch (2.54 cm) from an old site and never in areas that are tender, bruised, reddened, or hard.

• If injection-site reactions occur, a less concentrated solution (1 mg/mL) may be used.

ACTION

Disrupts intracellular homeostatic mechanisms by inhibiting the 26S proteasome, which regulates intracellular levels of certain proteins, causing cells to die.

Route	Onset	Peak	Duration
IV, subcut	Unknown	Unknown	Unknown

Half-life: 40 to 193 hours (1-mg/m^2 dose); 76 to 108 hours (1.3-mg/m^2 dose).

ADVERSE REACTIONS

CNS: anxiety, asthenia, dizziness, dysesthesia, fatigue, fever, headache, insomnia, paresthesia, peripheral neuropathy, neuralgia, rigors. **CV:** edema, hypotension. **EENT:** blurred vision. **GI:** abdominal pain, constipation, decreased appetite, diarrhea, dysgeusia, dyspepsia, nausea, vomiting. **Hematologic:** *neutropenia, thrombocytopenia,* anemia, leukopenia, lymphopenia. **Hepatic:** *acute liver failure, hepatitis,* hyperbilirubinemia, increased liver enzyme levels. **Metabolic:** anorexia. **Musculoskeletal:** arthralgia, back pain, bone pain, limb pain, muscle cramps, myalgia. **Respiratory:** cough, dyspnea, pneumonia, URI. **Skin:** pruritus, rash. **Other:** dehydration, herpes zoster.

INTERACTIONS

Drug-drug. *Antihypertensives:* May cause hypotension. Monitor patient's BP closely. *Drugs linked to peripheral neuropathy (amiodarone, antivirals, isoniazid, nitrofurantoin, statins):* May worsen neuropathy. Use together cautiously. *Drugs that prolong QT interval (antiarrhythmics [bretylium, disopyramide, dofetilide, procainamide, quinidine, sotalol],* *chlorpromazine, dolasetron, droperidol, mefloquine, mesoridazine, moxifloxacin, pentamidine, pimozide, tacrolimus, thioridazine, ziprasidone):* May prolong QT interval and increase risk of life-threatening ventricular arrhythmias. Use together with caution.

Inducers or inhibitors of CYP3A4: May increase risk of toxicity or may reduce drug's effects. Monitor patient closely.

Oral antidiabetics: May cause hypoglycemia or hyperglycemia. Monitor glucose level closely.

Drug-herb. *St. John's wort:* May decrease bortezomib exposure. Avoid concomitant use.

EFFECTS ON LAB TEST RESULTS
• May increase liver enzyme, bilirubin, and uric acid levels.
• May increase or decrease potassium, sodium, and glucose levels.
• May decrease calcium level.
• May decrease Hb level and neutrophil and platelet counts.

CONTRAINDICATIONS & CAUTIONS
• Contraindicated in patients hypersensitive to bortezomib, boron, or mannitol.
• Intrathecal administration is contraindicated.
• Use cautiously in patients with hepatic or renal impairment or with a history of syncope and in those who are dehydrated or receiving other drugs known to cause hypotension.
• Use cautiously in patients with risk factors for, or existing, heart disease. Closely monitor patients for acute development or exacerbation of HF and new-onset decreased LVEF.
Dialyzable drug: Yes.
⚠ *Overdose S&S:* Symptomatic hypotension, thrombocytopenia.

PREGNANCY-LACTATION-REPRODUCTION
• There are no adequate and well-controlled studies in pregnant women. Drug may cause fetal harm. Use during pregnancy isn't recommended.
• Women of childbearing potential should avoid becoming pregnant and should use effective contraception during treatment and for 2 months after final dose.
• It isn't known if drug appears in human milk. Women shouldn't breastfeed during treatment and for 2 months after final dose.

NURSING CONSIDERATIONS
• Monitor for evidence of neuropathy, such as a burning sensation, hyperesthesia, hypoesthesia, paresthesia, discomfort, or neuropathic pain.
• Consider subcut administration for patients at high risk for or with preexisting peripheral neuropathy.
• Be aware that the IV and subcut concentrations are different. Be sure to check that patient is receiving appropriate concentration of drug before administration.
• Monitor patient closely for posterior reversible encephalopathy syndrome (PRES)–associated symptoms (HTN, headache, visual disturbances, altered mental function, seizures), which may occur after starting drug. PRES can be confirmed only by MRI. If syndrome occurs, stop drug and provide supportive care.
• Monitor patient for signs and symptoms of TLS (hyperuricemia, hyperkalemia, hyperphosphatemia, hypocalcemia, acute renal failure).
• Monitor glucose levels in patients with diabetes who are taking oral hypoglycemics.
• Watch carefully for adverse effects, especially in elderly patients.
• Be sure patient has an order for an antiemetic, antidiarrheal, or both to treat drug-induced nausea, vomiting, or diarrhea.
• Provide fluid and electrolyte replacement to prevent dehydration.
• To manage orthostatic hypotension, adjust antihypertensive dosage, maintain hydration status, and give mineralocorticoids or sympathomimetics.
• Dialysis may reduce drug level; give after dialysis.
�альт *Alert:* Because thrombocytopenia is common, monitor patient's CBC and platelet counts carefully during treatment, before each dose, and especially on day 11.

PATIENT TEACHING
• Tell patient to notify prescriber about new or worsening peripheral neuropathy.

• Urge female patient to use effective contraception and not to breastfeed during treatment and for 2 months after final dose.

• Teach patient how to avoid dehydration, and stress the need to tell prescriber about dizziness, light-headedness, or fainting spells.

• Tell patient to use caution when driving or performing other hazardous activities because drug may cause fatigue, dizziness, faintness, light-headedness, and doubled or blurred vision.

bosentan
bow-SEN-tan

Tracleer

Therapeutic class: Vasodilators
Pharmacologic class: Endothelin-receptor antagonists

AVAILABLE FORMS
Tablets: 62.5 mg, 125 mg
Tablets (for suspension): 32 mg

INDICATIONS & DOSAGES
Black Box Warning Only prescribers and pharmacies registered with the Tracleer REMS Program (1-866-228-3546, option 1) may prescribe and distribute bosentan. ■
Adjust-a-dose (for all indications): Refer to manufacturer's instructions for toxicity-related dosage adjustments.
➤ **PAH (WHO Group 1) in patients with WHO/NYHA Class II to IV symptoms to improve exercise ability and decrease rate of clinical worsening**
Adults: 62.5 mg PO b.i.d., in the morning and evening, for 4 weeks. If patient weighs 40 kg or more, increase to maintenance dosage of 125 mg PO b.i.d., in the morning and evening. If patient weighs less than 40 kg, maintenance dosage is 62.5 mg PO b.i.d.
➤ **To improve pulmonary vascular resistance in PAH (idiopathic or congenital) in children age 3 and older**
Children older than age 12 weighing more than 40 kg: Initially, 62.5 mg PO b.i.d. After 4 weeks, increase to 125 mg PO b.i.d.

Children older than age 12 weighing less than 40 kg: Initial and maintenance dosage is 62.5 mg PO b.i.d.
Children age 12 and younger weighing more than 24 to 40 kg: Initial and maintenance dosage is 64 mg PO b.i.d.
Children age 12 and younger weighing more than 16 to 24 kg: Initial and maintenance dosage is 48 mg PO b.i.d.
Children age 12 and younger weighing more than 8 to 16 kg: Initial and maintenance dosage is 32 mg PO b.i.d.
Children age 12 and younger weighing 4 to 8 kg: Initial and maintenance dosage is 16 mg PO b.i.d.

ADMINISTRATION
PO
• Give drug in morning and evening without regard for meals.
• Disperse tablets for oral suspension, or dispersible tablet half, in a minimal amount of water immediately before administration.
• Store divided dispersible tablet pieces at 68° to 77° F (20° to 25° C) in opened blister for up to 7 days.

ACTION
Specific and competitive antagonist for endothelin-1 (ET-1). ET-1 levels are elevated in patients with PAH, suggesting a pathogenic role for ET-1 in this disease.

Route	Onset	Peak	Duration
PO	Unknown	3–5 hr	Unknown

Half-life: About 5 hours.

ADVERSE REACTIONS
CNS: headache, fatigue, syncope. **CV:** edema, flushing, hypotension, palpitations, chest pain. **EENT:** sinusitis. **Hematologic:** anemia. **Hepatic:** *hepatotoxicity.* **Musculoskeletal:** arthralgia. **Respiratory:** respiratory tract infection.

INTERACTIONS
Drug-drug. *Clarithromycin:* May increase risk of bosentan hepatotoxicity. Monitor patient closely. Stop one or both drugs if an interaction is suspected.
Cyclosporine: May increase bosentan level and decrease cyclosporine level. Use together is contraindicated.

CYP2C9 inhibitor (amiodarone, fluconazole) plus moderate CYP3A inhibitor (amprenavir, diltiazem, erythromycin, fluconazole) or strong CYP3A inhibitor (ketoconazole, itraconazole): May cause large increase in bosentan plasma concentration. Administration of bosentan with a CYP2C9 inhibitor plus a strong or moderate CYP3A inhibitor isn't recommended.

Glyburide: May increase risk of elevated LFT values and decrease levels of both drugs. Use together is contraindicated.

Hormonal contraceptives: May cause contraceptive failure. Patient should use two reliable methods of birth control.

Ketoconazole: May increase bosentan effect. Watch for adverse effects.

PDE5 inhibitors (sildenafil): May increase bosentan level and decrease sildenafil level. Use together with caution.

Rifampin: May alter bosentan level. Monitor hepatic function weekly for 4 weeks followed by routine monitoring.

Ritonavir: May increase risk of bosentan toxicity. Dosage adjustment may be needed. Discontinue bosentan at least 36 hours before start of ritonavir; at least 10 days after ritonavir start, resume bosentan at 62.5 mg once daily or every other day based on tolerability. If receiving ritonavir for at least 10 days, start bosentan at 62.5 mg once daily or every other day based on tolerability.

Simvastatin, other statins: May decrease levels of these drugs. Monitor cholesterol levels to assess need to adjust statin dose.

Tacrolimus: May increase bosentan levels. Use together cautiously.

Warfarin: May decrease warfarin level. Monitor coagulation tests and adjust warfarin dosage as needed.

EFFECTS ON LAB TEST RESULTS
`Black Box Warning` May increase AST, ALT, and bilirubin levels. ∎
• May decrease Hb level and hematocrit.

CONTRAINDICATIONS & CAUTIONS
• Contraindicated in patients hypersensitive to drug; reactions may include DRESS, anaphylaxis, rash, and angioedema.
• Contraindicated with concomitant use of cyclosporine or glyburide.

`Black Box Warning` Generally avoid using in patients with moderate to severe hepatic impairment or in those with elevated aminotransferase levels greater than 3 × ULN. ∎
• Use cautiously in patients with mild hepatic impairment.
Dialyzable drug: Unlikely.
⚠ *Overdose S&S:* Headache, nausea, vomiting, hypotension, dizziness, blurred vision.

PREGNANCY-LACTATION-REPRODUCTION
`Black Box Warning` Drug is likely to cause major birth defects. Contraindicated in pregnant women. Verify pregnancy status of women of childbearing potential before starting drug, monthly during treatment, and 1 month after final dose. ∎
`Black Box Warning` Females of childbearing potential must use one highly effective form of contraception (intrauterine device [IUD] or tubal sterilization) or a combination of methods (hormone method with a barrier method or two barrier methods). If a partner's vasectomy is the chosen method of contraception, a hormone or barrier method must be also used along with this method. Ensure contraception is continued until 1 month after completion of bosentan therapy. ∎
`Black Box Warning` There is a possibility of contraception failure when bosentan is administered with hormonal contraceptives; patient shouldn't use hormonal contraceptives alone when taking bosentan. ∎
• Decreased sperm counts have been observed in patients receiving drug.
• It isn't known if drug appears in human milk. Use isn't recommended in breastfeeding women.

NURSING CONSIDERATIONS
`Black Box Warning` Use of this drug can cause serious liver injury. AST and ALT level elevations may be dose dependent and reversible, so measure these levels before treatment and monthly thereafter, adjusting dosage accordingly. If elevations are accompanied by symptoms of liver injury (nausea, vomiting, fever, abdominal pain, jaundice, or unusual lethargy or fatigue) or if bilirubin level increases by 2 × ULN or greater, discontinue drug and notify prescriber immediately. ∎

Reactions in bold italics are *life-threatening*. Interactions may have a *rapid onset* or a *delayed onset*.

• Fluid retention and HF may occur. Patient may require diuretics, fluid management, or hospitalization for decompensating HF.
• Monitor Hb level after 1 and 3 months of therapy; then every 3 months.
• Gradually reduce dosage before stopping drug.

PATIENT TEACHING
• Advise patient to take doses in the morning and evening, with or without food.
Black Box Warning Warn patient to avoid becoming pregnant while taking this drug and for 1 month after final dose. Hormonal contraceptives, including oral, implantable, and injectable methods, may not be effective when used with this drug. Advise patient to use two acceptable methods of contraception during and for 1 month after treatment with bosentan. A monthly pregnancy test must be performed. ■
• Inform male patient of risk of low sperm count.
• Advise patient to have LFTs and blood counts performed regularly.

SAFETY ALERT!

brentuximab vedotin ☒
bren-TUX-eh-mab

Adcetris

Therapeutic class: Antineoplastics
Pharmacologic class: Antibodies

AVAILABLE FORMS
Powder for injection: 50-mg single-use vial

INDICATIONS & DOSAGES
Adjust-a-dose (for all indications): For severe renal impairment (CrCl less than 30 mL/minute), avoid use. For mild hepatic impairment (Child-Pugh class A), decrease starting dose to 1.2 mg/kg with a maximum dose of 120 mg. For moderate or severe hepatic impairment (Child-Pugh class B or C), avoid use.
   Refer to manufacturer's instructions for toxicity-related dosage adjustments.
➤ **Classic Hodgkin lymphoma (cHL) in patients at high risk for relapse or progression after autologous hematopoietic stem cell transplantation (auto-HSCT) consolidation**
Adults: 1.8 mg/kg IV every 3 weeks in 4 to 6 weeks after auto-HSCT or upon recovery from auto-HSCT for a maximum of 16 cycles or until disease progression or toxicities occur. Maximum dose is 180 mg.
➤ **Hodgkin lymphoma after failure of auto-HSCT or after failure of at least two multiagent chemotherapy regimens in patients who aren't auto-HSCT candidates; systemic anaplastic large cell lymphoma (ALCL) after failure of at least one multiagent chemotherapy regimen**
Adults: 1.8 mg/kg IV infusion every 3 weeks, or until disease progression or toxicities occur. Maximum dose is 180 mg.
➤ **Relapsed primary cutaneous ALCL or CD30-expressing mycosis fungoides**
Adults: 1.8 mg/kg IV infusion every 3 weeks for a maximum of 16 cycles or until disease progression or toxicities occur. Maximum dose is 180 mg.
➤ **Previously untreated stage III or IV cHL, in combination with chemotherapy**
Adults: 1.2 mg/kg IV infusion every 2 weeks until a maximum of 12 doses are given, or until disease progression or unacceptable toxicity occurs. Maximum dose is 120 mg.
✳ *NEW INDICATION:* **Previously untreated systemic ALCL or other CD30-expressing peripheral T-cell lymphomas (PTCL), including angioimmunoblastic T-cell lymphoma and PTCL not otherwise specified, in combination with cyclophosphamide, doxorubicin, and prednisone ☒**
Adults: 1.8 mg/kg IV infusion every 3 weeks, with each cycle of chemotherapy for six to eight doses. Maximum dose is 180 mg.

ADMINISTRATION
IV
▼ Drug is considered hazardous; use safe handling and disposal precautions.
▼ Reconstitute each 50-mg vial with 10.5 mL sterile water for injection to yield a single-use solution containing 5 mg/mL.
▼ Gently swirl contents; don't shake vial. Inspect for particulates and discoloration.

▼ Dilute further to yield 0.4 to 1.8 mg/mL in infusion bag of NSS injection, 5% dextrose injection, or lactated Ringer injection. Gently mix by inverting bag.

▼ After reconstitution, infuse immediately or store at 36° to 46° F (2° to 8° C) and use within 24 hours of reconstitution. Don't freeze. Discard unused portion left in vial.

▼ Administer drug only by IV infusion over 30 minutes; don't give by IV push or bolus.

▼ **Incompatibilities:** Don't mix or administer drug with other medications or fluids.

ACTION

Disrupts microtubule network of the cancer cell, which induces cell-cycle arrest and apoptotic death of the cells.

Route	Onset	Peak	Duration
IV	Rapid	1–3 days	Unknown

Half-life: 4 to 6 days.

ADVERSE REACTIONS

CNS: peripheral neuropathy (sensory, motor), headache, dizziness, fatigue, chills, insomnia, anxiety, pain, fever. **CV:** peripheral edema, *PE, supraventricular arrhythmia,* lymphadenopathy. **EENT:** oropharyngeal pain. **GI:** nausea, diarrhea, abdominal pain, vomiting, constipation, decreased appetite. **GU:** pyelonephritis, UTI. **Hematologic:** *neutropenia,* anemia, *thrombocytopenia.* **Metabolic:** decreased weight. **Musculoskeletal:** arthralgia, myalgia, back pain, extremity pain, muscle spasms. **Respiratory:** URI, cough, dyspnea, pneumonitis, pneumothorax. **Skin:** rash, pruritus, alopecia, night sweats, dry skin. **Other:** *septic shock, anaphylaxis,* immunogenicity.

INTERACTIONS

Drug-drug. *Bleomycin:* May increase risk of pulmonary toxicity. Concomitant use is contraindicated.

Inactivated-virus vaccines: Drug may diminish the therapeutic effect of vaccines. Complete all age-appropriate vaccinations at least 2 weeks before drug initiation. If patient is vaccinated during therapy, revaccinate at least 3 months after immunosuppressant is discontinued. Consider therapy modification.

Live-virus vaccines: Drug may enhance the adverse or toxic effects of vaccines. Avoid combination.

P-gp inhibitors: May increase brentuximab level. Monitor patient for increased adverse effects.

Strong CYP3A4 inducers (rifampin): May decrease brentuximab level. Monitor patient for brentuximab effectiveness.

Strong CYP3A4 inhibitors (ketoconazole): May increase brentuximab level. Monitor patient for increased adverse effects.

EFFECTS ON LAB TEST RESULTS

• May increase transaminase and bilirubin levels.

• May decrease RBC, WBC, platelet, and neutrophil counts.

CONTRAINDICATIONS & CAUTIONS

• Contraindicated in patients hypersensitive to drug and with concomitant bleomycin therapy due to pulmonary toxicity.

Black Box Warning John Cunningham (JC) virus infection resulting in progressive multifocal leukoencephalopathy (PML) and death can occur in patients receiving brentuximab. ■

⊘ *Alert:* Infusion-related reactions, including anaphylaxis, have occurred. If anaphylaxis occurs, discontinue drug immediately and permanently and initiate appropriate therapy. Interrupt infusion for other infusion-related reactions and treat appropriately. Patients with prior infusion-related reactions should be premedicated (acetaminophen, antihistamine, corticosteroid) for subsequent infusions.

• Avoid use in patients with severe renal impairment or moderate or severe hepatic impairment due to increased risk of grade 3 or greater adverse events.

• Serious infections (pneumonia, bacteremia, sepsis, fatal septic shock) have been reported.

Dialyzable drug: Unknown.

PREGNANCY-LACTATION-REPRODUCTION

• Drug may cause fetal harm if administered during pregnancy. Women of childbearing potential should avoid pregnancy during and for 6 months after therapy ends.

Reactions in bold italics are *life-threatening*. Interactions may have a *rapid onset* or a *delayed onset*.

• Drug may damage spermatozoa and testicular tissue, resulting in possible genetic abnormalities. Males with female sexual partners of childbearing potential should use effective contraception during therapy and for 6 months after therapy ends.

• Drug may compromise male fertility.

• It isn't known if drug appears in human milk. Breastfeeding isn't recommended during treatment.

NURSING CONSIDERATIONS

• Drug may cause severe peripheral neuropathy. Monitor patient for new or worsening signs and symptoms.

• Drug may cause hepatotoxicity, which can be fatal, especially in patients with preexisting liver disease or elevated baseline liver enzymes and in those taking concomitant medications. Monitor liver enzymes and bilirubin. Delay or reduce dose, or discontinue drug as clinically indicated for new, worsening, or recurrent hepatotoxicity.

• Monitor patient closely for infusion-related adverse effects; interrupt therapy and treat as necessary.

• Monitor patient for signs and symptoms of neutropenia. Monitor CBC before each dose, and more frequently if patient exhibits grade 3 or 4 neutropenia. Delay or reduce dose, or discontinue drug as required.

• Monitor patient for TLS, characterized by changes in electrolytes and kidney damage.

• Monitor patient for skin reactions, especially SJS. Discontinue drug if reactions occur.

Black Box Warning Monitor patient for vision loss, impaired speech, muscle weakness or paralysis, and cognitive deterioration, which may indicate PML. Hold drug for suspected PML and discontinue if diagnosis is confirmed. ▌

• Monitor patient for noninfectious pulmonary toxicity (pneumonitis, ILD, ARDS). Hold drug during evaluation of new or worsening pulmonary symptoms and until symptoms improve.

• Monitor patient for infection (bacterial, fungal, or viral) during treatment.

• Monitor patient for new or worsening GI signs and symptoms of perforation, hemorrhage, erosion, ulcer, intestinal obstruction, enterocolitis, neutropenic colitis, and ileus.

PATIENT TEACHING

• Tell patient to report muscle weakness or numbness or tingling of the hands or feet.

• Advise patient to report signs or symptoms of possible infection, including temperature of 100.5° F (38° C) or greater, chills, cough, or pain on urination.

• Warn patient to report signs or symptoms of possible infusion-related reactions, including fever, chills, rash, or breathing problems (wheezing, cough, chest tightness), blue skin color, and swelling of the face, lips, tongue, or throat.

• Caution female patient to avoid becoming pregnant during and for 6 months after therapy ends. Tell her to report possible pregnancy immediately.

• Breastfeeding isn't recommended during therapy.

• Caution male patient with female partner of childbearing potential to use effective contraception during and for 6 months after therapy ends.

brexpiprazole �
brex-PIP-ra-zole

Rexulti

Therapeutic class: Antipsychotics
Pharmacologic class: Atypical antipsychotics

AVAILABLE FORMS

Tablets: 0.25 mg, 0.5 mg, 1 mg, 2 mg, 3 mg, 4 mg

INDICATIONS & DOSAGES

Adjust-a-dose (for all indications): Refer to manufacturer's instructions for renal and hepatic impairment and drug-interaction dosage adjustments.

➤ **Adjunctive treatment of major depressive disorder**
Adults: Initially, 0.5 or 1 mg PO once daily. If starting at 0.5 mg, increase to 1 mg PO once daily after 1 week based on patient's response and tolerability. Then, increase to target dose of 2 mg PO once daily after 1 week. Maximum daily dose is 3 mg.

➤ **Schizophrenia**

Adults: Initially, 1 mg PO once daily on days 1 through 4; then titrate to 2 mg PO once daily on days 5 through 7; then increase to 4 mg PO once daily on day 8 based on patient's response and tolerability. Recommended target dose is 2 to 4 mg daily. Maximum daily dose is 4 mg.

ADMINISTRATION
PO
- Give without regard for food.
- If a dose is missed, give as soon as possible. If it's close to the time for next dose, skip missed dose and give next dose at the regular time. Don't double-dose.
- Store at 68° to 77° F (20° to 25° C).

ACTION
Exact mechanism unknown. Its effect may occur through partial agonist activity at serotonin 5-HT_{1A} and dopamine D_2 receptors, as well as antagonist activity at serotonin 5-HT_{2A} receptors.

Route	Onset	Peak	Duration
PO	Unknown	4 hr	Unknown

Half-life: 91 hours.

ADVERSE REACTIONS
CNS: fatigue, drowsiness, akathisia, headache, tremor, dizziness, anxiety, restlessness, somnolence, sedation, abnormal dreams, insomnia, extrapyramidal reactions. **EENT:** blurred vision, nasopharyngitis, dry mouth, sialorrhea. **GI:** constipation, dyspepsia, diarrhea, nausea, abdominal pain, flatulence. **GU:** UTI. **Metabolic:** weight gain, increased appetite. **Musculoskeletal:** myalgia. **Skin:** hyperhidrosis.

INTERACTIONS
Drug-drug. *Anticholinergics (diphenhydramine, meclizine, scopolamine):* May increase risk of body temperature dysregulation. Use together cautiously.
CNS depressants: May increase CNS depressant effects. Monitor therapy.
Strong CYP2D6 inhibitors (bupropion, fluoxetine, paroxetine, quinidine), strong CYP3A4 inhibitors (clarithromycin, itraconazole, ketoconazole, ritonavir): May increase brexpiprazole concentration. Reduce brexpiprazole dosage.
Strong CYP3A4 inducers (carbamazepine, phenytoin, rifampin): May decrease brexpiprazole concentration. Increase brexpiprazole dosage.
Drug-herb. *St. John's wort:* May decrease brexpiprazole concentration. Increase brexpiprazole dosage.
Drug-food. *Grapefruit juice:* May increase brexpiprazole concentration. Avoid use together.

EFFECTS ON LAB TEST RESULTS
- May increase CK, glucose, cortisol, triglyceride, and prolactin levels.
- May decrease WBC count.

CONTRAINDICATIONS & CAUTIONS
- Contraindicated in patients hypersensitive to drug or its components.
Black Box Warning Elderly patients with dementia-related psychosis treated with antipsychotics are at increased risk for death. Drug isn't approved for treatment of patients with dementia-related psychosis. ∎
Black Box Warning Antidepressants have increased the risk of suicidal thoughts and behaviors in patients younger than age 24. Safety and effectiveness in children haven't been studied. ∎
- Antipsychotics can cause NMS, which can be fatal.
- Antipsychotics can cause tardive dyskinesia, especially in elderly patients, most notably elderly women, and may be irreversible.
- Atypical antipsychotics are associated with metabolic changes, such as weight gain, dyslipidemia, hyperglycemia, and diabetes.
- Antipsychotics may increase the risk of seizures. Use cautiously in patients with a history of seizures or conditions that could lower the seizure threshold.
- Drug may alter the body's ability to lower the core temperature.
⚕ Use cautiously in patients who are poor metabolizers of CYP2D6, in patients with moderate to severe hepatic impairment (Child-Pugh score of 7 or more), and in those with moderate, severe, or end-stage renal impairment (CrCl less than 60 mL/minute); adjust dosage appropriately.

Reactions in bold italics are *life-threatening*. Interactions may have a *rapid onset* or a *delayed onset*.

• Use cautiously in patients with preexisting hypotension or who are taking other antihypertensives; drug can cause orthostatic hypotension or syncope.

• Use cautiously in patients at risk for aspiration pneumonia. Esophageal dysmotility and aspiration have been associated with antipsychotic use.

• Antipsychotics can impair thinking, judgment, and motor skills.

• Drug may cause intense impulsive or compulsive behavior urges, particularly for gambling, and the inability to control these urges. Other compulsive urges reported less frequently include sexual urges, shopping, and eating or binge eating.

• Drug may cause somnolence, orthostatic hypotension, and motor and sensory instability, which may lead to falls and, consequently, fractures or other injuries.

• Tablets may contain lactose; avoid use in patients with lactose-intolerant conditions.

• Use cautiously in elderly patients because of the increased risk of adverse events.

Dialyzable drug: Unlikely.

PREGNANCY-LACTATION-REPRODUCTION

• There are no adequate studies in pregnant women. Neonates exposed to antipsychotics during the third trimester are at risk for extrapyramidal or withdrawal signs and symptoms, which can vary in severity but may require prolonged hospitalization. Routine use during pregnancy isn't recommended; risks and benefits should be considered.

• Women exposed to drug during pregnancy should be enrolled in the National Pregnancy Registry for Atypical Antipsychotics (1-866-961-2388).

• It's unknown if drug appears in human milk. Consider risks and benefits before using in breastfeeding women.

NURSING CONSIDERATIONS

• Monitor patients for suicidal thoughts or behaviors, especially during the first few months of treatment and after dosage changes. Consider discontinuing drug in patients whose depression worsens or who experience suicidal thoughts or behaviors.

• Monitor patients for signs and symptoms of NMS (hyperpyrexia, muscle rigidity, change in mental status, tachycardia, change in BP or pulse, diaphoresis, arrhythmias, elevated CK level, rhabdomyolysis, acute renal failure). Discontinue drug if reactions appear, and treat appropriately.

• Monitor blood glucose, triglyceride, and lipid levels; observe for weight changes.

• Monitor patients for seizures, difficulty swallowing, and aspiration.

• Monitor patients with diabetes regularly for worsening of glucose control.

• Monitor patients at risk for diabetes (obesity, family history) before and periodically during treatment.

• Avoid exposing patients to extreme heat; make sure they are well hydrated.

• Monitor patients for tardive dyskinesia (involuntary, dyskinetic movements). Reassess need for continued treatment periodically. If tardive dyskinesia develops, consider discontinuing drug.

• Monitor patients with a history of significantly low WBC count or ANC or drug-induced neutropenia frequently during first few months of therapy. Consider discontinuing drug at first sign of significant decline in WBC count; monitor patients for fever or other signs or symptoms of infection. Discontinue drug in patients with severe neutropenia (ANC less than 1,000/mm^3).

• Monitor patients for orthostatic hypotension and syncope. Patients at increased risk include those with dehydration, hypovolemia, history of CV disease (HF, MI, ischemia, conduction abnormalities), or history of cerebrovascular disease; those taking antihypertensives; and patients who are antipsychotic-naive. Lower starting dose and slower titration may be needed in these patients.

• Complete fall risk assessments when initiating antipsychotic treatment and periodically for patients on long-term therapy, especially for patients who have diseases or conditions or are taking other medications that could exacerbate their fall risk.

• Monitor patients for impulsive or compulsive behavior urges; consider reducing dosage or stopping drug if they develop.

• Check with pharmacist regarding potential interactions with other drugs that are metabolized via the CYP450 enzyme system in the liver.

• *Look alike–sound alike:* Don't confuse Rexulti with Maxalt.

PATIENT TEACHING

❸ *Alert:* Counsel family members or caregivers to monitor for changes in behavior and to immediately report suicidal thoughts or behaviors to prescriber.

• Advise patient or caregivers to watch for and report new or intense gambling urges, compulsive sexual urges, compulsive shopping, binge or compulsive eating, or other urges.

• Explain the potential for dystonic or extrapyramidal symptoms (involuntary, abnormal movements). Instruct patient to immediately report symptoms to prescriber.

• Teach diabetic patient to monitor blood glucose level closely and to report changes in glucose level.

• Advise patient to report lactose intolerance before starting therapy.

• Educate patient about the risk of metabolic changes, how to recognize hyperglycemia, and the need for blood tests for glucose and lipid levels. Encourage patient to report weight gain.

• Caution patient about risk of orthostatic hypotension and syncope, especially at start of therapy and with dosage changes.

• Advise female patient to contact prescriber immediately if she is or plans to become pregnant or is breastfeeding.

• Remind patient to avoid strenuous exercise, dehydration, or exposure to extreme heat. Encourage patient to drink plenty of water while taking drug.

• Instruct patient to report muscle rigidity, increased sweating, changes in BP, or irregular heartbeats.

• Warn patient about potential for drug interactions and advise patient to report to prescriber all OTC drugs, prescription medications, and supplements being taken before start of therapy.

• Caution patient about risk of impaired judgment, thinking, or motor skills. Advise patient not to perform activities that require mental alertness, such as operating hazardous machinery, including motor vehicles, until drug's effects are known.

brimonidine tartrate
bri-MOE-ni-deen

Alphagan P, Lumify ◇, Mirvaso

Therapeutic class: Antiglaucoma drugs–dermatologic agents
Pharmacologic class: Selective alpha$_2$ agonists

AVAILABLE FORMS
Ophthalmic solution: 0.025% ◇, 0.1%, 0.15%, 0.2%
Topical gel: 0.33%

INDICATIONS & DOSAGES
➤ **To reduce IOP in open-angle glaucoma or ocular HTN**
Adults and children age 2 and older: 1 drop in affected eye t.i.d., about 8 hours apart.
➤ **Persistent erythema of rosacea (Mirvaso)**
Adults: Apply a pea-size amount to five areas of the face (central forehead, chin, nose, and each cheek) once daily.
✱ *NEW INDICATION:* **Relief of redness of the eye due to minor irritations**
Adults and children age 5 and older: Instill 1 drop in affected eye every 6 to 8 hours. Don't use more often than q.i.d.

ADMINISTRATION
Ophthalmic
• Don't touch tip of dropper to eye or surrounding tissue.
• If more than one ophthalmic product is being used, give them at least 5 minutes apart.
• Patient should remove contact lenses before administration and wait 10 minutes before reinserting or, if using products that contain benzalkonium chloride, wait 15 minutes.
Topical
• Apply a thin layer across the entire face, avoiding the lips and eyes.
• Don't apply to open wounds or irritated skin.
• Wash hands immediately after applying.

ACTION
Ophthalmic form reduces aqueous humor production and increases uveoscleral outflow.

Topical form may reduce erythema through direct vasoconstriction.

Route	Onset	Peak	Duration
Ophthalmic	Unknown	30 min–2½ hr	Unknown
Topical	Unknown	15 days	Unknown

Half-life: Ophthalmic, 2 hours; topical, unknown.

ADVERSE REACTIONS

CNS: asthenia, dizziness, headache, fatigue, somnolence. **CV:** HTN, hypotension. **EENT:** allergic conjunctivitis, ocular hyperemia, pruritus, abnormal vision, allergic reaction, blepharitis, burning; conjunctival edema, hemorrhage, or inflammation; dryness, eyelid edema or erythema, foreign body sensation, increased tearing, pain, photophobia, stinging (ophthalmic only). **GI:** dyspepsia, oral dryness. **Metabolic:** hypercholesterolemia. **Skin:** rash; acne rosacea, acne vulgaris, allergic contact dermatitis, dermatitis, erythema (topical only).

INTERACTIONS

Drug-drug. *Antihypertensives, beta blockers, cardiac glycosides:* May further decrease BP or pulse rate. Monitor vital signs.
Apraclonidine, dorzolamide, pilocarpine, timolol: May have additive IOP-lowering effects. Use cautiously together.
CNS depressants: May increase effects. Use cautiously together.
Linezolid, MAO inhibitors: May increase effects. Avoid using together.
TCAs: May interfere with brimonidine's effect. Use cautiously together.
Drug-lifestyle. *Alcohol use:* May increase CNS depressant effect. Avoid alcohol.

EFFECTS ON LAB TEST RESULTS

• May increase cholesterol level.

CONTRAINDICATIONS & CAUTIONS

• Ophthalmic form is contraindicated in patients hypersensitive to drug or its components, in those taking MAO inhibitors, and in neonates, infants, and children younger than age 2.
• Topical gel is contraindicated in patients hypersensitive to drug or its components; reactions have included angioedema, urticaria, and contact dermatitis.

• Use cautiously in patients with CV disease, cerebral or coronary insufficiency, hepatic or renal impairment, depression, Raynaud phenomenon, Sjögren syndrome, orthostatic hypotension, or thromboangiitis obliterans.
Dialyzable drug: Unknown.
⚠ Overdose S&S: Hypotension.

PREGNANCY-LACTATION-REPRODUCTION

• Use during pregnancy only if potential benefit justifies potential risk to the fetus.
• It isn't known if drug appears in human milk. Consider discontinuing breastfeeding or discontinuing drug.

NURSING CONSIDERATIONS

• Monitor IOP because drug effect may reverse after first month of therapy.
• Erythema, intermittent flushing, or pallor or excessive whitening may occur after topical application and may resolve when therapy is discontinued.
• Avoid applying gel to irritated skin or open wounds.

PATIENT TEACHING

• Tell patient to wait at least 15 minutes after instilling ophthalmic drug before wearing soft contact lenses.
• Caution patient to avoid hazardous activities because of risk of decreased mental alertness, fatigue, or drowsiness.
• Advise patient to avoid alcohol.
• Tell patient who's using more than one ophthalmic drug to apply them at least 5 minutes apart.
• Teach patient proper method of instilling eyedrops and to not touch tip of container to skin or surfaces.
• Instruct patient how to apply topical form. Caution patient that topical form is for external use only and shouldn't be used orally, intravaginally, or in the eyes.
• Instruct patient to use topical gel only for approved indications.

brivaracetam
BRIV-a-re-se-tam

Briviact

Therapeutic class: Anticonvulsants
Pharmacologic class: Anticonvulsants
Controlled substance schedule: V

AVAILABLE FORMS
Tablets ⊙ᴺᴱ: 10 mg, 25 mg, 50 mg, 75 mg, 100 mg
Injection: 50 mg/5 mL single-dose vial
Oral solution: 10 mg/mL

INDICATIONS & DOSAGES
➤ **Adjunctive therapy or monotherapy for partial-onset seizures in patients with epilepsy**
Adults and children age 16 and older: Initially, 50 mg PO or IV b.i.d. Titrate dosage to individual patient tolerability and therapeutic response to a minimum dose of 25 mg b.i.d. and a maximum dose of 100 mg b.i.d.
Children age 4 and older weighing 50 kg or more: 25 to 50 mg PO b.i.d. Adjust dosage based on clinical response and tolerability. Minimum dose, 25 mg b.i.d.; maximum dose, 100 mg b.i.d.
Children age 4 and older weighing 20 to less than 50 kg: 0.5 to 1 mg/kg PO b.i.d. Adjust dosage based on clinical response and tolerability. Minimum dose, 0.5 mg/kg b.i.d.; maximum dose, 2 mg/kg b.i.d.
Children age 4 and older weighing 11 to less than 20 kg: 0.5 to 1.25 mg/kg PO b.i.d. Adjust dosage based on clinical response and tolerability. Minimum dose, 0.5 mg/kg b.i.d.; maximum dose, 2.5 mg/kg b.i.d.
Adjust-a-dose: Refer to manufacturer's instructions for dosage adjustments in adults and children with hepatic impairment.
In patients also taking rifampin, increase brivaracetam dosage by up to 100% (double the dose).

ADMINISTRATION
PO
• May give with or without food.
• Patient should swallow tablets whole and not chew or crush them.

• Use a calibrated measuring device for measuring oral solution. Don't use a household teaspoon.
• May give oral solution via NG or gastrostomy tube.
• Discard any unused oral solution that remains 5 months after first opening the bottle.
• Store between 59° and 86° F (15° and 30° C). Don't freeze oral solution.

IV
▼ Visually inspect vial. Don't administer if particulate matter or discoloration is present.
▼ May give IV without further dilution.
▼ If further dilution is required, use NSS, lactated Ringer, or 5% dextrose solution.
▼ Administer IV over 2 to 15 minutes.
▼ Diluted solution shouldn't be stored for more than 4 hours at room temperature and may be stored in polyvinyl chloride bags. Don't freeze.
▼ Discard any unused portion of the injection vial contents.
▼ **Incompatibilities:** None listed by manufacturer. Consult a drug incompatibility reference for more information.

ACTION
Exact mechanism unknown. Anticonvulsant effect may be related to affinity for synaptic vesicle protein 2A in the brain.

Route	Onset	Peak	Duration
PO	Unknown	1 hr	Unknown
IV	Unknown	Unknown	Unknown

Half-life: About 9 hours.

ADVERSE REACTIONS
CNS: somnolence, sedation, ataxia, balance disorder, abnormal coordination, nystagmus, dizziness, fatigue, irritability, euphoric mood, feeling drunk, anxiety, nervousness, aggression, anger, agitation, restlessness, depression, apathy, mood swings, abnormal behavior, psychotic disorder (hallucination, paranoia, acute psychosis, psychotic behavior). **GI:** nausea, vomiting, constipation, dysgeusia. **Other:** infusion-site pain.

INTERACTIONS
Drug-drug. *Azelastine (nasal), orphenadrine, paraldehyde:* May increase CNS

Reactions in bold italics are *life-threatening*. Interactions may have a *rapid onset* or a *delayed onset*.

depressant effect of these drugs. Avoid use together.

Cannabis: May enhance CNS depressant effect. Monitor therapy.

Carbamazepine: May increase exposure to active metabolite carbamazepine-10,11-epoxide. Decrease carbamazepine dosage if intolerance occurs.

CNS depressants, magnesium sulfate: May enhance CNS depressant effects. Monitor therapy.

Orlistat: May decrease brivaracetam level. Monitor therapy.

Phenytoin: May increase phenytoin plasma concentration. Monitor phenytoin level when brivaracetam is started or stopped, and adjust dosage as needed.

Rifampin: May decrease brivaracetam level. Increase brivaracetam dosage by up to 100%.

Drug-herb. *Kava kava:* May enhance adverse effects of brivaracetam. Monitor therapy.

Drug-lifestyle. *Alcohol use:* May increase CNS depression. Monitor therapy.

EFFECTS ON LAB TEST RESULTS
• May decrease WBC count.

CONTRAINDICATIONS & CAUTIONS
• Contraindicated in patients hypersensitive to drug or its components.
• Hypersensitivity reactions, including bronchospasm and angioedema, and DRESS syndrome have been reported.
• Antiepileptics may increase risk of suicidal behavior and ideation. Consider risk before prescribing and administering.
• Use in patients with ESRD undergoing dialysis isn't recommended.
• Safety and effectiveness in children younger than age 4 haven't been established. Safety of injectable form in children younger than age 16 hasn't been established.
• Start elderly patients on low end of the dosing range, taking into consideration hepatic, kidney, or cardiac function and other concomitant disease and drugs.

Dialyzable drug: Unlikely.

⚠ *Overdose S&S:* Vertigo, balance disorder, fatigue, nausea, diplopia, anxiety, bradycardia.

PREGNANCY-LACTATION-REPRODUCTION
• There are no adequate and well-controlled studies in pregnant women. Use in pregnancy only if potential benefit justifies the risk to the fetus.
• Pregnant patients exposed to drug should enroll in the AED (Antiepileptic Drug) Pregnancy Registry (1-888-233-2334).
• It isn't known if drug appears in human milk. Patient should discontinue breastfeeding or discontinue drug.

NURSING CONSIDERATIONS
• Monitor patients for signs and symptoms of hypersensitivity reactions (bronchospasm, angioedema) and DRESS syndrome (fever, rash, eosinophilia, lymphadenopathy, hepatitis, nephritis, myocarditis). Discontinue drug and treat appropriately if signs and symptoms of hypersensitivity or DRESS syndrome occur.
• Abrupt withdrawal of drug may increase risk of increased seizure frequency and status epilepticus. Withdraw drug gradually.
• Monitor patients for new or worsening depression, suicidal thoughts or behaviors, or unusual changes in mood or behavior during therapy.
• Monitor patients for neurologic effects (somnolence, fatigue, asthenia, malaise, hypersomnia, sedation, lethargy, dizziness, vertigo, balance disorder, ataxia, nystagmus, gait disturbance, abnormal coordination). Patients shouldn't drive or operate machinery until drug's effects are known.

PATIENT TEACHING
• Counsel family member or caregivers to watch for changes in patient's behavior and to immediately report suicidal thoughts or behaviors, or thoughts about self-harm.
• Warn patient not to drive or operate machinery until drug's effects are known.
• Advise patient to report all adverse reactions and to immediately report behavioral changes, including irritability, depression, aggressive behavior, anxiety, and psychotic symptoms (hallucinations, paranoia).
• Warn patient to seek immediate medical care if signs or symptoms of hypersensitivity reactions, including bronchospasm and angioedema, occur.

• Instruct patient not to discontinue drug abruptly without first consulting prescriber.

brodalumab
broe-DAL-ue-mab

Siliq

Therapeutic class: Immunomodulators
Pharmacologic class: Interleukin receptor antagonists

AVAILABLE FORMS
Injection: 210 mg/1.5 mL in single-dose, prefilled syringe

INDICATIONS & DOSAGES
➤ **Moderate to severe plaque psoriasis in patients who are candidates for systemic therapy or phototherapy and have failed to respond or have lost response to other systemic therapies**
Adults: 210 mg subcut at weeks 0, 1, and 2, followed by 210 mg every 2 weeks. If adequate response hasn't been achieved after 12 to 16 weeks of treatment, consider discontinuing therapy as success is less likely.

ADMINISTRATION
Subcutaneous
• Allow syringe to reach room temperature (approximately 30 minutes) before injecting. Don't warm in any other way. Don't remove gray needle cap until ready to inject.
• Once syringe has reached room temperature, don't rerefrigerate.
• Don't use drug if cloudy or discolored or if foreign matter is present. A few translucent to white particles may be present.
• Inject full amount of 1.5 mL to administer a 210-mg dose.
• Don't inject into areas where skin is tender, bruised, red, hard, thick, scaly, or affected by psoriasis.
• Store drug refrigerated at 36° to 46° F (2° to 8° C) in original carton to protect from light and damage during storage. When necessary, may store drug at room temperature up to a maximum of 77° F (25° C) for a maximum single period of 14 days. Discard after 14 days at room temperature.

• Don't freeze or shake syringe or carton filled with syringes.

ACTION
A monoclonal antibody that binds to interleukin-17RA and inhibits proinflammatory cytokines and other inflammatory mediators, leading to decreased inflammation.

Route	Onset	Peak	Duration
Subcut	Unknown	3 days	Unknown

Half-life: Unknown.

ADVERSE REACTIONS
CNS: headache, fatigue. **EENT:** oropharyngeal pain. **GI:** diarrhea, nausea. **Hematologic:** *neutropenia.* **Musculoskeletal:** arthralgia, myalgia. **Skin:** injection-site reactions, tinea infections. **Other:** *suicidal ideation or behavior,* flulike symptoms, infections.

INTERACTIONS
Drug-drug. *Cyclosporine:* May decrease effect of cytokines on cyclosporine, a CYP450 substrate. Monitor cyclosporine level; adjust cyclosporine dosage as clinically indicated.
CYP450 substrates: May decrease effect of cytokines on CYP450 substrates. Adjust CYP450 substrate dosage as clinically indicated by drug concentration or therapeutic effect.
Live-virus vaccines: May affect ability to elicit immune response. Avoid use together.
Midazolam: Increases midazolam exposure. Monitor therapy.
Warfarin: May decrease effect of cytokines on warfarin, a CYP450 substrate. Monitor INR; adjust warfarin dosage as clinically indicated.

EFFECTS ON LAB TEST RESULTS
• May decrease ANC.

CONTRAINDICATIONS & CAUTIONS
• Contraindicated in patients with Crohn disease; drug may worsen disease.
Black Box Warning Suicidal ideation and behavior, including completed suicides, have occurred in patients treated with this drug. ∎
Black Box Warning Because of suicide risk, drug is available only through the restricted SILIQ REMS Program. ∎

Reactions in bold italics are *life-threatening*. Interactions may have a *rapid onset* or a *delayed onset*.

• Drug increases risk of infections, including serious infections.
• Drug increases risk of latent TB reactivation.
• Safety and effectiveness in children haven't been evaluated.
Dialyzable drug: Unknown.

PREGNANCY-LACTATION-REPRODUCTION
• There are no human data concerning use in pregnant women. Because human IgG antibodies cross the placental barrier, drug may be transmitted from mother to developing fetus.
• It isn't known if drug appears in human milk. Drug's effect on breastfed infants or on milk production is also unknown. Use only if benefit clearly outweighs risk to breastfed infant.

NURSING CONSIDERATIONS
• Discontinue drug if patient develops Crohn disease during therapy.
Black Box Warning Suicidal ideation and behavior, including completed suicides, have occurred in patients treated with this drug. Before therapy, consider potential risks and benefits in patients with a history of depression or suicidal ideation or behavior. ∎
Black Box Warning Because of suicide risk, drug is available only through the restricted SILIQ REMS Program. Information is available at 1-855-511-6135. ∎
Black Box Warning Assess for new or worsening suicidal thoughts and behavior, new-onset or worsening depression, anxiety, or other mood changes; refer patient to mental health professional, as appropriate. Reevaluate continued use of drug if changes occur. ∎
• Evaluate patients for TB before therapy begins. Consider anti-TB therapy before starting drug in patients with a history of latent TB or active TB when an adequate course of TB treatment can't be confirmed.
• Closely monitor patient for signs and symptoms of active TB during and after treatment.
• Consider risks and benefits before initiating drug in patients with a chronic infection or a history of recurrent infection.

• Monitor patient for signs and symptoms of infection (fever, malaise, cough, pain, skin changes, wound or rash with drainage). If a serious infection develops or patient isn't responding to standard treatment for the infection, discontinue drug until infection resolves.
• *Look alike–sound alike:* Don't confuse Siliq with Actiq.

PATIENT TEACHING
Black Box Warning Instruct patient and caregivers to watch for suicidal thoughts, new or worsening depression, anxiety, or other mood changes. Tell patient to carry provided Siliq patient wallet card and to call the National Suicide Prevention Lifeline (1-800-273-8255) if suicidal thoughts occur. ∎
• Provide patient with information (telephone number and website) on how to obtain drug, as it may be prescribed only by certified prescribers and is only available from certified pharmacies through the SILIQ REMS Program.
• Advise patient that signing a Patient-Prescriber Agreement Form is a necessary part of the SILIQ REMS Program.
• Explain that drug may lower the ability to fight infection. Tell patient to report signs and symptoms of infection.
• Teach patient to report signs and symptoms of Crohn disease (diarrhea, bloody stools, stomach pain or cramping, sudden or uncontrollable bowel movements, constipation, loss of appetite, weight loss, fever, fatigue).
• Show patient who plans to self-administer drug the injection technique per manufacturer's instructions.
• Tell patient not to use the syringe if it has been dropped on a hard surface because a break in the syringe (which may or may not be obvious) may have occurred. Instruct patient to use a new syringe and to call 1-800-321-4576.

bromocriptine mesylate
broe-moe-KRIP-teen

Cycloset, Parlodel

Therapeutic class: Antiparkinsonian drugs
Pharmacologic class: Dopamine receptor
agonists

AVAILABLE FORMS
Capsules: 5 mg
Tablets: 0.8 mg (Cycloset), 2.5 mg
(Parlodel)

INDICATIONS & DOSAGES
➤ **Parkinson disease (not Cycloset)**
Adults: 1.25 mg PO b.i.d. with meals. Increase dosage by 2.5 mg/day every 14 to
28 days, up to 100 mg daily.
➤ **Amenorrhea and galactorrhea from
hyperprolactinemia; hypogonadism, infertility (not Cycloset)**
Adults and adolescents age 16 and older:
1.25 to 2.5 mg PO daily, increased by 2.5 mg
daily at 2- to 7-day intervals until desired effect occurs. Usual therapeutic daily dose is
2.5 to 15 mg.
Children ages 11 to 15: 1.25 to 2.5 mg PO
daily. May increase as tolerated until therapeutic response is achieved. Range, 2.5 to
10 mg daily in children with prolactin-
secreting pituitary adenomas.
➤ **Acromegaly (not Cycloset)**
Adults: 1.25 to 2.5 mg PO with bedtime
snack for 3 days. Another 1.25 to 2.5 mg
may be added every 3 to 7 days until therapeutic benefit occurs. Maximum, 100 mg
daily. Usual therapeutic dose is 20 to 30 mg
daily.
➤ **Type 2 diabetes mellitus (Cycloset
only)**
Adults: Initially, 0.8 mg PO daily within
2 hours after waking in the morning. May
increase by 0.8 mg weekly until maximum
tolerated dosage of 1.6 to 4.8 mg daily is
achieved.
Adjust-a-dose: Dosage shouldn't exceed
1.6 mg once daily during concomitant use
of a moderate CYP3A4 inhibitor (erythromycin). Avoid use with strong CYP3A4
inhibitors (azole antimycotics, HIV protease
inhibitors).

ADMINISTRATION
PO
● Give drug in the evening with food to min-
imize adverse reactions (except Cycloset).
● For treatment of type 2 diabetes mellitus,
give Cycloset within 2 hours of patient's
waking in the morning.
● Protect Parlodel from light.

ACTION
Inhibits secretion of prolactin and acts as
a dopamine receptor agonist by activating
postsynaptic dopamine receptors; improves
glycemic control and is associated with increased insulin sensitivity.

Route	Onset	Peak	Duration
PO	2 hr	53–120 min	24 hr

Half-life: 5 hours (Parlodel); 6 hours (Cycloset).

ADVERSE REACTIONS
CNS: dizziness, headache, fatigue, *seizures,
stroke,* mania, light-headedness, drowsiness, delusions, hallucinations, nervousness, insomnia, depression. **CV:** orthostatic
hypotension, *acute MI.* **EENT:** blurred vision, nasal congestion, rhinitis, dry mouth.
GI: nausea, abdominal cramps, constipation, diarrhea, vomiting, anorexia. **GU:** urine
retention, urinary frequency. **Metabolic:**
hypoglycemia. **Skin:** coolness and pallor of
fingers and toes. **Other:** infection, flulike
symptoms.

INTERACTIONS
Drug-drug. *Amitriptyline, haloperidol,
imipramine, loxapine, MAO inhibitors,
methyldopa, phenothiazines, reserpine:*
May interfere with bromocriptine's effects.
Bromocriptine dosage may need to be increased.
Antihypertensives: May increase hypotensive effects. Adjust dosage of antihypertensive.
*Chloramphenicol, probenecid, salicylates,
sulfonamides:* May increase unbound fraction of other highly protein-bound drugs.
Monitor patient for increased adverse reactions.
CYP3A4 inhibitors or inducers: May increase or decrease circulating levels of Cycloset, respectively. Use together with caution. Limit Cycloset dose to 1.6 mg/day

---

Reactions in bold italics are *life-threatening*. Interactions may have a *rapid onset* or a *delayed onset*.

during concomitant use of moderate CYP3A4 inhibitors. Avoid concomitant use with strong CYP3A4 inhibitors and ensure washout of the strong CYP3A4 inhibitor before initiating Cycloset. May also interact with Parlodel; use together cautiously.

Dopamine receptor antagonists (butyrophenones, phenothiazines, thioxanthenes): May diminish effects of Cycloset. Concurrent use isn't recommended.

Ergot-related drugs: May increase occurrence of ergot-related adverse effects and reduce effectiveness of these therapies. Avoid concomitant use.

Estrogens, hormonal contraceptives, progestins: May interfere with effects of bromocriptine. Avoid using together.

Levodopa: May have additive effects. Adjust dosage of levodopa, if needed.

Macrolides (erythromycin): May increase bromocriptine level and risk of adverse reactions. Use together cautiously.

Triptans (sumatriptan): May have additive vasoconstrictive effects. Concomitant use is contraindicated; don't use within 24 hours of one another.

Drug-lifestyle. *Alcohol use:* May enhance toxic or adverse effects of alcohol. Discourage use together.

EFFECTS ON LAB TEST RESULTS
• May increase alkaline phosphatase, ALT, AST, BUN, CK, and uric acid levels.
• May decrease glucose level.

CONTRAINDICATIONS & CAUTIONS
• Contraindicated in patients hypersensitive to ergot derivatives and in those with uncontrolled HTN, toxemia of pregnancy, severe ischemic heart disease, hereditary galactose intolerance, lactase deficiency, glucose-galactose malabsorption, or PVD.
• Cycloset is also contraindicated in patients with syncopal migraines. Use isn't recommended in patients with severe psychotic disorders.
• Use cautiously in patients with impaired renal or hepatic function, history of MI with residual arrhythmias, or psychosis.
• Use cautiously in patients taking antihypertensives.
Dialyzable drug: Unlikely.

⚠ Overdose S&S: Nausea, vomiting, constipation, diaphoresis, dizziness, pallor, severe hypotension, malaise, confusion, lethargy, drowsiness, delusions, hallucinations, repetitive yawning.

PREGNANCY-LACTATION-REPRODUCTION
• Patient should be carefully observed throughout the pregnancy, including regular visual field checks, to monitor possible pituitary tumor expansion. Emergency pituitary surgery may be required.
• If hypertensive disorder of pregnancy occurs, weigh benefit of Parlodel against risk. A decision should be made whether therapy continues to be medically necessary or can be withdrawn.
• Patient should use contraceptive methods other than oral contraceptives or subdermal implants during treatment.
• Drug may lead to early postpartum conception. After menses resumes, patient should be tested for pregnancy every 4 weeks or as soon as a period is missed.
• Drug shouldn't be used in breastfeeding women. Product labeling for Cycloset specifically contraindicates use in breastfeeding women.

NURSING CONSIDERATIONS
• For Parkinson disease, bromocriptine usually is given with levodopa or levodopa–carbidopa. The levodopa–carbidopa dosage may need to be reduced.
❸ Alert: Monitor patient for adverse reactions, which occur in 68% of patients, particularly at start of therapy. Most reactions are mild to moderate; nausea is most common. Minimize adverse reactions by gradually adjusting dosages to effective levels. Adverse reactions are more common when drug is used for Parkinson disease.
• Baseline and periodic evaluations of cardiac, hepatic, renal, and hematopoietic function are recommended during prolonged therapy.
• Drug can cause orthostatic hypotension and syncope, particularly at start of therapy or when dosage is increased. Assess orthostatic vital signs before initiation of therapy and periodically thereafter.

- *Look alike–sound alike:* Don't confuse bromocriptine with benztropine or brimonidine. Don't confuse Parlodel with pindolol.

PATIENT TEACHING
- Instruct patient to take drug with meals.
- Tell patient to take Cycloset within 2 hours of waking in the morning.
- Advise patient to use contraceptive methods other than oral contraceptives or subdermal implants during treatment.
- Instruct patient to avoid dizziness and fainting by rising slowly to an upright position and avoiding sudden position changes.
- Inform patient that it may take 8 weeks or longer for menses to resume and excess production of milk to slow down.
- Advise patient to avoid alcohol while taking drug.
- Advise patient not to operate heavy machinery if somnolence occurs while taking drug.

budesonide (inhalation, intranasal)
byoo-DES-oh-nide

Pulmicort Flexhaler, Pulmicort Respules, Pulmicort Turbuhaler✸, Rhinocort Allergy ◇

Therapeutic class: Corticosteroids
Pharmacologic class: Corticosteroids

AVAILABLE FORMS
Dry powder inhaler: 90 mcg/dose, 100 mcg/dose✸, 180 mcg/dose, 200 mcg/dose✸, 400 mcg/dose✸
Inhalation suspension (Respules): 0.25 mg, 0.5 mg, 1 mg
Nasal spray: 32 mcg/metered spray

INDICATIONS & DOSAGES
➤ **As a preventative in maintenance of asthma**
All patients: Use lowest effective dose after stabilizing asthma.
Respules
Children ages 1 to 8 previously taking bronchodilator alone: 0.5 mg daily or 0.25 mg b.i.d. suspension via jet nebulizer. Maximum dose is 0.5 mg/day.

Children ages 1 to 8 previously taking inhaled corticosteroid: 0.5 mg daily or 0.25 mg b.i.d. suspension via jet nebulizer to maximum dose of 1 mg/day.
Children ages 1 to 8 previously taking oral corticosteroid: 1 mg daily or 0.5 mg b.i.d. via jet nebulizer. Maximum dose is 1 mg/day.
Adjust-a-dose: Symptomatic children not responding to nonsteroidal therapy may require starting dose of 0.25 mg daily.
Flexhaler
Adults: Initially, inhaled dose of 360 mcg b.i.d. to maximum of 720 mcg b.i.d. Starting dose of 180 mcg b.i.d. may be adequate in some adults.
Children ages 6 to 17: Initially, inhaled dose of 180 mcg b.i.d. to maximum of 360 mcg b.i.d. Starting dose of 360 mcg b.i.d. may be appropriate in some children.
Turbuhaler
Adults and children age 12 and older when treatment with inhaled glucocorticoids is started, during periods of severe asthma, and while oral glucocorticoids are being reduced or discontinued: Initially, inhaled dose of 400 to 2,400 mcg daily divided into two to four administrations. Maintenance dose is usually 200 to 400 mcg b.i.d. Individualize dose to the lowest possible to meet therapeutic objective.
Children ages 6 to 12 when beginning budesonide, during periods of severe asthma, and while oral corticosteroids are being reduced or discontinued: Initially, inhaled dose of 100 to 200 mcg b.i.d. For maintenance, use lowest dose necessary to control symptoms.
➤ **Symptoms of seasonal or perennial allergic rhinitis**
Adults and children age 6 and older: 1 spray in each nostril once daily. Maximum dose is 4 sprays per nostril once daily (256 mcg/day) for adults and children older than age 12 and 2 sprays per nostril once daily (128 mcg/day) for children age 6 to less than age 12.

ADMINISTRATION
Inhalational
- Give inhalation suspension at regular intervals daily or b.i.d., as directed.
- Give suspension with a jet nebulizer connected to a compressor with adequate

---

Reactions in bold italics are *life-threatening*. Interactions may have a *rapid onset* or a *delayed onset*.

airflow. Make sure that it's equipped with a mouthpiece or suitable face mask.
• Total daily dose may be increased or given as a divided dose to improve control if needed. Titrate dosage downward again after asthma is stabilized.
• When aluminum foil envelope has been opened, the shelf-life of unused ampules is 2 weeks when protected from light.
• Refer to manufacturer's instructions before use. Prime inhaler before first use. Have patient inhale deeply and forcefully each time unit is used. Remind patient to rinse mouth with water after inhalation.

Intranasal
• Prime pump by actuating eight times before first use. Reprime pump if not used for 2 or more days. Discard bottle after 120 sprays.
• If applicator hasn't been used for 14 days or more, rinse it and reprime with one spray or until a fine mist appears.
• Shake before each actuation.

ACTION
Exhibits potent glucocorticoid activity and weak mineralocorticoid activity. Drug inhibits mast cells, macrophages, and mediators (such as leukotrienes) involved in inflammation.

Route	Onset	Peak	Duration
Inhalation, powder	24 hr	1–2 wk	Unknown
Inhalation, Respules	2–8 days	4–6 wk	Unknown
Intranasal	10 hr	2 wk	Unknown

Half-life: Inhalation and intranasal, 2 to 3 hours.

ADVERSE REACTIONS
CNS: headache, asthenia, fever, hypertonia, insomnia, pain, syncope. **EENT:** sinusitis, pharyngitis, rhinitis, otitis media, voice alteration; epistaxis and nasal irritation (intranasal). **GI:** abdominal pain, dry mouth, dyspepsia, diarrhea, gastroenteritis, nausea, oral candidiasis, taste perversion, vomiting. **Metabolic:** weight gain. **Musculoskeletal:** back pain, fractures, myalgia. **Respiratory:** respiratory tract infection, *bronchospasm,* increased cough. **Skin:** ecchymoses, rash, dermatitis, pruritus. **Other:** flulike symptoms, hypersensitivity reactions, viral infection.

INTERACTIONS
Drug-drug. *Ketoconazole, other strong CYP3A4 inhibitors (atazanavir, clarithromycin, indinavir, itraconazole, nefazodone, nelfinavir, ritonavir, saquinavir, telithromycin):* May inhibit metabolism and increase level of budesonide. Monitor patient for adverse reactions and adjust dosage as needed.

EFFECTS ON LAB TEST RESULTS
None reported.

CONTRAINDICATIONS & CAUTIONS
• Contraindicated in patients hypersensitive to drug, in those with severe hypersensitivity to milk proteins (powder for inhalation), and in those with status asthmaticus or other acute asthma episodes.
• Use nasal formulation cautiously in patients with septal ulcers, nasal surgery, nasal trauma, or untreated localized nasal mucosa infections.
• Use cautiously, if at all, in patients with active or inactive TB, ocular HSV infections, or untreated systemic fungal, bacterial, viral, or parasitic infections.
Dialyzable drug: Unlikely.
⚠ Overdose S&S: Hyperadrenocorticism.

PREGNANCY-LACTATION-REPRODUCTION
• Hypoadrenalism may occur in infants of women who received corticosteroids during pregnancy. These infants should be carefully monitored.
• Studies of pregnant women using inhaled or intranasal form haven't demonstrated an increased risk of abnormalities. Inhaled corticosteroids are recommended for the treatment of asthma during pregnancy.
• Drug appears in human milk. Patient should use lowest possible dose immediately after breastfeeding to maximize time between dose and breastfeeding.

NURSING CONSIDERATIONS
⚠ Alert: When transferring from systemic corticosteroid to inhalation drug, use caution and gradually decrease corticosteroid dose to prevent adrenal insufficiency.
• Inhalation drug doesn't remove the need for systemic corticosteroid therapy in some situations.

• Systemic effects of corticosteroid therapy may occur if recommended daily dosage is exceeded.

• If bronchospasm occurs after inhalation use, stop therapy and treat with a bronchodilator.

• Lung function may improve within 24 hours of starting therapy, but maximum benefit may not be achieved for 1 to 2 weeks or longer.

• For Pulmicort Respules, lung function improves in 2 to 8 days, but maximum benefit may not be seen for 4 to 6 weeks.

• Watch for *Candida* infections of the mouth or pharynx.

 ☉ Alert: Corticosteroids may increase risk of developing serious or fatal infections in patients exposed to viral illnesses, such as chickenpox or measles.

• In rare cases, inhaled corticosteroids have been linked to increased IOP and cataract development. Stop drug if local irritation occurs.

• Monitor bone mineral density in patients at risk for decreased bone mineral content (prolonged immobilization, family history of osteoporosis, postmenopausal status).

• Monitor children for reduction in growth velocity. Use lowest effective dose.

• Monitor patients for hypercorticism and adrenal suppression and if they occur, reduce dosage slowly.

• Rare cases of eosinophilic conditions and Churg-Strauss syndrome have occurred when systemic corticosteroids have been reduced or withdrawn. Monitor patients for eosinophilia, vasculitic rash, worsening pulmonary symptoms, cardiac symptoms, and neuropathy.

PATIENT TEACHING

• Tell patient that budesonide inhaler isn't a bronchodilator and isn't intended to treat acute episodes of asthma.

• Instruct patient to use the inhaler according to manufacturer's instructions at regular intervals because effectiveness depends on twice-daily use on a regular basis.

• Tell patient that improvement in asthma control may be seen within 24 hours, although maximum benefit may not appear for 1 to 2 weeks. If signs or symptoms worsen

during this time, instruct patient to contact prescriber.

• Advise patient to avoid exposure to chickenpox or measles and to contact prescriber if exposure occurs.

• Instruct patient using inhaler to carry or wear medical identification indicating need for supplementary corticosteroids during periods of stress or an asthma attack.

• Advise patient that unused Respules are good for 2 weeks after the foil envelope has been opened; however, unused Respules should be returned to envelope to protect them from light.

• Tell patient to read and follow patient information leaflet contained in package.

• To instill intranasal drug, instruct patient to shake container before use, blow nose to clear nasal passages, tilt head slightly forward, and insert nozzle into nostril, pointing away from septum. Tell patient to hold other nostril closed and inhale gently while spraying. Next, have patient shake container and repeat in other nostril. Advise patient to avoid blowing nose for 15 minutes after use and to wipe spray tip clean with a tissue.

• Advise patient to store nasal canister with valve upward and away from extreme heat or cold. Caution patient not to incinerate or break canister because contents are under pressure.

• Advise patient using nasal formula to notify prescriber if signs or symptoms don't improve or if they worsen in 3 weeks.

• Teach patient good nasal and oral hygiene and not to share drug because this could spread infection.

budesonide (oral, rectal)
byoo-DES-oh-nide

Entocort EC, Uceris

Therapeutic class: Corticosteroids
Pharmacologic class: Glucocorticoids

AVAILABLE FORMS
Capsules (extended-release) ⓞⓃⓒ: 3 mg
Foam: 2 mg/actuation
Tablets (extended-release) ⓞⓃⓒ: 9 mg

INDICATIONS & DOSAGES

Adjust-a-dose (for all indications): In patients with moderate to severe liver disease who have increased signs or symptoms of hypercorticism, reduce dose.

➤ **Mild to moderate active Crohn disease involving the ileum, ascending colon, or both (capsules)**

Adults: 9 mg PO once daily in morning for up to 8 weeks. For recurrent episodes of active Crohn disease, a repeat 8-week course may be given.

Children ages 8 to 17 weighing more than 25 kg: 9 mg PO once daily in the morning for up to 8 weeks, followed by 6 mg once daily in the morning for 2 weeks.

➤ **To maintain remission in mild to moderate Crohn disease that involves the ileum or ascending colon (capsules)**

Adults: 6 mg PO daily in the morning for up to 3 months. Taper dosage to complete cessation after 3 months. Therapy for longer than 3 months doesn't have added benefit.

➤ **Induction of remission in active mild to moderate ulcerative colitis (tablets)**

Adults: 9 mg PO once daily in the morning for up to 8 weeks.

➤ **Induction of remission in mild to moderate distal ulcerative colitis (rectal foam)**

Adults: 2 mg (1 metered dose) PR b.i.d. for 2 weeks then 2 mg PR once daily for 4 weeks.

ADMINISTRATION

PO

• Give drug whole; don't break or crush capsule or tablet.

• For patients unable to swallow an intact capsule: open the capsule, mix the contents into 1 tablespoon of applesauce, and have patient consume within 30 minutes of mixing.

• Make sure patient avoids consuming grapefruit juice during therapy.

Rectal

• Wash hands before and after use.

• Attach applicator to canister nozzle. Warm canister in the hands while shaking it for 10 to 15 seconds.

• Unlock canister top; then turn it upside down and insert applicator tip into rectum.

• Push down on pump dome for 2 seconds and hold applicator in place for 10 to 15 seconds.

• Withdraw and discard used applicator.

ACTION

Significant glucocorticoid effects caused by drug's high affinity for glucocorticoid receptors.

Route	Onset	Peak	Duration
PO	Unknown	0.5–10 hr	Unknown
PO (extended-release)	Unknown	7.4–19.2 hr	Unknown
Rectal	Unknown	Unknown	Unknown

Half-life: 2 to 3.6 hours.

ADVERSE REACTIONS

CNS: headache, dizziness, asthenia, hyperkinesia, paresthesia, tremor, vertigo, fatigue, malaise, agitation, confusion, insomnia, nervousness, somnolence, pain, sleep disorder. **CV:** chest pain, HTN, palpitations, tachycardia, flushing. **EENT:** facial edema, ear infection, eye abnormality, abnormal vision, sinusitis. **GI:** nausea, diarrhea, dyspepsia, abdominal pain, flatulence, vomiting, anal disorder, aggravated Crohn disease, enteritis, epigastric pain, fistula, glossitis, hemorrhoids, intestinal obstruction, tongue edema, tooth disorder, increased appetite, abdominal distention, constipation. **GU:** dysuria, micturition frequency, nocturia, intermenstrual bleeding, menstrual disorder, hematuria, pyuria, UTI. **Hematologic:** leukocytosis, anemia. **Metabolic:** hypercorticism, dependent edema, hypokalemia, increased weight. **Musculoskeletal:** back pain, aggravated arthritis, cramps, arthralgia, myalgia. **Respiratory:** respiratory tract infection, bronchitis, dyspnea. **Skin:** acne, alopecia, dermatitis, eczema, skin disorder, increased sweating, purpura. **Other:** flulike disorder, candidiasis, viral infection.

INTERACTIONS

Drug-drug. *Barbiturates (phenobarbital), rifamycins (rifampin):* May decrease budesonide effects. Adjust budesonide dosage as clinically indicated.

CYP3A4 inhibitors (cyclosporine, erythromycin, indinavir, itraconazole, ketoconazole, ritonavir, saquinavir): May increase effects of budesonide. If use together is unavoidable, reduce budesonide dosage.

Gastric acid secretion inhibitors (antacids, H₂ blockers, PPIs): May affect dissolution of extended-release budesonide. Avoid use together or separate administration times by as much as possible and monitor clinical response to budesonide.

Quinolones (levofloxacin): May increase risk of tendon rupture when taken concomitantly with corticosteroids. Avoid use together.

Salicylates (aspirin): May decrease salicylate level and effectiveness and increase risk of GI bleeding. Monitor patient response and adjust salicylate dosage as needed.

Drug-food. *Grapefruit juice:* May increase drug effects. Discourage use together.

EFFECTS ON LAB TEST RESULTS
• May increase alkaline phosphatase and C-reactive protein levels. May decrease potassium, cortisol, and Hb levels.
• May increase erythrocyte sedimentation rate and WBC count.

CONTRAINDICATIONS & CAUTIONS
• Contraindicated in patients hypersensitive to drug.
• Use cautiously in patients with TB, HTN, diabetes mellitus, osteoporosis, hepatic impairment, peptic ulcer disease, glaucoma, or cataracts; those with a family history of diabetes or glaucoma; and those with any other condition in which glucocorticoids may have unwanted effects.
Dialyzable drug: Unlikely.
⚠ *Overdose S&S:* Hypercorticism, adrenal suppression.

PREGNANCY-LACTATION-REPRODUCTION
• Drug may be used cautiously for the induction of remission in pregnant women with inflammatory bowel disease. Use only if potential benefit justifies potential risk to the fetus.
• Monitor infants born of mothers receiving corticosteroids during pregnancy for signs and symptoms of hypoadrenalism, such as poor feeding, irritability, weakness, and vomiting.

• Glucocorticoids appear in human milk, and infants may have adverse reactions. Use cautiously in breastfeeding women and only if benefits outweigh risks.

NURSING CONSIDERATIONS
• Reduced liver function affects elimination of this drug; systemic availability of drug may increase in patients with liver cirrhosis. Consider dosage reduction.
• Patients undergoing surgery or other stressful situations may need systemic glucocorticoid supplementation in addition to budesonide therapy.
• Carefully monitor patients transferred from systemic glucocorticoid therapy to budesonide for signs and symptoms of corticosteroid withdrawal. Watch for immunosuppression, especially in patients who haven't had diseases such as chickenpox or measles; these can be fatal in patients who are immunosuppressed or receiving glucocorticoids.
• Replacement of systemic glucocorticoids with this drug may unmask allergies, such as eczema and rhinitis, which were previously controlled by systemic drug.
• Long-term use of drug may cause hypercorticism and adrenal suppression.

PATIENT TEACHING
• Tell patient to swallow capsules and tablets whole and not to chew, crush, or break them.
• Advise patient to avoid grapefruit juice while taking drug.
• Tell patient to notify prescriber immediately if patient is exposed to or develops chickenpox or measles or develops signs and symptoms of infection during treatment.
• Tell patient to keep container tightly closed.
• Teach patient how to administer rectal formulation and to keep it away from flame.

Reactions in bold italics are *life-threatening*. Interactions may have a *rapid onset* or a *delayed onset*.

B

bumetanide
byoo-MET-a-nide

Bumex⚘, Burinex✤

Therapeutic class: Diuretics
Pharmacologic class: Loop diuretics

AVAILABLE FORMS
Injection: 0.25 mg/mL
Tablets: 0.5 mg, 1 mg, 2 mg, 5 mg✤

INDICATIONS & DOSAGES
➤ **Edema caused by HF or hepatic or renal disease**
Adults: 0.5 to 2 mg PO once daily. If diuretic response isn't adequate, a second or third dose may be given at 4- to 5-hour intervals. Or (recommended as the safest and most effective method for the continued control of edema) give on an intermittent-dose schedule on alternate days or for 3 to 4 days with rest periods of 1 or 2 days in between. Maximum, 10 mg daily.

May give parenterally if oral route isn't possible. Usual first dose is 0.5 to 1 mg IV or IM. If response isn't adequate, may give a second or third dose at 2- to 3-hour intervals. Maximum, 10 mg daily.

ADMINISTRATION
PO
• To prevent nocturia, give drug in morning. If second dose is needed, give in early afternoon.
IV
▼ For direct injection, give drug over 1 to 2 minutes.
▼ For intermittent infusion, give diluted drug through an intermittent infusion device or piggyback into an IV line containing a free-flowing, compatible solution.
▼ Solutions should be freshly prepared and used within 24 hours. Protect from light.
▼ **Incompatibilities:** None listed by manufacturer. Consult a drug incompatibility reference for more information.
IM
• Document injection site.

ACTION
Inhibits sodium and chloride reabsorption in the ascending loop of Henle.

Route	Onset	Peak	Duration
PO	30–60 min	1–2 hr	4–6 hr
IV	Within min	15–30 min	2–3 hr
IM	40 min	Unknown	5–6 hr

Half-life: 1 to 1½ hours.

ADVERSE REACTIONS
CNS: dizziness, headache, vertigo. **CV:** orthostatic hypotension. **EENT:** deafness, tinnitus. **GU:** azotemia, oliguria. **Metabolic:** volume depletion and dehydration, hypokalemia, hypochloremic alkalosis, *hypomagnesemia,* asymptomatic hyperuricemia, hyponatremia, elevated blood glucose level. **Musculoskeletal:** muscle cramps. **Skin:** rash, pruritus.

INTERACTIONS
Drug-drug. *Aminoglycoside antibiotics:* May increase ototoxicity. Avoid using together if possible.
Antidiabetics: May decrease hypoglycemic effects. Monitor glucose level.
Antihypertensives: May increase hypotensive effects. Consider dosage adjustment.
Cardiac glycosides: May increase risk of digoxin toxicity from bumetanide-induced hypokalemia. Monitor potassium and digoxin levels.
Chlorothiazide, chlorthalidone, furosemide, hydrochlorothiazide, indapamide, metolazone: May cause excessive diuretic response, causing serious electrolyte abnormalities or dehydration. Adjust doses carefully, and monitor patient closely for signs and symptoms of excessive diuretic response.
Cisplatin: May increase risk of ototoxicity. Monitor patient closely.
Lithium: May decrease lithium clearance, increasing risk of lithium toxicity. Monitor lithium level.
Neuromuscular blockers: May prolong neuromuscular blockade. Monitor patient closely.
NSAIDs, probenecid: May inhibit diuretic response. Use together cautiously.
Other potassium-wasting drugs (amphotericin B, corticosteroids): May increase risk of hypokalemia. Use together cautiously.

Drug-herb. *Dandelion:* May increase diuresis. Discourage use together.
Licorice: May cause unexpected, rapid potassium loss. Discourage use together.

EFFECTS ON LAB TEST RESULTS
• May increase alkaline phosphatase, ALT, AST, bilirubin, cholesterol, creatinine, glucose, LDH, BUN, and urine urea levels.
• May decrease calcium, magnesium, potassium, sodium, and chloride levels.
• May decrease platelet count.

CONTRAINDICATIONS & CAUTIONS
• Contraindicated in patients hypersensitive to drug and in patients with anuria, hepatic coma, or severe electrolyte depletion.
• Patients allergic to sulfonamides may show hypersensitivity to bumetanide.
• Use cautiously in patients with hepatic cirrhosis and ascites, in elderly patients, and in those with decreased renal function.
Dialyzable drug: Unknown.
⚠ *Overdose S&S:* Electrolyte depletion, weakness, dizziness, confusion, anorexia, lethargy, vomiting, cramps, dehydration, circulatory collapse, vascular thrombosis, and embolism.

PREGNANCY-LACTATION-REPRODUCTION
• There are no adequate well-controlled studies in pregnant women. Use during pregnancy only if potential benefits justify potential risk to the fetus.
• Use in breastfeeding women isn't recommended.

NURSING CONSIDERATIONS
Black Box Warning Profound diuresis with electrolyte depletion can occur. Adjust dosage and dosing schedule to individual patient's needs; careful medical supervision is required. ∎
• Monitor fluid intake and output, weight, and electrolyte, BUN, creatinine, and carbon dioxide levels frequently, especially in elderly patients.
• Watch for evidence of hypokalemia, such as muscle weakness and cramps. Instruct patient to report these symptoms.
• Consult prescriber and dietitian about a high-potassium diet. Foods rich in potassium

include citrus fruits, tomatoes, bananas, dates, and apricots.
• Monitor glucose level in diabetic patients.
• Monitor uric acid level, especially in patients with history of gout.
• If oliguria or azotemia develops or increases, prescriber may stop drug.
• Drug can be safely used in patients allergic to furosemide; 1 mg of bumetanide equals about 40 mg of furosemide.
• Monitor patient for ototoxicity, especially when drug is given IV, at high doses, and in combination with other ototoxins.

PATIENT TEACHING
• Instruct patient to weigh self daily to monitor fluid status.
• Advise patient to take drug in morning to avoid need to urinate at night. Tell patient who needs second dose to take it in early afternoon.
• Advise patient to avoid sudden posture changes and to rise slowly to avoid dizziness upon standing quickly.
• Instruct patient to notify prescriber about extreme thirst, muscle weakness, cramps, nausea, or dizziness.

SAFETY ALERT!

buprenorphine
byoo-pre-NOR-feen

Butrans, Sublocade

buprenorphine hydrochloride
Belbuca, Buprenex, Probuphine

Therapeutic class: Opioid analgesics
Pharmacologic class: Opioid agonist-antagonists–opioid partial agonists
Controlled substance schedule: III

AVAILABLE FORMS
Buccal film: 75 mcg, 150 mcg, 300 mcg, 450 mcg, 600 mcg, 750 mcg, 900 mcg
Injection: 0.324 mg (equivalent to 0.3 mg base/mL)
Injection (extended-release): 100 mg/0.5 mL, 300 mg/1.5 mL prefilled syringes
Subdermal implant: 74.2 mg buprenorphine (equivalent to 80 mg of buprenorphine hydrochloride)

Sublingual tablets ⓓⓝⓒ: 2 mg, 8 mg (as base)
Transdermal patch: 5 mcg/hour, 7.5 mcg/
hour, 10 mcg/hour, 15 mcg/hour, 20 mcg/
hour

INDICATIONS & DOSAGES
➤ **Maintenance treatment of opioid dependence in patients who have achieved and sustained prolonged clinical stability on low to moderate doses (8 mg/day or less) of a transmucosal buprenorphine-containing product for 3 months or longer with no need for supplemental dosing or adjustments**
Adults: 1 dose (4 implants) inserted subdermally in the inner side of the upper arm and kept in place for 6 months. If continued treatment is desired, dose may be repeated once in the other arm for an additional 6 months.
➤ **Moderate to severe pain**
Adults and children age 13 and older: 0.3 mg IM or slow IV (over at least 2 minutes) every 6 hours p.r.n., or around the clock; repeat dose once (up to 0.3 mg), as needed, 30 to 60 minutes after first dose. May increase IM dosing to 0.6 mg/dose. *Children ages 2 to 12:* 2 to 6 mcg/kg IM or slow IV (over at least 2 minutes) every 4 to 6 hours.
Adjust-a-dose: In high-risk patients, such as debilitated or elderly patients, use minimum dose required.
➤ **Moderate to severe chronic pain in patients requiring continuous opioid analgesia for an extended period of time**
Adults (opioid-naive): 5 mcg/hour transdermal patch once every 7 days. To achieve adequate analgesia and minimize adverse effects, consider patient's tolerance, condition, and other medications and titrate dosage to maximum of 20 mcg/hour. Allow minimum of 72 hours between dosage increases. Or, 75 mcg buccal film once daily or, if tolerated, every 12 hours for at least 4 days; then increase to 150 mcg every 12 hours. Titrate dosage in increments of 150 mcg every 12 hours, no more frequently than every 4 days. Maximum, 450 mcg every 12 hours.
Adults (non–opioid-naive): Buprenorphine may precipitate withdrawal in patients already on opioids. For conversion from other

opioids to transdermal buprenorphine, taper patient's current around-the-clock opioids for up to 7 days to no more than morphine 30 mg or equivalent per day before beginning treatment with buprenorphine. Patients may use short-acting analgesics as needed until analgesic efficacy with buprenorphine is attained. For patients whose daily dose was less than morphine 30 mg PO or equivalent, initiate treatment with buprenorphine transdermal patch 5 mcg/hour. For patients whose daily dose was between 30 and 80 mg of morphine equivalents, initiate treatment with buprenorphine transdermal patch 10 mcg/hour.

For patients whose daily dose was greater than 80 mg of morphine equivalents, buprenorphine transdermal system 20 mcg/hour may not provide adequate analgesia for patients requiring greater than 80 mg/day oral morphine equivalents. Consider the use of an alternative analgesic.

To achieve adequate analgesia with tolerable adverse effects, consider patient's tolerance, condition, and other medications and titrate dosage to maximum of 20 mcg/hour transdermal patch once every 7 days. Allow minimum of 72 hours between dosage increases. If patch must be discontinued, taper dosage gradually every 7 days to prevent withdrawal in the physically dependent patient; consider initiating immediate-release opioids, if needed.

Or, for conversion from other opioids to buccal buprenorphine, taper dosage to no more than 30 mg PO morphine sulfate equivalents (MSE) per day. For patients taking less than 30 mg PO MSE per day, start treatment with 75 mcg buccal film once daily or every 12 hours. For patients taking between 30 and 89 mg PO MSE, start treatment with 150 mcg every 12 hours. For patients taking between 90 and 160 mg PO MSE, start treatment with 300 mg every 12 hours. Buccal buprenorphine may not provide adequate analgesia for patients requiring greater than 160 mg PO MSE per day. Consider using an alternative analgesic. Titrate dosage in increments of 150 mcg every 12 hours, no more frequently than every 4 days to a maximum dose of 900 mcg every 12 hours.

To discontinue buccal therapy, taper dosage gradually while monitoring patient carefully for signs and symptoms of withdrawal. If patient develops withdrawal signs or symptoms, increase dosage to previous level and taper more slowly by increasing the interval between decreases, decreasing the amount of change in dose, or both.

Adjust-a-dose: Transdermal buprenorphine hasn't been evaluated in patients with severe hepatic impairment. Consider use of an alternative analgesic that may permit more dosing flexibility in these patients.

Adjust-a-dose: In patients with severe hepatic impairment, reduce the buccal starting dose and reduce the buccal titration dose by half that of patients with normal liver function, from 150 to 75 mcg. In patients with known or suspected mucositis, reduce starting dosage and titration incremental dosage by half compared to patients without mucositis.

➤ **Opioid dependence**

Adults: 8 mg SL on day 1 and 16 mg SL on day 2. Titrate buprenorphine dosage in increments or decrements of 2 or 4 mg to a level that holds patient in treatment and suppresses opioid withdrawal signs and symptoms. Maintenance dose is generally in the range of 4 to 24 mg SL per day. Recommended target dosage is 16 mg as a single daily dose. Continue treatment for as long as patient is benefiting and the drug contributes to intended treatment goals.

➤ **Moderate to severe opioid use disorder in patients who have initiated treatment with a transmucosal buprenorphine-containing product, followed by dosage adjustment for a minimum of 7 days (Sublocade)**

Adults: 300 mg (extended-release) subcut monthly for first 2 months, followed by 100 mg (extended-release) subcut maintenance dose monthly. May increase maintenance dose to 300 mg monthly for patients who tolerate 100-mg dose but don't demonstrate a satisfactory clinical response. Administer drug with a minimum of 26 days between doses.

ADMINISTRATION
IV
▼ When mixed in a 1:1 volume ratio, drug is compatible with atropine sulfate, diphenhydramine hydrochloride, droperidol, glycopyrrolate, haloperidol lactate, hydroxyzine hydrochloride, promethazine hydrochloride, scopolamine hydrochloride, D_5W, 5% dextrose in NSS, NSS, lactated Ringer solution, and NSS injections.

▼ For direct injection, give slowly over at least 2 minutes into a vein or through tubing of a free-flowing, compatible IV solution.

▼ **Incompatibilities:** None listed by manufacturer. Consult a drug incompatibility reference for more information.

IM
● Refer to manufacturer's instructions.
● Give drug as deep IM injection.

Subcutaneous
Black Box Warning Sublocade may cause serious harm or death if given IV. Don't administer Sublocade IV or IM. ■
● Only health care providers should prepare and administer Sublocade.
● Use only syringe and safety needle supplied.
● Remove drug from refrigerator at least 15 minutes before use. Don't open foil pack until ready for use. Discard drug if left at room temperature for longer than 7 days.
● Don't use if particles are present.
● Remove excess air from syringe and inject drug subcut in abdomen only. Select a site between the transpyloric and transtubercular planes, avoiding areas where skin is irritated, red, bruised, infected, or scarred.
● Don't rub skin after injection. A lump may be felt for several weeks that will shrink over time.
● Rotate injection sites.
● Give a missed dose as soon as possible, with the next dose no sooner than 26 days later. Occasional dosing delays up to 2 weeks aren't expected to significantly impact treatment.

Sublingual
● Place all the tablets of the dose under the tongue until dissolved.
● Patient shouldn't eat or drink anything until the tablets are completely dissolved.

Subdermal

Black Box Warning Subdermal implant is only available through the Probuphine REMS Program. All health care providers must become certified before performing insertions or removals, or prescribing implants. ∎

• Each dose (4 implants) is inserted subdermally under local anesthesia in the inner side of the upper arm, remains in place for 6 months, then is removed at the end of the sixth month.

• At the time of implant removal, new implants may be inserted subdermally in an area of the inner side of either upper arm that hasn't been previously used, if continued treatment is desired. If new implants aren't inserted on the same day as implant removal, maintain patients on their previous dosage of transmucosal buprenorphine.

• After one insertion in each arm, most patients should be transitioned back to a transmucosal buprenorphine-containing product for continued treatment.

Transdermal

❸ *Alert:* Avoid exposing patch or surrounding area to direct external heat source or direct sunlight. Such exposure may increase amount of drug released, which can result in overdose and death.

❸ *Alert:* Transdermal patch is indicated only for moderate to severe chronic pain that requires around-the-clock analgesia for an extended period of time.

• Each patch is intended to be worn for 7 days. If patch falls off during 7-day dosing interval, apply new patch to different site.

• Don't use if pouch seal is broken or patch is cut, damaged, or altered. Apply patch to intact skin immediately after opening.

• Appropriate application sites are upper outer arm, upper chest, upper back, or side of the chest (eight total available sites).

• Application site should be hairless; clip hair if needed but don't shave site. If needed, clean selected site with water only and allow to dry completely before applying patch.

• Edges of patch may be taped to the skin if needed.

• After removing patch, fold it in half, seal it in patch-disposal unit, and place it in trash.

• Wait minimum of 3 weeks before applying new patch to same application site.

• Exposure of patch to water, such as while bathing or showering, is acceptable.

Buccal

• To administer, first have patient moisten inside of cheek with tongue or water.

• Apply film immediately after removal from sealed package. Place yellow side of film against inside of cheek and hold in place with dry fingers for 5 seconds; then leave in place until film fully dissolves (about 30 minutes).

• Make sure patient doesn't chew or swallow film and doesn't eat or drink until film has dissolved.

ACTION

Unknown. Binds with opioid receptors in the CNS, altering perception of and emotional response to pain.

Route	Onset	Peak	Duration
IV	Immediate	2 min	6 hr
IM	15 min	1 hr	6 hr
Subcut	Unknown	24 hr	Unknown
SL	Unknown	30–60 min	Unknown
Subdermal	Unknown	12 hr	24 wk
Transdermal	17 hr	3–6 days	7 days
Buccal	Unknown	½–4 hr	Unknown

Half-life: 1 to 7 hours; subcut, 43 to 60 days; subdermal, 24 to 48 hours; transdermal, 26 hours; buccal, 16 to 39 hours.

ADVERSE REACTIONS

CNS: dizziness, sedation, vertigo, *increased ICP,* asthenia (tablets only), confusion, depression, dreaming, euphoria, fatigue, headache, insomnia, nervousness, pain, paresthesia, psychosis, slurred speech, weakness, somnolence, fever. **CV:** *brady-cardia,* cyanosis, flushing, HTN, hypotension, tachycardia, peripheral edema. **EENT:** blurred vision, conjunctivitis, diplopia, visual abnormalities, miosis, tinnitus, rhinitis (tablets only), dry mouth (patch, buccal film), toothache, oropharyngeal pain. **GI:** nausea, abdominal pain (oral only), constipation, diarrhea (oral only), vomiting, anorexia, dry mouth, dyspepsia. **GU:** urine retention, UTI. **Musculoskeletal:** arthralgia, back pain (tablets only), joint swelling, extremity pain. **Respiratory:** *respiratory depression,* dyspnea, hypoventilation, URI. **Skin:** application-site rash or erythema (patch), diaphoresis, injection-site reactions, pruritus, sweating; implant-site pain, pruritus, erythema (Probuphine). **Other:** chills, infection (tablets only), withdrawal syndrome, flulike symptoms.

INTERACTIONS
Drug-drug. *Anticholinergics:* May increase risk of constipation and urine retention. Monitor therapy.

Black Box Warning *Benzodiazepines, CNS depressants:* May cause slow or difficult breathing, sedation, and death. Avoid use together. If use together is necessary, limit dosage and duration of each drug to the minimum necessary for desired effect. ■

Class IA or III antiarrhythmics: May increase risk of prolonged QT syndrome. Avoid use with transdermal patch.

CYP3A4 inducers (carbamazepine, phenobarbital, phenytoin, rifampin): May increase clearance of buprenorphine. Monitor patient for clinical effects of drug. If patient is taking Sublocade, patient may need to be transitioned back to a formulation that permits dosage adjustments.

CYP3A4 inhibitors (erythromycin, indinavir, ketoconazole, ritonavir, saquinavir): May decrease clearance of buprenorphine. Monitor patient for increased adverse effects.

Diuretics: May decrease therapeutic effects of diuretics. Monitor therapy.

MAO inhibitors: May cause additive effects. Avoid use together.

NNRTIs (delavirdine, efavirenz, etravirine, nevirapine): May increase or decrease therapeutic effects of Sublocade. Monitor therapy closely.

☉ Alert: *Serotonergic drugs (amoxapine, antiemetics [dolasetron, granisetron, ondansetron, palonosetron], antimigraine drugs, buspirone, cyclobenzaprine, dextromethorphan, linezolid, lithium, MAO inhibitors, maprotiline, methylene blue, mirtazapine, nefazodone, SSNRIs, SSRIs, TCAs, trazodone, tryptophan, vilazodone):* Can increase risk of serotonin syndrome. Use together cautiously; monitor patient for serotonin syndrome.

Skeletal muscle relaxants: May enhance neuromuscular blocking action and increase respiratory depression. Use together cautiously.

Drug-lifestyle. *Alcohol or illicit drug use:* May cause additive effects. Discourage use together.

EFFECTS ON LAB TEST RESULTS
• May increase amylase, ALT, AST, GGT, and CK levels.

CONTRAINDICATIONS & CAUTIONS
• Contraindicated in patients hypersensitive to drug and in those with paralytic ileus or GI obstruction.

Black Box Warning Serious, life-threatening, or fatal respiratory depression may occur, especially during drug initiation or after a dosage increase. Misuse or abuse of drug by chewing, swallowing, snorting, or injecting buprenorphine extracted from the transdermal system will result in the uncontrolled delivery of buprenorphine and will pose a significant risk of overdose and death. ■

Black Box Warning *Opioid class warning:* Opioids should only be prescribed with benzodiazepines or other CNS depressants to patients for whom alternative treatment options are inadequate. ■

Black Box Warning Rare but serious complications, including nerve damage and migration of the implant resulting in embolism and death, may result from improper insertion of implants inserted in the upper arm. Incomplete insertions or infections may lead to protrusion or expulsion. Because of the risks associated with insertion and removal, the buprenorphine implant is available only through the Probuphine REMS Program. All health care providers must be trained and certified before performing insertions or removals, or prescribing buprenorphine implants. ■

Black Box Warning Sublocade is only available through the Sublocade REMS Program. Health care settings and pharmacies that order and dispense this drug must be certified in this program and comply with the REMS requirements. ■

Black Box Warning Never inject Sublocade IV. Serious harm or death can occur as drug forms a solid mass upon contact with body fluids. If given IV, local tissue damage and thromboembolic events can occur. ■

◑ Alert: Don't exceed dose of one 20-mcg/hour transdermal patch every 7 days or 900 mcg every 12 hours for buccal film due to risk of prolonging QTc interval.

◑ Alert: Patients are at increased risk for oversedation and respiratory depression if they snore or have a history of sleep apnea, haven't used opioids recently or are first-time opioid users, have increased opioid dosage requirements or opioid habituation, received general anesthesia for longer lengths of time, received other sedating drugs, have thoracic or other surgical incisions that may impair breathing, or have preexisting pulmonary or cardiac disease. Monitor these patients carefully.

◑ Alert: Drug may lead to rare but serious decrease in adrenal gland cortisol production.

◑ Alert: Drug may cause decreased sex hormone levels with long-term use.

◑ Alert: Combined use of medication-assisted treatment (MAT) drugs methadone or buprenorphine with benzodiazepines or other CNS depressants increases risk of serious adverse effects; however, the harm caused by untreated opioid addiction may outweigh these risks. Patients may require MAT for opioid addiction indefinitely, and the use of these drugs should continue for as long as patients are benefiting and their use contributes to the intended treatment goals.

• Use cautiously in elderly or debilitated patients; patients who are opioid dependent; in those undergoing biliary tract surgery and those with biliary tract disease or pancreatitis; in those with head injury, intracranial lesions, and increased ICP; severe respiratory, liver, or kidney impairment; CNS depression or coma; those at risk for hypotension and circulatory shock; and in those with thyroid irregularities, adrenal insufficiency, prostatic hypertrophy, urethral stricture, acute alcoholism, delirium tremens, or kyphoscoliosis.

• The transdermal patch and buccal film are included in the REMS Program for extended-release and long-acting opioids. Prescribers are encouraged to undergo REMS training and counsel patients on safe drug use.

• Don't use Sublocade in patients with pre-existing moderate to severe hepatic impairment as buprenorphine levels can't be

rapidly adjusted. If patient develops moderate to severe hepatic impairment during treatment, and buprenorphine toxicity or overdose occurs within 2 weeks of drug administration, surgical removal of the depot may be needed.

Dialyzable drug: Unknown.

⚠ Overdose S&S: Respiratory depression, pinpoint pupils, sedation, hypotension, death, snoring, bradycardia, cool and clammy skin, partial or complete airway obstruction, skeletal muscle flaccidity, somnolence.

PREGNANCY-LACTATION-REPRODUCTION

• There are no adequate and controlled studies in pregnant women. Use during pregnancy only if potential benefits justify risk to the fetus.

Black Box Warning Prolonged use during pregnancy can result in neonatal opioid withdrawal syndrome, which may be life-threatening if not recognized and treated and requires management according to protocols developed by neonatology experts. If prolonged opioid use is required in a pregnant woman, advise patient of the risk of neonatal opioid withdrawal syndrome and ensure her that appropriate treatment will be available. ■

• Drug appears in human milk. Use in breastfeeding women isn't recommended.

• Breastfeeding infants exposed to large doses of opioids should be monitored for apnea and sedation. Withdrawal symptoms can occur in breastfed infants when maternal administration of drug is stopped or when breastfeeding is stopped.

NURSING CONSIDERATIONS

Black Box Warning Buprenorphine has potential for abuse similar to other opioids and is a controlled substance. Patients at risk for opioid abuse include those with personal or family history of substance abuse or mental illness. Assess for risk of abuse before prescribing, and monitor patients regularly. ■

Black Box Warning Accidental exposure to drug, especially in children, can cause a fatal overdose. ■

• Don't stop drug abruptly; withdraw slowly and individualize the gradual taper plan to prevent signs and symptoms of withdrawal, worsening pain, and psychological distress in physically dependent patients. Refer to manufacturer's label for specific tapering instructions.

• When tapering opioids, watch closely for signs and symptoms of opioid withdrawal. Such symptoms may indicate a need to taper more slowly. Also monitor patient for suicidal thoughts, use of other substances, and mood changes.

❸ *Alert:* Carefully monitor vital signs, pain level, respiratory status, and sedation level in patients receiving opioids, especially those receiving IV opioids postoperatively.

❸ *Alert:* If patient is taking opioids with serotonergic drugs, watch for signs and symptoms of serotonin syndrome (agitation, hallucinations, rapid HR, fever, excessive sweating, shivering or shaking, muscle twitching or stiffness, trouble with coordination, nausea, vomiting, diarrhea), especially when starting treatment or increasing dosages. Signs and symptoms may occur within several hours of coadministration but may also occur later, especially after dosage increase. Discontinue the opioid, serotonergic drug, or both if serotonin syndrome is suspected.

❸ *Alert:* Monitor patient for signs and symptoms of adrenal insufficiency (nausea, vomiting, loss of appetite, fatigue, weakness, dizziness, low BP). Perform diagnostic testing if adrenal insufficiency is suspected. If adrenal insufficiency is confirmed, treat with corticosteroids and wean patient off opioids if appropriate. Discontinue corticosteroids when clinically appropriate.

❸ *Alert:* Monitor patient for signs and symptoms of decreased sex hormone levels (low libido, erectile dysfunction, amenorrhea, infertility). If symptoms occur, evaluate patient and obtain additional laboratory testing.

❸ *Alert:* Monitor patient with subdermal implant for nerve damage; implant migration, protrusion, or expulsion; and infection.

❸ *Alert:* Work with patient to develop strategies to manage the use of prescribed or illicit benzodiazepines or other CNS depressants when starting MAT. Taper benzodiazepine or CNS depressant to discontinuation, if possible.

❸ *Alert:* If patient is receiving prescribed benzodiazepines or other CNS depressants

for anxiety or insomnia, verify diagnosis and consider other treatment options for these conditions, if possible.

❸ *Alert:* Coordinate care to ensure other prescribers are aware of patient's MAT.

❸ *Alert:* Monitor patient for illicit drug use, including urine or blood screening.

• Drug may prolong QT interval and increase risk of ventricular arrhythmias. Avoid use in patients with a personal or family history of long QT syndrome. Use caution and periodically monitor ECGs in patients with hypokalemia, hypomagnesemia, unstable cardiac disease including atrial fibrillation, unstable HF, or active myocardial ischemia.

• For patients at risk for hepatotoxicity, monitor LFTs before and during treatment.

• Drug should be used as part of a complete treatment program that includes counseling and psychosocial support.

• Taper dosage before discontinuing transdermal patch and buccal film. Monitor patients for signs and symptoms of withdrawal.

• Drug may worsen increased ICP and mask its signs and symptoms. Carefully monitor patient's pupillary reflexes and level of consciousness.

• Monitor patients with history of seizure disorders for worsening of condition.

• Monitor patients for signs and symptoms of hypotension after initiating therapy or increasing dosage.

• Monitor patients with fever or increased core body temperature after exertion; adjust dosage if signs or symptoms of respiratory or CNS depression occur.

• Watch for worsening of symptoms in patients with biliary tract disease, including acute pancreatitis; drug may cause spasm of sphincter of Oddi.

• Reassess patient's level of pain 15 and 30 minutes after parenteral administration.

• Buprenorphine 0.3 mg is equal to 10 mg of morphine and 75 mg of meperidine in analgesic potency. It has longer duration of action than morphine or meperidine.

❸ *Alert:* Naloxone won't completely reverse the respiratory depression caused by buprenorphine overdose; an overdose may require mechanical ventilation. Larger-than-usual doses of naloxone (more than 0.4 mg) and doxapram also may be indicated.

Reactions in bold italics are *life-threatening*. Interactions may have a *rapid onset* or a *delayed onset*.

• Treat accidental skin exposure by removing exposed clothing and rinsing skin with water.

• Drug may cause constipation. Assess bowel function and need for stool softeners and stimulant laxatives.

🜲 **Alert:** Drug's opioid antagonist properties may cause withdrawal syndrome in opioid-dependent patients.

• If dependence occurs, withdrawal symptoms may appear up to 14 days after drug is stopped.

• If Sublocade depot must be surgically removed, or treatment discontinued, monitor patient for signs and symptoms of withdrawal and treat appropriately.

• Regularly monitor Sublocade subcut injection site for evidence of tampering or attempted removal of the drug depot.

• Use cautiously in morbidly obese patients.

• In patients with oral mucositis using the buccal film, consider reducing dose; oral mucositis may lead to faster absorption and higher blood concentration of drug.

• **Look alike–sound alike:** Don't confuse Buprenex with Bumex. Don't confuse buprenorphine with bupropion.

PATIENT TEACHING

🜲 **Alert:** Encourage patient to report all medications being taken, including prescription and OTC drugs and supplements.

Black Box Warning *Opioid class warning:* Caution patient or caregiver of patient taking an opioid with a benzodiazepine, CNS depressant, or alcohol to seek immediate medical attention for dizziness, lightheadedness, extreme sleepiness, slowed or difficult breathing, or unresponsiveness. ∎

🜲 **Alert:** Caution patient to immediately report signs and symptoms of hypersensitivity reaction (rash, hives, itching, facial swelling, wheezing, dizziness), serotonin syndrome, adrenal insufficiency, decreased sex hormone levels, or liver impairment (yellowing of skin or eyes, dark urine, light-colored stools, abdominal pain, nausea).

🜲 **Alert:** Teach patient to avoid nonprescribed benzodiazepines, sedatives, or alcohol when taking MAT due to increased risk of overdose and death.

• Advise patient to notify all prescribers of MAT and not to stop MAT or other

prescribed drugs without first consulting prescriber to determine need for gradual tapering regimen.

• Tell patient and family to immediately report adverse reactions to prescriber.

• If an emergency occurs, advise patient and caregivers to report that patient is dependent on an opioid and to describe the specific treatment patient is receiving.

• Caution ambulatory patient about getting out of bed or chair quickly or walking, as hypotension can occur.

• Warn patient that drug can cause dependence, and withdrawal can occur when drug is discontinued.

• Teach patient not to drive, operate heavy machinery, or perform dangerous activities until drug's effects are known.

• When drug is used after surgery, encourage patient to turn, cough, and breathe deeply to prevent breathing problems.

• Explain assessment and monitoring process to patient and family. Instruct them to immediately report difficulty breathing or other signs or symptoms of potential adverse opioid-related reaction.

• Tell patient to place all tablets of dose under the tongue until dissolved. If this is uncomfortable, tell patient to take at least two at the same time. Warn patient not to eat or drink until all tablets are dissolved.

• Instruct patient in proper disposal of transdermal system.

• Teach patient proper patch application and to read package instructions.

• Warn patient not to apply heat to patch application site or to cut patch.

• Teach patient proper buccal film administration.

• Warn patient not to take other long-acting opioids while using transdermal system or buccal film.

• Teach patient that Sublocade may only be given by a health care provider and that the subcut depot may be felt as a lump for several weeks. Tell patient not to rub the injection site or wear restrictive clothing over it.

• Emphasize importance of counseling and psychosocial support to patient taking drug.

• Advise patient with subdermal implant to report signs and symptoms of infection or delayed wound healing, including evidence of implant extrusion from the skin.

• Tell patient that evaluation by the health care provider will be needed at least 1 week after implant insertion and monthly thereafter.

buPROPion hydrobromide
byoo-PROE-pee-on

Aplenzin

buPROPion hydrochloride
Forfivo XL, Wellbutrin SR✦, Wellbutrin XL, Zyban✦

Therapeutic class: Antidepressants
Pharmacologic class: Aminoketones

AVAILABLE FORMS
bupropion hydrobromide
Tablets (extended-release) ⒸⓅⒻ: 174 mg, 348 mg, 522 mg
bupropion hydrochloride
Tablets (extended-release 12-hour) ⒸⓅⒻ: 100 mg, 150 mg, 200 mg
Tablets (extended-release 24-hour) ⒸⓅⒻ: 150 mg, 300 mg, 450 mg
Tablets (immediate-release) ⒸⓅⒻ: 75 mg, 100 mg

INDICATIONS & DOSAGES
Adjust-a-dose (for all indications): In patients with renal impairment (GFR less than 90 mL/minute) or mild hepatic impairment (Child-Pugh score 5 to 6), consider reduced frequency or dosage. In patients with moderate to severe hepatic impairment (Child-Pugh score 7 to 15), don't exceed 174 mg every other day (Aplenzin); 100 mg per day or 150 mg every other day (sustained-release tablets); 150 mg every other day (extended-release tablets); 75 mg per day (immediate-release tablets); 150 mg every other day (Wellbutrin XL, Zyban). Forfivo XL isn't recommended in patients with renal or hepatic impairment.
➤ **Major depressive disorder (Aplenzin only)**
Adults: Initially, 174 mg PO (equivalent to 150 mg/day bupropion HCl) given as a single daily dose in the morning. If the 174-mg dose is adequately tolerated, increase to target dose of 348 mg once daily in the

morning as early as day 4 of dosing. The full antidepressant effect may not be evident for several months of treatment or longer. When switching patients from Wellbutrin SR or Wellbutrin XL to Aplenzin, give the equivalent total daily dose when possible (522 mg bupropion HBr is equivalent to 450 mg bupropion HCl; 348 mg bupropion HBr is equivalent to 300 mg bupropion HCl; 174 mg bupropion HBr is equivalent to 150 mg bupropion HCl).
➤ **Seasonal affective disorder**
Adults: Start treatment in autumn before depressive symptoms appear. Wellbutrin XL: Initially, 150 mg extended-release PO once daily in the morning. After 1 week, may increase to 300 mg once daily, if tolerated. Continue 300 mg daily during the autumn and winter and taper to 150 mg daily for 2 weeks before stopping the drug in the early spring. Aplenzin: 174 mg PO daily in the morning. May increase to 348 mg PO once daily after 7 days. Taper and discontinue drug in early spring.
➤ **Major depressive disorder (except Aplenzin)**
Adults: For immediate-release, initially, 100 mg PO b.i.d.; increase after 3 days to 100 mg PO t.i.d., if needed. If patient doesn't improve after several weeks of therapy, increase dosage to 150 mg t.i.d. No single dose should exceed 150 mg. Allow at least 6 hours between successive doses. Maximum dose is 450 mg daily. For sustained-release, initially, 150 mg PO every morning; increase to target dose of 150 mg PO b.i.d., as tolerated, as early as day 4 of dosing. Allow at least 8 hours between successive doses. Maximum dose is 400 mg daily. For extended-release, initially, 150 mg PO every morning; increase to target dosage of 300 mg PO daily, as tolerated, as early as day 4 of dosing. Allow at least 24 hours between successive doses. Maximum is 450 mg daily. Don't initiate treatment with Forfivo XL.
➤ **Aid to smoking-cessation treatment**
Adults: 150 mg Zyban PO daily for 3 days; increased to maximum of 300 mg daily in two divided doses at least 8 hours apart. Continue therapy for 7 to 12 weeks. Some patients may need continued treatment.

Reactions in bold italics are ***life-threatening***. Interactions may have a *rapid onset* or a ***delayed onset***.

ADMINISTRATION
PO
- Don't crush, split, or allow patients to chew tablets.
- Give with or without regard to meals.
- When switching patients from immediate-release or sustained-release tablets to extended-release tablets, give the same total daily dose (when possible) as the once-daily dosage provided.

ACTION
Unknown. Drug doesn't inhibit MAO, but it weakly inhibits norepinephrine, dopamine, and serotonin reuptake. Noradrenergic or dopaminergic mechanisms, or both, may cause drug's effect.

Route	Onset	Peak	Duration
PO (extended-release)	Unknown	5 hr	Unknown
PO (immediate-release)	Unknown	2 hr	Unknown
PO (sustained-release)	Unknown	3 hr	Unknown

Half-life: 8 to 24 hours.

ADVERSE REACTIONS
CNS: abnormal dreams, insomnia, headache, sedation, tremor, agitation, dizziness, *seizures, suicidal behavior,* anxiety, confusion, delusions, euphoria, fever, hostility, impaired concentration, impaired sleep quality, akinesia, akathisia, fatigue, syncope, somnolence. **CV:** tachycardia, *arrhythmias,* HTN, hypotension, palpitations, chest pain. **EENT:** blurred vision, rhinitis, auditory disturbances, epistaxis, pharyngitis, sinusitis, dry mouth. **GI:** constipation, nausea, vomiting, anorexia, taste disturbance, dyspepsia, diarrhea, abdominal pain, flatulence. **GU:** erectile dysfunction, menstrual complaints, urinary frequency, urine retention. **Metabolic:** increased appetite, weight loss, weight gain. **Musculoskeletal:** arthritis, myalgia, arthralgia, muscle spasm or twitch. **Respiratory:** upper respiratory complaints, increase in coughing. **Skin:** excessive sweating, pruritus, rash, cutaneous temperature disturbance, urticaria. **Other:** chills, decreased libido, accidental injury, hot flashes.

INTERACTIONS
Drug-drug. *Amantadine, levodopa:* May increase risk of adverse reactions. If used together, give small first doses of bupropion and increase dosage gradually.
Antidepressants (desipramine, fluoxetine, imipramine, nortriptyline, sertraline), antipsychotics (haloperidol, risperidone, thioridazine), systemic corticosteroids, theophylline: May lower seizure threshold. Use cautiously together.
Beta blockers, class IC antiarrhythmics: May increase levels of these drugs and adverse reactions. Use a reduced dose if used with bupropion.
Carbamazepine, phenobarbital, phenytoin: May enhance metabolism of bupropion and decrease its effect. Monitor patient closely.
CYP2B6 substrates or inhibitors (cyclophosphamide, orphenadrine, thiotepa), efavirenz, fluvoxamine, nelfinavir, norfluoxetine, paroxetine, ritonavir, sertraline: May increase bupropion activity. Monitor patient for expected therapeutic effects and adverse effects.
Linezolid, methylene blue: May increase hypertensive effect of bupropion. Use together is contraindicated.
MAO inhibitors: May increase hypertensive effect of bupropion. Don't use these drugs within 14 days of each other.
Nicotine replacement agents: May cause HTN. Monitor BP.
SSRIs: May increase risk of suicidal thinking and behavior in children, adolescents, and young adults with major depressive disorder. Use together cautiously.
Drug-lifestyle. *Alcohol use:* May alter seizure threshold. Discourage use together.
Sun exposure: May increase risk of photosensitivity reactions. Advise patient to avoid excessive sunlight exposure.

EFFECTS ON LAB TEST RESULTS
- May increase LFT values.
- May cause false-positive results for urine detection of amphetamines.

CONTRAINDICATIONS & CAUTIONS
- Contraindicated in patients hypersensitive to drug, in those who have taken MAO inhibitors within previous 14 days, and in those with seizure disorders or history of

bulimia or anorexia nervosa because of a higher risk of seizures.

❸ *Alert:* Concomitant use with SSRIs, linezolid, or methylene blue can cause serotonin syndrome (fever, mental status changes, muscle twitching, excessive sweating, shivering or shaking, diarrhea, loss of coordination). Use drug with SSRIs, linezolid, or methylene blue only for life-threatening or urgent conditions when the potential benefits outweigh the risks of toxicity.

• Hypersensitivity reactions, including anaphylaxis, pruritus, urticaria, angioedema, dyspnea, erythema multiforme, and SJS, have occurred.

• Contraindicated in patients abruptly stopping use of alcohol, sedatives (including benzodiazepines), or antiepileptics.

• Don't use with other drugs containing bupropion.

• Don't initiate therapy with Forfivo XL or taper Forfivo XL dosage; use another bupropion formulation for initial dosage titration and for tapering dosage before discontinuation.

❸ *Alert:* Bupropion hydrobromide (Aplenzin) isn't approved for smoking cessation treatment.

❸ *Alert:* Bupropion isn't approved for use in children.

• Use cautiously in patients with recent history of MI; unstable heart disease; renal or hepatic impairment; a history of seizures, head trauma, or other predisposition to seizures; and in those being treated with drugs that lower seizure threshold.

Dialyzable drug: Unknown.

⚠ *Overdose S&S:* Seizures, ECG changes, hallucinations, loss of consciousness, sinus tachycardia, coma, fever, hypotension, muscle rigidity, rhabdomyolysis, respiratory failure, stupor.

PREGNANCY-LACTATION-REPRODUCTION

• Use during pregnancy only when potential benefits justify potential risks to the fetus.

• Prescriber should be notified if patient plans to or becomes pregnant.

• Drug and its metabolites appear in human milk. Recommendations for breastfeeding vary by individual product; refer to manufacturer's labeling for recommendations.

NURSING CONSIDERATIONS

• Many patients experience a period of increased restlessness, including agitation, insomnia, and anxiety, especially at start of therapy.

❸ *Alert:* To minimize the risk of seizures, don't exceed maximum recommended dose.

❸ *Alert:* Patient with major depressive disorder may experience a worsening of depression and suicidal thoughts. Carefully monitor patient for worsening depression or suicidal thoughts, especially at the beginning of therapy and during dosage changes.

Black Box Warning Drug may increase the risk of suicidal thinking and behavior in children, adolescents, and young adults with major depressive disorder or other psychiatric disorder. ∎

❸ *Alert:* If SSRIs, linezolid, or methylene blue must be given, bupropion must be stopped and patient should be monitored for serotonin toxicity for 2 weeks or until 24 hours after the last dose of SSRIs, methylene blue, or linezolid, whichever comes first. Treatment with bupropion may be resumed 24 hours after last dose of SSRIs, methylene blue, or linezolid.

• Closely monitor patient with history of bipolar disorder. Antidepressants can cause manic episodes during the depressed phase of bipolar disorder. This may be less likely to occur with bupropion than with other antidepressants.

• Begin smoking-cessation treatment while patient is still smoking; about 1 week is needed to achieve steady-state drug levels.

• Stop smoking-cessation treatment if patient hasn't progressed toward abstinence by week 7. Treatment usually lasts up to 12 weeks. Patient can stop taking drug without tapering off.

• Monitor patients without iridectomy for narrow-angle glaucoma.

• Monitor BP for HTN before and periodically during treatment.

Black Box Warning Zyban isn't indicated for treatment of depression. ∎

• *Look alike–sound alike:* Don't confuse bupropion with buspirone. Don't confuse Zyban with Diovan. Don't confuse Wellbutrin SR with Wellbutrin XL.

Reactions in bold italics are *life-threatening*. Interactions may have a *rapid onset* or a *delayed onset*.

PATIENT TEACHING

Black Box Warning Advise families and caregivers to closely observe patient for increased suicidal thinking and behavior, as well as hostility, agitation, and depressed mood, and to contact health care provider immediately should these occur. ■

☼ Alert: Explain that excessive use of alcohol, abrupt withdrawal from alcohol or other sedatives, and addiction to cocaine, opiates, or stimulants during therapy may increase risk of seizures. Seizure risk is also increased in those using OTC stimulants, in anorectics, and in diabetic patients using oral antidiabetics or insulin.

☼ Alert: Teach patient to recognize and immediately report symptoms of serotonin toxicity (fever, mental status changes, muscle twitching, excessive sweating, shivering or shaking, diarrhea, loss of coordination).

• Tell patient not to chew, crush, or divide tablets.

• Advise patient to consult prescriber before taking other prescription or OTC drugs.

• Advise patient to avoid hazardous activities that require alertness and good psychomotor coordination until effects of drug are known.

• Tell patient that it may take 4 weeks or longer to reach full antidepressant effect.

☼ Alert: Advise patient to report mood swings or suicidal thoughts immediately.

• Inform patient that tablets may have an odor.

• Tell patient taking extended-release form that the empty shell may appear in stool.

---

burosumab-twza ⬚
bur-oh-SUE-mab

Crysvita

Therapeutic class: Metabolic agents
Pharmacologic class: Fibroblast growth factor inhibitors

AVAILABLE FORMS
Injection: 10 mg/mL, 20 mg/mL, 30 mg/mL in single-dose vials

INDICATIONS & DOSAGES
➤ **Treatment of X-linked hypophosphatemia** ⬚

Adults age 18 and older: 1 mg/kg body weight subcut rounded to the nearest 10 mg, to a maximum of 90 mg, every 4 weeks.

Adjust-a-dose: If serum phosphorus level increases above the normal range, withhold the next dose and reassess serum phosphorus level after 4 weeks. Once serum phosphorus level falls below the normal range, resume drug at approximately half the initial starting dose, up to a maximum of 40 mg, every 4 weeks. Reassess fasting serum phosphorus level 2 weeks after dosage change. Don't adjust dosage more frequently than every 4 weeks.

Children age 1 year to younger than age 18: 0.8 mg/kg body weight subcut rounded to the nearest 10 mg every 2 weeks. Minimum starting dose is 10 mg; maximum dose is 90 mg.

Adjust-a-dose: If serum phosphorus level is below the reference range for age, increase dosage stepwise up to approximately 2 mg/kg administered every 2 weeks (maximum dose of 90 mg). Refer to manufacturer's information for specific dosage adjustments. If serum phosphorus level is greater than 5 mg/dL, withhold the next dose and reassess fasting serum phosphorus level in 4 weeks. Once serum phosphorus level is below the reference range for age, reinitiate drug at decreased dosage according to manufacturer's information. Reassess fasting serum phosphorus level 4 weeks after dosage decrease. Don't adjust dosage more frequently than every 4 weeks.

ADMINISTRATION
Subcutaneous

• Visually inspect vial for particulate matter and discoloration before administration. Solution should be clear to slightly opalescent and colorless to pale brown-yellow. Don't use if discolored or cloudy or contains particles or foreign matter.

• Rotate injection site with each injection (upper arms, upper thighs, buttocks, or any quadrant of abdomen).

• Don't inject into moles, scars, or areas where the skin is tender, bruised, red, hard, or not intact.

• Maximum volume of drug per injection site is 1.5 mL. If more than 1.5 mL is required, divide the total volume into portions and administer at two different injection sites.

• Give missed dose as soon as possible.

• Store vials in original carton to protect from light. Keep refrigerated at 36° to 46° F (2° to 8° C) until time of use. Don't freeze or shake.

ACTION

A recombinant human IgG (IgG1), anti-human fibroblast growth factor 23 (FGF23) antibody that inhibits activity of excess FGF23 and restores renal phosphate reabsorption and increases serum concentrations of 1,25-dihydroxy vitamin D.

Route	Onset	Peak	Duration
Subcut	Unknown	8–11 days	Unknown

Half-life: 19 days.

ADVERSE REACTIONS

CNS: headache, fever, dizziness. **EENT:** toothache, tooth infection. **GI:** vomiting, constipation. **Metabolic:** decreased vitamin D level, hyperphosphatemia. **Musculoskeletal:** extremity pain, myalgia, back pain, restless legs syndrome. **Skin:** rash, injection-site reaction (injection-site urticaria, erythema, rash, swelling, bruising, pain, pruritus, hematoma), hypersensitivity.

INTERACTIONS

Drug-drug. *Active vitamin D analogues, oral phosphates:* May increase risk of hyperphosphatemia. Use together is contraindicated. Discontinue oral phosphate and active vitamin D analogues 1 week before initiation of treatment.

EFFECTS ON LAB TEST RESULTS

• May increase phosphorus and 1,25-dihydroxy vitamin D levels.

CONTRAINDICATIONS & CAUTIONS

• Contraindicated when serum phosphorus level is within or above the normal range for age.

• Contraindicated in patients with severe renal impairment or ESRD as these conditions are associated with abnormal mineral metabolism.

• Hypersensitivity reactions (rash, urticaria) have been reported.

• Local injection-site reactions can occur (injection-site urticaria, erythema, rash, swelling, bruising, pain, pruritus, hematoma).

• Hyperphosphatemia may increase the risk of nephrocalcinosis. Adjust dosage based on serum phosphorus level.

• Start drug at low end of the dosing range in elderly patients.

Dialyzable drug: Unknown.

PREGNANCY-LACTATION-REPRODUCTION

• Drug may cross the placental barrier. Risk to fetus is unknown.

• Report pregnancies to the Ultragenyx Adverse Event reporting line (1-888-756-8657).

• It isn't known if drug appears in human milk, affects human milk production, or has effects on the breastfed infant. Before use in breastfeeding patients, consider the benefits of breastfeeding and the potential risk to the breastfed infant.

NURSING CONSIDERATIONS

• Assess fasting serum phosphorus level before initiation of treatment.

• For adults, monitor fasting serum phosphorus level monthly, 2 weeks after a dose, for the first 3 months of treatment, and as appropriate thereafter. If serum phosphorus level is within the normal range, continue the same dosage.

• For children, monitor fasting serum phosphorus level every 4 weeks for the first 3 months, and as appropriate thereafter. If serum phosphorus level is above the lower limit of the reference range for age and less than 5 mg/dL, continue treatment with the same dosage. Adjust dosage to maintain serum phosphorus level within the reference range for age.

• If severe local injection-site reactions occur, discontinue drug and treat appropriately.

• If serious hypersensitivity reactions occur, discontinue drug and begin appropriate treatment.

Reactions in bold italics are *life-threatening*. Interactions may have a *rapid onset* or a *delayed onset*.

• Monitor adult patients for new-onset or worsening of existing restless legs syndrome.

PATIENT TEACHING
• Tell patient to report all adverse reactions.
• Tell patient that blood laboratory tests will be needed to monitor therapy.
• Caution patient to report hypersensitivity or injection-site reactions. Drug may need to be discontinued.
• Advise female patient of childbearing potential who is pregnant, plans to become pregnant, or is breastfeeding or plans to breastfeed to discuss risks with prescriber before starting therapy.
• Inform patient that drug may cause or worsen symptoms of restless legs syndrome and to report if symptoms occur or worsen.

busPIRone hydrochloride
byoo-SPYE-rone

Therapeutic class: Anxiolytics
Pharmacologic class: Azaspirodecane-dione derivatives

AVAILABLE FORMS
Tablets: 5 mg, 7.5 mg, 10 mg, 15 mg, 30 mg

INDICATIONS & DOSAGES
➤ **Anxiety disorders**
Adults: Initially, 7.5 mg PO b.i.d. Increase dosage by 5 mg daily at 2- to 3-day intervals. Usual maintenance dosage is 20 to 30 mg daily in divided doses. Don't exceed 60 mg daily.

ADMINISTRATION
PO
• Don't give drug with grapefruit juice.
• Give drug at the same times each day, and always with or always without food.

ACTION
May inhibit neuronal firing and reduce serotonin turnover in cortical, amygdaloid, and septohippocampal tissue.

Route	Onset	Peak	Duration
PO	Unknown	40–90 min	Unknown

Half-life: 2 to 3 hours.

ADVERSE REACTIONS
CNS: dizziness, drowsiness, headache, nervousness, insomnia, light-headedness, fatigue, numbness, excitement, confusion, depression, anger, decreased concentration, paresthesia, incoordination, tremor, hostility. **CV:** tachycardia, nonspecific chest pain. **EENT:** blurred vision. **GI:** dry mouth, nausea, diarrhea, abdominal distress, constipation, vomiting. **Musculoskeletal:** aches and pains. **Skin:** rash, sweating or clamminess.

INTERACTIONS
Drug-drug. *Azole antifungals:* May inhibit first-pass metabolism of buspirone. Monitor patient closely for adverse effects; adjust dosage as needed.
CNS depressants: May increase CNS depression. Use together cautiously.
CYP3A4 inducers (carbamazepine, dexamethasone, phenobarbital, phenytoin, rifabutin, rifampin): May decrease buspirone level. Adjust dosage as needed.
Drugs metabolized by CYP3A4 (clarithromycin, diltiazem, erythromycin, fluvoxamine, itraconazole, ketoconazole, nefazodone, ritonavir, verapamil): May increase buspirone level. Monitor patient; decrease buspirone dosage and adjust carefully.
Linezolid, methylene blue: May cause serotonin syndrome. Use extreme caution and monitor closely.
MAO inhibitors: May elevate BP and increase risk of serotonin syndrome. Avoid using together.
Nefazodone: May increase levels of both drugs. Use lower buspirone dosage if used together.
Sodium oxybate: May increase sleep duration and CNS depression. Use together is contraindicated.
Drug-food. *Grapefruit juice:* May increase drug level, increasing adverse effects. Give with liquid other than grapefruit juice.
Drug-lifestyle. *Alcohol use:* May increase CNS depression. Discourage use together.

EFFECTS ON LAB TEST RESULTS
• May interfere with urinary metanephrine/catecholamine assay testing for pheochromocytoma, resulting in a false-positive result.

CONTRAINDICATIONS & CAUTIONS
• Contraindicated in patients hypersensitive to drug and within 14 days of MAO inhibitor therapy.
❸ *Alert:* Concomitant use with linezolid or methylene blue can cause serotonin syndrome (fever, mental status changes, muscle twitching, excessive sweating, shivering or shaking, diarrhea, loss of coordination). Use drug with linezolid or methylene blue only for life-threatening or urgent conditions when the potential benefits outweigh the risks of toxicity.
• Drug isn't recommended for patients with severe hepatic or renal impairment.
Dialyzable drug: No.
⚠ *Overdose S&S:* Nausea, vomiting, dizziness, drowsiness, miosis, gastric distress.

PREGNANCY-LACTATION-REPRODUCTION
• Use in pregnant and breastfeeding women isn't recommended. Use during pregnancy only if clearly needed.

NURSING CONSIDERATIONS
• Monitor patient closely for adverse CNS reactions. Drug is less sedating than other anxiolytics, but CNS effects may be unpredictable.
❸ *Alert:* Before starting therapy, don't stop a previous benzodiazepine regimen abruptly because a withdrawal reaction may occur.
❸ *Alert:* If linezolid or methylene blue must be given, buspirone must be stopped and patient should be monitored for serotonin toxicity for 2 weeks or until 24 hours after the last dose of methylene blue or linezolid, whichever comes first. Treatment with buspirone may be resumed 24 hours after last dose of methylene blue or linezolid.
• Drug shows no potential for abuse and isn't classified as a controlled substance.
• *Look alike–sound alike:* Don't confuse buspirone with bupropion or risperidone.

PATIENT TEACHING
❸ *Alert:* Teach patient to recognize and immediately report symptoms of serotonin toxicity (fever, mental status changes, muscle twitching, excessive sweating, shivering or shaking, diarrhea, loss of coordination).

• Warn patient to avoid hazardous activities that require alertness and good coordination until effects of drug are known.
• Remind patient that drug effects may not be noticeable for several weeks.
• Warn patient not to abruptly stop a benzodiazepine because of risk of withdrawal symptoms.
• Tell patient to avoid use of alcohol and grapefruit juice during therapy.
• Advise patient to take consistently; that is, always with or always without food.

SAFETY ALERT!

butorphanol tartrate
byoo-TOR-fa-nole

Therapeutic class: Opioid analgesics
Pharmacologic class: Opioid agonist-antagonists–opioid partial agonists

AVAILABLE FORMS
Injection: 1 mg/mL, 2 mg/mL
Nasal spray: 10 mg/mL (1 mg/spray)

INDICATIONS & DOSAGES
➤ **Moderate to severe pain**
Adults: 1 to 4 mg IM every 3 to 4 hours p.r.n., or around the clock. Not to exceed 4 mg per dose. Or, 0.5 to 2 mg IV every 3 to 4 hours p.r.n., or around the clock. Or, 1 mg by nasal spray every 3 to 4 hours (1 spray in one nostril); repeat in 60 to 90 minutes if pain relief is inadequate. For severe pain, 2 mg (1 spray in each nostril) every 3 to 4 hours.
Adjust-a-dose: For patients with renal or hepatic impairment, increase dosage interval to 6 to 8 hours and give 50% of the normal dose. For elderly patients, give 1 mg IM or 0.5 mg IV; wait 6 hours before repeating dose. For nasal use, 1 mg (1 spray in one nostril). May give another 1 mg in 1.5 to 2 hours. Wait 6 hours before repeating sequence.
➤ **Labor for patients at full term; early labor (without signs of fetal distress)**
Adults: 1 or 2 mg IV or IM; repeat after 4 hours as needed. Don't give dose less than 4 hours before anticipated delivery.

Reactions in bold italics are *life-threatening*. Interactions may have a *rapid onset* or a *delayed onset*.

B

➤ **Preoperative anesthesia or preanes-thesia**
Adults: 2 mg IM 60 to 90 minutes before surgery.
➤ **Adjunct to balanced anesthesia**
Adults: 2 mg IV shortly before induction, or 0.5 to 1 mg IV in increments during anesthesia.
Elderly patients: One-half usual dose, with repeat doses determined by patient's response.

ADMINISTRATION
IV
▼ Compatible solutions include D₅W and NSS.
▼ Give by direct injection into a vein or into the tubing of a free-flowing IV solution.
▼ **Incompatibilities:** None listed by manufacturer. Consult a drug incompatibility reference for more information.
IM
• Give drug IM; don't give subcut.
Intranasal
• Watch for nasal congestion with nasal spray use.

ACTION
May bind with opioid receptors in the CNS, altering perception of and emotional response to pain.

Route	Onset	Peak	Duration
IV	1 min	30–60 min	3–4 hr
IM	10–30 min	30–60 min	3–4 hr
Nasal	15 min	1–2 hr	2½–5 hr

Half-life: About 2 to 9 hours.

ADVERSE REACTIONS
CNS: dizziness, insomnia, somnolence, anxiety, asthenia, confusion, euphoria, headache, lethargy, nervousness, paresthesia, tremor. **CV:** flushing, palpitations, vasodilation. **EENT:** nasal congestion, blurred vision, nasal irritation, pharyngitis, sinus congestion, sinusitis, rhinitis, tinnitus. **GI:** nausea, unpleasant taste, vomiting, anorexia, constipation, dry mouth, stomach pain. **Respiratory:** bronchitis, cough, dyspnea, URI, *respiratory depression.* **Skin:** clamminess, excessive diaphoresis, pruritus. **Other:** sensation of heat.

INTERACTIONS
Drug-drug. ▐ Black Box Warning ▌ *Benzodiazepines, CNS depressants:* May cause slow or difficult breathing, sedation, and death. Avoid use together. If use together is necessary, limit dosage and duration of each drug to the minimum necessary for desired effect. ▐
CNS depressants: May cause additive effects. Use together cautiously.
▐ Black Box Warning ▌ *CYP3A4 inducers (carbamazepine, phenytoin, rifampin):* May decrease level of intranasally administered drug, causing decreased effectiveness or drug withdrawal syndrome. Monitor patient closely. ▐
▐ Black Box Warning ▌ *CYP3A4 inhibitors (azole antifungals, macrolide antibiotics, protease inhibitors):* May increase level of intranasally administered drug, resulting in increased or prolonged adverse reactions; may cause potentially fatal respiratory depression. Avoid use together. ▐
🔆 *Alert: Serotonergic drugs:* May increase risk of serotonin syndrome. Use together cautiously; monitor patient for serotonin syndrome.
Drug-herb. 🔆 *Alert: St. John's wort:* May increase risk of serotonin syndrome. Use together cautiously; monitor patient for serotonin syndrome.
Drug-lifestyle. *Alcohol use:* May cause additive effects. Discourage use together.

EFFECTS ON LAB TEST RESULTS
None reported.

CONTRAINDICATIONS & CAUTIONS
• Contraindicated in patients hypersensitive to drug or to preservative, benzethonium chloride, and in those with opioid addiction; may cause withdrawal syndrome.
▐ Black Box Warning ▌ Drug exposes patients and other users to risks of opioid addiction, abuse, and misuse, which can lead to overdose and death. Assess each patient's risk before prescribing butorphanol tartrate injection, and monitor all patients regularly for development of these behaviors or conditions. ▐
▐ Black Box Warning ▌ Serious, life-threatening, or fatal respiratory depression may occur with use of butorphanol tartrate

injection. Monitor patients for respiratory depression, especially during drug initiation and after dosage increase. ▮

Black Box Warning Opioids should only be prescribed with benzodiazepines or other CNS depressants to patients for whom alternative treatment options are inadequate. ▮

❸ *Alert:* Drug may lead to rare but serious decrease in adrenal gland cortisol production.

❸ *Alert:* Drug may cause decreased sex hormone levels with long-term use.

• Use cautiously in patients with head injury, increased ICP, acute MI, ventricular dysfunction, coronary insufficiency, respiratory disease or depression, and renal or hepatic dysfunction.

• Use cautiously in patients who have recently received repeated doses of opioid analgesic.

• For patients who have been taking drug regularly, gradually taper dosage to prevent signs and symptoms of withdrawal.

• Safety and efficacy in patients younger than age 18 haven't been established.

• Patients age 65 and older may have increased sensitivity to drug. Use caution when selecting a dosage for such patients, and usually start at low end of dosing range.

Dialyzable drug: Unknown.

⚠ *Overdose S&S:* Respiratory depression, CNS depression, CV insufficiency, coma, death.

PREGNANCY-LACTATION-REPRODUCTION

• There are no adequate and well-controlled studies in pregnant women before 37 weeks' gestation. Use during pregnancy only if potential benefit justifies potential risk to the fetus.

• There have been rare reports of infant respiratory distress/apnea after butorphanol administration during labor. These reports have been associated with administration of a dose within 2 hours of delivery, use of multiple doses, use with additional analgesics or sedatives, or use in preterm pregnancies.

• If fetal HR pattern is abnormal, use butorphanol injection cautiously.

• The decision to continue therapy or discontinue breastfeeding should take into account risks versus benefits to the mother and infant.

❸ *Alert:* Monitor breastfeeding women and infants for psychomimetic reactions. Monitor breastfeeding infants for apnea and sedation. Withdrawal symptoms can occur in breastfed infants when maternal administration of an opioid analgesic is stopped, or when breastfeeding is stopped.

Black Box Warning Closely monitor neonates with prolonged opioid exposure during pregnancy for signs and symptoms of withdrawal, which may be life-threatening and may require management according to protocols developed by neonatology experts. ▮

NURSING CONSIDERATIONS

❸ *Alert:* If patient is taking opioids with serotonergic drugs, monitor for signs and symptoms of serotonin syndrome, especially when starting treatment or increasing dosages. Signs and symptoms may occur within several hours of coadministration but may also occur later, especially after dosage increase. Discontinue the opioid, serotonergic drug, or both if serotonin syndrome is suspected.

Black Box Warning For patients receiving the nasal spray, monitor the use of any coadministered CYP3A4 inhibitors or inducers. Using these agents with the nasal spray can cause an increase or decrease in drug levels, leading to fatal adverse effects. ▮

• Don't stop drug abruptly; withdraw slowly and individualize the gradual taper plan to prevent signs and symptoms of withdrawal, worsening pain, and psychological distress in physically dependent patients. Refer to manufacturer's label for specific tapering instructions.

• When tapering opioids, watch closely for signs and symptoms of opioid withdrawal. Such symptoms may indicate a need to taper more slowly. Monitor patient for suicidal thoughts, use of other substances, and mood changes.

❸ *Alert:* Monitor patient for signs and symptoms of adrenal insufficiency. Perform diagnostic testing if adrenal insufficiency is suspected. If adrenal insufficiency is confirmed, treat with corticosteroids and wean patient off opioids if appropriate. Discontinue corticosteroids when clinically appropriate.

Reactions in bold italics are *life-threatening*. Interactions may have a *rapid onset* or a *delayed onset*.

⚙ Alert: Monitor patient for signs and symptoms of decreased sex hormone levels. If signs and symptoms occur, evaluate patient and obtain laboratory testing.

• Reassess patient's level of pain 15 and 30 minutes after administration.

• Respiratory depression apparently doesn't increase with larger dosage.

• Drug may cause constipation. Assess bowel function and need for stool softener and stimulant laxatives.

Black Box Warning Psychological and physical addiction may occur. ■

• Periodically monitor postoperative vital signs and bladder function. Because drug decreases both rate and depth of respirations, monitor arterial oxygen saturation to help assess respiratory depression.

PATIENT TEACHING

⚙ Alert: Encourage patient to report all medications being taken, including prescription and OTC drugs and supplements.

Black Box Warning Caution patient or caregiver of patient taking an opioid with a benzodiazepine, CNS depressant, or alcohol to seek immediate medical attention for dizziness, light-headedness, extreme sleepiness, slowed or difficult breathing, or unresponsiveness. ■

• Counsel patient not to discontinue opioids without first discussing with prescriber the need for a gradual tapering regimen.

⚙ Alert: Caution patient to immediately report signs and symptoms of serotonin syndrome, adrenal insufficiency, and decreased sex hormone levels.

• Caution ambulatory patient about getting out of bed or walking. Warn outpatient to avoid driving and other hazardous activities that require mental alertness until it's clear how the drug affects the CNS.

⚙ Alert: Accidental ingestion of even one dose of nasal solution, especially by children, can result in a fatal overdose.

• Teach patient how to take nasal spray and how to store in child-resistant container.

• Instruct patient to avoid alcohol during therapy.

calcitonin salmon
kal-si-TOE-nin

Miacalcin

Therapeutic class: Antiosteoporotics
Pharmacologic class: Polypeptide
hormones

AVAILABLE FORMS
Injection: 200 units/mL in 2-mL ampules
Nasal spray: 200 units/activation

INDICATIONS & DOSAGES
➤ **Paget disease of bone (osteitis deformans)**
Adults: 100 units daily IM or subcut.
➤ **Hypercalcemia**
Adults: 4 units/kg every 12 hours IM or subcut. If response is inadequate after 1 or 2 days, increase dosage to 8 units/kg every 12 hours. If response remains unsatisfactory after 2 additional days, increase dosage to maximum of 8 units/kg every 6 hours.
➤ **Postmenopausal osteoporosis in women more than 5 years after menopause**
Adults: 200 units (one activation) daily intranasally, alternating nostrils daily. Or, 100 units IM or subcut daily. Patient should receive adequate vitamin D and calcium supplements (at least 1,000 mg elemental calcium and 600 units of vitamin D) daily.

ADMINISTRATION
IM
• IM route is preferred if volume of dose exceeds 2 mL; use multiple injection sites.
• Store in refrigerator between 36° and 46° F (2° and 8° C).
Intranasal
• Alternate nostrils daily.
• Allow bottle to reach room temperature and prime pump before first use by releasing at least 5 sprays until full spray is produced. Don't prime pump every day.
• Carefully insert nozzle into the nostril while patient's head is upright.
• Discard spray container after 30 doses.
• Keep bottle refrigerated between 36° and 46° F (2° and 8° C) while unopened; store in an upright position at room temperature after opening.

Subcutaneous
- Alternate injection sites.
- Store in refrigerator between 36° and 46° F (2° and 8° C).

ACTION

Decreases osteoclastic activity by inhibiting osteocytic osteolysis; decreases mineral release and matrix or collagen breakdown in bone.

Route	Onset	Peak	Duration
IM, subcut	2 hr	23 min	6–8 hr
Intranasal	Rapid	10–13 min	Unknown

Half-life: IM and subcut, 58 to 64 minutes; intranasal, 23 minutes.

ADVERSE REACTIONS

CNS: depression, headache, dizziness, paresthesia, fatigue. **CV:** flushing, edema of feet. **EENT:** eye pain, abnormal tearing, conjunctivitis, epistaxis, nasal congestion, rhinitis, sinusitis. **GI:** transient nausea, unusual taste, anorexia, nausea, abdominal pain. **GU:** increased urinary frequency, nocturia. **Hematologic:** infection, lymphadenopathy, *malignant neoplasm*. **Musculoskeletal:** arthrosis, myalgia. **Respiratory:** *bronchospasm,* URI, shortness of breath, sinusitis. **Skin:** rash, pruritus of ear lobes, injection-site reaction. **Other:** hypersensitivity reactions, *anaphylaxis,* chills, tender palms and soles, flulike symptoms.

INTERACTIONS

Drug-drug. *Lithium:* May reduce plasma lithium concentration due to increased urinary clearance of lithium. Monitor level and adjust lithium dosage as needed.
Zoledronic acid: May enhance hypocalcemic effect of zoledronic acid. Monitor therapy.

EFFECTS ON LAB TEST RESULTS

None reported.

CONTRAINDICATIONS & CAUTIONS

- Contraindicated in patients hypersensitive to drug.
Dialyzable drug: Unknown.
⚠ **Overdose S&S:** Hypocalcemic tetany (increased neuromuscular irritability, repetitive neuromuscular movements after a single stimulus).

PREGNANCY-LACTATION-REPRODUCTION

- Use during pregnancy only if potential benefits justify possible risks to patient and fetus.
- Nasal spray isn't indicated for use in females of childbearing potential.
- It isn't known if drug appears in human milk, but it has been shown to decrease milk production in animals. Before using in breastfeeding women, consider risk of infant exposure, benefits of breastfeeding to the infant, and benefits of treatment to the mother.

NURSING CONSIDERATIONS

- Skin test is usually done in patients with suspected drug sensitivity before therapy.
🔵 **Alert:** Systemic allergic reactions are possible because the hormone is a protein. Prepare for emergency treatment if needed.
🔵 **Alert:** Observe patient for signs of hypocalcemic tetany during therapy (muscle twitching, tetanic spasms, and seizures when hypocalcemia is severe).
🔵 **Alert:** Periodically reevaluate need for continued therapy because of the possible association between malignancy and long-term calcitonin salmon use.
- Monitor calcium level closely. Watch for symptoms of hypercalcemia relapse: bone pain, renal calculi, polyuria, anorexia, nausea, vomiting, thirst, constipation, lethargy, bradycardia, muscle hypotonicity, pathologic fracture, psychosis, and coma.
- Periodic examinations of urine sediment are recommended.
- Periodic nasal examination with visualization of nasal mucosa, turbinates, septum, and mucosal blood vessel status is recommended to assess for ulceration in patients using intranasal form.
- Monitor periodic alkaline phosphatase and 24-hour urine hydroxyproline levels to evaluate drug effect.
- In Paget disease, maximum reductions of alkaline phosphatase and urinary hydroxyproline excretion may take 6 to 24 months of continuous treatment.
- In patients with good first response to drug who have a relapse, expect to evaluate antibody response to the hormone protein.

Reactions in bold italics are *life-threatening*. Interactions may have a *rapid onset* or a *delayed onset*.

C

• If symptoms have been relieved after 6 months, treatment may be stopped until symptoms or radiologic signs recur.
• Nasal reactions occur more commonly in elderly patients.
• *Look alike–sound alike:* Don't confuse calcitonin with calcifediol or calcitriol.

PATIENT TEACHING
• When drug is given for postmenopausal osteoporosis, remind patient to take adequate calcium and vitamin D supplements.
• Teach patient how to prime pump before first dose. Patient shouldn't prime pump before each daily dose.
• If nasal spray is prescribed, tell patient to alternate nostrils daily, hold head upright while using, and report nasal irritation or evidence of an allergic response.
• Inform patient that local inflammatory reactions have been reported at subcut or IM injection sites in about 10% of patients and that facial flushing and warmth occur in 2% to 5% of patients within minutes of injection and usually last about 1 hour.
• Tell patient that nausea may occur at the onset of therapy.
• Tell patient to inform prescriber promptly if signs and symptoms of hypercalcemia occur.
• Advise breastfeeding patient that drug may inhibit lactation.

---

calcitriol (1,25-dihydroxycholecalciferol)
kal-SIH-trye-ol

Rocaltrol, Vectical

Therapeutic class: Antihypocalcemics
Pharmacologic class: Vitamin D analogues

AVAILABLE FORMS
Capsules: 0.25 mcg, 0.5 mcg
Injection: 1 mcg/mL
Oral solution: 1 mcg/mL
Topical ointment: 3 mcg/g

INDICATIONS & DOSAGES
➤ **Hypocalcemia in patients undergoing long-term dialysis (PO)**
Adults: Initially, 0.25 mcg PO daily. Increase by 0.25 mcg daily at 4- to 8-week intervals.

Maintenance oral dosage is 0.25 mcg every other day up to 1 mcg daily (most patients respond to doses between 0.5 and 1 mcg/day).
➤ **Hypocalcemia in patients undergoing long-term dialysis (IV)**
Adults and children age 13 and older: Usual IV dosage is 1 to 2 mcg IV three times weekly (approximately every other day). Increase dose by 0.5 to 1 mcg at 2- to 4-week intervals.
➤ **Hypoparathyroidism, pseudohypoparathyroidism**
Adults and children age 6 and older: Initially, 0.25 mcg PO daily in the morning. Dosage may be increased at 2- to 4-week intervals. Maintenance dosage is 0.5 to 2 mcg PO daily.
➤ **Hypoparathyroidism**
Children ages 1 to 5: Give 0.25 to 0.75 mcg PO daily.
➤ **To manage secondary hyperparathyroidism and resulting metabolic bone disease in predialysis patients (with CrCl of 15 to 55 mL/minute)**
Adults and children age 3 and older: Initially, 0.25 mcg PO daily. Dosage may be increased to 0.5 mcg/day if needed.
Children younger than age 3: Initially, 0.01 to 0.015 mcg/kg PO daily.
➤ **Mild to moderate plaque psoriasis**
Adults: Apply ointment topically to affected area b.i.d. in the morning and evening. Maximum weekly dosage is 200 g.

ADMINISTRATION
PO
• Give drug without regard for food.
• Don't give with magnesium-containing antacids.
IV
▼ For hypocalcemia in patient undergoing hemodialysis, give drug by rapid injection through catheter at end of hemodialysis session.

▼ **Incompatibilities:** None listed by manufacturer. Consult a drug incompatibility reference for more information.
Topical
• Topical form isn't for oral, ophthalmic, or intravaginal use.
• Gently rub into skin until no longer visible.

ACTION
Stimulates calcium absorption from the GI tract and promotes movement of calcium from bone to blood.

Route	Onset	Peak	Duration
PO	2–6 hr	3–6 hr	3–5 days
IV	Immediate	Unknown	3–5 days
Topical	Unknown	Unknown	Unknown

Half-life: 5 to 8 hours.

ADVERSE REACTIONS
CNS: headache, somnolence, weakness, irritability. **CV:** HTN, *arrhythmias.* **EENT:** conjunctivitis, photophobia, rhinorrhea. **GI:** nausea, vomiting, constipation, polydipsia, *pancreatitis,* metallic taste, dry mouth, anorexia. **GU:** polyuria, nocturia, nephrocalcinosis, hypercalciuria. **Metabolic:** weight loss. **Musculoskeletal:** bone and muscle pain. **Skin:** pruritus, skin discomfort at application area or injection site. **Other:** hyperthermia, decreased libido.

INTERACTIONS
Drug-drug. *Cardiac glycosides:* May increase risk of arrhythmias. Monitor therapy.
Cholestyramine, colestipol, excessive use of mineral oil: May decrease absorption of oral vitamin D analogues. Avoid using together.
Corticosteroids: May diminish vitamin D analogue effects. Monitor therapy.
Magnesium-containing antacids: May cause hypermagnesemia, especially in patients with chronic renal failure. Avoid using together.
Phenobarbital, phenytoin: May inhibit calcitriol synthesis. Dose may need to be increased.
Sucralfate: May increase serum concentrations of sucralfate and aluminum concentrations. Avoid using together.
Thiazide, thiazide-like diuretics: May cause hypercalcemia. Use together cautiously.

EFFECTS ON LAB TEST RESULTS
• May increase AST, ALT, BUN, creatinine, cholesterol, urine albumin, and calcium levels.

CONTRAINDICATIONS & CAUTIONS
• Contraindicated in patients with hypercalcemia or vitamin D toxicity. Withhold all preparations containing vitamin D.
• Use cautiously in patients receiving cardiac glycosides and in those with sarcoidosis or hyperparathyroidism.
Dialyzable drug: Unknown.
⚠ *Overdose S&S:* Hypercalcemia, hyperphosphatemia, hypercalciuria.

PREGNANCY-LACTATION-REPRODUCTION
• There are no adequate well-controlled studies in pregnant women. Use during pregnancy only if potential benefit justifies risk to the fetus.
• Ingested calcitriol may appear in human milk. Women shouldn't breastfeed while taking drug.

NURSING CONSIDERATIONS
• Effective therapy is dependent on adequate calcium intake.
• Monitor calcium level; this level times the phosphate level shouldn't exceed 70. During dose adjustment, determine calcium level twice weekly. If hypercalcemia occurs, stop drug and notify prescriber but resume after calcium level returns to normal. Patient should receive adequate daily intake of calcium. Observe for hypocalcemia, bone pain, and weakness before and during therapy.
• Monitor phosphorus level, especially in hypoparathyroid patients and dialysis patients.
• Reduce dose as parathyroid hormone levels decrease in response to therapy.
• Make sure patient taking calcitriol maintains adequate fluid status.
• The symptoms of vitamin D intoxication include headache, somnolence, weakness, irritability, HTN, arrhythmias, conjunctivitis, photophobia, rhinorrhea, nausea, vomiting, constipation, polydipsia, pancreatitis, metallic taste, dry mouth, anorexia, nephrocalcinosis, polyuria, nocturia, weight loss, bone and muscle pain, pruritus, hyperthermia, and decreased libido.
• Protect drug from heat and light.
• *Look alike–sound alike:* Don't confuse calcitriol with calcifediol or calcitonin.

C

PATIENT TEACHING
• Tell patient to report all adverse reactions and to immediately report early signs and symptoms of vitamin D intoxication: weakness, nausea, vomiting, dry mouth, constipation, muscle or bone pain, or metallic taste.
• Instruct patient to adhere to diet and calcium supplementation and to avoid OTC drugs and antacids that contain magnesium.
• Warn patient to avoid excessive exposure of topically treated areas to either artificial or natural sunlight, including phototherapy.
⚠ *Alert:* Tell patient that drug is the most potent form of vitamin D available and shouldn't be taken by anyone else.

---

calcium acetate
Calphron ◇, Phoslyra

calcium chloride

calcium citrate ◇
Citracal ◇, Cal-Citrate ◇, Cal-C-Cap ◇

calcium gluconate

calcium lactate
Cal-Lac ◇

Therapeutic class: Calcium supplements
Pharmacologic class: Calcium salts

AVAILABLE FORMS
calcium acetate
Contains 253 mg or 12.7 mEq of elemental calcium/g
Capsules: 667 mg
Gelcaps: 667 mg
Solution: 667 mg/5 mL
Tablets ⓞⓝⓒ: 667 mg, 668 mg ◇
calcium chloride
Contains 273 mg or 13.6 mEq of elemental calcium/g
Injection: 10% solution in 10-mL ampules, vials, and syringes
calcium citrate
Contains 211 mg or 10.6 mEq of elemental calcium/g
Capsules: 150 mg ◇, 180 mg ◇, 225 mg ◇
Granules for oral solution: 760 mg/3.5 g
Tablets: 200 mg ◇, 250 mg ◇, 950 mg ◇

calcium gluconate
Contains 93 mg or 4.7 mEq of elemental calcium/g
Capsules: 500 mg ◇
Injection: 100 mg/mL
Tablets: 50 mg ◇, 500 mg ◇
calcium lactate
Contains 130 mg or 6.5 mEq of elemental calcium/g
Capsules: 500 mg (96 mg elemental calcium) ◇
Tablets: 100 mg ◇, 648 mg ◇

INDICATIONS & DOSAGES
➤ **Hypocalcemia**
Adults: 7 to 14 mEq elemental calcium IV. May give as a 10% calcium chloride solution. Or, initially, 1 to 2 g calcium gluconate IV.
Children: 0.136 to 0.252 mEq elemental calcium/kg IV. Or, initially, 29 to 200 mg/kg calcium gluconate IV based on age.
➤ **Adjunctive treatment of magnesium intoxication**
Adults: Initially, 7 mEq IV. Base subsequent doses on patient's response.
➤ **During exchange transfusions**
Adults: 1.35 mEq IV with each 100 mL citrated blood.
Neonates: 0.45 mEq IV after each 100 mL citrated blood.
➤ **Hyperphosphatemia**
Adults: Initially, 2 capsules or tablets or 10 mL oral solution calcium PO t.i.d. with meals. Titrate dose every 2 to 3 weeks until an acceptable serum phosphorus level is reached; watch for hypercalcemia. Most dialysis patients need 3 to 4 capsules or tablets or 15 to 20 mL oral solution with each meal.
➤ **Dietary supplement**
Adults: 500 mg to 2 g PO daily.
➤ **Hyperkalemia with secondary cardiac toxicity ♦**
Adults: 2.25 to 14 mEq IV. Repeat dose after 1 to 2 minutes, if needed.

ADMINISTRATION
PO
• Give drug with a full glass of water.
• Give 1 to 1½ hours after meals if GI upset occurs.

IV

▼ Give calcium chloride and gluconate only by IV route.

▼ Dilute calcium gluconate before use in 5% dextrose or NSS per manufacturer's instructions and assess for potential drug or IV fluid incompatibilities.

▼ Monitor ECG when giving calcium IV. Stop drug and notify prescriber if patient complains of discomfort.

⚠ *Alert:* Extravasation may cause severe necrosis and tissue sloughing. Calcium gluconate is less irritating to veins and tissues than calcium chloride.

Direct injection

▼ Don't use scalp veins in children.

▼ Warm solution to body temperature before giving it.

▼ For calcium chloride, give at 0.5 to 1 mL/minute (1.36 mEq/minute). For calcium gluconate bolus injection, don't exceed an infusion rate of 200 mg/minute in adults or 100 mg/minute in children, including neonates.

▼ Give slowly through a small needle into a large vein or through an IV line containing a free-flowing, compatible solution.

▼ After injection, keep patient recumbent for 15 minutes.

Intermittent infusion

▼ Infuse diluted solution through an IV line containing a compatible solution.

▼ **Incompatibilities:** Calcium chloride: None listed by manufacturer. Consult a drug incompatibility reference for more information. Calcium gluconate: ceftriaxone, fluids containing bicarbonate or phosphate, minocycline.

ACTION

Replaces calcium and maintains calcium level.

Route	Onset	Peak	Duration
PO	Unknown	Unknown	Unknown
IV	Immediate	Immediate	30 min–2 hr

Half-life: Unknown.

ADVERSE REACTIONS

CNS: tingling sensations, sense of oppression or heat waves with IV use, syncope with rapid IV use. **CV:** *bradycardia, arrhythmias, cardiac arrest with rapid IV use,* mild drop in BP, vasodilation. **GI:** constipation, irritation, chalky taste, *hemorrhage,* nausea, vomiting, thirst, abdominal pain. **GU:** polyuria, renal calculi. **Metabolic:** hypercalcemia.

INTERACTIONS

Drug-drug. *Bisphosphonates:* May reduce absorption of bisphosphonate from GI tract. Give calcium salts at least 30 minutes after alendronate or risedronate, at least 60 minutes after ibandronate, and not within 2 hours of etidronate.

Calcium channel blockers: May diminish therapeutic effects of calcium channel blockers. Monitor therapy.

Cardiac glycosides: May increase digoxin toxicity. Give calcium cautiously, if at all, to digitalized patients.

Fluoroquinolones: Oral calcium may decrease absorption of oral quinolones. Consider therapy modification.

Iron supplements: May reduce iron absorption. Separate drug administration by 2 hours.

Sodium polystyrene sulfonate: May cause metabolic acidosis in patients with renal disease and a reduction of the resin's binding of potassium. Separate drugs by several hours.

Tetracyclines: May decrease serum concentration of tetracyclines. Avoid use together or, if concurrent use is absolutely necessary, consider separating administration of each agent by several hours.

Thiazide diuretics: May cause hypercalcemia. Avoid using together.

Drug-food. *Foods containing oxalic acid (rhubarb, spinach), phytic acid (bran, whole-grain cereals), or phosphorus (dairy products, milk):* May interfere with calcium absorption. Discourage use together.

EFFECTS ON LAB TEST RESULTS

• May increase calcium level.

CONTRAINDICATIONS & CAUTIONS

• Contraindicated in cancer patients with bone metastases and in those with ventricular fibrillation, hypercalcemia, hypophosphatemia, or renal calculi.

Dialyzable drug: Yes.

⚠ *Overdose S&S:* Hypercalcemia, confusion, delirium, stupor, coma.

Reactions in bold italics are *life-threatening*. Interactions may have a *rapid onset* or a *delayed onset*.

PREGNANCY-LACTATION-REPRODUCTION
• It isn't known if drug can cause fetal harm when used during pregnancy or if it can affect reproductive capacity. Use in pregnant women only if clearly needed.
• Calcium appears in human milk, but is thought to be compatible with breastfeeding. Monitor maternal serum calcium levels.

NURSING CONSIDERATIONS
• Use all calcium products with extreme caution in digitalized patients and patients with sarcoidosis, renal or cardiac disease, and electrolyte disturbances. Use calcium chloride cautiously in patients with cor pulmonale, respiratory acidosis, or respiratory failure.
◑ Alert: Double-check that you're giving the correct form of calcium; resuscitation cart may contain both calcium gluconate and calcium chloride.
• Monitor calcium levels frequently. Hypercalcemia may result after large doses in chronic renal failure. Report abnormalities.
• Signs and symptoms of severe hypercalcemia may include stupor, confusion, delirium, and coma. Signs and symptoms of mild hypercalcemia may include anorexia, nausea, and vomiting.
• Look alike–sound alike: Don't confuse calcium with calcitriol, calcium gluconate with calcium glubionate, or calcium chloride with calcium gluconate.

PATIENT TEACHING
• Tell patient to take oral calcium 1 to 1½ hours after meals if GI upset occurs.
• Tell patient to take oral calcium with a full glass of water.
• Tell patient to report anorexia, nausea, vomiting, constipation, abdominal pain, dry mouth, thirst, or polyuria.
• Advise patient to notify prescriber if taking OTC products such as iron.
• Warn patient not to eat rhubarb, spinach, bran and whole-grain cereals, or dairy products in the meal before taking calcium; these foods may interfere with calcium absorption.
• Inform patient that some products may contain phenylalanine or tartrazine.

canagliflozin
KAN-a-gli-FLOE-zin

Invokana

Therapeutic class: Antidiabetics
Pharmacologic class: Sodium-glucose cotransporter 2 inhibitors

AVAILABLE FORMS
Tablets: 100 mg, 300 mg

INDICATIONS & DOSAGES
Adjust-a-dose (for all indications): Refer to manufacturer's instructions for renal impairment and drug interaction dosage adjustments.
➤ **Adjunct to diet and exercise to improve glycemic control in patients with type 2 diabetes**
Adults: 100 mg PO once daily before first meal of the day. May increase to 300 mg/day.
✳ *NEW INDICATION:* **To reduce risk of major adverse CV events in patients with type 2 diabetes mellitus and established CV disease**
Adults: 100 mg PO once daily. May increase to 300 mg/day.

ADMINISTRATION
PO
• Give before first meal of the day.
• Store tablets at room temperature.

ACTION
Inhibits sodium-glucose cotransporter 2, which reabsorbs glucose filtered by the kidneys, increasing amount of urinary glucose that is excreted.

Route	Onset	Peak	Duration
PO	Unknown	1–2 hr	Unknown

Half-life: 10.6 hours for 100-mg dose; 13.1 hours for 300-mg dose.

ADVERSE REACTIONS
CNS: fatigue, asthenia, syncope, postural dizziness. **CV:** hypotension, orthostatic hypotension. **GI:** thirst, constipation, nausea, abdominal pain, dehydration, *pancreatitis.* **GU:** genital fungal infection, UTI,

increased urination, vulvovaginal pruritus, renal impairment. **Hematologic:** increased Hb level. **Metabolic:** *hypoglycemia, hyperkalemia,* hypercholesterolemia, hypermagnesemia, hyperphosphatemia. **Musculoskeletal:** bone fracture. **Other:** hypersensitivity reactions, falls.

INTERACTIONS

Drug-drug. *ACE inhibitors (enalapril, lisinopril, moexipril, quinapril), ARBs (candesartan, losartan, olmesartan, valsartan), eplerenone, potassium-sparing diuretics (amiloride, spironolactone):* May increase risk of hyperkalemia. Monitor potassium level closely.

Antihypertensives: May increase hypotension. Monitor patient closely.

Carbamazepine, efavirenz: May decrease canagliflozin serum concentration. Consider increasing canagliflozin dosage based on GFR.

Digoxin: May increase digoxin level. Monitor digoxin level periodically.

Insulin and insulin secretagogues (glipizide, repaglinide): May increase risk of hypoglycemia. Consider lower dosage of insulin or insulin secretagogue.

Lomitapide: May increase lomitapide level. Limit maximum adult dosage of lomitapide to 30 mg daily.

Loop diuretics: May cause hypotension and intravascular volume depletion. Consider alternative therapy.

Salicylates: May increase hypoglycemic effects. Monitor patient closely.

SSRIs (citalopram, fluoxetine, sertraline): May increase canagliflozin level. Monitor patient closely. Canagliflozin dosage may need adjustment if SSRI is discontinued.

UGT inducers (phenobarbital, phenytoin, rifampin, ritonavir): May decrease canagliflozin level. Adjust canagliflozin dosage based on estimated GFR.

Drug-herb. *St. John's wort:* May decrease canagliflozin serum concentration. Consider increasing canagliflozin dosage based on GFR.

EFFECTS ON LAB TEST RESULTS

• May increase serum creatinine, potassium, magnesium, phosphate, Hb, LDL cholesterol, non-HDL cholesterol, and urine glucose levels.

• May decrease GFR and serum glucose level.

• May cause positive test for glycosuria and interfere with assay 1,5-anhydroglucitol. Use other methods to monitor glycemic control.

CONTRAINDICATIONS & CAUTIONS

• Contraindicated in patients hypersensitive to drug or its components, in those with severe renal impairment (eGFR of <30 mL/minute/1.73 m^2) or ESRD, and in patients on dialysis.

• Drug isn't recommended in patients with type 1 diabetes mellitus or for treatment of diabetic ketoacidosis.

Black Box Warning Canagliflozin is associated with increased risk of lower limb amputations in patients with type 2 diabetes who have, or are at risk for, CV disease. Amputations of the toe and midfoot were most frequent; however, amputations involving the leg were also observed. Some patients had multiple amputations, some involving both limbs. Before drug is prescribed, consider factors that may increase the risk of amputation, such as a history of prior amputation, PVD, neuropathy, and diabetic foot ulcers. ∎

⊙ *Alert:* Drug may cause acidosis, which may require emergency department care or hospitalization.

⊙ *Alert:* Drug may cause hyperkalemia, especially in patients with renal impairment or who are taking potassium-sparing diuretics, ACE inhibitors, or ARBs.

⊙ *Alert:* Drug may increase risk of bone fracture as early as 12 weeks after start of treatment and has been linked to decreased bone mineral density. Consider factors that may contribute to bone fracture risk prior to prescribing.

⊙ *Alert:* Drug may increase risk of severe UTI, including urosepsis and pyelonephritis. Monitor patient and treat promptly if indicated.

⊙ *Alert:* Sodium-glucose cotransporter 2 inhibitors such as canagliflozin increase the risk of necrotizing fasciitis of the perineum (Fournier gangrene), a rare but serious and life-threatening infection requiring

---

Reactions in bold italics are *life-threatening*. Interactions may have a *rapid onset* or a *delayed onset*.

urgent surgical intervention that has been reported in both females and males. Serious outcomes have included hospitalization, multiple surgeries, and death.
• Drug isn't recommended for patients with severe hepatic disease (Child-Pugh class C).
• Drug increases serum creatinine level and decreases estimated GFR; patients with hypovolemia may be more susceptible to these changes. Renal function abnormalities can occur after drug initiation. More frequent renal function monitoring is recommended in patients with an eGFR of less than 60 mL/minute/1.73 m^2.
• Use cautiously in elderly patients and in patients with volume depletion, impaired renal function, chronic low systolic BP, or hypotension.
Dialyzable drug: No.

PREGNANCY-LACTATION-REPRODUCTION
• There are no adequate well-controlled studies in pregnant women. Use during pregnancy only if potential benefit justifies potential risk to the fetus.
• It isn't known if drug appears in human milk. Patient should discontinue breastfeeding or discontinue drug, taking into account importance of drug to the mother.

NURSING CONSIDERATIONS
Black Box Warning Monitor patients for infections, new pain or tenderness, and sores or ulcers of the lower limbs. Discontinue drug if these complications occur. ∎
🜂 Alert: Drug can increase risk of acute kidney injury. Before start of therapy, assess patient for factors that may predispose patient to acute kidney injury (decreased blood volume, chronic renal insufficiency, HF, concurrent use of other medications, such as diuretics, ACE inhibitors, ARBs, or NSAIDs). Assess renal function before starting drug and monitor patient periodically. If acute kidney injury occurs, drug should be discontinued and the kidney impairment treated.
• Correct volume depletion before initiating drug. Observe for hypotension during therapy.
🜂 Alert: Monitor patients for ketoacidosis, especially those with major illness, reduced food or fluid intake, or reduced insulin dose. Elevated urine or serum ketone

levels without associated very high glucose levels have occurred with sodium-glucose cotransporter-2 inhibitor use.
🜂 Alert: Assess patients with pain or tenderness, erythema, or swelling in the genital or perineal area, along with fever or malaise, for necrotizing fasciitis. If suspected, immediately discontinue drug because symptoms can worsen quickly, and start treatment with broad-spectrum antibiotics and, if necessary, surgical debridement. Monitor blood glucose levels and start alternative therapy for glycemic control.
• Monitor blood glucose level. Assess for signs and symptoms of hypoglycemia.
• Be aware that because of the drug's mechanism of action, urine test will be positive for glucose.
• Monitor electrolytes, such as potassium and magnesium. Correct levels as clinically indicated.
• Drug may increase lipid levels. Assess LDL cholesterol level periodically and treat as clinically indicated.
• Assess for genital mycotic (fungal) infections, especially in patients with a history of infection and in uncircumcised males. Treat appropriately.
• Monitor patient for hypersensitivity reaction (urticaria); reaction may occur hours to days after start of therapy. Discontinue drug and treat appropriately if hypersensitivity reaction occurs.

PATIENT TEACHING
Black Box Warning Counsel patient about the increased risk of lower limb amputations. Instruct patient about the importance of routine, preventive foot care and to immediately report infections, new pain or tenderness, and sores or ulcers involving the lower limbs. ∎
• Advise patient to discontinue drug and immediately report hypersensitivity reaction (generalized urticarial rash).
🜂 Alert: Teach patient the signs and symptoms of necrotizing fasciitis (temperature above 100.4° F [38° C], general feeling of being unwell, and tenderness, redness, or swelling of the genitals back to the rectum) and to seek immediate medical attention if any occur.

⟳ Alert: Instruct patient to seek medical attention immediately for signs and symptoms of ketoacidosis (difficulty breathing, hyperventilation, anorexia, nausea, vomiting, abdominal pain, confusion, unusual fatigue or sleepiness).

⟳ Alert: Instruct patient to seek medical attention for signs and symptoms of UTI (dysuria, frequency, pelvic pain, hematuria, urgency, fever, back pain, nausea, vomiting).

⟳ Alert: Advise patient to seek immediate medical attention for signs and symptoms of acute kidney injury (decreased urine output, swelling in legs or feet). Warn patient not to stop drug without first discussing with prescriber.

• Warn female patient of possible risks to fetus and infant during pregnancy or breastfeeding. Instruct breastfeeding patient that she should discontinue drug or discontinue breastfeeding.

• Caution patient to avoid dehydration, which can cause hypotension. Instruct patient regarding adequate fluid intake and to report signs and symptoms of hypotension (postural dizziness, weakness, syncope).

• Advise patient to use care during first few weeks of therapy because of an increased risk of falls.

• Instruct patient on general diabetes care, including importance of diet and exercise and monitoring blood glucose and HbA_{1c} levels; signs and management of hypoglycemia and hyperglycemia; and assessing for diabetes complications.

• Advise patient to seek medical advice promptly during periods of stress (such as fever, trauma, infection, or surgery) because medication requirements may change.

• Instruct patient that if a dose is missed, to take it as soon as it's remembered unless it's almost time for the next dose, in which case the patient should skip missed dose and take drug at the next regularly scheduled time. Advise patient not to take two doses of drug at the same time.

candesartan cilexetil
kan-dah-SAR-tan

Atacand◆

Therapeutic class: Antihypertensives
Pharmacologic class: ARBs

AVAILABLE FORMS
Tablets: 4 mg, 8 mg, 16 mg, 32 mg

INDICATIONS & DOSAGES
Adjust-a-dose (for all indications): If patient is taking a diuretic, especially a patient with impaired renal function, administer under close medical supervision and consider a lower starting dose.

➤ **HTN (used alone or with other antihypertensives)**
Adults: Initially, 16 mg PO once daily when used alone in patients who aren't volume-depleted; usual range is 8 to 32 mg PO daily as a single dose or in two divided doses. Double the dose about every 2 weeks, as tolerated, to target dose of 32 mg once daily.
Adjust-a-dose: In patients with moderate hepatic impairment, initially give 8 mg PO once daily.

➤ **Pediatric HTN (used alone or with other antihypertensives)**
⟳ Alert: Don't use in children with GFR less than 30 mL/minute/1.73 m^2.
Children ages 6 to younger than 17: Initially for patients weighing more than 50 kg, 8 to 16 mg PO once daily. May adjust dosage to between 4 and 32 mg PO as single dose or divided doses as indicated.

Initially for patients weighing less than 50 kg, 4 to 8 mg PO once daily. May adjust dosage to between 2 and 16 mg PO as single dose or divided doses as needed.
Children ages 1 to younger than 6: Initially, 0.2 mg/kg PO once daily. Dosage range is 0.05 to 0.4 mg/kg/day PO, given as single dose or divided doses.

➤ **HF (NYHA Class II to IV)**
Adults: Initially, 4 mg PO once daily. Double the dose about every 2 weeks as tolerated to a target dose of 32 mg once daily.

Reactions in bold italics are *life-threatening*. Interactions may have a *rapid onset* or a *delayed onset*.

ADMINISTRATION
PO
- Give drug without regard for food.
- Tablets may be made into suspension by pharmacist for patients unable to swallow pills.
- Suspension may be stored unopened at room temperature for 100 days.
- Shake suspension well before each use.
- Use suspension within 30 days of opening bottle.

ACTION
Inhibits vasoconstrictive action of angiotensin II by blocking angiotensin II receptor on the surface of vascular smooth muscle and other tissue cells.

Route	Onset	Peak	Duration
PO	Unknown	3–4 hr	24 hr

Half-life: 9 hours.

ADVERSE REACTIONS
CNS: dizziness, fatigue, headache. **CV:** chest pain, peripheral edema. **EENT:** pharyngitis, rhinitis, sinusitis. **GI:** abdominal pain, diarrhea, nausea, vomiting. **GU:** albuminuria. **Musculoskeletal:** arthralgia, back pain. **Respiratory:** coughing, bronchitis, URI. **Other:** *angioedema.*

INTERACTIONS
Drug-drug. *ACE inhibitors, other ARBs:* May increase risk of hypotension, hyperkalemia, and changes in renal function (including acute renal failure) when used with other drugs that cause blockade of the RAAS. Consider therapy modification.
Aliskiren: May increase risk of renal impairment, hypotension, and hyperkalemia in diabetic patients and those with moderate to severe renal impairment (GFR <60 mL/minute). Concomitant use is contraindicated in diabetic patients. Avoid concomitant use in those with moderate to severe renal impairment.
Canagliflozin: May enhance hyperkalemic and hypotensive effects. Monitor closely.
Lithium: May increase lithium concentration. Monitor lithium levels closely.
NSAIDs (celecoxib, ibuprofen): May decrease antihypertensive effect of candesartan. Coadministration in patients who are elderly, volume-depleted (including those taking diuretics), or with decreased renal function may result in deteriorating renal function. Monitor BP and renal function.
Potassium-sparing diuretics, potassium supplements: May cause hyperkalemia. Monitor patient closely.
Drug-herb. *Ma huang:* May decrease antihypertensive effects. Discourage use together.
Drug-food. *Salt substitutes containing potassium:* May cause hyperkalemia. Monitor patient closely.

EFFECTS ON LAB TEST RESULTS
- May increase potassium, BUN, and serum creatinine levels.
- May cause false-negative aldosterone-to-renin ratio.

CONTRAINDICATIONS & CAUTIONS
- Contraindicated in patients hypersensitive to drug or its components, in children with GFR of less than 30 mL/min/1.73 m^2, and in children younger than age 1.
- Use cautiously in patients whose renal function depends on the RAAS (such as patients with HF) because of risk of oliguria and progressive azotemia with acute renal failure or death.
- Use cautiously in patients who are volume or salt depleted; may cause symptoms of hypotension. Start therapy with a lower dosage range, and monitor BP carefully.
- Don't use for HTN in children younger than age 1 because of potential effects on the developing immature kidneys.
Dialyzable drug: No.
⚠ **Overdose S&S:** Hypotension, dizziness, tachycardia; possible bradycardia from parasympathetic stimulation.

PREGNANCY-LACTATION-REPRODUCTION
Black Box Warning Drugs such as candesartan that act directly on the RAAS can cause injury and death to the developing fetus. If pregnancy is detected, discontinue candesartan as soon as possible. ∎
- It isn't known if drug appears in human milk. Consider discontinuing breastfeeding or drug, taking into account importance of drug to the mother.

NURSING CONSIDERATIONS
• If hypotension occurs after a dose of candesartan, place patient in the supine position and treat appropriately.
• Most of drug's antihypertensive effect occurs within 2 weeks. Maximal effect may take 4 to 6 weeks. Diuretic may be added if BP isn't controlled by drug alone.
• Carefully monitor elderly patients and those with renal disease for therapeutic response and adverse reactions.

PATIENT TEACHING
• Inform female patient of childbearing potential of the consequences of exposure to drug during pregnancy and to notify prescriber immediately if pregnancy is suspected.
• Advise breastfeeding patient of the risk of adverse effects on the infant and the need to stop either breastfeeding or drug.
• Instruct patient to store drug at room temperature in tightly sealed container.
• Inform patient to report all adverse reactions without delay.
• Tell patient that drug may be taken without regard to meals.

SAFETY ALERT!

cangrelor
KAN-grel-or

Kengreal

Therapeutic class: Antiplatelet drugs
Pharmacologic class: Platelet aggregation inhibitors

AVAILABLE FORMS
Lyophilized powder for injection: 50 mg

INDICATIONS & DOSAGES
➤ **As an adjunct to PCI for reducing risk of periprocedural MI, repeat coronary revascularization, and stent thrombosis in patients who haven't been treated with a P2Y12 platelet inhibitor and aren't receiving a glycoprotein IIb/IIIa inhibitor**
Adults: 30 mcg/kg IV bolus before PCI followed immediately by a 4-mcg/kg/minute IV infusion continued for at least 2 hours or for duration of PCI, whichever is longer.

Transition patient to oral P2Y12 platelet inhibitor to maintain platelet inhibition. Recommended inhibitors include ticagrelor 180 mg PO at any time during infusion or immediately after discontinuation, or prasugrel 60 mg or clopidogrel 600 mg immediately after discontinuation of infusion, but not before.

ADMINISTRATION
IV
▼ For each 50-mg vial, reconstitute by adding 5 mL sterile water for injection. Swirl gently until all material is dissolved; avoid vigorous mixing. Ensure contents are fully dissolved, clear, colorless to pale yellow, and free from particulate matter.
▼ Dilute reconstituted drug immediately. Don't use without dilution.
▼ Further dilute each reconstituted vial by withdrawing contents from one reconstituted vial and adding to one 250-mL NSS or dextrose 5% bag. Mix bag thoroughly. This dilution will result in a concentration of 200 mcg/mL and should be sufficient for at least 2 hours of dosing. Patients weighing 100 kg or more will require a minimum of two bags.
▼ Discard any unused portion of reconstituted solution remaining in vial.
▼ Administer via a dedicated IV line.
▼ Administer bolus volume rapidly (less than 1 minute) from the diluted bag via manual IV push or pump. Ensure bolus is completely administered before start of PCI. Start infusion immediately after administration of bolus.
▼ Diluted drug is stable for up to 12 hours in 5% dextrose injection and 24 hours in NSS at room temperature.
▼ **Incompatibilities:** None listed by manufacturer. Consult a drug incompatibility reference for more information.

ACTION
A direct P2Y12 platelet receptor inhibitor that blocks ADP-induced platelet activation and aggregation. Binds selectively and reversibly to the P2Y12 platelet receptor to prevent further signaling and platelet activation.

Route	Onset	Peak	Duration
IV	2 min	2 min	1 hr after discontinuation of infusion

Half-life: 3 to 6 minutes.

ADVERSE REACTIONS

CNS: *intracranial hemorrhage.* **GU:** worsening renal function in patients with severe renal impairment. **Hematologic:** *bleeding.* **Respiratory:** dyspnea.

INTERACTIONS

Drug-drug. *Agents with antiplatelet properties (NSAIDs, P2Y12 platelet inhibitors, SSRIs):* May enhance antiplatelet effects. Monitor therapy.
Anticoagulants: May increase anticoagulant effects. Monitor therapy.
Glucosamine: May enhance antiplatelet effects. Monitor therapy.
Thienopyridines (clopidogrel, prasugrel): Negate antiplatelet effect. Don't give clopidogrel or prasugrel until the cangrelor infusion has been discontinued.
Drug-herb. *Alfalfa, anise, bilberry:* May increase risk of bleeding. Modify therapy.

EFFECTS ON LAB TEST RESULTS
None reported.

CONTRAINDICATIONS & CAUTIONS
• Contraindicated in patients hypersensitive to drug or its components and in those with significant active bleeding.
• Although rare, drug can cause serious hypersensitivity reactions, including anaphylaxis, bronchospasm, angioedema, and stridor.
• Safety and effectiveness in children haven't been established.
Dialyzable drug: Unknown.

PREGNANCY-LACTATION-REPRODUCTION
• There are no adequate studies in pregnant women. Some adverse effects were noted in animal studies.
• It isn't known if drug appears in human milk.

NURSING CONSIDERATIONS
• Monitor patients for hypersensitivity reactions, including anaphylactic reactions, anaphylactic shock, bronchospasm, angioedema, and stridor. Discontinue drug immediately and treat emergently.
• Monitor patients for signs of overt bleeding and symptoms of active bleeding.
• Platelet function will resume 1 hour after discontinuation of infusion.

PATIENT TEACHING
• Explain to patient that drug is used to inhibit platelet function during PCI and that platelet function and ability for clot formation will resume 1 hour after discontinuation of the infusion.
• Warn patient of the risk of bleeding; advise patient to immediately report signs and symptoms of bleeding (mental status changes, light-headedness, low BP, blood in stool or urine, bleeding from gums, joint pain and swelling, abnormal bruising, abdominal or chest pain).
• Caution patient that hypersensitivity reactions may occur and to immediately report difficulty breathing, swelling of throat and lips, feeling faint, hives, or rash.

SAFETY ALERT!

capecitabine ▨
kap-ah-SEAT-ah-been

Xeloda

Therapeutic class: Antineoplastics
Pharmacologic class: Pyrimidine analogues

AVAILABLE FORMS
Tablets ⓪⃝: 150 mg, 500 mg

INDICATIONS & DOSAGES
Adjust-a-dose (for all indications): Round to nearest dose that gives a whole tablet; don't cut tablets in half. Refer to manufacturer's instructions for toxicity-related dosage adjustments.
➤ **With docetaxel or alone, metastatic breast cancer resistant to both paclitaxel and an anthracycline-containing chemotherapy regimen or resistant to paclitaxel in patients for whom further anthracycline therapy isn't indicated; first-line treatment of metastatic colorectal cancer when fluoropyrimidine therapy**

alone is preferred; Dukes stage C colon cancer after complete resection of primary tumor when fluoropyrimidine alone is preferred

Adults: 1,250 mg/m^2 PO b.i.d. (morning and evening; equal to 2,500 mg/m^2 total daily dose) for 2 weeks, followed by a 1-week rest period; repeat every 3 weeks. Adjuvant treatment in patients with Dukes C colon cancer is recommended for a total of eight cycles (24 weeks). Maximum dose is 5,600 mg/day.

Adjust-a-dose: When used as monotherapy or in combination with docetaxel, reduce starting dose for patients with CrCl of 30 to 50 mL/minute to 75% of starting dose (from 1,250 to 950 mg/m^2 PO b.i.d.).

➤ **Breast cancer (adjuvant therapy) in patients with HER2-negative primary breast cancer who had residual invasive disease after neoadjuvant therapy (containing an anthracycline, taxane, or both) and surgery ◆**

Adults: 1,250 mg/m^2 PO b.i.d. on days 1 to 14 of a 21-day treatment cycle for six to eight cycles.

➤ **Pancreatic cancer (adjuvant therapy) after complete resection of pancreatic adenocarcinoma ◆**

Adults: 1,660 mg/m^2/day (in two divided doses) PO on days 1 to 21 every 28 days (in combination with gemcitabine) for six cycles beginning within 8 to 12 weeks of resection.

➤ **Pancreatic cancer (locally advanced or metastatic) ◆**

Adults: 1,250 mg/m^2 PO b.i.d. on days 1 to 14 of a 3-week cycle or 830 mg/m^2 b.i.d. (in combination with gemcitabine) on days 1 to 21 of a 4-week cycle until disease progression or unacceptable toxicity.

ADMINISTRATION
PO
• Give drug whole with water within 30 minutes after a meal.
• Don't cut or crush tablets.
• Use gloves and safety glasses to avoid exposure if tablets break.

ACTION
Converts to active 5-FU, which causes cellular injury by interfering with DNA synthesis to inhibit cell division and with RNA processing and protein synthesis.

Route	Onset	Peak	Duration
PO	Unknown	90–120 min	Unknown

Half-life: About 45 minutes.

ADVERSE REACTIONS
CNS: dizziness, fatigue, headache, insomnia, paresthesia, pyrexia, lethargy, peripheral neuropathy, asthenia, ataxia. **CV:** edema, chest pain, *venous thrombosis,* arrhythmias. **EENT:** eye irritation, epistaxis, increased lacrimation, rhinorrhea. **GI:** diarrhea, nausea, vomiting, stomatitis, abdominal pain, constipation, anorexia, dyspepsia, taste perversion. **Hematologic:** *neutropenia, thrombocytopenia,* anemia, *lymphopenia.* **Hepatic:** hyperbilirubinemia. **Metabolic:** dehydration. **Musculoskeletal:** myalgia, limb pain, back pain. **Respiratory:** dyspnea. **Skin:** hand-foot syndrome, dermatitis, nail disorder, alopecia, rash. **Other:** neutropenic fever.

INTERACTIONS
Drug-drug. *Antacids containing aluminum hydroxide or magnesium hydroxide:* May increase exposure to capecitabine and its metabolites. Monitor patient.
Fosphenytoin, phenytoin: May increase toxicity or fosphenytoin/phenytoin effect. Consider therapy modification or monitor phenytoin level.
Leucovorin: May increase cytotoxic effects of 5-FU with enhanced toxicity. Monitor patient carefully.
Black Box Warning *Warfarin:* May decrease clearance of warfarin and increase risk of bleeding. Monitor PT and INR frequently. ■
Drug-herb. *Echinacea:* May diminish therapeutic effects of 5-FU. Avoid concurrent use.

EFFECTS ON LAB TEST RESULTS
• May increase ALT and bilirubin levels. May decrease Hb level. May increase or decrease calcium level.
• May decrease neutrophil, platelet, and WBC counts.
Black Box Warning May prolong PT and increase INR (in patients taking warfarin concomitantly). ■

Reactions in bold italics are *life-threatening*. Interactions may have a *rapid onset* or a *delayed onset*.

CONTRAINDICATIONS & CAUTIONS

• Contraindicated in patients hypersensitive to 5-FU, patients with known dihydropyrimidine dehydrogenase deficiency, and in those with severe renal impairment (CrCl <30 mL/minute).

• Severe bone marrow suppression can occur and is more common when drug is used in combination therapy. Dosage adjustment may be needed.

• Use cautiously in elderly patients and those with history of CAD, mild to moderate hepatic dysfunction from liver metastases, hyperbilirubinemia, and renal insufficiency. Use cautiously in patients also taking warfarin.

⚝ Patients with certain homozygous or heterozygous mutations in dihydropyrimidine have increased risk of acute early-onset toxicity and severe, life-threatening, or fatal adverse reactions.

Dialyzable drug: Unknown.

⚠ *Overdose S&S:* Nausea, vomiting, diarrhea, GI irritation and bleeding, bone marrow depression.

PREGNANCY-LACTATION-REPRODUCTION

• Fetal harm may occur if drug is administered during pregnancy. Women of childbearing potential should use effective contraception during treatment and for 6 months after final dose.

• Male patients with female partners of childbearing potential should use effective contraception during treatment and for 3 months after final dose.

• It isn't known if drug appears in human milk. Women shouldn't breastfeed during treatment and for 2 weeks after final dose.

NURSING CONSIDERATIONS

• Elderly patients may have a greater risk of adverse GI effects.

• Assess patient for severe diarrhea, and notify prescriber if it occurs. Give fluid and electrolyte replacement if patient becomes dehydrated. Drug may need to be immediately interrupted until diarrhea resolves or becomes less intense.

• Discontinue drug for severe mucocutaneous reactions, such as SJS and toxic epidermal necrolysis.

• Monitor patient for hand-foot syndrome (numbness, paresthesia, painless or painful swelling, erythema, desquamation, blistering, and severe pain of hands or feet), hyperbilirubinemia, and severe nausea. Drug therapy must be immediately adjusted. Hand-foot syndrome is staged from 1 to 4; drug may be stopped if severe or recurrent episodes occur.

Black Box Warning Frequently monitor INR and PT of patients taking capecitabine and oral coumarin-derivative anticoagulant therapy; adjust anticoagulant dose accordingly. ∎

Black Box Warning Patients older than age 60 and those with a diagnosis of cancer are at increased risk of coagulopathy. ∎

⊙ *Alert:* Monitor patient carefully for toxicity, which may be managed by symptomatic treatment, dose interruptions, and dosage adjustments.

• *Look alike–sound alike:* Don't confuse Xeloda with Xenical.

PATIENT TEACHING

• Tell patient how to take drug. Drug is usually taken for 14 days, followed by 7-day rest period (no drug), as a 21-day cycle. Prescriber determines number of treatment cycles. Instruct patent to swallow tablets whole and not to cut or crush them.

⊙ *Alert:* Tell patient who also takes warfarin to report significant bleeding or bruising.

• Instruct patient to take drug with water within 30 minutes after a meal.

• If a combination of tablets is prescribed, teach patient importance of correctly identifying the tablets to avoid possible dosing error.

• For missed doses, instruct patient not to take the missed dose and not to double the next one. Instead, patient should continue with regular dosing schedule and check with prescriber.

• Inform patient and caregiver about expected adverse effects of drug (especially nausea, vomiting, diarrhea, and hand-foot syndrome [pain, swelling, or redness of hands or feet]) and that patient-specific dosage adaptations during therapy are expected and needed.

⊙ *Alert:* Instruct patient to stop taking drug and contact prescriber immediately if diarrhea (more than four bowel movements daily or diarrhea at night), vomiting (two to five episodes in 24 hours), nausea, appetite loss or decrease in amount of food eaten each day, stomatitis (pain, redness, swelling, or sores in mouth), hand-foot syndrome, temperature of 100.5° F (38° C) or higher, or other evidence of infection develops.

• Tell patient that most adverse effects improve within 2 to 3 days after stopping drug. Advise patient who doesn't improve to contact prescriber.

• Advise female patient of childbearing potential to avoid becoming pregnant during therapy.

• Advise breastfeeding patient to stop breastfeeding during therapy.

captopril ⌧
KAP-toe-pril

Therapeutic class: Antihypertensives
Pharmacologic class: ACE inhibitors

AVAILABLE FORMS
Tablets: 12.5 mg, 25 mg, 50 mg, 100 mg

INDICATIONS & DOSAGES
Adjust-a-dose (for all indications): Patients with impaired renal function may respond to smaller or less frequent doses. In patients with significant renal impairment, reduce initial daily dosage, and use smaller increments for a slow titration (1- to 2-week intervals). Slowly back-titrate dosage after desired therapeutic effect has been achieved to determine the minimal effective dose. A loop diuretic such as furosemide, rather than a thiazide diuretic, is preferred in patients with severe renal impairment when concomitant diuretic therapy is required.

➤ **HTN (alone or in combination with other antihypertensives)**
Adults: Initially, 25 mg PO b.i.d. or t.i.d. If dosage doesn't control BP satisfactorily in 1 or 2 weeks, increase it to 50 mg b.i.d. or t.i.d. If that dosage doesn't control BP satisfactorily after another 1 or 2 weeks, expect to add a diuretic. If patient needs further BP reduction, may increase dosage to 100 mg b.i.d. or t.i.d., then if necessary, to 150 mg b.i.d. or t.i.d. while continuing

diuretic. Usual dosage range is 25 to 150 mg b.i.d. or t.i.d. Maximum daily dosage is 450 mg.

➤ **Diabetic nephropathy**
Adults: 25 mg PO t.i.d.

➤ **HF**
Adults: Initially, 25 mg PO t.i.d. Patients with normal or low BP who have been vigorously treated with diuretics and who may be hyponatremic or hypovolemic may start with 6.25 or 12.5 mg PO t.i.d.; starting dosage may be adjusted over several days. Gradually increase dosage to 50 mg PO t.i.d.; once patient reaches this dosage, delay further dosage increases for at least 2 weeks to assess satisfactory response. Usual dosage is 50 to 100 mg PO t.i.d.; maximum dosage is 450 mg daily. Generally used in conjunction with a diuretic; may also add a cardiac glycoside in select patients.

➤ **Left ventricular dysfunction after acute MI**
Adults: Start therapy as early as 3 days after MI with 6.25 mg PO for one dose, followed by 12.5 mg PO t.i.d. Increase over several days to 25 mg PO t.i.d.; then increase to 50 mg PO t.i.d. over several weeks.

ADMINISTRATION
PO
• Give 1 hour before meals to enhance drug absorption.
• Drug may be compounded into a suspension if patient can't swallow tablets.
• Refrigerate suspension and shake well before use. Suspension is stable for 56 days if refrigerated.

ACTION
Inhibits ACE, preventing conversion of angiotensin I to angiotensin II, a potent vasoconstrictor. Less angiotensin II decreases peripheral arterial resistance, decreasing aldosterone secretion, which reduces sodium and water retention and lowers BP.

Route	Onset	Peak	Duration
PO	Within 15 min	60–90 min	Unknown

Half-life: Less than 2 hours.

ADVERSE REACTIONS
CNS: dizziness, fainting, headache, malaise, fatigue, fever, insomnia, paresthesia.

C

CV: tachycardia, hypotension, chest pain, angina pectoris, palpitations. **GI:** abdominal pain, anorexia, constipation, diarrhea, dry mouth, dysgeusia, nausea, vomiting. **Hematologic:** *leukopenia, agranulocytosis, thrombocytopenia, pancytopenia,* anemia. **Metabolic:** hyperkalemia. **Respiratory:** dry, persistent, nonproductive cough; dyspnea. **Skin:** urticarial rash, maculopapular rash, pruritus, alopecia. **Other:** *angioedema.*

INTERACTIONS

Drug-drug. *Aliskiren:* May increase risk of renal impairment, hypotension, and hyperkalemia in diabetic patients and those with moderate to severe renal impairment (GFR <60 mL/minute). Concomitant use is contraindicated in diabetic patients. Avoid concomitant use in those with moderate to severe renal impairment.

Antacids: May decrease captopril effect. Separate dosage times.

ARBs: May increase toxic effects of captopril. Consider alternative therapy.

Canagliflozin: May enhance hyperkalemic and hypotensive effects. Monitor potassium level and BP.

Diuretics, other antihypertensives: May cause excessive hypotension. May need to stop diuretic or reduce captopril dosage.

Insulin, oral antidiabetics: May cause hypoglycemia when captopril therapy is started. Monitor patient closely.

Lithium: May increase lithium level; symptoms of toxicity possible. Monitor lithium level and patient closely.

Neprilysin inhibitors (sacubitril–valsartan): May increase risk of angioedema. Separate administration by at least 36 hours. Use together is contraindicated.

NSAIDs: May reduce antihypertensive effect. Monitor BP.

Potassium-sparing diuretics, potassium supplements: May cause hyperkalemia. Avoid using together unless hypokalemia is confirmed.

Drug-herb. *Black catechu:* May cause additional hypotensive effect. Discourage use together.

Drug-food. *Salt substitutes containing potassium:* May cause hyperkalemia. Monitor patient closely.

EFFECTS ON LAB TEST RESULTS

• May increase alkaline phosphatase, bilirubin, BUN, serum creatinine, and potassium levels. May decrease sodium, glucose, and Hb levels and hematocrit.

• May decrease granulocyte, platelet, RBC, and WBC counts.

• May cause false-positive urine acetone test results.

CONTRAINDICATIONS & CAUTIONS

• Contraindicated in patients hypersensitive to drug or other ACE inhibitors and in patients who had angioedema related to previous treatment with an ACE inhibitor.

• Use cautiously in patients with impaired renal function or serious autoimmune disease, especially SLE, and in those who have been exposed to other drugs that affect WBC counts or immune response.

Dialyzable drug: Yes (hemodialysis in adults only).

⚠ *Overdose S&S:* Hypotension.

PREGNANCY-LACTATION-REPRODUCTION

Black Box Warning Use during pregnancy can cause injury and death to the developing fetus. When pregnancy is detected, stop drug as soon as possible. ∎

• Drug appears in human milk. Patient should discontinue breastfeeding or discontinue drug, taking into account importance of drug to the mother.

NURSING CONSIDERATIONS

⚏ Black patients who take ACE inhibitors as monotherapy for HTN have a smaller reduction in BP than nonblacks.

⚏ Black patients taking ACE inhibitors have a higher incidence of angioedema than nonblacks.

• Monitor patient's BP and pulse rate frequently.

◑ *Alert:* Elderly patients may be more sensitive to drug's hypotensive effects.

• Assess patient for signs of angioedema.

• Drug causes cough, most frequently of all ACE inhibitors.

• In patients with impaired renal function or collagen vascular disease, monitor WBC and differential counts before starting treatment, every 2 weeks for the first 3 months of therapy, and periodically thereafter.

• *Look alike–sound alike:* Don't confuse captopril with carvedilol.

PATIENT TEACHING
• Instruct patient to take drug 1 hour before meals; food in the GI tract may reduce absorption.
• Inform patient that light-headedness is possible, especially during first few days of therapy, and to rise slowly to minimize this effect and to report occurrence to prescriber. If fainting occurs, tell patient to stop drug and call prescriber immediately.
• Tell patient to use caution in hot weather and during exercise. Lack of fluids, vomiting, diarrhea, and excessive perspiration can lead to light-headedness and syncope.
• Advise patient to report signs and symptoms of infection, such as fever and sore throat.
• Tell female patient to notify prescriber if pregnancy occurs. Drug will need to be stopped.
• Urge patient to promptly report swelling of the face, lips, or mouth or difficulty breathing.
• Advise patient not to use potassium-sparing diuretics, potassium supplements, or potassium-containing salt substitutes without first consulting prescriber.

---

carBAMazepine ⌧
kar-ba-MAZ-e-peen

Carbatrol, Epitol, Equetro, TEGretol, TEGretol-XR

Therapeutic class: Anticonvulsants
Pharmacologic class: Iminostilbene derivatives

AVAILABLE FORMS
Capsules (extended-release) ⓞⓝⓒ: 100 mg, 200 mg, 300 mg
Oral suspension: 100 mg/5 mL
Tablets ⓞⓝⓒ: 100 mg, 200 mg, 300 mg, 400 mg
Tablets (chewable): 100 mg
Tablets (extended-release) ⓞⓝⓒ: 100 mg, 200 mg, 400 mg

INDICATIONS & DOSAGES
➤ **Generalized tonic-clonic and complex partial seizures, mixed seizure patterns**
Adults and children older than age 12: Initially, 200 mg PO b.i.d. (conventional or extended-release tablets or capsules), or 100 mg suspension PO q.i.d. with meals. May be increased weekly by 200 mg daily in divided doses at 12-hour intervals for extended-release tablets or capsules or 6- to 8-hour intervals for conventional tablets or suspension, adjusted to minimum effective level. Maximum, 1,000 mg daily in children ages 12 to 15 and 1,200 mg daily in patients older than age 15. Doses up to 1,600 mg daily have been used in adults in rare instances. Usual maintenance dosage is 800 to 1,200 mg daily.
Children younger than age 12 (Carbatrol): Children taking total daily dosages of immediate-release carbamazepine of 400 mg or greater may be converted to the same total daily dosage of Carbatrol extended-release capsules, using a twice-daily regimen. Usually, optimal clinical response is achieved at daily doses below 35 mg/kg.
Children ages 6 to 12: Initially, 100 mg PO b.i.d. (conventional or extended-release tablets) or 50 mg suspension PO q.i.d. with meals, increased at weekly intervals by up to 100 mg PO in three to four divided doses daily (in two divided doses for extended-release form). Maximum, 1,000 mg daily. Usual maintenance dosage is 400 to 800 mg daily or 20 to 30 mg/kg in three or four divided doses.
Children younger than age 6: 10 to 20 mg/kg/day in two to three divided doses (conventional tablets) or four divided doses (suspension). Maximum dosage is 35 mg/kg in 24 hours.
➤ **Acute manic and mixed episodes associated with bipolar I disorder (Equetro only)**
Adults: Initially, 200 mg Equetro PO b.i.d. Increase by 200 mg daily to achieve therapeutic response. Doses higher than 1,600 mg daily haven't been studied.
➤ **Trigeminal neuralgia**
Adults: Initially, 100 mg PO b.i.d. (conventional or extended-release tablets) or 50 mg suspension PO q.i.d. with meals, increased by 100 mg every 12 hours for tablets or

---

Reactions in bold italics are *life-threatening*. Interactions may have a *rapid onset* or a *delayed onset*.

C

50 mg q.i.d. for suspension until pain is relieved. Maximum, 1,200 mg daily. Maintenance dosage is usually 200 to 400 mg PO b.i.d.

Or, initially, 200-mg capsule PO daily. May increase daily dosage by up to 200 mg/day every 12 hours, only as needed to achieve freedom from pain. Don't exceed 1,200 mg daily.

ADMINISTRATION
PO

• Shake oral suspension well before measuring dose.

• When converting from tablets to suspension, administer the same number of milligrams per day in smaller, more frequent doses.

• Give chewable, immediate-release, and extended-release tablets with meals.

• Contents of extended-release capsules may be sprinkled over applesauce if patient has difficulty swallowing capsules. Extended-release capsules may be administered with or without food. Capsules and tablets shouldn't be crushed or chewed, unless labeled as chewable form.

• When giving by NG tube, mix dose with an equal volume of water, NSS, or D₅W. Flush tube with 100 mL of diluent after giving dose.

• Don't crush or split extended-release form or give broken or chipped tablets.

• Patients converting from immediate-release to extended-release form should receive the same total daily dosage.

ACTION
Thought to stabilize neuronal membranes and limit seizure activity by either increasing efflux or decreasing influx of sodium ions across cell membranes in the motor cortex during generation of nerve impulses.

Route	Onset	Peak	Duration
PO	Unknown	1½–12 hr	Unknown
PO (extended-release)	Unknown	4–8 hr	Unknown

Half-life: 25 to 65 hours with single dose; 8 to 29 hours with long-term use.

ADVERSE REACTIONS
CNS: ataxia, dizziness, drowsiness, somnolence, vertigo, *worsening of seizures,* confusion, fatigue, fever, headache, syncope, pain, depression including *suicidal ideation,* speech disorder. **CV:** *arrhythmias, AV block, HF,* aggravation of CAD, HTN, hypotension. **EENT:** blurred vision, conjunctivitis, diplopia, nystagmus, dry pharynx. **GI:** nausea, vomiting, abdominal pain, anorexia, diarrhea, dry mouth, dyspepsia, glossitis, stomatitis. **GU:** albuminuria, glycosuria, erectile dysfunction, urinary frequency, urine retention. **Hematologic:** *agranulocytosis, aplastic anemia, thrombocytopenia,* eosinophilia, leukocytosis. **Hepatic:** *hepatitis.* **Metabolic:** hyponatremia. **Musculoskeletal:** leg cramps. **Respiratory:** pulmonary hypersensitivity. **Skin:** *erythema multiforme,* SJS, excessive diaphoresis, rash, urticaria, pruritus. **Other:** SIADH, chills.

INTERACTIONS
Drug-drug. *Anticoagulants:* May reduce anticoagulant effect. Monitor PT when starting or stopping carbamazepine.

Aripiprazole: May decrease aripiprazole serum concentration. Double aripiprazole dose when carbamazepine is added, then base additional dosage increases on clinical evaluation. If carbamazepine is later withdrawn, reduce aripiprazole dose.

Atracurium, cisatracurium, pancuronium, rocuronium, vecuronium: May decrease the effects of nondepolarizing muscle relaxant, causing it to be less effective. May need to increase the dose of the nondepolarizing muscle relaxant.

Azole antifungals (itraconazole, ketoconazole): May increase carbamazepine level and decrease antifungal level. Monitor levels and effectiveness of drugs.

Cimetidine, danazol, diltiazem, fluoxetine, fluvoxamine, isoniazid, valproic acid, verapamil: May increase carbamazepine level. Use with isoniazid may increase risk of hepatotoxicity. Use together cautiously.

Clarithromycin, erythromycin: May inhibit metabolism of carbamazepine, increasing carbamazepine level and risk of toxicity. Avoid using together.

Cyclophosphamide: May increase risk of cyclophosphamide-related toxicities. Monitor carefully.

Doxycycline, felbamate, haloperidol, hormonal contraceptives, phenytoin, theophylline, tiagabine, topiramate, valproate: May decrease levels of these drugs. Watch for decreased effect.

Lamotrigine: May decrease lamotrigine level and increase carbamazepine level. Monitor patient for clinical effects and toxicity.

Lapatinib: May decrease lapatinib serum concentration; lapatinib dosage may need to be increased. Avoid use together when possible.

Lithium: May increase CNS toxicity of lithium. Avoid using together.

MAO inhibitors: May increase depressant and anticholinergic effects. Avoid using together. Discontinue MAO inhibitors at least 14 days before starting carbamazepine.

Nefazodone: May increase carbamazepine levels and toxicity while reducing nefazodone levels and therapeutic benefits. Use together is contraindicated.

Oral and other hormonal contraceptives: May cause breakthrough bleeding and reduced contraceptive effectiveness. Consider back-up method of birth control.

Phenobarbital, phenytoin, primidone: May decrease carbamazepine level. Watch for decreased effect.

SSRIs, TCAs: May increase carbamazepine level and decrease levels of antidepressant. Closely monitor patient and adjust dosage as needed.

Drug-food. *Grapefruit juice:* May increase carbamazepine level. Don't use together.

Drug-herb. *Plantains (psyllium seed):* May inhibit GI absorption of drug. Discourage use together.

EFFECTS ON LAB TEST RESULTS

• May increase BUN level and LFT values. May decrease sodium levels and thyroid function test values.

• May increase eosinophil and WBC counts. May decrease granulocyte and platelet counts.

• May interact with some pregnancy tests.

CONTRAINDICATIONS & CAUTIONS

• Contraindicated in patients hypersensitive to this drug or TCAs and in those with a history of bone marrow suppression; also contraindicated in those who have taken an MAO inhibitor within 14 days. Concomitant use with delavirdine or other NNRTIs or nefazodone is also contraindicated.

• Use cautiously in patients with mixed seizure disorders because they may experience an increased risk of seizures. Also, use cautiously in patients with renal and hepatic dysfunction. Avoid use in patients with porphyria.

• Serious and sometimes fatal DRESS syndrome can occur; drug may need to be stopped and patient converted to another therapy.

• Drug may cause AV heart block conduction abnormalities. Use cautiously in patients at risk for conduction abnormalities, in those with abnormal ECGs, and in patients with preexisting heart damage.

• Drug can cause hyponatremia. Risk appears dose-related and may be increased in elderly patients or patients taking diuretics. For symptomatic hyponatremia, drug may need to be discontinued.

• Safety and effectiveness of Equetro in children and adolescents haven't been established for indications other than epilepsy.

Dialyzable drug: Yes.

⚠ *Overdose S&S:* Conduction disorders, hypotension or HTN, impairment of consciousness, irregular breathing, respiratory depression, tachycardia, shock, seizures, adiadochokinesia, ataxia, athetoid movements, ballism, dizziness, drowsiness, dysmetria, motor restlessness, muscular twitching, mydriasis, nystagmus, opisthotonos, psychomotor disturbances, tremor; hyperreflexia followed by anuria or oliguria, hyporeflexia, nausea and vomiting, urine retention.

PREGNANCY-LACTATION-REPRODUCTION

• Drug can cause fetal harm, including major congenital malformations, when administered during pregnancy. Weigh benefits against the risks. If used in pregnant women, monotherapy, rather than use in combination with other anticonvulsants, is recommended to possibly reduce risk of teratogenic effects.

Reactions in bold italics are *life-threatening*. Interactions may have a *rapid onset* or a *delayed onset*.

C

• Consider tests to detect defects using currently accepted procedures as part of routine prenatal care in pregnant women receiving drug.

• Pregnant women taking carbamazepine should enroll themselves in the North American Antiepileptic Drug Pregnancy Registry by calling 1-888-233-2334 or by visiting www.aedpregnancyregistry.org.

• Drug and its metabolite appear in human milk. Patient should discontinue breastfeeding or discontinue drug, taking into account importance of drug to the mother.

NURSING CONSIDERATIONS

Black Box Warning Patients of Asian ancestry should be screened with blood tests to identify their genetic risk of rare, but serious skin reactions (toxic epidermal necrolysis, SJS). Screen for HLA-B*1502 allele before starting treatment with carbamazepine. ∎

• Watch for worsening of seizures, especially in patients with mixed seizure disorders, including atypical absence seizures.

⊕ **Alert:** Closely monitor all patients taking or starting AEDs for changes in behavior indicating worsening of suicidal thoughts or behavior or depression. Symptoms such as anxiety, agitation, hostility, mania, and hypomania may be precursors to emerging suicidality.

• Obtain baseline determinations of urinalysis, renal function, iron levels, electrolyte levels, liver function, CBC, and platelet and reticulocyte counts. Monitor these values periodically thereafter.

Black Box Warning Aplastic anemia and agranulocytosis have been reported in association with carbamazepine therapy. Obtain complete pretreatment hematologic testing as a baseline. If patient in the course of treatment exhibits low or decreased WBC or platelet counts, monitor patient closely. Consider discontinuing drug if significant bone marrow depression develops. ∎

• Never stop drug suddenly when treating seizures. Notify prescriber immediately if adverse reactions occur.

• Adverse reactions may be minimized by increasing dosages gradually.

• Therapeutic level is 4 to 12 mcg/mL. Monitor level and effects closely. Ask patient when last dose was taken to better evaluate drug level.

• When managing seizures, take appropriate precautions.

⊕ **Alert:** Watch for signs of anorexia or subtle appetite changes, which may indicate excessive drug level.

• **Look alike–sound alike:** Don't confuse carbamazepine with oxcarbazepine. Don't confuse Tegretol or Tegretol-XR with Trental, Topamax, Toprol-XL, or Toradol. Don't confuse Carbatrol with carvedilol.

PATIENT TEACHING

• Tell patient that genetic testing may be needed before start of therapy.

• Instruct patient to take drug with food to minimize GI distress. Tell patient taking suspension form to shake container well before measuring dose.

• Tell patient not to crush or chew tablets or capsules and not to take broken or chipped tablets.

• Tell patient that TEGretol-XR tablet coating may appear in stool because it isn't absorbed.

• Advise patient to keep tablets in the original container and to keep the container tightly closed and away from moisture. Some formulations may harden when exposed to excessive moisture, so that less is available in the body, decreasing seizure control.

• Inform patient that when drug is used for trigeminal neuralgia, an attempt to decrease dosage or withdraw drug is usually made every 3 months.

• Advise patient to report adverse reactions and to immediately report fever, sore throat, mouth ulcers, or easy bruising or bleeding.

• Tell patient that drug may cause mild to moderate dizziness and drowsiness when first taken and to avoid hazardous activities until effects disappear, usually within 3 to 4 days.

• Advise patient that periodic eye exams are recommended.

• Inform female patient of risks to fetus if pregnancy occurs while taking carbamazepine; advise her to enroll in the North American Antiepileptic Drug Pregnancy Registry.

• Advise female patient that breastfeeding isn't recommended during therapy.

CARBOplatin
KAR-bo-pla-tin

Therapeutic class: Antineoplastics
Pharmacologic class: Platinum-containing compounds

AVAILABLE FORMS
Aqueous solution for injection: 50 mg/5 mL, 150 mg/15 mL, 450 mg/45 mL, 600 mg/60 mL

INDICATIONS & DOSAGES
➤ **Advanced ovarian cancer**
Adults: 360 mg/m² IV on day 1 every 4 weeks. Or, 300 mg/m² on day 1 every 4 weeks for six cycles when used with other chemotherapy drugs. Or, use the Calvert formula to calculate initial dosage:

Total dose (mg) = (target AUC in mg/mL/minute)
$$\times \text{(GFR in mL/minute} + 25)$$

where *target AUC* (area under the curve) is usually 4 to 6 mg/mL/minute and *GFR* is measured in mL/minute.

Doses shouldn't be repeated until platelet count exceeds 100,000/mm³ and neutrophil count exceeds 2,000/mm³. Subsequent doses are based on blood counts: If platelet count is greater than 100,000/mm³ and neutrophil count is greater than 2,000/mm³, give 125% of prior dose. If platelet count is 50,000/mm³ to 100,000/mm³ and neutrophil count is 500/mm³ to 2,000/mm³, keep same dose. If platelet count is less than 50,000/mm³ and neutrophil count is less than 500/mm³, give 75% of dose.
Adjust-a-dose: If CrCl is 41 to 59 mL/minute, first dose is 250 mg/m². If CrCl is 16 to 40 mL/minute, first dose is 200 mg/m². Drug isn't recommended for patients with CrCl of 15 mL/minute or less.
➤ **Neuroblastoma, localized and unresectable**
Children weighing 10 kg or more: 200 mg/m²/day IV on days 1, 2, and 3 every 21 days for two cycles (in combination with etopo-

side for two cycles, then followed by cyclophosphamide, doxorubicin, and vincristine).
Children younger than age 1: 6.6 mg/kg/day IV on days 1, 2, and 3 (in combination with etoposide for two cycles, then followed by cyclophosphamide, doxorubicin, and vincristine).
➤ **Glioma**
Children and adolescents age 3 months and older: For induction, 175 mg/m² IV weekly for 4 weeks every 6 weeks for two cycles, with a 2-week recovery period between courses (in combination with vincristine).

For maintenance, 175 mg/m² IV weekly for 4 weeks (in combination with vincristine) for up to 12 cycles, with a 3-week recovery period between cycles.
➤ **Recurrent/refractory Ewing sarcoma and osteosarcoma**
Adults and children age 1 and older: 400 mg/m²/day IV for 2 days every 21 days (in combination with ifosfamide and etoposide).

ADMINISTRATION
IV

Black Box Warning Anaphylaxis may occur within minutes of administration. Keep epinephrine, corticosteroids, and antihistamines available when giving carboplatin. ■
▼ Hazardous agent; use safe handling and disposal precautions according to facility policy.
▼ Don't use aluminum needles or IV administration sets because drug may precipitate or lose potency.
▼ For premixed aqueous solution of 10 mg/mL, dilute for infusion with NSS or D₅W to a concentration as low as 0.5 mg/mL; however, most clinicians generally dilute dose in either 100 or 250 mL of NSS or D₅W.
▼ Give drug by continuous or intermittent infusion over at least 15 minutes.
▼ Store unopened vials at room temperature. Protect from light.
▼ Once diluted as directed, drug is stable at room temperature for 8 hours.
▼ Because drug contains no preservatives, discard after 8 hours.

▼ **Incompatibilities:** None listed by manufacturer. Consult a drug incompatibility reference for more information.

ACTION
May cross-link strands of cellular DNA and interfere with RNA transcription, causing an imbalance of growth that leads to cell death. Not specific to cell cycle.

Route	Onset	Peak	Duration
IV	Unknown	Unknown	Unknown

Half-life: Carboplatin, about 2½ to 6 hours; platinum, 5 or more days.

ADVERSE REACTIONS
CNS: dizziness, confusion, *stroke,* peripheral neuropathy, *central neurotoxicity,* pain, asthenia, fever. **CV:** *HF, embolism.* **EENT:** ototoxicity. **GI:** abdominal pain, constipation, diarrhea, nausea, vomiting, mucositis, change in taste, stomatitis. **GU:** renal toxicity. **Hematologic:** *thrombocytopenia, leukopenia, neutropenia,* anemia, *bone marrow suppression, bleeding.* **Skin:** alopecia. **Other:** hypersensitivity reactions.

INTERACTIONS
Drug-drug. *Bone marrow suppressants, including radiation therapy:* May increase hematologic toxicity. Monitor CBC with differential closely.
Live-virus vaccines: May diminish vaccine's effect. Don't give live-virus vaccines for 3 months after carboplatin.
Nephrotoxic drugs, especially aminoglycosides and amphotericin B: May enhance nephrotoxicity of carboplatin. Use together cautiously.
Phenytoin: May decrease phenytoin level. Monitor serum level and patient for decreased effectiveness.
Drug-herb. *Echinacea:* May diminish therapeutic effects of carboplatin. Avoid concurrent use.

EFFECTS ON LAB TEST RESULTS
• May increase alkaline phosphatase, AST, BUN, and creatinine levels. May decrease electrolyte and Hb levels and hematocrit.
• May decrease neutrophil, platelet, RBC, and WBC counts.

CONTRAINDICATIONS & CAUTIONS
• Contraindicated in patients with severe bone marrow suppression or bleeding and in patients with history of hypersensitivity to cisplatin, platinum-containing compounds, or mannitol.
Dialyzable drug: Yes.
⚠ *Overdose S&S:* Bone marrow suppression, hepatotoxicity.

PREGNANCY-LACTATION-REPRODUCTION
• There are no adequate well-controlled studies in pregnant women. Drug may cause fetal harm when administered to a pregnant woman. Avoid use in women of childbearing potential. Women shouldn't become pregnant during therapy.
• It's unknown if drug appears in human milk. Patient should discontinue breastfeeding during therapy.

NURSING CONSIDERATIONS
Black Box Warning Carboplatin should be administered under the supervision of a physician experienced in the use of chemotherapeutic agents. Appropriate management of therapy and complications is possible only when adequate treatment facilities are readily available. ■
• Determine electrolyte, creatinine, and BUN levels; CBC with differential; platelet count; and CrCl before first infusion and before each course of treatment.
⊕ *Alert:* When using the Calvert formula, the total dose is calculated in mg, not mg/m^2.
• Monitor CBC with differential and platelet count frequently during therapy and, when indicated, until recovery. Lowest WBC and platelet counts usually occur by day 21. Levels usually return to baseline by day 28. Don't repeat unless platelet count exceeds 100,000/mm^3.
Black Box Warning Bone marrow suppression is dose related and may be severe, resulting in infection or bleeding. ■
Black Box Warning Vomiting is another frequent drug-related side effect. ■
• Bone marrow suppression may be more severe in patients with CrCl below 60 mL/minute; adjust dosage.
⊕ *Alert:* Carefully check ordered dose against laboratory test results. Only one increase in dosage is recommended.

Subsequent doses shouldn't exceed 125% of starting dose.
• Therapeutic effects are commonly accompanied by toxicity.
• Drug has less nephrotoxicity and neurotoxicity than cisplatin, but it causes more severe myelosuppression.
• To prevent bleeding, avoid all IM injections when platelet count is below 50,000/mm^3.
• Monitor vital signs during infusion.
• Antiemetics are recommended to prevent nausea and vomiting.
Black Box Warning Anemia may be cumulative and may require transfusion support. ∎
• Patients older than age 65 are at greater risk for neurotoxicity.
• *Look alike–sound alike:* Don't confuse carboplatin with cisplatin.

PATIENT TEACHING
• Advise patient of most common adverse reactions: nausea, vomiting, bone marrow suppression, anemia, and reduction in blood platelets.
• Advise patient to watch for signs of infection (fever, sore throat, fatigue) and bleeding (easy bruising, nosebleeds, bleeding gums, tarry stools). Tell patient to take temperature daily.
• Instruct patient to avoid OTC products containing aspirin and NSAIDs.
• Advise female patient to stop breastfeeding during therapy because of risk of toxicity to infant.
• Because of risk of sterility and menstruation cessation, counsel both men and women of childbearing potential before starting therapy. Also recommend that women consult prescriber before becoming pregnant.

cariprazine hydrochloride
kar-IP-ra-zeen

Vraylar

Therapeutic class: Antipsychotics
Pharmacologic class: Atypical antipsychotics

AVAILABLE FORMS
Capsules: 1.5 mg, 3 mg, 4.5 mg, 6 mg

INDICATIONS & DOSAGES
Adjust-a-dose (for all indications): If a strong CYP3A4 inhibitor is initiated while patient is on a stable dose of cariprazine, reduce cariprazine dosage by half; if patient is taking 4.5 mg daily, reduce to 1.5 or 3 mg daily; if patient is taking 1.5 mg daily, give every other day. Adjust cariprazine dosage when CYP3A4 inhibitor is discontinued. If initiating cariprazine while patient is on a strong CYP3A4 inhibitor, give 1.5 mg on days 1 and 3 (with no dose on day 2); from day 4 onward, give 1.5 mg daily, and increase to a maximum dose of 3 mg daily. Adjust cariprazine dosage when CYP3A4 inhibitor is discontinued. Concomitant use of cariprazine and CYP3A4 inducers hasn't been studied and isn't recommended.
➤ **Schizophrenia; manic or mixed episodes associated with bipolar I disorder**
Adults: Initially, 1.5 mg PO once daily on day 1. May increase to 3 mg PO once daily on day 2. Based on patient's response and tolerability, may make further dosage adjustments in 1.5- or 3-mg increments. Recommended dosage range for schizophrenia is 1.5 to 6 mg once daily. Recommended dosage for bipolar I disorder is 3 to 6 mg once daily. Maximum, 6 mg daily.
➤ **Antidepressant augmentation in unipolar major depressive disorder ♦**
Adults: Initially, 0.5 mg/day. Beginning on day 3, increase based on response and tolerability in 0.5-mg increments to a goal dose of 2 mg/day by end of first week; may continue to increase based on response and tolerability in 0.5-mg/day increments up to 4.5 mg/day.
✳ *NEW INDICATION:* Treatment of depressive episodes associated with bipolar I disorder (bipolar depression)
Adults: Initially, 1.5 mg PO once daily. May increase to 3 mg PO once daily on day 15 based on patient's response and tolerability. Maximum dosage is 3 mg daily.

ADMINISTRATION
PO
• May give with or without food.
• Store at room temperature.
• Protect 3- and 4.5-mg capsules from light to prevent potential color fading.

Reactions in bold italics are *life-threatening*. Interactions may have a *rapid onset* or a *delayed onset*.

ACTION

Exact mechanism unknown. Action thought to occur through partial agonist activity at central dopamine D_2 and serotonin 5-HT$_{1A}$ receptors as well as antagonist activity at serotonin 5-HT$_{2A}$ receptors.

Route	Onset	Peak	Duration
PO	Unknown	3–6 hr	Unknown

Half-life: 48 to 96 hours (parent compound); 1 day to 3 weeks (major metabolites).

ADVERSE REACTIONS

CNS: fatigue, pyrexia, extrapyramidal symptoms, akathisia, headache, somnolence, dizziness, agitation, insomnia, restlessness, anxiety, dystonia, parkinsonism. **CV:** tachycardia, HTN. **EENT:** blurred vision, nasopharyngitis, toothache, oropharyngeal pain. **GI:** abdominal pain, constipation, diarrhea, dyspepsia, nausea, vomiting, dry mouth. **GU:** UTI. **Metabolic:** weight gain, decreased appetite. **Musculoskeletal:** arthralgia, back pain, extremity pain, stiffness. **Respiratory:** cough. **Skin:** rash.

INTERACTIONS

Drug-drug. *Antiparkinsonians (dopamine agonists):* May diminish therapeutic effect of dopamine agonists; when possible in patients with Parkinson disease, consider using an alternative antipsychotic, such as clozapine or quetiapine, which may convey the lowest interaction risk.
CNS depressants: May increase CNS depression. Monitor therapy.
CYP3A4 inducers (carbamazepine, rifampin): May increase or decrease cariprazine concentration. Use together isn't recommended.
Black Box Warning *Opioid class warning:* May cause slow or difficult breathing, sedation, and death. Avoid use together. If use together is necessary, limit dosage and duration of each drug to the minimum necessary for desired effect. ∎
Strong CYP3A4 inhibitors (itraconazole, ketoconazole): May increase cariprazine concentration. Reduce cariprazine dosage.
Drug-herb. *Kava kava:* May enhance adverse or toxic effects of cariprazine. Monitor concurrent use.

St. John's wort: May decrease cariprazine concentration. Discourage use together.
Drug-food. *Grapefruit juice (CYP3A4 inhibitor):* May increase cariprazine concentration. Discourage use together.

EFFECTS ON LAB TEST RESULTS
• May increase CK and liver enzyme levels.
• May decrease WBC count.

CONTRAINDICATIONS & CAUTIONS
• Contraindicated in patients hypersensitive to drug or its components.
Black Box Warning Antipsychotics increase the risk of death in elderly patients with dementia-related psychosis. Drug isn't approved to treat patients with dementia-related psychosis. ∎
Black Box Warning *Opioid class warning:* Opioids should only be prescribed with benzodiazepines or other CNS depressants to patients for whom alternative treatment options are inadequate. ∎
⚠ **Alert:** Antipsychotics can cause leukopenia and neutropenia, which can be fatal. Use cautiously in patients with preexisting low WBC count or ANC or history of drug-induced leukopenia or neutropenia.
• Antipsychotics can cause orthostatic hypotension and syncope. Drug hasn't been evaluated in patients with a recent history of MI or unstable CV disease.
• Antipsychotics can cause NMS, which can be fatal.
• Drug may cause irreversible tardive dyskinesia, especially in elderly patients, most notably elderly women.
• Antipsychotics can disrupt the body's ability to reduce core body temperature; impair judgment, thinking, or motor skills; and increase risk of metabolic changes (hyperglycemia, diabetes mellitus, dyslipidemia, weight gain), esophageal dysmotility, aspiration, aspiration pneumonia, and falls.
• Antipsychotics increase risk of seizures, especially in patients with a history of seizures or with conditions that lower the seizure threshold.
• Drug is associated with dystonia, especially in males and younger age-groups, most commonly during first few days of treatment.

- Use isn't recommended in patients with severe hepatic or renal impairment.
- Safety and effectiveness in children haven't been established.

Dialyzable drug: Unlikely.

⚠ *Overdose S&S:* Orthostasis, sedation.

PREGNANCY-LACTATION-REPRODUCTION

- Drug may cause fetal harm. Neonates exposed to antipsychotics during the third trimester are at risk for extrapyramidal and withdrawal signs and symptoms, which can vary in severity and require prolonged hospitalization.
- Encourage women exposed to drug during pregnancy to enroll in the National Pregnancy Registry for Atypical Antipsychotics (1-866-961-2388).
- It isn't known if drug appears in human milk. Consider risks and benefits before using in breastfeeding women.

NURSING CONSIDERATIONS

- Monitor patients for hypersensitivity reactions (rash, pruritus, urticaria, swollen tongue or lips, facial edema, pharyngeal edema).
- Monitor patients for signs and symptoms of NMS (hyperpyrexia, muscle rigidity, delirium, autonomic instability, elevated CK level, rhabdomyolysis, acute renal failure); discontinue drug immediately if reactions appear. Provide intensive symptomatic treatment and monitoring.
- Monitor patients for signs and symptoms of tardive dyskinesia (potentially irreversible, involuntary, dyskinetic movements). Drug may need to be discontinued.
- Monitor patients for signs and symptoms of dystonia (throat tightness, difficulty swallowing or breathing, tongue protrusion).
- Monitor blood glucose, triglyceride, and lipid levels and for changes in weight, waist circumference, and BMI.
- Monitor patients for clinically significant leukopenia, neutropenia, fever, or other signs and symptoms of infection; treat promptly. Agranulocytosis (sometimes fatal) has been reported with antipsychotic use. Discontinue drug for ANC less than 1,000/mm³ and monitor WBC count until abnormalities resolve.

- Monitor patients for orthostatic hypotension, especially in elderly patients and those with dehydration, hypovolemia, concomitant treatment with antihypertensives, and known CV or cerebrovascular disease. Complete fall risk assessments at baseline and periodically during treatment.
- Ask patients about a history of seizures and review patients' medications for those that might lower the seizure threshold, as drug may increase the risk of seizures.
- Monitor patients who are exposed to strenuous exercise or extreme heat, are dehydrated, or are taking anticholinergics for elevated core body temperature.
- Watch for abnormal, involuntary movements, which may indicate extrapyramidal reactions; drug may need to be stopped.
- *Look alike–sound alike:* Don't confuse Vraylar with Valchlor.

PATIENT TEACHING

Black Box Warning *Opioid class warning:* Caution patient or caregiver of patient taking an opioid with a benzodiazepine, CNS depressant, or alcohol to seek immediate medical attention for dizziness, lightheadedness, extreme sleepiness, slowed or difficult breathing, or unresponsiveness. ■

- Counsel patient on importance of following dosage escalation instructions.
- Explain potential for dystonic or extrapyramidal signs and symptoms (involuntary, abnormal movements). Advise patient to immediately report signs and symptoms to prescriber, as drug may need to be discontinued.
- Instruct patient to report signs and symptoms of NMS.
- Educate patient about risk of metabolic changes and how to recognize signs and symptoms of hyperglycemia and diabetes mellitus. Instruct patient that laboratory monitoring of blood glucose and lipid levels and monitoring weight for changes may be necessary.
- Advise patient to report fever or other signs or symptoms of infection, which may indicate blood dyscrasias.
- Remind patient to avoid strenuous exercise or exposure to extreme heat and to drink plenty of water, as drug may impair body temperature–regulating ability.

C

- Counsel patient on risk of orthostatic hypotension and syncope, especially during treatment initiation and dosage increases.
- Warn patient about potential for drug interactions and advise patient to report to prescriber all OTC and prescription drugs and natural supplements being taken.
- Caution patient about operating hazardous machinery, including motor vehicles, until drug's effects on cognitive and motor skills are known.
- Advise female patient who is pregnant, considering pregnancy, or is breastfeeding to discuss risks and benefits with prescriber.

carisoprodol
kar-eye-soe-PROE-dol

Soma✎

Therapeutic class: Skeletal muscle relaxants
Pharmacologic class: Carbamate
derivatives
Controlled substance schedule: IV

AVAILABLE FORMS
Tablets: 250 mg, 350 mg

INDICATIONS & DOSAGES
➤ **Adjunctive treatment for acute, painful musculoskeletal conditions**
Adults: 250 to 350 mg PO t.i.d. and at bedtime for a maximum of 2 to 3 weeks.

ADMINISTRATION
PO
- May give with or without food. Give with food or milk if GI upset occurs.

ACTION
May modify central perception of pain without modifying pain reflexes. Muscle relaxant effects may be related to sedative properties.

Route	Onset	Peak	Duration
PO	½ hr	1½–2 hr	4–6 hr

Half-life: 2 hours for carisoprodol, 10 hours for active metabolite.

ADVERSE REACTIONS
CNS: drowsiness, dizziness, headache.
Respiratory: *asthmatic episodes.* **Skin:**

erythema multiforme, pruritus, rash. **Other:**
angioedema, anaphylaxis.

INTERACTIONS
Drug-drug. *CNS depressants:* May increase CNS depression. Avoid using together.
CYP2C19 inducers (rifampin): May increase active metabolite (meprobamate) exposure and decrease available carisoprodol. Use cautiously together.
CYP2C19 inhibitors (fluvoxamine, omeprazole): May decrease metabolism of carisoprodol to meprobamate, increasing exposure to carisoprodol. Use cautiously together.
Meprobamate: May increase meprobamate level. Avoid use together.
Black Box Warning *Opioid class warning:* May cause slow or difficult breathing, sedation, and death. Avoid use together. If use together is necessary, limit dosage and duration of each drug to the minimum necessary for desired effect. ∎
Drug-herb. *Kava kava:* May enhance CNS adverse or toxic effects. Monitor therapy.
St. John's wort: May increase active metabolite (meprobamate) exposure and decrease available carisoprodol. Use cautiously together.
Drug-lifestyle. *Alcohol use:* May increase CNS depression. Discourage use together.

EFFECTS ON LAB TEST RESULTS
- May increase eosinophil count.

CONTRAINDICATIONS & CAUTIONS
- Contraindicated in patients hypersensitive to related compounds (such as meprobamate) and in those with intermittent porphyria.
Black Box Warning *Opioid class warning:* Opioids should only be prescribed with benzodiazepines or other CNS depressants to patients for whom alternative treatment options are inadequate. ∎
⊘ *Alert:* Drug is Schedule IV controlled substance; cases of dependence, withdrawal, and abuse have occurred.
- Use cautiously in patients with impaired hepatic or renal function.
- Safety and effectiveness in adults older than age 65 and children younger than age 16 haven't been established.

Dialyzable drug: Yes.

⚠ *Overdose S&S:* Stupor, coma, seizures, shock, respiratory depression, drowsiness, dizziness, headache, diplopia, nystagmus, delirium, dystonia, muscular incoordination.

PREGNANCY-LACTATION-REPRODUCTION
• Safe use during pregnancy hasn't been established. Use in pregnant women only if potential benefit justifies risk to the fetus.
• Drug appears in human milk. Use cautiously in breastfeeding women.

NURSING CONSIDERATIONS
❸ *Alert:* Watch for idiosyncratic reactions after first to fourth doses (weakness, ataxia, visual and speech difficulties, fever, skin eruptions, and mental status changes) and for severe reactions, including bronchospasm, hypotension, and anaphylactic shock. After unusual reactions, withhold dose and notify prescriber immediately.
• Record amount of relief to help prescriber determine whether dosage can be reduced.
• Don't stop drug abruptly, which may cause mild withdrawal effects, such as insomnia, headache, nausea, or abdominal cramps.
• Monitor patient for dependence and signs and symptoms of abuse and overdose.

PATIENT TEACHING
Black Box Warning *Opioid class warning:* Caution patient or caregiver of patient taking an opioid with a benzodiazepine, CNS depressant, or alcohol to seek immediate medical attention for dizziness, lightheadedness, extreme sleepiness, slowed or difficult breathing, or unresponsiveness. ∎
• Warn patient to avoid activities that require alertness until CNS effects of drug are known. Drowsiness is transient.
• Advise patient to avoid combining drug with alcohol or other CNS depressants.
• Tell patient to ask prescriber before using OTC cold or hay fever remedies.
• Instruct patient and family that drug can cause dependence.
• Advise patient to avoid sudden changes in posture if dizziness occurs.
• Tell patient to take drug with food or milk if GI upset occurs.

SAFETY ALERT!

carmustine (BCNU)
kar-MUS-teen

BiCNU, Gliadel Wafer

Therapeutic class: Antineoplastics
Pharmacologic class: Nitrosoureas

AVAILABLE FORMS
Injection: 100-mg vial (lyophilized), with a 3-mL vial of absolute alcohol supplied as a diluent
Wafer: 7.7 mg, for intracavitary use

INDICATIONS & DOSAGES
➤ **Brain tumor, Hodgkin lymphoma, malignant lymphoma, multiple myeloma**
Adults: 150 to 200 mg/m^2 IV by slow infusion every 6 weeks; may be divided into daily injections of 75 to 100 mg/m^2 on 2 successive days; repeat dose every 6 weeks if platelet count is greater than 100,000/mm^3 and WBC count is greater than 4,000/mm^3.
Adjust-a-dose: Dosage is reduced by 30% when WBC nadir is 2,000 to 2,999/mm^3 and platelet nadir is 25,000 to 74,999/mm^3. Dosage is reduced by 50% when WBC nadir is less than 2,000/mm^3 and platelet nadir is less than 25,000/mm^3.
➤ **Adjunct to surgery to prolong survival in patients with recurrent glioblastoma multiforme for whom surgical resection is indicated; adjunct to surgery and radiation in patients with newly diagnosed high-grade malignant glioma**
Adults: 8 wafers placed in the resection cavity if size and shape of cavity allow. If 8 wafers can't be accommodated, use maximum number of wafers allowed.

ADMINISTRATION
IV
▼ Preparing and giving parenteral form of drug may be mutagenic, teratogenic, or carcinogenic. Follow facility policy to reduce risks. Wear gloves when handling any form of drug.
▼ Prepare drug only in glass or polypropylene containers. Ensure the containers used are polyvinyl chloride (PVC) free and

---

Reactions in **bold italics** are *life-threatening*. Interactions may have a *rapid onset* or a ***delayed onset***.

DEHP free. Solution is unstable in PVC IV bags.

▼ If powder liquefies or appears oily, discard because decomposition has occurred.

▼ To reconstitute, dissolve 100 mg of drug in 3 mL of absolute alcohol provided by manufacturer.

▼ Dilute solution with 27 mL of sterile water for injection. Resulting solution should be clear and colorless to yellowish and contains 3.3 mg of carmustine/mL in 10% alcohol.

▼ For infusion, may further dilute in 500 mL D₅W or NSS in glass or polypropylene container to a concentration of 0.2 mg/mL.

▼ Don't use PVC IV tubing. May use polyethylene IV tubing.

▼ Don't mix with other drugs during administration.

▼ Give at least 250 mL over at least 2 hours.

▼ To reduce pain on infusion, dilute further or slow infusion rate.

▼ Reconstituted solution may be stored in refrigerator for 24 hours. Once further diluted in D₅W or NSS, store at room temperature and give within 8 hours. It may decompose at temperatures above 80° F (27° C). Solution is also stable for 24 hours refrigerated followed by 6 additional hours at room temperature. Protect from light.

▼ **Incompatibilities:** Sodium bicarbonate.

Intracavitary

• Unopened foil pouches of wafers may be kept at room temperature for a maximum of 6 hours. Open only in the operating room immediately before implantation.

• Wafers broken in half may be used; however, discard wafers as hazardous waste if broken into more than two pieces.

• Use double gloves when handling wafers. Discard outer gloves into a biohazard waste container after use.

ACTION

Inhibits enzymatic reactions involved with DNA synthesis, cross-links strands of cellular DNA, and interferes with RNA transcription, causing an imbalance of growth that leads to cell death. Not specific to cell cycle.

Route	Onset	Peak	Duration
IV, intra-cavitary	Unknown	Unknown	Unknown

Half-life: IV: Biphasic: initial, 1.4 minutes; secondary, 22 minutes (active metabolites: plasma half-life of 67 hours).

ADVERSE REACTIONS

IV and intracavitary wafer

CNS: ataxia, *brain edema, seizures.* **CV:** *hemorrhage.* **EENT:** visual disturbances. **GI:** nausea, vomiting, anorexia, diarrhea, dysphagia, *GI hemorrhage.* **GU:** *nephrotoxicity,* renal impairment. **Hematologic:** *cumulative bone marrow suppression, leukopenia, thrombocytopenia, acute leukemia or bone marrow dysplasia,* anemia. **Hepatic:** *hepatotoxicity.* **Metabolic:** hyperglycemia, *hypokalemia,* hyponatremia. **Respiratory:** *pulmonary fibrosis.* **Other:** intense pain at infusion site from venous spasm.

Intracavitary wafer only

CNS: headache, hemiplegia, confusion, aphasia, depression, somnolence, speech disorder, amnesia, *intracranial HTN,* personality disorder, anxiety, facial paralysis, neuropathy, hypoesthesia, abnormal thinking, abnormal gait, hallucinations, insomnia, incoordination, hypokinesia, pain, asthenia. **CV:** deep vein thrombophlebitis, *hemorrhage,* chest pain, *PE.* **GI:** constipation, abdominal pain. **GU:** UTI, urinary incontinence. **Musculoskeletal:** back pain. **Respiratory:** dyspnea, pneumonia. **Skin:** rash, facial edema, abscess. **Other:** fever, allergic reaction, accidental injury, abnormal healing.

INTERACTIONS

Drug-drug. *Cimetidine:* May increase carmustine's bone marrow toxicity. Avoid using together.

Clozapine: May increase risk of neutropenia. Monitor concurrent use.

Digoxin, phenytoin: May decrease levels of these drugs. Monitor patient.

Live-virus vaccines: May increase risk of infection in immunocompromised patients. Don't use together; don't give for at least 3 months after carmustine.

Myelosuppressants: May increase myelosuppression. Monitor patient.

Drug-herb. *Echinacea:* May diminish therapeutic effect of immunosuppressants. Consider therapy modification.

EFFECTS ON LAB TEST RESULTS
• May increase alkaline phosphatase, AST, bilirubin, Hb, and urine urea levels.
• May decrease platelet and WBC counts.

CONTRAINDICATIONS & CAUTIONS
• Contraindicated in patients hypersensitive to drug.
• Drug may increase risk of secondary malignancies.
Dialyzable drug: No.

PREGNANCY-LACTATION-REPRODUCTION
• Drug may cause fetal harm if used during pregnancy. Women of childbearing potential should use effective contraception during treatment.
• Drug may impair fertility.
• It isn't known if drug appears in human milk. Patient should discontinue breastfeeding during treatment.

NURSING CONSIDERATIONS
◑ *Alert:* Carmustine for injection should be administered under the supervision of a physician experienced in the use of cancer chemotherapeutic agents.
Black Box Warning Bone marrow suppression, notably thrombocytopenia and leukopenia, is the most common and severe of the toxic effects. It may contribute to bleeding and overwhelming infections in an already compromised patient. ■
Black Box Warning Pulmonary toxicity appears to be dose related. Patients receiving greater than 1,400 mg/m^2 cumulative dose are at higher risk. Pulmonary toxicity can occur years after treatment and can result in death, particularly in patients treated in childhood. ■
• Obtain pulmonary function tests before and during therapy.
Black Box Warning Bone marrow suppression is delayed with carmustine. Blood counts should be monitored weekly for at least 6 weeks after a dose and drug shouldn't be given more often than every 6 weeks. ■

Black Box Warning Bone marrow toxicity of carmustine for injection is cumulative; dosage adjustment must be considered on the basis of nadir blood cell counts from prior dose. Don't administer a repeat course of drug until blood counts recover. ■
• Drug is associated with a moderate to high emetic potential (dose-related); give antiemetic before drug to reduce nausea.
• If drug touches skin, wash off thoroughly. Avoid contact with skin because drug will stain skin brown.
• Perform liver, renal, and pulmonary function tests periodically.
• Monitor CBC with differential. The ANC may be used to better calculate patient's immunosuppressive state.
• Monitor uric acid level. To prevent hyperuricemia with resulting uric acid nephropathy, allopurinol may be used with adequate hydration.
• Therapeutic levels are commonly toxic.
• Acute leukemia or bone marrow dysplasia may occur after long-term use.
• Anticipate blood transfusions during treatment because of cumulative anemia.
• Monitor patient for secondary malignancies.

PATIENT TEACHING
• Advise patient about common adverse reactions to drug.
• Tell patient to watch for signs and symptoms of infection (fever, sore throat, fatigue) and bleeding (easy bruising, nosebleeds, bleeding gums, tarry stools) and to take temperature daily.
• Instruct patient to avoid OTC products containing aspirin and NSAIDs unless prescribed by health care provider.
• Advise female patient to stop breastfeeding during therapy because of possible risk of toxicity to infant.
• Caution female patient of childbearing potential to avoid becoming pregnant during therapy. Recommend that she consult prescriber before becoming pregnant.

Reactions in bold italics are *life-threatening*. Interactions may have a *rapid onset* or a ***delayed onset***.

carvedilol
kar-VAH-da-lol

Coreg

carvedilol phosphate
Coreg CR

Therapeutic class: Antihypertensives
Pharmacologic class: Alpha-nonselective
beta blockers

AVAILABLE FORMS
Capsules (extended-release) ⓪NC*: 10 mg,
20 mg, 40 mg, 80 mg
Tablets: 3.125 mg, 6.25 mg, 12.5 mg, 25 mg

INDICATIONS & DOSAGES
Adjust-a-dose (for all indications): In patients with pulse rate below 55 beats/minute,
reduce dosage.
➤ **HTN**
Adults: Dosage highly individualized. For
immediate-release tablets, initially, 6.25 mg
PO b.i.d. Measure standing BP 1 hour after
first dose. If tolerated, continue dosage for
7 to 14 days. May increase to 12.5 mg PO
b.i.d. for 7 to 14 days, following same BP
monitoring protocol as before. Maximum
dose is 25 mg PO b.i.d. as tolerated. May be
switched to extended-release capsule after
controlled on immediate-release tablets. Or,
for extended-release capsule, initially 20 mg
PO once daily. Measure standing BP 1 hour
after dose. May increase by 20 mg every
7 to 14 days to maximum of 80 mg PO once
daily if needed and tolerated, using standing systolic pressure 1 hour after dosing as a
guide for tolerance.
➤ **Left ventricular dysfunction after MI**
Adults: Dosage individualized. Start therapy after patient is hemodynamically
stable and fluid retention has been minimized. For immediate-release tablets, initially, 6.25 mg PO b.i.d. Increase after 3 to
10 days to 12.5 mg b.i.d., then again after
3 to 10 days to a target dose of 25 mg b.i.d.
Or start with 3.125 mg b.i.d., or adjust
dosage more slowly if indicated. May be
switched to extended-release capsule after
controlled on immediate-release tablets. Or,
10 to 20 mg extended-release capsules PO

once daily. May increase after 3 to 10 days to
20 to 40 mg PO once daily; continue increasing dose every 3 to 10 days until target dose
of 80 mg PO once daily based on tolerability
is reached.
➤ **Mild to severe HF**
Adults: Dosage highly individualized.
For immediate-release tablets, initially,
3.125 mg PO b.i.d. for 2 weeks; if tolerated,
may increase to 6.25 mg PO b.i.d. Dosage
may be doubled every 2 weeks, as tolerated.
Maximum dose for patients in severe HF
or who weigh less than 85 kg is 25 mg PO
b.i.d.; for those weighing more than 85 kg,
dose is 50 mg PO b.i.d. May be switched to
extended-release capsule after controlled
on immediate-release tablets. Or, 10-mg
extended-release capsule PO once daily for
2 weeks. May increase to 20, 40, and 80 mg
over successive intervals of at least 2 weeks
if tolerated.

ADMINISTRATION
PO
• Give drug with food.
• Make sure patient doesn't crush, chew, or
take capsules in divided doses.
• Capsules may be opened, contents sprinkled on cool applesauce, and taken immediately; don't store.
• Give capsules in the morning.
• Extended-release equivalent of 3.125 mg
immediate-release b.i.d. is 10 mg once daily,
6.25 mg immediate-release b.i.d. is 20 mg
once daily, 12.5 mg immediate-release b.i.d.
is 40 mg once daily, and 25 mg immediate-
release b.i.d. is 80 mg once daily. May
further titrate dosage based on clinical
response.
• Administer extended-release form and
drugs that contain alcohol 2 hours apart.

ACTION
Nonselective beta blocker with alpha-
blocking activity.

Route	Onset	Peak	Duration
PO	Rapid	1–2 hr	7–10 hr
PO (extended-release)	30 min	5 hr	Unknown

Half-life: Immediate-release, 7 to 10 hours;
extended-release, unknown.

ADVERSE REACTIONS
CNS: asthenia, dizziness, fatigue, *stroke,* pain, headache, malaise, fever, hypesthesia, vertigo, somnolence, depression, insomnia, syncope, paresthesia. **CV:** hypotension, orthostatic hypotension, *AV block, bradycardia,* edema, syncope, angina pectoris, peripheral edema, hypovolemia, fluid overload, HTN, palpitations, chest pain. **EENT:** abnormal vision, blurred vision. **GI:** diarrhea, vomiting, nausea, melena, periodontitis, abdominal pain, dyspepsia. **GU:** erectile dysfunction, abnormal renal function, albuminuria, hematuria, UTI. **Hematologic:** *thrombocytopenia,* purpura. **Metabolic:** hyperglycemia, weight gain, *hyperkalemia, hypoglycemia,* weight loss, hypercholesterolemia, hyperuricemia, hyponatremia, glycosuria, diabetes mellitus, gout. **Musculoskeletal:** arthralgia, muscle cramps. **Respiratory:** *lung edema,* cough, rales. **Other:** hypersensitivity reactions.

INTERACTIONS
Drug-drug. *Amiodarone:* May increase risk of bradycardia, AV block, and myocardial depression. Monitor patient's ECG and vital signs.
Catecholamine-depleting drugs (MAO inhibitors): May cause bradycardia or severe hypotension. Monitor patient closely.
Cimetidine: May increase bioavailability of carvedilol. Monitor vital signs closely.
Clonidine: May increase BP-lowering and HR-lowering effects. Monitor vital signs closely.
Cyclosporine: May increase cyclosporine level. Monitor cyclosporine level.
CYP4502D6 inhibitors (fluoxetine, paroxetine, propafenone, quinidine): May increase level of carvedilol. Monitor patient for hypotension and dizziness.
Digoxin: May increase digoxin level by about 15% when given together. Monitor digoxin level.
Diltiazem, verapamil: May cause isolated conduction disturbances. Monitor patient's heart rhythm and BP.
Insulin, oral antidiabetics: May enhance hypoglycemic properties. Monitor glucose level.
NSAIDs, salicylates: May decrease antihypertensive effects. Monitor BP.

Rifamycin (except rifabutin): May significantly reduce carvedilol level. Monitor vital signs closely.
Drug-herb. *Ma huang:* May decrease antihypertensive effects. Discourage use together.

EFFECTS ON LAB TEST RESULTS
• May increase alkaline phosphatase, ALT, AST, BUN, cholesterol, creatinine, GGT, nonprotein nitrogen, potassium, triglyceride, sodium, and uric acid levels. May increase or decrease glucose level.
• May shorten PT and decrease platelet count.

CONTRAINDICATIONS & CAUTIONS
• Contraindicated in patients hypersensitive to drug and in those with NYHA Class IV decompensated cardiac failure requiring IV inotropic therapy.
• Contraindicated in patients with bronchial asthma or related bronchospastic conditions, second- or third-degree AV block, sick sinus syndrome (unless a pacemaker is in place), cardiogenic shock, severe bradycardia, or severe hepatic impairment.
• Use cautiously in hypertensive patients with left-sided HF, perioperative patients who receive anesthetics that depress myocardial function, diabetic patients receiving insulin or oral antidiabetics, and in those subject to spontaneous hypoglycemia.
• Use cautiously in patients with thyroid disease (may mask hyperthyroidism; withdrawal may precipitate thyroid storm or exacerbation of hyperthyroidism), myasthenia gravis, pheochromocytoma, Prinzmetal or variant angina, bronchospastic disease (in those who can't tolerate other antihypertensives), or PVD (may precipitate or aggravate symptoms of arterial insufficiency).
• Safety and effectiveness in children younger than age 18 haven't been established.
Dialyzable drug: No.
⚠ *Overdose S&S:* Hypotension, bradycardia, cardiac insufficiency, cardiogenic shock, cardiac arrest, respiratory problems, bronchospasm, vomiting, lapses of consciousness, generalized seizures.

Reactions in bold italics are *life-threatening*. Interactions may have a *rapid onset* or a *delayed onset*.

PREGNANCY-LACTATION-REPRODUCTION

• There are no adequate well-controlled studies in pregnant women. Use during pregnancy only if potential benefit outweighs potential risk to the fetus.

• It's unknown if drug appears in human milk. Patient should discontinue breastfeeding or discontinue drug, taking into account importance of drug to the mother.

NURSING CONSIDERATIONS

⚠ *Alert:* Patients who have a history of severe anaphylactic reaction to several allergens may be more reactive to repeated challenge (accidental, diagnostic, or therapeutic). They may be unresponsive to dosages of epinephrine typically used to treat allergic reactions.

• Mild hepatocellular injury may occur during therapy. At first sign of hepatic dysfunction, perform tests for hepatic injury or jaundice; if present, stop drug.

• If drug must be stopped, do so gradually over 1 to 2 weeks, if possible.

• Monitor patient with HF for worsened condition, renal dysfunction, or fluid retention; diuretics may need to be increased.

• Monitor diabetic patient closely; drug may mask signs of hypoglycemia, or hyperglycemia may be worsened.

• Hypotension can occur. Observe patient for dizziness or light-headedness for 1 hour after giving each new dose.

• Monitor elderly patients carefully; drug levels are about 50% higher in elderly patients than in younger patients.

• *Look alike–sound alike:* Don't confuse carvedilol with carteolol or captopril.

PATIENT TEACHING

• Tell patient not to interrupt or stop drug without medical approval.

• Inform patient that improvement of HF symptoms might take several weeks of drug therapy.

• Advise patient with HF to call prescriber if weight gain or shortness of breath occurs.

• Inform patient that low BP when standing may occur. If patient feels dizzy or faint (rare), advise sitting or lying down and tell patient to notify prescriber if symptoms persist.

• Caution patient against performing hazardous tasks during start of therapy.

• Advise diabetic patient to promptly report changes in glucose level.

• Inform patient who wears contact lenses that eyes may feel dry.

• Tell patient to take drug with food. Extended-release capsule may be opened and contents sprinkled on cool applesauce and taken immediately. Advise patient not to store.

• Advise patient not to crush or chew capsules or divide their contents.

caspofungin acetate
KAS-po-fun-gin

Cancidas

Therapeutic class: Antifungals
Pharmacologic class: Echinocandins

AVAILABLE FORMS
Lyophilized powder for injection: 50 mg, 70 mg in single-use vials

INDICATIONS & DOSAGES
Adjust-a-dose (for all indications): For adults receiving rifampin, give 70 mg IV once daily. Adults receiving nevirapine, efavirenz, carbamazepine, dexamethasone, or phenytoin may also require 70 mg IV once daily. For children receiving rifampin, give 70 mg/m² IV once daily (not to exceed an actual daily dose of 70 mg). Also consider giving 70 mg/m² IV once daily (not to exceed 70 mg) for children receiving nevirapine, efavirenz, carbamazepine, dexamethasone, or phenytoin. For patients with Child-Pugh score of 7 to 9, after initial 70-mg loading dose (when indicated), give 35 mg/day. There's no clinical experience in adults with Child-Pugh score of more than 9 or in children with any degree of hepatic impairment.

➤ **Invasive aspergillosis in patients who are refractory to or intolerant of other therapies (amphotericin B, lipid forms of amphotericin B, itraconazole); candidemia and *Candida*-caused intra-abdominal abscesses, peritonitis, and pleural space infections**

Adults: Single 70-mg IV loading dose on day 1, followed by 50 mg IV over about 1 hour once daily. Base treatment duration on severity of patient's underlying disease, recovery from immunosuppression, and clinical response.

Children age 3 months to 17 years: Single 70 mg/m^2 IV loading dose over about 1 hour on day 1, followed by 50 mg/m^2 daily thereafter. May increase daily maintenance dose to 70 mg/m^2. Maximum loading dose and daily maintenance dose shouldn't exceed 70 mg.

➤ **Empirical treatment of presumed fungal infections in febrile, neutropenic patients**

Adults: Single 70-mg IV loading dose over about 1 hour on day 1, followed by 50 mg IV over 1 hour once daily thereafter. Continue empirical therapy until neutropenia resolves. If fungal infection is confirmed, treat for a minimum of 14 days and continue therapy for at least 7 days after neutropenia and symptoms resolve. May increase daily dose to 70 mg if the 50-mg dose is well tolerated but clinical response is suboptimal.

Children age 3 months to 17 years: Single 70 mg/m^2 IV loading dose over about 1 hour on day 1, followed by 50 mg/m^2 daily thereafter. May increase daily maintenance dose to 70 mg/m^2. Maximum loading dose and daily maintenance dose shouldn't exceed 70 mg.

➤ **Esophageal candidiasis**

Adults: 50 mg IV daily over about 1 hour for 7 to 14 days after symptoms resolve. Don't administer a loading dose.

Children age 3 months to 17 years: Single 70 mg/m^2 IV loading dose over about 1 hour on day 1, followed by 50 mg/m^2 daily thereafter. May increase daily maintenance dose to 70 mg/m^2. Maximum loading dose and daily maintenance dose shouldn't exceed 70 mg.

Adjust-a-dose: Consider suppressive oral therapy in adults with HIV infection due to the risk of oropharyngeal candidiasis relapse.

ADMINISTRATION

IV

▼ Let refrigerated vial warm to room temperature.

▼ Reconstitute drug by adding 10.8 mL of NSS, sterile water for injection, bacteriostatic water for injection with methylparaben and propylparaben, or bacteriostatic water for injection with benzyl alcohol 0.9% to the vial. Resulting solution will be clear.

▼ Reconstitution will lead to a concentration of 5 mg/mL for 50-mg vial and 7 mg/mL for 70-mg vial.

▼ Use reconstituted vials within 1 hour of reconstitution or discard. Vials are for single dose only. Discard unused portion.

▼ For patients on fluid restriction, dilute the 35-mg and 50-mg doses in 100 mL NSS or lactated Ringer solution. For other patients, dilute 35-mg, 50-mg, and 70-mg doses in 250 mL NSS or lactated Ringer solution. Don't exceed a final concentration of 0.5 mg/mL.

▼ Give drug by slow infusion over about 1 hour. Don't administer as an IV bolus.

▼ Monitor site carefully for phlebitis.

▼ The final product for infusion (solution in IV bag or bottle) can be stored at room temperature for 24 hours or at 36° to 46° F (2° to 8° C) for 48 hours.

▼ **Incompatibilities:** Don't mix or infuse with other drugs or dextrose solutions.

ACTION

Inhibits synthesis of 1,3-β-D-glucan, an essential component of the cell wall, in susceptible *Aspergillus* and *Candida* species. Drug is extensively distributed and has a prolonged half-life.

Route	Onset	Peak	Duration
IV	Unknown	Unknown	Unknown

Half-life: 9 to 11 hours; terminal, 40 to 50 hours.

ADVERSE REACTIONS

CNS: paresthesia, fever, headache. **CV:** tachycardia, phlebitis, infused vein complications, hypotension. **GI:** anorexia, nausea, vomiting, diarrhea, abdominal pain, mucosal inflammation. **GU:** proteinuria, hematuria. **Hematologic:** anemia, eosinophilia. **Metabolic:** hypokalemia. **Musculoskeletal:** pain, myalgia. **Respiratory:** dyspnea, crackles, cough, pneumonia, tachypnea. **Skin:** histamine-mediated symptoms, including rash, facial swelling,

---

Reactions in bold italics are *life-threatening*. Interactions may have a *rapid onset* or a *delayed onset*.

pruritus, sensation of warmth, sweating.
Other: chills.

INTERACTIONS
Drug-drug. *Cyclosporine:* May increase caspofungin level. May increase risk of elevated ALT level; avoid using together unless benefit outweighs risk.
Inducers of drug clearance or mixed inducer-inhibitors (carbamazepine, dexamethasone, efavirenz, nevirapine, phenytoin, rifampin): May reduce caspofungin level. May need to adjust dosage upward to 70 mg in patients who are clinically unresponsive.
Tacrolimus: May reduce tacrolimus level. Monitor tacrolimus level; expect to adjust dosage.

EFFECTS ON LAB TEST RESULTS
• May increase glucose, alkaline phosphatase, and liver enzyme levels. May decrease albumin, calcium, Hb, potassium, magnesium, and protein levels.
• May increase eosinophil count.

CONTRAINDICATIONS & CAUTIONS
• Contraindicated in patients hypersensitive to drug or its components.
• Anaphylaxis, other hypersensitivity reactions, and possible histamine-mediated adverse reactions, including rash, facial swelling, angioedema, pruritus, sensation of warmth, and bronchospasm, have been reported during administration.
• Cases of SJS and toxic epidermal necrolysis, some with a fatal outcome, have been reported.
• Safety and effectiveness in neonates and infants younger than age 3 months aren't known.
Dialyzable drug: No.

PREGNANCY-LACTATION-REPRODUCTION
• There are no adequate studies in pregnant women. Use during pregnancy only if potential benefit justifies potential risk to the fetus.
• It's unknown if drug appears in human milk. Use cautiously in breastfeeding women. Monitor infants for signs and symptoms of histamine release, such as facial swelling, rash, and GI symptoms.

NURSING CONSIDERATIONS
• Safety information is limited, but drug is well tolerated for therapy lasting longer than 2 weeks.
• Observe patients for histamine-mediated reactions, including rash, facial swelling, pruritus, and a sensation of warmth.
• Discontinue drug at first sign or symptom of a hypersensitivity reaction and administer appropriate treatment.
• Monitor patients who develop abnormal LFT values during therapy for evidence of worsening hepatic function and evaluate for the risks and benefits of continuing therapy.

PATIENT TEACHING
• Instruct patient to report signs and symptoms of phlebitis.
• Instruct patient to immediately report signs or symptoms of a hypersensitivity reaction, rash, or other skin reactions.

cefadroxil
sef-a-DROX-ill

Therapeutic class: Antibiotics
Pharmacologic class: First-generation cephalosporins

AVAILABLE FORMS
Capsules: 500 mg
Oral suspension: 250 mg/5 mL, 500 mg/5 mL
Tablets: 1 g

INDICATIONS & DOSAGES
➤ **UTIs caused by** *Escherichia coli,* ***Proteus mirabilis,* and** *Klebsiella* **species; skin and soft-tissue infections caused by staphylococci and streptococci; pharyngitis or tonsillitis caused by group A beta-hemolytic streptococci**
Adults: 1 to 2 g PO daily, depending on infection being treated. Usually given once daily or in two divided doses. For pharyngitis and tonsillitis, treat for 10 days.
Children: 30 mg/kg PO daily in a single dose or in two divided doses every 12 hours for tonsillitis, pharyngitis, and impetigo, and in two divided doses every 12 hours for other skin infections and UTIs. For beta-hemolytic strep infection, treat for at least 10 days.

Adjust-a-dose: In adult patient with renal impairment, give first dose of 1 g. Reduce additional doses based on CrCl. If CrCl is 25 to 50 mL/minute, give 500 mg PO every 12 hours. If CrCl is 10 to 25 mL/minute, give 500 mg PO every 24 hours; if CrCl is less than 10 mL/minute, give 500 mg PO every 36 hours.

ADMINISTRATION
PO
- Before administration, ensure patient isn't allergic to penicillins or cephalosporins.
- Obtain specimen for culture and sensitivity tests before giving first dose. Begin therapy while awaiting results.
- Administer without regard to meals but can give drug with food or milk to lessen GI discomfort.
- Keep oral suspension refrigerated and discard unused portion after 14 days. Shake well before using.

ACTION
Inhibits cell-wall synthesis, promoting osmotic instability; usually bactericidal.

Route	Onset	Peak	Duration
PO	Unknown	70–90 min	Unknown

Half-life: About 1 to 2 hours.

ADVERSE REACTIONS
CNS: *seizures,* fever. **GI:** *pseudomembranous colitis,* glossitis, abdominal cramps. **GU:** genital pruritus, candidiasis, vaginitis, renal dysfunction. **Hematologic:** *transient neutropenia, leukopenia, agranulocytosis, thrombocytopenia,* anemia, eosinophilia. **Musculoskeletal:** arthralgia. **Skin:** maculopapular and erythematous rashes, urticaria, pruritus. **Other:** *anaphylaxis, angioedema,* hypersensitivity reactions.

INTERACTIONS
Drug-drug. *Aminoglycosides:* May increase risk of nephrotoxicity. Avoid using together. *Estrogen-based contraceptives:* May decrease contraceptive absorption and effectiveness. Patient should avoid use together or use nonhormonal contraception for duration of antibiotic (or 14 days, whichever is longer) and for 7 days after completion of antibiotic.

Live-virus vaccines: May decrease vaccine effectiveness. Don't give together. *Probenecid:* May inhibit excretion and increase cefadroxil level. Use together cautiously. *Warfarin:* May enhance anticoagulant effects. Monitor therapy.

EFFECTS ON LAB TEST RESULTS
- May increase alkaline phosphatase, ALT, AST, bilirubin, GGT, and LDH levels. May decrease Hb level.
- May increase eosinophil count. May decrease granulocyte, neutrophil, platelet, and WBC counts.
- May falsely increase serum or urine creatinine level in tests using Jaffé reaction. May cause false-positive results of Coombs test and urine glucose tests that use cupric sulfate, such as Benedict reagent and Clinitest.

CONTRAINDICATIONS & CAUTIONS
- Contraindicated in patients hypersensitive to drug or other cephalosporins.
- Use cautiously in patients with a history of sensitivity to penicillin or GI diseases (colitis).
- Use cautiously in patients with impaired renal function; adjust dosage as needed.
- **Alert:** Seizures have occurred, particularly in patients with renal impairment when the dosage wasn't reduced. If seizures occur, discontinue drug and treat if clinically indicated.
- **Alert:** Drug can cause CDAD and pseudomembranous colitis ranging from mild to life-threatening that can occur more than 2 months after treatment.
Dialyzable drug: Yes.

PREGNANCY-LACTATION-REPRODUCTION
- There are no adequate studies in pregnant women. Use during pregnancy only if potential benefit justifies potential risk to the fetus.
- It isn't known if drug appears in human milk. Use cautiously in breastfeeding women.

NURSING CONSIDERATIONS
- If CrCl is less than 50 mL/minute, lengthen dosage interval so drug doesn't

---

Reactions in bold italics are *life-threatening*. Interactions may have a *rapid onset* or a *delayed onset*.

accumulate. Monitor renal function in patients with renal dysfunction.
• If large doses are given, therapy is prolonged, or patient is high risk, monitor patient for superinfection.
• Monitor patient for diarrhea and treat appropriately.
• *Look alike–sound alike:* Don't confuse drug with other cephalosporins that sound alike.

PATIENT TEACHING
• Instruct patient to take drug with food or milk to lessen GI discomfort.
• Tell patient to take entire amount of drug exactly as prescribed, even if feeling better.
• Advise patient to notify prescriber if rash develops or if signs and symptoms of superinfection appear, such as recurring fever, chills, and malaise.

ceFAZolin sodium
sef-AH-zoe-lin

Therapeutic class: Antibiotics
Pharmacologic class: First-generation cephalosporins

AVAILABLE FORMS
Infusion: 1 g/50 mL, 2 g/50 mL in 50-mL bag; 2 g/100 mL, 3 g/100 mL in 100-mL bag
Injection (parenteral): 500 mg, 1 g, 2 g

INDICATIONS & DOSAGES
Adjust-a-dose (for all indications): For adults with CrCl of 55 mL/minute or greater, give full dose every 6 to 8 hours; if CrCl is 35 to 54 mL/minute, give full dose every 8 hours or longer; if CrCl is 11 to 34 mL/minute, give 50% of usual dose every 12 hours; if CrCl is below 10 mL/minute, give 50% of usual dose every 18 to 24 hours.
➤ **Perioperative prevention in contaminated surgery**
Adults: 1 to 2 g IM or IV 30 to 60 minutes before surgery; then 0.5 to 1 g IM or IV every 6 to 8 hours for 24 hours. In operations lasting longer than 2 hours, give another 0.5- to 1-g dose IM or IV intraoperatively. Continue treatment for 3 to 5 days if life-threatening infection is likely.
➤ **Infections of respiratory, biliary, and GU tracts; skin, soft-tissue, bone, and**

joint infections; septicemia; endocarditis caused by *Escherichia coli*, Enterobacteriaceae, gonococci, *Haemophilus influenzae*, *Klebsiella* species, *Proteus mirabilis*, *Staphylococcus aureus*, *Streptococcus pneumoniae*, and group A beta-hemolytic streptococci
Adults: 250 to 500 mg IM or IV every 8 hours for mild infections or 500 mg to 1.5 g IM or IV every 6 to 8 hours for moderate to severe or life-threatening infections. Maximum, 12 g/day in life-threatening situations.
Children older than age 1 month: 25 to 50 mg/kg/day IM or IV in three or four divided doses. In severe infections, dose may be increased to 100 mg/kg/day.
Adjust-a-dose: For children with CrCl of 40 to 70 mL/minute, give 60% of normal daily dose divided every 12 hours; if CrCl is 20 to 40 mL/minute, give 25% of usual daily dose divided every 12 hours; if CrCl is 5 to 20 mL/minute, give 10% of usual dose every 24 hours.

ADMINISTRATION
IV
▼ Before giving first dose, obtain specimen for culture and sensitivity tests. Begin therapy while awaiting results.
▼ Before giving drug, ensure patient isn't allergic to penicillins or cephalosporins.
▼ Give commercially available frozen solutions in D_5W only by intermittent or continuous IV infusion.
▼ Reconstitute drug with sterile water, bacteriostatic water, or NSS as follows: Add 2 mL to 500-mg vial or 2.5 mL to 1-g vial, yielding 225 mg/mL or 330 mg/mL, respectively.
▼ Shake well until dissolved.
▼ For direct injection, further dilute with 5 mL of sterile water for injection.
▼ Inject into a large vein or into the tubing of a free-flowing IV solution over 3 to 5 minutes or as an intermittent infusion over 30 to 60 minutes.
▼ For intermittent infusion, add reconstituted drug to 50 to 100 mL of compatible solution or use premixed solution.
▼ If IV therapy lasts longer than 3 days, alternate injection sites. Use of small IV

needles in larger available veins may be preferable.

▼ Reconstituted drug is stable 24 hours at room temperature or 10 days refrigerated.

▼ **Incompatibilities:** None listed by manufacturer. Consult a drug incompatibility reference for more information.

IM

• Before giving first dose, obtain specimen for culture and sensitivity tests. Begin therapy while awaiting results.

• After reconstitution, inject drug IM without further dilution. This drug isn't as painful as other cephalosporins. Give injection deep into a large muscle.

ACTION

Inhibits cell-wall synthesis, promoting osmotic instability; usually bactericidal.

Route	Onset	Peak	Duration
IV	Immediate	Immediate	Unknown
IM	Unknown	½–2 hr	Unknown

Half-life: About 2 hours.

ADVERSE REACTIONS

CV: phlebitis, thrombophlebitis with IV injection. **GI:** diarrhea, *pseudomembranous colitis,* anorexia, glossitis, dyspepsia, abdominal cramps, anal pruritus, oral candidiasis. **GU:** genital pruritus, candidiasis, vaginitis. **Hematologic:** *neutropenia, leukopenia, thrombocytopenia,* eosinophilia. **Skin:** maculopapular and erythematous rashes, urticaria, pruritus, pain, induration, sterile abscesses, tissue sloughing at injection site, *SJS.* **Other:** *anaphylaxis,* hypersensitivity reactions, drug fever.

INTERACTIONS

Drug-drug. *Aminoglycosides:* May increase risk of nephrotoxicity. Avoid using together.

Anticoagulants: May increase anticoagulant effects. Monitor PT and INR.

Estrogen-based contraceptives: May decrease contraceptive absorption and effectiveness. Patient should avoid use together or use nonhormonal contraception for duration of antibiotic (or 14 days, whichever is longer) and for 7 days after completion of antibiotic.

Live-virus vaccines: May decrease effectiveness of live-virus vaccines. Concurrent use isn't recommended.

Phenytoin: May decrease protein binding of phenytoin. Monitor phenytoin level.

Probenecid: May inhibit excretion and increase cefazolin level. Use together isn't recommended.

Warfarin: May enhance anticoagulant effects. Monitor therapy.

EFFECTS ON LAB TEST RESULTS

• May increase alkaline phosphatase, ALT, AST, bilirubin, GGT, and LDH levels and prolong INR.

• May increase eosinophil count. May decrease neutrophil, platelet, and WBC counts.

• May falsely increase serum or urine creatinine level in tests using Jaffé reaction. May cause false-positive results of Coombs test and urine glucose tests that use cupric sulfate, such as Benedict reagent and Clinitest.

CONTRAINDICATIONS & CAUTIONS

• Contraindicated in patients hypersensitive to drug or other cephalosporins.

• Use cautiously in patients hypersensitive to penicillin because of the possibility of cross-sensitivity with other beta-lactam antibiotics.

• Use cautiously in patients with a history of colitis, seizure disorders, or renal insufficiency.

• Prolonged use may result in fungal or bacterial superinfection, including CDAD and pseudomembranous colitis, which can occur more than 2 months after treatment ends.

Dialyzable drug: Yes.

⚠ *Overdose S&S:* Pain, inflammation, and phlebitis at injection site; dizziness, paresthesia, headache, seizures; elevated creatinine, BUN, liver enzymes, and bilirubin levels; positive Coombs test; thrombocytosis, thrombocytopenia, eosinophilia; leukopenia; prolonged PT.

PREGNANCY-LACTATION-REPRODUCTION

• There are no adequate studies in pregnant women. Use during pregnancy only if clearly needed and potential benefit justifies potential risk to the fetus.

• Drug appears in very low concentrations in human milk. Use cautiously in breastfeeding women.

NURSING CONSIDERATIONS
• If CrCl falls below 55 mL/minute in adults or 70 mL/minute in children, adjust dosage.
• If large doses are given, therapy is prolonged, or patient is at high risk, monitor patient for signs and symptoms of superinfection.
• Monitor patient for diarrhea and treat appropriately.
• *Look alike–sound alike:* Don't confuse drug with other cephalosporins that sound alike.

PATIENT TEACHING
• Instruct patient to report adverse reactions promptly.
• Tell patient to report discomfort at IV injection site.
• Advise patient to notify prescriber if a rash develops or if signs and symptoms of superinfection, such as recurring fever, chills, and malaise, appear.

cefdinir
sef-DIN-er

Therapeutic class: Antibiotics
Pharmacologic class: Third-generation cephalosporins

AVAILABLE FORMS
Capsules: 300 mg
Suspension: 125 mg/5 mL, 250 mg/5 mL

INDICATIONS & DOSAGES
Adjust-a-dose (for all indications): If CrCl is less than 30 mL/minute, reduce dosage to 300 mg PO once daily for adults and 7 mg/kg (up to 300 mg) PO once daily for children ages 6 months to 12 years. In patients receiving long-term hemodialysis, give 300 mg or 7 mg/kg PO at end of each dialysis session and then every other day.
➤ **Mild to moderate infections caused by susceptible strains of microorganisms in community-acquired pneumonia, acute worsening of chronic bronchitis, acute maxillary sinusitis, acute bacterial otitis media, and uncomplicated skin and skin-structure infections**
Adults and children age 13 and older: 300 mg PO every 12 hours or 600 mg PO every 24 hours for 10 days. Give every 12 hours for pneumonia and skin infections.
Children ages 6 months to 12 years: 7 mg/kg PO every 12 hours or 14 mg/kg PO every 24 hours for 10 days, up to maximum dose of 600 mg daily. Give every 12 hours for skin infections.
➤ **Pharyngitis, tonsillitis**
Adults and children age 13 and older: 300 mg PO every 12 hours for 5 to 10 days or 600 mg PO every 24 hours for 10 days.
Children ages 6 months to 12 years: 7 mg/kg PO every 12 hours for 5 to 10 days; or 14 mg/kg PO every 24 hours for 10 days.

ADMINISTRATION
PO
• Before administration, ensure patient isn't allergic to penicillins or cephalosporins.
• Give antacids and iron supplements 2 hours before or after a dose of cefdinir.
• Give drug without regard for meals.
• Give twice-daily doses every 12 hours.
• Shake suspension well before use.
• Suspension can be stored at room temperature (68° to 77° F [20° to 25° C]) for 10 days.

ACTION
Inhibits cell-wall synthesis, promoting osmotic instability; usually bactericidal.

Route	Onset	Peak	Duration
PO	Unknown	2–4 hr	Unknown

Half-life: 1¾ hours.

ADVERSE REACTIONS
CNS: headache. **GI:** diarrhea, *pseudomembranous colitis,* abdominal pain, nausea. **GU:** vaginitis, increased urine proteins. **Hematologic:** increased WBC and RBC counts. **Other:** hypersensitivity reactions, *anaphylaxis.*

INTERACTIONS
Drug-drug. *Aminoglycosides:* May increase risk of nephrotoxicity. Avoid using together. *Antacids containing aluminum and magnesium, iron supplements, multivitamins*

containing iron: May decrease rate of absorption and bioavailability of cefdinir. Give such preparations 2 hours before or after cefdinir.

Estrogen-based contraceptives: May decrease contraceptive absorption and effectiveness. Patient should avoid use together or use nonhormonal contraception for duration of antibiotic (or 14 days, whichever is longer) and for 7 days after completion of antibiotic.

Live-virus vaccines: May decrease effectiveness of live-virus vaccines. Concurrent use isn't recommended.

Probenecid: May inhibit renal excretion of cefdinir. Monitor patient for adverse reactions.

Warfarin: May enhance anticoagulant effects. Monitor therapy.

EFFECTS ON LAB TEST RESULTS

• May increase alkaline phosphatase, GGT, and LDH levels. May decrease bicarbonate levels.

• May increase WBC, RBC, eosinophil, lymphocyte, and platelet counts.

• May falsely increase serum or urine creatinine level in tests using Jaffé reaction. May cause false-positive results of Coombs test and urine glucose tests that use cupric sulfate, such as Benedict reagent and Clinitest.

CONTRAINDICATIONS & CAUTIONS

• Contraindicated in patients hypersensitive to drug or other cephalosporins.

• Use cautiously in patients hypersensitive to penicillin because of the possibility of cross-sensitivity with other beta-lactam antibiotics.

• Use cautiously in patients with history of colitis or renal insufficiency.

Dialyzable drug: 63%.

PREGNANCY-LACTATION-REPRODUCTION

• There are no adequate studies in pregnant women. Use during pregnancy only if clearly needed and if potential benefit justifies potential risk to the fetus.

• It isn't known if drug appears in human milk. Use cautiously in breastfeeding women.

NURSING CONSIDERATIONS

• Prolonged drug treatment may result in emergence and overgrowth of resistant organisms. Monitor patient for signs and symptoms of superinfection.

• Pseudomembranous colitis and CDAD have been reported with cefdinir and can occur more than 2 months after therapy ends. Monitor for diarrhea in patients after antibiotic therapy and in those with history of colitis.

• *Look alike–sound alike:* Don't confuse drug with other cephalosporins that sound alike.

PATIENT TEACHING

• Instruct patient to take antacids and iron supplements 2 hours before or after a dose of cefdinir.

• Inform diabetic patient that each teaspoon of suspension contains 2.86 g of sucrose.

• Tell patient that drug may be taken without regard to meals.

• Tell patient to take drug as prescribed, even if feeling better.

• Advise patient to report severe diarrhea or diarrhea with abdominal pain.

• Tell patient to report all adverse reactions or signs and symptoms of superinfection promptly.

cefepime hydrochloride
SEF-ah-peem

Maxipime

Therapeutic class: Antibiotics
Pharmacologic class: Fourth-generation cephalosporins

AVAILABLE FORMS

Injection: 500-mg, 1-g, 2-g vials; 1 g/50 mL, 2 g/100 mL in Galaxy containers; 1-g, 2 g ADD-Vantage vials; 1 g/50 mL, 2 g/50 mL in duplex containers

INDICATIONS & DOSAGES

Adjust-a-dose (for all indications): Adjust adult dosage based on CrCl, as shown in the table below. For patients receiving hemodialysis, about 68% of drug is removed after a 3-hour dialysis session. Cefepime dosage

Adult dosage adjustments for renal impairment (cefepime hydrochloride)

CrCl (mL/min)	Recommended maintenance dosing schedule			
>60	500 mg every 12 hr	1 g every 12 hr	2 g every 12 hr	2 g every 8 hr
30–60	500 mg every 24 hr	1 g every 24 hr	2 g every 24 hr	2 g every 12 hr
11–29	500 mg every 24 hr	500 mg every 24 hr	1 g every 24 hr	2 g every 24 hr
<11	250 mg every 24 hr	250 mg every 24 hr	500 mg every 24 hr	1 g every 24 hr

for patients receiving hemodialysis is 1 g on day 1, followed by 500 mg every 24 hours for treatment of all infections except febrile neutropenia. For patients with febrile neutropenia, give 1 g every 24 hours. Give cefepime after hemodialysis and at the same time each day. For patients receiving continuous ambulatory peritoneal dialysis, give normal dose every 48 hours. Because pediatric and adult cefepime pharmacokinetics are similar, change the pediatric dosing regimen proportional to the adult regimen.

➤ **Mild to moderate UTI caused by *Escherichia coli*, *Klebsiella pneumoniae*, or *Proteus mirabilis*, including concurrent bacteremia with these microorganisms**
Adults and children age 16 and older: 0.5 to 1 g IM or IV over 30 minutes every 12 hours for 7 to 10 days. Use IM only for *E. coli* infection when IM route is considered more appropriate route of administration.

➤ **Severe UTI, including pyelonephritis, caused by *E. coli*, *P. mirabilis*, or *K. pneumoniae***
Adults and children age 16 and older: 2 g IV over 30 minutes every 12 hours for 10 days.

➤ **Moderate to severe pneumonia caused by *Streptococcus pneumoniae*, *Pseudomonas aeruginosa*, *K. pneumoniae*, or *Enterobacter* species**
Adults and children age 16 and older: 1 to 2 g IV over 30 minutes every 8 to 12 hours for 10 days. For *P. aeruginosa*, use 2 g IV every 8 hours for 10 days.

➤ **Moderate to severe skin infection, uncomplicated skin infection, and skin-structure infection caused by *Streptococcus pyogenes* or methicillin-susceptible strains of *Staphylococcus aureus***
Adults and children age 16 and older: 2 g IV over 30 minutes every 12 hours for 10 days.

➤ **Complicated intra-abdominal infection caused by *E. coli*, viridans group streptococci, *P. aeruginosa*, *K. pneumoniae*, *Enterobacter* species, or *Bacteroides fragilis***
Adults and children age 16 and older: 2 g IV over 30 minutes every 8 to 12 hours for 7 to 10 days. Give with metronidazole. For *P. aeruginosa*, give 2 g IV every 8 hours.

➤ **Empirical therapy for febrile neutropenia**
Adults and children age 16 and older: 2 g IV every 8 hours for 7 days or until neutropenia resolves. If fever resolves but patient remains neutropenic for more than 7 days, frequently reevaluate the need for continued antimicrobial therapy.

➤ **Uncomplicated and complicated UTI (including pyelonephritis), uncomplicated skin and skin-structure infection, pneumonia, empirical therapy for febrile neutropenic children**
Children ages 2 months to 16 years weighing up to 40 kg: 50 mg/kg/dose IV over 30 minutes every 12 hours for 7 to 10 days. For febrile neutropenia, give 50 mg/kg IV every 8 hours for 7 days or until neutropenia resolves. For UTI, treat for 7 to 10 days. Don't exceed 2 g/dose. May consider IM route only for mild to moderate, uncomplicated or complicated UTIs due to *E. coli*.

ADMINISTRATION

• Before giving, ensure patient isn't allergic to penicillins or cephalosporins.
• Obtain specimen for culture and sensitivity tests before giving. Start therapy while awaiting results.

IV
▼ Follow manufacturer's guidelines closely when reconstituting drug. They vary with concentration of drug ordered and how drug is packaged (duplex container, ADD-Vantage vial, or regular vial).
▼ The type of diluent varies with the product used. Use only solutions recommended by the manufacturer.
▼ Give intermittent IV infusion with a Y-type administration set and compatible solutions over 30 minutes.

▼ Interrupt flow of primary IV solution while drug is infusing.

▼ May also give by direct IV after vial reconstitution over 5 minutes.

▼ **Incompatibilities:** Aminophylline, ciprofloxacin, gentamicin, metronidazole, tobramycin, vancomycin.

IM

• Reconstitute drug using sterile water for injection, NSS for injection, D₅W injection, 0.5% or 1% lidocaine hydrochloride, or bacteriostatic water for injection with parabens or benzyl alcohol. Follow manufacturer's guidelines for quantity of diluent to use.

• Inspect solution for particulate matter before use. The powder and its solutions tend to darken, depending on storage conditions. If stored as recommended, potency isn't adversely affected.

• Pain may occur at injection site.

ACTION

Inhibits bacterial cell-wall synthesis, promotes osmotic instability, and destroys bacteria.

Route	Onset	Peak	Duration
IV	Unknown	30 min	Unknown
IM	Unknown	1–2 hr	Unknown

Half-life: Adults, 2 to 2½ hours.

ADVERSE REACTIONS

CNS: fever, headache. **CV:** phlebitis. **GI:** diarrhea, nausea, vomiting. **Skin:** rash, pruritus. **Other:** *anaphylaxis,* pain, inflammation, hypersensitivity reactions.

INTERACTIONS

Drug-drug. *Aminoglycosides:* May increase risk of nephrotoxicity. Monitor renal function closely.

Estrogen-based contraceptives: May decrease contraceptive absorption and effectiveness. Patient should avoid use together or use nonhormonal contraception for duration of antibiotic (or 14 days, whichever is longer) and for 7 days after completion of antibiotic.

Live-virus vaccines: May decrease effectiveness of live-virus vaccines. Concurrent use isn't recommended.

Potent diuretics: May increase risk of nephrotoxicity. Monitor renal function closely.

Probenecid: May inhibit renal excretion of cefepime. Monitor patient for adverse reactions.

Warfarin: May enhance anticoagulant effects. Monitor therapy.

EFFECTS ON LAB TEST RESULTS

• May increase ALT and AST levels. May decrease phosphorus level.

• May increase eosinophil count. May alter PT and PTT.

• May falsely increase serum or urine creatinine level in tests using Jaffé reaction. May cause false-positive results of Coombs test and urine glucose tests that use cupric sulfate, such as Benedict reagent and Clinitest.

CONTRAINDICATIONS & CAUTIONS

• Contraindicated in patients hypersensitive to drug, cephalosporins, beta-lactam antibiotics, or penicillins.

❸ *Alert:* Drug may increase risk of nonconvulsive status epilepticus (altered mental status, confusion, decreased responsiveness), especially in patients with renal impairment. To decrease risk, follow dosage adjustment guidelines for patients with CrCl of 60 mL/minute or less. Discontinue drug in patients with seizures associated with drug.

• Use cautiously in patients with history of colitis or renal insufficiency.

Dialyzable drug: 68%.

⚠ *Overdose S&S:* Encephalopathy, myoclonus, seizures, neuromuscular excitability.

PREGNANCY-LACTATION-REPRODUCTION

• There are no adequate studies in pregnant women. Use during pregnancy only if clearly needed and potential benefit justifies potential risk to the fetus.

• Drug appears in human milk in very low concentrations (0.5 mcg/mL). Use cautiously in breastfeeding women.

NURSING CONSIDERATIONS

• Monitor patient for superinfection, including CDAD and pseudomembranous colitis, which can occur more than 2 months after

---

Reactions in bold italics are *life-threatening*. Interactions may have a *rapid onset* or a *delayed onset*.

final dose. Drug may cause overgrowth of nonsusceptible bacteria or fungi.

• Drug may alter PT and increase bleeding risk. Patients at risk include those with renal or hepatic impairment or poor nutrition and those receiving prolonged therapy. Monitor PT and INR in these patients. Give vitamin K, as indicated.

• *Look alike–sound alike:* Don't confuse drug with other cephalosporins that sound alike.

PATIENT TEACHING

• Warn patient receiving drug IM that pain may occur at injection site.

• Advise patient to promptly report all adverse reactions, including rash, and signs and symptoms of superinfection (such as recurring fever, chills, malaise, and diarrhea).

cefotaxime sodium
sef-oh-TAKS-eem

Therapeutic class: Antibiotics
Pharmacologic class: Third-generation cephalosporins

AVAILABLE FORMS
Injection: 500 mg, 1 g, 2 g

INDICATIONS & DOSAGES

Adjust-a-dose (for all indications): For patients with CrCl less than 20 mL/minute/1.73 m^2, give half of usual dose at regular time interval. For patients receiving hemodialysis, give 0.5 to 2 g supplement after dialysis. For patients receiving continuous ambulatory peritoneal dialysis, give 1 g every 24 hours.

➤ **Perioperative prophylaxis in contaminated surgery**
Adults: 1 g IM or IV 30 to 90 minutes before surgery. In patients undergoing bowel surgery, provide preoperative mechanical bowel cleansing and give a nonabsorbable anti-infective, such as neomycin. In patients undergoing cesarean delivery, give 1 g IM or IV as soon as the umbilical cord is clamped; then 1 g IM or IV 6 and 12 hours later.

➤ **Uncomplicated gonorrhea caused by penicillinase-producing strains or non–penicillinase-producing strains of *Neisseria gonorrhoeae***

Adults and adolescents: 500 mg IM as a single dose.

➤ **Rectal gonorrhea**
Men: 1 g IM as a single dose.
Women: 500 mg IM as a single dose.

➤ **Serious infection of the lower respiratory and urinary tract, CNS, skin, bone, and joints; gynecologic and intra-abdominal infection; bacteremia; septicemia caused by susceptible microorganisms, such as streptococci (including *Streptococcus pneumoniae* and *Streptococcus pyogenes*, *Staphylococcus aureus* [penicillinase- and non–penicillinase-producing], and *Staphylococcus epidermidis*), *Escherichia coli*, *Klebsiella*, *Haemophilus influenzae*, *Serratia marcescens*, and species of *Pseudomonas* (including *P. aeruginosa*), *Enterobacter*, *Proteus*, and *Peptostreptococcus***
Adults and children weighing 50 kg or more: 1 to 2 g IV or IM every 6 to 8 hours. Up to 12 g daily can be given for life-threatening infections.
Children ages 1 month to 12 years weighing less than 50 kg: 50 to 180 mg/kg/day IM or IV in four to six divided doses.
Neonates ages 1 to 4 weeks: 50 mg/kg IV every 8 hours.
Neonates to age 1 week: 50 mg/kg IV every 12 hours.

ADMINISTRATION

• Before giving, ensure patient isn't allergic to penicillins or cephalosporins.

• Obtain specimen for culture and sensitivity tests before giving. Begin therapy while awaiting results.

IV

▼ For direct injection, reconstitute drug in 500-mg, 1-g, or 2-g vials with 10 mL of sterile water for injection. Solutions containing 1 g/14 mL are isotonic.

▼ Inject drug over 3 to 5 minutes into a large vein or into the tubing of a free-flowing IV solution. Potentially life-threatening arrhythmias have been reported with more rapid administration.

▼ For infusion, reconstitute drug in infusion vials with 50 to 100 mL of D$_5$W or NSS.

▼ Interrupt flow of primary IV solution, and infuse this drug over 15 to 30 minutes.

▼ **Incompatibilities:** Allopurinol, azithromycin, doxapram, filgrastim, fluconazole, hetastarch, pentamidine sodium bicarbonate injection, vancomycin.

IM
• Reconstitute 500-mg vial with 2 mL, 1-g vial with 3 mL, and 2-g vial with 5 mL sterile water for injection.
• For doses of 2 g, divide the dose and give at different sites.
• Inject deep into a large muscle, such as the gluteus maximus or the side of the thigh.

ACTION
Inhibits cell-wall synthesis, promoting osmotic instability; usually bactericidal.

Route	Onset	Peak	Duration
IV	Immediate	Immediate	Unknown
IM	Unknown	30 min	Unknown

Half-life: 1 to 2 hours.

ADVERSE REACTIONS
CNS: fever, headache. **CV:** phlebitis, thrombophlebitis. **GI:** diarrhea, *pseudomembranous colitis,* nausea, vomiting. **Hematologic:** *agranulocytosis, thrombocytopenia, transient neutropenia,* eosinophilia, hemolytic anemia. **Skin:** maculopapular and erythematous rashes, urticaria, pain, induration, sterile abscesses, temperature elevation, tissue sloughing at IM injection site. **Other:** *anaphylaxis,* hypersensitivity reactions, serum sickness.

INTERACTIONS
Drug-drug. *Aminoglycosides:* May increase risk of nephrotoxicity. Monitor patient's renal function tests.
Estrogen-based contraceptives: May decrease contraceptive absorption and effectiveness. Patient should avoid use together or use nonhormonal contraception for duration of antibiotic (or 14 days, whichever is longer) and for 7 days after completion of antibiotic.
Live-virus vaccines: May decrease effectiveness of live-virus vaccines. Concurrent use isn't recommended.
Probenecid: May inhibit excretion and increase cefotaxime level. Use together cautiously.

Warfarin: May enhance anticoagulant effects. Monitor therapy.

EFFECTS ON LAB TEST RESULTS
• May increase alkaline phosphatase, ALT, AST, bilirubin, GGT, and LDH levels. May decrease Hb level.
• May increase eosinophil count. May decrease granulocyte, neutrophil, and platelet counts.
• May cause positive Coombs test results.

CONTRAINDICATIONS & CAUTIONS
• Contraindicated in patients hypersensitive to drug or other cephalosporins.
• Use cautiously in patients hypersensitive to penicillin because of possibility of cross-sensitivity with other beta-lactam antibiotics.
• CDC guidelines for sexually transmitted diseases don't recommend cefotaxime as a treatment option for uncomplicated or rectal gonorrhea; ceftriaxone is preferred.
• Prolonged use may result in fungal or bacterial superinfection, including CDAD and pseudomembranous colitis, which can occur more than 2 months after treatment ends.
• Use cautiously in patients with history of colitis or renal insufficiency.
Dialyzable drug: Yes.
⚠ *Overdose S&S:* Elevated BUN and creatinine levels.

PREGNANCY-LACTATION-REPRODUCTION
• There are no adequate studies in pregnant women. Use during pregnancy only if clearly needed.
• Low concentrations of drug appear in human milk. Use cautiously in breastfeeding women.

NURSING CONSIDERATIONS
• If large doses are given, therapy is prolonged, or patient is at high risk, monitor patient for superinfection.
• Monitor patient for diarrhea and treat appropriately.
• *Look alike–sound alike:* Don't confuse drug with other cephalosporins that sound alike.

PATIENT TEACHING
• Tell patient to promptly report adverse reactions and signs and symptoms of superinfection, including diarrhea.

Reactions in bold italics are *life-threatening*. Interactions may have a *rapid onset* or a ***delayed onset***.

- Instruct patient to report discomfort at IV insertion site.

cefOXitin sodium
se-FOX-i-tin

Therapeutic class: Antibiotics
Pharmacologic class: Second-generation cephalosporins

AVAILABLE FORMS
Infusion: 1 g, 2 g in 50-mL duplex containers
Injection: 1 g, 2 g

INDICATIONS & DOSAGES
Adjust-a-dose (for all indications): For adults with renal insufficiency, give loading dose of 1 to 2 g. For adults with CrCl of 30 to 50 mL/minute, give 1 to 2 g every 8 to 12 hours; if CrCl is 10 to 29 mL/minute, 1 to 2 g every 12 to 24 hours; if CrCl is 5 to 9 mL/minute, 0.5 to 1 g every 12 to 24 hours; and if CrCl is less than 5 mL/minute, 0.5 to 1 g every 24 to 48 hours. For patients receiving hemodialysis, give a loading dose of 1 to 2 g after each hemodialysis session; then give the maintenance dose based on creatinine level. For patients receiving continuous ambulatory peritoneal dialysis, give 1 g every 24 hours.
➤ **Serious infection of the respiratory or GU tracts; skin, soft-tissue, bone, or joint infection; bloodstream or intra-abdominal infection caused by susceptible organisms (such as *Escherichia coli* and other coliform bacteria, penicillinase- and non–penicillinase-producing *Staphylococcus aureus, Staphylococcus epidermidis*, streptococci, *Klebsiella, Haemophilus influenzae*, and *Bacteroides*, including *B. fragilis*)**
Adults: 1 to 2 g IV every 6 to 8 hours for uncomplicated infections. Up to 12 g daily may be used in life-threatening infections.
Children older than age 3 months: 80 to 160 mg/kg daily IV, given in four to six equally divided doses. Maximum daily dose is 12 g.
➤ **Perioperative prophylaxis**
Adults: 2 g IV 30 to 60 minutes before surgery; then 2 g IV every 6 hours for up to 24 hours. For patients undergoing cesarean section, give 2 g IV as soon as the umbilical cord is clamped; may give additional 2-g doses 4 and 8 hours after initial dose.
Children age 3 months and older: 30 to 40 mg/kg IV 30 to 60 minutes before surgery; then 30 to 40 mg/kg every 6 hours for up to 24 hours.

ADMINISTRATION
IV
▼ Before giving drug, ensure patient isn't allergic to penicillins or cephalosporins.
▼ Obtain specimen for culture and sensitivity tests before giving. Begin therapy while awaiting results.
▼ Reconstitute 1 g with at least 10 mL of sterile water for injection and 2 g with 10 to 20 mL of sterile water for injection. Solutions of D_5W and NSS for injection also may be used.
▼ After reconstitution, drug may be stored for 6 hours at room temperature or 1 week under refrigeration.
▼ For direct injection, give drug over 3 to 5 minutes into a large vein or into the tubing of a free-flowing IV solution.
▼ For intermittent infusion, add reconstituted drug to 50 or 100 mL of D_5W or NSS for injection and administer over 10 to 60 minutes.
▼ Interrupt flow of primary solution during cefoxitin infusion.
▼ Assess site often to detect evidence of thrombophlebitis.
▼ **Incompatibilities:** Aminoglycosides, filgrastim, pantoprazole, pentamidine.

ACTION
Inhibits cell-wall synthesis, promoting osmotic instability; usually bactericidal.

Route	Onset	Peak	Duration
IV	Immediate	Immediate	Unknown

Half-life: About ½ to 1 hour.

ADVERSE REACTIONS
CNS: fever. **CV:** thrombophlebitis, hypotension. **GI:** diarrhea, *pseudomembranous colitis.* **GU:** *acute renal failure.* **Hematologic:** *thrombocytopenia, transient neutropenia,* eosinophilia, hemolytic anemia, anemia. **Respiratory:** dyspnea. **Skin:** maculopapular

and erythematous rashes, urticaria, pain, induration, sterile abscesses, tissue sloughing at injection site, exfoliative dermatitis.
Other: *anaphylaxis, angioedema,* hypersensitivity reactions, serum sickness.

INTERACTIONS
Drug-drug. *Aminoglycosides:* May increase risk of nephrotoxicity. Monitor patient's renal function tests.
Estrogen-based contraceptives: May decrease contraceptive absorption and effectiveness. Patient should avoid use together or use nonhormonal contraception for duration of antibiotic (or 14 days, whichever is longer) and for 7 days after completion of antibiotic.
Live-virus vaccines: May decrease effectiveness of live-virus vaccines. Concurrent use isn't recommended.
Probenecid: May inhibit excretion and increase cefoxitin level. Probenecid may be used for this effect.
Warfarin: May increase anticoagulation. Monitor PT, and adjust warfarin dosage as needed.

EFFECTS ON LAB TEST RESULTS
• May increase alkaline phosphatase, ALT, AST, bilirubin, and LDH levels. May decrease Hb level.
• May increase eosinophil count. May decrease neutrophil and platelet counts.
• May prolong PT.
• May falsely increase serum or urine creatinine level in tests using Jaffé reaction. May cause false-positive results of Coombs test and urine glucose tests that use cupric sulfate, such as Benedict reagent and Clinitest.

CONTRAINDICATIONS & CAUTIONS
• Contraindicated in patients hypersensitive to drug or other cephalosporins.
• Use cautiously in patients hypersensitive to penicillin because of possibility of cross-sensitivity with other beta-lactam antibiotics.
• Use cautiously in patients with history of colitis, renal insufficiency, or seizures.
• Drug can cause overgrowth of nonsusceptible organisms, including CDAD and pseudomembranous colitis, which can occur more than 2 months after treatment ends.

• Higher doses have been associated with risk of eosinophilia and elevated AST levels in children age 3 months and older.
Dialyzable drug: Yes.

PREGNANCY-LACTATION-REPRODUCTION
• There are no adequate studies in pregnant women. Use during pregnancy only if potential benefit justifies potential risk to the fetus.
• Drug appears in human milk in low concentrations. Use cautiously in breastfeeding women.

NURSING CONSIDERATIONS
• Monitor all patients for superinfection or diarrhea and treat appropriately, especially if large doses are given, therapy is prolonged, or patient is at high risk.
• *Look alike–sound alike:* Don't confuse drug with other cephalosporins that sound alike.

PATIENT TEACHING
• Tell patient to report adverse reactions and signs and symptoms of superinfection promptly.
• Instruct patient to report discomfort at IV site.
• Advise patient to report loose stools or diarrhea.

cefpodoxime proxetil
SEF-pod-OX-eem

Therapeutic class: Antibiotics
Pharmacologic class: Third-generation cephalosporins

AVAILABLE FORMS
Granules for oral suspension: 50 mg/5 mL or 100 mg/5 mL when reconstituted in 50- or 100-mL bottles
Tablets (film-coated): 100 mg, 200 mg

INDICATIONS & DOSAGES
Adjust-a-dose (for all indications): For patients with CrCl less than 30 mL/minute, increase dosage interval to every 24 hours. Give to hemodialysis patients three times weekly after hemodialysis.

Reactions in bold italics are *life-threatening*. Interactions may have a *rapid onset* or a *delayed onset*.

➤ **Acute community-acquired pneumonia caused by strains of *Haemophilus influenzae* or *Streptococcus pneumoniae***
Adults and children age 12 and older:
200 mg PO every 12 hours for 14 days.
➤ **Acute bacterial worsening of chronic bronchitis caused by *S. pneumoniae* or *H. influenzae* (strains that don't produce beta-lactamase only), or *Moraxella catarrhalis* (tablets only)**
Adults and children age 12 and older:
200 mg PO every 12 hours for 10 days.
➤ **Uncomplicated gonorrhea in men and women; rectal gonococcal infections in women**
Adults and children age 12 and older:
200 mg PO as a single dose.
➤ **Uncomplicated skin and skin-structure infections caused by *Staphylococcus aureus* or *Streptococcus pyogenes***
Adults and children age 12 and older:
400 mg PO every 12 hours for 7 to 14 days.
➤ **Acute otitis media caused by *S. pneumoniae* (penicillin-susceptible strains only), *S. pyogenes*, *H. influenzae*, or *M. catarrhalis***
Children ages 2 months to 12 years: 5 mg/kg oral suspension PO every 12 hours for 5 days. Don't exceed 200 mg per dose.
➤ **Pharyngitis or tonsillitis caused by *S. pyogenes***
Adults: 100 mg PO every 12 hours for 5 to 10 days.
Children ages 2 months to 12 years: 5 mg/kg PO every 12 hours for 5 to 10 days. Don't exceed 100 mg per dose.
➤ **Uncomplicated UTIs caused by *Escherichia coli*, *Klebsiella pneumoniae*, *Proteus mirabilis*, or *Staphylococcus saprophyticus***
Adults: 100 mg PO every 12 hours for 7 days.
➤ **Mild to moderate acute maxillary sinusitis caused by *H. influenzae*, *S. pneumoniae*, or *M. catarrhalis***
Adults and adolescents age 12 and older:
200 mg PO every 12 hours for 10 days.
Children ages 2 months to 12 years: 5 mg/kg PO every 12 hours for 10 to 14 days; maximum, 200 mg/dose.

ADMINISTRATION
PO
• Before administration, ensure patient isn't allergic to penicillins or cephalosporins.
• Obtain specimen for culture and sensitivity tests before giving. Begin therapy while awaiting results.
• Give tablets with food to enhance absorption. May give oral suspension without regard to food. Shake suspension well before using.
• Store suspension in the refrigerator (36° to 46° F [2° to 8° C]). Discard unused portion after 14 days.

ACTION
Inhibits cell-wall synthesis, promoting osmotic instability; usually bactericidal.

Route	Onset	Peak	Duration
PO	Unknown	2–3 hr	Unknown

Half-life: 2 to 3 hours.

ADVERSE REACTIONS
CNS: headache. **GI:** diarrhea, *pseudomembranous colitis,* nausea, vomiting, abdominal pain. **GU:** vaginal fungal infections. **Skin:** rash. **Other:** *anaphylaxis,* hypersensitivity reactions.

INTERACTIONS
Drug-drug. *Aminoglycosides:* May increase risk of nephrotoxicity. Monitor renal function tests closely.
Antacids, H$_2$-receptor antagonists: May decrease absorption of cefpodoxime. Separate H$_2$-receptor antagonist and cefpodoxime doses by at least 2 hours. Monitor therapy.
Estrogen-based contraceptives: May decrease contraceptive absorption and effectiveness. Patient should avoid use together or use nonhormonal contraception for duration of antibiotic (or 14 days, whichever is longer) and for 7 days after completion of antibiotic.
Live-virus vaccines: May decrease effectiveness of live-virus vaccines. Concurrent use isn't recommended.
Probenecid: May decrease excretion of cefpodoxime. Monitor patient for toxicity.
Warfarin: May prolong PT and increase INR. Monitor levels closely, and adjust warfarin dosage.

EFFECTS ON LAB TEST RESULTS

• May falsely increase serum or urine creatinine level in tests using Jaffé reaction.
• May decrease WBC, absolute neutrophil, platelet, and lymphocyte counts.
• May cause false-positive results of Coombs test and urine glucose tests that use cupric sulfate, such as Benedict reagent and Clinitest.

CONTRAINDICATIONS & CAUTIONS

• Contraindicated in patients hypersensitive to drug or other cephalosporins.
❸ *Alert:* Drug can cause CDAD and pseudomembranous colitis ranging from mild to life-threatening due to overgrowth of nonsusceptible bacteria or fungi.
• Use cautiously in patients with a history of penicillin hypersensitivity because of risk of cross-sensitivity.
• Use cautiously in patients receiving nephrotoxic drugs because other cephalosporins have been shown to have nephrotoxic potential.
• For children with otitis media, American Academy of Pediatrics guidelines recommend basing duration on patient age: For patients younger than age 2 or with severe symptoms (any age), 10-day course; for patients age 2 to 5 with mild to moderate symptoms, 7-day course; for patients age 6 and older with mild to moderate symptoms, 5- to 7-day course.
❸ *Alert:* Some dosage forms may contain benzoate, which is a metabolite of benzyl alcohol. Benzyl alcohol in large amounts has been linked to potentially fatal gasping syndrome in neonates. Avoid dosage forms with benzyl alcohol derivatives in neonates. Refer to manufacturer's labeling.
• Safety and effectiveness in children younger than age 2 months haven't been established.
Dialyzable drug: 23%.

PREGNANCY-LACTATION-REPRODUCTION

• There are no adequate studies in pregnant women. Use during pregnancy only if clearly needed.
• Drug appears in human milk. Patient should discontinue breastfeeding or discontinue drug, taking into account importance of drug to the mother.

NURSING CONSIDERATIONS

• Monitor renal function closely.
• Monitor patient for superinfection and diarrhea and treat appropriately. Use extreme caution when using drug in patients at increased risk for antibiotic-induced pseudomembranous colitis due to exposure to institutional settings (such as nursing homes or hospitals) with endemic *Clostridium difficile* infection.
• *Look alike–sound alike:* Don't confuse drug with other cephalosporins that sound alike.

PATIENT TEACHING

• Tell patient to take drug as prescribed, even if feeling better.
• Instruct patient to take tablets with food. Tell patient using suspension to shake container before measuring dose and to keep container refrigerated.
• Tell patient to report all adverse reactions, especially rash or signs and symptoms of superinfection.
• Instruct patient to promptly report loose stools or diarrhea.

cefprozil
sef-PRO-zil

Therapeutic class: Antibiotics
Pharmacologic class: Second-generation cephalosporins

AVAILABLE FORMS

Powder for oral suspension: 125 mg/5 mL, 250 mg/5 mL when reconstituted
Tablets: 250 mg, 500 mg

INDICATIONS & DOSAGES

Adjust-a-dose (for all indications): If CrCl is less than 30 mL/minute, give 50% of standard dose at standard intervals. If patient is receiving dialysis, give dose after hemodialysis is completed; drug is removed by hemodialysis.
➤ **Pharyngitis or tonsillitis caused by** *Streptococcus pyogenes*
Adults and children age 13 and older: 500 mg PO daily for at least 10 days.
Children ages 2 to 12: 7.5 mg/kg PO every 12 hours for 10 days. Don't exceed adult dosage of 500 mg/day.

➤ **Otitis media caused by *Streptococcus pneumoniae, Haemophilus influenzae,* or *Moraxella catarrhalis***
Infants and children ages 6 months to 12 years: 15 mg/kg PO every 12 hours for 10 days. Don't exceed adult dosage of 500 mg/dose or 1,000 mg/day.

➤ **Secondary bacterial infections of acute bronchitis and acute bacterial worsening of chronic bronchitis caused by *S. pneumoniae, H. influenzae,* or *M. catarrhalis***
Adults and children age 13 and older: 500 mg PO every 12 hours for 10 days.

➤ **Uncomplicated skin and skin-structure infections caused by *Staphylococcus aureus* or *S. pyogenes***
Adults and children age 13 and older: 250 or 500 mg PO every 12 hours or 500 mg PO daily for 10 days.
Children ages 2 to 12: 20 mg/kg PO every 24 hours for 10 days. Don't exceed adult dose.

ADMINISTRATION
PO
● Obtain specimen for culture and sensitivity tests before giving first dose. Start therapy while awaiting results.
● Before giving, ensure patient isn't allergic to penicillins or cephalosporins.
● Administer without regard to meals.
● Shake suspension well before using.

ACTION
Inhibits cell-wall synthesis, promoting osmotic instability; usually bactericidal.

Route	Onset	Peak	Duration
PO	Unknown	1½ hr	Unknown

Half-life: 1¼ hours in adults with normal renal function; 1½ hours in children; 2 hours in patients with impaired hepatic function; 5 to 6 hours in patients with renal impairment or ESRD.

ADVERSE REACTIONS
CNS: dizziness. **GI:** diarrhea, nausea, vomiting, abdominal pain. **GU:** genital pruritus, vaginitis. **Hematologic:** eosinophilia. **Skin:** rash. **Other:** *anaphylaxis,* superinfection, hypersensitivity reactions.

INTERACTIONS
Drug-drug. *Aminoglycosides:* May increase risk of nephrotoxicity. Monitor renal function tests closely.
Estrogen-based contraceptives: May decrease contraceptive absorption and effectiveness. Patient should avoid use together or use nonhormonal contraception for duration of antibiotic (or 14 days, whichever is longer) and for 7 days after completion of antibiotic.
Live-virus vaccines: May decrease effectiveness of live-virus vaccines. Concurrent use isn't recommended.
Probenecid: May inhibit excretion and increase cefprozil level. Use together cautiously.
Warfarin: May enhance anticoagulant effects. Monitor therapy.

EFFECTS ON LAB TEST RESULTS
● May increase alkaline phosphatase, ALT, AST, bilirubin, BUN, creatinine, and LDH levels.
● May increase eosinophil count. May decrease platelet and WBC counts.
● May prolong PT and PTT.
● May falsely increase serum or urine creatinine level in tests using Jaffé reaction. May cause false-positive results of Coombs test and urine glucose tests that use cupric sulfate, such as Benedict reagent and Clinitest.

CONTRAINDICATIONS & CAUTIONS
● Contraindicated in patients hypersensitive to drug or other cephalosporins.
● Use cautiously in patients hypersensitive to penicillin because of possibility of cross-sensitivity with other beta-lactam antibiotics.
● **Alert:** May cause mild to life-threatening CDAD and pseudomembranous colitis, which can occur even more than 2 months after therapy; drug may need to be discontinued and other treatment initiated. Use cautiously in patients with a history of GI disease, especially colitis.
● Use cautiously in patients with history of colitis and renal insufficiency.
Dialyzable drug: Yes.

PREGNANCY-LACTATION-REPRODUCTION
• There are no adequate studies in pregnant women. Use during pregnancy only if clearly needed and potential benefit justifies potential risk to the fetus.
• Small amounts of drug appear in human milk. Use cautiously in breastfeeding women.

NURSING CONSIDERATIONS
• Monitor renal function test and LFT results.
• Drug may cause overgrowth of nonsusceptible bacteria or fungi. Monitor patient for superinfection.
• Monitor patient for diarrhea and treat accordingly.
• *Look alike–sound alike:* Don't confuse drug with other cephalosporins that sound alike.

PATIENT TEACHING
• Advise patient to take drug as prescribed, even if feeling better.
• Tell patient to shake suspension well before measuring dose.
• Inform patient or parent that oral suspension is bubble gum–flavored to improve palatability and promote compliance in children. Tell patient to refrigerate reconstituted suspension and to discard unused drug after 14 days.
• Instruct patient to report all adverse reactions and to immediately report rash or signs and symptoms of superinfection, including diarrhea.

cefTAZidime
sef-TAZ-i-deem

Fortaz, Tazicef

Therapeutic class: Antibiotics
Pharmacologic class: Third-generation cephalosporins

AVAILABLE FORMS
Infusion: 1 g, 2 g in 50-mL and 100-mL vials (premixed)
Injection (with sodium carbonate): 500 mg, 1 g, 2 g

INDICATIONS & DOSAGES
Adjust-a-dose (for all indications): If CrCl is 31 to 50 mL/minute, give 1 g every 12 hours; if CrCl is 16 to 30 mL/minute, give 1 g every 24 hours; if CrCl is 6 to 15 mL/minute, give 500 mg every 24 hours; if CrCl is less than 5 mL/minute, give 500 mg every 48 hours. Ceftazidime is removed by hemodialysis; give a loading dose of 1 g, followed by 1 g after each hemodialysis period. If patient is receiving continuous ambulatory peritoneal dialysis, give a loading dose of 1 g, followed by 500 mg every 24 hours. Or, add 250 mg per 2 L of dialysis fluid.

➤ **Serious UTI and lower respiratory tract infection; skin, gynecologic, intra-abdominal, bone and joint, and CNS infection; bacteremia; and septicemia caused by susceptible microorganisms, such as streptococci (including *Streptococcus pneumoniae* and *Streptococcus pyogenes*), penicillinase- and non-penicillinase-producing *Staphylococcus aureus, Escherichia coli, Klebsiella, Proteus, Enterobacter, Haemophilus influenzae, Pseudomonas*, and some strains of *Bacteroides***
Adults and children age 12 and older: 1 to 2 g IV or IM every 8 to 12 hours. Route and dosage are determined by susceptibility of the organism, severity of infection, and condition of patient. Give up to 6 g daily in life-threatening infections.
Children ages 1 month to 12 years: 30 to 50 mg/kg IV every 8 hours. Maximum dose is 6 g/day.
Neonates up to age 4 weeks: 30 mg/kg IV every 12 hours.
➤ **Uncomplicated UTI**
Adults: 250 mg IV or IM every 12 hours.
➤ **Complicated UTI**
Adults and children age 12 and older: 500 mg to 1 g IV or IM every 8 to 12 hours.
➤ **Uncomplicated pneumonia**
Adults and children age 12 and older: 500 mg to 1 g IV or IM every 8 hours.
➤ **Lung infections caused by *Pseudomonas* in patients with cystic fibrosis with normal renal function**
Adults and children age 12 and older: 30 to 50 mg/kg IV every 8 hours. Maximum dose is 6 g/day.

➤ **Very severe life-threatening infections, especially in immunocompromised patients**
Adults and children older than age 12: 2 g IV every 8 hours.

ADMINISTRATION

IV
▼ Before administration, ensure patient isn't allergic to penicillins or cephalosporins.
▼ Obtain specimen for culture and sensitivity tests before giving. Begin therapy while awaiting results.
▼ Each brand of drug includes specific instructions for reconstitution. Read and follow them carefully.
▼ To reconstitute solution that contains sodium carbonate, add 5 mL sterile water for injection to a 500-mg vial, or add 10 mL to a 1-g or 2-g vial. Shake well to dissolve drug. Because carbon dioxide is released during dissolution, positive pressure will develop in vial.
▼ Infuse drug over 15 to 30 minutes.
▼ **Incompatibilities:** Aminophylline, amiodarone, azithromycin, clarithromycin, fluconazole, idarubicin, midazolam, pentamidine, ranitidine, sargramostim, vancomycin.

IM
• Before administration, ensure patient isn't allergic to penicillins or cephalosporins.
• Obtain specimen for culture and sensitivity tests before giving. Begin therapy while awaiting results.
• Inject deep into a large muscle, such as the gluteus maximus or the side of the thigh.

ACTION

Inhibits cell-wall synthesis, promoting osmotic instability; usually bactericidal.

Route	Onset	Peak	Duration
IV	Immediate	Immediate	Unknown
IM	Unknown	1 hr	Unknown

Half-life: 2 hours.

ADVERSE REACTIONS

CNS: *seizures.* **CV:** phlebitis, thrombophlebitis. **GI:** *pseudomembranous colitis,* nausea, vomiting, diarrhea, abdominal cramps. **Hematologic:**
agranulocytosis, leukopenia, thrombocytopenia, eosinophilia, thrombocytosis, hemolytic anemia. **Skin:** maculopapular and erythematous rashes, urticaria, pain, induration, sterile abscesses, tissue sloughing at injection site. **Other:** *anaphylaxis,* hypersensitivity reactions, serum sickness.

INTERACTIONS

Drug-drug. *Aminoglycosides:* May cause additive or synergistic effect against some strains of *Pseudomonas aeruginosa* and *Enterobacteriaceae;* may increase risk of nephrotoxicity. Monitor patient for effects and monitor renal function.
Chloramphenicol: May cause antagonistic effect. Avoid using together.
Estrogen-based contraceptives: May decrease contraceptive absorption and effectiveness. Patient should avoid use together or use nonhormonal contraception for duration of antibiotic (or 14 days, whichever is longer) and for 7 days after completion of antibiotic.
Live-virus vaccines: May decrease effectiveness of live-virus vaccines. Concurrent use isn't recommended.
Probenecid: May increase serum concentrations of cephalosporins. Monitor therapy.
Warfarin: May increase anticoagulation effect. Monitor PT and INR closely.

EFFECTS ON LAB TEST RESULTS

• May increase alkaline phosphatase, ALT, AST, bilirubin, and LDH levels. May decrease Hb level.
• May increase eosinophil count. May decrease granulocyte and WBC counts. May increase or decrease platelet count.
• May prolong PTT and PT, and increase INR.
• May falsely increase serum or urine creatinine level in tests using Jaffé reaction. May cause false-positive results of Coombs test and urine glucose tests that use cupric sulfate, such as Benedict reagent and Clinitest.

CONTRAINDICATIONS & CAUTIONS

• Contraindicated in patients hypersensitive to drug or other cephalosporins.
• Use cautiously in patients hypersensitive to penicillin; may cause cross-sensitivity with other beta-lactam antibiotics.

• Prolonged use can result in superinfection, including CDAD and pseudomembranous colitis, which can occur even more than 2 months after treatment ends.
• Use cautiously in patients with history of colitis, renal insufficiency, or seizures.
Dialyzable drug: Yes.
⚠ *Overdose S&S:* Seizures, encephalopathy, asterixis, neuromuscular excitability, coma (in patients with renal failure).

PREGNANCY-LACTATION-REPRODUCTION
• There are no adequate studies in pregnant women. Use during pregnancy only if clearly needed.
• Drug appears in human milk in low concentrations. Use caution in breastfeeding.

NURSING CONSIDERATIONS
• If large doses are given, therapy is prolonged, or patient is at high risk, monitor patient for superinfection.
• Monitor patient for diarrhea and treat appropriately.
• *Look alike–sound alike:* Don't confuse drug with other cephalosporins that sound alike.

PATIENT TEACHING
• Tell patient to report adverse reactions or signs of superinfection promptly.
• Instruct patient to report discomfort at IV insertion site.
• Advise patient to notify prescriber about loose stools or diarrhea.

cefTAZidime–avibactam sodium
sef-TAZ-i-deem/A-vi-BAK-tam sodium

Avycaz

Therapeutic class: Antibiotics
Pharmacologic class: Cephalosporins–beta-lactamase inhibitors

AVAILABLE FORMS
Injection (single-use vials): 2 g ceftazidime and 0.5 g avibactam per vial

INDICATIONS & DOSAGES
🔆 *Alert:* Dosage recommendations are expressed as total grams of the ceftazidime–avibactam combination.

Adjust-a-dose (for all indications): If CrCl is 31 to 50 mL/minute, give 1.25 g (1 g ceftazidime and 0.25 g avibactam) every 8 hours. If CrCl is 16 to 30 mL/minute, give 0.94 g (0.75 g ceftazidime and 0.19 g avibactam) every 12 hours. If CrCl is 6 to 15 mL/minute, give 0.94 g (0.75 g ceftazidime and 0.19 g avibactam) every 24 hours. If CrCl is 5 mL/minute or less, give 0.94 g (0.75 g ceftazidime and 0.19 g avibactam) every 48 hours. If patient is on hemodialysis, administer after hemodialysis on hemodialysis days.
➤ **Complicated intra-abdominal infections caused by susceptible microorganisms (*Escherichia coli, Klebsiella pneumoniae, Proteus mirabilis, Providencia stuartii, Enterobacter cloacae, Klebsiella oxytoca,* or *Pseudomonas aeruginosa*) in combination with metronidazole**
Adults: 2.5 g (2 g ceftazidime and 0.5 g avibactam) IV every 8 hours for 5 to 14 days.
➤ **Complicated UTI, including pyelonephritis, caused by susceptible microorganisms (*E. coli, K. pneumoniae, Citrobacter koseri, Enterobacter aerogenes, E. cloacae, Citrobacter freundii, Proteus* spp., or *P. aeruginosa*)**
Adults: 2.5 g (2 g ceftazidime and 0.5 g avibactam) IV every 8 hours for 7 to 14 days.
➤ **Hospital-acquired bacterial pneumonia and ventilator-associated bacterial pneumonia caused by susceptible microorganisms (*K. pneumoniae, E. cloacae, E. coli, Serratia marcescens, P. mirabilis, P. aeruginosa,* or *Haemophilus influenzae*)**
Adults: 2.5 g (2 g ceftazidime and 0.5 g avibactam) IV every 8 hours for 7 to 14 days.

ADMINISTRATION
IV
▼ Store unconstituted vials at 77° F (25° C); excursions permitted between 59° and 86° F (15° and 30° C). Protect from light.
▼ Reconstitute vial with 10 mL sterile water for injection, NSS, 5% dextrose, lactated Ringer solution, or all combinations of dextrose injection and sodium chloride injection containing up to 2.5% dextrose and 0.45% sodium chloride. Mix gently.
▼ Refer to package insert for specific information regarding volume to withdraw from

vial to dilute further to 50 or 250 mL to administer renal doses of drug.

▼ After reconstitution, transfer contents of vial within 30 minutes to an infusion bag for further dilution.

▼ Further dilute constituted solution with the same diluent used for constitution to achieve a total volume between 50 mL (40 and 10 mg/mL of ceftazidime and avibactam, respectively) and 250 mL (8 and 2 mg/mL of ceftazidime and avibactam, respectively). Mix gently. Inspect for particulate matter and discoloration (the color of solution ranges from clear to light yellow).

▼ Final admixed solution is stable for 12 hours at room temperature and for 24 hours if refrigerated at 36° to 46° F (2° to 8° C). Use final solution within 12 hours of subsequent storage at room temperature.

▼ Infuse final solution over 2 hours.

▼ **Incompatibilities:** Solutions other than those listed above. Refer to manufacturer's instructions for a list of compatible drugs or consult a drug incompatibility reference for more information.

ACTION
Ceftazidime is a bactericidal agent that inhibits cell-wall synthesis, promoting osmotic instability. Avibactam increases ceftazidime's effectiveness by inactivating certain beta-lactamases, which destroy ceftazidime.

Route	Onset	Peak	Duration
IV	Rapid	Unknown	Unknown

Half-life: Ceftazidime, about 3 hours; avibactam, about 2½ hours.

ADVERSE REACTIONS
CNS: dizziness, anxiety. **GI:** nausea, vomiting, constipation, abdominal pain, *CDAD.* **GU:** *acute renal failure,* renal impairment. **Hematologic:** eosinophilia, *thrombocytopenia.* **Hepatic:** increased alkaline phosphatase, ALT, and GGT levels. **Metabolic:** hypokalemia. **Skin:** rash. **Other:** hypersensitivity reaction, *drug-resistant bacterial infection.*

INTERACTIONS
Drug-drug. *Aminoglycosides:* May increase risk of nephrotoxicity. Monitor closely.
Estrogen-based contraceptives: May decrease contraceptive absorption and effectiveness. Patient should avoid use together or use nonhormonal contraception for duration of antibiotic (or 14 days, whichever is longer) and for 7 days after completion of antibiotic.
Live-virus vaccines: May decrease effectiveness of live-virus vaccines. Concurrent use isn't recommended.
Probenecid: May decrease ceftazidime–avibactam excretion. Avoid use together.
Vitamin K antagonists (warfarin): May enhance anticoagulation effects. Monitor therapy.

EFFECTS ON LAB TEST RESULTS
• May increase alkaline phosphatase, GGT, and ALT levels. May decrease potassium level.
• May prolong PT.
• May cause false-positive reaction for glucose in the urine with certain methods.
• May result in seroconversion from a negative to a positive direct Coombs test.

CONTRAINDICATIONS & CAUTIONS
• Contraindicated in patients hypersensitive to cephalosporins or avibactam.
• Use cautiously in patients with penicillin or other beta-lactam allergy because of cross-sensitivity.
⚠️ *Alert:* Drug may cause severe neurologic reactions, including encephalopathy, myoclonus, seizures, and nonconvulsive status epilepticus. Risk may increase in patients with renal impairment; ensure dosage adjustment for renal function. Discontinue drug if neurotoxicity occurs.
⚠️ *Alert:* Serious and fatal hypersensitivity reactions and anaphylaxis can occur.
• Use cautiously in patients with renal impairment.
• CDAD has been reported with the use of nearly all systemic antibacterial drugs, and may range in severity from mild diarrhea to fatal colitis. CDAD may occur more than 2 months after use of antibacterial drugs.
• Safety and effectiveness in children haven't been established.

- Use cautiously in elderly patients, who are more likely to have renal dysfunction.
Dialyzable drug: Yes.

PREGNANCY-LACTATION-REPRODUCTION
- Use cautiously in pregnant women and only if benefits outweigh risk to the fetus.
- Ceftazidime appears in human milk in low concentrations; it isn't known if avibactam appears in human milk. Use cautiously in breastfeeding women.

NURSING CONSIDERATIONS
- To reduce the development of drug-resistant bacteria and maintain the effectiveness of antibacterial drugs, ceftazidime–avibactam should be used only to treat infections that are proven or strongly suspected to be caused by susceptible bacteria.
- ❸ *Alert:* Monitor renal function at baseline and at least daily in patients with renal impairment.
- ❸ *Alert:* Monitor patients for CNS reactions (including seizures, nonconvulsive status epilepticus, encephalopathy, coma, asterixis, neuromuscular excitability, and myoclonia), particularly in those with renal impairment. Adjust dosage based on CrCl level or discontinue therapy as clinically indicated.
- ❸ *Alert:* Watch for CDAD in patients who develop diarrhea. If CDAD is suspected or confirmed, antibacterial drugs not directed against CDAD may need to be discontinued.
- Assess carefully for previous hypersensitivity reactions to cephalosporins, penicillins, or carbapenems.
- Monitor patient closely for hypersensitivity reaction. Discontinue drug if allergic reactions occur.
- Urine glucose tests based on enzymatic glucose oxidase reactions are recommended. False-positive reactions may occur with other methods.
- *Look alike–sound alike:* Don't confuse Avycaz with Fortaz or Avelox. Don't confuse avibactam with aztreonam.

PATIENT TEACHING
- Instruct patient to immediately report changes in CNS status (disturbance of consciousness, including confusion, hallucinations, stupor, and coma; myoclonus, seizures).

- Advise patient that diarrhea, including frequent watery or bloody diarrhea, may occur even months after antibacterial treatment ends and to consult health care provider for evaluation.
- Teach patient to report signs and symptoms of hypersensitivity reactions.
- Inform patient that blood tests to assess renal function will be needed during treatment.
- Counsel patient, family, or caregivers that antibacterial drugs should be used to treat bacterial infections only and aren't effective in treating viral infections (such as the common cold).
- Advise patient that it's common to feel better early in the course of therapy but to take the full course of the drug as prescribed. Skipping doses or not completing the full course of therapy may decrease the effectiveness of treatment and increase the likelihood that bacteria will develop resistance and won't be treatable in the future.
- Instruct female patient to inform prescriber if she is pregnant, plans to become pregnant, or is breastfeeding.

ceftolozane sulfate–tazobactam sodium
sef-TOL-oh-zane/TAZ-oh-BAK-tam

Zerbaxa

Therapeutic class: Antibiotics
Pharmacologic class: Cephalosporins–beta-lactamase inhibitors

AVAILABLE FORMS
Powder for injection: 1 g ceftolozane and 0.5 g tazobactam in single-dose vial

INDICATIONS & DOSAGES
❸ *Alert:* Dosage recommendations are expressed as total grams of the ceftolozane–tazobactam combination.
Adjust-a-dose (for all indications): If CrCl is 30 to 50 mL/minute, give 750 mg (500 mg ceftolozane and 250 mg tazobactam) IV every 8 hours; if CrCl is 15 to 29 mL/minute, give 375 mg (250 mg ceftolozane and 125 mg tazobactam) IV every 8 hours; if on hemodialysis or with ESRD, give single loading dose of 750 mg (500 mg ceftolozane and 250 mg tazobactam) IV followed by

maintenance dose of 150 mg (100 mg ceftolozane and 50 mg tazobactam) IV every 8 hours for remainder of treatment period. On hemodialysis days, give maintenance dose immediately after completion of dialysis. For patients with changing renal function, monitor CrCl at least daily and adjust dosage accordingly.

➤ **Complicated intra-abdominal infections caused by** *Enterobacter cloacae, Escherichia coli, Klebsiella oxytoca, Klebsiella pneumoniae, Proteus mirabilis, Pseudomonas aeruginosa, Bacteroides fragilis, Streptococcus anginosus, Streptococcus constellatus,* **or** *Streptococcus salivarius*
Adults: 1.5 g (1 g ceftolozane and 0.5 g tazobactam) IV every 8 hours for 4 to 14 days based on infection severity and clinical response. Give with metronidazole 500 mg IV every 8 hours.

➤ **Complicated UTIs, including pyelonephritis, caused by** *E. coli, K. pneumoniae, P. mirabilis,* **or** *P. aeruginosa*
Adults: 1.5 g (1 g ceftolozane and 0.5 g tazobactam) IV every 8 hours for 7 days.

✳ *NEW INDICATION:* **Treatment of hospital-acquired bacterial pneumonia and ventilator-associated bacterial pneumonia (HABP/VABP) caused by susceptible Gram-negative bacteria**
Adults: 3 g (2 g ceftolozane and 1 g tazobactam) IV infusion every 8 hours for 8 to 14 days based on infection severity and clinical response.

Adjust-a-dose: If CrCl is 30 to 50 mL/minute, give 1.5 g (1 g ceftolozane and 500 mg tazobactam) IV every 8 hours; if CrCl is 15 to 29 mL/minute, give 750 mg (500 mg ceftolozane and 250 mg tazobactam) IV every 8 hours; for ESRD on hemodialysis, give a single loading dose of 2.25 g (1.5 g ceftolozane and 750 mg tazobactam) followed by 450 mg (300 mg ceftolozane and 150 mg tazobactam) maintenance dose IV every 8 hours for the remainder of treatment. On hemodialysis days, give maintenance dose immediately after completion of dialysis.

ADMINISTRATION
IV
▼ Reconstitute vial with 10 mL sterile water for injection or NSS; gently shake to dissolve. The final volume is approximately

11.4 mL and must be added to a larger volume for infusion.
▼ To prepare required dose, withdraw appropriate volume from vial and add withdrawn volume to infusion bag containing 100 mL NSS or D_5W.
▼ Administer by infusion over 60 minutes.
▼ Once reconstituted, vials are stable for 1 hour; once placed in infusion bag, drug is stable for 24 hours at room temperature or 7 days under refrigeration. Don't freeze vials or infusion bags that contain drug.
▼ Infusions range from clear, colorless solutions to solutions that are clear and slightly yellow. Variations in color within this range don't affect product's potency.
▼ Vial doesn't contain a bacteriostatic preservative.
▼ **Incompatibilities:** Don't mix with other drugs or solutions except D_5W or NSS.

ACTION
Ceftolozane inhibits cell-wall synthesis by binding to penicillin-binding proteins. Tazobactam is an irreversible inhibitor of some beta-lactamases.

Route	Onset	Peak	Duration
IV	Unknown	1 hr	Unknown

Half-life: Ceftolozane, 3 hours; tazobactam, 1 hour.

ADVERSE REACTIONS
CNS: headache, insomnia, anxiety, dizziness, fever. **CV:** hypotension, atrial fibrillation. **GI:** nausea, diarrhea, CDAD, constipation, vomiting, abdominal pain. **Hematologic:** anemia, *thrombocytosis.* **Hepatic:** increased AST and ALT levels. **Metabolic:** *hypokalemia.* **Skin:** rash.

INTERACTIONS
Drug-drug. *Estrogen-based contraceptives:* May decrease contraceptive absorption and effectiveness. Patient should avoid use together or use nonhormonal contraception for duration of antibiotic (or 14 days, whichever is longer) and for 7 days after completion of antibiotic.
Live-virus vaccines: May decrease effectiveness of live-virus vaccines. Concurrent use isn't recommended.

Probenecid: May increase ceftolozane–tazobactam serum concentration. Monitor therapy.

Vitamin K antagonists (warfarin): May enhance anticoagulant effects. Monitor PT and INR.

EFFECTS ON LAB TEST RESULTS

• May increase ALT and AST levels. May decrease potassium level.
• May increase platelet count. May decrease Hb level, hematocrit, and RBC count.

CONTRAINDICATIONS & CAUTIONS

• Contraindicated in patients with serious hypersensitivity to ceftolozane–tazobactam, piperacillin–tazobactam, or other members of the beta-lactam class.
• Use cautiously in patients hypersensitive to cephalosporins or tazobactam.
• May cause fungal or bacterial superinfection, including CDAD and pseudomembranous colitis. Stop drug and take appropriate measures if diarrhea develops. CDAD has occurred more than 2 months after antibacterial treatment.
• Safety and effectiveness in children haven't been established.
Dialyzable drug: Ceftolozane, 66%; tazobactam, 56%.

PREGNANCY-LACTATION-REPRODUCTION

• Use in pregnant women hasn't been studied. Use cautiously and only if benefits outweigh potential risk to the fetus.
• It isn't known if drug appears in human milk. Use cautiously in breastfeeding women.

NURSING CONSIDERATIONS

• Obtain daily renal function tests. Adjust dosage as necessary based on CrCl.
• Monitor patient for signs and symptoms of hypersensitivity; institute appropriate therapy if needed.
• Monitor patient for development of superinfection, including diarrhea.
• *Look alike–sound alike:* Don't confuse Zerbaxa with Pradaxa.

PATIENT TEACHING

• Explain to patient that drug is used for presumed or actual serious bacterial infections.

• Teach patient that drug is given IV and to immediately report signs or symptoms of allergic reactions (wheezing, chest tightness, itching, or swelling of the face, lips, tongue, or throat).
• Advise patient not to skip doses, as this may decrease effectiveness of treatment.
• Counsel patient to report GI adverse effects such as severe watery or bloody diarrhea.

cefTRIAXone sodium
sef-try-AX-ohn

Therapeutic class: Antibiotics
Pharmacologic class: Third-generation cephalosporins

AVAILABLE FORMS

Infusion: 1 g, 2 g; 1 g/50 mL, 2 g/50 mL premixed
Injection: 250 mg, 500 mg, 1 g, 2 g

INDICATIONS & DOSAGES

Adjust-a-dose (for all indications): In patients with significant renal disease and hepatic dysfunction, maximum dose is 2 g/day. In patients receiving intermittent hemodialysis, give 1 to 2 g IV every 24 hours after dialysis session. This recommendation assumes patient is receiving standard intermittent hemodialysis three times a week and completes the full dialysis sessions.

➤ **Uncomplicated gonococcal vulvovaginitis**
Adults: 250 mg IM as a single dose, plus azithromycin 1 g PO as a single dose or doxycycline 100 mg PO b.i.d. for 7 days.

➤ **UTI; lower respiratory tract, gynecologic, bone or joint, intra-abdominal, skin, or skin-structure infection; septicemia**
Adults and children older than age 12: 1 to 2 g IM or IV daily or in equally divided doses every 12 hours. Total daily dose shouldn't exceed 4 g. Treat for 4 to 14 days. Complicated infections may require longer treatment.
Children age 12 and younger: 50 to 75 mg/kg IM or IV daily or in divided doses every 12 hours. Total daily dose not to exceed 2 g.

Reactions in bold italics are *life-threatening*. Interactions may have a *rapid onset* or a *delayed onset*.

C

➤ **Meningitis**
Adults: 1 to 2 g IV once daily or in two
equally divided doses. Usual duration of
therapy is 4 to 14 days; complicated infec-
tions may need longer therapy.
Children: Initially, 100 mg/kg IM or IV; then
100 mg/kg/day as a single dose or in divided
doses every 12 hours for 7 to 14 days. Maximum dose is 4 g/day.
➤ **Perioperative prophylaxis**
Adults: 1 g IV as a single dose 30 minutes to
2 hours before surgery.
➤ **Acute bacterial otitis media**
Adults: 1 to 2 g IM or IV once daily or in two
equally divided doses daily for 3 days.
Children: 50 mg/kg IM as a single dose.
Don't exceed 1 g.
➤ **Acute otitis media** ◆
Children: 50 mg/kg/day IV or IM for 1 to 3
consecutive days in patients unresponsive to
initial antibiotic therapy and in penicillin-
allergic patients.

ADMINISTRATION

IV
▼ Before giving drug, ensure patient isn't
allergic to penicillins or cephalosporins.
▼ Obtain specimen for culture and sensitivity tests before giving first dose. Begin
therapy while awaiting results.
▼ Reconstitute drug with sterile water for
injection, NSS for injection, D₅W, or a
combination of NSS and dextrose injection
and other compatible solutions.
▼ Add 2.4 mL of diluent to the 250-mg
vial, 4.8 mL to the 500-mg vial, 9.6 mL
to the 1-g vial, and 19.2 mL to the 2-g
vial. All reconstituted solutions average
100 mg/mL. For intermittent infusion, dilute further to achieve desired concentration, and give over 30 minutes.
▼ Diluted IV preparation is stable for
48 hours at room temperature or 10 days
if refrigerated.
☾ *Alert:* Don't mix or administer ceftriaxone with calcium-containing IV solutions,
including parenteral nutrition.
▼ **Incompatibilities:** Aminoglycosides,
aminophylline, azithromycin, calcium-
containing solutions, clindamycin phosphate, filgrastim, fluconazole, gentamicin,
labetalol, linezolid, pentamidine, theophylline, vancomycin, vinorelbine tartrate.

IM
● Before giving drug, ensure patient isn't
allergic to penicillins or cephalosporins.
● Obtain specimen for culture and sensitivity tests before giving first dose. Begin
therapy while awaiting results.
● Inject deep into a large muscle, such as the
gluteus maximus or the lateral aspect of the
thigh.

ACTION
Inhibits cell-wall synthesis, promoting
osmotic instability; usually bactericidal.

Route	Onset	Peak	Duration
IV	Immediate	Immediate	Unknown
IM	Unknown	2–3 hr	Unknown

Half-life: Adults with normal renal and hepatic
function, 5 to 9 hours.

ADVERSE REACTIONS
GI: *pseudomembranous colitis,* diarrhea.
Hematologic: eosinophilia, thrombocytosis, *leukopenia.* **Skin:** pain, induration,
tenderness at injection site, rash. **Other:**
hypersensitivity reactions, serum sickness,
anaphylaxis.

INTERACTIONS
Drug-drug. *Aminoglycosides:* May increase
nephrotoxicity and cause synergistic effect
against some strains of *Enterobacteriaceae*
species. Monitor patient.
Estrogen-based contraceptives: May decrease contraceptive absorption and effectiveness. Patient should avoid use together
or use nonhormonal contraception for duration of antibiotic (or 14 days, whichever
is longer) and for 7 days after completion of
antibiotic.
Live-virus vaccines: May decrease effectiveness of live-virus vaccines. Concurrent use
isn't recommended.
Probenecid: May increase ceftriaxone
concentration. Monitor therapy.
Warfarin: May increase anticoagulation
effect. Monitor PT and INR closely.

EFFECTS ON LAB TEST RESULTS
● May increase alkaline phosphatase, ALT,
AST, bilirubin, BUN, and LDH levels.
● May increase eosinophil and platelet
counts. May decrease WBC count.

• May prolong PTT and PT, and increase INR.
• May falsely increase serum or urine creatinine level in tests using Jaffé reaction. May cause false-positive results of Coombs test and urine glucose tests that use cupric sulfate, such as Benedict reagent and Clinitest.

CONTRAINDICATIONS & CAUTIONS
• Contraindicated in patients hypersensitive to drug or other cephalosporins.
• Use cautiously in patients hypersensitive to penicillin because of possibility of cross-sensitivity with other beta-lactam antibiotics.
❸ *Alert:* May cause superinfection and mild to fatal CDAD. If suspected, manage appropriately; discontinue drug if needed.
❸ *Alert:* May cause hemolytic anemia, which can be fatal. If anemia develops during therapy, stop drug until cause is determined.
• Use cautiously in patients with history of colitis, renal insufficiency, or GI or gallbladder disease.
Dialyzable drug: No.

PREGNANCY-LACTATION-REPRODUCTION
• There are no adequate studies in pregnant women. Use during pregnancy only if clearly needed and potential benefit justifies potential risk to the fetus.
• Drug appears in human milk in low concentrations. Use cautiously in breastfeeding women.

NURSING CONSIDERATIONS
• If large doses are given, therapy is prolonged, or patient is at high risk, monitor patient for signs and symptoms of superinfection.
• Monitor PT and INR in patients with impaired vitamin K synthesis or low vitamin K stores. Vitamin K therapy may be needed.
• Monitor patients for superinfection, diarrhea, and anemia and treat appropriately.
• *Look alike–sound alike:* Don't confuse drug with other cephalosporins that sound alike.

PATIENT TEACHING
• Tell patient to report adverse reactions promptly.
• Instruct patient to report discomfort at IV insertion site.
• If home care patient is diabetic and is testing urine for glucose, tell patient drug may

affect results of cupric sulfate tests and to use an enzymatic test instead.
• Tell patient to notify prescriber about loose stools or diarrhea.

cefuroxime axetil
se-fyoor-OX-eem

cefuroxime sodium
Zinacef

Therapeutic class: Antibiotics
Pharmacologic class: Second-generation cephalosporins

AVAILABLE FORMS
cefuroxime axetil
Suspension: 125 mg/5 mL, 250 mg/5 mL
Tablets: 125 mg, 250 mg, 500 mg
cefuroxime sodium
Infusion: 750-mg, 1.5-g vials, infusion packs, and ADD-Vantage vials
Injection: 750 mg, 1.5 g

INDICATIONS & DOSAGES
Adjust-a-dose (for all indications): For injectable form in adults with CrCl of 10 to 20 mL/minute, give 750 mg IV or IM every 12 hours; if CrCl is less than 10 mL/minute, give 750 mg IV or IM every 24 hours. Give patients on hemodialysis an additional dose after hemodialysis.
➤ **Serious lower respiratory tract infection, UTI, skin or skin-structure infections, bone or joint infection, septicemia, meningitis, and gonorrhea**
Adults and children age 13 and older: 750 mg to 1.5 g cefuroxime sodium IV or IM every 8 hours for 5 to 10 days. For life-threatening infections and infections caused by less susceptible organisms, 1.5 g IV or IM every 6 hours; for bacterial meningitis, up to 3 g IV every 8 hours.
Children ages 3 months to 12 years: 50 to 100 mg/kg/day cefuroxime sodium IV or IM in equally divided doses every 6 to 8 hours. Use higher dosage of 100 mg/kg/day, not to exceed maximum adult dosage, for more severe or serious infections. For bacterial meningitis, 200 to 240 mg/kg/day cefuroxime sodium IV in divided doses every 6 to 8 hours.

➤ **Perioperative prophylaxis**
Adults: 1.5 g IV 30 to 60 minutes before initial incision; in lengthy operations, 750 mg IV or IM every 8 hours. For open-heart surgery, 1.5 g IV at induction of anesthesia and then every 12 hours for a total dose of 6 g.

➤ **Mild to moderate acute bacterial exacerbations of chronic bronchitis**
Adults and children age 13 and older: 250 or 500 mg PO every 12 hours for 10 days.

➤ **Acute bacterial maxillary sinusitis**
Adults and children age 13 and older: 250 mg PO every 12 hours for 10 days.
Children ages 3 months to 12 years: 250 mg every 12 hours for 10 days. For children who can't swallow tablets whole, 30 mg/kg/day oral suspension in two divided doses for 10 days. Maximum daily dose for suspension is 1,000 mg.

➤ **Pharyngitis and tonsillitis**
Adults and children age 13 and older: 250 mg PO every 12 hours for 10 days.
Children ages 3 months to 12 years: 125 mg PO every 12 hours for 10 days. For children who can't swallow tablets whole, give 20 mg/kg daily of oral suspension in two divided doses for 10 days. Maximum daily dose for suspension is 500 mg.

➤ **Otitis media**
Children ages 3 months to 12 years: 250 mg PO every 12 hours for 10 days. For children who can't swallow tablets whole, give 30 mg/kg/day of oral suspension in two divided doses for 10 days. Maximum daily dose for suspension is 1,000 mg.

➤ **Uncomplicated skin and skin-structure infection**
Adults and children age 13 and older: 250 or 500 mg PO every 12 hours for 10 days.

➤ **Uncomplicated UTI**
Adults: 250 mg PO every 12 hours for 7 to 10 days.

➤ **Uncomplicated gonorrhea**
Adults: 1,000 mg PO as a single dose. Or, 1.5 g IM with 1 g probenecid PO for one dose.

➤ **Early Lyme disease**
Adults and children age 13 and older: 500 mg PO every 12 hours for 20 days.

➤ **Impetigo**
Children ages 3 months to 12 years: 30 mg/kg/day of oral suspension in two divided

doses for 10 days. Maximum daily dose, 1,000 mg.

ADMINISTRATION
• Obtain specimen for culture and sensitivity tests before giving first dose. May start therapy while awaiting results.
• Before giving drug, ensure patient isn't allergic to penicillins or cephalosporins.

PO
⊗ *Alert:* Tablets and oral suspension aren't bioequivalent and aren't substitutable on a milligram-per-milligram basis.
• Shake suspension well before each use.
• Give tablets without regard for meals; give oral suspension with food.
• Patients who can't swallow the tablet whole should receive the oral suspension. Don't crush tablets due to bitter taste.
• Store suspension at room temperature before reconstitution or under refrigeration after reconstitution. Discard reconstituted suspension after 10 days.

IV
▼ Reconstitute each 750-mg vial with 8 mL and each 1.5-g vial with 16 mL of sterile water for injection.
▼ Withdraw entire contents of vial for a dose.
▼ For direct injection, inject over 3 to 5 minutes into a large vein or into the tubing of a free-flowing IV solution.
▼ For intermittent infusion, add reconstituted drug to 100 mL D_5W, NSS for injection, or other compatible IV solution.
▼ Infuse over 15 to 60 minutes.
▼ **Incompatibilities:** Azithromycin, ciprofloxacin, cisatracurium, clarithromycin, doxapram, filgrastim, fluconazole, gentamicin, midazolam, ranitidine, sodium bicarbonate injection, vancomycin, vinorelbine tartrate.

IM
• Before giving drug, ensure patient isn't allergic to penicillins or cephalosporins.
• Obtain specimen for culture and sensitivity tests before giving first dose. Therapy may begin while awaiting results.
• Reconstitute 750-mg vial with 3 mL sterile water for injection.
• Inject deep into a large muscle, such as the gluteus maximus or the side of the thigh.

ACTION
Inhibits cell-wall synthesis, promoting osmotic instability; usually bactericidal.

Route	Onset	Peak	Duration
PO	Unknown	2–4 hr	Unknown
IV	Immediate	2–3 min	Unknown
IM	Unknown	15–60 min	Unknown

Half-life: 1 to 2 hours.

ADVERSE REACTIONS
CV: phlebitis, thrombophlebitis. **GI:** diarrhea, *pseudomembranous colitis,* nausea, anorexia, vomiting. **Hematologic:** hemolytic anemia, *thrombocytopenia, transient neutropenia,* eosinophilia. **Skin:** maculopapular and erythematous rashes, urticaria, pain, induration, sterile abscesses, temperature elevation, tissue sloughing at IM injection site. **Other:** *anaphylaxis,* hypersensitivity reactions, serum sickness.

INTERACTIONS
Drug-drug. *Aminoglycosides:* May cause synergistic activity against some organisms; may increase nephrotoxicity. Monitor patient's renal function closely.
Estrogen-based contraceptives: May decrease contraceptive absorption and effectiveness. Patient should avoid use together or use nonhormonal contraception for duration of antibiotic (or 14 days, whichever is longer) and for 7 days after completion of antibiotic.
Live-virus vaccines: May decrease effectiveness of live-virus vaccines. Concurrent use isn't recommended.
Loop diuretics: May increase risk of adverse renal reactions. Monitor renal function.
Probenecid: May inhibit excretion and increase cefuroxime level. Probenecid may be used for this effect.
Warfarin: May increase anticoagulation effects. Monitor PT and INR closely.

EFFECTS ON LAB TEST RESULTS
• May increase alkaline phosphatase, ALT, AST, bilirubin, and LDH levels. May decrease Hb level and hematocrit.
• May prolong PT and may increase INR and eosinophil count. May decrease neutrophil and platelet counts.

• May falsely increase serum or urine creatinine level in tests using Jaffé reaction. May cause false-positive results of Coombs test and urine glucose tests that use cupric sulfate, such as Benedict reagent and Clinitest.

CONTRAINDICATIONS & CAUTIONS
• Contraindicated in patients hypersensitive to drug or other cephalosporins.
• Use cautiously in patients hypersensitive to penicillin because of possibility of cross-sensitivity with other beta-lactam antibiotics.
• According to the CDC, oral cephalosporins aren't recommended to treat gonococcal infections.
• According to clinical practice guidelines, cefotaxime or ceftriaxone should be used to treat childhood bacterial meningitis and pneumococcal and meningococcal meningitis caused by penicillin-resistant strains and *Haemophilus influenzae* type b meningitis.
• Use cautiously in patients with history of colitis and in those with renal insufficiency.
🚯 Alert: Drug may cause CDAD and pseudomembranous colitis ranging from mild to life-threatening, which can occur even 2 months after therapy.
• Some cephalosporins have been associated with seizures in patients with renal impairment when the dosage wasn't reduced. If drug-associated seizures occur, discontinue drug and treat with anticonvulsant therapy if indicated.
Dialyzable drug: Yes.

PREGNANCY-LACTATION-REPRODUCTION
• There are no adequate studies in pregnant women. Use during pregnancy only if clearly needed and potential benefit justifies potential risk to the fetus.
• Drug appears in human milk. Patient should consider temporarily discontinuing breastfeeding during treatment.

NURSING CONSIDERATIONS
• Monitor patient for signs and symptoms of superinfection and diarrhea and treat appropriately.
• Drug may increase INR and risk of bleeding. Monitor patient.
• *Look alike–sound alike:* Don't confuse drug with other cephalosporins that sound alike.

Reactions in bold italics are *life-threatening*. Interactions may have a *rapid onset* or a *delayed onset*.

PATIENT TEACHING
• Tell patient to take drug as prescribed, even if feeling better.
• Advise patient who has difficulty swallowing tablets to ask prescriber for the suspension.
• Tell parent to shake suspension well before measuring dose. Suspension may be stored at room temperature or refrigerated, but must be discarded after 10 days.
• Instruct caregiver to give oral suspension with food.
• Instruct patient to notify prescriber about rash, loose stools, diarrhea, or evidence of superinfection.
• Advise patient receiving drug IV to report discomfort at IV insertion site.

celecoxib ☒
sell-ah-COCKS-ib

CeleBREX⚘

Therapeutic class: NSAIDs
Pharmacologic class: Cyclooxygenase-2 inhibitors

AVAILABLE FORMS
Capsules: 50 mg, 100 mg, 200 mg, 400 mg

INDICATIONS & DOSAGES
☒ *Adjust-a-dose (for all indications):* For elderly patients and those weighing less than 50 kg, start at lowest dosage. For patients with Child-Pugh class B hepatic impairment, reduce dosage by about 50%. Don't use in patients with severe renal or severe hepatic impairment. For patients who are poor metabolizers of CYP2C9, start treatment at half the lowest recommended dose.
➤ **To relieve signs and symptoms of osteoarthritis**
Adults: 200 mg PO daily as a single dose or in two equally divided doses.
➤ **To relieve signs and symptoms of RA**
Adults: 100 to 200 mg PO b.i.d.
➤ **To relieve signs and symptoms of ankylosing spondylitis**
Adults: 200 mg PO once daily or in two divided doses. If no response after 6 weeks, may increase dose to 400 mg daily. If no response after 6 more weeks, consider other treatment.

➤ **To relieve signs and symptoms of juvenile RA**
Children age 2 and older weighing 10 to 25 kg: 50 mg PO b.i.d.
Children age 2 and older weighing more than 25 kg: 100 mg PO b.i.d.
➤ **Acute pain and primary dysmenorrhea**
Adults: 400 mg PO, initially, followed by another 200-mg dose if needed on the first day. On subsequent days, 200 mg PO b.i.d. as needed.

ADMINISTRATION
PO
• May give dosages up to 200 mg b.i.d. without regard to food.
• For patients who have difficulty swallowing capsules, capsule contents can be added to applesauce. Carefully empty entire contents of capsule onto a level teaspoon of cool or room-temperature applesauce and give immediately with water. The capsule contents sprinkled on applesauce are stable for up to 6 hours under refrigeration.

ACTION
Thought to inhibit prostaglandin synthesis, impeding cyclooxygenase-2, to produce anti-inflammatory, analgesic, and antipyretic effects.

Route	Onset	Peak	Duration
PO	Unknown	3 hr	Unknown

Half-life: 11 hours.

ADVERSE REACTIONS
CNS: headache, dizziness, insomnia. **CV:** HTN, peripheral edema. **EENT:** pharyngitis, rhinitis, sinusitis. **GI:** abdominal pain, diarrhea, dyspepsia, flatulence, GI reflux, nausea. **Metabolic:** hyperchloremia. **Musculoskeletal:** back pain. **Respiratory:** dyspnea, URI. **Skin:** *erythema multiforme, exfoliative dermatitis, SJS, toxic epidermal necrolysis,* rash. **Other:** accidental injury.

INTERACTIONS
Drug-drug. *ACE inhibitors, ARBs:* May decrease antihypertensive effects. Monitor BP.
Antacids containing aluminum or magnesium: May decrease celecoxib level. Separate doses.

Anticoagulants, antiplatelets (clopidogrel, prasugrel): May increase bleeding risk. Use cautiously.

Aspirin: May increase risk of ulcers; low aspirin dosages can be used safely to reduce the risk of CV events. Monitor patient for signs and symptoms of GI bleeding.

Corticosteroids, SSRIs: May increase risk of GI bleeding. Use together cautiously.

CYP2C9 inhibitors (amiodarone, metronidazole, ritonavir, zafirlukast): May affect celecoxib metabolism. Use together cautiously.

Digoxin: May increase digoxin serum concentration. Monitor concurrent therapy.

Fluconazole, voriconazole: May increase celecoxib level. Reduce dosage of celecoxib to minimal effective dose.

Lithium: May increase lithium level. Consider therapy modification.

Loop and thiazide diuretics: May increase nephrotoxicity. Consider therapy modification.

Vancomycin: May increase vancomycin serum concentration. Monitor concurrent use.

Warfarin: May prolong PT and cause bleeding complications. Monitor PT and INR, and check for signs and symptoms of bleeding.

Drug-herb. *Alfalfa, anise:* May increase risk of bleeding. Discourage use together.

White willow: Herb and drug contain similar components. Discourage use together.

Drug-lifestyle. *Long-term alcohol use, smoking:* May cause GI irritation or bleeding. Check for signs and symptoms of bleeding.

EFFECTS ON LAB TEST RESULTS
• May increase ALT, AST, BUN, creatinine, and chloride levels.
• May decrease phosphate level.

CONTRAINDICATIONS & CAUTIONS
Black Box Warning Contraindicated for the treatment of perioperative pain after CABG. ∎
• Contraindicated in patients hypersensitive to drug, sulfonamides, aspirin, or other NSAIDs.
• Contraindicated in patients who experienced asthma, urticaria, or allergic-type reactions after taking aspirin or other NSAIDs

and in those who have demonstrated allergic-type reactions to sulfonamides.
• Serious skin reactions (SJS, toxic epidermal necrolysis) can occur. Discontinue drug at first sign of rash.
• Drug isn't recommended with any dose of a nonaspirin NSAID.

Black Box Warning NSAIDs can increase the risk of heart attack or stroke in patients with or without heart disease or risk factors for heart disease. ∎

☉ Alert: The risk of heart attack or stroke can occur as early as the first weeks of NSAID use. Risk appears greater at higher doses. Use lowest effective dose for shortest duration possible.

☉ Alert: NSAIDs increase the risk of HF.

⚕ Use cautiously in patients with history of ulcers or GI bleeding, advanced renal disease, dehydration, anemia, symptomatic liver disease, HTN, edema, HF, or asthma, and in poor CYP2C9 metabolizers.

⚕ Consider alternative therapies for treatment of juvenile RA in patients identified to be poor CYP2C9 metabolizers.

• Use cautiously in elderly or debilitated patients.

Black Box Warning Elderly patients and patients with a prior history of peptic ulcer disease or GI bleeding are at greater risk for serious GI events. ∎

Dialyzable drug: Unlikely.

⚠ Overdose S&S: Lethargy, drowsiness, nausea, vomiting, epigastric pain, GI bleeding, HTN, acute renal failure, respiratory depression, coma, anaphylaxis.

PREGNANCY-LACTATION-REPRODUCTION
• There are no adequate studies in pregnant women. Use during pregnancy isn't recommended because NSAID use close to conception may be associated with an increased risk of miscarriage, and use at 30 weeks' gestation and later may cause premature closure of the ductus arteriosus and other life-threatening fetal conditions.
• A registry is available for pregnant women exposed to autoimmune medications, including celecoxib. Contact the OTIS Autoimmune Diseases in Pregnancy Study at 1-877-311-8972.
• Drug appears in human milk. Use cautiously in breastfeeding women. Patient

---

should consider temporarily discontinuing breastfeeding during treatment.

• Long-term use of NSAIDs in women of reproductive age may be associated with infertility that's reversible on discontinuation of NSAID.

NURSING CONSIDERATIONS

◑ *Alert:* Patients allergic to or with a history of anaphylactic reactions to sulfonamides, aspirin, or other NSAIDs may be allergic to this drug.

Black Box Warning NSAIDs cause an increased risk of serious GI adverse events, including bleeding, ulceration, and perforation of the stomach or intestines, which can be fatal. ■

• Additional risk factors for GI bleeding include treatment with corticosteroids or anticoagulants, longer duration of NSAID treatment, smoking, alcoholism, older age, and poor overall health.

• Although drug may be used with low aspirin dosages, the combination may increase risk of GI bleeding.

• Watch for signs and symptoms of overt and occult bleeding and rash.

Black Box Warning NSAIDs may increase the risk of serious thrombotic events, MI, or stroke. The risk may be greater with longer use or in patients with CV disease or risk factors for CV disease. ■

◑ *Alert:* Watch for and immediately evaluate signs and symptoms of heart attack (chest pain, shortness of breath, trouble breathing) or stroke (weakness in one part or side of the body, slurred speech).

• Drug can cause fluid retention; monitor patient with HTN, edema, or HF.

• Assess patient for CV risk factors before therapy.

• Drug may be hepatotoxic; watch for signs and symptoms of liver toxicity.

• Before starting drug therapy, rehydrate dehydrated patient.

• Monitor patient's renal function; renal insufficiency is possible in patients with preexisting renal disease. Long-term administration may cause renal papillary necrosis and other renal injury.

• *Look alike–sound alike:* Don't confuse Celebrex with Cerebyx or Celexa.

PATIENT TEACHING

• Tell patient to report history of allergic reactions to sulfonamides, aspirin, or other NSAIDs before therapy.

• Instruct patient to promptly report signs of GI bleeding, such as blood in vomit, urine, or stool; or black, tarry stools.

◑ *Alert:* Advise patient to immediately report rash, unexplained weight gain, or swelling.

◑ *Alert:* Advise patient to seek medical attention immediately if chest pain, shortness of breath or trouble breathing, weakness in one part or side of the body, or slurred speech occurs.

• Tell female patient to notify prescriber if she becomes pregnant or is planning to become pregnant during drug therapy.

• Instruct patient to take drug with food if stomach upset occurs.

• Tell patient who has trouble swallowing capsule whole that contents of capsule may be taken with applesauce.

• Tell patient that drug may harm the liver. Advise patient to stop therapy and notify prescriber immediately if experiencing signs and symptoms of hepatotoxicity, including nausea, fatigue, lethargy, itching, yellowing of skin or eyes, right upper quadrant tenderness, and flulike syndrome.

• Inform patient that it may take several days before consistent pain relief occurs.

• Advise patient that using OTC NSAIDs with celecoxib may increase the risk of GI toxicity.

cephalexin
sef-a-LEX-in

Apo-Cephalex✦, Keflex🖉

Therapeutic class: Antibiotics
Pharmacologic class: First-generation cephalosporins

AVAILABLE FORMS
Capsules: 250 mg, 500 mg, 750 mg
Oral suspension: 125 mg/5 mL, 250 mg/ 5 mL
Tablets: 250 mg, 500 mg

INDICATIONS & DOSAGES

Adjust-a-dose (for all indications): For adults and children with CrCl of 30 to 59 mL/minute, no dosage adjustment is needed but maximum daily dose shouldn't exceed 1 g; for CrCl of 15 to 29 mL/minute, reduce dose to 250 mg every 8 or 12 hours; for CrCl of 5 to 14 mL/minute in patients not yet on dialysis, reduce dose to 250 mg every 24 hours; and for CrCl of 1 to 4 mL/minute in patients not yet on dialysis, reduce dose to 250 mg every 48 or 60 hours.

➤ **Respiratory tract infections caused by susceptible isolates of *Streptococcus pneumoniae* and *Streptococcus pyogenes*; GU tract infections caused by susceptible isolates of *Escherichia coli, Proteus mirabilis,* and *Klebsiella pneumoniae*; skin and skin-structure infections caused by susceptible isolates of *Staphylococcus aureus* or *S. pyogenes*; bone infections caused by susceptible isolates of *S. aureus* and *P. mirabilis*; and otitis media caused by susceptible isolates of *S. pneumoniae, Haemophilus influenzae, S. aureus, S. pyogenes,* and *Moraxella catarrhalis***

Adults and children age 15 and older: 250 mg to 1 g PO every 6 hours or 500 mg every 12 hours for 7 to 14 days. Maximum, 4 g daily.

Children older than age 1: 25 to 50 mg/kg/day PO in two to four equally divided doses for 7 to 14 days. For otitis media, 75 to 100 mg/kg PO in equally divided doses every 6 hours. For severe infections, 50 to 100 mg/kg PO in equally divided doses. Don't exceed recommended adult dosage.

ADMINISTRATION
PO

• Before giving, ensure patient isn't allergic to penicillins or cephalosporins.
• Obtain specimen for culture and sensitivity tests before giving. Begin therapy while awaiting results.
• To prepare oral suspension, add required amount of water to powder in two portions. Shake well after each addition. After mixing, store in refrigerator. Mixture will remain stable for 14 days. Keep tightly closed and shake well before using.

• May give without regard to meals but give drug with food or milk to lessen GI discomfort.

ACTION

Inhibits cell-wall synthesis, promoting osmotic instability; usually bactericidal.

Route	Onset	Peak	Duration
PO	Unknown	1 hr	Unknown

Half-life: Adults, 30 minutes to 1¼ hours; children ages 3 to 12 months, 2½ hours; neonates, 5 hours.

ADVERSE REACTIONS

CNS: dizziness, headache, fatigue, agitation, confusion, hallucinations. **GI:** anorexia, diarrhea, *pseudomembranous colitis,* gastritis, glossitis, dyspepsia, abdominal pain, anal pruritus, tenesmus, oral candidiasis. **GU:** genital pruritus, candidiasis, vaginitis, interstitial nephritis. **Hematologic:** *neutropenia, thrombocytopenia,* eosinophilia, anemia. **Musculoskeletal:** arthritis, arthralgia, joint pain. **Skin:** maculopapular and erythematous rashes, urticaria. **Other:** *anaphylaxis,* hypersensitivity reactions, serum sickness.

INTERACTIONS

Drug-drug. *Aminoglycosides:* May increase risk of nephrotoxicity. Avoid using together.
Estrogen-based contraceptives: May decrease contraceptive absorption and effectiveness. Patient should avoid use together or use nonhormonal contraception for duration of antibiotic (or 14 days, whichever is longer) and for 7 days after completion of antibiotic.
Live-virus vaccines: May decrease effectiveness of live-virus vaccines. Concurrent use isn't recommended.
Metformin: May increase metformin level. Monitor blood glucose level closely.
Multivitamins containing zinc: May decrease cephalexin absorption. Consider administering at least 3 hours after cephalexin. Consider therapy modification.
Probenecid: May increase cephalosporin level. Use together isn't recommended.
Warfarin: May enhance anticoagulant effects. Monitor therapy.

Reactions in bold italics are *life-threatening*. Interactions may have a *rapid onset* or a *delayed onset*.

EFFECTS ON LAB TEST RESULTS
• May increase alkaline phosphatase, ALT, AST, bilirubin, and LDH levels. May decrease Hb level and prolong PT.
• May increase eosinophil count. May decrease neutrophil and platelet counts.
• May falsely increase serum or urine creatinine level in tests using Jaffé reaction. May cause false-positive results of Coombs test and urine glucose tests that use cupric sulfate, such as Benedict reagent and Clinitest.

CONTRAINDICATIONS & CAUTIONS
• Contraindicated in patients hypersensitive to cephalosporins.
• Use cautiously in patients hypersensitive to penicillin because of possibility of cross-sensitivity with other beta-lactam antibiotics.
• Severe hypersensitivity reactions can occur. If an allergic reaction occurs, discontinue drug immediately and treat appropriately.
• Drug may increase risk of seizures. Use cautiously in patients with history of seizures.
• Use cautiously in patients with history of colitis and in those with renal insufficiency.
🔉 Alert: Drug can cause superinfection and CDAD and pseudomembranous colitis ranging from mild to life-threatening, which can occur even 2 months after therapy.
Dialyzable drug: Unknown.
⚠ Overdose S&S: Nausea, vomiting, epigastric distress, diarrhea, hematuria.

PREGNANCY-LACTATION-REPRODUCTION
• There are no adequate studies in pregnant women. Use during pregnancy only if clearly needed and potential benefit justifies potential risk to the fetus.
• Drug appears in human milk. Use cautiously in breastfeeding women.

NURSING CONSIDERATIONS
• If large doses are given or if therapy is prolonged, monitor patient for superinfection and diarrhea, especially if patient is high risk.
• Treat group A beta-hemolytic streptococcal infections for a minimum of 10 days.
• If anemia develops during or after cephalexin therapy, obtain a diagnostic work-up for drug-induced hemolytic anemia, discontinue drug, and institute appropriate therapy.
• *Look alike–sound alike:* Don't confuse Keflex with Keppra. Don't confuse drug with other cephalosporins that sound alike.

PATIENT TEACHING
• Tell patient to take drug exactly as prescribed, even if feeling better.
• Instruct patient to take drug with food or milk to lessen GI discomfort.
• Tell patient taking suspension form to shake container well before measuring dose and to store in refrigerator.
• Tell patient to report all adverse reactions and to immediately report rash and signs and symptoms of superinfection or diarrhea.

certolizumab pegol
SERT-oh-LIZ-u-mahb PEGH-ol

Cimzia

Therapeutic class: Immunomodulators
Pharmacologic class: TNF blockers

AVAILABLE FORMS
Lyophilized powder for injection: 200 mg
Prefilled syringe: 200 mg/mL

INDICATIONS & DOSAGES
➤ **Crohn disease when response to conventional therapy is inadequate**
Adults: Initially and at weeks 2 and 4, 400 mg subcut (given as two injections of 200 mg each), followed by a maintenance dose of 400 mg every 4 weeks, if adequate response.
➤ **RA**
Adults: Initially and at weeks 2 and 4, 400 mg subcut (given as two injections of 200 mg each), followed by maintenance dose of 200 mg every other week or 400 mg every 4 weeks.
➤ **Psoriatic arthritis; active ankylosing spondylitis**
Adults: 400 mg subcut (given as two injections of 200 mg each) initially; repeat dose at week 2 and then again at week 4. Maintenance dosage is 200 mg every other week, or 400 mg every 4 weeks.

➤ **Moderate-to-severe plaque psoriasis in patients who are candidates for systemic therapy or phototherapy**
Adults: 400 mg (given as 2 subcut injections of 200 mg each) every other week.
Adults weighing 90 kg or less: Consider initial dose of 400 mg (given as 2 subcut injections of 200 mg each) at weeks 0, 2 and 4, then 200 mg every other week.
✳ *NEW INDICATION:* **Non-radiographic axial spondyloarthritis (nr-axSpA), with objective signs of inflammation**
Adults: 400 mg subcut (given as two 200-mg injections) initially and at weeks 2 and 4. Maintenance dosage is 200 mg every other week, or 400 mg every 4 weeks.

ADMINISTRATION
Subcutaneous
● Bring drug to room temperature for 30 minutes before reconstituting.
● Each 400-mg dose requires two vials. Reconstitute each vial with 1 mL of sterile water for injection, using provided 20G needle. Gently swirl the vial without shaking. May take up to 30 minutes to fully reconstitute. Inspect vial for particulate matter and discoloration, and discard if present.
● Draw up each vial in its own syringe, switching each 20G needle to a 23G needle. Inject prepared or prefilled syringes into separate sites in the abdomen or thigh. Don't inject in areas where skin is tender, bruised, red, or hard. Discard unused portion of vial or syringe.
● Reconstituted drug is stable for 2 hours at room temperature or for up to 24 hours if refrigerated. Don't freeze.
● May store prefilled syringes at room temperature for up to 7 days; write date removed from refrigerator and discard if not used within 7 days. Store in original carton (to protect from light) and don't return to refrigerator.
● The needle shield inside removable cap of prefilled syringe contains natural rubber latex, which may cause an allergic reaction in latex-sensitive individuals.
● Give at room temperature.

ACTION
Selectively neutralizes TNFα, a proinflammatory cytokine responsible for stimulating the production of inflammatory mediators.

Route	Onset	Peak	Duration
Subcut	Unknown	54–171 hr	Unknown

Half-life: 14 days.

ADVERSE REACTIONS
CNS: anxiety, bipolar disorder, *suicide attempt,* fever, headache. **CV:** angina pectoris, *arrhythmias, HF,* HTN, *MI,* pericardial effusion and pericarditis, vasculitis, *stroke,* thrombophlebitis, hemorrhage. **EENT:** optic neuritis, retinal hemorrhage, uveitis, nasopharyngitis. **GI:** abdominal pain. **GU:** UTI, nephrotic syndrome. **Hematologic:** anemia, *leukopenia,* lymphadenopathy, *pancytopenia,* thrombophilia. **Hepatic:** elevated liver enzymes, *hepatitis.* **Musculoskeletal:** arthralgia, extremity pain. **Respiratory:** URI, TB, cough, bronchitis. **Skin:** alopecia, dermatitis, peripheral edema, erythema nodosum, urticaria, injection-site pain and erythema.

INTERACTIONS
Drug-drug. *Abatacept, anakinra, canakinumab, natalizumab, rilonacept, rituximab:* May increase risk of serious infection and neutropenia. Avoid using together.
Live-virus vaccines: May cause infection. Avoid using together.
Pimecrolimus, tacrolimus (topical), tofacitinib, tocilizumab, vedolizumab: May enhance adverse or toxic effects of immunosuppressants. Avoid using together.
Drug-herb. *Echinacea:* May diminish therapeutic effects. Consider therapy modification.

EFFECTS ON LAB TEST RESULTS
● May falsely prolong PTT.

CONTRAINDICATIONS & CAUTIONS
● Contraindicated in patients with a history of hypersensitivity reaction to drug or its components, including angioedema, anaphylactoid reaction, serum sickness, and urticaria.
● Use cautiously in patients with known hypersensitivity to other TNF blockers and those with underlying conditions that may increase the risk of infections.

Reactions in bold italics are *life-threatening.* Interactions may have a *rapid onset* or a *delayed onset.*

C

• Use cautiously in patients with underlying hematologic disorders because significant hematologic abnormalities have occurred.

• Don't use in combination with biological DMARDs or other TNF-blocker therapy.

Black Box Warning Patients treated with certolizumab are at increased risk for serious infections that may lead to hospitalization or death. Most patients who developed these infections were taking concomitant immunosuppressants, such as methotrexate or corticosteroids. ■

Black Box Warning Prophylactic antifungal therapy should be considered for patients at risk for invasive fungal infections who develop severe systemic illness. ■

• Use cautiously in patients with a history of recurrent infections or concomitant immunosuppressive therapy and in those who have resided in regions where TB and histoplasmosis are endemic. Don't begin drug in patients with active infections.

• Use cautiously in patients with a history of CNS demyelinating disorder, hematologic disorders, or HF.

• Rare reactivation of HBV infection can occur, usually in chronic carriers who are also receiving immunosuppressants. Evaluate patient for HBV infection before initiating treatment. Monitor HBV carriers for clinical signs and symptoms of active infection and altered laboratory values during and for several months after therapy ends.

Black Box Warning Certolizumab isn't indicated for use in children or adolescents because of the risk of lymphoma and other malignancies reported with the use of TNF blockers. ■

• Use cautiously in elderly patients because of increased risk of infection.

Dialyzable drug: Unknown.

PREGNANCY-LACTATION-REPRODUCTION

• Use during pregnancy only when clearly needed and benefits outweigh risks to the fetus. Enroll women exposed to certolizumab pegol during pregnancy in the Autoimmune Diseases in Pregnancy Study by contacting 1-877-311-8972.

• It isn't known if drug appears in human milk. For use during breastfeeding, prescriber should take into account importance of drug to the mother and potential adverse effects on the infant.

NURSING CONSIDERATIONS

Black Box Warning Carefully consider risks and benefits of treatment before initiating therapy in patients with chronic or recurrent infection. ■

Black Box Warning Monitor patient for signs and symptoms of invasive fungal infection and other opportunistic infections during and after treatment. Discontinue treatment if serious infection or sepsis develops. Fatal infections have occurred. ■

Black Box Warning Invasive fungal infections, including histoplasmosis, coccidioidomycosis, candidiasis, aspergillosis, blastomycosis, and pneumocystosis, may present with disseminated, rather than localized disease. Antigen and antibody testing for histoplasmosis may be negative in some patients with active infection. Consider empirical antifungal therapy in patients at risk for invasive fungal infections who develop severe systemic illness. ■

Black Box Warning Bacterial, viral, and other infections due to opportunistic pathogens, including *Legionella* and *Listeria*, have occurred. ■

Black Box Warning Test patient for latent TB before and during therapy; active TB, including reactivation of latent TB, has occurred. Initiate treatment for latent infection before starting therapy. ■

Black Box Warning Closely monitor patient for signs and symptoms of infection during and after treatment, including the possible development of TB in patients who tested negative for latent TB before starting therapy. ■

• Before therapy, evaluate patients at risk for HBV infection and test for previous HBV infection.

• Monitor patient for rash. Postmarketing reports indicate severe skin reactions have occurred.

PATIENT TEACHING

Black Box Warning Teach patient to seek prompt medical attention if persistent fever, cough, shortness of breath, or fatigue develops. ■

- Advise patient to seek immediate medical attention for signs and symptoms of infection or for unusual bruising or bleeding.
- Instruct patient to seek immediate medical attention if any symptoms of severe allergic reaction develop.
- Tell patient to report signs and symptoms of HF.

SAFETY ALERT!

cetuximab 🔏
seh-TUX-eh-mab

Erbitux

Therapeutic class: Antineoplastics
Pharmacologic class: Monoclonal antibodies

AVAILABLE FORMS
Injection: 2 mg/mL

INDICATIONS & DOSAGES
Adjust-a-dose (for all indications): If patient develops a grade 1 or 2 CTCAE infusion reaction, permanently reduce infusion rate by 50%. If patient develops a grade 3 or 4 CTCAE infusion reaction, stop drug immediately and permanently. Refer to manufacturer's instructions for dosage modifications for other toxicities.
➤ **Squamous cell carcinoma of the head and neck**
Adults: A loading dose of 400 mg/m^2 IV infusion followed by weekly maintenance dose of 250 mg/m^2 IV infusion. If used with radiation therapy, begin drug 1 week before radiation course or on day of initiation of platinum-based therapy with 5-FU. Complete administration 1 hour before radiation or platinum-based therapy with 5-FU. Continue for the duration (6 or 7 weeks) of radiation therapy or until disease progression or unacceptable toxicity occurs. If used as monotherapy for recurrent or metastatic disease after failure of platinum-based therapy, continue until disease progresses or unacceptable toxicity occurs.
➤ *KRAS* **mutation-negative (wild type), epidermal growth factor receptor (EGFR)–expressing, metastatic colorectal cancer as determined by FDA-approved tests in combination with FOLFIRI**
(irinotecan, 5-FU, leucovorin) **chemotherapy regimen for first-line treatment, or in combination with irinotecan in patients refractory to irinotecan-based chemotherapy, or as a single agent in patients who have failed oxaliplatin- and irinotecan-based chemotherapy or who are intolerant to irinotecan** 🔏
Adults: Loading dose of 400 mg/m^2 IV infusion. Complete drug administration 1 hour before initiating FOLFIRI regimen. Maintenance dosage is 250 mg/m^2 IV infusion weekly until disease progression or unacceptable toxicity occurs.

ADMINISTRATION
IV

▼ Drug is a potential teratogen. Follow safe handling procedures when preparing or administering.
▼ Premedicate with an H$_1$-antagonist such as diphenhydramine 50 mg IV 30 to 60 minutes before first dose. Premedication before subsequent doses should be based on clinical judgment and severity of prior infusion reactions.
▼ Solution should be clear and colorless and may contain a small amount of particulates.
▼ Don't shake or dilute.
▼ Drug can be given by infusion pump or syringe pump, piggybacked into patient's infusion line. Don't give drug by IV push or bolus.
▼ Give initial loading dose over 120 minutes and subsequent infusions over 60 minutes. Don't exceed infusion rate of 10 mg/minute.
▼ Give drug through a low–protein-binding 0.22-micron in-line filter.
▼ Flush line with NSS at the end of the infusion.
▼ Observe patient for 1 hour after administration.
▼ Store vials at 36° to 46° F (2° to 8° C). Don't freeze.
▼ Solution in infusion container is stable up to 12 hours at 36° to 46° F (2° to 8° C) and up to 8 hours at 68° to 77° F (20° to 25° C).
▼ **Incompatibilities:** Don't dilute with other solutions.

Reactions in bold italics are *life-threatening*. Interactions may have a *rapid onset* or a *delayed onset*.

ACTION
An EGFR antagonist that binds to the EGFR on normal and tumor cells.

Route	Onset	Peak	Duration
IV	Unknown	Unknown	Unknown

Half-life: 4.6 days.

ADVERSE REACTIONS
CNS: asthenia, depression, fever, headache, insomnia, pain, peripheral neuropathy. **CV:** edema, *cardiopulmonary arrest, PE.* **EENT:** conjunctivitis. **GI:** abdominal pain, anorexia, constipation, diarrhea, dyspepsia, dysphagia, mucositis, nausea, stomatitis, vomiting, xerostomia. **GU:** *acute renal failure.* **Hematologic:** anemia, *neutropenia, leukopenia.* **Metabolic:** dehydration, *hypomagnesemia,* weight loss. **Musculoskeletal:** back pain. **Respiratory:** cough, dyspnea. **Skin:** alopecia, maculopapular rash, pruritus, radiation dermatitis, acneiform rash, nail changes, hand-foot syndrome. **Other:** antibody development, chills, infection, infusion reaction, *sepsis.*

INTERACTIONS
Drug-lifestyle. *Sun exposure:* May worsen skin reactions. Advise patient to avoid excessive sun exposure.

EFFECTS ON LAB TEST RESULTS
• May increase LFT values.
• May decrease magnesium, calcium, and potassium levels.

CONTRAINDICATIONS & CAUTIONS
• Use cautiously in patients hypersensitive to drug, its components, or murine proteins. If used with radiation, use cautiously in patients with a history of CAD, arrhythmias, and HF.
• Risk of anaphylactic reactions may be increased in patients with a history of tick bites or red meat allergy, or in the presence of IgE antibodies directed against galactose-α-1,3-galactose (alpha-gal).
▒ Determine *RAS* mutation and EGFR-negative expression status using FDA-approved tests before initiating treatment for colorectal cancer. Drug isn't indicated for treatment of *RAS*-mutant colorectal cancer or when results of *RAS* mutation tests are

unknown; increased tumor progression, increased mortality, or lack of benefit may occur in patients with *RAS*-mutant metastatic colorectal cancer.
• Acneiform rash has been reported in up to 88% of patients. Rash usually develops in first 2 weeks of therapy and may require dosage modification and treatment with topical or oral antibiotics.
• Life-threatening and fatal bullous mucocutaneous disease with blisters, erosions, and skin sloughing has been observed in patients treated with cetuximab. It couldn't be determined if these mucocutaneous adverse reactions were directly related to EGFR inhibition or to idiosyncratic immune-related effects (such as SJS or toxic epidermal necrolysis).
Dialyzable drug: No.

PREGNANCY-LACTATION-REPRODUCTION
• There are no adequate studies in pregnant women. Drug may cause fetal harm and isn't recommended for use during pregnancy. Inform pregnant women of potential risk to a fetus.
• Women of childbearing potential should use effective contraception during treatment and for 2 months after final dose.
• Women shouldn't breastfeed during therapy and for at least 2 months after final dose.

NURSING CONSIDERATIONS
Black Box Warning Severe and fatal infusion reactions, including acute airway obstruction, urticaria, and hypotension, may occur, usually with the first infusion. If a severe infusion reaction occurs, stop drug immediately and permanently and provide symptomatic treatment. ▪
• Keep epinephrine, corticosteroids, IV antihistamines, bronchodilators, and oxygen available for severe infusion reactions.
• Manage mild to moderate infusion reactions by decreasing infusion rate and premedicating with an antihistamine for subsequent infusions.
• Monitor patient for infusion reactions for 1 hour after infusion ends.
• Verify pregnancy status in women of childbearing potential before starting drug.

• Assess patient for acute onset or worsening of pulmonary symptoms. If ILD is confirmed, stop drug.
• Monitor patient for skin toxicity, which starts most often during first 2 weeks of therapy. Treat with topical and oral antibiotics.
• Periodically monitor serum electrolyte levels during and for at least 8 weeks after therapy ends.
Black Box Warning In patients also receiving radiation therapy or platinum-based therapy with 5-FU, closely monitor electrolytes, especially magnesium, potassium, and calcium, during and after therapy. Cardiopulmonary arrest or sudden death has occurred. ∎

PATIENT TEACHING

• Tell patient to promptly report adverse reactions, including dyspnea, chills, and fever.
• Inform patient that skin reactions may occur, typically during the first 2 weeks of treatment.
• Advise patient to avoid prolonged or unprotected sun exposure during and 2 months after treatment.
• Instruct female patient not to breastfeed during therapy and for at least 2 months after final dose.
• Advise female patient of childbearing potential to use adequate contraception during therapy and for 2 months after final dose.

chloroquine phosphate ◪
KLO-ro-kwin

Therapeutic class: Antimalarials
Pharmacologic class: Aminoquinolines

AVAILABLE FORMS
Tablets: 250 mg (equivalent to 150 mg base), 500 mg (equivalent to 300 mg base)

INDICATIONS & DOSAGES
❸ *Alert:* Prescribers should be completely familiar with this drug before prescribing.
➤ **Acute malarial attacks caused by *Plasmodium vivax, Plasmodium malariae, Plasmodium ovale*, and susceptible strains of *Plasmodium falciparum***
Adults: Initially, 1 g (600 mg base) PO; then 500 mg (300 mg base) at 6, 24, and 48 hours.

Adults of low body weight and children: Initially, 16.6 mg/kg (10 mg/kg base) PO; then 8.3 mg/kg (5 mg/kg base) at 6, 24, and 48 hours. Don't exceed adult dose of 1,000 mg (600 mg base) for initial dosage and 500 mg (300 mg base) for subsequent doses.
Adjust-a-dose: For adults and children, for treatment of chloroquine-sensitive *P. vivax* and *P. malariae*, concomitant therapy with an 8-aminoquinoline is necessary.
➤ **To prevent malaria**
Adults: 500 mg (300 mg base) PO once weekly on the same day each week, for 1 to 2 weeks before entering a malaria-endemic area and continued for 8 weeks after leaving the area. If treatment begins after exposure, give 1 g (600 mg base) PO initially, in two divided doses 6 hours apart, followed by the usual dosing regimen.
Adults of low body weight and children: Initially, 8.3 mg/kg (5 mg/kg base) PO once weekly on the same day each week, for 1 to 2 weeks before entering a malaria-endemic area and continued for 8 weeks after leaving the area. Don't exceed 500 mg (300 mg base). If treatment begins after exposure, give 16.6 mg/kg (10 mg/kg base) PO initially, in two divided doses 6 hours apart, followed by the usual dosing regimen.
➤ **Extraintestinal amebiasis**
Adults: 1 g (600 mg base) PO once daily for 2 days; then 500 mg (300 mg base) daily for 2 to 3 weeks. Treatment is usually combined with an intestinal amebicide.

ADMINISTRATION
PO
❸ *Alert:* Drug dosage may be discussed in "mg" or "mg base"; be aware of the difference.
• To improve compliance when drug is used for prevention, advise patient to take drug immediately before or after a meal on the same day each week.
• An oral suspension can be prepared by pharmacist if patient can't swallow pills.

ACTION
May bind to and alter the properties of DNA in susceptible parasites.

Route	Onset	Peak	Duration
PO	Unknown	1–2 hr	Unknown

Half-life: 3 to 5 days.

ADVERSE REACTIONS

CNS: *seizures,* agitation, anxiety, confusion, mild and transient headache, psychic stimulation, neuropathy, acute extrapyramidal reactions, hallucinations. **CV:** hypotension, ECG changes, *cardiomyopathy.* **EENT:** blurred vision, difficulty in focusing, reversible corneal changes; typically irreversible, sometimes progressive or delayed retinal changes (such as narrowing of arterioles, macular lesions, pallor of optic disk, optic atrophy, and patchy retinal pigmentation, typically leading to blindness); ototoxicity, nerve deafness, vertigo, tinnitus. **GI:** anorexia, abdominal cramps, diarrhea, nausea, vomiting. **Hematologic:** *agranulocytosis, aplastic anemia, thrombocytopenia.* **Hepatic:** *hepatitis.* **Musculoskeletal:** myopathy or neuromyopathy leading to progressive weakness and atrophy of proximal muscle groups. **Skin:** pruritus, lichen planus eruptions, skin and mucosal pigmentary changes, pleomorphic skin eruptions, *erythema multiforme, SJS, toxic epidermal necrolysis,* exfoliative dermatitis, urticaria, DRESS syndrome (drug rash with eosinophilia and systemic symptoms), hair loss and bleaching of hair pigment. **Other:** *anaphylaxis, angioedema.*

INTERACTIONS

Drug-drug. *Aluminum salts (kaolin), antacids, magnesium:* May decrease GI absorption. Separate dose times by 4 hours.
Ampicillin: May significantly reduce bioavailability of ampicillin. Separate dose times by 2 hours.
Cimetidine: May decrease hepatic metabolism of chloroquine. Monitor patient for toxicity.
Cyclosporine: May cause a sudden increase in serum cyclosporine level. Monitor patient closely. If necessary, discontinue chloroquine.
Drugs that prolong QT interval: May have additive effects on QT interval and increase risk of life-threatening arrhythmias. Avoid concurrent use if possible.

Mefloquine: May increase seizure risk. Avoid concurrent use, and delay administration of mefloquine until at least 12 hours after the last dose of chloroquine when possible.
Drug-lifestyle. *Sun exposure:* May cause drug-induced dermatoses. Advise patient to avoid sun exposure.

EFFECTS ON LAB TEST RESULTS

• May increase liver enzyme levels.
• May decrease Hb level and granulocyte and platelet counts.

CONTRAINDICATIONS & CAUTIONS

• Contraindicated in patients hypersensitive to drug and in those with retinal or visual field changes or porphyria.
🧬 Use cautiously in patients with severe GI, neurologic, or blood disorders; hepatic disease or alcoholism; or G6PD deficiency or psoriasis.
• Don't use to treat *P. falciparum* acquired in an area of known chloroquine resistance or when chloroquine prophylaxis has failed. Use other antimalarials if patient has a resistant strain of plasmodia.
• Risk of toxic reactions may be greater in elderly patients and in those with impaired renal function because drug is substantially excreted by the kidneys. Monitor renal function closely.
Dialyzable drug: Unknown.
⚠ **Overdose S&S:** Headache, drowsiness, visual disturbances, nausea, vomiting, CV collapse, seizures, sudden and early respiratory and cardiac arrest; atrial standstill, nodal rhythm, prolonged intraventricular conduction time, progressive bradycardia leading to ventricular fibrillation or arrest.

PREGNANCY-LACTATION-REPRODUCTION

• Safety and effectiveness of chloroquine in pregnant women aren't known. Avoid use during pregnancy except in the suppression or treatment of malaria when benefit outweighs potential risk to the fetus.
• Serious adverse reactions may occur in breastfed infants. Patient should discontinue breastfeeding or discontinue drug, taking into account importance of drug to the mother.

NURSING CONSIDERATIONS
• Ensure that baseline and periodic ophthalmic examinations are performed. Check periodically for ocular muscle weakness after long-term use. Risk factors for development of retinopathy during treatment include advanced age, subnormal glomerular filtration, concurrent use of tamoxifen citrate or concurrent macular disease, duration of treatment, and high daily or accumulated dosage.
• Make sure patient is tested with an audiometer before, during, and after therapy, especially if therapy is long-term.
• Monitor CBC and LFTs periodically during long-term therapy. If a severe blood disorder—not caused by the disease—develops, drug may need to be stopped.
• For malaria prevention, the manufacturer's instructions state that patient take drug for 8 weeks after leaving a malaria-endemic area; the CDC recommends that patient take drug for 4 weeks after leaving the area.
⊙ **Alert:** Monitor patient for overdose, which can quickly lead to toxic symptoms. Children are extremely susceptible to toxicity; avoid long-term treatment.

PATIENT TEACHING
• To improve compliance when using drug for prevention, advise patient to take drug immediately before or after a meal on the same day each week.
• Instruct patient to avoid excessive sun exposure to prevent worsening of drug-induced dermatoses.
• Tell patient to report adverse reactions promptly, especially blurred vision, increased sensitivity to light, tinnitus, hearing loss, or muscle weakness.
• Instruct patient to keep drug out of reach of children. Overdose may be fatal.

cholestyramine
koe-LESS-tir-a-meen

Prevalite

Therapeutic class: Antilipemics
Pharmacologic class: Bile acid sequestrants

AVAILABLE FORMS
Powder: 210-g, 231-g, 378-g cans; 9-g single-dose packets; each scoop of powder or single-dose packet contains 4 g of cholestyramine resin

INDICATIONS & DOSAGES
➤ **Primary hyperlipidemia or pruritus caused by partial bile obstruction, adjunct for reduction of increased cholesterol level in patients with primary hypercholesterolemia**
Adults: 4 g PO once daily or b.i.d. Maintenance dose is 8 to 16 g daily divided into two doses. Maximum daily dose is 24 g.
Children: 240 mg/kg/day PO in two to three divided doses, not to exceed 8 g/day.

ADMINISTRATION
PO
• Mix thoroughly with 60 to 180 mL of water, other noncarbonated beverage, highly fluid soup, or pulpy fruit with high moisture content, such as applesauce or crushed pineapple.
• Give drug with a meal.
• Give other drugs 1 hour before or at least 4 hours after cholestyramine to avoid impeding their absorption.

ACTION
Binds bile acids in the intestinal tract, impeding their absorption and causing their elimination in feces. In response to this bile acid depletion, LDL cholesterol levels decrease as the liver uses LDL cholesterol to replenish reduced bile acid stores.

Route	Onset	Peak	Duration
PO	Unknown	Unknown	2–4 wk

Half-life: Unknown.

Reactions in bold italics are *life-threatening*. Interactions may have a *rapid onset* or a *delayed onset*.

ADVERSE REACTIONS

CNS: dizziness, headache, vertigo, anxiety, fatigue, insomnia, syncope, tinnitus. **GI:** abdominal discomfort, constipation, fecal impaction, nausea, anorexia, diarrhea, flatulence, *GI bleeding,* hemorrhoids, steatorrhea, vomiting. **GU:** dysuria, hematuria. **Hematologic:** anemia, bleeding tendencies, ecchymoses. **Metabolic:** hyperchloremic acidosis. **Musculoskeletal:** backache, muscle and joint pains, osteoporosis. **Skin:** rash; irritation of skin, tongue, and perianal area. **Other:** vitamin A, D, E, and K deficiencies from decreased absorption.

INTERACTIONS

Drug-drug. *Acetaminophen, beta blockers, cardiac glycosides, corticosteroids, estrogens, ezetimibe, fat-soluble vitamins (A, D, E, and K), iron preparations, niacin, penicillin G, phenobarbital, progestins, tetracycline, thiazide diuretics, thyroid hormones, warfarin and other coumarin derivatives:* May decrease absorption of these drugs. Give other drugs 1 to 2 hours before or 4 to 6 hours after cholestyramine.
Amiodarone: May decrease bioavailability of amiodarone. Consider therapy modification.
Mycophenolate: May decrease mycophenolate serum concentration. Avoid concurrent use.

EFFECTS ON LAB TEST RESULTS

• May increase alkaline phosphatase and triglyceride levels. May decrease Hb level and hematocrit.
• May prolong PT.
• May cause abnormal results in cholecystography that uses iopanoic acid because iopanoic acid is also bound by cholestyramine.

CONTRAINDICATIONS & CAUTIONS

• Contraindicated in patients hypersensitive to bile-acid sequestering resins and in those with complete biliary obstruction.
• Use cautiously in patients predisposed to constipation and in those with conditions aggravated by constipation, such as severe, symptomatic CAD.
Dialyzable drug: Unknown.
⚠ *Overdose S&S:* GI tract obstruction.

PREGNANCY-LACTATION-REPRODUCTION

• There are no adequate well-controlled studies in pregnant women. Drug may interfere with absorption of fat-soluble vitamins, causing fetal harm. Weigh potential benefit against potential risk to the fetus.
• Use cautiously in breastfeeding women. The possible lack of proper vitamin absorption may have an effect on breastfed infants.

NURSING CONSIDERATIONS

• Monitor cholesterol and triglyceride levels regularly during therapy.
• Monitor levels of cardiac glycosides in patients receiving cardiac glycosides and cholestyramine together. If cholestyramine therapy is stopped, adjust dosage of cardiac glycosides, if necessary, to avoid toxicity.
• Monitor bowel habits. Encourage a diet high in fiber and fluids. If severe constipation develops, decrease dosage, add a stool softener, or stop drug.
• Watch for hyperchloremic acidosis with long-term use or very high doses.
• Long-term use may lead to deficiencies of vitamins A, D, E, and K and folic acid.

PATIENT TEACHING

⚠ *Alert:* Tell patient never to take drug in its dry form because it may irritate the esophagus or cause severe constipation.
• Tell patient to prepare drug in a large glass containing water, milk, or juice (especially pulpy fruit juice) and to sprinkle powder on the surface of the beverage, let the mixture stand for a few minutes, and then stir thoroughly. Discourage mixing with carbonated beverages because of excessive foaming. After drinking preparation, patient should swirl a small additional amount of liquid in the same glass and then drink again to make sure entire dose has been taken.
• Tell patient to avoid sipping or holding the suspension in the mouth because drug may damage tooth surfaces. Advise patient to maintain good oral hygiene.
• Advise patient to take at mealtime, if possible.
• Advise patient to take all other drugs at least 1 to 2 hours before or 4 to 6 hours after cholestyramine to avoid blocking their absorption.

• Teach patient about proper dietary management of fats. When appropriate, recommend weight control, exercise, and smoking cessation programs.
• Tell patient that drug may deplete body stores of vitamins A, D, E, and K and folic acid. Patient should discuss need for supplements with prescriber.
• Inform patient with phenylketonuria that light form of drug contains 28.1 mg of phenylalanine per 6.4-g dose.

---

ciclesonide (inhalation, intranasal)
si-CLEH-son-ide

Alvesco, Omnaris, Zetonna

Therapeutic class: Corticosteroids
Pharmacologic class: Corticosteroids

AVAILABLE FORMS
Nasal aerosol solution: 37 mcg/metered spray
Nasal suspension: 50 mcg/metered spray
Oral inhalation aerosol: 80 mcg, 160 mcg

INDICATIONS & DOSAGES
➤ **Preventative during asthma maintenance (Alvesco)**
Adults and children age 12 and older who were previously taking bronchodilators alone: Initially, inhaled dose of 80 mcg b.i.d.; increase to maximum of 160 mcg b.i.d. after 4 weeks if not controlled.
Adults and children age 12 and older who were previously taking inhaled corticosteroids: Initially, 80 mcg b.i.d.; increase to maximum of 320 mcg b.i.d. after 4 weeks if not controlled.
Adults and children age 12 and older who were previously taking oral corticosteroids: 320 mcg b.i.d.
➤ **Signs and symptoms of perennial allergic rhinitis**
Adults and children age 12 and older: 2 sprays of Omnaris in each nostril once daily (200 mcg/day). Or, 1 actuation of Zetonna per nostril once daily.
➤ **Signs and symptoms of seasonal allergic rhinitis**
Adults and children age 12 and older: 1 actuation of Zetonna per nostril once daily.

Adults and children age 6 and older: 2 sprays of Omnaris in each nostril once daily (200 mcg/day).

ADMINISTRATION
Inhalational
• Patient should rinse mouth after inhalation.
Intranasal
• Before first use of Omnaris, gently shake container, then prime by spraying eight times. If not used for 4 consecutive days, gently shake and reprime with 1 spray or until a fine mist appears.
• Before first use of Zetonna, prime by actuating three times. If not used for 10 consecutive days, prime by actuating three times. If the product is dropped, the canister and actuator may become separated; if this happens, instruct patient to reassemble product and test spray once into the air before using.

ACTION
May decrease inflammation by inhibiting macrophages, eosinophils, and mediators such as leukotrienes involved in the asthmatic response.

Route	Onset	Peak	Duration
Inhalation	>4 wk	1 hr	Unknown
Intranasal	1–2 days	1–5 wk	Unknown

Half-life: Inhalation drug, less than 1 hour; inhalation drug's active metabolite, 6 to 7 hours; intranasal drug, unknown.

ADVERSE REACTIONS
CNS: headache, back pain. **EENT:** ear pain, nasopharyngitis, sinusitis, pharyngolaryngeal pain, nasal congestion or discomfort, epistaxis, URI. **Metabolic:** growth retardation. **Musculoskeletal:** arthralgia, pain in the extremities or back.

INTERACTIONS
Drug-drug. *Ceritinib:* May enhance hyperglycemic effect of ceritinib. Monitor blood glucose level.
Desmopressin: May enhance hyponatremic effect of desmopressin. Avoid concurrent use.
Ketoconazole, other inhibitors of CYP450: May increase ciclesonide level and adverse

---

effects. Use together cautiously; adjust ciclesonide dosage as needed.

EFFECTS ON LAB TEST RESULTS
None reported.

CONTRAINDICATIONS & CAUTIONS
• Contraindicated as primary treatment of status asthmaticus or other acute asthmatic episodes, and in patients hypersensitive to drug or its components.
• Intranasal form is contraindicated in patients who have had recent nasal septal ulcers, nasal surgery, or nasal trauma until healing has occurred.
• Use cautiously in patients who have changed from systemic to inhaled corticosteroids because renal insufficiency, steroid withdrawal (pain, lassitude, depression), or acute worsening of symptoms may occur.
• Use cautiously in immunosuppressed patients and in those with wounds; corticosteroids suppress the immune system.
• Use cautiously in children; may cause a decline in growth rate.
• Use cautiously, if at all, in patients with active or quiescent respiratory TB infection; untreated systemic fungal, bacterial, viral, or parasitic infections; or ocular HSV infection.
Dialyzable drug: Unknown.
⚠ *Overdose S&S:* Hyperadrenocorticism.

PREGNANCY-LACTATION-REPRODUCTION
• There are no adequate well-controlled studies in pregnant women. Use during pregnancy only if potential benefit justifies potential risk to the fetus.
• If a woman takes a corticosteroid during pregnancy, monitor neonate for hypoadrenalism.
• It isn't known if drug appears in human milk. Use cautiously in breastfeeding women.

NURSING CONSIDERATIONS
🔔 *Alert:* Don't use for acute bronchospasm or acute asthma.
• Assess patient for bone loss during long-term use.
• Watch for evidence of localized mouth infections, glaucoma, cataracts, and immunosuppression.

• Monitor infants born to mothers using drug during pregnancy for hypoadrenalism.
• Monitor patients who are switched from systemic to inhaled corticosteroids for worsening of signs and symptoms and other adverse effects of withdrawal.
• Monitor children for decline in growth rate; the potential to regain growth after drug is stopped hasn't been studied.
• Monitor patients for nasal adverse effects.
• For patients who don't respond adequately to starting dose after 4 weeks of therapy, higher doses may provide additional asthma control.
• After asthma stability has been achieved, titrate to lowest effective dosage to minimize systemic effects.

PATIENT TEACHING
• Teach patient how to use drug properly. Refer patient to manufacturer's instructions.
• Tell patient to discard Omnaris bottle after 120 actuations following initial priming or 4 months after removal from foil pouch, whichever occurs first.
• Tell patient to replace Zetonna nasal aerosol when indicator shows zero.
• Inform patient that drug isn't indicated for the relief of acute bronchospasm.
• Instruct patient to rinse mouth with water and spit out after inhalation.
• Advise patient to use drug at regular intervals or about the same time every day, as directed.
• Instruct patient using intranasal form to contact prescriber if there is no relief from symptoms after 1 week.
• Warn patient to avoid exposure to chickenpox, measles, or other infections and, if exposed, to consult prescriber immediately.
• Inform patient that asthma-related therapeutic results may take several weeks and to contact prescriber if symptoms don't improve after 4 weeks of treatment or if condition worsens.
• Advise parents of child receiving long-term therapy that child should have periodic growth measurements.

cidofovir
sye-DOE-fo-veer

Therapeutic class: Antivirals
Pharmacologic class: Nucleosides–nucleotides

AVAILABLE FORMS
Injection: 75 mg/mL in 5-mL vial

INDICATIONS & DOSAGES
Black Box Warning Cidofovir is indicated only for the treatment of CMV retinitis in patients with AIDS. █
➤ **CMV retinitis in patients with AIDS**
Adults: Initially, 5 mg/kg IV infused over 1 hour once weekly for 2 consecutive weeks; then maintenance dose of 5 mg/kg IV infused over 1 hour once every 2 weeks. Give probenecid and prehydration with IV NSS simultaneously to reduce risk of nephrotoxicity.
Adjust-a-dose: For patients with creatinine level of 0.3 to 0.4 mg/dL above baseline, reduce dosage to 3 mg/kg at same rate and frequency. If creatinine level reaches 0.5 mg/dL or more above baseline, or patient develops 3+ or higher proteinuria, stop drug.

Don't start drug if serum creatinine level is more than 1.5 mg/dL, CrCl is 55 mL/minute or less, or urine protein level is 100 mg/dL or more (at least 2+ proteinuria).

ADMINISTRATION
IV
▼ Drug has mutagenic effects; prepare it in a class II laminar flow biological safety cabinet and wear surgical gloves and a closed-front surgical gown with knit cuffs.
▼ If drug contacts skin, wash and flush thoroughly with water.
▼ Place excess drug and all materials used to prepare and give it in a leak-proof, puncture-proof container.
▼ Let drug reach room temperature before use.
▼ Using a syringe, withdraw prescribed dose and add to an IV bag containing 100 mL of NSS.
▼ Infuse over 1 hour using an infusion pump.

▼ Because of the risk of nephrotoxicity, don't exceed recommended dosages or frequency or rate of infusion.
▼ Discard any partially used vials.
▼ Give within 24 hours of preparing. Admixture may be refrigerated at 36° to 46° F (2° to 8° C) for up to 24 hours.
Black Box Warning Because of increased risk of nephrotoxicity, give 1 L NSS IV over 1 to 2 hours, immediately before giving drug. Also give probenecid with each cidofovir infusion. █
◑ *Alert:* If tolerated, a second liter of NSS may be administered over a 1- to 3-hour period at the start of or immediately after cidofovir infusion.
▼ Compatibility of admixture with Ringer, lactated Ringer, and bacteriostatic solutions hasn't been evaluated.
▼ **Incompatibilities:** Other drugs or supplements.

ACTION
Suppresses CMV replication by selective inhibition of viral DNA synthesis.

Route	Onset	Peak	Duration
IV	Unknown	Unknown	Unknown

Half-life: Unknown.

ADVERSE REACTIONS
CNS: asthenia, fever, headache, *seizures,* abnormal gait, amnesia, anxiety, confusion, depression, dizziness, hallucinations, insomnia, neuropathy, paresthesia, somnolence, malaise. **CV:** hypotension, orthostatic hypotension, pallor, syncope, tachycardia, vasodilation. **EENT:** ocular hypotony, abnormal vision, amblyopia, conjunctivitis, eye disorders, iritis, pharyngitis, retinal detachment, rhinitis, sinusitis, uveitis. **GI:** abdominal pain, anorexia, diarrhea, nausea, vomiting, aphthous stomatitis, colitis, constipation, dry mouth, dyspepsia, dysphagia, flatulence, gastritis, melena, mouth ulcers, oral candidiasis, rectal disorders, stomatitis, taste perversion, tongue discoloration. **GU:** proteinuria, *nephrotoxicity,* glycosuria, hematuria, urinary incontinence, UTI. **Hematologic:** anemia, *neutropenia, thrombocytopenia.* **Hepatic:** hepatomegaly. **Metabolic:** fluid imbalance, hyperglycemia, hyperlipidemia, hypocalcemia,

---

hypokalemia, weight loss. **Musculoskele-tal:** arthralgia, myalgia, myasthenia; pain in back, chest, or neck. **Respiratory:** dyspnea, asthma, bronchitis, coughing, hiccups, increased sputum, lung disorders, pneumonia. **Skin:** alopecia, rash, acne, dry skin, pruritus, skin discoloration, sweating, urticaria. **Other:** chills, infections, *sarcoma, sepsis,* allergic reactions, facial edema, HSV infection.

INTERACTIONS

Drug-drug. Black Box Warning *Nephrotoxic drugs (such as aminoglycosides, amphotericin B, foscarnet, IV pentamidine):* May increase nephrotoxicity. Don't use together. ▪

Tenofovir: May increase serum concentrations of both tenofovir and cidofovir. Monitor therapy.

Zidovudine: Stop zidovudine or reduce dosage by 50% on the days cidofovir is given; probenecid reduces metabolic clearance of zidovudine.

EFFECTS ON LAB TEST RESULTS

• May increase alkaline phosphatase, ALT, AST, BUN, creatinine, glucose, cholesterol, LDH, and urine protein levels.
• May decrease bicarbonate, calcium, potassium, and Hb levels.
• May decrease neutrophil and platelet counts.

CONTRAINDICATIONS & CAUTIONS

• Contraindicated in patients hypersensitive to drug, probenecid, and other sulfa drugs.
• Contraindicated in patients with creatinine level more than 1.5 mg/dL, CrCl of 55 mL/minute or less, or urine protein level of 100 mg/dL or more (equivalent to 2+ proteinuria or more).

Black Box Warning Renal failure has occurred with as few as one or two doses of cidofovir. Monitor renal function within 48 hours before each dose and modify dosage as needed. Contraindicated in patients receiving other drugs with nephrotoxic potential (stop such drugs at least 7 days before starting cidofovir therapy). ▪

• Use within 1 month of placement of a ganciclovir ocular implant may cause profound hypotony.

• Direct intraocular injection is contraindicated and is associated with iritis, ocular hypotony, and permanent vision impairment.
• Use cautiously in patients with renal impairment. Monitor renal function tests and patient's fluid balance.
• Safety and effectiveness in children haven't been established.

Dialyzable drug: 75% (high-flux hemodialysis only).

PREGNANCY-LACTATION-REPRODUCTION

• There are no adequate studies in pregnant women. Use during pregnancy only if potential benefit justifies potential risk to the fetus.

Black Box Warning In animal studies, cidofovir was carcinogenic and teratogenic and caused hypospermia. ▪

• Advise women of childbearing potential to use effective contraception during and for 1 month after treatment with cidofovir. Advise men to use barrier contraception methods during and for 3 months after treatment with cidofovir.
• It isn't known if drug appears in human milk. Because of potential for adverse reactions and potential for tumorigenicity as shown in animal studies, drug shouldn't be used in breastfeeding women. The CDC advises that HIV-infected women not breastfeed, to avoid postnatal transmission of HIV to an infant who may not yet be infected.

NURSING CONSIDERATIONS

Black Box Warning Due to increased risk of nephrotoxicity and bone marrow suppression, monitor creatinine and urine protein levels and WBC counts with differential before each dose. ▪

Black Box Warning Neutropenia has been observed in association with treatment. Monitor neutrophil count during therapy. ▪

• Drug may cause Fanconi syndrome and decreased bicarbonate level with renal tubular damage. Monitor patient closely.
• Drug may cause granulocytopenia.

Black Box Warning Give drug with adequate hydration and give probenecid with each cidofovir infusion. ▪

PATIENT TEACHING
• Inform patient that drug doesn't cure CMV retinitis and that regular ophthalmologic examinations are needed.
• Alert patient taking zidovudine to obtain dosage guidelines on days cidofovir is given.
• Tell patient that close monitoring of kidney function will be needed and that abnormalities may require a change in therapy.
• Stress importance of completing a full course of probenecid with each cidofovir dose. Tell patient to take probenecid after a meal to decrease nausea.
• Advise female patient of the limited enrollment of women in clinical trials and that cidofovir injection should be considered a potential carcinogen.
• Advise female patient of childbearing potential to use effective contraception, especially during treatment and for 1 month after final dose.
• Advise male patient to use barrier contraception during and for 3 months after treatment.

cilostazol
sill-AHS-tah-zoll

Therapeutic class: Antiplatelet drugs
Pharmacologic class: cAMP phosphodiesterase inhibitors

AVAILABLE FORMS
Tablets: 50 mg, 100 mg

INDICATIONS & DOSAGES
➤ **To reduce symptoms of intermittent claudication**
Adults: 100 mg PO b.i.d.
Adjust-a-dose: Decrease dose to 50 mg PO b.i.d. when giving with drugs that may interact to cause an increase in cilostazol level (such as fluconazole, omeprazole, ticlopidine, diltiazem, erythromycin, itraconazole, ketoconazole).

ADMINISTRATION
PO
• Give drug at least 30 minutes before or 2 hours after breakfast and dinner.
• Don't give with grapefruit juice.

ACTION
Thought to inhibit the enzyme phosphodiesterase III, thus inhibiting platelet aggregation and causing vasodilation.

Route	Onset	Peak	Duration
PO	Unknown	Unknown	Unknown

Half-life: 11 to 13 hours.

ADVERSE REACTIONS
CNS: dizziness, headache, vertigo. **CV:** palpitations, peripheral edema, tachycardia. **EENT:** pharyngitis, rhinitis. **GI:** abnormal stools, diarrhea, abdominal pain, dyspepsia, flatulence, nausea. **Hematologic:** bleeding. **Musculoskeletal:** back pain, myalgia. **Respiratory:** increased cough. **Other:** infection.

INTERACTIONS
Drug-drug. *Anticoagulants, antiplatelet agents:* May increase bleeding risk. Use together cautiously.
Fluconazole, omeprazole, ticlopidine: May increase cilostazol level. Reduce cilostazol dosage to 50 mg b.i.d.
Erythromycin, other macrolides, strong or moderate CYP3A4 inhibitors (diltiazem, itraconazole, ketoconazole): May increase level of cilostazol and its metabolites. Reduce cilostazol dosage to 50 mg b.i.d.
Drug-herb. *Herbs with anticoagulant properties (anise, bilberry):* May prolong bleeding time. Discourage use together.
Drug-lifestyle. *Smoking:* May decrease drug exposure. Discourage smoking.

EFFECTS ON LAB TEST RESULTS
• May reduce triglyceride levels. May increase HDL level.

CONTRAINDICATIONS & CAUTIONS
• Contraindicated in patients hypersensitive to drug or its components.
Black Box Warning Contraindicated in patients with HF of any severity. ▮
• Contraindicated in patients with hemostatic disorders or active bleeding, such as bleeding peptic ulcer and intracranial bleeding.
• Use cautiously in patients with severe underlying heart disease; also use cautiously with other drugs having antiplatelet activity.

Reactions in bold italics are *life-threatening*. Interactions may have a *rapid onset* or a ***delayed onset***.

• Use cautiously in patients with severe renal impairment (CrCl <25 mL/minute) and in those with moderate to severe hepatic impairment.
• Left ventricular outflow tract obstruction has been reported in patients with sigmoid-shaped interventricular septum.
Dialyzable drug: No.
⚠ **Overdose S&S:** Severe headache, diarrhea, hypotension, tachycardia, cardiac arrhythmias.

PREGNANCY-LACTATION-REPRODUCTION
• There are no adequate studies in pregnant women. Therefore, assessment of risk to the fetus isn't possible.
• Drug may appear in human milk. Patient should discontinue breastfeeding or discontinue drug, taking into account importance of drug to the mother.

NURSING CONSIDERATIONS
• Beneficial effects may not be seen for up to 12 weeks after therapy starts.
• Monitor patients for development of a new systolic murmur or cardiac signs or symptoms after drug initiation.
Black Box Warning Cilostazol and similar drugs that inhibit the enzyme phosphodiesterase decrease the likelihood of survival in patients with class III and IV HF. ∎
🔆 **Alert:** CV risk is unknown in patients who use drug on long-term basis and in those with severe underlying heart disease.
• Dosage can be reduced or stopped without such rebound effects as platelet hyperaggregation.
• If aspirin is added to drug therapy, monitor patient for aspirin-related adverse reactions.

PATIENT TEACHING
• Instruct patient to take drug on an empty stomach, at least 30 minutes before or 2 hours after breakfast and dinner.
• Tell patient that beneficial effect of drug on cramping pain isn't likely to be noticed for 2 to 4 weeks and that it may take as long as 12 weeks.
• Advise patient to avoid drinking grapefruit juice during drug therapy.
• Inform patient that CV risk is unknown in patients who use drug on a long-term basis

and in those with severe underlying heart disease.
• Tell patient that drug may cause dizziness. Caution patient not to drive or perform other activities that require alertness until response to drug is known.

cimetidine
sye-MET-i-deen

Tagamet HB ◇

cimetidine hydrochloride

Therapeutic class: Antiulcer drugs
Pharmacologic class: H_2-receptor antagonists

AVAILABLE FORMS
Oral liquid: 300 mg/5 mL*
Tablets: 200 mg ◇, 300 mg, 400 mg, 800 mg

INDICATIONS & DOSAGES
Adjust-a-dose (for all indications): In patients with renal impairment, decrease dosage to 300 mg PO every 12 hours, increasing frequency to every 8 hours with caution. A renally impaired patient who also has liver dysfunction may require even further dosage reduction. Schedule dose at the end of hemodialysis.
➤ **Short-term treatment of duodenal ulcer; maintenance therapy**
Adults and children age 16 and older: 800 mg PO at bedtime. Or, 400 mg PO b.i.d. or 300 mg PO q.i.d. (with meals and at bedtime). Or, 200 mg PO t.i.d. with a 400-mg bedtime dose. Treatment lasts 4 to 6 weeks unless endoscopy shows healing.
    Alternatively, higher doses of 1,600 mg at bedtime for 4 weeks may be beneficial for patients with larger duodenal ulcers (larger than 1 cm defined endoscopically) who are also heavy smokers (1 pack/day or more) when it's important to ensure healing within 4 weeks for this subpopulation.
    For maintenance therapy, 400 mg at bedtime.
➤ **Active benign gastric ulceration**
Adults: 800 mg PO at bedtime or 300 mg PO q.i.d. (with meals and at bedtime) for up to 8 weeks.

➤ **Pathologic hypersecretory conditions, such as Zollinger-Ellison syndrome, systemic mastocytosis, and multiple endocrine adenomas**
Adults and children age 16 and older:
300 mg PO q.i.d. with meals and at bedtime, adjusted to patient needs. Maximum oral amount, 2,400 mg daily.

➤ **GERD with erosive esophagitis**
Adults: 800 mg PO b.i.d. or 400 mg PO q.i.d. before meals and at bedtime for up to 12 weeks.

➤ **Heartburn**
Adults and children age 12 and older:
200 mg Tagamet HB PO with water as symptoms occur, or as directed, up to b.i.d. For prevention, 200 mg PO right before or up to 30 minutes before eating food or drinking beverages that cause heartburn. Maximum, 400 mg daily. Drug shouldn't be taken daily for longer than 2 weeks.

ADMINISTRATION
PO
• Give dose at end of hemodialysis.

ACTION
Competitively inhibits action of histamine on the H_2 receptor sites of parietal cells, decreasing gastric acid secretion.

Route	Onset	Peak	Duration
PO	1 hr	45–90 min	4–5 hr

Half-life: 2 hours.

ADVERSE REACTIONS
CNS: confusion, dizziness, hallucinations, headache, peripheral neuropathy, somnolence. **GI:** mild and transient diarrhea. **GU:** erectile dysfunction. **Musculoskeletal:** arthralgia, muscle pain. **Other:** mild gynecomastia if used longer than 1 month, hypersensitivity reactions.

INTERACTIONS
Drug-drug. *Amiodarone:* May increase amiodarone level. Avoid combination if possible. Monitor for increased amiodarone concentrations and effects. Consider therapy modification.
Antacids: May interfere with cimetidine absorption. Separate doses by at least 1 hour, if possible.

Atazanavir: May decrease atazanavir serum concentration. Refer to atazanavir prescribing information for management.
Carbamazepine: May transiently increase carbamazepine level. Monitor therapy.
Carmustine: May enhance the bone marrow suppressant effects of carmustine. Avoid use together.
Digoxin, fluconazole, indomethacin, iron salts, ketoconazole, tetracycline: May decrease drug absorption. Separate doses by at least 2 hours.
Escitalopram: May increase escitalopram-related toxicity. Consider alternative therapy.
Fosphenytoin, phenytoin, some benzodiazepines, theophylline: May inhibit hepatic microsomal enzyme metabolism of these drugs. Monitor drug level.
IV lidocaine: May decrease clearance of lidocaine, increasing the risk of toxicity. Consider using a different H_2 antagonist, if possible. Monitor lidocaine level closely.
Metoprolol, propranolol, timolol: May increase the effects of beta blocker. Consider another H_2 antagonist or decrease the dose of beta blocker.
Procainamide: May increase procainamide level. Avoid this combination, if possible. Monitor procainamide level closely and adjust the dose as necessary.
Warfarin-type anticoagulants: May increase blood levels of these drugs. Closely monitor PT and adjust anticoagulant dosage if necessary.
Drug-lifestyle. *Alcohol use:* May increase blood alcohol level. Discourage use together.
Smoking: May decrease drug's ability to inhibit nocturnal gastric secretion. Urge patient to quit smoking.

EFFECTS ON LAB TEST RESULTS
• May increase ALT, AST, and creatinine levels.
• May antagonize pentagastrin's effect during gastric acid secretion tests. May cause false-negative results in skin tests using allergen extracts. May impair interpretation of Hemoccult and Gastroccult test results on gastric content aspirate because of FD&C blue dye #2 used in tablets.

CONTRAINDICATIONS & CAUTIONS
• Contraindicated in patients hypersensitive to drug.
• Use cautiously in elderly or debilitated patients because they may be more susceptible to drug-induced confusion.
• Use cautiously in patients with renal or hepatic impairment.
• Prolonged treatment (2 years or more) increases risk of vitamin B_{12} malabsorption and deficiency, especially in women and patients younger than age 30.
• Drug may increase risk of acute gastroenteritis and community-acquired pneumonia in children.
Dialyzable drug: Yes.
⚠ *Overdose S&S:* Mental deterioration, unresponsiveness, death.

PREGNANCY-LACTATION-REPRODUCTION
• There are no adequate studies in pregnant women. Use during pregnancy only if clearly needed and potential benefit justifies potential risk to the fetus.
• Drug appears in human milk. As a general rule, women shouldn't breastfeed while taking drug.

NURSING CONSIDERATIONS
• Assess patient for abdominal pain. Note blood in emesis, stool, or gastric aspirate.
• Identify tablet strength when obtaining a drug history.
• Schedule dose at end of hemodialysis treatment because hemodialysis reduces drug levels.
• Wait at least 15 minutes after giving tablet before drawing sample for Hemoccult or Gastroccult test, and follow test manufacturer's instructions closely.
• Treatment of gastric ulcer isn't as effective as treatment of duodenal ulcer.
• *Look alike–sound alike:* Don't confuse cimetidine with simethicone.

PATIENT TEACHING
• Remind patient taking drug once daily to take it at bedtime and to take multiple daily doses with meals.
• Instruct patient taking Tagamet HB not to exceed recommended dosage and not to take daily for longer than 14 days.

• Urge patient to avoid cigarette smoking because it may increase gastric acid secretion and worsen disease.
• Advise patient to report all adverse reactions, including abdominal pain, blood in stools or emesis, black tarry stools, and coffee-ground emesis.
• Tell patient to check with prescriber or pharmacist before taking other drugs.

cinacalcet hydrochloride
sin-ah-KAL-set

Sensipar

Therapeutic class: Hyperparathyroidism drugs
Pharmacologic class: Calcimimetics

AVAILABLE FORMS
Tablets ⬤: 30 mg, 60 mg, 90 mg

INDICATIONS & DOSAGES
Adjust-a-dose (for all indications): Patients with moderate to severe hepatic impairment (Child-Pugh class B or C) may experience increased exposure to cinacalcet and increased half-life. Dosage adjustments may be necessary based on serum calcium, serum phosphorus, or intact parathyroid hormone (iPTH) level.
➤ **Primary hyperparathyroidism**
Adults: Initially, 30 mg PO b.i.d. Titrate every 2 to 4 weeks through sequential doses of 30 mg, 60 mg, and 90 mg PO b.i.d., and 90 mg PO t.i.d. or q.i.d. to normalize calcium levels.
➤ **Secondary hyperparathyroidism in patients with chronic kidney disease undergoing dialysis**
Adults: Initially, 30 mg PO once daily; adjust no more than every 2 to 4 weeks through sequential doses of 60 mg, 90 mg, 120 mg, and 180 mg PO once daily to reach target range of 150 to 300 picograms (pg)/mL for iPTH level.
➤ **Hypercalcemia in patients with parathyroid carcinoma**
Adults: Initially, 30 mg PO b.i.d.; adjust every 2 to 4 weeks through sequential doses of 30 mg, 60 mg, and 90 mg PO b.i.d., and 90 mg PO t.i.d. or q.i.d. daily if needed to normalize calcium level.

ADMINISTRATION
PO
• Don't break or crush tablets; give them whole, with food or shortly after a meal.

ACTION
Increases sensitivity of calcium-sensing receptor to extracellular calcium, letting calcium be absorbed despite decreased PTH.

Route	Onset	Peak	Duration
PO	Unknown	2–6 hr	Unknown

Half-life: Terminal half-life, 30 to 40 hours.

ADVERSE REACTIONS
CNS: dizziness, asthenia, *seizures,* depression, fatigue, headache, paresthesia. **CV:** chest pain, hypotension, HTN. **GI:** diarrhea, nausea, vomiting, anorexia, constipation, abdominal pain. **Hematologic:** anemia. **Metabolic:** hypocalcemia, dehydration, hypercalcemia, hypoparathyroidism. **Musculoskeletal:** myalgia, arthralgia, fracture, limb pain. **Respiratory:** URI, cough, dyspnea. **Other:** hypersensitivity reaction, dialysis access infection.

INTERACTIONS
Drug-drug. *Amitriptyline:* Amitriptyline and nortriptyline exposure increases by 20% in patients who are CYP2D6 extensive metabolizers. Avoid using together, if possible.
Drugs metabolized mainly by CYP2D6 with a narrow therapeutic index (flecainide, thioridazine, most TCAs, vinblastine): May strongly inhibit CYP2D6, decreasing metabolism and increasing levels of these drugs. Adjust dosage of other drugs, as needed.
Drugs that strongly inhibit CYP3A4 (erythromycin, itraconazole, ketoconazole): May increase cinacalcet level. Use together cautiously, monitoring PTH and calcium level closely and adjusting cinacalcet dosage, as needed.
Etelcalcetide: May enhance hypocalcemic effect of etelcalcetide. Avoid concurrent use.

EFFECTS ON LAB TEST RESULTS
• May decrease calcium, phosphorus, and testosterone levels.

CONTRAINDICATIONS & CAUTIONS
• Contraindicated in patients hypersensitive to drug or its components and in patients with calcium level less than 8.4 mg/dL.
• Use cautiously in patients with history of seizures and in those with moderate to severe hepatic impairment.
• If iPTH level is less than 150 pg/mL, reduce dosage of cinacalcet or vitamin D sterols or discontinue therapy.
• Isolated, idiosyncratic cases of hypotension, worsening HF, or arrhythmia have been reported in patients with impaired cardiac function.
Dialyzable drug: No.
⚠ *Overdose S&S:* Hypocalcemia.

PREGNANCY-LACTATION-REPRODUCTION
• There are no adequate studies in pregnant women. Use during pregnancy only if potential benefit justifies potential risk to the fetus.
• It isn't known if drug appears in human milk. Patient should discontinue breastfeeding or discontinue drug, taking into account importance of drug to the mother.

NURSING CONSIDERATIONS
❸ *Alert:* Monitor calcium level closely. Hypocalcemia can prolong QT interval, potentially resulting in ventricular arrhythmia, and lower the seizure threshold.
• Monitor patients for worsening of common GI adverse reactions (nausea and vomiting) and for signs and symptoms of GI bleeding and ulcerations. Patients with risk factors for upper GI bleeding (known gastritis, esophagitis, ulcers, severe vomiting) may be at increased risk. Promptly evaluate and treat suspected GI bleeding.
• Patients with moderate to severe hepatic impairment may need dosage adjustment based on PTH and calcium levels. Monitor these patients closely.
• Give drug alone or with vitamin D sterols, phosphate binders, or both.
• Measure calcium level within 1 week after starting therapy or adjusting dosage. After maintenance dose is established, measure calcium level monthly for patients with chronic kidney disease receiving dialysis and every 2 months for those with parathyroid carcinoma.

Reactions in bold italics are *life-threatening*. Interactions may have a *rapid onset* or a *delayed onset*.

• Watch carefully for evidence of hypocalcemia: paresthesia, myalgias, cramping, tetany, and seizures.
• For patients with secondary hyperparathyroidism: If calcium level is 7.5 to 8.4 mg/dL or patient develops symptoms of hypocalcemia, give calcium-containing phosphate binders, vitamin D sterols, or both, to raise calcium level. If calcium level is below 7.5 mg/dL or hypocalcemia symptoms persist and the vitamin D dose can't be increased, withhold drug until calcium level reaches 8.0 mg/dL, hypocalcemia symptoms resolve, or both. Resume therapy with the next lowest dose.
• Measure iPTH level 1 to 4 weeks after therapy starts or dosage changes. After the maintenance dose is established, monitor PTH level every 1 to 3 months. Levels in patients with chronic kidney disease receiving dialysis should be 150 to 300 pg/mL.
• Adynamic bone disease may develop if iPTH levels are suppressed below 100 pg/mL. If this occurs, notify prescriber.
❸ Alert: Don't use drug in patients with chronic kidney disease who aren't receiving dialysis because they have an increased risk of hypocalcemia.

PATIENT TEACHING
• Tell patient not to divide tablets but to take them whole, with food or shortly after a meal.
• Advise patient to report to prescriber adverse reactions and signs of hypocalcemia, which include paresthesia, muscle weakness, muscle cramping, and muscle spasm.
• Advise patient to immediately report signs or symptoms of GI bleeding, such as black or tarry stool, bright red blood in vomit, dark or bright red blood mixed with stool, and abdominal cramps.

---

ciprofloxacin
si-proe-FLOX-a-sin

Cipro✿

Therapeutic class: Antibiotics
Pharmacologic class: Fluoroquinolones

AVAILABLE FORMS
Infusion (premixed): 200 mg in 100 mL D₅W, 400 mg in 200 mL D₅W

Injection: 200 mg, 400 mg
Suspension (oral): 250 mg/5 mL (5%), 500 mg/5 mL (10%)
Tablets (extended-release, film-coated) 🚫: 500 mg, 1,000 mg
Tablets (film-coated): 100 mg, 250 mg, 500 mg, 750 mg

INDICATIONS & DOSAGES
Black Box Warning Use in patients with sinusitis, bronchitis, and uncomplicated UTI isn't recommended because of risk of serious adverse effects. Use in these patients only when there are no other treatment options. ■
Adjust-a-dose (for all indications): For patients with a CrCl of 30 to 50 mL/minute, give 250 to 500 mg PO every 12 hours or the usual IV dose; if CrCl is 5 to 29 mL/minute, give 250 to 500 mg PO every 18 hours or 200 to 400 mg IV every 18 to 24 hours. If patient is receiving hemodialysis or peritoneal dialysis, give 250 to 500 mg PO every 24 hours after dialysis.
➤ **Complicated intra-abdominal infection**
Adults: 500 mg PO or 400 mg IV every 12 hours for 7 to 14 days. Give with metronidazole.
➤ **Severe or complicated bone or joint infection, severe respiratory tract infection, severe skin or skin-structure infection**
Adults: 750 mg PO every 12 hours or 400 mg IV every 8 hours.
➤ **Severe or complicated UTI; mild to moderate bone or joint infection; mild to moderate respiratory infection; mild to moderate skin or skin-structure infection; infectious diarrhea; typhoid fever**
Adults: 500 mg PO or 400 mg IV every 12 hours. Or, 1,000 mg extended-release tablets PO every 24 hours.
➤ **Complicated UTI or pyelonephritis**
Adults: 500 mg PO every 12 hours for 7 to 14 days. Or 1,000 mg extended-release tablets PO every 24 hours for 7 to 14 days.
Children ages 1 to 17: 6 to 10 mg/kg IV every 8 hours for 10 to 21 days. Maximum IV dose, 400 mg. Or, 10 to 20 mg/kg PO every 12 hours. Maximum PO dose, 750 mg. Don't exceed maximum dose, even in patients who weigh more than 51 kg.
Adjust-a-dose: If CrCl is less than 30 mL/minute, reduce dosage of extended-release

---

form from 1,000 to 500 mg daily. Give 500 mg extended-release form after hemodialysis or peritoneal dialysis is completed.

➤ **Nosocomial pneumonia**
Adults: 400 mg IV every 8 hours for 10 to 14 days.

➤ **Mild to moderate UTI**
Adults: 250 mg PO or 200 mg IV every 12 hours for 7 to 14 days.

➤ **Uncomplicated UTI**
Adults: 500 mg extended-release tablet PO once daily for 3 days, or 250 mg PO every 12 hours for 3 days.

➤ **Chronic bacterial prostatitis**
Adults: 500 mg PO every 12 hours or 400 mg IV every 12 hours for 28 days.

➤ **Lower respiratory tract infections**
Adults: 500 to 750 mg PO every 12 hours or 400 mg IV every 8 to 12 hours for 7 to 14 days.

➤ **Mild to moderate acute sinusitis**
Adults: 500 mg PO or 400 mg IV every 12 hours for 10 days.

➤ **Empirical therapy in febrile neutropenic patients**
Adults: 400 mg IV every 8 hours used with piperacillin 50 mg/kg IV every 4 hours (not to exceed 24 g/day of piperacillin) for 7 to 14 days.

➤ **Inhalation anthrax (postexposure)**
Adults: 400 mg IV every 12 hours initially until susceptibility test results are known; then 500 mg PO every 12 hours. Give drug with one or two additional antimicrobials. Switch to oral therapy when appropriate. Treat for 60 days (IV and PO combined).
Children: 10 mg/kg IV every 12 hours; then 15 mg/kg PO every 12 hours. Don't exceed 800 mg/day IV or 1,000 mg/day PO. Give drug with one or two additional antimicrobials. Switch to oral therapy when appropriate. Treat for 60 days (IV and PO combined).

➤ **Plague due to *Yersinia pestis*; plague prophylaxis as soon as possible after suspected or confirmed exposure**
Adults: 400 mg IV every 8 to 12 hours or 500 to 750 mg PO every 12 hours for 14 days.
Children ages 1 to 17: 10 mg/kg IV or 15 mg/kg PO every 8 to 12 hours for 10 to 21 days. Maximum dosage, 500 mg/dose PO and 400 mg/dose IV.

ADMINISTRATION
PO
• Extended- and immediate-release oral forms aren't interchangeable.
• Obtain specimen for culture and sensitivity tests before giving first dose. Begin therapy while awaiting results.
• To avoid decreasing the effects of ciprofloxacin, give at least 2 hours before or 6 hours after certain drugs and vitamins. Food doesn't affect absorption but may delay peak levels.
• Caffeine should be avoided during therapy with this drug because of potential for increased caffeine effects.
• Give drug with plenty of fluids to reduce risk of urine crystals.
• Don't crush or split extended-release tablets.
• Shake oral suspension vigorously each time before use for approximately 15 seconds; don't give through feeding tube.

IV
▼ Obtain specimen for culture and sensitivity tests before giving first dose. Begin therapy while awaiting results.
▼ Dilute drug to 1 to 2 mg/mL using D_5W or NSS for injection.
▼ If giving drug through a Y-type set, stop the other IV solution while infusing.
▼ Infuse over 1 hour into a large vein to minimize discomfort and vein irritation.
▼ **Incompatibilities:** Aminophylline, ampicillin–sulbactam, azithromycin, cefepime, clindamycin phosphate, dexamethasone sodium phosphate, furosemide, heparin sodium, methylprednisolone sodium succinate, phenytoin sodium.

ACTION
Inhibits bacterial DNA synthesis, mainly by blocking DNA gyrase; bactericidal.

Route	Onset	Peak	Duration
PO	Unknown	30–120 min	Unknown
PO (extended-release)	Unknown	1–4 hr	Unknown
IV	Unknown	Immediate	Unknown

Half-life: 4 hours; extended-release, 6 hours in adults with normal renal function.

ADVERSE REACTIONS
CNS: *seizures,* confusion, headache, restlessness. **GI:** *pseudomembranous colitis,*

diarrhea, nausea, vomiting. **GU:** crystal-luria, interstitial nephritis. **Hematologic:** *leukopenia, neutropenia, thrombocytope-nia,* eosinophilia. **Musculoskeletal:** tendon rupture. **Skin:** rash, *SJS, toxic epidermal necrolysis.* **Other:** hypersensitivity reactions.

INTERACTIONS
Drug-drug. *Aluminum hydroxide, aluminum-magnesium hydroxide, calcium carbonate, didanosine (chewable tablets, buffered tablets, or pediatric powder for oral solution), magnesium hydroxide, products containing zinc:* May decrease ciprofloxacin absorption and effects. Give ciprofloxacin 2 hours before or 6 hours after these drugs.
Cyclosporine: May increase risk for cyclosporine toxicity. Monitor cyclosporine level.
Drugs primarily metabolized by CYP1A2 (caffeine, clozapine, methylxanthines, olanzapine, theophylline, tizanidine, ropinirole, zolpidem): May increase plasma concentrations of coadministered drug, leading to clinically significant adverse reactions of coadministered drug. Monitor patient for adverse reactions.
Drugs that prolong QT interval: May additionally increase QT interval and risk of life-threatening cardiac arrhythmias. Use together cautiously.
Iron salts: May decrease absorption of ciprofloxacin, reducing anti-infective response. Give at least 2 hours apart.
NSAIDs: May increase risk of CNS stimulation. Monitor patient closely.
Probenecid: May elevate level of ciprofloxacin. Monitor patient for toxicity.
Black Box Warning *Steroids:* May increase risk of tendinitis and tendon rupture. ∎
Sucralfate: May decrease ciprofloxacin absorption, reducing anti-infective response. If use together can't be avoided, give at least 6 hours apart.
Theophylline: May increase theophylline level and prolong theophylline half-life. Monitor level of theophylline and watch for adverse effects.
Tizanidine: Increases tizanidine levels, causing low BP, somnolence, dizziness, and slowed psychomotor skills. Use together is contraindicated.

Warfarin: May increase anticoagulant effects. Monitor PT and INR closely.
Drug-herb. *Dong quai, St. John's wort:* May cause photosensitivity. Advise patient to avoid excessive sunlight exposure.
Yerba maté: May decrease clearance of herb's methylxanthines and cause toxicity. Discourage use together.
Drug-food. *Caffeine:* May increase effect of caffeine. Monitor patient closely.
Dairy products, other foods: May delay peak drug levels. Advise patient to take drug on an empty stomach.
Orange juice fortified with calcium: May decrease GI absorption of drug, reducing its effects. Discourage use together.
Drug-lifestyle. *Sun exposure:* May cause photosensitivity reactions. Advise patient to avoid excessive sunlight exposure.

EFFECTS ON LAB TEST RESULTS
• May increase alkaline phosphatase, ALT, AST, bilirubin, BUN, creatinine, LDH, and GGT levels.
• May increase eosinophil count. May decrease WBC, neutrophil, and platelet counts.

CONTRAINDICATIONS & CAUTIONS
• Contraindicated in patients sensitive to fluoroquinolones.
⦿ *Alert:* Serious and occasionally fatal hypersensitivity reactions, some after first dose, have been reported. Emergency treatment for anaphylaxis may be necessary. Immediately discontinue drug at first appearance of rash, jaundice, or other signs and symptoms of hypersensitivity.
⦿ *Alert:* Cases of severe hepatotoxicity, including fatal events, have been reported. Acute liver injury can be rapid and is frequently associated with hypersensitivity. If signs and symptoms of hepatitis occur, discontinue drug immediately.
⦿ *Alert:* Patients receiving systemic drug have an increased risk of hyperglycemia and hypoglycemia, which can result in coma. Hypoglycemia has been reported more frequently in the elderly and in those with diabetes.
⦿ *Alert:* Drug may increase risk of aortic dissection or rupture when used systemically. Avoid use in patients with known aortic aneurysm or who are at risk for

aortic aneurysm, including those with peripheral atherosclerotic vascular diseases, HTN, or certain genetic conditions (Marfan syndrome, Ehlers-Danlos syndrome), and elderly patients. Drug should only be used in these patients if no other treatment options are available.

• Use cautiously in patients with CNS disorders, such as severe cerebral arteriosclerosis or seizure disorders, and in those at risk for seizures. Drug may cause CNS stimulation.

Black Box Warning Drug is associated with increased risk of tendinitis and tendon rupture, especially in patients older than age 60 and those with heart, kidney, or lung transplants. ■

Black Box Warning Drug may exacerbate muscle weakness in patients with myasthenia gravis. Avoid use of fluoroquinolones in patients with a known history of myasthenia gravis. ■

◆ *Alert:* Oral or parenteral fluoroquinolones may increase the risk of peripheral neuropathy of the arms or legs. Symptoms can occur anytime during treatment and can last for months to years or be permanent. Stop drug immediately if patient develops symptoms and switch to a nonfluoroquinolone antibacterial drug unless the benefits of continued treatment outweigh the risks.

Black Box Warning Fluoroquinolones have been associated with disabling and potentially irreversible serious adverse reactions that have occurred together, including tendinitis and tendon rupture, peripheral neuropathy, and CNS effects. Drug is associated with increased risk of serious adverse CNS reactions (seizures, toxic psychoses, increased ICP, pseudotumor cerebri, tremors, restlessness, anxiety, light-headedness, confusion, hallucinations, paranoia, depression, nightmares, insomnia, disturbances in attention, disorientation, agitation, memory impairment, delirium and, rarely, suicidal thoughts or acts). If any of these serious adverse reactions occur, discontinue drug immediately. ■

Black Box Warning Reserve drug for use in patients who have no alternative treatment options for acute exacerbation of chronic bronchitis and acute sinusitis. ■

• Drug may cause CDAD ranging in severity from mild diarrhea to fatal colitis and possibly occurring more than 2 months after therapy ends. Drug may need to be discontinued if CDAD develops during therapy.
Dialyzable drug: Less than 10%.

PREGNANCY-LACTATION-REPRODUCTION

• There are no adequate studies in pregnant women. Use during pregnancy only if potential benefit justifies potential risk to the fetus.

• Pregnant women and immunocompromised patients should receive the usual doses and regimens for anthrax postexposure prophylaxis.

• Drug appears in human milk, and the amount absorbed by a breastfeeding infant is unknown. Because of the risk of serious adverse reactions (including articular damage), a decision should be made to discontinue breastfeeding or discontinue drug, taking into account importance of drug to the mother.

NURSING CONSIDERATIONS

• Monitor patient's intake and output, and observe patient for signs of crystalluria.

Black Box Warning Tendon rupture may occur in patients receiving quinolones. If pain or inflammation occurs or if patient ruptures a tendon, stop drug. ■

◆ *Alert:* Monitor patients for signs and symptoms of aortic aneurysm, dissection, and rupture (sudden, severe, and constant pain in the stomach, chest, or back; throbbing in the stomach area, deep pain in the back or the side of the stomach; steady, gnawing pain in the stomach that lasts for hours or days; pain in the jaw, neck, back, or chest; coughing or hoarseness; shortness of breath, trouble swallowing). Discontinue drug immediately if any of these aortic disorders are suspected.

◆ *Alert:* Monitor patient for symptoms of peripheral neuropathy (pain, burning, tingling, numbness, weakness, or a change in sensation to light touch, pain, temperature, or sense of body position), and report them immediately to the practitioner.

◆ *Alert:* Immediately report signs and symptoms of hepatitis (anorexia, jaundice, dark urine, pruritus, abdominal tenderness) and discontinue drug.

- Long-term therapy may result in overgrowth of organisms resistant to drug.
- Cutaneous anthrax patients with signs of systemic involvement, extensive edema, or lesions on the head or neck need IV therapy and a multidrug approach.

❸ Alert: Monitor patients receiving systemic drug for symptoms of hypoglycemia (confusion, pounding or rapid heartbeat, dizziness, pale skin, shakiness, sweating, unusual hunger, trembling, headache, weakness, irritability, unusual anxiety). Immediately discontinue drug for blood glucose disturbances, and switch to a nonfluoroquinolone antibiotic if possible.

Black Box Warning Monitor patients receiving systemic drug for CNS (seizures, increased ICP, pseudotumor cerebri, dizziness, tremors) and psychiatric (disturbances in attention, disorientation, agitation, nervousness, memory impairment, delirium) adverse reactions. Discontinue drug for CNS adverse effects, including psychiatric adverse reactions. ■

- Additional antimicrobials for anthrax multidrug regimens can include rifampin, vancomycin, penicillin, ampicillin, chloramphenicol, imipenem, clindamycin, and clarithromycin.
- Steroids may be used as adjunctive therapy for anthrax patients with severe edema and for meningitis.
- Follow current CDC recommendations for anthrax.

PATIENT TEACHING
- Tell patient to take drug as prescribed, even after feeling better.
- Advise patient to drink plenty of fluids to reduce risk of urine crystals.
- Advise patient not to crush, split, or chew the extended-release tablets.

❸ Alert: Warn patient to seek immediate medical attention for signs or symptoms of aortic aneurysm, dissection, or rupture.

❸ Alert: Warn patient to immediately notify prescriber for signs and symptoms of serious adverse reactions, including unusual joint or tendon pain, muscle weakness, "pins and needles" tingling or pricking sensation, numbness in the arms or legs, confusion or hallucinations.

❸ Alert: Caution patients that significantly low blood sugar levels can occur. Instruct patients how to manage symptoms and to immediately report any occurrence to the prescriber.

❸ Alert: Advise patients with diabetes that they may need to monitor blood glucose levels more frequently during therapy.

❸ Alert: Inform patients to immediately report psychiatric adverse reactions and that these can occur after just one dose.

- Warn patient to avoid hazardous tasks that require alertness, such as driving, until effects of drug are known.
- Instruct patient to avoid caffeine while taking drug because of potential for increased caffeine effects.
- Advise patient that hypersensitivity reactions may occur even after first dose. If a rash or other allergic reaction occurs, tell patient to stop drug immediately and notify prescriber.
- Tell patient that tendon rupture can occur with drug and to notify prescriber if pain or inflammation occurs.
- Tell patient to avoid excessive sunlight or artificial ultraviolet light during therapy.

SAFETY ALERT!

cisatracurium besylate
sis-ah-trah-KYOO-ee-hum

Nimbex

Therapeutic class: Skeletal muscle relaxants
Pharmacologic class: Nondepolarizing neuromuscular blockers

AVAILABLE FORMS
Injection: 2 mg/mL, 10 mg/mL*

INDICATIONS & DOSAGES
➤ **Adjunct to general anesthesia to facilitate ET intubation and relax skeletal muscles during surgery**
Adults: First dose of 0.15 mg/kg IV; then maintenance dosages of 0.03 mg/kg IV every 40 to 50 minutes p.r.n. Or, first dose of 0.2 mg/kg IV; then maintenance dosages of 0.03 mg/kg IV every 50 to 60 minutes p.r.n. Or, as a continuous infusion in operating room, after an initial bolus dose, give a

maintenance infusion at 3 mcg/kg/minute and reduce to 1 to 2 mcg/kg/minute as needed. Initiate infusion only after early evidence of spontaneous recovery from initial bolus dose.

Children ages 2 to 12: 0.1 to 0.15 mg/kg IV over 5 to 10 seconds. After first dose, give a maintenance infusion of 3 mcg/kg/minute, then reduce to 1 to 2 mcg/kg/minute as needed.

Children ages 1 to 23 months: 0.15 mg/kg over 5 to 10 seconds. No information is available for continuous infusion.

Adjust-a-dose: During CABG surgery (adults) with induced hypothermia, reduce infusion rate by 50%. Patients with burns may need increased amount.

➤ **To maintain neuromuscular blockade during mechanical ventilation in ICU**
Adults: Principles for infusion in operating room apply to use in ICU. After first dose, give 3 mcg/kg/minute by IV infusion. Range, 0.5 to 10.2 mcg/kg/minute.

Adjust-a-dose: In patients with neuromuscular disease, such as myasthenia gravis or carcinomatosis, don't exceed 0.02 mg/kg. Patients with burns may need increased amount.

ADMINISTRATION

IV

🔴 *Alert:* Accidental administration of neuromuscular blockers may be fatal. Store drug with the cap and ferrule intact and in a manner that minimizes the possibility of selecting the wrong product.

▼ Drug is colorless to slightly yellow or green-yellow. Inspect vials for particulates and discoloration before use. Don't use unclear solutions or those with visible particulates.

🔴 *Alert:* The 20-mL vial is intended for use only in the ICU.

▼ Use only under direct supervision of medical staff skilled in using neuromuscular blockers and maintaining airway patency. Don't give drug unless resources for intubation, mechanical ventilation, and oxygen therapy are within reach.

▼ Keep refrigerated; don't freeze. After removal from refrigeration to room temperature (77° F [25° C]), use within 21 days, even if rerefrigerated.

▼ Use drug within 24 hours when diluted to a concentration of 0.1 mg/mL in D_5W, NSS, or 5% dextrose and NSS.

▼ **Incompatibilities:** Alkaline solutions with pH higher than 8.5, propofol, ketorolac.

ACTION

Binds to cholinergic receptors on the motor end plate, antagonizing acetylcholine and blocking neuromuscular transmission.

Route	Onset	Peak	Duration
IV	2–3 min	3–5 min	35–45 min

Half-life: 22 to 29 minutes; about 3 hours for laudanosine.

ADVERSE REACTIONS

CV: *bradycardia,* hypotension, flushing. **Respiratory:** *bronchospasm, prolonged apnea.* **Skin:** rash.

INTERACTIONS

Drug-drug. *Aminoglycosides, bacitracin, calcium channel blockers, clindamycin, colistimethate sodium, colistin, lithium, local anesthetics, magnesium salts, polymyxins, procainamide, quinidine, quinine, tetracyclines, vancomycin:* May enhance neuromuscular blocking action of cisatracurium. Use together cautiously.

Carbamazepine, phenytoin: May decrease the effects of cisatracurium. May need to increase cisatracurium dose.

Enflurane or isoflurane given with nitrous oxide or oxygen: May prolong cisatracurium duration of action. Patient may need less frequent maintenance doses, lower maintenance doses, or reduced infusion rate of cisatracurium. Effects are dependent on duration of volatile agent administration.

Succinylcholine: May shorten time to onset of maximal neuromuscular block. Monitor patient.

EFFECTS ON LAB TEST RESULTS

None reported.

CONTRAINDICATIONS & CAUTIONS

● Contraindicated in patients who are hypersensitive to drug, to other bisbenzylisoquinolinium drugs, or to benzyl alcohol (found in 10-mg/mL vial). Don't use

---

10-mL vials with benzyl alcohol in neonates and premature infants.

• Severe hypersensitivity reactions, including fatal and life-threatening anaphylactic reactions, have been reported. Wheezing, laryngospasm, bronchospasm, rash, and itching have been reported in children.

• Patients with renal or hepatic impairment receiving extended administration may be at higher risk for seizures.

Dialyzable drug: Unknown.

⚠ *Overdose S&S:* Prolonged neuromuscular blockade.

PREGNANCY-LACTATION-REPRODUCTION

• There are no adequate studies in pregnant women. Use during pregnancy only if clearly needed and potential benefit justifies potential risk to the fetus.

• It isn't known if drug appears in human milk. Use cautiously in breastfeeding women.

NURSING CONSIDERATIONS

• Drug isn't recommended for rapid-sequence ET intubation because of its intermediate onset.

• Consider extending interval between administering drug and attempting intubation by at least 1 minute to achieve adequate intubation conditions in elderly patients and patients with ESRD.

• Dosage requirements vary widely among patients. Base subsequent dosage on patient's response to initial doses.

• Drug has been associated with residual paralysis. To prevent complications resulting from drug-associated residual paralysis, extubation is recommended only after patient has recovered sufficiently from neuromuscular blockade. Consider using a reversal agent, especially in cases in which residual paralysis is more likely to occur.

• To reduce the risk of respiratory arrest and death, confirm proper selection and dose of intended product and avoid confusion with other injectable solutions present in critical care and other clinical settings.

⚠ *Alert:* Drug has no known effect on consciousness, pain threshold, or cerebration. To avoid patient distress, don't induce neuromuscular block before unconsciousness.

⚠ *Alert:* Never give by IM injection. Administer undiluted as bolus injection over 5 to 10 seconds. Continuous infusion requires use of an infusion pump.

• Monitor neuromuscular function with nerve stimulator during drug administration. If stimulation doesn't elicit a response, stop infusion until response returns.

⚠ *Alert:* Drug should only be given by clinicians experienced in its use. Don't give drug unless personnel and facilities for resuscitation, life-support, and drug antagonist are immediately available.

• To avoid inaccurate dosing, perform neuromuscular monitoring on a nonparetic arm or leg in patients with hemiparesis or paraparesis.

• Monitor acid-base balance and electrolyte levels. Abnormalities may potentiate or antagonize the action of cisatracurium.

• Monitor patient for malignant hyperthermia.

• Give analgesics, if indicated. Patient can feel pain but can't indicate its presence.

⚠ *Alert:* Careful dosage calculation is essential. Always verify dosage with another health care professional.

PATIENT TEACHING

• Explain purpose of drug.

• Assure patient that monitoring will be continuous.

• Explain all procedures and events because patient can still hear.

SAFETY ALERT!

CISplatin (CDDP)
SIS-pla-tin

Therapeutic class: Antineoplastics
Pharmacologic class: Platinum-containing compounds

AVAILABLE FORMS
Injection: 1 mg/mL

INDICATIONS & DOSAGES
Black Box Warning Confirm dosages greater than 100 mg/m^2/cycle with prescriber once every 3 to 4 weeks. Confirm that dose is total dose per cycle, not daily dose. ■

Adjust-a-dose (for all indications): Don't give repeat course of cisplatin until serum creatinine level is below 1.5 mg/dL or BUN level is below 25 mg/dL, platelets are 100,000/mm^3 or higher, WBCs are 4,000/mm^3 or higher, and audiometric analysis indicates that auditory acuity is within normal limits.

➤ **Adjunctive therapy in metastatic testicular cancer**
Adults: 20 mg/m^2 IV daily for 5 days. Repeat every 3 weeks for three cycles.

➤ **Adjunctive therapy in metastatic ovarian cancer**
Adults: 100 mg/m^2 IV; repeat every 4 weeks. Or, 75 to 100 mg/m^2 IV once every 4 weeks with cyclophosphamide.

➤ **Advanced bladder cancer**
Adults: 50 to 70 mg/m^2 IV every 3 to 4 weeks. Give 50 mg/m^2 every 4 weeks in patients who have received other antineoplastics or radiation therapy.

ADMINISTRATION

IV

▼ Preparing and giving parenteral form of drug may be mutagenic, teratogenic, or carcinogenic. Follow facility policy to reduce risks.

▼ Hydrate patient with 1 to 2 liters of NSS for 8 to 12 hours before giving drug and for 24 hours after administration. Maintain urine output of at least 100 mL/hour for 4 consecutive hours before therapy and for 24 hours after therapy.

Black Box Warning Anaphylactic-type reactions may occur within minutes of administration. Have emergency equipment available. ■

❸ *Alert:* Don't use needles or IV sets containing aluminum parts for preparation or administration.

▼ Infusions are most stable in solutions containing chloride (such as NSS or half-NSS and 0.22% sodium chloride). Don't use D$_5$W alone.

▼ Further dilute with dextrose 5% in 0.3% sodium chloride injection or dextrose 5% in half-NSS for injection with 37.5 g mannitol added.

▼ Administer over 6 to 8 hours.

▼ Solutions in vials that have been entered are stable for 7 days at room temperature under fluorescent light; if protected from light, stability is 28 days. Don't refrigerate.

▼ **Incompatibilities:** None listed by manufacturer. Consult a drug incompatibility reference for more information.

ACTION

May cross-link strands of cellular DNA and interfere with RNA transcription, causing an imbalance of growth that leads to cell death. Not specific to cell cycle.

Route	Onset	Peak	Duration
IV	Rapid	Unknown	Several days

Half-life: Initial phase, 14 to 49 minutes; beta, 0.7 to 4.6 hours; gamma, 24 to 127 hours.

ADVERSE REACTIONS

CNS: peripheral neuritis, *seizures.* **EENT:** tinnitus, hearing loss. **GI:** anorexia, diarrhea, loss of taste, nausea, vomiting. **GU:** *prolonged renal toxicity with repeated courses of therapy.* **Hematologic:** *myelosuppression, leukopenia, thrombocytopenia,* anemia. **Metabolic:** *hypomagnesemia, hypokalemia, hypocalcemia.* **Other:** *anaphylactoid reaction.*

INTERACTIONS

Drug-drug. *Aminoglycosides:* May increase nephrotoxicity. Carefully monitor renal function study results.
Aminoglycosides, bumetanide, ethacrynic acid, furosemide, torsemide: May increase ototoxicity. Avoid using together, if possible.
Aspirin, NSAIDs: May increase risk of bleeding. Avoid using together.
Fosphenytoin, phenytoin: May decrease phenytoin and fosphenytoin levels. Monitor levels.
Myelosuppressants: May increase myelosuppression. Monitor patient.

EFFECTS ON LAB TEST RESULTS

● May increase uric acid level. May decrease calcium, Hb, magnesium, phosphate, potassium, and sodium levels.
● May decrease platelet and WBC counts.

CONTRAINDICATIONS & CAUTIONS

Black Box Warning Anaphylaxis-like hypersensitivity reactions requiring emergency treatment have been reported. Facial edema,

---

Reactions in bold italics are *life-threatening*. Interactions may have a *rapid onset* or a *delayed onset*.

bronchoconstriction, tachycardia, and hypotension may occur within minutes of administration. Epinephrine, corticosteroids, and antihistamines have been used effectively to alleviate symptoms. ■

• Contraindicated in patients hypersensitive to drug or other platinum-containing compounds and in those with preexisting renal impairment, hearing impairment, or myelosuppression.

• Use cautiously in patients previously treated with radiation or cytotoxic drugs and in those with peripheral neuropathies; also use cautiously with other ototoxic and nephrotoxic drugs.

• Secondary malignancies have been reported.

• Drug can cause hyperuricemia requiring antihyperuricemia therapy to reduce uric acid levels, especially with dosages higher than 50 mg/m^2.

Dializable drug: No.

⚠ Overdose S&S: Renal failure, liver failure, deafness, ocular toxicity, significant myelosuppression, intractable nausea and vomiting, neuritis, death.

PREGNANCY-LACTATION-REPRODUCTION

• Drug can cause fetal harm when used during pregnancy. Women of childbearing potential should be advised to avoid pregnancy during treatment.

• Drug appears in human milk. Women shouldn't breastfeed during therapy.

NURSING CONSIDERATIONS

Black Box Warning Drug should be administered under the supervision of a physician experienced in the use of cancer chemotherapeutic agents. ■

Black Box Warning Myelosuppression is a major dose-related toxicity and occurs in approximately 30% of patients. Other dose-related toxicities include nausea and vomiting. ■

⚠ Alert: Cisplatin is considered a vesicant if more than 20 mL is administered or if it's given at a concentration of 0.5 mg/mL or more. Monitor infusion site; stop infusion immediately and notify prescriber if extravasation occurs. Don't flush the line.

• Monitor CBC, electrolyte levels (especially potassium and magnesium), platelet count, and renal function studies before initial and subsequent doses.

Black Box Warning Ototoxicity, which may be more pronounced in children, is manifested by tinnitus or loss of high-frequency hearing and, occasionally, deafness. ■

• To detect hearing loss, obtain audiometry tests before initial and subsequent doses.

• Prehydration and mannitol diuresis may significantly reduce renal toxicity and ototoxicity.

• Therapeutic effects are frequently accompanied by toxicity.

• Drug is highly emetogenic. Nausea and vomiting may occur immediately or may be delayed. Antiemetics are recommended. Monitor intake and output. Continue IV hydration until patient can tolerate adequate oral intake.

Black Box Warning Renal toxicity is cumulative; don't give next dose until renal function returns to normal. ■

• Don't repeat dose unless platelet count exceeds 100,000/mm^3, WBC count exceeds 4,000/mm^3, creatinine level is below 1.5 mg/dL, BUN level is below 25 mg/dL, and auditory acuity is within normal limits.

• To prevent bleeding, avoid all IM injections when platelet count is less than 50,000/mm^3.

• Anticipate need for blood transfusions during treatment because of cumulative anemia.

Black Box Warning Immediately give epinephrine, corticosteroids, or antihistamines for anaphylactoid reactions. ■

• Safe use in children hasn't been established.

• *Look alike–sound alike:* Don't confuse cisplatin with carboplatin; they aren't interchangeable.

PATIENT TEACHING

• Teach patient to report all adverse reactions, including nausea and vomiting and infusion-site discomfort.

• Advise patient to watch for signs and symptoms of infection (fever, sore throat, fatigue) and bleeding (easy bruising, nosebleeds, bleeding gums, tarry stools). Tell patient to take temperature daily.

- Tell patient to immediately report ringing in the ears or numbness in hands or feet.
- Instruct patient to avoid OTC products containing aspirin.
- Advise female patient to stop breastfeeding during therapy because of risk of toxicity to infant.
- Advise female patient of childbearing potential to avoid becoming pregnant during therapy because drug may cause fetal harm.

citalopram hydrobromide ℞
si-TAL-oh-pram

CeleXA⬦

Therapeutic class: Antidepressants
Pharmacologic class: SSRIs

AVAILABLE FORMS
Solution: 10 mg/5 mL
Tablets: 10 mg, 20 mg, 40 mg

INDICATIONS & DOSAGES
℞ *Adjust-a-dose (for all indications):* For patients with hepatic impairment and for those who are CYP2C19 poor metabolizers, are taking cimetidine or another CYP2C19 inhibitor, or are older than age 60, the maximum dosage is 20 mg/day.
➤ **Depression**
Adults: Initially, 20 mg PO once daily, increasing to 40 mg daily after no less than 1 week. Maximum recommended dose is 40 mg daily.
Patients older than age 60: 20 mg PO daily.

ADMINISTRATION
PO
- Give drug without regard for food.

ACTION
Probably linked to potentiation of serotonergic activity in the CNS resulting from inhibition of neuronal reuptake of serotonin.

Route	Onset	Peak	Duration
PO	1–4 wk	4 hr	1–2 days

Half-life: 35 hours.

ADVERSE REACTIONS
CNS: somnolence, insomnia, *suicide attempt*, anxiety, agitation, dizziness, paresthesia, migraine, impaired concentration, amnesia, depression, apathy, tremor, confusion, fatigue, fever. **CV:** tachycardia, orthostatic hypotension, hypotension, *prolonged QT interval.* **EENT:** rhinitis, sinusitis, abnormal accommodation. **GI:** dry mouth, nausea, diarrhea, anorexia, dyspepsia, vomiting, abdominal pain, taste perversion, increased saliva, flatulence, increased appetite. **GU:** dysmenorrhea, amenorrhea, ejaculation disorder, erectile dysfunction, anorgasmia, polyuria, decreased libido. **Metabolic:** decreased or increased weight. **Musculoskeletal:** arthralgia, myalgia. **Respiratory:** URI, coughing. **Skin:** rash, pruritus. **Other:** increased sweating, yawning, decreased libido.

INTERACTIONS
Drug-drug. *Amphetamines, antiemetics, antipsychotics, buspirone, dextromethorphan, dihydroergotamine, opioids, other SSRIs or SSNRIs (duloxetine, venlafaxine), TCAs,* **tramadol**, *trazodone, tryptophan:* May increase risk of serotonin syndrome. Avoid other drugs that increase the availability of serotonin in the CNS; monitor patient closely if used together.
Antiarrhythmics (Class IA [procainamide, quinidine], Class III [amiodarone, sotalol]), antibiotics (clarithromycin, erythromycin, levofloxacin, moxifloxacin), antipsychotics (chlorpromazine, thioridazine), drugs that prolong QTc interval (dolasetron, methadone, ondansetron, pentamidine): May cause QTc prolongation and increase risk of torsades de pointes. Use together isn't recommended.
Carbamazepine: May increase citalopram clearance. Monitor patient for effects.
CNS drugs: May cause additive effects. Use together cautiously.
Drugs that affect coagulation (aspirin, NSAIDs): May increase bleeding risk. Monitor patient closely.
Drugs that inhibit CYP3A4 and CYP2C19: May cause decreased clearance of citalopram. Monitor patient for increased adverse effects.

Reactions in bold italics are *life-threatening*. Interactions may have a *rapid onset* or a **delayed onset**.

C

Imipramine, other TCAs: May increase level of imipramine metabolite desipramine by about 50%. Use together cautiously.

Linezolid, methylene blue: May cause serotonin syndrome. Use together is contraindicated.

Lithium: May enhance serotonergic effect of citalopram. Use together cautiously, and monitor lithium level.

MAO inhibitors (phenelzine, selegiline, tranylcypromine): May cause serotonin syndrome or signs and symptoms resembling NMS. Avoid using within 14 days of MAO inhibitor therapy.

Sumatriptan: May cause weakness, hyperreflexia, and incoordination. Monitor patient closely.

Drug-lifestyle. *Alcohol use:* May increase CNS effects. Discourage use together.

EFFECTS ON LAB TEST RESULTS
None reported.

CONTRAINDICATIONS & CAUTIONS
• Contraindicated in patients hypersensitive to drug or its inactive components, within 14 days of MAO inhibitor therapy, and in patients taking pimozide.

🗴 ❶ *Alert:* Drug isn't recommended for patients with congenital long QT syndrome, bradycardia, hypokalemia, hypomagnesemia, recent acute MI, or uncompensated HF.

🗴 ❶ *Alert:* High doses can prolong the QT interval and cause torsades de pointes, a potentially fatal heart rhythm. Maximum dose is 40 mg/day in patients age 60 and younger. Maximum dose is 20 mg/day in patients older than age 60, patients with hepatic impairment, and CYP2C19 poor metabolizers or patients taking cimetidine or another CYP2C19 inhibitor.

❶ *Alert:* Discontinue drug in patients with persistent QTc interval measurement longer than 500 msec.

❶ *Alert:* Concomitant use with linezolid or methylene blue can cause serotonin syndrome (fever, mental status changes, muscle twitching, excessive sweating, shivering or shaking, diarrhea, loss of coordination). Use together is contraindicated.

• Use cautiously in patients with history of mania, seizures, suicidal thoughts, or hepatic or renal impairment.

Dialyzable drug: No.

⚠ *Overdose S&S:* Dizziness, sweating, nausea, vomiting, tremor, somnolence, sinus tachycardia, amnesia, confusion, coma, seizures, hyperventilation, cyanosis, rhabdomyolysis, ECG changes.

PREGNANCY-LACTATION-REPRODUCTION
• There are no adequate well-controlled studies in pregnant women. Use during pregnancy only if potential benefit justifies potential risk to the fetus.

• Use in third trimester may be linked to neonatal complications at birth requiring respiratory support and tube feeding. Consider risk versus benefit of treatment during this time.

• Drug appears in human milk. Patient should discontinue breastfeeding or discontinue drug, taking into account importance of drug to the mother.

NURSING CONSIDERATIONS
• Correct electrolyte disturbances before starting drug; monitor patients at high risk for electrolyte disturbances periodically during therapy.

• Although drug hasn't been shown to impair psychomotor performance, any psychoactive drug has the potential to impair judgment, thinking, or motor skills.

Black Box Warning The possibility of a suicide attempt is inherent in depression and may persist until significant remission occurs. Closely supervise all patients for clinical worsening, suicidality, or unusual changes in behavior at start of drug therapy. ∎

• Reduce risk of overdose by limiting amount of drug available per refill.

Black Box Warning Drug may increase the risk of suicidal thinking and behavior in children, adolescents, and young adults with major depressive disorder or other psychiatric disorders. Drug isn't approved for use in children. ∎

• At least 14 days should elapse between MAO inhibitor therapy and citalopram therapy.

⟁ Alert: Combining triptans with an SSRI or an SSNRI may cause serotonin syndrome or NMS-like reactions. Signs and symptoms of serotonin syndrome may include restlessness, hallucinations, loss of coordination, fast heartbeat, rapid changes in BP, increased body temperature, overactive reflexes, nausea, vomiting, and diarrhea. Serotonin syndrome may be more likely to occur when starting or increasing the dose of the triptan, SSRI, or SSNRI.

⟁ Alert: If linezolid or methylene blue must be given, stop drug and monitor patient for serotonin toxicity for 2 weeks, or until 24 hours after the last dose of methylene blue or linezolid, whichever comes first. Treatment may be resumed 24 hours after last dose of methylene blue or linezolid.

• Don't discontinue drug abruptly because a discontinuation syndrome can develop, with varying symptoms.

• **Look alike–sound alike:** Don't confuse CeleXA with Zyprexa, Celebrex, or Cerebyx.

PATIENT TEACHING

Black Box Warning Advise families and caregivers to closely observe patient for increased suicidal thinking and behavior. ∎

⟁ Alert: Teach patient to recognize and immediately report symptoms of serotonin toxicity (fever, mental status changes, muscle twitching, excessive sweating, shivering or shaking, diarrhea, loss of coordination).

• Caution patient against use of MAO inhibitors while taking citalopram.

• Although improvement may take 1 to 4 weeks, inform patient to continue therapy as prescribed.

• Advise patient not to stop drug abruptly.

• Tell patient that drug may be taken in the morning or evening without regard to meals. If drowsiness occurs, patient should take drug in evening.

• Instruct patient to exercise caution when driving or operating hazardous machinery; drug may impair judgment, thinking, and motor skills.

• Advise patient to consult prescriber before taking other prescription or OTC drugs.

• Advise female patient of childbearing potential to consult prescriber before breast-feeding.

• Warn patient to avoid alcohol during drug therapy.

• Instruct female patient of childbearing potential to use contraception during drug therapy and to notify prescriber immediately if pregnancy is suspected.

clarithromycin
klar-ITH-ro-my-sin

Therapeutic class: Antibiotics
Pharmacologic class: Macrolides

AVAILABLE FORMS
Suspension: 125 mg/5 mL, 250 mg/5 mL
Tablets (extended-release) ⓞⓡⓒ: 500 mg
Tablets (film-coated): 250 mg, 500 mg

INDICATIONS & DOSAGES
Adjust-a-dose (for all indications): In patients with CrCl of less than 30 mL/minute, reduce dosage by 50%. For concomitant use with atazanavir or ritonavir in patients with CrCl of 30 to 60 mL/minute, reduce dosage by 50%; if CrCl is less than 30 mL/minute, reduce dosage by 75%. In patients with normal renal function, decrease clarithromycin dose by 50% when administered with atazanavir.

➤ **Pharyngitis or tonsillitis caused by** *Streptococcus pyogenes*
Adults: 250 mg PO every 12 hours for 10 days.
Children age 6 months and older: 7.5 mg/kg PO every 12 hours for 10 days.

➤ **Acute maxillary sinusitis caused by** *Streptococcus pneumoniae, Haemophilus influenzae,* **or** *Moraxella catarrhalis*
Adults: 500 mg PO every 12 hours for 14 days. Or, if using extended-release form, give two 500-mg tablets PO daily for 14 days.
Children age 6 months and older: 7.5 mg/kg PO every 12 hours for 10 days.

➤ **Acute worsening of chronic bronchitis caused by** *M. catarrhalis* **or** *S. pneumoniae*
Adults: 250 mg PO every 12 hours for 7 to 14 days.

➤ **Acute worsening of chronic bronchitis caused by** *H. influenzae* **or** *Haemophilus parainfluenzae*
Adults: 500 mg PO every 12 hours for 7 days *(H. parainfluenzae)* or 7 to 14 days *(H. influenzae).*

➤ **Acute worsening of chronic bronchitis caused by *M. catarrhalis, S. pneumoniae, H. parainfluenzae,* or *H. influenzae***
Adults: Two 500-mg extended-release tablets PO daily for 7 days.

➤ **Mild to moderate community-acquired pneumonia caused by *H. influenzae, S. pneumoniae, Chlamydophila pneumoniae,* or *Mycoplasma pneumoniae***
Adults: 250 mg PO every 12 hours for 7 days (*H. influenzae*) or 7 to 14 days (other bacteria).

➤ **Mild to moderate community-acquired pneumonia caused by *H. influenzae, H. parainfluenzae, M. catarrhalis, S. pneumoniae, C. pneumoniae,* or *M. pneumoniae***
Adults: Two 500-mg extended-release tablets PO once daily for 7 days.

➤ **Mild to moderate community-acquired pneumonia caused by *S. pneumoniae, C. pneumoniae,* or *M. pneumoniae***
Children age 6 months and older: 7.5 mg/kg PO every 12 hours for 10 days.

➤ **Uncomplicated skin and skin-structure infections caused by *Staphylococcus aureus* or *S. pyogenes***
Adults: 250 mg PO every 12 hours for 7 to 14 days.
Children age 6 months and older: 7.5 mg/kg PO every 12 hours for 10 days.

➤ **Acute otitis media**
Children age 6 months and older: 7.5 mg/kg PO every 12 hours for 10 days.

➤ **To prevent and treat disseminated infection caused by *Mycobacterium avium* complex**
Adults: 500 mg PO b.i.d. Therapy should continue if clinical response is observed; can be discontinued when patient is considered at low risk for disseminated infection.
Children age 20 months and older: 7.5 mg/kg PO b.i.d., up to 500 mg b.i.d.

➤ **To reduce risk of duodenal ulcer recurrence in *Helicobacter pylori* infection**
Adults: 500 mg clarithromycin with 30 mg lansoprazole and 1 g amoxicillin, all given PO every 12 hours for 10 to 14 days. Or, 500 mg clarithromycin with 20 mg omeprazole and 1 g amoxicillin, all given PO every 12 hours for 10 days. Or, two-drug regimen with 500 mg clarithromycin PO every 8 hours and 40 mg omeprazole PO once

daily for 14 days. Continue omeprazole for 14 additional days.

ADMINISTRATION
PO
• There is resistance to macrolides in certain bacterial infections caused by *S. pneumoniae* and *S. aureus.* Obtain specimen for culture and sensitivity tests before giving. Begin therapy while awaiting results.
• Give immediate-release form with or without food; give extended-release tablets with food. Extended-release tablets should not be crushed.
• Don't refrigerate the suspension form; discard unused portion after 14 days.

ACTION
Binds to the 50S subunit of bacterial ribosomes, blocking protein synthesis; bacteriostatic or bactericidal, depending on concentration.

Route	Onset	Peak	Duration
PO	Unknown	2–3 hr	Unknown
PO (extended-release)	Unknown	5–8 hr	Unknown

Half-life: 3 to 7 hours.

ADVERSE REACTIONS
CNS: headache, insomnia. **GI:** *pseudomembranous colitis,* abdominal pain or discomfort, diarrhea, nausea, taste perversion, dyspepsia, flatulence, vomiting (in children). **Hematologic:** coagulation abnormalities. **Skin:** rash (in children).

INTERACTIONS
Drug-drug. *Alfuzosin, alprazolam, midazolam, triazolam:* May decrease clearance of these drugs, causing adverse reactions. Use together cautiously.
Almotriptan: May increase almotriptan serum concentration. Limit initial almotriptan adult dose to 6.25 mg and maximum adult dose to 12.5 mg/24 hours; avoid concurrent use in patients with impaired hepatic or renal function. Consider therapy modification.
Apixaban, dabigatran, edoxaban, rivaroxaban: May increase concentrations of these drugs. Apixaban, dabigatran, rivaroxaban, or edoxaban dosage reductions or avoidance

of combination may be necessary. Consider therapy modification.

Atazanavir, ritonavir: May increase clarithromycin level. Reduce clarithromycin dosage in renally impaired patients and in all patients taking atazanavir.

Carbamazepine, phenytoin: May inhibit metabolism of these drugs, increasing serum levels and risk of toxicity. Avoid using together.

Colchicine: May increase colchicine level. Concomitant use is contraindicated in patients with renal or hepatic impairment. In those with normal renal and hepatic function, reduce colchicine dose.

Cyclosporine: May increase cyclosporine levels. Monitor cyclosporine level.

CYP3A4 substrates (colchicine): May increase substrate concentration. Avoid use together or reduce substrate dosage.

Digoxin: May increase digoxin level. Monitor patient for digoxin toxicity.

Dihydroergotamine, ergotamine: May cause acute ergot toxicity. Use together is contraindicated.

Fluconazole: May increase clarithromycin level. Monitor patient closely.

HMG-CoA reductase inhibitors: Lovastatin and simvastatin are contraindicated. Use with other statins may increase levels of these drugs and may rarely cause rhabdomyolysis. Use together cautiously. For adults, limit atorvastatin to a maximum dose of 20 mg/day and pravastatin to 40 mg/day.

Other drugs that prolong QTc interval (amiodarone, antipsychotics, disopyramide, fluoroquinolones, fluoxetine, procainamide, quinidine, sotalol, TCAs): May have additive effects. Monitor ECG for QTc interval prolongation. Avoid using together if possible.

Pimozide: May cause torsades de pointes. Use together is contraindicated.

Rifamycin: May decrease therapeutic effects of clarithromycin while increasing adverse effects of rifamycin. Monitor patient.

Sildenafil: May prolong absorption of sildenafil. May need to reduce sildenafil dosage.

Theophylline: May increase theophylline level. Monitor drug level.

Warfarin: May prolong PT and increase INR. Monitor PT and INR carefully.

Zidovudine: May alter zidovudine level. Monitor patient closely.

Drug-herb. *St. John's wort:* May decrease clarithromycin level. Avoid use.

Drug-food. *Grapefruit juice:* May inhibit metabolism, increasing adverse effects. Don't take with grapefruit juice.

EFFECTS ON LAB TEST RESULTS
• May increase BUN level.
• May prolong PT and increase INR.

CONTRAINDICATIONS & CAUTIONS
❸ **Alert:** Use in patients with CAD has shown an increased risk of all-cause mortality 1 year or more after the end of treatment. Consider potential risk versus benefits before using in patients with suspected or confirmed heart disease. Use of an alternative antibiotic is recommended.

• Severe acute hypersensitivity reactions, including anaphylaxis, SJS, toxic epidermal necrolysis, drug rash with eosinophilia, and Henoch-Schönlein purpura, have been reported. Discontinue drug and begin immediate treatment if these occur.

• Contraindicated in patients hypersensitive to clarithromycin, erythromycin, or other macrolides and in those receiving pimozide or other drugs that prolong QT interval or cause cardiac arrhythmias.

• Contraindicated in patients with a history of cholestatic jaundice or hepatic impairment associated with prior use of clarithromycin.

• Avoid use in patients with ongoing proarrhythmic conditions, such as uncorrected hypokalemia or hypomagnesemia or clinically significant bradycardia, and in patients receiving Class IA or Class III antiarrhythmics. Elderly patients may be more susceptible to drug-associated effects on the QT interval.

• Use cautiously in patients with hepatic or renal impairment.

• Use cautiously when administered concurrently with medications that induce CYP3A4.

• May cause exacerbation of or new signs and symptoms in patients with myasthenia gravis. Use cautiously in these patients.

• Drug may cause CDAD and pseudomembranous colitis, which can occur more than 2 months after therapy ends.

Reactions in bold italics are *life-threatening*. Interactions may have a *rapid onset* or a *delayed onset*.

C

• Safety and effectiveness in children younger than age 6 months haven't been established.
Dialyzable drug: No.

PREGNANCY-LACTATION-REPRODUCTION
• There are no adequate well-controlled studies in pregnant women; animal studies show adverse pregnancy outcome and embryo-fetal risk. Use during pregnancy only in clinical circumstances in which no alternative therapy is appropriate. Inform patient of potential risk to the fetus.
• Drug appears in human milk. Use cautiously in breastfeeding women and weigh benefits against risks.

NURSING CONSIDERATIONS
🔆 *Alert:* Be sure to use extended-release form to only treat infections for which it is approved.
• Monitor patient for superinfection. Drug may cause overgrowth of nonsusceptible bacteria or fungi.

PATIENT TEACHING
• Tell patient to take drug as prescribed, even after feeling better.
• Advise patient to report all adverse reactions.
• Advise patient of the importance of taking immediate-release product every 12 hours.
• Inform patient that immediate-release form may be taken with or without food but extended-release form should be taken with food.
• Tell patient not to refrigerate the suspension form, but to discard unused portion after 14 days.

clevidipine
cle-VIH-deh-peen

Cleviprex

Therapeutic class: Antihypertensives
Pharmacologic class: Dihydropyridine calcium channel blockers

AVAILABLE FORMS
Injection: 0.5 mg/mL in 50- and 100-mL single-use vials

INDICATIONS & DOSAGES
➤ **To lower BP when oral therapy isn't feasible or desirable**
Adults: Begin infusion at 1 to 2 mg/hour and titrate by doubling the dose every 90 seconds. When BP approaches goal, titrate every 5 to 10 minutes at less than double the dose. Maintenance dose is usually 4 to 6 mg/hour. Maximum dose is 1,000 mL (average of 21 mg/hour) per 24-hour period. Drug isn't recommended for use beyond 72 hours.

ADMINISTRATION
IV
▼ Store vials in cartons in refrigerator because drug is photosensitive. May store at controlled room temperature (77° F [25° C]) for up to 2 months.
▼ Maintain aseptic technique when handling solution. Drug can support growth of microorganisms.
▼ Invert vial several times to mix emulsion before use.
▼ Inspect solution and discard if particulate matter or discoloration is present before use. Don't dilute.
▼ Use a continuous infusion pump to regulate flow.
▼ Discard unused portion within 12 hours after stopper puncture.
▼ **Incompatibilities:** Don't administer drug in same IV line with other medications.

ACTION
Inhibits calcium ion influx across cardiac and smooth-muscle cells, decreasing contractility and oxygen demand. Dilates coronary arteries and arterioles, decreasing systemic vascular resistance.

Route	Onset	Peak	Duration
IV	2–4 min	Unknown	5–15 min

Half-life: 15 minutes; metabolite, 9 hours.

ADVERSE REACTIONS
CNS: headache. **CV:** atrial fibrillation. **GI:** nausea, vomiting. **GU:** *acute renal failure.*

INTERACTIONS
None reported.

EFFECTS ON LAB TEST RESULTS
• May increase bilirubin, AST, and ALT levels.

CONTRAINDICATIONS & CAUTIONS
• Contraindicated in patients hypersensitive to soybeans, soy products, eggs, or egg products and in those with defective lipid metabolism or severe aortic stenosis.
• Use cautiously in patients with HF, and monitor for exacerbations.
• Safety and effectiveness in children younger than age 18 haven't been established.
Dialyzable drug: Unknown.
⚠ *Overdose S&S:* Hypotension, reflex tachycardia.

PREGNANCY-LACTATION-REPRODUCTION
• There are no adequate well-controlled studies in pregnant women. Use during pregnancy only if potential benefit justifies potential risk to the fetus.
• It isn't known if drug appears in human milk. Consider the possibility of infant exposure during breastfeeding, and monitor infant for adverse effects.

NURSING CONSIDERATIONS
• Monitor BP and HR continuously, especially when starting drug and during dosage adjustments.
• Drug may exacerbate HF; monitor patient closely.
• Titrate dose slowly; rapid titration may cause hypotension and reflex tachycardia. If either occurs, decrease clevidipine dosage.
• Monitor patient who received prolonged infusion for rebound HTN for at least 8 hours after infusion is stopped if no other antihypertensive is prescribed.
• To convert to oral therapy, discontinue or titrate drug downward while appropriate oral therapy is established. When an oral antihypertensive is started, consider the lag time of onset of the oral agent's effect and continue BP monitoring until desired effect is achieved.
• Drug isn't a beta-adrenergic blocker; if given with beta-adrenergic blocker, gradually reduce beta-adrenergic blocker dosage to avoid withdrawal symptoms.

PATIENT TEACHING
• Tell patient to report adverse reactions promptly.
• Advise patient to seek medical attention immediately if signs and symptoms of hypertensive emergency occur (visual changes, neurologic symptoms, HF).

clindamycin hydrochloride
klin-da-MYE-sin

Cleocin Hydrochloride, Dalacin C✦

clindamycin palmitate hydrochloride
Cleocin Pediatric, Dalacin C Flavored Granules✦

clindamycin phosphate (injection)
Cleocin Phosphate, Dalacin C Phosphate✦

Therapeutic class: Antibiotics
Pharmacologic class: Lincomycin derivatives

AVAILABLE FORMS
clindamycin hydrochloride
Capsules: 75 mg, 150 mg, 300 mg
clindamycin palmitate hydrochloride
Granules for oral solution: 75 mg/5 mL
clindamycin phosphate (injection)
Injectable infusion (in D$_5$W): 300 mg (50 mL), 600 mg (50 mL), 900 mg (50 mL)
Injection: 150 mg base/mL, 300 mg base/2 mL, 600 mg base/4 mL, 900 mg base/6 mL

INDICATIONS & DOSAGES
➤ **Infections caused by sensitive staphylococci, streptococci, pneumococci, *Bacteroides, Fusobacterium, Clostridium perfringens*, or other sensitive aerobic and anaerobic organisms**
Adults: 150 to 450 mg PO every 6 hours; or 300 to 600 mg IM or IV every 6, 8, or 12 hours. In more severe infections, dosage may be increased to 1,200 to 2,700 mg/day IM or IV in two, three, or four divided doses. In life-threatening infections, dosages as high as 4,800 mg daily can be given.

Children ages 1 month to 16 years: 20 to 40 mg/kg/day or 350 to 450 mg/kg/day IM or IV in three or four equal doses. In beta-hemolytic streptococcal infections, treatment should continue for at least 10 days.
Neonates younger than age 1 month: 15 to 20 mg/kg/day IM or IV in three or four equal doses. Consider 15 mg/kg/day for small premature infants.

ADMINISTRATION
PO
● Obtain specimen for culture and sensitivity tests before giving first dose. Begin therapy while awaiting results.
● Give capsule form with a full glass of water to prevent esophageal irritation.
● Don't refrigerate reconstituted oral solution because it will thicken. Drug is stable for 2 weeks at room temperature.
IV
▼ Obtain specimen for culture and sensitivity tests before giving first dose. Begin therapy while awaiting results.
▼ Never give undiluted as a bolus.
▼ For infusion, dilute each 300 mg in 50 mL solution and give over 10 to 60 minutes at no more than 30 mg/minute.
▼ Check site daily for phlebitis and irritation.
▼ Drug may contain benzyl alcohol. Benzyl alcohol has been associated with a fatal gasping syndrome in premature infants.
▼ **Incompatibilities:** Aminophylline, ampicillin, barbiturates, calcium gluconate, magnesium sulfate, phenytoin.
IM
● Obtain specimen for culture and sensitivity tests before giving first dose. Begin therapy while awaiting results.
● Inject deep into muscle. Rotate sites. Don't exceed 600 mg per injection.

ACTION
Inhibits bacterial protein synthesis by binding to the 50S subunit of the ribosome.

Route	Onset	Peak	Duration
PO	Unknown	45–60 min	Unknown
IV	Immediate	Immediate	Unknown
IM	Unknown	3 hr	Unknown

Half-life: 2½ to 3 hours.

ADVERSE REACTIONS
CV: thrombophlebitis. **GI:** nausea, *pseudomembranous colitis,* abdominal pain, diarrhea, vomiting. **Hematologic:** *thrombocytopenia, transient leukopenia,* eosinophilia. **Hepatic:** jaundice. **Skin:** maculopapular rash, urticaria. **Other:** *anaphylaxis.*

INTERACTIONS
Drug-drug. *Erythromycin:* May block access of clindamycin to its site of action. Avoid using together.
Live-virus vaccines: May decrease vaccine effectiveness. Don't give together.
Neuromuscular blockers: May increase neuromuscular blockade. Monitor patient closely.

EFFECTS ON LAB TEST RESULTS
● May increase alkaline phosphatase, AST, and bilirubin levels.
● May increase eosinophil count. May decrease platelet and WBC counts.

CONTRAINDICATIONS & CAUTIONS
● Contraindicated in patients hypersensitive to drug or lincomycin. Severe hypersensitivity reactions requiring emergency treatment have been reported. Severe skin reactions and DRESS syndrome have been reported. Discontinue drug if these occur.
● Clindamycin use may result in overgrowth of nonsusceptible organisms, particularly yeasts. Monitor patient for sign of superinfection.
● Use cautiously in neonates and patients with renal or hepatic disease, asthma, history of GI disease, or significant allergies.
● Severe or fatal reactions such as toxic epidermal necrolysis have been reported. Discontinue drug if severe skin reaction occurs.
Black Box Warning Clindamycin has been associated with development of CDAD, which may evolve into severe, possibly fatal, colitis; its use should be reserved for serious infections. If CDAD is suspected or confirmed, drug may need to be discontinued and appropriate treatment initiated. ■
Dialyzable drug: No.

PREGNANCY-LACTATION-REPRODUCTION
• There are no adequate studies in pregnant women. Use during pregnancy only if clearly needed and potential benefit justifies potential risk to the fetus.
• Drug appears in human milk. Use in breastfeeding women isn't recommended.

NURSING CONSIDERATIONS
• IM injection may raise CK level in response to muscle irritation.
• Monitor renal, hepatic, and hematopoietic functions during prolonged therapy.
• Observe patient for signs and symptoms of superinfection.
• **Alert:** Don't give opioid antidiarrheals to treat drug-induced diarrhea; they may prolong and worsen this condition.
Black Box Warning Diarrhea, colitis, and pseudomembranous colitis have developed up to 2 months after cessation of drug therapy. ∎
• Drug doesn't penetrate blood-brain barrier.

PATIENT TEACHING
• Advise patient to take capsule form with a full glass of water to prevent esophageal irritation.
• Warn patient that IM injection may be painful.
• Tell patient to report discomfort at IV insertion site.
• Instruct patient to report all adverse reactions (especially diarrhea and hypersensitivity reactions). Warn patient not to self-treat diarrhea because drug may cause life-threatening colitis.

clindamycin phosphate (intravaginal, topical)
klin-da-MYE-sin

Cleocin, Cleocin T, Clinda-Derm, Clindagel, Clinda-T✹, Clindesse, Clindets, Dalacin T✹, Evoclin

Therapeutic class: Antibiotics
Pharmacologic class: Lincomycin derivatives

AVAILABLE FORMS
Foam: 1%
Gel: 1%
Lotion: 1%
Pledget: 1%*
Topical cream: 1%, 2%
Topical solution: 1%*
Vaginal cream: 2%
Vaginal suppositories: 100 mg

INDICATIONS & DOSAGES
➤ **Inflammatory acne vulgaris**
Adults and children age 12 and older: Apply to skin b.i.d., morning and evening, or once daily if using Clindagel or Evoclin.
➤ **Bacterial vaginosis**
Adults: 1 applicatorful vaginally at bedtime for 3 to 7 days in nonpregnant women or 7 days in pregnant women, or 1 suppository vaginally at bedtime for 3 days, or 1 applicatorful of Clindesse vaginally as a single dose.

ADMINISTRATION
Topical
• Wash area with warm water and soap, rinse, pat dry, and wait 30 minutes after washing or shaving to apply.
• Avoid excessive washing of affected area.
• Apply to entire area, but avoid contact with eyes, nose, mouth, and other mucous membranes.
• Remove pledgets from foil just before use.
• Use pledgets only once and then discard; more than 1 pledget may be used per application.
• If using foam or Clindagel, discontinue use if there has been no improvement after 6 to 8 weeks, or if condition worsens.
Vaginal
• Make sure patient knows how to use applicators that come with drug.

ACTION
Bacteriostatic or bactericidal based on drug level and susceptibility of organism; suppresses growth of susceptible organisms in sebaceous glands by blocking protein synthesis.

Route	Onset	Peak	Duration
Topical, vaginal	Unknown	Unknown	Unknown

Half-life: Topical and vaginal cream, 1½ to 2½ hours; vaginal suppositories, 11 hours.

ADVERSE REACTIONS

CNS: headache. **EENT:** pharyngitis. **GI:** abdominal pain, bloody diarrhea, colitis including *pseudomembranous colitis*, constipation, diarrhea, GI upset. **GU:** *Candida albicans* overgrowth, cervicitis, vaginitis, vulvar irritation, UTI, vaginal discharge, vaginal candidiasis. **Skin:** dryness, redness, burning, contact dermatitis, irritation, rash, pruritus, swelling.

INTERACTIONS

Drug-drug. *Erythromycin (topical, vaginal):* May antagonize clindamycin's effect. Avoid combination.
Isotretinoin: May cause cumulative dryness, resulting in excessive skin irritation. Use together cautiously.
Neuromuscular blockers: May increase action of neuromuscular blocker. Use together cautiously.
Drug-lifestyle. *Abrasive or medicated soaps or cleansers, acne products, or other preparations containing peeling drugs (benzoyl peroxide, resorcinol, salicylic acid, sulfur, tretinoin), alcohol-containing products (aftershave, cosmetics, perfumed toiletries, shaving creams or lotions), astringent soaps or cosmetics, medicated cosmetics or cover-ups:* May cause cumulative dryness, resulting in excessive skin irritation. Urge caution.

EFFECTS ON LAB TEST RESULTS

• May increase liver enzyme levels.

CONTRAINDICATIONS & CAUTIONS

• Contraindicated in patients hypersensitive to clindamycin or lincomycin and in those with history of ulcerative colitis, regional enteritis, or antibiotic-related colitis.
• Intravaginal form can be absorbed systemically and cause CDAD even 2 months after therapy ends.
Dialyzable drug: No.
⚠ *Overdose S&S:* Systemic effects.

PREGNANCY-LACTATION-REPRODUCTION

• There are no adequate studies in pregnant women. Use during pregnancy only if clearly needed and potential benefit justifies potential risk to the fetus.
• Drug appears in human milk. Patient should discontinue breastfeeding or discontinue drug, taking into account importance of drug to the mother.

NURSING CONSIDERATIONS

• For treating acne, drug may be used with tretinoin or benzoyl peroxide, as well as systemic antibiotics.
• Drug can cause excessive dryness.
• Topical solution and pledgets contain alcohol base, which may irritate eyes.
• Monitor elderly patients for systemic effects.
• Monitor patients for diarrhea.

PATIENT TEACHING

• Tell patient to wash area with warm water and soap, rinse, pat dry, and wait 30 minutes after washing or shaving before applying topically.
• Warn patient to avoid excessive washing of area. Tell patient to cover entire affected area but to avoid contact with eyes, nose, mouth, and other mucous membranes.
• Instruct patient to use other prescribed acne medicines at a different time.
• Tell patient to use only as prescribed.
• Instruct patient to dab, not roll, applicator-tipped bottle. If tip becomes dry, patient should invert bottle and depress tip several times to moisten.
• Warn patient not to smoke while applying topical solution or foam.
• For vaginal treatment, instruct patient how to use vaginal applicators.
• Advise patient that the vaginal form contains mineral oil, which can weaken latex or rubber products, such as condoms and diaphragms, and that she should use another form of birth control during and within 3 days of therapy (Cleocin) or 5 days (Clindesse).
• Advise patient to avoid sexual intercourse and use of tampons or douches during vaginal treatment.
• Instruct patient to notify prescriber immediately if abdominal pain or diarrhea occurs. Inform patient that an antidiarrheal may worsen condition and should only be used as directed by prescriber.
• Tell patient to remove pledgets from foil before use.

- Advise patient to use pledgets only once and then discard. Also, more than 1 pledget may be used per application.
- Advise patient to complete entire course of therapy.

cloBAZam ⊠
KLOE-ba-zam

Onfi, Sympazan

Therapeutic class: Anticonvulsants
Pharmacologic class: Benzodiazepines
Controlled substance schedule: IV

AVAILABLE FORMS
Oral film: 5 mg, 10 mg, 20 mg
Oral suspension: 2.5 mg/mL
Tablets: 10 mg, 20 mg

INDICATIONS & DOSAGES
➤ **Adjunctive treatment of seizures associated with Lennox-Gastaut syndrome** ⊠
Adults and children age 2 and older weighing more than 30 kg: Initially, 5 mg PO b.i.d. for 6 days. On day 7, increase to 10 mg PO b.i.d.; on day 14, titrate to 20 mg PO b.i.d. as tolerated. Dosage escalation shouldn't proceed more rapidly than weekly. Maximum dose is 40 mg/day.
Adults and children age 2 and older weighing 30 kg or less: Initially, 5 mg PO once daily for 6 days. On day 7, increase to 5 mg PO b.i.d.; on day 14, titrate to 10 mg PO b.i.d. as tolerated. Dosage escalation shouldn't proceed more rapidly than weekly. Maximum dose is 20 mg/day.
⊠ *Adjust-a-dose:* For elderly patients, those with mild to moderate hepatic impairment (Child-Pugh score 5 to 9), and those who are poor CYP2C19 metabolizers, initially 5 mg PO daily for 1 week; then titrate according to weight but at half the recommended dose as tolerated. If necessary, may start an additional titration to the maximum dosage (20 or 40 mg/day depending on weight) on day 21. There are no dosage recommendations for patients with severe hepatic or renal impairment.

ADMINISTRATION
PO
- May give tablets whole, broken in half, or crushed and mixed in applesauce.
- May give with or without food.
- For daily dose greater than 5 mg, divide dose equally and give b.i.d.
- Shake oral suspension well before every dose and use only oral dosing syringe supplied with product.
- Use oral suspension within 90 days of first opening; discard any remaining product.
- For oral film: Immediately after opening foil pouch, apply one film on top of tongue, where it will dissolve. If a second film is needed, apply after the first film has completely dissolved.
- Don't administer film with liquids. As film dissolves, patient should swallow in a normal manner and not chew, spit, or talk.
- To discontinue drug, taper gradually by 5 to 10 mg/day on a weekly basis.

ACTION
Thought to involve potentiating GABA neurotransmission, which results from binding at the benzodiazepine site of the $GABA_A$ receptor.

Route	Onset	Peak	Duration
PO	Rapid	½–4 hr	Unknown

Half-life: 36 to 82 hours.

ADVERSE REACTIONS
CNS: somnolence, lethargy, pyrexia, irritability, fatigue, sedation, ataxia, psychomotor hyperactivity, insomnia, aggression.
EENT: drooling. **GI:** vomiting, constipation, dysphagia. **GU:** UTI. **Metabolic:** increased or decreased appetite. **Musculoskeletal:** dysarthria. **Respiratory:** URI, pneumonia, cough, bronchitis.

INTERACTIONS
Drug-drug. *CNS depressants (TCAs):* May increase sedation. Avoid use together.
CYP2C19 inhibitors (fluconazole, fluvoxamine, ketoconazole, omeprazole, ticlopidine): May increase levels of clobazam or its metabolite. Decrease clobazam dosage if needed.
Drugs metabolized by CYP2D6 inhibitors (dextromethorphan): May increase levels of

drugs metabolized by CYP2D6 inhibitors. Decreased dosages of these drugs may be needed.

Hormonal contraceptives: May diminish contraceptive effectiveness. Patient should use nonhormonal contraception as needed.

Black Box Warning *Opioids:* May cause slow or difficult breathing, sedation, and death. Avoid use together. If use together is necessary, limit dosage and duration of each drug to the minimum necessary for desired effect. ∎

Drug-lifestyle. *Alcohol use:* May increase clobazam level by up to 50% and increase CNS depression. Discourage alcohol use.

EFFECTS ON LAB TEST RESULTS
None reported.

CONTRAINDICATIONS & CAUTIONS
• Contraindicated in patients hypersensitive to drug or its components.
• Withdraw clobazam gradually to minimize risk of precipitating seizures, seizure exacerbation, status epilepticus, or withdrawal signs and symptoms (seizures, psychosis, hallucinations, behavioral disorder, tremor, anxiety).

Black Box Warning Opioids should only be prescribed with benzodiazepines or other CNS depressants to patients for whom alternative treatment options are inadequate. ∎
• Use cautiously in patients with history of dependence.
• Drug may increase risk of suicidal thoughts or behavior.

Dialyzable drug: Unknown.

⚠ **Overdose S&S:** Drowsiness, confusion, lethargy, respiratory depression, hypotension, ataxia, coma.

PREGNANCY-LACTATION-REPRODUCTION
• There are no adequate well-controlled studies in pregnant women. Use during pregnancy only if benefit to mother outweighs risk to the fetus.
• Neonatal flaccidity, respiratory and feeding difficulties, hypothermia, and withdrawal signs and symptoms have occurred in infants born to women who received benzodiazepines, including clobazam, late in pregnancy.

• Advise pregnant women to enroll in the North American AED Pregnancy Registry (1-888-233-2334).
• Drug appears in human milk. Patient should discontinue breastfeeding or discontinue drug, taking into account importance of drug to the mother.

NURSING CONSIDERATIONS
⊕ **Alert:** Monitor patients for skin reactions (rash, blistering or peeling skin, mouth sores, hives). Rare but serious skin reactions, including SJS and toxic epidermal necrolysis, have occurred with drug use, especially during first 8 weeks of treatment or when reintroducing therapy. Discontinue drug at first sign of reaction unless reaction is obviously not drug-related. Don't resume drug if rash is suggestive of SJS or toxic epidermal necrolysis.

⊕ **Alert:** Drug may increase risk of suicidal thoughts or behavior. Monitor patients treated with AEDs for indications of emergence or worsening of depression, suicidal thoughts or behavior, or unusual changes in mood or behavior.

Black Box Warning Monitor patient taking an opioid concomitantly with clobazam for signs and symptoms of respiratory depression and sedation. ∎
• Monitor patients for signs and symptoms of abuse or physical dependence.
• Monitor patients for somnolence. This can occur at all dosage ranges, is usually seen within the first month, and then may subside with continued therapy.
• Monitor patients for dependence. Dependence may occur at the recommended dosage range over only a few weeks. Risk increases with increasing dosage and duration of treatment. Risk is increased in those with a history of alcohol or drug abuse.

PATIENT TEACHING
Black Box Warning *Opioid class warning:* Caution patient or caregiver of patient taking an opioid with a benzodiazepine, CNS depressant, or alcohol to seek immediate medical attention for dizziness, lightheadedness, extreme sleepiness, slowed or difficult breathing, or unresponsiveness. ∎
• Advise patient and caregivers to notify health care providers before taking or giving

clobazam with other CNS depressants (other benzodiazepines, opioids, TCAs, sedating antihistamines, alcohol).
• Inform patient to use caution if operating heavy machinery, including cars, when taking drug until its effects are known.
• Caution patient and caregivers not to stop drug or change dosage without first discussing with prescriber.
• Advise women using hormonal contraception to use nonhormonal methods during therapy and to continue these methods for 28 days after stopping drug.
• Caution patient and caregivers that drug may increase risk of suicidal thoughts. Tell them to report signs and symptoms of depression or changes in mood or behavior.
• Instruct female patient to inform health care provider if she is pregnant, plans to become pregnant, or plans to breastfeed during therapy.
• Instruct patient or caregiver to discard any remaining oral suspension within 90 days of first opening the bottle.
• Teach patient or caregiver how to use the dosing syringe for the oral suspension.
• Teach patient or caregiver how to use oral film.

clobetasol propionate
kloe-BAY-ta-sol

Clobex, Clodan, Impoyz, Olux, Olux-E

Therapeutic class: Corticosteroids
Pharmacologic class: Corticosteroids

AVAILABLE FORMS
Cream: 0.025%, 0.05%
Foam: 0.05%*
Gel: 0.05%
Lotion: 0.05%
Ointment: 0.05%
Scalp application: 0.05%*
Shampoo: 0.05%*
Solution: 0.05%*
Spray: 0.05%*

INDICATIONS & DOSAGES
➤ **Short-term topical treatment for moderate to severe plaque-type psoriasis of**

nonscalp regions, excluding the face and intertriginous areas
Adults: Apply thin layer of lotion or cream to affected areas b.i.d., morning and evening, for up to 14 days. Or, apply spray directly onto affected areas b.i.d. and rub in gently and completely. For localized lesions (less than 10% of BSA) that haven't improved sufficiently, continue treatment for up to 2 more weeks. Total dose shouldn't exceed 50 g (50 mL) weekly.
Adolescents age 16 and older: Apply thin layer of emollient cream to affected areas b.i.d. and rub in gently and completely. If applied to 5% to 10% of BSA, can be used for up to 4 consecutive weeks. Total dosage shouldn't exceed 50 g (50 mL) weekly.
➤ **Inflammation and pruritus from corticosteroid-responsive dermatoses**
Adults: Apply thin layer of cream, emollient cream, foam, gel, lotion, solution, or ointment to affected areas b.i.d., morning and evening, for maximum of 14 days. Total dose shouldn't exceed 50 g (50 mL) weekly.
Children age 12 and older: Apply thin layer of cream, emollient cream, foam, gel, solution, or ointment to affected areas b.i.d., morning and evening, for maximum of 14 days. Total dose shouldn't exceed 50 g (50 mL) weekly.
➤ **Short-term topical treatment of mild to moderate plaque-type psoriasis of nonscalp regions, excluding the face and intertriginous areas**
Adults and children age 12 and older: Apply thin layer of foam to affected areas b.i.d., morning and evening, for maximum of 14 days. Total dose shouldn't exceed 50 g (21 capfuls) weekly.
➤ **Inflammation and pruritus of moderate to severe corticosteroid-responsive dermatoses of the scalp**
Adults and children age 12 and older: Apply thin layer of solution to the affected scalp area b.i.d., morning and evening. Massage into affected scalp area gently and completely. Limit treatment to 14 days, with no more than 50 g (50 mL) weekly.
➤ **Moderate to severe scalp psoriasis**
Adults: Apply thin film of shampoo to affected areas of dry scalp once daily. Leave in place for 15 minutes before lathering and rinsing. Limit treatment to 4 consecutive

weeks. If complete disease control isn't achieved after 4 weeks, substitute treatment with a less potent topical steroid. Maximum dose is 50 g (50 mL) weekly. Or, apply thin layer of foam to scalp b.i.d. for up to 2 weeks. Maximum dose is 50 g (21 capfuls) weekly.

Children age 12 and older: Apply thin layer of foam to scalp b.i.d. for up to 2 weeks. Maximum dose is 50 g (21 capfuls) weekly.

ADMINISTRATION
Topical
• Apply the smallest amount that will cover affected area.
• Gently wash skin before applying. To prevent skin damage, rub medication in gently and completely. When treating hairy sites, part hair and apply directly to lesions.
• To dispense foam, hold the can upside down and depress the actuator.
• Avoid applying near eyes or mucous membranes or in ear canal.
• **Alert:** Don't use occlusive dressings or bandages. Don't cover or wrap treated areas unless directed by prescriber.

ACTION
Unclear. Diffuses across cell membranes to form complexes with receptors, showing anti-inflammatory, antipruritic, vasoconstrictive, and antiproliferative activity. Considered a very-high-potency to high-potency drug, according to vasoconstrictive properties.

Route	Onset	Peak	Duration
Topical	Unknown	Unknown	Unknown

Half-life: Unknown.

ADVERSE REACTIONS
GU: glycosuria. **Metabolic:** hyperglycemia. **Skin:** burning, pruritus, irritation, dryness, erythema, folliculitis, perioral dermatitis, allergic contact dermatitis, hypopigmentation, hypertrichosis, acneiform eruptions, skin atrophy, telangiectasia. **Other:** *HPA axis suppression,* Cushing syndrome, finger numbness.

INTERACTIONS
None significant.

EFFECTS ON LAB TEST RESULTS
• May increase glucose level.

CONTRAINDICATIONS & CAUTIONS
• Contraindicated in patients hypersensitive to corticosteroids and in those with primary scalp infections (scalp solution only).
• Topical corticosteroids may be absorbed and cause hyperadrenocorticism or suppression of the HPA axis, particularly in younger children and in patients receiving high doses for prolonged periods.
• Rarely, prolonged treatment with corticosteroids is associated with development of Kaposi sarcoma.
• Don't use as monotherapy for primary bacterial infections (impetigo, paronychia, erysipelas, cellulitis, angular cheilitis, erythrasma), rosacea, perioral dermatitis, or acne.
• Don't use very-high-potency or high-potency agents on the face, groin, or axilla areas.
• Drug isn't for ophthalmic use.
• Use cautiously in children. Use in children younger than age 12 isn't recommended. Lotion, shampoo, and spray formulations aren't recommended for use in children age 17 and younger.
Dialyzable drug: Unknown.
⚠ Overdose S&S: Systemic effects.

PREGNANCY-LACTATION-REPRODUCTION
• There are no adequate studies in pregnant women. Use during pregnancy only if potential benefit justifies potential risk to the fetus. Extensive use during pregnancy isn't recommended.
• It isn't known if drug appears in human milk. Use cautiously in breastfeeding women.

NURSING CONSIDERATIONS
• If antifungal or antibiotic combined with corticosteroid fails to provide prompt improvement, stop corticosteroid until infection is controlled.
• Stop drug and notify prescriber if skin infection, striae, or atrophy occurs.
• HPA axis suppression occurs at doses as low as 2 g daily.

PATIENT TEACHING

• Teach patient how to apply drug, to avoid contact with eyes, and to wash hands after application.

• Tell patient to stop drug and report signs of systemic absorption, skin irritation or ulceration, hypersensitivity, or infection.

• Warn patient to use drug for no longer than 14 consecutive days, except shampoo, which can be used for 4 consecutive weeks.

• Tell patient using the foam to invert can and dispense a small amount of Olux foam (up to a golf ball-size dollop) into the cap of the can, onto a saucer or other cool surface, or directly on the lesion, taking care to avoid contact with the eyes. Dispensing directly onto hands isn't recommended because foam will melt immediately on contact with warm skin. Tell patient to move hair away from affected area of scalp so that foam can be applied to each affected area.

• Tell patient using foam that contents are flammable and under pressure, and to avoid smoking during and immediately after application and to keep can away from flames. Also tell patient not to puncture or incinerate container.

SAFETY ALERT!

clonazePAM
kloe-NAZ-e-pam

KlonoPIN⬦

Therapeutic class: Anticonvulsants
Pharmacologic class: Benzodiazepines
Controlled substance schedule: IV

AVAILABLE FORMS

Tablets: 0.5 mg, 1 mg, 2 mg
Tablets (ODTs): 0.125 mg, 0.25 mg, 0.5 mg, 1 mg, 2 mg

INDICATIONS & DOSAGES

➤ **Lennox-Gastaut syndrome, atypical absence seizures, akinetic and myoclonic seizures**
Adults and children older than age 10 or weighing more than 30 kg: Initially, no more than 1.5 mg/day PO in three divided doses. May be increased by 0.5 to 1 mg every 3 days until seizures are controlled or

adverse effects prevent further increases. If given in unequal doses, give largest dose at bedtime. Maximum recommended daily dose is 20 mg.
Children age 10 and younger or weighing 30 kg or less: Initially, 0.01 to 0.03 mg/kg PO daily (not to exceed 0.05 mg/kg daily) in two or three divided doses. Increase by 0.25 to 0.5 mg every third day to maximum maintenance dose of 0.1 to 0.2 mg/kg PO daily divided into three equal doses, as needed.
➤ **Panic disorder**
Adults: Initially, 0.25 mg PO b.i.d.; increase to target dose of 1 mg daily after 3 days. Some patients may benefit from dosages up to maximum of 4 mg daily. To achieve 4 mg daily, increase dosage in increments of 0.125 to 0.25 mg b.i.d. every 3 days, as tolerated, until panic disorder is controlled or adverse effects make further increases undesired. Taper drug with decrease of 0.125 mg b.i.d. every 3 days until drug is stopped.

ADMINISTRATION
PO

• Have patient swallow tablets whole with water. Give ODT to patient with or without water.

• Peel back the foil of the ODT pouch carefully. Don't push ODT through foil.

• Pharmacist can prepare oral suspension from tablets if necessary for younger patients.

ACTION

Unknown. Probably acts by facilitating the effects of the inhibitory neurotransmitter GABA.

Route	Onset	Peak	Duration
PO	20–40 min	1–4 hr	6–12 hr

Half-life: Adults, 17 to 60 hours; children, 22 to 33 hours.

ADVERSE REACTIONS

CNS: amnesia, aphonia, choreiform movements, coma, confusion, depression, dysarthria, dysdiadochokinesis, "glassy-eyed" appearance, hallucinations, headache, hemiparesis, hypotonia, hysteria, increased libido, insomnia, psychosis, slurred speech, tremor, vertigo, paradoxical reactions

---

Reactions in bold italics are *life-threatening*. Interactions may have a *rapid onset* or a ***delayed onset***.

(aggressive behavior, agitation, anxiety, excitability, hostility, irritability, nervousness, nightmares and vivid dreams, sleep disturbances), fever, ataxia, abnormal coordination, somnolence, dizziness, nervousness, reduced intellectual ability. **CV:** palpitations. **EENT:** abnormal eye movements, diplopia, nystagmus, blurred vision, pharyngitis, rhinitis, sinusitis. **GI:** anorexia, coated tongue, constipation, diarrhea, dry mouth, encopresis, gastritis, increased or decreased appetite, nausea, sore gums, abdominal pain. **GU:** dysuria, enuresis, nocturia, urine retention, colpitis, dysmenorrhea, delayed ejaculation, erectile dysfunction, urinary frequency, UTI. **Hematologic:** anemia, eosinophilia, *leukopenia, thrombocytopenia.* **Hepatic:** hepatomegaly, transient elevations of serum transaminases and alkaline phosphatase. **Metabolic:** dehydration, weight loss or gain. **Musculoskeletal:** muscle weakness, muscle pains. **Respiratory:** chest congestion, hypersecretion in upper respiratory tract passages, respiratory depression, rhinorrhea, shortness of breath, bronchitis, URI, cough. **Skin:** hair loss, hirsutism, rash. **Other:** ankle and facial edema, general deterioration, lymphadenopathy, allergic reaction, influenza.

INTERACTIONS
Drug-drug. *Carbamazepine, phenobarbital, phenytoin:* May lower clonazepam levels. Monitor patient closely.
Clozapine: May increase clozapine-related toxicities. Consider therapy modification.
CNS depressants: May increase CNS depression. Avoid using together.
Digoxin: May increase digoxin level and toxicity. Monitor digoxin level.
Fluconazole, itraconazole, ketoconazole, miconazole: May increase and prolong drug levels, CNS depression, and psychomotor impairment. Avoid using together.
Methadone: May increase potential for fatal respiratory depression. Use cautiously.
Olanzapine: May enhance clonazepam-related toxicity. Avoid concomitant use with IM olanzapine due to risks of additive adverse events.
Black Box Warning *Opioids:* May cause slow or difficult breathing, sedation, and death. Avoid use together. If use together is

necessary, limit dosage and duration of each drug to the minimum necessary for desired effect. ▮
Protease inhibitors (nelfinavir, ritonavir): May cause severe respiratory depression. Monitor patient carefully.
SSRIs: May enhance adverse/toxic effects of SSRIs and increase risk of psychomotor impairment. Monitor patient closely.
Thalidomide: May enhance CNS depressant effect of thalidomide. Avoid concurrent use.
Theophylline: May decrease clonazepam effects. Monitor patient closely.
Valproic acid: May increase clonazepam toxicity and absence status and increase seizure risk and teratogenic effects of both drugs in first trimester. Use cautiously.
Drug-herb. *St. John's wort:* May decrease clonazepam serum concentration, resulting in decreased drug effects. Consider therapy modification.
Drug-lifestyle. *Alcohol use:* May cause additive CNS effects. Discourage use together.

EFFECTS ON LAB TEST RESULTS
• May increase LFT values and eosinophil count. May decrease platelet and WBC counts.

CONTRAINDICATIONS & CAUTIONS
Black Box Warning *Opioid class warning:* Opioids should only be prescribed with benzodiazepines or other CNS depressants to patients for whom alternative treatment options are inadequate. ▮
• Contraindicated in patients hypersensitive to benzodiazepines and in those with significant hepatic disease or acute angle-closure glaucoma.
• Use cautiously in patients with mixed-type seizures because drug may cause generalized tonic-clonic seizures.
• Use cautiously in children; in patients with chronic respiratory disease, open-angle glaucoma, porphyria, or a history of drug or alcohol addiction; and in those at risk for falls.
• Use cautiously in elderly patients. Drug may accumulate due to potential decrease in hepatic and renal function.
Dialyzable drug: No.
⚠ **Overdose S&S:** Somnolence, confusion, coma, diminished reflexes.

PREGNANCY-LACTATION-REPRODUCTION

• Drug may cause fetal harm. Use during pregnancy only if clearly needed and potential benefit justifies potential risk to the fetus.

• Drug may cause neonatal flaccidity, respiratory and feeding difficulties, and hypothermia in infants born to women who received benzodiazepines late in pregnancy. In addition, neonates born to women who received benzodiazepines late in pregnancy may be at some risk for experiencing withdrawal symptoms during the postnatal period.

• Encourage women who are taking drug during pregnancy to register in the North American AED Pregnancy Registry (1-888-233-2334 or www.aedpregnancyregistry. org); registration must be done by patients themselves.

• Drug appears in human milk. Patient should discontinue breastfeeding or discontinue drug, taking into account importance of drug to the mother.

NURSING CONSIDERATIONS

❸ Alert: Closely monitor all patients for changes in behavior that may indicate worsening of suicidal thoughts or behavior or depression.

• Don't stop drug abruptly because this may worsen seizures. Notify prescriber at once if adverse reactions develop.

• Assess elderly patient's response closely. Elderly patients are more sensitive to drug's CNS effects.

• Monitor patient for oversedation.

• Monitor CBC and LFTs.

• Withdrawal symptoms are similar to those of barbiturates.

• To reduce inconvenience of somnolence when drug is used for panic disorder, giving one dose at bedtime may be desirable.

Black Box Warning Monitor patient taking an opioid concomitantly with clonazepam for signs and symptoms of respiratory depression and sedation. ∎

• **Look alike–sound alike:** Don't confuse clonazepam with clonidine, clozapine, or lorazepam. Don't confuse Klonopin with clonidine.

PATIENT TEACHING

Black Box Warning Caution patient or caregiver of patient taking an opioid with a benzodiazepine, CNS depressant, or alcohol to seek immediate medical attention for dizziness, light-headedness, extreme sleepiness, slowed or difficult breathing, or unresponsiveness. ∎

• Advise patient to avoid driving and other hazardous activities that require mental alertness until drug's CNS effects are known.

• Instruct parent to monitor child's school performance because drug may interfere with attentiveness.

• Warn patient and parents not to stop drug abruptly because seizures may occur.

• Advise patient that drug isn't for use during pregnancy or breastfeeding.

• Tell patient to open pouch of ODTs and peel back the foil. Advise patient not to push the tablet *through* the foil.

• Tell patient to use dry hands when removing the ODT.

• Tell patient that ODTs can be taken with or without water but that regular tablets should be swallowed whole with water.

cloNIDine
KLOE-ni-deen

cloNIDine hydrochloride
Catapres, Catapres-TTS, Duraclon, Kapvay

Therapeutic class: Antihypertensives
Pharmacologic class: Centrally acting alpha agonists

AVAILABLE FORMS
Injection for epidural use: 100 mcg/mL
Injection for epidural use, concentrate: 500 mcg/mL
Tablets: 0.1 mg, 0.2 mg, 0.3 mg
Tablets (extended-release) ⓄⓃⒼ: 0.1 mg
Transdermal: 0.1 mg/24 hours, 0.2 mg/ 24 hours, 0.3 mg/24 hours

INDICATIONS & DOSAGES
➤ **Essential and renal HTN**
Adults: Initially, 0.1 mg PO b.i.d.; then increased by 0.1 mg daily on a weekly basis.

Reactions in bold italics are *life-threatening*. Interactions may have a *rapid onset* or a ***delayed onset***.

Usual range is 0.2 to 0.6 mg daily in divided doses; infrequently, dosages as high as 2.4 mg daily are used.

Or, apply transdermal patch once every 7 days, starting with 0.1-mg system and adjusted with another 0.1-mg or larger system after 1 or 2 weeks if desired BP reduction isn't achieved. Don't exceed concurrent use of two clonidine 0.3-mg transdermal systems.

➤ **Severe cancer pain that is unresponsive to epidural or spinal opiate analgesia or other more conventional methods of analgesia**

Adults: Initially, 30 mcg/hour by continuous epidural infusion. Experience with rates greater than 40 mcg/hour is limited.

Children old enough to tolerate placement and management of an epidural catheter: Initially, 0.5 mcg/kg/hour by epidural infusion. Dosage should be cautiously adjusted, based on response.

➤ **ADHD as monotherapy or as adjunctive therapy to stimulant medications**

Children ages 6 to 17: Initially, 0.1 mg extended-release tablet (Kapvay) PO at bedtime. Adjust by 0.1 mg/day at weekly intervals to desired response. With first dosage increase, give tablets b.i.d., with equal or higher dose given at bedtime. Maximum dose is 0.4 mg/day.

ADMINISTRATION

PO
• Don't crush, break, or allow patient to chew extended-release tablets.
• Immediate-release and extended-release forms can't be substituted on a milligram-per-milligram basis.
• Give last dose immediately before bedtime.
• Reduce dosage gradually over 2 to 4 days before discontinuing. Decrease dosage of extended-release form by no more than 0.1 mg every 3 to 7 days.

Transdermal
• Apply patch to nonhairy area of intact skin on upper arm or torso.
• When converting from oral to patch form, place patch on patient and gradually decrease oral dose over several days. Antihypertensive effect of patch takes 2 to 3 days to appear.

Epidural
Black Box Warning The injection form concentrate, containing 500 mcg/mL, must be diluted in NSS injection before use to yield 100 mcg/mL. ■
❸ Alert: The injection form must not be used with a preservative.

ACTION

Unknown. Thought to stimulate alpha$_2$ receptors and inhibit the central vasomotor centers, decreasing sympathetic outflow to the heart, kidneys, and peripheral vasculature and lowering peripheral vascular resistance, BP, and HR.

Route	Onset	Peak	Duration
PO (immediate-release)	30–60 min	1–3 hr	6–10 hr
PO (extended-release)	1–2 wk	7–8 hr	Unknown
Transdermal	2–3 days	3 days	7 days
Epidural	Unknown	30–60 min	Unknown

Half-life: Immediate- and extended-release, 12 to 16 hours; transdermal, 20 hours; epidural, 1 to 2 hours.

ADVERSE REACTIONS

CNS: drowsiness, dizziness, sedation, weakness, fatigue, malaise, agitation, depression.
CV: *bradycardia, severe rebound HTN,* orthostatic hypotension. **GI:** constipation, dry mouth, nausea, vomiting, anorexia.
GU: urine retention, erectile dysfunction.
Metabolic: weight gain. **Skin:** pruritus, dermatitis with transdermal patch, rash. **Other:** loss of libido.

INTERACTIONS

Drug-drug. *Amitriptyline, amoxapine, clomipramine, desipramine, doxepin, imipramine, mirtazapine, nortriptyline, protriptyline, trimipramine:* May cause loss of BP control with life-threatening elevations in BP. Avoid using together.
Beta blockers: May cause life-threatening HTN. Closely monitor BP.
CNS depressants: May increase CNS depression. Use together cautiously.
Digoxin, verapamil: May cause AV block and severe hypotension. Monitor BP and ECG.

♣Canada   ◇OTC   ◆ Off-label use   𝒫 Photoguide   ⓓ Do not crush   *Liquid contains alcohol   ✺ Genetic

Diuretics, other antihypertensives: May increase hypotensive effect. Monitor patient closely.

Levodopa: May reduce effectiveness of levodopa. Monitor patient.

Drug-herb. *Capsicum:* May reduce antihypertensive effectiveness. Discourage use together.

Ma huang: May decrease antihypertensive effects. Discourage use together.

EFFECTS ON LAB TEST RESULTS

• May decrease urinary excretion of vanillylmandelic acid and catecholamines. May cause a weakly positive Coombs test result.

CONTRAINDICATIONS & CAUTIONS

• Contraindicated in patients hypersensitive to drug.

• Transdermal form is contraindicated in patients hypersensitive to any component of the adhesive layer of transdermal system.

• Epidural form is contraindicated in patients receiving anticoagulant therapy, in those with bleeding diathesis, in those with an injection-site infection, and in those who are hemodynamically unstable or have severe CV disease.

• Use cautiously in patients with severe coronary insufficiency, conduction disturbances, recent MI, cerebrovascular disease, chronic renal failure, or impaired liver function.

• Safety and effectiveness in children for essential and renal HTN haven't been established in adequate and well-controlled trials.

Dialyzable drug: No.

⚠ **Overdose S&S:** Early HTN, then hypotension; bradycardia; respiratory and CNS depression; hypothermia; drowsiness; decreased or absent reflexes; weakness; irritability; miosis. With large overdoses: Reversible cardiac conduction defects or arrhythmias, apnea, coma, seizures.

PREGNANCY-LACTATION-REPRODUCTION

• There are no adequate well-controlled studies in pregnant women. Use during pregnancy only if clearly needed and potential benefit justifies potential risk to the fetus.

Black Box Warning Epidural clonidine isn't recommended for obstetric, postpartum, or perioperative pain management due to the risk of hemodynamic instability, especially hypotension and bradycardia, except in rare cases in which the potential benefits outweigh the risks. ■

• Drug appears in human milk. Patient should discontinue breastfeeding or discontinue drug, taking into account importance of drug to the mother.

NURSING CONSIDERATIONS

• Drug may be given to lower BP rapidly in some hypertensive emergencies.

• Monitor BP and pulse rate frequently. Dosage is usually adjusted to patient's BP and tolerance.

• Elderly patients may be more sensitive than younger ones to drug's hypotensive effects.

• Observe patient for tolerance to drug's therapeutic effects, which may require increased dosage.

• Noticeable antihypertensive effects of transdermal clonidine may take 2 to 3 days. Oral antihypertensive therapy may have to be continued in the interim; wean patient from oral dose in the 2 to 3 days after first patch is applied.

⚠ **Alert:** Remove transdermal patch before defibrillation or cardioversion to prevent arcing.

• Stop drug gradually by reducing dosage over 2 to 4 days to avoid rapid rise in BP, agitation, headache, and tremor. When stopping therapy in patients receiving both clonidine and a beta blocker, gradually withdraw the beta blocker several days before gradually stopping clonidine to minimize adverse reactions.

• Don't stop drug before surgery.

• When drug is given epidurally, carefully monitor infusion pump, and inspect catheter tubing for obstruction or dislodgment.

• *Look alike–sound alike:* Don't confuse clonidine with clonazepam, clozapine, Klonopin, quinidine, or clomiphene.

PATIENT TEACHING

• Instruct patient to take drug exactly as prescribed and to report adverse reactions.

• Advise patient that stopping drug abruptly may cause severe high rebound BP; dosage must be reduced gradually over 2 to 4 days, as instructed by prescriber.

Reactions in bold italics are *life-threatening*. Interactions may have a *rapid onset* or a *delayed onset*.

• Tell patient to take the last dose immediately before bedtime.
• Reassure patient that the transdermal patch usually remains attached despite showering and other routine daily activities. Instruct patient on the use of the adhesive overlay to provide additional skin adherence, if needed. Also tell patient to place patch at a different site each week.
• Caution patient that drug may cause drowsiness but that this adverse effect usually diminishes over 4 to 6 weeks.
• Inform patient that dizziness upon standing can be minimized by rising slowly from a sitting or lying position and avoiding sudden position changes.
• Advise patient that, if an MRI is scheduled, to alert the facility about wearing a transdermal patch.

---

clopidogrel bisulfate 🔯
cloe-PID-oh-grel

Plavix⬙

Therapeutic class: Antiplatelet drugs
Pharmacologic class: Platelet aggregation inhibitors

AVAILABLE FORMS
Tablets: 75 mg, 300 mg

INDICATIONS & DOSAGES
➤ **To reduce rate of MI and stroke in patients with established peripheral arterial disease or history of recent MI or stroke**
Adults: 75 mg PO daily.
➤ **To reduce rate of MI and stroke in patients with unstable angina/non-ST-elevation MI (NSTEMI), including those managed medically and those managed with coronary revascularization; to reduce rate of MI and stroke in patients with acute ST-elevation MI (STEMI) who are to be managed medically**
Adults: Initially, a single 300-mg PO loading dose; then 75 mg PO once daily. Start and continue aspirin with clopidogrel. Initiating clopidogrel without a loading dose will delay (by several days) establishing antiplatelet effects.

ADMINISTRATION
PO
• Give drug without regard to meals.
• Patient shouldn't consume grapefruit or grapefruit juice.

ACTION
Inhibits the binding of the P2Y12 component of ADP to its platelet receptor, impeding ADP-mediated activation and subsequent platelet aggregation, and irreversibly modifies the platelet ADP receptor.

Route	Onset	Peak	Duration
PO	2 hr	45 min	5 days

Half-life: 6 hours.

ADVERSE REACTIONS
CNS: confusion, *fatal intracranial bleeding,* hallucinations, headache. **CV:** hypotension, *hemorrhage at any site.* **EENT:** epistaxis, rhinitis, taste disorder. **GI:** *hemorrhage,* abdominal pain, constipation, diarrhea, dyspepsia, gastritis, ulcers. **GU:** UTI, hematuria. **Hematologic:** *thrombotic thrombocytopenic purpura.* **Musculoskeletal:** arthralgia, myalgia, arthritis. **Respiratory:** *bronchospasm,* interstitial pneumonitis, respiratory tract bleeding. **Skin:** rash, pruritus, bruising, eczema, *erythema multiforme,* urticaria, *SJS, toxic epidermal necrolysis.* **Other:** flulike syndrome, *angioedema, anaphylaxis,* serum sickness.

INTERACTIONS
Drug-drug. *Apixaban, dabigatran, edoxaban, rivaroxaban:* May increase risk of bleeding. Use together cautiously.
Aspirin, NSAIDs: May increase risk of GI bleeding. Monitor patient.
Bupropion: May elevate bupropion plasma concentration. Closely monitor patient and adjust bupropion dosage as needed when clopidogrel is started or stopped.
Macrolides: May inhibit antiplatelet effect. Adjust clopidogrel dosage as needed. Consider using azithromycin if a macrolide is necessary.
Repaglinide: May increase repaglinide serum concentration. Avoid use together.
Rifamycins: May increase antiplatelet effect. Carefully monitor platelet function when starting, stopping, or changing

---

rifamycin dosage. Adjust clopidogrel dosage as needed.

Salicylates: May increase the risk of serious bleeding in patients with TIA or ischemic stroke. Avoid use together.

Strong or moderate CYP2C19 inhibitors (cimetidine, esomeprazole, etravirine, felbamate, fluconazole, fluoxetine, fluvoxamine, ketoconazole, omeprazole, ticlopidine, voriconazole), PPIs: May decrease effects of clopidogrel. Avoid use together.

Warfarin: May increase risk of bleeding. Use together cautiously.

Drug-herb. *Herbs with antiplatelet activity (capsicum, fenugreek, garlic, ginkgo biloba, turmeric, many others):* May increase risk of bleeding. Discourage use together.

Drug-food. *Grapefruit, grapefruit juice:* May reduce drug's antiplatelet effects. Avoid use together.

EFFECTS ON LAB TEST RESULTS
• May decrease platelet count.

CONTRAINDICATIONS & CAUTIONS
• Contraindicated in patients hypersensitive to drug or its components, in those with a history of hypersensitivity or hematologic reaction to other thienopyridines, and in those with pathologic bleeding (such as peptic ulcer or intracranial hemorrhage).
• Hypersensitivity reactions, including rash, angioedema, and hematologic reactions, have been reported.
• Consider discontinuing drug 5 days before elective surgery, including elective CABG. Platelet aggregation won't return to normal for at least 5 days after drug has been stopped.
• Premature interruption of therapy may result in stent thrombosis with subsequent fatal or nonfatal MI. Duration of therapy, in general, is determined by type of stent placed (bare metal or drug eluting) and whether an ACS event was ongoing at the time of placement.
• Use cautiously in patients at risk for increased bleeding from trauma, surgery, or other pathologic conditions and in those with renal or hepatic impairment.

Dialyzable drug: Unknown.

⚠ *Overdose S&S:* Prolonged bleeding time, bleeding complications.

PREGNANCY-LACTATION-REPRODUCTION
• Information related to use during pregnancy is limited. Use cautiously in pregnant women and only if clearly needed.
• It isn't known if drug appears in human milk. Patient should discontinue breastfeeding or discontinue drug, taking into account importance of drug to the mother.

NURSING CONSIDERATIONS
▧ **Black Box Warning** Drug effectiveness depends on the drug's activation to an active metabolite by the cytochrome P450 system, principally CYP2C19. Patients who are poor metabolizers form less of the active metabolite and the effects of the drug on platelet activity are reduced. Tests are available to assess a patient's CYP2C19 genotype. Consider alternative treatment for patients identified as poor metabolizers. ▮
▧ Approximately 2% of White patients and 4% of Black patients are poor metabolizers of CYP2C19 and the prevalence is higher in Asian patients (14% of Chinese patients).
❸ *Alert:* Drug may cause fatal thrombotic thrombocytopenic purpura (thrombocytopenia, hemolytic anemia, neurologic findings, renal dysfunction, and fever) that requires urgent treatment, including plasmapheresis.
• *Look alike–sound alike:* Don't confuse Plavix with Paxil.

PATIENT TEACHING
• Advise patient that it may take longer than usual to stop bleeding and to refrain from activities in which trauma and bleeding may occur. Encourage patient to wear a seat belt when in a car.
• Instruct patient to notify prescriber if unusual bleeding or bruising occurs.
• Tell patient to inform all health care providers, including dentists, before undergoing procedures or starting new drug therapy, about taking drug.
• Inform patient that drug may be taken without regard to meals.

Reactions in bold italics are *life-threatening*. Interactions may have a *rapid onset* or a *delayed onset*.

clotrimazole
kloe-TRIM-a-zole

Canesten❋, Clotrimaderm❋, Cruex ◇, Desenex ◇, Lotrimin AF Cream ◇, Trivagizole 3 ◇

Therapeutic class: Antifungals
Pharmacologic class: Imidazole derivatives

AVAILABLE FORMS
Combination pack: Vaginal suppositories 100 mg and vulvar cream 1% ◇, vaginal tablets 200 mg and vulvar cream 1% ◇
Topical cream: 1%
Topical lotion: 1%
Topical solution: 1%
Troches (lozenges) ⓪: 10 mg
Vaginal cream: 1% ◇, 2% ◇
Vaginal suppositories: 100 mg ◇, 200 mg ◇
Vaginal tablets: 100 mg ◇, 200 mg❋ ◇, 500 mg❋ ◇

INDICATIONS & DOSAGES
➤ **Superficial fungal infections (tinea corporis, tinea cruris, tinea pedis, tinea versicolor, candidiasis)**
Adults and children age 2 and older: Apply thin film and massage into affected and surrounding area b.i.d., morning and evening, for 2 to 4 weeks. If improvement doesn't occur after 4 weeks, reevaluate patient.
➤ **Vulvovaginal candidiasis**
Adults and children age 12 and older: One 100-mg vaginal suppository inserted daily at bedtime for 7 consecutive days. Or, one 200-mg vaginal suppository at bedtime for 3 days. Or, 1 applicatorful of vaginal cream daily at bedtime for 3 days (2%) or 7 days (1%).
➤ **Oropharyngeal candidiasis**
Adults and children age 3 and older: Patient should dissolve lozenge in mouth over 15 to 30 minutes five times daily for 14 consecutive days. When drug is used for initial treatment in patients with HIV-1 infection, duration of therapy is 7 to 14 days.
➤ **To prevent oropharyngeal candidiasis in patients immunocompromised by chemotherapy, radiotherapy, or corticosteroid therapy in the treatment of leukemia, solid tumors, or renal transplantation**
Adults: Patient should dissolve lozenge in mouth over 15 to 30 minutes t.i.d. for duration of chemotherapy or until corticosteroid is reduced to maintenance levels.

ADMINISTRATION
PO
• Lozenges should dissolve in mouth and not be chewed, for full benefit.
Topical
• Clean and dry area before applying drug.
• Don't use occlusive wrappings or dressings.
Vaginal
• Insert suppository high into vagina.
• Applicators for cream and some suppositories are disposable. If not disposable, wash applicator with soap and warm water immediately after use. Rinse thoroughly and dry.

ACTION
Fungistatic or fungicidal, depending on level. Alters fungal cell-wall permeability and produces osmotic instability.

Route	Onset	Peak	Duration
PO	Unknown	Unknown	3 hr
Topical, vaginal	Unknown	Unknown	Unknown

Half-life: Unknown.

ADVERSE REACTIONS
GI: lower abdominal cramps, nausea and vomiting with lozenges. **GU:** mild vaginal burning or irritation, urinary frequency. **Skin:** erythema, blistering, burning, edema, general irritation, peeling, pruritus, skin fissures, stinging, urticaria.

INTERACTIONS
None significant.

EFFECTS ON LAB TEST RESULTS
• May increase liver enzyme levels.

CONTRAINDICATIONS & CAUTIONS
• Contraindicated in patients hypersensitive to drug.
• Contraindicated for ophthalmic use.
Dialyzable drug: Unknown.

PREGNANCY-LACTATION-REPRODUCTION
• There are no adequate studies in pregnant women. Use lozenges during pregnancy only if potential benefit justifies potential risk to the fetus.
• Use topical clotrimazole during first trimester only if clearly indicated.
• Manual insertion may be preferred over use of vaginal applicator. Use only on advice of physician.
• It's unknown if drug appears in human milk. Use cautiously in breastfeeding women. Patient should consider discontinuing breastfeeding.

NURSING CONSIDERATIONS
• Consult prescriber before using topical preparations in children younger than age 2. Don't use troches in children younger than age 3; don't use vaginal preparations in children younger than age 12.
• Watch for irritation or sensitivity; stop if irritation occurs, and notify prescriber.
• Improvement usually occurs within 1 week; if no improvement is seen within 4 weeks, review diagnosis.

PATIENT TEACHING
• Reassure patient that hypopigmentation from tinea versicolor will resolve gradually.
• Warn patient not to use occlusive wrappings or dressings.
• Warn patient to avoid contact with eyes.
• Caution patient that frequent or persistent yeast infections may suggest a more serious medical problem.
• Tell patient to refrain from sexual intercourse during vaginal treatment.
• Warn patient that topical preparation may stain clothing.
• Tell patient that using a sanitary napkin protects clothing when using vaginal preparation.
• Stress need to continue use of vaginal preparations, as prescribed, even if menstruation begins.
• Tell patient with athlete's foot to change shoes and cotton socks daily and to dry between the toes after bathing.
• Tell patient to allow lozenges to dissolve in mouth and not to chew, for full benefit.

• Stress need to continue treatment for full course and to notify prescriber if no improvement occurs after 4 weeks.

SAFETY ALERT!

cloZAPine ⌧
KLOE-za-peen

Clozaril⧸, FazaClo ODT, Versacloz

Therapeutic class: Antipsychotics
Pharmacologic class: Dibenzapine derivatives

AVAILABLE FORMS
Oral suspension: 50 mg/mL
Tablets: 25 mg, 50 mg, 100 mg, 200 mg
Tablets (ODTs): 12.5 mg, 25 mg, 100 mg, 150 mg, 200 mg

INDICATIONS & DOSAGES
➤ **Schizophrenia in severely ill patients unresponsive to other therapies; to reduce risk of recurrent suicidal behavior in schizophrenia or schizoaffective disorders**
Adults: Initially, 12.5 mg PO once daily or b.i.d. Adjust dose upward by 25 to 50 mg daily (if tolerated) to 300 to 450 mg daily by end of 2 weeks. Individual dosage is based on clinical response, patient tolerance, and adverse reactions. Subsequent dosage shouldn't be increased more than once or twice weekly and shouldn't exceed 100-mg increments. Don't exceed 900 mg daily. For the general population, if ANC is 1,500/mm^3 or greater (normal baseline range), treatment may be initiated. Confirm all initial reports of ANC less than 1,500/mm^3 with a repeat ANC within 24 hours. For patients with benign ethnic neutropenia (BEN), obtain two baseline ANC levels before initiating treatment (normal ANC range for those with BEN is 1,000/mm^3 or greater). For patients with BEN, if ANC is 1,000/mm^3 or greater, treatment may be initiated. When restarting drug in those who have discontinued clozapine for 2 days or more, re-initiate at 12.5 mg once daily or b.i.d. to minimize the risk of hypotension, bradycardia, and syncope. If that dose is well tolerated, the dose may be increased to the previously therapeutic dose

more quickly than recommended for initial treatment.

𝕾 *Adjust-a-dose:* Refer to manufacturer's instructions for ANC monitoring and dosage interruption for neutropenia, and for concurrent use with CYP1A2, CYP2D6, or CYP3A4 inhibitors or CYP1A2 or CYP3A4 inducers. Reduce dosages in those with significant renal or hepatic impairment and in those who are poor metabolizers of CYP2D6.

Discontinue drug in those with QT interval greater than 500 msec, those with symptoms of ventricular arrhythmias, or those with cardiomyopathy/myocarditis or NMS.

ADMINISTRATION
PO
• Give with or without food.
• May divide total daily dose into uneven doses, with larger dose given at bedtime.
• Peel the foil from the ODT blister and gently remove the tablet immediately before giving. Don't push tablet through foil.
• Give ODT with or without water.
• Shake bottle for 10 seconds before withdrawing suspension using provided oral syringe and syringe adaptor.

ACTION
Unknown. Binds selectively to dopaminergic receptors in the CNS and may interfere with adrenergic, cholinergic, histaminergic, and serotonergic receptors.

Route	Onset	Peak	Duration
PO	Unknown	1–6 hr	4–12 hr

Half-life: Proportional to dose; may range from 4 to 66 hours.

ADVERSE REACTIONS
CNS: drowsiness, sedation, dizziness, vertigo, headache, *seizures,* syncope, tremor, disturbed sleep or nightmares, restlessness, hypokinesia or akinesia, agitation, rigidity, akathisia, confusion, fatigue, insomnia, hyperkinesia, weakness, lethargy, ataxia, slurred speech, depression, myoclonus, anxiety, fever. **CV:** tachycardia, hypotension, HTN, chest pain, ECG changes, orthostatic hypotension. **EENT:** visual disturbances. **GI:** constipation, excessive salivation, dry mouth, nausea, vomiting, heartburn,

diarrhea. **GU:** urinary frequency or urgency, urine retention, incontinence, abnormal ejaculation. **Hematologic:** *leukopenia, neutropenia,* eosinophilia. **Metabolic:** hyperglycemia, weight gain, hypercholesterolemia, hypertriglyceridemia. **Musculoskeletal:** muscle pain or spasm, muscle weakness. **Respiratory:** *respiratory arrest.* **Skin:** rash, diaphoresis.

INTERACTIONS
Drug-drug. *Anticholinergics:* May potentiate anticholinergic effects of clozapine. Use together cautiously.
Antihypertensives: May potentiate hypotensive effects. Monitor BP.
❶ *Alert: Benzodiazepines, other psychotropic drugs:* May increase risk of sedation and CV and respiratory arrest. Use together cautiously.
Bone marrow suppressants: May increase bone marrow toxicity. Avoid using together.
Citalopram, *fluoroquinolones,* **fluoxetine, fluvoxamine,** *paroxetine,* **sertraline:** May increase clozapine levels and toxicity. Adjust clozapine dose as needed.
CYP1A2 inducers (tobacco smoking): May decrease clozapine effectiveness. Increase clozapine dosage as necessary.
CYP2D6 or CYP3A4 inhibitors (bupropion, cimetidine, duloxetine, erythromycin, escitalopram, fluoxetine, paroxetine, quinidine, sertraline, terbinafine); moderate or weak CYP1A2 inhibitors (caffeine, oral contraceptives): Monitor patient for adverse reactions. Reduce clozapine oral dosage if necessary.
Digoxin, other highly protein-bound drugs, warfarin: May increase levels of these drugs. Monitor patient closely for adverse reactions.
Drugs that prolong the QT interval (antiarrhythmics, citalopram, ziprasidone): May increase risk of prolonged QT interval and ventricular arrhythmias. Avoid use together.
Black Box Warning *Opioid class warning:* May cause slow or difficult breathing, sedation, and death. Avoid use together. If use together is necessary, limit dosage and duration of each drug to the minimum necessary for desired effect. ■
Phenytoin: May decrease clozapine level and cause breakthrough psychosis. Monitor

patient for psychosis and adjust clozapine dosage.

Psychoactive drugs: May cause additive effects. Use together cautiously.

Ritonavir: May increase clozapine levels and toxicity. Avoid using together.

Strong CYP3A4 inducers (carbamazepine, phenytoin, rifampin): May decrease clozapine effectiveness. Use together isn't recommended. If coadministration is necessary, consider increasing clozapine dosage.

Strong CYP1A2 inhibitors (ciprofloxacin, fluvoxamine): May increase clozapine level. Reduce clozapine dosage to ⅓ during coadministration.

Drug-herb. *St. John's wort:* May decrease drug level. Discourage use together.

Drug-lifestyle. *Alcohol use:* May increase CNS depression. Discourage use together.

Smoking: May decrease drug level. Urge patient to quit smoking. Monitor patient for effectiveness and adjust dosage.

EFFECTS ON LAB TEST RESULTS
• May increase glucose, cholesterol, and triglyceride levels.
• May increase eosinophil count. May decrease granulocyte, WBC counts, and ANC.

CONTRAINDICATIONS & CAUTIONS
Black Box Warning Because of risk of severe neutropenia, which can lead to fatal infections, drug is available only through the Clozapine REMS Program. Prescribers, patients, and dispensing pharmacists must enroll in the program and be certified. More information is available at www.clozapinerems.com or by calling 1-844-267-8678. ∎

Black Box Warning Obtain CBC with differential before initiating treatment: ANC must be at least 1,500/mm³ for the general population and must be at least 1,000/mm³ for patients with documented BEN. Monitor ANC regularly during treatment. ∎

Black Box Warning *Opioid class warning:* Opioids should only be prescribed with benzodiazepines or other CNS depressants to patients for whom alternative treatment options are inadequate. ∎

• Contraindicated in patients with a history of serious hypersensitivity to drug or its components, in patients who experienced clozapine-induced agranulocytosis or severe granulocytopenia, and in patients with uncontrolled epilepsy.

• Closely monitor patients taking other drugs that suppress bone marrow function.

• Use cautiously in patients with prostatic hyperplasia or angle-closure glaucoma because drug has potent anticholinergic effects. Severe GI reactions (constipation, intestinal obstruction, fecal impaction, paralytic ileus) can also occur.

Black Box Warning Fatal myocarditis and cardiomyopathy may occur at any time during treatment. If signs or symptoms (chest pain, tachycardia, palpitations, dyspnea, fever, flulike symptoms, hypotension, ECG changes) occur, obtain a cardiac evaluation, and discontinue drug. Generally, patients with clozapine-related myocarditis or cardiomyopathy shouldn't be re-challenged with the drug. ∎

• Drug is associated with development of eosinophilia, which usually occurs during the first month of treatment. Eosinophilia has been associated with organ involvement (myocarditis, pancreatitis, hepatitis, colitis, nephritis) and could be consistent with a drug-induced hypersensitivity syndrome. If eosinophilia develops, evaluate for signs and symptoms of systemic reactions and, if clozapine-related disease is suspected, discontinue drug immediately. If a cause for eosinophilia unrelated to clozapine is identified, the underlying cause should be treated and clozapine may be continued.

• Drug is associated with QT-interval prolongation and life-threatening ventricular arrhythmias. Use caution in those with risk factors for QT-interval prolongation or serious CV reactions and in those taking drugs known to prolong the QT interval. Consider obtaining a baseline ECG and serum chemistry panel, and correct electrolyte abnormalities before starting treatment. Discontinue clozapine if QTc interval is greater than 500 msec. Obtain a cardiac evaluation and discontinue drug if patient has symptoms of torsades de pointes or other arrhythmias (syncope, presyncope, dizziness, palpitations).

• Drug can cause NMS, which can be fatal. If signs and symptoms of NMS (hyperpyrexia, muscle rigidity, altered mental

---

status, irregular pulse, fluctuating BP, tachycardia, diaphoresis, cardiac arrhythmias, elevated CK level, myoglobinuria, rhabdomyolysis, acute renal failure) occur, discontinue drug and begin appropriate treatment and monitoring.

• Tardive dyskinesia (TD), a syndrome of potentially irreversible, involuntary dyskinetic movements, has occurred in patients taking antipsychotics. Use the lowest effective dosage for the shortest duration possible. Consider discontinuing drug if TD occurs. (*Note:* Some patients may require treatment despite TD.)

• Somnolence, orthostatic hypotension, and motor and sensory instability have been reported, which may lead to falls and, consequently, fractures or other fall-related injuries.

• Elderly patients may have an increased sensitivity to anticholinergic effects of drug; sedating effects of drug may increase the risk of falls in this population.

• Safe and effective use in children hasn't been established.

Dialyzable drug: No.

⚠ *Overdose S&S:* Altered state of consciousness, drowsiness, delirium, coma, tachycardia, hypotension, respiratory depression or failure, hypersalivation, aspiration pneumonia, cardiac arrhythmias, seizures.

PREGNANCY-LACTATION-REPRODUCTION

• There are no adequate studies in pregnant women. Use during pregnancy only if clearly needed and potential benefit justifies potential risk to the fetus.

🖲 *Alert:* Neonates exposed to antipsychotics during the third trimester of pregnancy are at risk for developing extrapyramidal signs and symptoms (repetitive muscle movements of the face and body) and withdrawal symptoms (agitation, abnormally increased or decreased muscle tone, tremors, sleepiness, severe difficulty breathing, and difficulty feeding) after delivery.

• Drug appears in human milk. Women receiving drug shouldn't breastfeed.

NURSING CONSIDERATIONS

🖲 *Alert:* Drug may cause hyperglycemia. Monitor patients with diabetes regularly. In patients with risk factors for diabetes, obtain fasting blood glucose test results at baseline and periodically.

🖲 *Alert:* Monitor patient for metabolic syndrome, including significant weight gain and increased BMI, HTN, hyperglycemia, hypercholesterolemia, and hypertriglyceridemia.

• Monitor patient for signs and symptoms of myocarditis and cardiomyopathy.

Black Box Warning Orthostatic hypotension, with or without syncope and bradycardia, can occur. Rarely, collapse can be profound and be accompanied by respiratory or cardiac arrest. Orthostatic hypotension is more likely to occur during initial titration with rapid dose escalation and can occur with the first dose and with doses as low as 12.5 mg. Start treatment with 12.5 mg once daily or b.i.d. and titrate slowly using divided dosages. Use caution in patients with CV or cerebrovascular disease or conditions that may cause hypotension. ∎

Black Box Warning Seizures may occur, especially in patients receiving high doses. Begin treatment at 12.5 mg, titrate gradually, and use divided dosing. Use caution with patients with a history of seizures or risk factors for seizures (CNS pathology, drugs that lower the seizure threshold, alcohol abuse). ∎

• Some patients experience transient fever with temperature higher than 100.4° F (38° C), especially in the first 3 weeks of therapy. Monitor these patients closely.

Black Box Warning Drug isn't indicated for use in elderly patients with dementia-related psychoses because of an increased risk for death from CV disease or infection. ∎

🖲 *Alert:* Fever may be the first sign of neutropenic infection. Interrupt therapy and obtain ANC level in any patient who develops fever (temperature 101.3° F [38.5° C]). If fever occurs in any patient with ANC less than 1,000/mm^3, initiate appropriate workup and treatment and monitor/manage patient appropriately.

• If drug is to be discontinued and patient doesn't have moderate to severe neutropenia, reduce dose gradually over 1 to 2 weeks. To discontinue the drug abruptly for a reason unrelated to neutropenia, continue to monitor ANC until it is 1,500/mm^3 or greater (for the general population), or until ANC is 1,000/mm^3 or greater or above patient's baseline (for those with BEN).

• If patient reports onset of fever (temperature 101.3° F or greater) while discontinuing drug, continue to monitor ANC for an additional 2 weeks after drug is discontinued.

• When discontinuing drug, monitor patients carefully for recurrence of psychotic symptoms and symptoms related to cholinergic rebound (profuse sweating, headache, nausea, vomiting, diarrhea).

• PE and DVT have occurred in patients taking clozapine. It isn't known whether these can be attributed to the drug or to some other patient characteristic. Monitor for PE if patient develops DVT, acute dyspnea, chest pain, or other respiratory signs and symptoms.

• Drug can cause sedation and impair cognitive and motor performance. Monitor patient carefully for CNS changes.

• Complete fall risk assessments when initiating therapy and recurrently for patients on long-term therapy, especially elderly patients and patients with diseases or conditions or who are taking other medications that could exacerbate fall risk.

• *Look alike–sound alike:* Don't confuse clozapine with clonidine, clonazepam, or Klonopin. Don't confuse Clozaril with Colazal.

PATIENT TEACHING

Black Box Warning Tell patient about need for regular blood tests to check for low ANC. Advise patient to report flulike symptoms, fever, sore throat, lethargy, weakness, malaise, or other signs of neutropenia or infection. ∎

Black Box Warning Warn patient taking drug to avoid hazardous activities that require alertness and good coordination and where sudden loss of consciousness and falls could cause serious risk to patient or others. ∎

• Tell patient to check with prescriber before taking alcohol or OTC drugs.

• Advise patient that smoking may decrease drug effectiveness.

• Advise patient to rise slowly to avoid dizziness and to immediately report feeling faint, loss of consciousness, or irregular or slow heartbeat.

• Advise patient that drug may cause somnolence, orthostatic hypotension, and motor and sensory instability, which may lead to falls and, consequently, fractures or other injuries.

• Tell patient to keep ODTs in the blister package until patient is ready to take them.

• Inform patient about risk for metabolic changes, seizures, and TD.

• Caution patient not to restart drug and to notify prescriber if more than 2 days of treatment have been missed.

SAFETY ALERT!

codeine phosphate–acetaminophen ⚠
koe-DEEN/a-seet-a-MIN-a-fen

Tylenol with Codeine #3✷,
Tylenol with Codeine #4

Therapeutic class: Opioid analgesics
Pharmacologic class: Opioids–para-aminophenol derivatives
Controlled substance schedule:
III (tablets); V (liquid)

AVAILABLE FORMS
Oral solution or suspension: 12 mg codeine and 120 mg acetaminophen/5 mL*
Tablets: 15 mg codeine and 300 mg acetaminophen, 30 mg codeine and 300 mg acetaminophen, 60 mg codeine and 300 mg acetaminophen

INDICATIONS & DOSAGES
Adjust-a-dose (for all indications): Consider decreased dosage in patients with renal impairment, elderly patients, and patients overly sensitive to effects of opioids. For patients with hepatic impairment, maximum total daily acetaminophen dose is 2,000 mg.

➤ **Mild to moderately severe pain**
Adults: Codeine 15 to 60 mg and acetaminophen 300 to 1,000 mg PO every 4 hours as needed for pain; adjust dosage based on pain severity and patient response. Maximum total daily dosage: acetaminophen 4,000 mg and codeine 360 mg.

Reactions in bold italics are *life-threatening*. Interactions may have a *rapid onset* or a *delayed onset*.

ADMINISTRATION
PO
• Initiate dosing regimen for each patient individually, taking into account patient's severity of pain, patient response, prior analgesic treatment experience, and risk factors for addiction, abuse, and misuse.
• Store tablets at room temperature.
• Give with milk or meals to avoid GI upset.
• For oral solution/suspension, be sure to use a calibrated measuring device.

ACTION
Codeine may bind with opioid receptors in the CNS, altering perception and emotional response to pain. Acetaminophen is thought to produce analgesia by inhibiting prostaglandin and other substances that sensitize pain receptors.

Route	Onset	Peak	Duration
PO (codeine)	30–45 min	1–2 hr	4–6 hr
PO (aceta-minophen)	Rapid	½–2 hr	3–4 hr

Half-life: Codeine, 2.9 hours; acetaminophen, 1.25 to 3 hours.

ADVERSE REACTIONS
CNS: drowsiness, light-headedness, dizziness, sedation, euphoria, dysphoria. **GI:** nausea, vomiting, constipation, abdominal pain. **Hematologic:** *thrombocytopenia, agranulocytosis.* **Respiratory:** shortness of breath, *respiratory depression.* **Skin:** pruritus, rash, sweating. **Other:** allergic reactions.

INTERACTIONS
Drug-drug. *Antipsychotics, general anesthetics, opioid analgesics, sedative-hypnotics, tranquilizers, other CNS depressants:* May increase CNS depression. Use together cautiously.
Black Box Warning *Benzodiazepines, CNS depressants:* May cause slow or difficult breathing, sedation, and death. Avoid use together. If use together is necessary, limit dosage and duration of each drug to the minimum necessary for desired effect. ∎
Cimetidine: May enhance effects of codeine, increasing toxicity. Monitor patient carefully.
Black Box Warning *CYP2D6 inducers:* May decrease analgesic effects or result in opioid withdrawal. Use cautiously. ∎

Black Box Warning *CYP3A4 inducers and inhibitors, CYP2D6 inhibitors:* Effects of concomitant use or discontinuation of these drugs with codeine are complex. Their use with codeine requires careful consideration of the effects on the parent drug, codeine, and the active metabolite, morphine. ∎
Black Box Warning *CYP3A4 inhibitors:* May increase codeine concentration and increase adverse reactions, including fatal respiratory depression. Use cautiously. ∎
MAO inhibitors: May cause serotonin syndrome or opioid toxicity (respiratory depression, coma). Use together or within 14 days is contraindicated. If urgent use of an opioid is necessary, use test doses and frequent titration of small doses of other opioids (such as oxycodone, hydrocodone, oxymorphone, or buprenorphine) to treat pain while closely monitoring BP and signs and symptoms of CNS and respiratory depression.
❸ *Alert:* Serotonergic drugs (amoxapine, antiemetics [dolasetron, granisetron, ondansetron, palonosetron], antimigraine drugs, buspirone, cyclobenzaprine, dextromethorphan, lithium, maprotiline, methylene blue, mirtazapine, nefazodone, SSNRIs, SSRIs, TCAs, trazodone, tryptophan, vilazodone): May increase risk of serotonin syndrome. Use together cautiously and monitor patient for serotonin syndrome.
Drug-herb. ❸ *Alert: St. John's wort:* May increase risk of serotonin syndrome. Use together cautiously.
Drug-lifestyle. **Black Box Warning** *Alcohol use:* May cause slow or difficult breathing, sedation, and death. Avoid use together. ∎

EFFECTS ON LAB TEST RESULTS
• May increase serum amylase level.
• May cause false-positive results for urinary 5-hydroxyindoleacetic acid.
• May cause urine drug screen to be positive for morphine.

CONTRAINDICATIONS & CAUTIONS
• Contraindicated in patients hypersensitive to codeine or acetaminophen and in patients with significant respiratory depression, acute or severe bronchial asthma in an unmonitored setting or in the absence of

resuscitative equipment, and in those with known or suspected GI obstruction, including paralytic ileus.

Black Box Warning Use exposes patient and others to the risk of opioid addiction, abuse, and misuse. To ensure that the benefits of opioid analgesics outweigh the risks of addiction, abuse, and misuse, the FDA has required a REMS program for these products. Assess each patient's risk before prescribing; monitor all patients for these behaviors. ▪

Black Box Warning *Opioid class warning:* Opioids should only be prescribed with benzodiazepines or other CNS depressants to patients for whom alternative treatment options are inadequate. ▪

Black Box Warning *Opioid class warning:* Life-threatening respiratory depression and death have occurred in children who received codeine. Most of the reported cases occurred after tonsillectomy or adenoidectomy, and many of the children had evidence of being an ultrarapid metabolizer of codeine due to a CYP2D6 polymorphism. Codeine phosphate–acetaminophen is contraindicated in children younger than age 12 and in children younger than age 18 after tonsillectomy or adenoidectomy. Avoid using drug in adolescents ages 12 to 18 who have other risk factors that may increase their sensitivity to the respiratory depressant effects of codeine unless benefits outweigh risks. Risk factors include conditions associated with hypoventilation, such as postoperative status, obstructive sleep apnea, obesity, severe pulmonary disease, neuromuscular disease, and concomitant use of other drugs that cause respiratory depression. ▪

Black Box Warning Accidental ingestion of even one dose of codeine–acetaminophen, especially by children, can result in a fatal overdose. ▪

Black Box Warning May cause life-threatening or fatal respiratory depression. Monitor carefully when starting or increasing dosages. ▪

۞ Alert: For managing pain (not associated with tonsillectomy or adenoidectomy), codeine should be used in children only if benefits outweigh risks.

۞ Alert: Safety and effectiveness in children younger than age 18 haven't been established.

۞ Alert: Drug may lead to a rare but serious decrease in adrenal gland cortisol production.

۞ Alert: Drug may decrease sex hormone levels with long-term use.

۞ Alert: Patients are at increased risk for oversedation and respiratory depression if they snore or have a history of sleep apnea, no recent history of opioid use or are first-time opioid users, have increased opioid dose requirements or opioid habituation, received general anesthesia for longer lengths of time, received other sedating drugs, have preexisting pulmonary or cardiac disease, or have thoracic or other surgical incisions that may impair breathing. Monitor patients carefully.

• Use cautiously in patients with head injury, intracranial lesions, increased ICP, or acute abdominal conditions.

Black Box Warning Acetaminophen has been associated with acute liver failure, usually at doses greater than 4,000 mg/day and often when more than one acetaminophen-containing product is used. Liver failure may result in liver transplant or death. ▪

۞ Alert: May cause serious, potentially fatal skin reactions, including SJS, toxic epidermal necrolysis, and acute generalized exanthematous pustulosis. Reaction may occur with first or subsequent use when acetaminophen is used as monotherapy or when it is one component of combination drug therapy. Monitor for reddening of the skin, rash, blisters, and detachment of the upper surface of the skin. Stop drug immediately if skin reaction is suspected.

• Use cautiously in patients with asthma or sulfite sensitivity because allergy-type reactions, anaphylaxis, and asthmatic episodes may occur.

▨ Use cautiously in elderly or debilitated patients; in those with severe renal or hepatic impairment, hypothyroidism, urethral stricture, Addison disease, or prostatic hypertrophy; in patients identified as ultra-rapid metabolizers of codeine; and in those with identified polymorphism of CYP2D6 genotype.

Dializable drug: Unknown.

⚠ Overdose S&S: Extreme sleepiness, confusion, shallow breathing. Codeine: Pinpoint pupils, respiratory depression, loss of consciousness, seizures. Acetaminophen: Hepatic necrosis, nausea, vomiting, diaphoresis, malaise, renal tubular necrosis, hypoglycemia, coma, coagulation defects.

PREGNANCY-LACTATION-REPRODUCTION

Black Box Warning Prolonged use during pregnancy can result in neonatal opioid withdrawal syndrome, which may be life-threatening and requires management according to expert neonatology protocols. If prolonged use is needed, advise patient of the risks and ensure appropriate treatment will be available. ■

◑ *Alert:* There are no adequate studies in pregnant women. Use during pregnancy only if potential benefit justifies potential risk to the fetus; dependence and withdrawal in newborns may occur.

• Don't administer drug during labor when delivery of a premature infant is anticipated.

◑ *Alert:* Codeine and its metabolites and acetaminophen appear in human milk. Breastfeeding isn't recommended for patients taking codeine due to risk of serious adverse reactions in breastfed infants, such as excess sleepiness, difficulty breastfeeding, or serious breathing problems that could result in death.

NURSING CONSIDERATIONS

Black Box Warning Serious, life-threatening, or fatal respiratory depression may occur with use of codeine–acetaminophen. Monitor patients for respiratory depression, especially during initiation or after a dosage increase. ■

Black Box Warning Monitor all patients regularly for development of opioid addiction, abuse, and misuse, which can lead to overdose and death. ■

• Prescribe lowest effective dosage for shortest period of time and inform patients of risks and signs and symptoms of acetaminophen and codeine toxicity.

Black Box Warning Ensure accuracy when prescribing, dispensing, and administering codeine 12 mg–acetaminophen 120 mg/ 5 mL. Dosing errors due to confusion between mg and mL and other codeine–acetaminophen oral suspensions of different concentrations can result in accidental overdose and death. ■

◑ *Alert:* If patient is taking opioids with serotonergic drugs, watch for signs and symptoms of serotonin syndrome (agitation, hallucinations, rapid HR, fever, excessive sweating, shivering or shaking, muscle twitching or stiffness, trouble with coordination, nausea, vomiting, diarrhea), especially when at start of treatment or after dosage increases. Signs and symptoms may occur within several hours of coadministration but may occur later, especially after dosage increase. Discontinue opioid, serotonergic drug, or both if serotonin syndrome is suspected.

◑ *Alert:* Monitor patient for signs and symptoms of adrenal insufficiency (nausea, vomiting, loss of appetite, fatigue, weakness, dizziness, low BP). Perform diagnostic testing if adrenal insufficiency is suspected. If adrenal insufficiency is confirmed, treat with corticosteroids and wean patient off opioids if appropriate. Discontinue corticosteroids when clinically appropriate.

◑ *Alert:* Monitor patient for signs and symptoms of decreased sex hormone levels (low libido, erectile dysfunction, amenorrhea, infertility). If signs and symptoms occur, evaluate patient and obtain laboratory testing.

• When patient who has been taking codeine–acetaminophen regularly and who may be physically dependent no longer requires therapy, taper dosage gradually, by 25% to 50% every 2 to 4 days, while monitoring patient carefully for signs and symptoms of withdrawal. If patient develops withdrawal signs or symptoms, raise the dosage to previous level and taper more slowly, either by increasing the interval between decreases, decreasing the amount of change in dosage, or both. Don't abruptly discontinue drug in a physically dependent patient.

◑ *Alert:* Carefully monitor vital signs, pain level, respiratory status, and sedation level in all patients receiving opioids, especially those receiving IV drugs, even those given postoperatively.

▓ Carefully monitor patients identified as ultrarapid metabolizers of codeine and those with identified polymorphism of CYP2D6 genotype. Overdose signs and symptoms and exaggerated adverse effects may occur at normal doses in these patients.

• Monitor serial renal function tests or LFTs in patients with severe hepatic or renal disease.

❸ *Alert:* Don't stop drug abruptly; withdraw slowly and individualize the gradual taper plan to prevent signs and symptoms of withdrawal, worsening pain, and psychological distress in physically dependent patients. Refer to manufacturer's label for specific tapering instructions.

❸ *Alert:* When tapering opioids, monitor patient closely for signs and symptoms of opioid withdrawal (restlessness, lacrimation, rhinorrhea, yawning, perspiration, chills, myalgia, mydriasis, irritability, anxiety, insomnia, backache, joint pain, weakness, abdominal cramps, anorexia, nausea, vomiting, diarrhea, increased BP or HR, increased respiratory rate). Such symptoms may indicate a need to taper more slowly. Also monitor patient for suicidal thoughts, use of other substances, and mood changes.

PATIENT TEACHING

Black Box Warning Caution patient or caregiver of patient taking an opioid with a benzodiazepine, CNS depressant, or alcohol to seek immediate medical attention for dizziness, light-headedness, extreme sleepiness, slowed or difficult breathing, or unresponsiveness. ∎

❸ *Alert:* Warn patient and caregiver of patient taking codeine to watch for slow or shallow breathing, difficult or noisy breathing, confusion, excessive sleepiness, or trouble breastfeeding or limpness (in infant). If any of these signs occur, tell patient to stop drug and immediately seek emergency medical attention.

❸ *Alert:* Warn patient to stop drug and seek medical attention immediately if skin rash or reaction occurs while using acetaminophen.

❸ *Alert:* Encourage patient to report all medications being taken, including prescriptions and OTC medications and supplements.

❸ *Alert:* Caution patient to immediately report signs and symptoms of serotonin syndrome, adrenal insufficiency, and decreased sex hormone levels.

❸ *Alert:* Counsel patient not to discontinue opioids without first discussing the need for gradual tapering of the regimen with prescriber.

• Explain the assessment and monitoring process to patient and family. Instruct them to immediately report if patient has any difficulty breathing or any other signs of a potential adverse opioid-related reaction.

• Inform patient with severe hepatic or renal disease that serial renal function tests or LFTs will be needed.

• Caution patient not to drive a car or operate heavy machinery while taking this drug.

• Warn patient about alcohol use during therapy.

• Warn patient that codeine may be habit-forming and to take only as long as it's prescribed and in the amounts prescribed.

▨ Advise breastfeeding patient who is an ultrarapid metabolizer to obtain emergency treatment if the infant shows signs and symptoms of codeine toxicity (sleepiness, difficulty breastfeeding or breathing, limpness).

SAFETY ALERT!

codeine sulfate ▨

Therapeutic class: Opioid analgesics
Pharmacologic class: Opioids
Controlled substance schedule: II

AVAILABLE FORMS
Tablets: 15 mg, 30 mg, 60 mg

INDICATIONS & DOSAGES
➤ **Mild to moderately severe pain**
Adults: 15 to 60 mg PO up to every 4 hours as needed for pain. Adjust dosage to obtain appropriate balance between pain management and opioid-related adverse reactions. Maximum is 360 mg/24 hours.
Adjust-a-dose: For patients with renal or hepatic impairment, begin with lower-than-normal dosages or with longer dosing intervals and titrate slowly while monitoring for respiratory depression, sedation, and hypotension.

ADMINISTRATION
PO
• Give drug with milk or meals to avoid GI upset.
• Initiate dosing regimen for each patient individually, taking into account patient's

severity of pain, patient response, prior analgesic treatment experience, and risk factors for addiction, abuse, and misuse.

ACTION

May bind with opioid receptors in the CNS, altering perception of and emotional response to pain. Also suppresses the cough reflex by direct action on the cough center in the medulla.

Route	Onset	Peak	Duration
PO	30–60 min	1–2 hr	4–6 hr

Half-life: 2½ to 3½ hours.

ADVERSE REACTIONS

CNS: clouded sensorium, sedation, dizziness, euphoria, light-headedness, physical dependence. **CV:** *bradycardia,* flushing, hypotension. **GI:** constipation, dry mouth, ileus, nausea, vomiting. **GU:** urine retention. **Respiratory:** *respiratory depression.* **Skin:** diaphoresis, pruritus.

INTERACTIONS

Drug-drug. Black Box Warning *Benzodiazepines, CNS depressants:* May cause slow or difficult breathing, sedation, and death. Avoid use together. If use together is necessary, limit dosage and duration of each drug to the minimum necessary for desired effect. ▪

Cimetidine: May lead to increased effect or toxicity. Monitor patient response.

CNS depressants, general anesthetics, hypnotics, other opioid analgesics, sedatives, TCAs, tranquilizers: May cause additive effects. Use together cautiously; monitor patient response.

Black Box Warning *CYP3A4 inducers and inhibitors, CYP2D6 inhibitors:* Effects of concomitant use or discontinuation of these drugs with codeine are complex. Their use with codeine sulfate requires careful consideration of the effects on the parent drug, codeine, and the active metabolite, morphine. ▪

MAO inhibitors: May cause serotonin syndrome or opioid toxicity (respiratory depression, coma). Use together or within 14 days is contraindicated. If urgent use of an opioid is necessary, use test doses and frequent titration of small doses of other

opioids (such as oxycodone, hydrocodone, oxymorphone, or buprenorphine) to treat pain while closely monitoring BP and signs and symptoms of CNS and respiratory depression.

Opioid antagonists: May reduce analgesic effect or precipitate withdrawal symptoms. Consider therapy modification.

❸ *Alert:* *Serotonergic drugs (amoxapine, antiemetics [dolasetron, granisetron, ondansetron, palonosetron], antimigraine drugs, buspirone, cyclobenzaprine, dextromethorphan, lithium, maprotiline, methylene blue, mirtazapine, nefazodone, SSNRIs, SSRIs, TCAs, trazodone, tryptophan, vilazodone):* May increase risk of serotonin syndrome. Use together cautiously and monitor patient for serotonin syndrome.

Drug-lifestyle. Black Box Warning *Alcohol use:* May cause slow or difficult breathing, sedation, and death. Avoid use together. ▪

EFFECTS ON LAB TEST RESULTS

• May increase amylase and lipase levels.
• May cause urine drug screen to be positive for morphine.

CONTRAINDICATIONS & CAUTIONS

Black Box Warning Contraindicated in children younger than age 12, and for postoperative management in children younger than age 18 after tonsillectomy or adenoidectomy. ▪

• Contraindicated in patients hypersensitive to drug and in patients with significant respiratory depression, acute or severe bronchial asthma in an unmonitored setting or in the absence of resuscitative equipment, and in those with known or suspected GI obstruction, including paralytic ileus.

Black Box Warning Opioids should only be prescribed with benzodiazepines or other CNS depressants to patients for whom alternative treatment options are inadequate. ▪

Black Box Warning Drug exposes users to the risks of opioid addiction, abuse, and misuse, which can lead to overdose and death. To ensure that the benefits of opioid analgesics outweigh the risks of addiction, abuse, and misuse, the FDA has required a REMS program for these products. Assess each patient's risk (previous substance use disorder, younger age, major depression, psychotropic drug use) before prescribing drug. ▮

◑ Alert: Safety and effectiveness and pharmacokinetics of codeine in children younger than age 18 haven't been established.

▨ Black Box Warning Children who receive codeine for pain relief after a tonsillectomy or adenoidectomy and are ultrarapid metabolizers due to a CYP2D6 polymorphism have an increased risk of death. Codeine is contraindicated for pain management after these surgeries. ▮

◑ Alert: Drug may lead to a rare but serious decrease in adrenal gland cortisol production.

◑ Alert: Drug may decrease sex hormone levels with long-term use.

◑ Alert: Patients are at increased risk of oversedation and respiratory depression if they have snoring or history of sleep apnea, no recent opioid use or are first-time opioid users, increased opioid dose requirements or opioid habituation, received general anesthesia for longer lengths of time, received other sedating drugs, preexisting pulmonary or cardiac disease, or have thoracic or other surgical incisions that may impair breathing. Monitor patients carefully.

Black Box Warning Accidental ingestion of even one dose of codeine sulfate tablets, especially by children, can result in a fatal overdose. ▮

• Use cautiously in elderly or debilitated patients and in those with head injury, increased ICP, increased CSF pressure, hepatic or renal disease, hypothyroidism, Addison disease, acute alcoholism, seizures, severe CNS depression, bronchial asthma, COPD, respiratory depression, and shock.

Dialyzable drug: Unknown.

⚠ Overdose S&S: CNS depression, respiratory depression, apnea, flaccid skeletal muscles, bradycardia, hypotension, circulatory collapse, death.

PREGNANCY-LACTATION-REPRODUCTION

◑ Alert: There are no adequate well-controlled studies in pregnant women. Use during pregnancy only if potential benefit justifies potential risk to the fetus.

Black Box Warning Prolonged use during pregnancy can cause neonatal withdrawal syndrome, which can be life-threatening and requires management according to protocols developed by neonatology experts. If used during pregnancy, advise patient of risks and ensure appropriate treatment is available. ▮

• Don't administer drug during labor when delivery of a premature infant is anticipated. ▮

◑ Alert: Breastfeeding isn't recommended for patients taking codeine because of the risk of serious adverse reactions in breastfed infants, such as excess sleepiness, difficulty breastfeeding, or serious breathing problems that could result in death.

NURSING CONSIDERATIONS

Black Box Warning Serious, life-threatening, or fatal respiratory depression may occur with use of codeine sulfate tablets. Monitor patients for respiratory depression, especially during initiation or after a dosage increase. ▮

Black Box Warning Monitor all patients regularly for development of opioid addiction, abuse, and misuse, which can lead to overdose and death. ▮

◑ Alert: If patient is taking opioids with serotonergic drugs, watch for signs and symptoms of serotonin syndrome (agitation, hallucinations, rapid HR, fever, excessive sweating, shivering or shaking, muscle twitching or stiffness, trouble with coordination, nausea, vomiting, diarrhea), especially at start of treatment or after dosage increases. Signs and symptoms may occur within several hours of coadministration but may occur later, especially after dosage increase. Discontinue opioid, serotonergic drug, or both if serotonin syndrome is suspected.

◑ Alert: Monitor patient for signs and symptoms of adrenal insufficiency (nausea, vomiting, loss of appetite, fatigue, weakness, dizziness, low BP). Perform diagnostic testing if adrenal insufficiency is suspected. If adrenal insufficiency is confirmed, treat with corticosteroids and wean patient off opioids if appropriate. Discontinue corticosteroids when clinically appropriate.

◑ Alert: Monitor patient for signs and symptoms of decreased sex hormone levels (low libido, erectile dysfunction, amenorrhea, infertility). If signs and symptoms occur, evaluate patient and obtain laboratory testing.

Reactions in bold italics are *life-threatening*. Interactions may have a *rapid onset* or a *delayed onset*.

C

⟳ *Alert:* Don't stop drug abruptly; withdraw slowly and individualize the gradual taper plan to prevent signs and symptoms of withdrawal, worsening pain, and psychological distress in physically dependent patients. Refer to manufacturer's label for specific tapering instructions.

⟳ *Alert:* When tapering opioids, monitor patient closely for signs and symptoms of opioid withdrawal (restlessness, lacrimation, rhinorrhea, yawning, perspiration, chills, myalgia, mydriasis, irritability, anxiety, insomnia, backache, joint pain, weakness, abdominal cramps, anorexia, nausea, vomiting, diarrhea, increased BP or HR, increased respiratory rate). Such symptoms may indicate a need to taper more slowly. Also monitor patient for suicidal thoughts, use of other substances, and mood changes.

• Reassess patient's level of pain at least 15 and 30 minutes after use.

• For full analgesic effect, give drug before patient has intense pain.

• Drug is an antitussive and shouldn't be used when cough is a valuable diagnostic sign or is beneficial (as after thoracic surgery). Monitor cough type and frequency.

• Monitor respiratory and circulatory status.

• Opioids may cause constipation. Assess bowel function and need for stool softeners and stimulant laxatives.

• Codeine may delay gastric emptying, increase biliary tract pressure from contraction of the sphincter of Oddi, and interfere with hepatobiliary imaging studies.

• When patient who has been taking codeine sulfate regularly and who may be physically dependent no longer requires codeine sulfate, taper dosage gradually, by 25% to 50% every 2 to 4 days, while monitoring carefully for signs and symptoms of withdrawal. If patient develops withdrawal signs or symptoms, raise dosage to previous level and taper more slowly, either by increasing the interval between decreases, decreasing the amount of change in dosage, or both. Don't abruptly discontinue drug in a physically dependent patient.

• *Look alike–sound alike:* Don't confuse codeine with Cardene or Cordran.

PATIENT TEACHING

Black Box Warning Caution patient or caregiver of patient taking an opioid with a benzodiazepine, CNS depressant, or alcohol to seek immediate medical attention for dizziness, light-headedness, extreme sleepiness, slowed or difficult breathing, or unresponsiveness. ■

⟳ *Alert:* Warn patient and caregiver of patient taking codeine to watch for slow or shallow breathing, difficult or noisy breathing, confusion, excessive sleepiness, or trouble breastfeeding or limpness (in infant). If any of these signs occur, tell patient or caregiver to stop drug and immediately seek emergency medical attention.

⟳ *Alert:* Encourage patient to report all medications being taken, including prescriptions and OTC medications and supplements.

⟳ *Alert:* Caution patient to immediately report signs and symptoms of serotonin syndrome, adrenal insufficiency, and or decreased sex hormone levels.

⟳ *Alert:* Counsel patient not to discontinue opioids without first discussing the need for a gradual tapering regimen with prescriber.

• Explain the assessment and monitoring process to patient and family. Instruct them to immediately report if patient has any difficulty breathing or any other signs of a potential adverse opioid-related reaction.

• Advise patient that GI distress caused by taking drug orally can be eased by taking drug with milk or meals.

• Instruct patient to ask for or to take drug before pain is intense.

• Caution ambulatory patient about getting out of bed or walking. Warn outpatient to avoid driving and other hazardous activities that require mental alertness until drug's effects on the CNS are known.

• Advise patient to avoid alcohol during therapy.

Black Box Warning Warn patient that accidental ingestion of even one dose of codeine sulfate, especially by children, can result in a fatal overdose of codeine. ■

• Warn breastfeeding patient to watch for increased sleepiness, difficulty breastfeeding or breathing, or limpness (in infant). Tell her to immediately seek medical attention if this occurs.

✽ Canada ◇ OTC ◆ Off-label use ✔ Photoguide ⊕ Do not crush *Liquid contains alcohol ✕ Genetic

colchicine ⚗
KOL-chih-seen

Colcrys✦, Gloperba, Mitigare

Therapeutic class: Antigout drugs
Pharmacologic class: Colchicum autumnale alkaloids

AVAILABLE FORMS
Capsules: 0.6 mg
Oral solution: 0.6 mg/5 mL
Tablets: 0.6 mg

INDICATIONS & DOSAGES
Adjust-a-dose (for all indications): Coadministration of CYP3A4 or P-gp inhibitors or inhibitors of both CYP3A4 and P-gp has been reported to lead to colchicine toxicity. Consider the potential for drug-drug interactions before and during therapy. If coadministration is required, patient's colchicine dose may need to be reduced or therapy interrupted; monitor patient carefully for colchicine toxicity.

➤ **Prevention of gout flares**
Adults: 0.6 mg PO once daily or b.i.d. Maximum daily dose is 1.2 mg.
Adjust-a-dose: For patients taking Colcrys with CrCl of less than 30 mL/minute, give 0.3 mg/day. Closely monitor patient after dosage increases. For patients on dialysis, starting doses should be 0.3 mg twice a week with close monitoring. Closely monitor patients with mild to moderate hepatic impairment; no dosage adjustment is required. Consider dosage reduction in patients with severe hepatic impairment.

For patients taking Mitigare or Gloperba, consider dosage reduction or alternative drug in patients with severe renal impairment; closely monitor patients undergoing hemodialysis for toxicity. Consider dosage reduction or alternative drug in patients with severe hepatic impairment. Mitigare and Gloperba are contraindicated in patients with renal impairment with concomitant hepatic impairment.

➤ **Gout flares (Colcrys)**
Adults: 1.2 mg PO at first sign of a flare, followed by 0.6 mg 1 hour later; maximum dosage is 1.8 mg over a 1-hour period.

Adjust-a-dose: For patients with CrCl of less than 30 mL/minute or severe hepatic impairment, no dosage adjustment is needed but treatment course should be repeated no more than once every 2 weeks. For patients with severe renal or hepatic impairment requiring repeated courses for the treatment of gout flares, consider alternative therapy. For patients on dialysis, reduce total recommended dose for treatment of gout flares to a single dose of 0.6 mg (one tablet). For these patients, treatment course shouldn't be repeated more than once every 2 weeks.

➤ **Familial Mediterranean fever (Colcrys)** ⚗
Adults: 1.2 to 2.4 mg PO daily; may increase by 0.3 mg/day to maximum daily dosage given once daily or in two divided doses.
Adolescents age 13 and older: 1.2 to 2.4 mg PO once daily or in two divided doses.
Children ages 6 to 12: 0.9 to 1.8 mg PO once daily or in two divided doses.
Children ages 4 to 6: 0.3 to 1.8 mg PO once daily or in two divided doses.
Adjust-a-dose: For patients with CrCl of less than 30 mL/minute or ESRD requiring dialysis, initially 0.3 mg/day, carefully increasing dosage as needed. In patients with severe hepatic disease, consider dosage reduction with careful monitoring.

➤ **Behçet syndrome with arthritis, cutaneous lesions, or mucocutaneous ulcers** ◆
Adults: 1.2 to 1.8 mg/day in two to three divided doses.

➤ **Pericarditis, acute and recurrent, in combination with aspirin or NSAIDs** ◆
Adults: For maintenance, with or without loading dose: In patients weighing 70 kg or more, give 0.6 mg b.i.d.; for those weighing less than 70 kg or unable to tolerate higher dosing regimen, give 0.6 mg once daily.

ADMINISTRATION
PO
• Hazardous drug; use safe handling and disposal precautions.
• Give drug with or without food.

ACTION
Exact mechanism of action is not fully known; thought to involve a reduction in lactic acid produced by leukocytes, reducing

---

uric acid deposits and phagocytosis, thereby decreasing the inflammatory process.

Route	Onset	Peak	Duration
PO	Unknown	30–180 min	Unknown

Half-life: 27 to 31 hours.

ADVERSE REACTIONS

CNS: fatigue, headache. **EENT:** pharyngolaryngeal pain. **GI:** diarrhea, nausea, vomiting, abdominal pain. **Hematologic:** *aplastic anemia, granulocytopenia, leukopenia, pancytopenia, thrombocytopenia.* **Other:** gout.

INTERACTIONS

Drug-drug. *Acidifying agents:* May inhibit action of colchicine. Avoid use together.
Alkalinizing agents: May increase action of colchicine. Avoid use together.
CNS depressants, sympathomimetics (such as phenylephrine): May increase sensitivity to these drugs. Monitor patient closely and adjust dosage as needed.
Digoxin, HMG-CoA reductase inhibitors (atorvastatin, simvastatin): May increase risk of myopathy or rhabdomyolysis. Avoid use together. If coadministration can't be avoided, monitor patient carefully. Discontinue colchicine if signs or symptoms occur.
Moderate CYP3A4 inhibitors (amprenavir, aprepitant, diltiazem, erythromycin, fluconazole, fosamprenavir, verapamil), P-gp inhibitors (cyclosporine, ranolazine), strong CYP3A4 inhibitors (atazanavir, clarithromycin, indinavir, itraconazole, ketoconazole, lopinavir–ritonavir, nefazodone, nelfinavir, ritonavir, ritonavir-boosted darunavir, ritonavir-boosted fosamprenavir, ritonavir-boosted tipranavir, saquinavir; the fixed combination of elvitegravir–cobicistat–emtricitabine–tenofovir): May increase colchicine level, increasing the risk of toxic effects. Reduce colchicine dosage if alternative treatment isn't available. Concurrent use in patients with renal or hepatic impairment is contraindicated.
Drug-food. *Grapefruit, grapefruit juice:* May increase drug level. Discourage use together.

EFFECTS ON LAB TEST RESULTS

• May increase AST, ALT, and CK levels.
• May decrease Hb level and hematocrit.
• May decrease leukocyte, granulocyte, and platelet counts.
• May cause false-positive results when urine is tested for RBCs or Hb.

CONTRAINDICATIONS & CAUTIONS

• Contraindicated in patients with serious CV, renal, hepatic, or GI impairment and in those taking P-gp inhibitors or strong CYP3A4 inhibitors.
• Don't give Mitigare or Gloperba to patients with both renal and hepatic impairment.
• Myelosuppression has been reported. Use cautiously in patients with hematologic disorders.
🔆 *Alert:* Fatal overdoses, both accidental and intentional, have been reported in adults and children who have ingested colchicine.
Dialyzable drug: No.
⚠ *Overdose S&S:* Abdominal pain, nausea, vomiting, diarrhea, hypovolemia, multiorgan failure, death.

PREGNANCY-LACTATION-REPRODUCTION

• There are no adequate studies in pregnant women. Use during pregnancy only if potential benefit justifies potential risk to the fetus.
• Drug isn't expected to appear in human milk. Use cautiously in breastfeeding women and observe breastfed infants for adverse effects related to vitamin absorption.

NURSING CONSIDERATIONS

• Safety and effectiveness of repeat treatment for gout flares haven't been established.
🔆 *Alert:* Colcrys, Gloperba, and Mitigare are the only FDA-approved single-ingredient colchicine products.
• Drug isn't an analgesic and shouldn't be used to treat pain from other causes.
• Obtain baseline laboratory studies, including CBC, before starting therapy and periodically thereafter; watch for myelosuppression, leukopenia, granulocytopenia, thrombocytopenia, pancytopenia, and aplastic anemia.

• Monitor patient who has used drug for a prolonged period for neuromuscular toxicity and rhabdomyolysis.
• If nausea, vomiting, or diarrhea occurs, discontinue drug.
• Drug may increase risk of malignancy.
• When used for gout prophylaxis, colchicine must be given with allopurinol or a uricosuric drug (such as probenecid) to decrease serum uric acid level. However, colchicine should be started before the other agent because a sudden change in uric acid level may cause a gout attack.
• *Look alike–sound alike:* Don't confuse colchicine with Cortrosyn.

PATIENT TEACHING
• Explain to patient that drug can be taken without regard to food but to avoid grapefruit and grapefruit juice.
• Tell patient to keep drug out of the reach of children due to risk of fatal overdose.
• Advise patient to report all adverse reactions, including muscle pain or weakness, tingling or numbness in fingers or toes, unusual bleeding or bruising, increased infections, weakness, tiredness, cyanosis, nausea, vomiting, or diarrhea; advise patient to discontinue drug.

---

colesevelam hydrochloride
koe-leh-SEVE-eh-lam

Welchol

Therapeutic class: Antilipemics
Pharmacologic class: Bile acid sequestrants

AVAILABLE FORMS
Oral suspension: 3.75-g packets
Tablets: 625 mg

INDICATIONS & DOSAGES
➤ **Adjunct to diet and exercise, either alone or with an HMG-CoA reductase inhibitor, to reduce elevated LDL cholesterol (LDL-C) in patients with primary hypercholesterolemia (Fredrickson type IIa); in boys and postmenarchal girls, ages 10 to 17, with heterozygous familial hypercholesterolemia if, after an adequate trial of diet therapy, LDL-C is 190 mg/dL or higher or LDL-C is 160 mg/dL or higher and patient has a positive family history of premature CV disease or two or more other CV disease risk factors**
Adults: 3 tablets (1,875 mg) PO b.i.d. or 6 tablets (3,750 mg) PO once daily. Or, one 3.75-g packet PO once daily.
Children ages 10 to 17: One 3.75-g packet PO once daily.
➤ **Adjunct to diet and exercise to improve glycemic control in type 2 diabetes mellitus**
Adults: 3 tablets (1,875 mg) PO b.i.d. or 6 tablets (3,750 mg) PO once daily. Or, one 3.75-g packet PO once daily.

ADMINISTRATION
PO
• Give drug with a meal and plenty of fluids.
• Store tablets at room temperature and protect them from moisture.
• Empty entire contents of one packet into glass and add 8 oz of water, fruit juice, or diet soft drink. Stir well and give immediately with a meal.

ACTION
Binds bile acids in the intestinal tract, impeding their absorption and causing their elimination in feces. In response to this bile acid depletion, LDL-C levels decrease as the liver uses LDL-C to replenish reduced bile acid stores.

Route	Onset	Peak	Duration
PO	Unknown	2 wk	Unknown

Half-life: Unknown.

ADVERSE REACTIONS
CNS: headache, asthenia, pain. **EENT:** pharyngitis, rhinitis, sinusitis. **GI:** constipation, flatulence, abdominal pain, diarrhea, dyspepsia, nausea. **Musculoskeletal:** back pain, myalgia. **Respiratory:** increased cough. **Other:** infection, accidental injury, flulike syndrome.

INTERACTIONS
Drug-drug. *Amiodarone:* May decrease amiodarone bioavailability. Consider therapy modification.

Reactions in bold italics are *life-threatening*. Interactions may have a *rapid onset* or a *delayed onset*.

Cyclosporine: May decrease cyclosporine level. Give cyclosporine at least 4 hours before colesevelam; monitor patient for decreased cyclosporine concentration during concomitant therapy.

Glimepiride, glipizide, glyburide: May decrease level of antidiabetic drug. Administer antidiabetic drug at least 4 hours before colesevelam.

Hormonal contraceptives (estrogens, progestins): May decrease levels of these contraceptives. Administer hormonal contraceptive at least 4 hours before or 4 to 6 hours after colesevelam dose.

Multivitamins: May decrease serum concentration of vitamins and minerals by impairing absorption of fat-soluble vitamins. Separate administration by several hours.

Mycophenolate: May decrease mycophenolate serum concentration. Avoid concurrent use.

Phenytoin: May decrease phenytoin level and increase seizure activity. Administer phenytoin 4 hours before colesevelam dose and monitor phenytoin level.

Thyroid hormones: Coadministration may increase TSH level. Administer thyroid hormone replacement 4 hours before colesevelam dose.

Warfarin: May decrease INR. Monitor INR and patient closely and give warfarin 4 hours before colesevelam.

EFFECTS ON LAB TEST RESULTS
• May increase triglyceride levels.

CONTRAINDICATIONS & CAUTIONS
• Contraindicated in patients hypersensitive to drug or its components and in those with a history of hypertriglyceridemia-induced pancreatitis, triglyceride levels greater than 500 mg/dL, or bowel obstruction.
• Contraindicated for glycemic control in patients with type 1 diabetes and for the treatment of diabetic ketoacidosis.
• Use cautiously in patients susceptible to vitamin K or fat-soluble vitamin deficiencies and in patients with swallowing disorders, severe GI motility disorders, or major GI tract surgery.
• Use cautiously in patients with triglyceride levels greater than 300 mg/dL.

• Don't use tablets in younger patients due to tablet size.
• Oral suspension contains 27 mg phenylalanine/3.75-g packet.
Dialyzable drug: Unknown.
⚠ **Overdose S&S:** Severe local GI reactions, especially constipation.

PREGNANCY-LACTATION-REPRODUCTION
• There are no adequate studies in pregnant women. Use during pregnancy may interfere with vitamin absorption. Use only if needed.
• Drug doesn't appear in human milk but may interfere with vitamin absorption and affect breastfeeding infants. Use cautiously in breastfeeding women.

NURSING CONSIDERATIONS
• Before starting drug, assess patient for underlying causes of hypercholesterolemia, such as poorly controlled diabetes, hypothyroidism, nephrotic syndrome, dysproteinemias, obstructive liver disease, other drug therapy, and alcoholism.
• Monitor patient's bowel habits. If severe constipation develops, decrease dosage, add a stool softener, or stop drug.
• Monitor the effects of patient's other drugs to identify drug interactions.
• Monitor INR, total cholesterol, and LDL-C and triglyceride levels periodically.

PATIENT TEACHING
• Instruct patient to take drug with a meal and plenty of fluids.
• Teach patient to monitor bowel habits. Encourage a diet high in fiber and fluids. Instruct patient to notify prescriber promptly if severe constipation develops.
• Encourage patient to follow prescribed diet, exercise, and monitoring of cholesterol and triglyceride levels.
• Tell patient to notify prescriber if she's pregnant or breastfeeding.

conivaptan hydrochloride
kah-nih-VAP-tan

Vaprisol

Therapeutic class: Vasopressin antagonists
Pharmacologic class: Arginine vasopressin receptor antagonists

AVAILABLE FORMS
Injection (premixed): 0.2 mg/mL in 100 mL D₅W

INDICATIONS & DOSAGES
➤ **Euvolemic hyponatremia (as from SIADH, hypothyroidism, adrenal insufficiency, pulmonary disorders) and hypervolemic hyponatremia in hospitalized patients**
Adults: Loading dose of 20 mg IV over 30 minutes; then 20 mg IV by continuous infusion over 24 hours for an additional 1 to 3 days. If sodium level isn't rising at desired rate, increase to maximum dose of 40 mg over 24 hours by continuous infusion. Total duration of infusion shouldn't exceed 4 days.
Adjust-a-dose: If sodium level rises more than 12 mEq/L in 24 hours, stop infusion. If hyponatremia persists or recurs and patient has had no adverse neurologic effects from the rapid rise in sodium level, restart infusion at a reduced dose. If patient develops hypotension or hypovolemia, stop infusion. Monitor vital signs and volume status often. If hyponatremia persists once patient is no longer hypotensive and volume returns to normal, restart infusion at a reduced dose. In patients with hepatic impairment (Child-Pugh class A, B, or C), give a loading dose of 10 mg over 30 minutes followed by a continuous infusion of 10 mg over 24 hours for 2 to 4 days. If serum sodium level isn't rising at desired rate, drug may be titrated upward to 20 mg over 24 hours. Don't use if CrCl is less than 30 mL/minute.

ADMINISTRATION
IV
▼ Give via a large vein, and change infusion site every 24 hours.
▼ Protect premixed solution from light until ready to use.

▼ **Incompatibilities:** Furosemide, lactated Ringer solution, NSS. Don't mix or infuse with other IV drugs.

ACTION
Increases free water eliminated by kidneys, inhibiting inappropriate or excessive arginine vasopressin (ADH) secretion. Typically, this causes increased net fluid loss, increased urine output, and decreased urine osmolality.

Route	Onset	Peak	Duration
IV	Unknown	Unknown	12 hr

Half-life: 5 hours.

ADVERSE REACTIONS
CNS: headache, confusion, fever, insomnia.
CV: atrial fibrillation, HTN, hypotension, orthostatic hypotension. **EENT:** pharyngolaryngeal pain. **GI:** constipation, diarrhea, dry mouth, nausea, oral candidiasis, vomiting.
GU: frequency, hematuria, polyuria, UTI.
Hematologic: anemia. **Metabolic:** *hypoglycemia,* hypokalemia, dehydration, hyperglycemia, *hypomagnesemia,* hyponatremia.
Respiratory: pneumonia. **Skin:** erythema.
Other: infusion-site reactions, thirst.

INTERACTIONS
Drug-drug. *Amlodipine:* May increase amlodipine level and half-life. Monitor BP.
Digoxin: May increase digoxin level. Monitor patient, and adjust digoxin dose, as needed.
Midazolam: May increase midazolam level. Monitor patient for respiratory depression and hypotension.
Potent CYP3A4 inhibitors (clarithromycin, indinavir, itraconazole, ketoconazole, ritonavir): May seriously increase levels and toxic effects. Use together is contraindicated. Allow an interval of at least 1 week to elapse after discontinuing conivaptan and initiating treatment with a drug metabolized by CYP3A.
Simvastatin: May increase simvastatin level. Monitor patient for signs of rhabdomyolysis, including muscle pain, weakness, and tenderness.
Drug-herb. *St John's wort:* May decrease conivaptan serum concentration. Don't use together.

Reactions in bold italics are *life-threatening*. Interactions may have a *rapid onset* or a *delayed onset*.

EFFECTS ON LAB TEST RESULTS
• May decrease potassium, magnesium, sodium, and Hb levels and hematocrit. May increase or decrease blood glucose level.

CONTRAINDICATIONS & CAUTIONS
• Contraindicated in patients with hypovolemic hyponatremia or anuria; patients hypersensitive to drug or its components, corn, or corn products; and those taking potent CYP3A4 inhibitors, such as clarithromycin, indinavir, itraconazole, ketoconazole, or ritonavir.
• Use cautiously in hyponatremic patients with underlying HF and patients with hepatic or renal impairment.
• Drug isn't approved for treatment of HF.
Dialyzable drug: Unknown.
⚠ *Overdose S&S:* Hypotension, thirst.

PREGNANCY-LACTATION-REPRODUCTION
• Although there are no adequate well-controlled studies in pregnant women, drug may cause fetal harm. Use during pregnancy only if potential benefit justifies potential risk to the fetus.
• It isn't known if drug appears in human milk. Patient should discontinue breastfeeding or discontinue drug, taking into account importance of drug to the mother.

NURSING CONSIDERATIONS
• Monitor sodium level and neurologic status regularly during therapy.
✪ *Alert:* Rapid correction of sodium level may cause osmotic demyelination syndrome. Monitor sodium level and volume status. Don't exceed a rise in serum sodium level greater than 12 mEq/L/24 hours.
• Drug may cause significant infusion-site reactions, even with proper dilution and administration. Rotate infusion site every 24 hours to reduce risk of reaction.

PATIENT TEACHING
• Inform patient that low BP when standing may occur. Advise patient who may feel dizzy or faint to sit or lie down.
• Advise patient to promptly report signs and symptoms of hypoglycemia, such as feeling shaky, nervous, tired, sweaty, cold, hungry, confused, or irritable.

• Emphasize the importance of reporting an unusually fast heartbeat or weakness.

crisaborole
kris-a-BOR-ole

Eucrisa

Therapeutic class: Dermatologic agents
Pharmacologic class: Phosphodiesterase 4 inhibitors

AVAILABLE FORMS
Topical ointment: 2%

INDICATIONS & DOSAGES
➤ **Mild to moderate atopic dermatitis**
Adults and children age 2 and older: Apply a thin film to affected areas b.i.d.

ADMINISTRATION
Topical
• Drug is for external use only; not for ophthalmic, oral, or intravaginal use.
• Store at room temperature; excursions permitted to 59° to 86° F (15° to 30° C).
• Keep tube tightly closed.

ACTION
Exact mechanism unknown. Drug is a phosphodiesterase 4 inhibitor that increases intracellular cAMP levels.

Route	Onset	Peak	Duration
Topical	Unknown	Unknown	Unknown

Half-life: Unknown.

ADVERSE REACTIONS
Skin: application-site pain, burning, or stinging.

INTERACTIONS
None reported.

EFFECTS ON LAB TEST RESULTS
None reported.

CONTRAINDICATIONS & CAUTIONS
• Contraindicated in patients hypersensitive to drug or its components.
• Hypersensitivity reactions have been reported, including contact urticaria.

• Safety and effectiveness in children younger than age 2 haven't been established.
Dialyzable drug: Unlikely.

PREGNANCY-LACTATION-REPRODUCTION

• Drug hasn't been studied in pregnant women. In animal studies, there were no adverse developmental effects.
• Drug is systemically absorbed; risk of harm in breastfed infants is unknown. Consider benefits to mother and risks to infant before using.

NURSING CONSIDERATIONS

• Monitor patient for severe pruritus, swelling, and erythema, which may indicate hypersensitivity. If these occur, discontinue drug.

PATIENT TEACHING

• Advise patient to discontinue drug and immediately report signs or symptoms of hypersensitivity reactions, such as hives, itching, swelling, and redness.
• Warn patient that effects of drug in pregnant or breastfeeding women are unknown.
• Remind patient or caregivers to wash hands after applying drug unless patient's hands are being treated.
• Caution patient or caregivers that drug is for external use only and not for ophthalmic, oral, or intravaginal use.

cyclobenzaprine hydrochloride
sye-kloe-BEN-za-preen

Amrix

Therapeutic class: Skeletal muscle relaxants
Pharmacologic class: TCA derivatives

AVAILABLE FORMS
Capsules (extended-release) ⊙*:* 15 mg, 30 mg
Tablets: 5 mg, 7.5 mg, 10 mg

INDICATIONS & DOSAGES
➤ **Adjunct to rest and physical therapy to relieve muscle spasm from acute, painful musculoskeletal conditions**

Adults and children age 15 and older:
5 mg PO t.i.d. Based on response, dose may be increased to 10 mg t.i.d. Don't exceed 30 mg/day. Or, 15 to 30 mg extended-release capsule PO once daily (adults only). Use for longer than 2 or 3 weeks isn't recommended.
Adjust-a-dose: In elderly patients and in those with mild hepatic impairment, start with 5-mg conventional tablets and adjust slowly upward; consider less frequent dosing. Drug isn't recommended in patients with moderate to severe hepatic impairment. Don't use extended-release capsules in children, elderly patients, or those with impaired hepatic function.

ADMINISTRATION
PO
• Don't split the generic 10-mg tablets because of the high risk of inconsistent doses.
• Give extended-release capsules whole; don't crush or break.
• In patients able to reliably swallow applesauce without chewing, sprinkle capsule contents onto a tablespoon of applesauce; have patient consume immediately without chewing then rinse the mouth to ensure all of the contents have been swallowed.

ACTION
Unknown. Relieves skeletal muscle spasm of local origin without disrupting muscle function.

Route	Onset	Peak	Duration
PO	1 hr	4 hr	12–24 hr
PO (extended-release)	1½ hr	7–8 hr	Unknown

Half-life: Tablets, 18 hours; extended-release capsules, 32 hours.

ADVERSE REACTIONS
CNS: dizziness, drowsiness, *seizures,* headache, tremor, insomnia, fatigue, asthenia, nervousness, confusion, paresthesia, depression, attention disturbances, dysarthria, ataxia, syncope. **CV:** *arrhythmias,* palpitations, hypotension, tachycardia. **EENT:** visual disturbances, blurred vision. **GI:** dry mouth, dyspepsia, abnormal taste, constipation, nausea. **Skin:** rash, pruritus, acne.

INTERACTIONS

Drug-drug. *CNS depressants:* May increase CNS depression. Avoid using together.
MAO inhibitors: May cause hyperpyretic crisis, seizures, and death when MAO inhibitors are used with TCAs; may also occur with cyclobenzaprine. Avoid using within 2 weeks of MAO inhibitor therapy.

Black Box Warning *Opioid class warning:* Use with opioids may cause slow or difficult breathing sedation and death. Avoid use together. If use together is necessary, limit dosage and duration of each drug to the minimum necessary for desired effect. ▌

Naproxen: May increase drowsiness. Make patient aware of this interaction.
Tramadol: May increase risk of seizures. Use together cautiously.

Drug-lifestyle. *Alcohol use:* May increase CNS depression. Discourage use together.

EFFECTS ON LAB TEST RESULTS

• May cause false-positive serum TCA screen.

CONTRAINDICATIONS & CAUTIONS

• Contraindicated in patients hypersensitive to drug; in those with hyperthyroidism, heart block, arrhythmias, conduction disturbances, or HF; in those who have received MAO inhibitors within 14 days; and in those in the acute recovery phase of an MI.
• There is increased risk of potentially life-threatening serotonin syndrome when drug is used in combination with SSRIs, SSNRIs, other TCAs, tramadol, bupropion, meperidine, or verapamil.
• Use cautiously in elderly or debilitated patients and in those with a history of urine retention, acute angle-closure glaucoma, or increased IOP.
• Safety and effectiveness in children younger than age 15 haven't been established.

Dialyzable drug: Unknown.

⚠ *Overdose S&S:* Drowsiness, tachycardia, tremor, agitation, coma, ataxia, HTN, slurred speech, confusion, dizziness, nausea, vomiting, hallucinations, cardiac arrest, chest pain, cardiac arrhythmias, ECG changes (changes in QRS axis or width).

PREGNANCY-LACTATION-REPRODUCTION

• There are no adequate well-controlled studies in pregnant women. Use during pregnancy only if clearly needed.
• It isn't known if drug appears in human milk. Use cautiously in breastfeeding women.

NURSING CONSIDERATIONS

• Drug may cause toxic reactions similar to those caused by TCAs. Observe same precautions as when giving TCAs.
• Monitor patient for nausea, headache, and malaise, which may occur if drug is stopped abruptly after long-term use.
🔔 *Alert:* Notify prescriber immediately of signs and symptoms of overdose, including cardiac toxicity.

PATIENT TEACHING

Black Box Warning Caution patient or caregiver of patient taking an opioid with a benzodiazepine, CNS depressant, or alcohol to seek immediate medical attention for dizziness, light-headedness, extreme sleepiness, slowed or difficult breathing, or unresponsiveness. ▌

• Advise patient to report urinary hesitancy or urine retention. If constipation is a problem, suggest that patient increase fluid intake and use a stool softener.
• Warn patient to avoid activities that require alertness until CNS effects of drug are known.
• Warn patient not to combine with alcohol or other CNS depressants, including OTC cold or allergy remedies.
• Instruct patient not to split the generic 10-mg tablets because of the high risk of inconsistent doses and not to crush or break capsules.
• Teach patient that capsule may be opened, contents sprinkled on a tablespoon of applesauce, and swallowed immediately (if patient is able to reliably swallow it without chewing). Instruct patient to then rinse mouth to ensure all of the contents were swallowed.
• Advise patient that using drug for longer than 2 to 3 weeks isn't recommended.

SAFETY ALERT!

cyclophosphamide
sye-kloe-FOSS-fa-mide

Procytox ✤

Therapeutic class: Antineoplastics
Pharmacologic class: Nitrogen mustards

AVAILABLE FORMS
Capsules ⊙℞ℂ: 25 mg, 50 mg
Injection: 200-mg ✤, 500-mg, 1-g, 2-g vials

INDICATIONS & DOSAGES
Adjust-a-dose (for all indications): Consider dosage reduction to 75% of usual dosage in patients with severe renal failure (CrCl of 0 to 10 mL/minute). Adjust dosage for patients with hepatic dysfunction as follows: If bilirubin level is 3.1 to 5 mg/dL or transaminase levels are greater than $3 \times$ ULN, give 75% of dose. Don't give if bilirubin level is greater than 5 mg/dL.
➤ **Breast or ovarian cancer, Hodgkin lymphoma, chronic lymphocytic leukemia, chronic myelocytic leukemia, acute lymphoblastic leukemia, acute myelocytic and monocytic leukemia, neuroblastoma, retinoblastoma, malignant lymphoma, multiple myeloma, mycosis fungoides**
Adults and children: Initially for induction, 40 to 50 mg/kg IV in divided doses over 2 to 5 days. Or, 10 to 15 mg/kg IV every 7 to 10 days, 3 to 5 mg/kg IV twice weekly, or 1 to 5 mg/kg PO daily, based on patient tolerance. Adjust subsequent doses according to evidence of antitumor activity or leukopenia.
➤ **Minimal-change nephrotic syndrome in patients who failed to adequately respond to or are unable to tolerate adrenocorticosteroid therapy**
Children: 2 mg/kg PO daily for 8 to 12 weeks. Maximum cumulative dose, 168 mg/kg.

ADMINISTRATION
• Preparing and administering drug may be mutagenic, teratogenic, or carcinogenic. Follow facility policy to reduce risks. Always wear gloves.

PO
• Give oral form in the morning; infrequent urination during the night may increase possibility of cystitis.
• Make sure patient receives adequate fluids or is infused to force diuresis to reduce risk of urinary tract toxicity.
• Don't open, cut, crush, or allow patient to chew capsules.

IV
▼ For direct IV injection, reconstitute powder with NSS for injection only.
▼ For IV infusion, first reconstitute powder using NSS for injection or sterile water for injection.
▼ Add 25 mL to 500-mg vial, 50 mL to 1-g vial, or 100 mL to 2-g vial to produce a solution containing 20 mg/mL. Shake vigorously to dissolve. If powder doesn't dissolve completely, let vial stand for a few minutes.
▼ Check reconstituted solution for small particles. Filter solution, if needed.
▼ For infusion, further dilute with D_5W, dextrose 5% in NSS for injection, or half-NSS for injection to minimum concentration of 2 mg/mL.
▼ Give by direct IV injection slowly or IV infusion over 1 to 2 hours.
▼ Without further dilution, solution reconstituted in NSS for injection is stable for 6 days if refrigerated or 24 hours at room temperature. Solution reconstituted in sterile water for injection must be used immediately.
▼ Reconstituted solutions further diluted in half-NSS for injection are stable for 24 hours at room temperature or 6 days if refrigerated; those diluted in D_5W or dextrose 5% in NSS for injection are stable for 24 hours at room temperature or 36 hours if refrigerated.
▼ Use stored solutions cautiously because drug contains no preservatives.
▼ **Incompatibilities:** None listed by manufacturer. Consult a drug incompatibility reference for more information.

ACTION
Cross-links strands of cellular DNA and interferes with RNA transcription, causing an imbalance of growth that leads to cell death. Not specific to cell cycle.

Reactions in bold italics are *life-threatening*. Interactions may have a *rapid onset* or a *delayed onset*.

Route	Onset	Peak	Duration
PO	Unknown	Unknown	Unknown
IV	Unknown	2–3 hr	Unknown

Half-life: 3 to 12 hours.

ADVERSE REACTIONS

CV: *cardiotoxicity with very high doses and with doxorubicin.* **GI:** nausea and vomiting, anorexia, stomatitis. **GU:** *hemorrhagic cystitis,* impaired fertility. **Hematologic:** *leukopenia, thrombocytopenia,* anemia. **Hepatic:** *hepatotoxicity.* **Metabolic:** hyperuricemia, SIADH. **Respiratory:** *pulmonary fibrosis with high doses.* **Skin:** alopecia. **Other:** *secondary malignant disease, anaphylaxis,* hypersensitivity reactions.

INTERACTIONS

Drug-drug. *ACE inhibitors, allopurinol, clozapine, natalizumab, paclitaxel, thiazide diuretics, zidovudine:* May increase hematotoxicity and immunosuppression. Monitor therapy.
Amiodarone, G-CSF drugs: May increase risk of pulmonary toxicity. Monitor therapy.
Amphotericin B, indomethacin: May increase risk of nephrotoxicity. Monitor patient closely.
Azathioprine: May increase risk of hepatotoxicity (liver necrosis). Monitor patient closely.
Busulfan: May increase risk of hepatic veno-occlusive disease. Monitor patient closely.
Cardiotoxic drugs (anthracyclines), cytarabine, pentostatin, trastuzumab: May increase adverse cardiac effects. Monitor patient for toxicity.
Cyclosporine: May decrease cyclosporine concentration and increase risk of GVHD. Monitor patient closely.
Etanercept: May increase risk of malignant solid tumors in patients with Wegener granulomatosis. Use cautiously.
Live-virus vaccines: May increase vaccine-induced adverse reactions. Don't give together.
Protease inhibitors: May increase cyclophosphamide-related toxicities and mucositis. Monitor therapy.
Succinylcholine: May prolong neuromuscular blockade and cause apnea. Avoid using together and alert anesthesiologist if drug has been given within 10 days of general anesthesia.
Tamoxifen: May increase risk of thromboembolism. Monitor patient closely.
Warfarin: May increase or decrease warfarin effects. Monitor patient closely.

EFFECTS ON LAB TEST RESULTS

• May increase uric acid level. May decrease Hb and pseudocholinesterase levels.
• May decrease platelet, RBC, and WBC counts.
• May suppress positive reaction to *Candida,* mumps, *Trichophyton,* and tuberculin skin test results. May cause a false-positive Papanicolaou test result.

CONTRAINDICATIONS & CAUTIONS

• Contraindicated in patients hypersensitive to drug and in those with severe bone marrow suppression or urinary outflow obstruction.
• Use cautiously in patients with leukopenia, thrombocytopenia, malignant cell infiltration of bone marrow, or hepatic, cardiac, or renal disease and in those who have recently undergone radiation therapy or chemotherapy.
Dialyzable drug: Yes.
⚠ Overdose S&S: Infection, myelosuppression, cardiotoxicity.

PREGNANCY-LACTATION-REPRODUCTION

• Drug may cause fetal harm if used during pregnancy. Women of childbearing potential should avoid pregnancy while receiving cyclophosphamide and for up to 1 year after completion of treatment. Male patients who are sexually active with female partners who are or may become pregnant should use a condom during and for at least 4 months after treatment.
• Amenorrhea, transient or permanent, develops in a proportion of women treated with drug. The risk of premature menopause increases with age.
• Men treated with drug may develop oligospermia or azoospermia. Development of sterility appears to depend on dose, duration of therapy, and state of gonadal function at time of treatment. Sterility may be irreversible in some patients. Treatment for

nephrotic syndrome beyond 90 days in boys increases the probability of sterility.
• Drug appears in human milk. Patient should discontinue breastfeeding or discontinue drug, taking into account importance of drug to the mother.

NURSING CONSIDERATIONS
• If cystitis occurs, stop drug and notify prescriber. Cystitis can occur months after therapy ends. Mesna may be given to reduce frequency and severity of bladder toxicity. Test urine for blood.
• Adequately hydrate patients before and after dose to decrease risk of cystitis.
• Use caution to ensure correct dose to decrease risk of cardiac toxicity.
• Monitor CBC and renal function tests and LFT results.
• Monitor patient closely for leukopenia (nadir between days 8 and 15, recovery in 17 to 28 days). Withhold drug for ANC less than 1,500/mm^3.
• Monitor uric acid level. To prevent hyperuricemia with resulting uric acid nephropathy, allopurinol may be used with adequate hydration.
• To prevent bleeding, avoid all IM injections when platelet count is less than 50,000/mm^3.
• Monitor patients for renal, pulmonary, and cardiac toxicities, veno-occlusive liver disease, secondary malignancies, impaired wound healing, and hyponatremia.
• Anticipate blood transfusions because of cumulative anemia.
• Therapeutic effects are often accompanied by toxicity.
• Drug is associated with a moderate to high emetic potential (depending on dose, regimen, or administration route); antiemetics are recommended to prevent nausea and vomiting.

PATIENT TEACHING
• Warn patient that hair loss is likely to occur but is reversible.
• Advise patient to report all adverse reactions, especially signs and symptoms of infection (fever, sore throat, fatigue) and bleeding (easy bruising, nosebleeds, bleeding gums, tarry stools, bloody urine),

dyspnea, cough, edema, and dizziness. Tell patient to take temperature daily.
• Instruct patient to avoid OTC products that contain aspirin.
• To minimize risk of hemorrhagic cystitis, encourage patient to urinate every 1 to 2 hours while awake and to drink at least 3 L of fluid daily.
• Tell patient taking capsules to take them in the morning because infrequent urination during night increases risk of cystitis.
• Advise patient that drug is associated with a moderate to high emetic potential and that antiemetics are recommended.
• Advise both male and female patients to practice contraception during therapy and for 4 months afterward for men and 12 months for women; drug may cause birth defects.
• Advise female patient to stop breastfeeding during therapy because of risk of toxicity to infant.
• Drug can cause irreversible sterility in both males and females. Before therapy, counsel patient who is considering parenthood. Also recommend that female patient consult prescriber before becoming pregnant.

cycloSPORINE
sye-kloe-SPOR-een

Sandimmune

cycloSPORINE (modified)
Gengraf, Neoral

Therapeutic class: Immunosuppressants
Pharmacologic class: Immunosuppressants

AVAILABLE FORMS
Capsules for microemulsion (modified)*: 25 mg, 50 mg, 100 mg
Capsules (nonmodified): 25 mg, 50 mg, 100 mg
Injection: 50 mg/mL
Oral solution (modified and nonmodified): 100 mg/mL*

INDICATIONS & DOSAGES
➤ **To prevent organ rejection in renal, hepatic, or cardiac transplantation**

Adults and children: 15 mg/kg PO 4 to 12 hours before transplantation, continued daily for 1 to 2 weeks postoperatively. Then reduce dosage by 5% each week to maintenance level of 5 to 10 mg/kg daily. Or, 5 to 6 mg/kg IV concentrate 4 to 12 hours before transplantation as a slow IV infusion over 2 to 6 hours. Postoperatively, repeat dose daily until patient can tolerate oral forms.

For conversion from Sandimmune to Gengraf or Neoral, use same daily dose as previously used for Sandimmune. Monitor blood levels every 4 to 7 days after conversion, and monitor BP and creatinine level every 2 weeks during the first 2 months.

➤ **Severe, active RA that hasn't adequately responded to methotrexate (Gengraf or Neoral)**
Adults: 1.25 mg/kg PO b.i.d. Onset of action generally occurs between 4 and 8 weeks. Dosage may be increased by 0.5 to 0.75 mg/kg daily after 8 weeks and again after 12 weeks to a maximum of 4 mg/kg daily. If no response is seen after 16 weeks, stop therapy.
Adjust-a-dose: Decrease dosage by 25% to 50% to control adverse reactions (such as HTN, serum creatinine elevations [30% above patient's pretreatment level], or clinically significant laboratory abnormalities). If dosage reduction doesn't control abnormalities, or if adverse reaction or abnormality is severe, discontinue drug.

➤ **Psoriasis (Gengraf or Neoral)**
Adults: 1.25 mg/kg daily PO b.i.d. for at least 4 weeks. Increase dosage by 0.5 mg/kg daily once every 2 weeks as needed to a maximum of 4 mg/kg daily.
Adjust-a-dose: Decrease dosage by 25% to 50% to control adverse reactions (such as HTN, serum creatinine elevations [30% above patient's pretreatment level], or clinically significant laboratory abnormalities). If dosage reduction doesn't control abnormalities, or if adverse reaction or abnormality is severe, discontinue drug.

ADMINISTRATION

● Hazardous drug; follow safe handling procedures when preparing, administering, or dispensing.

PO
● Give Neoral or Gengraf on an empty stomach in two divided doses.
● Measure oral solution doses carefully in an oral syringe. Don't rinse dosing syringe with water. If syringe is cleaned, it must be completely dry before reuse.
● To improve the taste of Sandimmune oral solution, mix it with milk, chocolate milk, or orange juice. Gengraf or Neoral oral solution may be mixed with orange or apple juice (not grapefruit juice); it's less palatable when mixed with milk.
● Use a glass container to mix, and have patient drink at once.

IV
▼ This form is usually reserved for patients who can't tolerate oral drugs.
▼ Immediately before use, dilute each milliliter of concentrate in 20 to 100 mL of D₅W or NSS for injection. Give at ⅓ the oral dose.
▼ Infuse over 2 to 6 hours.
▼ Protect diluted drug from light.
▼ **Incompatibilities:** Amphotericin B cholesteryl sulfate complex, magnesium sulfate.

ACTION

May inhibit proliferation and function of T lymphocytes and inhibit production and release of lymphokines.

Route	Onset	Peak	Duration
PO	Unknown	90 min–3 hr	Unknown
IV	Unknown	Unknown	Unknown

Half-life: Initial phase, about 1 hour; terminal phase, 8½ to 27 hours.

ADVERSE REACTIONS

CNS: tremor, headache, confusion, paresthesia, *seizures.* **CV:** HTN, flushing. **EENT:** gum hyperplasia, sinusitis. **GI:** nausea, vomiting, diarrhea, abdominal discomfort. **GU:** *nephrotoxicity.* **Hematologic:** anemia, *leukopenia, thrombocytopenia.* **Hepatic:** *hepatotoxicity.* **Metabolic:** hyperglycemia. **Skin:** hirsutism, acne. **Other:** infections, *anaphylaxis.*

INTERACTIONS

Drug-drug. *Acyclovir, aminoglycosides, amphotericin B, cimetidine, diclofenac,* *gentamicin, ketoconazole, melphalan, NSAIDs, ranitidine, sulfamethoxazole–trimethoprim, tacrolimus, tobramycin, vancomycin:* May increase risk of nephrotoxicity. Avoid using together.

*Allopurinol, **azole antifungals**, bromocriptine, **caspofungin**, cimetidine, clarithromycin, danazol, diltiazem, erythromycin, imipenem–cilastatin, methylprednisolone, metoclopramide, **micafungin**, nicardipine, prednisolone, verapamil:* May increase cyclosporine level. Monitor patient for increased toxicity.

Azathioprine, corticosteroids, cyclophosphamide, verapamil: May increase immunosuppression. Monitor patient closely.

*Carbamazepine, isoniazid, nafcillin, octreotide, **orlistat**, phenobarbital, **phenytoin, rifabutin, rifampin**, ticlopidine:* May decrease immunosuppressant effect from low cyclosporine level. Cyclosporine dosage may need to be increased.

Digoxin, HMG-CoA reductase inhibitors (lovastatin), prednisolone: May decrease clearance of these drugs. Use together cautiously.

Mycophenolate mofetil: May decrease mycophenolate level. Monitor patient closely when cyclosporine is added to or removed from therapy.

Potassium-sparing diuretics: May induce hyperkalemia. Monitor patient closely.

Sirolimus: May increase sirolimus level. Take sirolimus at least 4 hours after cyclosporine dose. If separating doses isn't possible, monitor patient for increased adverse effects.

Vaccines: May decrease immune response. Delay routine immunization.

Drug-herb. *Astragalus, echinacea, licorice:* May interfere with drug's effect. Discourage use together.

St. John's wort: May reduce drug level, resulting in transplant failure. Discourage use together.

Drug-food. *Alfalfa sprouts:* May interfere with drug's effect. Discourage use together.

Grapefruit and grapefruit juice: May increase drug level and cause toxicity. Advise patient to avoid use together.

Drug-lifestyle. *Sun exposure:* May increase risk of sensitivity to sunlight. Advise patient to avoid excessive sun exposure.

EFFECTS ON LAB TEST RESULTS
• May increase ALT, AST, bilirubin, BUN, creatinine, glucose, and LDL levels.
• May decrease Hb and magnesium levels.
• May decrease platelet and WBC counts.

CONTRAINDICATIONS & CAUTIONS
• Contraindicated in patients hypersensitive to drug or polyoxyethylated castor oil (found in injectable form).
• Contraindicated in patients with RA or psoriasis with abnormal renal function, uncontrolled HTN, or malignancies (Neoral or Gengraf).
• Contraindicated with psoralen and ultraviolet A light (PUVA), methotrexate or other immunosuppressive agents, ultraviolet B light (UVB), coal tar, or radiation therapy in psoriasis patients (Neoral or Gengraf).

Black Box Warning Manage patients receiving drug in facilities equipped and staffed with adequate laboratory and supportive medical resources. ∎
Dialyzable drug: No.

PREGNANCY-LACTATION-REPRODUCTION
• There are no adequate studies in pregnant women; use during pregnancy isn't recommended. If drug is needed during pregnancy, use only if potential benefit justifies potential risk to the fetus.
• Alcohol is present in cyclosporine preparations; this fact should be considered when using drug in pregnant women.
• Drug and ethanol present in cyclosporine preparations appear in human milk. Patient should discontinue breastfeeding or discontinue drug, taking into account importance of drug to the mother.

NURSING CONSIDERATIONS
Black Box Warning Only experienced physicians should prescribe this drug. ∎
Black Box Warning Psoriasis patients previously treated with PUVA, methotrexate or other immunosuppressive agents, UVB, coal tar, or radiation therapy are at an increased risk for skin malignancies when taking Neoral or Gengraf. ∎
• Drug can cause hepatotoxicity.
Black Box Warning Neoral and Gengraf may increase the patient's susceptibility to infection and the development of neoplasia. ∎

Reactions in bold italics are *life-threatening*. Interactions may have a *rapid onset* or a *delayed onset*.

◑ Alert: Drugs causing immunosuppression increase the risk of opportunistic infections, including activation of latent viral infections such as BK virus–associated neuropathy, which may lead to serious outcomes, including kidney graft loss.

Black Box Warning Monitor patient's renal function. ■

Black Box Warning Monitor cyclosporine level at regular intervals with prolonged Sandimmune use. Absorption of capsules and oral solution can be erratic during long-term use. ■

Black Box Warning Neoral and Gengraf have greater bioavailability than Sandimmune. A lower dose of Neoral or Gengraf may be needed to provide blood level similar to that achieved with Sandimmune. Monitor blood level when switching patients between these two brands. ■

Black Box Warning Gengraf is bioequivalent to and interchangeable with Neoral capsules, but neither is interchangeable with Sandimmune. ■

Black Box Warning Always give Sandimmune with corticosteroids; however, don't give Sandimmune with other immunosuppressants. ■

Black Box Warning Drug can cause systemic HTN and nephrotoxicity; risk increases with increasing dosage and duration of therapy. ■

• Use Neoral or Gengraf to treat RA or psoriasis.

RA

• Before starting treatment, measure BP at least twice and obtain two creatinine levels to estimate baseline.

• Evaluate BP and creatinine level every 2 weeks during first 3 months and then monthly if patient is stable.

• Monitor BP and creatinine level after an increase in NSAID dosage or introduction of a new NSAID. Monitor CBC and LFTs monthly if patient also receives methotrexate.

Psoriasis

• Measure BP at least twice to determine a baseline. Monitor BP after dosage changes.

• Evaluate patient for occult infection and tumors initially and throughout treatment.

• Obtain baseline creatinine level (on two occasions), CBC, and BUN, magnesium, uric acid, potassium, and lipid levels.

• Evaluate BP, CBC, and uric acid, potassium, lipid, magnesium, creatinine, and BUN levels every 2 weeks during first 3 months and then monthly thereafter if patient is stable.

• Monitor creatinine level after increasing NSAID dose or starting a new NSAID.

• Improvement in psoriasis takes 12 to 16 weeks of therapy.

• **Look alike–sound alike:** Don't confuse cyclosporine with cyclophosphamide or cycloserine. Don't confuse Sandimmune with Sandostatin.

PATIENT TEACHING

• Encourage patient to take drug at same time each day and to be consistent with relation to meals.

• Teach patient how to measure dosage and mask taste of oral solution. Tell patient not to take drug with grapefruit juice.

• Instruct patient to fill glass with water after dose and drink it to make sure all of drug has been consumed.

• Advise patient to take drug with meals if nausea occurs.

• Advise patient to take Neoral or Gengraf on an empty stomach.

• Tell patient being treated for psoriasis that improvement may not occur until after 12 to 16 weeks of therapy.

• Stress that drug shouldn't be stopped without prescriber's approval.

• Explain to patient the importance of frequent laboratory monitoring while receiving therapy.

• Tell patient to avoid people with infections because drug lowers resistance to infection.

• Advise patient to perform careful oral care and to see a dentist regularly because drug can cause gum disease.

• Advise female patient to use barrier contraception, not hormonal contraceptives, during therapy. Advise patient of the potential risk during pregnancy and the increased risk of tumors, high BP, and renal problems.

• Warn patient to wear protection in the sun and to avoid excessive sun exposure.

cytarabine (ara-C, cytosine arabinoside)
sye-TARE-a-been

Cytosar♦

Therapeutic class: Antineoplastics
Pharmacologic class: Pyrimidine analogues

AVAILABLE FORMS
Injection: 20 mg/mL, 100 mg/mL

INDICATIONS & DOSAGES
Adjust-a-dose (for all indications): Consider dosage reduction in patients with poor renal function.
➤ **Acute nonlymphocytic leukemia**
Adults and children: 100 mg/m^2 IV daily by continuous IV infusion or 100 mg/m^2 IV every 12 hours by rapid IV injection or IV infusion on days 1 to 7 in a course of therapy or daily until remission is attained.
➤ **Acute lymphocytic leukemia**
Consult literature for current recommendations.
➤ **Meningeal leukemia**
Adults and children: Varies from 5 to 75 mg/m^2 intrathecally. Frequency varies from once daily for 4 days to once every 4 days. The most frequently used dose is 30 mg/m^2 every 4 days until CSF is normal; then one additional dose.
➤ **Acute promyelocytic leukemia (induction)** ◆
Adults: 200 mg/m^2 IV daily by continuous IV infusion for 7 days beginning on day 3 of treatment (in combination with tretinoin and daunorubicin).

ADMINISTRATION
• Hazardous drug; use safe handling and disposal precautions.

IV
▼ To reduce nausea, give antiemetic before drug. Nausea and vomiting are more likely with large doses given by IV push. Dizziness may occur with rapid infusion.
▼ For IV infusion, dilute solution in vial using NSS for injection or D$_5$W and administer as a continuous infusion.

▼ **Incompatibilities:** None listed by manufacturer. Consult a drug incompatibility reference for more information.

Intrathecal
• The single-use vial doesn't contain any preservative; drug should be used as soon as possible after preparation. Discard unused portions of each vial properly.
• After drug administration by lumbar puncture, instruct patient to lie flat for 1 hour.
• Patients should be observed by physician for immediate toxic reactions.

ACTION
Inhibits DNA synthesis.

Route	Onset	Peak	Duration
IV, intrathecal	Unknown	Unknown	Unknown

Half-life: Initial, 8 minutes; terminal, 1 to 3 hours; in CSF, 2 hours.

ADVERSE REACTIONS
CNS: *neurotoxicity,* malaise, dizziness, headache, cerebellar syndrome, fever. **CV:** thrombophlebitis, edema. **EENT:** conjunctivitis. **GI:** nausea, vomiting, diarrhea, anorexia, anal ulceration, abdominal pain, oral ulcers in 5 to 10 days, projectile vomiting, *bowel necrosis with high doses given by rapid IV.* **GU:** urine retention, renal dysfunction. **Hematologic:** *leukopenia,* anemia, reticulocytopenia, *thrombocytopenia,* megaloblastosis. **Hepatic:** *hepatotoxicity,* jaundice. **Metabolic:** hyperuricemia. **Musculoskeletal:** myalgia, bone pain. **Respiratory:** *pulmonary edema,* shortness of breath, pulmonary hypersensitivity. **Skin:** rash, pruritus, alopecia, freckling. **Other:** flulike syndrome, infection, *anaphylaxis.*

INTERACTIONS
Drug-drug. *Digoxin, except oral liquid:* May decrease oral digoxin absorption. Monitor digoxin level closely.
Flucytosine: May decrease flucytosine activity. Avoid using together.

EFFECTS ON LAB TEST RESULTS
• May increase bilirubin, phosphorus, potassium, and uric acid levels. May decrease Hb level.

Reactions in bold italics are *life-threatening*. Interactions may have a *rapid onset* or a ***delayed onset***.

• May increase megaloblast count. May decrease platelet, RBC, reticulocyte, and WBC counts.

CONTRAINDICATIONS & CAUTIONS
• Contraindicated in patients hypersensitive to drug. Anaphylaxis has been reported (rare).
• Use cautiously in patients with hepatic or renal impairment, gout, or myelosuppression.
• TLS may occur. Consider antihyperuricemic therapy and ensure adequate hydration.
❶ *Alert:* With high-dose therapy, drug is associated with sudden respiratory distress syndrome, which can be fatal.
Dialyzable drug: Yes.
⚠ *Overdose S&S:* Irreversible CNS toxicity, death.

PREGNANCY-LACTATION-REPRODUCTION
• Drug can cause fetal harm if a pregnant woman is exposed to drug systemically. Advise women of childbearing potential to avoid becoming pregnant during therapy. If drug is used during pregnancy or if patient becomes pregnant while taking drug, patient should be apprised of the potential harm to the fetus.
• It isn't known if drug appears in human milk. Patient should discontinue breastfeeding or discontinue drug, taking into account importance of drug to the mother.

NURSING CONSIDERATIONS
Black Box Warning Cytarabine should be administered by physicians experienced in cancer chemotherapy. For induction therapy, patients should be treated in a facility with laboratory and supportive resources sufficient to monitor drug tolerance and protect and maintain a patient compromised by drug toxicity. The physician must judge possible benefit to patient against known toxic effects of cytarabine. ∎
• Drug is an irritant. If extravasation occurs, stop the infusion immediately and follow facility policy for monitoring and treatment.
• Monitor fluid intake and output carefully. Maintain high fluid intake and give allopurinol to avoid urate nephropathy in leukemia-induction therapy. Monitor uric acid level.

• Monitor renal function studies, LFTs, and CBC with differential.
• Therapy may be modified or stopped if granulocyte count is below 1,000/mm^3 or platelet count is below 50,000/mm^3.
• Corticosteroid eye drops help prevent drug-induced conjunctivitis.
• Provide diligent mouth care to help minimize stomatitis.
❶ *Alert:* Assess patient receiving high doses for neurotoxicity, which may first appear as nystagmus but can progress to ataxia and cerebellar dysfunction.
• To prevent bleeding, avoid all IM injections when platelet count is below 50,000/mm^3.
• Anticipate blood transfusions because of cumulative anemia. Patient may receive RBC colony-stimulating factors to promote RBC production and decrease need for blood transfusions.
Black Box Warning Monitor patient for toxic effects, including bone marrow suppression, nausea, vomiting, diarrhea, oral ulceration, and hepatic dysfunction. ∎
• In leukopenia, initial WBC count nadir occurs 7 to 9 days after drug is stopped. A second, more severe nadir occurs 15 to 24 days after drug is stopped. In thrombocytopenia, platelet count nadir occurs on days 12 to 15.
❶ *Alert:* A cytarabine syndrome has been described and is characterized by fever, myalgia, bone pain, occasionally chest pain, maculopapular rash, conjunctivitis, and malaise. It usually occurs 6 to 12 hours after drug administration. Corticosteroids have been shown to be beneficial in the treatment or prevention of this syndrome.
• *Look alike–sound alike:* Don't confuse cytarabine with clofarabine or vidarabine.

PATIENT TEACHING
• Instruct patient to watch for signs and symptoms of infection (fever, sore throat, fatigue) and bleeding (easy bruising, nosebleeds, bleeding gums, tarry stools). Tell patient to take temperature daily.
• Advise patient to report vision changes, blurred vision, or eye pain to prescriber.
• Advise breastfeeding patient to stop breastfeeding during therapy because of risk of toxicity in infant.

• Caution female patient of childbearing potential to consult prescriber before becoming pregnant because drug may harm fetus.

dabigatran etexilate mesylate
da-BIG-a-tran e-TEX-i-late

Pradaxa⏑

Therapeutic class: Anticoagulants
Pharmacologic class: Direct thrombin inhibitors

AVAILABLE FORMS
Capsules ⓞⓝⓒ: 75 mg, 110 mg, 150 mg

INDICATIONS & DOSAGES
➤ **To reduce risk of stroke and systemic embolism in patients with nonvalvular atrial fibrillation**
Adults: 150 mg PO b.i.d. if CrCl is greater than 30 mL/minute. Refer to manufacturer's instructions when converting to and from warfarin or parenteral anticoagulants.
Adjust-a-dose: For patients with CrCl of 15 to 30 mL/minute or for those with CrCl of 30 to 50 mL/minute who are taking dronedarone or oral ketoconazole concurrently, give 75 mg PO b.i.d. Avoid use in patients with CrCl of less than 30 mL/minute also taking P-gp inhibitors. Don't use in patients on dialysis or in those with CrCl of less than 15 mL/minute.
➤ **To treat DVT and PE in patients with CrCl greater than 30 mL/minute who have been treated with a parenteral anticoagulant for 5 to 10 days; to reduce risk of recurrence of DVT and PE in patients with CrCl greater than 30 mL/minute who have been previously treated**
Adults: 150 mg PO b.i.d.
Adjust-a-dose: There are no dosing recommendations for patients with CrCl of 30 mL/minute or less or for those on dialysis. Avoid use in patients with CrCl of less than 50 mL/minute also taking P-gp inhibitors.
➤ **Prophylaxis of DVT and PE after hip replacement surgery**

Adults: 110 mg PO 1 to 4 hours after surgery and after hemostasis has been achieved, then 220 mg once daily for 28 to 35 days. If drug isn't started on day of surgery, after hemostasis has been achieved, start treatment with 220 mg once daily.
Adjust-a-dose: There are no dosing recommendations for patients with CrCl of less than 30 mL/minute or for those on dialysis. Avoid use in patients with CrCl of less than 50 mL/minute also taking P-gp inhibitors.

ADMINISTRATION
PO
• Give without regard to food.
• Don't crush capsule, empty its contents, or allow patient to chew capsule. Patient must swallow capsule whole with full glass of water.
• Temporarily discontinue drug before invasive or surgical procedures. Restart drug promptly after procedure.

ACTION
Reversible, direct thrombin inhibitor that prevents development of a thrombus.

Route	Onset	Peak	Duration
PO	Unknown	1–2 hr	Unknown

Half-life: 12 to 17 hours.

ADVERSE REACTIONS
GI: dyspepsia, abdominal pain, abdominal discomfort, gastritis-like symptoms, GERD, esophagitis, erosive gastritis, *gastric hemorrhage, hemorrhagic erosive gastritis,* GI ulcer, diarrhea, nausea, *GI bleeding.* **Hematologic:** *life-threatening bleeding,* major bleeding, any bleeding.

INTERACTIONS
Drug-drug. *Antiplatelet drugs, aspirin, fibrinolytic therapy, heparin, NSAIDs:* May increase risk of bleeding. Carefully consider risks and benefits of using together, monitor closely, and consider therapy modification.
P-gp inducers (rifampin): May reduce dabigatran level. Avoid use together.
P-gp inhibitors (dronedarone, systemic ketoconazole): May increase effectiveness of dabigatran; dosage reductions may be needed. Refer to indication-specific dosage

---

Reactions in bold italics are *life-threatening*. Interactions may have a *rapid onset* or a *delayed onset*.

adjustments above and manufacturer's instructions for additional information.
Drug-herb. *Herbs with anticoagulant/antiplatelet properties (alfalfa, anise, bilberry):* May increase risk of bleeding. Consider therapy modification.

EFFECTS ON LAB TEST RESULTS
• May increase aPTT, ecarin clotting time (ECT), and thrombin time.

CONTRAINDICATIONS & CAUTIONS
Black Box Warning Consider potential risk of epidural or spinal hematoma versus potential benefit in patients scheduled for spinal procedures, such as spinal or epidural anesthesia or spinal puncture. Hematomas may result in long-term or permanent paralysis. Increased risk may occur with use of indwelling epidural catheters, concomitant use of drugs that affect hemostasis (NSAIDs, platelet inhibitors, anticoagulants), history of traumatic or repeated epidural or spinal punctures, or history of spinal deformity or surgery. Optimal timing between administration of drug and spinal or epidural procedure isn't known. ∎
• Contraindicated in patients hypersensitive to drug and in those with active pathologic bleeding.
• Contraindicated in patients with mechanical prosthetic valves. Use in patients with atrial fibrillation in the setting of other forms of valvular heart disease, including the presence of a bioprosthetic heart valve, isn't recommended.
• Use cautiously in elderly patients, in patients with a history of bleeding, and when used with other drugs that increase the risk of bleeding.
• Because of risk of clot formation and stroke, avoid lapses in therapy when possible. Restart therapy as soon as possible.
Black Box Warning Discontinuing drug prematurely increases risk of thrombotic events. If drug must be discontinued for a reason other than pathologic bleeding or completion of a course of therapy, consider coverage with another anticoagulant. ∎
Dialyzable drug: Approximately 57%.
⚠ *Overdose S&S:* Hemorrhagic complications.

PREGNANCY-LACTATION-REPRODUCTION
• There are no adequate well-controlled studies in pregnant women. Consider risks of bleeding and stroke if drug is used during pregnancy.
• Drug may increase bleeding risk in the fetus and neonate. Monitor neonates for bleeding.
• It isn't known if drug appears in human milk. Patient should discontinue breastfeeding or discontinue drug, taking into account importance of drug to the mother.

NURSING CONSIDERATIONS
• Monitor patient for signs of bleeding. If bleeding occurs, stop drug, investigate cause, and provide supportive measures.
• A specific reversal agent (idarucizumab) is available. Refer to the idarucizumab prescribing information for additional information.
• Monitor ECT or aPPT to assess treatment effectiveness.
Black Box Warning Monitor patient for neurologic impairment (midline back pain, sensory or motor deficits such as numbness or weakness in lower limbs, bowel or bladder dysfunction). Treat impairment urgently. ∎
• Discontinue dabigatran 1 to 2 days before invasive or surgical procedures in patients with CrCl of 50 mL/minute or more and 3 to 5 days in patients with CrCl of less than 50 mL/minute. Consider longer times for patients undergoing major surgery, spinal puncture, or placement of a spinal or epidural catheter or port, in whom complete hemostasis may be required.

PATIENT TEACHING
⊙ *Alert:* Advise patient to keep drug in original bottle to protect from moisture, to remove only one capsule from the opened bottle at the time of use, to tightly close the bottle immediately after removing drug, and not to put drug in pill boxes or pill organizers.
• Tell patient that drug may be taken without regard to food.
• Advise patient to take dabigatran at approximately the same times each day. A missed dose may be skipped only if it can't be taken at least 6 hours before the next scheduled dose.

• Teach patient to swallow the capsule whole with a full glass of water and not to open, crush, or chew it.

• Caution patient to take drug as prescribed and not to stop or change dosage without first consulting prescriber.

• Advise patient to tell all health care providers about taking drug.

• Tell patient to inform prescriber about use of other drugs, including OTCs, vitamins, and herbs.

• Warn patient that bruising may occur more easily and bleeding may last longer during therapy.

• Instruct patient to report bleeding when brushing teeth or shaving; blood in vomit, urine, or stool; heavier menstrual bleeding; or nosebleeds.

• Tell patient regular blood tests to monitor drug's effects will be needed.

• Instruct patient to inform health care provider of scheduled invasive procedures, including dental work. Drug may need to be stopped temporarily.

SAFETY ALERT!

dacarbazine (DTIC)
da-KAR-ba-zeen

Therapeutic class: Antineoplastics
Pharmacologic class: Triazenes

AVAILABLE FORMS
Injection: 200-mg vials

INDICATIONS & DOSAGES
➤ **Metastatic malignant melanoma**
Adults: 2 to 4.5 mg/kg IV daily for 10 days; repeat every 4 weeks as tolerated. Or, 250 mg/m^2 IV daily for 5 days; repeat every 3 weeks.
➤ **Hodgkin lymphoma**
Adults: 150 mg/m^2 IV daily (with other drugs) for 5 days; repeat every 4 weeks. Or, 375 mg/m^2 on first day of combination regimen; repeat every 15 days.
➤ **Advanced soft-tissue sarcomas ◆**
Adults: 250 mg/m^2 daily by continuous IV infusion for 4 days every 3 weeks (total dacarbazine dose is 1,000 mg/m^2 over 96 hours) (MAID regimen; in combination with mesna, doxorubicin, and ifosfamide).

ADMINISTRATION
IV
▼ Preparing and giving parenteral drug may be mutagenic, teratogenic, or carcinogenic. Follow facility policy to reduce risks.
▼ Reconstitute drug using sterile water for injection. Add 19.7 mL to 200-mg vial to yield a concentration of 10 mg/mL.
▼ For infusion, dilute further with NSS or D$_5$W.
▼ Infuse over 15 to 60 minutes. To decrease pain at insertion site, dilute drug further or decrease infusion rate.
▼ Watch for irritation and infiltration during infusion; extravasation can cause severe pain, tissue damage, and necrosis. If solution infiltrates, notify prescriber and follow facility protocol.
▼ Reconstituted solutions in the vial are stable 8 hours at room temperature and with normal lighting conditions, or up to 3 days if refrigerated.
▼ Solution should be colorless to clear yellow. If solution turns pink, it has decomposed. Discard it.
▼ Diluted solutions are stable 8 hours at room temperature and with normal lighting, or up to 24 hours if refrigerated.
▼ **Incompatibilities:** Allopurinol sodium, cefepime, piperacillin–tazobactam. Consult a drug incompatibility reference for more information.

ACTION
Alkylating agent that binds to DNA, breaking the strands, and interferes with protein synthesis. Not cell-cycle specific.

Route	Onset	Peak	Duration
IV	Unknown	Unknown	Unknown

Half-life: Initial phase, 19 minutes; terminal phase, 5 hours.

ADVERSE REACTIONS
GI: anorexia, severe nausea and vomiting, stomatitis. **Hematologic:** *leukopenia, thrombocytopenia.* **Skin:** alopecia. **Other:** *anaphylaxis,* severe pain with infiltration or a too-concentrated solution, tissue damage.

Reactions in bold italics are *life-threatening*. Interactions may have a *rapid onset* or a ***delayed onset***.

INTERACTIONS
Drug-lifestyle. *Sun exposure:* May cause photosensitivity reaction. Advise patient to avoid excessive sunlight exposure.

EFFECTS ON LAB TEST RESULTS
• May increase BUN and liver enzyme levels.
• May decrease platelet, RBC, and WBC counts.

CONTRAINDICATIONS & CAUTIONS
• Contraindicated in hypersensitivity to drug.
• Use cautiously in patients with impaired bone marrow function and those with severe renal or hepatic dysfunction.
Dialyzable drug: Unknown.

PREGNANCY-LACTATION-REPRODUCTION
Black Box Warning Studies have demonstrated this agent to have a carcinogenic and teratogenic effect when used in animals. ■
• There are no adequate well-controlled studies in pregnant women. Use during pregnancy only if potential benefit justifies potential risk to the fetus.
• It isn't known if drug appears in human milk. Patient should discontinue breastfeeding or discontinue drug, taking into account importance of drug to the mother.

NURSING CONSIDERATIONS
Black Box Warning Dacarbazine should be administered under the supervision of a physician experienced in the use of cancer chemotherapeutic agents. The physician must carefully weigh the possibility of therapeutic benefit against the risk of toxicity for each patient. ■
• Give antiemetics before giving this drug. Nausea and vomiting may subside after several doses.
• To prevent bleeding, avoid all IM injections when platelet count is below 50,000/mm^3.
Black Box Warning Hematopoietic depression is the most common toxicity. ■
• Anticipate need for blood transfusions to combat anemia.
• Therapeutic effects commonly occur with toxicity. Monitor CBC and platelet count.

Black Box Warning Hepatic necrosis may occur. Monitor LFTs. ■
• For Hodgkin lymphoma, drug is usually given in combination with other antineoplastics.
• *Look alike–sound alike:* Don't confuse dacarbazine with procarbazine.

PATIENT TEACHING
• Tell patient to watch for signs of infection (fever, sore throat, fatigue) and bleeding (easy bruising, nosebleeds, bleeding gums, tarry stools) and to take temperature daily.
• Tell patient to avoid people with URIs.
• Advise patient to avoid sunlight.
• Reassure patient that fever, malaise, and muscle pain, beginning 7 days after treatment ends and possibly lasting 7 to 21 days, may be treated with mild fever reducers such as acetaminophen.
• Tell patient that restricting food intake for 4 to 6 hours before dose may help to decrease adverse GI effects.
• Reassure patient that hair loss is reversible.
• Advise female patient to avoid pregnancy and breastfeeding during therapy.

daclatasvir dihydrochloride ⬚
dak-LAT-as-vir

Daklinza

Therapeutic class: Antivirals
Pharmacologic class: HCV NS5A replication complex inhibitors

AVAILABLE FORMS
Tablets: 30 mg, 60 mg

INDICATIONS & DOSAGES
➤ **Treatment of HCV genotype 1 or 3 infection in combination with sofosbuvir and with or without ribavirin** ⬚
Adults: 60 mg PO once daily for 12 weeks in combination with sofosbuvir.
Adjust-a-dose: When given with strong CYP3A inhibitors, reduce dosage to 30 mg once daily. When given with moderate CYP3A inducers, increase dosage to 90 mg once daily.

For patients with HCV genotype 1 or 3 infection with Child-Pugh class B or C decompensated cirrhosis and posttransplantation patients, give drug with sofosbuvir and ribavirin for 12 weeks. Starting dose of ribavirin is 600 mg PO daily, increasing up to 1,000 mg PO daily as tolerated. May decrease starting dose and on-treatment dose of ribavirin based on Hb level and CrCl.

For patients with HCV genotype 3 infection with compensated cirrhosis (Child-Pugh class A), give drug with sofosbuvir and ribavirin for 12 weeks. Recommended ribavirin dosage is based on weight (1,000 mg PO for patients weighing less than 75 kg and 1,200 mg PO for those weighing at least 75 kg administered in two divided doses with food).

ADMINISTRATION
PO
• May give with or without food.
• If a dose is missed, give as soon as possible within the same day. If missed dose isn't within the same day, give next scheduled dose at the appropriate time.
• Store at room temperature.

ACTION
Inhibits both viral RNA replication and virion assembly.

Route	Onset	Peak	Duration
PO	Unknown	2 hr	Unknown

Half-life: 12 to 15 hours.

ADVERSE REACTIONS
CNS: fatigue, headache, insomnia, somnolence. **Hematologic:** anemia. **GI:** diarrhea, nausea. **Metabolic:** elevated lipase level. **Skin:** rash.

INTERACTIONS
Drug-drug. ◑ *Alert: Amiodarone:* May cause serious symptomatic bradycardia. Use together isn't recommended. If use together is required, use cardiac monitoring.
Dabigatran: May increase dabigatran level. Use together isn't recommended in some patients with renal impairment. Refer to dabigatran manufacturer's instructions for specific recommendations.

Digoxin: May increase digoxin level. For patients already taking daclatasvir, initiate digoxin using lowest appropriate dosage; monitor and adjust digoxin dosage as needed. For those already taking digoxin, measure serum digoxin level before initiating daclatasvir. Reduce digoxin concentration by decreasing digoxin dosage by approximately 15% to 30% or by modifying dosing frequency; continue monitoring.
HMG-CoA reductase inhibitors (atorvastatin, fluvastatin, pitavastatin, pravastatin, rosuvastatin, simvastatin): May increase HMG-CoA reductase inhibitor level. Monitor for HMG-CoA reductase inhibitor–related adverse events such as myopathy.
Moderate CYP3A inducers (bosentan, dexamethasone, efavirenz, etravirine, modafinil, nafcillin, rifapentine): May reduce daclatasvir level. Increase daclatasvir dose to 90 mg once daily.
Moderate CYP3A inhibitors (atazanavir, ciprofloxacin, darunavir/ritonavir, diltiazem, erythromycin, fluconazole, fosamprenavir, verapamil): May increase daclatasvir level. Monitor patient for daclatasvir-related adverse events.
Strong CYP3A inducers (carbamazepine, phenytoin, rifampin): May reduce daclatasvir level. Use together is contraindicated.
Strong CYP3A inhibitors (atazanavir/ritonavir, clarithromycin, indinavir, itraconazole, ketoconazole, nefazodone, nelfinavir, posaconazole, ritonavir, saquinavir, telithromycin, voriconazole): May increase daclatasvir level. Reduce daclatasvir dosage to 30 mg once daily.
Drug-herb. *St. John's wort:* May diminish daclatasvir effectiveness. Use together is contraindicated.

EFFECTS ON LAB TEST RESULTS
• May increase lipase level.

CONTRAINDICATIONS & CAUTIONS
• Contraindicated in combination with drugs or herbs that strongly induce CYP3A (such as carbamazepine, phenytoin, rifampin, St. John's wort) because of loss of efficacy of daclatasvir.
◑ *Alert:* May cause serious symptomatic bradycardia when given with amiodarone.

Reactions in bold italics are *life-threatening*. Interactions may have a *rapid onset* or a *delayed onset*.

Bradycardia can occur hours after administration or up to 2 weeks after treatment initiation. Inpatient cardiac monitoring is recommended for first 48 hours if daclatasvir is used with amiodarone. Outpatient or self-monitoring of HR should occur daily for at least first 2 weeks of treatment.

• Patients who have recently discontinued amiodarone should undergo cardiac monitoring when beginning daclatasvir because of amiodarone's long half-life.

• Patients receiving beta blockers or with underlying cardiac comorbidities or advanced liver disease may be at increased risk for symptomatic bradycardia. Bradycardia usually resolves after daclatasvir is discontinued.

• If daclatasvir and sofosbuvir are administered with ribavirin, the warnings and precautions for ribavirin, in particular the pregnancy avoidance warning, apply to this combination regimen. Refer to the ribavirin prescribing information for a full list of the warnings and precautions for ribavirin.

• Safe use in children hasn't been established.

Dialyzable drug: Unlikely.

PREGNANCY-LACTATION-REPRODUCTION
• There are no adequate studies in pregnant women. Consider risks and benefits before use during pregnancy.

• If daclatasvir and sofosbuvir are administered with ribavirin, the combination regimen is contraindicated in pregnant women and in men whose female partners are pregnant.

• It isn't known if drug appears in human milk. Use cautiously and consider risks and benefits to mother and infant. If given with ribavirin, refer to ribavirin prescribing information for additional recommendations.

NURSING CONSIDERATIONS
▓ Before treatment initiation in patients with genotype 1a, consider screening for the presence of *NS5A* polymorphisms at amino acid positions M28, Q30, L31, and Y93 in patients with cirrhosis.

Black Box Warning Test all patients for evidence of current or prior HBV infection by measuring HbsAg and hepatitis B core antibody before initiating treatment. Initiate

appropriate treatment for HBV infection as clinically indicated. ▋

• Drug must be taken in combination with sofosbuvir. If sofosbuvir is permanently discontinued, daclatasvir should be discontinued.

• Dosage reduction for adverse reactions isn't recommended. Lower dosage may cause loss of therapeutic effect and possible development of resistance.

• Review concomitant medications during therapy and monitor patients for adverse reactions associated with those drugs.

• Monitor patients for bradycardia (HR less than 60 beats/minute, syncope, near-syncope, dizziness, light-headedness, malaise, weakness, tiredness, dyspnea, chest pain, confusion, memory problems). Report signs and symptoms immediately.

• *Look alike–sound alike:* Don't confuse daclatasvir with ledipasvir or entecavir.

PATIENT TEACHING
• Counsel patient on importance of reporting to prescriber all other drugs and supplements being taken before beginning treatment, as some are contraindicated during daclatasvir therapy.

• Advise patient to immediately report signs and symptoms of serious bradycardia (slow heartbeat, near fainting, dizziness, weakness, chest pain, confusion, dyspnea).

• Instruct patient that if a dose is missed to take dose as soon as possible if it's within the same day. If missed dose isn't remembered within the same day, patient should skip missed dose and should take next dose at the appropriate time.

• Teach patient appropriate precautions to prevent transmission of HCV during therapy.

dalbavancin hydrochloride
dal-ba-VAN-sin

Dalvance

Therapeutic class: Antibiotics
Pharmacologic class: Lipoglycopeptides

AVAILABLE FORMS
Injection: 500-mg single-use vial

INDICATIONS & DOSAGES
➤ Acute bacterial skin and skin-structure infections caused by susceptible strains of gram-positive microorganisms (*Staphylococcus aureus* [including MRSA], *Streptococcus pyogenes*, *Streptococcus agalactiae*, *Streptococcus dysgalactiae*, *Streptococcus anginosus* group [*S. anginosus, S. intermedius, S. constellatus*]), *Enterococcus faecalis* (vancomycin-susceptible strains)

Adults: 1,500 mg IV infusion as a single dose, or 1,000 mg IV infusion followed by a second dose of 500 mg IV infusion 1 week later.

Adjust-a-dose: For patients with CrCl of less than 30 mL/minute who aren't receiving hemodialysis, give 1,125 mg IV infusion as a single dose, or 750 mg IV infusion followed by a second dose of 375 mg IV infusion 1 week later. No dosage adjustment is necessary for patients on regularly scheduled hemodialysis; give without regard to hemodialysis timing.

ADMINISTRATION

IV

▼ Reconstitute each vial with 25 mL sterile water for injection or 5% dextrose injection. Swirl gently, and invert vial until vial contents are completely dissolved. Don't shake. Reconstituted vial contains a concentration of 20 mg/mL. Dilute further with dextrose 5% to a final concentration of 1 to 5 mg/mL.

▼ Inspect for particulate matter before infusion. Don't infuse if particulate matter is identified.

▼ To reduce risk of infusion-related reactions, infuse drug over 30 minutes.

▼ Flush IV line before and after each dalbavancin infusion with 5% dextrose injection if line is used to administer other drugs in addition to dalbavancin.

▼ Store reconstituted vials or final IV bags or bottles in refrigerator or at room temperature. Use within 48 hours.

▼ **Incompatibilities:** Other medications, electrolytes, saline-based solutions.

ACTION
Bactericidal; interferes with cell-wall synthesis within the bacteria.

Route	Onset	Peak	Duration
IV	Unknown	Unknown	7 days

Half-life: 8½ days.

ADVERSE REACTIONS
CNS: headache, dizziness. **CV:** flushing, phlebitis, spontaneous hematoma. **EENT:** oral candidiasis. **GI:** nausea, vomiting, diarrhea, *GI hemorrhage,* melena, hematochezia, abdominal pain, *C. difficile colitis.* **GU:** vulvovaginal mycotic infection. **Hematologic:** anemia, *hemorrhagic anemia, leukopenia, neutropenia, thrombocytopenia,* eosinophilia, *thrombocytosis.* **Hepatic:** *hepatotoxicity.* **Metabolic:** *hypoglycemia.* **Respiratory:** *bronchospasm.* **Skin:** rash, pruritus, urticaria, petechiae. **Other:** infusion-site reactions, *anaphylactoid reaction, wound hemorrhage.*

INTERACTIONS
None reported.

EFFECTS ON LAB TEST RESULTS
• May increase INR and LDH, GGT, ALT, AST, and alkaline phosphatase levels.
• May decrease Hb level and platelet and WBC counts.

CONTRAINDICATIONS & CAUTIONS
• Contraindicated in patients hypersensitive to drug or its components.
• Don't use unless proven or strongly suspected bacterial infection exists.
• Use cautiously in patients with known hypersensitivity to glycopeptides.
• Use cautiously in patients with moderate to severe hepatic impairment (Child-Pugh class B or C).
• Safety and effectiveness in children haven't been established.
• Use cautiously in elderly patients. Drug is substantially excreted by the kidneys.
Dialyzable drug: No.

PREGNANCY-LACTATION-REPRODUCTION
• There are no adequate well-controlled studies in pregnant women. Use during pregnancy only if clearly needed and potential benefit justifies potential risk to the fetus.
• It isn't known if drug appears in human milk. Use cautiously in breastfeeding women.

NURSING CONSIDERATIONS

❶ *Alert:* Monitor patient for development of CDAD, which can range from mild to fatal colitis and can occur more than 2 months after treatment ends.

• Ensure a suspected or confirmed serious bacterial infection exists before administering drug.

• Monitor patient for infusion reactions or hypersensitivity. Discontinue drug if reaction occurs.

• Rapid infusion (less than 30 minutes) may result in "red man syndrome" (upper body flushing, urticaria, pruritus, rash). Stopping or slowing infusion may stop this reaction.

PATIENT TEACHING

• Instruct patient to notify prescriber of allergy or hypersensitivity to other glycopeptides such as vancomycin before treatment.

• Explain to patient that drug is used only for presumed or actual serious bacterial infections.

• Teach patient that drug will be given intravenously, and to immediately report signs or symptoms of reactions.

• Advise patient not to skip any doses of antibacterial drugs as this may decrease effectiveness of treatment.

• Tell patient to report GI side effects such as diarrhea, which is common and may be serious. Tell patient to contact prescriber if severe watery or bloody diarrhea occurs.

• Warn female patient to alert prescriber if she is pregnant or breastfeeding.

SAFETY ALERT!

dalteparin sodium
DAHL-tep-ah-rin

Fragmin

Therapeutic class: Anticoagulants
Pharmacologic class: Low-molecular-weight heparins

AVAILABLE FORMS

Injection: 2,500 antifactor Xa international units/0.2-mL syringe, 5,000 antifactor Xa international units/0.2-mL syringe, 7,500 antifactor Xa international units/0.3-mL syringe, 10,000 antifactor Xa international units/1-mL syringe, 12,500 antifactor Xa international units/0.5-mL syringe, 15,000 antifactor Xa international units/0.6-mL syringe, 18,000 antifactor Xa international units/0.72-mL syringe, 95,000 antifactor Xa international units/3.8-mL vial*

INDICATIONS & DOSAGES

➤ **To prevent DVT in patients undergoing abdominal surgery who are at moderate to high risk for thromboembolic complications**

Adults: 2,500 international units subcut daily, starting 1 to 2 hours before surgery and repeated once daily for 5 to 10 days postoperatively. Or, for patients at high risk, give 5,000 international units subcut the evening before surgery, then once daily postoperatively for 5 to 10 days. Or, in patients with malignancy, give 2,500 international units subcut 1 to 2 hours before surgery followed by 2,500 international units subcut 12 hours later, then 5,000 international units subcut once daily for 5 to 10 days postoperatively.

➤ **To prevent DVT in patients undergoing hip replacement surgery**

Adults: 2,500 international units subcut within 2 hours before surgery and second dose of 2,500 international units subcut in the evening after surgery (4 to 8 hours after surgery or later if hemostasis hasn't been achieved). Starting on first postoperative day, allowing a minimum of 6 hours after postoperative dose, give 5,000 international units subcut once daily for 5 to 10 days. Or, give 5,000 international units subcut 10 to 14 hours before surgery; then 5,000 international units subcut once daily starting 4 to 8 hours after surgery for 5 to 10 days postoperatively. Allow approximately 24 hours between preoperative and first postoperative doses.

If starting postoperatively, give 2,500 international units subcut in the evening after surgery (4 to 8 hours after surgery, or later if hemostasis hasn't been achieved). Starting on first postoperative day, allowing a minimum of 6 hours after postoperative dose, give 5,000 international units subcut once daily for 5 to 10 days.

➤ **Prophylaxis of ischemic complications in patients with unstable angina; non-Q-wave MI**
Adults: 120 international units/kg subcut every 12 hours with aspirin (75 to 165 mg daily) PO, unless contraindicated. Maximum dose, 10,000 international units. Treatment usually lasts 5 to 8 days.

➤ **To prevent DVT in patients at risk for thromboembolic complications because of severely restricted mobility during acute illness**
Adults: 5,000 international units subcut once daily for 12 to 14 days.

➤ **Symptomatic venous thromboembolism (VTE) in cancer patients**
Adults: Initially, 200 international units/kg (maximum, 18,000 international units) subcut daily for 30 days; then 150 international units/kg (maximum, 18,000 international units) subcut daily months 2 through 6.
Adjust-a-dose: In patients with platelet count 50,000 to 100,000/mm^3, reduce dose by 2,500 international units until platelet count exceeds 100,000/mm^3. In patients with platelet count less than 50,000/mm^3, stop drug until platelet count exceeds 50,000/mm^3. In patients with CrCl of 30 mL/minute or less, monitor anti-Xa levels to determine appropriate dose. Target anti-Xa range is 0.5 to 1.5 international units/mL. Draw anti-Xa 4 to 6 hours after dose and only after patient has received three to four doses.

➤ **Acute symptomatic superficial lower extremity vein thrombosis 5 cm or greater in length ◆**
Adults: 5,000 units subcut every 12 hours for 45 days.
Adjust-a-dose: Recurrence risk is high if anticoagulation is discontinued earlier than 45 days. Monitor D-dimer at baseline and again at 45 days; if D-dimer remains elevated, a longer course may be necessary.
✷ *NEW INDICATION:* **Reduced recurrence of symptomatic venous thromboembolism (VTE) in pediatric patients**
Refer to manufacturer's instructions.

ADMINISTRATION
Subcutaneous
● Have patient sit or lie supine when giving drug.

● Injection sites include a U-shaped area around the navel, upper outer side of thigh, and upper outer quadrangle of buttock. Rotate sites daily.
● When area around the navel or thigh is used, use thumb and forefinger to lift up a fold of skin while giving injection.
● Give subcut injection deeply, inserting entire length of needle at a 45- to 90-degree angle.
● After first penetration of rubber stopper, store multidose vial at room temperature for up to 2 weeks. Discard any unused solution after 2 weeks.

ACTION
Enhances inhibition of factor Xa and thrombin by antithrombin.

Route	Onset	Peak	Duration
Subcut	1–2 hr	4 hr	>12 hr

Half-life: 2 to 5 hours.

ADVERSE REACTIONS
CNS: fever. **GU:** hematuria. **Hematologic:** *thrombocytopenia, hemorrhage,* ecchymoses, bleeding complications. **Skin:** pruritus, rash, hematoma at injection site, injection-site pain. **Other:** *anaphylaxis.*

INTERACTIONS
Drug-drug. *Antiplatelet drugs (aspirin, NSAIDs, clopidogrel, dipyridamole, ticlopidine), oral anticoagulants, SSRIs (fluoxetine), thrombolytics:* May increase risk of bleeding. Use together cautiously.
Drug-herb. *Herbs with anticoagulant/antiplatelet properties (alfalfa, anise, bilberry, willow):* May increase risk of bleeding. Discourage use together.

EFFECTS ON LAB TEST RESULTS
● May increase ALT and AST levels.
● May decrease platelet count.

CONTRAINDICATIONS & CAUTIONS
● Contraindicated in patients hypersensitive to drug, heparin, or pork products; in those with active major bleeding; and in those with thrombocytopenia and antiplatelet antibodies in the presence of the drug.
● Contraindicated in patients with unstable angina or non-Q-wave MI or prolonged

VTE prophylaxis who are undergoing epidural/neuraxial anesthesia.
• Use cautiously in patients with history of heparin-induced thrombocytopenia and in patients at increased risk for hemorrhage, such as those with severe uncontrolled HTN, bacterial endocarditis, congenital or acquired bleeding disorders, active ulceration, angiodysplastic GI disease, or hemorrhagic stroke; also use with caution shortly after brain, spinal, or ophthalmic surgery. Monitor vital signs.
• Use cautiously in patients with bleeding diathesis, thrombocytopenia, platelet defects, severe hepatic or renal insufficiency, hypertensive or diabetic retinopathy, or recent GI bleeding.
• Use preservative-free dalteparin in neonates and infants because serious and fatal adverse reactions, including "gasping syndrome," can occur in neonates and low-birth-weight infants treated with medications containing benzyl alcohol.
Dialyzable drug: Unknown.
⚠ *Overdose S&S:* Hemorrhagic complications.

PREGNANCY-LACTATION-REPRODUCTION
• There are no adequate well-controlled studies in pregnant women. Use during pregnancy only if clearly needed.
• Use preservative-free formulations without benzyl alcohol (not multidose vial) when possible during pregnancy and only if clearly needed. Benzyl alcohol may cross the placental barrier.
• Small amounts of anti-Xa activity have been detected in human milk; clinical implications, if any, for a breastfeeding infant are unknown. Use cautiously in breastfeeding women.

NURSING CONSIDERATIONS
Black Box Warning Patients who have received epidural or spinal anesthesia or spinal puncture are at increased risk for developing an epidural or spinal hematoma, which may result in long-term or permanent paralysis. Increased risk may occur with use of indwelling epidural catheters, concomitant use of drugs that affect hemostasis (NSAIDs, platelet inhibitors, anticoagulants), history

of traumatic or repeated epidural or spinal punctures, or history of spinal deformity or surgery. Monitor these patients closely for neurologic impairment and treat urgently. ▮
Black Box Warning Monitor patients for neurologic impairment (midline back pain, sensory or motor deficits such as numbness or weakness in lower limbs, bowel or bladder dysfunction). Treat impairment urgently. ▮
Black Box Warning Optimal timing between administration of drug and neuraxial procedures isn't known. Consider benefits and risks before neuraxial intervention in patients anticoagulated or to be anticoagulated for thromboprophylaxis. ▮
• DVT is a risk factor in patients who are candidates for therapy, including those older than age 40, those who are obese, those undergoing surgery under general anesthesia lasting longer than 30 minutes, and those who have additional risk factors (such as malignancy or history of DVT or PE).
• Never give drug IM.
• Don't mix with other injections or infusions unless specific compatibility data support such mixing.
⊘ *Alert:* Drug isn't interchangeable (unit for unit) with unfractionated heparin or other low–molecular-weight heparin.
• Periodic, routine CBC and fecal occult blood tests are recommended during therapy. Patients don't need regular monitoring of PT or aPTT.
• Monitor patient closely for thrombocytopenia and hyperkalemia.
• Stop drug if a thromboembolic event occurs despite dalteparin prophylaxis.
• Obtain a complete list of patient's prescription and OTC drugs and supplements, including herbs.

PATIENT TEACHING
• Instruct patient and family to watch for and report signs of bleeding (bruising and blood in stools) and to report all adverse reactions promptly.
• Tell patient to avoid OTC drugs containing aspirin or other salicylates unless ordered by prescriber.
• Advise patient to consult with prescriber before initiating any herbal therapy; many

herbs have anticoagulant, antiplatelet, and fibrinolytic properties.

• Tell patient to use a soft toothbrush and electric razor during treatment.

dapagliflozin
DAP-a-gli-FLOE-zin

Farxiga

Therapeutic class: Antidiabetics
Pharmacologic class: Sodium-glucose cotransporter 2 inhibitors

AVAILABLE FORMS
Tablets: 5 mg, 10 mg

INDICATIONS & DOSAGES
➤ **Adjunct to diet and exercise to improve glycemic control in patients with type 2 diabetes**
Adults with eGFR of 45 mL/minute/1.73 m² or greater: Initially, 5 mg PO once daily; may increase to 10 mg daily for patients who require additional glycemic control.
Adjust-a-dose: Drug isn't recommended when eGFR is less than 45 mL/minute/1.73 m², and is contraindicated in patients with eGFR less than 30 mL/minute/1.73 m². Drug hasn't been studied in severe hepatic impairment.

ADMINISTRATION
PO
• Give dose in the morning.
• May give without regard for food.
• Store at room temperature.

ACTION
Reduces reabsorption of filtered glucose from the proximal renal tubule and lowers the renal threshold for glucose, resulting in increased urinary glucose excretion.

Route	Onset	Peak	Duration
PO	Unknown	2 hr	Unknown

Half-life: About 12.9 hours.

ADVERSE REACTIONS
CV: volume depletion (dehydration, hypovolemia, orthostatic hypotension,

hypotension). **EENT:** nasopharyngitis. **GI:** nausea, constipation. **GU:** genital mycotic infection, UTI, increased urination, dysuria. **Metabolic:** dyslipidemia, *hypoglycemia.* **Musculoskeletal:** back pain, extremity pain. **Other:** influenza.

INTERACTIONS
Drug-drug. *Insulin, insulin secretagogues:* May increase risk of hypoglycemia. Monitor patient closely and adjust insulin and secretagogue dosages as necessary.
Loop diuretics: May increase risk of hypotension. Monitor patient closely.

EFFECTS ON LAB TEST RESULTS
• May increase hematocrit and serum phosphorus, creatinine, and LDL cholesterol levels. May decrease eGFR level.
• May cause positive urine glucose test.
• May interfere with 1,5-AG assay. Use alternative methods to monitor glycemic control.

CONTRAINDICATIONS & CAUTIONS
• Contraindicated in patients with severe renal impairment (eGFR less than 30 mL/minute/1.73 m²) or ESRD, patients on dialysis, and patients with history of serious hypersensitivity reactions (anaphylaxis, angioedema, or severe cutaneous reactions) to dapagliflozin-containing products.
• Use isn't recommended in patients with an eGFR less than 45 mL/minute/1.73 m².
• Not recommended for use in patients with type 1 diabetes or for treatment of diabetic ketoacidosis.
• Use cautiously in elderly patients because of increased risk of adverse events.
• Drug increases serum creatinine level and decreases eGFR; elderly patients and patients with hypovolemia may be more susceptible to these changes.
• Don't use in patients with active bladder cancer; use cautiously in patients with history of bladder cancer. Drug may increase risk of cancer reactivation.
⚠ *Alert:* Sodium-glucose cotransporter 2 inhibitors such as dapagliflozin increase the risk of necrotizing fasciitis of the perineum (Fournier gangrene), a rare but serious and life-threatening infection requiring urgent surgical intervention, that has been

---

Reactions in bold italics are *life-threatening*. Interactions may have a *rapid onset* or a *delayed onset*.

reported in both females and males. Serious outcomes have included hospitalization, multiple surgeries, and death.

⟲ Alert: Drug may cause acidosis, which may require emergency department care or hospitalization. Monitor patients for ketoacidosis, especially those with major illness, reduced food or fluid intake, or reduced insulin dosage. Elevated urine or serum ketone levels without associated very high glucose levels have occurred with sodium-glucose cotransporter 2 inhibitor use.

Dialyzable drug: Unknown.

PREGNANCY-LACTATION-REPRODUCTION

• There are no adequate studies in pregnant women. Use during pregnancy, especially during the second and third trimesters, isn't recommended. If needed during pregnancy, use only if potential benefit justifies potential risk to the fetus.

• It isn't known if drug appears in human milk. Use while breastfeeding isn't recommended. Patient should discontinue breastfeeding or discontinue drug.

NURSING CONSIDERATIONS

⟲ Alert: Drug can increase risk of acute kidney injury. Before starting therapy, assess patient for factors that may predispose to acute kidney injury (decreased blood volume, chronic renal insufficiency, HF, concurrent use of other medications such as diuretics, ACE inhibitors, ARBs, and NSAIDs). Assess renal function before start of therapy and monitor periodically. Correct volume depletion before starting drug. If acute kidney injury occurs, drug should be discontinued and the kidney impairment treated.

⟲ Alert: Drug may increase risk of severe UTI, including urosepsis and pyelonephritis. Monitor patient and treat promptly if indicated.

⟲ Alert: Assess patients with pain or tenderness, erythema, or swelling in the genital or perineal area, along with fever or malaise, for necrotizing fasciitis. If suspected, immediately discontinue drug because symptoms can worsen quickly, and start treatment with broad-spectrum antibiotics and, if necessary, surgical debridement. Monitor blood glucose level and start alternative therapy for glycemic control.

• Monitor glucose level closely, especially if patient is taking antidiabetic agents concurrently. Adjust hypoglycemic dosages if needed.

• Monitor patient for mycotic infections.

• Stop drug immediately if hypersensitivity, reduced renal function, or bladder cancer is suspected.

• Monitor volume status and watch for signs and symptoms of hypotension, particularly in patients with impaired renal function (eGFR less than 60 mL/minute/1.73 m²), elderly patients, and patients taking loop diuretics. Increased urinary glucose excretion also results in increased urine volume.

PATIENT TEACHING

• Warn patient to use drug only as directed. If a dose is missed, patient should take the missed dose as soon as it's remembered unless it is almost time for the next dose. Caution patient not to double a dose.

⟲ Alert: Advise patient to seek immediate medical attention for signs and symptoms of acute kidney injury (decreased urine output, swelling in legs or feet). Warn patient not to stop taking drug without first discussing with prescriber.

⟲ Alert: Teach patient signs and symptoms of necrotizing fasciitis (temperature above 100.4° F [38° C], general feeling of being unwell, and tenderness, redness, or swelling of the genitals back to the rectum) and to seek immediate medical attention if any occur.

• Inform patient of increased risk of UTI. Teach patient to report painful urination or discolored urine.

• Instruct patient to report signs and symptoms of yeast infections (itching, burning, discharge) promptly. Counsel patient on importance of diet and exercise in addition to medication for diabetes control.

• Teach patient to obtain periodic blood testing as requested by prescriber.

⟲ Alert: Instruct patient to seek medical attention immediately for signs and symptoms of ketoacidosis (difficulty breathing, hyperventilation, anorexia, nausea, vomiting, abdominal pain, confusion, unusual fatigue or sleepiness).

⟲ Alert: Instruct patient to seek medical attention for signs and symptoms of UTI

(painful urination, urinary frequency, blood in urine, urgency, pelvic pain, fever, back pain, nausea, vomiting).
• Advise patient to watch for signs and symptoms of hypoglycemia (fatigue, weakness, confusion, headache, pallor, or profuse sweating).
• Caution patient to maintain adequate fluid intake to decrease risk of hypotension.
• Warn patient to contact prescriber for signs and symptoms of hypotension, such as light-headedness (especially with position change) and weakness.
• Advise patient to seek medical attention promptly for fever, trauma, infection, or when surgery is needed; dosage adjustment may be needed owing to stress.

DAPTOmycin
dap-toe-MYE-sin

Cubicin, Cubicin RF

Therapeutic class: Antibiotics
Pharmacologic class: Cyclic lipopeptides

AVAILABLE FORMS
Powder for injection: 500-mg vial

INDICATIONS & DOSAGES
➤ **Bacteremia caused by *Staphylococcus aureus* (including right-sided endocarditis caused by methicillin-susceptible and methicillin-resistant strains)**
Adults: 6 mg/kg IV infusion over 30 minutes or IV injection over 2 minutes every 24 hours for at least 2 to 6 weeks based on patient response.
Adjust-a-dose: For bacteremic patients with CrCl of less than 30 mL/minute, including those on hemodialysis or continuous ambulatory peritoneal dialysis, give 6 mg/kg IV every 48 hours. When possible, give drug after hemodialysis on hemodialysis days.
➤ **Bacteremia caused by *S. aureus* in children with normal renal function**
Children ages 12 to 17: 7 mg/kg IV infusion over 30 minutes once every 24 hours for up to 42 days.
Children ages 7 to 11: 9 mg/kg IV infusion over 30 minutes once every 24 hours for up to 42 days.

Children ages 1 to 6: 12 mg/kg IV infusion over 60 minutes once every 24 hours for up to 42 days.
➤ **Complicated skin or skin-structure infection (cSSSI) caused by susceptible strains of *S. aureus* (including MRSA), *Streptococcus pyogenes*, *Streptococcus agalactiae*, *Streptococcus dysgalactiae*, and *Enterococcus faecalis* (vancomycin-susceptible strains only)**
Adults: 4 mg/kg IV infusion over 30 minutes or IV injection over 2 minutes every 24 hours for 7 to 14 days.
Children ages 12 to 17 with normal renal function: 5 mg/kg IV infusion over 30 minutes once every 24 hours for up to 14 days.
Children ages 7 to 11 with normal renal function: 7 mg/kg IV infusion over 30 minutes once every 24 hours for up to 14 days.
Children ages 2 to 6 with normal renal function: 9 mg/kg IV infusion over 60 minutes once every 24 hours for up to 14 days.
Children ages 1 to less than 2 with normal renal function: 10 mg/kg IV infusion over 60 minutes once every 24 hours for up to 14 days.
Adjust-a-dose: In adult patients with cSSSI and CrCl of less than 30 mL/minute, including those on hemodialysis or continuous ambulatory peritoneal dialysis, give 4 mg/kg IV every 48 hours. When possible, give drug after hemodialysis on hemodialysis days.

ADMINISTRATION
IV
▼ Obtain specimen for culture and sensitivity tests before giving first dose. Begin therapy while awaiting results.
🌓 *Alert:* The two formulations of daptomycin, Cubicin and Cubicin RF, differ concerning storage and reconstitution. Refer to, and carefully follow, the manufacturer's instructions for reconstituting and storing each drug when preparing these drugs for administration.
▼ Infuse over 30 minutes in adults and children age 7 and older. For children ages 1 to 6, infuse over 60 minutes.
▼ For IV injection over 2 minutes, give at a concentration of 50 mg/mL (adults only).
▼ Vials are for single use; discard excess.
▼ Don't use drug with ReadyMED elastomeric infusion pumps (Cardinal Health);

an impurity may leach from the pump into the solution.

▼ **Incompatibilities:** Dextrose-containing solutions and other IV drugs. If an IV line is used for several drugs, flush the line with NSS or lactated Ringer solution injection between drugs.

ACTION

Bactericidal; binds to and depolarizes susceptible bacterial membranes to inhibit protein, DNA, and RNA synthesis.

Route	Onset	Peak	Duration
IV	Rapid	<1 hr	Unknown

Half-life: About 8 hours.

ADVERSE REACTIONS

CNS: anxiety, confusion, dizziness, fever, headache, insomnia. **CV:** *cardiac failure,* chest pain, edema, HTN, hypotension. **EENT:** sore throat. **GI:** *pseudomembranous colitis,* abdominal pain, constipation, decreased appetite, diarrhea, nausea, vomiting. **GU:** *renal failure,* UTI. **Hematologic:** anemia. **Musculoskeletal:** limb and back pain, myopathy. **Respiratory:** cough, dyspnea, eosinophilic pneumonia. **Skin:** cellulitis, injection-site reactions, pruritus, rash, diaphoresis. **Other:** fungal infections, bacteremia, sepsis.

INTERACTIONS

Drug-drug. *HMG-CoA reductase inhibitors:* May increase risk of myopathy. Consider stopping these drugs while giving daptomycin.
Warfarin: May alter anticoagulant activity. Monitor PT and INR for the first several days of daptomycin therapy.

EFFECTS ON LAB TEST RESULTS

• May increase alkaline phosphatase and CK levels.
• May increase LFT values.
• May decrease Hb level and hematocrit. May cause false elevation of INR and false prolongation of PT.

CONTRAINDICATIONS & CAUTIONS

• Contraindicated in patients hypersensitive to drug.

• Use cautiously in those with renal insufficiency and those older than age 65.
• Drug isn't indicated in children with renal impairment because dosage hasn't been established in these patients.
• Safety and effectiveness haven't been established in children younger than age 12 months. Avoid use in children younger than age 12 months because of risk of potential effects on muscular, neuromuscular, or nervous systems (peripheral or central).
Dialyzable drug: Yes.

PREGNANCY-LACTATION-REPRODUCTION

• There are no adequate well-controlled studies in pregnant women. Use during pregnancy only if potential benefit justifies potential risk to the fetus.
• Drug appears in human milk in low amounts. Use cautiously if breastfeeding.

NURSING CONSIDERATIONS

• Monitor CBC, renal function tests, and LFTs periodically.
⚠ *Alert:* Because drug may increase the risk of myopathy, monitor CK level weekly or more frequently with renal impairment. If CK level rises, monitor it more often. In patients with unexplained signs and symptoms of myopathy with CK level greater than 1,000 units/L (approximately 5 × ULN) and in patients without reported signs and symptoms with CK level greater than 2,000 units/L (10 × ULN or greater), stop drug. Consider stopping all other drugs linked with myopathy (such as HMG-CoA reductase inhibitors) during therapy.
• Monitor patient for superinfection because drug may cause overgrowth of nonsusceptible organisms.
⚠ *Alert:* Drug may cause eosinophilic pneumonia, a rare type of pneumonia in which eosinophil-type WBCs fill the lungs, causing fever, cough, shortness of breath, and difficulty breathing. Monitor patient closely.
• Monitor patient for signs and symptoms of neuropathy; consider stopping drug if neuropathy occurs.
• Watch for evidence of CDAD, which can occur more than 2 months after therapy.
• Monitor patient for muscle pain or weakness, particularly of the distal extremities.

• *Look alike–sound alike:* Don't confuse daptomycin with dactinomycin.

PATIENT TEACHING
• Advise patient to immediately report muscle weakness and infusion-site irritation.
• Tell patient to report all adverse reactions, especially severe diarrhea, rash, and infection.
• Inform patient about possible adverse reactions.

SAFETY ALERT!

daratumumab
dar-a-TOOM-ue-mab

Darzalex

Therapeutic class: Antineoplastics
Pharmacologic class: Monoclonal antibodies

AVAILABLE FORMS
Injection: 100 mg/5 mL, 400 mg/20 mL in single-dose vials

INDICATIONS & DOSAGES
Adjust-a-dose (for all indications): Refer to manufacturer's instructions for toxicity-related and infusion reaction adjustments. No dosage reductions of daratumumab are recommended.
➤ **Multiple myeloma monotherapy in patients who received at least three prior lines of therapy, including a proteasome inhibitor (PI) and an immunomodulatory agent or who are double refractory to a PI and an immunomodulatory agent; multiple myeloma in combination with lenalidomide and low-dose dexamethasone in patients who have received at least one prior therapy**
Adults: Initially, 16 mg/kg (actual body weight) IV infusion once weekly for weeks 1 through 8 (total of eight doses); then for weeks 9 through 24, give 16 mg/kg IV infusion every 2 weeks (total of eight doses). Then, beginning week 25 onwards, give 16 mg/kg IV infusion every 4 weeks until disease progression. Refer to manufacturer's instructions for dosing instructions for combination agents.

➤ **Multiple myeloma in combination with bortezomib and dexamethasone in patients who have received at least one prior therapy**
Adults: Initially, 16 mg/kg (actual body weight) IV infusion once weekly for weeks 1 through 9 (total of nine doses); then give 16 mg/kg IV infusion every 3 weeks beginning week 10 through week 24 (total of five doses); then give 16 mg/kg IV infusion every 4 weeks beginning week 25 onwards until disease progression. Refer to manufacturer's instructions for dosing instructions for combination agents.
➤ **Multiple myeloma given in combination with pomalidomide and dexamethasone for patients who have received at least 2 prior therapies, including lenalidomide and a PI**
Adults: Initially, 16 mg/kg (actual body weight) IV infusion once weekly for weeks 1 through 8 (total of eight doses); then for weeks 9 through 24, give 16 mg/kg IV infusion every 2 weeks (total of eight doses). Then, beginning week 25 onward, give 16 mg/kg IV infusion every 4 weeks until disease progresses. Refer to manufacturer's dosing instructions for combination agents.
➤ **Newly diagnosed multiple myeloma in patients ineligible for autologous stem cell transplant, given in combination with bortezomib, melphalan, and prednisone**
Adults: Initially, 16 mg/kg (actual body weight) IV infusion once weekly for weeks 1 through 6 (total of six doses); then, for weeks 7 through 54, give 16 mg/kg IV infusion every 3 weeks (total of 16 doses). Then, beginning on week 55 and onward, give 16 mg/kg IV infusion every 4 weeks until disease progresses. Refer to manufacturer's dosing instructions for bortezomib, melphalan, and prednisone.

ADMINISTRATION
IV
▼ One to three hours before each infusion, premedicate with IV corticosteroid (methylprednisolone 100 mg or equivalent dose of an intermediate- or long-acting corticosteroid for monotherapy or 20 mg dexamethasone for combination therapy), an oral antipyretic (acetaminophen 650 to 1,000 mg), and an oral or IV antihistamine

(diphenhydramine 25 to 50 mg or equivalent). After second monotherapy infusion, may reduce methylprednisolone dose to 60 mg PO or IV. In combination therapy, after first infusion, may consider dexamethasone 20 mg PO before subsequent infusions.

▼ On first and second day after monotherapy infusions, administer an oral corticosteroid (20 mg methylprednisolone or equivalent dose of an intermediate- or long-acting corticosteroid). For combination therapy, may consider methylprednisolone 20 mg or less PO or equivalent the day after infusion.

▼ For patients with a history of obstructive pulmonary disorder, postinfusion medications, such as short- and long-acting bronchodilators and inhaled corticosteroids, may be indicated. After first four infusions, if patient has no major infusion reactions, the additional postinfusion drugs may be discontinued.

▼ Solution should be colorless to pale yellow; don't use if vials contain opaque particles, discoloration, or other foreign particles.

▼ Remove volume of NSS from infusion bag that's equal to the volume of drug. Infusion bags should be made of polyvinyl chloride (PVC), polypropylene (PP), polyethylene (PE), or polyolefin blend.

▼ Withdraw medication from vial and add to infusion bag. Discard unused solution.

▼ Gently invert bag; don't shake.

▼ May keep diluted solution at room temperature for a maximum of 15 hours (including infusion time). May store infusion bag up to 24 hours in refrigerator at 36° to 46° F (2° to 8° C). Protect from light; don't freeze.

▼ Allow infusion bag to come to room temperature; then use immediately, as the solution doesn't contain a preservative.

▼ Administer with infusion set with flow regulator and in-line, sterile, nonpyrogenic, low-protein-binding polyethersulfone filter (pore size 0.22 or 0.2 micron). Polyurethane, polybutadiene, PVC, PP, or PE administration sets must be used.

▼ Give first infusion of 1,000 mL initially at 50 mL/hour; may increase by 50 mL/hour every hour to maximum rate of 200 mL/hour. Consider escalating infusion rate only in the absence of infusion reactions. If there are no grade 1 or greater infusion reactions during first 3 hours of first infusion, may decrease second infusion dilution volume to 500 mL and begin infusion at 50 mL/hour and increase by 50 mL/hour to a maximum of 200 mL/hour. Otherwise, continue the dilution volume of 1,000 mL and instructions for the first infusion. If there are no grade 1 or greater infusion reactions during final infusion rate of 100 mL/hour or more in first two infusions, may give subsequent infusions in 500 mL at an initial rate of 100 mL/hour; may increase by 50 mL/hour every hour to maximum rate of 200 mL/hour. Otherwise, continue to use instructions for the second infusion.

▼ Complete infusion within 15 hours.

▼ Give missed dose as soon as possible and adjust dosing schedule accordingly to maintain treatment interval.

▼ **Incompatibilities:** Don't infuse in same IV line with other agents.

ACTION

An IgG1kappa human monoclonal antibody that binds to CD38 and inhibits growth of CD38-expressing tumor cells by inducing apoptosis.

Route	Onset	Peak	Duration
IV	Unknown	Unknown	Unknown

Half-life: Monotherapy, 9 to 27 days; combination therapy, 22 to 23 days.

ADVERSE REACTIONS

CNS: fatigue, pyrexia, headache. **CV:** HTN. **EENT:** nasal congestion, nasopharyngitis. **GI:** nausea, vomiting, diarrhea, constipation, decreased appetite. **Hematologic:** anemia, *thrombocytopenia, neutropenia, lymphopenia.* **Musculoskeletal:** back pain, arthralgia, extremity pain, musculoskeletal chest pain. **Respiratory:** cough, dyspnea, URI, pneumonia. **Other:** infusion reactions, chills, herpes zoster reactivation.

INTERACTIONS
None reported.

EFFECTS ON LAB TEST RESULTS
• May decrease RBC, platelet, neutrophil, and lymphocyte counts.
• May cause positive indirect antiglobulin tests (Coombs test), interfering with cross-matching and RBC antibody screening that may persist for up to 6 months after last daratumumab infusion.
• May cause false-positive serum protein electrophoresis and immunofixation assay results in patients with IgG kappa myeloma protein affecting assessment of complete response by International Myeloma Working Group criteria.

CONTRAINDICATIONS & CAUTIONS
◑ Alert: Drug should only be given by health care professional with immediate access to emergency equipment and medical support to manage severe infusion reactions. Approximately half of all patients may experience an infusion reaction, and most occur during the first infusion. Infusion reactions can occur with subsequent infusions and within 4 hours of completing an infusion.
• Drug may increase risk of herpes zoster reactivation. Initiate antiviral prophylaxis within 1 week of starting treatment and continue for 3 months after treatment ends.
• Safety and effectiveness in children haven't been established.
Dialyzable drug: Unknown.

PREGNANCY-LACTATION-REPRODUCTION
• Risk during pregnancy is unknown. Patient should use contraception during therapy and for up to 3 months after therapy ends.
• Based on the mechanism of action, drug may cause fetal myeloid- or lymphoid-cell depletion and decrease bone density with in utero exposure. Delay administering live-virus vaccines to neonates and infants exposed to drug in utero until hematology evaluation is completed.
• It isn't known if drug appears in human milk. Discuss risk and benefits with patient who plans to breastfeed.

NURSING CONSIDERATIONS
◑ Alert: Be sure to premedicate patient and frequently monitor for signs and symptoms of infusion reaction (bronchospasm,

hypoxia, dyspnea, HTN or hypotension, cough, wheezing, larynx and throat tightness or irritation, laryngeal edema, pulmonary edema, nasal congestion, allergic rhinitis, headache, rash, urticaria, pruritus, nausea, vomiting, chills). Emergency treatment may be needed for severe infusion reactions.
• There is increased risk of neutropenia and thrombocytopenia, especially when drug is used in combination with other chemotherapy agents. Monitor CBC periodically. Growth factors or platelet transfusion may be needed.
• Patients should be typed and screened for blood transfusions before start of therapy because drug can interfere with cross-matching and antibody screening. Inform blood bank that patient is taking drug if typed and screened after initiating therapy.

PATIENT TEACHING
• Advise patient to immediately report signs and symptoms of infusion reaction.
• Explain to patient that blood test results to match blood type for transfusions may be affected for up to 6 months after last dose. Advise patient to inform all health care providers about taking daratumumab in the event of a planned transfusion.
• Inform patient that drug may occasionally affect results of some tests used to determine complete response and additional tests may be needed.
• Advise patient to report all adverse reactions and to immediately report fever or signs and symptoms of bruising or bleeding.
• Instruct female patient to avoid pregnancy and to use effective contraception during therapy and for up to 3 months after last dose.
• Warn female patient who wants to breast-feed that it isn't known if drug appears in human milk.
• Caution patient to take postinfusion medications and antiviral prophylaxis, as prescribed.

---

darbepoetin alfa
dar-bah-poe-E-tin

Aranesp

Therapeutic class: Colony stimulating factors
Pharmacologic class: Recombinant human erythropoietins

AVAILABLE FORMS
Injection (with polysorbate solution):
25 mcg/mL, 40 mcg/mL, 60 mcg/mL, 100 mcg/mL, 200 mcg/mL, 300 mcg/mL in single-dose vials
Prefilled syringe or autoinjector (with polysorbate solution): 10 mcg/0.4 mL, 25 mcg/0.42 mL, 40 mcg/0.4 mL, 60 mcg/0.3 mL, 100 mcg/0.5 mL, 150 mcg/0.3 mL, 200 mcg/0.4 mL, 300 mcg/0.6 mL, 500 mcg/mL

INDICATIONS & DOSAGES
➤ **Anemia due to chronic kidney disease**
Adults: The IV route is preferred for patients on dialysis. For patients on dialysis, give 0.45 mcg/kg IV or subcut once weekly. Or, give 0.75 mcg/kg IV or subcut once every 2 weeks. For patients not on dialysis, give 0.45 mcg/kg IV or subcut at 4-week intervals. Give the lowest effective dose to gradually increase Hb to a level at which blood transfusion isn't necessary. Refer to manufacturer's instructions for specific dosing. Don't increase dose more often than once a month.
Children younger than age 18: For patients on dialysis, give 0.45 mcg/kg IV or subcut once weekly. For patients not on dialysis, give 0.75 mcg/kg IV or subcut once every 2 weeks.
Adults and children older than age 1 who are on dialysis and converting from epoetin alfa: Refer to manufacturer's instructions.
Adjust-a-dose: For patients with chronic renal disease who aren't on dialysis, if the Hb level exceeds 10 g/dL, reduce dosage or interrupt therapy; use the lowest dosage sufficient to reduce the need for RBC transfusions. For patients with chronic renal disease who are on dialysis, if the Hb level

approaches or exceeds 11 g/dL, reduce dosage or interrupt therapy.
➤ **Anemia due to chemotherapy in patients with nonmyeloid malignancies**
Adults: Initiate drug only if Hb level is less than 10 g/dL and if there is a minimum of 2 additional months of planned chemotherapy; 2.25 mcg/kg subcut once weekly or 500 mcg subcut once every 3 weeks.
Adjust-a-dose: For either dosing schedule, adjust dose to maintain a target Hb level necessary to avoid RBC transfusions. Give the lowest effective dose to gradually increase Hb to a level at which blood transfusion isn't necessary. Refer to manufacturer's instructions for dosing adjustment.
  If after 8 weeks of therapy there is no response as measured by Hb levels or if transfusions are still required, discontinue drug. Discontinue drug after completion of chemotherapy course.

ADMINISTRATION
IV
🔸 *Alert:* The needle cover of the prefilled syringe contains dry natural rubber (a derivative of latex). Assess patient for a history of latex allergy.
▼ Don't shake. Shaking can denature drug.
▼ If drug contains particles or is discolored, don't use.
▼ Give undiluted by IV injection.
▼ Single-dose vials contain no preservatives; don't pool unused portions.
▼ Store drug in refrigerator; don't freeze. Don't use if drug has been frozen. Protect drug from light.
▼ **Incompatibilities:** Other IV drugs or solutions.
Subcutaneous
🔸 *Alert:* The needle cover of the prefilled syringe contains dry natural rubber (a derivative of latex). Assess patient for a history of latex allergy.
● Don't give subcutaneously in patients with chronic renal failure on dialysis.
● Don't shake. Shaking can denature drug.
● Store drug in refrigerator; don't freeze. Protect drug from light.

ACTION
Induces erythropoiesis. Functions as a growth factor and as a differentiating factor, enhancing RBC production.

Route	Onset	Peak	Duration
IV	Unknown	Unknown	Unknown
Subcut	Slow	48 hr	Unknown

Half-life: IV: 21 hours. Subcut: patients with chronic kidney disease (CKD) on dialysis, 46 hours; patients with CKD not on dialysis, 70 hours.

ADVERSE REACTIONS
CNS: *seizures,* dizziness, fatigue, TIA, *stroke.* **CV:** *cardiac arrest, cardiac arrhythmia,* edema, HTN, hypotension, peripheral edema, *PE, acute MI, HF, thrombosis,* angina, chest pain, vascular access thrombosis. **GI:** abdominal pain. **Respiratory:** cough, dyspnea. **Skin:** pruritus, rash, erythema. **Other:** infection, *sepsis,* abscess, access infection, fluid overload, injection-site pain, hypersensitivity reactions.

INTERACTIONS
Drug-drug. *Lenalidomide, pomalidomide, thalidomide:* May increase thrombogenic effects. Monitor therapy.

EFFECTS ON LAB TEST RESULTS
• May increase Hb level.

CONTRAINDICATIONS & CAUTIONS
• Contraindicated in patients hypersensitive to drug or its components, in those with uncontrolled HTN, and in patients with pure red cell aplasia that begins after treatment with Aranesp or other erythropoietin protein drugs.
• Not indicated for use in patients with cancer receiving hormonal agents, biologic products, or radiotherapy unless patients are also receiving concomitant myelosuppressive chemotherapy; in those receiving myelosuppressive chemotherapy when the anemia can be managed by transfusion; or as a substitute for RBC transfusions in patients who require immediate correction of anemia.
Black Box Warning Drug isn't indicated for patients receiving myelosuppressive therapy when the anticipated outcome is cure. ∎

• Blistering and skin exfoliation reactions, including erythema multiforme and SJS syndrome/toxic epidermal necrolysis, have been reported. Discontinue therapy immediately if a severe cutaneous reaction is suspected.
• Safety and effectiveness in children with cancer haven't been established.
Dialyzable drug: No.
⚠ *Overdose S&S:* CV and thrombotic reactions, polycythemia.

PREGNANCY-LACTATION-REPRODUCTION
• There are no adequate well-controlled studies in pregnant women; animal studies show that drug may cause fetal harm. Use during pregnancy only if potential benefit justifies potential risk to the fetus.
• It isn't known if drug appears in human milk. Use cautiously in breastfeeding women.

NURSING CONSIDERATIONS
Black Box Warning Erythropoiesis-stimulating agents increase risk of death, MI, stroke, venous thromboembolism, vascular access thrombosis, and tumor progression or recurrence. No trial has identified an Hb target level, drug dose, or dosing strategy that doesn't increase these risks. ∎
Black Box Warning Patients with chronic renal disease have an increased risk of death and serious CV events, including stroke, when erythropoiesis-stimulating agents are used to increase Hb level to greater than 11 g/dL. Therapy should be individualized for each patient; the lowest possible dose sufficient to reduce the need for RBC transfusions should be used. ∎
Black Box Warning In patients with NSCLC and breast, head and neck, lymphoid, and cervical cancers, there is a risk of tumor growth and shortened survival when Hb levels exceed the lowest dose needed to avoid RBC transfusion. Target for the lowest dosage needed to avoid RBC transfusions. Use only for treatment of anemia due to concomitant myelosuppressive chemotherapy, and discontinue drug after chemotherapy course. ∎
• Evaluate iron status in all patients before and during treatment. Administer supplemental iron when serum ferritin level is less than 100 mcg/L or when serum transferrin

---

saturation is less than 20%. The majority of patients with chronic kidney disease will require supplemental iron during the course of erythropoietin-stimulating agent therapy.

• When initiating therapy or adjusting dosage, monitor Hb level at least weekly until stable; then, at least monthly.

• Hb level may not increase until 2 to 6 weeks after starting therapy.

• If patient has a minimal response or lack of response at recommended dose, check for deficiencies in folic acid, iron, or vitamin B_{12}. Other contributing factors include infection, malignancy, and occult blood loss.

❸ Alert: If patient develops a sudden loss of response with severe anemia and low reticulocyte count, withhold drug and test patient for antierythropoietin antibodies. If antibodies are present, stop treatment. Don't switch to another erythropoietic protein because a cross-reaction is possible.

• Control BP and monitor it carefully.

• Monitor renal function and electrolytes in predialysis patients.

• Monitor patency of vascular and dialysis access and report problems immediately.

• Patients who are marginally dialyzed may need adjustments in dialysis prescriptions.

• Serious allergic reactions, including skin rash and urticaria, may occur. If an anaphylactic reaction occurs, stop the drug and give appropriate therapy.

PATIENT TEACHING

• Instruct patients on proper administration and on proper use and disposal of needles.

• Advise patient of possible side effects and allergic reactions.

• Inform patient of the need for frequent monitoring of BP and Hb level; stress compliance with treatment for high BP.

• Instruct patient how to take drug correctly at home, including how to store drug and dispose of supplies properly.

darifenacin hydrobromide
dar-i-FEN-a-sin

Enablex✔

Therapeutic class: Antispasmodics
Pharmacologic class: Anticholinergics

AVAILABLE FORMS
Tablets (extended-release) ⓓⓝⓒ: 7.5 mg, 15 mg

INDICATIONS & DOSAGES
➤ **Urge incontinence, urgency, and frequency from an overactive bladder**
Adults: Initially, 7.5 mg PO once daily. After 2 weeks, may increase to 15 mg PO once daily if needed.

Adjust-a-dose: If patient has moderate hepatic impairment (Child-Pugh class B) or when drug is administered with potent CYP3A4 inhibitors (ketoconazole, itraconazole, ritonavir, nelfinavir, clarithromycin, nefazodone), don't exceed 7.5 mg PO once daily. Drug isn't recommended for use in patients with severe hepatic impairment (Child-Pugh class C).

ADMINISTRATION
PO
• Don't crush, divide, or allow patient to chew tablet; patient should swallow tablet whole with water.

• Give drug without regard for food.

ACTION
Relaxes smooth muscle of bladder by antagonizing muscarinic receptors.

Route	Onset	Peak	Duration
PO	Unknown	7 hr	Unknown

Half-life: 13 to 19 hours.

ADVERSE REACTIONS
CNS: asthenia, dizziness, pain, headache, somnolence. **CV:** HTN, peripheral edema. **EENT:** abnormal vision, dry eyes, pharyngitis, rhinitis, sinusitis. **GI:** dry mouth, constipation, abdominal pain, diarrhea, dyspepsia, nausea, vomiting. **GU:** urinary tract disorder, UTI, vaginitis, urine retention. **Metabolic:** weight gain. **Musculoskeletal:** arthralgia, back pain. **Respiratory:** bronchitis. **Skin:**

---

dry skin, pruritus, rash. **Other:** accidental injury, flulike syndrome.

INTERACTIONS
Drug-drug. *Anticholinergics:* May increase anticholinergic effects, such as dry mouth, blurred vision, and constipation. Monitor patient closely.
Digoxin: May increase digoxin level. Monitor digoxin level.
Drugs metabolized by CYP2D6 (flecainide, TCAs, thioridazine): May increase levels of these drugs. Use together cautiously.
Midazolam: May increase midazolam level. Monitor patient carefully.
Potent CYP3A4 inhibitors (clarithromycin, itraconazole, ketoconazole, nefazodone, nelfinavir, ritonavir): May increase darifenacin level. Maintain dosage no higher than 7.5 mg PO daily.
Drug-lifestyle. *Hot weather:* May cause heat prostration from decreased sweating. Urge caution.

EFFECTS ON LAB TEST RESULTS
None reported.

CONTRAINDICATIONS & CAUTIONS
• Contraindicated in patients hypersensitive to drug or its components. Angioedema can be life-threatening and has been reported after the first dose. If angioedema occurs, discontinue drug, start appropriate therapy, and ensure patent airway.
• Contraindicated in those with or at risk for urine retention, gastric retention, or uncontrolled angle-closure glaucoma.
• Use cautiously in patients with bladder outflow or GI obstruction, ulcerative colitis, myasthenia gravis, severe constipation, controlled angle-closure glaucoma, decreased GI motility, or Child-Pugh class B hepatic impairment.
Dialyzable drug: Unknown.
⚠ *Overdose S&S:* Severe antimuscarinic effects (mydriasis, decreased secretions, ileus, urine retention, tachycardia, altered mental status).

PREGNANCY-LACTATION-REPRODUCTION
• There are no studies in pregnant women. Use only if potential benefit justifies potential risk to the fetus.

• It isn't known if drug appears in human milk. Use cautiously if breastfeeding.

NURSING CONSIDERATIONS
• Assess bladder function, and monitor drug effects.
• If patient has bladder outlet obstruction, watch for urine retention.
• Assess patient for decreased gastric motility and constipation.

PATIENT TEACHING
• Tell patient to swallow tablet whole with water; caution against crushing, dividing, or chewing tablet.
• Inform patient that drug may be taken with or without food.
• Tell patient to use caution, especially when performing hazardous tasks, until drug effects are known.
• Tell patient to report blurred vision, constipation, and urine retention and to immediately report swelling of the face, lips, or tongue or difficulty speaking.
• Discourage use of other drugs that may cause dry mouth, constipation, urine retention, or blurred vision.
• Tell patient that drug decreases sweating, and advise cautious use in hot environments and during strenuous activity.

SAFETY ALERT!

degarelix acetate
deg-a-REL-ix

Firmagon

Therapeutic class: Antineoplastics
Pharmacologic class: Gonadotropin-releasing hormone receptor antagonists

AVAILABLE FORMS
Injection: 80-mg, 120-mg vial

INDICATIONS & DOSAGES
➤ **Advanced prostate cancer**
Adult men: Initially, 240 mg subcut, administered as two 120-mg injections at a concentration of 40 mg/mL. Maintenance dose is 80 mg subcut given as one injection at a concentration of 20 mg/mL every 28 days starting 28 days after first dose.

Reactions in bold italics are *life-threatening*. Interactions may have a *rapid onset* or a *delayed onset*.

ADMINISTRATION
Subcutaneous
• Drug is considered hazardous; use safe handling and disposal precautions.
• Give drug within 1 hour of reconstitution.
• Attach vial adaptor and reconstitute with provided prefilled syringe containing preservative-free sterile water for injection (reconstitute each 120-mg vial with 3 mL; reconstitute 80-mg vial with 4.2 mL). Leave syringe in place.
• Keeping vial in an upright position, swirl it very gently until liquid looks clear and has no undissolved powder or particles. If powder adheres to vial over the liquid surface, vial can be tilted slightly to dissolve powder. Avoid shaking, to prevent foam formation. A ring of small air bubbles on surface of liquid is acceptable. The reconstitution procedure may take up to 15 minutes.
• To withdraw for administration, turn vial completely upside down and pull down on the plunger to withdraw all of the reconstituted solution from vial to the syringe; expel all air bubbles. Detach the syringe by unscrewing it from vial adaptor.
• While holding the syringe with the tip pointing up, screw the injection needle clockwise onto the syringe.
• Inject drug only in areas of the abdomen that won't be exposed to pressure, for example, not close to waistband or belt nor close to the ribs.
• Inject degarelix subcut immediately after reconstitution. Pinch skin of abdomen, and elevate subcutaneous tissue. Insert needle deeply at angle of not less than 45 degrees. Gently pull back plunger to check if blood is aspirated. If blood appears in syringe, reconstituted product can no longer be used. Discontinue procedure and discard syringe and needle. Reconstitute new dose.
• Repeat reconstitution procedure for second 120-mg initial dose. Choose different injection site and inject.

ACTION
Gonadotropin-releasing hormone (GnRH) antagonist that binds to GnRH receptors and reduces the release of gonadotropins and, consequently, testosterone.

Route	Onset	Peak	Duration
Subcut	Unknown	2 days	Unknown

Half-life: Loading dose, about 53 days; maintenance dose, about 31 days.

ADVERSE REACTIONS
CNS: asthenia, dizziness, fatigue, fever, headache, insomnia. **CV:** HTN, hot flashes. **GI:** constipation, diarrhea, nausea. **GU:** erectile dysfunction, UTI, testicular atrophy. **Hepatic:** increased transaminase levels. **Metabolic:** weight gain, weight loss, increased GGT. **Musculoskeletal:** arthralgia, back pain, decrease in bone density. **Skin:** injection-site reactions (including pain, erythema, swelling, induration, and nodule formation), night sweats, hyperhidrosis. **Other:** chills, gynecomastia.

INTERACTIONS
Drug-drug. *Class IA, Class III antiarrhythmics (amiodarone, procainamide, quinidine, sotalol):* May prolong QT interval. Avoid use together.

EFFECTS ON LAB TEST RESULTS
• May increase PSA, AST, ALT, and GGT levels.

CONTRAINDICATIONS & CAUTIONS
• Contraindicated in patients hypersensitive to drug or its components. Discontinue drug for serious hypersensitivity reactions and don't rechallenge.
• Drug may increase risk of CV disease, anemia, and diabetes.
• Androgen deprivation therapy may prolong the QT interval. Prescribers should consider whether benefits of therapy outweigh potential risks. Use cautiously in patients with congenital long QT syndrome, electrolyte abnormalities, or HF and in those taking Class IA or Class III antiarrhythmics.
• Use cautiously in patients with CrCl of less than 50 mL/minute or severe hepatic impairment.
Dialyzable drug: Unknown.

PREGNANCY-LACTATION-REPRODUCTION
• Drug isn't indicated for use in women and is contraindicated in women who are or may become pregnant or are breastfeeding.

NURSING CONSIDERATIONS
• Monitor QT interval and electrolyte levels in patients with congenital long QT syndrome, electrolyte abnormalities, or HF, and in those taking Class IA or Class III antiarrhythmics.
• Monitor PSA level; if level is elevated, monitor testosterone level.
• Monitor bone density tests periodically.
• Monitor LFT values, CBC, and glucose levels.

PATIENT TEACHING
• Teach injection technique and methods of record-keeping to patient or family if they will be giving drug.
• Advise patient about possible adverse effects, including hot flashes, flushing of the skin, weight gain, decreased sex drive, and difficulties with erectile function. Injection-site reactions are usually mild, self-limiting, and decrease within 3 days.
• Emphasize to patient the importance of notifying health care provider of heart problems, such as HF, irregular heart rhythm, or salt imbalance, before taking drug.
• Advise patient to inform all health care providers about taking drug.

delafloxacin meglumine
del-a-FLOKS-a-sin

Baxdela

Therapeutic class: Antibiotics
Pharmacologic class: Fluoroquinolones

AVAILABLE FORMS
Injection: 300 mg in single-dose vial
Tablets: 450 mg

INDICATIONS & DOSAGES
➤ **Acute bacterial skin and skin-structure infections caused by susceptible bacteria, including gram-positive organisms (*Staphylococcus aureus* [including MRSA and methicillin-susceptible isolates], *Staphylococcus haemolyticus, Staphylococcus lugdunensis, Streptococcus agalactiae, Streptococcus anginosus* group [including *S. anginosus, Streptococcus intermedius,* and *Streptococcus constellatus*],** *Streptococcus pyogenes,* **and** *Enterococcus faecalis*) **and gram-negative organisms (*Escherichia coli, Enterobacter cloacae, Klebsiella pneumoniae,* and *Pseudomonas aeruginosa*)**
Adults: 300 mg IV infusion or 450 mg PO every 12 hours for 5 to 14 days. May switch from IV to PO dosing at prescriber's discretion.
Adjust-a-dose: If eGFR is between 15 and 29 mL/minute/1.73 m^2, no dosage adjustment is needed for tablets but decrease IV dosage to 200 mg every 12 hours, or give 200 mg IV every 12 hours, then switch to 450 mg PO every 12 hours at prescriber's discretion.

ADMINISTRATION
PO
• May give with or without food.
• Administer at least 2 hours before or 6 hours after antacids containing magnesium or aluminum, sucralfate, metal cations such as iron, multivitamin preparations containing zinc or iron, or didanosine buffered tablets for oral suspension or didanosine pediatric powder for oral solution.
• May give missed dose any time up to 8 hours before the next scheduled dose.
IV
▼ Reconstitute vial using 10.5 mL of D$_5$W or NSS for each 300-mg vial.
▼ Shake vial vigorously until contents are completely dissolved. Final concentration is 300 mg/12 mL (25 mg/mL) as a clear yellow to amber solution.
▼ Withdraw 12 mL from reconstituted vial for a 300-mg dose and 8 mL for a 200-mg dose. Add volume withdrawn to a total volume of 250 mL using either NSS or D$_5$W to achieve a final concentration of 1.2 mg/mL before administration.
▼ Infuse over 60 minutes. If a common IV line is used to administer other drugs, flush line before and after infusion with NSS or D$_5$W.
▼ Inspect for particulate matter and discoloration before administration.
▼ Store unopened vials at room temperature (68° to 77° F [20° to 25° C]).
▼ Reconstituted vials or diluted IV bag may be stored either refrigerated at 36° to 46° F (2° to 8° C) or at room

temperature (68° to 77° F [20° to 25° C]) for up to 24 hours; don't freeze.
▼ **Incompatibilities:** Magnesium, other multivalent cations given through same IV line, and other drugs.

ACTION
A fluoroquinolone that inhibits bacterial DNA replication, transcription, repair, and recombination; bactericidal.

Route	Onset	Peak	Duration
PO	Unknown	¾–1 hr	Unknown
IV	Unknown	1 hr	Unknown

Half-life: Oral, 4 to 8½ hours; IV, 3.7 hours.

ADVERSE REACTIONS
CNS: headache, dizziness, hypoesthesia, paresthesia, presyncope, syncope, anxiety, insomnia, abnormal dreams. **CV:** sinus tachycardia, palpitations, bradycardia, hypotension, HTN, flushing. **EENT:** blurred vision, tinnitus, vertigo, oral candidiasis. **GI:** nausea, diarrhea, vomiting, abdominal pain, dyspepsia, dysgeusia, CDAD. **GU:** vulvovaginal candidiasis, renal impairment, *renal failure.* **Hepatic:** elevated transaminase levels. **Metabolic:** *hypoglycemia,* hyperglycemia. **Musculoskeletal:** myalgia. **Skin:** infusion-site extravasation, infusion-site reactions (bruising, discomfort, edema, erythema, irritation, pain, phlebitis, swelling, thrombosis), pruritus, urticaria, dermatitis, rash. **Other:** hypersensitivity reaction, fungal infection.

INTERACTIONS
Drug-drug. *Antacids containing aluminum or magnesium, didanosine, iron, multivitamins containing iron or zinc, sucralfate:* May lower delafloxacin level when taken with PO formulation. Separate delafloxacin dose by at least 2 hours before or 6 hours after these drugs.
Corticosteroids: May increase risk of tendon injury. Avoid concurrent use.

EFFECTS ON LAB TEST RESULTS
• May increase liver transaminase, alkaline phosphatase, creatinine, and CK levels.
• May increase or decrease blood glucose level.

CONTRAINDICATIONS & CAUTIONS
• Contraindicated in patients hypersensitive to drug, its components, or other fluoroquinolones.
🛈 *Alert:* Patients receiving systemic drug have an increased risk of hyperglycemia and hypoglycemia, which can result in coma. Hypoglycemia has been reported more frequently in elderly patients and in those with diabetes.
🛈 *Alert:* Drug may increase risk of aortic dissection or rupture when used systemically. Avoid use in patients with known aortic aneurysm, in patients at risk for an aortic aneurysm, including those with peripheral atherosclerotic vascular diseases, HTN, or certain genetic conditions (Marfan syndrome, Ehlers-Danlos syndrome), and in elderly patients. Drug should only be used in these patients if no other treatment options are available.
• Use should be limited to infections that are proven or strongly suspected to be caused by susceptible bacteria to reduce risk of drug-resistant bacteria and to maintain drug's effectiveness.
Black Box Warning Fluoroquinolones have been associated with disabling and potentially irreversible serious adverse reactions that have occurred together, including tendinitis and tendon rupture, peripheral neuropathy, and CNS effects. Discontinue immediately if signs and symptoms occur; avoid using fluoroquinolones in patients who experience any of these serious adverse reactions. ▪
Black Box Warning Fluoroquinolones may exacerbate muscle weakness in patients with myasthenia gravis. Avoid using fluoroquinolones in patients with known history of myasthenia gravis. ▪
Black Box Warning Oral or parenteral fluoroquinolones may increase risk of peripheral neuropathy of the arms or legs. Signs or symptoms can occur anytime during treatment and can last for months to years or be permanent. Stop drug immediately if patient develops signs or symptoms. Avoid use in patients who have previously experienced peripheral neuropathy. ▪
Black Box Warning Use cautiously in patients with a history of known or suspected CNS disorders (severe cerebral

arteriosclerosis, epilepsy) or other risk factors that increase the risk of seizures or lower the seizure threshold. Drug may increase risk of CNS reactions, including seizures, increased ICP (including pseudotumor cerebri), dizziness, and tremors. If these reactions occur, discontinue drug immediately and institute appropriate measures. ■

• Fluoroquinolones have been associated with an increased risk of psychiatric adverse reactions, including toxic psychosis; hallucinations or paranoia; depression or suicidal thoughts or acts; delirium, disorientation, confusion, or disturbances in attention; anxiety, agitation, or nervousness; insomnia or nightmares; and memory impairment. These adverse reactions may occur after first dose. Stop drug immediately and institute appropriate measures if patient develops any of these reactions.

• Drug isn't indicated for patients with eGFR of less than 15 mL/minute/1.73 m², including hemodialysis patients.

• Drug may cause CDAD ranging in severity from mild diarrhea to fatal colitis and possibly occurring more than 2 months after therapy ends. Drug may need to be discontinued if CDAD develops during therapy.

• Use cautiously in patients older than age 60; patients taking corticosteroids; patients with kidney, heart, or lung transplant; patients with renal impairment; patients with previous tendon disorders, including RA; and those participating in strenuous physical activity as risk of tendinitis or tendon rupture may be increased.

• Drug isn't approved for children younger than age 18.

Dialyzable drug: Yes.

PREGNANCY-LACTATION-REPRODUCTION
• Data are limited on the safety of delafloxacin in pregnant women. Use cautiously and only if benefits outweigh risk to the fetus.

• It isn't known if drug appears in human milk. Consider benefits of therapy and risks of breastfeeding in the infant.

NURSING CONSIDERATIONS
• Whenever possible, obtain specimen for culture and sensitivity testing before first dose. Begin therapy while awaiting results.

🛈 *Alert:* Monitor patients for signs and symptoms of aortic aneurysm, dissection, or rupture (sudden, severe, and constant pain in the stomach, chest, or back; throbbing in the stomach area; deep pain in the back or the side of the stomach; steady, gnawing pain in the stomach that lasts for hours or days; pain in the jaw, neck, back, or chest; coughing or hoarseness; shortness of breath or trouble swallowing). Discontinue drug immediately if any of these aortic disorders are suspected.

• Monitor patient for tendinitis (pain, swelling, inflammation), tendon rupture, arthralgia, and myalgia. Tendinitis or tendon rupture frequently involves the Achilles but may also occur in the hand, shoulder, or other tendons. Symptoms may occur hours after starting drug to several months after therapy ends. Discontinue drug immediately if symptoms occur.

• Monitor patient for peripheral neuropathy (pain; burning; tingling; numbness; weakness; alterations in light touch, pain, temperature, position sense, and vibratory sensation; and motor strength) and CNS effects (seizures, increased ICP, pseudotumor cerebri, severe headaches, dizziness, tremors). Signs and symptoms may occur hours or weeks after initial dose. Discontinue drug if these reactions occur.

• Monitor patients with myasthenia gravis for exacerbation of muscle weakness; discontinue drug immediately if symptoms occur.

• Monitor patients for rash or other signs and symptoms of hypersensitivity. Discontinue drug at first appearance of reaction.

• Monitor patients for CDAD, which has been reported in users of nearly all systemic antibacterial drugs. Stop drug and provide appropriate therapy if CDAD occurs.

🛈 *Alert:* Monitor patients receiving systemic drug for symptoms of hypoglycemia (confusion, pounding or rapid heartbeat, dizziness, pale skin, shakiness, sweating, unusual hunger, trembling, headache, weakness, irritability, unusual anxiety). Immediately discontinue drug for blood glucose disturbances, and switch to a nonfluoroquinolone antibiotic if possible.

🛈 *Alert:* Monitor patients receiving systemic drug for psychiatric adverse reactions (toxic psychosis, hallucinations, paranoia,

---

depression, suicidal thoughts or acts, confusion, insomnia or nightmares, disturbances in attention, disorientation, agitation, nervousness, memory impairment, delirium). Discontinue drug if these reactions occur.

PATIENT TEACHING
• Discuss importance of taking every dose and of completing a full treatment course to prevent antibacterial resistance and to avoid decreasing drug's effectiveness. If drug is stopped because of adverse effects, patient should discuss with prescriber completing treatment with another antibacterial drug.
⊙ *Alert:* Warn patient to seek immediate medical attention for signs or symptoms of aortic aneurysm, dissection, or rupture.
Black Box Warning Tell patient that tendon rupture can occur during therapy and to notify prescriber if pain, swelling or inflammation of tendon, or weakness or inability to use a joint occurs. Advise patient to stop drug and to rest and refrain from exercise. ∎
Black Box Warning Inform patient with myasthenia gravis that drug may exacerbate signs and symptoms of muscle weakness, including respiratory difficulties, and to immediately report worsening. ∎
Black Box Warning Caution patient to immediately report signs and symptoms of peripheral neuropathy (pain, tingling, burning, numbness, weakness) to prescriber and to stop drug. ∎
Black Box Warning Explain risk of CNS adverse effects (seizures, dizziness, lightheadedness, increased ICP, headache with or without blurred vision) with use of drug and advise patient to notify prescriber immediately if these occur. ∎
• Warn patient to avoid hazardous tasks that require alertness such as driving until drug's effects are known.
• Advise patient to report all adverse reactions and to immediately report hypersensitivity reactions (rash, hives, other skin reactions, tachycardia, difficulty swallowing or breathing, tightness of the throat, hoarseness, and swelling of the lips, tongue, or face), which can occur even after a single dose.
⊙ *Alert:* Caution patients that significantly low blood sugar levels can occur. Instruct patients how to manage symptoms and to

immediately report any occurrence to the prescriber.
⊙ *Alert:* Advise patients with diabetes that they may need to monitor blood glucose levels more frequently during therapy.
⊙ *Alert:* Inform patients to immediately report psychiatric adverse reactions and that these can occur after just one dose.
• Caution patient to immediately report watery or bloody stools with or without abdominal cramping and fever. Diarrhea may occur during therapy or 2 months or more after last dose.

---

delavirdine mesylate
dell-ah-VIR-deen

Rescriptor

Therapeutic class: Antiretrovirals
Pharmacologic class: NNRTIs

AVAILABLE FORMS
Tablets: 100 mg, 200 mg

INDICATIONS & DOSAGES
➤ **HIV-1 infection in combination with at least two other active antiretrovirals**
Adults and adolescents age 16 and older: 400 mg PO t.i.d.
   Resistant virus emerges rapidly when delavirdine is administered as monotherapy. Always administer with appropriate antiretroviral therapy.

ADMINISTRATION
PO
• Patient may take drug with or without food.
• For patient with achlorhydria (absence of gastric acid in the stomach), drug should be taken with an acidic beverage, such as orange juice or cranberry juice.
• Patient should separate doses of delavirdine and antacid by at least 1 hour.
• May disperse 100-mg tablets in water before ingestion. Add four 100-mg tablets to at least 90 mL of water, allow to stand for a few minutes, and stir until a uniform dispersion occurs. Tell patient to drink dispersion promptly, rinse glass, and swallow the rinse to ensure that entire dose is consumed.

Don't try to disperse 200-mg tablets because they don't disperse well; take 200-mg tablets intact.

ACTION

A nonnucleoside reverse transcriptase inhibitor of HIV-1 that binds directly to reverse transcriptase and blocks RNA- and DNA-dependent DNA polymerase activities.

Route	Onset	Peak	Duration
PO	Unknown	1 hr	Unknown

Half-life: 2 to 11 hours.

ADVERSE REACTIONS

CNS: anxiety, asthenia, fatigue, headache, depression, fever, insomnia, pain. **EENT:** pharyngitis, sinusitis. **GI:** nausea, abdominal cramps, diarrhea, abdominal distention or pain, vomiting. **Respiratory:** bronchitis, cough, URI. **Skin:** rash. **Other:** flulike syndrome.

INTERACTIONS

Drug-drug. *Amphetamines:* May increase amphetamine level. Use cautiously.

Antacids: May reduce delavirdine absorption. Separate doses by at least 1 hour.

Antiarrhythmics (flecainide, quinidine, propafenone, systemic lidocaine): May affect antiarrhythmic levels. Use cautiously and monitor antiarrhythmic therapeutic concentrations.

Anticonvulsants (carbamazepine, phenytoin), antimycobacterials (rifabutin, rifampin): May cause loss of virologic response. Use together is contraindicated.

Antihistamines (astemizole, terfenadine), bepridil, ergot derivatives, lovastatin, pimozide, sedative/hypnotics (alprazolam, midazolam, triazolam), simvastatin: May cause life-threatening arrhythmias or adverse reactions. Use together is contraindicated.

Atorvastatin, fluvastatin: May increase atorvastatin or fluvastatin level. Carefully monitor patient; consider another drug such as pravastatin.

Calcium channel blockers: May increase calcium channel blocker level. Use cautiously and monitor patient closely.

Clarithromycin: May increase clarithromycin level. When used together in patients with CrCl of 30 to 60 mL/minute, reduce clarithromycin dose by 50%. For patients with CrCl of less than 30 mL/minute, reduce dose by 75%.

Corticosteroids (dexamethasone): May decrease delavirdine level and reduce therapeutic effect. Use cautiously.

Cyclosporine, rapamycin, tacrolimus: May increase immunosuppressant levels. Monitor immunosuppressant therapeutic concentrations.

Didanosine: May decrease concentration levels of both drugs. Separate doses by at least 1 hour.

Fluticasone: May increase fluticasone concentration. Use cautiously; consider alternative drug for long-term use.

H_2-receptor antagonists (cimetidine, famotidine, nizatidine, ranitidine), PPIs: May decrease delavirdine absorption. Prolonged use together isn't recommended.

Indinavir: May increase indinavir level. Consider reducing indinavir dosage to 600 mg t.i.d.

Maraviroc: May increase maraviroc level. Reduce maraviroc dosage.

Methadone: May increase methadone level. Methadone dosage may need to be decreased.

Sildenafil: May increase sildenafil level. Don't exceed single dose of sildenafil 25 mg in a 48-hour period.

Trazodone: May increase trazodone level. Use cautiously; consider lower trazodone dosage.

Warfarin: May increase warfarin level. Monitor INR.

Drug-herb. *St. John's wort:* May lead to loss of virologic response. Use together is contraindicated.

EFFECTS ON LAB TEST RESULTS

• May increase alkaline phosphatase, ALT, amylase, AST, bilirubin level, CK, creatinine, GGT, and lipase levels. May decrease glucose and Hb levels and hematocrit.

• May increase eosinophil count; may prolong PT and PTT. May decrease granulocyte, neutrophil, platelet, RBC, and WBC counts.

Reactions in bold italics are *life-threatening*. Interactions may have a *rapid onset* or a *delayed onset*.

CONTRAINDICATIONS & CAUTIONS
• Contraindicated in patients hypersensitive to drug or its components and in those taking drugs that are highly dependent on CYP3A metabolism (antihistamines, ergot derivatives, sedative/hypnotics).
• Immune reconstitution syndrome has been reported. Inflammatory response to indolent or residual opportunistic infections (*Mycobacterium avium* infection, cytomegalovirus, *Pneumocystis jiroveci* pneumonia, TB) can occur that may need evaluation and treatment. Autoimmune disorders (Graves disease, polymyositis, Guillain-Barré syndrome) have been reported in the setting of immune reconstitution; time to onset is variable and can occur months after therapy begins.
• Rare but severe rash (erythema multiforme, SJS) has been reported. Most cases didn't require dosage reduction or drug discontinuation.
• Use cautiously in elderly patients and in patients with impaired hepatic function.
Dialyzable drug: Unlikely.

PREGNANCY-LACTATION-REPRODUCTION
• There are no adequate well-controlled studies in pregnant women. Use during pregnancy only if potential benefit justifies potential risk to the fetus.
• HIV-positive women shouldn't breastfeed, to avoid postnatal HIV transmission and possible adverse reactions in breastfed infants.
• Encourage pregnant patients to enroll in the Antiretroviral Pregnancy Registry (1-800-258-4263).

NURSING CONSIDERATIONS
• Because drug's effects in patients with hepatic or renal impairment haven't been studied, monitor renal function test results and LFTs carefully.
• Drug-induced diffuse, maculopapular, erythematous, pruritic rash occurs most commonly on upper body and arms of patients with lower CD4 cell counts, usually within first 3 weeks of treatment. Dosage adjustment doesn't seem to affect rash. Treat symptoms with diphenhydramine, hydroxyzine, or topical corticosteroids.

• Drug doesn't reduce risk of transmission of HIV-1.
• Monitor patient's fluid balance and weight.

PATIENT TEACHING
• Tell patient to stop drug and call prescriber if severe rash or such symptoms as fever, fatigue, headache, nausea, abdominal pain, or cough occur.
• Inform patient that drug doesn't cure HIV-1 infection and that illnesses may continue to occur, including opportunistic infections related to HIV-1 infection. Therapy hasn't been shown to reduce the risk or frequency of such illnesses. Drug hasn't been shown to reduce transmission of HIV.
• Advise patient to remain under medical supervision when taking drug because the long-term effects aren't known.
• Tell patient to take drug as prescribed and not to alter doses without prescriber's approval. If a dose is missed, tell patient to take the next dose as soon as possible and not to double the next dose.
• Inform patient that 100-mg form of drug may be dispersed in water before ingestion. Add four 100-mg tablets to at least 3 oz (90 mL) of water, allow to stand for a few minutes, and stir until a uniform dispersion occurs. Tell patient to drink dispersion promptly, rinse glass, and swallow the rinse to ensure that entire dose is consumed.
• Instruct patient to take 200-mg tablets whole; 200-mg tablets don't disperse well in water.
• Tell patient that drug may be taken with or without food.
• Tell patient with achlorhydria to take drug with an acidic beverage, such as orange or cranberry juice.
• Instruct patient to take drug and antacids at least 1 hour apart.
• Advise patient to report use of other prescription or nonprescription drugs, including herbal remedies.
• Advise patient taking sildenafil about an increased risk of sildenafil-related adverse events, including low BP, visual changes, and painful penile erection. Tell patient to promptly report any symptoms to prescriber. Tell patient not to exceed 25 mg of sildenafil in 48 hours.

denosumab
deh-KNOW-sue-mab

Prolia, Xgeva

Therapeutic class: Antiosteoporotics–antiresorptives
Pharmacologic class: Monoclonal antibodies

AVAILABLE FORMS
Injection: 60 mg/mL in prefilled syringe (Prolia); 120 mg/1.7 mL (70 mg/mL) in single-use vial (Xgeva)

INDICATIONS & DOSAGES
➤ **Osteoporosis in men and post-menopausal women at risk for fracture (Prolia only)**
Adults: 60 mg subcut every 6 months. All patients should receive 1,000 mg of calcium daily and at least 400 international units of vitamin D daily.
➤ **To increase bone mass in men at high risk for fracture who are receiving androgen deprivation therapy for nonmetastatic prostate cancer and in women who are receiving adjuvant aromatase inhibitor therapy for breast cancer (Prolia only)**
Adults: 60 mg subcut once every 6 months. All patients should receive calcium 1,000 mg daily and at least 400 international units of vitamin D daily.
✳ *NEW INDICATION:* **Glucocorticoid-induced osteoporosis in men and women at high risk for fracture who are either initiating or continuing systemic glucocorticoids in a daily dosage equivalent to 7.5 mg or greater of prednisone and expected to remain on glucocorticoids for at least 6 months (Prolia only)**
Adults: 60 mg subcut once every 6 months. All patients should receive calcium 1,000 mg daily and at least 400 international units of vitamin D daily.
➤ **Giant cell tumor of bone (Xgeva only)**
Adults and skeletally mature adolescents age 13 and older: 120 mg subcut every 4 weeks with additional 120-mg doses on days 8 and 15 of first month of therapy. Administer calcium and vitamin D as necessary to prevent or treat hypocalcemia.

➤ **Hypercalcemia of malignancy refractory to bisphosphonate therapy (Xgeva only)**
Adults: 120 mg subcut every 4 weeks with additional 120-mg doses on days 8 and 15 of first month of therapy.
➤ **Bone metastases from solid tumors; prevention of skeletal-related events in patients with multiple myeloma (Xgeva only)**
Adults: 120 mg subcut every 4 weeks, with calcium and vitamin D as necessary to prevent or treat hypocalcemia.

ADMINISTRATION
Subcutaneous
• Don't use if solution is discolored or cloudy or contains many particles or foreign particulate matter.
• Before administration, drug may be removed from refrigerator and brought to room temperature (up to 77° F [25° C]) by letting stand in original container. This generally takes 15 to 30 minutes. Don't warm drug in any other way. Avoid vigorous shaking of drug. Once removed from refrigerator, maintain at 77° F or lower and use within 14 days. Discard after 14 days if not used.
• Protect from direct light and heat.
• Use 27G needle to withdraw drug from single-use vial, and inject entire contents of vial. Don't reenter vial.
• Administer via subcut injection in upper arm, upper thigh, or abdomen.
• Drug is intended for subcut route only and shouldn't be administered IV, IM, or intradermally.

ACTION
Inhibits osteoclast activity, thereby decreasing bone resorption and increasing bone mass and strength.

Route	Onset	Peak	Duration
Subcut	Unknown	10 days	4–5 mo

Half-life: About 25 to 28 days.

ADVERSE REACTIONS
CNS: asthenia, insomnia, sciatica, vertigo, headache, fatigue. **CV:** angina, atrial fibrillation, peripheral edema. **EENT:** pharyngitis. **GI:** flatulence, GERD, upper abdominal pain, nausea, decreased appetite, vomiting, constipation, diarrhea. **GU:** cystitis.

Reactions in bold italics are *life-threatening*. Interactions may have a *rapid onset* or a *delayed onset*.

Hematologic: anemia. **Metabolic:** hypercholesterolemia, *hypocalcemia,* hypophosphatemia. **Musculoskeletal:** back pain, bone pain, extremity pain, musculoskeletal pain, myalgia, spinal osteoarthritis. **Respiratory:** pneumonia, URI, dyspnea. **Skin:** pruritus, rash, dermatitis. **Other:** *anaphylaxis,* facial swelling, herpes zoster, *osteonecrosis of the jaw.*

INTERACTIONS
Drug-drug. *Immunosuppressants (except cytarabine [liposomal]):* May enhance adverse/toxic effect of immunosuppressants and increase risk of serious infections. Monitor patient closely.
Drug-lifestyle. *Alcohol use:* May increase risk of osteoporosis. Avoid use together.

EFFECTS ON LAB TEST RESULTS
• May increase cholesterol level. May decrease calcium, magnesium, and phosphate levels.

CONTRAINDICATIONS & CAUTIONS
• Contraindicated in patients with a history of systemic hypersensitivity to components of the product. Reactions have included anaphylaxis, facial swelling, and urticaria.
• Contraindicated in patients with hypocalcemia.
• Discontinue use if severe bone, joint, or muscle pain occurs.
• Use cautiously in patients with history of hypoparathyroidism, thyroid surgery, parathyroid surgery, malabsorption syndromes, excision of small intestine, or severe renal impairment.
• Clinically significant hypercalcemia requiring hospitalization and complicated by acute renal injury has been reported within the first year after treatment discontinuation in Xgeva-treated patients with giant cell tumor of bone and in patients with growing skeletons.
• Use cautiously in patients taking immunosuppressants and in those with an impaired immune system.
Dialyzable drug: Unknown.

PREGNANCY-LACTATION-REPRODUCTION
• Drug may cause fetal harm; Prolia is contraindicated in pregnant women. Verify pregnancy status of women of childbearing potential before starting drug. There are no adequate studies of Xgeva in pregnant women. If drug is used during pregnancy, or if patient becomes pregnant while taking drug, inform patient of potential fetal hazard.
• Caution women of childbearing potential to use highly effective contraception during therapy and for at least 5 months after last dose.
• It isn't known if drug appears in human milk. Patient should discontinue breastfeeding or discontinue drug, taking into account importance of drug to the mother.

NURSING CONSIDERATIONS
• Make sure patient has adequate intake of calcium and vitamin D.
• Monitor calcium (especially in first weeks of therapy), vitamin D, magnesium, and phosphorus levels before and during therapy. Administer calcium, magnesium, and vitamin D as needed.
• Drug can cause severe symptomatic hypocalcemia; fatal cases have been reported. Correct hypocalcemia before starting drug.
• Multiple vertebral fractures have been reported after treatment ends. Evaluate patient's individual risk of vertebral fractures and consider transitioning to an alternative antiresorptive therapy.
• Drug may cause osteonecrosis of the jaw, which can occur spontaneously and is commonly associated with tooth extraction, local infection with delayed healing, or both. Monitor patients for signs and symptoms and perform an oral examination and ensure appropriate preventive dentistry before starting drug and periodically during therapy.
• Consider stopping drug if severe skin reactions occur.
• When treatment is discontinued, monitor patients for signs and symptoms of hypercalcemia (nausea, vomiting, headache, decreased alertness), assess serum calcium level periodically, reevaluate patient's calcium and vitamin D supplementation requirements, and treat appropriately.
◊ *Alert:* Needle cap on single-use syringe contains latex; keep away from those with latex allergy.

D

◑ *Alert:* Prolia and Xgeva contain the same active ingredient, denosumab. Patients receiving Prolia should not receive Xgeva.

PATIENT TEACHING
• Caution patient to read medication guide that comes with prescription before starting treatment and at every prescription refill.
• Warn patient to immediately report signs and symptoms of low calcium (spasms, twitching or muscle cramps, and numbness or tingling of fingers or toes or around mouth); emphasize the importance of maintaining normal calcium levels.
• Advise patient to have a dental exam before treatment and to follow good oral hygiene practices during therapy.
• Instruct patient to tell dentist before dental procedures about taking drug, and to inform dentist or prescriber if persistent pain or slow healing of mouth or jaw occurs after dental surgery.
• Tell patient to report jaw pain, swelling, or numbness; loose teeth; or dramatic gum loss.
• Advise patient to seek prompt medical care if signs and symptoms of severe infection occur, including cellulitis or skin reactions (such as dermatitis, rash, or eczema).
• Advise patient to contact health care provider if severe bone, joint, or muscle pain occurs.
• Instruct patient with severe renal impairment about signs and symptoms of hypocalcemia and the importance of maintaining normal calcium levels.
• Tell patient to take calcium and vitamin D supplement, as directed by prescriber.

desipramine hydrochloride
des-IP-ra-meen

Norpramin

Therapeutic class: Antidepressants
Pharmacologic class: TCAs

AVAILABLE FORMS
Tablets: 10 mg, 25 mg, 50 mg, 75 mg, 100 mg, 150 mg

INDICATIONS & DOSAGES
➤ **Depression**
Adults: 100 to 200 mg PO daily in divided doses; increase to maximum of 300 mg daily. Or, give entire dose at bedtime.
Adolescents and elderly patients: 25 to 100 mg PO daily in divided doses; increase gradually to maximum of 150 mg daily, if needed.

ADMINISTRATION
PO
• Give drug without regard for food.

ACTION
Unknown. Increases the amount of norepinephrine, serotonin, or both in the CNS by blocking their reuptake by the presynaptic neurons.

Route	Onset	Peak	Duration
PO	Unknown	About 6 hr	Unknown

Half-life: 15 to 24 hours.

ADVERSE REACTIONS
CNS: drowsiness, dizziness, *seizures,* excitation, tremor, weakness, confusion, anxiety, restlessness, agitation, headache, nervousness, EEG changes, extrapyramidal reactions, ataxia, delusions, insomnia, fatigue, peripheral neuropathy, *stroke.* **CV:** tachycardia, orthostatic hypotension, ECG changes, HTN, *MI.* **EENT:** blurred vision, mydriasis, tinnitus. **GI:** dry mouth, constipation, nausea, vomiting, anorexia, paralytic ileus, diarrhea. **GU:** urine retention, erectile dysfunction, nocturia, decreased libido, painful ejaculation, testicular swelling, urinary hesitancy. **Hematologic:** *agranulocytosis, thrombocytopenia,* eosinophilia, purpura. **Metabolic:** *hypoglycemia,* hyperglycemia, weight loss or gain. **Skin:** rash, urticaria, photosensitivity reactions, diaphoresis, alopecia. **Other:** *sudden death in children,* hypersensitivity reactions.

INTERACTIONS
Drug-drug. *Barbiturates, CNS depressants:* May enhance CNS depression. Avoid using together.
Cimetidine, **fluoxetine, fluvoxamine, paroxetine, sertraline:** May increase desipramine

---

level. Monitor drug levels and patient for signs of toxicity.

Clonidine: May cause life-threatening BP elevations. Avoid using together.

Drugs that prolong QT interval (antiarrhythmics, clarithromycin, droperidol, fluoroquinolones, pimozide, ziprasidone): May increase QT-interval prolongation and risk of ventricular arrhythmias. Avoid combination if possible.

Epinephrine, norepinephrine: May increase hypertensive effect. Use together cautiously.

Linezolid, methylene blue: May cause serotonin syndrome. Use with extreme caution and monitor closely.

MAO inhibitors: May cause severe excitation, hyperpyrexia, or seizures, usually with high doses. Avoid using within 14 days of MAO inhibitor therapy.

Quinolones: May increase the risk of life-threatening arrhythmias. Avoid using together.

Serotonergic drugs (buspirone, fentanyl, lithium, tramadol, triptans, tryptophan): Increase risk of serotonin syndrome. Monitor closely if use together is clinically warranted. Discontinue desipramine and other serotonergic drugs if syndrome occurs, and initiate supportive treatment.

Drug-herb. *Evening primrose oil:* May cause additive or synergistic effect, resulting in lower seizure threshold and increasing the risk of seizure. Discourage use together.

St. John's wort, *SAM-e, yohimbe:* May cause serotonin syndrome. Discourage use together.

Drug-food. *Grapefruit juice:* May increase desipramine level, increasing pharmacologic effects and risk of adverse reactions. Avoid use together.

Drug-lifestyle. *Alcohol use:* May enhance CNS depression. Discourage use together.

Smoking: May lower drug level. Monitor patient for lack of effect.

Sun exposure: May increase risk of photosensitivity reactions. Advise patient to avoid excessive sunlight exposure.

EFFECTS ON LAB TEST RESULTS

• May increase or decrease glucose level.
• May increase LFT values.
• May cause false-positive urine detection of amphetamines or methamphetamines.

CONTRAINDICATIONS & CAUTIONS

• Contraindicated in patients hypersensitive to drug and in those who have taken MAO inhibitors within previous 14 days.

⚠ *Alert:* Concomitant use with linezolid or methylene blue can cause serotonin syndrome (fever, mental status changes, muscle twitching, excessive sweating, shivering or shaking, diarrhea, loss of coordination) and is contraindicated.

• Contraindicated during acute recovery phase after MI.

Black Box Warning Drug isn't approved for use in children. ▮

• Use with extreme caution in patients with CV disease; in those with a family history of sudden death, cardiac arrhythmias, or cardiac conduction disturbances; in those with history of urine retention, glaucoma, seizure disorders, or thyroid disease; and in those taking thyroid drug.

⚠ *Alert:* Treatment of patients who require as much as 300 mg desipramine should be initiated in hospitals where access to skilled health care providers and frequent ECGs is available. High doses may cause prolongation of the QRS or QT interval.

Dialyzable drug: No.

⚠ *Overdose S&S:* Cardiac arrhythmias, severe hypotension, seizures, CNS depression, coma, ECG changes, confusion, disturbed concentration, transient visual hallucinations, dilated pupils, agitation, hyperactive reflexes, stupor, drowsiness, muscle rigidity, vomiting, hypothermia, hyperpyrexia.

PREGNANCY-LACTATION-REPRODUCTION

• Safe use in pregnant women hasn't been established. Use during pregnancy only if clearly needed and potential benefit justifies potential risk to the fetus.

• Drug appears in human milk. Patient should discontinue breastfeeding or discontinue drug, taking into account importance of drug to the mother.

NURSING CONSIDERATIONS

⚠ *Alert:* Drug has been shown to lower the seizure threshold. Seizures precede cardiac arrhythmias and death in some patients.

• Monitor patient for nausea, headache, and malaise after abrupt withdrawal of long-term

therapy; these symptoms don't indicate addiction.
- Don't withdraw drug abruptly.
- Because patients may experience hypertensive episodes, cardiac arrhythmias, or drug interactions with anesthesia during surgery, stop drug gradually several days before elective surgery.

☹ *Alert:* If linezolid or methylene blue must be given, stop drug and monitor patient for serotonin toxicity for 2 weeks or until 24 hours after the last dose of methylene blue or linezolid, whichever comes first. Treatment may be resumed 24 hours after last dose of methylene blue or linezolid.
- If signs or symptoms of psychosis occur or increase, notify prescriber. Record mood changes. Monitor patient for suicidal tendencies.

Black Box Warning Drug may increase risk of suicidal thinking and behavior in children, adolescents, and young adults ages 18 to 24, especially during the first few months of treatment, especially in those with major depressive disorder or other psychiatric disorder. ∎

☹ *Alert:* Norpramin may contain tartrazine.
- *Look alike–sound alike:* Don't confuse desipramine with disopyramide or imipramine.

PATIENT TEACHING
Black Box Warning Advise families and caregivers to observe patient closely for increased suicidal thinking and behavior. ∎
- Advise patient to take full dose at bedtime to avoid daytime sedation; if insomnia occurs, tell patient to take drug in the morning.
- Warn patient to avoid hazardous activities that require alertness and good coordination until effects of drug are known. Drowsiness and dizziness usually subside after a few weeks.

☹ *Alert:* Teach patient to recognize and immediately report symptoms of serotonin toxicity (fever, mental status changes, muscle twitching, excessive sweating, shivering or shaking, diarrhea, loss of coordination).
- Advise patient to call prescriber if fever and sore throat occur. Blood counts may need to be obtained.
- Tell patient to avoid alcohol during therapy because it may antagonize effects of drug.

- Tell patient to consult prescriber before taking other prescription or OTC drugs.
- Warn patient not to stop drug suddenly.
- To prevent sensitivity to the sun, advise patient to use sunblock, wear protective clothing, and avoid prolonged exposure to strong sunlight.

desloratadine
dess-lor-AT-a-deen

Clarinex✐

Therapeutic class: Antihistamines
Pharmacologic class: Piperidines

AVAILABLE FORMS
Oral solution: 0.5 mg/mL
Tablets: 5 mg
Tablets (ODTs): 2.5 mg, 5 mg

INDICATIONS & DOSAGES
➤ **Seasonal allergic rhinitis (patients age 2 and older); perennial allergic rhinitis and chronic idiopathic urticaria (patients age 6 months and older)**
Adults and children age 12 and older: 5 mg tablets or solution PO once daily.
Children ages 6 to 11: 2.5 mg ODT or solution PO once daily.
Children ages 12 months to 5 years: 1.25 mg ODT or solution PO once daily.
Infants ages 6 to 11 months: 1 mg solution PO once daily.
Adjust-a-dose: In adults with hepatic or renal impairment, start dosage at 5 mg PO every other day.

ADMINISTRATION
PO
- Give drug without regard for meals.
- Place ODTs on tongue immediately after opening blister pack.
- Give ODTs with or without water.
- Administer oral solution with a commercially available measuring dropper or syringe that's calibrated to deliver 2 mL and 2.5 mL.

ACTION
Long-acting tricyclic antihistamine with selective H_1-receptor antagonist activity. It

inhibits histamine release from human mast cells in vitro.

Route	Onset	Peak	Duration
PO	<1 hr	3 hr	Up to 24 hr

Half-life: 27 hours.

ADVERSE REACTIONS
CNS: headache, somnolence, fatigue, dizziness, irritability, fever, drowsiness. **EENT:** pharyngitis, dry throat, rhinorrhea, epistaxis. **GI:** nausea, diarrhea, dry mouth, dyspepsia. **GU:** dysmenorrhea. **Musculoskeletal:** myalgia. **Respiratory:** bronchitis, cough, URI.

INTERACTIONS
Drug-drug. *CNS depressants:* May increase CNS depression. Monitor therapy.
Drug-lifestyle. *Alcohol use:* May increase CNS depression. Avoid use together.

EFFECTS ON LAB TEST RESULTS
• May prevent, reduce, or mask positive result in diagnostic skin test.

CONTRAINDICATIONS & CAUTIONS
• Contraindicated in patients hypersensitive to drug or its components, or to loratadine.
• Hypersensitivity reactions, including rash, pruritus, urticaria, edema, dyspnea, and anaphylaxis, have been reported. If these occur, stop drug immediately and consider alternative treatments.
• Use cautiously in elderly patients because of the greater likelihood of decreased hepatic, renal, or cardiac function and concomitant disease or other drug therapy.
Dialyzable drug: No.
⚠ *Overdose S&S:* Somnolence, increased QTc interval.

PREGNANCY-LACTATION-REPRODUCTION
• There are no adequate well-controlled studies in pregnant women. Use during pregnancy only if clearly needed and potential benefit justifies potential risk to the fetus.
• Drug appears in human milk. Patient should discontinue breastfeeding or discontinue drug, taking into account importance of drug to the mother.

NURSING CONSIDERATIONS
• Stop drug 4 days before diagnostic skin testing because antihistamines can prevent, reduce, or mask positive skin test response.

PATIENT TEACHING
• Advise patient not to exceed recommended dosage. Higher doses don't increase effectiveness and may cause somnolence.
• Tell patient that drug can be taken without regard to meals.
• Instruct patient to remove ODTs from blister pack and place on tongue immediately to dissolve.
• ODTs may be taken with or without water.
• Tell patient to report adverse effects.
• Advise patient with phenylketonuria that ODTs contain phenylalanine.

desmopressin acetate ▒
des-moe-PRESS-in

DDAVP, Nocdurna, Noctiva, Stimate

Therapeutic class: Hemostatics
Pharmacologic class: Posterior pituitary hormones

AVAILABLE FORMS
Injection: 4 mcg/mL
Metered nasal spray: 0.83 mcg/spray, 1.66 mcg/spray, 10 mcg/spray, 150 mcg/spray
Nasal solution: 0.1 mg/mL, 1.5 mg/mL
Tablets: 0.1 mg, 0.2 mg
Tablets (SL): 27.7 mcg, 55.3 mcg

INDICATIONS & DOSAGES
➤ **Nonnephrogenic diabetes insipidus, temporary polyuria, and polydipsia related to pituitary trauma**
Intranasal, IV, or subcutaneous
Adults and children older than age 12: 10 to 40 mcg (0.1 to 0.4 mL) intranasally daily in one to three doses. Most adults need 0.2 mL (20 mcg) daily in two divided doses. Or, give 2 to 4 mcg (0.5 to 1 mL) IV or subcut daily, usually in two divided doses.
PO
Adults and children older than age 4: Initially, 0.05 mg (half of the 0.1-mg tablet)

PO b.i.d.; adjust dosage to patient response. If patient previously received the drug intranasally, begin oral therapy 12 hours after last intranasal dose. Maximum dose is 1.2 mg/day (divided into two or three doses) for patients with diabetes insipidus.

Intranasal

Children ages 3 months to 12 years: 5 to 30 mcg (0.05 to 0.3 mL) intranasally daily in one or two doses.

➤ **Hemophilia A and von Willebrand disease** ⚕

Adults and children age 3 months and older: 0.3 mcg/kg diluted in NSS and infused IV over 15 to 30 minutes. Repeat dose, if needed, as indicated by laboratory response and patient's condition. If used preoperatively, give 30 minutes before the scheduled procedure.

Adults and children age 11 months and older: A total dose of 300 mcg (one spray [150 mcg] of solution containing 1.5 mg/mL in each nostril). Dose of 150 mcg (one spray of solution containing 1.5 mg/mL into a single nostril) may be adequate for patients weighing less than 50 kg. If used preoperatively, give drug 2 hours before surgery.

➤ **Primary nocturnal enuresis**

Adults and children age 6 and older: Initially, 0.2 mg PO at bedtime; adjust dose up to 0.6 mg to achieve desired response.

➤ **Nocturnal polyuria in adults who awaken at least two times per night to void (Noctiva, Nocdurna)**

Adults younger than age 65 who aren't at increased risk for hyponatremia: One spray of 1.66 mcg in either the left or right nostril approximately 30 minutes before bedtime.

Adults age 65 and older or younger patients at increased risk for hyponatremia: Initially, one spray of 0.83 mcg in either the left or right nostril approximately 30 minutes before bedtime. After at least 7 days of treatment, can increase dose to 1.66 mcg, if needed, provided the serum sodium level is within the normal range during treatment with the 0.83-mcg dose.

Women: 27.7 mcg SL daily without water, 1 hour before bedtime.

Men: 55.3 mcg SL daily without water, 1 hour before bedtime.

➤ **Prevention of surgical bleeding in patients with uremia** ◆

Adults: 0.3 mcg/kg IV over 30 minutes.

ADMINISTRATION

PO

• Discontinue in patient with acute illness that may result in fluid or electrolyte imbalance.

• Store at controlled room temperature.

IV

▼ Don't give injection to patients with hemophilia A with factor VIII activity of up to 5% or with severe von Willebrand disease.

▼ For adults and children weighing more than 10 kg, dilute with 50 mL sterile physiologic saline solution. For children weighing 10 kg or less, 10 mL of diluent is recommended.

▼ Inspect drug for particulates and discoloration before infusing.

▼ Monitor BP and pulse rate during infusion.

▼ The comparable antidiuretic dose of the injection is about one-tenth of the intranasal dose.

▼ Solution and injection must be refrigerated.

▼ **Incompatibilities:** None listed by manufacturer. Consult a drug incompatibility reference for more information.

Intranasal

• Ensure nasal passages are intact, clean, and free of obstruction before giving intranasally.

• For Noctiva, don't shake bottle. Prime before first use by pumping 5 actuations into the air away from face. Reprime by pumping 2 actuations into the air if the product isn't used for more than 3 days. If a dose is missed, don't double the dose at next use.

• Two sprays of Noctiva 0.83 mcg aren't interchangeable with 1 spray of 1.66 mcg form.

• Store Noctiva upright in refrigerator before opening and upright at room temperature after opening. Discard 60 days after opening.

• Nasal spray pump delivers only doses of 10 mcg DDAVP (per 0.1-mL dose) or 150 mcg Stimate (per 0.1-mL dose). If doses

other than these are required, use the nasal tube delivery system or injection.
• The spray pump must be primed before first use. To prime pump, press down four times. Discard bottle after 25 doses (150 mcg/spray) or 50 doses (10 mcg/spray), depending on the strength, since the amount delivered thereafter per spray may be substantially less than the required dose.
• Nasal spray may be stored at room temperature.

Sublingual
• Patient should empty bladder immediately before bedtime and limit fluid intake to a minimum from 1 hour before until 8 hours after administration.
• Patient should keep tablet under tongue until it has fully dissolved.

Subcutaneous
• Teach patient to rotate injection sites to prevent tissue damage.

ACTION

Synthetic analogue of ADH that increases the permeability of renal tubular epithelium to adenosine monophosphate and water, enabling the epithelium to promote reabsorption of water and produce a concentrated urine. Also increases factor VIII activity by releasing endogenous factor VIII from plasma storage sites.

Route	Onset	Peak	Duration
PO	1 hr	1–1½ hr	6–14 hr
IV	30 min	1½–2 hr	6–14 hr
Intranasal	15–30 min	¼–1½ hr	6–14 hr
Subcut	Unknown	Unknown	Unknown
SL	30 min	Unknown	6 hr

Half-life: PO, 1½ to 2½ hours; IV, 3 hours; intranasal (DDAVP), 7.8 minutes (initial phase) and 75.5 minutes (terminal phase); intranasal (Stimate), 3.3 to 3.5 hours; intranasal (Noctiva), 1.4 to 3.8 hours; SL (Nocdurna), 2.8 hours.

ADVERSE REACTIONS

CNS: headache, *seizures;* dizziness (Noctiva). **CV:** flushing, slight rise in BP; fluid retention, HTN (Noctiva). **EENT:** rhinitis, epistaxis, sore throat, conjunctivitis, edema around eyes; nasal discomfort or congestion, nasopharyngitis, sneezing (Noctiva). **GI:** nausea, abdominal cramps. **GU:** vulvar pain. **Metabolic:** hyponatremia. **Musculoskeletal:** back pain (Noctiva). **Respira-**

tory: cough; bronchitis (Noctiva). **Skin:** local erythema, swelling, or burning after injection.

INTERACTIONS

Drug-drug. *Carbamazepine, chlorpropamide:* May increase ADH; may increase desmopressin effect. Avoid using together.
Chlorpromazine, demeclocycline, epinephrine, heparin, lamotrigine, lithium, NSAIDs, opioid analgesics, SSRIs, TCAs: May increase risk of adverse effects. Monitor patient closely.
Clofibrate: May enhance and prolong effects of desmopressin. Monitor patient closely.
Black Box Warning *Loop diuretics, systemic or inhaled glucocorticoids:* May increase risk of hyponatremia. Use with Noctiva or Nocdurna is contraindicated. Drug can be started or resumed 3 days or 5 half-lives after the glucocorticoid is discontinued, whichever is longer. ■
Pressor agents: May enhance pressor effects with large doses of desmopressin. Monitor patient closely.
Drug-lifestyle. *Alcohol use:* May increase risk of adverse effects. Discourage use together.

EFFECTS ON LAB TEST RESULTS
• May decrease sodium level.

CONTRAINDICATIONS & CAUTIONS

⚕ Contraindicated in patients hypersensitive to drug and in those with type IIB von Willebrand disease, moderate to severe renal impairment, hyponatremia, or a history of hyponatremia.
Black Box Warning Noctiva and Nocdurna are contraindicated in patients at increased risk for severe hyponatremia, such as patients with excessive fluid intake or illnesses that can cause fluid or electrolyte imbalances (e.g., gastroenteritis, salt-wasting nephropathies, systemic infection) and in those using loop diuretics or systemic or inhaled glucocorticoids. ■
• Noctiva and Nocdurna are contraindicated in patients with HF (NYHA Class II to IV), uncontrolled HTN, hyponatremia or a history of hyponatremia, polydipsia, primary nocturnal enuresis, renal impairment with an

eGFR less than 50 mL/minute/1.73 m^2, and known or suspected SIADH secretion due to an increased risk of severe hyponatremia.

Black Box Warning Noctiva and Nocdurna can cause hyponatremia. Severe hyponatremia can be life-threatening, leading to seizures, coma, respiratory arrest, or death. ∎

• Use cautiously in patients with coronary artery insufficiency, hypertensive CV disease, and conditions linked to fluid and electrolyte imbalances, such as cystic fibrosis, because these patients are susceptible to hyponatremia.

• Use cautiously in patients at risk for water intoxication with hyponatremia.

Dialyzable drug: Unknown.

⚠ Overdose S&S: Confusion, drowsiness, continuing headache, problems passing urine, rapid weight gain due to fluid retention.

PREGNANCY-LACTATION-REPRODUCTION

• There are no adequate well-controlled studies in pregnant women. Use during pregnancy only if clearly needed and potential benefit justifies potential risk to the fetus.

• Drug appears in small amounts in human milk, and is poorly absorbed orally by infants. Use cautiously in breastfeeding women.

NURSING CONSIDERATIONS

• Before starting Noctiva or Nocdurna, evaluate patient for possible causes of nocturia, including excessive fluid intake before bedtime, and optimize the treatment of underlying conditions that may be contributing to nocturia. Confirm the diagnosis of nocturnal polyuria with a 24-hour urine collection, if one hasn't been obtained previously.

Black Box Warning Ensure serum sodium concentrations are normal before starting or resuming Noctiva or Nocdurna or increasing the dosage. Measure serum sodium level within 7 days and approximately 1 month after initiating therapy or increasing the dosage, and periodically during treatment. Monitor serum sodium level more frequently in patients age 65 and older and in patients at increased risk for hyponatremia. ∎

Black Box Warning If hyponatremia occurs, Noctiva and Nocdurna may need to be temporarily or permanently discontinued. ∎

• Discontinue Noctiva in patients with concurrent nasal conditions that may increase systemic absorption (atrophy of nasal mucosa, acute or chronic rhinitis), because the increased absorption may increase the risk of hyponatremia. Resume drug when these conditions resolve.

• Noctiva isn't recommended for use in patients who require treatment with other drugs via the intranasal route.

• Morning and evening doses are adjusted separately for adequate diurnal rhythm of water turnover.

• Intranasal use can cause changes in the nasal mucosa, resulting in erratic, unreliable absorption. Report worsening condition to prescriber, who may recommend injectable DDAVP.

• Restrict fluid intake to reduce risk of water intoxication and sodium depletion, especially in children or elderly patients.

❸ Alert: Overdose may cause oxytocic or vasopressor activity. Withhold drug and notify prescriber. If fluid retention is excessive, give furosemide.

• **Look alike–sound alike:** Don't confuse desmopressin with vasopressin.

PATIENT TEACHING

• Advise patient taking Noctiva or Nocdurna to moderate fluid intake in the evening and nighttime hours to decrease the risk of hyponatremia.

• Teach patient to immediately report signs or symptoms associated with hyponatremia (headache, nausea/vomiting, weight gain, restlessness, fatigue, lethargy, disorientation, depressed reflexes, loss of appetite, irritability, muscle weakness, muscle spasms or cramps, abnormal mental status, such as hallucinations, decreased consciousness, and confusion). Severe symptoms may include one or a combination of the following: seizure, coma, or respiratory arrest.

• Some patients may have trouble measuring and inhaling drug into nostrils. Teach patient and caregivers correct administration method.

• Instruct patient to clear nasal passages before giving drug.

• Instruct patient to prime Noctiva before first use by pumping 5 sprays into the air away from the face and to reprime it by

---

pumping 2 sprays into the air if the bottle hasn't been used in more than 3 days.
• Tell patient to store Noctiva upright in refrigerator before opening and upright at room temperature after opening and to discard 60 days after opening.
• Instruct patient not to administer 2 sprays of Noctiva 0.83-mcg dose.
• Instruct patient to press down four times to prime pump and to discard the bottle after 25 doses (150 mcg/spray) or 50 doses (10 mcg/spray), depending on the strength, because the amount left may be less than desired dose.
• Advise patient to report nasal congestion, allergic rhinitis, or URI to prescriber; dosage adjustment may be needed.
• Teach patient using subcut drug to rotate injection sites to prevent tissue damage.
• Warn patient to drink only enough water to satisfy thirst.
🎗 Inform patient with hemophilia A or von Willebrand disease that taking desmopressin may prevent hazards of using blood products.
• Advise patient to carry medical identification indicating use of drug.
• Instruct patient to keep Nocdurna SL tablet under tongue until it has fully dissolved.

---

desoximetasone
dess-OX-ee-MET-ah-sone

Topicort

Therapeutic class: Corticosteroids
Pharmacologic class: Corticosteroids

AVAILABLE FORMS
Cream: 0.05%, 0.25%
Gel: 0.05%*
Ointment: 0.05%, 0.25%
Spray: 0.25%

INDICATIONS & DOSAGES
➤ **Inflammation from corticosteroid-responsive dermatoses (except spray)**
Adults and children: Clean area; apply a thin film and rub in gently b.i.d. Don't use 0.25% ointment on children younger than age 10.

➤ **Plaque psoriasis (spray only)**
Adults: Apply a thin film to affected areas and rub in gently b.i.d. Treatment beyond 4 weeks isn't recommended.

ADMINISTRATION
Topical
• Gently wash skin before applying. To prevent skin damage, rub in gently, leaving thin coat. When treating hairy sites, part hair and apply directly to lesions.
• Avoid applying near eyes, mucous membranes, or in ear canal.
⚠ *Alert:* Don't bandage, cover, or wrap the treated skin area unless ordered.
• Stop drug and notify prescriber if skin infection, striae, or atrophy occur.
• Continue drug for a few days after lesions clear.
• Avoid using spray on face, axilla, or groin or if atrophy is present.
• Discard unused portion after 30 days.

ACTION
Diffuses across cell membranes to form complexes with receptors, showing anti-inflammatory, antipruritic, vasoconstrictive, and antiproliferative activity.

Route	Onset	Peak	Duration
Topical	Unknown	Unknown	Unknown

Half-life: 13 to 17 hours (urine).

ADVERSE REACTIONS
GU: glycosuria. **Metabolic:** hyperglycemia. **Skin:** burning, pruritus, irritation, dryness, erythema, folliculitis, hypertrichosis, acneiform eruptions, perioral dermatitis, hypopigmentation, allergic contact dermatitis, maceration, secondary infection, atrophy, striae, miliaria with occlusive dressings. **Other:** *HPA axis suppression,* Cushing syndrome.

INTERACTIONS
None significant.

EFFECTS ON LAB TEST RESULTS
• May increase glucose level.

CONTRAINDICATIONS & CAUTIONS
• Contraindicated in patients hypersensitive to drug or its components.

- Don't use as monotherapy in primary bacterial infections (impetigo, paronychia, erysipelas, cellulitis, angular cheilitis), treatment of rosacea, perioral dermatitis, or acne.
- Don't use very-high-potency or high-potency agents on the face, groin, or axillae.
- Don't use spray if atrophy is present at treatment site.
- Drug isn't for ophthalmic use.
- Use cautiously in children. Spray isn't recommended for use in children.

Dialyzable drug: Unknown.

⚠ *Overdose S&S:* Systemic effects.

PREGNANCY-LACTATION-REPRODUCTION
- There are no adequate well-controlled studies in pregnant women. Use during pregnancy only if potential benefit justifies potential risk to the fetus.
- Don't use extensively, in large amounts, or for prolonged periods in pregnant patients.
- It isn't known if topical corticosteroids are sufficiently absorbed systemically to produce detectable quantities in human milk. Use cautiously in breastfeeding women. If used during breastfeeding, don't apply on the chest, to avoid accidental ingestion by the infant.

NURSING CONSIDERATIONS
- If fever develops and occlusive dressing is in place, notify prescriber and remove occlusive dressing.
- If antifungal or antibiotic combined with corticosteroid fails to provide prompt improvement, stop corticosteroid until infection is controlled.
- Systemic absorption is likely with use of occlusive dressings, prolonged treatment, or extensive body surface treatment. Watch for symptoms of HPA axis suppression, Cushing syndrome, hyperglycemia, and glycosuria.
- Avoid using plastic pants or tight-fitting diapers on treated areas in young children. Children may absorb larger amounts of drug and be more susceptible to systemic toxicity.
- Gel contains alcohol and may cause burning or irritation in open lesions.
- *Look alike–sound alike:* Don't confuse desoximetasone with dexamethasone.

PATIENT TEACHING
- Teach patient how to apply drug and to report all adverse reactions.
- Tell patient this drug is for external use only and to avoid contact with the eyes.
- If an occlusive dressing is ordered, advise patient to leave it in place for no longer than 12 hours each day and not to use the dressing on infected or weeping lesions.
- Tell patient to stop drug and report signs of systemic absorption, skin irritation or ulceration, hypersensitivity, or infection.

---

desvenlafaxine
des-ven-lah-FAX-in

Khedezla

desvenlafaxine succinate
Pristiq⌀

Therapeutic class: Antidepressants
Pharmacologic class: SSNRIs

AVAILABLE FORMS
desvenlafaxine
Tablets (extended-release) ⦿*:* 50 mg, 100 mg
desvenlafaxine succinate
Tablets (extended-release) ⦿*:* 25 mg, 50 mg, 100 mg

INDICATIONS & DOSAGES
Adjust-a-dose (for all indications): For patients with CrCl of 30 to 50 mL/minute, give 50 mg PO once daily. For patients with CrCl of less than 30 mL/minute or ESRD, give 25 mg PO daily or 50 mg PO every other day. Don't give supplemental doses after dialysis. For patients with moderate to severe hepatic impairment, give 50 mg PO daily; dosage escalation above 100 mg/day isn't recommended.
➤ **Major depressive disorder**
Adults: 50 mg PO once daily.
➤ **Reduction of hot flash frequency or severity in women with natural or medically induced menopause** ◆
Adults: 100 to 150 mg PO once daily; titration during first 1 to 2 weeks of therapy may help manage adverse effects at therapy initiation.

Reactions in bold italics are *life-threatening*. Interactions may have a *rapid onset* or a *delayed onset*.

ADMINISTRATION
PO
• Administer at approximately the same time each day with or without food.
• Patient must swallow tablets whole with fluid and not divide, crush, chew, or dissolve them.
• Use 25-mg/day dose for gradual reduction when discontinuing treatment, to minimize discontinuation symptoms.

ACTION
Thought to stimulate receptors, increasing the release of serotonin and norepinephrine.

Route	Onset	Peak	Duration
PO	Unknown	7½ hr	Unknown

Half-life: About 11 hours.

ADVERSE REACTIONS
CNS: abnormal dreams, anxiety, asthenia, chills, dizziness, fatigue, jittery feeling, headache, insomnia, irritability, paresthesia, somnolence, tremor. **CV:** hot flashes, HTN, palpitations, tachycardia. **EENT:** blurred vision, mydriasis, tinnitus. **GI:** constipation, diarrhea, dry mouth, dysgeusia, *GI bleeding,* nausea, vomiting. **GU:** proteinuria, sexual dysfunction. **Metabolic:** decreased appetite, weight loss. **Skin:** hyperhidrosis, rash. **Other:** yawning.

INTERACTIONS
Drug-drug. *Aspirin, NSAIDs, warfarin, other drugs that affect coagulation:* May increase risk of bleeding. Use together cautiously.
CNS drugs: Drug may cause additive CNS effects. Avoid using together.
CYP3A4 inhibitors (ketoconazole): May increase desvenlafaxine levels. Use together cautiously.
Desipramine, other drugs metabolized by CYP2D6: May increase levels of these drugs. Use together cautiously.
Linezolid, methylene blue: Increases risk of serotonin syndrome. Use together is contraindicated. If urgent treatment with either of these drugs is needed, stop desvenlafaxine immediately; then administer linezolid or methylene blue. Watch for signs and symptoms of serotonin syndrome for 7 days or until 24 hours after last dose of linezolid

or methylene blue. Restart desvenlafaxine 24 hours after last dose of linezolid or methylene blue.
MAO inhibitors: May cause serotonin syndrome or signs and symptoms resembling NMS. Allow at least 14 days between discontinuation of an MAO inhibitor and starting desvenlafaxine, and 7 days after stopping desvenlafaxine before starting an MAO inhibitor.
Midazolam, other drugs metabolized by CYP3A4: May decrease levels of these drugs. Use together cautiously.
SSNRIs, SSRIs: May increase risk of serotonin syndrome. Monitor patient closely if used together.
Venlafaxine: Drug is a major active metabolite of venlafaxine. Avoid using together.
Drug-lifestyle. *Alcohol use:* May enhance CNS depression. Discourage use together.

EFFECTS ON LAB TEST RESULTS
• May increase total cholesterol, LDL, and triglyceride levels. May decrease sodium level.
• May cause false-positive test for phencyclidine and amphetamines.

CONTRAINDICATIONS & CAUTIONS
• Contraindicated in patients hypersensitive to drug or within 14 days of MAO inhibitor therapy.
❸ *Alert:* Concomitant use with linezolid or methylene blue can cause serotonin syndrome (fever, mental status changes, muscle twitching, excessive sweating, shivering or shaking, diarrhea, loss of coordination). Use with linezolid or methylene blue is contraindicated. Stop drug when linezolid or methylene blue is started and restart 24 hours after last dose of linezolid or methylene blue.
• Use cautiously in elderly patients and in patients with renal impairment, diseases or conditions that could affect hemodynamic responses or metabolism, and in those with a history of mania or seizures.
• Potentially life-threatening serotonin syndrome has been reported with desvenlafaxine alone, but particularly with concomitant use of other serotonergic drugs and with drugs that impair serotonin metabolism.

• Angle-closure glaucoma has occurred in patients with untreated anatomically narrow angles who have taken antidepressants.

Black Box Warning Desvenlafaxine isn't approved for use in children. ∎

Dialyzable drug: No.

⚠ *Overdose S&S:* Headache, vomiting, agitation, dizziness, nausea, constipation, diarrhea, dry mouth, paresthesia, tachycardia, change in level of consciousness, mydriasis, seizures, ECG changes.

PREGNANCY-LACTATION-REPRODUCTION

• There are no adequate well-controlled studies in pregnant women. Use during pregnancy only if clearly needed and potential benefit justifies potential risk to the fetus.

• Drug appears in human milk. Patient should discontinue breastfeeding or discontinue drug, taking into account importance of drug to the mother.

NURSING CONSIDERATIONS

Black Box Warning Closely monitor all patients being treated for depression for signs and symptoms of clinical worsening and suicidal ideation, especially at the beginning of therapy and with dosage adjustments. Symptoms may include agitation, insomnia, anxiety, aggressiveness, or panic attacks. ∎

☕ *Alert:* If linezolid or methylene blue must be given, stop drug and monitor patient for serotonin toxicity for 7 days, or until 24 hours after the last dose of methylene blue or linezolid, whichever comes first. Treatment may be resumed 24 hours after last dose of methylene blue or linezolid.

• Carefully monitor BP. Drug may cause dose-related increases in BP.

• Monitor IOP in patients at risk for angle-closure glaucoma.

• Record mood changes. Monitor patient for suicidal tendencies and allow patient only a minimal supply of the drug.

• Monitor patient for signs and symptoms of bleeding.

• Monitor lipid and sodium levels before and during therapy.

• Hyponatremia can occur with desvenlafaxine use. Consider stopping drug in patients with symptomatic hyponatremia; institute appropriate medical intervention.

☕ *Alert:* Don't stop drug abruptly. Withdrawal or discontinuation syndrome may occur if drug is stopped abruptly. Signs and symptoms of withdrawal syndrome include dizziness, nausea, headache, irritability, insomnia, diarrhea, anxiety, fatigue, abnormal dreams, and hyperhidrosis. Taper drug slowly.

• Monitor respiratory status. Drug may cause ILD or eosinophilic pneumonia. If patient develops dyspnea, cough, or chest discomfort, discontinue drug.

• Monitor patient for signs and symptoms of serotonin syndrome, including mental status changes, autonomic instability, neuromuscular symptoms, seizures, and GI symptoms.

PATIENT TEACHING

Black Box Warning Warn family members to closely monitor patient for signs and symptoms of worsening condition or suicidal ideation. ∎

☕ *Alert:* Teach patient to recognize and immediately report symptoms of serotonin toxicity (fever, mental status changes, muscle twitching, excessive sweating, shivering or shaking, diarrhea, loss of coordination).

• Tell patient to avoid alcohol and to consult prescriber before taking other prescription or OTC drugs.

• Teach patient to report all adverse reactions, including abnormal bleeding.

• Warn patient to avoid hazardous activities that require alertness and good coordination until effects of drug are known.

• If medication is to be stopped, tell patient to stop drug gradually by tapering the dosage as instructed by prescriber and not to abruptly stop taking drug.

• Tell patient not to divide, crush, chew, or dissolve tablets.

• Advise female patient of childbearing potential to contact prescriber if she becomes pregnant, intends to become pregnant during therapy, or is breastfeeding.

Reactions in bold italics are *life-threatening*. Interactions may have a *rapid onset* or a *delayed onset*.

dexamethasone (oral)
dex-a-METH-a-sone

Dexamethasone Intensol*

dexamethasone sodium phosphate injection

Therapeutic class: Corticosteroids
Pharmacologic class: Glucocorticoids

AVAILABLE FORMS
dexamethasone
Elixir: 0.5 mg/5 mL*
Oral concentrate: 1 mg/mL*
Oral solution: 0.5 mg/5 mL
Tablets: 0.5 mg, 0.75 mg, 1 mg, 1.5 mg, 2 mg, 4 mg, 6 mg
dexamethasone sodium phosphate
Injection: 4 mg/mL, 10 mg/mL

INDICATIONS & DOSAGES
➤ **Cerebral edema**
Adults: Initially, 10 mg phosphate IV; then 4 mg IM every 6 hours until symptoms subside (usually 2 to 4 days); then taper over 5 to 7 days. Oral therapy (1 to 3 mg t.i.d.) should replace IM dosing as soon as possible.
➤ **Palliative management of recurrent or inoperable brain tumors**
Adults: 2 mg PO, IM, or IV b.i.d. to t.i.d. for maintenance therapy.
➤ **Inflammatory conditions, neoplasias**
Adults: 0.75 to 9 mg/day PO or 0.5 to 9 mg/day phosphate IM or IV, depending on size and location of affected area.
➤ **Acute, self-limited allergic disorders; acute exacerbations of chronic allergic disorders**
Adults: On day one, give 4 or 8 mg IM (using 4 mg/mL preparation). On days two and three, give four 0.75-mg tablets PO in two divided doses. On day four, give two 0.75-mg tablets PO in two divided doses. On days five and six, give one 0.75-mg tablet PO. A follow-up visit should take place on day eight.
➤ **Shock**
Adults: 1 to 6 mg/kg phosphate IV as single dose. Or, 40 mg phosphate IV every 2 to 6 hours, as needed, while shock persists.

➤ **Dexamethasone suppression test for Cushing syndrome**
Adults: Determine baseline 24-hour urine levels of 17-hydroxycorticosteroids; then, give 0.5 mg PO every 6 hours for 48 hours. Repeat 24-hour urine collection to determine 17-hydroxycorticosteroid excretion during second 24 hours of dexamethasone administration. Or, 1 mg PO as single dose at 11:00 p.m. with determination of plasma cortisol at 8 a.m. the next morning.
➤ **Adrenocortical insufficiency**
Children: 0.02 to 0.3 mg/kg/day or 0.6 to 9 mg/m²/day PO in three or four divided doses.
➤ **Acute exacerbation of MS**
Adults: 30 mg PO daily for 1 week, followed by 4 to 12 mg every other day for 1 month.
➤ **Adjunctive therapy for short-term administration in synovitis of osteoarthritis, RA, bursitis, acute gouty arthritis, epicondylitis, acute nonspecific tenosynovitis, posttraumatic osteoarthritis; lesions (keloids; localized, hypertrophic, infiltrated, inflammatory lesions of lichen planus, psoriatic plaques, granuloma annulare, or lichen simplex chronicus; discoid lupus erythematosus; necrobiosis lipoidica diabeticorum; alopecia areata; cystic tumors of an aponeurosis or tendon [ganglia])**
Adults: 0.2 to 6 mg intra-articular or intralesional injection ranging from one single injection to injection every 3 to 5 days to once every 2 to 3 weeks. Dosage and frequency of injection vary depending on condition and site of injection.

ADMINISTRATION
PO
• Give oral dose with food when possible. Patient may need measures to prevent GI irritation.
• Only give concentrated oral solution using calibrated dropper supplied with product. Discard opened bottle after 90 days.
IV
▼ For direct injection, inject undiluted over at least 1 minute (doses 10 mg or less).
▼ For intermittent or continuous infusion, dilute solution according to manufacturer's instructions and give over prescribed duration.

▼ During continuous infusion, change solution every 24 hours.
▼ **Incompatibilities:** Ciprofloxacin, diphenhydramine, doxapram, glycopyrrolate, idarubicin, midazolam, vancomycin.

IM
• Give IM injection deep into gluteal muscle. Rotate injection sites to prevent muscle atrophy. Avoid subcut injection because atrophy and sterile abscesses may occur.

Intra-articular, intralesional
• Frequent intra-articular injection may damage joint tissues.

ACTION

Unclear. Decreases inflammation, mainly by stabilizing leukocyte lysosomal membranes; suppresses immune response; stimulates bone marrow; and influences protein, fat, and carbohydrate metabolism.

Route	Onset	Peak	Duration
PO	1–2 hr	1–2 hr	2½ days
IV	1 hr	1 hr	Variable
IM	1 hr	1 hr	6 days
Intra-articular, intralesional	Unknown	Unknown	Unknown

Half-life: About 1 to 2 days.

ADVERSE REACTIONS

CNS: euphoria, insomnia, psychotic behavior, *pseudotumor cerebri,* vertigo, headache, paresthesia, *seizures,* depression. **CV:** *HF,* HTN, edema, *arrhythmias,* thrombophlebitis, *thromboembolism.* **EENT:** cataracts, glaucoma. **GI:** peptic ulceration, GI irritation, increased appetite, *pancreatitis,* nausea, vomiting. **GU:** menstrual irregularities, increased urine glucose and calcium levels. **Metabolic:** *hypokalemia,* hyperglycemia, carbohydrate intolerance, hypercholesterolemia, *hypocalcemia,* sodium retention, weight gain. **Musculoskeletal:** growth suppression in children, muscle weakness, osteoporosis, tendon rupture, myopathy. **Skin:** hirsutism, delayed wound healing, acne, various skin eruptions, atrophy at IM injection site, thin fragile skin. **Other:** cushingoid state, susceptibility to infections, acute adrenal insufficiency after increased stress or abrupt withdrawal after long-term therapy, *angioedema.* **After abrupt withdrawal:** rebound inflammation, fatigue, weakness, arthralgia, fever, dizziness, lethargy, fainting, orthostatic hypotension, dyspnea, anorexia, *hypoglycemia. After prolonged use, sudden withdrawal may be fatal.*

INTERACTIONS

Drug-drug. *Antidiabetics, including insulin:* May decrease response. May need dosage adjustment.
Aspirin, indomethacin, other NSAIDs: May increase risk of GI distress and bleeding. Use together cautiously.
Barbiturates, carbamazepine, phenytoin, rifampin: May decrease corticosteroid effect. Increase corticosteroid dosage.
Cardiac glycosides: May increase risk of arrhythmia resulting from hypokalemia. May need dosage adjustment.
Cyclosporine: May increase toxicity. Monitor patient closely.
Ketoconazole: May decrease metabolism of dexamethasone and increase risk of corticosteroid-related adverse effects. Consider therapy modification.
Oral anticoagulants: May alter dosage requirements. Monitor PT and INR closely.
Potassium-depleting drugs such as thiazide diuretics: May enhance potassium-wasting effects of dexamethasone. Monitor potassium level.
Salicylates: May decrease salicylate level. Monitor patient for lack of salicylate effectiveness.
Skin-test antigens: May decrease response. Postpone skin testing until therapy is completed.
Toxoids, vaccines: May decrease antibody response and may increase risk of neurologic complications. Avoid using together.
Drug-herb. *Echinacea:* May reduce drug's therapeutic effects. Don't use together.
Drug-lifestyle. *Alcohol use:* May increase risk of gastric irritation and GI ulceration. Discourage use together.

EFFECTS ON LAB TEST RESULTS

• May increase cholesterol and glucose levels. May decrease calcium, potassium, T_3, and T_4 levels.
• May decrease ^{131}I uptake and protein-bound iodine levels in thyroid function tests.

Reactions in bold italics are *life-threatening*. Interactions may have a *rapid onset* or a *delayed onset*.

D

• May cause false-negative results in nitro blue tetrazolium test for systemic bacterial infections. May alter reactions to skin tests.

CONTRAINDICATIONS & CAUTIONS
• Contraindicated in patients hypersensitive to drug or its ingredients, in those with systemic fungal infections, and in those receiving immunosuppressive doses together with live-virus vaccines. IM administration is contraindicated in patients with ITP.
• Use cautiously in patients with recent MI.
• Use cautiously in patients with GI ulcer, renal disease, HTN, osteoporosis, diabetes mellitus, hypothyroidism, cirrhosis, diverticulitis, nonspecific ulcerative colitis, recent intestinal anastomoses, thromboembolic disorders, seizures, myasthenia gravis, HF, TB, active hepatitis, ocular HSV infection, emotional instability, or psychotic tendencies.
• Because some forms contain sulfite preservatives, also use cautiously in patients sensitive to sulfites.
Dialyzable drug: No.

PREGNANCY-LACTATION-REPRODUCTION
• Use in pregnant women only if potential benefit justifies potential risk to the fetus. When systemic corticosteroids are needed during pregnancy, it's generally recommended to use lowest effective dose for shortest duration of time, avoiding high doses during first trimester.
• Drug appears in human milk. Patient should discontinue breastfeeding or discontinue drug, taking into account importance of drug to the mother.

NURSING CONSIDERATIONS
❸ *Alert:* Epidural corticosteroid injections to treat neck and back pain and radiating pain in the arms and legs may result in rare but serious adverse events (vision loss, stroke, paralysis, death). The use of epidural corticosteroid injections isn't approved by the FDA.
• Most adverse reactions to corticosteroids are dose- or duration-dependent.
• For better results and less toxicity, give once-daily dose in morning.
• Always adjust to lowest effective dose.
• Monitor patient's weight, BP, and electrolyte levels.

• Monitor patient for cushingoid effects, including moon face, buffalo hump, central obesity, thinning hair, HTN, and increased susceptibility to infection.
• Watch for depression or psychotic episodes, especially in high-dose therapy.
• Diabetic patient may need increased insulin; monitor glucose levels.
• Drug may mask or worsen infections, including latent amebiasis.
• Elderly patients may be more susceptible to osteoporosis with long-term use.
• Inspect patient's skin for petechiae.
• Gradually reduce dosage after long-term therapy.
• *Look alike–sound alike:* Don't confuse dexamethasone with desoximetasone.

PATIENT TEACHING
• Instruct patient to take drug with food or milk.
❸ *Alert:* Counsel patient receiving epidural corticosteroid injections to seek immediate medical attention for loss of vision or vision changes; tingling in the arms or legs; sudden weakness or numbness of the face, arm, or leg on one or both sides of the body; dizziness; severe headache; or seizures.
• Tell patient not to stop drug abruptly or without prescriber's consent.
• Teach patient signs and symptoms of early adrenal insufficiency: fatigue, muscle weakness, joint pain, fever, anorexia, nausea, shortness of breath, dizziness, and fainting.
• Instruct patient to carry medical identification indicating the need for supplemental systemic glucocorticoids during stress, especially when dosage is decreased. This card should contain prescriber's name, drug name, and drug dosage.
• Warn patient on long-term therapy about cushingoid effects (moon face, buffalo hump) and the need to notify prescriber about sudden weight gain or swelling.
• Warn patient about easy bruising.
• Advise patient receiving long-term therapy to consider exercise or physical therapy. Tell patient to ask prescriber about vitamin D or calcium supplement.
• Instruct patient receiving long-term therapy to have periodic eye examinations.
• Advise patient to avoid exposure to infections (such as measles and chickenpox)

and to notify prescriber if such exposure occurs.
- Tell patient to avoid alcohol.

⚠ **Alert:** Counsel patient to discuss benefits and risks along with other possible treatments with health care provider before undergoing epidural corticosteroid injection.

dexlansoprazole
deks-lan-SOE-pra-zole

Dexilant⬦

Therapeutic class: Antiulcer drugs
Pharmacologic class: PPIs

AVAILABLE FORMS
Capsules ⒹⓃⒸ: 30 mg, 60 mg

INDICATIONS & DOSAGES
➤ **Healing of erosive esophagitis**
Adults and children age 12 and older: Initially, 60-mg capsule PO once daily for up to 8 weeks.
Adjust-a-dose: For patients with moderate hepatic impairment (Child-Pugh class B), maximum dose is 30-mg capsule PO daily for up to 8 weeks.
➤ **Maintenance of healed erosive esophagitis; heartburn relief**
Adults and children age 12 and older: One 30-mg capsule PO once daily for up to 6 months in adults and 16 weeks in patients ages 12 to 17.
➤ **Symptomatic nonerosive GERD**
Adults and children age 12 and older: 30-mg capsule PO once daily for 4 weeks.

ADMINISTRATION
PO
- Give capsule with or without food.
- Patient should swallow capsules whole. Or, capsules can be opened and the intact granules sprinkled on 1 tablespoon of applesauce and swallowed immediately. Or, give capsules with water via oral syringe or NG tube. Refer to manufacturer's instructions for administration via NG tube.
- If a dose is missed, give as soon as possible. Don't give missed dose if next scheduled dose is due; give the next dose on time. Don't give two doses at one time.

ACTION
Inhibits proton pump activity by binding to hydrogen–potassium adenosine triphosphatase, located at the secretory surface of the gastric parietal cells, to suppress gastric acid secretion.

Route	Onset	Peak	Duration
PO	Unknown	4 hr	Unknown

Half-life: 1 to 2 hours.

ADVERSE REACTIONS
CNS: headache. **GI:** abdominal discomfort, abdominal tenderness, diarrhea, flatulence, nausea, vomiting. **Respiratory:** URI.

INTERACTIONS
Drug-drug. *Atazanavir, nelfinavir:* May decrease antiviral effect and promote development of drug resistance. Don't use together.
Azole antifungals (itraconazole, ketoconazole): May decrease antifungal level. Avoid concomitant use if possible.
Clopidogrel: May reduce clopidogrel's plasma concentration and clinical effect. Avoid use together.
Drugs with pH-dependent absorption (ampicillin, digoxin, ketoconazole, iron): May decrease absorption of these drugs. Use together cautiously.
Methotrexate: May increase methotrexate toxicity, especially with high doses. Consider discontinuing dexlansoprazole.
Rifampin: May decrease dexlansoprazole exposure. Avoid concomitant use.
Saquinavir: May increase saquinavir toxicity. Monitor for potential toxicity.
Tacrolimus (systemic): May increase tacrolimus level. Monitor blood trough concentrations and adjust dosage to maintain therapeutic levels.
Warfarin: May increase INR and the risk of bleeding. Monitor patient closely.
Drug-herb. *St. John's wort:* May decrease dexlansoprazole exposure. Avoid concomitant use.
Drug-lifestyle. *Alcohol use:* May decrease dexlansoprazole serum concentration. Avoid combination.

EFFECTS ON LAB TEST RESULTS
- May increase alkaline phosphatase, ALT, and AST levels. May increase creatinine,

gastrin, protein, glucose, and potassium levels.
• May increase or decrease bilirubin level. May decrease magnesium level.
• May decrease platelet count.
• May alter secretin stimulation test result.
• May cause false-positive urine drug screen for tetrahydrocannabinol.

CONTRAINDICATIONS & CAUTIONS
• Contraindicated in patients hypersensitive to drug or its components and with rilpivirine-containing products.
❶ Alert: There may be an increased risk of hip, wrist, and spine fractures associated with PPIs.
• Use cautiously in patients with suspected gastric malignancy. Response to treatment doesn't eliminate the possibility of malignancy.
• Prolonged treatment (2 years or more) can lead to vitamin B₁₂ malabsorption and deficiency, especially in women and those younger than age 30.
• May increase risk of GI infections.
• PPI use is associated with an increased risk of fundic gland polyps that increases with long-term use, especially beyond 1 year. Use shortest duration of therapy appropriate to condition being treated.
• Acute interstitial nephritis has been observed in patients taking PPIs, may occur at any point during therapy, and is generally attributed to an idiopathic hypersensitivity reaction. Discontinue drug if acute interstitial nephritis develops.
• Drug isn't recommended in patients with severe hepatic impairment (Child-Pugh class C).
• Safety and effectiveness in children younger than age 12 haven't been established.
Dialyzable drug: No.

PREGNANCY-LACTATION-REPRODUCTION
• There are no adequate well-controlled studies in pregnant women. Use during pregnancy only if clearly needed.
• It isn't known if drug appears in human milk. Patient should discontinue breastfeeding or discontinue drug, taking into account importance of drug to the mother.

NURSING CONSIDERATIONS
• Monitor patient periodically for improvement in the signs and symptoms of GERD and erosive esophagitis to assess success of therapy.
• Monitor LFT results and glucose and electrolyte levels periodically during therapy.
• Monitor patient for bleeding during therapy.
• May cause false-positive results in diagnostic investigations for neuroendocrine tumors. Temporarily stop drug at least 14 days before assessing serum chromogranin A (CgA) levels and consider repeating test if initial CgA levels are high. If serial tests are performed (for example, for monitoring), use the same commercial laboratory for testing, as reference ranges among tests may vary.
❶ Alert: Prolonged use of PPIs may cause low magnesium levels (rare). Monitor magnesium levels before starting treatment and periodically thereafter.
❶ Alert: Monitor patient for symptoms of low magnesium, such as abnormal HR or rhythm, palpitations, muscle spasms, tremor, or seizures. In children, abnormal HR may present as fatigue, upset stomach, dizziness, and light-headedness. Magnesium supplementation or drug discontinuation may be required.
❶ Alert: Drug may cause CDAD. Evaluate for CDAD in patients who develop diarrhea that doesn't improve.

PATIENT TEACHING
• Tell patient to report hypersensitivity reactions immediately.
• Tell patient to swallow capsule whole and not to crush, split, or chew it. Capsule may be opened and its contents sprinkled on applesauce if desired.
• Advise patient that drug can be taken without regard to meals.
• Advise female patient to notify prescriber if she is pregnant, plans to become pregnant, or is breastfeeding.
• Tell patient to report all adverse reactions, including diarrhea.
• Teach patient to recognize and report signs and symptoms of low magnesium level.
• Advise patient to avoid alcohol use.

dexmethylphenidate hydrochloride
dex-meth-il-FEN-i-date

Focalin, Focalin XR✔

Therapeutic class: CNS stimulants
Pharmacologic class: Methylphenidate derivatives
Controlled substance schedule: II

AVAILABLE FORMS
Capsules (extended-release) ⓄⒷⒸ: 5 mg, 10 mg, 15 mg, 20 mg, 25 mg, 30 mg, 35 mg, 40 mg
Tablets: 2.5 mg, 5 mg, 10 mg

INDICATIONS & DOSAGES
➤ ADHD
Immediate-release tablets
Adults and children age 6 and older:
For patients who aren't currently taking methylphenidate, initially, 2.5 mg PO b.i.d., given at least 4 hours apart. Increase weekly by 2.5 to 5 mg daily, up to a maximum of 20 mg daily in divided doses.

For patients who are currently taking methylphenidate, initially give half the current methylphenidate dosage, up to a maximum of 20 mg PO daily in divided doses at least 4 hours apart.

Extended-release capsules
Adults: For patients who aren't currently taking dexmethylphenidate or methylphenidate, or who are on stimulants other than methylphenidate, give 10 mg PO once daily in the morning. May adjust in weekly increments of 10 mg to a maximum dose of 40 mg daily.

For patients who are currently taking methylphenidate, initially give half the total daily dose of methylphenidate. Patients who are currently taking the immediate-release form of dexmethylphenidate may be switched to the same daily dose of extended-release form. Maximum daily dose is 40 mg.
Children age 6 and older: For patients who aren't currently taking dexmethylphenidate or methylphenidate, or who are on stimulants other than methylphenidate, give 5 mg PO daily in the morning. May adjust

in weekly increments of 5 mg to a maximum daily dose of 30 mg.

For patients who aren't currently taking methylphenidate, initially give half the total daily dose of methylphenidate. Patients who are currently taking the immediate-release form of dexmethylphenidate may be switched to the same daily dose of extended-release form. Maximum daily dose is 30 mg.

ADMINISTRATION
PO
• Capsules may be swallowed whole with or without food or the contents sprinkled on a small amount of applesauce and eaten immediately.
• Don't crush or divide the capsule or its contents.

ACTION
Blocks presynaptic reuptake of norepinephrine and dopamine and increases their release, increasing concentration in the synapse.

Route	Onset	Peak	Duration
PO (immediate-release)	Unknown	1–1½ hr	Unknown
PO (extended-release)	Unknown	1–4 hr; 4½–7 hr	Unknown

Half-life: 2 to 7 hours (adults); 2 to 3 hours (children).

ADVERSE REACTIONS
CNS: headache, anxiety, feeling jittery, nervousness, insomnia, fever, dizziness. **CV:** tachycardia. **GI:** anorexia, abdominal pain, nausea, dyspepsia, dry mouth, decreased appetite, vomiting. **Musculoskeletal:** twitching (motor or vocal tics). **Other:** hypersensitivity reactions.

INTERACTIONS
Drug-drug. *Antacids, acid suppressants:* May alter the release of extended-release form. Avoid using together.
Anticoagulants, phenobarbital, phenytoin, primidone, TCAs: May inhibit metabolism of these drugs. May need to decrease dosage of these drugs; monitor drug levels.
Antihypertensives: May decrease effectiveness of these drugs. Use together cautiously; monitor BP.

Clonidine, other centrally acting alpha agonists: May cause serious adverse effects. Use together cautiously.

MAO inhibitors: May increase risk of hypertensive crisis. Using together within 14 days of MAO inhibitor therapy is contraindicated.

EFFECTS ON LAB TEST RESULTS
None reported.

CONTRAINDICATIONS & CAUTIONS
• Contraindicated in patients hypersensitive to methylphenidate or other components or within 14 days of MAO inhibitor therapy.

◑ Alert: Avoid use in patients with known serious structural cardiac abnormalities, cardiomyopathy, serious heart rhythm abnormalities, CAD, and other serious heart problems.

Black Box Warning Use cautiously in patients with a history of substance abuse, including alcoholism. Chronic abuse can lead to marked tolerance and psychological dependence. Psychotic episodes can occur. Withdraw patient carefully from abusive use because severe depression can occur. Withdrawal after long-term use may unmask signs and symptoms of an underlying disorder that may require follow-up. ▪

• Use cautiously in patients with a psychiatric illness, bipolar disorder, depression, or family history of suicide, and in patients with seizures, HTN, hyperthyroidism, HF, stroke, or recent MI.

• Rare cases of priapism have been reported.

Dialyzable drug: Unknown.

⚠ Overdose S&S: Agitation, cardiac arrhythmias, confusion, seizures, delirium, dryness of mucous membranes, euphoria, flushing, hallucinations, headache, hyperpyrexia, hyperreflexia, HTN, muscle twitching, mydriasis, palpitations, sweating, tachycardia, tremors, vomiting.

PREGNANCY-LACTATION-REPRODUCTION
• There are no adequate well-controlled studies in pregnant women. Use during pregnancy only if clearly needed and potential benefit justifies potential risk to the fetus.

• It isn't known if drug appears in human milk. Use cautiously in breastfeeding women.

NURSING CONSIDERATIONS
• Diagnosis of ADHD must be based on complete history and evaluation of patient by psychological and educational experts.

• Obtain a detailed patient history, including a family history for mental disorders, family suicide, ventricular arrhythmias, or sudden death.

• Refer patient for psychological, educational, and social support.

• Periodically reevaluate the long-term usefulness of the drug.

• Monitor CBC and differential and platelet counts during prolonged therapy.

• Don't use for severe depression or normal fatigue states.

• Stop treatment or reduce dosage if symptoms worsen or adverse reactions occur.

• Long-term stimulant use may temporarily suppress growth. Monitor children for growth and weight gain. If growth slows or weight gain is lower than expected, stop drug.

◑ Alert: Periodically monitor patient for changes in HR or BP. Promptly evaluate patients with chest pain, unexplained syncope, or other signs or symptoms of cardiac disease.

• Monitor patient for signs of drug dependence or abuse.

• If seizures occur, stop drug.

• *Look alike–sound alike:* Don't confuse dexmethylphenidate with methadone, methylphenidate, or dextroamphetamine.

PATIENT TEACHING
• Stress the importance of taking the correct dose of drug at the same time every day. Report accidental overdose immediately.

◑ Alert: Warn patient that the misuse of amphetamines can have serious effects, including sudden death.

• Advise patient unable to swallow capsules to empty the contents of the capsule onto a spoonful of applesauce and eat immediately.

◑ Alert: Tell patient not to cut, crush, or chew contents of the extended-release beaded capsule.

• Advise parents to monitor child for medication abuse or sharing. Also inform parents to watch for increased aggression or hostility and to report worsening behavior.

◑ *Alert:* Instruct patient to immediately report chest pain, shortness of breath, or fainting.
• Advise patient to seek immediate medical attention for prolonged or painful erections.
• Advise parents to monitor child's height and weight and to tell prescriber if they suspect growth is slowing.
• Instruct patient or caregivers to report new numbness, pain, skin color change, or sensitivity to temperature in fingers or toes, because of the risk of peripheral vasculopathy, including Raynaud phenomenon.
• Caution patient that blurred vision or difficulty with accommodation may occur and to exercise caution while performing activities that require a clear visual field. Advise patient to report blurred vision to prescriber.

dextroamphetamine sulfate
dex-troe-am-FET-a-meen

Dexedrine, ProCentra, Zenzedi

Therapeutic class: CNS stimulants
Pharmacologic class: Amphetamines
Controlled substance schedule: II

AVAILABLE FORMS
Capsules (extended-release) ⒪ⓃⒸ: 5 mg, 10 mg, 15 mg
Oral solution: 5 mg/5 mL
Tablets: 2.5 mg, 5 mg, 7.5 mg, 10 mg, 15 mg, 20 mg, 30 mg

INDICATIONS & DOSAGES
➤ **Narcolepsy**
Adults: 5 to 60 mg PO daily in divided doses.
Children age 12 and older: 10 mg PO daily. Increase by 10 mg at weekly intervals, as needed. Give first dose on awakening; give additional doses (one or two) at intervals of 4 to 6 hours.
Children ages 6 to 12: 5 mg PO daily. Increase by 5 mg at weekly intervals as needed.
➤ **ADHD**
Children age 6 and older: 5 mg PO once daily or b.i.d. Increase by 5 mg at weekly intervals, as needed. It's rarely necessary to exceed 40 mg/day.

Children ages 3 to 5: Initially, 2.5 mg immediate-release tablets or solution PO daily. May increase daily dosage in increments of 2.5 mg at weekly intervals until optimal response is obtained.

ADMINISTRATION
PO
• Avoid late-evening doses, particularly with extended-release capsules, due to resulting insomnia. Give initial dose upon awakening.
• Some formulations may contain tartrazine (immediate-release tablets) or benzoic acid, which is a derivative of benzyl alcohol (oral solution). Derivatives of benzyl alcohol are associated with potentially fatal "gasping syndrome" in neonates.
• Make sure patient doesn't chew or crush extended-release capsules.

ACTION
Promotes release of dopamine and norepinephrine from nerve terminals in the brain and, to a lesser extent, the reuptake of catecholamines.

Route	Onset	Peak	Duration
PO	Unknown	3 hr	4–6 hr
PO (extended-release)	Unknown	8 hr	8 hr

Half-life: 10 to 12 hours.

ADVERSE REACTIONS
CNS: insomnia, nervousness, restlessness, tremor, dizziness, headache, chills, overstimulation, dysphoria, euphoria, dyskinesia, aggressive behavior. **CV:** tachycardia, palpitations, *arrhythmias,* HTN. **EENT:** blurred vision. **GI:** dry mouth, taste perversion, diarrhea, constipation, anorexia, other GI disturbances. **GU:** erectile dysfunction. **Metabolic:** weight loss. **Musculoskeletal:** *rhabdomyolysis.* **Skin:** urticaria. **Other:** increased libido.

INTERACTIONS
Drug-drug. *Acetazolamide, alkalizing drugs, antacids, sodium bicarbonate:* May increase renal reabsorption. Monitor patient for enhanced amphetamine effects.
Acidifying drugs, ammonium chloride, ascorbic acid: May decrease level and

---

Reactions in bold italics are *life-threatening*. Interactions may have a *rapid onset* or a *delayed onset*.

increase renal clearance of dextroamphetamine. Monitor patient for decreased amphetamine effects.

Adrenergic blockers: May inhibit adrenergic blocking effects. Avoid using together.

Antihypertensives: May diminish antihypertensive effects. Monitor BP.

Lithium: May inhibit central stimulant effects of amphetamines. Monitor therapy.

MAO inhibitors: May cause severe HTN or hypertensive crisis. Avoid using within 14 days of MAO inhibitor therapy.

Meperidine: May potentiate analgesic effect. Use together cautiously.

Methenamine: May increase urinary excretion of amphetamines and reduce effectiveness. Monitor drug effects.

Norepinephrine: May enhance adrenergic effect of norepinephrine. Monitor patient.

Phenobarbital, phenytoin: May delay absorption of these drugs. Monitor patient closely.

Drug-food. *Acidic foods, fruit juice:* Decreases amphetamine absorption. May decrease effectiveness of oral solution. Avoid giving together.

EFFECTS ON LAB TEST RESULTS

• May increase corticosteroid levels.
• May interfere with urinary steroid determinations.

CONTRAINDICATIONS & CAUTIONS

• Contraindicated in patients hypersensitive to or with idiosyncratic reactions to sympathomimetic amines and in those with hyperthyroidism, moderate to severe HTN, symptomatic CV disease, glaucoma, advanced arteriosclerosis, and history of drug abuse. Also contraindicated during or within 14 days after MAO inhibitor therapy.

۞ Alert: Use cautiously in agitated patients and patients with motor tics, phonic tics, or Tourette syndrome. Also use cautiously in patients whose underlying condition may be worsened by an increase in BP or HR (preexisting HTN, HF, recent MI); patients with a psychiatric illness, bipolar disorder, depression, or family history of suicide; and those with a seizure disorder.

• Don't use in children or adolescents with structural cardiac abnormalities or other serious heart problems.

Dialyzable drug: Unknown.

⚠ Overdose S&S: Assaultiveness, confusion, hallucinations, hyperreflexia, rapid respiration, restlessness, rhabdomyolysis, tremor, hyperpyrexia, panic states, fatigue, depression, arrhythmias, HTN, hypotension, circulatory collapse, nausea, vomiting, diarrhea, abdominal cramps, seizures, coma.

PREGNANCY-LACTATION-REPRODUCTION

• There are no adequate well-controlled studies in pregnant women. Use during pregnancy only if potential benefit justifies potential risk to the fetus.
• Infants born to mothers dependent on amphetamines have an increased risk of premature delivery and low birth weight, and may experience signs and symptoms of withdrawal as demonstrated by dysphoria, including agitation, and significant lassitude.
• Drug appears in human milk. Use in breastfeeding women isn't recommended.

NURSING CONSIDERATIONS

• Obtain a detailed patient history, including a family history for mental disorders, family suicide, ventricular arrhythmias, or sudden death.
• Monitor patients beginning treatment for ADHD for aggressive behavior or hostility.
• Drug shouldn't be used to prevent fatigue.
Black Box Warning Drug has a high abuse potential and may cause dependence. Monitor patient closely. Pay particular attention to the possibility of patients obtaining amphetamines for nontherapeutic use or distribution to others. ∎
۞ Alert: Periodically monitor patient for changes in HR or BP.
• Monitor for growth retardation in children.
• Don't crush extended-release capsules.
• **Look alike–sound alike:** Don't confuse Dexedrine with dextran or Excedrin.

PATIENT TEACHING

Black Box Warning Warn patient that the misuse of amphetamines can cause serious CV adverse events, including sudden death. ∎
• Tell patient not to chew or crush extended-release capsules.
۞ Alert: Instruct patient to immediately report chest pain, shortness of breath, or fainting.

- Warn patient to avoid activities that require alertness, a clear visual field, or good coordination until CNS effects of drug are known.
- Tell patient fatigue may occur as drug effects wear off.
- Ask patient to report signs and symptoms of excessive stimulation.
- Inform parents that children may show increased aggression or hostility and to report worsening of behavior.
- Tell patient not to drink fruit juice at same time as oral solution.
- Warn patient with a seizure disorder that drug may decrease seizure threshold and to notify prescriber if seizures occur.

dextroamphetamine sulfate–dextroamphetamine saccharate–amphetamine aspartate–amphetamine sulfate
dex-tro-am-PHET-ta-meen/
am-PHET-ta-meen

Adderall XR, Mydayis

Therapeutic class: CNS stimulants
Pharmacologic class: Amphetamines
Controlled substance schedule: II

AVAILABLE FORMS
Capsules (extended-release) ⓄⒼ: 5 mg: 1.25 mg dextroamphetamine sulfate, 1.25 mg dextroamphetamine saccharate, 1.25 mg amphetamine aspartate, and 1.25 mg amphetamine sulfate; 10 mg: 2.5 mg dextroamphetamine sulfate, 2.5 mg dextroamphetamine saccharate, 2.5 mg amphetamine aspartate, and 2.5 mg amphetamine sulfate; 12.5 mg (Mydayis): 3.125 mg dextroamphetamine sulfate, 3.125 mg dextroamphetamine saccharate, 3.125 mg amphetamine aspartate, and 3.125 mg amphetamine sulfate; 15 mg: 3.75 mg dextroamphetamine sulfate, 3.75 mg dextroamphetamine saccharate, 3.75 mg amphetamine aspartate, and 3.75 mg amphetamine sulfate; 20 mg: 5 mg dextroamphetamine sulfate, 5 mg dextroamphetamine saccharate, 5 mg amphetamine aspartate, and 5 mg amphetamine sulfate;

25 mg: 6.25 mg dextroamphetamine sulfate, 6.25 mg dextroamphetamine saccharate, 6.25 mg amphetamine aspartate, and 6.25 mg amphetamine sulfate; 25 mg (Mydayis): 6.25 mg dextroamphetamine sulfate, 6.25 mg dextroamphetamine saccharate, 6.25 mg amphetamine aspartate, and 6.25 mg amphetamine sulfate; 30 mg: 7.5 mg dextroamphetamine sulfate, 7.5 mg dextroamphetamine saccharate, 7.5 mg amphetamine aspartate, and 7.5 mg amphetamine sulfate; 37.5 mg (Mydayis): 9.375 mg dextroamphetamine sulfate, 9.375 mg dextroamphetamine saccharate, 9.375 mg amphetamine aspartate, and 9.375 mg amphetamine sulfate; 50 mg (Mydayis): 12.5 mg dextroamphetamine sulfate, 12.5 mg dextroamphetamine saccharate, 12.5 mg amphetamine aspartate, and 12.5 mg amphetamine sulfate
Tablets: 5 mg: 1.25 mg dextroamphetamine sulfate, 1.25 mg dextroamphetamine saccharate, 1.25 mg amphetamine aspartate, and 1.25 mg amphetamine sulfate; 7.5 mg: 1.875 mg dextroamphetamine sulfate, 1.875 mg dextroamphetamine saccharate, 1.875 mg amphetamine aspartate, and 1.875 mg amphetamine sulfate; 10 mg: 2.5 mg dextroamphetamine sulfate, 2.5 mg dextroamphetamine saccharate, and 2.5 mg amphetamine aspartate, and 2.5 mg amphetamine sulfate; 12.5 mg: 3.125 mg dextroamphetamine sulfate, 3.125 mg dextroamphetamine saccharate, 3.125 mg amphetamine aspartate, and 3.125 mg amphetamine sulfate; 15 mg: 3.75 mg dextroamphetamine sulfate, 3.75 mg dextroamphetamine saccharate, 3.75 mg amphetamine aspartate, and 3.75 mg amphetamine sulfate; 20 mg: 5 mg dextroamphetamine sulfate, 5 mg dextroamphetamine saccharate, 5 mg amphetamine aspartate, and 5 mg amphetamine sulfate; 30 mg: 7.5 mg dextroamphetamine sulfate, 7.5 mg dextroamphetamine saccharate, 7.5 mg amphetamine aspartate, and 7.5 mg amphetamine sulfate

INDICATIONS & DOSAGES
➤ **Narcolepsy**
Adults and children age 12 and older: Initially, 10 mg (immediate-release) tablet PO daily. May increase daily dose by 10 mg at

weekly intervals to maximum of 60 mg/day. Give in one to three divided doses per day.
Children ages 6 to younger than 12: Initially, 5 mg (immediate-release) tablet PO daily. May increase daily dose by 5 mg at weekly intervals until optimal response is achieved. Give in one to three divided doses per day.
Adjust-a-dose: For adverse reactions (insomnia or anorexia), reduce dosage.

➤ **ADHD**
Adults: Initially, 5 mg (immediate-release) tablet PO once daily or b.i.d. May increase daily dose by 5 mg at weekly intervals until optimal response achieved; maximum dose, 40 mg/day. Or, 20-mg extended-release capsule PO once daily in morning. Maximum dose, 30 mg/day. Or, in adults ages 18 to 55, 12.5 to 25 mg Mydayis PO once daily in the morning. May increase daily dose by 12.5 mg at weekly intervals until optimal response achieved; maximum dose, 50 mg/day.
Adolescents ages 13 to 17 (extended-release): Initially, 10 mg PO daily in morning. May increase to 20 mg/day after 1 week if symptoms aren't controlled. Or, 12.5 mg Mydayis PO daily in the morning. May increase to maximum of 25 mg/day after 1 week if symptoms aren't controlled.
Children age 6 and older (immediate-release): Initially, 5 mg PO once daily or b.i.d. May increase daily dose by 5 mg at weekly intervals until optimal response is achieved. Give in one to three divided doses per day. Rarely necessary to exceed a total of 40 mg/day.
Children ages 6 to 12 (extended-release): Initially, 5 to 10 mg PO once daily in morning. May increase daily dose by 5 or 10 mg at weekly intervals. Maximum dose, 30 mg/day.
Children ages 3 to 5 (immediate-release): Initially, 2.5 mg PO daily. May increase daily dose by 2.5 mg at weekly intervals until optimal response is achieved. Give in one to three divided doses per day.
Adjust-a-dose: In adults with severe renal impairment, dosages may need to be reduced. Refer to manufacturer's instructions.

ADMINISTRATION
PO
● May give with or without food. Give Mydayis consistently either with or without food.
● Give first dose upon awakening to avoid insomnia.
● Make sure patient takes extended-release capsules whole, or open the capsules and sprinkle entire contents on applesauce and have patient consume immediately without chewing.

ACTION
Promotes release of dopamine and norepinephrine from nerve terminals in the brain and, to a lesser extent, the reuptake of catecholamines.

Route	Onset	Peak	Duration
PO (immediate-release)	Unknown	3 hr	4–6 hr
PO (extended-release)	Unknown	7–8 hr	Unknown

Half-life: Immediate-release, 9 to 14 hours; extended-release, 10 to 14 hours.

ADVERSE REACTIONS
CNS: headache, insomnia, agitation, anxiety, dizziness, drowsiness, emotional lability, fatigue, speech disturbance, twitching, fever.
CV: systolic HTN, palpitations, tachycardia. **EENT:** dry mouth, teeth clenching, tooth infection. **GI:** abdominal pain, decreased appetite, anorexia, constipation, diarrhea, dyspepsia, nausea, vomiting. **GU:** decreased libido, erectile dysfunction, UTI.
Metabolic: weight loss. **Respiratory:** dyspnea. **Skin:** diaphoresis, skin photosensitivity.
Other: infection.

INTERACTIONS
Drug-drug. *Acetazolamide, thiazides:* May increase amphetamine concentration through decreased urine excretion. Monitor patient response.
Adrenergic blockers, antihistamines, antihypertensives, ethosuximide, phenobarbital, phenytoin: Amphetamines may reduce therapeutic effects of these drugs. Monitor patient response.
Ammonium chloride, ascorbic acid, glutamic acid, guanethidine, methenamine, reserpine, sodium acid phosphate: May lower

amphetamine blood level and absorption. Don't use together.

Antacids, MAO inhibitors, sodium bicarbonate: May increase amphetamine concentrations and risk of adverse reactions. Avoid concurrent use, and don't give drug within 14 days of MAO inhibitors.

Lithium carbonate: May reduce therapeutic effects of amphetamines. Monitor patient response.

PPIs: May increase amphetamine absorption rate. Monitor therapy.

Serotonergic agents: Amphetamines may increase effects of these drugs and risk of adverse reactions related to these drugs. Monitor patient response.

Drug-herb. *Ephedra:* May cause HTN or arrhythmias. Don't use together.

St. John's wort: May increase risk of serotonin syndrome. Use together cautiously.

Drug-lifestyle. *Alcohol use:* May increase risk of drug dependency. Concurrent use is contraindicated in patients with a history of ethanol or drug dependency.

EFFECTS ON LAB TEST RESULTS
• May increase plasma corticosteroid level.
• May interfere with urinary steroid testing.

CONTRAINDICATIONS & CAUTIONS
Black Box Warning Amphetamines have a high potential for abuse. Administration of amphetamines for prolonged periods of time may lead to drug dependence and must be avoided. Particular attention should be paid to the possibility of persons obtaining amphetamines for nontherapeutic use or distribution to others, and the drugs should be prescribed or dispensed sparingly. ∎
Black Box Warning Misuse of amphetamines may cause sudden death and serious CV adverse events. ∎
• Contraindicated in patients with advanced arteriosclerosis, symptomatic CV disease, moderate to severe HTN, hyperthyroidism, known hypersensitivity or idiosyncrasy to sympathomimetic amines, glaucoma, agitated states, or history of drug abuse. Also contraindicated during or within 14 days after administration of MAO inhibitors.
◑ *Alert:* Sudden death has been reported at usual doses in patients with structural cardiac abnormalities and other serious heart

problems. Stimulants generally should not be used in adults, children, or adolescents with structural cardiac abnormalities, cardiomyopathy, serious heart rhythm abnormalities, or other serious cardiac problems.
• Drug can increase BP. Use cautiously in patients with underlying medical conditions (preexisting HTN, HF, recent MI, ventricular arrhythmia) that might be compromised by increases in BP or HR.
• Use cautiously in patients with a history of seizures, tics or Tourette syndrome, or mental problems, including psychosis, bipolar illness, mania, or depression.
• Drug may cause peripheral vasculopathy, including Raynaud phenomenon, which may improve after dosage reduction or drug discontinuation.
• Drug hasn't been studied in elderly patients.
• Immediate-release tablets aren't recommended for children with ADHD younger than age 3 or for children with narcolepsy younger than age 6. Use of extended-release capsules in children younger than age 6 hasn't been studied.
• Safety and effectiveness of Mydayis in children age 12 and younger haven't been established.
Dialyzable drug: Unknown.
⚠ *Overdose S&S:* Restlessness, tremor, hyperreflexia, rapid respiration, confusion, assaultiveness, hallucinations, panic states, hyperpyrexia, rhabdomyolysis; fatigue, depression (usually follow central stimulation); arrhythmias, HTN or hypotension, circulatory collapse; nausea, vomiting, diarrhea, abdominal cramps; seizures, coma (usually precede fatal poisoning).

PREGNANCY-LACTATION-REPRODUCTION
• There are no adequate well-controlled studies in pregnant women. Infants born to mothers dependent on amphetamines have an increased risk of premature delivery and low birth weight. These infants may also experience signs and symptoms of withdrawal, such as dysphoria, including agitation, and significant lassitude. Use during pregnancy only if potential benefit justifies potential risk to the fetus.
• Drug appears in human milk. Breastfeeding women shouldn't use drug.

NURSING CONSIDERATIONS
• Administer drug upon awakening to prevent insomnia.
• Interrupt therapy occasionally to assess if behavioral symptoms warrant continued therapy.
• Perform a careful history and physical examination in all patients to assess for the presence of cardiac disease. Further cardiac evaluation may be needed. All patients who develop cardiac signs and symptoms (chest pain, syncope) during therapy should have a prompt cardiac evaluation.
• Evaluate patient for dependence on other prescription drugs, illicit drugs, or alcohol before start of therapy.
• Monitor BP during therapy.
• Screen patient for a family history of suicide, bipolar disorder, and depression before use. Monitor patient for increased aggression, worsening of existing psychiatric signs and symptoms, or psychosis.
• When used long term, drug may slow growth rate in children. Monitor growth rate; interrupt treatment for children not growing or gaining weight as expected.
• Monitor patient for risk of vasculopathies, including Raynaud phenomenon, and evaluate unexplained wounds on fingers and toes.
• Single doses of 20 mg extended-release capsules and 10 mg immediate-release tablets given b.i.d. (4 hours apart) have been shown to produce comparable plasma amphetamine concentrations.
• When switching from other dextroamphetamine/amphetamine preparations to Mydayis, discontinue previous formation and titrate per package labeling. Don't substitute on a milligram-per-milligram basis.
• *Look alike–sound alike:* Don't confuse Adderall XR with Inderal.

PATIENT TEACHING
• Tell patient to report all drugs and supplements being taken before start of therapy, especially if patient has taken an MAO inhibitor within the past 2 weeks.
• Explain that serious cardiac effects are possible during therapy. Advise patient to immediately report chest pain, shortness of breath, or fainting.

• Advise patient to report development of such conditions as glaucoma, high BP, or hyperthyroidism.
• Advise patient to keep regular follow-up appointments for monitoring of HR and BP, and for growth checks in children.
• Advise patient to report worsening of psychiatric signs and symptoms or behavioral changes during therapy.
• Explain that drug may cause circulatory problems. Advise patient to immediately report unexplained wounds on fingers or toes.
• Instruct patient to take drug in early part of day (preferably upon awakening) to avoid insomnia.
• Tell patient who misses a dose of Mydayis not to take the dose later in the day because the effects may last up to 16 hours.
• Advise patient to swallow capsules and tablets whole, but that extended-release capsules can be opened, the contents sprinkled on applesauce, and then the applesauce swallowed immediately without chewing.

SAFETY ALERT!

diazePAM
dye-AZ-e-pam

Diastat*, Diastat AcuDial*, Diazepam Intensol*, Valium✔

Therapeutic class: Anxiolytics
Pharmacologic class: Benzodiazepines
Controlled substance schedule: IV

AVAILABLE FORMS
Injection: 5 mg/mL
Oral solution: 5 mg/5 mL, 5 mg/mL*
Rectal gel twin packs: 2.5 mg (pediatric); 10 mg, 20 mg (adult)
Tablets: 2 mg, 5 mg, 10 mg

INDICATIONS & DOSAGES
Adjust-a-dose (for all indications): For elderly or debilitated patients, give 2 to 2.5 mg PO daily or b.i.d. initially; increase gradually as needed and tolerated. Or, when using injection, use lower doses (2 to 5 mg) and increase dosage more gradually.

➤ **Anxiety**
Adults: Depending on severity, 2 to 10 mg PO b.i.d. to q.i.d. Or, 2 to 10 mg IM or IV. May repeat in 3 to 4 hours if needed.
Children age 6 months and older: 1 to 2.5 mg PO t.i.d. or q.i.d., increased gradually, as needed and tolerated.

➤ **Acute alcohol withdrawal**
Adults: 10 mg PO t.i.d. or q.i.d. during first 24 hours; reduce to 5 mg PO t.i.d. or q.i.d., p.r.n. Or, 10 mg IV or IM initially; then 5 to 10 mg IV or IM again in 3 to 4 hours if needed.

➤ **Before endoscopic procedures**
Adults: Adjust IV dose to desired sedative response (up to 20 mg). If IV can't be used, give 5 to 10 mg IM 30 minutes before procedure.

➤ **Muscle spasm**
Adults: 2 to 10 mg PO b.i.d. to q.i.d. as an adjunct. Or, 5 to 10 mg IV or IM initially; then 5 to 10 mg IV or IM again in 3 to 4 hours if needed.

➤ **Preoperative sedation**
Adults: 10 mg IM or IV before surgery.

➤ **Adjunctive treatment for seizure disorders**
Adults: 2 to 10 mg PO b.i.d. to q.i.d.
Children age 6 months and older:
1 to 2.5 mg PO t.i.d. or q.i.d. initially; increase as needed and as tolerated.

➤ **Status epilepticus, severe recurrent seizures**
Adults: 10 mg IV or IM initially. Use IM route only if IV access is unavailable. Repeat every 10 to 15 minutes, p.r.n., up to maximum dose of 30 mg. Repeat every 2 to 4 hours, if needed.
Children age 5 and older: 1 mg IV slowly every 2 to 5 minutes to a maximum of 10 mg (IV preferred). Repeat in 2 to 4 hours if necessary.
Children ages 30 days to younger than 5 years: 0.2 to 0.5 mg IV slowly every 2 to 5 minutes up to a maximum of 5 mg (IV preferred).

➤ **Patients on stable regimens of antiepileptic drugs who need diazepam intermittently to control bouts of increased seizure activity**
Adults and children age 12 and older: 0.2 mg/kg PR, rounding up to the nearest

available dose form. A second dose may be given 4 to 12 hours later.
Children ages 6 to 11: 0.3 mg/kg PR, rounding up to the nearest available dose form. A second dose may be given 4 to 12 hours later.
Children ages 2 to 5: 0.5 mg/kg PR, rounding up to the nearest available dose form. A second dose may be given 4 to 12 hours later.

➤ **Tetanus**
Adults: Initially, 10 mg IV or IM then 10 mg in 3 to 4 hours if needed. Larger doses may be required.
Children age 5 and older: 5 to 10 mg IM or IV repeated every 3 to 4 hours, p.r.n.
Children ages 30 days to younger than 5 years: 1 to 2 mg IM or IV slowly repeated every 3 to 4 hours, p.r.n.

ADMINISTRATION
PO
- When using oral solution, dilute dose just before giving with liquid or semisolid food, such as water, juices, soda or sodalike beverages, applesauce, or pudding.
- Discard opened bottle of concentrated solution after 90 days.

IV
▼ Keep emergency resuscitation equipment and oxygen at bedside.
▼ For adults, give at no more than 5 mg/minute.
▼ For children, administer slowly over 3 minutes. Don't exceed 0.25 mg/kg.
▼ Avoid infusion sets or containers made from polyvinyl chloride.
▼ If possible, inject directly into a large vein. If not, inject slowly through infusion tubing as near to the insertion site as possible. Watch closely for phlebitis at injection site.
▼ Monitor respirations every 5 to 15 minutes and before each dose.
▼ Don't store parenteral solution in plastic syringes.
▼ **Incompatibilities:** All other IV drugs, most IV solutions.

IM
- Use the IM route if IV administration is impossible.

Reactions in bold italics are *life-threatening*. Interactions may have a *rapid onset* or a ***delayed onset***.

Rectal

• Use Diastat rectal gel to treat no more than five episodes per month and no more than one episode every 5 days.

⊕ **Alert:** Only caregivers who can distinguish the distinct cluster of seizures or events from patient's ordinary seizure activity, who have been instructed and can give the treatment competently, who understand which seizures may be treated with Diastat, and who can monitor the clinical response and recognize when immediate professional medical evaluation is needed should give Diastat rectal gel.

ACTION

A benzodiazepine that potentiates the effects of GABA, depresses the CNS, and suppresses the spread of seizure activity.

Route	Onset	Peak	Duration
PO	30 min	¼–2½ hr	20–80 hr
IV	1–5 min	1–5 min	15–60 min
IM	Unknown	1 hr	Unknown
PR	Unknown	90 min	Unknown

Half-life: About 1 to 12 days. Varies with route and patient age.

ADVERSE REACTIONS

CNS: drowsiness, dysarthria, slurred speech, tremor, transient amnesia, fatigue, ataxia, headache, insomnia, paradoxical anxiety, hallucinations, minor changes in EEG patterns, pain, vertigo, confusion, depression. **CV:** *CV collapse, bradycardia,* hypotension. **EENT:** diplopia, blurred vision, nystagmus. **GI:** nausea, constipation, diarrhea with rectal form, dry mouth. **GU:** incontinence, urine retention. **Hematologic:** *neutropenia.* **Hepatic:** jaundice. **Respiratory:** *respiratory depression, apnea,* hiccups. **Skin:** rash, phlebitis at injection site. **Other:** altered libido, physical or psychological dependence.

INTERACTIONS

Drug-drug. *Cimetidine, disulfiram, fluoxetine, fluvoxamine, hormonal contraceptives, isoniazid, metoprolol, propranolol, valproic acid:* May decrease clearance of diazepam and increase risk of adverse effects. Monitor patient for excessive sedation and impaired psychomotor function.
CNS depressants: May increase CNS depression. Use together cautiously.

Digoxin: May increase digoxin level and risk of toxicity. Monitor patient and digoxin level closely.
Diltiazem: May increase CNS depression and prolong effects of diazepam. Reduce dose of diazepam.
Fluconazole, itraconazole, ketoconazole, miconazole: May increase and prolong diazepam level, CNS depression, and psychomotor impairment. Avoid using together.
Levodopa: May decrease levodopa effectiveness. Monitor patient.
Black Box Warning *Opioids:* May cause slow or difficult breathing, sedation, and death. Avoid use together. If use together is necessary, limit dosage and duration of each drug to the minimum necessary for desired effect. ▪
Phenobarbital: May increase effects of both drugs. Use together cautiously.
Drug-herb. *Kava:* May increase sedation. Discourage use together.
Drug-lifestyle. Black Box Warning *Alcohol use:* May cause additive CNS effects. Don't use together. ▪
Smoking: May decrease effectiveness of drug. Monitor patient closely.

EFFECTS ON LAB TEST RESULTS

• May increase LFT values.
• May decrease neutrophil count.

CONTRAINDICATIONS & CAUTIONS

Black Box Warning Opioids should only be prescribed with benzodiazepines or other CNS depressants to patients for whom alternative treatment options are inadequate. ▪
• Contraindicated in patients hypersensitive to drug and in infants younger than age 6 months (oral form).
• Diazepam (oral form) is contraindicated in patients with myasthenia gravis, severe respiratory insufficiency, severe hepatic insufficiency, or sleep apnea syndrome.
• Diazepam is contraindicated in patients with acute angle-closure glaucoma.
• Use cautiously in patients experiencing shock, coma, or acute alcohol intoxication (parenteral form).
• Use cautiously in elderly and debilitated patients and in patients with hepatic or renal impairment, depression, history of substance abuse, impaired gag reflex, or chronic

open-angle glaucoma (who are receiving appropriate therapy) and in those at risk for falls.
• Some injectable forms may contain propylene glycol; large amounts are potentially toxic and have been associated with hyperosmolality, lactic acidosis, seizures, and respiratory depression.
Dialyzable drug: No.
⚠ *Overdose S&S:* Somnolence, confusion, coma, diminished reflexes.

PREGNANCY-LACTATION-REPRODUCTION
• Use during pregnancy isn't recommended, especially during first and third trimesters. If drug is needed during pregnancy, use only if potential benefit justifies potential risk to the fetus.
• Neonatal flaccidity, respiratory and feeding difficulties, hypothermia, and withdrawal symptoms have been reported in infants born to mothers who received benzodiazepines late in pregnancy.
• Drug appears in human milk. Use in breastfeeding women isn't recommended.

NURSING CONSIDERATIONS
• Periodically monitor LFTs, CBC, and renal function in patients receiving repeated or prolonged therapy.
• Monitor HR, BP, and mental status changes. Patients are at an increased risk for falls.
☉ *Alert:* Use of drug may lead to abuse and addiction. Don't withdraw drug abruptly after long-term use because withdrawal symptoms may occur; taper gradually.
• *Look alike–sound alike:* Don't confuse diazepam with diazoxide or Ditropan. Don't confuse Valium with Valcyte.

PATIENT TEACHING
Black Box Warning Caution patient or caregiver of a patient taking an opioid with a benzodiazepine, CNS depressant, or alcohol to seek immediate medical attention for dizziness, light-headedness, extreme sleepiness, slowed or difficult breathing, or unresponsiveness. ▪
• Warn patient to report all adverse reactions and to avoid activities that require alertness and good coordination until effects of drug are known.

• Tell patient to avoid alcohol while taking drug.
• Warn patient not to abruptly stop drug because withdrawal symptoms may occur.
• Advise female patient to avoid use during pregnancy; inform her of the potential hazard to the fetus if drug is used during pregnancy or if patient becomes pregnant while taking drug.
• Instruct patient's caregiver on the proper use of Diastat rectal gel.

diclofenac (oral)
dye-KLOE-fen-ak

Zorvolex

diclofenac potassium
Apo-Diclo Rapide♣, Cambia, Voltaren Rapide♣, Zipsor

diclofenac sodium (oral)
Apo-Diclo♣, Voltaren SR♣

Therapeutic class: NSAIDs
Pharmacologic class: NSAIDs

AVAILABLE FORMS
diclofenac (oral)
Capsules: 18 mg, 35 mg
diclofenac potassium
Capsules: 25 mg*
Powder for solution: 50 mg/packet
Tablets: 50 mg
diclofenac sodium (oral)
Tablets (delayed-release) ⊙: 25 mg, 50 mg, 75 mg, 100 mg
Tablets (extended-release) ⊙: 100 mg

INDICATIONS & DOSAGES
Adjust-a-dose (for all indications): Patients with hepatic impairment may require lower initial dosages. Discontinue immediately if hepatic impairment occurs during therapy, including persistent or worsening abnormal LFT values, clinical signs or symptoms consistent with liver disease, or systemic manifestations of liver disease. Use Cambia in patients with hepatic impairment only if benefits outweigh risks. Initiate treatment with Zorvolex or Zipsor at the lowest

---

Reactions in bold italics are *life-threatening*. Interactions may have a *rapid onset* or a *delayed onset*.

dosage; if efficacy isn't achieved with the lowest dosage, discontinue drug.

➤ **Ankylosing spondylitis**
Adults: 25 mg delayed-release diclofenac sodium PO q.i.d.; may add another 25-mg dose at bedtime if needed.

➤ **Osteoarthritis**
Adults: 50 mg diclofenac potassium or delayed-release diclofenac sodium PO b.i.d. or t.i.d., or 75 mg delayed-release diclofenac sodium PO b.i.d. Or, 35 mg Zorvolex PO t.i.d. Or, 100 mg extended-release diclofenac sodium PO daily.

➤ **RA**
Adults: 50 mg diclofenac potassium or delayed-release diclofenac sodium PO t.i.d. or q.i.d., or 75 mg delayed-release diclofenac sodium PO b.i.d. Or, 100 mg extended-release diclofenac sodium PO daily or b.i.d.

➤ **Analgesia**
Adults: 50 mg diclofenac potassium PO t.i.d. For some patients, the first dose on the first day may be 100 mg, followed by 50 mg for the second and third doses; maximum dose for first day is 200 mg. Don't exceed 150 mg daily after the first day. Or, 25 mg Zipsor PO q.i.d. or 18 or 35 mg Zorvolex PO t.i.d.

➤ **Primary dysmenorrhea**
Adults: 50 mg diclofenac potassium PO t.i.d. For some patients, the first dose on the first day may be 100 mg, followed by 50 mg for the second and third doses; maximum dose for first day is 200 mg. Don't exceed 150 mg daily after the first day.

➤ **Migraine**
Adults: 50 mg (1 packet) PO as a single dose.

ADMINISTRATION
PO
• Give drug (except Cambia) with milk, meals, or antacids.
• Don't crush or break delayed- or extended-release tablets.
• Mix powder (Cambia) in 30 to 60 mL water only. Use no other liquid.
• Mix solution well and have patient drink immediately.
• Powder (Cambia) and Zorvolex may be less effective if taken with food.
• Cambia, Zorvolex, and Zipsor aren't interchangeable with other formulations of oral

diclofenac even if the milligram strength is the same.

ACTION
Reversibly inhibits cyclooxygenase 1 and 2 enzymes, which decreases proinflammatory processes. Has analgesic, anti-inflammatory, and antipyretic properties.

Route	Onset	Peak	Duration
PO (delayed-release)	30 min	2–3 hr	8 hr
PO (extended-release)	Unknown	5–6 hr	Unknown
PO	10 min	1 hr	8 hr

Half-life: 1 to 2 hours.

ADVERSE REACTIONS
CNS: anxiety, dizziness, drowsiness, headache, irritability. **CV:** *HF,* edema, fluid retention, HTN. **EENT:** blurred vision, epistaxis, eye pain, night blindness, reversible hearing loss, swelling of the lips and tongue, tinnitus. **GI:** abdominal distention, abdominal pain or cramps, *bleeding,* constipation, diarrhea, flatulence, indigestion, melena, nausea, peptic ulceration, taste disorder, bloody diarrhea, appetite change, colitis, vomiting. **GU:** nephrotic syndrome, *acute renal failure,* fluid retention, interstitial nephritis, oliguria, papillary necrosis, proteinuria. **Hepatic:** jaundice, *hepatitis, hepatotoxicity.* **Metabolic:** *hypoglycemia,* hyperglycemia. **Musculoskeletal:** back, leg, or joint pain. **Respiratory:** *asthma, laryngeal edema.* **Skin:** *SJS,* allergic purpura, alopecia, bullous eruption, dermatitis, eczema, photosensitivity reactions, pruritus, rash, urticaria. **Other:** *anaphylactoid reactions, anaphylaxis, angioedema.*

INTERACTIONS
Drug-drug. *ACE inhibitors, ARBs:* May enhance adverse or toxic effect of NSAIDs and result in a significant decrease in renal function. May diminish antihypertensive effect of ACE inhibitors and ARBs. Monitor therapy.
Anticoagulants, antiplatelet agents, SSNRIs, SSRIs, warfarin: May cause bleeding. Monitor patient closely.
Aspirin: May decrease effectiveness of diclofenac and increase GI toxicity. Avoid using together.

Beta blockers: May decrease antihypertensive effects. Monitor patient closely.

Cyclosporine, digoxin, lithium, methotrexate: May reduce renal clearance of these drugs and increase risk of toxicity. Monitor patient closely.

Diuretics: May decrease effectiveness of diuretics. Avoid using together.

Insulin, oral antidiabetics: May alter requirements for antidiabetics. Monitor patient closely.

Potassium-sparing diuretics: May enhance retention and increase level of potassium. Monitor potassium level.

Drug-herb. *Alfalfa, anise, bilberry, willow:* May cause bleeding. Don't use together.

Drug-lifestyle. *Sun exposure:* May cause photosensitivity reactions. Advise patient to avoid excessive sunlight exposure.

EFFECTS ON LAB TEST RESULTS
• May increase ALT, AST, bilirubin, BUN, and creatinine levels.
• May increase or decrease glucose level.

CONTRAINDICATIONS & CAUTIONS
Black Box Warning Contraindicated for the treatment of pain after CABG surgery. ∎
• Contraindicated in patients hypersensitive to drug and in those with hepatic porphyria or history of asthma, urticaria, or other allergic reactions after taking aspirin or other NSAIDs. Zipsor is contraindicated in patients hypersensitive to bovine protein.

⊕ Alert: NSAIDs can increase the risk of MI or stroke in patients with or without heart disease or risk factors for heart disease. The risk of MI or stroke can occur as early as the first weeks of NSAID use. Risk appears greater at higher doses. Use lowest effective dose for shortest duration possible.

⊕ Alert: NSAIDs increase the risk of HF. Don't use in patients with severe HF unless the benefits are expected to outweigh risks.
• Use cautiously in patients with history of peptic ulcer disease, hepatic dysfunction, cardiac disease, HTN, fluid retention, or impaired renal function.
• Drug may cause photosensitivity as well as serious skin adverse events, including exfoliative dermatitis, SJS, and toxic epidermal necrolysis, which can be fatal. Discontinue at first sign of rash or hypersensitivity.

Dialyzable drug: Unknown.

⚠ Overdose S&S: Drowsiness, confusion, GI bleeding, hypotonia, loss of consciousness, vomiting, aspiration, pneumonitis, increased ICP.

PREGNANCY-LACTATION-REPRODUCTION
⊕ Alert: Drug can cause fetal harm when administered at 30 weeks' gestation or later. Use during pregnancy before 30 weeks' gestation only if potential benefit justifies potential risk to the fetus.

⊕ Alert: NSAIDs can cause premature closure of the ductus arteriosus. Avoid use during pregnancy, particularly late pregnancy.
• Drug may appear in human milk. Patient should discontinue breastfeeding or discontinue drug, taking into account importance of drug to the mother.

NURSING CONSIDERATIONS
⊕ Alert: Monitor patient and immediately evaluate signs and symptoms of heart attack (chest pain, shortness of breath, trouble breathing) or stroke (weakness in one part or side of the body, slurred speech).
• Because NSAIDs impair the synthesis of renal prostaglandins, they can decrease renal blood flow and lead to reversible renal impairment, especially in patients with renal failure, HF, or liver dysfunction; in elderly patients; and in those taking diuretics. Monitor these patients closely.
• LFT values may increase during therapy. Monitor transaminase, especially ALT, levels periodically in patients undergoing long-term therapy. Make first transaminase measurement no later than 8 weeks after therapy begins.
Black Box Warning NSAIDs cause an increased risk of serious GI adverse events, including bleeding, ulceration, and perforation of the stomach or intestines, which can be fatal. Elderly patients are at greater risk. ∎
Black Box Warning NSAIDs may increase the risk of serious thrombotic events, MI, or stroke, which can be fatal. The risk may be greater with longer use or in patients with CV disease or risk factors for CV disease. ∎
⊕ Alert: Different formulations of oral diclofenac are not bioequivalent even if the milligram strength is the same.

Reactions in bold italics are *life-threatening*. Interactions may have a *rapid onset* or a *delayed onset*.

- Because of their antipyretic and anti-inflammatory actions, NSAIDs may mask the signs and symptoms of infection.
- Consider periodic CBC and chemistry profile monitoring with long-term NSAID treatment because serious GI bleeding, hepatotoxicity, and renal injury can occur without warning.
- *Look alike–sound alike:* Don't confuse diclofenac with Diflucan.

PATIENT TEACHING
- Tell patient to take tablets or capsules with milk, meals, or antacids to minimize GI distress; however, taking Cambia or Zorvolex with food may reduce its effectiveness.
- Instruct patient not to crush, break, or chew delayed- or extended-release tablets.
- ⓘ *Alert:* Advise patient to seek medical attention immediately if chest pain, shortness of breath or trouble breathing, weakness in one part or side of the body, or slurred speech occurs.
- Tell patient to mix powder form well in 30 to 60 mL of water only and to drink immediately.
- Advise patient not to take this drug with other diclofenac-containing products (such as Arthrotec), other NSAIDs, or salicylates (salsalate, diflunisal).
- Teach patient signs and symptoms of GI bleeding (blood in vomit, urine, or stool; coffee-ground vomit; black, tarry stools) and to notify prescriber immediately if any of these occur.
- Teach patient the signs and symptoms of damage to the liver, including nausea, fatigue, lethargy, itching, yellowed skin or eyes, right upper quadrant tenderness, and flulike symptoms. Tell patient to contact prescriber immediately if these symptoms occur.
- Advise patient to avoid drinking alcohol or taking aspirin during drug therapy.
- Tell patient to wear sunscreen or protective clothing because drug may cause sensitivity to sunlight.
- Warn patient to avoid hazardous activities that require alertness until it is known whether the drug causes CNS symptoms.
- Tell female patient who is pregnant to avoid use of drug during last trimester.

- Advise patient that use of OTC NSAIDs (which may be present in OTC medications for treatment of colds, fever, or insomnia) and diclofenac may increase risk of GI toxicity.

diclofenac epolamine
dye-KLOE-fen-ak

Flector

diclofenac sodium (topical)
Pennsaid, Voltaren

Therapeutic class: NSAIDs
Pharmacologic class: NSAIDs

AVAILABLE FORMS
Topical gel: 1%, 3%
Topical solution: 1.5%, 2%
Transdermal patch: 1.3%

INDICATIONS & DOSAGES
➤ **Actinic keratosis (3% gel only)**
Adults: Apply gel to lesion b.i.d. for 60 to 90 days.
➤ **Osteoarthritis (Voltaren only)**
Adults: Apply 4 g of 1% gel to affected foot, knee, or ankle q.i.d. Maximum dose of 16 g to any single joint of the lower extremities. Or apply 2 g of 1% gel to affected hand, elbow, or wrist q.i.d. Maximum dose of 8 g to any single joint of the upper extremities. Total dose shouldn't exceed 32 g daily for all affected joints.
➤ **Acute pain due to minor strains, sprains, and contusions**
Adults: Apply 1 patch to most painful area b.i.d.
➤ **Osteoarthritis of the knee**
Adults: Count 10 drops at a time of 1.5% topical solution onto hand or directly onto knee. Apply to each side, front and back, spreading evenly, using a total of 40 drops q.i.d. Or, 2 pump actuations (40 mg) of 2% topical solution on each painful knee b.i.d. Dispense solution directly onto the knee or first into the hand and then onto the knee. Spread evenly around front, back, and sides of the knee.

ADMINISTRATION
Topical
• Apply to clean, dry skin.
• Don't apply to open wounds or broken skin.
• Avoid contact with eyes.
• Use enough gel to cover the lesion; for example, use 0.5 g of gel on a 5 × 5-cm lesion.
• Don't apply Flector patch to nonintact or damaged skin, including from exudative dermatitis, eczema, infected lesions, burns, or wounds.
• Patient shouldn't wear patch while bathing or showering.
• Measure gel using supplied dosing cards in package.
• Wear gloves to gently massage Voltaren into skin of entire joint.
• Wash hands after applying. If treatment area is the hands, patient should wait at least 1 hour before washing hands.
• Pump for 2% topical solution must be primed before first use. Depress pump four times while holding bottle upright; discard solution obtained during priming.

ACTION
Unknown. May produce anti-inflammatory and analgesic effects by ability to inhibit prostaglandin synthesis.

Route	Onset	Peak	Duration
Topical	Unknown	4–12 hr	Unknown
Transdermal	Unknown	10–20 hr	Unknown

Half-life: 1 to 3 hours; 12 hours for patch.

ADVERSE REACTIONS
CNS: paresthesia, headache, pain, asthenia, migraine, hypokinesia. **CV:** chest pain, HTN. **EENT:** sinusitis, pharyngitis, rhinitis, conjunctivitis, eye pain. **GI:** diarrhea, dyspepsia, abdominal pain, flatulence, nausea. **GU:** hematuria, renal impairment. **Hepatic:** liver impairment. **Metabolic:** hypercholesterolemia, hyperglycemia. **Musculoskeletal:** arthralgia, arthrosis, back pain, myalgia, neck pain. **Respiratory:** *asthma,* dyspnea, pneumonia. **Skin:** reaction at application site, contact dermatitis, dry skin, exfoliation, localized pain, pruritus, rash, localized edema, acne, alopecia, photosensitivity reactions, skin ulcer. **Other:** *anaphylaxis,* flulike syndrome, infection, allergic reaction.

INTERACTIONS
Drug-drug. *ACE inhibitors, ARBs:* May enhance adverse or toxic effect of NSAIDs and result in a significant decrease in renal function. May diminish antihypertensive effect of ACE inhibitors and ARBs. Monitor therapy.
Anticoagulants, antiplatelet agents, SSNRIs, SSRIs, warfarin: May cause bleeding. Monitor patient closely.
Aspirin: May decrease effectiveness of diclofenac and increase GI toxicity. Avoid using together.
Beta blockers: May decrease antihypertensive effects. Monitor patient closely.
Cyclosporine, digoxin, lithium, methotrexate: May reduce renal clearance of these drugs and increase risk of toxicity. Monitor patient closely.
Diuretics: May decrease effectiveness of diuretics. Avoid using together.
Insulin, oral antidiabetics: May alter requirements for antidiabetics. Monitor patient closely.
Oral NSAIDs: May increase diclofenac effects. Minimize use together.
Potassium-sparing diuretics: May enhance retention and increase potassium level. Monitor potassium level.
Herb-drug. *Alfalfa, anise, bilberry, willow:* May cause bleeding. Don't use together.
Drug-lifestyle. *Sun exposure:* May increase risk of photosensitivity reactions. Advise patient to avoid excessive sun exposure.

EFFECTS ON LAB TEST RESULTS
• May increase ALT, AST, cholesterol, creatinine, glucose, and transaminase levels.

CONTRAINDICATIONS & CAUTIONS
• Contraindicated in patients hypersensitive to diclofenac. Diclofenac 3% sodium gel is also contraindicated in patients with a known hypersensitivity to benzyl alcohol, polyethylene glycol monomethyl ether 350, or hyaluronate sodium.
• Contraindicated in patients with a history of asthma, urticaria, or other allergic reactions after taking aspirin or other NSAIDs.
• Flector patch is contraindicated for use on nonintact or damaged skin, including from exudative dermatitis, eczema, infected lesions, burns, or wounds.

Black Box Warning Contraindicated for perioperative pain for CABG surgery. ∎

🕃 *Alert:* NSAIDs can increase risk of MI or stroke in patients with or without heart disease or risk factors for heart disease.

🕃 *Alert:* Risk of MI or stroke can occur as early as the first weeks of NSAID use. Risk appears greater at higher doses. Use lowest effective dose for shortest duration possible.

🕃 *Alert:* NSAIDs increase risk of HF. Don't use in patients with severe HF unless benefits are expected to outweigh risks.

• Use cautiously in patients with the aspirin triad; these patients are usually asthmatics who develop rhinitis, with or without nasal polyps, after taking aspirin or other NSAIDs.

• Use cautiously in patients with active GI bleeding or ulceration and in those with severe renal or hepatic impairment.

• May cause serious adverse skin events, including exfoliative dermatitis, SJS, and toxic epidermal necrolysis, which can be fatal. Discontinue use at first sign of rash or hypersensitivity.

Dialyzable drug: Unknown.

PREGNANCY-LACTATION-REPRODUCTION

🕃 *Alert:* Drug can cause fetal harm when administered at 30 weeks' gestation or later. Use during pregnancy before 30 weeks' gestation only if potential benefit justifies potential risk to the fetus.

• Drug may cause constriction of ductus arteriosus. Avoid use in late pregnancy.

• Drug may appear in human milk. Patient should discontinue breastfeeding or discontinue drug, taking into account importance of drug to the mother.

NURSING CONSIDERATIONS

Black Box Warning NSAIDs may increase the risk of serious CV thrombotic events. The risk may increase with duration of use. Patients with CV disease or risk factors for CV disease may be at greater risk. ∎

Black Box Warning NSAIDs increase the risk of serious GI adverse reactions, including bleeding, ulceration, and perforation of the stomach or intestines, which can be fatal. These reactions can occur at any time and without warning. Elderly patients are at greater risk. ∎

🕃 *Alert:* Monitor patient and immediately evaluate signs and symptoms of MI (chest pain, shortness of breath, trouble breathing) or stroke (weakness in one part or side of the body, slurred speech).

• Avoid use in patients with recent MI unless benefits are expected to outweigh risk of recurrent CV thrombotic events. If used in patients with recent MI, watch for signs and symptoms of cardiac ischemia.

• Avoid use in patients with severe HF unless benefits are expected to outweigh risk of worsening HF. If used in patients with severe HF, watch for signs and symptoms of worsening HF.

• Evaluate patient with signs or symptoms of liver dysfunction or with abnormal LFT results for development of more severe hepatic reaction while taking drug.

• If clinical signs or symptoms of liver disease develop, or if systemic manifestation (eosinophilia, rash) occurs, discontinue drug.

• Safety and effectiveness of sunscreens, cosmetics, or other topical medications used with drug are unknown.

• Complete healing or optimal therapeutic effect may not be seen until 30 days after therapy is complete.

• Reevaluate lesions that don't respond to therapy.

PATIENT TEACHING

• Inform patient about risk of skin reactions (rash, itchiness, pain, irritation) at the application site. Urge patient to seek medical attention if adverse reactions occur.

🕃 *Alert:* Advise patient to seek medical attention immediately if chest pain, shortness of breath or trouble breathing, weakness in one part or side of the body, or slurred speech occurs.

• Instruct patient that pump solution must be primed (four pumps) before first use.

• Encourage patient to minimize sun exposure during therapy. Explain that sunscreen may be helpful but that the safety of using sunscreen with drug is unknown.

• Advise patient needing an MRI to inform the facility about wearing a transdermal patch.

• Tell patient using diclofenac 3% sodium gel that complete healing or optimal

---

♣ Canada   ◇ OTC   ♦ Off-label use   ✐ Photoguide   ⊞ Do not crush   *Liquid contains alcohol   ⊠ Genetic

therapeutic effect may not occur for up to 30 days after stopping therapy.
• Caution patient not to apply gel to open wounds or broken skin.
• Instruct patient to avoid contact with eyes.
• Instruct patient not to apply other topical drugs or cosmetics to affected area while using drug, unless directed.
• Advise patient to use only on intact skin unless otherwise directed.
• Inform patient that if Flector patch begins to peel off, the edges may be taped down. Instruct patient not to wear Flector patch during bathing or showering. Bathing should take place in between scheduled patch removal and application.
• Tell patient to wash hands after applying gel unless the hands are the treated area and to wait at least 1 hour after application before washing hands.
• Instruct patient not to cover area with clothing for at least 10 minutes after applying gel and to wait at least 1 hour before showering or bathing.
• Tell female patient to notify prescriber if she is pregnant or breastfeeding.

dicyclomine hydrochloride
dye-SYE-kloe-meen

Bentyl, Protylol ✤

Therapeutic class: Antispasmodics
Pharmacologic class: Anticholinergics–antimuscarinics

AVAILABLE FORMS
Capsules: 10 mg
Injection: 10 mg/mL
Syrup: 10 mg/5 mL
Tablets: 10 mg ✤, 20 mg

INDICATIONS & DOSAGES
➤ **IBS, other functional GI disorders**
Adults: Initially, 20 mg PO q.i.d.; may increase to 40 mg PO q.i.d. after 1 week unless adverse effects limit dosage escalation. Or, 10 to 20 mg IM q.i.d. Don't use IM form for longer than 1 to 2 days.

ADMINISTRATION
PO
• Store in light-resistant container.
• Protect from excessive heat.
IM
❸ *Alert:* Don't give subcut or IV.
• Aspirate syringe before injecting to avoid IV injection; thrombosis and injection-site reaction may occur if drug is inadvertently injected IV.
❸ *Alert:* Injection concentration is 10 mg/mL. Carefully calculate appropriate amount of solution for administering correct dose.

ACTION
Inhibits action of acetylcholine on postganglionic, parasympathetic muscarinic receptors, decreasing GI motility. Drug possesses local anesthetic properties that may be partly responsible for spasmolysis.

Route	Onset	Peak	Duration
PO, IM	Unknown	1–1½ hr	Unknown

Half-life: Initially, about 1.8 hours.

ADVERSE REACTIONS
CNS: asthenia, headache, dizziness, fever, insomnia, light-headedness, drowsiness, nervousness, confusion, excitement (in elderly patients), somnolence, tingling, dyskinesia, lethargy, weakness, numbness. **CV:** palpitations, tachycardia. **EENT:** blurred vision, increased IOP, mydriasis, photophobia, diplopia. **GI:** constipation, dry mouth, thirst, vomiting, nausea, abdominal distention, heartburn, paralytic ileus. **GU:** urinary hesitancy, urine retention, erectile dysfunction. **Skin:** urticaria, decreased sweating or inability to sweat, local irritation, rash. **Other:** allergic reactions, heat prostration.

INTERACTIONS
Drug-drug. *Amantadine, antihistamines, antiparkinsonians, disopyramide, glutethimide, meperidine, phenothiazines, procainamide, quinidine, TCAs:* May have additive adverse effects. Avoid using together.
Antacids: May interfere with dicyclomine absorption. Give dicyclomine at least 1 hour before antacid.

Reactions in bold italics are *life-threatening*. Interactions may have a *rapid onset* or a ***delayed onset***.

Antiglaucoma drugs: May decrease therapeutic effect of these drugs. Use together is contraindicated.

GI motility agents (metoclopramide): May decrease effectiveness of motility agents. Monitor therapy.

EFFECTS ON LAB TEST RESULTS
None reported.

CONTRAINDICATIONS & CAUTIONS
• Contraindicated in patients hypersensitive to anticholinergics, in children younger than age 6 months, and in those with obstructive uropathy, obstructive disease of the GI tract, reflux esophagitis, severe ulcerative colitis, toxic megacolon, myasthenia gravis, unstable CV status in acute hemorrhage, or glaucoma.
• Use cautiously in patients with tachycardia secondary to cardiac insufficiency or thyrotoxicosis.
• Don't use in patients with myasthenia gravis except to reduce adverse muscarinic effects of an anticholinesterase.
• Use cautiously in patients with autonomic neuropathy, hyperthyroidism, CAD, arrhythmias, HF, HTN, hiatal hernia, hepatic or renal disease, prostatic hyperplasia, known or suspected GI infection, and ulcerative colitis.
• Use cautiously in patients in hot or humid environments; drug can cause heatstroke.
• May affect GI absorption of various drugs (such as slowly dissolving dosage forms of digoxin) by affecting GI motility, which may increase serum concentrations.
⊙ Alert: Use cautiously in patients sensitive to anticholinergic drugs, especially elderly patients and those with mental illness, because of the risk of psychosis and delirium. When present, these signs and symptoms usually resolve within 12 to 24 hours after discontinuation of drug.
• Safety and effectiveness in children haven't been established.
Dialyzable drug: Unknown.
⚠ Overdose S&S: Headache; nausea; vomiting; blurred vision; dilated pupils; hot, dry skin; dry mouth; dysphagia; CNS stimulation; muscle weakness; paralysis.

PREGNANCY-LACTATION-REPRODUCTION
• There are no adequate well-controlled studies in pregnant women. Use during pregnancy only if clearly needed.
• Drug appears in human milk. Contraindicated in breastfeeding women. Patient should discontinue breastfeeding or drug, taking into account importance of drug to the mother.

NURSING CONSIDERATIONS
• Adjust dosage based on patient's needs and response. Dosages up to 40 mg PO q.i.d. have been used in adults, but safety and effectiveness for longer than 2 weeks haven't been established.
• Dicyclomine may have atropine-like adverse reactions.
⊙ Alert: Overdose may cause curare-like effects, such as respiratory paralysis. Keep emergency equipment available.
• Monitor patient's vital signs and urine output carefully.
Look alike–sound alike: Don't confuse dicyclomine with dyclonine or doxycycline. Don't confuse Bentyl with Benadryl.

PATIENT TEACHING
• Tell patient when to take drug, and stress importance of doing so on time and at evenly spaced intervals and to report all adverse reactions.
• Advise patient to avoid driving and other hazardous activities if drowsiness, dizziness, or blurred vision occurs; to drink plenty of fluids to help prevent constipation; and to report rash or other skin eruption.
• Warn patient that heat prostration may occur during therapy when environmental temperatures are high. If signs and symptoms (fever, decreased sweating) occur, instruct patient to stop drug and contact prescriber.
• Advise female patient not to breastfeed during therapy.

---

didanosine
(ddI, dideoxyinosine)
dye-DAN-oh-seen

Videx, Videx EC

Therapeutic class: Antiretrovirals
Pharmacologic class: Nucleoside–
nucleotide reverse transcriptase inhibitors

AVAILABLE FORMS
Capsules (delayed-release) ⓄⓃⒸ: 125 mg,
200 mg, 250 mg, 400 mg
Powder for oral solution (pediatric):
10 mg/mL

INDICATIONS & DOSAGES
➤ **HIV infection**
Delayed-release capsules
Adults and children age 6 and older weighing 60 kg or more: 400-mg capsule PO daily.
Adults and children age 6 and older weighing 25 kg to less than 60 kg: 250-mg capsule PO daily.
Adults and children age 6 and older weighing 20 kg to less than 25 kg: 200-mg capsule PO daily.
Powder for oral solution
Adults weighing 60 kg or more: 200 mg PO b.i.d. (preferred) or 400 mg PO daily.
Adults weighing less than 60 kg: 125 mg PO b.i.d. (preferred) or 250 mg PO daily.
Children older than age 8 months to 18 years: 120 mg/m² PO b.i.d. Maximum dose is 200 mg PO b.i.d.
Children ages 2 weeks to 8 months: 100 mg/m² PO b.i.d. Maximum dose is 200 mg PO b.i.d.
Adjust-a-dose: Refer to manufacturer's instructions for renal impairment dosage adjustments according to patient weight, CrCl, and dosage form. For adults taking tenofovir who weigh 60 kg or more with a CrCl of 60 mL/minute or more, reduce didanosine dose to 250 mg once daily. For adults taking tenofovir who weigh less than 60 kg with a CrCl of 60 mL/minute or more, reduce didanosine dose to 200 mg once daily. Avoid concomitant therapy in patients with CrCl less than 60 mL/minute.

ADMINISTRATION
PO
• Give drug on an empty stomach, at least 30 minutes before or 2 hours after eating; giving drug with meals can decrease absorption by 50%.
• Store capsules in tightly closed containers at 77° F (25° C).
⚠ *Alert:* The pediatric powder for oral solution must be prepared by a pharmacist before dispensing. It must be constituted with purified USP water to an initial concentration of 20 mg/mL, then immediately diluted with an antacid to a final concentration of 10 mg/mL. The admixture is stable for 30 days at 36° to 46° F (2° to 8° C). Shake solution well before measuring dose. Discard unused portion after 30 days.

ACTION
Inhibits the enzyme HIV-RNA–dependent DNA polymerase (reverse transcriptase) and terminates DNA chain growth.

Route	Onset	Peak	Duration
PO	Unknown	15–90 min	Unknown
PO (delayed-release)	Unknown	0.25–2 hr	Unknown

Half-life: Adults, 1½ hours; children, about 1 hour.

ADVERSE REACTIONS
CNS: dizziness, fever, headache, peripheral neuropathy. **EENT:** optic neuritis, retinal changes. **GI:** abdominal pain, diarrhea, nausea, vomiting, *pancreatitis,* anorexia, dry mouth. **Hepatic:** *hepatic failure.*
Metabolic: hyperuricemia. **Skin:** alopecia, pruritus, rash.

INTERACTIONS
Drug-drug. *Allopurinol:* Increases didanosine level. Use together is contraindicated.
Amprenavir, atazanavir, darunavir, delavirdine, indinavir, lopinavir, nelfinavir, rilpivirine, ritonavir, saquinavir, tipranavir: May alter pharmacokinetics of didanosine or these drugs. Give didanosine at least 1 hour after these drugs.
Antacids containing magnesium or aluminum hydroxides: May enhance adverse effects of the antacid component (including diarrhea or constipation) when given with

---

Reactions in bold italics are *life-threatening*. Interactions may have a *rapid onset* or a *delayed onset*.

didanosine tablets or pediatric suspension. Avoid using together.

Dapsone, drugs that require gastric acid for adequate absorption, ketoconazole: May decrease absorption from buffering action. Give these drugs 2 hours before didanosine.

Fluoroquinolones, tetracyclines: May decrease absorption from buffering products in didanosine tablets or antacids in pediatric suspension. Give oral quinolones at least 2 hours before or 6 hours after didanosine.

Hydroxyurea: Enhances toxic effects of didanosine. Avoid combination.

Itraconazole: May decrease itraconazole level. Avoid using together.

Methadone: Increases didanosine concentration (with pediatric powder for oral solution). Give delayed-release capsule if methadone is required. Monitor clinical response closely, including changes in HIV-RNA viral load.

Ribavirin: Increases risk of fatal hepatic failure, peripheral neuropathy, pancreatitis, and systematic hyperlactemia/lactic acidosis. Use together is contraindicated.

Black Box Warning *Stavudine with other antiretrovirals:* Fatal lactic acidosis has been reported in pregnant women taking didanosine. Use together is contraindicated. ∎

Sulfamethoxazole–trimethoprim, pentamidine, other drugs linked to pancreatitis: May increase risk of pancreatic toxicity. Use together cautiously; consider temporarily stopping didanosine during administration of these drugs.

Tenofovir: May increase didanosine levels and risk of life-threatening adverse effects, including lactic acidosis and pancreatitis. Adjust didanosine dosage.

Drug-food. *Any food:* May decrease rate of absorption. Advise patient to take drug on an empty stomach at least 30 minutes before a meal or 2 hours after eating.

Drug-lifestyle. *Alcohol use:* Increases risk of pancreatitis. Avoid use together.

EFFECTS ON LAB TEST RESULTS

• May increase alkaline phosphatase, ALT, AST, bilirubin, and uric acid levels. May decrease Hb level.
• May decrease granulocyte, platelet, and WBC counts.

CONTRAINDICATIONS & CAUTIONS

• Contraindicated in patients hypersensitive to drug or its components.

🜄 *Alert:* Administration with stavudine, allopurinol, or ribavirin is contraindicated.

Black Box Warning Contraindicated in patients with confirmed pancreatitis. Use cautiously in patients with history of pancreatitis; deaths have occurred. ∎

Black Box Warning Lactic acidosis and severe hepatomegaly with steatosis, including fatal cases, have been reported. ∎

• Suspend treatment in patients who develop clinical signs or symptoms with or without laboratory findings consistent with symptomatic hyperlactatemia, lactic acidosis, or pronounced hepatotoxicity.

• Retinal changes and optic neuritis have been reported in patients taking drug. Consider periodic retinal exams.

• Use cautiously in patients with peripheral neuropathy, renal or hepatic impairment, or hyperuricemia. Monitor LFTs and renal function tests.

Dialyzable drug: 7% or less.

⚠ **Overdose S&S:** Pancreatitis, peripheral neuropathy, diarrhea, hyperuricemia, hepatic dysfunction.

PREGNANCY-LACTATION-REPRODUCTION

Black Box Warning Fatal lactic acidosis has been reported in pregnant women using didanosine and stavudine in combination with other antiretrovirals. ∎

• There are no adequate well-controlled studies in pregnant women. Use during pregnancy only in special circumstances and only if potential benefit justifies potential risk to the fetus.

• Not recommended for initial therapy in antiretroviral-naive pregnant women due to toxicity.

• It isn't known if drug appears in human milk. Because of the potential for HIV transmission and for serious adverse reactions in breastfeeding infants, women shouldn't breastfeed during therapy.

• Enroll pregnant women exposed to antiretrovirals in the Antiretroviral Pregnancy Registry (1-800-258-4263 or www.apregistry.com).

NURSING CONSIDERATIONS

• Using drug in patients with advanced HIV disease or history of peripheral neuropathy or use with neurotoxic drugs may cause numbness, tingling, or pain in the hands and feet. Discontinue drug if neuropathy occurs.
• Patients may tolerate a reduced dose of Videx after symptoms of peripheral neuropathy resolve; if symptoms recur, consider permanently stopping drug.
• Because of a high rate of early virologic failure and emergence of resistance, using tenofovir with didanosine and lamivudine isn't recommended as a new treatment regimen for therapy-naive or therapy-experienced patients with HIV infection. Patients on this regimen should be considered for treatment modification.
• *Look alike–sound alike:* Don't confuse drug with other antiretrovirals that use abbreviations for identification.

PATIENT TEACHING

• Instruct patient to take drug on an empty stomach, 30 minutes before or 2 hours after eating.
• Inform patient that drug doesn't cure HIV infection, that opportunistic infections and other complications of HIV infection may continue to occur, and that transmission of HIV to others through sexual contact or blood contamination is still possible.
• Tell patient to report all adverse reactions and to immediately report signs and symptoms of inflammation of the pancreas (abdominal pain, nausea, vomiting, diarrhea) and signs and symptoms of peripheral neuropathy (numbness, tingling, or pain in hands or feet).

SAFETY ALERT!

digoxin
di-JOX-in

Lanoxin*, Lanoxin Pediatric, Toloxin✹

Therapeutic class: Inotropes
Pharmacologic class: Cardiac glycosides

AVAILABLE FORMS

Oral solution: 0.05 mg/mL (pediatric)

Injection*: 0.1 mg/mL (pediatric), 0.25 mg/mL
Tablets: 0.0625 mg, 0.125 mg, 0.25 mg

INDICATIONS & DOSAGES

❸ Alert: Factors to consider when a digoxin dosing regimen is selected include body weight, age, renal function, concomitant drugs, and disease. Toxic levels of digoxin are only slightly higher than therapeutic levels.

Adjust-a-dose (for all indications): Refer to manufacturer's information for recommended dosage adjustments based on renal function and weight.

➤ **HF, rapid digitalization**
Tablets
Adults and children older than age 10: Total loading dose is 10 to 15 mcg/kg PO. Initially, give half the total loading dose followed by one-quarter of the loading dose every 6 to 8 hours twice. Carefully assess clinical response and toxicity before each dose. Recommended starting maintenance dose for patients with normal renal function is 3.4 to 5.1 mcg/kg/day PO once daily. May increase every 2 weeks based on clinical response, serum drug levels, and toxicity. Refer to manufacturer's instructions for once-daily maintenance dose recommendations based on renal function and lean body weight.
Children ages 5 to 10: Total loading dose is 20 to 45 mcg/kg PO. Initially, give half the total loading dose followed by one-quarter of the loading dose every 6 to 8 hours twice. Carefully assess clinical response and toxicity before each dose. Recommended starting maintenance dosage for patients with normal renal function is 3.2 to 6.4 mcg/kg PO b.i.d. Refer to manufacturer's instructions for daily maintenance dose recommendations based on renal function and lean body weight.
Oral solution
In children, if a loading dose is needed, it can be administered with roughly half the total given as the first dose. Additional fractions of this planned total dose may be given at 4- to 8-hour intervals, with careful assessment of clinical response before each additional dose. If patient's clinical response necessitates a change from the calculated loading dose of digoxin, base the calculation of

the maintenance dose on the amount actually given as the loading dose.

Children older than age 10: Loading dose is 10 to 15 mcg/kg PO given in divided doses, followed by maintenance dose of 3 to 4.5 mcg/kg PO once daily.

Children ages 5 to 10: Loading dose is 20 to 35 mcg/kg PO given in divided doses, followed by maintenance dose of 2.8 to 5.6 mcg/kg/dose PO b.i.d.

Children ages 2 to 5: Loading dose is 30 to 45 mcg/kg PO given in divided doses, followed by maintenance dose of 4.7 to 6.6 mcg/kg/dose PO b.i.d.

Infants ages 1 to 24 months: Loading dose is 35 to 60 mcg/kg PO given in divided doses, followed by maintenance dose of 5.6 to 9.4 mcg/kg/dose PO b.i.d.

Full-term infants: Loading dose is 25 to 35 mcg/kg PO in divided doses, followed by maintenance dose of 3.8 to 5.6 mcg/kg/dose PO b.i.d.

Preterm infants: Loading dose is 20 to 30 mcg/kg PO given in divided doses, followed by maintenance dose of 2.3 to 3.9 mcg/kg/dose PO b.i.d.

IV

Initially for all patients, give half the total loading dose followed by one-quarter of the loading dose every 6 to 8 hours twice. Carefully assess clinical response and toxicity before each dose. Recommended starting maintenance doses assume the presence of normal renal function. May increase every 2 weeks based on clinical response, serum drug levels, and toxicity. Refer to manufacturer's instructions for maintenance dose recommendations based on renal function and lean body weight.

Adults and children older than age 10: Total loading dose is 8 to 12 mcg/kg IV in divided doses, followed by a starting maintenance dose of 2.4 to 3.6 mcg/kg IV once daily.

Children ages 5 to 10: Total loading dose is 15 to 30 mcg/kg IV in divided doses, followed by a starting maintenance dose of 2.3 to 4.5 mcg/kg/dose IV b.i.d.

Children ages 2 to 5: Total loading dose is 25 to 35 mcg/kg IV in divided doses, followed by a starting maintenance dose of 3.8 to 5.3 mcg/kg/dose IV b.i.d.

Infants ages 1 to 24 months: Total loading dose is 30 to 50 mcg/kg IV in divided doses,

followed by a starting maintenance dose of 4.5 to 7.5 mcg/kg/dose IV b.i.d.

Full-term infants: Total loading dose is 20 to 30 mcg/kg IV in divided doses, followed by a starting maintenance dose of 3 to 4.5 mcg/kg/dose IV b.i.d.

Preterm infants: Total loading dose is 15 to 25 mcg/kg IV in divided doses, followed by a starting maintenance dose of 1.9 to 3.1 mcg/kg/dose IV b.i.d.

➤ **HF, gradual digitalization**

Tablets

More gradual attainment of digoxin levels can also be accomplished by beginning an appropriate maintenance dosage without a loading dose in patients with normal renal function.

Adults and children older than age 10: Give starting maintenance dose of 3.4 to 5.1 mcg/kg PO once daily.

Children ages 5 to 10: Give starting maintenance dose of 3.2 to 6.4 mcg/kg/dose PO b.i.d.

Adjust-a-dose: Refer to manufacturer's instructions for dosage adjustment based on renal function and lean body weight.

Oral solution

More gradual attainment of digoxin levels can also be accomplished by beginning an appropriate maintenance dosage without a loading dose in patients with normal renal function. In general, divided daily dosing is recommended for infants and children younger than age 10. In newborns, renal clearance of digoxin is diminished and suitable dosage adjustments must be observed, especially in preterm infants. Beyond the immediate newborn period, children generally require proportionally larger doses than adults on the basis of body weight or surface area. Children older than age 10 require adult dosages in proportion to their body weight.

Adults and children older than age 10: 3 to 4.5 mcg/kg PO once daily.

Children ages 5 to 10: 2.8 to 5.6 mcg/kg/dose PO b.i.d.

Children ages 2 to 5: 4.7 to 6.6 mcg/kg/dose PO b.i.d.

Infants ages 1 to 24 months: 5.6 to 9.4 mcg/kg/dose PO b.i.d.

Full-term infants: 3.8 to 5.6 mcg/kg/dose PO b.i.d.

Preterm infants: 2.3 to 3.9 mcg/kg/dose PO b.i.d.

Adjust-a-dose: Refer to manufacturer's instructions for dosage adjustment based on renal function and lean body weight.

IV

Gradual digitalization can be accomplished by beginning an appropriate maintenance dose. Recommended starting doses assume the presence of normal renal function. May increase every 2 weeks based on clinical response, serum drug levels, and toxicity. Refer to manufacturer's instructions for dose recommendations based on renal function and lean body weight.

Adults and children older than age 10: Give a starting dose of 2.4 to 3.6 mcg/kg IV once daily.

Children ages 5 to 10: Give a starting dose of 2.3 to 4.5 mcg/kg/dose IV b.i.d.

Children ages 2 to 5: Give a starting dose of 3.8 to 5.3 mcg/kg/dose IV b.i.d.

Infants ages 1 to 24 months: Give a starting dose of 4.5 to 7.5 mcg/kg/dose IV b.i.d.

Full-term infants: Give a starting dose of 3 to 4.5 mcg/kg/dose IV b.i.d.

Preterm infants: Give a starting dose of 1.9 to 3.1 mcg/kg/dose IV b.i.d.

➤ **Atrial fibrillation (chronic)**

PO, IV

Adults: If a loading dose is used, total loading dose is 10 to 15 mcg/kg PO (tablets, elixir). Initially, give half the total loading dose followed by one-quarter of the loading dose every 6 to 8 hours twice. Carefully assess clinical response and toxicity before each dose. Recommended starting maintenance dosage for patients with normal renal function is 3.4 to 5.1 mcg/kg (tablets) PO once daily or 3 to 4.5 mcg/kg (elixir) PO once daily.

Or, for more gradual PO digitalization in patients with normal renal function, begin with the starting maintenance dosage of 3.4 to 5.1 mcg/kg (tablets) PO once daily or 3 to 4.5 mcg/kg (oral solution) PO once daily. May increase every 2 weeks based on clinical response, serum drug levels, and toxicity. Refer to manufacturer's instructions for once-daily maintenance dose recommendations based on renal function and lean body weight.

Or, if using an IV loading dose, give a total loading dose of 8 to 12 mcg/kg IV by initially giving half the total loading dose followed by one-quarter of the loading dose every 6 to 8 hours twice. Carefully assess clinical response and toxicity before each dose. Recommended starting maintenance dosage for patients with normal renal function is 2.4 to 3.6 mcg/kg IV once daily.

Or, for more gradual IV digitalization in patients with normal renal function, begin with the starting maintenance dosage of 2.4 to 3.6 mcg/kg IV once daily. Increase every 2 weeks according to clinical response, serum drug levels, and toxicity. Refer to manufacturer's instructions for dosage recommendations based on renal function and lean body weight.

ADMINISTRATION

PO

• Before giving loading dose, obtain baseline data (HR and rhythm, BP, and electrolyte levels) and ask patient about use of cardiac glycosides within the previous 2 to 3 weeks.

• Before giving drug, take apical-radial pulse for 1 minute. Record and notify prescriber of significant changes (sudden increase or decrease in pulse rate, pulse deficit, irregular beats and, particularly, regularization of a previously irregular rhythm). If these occur, check BP and obtain a 12-lead ECG.

IV

▼ Before giving loading dose, obtain baseline data (HR and rhythm, BP, and electrolyte levels) and ask patient about use of cardiac glycosides within the previous 2 to 3 weeks.

▼ Before giving drug, take apical-radial pulse for 1 minute. Record and notify prescriber of significant changes (sudden increase or decrease in pulse rate, pulse deficit, irregular beats and, particularly, regularization of a previously irregular rhythm). If these occur, check BP and obtain a 12-lead ECG.

▼ May administer undiluted or diluted with a fourfold or greater volume of D_5W, NSS, or sterile water for injection; use immediately. Using less than a fourfold volume of

D

diluent could lead to precipitation of the digoxin.

▼ Infuse drug slowly over at least 5 minutes or longer.

▼ Protect solution from light.

▼ **Incompatibilities:** Other IV drugs.

ACTION

Inhibits sodium-potassium–activated adenosine triphosphatase, promoting movement of calcium from extracellular to intracellular cytoplasm and strengthening myocardial contraction. Also acts on CNS to enhance vagal tone, slowing conduction through the SA and AV nodes.

Route	Onset	Peak	Duration
PO	30–120 min	2–6 hr	3–4 days
IV	5–30 min	1–4 hr	3–4 days

Half-life: With normal renal function: adults, 36 to 48 hours; children, 18 to 36 hours.

ADVERSE REACTIONS

CNS: agitation, fatigue, generalized muscle weakness, hallucinations, dizziness, headache, malaise, paresthesia, stupor, vertigo. **CV:** *arrhythmias, heart block.* **EENT:** blurred vision, diplopia, light flashes, photophobia, yellow-green halos around visual images. **GI:** anorexia, nausea, diarrhea, vomiting.

INTERACTIONS

Drug-drug. *Amiloride:* May decrease digoxin effect and increase renal clearance of digoxin. Monitor patient for altered digoxin effect.

Amiodarone, diltiazem, dronedarone, indomethacin, nifedipine, protease inhibitors, quinidine, verapamil: May increase digoxin level. Monitor patient for toxicity.

Amphotericin B, carbenicillin, corticosteroids, diuretics (chlorthalidone, loop diuretics, metolazone), ticarcillin: May cause hypokalemia and hypomagnesemia, predisposing patient to cardiac glycoside toxicity. Monitor electrolyte levels.

Antacids: May decrease absorption of oral digoxin. Separate doses as much as possible.

Antibiotics (azole antifungals, macrolides, telithromycin, tetracyclines), propafenone, ritonavir: May increase risk of cardiac

glycoside toxicity. Monitor patient for toxicity.

Beta blockers, calcium channel blockers: May have additive effects on AV node conduction, causing advanced or complete heart block. Use cautiously.

Cholestyramine, colestipol, metoclopramide: May decrease absorption of oral digoxin. Monitor patient for decreased digoxin level and effect. Give digoxin 1½ hours before or 2 hours after other drugs.

Parenteral calcium, thiazides: May cause hypercalcemia and hypomagnesemia, predisposing patient to digitalis toxicity. Monitor calcium and magnesium levels.

Drug-herb. *Foxglove, fumitory, goldenseal, hawthorn:* May increase cardiac effects. Discourage use together.

Licorice, Siberian ginseng: May increase toxicity. Monitor patient closely.

St. John's wort: May decrease digoxin serum concentration. Monitor therapy.

EFFECTS ON LAB TEST RESULTS

• May prolong PR interval or depress ST segment.

CONTRAINDICATIONS & CAUTIONS

• Contraindicated in patients hypersensitive to drug and in those with digitalis-induced toxicity, ventricular fibrillation, or ventricular tachycardia unless caused by HF.

• Don't use in patients with Wolff-Parkinson-White syndrome unless the conduction accessory pathway has been pharmacologically or surgically disabled.

• Use with extreme caution in elderly patients and in those with acute MI, incomplete AV block, sinus bradycardia, PVCs, chronic constrictive pericarditis, hypertrophic cardiomyopathy, renal insufficiency, severe pulmonary disease, or hypothyroidism.

Dialyzable drug: No.

⚠ **Overdose S&S:** Ventricular tachycardia, ventricular fibrillation, bradycardia, heart block, cardiac arrest, hyperkalemia.

PREGNANCY-LACTATION-REPRODUCTION

• It isn't known if drug can cause fetal harm when used during pregnancy or if drug can affect reproductive capacity. Use during pregnancy only if clearly needed.

✦Canada ◇OTC ◆Off-label use ℗Photoguide ⓓⓝⓒDo not crush *Liquid contains alcohol ▓Genetic

• Drug appears in human milk; however, a breastfeeding infant is exposed to an amount estimated to be far below the usual infant maintenance dose. Use cautiously, but the amount should have no pharmacologic effect on a breastfeeding infant.

NURSING CONSIDERATIONS

• Drug-induced arrhythmias may increase the severity of HF and hypotension.
• In children, cardiac arrhythmias, including sinus bradycardia, are usually early signs of toxicity.
• Patients with hypothyroidism are extremely sensitive to cardiac glycosides and may need lower doses.
• According to the 2013 guideline for the management of HF (American College of Cardiology Foundation/American Heart Association), there is no reason to use loading doses to initiate digoxin therapy in patients with HF. The guideline indicates that digoxin therapy is usually initiated and maintained at 0.125 to 0.25 mg PO once daily; higher daily doses (up to 0.5 mg/day) are rarely necessary. If patient is older than age 70, has impaired renal function, or has a low lean body mass, initially use low doses (0.125 mg daily or every other day).
• Monitor patient for toxicity. Toxic effects on the heart may be life-threatening and require immediate attention. Signs and symptoms of toxicity include anorexia, nausea, vomiting, visual changes, and cardiac arrhythmias. Patients with low body weight, advanced age, renal impairment, and electrolyte disturbances are at increased risk.
• Monitor digoxin level. Therapeutic level ranges from 0.5 to 2 nanograms/mL. Obtain blood for digoxin level at least 6 to 8 hours after last oral dose, preferably just before next scheduled dose.

Alert: Excessively slow pulse rate (60 beats/minute [bpm] or less) may be a sign of digitalis toxicity. Withhold drug and notify prescriber.

• Monitor potassium level carefully. Take corrective action before hypokalemia occurs. Hyperkalemia may result from digoxin toxicity.
• Reduce dose or discontinue drug for 1 or 2 days before elective cardioversion. Adjust dosage after cardioversion.
• ***Look alike–sound alike:*** Don't confuse digoxin with doxepin.

PATIENT TEACHING

• Teach patient and a responsible family member about drug action, dosage regimen, how to take pulse, reportable signs, and follow-up care.
• Tell patient to report pulse rate less than 60 bpm or more than 110 bpm or skipped beats or other rhythm changes.
• Instruct patient to report all adverse reactions promptly. Nausea, vomiting, diarrhea, appetite loss, and visual disturbances may indicate toxicity.
• Encourage patient to eat a consistent amount of potassium-rich foods.
• Tell patient not to substitute one brand for another.
• Advise patient to avoid using herbal supplements and to consult prescriber before taking one.

dilTIAZem hydrochloride

dil-TYE-a-zem

Apo-Diltiaz, Cardizem, Cardizem CD, Cardizem LA, Cartia XT, Dilt XR, Matzim LA, Taztia XT, Tiazac, Tiazac XC

Therapeutic class: Antihypertensives
Pharmacologic class: Calcium channel blockers

AVAILABLE FORMS

Capsules (extended-release) DNC: 60 mg, 90 mg, 120 mg, 180 mg, 240 mg, 300 mg, 360 mg, 420 mg
Injection: 5 mg/mL in 5-, 10-, and 25-mL vials
Powder for injection: 100 mg
Tablets: 30 mg, 60 mg, 90 mg, 120 mg
Tablets (extended-release) DNC: 120 mg, 180 mg, 240 mg, 300 mg, 360 mg, 420 mg

INDICATIONS & DOSAGES

➤ **To manage Prinzmetal or variant angina or chronic stable angina pectoris**
Adults: 30 mg PO q.i.d. (immediate-release tablets) before meals and at bedtime. Increase dose gradually to maximum of 360 mg/day divided into three or

four doses, as indicated. Or, give 120- or 180-mg extended-release capsule or 180-mg extended-release tablet PO once daily. Adjust over a 7- to 14-day period as needed and tolerated up to a maximum dose of 360 mg/day (Cardizem LA, Matzim LA), 480 mg/day (Cardizem CD, Cartia XT), or 540 mg/day (Tiazac, Taztia XT).

➤ **HTN, alone or as combination therapy**
Adults: Initially 180 to 240 mg extended-release capsules PO once daily. Adjust dosage based on patient response to a maximum dose of 480 mg/day (Cardizem CD, Cartia XT). Or, 120 to 240 mg extended-release capsules PO once daily. Adjust dosage based on patient response to a maximum dose of 540 mg/day (Tiazac, Taztia XT). Or, 180 to 240 mg extended-release tablet PO once daily. Dosage can be adjusted approximately every 14 days to a maximum of 540 mg daily.

➤ **Atrial fibrillation or flutter; paroxysmal supraventricular tachycardia**
Adults: 0.25 mg/kg IV as a bolus injection over 2 minutes. Repeat after 15 minutes if response isn't adequate with a dose of 0.35 mg/kg IV over 2 minutes. Follow bolus with continuous IV infusion at 5 to 15 mg/hour (for up to 24 hours).

➤ **Improvement of exercise tolerance in patients with chronic stable angina (Cardizem LA)**
Adults: Initially, 180 mg extended-release tablets PO once daily; increase dose at intervals of 7 to 14 days until adequate response is obtained. Maximum dosage is 360 mg.

ADMINISTRATION
PO
• Don't crush or allow patient to chew extended-release tablets or capsules; they should be swallowed whole.
• Tiazac and Taztia extended-release capsules can be opened and the contents sprinkled onto a spoonful of applesauce. The applesauce must be eaten immediately and without chewing, followed by a glass of cool water.

IV
▼ For direct injection, you need not dilute the 5 mg/mL injection.
▼ For continuous infusion, refer to manufacturer's instructions for dilution and ad-

ministration. Compatible solutions include NSS, D$_5$W, or 5% dextrose and half-NSS.
▼ Continuous infusion rate ranges from 5 to 15 mg/hour.
▼ For direct injection or continuous infusion, give slowly while monitoring ECG and BP continuously.
▼ Don't infuse for longer than 24 hours.
▼ **Incompatibilities:** Acetazolamide, acyclovir, aminophylline, ampicillin, ampicillin sodium–sulbactam sodium, diazepam, furosemide, heparin, hydrocortisone, insulin, methylprednisolone, nafcillin, phenytoin, rifampin, sodium bicarbonate, thiopental.

ACTION
A calcium channel blocker that inhibits calcium ion influx across cardiac and smooth-muscle cells, decreasing myocardial contractility and oxygen demand. Drug also dilates coronary arteries and arterioles.

Route	Onset	Peak	Duration
PO	30–60 min	2–3 hr	6–8 hr
PO (extended-release capsule)	2–3 hr	10–14 hr	12–24 hr
PO (Cardizem LA, Matzim LA)	3–4 hr	11–18 hr	6–9 hr
IV	<3 min	2–7 min	1–10 hr

Half-life: 3 to 9 hours.

ADVERSE REACTIONS
CNS: headache, dizziness, asthenia, somnolence. **CV:** edema, *arrhythmias, AV block, bradycardia, HF,* flushing, hypotension, conduction abnormalities, abnormal ECG. **GI:** nausea, constipation, abdominal discomfort. **Hepatic:** *acute hepatic injury.* **Skin:** rash.

INTERACTIONS
Drug-drug. *Anesthetics:* May increase effects of anesthetics. Monitor patient.
Atazanavir, cimetidine: May inhibit diltiazem metabolism, increasing additive AV node conduction slowing. Monitor patient for toxicity.
Buspirone, quinidine, sirolimus, tacrolimus: May increase level of these drugs. Monitor drug levels and patient for toxicity.
Carbamazepine: May increase level of carbamazepine. Monitor carbamazepine

level, and watch for signs and symptoms of toxicity.

Cyclosporine: May increase cyclosporine level. Monitor cyclosporine level with each dosage change.

Diazepam, midazolam, triazolam: May increase CNS depression and prolonged effects of these drugs. Use lower dose of these benzodiazepines.

Digoxin: May increase digoxin level. Monitor patient for digoxin toxicity.

HMG-CoA reductase inhibitors (lovastatin, simvastatin): May increase risk of myopathy, rhabdomyolysis, and kidney failure. Use lower starting and maintenance doses of diltiazem and statins.

Lithium: May reduce lithium level, causing loss of mania control. May also enhance lithium's neurotoxic effects. Monitor therapy.

Propranolol, other beta blockers: May precipitate HF or prolong conduction time. Use together cautiously.

Rifampin: May lower diltiazem level significantly. Avoid use together.

Theophylline: May enhance action of theophylline, causing intoxication. Monitor theophylline levels.

EFFECTS ON LAB TEST RESULTS
• May increase ALT, AST, LDH, bilirubin, and alkaline phosphatase levels.

CONTRAINDICATIONS & CAUTIONS
• Contraindicated in patients hypersensitive to drug and in those with sick sinus syndrome or second- or third-degree AV block in the absence of an artificial pacemaker, hypotension (systolic less than 90 mm Hg), acute MI, and pulmonary congestion.

• Additional contraindications for IV form include patients who have atrial fibrillation or flutter with an accessory bypass tract, as in Wolff-Parkinson-White syndrome or short PR interval syndrome, cardiogenic shock, and ventricular tachycardia, and within a few hours of IV beta-blocker therapy.

• Use cautiously in elderly patients and in those with HF, hypertrophic obstructive cardiomyopathy, or impaired hepatic or renal function.

Dialyzable drug: No.

⚠ *Overdose S&S:* Bradycardia, hypotension, heart block, cardiac failure.

PREGNANCY-LACTATION-REPRODUCTION
• There are no adequate well-controlled studies in pregnant women. Use during pregnancy only if clearly needed and potential benefit justifies potential risk to the fetus.

• Drug appears in human milk. Patient should discontinue breastfeeding or discontinue drug, taking into account importance of drug to the mother.

NURSING CONSIDERATIONS
• Patients controlled on drug alone or with other drugs may be switched to Cardizem LA tablets once a day at the nearest equivalent total daily dose.

• Monitor BP and HR when starting therapy and during dosage adjustments.

• Maximal antihypertensive effect may not be seen for 14 days.

• If systolic BP is below 90 mm Hg or HR is below 60 beats/minute, withhold dose and notify prescriber.

• *Look alike–sound alike:* Don't confuse Tiazac with Ziac.

PATIENT TEACHING
• Instruct patient to take drug as prescribed, even when feeling better, and to report all adverse reactions.

• Advise patient to avoid hazardous activities during start of therapy.

• If nitrate therapy is prescribed during dosage adjustment, stress patient compliance. Tell patient that SL nitroglycerin may be taken with drug, as needed, when angina symptoms are acute.

⚠ *Alert:* Tell patient to swallow extended-release tablets whole, and not to crush or chew them.

• Inform patient taking Tiazac or Taztia extended-release capsules that these capsules can be opened and the contents sprinkled on a spoonful of applesauce. Advise patient to eat the applesauce immediately and without chewing, and then drink a glass of cool water.

Reactions in bold italics are *life-threatening*. Interactions may have a *rapid onset* or a *delayed onset*.

diphenhydrAMINE hydrochloride

dye-fen-HYE-drah-meen

Banophen ◊, Benadryl ◊, Children's Benadryl Allergy ◊, Sominex ◊, Unisom SleepMelts ◊

Therapeutic class: Antihistamines
Pharmacologic class: Ethanolamines

AVAILABLE FORMS

Capsules: 25 mg ◊, 50 mg ◊
Elixir: 12.5 mg/5 mL ◊*
Injection: 50 mg/mL
Syrup: 12.5 mg/5 mL ◊*
Tablets: 25 mg ◊, 50 mg ◊
Tablets (chewable): 12.5 mg ◊
Tablets (ODTs): 12.5 mg ◊, 25 mg ◊

INDICATIONS & DOSAGES

➤ **Rhinitis, allergy symptoms, motion sickness, Parkinson disease**
Adults and children age 12 and older: 25 to 50 mg PO every 4 to 6 hours. Maximum, 300 mg PO daily. Or, 10 to 50 mg IV or deep IM. Maximum IV or IM dosage, 400 mg daily. Don't exceed 25 mg/minute when giving IV.
Children ages 6 to 11: 12.5 to 25 mg PO every 4 to 6 hours. Maximum dose is 150 mg daily.
Children other than premature infants and neonates: 5 mg/kg/24 hours deep IM or IV divided into four doses. Don't exceed 25 mg/minute when giving IV. Maximum dose is 300 mg daily.

➤ **Nighttime sleep aid**
Adults and children age 12 and older: 50 mg PO at bedtime.

➤ **Nonproductive cough**
Adults and children age 12 and older: 25 mg (syrup) PO every 4 hours. Don't exceed 150 mg daily. Or, 25 to 50 mg (liquid) PO every 4 hours. Don't exceed 300 mg daily.

ADMINISTRATION

PO
• Give drug with food or milk to reduce GI distress.

IV
▼ For injection, don't exceed 25 mg/minute.
▼ **Incompatibilities:** Allopurinol, amobarbital, amphotericin B, cefepime, dexamethasone, foscarnet, haloperidol, pentobarbital, phenobarbital, phenytoin, thiopental.
IM
• Give IM injection deep into large muscle; alternate injection sites to prevent irritation.

ACTION

Competes with histamine for H_1-receptor sites. Prevents, but doesn't reverse, histamine-mediated responses, particularly those of the bronchial tubes, GI tract, uterus, and blood vessels.

Route	Onset	Peak	Duration
PO	15 min	1–4 hr	3–6 hr
IV	Immediate	1–4 hr	3–6 hr
IM	Unknown	1–4 hr	3–6 hr

Half-life: About 4 to 18 hours.

ADVERSE REACTIONS

CNS: drowsiness, sedation, sleepiness, dizziness, incoordination, *seizures,* confusion, insomnia, headache, vertigo, fatigue, restlessness, tremor, nervousness. **CV:** palpitations, hypotension, tachycardia. **EENT:** diplopia, blurred vision, nasal congestion, tinnitus. **GI:** dry mouth, nausea, epigastric distress, vomiting, diarrhea, constipation, anorexia. **GU:** dysuria, urine retention, urinary frequency, early menses. **Hematologic:** *thrombocytopenia, agranulocytosis,* hemolytic anemia. **Respiratory:** thickening of bronchial secretions. **Skin:** urticaria, photosensitivity, rash. **Other:** *anaphylactic shock.*

INTERACTIONS

Drug-drug. *CNS depressants:* May increase sedation. Use together cautiously.
MAO inhibitors: May increase anticholinergic effects. Avoid using together.
Other products that contain diphenhydramine (including topical therapy): May increase risk of adverse reactions. Avoid using together.
Drug-lifestyle. *Alcohol use:* May increase CNS depression. Discourage use together.

Sun exposure: May cause photosensitivity reactions. Advise patient to avoid extensive sunlight exposure.

EFFECTS ON LAB TEST RESULTS
• May decrease Hb level and hematocrit.
• May decrease granulocyte and platelet counts.
• May prevent, reduce, or mask positive result in diagnostic skin test.
• May produce false-positives in urine detection of methadone and phencyclidine and in serum TCA screens.

CONTRAINDICATIONS & CAUTIONS
• Contraindicated in patients hypersensitive to drug and other similar antihistamines, in newborns, and in premature neonates.
• Use cautiously in patients with angle-closure glaucoma, stenosing peptic ulcer, symptomatic prostatic hyperplasia, bladder neck obstruction, pyloroduodenal obstruction, or asthma.
• Avoid use in patients taking MAO inhibitors.
• Use with caution in patients with prostatic hyperplasia, asthma, COPD, increased IOP, hyperthyroidism, CV disease, and HTN.
• Children younger than age 12 should use drug only as directed by prescriber.
Dialyzable drug: Unlikely.
⚠ *Overdose S&S:* Dry mouth, fixed or dilated pupils, flushing, GI symptoms.

PREGNANCY-LACTATION-REPRODUCTION
• There are no adequate well-controlled studies in pregnant women. Use during pregnancy only if clearly needed.
• Drug appears in human milk. Contraindicated in breastfeeding women.

NURSING CONSIDERATIONS
• Stop drug 4 days before diagnostic skin testing.
• Injection form is for IV or IM administration only.
• Dizziness, excessive sedation, syncope, toxicity, paradoxical stimulation, and hypotension are more likely to occur in elderly patients.
• *Look alike–sound alike:* Don't confuse diphenhydramine with dimenhydrinate.

Don't confuse Benadryl with Bentyl or benazepril.

PATIENT TEACHING
• Warn patient not to take this drug with any other products that contain diphenhydramine (including topical therapy) because of increased adverse reactions.
• Instruct patient to take drug 30 minutes before travel to prevent motion sickness.
• Tell patient to take diphenhydramine with food or milk to reduce GI distress.
• Warn patient to avoid alcohol and hazardous activities that require alertness until CNS effects of drug are known.
• Tell patient to notify prescriber if tolerance develops because a different antihistamine may need to be prescribed.
• Drug is in many OTC sleep and cold products. Advise patient to consult prescriber before using these products.
• Warn patient of possible photosensitivity reactions. Advise use of a sunblock.

dipyridamole
dye-peer-IH-duh-mohl

Persantine

Therapeutic class: Antiplatelet drugs
Pharmacologic class: Pyrimidine analogues

AVAILABLE FORMS
Injection: 5 mg/mL in 2-mL and 10-mL vials
Tablets: 25 mg, 50 mg, 75 mg

INDICATIONS & DOSAGES
➤ **To inhibit platelet adhesion in prosthetic heart valves (given together with warfarin)**
Adults and children age 12 and older: 75 to 100 mg PO q.i.d.
➤ **Alternative to exercise in evaluation of CAD during thallium myocardial perfusion scintigraphy**
Adults: 0.57 mg/kg (total dose) as an IV infusion at a constant rate over 4 minutes (0.142 mg/kg/minute).

ADMINISTRATION
PO
• If GI distress develops, give drug 1 hour before meals or with meals.
IV
▼ For use as a diagnostic drug, dilute in half-NSS, NSS, or D₅W in at least a 1:2 ratio for a total volume of 20 to 50 mL.

▼ Inject thallium-201 within 5 minutes after completing the 4-minute dipyridamole infusion.

▼ Don't mix in same syringe or infusion container with other drugs.

▼ **Incompatibilities:** Other drugs.

ACTION
Inhibits adenosine deaminase and phosphodiesterase, which increases adenosine, a coronary vasodilator and platelet aggregation inhibitor.

Route	Onset	Peak	Duration
PO	Unknown	75 min	Unknown
IV	Unknown	2 min	Unknown

Half-life: 1 to 12 hours; alpha half-life of oral form, 40 minutes; beta half-life of oral form, 10 hours.

ADVERSE REACTIONS
CNS: dizziness, headache, fatigue. **CV:** angina pectoris, chest pain, *ECG abnormalities,* flushing, hypotension, HTN. **GI:** nausea, abdominal distress, diarrhea, vomiting. **Skin:** rash, pruritus.

INTERACTIONS
Drug-drug. *Adenosine:* May increase levels and cardiac effects of adenosine. Adjust adenosine dose as needed.

Anticoagulants, apixaban, dabigatran, drugs with antiplatelet properties (NSAIDs, P2Y12 inhibitors, SSRIs), edoxaban, heparin, rivaroxaban, salicylates, thrombolytics: May increase bleeding risks. Monitor therapy.

Cholinesterase inhibitors: May counteract anticholinesterase effects and aggravate myasthenia gravis. Monitor patient.

Theophylline, other xanthine derivatives: May prevent coronary vasodilation by IV dipyridamole, causing a false-negative thallium-imaging result. Avoid using together.

EFFECTS ON LAB TEST RESULTS
• May increase liver enzyme levels.

CONTRAINDICATIONS & CAUTIONS
• Contraindicated in patients hypersensitive to drug.

• Use cautiously in patients with hypotension or severe CAD.

🜂 *Alert:* IV drug is associated with cardiac death, fatal and nonfatal MI, ventricular fibrillation, symptomatic ventricular tachycardia, stroke, transient cerebral ischemia, seizures, anaphylactoid reaction, and bronchospasm.

• Patients with myasthenia gravis who are receiving cholinesterase inhibitors may experience worsening of their disease when exposed to the IV drug.

• Safety and effectiveness in children younger than age 12 haven't been established.

Dialyzable drug: Unlikely.

⚠ *Overdose S&S:* Hypotension, warm feeling, flushes, sweating, restlessness, weakness, dizziness, tachycardia.

PREGNANCY-LACTATION-REPRODUCTION
• There are no adequate well-controlled studies in pregnant women. Use during pregnancy only if clearly needed.

• Drug appears in human milk. Use cautiously in breastfeeding women.

NURSING CONSIDERATIONS
• Observe for adverse reactions, especially with large doses. Monitor BP.

• Observe for signs and symptoms of bleeding.

• Dipyridamole injection may contain tartrazine, which may cause allergic reactions in some patients.

• *Look alike–sound alike:* Don't confuse dipyridamole with disopyramide.

PATIENT TEACHING
• Instruct patient to take drug exactly as prescribed.

• Tell patient to report adverse reactions promptly.

• Tell patient receiving drug IV to report discomfort at IV insertion site.

SAFETY ALERT!

DOBUTamine hydrochloride
DOE-byoo-ta-meen

Therapeutic class: Inotropes
Pharmacologic class: Adrenergics–beta$_1$ agonists

AVAILABLE FORMS
Dobutamine in 5% dextrose: 1 mg/mL (250 or 500 mg); 2 mg/mL (500 mg); 4 mg/mL (1,000 mg)
Injection: 12.5 mg/mL in 20-mL and 40-mL vials (parenteral)

INDICATIONS & DOSAGES
➤ **To increase cardiac output during short-term treatment of cardiac decompensation caused by depressed contractility, such as during refractory HF; adjunctive therapy in cardiac surgery**
Adults: 0.5 to 1 mcg/kg/minute IV infusion, titrating to optimum dosage of 2 to 20 mcg/kg/minute. Usual effective range to increase cardiac output is 2.5 to 15 mcg/kg/minute. Usual maximum dosage is 20 mcg/minute and, rarely, rates up to 40 mcg/kg/minute may be needed.

ADMINISTRATION
IV
▼ Before starting therapy, give a plasma volume expander to correct hypovolemia and, in patients who have atrial fibrillation with rapid ventricular response, a cardiac glycoside.
▼ Dilute concentrate before injecting. Compatible solutions include D_5W, $D_{10}W$, D_5W and NSS injection, D_5W and half-NSS injection, D_5W in lactated Ringer injection, NSS for injection, lactated Ringer solution for injection, Isolyte-M with D_5W, Normosol-M in D_5W, 20% mannitol in water for injection, and sodium lactate injection.
▼ Oxidation may slightly discolor admixture. This doesn't indicate a significant loss of potency, provided drug is used within 24 hours of reconstitution.
▼ Don't administer unless solution is clear and container is undamaged.

▼ Give through a CVAD or large peripheral vein using an infusion pump.
▼ Titrate rate according to patient's condition.
▼ Infusions lasting up to 72 hours produce no more adverse effects than shorter infusions.
▼ Watch for irritation and infiltration; extravasation can cause tissue damage and necrosis. Change IV sites regularly to avoid phlebitis.
▼ Solution remains stable for 24 hours. Don't freeze.
▼ **Incompatibilities:** Diluents containing both sodium bisulfite and ethanol and other drugs, 5% sodium bicarbonate injection and other strongly alkaline solutions.

ACTION
Stimulates heart's beta$_1$ receptors to increase myocardial contractility and stroke volume. At therapeutic dosages, drug increases cardiac output by decreasing peripheral vascular resistance, reducing ventricular filling pressure, and facilitating AV node conduction.

Route	Onset	Peak	Duration
IV	1–2 min	10 min	<5 min after infusion

Half-life: 2 minutes.

ADVERSE REACTIONS
CNS: headache. **CV:** HTN, increased HR, angina, PVCs, phlebitis, nonspecific chest pain, palpitations, ventricular ectopy, hypotension. **GI:** nausea, vomiting. **Respiratory:** *asthma attack,* shortness of breath. **Other:** *anaphylaxis,* hypersensitivity reactions.

INTERACTIONS
Drug-drug. *Beta blockers:* May antagonize dobutamine effects. Avoid using together.
Guanethidine, oxytocic drugs: May increase pressor response, causing severe HTN. Monitor BP closely.
Linezolid: May increase hypertensive effect of sympathomimetics. May need to decrease initial doses of dobutamine and titrate to effect.
TCAs: May potentiate pressor response and cause arrhythmias. Use together cautiously.

Reactions in bold italics are *life-threatening*. Interactions may have a *rapid onset* or a *delayed onset*.

Drug-herb. *Rue:* May increase inotropic potential. Discourage use together.

EFFECTS ON LAB TEST RESULTS
• May decrease potassium level.
• May decrease platelet count.

CONTRAINDICATIONS & CAUTIONS
• Contraindicated in patients hypersensitive to drug or its components and in those with idiopathic hypertrophic subaortic stenosis.
• Use cautiously in patients with history of HTN because drug may increase pressor response.
• Use cautiously after acute MI.
• Use cautiously in patients with history of sulfite sensitivity. Anaphylaxis or asthmatic episodes can occur.
• May precipitate or exacerbate ventricular ectopic activity, but rarely has caused ventricular tachycardia.
Dialyzable drug: Unknown.
⚠ **Overdose S&S:** Anorexia, nausea, vomiting, tremor, anxiety, palpitations, headache, shortness of breath, anginal and nonspecific chest pain, HTN, tachyarrhythmias, myocardial ischemia, ventricular fibrillation, hypotension.

PREGNANCY-LACTATION-REPRODUCTION
• There are no adequate well-controlled studies in pregnant women. Use during pregnancy only if clearly needed and potential benefit justifies potential risk to the fetus.
• It isn't known if drug appears in human milk. Use cautiously in breastfeeding women or discontinue breastfeeding during therapy.

NURSING CONSIDERATIONS
⊕ *Alert:* Because drug increases AV node conduction, patients with atrial fibrillation may develop a rapid ventricular rate.
• Continuously monitor ECG, BP, pulmonary artery wedge pressure, cardiac output, and urine output during therapy.
• Correct hypovolemia before therapy.
• Monitor electrolyte levels. Drug may lower potassium level.
• *Look alike–sound alike:* Don't confuse dobutamine with dopamine.

PATIENT TEACHING
• Tell patient to report all adverse reactions promptly, especially labored breathing, angina, palpitations, dizziness, and drug-induced headache.
• Instruct patient to report discomfort at IV insertion site.

SAFETY ALERT!

DOCEtaxel
dohs-eh-TAX-ell

Taxotere*

Therapeutic class: Antineoplastics
Pharmacologic class: Taxoids

AVAILABLE FORMS
Injection concentrate:* 20 mg/0.5 mL, 20 mg/mL, 80 mg/2 mL, 80 mg/4 mL, 160 mg/8 mL, 200 mg/10 mL
Injection solution: 20 mg/mL, 20 mg/2 mL*, 80 mg/4 mL, 80 mg/8 mL*, 160 mg/8 mL, 160 mg/16 mL*

INDICATIONS & DOSAGES
Adjust-a-dose (for all indications): Refer to manufacturer's instructions for toxicity-related dosage adjustments and treatment.
➤ **Locally advanced or metastatic breast cancer after failure of previous chemotherapy**
Adults: 60 to 100 mg/m^2 IV over 1 hour every 3 weeks.
➤ **Adjuvant postsurgery treatment of operable, node-positive breast cancer**
Adults: 75 mg/m^2 IV as a 1-hour infusion given 1 hour after doxorubicin 50 mg/m^2 and cyclophosphamide 500 mg/m^2 every 3 weeks for six cycles. May use prophylactic G-CSF therapy to decrease risk of hematologic toxicities.
➤ **Locally advanced or metastatic NSCLC after failure of previous cisplatin-based chemotherapy**
Adults: 75 mg/m^2 IV over 1 hour every 3 weeks.
➤ **With cisplatin, unresectable, locally advanced, or metastatic NSCLC not previously treated with chemotherapy**

Adults: 75 mg/m^2 docetaxel IV over 1 hour, immediately followed by cisplatin 75 mg/m^2 IV over 30 to 60 minutes every 3 weeks.

➤ **Metastatic castration-resistant prostate cancer, with prednisone**

Adults: 75 mg/m^2 IV, as a 1-hour infusion every 3 weeks, given with 5 mg prednisone PO b.i.d. continuously. Premedicate with dexamethasone 8 mg PO at 12 hours, 3 hours, and 1 hour before docetaxel infusion.

➤ **Advanced gastric adenocarcinoma, in combination with cisplatin and 5-FU**

Adults: Premedicate with antiemetics and hydration per cisplatin recommendations. Give 75 mg/m^2 docetaxel IV over 1 hour, followed by cisplatin 75 mg/m^2 IV over 1 to 3 hours both on day 1 only, then 5-FU 750 mg/m^2 IV daily as a 24-hour continuous infusion for 5 days beginning at the end of cisplatin infusion. Repeat cycle every 3 weeks.

➤ **Induction treatment of inoperable locally advanced squamous cell cancer of the head and neck (SCCHN), with cisplatin and 5-FU**

Adults: Premedicate with antiemetics and hydration per cisplatin recommendations. Use prophylaxis for neutropenic infections. Give 75 mg/m^2 IV infusion over 1 hour, followed by cisplatin 75 mg/m^2 IV infusion over 1 hour, on day 1, followed by 5-FU 750 mg/m^2 daily as a continuous IV infusion for 5 days. Repeat this regimen every 3 weeks for four cycles. After chemotherapy, patients should receive radiotherapy.

➤ **Induction treatment for locally advanced (unresectable, low surgical cure, or organ preservation) SCCHN with cisplatin and 5-FU before chemoradiotherapy**

Adults: Premedicate with antiemetics and hydration per cisplatin recommendations. Give 75 mg/m^2 IV infusion over 1 hour, followed by cisplatin 100 mg/m^2 IV infusion over 30 minutes to 3 hours on day 1, followed by 5-FU 1,000 mg/m^2 daily as a continuous IV infusion from day 1 to day 4. Repeat this regimen every 3 weeks for three cycles. After chemotherapy, patients should receive chemoradiotherapy.

ADMINISTRATION

IV

▼ Give oral corticosteroid such as dexamethasone 16 mg PO (8 mg b.i.d.) daily for 3 days, starting 1 day before docetaxel administration, to reduce risk or severity of fluid retention and hypersensitivity reactions.

▼ Wear gloves to prepare and give drug. If solution contacts skin, wash immediately and thoroughly with soap and water. If solution contacts mucous membranes, flush thoroughly with water.

🕄 *Alert:* Carefully read package instructions and confirm concentration being used; admixture errors have occurred due to the availability of various concentrations.

▼ If using the 2-vial formulation, dilute using supplied diluent. Let drug and diluent stand at room temperature for 5 minutes before mixing. After adding all the diluent to drug vial, gently rotate vial for about 45 seconds. Let solution stand for a few minutes so foam dissipates. All foam need not dissipate before preparing infusion solution.

▼ If using the 1-vial formulation, no dilution is needed. The product comes ready to add to the infusion solution.

▼ Prepare infusion solution by withdrawing needed amount of premixed solution from vial and injecting it into 250 mL NSS or D$_5$W to yield 0.3 to 0.74 mg/mL. Doses of more than 200 mg need a larger volume to stay below 0.74 mg/mL of drug. Mix infusion thoroughly by manual rotation.

▼ Prepare and store infusion solution in bottles (glass, polyolefin, or polypropylene) or plastic bags, and give through polyethylene-lined administration sets.

▼ Contact between undiluted concentrate and polyvinyl chloride equipment or devices isn't recommended.

▼ If solution isn't clear or if it contains precipitate, discard.

▼ The first dilution is stable for 8 hours. Use infusion solution within 4 hours.

▼ Infuse over 1 hour.

▼ Store unopened vials between 36° and 77° F (2° and 25° C).

🕄 *Alert:* Mark all waste materials with CHEMOTHERAPY HAZARD labels.

Reactions in bold italics are *life-threatening*. Interactions may have a *rapid onset* or a *delayed onset*.

▼ **Incompatibilities:** None listed by manufacturer. Consult a drug incompatibility reference for more information.

ACTION
Promotes formation and stabilization of nonfunctional microtubules. This prevents mitosis and leads to cell death.

Route	Onset	Peak	Duration
IV	Rapid	Unknown	Unknown

Half-life: Terminal phase, 11 hours.

ADVERSE REACTIONS
CNS: asthenia, paresthesia, dysesthesia, peripheral neuropathy, weakness. **CV:** fluid retention, peripheral edema, *arrhythmias,* chest tightness, flushing, hypotension. **EENT:** altered hearing, tearing. **GI:** anorexia, diarrhea, dysphagia, esophagitis, nausea, stomatitis, vomiting, dysgeusia. **Hematologic:** *febrile neutropenia, leukopenia, myelosuppression, neutropenia, thrombocytopenia,* anemia. **Hepatic:** *hepatotoxicity.* **Musculoskeletal:** myalgia, arthralgia, back pain. **Respiratory:** dyspnea, *pulmonary edema.* **Skin:** alopecia, desquamation, skin eruptions, nail pigmentation alterations, nail pain, rash, reaction at injection site. **Other:** infection, chills, drug fever, hypersensitivity reactions.

INTERACTIONS
Drug-drug. *Compounds that induce, inhibit, or are metabolized by CYP3A4 (cyclosporine, erythromycin, ketoconazole, troleandomycin):* May modify metabolism of docetaxel. Use together cautiously.
Ketoconazole or other CYP3A4 inhibitors: May increase docetaxel level and toxicity, including neutropenia. Monitor patient closely. Consider docetaxel dosage reduction if administration with strong CYP3A4 inhibitors can't be avoided.

EFFECTS ON LAB TEST RESULTS
• May increase alkaline phosphatase, ALT, AST, and bilirubin levels. May decrease Hb level.
• May decrease platelet and WBC counts.

CONTRAINDICATIONS & CAUTIONS
Black Box Warning Contraindicated in patients with neutrophil counts less than 1,500/mm^3. Perform frequent blood cell counts during therapy. ■
Black Box Warning Treatment-related mortality increases in patients with abnormal liver function, those receiving higher doses, and patients with NSCLC and a history of prior treatment with platinum-based chemotherapy who receive docetaxel as a single agent at a dose of 100 mg/m^2. ■
Black Box Warning Patients with severe hepatic impairment shouldn't receive this drug. Don't give drug to patients with bilirubin levels exceeding the ULN, or those with ALT or AST levels above 1.5 × ULN and alkaline phosphatase levels above 2.5 × ULN. Obtain bilirubin, AST or ALT, and alkaline phosphatase levels before each therapy cycle. ■
Black Box Warning Contraindicated in patients severely hypersensitive to drug or with a history of hypersensitivity to polysorbate 80. Some dosage forms may contain polysorbate 80. ■
• Safety and effectiveness in children haven't been established.
• Discontinue treatment if cystoid macular edema develops.
• **Alert:** Some drug formulations may contain alcohol. Use cautiously in patients with hepatic impairment and in those in whom ethanol intake should be avoided or minimized. Some medications, such as pain relievers and sleep aids, may interact with the alcohol in the docetaxel infusion and worsen the intoxicating effects. A generic, nonalcoholic form of docetaxel is available.
Dialyzable drug: No.
⚠ *Overdose S&S:* Severe neutropenia, mild asthenia, cutaneous reactions, mild paresthesia, bone marrow suppression, peripheral neurotoxicity, mucositis.

PREGNANCY-LACTATION-REPRODUCTION
• Drug can cause fetal harm when used during pregnancy. Advise women of childbearing potential to avoid becoming pregnant during therapy.
• It isn't known if drug appears in human milk. Patient should discontinue breastfeeding

or discontinue drug, taking into account importance of drug to the mother.

NURSING CONSIDERATIONS

❸ *Alert:* Drug should be administered only under the supervision of a physician experienced with antineoplastics and in a facility equipped to handle anaphylaxis.

• Bone marrow toxicity is the most frequent and dose-limiting toxicity. Frequent blood count monitoring is needed during therapy.

Black Box Warning Monitor patient closely for hypersensitivity reactions, especially during first and second infusions. Severe and even fatal reactions have occurred in patients who have received recommended 3-day dexamethasone premedication. For severe reactions, discontinue docetaxel immediately and administer appropriate therapy. ▌

Black Box Warning Fluid retention is dose related and may be severe. Monitor patient closely. ▌

• Patients who have previously experienced a hypersensitivity reaction to paclitaxel may develop a hypersensitivity reaction to docetaxel that may include severe or fatal reactions such as anaphylaxis. Monitor patients with a previous history of hypersensitivity to paclitaxel closely during initiation of therapy. Hypersensitivity reactions may occur within a few minutes after infusion is started. If minor reactions, such as flushing or localized skin reactions, occur, therapy interruption isn't required.

• Enterocolitis and neutropenic colitis (typhlitis) have occurred in patients treated with docetaxel alone and in combination with other chemotherapeutic agents, despite the coadministration of G-CSF. Use cautiously in patients with neutropenia, particularly those at risk for developing GI complications. Enterocolitis and neutropenic colitis may develop at any time, and could lead to death as early as the first day of symptom onset. Monitor patients closely from onset of signs and symptoms of GI toxicity.

❸ *Alert:* Evaluate patients for history of problems with alcohol or drinking, liver disease, or other conditions that may be affected by alcohol intake.

❸ *Alert:* Monitor patients for signs and symptoms of alcohol intoxication during and after treatment (appearance of being drunk,

confusion, stumbling, somnolence). Consider using formulation with lowest alcohol content for patients who experience adverse reactions. Slowing infusion rate during administration may help resolve signs and symptoms of alcohol intoxication.

❸ *Alert:* When indicated, cisplatin dose should follow docetaxel dose.

• Monitor patient for vision changes. If they occur, patient should have a prompt, comprehensive eye examination.

• Monitor patient who received docetaxel, doxorubicin, and cyclophosphamide for delayed myelodysplasia or myeloid leukemia.

• *Look alike–sound alike:* Don't confuse docetaxel with paclitaxel. Don't confuse Taxotere with Taxol.

PATIENT TEACHING

❸ *Alert:* Caution patient to avoid driving, operating machinery, or performing other hazardous activities for 1 to 2 hours after treatment.

❸ *Alert:* Instruct patient to immediately report signs and symptoms of alcohol intoxication that may occur during or 1 to 2 hours after treatment.

• Caution female patient of childbearing potential to avoid pregnancy or breastfeeding during therapy.

• Inform female patient of potential hazard to the fetus if drug is used during pregnancy, or if patient becomes pregnant during therapy.

• Advise patient that premedication with dexamethasone will be needed.

• Advise patient to report any pain or burning at injection site during or after administration.

• Warn patient that hair loss occurs in almost 80% of patients and usually reverses when treatment stops; cases of permanent hair loss have been reported.

• Tell patient to report all adverse reactions and to promptly report sore throat, fever, or unusual bruising or bleeding, as well as signs and symptoms of fluid retention, such as swelling or shortness of breath.

• Tell patient to report new or worsening signs or symptoms of GI toxicity.

---

dofetilide
doe-FE-ti-lyed

Tikosyn

Therapeutic class: Antiarrhythmics
Pharmacologic class: Antiarrhythmics

AVAILABLE FORMS
Capsules: 125 mcg, 250 mcg, 500 mcg

INDICATIONS & DOSAGES
➤ **To maintain normal sinus rhythm in patients with symptomatic atrial fibrillation or atrial flutter lasting longer than 1 week who have been converted to normal sinus rhythm; to convert atrial fibrillation and atrial flutter to normal sinus rhythm**
Adults: Individualized dosage based on CrCl and baseline QTc interval (or QT interval if HR is below 60 beats/minute), determined before first dose; usually 500 mcg PO b.i.d. for patients with CrCl greater than 60 mL/minute.
Adjust-a-dose: If CrCl is 40 to 60 mL/minute, starting dose is 250 mcg PO b.i.d.; if CrCl is 20 to 39 mL/minute, starting dose is 125 mcg PO b.i.d. Don't use drug at all if CrCl is less than 20 mL/minute.

Determine QTc interval 2 to 3 hours after first dose. If QTc interval has increased by more than 15% above baseline or if it's more than 500 msec (550 msec in patients with ventricular conduction abnormalities), adjust dosage as follows: If starting dose based on CrCl was 500 mcg PO b.i.d., give 250 mcg PO b.i.d. If starting dose based on CrCl was 250 mcg b.i.d., give 125 mcg b.i.d. If starting dose based on CrCl was 125 mcg b.i.d., give 125 mcg once a day.

Determine QTc interval 2 to 3 hours after each subsequent dose while patient is in hospital. If at any time after second dose the QTc interval exceeds 500 msec (550 msec in patients with ventricular conduction abnormalities), stop drug.

ADMINISTRATION
PO
• Give drug without regard for food or antacid administration.
• Don't give drug with grapefruit juice.

ACTION
Prolongs repolarization without affecting conduction velocity (Vaughan-Williams Class III antiarrhythmic). Drug doesn't affect sodium channels, alpha-adrenergic receptors, or beta-adrenergic receptors.

Route	Onset	Peak	Duration
PO	Unknown	2–3 hr	Unknown

Half-life: 10 hours.

ADVERSE REACTIONS
CNS: headache, *stroke,* dizziness, insomnia, anxiety, migraine, cerebral ischemia, asthenia, paresthesia, syncope. **CV:** chest pain, *ventricular fibrillation, ventricular tachycardia, torsades de pointes, AV block, heart block, bradycardia, cardiac arrest, MI,* bundle-branch block, angina, atrial fibrillation, HTN, palpitations, peripheral edema. **GI:** nausea, diarrhea, abdominal pain. **GU:** UTI. **Hepatic:** liver damage. **Musculoskeletal:** back pain, arthralgia, facial paralysis. **Respiratory:** respiratory tract infection, dyspnea, increased cough. **Skin:** rash, sweating. **Other:** *angioedema,* flulike syndrome.

INTERACTIONS
Drug-drug. *Antiarrhythmics (Class I and III):* May increase dofetilide level. Withhold other antiarrhythmics for at least three plasma half-lives before giving dofetilide. *CYP3A4 inhibitors (amiodarone, **azole antifungals,** cannabinoids, diltiazem, **macrolides,** nefazodone, norfloxacin, protease inhibitors, quinine, SSRIs, zafirlukast):* May decrease metabolism and increase dofetilide level. Use together cautiously. *Drugs secreted by renal tubular cationic transport (amiloride, metformin, triamterene):* May increase dofetilide level. Use together cautiously; monitor patient for adverse effects. *Drugs that prolong QT interval:* May increase risk of QT interval prolongation. Avoid using together. ***Inhibitors of renal cationic secretion (cimetidine, ketoconazole, megestrol, prochlorperazine, sulfamethoxazole–trimethoprim), trimethoprim, verapamil:*** May increase dofetilide level. Use together is contraindicated.

♣Canada   ◇OTC   ◆Off-label use   ✐Photoguide   ⊛Do not crush   *Liquid contains alcohol   ✇Genetic

Potassium-depleting diuretics: May increase risk of hypokalemia or hypomagnesemia. Monitor potassium and magnesium levels.

Thiazide diuretics: May cause hypokalemia and arrhythmias. Use together is contraindicated.

Drug-food. *Grapefruit juice:* May decrease hepatic metabolism and increase drug level. Discourage use together.

EFFECTS ON LAB TEST RESULTS
None reported.

CONTRAINDICATIONS & CAUTIONS
• Contraindicated in patients hypersensitive to drug, in those with congenital or acquired long QT interval syndromes or with baseline QTc interval greater than 440 msec (500 msec in patients with ventricular conduction abnormalities), and in those with CrCl less than 20 mL/minute.
• Use cautiously in patients with severe hepatic impairment.
• Safety and effectiveness in children haven't been studied.

Dialyzable drug: Unknown.

⚠ **Overdose S&S:** Prolonged QT interval, ventricular fibrillation, torsades de pointes, cardiac arrest.

PREGNANCY-LACTATION-REPRODUCTION
• There are no adequate well-controlled studies in pregnant women. Use during pregnancy only if clearly needed and potential benefit justifies potential risk to the fetus.
• It isn't known if drug appears in human milk. Women shouldn't breastfeed while taking drug.

NURSING CONSIDERATIONS
Black Box Warning When dofetilide is initiated or reinitiated, patients should be hospitalized for a minimum of 3 days in a facility that can provide calculations of CrCl, continuous ECG monitoring, and cardiac resuscitation. ∎
• Don't discharge patient within 12 hours of conversion to normal sinus rhythm.
• Before discharge, ensure patient has an adequate supply of medication to allow uninterrupted dosing until patient can fill a prescription as an outpatient.

• Monitor patient for prolonged diarrhea, sweating, and vomiting. Report these signs to prescriber because electrolyte imbalance may increase potential for arrhythmia development.
• Monitor renal function and QTc interval every 3 months. Drug can cause torsades de pointes ventricular arrhythmia.
• Use of potassium-depleting diuretics may cause hypokalemia and hypomagnesemia, increasing the risk of torsades de pointes. Give dofetilide after potassium level reaches and stays in normal range.
• Before starting dofetilide, stop previous antiarrhythmics while carefully monitoring patient for a minimum of three plasma half-lives. Don't give drug after amiodarone therapy until amiodarone level falls below 0.3 mcg/mL or until amiodarone has been stopped for at least 3 months.
• If dofetilide must be stopped to allow dosing with interacting drugs, allow at least 2 days before starting other drug therapy.

PATIENT TEACHING
• Tell patient to report any change in OTC drug, prescription drug, supplement, or herb use.
• Inform patient that drug can be taken without regard to meals or antacid administration.
• Tell patient to immediately report chest pain, dyspnea, palpitations, excessive or prolonged diarrhea, sweating, vomiting, or loss of appetite or thirst.
• If a dose is missed, tell patient not to double a dose but to skip that dose and take the next regularly scheduled dose.
• Advise patient not to take drug with grapefruit juice.
• If antiulcer therapy is needed, tell patient that omeprazole, ranitidine, or antacids (aluminum and magnesium hydroxides) will be prescribed.
• Instruct patient to tell prescriber if she becomes pregnant.
• Advise patient not to breastfeed while taking dofetilide.

D

dolutegravir–rilpivirine
doe-loo-TEG-ra-vir/ril-pi-VIR-een

Juluca

Therapeutic class: Antiretrovirals
Pharmacologic class: Integrase strand
transfer inhibitors–NNRTIs

AVAILABLE FORMS
Tablets: 50 mg dolutegravir base/25 mg
rilpivirine base

INDICATIONS & DOSAGES
➤ HIV-1 infection in patients who are virologically suppressed (HIV-1 RNA less
than 50 copies/mL) on a stable antiretroviral regimen for at least 6 months with
no history of treatment failure and no
known substitutions associated with resistance to the individual components of
the drug
Adults: 50 mg dolutegravir/25 mg rilpivirine
(1 tablet) PO once daily.
Adjust-a-dose: If administered with rifabutin,
give an additional 25-mg rilpivirine tablet
once daily for the duration of rifabutin coadministration.

ADMINISTRATION
PO
• Give with a meal.
• If a dose is missed, give it as soon as possi-
ble. Don't double the next dose.
• Store in original bottle; don't remove
desiccant. Protect from moisture.
• Store at 59° to 86° F (15° to 30° C).

ACTION
Dolutegravir inhibits HIV integrase by binding to the integrase active site and blocking retroviral DNA integration essential for
HIV replication. Rilpivirine inhibits HIV-1
replication by noncompetitive inhibition of
HIV-1 reverse transcriptase.

Route	Onset	Peak	Duration
PO (dolutegravir)	Unknown	3 hr	Unknown
PO (rilpivirine)	Unknown	4 hr	Unknown

Half-life: Dolutegravir, 14 hours; rilpivirine,
50 hours.

ADVERSE REACTIONS
CNS: headache, depressive disorders (including *suicidal ideation, behavior, or completion*), fatigue, dizziness, somnolence,
anxiety, insomnia, sleep disorders, abnormal dreams. **GI:** diarrhea, abdominal pain
or discomfort, flatulence, nausea, vomiting, decreased appetite. **GU:** membranous
glomerulonephritis, mesangioproliferative
glomerulonephritis, nephrolithiasis, renal
impairment. **Hepatic:** *hepatotoxicity,* cholecystitis, cholelithiasis, *hepatitis.* **Metabolic:**
hyperglycemia. **Musculoskeletal:** myositis,
decreased bone mineral density. **Skin:** rash,
pruritus. **Other:** immune reconstitution syndrome.

INTERACTIONS
Drug-drug. *Antacids (aluminum hydroxide,
magnesium hydroxide, calcium carbonate):*
May decrease rilpivirine level. Administer
drug 4 hours before or 6 hours after antacids.
*Anticonvulsants (carbamazepine, oxcar-
bazepine, phenobarbital, phenytoin):* May
decrease dolutegravir and rilpivirine levels,
resulting in loss of virologic response. Use
together is contraindicated.
*Calcium and iron supplements (oral), multi-
vitamins containing calcium or iron:* May
decrease dolutegravir level. Administer
supplements and dolutegravir–rilpivirine
together with a meal or give supplements
4 hours before or 6 hours after dolutegravir–
rilpivirine.
Clarithromycin, erythromycin: May increase
rilpivirine level. Consider alternative antibiotics such as azithromycin.
Dexamethasone (systemic): May decrease
rilpivirine level when dexamethasone is
given as more than a single-dose treatment,
resulting in loss of virologic response. Use
together is contraindicated except for a single dose of dexamethasone.
Dofetilide: May increase dofetilide level,
causing serious or life-threatening events.
Use together is contraindicated.
*Drugs containing polyvalent cations (alu-
minum, magnesium), such as buffered drugs,
cation-containing products or laxatives, sucralfate:* May decrease dolutegravir level.
Administer dolutegravir–rilpivirine 4 hours
before or 6 hours after drugs containing
polyvalent cations.

Drugs known to prolong QTc interval and increase risk of torsades de pointes (amiodarone, erythromycin, haloperidol, oxycodone): May increase risk of QT-interval prolongation and torsades de pointes. Avoid use together.

H₂-receptor antagonists (cimetidine, famotidine, nizatidine, ranitidine): May decrease rilpivirine level. Give dolutegravir–rilpivirine at least 4 hours before or 12 hours after H₂-receptor antagonist.

Metformin: May increase metformin level. When used together, limit metformin to 1,000 mg daily when starting metformin or dolutegravir–rilpivirine. When starting or stopping dolutegravir–rilpivirine, monitor glucose level and adjust metformin dosage. Monitor glucose level when initiating concomitant use and after withdrawal of dolutegravir–rilpivirine.

Methadone: May decrease methadone level. No dosage adjustments are required when starting administration of methadone with dolutegravir–rilpivirine. Monitor patients on methadone maintenance therapy, as dosage adjustments may be needed.

Other antiretrovirals to treat HIV-1: Dolutegravir–rilpivirine is a complete regimen. Use with other antiretrovirals isn't recommended.

PPIs (esomeprazole, lansoprazole, omeprazole, pantoprazole, rabeprazole): May decrease rilpivirine level due to gastric pH increase, which may result in loss of virologic response. Use together is contraindicated.

Rifabutin: May decrease rilpivirine level. Give an additional 25-mg tablet of rilpivirine once daily for duration of the rifabutin coadministration.

Rifampin, rifapentine: May decrease dolutegravir and rilpivirine levels, resulting in loss of virologic response. Use together is contraindicated.

Drug-herb. *St. John's wort:* May decrease dolutegravir and rilpivirine levels, resulting in loss of virologic response. Use together is contraindicated.

EFFECTS ON LAB TEST RESULTS
• May increase ALT, AST, total bilirubin, CK, lipase, and glucose levels.
• May decrease cortisol level.

CONTRAINDICATIONS & CAUTIONS
• Contraindicated in patients hypersensitive to dolutegravir, rilpivirine, or other components of the tablet.
• Contraindicated with concomitant administration of dofetilide, some anticonvulsants, rifampin, rifapentine, multidose dexamethasone, PPIs, and St. John's wort.
• Use cautiously in patients with underlying HBV or HCV infection or marked elevations in transaminase levels before treatment. Drug may increase risk of worsening or development of transaminase elevations, immune reconstitution syndrome, or HBV reactivation.
• Use cautiously in elderly patients and in patients with severe ESRD or severe hepatic impairment (Child-Pugh class C).
• Safety and effectiveness in children haven't been established.
Dialyzable drug: Unlikely.

PREGNANCY-LACTATION-REPRODUCTION
۞ Alert: Dolutegravir may increase risk of neural tube birth defects, especially when taken during the first trimester. Prescribers should weigh the risks and benefits of the drug and consider the use of alternative antiretrovirals before prescribing dolutegravir–rilpivirine to women of childbearing potential.
۞ Alert: Testing to exclude pregnancy should be performed before start of therapy.
۞ Alert: Adolescents and adults of childbearing potential using drug should use consistent, effective contraception.
• Enroll women exposed to drug during pregnancy in the Antiretroviral Pregnancy Registry (1-800-258-4263).
• The CDC recommends that women infected with HIV-1 shouldn't breastfeed due to the potential risk of HIV-1 transmission to the infant.

NURSING CONSIDERATIONS
۞ Alert: Drug may cause severe skin reactions and severe hypersensitivity reactions such as DRESS syndrome with organ dysfunction, including liver injury. Monitor LFT values and initiate appropriate therapy.
۞ Alert: Monitor patient for severe rash (or rash accompanied by fever, general malaise, skin blisters or skin peeling, oral blisters

---

or lesions, conjunctivitis, facial edema, hepatitis, eosinophilia, angioedema, or difficulty breathing). Discontinue drug immediately if these signs or symptoms occur; delay in stopping drug may result in a life-threatening reaction.

• Monitor patient for severe depressive symptoms (depressed mood, depression, dysphoria, major depression, altered mood, negative thoughts, suicide attempt, suicidal ideation). Promptly evaluate depressive symptoms to assess whether the symptoms are related to the drug and to determine whether the risks of continued therapy outweigh the benefits.

• Monitor patient for signs and symptoms of hepatotoxicity (elevated LFT values, yellowing of the skin or whites of the eyes, dark urine, pale-colored stools, nausea, vomiting, loss of appetite, right-sided abdominal pain or tenderness), especially in patients with HBV or HCV infection, who may be at increased risk. Hepatotoxicity has also occurred in patients without preexisting hepatic disease or identifiable risk factors.

• *Look alike–sound alike:* Don't confuse rilpivirine with ritonavir. Don't confuse Juluca with Jublia or Januvia.

PATIENT TEACHING
• Teach patient to report all adverse reactions and to stop drug and immediately report a rash with signs or symptoms of hypersensitivity, DRESS syndrome, or hepatotoxicity.
• Tell patient to report all drugs and supplements being taken before start of therapy, as drug interactions may lead to loss of therapeutic effect, development of resistance, and an increase in adverse reactions.
• Advise patient that drug isn't a cure for HIV or AIDS. Stress the importance of taking drug as directed and staying on continuous antiretroviral therapy to control HIV infection and prevent resistance to therapy.
• Instruct patient to take tablet with a meal.
• Caution patient and caregiver to immediately report depressive symptoms (depressed mood, depression, dysphoria, major depression, altered mood, negative thoughts, suicide attempt, suicidal ideation).
• Instruct female patient to immediately report if she is pregnant. Inform patient there

is an antiretroviral registry to monitor fetal outcomes if she is exposed to drug during pregnancy.
• Caution female patient not to breastfeed during therapy.

donepezil hydrochloride
doe-NEP-eh-zill

Aricept✐, Aricept ODT

Therapeutic class: Anti-Alzheimer drugs
Pharmacologic class: Acetylcholinesterase inhibitors

AVAILABLE FORMS
Tablets ⓓ: 5 mg, 10 mg, 23 mg
Tablets (ODTs) ⓓ: 5 mg, 10 mg

INDICATIONS & DOSAGES
➤ **Mild to moderate Alzheimer dementia**
Adults: 5 mg PO once daily for 4 to 6 weeks; may then increase dosage to 10 mg PO once daily.
➤ **Moderate to severe Alzheimer disease**
Adults: Initially, 5 mg PO once daily for 4 to 6 weeks; dose may then be increased to 10 mg PO once daily. The dose may be increased to 23 mg PO once daily after patient has been taking 10 mg daily for 3 months.

ADMINISTRATION
PO
• Allow ODT to dissolve on tongue; then follow with water.
• Give drug at bedtime, without regard for food.
• Don't split or crush tablets.

ACTION
Inhibits acetylcholinesterase, the enzyme that causes acetylcholine hydrolysis, resulting in increased acetylcholine available for synaptic transmission in the CNS.

Route	Onset	Peak	Duration
PO	Unknown	3–8 hr	Unknown

Half-life: 70 hours.

ADVERSE REACTIONS
CNS: headache, insomnia, *seizures,* dizziness, fatigue, depression, somnolence,

syncope, pain, hallucinations, abnormal dreams. **CV:** chest pain, HTN, atrial fibrillation, edema, hypotension, *bradycardia, heart block.* **EENT:** cataract, blurred vision, eye irritation, sore throat. **GI:** nausea, diarrhea, vomiting, anorexia, fecal incontinence, *GI bleeding,* weight loss. **GU:** urinary incontinence, urinary frequency. **Metabolic:** weight loss, dehydration. **Musculoskeletal:** muscle cramps, arthritis, bone fracture. **Respiratory:** dyspnea, bronchitis. **Skin:** pruritus, urticaria, diaphoresis, ecchymoses. **Other:** toothache, influenza, increased libido.

INTERACTIONS
Drug-drug. *Anticholinergics:* May decrease donepezil effects. Avoid using together.
Anticholinesterases, bethanechol, cholinomimetics, succinylcholine: May have synergistic effect. Monitor patient closely.
Carbamazepine, dexamethasone, phenobarbital, phenytoin, rifampin: May increase rate of donepezil elimination. Monitor patient.
Drugs that prolong QT interval: May increase risk of QT-interval prolongation. Monitor patient; consider therapy modification.
NSAIDs: May increase gastric acid secretions. Monitor for active or occult GI bleeding.

EFFECTS ON LAB TEST RESULTS
• May increase CK level.

CONTRAINDICATIONS & CAUTIONS
• Contraindicated in patients hypersensitive to drug or piperidine derivatives.
• Use cautiously in patients who take NSAIDs or have CV disease, are at risk for rhabdomyolysis and renal failure, or have asthma, obstructive pulmonary disease, seizure disorders, urinary outflow impairment, GI bleeding, or history of ulcer disease.
Dialyzable drug: Unknown.
⚠ *Overdose S&S:* Severe nausea, vomiting, salivation, sweating, bradycardia, hypotension, respiratory depression, collapse, seizures, increasing muscle weakness.

PREGNANCY-LACTATION-REPRODUCTION
• There are no adequate well-controlled studies in pregnant women. Use during pregnancy only if clearly needed and potential benefit justifies potential risk to the fetus.
• It isn't known if drug appears in human milk. Use cautiously in breastfeeding women.

NURSING CONSIDERATIONS
• Monitor patient for evidence of active or occult GI bleeding.
• Monitor patient for bradycardia because of potential for vagotonic effects.
• *Look alike–sound alike:* Don't confuse Aricept with Ascriptin, Aciphex, or Azilect.

PATIENT TEACHING
• Stress that drug doesn't alter underlying degenerative disease but can temporarily stabilize or relieve symptoms. Effectiveness depends on taking drug at regular intervals.
• Tell caregiver to give drug just before patient's bedtime.
• Tell patient and caregiver not to break or crush tablets.
• ODTs may be taken with or without food. Advise patient to allow tablet to dissolve on tongue, then swallow with a sip of water.
• Advise patient and caregiver to report significant adverse effects or changes in overall health status immediately and to inform health care team that patient is taking drug before patient receives anesthesia.
• Tell patient to avoid OTC cold or sleep remedies because of risk of increased anticholinergic effects.

SAFETY ALERT!

DOPamine hydrochloride
DOE-pa-meen

Therapeutic class: Vasopressors
Pharmacologic class: Adrenergics

AVAILABLE FORMS
Injection: 40 mg/mL, 80 mg/mL, 160 mg/mL parenteral concentrate for injection for IV infusion; 0.8 mg/mL (200 or 400 mg) in D_5W; 1.6 mg/mL (400 or 800 mg) in D_5W; 3.2 mg/mL (800 mg) in D_5W parenteral injection for IV infusion

INDICATIONS & DOSAGES
➤ **To treat shock and correct hemodynamic imbalances; to improve perfusion to vital organs; to increase cardiac output; to correct hypotension**
Adults: Initially, 2 to 5 mcg/kg/minute by IV infusion. Titrate dosage to desired hemodynamic or renal response. In seriously ill patients, start with 5 mcg/kg/minute and increase gradually in increments of 5 to 10 mcg/kg/minute to a rate of 20 to 50 mcg/kg/minute, as needed.
Adjust-a-dose: In patients with occlusive vascular disease, initial dose is 1 mcg/kg/minute or less. Initial dopamine dosages shouldn't exceed one-tenth of the usual dosage in patients who have received MAO inhibitors within the prior 2 to 3 weeks.

ADMINISTRATION
IV
▼ Dilute with D₅W, NSS, D₅W in NSS or half-NSS, lactated Ringer solution, D₅W in lactated Ringer solution, or sodium lactate injection. Mix just before use.
▼ Use a central line or large vein, as in the antecubital fossa, to minimize risk of extravasation.
▼ Use a continuous infusion pump to regulate flow rate. Avoid inadvertent administration of a bolus of the drug.
Black Box Warning Watch infusion site carefully for extravasation; if it occurs, stop infusion immediately and call prescriber. To prevent sloughing and necrosis in ischemic areas, infiltrate the area with 5 to 10 mg phentolamine in 10 to 15 mL NSS as soon as possible. ■
▼ Because solution will deteriorate rapidly, discard after 24 hours or earlier if it's discolored.
▼ Don't use product if it's darker than slightly yellow or discolored in another way.
▼ **Incompatibilities:** Alkalies (including sodium bicarbonate), oxidizing agents, iron salts.

ACTION
Stimulates dopaminergic and alpha and beta receptors of the sympathetic nervous system, resulting in a positive inotropic effect and increased cardiac output. Action is

dose-related; large doses cause mainly alpha stimulation.

Route	Onset	Peak	Duration
IV	5 min	Unknown	<10 min after infusion

Half-life: 2 minutes.

ADVERSE REACTIONS
CNS: headache, anxiety. **CV:** hypotension, *ventricular arrhythmias (high doses),* ectopic beats, tachycardia, angina, palpitations, vasoconstriction. **GI:** nausea, vomiting. **Metabolic:** azotemia, hyperglycemia. **Respiratory:** *asthmatic episodes,* dyspnea. **Skin:** necrosis and tissue sloughing with extravasation, piloerection. **Other:** *anaphylactic reactions.*

INTERACTIONS
Drug-drug. *Alpha and beta blockers:* May antagonize dopamine effects. Monitor patient closely.
Diuretics (furosemide): May potentiate diuresis. Use together cautiously and monitor fluid volume closely.
Ergot alkaloids: May cause extremely high BP. Avoid using together.
Inhaled anesthetics: May increase risk of arrhythmias or HTN. Monitor patient closely.
🟢 *Alert: MAO inhibitors (phenelzine, tranylcypromine):* May cause fever, hypertensive crisis, or severe headache. Avoid using together; if patient received an MAO inhibitor in the past 2 to 3 weeks, initial dopamine dose is less than or equal to 10% of the usual dose.
Oxytocics: May cause severe, persistent HTN. Use together cautiously.
Phenytoin: May cause severe hypotension, bradycardia, and cardiac arrest. Monitor patient carefully.
TCAs: May decrease pressor response. Monitor patient closely.

EFFECTS ON LAB TEST RESULTS
● May increase catecholamine, glucose, and BUN levels.

CONTRAINDICATIONS & CAUTIONS
● Contraindicated in patients with uncorrected tachyarrhythmias, pheochromocytoma, or ventricular fibrillation.

• Use cautiously in patients with occlusive vascular disease, cold injuries, diabetic endarteritis, and arterial embolism; in those with a history of sulfite sensitivity; and in those taking MAO inhibitors.
Dialyzable drug: Unlikely.
⚠ *Overdose S&S:* Excessive BP elevation.

PREGNANCY-LACTATION-REPRODUCTION
• There are no adequate well-controlled studies in pregnant women. Use during pregnancy only if potential benefit justifies potential risk to the fetus.
• If vasopressors are used to correct hypotension or are added to a local anesthetic solution during labor or delivery, some oxytocics may cause severe persistent HTN. Monitor patient closely.
• It isn't known if drug appears in human milk. Use cautiously in breastfeeding women.

NURSING CONSIDERATIONS
• Most patients receive less than 20 mcg/kg/minute. Doses of 0.5 to 2 mcg/kg/minute mainly stimulate dopamine receptors and dilate the renal vasculature. Doses of 2 to 10 mcg/kg/minute stimulate beta receptors for a positive inotropic effect. Higher doses also stimulate alpha receptors, constricting blood vessels and increasing BP.
• Drug isn't a substitute for blood or fluid volume deficit. If deficit exists, replace fluid before giving vasopressors.
• During infusion, frequently monitor ECG, BP, cardiac output, central venous pressure, pulmonary artery wedge pressure, pulse rate, urine output, and color and temperature of limbs.
• If diastolic pressure rises disproportionately with a significant decrease in pulse pressure, decrease infusion rate and watch carefully for further evidence of predominant vasoconstrictor activity, unless such an effect is desired.
• Observe patient closely for adverse reactions; dosage may need to be adjusted or drug stopped.
• Check urine output often. If urine flow decreases without hypotension, notify prescriber because dosage may need to be reduced.

◑ *Alert:* After drug is stopped, watch closely for sudden drop in BP. Taper dosage slowly to evaluate stability of BP, and provide IV fluids as clinically indicated to expand blood volume.
• Acidosis decreases effectiveness of drug. Correct before or during dopamine infusion.
• *Look alike–sound alike:* Don't confuse dopamine with dobutamine.

PATIENT TEACHING
• Tell patient to report adverse reactions promptly.
• Instruct patient to immediately report discomfort at IV insertion site.

doxazosin mesylate
dox-AY-zo-sin

Cardura◆, Cardura XL

Therapeutic class: Antihypertensives
Pharmacologic class: Alpha blockers

AVAILABLE FORMS
Tablets (immediate-release): 1 mg, 2 mg, 4 mg, 8 mg
Tablets (extended-release) ⒪ⓃⒼ: 4 mg, 8 mg

INDICATIONS & DOSAGES
➤ **Essential HTN**
Adults: Initially, 1 mg immediate-release tablet PO daily. After the initial dose and with each dosage increase, monitor BP for at least 6 hours. May increase to 2 mg and thereafter 4 mg and 8 mg once daily, if needed. Maximum daily dose is 16 mg, but doses over 4 mg daily increase the risk of adverse reactions. Don't use extended-release formulation to treat HTN.
➤ **BPH**
Adults: Initially, 1 mg immediate-release tablet PO once daily in the morning or evening; may increase at 1- or 2-week intervals to 2 mg and, thereafter, 4 mg and 8 mg once daily, if needed. Or, one 4-mg extended-release tablet once daily with breakfast. May increase to 8 mg in 3 to 4 weeks.

Reactions in bold italics are *life-threatening*. Interactions may have a *rapid onset* or a *delayed onset*.

ADMINISTRATION
PO
• Patient should swallow extended-release tablets whole and not chew, divide, cut, or crush them.
• Give extended-release tablet with breakfast.
• Don't give evening dose the night before switching to extended-release tablets from immediate-release formula. Start extended-release tablets at lowest dose (4 mg once daily) the next morning.
• If therapy is interrupted for several days, restart drug at 4 mg once daily.

ACTION
An alpha₁ blocker that acts on the peripheral vasculature to reduce peripheral vascular resistance and produce vasodilation. Drug also decreases smooth muscle tone in the prostate and bladder neck.

Route	Onset	Peak	Duration
PO	1–2 hr	2–13.5 hr	24 hr

Half-life: Extended-release, 15 to 19 hours; immediate-release, 22 hours.

ADVERSE REACTIONS
CNS: dizziness, asthenia, headache, vertigo, somnolence, malaise, drowsiness, pain, fatigue. **CV:** orthostatic hypotension, *arrhythmias,* hypotension, edema, palpitations, tachycardia. **EENT:** rhinitis, abnormal vision, dry mouth. **GI:** abdominal pain, nausea, vomiting, diarrhea, constipation. **GU:** erectile dysfunction, polyuria. **Hematologic:** *leukopenia, neutropenia.* **Musculoskeletal:** arthralgia, myalgia, back pain. **Respiratory:** dyspnea. **Skin:** rash, pruritus.

INTERACTIONS
Drug-drug. *Antihypertensives, diuretics:* May increase hypotensive effects. Adjust dosages as necessary.
Midodrine: May decrease the effectiveness of midodrine. Monitor patient for therapeutic effect.
PDE5 inhibitors (sildenafil, tadalafil, vardenafil): May cause additive hypotensive effects and symptomatic hypotension. Initiate PDE5 therapy at lowest possible dosage.
Strong CYP3A4 inhibitors (atazanavir, clarithromycin, ketoconazole, ritonavir): May

increase doxazosin level. Use together with caution; monitor BP and watch for hypotension signs and symptoms.
Drug-herb. *Ma huang:* May decrease antihypertensive effects. Discourage use together.

EFFECTS ON LAB TEST RESULTS
• May decrease WBC and neutrophil counts.

CONTRAINDICATIONS & CAUTIONS
• Contraindicated in patients hypersensitive to drug and quinazoline derivatives (including prazosin and terazosin).
• Use cautiously in patients with impaired hepatic function.
• Intraoperative floppy iris syndrome has been observed during cataract surgery in some patients on or previously treated with alpha₁ blockers.
• Rarely, drug has been associated with priapism (painful penile erection, sustained for hours and unrelieved by sexual intercourse or masturbation), which can lead to permanent erectile dysfunction if not promptly treated.
Dialyzable drug: No.
△ *Overdose S&S:* Hypotension.

PREGNANCY-LACTATION-REPRODUCTION
• There are no adequate well-controlled studies in pregnant women. Use immediate-release form during pregnancy only if clearly needed; extended-release form isn't indicated.
• Drug may appear in human milk. Use of extended-release form in women isn't recommended. Use immediate-release form cautiously.

NURSING CONSIDERATIONS
• Monitor BP closely.
• If syncope occurs, place patient in a recumbent position and treat supportively. A transient hypotensive response isn't considered a contraindication to continued therapy.
• Rule out prostate cancer before starting treatment for BPH.
• Initial extended-release dose is 4 mg. If patient stops medication briefly, patient should resume at 4-mg dose and titrate back to 8 mg if appropriate.

• Wait 3 to 4 weeks before increasing extended-release dose.
• *Look alike–sound alike:* Don't confuse doxazosin with doxapram, doxorubicin, or doxepin. Don't confuse Cardura with Coumadin, K-Dur, Cardene, or Cordarone.

PATIENT TEACHING
• Instruct patient to take drug exactly as prescribed.
🜚 *Alert:* Advise patient that a first-dose effect (marked low BP on standing up, with dizziness or fainting) may occur. This is most common after first dose but also can occur during dosage adjustment or interruption of therapy.
• Advise patient to consult prescriber if dizziness or palpitations are bothersome.
• Advise patient to rise slowly from sitting or lying position.
• Advise patient to avoid driving and other hazardous activities until drug's effects are known.
• Advise patient to inform surgeon of alpha$_1$-blocker therapy before having cataract surgery.
• Inform male patient that drug has been associated with rare, but serious, priapism. Tell him to seek immediate medical treatment for a painful penile erection lasting longer than 4 hours.

doxepin hydrochloride
DOKS-eh-pin

Silenor

Therapeutic class: Antidepressants
Pharmacologic class: TCAs

AVAILABLE FORMS
Capsules: 10 mg, 25 mg, 50 mg, 75 mg, 100 mg, 150 mg
Oral concentrate: 10 mg/mL
Tablets: 3 mg, 6 mg

INDICATIONS & DOSAGES
➤ **Depression; anxiety**
Adults: Initially, 75 mg PO daily. Usual dosage range is 75 to 150 mg daily to maximum of 300 mg daily in divided doses. Mild symptoms may require only 25 to 50 mg/day.

Or, may give entire maintenance dose once daily to a maximum dose of 150 mg/day.
➤ **Insomnia (Silenor only)**
Adults: 3 to 6 mg PO once daily within 30 minutes of bedtime.
Adjust-a-dose: For patients age 65 and older, give 3 mg PO once daily within 30 minutes of bedtime. May increase daily dose to 6 mg if indicated. For patients with hepatic impairment, initial dose is 3 mg PO once daily. For administration with cimetidine, give maximum dose of 3 mg once daily.

ADMINISTRATION
PO
• Dilute oral concentrate with 4 oz (120 mL) of water, milk, or juice (orange, grapefruit, tomato, prune, or pineapple, but not grape); don't mix preparation with carbonated beverages.
• Give at bedtime, if possible, because it may cause drowsiness and dizziness.
• Don't give Silenor within 3 hours of a meal.

ACTION
Increases amount of norepinephrine, serotonin, or both in the CNS by blocking their reuptake by the presynaptic neurons.

Route	Onset	Peak	Duration
PO	Unknown	3½ hr	Unknown

Half-life: About 15 hours.

ADVERSE REACTIONS
CNS: drowsiness, dizziness, *seizures,* confusion, numbness, hallucinations, paresthesia, ataxia, weakness, headache, extrapyramidal reactions. **CV:** orthostatic hypotension, tachycardia, ECG changes. **EENT:** blurred vision, tinnitus. **GI:** dry mouth, constipation, nausea, vomiting, anorexia. **GU:** urine retention, change in libido. **Metabolic:** *hypoglycemia,* hyperglycemia. **Skin:** diaphoresis, rash, urticaria, photosensitivity reactions. **Other:** hypersensitivity reactions, breast enlargement.

INTERACTIONS
Drug-drug. *Barbiturates, CNS depressants:* May enhance CNS depression. Avoid using together.

Reactions in bold italics are *life-threatening*. Interactions may have a *rapid onset* or a *delayed onset*.

Clonidine: May cause life-threatening HTN. Avoid using together.

*Drugs metabolized by CYP2D6 (cimetidine, flecainide, phenothiazines, propafenone, quinidine, SSRIs [**fluoxetine, fluvoxamine, paroxetine, sertraline**]):* May increase doxepin level. Monitor drug levels and watch for signs and symptoms of toxicity.

Epinephrine, norepinephrine: May increase hypertensive effect. Use together cautiously.

Linezolid, methylene blue: May cause serotonin syndrome. Use with extreme caution and monitor closely.

MAO inhibitors: May cause severe excitation, hyperpyrexia, or seizures. Avoid using within 14 days of MAO inhibitor therapy.

Quinolones: May increase risk of life-threatening arrhythmias. Avoid use together.

Drug-herb. *Evening primrose oil:* May cause additive or synergistic effect, resulting in lower seizure threshold and increasing the risk of seizure. Discourage use together.

St. John's wort, SAM-e, yohimbe: May cause serotonin syndrome. Discourage use together.

Drug-lifestyle. *Alcohol use:* May enhance CNS depression. Discourage use together.

Sun exposure: May increase risk of photosensitivity reactions. Advise patient to avoid excessive sunlight exposure.

EFFECTS ON LAB TEST RESULTS
• May increase or decrease glucose level.
• May increase LFT values.

CONTRAINDICATIONS & CAUTIONS
• Contraindicated in patients hypersensitive to drug and in those with glaucoma or tendency toward urine retention; also contraindicated in those who have received an MAO inhibitor within past 14 days and during acute recovery phase of an MI.

Black Box Warning Doxepin isn't approved for use in children. Clinicians considering the use of doxepin in a child, adolescent, or young adult must balance risk with clinical need. ∎

☉ Alert: Concomitant use with linezolid or methylene blue can cause serotonin syndrome (fever, mental status changes, muscle twitching, excessive sweating, shivering or shaking, diarrhea, loss of coordination). Use with linezolid or methylene blue only for life-threatening or urgent conditions when the potential benefits outweigh the risks of toxicity.

• Avoid use in patients with bipolar disorder. Drug isn't approved to treat bipolar depression.

Dialyzable drug: No.

⚠ Overdose S&S: Cardiac arrhythmias, severe hypotension, seizures, CNS depression, coma, confusion, disturbed concentration, transient visual hallucinations, dilated pupils, agitation, hyperactive reflexes, stupor, drowsiness, muscle rigidity, vomiting, hypothermia, hyperpyrexia.

PREGNANCY-LACTATION-REPRODUCTION
• There are no adequate well-controlled studies in pregnant women. Use during pregnancy only if clearly needed and potential benefit justifies potential risk to the fetus.

• Drug appears in human milk. Apnea and drowsiness have been reported in breastfeeding infant whose mother was taking doxepin. Use cautiously in breastfeeding women.

NURSING CONSIDERATIONS
• Don't withdraw drug abruptly; gradually taper dosage to minimize withdrawal symptoms.

• Monitor patient for nausea, headache, and malaise after abrupt withdrawal of long-term therapy; these symptoms don't indicate addiction.

☉ Alert: If linezolid or methylene blue must be given, stop drug and monitor patient for serotonin toxicity for 2 weeks, or until 24 hours after the last dose of methylene blue or linezolid, whichever comes first. Treatment may be resumed 24 hours after last dose of methylene blue or linezolid.

• If signs or symptoms of psychosis occur or increase, expect prescriber to reduce dosage. Record mood changes. Monitor patient for suicidal tendencies, and allow only a minimum supply of drug.

Black Box Warning Drug may increase risk of suicidal thinking and behavior in children, adolescents, and young adults ages 18 to 24, especially during the first few months of treatment, especially in those with major depressive disorder or other psychiatric disorder. ∎

• Drug has strong anticholinergic effects and is one of the most sedating TCAs. Adverse anticholinergic effects can occur rapidly.

• Recommend use of sugarless hard candy or gum to relieve dry mouth.

• *Look alike–sound alike:* Don't confuse doxepin with doxazosin, digoxin, doxapram, or Doxidan.

PATIENT TEACHING

۞ *Alert:* Teach patient to recognize and immediately report symptoms of serotonin toxicity (fever, mental status changes, muscle twitching, excessive sweating, shivering or shaking, diarrhea, loss of coordination).

• Tell patient to dilute oral concentrate with 4 oz (120 mL) of water, milk, or juice (orange, grapefruit, tomato, prune, or pineapple, but not grape); preparation shouldn't be mixed with carbonated beverages.

Black Box Warning Advise families and caregivers to closely observe patient for increased suicidal thinking and behavior. ∎

• Tell patient to take full dose at bedtime whenever possible but to watch for possible morning dizziness on standing up quickly.

• Tell patient to avoid taking Silenor within 3 hours of a meal, to minimize the potential for next-day effect.

• Advise patient to consult prescriber before taking other prescription or OTC drugs.

• Warn patient to avoid hazardous activities that require alertness and good psychomotor coordination until effects of drug are known. Drowsiness and dizziness usually subside after a few weeks.

• Tell patient to avoid alcohol during drug therapy.

• Tell patient that antianxiety effect is apparent before antidepressant effect; maximal effect may not be evident for 2 to 3 weeks.

• Warn patient not to stop drug suddenly.

• To prevent sensitivity to the sun, advise patient to use sunblock, wear protective clothing, and avoid prolonged exposure to strong sunlight.

SAFETY ALERT!

DOXOrubicin hydrochloride
dox-oh-ROO-bi-sin

Therapeutic class: Antineoplastics
Pharmacologic class: Anthracycline glycoside antibiotics

AVAILABLE FORMS
Injection (preservative-free): 2 mg/mL
Powder for injection: 10 mg, 20 mg, 50 mg

INDICATIONS & DOSAGES
Adjust-a-dose (for all indications): Refer to manufacturer's instructions for toxicity-related dosage adjustments.

➤ **Bladder, breast, lung, ovarian, stomach, and thyroid cancers; non-Hodgkin lymphoma; Hodgkin lymphoma; acute lymphoblastic and myeloblastic leukemia; Wilms tumor; neuroblastoma; lymphoma; soft-tissue and bone sarcomas**
Adults and children: 60 to 75 mg/m^2 IV as single dose every 21 days, or when used in combination with other chemotherapy drugs, 40 to 75 mg/m^2 IV every 21 to 28 days.

➤ **Adjuvant treatment in combination with cyclophosphamide in women with evidence of axillary lymph node involvement after resection of primary breast cancer**
Women: 60 mg/m^2 IV bolus on day 1 of each 21-day treatment cycle for a total of four cycles.

➤ **Endometrial carcinoma ♦**
Women: 60 mg/m^2 IV on day 1 of each 21-day treatment cycle for eight cycles in combination with cisplatin.

➤ **Multiple myeloma ♦**
Adults: In combination with other chemotherapy drugs, 9 mg/m^2/day IV on days 1 to 4 for three cycles or 10 mg/m^2/day IV as a continuous infusion on days 1 to 4 of each cycle.

➤ **Uterine sarcoma ♦**
Women: 60 mg/m^2 IV on day 1 every 21 days; maximum cumulative dose, 480 mg/m^2. Or, 50 mg/m^2 IV (over 15 minutes) on day 1 every 21 days in combination with ifosfamide/mesna; maximum cumulative dose, 450 mg/m^2.

Reactions in bold italics are *life-threatening*. Interactions may have a *rapid onset* or a *delayed onset*.

➤ **Waldenström macroglobulinemia** ◆
Adults: 50 mg/m² IV on day 1 of each
21-day treatment cycle for four to eight
cycles in combination with other chemotherapy drugs.

ADMINISTRATION

IV

Black Box Warning Never give drug IM
or subcut. ∎

Black Box Warning If extravasation occurs, stop infusion immediately, apply ice
to affected area, and notify prescriber. Extravasation can result in severe local tissue
injury and necrosis requiring wide excision
and skin grafting. ∎

▼ Preparing and giving parenteral drug
may be mutagenic, teratogenic, or carcinogenic. Follow facility policy to reduce
risks.

▼ Reconstitute with preservative-free NSS
for injection to yield 2 mg/mL; add 5 mL to
10-mg vial, 10 mL to 20-mg vial, or 25 mL
to 50-mg vial. Shake vial to dissolve drug.

▼ Don't place IV catheter over joints or
in limbs with poor venous or lymphatic
drainage.

▼ Give by direct injection over 3 to 10 minutes into the tubing of a free-flowing IV
solution containing D₅W or NSS for
injection.

▼ Some protocols give doxorubicin as a
prolonged infusion, which requires central
venous access.

▼ If vein streaking proximal to the site of
infusion or facial flushing occurs, slow administration rate. If welts appear, stop drug
and notify prescriber.

▼ Refrigerated, reconstituted solution is
stable 15 days; at room temperature, it's
stable 7 days.

▼ **Incompatibilities:** Other drugs and
alkaline solutions.

ACTION

Interferes with DNA-dependent RNA synthesis by intercalation.

Route	Onset	Peak	Duration
IV	Unknown	Unknown	Unknown

Half-life: Initial, 5 minutes; terminal, 20 to
48 hours.

ADVERSE REACTIONS

CV: cardiac depression, *arrhythmias, acute
left ventricular failure, irreversible cardiomyopathy.* **GI:** nausea, vomiting, diarrhea, stomatitis, esophagitis, anorexia. **GU:**
transient red urine. **Hematologic:** *leukopenia, thrombocytopenia, myelosuppression.*
Metabolic: hyperuricemia, weight loss,
weight gain. **Skin:** severe cellulitis and tissue sloughing with drug extravasation, urticaria, facial flushing, complete alopecia
within 3 to 4 weeks, hyperpigmentation of
nail beds and dermal creases, radiation recall effect. **Other:** chills, *anaphylaxis, secondary malignancy (acute myelogenous
leukemia [AML], myelodysplastic syndrome).*

INTERACTIONS

Drug-drug. *Calcium channel blockers:* May
increase cardiotoxic effects. Monitor patient's ECG closely.

Cyclosporine: May increase doxorubicin
concentration. Monitor patient for toxicity.

Digoxin: May decrease digoxin level. Monitor digoxin level closely.

Fosphenytoin, phenytoin: May decrease
level of phenytoin or fosphenytoin. Monitor
drug level.

Paclitaxel: May decrease doxorubicin clearance. Give doxorubicin before paclitaxel if
used together.

Phenobarbital: May increase doxorubicin
clearance. Monitor patient closely.

Progesterone: May enhance neutropenia and
thrombocytopenia. Monitor patient and laboratory values closely.

Streptozocin: May increase and prolong
doxorubicin level. Doxorubicin dosage may
have to be adjusted.

Trastuzumab: May increase risk of cardiac
abnormalities. Consider therapy modification.

Vaccines (inactivated): May diminish therapeutic effect of vaccines. If patient is vaccinated during therapy, revaccinate 3 months
after stopping immunosuppressant.

Vaccines (live-virus): May increase vaccine-related toxicities and decrease vaccine's
therapeutic effects. Avoid use of live-virus
vaccines with immunosuppressants.

Drug-herb. *St. John's wort:* May decrease doxorubicin serum concentration. Avoid combination.

EFFECTS ON LAB TEST RESULTS
• May increase transaminase, bilirubin, and uric acid levels.
• May decrease platelet and WBC counts.

CONTRAINDICATIONS & CAUTIONS
• Contraindicated in patients with a history of sensitivity reactions to drug or its components.
• Contraindicated in patients with severe myocardial insufficiency, recent (past 4 to 6 weeks) MI, severe persistent drug-induced myelosuppression, baseline neutrophil count less than 1,500 cells/mm^3, or severe hepatic impairment (Child-Pugh class C or serum bilirubin level above 5 mg/dL).
• Don't use in patients who had previous treatment with complete cumulative doses of doxorubicin, daunorubicin, idarubicin, or other anthracyclines or anthracenediones.
Dialyzable drug: No.

PREGNANCY-LACTATION-REPRODUCTION
• May cause fetal harm if used during pregnancy. Female patients of reproductive potential and male patients with female partners of reproductive potential should avoid pregnancy.
• Advise female patients of reproductive potential and male patients with female partners of reproductive potential to use effective nonhormonal contraception during and for 6 months after therapy ends.
• Drug appears in human milk. Women shouldn't breastfeed during therapy.

NURSING CONSIDERATIONS
Black Box Warning Drug should be administered under the supervision of a physician experienced with cancer chemotherapeutic agents. ∎
• Perform cardiac function studies, including a MUGA or echocardiogram, ECG, and LVEF, before treatment, periodically throughout therapy, and after therapy is completed.
• Take preventive measures, including adequate hydration of patient, before starting treatment. Rapid lysis of leukemic cells may

cause hyperuricemia. Allopurinol may be ordered.
• Premedicate with antiemetic to reduce nausea.
• If skin or mucosal contact occurs, immediately wash with soap and water.
Black Box Warning Reduce dosage in patients with hepatic impairment. ∎
Black Box Warning Severe myelosuppression may occur, possibly resulting in hospitalization or death. ∎
Black Box Warning Risk of secondary AML or myelodysplastic syndrome increases with doxorubicin use, especially when given with DNA-damaging antineoplastics or radiotherapy, when patients have been heavily pretreated with cytotoxic drugs, when doses have been escalated, or when patients age 50 and older had an existing increased risk of secondary AML or myelodysplastic syndrome. Children are also at risk for developing secondary AML. ∎
• Monitor CBC with differential, electrolyte levels, renal function, and LFT values; monitor ECG during therapy.
• Monitor ECG for changes, such as sinus tachycardia, T-wave flattening, ST-segment depression, and voltage reduction.
• Leukopenia may occur during days 10 to 14, with recovery by day 21.
Black Box Warning Cardiomyopathy risk is proportional to the cumulative exposure, with incidence rates of 1% to 20% for cumulative doses ranging from 300 to 500 mg/m^2 when drug is given every 3 weeks. Cardiomyopathy risk is further increased with concomitant cardiotoxic therapy. Assess LVEF before, regularly during, and after doxorubicin treatment. ∎
• If tachycardia develops, stop drug or slow rate of infusion, and notify prescriber.
Black Box Warning Myocardial toxicity, including acute left ventricular failure, may occur during therapy or months to years after termination of therapy. Assess LVEF regularly, during, and after treatment with doxorubicin. Children are at increased risk for developing delayed cardiotoxicity. ∎
🔹 *Alert:* If signs of HF develop, stop drug and notify prescriber. HF can often be prevented by increasing frequency of ECG assessments or multigated radionuclide

angiography as the cumulative dose exceeds 300 mg/m^2 when patient is also receiving or has received cyclophosphamide, trastuzumab, or radiation therapy to cardiac area.

◆ **Alert:** Reddish color of drug is similar to that of daunorubicin; don't confuse the two drugs.

• Esophagitis is common in patients who also have received radiation therapy.

◆ **Alert:** Patient who has previously received radiation therapy is susceptible to radiation recall effect.

• **Look alike–sound alike:** Don't confuse doxorubicin with doxorubicin liposomal, daunorubicin, or idarubicin.

PATIENT TEACHING

◆ **Alert:** Advise patient to immediately report pain or burning at injection site during or after administration.

• Advise patient to watch for signs and symptoms of infection (fever, sore throat, fatigue) and bleeding (easy bruising, nosebleeds, bleeding gums, tarry stools) and to take temperature daily.

• Advise patient that orange to red urine for 1 to 2 days is normal and doesn't indicate presence of blood.

• Inform patient that hair loss may occur but that it's usually reversible. Hair may regrow 2 to 5 months after drug is stopped.

• Advise patient to take antiemetics on a regular basis to avoid nausea and vomiting.

SAFETY ALERT!

DOXOrubicin hydrochloride liposomal
dox-oh-ROO-bi-sin

Doxil

Therapeutic class: Antineoplastics
Pharmacologic class: Anthracycline glycoside antibiotics

AVAILABLE FORMS
Injection: 20 mg/10 mL, 50 mg/25 mL

INDICATIONS & DOSAGES
Adjust-a-dose (for all indications): Refer to manufacturer's instructions for toxicity-related dosage adjustments.

➤ **Ovarian cancer that has progressed or recurred after platinum-based chemotherapy**
Women: 50 mg/m^2 IV. Repeat treatment once every 28 days until disease progression or unacceptable toxicity.

➤ **AIDS-related Kaposi sarcoma after failure of prior systemic chemotherapy or intolerance to such therapy**
Adults: 20 mg/m^2 IV every 21 days until disease progression or unacceptable toxicity.

➤ **Multiple myeloma in patients who haven't previously received bortezomib and have received at least one prior therapy**
Adults: 30 mg/m^2 IV on day 4 of every 21-day cycle (administer after bortezomib) for eight cycles or until disease progression or unacceptable toxicity.

➤ **Refractory metastatic breast cancer ◆**
Adults: 50 mg/m^2 IV every 4 weeks.

ADMINISTRATION
IV

▼ Follow safe handling and disposal procedures for antineoplastics.

▼ Don't give as an undiluted suspension or as an IV bolus. Don't give IM or subcut.

▼ Dilute doses up to 90 mg in 250 mL D$_5$W using aseptic technique. Dilute doses exceeding 90 mg in 500 mL D$_5$W.

◆ **Alert:** Carefully check label on IV bag before giving drug. Accidentally substituting doxorubicin hydrochloride liposomal for conventional doxorubicin hydrochloride may cause severe adverse reactions. The two products can't be substituted on a milligram-per-milligram basis.

▼ Don't use an in-line filter.

▼ Inspect product visually for particulate matter and discoloration before administration; don't use if a precipitate or foreign matter is present.

▼ Initiate infusion at 1 mg/minute and if no infusion-related reactions occur, increase rate to complete administration over 60 minutes. Monitor patient carefully during infusion. Never give as bolus injection.

Black Box Warning Serious, sometimes fatal, allergic infusion reactions can occur. Make sure emergency equipment and medications are available. Acute infusion-related reactions include flushing, shortness of breath, facial swelling, headache, chills, back pain, tightness in chest or throat, and hypotension. ■

▼ If extravasation occurs, stop infusion immediately and attempt to aspirate extravasated fluid before removing needle. Don't flush line or apply pressure to the site. Apply ice to the site intermittently for 15 minutes four times a day for 3 days. If extravasation is in an extremity, elevate the extremity. Restart infusion in another vein.

▼ Refrigerate diluted solution at 36° to 46° F (2° to 8° C) and give within 24 hours.

▼ **Incompatibilities:** Other IV drugs.

ACTION

Consists of doxorubicin hydrochloride encapsulated in liposomes. Inhibits DNA and RNA synthesis through intercalation.

Route	Onset	Peak	Duration
IV	Unknown	Unknown	Unknown

Half-life: 3.6 to 6.6 hours in first phase; 46.7 to 59.8 hours in second phase with doses of 10 to 20 mg/m^2.

ADVERSE REACTIONS

CNS: asthenia, paresthesia, headache, somnolence, dizziness, depression, insomnia, anxiety, malaise, emotional lability, fatigue, fever. **CV:** chest pain, hypotension, tachycardia, flushing, peripheral edema, *cardiomyopathy, HF, arrhythmias,* pericardial effusion, *cardiac arrest.* **EENT:** conjunctivitis, optic neuritis, retinitis, epistaxis, rhinitis, pharyngitis, sinusitis. **GI:** nausea, vomiting, constipation, anorexia, diarrhea, abdominal pain, dyspepsia, oral candidiasis, enlarged abdomen, esophagitis, dysphagia, stomatitis, taste perversion, glossitis, secondary oral cancers. **GU:** UTI, hematuria, vaginal candidiasis. **Hematologic:** *leukopenia, neutropenia, thrombocytopenia,* anemia. **Hepatic:** hyperbilirubinemia. **Metabolic:** dehydration, weight loss, hypercalcemia, *hypokalemia,* hyponatremia, hyperglycemia. **Musculoskeletal:** myalgia, back pain. **Respiratory:** dyspnea, increased cough, pneumonia. **Skin:** rash, alopecia, dry skin, pruritus, skin discoloration, skin disorder, exfoliative dermatitis, sweating, palmar–plantar erythrodysesthesia. **Other:** allergic reaction, chills, herpes zoster, infection, *infusion-related reactions.*

INTERACTIONS

No formal drug interaction studies have been conducted. However, doxorubicin hydrochloride liposomal may interact with drugs that interact with the conventional form of doxorubicin hydrochloride.

EFFECTS ON LAB TEST RESULTS

• May increase bilirubin, calcium, ALT, alkaline phosphatase, bilirubin, and glucose levels. May decrease potassium, sodium, and Hb levels.

• May prolong PT and increase INR. May decrease neutrophil, platelet, and WBC counts.

CONTRAINDICATIONS & CAUTIONS

• Contraindicated in patients hypersensitive to conventional formulation of doxorubicin hydrochloride or any component of the liposomal form.

Black Box Warning May cause myocardial damage, including HF, as the total cumulative doxorubicin dose approaches 550 mg/m^2. Risk of cardiomyopathy may be increased at lower cumulative doses in patients with prior mediastinal irradiation. Prior use of other anthracyclines or anthracenediones should be included in calculations of total cumulative dosage. ■

• Risk of cardiomyopathy with doxorubicin is generally proportional to the cumulative exposure, although the relationship between cumulative doxorubicin liposomal dose and risk of cardiotoxicity isn't known. Anthracycline-induced cardiotoxicity may be delayed (after discontinuation of anthracycline treatment).

Dialyzable drug: Unknown.

⚠ *Overdose S&S:* Leukopenia, mucositis, thrombocytopenia.

PREGNANCY-LACTATION-REPRODUCTION

• Drug may cause fetal harm if used during pregnancy. Female patients of childbearing potential and male patients with female partners of childbearing potential should use effective contraception during therapy and for 6 months after final dose.

Reactions in bold italics are *life-threatening*. Interactions may have a *rapid onset* or a *delayed onset*.

• It isn't known if drug appears in human milk. Patient should discontinue breastfeeding during treatment.

• Drug may damage spermatozoa and testicular tissue in males and may result in oligospermia, azoospermia, and permanent loss of fertility.

• Drug may cause amenorrhea, infertility, and premature menopause in females. Recovery of menses and ovulation is related to age at time of treatment.

NURSING CONSIDERATIONS

• Consider previous or current therapy with related compounds such as daunorubicin when calculating total dose of drug to be given. HF and cardiomyopathy may occur after therapy ends.

• Assess left ventricular cardiac function (multigated radionuclide angiogram scan or echocardiogram) before drug initiation, during treatment to detect acute changes, and after treatment to detect delayed cardiotoxicity.

• Give drug to patient with history of CV disease only when benefit outweighs risk to patient.

❸ Alert: Monitor patient for signs and symptoms of hand-foot syndrome, hematologic toxicity, and stomatitis. These adverse reactions may be managed with dosage delays and adjustments.

❸ Alert: If an infusion-related reaction occurs, temporarily stop drug until resolution, then resume at a reduced infusion rate. Discontinue infusion for serious or life-threatening reactions.

• Evaluate patient's hepatic function before therapy, and reduce dosage for serum bilirubin level of 1.2 mg/dL or higher.

• Drug may increase toxicity of other antineoplastics.

• Closely monitor cardiac function by endomyocardial biopsy, echocardiography, or gated radionuclide scans. If results indicate possible cardiac injury, the benefit of continued therapy must be weighed against the risk of myocardial injury.

• Severe myelosuppression may occur.

• Monitor CBC, including platelets, before each dose and frequently throughout therapy. Leukopenia is usually transient. Persistent severe myelosuppression may result in

superinfection or hemorrhage. Patient may need G-CSF to support blood counts.

• Secondary oral cancers, primarily squamous cell carcinoma, have been reported during treatment and for up to 6 years after last dose in patients with long-term (more than 1 year) exposure to drug. Assess patients at regular intervals for the presence of oral ulceration or any oral discomfort that may indicate secondary oral cancer.

• Drug is cytotoxic. Follow applicable special handling and disposal procedures. Immediately wash thoroughly with soap and water if drug contacts skin or mucosa.

• *Look alike–sound alike:* Don't confuse doxorubicin with daunorubicin. Don't confuse Doxil with Paxil. Don't confuse regular formulation of doxorubicin with liposomal formulation.

PATIENT TEACHING

• Tell patient to notify prescriber of all adverse reactions, including signs and symptoms of hand-foot syndrome (such as tingling or burning, redness, flaking, bothersome swelling, small blisters, or small sores on palms of hands or soles of feet).

• To reduce the risk of hand-foot syndrome, advise patient to follow these guidelines at least 1 day before and for 3 to 5 days after treatment:
  – Avoid direct sunlight and use sunblock SPF 15 or higher on all exposed skin.
  – Wear loose clothing and comfortable, well-ventilated, low-heeled shoes.
  – Avoid contact with hot water and take cool, short showers or baths.
  – Don't put pressure on your skin. (Avoid kneeling, leaning on your elbows, wearing tight jewelry or undergarments, and chopping hard foods.)

• Advise patient to report signs and symptoms of stomatitis (such as painful redness, swelling, or sores in mouth).

• Warn patient to avoid exposure to people with infections. Tell patient to report temperature of 100.5° F (38° C) or higher.

• Tell patient to report nausea, vomiting, tiredness, weakness, rash, or mild hair loss.

• Advise female patient of childbearing potential to avoid pregnancy and to use effective contraception during treatment and for

6 months after final dose. Discontinue breastfeeding during therapy.
• Advise male patient with female partner of childbearing potential to use effective contraception during treatment and for 6 months after final dose.

doxycycline
dox-i-SYE-kleen

Oracea

doxycycline calcium
Vibramycin

doxycycline hyclate
Acticlate, Acticlate Cap, Atridox, Doryx, Doryx MPC, Doxy 100, Morgidox, Vibramycin

doxycycline monohydrate
Apprilon✹, Monodox, Vibramycin

Therapeutic class: Antibiotics
Pharmacologic class: Tetracyclines

AVAILABLE FORMS
doxycycline
Capsules: 40 mg, 50 mg, 75 mg, 100 mg, 150 mg
Injection: 100-mg vial
Oral suspension: 25 mg/5 mL
Tablets: 50 mg, 75 mg, 100 mg, 150 mg
doxycycline calcium
Syrup: 50 mg/5 mL
doxycycline hyclate
Capsules: 50 mg, 100 mg
Injection: 100 mg, 200 mg
Periodontal system: 50 mg
Tablets: 20 mg, 75 mg, 100 mg, 150 mg
Tablets (delayed-release) ⓞⓝⓒ: 50 mg, 75 mg, 100 mg, 120 mg, 150 mg, 200 mg
doxycycline monohydrate
Capsules: 40 mg, 50 mg, 75 mg, 100 mg, 150 mg
Oral suspension: 25 mg/5 mL
Tablets: 50 mg, 75 mg, 100 mg, 150 mg

INDICATIONS & DOSAGES
➤ **Infections caused by susceptible gram-positive and gram-negative organisms (including *Haemophilus ducreyi,***

***Yersinia pestis, Francisella tularensis,* and *Campylobacter fetus*), *Rickettsiae* species, *Mycoplasma pneumoniae, Chlamydia trachomatis,* or *Borrelia burgdorferi* (Lyme disease); *Chlamydophila* psittacosis; granuloma inguinale**
Adults and children older than age 8 weighing 45 kg or more: 100 mg PO or 120 mg (Doryx MPC) PO every 12 hours on first day; then 100 mg PO or 120 mg Doryx MPC daily as a single dose or in two divided doses. Or, 200 mg IV on first day in one or two infusions; then 100 to 200 mg IV daily. Daily doses of 200 mg IV can be given as a single dose or in two divided doses.
Children older than age 8 weighing less than 45 kg for severe or life-threatening infections: 2.2 mg/kg PO or IV or 2.6 mg/kg Doryx MPC PO every 12 hours.
Children older than age 8 weighing less than 45 kg for less severe infections: 4.4 mg/kg PO or IV divided into two doses on first day of treatment, followed by maintenance dose of 2.2 mg/kg PO given as a single daily dose or divided into twice-daily doses or 2.2 to 4.4 mg/kg/day IV given as one or two infusions, depending on the severity of the infection. Or, 5.3 mg/kg Doryx MPC PO divided into two doses on first day of treatment, followed by maintenance dose of 2.6 mg/kg given as a single daily dose or divided into twice-daily doses.

Give IV infusion slowly (minimum 1 hour). Refer to manufacturer's instructions for duration of therapy.
➤ **Gonorrhea in patients allergic to penicillin**
Adults: 100 mg PO b.i.d. for 7 days. Or, 300 mg PO once, followed in 1 hour with a second 300-mg PO dose.
➤ **Uncomplicated gonococcal infections (except anorectal infections in men)**
Adults: 120 mg Doryx MPC PO b.i.d. for 7 days. Or, 360 mg Doryx MPC PO followed by 360 mg PO in 1 hour.
➤ **Acute epididymo-orchitis caused by *Neisseria gonorrhoeae* or *C. trachomatis* (Doryx MPC)**
Adults: 120 mg PO b.i.d. for at least 10 days.
➤ **Syphilis in patients allergic to penicillin**
Adults: 100 mg PO or 120 mg Doryx MPC PO b.i.d. for 14 days (early). If more than

---

Reactions in bold italics are *life-threatening*. Interactions may have a *rapid onset* or a *delayed onset*.

1-year duration, 100 mg PO or 120 mg Doryx MPC PO b.i.d. for 4 weeks.

➤ **Primary or secondary syphilis in patients allergic to penicillin**
Adults: 300 mg PO daily in divided doses for 14 days.

➤ **Uncomplicated urethral, endocervical, or rectal infections caused by *C. trachomatis* or *Ureaplasma urealyticum***
Adults: 100 mg PO or 120 mg Doryx MPC b.i.d. for at least 7 days.

➤ **To prevent malaria**
Adults: 100 mg PO or 120 mg Doryx MPC PO daily beginning 1 to 2 days before travel to endemic area and continued for 4 weeks after travel.
Children older than age 8: Give 2 mg/kg (2.4 mg/kg for Doryx MPC) PO once daily beginning 1 to 2 days before travel to endemic area and continued for 4 weeks after travel. Don't exceed daily dose of 100 mg (excluding Doryx MPC).

➤ **Adjunct to other antibiotics for inhalation, GI, and oropharyngeal anthrax**
Adults: 100 mg every 12 hours IV initially until susceptibility test results are known. Switch to 100 mg PO or 120 mg Doryx MPC PO b.i.d. when appropriate. Treat for 60 days total.
Children older than age 8 weighing more than 45 kg: 100 mg every 12 hours IV; then switch to 100 mg PO b.i.d. when appropriate. Treat for 60 days total.
Children older than age 8 weighing 45 kg or less: 2.2 mg/kg every 12 hours IV; then switch to 2.2 mg/kg (up to 100 mg) PO b.i.d. when appropriate. Treat for 60 days total.
Children age 8 and younger: 2.2 mg/kg IV every 12 hours; then switch to 2.2 mg/kg (up to 100 mg) PO b.i.d. when appropriate. Treat for 60 days total.

➤ **Inhalational anthrax (postexposure) (Doryx MPC)**
Adults and children weighing 45 kg or more: 120 mg PO b.i.d. for 60 days.
Children weighing less than 45 kg: 2.6 mg/kg PO b.i.d. for 60 days.

➤ **Cutaneous anthrax**
Adults: 100 mg PO every 12 hours for 60 days.
Children older than age 8 weighing more than 45 kg: 100 mg PO every 12 hours for 60 days.

Children older than age 8 weighing 45 kg or less: 2.2 mg/kg (up to 100 mg) PO every 12 hours for 60 days.
Children age 8 and younger: 2.2 mg/kg (up to 100 mg) PO every 12 hours for 60 days.

➤ **Adjunct to scaling and root planing to improve attachment and reduce pocket depth in periodontitis**
Adults: 20 mg PO b.i.d., more than 1 hour before or 2 hours after the morning and evening meals and after scaling and root planing. Effective for up to 9 months.

➤ **Inflammatory lesions of rosacea**
Adults: 40 mg Oracea PO once daily in the morning, 1 hour before or 2 hours after a meal. Give with a full glass of water. Reevaluate treatment after 16 weeks.

ADMINISTRATION
PO
• Obtain specimen for culture and sensitivity tests before giving. Begin therapy while awaiting results.
• Doryx MPC can't be substituted on a milligram-per-milligram basis with other oral doxycyclines.
🔾 *Alert:* Check expiration date. Outdated or deteriorated tetracyclines may cause reversible nephrotoxicity (Fanconi syndrome).
• Give drug with food or milk if stomach upset occurs.
• Increase fluid intake and don't administer tablets or capsules within 1 hour of bedtime because of possible esophageal irritation or ulceration.
• Give Oracea with a full glass of water.
• Don't crush delayed-release tablets or capsules. Delayed-released tablets and capsules can be carefully broken apart and their contents sprinkled onto a spoonful of applesauce and swallowed without chewing.
• Immediate-release tablets may be crushed and mixed with low-fat or chocolate milk, chocolate pudding, or apple juice mixed equally with sugar. Store mixtures in refrigerator (except apple juice mixture, which can be stored at room temperature) and discard after 24 hours.

IV
▼ Obtain specimen for culture and sensitivity tests before giving. Begin therapy while awaiting results.

▼ Reconstitute powder for injection with sterile water for injection. Use 10 mL in 100-mg vial and 20 mL in 200-mg vial. Further dilute solution to a concentration of 0.1 mg/mL to 1 mg/mL; don't infuse solution that contains more than 1 mg/mL. Refer to manufacturer's instructions for compatible solutions.

▼ Don't expose drug to light or heat. Protect it from sunlight during infusion.

▼ Infusion time varies with dose but usually ranges from 1 to 4 hours. Infusion must be completed within 12 hours or within 6 hours in lactated Ringer solution or dextrose 5% in lactated Ringer solution.

▼ Monitor infusion site for evidence of thrombophlebitis.

▼ Reconstituted injectable solution is stable 72 hours if refrigerated and protected from light.

▼ **Incompatibilities:** Allopurinol, drugs that are unstable in acidic solutions (such as barbiturates), erythromycin lactobionate, heparin, meropenem, nafcillin, penicillin G potassium, piperacillin–tazobactam, riboflavin, sulfonamides.

ACTION

Exerts bacteriostatic effect by binding to the 30S and possibly 50S ribosomal subunits of microorganisms and inhibiting protein synthesis.

Route	Onset	Peak	Duration
PO	Unknown	1½–4 hr	Unknown
PO (delayed-release)	Unknown	2–4 hr	Unknown
IV	Immediate	Unknown	Unknown

Half-life: About 1 day after multiple dosing.

ADVERSE REACTIONS

CNS: *intracranial HTN,* headache. **CV:** pericarditis, thrombophlebitis. **GI:** diarrhea, epigastric distress, nausea, anorexia, glossitis, dysphagia, vomiting, oral candidiasis, enterocolitis, anogenital inflammation. **GU:** vaginitis. **Hematologic:** *neutropenia, thrombocytopenia,* eosinophilia, hemolytic anemia. **Musculoskeletal:** bone growth retardation in children younger than age 8. **Skin:** maculopapular and erythematous rashes, photosensitivity reactions, increased pigmentation, urticaria. **Other:**

anaphylaxis, hypersensitivity reactions, superinfection, permanent discoloration of teeth, enamel defects.

INTERACTIONS

Drug-drug. *Antacids and laxatives containing aluminum, magnesium, or calcium; antidiarrheals:* May decrease antibiotic absorption. Give antibiotic 1 hour before or 2 hours after these drugs.

Anticoagulants: May decrease thrombin activity. Reduced anticoagulant dosages may be needed.

Barbiturates, carbamazepine, phenobarbital, phenytoin, rifamycins: May decrease antibiotic effect. Consider therapy modification.

Ferrous sulfate and other iron products, zinc: May decrease antibiotic absorption. Give drug 2 hours before or 3 hours after iron.

Hormonal contraceptives: May decrease contraceptive effectiveness and increase risk of breakthrough bleeding. Advise use of a nonhormonal contraceptive.

Isotretinoin: May increase risk of pseudotumor cerebri. Avoid using together.

Methoxyflurane: May cause nephrotoxicity with tetracyclines. Avoid using together.

Penicillins: May interfere with bactericidal action of penicillins. Avoid using together.

Warfarin: May increase anticoagulant effect. Monitor PT and INR; adjust dosage.

Drug-lifestyle. *Alcohol use:* May decrease drug's effect. Discourage use together.

Sun exposure: May cause photosensitivity reactions. Advise patient to avoid excessive sunlight exposure.

EFFECTS ON LAB TEST RESULTS

• May increase BUN and liver enzyme levels. May decrease Hb level.

• May increase eosinophil count. May decrease platelet, neutrophil, and WBC counts.

• May falsely elevate fluorometric tests for urine catecholamines. May cause false-negative results in urine glucose tests using glucose oxidase reagent (Diastix or Chemstrip uG). Parenteral form may cause false-positive Clinitest results.

Reactions in bold italics are *life-threatening.* Interactions may have a *rapid onset* or a *delayed onset*.

CONTRAINDICATIONS & CAUTIONS

• Contraindicated in patients hypersensitive to drug or other tetracyclines.

• Use cautiously in patients with impaired renal or hepatic function.

• CDAD has been reported and may range in severity from mild diarrhea to fatal colitis. If CDAD is suspected or confirmed, ongoing antibiotic use not directed against *Clostridium difficile* may need to be discontinued. Institute appropriate treatment.

• In a fetus in the last half of gestation or in a child younger than age 8, drug may cause permanently discolored teeth, enamel defects, and bone growth retardation. Drug shouldn't be used in this age-group unless other drugs aren't likely to be effective or are contraindicated.

• Use in patients age 8 and younger only when potential benefits are expected to outweigh risks in severe or life-threatening conditions, such as anthrax or Rocky Mountain spotted fever, particularly when there are no alternative therapies.

Dialyzable drug: No.

⚠ Overdose S&S: Dizziness, nausea, vomiting.

PREGNANCY-LACTATION-REPRODUCTION

• Drug is generally considered a second-line antibiotic in pregnant women and use should be avoided. Use during pregnancy only when other drugs are contraindicated or ineffective. Contraindicated in second and third trimesters.

• In pregnant women and immunocompromised patients, use the usual dosage schedule for anthrax.

• Drug appears in human milk. Patient should take into account benefits of breastfeeding versus risk of exposure to the infant.

NURSING CONSIDERATIONS

• If patient receives large doses or prolonged therapy or if patient is at high risk, watch for signs and symptoms of superinfection. If superinfection occurs, drug should be discontinued and appropriate therapy instituted.

• Cutaneous anthrax with signs of systemic involvement, extensive edema, or lesions on the head or neck requires IV therapy and a multidrug approach.

• Ciprofloxacin and doxycycline are first-line therapies for anthrax. If anthrax patient also has meningitis, ciprofloxacin is preferred because of better distribution to the CNS.

• Drug may increase risk of intracranial HTN (IH) and pseudotumor cerebri, especially in women who are overweight or have a history of IH. Monitor patient for headache, blurred vision, diplopia, and vision loss. If visual changes occur, prompt ophthalmic evaluation is needed.

• Check patient's tongue for signs of fungal infection. Emphasize good oral hygiene.

• Photosensitivity reactions may occur within a few minutes to several hours after exposure and may last after therapy ends. Discontinue drug at first evidence of skin erythema.

• *Look alike–sound alike:* Don't confuse doxycycline with doxylamine or dicyclomine. Don't confuse Oracea with Orencia.

PATIENT TEACHING

• Tell patient to take entire amount of drug exactly as prescribed, even if feeling better.

• Instruct patient to report adverse reactions promptly, especially signs or symptoms of hypersensitivity or IH. If drug is being given IV, tell patient to report discomfort at IV site.

• Advise patient to take oral form of drug with food or milk if stomach upset occurs.

• Advise patient to increase fluid intake and not to take oral tablets or capsules within 1 hour of bedtime because of possible esophageal irritation or ulceration.

• Advise parent giving drug to a child that delayed-release tablets may not be crushed; however, immediate-release tablets may be crushed and mixed with low-fat or chocolate milk, chocolate pudding, or apple juice mixed equally with sugar. Tell parent to store mixtures in refrigerator (except apple juice mixture, which can be stored at room temperature) and to discard after 24 hours.

• Warn patient to avoid direct sunlight and ultraviolet light, wear protective clothing, and use sunscreen.

• Tell patient to report signs and symptoms of superinfection to prescriber.

• Tell patient taking Oracea to take drug with a full glass of water.

doxylamine succinate–pyridoxine hydrochloride
docks-ILL-ah-meen/peer-reh-DOCK-seen

Bonjesta, Diclectin✤, Diclegis

Therapeutic class: Antiemetics
Pharmacologic class: Antihistamines–vitamin B_6 analogues

AVAILABLE FORMS
Tablets (delayed-release) ⓄⓃⒸ: doxylamine succinate 10 mg/pyridoxine hydrochloride 10 mg
Tablets (extended-release) ⓄⓃⒸ: doxylamine succinate 20 mg/pyridoxine hydrochloride 20 mg

INDICATIONS & DOSAGES
➤ **Nausea and vomiting of pregnancy in women who don't respond to conservative management**
Adults (Diclegis): 2 tablets at bedtime on day 1. If that dosage adequately controls symptoms the next day, continue taking at bedtime. If symptoms persist into the afternoon of day 2, patients should take 2 tablets at bedtime that night, then take 1 tablet in the morning and 2 tablets at bedtime on day 3. If that dosage adequately controls symptoms on day 4, patients should continue taking 1 tablet in the morning and 2 tablets at bedtime. Otherwise, they should take 1 tablet in the morning, 1 tablet in the midafternoon, 2 tablets at bedtime on day 4.
Adults (Bonjesta): Initially, 1 tablet at bedtime on day 1. If symptoms aren't adequately controlled on day 2, increase dose to 1 tablet in the morning and 1 tablet at bedtime. Maximum dose is 1 tablet in the morning and 1 tablet at bedtime.

ADMINISTRATION
PO
• Give tablets whole on an empty stomach with a glass of water. Don't crush, split, or allow patient to chew tablets.
• Patient should take tablets daily and not p.r.n.
• Store bottle at room temperature. Keep bottle tightly closed and protect from moisture. Don't remove desiccant canister from bottle.

ACTION
Unknown. The combination of antihistamine and vitamin B_6 may cause anticholinergic effects, decreasing nausea.

Route	Onset	Peak	Duration
PO (doxylamine)	Unknown	1.7–8½ hr	Unknown
PO (pyridoxine)	Unknown	½–4.7 hr	Unknown

Half-life: Doxylamine, 12½ hours; pyridoxine, ½ hour.

ADVERSE REACTIONS
CNS: somnolence.

INTERACTIONS
Drug-drug. *CNS depressants (hypnotic sedatives and tranquilizers):* May have additive effects. Don't use together.
MAO inhibitors (selegiline, tranylcypromine): May prolong and intensify CNS anticholinergic effects. Use together is contraindicated.
Other ethanolamine derivative antihistamines (diphenhydramine): May have additive effects. Avoid use together.
Drug-food. *Any food:* May delay onset and reduce absorption if taken with food. Patient should take drug on an empty stomach.
Drug-lifestyle. *Alcohol use:* May cause additive CNS depression. Alcohol isn't recommended during pregnancy.

EFFECTS ON LAB TEST RESULTS
• May cause false-positive urine screening tests for methadone, opiates, and phencyclidine.

CONTRAINDICATIONS & CAUTIONS
• Contraindicated in women hypersensitive to drug or its components.
• Contraindicated with MAO inhibitors.
• Use cautiously in patients with asthma, increased IOP, angle-closure glaucoma, stenosing peptic ulcer, or pyloroduodenal or urinary bladder neck obstruction because of anticholinergic effects.
Dialyzable drug: Unknown.
⚠ *Overdose S&S:* Restlessness, dry mouth, dilated pupils, sleepiness, vertigo, mental

---

Reactions in bold italics are *life-threatening*. Interactions may have a *rapid onset* or a *delayed onset*.

confusion, tachycardia, seizures, rhabdomyolysis, acute renal failure, death.

PREGNANCY-LACTATION-REPRODUCTION
• Drug is intended for use in pregnant women. Drug hasn't been studied in women with hyperemesis gravidarum.
• Drug appears in human milk. Women shouldn't breastfeed while taking drug.

NURSING CONSIDERATIONS
• Reassess for continued need for drug as the pregnancy progresses.
• Monitor patient for anticholinergic effects (dry mouth, tachycardia, urine retention, constipation, ataxia).
• Monitor patient for somnolence, increased falls, and other CNS depressant effects.

PATIENT TEACHING
• Warn patient about adverse reactions, including somnolence, increased falls, other CNS depressant effects, dry mouth, dilated pupils, dizziness, confusion, fast heartbeat, and fluid retention.
• Teach patient to take drug as prescribed and that drug isn't to be used on an as-needed basis.
• Advise patient to avoid alcohol and sedating medications, including antihistamine cough and cold products, opioids, and sleep aids, while taking this drug because of increased risk of additive effects.
• Caution patient to avoid driving and operating heavy equipment or other activities that require complete mental alertness.

---

dronabinol (delta-9-tetrahydrocannabinol) ✄
droe-NAB-i-nol

Marinol, Syndros

Therapeutic class: Antiemetics
Pharmacologic class: Cannabinoids
Controlled substance schedule: III (Marinol); II (Syndros)

AVAILABLE FORMS
Capsules: 2.5 mg, 5 mg, 10 mg
Oral solution: 5 mg/mL*

INDICATIONS & DOSAGES
➤ **Nausea and vomiting from cancer chemotherapy after failure of conventional antiemetics**
Adults and children: 5 mg/m² (capsules) PO 1 to 3 hours before chemotherapy session. Then, 5 mg/m² (capsules) PO every 2 to 4 hours after chemotherapy, for total of four to six doses per day. If needed, increase dosage in 2.5-mg/m² increments to maximum of 15 mg/m² (capsules) per dose. Or, for adults only, 4.2 mg/m² (oral solution) 1 to 3 hours before chemotherapy, then every 2 to 4 hours after chemotherapy for a total of four to six doses per day. If needed, increase oral solution dosage as tolerated in increments of 2.1 mg/m². Maximum dosage is 12.6 mg/m² (oral solution)/dose.
Adjust-a-dose: For elderly patients: Initiate capsules at low end of dosing range; may initiate oral solution at 2.1 mg/m² once daily before chemotherapy to reduce risk of CNS symptoms.
➤ **Anorexia and weight loss in patients with AIDS**
Adults: 2.5 mg (capsules) PO b.i.d. 1 hour before lunch and dinner. If patient can't tolerate twice-daily dosing, decrease to 2.5 mg (capsules) PO given as a single dose daily before dinner or at bedtime. May gradually increase to maximum of 20 mg (capsules) daily given in divided doses. Or, 2.1 mg (oral solution) PO b.i.d. 1 hour before lunch and dinner. If needed, may increase dosage gradually to 2.1 mg (oral solution) PO 1 hour before lunch and 4.2 mg 1 hour before dinner. If needed, may further increase dosage to 4.2 mg (oral solution) PO 1 hour before lunch and 4.2 mg 1 hour before dinner. Maximum dosage is 8.4 mg b.i.d.
Adjust-a-dose: For elderly patients, initiate capsules at low end of dosing range; may initiate at 2.1 mg (oral solution) PO once daily 1 hour before dinner or at bedtime to reduce risk of CNS symptoms. For patients with severe or persistent CNS symptoms, may reduce dosage to 2.5 mg (capsules) PO or 2.1 mg (oral solution) PO once daily 1 hour before dinner or at bedtime.

ADMINISTRATION
PO
• Give 1 to 3 hours before chemotherapy.

- Give first dose on an empty stomach at least 30 minutes before patient eats; can give subsequent doses without regard to meals.
- Dosing later in the day may reduce frequency of CNS adverse reactions.
- Always use the calibrated oral dosing syringe when administering oral solution. Patient should take each dose with 180 to 240 mL of water.
- Can give Syndros via a silicone enteral feeding tube, #14 French or greater. Don't use tubes made of polyurethane. Flush the feeding tube with 30 mL of water after administration.
- Store capsules in cool environment, but protect from freezing. May store opened bottle of oral solution at 77° F (25° C); discard unused oral solution 42 days after opening.

ACTION
Cannabinoid that potentiates the activity of CB-1 and CB-2 receptors.

Route	Onset	Peak	Duration
PO	30–60 min	½–4 hr	4–6 hr (psychoactive effect); >24 hr (appetite stimulation)

Half-life: 1 to 1½ days (terminal).

ADVERSE REACTIONS
CNS: ataxia, dizziness, drowsiness, euphoria, paranoia, amnesia, asthenia, confusion, depersonalization, hallucinations, muddled thinking, somnolence, anxiety, nervousness, headache, malaise, depression, nightmares, speech difficulty. **CV:** orthostatic hypotension, palpitations, tachycardia, vasodilation, facial flushing. **EENT:** visual disturbances, tinnitus. **GI:** abdominal pain, dry mouth, nausea, vomiting, diarrhea, fecal incontinence. **Musculoskeletal:** myalgia. **Other:** chills.

INTERACTIONS
Drug-drug. *CNS depressants, psychomimetic substances, sedatives, TCAs:* May cause additive CNS depression. Avoid using together.
CYP2C9 inhibitors (amiodarone, fluconazole), CYP3A4 inhibitors (clarithromycin, erythromycin, itraconazole, ketoconazole, ritonavir): May increase dronabinol-related adverse reactions. Monitor carefully.

Disulfiram, metronidazole (Syndros only): May cause disulfiram-like reaction. Discontinue products containing disulfiram or metronidazole at least 14 days before starting treatment and don't give them within 7 days of completing treatment.
Drug-food. *Grapefruit juice:* May increase dronabinol-related adverse reactions. Avoid use.
Drug-lifestyle. *Alcohol use:* May cause additive CNS depression. Discourage use together.

EFFECTS ON LAB TEST RESULTS
- May increase LFT values.

CONTRAINDICATIONS & CAUTIONS
- Contraindicated in patients hypersensitive to sesame oil or cannabinoids.
- Oral solution is contraindicated in patients hypersensitive to alcohol and within 14 days of products containing disulfiram or metronidazole.
- Oral solution contains propylene glycol; large amounts are toxic and are associated with hyperosmolarity, lactic acidosis, renal toxicity, CNS depression, seizures, cardiac arrhythmias, ECG changes, and hemolysis. Use caution.
- Use cautiously in children, elderly patients, and in those with heart disease, seizure disorders, or history of substance abuse.
- Safety and effectiveness of oral solution in children haven't been established.
Dialyzable drug: Unknown.
⚠ *Overdose S&S:* Mild—drowsiness, euphoria, heightened sensory awareness, altered time perception, reddened conjunctiva, dry mouth, tachycardia; moderate—memory impairment, depersonalization, mood alteration, urine retention, decreased bowel motility; severe—decreased motor coordination, lethargy, slurred speech, orthostatic hypotension; lactic acidosis, hypoglycemia, CNS depression, coma, seizures (oral solution).

PREGNANCY-LACTATION-REPRODUCTION
- Drug may cause fetal harm. Avoid use in pregnant women.
- Data are limited on the presence of dronabinol in human milk and its effects on

---

the breastfed infant or on milk production. Women with HIV shouldn't breastfeed due to the risk of postnatal HIV transmission. Because of the possible adverse effects on the breastfed infant, women with nausea and vomiting associated with cancer chemotherapy shouldn't breastfeed during treatment and for 9 days after final dose.

NURSING CONSIDERATIONS

- Expect drug to be prescribed only for patients who haven't responded satisfactorily to other antiemetics.
- ☻ *Alert:* Drug is the principal active substance in *Cannabis sativa* (marijuana), which can produce both physiologic and psychological dependence and has a high risk of abuse. Use cautiously in patients receiving sedatives, hypnotics, or other psychoactive drugs.
- Assess patient's risk of abuse or misuse before drug is prescribed. Monitor patients with a history of substance abuse for abuse or misuse behaviors during treatment.
- ☒ Patients who are known to carry genetic variants associated with CYP2C9 function (CYP2C9 polymorphism) have increased risk of adverse drug-related effects.
- Monitor patient for hypotension, HTN, syncope, and tachycardia.
- Drug can exacerbate mania, depression, and schizophrenia. Screen patients for these illnesses before giving drug. If drug must be used, monitor patient for worsening signs and symptoms of psychiatric illness. Elderly patients may be more sensitive to drug's effects.
- CNS effects are intensified at higher dosages.
- Drug effects may persist for days after treatment ends.
- New or worsening nausea, vomiting, or abdominal pain can occur during treatment. Ask patients about these symptoms as they may not recognize them as abnormal.
- *Look alike–sound alike:* Don't confuse dronabinol with droperidol.

PATIENT TEACHING

- Tell patient to report all adverse reactions; tell patient that drug may induce unusual changes in mood or other adverse behavioral effects.

- Advise patient to report new or worsening nausea, vomiting, or abdominal pain.
- Caution patient that oral solution can't be taken within 14 days of disulfiram or metronidazole.
- Advise patient against performing activities that require alertness until CNS effects of drug are known.
- Warn caregivers to supervise patient during and immediately after treatment.
- Advise patient to store drug securely.
- Advise patient not to breastfeed during therapy and for 9 days after final dose.

---

dronedarone
dro-neh-DAR-rone

Multaq

Therapeutic class: Antiarrhythmics
Pharmacologic class: Benzofuran derivatives

AVAILABLE FORMS
Tablets: 400 mg

INDICATIONS & DOSAGES
➤ **To reduce risk of hospitalization for atrial fibrillation in patients in sinus rhythm with a history of paroxysmal or persistent atrial fibrillation**
Adults: 400 mg PO b.i.d.

ADMINISTRATION
PO
- Give drug with morning and evening meals.
- Don't give grapefruit juice to patient taking this drug.

ACTION
Unknown. Exhibits properties of all four Vaughan-Williams antiarrhythmic classes; it's unclear which of these is important in producing drug's clinical effects.

Route	Onset	Peak	Duration
PO	Unknown	3–6 hr	Unknown

Half-life: 13 to 19 hours.

ADVERSE REACTIONS

CNS: asthenia. **CV:** *bradycardia, HF, QT-interval prolongation.* **GI:** abdominal pain, diarrhea, dyspepsia, nausea, vomiting. **GU:** prerenal azotemia, *acute renal failure,* elevated creatinine level. **Metabolic:** hypovolemia. **Skin:** allergic dermatitis, dermatitis, eczema, pruritus, rash.

INTERACTIONS

Drug-drug. *Beta blockers:* May cause bradycardia. Initially, give low dose of beta blocker and increase dosage only after monitoring ECG for tolerance.

Calcium channel blockers: May cause additive AV-blocking effects. Reduce initial dosage of calcium channel blocker; increase dosage only after monitoring ECG for tolerance.

CYP2C9 substrates (losartan, warfarin): May increase metabolite levels. Monitor patient closely; monitor INR in patient taking warfarin.

CYP3A inducers (carbamazepine, phenobarbital, phenytoin, rifampin): May decrease dronedarone level. Use together is contraindicated.

CYP3A inhibitors (clarithromycin, erythromycin, itraconazole, ketoconazole, ritonavir, voriconazole): May increase dronedarone level. Use together is contraindicated.

CYP3A substrates (sirolimus, tacrolimus): May increase levels of these drugs. Monitor drug levels.

Digoxin: May increase digoxin level and electrophysiologic effects of dronedarone. Avoid use together; if necessary to use together, decrease digoxin dosage by 50%, monitor levels, and observe for toxicity.

Drugs that prolong QT interval (Class I and III antiarrhythmics, macrolide antibiotics, phenothiazines, TCAs): May further increase QT interval, leading to torsades de pointes. Use together is contraindicated.

Statins: May increase statin level. Use together cautiously.

Drug-herb. *St John's wort:* May decrease drug level. Discourage use together.

Drug-lifestyle. *Grapefruit juice:* May increase drug level. Don't use together.

EFFECTS ON LAB TEST RESULTS

• May increase serum creatinine level.
• May decrease potassium and magnesium levels (in patients taking potassium-depleting diuretics).

CONTRAINDICATIONS & CAUTIONS

Black Box Warning Contraindicated in patients with NYHA Class IV HF or Class II to III HF with recent decompensation requiring hospitalization or referral to an HF clinic. ∎

Black Box Warning Contraindicated in patients with atrial fibrillation who won't or can't be restored to normal sinus rhythm. Drug doubles risk of death, stroke, and hospitalization for HF in patients with permanent atrial fibrillation. ∎

• Contraindicated in patients hypersensitive to drug or its components.
• Contraindicated in patients with second- or third-degree AV block or sick sinus syndrome (unless a functioning pacemaker is in place), bradycardia (less than 50 beats/minute), severe hepatic impairment, QTc interval of 500 msec or greater, or PR interval greater than 280 msec.
• Contraindicated with concomitant use of strong CYP3A inhibitors and drugs or herbal preparations that prolong QT interval.
• Contraindicated in patients with previous pulmonary toxicity with amiodarone use.

۞ Alert: Discontinue Class I or III antiarrhythmics, such as amiodarone, flecainide, propafenone, quinidine, disopyramide, dofetilide, and sotalol, and strong CYP3A inhibitors before starting drug.

۞ Alert: Drug may increase risk of severe hepatic injury or failure.

• Use cautiously in patients with new or worsening HF.
• ILD has been reported. Discontinue drug if pulmonary toxicity is confirmed.
• Marked increase in serum creatinine level, prerenal azotemia, and acute renal failure, frequently in the setting of HF or hypovolemia, have been reported. Effects appear to be reversible upon drug discontinuation and with appropriate medical treatment. Monitor renal function periodically.

Dialyzable drug: Unknown.

⚠ Overdose S&S: QTc-interval prolongation.

Reactions in bold italics are *life-threatening*. Interactions may have a *rapid onset* or a *delayed onset*.

PREGNANCY-LACTATION-REPRODUCTION
• Drug may cause fetal harm, and use in pregnant women is contraindicated. Women of childbearing potential should use effective birth control during therapy.
• Drug is contraindicated in breastfeeding women; it isn't known if drug appears in human milk. Women should discontinue breastfeeding or discontinue drug.

NURSING CONSIDERATIONS
• Potassium-depleting diuretics may cause hypokalemia and hypomagnesemia, increasing the risk of torsades de pointes. Initiate dronedarone therapy after potassium and magnesium levels reach and stay within normal range.
• Ensure that patients discontinue Class I or III antiarrhythmics or drugs that are strong inhibitors of CYP3A before starting drug.
• Monitor CV status, ECG, electrolyte levels, and QTc interval routinely.
• Monitor renal function regularly. Renal impairment can occur.
• Monitor hepatic serum enzyme levels, especially during the first 6 months of therapy. Discontinue drug if hepatic injury is suspected.

PATIENT TEACHING
• Instruct patient to take drug with morning and evening meals.
• Tell patient to avoid grapefruit juice.
• Advise patient to report weight gain, dyspnea, fatigue, and peripheral edema, which may indicate worsening HF.
• Tell patient to report changes in OTC or prescription drug use, or in supplement or herb use.
• If patient misses a dose, tell patient not to double the dose but to skip that dose and take the next regularly scheduled dose.
• Instruct patient to report slowed heartbeat, diarrhea, nausea, vomiting, abdominal pain, indigestion, fatigue, or rash.
• Advise female patient of childbearing potential to use an effective method of birth control while taking drug and to notify prescriber if becoming pregnant or thinking of becoming pregnant.
• Advise female patient not to breastfeed while taking dronedarone because drug may appear in human milk.

drospirenone–ethinyl estradiol
droh-SPYE-re-none/ETH-i-nill es-tra-DYE-ole

Gianvi, Loryna, Mya✿, Nikki, Ocella, Syeda, Vestura, Yasmin, Yaz, Zamine 21✿, Zamine 28✿, Zarah

Therapeutic class: Contraceptives
Pharmacologic class: Estrogen–progestin combinations

AVAILABLE FORMS
Tablets: 3 mg drospirenone and 0.03 mg ethinyl estradiol as 21 active tablets (Zamine 21) and 7 inert tablets (Ocella, Syeda, Yasmin, Zamine 28, Zarah); 3 mg drospirenone and 0.02 mg ethinyl estradiol as 24 active tablets and 4 inert tablets (Gianvi, Loryna, Mya, Nikki, Vestura, Yaz)

INDICATIONS & DOSAGES
➤ **Contraception**
Women: 1 active tablet PO daily for 21 days beginning on day 1 of menstrual cycle or first Sunday after onset of menstruation. Then 1 inert tablet PO daily on days 22 through 28. Or 1 active tablet PO daily for 24 days beginning on day 1 of menstrual cycle or first Sunday after onset of menstruation. Then 1 inert tablet PO daily on days 25 through 28. Begin next and all subsequent 28-day regimens on same day of week that first regimen began, following same schedule. Restart active tablets on next day after last inert tablet.
➤ **Premenstrual dysphoric disorder (Gianvi, Vestura, Yaz)**
Women: 1 active tablet PO daily for 24 days beginning on day 1 of menstrual cycle or first Sunday after menstruation begins. Then 1 inert tablet PO daily on days 25 through 28. Begin next and all subsequent 28-day regimens on same day of week that first regimen began, following same schedule. Restart active tablets on next day after last inert tablet.
➤ **Acne in women at least age 14 and only if patient desires an oral contraceptive for birth control (Gianvi, Loryna, Nikki, Vestura, Yaz)**

Women: Follow guidelines of use for contraception. The 28-day dosing regimen consists of 1 active tablet PO for 24 consecutive days followed by 1 inert tablet PO daily for 4 days. After 28 tablets are taken, new course is started next day.

ADMINISTRATION
PO
• Give at same time each day.

ACTION
Reduces chance of conception by inhibiting ovulation, inhibiting sperm progression, and reducing chance of implantation.

Route	Onset	Peak	Duration
PO	Unknown	1–2 hr	Unknown

Half-life: Drospirenone, 30 hours; ethinyl estradiol, 24 hours.

ADVERSE REACTIONS
CNS: *cerebral hemorrhage, cerebral thrombosis,* asthenia, depression, dizziness, emotional lability, headache, migraine, nervousness. **CV:** *arterial thromboembolism, mesenteric thrombosis, MI, PE,* HTN, thrombophlebitis, fluid retention, edema. **EENT:** cataracts, steepening of corneal curvature, intolerance to contact lenses, pharyngitis, retinal thrombosis, sinusitis. **GI:** abdominal pain, abdominal cramping, bloating, changes in appetite, colitis, diarrhea, gastroenteritis, nausea, vomiting, gallbladder disease. **GU:** amenorrhea, breakthrough bleeding, change in cervical erosion and secretion, change in menstrual flow, cystitis, cystitis-like syndrome, dysmenorrhea, impaired renal function, leukorrhea, menstrual disorder, premenstrual syndrome, spotting, temporary infertility after discontinuing treatment, UTI, vaginal candidiasis, vaginitis. **Hepatic:** *Budd-Chiari syndrome, hepatic adenomas,* cholestatic jaundice, benign liver tumors. **Metabolic:** reduced glucose tolerance, porphyria, weight change, *hyperkalemia.* **Musculoskeletal:** back pain. **Respiratory:** bronchitis, URI. **Skin:** *erythema multiforme,* acne, erythema nodosum, hemorrhagic eruption, hirsutism, loss of scalp hair, melasma, pruritus, rash. **Other:** changes in libido, breast tenderness.

INTERACTIONS
Drug-drug. *ACE inhibitors, aldosterone antagonists, ARBs, NSAIDs, potassium-sparing diuretics:* May increase risk of hyperkalemia. Monitor potassium level.
Acetaminophen: May increase level of contraceptive and decrease effectiveness of acetaminophen. Monitor patient for adverse effects. Adjust acetaminophen dose as needed.
Antibiotics, griseofulvin, penicillins, tetracycline: May decrease contraceptive effect. Advise patient to use additional method of birth control while taking the antibiotic.
Ascorbic acid, atorvastatin: May increase level of contraceptive. Monitor patient for adverse effects.
Carbamazepine, modafinil, oxcarbazepine, phenobarbital, phenytoin, protease inhibitors: May increase metabolism of ethinyl estradiol and decrease contraceptive effectiveness. Advise patient to use another method of birth control.
Clofibrate, morphine, salicylic acid, temazepam: May decrease levels and increase clearance of these drugs. Monitor patient for effectiveness.
Cyclosporine, prednisolone, theophylline: May increase levels of these drugs. Monitor patient for adverse effects and toxicity.
Lamotrigine: May decrease lamotrigine level and reduce seizure control. Dosage adjustment may be necessary.
Rifampin: May decrease contraceptive effectiveness and increase menstrual irregularities. Advise patient to use another method of birth control.
Troleandomycin: May increase risk of intrahepatic cholestasis and decrease contraceptive effect. Advise patient to use an alternative method of birth control.
Warfarin, other anticoagulants: May increase or decrease anticoagulation effect. Monitor INR or consider therapy modification.
Drug-herb. *St. John's wort:* May decrease contraceptive effectiveness and increase breakthrough bleeding. Discourage use together, or advise use of additional method of birth control.
Drug-lifestyle. *Smoking:* May increase risk of adverse CV effects. Advise patient to avoid smoking.

Reactions in bold italics are *life-threatening*. Interactions may have a *rapid onset* or a *delayed onset*.

EFFECTS ON LAB TEST RESULTS
• May increase potassium, corticoid, prothrombin, thyroid-binding globulin, total circulating sex steroid, total thyroid hormone, triglyceride, amylase, GGT, transferrin, prolactin, renin activity, vitamin A, and factor VII, VIII, IX, and X levels, as well as iron-binding capacity.
• May decrease antithrombin III level, folate, albumin, zinc, and vitamin B_{12}.
• May increase norepinephrine-induced platelet aggregation. May decrease glucose tolerance and free T_3 resin uptake.

CONTRAINDICATIONS & CAUTIONS
• Contraindicated in women with hepatic dysfunction, tumor, or disease; renal or adrenal insufficiency; thrombophlebitis, thromboembolic disorders, or history of DVT or thromboembolic disorders, inherited hypercoagulopathies; cerebrovascular disease or CAD, uncontrolled HTN, diabetes with vascular disease; headaches with focal neurologic symptoms; known or suspected breast cancer, endometrial cancer, or other estrogen-dependent neoplasia; undiagnosed abnormal uterine bleeding; or cholestatic jaundice of pregnancy or jaundice with other hormonal contraceptive use; and in patients older than age 35 who smoke and in those who smoke 15 or more cigarettes daily.
• Contraindicated in women age 65 or older.
• Use cautiously in patients with CV risk factors such as HTN, hyperlipidemias, obesity, and diabetes.
• Don't use in patients predisposed to hyperkalemia; drug may increase potassium level.
• Use cautiously in patients with conditions aggravated by fluid retention.
Dialyzable drug: Unknown.
⚠ Overdose S&S: Nausea, withdrawal uterine bleeding.

PREGNANCY-LACTATION-REPRODUCTION
• Contraindicated in women who are or may become pregnant. There is little or no increased risk of birth defects in women who inadvertently use combined oral contraceptives during early pregnancy.
• Small amounts of hormonal contraceptives appear in human milk. Use of drug in breastfeeding women isn't recommended; may reduce milk production.

NURSING CONSIDERATIONS
❸ Alert: The use of contraceptives causes increased risk of MI, thromboembolism, stroke, hepatic neoplasia, gallbladder disease, and HTN. Risk increases in patients with HTN, diabetes, hyperlipidemia, and obesity.

Black Box Warning Smoking increases the risk of serious CV adverse effects. The risk increases with age (especially age older than 35) and in patients who smoke 15 or more cigarettes daily. ▮
• The relationship between the use of hormonal contraceptives and breast and cervical cancers is unclear. Encourage women to schedule a complete gynecologic examination at least yearly and to perform breast self-examinations monthly.
• In patients scheduled to have elective surgery that may increase the risk of thromboembolism, stop contraceptive use from at least 4 weeks before until 2 weeks after surgery. Also stop use during and after prolonged immobilization.
• Because of increased risk of thromboembolism in the postpartum period, don't start contraceptive earlier than 4 to 6 weeks after delivery.
• Stop use and evaluate patient if loss of vision, proptosis, diplopia, papilledema, or retinal vascular lesions occur. Recommend that contact lens wearers be evaluated by an ophthalmologist if visual changes or lens intolerance occurs.
• If patient misses two consecutive periods, she should obtain a negative pregnancy test result before continuing use of contraceptive.
• Immediately stop use if pregnancy is confirmed.
• Closely monitor patient with diabetes. Glucose intolerance may occur.
• Closely monitor patient with HTN or a history of depression. Stop drug if these events occur.
• In patient at high risk for hyperkalemia and patient taking medications that may increase potassium, check potassium level during the first treatment cycle.
• Stop drug and evaluate patient if persistent, severe headaches occur or if migraines occur or are worsened.

- Evaluate patient for malignancy or pregnancy if she experiences breakthrough bleeding or spotting.
- Closely monitor patient with hyperlipidemias.
- Stop use if jaundice occurs.
- In patients being treated for HCV infection with a combination drug regimen that contains ombitasvir/paritaprevir/ritonavir, with or without dasabuvir, discontinue drospirenone–ethinyl estradiol before starting therapy due to the risk of significant increases in liver enzyme levels. May restart approximately 2 weeks after completion of the combination drug regimen.
- **_Look alike–sound alike:_** Don't confuse Yaz with Yasmin.

PATIENT TEACHING

- Advise patient to use additional method of birth control during the first 7 days of the first cycle of hormonal contraceptive.
- Inform patient that pills don't protect against sexually transmitted diseases such as HIV.
- Advise patient of the dangers of smoking while taking hormonal contraceptives. Suggest smokers choose a different form of birth control.
- Tell patient to schedule gynecologic examinations yearly and to perform breast self-examination monthly.
- Inform patient that spotting, light bleeding, or stomach upset may occur while she is taking the first one to three packs of pills. Tell her to continue taking the pills and to notify health care provider if these symptoms persist.
- Tell patient to take the pill at the same time each day.
- Tell patient to immediately report sharp chest pain, coughing of blood or sudden shortness of breath, calf pain, crushing chest pain or chest heaviness, sudden severe headache or vomiting, dizziness or fainting, visual or speech disturbances, weakness or numbness in an arm or leg, vision loss, breast lumps, severe stomach pain or tenderness, difficulty sleeping, lack of energy, fatigue, change in mood, or jaundice with fever, fatigue, loss of appetite, dark urine, or light-colored bowel movements.

- Tell patient to notify health care provider if she wears contact lenses and notices a change in vision or has trouble wearing the lenses.
- Tell patient that risk of pregnancy increases with each active tablet she forgets to take. Inform patient what to do if she misses pills.
- Tell patient to use an additional method of birth control and to notify health care provider if she isn't sure what to do about missed pills.
- Advise patient that amenorrhea may occur. Rule out pregnancy if amenorrhea occurs in two or more consecutive cycles.
- Advise patient who is breastfeeding to use an alternative method of birth control until infant is completely weaned. Quality and quantity of human milk may be decreased. Yellowing of skin and eyes (jaundice) and breast enlargement may occur in breastfed neonates.

droxidopa
droks-eye-DOE-pa

Northera

Therapeutic class: Vasopressors
Pharmacologic class: Norepinephrine precursors

AVAILABLE FORMS
Capsules ⊙: 100 mg, 200 mg, 300 mg

INDICATIONS & DOSAGES
➤ **Symptomatic neurogenic orthostatic hypotension caused by primary autonomic failure (Parkinson disease, multiple system atrophy, and pure autonomic failure), dopamine beta-hydroxylase deficiency, nondiabetic autonomic neuropathy**
Adults: Initially, 100 mg PO t.i.d. Titrate to symptomatic response in increments of 100 mg t.i.d. every 24 to 48 hours. Maximum dose is 600 mg t.i.d.

ADMINISTRATION
PO
- Give when patient arises in morning, at midday, and in late afternoon at least 3 hours before bedtime.

- Monitor supine BP before initiating drug and after dosage increase.
- Give consistently with or without food.
- Ensure patient swallows capsule whole.
- Store capsules at room temperature.

ACTION
Metabolized to norepinephrine, which induces peripheral arterial and venous vasoconstriction, causing increased BP.

Route	Onset	Peak	Duration
PO	Rapid	1–4 hr	Unknown

Half-life: 2½ hours.

ADVERSE REACTIONS
CNS: headache, dizziness, syncope. **CV:** HTN. **GI:** nausea. **GU:** UTI. **Other:** falls.

INTERACTIONS
Drug-drug. *Carbidopa, dopa-decarboxylase inhibitors:* May decrease clearance of droxidopa. Monitor clinical effectiveness of droxidopa and adjust dosage as needed.
Drugs that increase BP (ephedrine, midodrine, norepinephrine, triptans [migraine indications]): May increase risk of supine HTN. Monitor BP closely.
Linezolid, nonselective MAO inhibitors: Based on mechanism of action, may increase BP. Avoid use together.
Serotonin 5-HT$_{1D}$ receptor agonists: May enhance hypertensive effects. Monitor therapy.
Drug-herb. *Ephedra, ma huang:* May increase BP. Don't use together.

EFFECTS ON LAB TEST RESULTS
None reported.

CONTRAINDICATIONS & CAUTIONS
- Contraindicated in patients hypersensitive to drug or its components.
Black Box Warning Droxidopa may cause or exacerbate supine HTN, increasing risk of stroke, MI, or death if not well managed. ■
- Use cautiously in patients with ischemic heart disease, arrhythmias, or HF.
- Use cautiously in patients with hypersensitivity to FD + C Yellow No. 5 (tartrazine) or aspirin. Risk of allergic reaction to droxidopa may be increased in these patients.

- Safe use in children hasn't been established.
Dialyzable drug: Unknown.
⚠ *Overdose S&S:* Hypertensive crisis.

PREGNANCY-LACTATION-REPRODUCTION
- There are no adequate well-controlled studies in pregnant women.
- Drug may appear in human milk. Consider discontinuing breastfeeding or drug.

NURSING CONSIDERATIONS
- Periodically assess patient for continued effectiveness of drug. Effectiveness beyond 2 weeks hasn't been established.
Black Box Warning Monitor supine BP before starting drug, periodically during treatment, and after dosage increases. Have patient elevate the head of the bed to reduce risk of supine HTN when resting or sleeping. If elevating head of bed doesn't manage supine HTN, reduce dosage or discontinue drug. ■
- Monitor BP in both supine and head-elevated sleeping positions. Monitor BP before starting drug and after dosage increase.
- Monitor patient for worsening of existing ischemic heart disease, arrhythmias, or HF.
- Monitor patient when droxidopa dosage is changed or when concomitant levodopa dosage is reduced abruptly or when levodopa is discontinued, especially if patient is receiving neuroleptics, for a symptom complex resembling NMS (fever, hyperthermia, muscle rigidity, involuntary movements, altered consciousness, mental status changes).

PATIENT TEACHING
- Tell patient to take droxidopa consistently, either with food or without food.
- Instruct patient to take last dose each day at least 3 hours before bedtime to reduce risk of supine HTN.
Black Box Warning Educate patient to monitor supine BP regularly. ■
Black Box Warning Advise patient to elevate the head of the bed to reduce risk of supine HTN. ■
- Caution patient to wait to take next scheduled dose if a dose is missed and never to double a dose to make up for missed dose.

SAFETY ALERT!

dulaglutide
DOO-la-gloo-tide

Trulicity

Therapeutic class: Antidiabetics
Pharmacologic class: Glucagon-like
peptide-1 receptor agonists

AVAILABLE FORMS
Injection: 0.75 mg/0.5 mL, 1.5 mg/0.5 mL
in single-dose pens or single-dose prefilled
syringes

INDICATIONS & DOSAGES
➤ **Adjunct to diet and exercise to improve
glycemic control in patients with type 2
diabetes mellitus**
Adults: 0.75 mg subcut once weekly. May
titrate to a maximum of 1.5 mg weekly.

ADMINISTRATION
Subcutaneous
• Inject into abdomen, thigh, or upper arm
once weekly any time of day. Use a different
injection site each week.
• May give without regard to meals.
❸ *Alert:* Don't mix dulaglutide with insulin.
Give as separate injections in nonadjacent
areas.
• Don't give IM or IV.
• Inspect for particulate matter and discoloration before administration. Don't give if
present.
• Refrigerate at 36° to 46° F (2° to 8° C).
May store at room temperature for a total of
14 days if temperature doesn't exceed 86° F
(30° C).
• Don't freeze. Don't use drug if it has been
frozen.
• Protect from light by storing in original
carton until time of administration.
• Discard injection device after each use in
puncture-resistant container.
• If a dose is missed, give within 3 days of
missed dose; then resume prior schedule. If
less than 3 days remain until next scheduled
dose, skip the missed dose and give the next
dose on schedule.

• The day of weekly administration may be
changed if necessary as long as the last dose
was 3 or more days before the new day.

ACTION
A human glucagon-like peptide-1 (GLP-1)
receptor agonist that, like endogenous GLP-
1, binds to and activates the GLP-1 receptor in the pancreatic beta cells, leading to
glucose-dependent insulin release. Also decreases glucagon secretion and slows gastric
emptying.

Route	Onset	Peak	Duration
Subcut	Unknown	24–72 hr	Unknown

Half-life: About 5 days.

ADVERSE REACTIONS
CNS: fatigue, asthenia, malaise. **CV:** tachycardia, increased PR interval, first-degree
AV block. **GI:** *pancreatitis,* nausea, diarrhea,
vomiting, decreased appetite, dyspepsia,
constipation, flatulence, GERD, eructation;
abdominal pain, tenderness, or distention.
GU: renal impairment. **Hepatic:** elevated
lipase and amylase levels. **Metabolic:** *hypoglycemia.* **Other:** *hypersensitivity reactions, thyroid C-cell tumors (adenomas and
carcinomas),* antidrug antibody formation.

INTERACTIONS
Drug-drug. *Insulin, insulin secretagogues
(meglitinides, sulfonylureas):* May increase
risk of hypoglycemia. Consider reducing insulin or insulin secretagogue dosage; monitor blood glucose level closely.
Oral medications: May affect absorption of
oral medications since dulaglutide delays
gastric emptying. Monitor effects, especially
when given with other drugs with a narrow
therapeutic index.

EFFECTS ON LAB TEST RESULTS
• May increase lipase and amylase levels.
May decrease glucose level.

CONTRAINDICATIONS & CAUTIONS
Black Box Warning Contraindicated in patients with a personal or family history of
medullary thyroid carcinoma (MTC) and in
patients with multiple endocrine neoplasia
syndrome type 2. ■

Reactions in bold italics are *life-threatening*. Interactions may have a *rapid onset* or a *delayed onset*.

D

Black Box Warning Thyroid C-cell adenomas and carcinomas occurred in animal studies. It isn't known if dulaglutide causes thyroid C-cell tumors, including MTC, in humans. ■

• Contraindicated in patients with a serious hypersensitivity reaction to drug or its components.

• Hypersensitivity reactions (including anaphylaxis and angioedema) have been reported with other GLP-1 receptor agonists. Use cautiously in patients with a history of angioedema or anaphylaxis with another GLP-1 receptor agonist.

• Drug hasn't been studied in patients with a history of pancreatitis. Consider alternatives.

• Drug isn't recommended as first-line therapy in patients who have inadequate response to diet and exercise.

• Drug shouldn't be used in patients with type 1 diabetes mellitus or for treatment of diabetic ketoacidosis. Drug isn't a substitute for insulin.

• To reduce risk of hypoglycemia, consider dosage reduction of concomitantly administered secretagogues or insulin when initiating dulaglutide.

• Avoid use in patients with severe GI disease, including severe gastroparesis; drug slows gastric emptying and hasn't been studied in this population.

• Use cautiously in patients with hepatic or renal insufficiency or heart disease.

• Safety and effectiveness in children haven't been established.

Dialyzable drug: Unknown.

⚠ *Overdose S&S:* Mild or moderate GI symptoms, nonsevere hypoglycemia.

PREGNANCY-LACTATION-REPRODUCTION

• There are no adequate studies in pregnant women. Use cautiously during pregnancy and only if potential benefit justifies potential risk to the fetus.

• It isn't known if drug appears in human milk. Patient should discontinue breastfeeding or discontinue drug.

NURSING CONSIDERATIONS

• Use caution when initiating dulaglutide therapy or escalating dosage in patients with renal insufficiency. Monitor renal function, especially in patients who report severe GI

adverse reactions (nausea, vomiting, diarrhea, dehydration).

• Monitor patients for signs and symptoms of pancreatitis (including persistent severe abdominal pain, sometimes radiating to the back, which may or may not be accompanied by vomiting). Discontinue drug if pancreatitis is suspected. Don't restart drug if pancreatitis is confirmed.

• Monitor patient for tachycardia; monitor ECG for PR-interval prolongation.

• Refer patients with elevated serum calcitonin level or thyroid nodules on examination or neck imaging to an endocrinologist.

• *Look alike–sound alike:* Don't confuse dulaglutide with duloxetine or dutasteride.

PATIENT TEACHING

• Explain to patient that dulaglutide isn't a substitute for insulin. Educate patient on general diabetes care, including the need to monitor glucose and HbA_{1c} levels, how to recognize the signs and symptoms of hypoglycemia or hyperglycemia, the importance of diet and exercise, and the impact stress or trauma may have on glucose levels.

• Warn patient to immediately discontinue drug and inform prescriber if hypersensitivity reactions occur.

• Advise patient to report heart palpitations or feelings of a racing heartbeat while at rest.

• Teach patient of risk of dehydration due to GI adverse reactions, including the associated risk of worsening renal function. Counsel patient to take precautions to avoid fluid depletion.

• Teach patient signs and symptoms of acute pancreatitis (persistent severe abdominal pain, sometimes radiating to the back, which may or may not be accompanied by vomiting) and to discontinue drug promptly and contact prescriber if any of these signs and symptoms occur.

Black Box Warning Inform patient of risk of MTC. Teach the signs and symptoms of thyroid tumors (a mass in the neck, dysphagia, dyspnea, persistent hoarseness). ■

• Instruct patient on the proper use of drug (rotating sites, inspecting solution for particles, discarding needles, storing pens and syringes, handling a missed dose).

• Caution patient never to mix insulin and dulaglutide but to give as separate injections.

Although dulaglutide and insulin may be injected in the same body area, they shouldn't be injected adjacent to each other.

• Instruct female patient to tell prescriber if she is or plans to become pregnant or is breastfeeding.

DULoxetine hydrochloride
doo-LOX-ah-teen

Cymbalta♦

Therapeutic class: Antidepressants
Pharmacologic class: SSNRIs

AVAILABLE FORMS
Capsules (delayed-release) ⦿: 20 mg, 30 mg, 40 mg, 60 mg

INDICATIONS & DOSAGES
Adjust-a-dose (for all indications): Duloxetine isn't recommended for patients with ESRD, severe renal dysfunction (CrCl of less than 30 mL/minute), or hepatic dysfunction.

➤ **Major depressive disorder**
Adults: Initially, 20 mg PO b.i.d. to 60 mg PO once daily or divided in two equal doses. May also start at 30 mg/day for 1 week to allow patients to adjust to medication. Maximum, 120 mg daily.

➤ **Generalized anxiety disorder**
Adults: 60 mg PO daily. Or, 30 mg PO daily for 1 week; then increase to 60 mg PO daily. May increase in increments of 30 mg daily to 120 mg PO once daily.
Children ages 7 to 17: 30 mg PO once daily for 2 weeks; may increase to 60 mg once daily. For doses greater than 60 mg/day, increase dosage in increments of 30 mg/day. Maximum, 120 mg daily.
Adjust-a-dose: In elderly patients, initially, 30 mg PO once daily for 2 weeks before considering an increase to target dose of 60 mg once daily. If needed, increase dosage further in increments of 30 mg once daily. Maximum, 120 mg daily.

➤ **Fibromyalgia**
Adults: Initially, 30 mg PO once daily for 1 week; increase to 60 mg PO once daily after a week. Some patients may respond to the starting dose. Maximum dose is 60 mg/day. Base continued treatment on individual patient response.

➤ **Neuropathic pain related to diabetic peripheral neuropathy**
Adults: 60 mg PO once daily.
Adjust-a-dose: Consider a lower starting dose and a gradual increase in dose for patients with renal impairment.

➤ **Chronic musculoskeletal pain**
Adults: Initially, 30 mg PO once daily for 1 week; then increase to 60 mg PO once daily.

ADMINISTRATION
PO
• Give whole; don't crush or open capsules.
• Give without regard to meals.

ACTION
Inhibits serotonin and norepinephrine reuptake and is a weak inhibitor of dopamine reuptake in the CNS.

Route	Onset	Peak	Duration
PO	Unknown	6 hr (fasting)	Unknown

Half-life: 12 hours.

ADVERSE REACTIONS
CNS: dizziness, fatigue, headache, insomnia, somnolence, *suicidal thoughts,* fever, hypoesthesia, irritability, lethargy, nervousness, nightmares, restlessness, sleep disorder, anxiety, asthenia, tremor, agitation. **CV:** hot flashes, HTN, increased HR, palpitations. **EENT:** blurred vision, nasopharyngitis, pharyngolaryngeal pain. **GI:** constipation, diarrhea, dry mouth, nausea, dyspepsia, gastritis, vomiting, flatulence. **GU:** abnormal orgasm, abnormally increased frequency of urinating, delayed or dysfunctional ejaculation, dysuria, erectile dysfunction, urinary hesitation. **Metabolic:** decreased appetite, *hypoglycemia,* increased appetite, weight gain or loss, hyponatremia. **Musculoskeletal:** muscle cramps, myalgia. **Respiratory:** cough. **Skin:** increased sweating, night sweats, pruritus, rash. **Other:** decreased libido, rigors, yawning.

INTERACTIONS
Drug-drug. *Anticoagulants (aspirin, NSAIDs, warfarin):* May increase bleeding risk. Monitor patient closely.

Reactions in bold italics are *life-threatening*. Interactions may have a *rapid onset* or a *delayed onset*.

Class IC antiarrhythmics (flecainide, propafenone), phenothiazines: May increase levels of these drugs. Use together cautiously.

CNS drugs: May increase adverse effects. Use together cautiously.

CYP1A2 inhibitors (cimetidine, fluvoxamine, certain quinolones): May increase duloxetine level. Avoid using together.

CYP2D6 inhibitors (fluoxetine, paroxetine, quinidine): May increase duloxetine level. Use together cautiously.

Drugs that reduce gastric acidity: May cause premature breakdown of duloxetine's protective coating and early release of the drug. Monitor patient for effects.

Linezolid, methylene blue: May cause serotonin syndrome. Don't use together.

Lithium, SSNRIs, SSRIs, tramadol: May increase risk of serotonin syndrome. Avoid use together.

◑ Alert: *MAO inhibitors (phenelzine, rasagiline, selegiline):* May cause hyperthermia, rigidity, myoclonus, autonomic instability, rapid fluctuations of vital signs, agitation, delirium, and coma. Avoid use within 2 weeks after MAO inhibitor therapy; wait at least 5 days after stopping duloxetine before starting MAO inhibitor.

TCAs (amitriptyline, imipramine, nortriptyline): May increase levels of these drugs. Reduce TCA dose, and monitor drug levels closely.

Thioridazine: May prolong the QT interval and increase risk of serious ventricular arrhythmias and sudden death. Avoid using together.

Triptans: May cause serotonin syndrome (restlessness, hallucinations, loss of coordination, fast heartbeat, rapid changes in BP, increased body temperature, hyperreflexia, nausea, vomiting, and diarrhea) or NMS. Use cautiously and with increased monitoring, especially when starting or increasing dosages.

Drug-herb. *St. John's wort:* May increase risk of serotonin syndrome. Discourage use together.

Drug-lifestyle. *Alcohol use:* May increase risk of liver damage. Discourage use together.

EFFECTS ON LAB TEST RESULTS
• May increase alkaline phosphatase, ALT, AST, bilirubin, and CK levels.

CONTRAINDICATIONS & CAUTIONS
• Contraindicated in patients hypersensitive to drug or its ingredients, patients taking MAO inhibitors, and patients with a CrCl less than 30 mL/minute. Drug isn't recommended for patients with hepatic dysfunction or ESRD.

◑ Alert: Before using duloxetine in a child or adolescent, balance potential risks with clinical need.

• Safety and effectiveness in children younger than age 7 haven't been established.

• Don't begin duloxetine in patients receiving linezolid or methylene blue. If urgent treatment with linezolid or methylene blue is needed in patient already receiving duloxetine, discontinue duloxetine; then administer linezolid or methylene blue.

• Monitor for serotonin syndrome for 5 days or until 24 hours after last dose of linezolid or methylene blue, whichever comes first. May resume duloxetine 24 hours after last dose of linezolid or methylene blue.

• Use cautiously in patients with a history of mania or seizures, patients who drink substantial amounts of alcohol, patients with HTN, patients with controlled angle-closure glaucoma, and those with conditions that slow gastric emptying.

• Pupil dilation that occurs after duloxetine use may trigger an angle-closure attack in a patient with anatomically narrow angles who doesn't have a patent iridectomy.

• Drug may increase risk of bleeding events.

• Orthostatic hypotension, falls, and syncope have been reported with therapeutic doses and tend to occur within first week of therapy but can occur at any time during treatment, particularly after dosage increases. Fall risk appears to increase steadily with age and be related to degree of orthostatic decrease in BP as well as other factors that may increase the underlying risk of falls. Consider dosage reduction or discontinuing drug if falls occur.

Dialyzable drug: Unlikely.

⚠ Overdose S&S: Coma, hypotension, HTN, seizures, serotonin syndrome, somnolence, syncope, tachycardia, vomiting.

PREGNANCY-LACTATION-REPRODUCTION

• There are no adequate well-controlled studies in pregnant women. Use during pregnancy only if potential benefit justifies potential risk to the fetus.

• To monitor pregnancy outcomes, enroll women exposed to drug during pregnancy in the Cymbalta Pregnancy Registry (1-866-814-6975).

• Use during the third trimester may cause neonatal complications, including respiratory distress, cyanosis, apnea, seizures, vomiting, hypoglycemia, hypotonia, and hyperreflexia, which may require prolonged hospitalization, respiratory support, and tube feeding.

• Drug appears in human milk. Use cautiously in breastfeeding women and only when benefits outweigh potential risks.

NURSING CONSIDERATIONS

Black Box Warning Drug may increase risk of suicidal thinking and behavior in children, adolescents, and young adults ages 18 to 24, especially during the first few months of treatment, and in those with major depressive disorder or other psychiatric disorder. ∎

Black Box Warning Monitor all patients for worsening of depression or emergence of suicidal thoughts or behavior, especially when therapy starts or dosage changes. ∎

⚠ **Alert:** Concomitant use with linezolid or methylene blue can cause serotonin syndrome (fever, mental status changes, muscle twitching, excessive sweating, shivering or shaking, diarrhea, loss of coordination). If linezolid or methylene blue must be given, stop drug and monitor patient for serotonin toxicity for 5 days or until 24 hours after last dose of methylene blue or linezolid, whichever comes first. May resume treatment 24 hours after last dose of methylene blue or linezolid.

• Treatment of overdose is symptomatic. Don't induce emesis; gastric lavage or activated charcoal may be performed soon after ingestion or if patient is still symptomatic. Because drug undergoes extensive distribution, forced diuresis, dialysis, hemoperfusion, and exchange transfusion aren't useful. Contact a poison control center for information.

• If taken with TCAs, duloxetine metabolism will be prolonged, and patient will need extended monitoring.

• Severe skin reactions, including erythema multiforme and SJS, can occur. Discontinue at first sign of blisters, peeling rash, mucosal erosions, or other signs or symptoms of hypersensitivity if no other etiology can be identified.

• Periodically reassess patient to determine the need for continued therapy.

• Don't stop drug abruptly. Decrease dosage gradually, and watch for symptoms that may arise when drug is stopped, such as dizziness, nausea, headache, paresthesia, vomiting, irritability, and nightmares.

• If intolerable symptoms arise when decreasing or stopping drug, restart at previous dose and decrease even more gradually.

• Monitor BP periodically during treatment.

• Older patients may be more sensitive to drug effects than younger adults.

⚠ **Alert:** Combining triptans with an SSRI or an SSNRI may cause serotonin syndrome or NMS-like reactions. Signs and symptoms of serotonin syndrome may include restlessness, hallucinations, loss of coordination, fast heartbeat, rapid changes in BP, increased body temperature, overactive reflexes, nausea, vomiting, and diarrhea. Serotonin syndrome may be more likely to occur when starting or increasing the dose of triptan, SSRI, or SSNRI.

• May worsen glycemic control in patients with diabetes. Monitor blood glucose levels.

• *Look alike–sound alike:* Don't confuse duloxetine with fluoxetine or paroxetine. Don't confuse Cymbalta with Symbyax.

PATIENT TEACHING

Black Box Warning Warn families or caregivers to report signs of worsening depression (such as agitation, irritability, insomnia, hostility, impulsivity) and signs of suicidal behavior to prescriber immediately. ∎

⚠ **Alert:** Teach patient to recognize and immediately report signs and symptoms of serotonin toxicity (fever, mental status changes, muscle twitching, excessive sweating, shivering or shaking, diarrhea, loss of coordination).

• Tell patient to contact prescriber immediately and to discontinue drug at first sign of hypersensitivity (including blisters, peeling rash, or mucosal erosions).
• Tell patient to not stop drug abruptly; dosage must be gradually reduced to avoid adverse effects.
• Tell patient to consult prescriber or pharmacist before taking other prescription or OTC drugs or herbal or other dietary supplements.
• Instruct patient to swallow capsules whole and not to chew, crush, or open them because they have an enteric coating.
• Urge patient to avoid activities that are hazardous or require mental alertness until drug's effects are known.
• Warn against drinking alcohol during therapy.
• If patient takes drug for depression, explain that it may take 1 to 4 weeks to notice an effect.
• Advise patients with diabetes to closely monitor blood glucose level.

dutasteride
doo-TAS-teh-ride

Avodart✐

Therapeutic class: BPH drugs
Pharmacologic class: 5-alpha-reductase enzyme inhibitors

AVAILABLE FORMS
Capsules ⓐ: 0.5 mg

INDICATIONS & DOSAGES
➤ **To treat and improve the symptoms of BPH, reduce the risk of acute urine retention, and reduce the need for BPH-related surgery**
Men: 0.5 mg PO once daily as monotherapy. May be given with tamsulosin 0.4 mg PO once daily as combination therapy.

ADMINISTRATION
PO
🜲 *Alert:* Drug is considered a teratogen. Follow safe handling and disposal procedures.

• Don't crush, break, or allow patient to chew capsules; contact with contents may cause oropharyngeal irritation.
• Give drug without regard for food.

ACTION
Inhibits conversion of testosterone to dihydrotestosterone, the androgen primarily responsible for the initial development and subsequent enlargement of the prostate gland.

Route	Onset	Peak	Duration
PO	Unknown	2–3 hr	Unknown

Half-life: About 5 weeks.

ADVERSE REACTIONS
GU: erectile dysfunction, decreased libido, ejaculation disorder. **Other:** gynecomastia.

INTERACTIONS
Drug-drug. *CYP3A4 inhibitors (cimetidine, ciprofloxacin, diltiazem, ketoconazole, ritonavir, verapamil):* May increase dutasteride level. Use together cautiously and monitor therapy.

EFFECTS ON LAB TEST RESULTS
• May increase total testosterone and TSH levels.
• May lower PSA level.

CONTRAINDICATIONS & CAUTIONS
• Contraindicated in women and children and in patients hypersensitive to dutasteride or its ingredients or to other 5-alpha-reductase inhibitors.
🜲 *Alert:* 5-Alpha-reductase inhibitors may increase the risk of high-grade prostate cancer. Before start of therapy, evaluate patients to rule out other urologic conditions, including prostate cancer that might mimic BPH. Any increase in PSA level in patient receiving dutasteride should be considered significant; evaluate patient for prostate cancer.
• Use cautiously in patients with hepatic disease and in those taking long-term potent CYP450 inhibitors.
Dialyzable drug: Unknown.

PREGNANCY-LACTATION-REPRODUCTION
• Drug isn't indicated for use in women. Contraindicated in women of childbearing potential and during pregnancy.

◑ *Alert:* Because drug may be absorbed through the skin, women who are or may become pregnant shouldn't handle drug, especially avoiding contact with crushed or broken tablets. If contact occurs, wash contact area immediately with soap and water.
• It isn't known if drug appears in human milk. Contraindicated for use in breastfeeding women.
• Drug appears in semen.

NURSING CONSIDERATIONS
• If contact is made with a leaking capsule, wash the contact area immediately with soap and water.
• Carefully monitor patients with a large residual urine volume or severely diminished urine flow, or both, for obstructive uropathy.
• Patients should wait at least 6 months after their last dose before donating blood.
• Establish a new baseline PSA level at least 3 months after start of treatment, and use it to assess potentially cancer-related changes in PSA level.
• To interpret PSA values in men treated for 3 months or more, double the PSA value for comparison with normal values in untreated men.
• Evaluate patients for prostate cancer and other urologic conditions that may cause similar signs and symptoms before initiating therapy and periodically thereafter.

PATIENT TEACHING
• Tell patient to swallow the capsule whole.
• Inform patient that ejaculate volume may decrease but that sexual function should remain normal.
• Teach women who are pregnant or may become pregnant not to handle drug. A male fetus exposed to drug by the mother's swallowing or absorbing the drug through her skin may be born with abnormal sex organs.
◑ *Alert:* Tell patient not to donate blood for at least 6 months after final dose to prevent drug administration to a pregnant female transfusion recipient.
• Advise patient that drug is present in semen.
• Counsel patient to avoid contact with pregnant females and those of childbearing potential.

• Tell patient periodic blood tests will be needed to monitor therapeutic effects.

SAFETY ALERT!

edoxaban tosylate
e-DOX-a-ban

Savaysa

Therapeutic class: Factor Xa inhibitors
Pharmacologic class: Anticoagulants

AVAILABLE FORMS
Tablets: 15 mg, 30 mg, 60 mg

INDICATIONS & DOSAGES
Adjust-a-dose (for all indications): If CrCl is 15 to 50 mL/minute, decrease dosage to 30 mg PO once daily.
➤ **To reduce risk of stroke and systemic embolism in patients with nonvalvular atrial fibrillation (NVAF)**
Adults: 60 mg PO once daily. Refer to manufacturer's instructions for transitioning to or from other anticoagulants.
Black Box Warning Don't use for treatment of NVAF in patients with CrCl greater than 95 mL/minute because of increased risk of ischemic stroke. ▮
➤ **Treatment of DVT and PE**
Adults: In patients weighing more than 60 kg, give 60 mg PO once daily after 5 to 10 days of therapy with a parenteral anticoagulant. Refer to manufacturer's instructions for transitioning to or from other anticoagulants.
Adjust-a-dose: If patient weighs 60 kg or less or is taking concomitant P-gp inhibitors, decrease dosage to 30 mg PO once daily.

ADMINISTRATION
PO
• Give without regard to meals.
• For patients who can't swallow whole tablets, crush tablets and mix with applesauce or 60 to 90 mL water; give immediately. For patients with a gastric tube, mix crushed tablets with 60 to 90 mL water and give immediately.
• If a dose is missed, give as soon as possible on the same day. Resume normal schedule the following day. Don't double the dose to make up for missed dose.

Reactions in bold italics are *life-threatening*. Interactions may have a *rapid onset* or a *delayed onset*.

ACTION

Inhibits free factor Xa, prothrombinase activity, and thrombin-induced platelet aggregation. Inhibition of factor Xa in the coagulation cascade reduces thrombin generation and thrombus formation.

Route	Onset	Peak	Duration
PO	Unknown	1–2 hr	Unknown

Half-life: 10 to 14 hours.

ADVERSE REACTIONS

CNS: *intracranial hemorrhage, hemorrhagic stroke, epidural or spinal hematoma.* **EENT:** epistaxis, *oral hemorrhage.* **GI:** *GI hemorrhage.* **GU:** *vaginal hemorrhage,* hematuria. **Hematologic:** *hemorrhage,* anemia, bruising. **Hepatic:** abnormal LFT values. **Skin:** rash, puncture-site bleeding.

INTERACTIONS

Drug-drug. *Anticoagulants, antiplatelet drugs (aspirin, P2Y12 inhibitors), NSAIDs, omega-3-fatty acids, thrombolytics, vitamin E, vorapaxar:* May increase risk of bleeding. Avoid concomitant use.
Aspirin: May cause bleeding. Monitor patients on long-term low-dose aspirin therapy for signs and symptoms of bleeding.
Digoxin: May increase digoxin level. Monitor digoxin level closely to determine if dosage adjustments are needed.
P-gp inducers (rifampin): May increase P-gp inducer exposure and decrease edoxaban serum concentration. Avoid concomitant use.
Verapamil: May decrease verapamil level. Monitor effects of verapamil and titrate dosage as necessary.
Drug-herb. *Alfalfa, anise, bilberry:* May increase bleeding risk. Don't use together.

EFFECTS ON LAB TEST RESULTS

• May increase LFT values.
• May increase PT, aPTT, and INR.
• May decrease RBC count.

CONTRAINDICATIONS & CAUTIONS

• Contraindicated in patients hypersensitive to drug or its components and in those with active pathological bleeding.

Black Box Warning Contraindicated in patients with CrCl greater than 95 mL/minute. Efficacy is reduced in patients with NVAF with CrCl greater than 95 mL/minute, increasing the risk of stroke. There is an increased risk of ischemic stroke in patients with NVAF if their renal function improves and edoxaban blood level decreases. ∎

• Drug hasn't been studied in patients with mechanical heart valves or moderate to severe mitral stenosis or when CrCl is less than 15 mL/minute. Use isn't recommended in these patients.
• Use isn't recommended in patients with moderate to severe hepatic impairment (Child-Pugh classes B and C) because of possible intrinsic coagulation abnormalities.
Black Box Warning Epidural or spinal hematomas may occur in patients treated with edoxaban who are receiving neuraxial anesthesia or undergoing spinal puncture. Risk increases with indwelling epidural catheters, concomitant drugs that affect hemostasis (NSAIDs, platelet inhibitors, anticoagulants), spinal surgery or deformity, or a history of traumatic or repeated epidural or spinal punctures. The optimal timing between edoxaban administration and neuraxial procedures isn't known. Weigh risks and benefits before neuraxial intervention in patients who are or will be anticoagulated. ∎

• Safety and effectiveness in children haven't been established.
Dialyzable drug: 7%.
⚠ Overdose S&S: Bleeding.

PREGNANCY-LACTATION-REPRODUCTION

• There are no adequate studies in pregnant women. It isn't known if drug causes fetal harm. Use during pregnancy only if benefit outweighs risk to the fetus.
• It isn't known if drug appears in human milk. Patient should discontinue breastfeeding or discontinue drug.

NURSING CONSIDERATIONS

Black Box Warning Premature discontinuation of drug increases risk of ischemic events. If drug is stopped for a reason other than pathological bleeding or completion of treatment, consider transitioning to an alternative anticoagulant. ∎

• Monitor patient for bleeding. Immediately evaluate signs or symptoms of blood loss; discontinue drug if acute pathological bleeding occurs. Drug can cause serious and potentially fatal bleeding.
• Discontinue edoxaban at least 24 hours before invasive or surgical procedures. If surgery can't be delayed, weigh risk of bleeding against urgency of intervention.
• After surgery or other procedure, may restart edoxaban as soon as hemostasis has been achieved and patient can take oral medication.
❸ **Alert:** Don't remove indwelling epidural or intrathecal catheters earlier than 12 hours after last dose of edoxaban. Don't give next dose earlier than 2 hours after removal of the catheter.
Black Box Warning Monitor patients frequently after spinal or epidural anesthesia or puncture for signs and symptoms of neurologic impairment (numbness or weakness of the legs, bowel or bladder dysfunction). Evaluate impairment urgently. ▪
• Be aware that vitamin K, protamine, tranexamic acid, and dialysis aren't expected to reverse the effects of edoxaban.

PATIENT TEACHING
• Warn patient that bruising and bleeding may occur more easily and that bleeding may last longer during therapy.
• Instruct patient to immediately report unusual bleeding to prescriber.
• Instruct patient to take drug exactly as prescribed and, if a dose is missed, to take the next dose as soon as possible the same day and resume the normal dosing schedule the following day. Caution patient not to double a dose to make up for a missed dose.
• Advise patient not to discontinue drug without first consulting prescriber.
• Instruct patient to inform health care providers about taking edoxaban before scheduling surgery or medical or dental procedures.
• Instruct patient to inform health care providers and dentists about prescription medications, OTC drugs, or herbal products currently being taken or that may be taken.
• Advise female patient to immediately report if she is pregnant, plans to become

pregnant, is breastfeeding, or intends to breastfeed during treatment.
• Warn patient having neuraxial anesthesia or spinal puncture to watch for signs and symptoms of spinal or epidural hematoma, such as back pain, tingling, numbness (especially in the lower limbs), muscle weakness, and stool or urine incontinence. If any of these symptoms occur, advise patient to immediately contact health care provider.
• Warn patient to immediately report signs and symptoms of hemorrhage or adverse reactions, such as one-sided weakness, problems thinking or speaking, dizziness, balance changes, blurred vision, severe headache, and pale skin.

efavirenz
eff-ah-VYE-renz

Sustiva

Therapeutic class: Antiretrovirals
Pharmacologic class: NNRTIs

AVAILABLE FORMS
Capsules ⓄⓃⒸ: 50 mg, 200 mg
Tablets ⓄⓃⒸ: 600 mg

INDICATIONS & DOSAGES
➤ **Treatment of HIV-1 infection, with a protease inhibitor with or without NRTIs**
Adults and children age 3 months and older weighing 40 kg or more: 600 mg (three 200-mg capsules or one 600-mg tablet) PO once daily on an empty stomach, preferably at bedtime.
Children age 3 months and older weighing 32.5 to less than 40 kg: 400 mg PO once daily, preferably at bedtime.
Children age 3 months and older weighing 25 to less than 32.5 kg: 350 mg PO once daily, preferably at bedtime.
Children age 3 months and older weighing 20 to less than 25 kg: 300 mg PO once daily, preferably at bedtime.
Children age 3 months and older weighing 15 to less than 20 kg: 250 mg PO once daily, preferably at bedtime.
Children age 3 months and older weighing 7.5 to less than 15 kg: 200 mg PO once daily, preferably at bedtime.

Reactions in bold italics are *life-threatening*. Interactions may have a *rapid onset* or a *delayed onset*.

Children age 3 months and older weighing 5 to less than 7.5 kg: 150 mg PO once daily, preferably at bedtime.

Children age 3 months and older weighing 3.5 to less than 5 kg: 100 mg PO once daily, preferably at bedtime.

Adjust-a-dose: For adults also taking voriconazole, increase voriconazole maintenance dose to 400 mg every 12 hours and decrease efavirenz dose to 300 mg once daily using capsule formulation. For adults and children weighing 50 kg or more who are also taking rifampin, recommended efavirenz dosage is 800 mg once daily.

ADMINISTRATION
PO
- Drug must be given in combination with other antiretrovirals.
- Give drug at bedtime to decrease CNS adverse effects.
- In children, consider prophylaxis with antihistamines before initiating therapy, to prevent rash.
- Don't break or crush tablets. Don't crush capsules.
- Give once daily on an empty stomach.
- For patients who can't swallow capsules or tablets, capsule contents may be sprinkled over a small amount (1 or 2 tsp) of food and mixed gently. For patients who can tolerate solid foods, mix with soft food, such as applesauce, grape jelly, or yogurt.
- For young infants, dose can be gently mixed into 10 mL of reconstituted room-temperature infant formula in a medicine cup. Draw up dose mixture into a 10-mL dosing syringe to administer; then add an additional 10 mL to mixing cup and stir to disperse any remaining residue. Administer to infant.
- Give efavirenz mixture within 30 minutes of mixing. Patient shouldn't consume any additional food or additional formula for 2 hours after administration.

ACTION
Inhibits the transcription of HIV-1 RNA to DNA, a critical step in the viral replication process, suppressing viral replication.

Route	Onset	Peak	Duration
PO	Unknown	3–5 hr	Unknown

Half-life: Single dose, 52 to 76 hours; multiple doses, 40 to 55 hours.

ADVERSE REACTIONS
CNS: dizziness, abnormal dreams or thinking, agitation, amnesia, confusion, depersonalization, depression, euphoria, fever, fatigue, hallucinations, headache, hypoesthesia, impaired concentration, insomnia, nervousness, somnolence. **GI:** diarrhea, nausea, abdominal pain, anorexia, dyspepsia, vomiting. **Skin:** rash, *erythema multiforme, SJS, toxic epidermal necrolysis,* increased sweating, pruritus.

INTERACTIONS
Drug-drug. *Amprenavir, clarithromycin, indinavir, lopinavir:* May decrease levels of these drugs. Consider alternative therapy or dosage adjustment.

Atorvastatin, calcium channel blockers, itraconazole, pravastatin, rifampin, simvastatin: May decrease levels of these drugs. Dosage adjustments may be necessary.

Axitinib, bortezomib, bosutinib, cabazitaxel: May decrease pharmacologic effects of these drugs. Avoid concurrent use.

Bepridil, ergot derivatives, midazolam, pimozide, triazolam: May inhibit metabolism of these drugs and cause serious or life-threatening adverse events (such as arrhythmias, prolonged sedation, or respiratory depression). Avoid using together.

Bupropion: May decrease plasma concentrations and clinical effects of bupropion. Guide bupropion dosage by clinical response.

Carbamazepine: May decrease both carbamazepine and efavirenz levels. Avoid using together.

CYP2B6 inducers (strong): May increase metabolism of CYP2B6 substrates. Consider an alternative for one of the interacting drugs. Some combinations may be specifically contraindicated. Consult appropriate manufacturer labeling. Consider therapy modification.

CYP2B6 inhibitors (moderate): May decrease metabolism of CYP2B6 substrates. Monitor therapy.

CYP2B6 inhibitors (strong): May decrease metabolism of CYP2B6 substrates. Consider therapy modification.

CYP2C19 substrates: CYP2C19 moderate inhibitors may decrease metabolism of CYP2C19 substrates. Monitor therapy.

CYP3A4 inducers (strong): May increase metabolism of CYP3A4 substrates. Consider an alternative for one of the interacting drugs. Some combinations may be specifically contraindicated. Consult appropriate manufacturer labeling. Consider therapy modification.

CYP3A4 substrates: CYP3A4 moderate inhibitors may decrease metabolism of CYP3A4 substrates. Monitor therapy.

Drugs that induce the CYP3A enzyme system (phenobarbital, phenytoin, rifampin): May decrease efavirenz level. Avoid using together. Refer to manufacturer's instructions for contraindications.

Estrogens, ritonavir: May increase drug levels. Monitor patient.

Hormonal contraceptives (ethinyl estradiol–norgestimate, etonogestrel): May decrease norgestimate and etonogestrel levels. Advise use of a reliable method of barrier contraception in addition to use of hormonal contraceptives.

Nevirapine: May decrease efavirenz clinical effectiveness and increase risk of adverse reactions. Avoid using together.

Psychoactive drugs: May cause additive CNS effects. Avoid using together.

Rifabutin: May decrease rifabutin level. Increase daily rifabutin dosage by 50%. Consider doubling rifabutin dosage when rifabutin is given two to three times per week.

Rifampin: May decrease efavirenz concentration. Monitor therapy.

Ritonavir: May increase levels of both drugs. Monitor patient and liver function closely.

Saquinavir: May decrease saquinavir level and efavirenz exposure to the body. Don't use with saquinavir as sole protease inhibitor.

Voriconazole (in standard doses): Decreases voriconazole level significantly, while efavirenz level significantly increases. Avoid using together unless doses of each are adjusted.

Warfarin: May increase or decrease level and effects of warfarin. Monitor INR.

Drug-herb. *St. John's wort:* May decrease response and lead to possible resistance to efavirenz or all same-class drugs. Don't use together.

Ginkgo biloba: May decrease efavirenz concentration. Monitor concurrent use.

Kava kava: May enhance adverse/toxic effect of CNS depressants. Monitor therapy.

Drug-food. *High-fat meals:* May increase absorption of drug. Instruct patient to maintain a proper low-fat diet.

Drug-lifestyle. *Alcohol use:* May enhance CNS effects. Discourage use together.

EFFECTS ON LAB TEST RESULTS

- May increase ALT, AST, triglyceride, glucose, and cholesterol levels.
- May cause false-positive urine cannabinoid test results.

CONTRAINDICATIONS & CAUTIONS

- Contraindicated in patients hypersensitive to drug or its components and when used concomitantly with elbasvir or grazoprevir.
- Use in patients with moderate or severe hepatic impairment (Child-Pugh class B or C) isn't recommended.
- Don't give as a single agent or add on as a sole agent to a failing regimen.
- Administration with Atripla (efavirenz 600 mg/emtricitabine 200 mg/tenofovir disoproxil fumarate 300 mg) isn't recommended unless needed for dosage adjustment (e.g., with rifampin), because efavirenz is one of its active ingredients.
- Use cautiously in patients with mild hepatic impairment (Child-Pugh class A) and in those receiving hepatotoxic drugs. Monitor LFT values in patients with history of hepatitis B or C and in those taking ritonavir.
- Serious psychiatric adverse reactions have been reported, including aggressive behavior, severe depression, suicidal ideation, nonfatal suicide attempts, paranoia, and mania. Use cautiously in patients with a history of mental illness or substance abuse.
- Drug may prolong QT interval. Avoid use with other drugs with known risk of torsades de pointes. Consider an alternative to efavirenz.

Reactions in bold italics are *life-threatening*. Interactions may have a *rapid onset* or a *delayed onset*.

• Use cautiously in patients with a history of seizures.
• Immune reconstitution syndrome has been reported in patients treated with combination antiretroviral therapy.
• Drug frequently affects the nervous system. Signs and symptoms usually begin 1 to 2 days after start of therapy and resolve in 2 to 4 weeks but don't indicate onset of psychiatric signs and symptoms. Giving dose at bedtime may improve tolerability.
• Rash usually begins within 1 to 2 weeks after start of therapy and resolves within 4 weeks. Discontinue drug if severe rash develops.
Dialyzable drug: No.
⚠ *Overdose S&S:* Increased nervous system symptoms, involuntary muscle contractions.

PREGNANCY-LACTATION-REPRODUCTION
• Because of the risk of neural tube defects, drug shouldn't be used in the first trimester. Advise pregnant women of the risk to a fetus. Other antiretrovirals should strongly be considered.
• Register pregnant women in the Antiretroviral Pregnancy Registry at 1-800-258-4263.
• Advise women not to breastfeed because of the risk of HIV transmission.
• Women of childbearing potential should undergo pregnancy testing before therapy starts and should use barrier contraception in combination with other (hormonal) contraception methods during therapy and for 12 weeks after therapy ends.

NURSING CONSIDERATIONS
❸ *Alert:* Drug shouldn't be used as monotherapy or added on as a single drug to a regimen failing because of viral resistance.
• Using drug with ritonavir may increase liver enzyme levels and adverse effects (such as dizziness, nausea, and paresthesia).
• Monitor LFT values before and during treatment in all patients. Consider discontinuing drug in patients with persistent elevations of serum transaminase levels greater than 5 × ULN. Discontinue drug if elevation is accompanied by clinical signs or symptoms of hepatitis or hepatic decompensation.
• Children may be more prone to adverse reactions, especially diarrhea, nausea, vomiting, and rash. Consider prophylaxis with

antihistamines before initiating therapy, to prevent rash in this population.
• Discontinue drug if patient develops severe rash associated with blistering, desquamation, mucosal involvement, or fever.
• Monitor patients for elevated triglyceride and cholesterol levels before therapy and periodically during treatment.

PATIENT TEACHING
• Tell patient to immediately report signs and symptoms of serious psychiatric adverse effects.
• Instruct patient to take drug with water, preferably at bedtime and on an empty stomach. Tell patient not to break or crush tablets.
• Inform patient about need for blood tests to monitor LFT values and triglyceride levels.
• Tell patient to use a barrier contraceptive with a hormonal contraceptive during therapy and for 12 weeks after therapy ends and to notify prescriber immediately if pregnancy is suspected; drug is a known risk to the fetus. Hormonal methods that contain progesterone may have decreased effectiveness.
• Inform patient that drug doesn't cure HIV infection, that opportunistic infections and other complications of HIV infection may continue to occur, and that transmission of HIV to others through sexual contact or blood contamination is still possible.
• Instruct patient to take drug at the same time every day and always with other antiretrovirals.
• Tell patient to take drug exactly as prescribed and not to stop it without medical approval. Also instruct patient to report adverse reactions.
• Inform patient that rash is the most common adverse effect. Tell patient to report rash immediately because it may be serious in rare cases.
• Advise patient to report use of other drugs, including OTC drugs and herbal supplements.
• Advise patient that dizziness, difficulty sleeping or concentrating, drowsiness, or unusual dreams may occur during the first few days of therapy. Reassure patient that these symptoms typically resolve after 2 to 4 weeks and may be less problematic if drug is taken at bedtime.

- Tell patient to avoid alcohol, driving, or operating machinery until the drug's effects are known.

elagolix
el-a-GOE-lix

Orilissa

Therapeutic class: Endocrine drugs
Pharmacologic class: Gonadotropin-releasing hormone receptor antagonists

AVAILABLE FORMS
Tablets: 150 mg, 200 mg

INDICATIONS & DOSAGES
Adjust-a-dose (for all indications): For patients with moderate hepatic impairment (Child-Pugh class B), give 150 mg PO once daily for up to 6 months.

➤ **Management of moderate to severe pain associated with endometriosis**
Women age 18 and older: 150 mg PO once daily for up to 24 months.

➤ **Management of moderate to severe pain associated with endometriosis with dyspareunia**
Women age 18 and older: 200 mg PO b.i.d. for up to 6 months.

ADMINISTRATION
PO
- Exclude pregnancy before starting drug or start drug within 7 days from the onset of menses.
- Give at approximately the same time each day, with or without food.
- Give missed dose on the same day as soon as possible; then resume regular dosing schedule.
- Store at 36° to 86° F (2° to 30° C).

ACTION
A gonadotropin-releasing hormone receptor antagonist that suppresses the pituitary gland and decreases concentrations of the ovarian sex hormones, estradiol and progesterone.

Route	Onset	Peak	Duration
PO	Unknown	1 hr	Unknown

Half-life: 4 to 6 hours.

ADVERSE REACTIONS
CNS: headache, insomnia, anxiety, depression, mood changes, exacerbation of mood disorders, dizziness, irritability. **GI:** nausea, diarrhea, abdominal pain, constipation. **GU:** changes in menstrual bleeding pattern, amenorrhea, decreased libido. **Hepatic:** elevated transaminase levels. **Metabolic:** hot flashes, night sweats, weight gain. **Musculoskeletal:** arthralgia, bone loss. **Skin:** rash. **Other:** hypersensitivity reactions.

INTERACTIONS
Drug-drug. *CYP3A inducers (carbamazepine, phenytoin):* May decrease elagolix level. Don't use together.
Hormonal contraceptives: May reduce efficacy of elagolix if contraceptive contains estrogen. Use of nonhormonal contraception is recommended.
Midazolam: May decrease midazolam level. Monitor patient for effectiveness; adjust midazolam dosage as clinically indicated.
Rifampin: May increase elagolix level. Limit elagolix dosage to 150 mg once daily and concomitant use to 6 months.
Rosuvastatin: May decrease rosuvastatin level. Consider increasing rosuvastatin dosage.
Strong CYP3A inhibitors (cobicistat, conivaptan, danoprevir, elvitegravir, indinavir, itraconazole, ketoconazole, lopinavir, posaconazole, ritonavir, saquinavir, tipranavir, voriconazole): May increase elagolix concentration. Limit 200-mg b.i.d. regimen to 1 month and limit concomitant use of 150-mg once-daily regimen to 6 months.
Strong OATP1B1 inhibitors (cyclosporine, gemfibrozil): May decrease elagolix concentration. Use together is contraindicated.
Substrates of CYP3A (alprazolam, atorvastatin, buspirone, colchicine, darunavir, rivaroxaban, saquinavir, simvastatin, tipranavir, triazolam): May decrease concentrations of these drugs. Monitor patient for therapeutic effect; adjust substrate dosage as clinically indicated.

Reactions in bold italics are *life-threatening*. Interactions may have a *rapid onset* or a *delayed onset*.

Substrates of P-gp (digoxin): May increase digoxin concentration. Monitor digoxin level; adjust dosage as indicated.

EFFECTS ON LAB TEST RESULTS
• May increase hepatic transaminase, total cholesterol, LDL-C, HDL-C, and triglyceride levels.

CONTRAINDICATIONS & CAUTIONS
• Contraindicated in patients hypersensitive to drug and in those with severe hepatic impairment (Child-Pugh class C) or known osteoporosis.
❸ Alert: Use cautiously in patients with a history of suicidality or depression. Drug may increase risk of suicidal ideation and mood disorders.
• Drug can cause liver impairment and should be used at the lowest effective dose.
• Drug may cause bone loss, which may not be completely reversible. Assess bone mineral density in women with additional risk factors for osteoporosis. Limit duration of use in all patients.
• Safety and effectiveness in women younger than age 18 haven't been studied.
Dialyzable drug: No.

PREGNANCY-LACTATION-REPRODUCTION
• Use is contraindicated in pregnant women. Drug may increase risk of early pregnancy loss. Discontinue drug if pregnancy occurs during treatment.
• Exclude pregnancy before start of treatment and obtain pregnancy test if pregnancy is suspected during treatment.
• Women should use nonhormonal contraception during treatment and for 1 week after final dose.
• There are no data on the presence of drug or its metabolites in human milk or on the effects on the breastfed infant or on milk production. Consider benefits of treatment and risks to the breastfed infant before use.

NURSING CONSIDERATIONS
❸ Alert: Monitor patient for suicidal ideation, suicidal behavior, and exacerbation of existing mood disorders.
❸ Alert: Promptly evaluate patient with depressive symptoms to determine whether risks of continued therapy outweigh benefits.

❸ Alert: Refer patients with new or worsening depression, anxiety, or other mood changes to a mental health professional for assessment.
• Monitor bone mineral density in patients with a history of low-trauma fracture or other risk factors for osteoporosis or bone loss.
• Consider supplementation with calcium and vitamin D. The benefit of patients taking these supplements during treatment with elagolix hasn't been studied, but supplements may be beneficial for all patients.
• Monitor patient for changes in menstrual bleeding (reduction in amount, intensity, or duration). These changes can make it difficult to recognize pregnancy. Perform pregnancy testing if pregnancy is suspected.
• Monitor patient for signs and symptoms of liver injury (jaundice, abdominal pain, dark amber–colored urine, fatigue, nausea, vomiting, generalized swelling, easy bruising). Obtain LFT values if signs and symptoms occur.

PATIENT TEACHING
❸ Alert: Advise patient to seek immediate medical attention for suicidal ideation and behavior, new-onset or worsening depression, anxiety, or other mood changes.
❸ Alert: Counsel family member or caregivers to watch for changes in behavior and to immediately report suicidal thoughts or behaviors to prescriber.
• Advise patient that drug may cause menstrual changes, which can make it difficult to detect an early pregnancy. Counsel patient to obtain a pregnancy test if pregnancy is suspected and to discontinue drug if pregnancy is confirmed.
• Caution patient to avoid pregnancy while using drug and to use nonhormonal contraceptives during and for 1 week after treatment, even if taking oral contraceptives.
• Inform patient that estrogen-containing contraceptives are expected to reduce drug's efficacy.
• Inform patient about the risk of bone loss. Advise adequate intake of calcium and vitamin D and supplementation if prescribed.
• Counsel patient to immediately report signs and symptoms of liver injury.

• Instruct patient who misses a dose to take the missed dose on the same day as soon as she remembers and then resume regular dosing schedule.

• Instruct patient to dispose of unused drug via a take-back option if available or to otherwise follow FDA instructions for disposing of drug in the household trash (www.fda.gov/drugdisposal) and not to flush drug down the toilet.

elbasvir–grazoprevir ⚕
EL-bas-vir/graz-OH-pre-vir

Zepatier

Therapeutic class: Antivirals
Pharmacologic class: HCV NS5A inhibitors/HCV NS3/4A protease inhibitors

AVAILABLE FORMS
Tablets: elbasvir 50 mg/grazoprevir 100 mg

INDICATIONS & DOSAGES
➤ **Chronic HCV genotypes 1 or 4 infection, with or without ribavirin** ⚕
Adults: 1 tablet PO once daily. See manufacturer's instructions for information on recommended dosing regimens and durations for treatment of HCV genotype 1 or 4 in patients with or without cirrhosis.
Adjust-a-dose: If ALT level is greater than 10 × ULN, consider discontinuing drug. If ALT level is elevated and accompanied by signs or symptoms of liver inflammation, increased conjugated bilirubin or alkaline phosphatase level, or increased INR, discontinue drug. If CrCl is 50 mL/minute or less and ribavirin is used, refer to ribavirin prescribing information for ribavirin dosage adjustment.

ADMINISTRATION
PO
• May give without regard for food.
• Store at 68° to 77° F (20° to 25° C).
• Store in original container. Protect from moisture.

ACTION
Elbasvir inhibits HCV NS5A, which is an enzyme needed for viral RNA replication and assembly of virions. Grazoprevir inhibits HCV NS3/4A protease, which is an enzyme that is essential for viral replication and is responsible for HCV protein cleavage.

Route	Onset	Peak	Duration
PO (elbasvir)	Unknown	3 hr	Unknown
PO (grazoprevir)	Unknown	2 hr	Unknown

Half-life: Elbasvir, 24 hours; grazoprevir, 31 hours.

ADVERSE REACTIONS
CNS: headache, fatigue, insomnia, irritability, depression. **GI:** nausea, diarrhea, abdominal pain (with ribavirin). **Hematologic:** anemia. **Hepatic:** ALT elevations, bilirubin elevations. **Musculoskeletal:** arthralgia (with ribavirin). **Respiratory:** dyspnea (with ribavirin). **Skin:** rash, pruritus (with ribavirin).

INTERACTIONS
Drug-drug. *Antibiotics (nafcillin):* May decrease concentrations of elbasvir and grazoprevir and therapeutic effects. Use together isn't recommended.
HIV medications (cobicistat, elvitegravir, emtricitabine, etravirine, tenofovir): May increase elbasvir–grazoprevir concentrations. Use together isn't recommended. Etravirine may decrease elbasvir–grazoprevir concentrations and lead to decreased effectiveness. Use together isn't recommended.
HMG-CoA reductase inhibitors (atorvastatin, rosuvastatin): May increase atorvastatin and rosuvastatin concentrations. Maximum recommended doses are atorvastatin 20 mg/day and rosuvastatin 10 mg/day.
HMG-CoA reductase inhibitors (fluvastatin, lovastatin, simvastatin): May increase concentrations of HMG-CoA reductase inhibitors. Use lowest necessary statin dosage and monitor patient closely for statin-associated adverse effects such as myopathy.
Immunosuppressants (tacrolimus): May increase tacrolimus concentration. Frequently monitor renal function and tacrolimus level, and watch for tacrolimus-associated adverse effects.
Moderate CYP3A inducers (bosentan, modafinil): May decrease elbasvir–grazoprevir plasma concentrations. Use together isn't recommended.

Reactions in bold italics are **life-threatening**. Interactions may have a *rapid onset* or a **delayed onset**.

OATP1B1/3 inhibitors (atazanavir, cyclosporine, darunavir, lopinavir, saquinavir, tipranavir): May increase risk of ALT elevation. Use together is contraindicated.

Strong CYP3A inducers (carbamazepine, efavirenz, phenytoin, rifampin): May cause loss of virologic response. Use together is contraindicated.

Strong CYP3A inhibitors (clarithromycin, indinavir, itraconazole, ketoconazole, nefazodone, nelfinavir, ritonavir, telithromycin): May increase elbasvir or grazoprevir concentrations. Use together isn't recommended.

Drug-herb. *St. John's wort:* May decrease elbasvir–grazoprevir concentrations and cause loss of virologic response. Use together is contraindicated.

EFFECTS ON LAB TEST RESULTS
• May increase ALT and bilirubin levels. May decrease Hb level.

CONTRAINDICATIONS & CAUTIONS
▨ Patients with HCV genotype 1a infection should undergo testing for NS5A resistance-associated polymorphisms before starting treatment, to determine the need for ribavirin and treatment duration.
• If elbasvir–grazoprevir is administered with ribavirin, the contraindications with ribavirin also apply.
Black Box Warning Reactivation of HBV may occur in HCV coinfected patients, and result in fulminant hepatitis, hepatic failure, and death. Screen all patients for current or prior HBV infection before treatment and if positive for HBV infection, assess baseline HBV DNA. ∎
• Contraindicated in patients with moderate or severe hepatic impairment (Child-Pugh class B or C).
▨ Female patients, Asian patients, and patients age 65 and older are at increased risk for elevated ALT level.
• Safe use in children, liver transplant recipients, and patients with HBV/HCV coinfection hasn't been established.
Dialyzable drug: No.

PREGNANCY-LACTATION-REPRODUCTION
• There are no human data regarding use in pregnant women, and safe use during

pregnancy hasn't been established. If drug is used with ribavirin, the combination regimen is contraindicated in pregnant women and in men whose female partners are pregnant.
• If drug is given with ribavirin, a negative pregnancy test is required immediately before initiation, monthly during therapy, and for 6 months after treatment ends.
• It isn't known if elbasvir or grazoprevir appears in human milk. Use cautiously in breastfeeding women.

NURSING CONSIDERATIONS
Black Box Warning Monitor patient with current or prior HBV infection for hepatitis flare or HBV reactivation with laboratory testing and watch for signs and symptoms of liver injury during active and posttreatment follow-up. ∎
• Obtain LFT values before start of therapy, at treatment week 8, at week 12 in patients receiving 16 weeks of treatment, and as clinically indicated.
• Drug is approved for patients with or without cirrhosis.
• Monitor patients for signs and symptoms of liver inflammation (fatigue, weakness, lack of appetite, abdominal pain, nausea, vomiting, jaundice, and discolored feces).

PATIENT TEACHING
Black Box Warning Warn patient to immediately report signs and symptoms of liver injury (fatigue, weakness, loss of appetite, nausea, vomiting, yellowing of skin or eyes, light-colored stool). ∎
• Instruct patient to report current or new prescription or OTC medications or supplements being taken before starting therapy because of possible interactions.
• Explain importance of taking drug around the same time every day, without missing or skipping doses. Advise patient to contact prescriber if a dose is missed and not to double a dose.
• Teach patient importance of adherence and regular follow-up with prescriber during therapy.
• Advise female patient to avoid pregnancy during and for 6 months after final dose when drug is used concomitantly with ribavirin.

• Warn patient to watch for and immediately report signs and symptoms of hepatotoxicity (tiredness, nausea and vomiting, lack of appetite, jaundice, discolored stools).

eletriptan hydrobromide
ell-ah-TRIP-tan

Relpax✔

Therapeutic class: Antimigraine drugs
Pharmacologic class: Serotonin 5-HT$_1$ receptor agonists

AVAILABLE FORMS
Tablets ⓄⓉⒸ: 20 mg, 40 mg

INDICATIONS & DOSAGES
➤ **Acute migraine with or without aura**
Adults: 20 to 40 mg PO at first migraine symptom. If headache recurs, dose may be repeated at least 2 hours later to a maximum of 80 mg in any 24-hour period.

ADMINISTRATION
PO
• Give drug without regard for food.
• Give drug whole; don't crush or break tablet.
• Give drug with a full glass of water.

ACTION
Binds to 5-HT$_{1B/1D}$ receptors and may constrict intracranial blood vessels and inhibit proinflammatory neuropeptide release.

Route	Onset	Peak	Duration
PO	½ hr	1½–2 hr	Unknown

Half-life: About 4 hours.

ADVERSE REACTIONS
CNS: asthenia, dizziness, drowsiness, headache, hypertonia, hypoesthesia, pain, paresthesia, somnolence, vertigo. **CV:** chest tightness, pain, and pressure; flushing, palpitations. **EENT:** pharyngitis. **GI:** abdominal pain, discomfort, or cramps; dry mouth, dyspepsia, dysphagia, nausea. **Musculoskeletal:** back pain. **Skin:** diaphoresis. **Other:** chills.

INTERACTIONS
Drug-drug. *CYP3A4 inhibitors (clarithromycin, itraconazole, ketoconazole, nefazodone, nelfinavir, ritonavir):* May increase eletriptan metabolism. Avoid use within 72 hours of these drugs.
Ergotamine-containing or ergot-type drugs (dihydroergotamine, methysergide), other triptans: May prolong vasospastic reactions. Avoid use within 24 hours of these drugs.
Linezolid: May enhance serotonergic effect of eletriptan, possibly resulting in serotonin syndrome. Discontinue eletriptan 2 weeks before starting linezolid, but if urgent initiation of linezolid is needed, discontinue eletriptan immediately and monitor patient.
MAO inhibitors, SSNRIs, SSRIs, TCAs: May increase the risk of serotonin syndrome (weakness, hyperreflexia, and incoordination). Monitor patient closely.
Methylene blue: May increase risk of serotonin syndrome. Avoid concurrent use.
Other 5-HT$_1$ antagonists: Concomitant use is contraindicated. Avoid concurrent use.

EFFECTS ON LAB TEST RESULTS
• None known.

CONTRAINDICATIONS & CAUTIONS
• Contraindicated in patients hypersensitive to drug or its components. Serious and fatal hypersensitivity reactions have been reported. Anaphylactic reactions are more likely in patients with a history of sensitivity to multiple allergens.
• Contraindicated in patients with severe hepatic impairment, ischemic heart disease, history of MI, or silent ischemia; coronary artery vasospasm, including Prinzmetal variant angina; Wolff-Parkinson-White syndrome or arrhythmias associated with other cardiac accessory conduction pathway disorders; and other significant CV conditions.
• Contraindicated within 24 hours of treatment with another 5-HT$_1$ agonist or ergot-containing drug or within 72 hours of ketoconazole, itraconazole, nefazodone, clarithromycin, ritonavir, or nelfinavir.
• Contraindicated in patients with cerebrovascular syndromes, such as stroke or TIA; PVD, including ischemic bowel disease; uncontrolled HTN; or hemiplegic or basilar migraine.

Reactions in bold italics are *life-threatening*. Interactions may have a *rapid onset* or a *delayed onset*.

- Contraindicated in patients with risk factors for CAD, such as HTN, hypercholesterolemia, smoking, obesity, diabetes, strong family history of CAD, postmenopausal women, or men older than age 40, unless patient is free from cardiac disease. Monitor patient closely after first dose.
- Safety of treating more than three migraine headaches in 30 days hasn't been established.

Dialyzable drug: Unknown.

⚠ *Overdose S&S:* HTN, serious CV reactions.

PREGNANCY-LACTATION-REPRODUCTION
- Use cautiously in pregnant women and only if benefit outweighs possible risk to the fetus.
- Drug appears in human milk. Use cautiously in breastfeeding women.

NURSING CONSIDERATIONS
- Drug isn't intended for migraine prevention.

🔔 *Alert:* Combining a triptan with an SSRI or SSNRI, TCAs, linezolid, methylene blue, or MAO inhibitors may cause serotonin syndrome. Signs and symptoms, which may include restlessness, hallucinations, loss of coordination, fast heartbeat, rapid changes in BP, increased body temperature, hyperreflexia, nausea, vomiting, and diarrhea, occur within minutes to hours of patient receiving a new or increased dosage of the serotonergic drug; signs and symptoms may be more likely to occur at start of therapy or when serotonergic drug dosage is increased.
- Use drug only when patient has a clear diagnosis of migraine. If the first use produces no response, reconsider the migraine diagnosis.

🔔 *Alert:* Serious cardiac events, including acute MI, arrhythmias, and death, occur rarely within a few hours after use of 5-HT$_1$ agonists. Don't use in patients with a history of CV disease.
- Ophthalmologic effects may occur with long-term use.
- Significant HTN can occur even in patients with no history of HTN. Monitor BP closely.

PATIENT TEACHING
- Instruct patient to take dose at first sign of a migraine headache. If the headache comes back after the first dose, patient may take a second dose after 2 hours. Caution patient not to take more than 80 mg in 24 hours.
- Warn patient to avoid driving and operating machinery if dizziness or fatigue occurs.
- Tell patient to immediately report pain, tightness, heaviness, or pressure in the chest, throat, neck, or jaw.
- Tell patient to swallow tablet whole with a full glass of water and not to split, crush, or chew it.

SAFETY ALERT!

elotuzumab
el-oh-TOOZ-ue-mab

Empliciti

Therapeutic class: Antineoplastics
Pharmacologic class: Monoclonal antibodies

AVAILABLE FORMS
Injection: 300-mg, 400-mg single-dose vials

INDICATIONS & DOSAGES
➤ **Multiple myeloma in combination with lenalidomide and dexamethasone in patients who have received one to three prior therapies**
Adults: 10 mg/kg IV every week for first two 28-day cycles, then every 2 weeks thereafter in combination with lenalidomide 25 mg PO on days 1 through 21 of every cycle until disease progression or unacceptable toxicity. Between 3 and 24 hours before elotuzumab is given, administer dexamethasone 28 mg PO. Additionally, give dexamethasone 8 mg IV between 45 and 90 minutes before elotuzumab is administered. On days that elotuzumab isn't administered (days 8 and 22 of cycle 3 and all subsequent cycles), give dexamethasone 40 mg PO. Elotuzumab must be given with premedications (dexamethasone, diphenhydramine, ranitidine, and acetaminophen).
➤ **Treatment of multiple myeloma in combination with pomalidomide and dexamethasone in patients who have received**

at least two prior therapies including lenalidomide and a proteasome inhibitor

Adults age 75 and older: 10 mg/kg IV once every week for the first two 28-day cycles; then starting at cycle 3, give 20 mg/kg every 4 weeks thereafter. Use in combination with pomalidomide 4 mg PO on days 1 through 21 of every cycle. Between 3 and 24 hours before elotuzumab is given, administer dexamethasone 8 mg PO. Additionally, give dexamethasone 8 mg IV between 45 and 90 minutes before elotuzumab is administered. On days that elotuzumab isn't administered (days 8, 15, and 22 of cycle 3 and all subsequent cycles), give dexamethasone 20 mg PO. Continue treatment until disease progression or unacceptable toxicity.

Adults age 75 and younger: 10 mg/kg IV once every week for the first two 28-day cycles; then starting at cycle 3, give 20 mg/kg every 4 weeks thereafter. Use in combination with pomalidomide 4 mg PO on days 1 through 21 of every cycle. Between 3 and 24 hours before elotuzumab is given, administer dexamethasone 28 mg PO. Additionally, give dexamethasone 8 mg IV between 45 and 90 minutes before elotuzumab is administered. On days that elotuzumab isn't administered (days 8, 15, and 22 of cycle 3 and all subsequent cycles), give dexamethasone 40 mg PO. Continue treatment until disease progression or unacceptable toxicity.

Adjust-a-dose: If the dose of one drug in the regimen is delayed or interrupted or the drug is discontinued, treatment with the other drugs may continue as scheduled. However, if dexamethasone is delayed or discontinued, base the decision whether to administer drug on clinical judgment for the risk of hypersensitivity. For grade 2 or higher infusion reaction, interrupt infusion and institute appropriate medical and supportive measures; upon resolution to grade 1 or lower, restart drug at 0.5 mL/minute and gradually increase at a rate of 0.5 mL/minute every 30 minutes as tolerated to rate at which the infusion reaction occurred. Resume the escalation regimen if there's no recurrence of the infusion reaction. If an infusion reaction recurs, stop infusion and don't restart on that day; severe infusion reactions may require permanent discontinuation of drug and emergency treatment.

Delay and modify dosage of dexamethasone and lenalidomide as recommended in their prescribing information. Delay and modify dosage of dexamethasone and pomalidomide as recommended in their prescribing information.

ADMINISTRATION
IV

▼ Premedicate patient 45 to 90 minutes before infusion with diphenhydramine 25 to 50 mg PO or IV, or equivalent H_1 blocker; ranitidine 50 mg IV or 150 mg PO, or equivalent H_2 blocker; and acetaminophen 650 to 1,000 mg PO.

▼ Reconstitute each vial with sterile water for injection; 13 mL for 300-mg vial and 17 mL for 400-mg vial for a final concentration in either vial of 25 mg/mL.

▼ Hold vial upright and swirl solution by rotating vial to dissolve the lyophilized cake. Invert vial a few times to dissolve any powder that may be present on top of vial or stopper; don't shake. Powder should dissolve in less than 10 minutes. After dissolution, allow reconstituted solution to stand for 5 to 10 minutes.

▼ Solution should be colorless to slightly yellow, clear to slightly opalescent. Discard solution if particulate matter or discoloration is observed.

▼ After reconstitution, withdraw necessary volume for the calculated dose from each vial, up to a maximum of 16 mL from 400-mg vial and 12 mL from 300-mg vial and further dilute with 230 mL of either NSS or D_5W into an infusion bag made of polyvinyl chloride or polyolefin. Volume of NSS or D_5W can be adjusted so as not to exceed 5 mL/kg of patient weight at any given dose of drug.

▼ Complete infusion within 24 hours of reconstitution. If not used immediately, store under refrigeration at 36° to 46° F (2° to 8° C) and protected from light for up to 24 hours. A maximum of 8 hours of the total 24 hours can be at room temperature and room light.

▼ Administer infusion through a nonpyrogenic low-protein-binding filter (with a

---

pore size of 0.2 to 1.2 microns) using an automated infusion pump.

▼ Initiate infusion at a rate of 0.5 mL/minute and increase in stepwise fashion as follows if no infusion reactions develop: For cycle 1/dose 1, infuse at 0.5 mL/minute for first 30 minutes, then increase to 1 mL/minute for next 30 minutes, then increase to 2 mL/minute until infusion is completed. For cycle 1/dose 2, for first 30 minutes, infuse at 3 mL/minute, then 4 mL/minute from 30 minutes until finished; all infusions after this may be infused at 5 mL/minute. Maximum infusion rate shouldn't exceed 5 mL/minute. Adjust infusion rate after any grade 2 or higher infusion reaction.

▼ Keep unopened vials under refrigeration.

▼ **Incompatibilities:** Administer alone; don't mix or infuse in same line with other drugs.

ACTION

A humanized IgG1 monoclonal antibody that specifically targets the SLAMF7 signaling protein, activating natural killer cells and targeting the SLAMF7 protein on myeloma cells to kill the cells.

Route	Onset	Peak	Duration
IV	Unknown	Unknown	Unknown

Half-life: Unknown.

ADVERSE REACTIONS

CNS: peripheral neuropathy, headache, hypoesthesia, fatigue, pyrexia, altered mood. **CV:** chest pain, HTN, hypotension, tachycardia, *bradycardia.* **EENT:** cataracts, nasopharyngitis, oropharyngeal pain. **GI:** diarrhea, constipation, vomiting, decreased appetite. **GU:** *acute renal failure.* **Hematologic:** anemia, *leukopenia, thrombocytopenia.* **Hepatic:** *hepatotoxicity.* **Metabolic:** decreased weight, hyperglycemia, *hyperkalemia,* hypoalbuminemia, elevated alkaline phosphatase level, *hypocalcemia.* **Musculoskeletal:** pain in extremities. **Respiratory:** cough, URI, pneumonia, *PE.* **Skin:** night sweats. **Other:** hypersensitivity, infusion reactions.

INTERACTIONS

Drug-drug. *Immunosuppressants:* May enhance infection risk or toxic effects. Monitor patient response.

Live-virus vaccines: May enhance adverse/toxic effect of vaccines. Don't give live-virus vaccines for at least 3 months after elotuzumab.

Drug-herb. *Echinacea:* May diminish therapeutic effect of elotuzumab. Avoid concurrent use.

EFFECTS ON LAB TEST RESULTS

• May increase transaminase, bilirubin, alkaline phosphatase, glucose, and potassium levels. May decrease albumin, calcium, and bicarbonate levels.

• May decrease lymphocyte, leukocyte, and platelet counts.

• May interfere with gamma region serum protein electrophoresis and immunofixation assay results.

CONTRAINDICATIONS & CAUTIONS

• May cause hypersensitivity reactions. Patient must be premedicated with dexamethasone, diphenhydramine, ranitidine, and acetaminophen.

• Infections can occur. Monitor patients for fever and other signs and symptoms of infection; treat promptly.

• Second primary malignancies can occur.

• Drug can interfere with assays used to monitor M-protein, which can impact the determination of complete response.

• Safety and effectiveness in children haven't been established.

Dialyzable drug: No.

PREGNANCY-LACTATION-REPRODUCTION

• There are no studies of elotuzumab use in pregnant women. Drug may cause fetal harm. Lenalidomide is contraindicated for use during pregnancy.

• Males and females of reproductive potential must use effective contraception during treatment and for a significant amount of time after final dose. Follow lenalidomide prescribing information for specific details on pregnancy testing and contraception.

• It isn't known if drug appears in human milk. Breastfeeding isn't recommended.

E

NURSING CONSIDERATIONS
• Monitor patients for development of infusion reactions (fever, chills, HTN or hypotension, bradycardia). Interrupt infusion for grade 2 or higher infusion reactions and treat appropriately.
• In patients who experience an infusion reaction, monitor vital signs every 30 minutes for 2 hours after end of infusion.
• Ensure patient has taken premedications before infusion.
• Monitor patients for development of infection, which can be fatal, and treat promptly.
• Monitor patients for second primary malignancies.
• Obtain baseline liver enzyme levels and monitor periodically during treatment. Stop drug for grade 3 or higher liver enzyme elevations. May consider continuing treatment after results return to baseline.

PATIENT TEACHING
• Advise patient that lenalidomide used in combination with elotuzumab can cause fetal harm and has specific requirements regarding contraception, pregnancy testing, blood and sperm donation, and transmission in sperm.
• Inform patient of risk of liver toxicity during treatment; tell patient to report signs and symptoms of toxicity (tiredness, weakness, loss of appetite, confusion, jaundice, change in stool color, abdominal pain, swelling of stomach area).
• Advise patient to immediately report signs and symptoms of infusion reactions (fever, chills, rash, breathing problems, dizziness, light-headedness) that could occur within 24 hours of infusion.
• Instruct patient that oral dexamethasone, an H_1 blocker, an H_2 blocker, and acetaminophen will be required before infusions to reduce risk of infusion reactions.
• Caution patient about risk of developing infections during treatment; teach patient to report signs and symptoms of infection (fever, flulike symptoms, cough, shortness of breath, burning with urination, painful rash).
• Warn patient of risk of developing second primary malignancies during treatment.
• Advise patient that laboratory testing will be needed to monitor treatment.

SAFETY ALERT!

eluxadoline
el-ux-AD-oh-leen

Viberzi

Therapeutic class: Anti–IBS drugs
Pharmacologic class: Mu-opioid receptor agonists, delta-opioid receptor agonists, kappa-opioid receptor agonists
Controlled substance schedule: IV

AVAILABLE FORMS
Tablets: 75 mg, 100 mg

INDICATIONS & DOSAGES
➤ **IBS with diarrhea (IBS-D)**
Adults: 100 mg PO b.i.d.
Adjust-a-dose: Reduce dosage to 75 mg b.i.d. in patients who are unable to tolerate the 100-mg dose, are receiving concomitant OATP1B1 inhibitors (cyclosporine, gemfibrozil, atazanavir, lopinavir, ritonavir, saquinavir, tipranavir, rifampin, eltrombopag), or have mild to moderate (Child-Pugh class A or B) hepatic impairment.

ADMINISTRATION
PO
• Give with food.
• If a dose is missed, give next dose at the regular time. Don't give two doses at the same time to make up for a missed dose.
• Store at room temperature.

ACTION
Mu-opioid receptor agonist, delta-opioid receptor antagonist, and kappa-opioid receptor agonist that decreases peristaltic action of the intestines. Acts locally to reduce abdominal pain and IBS-D without constipating adverse effects.

Route	Onset	Peak	Duration
PO (with food)	Unknown	1½ hr (range, 1–8 hr)	Unknown

Half-life: 3.7 to 6 hours.

ADVERSE REACTIONS
CNS: dizziness, fatigue, drowsiness, euphoria, intoxicated feeling, sedation. **EENT:** nasopharyngitis. **GI:** constipation, nausea,

---

Reactions in bold italics are *life-threatening*. Interactions may have a *rapid onset* or a ***delayed onset***.

vomiting, abdominal pain, abdominal distention, flatulence, viral gastroenteritis, gastroesophageal reflux. **Hepatic:** elevated ALT and AST levels. **Respiratory:** URI, bronchitis, *asthma*. **Skin:** rash.

INTERACTIONS

Drug-drug. *CYP3A substrates with narrow therapeutic index (alfentanil, ergotamine, fentanyl, pimozide, quinidine, sirolimus, tacrolimus):* May increase concentration of CYP3A substrates. Monitor drug concentrations or other pharmacodynamic markers of drug effect when use with eluxadoline is initiated or discontinued.

Drugs that cause constipation (alosetron, anticholinergics, opioids): May increase risk of constipation-related adverse reactions. Avoid use together.

OATP1B1 inhibitors (atazanavir, cyclosporine, eltrombopag, gemfibrozil, lopinavir, rifampin, ritonavir, saquinavir, tipranavir): May increase eluxadoline concentration. Give eluxadoline at a dose of 75 mg b.i.d.; monitor patient for eluxadoline-related adverse reactions.

Rosuvastatin: May increase rosuvastatin concentration and risk of myopathy/rhabdomyolysis. Use lowest effective rosuvastatin dose.

Strong CYP inhibitors (ciprofloxacin [CYP1A2], clarithromycin [CYP3A4], fluconazole [CYP2C19], gemfibrozil [CYP2C8], paroxetine and bupropion [CYP2D6]): May increase eluxadoline concentration. Monitor patient for eluxadoline-related adverse reactions.

Drug-lifestyle. *Alcohol use:* May increase risk of acute pancreatitis. Patient should avoid prolonged or acute excessive alcohol use while taking drug. Monitor patient closely.

EFFECTS ON LAB TEST RESULTS

• May increase ALT and AST levels.

CONTRAINDICATIONS & CAUTIONS

• Contraindicated in patients hypersensitive to drug or its components.
• Contraindicated in patients without a gallbladder, with known or suspected biliary duct obstruction or sphincter of Oddi disease or dysfunction. Permanently discontinue

drug in patients who develop biliary duct obstruction or sphincter of Oddi spasm while taking eluxadoline.
• Contraindicated in patients with alcohol abuse, alcohol addiction, alcoholism, or consumption of more than three alcoholic beverages each day; history of pancreatitis or structural diseases of the pancreas or suspected pancreatic duct obstruction with severe hepatic impairment (Child-Pugh class C); history of chronic or severe constipation or sequelae from constipation; or known or suspected mechanical GI obstruction.
• Drug has potential for abuse and psychological dependence. Consider naloxone in the event of overdose.
• Safety and effectiveness in children haven't been established.
• Use cautiously in elderly patients, for whom the same effectiveness was observed but with a higher incidence of adverse reactions.

Dialyzable drug: Unlikely.

PREGNANCY-LACTATION-REPRODUCTION

• Use cautiously in pregnant women. Risk to fetus is unknown.
• It isn't known if drug appears in human milk. Use cautiously in breastfeeding women, taking into account maternal benefits and risk to the fetus.

NURSING CONSIDERATIONS

• Monitor patients with hepatic impairment for impaired mental or physical abilities needed to perform potentially hazardous activities, such as driving or operating machinery.
• Monitor patients for sphincter of Oddi spasm (unusual or severe epigastric or upper right quadrant abdominal pain that may radiate to the back or shoulder, with or without nausea and vomiting, and with liver or pancreatic enzyme elevations). Discontinue drug if signs or symptoms develop.
• Monitor patients, especially those with excessive alcohol intake, for pancreatitis (new or worsening abdominal or epigastric pain that may radiate to the back, associated with elevated pancreatic enzyme levels). Discontinue drug if signs and symptoms occur.

• Monitor patients for constipation. Discontinue drug if severe constipation lasting more than 4 days develops.
• Watch for signs and symptoms of abuse of drug, including psychological dependence.

PATIENT TEACHING
• Advise patient to read the FDA-approved medication guide.
• Warn patient to stop drug and seek medical attention for new or worsening upper right quadrant abdominal pain that radiates to the shoulder or back or if nausea or vomiting occurs.
• Advise patient to avoid prolonged and acute excessive alcohol use while taking drug.
• Advise patient to discontinue drug and contact prescriber for constipation lasting more than 4 days.
• Instruct patient to avoid taking drug with other medications that may cause constipation and to ask prescriber for a list of these medications.
• Inform patient that loperamide may occasionally be used with eluxadoline but must be stopped if constipation develops.
• Caution patient with hepatic impairment not to drive, operate machinery, or perform other dangerous activities until effects of drug are known.
• Advise patient that if a dose is missed to take the next dose at the regular time and not to take two doses at the same time to make up for the missed dose.

---

elvitegravir–cobicistat–emtricitabine–tenofovir disoproxil fumarate
el-vye-TEG-ra-veer/koe-BIK-i-stat/em-tra-SYE-tah-ben/te-NOE-fo-veer

Stribild

Therapeutic class: Antiretrovirals
Pharmacologic class: Antivirals

AVAILABLE FORMS
Tablet: Each tablet contains 150 mg elvitegravir, 150 mg cobicistat, 200 mg emtricitabine, and 300 mg tenofovir disoproxil fumarate

INDICATIONS & DOSAGES
➤ **HIV-1 infection in adults and children age 12 and older weighing at least 35 kg who are antiretroviral treatment–naive; to replace current antiretroviral regimen in adults and children age 12 and older weighing at least 35 kg who are virologically suppressed (HIV-1 RNA <50 copies/mL) on a stable regimen for at least 6 months with no history of treatment failure and no known substitutions associated with resistance to individual components**
Adults and children age 12 and older weighing at least 35 kg and with CrCl of 70 mL/minute or more: 1 tablet PO once daily.
Adjust-a-dose: Initiation of drug in patients with estimated CrCl below 70 mL/minute isn't recommended. Discontinue drug in patients with estimated CrCl of less than 50 mL/minute and patients with Child-Pugh class C hepatic impairment.

ADMINISTRATION
PO
• Give with food.
• Drug is used as a complete treatment; don't give with other antiretrovirals.

ACTION
Combination of agents with differing mechanisms of action (integrase strand transfer inhibition, pharmacokinetic enhancement, nucleoside analogue HIV-1 reverse transcriptase inhibition) working together to inhibit HIV replication.

Route	Onset	Peak	Duration
PO (elvitegravir)	Unknown	4 hr	Unknown
PO (cobicistat, emtricitabine)	Unknown	3 hr	Unknown
PO (tenofovir)	Unknown	2 hr	Unknown

Half-life: Elvitegravir, 13 hours; cobicistat, 4 hours; emtricitabine, 10 hours; tenofovir, 12 to 18 hours.

ADVERSE REACTIONS
CNS: anxiety, headache, dizziness, insomnia, abnormal dreams, fatigue, somnolence, depression, fever, pain. **GI:** diarrhea, nausea, flatulence. **GU:** proteinuria, hematuria. **Musculoskeletal:** arthralgia, back pain, bone fracture, myalgia. **Respiratory:** cough, pneumonia. **Skin:** rash.

Reactions in bold italics are *life-threatening*. Interactions may have a *rapid onset* or a *delayed onset*.

INTERACTIONS
Drug-drug. *Acyclovir, cidofovir, ganciclovir, valacyclovir, valganciclovir:* May increase concentrations of these drugs, emtricitabine, and tenofovir due to competition for renal excretion. Use together carefully.

Additional antiretrovirals: May increase risk of drug interactions and altered pharmacokinetics of drug components. Use together is contraindicated.

Alfuzosin: May increase alfuzosin level and risk of severe hypotension. Use together is contraindicated.

Antacids: May decrease elvitegravir concentration. Separate administration times by 2 hours.

Antiarrhythmics, digoxin: May increase levels of these drugs. Use together cautiously and monitor drug levels if possible.

Antidepressants (SSRIs, TCAs, trazodone): May increase levels of these drugs. Use together cautiously and titrate antidepressant according to response.

Antifungals (itraconazole, ketoconazole, voriconazole): May increase levels of these drugs, elvitegravir, and cobicistat. Use together cautiously. Don't exceed 200 mg/day of ketoconazole or itraconazole.

Beta blockers (metoprolol, timolol): May increase beta blocker concentration. Monitor patient carefully and decrease beta blocker dosage as necessary.

Bosentan: May increase bosentan level. Give bosentan dose based on manufacturer's instructions and adjust according to patient tolerance.

Calcium channel blockers (amlodipine, diltiazem, felodipine, nicardipine, nifedipine, verapamil): May increase level of calcium channel blocker. Use together cautiously and monitor patient closely.

Carbamazepine, oxcarbazepine, phenobarbital, phenytoin: May significantly decrease elvitegravir and cobicistat levels; may increase carbamazepine level. Use together is contraindicated.

Clarithromycin, telithromycin: May increase level of clarithromycin, telithromycin, and cobicistat. Use together cautiously. Decrease clarithromycin dosage by 50% if CrCl is between 50 and 60 mL/minute.

Clonazepam, ethosuximide: May increase levels of these drugs. Use together cautiously.

Colchicine: May increase colchicine concentration. Adjust dosage according to manufacturer's instructions. Use together is contraindicated in patients with renal or hepatic impairment.

CYP2D6, CYP3A, P-gp substrates: May alter plasma concentrations of the four drug components (elvitegravir, cobicistat, emtricitabine, and tenofovir). Use together cautiously.

Dexamethasone: May significantly decrease cobicistat and elvitegravir levels. Monitor patient carefully for loss of therapeutic effect (elvitegravir, cobicistat) and development of resistance.

Ergot derivatives (dihydroergotamine, ergotamine, methylergonovine): May increase levels of these drugs. Use together is contraindicated.

Fluticasone: May increase fluticasone level. Choose an alternative corticosteroid.

HMG-CoA reductase inhibitors (atorvastatin): May increase statin drug level and risk of myopathy. Start statin at lowest dosage and titrate carefully.

Hormonal contraceptives: May alter levels of these drugs. Consider nonhormonal forms of birth control.

Immunosuppressants (cyclosporine, sirolimus, tacrolimus): May increase immunosuppressant level. Use together cautiously.

Lovastatin, simvastatin: May increase statin level and risk of myopathy. Use together is contraindicated.

Lurasidone, pimozide: May increase risk of cardiac adverse effects. Use together is contraindicated.

Midazolam: May increase midazolam level. Use with oral midazolam is contraindicated. Use parenteral form cautiously and monitor patient closely.

Neuroleptics (perphenazine, quetiapine, risperidone, thioridazine): May increase neuroleptic drug level. Decrease neuroleptic dosage as needed.

PDE5 inhibitors (sildenafil, tadalafil, vardenafil): May increase effects of PDE5 inhibitors. Adjust dosage according to

E

manufacturer's instructions. Use with sildenafil for PAH is contraindicated.

Rifabutin, rifapentine: May decrease cobicistat and elvitegravir levels. Avoid use together.

Rifampin: May decrease elvitegravir and cobicistat concentrations, decreasing therapeutic effect. Use together is contraindicated.

Salmeterol: May increase risk of CV effects of salmeterol, including QT-interval prolongation, palpitations, and tachycardia. Avoid use together.

Sedative/hypnotics (buspirone, clorazepate, diazepam, estazolam, flurazepam, zolpidem): May increase concentrations of sedative/hypnotics. Use cautiously together and monitor patient carefully.

Triazolam: May increase triazolam concentration. Use together is contraindicated.

Warfarin: Effect on warfarin concentration isn't known. Monitor INR carefully.

Drug-herb. *St. John's wort:* May reduce concentrations of drug components and decrease therapeutic effect. Use together is contraindicated.

EFFECTS ON LAB TEST RESULTS

• May increase AST, amylase, CK, total cholesterol, HDL, LDL, and triglyceride levels.

• May increase urine RBC count.

CONTRAINDICATIONS & CAUTIONS

• Contraindicated in patients hypersensitive to drugs or their components and in those with CrCl of less than 70 mL/minute or severe hepatic impairment (Child-Pugh class C).

• Contraindicated with drugs that are highly dependent on CYP3A for clearance or strongly induce CYP3A: alfuzosin, carbamazepine, phenobarbital, phenytoin, rifampin, dihydroergotamine, ergotamine, methylergonovine, St. John's wort, lovastatin, simvastatin, lurasidone, pimozide, sildenafil (for PAH), triazolam, and oral midazolam.

• Use cautiously in new-onset or worsening renal impairment, including acute renal failure and Fanconi syndrome. Avoid administering with other nephrotoxic agents.

• Use cautiously in patients with a history of pathologic fracture or other risk factors for osteoporosis or bone loss. Consider calcium and vitamin D supplementation.

Black Box Warning Drug isn't approved for the treatment of chronic HBV infection; safety and effectiveness of drug haven't been established in patients infected with both HBV and HIV-1. Severe acute exacerbations of hepatitis B have been reported in patients who are infected with both HBV and HIV-1 and who have discontinued emtricitabine (Emtriva) or tenofovir (Viread), which are components of this drug. Monitor hepatic function closely with both clinical and laboratory follow-up for at least several months in patients who are infected with both HBV and HIV-1 and who discontinue this drug. If appropriate, initiation of anti–hepatitis B therapy may be warranted. ■

• Lactic acidosis and severe hepatomegaly with steatosis, including fatal cases, have been reported with use of nucleoside analogues, including tenofovir and emtricitabine, in combination with other antiretrovirals.

• Drug may increase risk of pancreatitis. Use cautiously in patients at risk for or with a history of pancreatitis.

• Drug may cause immune reconstitution syndrome.

Dialyzable drug: Elvitegravir, unlikely; cobicistat, unlikely; emtricitabine, 30% hemodialysis; tenofovir, 10% hemodialysis.

PREGNANCY-LACTATION-REPRODUCTION

• Register pregnant women in the Antiretroviral Pregnancy Registry at 1-800-258-4263.

• Not recommended for use during pregnancy. Don't initiate in pregnant women.

• Drug (emtricitabine, tenofovir) appears in human milk. Because of risk of HIV transmission, women shouldn't breastfeed.

NURSING CONSIDERATIONS

• Suspend treatment in patients who develop signs and symptoms or laboratory findings suggestive of lactic acidosis or pronounced hepatotoxicity (including nausea, vomiting, unusual or unexpected stomach discomfort, and weakness).

• Test for HBV before starting therapy; severe acute exacerbations of hepatitis B have been reported in patients infected with both HBV and HIV-1.

Reactions in bold italics are *life-threatening*. Interactions may have a *rapid onset* or a *delayed onset*.

- Avoid concurrent or recent use of a nephrotoxic agent because renal impairment is possible.
- Assess CrCl, urine glucose, and urine protein before initiating and periodically during treatment.
- Monitor serum phosphorus level in patients at risk for renal impairment.
- Closely monitor patients with a confirmed increase in serum creatinine level of greater than 0.4 mg/dL from baseline for renal safety.
- Consider assessing bone mineral density (BMD) in patients with a history of pathologic bone fracture or other risk factors for osteoporosis or bone loss because of risk of drug-related decreased BMD.
- Monitor patients for infection and development of immune reconstitution syndrome (inflammatory response to indolent or residual opportunistic infections, such as *Mycobacterium avium* infection, CMV, *Pneumocystis jiroveci* pneumonia, or TB), which may necessitate further evaluation and treatment.
- Autoimmune disorders (such as Graves disease, polymyositis, and Guillain-Barré syndrome) have also been reported in the setting of immune reconstitution; however, the time to onset is more variable, and the disorder can occur many months after initiation of treatment.

PATIENT TEACHING
- Caution patient to remain under the care of a health care provider and to comply with routine monitoring to decrease risk of adverse events.
- Inform patient that this drug isn't a cure for HIV-1 infection; patient must stay on continuous HIV therapy to control HIV-1 infection and decrease HIV-related illnesses.
- Instruct patient to avoid behaviors that can spread HIV-1 infection to others (such as sharing needles or other injection equipment; sharing personal items that may have blood or body fluids on them, such as toothbrushes and razor blades; or having sex without the protection of a latex or polyurethane condom).
- Warn female patient not to breastfeed because HIV-1 can be passed to the infant in human milk.

- Teach patient to take drug on a regular dosing schedule with food and not to miss doses.
- Advise patient to immediately report nausea, vomiting, unusual or unexpected stomach discomfort, and weakness.
- Instruct patient not to change dose or stop drug without first consulting health care provider.
- Caution patient to report signs and symptoms of infection.
- Teach patient to report yellowing of skin or sclera, dark urine, light-colored stools, loss of appetite, or nausea.

SAFETY ALERT!

empagliflozin
EM-pa-gli-FLOE-zin

Jardiance

Therapeutic class: Antidiabetics
Pharmacologic class: Sodium-glucose cotransporter 2 inhibitors

AVAILABLE FORMS
Tablets: 10 mg, 25 mg

INDICATIONS & DOSAGES
Adjust-a-dose (for all indications): Discontinue drug if GFR is less than 45 mL/minute/1.73 m^2.
➤ **As adjunct to diet and exercise to improve glycemic control in patients with type 2 diabetes mellitus**
Adults: 10 mg PO daily in the morning. May increase to 25 mg daily.
➤ **To reduce risk of CV death in patients with type 2 diabetes mellitus and established CV disease**
Adults: 10 mg PO daily in the morning. May increase to 25 mg daily.

ADMINISTRATION
PO
- May give without regard for food.
- Store at room temperature.

ACTION
Inhibits renal reabsorption of glucose and lowers renal threshold for glucose, resulting in increased urinary excretion of glucose.

Route	Onset	Peak	Duration
PO	Unknown	1½ hr	Unknown

Half-life: 12.4 hours.

ADVERSE REACTIONS
GI: nausea, thirst. **GU:** genital mycotic infections, UTI, renal impairment, increased urination. **Metabolic:** dyslipidemia, *hypoglycemia.* **Musculoskeletal:** arthralgia. **Respiratory:** URI.

INTERACTIONS
Drug-drug. *Diuretics:* May enhance diuretic effect. Closely monitor patient for volume depletion.
Insulin, insulin secretagogues, sulfonylureas, other antidiabetic agents: May increase hypoglycemic risk. Monitor patient closely.

EFFECTS ON LAB TEST RESULTS
• May increase hematocrit and LDL and serum creatinine levels. May decrease GFR.
• May cause false-positive urine glucose tests.
• Interferes with 1,5-anhydroglucitol assay.

CONTRAINDICATIONS & CAUTIONS
• Contraindicated in patients with history of serious hypersensitivity reaction to drug or its components.
• Contraindicated in patients with severe renal impairment or ESRD and in those on dialysis.
• Don't use in patients with GFR of less than 45 mL/minute.
• Serious hypersensitivity reactions, including angioedema, have been reported in patients treated with empagliflozin. Discontinue drug if a hypersensitivity reaction occurs, treat promptly per standard of care, and monitor patients until signs and symptoms resolve.
۞ Alert: Drug may cause ketoacidosis, which may require emergency department care or hospitalization for treatment. Monitor for ketoacidosis, especially in patients with major illness, reduced food or fluid intake, or reduced insulin dose. Elevated urine or serum ketone level without associated very high glucose levels has occurred with

sodium-glucose cotransporter 2 inhibitor use.
• Drug isn't recommended for type 1 diabetes or for the treatment of diabetic ketoacidosis.
• Use cautiously in patients with low BP or moderate renal impairment and in those taking diuretics; drug may increase risk of hypotension.
• Drug may increase risk of adverse events related to volume depletion and reduced renal function, especially in elderly patients and those with renal impairment.
• Drug may increase incidence of bone fractures. Per American Diabetes Association guidelines, sodium-glucose cotransporter 2 inhibitors should be avoided in patients with fracture risk factors.
• Use cautiously in patients with elevated hematocrit at baseline, as value may increase.
• Safety and effectiveness in children haven't been established.
Dialyzable drug: Unknown.

PREGNANCY-LACTATION-REPRODUCTION
• Drug hasn't been studied in pregnant women. Drug isn't recommended during the second and third trimesters. Use in pregnant women only if benefit justifies risk to the fetus.
• It isn't known if drug appears in human milk. Patient should discontinue breastfeeding or discontinue drug.

NURSING CONSIDERATIONS
• Assess renal function before initiating therapy and periodically during treatment. Don't start therapy if GFR is less than 45 mL/minute. Closely monitor patients with GFR of less than 60 mL/minute.
• Assess fluid status. Correct volume depletion before starting therapy.
• Monitor patients for signs and symptoms of hypotension (fatigue, dizziness, blurred vision, clammy skin) during therapy. Drug may increase risk of hypotension due to intravascular volume contraction.
• Monitor glucose level closely during drug initiation. Concomitant use of insulin and other antidiabetic agents may increase risk of hypoglycemia.

Reactions in bold italics are *life-threatening*. Interactions may have a *rapid onset* or a *delayed onset*.

• Watch for genital mycotic infections and treat appropriately.

⚠ *Alert:* Drug may increase risk of severe UTI, including urosepsis and pyelonephritis. Monitor patient and treat promptly if indicated.

• Monitor LDL cholesterol periodically; treat appropriately.

• Drug causes positive urine glucose tests. Avoid urine glucose testing for glycemic control monitoring.

• *Look alike–sound alike:* Don't confuse empagliflozin with canagliflozin or dapagliflozin. Don't confuse Jardiance with Januvia, Jantoven, or Janumet.

PATIENT TEACHING

• Instruct patient to take drug in the morning, with or without food.

• Advise patient that if a dose is missed, to take missed dose as soon as remembered and not to double a dose.

• Stress importance of adhering to diet, weight reduction, exercise, personal hygiene, and blood glucose monitoring while on therapy.

• Teach patient to report all adverse reactions and how to identify and manage signs and symptoms of hypoglycemia (dizziness, weakness, shaking, fast heartbeat).

• Teach patient how to identify and manage signs and symptoms of hypotension (fatigue, dizziness, blurred vision, clammy skin). Encourage patient to maintain adequate fluid intake.

⚠ *Alert:* Instruct patient to seek medical attention immediately for signs and symptoms of ketoacidosis (difficulty breathing, hyperventilation, anorexia, nausea, vomiting, abdominal pain, confusion, unusual fatigue or sleepiness).

• Instruct patient to seek medical advice during periods of stress or illness because medication requirements may change.

⚠ *Alert:* Instruct patient to seek medical attention for signs and symptoms of UTI (difficulty urinating, frequency, urgency, pelvic pain, blood in urine, fever, back pain, nausea, vomiting).

• Inform patient that periodic monitoring of blood glucose and HbA$_{1c}$ levels and renal function will be needed.

• Advise patient that urine glucose tests will be falsely positive because drug increases glucose excretion, and recommend alternative methods to monitor glycemic control.

• Counsel patient to consult prescriber before starting new prescription or OTC medications or supplements.

• Advise patient to inform prescriber if she becomes pregnant, intends to become pregnant, or is breastfeeding.

E

emtricitabine
em-tra-SYE-tah-ben

Emtriva

Therapeutic class: Antiretrovirals
Pharmacologic class: NRTIs

AVAILABLE FORMS
Capsules: 200 mg
Oral solution: 10 mg/mL

INDICATIONS & DOSAGES
➤ **HIV-1 infection, with other antiretrovirals**
Adults: One 200-mg capsule or 240 mg (24 mL) oral solution PO once daily.
Children ages 3 months to 17 years: For children weighing more than 33 kg who can swallow intact capsules, give one 200-mg capsule PO once daily. Otherwise, give 6 mg/kg, up to a maximum dose of 240 mg (24 mL) oral solution PO once daily.
Children younger than age 3 months: 3 mg/kg oral solution PO once daily.
Adjust-a-dose: In adults with CrCl of 30 to 49 mL/minute, give one 200-mg capsule every 48 hours or 120 mg oral solution every 24 hours; if CrCl is 15 to 29 mL/minute, give one 200-mg capsule every 72 hours or 80 mg oral solution every 24 hours; if CrCl is less than 15 mL/minute or patient is receiving hemodialysis, give one 200-mg capsule every 96 hours or 60 mg oral solution every 24 hours. Give dose after hemodialysis session. In children with renal insufficiency, consider a dose reduction or increased dosing interval.

ADMINISTRATION
PO
• Give drug with or without food.
• Refrigerate oral solution; if stored at room temperature, use within 3 months.
• Dispense in original containers; keep containers tightly closed.

ACTION
Inhibits replication of HIV by blocking viral DNA synthesis and inhibits reverse transcriptase by acting as an alternative for the enzyme's substrate, deoxycytidine triphosphate.

Route	Onset	Peak	Duration
PO	Unknown	1–2 hr	Unknown

Half-life: About 10 hours.

ADVERSE REACTIONS
CNS: abnormal dreams, asthenia, dizziness, headache, insomnia, depression, fatigue, neuritis, paresthesia, peripheral neuropathy. **EENT:** rhinitis. **GI:** abdominal pain, diarrhea, nausea, dyspepsia, vomiting. **Hepatic:** *hepatotoxicity.* **Musculoskeletal:** arthralgia, myalgia. **Respiratory:** increased cough. **Skin:** allergic skin reaction, discoloration, maculopapular rash, pruritus, urticarial and purpuric lesions, vesiculobullous rash.

INTERACTIONS
Drug-drug. *Lamivudine:* May enhance adverse/toxic effect of emtricitabine. Avoid concurrent use.
Orlistat: May decrease serum concentration of antiretrovirals. Monitor concurrent use.

EFFECTS ON LAB TEST RESULTS
• May increase ALT, amylase, AST, bilirubin, CK, lipase, glucose, and triglyceride levels.
• May decrease neutrophil count.

CONTRAINDICATIONS & CAUTIONS
• Contraindicated in patients hypersensitive to drug or its ingredients.
• In elderly patients, use cautiously because of the potential for other diseases and drug therapies and for decreased hepatic, renal, or cardiac function.

• Use cautiously in patients with impaired renal function.
Black Box Warning Drug isn't approved for treatment of chronic HBV infection; safety and effectiveness haven't been established in patients infected with both HBV and HIV-1. Severe acute exacerbations of HBV infection have been reported in patients infected with both HBV and HIV-1 who have discontinued emtricitabine or tenofovir, which are components of this drug. Monitor hepatic function closely with both clinical and laboratory follow-up for at least several months in patients infected with both HIV-1 and HBV who discontinue this drug. If appropriate, initiation of anti–HBV therapy may be warranted. ∎
• Lactic acidosis and severe hepatomegaly with steatosis, including fatal cases, have been reported with use of nucleoside analogues, alone or in combination with other antiretrovirals.
• Don't give drug with other emtricitabine- or lamivudine-containing drugs.
Dialyzable drug: 30% over 3-hour hemodialysis period.

PREGNANCY-LACTATION-REPRODUCTION
• Use drug during pregnancy only if clearly needed.
• Register pregnant women in the Antiretroviral Pregnancy Registry at 1-800-258-4263.
• Patients should avoid breastfeeding because of potential for HIV-1 transmission and serious adverse reactions in breastfed infants.

NURSING CONSIDERATIONS
• Test all patients for HBV before starting drug.
• Suspend treatment in patients who develop signs and symptoms or laboratory findings suggestive of lactic acidosis or pronounced hepatotoxicity (including nausea, vomiting, unusual or unexpected stomach discomfort, and weakness).
Black Box Warning Monitor hepatic function closely with both clinical and laboratory follow-up for at least several months in patients infected with both HIV-1 and HBV who discontinue this drug. Severe acute exacerbations of hepatitis B have been reported. ∎

Reactions in bold italics are *life-threatening*. Interactions may have a *rapid onset* or a *delayed onset*.

• Don't use drug with combination drugs containing emtricitabine or lamivudine.
• Monitor patients for infection and development of immune reconstitution syndrome (inflammatory response to indolent or residual opportunistic infections, such as *Mycobacterium avium* infection, CMV, *Pneumocystis jiroveci* pneumonia, or TB), which may necessitate further evaluation and treatment.
• Hyperpigmentation occurs more frequently in children.

PATIENT TEACHING
• Remind patient that anti-HIV medicine must be taken for life.
• Inform patient that drug doesn't cure HIV infection, that opportunistic infections and other complications of HIV infection may continue to occur, and that transmission of HIV to others through sexual contact or blood contamination is still possible.
• Explain possible adverse reactions, including lactic acidosis and hepatotoxicity; advise patient to report all adverse reactions.
• Tell female patient to notify prescriber immediately if she is or could be pregnant.
• Warn female patient against breastfeeding.
• Inform patient that the drug may be taken with or without food.
• Tell patient to refrigerate oral solution and, if stored at room temperature, to use solution within 3 months.

emtricitabine–rilpivirine–tenofovir alafenamide fumarate
em-tra-SYE-ta-ben/ril-pi-VIR-een/ te-NOE-fo-veer

Odefsey

Therapeutic class: Antiretrovirals
Pharmacologic class: NRTIs–NNRTIs

AVAILABLE FORMS
Tablets: 200 mg emtricitabine, 25 mg rilpivirine, and 25 mg tenofovir alafenamide fumarate

INDICATIONS & DOSAGES
➤ **HIV-1 infection as initial therapy in patients with no antiretroviral treatment**
history and HIV-1 RNA 100,000 copies/mL or less; or to replace a stable antiretroviral regimen in patients who are virologically suppressed (HIV-1 RNA less than 50 copies/mL) for at least 6 months with no history of treatment failure and no known substitutions associated with resistance to the individual components
Adults and children weighing 35 kg or more with CrCl of 30 mL/minute or more: 1 tablet PO once daily with a meal.

ADMINISTRATION
PO
• Give drug once daily with a meal.
• Store below 86° F (30° C).
• Keep only in tightly closed, original container.

ACTION
Each drug interferes with HIV viral RNA-dependent DNA polymerase activities, resulting in inhibition of viral replication.

Route	Onset	Peak	Duration
PO (emtricitabine)	Unknown	3 hr	Unknown
PO (rilpivirine)	Unknown	4 hr	Unknown
PO (tenofovir)	Unknown	1 hr	Unknown

Half-life: Emtricitabine, 10 hours; rilpivirine, 50 hours; tenofovir, 0.51 hour.

ADVERSE REACTIONS
CNS: headache, insomnia, sleep disturbances, depression, somnolence, dizziness. **GI:** nausea, vomiting, abdominal pain. **GU:** *acute renal failure,* Fanconi syndrome, nephrotic syndrome. **Hepatic:** *lactic acidosis, severe hepatomegaly with steatosis.* **Metabolic:** weight gain, hypophosphatemia. **Skin:** rash. **Other:** hypersensitivity reaction, DRESS syndrome, autoimmune disorders, opportunistic infections.

INTERACTIONS
Drug-drug. *Acyclovir, aminoglycosides, cidofovir, ganciclovir, valacyclovir, valganciclovir:* May increase Odefsey (specifically tenofovir) concentration. Monitor patient for Odefsey-related increased adverse effects. Tenofovir products may increase ganciclovir or valganciclovir serum concentration. Monitor therapy.

Antacids (aluminum, magnesium hydroxide, calcium carbonate): May decrease Odefsey (specifically rilpivirine) serum concentration. Give antacids at least 2 hours before or at least 4 hours after Odefsey.

Anticonvulsants (carbamazepine, oxcarbazepine, phenobarbital, phenytoin): May decrease Odefsey (specifically tenofovir and rilpivirine) serum concentration, resulting in loss of virologic response and possible drug resistance. Use together is contraindicated.

Antimycobacterial drugs (rifabutin, rifampin, rifapentine): May decrease Odefsey (specifically tenofovir) serum concentration, resulting in loss of virologic response and possible drug resistance. Use together is contraindicated.

Azole antifungals (fluconazole, itraconazole, ketoconazole): May decrease azole level. Monitor patient for breakthrough fungal infections.

CYP3A inducers: May decrease Odefsey serum concentration, resulting in loss of virologic response and possible drug resistance. Use together is contraindicated.

CYP3A inhibitors: May increase Odefsey plasma concentration and possible Odefsey-related adverse events. Monitor therapy.

Dexamethasone (systemic): May decrease Odefsey (specifically rilpivirine) serum concentration, resulting in loss of virologic response and possible drug resistance. Use of more than a single dose of dexamethasone with Odefsey is contraindicated.

Didanosine: May decrease didanosine serum concentration. Give didanosine on an empty stomach at least 2 hours before or 4 hours after Odefsey due to the requirement that rilpivirine be administered with food.

H₂-receptor antagonists (cimetidine, famotidine, nizatidine, ranitidine): May decrease Odefsey (specifically rilpivirine) serum concentration. Administer H₂-receptor antagonist at least 12 hours before or 4 hours after Odefsey. Consider therapy modification.

Ketolide or macrolide antibiotics (clarithromycin, erythromycin, telithromycin): May increase Odefsey (specifically rilpivirine) serum concentration. Consider using an alternative antibiotic.

Methadone: May increase methadone metabolism. Adjust methadone dosage as clinically indicated.

NSAIDs: May increase risk of nephrotoxicity and adverse effects, especially at high doses. Use alternatives to these combinations if possible.

P-gp inducers: May decrease Odefsey absorption and plasma concentration, which may lead to loss of therapeutic effect and resistance. Monitor patient closely.

P-gp inhibitors: May increase Odefsey absorption and plasma concentration. Monitor patient for increased Odefsey-related adverse effects.

PPIs (dexlansoprazole, esomeprazole, lansoprazole, omeprazole, pantoprazole, rabeprazole): May decrease Odefsey serum concentration, resulting in loss of virologic response and possible drug resistance. Use together is contraindicated.

QTc interval–prolonging agents: May enhance QTc interval–prolonging effect. Consider alternative medications to Odefsey in patients with known risk of torsades de pointes.

Drug-herb. *St. John's wort:* May decrease Odefsey serum concentration, resulting in loss of virologic response and possible resistance to drug combination. Don't use together.

EFFECTS ON LAB TEST RESULTS
• May increase triglyceride and lipid levels.
• May increase serum lactate level.
• May decrease urine protein-to-creatinine ratio.

CONTRAINDICATIONS & CAUTIONS
• Drug may cause lactic acidosis and hepatomegaly with steatosis, including fatal cases. These effects may occur without elevated transaminase levels and in patients with no known risk factors. Risk factors include long-term antiretroviral use, obesity, and being female. Monitor all patients closely.
• Use very cautiously in patients with risk factors for liver disease. Hepatic adverse events have been reported.
Black Box Warning Odefsey isn't approved for treatment of chronic HBV infection, and safety and effectiveness haven't been established in patients coinfected with HIV-1 and HBV. Severe acute exacerbations of HBV infection have been reported in patients

---

Reactions in bold italics are *life-threatening*. Interactions may have a *rapid onset* or a *delayed onset*.

coinfected with HIV-1 and HBV after discontinuation of antiretroviral therapy. Monitor hepatic function during and for several months after discontinuation of treatment. If appropriate, initiate anti-HBV therapy. ■

• Contraindicated in patients hypersensitive to drug or its components.

• Consider alternative therapy in patients at high risk for torsades de pointes or when administered with medications known to increase risk of torsades de pointes. Supratherapeutic dosages of Odefsey have been shown to prolong QTc interval and may increase risk of ventricular arrhythmias.

• May increase risk of immune reconstitution syndrome, resulting in an inflammatory response to an indolent or opportunistic infection or activation of autoimmune disorders (*Mycobacterium avium* infection, CMV, *Pneumocystis jiroveci* pneumonia, TB, Graves disease, polymyositis, Guillain-Barré syndrome).

• Use isn't recommended in patients with CrCl of less than 30 mL/minute.

• Use cautiously in patients at risk for renal dysfunction. Hypophosphatemia has been reported secondary to proximal renal tubulopathy.

• Use in patients with severe hepatic impairment hasn't been studied.

Dialyzable drug: Emtricitabine, 30%; rilpivirine, unlikely; tenofovir, 54%.

PREGNANCY-LACTATION-REPRODUCTION

• There are no well-controlled studies in pregnant women. Use cautiously during pregnancy. Patients who become pregnant during therapy may continue drug.

• Some components of drug appear in human milk. It isn't known if Odefsey affects lactation or has effects on an infant. The CDC recommends that HIV-infected mothers not breastfeed, to avoid HIV transmission to the infant.

• To monitor pregnancy outcomes, health care providers are encouraged to register patients in the Antiretroviral Pregnancy Registry (1-800-258-4263).

NURSING CONSIDERATIONS

• Discontinue Odefsey if clinical or laboratory findings suggestive of lactic acidosis or hepatotoxicity develop.

• Test for HBV before initiation of antiretroviral therapy in all patients.

• Assess CD4 count, HIV-1 RNA plasma levels, LFT values, serum creatinine, urine glucose, and urine protein before initiation and during therapy.

• In virologically suppressed patients, additional monitoring of HIV-1 RNA and regimen tolerability is recommended after replacing therapy to assess for potential virologic failure or rebound.

• Monitor patient for hypersensitivity, rash, and severe skin reactions, including DRESS syndrome (severe rash or rash accompanied by fever, blisters, mucosal involvement, conjunctivitis, facial edema, angioedema, hepatitis, eosinophilia). Most rashes occur within first 4 to 6 weeks of therapy. Monitor laboratory parameters and clinical status. Stop drug immediately if hypersensitivity or rash develops.

• Monitor serum phosphorus level in patients with chronic kidney disease. Odefsey may increase risk of Fanconi syndrome. Discontinue drug for significantly decreased renal function or evidence of Fanconi syndrome.

• Calcium and vitamin D supplementation may be beneficial for all patients.

• Monitor patient for depression, dysphoria, mood changes, negative thoughts, suicide attempts, or suicidal ideation. Patients who develop these symptoms should be promptly evaluated; consider risks versus benefits of continued treatment.

PATIENT TEACHING

🛈 *Alert:* Counsel patient, family members, or caregivers to watch for signs and symptoms of depression and to immediately report depression, negative thoughts, dysphoria, or suicidal thoughts or behaviors to prescriber.

• Advise patient that Odefsey can cause buildup of lactic acid in the blood. Instruct patient to seek immediate medical attention for weakness, fatigue, muscle pain, trouble breathing, stomachache with nausea and vomiting, dizziness, chills, or fast or irregular heartbeat.

• Caution patient that Odefsey may cause liver problems. Instruct patient to seek immediate medical attention for yellowing of the skin or eyes, dark-colored urine, loss of appetite, light-colored stool, nausea, or pain or tenderness on right side of the stomach.

❸ **Alert:** Warn patient to stop taking drug and immediately seek medical attention for allergic reactions (rash, fever, blisters, mucosal involvement, eye inflammation; swelling of the face eyes, lips, mouth, tongue, or throat, which may lead to difficulty swallowing or breathing).

• Caution patient not to discontinue drug combination without first discussing with prescriber. Advise patient of the importance of not running out of the medications and of not missing doses. Severe acute exacerbations of hepatitis B have been reported in coinfected patients.

• Remind patient to notify prescriber about other prescription or OTC drugs, including herbal and vitamin supplements, patient is taking or plans to take.

• Inform patient that blood tests will be needed to check for effectiveness and adverse effects of therapy.

• Advise patient to immediately report signs and symptoms of infection.

• Tell female patient of childbearing potential to notify prescriber about planned, suspected, or known pregnancy and that there is a pregnancy registry for women who take antivirals during pregnancy.

• Advise female patient not to breastfeed during therapy.

emtricitabine–tenofovir alafenamide fumarate
em-tra-SYE-tah-ben/te-NOE-fo-veer

Descovy

Therapeutic class: Antiretrovirals
Pharmacologic class: NNRTIs

AVAILABLE FORMS
Tablets: 200 mg emtricitabine and 25 mg tenofovir alafenamide fumarate

INDICATIONS & DOSAGES
➤ **Treatment of HIV-1 infection in combination with other antiretrovirals**
Adults and children weighing 35 kg or more, with CrCl of 30 mL/minute or more: 1 tablet PO once daily.

➤ **Treatment of HIV-1 infection in combination with other antiretrovirals other than protease inhibitors that require a CYP3A inhibitor**
Children weighing at least 25 to less than 35 kg with CrCl of 30 mL/minute or more: 1 tablet PO once daily.

ADMINISTRATION
PO
• May give with or without food.
• Store below 86° F (30° C). Keep container tightly closed.
• Give a missed dose as soon possible. If it's close to the time for the next dose, skip missed dose. Don't give two doses at the same time or extra doses.

ACTION
Interferes with HIV viral RNA-dependent DNA polymerase activities, resulting in inhibition of viral replication.

Route	Onset	Peak	Duration
PO (emtricitabine)	Unknown	3 hr	Unknown
PO (tenofovir)	Unknown	1 hr	Unknown

Half-life: Emtricitabine, 10 hours; tenofovir, ½ hour.

ADVERSE REACTIONS
CNS: dizziness, asthenia, headache, pain, fever, peripheral neuropathy, neuritis, paresthesia, insomnia, abnormal dreams, depression, anxiety, fatigue. **CV:** chest pain. **EENT:** otitis media, rhinitis, sinusitis, pharyngitis. **GI:** nausea, diarrhea, vomiting, abdominal pain, dyspepsia, flatulence, gastroenteritis. **GU:** *acute renal failure, Fanconi syndrome, nephrotic syndrome,* hematuria. **Hematologic:** *neutropenia,* anemia. **Hepatic:** *lactic acidosis, severe hepatomegaly with steatosis.* **Metabolic:** hyperglycemia, hypercholesterolemia, hypertriglyceridemia. **Musculoskeletal:** arthralgia, myalgia, increased CK level, back pain, decreased bone mineral density. **Respiratory:** cough, pneumonia, URI. **Skin:** hyperpigmentation, rash, allergic skin reaction, pruritus.

INTERACTIONS
Drug-drug. *Acyclovir, valacyclovir:* May increase serum concentration of tenofovir products. Tenofovir products may increase

---

serum concentration of acyclovir or valacy-clovir. Monitor therapy.

Adefovir: May diminish therapeutic effect of tenofovir products. Adefovir may increase serum concentration of tenofovir products. Tenofovir products may increase adefovir serum concentration. Avoid use together.

Aminoglycosides: May increase serum concentration of tenofovir products. Tenofovir products may increase serum concentration of aminoglycosides. Monitor therapy.

Anticonvulsants (carbamazepine, oxcarbazepine, phenobarbital, phenytoin): May decrease tenofovir serum concentration. Consider alternative anticonvulsant.

Antimycobacterial drugs (rifabutin, rifampin, rifapentine): May decrease tenofovir level. Use together isn't recommended.

Cidofovir: May increase serum concentration of tenofovir products. Tenofovir products may increase cidofovir serum concentration. Monitor therapy.

Cobicistat: May increase risk of adverse effects of tenofovir. Monitor therapy.

Ganciclovir, valganciclovir: May increase tenofovir serum concentration and risk of adverse effects. Tenofovir may also increase ganciclovir or valganciclovir concentration. Monitor patient closely for increased adverse effects.

Lamivudine: May increase risk of adverse effects of emtricitabine. Avoid use together.

NSAIDs: May enhance nephrotoxic effect of tenofovir. Seek alternatives to this combination whenever possible. Avoid use of tenofovir with multiple NSAIDs or with any NSAID given at a high dose.

P-gp inducers: May decrease tenofovir absorption, causing loss of therapeutic effect and development of resistance.

P-gp inhibitors: May increase tenofovir level. Use cautiously together.

Primidone: May decrease tenofovir serum concentration. Avoid combination.

Protease inhibitors (ritonavir, tipranavir): May decrease tenofovir serum concentration. Use together isn't recommended.

Ribavirin (oral inhalation, systemic): May increase risk of hepatotoxicity. Use together cautiously.

Drug-herb. *St. John's wort:* May decrease tenofovir serum concentration. Use together isn't recommended.

EFFECTS ON LAB TEST RESULTS

• May increase total cholesterol, LDL, HDL, triglyceride, ALT, amylase, AST, bilirubin, CK, lipase, serum creatinine, and glucose levels. May decrease phosphate level.

• May decrease neutrophil count.

CONTRAINDICATIONS & CAUTIONS

ⓘ Alert: Lactic acidosis and severe hepatomegaly with steatosis, including fatal cases, have been reported with nucleoside analogues (tenofovir) in combination with other antiretrovirals. Interrupt treatment in patients who develop clinical or laboratory findings suggestive of lactic acidosis or hepatotoxicity (hepatomegaly and steatosis with or without transaminase elevations). Some cases of hepatotoxicity have occurred in patients with no hepatic disease before treatment.

• Use cautiously in women, obese patients, patients with risk factors for liver disease, and those with prolonged nucleoside exposure.

Black Box Warning Drug isn't approved for treatment of chronic HBV infection. Safety and effectiveness haven't been established for patients coinfected with HIV and HBV; acute, severe exacerbations of HBV infection (liver decompensation and liver failure) have been reported after discontinuation of antiretroviral therapy. ▮

• Descovy isn't indicated for preexposure prophylaxis to reduce risk of sexually acquired HIV-1 in high-risk adults.

• Descovy isn't recommended for patients with CrCl of less than 30 mL/minute.

• Immune reconstitution syndrome may occur, resulting in an inflammatory response to an indolent or residual opportunistic infection (*Mycobacterium avium* infection, CMV, *Pneumocystis jiroveci* pneumonia, TB) or an autoimmune disorder (Graves disease, polymyositis, Guillain-Barré syndrome); evaluate and treat appropriately.

• Use cautiously in patients at risk for renal dysfunction. Evaluate patients with persistent or worsening bone or muscle symptoms for renal dysfunction (including Fanconi syndrome), hypophosphatemia, and osteomalacia.

- Drug may increase risk of acute renal failure and Fanconi syndrome. Patients with preexisting renal impairment and those taking nephrotoxic agents (including NSAIDs) are at increased risk.
- Use in patients with severe hepatic impairment (Child-Pugh class C) hasn't been studied.
- Calcium and vitamin D supplements may be beneficial for all patients.
- Safety and effectiveness when administered with an HIV-1 protease inhibitor that's given with either ritonavir or cobicistat haven't been established in children weighing less than 35 kg.
- Safety and effectiveness in children weighing less than 25 kg haven't been established.
- Drug may cause immune reconstitution syndrome.

Dialyzable drug: Emtricitabine, 30%; tenofovir alafenamide, 54%.

PREGNANCY-LACTATION-REPRODUCTION

- If indicated, drug shouldn't be withheld because of pregnancy.
- Emtricitabine and tenofovir appear in human milk. Both drugs are contraindicated in breastfeeding women.
- The CDC recommends that HIV-infected mothers shouldn't breastfeed, to avoid risking postnatal transmission of HIV.
- To monitor pregnancy outcomes, health care providers are encouraged to register patients in the Antiretroviral Pregnancy Registry (1-800-258-4263).

NURSING CONSIDERATIONS

- Test for HBV before initiation of antiretroviral therapy. Drug isn't approved for the treatment of chronic HBV infection.
- Descovy must be given as part of a regimen with other antiretrovirals.
- Monitor CD4 counts and HIV RNA plasma levels to evaluate effectiveness of treatment.
- Assess estimated CrCl, urine protein, and urine glucose before initiation and during therapy. Monitor serum phosphorus level in patients with chronic kidney disease due to increased risk of developing Fanconi syndrome. Discontinue drug in patients who develop clinically significant decreases in renal function or evidence of Fanconi syndrome.

- Monitor lipid levels periodically.
- **Black Box Warning** Monitor patients with HIV and HBV coinfection for several months after therapy discontinuation for acute exacerbations of HBV infection. Monitor hepatic function by clinical assessment and laboratory testing. Start anti–hepatitis B therapy as clinically indicated, especially in patients with advanced liver disease or cirrhosis. ■

PATIENT TEACHING

- Caution patient that drug may cause liver enlargement and increased acid in the blood; risk may be higher in women, overweight people, and in people who have taken similar drugs for a long time.
- Advise patient that hepatitis B sometimes worsened when drug was stopped in patients with hepatitis B and that close follow-up for a few months is needed when therapy is stopped.
- Caution patient not to stop drug without first discussing with prescriber.
- Advise patient of importance of taking drug without missing doses, to avoid loss of treatment effectiveness.
- Warn patient to report signs and symptoms of kidney problems (inability to pass urine, change in how much urine is passed, blood in the urine, weight gain).
- **Black Box Warning** Instruct patient to report signs and symptoms of liver problems (dark urine, loss of appetite, nausea, right upper quadrant abdominal pain, achiness or tenderness, light-colored stools, vomiting, yellowing of skin or eyes). ■
- Advise patient to report signs and symptoms of lactic acidosis (trouble breathing, fast or irregular heartbeat, stomach pain with nausea or vomiting, fatigue, shortness of breath, weakness, dizziness or lightheadedness, feeling cold, muscle pain or cramps).
- Instruct patient to report signs and symptoms of infection (fever, sore throat, weakness, cough, shortness of breath).
- Teach patient to avoid behaviors that can spread HIV-1 infection to others, including sharing or reusing needles, sharing razors or toothbrushes, or having sex without using a latex or polyurethane condom.

Reactions in bold italics are *life-threatening*. Interactions may have a *rapid onset* or a *delayed onset*.

- Caution female patient not to breastfeed, to avoid transmitting HIV-1 to infant.
- Inform patient that there is an antiretroviral pregnancy registry to monitor fetal outcomes of pregnant women exposed to Descovy.

enalaprilat ☒
eh-NAH-leh-prel-at

enalapril maleate ☒
Epaned, Epaned Kit, Vasotec✿

Therapeutic class: Antihypertensives
Pharmacologic class: ACE inhibitors

AVAILABLE FORMS
enalaprilat
Injection: 1.25 mg/mL
enalapril maleate
Oral solution: 1 mg/mL
Powder for oral solution: 150 mg/150 mL bottle
Tablets: 2.5 mg, 5 mg, 10 mg, 20 mg

INDICATIONS & DOSAGES
➤ **HTN**
Adults: In patients not taking diuretics, initially, 5 mg PO once daily; then adjusted based on response. Usual dosage range is 10 to 40 mg daily as a single dose or two divided doses. Or, 1.25 mg IV infusion over 5 minutes every 6 hours.
Children ages 1 month to 16 years: 0.08 mg/kg (up to 5 mg) PO once daily; dosage should be adjusted as needed up to 0.58 mg/kg (maximum 40 mg). Don't use if CrCl is less than 30 mL/minute/1.73 m².
Adjust-a-dose: If patient is taking diuretics or CrCl is 30 mL/minute or less, initially, 2.5 mg PO once daily and titrate to a maximum dose of 40 mg daily. Or, 0.625 mg IV over 5 minutes, and repeat in 1 hour, if needed; then 1.25 mg IV every 6 hours. For dialysis patients, give 2.5 mg PO on dialysis days; adjust dosage on dialysis days based on BP response.
➤ **To convert from IV therapy to oral therapy in patients receiving diuretics**
Adults: Initially, 2.5 mg PO once daily; if patient was receiving 0.625 mg IV every

6 hours, then 2.5 mg PO once daily. Adjust dosage based on response.
➤ **To convert from oral therapy to IV therapy**
Adults: 1.25 mg IV over 5 minutes every 6 hours.
➤ **To convert from IV therapy to oral therapy**
Adults: 5 mg PO once daily.
Adjust-a-dose: For patients with CrCl of 30 mL/minute or less, give 2.5 mg PO once daily.
➤ **To manage symptomatic HF**
Adults: Initially, 2.5 mg PO b.i.d., increased gradually over several weeks. Maintenance is 5 to 40 mg daily in two divided doses. Maximum daily dose is 40 mg in two divided doses.
Adjust-a-dose: For patients with hyponatremia (serum sodium level of less than 130 mEq/L) or serum creatinine level greater than 1.6 mg/dL, recommended initial dose is 2.5 mg once daily.
➤ **Asymptomatic left ventricular dysfunction**
Adults: Initially, 2.5 mg PO b.i.d. Increase as tolerated to target daily dose of 20 mg PO in divided doses.

ADMINISTRATION
PO
- Give drug without regard for food.
- Request oral suspension for patient who has difficulty swallowing.
IV
▼ Inspect solution for particulate matter and discoloration before administration.
▼ Compatible solutions include D₅W, NSS for injection, dextrose 5% in lactated Ringer injection, dextrose 5% in NSS for injection, and Isolyte E.
▼ Inject drug slowly over at least 5 minutes, or dilute in 50 mL of a compatible solution and infuse over 15 minutes.
▼ **Incompatibilities:** Amphotericin B, cefepime, phenytoin.

ACTION
Inhibits ACE, preventing conversion of angiotensin I to angiotensin II, a potent vasoconstrictor. Less angiotensin II decreases peripheral arterial resistance, decreasing

aldosterone secretion, reducing sodium and water retention, and lowering BP.

Route	Onset	Peak	Duration
PO	1 hr	3–4 hr	24 hr
IV	15 min	1–4 hr	6 hr

Half-life: 11 hours.

ADVERSE REACTIONS
CNS: asthenia, headache, dizziness, fatigue, vertigo, syncope, weakness. **CV:** hypotension, chest pain, angina. **GI:** anorexia, diarrhea, nausea, abdominal pain, vomiting. **GU:** decreased renal function (especially in patients with bilateral renal artery stenosis or HF). **Hematologic:** bone marrow depression. **Respiratory:** bronchitis; dry, persistent, tickling, nonproductive cough; dyspnea. **Skin:** rash. **Other:** *angioedema, anaphylaxis.*

INTERACTIONS
Drug-drug. *Aldosterone blockers (eplerenone), aliskiren, ARBs (candesartan, telmisartan), trimethoprim:* May increase risk of hyperkalemia. Monitor potassium level and clinical response. Drug is contraindicated for use with aliskiren in patients with diabetes.
Azathioprine: May increase risk of anemia or leukopenia. Monitor hematologic study results if used together.
Diuretics: May excessively reduce BP. Use together cautiously.
Insulin, oral antidiabetics: May cause hypoglycemia, especially at start of enalapril therapy. Monitor patient closely.
Lithium: May cause lithium toxicity. Monitor lithium level.
mTOR inhibitors (sirolimus, temsirolimus): May increase risk of angioedema. Monitor patient closely.
Neprilysin inhibitors (sacubitril): May increase risk of angioedema. Use together is contraindicated. Don't give within 36 hours of switching to or from sacubitril–valsartan, a neprilysin inhibitor.
NSAIDs: May reduce antihypertensive effect. Monitor BP.
Potassium-sparing diuretics, potassium supplements: May cause hyperkalemia. Avoid using together unless hypokalemia is confirmed.

Drug-herb. *Capsaicin:* May cause cough. Discourage use together.
Ma huang: May decrease antihypertensive effects. Discourage use together.
Drug-food. *Salt substitutes containing potassium:* May cause hyperkalemia. Monitor patient closely.

EFFECTS ON LAB TEST RESULTS
• May increase bilirubin, BUN, creatinine, and potassium levels. May decrease sodium and Hb levels and hematocrit.
• May increase LFT values.

CONTRAINDICATIONS & CAUTIONS
⚕ Contraindicated in patients hypersensitive to drug, in those with a history of angioedema related to previous treatment with an ACE inhibitor, and in patients with hereditary or idiopathic angioedema.
• Contraindicated in combination with aliskiren in patients with diabetes and with neprilysin inhibitors (e.g., sacubitril). Don't give within 36 hours of switching to or from sacubitril–valsartan, a neprilysin inhibitor, due to increased risk of angioedema.
• Safety and effectiveness of IV use in children haven't been established.
• Oral drug isn't recommended in neonates (younger than age 1 month), preterm infants who haven't reached a corrected postconceptual age of 44 weeks, and in children with GFR of less than 30 mL/minute/1.73 m^2.
• Use cautiously in renally impaired patients or those with aortic stenosis or hypertrophic cardiomyopathy.
Dialyzable drug: Yes.
⚠ *Overdose S&S:* Hypotension.

PREGNANCY-LACTATION-REPRODUCTION
Black Box Warning Use during pregnancy can cause injury and death to the developing fetus. If pregnancy is detected, stop drug as soon as possible. ∎
• Drug appears in human milk. Breastfeeding isn't recommended.

NURSING CONSIDERATIONS
• Closely monitor BP response to drug.
• Monitor CBC with differential counts before and during therapy.
• Diabetic patients, those with impaired renal function or HF, and those receiving drugs

that can increase potassium level may develop hyperkalemia. Monitor potassium intake and potassium level.

⬚ Black patients who take ACE inhibitors as monotherapy for HTN have a smaller reduction in BP than non-Black patients. Black patients taking ACE inhibitors have a higher incidence of angioedema than non-Blacks.

• **Look alike–sound alike:** Don't confuse enalapril with Anafranil or Eldepryl.

PATIENT TEACHING

• Instruct patient to report breathing difficulty or swelling of face, eyes, lips, or tongue. Swelling of the face and throat (including swelling of the larynx) may occur, especially after first dose.

• Advise patient to report signs of infection, such as fever and sore throat.

• Inform patient that light-headedness can occur, especially during first few days of therapy. Tell patient to rise slowly to minimize this effect and to notify prescriber if symptoms develop. If fainting occurs, advise patient to stop drug and call prescriber immediately.

• Tell patient to use caution in hot weather and during exercise. Inadequate fluid intake, vomiting, diarrhea, and excessive perspiration can lead to light-headedness and fainting.

• Advise patient to avoid salt substitutes; these products may contain potassium, which can cause high potassium levels in patients taking this drug.

Black Box Warning Tell female patient of childbearing potential to notify prescriber if pregnancy occurs. Drug will need to be stopped. ■

SAFETY ALERT!

enfuvirtide
en-foo-VEER-tide

Fuzeon

Therapeutic class: Antiretrovirals
Pharmacologic class: Fusion inhibitors

AVAILABLE FORMS
Powder for injection: 108-mg single-use vials (90 mg/mL after reconstitution)

INDICATIONS & DOSAGES
➤ **To help control HIV-1 infection, with other antiretrovirals, in patients who have continued HIV-1 replication despite antiretroviral therapy**
Adults: 90 mg subcut b.i.d.
Children weighing at least 11 kg: 2 mg/kg subcut b.i.d. Maximum, 90 mg/dose.

ADMINISTRATION
Subcutaneous
• Reconstitute vial with 1 mL sterile water for injection. Tap vial for 10 seconds and then gently roll to prevent foaming. Let drug stand for up to 45 minutes to ensure reconstitution but allow more time if solution is foamy or jelled. Or, gently roll vial between hands until product is completely dissolved. When completely mixed the solution should be clear, colorless and without bubbles or particulate matter. If the solution is foamy or jelled, allow more time for it to dissolve. Then draw up correct dose and inject drug.
• If drug isn't used immediately after reconstitution, refrigerate in original vial and use within 24 hours. Don't inject drug until it's at room temperature.
• Vial is for single use; discard unused portion.
• Inject into upper arm, anterior thigh, or abdomen. Rotate injection sites. Don't inject into same site for two consecutive doses, and don't inject into moles, scar tissue, bruises, tattoos, or the navel, where large nerves course close to the skin.
• Store unreconstituted vials at room temperature.

ACTION
Interferes with entry of HIV-1 into cells by inhibiting fusion of HIV-1 to CD4 cell membranes.

Route	Onset	Peak	Duration
Subcut	Unknown	4–8 hr	Unknown

Half-life: 3.8 hours.

ADVERSE REACTIONS
CNS: fatigue, insomnia, anxiety, asthenia, depression, peripheral neuropathy.
EENT: conjunctivitis, sinusitis, taste disturbance. **GI:** diarrhea, nausea, *pancreatitis,* abdominal pain, constipation, dry

mouth. **Metabolic:** anorexia, weight decrease. **Musculoskeletal:** myalgia. **Respiratory:** *bacterial pneumonia*, cough. **Skin:** injection-site reactions, pruritus, skin papilloma. **Other:** herpes simplex, influenza, influenza-like illness, lymphadenopathy.

INTERACTIONS
Drug-drug. *Orlistat:* May decrease enfuvirtide serum concentration. Monitor therapeutic response.
Protease inhibitors: May increase concentrations of either drug. Monitor therapy.

EFFECTS ON LAB TEST RESULTS
• May increase ALT, amylase, AST, CK, GGT, lipase, and triglyceride levels.
• May increase eosinophil count. May decrease Hb level.

CONTRAINDICATIONS & CAUTIONS
• Contraindicated in patients hypersensitive to drug and in those not infected with HIV.
Dialyzable drug: Unlikely.

PREGNANCY-LACTATION-REPRODUCTION
• There are no well-controlled studies in pregnant women. Use during pregnancy only if clearly needed.
• Register pregnant women in the Antiretroviral Pregnancy Registry at 1-800-258-4263.
• Because of the potential for HIV transmission, women shouldn't breastfeed.

NURSING CONSIDERATIONS
• Injection-site reactions (pain, discomfort, induration, erythema, pruritus, nodules, cysts, ecchymosis) are common and may require analgesics or rest.
• Monitor patients for infection and development of immune reconstitution syndrome (inflammatory response to indolent or residual opportunistic infections, such as *Mycobacterium avium* infection, CMV, *Pneumocystis jiroveci* pneumonia, or TB), which may necessitate further evaluation and treatment. Autoimmune disorders (such as Graves disease, polymyositis, and Guillain-Barré syndrome) have also been reported in the setting of immune reconstitution; however, the time to onset is more variable, and can occur many months after initiation of treatment.

• Nerve pain (neuralgia or paresthesia) lasting up to 6 months and associated with administration at sites where large nerves course close to the skin, bruising, and hematomas have occurred. Patients receiving anticoagulants and those with hemophilia or other coagulation disorders may have a higher risk of postinjection bleeding.
❸ *Alert:* Monitor patient closely for evidence of bacterial pneumonia. Patients at high risk include those with a low initial CD4 count or high initial viral load, those who use IV drugs or smoke, and those with history of lung disease.
• Hypersensitivity may occur with first dose or later doses. If systemic symptoms occur, stop drug and don't rechallenge.

PATIENT TEACHING
• Teach patient how to prepare and give drug and how to safely dispose of used needles and syringes.
• Tell patient to rotate injection sites and to watch for cellulitis or local infection.
• Urge patient to immediately report evidence of pneumonia, such as cough with fever, rapid breathing, or shortness of breath.
• Tell patient to stop taking drug and seek medical attention if evidence of hypersensitivity develops, such as rash, fever, nausea, vomiting, chills, rigors, and hypotension.
• Teach patient that drug doesn't cure HIV infection and that it must be taken with other antiretrovirals.
• Tell patient to inform prescriber if she's pregnant, plans to become pregnant, or is breastfeeding while taking drug. Because HIV could be transmitted to the infant, HIV-infected mothers shouldn't breastfeed.
• Tell patient that drug may affect the ability to drive or operate machinery.
• Tell patient that information on self-administration is available (1-877-4FUZEON [1-877-438-9366]).

Reactions in bold italics are *life-threatening*. Interactions may have a *rapid onset* or a *delayed onset*.

enoxaparin sodium
en-OCKS-a-par-in

Lovenox

Therapeutic class: Anticoagulants
Pharmacologic class: Low–molecular-
weight heparins

E

AVAILABLE FORMS
Syringes (graduated prefilled): 60 mg/
0.6 mL, 80 mg/0.8 mL, 100 mg/mL,
120 mg/0.8 mL, 150 mg/mL
Syringes (prefilled): 30 mg/0.3 mL, 40 mg/
0.4 mL

INDICATIONS & DOSAGES
➤ **To prevent PE and DVT after hip or
knee replacement surgery**
Adults: 30 mg subcut every 12 hours for 7
to 10 days. Treatment for up to 14 days has
been well tolerated. Give initial dose between 12 and 24 hours postoperatively, as
long as hemostasis has been established.
Continue treatment during postoperative
period until risk of DVT has diminished.
Hip replacement patients may receive 40 mg
subcut given 12 hours (range, 9 to 15 hours)
preoperatively. After initial phase of therapy,
hip replacement patients should continue
with 40 mg subcut daily for 3 weeks.
Adjust-a-dose: In patients with CrCl of less
than 30 mL/minute, give 30 mg subcut once
daily.
➤ **To prevent PE and DVT after abdominal surgery**
Adults: 40 mg subcut daily with initial dose
2 hours before surgery. Give subsequent
dose, as long as hemostasis has been established, 24 hours after initial preoperative dose, and continue once daily for 7 to
10 days. Treatment for up to 12 days has
been well tolerated. Continue treatment during postoperative period until risk of DVT
has diminished.
Adjust-a-dose: In patients with CrCl of less
than 30 mL/minute, give 30 mg subcut once
daily.
➤ **To prevent PE and DVT in patients
with acute illness who are at increased
risk because of decreased mobility**

Adults: 40 mg subcut once daily for 6 to
11 days. Treatment for up to 14 days has
been well tolerated.
Adjust-a-dose: In patients with CrCl of less
than 30 mL/minute, give 30 mg subcut once
daily.
➤ **To prevent ischemic complications of
unstable angina and non–Q-wave MI with
oral aspirin therapy**
Adults: 1 mg/kg subcut every 12 hours until
clinical stabilization (minimum 2 days) with
aspirin 100 to 325 mg PO once daily. Usual
duration of treatment is 2 to 8 days.
Adjust-a-dose: In patients with CrCl of less
than 30 mL/minute, give 1 mg/kg subcut
once daily.
➤ **Acute ST-segment elevation MI**
Adults younger than age 75: 30 mg single
IV bolus plus 1 mg/kg subcut followed by
1 mg/kg subcut every 12 hours (maximum
of 100 mg for the first two doses only) with
aspirin 75 to 325 mg PO once daily. When
given with a thrombolytic, give enoxaparin
from 15 minutes before to 30 minutes after
the start of fibrinolytic therapy. For patients
undergoing PCI, if the last subcut dose was
given less than 8 hours before balloon inflation, no additional dose is needed. If the
last dose was given more than 8 hours before
balloon inflation, give 0.3 mg/kg IV bolus.
Adults age 75 and older: Don't use an initial IV bolus. Give 0.75 mg/kg subcut every
12 hours (maximum 75 mg for the first two
doses only).
Adjust-a-dose: In adults younger than age 75
with severe renal impairment (CrCl of less
than 30 mL/minute), 30 mg single IV bolus
plus 1 mg/kg subcut followed by 1 mg/kg
subcut once daily. In adults age 75 and older
with severe renal impairment, 1 mg/kg subcut once daily with no initial bolus. Give
with aspirin.
➤ **Inpatient treatment of acute DVT with
and without PE when given with warfarin
sodium**
Adults: 1 mg/kg subcut every 12 hours.
Or, 1.5 mg/kg subcut once daily (at same
time daily) for 5 to 7 days until therapeutic
oral anticoagulant effect (INR 2.0 to 3.0) is
achieved. Warfarin sodium therapy is usually started within 72 hours of enoxaparin
injection.

Adjust-a-dose: In patients with CrCl of less than 30 mL/minute, give 1 mg/kg subcut once daily.

➤ **Outpatient treatment of acute DVT without PE when given with warfarin sodium**

Adults: 1 mg/kg subcut every 12 hours for 5 to 7 days until therapeutic oral anticoagulant effect (INR 2.0 to 3.0) is achieved. Warfarin sodium therapy usually is started within 72 hours of enoxaparin injection.

Adjust-a-dose: In patients with CrCl of less than 30 mL/minute, give 1 mg/kg subcut once daily.

➤ **To prevent PE and DVT in general surgery patients**

Adults: 40 mg subcut once daily, with initial dose given 2 hours before surgery. Usual duration of administration is until hospital discharge or up to 7 to 10 days; for selected high-risk general surgery patients, including those who have undergone major cancer surgery or have previously experienced a venous thrombotic event, consider continuation for up to 28 days after hospital discharge.

Adjust-a-dose: In patients with CrCl of less than 30 mL/minute, give 30 mg subcut once daily.

ADMINISTRATION

IV

▼ Flush IV access with sufficient amount of saline or dextrose solution before and after IV bolus administration.

▼ **Incompatibilities:** Don't mix or administer with other IV drugs.

Subcutaneous

• With patient lying down, give by deep subcut injection, alternating doses between left and right anterolateral and posterolateral abdominal walls. Hold skin fold between thumb and forefinger and insert entire length of needle. Push plunger to bottom of syringe. Don't expel air bubble from prefilled syringes before injection.

• Don't massage after subcut injection. Watch for signs of bleeding at site. Rotate sites and keep record.

ACTION

Accelerates formation of antithrombin III–thrombin complex and deactivates thrombin,

preventing conversion of fibrinogen to fibrin. Drug has a higher antifactor-Xa-to-antifactor-IIa activity ratio than heparin.

Route	Onset	Peak	Duration
IV	Unknown	Unknown	Unknown
Subcut	Unknown	4 hr	Unknown

Half-life: 4½ hours after a single dose; 7 hours after repeated dosing.

ADVERSE REACTIONS

CNS: confusion, fever, pain. **CV:** edema, peripheral edema. **GI:** nausea, diarrhea. **Hematologic:** *thrombocytopenia, hemorrhage,* ecchymoses, bleeding complications, hypochromic anemia. **Respiratory:** dyspnea. **Skin:** irritation, pain, hematoma, and erythema at injection site; rash; urticaria. **Other:** *angioedema, anaphylaxis.*

INTERACTIONS

Drug-drug. *Anticoagulants, antiplatelet drugs, NSAIDs:* May increase risk of bleeding. Use together cautiously and monitor patient for bleeding.
SSRIs: May increase risk of severe bleeding. Monitor patient for bleeding. Adjust therapy as needed.
Drug-herb. *Alfalfa, anise, bilberry:* May increase risk of bleeding. Discourage use together.

EFFECTS ON LAB TEST RESULTS

• May increase potassium, ALT, and AST levels.
• May decrease Hb level and platelet count.

CONTRAINDICATIONS & CAUTIONS

• Contraindicated in patients hypersensitive to drug, heparin, pork products, or benzyl alcohol; in those with active major bleeding; and in those with history of immune-mediated heparin-induced thrombocytopenia (HIT) within the past 100 days or in the presence of circulating antibodies.

Black Box Warning Monitor patients frequently for signs and symptoms of neurologic impairment. If neurologic compromise is noted, urgent treatment is necessary. ∎

• Use drug in patients with a history of HIT only if more than 100 days have elapsed since the prior HIT episode and no circulating antibodies are present. Because HIT may still occur in these circumstances, the decision to use enoxaparin in such a case must be made only after a careful benefit-risk assessment and after nonheparin alternative treatments have been considered.

• Use cautiously in patients with history of aneurysms, cerebrovascular hemorrhage, spinal or epidural punctures (as with anesthesia), uncontrolled HTN, or threatened abortion.

• Use cautiously in elderly patients and in those with conditions that place them at increased risk for hemorrhage, such as bacterial endocarditis, congenital or acquired bleeding disorders, ulcer disease, angiodysplastic GI disease, hemorrhagic stroke, or recent spinal, eye, or brain surgery.

• Use cautiously in patients with prosthetic heart valves, with regional or lumbar block anesthesia, blood dyscrasias, recent childbirth, pericarditis or pericardial effusion, renal insufficiency, or severe CNS trauma.

• Multidose vials aren't approved for use in neonates or infants due to the risk of "gasping syndrome" caused by the benzyl alcohol preservative.

Dialyzable drug: No.

⚠ Overdose S&S: Hemorrhagic complications.

PREGNANCY-LACTATION-REPRODUCTION

• There are no well-controlled studies in pregnant women. Monitor pregnant women closely for evidence of bleeding or excessive coagulation. Warn pregnant women and women of childbearing potential about potential risk of therapy.

• Consider using a shorter-acting anticoagulant as delivery approaches.

• Multidose vial shouldn't be used in pregnant women because of benzyl alcohol content.

• It isn't known if drug appears in human milk. Patient should discontinue breastfeeding or discontinue drug.

NURSING CONSIDERATIONS

• It's important to achieve hemostasis at the puncture site after PCI. The vascular access sheath for instrumentation should remain in place for 6 hours after enoxaparin dose if manual compression method is used; give next dose no sooner than 6 to 8 hours after

sheath removal. Monitor vital signs and site for hematoma and bleeding.

• Monitor anti-Xa levels in pregnant women with mechanical heart valves and in patients with significant renal impairment.

Black Box Warning Patients who receive epidural or spinal anesthesia or spinal puncture during therapy are at increased risk for developing an epidural or spinal hematoma, which may result in long-term or permanent paralysis. Factors that can increase these risks include use of indwelling epidural catheters, concurrent use of other drugs that affect hemostasis, history of traumatic or repeated epidural or spinal puncture, and history of spinal deformity or spinal surgery. Monitor these patients closely for neurologic impairment, as urgent treatment is necessary. ∎

Black Box Warning Optimal timing between administration of enoxaparin and spinal procedures isn't known. ∎

ⓘ Alert: For spinal procedures, consider both dose and elimination half-life of drug. Delay placement or removal of a spinal catheter for at least 12 hours after prophylactic doses or for 24 hours for higher therapeutic doses of 1 mg/kg b.i.d. or 1.5 mg/kg daily. Give postprocedure doses no sooner than 4 hours after catheter removal.

• Draw blood to establish baseline coagulation parameters before therapy.

• Never give drug IM.

ⓘ Alert: Don't try to expel the air bubble from the 30- or 40-mg prefilled syringes. This may lead to loss of drug and an incorrect dose.

• Avoid IM injections of other drugs to prevent or minimize hematoma.

• Monitor platelet counts regularly. Patients with normal coagulation won't need close monitoring of PT or PTT.

• Regularly inspect patient for bleeding gums, bruises on arms or legs, petechiae, nosebleeds, melena, tarry stools, hematuria, and hematemesis.

• To treat severe overdose, give protamine sulfate (a heparin antagonist) by slow IV injection. Refer to manufacturer's instructions for protamine use.

ⓘ Alert: Drug isn't interchangeable with heparin or other low-molecular-weight heparins.

PATIENT TEACHING

- Instruct patient and family to watch for signs of bleeding or abnormal bruising and to notify prescriber immediately.

Black Box Warning Tell patient to immediately report signs and symptoms of spinal or epidural hematoma, such as numbness (especially of the lower limbs) and muscle weakness. ∎

- Tell patient to avoid OTC drugs containing aspirin or other salicylates unless ordered by prescriber.
- Advise patient to consult prescriber before initiating herbal therapy; many herbs have anticoagulant, antiplatelet, or fibrinolytic properties.
- Show patient how to properly administer subcut injection.
- Inform patient that a longer-than-usual time may be needed to stop bleeding and that bruising or bleeding may occur more easily.
- Instruct patient to inform physicians and dentists of all medications being taken, including OTC products, such as aspirin or other NSAIDs.

entecavir
en-TEK-ah-veer

Baraclude

Therapeutic class: Antivirals
Pharmacologic class: Nucleosides–nucleotides

AVAILABLE FORMS
Oral solution: 0.05 mg/mL
Tablets: 0.5 mg, 1 mg

INDICATIONS & DOSAGES
➤ **Chronic HBV infection in patients with active viral replication and either persistently increased aminotransferase levels or histologically active disease**
Adults and adolescents age 16 and older with no previous nucleoside treatment and with compensated liver disease: 0.5 mg PO once daily at least 2 hours before or after a meal.
Adjust-a-dose: If CrCl is 30 to less than 50 mL/minute, give 0.25 mg PO once daily

or 0.5 mg PO every 48 hours. If CrCl is 10 to less than 30 mL/minute, give 0.15 mg PO once daily or 0.5 mg PO every 72 hours. If CrCl is less than 10 mL/minute or patient is undergoing hemodialysis or continuous ambulatory peritoneal dialysis (CAPD), give 0.05 mg PO once daily or 0.5 mg PO every 7 days.
Children age 2 to younger than age 16 and weighing at least 10 kg who have had no previous nucleoside treatment: For children weighing more than 30 kg, 10 mL (0.5 mg) oral solution or one 0.5-mg tablet PO once daily. For children weighing more than 26 to 30 kg, 9 mL (0.45 mg) oral solution PO once daily. For children weighing more than 23 to 26 kg, 8 mL (0.4 mg) oral solution PO once daily. For children weighing more than 20 to 23 kg, 7 mL (0.35 mg) oral solution PO once daily. For children weighing more than 17 to 20 kg, 6 mL (0.3 mg) oral solution PO once daily. For children weighing more than 14 to 17 kg, 5 mL (0.25 mg) oral solution PO once daily. For children weighing more than 11 to 14 kg, 4 mL (0.2 mg) oral solution PO once daily. For children weighing more than 10 to 11 kg, 3 mL (0.15 mg) oral solution PO once daily.
Adjust-a-dose: Insufficient data are available for specific dosage adjustments in children with renal impairment. Consider reducing dosage or increasing dosing interval similar to adjustments for adults.
Adults and adolescents age 16 and older with a history of hepatitis B viremia and who are taking lamivudine or telbivudine or have resistance mutations, or patients with decompensated liver disease: 1 mg PO once daily at least 2 hours before or after a meal.
Adjust-a-dose: If CrCl is 30 to less than 50 mL/minute, give 0.5 mg PO once daily or 1 mg PO every 48 hours. If CrCl is 10 to less than 30 mL/minute, give 0.3 mg PO once daily or 1 mg PO every 72 hours. If CrCl is less than 10 mL/minute or patient is undergoing hemodialysis or CAPD, give 0.1 mg PO once daily or 1 mg PO every 7 days.
Children age 2 to younger than age 16 and weighing at least 10 kg who are lamivudine-experienced: For children weighing more than 30 kg, 20 mL (1 mg) oral solution or one 1-mg tablet PO once daily. For children weighing more than 26 to 30 kg, 18 mL

(0.9 mg) oral solution PO once daily. For children weighing more than 23 to 26 kg, 16 mL (0.8 mg) oral solution PO once daily. For children weighing more than 20 to 23 kg, 14 mL (0.7 mg) oral solution PO once daily. For children weighing more than 17 to 20 kg, 12 mL (0.6 mg) oral solution PO once daily. For children weighing more than 14 to 17 kg, 10 mL (0.5 mg) oral solution PO once daily. For children weighing more than 11 to 14 kg, 8 mL (0.4 mg) oral solution PO once daily. For children weighing more than 10 to 11 kg, 6 mL (0.3 mg) oral solution PO once daily.

Adjust-a-dose: Insufficient data are available for specific dosage adjustments in children with renal impairment. Consider reducing dosage or increasing dosing interval similar to adjustments for adults.

ADMINISTRATION
PO
• Hazardous drug; use safe handling and disposal procedures.
• Drug should be taken on an empty stomach at least 2 hours before or after a meal to increase absorption.
• Store tablets at room temperature in tightly closed container.
• Protect oral solution from light by storing in the outer carton.
• After oral solution has been opened, it can be used up to expiration date on the bottle.

ACTION
Inhibits HBV polymerase and reduces viral DNA levels.

Route	Onset	Peak	Duration
PO	Unknown	½–1½ hr	Unknown

Half-life: About 5 to 6 days.

ADVERSE REACTIONS
CNS: dizziness, fatigue, headache. **GI:** diarrhea, dyspepsia, nausea. **GU:** glycosuria, hematuria. **Hepatic:** hepatomegaly. **Metabolic:** *lactic acidosis.*

INTERACTIONS
Drug-drug. *Drugs that reduce renal function or compete for active tubular secretion:* May increase level of either drug. Monitor renal function, and watch for adverse effects.

Orlistat: May increase entecavir serum concentration. Monitor therapy.
Drug-food. *All foods:* Delays absorption and decreases drug level. Give drug at least 2 hours before or after a meal.

EFFECTS ON LAB TEST RESULTS
• May increase ALT, amylase, AST, blood glucose, creatinine, lipase, and total bilirubin levels.
• May decrease platelet count.

CONTRAINDICATIONS & CAUTIONS
• Contraindicated in patients hypersensitive to drug or its components.
Black Box Warning Don't use in patients infected with both HIV and HBV who aren't also receiving highly active antiretroviral therapy (HAART). ▊
• Use cautiously in patients with renal impairment and in patients who have had a liver transplant.
Dialyzable drug: 13% after 4-hour hemodialysis.

PREGNANCY-LACTATION-REPRODUCTION
• Use cautiously in pregnant women and only if benefit outweighs risk to the fetus.
• Register pregnant women in the Antiretroviral Pregnancy Registry at 1-800-258-4263.
• It isn't known if drug appears in human milk. Patient should discontinue breastfeeding or discontinue drug.

NURSING CONSIDERATIONS
Black Box Warning Drug may cause life-threatening lactic acidosis and severe hepatomegaly with steatosis when used alone or in combination with antiretrovirals. ▊
Black Box Warning HBV infection may worsen severely after therapy stops. Monitor hepatic function for several months in patients who stop therapy. If appropriate, start therapy for HBV infection. ▊
• Closely monitor patients with renal impairment and patients who have had a liver transplant.
• Oral solution should be used for patients weighing up to 30 kg and for doses less than 0.5 mg.
• In elderly patients, adjust dosage for age-related decrease in renal function.

PATIENT TEACHING
• Tell patient to take drug on an empty stomach at least 2 hours before or after a meal.
• Caution against mixing or diluting oral solution with any other substance. Teach proper use of dosing spoon.
• Tell patient to report all adverse effects of this drug and any new drugs being taken.
• Explain that drug doesn't reduce the risk of HBV transmission to others.
• Teach patient the signs and symptoms of lactic acidosis, such as muscle pain, weakness, dyspnea, GI distress, cold hands and feet, dizziness, or fast or irregular heartbeat.
• Teach patient the signs and symptoms of hepatotoxicity, such as jaundice, dark urine, light-colored stool, loss of appetite, nausea, and stomach pain.
• Warn patient not to stop drug abruptly.

SAFETY ALERT!

EPINEPHrine (adrenaline)
ep-i-NEF-rin

EPINEPHrine hydrochloride
Adrenalin, Auvi-Q, EpiPen, EpiPen Jr

Therapeutic class: Vasopressors
Pharmacologic class: Adrenergics

AVAILABLE FORMS
Injection: 0.1 mg/mL, 1 mg/mL
Injection device: 0.15 mg/0.15 mL, 0.3 mg/0.3 mL

INDICATIONS & DOSAGES
➤ **Anaphylaxis**
Adults and children weighing 30 kg or more:
0.3 to 0.5 mg IM or subcut, repeated every 5 to 10 minutes as needed. Maximum single dose is 0.5 mg. Or, 0.3 mg IM or subcut with autoinjector into anterolateral aspect of thigh, through clothing if necessary. Repeat once as needed. More than two sequential doses should only be administered under direct medical supervision.
Children weighing less than 30 kg:
0.01 mg/kg IM or subcut up to a maximum of 0.3 mg per injection, repeated every 5 to 10 minutes as needed. Or, for patients weighing 15 to less than 30 kg, give 0.15 mg IM or subcut with autoinjector into the anterolateral thigh, through clothing if necessary. Repeat once as needed. More than two sequential doses should only be administered under direct medical supervision.
➤ **Hypotension associated with septic shock**
Adults: 0.05 to 2 mcg/kg/minute IV infusion titrated to achieve desired mean arterial pressure. May adjust dosage every 10 to 15 minutes in increments of 0.05 to 0.2 mcg/kg/minute to achieve desired BP goal. After hemodynamic stabilization, wean incrementally over time, such as by decreasing epinephrine dosages every 30 minutes over a 12- to 24-hour period.
➤ **Asthma**
Adults and children older than age 12:
0.01 mg/kg divided into three doses of approximately 0.3 mg subcut every 20 minutes as needed. Start with small dose and increase if needed. Use product with 1 mg/mL concentration.
➤ **Cardiac resuscitation**
Adults: 1 mg IV or intraosseously every 3 to 5 minutes until return of spontaneous circulation.
Children: 0.01 mg/kg IV or intraosseously, up to 1 mg, repeated every 3 to 5 minutes until return of spontaneous circulation.

ADMINISTRATION
IV
▼ Keep solution in light-resistant container, and don't remove before use.
▼ Just before use, mix with D_5W or combinations of dextrose in saline solution.
▼ Monitor BP, HR, and ECG when therapy starts and frequently thereafter.
▼ Discard solution if it's discolored or contains precipitate or after 24 hours.
▼ When giving as a continuous infusion, use a central line with an infusion pump. Extravasation can cause tissue necrosis.
▼ Don't give autoinjectors IV.
▼ **Incompatibilities:** Don't mix with alkaline solutions. Consult a drug incompatibility reference for more information.
IM
• Give into the anterolateral aspect of the thigh through clothing if necessary. May

---

Reactions in bold italics are *life-threatening*. Interactions may have a *rapid onset* or a ***delayed onset***.

repeat injection every 5 to 10 minutes if necessary.
• Massage site after IM injection to counteract vasoconstriction. Repeated local injection can cause necrosis at injection site.
• Don't give if solution is discolored or contains precipitate.
• Don't give autoinjectors IV.
Subcutaneous
• Don't give if solution is discolored or contains precipitate.
• Don't give autoinjectors IV.
• Don't inject deeply into the muscle.
• Protect from light and freezing; store between 68° and 77° F (20° and 25° C).

ACTION

Relaxes bronchial smooth muscle by stimulating beta$_2$ receptors and alpha and beta receptors in the sympathetic nervous system.

Route	Onset	Peak	Duration
IV	Immediate	5 min	Short
IM	Variable	Unknown	1–4 hr
Subcut	5–15 min	30 min	1–4 hr

Half-life: Unknown.

ADVERSE REACTIONS

CNS: drowsiness, headache, nervousness, tremor, *cerebral hemorrhage, stroke,* vertigo, pain, disorientation, agitation, anxiety, apprehensiveness, fear, restlessness, dizziness, weakness, *subarachnoid hemorrhage.*
CV: palpitations, *ventricular fibrillation, shock,* widened pulse pressure, HTN, tachycardia, anginal pain, cardiac arrhythmias, altered ECG (including decreased T-wave amplitude). **GI:** nausea, vomiting. **Respiratory:** dyspnea, respiratory difficulties. **Skin:** urticaria, hemorrhage at injection site, pallor, sweating. **Other:** tissue necrosis.

INTERACTIONS

Drug-drug. *Alpha blockers:* May cause hypotension from unopposed beta-adrenergic effects. Avoid using together.
Antihistamines, thyroid hormones: When given with sympathomimetics, may cause severe adverse cardiac effects. Avoid using together.
Cardiac glycosides, diuretics, general anesthetics (halogenated hydrocarbons): May

increase risk of ventricular arrhythmias. Monitor ECG closely.
Carteolol, nadolol, penbutolol, pindolol, propranolol, timolol: May cause HTN followed by bradycardia. Stop beta blocker 3 days before starting epinephrine.
Doxapram, methylphenidate: May enhance CNS stimulation or pressor effects. Monitor patient closely.
Ergot alkaloids: May decrease vasoconstrictor activity. Monitor patient closely.
Levodopa: May enhance risk of arrhythmias. Monitor ECG closely.
MAO inhibitors: May increase risk of hypertensive crisis. Monitor BP closely.
TCAs: May potentiate the pressor response and cause arrhythmias. Use together cautiously.

EFFECTS ON LAB TEST RESULTS

• May increase BUN, glucose, and lactic acid levels.

CONTRAINDICATIONS & CAUTIONS

• Contraindicated in patients with angle-closure glaucoma, shock (other than anaphylactic shock), organic brain damage, HF, cardiac dilation, arrhythmias, coronary insufficiency, or cerebral arteriosclerosis.
• Contraindicated in patients receiving general anesthesia with halogenated hydrocarbons or cyclopropane and in patients in labor (may delay second stage).
• Commercial products containing sulfites (including epinephrine) are contraindicated in patients with sulfite allergies, except when epinephrine is used to treat serious allergic reactions or other emergency situations.
• Do not use epinephrine with local anesthetic in fingers, toes, ears, nose or genitalia.
• Use cautiously in patients with longstanding bronchial asthma or emphysema who have developed degenerative heart disease.
• Use cautiously in elderly patients and in those with hyperthyroidism, CV disease, HTN, psychoneurosis, and diabetes.
Dialyzable drug: Unknown.
⚠ **Overdose S&S:** Precordial distress, vomiting, headache, dyspnea, HTN, peripheral vascular constriction, pulmonary edema, cerebral hemorrhage, arrhythmias, extreme

pallor and coldness of the skin, metabolic acidosis, kidney failure.

PREGNANCY-LACTATION-REPRODUCTION
• Use during pregnancy only if potential benefit justifies potential risk to the fetus.
• Parenteral administration of epinephrine, if used to support BP during low or other spinal anesthesia for delivery, can cause accelerated fetal HR and shouldn't be used in obstetrics when maternal BP exceeds 130/80 mm Hg.
• It isn't known if drug appears in human milk. Use cautiously in breastfeeding women.

NURSING CONSIDERATIONS
• In patients with Parkinson disease, drug increases rigidity and tremor.
• Drug interferes with tests for urinary catecholamines.
• **Alert:** In 2016, the USP labeling standard for single-entity drug products changed to prohibit use of ratios to express drug concentrations. Concentrations of epinephrine preparations expressed in ratios (e.g., 1:1,000 or 1:10,000) are no longer acceptable because of the risk of dosing errors. Labels with ratio expression may remain in inventory until replaced by products with revised labeling.
• Epinephrine is drug of choice in emergency treatment of acute anaphylactic reactions.
• Observe patient closely for adverse reactions. Notify prescriber if adverse reactions develop; adjusting dosage or stopping drug may be necessary.
• If BP increases sharply, give rapid-acting vasodilators, such as nitrates and alpha blockers, to counteract the marked pressor effect of large doses.
• Drug is rapidly destroyed by oxidizing products, such as iodine, chromates, nitrites, oxygen, and salts of easily reducible metals (such as iron).
• When treating patient with reactions caused by other drugs given IM or subcut, inject this drug into the site where the other drug was given to minimize further absorption.

• *Look alike–sound alike:* Don't confuse epinephrine with ephedrine or norepinephrine.

PATIENT TEACHING
• If patient has acute hypersensitivity reactions (such as to bee stings), it may be necessary to teach patient how to self-inject.
• Instruct patient in autoinjector use. Tell patient to give autoinjector in outer thigh and not into buttock.
• Caution patient or caregiver to only give two sequential doses unless under direct medical supervision. Patient should seek immediate medical care for acute hypersensitivity reactions.
• Tell patient to promptly report all adverse reactions.

SAFETY ALERT!

epiRUBicin hydrochloride
ep-uh-ROO-bi-sin

Ellence

Therapeutic class: Antineoplastics
Pharmacologic class: Anthracycline glycoside antibiotics

AVAILABLE FORMS
Injection: 50 mg/25 mL, 200 mg/100 mL

INDICATIONS & DOSAGES
➤ **Adjuvant therapy in patients with evidence of axillary node tumor involvement after resection of primary breast cancer**
Adults: 100 to 120 mg/m^2 IV infusion over 3 to 20 minutes, depending on dosage and infusion volume, through a free-flowing IV solution on day 1 of each cycle, or divided equally in two doses on days 1 and 8 of each cycle; cycle repeated every 3 to 4 weeks for six cycles; used with regimens containing cyclophosphamide and 5-FU. CEF-120 regimen: 60 mg/m^2 IV on days 1 and 8 every 28 days; FEC-100 regimen: 100 mg/m^2 repeated every 21 days for six cycles. Don't exceed cumulative lifetime dose of 900 mg/m^2.

Dosage modification after first cycle is based on toxicity. For patients with platelet count nadir below 50,000/mm^3, ANC below

---

250/mm³, neutropenic fever, or grade 3 or 4 nonhematologic toxicity, reduce day 1 dose in subsequent cycles to 75% of day 1 dose given in current cycle. Delay day 1 therapy in subsequent cycles until platelet count is at least 100,000/mm³, ANC is at least 1,500/mm³, and nonhematologic toxicities recover to grade 1 or less.

For patients receiving divided doses (days 1 and 8), day 8 dose should be 75% of day 1 dose if platelet count is 75,000 to 100,000/mm³ and ANC is 1,000 to 1,499/mm³. If day 8 platelet count is below 75,000/mm³, ANC is below 1,000/mm³, or grade 3 or 4 nonhematologic toxicity has occurred, omit day 8 dose.

Adjust-a-dose: For patients with bone marrow dysfunction (heavily pretreated patients, patients with bone marrow depression, or those with neoplastic bone marrow infiltration), start at lower doses of 75 to 90 mg/m².

For patients with hepatic dysfunction, if bilirubin is 1.2 to 3 mg/dL or AST is 2 to 4 × ULN, give half recommended starting dose. If bilirubin level is above 3 mg/dL or AST is more than 4 × ULN, give one-quarter the recommended starting dose.

For patients with severe renal dysfunction (creatinine level over 5 mg/dL), consider lower doses.

➤ **Esophageal cancer; gastric cancer ◆**
Adults: 50 mg/m² IV on day 1 every 21 days for up to eight cycles, in combination with cisplatin, oxaliplatin, 5-FU, or capecitabine.

ADMINISTRATION

IV

▼ Wear protective clothing (goggles, gown, disposable gloves) when handling drug, which is a vesicant.

Black Box Warning Never give drug IM or subcut; severe tissue necrosis may result. Always give IV in free-flowing NSS or D₅W over 3 to 20 minutes depending on dosage and volume of infusion solution. ∎

Black Box Warning Avoid veins over joints or in limbs with compromised venous or lymphatic drainage. ∎

▼ Avoid repeated injection into the same vein.

▼ Facial flushing and erythematous streaking along vein may indicate overly rapid delivery.

Black Box Warning If burning or stinging occurs, stop infusion immediately and restart in another vein. ∎

▼ After vial has been penetrated, discard unused solution after 24 hours.

▼ Store refrigerated solution between 36° and 46° F (2° and 8° C). Don't freeze. Protect from light.

▼ **Incompatibilities:** 5-FU, heparin, any alkaline pH solutions, other IV drugs.

ACTION

May form a complex with DNA by getting between nucleotide base pairs, inhibiting DNA, RNA, and protein synthesis; DNA cleavage occurs, resulting in cytocidal activity. Drug may also interfere with replication and transcription of DNA and may generate cytotoxic free radicals.

Route	Onset	Peak	Duration
IV	Unknown	Unknown	Unknown

Half-life: 31 to 35 hours.

ADVERSE REACTIONS

CNS: lethargy, fever. **CV:** *cardiomyopathy, HF.* **EENT:** conjunctivitis, keratitis. **GI:** nausea, vomiting, diarrhea, anorexia, mucositis. **GU:** amenorrhea, red urine. **Hematologic:** *leukopenia, neutropenia, febrile neutropenia,* anemia. **Skin:** alopecia, rash, pruritus, skin changes, local toxicity.

INTERACTIONS

Drug-drug. *Calcium channel blockers, other cardioactive compounds:* May increase risk of HF. Monitor cardiac function closely.

Cimetidine: May increase epirubicin level by 50%. Don't use together.

Cytotoxic drugs: May cause additive toxicities (especially hematologic and GI). Monitor patient closely.

Live-virus vaccines: May increase risk of vaccine-induced adverse reactions. Avoid concomitant use; don't give for at least 3 months after drug.

EFFECTS ON LAB TEST RESULTS

• May decrease Hb level.
• May decrease neutrophil, platelet, and WBC counts.

CONTRAINDICATIONS & CAUTIONS

• Contraindicated in patients hypersensitive to drug, other anthracyclines, or anthracenediones, and in patients with baseline neutrophil counts below 1,500/mm^3, severe myocardial insufficiency, recent MI, cardiomyopathy or HF, serious arrhythmias, previous treatment with anthracyclines up to the maximum cumulative dose, or severe hepatic dysfunction.

• Use cautiously in patients with active or dormant cardiac disease, previous or current radiotherapy to mediastinal and pericardial areas, or previous therapy with other anthracyclines or anthracenediones.

• Use cautiously in patients receiving other cardiotoxic drugs.

Dialyzable drug: Unknown.

⚠ *Overdose S&S:* Bone marrow aplasia, grade 4 mucositis, GI bleeding, hyperthermia, multiple organ failure, lactic acidosis, increased LDH level, anuria, death.

PREGNANCY-LACTATION-REPRODUCTION

• Drug can cause fetal harm. If drug is used during pregnancy, or if patient becomes pregnant during therapy, apprise patient of potential fetal hazard. Women of childbearing potential should be advised to avoid becoming pregnant; men taking drug should use effective contraception.

• It isn't known if drug appears in human milk. Patient should discontinue breastfeeding or discontinue drug.

NURSING CONSIDERATIONS

Black Box Warning Give drug under supervision of prescriber experienced in cancer chemotherapy. ▮

• Don't handle drug if you are pregnant.

• For patients taking 120 mg/m^2 regimen, give prophylactic antibiotic therapy.

• Drug is considered moderately to highly emetogenic; give antiemetic before drug to reduce nausea and vomiting.

• Before therapy, obtain total bilirubin, AST, and creatinine levels; CBC including ANC; and LVEF.

• Monitor LVEF regularly during therapy. Stop drug at first sign of impaired cardiac function. Early signs of cardiac toxicity include sinus tachycardia, ECG abnormalities,

tachyarrhythmias, bradycardia, AV block, and bundle-branch block.

Black Box Warning Cardiac toxicity may occur during therapy or months to years after treatment ends; indications include reduced LVEF and signs and symptoms of HF (tachycardia, dyspnea, pulmonary edema, dependent edema, hepatomegaly, ascites, pleural effusion, and gallop rhythm). Delayed cardiac toxicity depends on cumulative dose of epirubicin. Don't exceed cumulative lifetime dose of 900 mg/m^2. ▮

Black Box Warning Severe myelosuppression may occur. ▮

• Obtain total and differential WBC, CBC, platelet count, and LFTs before and during each cycle of therapy.

• WBC nadir is usually reached 10 to 14 days after drug administration, and WBC count returns to normal by day 21.

• Monitor uric acid, potassium, calcium, phosphate, and creatinine levels immediately after initial chemotherapy administration in patients susceptible to TLS. Hydration, urine alkalinization, and prophylaxis with allopurinol may prevent hyperuricemia and minimize potential complications of TLS.

• Drug may enhance the effects of radiation therapy or cause an inflammatory cell reaction at irradiation site. Monitor patient closely.

Black Box Warning Secondary acute myeloid leukemia has been reported in patients with breast cancer treated with anthracyclines, including epirubicin. ▮

PATIENT TEACHING

• Advise patient to report any pain or burning at injection site during or after administration.

• Advise patient to report nausea, vomiting, mouth inflammation, dehydration, fever, evidence of infection, or symptoms of HF (rapid heartbeat, labored breathing, swelling).

• Tell patient that urine will be reddish pink for 1 to 2 days after treatment.

• Inform patient of risk of heart damage and treatment-related leukemia with use of drug.

• Advise male patient to use effective contraception during treatment.

Reactions in bold italics are *life-threatening*. Interactions may have a *rapid onset* or a *delayed onset*.

• Advise female patient that irreversible, premature menopause may occur.
• Tell patient that hair usually regrows within 2 to 3 months after final dose.

eplerenone
ep-LER-eh-nown

Inspra

Therapeutic class: Antihypertensives
Pharmacologic class: Selective aldosterone receptor antagonists

AVAILABLE FORMS
Tablets: 25 mg, 50 mg

INDICATIONS & DOSAGES
➤ **HTN**
Adults: 50 mg PO once daily. If response is inadequate after 4 weeks, increase dosage to 50 mg PO b.i.d. Maximum daily dose, 100 mg/day.
Adjust-a-dose: In patients taking moderate CYP3A4 inhibitors (erythromycin, fluconazole, saquinavir, verapamil), reduce eplerenone starting dose to 25 mg PO once daily. If BP response is inadequate, may increase dosage to a maximum of 25 mg b.i.d.
➤ **HF after an MI**
Adults: Initially, 25 mg PO once daily. Increase within 4 weeks, as tolerated and according to potassium level, to 50 mg PO once daily.
Adjust-a-dose: Once treatment begins, if potassium level is less than 5 mEq/L, increase dosage from 25 mg every other day to 25 mg daily; or increase dosage from 25 mg daily to 50 mg daily. If potassium level is 5 to 5.4 mEq/L, don't adjust dosage. If potassium level is 5.5 to 5.9 mEq/L, decrease dosage from 50 mg daily to 25 mg daily; or decrease dosage from 25 mg daily to 25 mg every other day; or if dosage was 25 mg every other day, withhold drug. If potassium level is 6 mEq/L or greater, withhold drug. May restart drug at 25 mg every other day when potassium level is less than 5.5 mEq/L. In patients receiving a moderate CYP3A inhibitor (erythromycin, saquinavir, verapamil, fluconazole), don't exceed 25 mg once daily.

ADMINISTRATION
PO
• Give drug without regard for meals.
• Don't give with grapefruit juice.

ACTION
Binds to mineralocorticoid receptors and blocks aldosterone, which increases BP through induction of sodium reabsorption and possibly other mechanisms.

Route	Onset	Peak	Duration
PO	Unknown	1½ –2 hr	Unknown

Half-life: 3 to 6 hours.

ADVERSE REACTIONS
CNS: dizziness, fatigue. **GI:** diarrhea, abdominal pain. **GU:** albuminuria, abnormal vaginal bleeding. **Metabolic:** *hyperkalemia.* **Respiratory:** cough. **Other:** flu-like syndrome.

INTERACTIONS
Drug-drug. *ACE inhibitors, ARBs:* May increase risk of hyperkalemia. Use together cautiously.
Azole antifungals (fluconazole, itraconazole, ketoconazole), macrolides (clarithromycin), nefazodone, protease inhibitors (nelfinavir, ritonavir): Inhibits the CYP3A4 metabolism of eplerenone. Use together is contraindicated.
Canagliflozin: May increase risk of hyperkalemia. Monitor therapy.
Lithium: May increase risk of lithium toxicity. Monitor lithium level.
Moderate CYP3A4 inhibitors (erythromycin, fluconazole, saquinavir, verapamil): May increase eplerenone level. Reduce eplerenone starting dose to 25 mg PO once daily.
NSAIDs: May reduce the antihypertensive effect and cause severe hyperkalemia in patients with impaired renal function. Monitor BP and potassium level.
Potassium supplements, potassium-sparing diuretics (amiloride, spironolactone, triamterene): May increase risk of hyperkalemia and sometimes-fatal arrhythmias. Use together is contraindicated.
Drug-herb. *St. John's wort:* May decrease eplerenone level over time. Discourage use together.

Drug-food. *Grapefruit juice:* May increase eplerenone level by about 25%.

EFFECTS ON LAB TEST RESULTS
• May increase ALT, BUN, cholesterol, creatinine, GGT, potassium, triglyceride, and uric acid levels. May decrease sodium level.

CONTRAINDICATIONS & CAUTIONS
• When used for HTN, contraindicated in patients with type 2 diabetes with microalbuminuria, creatinine level greater than 2 mg/dL in men or greater than 1.8 mg/dL in women, or CrCl less than 50 mL/minute and in patients taking potassium supplements or potassium-sparing diuretics (amiloride, spironolactone, triamterene).
• Contraindicated in patients with potassium level greater than 5.5 mEq/mL at initiation or CrCl of 30 mL/minute or less and in patients taking strong CYP3A4 inhibitors, such as ketoconazole, clarithromycin, ritonavir, nelfinavir, nefazodone, and itraconazole.
• Use cautiously in patients with mild to moderate hepatic impairment.
Dialyzable drug: No.
⚠ **Overdose S&S:** Hypotension, hyperkalemia.

PREGNANCY-LACTATION-REPRODUCTION
• Use in pregnant women only if potential benefits justify potential risk to the fetus.
• It isn't known if drug appears in human milk. Patient should discontinue breastfeeding or discontinue drug.

NURSING CONSIDERATIONS
• Drug may be used alone or with other antihypertensives.
• Full therapeutic effect of the drug occurs in 4 weeks.
• Measure potassium level at baseline, within first week or after dosage adjustment, at 1 month after starting therapy, and periodically thereafter.
• Monitor patient for signs and symptoms of hyperkalemia.
• *Look alike–sound alike:* Don't confuse Inspra with Spiriva.

PATIENT TEACHING
• Inform patient that drug may be taken with or without food.

• Advise patient to avoid potassium supplements and salt substitutes during treatment.
• Tell patient to report adverse reactions.

SAFETY ALERT!
BIOSIMILAR DRUG

epoetin alfa (erythropoietin)
i-POE-i-tin

Epogen, Eprex✦, Procrit

epoetin alfa-epbx
Retacrit

Therapeutic class: Colony-stimulating factors
Pharmacologic class: Recombinant human erythropoietins

AVAILABLE FORMS
Injection (single-use vial): 2,000 units/mL, 3,000 units/mL, 4,000 units/mL, 10,000 units/mL, 40,000 units/mL
Injection (multidose vial)*(Epogen, Procrit): 20,000 units/mL, 20,000 units/2 mL

INDICATIONS & DOSAGES
➤ **Anemia caused by chronic renal disease**
Adults: Dosage is individualized. For patients on hemodialysis, start treatment only if Hb level is less than 10 g/dL. For patients not on hemodialysis, start treatment only if Hb level is less than 10 g/dL, the rate of decline of Hb level indicates that patient will require an RBC transfusion, and reducing the risk of alloimmunization and other RBC transfusion–related risks is a treatment goal. Starting dose is 50 to 100 units/kg subcut or IV three times weekly. IV route is preferred for patients receiving hemodialysis.
Maintenance dosage is highly individualized. Give the lowest effective dose to gradually increase Hb to a level at which blood transfusion isn't necessary.
Children age 1 month and older: Initially, 50 units/kg IV or subcut three times weekly. Start treatment only if Hb level is less than 10 g/dL. IV route is preferred for patients receiving hemodialysis.
Maintenance dosage is highly individualized to keep Hb level within target range. Give the lowest effective dose to gradually

---

Reactions in bold italics are *life-threatening*. Interactions may have a *rapid onset* or a *delayed onset*.

increase Hb to a level at which blood transfusion isn't necessary.

Adjust-a-dose: For all patients, don't increase dosage more frequently than every 4 weeks. Reduce dosage by 25% or more as needed to reduce rapid responses if Hb level rises more than 1 g/dL in any 2-week period. Increase dosage by 25% if Hb level is less than 10 g/dL and hasn't increased by 1 g/dL after 4 weeks or if Hb level falls below 10 g/dL. For adults on dialysis, if Hb level approaches or exceeds 11 g/dL, reduce dosage or interrupt therapy. For adults not on dialysis, if Hb level exceeds 10 g/dL, reduce dosage or interrupt therapy. For children, if Hb level approaches or exceeds 12 g/dL, reduce dosage or interrupt therapy.

➤ **Anemia from zidovudine therapy (4,200 mg/week or less) in HIV-infected patients**
Adults: Initially, 100 units/kg IV or subcut three times weekly for 8 weeks or until target Hb level is reached. If response isn't satisfactory after 8 weeks, increase dosage by 50 to 100 units/kg IV or subcut three times weekly. Evaluate response every 4 to 8 weeks thereafter; further increase dosage in increments of 50 to 100 units/kg three times weekly, up to maximum of 300 units/kg IV or subcut. Give the lowest effective dose to gradually increase Hb to a level where blood transfusion isn't necessary. Withhold drug if Hb level exceeds 12 g/dL. Restart drug at 25% below the previous dosage if Hb level declines to less than 11 g/dL. Discontinue if an increase in Hb isn't achieved at 300 units/kg for 8 weeks.

➤ **Anemia from chemotherapy**
Adults: Start therapy if Hb level is less than 10 g/dL and a minimum of 2 additional months of chemotherapy is planned. Initially, 150 units/kg subcut three times weekly. Or, 40,000 units subcut weekly until completion of a chemotherapy course. If Hb level hasn't increased by at least 1 g/dL (in the absence of RBC transfusion) and remains below 10 g/dL after initial 4 weeks of therapy, increase dosage up to 300 units/kg subcut three times weekly or 60,000 units weekly. Give the lowest effective dose to gradually increase Hb to a level at which blood transfusion isn't necessary. Discontinue drug after 8 weeks if no response, as

measured by Hb level or if transfusions are still required.

Children ages 5 to 18: 600 units/kg IV once weekly until completion of a chemotherapy course. If Hb level hasn't increased by at least 1 g/dL (in the absence of RBC transfusion) and remains below 10 g/dL after initial 4 weeks of therapy, increase dosage to 900 units/kg IV (maximum, 60,000 units). Discontinue drug after 8 weeks if no response, as measured by Hb level or if transfusions are still required.

Adjust-a-dose: Withhold drug if Hb level exceeds level needed to avoid an RBC transfusion. Restart drug at dosage 25% below previous dosage when Hb level approaches a level at which an RBC transfusion may be required. Reduce dosage by 25% if Hb level increases more than 1 g/dL in a 2-week period or reaches a level needed to avoid an RBC transfusion.

➤ **To reduce need for allogenic blood transfusion in anemic patients scheduled to have elective, noncardiac, nonvascular surgery**
Adults: 300 units/kg subcut daily for 10 days before surgery, on day of surgery, and for 4 days after surgery. Or, 600 units/kg subcut in once-weekly doses (21, 14, and 7 days before surgery), plus a fourth dose on day of surgery. DVT prophylaxis is recommended for surgery patients during epoetin therapy.

➤ **Symptomatic anemia in myelodysplastic syndromes** ◆
Adults: 150 to 300 units/kg subcut once daily or 450 to 1,000 units/kg/week in divided doses, three to seven times a week or 60,000 units once weekly.

ADMINISTRATION

IV
▼ Store solution in refrigerator; don't freeze.
▼ Protect from light.
▼ Don't shake.
▼ Give by direct injection without dilution.
▼ If patient is having dialysis, drug may be given into venous return line after dialysis session. To keep drug from adhering to tubing, inject drug with blood still in the line. Then flush with NSS.

▼ Single-dose vials contain no preservatives. Discard unused portion. Don't reenter preservative-free vials.

▼ Store unused portions of multidose vials at 36° to 46° F (2° to 8° C). Discard 21 days after initial entry.

◑ *Alert:* Multidose vials contain benzyl alcohol, which has been associated with sometimes fatal neurologic and other complications in premature infants.

▼ **Incompatibilities:** Other IV drugs.

Subcutaneous

• Store solution in refrigerator; don't freeze.

• Protect from light.

• Don't shake.

• Don't use if solution is discolored or has particulate matter.

• Give in upper arm, abdomen, mid-thigh, or outer buttocks.

• Single-use vial without preservative may be admixed in a syringe with bacteriostatic NSS for injection with benzyl alcohol 0.9% (bacteriostatic saline) at a 1:1 ratio to provide local anesthetic.

• Rotate injection sites and document.

ACTION

Mimics effects of erythropoietin. Functions as a growth factor and as a differentiating factor, enhancing RBC production.

Route	Onset	Peak	Duration
IV	Immediate	Immediate	Unknown
Subcut	Unknown	5–24 hr	Unknown

Half-life: 4 to 13 hours.

ADVERSE REACTIONS

CNS: asthenia, dizziness, depression, fatigue, headache, insomnia, paresthesia, pyrexia, chills, *seizures.* **CV:** edema, HTN, increased clotting of arteriovenous grafts, vascular occlusion, DVT. **EENT:** pharyngitis. **GI:** diarrhea, nausea, vomiting, stomatitis. **Metabolic:** hyperglycemia, *hypokalemia,* hyperphosphatemia, hyperuricemia, weight loss. **Musculoskeletal:** arthralgia, myalgia, bone pain, muscle spasm. **Respiratory:** cough, shortness of breath, URI. **Skin:** injection-site reactions, rash, urticaria, pruritus. **Other:** medical device malfunction.

INTERACTIONS

Drug-drug. *Lenalidomide, pomalidomide, thalidomide:* May enhance thrombogenic effects of these drugs. Monitor therapeutic response.

EFFECTS ON LAB TEST RESULTS

• May increase BUN, creatinine, phosphate, potassium, Hb, and uric acid levels.

CONTRAINDICATIONS & CAUTIONS

• Contraindicated in patients hypersensitive to products derived from mammal cells or albumin (human) and in those with uncontrolled HTN or pure RBC aplasia that begins after treatment with epoetin.

Dialyzable drug: Unknown.

⚠ *Overdose S&S:* Severe HTN.

PREGNANCY-LACTATION-REPRODUCTION

• Use single-dose formulations during pregnancy only if potential benefit justifies potential risk to the fetus.

• Use of multidose vials (which contain benzyl alcohol) is contraindicated in pregnant women, neonates, infants, and breastfeeding women.

• Women who become pregnant during treatment should enroll in Amgen's Pregnancy Surveillance Program. Patients or their physicians should call 1-800-772-6436.

• It isn't known if drug appears in human milk. Use single-dose vials cautiously in breastfeeding women.

NURSING CONSIDERATIONS

Black Box Warning Patients with chronic renal disease have an increased risk of death, serious adverse CV events, and stroke when erythropoiesis-stimulating agents are used to increase Hb level to more than 11 g/dL. Individualize therapy and use the lowest dosage needed to reduce the need for RBC transfusion. ▌

• Before starting therapy, evaluate patient's iron status. Patient should receive adequate iron supplementation beginning no later than when epoetin alfa treatment starts and continuing throughout therapy. Patient also may need vitamin B_{12} and folic acid.

• Monitor BP before therapy. Most patients with chronic renal failure have HTN. BP

Reactions in bold italics are *life-threatening.* Interactions may have a *rapid onset* or a *delayed onset.*

may increase, especially when hematocrit increases in the early part of therapy.

Black Box Warning In patients with NSCLC and breast, head and neck, lymphoid, and cervical cancers, there is a risk of tumor growth and shortened survival. Use the lowest dosage needed to avoid RBC transfusions. Use only for treatment of anemia due to concomitant myelosuppressive chemotherapy and discontinue drug following chemotherapy course. Erythropoiesis-stimulating agents (ESAs) aren't indicated for patients receiving myelosuppressive therapy when the anticipated outcome is cure. ∎

• Institute diet restrictions or drug therapy to control BP.

• Monitor Hb level twice weekly until it stabilizes in the target range and maintenance dose is established, then continue to monitor at least monthly. Resume twice-weekly testing after any dosage adjustments.

• When used in HIV-infected adults, dosage recommendations are for those with endogenous erythropoietin levels of 500 milliunits/mL or less and cumulative zidovudine doses of 4.2 g/week or less.

• Monitor blood counts; elevated hematocrit may cause excessive clotting. For patients with chronic renal disease, monitor Hb level weekly until stable and then at least monthly.

• For patients who don't respond adequately over a 12-week escalation period, increasing dosage further is unlikely to improve response and may increase risks. Evaluate other causes of anemia and discontinue drug if responsiveness doesn't improve.

• Patient may need additional heparin to prevent clotting during dialysis treatments.

• Drug increases risk of seizures in patients with chronic kidney disease. Monitor patients closely for neurologic signs and symptoms.

Black Box Warning Due to increased risk of DVT, consider prophylaxis. ∎

🜂 *Alert:* Evaluate patient who experiences a lack or loss of effect for pure red cell aplasia.

• *Look alike–sound alike:* Don't confuse Epogen with Neupogen.

PATIENT TEACHING

• Inform patient that pain or discomfort in limbs (long bones) and pelvis, feelings of cold, and sweating may occur after injection (usually within 2 hours). Symptoms may last for 12 hours and then disappear.

• Advise patient to avoid driving or operating heavy machinery at start of therapy. There may be a relationship between too-rapid increase in hematocrit and seizures.

• Tell patient to monitor BP at home and to adhere to dietary restrictions.

• Advise female patient that she may resume menstruating after therapy and to consider the need for contraception.

SAFETY ALERT!

eptifibatide
ep-tiff-IB-ah-tide

Integrilin

Therapeutic class: Antiplatelet drugs
Pharmacologic class: Glycoprotein IIb/IIIa inhibitors

AVAILABLE FORMS
Injection: 20 mg/10 mL (2 mg/mL), 75 mg/100 mL (0.75 mg/mL), 200 mg/100 mL (2 mg/mL) vials

INDICATIONS & DOSAGES
➤ **ACS (unstable angina or non–ST-segment elevation MI) in patients receiving drug therapy and in those undergoing a PCI**
Adults: 180 mcg/kg IV bolus as soon as possible after diagnosis, followed by a continuous IV infusion at a rate of 2 mcg/kg/minute until hospital discharge or start of CABG surgery, for up to 72 hours. Give aspirin (160 to 325 mg) and heparin (target aPTT, 50 to 70 sec) daily.
Adjust-a-dose: If CrCl is less than 50 mL/minute, give 180 mcg/kg IV bolus as soon as possible after diagnosis, followed by a continuous IV infusion at 1 mcg/kg/minute.
➤ **PCI**
Adults: 180 mcg/kg IV bolus given just before the procedure, immediately followed by an infusion of 2 mcg/kg/minute and a second IV bolus of 180 mcg/kg given 10 minutes after the first bolus. Continue infusion until hospital discharge or for 18 to 24 hours, whichever comes first. Minimum duration of infusion is 12 hours; maximum duration is

96 hours. Give aspirin 160 to 325 mg PO 1 to 24 hours before PCI and daily thereafter; give heparin before PCI (but not after). *Adjust-a-dose:* If CrCl is less than 50 mL/minute, give 180 mcg/kg IV bolus just before the procedure, immediately followed by a continuous IV infusion at 1 mcg/kg/minute and a second bolus of 180 mcg/kg given 10 minutes after the first bolus.

ADMINISTRATION

IV

▼ Inspect solution for particles before use; if they appear, drug may not be sterile. Discard it.

▼ Protect drug from light before giving.

▼ Drug may be given in same line with NSS, D₅W, alteplase, atropine, dobutamine, heparin, lidocaine, meperidine, metoprolol, midazolam, morphine, nitroglycerin, or verapamil. Main infusion may also contain up to 60 mEq/L of potassium chloride.

▼ For IV push, withdraw bolus dose from 10-mL vial into a syringe and give over 1 or 2 minutes.

▼ For infusion, give undiluted drug directly from 100-mL vial using an infusion pump.

▼ Administer drug with heparin titrated to dosing parameters.

▼ If patient needs thrombolytics, stop infusion.

▼ Refrigerate vials at 36° to 46° F (2° to 8° C). Store vials at room temperature for no longer than 2 months; afterward, discard them.

▼ **Incompatibilities:** Furosemide.

ACTION

Reversibly binds to the glycoprotein IIb/IIIa (GPIIb/IIIa) receptor on human platelets and inhibits platelet aggregation.

Route	Onset	Peak	Duration
IV	Immediate	Immediate	4–8 hr

Half-life: 2½ hours.

ADVERSE REACTIONS

CV: hypotension. **GU:** hematuria. **Hematologic:** *thrombocytopenia, major bleeding,* minor bleeding. **Other:** bleeding at femoral artery access site.

INTERACTIONS

Drug-drug. *Apixaban, clopidogrel, dabigatran, dipyridamole, edoxaban, NSAIDs, oral anticoagulants (warfarin), rivaroxaban, SSRIs, thrombolytics, ticlopidine:* May increase risk of bleeding. Monitor patient closely for signs of bleeding.

Other inhibitors of GPIIb/IIIa: May cause serious bleeding. Avoid using together.

EFFECTS ON LAB TEST RESULTS

• May decrease platelet count.

CONTRAINDICATIONS & CAUTIONS

• Contraindicated in patients hypersensitive to drug or its components and in those with history of bleeding diathesis or evidence of active abnormal bleeding within previous 30 days; severe HTN (systolic BP higher than 200 mm Hg or diastolic BP higher than 110 mm Hg) not adequately controlled with antihypertensives; major surgery within previous 6 weeks; history of stroke within 30 days or history of hemorrhagic stroke; current or planned use of another parenteral GPIIb/IIIa inhibitor; or platelet count less than 100,000/mm³.

• Contraindicated in patients with creatinine level of 4 mg/dL or higher and in patients dependent on hemodialysis.

• Use cautiously in patients at increased risk for bleeding, in those with hemorrhagic retinopathy, and in those weighing more than 143 kg.

Dialyzable drug: Yes.

PREGNANCY-LACTATION-REPRODUCTION

• Use during pregnancy only if clearly needed.

• It isn't known if drug appears in human milk. Use cautiously in breastfeeding women.

NURSING CONSIDERATIONS

• Drug is intended for use with heparin and aspirin.

• At least 4 hours before hospital discharge, stop this drug and heparin and achieve sheath hemostasis by standard compressive techniques.

• Remove sheath during infusion only after heparin has been stopped and its effects largely reversed.

Reactions in bold italics are *life-threatening*. Interactions may have a *rapid onset* or a *delayed onset*.

• If patient is to undergo CABG, stop infusion at least 2 to 4 hours before surgery.
• Minimize use of arterial and venous punctures, IM injections, urinary catheters, and nasotracheal and NG tubes.
• When obtaining IV access, avoid use of noncompressible sites (such as subclavian or jugular veins).
• Monitor patient for bleeding.
🛇 *Alert:* If platelet count is less than 100,000/mm³, stop this drug and heparin.
• Perform baseline laboratory tests before start of drug therapy; also determine Hb level, hematocrit, PT, INR, aPTT, platelet count, and creatinine level.

PATIENT TEACHING
• Advise patient to inform health care provider of all drugs and supplements being taken.
• Explain that drug inhibits blood clotting and is used to prevent chest pain and heart attack.
• Explain that benefits of drug outweigh risk of serious bleeding.
• Tell patient to report chest discomfort or other adverse effects to prescriber immediately.
• Tell patient to report unusual bleeding, bruising, or blood in stools.

---

erenumab-aooe
e-REN-ue-mab

Aimovig

Therapeutic class: Antimigraine drugs
Pharmacologic class: Monoclonal antibodies

AVAILABLE FORMS
Injection: 70 mg/mL prefilled autoinjector or syringes

INDICATIONS & DOSAGES
➤ **Migraine prevention**
Adults: 70 mg subcut once monthly. If ineffective, 140 mg subcut monthly.

ADMINISTRATION
Subcutaneous
🛇 *Alert:* The needle shield of the autoinjector and the needle cap of the syringe contain dry natural rubber (a derivative of latex) and may cause allergic reactions in patients sensitive to latex.
• Before administration, allow product to sit at room temperature for at least 30 minutes protected from direct sunlight. Don't warm by using a heat source, such as hot water or microwave.
• Don't shake product.
• Visually inspect solution for discoloration or particulate matter. Don't use if solution is cloudy, discolored, or contains flakes or particles.
• Products are for single use; give entire contents.
• Administer subcut in the abdomen, thigh, or upper arm. Don't inject into areas where skin is tender, bruised, red, or hard.
• Give missed dose as soon as possible; then schedule monthly from the date of the last dose.
• Store product refrigerated at 36° to 46° F (2° to 8° C) in original carton to protect from light until time of use. Don't freeze.
• If removed from the refrigerator, store at room temperature (up to 77° F [25° C]) in original carton and use within 7 days. Don't return product to the refrigerator after it has been warmed. Discard product if left at room temperature for more than 7 days.

ACTION
Human monoclonal antibody that binds to the calcitonin gene-related peptide (CGRP) receptor and antagonizes CGRP receptor function.

Route	Onset	Peak	Duration
Subcut	Unknown	6 days	Unknown

Half-life: 28 days.

ADVERSE REACTIONS
GI: constipation. **Musculoskeletal:** muscle spasms, cramps. **Skin:** injection-site reaction (pain, erythema, pruritus). **Other:** antibody development.

EFFECTS ON LAB TEST RESULTS
None reported.

CONTRAINDICATIONS & CAUTIONS
• Safety and effectiveness in children haven't been established.

• Use cautiously in patients age 65 and older. Begin at lowest dosage and consider how hepatic, renal, and cardiac function; other disease states; or other drug therapy may affect drug effectiveness.
Dialyzable drug: Unknown.

PREGNANCY-LACTATION-REPRODUCTION
• There are no data regarding drug's use in pregnant women. Data suggest that women with migraine may be at increased risk for preeclampsia during pregnancy.
• It isn't known if drug appears in human milk or how drug affects a breastfed infant. Before use in breastfeeding patients, consider the mother's need for the drug and potential adverse effects on the infant.

NURSING CONSIDERATIONS
❸ *Alert:* The needle shield of the autoinjector and the needle cap of the syringe contain dry natural rubber (a derivative of latex) and may cause allergic reactions in patients sensitive to latex.
• Monitor patients for injection-site and other adverse reactions.
• *Look alike–sound alike:* Don't confuse Aimovig with Amerge.

PATIENT TEACHING
• Advise patient to read the Patient Information leaflet enclosed with drug.
❸ *Alert:* Warn latex-sensitive patient about the risk of allergic reaction since the needle shield of the autoinjector and the needle cap of the syringe contain dry natural rubber.
• Teach patient how to properly administer and store drug according to manufacturer's instructions.
• Educate patient that if a dose is missed, to administer it as soon as possible and to administer subsequent doses a month from the last dose.
• Advise patient to report injection-site reactions or other adverse effects.
• Warn patient not to use an autoinjector or syringe that has been dropped on a hard surface as it may have broken, even if no visible damage is seen. Tell patient to use a new autoinjector or syringe and to call 1-800-77-AMGEN (1-800-772-6436).

eriBULin mesylate
er-ih-BYOO-lin

Halaven

Therapeutic class: Antineoplastics
Pharmacologic class: Microtubule inhibitors

AVAILABLE FORMS
Injection: 1 mg/2 mL vial

INDICATIONS & DOSAGES
➤ **To treat metastatic breast cancer in patients who have received at least two chemotherapeutic regimens for the treatment of metastatic disease, and whose treatments have included an anthracycline and a taxane in either the adjuvant or metastatic setting; unresectable or metastatic liposarcoma in patients who have received a prior anthracycline-containing regimen**
Adults: 1.4 mg/m^2 IV on days 1 and 8 of a 21-day cycle. Assess for peripheral neuropathy and obtain CBCs before each dose. Don't administer drug on day 1 or 8 if ANC is less than 1,000/mm^3, platelet count is less than 75,000/mm^3, or grade 3 or 4 nonhematologic toxicities exist. May delay day-8 dose for a maximum of 1 week.

If toxicities don't resolve or improve to grade 2 or less by day 15, omit dose. If toxicities resolve or improve to grade 2 or less by day 15, give eribulin at a reduced dose and initiate next cycle no sooner than 2 weeks later. Don't reescalate eribulin dose after it has been reduced.
Adjust-a-dose: In mild hepatic impairment (Child-Pugh class A) and in patients with moderate or severe renal impairment (CrCl of 15 to 49 mL/minute), give 1.1 mg/m^2 IV over 2 to 5 minutes on days 1 and 8 of a 21-day cycle. In moderate hepatic impairment (Child-Pugh class B), give 0.7 mg/m^2 IV over 2 to 5 minutes on days 1 and 8 of a 21-day cycle. If toxicities occur, refer to manufacturer's instructions for dosage adjustments. Don't reescalate dosage after it has been reduced. Discontinue drug for any event requiring permanent dosage reduction while patient is receiving 0.7 mg/m^2.

Reactions in bold italics are *life-threatening*. Interactions may have a *rapid onset* or a *delayed onset*.

ADMINISTRATION
IV

▼ Hazardous drug; use safe handling and disposal precautions.

▼ Draw up required amount from vial and administer undiluted, or dilute in 100 mL NSS. Don't use dextrose.

▼ Administer IV over 2 to 5 minutes.

▼ May store undiluted drug in a syringe or diluted solutions for 4 hours at room temperature or 24 hours if refrigerated.

▼ Discard unused portion of vial.

▼ **Incompatibilities:** Dextrose, other IV drugs.

ACTION
Causes cell death by inhibiting cell division.

Route	Onset	Peak	Duration
IV	Unknown	Unknown	Unknown

Half-life: About 40 hours.

ADVERSE REACTIONS
CNS: dizziness, depression, peripheral neuropathy, headache, insomnia, asthenia, fatigue, pyrexia. **CV:** *QT-interval prolongation,* peripheral edema. **EENT:** increased lacrimation, mucosal inflammation. **GI:** anorexia, dysgeusia, dyspepsia, abdominal pain, stomatitis, dry mouth, constipation, diarrhea, nausea, vomiting. **GU:** UTI. **Hematologic:** *neutropenia,* anemia, *thrombocytopenia.* **Metabolic:** weight loss, *hypokalemia,* hypocalcemia. **Musculoskeletal:** muscle spasms, muscle weakness, arthralgia, myalgia, back pain, bone pain, pain in extremity. **Respiratory:** URI, cough, dyspnea. **Skin:** rash, alopecia.

INTERACTIONS
Drug-drug. *Class IA and III antiarrhythmics, other drugs known to prolong QT interval:* May further prolong QT interval. Use together cautiously and monitor patient carefully.

EFFECTS ON LAB TEST RESULTS
• May increase ALT and bilirubin levels. May decrease potassium level.

• May decrease Hb level and neutrophil and platelet counts.

CONTRAINDICATIONS & CAUTIONS
• Contraindicated in patients hypersensitive to drug or its components.

• Avoid use in patients with existing congenital long QT syndrome.

• Use cautiously in patients with liver or renal insufficiency and in those at risk for neutropenia or peripheral motor or sensory neuropathy.

• Use cautiously in patients with HF, bradyarrhythmias, or electrolyte imbalance and in those taking drugs known to prolong QT interval or with a history of prolonged QT interval.

• Safety and effectiveness in children haven't been established.

Dialyzable drug: Unknown.

⚠ *Overdose S&S:* Neutropenia, hypersensitivity reaction.

PREGNANCY-LACTATION-REPRODUCTION
• There are no well-controlled studies in pregnant women, but drug is expected to cause fetal harm. Use during pregnancy only if benefits outweigh risk and patient is aware of potential fetal hazard.

• It isn't known if drug appears in human milk. Patient should discontinue breastfeeding or discontinue drug.

NURSING CONSIDERATIONS
• Assess patient for peripheral neuropathy before each dose.

• Monitor patient for hypokalemia and hypomagnesemia before and periodically during therapy.

• Monitor patient for signs and symptoms of infection.

• Monitor blood counts and obtain CBC before each dose.

• Monitor LFTs and renal function tests during therapy.

• Monitor ECG for changes, especially QT-interval prolongation.

• Consider prophylactic antiemetics for nausea and vomiting.

• Day-8 dose may be delayed for a maximum of 1 week. If toxicities don't resolve or improve to grade 2 or less by day 15, omit dose. If toxicities resolve or improve to grade 2 or less by day 15, administer Halaven at a reduced dose and initiate the next cycle no sooner than 2 weeks later.

PATIENT TEACHING

• Tell patient to report a temperature of 100.4° F (38° C) or greater and other signs or symptoms of infection, such as chills, cough, or burning or pain on urination.

• Advise patient that drug may cause nerve damage and to contact prescriber if burning, tingling, or radiating pain occurs in any extremity.

• Caution patient to immediately report irregular heartbeat.

• Warn patient to avoid pregnancy and to use effective contraception during treatment.

• Tell patient to consult prescriber before breastfeeding.

SAFETY ALERT!

erlotinib ☒
ur-LOE-tih-nib

Tarceva

Therapeutic class: Antineoplastics
Pharmacologic class: Epidermal growth factor receptor inhibitors

AVAILABLE FORMS
Tablets ⓪*:* 25 mg, 100 mg, 150 mg

INDICATIONS & DOSAGES
Adjust-a-dose (for all indications): Refer to manufacturer's instructions for toxicity-related dosage adjustments.

➤ **With gemcitabine, first-line treatment of locally advanced, unresectable, or metastatic pancreatic cancer**
Adults: 100 mg PO once daily taken at least 1 hour before or 2 hours after meals. Continue until disease progresses or intolerable toxicity occurs.

➤ **Maintenance therapy for locally advanced or metastatic NSCLC in patients whose disease hasn't progressed after four cycles of platinum-based, first-line chemotherapy; locally advanced or metastatic NSCLC after failure of at least one chemotherapy regimen**
Adults: 150 mg PO once daily at least 1 hour before or 2 hours after meals. Continue until disease progresses or intolerable toxicity occurs.

➤ **Metastatic NSCLC in patients with tumors with epidermal growth factor receptor (*EGFR*) exon 19 deletions or exon 21 (L858R) substitution mutations as detected by an FDA-approved test receiving first-line, maintenance, or second or greater line treatment after progression following at least one prior chemotherapy regimen** ☒
Adults: 150 mg PO once daily at least 1 hour before or 2 hours after a meal. Continue until disease progresses or intolerable toxicity occurs.

ADMINISTRATION
PO
• Hazardous drug; use appropriate precautions for handling and disposal.

• Give drug 1 hour before or 2 hours after a meal.

• For patients unable to swallow tablets whole, tablets may be dissolved in 100 mL water and given orally or via feeding tube (silicone-based). To ensure full dose is received, rinse container with 40 mL water, administer residue, and repeat rinse.

ACTION
Inhibits tyrosine kinase activity in EGFRs, which are expressed on the surface of normal and cancer cells.

Route	Onset	Peak	Duration
PO	Unknown	4 hr	Unknown

Half-life: About 36 hours.

ADVERSE REACTIONS
CNS: fatigue, syncope, *stroke,* anxiety, depression, dizziness, headache, insomnia, neuropathies, pyrexia, rigors. **CV:** chest pain, arrhythmias, edema, *MI, DVT.* **EENT:** conjunctivitis, keratoconjunctivitis sicca, decreased tear production, abnormal eyelash growth. **GI:** abdominal pain, anorexia, diarrhea, decreased appetite, nausea, stomatitis, vomiting, constipation, dyspepsia, flatulence, *pancreatitis.* **GU:** renal insufficiency. **Hematologic:** hemolytic anemia. **Metabolic:** decreased weight. **Musculoskeletal:** bone pain, myalgia. **Respiratory:** cough, dyspnea, *pulmonary toxicity.* **Skin:** acne, dry skin, pruritus, rash, alopecia, paronychia. **Other:** infection.

Reactions in bold italics are *life-threatening*. Interactions may have a *rapid onset* or a *delayed onset*.

INTERACTIONS

Drug-drug. *Antacids:* May reduce bioavailability of drug. Separate doses by several hours if an antacid is necessary.

Anticoagulants, such as warfarin: May increase risk of bleeding. Monitor PT and INR.

Ciprofloxacin: May increase erlotinib plasma concentration. Consider reducing erlotinib dosage if severe adverse reactions occur; avoid use together if possible.

CYP3A4 inducers (carbamazepine, phenobarbital, phenytoin, rifabutin, rifampin): May increase erlotinib metabolism. Avoid use if possible or increase erlotinib dosage by 50-mg increments at 2-week intervals to a maximum of 450 mg as tolerated.

H₂-receptor antagonists: May reduce bioavailability of drug. Give erlotinib 10 hours after and at least 2 hours before H₂-antagonist dosing.

PPIs: May reduce bioavailability of drug. Dose separation may not eliminate interaction; avoid use together if possible.

Strong CYP3A4 inhibitors (atazanavir, clarithromycin, indinavir, itraconazole, ketoconazole, nefazodone, nelfinavir, ritonavir, saquinavir, telithromycin, voriconazole): May decrease erlotinib metabolism. Avoid use together if possible or reduce erlotinib dosage by 50-mg decrements.

Drug-herb. *St. John's wort:* May increase drug metabolism. Drug dosage may need to be increased. Discourage use together.

Drug-food. *Any food:* May increase bioavailability of drug. Give drug 1 hour before or 2 hours after meals.

Grapefruit or grapefruit juice: May increase drug level. Avoid use together.

Drug-lifestyle. *Cigarette smoking:* May decrease drug level. Increase drug dosage by 50-mg increments at 2-week intervals to a maximum of 300 mg. Immediately reduce dosage to recommended dose (100 or 150 mg daily) upon smoking cessation.

Sun exposure: May cause photosensitivity reactions. Patient should use alcohol-free emollient cream and sunscreen and avoid sun exposure.

EFFECTS ON LAB TEST RESULTS

• May increase ALT, AST, bilirubin, BUN, and creatinine levels.
• May increase INR and prolong PT.

CONTRAINDICATIONS & CAUTIONS

• Use cautiously in patients with pulmonary disease or liver impairment. Also use cautiously in patients who have received or are receiving chemotherapy because it may worsen adverse pulmonary effects.

• Withhold drug for acute onset of new or progressive unexplained pulmonary signs and symptoms, such as dyspnea, cough, and fever (pending diagnostic evaluation), and for grade 3 or 4 keratitis lasting more than 2 weeks. Withhold drug for acute or worsening ocular disorders such as eye pain, and consider discontinuation.

• Use cautiously in patients receiving other antiangiogenic agents, corticosteroids, NSAIDs, or taxane-based chemotherapy, and in those with a history of peptic ulcer disease because of increased risk of GI perforation.

• Interrupt therapy or discontinue drug in patients with dehydration at risk for renal failure.

• Discontinue if severe bullous, blistering, or exfoliating skin conditions develop.

Dialyzable drug: Unknown.

⚠ *Overdose S&S:* Severe adverse reactions (diarrhea, ALT or AST elevation, rash).

PREGNANCY-LACTATION-REPRODUCTION

• Drug may cause fetal harm. If drug is used during pregnancy, or if patient becomes pregnant during therapy, apprise patient of potential hazard to fetus.

• Women of childbearing potential should use effective contraception during therapy and for 1 month after final dose.

• It isn't known if drug appears in human milk. Patient should discontinue breastfeeding until 2 weeks after final dose or discontinue drug.

NURSING CONSIDERATIONS

• Monitor renal function tests and LFTs periodically during therapy.

🔵 *Alert:* GI perforation with fatalities has been reported. Permanently discontinue drug if GI perforation occurs.

🔵 *Alert:* Rarely, serious ILD may occur. If patient develops dyspnea, cough, and fever, notify prescriber. Therapy may need to be interrupted or stopped.

E

• Monitor patient for severe diarrhea, and give loperamide if needed.
• Monitor patient for eye ulcers, bullous blistering, and exfoliative skin conditions.

PATIENT TEACHING

🚯 *Alert:* Tell patient to immediately report new or worsened cough, shortness of breath, eye irritation or pain, or severe or persistent diarrhea, nausea, anorexia, or vomiting.
• Instruct patient to take drug 1 hour before or 2 hours after food.
• Explain the likelihood of serious interactions with other drugs and herbal supplements and the need to tell prescriber about any change in drugs and supplements taken.
• Counsel patient about smoking cessation, as smoking may decrease drug level and effectiveness.

ertapenem sodium
er-tah-PEN-em

INVanz

Therapeutic class: Antibiotics
Pharmacologic class: Carbapenems

AVAILABLE FORMS
Injection: 1 g

INDICATIONS & DOSAGES

Adjust-a-dose (for all indications): In adults with CrCl of 30 mL/minute/1.73 m² or less, give 500 mg/day. In hemodialysis patients receiving daily 500-mg dose less than 6 hours before hemodialysis, give supplementary 150-mg dose afterward. In hemodialysis patients receiving dose 6 hours or more before hemodialysis, no supplementary dose is needed.

➤ **Complicated intra-abdominal infection caused by** *Escherichia coli, Clostridium clostridioforme, Eubacterium lentum, Peptostreptococcus* **species,** *Bacteroides fragilis, Bacteroides distasonis, Bacteroides ovatus, Bacteroides thetaiotaomicron,* **or** *Bacteroides uniformis*
Adults and children age 13 and older: 1 g IV or IM once daily for 5 to 14 days.
Infants and children ages 3 months to 12 years: 15 mg/kg IV or IM every 12 hours for 5 to 14 days. Don't exceed 1 g daily.

➤ **Complicated skin or skin-structure infection, including diabetic foot infections without osteomyelitis, caused by** *Staphylococcus aureus* **(methicillin-susceptible strains),** *Streptococcus agalactiae, Streptococcus pyogenes, E. coli, Klebsiella pneumoniae, Proteus mirabilis, B. fragilis, Peptostreptococcus* **species,** *Porphyromonas asaccharolytica,* **or** *Prevotella bivia*
Adults and children age 13 and older: 1 g IV or IM once daily for 7 to 14 days. Diabetic foot infections may need up to 28 days of treatment.
Infants and children ages 3 months to 12 years: 15 mg/kg IV or IM every 12 hours for 7 to 14 days. Don't exceed 1 g daily.

➤ **Community-acquired pneumonia from** *S. pneumoniae* **(penicillin-susceptible strains),** *Haemophilus influenzae* **(beta-lactamase–negative strains), or** *Moraxella catarrhalis;* **complicated UTI, including pyelonephritis caused by** *E. coli* **or** *K. pneumoniae*
Adults and children age 13 and older: 1 g IV or IM once daily for 10 to 14 days. If patient improves after at least 3 days of treatment, use appropriate oral therapy to complete the full course of therapy.
Infants and children ages 3 months to 12 years: 15 mg/kg IV or IM every 12 hours for 10 to 14 days. Don't exceed 1 g daily. If patient improves after at least 3 days of treatment, use appropriate oral therapy to complete the full course of therapy.

➤ **Acute pelvic infection, including postpartum endomyometritis, septic abortion, and postsurgical gynecologic infection caused by** *S. agalactiae, E. coli, B. fragilis, P. asaccharolytica, Peptostreptococcus* **species, or** *P. bivia*
Adults and children age 13 and older: 1 g IV or IM once daily for 3 to 10 days.
Infants and children ages 3 months to 12 years: 15 mg/kg IV or IM every 12 hours for 3 to 10 days. Don't exceed 1 g daily.

➤ **Prevention of surgical site infection after elective colorectal surgery**
Adults: 1 g IV 1 hour before surgical incision.

➤ **Complicated urinary tract infections, including pyelonephritis**
Adults and children age 13 and older: 1 g IV or IM once daily for 10 to 14 days.

Reactions in bold italics are *life-threatening*. Interactions may have a *rapid onset* or a ***delayed onset***.

Infants and children ages 3 months to 12 years: 15 mg/kg IV or IM every 12 hours for 10 to 14 days. Don't exceed 1 g daily.

ADMINISTRATION

IV

▼ Obtain specimens for culture and sensitivity testing before giving. Begin therapy while awaiting results.

▼ Before giving first dose, check for previous hypersensitivity to penicillin, cephalosporin, beta-lactam, or local amide-type anesthetics.

▼ Reconstitute 1-g vial with 10 mL of sterile water for injection, NSS for injection, or bacteriostatic water for injection.

▼ Shake well to dissolve, and then immediately transfer contents to 50 mL of NSS.

▼ For children ages 3 months to 12 years, immediately withdraw a volume equal to 15 mg/kg (not to exceed 1 g/day); dilute in NSS to a final concentration of 20 mg/mL or less.

▼ Infuse over 30 minutes.

▼ Complete the infusion within 6 hours of reconstitution or refrigerate for up to 24 hours. Infuse within 4 hours once removed from refrigeration. Don't freeze.

▼ **Incompatibilities:** Diluents containing dextrose, other IV drugs.

IM

• Obtain specimens for culture and sensitivity testing before giving. Begin therapy while awaiting results.

• Before giving first dose, check for previous hypersensitivity to penicillin, cephalosporin, beta-lactam, or local amide-type anesthetics.

• Reconstitute 1-g vial with 3.2 mL of 1% lidocaine hydrochloride injection (without epinephrine). Shake vial thoroughly to form solution. Immediately withdraw volume equal to 15 mg/kg of body weight (not to exceed 1 g/day) and give by deep IM injection into a large muscle, such as the gluteal muscles or lateral part of the thigh. Use the reconstituted IM solution within 1 hour after preparation. Don't give reconstituted solution IV.

ACTION

Inhibits cell-wall synthesis through penicillin-binding proteins.

Route	Onset	Peak	Duration
IV	Immediate	30 min	24 hr
IM	Unknown	2 hr	24 hr

Half-life: 4 hours.

ADVERSE REACTIONS

CNS: altered mental status, anxiety, asthenia, dizziness, fatigue, fever, headache, insomnia. **CV:** chest pain, edema, HTN, hypotension, phlebitis, swelling, tachycardia, thrombophlebitis. **EENT:** pharyngitis. **GI:** diarrhea, abdominal pain, acid regurgitation, constipation, dyspepsia, nausea, oral candidiasis, vomiting. **GU:** renal dysfunction, vaginitis. **Hematologic:** *leukopenia, neutropenia, thrombocytopenia,* anemia, coagulation abnormalities, eosinophilia, *thrombocytosis.* **Hepatic:** jaundice. **Metabolic:** *hyperkalemia, hypokalemia,* hyperglycemia. **Musculoskeletal:** leg pain. **Respiratory:** cough, dyspnea, rales, *respiratory distress,* rhonchi. **Skin:** erythema, extravasation, infusion-site pain and redness, pruritus, rash. **Other:** hypersensitivity reactions, infused vein complications.

INTERACTIONS

Drug-drug. *Probenecid:* May reduce renal clearance and may increase half-life. Don't give together with probenecid to extend half-life.

Valproic acid: May decrease valproic acid level, leading to loss of seizure control. Monitor valproic acid level, and observe patient for signs of seizure activity. Use of carbapenems with valproic acid/divalproex sodium is generally not recommended.

EFFECTS ON LAB TEST RESULTS

• May increase albumin, ALT, alkaline phosphatase, AST, bilirubin, creatinine, glucose, and potassium levels. May decrease Hb level and hematocrit.

• May increase eosinophil count, urine RBC count, or urine WBC count. May prolong PT. May decrease segmented neutrophil and serum WBC counts. May increase or decrease platelet count.

E

CONTRAINDICATIONS & CAUTIONS
• Contraindicated in patients hypersensitive to components of the drug or to other drugs in the same class and in patients who have had anaphylactic reactions to beta-lactams.
• IM use is contraindicated in patients hypersensitive to local anesthetics of the amide type because of the use of lidocaine as the diluent.
• Drug may cause CDAD, ranging in severity from mild to fatal colitis, which may occur during treatment or more than 2 months after treatment. Drug may need to be discontinued if CDAD is suspected.
• Use cautiously in patients with CNS disorders, elderly patients, and those with compromised renal function, as toxic reactions may occur in these patients.
Dialyzable drug: Yes.
⚠ *Overdose S&S:* Nausea, diarrhea, dizziness.

PREGNANCY-LACTATION-REPRODUCTION
• There are no well-controlled studies in pregnant women. Use during pregnancy only if clearly needed.
• Drug appears in human milk. Use cautiously and only when expected benefit outweighs risk.

NURSING CONSIDERATIONS
• If patient has diarrhea during therapy, notify prescriber and collect stool specimen for culture to rule out CDAD.
• Vomiting occurs more frequently in children than adults. Monitor children closely for signs and symptoms of dehydration and electrolyte imbalance.
• If allergic reaction occurs, stop drug immediately.
• Anaphylactic reactions require immediate emergency treatment with epinephrine, oxygen, IV steroids, and airway management.
• Anticonvulsants may continue in patients with seizure disorders. If focal tremors, myoclonus, or seizures occur, notify prescriber. Drug may need to be decreased or stopped.
• Monitor renal, hepatic, and hematopoietic function during prolonged therapy.
• MRSA and *Enterococcus* species are resistant to drug.
• *Look alike–sound alike:* Don't confuse INVanz with AVINza.

PATIENT TEACHING
• Tell patient to report all adverse reactions.
• Tell patient to alert nurse if discomfort occurs at injection site.
• Tell patient to report diarrhea as soon as possible.

SAFETY ALERT!

ertugliflozin
er-too-gli-FLOE-zin

Steglatro

Therapeutic class: Antidiabetics
Pharmacologic class: Sodium-glucose cotransporter 2 inhibitors

AVAILABLE FORMS
Tablets: 5 mg, 15 mg

INDICATIONS & DOSAGES
➤ **Adjunct to diet and exercise to improve glycemic control in patients with type 2 diabetes mellitus**
Adults: 5 mg PO once daily in the morning. May increase to 15 mg once daily.
Adjust-a-dose: Initiation of therapy and continued use isn't recommended in patients with an eGFR persistently 30 to less than 60 mL/minute/1.73 m^2.

ADMINISTRATION
PO
• May give with or without food.
• If a dose is missed, give it as soon as possible. If it's almost time for the next dose, skip the missed dose and give at the next regularly scheduled time. Don't give two doses at the same time.
• Store in a dry place at controlled room temperature (68° to 77° F [20° to 25° C]).

ACTION
Increases the amount of urinary glucose excreted by inhibiting sodium-glucose cotransporter 2 (SGLT2), which reabsorbs glucose through the kidneys.

Route	Onset	Peak	Duration
PO	Unknown	1–2 hr	Unknown

Half-life: 16.6 hours.

Reactions in bold italics are *life-threatening*. Interactions may have a *rapid onset* or a *delayed onset*.

ADVERSE REACTIONS

CNS: headache, postural dizziness, presyncope, syncope. **EENT:** nasopharyngitis.
CV: hypotension, orthostatic hypotension.
GI: thirst. **GU:** genital fungal infections, UTI, vaginal pruritus, increased urination, renal impairment, acute kidney injury, acute prerenal failure. **Hematologic:** volume depletion, increased Hb level. **Metabolic:** weight loss, *hypoglycemia*. **Musculoskeletal:** back pain.

INTERACTIONS

Drug-drug. *ACE inhibitors (enalapril, lisinopril), ARBs (candesartan, losartan, valsartan), diuretics, NSAIDs:* May increase risk of acute kidney injury. Monitor patient closely and use together cautiously.
Insulin, insulin secretagogues (glipizide, repaglinide): May increase risk of hypoglycemia. Consider lower dosage of insulin or insulin secretagogue.

EFFECTS ON LAB TEST RESULTS

• May increase serum creatinine, LDL-C, phosphate, and Hb levels.
• Causes false-positive urine glucose tests. Use alternative methods to monitor glycemic control.
• May cause unreliable 1,5-AG assay results. Use alternative methods to monitor glycemic control.

CONTRAINDICATIONS & CAUTIONS

• Contraindicated in patients hypersensitive to drug or its components and in patients with severe renal impairment (eGFR less than 30 mL/minute/1.73 m^2) or ESRD, or on dialysis.
• Drug isn't indicated in patients with type 1 diabetes mellitus or for the treatment of ketoacidosis.
• Use in patients with severe hepatic impairment isn't recommended.
• Use cautiously in patients with an eGFR less than 60 mL/minute/1.73 m^2, in patients with low systolic BP, and in patients on diuretics as these patients are at increased risk for hypotension due to the intravascular volume contraction effect of drug.
• Drug isn't recommended in patients whose eGFR is persistently 30 to 60 mL/minute/1.73 m^2. Drug increases serum

creatinine level and decreases eGFR. More frequent renal function monitoring is recommended if drug is used in these patients.
• Use cautiously in patients with pancreatic insulin deficiency, calorie-restricted individuals, and patients with a history of alcohol abuse as ketoacidosis is more likely to occur in these individuals.
• Use cautiously in patients with hypovolemia, chronic renal insufficiency, or HF as renal impairment and acute kidney injury can occur.
• Drug may increase risk of serious UTIs, including urosepsis and pyelonephritis.
• Use cautiously in patients with a history of prior amputation, peripheral vascular disease, neuropathy, and diabetic foot ulcers as studies have shown an increased risk of lower limb amputation with another SGLT2 inhibitor.
• Safety and effectiveness in children haven't been established.
• Use cautiously in elderly patients, who may be more at risk for hypovolemia and hypotension.
⚠ Alert: SGLT2 inhibitors increase risk of a rare but serious necrotizing fasciitis of the perineum, also known as Fournier gangrene. If necrotizing fasciitis is suspected, immediately discontinue the SGLT2 inhibitor and begin broad-spectrum antibiotics. Surgical debridement may be necessary. Monitor blood glucose levels and start alternative therapy for glycemic control.
Dialyzable drug: Unknown.

PREGNANCY-LACTATION-REPRODUCTION

• Drug may cause adverse renal effects; use isn't recommended during second and third trimesters.
• There are no data regarding the presence of drug in human milk, the effects on the breastfed infant, or the effects on milk production. Because of the potential for serious adverse reactions in breastfed infants, patients shouldn't breastfeed during therapy.

NURSING CONSIDERATIONS

• Correct fluid volume depletion before starting drug, if clinically indicated.
• Monitor patients for signs and symptoms of acute kidney injury. Assess renal function

at baseline and periodically throughout therapy.

• Monitor patients for hypotension during therapy.

• Monitor patients for signs and symptoms of UTI and treat promptly if indicated.

• Monitor patients for signs and symptoms of genital mycotic infections, especially uncircumcised males and patients with a history of genital mycotic infections. Treat promptly.

❸ Alert: Watch for and immediately report signs and symptoms of necrotizing fasciitis of the perineum (temperature above 100.4° F [38° C], general feeling of being unwell, tenderness, redness, or swelling of the genitals back to the rectum). Signs and symptoms can worsen quickly. Immediately discontinue drug and prepare to administer broad-spectrum antibiotics.

• Monitor blood glucose level. Assess for signs and symptoms of hypoglycemia.

• Monitor patients for ketoacidosis (dehydration, severe metabolic acidosis, nausea, vomiting, abdominal pain, generalized malaise, shortness of breath), even patients with glucose levels less than 250 mg/dL. Discontinue drug if ketoacidosis is suspected and treat appropriately.

• Consider temporarily discontinuing therapy in patients with reduced oral intake (such as acute illness or prolonged fasting for surgery) or fluid losses (such as GI illness or excessive heat exposure), as renal impairment and acute kidney injury can occur.

• Because of drug's mechanism of action, urinary glucose tests will be positive.

• Drug may increase LDL-C. Assess periodically and treat if clinically indicated.

• Monitor patients for signs and symptoms of infection, new pain or tenderness, and sores or ulcers of the lower limbs. Treat as indicated; discontinue drug if these complications occur.

• **Look alike–sound alike:** Don't confuse ertugliflozin with canagliflozin, dapagliflozin, or empagliflozin. Don't confuse Steglatro with Segluromet or Steglujan.

PATIENT TEACHING

• Stress importance of adherence to dietary instructions, regular physical activity,

periodic blood glucose monitoring, and HbA$_{1c}$ testing.

• Advise patient to report all adverse reactions.

• Teach patient how to recognize and manage hypoglycemia and hyperglycemia, and to watch for diabetic complications.

• Advise patient to seek medical advice promptly during periods of stress, such as fever, trauma, infection, or surgery, as drug requirements may change.

• Instruct patient that if a dose is missed, to take it as soon as it's remembered unless it's almost time for the next dose, in which case patient should skip the missed dose and take drug at the next regularly scheduled time. Advise patient not to take two doses at the same time.

• Caution patient to avoid dehydration, which can cause hypotension. Instruct patient to maintain adequate fluid intake and to report signs and symptoms of hypotension (postural dizziness, weakness, syncope).

• Warn patient to immediately report signs and symptoms of ketoacidosis (nausea, vomiting, abdominal pain, tiredness, and labored breathing).

• Inform patient that acute kidney injury has been reported and to immediately report reduced oral intake (due to acute illness or fasting) or increased fluid losses (due to vomiting, diarrhea, or excessive heat exposure), as ertugliflozin may need to be temporarily discontinued.

• Advise patient that laboratory monitoring of renal function will be needed.

• Teach patient signs and symptoms of UTIs (changes in urination, frequent urination, burning with urination) and to seek medical attention if they occur.

• Inform patient of the increased risk of amputation. Counsel patient about the importance of routine preventive foot care.

• Instruct patient to watch for and immediately report new pain or tenderness, sores or ulcers, or infections involving the leg or foot.

• Teach patient to recognize and report signs and symptoms of genital yeast infections (redness or rash of the glans or foreskin of the penis or vulva, burning with urination, discharge).

Reactions in bold italics are *life-threatening*. Interactions may have a *rapid onset* or a *delayed onset*.

◑ *Alert:* Teach patient signs and symptoms of necrotizing fasciitis and to seek immediate medical attention if any of these signs and symptoms occur.

• Advise pregnant patient of the potential risk to a fetus and to immediately inform prescriber if she becomes pregnant or is planning to become pregnant.

• Advise female patient not to breastfeed during therapy.

• Inform patient that urine will test positive for glucose during therapy.

SAFETY ALERT!

ertugliflozin–metformin hydrochloride
er-too-gli-FLOE-zin/met-FORE-min

Segluromet

Therapeutic class: Antidiabetics
Pharmacologic class: Sodium-glucose cotransporter 2 inhibitors–biguanides

AVAILABLE FORMS
Tablets: 2.5 mg ertugliflozin/500 mg metformin hydrochloride; 2.5 mg ertugliflozin/1,000 mg metformin hydrochloride; 7.5 mg ertugliflozin/500 mg metformin hydrochloride; 7.5 mg ertugliflozin/1,000 mg metformin hydrochloride

INDICATIONS & DOSAGES
➤ **Adjunct to diet and exercise to improve glycemic control in patients with type 2 diabetes mellitus who aren't adequately controlled on a regimen containing ertugliflozin or metformin, or in patients who are already treated with both ertugliflozin and metformin**
Adults: In patients taking metformin, switch to tablets containing 2.5 mg ertugliflozin with a similar total daily dose of current metformin regimen and give PO in divided doses b.i.d. In patients taking ertugliflozin, switch to tablets containing 500 mg metformin with a similar total daily dose of current ertugliflozin regimen and give PO in divided doses b.i.d. In patients taking ertugliflozin and metformin, switch to tablets containing the same total daily dose of current ertugliflozin regimen and a similar daily dose of current metformin regimen and give PO in divided doses b.i.d. Gradually escalate dose based on effectiveness and tolerability to a maximum daily dose of 15 mg ertugliflozin and 2,000 mg metformin.

ADMINISTRATION
PO
• Give with meals.

• If a dose is missed, give dose as soon as it's remembered. If it's almost time for the next dose, skip the missed dose and give drug at the next regularly scheduled time. Don't give two doses at the same time.

• Store at controlled room temperature (68° to 77° F [20° to 25° C]). Excursions to 59° to 86° F (15° to 30° C) are allowed.

• Protect from moisture; store in a dry place.

ACTION
Ertugliflozin increases the amount of urinary glucose excreted by inhibiting sodium-glucose cotransporter 2 (SGLT2), which reabsorbs glucose through the kidneys. Metformin decreases hepatic glucose production and intestinal absorption of glucose and improves insulin sensitivity by increasing peripheral glucose uptake and utilization.

Route	Onset	Peak	Duration
PO (ertugliflozin)	Unknown	1–2 hr	Unknown
PO (metformin hydrochloride)	Unknown	2–3 hr	Unknown

Half-life: Ertugliflozin, 16.6 hours; metformin hydrochloride, 6.2 hours.

ADVERSE REACTIONS
CNS: headache, asthenia. **CV:** hypotension. **EENT:** nasopharyngitis. **GI:** thirst, diarrhea, nausea, vomiting, flatulence, abdominal discomfort, indigestion. **GU:** genital fungal infections, UTI, vaginal pruritus, increased urination, renal impairment. **Metabolic:** volume depletion, weight loss, increased LDL level, *hypoglycemia, lactic acidosis.* **Musculoskeletal:** back pain.

INTERACTIONS
Drug-drug. *Calcium channel blockers, corticosteroids, estrogens, isoniazid, nicotinic acid, oral contraceptives, phenothiazines, phenytoin, sympathomimetics, thiazides and other diuretics, thyroid products:* May

increase hyperglycemia and lead to loss of glycemic control. Closely monitor glycemic control.

Black Box Warning *Carbonic anhydrase inhibitors (acetazolamide, dichlorphenamide, topiramate, zonisamide):* May increase risk of lactic acidosis. Consider more frequent monitoring of patient. ▪

Drugs that reduce metformin clearance (cimetidine, dolutegravir, ranolazine, vandetanib): May increase systemic exposure to metformin and risk of lactic acidosis. Consider benefits and risks of concomitant use.

Insulin, insulin secretagogues (sulfonylurea): May increase risk of hypoglycemia. Lower insulin or insulin secretagogue dosages may be needed.

Black Box Warning *Radiologic contrast dye:* May cause acute decrease in renal function and increase risk of lactic acidosis. Stop drug at the time of, or before, an iodinated contrast imaging procedure in patients with an eGFR of less than 60 mL/minute/1.73 m^2. Reevaluate eGFR 48 hours after imaging procedure. May restart drug if renal function is stable. ▪

Drug-lifestyle. **Black Box Warning** *Alcohol use (excessive):* May increase risk of lactic acidosis. Discourage use together. ▪

EFFECTS ON LAB TEST RESULTS

• May increase serum creatinine, LDL-C, phosphate, and Hb levels.

• May decrease vitamin B_{12} level and eGFR.

• May cause unreliable 1,5-AG assay results and false-positive urine glucose test results.

CONTRAINDICATIONS & CAUTIONS

Black Box Warning Metformin-containing drugs increase the risk of lactic acidosis and can result in hypothermia, hypotension, resistant bradyarrhythmias, and death. If metformin-associated lactic acidosis is suspected, immediately discontinue drug. Prompt hemodialysis is recommended. ▪

Black Box Warning Risk factors for metformin-associated lactic acidosis include renal impairment, use of carbonic anhydrase inhibitors, age 65 and older, radiologic study with contrast, surgery or other procedures, and hypoxic states (HF, MI, sepsis, shock). ▪

Black Box Warning Patients with hepatic impairment are at increased risk for developing metformin-associated lactic acidosis. Avoid use in patients with hepatic disease. ▪

• Contraindicated in patients hypersensitive to ertugliflozin or metformin or its components, in those with severe renal impairment or ESRD, and in patients on dialysis.

• Contraindicated in patients with an eGFR of less than 30 mL/minute/1.73 m^2. Use isn't recommended in patients with an eGFR persistently between 30 and 60 mL/minute/ 1.73 m^2.

• Contraindicated in patients with acute or chronic metabolic acidosis, including diabetic ketoacidosis, with or without coma.

• Drug isn't indicated for patients with type 1 diabetes or for treatment of diabetic ketoacidosis.

• Use cautiously in patients with an eGFR of less than 60 mL/minute/1.73 m^2, in patients age 65 or older, in patients with low systolic BP, and in patients on diuretics, as intravascular volume contraction and hypotension can occur. Correct hypovolemia before starting drug.

• Use cautiously in patients with pancreatic insulin deficiency, calorie-restricted patients, and patients with a history of alcohol abuse, as ketoacidosis is more likely to occur.

• Use cautiously in patients with hypovolemia, chronic renal insufficiency, or congestive HF and in those receiving concomitant diuretic, ACE inhibitor, ARB, or NSAID therapy, as renal impairment and acute kidney injury can occur.

• If acute kidney injury occurs, discontinue drug and begin treatment.

• Use cautiously in patients with a history of prior amputation, peripheral vascular disease, neuropathy, and diabetic foot ulcers, as an increased risk of lower limb amputation (primarily of the toe) was observed in clinical studies with another SGLT2 inhibitor.

• Use cautiously in patients with a history of genital mycotic infections and in uncircumcised patients, as they are more likely to develop genital mycotic infections.

🔴 *Alert:* SGLT2 inhibitors increase risk of a rare but serious necrotizing fasciitis of the perineum, also known as Fournier gangrene.

Reactions in bold italics are *life-threatening*. Interactions may have a *rapid onset* or a *delayed onset*.

If necrotizing fasciitis is suspected, immediately discontinue the SGLT2 drug and begin broad-spectrum antibiotics. Surgical debridement may be necessary. Monitor blood glucose levels and start alternative therapy for glycemic control.

• Use cautiously in patients with inadequate vitamin B_{12} or calcium intake or absorption. Drug may decrease vitamin B_{12} level. Monitor vitamin B_{12} levels every 2 to 3 years in these high-risk patients; monitor hematologic parameters annually in all patients to assess for anemia.

• Safety and effectiveness in children haven't been established.

Dialyzable drug: Ertugliflozin, unknown; metformin hydrochloride, yes.

⚠ *Overdose S&S:* Hypoglycemia, lactic acidosis.

PREGNANCY-LACTATION-REPRODUCTION

• Drug isn't recommended during the second and third trimesters, as animal studies suggest increased risk of adverse renal effects from ertugliflozin.

• It isn't known if ertugliflozin appears in human milk or how drug affects the breastfed infant or milk production. Metformin is present in human milk. Because of the potential for serious adverse reactions in infants, patients shouldn't breastfeed.

• Metformin may cause ovulation in some premenopausal anovulatory women. Advise women of the potential for unintended pregnancy.

NURSING CONSIDERATIONS

• Correct volume depletion before start of treatment. Monitor patients for signs and symptoms of hypotension after initiating therapy.

• Monitor patients for signs and symptoms of acute kidney injury, and assess renal function, including eGFR, at baseline and periodically throughout therapy.

• Monitor patients for signs and symptoms of genital mycotic infections; treat promptly if indicated.

❸ *Alert:* Watch for and immediately report signs and symptoms of necrotizing fasciitis of the perineum (temperature above 100.4° F [38° C], general feeling of being unwell, tenderness, redness, or swelling of

the genitals back to the rectum). Signs and symptoms can worsen quickly. Immediately discontinue drug and prepare to administer broad-spectrum antibiotics.

• Monitor blood glucose level. Assess for signs and symptoms of hypoglycemia.

• Drug may increase LDL-C level. Assess periodically and treat if clinically indicated.

• Monitor patients for signs and symptoms of infection, osteomyelitis, new pain, and ulcers of the lower limbs. Discontinue drug if these occur.

• Monitor patients for peripheral vascular disease, neuropathy, and diabetic foot ulcers. Treat as indicated.

• Postmarketing reports of serious UTIs and urosepsis have occurred. Monitor patients for signs and symptoms of UTIs and treat promptly.

Black Box Warning Monitor patients for signs and symptoms of metformin-associated lactic acidosis (hypothermia, hypotension, resistant bradyarrhythmias), including subtle, nonspecific signs and symptoms (dehydration, nausea, vomiting, malaise, myalgia, abdominal pain, respiratory distress, increased somnolence) and laboratory abnormalities (elevated blood lactate levels, anion gap acidosis, increased lactate/pyruvate ratios, metformin level greater than 5 mcg/mL). Treat suspected lactic acidosis as clinically indicated and immediately discontinue drug. Hemodialysis may reverse symptoms and lead to recovery. ■

❸ *Alert:* Drug may need to be temporarily discontinued during times of reduced oral intake of food and fluids (such as surgery, acute illness or fasting, fluid losses from GI illness or excessive heat exposure). Renal impairment and acute kidney injury can occur.

• Don't use urine tests to monitor glycemic control.

• *Look alike–sound alike:* Don't confuse ertugliflozin with canagliflozin, dapagliflozin, or empagliflozin. Don't confuse Segluromet with Steglatro or Steglujan.

PATIENT TEACHING

Black Box Warning Inform patient of the risks of lactic acidosis due to the metformin component. Teach patient the signs and symptoms of lactic acidosis and conditions that predispose to lactic acidosis. Advise patient to discontinue drug immediately and report unexplained hyperventilation, malaise, myalgia, unusual somnolence, slow or irregular heartbeat, sensation of feeling cold (especially in the extremities), or other nonspecific symptoms. Stress importance of adhering to dietary instructions, regular physical activity, periodic blood glucose and HbA_{1c} monitoring, and renal function testing. ■

• Teach patient to report all adverse reactions.

• Teach patient how to recognize and manage hypoglycemia and hyperglycemia, and to watch for diabetic complications.

• Advise patient to promptly seek medical advice during periods of stress (such as fever, trauma, infection, or surgery), as drug requirements may change.

• Caution patient to avoid dehydration, which can cause hypotension. Instruct patient to maintain adequate fluid intake and to immediately report signs and symptoms of hypotension (postural dizziness, weakness, temporary loss of consciousness).

• Instruct patient to seek immediate medical advice if signs and symptoms of ketoacidosis (nausea, vomiting, abdominal pain, tiredness, labored breathing) occur.

• Inform patient that acute kidney injury has been reported and to seek medical advice immediately if reduced oral intake (due to acute illness or fasting) or increased fluid losses (due to vomiting, diarrhea, or excessive heat exposure) occur, as drug may need to be temporarily discontinued.

• Instruct patient to recognize and immediately report signs and symptoms of UTIs (abdominal, pelvic, or back pain; frequent urination; burning with urination; fever; nausea; vomiting).

• Inform patient that drug may increase the risk of amputations. Stress importance of routine preventive foot care. Instruct patient to watch for and immediately report new pain or tenderness, sores or ulcers, or infections involving the leg or foot.

• Tell patient to report signs and symptoms of genital yeast infections (itching, redness, rash, discharge, genital pain).

◗ **Alert:** Teach patient signs and symptoms of necrotizing fasciitis and to seek immediate medical attention if any of these signs and symptoms occur.

• Inform patient that urine glucose tests shouldn't be used for monitoring glycemic control during therapy because patient's urine will test positive for glucose.

• Advise female patient of the potential risk to a fetus and to immediately tell prescriber if she is pregnant or plans to become pregnant.

• Advise female patient not to breastfeed during therapy.

• Inform premenopausal patient who is anovulatory that metformin therapy may result in ovulation.

SAFETY ALERT!

ertugliflozin–sitagliptin
er-TOO-gli-FLOE-zin/sit-a-GLIP-tin

Steglujan

Therapeutic class: Antidiabetics
Pharmacologic class: Sodium-glucose cotransporter 2 inhibitors–DPP-4 enzyme inhibitors

AVAILABLE FORMS
Tablets: 5 mg ertugliflozin/100 mg sitagliptin; 15 mg ertugliflozin/100 mg sitagliptin

INDICATIONS & DOSAGES
➤ **Adjunct to diet and exercise to improve glycemic control in adults with type 2 diabetes mellitus when treatment with both ertugliflozin and sitagliptin is appropriate**
Adults: Initially, 5 mg ertugliflozin/100 mg sitagliptin PO once daily in the morning. May increase to a maximum dose of 15 mg/100 mg PO once daily if drug is tolerated and additional glycemic control is needed. For patients already treated with ertugliflozin, maintain current ertugliflozin dose when switching to combination product.

ADMINISTRATION
PO
• May give with or without food.

E

• If a dose is missed, give it as soon as it's remembered. If it's almost time for the next dose, skip the missed dose and give drug at the next regularly scheduled time. Don't give two doses at the same time.
• Store at room temperature 68° to 77° F (20° to 25° C).

ACTION
Ertugliflozin increases the amount of urinary glucose excreted by inhibiting sodium-glucose cotransporter 2 (SGLT2), which reabsorbs glucose through the kidneys. Sitagliptin inhibits DPP-4. By increasing and prolonging active incretin levels, sitagliptin helps increase insulin release and decrease circulating glucose.

Route	Onset	Peak	Duration
PO (ertugliflozin)	Unknown	1–2 hr	Unknown
PO (sitagliptin)	Rapid	1–4 hr	Unknown

Half-life: Ertugliflozin, 16.6 hours; sitagliptin, 12.4 hours.

ADVERSE REACTIONS
CNS: headache, dizziness, presyncope, syncope. **CV:** peripheral edema, hypotension. **EENT:** nasopharyngitis. **GI:** thirst, abdominal pain, nausea, diarrhea. **GU:** genital fungal infections, UTI, vaginal pruritus, increased urination, renal impairment. **Hematologic:** volume depletion, increased Hb level. **Metabolic:** weight loss, increased LDL-C level, *hypoglycemia,* hyperphosphatemia. **Musculoskeletal:** back pain. **Respiratory:** URI.

INTERACTIONS
Drug-drug. *ACE inhibitors, ARBs, diuretics, NSAIDs:* May increase risk of renal impairment and acute kidney injury. Use cautiously together.
Digoxin: May increase digoxin concentration. Monitor digoxin level.
Insulin, insulin secretagogues: May increase risk of hypoglycemia. Consider lower insulin or insulin secretagogue dosage.

EFFECTS ON LAB TEST RESULTS
• May increase serum creatinine, LDL-C, phosphate, digoxin, and Hb levels.
• May decrease eGFR.

• May cause false-positive urine glucose tests and unreliable 1,5-AG assay results.

CONTRAINDICATIONS & CAUTIONS
• Contraindicated in patients hypersensitive to sitagliptin, ertugliflozin, or components of product, in patients with severe renal impairment (eGFR less than 30 mL/minute/1.73 m^2) or ESRD, and in patients on dialysis.
• Rare but serious allergic and hypersensitivity reactions, such as anaphylaxis, angioedema, and exfoliative skin conditions including SJS, have been reported with sitagliptin and other DPP-4 inhibitors. If reactions occur, discontinue drug and begin appropriate monitoring and treatment.
• Drug isn't for treatment of patients with type 1 diabetes mellitus or diabetic ketoacidosis.
• Drug hasn't been studied in patients with a history of pancreatitis. There are postmarketing reports of acute pancreatitis, including fatal and nonfatal hemorrhagic or necrotizing pancreatitis, in patients taking sitagliptin. It's unknown if a history of pancreatitis increases risk of sitagliptin-related pancreatitis.
• Drug may increase risk of symptomatic hypotension from intravascular volume contraction. Use cautiously in patients with impaired renal function (eGFR less than 60 mL/minute/1.73 m^2) or preexisting hypotension and in those age 65 and older.
• Drug isn't recommended in patients with eGFR persistently between 30 and 60 mL/minute/1.73 m^2. Drug increases serum creatinine level and decreases eGFR. More frequent monitoring is recommended in these patients.
• HF has occurred with other DPP-4 inhibitors. Before starting drug, consider risks and benefits of therapy in patients with known risk factors for HF.
• Serious and life-threatening ketoacidosis has been reported in patients taking SGLT2 inhibitors and in patients taking ertugliflozin. If ketoacidosis is suspected, discontinue drug, evaluate patient, and treated promptly. In some cases, risk factors for ketoacidosis (insulin dosage reduction, acute febrile illness, reduced calorie intake due to illness or surgery, pancreatic insulin deficiency, or alcohol abuse) were identified.

• Use cautiously in patients with hypovolemia, chronic renal insufficiency, and congestive HF as drug may increase risk of renal impairment and acute kidney injury.

• Use cautiously in patients with a history of prior amputation, peripheral vascular disease, neuropathy, and diabetic foot ulcers as an increased risk of lower limb amputation (primarily of the toe) was observed in clinical studies with another SGLT2 inhibitor.

• Use cautiously in patients with a history of genital mycotic infections and in uncircumcised male patients as they are more likely to develop genital mycotic infections.

❸ *Alert:* SGLT2 inhibitors increase risk of a rare but serious necrotizing fasciitis of the perineum, also known as Fournier gangrene. If necrotizing fasciitis is suspected, immediately discontinue the drug and begin broad-spectrum antibiotics. Surgical debridement may be necessary. Monitor blood glucose levels and start alternative therapy for glycemic control.

• Drug may increase risk of severe and disabling arthralgia, which may occur soon after therapy begins or years later. If disabling joint pain occurs, discontinue drug if appropriate.

• Postmarketing cases of bullous pemphigoid requiring hospitalization have been reported.

• Safety and effectiveness in children haven't been determined.

Dialyzable drug: Ertugliflozin, unknown; sitagliptin, 13.5%.

PREGNANCY-LACTATION-REPRODUCTION

• Drug isn't recommended during the second and third trimesters, as animal studies suggest increased risk of adverse renal effects from ertugliflozin.

• Report prenatal exposure to drug to the Merck Pregnancy Registry (1-800-986-8999).

• It isn't known if drug appears in human milk or how drug affects the breastfed infant or milk production. Because of the potential for serious adverse reactions in breastfed infants, patient shouldn't breastfeed during therapy.

NURSING CONSIDERATIONS

• Assess for volume depletion at baseline and correct fluid balance before initiating therapy.

• Monitor patients for signs and symptoms of acute kidney injury. Assess renal function at baseline and periodically during therapy.

• Monitor patients for symptomatic hypotension.

• Monitor patients for HF.

• Postmarketing reports of serious UTIs and urosepsis have occurred. Monitor patients for signs and symptoms of UTIs and treat promptly.

❸ *Alert:* Drug may need to be temporarily discontinued during times of reduced oral intake of food or fluids (such as acute illness or fasting, fluid losses due to GI illness or excessive heat exposure), as renal impairment and acute kidney injury can occur.

• Monitor patients for signs and symptoms of UTIs, urosepsis, and pyelonephritis; treat promptly if indicated.

• Monitor patients for signs and symptoms of genital mycotic infections; treat promptly if indicated.

❸ *Alert:* Watch for and immediately report signs and symptoms of necrotizing fasciitis of the perineum (temperature above 100.4° F [38° C], general feeling of being unwell, tenderness, redness, or swelling of the genitals back to the rectum). Signs and symptoms can worsen quickly. Immediately discontinue drug and prepare to administer broad-spectrum antibiotics.

• Monitor blood glucose level. Assess for signs and symptoms of hypoglycemia.

• Drug may increase LDL-C level. Assess periodically and treat if clinically indicated.

• Monitor patients for signs and symptoms of infection, osteomyelitis, new pain, and ulcers of the lower limbs. Discontinue drug if these occur.

• Monitor patients for PVD, neuropathy, and diabetic foot ulcers. Treat as indicated.

• Monitor patients for acute pancreatitis. If pancreatitis is suspected, promptly discontinue drug and treat appropriately.

• Monitor patients for signs and symptoms of HF. If HF develops, treat as clinically indicated; drug may need to be discontinued.

• Monitor patients for serious allergic and hypersensitivity reactions. If reactions occur,

---

discontinue drug and institute appropriate monitoring and treatment.

• Monitor patients for arthralgia. If severe joint pain occurs, drug may need to be discontinued.

• Monitor patients for blisters or erosions, as this may indicate bullous pemphigoid. If bullous pemphigoid is suspected, discontinue drug and refer patient to a dermatologist for diagnosis and treatment.

• Urine tests shouldn't be used to monitor glycemic control.

• *Look alike–sound alike:* Don't confuse ertugliflozin with canagliflozin, dapagliflozin, or empagliflozin. Don't confuse sitagliptin with saxagliptin, linagliptin, or alogliptin. Don't confuse Steglujan with Steglatro or Segluromet.

PATIENT TEACHING

• Advise patient to report all adverse reactions.

• Stress importance of adhering to dietary instructions, regular physical activity, periodic blood glucose and HbA$_{1c}$ monitoring, and renal function testing.

• Teach patient how to recognize and manage hypoglycemia and hyperglycemia, and to watch for diabetic complications. Caution patient that use with insulin and insulin secretagogues may increase the risk of hypoglycemia.

• Advise patient to discontinue drug and seek immediate medical attention for allergic reactions (rash; hives; swelling of the face, lips, tongue, and throat; difficulty swallowing or breathing).

• Advise patient to promptly seek medical advice during periods of stress (such as fever, trauma, infection, or surgery), as drug requirements may change.

• Caution patient to avoid dehydration, which can cause hypotension. Instruct patient regarding adequate fluid intake and to report signs and symptoms of hypotension (postural dizziness, weakness, temporary loss of consciousness).

• Instruct patient to immediately seek medical advice if signs and symptoms of ketoacidosis (nausea, vomiting, abdominal pain, tiredness, and labored breathing) occur.

• Inform patient that acute kidney injury has been reported and to immediately seek

medical advice if reduced oral intake (due to acute illness or fasting) or increased fluid losses (due to vomiting, diarrhea, or excessive heat exposure) occur, as drug may need to be temporarily discontinued.

• Advise patient to immediately report symptoms of HF (increasing shortness of breath, rapid increase in weight, or swelling of the feet).

• Advise patient that acute pancreatitis can occur. Tell patient to discontinue drug and immediately report severe, persistent abdominal pain that may radiate to the back, with or without vomiting.

• Instruct patient to recognize and immediately report signs and symptoms of UTIs (abdominal, pelvic, or back pain; frequent urination; burning with urination; fever; nausea; vomiting).

• Inform patient of the increased risk of amputations. Counsel patient about the importance of routine preventive foot care.

• Instruct patient to watch for and immediately report new pain or tenderness, sores or ulcers, or infections involving the leg or foot.

• Advise patient that arthralgia can occur at any time during treatment and to report severe joint pain to prescriber.

• Advise patient that bullous pemphigoid requiring hospitalization can occur and to immediately report blisters or skin erosions.

• Tell patient to report signs and symptoms of genital yeast infections (itching, redness, rash, discharge, genital pain).

🔵 *Alert:* Teach patient signs and symptoms of necrotizing fasciitis and to seek immediate medical attention if any of these signs and symptoms occur.

• Inform patient that urine glucose tests shouldn't be used for monitoring glycemic control during therapy because patient's urine will test positive for glucose.

• Advise female patient of the potential risk to a fetus and to immediately tell prescriber if she is pregnant or plans to become pregnant.

• Advise female patient not to breastfeed during therapy.

erythromycin (ophthalmic, topical)
er-ith-roe-MYE-sin

Erygel, Ery 2% Pads

Therapeutic class: Antibiotics
Pharmacologic class: Macrolides

AVAILABLE FORMS
Ointment: 2%
Ophthalmic ointment: 0.5%
Topical gel: 2%
Topical pad: 2%
Topical solution: 2%*

INDICATIONS & DOSAGES
➤ **Acute and chronic conjunctivitis, other eye infections (ophthalmic ointment)**
Adults and children: Apply a ribbon of ointment about 1 cm long directly to infected eye up to six times daily, depending on severity of infection.
➤ **To prevent ophthalmia neonatorum caused by** *Neisseria gonorrhoeae* **or** *Chlamydia trachomatis* **(ophthalmic ointment)**
Neonates: Apply a ribbon of ointment about 1 cm long in lower conjunctival sac of each eye shortly after birth.
➤ **Inflammatory acne vulgaris (topical gel, topical pads, topical solution)**
Adults and children: Apply to affected areas b.i.d., morning and evening. If no improvement in 6 to 8 weeks, discontinue drug; prescriber should reevaluate treatment.

ADMINISTRATION
Ophthalmic
• Don't use for infection unless causative organism has been identified.
• To prevent ophthalmia neonatorum, apply ointment no later than 1 hour after birth. Use drug in neonates born either vaginally or by cesarean birth. Gently massage eyelids for 1 minute to spread ointment. Use new tube for each neonate.
Topical
• Wash, rinse, and pat affected areas dry before application.
• Wash hands after each application.

• Avoid contact with eyes, nose, mouth, other mucous membranes, and broken skin.

ACTION
Inhibits protein synthesis; usually bacteriostatic, but may be bactericidal in high concentrations or against highly susceptible organisms.

Route	Onset	Peak	Duration
Ophthalmic, topical	Unknown	Unknown	Unknown

Half-life: Unknown.

ADVERSE REACTIONS
EENT: minor ocular irritations, redness.
Skin: burning, dryness, pruritus, erythema, irritation, oily skin, peeling, sensitivity reactions. **Other:** hypersensitivity reactions.

INTERACTIONS
Drug-drug. *Clindamycin (topical):* Topical erythromycin may antagonize clindamycin's effect. Avoid using together.
Drug-lifestyle. *Abrasive or medicated soaps or cleansers, acne products or other preparations containing peeling drugs (benzoyl peroxide, resorcinol, salicylic acid, sulfur, tretinoin), alcohol-containing products (aftershave, cosmetics, perfumed toiletries, shaving creams or lotions), astringent soaps or cosmetics, medicated cosmetics or coverups:* May cause cumulative dryness, resulting in excessive skin irritation. Urge caution.

EFFECTS ON LAB TEST RESULTS
None reported.

CONTRAINDICATIONS & CAUTIONS
• Contraindicated in patients hypersensitive to drug.
• Safety and effectiveness of topical drug in children haven't been established.
Dialyzable drug: Unknown.

PREGNANCY-LACTATION-REPRODUCTION
• Use during pregnancy only if clearly needed. Topical drug may be used to treat acne during pregnancy.
• It isn't known if drug appears in human milk after topical application. Use cautiously in breastfeeding women.

---

*Reactions in bold italics are **life-threatening**. Interactions may have a rapid onset or a delayed onset.*

NURSING CONSIDERATIONS
• Ointment and pads are intended only for treatment of inflammatory acne and not for treatment of superficial skin infections.
• Store ophthalmic drug at room temperature in tightly closed, light-resistant container.
❸ **Alert:** Prolonged topical use may result in fungal or bacterial superinfection, including pseudomembranous colitis and CDAD, during and even 2 months after treatment. Consider these diagnoses in patients who present with diarrhea; stop drug for significant diarrhea, abdominal cramps, or passage of blood or mucus.
• Topical drug may be flammable; keep away from heat and flame.

PATIENT TEACHING
• Tell patient to clean eye area of excessive discharge before ophthalmic application.
• Teach patient how to apply drug and to wash hands before and after applying ointment. Warn patient not to touch tip of applicator to eye or surrounding tissue.
• Tell patient that vision may be blurred for a few minutes after applying ophthalmic ointment. Instruct patient to keep eyes closed for 1 to 2 minutes after applying drug.
• Advise patient to watch for and report signs and symptoms of sensitivity (itching lids, redness, swelling, or constant burning of eyes or skin).
• Tell patient not to share drug, washcloths, or towels with family members and to notify prescriber if anyone develops same signs or symptoms.
• Tell patient to wash hands after each application.
• Stress importance of compliance with recommended therapy.
• Advise patient to wash, rinse, and dry face thoroughly before each topical use.
• Advise patient to avoid topical use near eyes, nose, mouth, or other mucous membranes.
• Tell patient to stop using drug and notify prescriber if condition worsens, or if there is no improvement.
• Caution patient to keep topical drug away from heat and open flame.
• Advise patient to report diarrhea immediately.

erythromycin base
er-ith-roe-MYE-sin

Eryc♦, Ery-Tab♦

erythromycin ethylsuccinate
E.E.S. Granules, EryPed

erythromycin lactobionate
Erythrocin

erythromycin stearate
Erythrocin Stearate

Therapeutic class: Antibiotics
Pharmacologic class: Macrolides

AVAILABLE FORMS
erythromycin base
Capsules (delayed-release): 250 mg
Tablets (delayed-release): 250 mg, 333 mg, 500 mg
Tablets (enteric-coated): 250 mg, 333 mg, 500 mg
erythromycin ethylsuccinate
Oral suspension: 200 mg/5 mL, 400 mg/5 mL
Powder for oral suspension: 200 mg/5 mL, 400 mg/5 mL
Tablets: 400 mg
erythromycin lactobionate
Injection: 500 mg
erythromycin stearate
Tablets (film-coated): 250 mg

INDICATIONS & DOSAGES
➤ **Acute pelvic inflammatory disease caused by *Neisseria gonorrhoeae* in women with a history of penicillin sensitivity**
Adults: 500 mg IV every 6 hours for 3 days; then 500 mg (base) PO every 12 hours, or 333 mg (base) PO every 8 hours, or 250 mg (base) PO every 6 hours for 7 days.
➤ **Intestinal amebiasis caused by *Entamoeba histolytica***
Adults: 500 mg (base or stearate) PO every 12 hours, or 333 mg (base) PO every 8 hours, or 250 mg (base or stearate) PO every 6 hours, or 400 mg (ethylsuccinate) q.i.d. for 10 to 14 days.

Children: 30 to 50 mg/kg PO daily, in divided doses, for 10 to 14 days.

➤ **To prevent rheumatic fever recurrence in patients allergic to penicillin and sulfonamides**

Adults: 250 mg (base or stearate) PO b.i.d., or 400 mg (ethylsuccinate) PO b.i.d.

➤ **Mild to moderately severe respiratory tract, skin, or soft-tissue infection from sensitive group A beta-hemolytic streptococci, *Streptococcus pneumoniae*, *Mycoplasma pneumoniae*, *Corynebacterium diphtheriae*, or *Bordetella pertussis*; *Listeria monocytogenes* infection**

Adults: 250 mg PO every 6 hours, 333 mg PO every 8 hours, or 500 mg PO every 12 hours. Maximum dose is 4 g daily. Or 15 to 20 mg/kg IV daily, as continuous infusion or in divided doses every 6 hours for 10 days (3 weeks for *Mycoplasma* species infection). Maximum dosage is 4 g/day.

Children: 30 to 50 mg/kg PO daily, in divided doses every 6 hours; or 15 to 20 mg/kg IV daily, in divided doses every 4 to 6 hours for 10 days (3 weeks for *Mycoplasma* species infection).

➤ **Nongonococcal urethritis caused by *Ureaplasma urealyticum* when tetracycline is contraindicated or not tolerated**

Adults: 500 mg (base or stearate) PO every 6 hours, or 666 mg (base) PO every 8 hours, or 800 mg (ethylsuccinate) PO every 8 hours for at least 7 days.

➤ **Legionnaires disease**

Adults: 1 to 4 g (base or stearate) or 1.6 to 4 g (ethylsuccinate) PO daily in divided doses for 10 to 14 days alone or with rifampin. IV route may be used initially in severe cases.

➤ **Uncomplicated urethral, endocervical, or rectal infection caused by *Chlamydia trachomatis*, when tetracyclines are contraindicated**

Adults: 500 mg base PO q.i.d. for at least 7 days, or 666 mg PO every 8 hours for at least 7 days, or 250 mg PO q.i.d. for 14 days if patient can't tolerate higher doses.

➤ **Urogenital *C. trachomatis* infection during pregnancy**

Women: 500 mg (base or stearate) PO q.i.d. or 666 mg (base) PO every 8 hours for at least 7 days. Women who can't tolerate this regimen may receive 500 mg (base or stearate) PO every 12 hours, or 333 mg (base) PO every 8 hours, or 250 mg (base or stearate) PO q.i.d. for at least 14 days.

➤ **Conjunctivitis of the newborn caused by *C. trachomatis***

Neonates: 50 mg/kg/day PO in divided doses for at least 2 weeks.

➤ **Pneumonia in infants caused by *C. trachomatis***

Infants: 50 mg/kg/day (base or stearate) PO in four divided doses for 21 days, or 15 to 20 mg/kg/day (lactobionate) IV as a continuous infusion or in four divided doses.

➤ **Pertussis**

Adults: 40 to 50 mg/kg/day PO in divided doses for 5 to 14 days.

➤ **Preoperative prophylaxis for elective colorectal surgery**

Adults: Two 500-mg tablets, three 333-mg tablets, or four 250-mg tablets PO at 1 p.m., 2 p.m., and 11 p.m. on preoperative day 1 before 8 a.m. surgery.

➤ **Primary syphilis**

Adults: 30 to 40 g (base or stearate) PO or 48 to 64 g (ethylsuccinate) PO in divided doses for 10 to 15 days. (CDC guidelines don't recommend erythromycin for this indication.)

ADMINISTRATION
PO

• Obtain specimen for culture and sensitivity tests before giving. Begin therapy while awaiting results.

• When giving suspension, note the concentration.

• Give drug with full glass of water 2 hours before or 2 hours after meals for best absorption.

• Give drug with food if GI upset occurs. Don't give drug with fruit juice. Make sure patient doesn't swallow chewable tablets whole.

• Coated tablets or encapsulated pellets cause less GI upset, so they may be better tolerated by patients who have trouble tolerating drug.

• Protect capsules from moisture and excessive heat.

IV

▼ Obtain specimen for culture and sensitivity tests before giving. Begin therapy while awaiting results.

▼ Reconstitute drug according to manufacturer's directions.

▼ Dilute each 250 mg in at least 100 mL of NSS.

▼ Infuse over 1 hour.

▼ **Incompatibilities:** None listed by manufacturer. Consult a drug incompatibility reference for more information.

ACTION

Inhibits bacterial protein synthesis by binding to the 50S subunit of the ribosome. Bacteriostatic or bactericidal, depending on concentration.

Route	Onset	Peak	Duration
PO	Unknown	½ –4 hr	Unknown
IV	Immediate	2½ hr	Unknown

Half-life: 1½ to 2 hours.

ADVERSE REACTIONS

CNS: fever. **CV:** vein irritation or thrombophlebitis after IV injection, *ventricular arrhythmias.* **GI:** *pseudomembranous colitis,* abdominal pain and cramping, diarrhea, nausea, vomiting. **Hepatic:** hepatic dysfunction. **Skin:** eczema, rash, urticaria. **Other:** *anaphylaxis,* overgrowth of nonsusceptible bacteria or fungi.

INTERACTIONS

Drug-drug. *Azole antifungals (ketoconazole):* May increase erythromycin and antifungal concentrations, leading to increased risk of adverse reactions, including sudden death from cardiac causes. Avoid use together.

Carbamazepine: May inhibit metabolism of carbamazepine, increasing blood level and risk of toxicity. Avoid using together.

Clindamycin, lincomycin: May be antagonistic. Avoid using together.

Clarithromycin: May increase QTc interval and risk of arrhythmias. Avoid use together.

Clopidogrel: May inhibit antiplatelet effect of clopidogrel. Monitor platelet function when starting or stopping erythromycin. Adjust clopidogrel dosage as needed.

Colchicine: May increase colchicine level and risk of colchicine-related adverse reactions. Use cautiously and monitor patient for colchicine-related toxicity.

Cyclosporine: May increase cyclosporine level. Monitor drug level.

Digoxin: May increase digoxin level. Monitor patient for digoxin toxicity.

Dihydroergotamine, ergotamine, pimozide: May increase QTc interval and risk of ventricular arrhythmias. Use together is contraindicated.

Disopyramide: May increase disopyramide level, which may cause arrhythmias and prolonged QT intervals. Monitor ECG.

Fluoroquinolones, *other drugs that prolong the QTc interval (amiodarone, antipsychotics, procainamide, quinidine, sotalol, TCAs):* May have additive effects. Monitor ECG for QTc interval prolongation. Avoid using together, if possible.

HMG-CoA reductase inhibitors (lovastatin, simvastatin): May increase concentrations of HMG-CoA reductase inhibitors; rhabdomyolysis has occurred rarely. Monitor CK and serum transaminase levels.

Midazolam, triazolam: May increase effects of these drugs. Monitor patient closely.

Oral anticoagulants: May increase anticoagulant effect. Monitor PT and INR closely.

Rifamycins (rifabutin, rifampin, rifapentine): May decrease therapeutic effects of erythromycin while increasing adverse effects of rifamycin. Monitor patient.

Strong CYP3A inhibitors (diltiazem, verapamil): May increase the risk of sudden death from cardiac causes. Don't use together.

Theophylline: May decrease erythromycin level and increase theophylline toxicity. Use together cautiously.

Drug-food. *Grapefruit juice:* May inhibit drug's metabolism; caution patient to avoid grapefruit juice during therapy.

EFFECTS ON LAB TEST RESULTS

• May increase alkaline phosphatase, ALT, AST, and bilirubin levels.

• May interfere with fluorometric determination of urine catecholamines and with colorimetric assays.

CONTRAINDICATIONS & CAUTIONS

• Contraindicated in patients hypersensitive to drug or other macrolides.

🕒 *Alert:* Drug has been associated with prolonged QT interval and infrequent cases of

E

arrhythmia, including torsades de pointes. Avoid drug in patients with known prolonged QT interval, proarrhythmic conditions, or clinically significant bradycardia, and in those receiving class IA (quinidine, procainamide) or class III (dofetilide, amiodarone, sotalol) antiarrhythmics.

• Use erythromycin salts cautiously in patients with impaired hepatic function.

• May cause infantile hypertrophic pyloric stenosis (HPS) requiring surgery. Benefit of therapy needs to be weighed against risk of developing HPS.

• Prolonged or repeated use may result in superinfection. If superinfection occurs, discontinue drug.

• Drug may cause CDAD, ranging in severity from mild to life-threatening colitis, during treatment and for up to 2 months after treatment. Drug may need to be discontinued if CDAD is suspected or confirmed.

• Don't use drug to treat neurosyphilis.
Dialyzable drug: No.

PREGNANCY-LACTATION-REPRODUCTION

• Use drug during pregnancy only if clearly needed.

• Drug appears in human milk. Use cautiously in breastfeeding women.

NURSING CONSIDERATIONS

• Monitor patient for superinfection and diarrhea. Drug may cause overgrowth of non-susceptible bacteria or fungi.

• Monitor hepatic function. Drug may cause hepatotoxicity.

• Elderly patients may be more at risk for developing drug-induced hearing loss. Monitor patient for new hearing loss.

PATIENT TEACHING

• Tell patient to take drug as prescribed, even after feeling better.

• Instruct patient to take oral form of drug with full glass of water 2 hours before or 2 hours after meals for best absorption.

• Drug may be taken with food if GI upset occurs. Tell patient not to take drug with fruit juice or to swallow the chewable tablets whole.

• Instruct patient to report all adverse reactions, especially diarrhea, nausea, abdominal pain, vomiting, and fever.

• Instruct parents or caregivers to report vomiting or irritability immediately.

escitalopram oxalate
ess-si-TAL-oh-pram

Lexapro⬦

Therapeutic class: Antidepressants
Pharmacologic class: SSRIs

AVAILABLE FORMS
Oral solution: 5 mg/5 mL
Tablets: 5 mg, 10 mg, 20 mg

INDICATIONS & DOSAGES
Adjust-a-dose (for all indications): For elderly patients and those with hepatic impairment, 10 mg PO daily, initially and as maintenance dosages.

➤ **Treatment and maintenance therapy for patients with major depressive disorder**
Adults and adolescents age 12 and older: Initially, 10 mg PO once daily, increasing to 20 mg if needed after at least 1 week in adults and 3 weeks in adolescents.

➤ **Generalized anxiety disorder**
Adults: Initially, 10 mg PO once daily, increasing to 20 mg if needed after at least 1 week.

➤ **Obsessive-compulsive disorder** ⬦
Adults and adolescents age 12 and older: Initially, 10 mg PO once daily. May increase dose in 10-mg increments at 1-week or greater intervals up to 40 mg once daily.

➤ **Premenstrual dysphoric disorder** ⬦
Adult women: Continuous daily dosing regimen: Initially, 5 to 10 mg PO once daily. Over the first month, may increase dose, based on response and tolerability, to 20 mg once daily.
Luteal phase dosing regimen: 5 to 10 mg PO once daily, starting 14 days before anticipated onset of menstruation and continuing to the onset of menses. Over the first month, may increase dose to 20 mg once daily during the luteal phase.
Symptom-onset dosing regimen: 5 to 10 mg PO once daily from the day of symptom onset until a few days after start of menses. Over the first month, may increase dose,

based on response and tolerability, to 20 mg once daily.

ADMINISTRATION
PO
- Give without regard for food.
- Give in the morning or evening.

ACTION
Action may be linked to increase of serotonergic activity in the CNS from inhibition of neuronal reuptake of serotonin. Drug is closely related to citalopram, which may be the active component.

Route	Onset	Peak	Duration
PO	Unknown	5 hr	Unknown

Half-life: 27 to 32 hours.

ADVERSE REACTIONS
CNS: *suicidal behavior,* fever, insomnia, dizziness, somnolence, paresthesia, lightheadedness, migraine, tremor, vertigo, abnormal dreams, irritability, impaired concentration, fatigue, lethargy. **CV:** palpitations, HTN, flushing, chest pain. **EENT:** rhinitis, sinusitis, blurred vision, tinnitus, earache. **GI:** nausea, diarrhea, constipation, indigestion, abdominal pain, vomiting, increased or decreased appetite, dry mouth, flatulence, heartburn, cramps, gastroesophageal reflux. **GU:** ejaculation disorder, erectile dysfunction, anorgasmia, menstrual cramps, UTI, urinary frequency. **Metabolic:** weight gain or loss, hyponatremia. **Musculoskeletal:** arthralgia, myalgia, muscle cramps, pain in arms or legs. **Respiratory:** bronchitis, cough. **Skin:** rash, increased sweating. **Other:** decreased libido, yawning, flulike symptoms.

INTERACTIONS
Drug-drug. *Antiparkinsonians (rasagiline, selegiline):* May cause serotonin syndrome. Avoid use together.
Aspirin, NSAIDs, other drugs known to affect coagulation: May increase the risk of bleeding. Use together cautiously.
Beta blockers: May cause bradycardia and increase risk of CNS toxicity. Monitor patient closely.

Buspirone, methylphenidate: May increase risk of serotonin syndrome. Monitor patient closely.
Carbamazepine: May increase escitalopram clearance. Monitor patient for expected antidepressant effect and adjust dose as needed.
Cimetidine: May increase escitalopram level. Monitor patient for increased adverse reactions to escitalopram.
Citalopram: May cause additive effects. Using together is contraindicated.
CNS drugs: May cause additive effects. Use together cautiously.
Desipramine, other drugs metabolized by CYP2D6: May increase levels of these drugs. Use together cautiously.
Linezolid, methylene blue: May cause serotonin syndrome. Avoid use together.
Lithium: May enhance serotonergic effect of escitalopram. Use together very cautiously.
MAO inhibitors: May cause fatal serotonin syndrome or signs and symptoms resembling NMS. Avoid using within 14 days of MAO inhibitor therapy.
Triptans: May increase serotonergic effects. Use together cautiously, especially at the start of therapy or at dosage increases.
Tramadol: May cause serotonin syndrome. Monitor patient closely.
Drug-herb. *St. John's wort:* May cause serotonin syndrome. Use with caution.
Drug-lifestyle. *Alcohol use:* May increase CNS effects. Discourage use together.

EFFECTS ON LAB TEST RESULTS
- May increase bilirubin and cholesterol levels, LFT values, and INR.
- May decrease serum potassium and sodium levels.
- May increase or decrease glucose level.

CONTRAINDICATIONS & CAUTIONS
- Contraindicated in patients taking pimozide, MAO inhibitors, or within 14 days of MAO inhibitor therapy and in those hypersensitive to escitalopram, citalopram, or any of its inactive ingredients.
- **Black Box Warning** Escitalopram isn't approved for use in children younger than age 12. ■
- **Alert:** Concomitant use with methylene blue or linezolid can cause serotonin

---

syndrome (fever, mental status changes, muscle twitching, sweating, shivering, shaking, diarrhea, loss of coordination). Don't start drug in patients receiving methylene blue or linezolid.

🕚 *Alert:* If linezolid or methylene blue must be given, escitalopram must be stopped and patient should be monitored for serotonin toxicity for 2 weeks or until 24 hours after the last dose of methylene blue or linezolid, whichever comes first. Treatment with escitalopram may be resumed 24 hours after the last dose of methylene blue or linezolid.

• Use cautiously in patients with a history of mania, seizure disorders, suicidal thoughts, or renal or hepatic impairment.

• Use cautiously in patients with diseases that produce altered metabolism or hemodynamic responses.

• Use with caution in elderly patients because they may have greater sensitivity to drug.

Dialyzable drug: Unknown.

⚠ *Overdose S&S:* Seizures, coma, dizziness, ECG changes, hypotension, insomnia, nausea, sinus tachycardia, somnolence, vomiting, acute renal failure.

PREGNANCY-LACTATION-REPRODUCTION

• Use in pregnant women only if potential benefit justifies potential risk to the fetus.

• Prescriber should consider tapering dosage in the third trimester by carefully weighing established benefit of treating depression with an antidepressant against potential risks; decision can only be made on a case-by-case basis.

• Drug appears in human milk. Use cautiously in breastfeeding women; monitor infants for adverse reactions.

NURSING CONSIDERATIONS

Black Box Warning Drug may increase risk of suicidal thinking and behavior in children, adolescents, and young adults ages 18 to 24, especially during the first few months of treatment, especially in those with major depressive disorder or other psychiatric disorder. ∎

• Closely monitor patients at high risk for suicide.

• Evaluate patient for history of drug abuse, and observe for signs of misuse or abuse.

• When discontinuing drug, taper gradually and monitor patient for reemerging signs and symptoms.

• Periodically reassess patient to determine need for maintenance treatment and appropriate dosing.

🕚 *Alert:* Combining triptans with an SSRI or an SSNRI may cause serotonin syndrome or NMS-like reactions. Serotonin syndrome may be more likely to occur when starting or increasing the dose of triptan, SSRI, or SSNRI.

• *Look alike–sound alike:* Don't confuse escitalopram with estazolam.

PATIENT TEACHING

• Inform patient that symptoms should improve gradually over several weeks, rather than immediately.

• Tell patient that although improvement may occur within 1 to 4 weeks, to continue drug as prescribed.

Black Box Warning Caution patient and patient's family to report signs of worsening depression (such as agitation, irritability, insomnia, hostility, impulsivity) and signs of suicidal behavior to prescriber immediately. ∎

🕚 *Alert:* Teach patient to recognize and immediately report symptoms of serotonin toxicity (fever, mental status changes, muscle twitching, excessive sweating, shivering or shaking, diarrhea, loss of coordination).

• Tell patient to use caution while driving or operating hazardous machinery because of drug's potential to impair judgment, thinking, and motor skills.

• Advise patient to consult health care provider before taking other prescription or OTC drugs.

• Tell patient that drug may be taken in the morning or evening without regard to meals.

• Encourage patient to avoid alcohol while taking drug.

• Advise female patient to notify health care provider if she is pregnant or breastfeeding before starting therapy.

Reactions in bold italics are *life-threatening*. Interactions may have a *rapid onset* or a *delayed onset*.

eslicarbazepine acetate
ES-lye-kar-BAY-ze-peen

Aptiom

Therapeutic class: Anticonvulsants
Pharmacologic class: Carboxamide
derivatives

AVAILABLE FORMS
Tablets: 200 mg, 400 mg, 600 mg, 800 mg

INDICATIONS & DOSAGES
➤ **Monotherapy or adjunctive treatment for partial-onset seizures**
Adults: Initially, 400 mg PO once daily; may initiate treatment at 800 mg daily if need for additional seizure reduction outweighs an increased risk of adverse reactions. After 1 week at 400-mg daily dose, increase to recommended maintenance dosage of 800 mg PO once daily. May increase in weekly increments of 400 to 600 mg once daily to a recommended maintenance dose of 800 to 1,600 mg once daily. For monotherapy, consider the 800-mg once-daily maintenance dose in patients unable to tolerate 1,200-mg daily dose. For adjunctive therapy, consider the 1,600-mg daily dose in patients who didn't achieve a satisfactory response with a 1,200-mg daily dose.
Children ages 4 to 17: Dosage is based on body weight; increase based on clinical response and tolerability, but no more frequently than once per week.

For patients weighing 11 to 21 kg, initially 200 mg PO once daily; titrate in 200-mg increments to 400 to 600 mg PO once daily. For those weighing 22 to 31 kg, initially 300 mg PO once daily; titrate in 300-mg increments to 500 to 800 mg PO once daily. For those weighing 32 to 38 kg, initially 300 mg PO once daily; titrate in 300-mg increments to 600 to 900 mg PO once daily. For those weighing more than 38 kg, initially 400 mg PO once daily; titrate in 400-mg increments to 800 to 1,200 mg PO once daily.
Adjust-a-dose: For patients with moderate to severe renal impairment (CrCl of less than 50 mL/minute), the initial, titration, and maintenance doses should generally be reduced by 50%. Maintenance doses may be adjusted according to clinical response. Consider adjusting dosages of both eslicarbazepine and carbamazepine if given concurrently. Consider increasing eslicarbazepine dosage if given with enzyme-inducing AEDs, such as phenobarbital, primidone, or phenytoin.

ADMINISTRATION
PO
• Hazardous drug; use safe handling and disposal precautions.
• Give without regard for food.
• Patient may swallow tablet whole or crushed.

ACTION
Unknown. Thought to inhibit voltage-gated sodium channels, resulting in decreased seizure activity.

Route	Onset	Peak	Duration
PO	Rapid	1–4 hr	Unknown

Half-life: 13 to 20 hours.

ADVERSE REACTIONS
CNS: asthenia, gait disturbance, dizziness, drowsiness, somnolence, headache, ataxia, balance disorder, tremor, dysarthria, memory impairment, depression, insomnia, fatigue, vertigo. **CV:** HTN, peripheral edema. **EENT:** diplopia, blurred vision, visual impairment, nystagmus. **GI:** nausea, vomiting, diarrhea, constipation, abdominal pain, gastritis. **GU:** UTI. **Metabolic:** hyponatremia. **Respiratory:** cough. **Skin:** rash. **Other:** falls.

INTERACTIONS
Drug-drug. *Carbamazepine, phenobarbital, primidone:* May decrease eslicarbazepine concentration. Consider higher eslicarbazepine dosage.
Clobazam, omeprazole: May increase concentrations of these drugs. Monitor patient accordingly.
Ethinyl estradiol, levonorgestrel: May decrease hormone concentrations. Patient should use additional or alternative nonhormonal contraception.
Phenytoin: May increase phenytoin concentration. Monitor phenytoin level and adjust

E

dosage accordingly. May decrease eslicarbazepine concentration. Consider higher eslicarbazepine dosage.

Rosuvastatin, simvastatin: May lower statin level. Adjust statin dosage if significant change in lipids occur.

Warfarin: May decrease warfarin effect. Monitor INR and adjust dosage accordingly.

Drug-herb. *Evening primrose:* May decrease seizure threshold. Don't use together.

Drug-lifestyle. *Alcohol use:* May increase CNS depression. Avoid use together.

EFFECTS ON LAB TEST RESULTS

• May increase bilirubin, AST, ALT, total cholesterol, triglyceride, LDL, and CK levels.

• May decrease sodium, chloride, T_3, T_4, and Hb levels and hematocrit.

CONTRAINDICATIONS & CAUTIONS

❸ *Alert:* Contraindicated in patients hypersensitive to drug or its components. Rare cases of anaphylaxis and angioedema have been reported. Anaphylaxis and angioedema associated with laryngeal edema can be fatal. If patient develops any of these reactions after treatment, discontinue drug.

❸ *Alert:* Contraindicated in patients who have experienced dermatologic reaction, DRESS syndrome, anaphylactic reactions, or angioedema while taking oxcarbazepine.

• Don't give oxcarbazepine to patients also taking eslicarbazepine. Drugs are chemically related.

• Use in patients with severe hepatic impairment hasn't been evaluated and isn't recommended.

• Use cautiously in patients at risk for suicidal thoughts and behavior.

• Safety and effectiveness in children younger than age 4 haven't been established.

Dialyzable drug: Yes.

⚠ *Overdose S&S:* Hyponatremia, dizziness, nausea, vomiting, somnolence, euphoria, oral paresthesia, ataxia, walking difficulty, diplopia.

PREGNANCY-LACTATION-REPRODUCTION

• Use in pregnancy only if potential benefit justifies potential risk to the fetus. Recommend that pregnant patients enroll in the North American AED Pregnancy Registry at 1-888-233-2334.

• Women of childbearing potential who use hormonal contraceptives containing ethinyl estradiol or levonorgestrel should also use additional or alternative forms of nonhormonal contraception.

• Drug appears in human milk. Patient should discontinue breastfeeding or discontinue drug.

NURSING CONSIDERATIONS

• To discontinue drug, reduce dosage gradually; avoid abrupt discontinuation.

❸ *Alert:* Anticonvulsants can increase risk of suicidal thoughts or behavior in patients taking these drugs for any indication. Monitor patients for new or worsening depression, development of suicidal thoughts and behavior, or unusual change in mood or behavior.

• Monitor sodium and chloride levels initially and periodically during treatment, especially in patients taking drugs known to decrease serum sodium level. Reduce dosage or discontinue drug as clinically indicated.

• Monitor patients for signs and symptoms of hyponatremia (nausea, vomiting, malaise, headache, lethargy, confusion, irritability, muscle weakness, spasms, obtundation, and increased seizure frequency or severity).

• Obtain thyroid function tests at baseline and periodically during treatment.

• Obtain LFTs at baseline and periodically during therapy. Discontinue drug if jaundice, liver injury, or laboratory results suggestive of liver injury occur.

• Discontinue drug if hematologic adverse reactions occur.

• Monitor patient for dermatologic conditions, such as SJS and toxic epidermal necrolysis; discontinue drug if serious dermatologic changes occur.

❸ *Alert:* Monitor patient for DRESS syndrome or multiorgan hypersensitivity (fever, rash, lymphadenopathy, hepatitis, nephritis, hematologic abnormalities, myocarditis, or myositis). Discontinue drug if DRESS syndrome occurs.

• Monitor patient for development of dizziness or disturbances in gait and coordination (ataxia, vertigo, balance disorder, nystagmus), especially during dosage titration

---

and in patients age 60 and older. Consider dosage modification.

• Monitor patient for dose-dependent somnolence or fatigue, cognitive dysfunction (memory impairment, disturbance in attention, amnesia, confusion, aphasia, speech disorder, slowness of thought, disorientation, or psychomotor retardation), or visual changes (diplopia, blurred vision, impaired vision).

PATIENT TEACHING

• Advise patient not to operate motor vehicles or hazardous machinery while taking drug until drug's effects are known.

• Tell patient to report CNS signs and symptoms, such as dizziness or disturbances in gait and coordination (ataxia, vertigo, balance disorder, nystagmus).

• Advise patient that laboratory monitoring will be needed during therapy.

• Inform patient and caregivers of increased risk of suicidal thoughts and behavior. Advise them to immediately report new or worsening depression, unusual changes in mood or behavior, thoughts of suicide, or thoughts about self-harm.

• Counsel patient to report rash or other skin reactions.

• Advise patient to report signs and symptoms of hyponatremia (nausea, vomiting, malaise, headache, lethargy, confusion, irritability, muscle weakness, spasms, obtundation, increased seizure frequency or severity).

• Caution patient not to stop drug without first discussing with prescriber. If drug needs to be stopped, it must be tapered gradually to minimize risk of increased seizures.

SAFETY ALERT!

esmolol hydrochloride
ESS-moe-lol

Brevibloc

Therapeutic class: Antiarrhythmics
Pharmacologic class: Selective beta blockers

AVAILABLE FORMS
Injection: 10 mg/mL vial

Premixed bags in sodium chloride: 10 mg/mL in 250-mL bags; 20 mg/mL in 100-mL bags

INDICATIONS & DOSAGES
➤ **Supraventricular tachycardia; noncompensatory sinus tachycardias**
Adults: 500 mcg/kg as loading dose by IV infusion over 1 minute; then 4-minute maintenance infusion of 50 mcg/kg/minute. If adequate response doesn't occur within 5 minutes, may repeat loading dose and follow with maintenance infusion of 100 mcg/kg/minute for 4 minutes. May repeat loading dose and increase maintenance infusion by increments of 50 mcg/kg/minute. Range of maintenance dose is generally 50 to 200 mcg/kg/minute. Maximum maintenance infusion for tachycardia is 200 mcg/kg/minute. May continue maintenance infusions for up to 48 hours.

➤ **Intraoperative and postoperative tachycardia or HTN**
Adults: For immediate control: 1 mg/kg as a bolus dose over 30 seconds, followed by 150 mcg/kg/minute IV infusion, if needed. For gradual control (stepwise dosing): Loading dose is 500 mcg/kg over 1 minute, then 50 mcg/kg/minute for 4 minutes. Optional loading dose if needed, then 100 mcg/kg/minute for 4 minutes. Optional loading dose if needed, then 150 mcg/kg/minute for 4 minutes. If necessary, may increase to 200 mcg/kg/minute. Maximum doses are 200 mcg/kg/minute for tachycardia and 300 mcg/kg/minute for HTN.

ADMINISTRATION
IV

▼ Don't dilute single-dose vials or premixed containers.

▼ Give with an infusion-control device rather than by IV push. Administer by continuous IV infusion with or without a loading dose and titrate based on ventricular rate or BP at 4-minute or more intervals. Avoid infusing into small veins or through a butterfly catheter.

▼ If concentration exceeds 10 mg/mL, give drug through a central line.

▼ Don't use for longer than 48 hours. Watch infusion site carefully for signs of extravasation; if they occur, stop infusion immediately and call prescriber.

E

▼ **Incompatibilities:** Amphotericin B cholesteryl sulfate complex, diazepam, furosemide, procainamide, sodium bicarbonate 5%.

ACTION

A class II antiarrhythmic and ultra-short-acting selective beta blocker that decreases HR, contractility, and BP.

Route	Onset	Peak	Duration
IV	Immediate	5 min (with loading dose); 30 min (without loading dose)	30 min after discontinuation of infusion

Half-life: About 9 minutes.

ADVERSE REACTIONS

CNS: dizziness, somnolence, headache, agitation, confusion. **CV:** hypotension, peripheral ischemia. **GI:** nausea, vomiting. **Skin:** inflammation or induration at infusion site, hyperhidrosis.

INTERACTIONS

Drug-drug. *Antidiabetic agents:* May increase blood glucose-lowering effect of antidiabetic agent. Closely monitor blood glucose concentration.

Calcium channel blockers (diltiazem, nicardipine, nifedipine, verapamil), flecainide: May potentiate pharmacologic effects of both drugs. IV administration in close proximity is contraindicated. Monitor cardiac function closely and adjust therapy as needed.

Clonidine: May cause life-threatening BP increases. Closely monitor BP. Discontinue either agent gradually, preferably esmolol first.

Digoxin: May increase digoxin level by 10% to 20%. May increase bradycardia. Monitor digoxin level.

Lidocaine: May increase lidocaine concentration. Monitor patient closely and adjust dosage as needed.

MAO inhibitors: May worsen bradycardia or HTN. Discontinue esmolol or reduce esmolol dosage if needed.

Morphine: May increase esmolol level. Adjust esmolol dosage carefully.

NSAIDs: May impair antihypertensive effect of esmolol. Monitor BP and adjust esmolol dosage as needed.

Prazosin: May increase risk of orthostatic HTN. Help patient to stand slowly until effects are known.

Salicylates (aspirin): May impair antihypertensive effect of esmolol. Monitor patient and consider alternative therapy as needed.

Succinylcholine: May prolong neuromuscular blockade. Monitor patient closely.

Vasoconstrictive and positive inotropic agents (dopamine, epinephrine, norepinephrine): May increase risk of reduced cardiac contractility in presence of high systemic vascular resistance. Don't use together.

EFFECTS ON LAB TEST RESULTS

None reported.

CONTRAINDICATIONS & CAUTIONS

• Contraindicated in patients hypersensitive to drug or its components, in those with severe sinus bradycardia, second- or third-degree heart block, sick sinus syndrome, cardiogenic shock, decompensated HF, and pulmonary HTN, and in patients taking verapamil and diltiazem.

• Use cautiously in patients with renal impairment, diabetes, or bronchospasm.

• May cause myocardial ischemia when abruptly discontinued in patients with CAD.

⚠ *Alert:* Don't withdraw drug abruptly, as angina, MI, and ventricular arrhythmias can occur.

Dialyzable drug: Unknown.

⚠ *Overdose S&S:* Bradycardia, hypotension, loss of consciousness, cardiac arrest, pulseless electrical activity.

PREGNANCY-LACTATION-REPRODUCTION

• Use during the third trimester can cause fetal bradycardia. Use in pregnant women only if potential benefit justifies potential risk to the fetus.

• It isn't known if drug appears in human milk. Patient should discontinue breastfeeding or discontinue drug.

NURSING CONSIDERATIONS

⚠ *Alert:* Monitor ECG and BP continuously during infusion. Nearly half of patients will develop hypotension. Diaphoresis and dizziness may accompany hypotension. Monitor patient closely, especially if patient had low BP before treatment.

• Hypotension can usually be reversed within 30 minutes by decreasing the dose or, if needed, by stopping the infusion. Notify prescriber if this becomes necessary.

• If a local reaction develops at the infusion site, change to another site.

• When HR stabilizes, replace IV drug with an alternative antiarrhythmic. Reduce infusion rate by half 30 minutes after first dose of the new drug. Monitor patient response and, if HR is controlled for 1 hour after administration of second dose of the replacement drug, stop esmolol infusion.

• Monitor serum electrolyte levels, as hyperkalemia can occur, especially in patients with renal impairment.

• Drug can mask signs and symptoms of hyperthyroidism. Monitor patient for thyrotoxicosis when withdrawing drug.

PATIENT TEACHING
• Instruct patient to report all adverse reactions promptly.
• Tell patient to report discomfort at IV site.

---

esomeprazole magnesium
ess-oh-ME-pray-zol

Nexium✐, Nexium 24 HR ◇

esomeprazole sodium
Nexium IV

esomeprazole strontium

Therapeutic class: Antiulcer drugs
Pharmacologic class: PPIs

AVAILABLE FORMS
esomeprazole magnesium
Capsules (delayed-release) ⓘ: 20 mg, 40 mg
Powder for suspension (delayed-release): 2.5 mg, 5 mg, 10 mg, 20 mg, 40 mg
Tablets (delayed-release): 20 mg ◇
esomeprazole sodium
Powder for injection: 20-mg, 40-mg single-use vials

esomeprazole strontium
Capsules (delayed-release) ⓘ: 24.65 mg (equivalent to 20 mg esomeprazole), 49.3 mg (equivalent to 40 mg esomeprazole)

INDICATIONS & DOSAGES
Adjust-a-dose (for all indications): For patients with severe hepatic failure (Child-Pugh class C), maximum daily dose is 20 mg.
➤ **GERD; to heal erosive esophagitis**
Adults: 20 or 40 mg or 24.75 or 49.3 mg (strontium) PO daily for 4 to 8 weeks. Maintenance dose for healing erosive esophagitis is 20 mg PO daily for up to 6 months.
Children ages 1 to 11 weighing 20 kg or more: 10 or 20 mg PO once daily for up to 8 weeks.
Children ages 1 to 11 weighing less than 20 kg: 10 mg PO once daily for up to 8 weeks.
➤ **Symptomatic GERD**
Adults: 20 mg or 24.65 mg (strontium) PO daily for 4 weeks. If symptoms are unresolved, may continue treatment for 4 more weeks.
Children and adolescents ages 12 to 17: 20 mg PO once daily for up to 4 weeks.
Children ages 1 to 11: 10 mg PO once daily for up to 8 weeks.
➤ **Erosive esophagitis due to acid-mediated GERD only**
Infants ages 1 to 11 months weighing more than 7.5 to 12 kg: 10 mg PO once daily for up to 6 weeks.
Infants ages 1 to 11 months weighing more than 5 to 7.5 kg: 5 mg PO once daily for up to 6 weeks.
Infants ages 1 to 11 months weighing 3 to 5 kg: 2.5 mg PO once daily for up to 6 weeks.
➤ **Short-term treatment (up to 10 days) of GERD in patients with a history of erosive esophagitis who can't take drug orally**
Adults: Reconstitute 20 or 40 mg with 5 mL of D₅W, NSS, or lactated Ringer injection and give by IV bolus over 3 minutes. Or, further dilute to a total volume of 50 mL and give IV over 10 to 30 minutes. Switch patient to oral therapy as soon as tolerated.
Children ages 1 to 17 weighing 55 kg or more: 20 mg IV infusion once daily over 10 to 30 minutes.

E

Children ages 1 to 17 weighing less than 55 kg: 10 mg IV infusion once daily over 10 to 30 minutes.

Children ages 1 month to younger than 1 year: 0.5 mg/kg IV infusion once daily over 10 to 30 minutes.

➤ **To reduce the risk of gastric ulcers in patients receiving continuous NSAID therapy**

Adults: 20 or 40 mg or 24.65 or 49.3 mg (strontium) PO once daily for up to 6 months.

➤ **Long-term treatment of pathologic hypersecretory conditions, including Zollinger-Ellison syndrome**

Adults: 40 mg or 49.3 mg (strontium) PO b.i.d. Adjust dosage based on patient response.

➤ **To eliminate *Helicobacter pylori***

Adults: 40 mg (magnesium) or 49.3 mg (strontium) PO daily, 1,000 mg amoxicillin PO b.i.d., and 500 mg clarithromycin PO b.i.d., given together for 10 days to reduce duodenal ulcer recurrence.

➤ **Reduction of risk of rebleeding of gastric or duodenal ulcers after therapeutic endoscopy**

Adults: 80 mg IV over 30 minutes, followed by continuous infusion of 8 mg/hour for a total IV treatment duration of 72 hours, followed by oral acid-suppressive therapy.

Adjust-a-dose: In patients with mild to moderate hepatic impairment (Child-Pugh classes A and B), maximum continuous infusion rate is 6 mg/hour. In patients with severe hepatic impairment (Child-Pugh class C), maximum continuous infusion rate is 4 mg/hour.

➤ **Dyspepsia ◆**

Adults: 40 mg PO daily for up to 8 weeks.

ADMINISTRATION

PO

• Give drug at least 1 hour before meals. If patient has difficulty swallowing the capsule, contents of the capsule can be emptied and mixed with 1 tablespoon of applesauce and swallowed (without chewing the enteric-coated pellets).

• If giving capsule via NG tube, open capsule and empty the granules into a 60-mL syringe. Mix with 50 mL of water. Replace the plunger and shake vigorously for

15 seconds. Flush NG tube with additional water after use. Don't give if pellets have dissolved or disintegrated.

• For oral suspension, mix contents of a 2.5- or 5-mg packet with 5 mL of water; mix contents of a 10-, 20-, or 40-mg packet with 15 mL of water. Then let it sit for 2 to 3 minutes to thicken. Stir the suspension and drink within 30 minutes.

• To give oral suspension via NG tube, add 5 mL of water to a syringe, then add contents of 2.5- or 5-mg packet; or add 15 mL of water to a syringe, then add contents of 10-, 20-, or 40-mg packet. Shake syringe and leave for 2 to 3 minutes to thicken. Shake syringe again and inject through NG or gastric tube within 30 minutes. Flush any remaining contents into the stomach with additional water.

IV

▼ Flush IV line with D_5W, NSS, or lactated Ringer injection before and after administration.

▼ Use reconstituted powder within 12 hours.

▼ Use admixture diluted with D_5W within 6 hours.

▼ If diluted with NSS or lactated Ringer injection, use within 12 hours.

▼ Store reconstituted solution and admixture at room temperature.

▼ **Incompatibilities:** Other IV drugs.

ACTION

Reduces gastric acid secretion and decreases gastric acidity.

Route	Onset	Peak	Duration
PO	Unknown	1½ hr	13–17 hr
IV	Unknown	Unknown	Unknown

Half-life: 1 to 1½ hours.

ADVERSE REACTIONS

CNS: headache, dizziness. **GI:** abdominal pain, constipation, diarrhea, dry mouth, flatulence, nausea, vomiting. **Skin:** pruritus.

INTERACTIONS

Drug-drug. *Calcium salts (calcium carbonate):* May interfere with GI absorption of calcium salts. Closely monitor clinical response to calcium; larger dosages of calcium may be needed.

Reactions in bold italics are *life-threatening*. Interactions may have a *rapid onset* or a *delayed onset*.

Cilostazol: May increase concentrations of cilostazol and its active metabolite. Consider a cilostazol dose reduction when esomeprazole is given concurrently.

Clopidogrel: May decrease antiplatelet activity. Use esomeprazole magnesium or esomeprazole sodium cautiously with clopidogrel.

Dabigatran: May decrease concentration of active metabolite of dabigatran. Monitor patient closely.

Diazepam: May decrease clearance of diazepam. Monitor patient for diazepam toxicity.

Digoxin: May increase serum digoxin level. Monitor digoxin concentration and clinical response. If an interaction is suspected, adjust digoxin dosage as needed.

Drugs metabolized by CYP2C19: May alter clearance of esomeprazole, especially in elderly patients or patients with hepatic insufficiency. Monitor patient for toxicity.

Fluvoxamine: May increase risk of adverse reactions. Use cautiously.

Iron salts (ferrous sulfate): May interfere with absorption of iron salts. Temporary cessation of esomeprazole may be required to achieve appropriate clinical response to oral iron. If stopping esomeprazole isn't an option, parenteral iron may be a suitable alternative.

Ketoconazole, voriconazole: May increase esomeprazole concentration. Monitor therapy.

Methotrexate: May increase methotrexate concentration and risk of toxicity. Monitor patient closely.

Mycophenolate: May decrease mycophenolate plasma concentration and pharmacologic effects. Monitor clinical response and adjust mycophenolate dosage as needed.

Protease inhibitors (atazanavir, nelfinavir, saquinavir): May reduce plasma levels of atazanavir or nelfinavir. Use together isn't recommended. May increase saquinavir levels. Monitor carefully and reduce dosage if needed.

Rifampin: May decrease esomeprazole levels. Avoid using together.

Rilpivirine: May cause loss of virologic response or resistance. Use together is contraindicated.

Tacrolimus: May increase pharmacologic effects of tacrolimus and risk of adverse reactions. Closely monitor tacrolimus trough concentration when starting or stopping esomeprazole. Adjust tacrolimus dosage as needed.

Warfarin: May prolong PT and increase INR, causing abnormal bleeding. Monitor patient and PT and INR.

Drug-herb. *St. John's wort:* May decrease esomeprazole level. Avoid use together.

Drug-food. *Any food:* May reduce drug level. Advise patient to take drug 1 hour before food.

EFFECTS ON LAB TEST RESULTS
• May decrease magnesium level.

CONTRAINDICATIONS & CAUTIONS
• Contraindicated in patients hypersensitive to drug or components of esomeprazole or omeprazole (a drug similar to this one).

◑ *Alert:* There may be an increased risk of osteoporosis-related hip, wrist, and spine fractures associated with PPIs. Risk is increased in patients who received high-dose and long-term (longer than 1 year) therapy. The lowest dosage for the shortest duration should be used.

• Use cautiously in patients receiving continuous NSAID therapy who are at increased risk for gastric ulcers (those age 60 and older and those with a history of gastric ulcers).

• Drug-induced decreases in gastric acidity may increase serum chromogranin A (CgA) level, possibly causing false-positive results in diagnostic investigations for neuroendocrine tumors. Temporarily stop esomeprazole at least 14 days before assessing CgA level; consider repeating the test if initial CgA level is high.

• If cutaneous lupus or SLE occurs, discontinue drug.

• American College of Gastroenterology Clinical Guideline 2017 recommends avoiding use of clarithromycin triple therapy (a PPI, clarithromycin, and amoxicillin or metronidazole) to eliminate *H. pylori* in patients with risk factors for macrolide resistance (prior macrolide exposure, local clarithromycin resistance rates of 15% or higher, eradication rates with clarithromycin-based regimens of 85% or lower).

Dialyzable drug: Unlikely.
⚠ *Overdose S&S:* Blurred vision, confusion, tremor, ataxia, intermittent clonic seizures, diaphoresis, drowsiness, flushing, headache, nausea, tachycardia.

PREGNANCY-LACTATION-REPRODUCTION
• Use during pregnancy only if potential benefit justifies potential risk to the fetus.
• It isn't known if drug appears in human milk, but omeprazole does. Use cautiously in breastfeeding women.

NURSING CONSIDERATIONS
• Antacids can be used while taking drug, unless otherwise directed by prescriber.
• Monitor patient for rash or signs and symptoms of hypersensitivity. Monitor GI symptoms for improvement or worsening. Monitor LFTs, especially in patients with preexisting hepatic disease.
◑ *Alert:* Prolonged use may cause low magnesium levels that require magnesium supplementation and possibly discontinuation of drug. Monitor magnesium level before treatment and periodically during treatment. Monitor patient for signs and symptoms of low magnesium level, such as abnormal HR or heart rhythm, palpitations, muscle spasms, tremor, and seizures. In children, abnormal HR may present as fatigue, upset stomach, dizziness, and light-headedness.
◑ *Alert:* May increase risk of CDAD. Evaluate for CDAD in patients who develop diarrhea that doesn't improve.
◑ *Alert:* Prolonged treatment (at least 3 years or more) may lead to vitamin B$_{12}$ malabsorption and subsequent vitamin B$_{12}$ deficiency, which is dose-related and more severe in women and those younger than age 30; prevalence decreases after discontinuation of therapy.
• *Look alike–sound alike:* Don't confuse Nexium with Nexavar.

PATIENT TEACHING
• Instruct patient to take drug exactly as prescribed.
• Tell patient to take drug at least 1 hour before a meal.
• Advise patient that antacids can be used while taking drug unless otherwise directed by prescriber.

• Warn patient not to chew or crush drug pellets because this inactivates the drug.
• Tell patient who has difficulty swallowing capsule to mix contents of capsule with 1 tablespoon of soft applesauce and swallow immediately.
• Advise patient to store capsules at room temperature in a tight container.
• Tell patient to inform prescriber of worsening signs and symptoms, pain, or diarrhea that doesn't improve.
• Instruct patient to alert prescriber if rash or other signs and symptoms of allergy occur.
• Warn patient to immediately report symptoms of low magnesium level, such as involuntary muscle movements or seizures.

esterified estrogens
ESS-tehr-eh-fide ESS-troe-jenz

Menest

Therapeutic class: Estrogens
Pharmacologic class: Estrogens

AVAILABLE FORMS
Tablets (film-coated): 0.3 mg, 0.625 mg, 1.25 mg, 2.5 mg

INDICATIONS & DOSAGES
➤ **Inoperable progressing prostate cancer**
Men: 1.25 to 2.5 mg PO t.i.d.
➤ **Palliative treatment for metastatic breast cancer**
Men and postmenopausal women: 10 mg PO t.i.d. for 3 or more months.
➤ **Hypogonadism**
Women: 2.5 to 7.5 mg PO daily in divided doses in cycles of 20 days on, 10 days off.
➤ **Castration, primary ovarian failure**
Women: 1.25 mg PO daily in cycles of 3 weeks on, 1 week off. Adjust for symptoms. Can be given continuously.
➤ **Vasomotor menopausal symptoms**
Women: 1.25 mg PO daily in cycles of 3 weeks on, 1 week off. If patient is menstruating, cyclic administration is started on day 5 of bleeding.
➤ **Moderate to severe menopausal vulvar and vaginal atrophy**
Women: 0.3 to 1.25 mg or more PO daily, depending on tissue response of individual patient, in cycles of 3 weeks on, 1 week off.

Reactions in bold italics are *life-threatening*. Interactions may have a *rapid onset* or a *delayed onset*.

ADMINISTRATION
PO
• Use lowest effective dose needed for specific indication.
• Reevaluate at 3- to 6-month intervals for tapering or discontinuation of therapy.
• Give without regard to food.

ACTION
Mimics the actions of endogenous estrogens; increases synthesis of DNA, RNA, and protein in responsive tissues; reduces release of FSH and luteinizing hormone from pituitary gland.

Route	Onset	Peak	Duration
PO	Unknown	Unknown	Unknown

Half-life: Unknown.

ADVERSE REACTIONS
CNS: headache, dizziness, chorea, depression, nervousness, mood disturbance, irritability, exacerbation of epilepsy, dementia, *stroke, seizures.* **CV:** thrombophlebitis, *thromboembolism,* HTN, edema, *PE, MI.*
EENT: worsening myopia or astigmatism, intolerance of contact lenses. **GI:** nausea, vomiting, abdominal cramps, bloating, anorexia, increased appetite, *pancreatitis,* increased risk of gallbladder disease. **GU:** breakthrough bleeding, altered menstrual flow, dysmenorrhea, amenorrhea, *increased risk of endometrial cancer,* cervical erosion, altered cervical secretions, enlargement of uterine fibromas, vaginal candidiasis, testicular atrophy, impotence. **Hepatic:** cholestatic jaundice, *hepatic adenoma.*
Metabolic: hypercalcemia, weight changes, hypertriglyceridemia. **Skin:** melasma, rash, hirsutism or hair loss, erythema nodosum, *erythema multiforme,* dermatitis. **Other:** breast tenderness, enlargement, or secretion; gynecomastia; *increased risk of breast cancer.*

INTERACTIONS
Drug-drug. *Anastrozole:* May interfere with anastrozole effectiveness. Avoid use together.
Carbamazepine, fosphenytoin, phenobarbital, phenytoin, rifampin: May decrease effectiveness of estrogen therapy. Monitor patient closely.

Clarithromycin, erythromycin, itraconazole, ketoconazole, ritonavir: May increase estrogen plasma levels and side effects. Monitor patient.
Corticosteroids: May increase corticosteroid effects. Monitor patient closely.
Dantrolene, hepatotoxic drugs: May increase risk of hepatotoxicity. Monitor liver function closely.
Exemestane: May interfere with exemestane effectiveness. Avoid use together.
Oral anticoagulants: May decrease anticoagulant effects. Adjust dosage if needed. Monitor PT and INR.
Ospemifene: May enhance adverse/toxic effect of and interfere with effectiveness of ospemifene. Avoid use together.
Tamoxifen: May interfere with tamoxifen effectiveness. Avoid using together.
Thyroid replacement therapy: May decrease thyroid hormone levels. Higher doses of thyroid hormone may be required.
Drug-herb. *Red clover:* May increase estrogen effects. Discourage use together.
St. John's wort: May decrease effects of drug. Discourage use together.
Drug-food. *Grapefruit, grapefruit juice:* May increase risk of adverse effects. Discourage use together.
Drug-lifestyle. *Smoking:* May increase risk of CV effects. If smoking continues, may need another form of therapy.

EFFECTS ON LAB TEST RESULTS
• May increase calcium, thyroid-binding globulin, circulating thyroid hormone, serum triglyceride, HDL, and serum phospholipid levels.
• May decrease LDL level.
• May alter clotting factors.
• May increase norepinephrine-induced platelet aggregation and may prolong PT.
• May reduce response to metyrapone test. May cause impaired glucose tolerance.

CONTRAINDICATIONS & CAUTIONS
• Contraindicated in patients hypersensitive to drug and in patients with breast cancer (except metastatic disease), estrogen-dependent neoplasia, active thrombophlebitis, thromboembolic disorders, undiagnosed abnormal genital bleeding, or history of thromboembolic disease.

• Use cautiously in patients with history of HTN, mental depression, cardiac or renal dysfunction, liver impairment, gallbladder disease, bone disease, migraine, seizures, or diabetes.

Black Box Warning Drug shouldn't be used for prevention of CV disease. Drug is associated with development of dementia in postmenopausal women age 65 and older. Estrogens with or without progestins should be prescribed at the lowest effective doses for the shortest duration consistent with treatment goals. ∎

Dialyzable drug: Unknown.

⚠ *Overdose S&S:* Nausea, withdrawal bleeding in females.

PREGNANCY-LACTATION-REPRODUCTION

• Estrogens shouldn't be used during pregnancy.

• There is no indication for use in pregnancy. There appears to be little or no increased risk of birth defects in children born to women who have used estrogens and progestins from oral contraceptives inadvertently during early pregnancy.

• Estrogens have been shown to decrease the quantity and quality of human milk. Use only if clearly needed; monitor infant's growth closely.

NURSING CONSIDERATIONS

❸ *Alert:* Drug is considered a high-risk medication for elderly patients.

Black Box Warning Close clinical surveillance of all women taking estrogens is important. Adequate diagnostic measures, including endometrial sampling when indicated, should be undertaken to rule out malignancy in all cases of undiagnosed persistent or recurring abnormal vaginal bleeding. ∎

• When given cyclically for short-term use, administration should be cyclic and attempts to discontinue or taper the medication should be made at 3- to 6-month intervals.

• Make sure patient has thorough physical examination before starting estrogen therapy. Patients receiving long-term estrogen therapy should have annual examinations. Periodically monitor body weight, BP, lipid levels, and hepatic function.

• Notify pathologist about patient's estrogen therapy when sending specimens to laboratory for evaluation.

❸ *Alert:* Because of risk of thromboembolism, stop therapy at least 4 to 6 weeks before procedures that cause prolonged immobilization or increased risk of thromboembolism, such as knee or hip surgery.

Black Box Warning Estrogens have been reported to increase the risk of endometrial carcinoma. ∎

• Glucose tolerance may be impaired. Monitor glucose level closely in patients with diabetes.

PATIENT TEACHING

• Advise patient to report all adverse reactions promptly.

• Emphasize importance of regular physical examinations. Postmenopausal women who use estrogen replacement for longer than 5 years to treat menopausal symptoms may be at increased risk for endometrial cancer. This risk is reduced by using cyclic rather than continuous therapy and the lowest possible estrogen dosage. Adding progestins to the regimen decreases risk of endometrial hyperplasia, but it's unknown whether progestins affect risk of endometrial cancer.

❸ *Alert:* Warn patient to immediately report abdominal pain; pain, numbness, or stiffness in legs or buttocks; pressure or pain in chest or shortness of breath; severe headaches; visual disturbances, such as blind spots, flashing lights, or blurriness; vaginal bleeding or discharge; breast lumps; swelling of hands or feet; yellow skin or sclera; dark urine; or light-colored stools.

• Tell diabetic patient to report elevated glucose level so that antidiabetic dosage can be adjusted.

• Explain to female patient receiving cyclic therapy for postmenopausal symptoms that she may experience withdrawal bleeding during week off drug. Tell her to report unusual vaginal bleeding.

• Teach female patient to perform routine breast self-examination.

• Advise female patient of childbearing potential to consult prescriber before taking drug and to advise prescriber immediately if she becomes pregnant.

Reactions in bold italics are *life-threatening*. Interactions may have a *rapid onset* or a *delayed onset*.

E

- Teach patient methods to decrease risk of blood clots.
- Encourage patient to stop smoking or reduce number of cigarettes smoked because of the risk of CV complications.

estradiol ⌧
ess-tra-DYE-ole

Alora, Climara, Estrace Vaginal Cream, Estring Vaginal Ring, Evamist, Menostar, Minivelle, Vagifem, Vivelle, Vivelle-Dot, Yuvafem

estradiol acetate
Femring

estradiol cypionate
Depo-Estradiol

estradiol gel
Divigel, Elestrin, EstroGel

estradiol valerate
Delestrogen

Therapeutic class: Estrogens
Pharmacologic class: Estrogens

AVAILABLE FORMS
estradiol
Spray, topical solution: 1.53 mg/spray
Tablets (micronized): 0.5 mg, 1 mg, 2 mg
Transdermal: 0.014 mg/24 hours, 0.025 mg/24 hours, 0.0375 mg/24 hours, 0.05 mg/24 hours, 0.06 mg/24 hours, 0.075 mg/24 hours, 0.1 mg/24 hours
Vaginal cream (in nonliquefying base): 0.1 mg/g
Vaginal ring (extended-release): 2 mg (0.0075 mg/24 hours)
Vaginal tablets: 10 mcg
estradiol acetate
Vaginal ring: 0.05 mg/24 hours; 0.1 mg/24 hours
estradiol cypionate
Injection (in oil): 5 mg/mL
estradiol gel
Transdermal gel: 0.06% (1.25 g/metered dose), 0.06% (0.87 g/activation), 0.1% (in 0.25-, 0.5-, and 1-g single-dose packets)

estradiol valerate
Injection (in oil): 10 mg/mL, 20 mg/mL, 40 mg/mL

INDICATIONS & DOSAGES
➤ **Vasomotor menopausal symptoms, female hypogonadism, female castration, primary ovarian failure**
Women: 1 to 2 mg PO estradiol daily. Or, for vasomotor symptoms, 1 to 5 mg cypionate IM once every 3 to 4 weeks; for female hypogonadism, 1.5 to 2 mg cypionate IM once every month.
Transdermal patch
Women: Apply patch according to manufacturer's instructions. Alora, Vivelle, and Vivelle-Dot are applied twice weekly. Climara and Menostar are applied once a week. Apply to clean, dry area of the trunk. Adjust dose, if necessary, after the first 2 or 3 weeks of therapy; then every 3 to 6 months as needed. Rotate application sites weekly with an interval of at least 1 week between particular sites used. Adjust dosage as needed.
➤ **Postmenopausal urogenital symptoms**
Women: One ring inserted into the upper third of the vagina. Ring is kept in place for 3 months.
➤ **Vulvar and vaginal atrophy**
Women: 0.05 mg/24 hours applied twice weekly in a cyclic regimen. Or, 0.05 mg/24 hours Climara applied weekly in a cyclic regimen. Or, 2 to 4 g vaginal applications of cream daily for 1 to 2 weeks; then gradually reduce to one-half initial dosage for 1 to 2 weeks. When vaginal mucosa is restored, maintenance dose is 1 g one to three times weekly in a cyclic regimen. Attempt to taper or discontinue at 3- to 6-month intervals. If using Vagifem or Yuvafem for atrophic vaginitis, give 1 tablet vaginally once daily for 2 weeks. Maintenance dose is 1 tablet inserted vaginally twice weekly. Or, 10 to 20 mg valerate IM every 4 weeks as needed. Or, 1 to 5 mg cypionate IM once every 3 to 4 weeks. Or, 0.05 to 0.1 mg daily by vaginal ring. Replace vaginal ring every 3 months. Or, 1.25 g EstroGel applied once daily to skin.
➤ **Palliative treatment of advanced, inoperable breast cancer**
Men and postmenopausal women: 10 mg PO estradiol t.i.d. for 3 months.

➤ **Palliative treatment of advanced, inoperable prostate cancer**

Men: 30 mg valerate IM every 1 to 2 weeks, or 1 to 2 mg estradiol PO t.i.d.

➤ **To prevent postmenopausal osteoporosis**

Women: Place a 6.5-cm^2 (0.025 mg/24 hours) Climara patch once weekly on clean, dry skin of lower abdomen or upper quadrant of buttock. Or, place a 3.25-cm^2 (0.014 mg/24 hours) Menostar patch once weekly to clean, dry area of the lower abdomen. Or, place a 0.5 mg/24 hours patch twice weekly in a cyclic regimen in women with an intact uterus. In women with a hysterectomy, apply one patch twice weekly in a continuous regimen. For each system, press firmly in place for about 10 seconds; ensure complete contact, especially around edges. Or, 0.025-mg/24 hours Vivelle, Vivelle-Dot, or Alora system applied to a clean, dry area of the trunk twice weekly. Or, 0.5 mg PO daily for 23 days, followed by 5 days without drug.

➤ **Moderate to severe vasomotor symptoms from menopause**

Women: Divigel 0.1% at dose of 0.25, 0.5, or 1 g/day. Start with Divigel 0.25 g daily and adjust dosage based on patient response (range, up to 1 g/day). Or, 1 pump per day of Elestrin applied to the upper arm. Or, Evamist 1 spray per day initially; may adjust dose based on clinical response (1 to 3 sprays/day). Or, 0.05 to 0.1 mg daily by vaginal ring. Replace vaginal ring every 3 months. Or, 1.25 g EstroGel applied once daily to skin.

ADMINISTRATION

PO

• Give without regard for food. If stomach upset occurs, give with food.
• Don't give drug with grapefruit juice.
• Store at controlled room temperature.

IM

• To give IM injection, make sure drug is well dispersed by rolling vial between palms. Inject deep into large muscle. Rotate injection sites to prevent muscle atrophy. Never give drug IV.

Transdermal

• Apply Elestrin once daily to the upper arm.
• Apply EstroGel over the entire area of one arm on the inside and outside from wrist to shoulder. Don't massage or rub EstroGel. Patient should allow gel to dry for 5 minutes before getting dressed.
• Apply Evamist each morning to adjacent, nonoverlapping areas on the inner surface of the forearm, starting near the elbow. Allow to dry for 2 minutes and do not wash the site for 30 minutes.
• Apply Divigel once daily on skin of either right or left upper thigh. Application surface area should be about 5 by 7 inches (about 12.5 by 18 cm; about the size of two palm prints). Apply entire contents of a unit-dose packet each day. To avoid potential skin irritation, apply Divigel to right or left upper thigh on alternating days. Don't apply Divigel on face, breasts, or irritated skin, or in or around the vagina. After application, allow gel to dry before dressing. Don't wash application site within 1 hour after applying Divigel. Avoid contact of gel with eyes. Wash hands after application.
• Apply transdermal patch to clean, dry, hairless, intact skin on abdomen or buttock. Don't apply to breasts, waistline, or other areas where clothing can loosen patch. When applying, ensure thorough contact between patch and skin, especially around edges, and hold in place for about 10 seconds. Apply patch immediately after opening and removing protective cover. Rotate application sites.

Vaginal

• Using the applicator, insert vaginal tablet as far into vagina as it can comfortably go, without using force.
• Remove vaginal ring from its pouch. Squeeze sides together and insert ring into vagina where comfortable.

ACTION

Increases synthesis of DNA, RNA, and protein in responsive tissues; reduces release of FSH and luteinizing hormone from the pituitary gland.

Route	Onset	Peak	Duration
PO, IM, vaginal	Unknown	Unknown	Unknown
Transdermal gel (EstroGel)	Immediate	1 hr	24–36 hr

Half-life: Alora transdermal patch, 1.75 ± 2.87 hours; Vivelle transdermal patch, 4.4 ± 2.3 hours; Vivelle-Dot transdermal patch, 5.9 to 7.7 hours; other forms, unknown.

ADVERSE REACTIONS

CNS: *stroke,* headache, dizziness, chorea, depression, *seizures,* insomnia. **CV:** thrombophlebitis, *thromboembolism,* HTN, edema, *PE, MI.* **EENT:** worsening myopia or astigmatism, intolerance of contact lenses, sinusitis (Vagifem). **GI:** nausea, vomiting, abdominal cramps, bloating, increased appetite, *pancreatitis,* anorexia, gallbladder disease, dyspepsia (Vagifem). **GU:** breakthrough bleeding, altered menstrual flow, dysmenorrhea, amenorrhea, *increased risk of endometrial cancer,* cervical erosion, abnormal Pap smear, altered cervical secretions, enlargement of uterine fibromas, vaginal candidiasis in women, testicular atrophy, erectile dysfunction, genital pruritus, hematuria, vaginal discomfort, vaginitis. **Hepatic:** cholestatic jaundice, *hepatic adenoma.* **Metabolic:** weight changes, hypothyroidism, hypercalcemia (in patients with breast cancer and bone metastases). **Respiratory:** URI, allergy, bronchitis (Vagifem). **Skin:** melasma, urticaria, erythema nodosum, dermatitis, hair loss, pruritus. **Other:** gynecomastia; *increased risk of breast cancer;* hot flashes; pain (Vagifem); breast tenderness, enlargement, or secretion; flulike syndrome.

INTERACTIONS

Drug-drug. *Anastrozole:* May interfere with anastrozole effectiveness. Avoid use together.

Carbamazepine, fosphenytoin, phenobarbital, phenytoin, rifampin: May decrease effectiveness of estrogen therapy. Monitor patient closely.

Clarithromycin, erythromycin, itraconazole, ketoconazole, ritonavir: May increase estrogen plasma levels and side effects. Monitor patient.

Corticosteroids: May enhance effects of corticosteroids. Monitor patient closely.

Cyclosporine: May increase risk of toxicity. Use together with caution, and monitor cyclosporine level frequently.

Dantrolene, other hepatotoxic drugs: May increase risk of hepatotoxicity. Monitor liver function closely.

Exemestane: May interfere with exemestane effectiveness. Avoid use together.

Oral anticoagulants: May decrease anticoagulant effect. Dosage adjustments may be needed. Monitor PT and INR.

Ospemifene: May enhance adverse/toxic effects of ospemifene and interfere with its effectiveness. Avoid use together.

Tamoxifen: May interfere with tamoxifen effectiveness. Avoid using together.

Thyroid hormones: May change thyroid hormone concentrations. May increase thyroid hormone requirements.

Drug-herb. *Red clover:* May increase estrogen effects. Discourage use together.

Saw palmetto: May negate drug's effects. Discourage use together.

St. John's wort: May decrease effects of drug. Discourage use together.

Drug-food. *Caffeine:* May increase caffeine level. Advise patient to avoid or minimize use of caffeine.

Grapefruit juice: May elevate drug level. Tell patient to take drug with liquid other than grapefruit juice.

Drug-lifestyle. *Smoking:* May increase risk of adverse CV effects. If smoking continues, may need another therapy.

EFFECTS ON LAB TEST RESULTS

• May increase total T_4, thyroid-binding globulin, and triglyceride levels. May increase LFT values.

• May alter clotting factors.

• May increase norepinephrine-induced platelet aggregation and prolong PT.

• May decrease metyrapone test results. May impair glucose tolerance.

CONTRAINDICATIONS & CAUTIONS

• Contraindicated in patients with thrombophlebitis or thromboembolic disorders, estrogen-dependent neoplasia, breast or reproductive organ cancer (except for palliative treatment), undiagnosed abnormal genital bleeding, or history of thrombophlebitis or thromboembolic disorders linked to previous estrogen use (except for palliative treatment of breast and prostate cancer).

• Contraindicated in patients with liver dysfunction or disease.

⚗ Contraindicated in patients with known anaphylactic reaction or angioedema caused by drug. Exogenous estrogens may exacerbate

E

signs and symptoms of angioedema in women with hereditary angioedema.
• Use cautiously in patients with cerebrovascular disease or CAD, asthma, bone disease, migraine, seizures, or cardiac or renal dysfunction.
⚡ Use cautiously in women who have a strong family history (grandmother, mother, sister) of breast cancer, breast nodules, fibrocystic breasts, or abnormal mammogram findings.
◑ *Alert:* Postmenopausal women ages 50 to 79 who are taking estrogen and progestin have an increased risk of MI, stroke, invasive breast cancer, PE, and thrombosis. Postmenopausal women age 65 or older also have an increased risk of dementia.
Dialyzable drug: Unknown.
⚠ *Overdose S&S:* Nausea, vomiting, withdrawal uterine bleeding.

PREGNANCY-LACTATION-REPRODUCTION
• Drug is contraindicated in pregnancy.
• Use of estrogen and progestin as in combination hormonal contraceptives hasn't been associated with teratogenic effects when inadvertently taken early in pregnancy.
• Estrogens have been shown to decrease the quantity and quality of human milk. Use only if clearly needed; monitor infant's growth closely.

NURSING CONSIDERATIONS
• Ensure that patient has physical examination before starting therapy. Patients receiving long-term therapy should have yearly examinations. Monitor lipid levels, BP, body weight, and hepatic function.
`Black Box Warning` Estrogen increases the risk of endometrial cancer. Use adequate diagnostic measures, including endometrial sampling when indicated, to rule out malignancy in all cases of undiagnosed persistent or recurring abnormal vaginal bleeding. ∎
`Black Box Warning` Don't use estrogens with or without progestins to prevent CV disease or dementia. Use the lowest effective doses and for the shortest duration consistent with treatment goals. ∎
• When estrogen is prescribed for a postmenopausal woman with a uterus, also initiate a progestin to reduce the risk of endometrial cancer.

◑ *Alert:* EstroGel contains alcohol. Avoid fire, flame, or smoking until area dries in 2 to 5 minutes.
• In women also taking oral estrogen, treatment with the transdermal patch can begin 1 week after withdrawal of oral therapy, or sooner if menopausal symptoms appear before the end of the week.
• Transdermal systems may be used continually rather than cyclically in patients without an intact uterus. Other alternative regimens are 1 to 5 mg cypionate IM every 3 to 4 weeks and 10 to 20 mg valerate IM every 4 weeks, as needed.
• Instruct patients using Vagifem who have severely atrophic vaginal mucosa to be careful when inserting the applicator. After gynecologic surgery, tell patient to use any vaginal applicator cautiously and only if clearly indicated.
• The prescriber should assess patient's need to continue estradiol therapy. Make attempts to stop or taper at 3- to 6-month intervals.
• Because of risk of thromboembolism, stop therapy at least 1 month before high-risk procedures or those that cause prolonged immobilization, such as knee or hip surgery.
• Glucose tolerance may be impaired. Monitor glucose level closely in patients with diabetes.
• Notify pathologist about estrogen therapy when sending specimens to laboratory for evaluation.

PATIENT TEACHING
• Tell patient to read package insert describing estrogen's adverse effects and give her a verbal explanation of those effects.
• Emphasize importance of regular physical examinations. Postmenopausal women who use estrogen replacement for longer than 5 years may be at increased risk for endometrial cancer. Risk is reduced by using cyclic rather than continuous therapy and the lowest possible dosages of estrogen. Adding progestins to the regimen decreases risk of endometrial hyperplasia; however, it isn't known whether progestins affect risk of endometrial cancer. No increased risk of breast cancer has been reported.
`Black Box Warning` Advise patient not to allow contact between children and Evamist application site. Accidental exposure may

---

Reactions in bold italics are *life-threatening*. Interactions may have a *rapid onset* or a *delayed onset*.

cause breast budding and breast masses in prepubertal females and gynecomastia and breast masses in prepubertal males. Ensure children don't come in contact with application site. ■

• Teach patient how to use vaginal cream. She should wash vaginal area with soap and water before applying and should insert cream high into the vagina (about two-thirds the length of the applicator). She should take drug at bedtime or lie flat for 30 minutes after instillation to minimize drug loss.

• Tell patient using topical emulsion, gel, or mist not to apply it with sunscreen.

• Tell patient to use transdermal system correctly, to rotate sites, to avoid breasts and waistline, and to reapply patch if it falls off.

• Teach patient using transdermal gel (EstroGel) to apply in a thin layer on one arm and allow to dry before smoking, getting near flames, dressing, or touching the arm. Recommend bathing before application to maintain full dosage.

• Tell patient that estradiol gel should never be applied directly to the breast.

• Tell patient to insert Vagifem or Yuvafem by the applicator as far into vagina as it can comfortably go, without using force.

• **Alert:** Warn patient to immediately report abdominal pain, pressure or pain in chest, shortness of breath, severe headaches, visual disturbances, vaginal bleeding or discharge, breast lumps, swelling of hands or feet, yellow skin or sclera, dark urine, light-colored stools, and pain, numbness, or stiffness in legs or buttocks.

• Explain to patient receiving cyclic therapy for postmenopausal symptoms that withdrawal bleeding may occur during week off drug. Tell her to report unusual vaginal bleeding.

• Tell diabetic patient to report elevated glucose level so that antidiabetic dosage can be adjusted.

• Teach patient how to perform routine breast self-examination.

• Teach patient methods to decrease risk of blood clots.

• Advise patient not to become pregnant during estrogen therapy.

• Encourage patient to stop or reduce smoking because of the risk of CV complications.

• Advise patient not to allow pets to lick or touch Evamist application site. If signs of illness occur, patient should contact pet's veterinarian.

---

estradiol–norethindrone acetate transdermal system ※

ess-tra-DYE-ole/nor-ETH-in-drone

CombiPatch

Therapeutic class: Estrogens
Pharmacologic class: Estrogen–progestin combinations

E

AVAILABLE FORMS

Transdermal: 9-cm^2 system releasing 0.05 mg estradiol and 0.14 mg norethindrone acetate daily; 16-cm^2 system releasing 0.05 mg estradiol and 0.25 mg norethindrone acetate daily

INDICATIONS & DOSAGES

➤ **Moderate to severe vasomotor symptoms from menopause; vulval and vaginal atrophy; hypoestrogenemia from hypogonadism, castration, or primary ovarian failure in woman with intact uterus**
Continuous combined regimen
Women: Wear 9-cm^2 patch system continuously on lower abdomen. Replace system twice weekly during 28-day cycle. May increase to 16-cm^2 patch.

➤ **Continuous sequential regimen**
Women: For use in sequential regimen with an estradiol transdermal system (such as Alora, Vivelle), wear 0.05-mg estradiol transdermal patch for first 14 days of 28-day cycle; replace system twice weekly. Wear 9-cm^2 patch system on lower abdomen for rest of 28-day cycle; replace system according to product directions. May increase to 16-cm^2 patch.

ADMINISTRATION
Transdermal

• Apply patch system to a smooth (fold-free), clean, dry, nonirritated area of skin on lower abdomen, avoiding the waistline. Rotate application sites, with an interval of at

---

least 1 week between applications to same site.
• Don't apply patch on or near breasts.
• Avoid applying to areas that may get prolonged sun exposure.
• Reapply patch, if needed, to another area of lower abdomen. If patch fails to adhere, replace with a new one.

ACTION

A matrix transdermal system in which estradiol and norethindrone are released continuously. Estrogen replacement therapy can reduce menopausal symptoms and release of FSH and luteinizing hormone in postmenopausal women.

Route	Onset	Peak	Duration
Transdermal	12–24 hr	Unknown	Unknown

Half-life: Estradiol, 2 to 3 hours; norethindrone, 6 to 8 hours.

ADVERSE REACTIONS

CNS: asthenia, *stroke,* depression, insomnia, nervousness, dizziness, headache, weakness, pain. **CV:** *thromboembolism,* thrombophlebitis, HTN, edema, *PE, MI.* **EENT:** pharyngitis, rhinitis, sinusitis, retinal vascular thrombosis, intolerance to contact lenses. **GI:** abdominal pain, diarrhea, dyspepsia, changes in appetite, flatulence, nausea, constipation, gallbladder disease. **GU:** dysmenorrhea, leukorrhea, menstrual disorder, suspicious Papanicolaou smears, vaginitis, menorrhagia, *vaginal hemorrhage.* **Hepatic:** cholestatic jaundice. **Metabolic:** weight changes, hypercalcemia, hypertriglyceridemia. **Musculoskeletal:** arthralgia, back pain. **Respiratory:** respiratory disorder, bronchitis, URI. **Skin:** application-site reactions, acne, melasma, chloasma. **Other:** accidental injury, flulike syndrome, breast pain, tooth disorder, breast enlargement, infection, changes in libido.

INTERACTIONS

Drug-drug. *Anastrozole:* May interfere with anastrozole effectiveness. Avoid using together.
Carbamazepine, fosphenytoin, phenobarbital, phenytoin, rifampin: May decrease estrogen therapy effectiveness. Monitor patient closely.

Clarithromycin, erythromycin, itraconazole, ketoconazole, ritonavir: May increase estrogen plasma levels and side effects. Monitor patient.
Corticosteroids: May enhance effects of corticosteroids. Monitor patient closely.
Cyclosporine: May increase risk of toxicity. Use together with caution; monitor cyclosporine level frequently.
Dantrolene, hepatotoxic drugs: May increase risk of hepatotoxicity. Monitor liver function closely.
Exemestane: May interfere with exemestane effectiveness. Avoid use together.
Oral anticoagulants: May decrease effect of anticoagulant. May need to adjust dose. Monitor PT and INR.
Ospemifene: May enhance adverse/toxic effects of ospemifene and interfere with its effectiveness. Avoid use together.
Tamoxifen: May interfere with tamoxifen effectiveness. Avoid using together.
Drug-herb. *Red clover:* May increase estrogen effects. Discourage use together.
Saw palmetto: May cause antiestrogenic effects. Discourage use together.
St. John's wort: May decrease effects of drug. Discourage use together.
Drug-food. *Caffeine:* May increase caffeine level. Advise patient to avoid or minimize use of caffeine.
Grapefruit juice: May elevate estrogen level. Advise patient to take with liquid other than grapefruit juice.
Drug-lifestyle. *Smoking:* May increase risk of adverse CV effects. If smoking continues, may need alternative therapy.
Sun exposure: May cause photosensitivity reactions. Don't expose patch to the sun for long periods of time.

EFFECTS ON LAB TEST RESULTS

• May increase T_3 and T_4, HDL, and triglyceride levels. May decrease LDL levels.
• May increase fibrinogen activity and platelet count. May decrease T_3 resin uptake. May alter aPTT, INR, and platelet aggregation times.
• May reduce response to metyrapone test. May alter glucose tolerance test results.

Reactions in bold italics are *life-threatening.* Interactions may have a *rapid onset* or a *delayed onset.*

CONTRAINDICATIONS & CAUTIONS

• Contraindicated in women hypersensitive to estrogen, progestin, or any component of the patch and in patients with known or suspected breast cancer, known or suspected estrogen-dependent neoplasia, known anaphylactic reaction or angioedema, known hepatic impairment or disease, thrombophilic disorders, known or suspected pregnancy, undiagnosed abnormal genital bleeding, active thrombophlebitis, thromboembolic disorders, including MI, PE, or stroke.

🜛 Exogenous estrogens may exacerbate signs and symptoms of angioedema in women with hereditary angioedema.

• Use cautiously in patients with impaired liver function, asthma, epilepsy, migraine, or cardiac or renal dysfunction.

Dialyzable drug: Unknown.

⚠ *Overdose S&S:* Nausea, withdrawal bleeding.

PREGNANCY-LACTATION-REPRODUCTION

• Don't give to pregnant women.
• Estrogen has been shown to decrease the quantity and quality of human milk. Use cautiously in breastfeeding women.

NURSING CONSIDERATIONS

Black Box Warning Don't use estrogens, with or without progestins, to prevent CV disease or dementia. Use drug with or without progestins at the lowest effective doses and for the shortest duration consistent with treatment goals. ▮

Black Box Warning Postmenopausal women treated for 5 years have an increased risk of MI, stroke, invasive breast cancer, PE, and DVT. ▮

• Treatment of postmenopausal symptoms usually starts during menopausal stage when vasomotor symptoms occur.

• A combined estrogen–progestin regimen is indicated for a woman with an intact uterus. Progestins taken with estrogen significantly reduce, but don't eliminate, risk of endometrial cancer linked to use of estrogen alone.

• Women not receiving continuous estrogen or combined estrogen–progestin therapy may start therapy at any time.

• Women receiving continuous hormone replacement therapy should complete the current cycle before starting therapy. Women commonly have withdrawal bleeding at completion of cycle; first day of withdrawal bleeding is an appropriate time to start therapy.

• Reevaluate therapy at 3- to 6-month intervals.

• Because of risk of thromboembolism, stop therapy at least 4 to 6 weeks before surgery associated with an increased risk of thromboembolism, or during periods of prolonged immobilization.

• BP increases have been linked to estrogen use. Monitor patient's BP regularly.

• Monitor glucose level closely in patients with diabetes.

🛈 *Alert:* Don't interchange CombiPatch with other estrogen patches. Verify therapy before application.

PATIENT TEACHING

• Teach patient how to apply patch properly. She should wear only one patch at any time during therapy. Tell her to apply patch immediately after opening protective cover.

• Tell patient that an oil-based cream or lotion may help remove adhesive from the skin after patch has been removed and the area allowed to dry for 15 minutes.

• Advise patient not to use patch if she's pregnant or plans to become pregnant.

• Urge patient of childbearing potential to consult prescriber before applying patch and to advise prescriber immediately if she becomes pregnant.

• Instruct patient that the continuous combined regimen may lead to irregular bleeding, particularly in the first 6 months, but that it usually decreases with time and often stops completely.

• Tell patient that, for the continuous sequential regimen, monthly withdrawal bleeding is common.

• Advise patient to alert prescriber and remove patch at first sign of clotting disorders (thrombophlebitis, cerebrovascular disorders, PE).

• Instruct patient to stop using patch and call prescriber about any loss of vision, sudden onset of protrusion of the eyeball (proptosis), double vision, or migraine.

• Encourage patient to stop or reduce smoking because of the risk of CV complications.

• Tell patient to perform monthly breast self-examinations and to have annual gynecologic and breast examinations by a health care provider.
• Advise patient not to store patches where extreme temperatures can occur.
• Tell patient undergoing an MRI to alert facility that she's using a transdermal patch.

estradiol–progesterone
ES-tra-dye-ole/proe-JES-te-rone

Bijuva

Therapeutic class: Menopause drugs
Pharmacologic class: Estrogen–progestin combinations

AVAILABLE FORMS
Capsules: 1 mg estradiol/100 mg progesterone

INDICATIONS & DOSAGES
➤ **Moderate to severe vasomotor symptoms due to menopause**
Women with intact uterus: 1 capsule PO once daily in the evening.

ADMINISTRATION
PO
• Give with food.
• If a dose is missed, give as soon as possible unless it's within 2 hours of the next dose.
• Store at 68° to 77° F (20° to 25° C).

ACTION
Circulating estrogens modulate the pituitary secretion of the gonadotropins luteinizing hormone and FSH through a negative feedback mechanism. Estrogens reduce the elevated levels of these hormones seen in postmenopausal women. Progesterone opposes the action of estrogen by decreasing estrogen receptor levels, increasing the metabolism of estrogen to less active metabolites, or blunting the response to estrogen at the cellular level.

Route	Onset	Peak	Duration
PO	Unknown	Estradiol, 5 hr; progesterone, 3 hr	Unknown

Half-life: Estradiol, 26 hours; progesterone, 10 hours.

ADVERSE REACTIONS
CNS: headache. **GU:** vaginal bleeding, vaginal discharge, pelvic pain. **Other:** breast tenderness.

INTERACTIONS
Drug-drug. *CYP3A4 inducers (carbamazepine, phenobarbital, rifampin):* May decrease estrogen and progestin levels, decreasing therapeutic effect and causing changes in uterine bleeding. Monitor patient closely.
CYP3A4 inhibitors (erythromycin, ketoconazole, ritonavir): May increase estrogen and progestin levels and increase adverse effects. Monitor patient closely.
Drug-herb. *St. John's wort:* May decrease estrogen and progestin levels, decreasing therapeutic effect and causing changes in uterine bleeding. Monitor patient closely.
Drug-food. *Grapefruit juice:* May increase plasma concentrations of estrogens and progestins. Discourage use together.
Drug-lifestyle. *Smoking:* May increase risk of adverse CV effects. Discourage use together. If smoking continues, consider alternative therapy.

EFFECTS ON LAB TEST RESULTS
• May increase HDL and triglyceride levels.
• May decrease LDL level.
• May increase or decrease calcium level.
• May accelerate PT, PTT, and platelet aggregation time. May increase platelet count and clotting factors.
• May decrease antifactor Xa and antithrombin III levels.
• May increase fibrinogen level and fibrinogen activity. May increase plasminogen antigen level and activity.
• May increase circulating total thyroid hormone levels, corticosteroid binding globulin levels, sex hormone-binding globulin levels, free testosterone levels, free estradiol levels, and other plasma protein tests.
• May impair glucose tolerance.

CONTRAINDICATIONS & CAUTIONS
• Contraindicated in women with undiagnosed abnormal genital bleeding; known, suspected, or history of breast cancer; known or suspected estrogen-dependent neoplasia; active DVT, PE, arterial thromboembolic

disease, or history of these conditions; known anaphylactic reaction, angioedema, or hypersensitivity to estrogen or progesterone or capsule ingredients; known liver impairment or disease; or known protein C, protein S, or antithrombin deficiency, or other known thrombophilic disorders.

Black Box Warning Postmenopausal women ages 50 to 79 who are taking estrogen and progestin have an increased risk of DVT, PE, stroke, MI, and invasive breast cancer. Postmenopausal women age 65 and older also have an increased risk of developing probable dementia. ∎

Black Box Warning There is an increased risk of endometrial cancer in women with a uterus who use unopposed estrogen. Adding a progestin to estrogen therapy has been shown to reduce the risk of endometrial hyperplasia, which may be a precursor to endometrial cancer. ∎

Black Box Warning Estrogen plus progestin therapy should not be used for the prevention of CV disease or dementia. ∎

Black Box Warning Use the lowest effective dose and for the shortest duration consistent with treatment goals and individual risks. Reevaluate patients periodically as clinically appropriate to determine if treatment is still necessary. ∎

• Estrogen therapy may cause retinal vascular thrombosis.

• Drug may increase risk of gallbladder disease in postmenopausal women.

• Drug may increase risk of pancreatitis in patients with preexisting hypertriglyceridemia. If pancreatitis occurs, consider discontinuing drug.

• Drug may be poorly metabolized by patients with impaired liver function. Use cautiously in patients with a history of cholestatic jaundice associated with estrogen use or with pregnancy. If cholestatic jaundice recurs, discontinue drug.

• Use cautiously in patients with a history of asthma, diabetes, cardiac or renal dysfunction, epilepsy, migraine headaches, porphyria, SLE, hepatic hemangiomas, or hereditary angioedema, as estrogen therapy may exacerbate these conditions.

• Drug isn't indicated for use in children.

Dialyzable drug: Unknown.

⚠ *Overdose S&S:* Nausea, vomiting, breast tenderness, abdominal pain, drowsiness, fatigue, withdrawal bleeding.

PREGNANCY-LACTATION-REPRODUCTION

• Drug isn't indicated for use in pregnancy or in women of childbearing potential.

• Estrogens appear in human milk and can decrease milk production in breastfeeding women.

NURSING CONSIDERATIONS

Black Box Warning Assess postmenopausal women with undiagnosed persistent or recurring abnormal genital bleeding to rule out malignancy. ∎

• Assess baseline risk of breast cancer and CV disease before starting drug.

• Monitor BP, fluid status, lipid levels, LFT values, and thyroid function during therapy as clinically indicated. Women on thyroid replacement therapy may require a higher dose of thyroid hormone.

• Monitor calcium level in women with breast cancer and bone metastases. Discontinue drug for hypercalcemia and treat calcium level as appropriate.

• Ensure patient receives age-appropriate breast and pelvic exams.

• Monitor patient for vision abnormalities. If sudden partial or complete loss of vision, or a sudden onset of proptosis, diplopia, or migraine occurs, discontinue drug and obtain eye exam. If eye exam reveals papilledema or retinal vascular lesions, permanently discontinue drug.

• Discontinue estrogen therapy at least 4 to 6 weeks before surgery when there is an increased risk of thromboembolism, or during periods of prolonged immobilization.

• *Look alike–sound alike:* Don't confuse this product with other estrogen or progesterone products.

PATIENT TEACHING

• Teach patient safe drug administration and to report all adverse reactions.

Black Box Warning Warn patient of possible serious adverse reactions related to drug, including CV disorders, malignant neoplasms, and age-related probable dementia. ∎

• Instruct patient to immediately report abnormal vaginal bleeding; new breast lumps; changes in vision or speech; sudden, new headaches; severe chest or leg pain with or without shortness of breath; weakness and fatigue; or vomiting.

• Instruct patient that drug may need to be stopped before surgery or if patient will be on bed rest.

• Tell patient that prescriber will evaluate continued need for treatment every 3 to 6 months.

• Teach patient that she should have yearly pelvic and breast exams and mammograms unless otherwise directed by prescriber.

estradiol valerate–estradiol valerate with dienogest ℞
ess-tra-DYE-ole VAL-er-ate/
dye-EN-oh-jest

Natazia

Therapeutic class: Estrogens
Pharmacologic class: Estrogen–progestin combinations

AVAILABLE FORMS
Tablets: 28-day blister pack containing two 3-mg estradiol valerate, five 2-mg estradiol valerate with 2-mg dienogest, seventeen 2-mg estradiol valerate with 3-mg dienogest, two 1-mg estradiol valerate, and two inert tablets

INDICATIONS & DOSAGES
➤ **Contraception; treatment of heavy menstrual bleeding in women without organic pathology who choose to use an oral contraceptive as their method of contraception**
Women: 1 tablet PO daily beginning on first day of menstrual cycle (first day of menstrual bleeding) as directed on blister pack at same time each day. When changing from another combination hormonal contraceptive, begin on first day of withdrawal bleeding. When changing from combination hormonal vaginal ring or transdermal patch, begin on day vaginal ring or transdermal patch is removed. When changing from progestin-only contraceptive, begin next day. When changing from implant contraceptive or intrauterine system, begin day of implant or intrauterine system removal. When changing from injection contraceptive, begin day next injection is due.

ADMINISTRATION
PO
• Give at same time each day; don't skip or delay intake by more than 12 hours.

• Follow manufacturer's detailed instructions if 1 or 2 tablets are missed; patient should use additional backup nonhormonal forms of contraception if necessary.

• Must give tablets in order indicated on blister pack.

ACTION
Prevents pregnancy by suppressing ovulation. May also cause changes in endometrium and cervical mucus, inhibiting sperm penetration and reducing likelihood of implantation.

Route	Onset	Peak	Duration
PO	Unknown	3 hr (estradiol); 1½ hr (dienogest)	Unknown

Half-life: Estradiol, 14 hours; dienogest, 11 hours.

ADVERSE REACTIONS
CNS: depression, headache, migraine. **CV:** *MI, DVT,* HTN. **GI:** nausea, vomiting. **GU:** menstrual disorder, amenorrhea, irregular uterine bleeding, metrorrhagia, oligomenorrhea, *uterine leiomyoma, ruptured ovarian cyst.* **Metabolic:** weight gain, hyperglycemia. **Skin:** acne. **Other:** breast pain, tenderness, or discomfort; mood change.

INTERACTIONS
Drug-drug. *Antibiotics:* May reduce contraceptive effectiveness. Advise use of backup contraception during therapy.
HIV protease inhibitors: May either increase or decrease estrogen and progesterone levels. Use together cautiously and monitor patient for effectiveness of hormone treatment.
Lamotrigine: May decrease lamotrigine serum level, reducing seizure control. Adjust lamotrigine dosage as necessary.
Strong CYP3A4 inducers (barbiturates, carbamazepine, felbamate, griseofulvin, oxcarbazepine, phenytoin, rifampin,

topiramate): May reduce contraceptive effectiveness or increase breakthrough bleeding. An alternative method of birth control should be used.

Strong and moderate inhibitors of CYP3A4 (cimetidine, erythromycin, ketoconazole, SSRIs, verapamil): May increase levels of hormones. Avoid use together. If drugs must be used together, monitor patient for adverse effects.

Thyroid hormone: May increase serum concentration of thyroid-binding globulin, leading to decreased effectiveness of thyroid replacement therapy. Monitor patient; thyroid hormone dosage may need adjustment.

Drug-herb. *Red clover:* May increase estrogen effects. Discourage use together.

St. John's wort: May reduce contraceptive effectiveness or increase breakthrough bleeding. Recommend alternative method of birth control.

Drug-food. *Grapefruit juice:* May increase levels of hormones. Avoid use together.

Drug-lifestyle. ▇Black Box Warning▇ *Smoking:* Increases risk of medical problems, such as stroke, emboli, or heart disease. Recommend smoking cessation. ■

EFFECTS ON LAB TEST RESULTS
• May increase thyroid-binding globulin, glucose, cholesterol, and lipid levels.
• May alter clotting factors.

CONTRAINDICATIONS & CAUTIONS
• Contraindicated in patients with benign or malignant liver tumors; liver disease; current or history of breast cancer or other estrogen- or progestin-sensitive cancer; undiagnosed abnormal uterine bleeding; headaches with focal neurologic symptoms or migraine headaches with or without aura if older than age 35; diabetes with vascular disease; uncontrolled HTN; HTN with vascular disease; inherited or acquired hypercoagulopathies; thrombogenic valvular or thrombogenic rhythm disease of heart, such as endocarditis or atrial fibrillation; CAD; cerebrovascular disease; and current or past DVT or PE.
▇Black Box Warning▇ Contraindicated in women who smoke and who are older than age 35. ■
• Use cautiously in women with CV disease risk factors, history of cholestasis,

history of well-controlled HTN, prediabetes or well-controlled diabetes, history of hyperlipidemia, new-onset headaches, history of bleeding irregularities, history of emotional disorders, angioedema, or chloasma.

▧ Exogenous estrogens may exacerbate signs and symptoms of angioedema in women with hereditary angioedema.
• Safety and effectiveness in women with BMI greater than 30 kg/m^2 haven't been evaluated.
• Drug hasn't been studied in postmenopausal women and isn't indicated in this population.

Dialyzable drug: Unknown.
⚠ ***Overdose S&S:*** Nausea, withdrawal bleeding.

PREGNANCY-LACTATION-REPRODUCTION
• Don't give to pregnant women.
• There is little or no increased risk of birth defects in women who inadvertently use combined oral contraceptives during early pregnancy.
• Estrogen has been shown to decrease the quantity and quality of human milk. Drug shouldn't be used in breastfeeding women.
• Use before menarche isn't indicated.

NURSING CONSIDERATIONS
• Start drug no earlier than 4 weeks after delivery in women who aren't breastfeeding. Risk of postpartum venous thromboembolic event (VTE) decreases and ovulation risk increases after third postpartum week.
• Monitor BP; elevations are possible in nonhypertensive women.
• Monitor coagulation factors as appropriate.
• Monitor glucose and cholesterol levels regularly, especially in women who are prediabetic and in those with history of elevated lipid levels.
• Monitor women for headache. New-onset headaches may require discontinuing oral contraceptives.
• Carefully monitor women with history of depression for recurrence or exacerbation.
• Stop drug if arterial or deep VTE occurs. Highest risk of VTE is during first year of contraceptive use. If feasible, stop tablets at least 4 weeks before and for 2 weeks after major surgery.

• Oral contraceptives are associated with increased risk of thrombotic and hemorrhagic strokes, especially in women older than age 35, in those with HTN, and in smokers. Stop drug if unexplained vision loss, proptosis, diplopia, papilledema, or retinal vascular changes occur. Evaluate retinal vein thrombosis immediately.

• Risk of drug causing breast cancer or cervical or endometrial cancer is controversial and uncertain. As a precaution, women should have regular Papanicolaou tests, breast examinations, and mammograms.

• Discontinue drug if jaundice develops. Women who take oral contraceptives are at slightly higher risk for developing liver tumors and gallstones. Monitor patient for skin color changes and pain in right upper quadrant.

• Ensure that patient uses a nonhormonal contraceptive method, such as a condom or spermicide, for the first 9 days.

PATIENT TEACHING

• Teach patient to take tablet once daily and not to skip doses or delay taking tablet by more than 12 hours. Advise patient that tablets should be taken in the order marked on each pack.

• Instruct patient to read patient guide for using Natazia for information on missed tablets and when to contact her pharmacist or prescriber; tell her that backup contraception must be used.

• Tell patient starting drug for first time to begin taking tablets on day 1 of her period and to use backup contraceptive method for first 9 days.

• Instruct patient that spotting or light bleeding is normal at first.

• Advise patient that she may feel nauseous, especially during first few months, but that this symptom usually disappears and she shouldn't stop taking tablets. Tell patient to report to prescriber if nausea doesn't resolve.

• Warn patient to start drug no earlier than 4 weeks after giving birth.

• Advise patient to notify prescriber if she is pregnant before taking drug.

• Tell patient that breastfeeding while taking tablets isn't recommended because milk production may be reduced and small amounts of drug appear in human milk.

• Inform patient taking tablets that blood tests may be needed to check blood glucose and cholesterol levels, as well as how her blood is clotting, and that her BP may also be checked.

• Tell patient to inform prescriber of all prescription, over-the-counter, and herbal supplements she is taking.

• Advise patient, if appropriate, to quit smoking before taking drug.

Black Box Warning Advise patient who smokes that she is at increased risk for serious CV events from combination oral contraceptive use. Risk increases with age, especially after age 35, and with number of cigarettes smoked. ■

• Warn patient that contraceptive use doesn't protect against HIV infection or other sexually transmitted diseases.

• Tell patient that a missed period may occur but that pregnancy should be ruled out if she misses two or more consecutive menstrual cycles.

• Warn patient to call prescriber immediately if she experiences persistent leg pain; sudden shortness of breath; sudden blindness (partial or complete); severe chest pain; sudden, severe headache; weakness or numbness in an arm or leg; trouble speaking; or yellowing of skin or eyes.

• Advise patient with tendency to chloasma to avoid sun exposure and ultraviolet radiation.

• Advise patient to stop smoking while taking oral contraceptive because of increased risk of stroke and other thromboembolic events.

• Tell patient who experiences vomiting or diarrhea within 3 to 4 hours after taking a colored tablet to regard it as a missed tablet.

---

estrogens (conjugated) (estrogenic substances, conjugated; oestrogens, conjugated) ▨
Premarin✒

Therapeutic class: Estrogens
Pharmacologic class: Estrogens

AVAILABLE FORMS
Injection: 25-mg vial

Reactions in bold italics are *life-threatening*. Interactions may have a *rapid onset* or a *delayed onset*.

Tablets: 0.3 mg, 0.45 mg, 0.625 mg, 0.9 mg, 1.25 mg
Vaginal cream: 0.625 mg/g

INDICATIONS & DOSAGES

➤ **Abnormal uterine bleeding (hormonal imbalance)**
Women: 25 mg slow IV (preferred) or IM. Repeat dose in 6 to 12 hours, if necessary.
➤ **Vulvar or vaginal atrophy; kraurosis vulvae**
Women: 0.5 to 2 g cream intravaginally once daily in cycles of 21 days on, 7 days off.
➤ **Moderate to severe dyspareunia due to menopause-related vulvar and vaginal atrophy**
Women: 0.5 g cream intravaginally twice weekly as a continuous regimen. Or, 0.5 g intravaginally once daily for 21 days followed by 7 days off.
➤ **Castration and primary ovarian failure**
Women: Initially, 1.25 mg Premarin PO daily in cycles of 3 weeks on, 1 week off. Adjust dose as needed.
➤ **Female hypogonadism**
Women: 0.3 to 0.625 mg Premarin PO daily, given cyclically 3 weeks on, 1 week off. Adjust dose depending on symptom severity and responsiveness of the endometrium.
➤ **Moderate to severe vasomotor symptoms with or without moderate to severe symptoms of vulvar and vaginal atrophy associated with menopause**
Women: Initially, 0.3 mg Premarin PO daily. Premarin may also be given cyclically 25 days on, 5 days off. Adjust dosage based on patient response.
➤ **To prevent osteoporosis**
Women: 0.3 mg Premarin PO daily, or cyclically 25 days on, 5 days off. Adjust dose based on response of bone mineral density testing.
➤ **Palliative treatment of inoperable prostatic cancer**
Men: 1.25 to 2.5 mg Premarin PO t.i.d. Judge effectiveness based on phosphatase determinations and symptomatic improvement.
➤ **Palliative treatment of breast cancer**
Adults (men and women): 10 mg Premarin PO t.i.d. for at least 3 months.

ADMINISTRATION

PO
• Give drug at same time each day.
• May give with or without food.
• Store tablets at controlled room temperature.

IV
▼ IV use is preferred over IM because a more rapid response can be expected.
▼ Refrigerate before reconstituting.
▼ Store injection in refrigerator (36° to 46° F [2° to 8° C]).
▼ Reconstitute slowly with 5 mL sterile water for injection. Don't shake.
▼ Drug is compatible with NSS and dextrose and invert sugar solutions.
▼ Use solutions immediately after reconstitution.
▼ Give direct injection slowly to avoid flushing reaction.
▼ **Incompatibilities:** Acidic solutions, ascorbic acid, protein hydrolysate.

IM
• Reconstitute with sterile water for injection. Agitate gently after adding diluent.
• Inject deep into large muscle. Rotate injection sites to prevent muscle atrophy.

Vaginal
• Wash the vaginal area with soap and water, insert about two-thirds the length of the applicator into the vagina, and release drug.
• Give drug at bedtime or when patient will lie flat for 30 minutes after use to minimize drug loss.
• Store cream at controlled room temperature.

ACTION

Increases synthesis of DNA, RNA, and protein in responsive tissues. Also reduces release of FSH and luteinizing hormone from the pituitary gland.

Route	Onset	Peak	Duration
PO, IV, IM, vaginal	Unknown	7 hr	Unknown

Half-life: 27 hours.

ADVERSE REACTIONS

CNS: headache, dizziness, chorea, migraine, depression, asthenia, insomnia, nervousness, *stroke, seizures.* **CV:** flushing with rapid IV administration; thrombophlebitis,

thromboembolism, HTN, edema, *PE, MI.*
EENT: worsening myopia or astigmatism, intolerance of contact lenses. **GI:** nausea, vomiting, abdominal cramps, bloating, anorexia, increased appetite, dyspepsia, flatulence, diarrhea, *pancreatitis,* gallbladder disease. **GU:** breakthrough bleeding, altered menstrual flow, dysmenorrhea, amenorrhea, *increased risk of endometrial cancer,* cervical erosion, altered cervical secretions, enlargement of uterine fibromas, vaginal candidiasis, testicular atrophy, impotence. **Hepatic:** cholestatic jaundice, *hepatic adenoma.* **Metabolic:** weight changes, hypercalcemia, hypertriglyceridemia. **Musculoskeletal:** arthralgia, back pain, leg cramps, myalgia. **Respiratory:** URI. **Skin:** melasma, chloasma, urticaria, hirsutism or hair loss, erythema nodosum, dermatitis. **Other:** breast tenderness, enlargement, or secretion; gynecomastia; increased risk of breast cancer; changes in libido.

INTERACTIONS
Drug-drug. *Anastrozole:* May interfere with anastrozole effectiveness. Avoid use together.
Carbamazepine, fosphenytoin, phenobarbital, phenytoin, rifampin: May decrease effectiveness of estrogen therapy. Monitor patient closely.
Corticosteroids: May enhance corticosteroid effects. Monitor patient closely.
Cyclosporine: May increase risk of toxicity. Use together with caution, and monitor cyclosporine level frequently.
Dantrolene, other hepatotoxic drugs: May increase risk of hepatotoxicity. Monitor liver function closely.
Exemestane: May interfere with exemestane effectiveness. Avoid use together.
Itraconazole, ketoconazole, macrolide antibiotics, ritonavir: May increase estrogen plasma levels and risk of adverse effects. Monitor patient.
Oral anticoagulants: May decrease anticoagulant effects. May need to adjust dosage. Monitor PT and INR.
Ospemifene: May enhance adverse/toxic effects of ospemifene and interfere with its effectiveness. Avoid use together.
Tamoxifen: May interfere with tamoxifen effectiveness. Avoid using together.

Thyroid hormones: May increase serum thyroxine-binding globulin levels, which may increase thyroid hormone requirements.
Drug-herb. *Red clover:* May increase estrogen effects. Discourage use together.
Saw palmetto: May have antiestrogenic effects. Discourage use together.
St. John's wort: May decrease effects of drug. Discourage use together.
Drug-food. *Caffeine:* May increase caffeine level. Advise caution.
Grapefruit juice: May increase concentration of estrogen. Avoid using together.
Drug-lifestyle. *Smoking:* May increase risk of adverse CV effects. If smoking continues, recommend nonhormonal contraception.

EFFECTS ON LAB TEST RESULTS
• May increase HDL and triglyceride levels. May decrease LDL level.
• May increase T_3 and total T_4, phospholipid, and thyroid-binding globulin levels.
• May alter clotting factors.
• May increase norepinephrine-induced platelet aggregation and PT.
• May cause a false-positive metyrapone test result.
• May interfere with glucose tolerance test.

CONTRAINDICATIONS & CAUTIONS
• Contraindicated in patients with liver dysfunction; known or suspected pregnancy; thrombophlebitis, thromboembolic disorders; known protein C, protein S, or antithrombin deficiency or other thrombophilic disorders (active DVT/PE); estrogen-dependent neoplasia; breast or reproductive cancer (except for palliative treatment); undiagnosed abnormal genital bleeding; and known anaphylactic reaction or angioedema to conjugated estrogens.
• Use cautiously in patients with cerebrovascular disease or CAD, asthma, bone disease, migraine, seizures, or cardiac, hepatic, or renal dysfunction.
🜨 Use cautiously in women who have a strong family history (mother, grandmother, sister) of breast or reproductive tract cancer, breast nodules, fibrocystic breasts, or abnormal mammogram findings.
🜨 Exogenous estrogens may exacerbate signs and symptoms of angioedema in women with hereditary angioedema.

Reactions in bold italics are *life-threatening*. Interactions may have a *rapid onset* or a *delayed onset*.

Dialyzable drug: Unknown.

⚠ *Overdose S&S:* Nausea, vomiting, breast tenderness, abdominal pain, drowsiness or fatigue, withdrawal uterine bleeding.

PREGNANCY-LACTATION-REPRODUCTION
• Contraindicated during pregnancy.
• Drug shouldn't be used during breastfeeding. Estrogen has been shown to decrease the quantity and quality of human milk.

NURSING CONSIDERATIONS
• Make sure patient has thorough physical examination before starting therapy; patients receiving long-term therapy should have yearly examinations. Periodically monitor lipid levels, BP, body weight, and hepatic function.
• Rapid treatment of dysfunctional uterine bleeding or reduction of surgical bleeding usually requires delivery by IV or IM route.

Black Box Warning Don't use to prevent CV disease. In postmenopausal women receiving therapy for more than 5 years, drug may increase risks of MI, stroke, invasive breast cancer, PE, and DVT. Use the lowest effective doses for the shortest time, considering the benefits and risks. ■

Black Box Warning In postmenopausal women receiving therapy for more than 5 years, drug may increase risk of endometrial cancer. Cyclic therapy and the lowest possible dose reduce risk. Adding progestins decreases risk of endometrial hyperplasia, but it's unknown whether they affect risk of endometrial cancer. ■

Black Box Warning In postmenopausal women age 65 or older receiving 4 years of treatment with conjugated estrogens plus medroxyprogesterone acetate, drug may increase the risk of dementia. ■

• Periodically reevaluate need for therapy.
• When used solely for the treatment of vulval and vaginal atrophy, consider topical products.
• Because of thromboembolism risk, stop therapy at least 4 to 6 weeks before procedures that prolong immobilization or raise risk of thromboembolism, such as knee or hip surgery.
• Notify pathologist about estrogen therapy when sending specimens to laboratory for evaluation.

• Glucose tolerance may be impaired. Monitor glucose level closely in patients with diabetes.
• *Look alike–sound alike:* Don't confuse Premarin with Primaxin, Provera, or Remeron.

PATIENT TEACHING
• Teach patient about adverse effects and advise her to report them promptly.
• Emphasize importance of regular physical examinations.
• Teach female patient how to use vaginal cream. Tell patient to wash the vaginal area with soap and water, insert about two-thirds the length of the applicator into the vagina, and release drug. Tell her to use drug at bedtime or to lie flat for 30 minutes after use to minimize drug loss.
• Explain to patient that cyclic therapy for postmenopausal symptoms may cause withdrawal bleeding during week off drug. Tell her to report unusual vaginal bleeding.
• *Alert:* Warn patient to immediately report abdominal pain; pain, numbness, or stiffness in legs or buttocks; pressure or pain in chest; shortness of breath; severe headaches; visual disturbances, such as blind spots, flashing lights, or blurriness; vaginal bleeding or discharge; breast lumps; swelling of hands or feet; yellow skin or sclera; dark urine; and light-colored stools.
• Tell diabetic patient to report elevated glucose level so that antidiabetic dosage can be adjusted.
• Teach female patient how to perform routine breast self-examination.
• Advise female patient not to become pregnant during estrogen therapy.
• Advise female patient of childbearing potential to consult prescriber before taking drug and to advise prescriber immediately if she becomes pregnant.
• Encourage patient to stop smoking or reduce number of cigarettes smoked because of the risk of CV complications.
• Tell patient using drug for osteoporosis prevention to ensure adequate intake of calcium and vitamin D.
• Inform patient that vaginal cream has been reported to weaken latex condoms and to use an alternative method of birth control.

estropipate ⚕
ess-troe-PIH-pate

Ogen 5

Therapeutic class: Estrogens
Pharmacologic class: Estrogens

AVAILABLE FORMS
Tablets: 0.75 mg, 1.5 mg

INDICATIONS & DOSAGES
➤ **Vulval and vaginal atrophy**
Women: 0.75 to 6 mg PO daily, 3 weeks on and 1 week off. If patient is menstruating, start cyclic administration on day 5 of bleeding.
➤ **Primary ovarian failure, female castration, female hypogonadism**
Women: 1.5 to 9 mg PO daily for first 3 weeks; then a rest period of 8 to 10 days. If bleeding doesn't occur by end of rest period, cycle is repeated.
➤ **Moderate to severe vasomotor menopausal symptoms**
Women: 0.75 to 6 mg PO daily in cyclic method, 3 weeks on and 1 week off. Can be given continuously. If patient is menstruating, start cyclic administration on day 5 of bleeding.
➤ **To prevent osteoporosis**
Women: 0.75 mg PO daily for 25 consecutive days of a 31-day cycle, followed by 6 days without drug. Repeat regimen as indicated.

ADMINISTRATION
PO
• Give with or without food.
• Store below 77° F (25° C).

ACTION
Increases synthesis of DNA, RNA, and proteins in responsive tissues; reduces FSH and luteinizing hormone levels.

Route	Onset	Peak	Duration
PO	Unknown	Unknown	Unknown

Half-life: Unknown.

ADVERSE REACTIONS
CNS: depression, headache, dizziness, migraine, chorea, nervousness, mood disturbances, irritability, epilepsy exacerbation, *seizures, stroke.* **CV:** edema, thrombophlebitis, HTN, *PE, MI, thromboembolism.* **EENT:** steepening of corneal curvature, intolerance to contact lenses. **GI:** nausea, vomiting, gallbladder disease, abdominal cramps, bloating, pancreatitis, diarrhea. **GU:** increased size of uterine fibromas, *endometrial cancer,* vaginal candidiasis, cystitis-like syndrome, dysmenorrhea, amenorrhea, breakthrough bleeding, condition resembling premenstrual syndrome, enlargement of uterine leiomyomata, vaginitis, change in amount of cervical secretion, vaginal candidiasis. **Hepatic:** cholestatic jaundice, *hepatic adenoma,* enlargement of hepatic hemangiomas. **Metabolic:** weight changes, hypocalcemia, hypertriglyceridemia. **Skin:** hemorrhagic eruption, erythema nodosum, *erythema multiforme,* hirsutism or hair loss, melasma, pruritus, rash. **Other:** breast engorgement or enlargement, *breast cancer,* breast tenderness, changes in libido, leg cramps, nipple discharge.

INTERACTIONS
Drug-drug. *Anastrozole:* May interfere with anastrozole effectiveness. Avoid use together.
Carbamazepine, fosphenytoin, phenobarbital, phenytoin, rifampin: May decrease estropipate effect. Monitor patient closely.
Clarithromycin, erythromycin, itraconazole, ketoconazole, ritonavir: May increase estropipate plasma levels and side effects. Monitor patient.
Corticosteroids: May enhance corticosteroid effect. Monitor patient closely.
Cyclosporine: May increase risk of toxicity. Use together with caution; frequently monitor cyclosporine level.
Dantrolene, other hepatotoxic drugs: May increase risk of hepatotoxicity. Monitor liver function closely.
Exemestane: May interfere with exemestane effectiveness. Avoid use together.
Oral anticoagulants: May decrease anticoagulant effect. Dosage adjustments may be needed. Monitor PT and INR.

Reactions in bold italics are *life-threatening*. Interactions may have a *rapid onset* or a *delayed onset*.

Ospemifene: May enhance adverse/toxic effects of ospemifene and interfere with its effectiveness. Avoid use together.

Tamoxifen: May interfere with tamoxifen effect. Avoid using together.

Drug-herb. *Red clover:* May increase estrogen effects. Discourage use together.

St. John's wort: May decrease estrogen effect. Discourage use together.

Drug-food. *Caffeine:* May increase caffeine level. Advise caution.

Grapefruit juice: May increase concentration of drug and risk of adverse effects. Avoid use together.

Drug-lifestyle. *Smoking:* May increase risk of adverse CV effects. If smoking continues, may need alternative therapy.

EFFECTS ON LAB TEST RESULTS

• May increase HDL and triglyceride levels.
• May decrease LDL and serum folate levels.
• May increase total T_4, phospholipid, and thyroid-binding globulin levels.
• May alter clotting factors.
• May increase norepinephrine-induced platelet aggregation and prolong PT.
• May reduce response to metyrapone test. May impair glucose tolerance.

CONTRAINDICATIONS & CAUTIONS

• Contraindicated in patients with known hypersensitivity to drug and in those with liver dysfunction, known or suspected pregnancy, active thrombophlebitis, arterial thromboembolic disorders, estrogen-dependent neoplasia, undiagnosed genital bleeding, and breast, reproductive organ, or genital cancer.
• Use cautiously in patients with cerebrovascular disease or CAD; asthma; mental depression; bone disease; migraine; seizures; or cardiac, hepatic, or renal dysfunction.
🦰 Use cautiously in women who have a family history (mother, grandmother, sister) of breast or genital tract cancer, breast nodules, fibrocystic breasts, or abnormal mammogram findings.

Dialyzable drug: Unknown.

⚠ **Overdose S&S:** Nausea, vomiting, withdrawal uterine bleeding.

PREGNANCY-LACTATION-REPRODUCTION

• There is no indication for use during pregnancy. Use is contraindicated.
• Estrogens can be detected in human milk and have been shown to decrease the quantity and quality of milk. Use cautiously in breastfeeding women.

NURSING CONSIDERATIONS

• Make sure patient has thorough physical exam before starting estrogen therapy. Patients receiving long-term therapy should have examinations yearly. Periodically monitor lipid levels, BP, body weight, and hepatic function.

Black Box Warning Estrogens and progestins shouldn't be used to prevent CV disease. The Women's Health Initiative study reported increased risks of MI, stroke, invasive breast cancer, PE, and DVT in postmenopausal women during 5 years of combination therapy. Because of these risks, estrogens and progestins should be prescribed at the lowest effective doses and for the shortest duration consistent with treatment goals and risks for the individual woman. The Women's Health Initiative study also reported increased risk of the development of dementia in postmenopausal women age 65 and older during 4 years of treatment with oral conjugated estrogens plus medroxyprogesterone. It isn't known if this finding also applies to younger postmenopausal women or to women taking estrogen alone. ∎

Black Box Warning Estrogens may increase the risk of endometrial cancer in postmenopausal women. ∎

Black Box Warning Close clinical surveillance of all women taking estrogens is important. Adequate diagnostic measures, including endometrial sampling when indicated, should be undertaken to rule out malignancy in all cases of undiagnosed persistent or recurring abnormal vaginal bleeding. ∎

• When used to treat hypogonadism, duration of therapy needed to produce withdrawal bleeding depends on patient's endometrial response to drug. If satisfactory withdrawal bleeding doesn't occur, an oral progestin is added to the regimen. Explain to patient that, despite return of withdrawal

E

bleeding, pregnancy can't occur because she doesn't ovulate.

• Because of risk of thromboembolism, stop therapy at least 4 to 6 weeks before procedures that prolong immobilization or raise the risk of thromboembolism, such as knee or hip surgery.

• Glucose tolerance may be impaired. Monitor glucose level closely in patients with diabetes.

PATIENT TEACHING

• Tell patient to report all adverse effects; explain effects verbally.

• Tell diabetic patient to report elevated glucose level to prescriber.

• Stress importance of regular physical examinations. Postmenopausal women who use estrogen replacement for longer than 5 years may have increased risk of endometrial cancer. Using cyclic therapy and lowest possible estrogen dosage reduces risk. Adding progestins to regimen decreases risk of endometrial hyperplasia; however, it isn't known whether progestins affect risk of endometrial cancer.

◐ **Alert:** Warn patient to immediately report abdominal pain; pain, stiffness, or numbness in legs or buttocks; pressure or pain in chest; shortness of breath; severe headaches; visual disturbances, such as blind spots or flashing lights; vaginal bleeding or discharge; breast lumps; swelling of hands or feet; yellow skin or sclera; dark urine; and light-colored stools.

• Teach female patient how to perform routine breast self-examination.

• Advise female patient not to become pregnant while on estrogen therapy.

• Encourage patient to stop or reduce smoking because of the risk of CV complications.

• Advise female patient of childbearing potential to consult prescriber before taking drug and to tell prescriber immediately if she becomes pregnant.

• Teach patient at risk for osteoporosis about the importance of adequate calcium and vitamin D intake.

SAFETY ALERT!

eszopiclone
ess-ZOP-ah-klone

Lunesta✐

Therapeutic class: Hypnotics
Pharmacologic class: Pyrrolopyrazine derivatives
Controlled substance schedule: IV

AVAILABLE FORMS
Tablets: 1 mg, 2 mg, 3 mg

INDICATIONS & DOSAGES
➤ **Insomnia**
Adults: 1 mg PO immediately before bedtime. Increase to 2 or 3 mg as needed.
Elderly and debilitated patients: 1 mg PO immediately before bedtime. Increase to 2 mg as needed. Maximum dose is 2 mg.
Adjust-a-dose: In patients with severe hepatic impairment and in those also taking a potent CYP3A4 inhibitor, start with 1 mg PO and increase to 2 mg as needed. Maximum dose is 2 mg. In elderly or debilitated patients, don't exceed 2 mg.

ADMINISTRATION
PO
• Avoid giving drug after a high-fat meal.
• Give drug immediately before bedtime because drug may cause dizziness or lightheadedness.

ACTION
Probably interacts with GABA receptors at binding sites close to or connected to benzodiazepine receptors.

Route	Onset	Peak	Duration
PO	Rapid	1 hr	Unknown

Half-life: 6 hours.

ADVERSE REACTIONS
CNS: abnormal dreams, anxiety, complex sleep-related behavior, confusion, depression, dizziness, hallucinations, headache, nervousness, pain, somnolence, neuralgia. **GI:** diarrhea, dry mouth, dyspepsia, nausea, vomiting, unpleasant taste. **GU:** dysmenorrhea, UTI, decreased libido, gynecomastia.

Respiratory: URI. **Skin:** pruritus, rash.
Other: accidental injury, viral infection.

INTERACTIONS
Drug-drug. *CNS depressants:* May have additive CNS effects. Adjust dosage of either drug as needed.
CYP3A4 inhibitors (clarithromycin, itraconazole, ketoconazole, nefazodone, nelfinavir, ritonavir, troleandomycin): May decrease eszopiclone elimination, increasing the risk of toxicity. Use together cautiously. Limit eszopiclone dose to maximum of 2 mg.
Olanzapine: May impair cognitive function or memory. Use together cautiously.

Black Box Warning *Opioid class warning:* May cause slow or difficult breathing, sedation, and death. Avoid use together. If use together is necessary, limit dosage and duration of each drug to minimum necessary for desired effect. ∎
Rifampin: May decrease eszopiclone activity. Don't use together.
Drug-herb. *St. John's wort:* May decrease eszopiclone serum concentration. Discourage concurrent use.
Drug-food. *High-fat meals:* May delay drug's effects. Discourage high-fat meals with or just before taking drug.
Drug-lifestyle. *Alcohol use:* May decrease psychomotor ability. Discourage taking drug if patient drank alcohol that evening or before bed.

EFFECTS ON LAB TEST RESULTS
None reported.

CONTRAINDICATIONS & CAUTIONS
• Contraindicated in patients with known hypersensitivity to eszopiclone.
• Rarely, drug may cause angioedema and anaphylaxis that require emergency treatment and can be fatal. Don't rechallenge patients who develop angioedema after treatment with drug.

Black Box Warning *Opioid class warning:* Opioids should only be prescribed with benzodiazepines or other CNS depressants when alternative treatment options are inadequate. ∎
• Use cautiously in elderly and debilitated patients, in patients with diseases or conditions that could affect metabolism or hemodynamic responses, and in patients with compromised respiratory function or severe hepatic impairment. Also use cautiously in patients with signs and symptoms of depression because of the increased risk of suicide.
• Dosage adjustments may be needed when drug is combined with other CNS depressants because of potentially additive effects.
• Impaired alertness and motor coordination can occur; risk increases with dose. Patient taking 3-mg dose shouldn't drive or perform activities requiring complete mental alertness during the morning after use.
⚠ **Overdose S&S:** CNS depression.

PREGNANCY-LACTATION-REPRODUCTION
• Use during pregnancy only if potential benefit justifies potential risk to the fetus.
• It isn't known if drug appears in human milk. Breastfeeding isn't recommended.

NURSING CONSIDERATIONS
🔆 *Alert:* Anaphylaxis and angioedema may occur as early as the first dose; monitor patient closely.
🔆 *Alert:* Drug may increase risk of next-day impairment of driving and other activities that require full alertness. Recommended starting dose for all patients is 1 mg.
• Evaluate patient for physical and psychiatric disorders before treatment.
• Use the lowest effective dose.
🔆 *Alert:* Give drug immediately before patient goes to bed or after patient has gone to bed and has trouble falling asleep.
• Use only for short periods (for example, 7 to 10 days). If patient still has trouble sleeping, check for other psychological disorders.
• Risk of abuse and dependence increases with the dose and duration of treatment and the concurrent use of other psychoactive drugs. Abrupt discontinuation may cause withdrawal symptoms.
• Monitor patient for changes in behavior, such as decreased inhibition, aggression, and agitation, and including those that suggest depression or suicidal thinking. Amnesia and other neuropsychiatric symptoms may occur unpredictably.

PATIENT TEACHING

Black Box Warning *Opioid class warning:* Caution patient or caregiver of patient taking an opioid with a benzodiazepine, CNS depressant, or alcohol to seek immediate medical attention for dizziness, lightheadedness, extreme sleepiness, slowed or difficult breathing, or unresponsiveness. ■

◑ **Alert:** Warn patient that drug may cause allergic reactions, facial swelling, and complex sleep-related behaviors, such as driving, eating, and making phone calls while asleep. Advise patient to report these adverse effects.

◑ **Alert:** Caution patient taking 3 mg of eszopiclone not to drive or engage in activities that are hazardous or require complete mental alertness the day after use.

• Urge patient to take drug immediately before going to bed because drug may cause dizziness or light-headedness.

• Caution patient not to take drug unless a full night's sleep is possible.

• Advise patient to avoid taking drug after a high-fat meal and to avoid alcohol.

• Tell patient to avoid activities that require mental alertness until the drug's effects are known.

• Urge patient to immediately report changes in behavior and thinking.

• Warn patient not to stop drug abruptly or change dose without consulting the prescriber.

• Inform patient that tolerance or dependence may develop if drug is taken for a prolonged period.

BIOSIMILAR DRUG

etanercept
ee-TAN-er-sept

Enbrel, Enbrel SureClick

etanercept-szzs
Erelzi

Therapeutic class: Antiarthritics
Pharmacologic class: TNF blockers

AVAILABLE FORMS
Injection: 25-mg multiuse vial
Prefilled autoinjector: 50 mg/mL

Prefilled single-dose Sensoready pen: 50 mg/mL
Prefilled single-dose syringe: 25 mg/0.5 mL, 50 mg/mL

INDICATIONS & DOSAGES
➤ **To reduce signs and symptoms of moderately to severely active polyarticular juvenile idiopathic arthritis in patients whose response to one or more DMARDs has been inadequate**
Children ages 2 to 17: For children weighing 63 kg or more, 50 mg subcut once weekly. For children weighing less than 63 kg (Enbrel only), 0.8 mg/kg subcut once weekly as two injections, either on the same day or 3 or 4 days apart using the multiuse vial. Maximum dosage is 50 mg/week. Glucocorticoids, NSAIDs, or analgesics may be continued during treatment. Use with methotrexate hasn't been studied in children.
➤ **RA, ankylosing spondylitis**
Adults: 50 mg subcut once weekly. Methotrexate, glucocorticoids, salicylates, NSAIDs, and analgesics may be continued during treatment.
➤ **Psoriatic arthritis (Enbrel only)**
Adults: 50 mg subcut once weekly. May continue methotrexate, glucocorticoids, salicylates, NSAIDs, and analgesics during treatment.
➤ **Chronic moderate to severe plaque psoriasis in patients who are candidates for systemic therapy or phototherapy**
Adults: 50 mg (Enbrel) subcut twice weekly, 3 to 4 days apart, for 3 months. Then, reduce dosage to 50 mg subcut once weekly. Or, initially, 50 mg (Erelzi) subcut twice weekly for 3 months; then 50 mg subcut once weekly.
Children age 4 and older: For patients weighing 63 kg or more, 50 mg subcut once weekly. For patients weighing less than 63 kg, 0.8 mg/kg subcut once weekly. Maximum dosage is 50 mg/week.

ADMINISTRATION
Subcutaneous
• Give 50-mg dose as one subcut injection using a 50-mg/mL single-use prefilled syringe or prefilled autoinjector or pen or as two 25-mg subcut injections using multiuse vial. Give the two 25-mg injections on the same day or 3 to 4 days apart.

Reactions in bold italics are *life-threatening*. Interactions may have a *rapid* onset or a ***delayed onset***.

- There is no dosage form for Erelzi that allows weight-based dosing for children weighing less than 63 kg.
- Store prefilled syringe or pen refrigerated at 36° to 46° F (2° to 8° C), but let it reach room temperature (15 to 30 minutes) before use. Don't remove needle cover while allowing syringe to reach room temperature.
- Store prefilled autoinjector refrigerated at 36° to 46° F (2° to 8° C) but let it reach room temperature before use. Don't remove the needle cover while allowing syringe to reach room temperature.
- Don't return an autoinjector, prefilled syringe, dose tray, or prefilled pen to the refrigerator after it has reached room temperature. Protect from light and heat and discard after 14 days (Enbrel) or 28 days (Erelzi).
- Reconstitute multiple-use vial aseptically with 1 mL of supplied sterile bacteriostatic water for injection (0.9% benzyl alcohol). Use a 25G needle rather than the supplied vial adapter if the vial will be used for multiple doses, but use a 27G needle for injection. Don't filter reconstituted solution when preparing or giving drug. Inject diluent slowly into vial. Refrigerate reconstituted vial for up to 14 days at 36° to 46° F (2° to 8° C) and discard 14 days after reconstitution.
- Minimize foaming by gently swirling during dissolution rather than shaking. Dissolution takes less than 10 minutes.
- Don't use solution if it's discolored or cloudy, or if it contains particulate matter.
- Separate injection sites by at least 1 inch (2.5 cm), rotate regularly, and never use areas where skin is tender, bruised, red, or hard. Use sites on the thigh, abdomen, and upper arm.
- ☉ *Alert:* Needle covers of diluent syringe and prefilled syringe and internal needle cover within cap of the pen contain latex and shouldn't be handled by persons sensitive to latex.

ACTION

Binds specifically to TNF and blocks its action with cell-surface TNF receptors, reducing inflammatory and immune responses found in RA.

Route	Onset	Peak	Duration
Subcut	Unknown	72 hr	Unknown

Half-life: About 5 days.

ADVERSE REACTIONS

CNS: headache, asthenia, dizziness, fever. **CV:** peripheral edema. **EENT:** rhinitis, pharyngitis, sinusitis, mouth ulcers. **GI:** abdominal pain, dyspepsia, nausea, vomiting, diarrhea. **Respiratory:** URI, cough, respiratory disorder, pneumonia (Erelzi). **Skin:** injection-site reaction, rash, alopecia, urticaria, pruritus. **Other:** infections, antibody development, *malignancies.*

INTERACTIONS

Drug-drug. *Abatacept, anakinra, belimumab, canakinumab, certolizumab pegol, infliximab, natalizumab, vedolizumab:* Increases rate of serious infection. Use together isn't recommended.
Antidiabetics: Increase risk of hypoglycemia. Antidiabetic dosage reduction may be needed.
Cyclophosphamide: May increase risk of solid malignancies. Concurrent use not recommended.
Sulfasalazine: May cause decreased neutrophil count. Monitor patient carefully.
Vaccines (inactivated): May reduce vaccine effectiveness. Complete all age-appropriate vaccinations at least 2 weeks before start of immunosuppressive therapy.
Vaccines (live-virus): May affect normal immune response. Postpone live-virus vaccination until 3 months after etanercept discontinuation.

EFFECTS ON LAB TEST RESULTS
None reported.

CONTRAINDICATIONS & CAUTIONS

- Contraindicated in patients hypersensitive to drug or its components, in those with sepsis, and in those receiving a live-virus vaccine.
- Use cautiously in patients age 65 and older and in patients with underlying diseases that predispose them to infection, such as diabetes, HF, or history of active or chronic infections.

• Rare cases of new-onset or exacerbations of CNS and peripheral nervous system demyelinating disorders (transverse myelitis, optic neuritis, MS, Guillain-Barré syndrome) and seizure disorders have occurred.

• Use cautiously in patients with a history of HF and moderate to severe alcoholic hepatitis.

• Don't start drug in patients with an active infection, patients who have been exposed to TB, or patients with a history of an opportunistic infection, including clinically important localized infections, because of the increased risk of the development of serious infections that may lead to hospitalizations or death.

• Use cautiously in patients who have resided or traveled in areas of endemic TB or endemic mycoses, such as histoplasmosis, coccidioidomycosis, or blastomycosis.

• Use cautiously in patients previously infected with HBV. Evaluate patients at increased risk for HBV infection before treatment and monitor patients for reactivation during and for several months after therapy ends. If reactivation occurs, drug may need to be stopped and antiviral therapy begun.

• Avoid use in patients with Wegener granulomatosis who are receiving immunosuppressants; drug may increase risk of malignancy.

• Temporarily interrupt treatment in patients with varicella virus exposure; consider prophylactic treatment with varicella zoster immune globulin.

• Children should be up to date with all immunizations before start of therapy.
Dialyzable drug: Unknown.

PREGNANCY-LACTATION-REPRODUCTION

• Use during pregnancy only if clearly needed.

• Drug is present in low levels in human milk and is minimally absorbed by a breastfed infant. Use cautiously if breastfeeding.

NURSING CONSIDERATIONS

• Etanercept-szzs (Erelzi) is biosimilar to the FDA-approved reference product etanercept (Enbrel). There are no clinically meaningful differences between the biosimilar product and the reference product based on

the conditions of their use. However, they aren't considered to be interchangeable.

• Methotrexate, glucocorticoids, salicylates, NSAIDs, or analgesics may be continued during treatment in adults.

Black Box Warning Patients treated with anti-TNF therapies are at increased risk for developing serious, sometimes fatal, infections (TB; invasive fungal infections; bacterial, viral, and other infections). Most patients who developed serious infections were also receiving immunosuppressants, such as methotrexate or corticosteroids. Monitor patient carefully; if serious infection occurs, stop therapy and notify prescriber. ∎

Black Box Warning Infections, including bacterial sepsis and TB, have been reported. Evaluate patient's risk factors and test for latent TB. Begin treatment for latent TB before therapy with etanercept. ∎

۞ *Alert:* Don't give live-virus vaccines during therapy.

Black Box Warning Histoplasmosis, coccidioidomycosis, blastomycosis, and other opportunistic infections may develop with use of this drug. Consider empirical antifungal therapy in patients at risk for invasive fungal infections who develop severe systemic illness. ∎

Black Box Warning Lymphoma and other malignancies, sometimes fatal, have been reported in children and adolescents. ∎

• *Look alike–sound alike:* Don't confuse etanercept-szzs (Erelzi) with the reference drug etanercept (Enbrel).

PATIENT TEACHING

• Teach patient who is self-administering drug about mixing and injection techniques, including rotating injection sites.

• Tell patient that injection-site reactions usually disappear in 3 to 5 days but to contact prescriber if they persist beyond that.

• Inform patient about avoiding live-virus vaccine administration during therapy.

• Advise patient to report signs or symptoms of pancytopenia, such as bruising, bleeding, persistent fever, or pallor.

• Advise patient to report signs or symptoms of new or worsening medical conditions, such as CNS demyelinating disorders (numbness, tingling, vision changes,

---

weakness of arms and legs, dizziness), seizures, or HF.
• Stress importance of alerting other health care providers about this therapy.
• Instruct patient to promptly report signs of infection, including persistent fever, cough, shortness of breath, or fatigue.
• Advise female patient to stop breastfeeding.

ethacrynate sodium
eth-uh-KRIH-nayt

Edecrin

ethacrynic acid
Edecrin

Therapeutic class: Diuretics
Pharmacologic class: Loop diuretics

AVAILABLE FORMS
ethacrynate sodium
Injection: 50 mg/vial
ethacrynic acid
Tablets: 25 mg

INDICATIONS & DOSAGES
➤ **Edema (rapid diuresis)**
Adults: 50 mg or 0.5 to 1 mg/kg IV. Usually only one dose is needed, although a second dose may be needed.
➤ **Edema**
Adults: 50 to 200 mg PO daily. May increase to 200 mg b.i.d. if needed for desired effect in 25- to 50-mg increments.
Children age 13 months and older: First dose is 25 mg PO, increased cautiously by 25 mg daily until desired effect is achieved.
Adjust-a-dose: If added to an existing diuretic regimen, first dose is 25 mg and dosage adjustments are made in 25-mg increments.

ADMINISTRATION
PO
• Give in morning to prevent nocturia.
• Give after meals.
IV
▼ Add 50 mL of D₅W or NSS to vial.
▼ Don't use cloudy or opalescent solution.
▼ Give over several minutes through tubing of running infusion.

▼ If more than one IV dose is needed, use a new injection site to avoid thrombophlebitis.
▼ Discard unused solution after 24 hours.
▼ **Incompatibilities:** Hydralazine, Normosol-M, procainamide, ranitidine, reserpine, solutions or drugs with pH below 5, whole blood and its derivatives.

ACTION
Potent loop diuretic; inhibits sodium and chloride reabsorption at the proximal and distal tubules and the ascending loop of Henle.

Route	Onset	Peak	Duration
PO	30 min	2 hr	6–8 hr
IV	5 min	15–30 min	2 hr

Half-life: 2 to 4 hours.

ADVERSE REACTIONS
CNS: malaise, confusion, fatigue, apprehension, vertigo, headache, fever. **CV:** orthostatic hypotension. **EENT:** transient or permanent deafness with over-rapid IV injection, blurred vision, tinnitus, hearing loss. **GI:** cramping, diarrhea, anorexia, nausea, vomiting, abdominal discomfort, dysphagia, *GI bleeding, pancreatitis.* **GU:** oliguria, hematuria, nocturia, polyuria, frequent urination, azotemia. **Hematologic:** *agranulocytosis, neutropenia, thrombocytopenia, Henoch-Schönlein purpura.* **Metabolic:** asymptomatic hyperuricemia; hypokalemia; hypochloremic alkalosis; fluid and electrolyte imbalances, including dilutional hyponatremia, hypocalcemia, and hypomagnesemia; hyperglycemia and impaired glucose tolerance; volume depletion and dehydration. **Skin:** rash. **Other:** chills.

INTERACTIONS
Drug-drug. *Aminoglycoside antibiotics:* May increase ototoxic adverse reactions to both drugs. Use together cautiously.
Antidiabetics: May decrease hypoglycemic effects. Monitor glucose level.
Antihypertensives: May increase risk of hypotension. Use together cautiously.
Cardiac glycosides: May increase risk of digoxin toxicity from ethacrynate-induced hypokalemia. Monitor potassium and digoxin levels.

✚ Canada   ◇ OTC   ◆ Off-label use   ✐ Photoguide   ⊙ Do not crush   *Liquid contains alcohol   ▒ Genetic

Chlorothiazide, chlorthalidone, hydrochloro-thiazide, indapamide, metolazone: May cause excessive diuretic response, causing serious electrolyte abnormalities or dehydration. Adjust doses carefully, and monitor patient closely for signs and symptoms of excessive diuretic response.

Cisplatin: May increase risk of ototoxicity. Avoid using together.

Lithium: May decrease lithium clearance, increasing risk of lithium toxicity. Monitor lithium level.

Neuromuscular blockers: May enhance neuromuscular blockade. Monitor patient closely.

NSAIDs: May decrease diuretic effect. Use together cautiously.

Other potassium-wasting drugs (amphotericin B, corticosteroids): May increase risk of hypokalemia and hypocalcemia. Use cautiously.

Probenecid: May decrease diuretic effect. Avoid using together.

Risperidone: May enhance adverse or toxic effect of risperidone. Consider therapy modification and maintain adequate hydration.

Warfarin: May increase anticoagulant effect. Use together cautiously.

Drug-herb. *Dandelion:* May increase diuresis. Discourage use together.

Licorice: May cause unexpected rapid potassium loss. Discourage use together.

EFFECTS ON LAB TEST RESULTS
• May increase glucose and uric acid levels. May decrease calcium, magnesium, potassium, and sodium levels.
• May decrease granulocyte, neutrophil, and platelet counts.

CONTRAINDICATIONS & CAUTIONS
• Contraindicated in infants, patients hypersensitive to drug, and patients with anuria.
❸ *Alert:* Drug is potent diuretic and can cause severe diuresis with water and electrolyte depletion. Monitor patient closely.
• Use cautiously in patients with electrolyte abnormalities or hepatic impairment.
• Ototoxicity has been reported, most often with IV use and with excessive doses.
Dialyzable drug: Unknown.
⚠ *Overdose S&S:* Dehydration, electrolyte depletion.

PREGNANCY-LACTATION-REPRODUCTION
• Use in pregnancy only if clearly needed.
• It isn't known if drug appears in human milk. Patient should discontinue breastfeeding or discontinue drug.

NURSING CONSIDERATIONS
• Monitor fluid intake and output, weight, BP, and electrolyte levels.
• Watch for signs and symptoms of orthostatic hypotension (dizziness, vertigo, syncope) and hypokalemia (muscle weakness and cramps).
• Monitor glucose level in diabetic patients.
• Consult prescriber and dietitian about providing a high-potassium diet. Potassium chloride and sodium supplements may be needed.
• Dosage may be on an alternate-day schedule, or more prolonged periods of diuretic therapy may be interspersed with rest periods. Intermittent dosage schedule allows time to correct electrolyte imbalance and may provide a more efficient diuretic response.
• Drug may increase risk of gastric hemorrhage caused by steroid treatment.
• Monitor elderly patients, who are especially susceptible to hypotension and other effects of excessive diuresis.
• Monitor uric acid level, especially in patients with history of gout.
❸ *Alert:* If patient develops severe diarrhea, stop drug. Patient shouldn't receive drug again after diarrhea has resolved.

PATIENT TEACHING
• Instruct patient to take drug with food to minimize GI upset.
• Advise patient to take drug in morning to avoid need to urinate at night. If a second dose is needed, tell patient to take it in early afternoon.
• Advise patient to avoid sudden posture changes and to rise slowly to avoid dizziness upon standing quickly.
• Tell patient to notify prescriber about muscle weakness, cramps, nausea, diarrhea, or dizziness.
• Caution patient not to perform hazardous activities if drug causes drowsiness.
• Advise diabetic patient to closely monitor glucose level.

ethambutol hydrochloride
e-THAM-byoo-tole

Etibi✤, Myambutol

Therapeutic class: Antituberculotics
Pharmacologic class: Synthetic
antituberculotics

E

AVAILABLE FORMS
Tablets: 100 mg, 400 mg

INDICATIONS & DOSAGES
➤ **Adjunctive treatment for pulmonary TB**
Adults and children age 13 and older: In patients who haven't received prior antituberculotics, 15 mg/kg PO daily as a single dose once every 24 hours, combined with other antituberculous therapy. For retreatment, 25 mg/kg PO every 24 hours as a single dose for 60 days (or until bacteriologic smears and cultures become negative) with at least one other antituberculotic; after 60 days, decrease to 15 mg/kg/day as a single dose every 24 hours.

ADMINISTRATION
PO
• Always give with other antituberculotics to prevent development of resistant organisms.
• Giving with food doesn't significantly alter absorption.
• Give on a once-every-24-hour basis only.

ACTION
May inhibit synthesis of one or more metabolites of susceptible bacteria, changing cell metabolism during cell division; bacteriostatic.

Route	Onset	Peak	Duration
PO	Unknown	2–4 hr	Unknown

Half-life: About 3½ hours.

ADVERSE REACTIONS
CNS: dizziness, fever, hallucinations, headache, malaise, mental confusion, peripheral neuritis. **EENT:** optic neuritis, irreversible blindness, decreased visual acuity. **GI:** abdominal pain, anorexia, GI upset, nausea, vomiting. **Hematologic:** *thrombocytopenia, leukopenia, neutropenia.* **Metabolic:** hyperuricemia. **Musculoskeletal:** joint pain. **Skin:** *toxic epidermal necrolysis,* dermatitis, pruritus. **Other:** *anaphylactoid reactions,* precipitation of acute gout.

INTERACTIONS
Drug-drug. *Aluminum salts:* May delay and reduce ethambutol absorption. Separate doses by at least 4 hours.

EFFECTS ON LAB TEST RESULTS
• May increase ALT, AST, bilirubin, and uric acid levels. May decrease glucose level.
• May decrease WBC and platelet counts.

CONTRAINDICATIONS & CAUTIONS
• Contraindicated in children younger than age 13, patients hypersensitive to drug, and patients with optic neuritis.
• Use cautiously in patients with impaired renal function, cataracts, recurrent eye inflammation, gout, or diabetic retinopathy. Irreversible blindness has occurred.
• Liver toxicities, including fatalities, have been reported. Obtain baseline and periodic assessment of hepatic function.
Dialyzable drug: Unknown.

PREGNANCY-LACTATION-REPRODUCTION
• Use during pregnancy only if benefit justifies potential risk to the fetus.
• Drug appears in human milk. Use only if expected benefit to the mother outweighs potential risk to the infant.

NURSING CONSIDERATIONS
• Perform visual acuity and color discrimination tests before and during therapy. Patients taking more than 15 mg/kg/day should have monthly eye examinations.
• Ensure that any changes in vision don't result from an underlying condition.
• Obtain AST and ALT levels before therapy, and monitor these levels every 3 to 4 weeks.
• In patients with impaired renal function, base dosage on drug level.
• Monitor uric acid level; observe patient for signs and symptoms of gout.

PATIENT TEACHING
• Tell patient to report all vision changes immediately; explain that eye examinations will be necessary. Advise patient that visual disturbances usually disappear several weeks to months after drug is stopped. Inflammation of the optic nerve is related to dosage and duration of treatment.
• Inform patient that drug is given with other antituberculotics.
• Stress importance of compliance with drug therapy.
• Advise patient to report adverse reactions to prescriber.

ethinyl estradiol–desogestrel
ETH-i-nill/DAY-so-jest-rul

Monophasic
Desogen, Emoquette

Biphasic
Kariva, Pimtrea, Viorele

Triphasic
Cyclessa, Velivet

ethinyl estradiol–ethynodiol diacetate
Monophasic
Kelnor 1/35, Zovia 1/35E-28, Zovia 1/50E-28

ethinyl estradiol–levonorgestrel
Monophasic
Altavera, Aviane-28, Falmina, Introvale, Lessina-28, Levora 0.15/30-28, Marlissa, Orsythia, Portia-28, Quasense, Seasonale

Biphasic
Daysee, Lo Seasonique, Seasonique

Triphasic
Enpresse-28, Levonest, Myzilra, Trivora-28

ethinyl estradiol–norethindrone
Monophasic
Alyacen 1/35, Alyacen 777, Aranelle, Balziva-28, Brevicon 28-Day, Briellyn, Cyclafem 1/35, Dasetta 1/35, Norinyl 1 + 35, Nortrel 0.5/35-28, Nortrel 1/35, Ortho-Novum 1/35-28, Philith, Wera

Triphasic
Alyacen 7/7/7, Aranelle, Cyclafem 7/7/7, Dasetta 7/7/7, Nortrel 7/7/7, Ortho-Novum 7/7/7-28, Tri-Norinyl 28-day

ethinyl estradiol–norethindrone acetate
Monophasic
Activella, Femhrt, Junel 1/20, Junel 1.5/30, Junel Fe 1/20, Junel Fe 1.5/30, Larin 1/20, Larin 1.5/30, Loestrin 21 1/20, Loestrin 21 1.5/30, Microgestin 1/20, Microgestin 1.5/30

ethinyl estradiol–norgestimate
Monophasic
Mono-Linyah, Ortho-Cyclen-28, Previfem, Sprintec

Triphasic
Ortho Tri-Cyclen, Ortho Tri-Cyclen Lo, Tri-Linyah, Tri-Previfem, Tri-Sprintec

ethinyl estradiol–norgestrel
Monophasic
Cryselle, Elinest, Ogestrel 0.5/50-28

ethinyl estradiol–norethindrone acetate–ferrous fumarate
Monophasic
Blisovi 24 Fe, Blisovi Fe 1.5/30, Blisovi Fe 1/20, Femcon Fe, Gildess Fe 1/20, Gildess Fe 1.5/30, Junel Fe 1/20, Junel Fe 1.5/30, Larin 24 Fe, Larin Fe 1/20, Larin Fe 1.5/30, Loestrin 24 Fe, Loestrin Fe 1/20, Loestrin Fe 1.5/30, Lo Loestrin Fe, Microgestin Fe 1/20, Microgestin Fe 1.5/30

Triphasic
Estrostep Fe, Tri-Legest Fe

Reactions in bold italics are *life-threatening*. Interactions may have a *rapid onset* or a *delayed onset*.

mestranol–norethindrone
Monophasic
Norinyl 1 + 50 28 Day

Therapeutic class: Contraceptives
Pharmacologic class: Estrogen–progestin
combinations

E

AVAILABLE FORMS
Monophasic hormonal contraceptives
ethinyl estradiol–desogestrel
Tablets: ethinyl estradiol 30 mcg and desogestrel 0.15 mg (Desogen, Emoquette)
ethinyl estradiol–ethynodiol diacetate
Tablets: ethinyl estradiol 35 mcg and ethynodiol diacetate 1 mg (Kelnor 1/35, Zovia
1/35E-28); ethinyl estradiol 50 mcg and
ethynodiol diacetate 1 mg (Zovia 1/50E-28)
ethinyl estradiol–levonorgestrel
Tablets: ethinyl estradiol 20 mcg and levonorgestrel 0.1 mg (Aviane-28, Falmina,
Lessina-28, Orsythia); ethinyl estradiol
30 mcg and levonorgestrel 0.15 mg
(Altavera, Introvale, Levora 0.15/30-28,
Marlissa, Portia-28, Quasense, Seasonale);
ethinyl estradiol 30 mcg and 0.15 mg levonorgestrel (84 tablets), and 10 mcg ethinyl
estradiol (7 tablets) (Seasonale)
ethinyl estradiol–norethindrone
Tablets: ethinyl estradiol 35 mcg and
norethindrone 0.4 mg (Balziva-28, Briellyn, Philith); ethinyl estradiol 35 mcg and
norethindrone 0.5 mg (Aranelle, Brevicon
28-Day, Nortrel 0.5/35-28, Wera); ethinyl
estradiol 35 mcg and norethindrone 0.75 mg
(Alyacen 777); ethinyl estradiol 35 mcg
and norethindrone 1 mg (Alyacen 1/35,
Alyacen 777, Cyclafem 1/35, Dasetta 1/35,
Norinyl 1 + 35, Nortrel 1/35, Ortho-Novum
1/35-28)
**ethinyl estradiol–norethindrone
acetate**
Tablets: ethinyl estradiol 2.5 mcg and
norethindrone acetate 0.5 mg; ethinyl
estradiol 5 mcg and norethindrone acetate
1 mg; ethinyl estradiol 20 mcg and norethindrone acetate 1 mg (Junel 1/20, Larin 1/20,
Loestrin 21 1/20, Microgestin 1/20); ethinyl
estradiol 30 mcg and norethindrone acetate
1.5 mg (Junel 1.5/30, Larin 1.5/30, Loestrin
21 1.5/30, Microgestin 1.5/30); ethinyl
estradiol 0.5 mg and norethindrone acetate

0.1 mg; ethinyl estradiol 1 mg and norethindrone acetate 0.5 mg
ethinyl estradiol–norgestimate
Tablets: ethinyl estradiol 35 mcg and norgestimate 0.25 mg (Mono-Linyah, Ortho-
Cyclen-28, Previfem, Sprintec)
ethinyl estradiol–norgestrel
Tablets: ethinyl estradiol 30 mcg and
norgestrel 0.3 mg (Cryselle, Elinest); ethinyl
estradiol 50 mcg and norgestrel 0.5 mg
(Ogestrel 0.5/50-28)
**ethinyl estradiol–norethindrone
acetate–ferrous fumarate**
Chewable tablets: norethindrone 0.4 mg and
ethinyl estradiol 35 mcg; inactive tablets
contain ferrous fumarate 75 mg
Tablets: ethinyl estradiol 10 mcg, norethindrone acetate 1 mg, and ferrous fumarate
75 mg (Lo Loestrin Fe); ethinyl estradiol
20 mcg, norethindrone acetate 1 mg, and ferrous fumarate 75 mg (Blisovi 24 Fe, Blisovi
Fe 1/20, Gildess Fe 1/20, Junel Fe 1/20,
Larin 24 Fe, Larin Fe 1/20, Loestrin Fe 1/20,
Loestrin 24 Fe, Microgestin Fe 1/20); ethinyl
estradiol 30 mcg, norethindrone acetate
1.5 mg, and ferrous fumarate 75 mg (Blisovi
Fe 1.5/30, Gildess Fe 1.5/30, Junel Fe 1.5/30,
Larin Fe 1.5/30, Loestrin Fe 1.5/30, Microgestin Fe 1.5/30)
mestranol–norethindrone
Tablets: mestranol 50 mcg and norethindrone 1 mg (Norinyl 1 + 50 28 Day)
Biphasic hormonal contraceptives
ethinyl estradiol–desogestrel
Tablets: ethinyl estradiol 20 mcg and desogestrel 0.15 mg (21 days), then inert tablets
(2 days), then ethinyl estradiol 10 mcg
(5 days) (Kariva, Pimtrea, Viorele)
ethinyl estradiol–levonorgestrel
Tablets: ethinyl estradiol 0.02 mg and levonorgestrel 0.1 mg (84 days), then ethinyl
estradiol 0.01 mg (7 days) (Lo Seasonique);
ethinyl estradiol 30 mcg and levonorgestrel
0.15 mg (84 days), then ethinyl estradiol
10 mcg (7 days) (Daysee, Seasonique)
Triphasic hormonal contraceptives
ethinyl estradiol–desogestrel
Tablets: 0.1 mg desogestrel and 25 mcg
ethinyl estradiol (7 tablets); 0.125 mg
desogestrel and 25 mcg ethinyl estradiol
(7 tablets); 0.15 mg desogestrel and 25 mcg
ethinyl estradiol (7 tablets) (Cyclessa,
Velivet)

ethinyl estradiol–levonorgestrel
Tablets: ethinyl estradiol 30 mcg and levonorgestrel 0.05 mg (6 days); ethinyl estradiol 40 mcg and levonorgestrel 0.075 mg (5 days); ethinyl estradiol 30 mcg and levonorgestrel 0.125 mg (10 days) (Enpresse-28, Levonest, Myzilra, Trivora-28)
ethinyl estradiol–norethindrone
Tablets: ethinyl estradiol 30 mcg and norethindrone 0.5 mg (7 days); ethinyl estradiol 35 mcg and norethindrone 1 mg (9 days); ethinyl estradiol 35 mcg and norethindrone 0.5 mg (5 days) (Aranelle, Tri-Norinyl 28-day); ethinyl estradiol 35 mcg and norethindrone 0.5 mg (7 days); ethinyl estradiol 35 mcg and norethindrone 0.75 mg (7 days); ethinyl estradiol 35 mcg and norethindrone 1 mg (7 days) (Alyacen 7/7/7, Cyclafem 7/7/7, Dasetta 7/7/7, Nortrel 7/7/7, Ortho-Novum 7/7/7-28)
ethinyl estradiol–norgestimate
Tablets: ethinyl estradiol 25 mcg and norgestimate 0.18 mg (7 days); ethinyl estradiol 25 mcg and norgestimate 0.215 mg (7 days); ethinyl estradiol 25 mcg and norgestimate 0.25 mg (7 days) (Ortho Tri-Cyclen Lo); ethinyl estradiol 35 mcg and norgestimate 0.18 mg (7 days); ethinyl estradiol 35 mcg and norgestimate 0.215 mg (7 days); ethinyl estradiol 35 mcg and norgestimate 0.25 mg (7 days) (Ortho Tri-Cyclen, Tri-Linyah, Tri-Previfem, Tri-Sprintec)
ethinyl estradiol–norethindrone acetate–ferrous fumarate
Tablets: ethinyl estradiol 20 mcg and norethindrone acetate 1 mg (5 days); ethinyl estradiol 30 mcg and norethindrone acetate 1 mg (7 days); ethinyl estradiol 35 mcg and norethindrone acetate 1 mg (9 days); 75-mg ferrous fumarate tablets (7 days) (Estrostep Fe, Tri-Legest Fe)

INDICATIONS & DOSAGES
➤ **Contraception**
Monophasic hormonal contraceptives
Women: 1 tablet PO daily beginning on first day of menstrual cycle or first Sunday after menstrual cycle begins. With 20- and 21-tablet package, new cycle begins 7 days after last tablet taken. With 28-tablet package, dosage is 1 tablet daily without interruption; extra tablets taken on days 22 to 28 are placebos or contain iron. Or, for

Seasonale, 1 pink tablet PO daily beginning on first Sunday after menstrual cycle begins, for 84 consecutive days, followed by 7 days of white (inert) tablets.

When changing from 21-day or 28-day combination oral contraceptive, begin on first day of withdrawal bleeding, at the latest 7 days after last active tablet. When changing from progestin-only pill, begin the next day. When changing from implant contraceptive, begin the day of implant removal. When changing from injection contraceptive, begin the day when next injection is due.
Biphasic hormonal contraceptives
Women: 1 color tablet PO daily for 10 days; then next color tablet for 11 days. With 21-tablet packages, new cycle begins 7 days after last tablet taken. With 28-tablet packages, dosage is 1 tablet daily without interruption. Or, for Seasonique, 1 light blue-green tablet PO once daily for 84 consecutive days followed by 1 yellow tablet for 7 consecutive days; then repeat cycle.
Triphasic hormonal contraceptives
Women: 1 tablet PO daily in the sequence specified by the brand. With 21-tablet packages, new dosing cycle begins 7 days after last tablet taken. With 28-tablet packages, dosage is 1 tablet daily without interruption.
➤ **Moderate acne vulgaris in women age 15 and older who have no known contraindications to hormonal contraceptive therapy, who want oral contraception for at least 6 months, who have reached menarche, and who are unresponsive to topical antiacne drugs**
Women age 15 and older: 1 tablet Ortho Tri-Cyclen or Estrostep Fe PO daily (21 tablets contain active ingredients and 7 are inert).
➤ **Menopausal signs and symptoms; to prevent osteoporosis (Activella, Femhrt)**
Women with intact uterus: 1 tablet PO daily.

ADMINISTRATION
PO
• Give drug at the same time each day; give at night to reduce nausea and headaches.
• Chewable tablet may be swallowed whole or chewed and followed with a full glass of liquid.

Reactions in bold italics are *life-threatening*. Interactions may have a *rapid onset* or a *delayed onset*.

ACTION

Inhibits ovulation and may prevent transport of the ovum (if ovulation should occur) through the fallopian tubes.

Estrogen suppresses FSH, blocking follicular development and ovulation.

Progestin suppresses luteinizing hormone so that ovulation can't occur even if the follicle develops; it also thickens cervical mucus, interfering with sperm migration, and prevents implantation of the fertilized ovum.

Route	Onset	Peak	Duration
PO	Unknown	2 hr (ethinyl estradiol), ½–4 hr (varies by progestin)	Unknown

Half-life: 6 to 20 hours (ethinyl estradiol); 5 to 45 hours (varies by progestin).

ADVERSE REACTIONS

CNS: headache, dizziness, depression, lethargy, migraine, *stroke, cerebral hemorrhage.* **CV:** *thromboembolism,* HTN, edema, *PE, MI.* **EENT:** worsening myopia or astigmatism, intolerance of contact lenses, exophthalmos, diplopia. **GI:** nausea, vomiting, abdominal cramps, bloating, anorexia, changes in appetite, gallbladder disease, *pancreatitis.* **GU:** breakthrough bleeding, spotting, granulomatous colitis, dysmenorrhea, amenorrhea, cervical erosion or abnormal secretions, enlargement of uterine fibromas, vaginal candidiasis. **Hepatic:** cholestatic jaundice, *liver tumors,* gallbladder disease. **Metabolic:** weight change, additive insulin resistance in diabetics. **Skin:** rash, acne, *erythema multiforme,* melasma, hirsutism. **Other:** breast tenderness, enlargement, or secretion; *anaphylaxis; hemolytic-uremic syndrome.*

INTERACTIONS

Drug-drug. *Anastrozole:* May inhibit anastrozole effect. Avoid use together.

Anti-infectives (chloramphenicol, fluconazole, griseofulvin, neomycin, nitrofurantoin, penicillins, sulfonamides, tetracyclines): May decrease contraceptive effect. Advise patient to use another method of contraception.

Atorvastatin: May increase norethindrone and ethinyl estradiol levels. Monitor patient for adverse effects.

Benzodiazepines: May decrease or increase benzodiazepine levels. Adjust dosage, if necessary.

Beta blockers: May increase beta blocker level. Dosage adjustment may be necessary.

Carbamazepine, fosphenytoin, phenobarbital, phenytoin, rifampin: May decrease estrogen effect. Use together cautiously.

Corticosteroids: May enhance corticosteroid effect. Monitor patient closely.

Exemestane: May interfere with exemestane effectiveness. Avoid use together.

Insulin, sulfonylureas: Glucose intolerance may decrease antidiabetic effects. Monitor these effects.

Iron supplements: Increase risk of iron-related toxicity if blister card contains iron. Don't use together.

NNRTIs, protease inhibitors: May decrease hormonal contraceptive effect. Avoid using together, if possible.

Oral anticoagulants: May decrease anticoagulant effect. Dosage adjustments may be needed. Monitor PT and INR.

Ospemifene: May enhance adverse/toxic effects of ospemifene and interfere with its effectiveness. Avoid use together.

Tamoxifen: May inhibit tamoxifen effect. Avoid using together.

Drug-herb. *Red clover:* May interfere with drug. Discourage use together.

St. John's wort: May decrease drug effect because of increased hepatic metabolism. Discourage use together, or advise patient to use an additional method of contraception.

Drug-food. *Caffeine:* May increase caffeine level. Urge caution.

Grapefruit juice: May increase estrogen level. Advise patient to take with liquid other than grapefruit juice.

Drug-lifestyle. *Smoking:* May increase risk of adverse CV effects. If smoking continues, may need alternative therapy.

EFFECTS ON LAB TEST RESULTS

- May increase phospholipid, plasminogen, thyroid-binding globulin, total T_4, and triglyceride levels.
- May alter clotting factors.
- May increase norepinephrine-induced platelet aggregation and prolong PT.
- May reduce response to metyrapone test.

• May cause false-positive result in nitro-blue tetrazolium test.

CONTRAINDICATIONS & CAUTIONS
• Contraindicated in patients with thromboembolic disorders, cerebrovascular disease or CAD, diplopia or ocular lesions arising from ophthalmic vascular disease, classic migraine, MI, known or suspected breast cancer, known or suspected estrogen-dependent neoplasia, benign or malignant liver tumors, active liver disease or history of cholestatic jaundice with pregnancy or previous use of hormonal contraceptives, or undiagnosed abnormal vaginal bleeding. Also contraindicated in patients receiving hepatitis C drug combinations containing ombitasvir/paritaprevir/ritonavir, with or without dasabuvir.
• Use cautiously in patients with hyperlipidemia, HTN, migraines, seizure disorders, asthma, bleeding irregularities, gallbladder disease, ocular disease, diabetes, emotional disorders, and cardiac, renal, or hepatic insufficiency.
Dialyzable drug: Unknown.
⚠ *Overdose S&S:* Nausea, withdrawal uterine bleeding.

PREGNANCY-LACTATION-REPRODUCTION
• Use during pregnancy isn't indicated. Discontinue if pregnancy is confirmed. There is little or no increased risk of birth defects in women who accidently use drug during early pregnancy.
• Estrogens can reduce the quantity and quality of human milk. Breastfeeding women should use other forms of contraception while breastfeeding. Those not breastfeeding may start oral contraceptives 4 to 6 weeks postpartum.

NURSING CONSIDERATIONS
Black Box Warning Cigarette smoking increases the risk of serious CV adverse effects from oral contraceptives. Women who use oral contraceptives shouldn't smoke. ∎
• Triphasic hormonal contraceptives may cause fewer adverse reactions, such as breakthrough bleeding and spotting.
• The CDC reports that use of hormonal contraceptives may decrease risk of ovarian and endometrial cancers and doesn't seem to increase risk of breast cancer. However, the FDA reports that some studies suggest that hormonal contraceptives may be linked to an increase in cervical cancer.
• Monitor lipid levels, BP, body weight, and hepatic function.
🜚 *Alert:* Many hormonal contraceptives share similar names. Make sure to check the hormone strength for verification.
• Estrogens and progestins may alter glucose tolerance, thus changing dosage requirements for antidiabetics. Monitor glucose level.
• Stop hormonal contraceptives for a few weeks before adrenal function tests.
• Stop hormonal contraceptive and notify prescriber if patient develops granulomatous colitis.
• Stop drug at least 1 week before surgery to decrease risk of thromboembolism. Tell patient to use an alternative method of birth control.
• Women who are nonlactating mothers or those who have had second-trimester abortion must wait 28 days before starting oral contraception.

PATIENT TEACHING
• Tell patient to take tablets at same time each day; nighttime doses may reduce nausea and headaches.
• Advise patient to use additional method of birth control, such as condom or diaphragm with spermicide, for first week of first cycle.
• Tell patient that missing doses in midcycle greatly increases likelihood of pregnancy.
• Tell patient that missing a dose may cause spotting or light bleeding.
• Tell patient that hormonal contraceptives don't protect against HIV or other sexually transmitted diseases.
• Tell patient using Daysee or Seasonale that there will be four planned menses per year, but spotting or bleeding between menses may occur.
• If 1 pill is missed, tell patient to take it as soon as possible (2 pills if remembered on the next day) and then to continue regular schedule. Advise an additional method of contraception for remainder of cycle. If 2 consecutive pills are missed, tell patient to take 2 pills a day for next 2 days and then resume regular schedule. Advise an additional

---

Reactions in bold italics are *life-threatening*. Interactions may have a *rapid onset* or a *delayed onset*.

method of contraception for the next 7 days or preferably for the remainder of cycle. If 2 consecutive pills are missed in the 3rd or 4th week or if patient misses 3 consecutive pills, tell patient to contact prescriber for instructions.

• Warn patient of common adverse effects, such as headache, nausea, dizziness, breast tenderness, spotting, and breakthrough bleeding, which usually diminish after 3 to 6 months.

• Instruct patient to weigh herself at least twice a week and to report any sudden weight gain or swelling to prescriber.

• Warn patient to avoid exposure to ultraviolet light or prolonged exposure to sunlight.

❸ *Alert:* Warn patient to immediately report abdominal pain; numbness, stiffness, or pain in legs or buttocks; pressure or pain in chest; shortness of breath; severe headache; visual disturbances, such as blind spots, blurriness, or flashing lights; undiagnosed vaginal bleeding or discharge; two consecutive missed menstrual periods; lumps in the breast; swelling of hands or feet; or severe pain in the abdomen (tumor rupture in liver).

• Advise patient of increased risks created by simultaneous use of cigarettes and hormonal contraceptives.

• If one menstrual period is missed and tablets have been taken on schedule, tell patient to continue taking them. If two consecutive menstrual periods are missed, tell patient to stop drug and have pregnancy test. Progestins may cause birth defects if taken early in pregnancy.

• Tell patient to chew chewable tablet and follow with a full glass of liquid or swallow whole.

• Advise patient not to take same drug for longer than 12 months without consulting prescriber. Stress importance of Papanicolaou tests and annual gynecologic examinations.

• Advise patient to check with prescriber about how soon pregnancy may be attempted after hormonal therapy is stopped. Many prescribers recommend that women not become pregnant within 2 months after stopping drug.

• Warn patient of possible delay in achieving pregnancy when drug is stopped.

• Warn patient that hormonal contraceptives don't protect against HIV infection or other sexually transmitted diseases.

• Teach patient methods to decrease risk of thromboembolism.

• Advise patient taking hormonal contraceptives to use additional form of birth control during concurrent treatment with certain antibiotics.

• Advise patient that hormonal contraceptives may change the fit of contact lenses.

etonogestrel–ethinyl estradiol vaginal ring
e-toe-noe-JES-trel/ETH-i-nill

NuvaRing

Therapeutic class: Contraceptives
Pharmacologic class: Progestin–estrogen combinations

AVAILABLE FORMS
Vaginal ring: Delivers 0.12 mg/day etonogestrel and 0.015 mg/day ethinyl estradiol

INDICATIONS & DOSAGES
➤ **Contraception**
Women: Insert 1 ring into the vagina and leave in place for 3 weeks. Insert new ring 1 week after the previous ring is removed.

ADMINISTRATION
Vaginal
• In women who did not use hormonal contraception during the previous month, therapy should be initiated on the first day of the menstrual cycle. A woman using a combination oral contraceptive may switch to NuvaRing on any day, but at the latest on the day following the usual hormone-free interval.

• Leave ring in place continuously for a full 3 weeks to maintain effect. It's then removed for 1 week. During this time, withdrawal bleeding occurs (usually starting 2 or 3 days after removal). Insert a new ring 1 week after removal of the previous one, at approximately the same time of day, regardless of whether patient is still menstruating.

• Before dispensing to user, store refrigerated (36° to 46° F [2° to 8° C]). After dispensing, can be stored for up to 4 months at 77° F (25° C); excursions permitted to 59° to 86° F (15° to 30° C).

ACTION

Suppresses gonadotropins, which inhibits ovulation, increases the viscosity of cervical mucus (decreasing the ability of sperm to enter the uterus), and alters the endometrial lining (reducing potential for implantation).

Route	Onset	Peak	Duration
Vaginal	Rapid	200 hr (etono-gestrel); 60 hr (ethinyl estradiol)	Unknown

Half-life: Etonogestrel, 29 hours; ethinyl estradiol, 45 hours.

ADVERSE REACTIONS

CNS: headache, emotional lability, mood changes, depression, migraine, *cerebral thrombosis, cerebral hemorrhage.* **CV:** HTN, edema, *thromboembolic events, MI.* **EENT:** sinusitis, changes in corneal curvature, intolerance to contact lenses. **GI:** nausea, vomiting, abdominal pain. **GU:** vaginitis, leukorrhea, device-related events (for example, foreign body sensation, coital difficulties, device expulsion), vaginal discomfort, breakthrough bleeding, vaginal discharge, dysmenorrhea. **Hematologic:** *coagulation abnormalities.* **Hepatic:** *hepatic adenomas,* benign liver tumors, cholestatic jaundice. **Metabolic:** weight gain. **Respiratory:** URI. **Skin:** melasma, acne. **Other:** breast pain/tenderness, decreased libido.

INTERACTIONS

Drug-drug. *Acetaminophen:* May decrease acetaminophen level and increase ethinyl estradiol level. Monitor patient for effects.
Ampicillin, barbiturates, carbamazepine, felbamate, griseofulvin, oxcarbazepine, phenytoin, rifampin, tetracyclines, topiramate: May decrease contraceptive effect and increase risk of pregnancy, breakthrough bleeding, or both. Tell patient to use an additional form of contraception while taking these drugs.
Anastrozole: May diminish therapeutic effect of anastrozole. Avoid use together.
Ascorbic acid, atorvastatin, itraconazole: May increase ethinyl estradiol level. Monitor patient for adverse effects.

Clofibrate, morphine, salicylic acid, temazepam: May increase clearance of these drugs. Monitor patient for effectiveness.
Cyclosporine, prednisolone, theophylline: May increase levels of these drugs. Monitor levels if appropriate and adjust dosage.
Exemestane: May interfere with exemestane effectiveness. Avoid use together.
HIV protease inhibitors: May affect contraceptive effect. Refer to the specific protease inhibitor drug literature. May need to use a backup method of contraception.
Miconazole (oil-based vaginal capsule): May increase serum concentrations of etonogestrel and ethinyl estradiol. Monitor patient for adverse effects.
Ospemifene: May enhance adverse/toxic effects of ospemifene and interfere with its effectiveness. Avoid use together.
Drug-herb. *St. John's wort:* May reduce drug effectiveness and increase the risk of breakthrough bleeding and pregnancy. Discourage use together.
Drug-lifestyle. **Black Box Warning** *Smoking:* May increase risk of serious CV adverse effects, especially in patients older than age 35 who smoke. Drug shouldn't be used in those older than age 35 who smoke. Urge patient to avoid smoking. ∎

EFFECTS ON LAB TEST RESULTS

• May increase coagulation factors, thyroid-binding globulin (leading to increased circulating total thyroid hormone levels), sex hormone-binding globulin (and other binding proteins), and triglyceride levels. May decrease antithrombin III and folate levels.
• May increase norepinephrine-induced platelet aggregation. May decrease T_3 resin uptake and glucose tolerance.

CONTRAINDICATIONS & CAUTIONS

• Contraindicated in patients hypersensitive to components of drug and in patients older than age 35 who smoke 15 or more cigarettes daily.
• Contraindicated in patients with thrombophlebitis, thromboembolic disorder, history of deep vein thrombophlebitis, cerebrovascular disease or CAD (current or previous), valvular heart disease with complications, severe HTN, diabetes with vascular complications, headache with focal

---

Reactions in bold italics are *life-threatening*. Interactions may have a *rapid onset* or a *delayed onset*.

neurologic symptoms or migraine headaches with aura, known or suspected cancer of the endometrium or breast; estrogen-dependent neoplasia, abnormal undiagnosed genital bleeding, jaundice related to pregnancy or previous use of hormonal contraceptives, active liver disease, or benign or malignant hepatic tumors.
• Contraindicated in women older than age 35 with migraine headaches and in those undergoing major surgery with prolonged immobilization.
• Contraindicated in patients receiving hepatitis C drug combinations containing ombitasvir/paritaprevir/ritonavir, with or without dasabuvir.
• Use cautiously in patients with HTN, hyperlipidemias, obesity, or diabetes.
• Use cautiously in patients with conditions that could be aggravated by fluid retention, and in patients with a history of depression.
• Ring may not be suitable for women with conditions that make the vagina more susceptible to vaginal irritation or ulceration. Vaginal/cervical erosion or ulceration has been reported.
• Ring may interfere with the correct placement and position of barrier contraceptive methods, such as a diaphragm, cervical cap, or female condom. These methods aren't recommended as backup methods with ring use.
Dialyzable drug: Unknown.

PREGNANCY-LACTATION-REPRODUCTION
• Not indicated for use in pregnancy; drug is contraindicated. Discontinue drug if pregnancy is confirmed.
• There is little or no increased risk of birth defects in women who accidently use combined hormonal contraceptives during early pregnancy.
• Drug may appear in human milk and may decrease the quantity and quality of milk. Breastfeeding women should use other forms of contraception while breastfeeding.

NURSING CONSIDERATIONS
❸ *Alert:* Drug may increase the risk of MI, thromboembolism, stroke, hepatic neoplasia, and gallbladder disease.
Black Box Warning Cigarette smoking increases the risk of serious adverse cardiac

effects. The risk increases with age and in patients who smoke 15 or more cigarettes daily. ∎
• Stop drug at least 4 weeks before and for 2 weeks after procedures that may increase the risk of thromboembolism, and during and after prolonged immobilization.
• Stop drug and notify prescriber if patient develops unexplained partial or complete loss of vision, proptosis, diplopia, papilledema, retinal vascular lesions, migraines, depression, or jaundice.
• Monitor BP closely if patient has HTN or renal disease.
• Rule out pregnancy if woman hasn't adhered to the prescribed regimen and a period is missed, if prescribed regimen has been adhered to and two periods are missed, or if patient has retained the ring for longer than 4 weeks.

PATIENT TEACHING
• Stress importance of having regular annual physical examinations to check for adverse effects or developing contraindications.
• Tell patient that drug doesn't protect against HIV and other sexually transmitted diseases.
• Advise patient not to smoke while using contraceptive.
• Tell patient to use backup method of contraception until ring has been used continuously for 7 days. Tell patient not to use diaphragm, cervical cap, or female condom if backup method is needed.
• Tell patient who wears contact lenses to contact an ophthalmologist if vision or lens tolerance changes.
• Advise patient to follow manufacturer's instructions for use if switching from different form of hormonal contraceptive.
• Tell patient to insert ring into vagina (using fingers) and keep it in place continuously for 3 weeks to maintain effect, saving foil package for later disposal. Explain that it is then removed for 1 full week and that, during this time, withdrawal bleeding occurs (usually starting 2 or 3 days after removal). Tell patient to insert new ring 1 week after removing previous one at approximately the same time of day, regardless of menstrual bleeding. Tell patient to reseal ring in the package after removing it from vagina.

- Advise patient to regularly check for presence of ring in the vagina and not to deviate from the recommended regimen.
- Advise patient that, if the ring is removed or expelled (such as while removing a tampon, straining, or moving bowels), it should be washed with cool to lukewarm (not hot) water and reinserted immediately. Stress that contraceptive effect may be compromised if the ring stays out for longer than 3 hours and that she should use a backup method of contraception until the newly reinserted ring has been used continuously for 7 days.
- Tell patient that there's no danger of the vaginal ring being pushed too far up in the vagina or getting lost.

SAFETY ALERT!

etoposide
e-toe-POE-side

etoposide phosphate
Etopophos

Therapeutic class: Antineoplastics
Pharmacologic class: Podophyllotoxin derivatives

AVAILABLE FORMS
etoposide
Capsules: 50 mg
Injection: 20 mg/mL in 5-mL, 25-mL, 50-mL vials
etoposide phosphate
Injection: 114-mg vials equivalent to 100 mg etoposide

INDICATIONS & DOSAGES
Adjust-a-dose (for all indications): For patients with CrCl of 15 to 50 mL/minute, reduce dose by 25%. For patients with CrCl of less than 15 mL/minute, consider dosage reduction.

➤ **Refractory testicular cancer in combination with other chemotherapeutic agents**
Adults: 50 to 100 mg/m^2 daily IV on 5 consecutive days every 3 to 4 weeks. Or, 100 mg/m^2 daily IV on days 1, 3, and 5 every 3 to 4 weeks for three or four courses of therapy.

➤ **Small-cell carcinoma of the lung in combination with other chemotherapeutic agents**
Adults: 35 mg/m^2 daily IV for 4 days. Or, 50 mg/m^2 daily IV for 5 days. Repeat cycles every 3 to 4 weeks. Oral dose is two times IV dose (two times 35 mg/m^2 for 4 days to 50 mg/m^2 for 5 days), rounded to nearest 50 mg.
Adjust-a-dose: Adjust dose to account for myelosuppressive effects of coadministered drugs or effects of prior radiation therapy or chemotherapy.

ADMINISTRATION
PO
- Hazardous drug; use appropriate handling and disposal precautions.
- Give drug without regard for food.
- Don't give drug with grapefruit juice.
- Refrigerate capsules at 36° to 46° F (2° to 8° C). Don't freeze. Capsules are stable for 36 months under refrigeration.

IV
▼ Preparing and giving parenteral drug may be mutagenic, teratogenic, or carcinogenic. Follow facility policy to reduce risks. Use gloves.
▼ Plastic devices made of acrylic or ABS (acrylonitrile butadiene styrene) have been reported to crack and leak when used with undiluted etoposide injection.
▼ For etoposide infusion, dilute to 0.2 or 0.4 mg/mL in either D$_5$W or NSS. Higher concentrations may crystallize.
▼ Give etoposide by slow infusion over at least 30 to 60 minutes to prevent severe hypotension. Never give by rapid injection.
▼ For etoposide phosphate, reconstitute each vial with sterile water for injection, D$_5$W, NSS, bacteriostatic water for injection with benzyl alcohol, or bacteriostatic sodium chloride for injection with benzyl alcohol to a concentration of 20 mg/mL or 10 mg/mL. After reconstitution, give without further dilution or dilute to as low as 0.1 mg/mL in either D$_5$W or NSS.
▼ Give etoposide phosphate over 5 minutes to 3.5 hours.
▼ Check BP every 15 minutes during infusion. Hypotension may occur if infusion is too rapid. If systolic pressure falls below

90 mm Hg, stop infusion and notify prescriber.

▼ Etoposide diluted to 0.2 mg/mL is stable for 96 hours at room temperature in plastic or glass, unprotected from light; at 0.4 mg/mL, it's stable for 24 hours under same conditions. Diluted etoposide phosphate solution stored in glass or plastic containers is stable under refrigeration for 7 days or for 24 to 48 hours at room temperature, depending on diluent. Further diluted solutions are stable under refrigeration or at room temperature for 24 hours.

▼ **Incompatibilities:** Cefepime, filgrastim, gallium nitrate, idarubicin.

ACTION
Inhibits topoisomerase II enzyme, causing inability to repair DNA strand breaks, which leads to cell death. Cell-cycle specific to G_2 portion of cell cycle.

Route	Onset	Peak	Duration
PO, IV	Unknown	Unknown	Unknown

Half-life: Terminal phase, 4 to 11 hours.

ADVERSE REACTIONS
CNS: peripheral neuropathy, fever, *seizures.* **CV:** hypotension. **EENT:** transient cortical blindness, optic neuritis. **GI:** anorexia, diarrhea, nausea, vomiting, abdominal pain, stomatitis, mucositis, constipation, dysphagia. **Hematologic:** *leukopenia, neutropenia, thrombocytopenia, secondary leukemia,* anemia, *myelosuppression.* **Hepatic:** *hepatotoxicity.* **Respiratory:** interstitial pneumonitis/pulmonary fibrosis. **Skin:** reversible alopecia, rash, pigmentation, *SJS.* **Other:** *anaphylaxis,* hypersensitivity reactions.

INTERACTIONS
Drug-drug. *Cyclosporine:* May increase etoposide level and toxicity. Monitor CBC and adjust etoposide dose.
Live-virus vaccines: May increase risk of adverse reactions to live-virus vaccine. Concurrent use isn't recommended.
Phosphatase inhibitors: May decrease etoposide effectiveness. Monitor drug effects.
Warfarin: May further prolong PT. Monitor PT and INR closely.

Drug-food. *Grapefruit juice:* May reduce etoposide concentrations. Avoid using together.

EFFECTS ON LAB TEST RESULTS
• May decrease Hb level.
• May decrease neutrophil, platelet, RBC, and WBC counts.

CONTRAINDICATIONS & CAUTIONS
• Contraindicated in patients hypersensitive to drug.
• Use cautiously in patients who have had cytotoxic or radiation therapy and in those with hepatic impairment.
Dialyzable drug: No.

PREGNANCY-LACTATION-REPRODUCTION
• Drug can cause fetal harm if used during pregnancy. Advise women of childbearing potential to avoid becoming pregnant. If drug is used during pregnancy, or if patient becomes pregnant during therapy, patient should be apprised of potential fetal hazard.
• Drug appears in human milk. Patient should discontinue breastfeeding or discontinue drug.

NURSING CONSIDERATIONS
Black Box Warning Give drug under the supervision of a physician experienced in the use of cancer chemotherapy. Severe myelosuppression with infection or bleeding may occur. ∎
• Obtain baseline BP before starting therapy.
• Anticipate need for antiemetics.
• Have diphenhydramine, hydrocortisone, epinephrine, and emergency equipment available to establish an airway in case anaphylaxis occurs.
• Store capsules in refrigerator.
Black Box Warning Monitor CBC. Watch for evidence of bone marrow suppression, which could lead to infection or bleeding. ∎
• Observe patient's mouth for signs of ulceration.
• To prevent bleeding, avoid all IM injections when platelet count is below 50,000/mm^3.
• Etoposide phosphate dose is expressed as etoposide equivalents; 114 mg of etoposide phosphate is equivalent to 100 mg of etoposide.

PATIENT TEACHING
• Tell patient to report all adverse reactions and to watch for signs and symptoms of infection (fever, sore throat, fatigue) and bleeding (easy bruising, nosebleeds, bleeding gums, tarry stools). Tell patient to take temperature daily.
• Inform patient of need for frequent BP readings during IV administration.
• Inform patient of the risk of secondary cancers with long-term use.
• Caution female patient of childbearing potential to avoid pregnancy and breastfeeding during therapy.
• Advise male patient to use effective contraception for 4 months after final dose.

---

etravirine
eh-trah-VIGH-reen

Intelence

Therapeutic class: Antiretrovirals
Pharmacologic class: NNRTIs

AVAILABLE FORMS
Tablets ⓞ: 25 mg, 100 mg, 200 mg

INDICATIONS & DOSAGES
➤ **HIV-1 in treatment-experienced patients with evidence of viral replication and HIV-1 strains resistant to an NNRTI and other antiretrovirals**
Adults: 200 mg PO b.i.d., given with other antiretrovirals.
Children age 2 and older weighing 30 kg or more: 200 mg PO b.i.d.
Children age 2 and older weighing 25 to less than 30 kg: 150 mg PO b.i.d.
Children age 2 and older weighing 20 to less than 25 kg: 125 mg PO b.i.d.
Children age 2 and older weighing 10 to less than 20 kg: 100 mg PO b.i.d.

ADMINISTRATION
PO
• Give drug after meals.
• Have patient swallow tablets whole with a liquid such as water.
• If patient can't swallow whole tablets, place tablets in a glass with 5 mL of water.

Stir water well until it looks milky. May add 15 mL more water, orange juice, or milk to glass (avoid grapefruit juice, fluids warmer than 104° F [40° C], or carbonated beverages) and have patient drink immediately. Rinse glass with water several times and have patient swallow each rinse completely.

ACTION
Binds to reverse transcriptase, an enzyme that replicates HIV.

Route	Onset	Peak	Duration
PO	Unknown	2½–4 hr	Unknown

Half-life: About 41 ± 20 hours.

ADVERSE REACTIONS
CNS: abnormal dreams, amnesia, anxiety, confusion, disorientation, fatigue, headache, hypoesthesia, insomnia, paresthesia, peripheral neuropathy, *seizures,* sluggishness, syncope, tremors. **CV:** angina, *atrial fibrillation,* HTN, *MI.* **EENT:** blurred vision, vertigo. **GI:** abdominal distension, abdominal pain, anorexia, constipation, diarrhea, dry mouth, flatulence, gastritis, GERD, hematemesis, nausea, *pancreatitis,* retching, stomatitis, vomiting. **GU:** *renal failure.* **Hepatic:** *hepatitis,* hepatomegaly, increased liver enzyme levels. **Hematologic:** anemia, hemolytic anemia. **Metabolic:** *diabetes,* dyslipidemia. **Respiratory:** *bronchospasm,* dyspnea. **Skin:** rash.

INTERACTIONS
Drug-drug. *Amiodarone, bepridil, disopyramide, flecainide, lidocaine, mexiletine, propafenone, quinidine:* May decrease levels of these drugs. Use caution, and monitor patient closely.
Atazanavir with ritonavir: May decrease atazanavir level and increase etravirine level. Avoid use together.
Atorvastatin, lovastatin, simvastatin: May decrease levels of these drugs. Adjust dosage, if needed.
Clarithromycin: May decrease clarithromycin level and increase etravirine level. Consider using azithromycin for treating *Mycobacterium avium* complex.
CYP3A4 inhibitors (itraconazole, ketoconazole): May decrease levels of these drugs.

Reactions in bold italics are *life-threatening*. Interactions may have a *rapid onset* or a *delayed onset*.

May increase etravirine level. Adjust dosage, if needed.

CYP450 inducers (carbamazepine, phenobarbital, phenytoin): May decrease etravirine level. Avoid use together.

Delavirdine: May increase etravirine level. Avoid use together.

Dexamethasone: May decrease etravirine level. Avoid use together.

Diazepam: May increase diazepam level. Reduce diazepam dose, as needed.

Efavirenz, nevirapine: May decrease etravirine level. Avoid use together.

Fluconazole, posaconazole: May increase etravirine level. Use together cautiously.

Fluvastatin: May increase fluvastatin level. Adjust dosage, if needed.

Immunosuppressants (cyclosporine, sirolimus, tacrolimus): May decrease levels of these drugs. Use together cautiously, and monitor patient closely.

Lopinavir–ritonavir: May decrease etravirine level. Use together cautiously.

Methadone: May cause withdrawal symptoms. Monitor patient, and consider increasing methadone dosage.

PDE5 inhibitors (sildenafil, tadalafil, vardenafil): May decrease effectiveness of these drugs. Adjust dosage, as needed.

Protease inhibitors (atazanavir, fosamprenavir, indinavir, nelfinavir): May alter protease inhibitor level if given without ritonavir. Avoid use together unless given with low-dose ritonavir.

Rifabutin: May decrease etravirine and rifabutin levels. If etravirine isn't given with a protease inhibitor and ritonavir, give rifabutin 300 mg daily. If etravirine is given with darunavir and ritonavir or with saquinavir and ritonavir, avoid rifabutin.

Rifampin, rifapentine: May decrease etravirine level. Avoid use together.

Ritonavir: May decrease etravirine level. Avoid use together.

Ritonavir and tipranavir: May decrease etravirine level. Avoid use together.

Warfarin: May increase warfarin level. Monitor INR closely, and adjust warfarin dosage if needed.

Drug-herb. *St. John's wort:* May decrease etravirine level. Avoid use together.

EFFECTS ON LAB TEST RESULTS
• May increase amylase, lipase, creatinine, total cholesterol, LDL, triglyceride, AST, ALT, and glucose levels.
• May decrease Hb level and WBC, neutrophil, and platelet counts.

CONTRAINDICATIONS & CAUTIONS
• Contraindicated in patients hypersensitive to etravirine or its components.
• Hypersensitivity reactions, including DRESS syndrome (drug rash with eosinophilia and systemic symptoms), ranging from rash to organ dysfunction, and severe, potentially life-threatening and fatal skin reactions (SJS, toxic epidermal necrolysis, erythema multiforme) have been reported. Discontinue drug immediately if signs or symptoms of hypersensitivity reactions or severe skin reactions develop.
• Concomitant use with other drugs may result in potentially significant drug interactions, some of which may lead to loss of therapeutic effect and possible resistance. See manufacturer's recommendations for dosage adjustments.
• Use cautiously in elderly patients and patients with hepatic impairment or HBV or HCV infection.
• For children, don't exceed adult dosage or give to children younger than age 2.
Dialyzable drug: Unlikely.

PREGNANCY-LACTATION-REPRODUCTION
• Use only if potential benefit outweighs risk to the fetus.
• Register pregnant patients in the Antiretroviral Pregnancy Registry at 1-800-258-4263.
• It isn't known if drug appears in human milk. Women with HIV infection shouldn't breastfeed.

NURSING CONSIDERATIONS
❸ *Alert:* Etravirine may interact with many drugs. Review patient's complete drug regimen.
• If patient can't swallow the tablet whole, dissolve it in water and have patient drink it immediately. To make sure patient receives entire dose, refill the glass several times and have patient drink.

❸ *Alert:* Monitor patient closely for skin reactions. Fatalities have occurred due to toxic epidermal necrolysis, SJS, or erythema multiforme, and hypersensitivity reactions that may be accompanied by hepatic failure. Discontinue drug if severe skin or hypersensitivity reactions develop.

• Monitor patient for signs of fat redistribution (central obesity, buffalo hump, peripheral wasting, breast enlargement, cushingoid appearance).

• Immune reconstitution syndrome can occur. Monitor patient for inflammatory response to indolent or residual infections or autoimmune disorders.

• Notify prescriber if signs, symptoms, or laboratory abnormalities suggest pancreatitis. Monitor amylase and lipase levels.

• Monitor patient's CBC, platelet count, LFTs, and renal function studies. Report abnormalities.

PATIENT TEACHING

• Advise patient to take etravirine after a meal.

• Warn patient to tell prescriber about any other prescription drugs, OTC drugs, and herbal supplements being taken.

• Advise patient to report adverse effects to prescriber.

• Inform patient that drug doesn't cure HIV infection, that opportunistic infections and other complications of HIV infection may still occur, and that HIV may still be transmitted to others through sexual contact or blood contamination.

• Advise patient to take drug as prescribed and not to alter dose or stop drug without medical approval.

• If patient misses a dose, tell patient to take it as soon as possible and then return to normal schedule. Advise patient not to double the dose.

• Tell patient that routine blood tests will be needed to assess tolerance of drug therapy.

SAFETY ALERT!

everolimus ℞
eh-ver-OH-lih-mus

Afinitor, Afinitor Disperz, Zortress

Therapeutic class: Antineoplastics
Pharmacologic class: Kinase inhibitors

AVAILABLE FORMS

Tablets (Afinitor) ⓞ: 2.5 mg, 5 mg, 7.5 mg, 10 mg
Tablets (Zortress) ⓞ: 0.25 mg, 0.5 mg, 0.75 mg
Tablets for oral suspension (Afinitor Disperz) ⓞ: 2 mg, 3 mg, 5 mg

INDICATIONS & DOSAGES

➤ **Advanced renal cell carcinoma after treatment with sunitinib or sorafenib fails; renal angiomyolipoma with tuberous sclerosis complex; advanced hormone-receptor positive, HER2-negative breast cancer in postmenopausal women in combination with exemestane for recurrence or progression after treatment with letrozole or anastrozole; progressive neuroendocrine tumors of pancreatic origin (unresectable, locally advanced, or metastatic); progressive, well-differentiated, nonfunctional neuroendocrine tumors of GI or lung origin (locally advanced or metastatic) (Afinitor)**
Adults: 10 mg PO once daily. Continue until disease progression or unacceptable toxicity occurs.
Adjust-a-dose: Refer to manufacturer's instructions for dosage modifications for adverse effects, for patients with hepatic impairment, and for those taking drugs that inhibit or induce P-gp and CYP3A4.
➤ **Prevention of organ rejection in liver transplantation (Zortress only)**
Adults: 1 mg PO b.i.d. starting at least 30 days after transplant in combination with reduced-dose tacrolimus and corticosteroids. Adjust dosage based on trough concentrations obtained 4 to 5 days after previous dosing.
Adjust-a-dose: In patients with mild hepatic impairment, reduce initial dose by a third. In patients with moderate to severe hepatic

---

Reactions in bold italics are *life-threatening*. Interactions may have a *rapid onset* or a *delayed onset*.

impairment, reduce initial dose by half and monitor blood concentrations.

► **Prevention of kidney transplant rejection in patients at low to moderate immunologic risk (Zortress only)**

Adults: Initially, 0.75 mg PO b.i.d. in combination with basiliximab induction and a reduced dose of cyclosporine and corticosteroids as soon as possible after transplantation. Dosage adjustments may be made at 4- to 5-day intervals based on patient response and clinical situation.

Adjust-a-dose: In patients with mild hepatic impairment (Child-Pugh class A), reduce initial dose by a third. In patients with moderate to severe hepatic impairment (Child-Pugh class B or C), reduce initial dose by half and monitor blood concentrations.

► **Subependymal giant cell astrocytoma with tuberous sclerosis in patients who aren't surgical candidates (Afinitor or Afinitor Disperz)**

Adults and children age 1 and older: Initially, 4.5 mg/m^2 PO once daily until disease progression or unacceptable toxicity; round dose to nearest strength. Adjust dosage per manufacturer's instructions in 1- to 2-week intervals to trough concentration of 5 to 15 ng/mL. Maximum dose increment at any titration must not exceed 5 mg. Don't combine the two dosage forms (Afinitor tablets and Afinitor Disperz tablets) to achieve the desired dose. Use one dosage form or the other. Once a stable dose is attained, monitor trough concentrations every 3 to 6 months in patients with changing BSA or every 6 to 12 months in patients with stable BSA for duration of treatment.

Adjust-a-dose: Refer to manufacturer's instructions for dosage modifications for adverse effects, for patients with hepatic impairment, and for those taking drugs that inhibit or induce P-gp and CYP3A4.

► **Adjunctive treatment of patients with tuberous sclerosis complex (TSC)–associated partial-onset seizures (Afinitor Disperz)** 🗒

Adults and children age 2 and older: Initially, 5 mg/m^2 PO once daily. Titrate dosage to attain trough concentration of 5 to 15 ng/mL. Maximum dose increase is 5 mg every 1 to 2 weeks. Once a stable dose is attained, monitor trough concentrations every

3 to 6 months in patients with changing BSA or every 6 to 12 months in patients with stable BSA for duration of treatment.

Adjust-a-dose: For patients with severe hepatic impairment (Child-Pugh class C), initially, 2.5 mg/m^2 once daily; adjust dosage based on trough concentrations as recommended. Refer to manufacturer's instructions for toxicity-related dosage adjustments and for dosage adjustments when drug is used concurrently with P-gp and CYP3A4 inhibitors and P-gp and CYP3A4 inducers.

ADMINISTRATION
PO
Afinitor, Zortress
• Give drug at same time(s) each day, consistently with or without food.
• Have patient swallow tablets whole with a glass of water. Tablets shouldn't be chewed or crushed.
• Patient should avoid grapefruit or grapefruit juice while taking drug.

Afinitor Disperz
• Wear gloves to avoid possible contact with everolimus when preparing suspension.
• Give as a suspension only.
• Give drug orally once daily at the same time every day, either consistently with or without food.
• Administer suspension immediately after preparation. Discard suspension if not administered within 60 minutes after preparation. Prepare suspension in water only.
• To administer drug using an oral syringe, place the prescribed dose into a 10-mL syringe. Don't exceed a total of 10 mg per syringe. If higher doses are required, prepare an additional syringe. Don't break or crush tablets. Draw approximately 5 mL of water and 4 mL of air into the syringe. Place the filled syringe into a container (tip up) for 3 minutes, until the tablets are in suspension. Gently invert the syringe five times immediately before administration. After administration of prepared suspension, draw approximately 5 mL of water and 4 mL of air into the same syringe, and swirl contents to suspend remaining particles. Administer the entire contents of the syringe.
• To administer using a small drinking glass, place the prescribed dose into a small drinking glass (maximum size 100 mL)

containing approximately 25 mL of water. Don't exceed a total of 10 mg per glass. If higher doses are required, prepare an additional glass. Don't break or crush tablets. Allow 3 minutes for suspension to occur. Stir the contents gently with a spoon, immediately prior to drinking. After administration of the prepared suspension, add 25 mL of water and stir with the same spoon to resuspend remaining particles. Administer the entire contents of the glass.

ACTION

Binds to an intracellular protein, thereby inhibiting mammalian target rapamycin (mTOR), a kinase. Inhibiting mTOR reduces cancer cell proliferation, angiogenesis, and glucose uptake.

Route	Onset	Peak	Duration
PO	Unknown	1–2 hr	Unknown

Half-life: 30 hours.

ADVERSE REACTIONS

CNS: asthenia, dizziness, headache, insomnia, paresthesia, fever, fatigue, *seizures.* **CV:** chest pain, *HF,* HTN, tachycardia, edema, *hemorrhage.* **EENT:** conjunctivitis, eyelid edema, epistaxis, mucosal inflammation, nasopharyngitis, pharyngolaryngeal pain, rhinorrhea, sinusitis. **GI:** abdominal pain, anorexia, diarrhea, dry mouth, dysgeusia, dysphagia, hemorrhoids, nausea, stomatitis, vomiting, mouth ulcers, oral mucositis. **GU:** renal failure, UTI, menstrual irregularities. **Hematologic:** anemia, *leukopenia, neutropenia, thrombocytopenia.* **Hepatic:** elevated alkaline phosphatase, AST, ALT levels. **Metabolic:** exacerbation of diabetes mellitus, weight loss, fasting hyperglycemia, hypercholesterolemia, hypertriglyceridemia, hypophosphatemia, decreased appetite. **Musculoskeletal:** extremity pain, jaw pain, arthralgia. **Respiratory:** bronchitis, cough, dyspnea, pleural effusion, URI, pneumonia, *pneumonitis, bronchospasm.* **Skin:** acneiform dermatitis, dry skin, erythema, hand-foot syndrome, nail disorder, pruritus, onychoclasis, rash, skin lesion. **Other:** chills, peripheral edema, infection, hypersensitivity reactions, *angioedema.*

INTERACTIONS

Drug-drug. *Clozapine:* May enhance risk of neutropenia. Monitor patient response.

⬛ **Black Box Warning** *Cyclosporine:* Increased nephrotoxicity can occur with standard cyclosporine dosing in combination with Zortress. Decrease cyclosporine dosage, and monitor serum cyclosporine and everolimus levels. ∎

Strong CYP3A4 inducers (carbamazepine, dexamethasone, phenobarbital, phenytoin, rifabutin, rifampin): May decrease everolimus level. Avoid using together; if drugs must be used together, increase everolimus dosage per manufacturer's instructions.

Strong or moderate CYP3A4 inhibitors (amprenavir, aprepitant, atazanavir, clarithromycin, delavirdine, diltiazem, erythromycin, fluconazole, fosamprenavir, indinavir, itraconazole, ketoconazole, nefazodone, nelfinavir, ritonavir, saquinavir, telithromycin, verapamil, voriconazole) and P-gp inhibitors (amiodarone, spironolactone): May increase everolimus level. Avoid using together; if drugs must be used together, reduce everolimus dosage per manufacturer's instructions.

Vaccines (live-virus): Toxic effects of vaccines may increase and drug's therapeutic effects diminish. Avoid use together.

Drug-herb. *St. John's wort:* May alter drug level. Don't use together.

Drug-food. *Grapefruit, grapefruit juice:* May increase drug level. Don't use together.

EFFECTS ON LAB TEST RESULTS

• May increase urinary protein and creatinine, cholesterol, triglyceride, and glucose levels.

• May decrease Hb level and lymphocyte, neutrophil, and platelet counts.

CONTRAINDICATIONS & CAUTIONS

⬛ **Black Box Warning** Use of Zortress has been shown to increase mortality in a heart transplant clinical trial. Use in heart transplant patients isn't recommended. ∎

• Contraindicated in patients hypersensitive to drug, its components, or other rapamycin derivatives.

• Afinitor isn't indicated to treat functional carcinoid tumors.

Reactions in bold italics are *life-threatening*. Interactions may have a *rapid onset* or a *delayed onset*.

E

• Avoid use in patients with severe hepatic impairment or severe infection.
Dialyzable drug: No.

PREGNANCY-LACTATION-REPRODUCTION
• Avoid use during pregnancy because of potential hazards to fetus.
• Women of reproductive potential should avoid pregnancy and use highly effective contraception during treatment and for up to 8 weeks after last dose.
• The National Transplantation Pregnancy Registry (NTPR) follows pregnant women taking immunosuppressants after any solid organ transplant. The NTPR encourages reporting all immunosuppressant exposures during pregnancy in transplant recipients at 1-877-955-6877.
• Drug may cause male and female infertility.
• It isn't known if drug appears in human milk.

NURSING CONSIDERATIONS
Black Box Warning Zortress should only be prescribed by providers experienced in immunosuppressive therapy and management of transplant patients. ∎
• Don't crush tablets. Avoid direct contact with skin or mucous membranes. If contact occurs, wash area thoroughly.
Black Box Warning Zortress increases risk of infection and malignancies, such as lymphoma and skin cancer, due to immunosuppression. ∎
⚠ Alert: Drug may cause immunosuppression, predisposing patients to bacterial, fungal, viral, or protozoal infections, including reactivation of hepatitis B virus. Infections may be severe or even fatal. Complete treatment of preexisting invasive fungal infections before starting therapy. Consider holding or stopping everolimus if infection occurs. Discontinue drug if invasive systemic fungal infection is diagnosed, and treat infection appropriately. Incidence of serious infections was reported at a higher frequency in patients younger than age 6.
• Monitor patient for signs of infection (fever, chills, sore throat, fatigue).
Black Box Warning There is an increased risk of arterial and venous renal thrombosis leading to graft loss in patients taking

Zortress, mostly in first 30 days after transplant. ∎
Black Box Warning When drug is used with cyclosporine, increased nephrotoxicity can occur and reduced dosages of everolimus are needed. Monitor cyclosporine and everolimus whole blood trough concentrations. ∎
• Hyperglycemia, hypercholesterolemia, and hypertriglyceridemia have been reported. Withhold or permanently discontinue drug based on severity.
• Monitor renal function studies, glucose and lipid levels, and CBC before and during therapy.
• Monitor respiratory status for signs and symptoms of noninfectious pneumonitis (hypoxia, pleural effusion, cough, dyspnea). For severe cases, discontinue therapy and administer corticosteroids.

PATIENT TEACHING
• Advise female patient of childbearing potential to use an effective method of contraception during therapy and for 4 weeks after therapy with Afinitor or Afinitor Disperz or 8 weeks after therapy with Zortress.
• Advise male and female patient that use may impair fertility.
• Tell patient to swallow the Afinitor or Zortress tablets whole with a glass of water.
• Tell patient to take drug at the same time each day, consistently with or without food.
• Instruct caregiver how to prepare and administer Afinitor Disperz.
• Instruct patient that if a dose of Afinitor is missed, the missed dose may still be taken up to 6 hours after the normal time. If more than 6 hours have elapsed, tell patient to skip that day's dose and take it at the usual time the next day.
• Advise patient to limit sun exposure.
• Advise patient to report mouth ulcers, fever, shortness of breath, cough, rash, headache, loss of appetite, nausea, vomiting, diarrhea, swelling of the extremities or face, weakness, tiredness, or nosebleeds.
• Tell patient not to receive live-virus vaccines and to avoid close contact with anyone who has received a live-virus vaccine.

exenatide ℞
eks-EHN-uh-tyde

Bydureon, Bydureon BCise, Byetta

Therapeutic class: Antidiabetics
Pharmacologic class: Incretin mimetics

AVAILABLE FORMS
Injection: 5 mcg/dose in 1.2-mL prefilled pen (60 doses); 10 mcg/dose in 2.4-mL prefilled pen (60 doses)
Injection (extended-release): 2 mg/dose in single-use vial, 2 mg/dose in single-dose pen

INDICATIONS & DOSAGES
➤ **Adjunct to diet and exercise to improve glycemic control in patients with type 2 diabetes**
Adults: 5 mcg (immediate release) subcut b.i.d. within 60 minutes before morning and evening meals. Give doses at least 6 hours apart. If needed, increase to 10 mcg b.i.d. after 1 month. Or, 2 mg (extended-release) subcut any time of day, with or without a meal, once every 7 days.
Adjust-a-dose: Use caution when escalating doses of Byetta (injection) from 5 to 10 mcg in patients with moderate renal impairment (CrCl of 50 to 80 mL/minute). Drug isn't recommended for patients with ESRD or severe renal impairment (CrCl of less than 30 mL/minute). Use cautiously in patients with renal transplantation or moderate renal impairment.

When converting from Byetta immediate-release to Bydureon or Bydureon BCise extended-release formulation, initiate weekly administration of extended-release exenatide the day after discontinuing exenatide immediate-release. Patient may experience increased blood glucose levels for approximately 2 to 4 weeks after conversion. Pretreatment with exenatide immediate-release isn't required before initiating extended-release exenatide.

ADMINISTRATION
Subcutaneous
۞ Alert: Multidose pens are for single patient use only. Pens should never be shared even if the needle is changed. Clearly label with patient identifying information where it will not obstruct the dosing window, warning, or other product information.

• If patient misses a dose of extended-release form, give as soon as noticed, provided the next regularly scheduled dose is due 3 or more days later. Then, resume the usual dosing schedule of once every 7 days (weekly). If a dose is missed and the next regularly scheduled dose is due 1 or 2 days later, don't give the missed dose; instead, resume treatment with the next regularly scheduled dose.

Bydureon
• Give Bydureon at any time during the day and without regard to meals.
• To administer: Attach vial connector to vial.
— Connect prefilled diluent syringe to vial.
— Push on syringe's plunger to inject diluent into vial. Continue to push on plunger while shaking vial to thoroughly mix powder and diluent. Solution will be cloudy.
— Invert vial and withdraw solution to the black-dashed dose line on syringe.
— Remove vial connector and attach needle.
— Give immediately as a subcut injection in the thigh, abdomen, or back of upper arm. Rotate injection sites each week.
• Store in refrigerator at 36° to 46° F (2° to 8° C). May store at room temperature (68° to 77° F [20° to 25° C]) for up to 4 weeks. Don't freeze, and don't use drug if it has been frozen. Protect from light.

Bydureon BCise
• Give Bydureon BCise at any time during the day and without regard to meals.
• Remove autoinjector from refrigerator 15 minutes before mixing the injection, to reach room temperature.
• Mix by shaking vigorously for at least 15 seconds. After mixing, Bydureon BCise should appear as an opaque, white to off-white suspension, evenly mixed with no residual medicine along the side, bottom, or top of the inspection window.
• Inspect visually for particulate matter and discoloration before administration; drug contains microspheres that appear as white to off-white particles. Don't use if foreign particulate matter or discoloration is observed.

Reactions in bold italics are *life-threatening*. Interactions may have a *rapid onset* or a *delayed onset*.

• Give immediately as a subcut injection in thigh, abdomen, or back of upper arm. Rotate injection sites each week.
• Hold autoinjector straight up with the orange cap toward the ceiling. Turn the knob on bottom from the lock to unlock position until you hear a click; then unscrew and discard the orange cap.
• Push autoinjector against the skin. You will hear a click when the injection begins.
• Keep holding autoinjector against the skin for 15 seconds and until an orange rod appears in the window, to make sure the full dose is delivered.
• Store flat in the refrigerator between 36° and 46° F (2° and 8° C). Can keep at room temperature not to exceed 86° F (30° C) for no more than a total of 4 weeks, if needed.

Byetta
• Drug comes in two strengths; check cartridge carefully before use.
• Don't give after a meal.
• Give as a subcut injection in the thigh, abdomen, or upper arm.
• Inject subcut within 60 minutes before morning and evening meals or before the two main meals of the day approximately 6 hours or more apart.
• Before first use, store drug in refrigerator at 36° to 46° F (2° to 8° C). After first use, drug can be kept at room temperature up to 77° F (25° C). Don't freeze, and don't use drug if it has been frozen. Protect drug from light. Discard pen 30 days after first use, even if some drug remains.
• Don't mix with insulin.

ACTION
Reduces fasting and postprandial glucose levels in type 2 diabetes by stimulating insulin production in response to elevated glucose levels, inhibiting glucagon release after meals, and slowing gastric emptying.

Route	Onset	Peak	Duration
Subcut	Unknown	2 hr	Unknown
Subcut (extended-release)	Unknown	2 wk, 6–7 wk	10 wk

Half-life: 2½ hours; extended-release, unknown.

ADVERSE REACTIONS
CNS: dizziness, headache, fatigue, jittery feeling, nervousness. **GI:** anorexia, constipation, decreased appetite, diarrhea, dyspepsia, nausea, *pancreatitis,* vomiting, GERD. **Metabolic:** *hypoglycemia.* **Musculoskeletal:** asthenia. **Skin:** excessive sweating.

INTERACTIONS
Drug-drug. *Acetaminophen:* May decrease acetaminophen concentration. Give acetaminophen at least 1 hour before or 4 hours after exenatide injection.
Digoxin, lovastatin: May decrease concentrations of these drugs. Monitor patient.
Drugs that are rapidly absorbed: May slow gastric emptying and reduce absorption of some oral drugs. Separate administration by 1 hour.
Oral drugs that need to maintain a threshold concentration to maintain effectiveness (antibiotics, hormonal contraceptives): May reduce rate and extent of absorption of these drugs. Give these drugs at least 1 hour before giving exenatide.
Other antidiabetic agents (insulin, meglitinides [repaglinide]): May increase risk of hypoglycemia. Closely monitor blood glucose concentrations when exenatide is started or stopped, and reinforce patient instructions for hypoglycemia management, especially in patients receiving insulin.
Sulfonylureas: May increase the risk of hypoglycemia. Reduce sulfonylurea dose as needed, and monitor patient closely.
Warfarin: May increase INR and increase bleeding risk when administered together. Monitor INR frequently, especially when starting drug or changing dosage.

EFFECTS ON LAB TEST RESULTS
• Decreases glucose level.
• May increase INR.

CONTRAINDICATIONS & CAUTIONS
Black Box Warning Extended-release form is contraindicated in patients with personal or family history of medullary thyroid carcinoma (MTC) and in patients with multiple endocrine neoplasia syndrome type 2. ■
• Contraindicated in patients hypersensitive to drug or its components. Serious reactions (anaphylaxis, angioedema) have been reported. If hypersensitivity occurs, discontinue drug.

Black Box Warning Exenatide extended-release causes an increased incidence in thyroid C-cell tumors at clinically relevant exposures in rats compared to controls. It's unknown whether it causes thyroid C-cell tumors, including MTC, in humans, as the human relevance of exenatide extended-release–induced rodent thyroid C-cell tumors hasn't been determined. ■

• Exenatide extended-release isn't recommended as first-line therapy for patients with inadequate glycemic control on diet and exercise because of the uncertain relevance of the rat thyroid C-cell tumor findings to humans.

• Drug has been associated with acute pancreatitis, including fatal and nonfatal hemorrhagic or necrotizing pancreatitis. Discontinue immediately if pancreatitis is suspected. Don't restart if pancreatitis is confirmed.

• Don't use in patients with type 1 diabetes or diabetic ketoacidosis.

• Don't use in patients with ESRD, CrCl less than 30 mL/minute, or severe GI disease (including gastroparesis).

• Use cautiously in patients with renal transplant.

• Risk of hypoglycemia increases when drug is used in combination with other drugs that can lower blood glucose level (e.g., insulin, insulin secretagogues). Dosage reductions may be necessary.

• Drug hasn't been shown to reduce macrovascular outcomes.

Dialyzable drug: Unknown.

⚠ *Overdose S&S:* Severe nausea, severe vomiting, hypoglycemia.

PREGNANCY-LACTATION-REPRODUCTION

• Use only if potential benefit justifies potential risk to the fetus.

• Prescribers are encouraged to register patients in the Exenatide Pregnancy Registry (1-800-633-9081).

• It isn't known if drug appears in human milk. Patient should discontinue breastfeeding or discontinue drug.

NURSING CONSIDERATIONS

• Assess GI and renal function before and during treatment.

Black Box Warning Routine monitoring of serum calcitonin level or the use of thyroid ultrasound is of uncertain value for detection of MTC in patients treated with exenatide extended-release. ■

❸ *Alert:* Drug-related nausea, vomiting, and diarrhea resulting in dehydration have led to increased serum creatinine levels and acute renal failure.

• Monitor patient receiving extended-release form for serious injection-site reactions, such as abscess, cellulitis, and necrosis, with or without subcutaneous nodules.

• Monitor glucose level regularly and HbA$_{1c}$ level periodically.

❸ *Alert:* Stop drug if pancreatitis is suspected. Initiate appropriate treatment, and monitor patient carefully. Drug shouldn't be readministered.

• *Look alike–sound alike:* Don't confuse exenatide with ezetimibe.

PATIENT TEACHING

Black Box Warning Explain to patient taking extended-release exenatide the risk and signs and symptoms of thyroid tumors (mass in the neck, dysphagia, dyspnea, persistent hoarseness). ■

• Explain the risks of drug.

• Review proper use and storage of medication, particularly the one-time setup for each new pen or reconstitution procedure for powder.

• Instruct patient in the proper use of autoinjector.

• Inform patient that prefilled pen doesn't include a needle; the prescriber will indicate which needle length and gauge is appropriate.

• Instruct patient to inject Byetta in the thigh, abdomen, or upper arm within 60 minutes before morning and evening meals. Caution against injecting drug after a meal.

• Instruct patient to inject extended-release form in the thigh, abdomen, or back of upper arm immediately after mixing.

❸ *Alert:* Warn patient not to share the multi-dose pen device with other people, even if the needle is changed due to the risk of transmission of blood-borne pathogens, including HIV and hepatitis viruses.

Reactions in bold italics are *life-threatening*. Interactions may have a *rapid onset* or a *delayed onset*.

E

• Advise patient that drug may decrease appetite, food intake, and body weight, and that these changes don't warrant a change in dosage.

• Advise patient to seek immediate medical care if unexplained, persistent, severe abdominal pain, with or without vomiting, occurs.

• Inform patient receiving extended-release form about risk of serious injection-site reactions and to report signs and symptoms (erythema, pain, drainage, skin color changes) immediately.

• Review steps for managing hypoglycemia, especially if patient takes a sulfonylurea or insulin.

• Inform patient of potential risk of worsening renal function and signs and symptoms of renal dysfunction.

• Tell patient changing from immediate-release to extended-release form that transient blood glucose elevations are possible during the first 2 to 4 weeks of therapy.

• Stress importance of proper storage (refrigeration), infection prevention, and timing of exenatide dose in relation to other oral drugs.

• Tell patient that if a dose of Byetta is missed to resume treatment as prescribed with the next scheduled dose.

• Tell patient that if a dose of extended-release form is missed to administer it as soon as noticed, provided the next regularly scheduled dose is due at least 3 days later, and then to resume once-every-7-days dosing schedule. If a dose is missed and the next regularly scheduled dose is due in 1 to 2 days, tell patient not to administer the missed dose and instead to resume therapy with next regularly scheduled dose.

ezetimibe ☒
ee-ZET-ah-mibe

Zetia❧

Therapeutic class: Antilipemics
Pharmacologic class: Selective cholesterol absorption inhibitors

AVAILABLE FORMS
Tablets: 10 mg

INDICATIONS & DOSAGES
➤ **Adjunct to diet and exercise to reduce total cholesterol, LDL cholesterol (LDL-C), and apolipoprotein B (apo B) levels in patients with primary hypercholesterolemia, alone or combined with HMG-CoA reductase inhibitors (statins); adjunct to other lipid-lowering drugs (combined with atorvastatin or simvastatin) to reduce total cholesterol and LDL-C levels in patients with homozygous familial hypercholesterolemia; adjunct to diet in patients with homozygous sitosterolemia to reduce sitosterol and campesterol levels; adjunct to fenofibrate and diet to reduce total cholesterol, LDL-C, apo B, and non-HDL-C levels in patients with mixed hyperlipidemia** ☒
Adults and children age 10 and older: 10 mg PO daily.

ADMINISTRATION
PO
• Give drug without regard for meals.
• May give dose at same time as an HMG-CoA reductase inhibitor or fenofibrate.
• Give at least 2 hours before or at least 4 hours after administration of a bile acid sequestrant.

ACTION
Inhibits absorption of cholesterol by the small intestine, unlike other drugs used for cholesterol reduction; causes reduced hepatic cholesterol stores and increased cholesterol clearance from the blood.

Route	Onset	Peak	Duration
PO	Unknown	4–12 hr	Unknown

Half-life: 22 hours.

ADVERSE REACTIONS
CNS: dizziness, fatigue. **EENT:** nasopharyngitis, sinusitis. **GI:** diarrhea. **Musculoskeletal:** arthralgia, back pain, pain in extremity, myalgia. **Respiratory:** URI. **Other:** viral infection, flulike symptoms.

INTERACTIONS
Drug-drug. *Bile acid sequestrant (cholestyramine):* May decrease ezetimibe level. Give ezetimibe at least 2 hours before or 4 hours after cholestyramine.

✛Canada   ◇OTC   ◆Off-label use   ✐Photoguide   ⊞Do not crush   *Liquid contains alcohol   ☒Genetic

Cyclosporine, fenofibrate: May increase ezetimibe level. Monitor patient for adverse reactions.

Fibrates: May increase excretion of cholesterol into the gallbladder bile. Avoid using together.

Gemfibrozil: May increase risk of myopathy and cholelithiasis. Avoid use together.

EFFECTS ON LAB TEST RESULTS
• May increase LFT values and CK level.

CONTRAINDICATIONS & CAUTIONS
• Contraindicated in patients hypersensitive to components of drug.
• Contraindicated in combination with HMG-CoA reductase inhibitors in patients with active liver disease or unexplained increased transaminase levels.
• Rarely, myopathy, including rhabdomyolysis, has been reported. Risk may increase with concurrent use of fibrate drugs or high-dose statins, age greater than 65, hypothyroidism, or renal impairment. Discontinue ezetimibe and statin or fibrate immediately if myopathy is suspected or confirmed.
Dialyzable drug: Unknown.

PREGNANCY-LACTATION-REPRODUCTION
• Use only if potential benefit justifies potential risk to the fetus.
• When drug is used with a statin in a woman of childbearing potential, refer to pregnancy information and product labeling for the statin. All statins are contraindicated in pregnant and breastfeeding women.
• It isn't known if drug appears in human milk. Use drug only if potential benefit justifies potential risk to the infant.

NURSING CONSIDERATIONS
• Before starting treatment, assess patient for underlying causes of dyslipidemia.
• Obtain baseline triglyceride and total cholesterol, LDL-C, and HDL-C levels.
• Using drug with an HMG-CoA reductase inhibitor significantly decreases total cholesterol and LDL-C, apo B, and triglyceride levels and (except with pravastatin) increases HDL-C level more than use of an HMG-CoA reductase inhibitor alone. Check LFT values when therapy starts and thereafter according to the HMG-CoA

reductase inhibitor manufacturer's recommendations.
• Patient should maintain a cholesterol-lowering diet during treatment.
• Monitor patient for muscle pain, weakness, or tenderness. Discontinue drug if signs or symptoms of myopathy occur with CK more than 10 × ULN.

PATIENT TEACHING
• Emphasize importance of following a cholesterol-lowering diet during drug therapy.
• Inform patient that drug may be taken with or without food.
• Advise patient to report unexplained muscle pain, weakness, or tenderness.
• Urge patient to tell prescriber about any herbal or dietary supplements being taken.
• Advise patient to visit prescriber for routine follow-ups and blood tests.
• Tell female patient to notify prescriber if she becomes pregnant.

famciclovir
fam-SYE-kloe-vir

Therapeutic class: Antivirals
Pharmacologic class: Nucleosides–nucleotides

AVAILABLE FORMS
Tablets: 125 mg, 250 mg, 500 mg

INDICATIONS & DOSAGES
➤ **Acute herpes zoster infection (shingles)**
Adults: 500 mg PO every 8 hours for 7 days.
Adjust-a-dose: For patients with CrCl of 40 to 59 mL/minute, give 500 mg PO every 12 hours; if CrCl is 20 to 39 mL/minute, give 500 mg PO every 24 hours; if CrCl is less than 20 mL/minute, give 250 mg PO every 24 hours. For hemodialysis patients, give 250 mg PO after each hemodialysis session.
➤ **Recurrent genital herpes**
Adults: 1,000 mg PO b.i.d. for a single day. Begin therapy at the first sign or symptom.
Adjust-a-dose: For patients with CrCl of 40 to 59 mL/minute, give 500 mg every

12 hours for 1 day; for CrCl of 20 to 39 mL/minute, give 500 mg PO as a single dose; if CrCl is less than 20 mL/minute, give 250 mg as a single dose. For hemodialysis patient, give 250 mg single dose after hemodialysis session.

➤ **Suppression of recurrent genital herpes**
Adults: 250 mg PO b.i.d. for up to 1 year.
Adjust-a-dose: For patients with CrCl of 20 to 39 mL/minute, give 125 mg PO every 12 hours; if CrCl is less than 20 mL/minute, give 125 mg PO every 24 hours. For hemodialysis patients, give 125 mg PO after each hemodialysis session.

➤ **Recurrent mucocutaneous (orolabial/genital) herpes simplex infections in HIV-infected patients**
Adults: 500 mg PO b.i.d. for 7 days.
Adjust-a-dose: For patients with CrCl of 20 to 39 mL/minute, give 500 mg PO every 24 hours; if CrCl is less than 20 mL/minute, give 250 mg PO every 24 hours. For hemodialysis patients, give 250 mg PO after each hemodialysis session.

➤ **Recurrent herpes labialis (cold sores)**
Adults: 1,500 mg PO for one dose. Give at the first sign or symptom of cold sore.
Adjust-a-dose: For patients with CrCl of 40 to 59 mL/minute, give 750 mg as a single dose; for CrCl of 20 to 39 mL/minute, give 500 mg PO as a single dose; if CrCl is less than 20 mL/minute, give 250 mg as a single dose. For hemodialysis patient, give 250 mg single dose after hemodialysis session.

ADMINISTRATION
PO
• Give drug without regard for meals.
• Store at 77° F (25° C); excursions permitted to 59° to 86° F (15° to 30° C).

ACTION
A guanosine nucleoside that is converted to penciclovir, which enters viral cells and inhibits DNA polymerase and viral DNA synthesis.

Route	Onset	Peak	Duration
PO	Unknown	1 hr	Unknown

Half-life: Penciclovir, 2 to 4 hours.

ADVERSE REACTIONS
CNS: headache, fatigue, dizziness, paresthesia, somnolence. **GI:** nausea, abdominal pain, diarrhea, vomiting, flatulence. **GU:** dysmenorrhea. **Hematologic:** *leukopenia, neutropenia.* **Hepatic:** elevated AST and ALT levels, bilirubinemia. **Skin:** pruritus, rash. **Other:** zoster-related signs, symptoms, and complications.

INTERACTIONS
Drug-drug. *Varicella virus vaccine, zoster vaccine (live, attenuated):* May diminish effect of vaccines. When possible, discontinue famciclovir for at least 24 hours before and 14 days after vaccinations.

EFFECTS ON LAB TEST RESULTS
• May increase AST, ALT, amylase, lipase, and bilirubin levels.

CONTRAINDICATIONS & CAUTIONS
• Contraindicated in patients hypersensitive to drug, its components, or penciclovir.
• Use cautiously in patients with renal or hepatic impairment and in elderly patients.
Dialyzable drug: Yes.

PREGNANCY-LACTATION-REPRODUCTION
• Use drug during pregnancy only if benefit clearly outweighs potential risk to the fetus.
• Women exposed to drug during pregnancy should be enrolled in the Famvir Pregnancy Reporting system (1-888-669-6682).
• It isn't known if drug appears in human milk. Use only if benefits outweigh risk to the infant.

NURSING CONSIDERATIONS
• In patients with renal or hepatic impairment, adjust dosage as needed.
• Monitor LFTs and renal function tests.
• Periodically monitor CBC during long-term therapy.

PATIENT TEACHING
• Inform patient that drug doesn't cure herpes but can decrease the duration and severity of symptoms.
• Teach patient how to avoid spreading infection to others.

- Urge patient to recognize the early signs and symptoms of herpes infection, such as tingling, itching, burning, pain, or lesion and to report them. Therapy is more effective if started within 48 hours of rash onset.
- Drug may contain lactose. If patient is lactose-intolerant, advise patient to notify prescriber before taking drug.

famotidine
fa-MOE-ti-deen

Pepcid�, Pepcid AC ◊

Therapeutic class: Antiulcer drugs
Pharmacologic class: H_2-receptor antagonists

AVAILABLE FORMS
Injection: 0.4 mg/mL in NSS (premixed), 10 mg/mL
Powder for oral suspension: 40 mg/5 mL after reconstitution
Tablets: 10 mg ◊, 20 mg ◊, 40 mg
Tablets (chewable): 10 mg ◊, 20 mg ◊

INDICATIONS & DOSAGES
Adjust-a-dose (for all indications): For patients with CrCl below 50 mL/minute, give half the dose, or increase dosing interval to every 36 to 48 hours.
➤ **Short-term treatment for duodenal ulcer**
Adults, children, and adolescents weighing more than 40 kg: For acute therapy, 40 mg PO once daily at bedtime or 20 mg PO b.i.d. for up to 4 to 8 weeks. Healing usually occurs within 4 weeks.

For maintenance therapy (adults), 20 mg PO once daily at bedtime for 1 year or as clinically indicated.
Children ages 1 to 16: 0.5 mg/kg/day oral suspension PO at bedtime or divided b.i.d. (maximum dose, 40 mg/day); doses up to 1 mg/kg/day have been used.
➤ **Short-term treatment for benign gastric ulcer**
Adults, children, and adolescents weighing more than 40 kg: 40 mg PO daily at bedtime or 20 mg PO b.i.d. for up to 8 weeks.

Children ages 1 to 16: 0.5 mg/kg/day PO at bedtime or in two divided doses, up to 40 mg daily; doses up to 1 mg/kg/day have been used.
➤ **Pathologic hypersecretory conditions (such as Zollinger-Ellison syndrome)**
Adults: 20 mg PO every 6 hours, up to 160 mg every 6 hours. Maximum, 640 mg/day.
➤ **Hospitalized patients who can't take oral drug or who have intractable ulcers or hypersecretory conditions**
Adults: 20 mg IV every 12 hours.
Children ages 1 to 16: 0.25 mg/kg IV every 12 hours (maximum dose, 40 mg/day); doses up to 0.5 mg/kg every 12 hours have been used.
➤ **GERD**
Adults, children, and adolescents weighing more than 40 kg: Short-term therapy: 20 mg PO b.i.d. for up to 6 weeks. For esophagitis caused by GERD, 20 to 40 mg b.i.d. for up to 12 weeks.
Children ages 1 to 16: Short-term therapy: 0.5 mg/kg/dose PO b.i.d. (maximum dose, 40 mg b.i.d.). Up to 1 mg/kg/dose b.i.d. has been used.
Children ages 3 months to younger than 1 year: Short-term therapy: 0.5 mg/kg/dose oral suspension PO b.i.d. for up to 8 weeks.
Children younger than age 3 months: Short-term therapy: 0.5 mg/kg/dose oral suspension once daily for up to 8 weeks.
➤ **To prevent or treat heartburn (OTC only)**
Adults and children older than age 12: 10 to 20 mg up to b.i.d. for maximum of 40 mg/day.

ADMINISTRATION
PO
- Give without regard to meals.
- May give with antacids.
- Reconstitute and shake oral suspension before use.
- Store reconstituted oral suspension below 86° F (30° C). Discard after 30 days.
- Store tablets at 77° F (25° C); excursions permitted to 59° to 86° F (15° to 30° C). Protect from light.

IV

▼ Compatible solutions include sterile water for injection, NSS for injection, D_5W or dextrose 10% in water for injection, 5% sodium bicarbonate injection, and lactated Ringer injection. Drug also can be added to total parenteral nutrition solutions.

▼ Before use, store at 36° to 46° F (2° to 8° C). If solution freezes, allow to solubilize at room temperature. Protect from light.

▼ For direct injection, dilute 2 mL (20 mg) with compatible solution to a total volume of either 5 or 10 mL. Inject over at least 2 minutes.

▼ For intermittent infusion, dilute 20 mg (2 mL) in 100-mL compatible solution. The premixed 50-mL solution doesn't need further dilution. Infuse over 15 to 30 minutes.

▼ After dilution, solution is stable 48 hours at 36° to 46° F (2° to 8° C).

▼ **Incompatibilities:** Amphotericin B cholesteryl sulfate complex, azathioprine, cefepime, chloramphenicol, dantrolene, diazepam, ganciclovir, gemtuzumab, lansoprazole, mitomycin, pantoprazole, piperacillin–tazobactam, trimethoprim–sulfamethoxazole.

ACTION

Competitively inhibits action of histamine on the H_2-receptor sites of parietal cells, decreasing gastric acid secretion.

Route	Onset	Peak	Duration
PO	1 hr	1–3 hr	10–20 hr
IV	1 hr	1–4 hr	10–20 hr

Half-life: 2½ to 3½ hours.

ADVERSE REACTIONS

CNS: headache, dizziness; irritability, agitation (younger than age 1). **GI:** constipation, diarrhea; vomiting (younger than age 1).

INTERACTIONS

Cefuroxime: May decrease cefuroxime absorption. Separate oral doses by at least 2 hours. Avoid combination.
Delavirdine: May decrease delavirdine serum concentration. Avoid long-term famotidine therapy in patients taking delavirdine.

Neratinib: May decrease neratinib absorption and serum concentration. Administer neratinib at least 2 hours before or 10 hours after famotidine. Avoid combination.
Risedronate: May increase risedronate serum concentration, specifically delayed-release risedronate. Avoid combination.

EFFECTS ON LAB TEST RESULTS

• May increase BUN, creatinine, and liver enzyme levels.

• May cause false-negative results in skin tests using allergen extracts. May antagonize pentagastrin in gastric acid secretion tests.

CONTRAINDICATIONS & CAUTIONS

• Contraindicated in patients hypersensitive to drug or its components.

• Drug may cause reversible confusional states that clear within 3 to 4 days after discontinuation. Patients older than age 50 and those with renal or hepatic impairment may be more at risk.

⚠ **Alert:** QT-interval prolongation and torsades de pointes have been reported rarely in patients with renal dysfunction.

• Treatment lasting 2 years can cause vitamin B_{12} deficiency, which is dose-related and more likely to occur in women and those younger than age 30.

⚠ **Alert:** Some forms may contain benzyl alcohol, which is linked to "gasping syndrome" (metabolic acidosis, respiratory distress, CNS dysfunction, hypotension, CV collapse) in neonates.
Dialyzable drug: No.

PREGNANCY-LACTATION-REPRODUCTION

• Drug crosses placental barrier and appears in human milk. Use cautiously in pregnant and breastfeeding women.

NURSING CONSIDERATIONS

• Assess patient for abdominal pain.
• Look for blood in emesis, stool, or gastric aspirate.
• Monitor patients with renal dysfunction for QT-interval prolongation.

PATIENT TEACHING

• Instruct patient in proper use of OTC product, if appropriate.

• Tell patient to take prescription drug with a snack, if desired.

• Advise patient to limit use of prescription drug to no longer than 8 weeks, unless ordered by prescriber, and OTC drug to no longer than 2 weeks.

• With prescriber's knowledge, let patient take antacids together, especially at beginning of therapy when pain is severe.

• Urge patient to avoid cigarette smoking because it may increase gastric acid secretion and worsen disease.

• Advise patient to report abdominal pain, blood in stools or vomit, black tarry stools, or coffee-ground emesis.

febuxostat
feb-UX-oh-stat

Uloric

Therapeutic class: Antigout drugs
Pharmacologic class: Xanthine oxidase inhibitors

AVAILABLE FORMS
Tablets: 40 mg, 80 mg

INDICATIONS & DOSAGES
Black Box Warning Only use drug in patients who have an inadequate response to a maximally titrated dose of allopurinol, who are intolerant to allopurinol, or for whom treatment with allopurinol isn't advisable. ∎

➤ **Chronic management of hyperuricemia associated with gout**
Adults: 40 mg PO daily. May increase dosage to 80 mg after 2 weeks if uric acid level remains above 6 mg/dL.
Adjust-a-dose: Maximum dose in patients with severe renal impairment (CrCl of less than 30 mL/minute) is 40 mg/day.

ADMINISTRATION
PO
• Give drug without regard to food or antacid use.

ACTION
Reduces uric acid production by inhibiting xanthine oxidase.

Route	Onset	Peak	Duration
PO	Rapid	1–1½ hr	Unknown

Half-life: 5 to 8 hours.

ADVERSE REACTIONS
CNS: dizziness. **GI:** nausea. **Hepatic:** liver function abnormalities. **Musculoskeletal:** arthralgia. **Skin:** rash.

INTERACTIONS
Drug-drug. *Azathioprine, didanosine, mercaptopurine:* May increase levels of these drugs, leading to toxicity. Use together is contraindicated.
Pegloticase: May increase toxic effects of pegloticase. Avoid use together.
Theophylline: May increase theophylline level. Use cautiously together.

EFFECTS ON LAB TEST RESULTS
• May increase alkaline phosphatase, AST, and ALT levels.

CONTRAINDICATIONS & CAUTIONS
• Contraindicated in patients hypersensitive to drug or its components and in those taking azathioprine, mercaptopurine, or didanosine.
Black Box Warning Drug may increase risk of CV death in patients with CV disease compared to those treated with allopurinol, based on a CV outcomes study. Consider the risks and benefits of drug when deciding to prescribe or continue patients on febuxostat. Consider use of prophylactic low-dose aspirin in patients with a history of CV disease. ∎

• Use cautiously in patients with severe hepatic impairment (Child-Pugh class C) or renal impairment (CrCl of less than 30 mL/minute).

• Not recommended for the treatment of asymptomatic hyperuricemia.

• Safety and effectiveness in children haven't been established.
Dialyzable drug: Unlikely.

PREGNANCY-LACTATION-REPRODUCTION
• It isn't known if drug crosses the placental barrier. Use during pregnancy only if potential benefit justifies potential risk to the fetus.

Reactions in bold italics are *life-threatening*. Interactions may have a *rapid onset* or a *delayed onset*.

• It isn't known if drug appears in human milk. Use cautiously in breastfeeding women.

NURSING CONSIDERATIONS

Black Box Warning Monitor all patients for signs and symptoms of CV events. ∎

• Acute gout flares may occur during first 6 weeks of therapy; colchicine or another anti-inflammatory may be added prophylactically and drug should be continued.

• Monitor hepatic function at baseline, 2 months and 4 months after starting therapy, and periodically thereafter.

❸ *Alert:* Patients with unexplained serum ALT level greater than 3 × ULN with total bilirubin level greater than 2 × ULN are at risk for severe drug-induced liver injury. Stop drug in these patients and don't restart.

• Monitor uric acid level.

• Patient taking drug may be at risk for thromboembolic events, such as MI and stroke. Monitor patient closely.

PATIENT TEACHING

Black Box Warning Advise patient of the risk of CV events. Teach patient to seek immediate emergency medical care for chest pain, shortness of breath, dizziness, fainting, light-headedness, fast or irregular heartbeat, numbness or weakness on one side of the body, slurred speech, blurred vision, or sudden severe headache. ∎

• Warn patient about the risk of gout flares and the importance of taking an NSAID or colchicine during the first 6 weeks of treatment.

• Inform patient that drug may increase risk of MI or stroke. Advise patient to report all adverse reactions, including abnormal bleeding, nausea, malaise, light-colored stools, yellowing of eyes or skin, rash, chest pain, dyspnea, or neurologic symptoms of a stroke.

• Instruct patient to report signs or symptoms of severe skin reactions immediately.

felodipine
fe-LOE-di-peen

Plendil✦

Therapeutic class: Antihypertensives
Pharmacologic class: Calcium channel blockers

AVAILABLE FORMS

Tablets (extended-release) ⓞⓝⓒ: 2.5 mg, 5 mg, 10 mg

INDICATIONS & DOSAGES

➤ **HTN**

Adults: Initially, 2.5 to 5 mg PO daily. Adjust dosage based on patient response, usually at intervals of not less than 2 weeks. Usual dosage is 2.5 to 10 mg daily; maximum dosage is 10 mg daily.

Elderly patients: 2.5 mg PO daily; adjust dosage as for adults. Maximum dosage is 10 mg daily.

Adjust-a-dose: Patients with impaired hepatic function may respond to lower doses. Monitor BP during dosage adjustments.

ADMINISTRATION

PO

• Give drug whole; don't crush or cut tablets.

• Give drug without food or with a light meal low in fat and carbohydrates.

• Don't give drug with grapefruit juice.

• Store below 86° F (30° C). Protect from light.

ACTION

A dihydropyridine-derivative calcium channel blocker that prevents entry of calcium ions into vascular smooth muscle and cardiac cells; shows some selectivity for smooth muscle compared with cardiac muscle.

Route	Onset	Peak	Duration
PO	2–5 hr	2½–5 hr	24 hr

Half-life: 11 to 16 hours.

ADVERSE REACTIONS

CNS: headache, dizziness, paresthesia, asthenia. **CV:** peripheral edema, chest pain, palpitations, flushing. **EENT:** rhinorrhea, pharyngitis. **GI:** abdominal pain, nausea, constipation, diarrhea, dyspepsia. **Musculoskeletal:** muscle cramps, back pain. **Respiratory:** URI, cough, sneezing. **Skin:** rash.

INTERACTIONS
Drug-drug. *Anticonvulsants (long term):* May decrease felodipine level. Avoid using together.
Antipsychotics (atypical second-generation): May enhance hypotensive effects. Monitor therapy.
CYP3A4 inhibitors (azole antifungals, cimetidine, erythromycin): May decrease clearance of felodipine. Reduce doses of felodipine; monitor patient for toxicity.
Metoprolol: May alter pharmacokinetics of metoprolol. Monitor patient for adverse reactions.
Tacrolimus: May increase tacrolimus level. Monitor patient closely.
Drug-herb. *Herbs with hypertensive or hypotensive properties:* May increase or decrease antihypertensive effects. Discourage use together.
Drug-food. *Grapefruit:* May increase drug level and adverse effects. Discourage use together.

EFFECTS ON LAB TEST RESULTS
None reported.

CONTRAINDICATIONS & CAUTIONS
• Contraindicated in patients hypersensitive to drug.
• Drug may cause significant hypotension and rarely syncope.
• Safe use in patients with HF hasn't been established.
• Use cautiously and in lower doses in elderly patients and in those with hepatic impairment.
Dialyzable drug: Unlikely.
⚠ **Overdose S&S:** Peripheral vasodilation, hypotension, bradycardia.

PREGNANCY-LACTATION-REPRODUCTION
• There are no well-controlled studies in pregnant women, but animal studies show potential fetal hazards. If treatment for HTN during pregnancy is needed, other agents are preferred.

• It isn't known if drug appears in human milk. Patient should discontinue breastfeeding or discontinue drug.

NURSING CONSIDERATIONS
• Monitor BP and HR for response.
• Monitor patient for peripheral edema, which appears to be both dose- and age-related. It's more common in patients taking higher doses, especially those older than age 60.

PATIENT TEACHING
• Tell patient to swallow tablets whole and not to crush or chew them.
• Tell patient to take drug without food or with a light meal.
• Advise patient not to take drug with grapefruit juice.
• Advise patient to continue taking drug even when feeling better, to watch diet, and to check with prescriber or pharmacist before taking other drugs, including OTC drugs, nutritional supplements, or herbal remedies.
• Teach patient to report all adverse reactions.
• Advise patient to observe good oral hygiene and to see a dentist regularly; use of drug may cause mild gum problems.

fenofibrate
fee-no-FYE-brate

Antara, Fenoglide, Lipofen, TriCor♥, Triglide

fenofibrate (choline)
Trilipix

fenofibric acid
Fibricor

Therapeutic class: Antilipemics
Pharmacologic class: Fibric acid derivatives

AVAILABLE FORMS
fenofibrate
Capsules ⓞⓝⓒ: 50 mg, 150 mg
Capsules (micronized) ⓞⓝⓒ: 30 mg, 43 mg, 67 mg, 90 mg, 130 mg, 134 mg, 200 mg
Tablets ⓞⓝⓒ: 40 mg, 48 mg, 54 mg, 107 mg, 120 mg, 145 mg, 160 mg

---

fenofibrate (choline)
Capsules (delayed-release) ⓓⓝⓒ*:* 45 mg,
135 mg
fenofibric acid
Tablets: 35 mg, 105 mg

INDICATIONS & DOSAGES

Adjust-a-dose (for all indications): Refer to
specific product information for guidelines
regarding dosing for patients with renal impairment.

➤ **Hypertriglyceridemia (Fredrickson
types IV and V hyperlipidemia) in patients who don't respond adequately to
diet alone**
Adults: For Antara, initial dose is 30 to
90 mg PO daily, with maximum dose of
90 mg daily. For Fibricor, initial dose is
35 to 105 mg daily, with maximum dose of
105 mg daily. For fenofibrate (micronized),
initial dose is 43 to 130 mg once daily,
with maximum dose of 130 mg daily. For
Fenoglide, initial dose is 40 to 120 mg/day,
with maximum dose of 120 mg daily. For
Lipofen, initial dose is 50 to 150 mg daily,
with maximum dose of 150 mg daily. For
TriCor, initial dose is 48 to 145 mg daily,
with maximum dose of 145 mg daily. For
Triglide, initial dose is 160 mg daily, with
maximum dose of 160 mg daily. For Trilipix,
initial dose is 45 to 135 mg once daily, with
maximum dose of 135 mg once daily. For all
forms, adjust dose based on patient response
and repeat lipid determinations every 4 to
8 weeks.

➤ **Primary hypercholesterolemia or
mixed dyslipidemia (Fredrickson types
IIa and IIb) in patients who don't respond
adequately to diet alone**
Adults: For Antara, initial dose is 90 mg
PO daily. For Fenoglide, initial dose is
120 mg/day. For fenofibrate (micronized),
initial dose is 130 mg once daily. For Fib-
ricor, the dose is 105 mg PO daily. For
Lipofen, initial dose is 150 mg daily.
For TriCor, initial dose is 145 mg daily.
For Triglide, initial dose is 160 mg daily. For
Trilipix, initial dose is 135 mg once daily.
May reduce dose if lipid levels fall signifi-
cantly below the target range.

ADMINISTRATION
PO
- Administer Fenoglide and Lipofen with
meals.
- Administer Antara, Tricor, Triglide, and
Trilipix with or without food.
- Ensure patient swallows capsules and
tablets whole. Don't open capsules or crush,
dissolve, or allow patient to chew capsules
or tablets.
- Protect Fibricor, Lipofen, and Triglide
from light.

ACTION
May lower triglyceride levels by inhibiting
triglyceride synthesis with less VLDL released into circulation. Drug may also stimulate breakdown of triglyceride-rich protein.

Route	Onset	Peak	Duration
PO	Unknown	2–8 hr	Unknown

Half-life: 20 hours.

ADVERSE REACTIONS
CNS: dizziness, headache, localized pain.
CV: *PE,* thrombophlebitis. **EENT:** rhinitis, sinusitis, nasopharyngitis. **GI:** abdominal pain, constipation, diarrhea, dyspepsia.
Hepatic: elevated AST and ALT levels.
Musculoskeletal: arthralgia, back pain,
myalgia. **Respiratory:** URI. **Skin:** pruritus,
rash.

INTERACTIONS
Drug-drug. *Bile acid sequestrants:* May
bind and inhibit absorption of fenofibrate.
Separate doses by at least 2 hours; for
fenofibric acid, give drug 1 hour before or
4 to 6 hours after bile acid sequestrants.
Coumarin-type anticoagulants: May potentiate anticoagulant effect, prolonging PT and
INR. Monitor PT and INR closely. May need
to reduce anticoagulant dosage.
*Cyclosporine, immunosuppressants, nephro-
toxic drugs:* May induce renal dysfunction
that may affect fenofibrate elimination. Use
together cautiously.
HMG-CoA reductase inhibitors: May increase risk of adverse musculoskeletal effects. Avoid using together, unless potential
benefit outweighs risk.
Drug-food. *Any food:* May increase capsule
absorption. Advise patient to take capsule

with meals. Refer to specific product for more information.

Drug-lifestyle. *Alcohol use:* May increase triglyceride levels. Discourage use together.

EFFECTS ON LAB TEST RESULTS
• May increase ALT, AST, BUN, CK, and creatinine levels. May decrease uric acid and Hb levels and hematocrit.
• May decrease WBC count.

CONTRAINDICATIONS & CAUTIONS
• Contraindicated in patients hypersensitive to drug and in those with gallbladder disease, hepatic dysfunction, primary biliary cirrhosis, severe renal dysfunction or ESRD (including those receiving hemodialysis), or unexplained persistent liver function abnormalities.
• Some formulations may contain peanut oil or soya lecithin and are contraindicated in patients with these allergies. Refer to individual products.
• Use cautiously in patients with a history of pancreatitis.
• Anaphylaxis and angioedema have been reported with fenofibrate. In some cases, reactions were life-threatening and required emergency treatment.
• Select Trilipix dosage cautiously for elderly patients and those with renal impairment because of the increased risk of adverse reactions.

Dialyzable drug: No.

PREGNANCY-LACTATION-REPRODUCTION
• Safe use in pregnant women hasn't been established for all products. Refer to individual manufacturer's instructions for use during pregnancy.
• Contraindicated in breastfeeding women.

NURSING CONSIDERATIONS
• Obtain baseline lipid levels and LFT results before therapy, and monitor liver function periodically during therapy. Stop drug if enzyme levels persist above 3 × ULN.
• **Alert:** Watch for signs and symptoms of pancreatitis, myositis, rhabdomyolysis, hepatic impairment, cholelithiasis, and renal failure. Monitor patient for muscle pain, tenderness, or weakness, especially with malaise or fever.

• Severe cutaneous adverse reactions, including SJS, toxic epidermal necrolysis, and DRESS syndrome, have been reported, occurring days to weeks after drug initiation. Discontinue drug and treat appropriately.
• If an adequate response isn't obtained after 2 to 3 months of treatment with maximum daily dose, stop therapy.
• Drug lowers uric acid level by increasing uric acid excretion in patients with or without hyperuricemia.
• Beta blockers, estrogens, and thiazide diuretics may increase triglyceride levels; evaluate need for continued use of these drugs.
• Hb level, hematocrit, and WBC count may decrease when therapy starts but will stabilize with long-term administration.
• Discontinue if gallstones are found upon gallbladder studies.
• Discontinue if patient develops markedly elevated CK concentration or if myopathy/myositis is suspected or diagnosed.
• Permanently discontinue if high-density lipoprotein cholesterol (HDL-C) becomes severely depressed; monitor HDL-C level.

PATIENT TEACHING
• Inform patient that drug therapy doesn't reduce need for following a triglyceride-lowering diet.
• Advise patient to promptly report all adverse reactions, especially unexplained muscle weakness, pain, or tenderness, abdominal pain, and yellowing of skin or eyes, particularly with malaise or fever.
• Advise patient to immediately report development of skin reactions, such as a rash or exfoliative dermatitis.
• Teach patient which capsules should be taken with meals for best absorption.
• Advise patient to swallow capsules and tablets whole and not to open capsules or crush, dissolve, or chew capsules or tablets.
• Advise patient to continue weight control measures, including diet and exercise, and to limit alcohol before therapy.
• Instruct patient who is also taking a bile acid sequestrant to take fenofibrate 1 hour before or 4 to 6 hours after the bile acid sequestrant.

Reactions in bold italics are *life-threatening*. Interactions may have a *rapid onset* or a *delayed onset*.

SAFETY ALERT!

fentaNYL citrate
FEN-ta-nil

Sublimaze

fentaNYL nasal spray
Lazanda

fentaNYL sublingual spray
SUBSYS

fentaNYL transdermal system
Duragesic-12, Duragesic-25,
Duragesic-50, Duragesic-75,
Duragesic-100

fentaNYL transmucosal
Abstral, Actiq, Fentora

Therapeutic class: Opioid analgesics
Pharmacologic class: Opioid agonists
Controlled substance schedule: II

AVAILABLE FORMS
Injection: 50 mcg/mL
Nasal spray: 100 mcg, 300 mcg, 400 mcg
Transdermal system: Patches that release
12.5 mcg, 25 mcg, 37.5 mcg, 50 mcg,
62.5 mcg, 75 mcg, 87.5 mcg, or 100 mcg of
drug per hour
Transmucosal (buccal tablet): 100 mcg,
200 mcg, 400 mcg, 600 mcg, 800 mcg
Transmucosal (lozenge): 200 mcg, 400 mcg,
600 mcg, 800 mcg, 1,200 mcg, 1,600 mcg
Transmucosal (sublingual spray): 100 mcg,
200 mcg, 400 mcg, 600 mcg, 800 mcg,
1,200 mcg, 1,600 mcg
Transmucosal (sublingual tablet): 100 mcg,
200 mcg, 300 mcg, 400 mcg, 600 mcg,
800 mcg

INDICATIONS & DOSAGES
➤ **Adjunct to general anesthetic**
Adults: For low-dose therapy, 1 to 2 mcg/kg
IV. For moderate-dose therapy, 2 to 20 mcg/
kg IV; then 25 to 100 mcg IV or IM p.r.n. For
high-dose therapy, 20 to 50 mcg/kg IV; then
25 mcg to one-half initial loading dose IV
p.r.n.

➤ **Adjunct to regional anesthesia**
Adults: 50 to 100 mcg IM or slowly IV over
1 to 2 minutes p.r.n.
➤ **To induce and maintain anesthesia**
Children ages 2 and older: 2 to 3 mcg/kg IV
every 1 to 2 hours as needed.
➤ **Postoperative pain, restlessness,
tachypnea, and emergence delirium**
Adults: 50 to 100 mcg IM or IV every 1 to
2 hours p.r.n.
➤ **Preoperative medication**
Adults: 50 to 100 mcg IM 30 to 60 minutes
before surgery.
➤ **To manage persistent, moderate to
severe chronic pain in opioid-tolerant
patients who require around-the-clock
opioid analgesics for an extended time**
Adults and children age 2 and older: When
converting to transdermal system, base the
first dose on the daily dose, potency, and
characteristics of the current opioid therapy; the reliability of the relative potency
estimates used to calculate the needed dose;
the degree of opioid tolerance; and patient's
condition. Each patch may be worn for
72 hours, although some adult patients may
need a patch to be applied every 48 hours
during the first dosage period. May increase
dose 3 days after the first dose, then every
6 days thereafter.
Adjust-a-dose: For elderly, cachectic, or debilitated patients, start transdermal system
doses at no higher than 25 mcg/hr unless
these patients are already tolerating around-
the-clock opioid at a dose and potency comparable to fentanyl 25 mcg/hr transdermal
system.
➤ **To manage breakthrough cancer pain
in patients already receiving and tolerating an opioid**
Adults: 200 mcg Actiq initially; may give
second dose 15 minutes after completing the
first (30 minutes after first lozenge is placed
in mouth). Maximum dose is 2 lozenges per
breakthrough episode. If several episodes of
breakthrough pain requiring 2 lozenges occur, dose may be increased to the next available strength. After a successful dosage has
been reached, patient should limit use to no
more than 4 lozenges daily.

Or, initially 100 mcg buccal tablet between the upper cheek and gum. May repeat
same dose once per breakthrough episode

F

after at least 30 minutes. Adjust in 100-mcg increments. Doses above 400 mcg can be increased by 200 mcg. Generally, dosage should be increased when patient requires more than one dose per breakthrough episode. Once a successful maintenance dose has been established, reevaluate if patient experiences more than four breakthrough episodes per day.

Or, initially 100 mcg sublingual tablet. If adequate analgesia is obtained within 30 minutes, continue to treat subsequent episodes with this dose. If adequate analgesia isn't obtained, may give a second sublingual tablet after 30 minutes. Use no more than two doses per episode of breakthrough pain; it's essential to wait at least 2 hours before treating another episode. Dosage escalation may be performed in a stepwise manner over consecutive breakthrough episodes until adequate analgesia with tolerable adverse effects is achieved. Limit drug consumption to treat four or fewer breakthrough pain episodes per day once a successful dose is found.

Or, initially 100 mcg nasal spray. Titrate as needed to an effective dosage (from 100 to 200, to 300, to 400, to 600 mcg, up to maximum of 800 mcg) that gives adequate analgesia with tolerable adverse effects. Dose is a single spray into one nostril or single spray into each nostril per episode. Don't give more than four doses per 24 hours. Wait at least 2 hours before treating another episode. During an episode, if analgesia isn't achieved within 30 minutes, patient may use a rescue medication as directed by the health care provider.

Or, initially 100 mcg sublingual spray. If pain isn't relieved after 30 minutes during each breakthrough pain episode treated, one additional dose of the same strength may be given for that episode. May use a maximum of two doses for any breakthrough pain episode, and 4 hours must elapse before treating another episode of breakthrough pain with a higher dose. Titrate dosage level as needed to an effective dosage (from 100 to 200, to 400, to 600, to 800, to 1,200, to 1,600 mcg) that gives adequate analgesia with tolerable adverse effects using a single dose per breakthrough cancer pain episode. When drug has been titrated to an effective

dosage, patients should generally use only one dose of the appropriate strength per breakthrough pain episode.

➤ **Switching from Actiq to Fentora to manage breakthrough cancer pain in opioid-tolerant patients**
Adults: If current Actiq dose is 200 to 400 mcg, start with 100 mcg Fentora; if current Actiq dose is 600 to 800 mcg, use 200 mcg Fentora; if current Actiq dose is 1,200 to 1,600 mcg, use 400 mcg Fentora. Actiq and Fentora aren't bioequivalent.
Adjust-a-dose: For patients with renal or hepatic impairment, use lowest possible dose.

ADMINISTRATION
IV
▼ Only those trained to give IV anesthetics and manage adverse effects should give this form.
▼ Keep opioid antagonist (naloxone) and resuscitation equipment available.
▼ IV form often used with droperidol to produce neuroleptanalgesia.
▼ Inject slowly over 1 to 2 minutes.
▼ **Incompatibilities:** Azithromycin, dantrolene, gemtuzumab ozogamicin, pantoprazole, phenytoin, sulfamethoxazole–trimethoprim. Compatibility of many other drugs is undetermined.
IM
• Document administration site.
Intranasal
• Prime the device by spraying into the pouch (4 sprays in total).
• Insert the nozzle about ½ inch (1.25 cm) into the nose and point toward the bridge of the nose, tilting the bottle slightly.
• Press down firmly until a click is heard and the number in the counting window advances by one.
Transdermal
• Dosage equivalent charts are available to calculate the fentanyl transdermal dose based on the daily morphine intake; for example, for every 90 mg of oral morphine or 15 mg of IM morphine per 24 hours, 25 mcg/hour of transdermal fentanyl is needed.
• Clip hair at application site but don't use a razor, which may irritate skin. Wash area with clear water, if needed, but not with

soaps, oils, lotions, alcohol, or other substances that may irritate skin or prevent adhesion. Dry area completely before application.

• Remove transdermal system from package just before applying, hold in place for 30 seconds, and be sure edges of patch stick to skin.

• Don't cut or otherwise alter transdermal patch before applying.

• Place transdermal patch on the upper back for a child or patient who's cognitively impaired to reduce the chance the patch will be removed and placed in the mouth.

Black Box Warning Heat from fever or heating pads, electric blankets, heat lamps, hot tubs, or water beds may increase transdermal delivery and cause toxicity. ∎

• Always wear gloves when handling transdermal system.

• Make sure patient knows to avoid exposing device to electronic security systems.

Route	Onset	Peak	Duration
IV	1–2 min	3–5 min	30–60 min
IM	7–15 min	20–30 min	1–2 hr
Intranasal	15–21 min	25–35 min	Unknown
Transdermal	12–24 hr	1–3 days	Variable
Transmucosal	5–15 min	20–30 min	Unknown

Half-life: Parenteral, 3½ hours; intranasal, 15 to 24.9 hours; transmucosal, 5 to 15 hours; transdermal, 18 hours.

ADVERSE REACTIONS

CNS: asthenia, clouded sensorium, confusion, euphoria, sedation, somnolence, *seizures,* anxiety, depression, dizziness, hallucinations, headache, nervousness. **CV:** *arrhythmias,* chest pain, HTN, hypotension, *DVT, PE.* **EENT:** pharyngitis, dry eyes, swelling, strabismus, ptosis, epistaxis, nasal discomfort, rhinorrhea, nasal congestion, postnasal drip, rhinitis (intranasal). **GI:** constipation, abdominal pain, anorexia, diarrhea, dyspepsia, dry mouth, ileus, nausea, vomiting. **GU:** urine retention. **Musculoskeletal:** skeletal muscle rigidity (dose-related). **Respiratory:** *apnea, hypoventilation, respiratory depression,* dyspnea, cough, URI, bronchitis. **Skin:** diaphoresis, pruritus, erythema at application site (transdermal). **Other:** physical dependence.

INTERACTIONS

Drug-drug. *Amiodarone:* May cause hypotension, bradycardia, and decreased cardiac output. Monitor patient closely.

Black Box Warning *Benzodiazepines, CNS depressants:* May cause slow or difficult breathing, sedation, and death. Avoid use together. If use together is necessary, limit dosage and duration of each drug to the minimum necessary for desired effect. ∎

Black Box Warning *CYP3A4 inducers (carbamazepine, phenytoin, rifampin):* May decrease fentanyl level and result in decreased efficacy or precipitate a withdrawal syndrome in patients with a physical dependence on fentanyl. If CYP3A4 inducer is discontinued, fentanyl level may increase and cause fentanyl-related adverse reactions. Taper CYP3A4 inducers cautiously and adjust fentanyl dosage as needed. ∎

Black Box Warning *CYP3A4 inhibitors (erythromycin, ketoconazole, ritonavir):* May increase fentanyl level and increase risk of potentially fatal respiratory depression. Use together cautiously and monitor patient closely. ∎

Diazepam: May cause CV depression when given with high doses of fentanyl. Monitor patient closely.

Droperidol: May cause hypotension and decrease pulmonary arterial pressure. Use together cautiously.

General anesthetics, hypnotics, other opioid analgesics, sedatives, TCAs: May cause additive effects. Use together cautiously. Consider dosage reduction of one or both drugs if adverse effects occur.

Protease inhibitors: May increase fentanyl levels and adverse effects. Monitor patient closely for respiratory depression.

🌓 *Alert:* Serotonergic drugs (antiemetics [dolasetron, granisetron, ondansetron, palonosetron], amoxapine, antimigraine drugs, buspirone, cyclobenzaprine, dextromethorphan, linezolid, lithium, MAO inhibitors, maprotiline, methylene blue, mirtazapine, nefazodone, SSNRIs, SSRIs, TCAs, trazodone, tryptophan, vilazodone): May increase risk of serotonin syndrome. Use together cautiously; monitor for serotonin syndrome. Don't use fentanyl while patient is taking an MAO inhibitor or within 14 days of stopping one.

Drug-herb. ◑ Alert: *St. John's wort:* May increase risk of serotonin syndrome. Use together cautiously; monitor for serotonin syndrome.

Drug-lifestyle. *Alcohol use:* May cause additive effects. Discourage use together.

EFFECTS ON LAB TEST RESULTS
• May increase amylase and lipase levels.

CONTRAINDICATIONS & CAUTIONS
• Contraindicated in patients intolerant to drug.

`Black Box Warning` Opioids should only be prescribed with benzodiazepines or other CNS depressants to patients for whom alternative treatment options are inadequate. ▪

`Black Box Warning` Transdermal form contraindicated in patients hypersensitive to adhesives, those who are opioid-naive, those who need postoperative pain management, and those with acute, mild, or intermittent pain that can be managed with nonopioids. Don't use in patients with increased intracranial pressure, head injury, impaired consciousness, or coma. ▪

`Black Box Warning` Transmucosal forms contraindicated in those who need acute or postoperative pain management. ▪

`Black Box Warning` Nasal spray is contraindicated in opioid-nontolerant patients and in those who need acute or postoperative pain management. ▪

`Black Box Warning` Drug may increase risks of opioid addiction, abuse, and misuse, which can lead to overdose and death. Risks increase in patients with a personal or family history of substance abuse or mental illness. Assess risks before drug is prescribed. ▪

• Transdermal form is contraindicated in patients with acute or severe bronchial asthma, known or suspected paralytic ileus, and GI obstruction.

`Black Box Warning` Refer to manufacturer's instructions for REMS requirements. ▪

◑ **Alert:** Drug may lead to rare but serious decrease in adrenal gland cortisol production.

◑ **Alert:** Drug may cause decreased sex hormone levels with long-term use.

• Fentora contraindicated in patients with mucositis more severe than grade 1.

• Use with caution in patients with brain tumors, COPD, decreased respiratory reserve, potentially compromised respirations, hepatic or renal disease, or cardiac bradyarrhythmias.

• Use with caution in elderly or debilitated patients.

Dialyzable drug: Unknown.

⚠ **Overdose S&S:** CNS depression, respiratory depression, apnea, flaccid skeletal muscles, bradycardia, hypotension, circulatory collapse.

PREGNANCY-LACTATION-REPRODUCTION
• There are no well-controlled studies in pregnant women. Use during pregnancy only if potential benefit justifies potential risk to the fetus.

`Black Box Warning` Prolonged maternal use of opioids during pregnancy can cause neonatal withdrawal syndrome, which may be life-threatening and requires management by neonatology experts. Advise patient of the risk of neonatal withdrawal syndrome. ▪

• Drug appears in human milk. Refer to individual manufacturer's instructions for use in breastfeeding women.

NURSING CONSIDERATIONS
`Black Box Warning` Respiratory depression or death can occur even when transdermal drug has been used as recommended and has not been misused or abused. Drug should only be prescribed by health care providers knowledgeable in the use of potent opioids for management of long-term pain. Drug is contraindicated for use in conditions in which the risk of life-threatening respiratory depression is significantly increased. Transdermal patch is for hospital use only. ▪

`Black Box Warning` Regularly monitor patients for development of opioid addiction, abuse, and misuse. ▪

`Black Box Warning` Serious, life-threatening or fatal respiratory depression can occur. Monitor patient closely, especially within first 24 to 72 hours of drug initiation and after dosage increase. ▪

◑ **Alert:** If patient is taking opioids with serotonergic drugs, monitor for signs and symptoms of serotonin syndrome (agitation, hallucinations, rapid HR, fever, excessive sweating, shivering or shaking, muscle twitching or stiffness, trouble with coordination, nausea, vomiting, diarrhea), especially when starting treatment or increasing dosage. Symptoms may occur within several hours of coadministration but may also occur later, especially after dosage increase. Discontinue the opioid, serotonergic drug, or both if serotonin syndrome is suspected.

🟡 *Alert:* Monitor patient for signs and symptoms of adrenal insufficiency (nausea, vomiting, loss of appetite, fatigue, weakness, dizziness, low BP). Perform diagnostic testing if adrenal insufficiency is suspected. If adrenal insufficiency is confirmed, treat with corticosteroids and wean patient off opioids if appropriate. Discontinue corticosteroids when clinically appropriate.

🟡 *Alert:* Monitor patient for signs and symptoms of decreased sex hormone levels (low libido, erectile dysfunction, amenorrhea, infertility). If signs and symptoms occur, evaluate patient and obtain laboratory testing.

• For better analgesic effect, give drug before patient has intense pain.

🟡 *Alert:* High doses can produce muscle rigidity, which can be reversed with neuromuscular blockers; however, patient must be artificially ventilated.

🟡 *Alert:* Avoid use in patients at risk for increased ICP.

• Monitor circulatory and respiratory status and urinary function carefully. Drug may cause respiratory depression, hypotension, urine retention, nausea, vomiting, ileus, or altered level of consciousness, no matter how it's given.

• Periodically monitor postoperative vital signs and bladder function. Because drug decreases both rate and depth of respirations, monitoring of arterial oxygen saturation (SaO_2) may help assess respiratory depression. Immediately report respiratory rate below 12 breaths/minute, decreased respiratory volume, or decreased SaO_2.

• Drug may cause constipation. Assess bowel function and need for stool softeners and stimulant laxatives.

Black Box Warning Fentanyl is an opioid agonist and schedule II controlled substance with potential for abuse. Be alert for signs of misuse, abuse, or diversion. ∎

Transdermal form

Black Box Warning Transdermal drug levels peak between 24 and 72 hours after initial application and dose increases. Monitor patients for life-threatening hypoventilation, especially during these times. ∎

• Fentanyl patches should be used only in patients age 2 or older who are opioid tolerant, who have chronic moderate to severe pain poorly controlled by other drugs, and who need a total daily opioid dose at least equivalent to the 25-mcg/hour fentanyl patch.

• When converting patient from another opioid, determine the initial fentanyl dosage with great care; overestimating the dosage could be dangerous or fatal.

• Identify all daily drugs, particularly CYP3A4 inhibitors, which may increase fentanyl levels.

• Monitor patients closely, and provide immediate care for evidence of overdose, such as slow or shallow breathing, a slow heartbeat, severe sleepiness, cold and clammy skin, trouble walking and talking, and feeling faint, dizzy, or confused.

• Give patients detailed instructions for using fentanyl patches correctly and safely.

• Make dosage adjustments gradually in patient using the transdermal system. Reaching steady-state level of a new dosage may take up to 6 days; delay dosage adjustment until after at least two applications.

• Monitor patient who develops adverse reactions to the transdermal system for at least 12 hours after removal. Drug level drops gradually; it may take as long as 17 hours to decline by 50%.

• Most patients experience good control of pain for 3 days while wearing the transdermal system, but a few may need a new application after 48 hours.

• Because the drug level rises for the first 24 hours after application, analgesic effect can't be evaluated on the first day. Make sure patient has adequate supplemental analgesic to prevent breakthrough pain.

• When reducing opioid therapy or switching to a different analgesic, withdraw the transdermal system gradually. Because the drug level drops gradually after removal, give half the equianalgesic dose of the new analgesic 12 to 18 hours after removal.

☼ Alert: Transdermal patches must be stored, used, and disposed of properly to prevent poisonings or other harm, especially to children and pets. A patch that has been worn for 3 days may still contain enough fentanyl to cause harm, or even kill a child or pet. Patches should only be handled by patient or patient's caregivers.

Intranasal and transmucosal forms

`Black Box Warning` Intranasal and transmucosal forms are used only to manage breakthrough cancer pain in patients who are already receiving and tolerating opioids. ∎

`Black Box Warning` Intranasal and transmucosal forms aren't bioequivalent and can't be substituted on a microgram-per-microgram basis. ∎

• **Look alike–sound alike:** Don't confuse fentanyl with alfentanil.

PATIENT TEACHING

`Black Box Warning` Caution patient or caregiver of patient taking an opioid with a benzodiazepine, CNS depressant, or alcohol to seek immediate medical attention for dizziness, light-headedness, extreme sleepiness, slowed or difficult breathing, or unresponsiveness. ∎

`Black Box Warning` Advise patient that drug increases risk of opioid addiction, abuse, and misuse, which can lead to overdose and death. Teach patient proper use of drug. ∎

• When drug is used for pain control, instruct patient to request drug before pain becomes intense.

• **☼ Alert:** Encourage patient to report all medications being taken, including prescription and OTC medications and supplements.

• **☼ Alert:** Caution patient to immediately report signs and symptoms of serotonin syndrome, adrenal insufficiency, and decreased sex hormone levels to health care provider.

• When drug is used after surgery, encourage patient to turn, cough, and breathe deeply to prevent lung problems.

• Instruct patient to avoid hazardous activities until CNS effects subside.

• Tell home care patient to avoid drinking alcohol or taking other CNS-type drugs, unless specifically prescribed by practitioner, because additive effects can occur.

• Advise patient not to stop drug abruptly.

• Teach patient about proper application of transdermal patch. Tell patient to clip hair at application site but not to use a razor, which may irritate skin. Wash area with clear water, if needed, but not with soaps, oils, lotions, alcohol, or other substances that may irritate skin or prevent adhesion. Dry area completely before application.

• Tell patient to remove transdermal system from package just before applying, hold in place for 30 seconds, and be sure the edges of patch stick to skin.

• **☼ Alert:** Teach patient not to alter the transdermal patch (such as by cutting it) before applying.

• Advise parent or caregiver to place transdermal patch on the upper back for child or patient who's cognitively impaired, to reduce chance the patch will be removed and placed in the mouth.

• Teach patient to dispose of the transdermal patch by folding it so the adhesive side adheres to itself and then flushing it down the toilet.

• Tell patient that, if another patch is needed after 48 to 72 hours, to apply it to a different skin site.

• Tell patient that pain relief with the patch may not occur for several hours after the patch is applied. Oral, immediate-release opioids may be needed for initial pain relief.

`Black Box Warning` Inform patient that heat from fever or environment, such as from heating pads, electric blankets, heat lamps, hot tubs, or water beds, may increase transdermal delivery and cause toxicity requiring dosage adjustment. Instruct patient to notify prescriber if fever occurs or if patient will be spending time in a hot climate. ∎

• **☼ Alert:** Instruct patient that if an MRI is required, to inform the facility that patient is wearing a transdermal patch.

• Teach patient proper administration of transmucosal forms.

• Advise patient that transmucosal lozenge contains 2 g sugar per unit.

• Teach patient proper administration of the nasal spray, and explain that a fine mist isn't always felt and to rely on the audible click and advancement of the dose counter.

`Black Box Warning` Warn patient and patient's family that the amount of drug in transmucosal and intranasal forms can

---

Reactions in bold italics are **life-threatening**. Interactions may have a *rapid onset* or a **delayed onset**.

be fatal to a child. Advise patient to keep medicine well secured and out of children's reach. ∎

ferric carboxymaltose
FER-ik car-box-ee-MAL-tose

Injectafer

Therapeutic class: Iron supplements
Pharmacologic class: Hematinics

AVAILABLE FORMS
Injection: 750 mg of elemental iron in 15-mL single-dose vial

INDICATIONS & DOSAGES
➤ **Iron deficiency anemia in patients intolerant to or who have had unsatisfactory response to oral iron and in those with non-dialysis-dependent chronic kidney disease**
Adults: For patients weighing at least 50 kg, 750 mg IV on day 1; repeat dose after at least 7 days. May repeat course of therapy if anemia recurs. For patients weighing less than 50 kg, give 15 mg/kg body weight on day 1; repeat dose after at least 7 days. May repeat course of therapy if anemia recurs. Maximum cumulative dose is 1,500 mg per treatment course.

ADMINISTRATION
IV
▼ Inspect vial for particulate matter and discoloration before administration.
▼ Give either as an undiluted slow IV push (at 100 mg [2 mL]/minute) or as an infusion. To administer by infusion, dilute up to 750 mg iron in maximum of 250 mL sterile NSS injection. Infusion concentration must be not less than 2 mg iron/mL.
▼ Give infusion over at least 15 minutes.
▼ Infusion is stable for 72 hours at room temperature at 2- to 4-mg/mL concentrations.
▼ Store vials at 68° to 77° F (20° to 25° C), with excursions permitted to 59° to 86° F (15° to 30° C). Don't freeze vials.
▼ Vials are single-use and have no preservative. Discard any excess drug remaining in vial.

▼ **Incompatibilities:** None listed by manufacturer. Consult a drug incompatibility reference for more information.

ACTION
Colloidal iron (III) hydroxide acts in complex with carboxymaltose, a carbohydrate polymer that releases iron, an essential component in the formulation of Hb.

Route	Onset	Peak	Duration
IV	Unknown	15 min–1.21 hr	Unknown

Half-life: 7 to 12 hours.

ADVERSE REACTIONS
CNS: dizziness, headache, pyrexia, chills, syncope. **CV:** HTN, hypotension, flushing, tachycardia, chest discomfort. **GI:** nausea, vomiting, constipation, dysgeusia. **Skin:** injection-site discoloration, urticaria, pruritus, erythema.

INTERACTIONS
Drug-drug. *Baloxavir marboxil:* May decrease baloxavir marboxil serum concentration. Avoid combination.
Dimercaprol: May enhance nephrotoxic effect of iron salts. Avoid combination.

EFFECTS ON LAB TEST RESULTS
• May increase ALT and GGT levels.
• May decrease phosphorus level.
• May falsely elevate serum iron and transferrin-bound iron levels in the 24 hours after administration.

CONTRAINDICATIONS & CAUTIONS
• Contraindicated in patients hypersensitive to drug or its components, in patients with evidence of iron overload, and in those with anemia not caused by iron deficiency.
• Serious hypersensitivity reactions, including anaphylaxis, have been reported.
• Safety and effectiveness in children haven't been established.
Dialyzable drug: No.
⚠ *Overdose S&S:* Hemosiderosis, hypophosphatemic osteomalacia.

PREGNANCY-LACTATION-REPRODUCTION
• Use during pregnancy only if potential benefit justifies potential risk to the fetus.
• Drug appears in human milk.

✚Canada ◇OTC ◆Off-label use ✐Photoguide ⦿Do not crush *Liquid contains alcohol ⧰Genetic

NURSING CONSIDERATIONS
• Before administering, assess patient for prior history of reactions to parenteral iron products.
• Monitor patient for extravasation during administration. Extravasation may cause persistent discoloration. If extravasation occurs, discontinue infusion at that site.
• Monitor vital signs before and after each dose. Monitor patient for HTN after each dose.
• Monitor patient for hypersensitivity reactions during infusion and for at least 30 minutes after infusion or until patient is clinically stable. Only administer drug when personnel and therapies are immediately available for treatment of serious hypersensitivity reactions.
• Monitor iron status (Hb level and hematocrit, serum ferritin level, iron saturation) frequently during therapy.

PATIENT TEACHING
• Advise patient to report signs and symptoms of hypersensitivity reactions, such as rash, itching, dizziness, light-headedness, swelling, and breathing problems.
• Caution patient not to take oral iron supplements while receiving iron by infusion.
• Advise female patient to report pregnancy or intent to become pregnant to her practitioner.

fesoterodine fumarate
fezz-oh-TER-ah-deen

Toviaz

Therapeutic class: Antispasmodics
Pharmacologic class: Muscarinic receptor antagonists

AVAILABLE FORMS
Tablets (extended-release) ⒹⓃⒼ: 4 mg, 8 mg

INDICATIONS & DOSAGES
➤ **Urge incontinence, urinary urgency, and urinary frequency from overactive bladder**
Adults: 4 mg PO once daily; increase to 8 mg once daily if needed.

Adjust-a-dose: Don't exceed 4 mg daily in patients with CrCl of less than 30 mL/minute and in those taking CYP3A4 inhibitors.

ADMINISTRATION
PO
• Give drug with or without food.
• Don't divide or crush tablets. Give with liquid and have patient swallow whole.

ACTION
Antagonizes muscarinic (M3) receptors, increasing bladder capacity and decreasing unstable detrusor contractions.

Route	Onset	Peak	Duration
PO	Unknown	5 hr	Unknown

Half-life: 7 hours.

ADVERSE REACTIONS
CNS: headache, dizziness, insomnia. **CV:** peripheral edema. **EENT:** dry eyes. **GI:** dry mouth, constipation, dyspepsia, nausea, abdominal pain. **GU:** UTI, dysuria, urine retention. **Musculoskeletal:** back pain. **Respiratory:** URI, dry throat, cough. **Skin:** rash.

INTERACTIONS
Drug-drug. *Anticholinergics, antimuscarinics:* May increase risk of anticholinergic effects (such as constipation, blurred vision, urine retention). Use together cautiously.
Potassium preparations: May slow GI motility, arresting or delaying transport of solid dosage forms of potassium. Avoid use together.
Strong CYP3A4 inhibitors (clarithromycin, itraconazole, ketoconazole): May increase fesoterodine concentration. Fesoterodine doses of more than 4 mg aren't recommended when fesoterodine is used with strong CYP3A4 inhibitors.
Drug-lifestyle. *Alcohol use:* May cause additive CNS depression. Discourage use together.

EFFECTS ON LAB TEST RESULTS
• May increase ALT and GGT levels.

Reactions in bold italics are *life-threatening*. Interactions may have a *rapid onset* or a *delayed onset*.

CONTRAINDICATIONS & CAUTIONS

• Contraindicated in patients with hypersensitivity to drug or its components and in those with urine retention, gastric retention, or uncontrolled angle-closure glaucoma.

• Life-threatening angioedema with upper airway swelling can occur after first dose. Ensure a patent airway and discontinue drug if this occurs.

• Avoid use in patients with severe hepatic impairment.

• Use cautiously in patients with bladder outlet obstruction, decreased GI motility, myasthenia gravis, or controlled angle-closure glaucoma.

Dialyzable drug: Unknown.

⚠ *Overdose S&S:* Confusion, blurred vision, tachycardia, constipation, dry mouth, lightheadedness, difficulty starting and continuing urination, urinary incontinence.

PREGNANCY-LACTATION-REPRODUCTION

• Use during pregnancy and breastfeeding only if potential benefits outweigh potential risk to the fetus or neonate.

NURSING CONSIDERATIONS

• Give drug without regard to food.

• Monitor patient for urinary symptoms and adverse reactions.

• Monitor postvoid residual urine volume and assess for UTI before start of therapy.

PATIENT TEACHING

• Warn patient to avoid hot environments because drug may decrease sweating, causing severe heat illness.

• Advise patient to avoid driving, operating machinery, and other dangerous activities until drug's effects are known.

• Tell patient to avoid alcohol as it may cause drowsiness.

• Tell patient to report all adverse reactions (especially swelling of the face, lips, or tongue), stomach or intestinal problems, constipation, difficulty emptying the bladder, weak urine stream, glaucoma, kidney or liver problems, or myasthenia gravis.

• Tell patient to take drug with water and to swallow tablet whole. Warn patient not to chew, crush, or divide tablet.

fidaxomicin
fye-DAX-oh-MYE sin

Dificid

Therapeutic class: Antibiotics
Pharmacologic class: Macrolides

AVAILABLE FORMS
Tablets: 200 mg

INDICATIONS & DOSAGES
➤ CDAD
Adults: 200 mg PO b.i.d. for 10 days.

ADMINISTRATION
PO
• May give without regard for food.
• Store at room temperature.

ACTION
Acts on *Clostridium difficile* locally in the GI tract by inhibiting RNA synthesis through RNA polymerases.

Route	Onset	Peak	Duration
PO	<1 hr	1–5 hr	Unknown

Half-life: About 12 hours.

ADVERSE REACTIONS
GI: nausea, vomiting, abdominal pain or discomfort, *GI bleeding,* dyspepsia, flatulence, intestinal obstruction, megacolon. **Hematologic:** anemia, *neutropenia.* **Metabolic:** hyperglycemia, *metabolic acidosis.* **Skin:** drug eruption, rash, pruritus.

INTERACTIONS
None reported.

EFFECTS ON LAB TEST RESULTS
• May increase alkaline phosphatase, liver enzyme, and blood glucose levels.
• May decrease serum bicarbonate level and WBC, RBC, and platelet counts.

CONTRAINDICATIONS & CAUTIONS
• Contraindicated in patients hypersensitive to drug.
• Acute hypersensitivity reactions have been reported. Discontinue drug and treat

appropriately. Patients with known macrolide allergies may have increased risk.

• Drug isn't an effective treatment for systemic *Clostridium* infections. Don't prescribe fidaxomicin unless a *C. difficile* infection has been proven or is strongly suspected because this may lead to the development of drug-resistant bacteria.

Dialyzable drug: Unknown.

PREGNANCY-LACTATION-REPRODUCTION

• Use drug in pregnant women only if clearly needed.

• It isn't known if drug appears in human milk. Use cautiously if breastfeeding.

NURSING CONSIDERATIONS

• Obtain specimen for culture before start of treatment. Monitor response to treatment.

• Monitor glucose level, especially in diabetic patients.

• Monitor patient for abdominal pain or bleeding.

• Monitor patient for acute hypersensitivity.

PATIENT TEACHING

• Inform patient that drug can be taken with or without food.

• Advise patient that drug is used to treat CDAD only and shouldn't be used to treat other infections.

• Counsel patient to take the drug exactly as directed. Missing or skipping doses, or not completing the full course of therapy, may lead to reinfection, continued infection, or bacterial resistance.

BIOSIMILAR DRUG

filgrastim (G-CSF)
fill-GRASS-tim

Grastofil✳, Neupogen

filgrastim-aafi
Nivestym

filgrastim-sndz
Zarxio

tbo-filgrastim
Granix

Therapeutic class: Colony-stimulating factors
Pharmacologic class: Hematopoietics

AVAILABLE FORMS

Injection: 300 mcg/mL, 480 mcg/1.6 mL vials; 300 mcg/0.5 mL, 480 mcg/0.8 mL prefilled syringes

INDICATIONS & DOSAGES

➤ **Acute exposure to myelosuppressive doses of radiation (hematopoietic syndrome of acute radiation syndrome) (Neupogen)**

Adults and children: 10 mcg/kg subcut as soon as possible after suspected or confirmed exposure to radiation doses greater than 2 gray (Gy). Continue daily administration until ANC remains greater than 1,000/mm^3 for three consecutive CBCs or exceeds 10,000/mm^3 after a radiation-induced nadir.

➤ **To decrease incidence of infection in patients with nonmyeloid malignancies receiving myelosuppressive chemotherapy associated with risk of severe febrile neutropenia; to reduce time to neutrophil recovery and duration of fever after induction or consolidation chemotherapy for acute myeloid leukemia (Neupogen, Nivestym, Zarxio)**

Adults and children: 5 mcg/kg by a single subcut injection or short IV infusion (15 to 30 minutes), or continuous IV infusion once daily at least 24 hours after chemotherapy. Give daily for up to 2 weeks, until ANC reaches 10,000/mm^3.

Adjust-a-dose: May increase dosage by increments of 5 mcg/kg for each chemotherapy cycle, depending on duration and severity of ANC nadir.

➤ **To decrease risk of infection in patients with nonmyeloid malignant disease receiving myelosuppressive antineoplastics followed by bone marrow transplantation**

Adults and children: Neupogen, Nivestym, Zarxio: 10 mcg/kg daily IV infusion for no longer than 24 hours or as continuous 24-hour subcut infusion at least 24 hours after cytotoxic chemotherapy and bone marrow infusion. Adjust subsequent dosages based on neutrophil response.

Adjust-a-dose: For patients with ANC above 1,000/mm³ for 3 consecutive days, reduce dosage to 5 mcg/kg/day. If ANC decreases to less than 1,000/mm³ with 5-mcg/kg/day dose, increase dosage to 10 mcg/kg/day. If ANC remains above 1,000/mm³ for 3 more consecutive days, stop drug. If ANC decreases to below 1,000/mm³, resume therapy at 5 mcg/kg daily.

Granix: 5 mcg/kg/day subcut. Continue until anticipated nadir has passed and neutrophil count has recovered to normal range.

➤ **Chronic severe neutropenia (Neupogen, Nivestym, Zarxio)**
Adults and children: For patients with congenital neutropenia, starting dose is 6 mcg/kg subcut b.i.d. For patients with idiopathic or cyclic neutropenia, starting dose is 5 mcg/kg as a single daily subcut injection. Adjust dosage based on patient response.

➤ **Peripheral blood progenitor cell collection and therapy in cancer patients (Neupogen, Nivestym, Zarxio)**
Adults and children: 10 mcg/kg/day subcut (as bolus or continuous infusion). Begin treatment at least 4 days before leukapheresis and continue until last leukapheresis.

Adjust-a-dose: Monitor daily neutrophil count after 4 days of treatment; discontinue drug for WBC count above 100,000/mm³.

➤ **Hematopoietic stem cell mobilization in autologous transplantation in patients with non-Hodgkin lymphoma or multiple myeloma (in combination with plerixafor) (Neupogen)** ◆
Adults: 10 mcg/kg subcut daily; begin 4 days before plerixafor initiation and continue on each day before apheresis for up to 8 days.

ADMINISTRATION
• Give at least 24 hours after cytotoxic chemotherapy.
🔴 **Alert:** Direct administration of less than 0.3 mL isn't recommended because of potential for dosing errors.
🔴 **Alert:** Removable needle cap in prefilled syringes contains natural rubber latex. Don't use in patients with latex allergies.
• Store in refrigerator at 36° to 46° F (2° to 8° C) in original pack to protect from light. Don't shake.

• Before use, allow drug to reach room temperature for at least 30 minutes to a maximum of 24 hours. (If beyond 24 hours, discard drug.)
• Solution should be clear and colorless to slightly yellow. Discard if solution is discolored or contains particulate matter.
• Avoid freezing; if frozen, thaw in refrigerator before administering. Discard drug if frozen more than once.
• Discard unused portion of prefilled syringes.
• Refer to manufacturer's instructions for further administration details.

IV
▼ Dilute in 50 to 100 mL of D₅W. Dilution to less than 5 mcg/mL isn't recommended.
▼ Don't dilute with NSS; product may precipitate.
▼ If drug yield is 5 to 15 mcg/mL, add albumin at 2 mg/mL (0.2%) to minimize binding of drug to plastic containers or tubing.
▼ Give by intermittent infusion over 15 to 30 minutes or by continuous infusion over 24 hours.
▼ Once a dose is withdrawn, don't reuse vial. Discard unused portion. Vials are for single-dose use only.
▼ **Incompatibilities:** Sodium solutions. No other incompatibilities are listed by manufacturer. Consult a drug incompatibility reference for more information.

Subcutaneous
• Rotate administration sites and record.
• Administer in outer upper arms, abdomen, thighs, or upper outer areas of the buttock.
• Don't inject into areas that are tender, red, bruised, hardened, or scarred or into sites with stretch marks.

ACTION
Binds cell receptors to stimulate proliferation, differentiation, commitment, and end-cell function of neutrophils.

Route	Onset	Peak	Duration
IV	1–2 days	Unknown	4 days
Subcut	1–2 days	2–8 hr	4 days
Subcut (tbo-filgrastim)	3–5 days to max ANC	4–6 hr	21 days to baseline ANC return after chemotherapy completion

Half-life: 3 to 3½ hours.

ADVERSE REACTIONS

CNS: fever, headache, weakness, fatigue, dizziness, insomnia, pain, hypoesthesia. **CV:** *MI, arrhythmias,* chest pain, HTN, peripheral edema. **EENT:** epistaxis, sore throat. **GI:** nausea, vomiting, diarrhea, decreased appetite, constipation. **GU:** UTI. **Hematologic:** *thrombocytopenia,* anemia, leukocytosis, *neutropenic fever.* **Musculoskeletal:** bone pain, back pain, extremity pain, arthralgia, muscle spasms. **Respiratory:** dyspnea, cough, bronchitis, URI. **Skin:** alopecia, rash, cutaneous vasculitis. **Other:** hypersensitivity reactions, transfusion reaction, *sepsis,* splenomegaly, antibody development.

INTERACTIONS

Drug-drug. *Bleomycin, cyclophosphamide:* May increase pulmonary toxicity. Monitor therapy.

Chemotherapeutic drugs: Rapidly dividing myeloid cells may be sensitive to cytotoxic drugs. Don't use within 24 hours before or after a dose of one of these drugs.

EFFECTS ON LAB TEST RESULTS

• May increase alkaline phosphatase, creatinine, LDH, and uric acid levels.
• May increase WBC count. May decrease Hb level and platelet count.

CONTRAINDICATIONS & CAUTIONS

• Contraindicated in patients hypersensitive to drug or its components or to proteins derived from *Escherichia coli.*
• Severe allergic reactions, including anaphylaxis, can occur. Permanently discontinue drug for serious allergic reactions.
• Splenic rupture (including fatal cases), sickle cell crisis (including fatal cases), ARDS, cutaneous vasculitis, and capillary leak syndrome, which may be life-threatening, have been reported.
• Use cautiously in severe chronic neutropenia; confirm diagnosis before initiating drug. Drug may increase risk of myelodysplastic syndrome and acute myelogenous leukemia.
• G-CSF drugs may act as a growth factor on any type of tumor. Transmission of tumor cells by peripheral blood progenitor cell therapy infusion may occur and hasn't been well studied.

• Use cautiously in children as studies regarding safety and effectiveness in children are limited.
Dialyzable drug: Unknown.
⚠ Overdose S&S: Excessive leukocytosis.

PREGNANCY-LACTATION-REPRODUCTION

• Adverse effects have been seen in animal studies. Use during pregnancy only if potential benefit justifies potential risk to the fetus.
• It isn't known if drug appears in human milk. Use with extreme caution in breastfeeding women.

NURSING CONSIDERATIONS

• Filgrastim-sndz (Zarxio) is biosimilar to the FDA-approved reference product filgrastim (Neupogen).
⊙ Alert: Obtain baseline CBC after exposure to myelosuppressive doses of radiation; don't delay administration if CBC isn't readily available. Monitor CBC every third day until ANC remains greater than 1,000/mm³ for three consecutive CBCs.
• Obtain baseline CBC and platelet count before therapy.
• Obtain CBC and platelet count two to three times weekly during therapy. Patients who receive drug also may receive high doses of chemotherapy, which may increase risk of toxicities.
• A transiently increased neutrophil count is common 1 or 2 days after therapy starts. Give daily for up to 2 weeks or until ANC has returned to 10,000/mm³ after the expected chemotherapy-induced neutrophil nadir.
• Obtain CBC and platelet count at baseline, then twice weekly during cytotoxic chemotherapy.
• For severe chronic neutropenia, monitor CBC with differential and platelet count during initial 4 weeks of treatment and during the 2 weeks after dosage adjustments. Once patient is clinically stable, monitor monthly during first year of treatment, then as clinically indicated. Consider risks and benefits of continued treatment if abnormal cytogenetics or myelodysplasia occurs.
• Glomerulonephritis can occur; dosage reduction or drug discontinuation may be necessary.

• Monitor patients with left upper abdominal or shoulder pain for enlarged spleen or splenic rupture.

• Monitor patients for capillary leak syndrome (hypotension, hypoalbuminemia, edema, hemoconcentration), which can be life-threatening. Monitor patients closely; intensive care may be needed.

• Assess patients with fever, lung infiltrates, or respiratory distress for ARDS. Discontinue drug if ARDS is confirmed.

• Watch for sickle cell crisis in patients with sickle cell trait or sickle cell disease.

• Monitor patients for signs and symptoms of cutaneous vasculitis (purpura, erythema), especially patients on long-term therapy. Withhold drug if cutaneous vasculitis develops. Consider restarting drug at a reduced dosage when signs and symptoms have resolved and ANC has decreased.

• **Look alike–sound alike:** Don't confuse Neupogen with Epogen or Neumega. Don't confuse filgrastim-sndz with filgrastim.

PATIENT TEACHING
• Instruct patient and caregivers on proper timing, administration, and disposal of subcut self-administered drug.

• Patient with latex allergy shouldn't administer or receive drug in prefilled syringes.

• Instruct patient to report all adverse reactions promptly.

• Teach patient signs and symptoms of allergic reaction (rash, facial edema, wheezing, dyspnea, hypotension, rapid HR); advise patient to seek immediate medical attention if they occur.

• Advise patient to immediately report purpura or erythema.

• Warn patient to seek immediate medical attention if swelling, decreased urination, shortness of breath, abdominal swelling or feeling of fullness, dizziness, or fatigue occurs.

• **Alert:** Rarely, splenic rupture may occur. Advise patient to immediately report left upper abdominal or shoulder tip pain.

• Tell patient that routine blood tests will be needed before and during treatment to monitor for effectiveness and safe use.

• Warn female patient who is pregnant or breastfeeding about drug's risks.

finasteride
fin-AS-teh-ride

Propecia, Proscar🅿

Therapeutic class: BPH drugs
Pharmacologic class: 5-alpha reductase inhibitors

AVAILABLE FORMS
Tablets: 1 mg, 5 mg

INDICATIONS & DOSAGES
➤ **To improve symptoms of BPH and reduce risk of acute urine retention and need for surgery, including transurethral resection of prostate and prostatectomy; to reduce risk of BPH, with or without doxazosin (Proscar)**
Men: 5 mg PO daily.
➤ **Male pattern hair loss (androgenetic alopecia) in men only (Propecia)**
Men: 1 mg PO daily.

ADMINISTRATION
PO
• Give drug without regard for food.
• Store at room temperature. Protect from moisture and light.
• **Alert:** Drug is a potential teratogen. Follow safe handling procedures.

ACTION
Inhibits 5-alpha reductase, resulting in inhibition of the conversion of testosterone to dihydrotestosterone (DHT), the androgen primarily responsible for the initial development and subsequent enlargement of the prostate gland. In male pattern baldness, the scalp contains miniaturized hair follicles and increased DHT level; drug decreases scalp DHT level in such cases.

Route	Onset	Peak	Duration
PO	Unknown	1–2 hr	24 hr

Half-life: 6 hours; 8 hours in elderly patients.

ADVERSE REACTIONS
CNS: dizziness, drowsiness. **CV:** hypotension, orthostatic hypotension, peripheral edema. **EENT:** rhinitis. **GU:** erectile dysfunction, decreased volume of ejaculate,

decreased libido, erectile dysfunction, breast tenderness. **Respiratory:** dyspnea. **Other:** gynecomastia, rash.

INTERACTIONS
None reported.

EFFECTS ON LAB TEST RESULTS
• May decrease PSA level.

CONTRAINDICATIONS & CAUTIONS
• Contraindicated in patients hypersensitive to drug or to other 5-alpha reductase inhibitors, such as dutasteride.
❶ *Alert:* Drug may increase the risk of high-grade prostate cancer. Before starting drug, patient should be evaluated to rule out other urologic conditions, including prostate cancer, that might mimic BPH. An increase in PSA level during therapy should be considered significant and patient should be evaluated for prostate cancer.
• Use cautiously in patients with liver dysfunction.
Dialyzable drug: Unknown.

PREGNANCY-LACTATION-REPRODUCTION
• Use isn't indicated in women. Contraindicated in pregnant women and women of childbearing potential.
• Pregnant women should avoid contact with drug and with semen from a male partner taking drug.
• It isn't known if drug appears in human milk.

NURSING CONSIDERATIONS
• Before therapy, evaluate patient for conditions that mimic BPH, including hypotonic bladder, prostate cancer, infection, or stricture.
• Carefully monitor patients who have a large residual urine volume or severely diminished urine flow.
• Sustained increase in PSA level could indicate noncompliance with therapy.
• A minimum of 6 months of therapy may be needed for treatment of BPH.

PATIENT TEACHING
• Tell patient that drug may be taken with or without meals.

• Warn female patient who is or may become pregnant not to handle crushed or broken tablets because of risk of adverse effects on male fetus and to avoid contact with semen from a male partner exposed to finasteride.
• Inform patient that signs of improvement may require at least 3 months of daily use when drug is used to treat hair loss or at least 6 months when taken for BPH.
• Reassure patient that drug may decrease volume of ejaculate without impairing normal sexual function.
• Instruct patient to report breast changes, such as lumps, pain, or nipple discharge.

fingolimod
fin-GOL-ih-mod

Gilenya

Therapeutic class: Immunomodulators
Pharmacologic class: Sphingosine 1-phosphate receptor modulators

AVAILABLE FORMS
Capsules: 0.25 mg, 0.5 mg

INDICATIONS & DOSAGES
➤ **To reduce frequency of clinical exacerbations and to delay accumulation of physical disability in relapsing forms of MS**
Adults and children age 10 and older weighing more than 40 kg: 0.5 mg PO once daily.
Children age 10 and older weighing 40 kg or less: 0.25 mg PO once daily.

ADMINISTRATION
PO
• Hazardous drug; use appropriate handling and disposal precautions.
• May give without regard for food.
• Store at room temperature. Protect from moisture.

ACTION
Blocks activity of lymphocytes leaving lymph nodes, which reduces number of lymphocytes in the peripheral blood.

Route	Onset	Peak	Duration
PO	Unknown	12–16 hr	Unknown

Half-life: 6 to 9 days.

ADVERSE REACTIONS
CNS: asthenia, depression, dizziness, paresthesia, headache, migraine. **CV:** *bradycardia,* HTN. **EENT:** sinusitis, blurred vision, eye pain. **GI:** abdominal pain, gastroenteritis, diarrhea, nausea. **Hematologic:** *lymphopenia, leukopenia.* **Hepatic:** *hepatotoxicity.* **Metabolic:** hypertriglyceridemia, weight loss. **Musculoskeletal:** back pain, extremity pain. **Respiratory:** bronchitis, cough, dyspnea. **Skin:** tinea infections, alopecia, eczema, pruritus. **Other:** flulike symptoms, herpes viral infections.

INTERACTIONS
Drug-drug. *Antineoplastics, immunomodulators, immunosuppressants:* May increase risk of immunosuppression. Use cautiously together.

⊘ Alert: *Beta blockers, HR-lowering calcium channel blockers (diltiazem, verapamil), digoxin:* May increase risk of severe bradycardia or heart block. If possible, switch patient to cardiac drug that doesn't cause bradycardia before starting fingolimod. If change isn't possible, monitor patient with continuous ECG overnight after first dose to determine effects.

Class IA or III antiarrhythmics (amiodarone, procainamide, quinidine, sotalol): May increase risk of bradycardia or torsades de pointes. Contraindicated together.

Ketoconazole: May increase fingolimod level and risk of adverse effects. Use cautiously and monitor patient closely.

Live attenuated virus vaccines: May decrease vaccination effects or increase infection risk. Don't use together or give vaccine within 60 days of prior fingolimod use.

Drug-lifestyle. *Sun exposure:* May cause photosensitivity reactions. Advise patient to wear protective clothing and use a sunscreen with a high protection factor.

EFFECTS ON LAB TEST RESULTS
• May increase ALT, AST, GGT, and triglyceride levels.

• May decrease lymphocyte and neutrophil counts.

CONTRAINDICATIONS & CAUTIONS
• Contraindicated in patients hypersensitive to drug and in those with active acute or chronic infection.

⊘ Alert: Contraindicated in patients with MI, unstable angina, stroke, TIA, decompensated HF requiring hospitalization, or class III/IV HF within the past 6 months; in those with history or presence of Mobitz Type II second- or third-degree AV block or sick sinus syndrome unless patient has a functioning pacemaker; and in those with baseline QTc interval of 500 msec or greater.

⊘ Alert: Use cautiously after cardiac evaluation in patients with ischemic heart disease, history of MI, HF, history of cardiac arrest, cerebrovascular disease, history of symptomatic bradycardia, recurrent syncope, severe untreated sleep apnea, AV block, or SA heart block. Monitor patient in a setting with resources and personnel capable of managing symptomatic bradycardia.

• Use cautiously in patients with sick sinus syndrome and in patients taking Class IA or III antiarrhythmics, beta blockers, or calcium channel blockers.

• Use cautiously in patients with history of infection, macular edema, decreased pulmonary function test results, or liver disease.

• Use cautiously in patients older than age 65 who have concomitant disease or are taking other drugs.

• Safety and effectiveness in children haven't been established.

Dialyzable drug: No.

⚠ Overdose S&S: Chest tightness or discomfort.

PREGNANCY-LACTATION-REPRODUCTION
• Drug may cause fetal harm. Use in pregnant women only if benefit justifies risk to the fetus.

• Pregnant women should enroll in the Gilenya Pregnancy Registry at 1-877-598-7237.

• Women of childbearing potential should use effective contraception during therapy and for 2 months after final dose.

• It isn't known if drug appears in human milk. Patient should discontinue breastfeeding or discontinue drug.

NURSING CONSIDERATIONS

❸ *Alert:* Monitor HR and BP hourly for at least 6 hours after first dose in all patients. Obtain ECG before first dose and at the end of the observation period. Monitor BP routinely during treatment.

❸ *Alert:* Monitor high-risk patients and those who may not tolerate bradycardia with continuous ECG overnight. High-risk patients include those who develop severe bradycardia after receiving the first dose, those with preexisting conditions who may not tolerate bradycardia, those receiving other drugs that slow the HR or AV conduction, those with QT-interval prolongation before taking fingolimod or prolonged QT interval that occurs during monitoring period, those receiving other drugs that prolong QT interval, and those at risk for QT-interval prolongation due to hypokalemia, hypomagnesemia, or congenital long-QT syndrome.

❸ *Alert:* If CV symptoms occur (HR less than 45 beats/minute or at its lowest value 6 hours after dose, or new-onset second-degree or higher AV block 6 hours after dose), continue monitoring until symptoms resolve.

❸ *Alert:* Repeat first-dose monitoring guidelines after second dose in patients who required pharmacologic intervention for symptomatic bradycardia after first dose.

• Obtain baseline ECG if one wasn't done within 6 months before start of therapy, especially in patients receiving antiarrhythmics, beta blockers, or calcium channel blockers and in those with cardiac risk factors or slow or irregular HR on physical examination.

❸ *Alert:* Drug may cause progressive multifocal leukoencephalopathy (PML), which can cause severe disability or death. Monitor patient for progressive and diverse symptoms of PML (progressive weakness on one side of the body, clumsiness, vision problems, confusion, and changes in thinking, personality, memory, and orientation). Stop drug and perform diagnostic evaluation, including MRI, if PML is suspected.

• Test for varicella antibodies before treatment initiation, especially if patient has no history of chickenpox or immunization; consider vaccination against varicella zoster 1 month before start of fingolimod therapy.

• Obtain baseline ophthalmic examination and monitor patient for macular edema at 3 to 4 months after treatment initiation and if patient complains of visual disturbances. Although macular edema is a rare adverse reaction, patients with uveitis and diabetes are at increased risk.

• Drug may increase risk of infections. Monitor patient for signs and symptoms of infection during treatment and for 2 months after therapy ends. Obtain baseline CBC with differential within 6 months of beginning therapy. Stop treatment if patient has active infection.

• Monitor patient for hepatic impairment (unexplained nausea, vomiting, abdominal pain, fatigue, anorexia, jaundice, dark urine). Obtain LFTs at baseline and as needed during therapy. Most enzyme elevations occur within 3 to 4 months of treatment initiation. Drug may need to be discontinued if severe liver injury occurs.

• Monitor patient for respiratory changes. Obtain spirometry and diffusion lung capacity tests if clinically indicated.

• Drug is associated with basal cell carcinoma and melanoma. Monitor patient for suspicious skin lesions and evaluate promptly.

• Restart therapy as at initiation if patient discontinues treatment for more than 2 weeks.

PATIENT TEACHING

❸ *Alert:* Teach patient to immediately contact the health care provider if signs and symptoms of a slowing HR, such as dizziness, tiredness, irregular heartbeat, or palpitations, occur.

❸ *Alert:* Advise patient to immediately report symptoms of PML (new or worsening weakness; trouble using arms or legs; changes in thinking, eyesight, strength, or balance). Tell patient not to stop drug without first discussing with prescriber.

• Instruct patient to report visual disturbances, trouble breathing, changes in HR (low HR, dizziness, fatigue, chest pain) or

---

Reactions in bold italics are *life-threatening*. Interactions may have a *rapid onset* or a *delayed onset*.

rhythm (palpitations), infection (pain, fever, malaise), or suspicious skin lesions.
• Tell patient to immediately report unexplained nausea, vomiting, abdominal pain, fatigue, anorexia, jaundice, or dark urine.
• Advise patient to notify prescriber of any medication changes.
• Warn female patient of childbearing potential about possible risk to fetus; advise her to use effective contraception during treatment and for 2 months after treatment ends.
• Advise female patient to notify prescriber immediately if she is or plans to become pregnant.
• Advise patient to promptly report suspicious skin lesions and to limit exposure to sun and ultraviolet light by wearing protective clothing and using a sunscreen with a high protection factor.

flecainide acetate
FLEH-kay-nide

Tambocor

Therapeutic class: Antiarrhythmics
Pharmacologic class: Benzamide derivatives

AVAILABLE FORMS
Tablets: 50 mg, 100 mg, 150 mg

INDICATIONS & DOSAGES
➤ **Prevention of paroxysmal supraventricular tachycardia, including AV nodal reentrant tachycardia and AV reentrant tachycardia or paroxysmal atrial fibrillation or flutter in patients without structural heart disease; life-threatening ventricular arrhythmias such as sustained ventricular tachycardia**
Adults: For paroxysmal supraventricular tachycardia or paroxysmal atrial fibrillation or flutter, 50 mg PO every 12 hours. Increase in increments of 50 mg b.i.d. every 4 days. Maximum dose is 300 mg/day. For life-threatening ventricular arrhythmias, 50 to 100 mg PO every 12 hours. Increase in increments of 50 mg b.i.d. every 4 days until desired effect occurs. Maximum dose for most patients is 400 mg/day.

Children older than age 6 months: Initially, 100 mg/m²/day in divided doses every 8 to 12 hours. May titrate dosage at 4-day intervals. Maximum dosage is 200 mg/m²/day.
Children age 6 months and younger: 50 mg/m²/day in divided doses every 8 to 12 hours. May titrate dosage at 4-day intervals. Maximum dosage is 200 mg/m²/day.
Adjust-a-dose: For adults, if CrCl is 35 mL/minute or less, first dose is 100 mg PO once daily or 50 mg PO b.i.d.

ADMINISTRATION
PO
• Give drug without regard for food.

ACTION
A Class IC antiarrhythmic that decreases excitability, conduction velocity, and automaticity by slowing atrial, AV node, His-Purkinje system, and intraventricular conduction; prolongs refractory periods in these tissues.

Route	Onset	Peak	Duration
PO	Unknown	1–6 hr	Unknown

Half-life: 12 to 27 hours (adults); 11 to 12 hours (adolescents age 12 to 15); 8 hours (children); 6 hours (12 months [infants]); 11 to 12 hours (3 months [infants]); 29 hours or less (newborns).

ADVERSE REACTIONS
CNS: dizziness, headache, light-headedness, syncope, fatigue, fever, tremor, anxiety, insomnia, depression, malaise, paresthesia, ataxia, vertigo, asthenia, somnolence. **CV:** *new or worsened arrhythmias, HF, cardiac arrest,* chest pain, palpitations, edema, flushing. **EENT:** blurred vision and other visual disturbances, eye pain, eye irritation, dry mouth. **GI:** nausea, constipation, abdominal pain, dyspepsia, vomiting, diarrhea, anorexia. **Respiratory:** dyspnea. **Skin:** rash.

INTERACTIONS
Drug-drug. *Amiodarone, cimetidine, CYP2D6 inhibitors (clozapine, quinidine):* May increase level of flecainide. Watch for toxicity. In the presence of amiodarone, reduce usual flecainide dose by 50% and monitor patient for adverse effects.

Digoxin: May increase digoxin level. Monitor digoxin level.

Disopyramide, verapamil: May increase negative inotropic properties. Avoid using together.

Propranolol, other beta blockers: May increase flecainide and propranolol levels. Watch for propranolol and flecainide toxicity (negative inotropic effects).

QTc interval–prolonging drugs (fluoroquinolones, ondansetron, posaconazole): May increase risk of cardiotoxicity and arrhythmias. Consider therapy modification.

Ritonavir: May significantly increase flecainide levels and toxicity. Use together is contraindicated.

Drug-food. *Milk:* May interfere with drug absorption. Monitor trough drug levels during major changes in dietary milk intake.

EFFECTS ON LAB TEST RESULTS
None reported.

CONTRAINDICATIONS & CAUTIONS
• Contraindicated in hypersensitivity to drug and in those with second- or third-degree AV block or right bundle-branch block with left hemiblock (in the absence of an artificial pacemaker), recent MI, structural heart disease, or cardiogenic shock, and in those taking ritonavir.

Black Box Warning Patients who received flecainide for atrial fibrillation or flutter were at increased risk for ventricular tachycardia and ventricular fibrillation. Its use for these conditions isn't recommended. ∎

• Use cautiously in patients with severe renal disease, prolonged QT interval, sick sinus syndrome, or blood dyscrasia. Avoid use in HF.

• In patients with hepatic disease, use drug only if potential benefits outweigh risk, and use frequent and early drug-level monitoring to guide dosage.

• When transferring patient from another antiarrhythmic to flecainide, allow two to four plasma half-lives to elapse for the drug being discontinued before starting flecainide at the usual dosage. Consider hospitalizing patients in whom withdrawal of a previous antiarrhythmic produced life-threatening arrhythmias.

Dialyzable drug: No.

PREGNANCY-LACTATION-REPRODUCTION
• Use during pregnancy only if potential benefit justifies potential risk to the fetus.
• Drug appears in human milk. Consider discontinuing breastfeeding or drug.

NURSING CONSIDERATIONS
Black Box Warning When used to prevent ventricular arrhythmias, reserve drug for patients with documented life-threatening arrhythmias. For patients with sustained ventricular tachycardia, initiate therapy in the hospital and monitor rhythm. ∎

Black Box Warning Patients treated with flecainide for atrial flutter have a 1:1 AV conduction due to slowing of the atrial rate. A paradoxical increase in the ventricular rate may occur. Concomitant negative chronotropic therapy with digoxin or beta blockers may lower the risk of this complication. ∎

• Due to safety risks, flecainide should be reserved for symptomatic supraventricular tachycardia in patients without structural or ischemic heart disease who aren't candidates for, or prefer not to undergo, catheter ablation and in whom other therapies have failed or are contraindicated.

• Flecainide is an appropriate adjunctive therapy in patients with type 3 long QT syndrome or catecholaminergic polymorphic ventricular tachycardia who are already taking a maximally tolerated beta blocker but are still experiencing symptoms.

• Check that pacing threshold was determined 1 week before and after starting therapy in patient with a pacemaker; flecainide can alter endocardial pacing thresholds.

• Correct hypokalemia or hyperkalemia before giving flecainide; these electrolyte disturbances may alter drug's effect.

• Monitor ECG for proarrhythmic effects.

• Most patients can be maintained on an every-12-hours dosing schedule; some need to receive flecainide every 8 hours.

• Monitor flecainide level, especially if patient has renal failure or HF. Therapeutic flecainide levels range from 0.2 to 1 mcg/mL. Risk of adverse effects increases when trough blood level exceeds 1 mcg/mL.

Reactions in bold italics are *life-threatening*. Interactions may have a *rapid onset* or a *delayed onset*.

PATIENT TEACHING

• Stress importance of taking drug exactly as prescribed.

• Instruct patient to report adverse reactions promptly and to limit fluid and sodium intake to minimize fluid retention.

fluconazole ⚕

floo-KON-a-zole

Diflucan◆

Therapeutic class: Antifungals
Pharmacologic class: Triazoles

F

AVAILABLE FORMS

Injection: 100 mg/50 mL, 200 mg/100 mL, 400 mg/200 mL
Powder for oral suspension: 50 mg/5 mL, 200 mg/5 mL
Tablets: 50 mg, 100 mg, 150 mg, 200 mg

INDICATIONS & DOSAGES

Adjust-a-dose (for all indications except vulvovaginal candidiasis): If CrCl is less than 50 mL/minute and patient isn't receiving dialysis, give initial loading dose of 50 to 400 mg for patients about to receive multiple doses; then reduce dosage by 50%. Patients receiving regular hemodialysis treatment should receive usual dose after each dialysis session.

➤ **Oropharyngeal candidiasis**
Adults: 200 mg PO or IV on first day, then 100 mg once daily for at least 2 weeks.
Children: 6 mg/kg PO or IV on first day, then 3 mg/kg daily for 2 weeks.
Adjust-a-dose (for premature neonates [gestational age, 26 to 29 weeks]): For first 2 weeks of life, give same dosage as for older children every 72 hours. After first 2 weeks, give dose once daily. Maximum daily dose 600 mg.

➤ **Esophageal candidiasis**
Adults: 200 mg PO or IV on first day, then 100 mg once daily. Up to 400 mg daily has been used, depending on patient's condition and tolerance of treatment. Patients should receive drug for at least 3 weeks and for 2 weeks after symptoms resolve.
Children: 6 mg/kg PO or IV on first day, then 3 to 12 mg/kg daily for at least 3 weeks

and for at least 2 weeks after symptoms resolve. Maximum daily dose, 12 mg/kg (or 600 mg).
Adjust-a-dose (for premature neonates [gestational age, 26 to 29 weeks]): For first 2 weeks of life, give same dosage as for older children every 72 hours. After first 2 weeks, give dose once daily.

➤ **Vulvovaginal candidiasis**
Adults: 150 mg PO for one dose only.

➤ **Systemic candidiasis**
Adults: Optimal therapeutic dosage and duration of therapy haven't been established; doses of up to 400 mg PO or IV daily have been used.
Children: 6 to 12 mg/kg/day PO or IV. Maximum daily dose, 600 mg.
Adjust-a-dose (for premature neonates [gestational age, 26 to 29 weeks]): For first 2 weeks of life, give same dosage as for older children every 72 hours. After first 2 weeks, give dose once daily.

➤ **Cryptococcal meningitis**
Adults: 400 mg PO or IV on first day, then 200 mg once daily for 10 to 12 weeks after CSF culture result is negative. Doses up to 400 mg/day may be used.
Children: 12 mg/kg/day PO or IV on first day, then 6 to 12 mg/kg/day for 10 to 12 weeks after CSF culture result is negative. Maximum daily dose, 600 mg.
Adjust-a-dose (for premature neonates [gestational age, 26 to 29 weeks]): For the first 2 weeks of life, administer the same dosage as older children every 72 hours. After the first 2 weeks, administer dose once daily.

➤ **To prevent candidiasis in bone marrow transplant and cancer patients**
Adults: 400 mg PO or IV once daily. Start treatment several days before anticipated agranulocytosis, and continue for 7 days after neutrophil count exceeds 1,000/mm³.

➤ **To suppress relapse of cryptococcal meningitis in patients with AIDS**
Adults: 200 mg PO or IV daily.
Children: 6 mg/kg/day PO or IV once daily.
Adjust-a-dose (for premature neonates [gestational age, 26 to 29 weeks]): For first 2 weeks of life, give same dosage as for older children every 72 hours. After first 2 weeks, give dose once daily.

➤ ***Candida*-related peritonitis; UTI**
Adults: 50 to 200 mg PO or IV once daily.

ADMINISTRATION

PO

• Drug is considered hazardous; use safe handling and disposal precautions.

• Give drug without regard for food.

• Add 24 mL of distilled or purified water to the bottle and shake oral suspension well before giving.

• Store tablets and powder for oral suspension below 86° F (30° C). Store reconstituted suspension between 41° and 86° F (5° and 30° C). Discard unused portion after 2 weeks.

• Protect from freezing.

IV

▼ Drug is considered hazardous; use safe handling and disposal precautions.

▼ To ensure product sterility, don't remove protective wrap from IV bag until just before use.

▼ The plastic container may show some opacity from moisture absorbed during sterilization. This doesn't affect drug and diminishes over time.

▼ To prevent air embolism, don't connect in series with other infusions.

▼ Use an infusion pump.

▼ Give by continuous infusion at no more than 200 mg/hour.

▼ Don't use if solution is cloudy or precipitated.

▼ **Incompatibilities:** Many other IV drugs are incompatible. Consult a drug incompatibility reference for more information. Don't add other drugs to IV bag.

ACTION

Inhibits fungal CYP450 (responsible for fungal sterol synthesis); weakens fungal cell walls.

Route	Onset	Peak	Duration
PO	Rapid	1–2 hr	30 hr
IV	Immediate	Immediate	Unknown

Half-life: 20 to 50 hours.

ADVERSE REACTIONS

CNS: headache, dizziness, seizures. **GI:** nausea, vomiting, abdominal pain, diarrhea, dyspepsia, taste perversion. **Skin:** rash.

INTERACTIONS

Drug-drug. *Alprazolam, chlordiazepoxide, clonazepam, clorazepate, diazepam, estazolam, flurazepam, midazolam, quazepam, triazolam:* Fluconazole may increase levels of these drugs and may cause increased CNS depression and psychomotor impairment. Avoid using together.

Carbamazepine, celecoxib, cyclosporine, phenytoin, theophylline: May increase levels of these drugs. Monitor carbamazepine, cyclosporine, phenytoin, and theophylline levels. Consider reducing celecoxib dosage by half when using with fluconazole.

Cimetidine: May decrease fluconazole level. Monitor patient's response to fluconazole.

Erythromycin, quinidine: May cause prolonged QT interval and sudden death. Don't use together.

HMG-CoA reductase inhibitors (atorvastatin, fluvastatin, lovastatin, pravastatin, simvastatin): May increase levels and adverse effects of these drugs. Avoid using together or reduce dosage of HMG-CoA reductase inhibitor.

Isoniazid, oral sulfonylureas, phenytoin, rifampin, valproic acid: May increase hepatic transaminase level. Monitor LFT results closely.

Oral sulfonylureas (glipizide, glyburide): May increase levels of these drugs. Monitor patient for enhanced hypoglycemic effect.

Rifampin: May enhance fluconazole metabolism. Monitor patient for lack of response to fluconazole.

Tacrolimus: May increase tacrolimus level and nephrotoxicity. Monitor patient carefully.

Warfarin: May increase risk of bleeding. Monitor PT and INR.

Zidovudine: May increase zidovudine-related toxicities. Monitor patient closely; zidovudine dosage decrease may be needed.

Zolpidem: May increase therapeutic effects of zolpidem. Monitor patient closely. A decrease in dosage may be needed.

EFFECTS ON LAB TEST RESULTS

• May increase alkaline phosphatase, ALT, AST, bilirubin, and GGT levels.

• May decrease platelet and WBC counts.

Reactions in bold italics are *life-threatening*. Interactions may have a *rapid onset* or a *delayed onset*.

CONTRAINDICATIONS & CAUTIONS
• Rarely, anaphylaxis has been reported.
• Contraindicated in patients hypersensitive to drug.
• Contraindicated with CYP3A4 substrates that may lead to QT-interval prolongation (astemizole, erythromycin, pimozide, quinidine).
• Use dosage forms containing benzyl alcohol derivatives cautiously in neonates or avoid use.
• Use cautiously in patients hypersensitive to other antifungal azole compounds.
🧬 Oral suspension contains sucrose and shouldn't be used in patients with hereditary fructose, glucose, or galactose malabsorption or sucrase-isomaltase deficiency.
Dialyzable drug: 50%.
⚠ *Overdose S&S:* Hallucinations, paranoid behavior.

PREGNANCY-LACTATION-REPRODUCTION
• Contraindicated in pregnant women for most indications. Long-term treatment with high doses (400 to 800 mg/day) during the first trimester of pregnancy may be associated with birth defects.
• Drug appears in human milk. Use cautiously in breastfeeding women.

NURSING CONSIDERATIONS
🔴 *Alert:* Serious hepatotoxicity has occurred in patients with underlying medical conditions. Monitor LFTs and discontinue drug if hepatic dysfunction develops.
• Rare cases of exfoliative skin disorders have been reported. Closely monitor patients who develop mild rash. Stop drug if lesions progress.
• Use cautiously in patients with renal impairment. Monitor renal function during treatment; dosage adjustment may be necessary.
• Monitor potassium level.
• Likelihood of adverse reactions may be greater in HIV-infected patients.

PATIENT TEACHING
• Tell patient to take drug as directed, even after feeling better.
• Instruct patient to report all adverse reactions promptly.

---

fludarabine phosphate
floo-DAR-a-been

Therapeutic class: Antineoplastics
Pharmacologic class: Purine antagonists

F

AVAILABLE FORMS
Powder for injection: 50 mg
Solution for injection: 50 mg/2 mL

INDICATIONS & DOSAGES
➤ **B-cell chronic lymphocytic leukemia in patients with no or inadequate response to at least one standard alkylating drug regimen**
Adults: 25 mg/m^2 IV daily for 5 consecutive days. Repeat cycle every 28 days. The optimal duration of treatment hasn't been established, but it's recommended to give three additional cycles after maximal response is obtained.
➤ **Newly diagnosed pediatric acute myeloid leukemia as part of a multiagent chemotherapy regimen, in combination with cytarabine and idarubicin during consolidation phase of treatment ◆**
Children: 10.5 mg/m^2 IV over 15 minutes as a single dose, followed by a continuous IV infusion of 30.5 mg/m^2/day for 48 hours during consolidation phase of treatment.
➤ **Allogeneic hematopoietic stem cell transplantation in older adults as a myeloablative conditioning regimen, in combination with busulfan ◆**
Adults: 40 mg/m^2/day IV for 4 days (in combination with busulfan) beginning 6 days before transplantation.
Adjust-a-dose: In patients with CrCl of 50 to 79 mL/minute, starting dose is 20 mg/m^2. In patients with CrCl of 30 to 49 mL/minute, starting dose is 15 mg/m^2. If CrCl is less than 30 mL/minute, don't give drug.

ADMINISTRATION
IV
▼ Preparing and giving parenteral drug may be mutagenic, teratogenic, or carcinogenic. Follow facility policy to reduce risks.
▼ To prepare, add 2 mL of sterile water for injection to the vial. If using powder for

---

injection, dissolution should occur within 15 seconds.

▼ Each milliliter contains 25 mg of fludarabine phosphate and 25 mg of mannitol.

▼ Dilute further in 100 or 125 mL of D₅W or NSS for injection.

▼ Use within 8 hours of reconstitution. Administer over approximately 30 minutes.

▼ Store drug in refrigerator at 36° to 46° F (2° to 8° C) or at room temperature, as specified according to each manufacturer's labeling.

▼ Protect from light.

▼ **Incompatibilities:** Don't mix with other drugs.

ACTION

After conversion to its active metabolite, drug interferes with DNA synthesis by inhibiting DNA polymerase alpha, ribonucleotide reductase, and DNA primase, thus inhibiting DNA synthesis.

Route	Onset	Peak	Duration
IV	Unknown	Unknown	Unknown

Half-life: About 20 hours.

ADVERSE REACTIONS

CNS: fatigue, malaise, weakness, paresthesia, peripheral neuropathy, *stroke,* headache, sleep disorder, depression, cerebellar syndrome, *TIA, agitation, confusion, fever, coma, pain.* **CV:** edema, angina, phlebitis, *arrhythmias, HF, MI,* supraventricular tachycardia, *DVT, aneurysm, hemorrhage.* **EENT:** visual disturbances, delayed blindness, optic neuritis, optic neuropathy, hearing loss, epistaxis, sinusitis, pharyngitis. **GI:** nausea, vomiting, diarrhea, constipation, anorexia, stomatitis, *GI bleeding,* esophagitis, mucositis. **GU:** dysuria, UTI, urinary hesitancy, proteinuria, hematuria, *renal failure.* **Hematologic:** hemolytic anemia, *myelosuppression.* **Hepatic:** *liver failure,* cholelithiasis. **Metabolic:** hypocalcemia, hyperkalemia, hyperglycemia, dehydration, hyperuricemia, hyperphosphatemia. **Musculoskeletal:** myalgia. **Respiratory:** cough, pneumonia, dyspnea, URI, allergic pneumonitis, hemoptysis, hypoxia, bronchitis. **Skin:** rash, pruritus, alopecia, seborrhea, diaphoresis. **Other:** chills, *TLS, infection, anaphylaxis.*

INTERACTIONS

Drug-drug. *Live-virus vaccines:* May increase risk of vaccine-related reactions. Avoid vaccines during and after fludarabine therapy.

Myelosuppressive agents: May increase toxicity. Avoid using together, if possible.

Black Box Warning *Pentostatin:* May increase risk of pulmonary toxicity, which can be fatal. Avoid using together. ∎

EFFECTS ON LAB TEST RESULTS

● May increase glucose, phosphate, potassium, and uric acid levels.

● May decrease calcium and Hb levels. May decrease platelet, RBC, and WBC counts.

CONTRAINDICATIONS & CAUTIONS

● Contraindicated in patients hypersensitive to drug or its components.

● Use cautiously in patients with renal insufficiency.

Black Box Warning May cause life-threatening and fatal autoimmune phenomena, such as acquired hemophilia, thrombocytopenia or thrombocytopenic purpura, Evans syndrome, and hemolytic anemia, after one or more cycles. ∎

Dialyzable drug: Yes.

⚠ *Overdose S&S:* Delayed blindness, coma, thrombocytopenia, neutropenia, death.

PREGNANCY-LACTATION-REPRODUCTION

● May cause fetal harm. If used in pregnancy, apprise patient of potential fetal hazard.

● Women of childbearing potential and men with sexual partners of childbearing potential must use contraceptives during therapy and for at least 6 months after therapy ends.

● Drug may damage testicular tissue and spermatozoa.

● It isn't known if drug appears in human milk. Patient should discontinue breastfeeding or discontinue drug.

NURSING CONSIDERATIONS

Black Box Warning Administer under the supervision of a physician experienced in the use of antineoplastic therapy. ∎

Black Box Warning Higher than recommended doses are associated with severe neurologic toxicity, including blindness, coma, and death. ∎

Reactions in bold italics are *life-threatening*. Interactions may have a *rapid onset* or a *delayed onset*.

🜂 *Alert:* Monitor patient closely and expect modified dosage based on toxicity. Most toxic effects are dose dependent. Advanced age, renal insufficiency, and bone marrow impairment may predispose patients to increased or excessive toxicity.

Black Box Warning Careful hematologic monitoring, especially of neutrophil and platelet counts, is needed. Bone marrow suppression can be severe. ■

Black Box Warning Instances of life-threatening and sometimes fatal autoimmune phenomena have been reported. Monitor patient for development of hemolysis. ■

• To prevent bleeding, avoid all IM injections when platelet count is below 50,000/mm^3.

• Give blood transfusions because of cumulative anemia. Patients should be given irradiated blood only, to minimize transfusion-associated GVHD.

• Hyperuricemia, hypocalcemia, hyperkalemia, and renal failure may result from rapid lysis of tumor cells. Take preventive measures against TLS, such as IV hydration, alkalinization of urine, and treatment with allopurinol as appropriate.

• *Look alike–sound alike:* Don't confuse fludarabine with floxuridine, fluorouracil, or flucytosine.

PATIENT TEACHING

• Instruct patient to report all adverse reactions, especially signs and symptoms of infection (fever, sore throat, fatigue) and bleeding (easy bruising, nosebleeds, bleeding gums, tarry stools). Tell patient to take temperature daily.

flumazenil
floo-MAZ-eh-nill

Therapeutic class: Benzodiazepine antagonists
Pharmacologic class: Antidotes

AVAILABLE FORMS
Injection: 0.1 mg/mL in 5-mL and 10-mL multiple-dose vials

INDICATIONS & DOSAGES
➤ **Complete or partial reversal of sedative effects of benzodiazepines after anesthesia (adults) or conscious sedation (adults and children)**

Adults: Initially, 0.2 mg IV over 15 seconds. If patient doesn't reach desired level of consciousness after 45 seconds, repeat dose. Repeat at 1-minute intervals, if needed, until cumulative dose of 1 mg has been given (first dose plus four more doses). Most patients respond after 0.6 to 1 mg of drug. In case of resedation, dosage may be repeated after 20 minutes, but never give more than 1 mg at any one time or exceed 3 mg in any 1 hour.

Children age 1 year and older: 0.01 mg/kg (up to 0.2 mg) IV over 15 seconds. If patient doesn't reach desired level of consciousness after 45 seconds, repeat dose. Repeat at 1-minute intervals, if needed, until cumulative dose of 0.05 mg/kg or 1 mg, whichever is lower, has been given (first dose plus four more doses).

➤ **Suspected benzodiazepine overdose**
Adults: Initially, 0.2 mg IV over 30 seconds. If patient doesn't reach desired level of consciousness after 30 seconds, give 0.3 mg over 30 seconds. If patient still doesn't respond adequately, give 0.5 mg over 30 seconds. Repeat 0.5-mg doses, as needed, at 1-minute intervals until cumulative dose of 3 mg has been given. Most patients with benzodiazepine overdose respond to cumulative doses between 1 and 3 mg; rarely, patients who respond partially after 3 mg may need additional doses, up to 5 mg total. If patient doesn't respond in 5 minutes after receiving 5 mg, sedation is unlikely to be caused by benzodiazepines. In case of resedation, may repeat dose after 20 minutes, but never give more than 1 mg (give as 0.5 mg/minute) at any one time or exceed 3 mg in any 1 hour.

ADMINISTRATION
IV
▼ Store drug in vial until use.
▼ Make sure airway is secure and patent.
▼ Compatible solutions include D$_5$W, lactated Ringer injection, and NSS.
▼ To minimize pain at injection site, inject drug over 15 to 30 seconds into large vein through free-flowing solution.
▼ Monitor patient for signs and symptoms of extravasation.

▼ Drug is stable in a syringe for 24 hours.

▼ **Incompatibilities:** None listed by manufacturer. Consult a drug incompatibility reference for more information.

ACTION

Competitively inhibits the actions of benzodiazepines on the GABA–benzodiazepine receptor complex.

Route	Onset	Peak	Duration
IV	1–2 min	6–10 min	1 hr (variable range: 19–50 min)

Half-life: Adults: 40 to 80 minutes (terminal); children: 20 to 75 minutes (terminal).

ADVERSE REACTIONS

CNS: dizziness, headache, *seizures,* agitation, emotional lability, anxiety, nervousness, tremor, insomnia, vertigo, fatigue, malaise, paresthesia. **CV:** *arrhythmias,* cutaneous vasodilation, palpitations, flushing. **EENT:** abnormal or blurred vision, lacrimation, dry mouth. **GI:** nausea, vomiting. **Respiratory:** dyspnea, hyperventilation. **Skin:** diaphoresis. **Other:** pain at injection site.

INTERACTIONS

Drug-drug. *Antidepressants, drugs that may cause seizures or arrhythmias:* May increase risk of seizures or arrhythmias. Don't use flumazenil when overdose involves more than one drug, especially when seizures (from any cause) are likely.

EFFECTS ON LAB TEST RESULTS

None reported.

CONTRAINDICATIONS & CAUTIONS

• Contraindicated in patients hypersensitive to flumazenil or benzodiazepines, in those with evidence of serious TCA overdose, and in those who have received benzodiazepines to treat a potentially life-threatening condition such as status epilepticus.

• Use cautiously in patients with head injury, psychiatric disorders, or alcohol dependence.

• Use cautiously in patients at high risk for developing seizures and in those who have recently received multiple doses of a parenteral benzodiazepine, who display signs of seizure activity, or who may be at risk for benzodiazepine dependence, such as ICU patients.

Dialyzable drug: No.

⚠ *Overdose S&S:* Anxiety, agitation, increased muscle tone, hyperesthesia, seizures.

PREGNANCY-LACTATION-REPRODUCTION

• There are no adequate and well-controlled studies in pregnant women. Use during pregnancy only if benefit outweighs risk to the fetus.

• It isn't known if drug appears in human milk. Use cautiously in breastfeeding women.

NURSING CONSIDERATIONS

• Monitor patient closely for resedation, respiratory depression, or other residual effects that may occur after reversal of benzodiazepine effects; drug's duration of action is the shortest of all benzodiazepines. Length of monitoring period depends on specific drug being reversed. Monitor patient closely after doses of long-acting benzodiazepines such as diazepam, or after high doses of short-acting benzodiazepines such as 10 mg of midazolam. In most cases, severe resedation and respiratory depression are unlikely in patients who fail to show signs of resedation 2 hours after a 1-mg dose.

• Repeat doses of flumazenil in patients with liver disease should be reduced in size or frequency because flumazenil clearance is reduced to 40% to 60% of normal in patients with mild to moderate hepatic disease and to 25% of normal in patients with severe hepatic dysfunction; dose of flumazenil used for initial reversal of benzodiazepine effects isn't affected.

Black Box Warning Monitor patients for seizures, especially those who have been on benzodiazepines for long-term sedation or in overdose cases in which patients are showing signs of serious TCA overdose. Practitioners should individualize flumazenil dosage and be prepared to manage seizures. ∎

PATIENT TEACHING

• Warn patient not to perform hazardous activities within 24 hours of procedure because of the risk of residual sedative effects of the benzodiazepine.

Reactions in bold italics are *life-threatening.* Interactions may have a *rapid onset* or a *delayed onset.*

• Tell patient to avoid alcohol, CNS depressants, and OTC drugs for 24 hours and to report all adverse reactions.

• Give family necessary instructions and provide patient with written instructions. Patient may not be able to recall information given after the procedure; drug doesn't reverse amnesic effects of benzodiazepines.

flunisolide (inhalation, intranasal)
floo-NISS-oh-lide

AeroSpan

Therapeutic class: Corticosteroids
Pharmacologic class: Corticosteroids

AVAILABLE FORMS
Oral inhalant in a hydrofluoroalkane inhaler: 80 mcg/metered dose (AeroSpan)
Nasal spray: 25 mcg/spray

INDICATIONS & DOSAGES
➤ **Chronic asthma (inhalation)**
Adults and children age 12 and older: 2 inhalations (160 mcg) with AeroSpan inhaler b.i.d. May increase dose after 2 weeks in patients who aren't adequately controlled. Titrate to lowest effective dose once asthma stability is achieved. Don't exceed 320 mcg b.i.d.
Children ages 6 to 11: 1 inhalation (80 mcg) with AeroSpan inhaler b.i.d. May increase dose after 2 weeks in patients who are not adequately controlled. Titrate to lowest effective dose once asthma stability is achieved. Don't exceed 160 mcg b.i.d.
➤ **Symptoms of seasonal or perennial allergic rhinitis (nasal spray)**
Adults and children age 15 and older: Starting dose is 2 sprays in each nostril b.i.d. If needed, may increase dosage to 2 sprays in each nostril t.i.d. Maximum total daily dose is 8 sprays in each nostril per day.
Children ages 6 to 14: Starting dose is 1 spray in each nostril t.i.d. or 2 sprays in each nostril b.i.d. Maximum total daily dose is 4 sprays in each nostril per day.

ADMINISTRATION
Inhalational
• For best results, the canister should be at room temperature before use.
• Allow at least 20 seconds between inhalations.
• Shake well before use. Prime before using for the first time by releasing two test sprays into the air away from the face. If the inhaler hasn't been used for more than 2 weeks, prime the inhaler again by releasing two test sprays into the air away from the face.
Intranasal
• Shake well before each use.
• Before first use, prime nasal spray by pushing down on pump five or six times until a fine mist appears. If pump hasn't been used for 5 days or more, it must be primed again.

ACTION
A corticosteroid that may decrease inflammation by inhibiting macrophages, T cells, eosinophils, and mediators such as leukotrienes while reducing the number of mast cells within the airway.

Route	Onset	Peak	Duration
Inhalation	1–4 wk	Unknown	Unknown
Intranasal	Unknown	Unknown	Unknown

Half-life: Inhalation, about 1¾ hours; intranasal, 1 to 2 hours.

ADVERSE REACTIONS
CNS: headache, dizziness, insomnia, migraine, pain, anxiety, depression, fatigue, vertigo. **CV:** chest pain, edema, HTN, tachycardia, palpitations. **EENT:** conjunctivitis, ear pain, nasal dryness, nasal congestion, loss of smell, epistaxis, rhinitis, laryngitis, voice alteration, taste perversion, pharyngitis, sinusitis. **GI:** dyspepsia, vomiting, diarrhea, gastroenteritis, nausea, oral moniliasis, abdominal pain, constipation, flatulence, decreased appetite, heartburn. **GU:** UTI, dysmenorrhea, vaginitis. **Metabolic:** weight gain. **Musculoskeletal:** neck pain, myalgia. **Respiratory:** cough, bronchitis. **Skin:** *erythema multiforme,* rash, pruritus, urticaria, acne vulgaris. **Other:** infection, allergic reaction.

INTERACTIONS
Inhalation
Drug-drug. *Aldesleukin:* May diminish antineoplastic effect of aldesleukin. Avoid using together.

Amphotericin B: May enhance hypokalemic effect of amphotericin B. Monitor patient.

Corticorelin: May diminish therapeutic effect of corticorelin. Monitor therapy.

CYP3A4 inhibitors (strong): May increase serum concentration of corticosteroids. Use with oral inhalation isn't recommended.

Deferasirox: May enhance adverse effects of deferasirox. Monitor patient.

Loop diuretics, thiazide diuretics: May enhance hypokalemic effect of these drugs. Monitor patient.

Drug-herb. *Echinacea:* May diminish therapeutic effect of immunosuppressants. Consider therapy modification.

Intranasal. None significant.

EFFECTS ON LAB TEST RESULTS
• May decrease bone mineral density.

CONTRAINDICATIONS & CAUTIONS
• Contraindicated in patients hypersensitive to drug. Inhalation formulation is contraindicated in patients for primary treatment of status asthmaticus or acute asthma episodes.

• Inhalational drug isn't recommended in patients with nonasthmatic bronchial diseases or with asthma controlled by bronchodilator or other noncorticosteroid alone.

• Use cautiously, if at all, in patients with active or quiescent respiratory tract TB infections or untreated fungal, bacterial, or systemic viral or ocular herpes simplex infections.

❸ *Alert:* Drug is absorbed into the circulation, and excessive doses may suppress HPA axis function.

• Use intranasal form cautiously in patients who have recently had nasal septal ulcers, nasal surgery, or nasal trauma.

Dialyzable drug: Unknown.

PREGNANCY-LACTATION-REPRODUCTION
• Use during pregnancy only if potential benefit justifies potential risk to the fetus.

• Inhaled corticosteroids are likely acceptable to use in pregnant and breastfeeding women when weighed against patient's risk of asthma exacerbation(s).

• Use intranasal form cautiously during pregnancy and breastfeeding and at lowest effective dose.

NURSING CONSIDERATIONS
❸ *Alert:* All patients with asthma should have routine tests of adrenal cortical function, including measurement of early-morning resting cortisol levels to establish a baseline in the event of an emergency.

❸ *Alert:* There is an increased risk of death due to adrenal insufficiency in patients transferred from systemically active corticosteroids to flunisolide inhaler. Monitor patient carefully.

❸ *Alert:* Withdraw drug slowly in patients who have received long-term oral corticosteroid therapy.

❸ *Alert:* After withdrawing systemic corticosteroids, patient may need supplemental systemic corticosteroids if stress (trauma, surgery, or infection) causes adrenal insufficiency.

• If patient develops paradoxical bronchospasm immediately after using inhalational drug, treat immediately with a fast-acting bronchodilator and discontinue drug.

• Assess bone mineral density initially and periodically in patients at risk for osteoporosis who are using inhalational drug.

• Inhalational drug may increase risk of cataracts and increased IOP. Monitor patient closely.

• Intranasal drug isn't effective for acute exacerbations of rhinitis. Decongestants or antihistamines may be needed.

• Don't give intranasal drug for more than 3 weeks unless there is significant symptom improvement.

• *Look alike–sound alike:* Don't confuse flunisolide with fluocinonide.

PATIENT TEACHING
• Warn patient that drug shouldn't be used to relieve acute asthma attacks.

❸ *Alert:* Instruct patient to immediately contact prescriber if asthma episodes unresponsive to bronchodilators occur during treatment.

• Advise patient to ensure delivery of proper dose by gently warming the inhalation canister to room temperature before using.
• Children should administer drug under adult supervision.
• Tell patient who also uses a bronchodilator to use it several minutes before beginning inhalational flunisolide treatment.
• Instruct patient to begin inhaling immediately before activating the canister to get the full dose.
• Instruct patient to allow 20 seconds to elapse before repeating inhalations and to hold breath for a few seconds to enhance drug action.
• Teach patient to keep inhaler clean and unobstructed. The inhaler doesn't need cleaning during normal use.
• Advise patient that the contents are under pressure and that inhaler shouldn't be punctured or used or stored near heat or open flame.
• Tell patient to protect inhaler from freezing temperatures and prolonged exposure to sunlight. Exposure to temperatures above 120° F (49° C) may cause bursting. Caution patient never to throw into fire or incinerator.
• Advise patient to prevent oral fungal infections by gargling or rinsing mouth with water after each inhaler use. Caution patient not to swallow the water.
• Instruct patient to shake intranasal container before use, blow nose to clear nasal passages, tilt head slightly forward, and insert nozzle into nostril, pointing away from septum. Tell patient to hold other nostril closed and inhale gently while spraying and then to repeat procedure in other nostril. Advise patient to clean nosepiece with warm water daily.
• Caution patient using intranasal container not to spray in eyes.
• Explain that intranasal drug doesn't work right away. Most patients notice improvement within a few days, but some may need 2 to 3 weeks.
• Tell patient to stop intranasal drug and notify prescriber if signs and symptoms don't diminish in 3 weeks or if nasal irritation persists.
• Teach patient to check mucous membranes frequently for signs and symptoms of fungal infection.

• Warn patient to avoid exposure to chickenpox or measles. If exposed, contact prescriber immediately.
• Advise parents of a child receiving long-term therapy that the child should have periodic growth measurements and be checked for evidence of HPA axis suppression.

fluocinolone acetonide
floo-oh-SIN-oh-lone

Capex, Derma-Smoothe/FS, Dermotic, Synalar, Synalar TS, Xilapak

Therapeutic class: Corticosteroids
Pharmacologic class: Corticosteroids

AVAILABLE FORMS
Cream: 0.01%, 0.025%
Oil: 0.01%
Oil/drops (otic): 0.01%
Ointment: 0.025%
Shampoo: 0.01%
Topical solution: 0.01%

INDICATIONS & DOSAGES
➤ **Inflammation from corticosteroid-responsive dermatoses (cream, ointment, solution)**
Adults and children: Clean area; apply product sparingly b.i.d. to q.i.d.
➤ **Atopic dermatitis**
Adults: Apply thin film of body oil t.i.d.
Children age 3 months and older: Moisten skin then apply thin film of body oil b.i.d. for maximum of 4 weeks. Avoid face and diaper area.
➤ **Scalp psoriasis**
Adults: Wet or dampen hair and scalp thoroughly. Apply a thin film of scalp oil and massage into scalp. Cover with supplied shower cap overnight or for a minimum of 4 hours before washing thoroughly with regular shampoo and then rinsing thoroughly with water.
➤ **Seborrheic dermatitis of the scalp**
Adults: Apply no more than 30 mL of 0.01% shampoo to the scalp once daily, lather, and rinse thoroughly with water after 5 minutes.

➤ **Eczematous external otitis**
Adults and children age 2 and older: Apply 5 drops of oil (otic) into affected ear b.i.d. for 7 to 14 days.

ADMINISTRATION
Otic
• Tilt head to one side so the affected ear is facing up. Gently pull earlobe backward and upward and apply 5 drops of oil into the ear. Keep head tilted for at least 1 minute.
• Gently pat excess material dripping out of ear using a clean cotton ball.
Topical
• Gently wash skin before applying. To prevent skin damage, rub in gently, leaving a thin coat. When treating hairy sites, part hair and apply directly to lesions.
• Avoid application near eyes or mucous membranes; in armpits, groin, or rectal area; or in ear canal if eardrum is perforated.
• Do not use occlusive dressing unless ordered.
• For patients with eczematous dermatitis whose skin may be irritated by adhesive material, hold dressing in place with gauze, elastic bandages, stockings, or stockinette.
• Change dressing as prescribed. Stop drug and notify prescriber if skin infection, striae, or atrophy occur.
• Shake shampoo well before use. Discard shampoo after 2 months.

ACTION
Unclear. Is diffused across cell membranes to form complexes with receptors, resulting in decreased formation, release, and activity of inflammatory mediators.

Route	Onset	Peak	Duration
Otic, topical	Unknown	Unknown	Unknown

Half-life: Unknown.

ADVERSE REACTIONS
GI: diarrhea, vomiting. **GU:** glycosuria. **Metabolic:** hyperglycemia. **Respiratory:** cough. **Skin:** burning, pruritus, irritation, dryness, erythema, folliculitis, hypertrichosis, hypopigmentation, hyperpigmentation, acneiform eruptions, perioral dermatitis, allergic contact dermatitis, maceration, secondary infection, atrophy, striae, miliaria with occlusive dressings, abscess.

INTERACTIONS
None significant.

EFFECTS ON LAB TEST RESULTS
• May increase glucose level.

CONTRAINDICATIONS & CAUTIONS
• Contraindicated in patients hypersensitive to drug or its components.
• Don't use as monotherapy in primary bacterial infections (impetigo, paronychia, erysipelas, cellulitis, angular cheilitis), treatment of rosacea, perioral dermatitis, or acne.
• Drug isn't for ophthalmic use.
Dialyzable drug: Unknown.
⚠ *Overdose S&S:* Systemic effects.

PREGNANCY-LACTATION-REPRODUCTION
• Use cautiously in pregnant and breastfeeding women at lowest effective dose.

NURSING CONSIDERATIONS
• If an occlusive dressing has been applied and a fever develops, notify prescriber and remove dressing.
• If antifungal or antibiotic combined with corticosteroid fails to provide prompt improvement, stop corticosteroid until infection is controlled.
• Systemic absorption is likely with use of occlusive dressings, prolonged treatment, or extensive body surface treatment. Watch for symptoms, such as hyperglycemia, glycosuria, HPA axis suppression, or Cushing syndrome.
• Avoid using plastic pants or tight-fitting diapers on treated areas in young children. Children may absorb larger amounts of drug and be more susceptible to systemic toxicity.
🕭 *Alert:* Body oil and scalp oil formulations contain peanut oil.
• *Look alike–sound alike:* Don't confuse fluocinolone with fluocinonide or fluticasone.

PATIENT TEACHING
• Teach patient or family how to apply drug using gloves or sterile applicator.
• Tell patient to wash hands after application.
• If an occlusive dressing is used, advise patient to leave it in place for no longer than 12 hours each day and not to use dressing on infected or weeping lesions.

- Tell patient to stop using solution and notify prescriber if signs of systemic absorption, skin irritation or ulceration, hypersensitivity, or infection develop.
- Advise patient using the shampoo not to bandage, cover, or wrap the treated scalp area unless directed.

fluocinonide
floo-oh-SIN-oh-nide

Lidex, Vanos

Therapeutic class: Corticosteroids
Pharmacologic class: Corticosteroids

AVAILABLE FORMS
Cream: 0.05%, 0.1%
Gel: 0.05%
Ointment: 0.05%
Topical solution: 0.05%

INDICATIONS & DOSAGES
➤ **Inflammation from corticosteroid-responsive dermatoses**
Adults and children age 12 and older: Clean area; apply cream, gel, ointment, or topical solution sparingly b.i.d. to q.i.d. In children, use lowest dosage that promotes healing. If using Vanos 0.1% cream in adults and children age 12 and older, apply a thin layer once daily or b.i.d. for up to 2 weeks. Maximum, 60 g/week.

ADMINISTRATION
Topical
- Gently wash skin before applying. To prevent skin damage, rub in gently, leaving a thin coat. When treating hairy sites, part hair and apply directly to lesion.
- Avoid applying near eyes or mucous membranes or in ear canal.
- Occlusive dressings may be used in severe or resistant dermatoses.
- For patients with eczematous dermatitis whose skin may be irritated by adhesive material, hold dressing in place with gauze, elastic bandages, stockings, or stockinette.
- Change dressing as prescribed. Stop drug and notify prescriber if skin infection, striae, or atrophy occur.

- Continue treatment for a few days after lesions clear.

ACTION
Diffuses across cell membranes to form complexes with cytoplasmic receptors.

Route	Onset	Peak	Duration
Topical	Unknown	Unknown	Unknown

Half-life: Unknown.

ADVERSE REACTIONS
GU: glycosuria. **Metabolic:** hyperglycemia. **Skin:** burning, pruritus, irritation, dryness, erythema, folliculitis, hypertrichosis, hypopigmentation, acneiform eruptions, perioral dermatitis, allergic contact dermatitis, maceration, secondary infection, atrophy, striae, miliaria with occlusive dressings.

INTERACTIONS
None significant.

EFFECTS ON LAB TEST RESULTS
- May increase glucose level.

CONTRAINDICATIONS & CAUTIONS
- Contraindicated in patients hypersensitive to drug or its components.
- Don't use as monotherapy in primary bacterial infections (impetigo, paronychia, erysipelas, cellulitis, angular cheilitis), treatment of rosacea, perioral dermatitis, or acne.
- Don't use very-high-potency or high-potency agents on the face, groin, or armpits.
- Drug isn't for ophthalmic use.
Dialyzable drug: Unknown.
⚠ **Overdose S&S:** Systemic effects.

PREGNANCY-LACTATION-REPRODUCTION
- Use cautiously in pregnant and breastfeeding women at lowest effective dose.

NURSING CONSIDERATIONS
- If an occlusive dressing has been applied and a fever develops, notify prescriber and remove dressing.
- If antifungal or antibiotic combined with corticosteroid fails to provide prompt improvement, stop corticosteroid until infection is controlled.

• Systemic absorption is likely with use of occlusive dressings, prolonged treatment, or extensive body surface treatment. Watch for such symptoms as hyperglycemia, glycosuria, and HPA axis suppression.

• Avoid using plastic pants or tight-fitting diapers on treated areas in young children. Children may absorb larger amounts of drug and be more susceptible to systemic toxicity.

• *Look alike–sound alike:* Don't confuse fluocinonide with fluocinolone or fluticasone.

PATIENT TEACHING

• Teach patient and family how to apply drug using careful hand washing and gloves or sterile applicator.

• If an occlusive dressing is ordered, advise patient to leave it in place no more than 12 hours each day and not to use the dressing on infected or weeping lesions.

• Tell patient to stop drug and report signs of systemic absorption, skin irritation or ulceration, hypersensitivity, or infection.

SAFETY ALERT!

fluorouracil (5-FU)
flure-oh-YOOR-a-sill

Carac, Efudex, Fluoroplex, Tolak

Therapeutic class: Antineoplastics
Pharmacologic class: Pyrimidine analogues

AVAILABLE FORMS
Cream: 0.5%, 1%, 4%, 5%
Injection: 50 mg/mL
Topical solution: 2%, 5%

INDICATIONS & DOSAGES
Adjust-a-dose (for all IV indications): Individualize 5-FU dosage and dosing schedule based on tumor type, specific regimen administered, disease state, response to treatment, and patient risk factors. Refer to manufacturer's instructions for toxicity-related dosage adjustments.

➤ **Colon and rectal adenocarcinoma**
Adults (infusional regimen in combination with leucovorin alone, or in combination with leucovorin and oxaliplatin or irinotecan): 400 mg/m^2 by IV bolus on day 1, followed by 1,200 to 1,500 mg/m^2 IV as a continuous infusion over 46 hours every 2 weeks.

Adults (bolus dosing regimen in combination with leucovorin): 500 mg/m^2 by IV bolus on days 1, 8, 15, 22, 29, and 36 in 8-week cycles for four cycles.

➤ **Breast adenocarcinoma as part of a cyclophosphamide-based multidrug regimen**
Adults: 500 or 600 mg/m^2 IV on days 1 and 8 every 28 days for six cycles.

➤ **Gastric adenocarcinoma as part of a platinum-containing multidrug chemotherapy regimen**
Adults: 200 to 1,000 mg/m^2 IV as a continuous infusion over 24 hours. Frequency of dosing in each cycle and length of each cycle will depend on the dose of 5-FU injection and the specific regimen administered.

➤ **Pancreatic adenocarcinoma in combination with leucovorin or as a component of a multidrug chemotherapy regimen that includes leucovorin**
Adults: 400 mg/m^2 IV bolus on day 1, followed by 1,200 mg/m^2 IV as a continuous infusion over 46 hours every 2 weeks.

➤ **Multiple actinic (solar) keratoses**
Adults: Apply Carac cream (0.5%) once daily for up to 4 weeks. Apply Tolak cream (4%) once daily for 4 weeks. Or, apply Efudex (5%) cream or topical solution or Fluoroplex cream (1%) b.i.d. for 2 to 6 weeks.

➤ **Superficial basal cell carcinoma**
Adults: Apply 5% Efudex cream or topical solution b.i.d. usually for 3 to 6 weeks; maximum, 12 weeks.

➤ **Anal carcinoma, in combination with mitomycin and radiation ◆**
Adults: 1,000 mg/m^2/day continuous IV infusion days 1 to 4 and days 29 to 32.

➤ **Muscle-invasive bladder cancer, in combination with mitomycin and radiation ◆**
Adults: 500 mg/m^2/day continuous IV infusion during radiation therapy fractions 1 to 5 and 16 to 20.

➤ **Cervical cancer, in combination with cisplatin and radiation ◆**
Adults: 1,000 mg/m^2/day continuous IV infusion days 1 to 4 every 3 weeks for three cycles.

➤ **Advanced esophageal cancer, in combination with mitomycin and cisplatin ◆**

Adults: 300 mg/m²/day continuous IV infusion for up to 6 months.

➤ **Preoperatively and postoperatively for management of adenocarcinoma of the stomach, esophagogastric junction, or lower esophagus, in combination with epirubicin and cisplatin ◆**

Adults: 200 mg/m²/day continuous IV infusion days 1 to 21 every 3 weeks for six cycles (three cycles preoperatively and three cycles postoperatively).

➤ **Gastric and gastroesophageal cancer, in combination with cisplatin and docetaxel ◆**

Adults: 750 mg/m²/day continuous IV infusion days 1 to 5 every 3 weeks until disease progression or unacceptable toxicity occurs.

➤ **Advanced esophagogastric cancer, in combination with epirubicin and either cisplatin or oxaliplatin ◆**

Adults: 200 mg/m²/day continuous IV infusion days 1 to 21 every 3 weeks for a planned duration of 24 weeks.

➤ **Preoperative esophageal cancer, in combination with cisplatin and radiation ◆**

Adults: 1,000 mg/m²/day continuous IV infusion days 1 to 4 and days 29 to 32 of a 35-day treatment cycle.

➤ **Head and neck cancer ◆**

Adults: 1,000 mg/m²/day continuous IV infusion days 1 to 4 every 3 weeks (in combination with cisplatin) for at least six cycles, or 1,000 mg/m²/day continuous IV infusion days 1 to 4 every 4 weeks (in combination with carboplatin), or 600 mg/m²/day continuous IV infusion days 1 to 4, 22 to 25, and 43 to 46 (in combination with carboplatin and radiation).

Or, 1,000 mg/m²/day continuous IV infusion days 1 to 4 every 3 weeks (in combination with docetaxel and cisplatin) for three cycles, followed by chemoradiotherapy, or 750 mg/m²/day continuous IV infusion days 1 to 5 every 3 weeks (in combination with docetaxel and cisplatin) for up to four cycles, followed by radiation in patients without progressive disease.

Or, 1,000 mg/m²/day continuous IV infusion days 1 to 4 every 3 weeks (in combination with cetuximab and either cisplatin or carboplatin) for a total of up to six cycles.

ADMINISTRATION

IV

▼ Preparing and giving parenteral drug may be mutagenic, teratogenic, or carcinogenic. Follow facility policy to reduce risks.

▼ To reduce nausea, give antiemetic before 5-FU.

▼ Don't use cloudy solution. If crystals form, redissolve by warming and shaking vigorously. Allow solution to cool to body temperature before administration.

▼ May give drug by direct injection without dilution or as a continuous infusion. IV administration rates vary by protocol. Refer to specific reference for protocol.

▼ For infusion, dilute drug with D₅W, sterile water for injection, or NSS for injection.

▼ For continuous infusion, use plastic IV containers. Solution is more stable in plastic than in glass bottles.

▼ For IV infusion regimens, administer through CVAD using an infusion pump.

⚠️ **Alert:** Serious dosing errors involving continuous ambulatory infusion pumps have occurred. Carefully select the device and double-check flow rate. Drug should be prescribed in single daily doses (not course doses) and include instructions to infuse over a specific time period. Utilize independent double-checks during administration.

▼ Don't refrigerate. Protect drug from sunlight.

▼ Can store diluted solutions and syringes (nondiluted) at room temperature for up to 4 hours.

▼ **Incompatibilities:** Don't administer in same IV line concomitantly with other medicinal products.

Topical

• Use appropriate precautions for receiving, handling, administering, and disposing of drug. Wear gloves (single) during receiving, unpacking, and placing in storage.

• Apply topical form cautiously near patient's eyes, nose, and mouth.

• Not for vaginal use.

- Apply 10 minutes after washing, rinsing, and drying affected area.
- Avoid occlusive dressings with topical form because they increase risk of inflammatory reactions in adjacent normal skin.
- Apply topical form with nonmetal applicator or suitable gloves. Wash hands immediately after handling topical form.
- The 1% topical strength is used on patient's face. Higher strengths, such as 5%, are used for thicker skinned areas or resistant lesions, such as superficial basal cell carcinoma.

ACTION

Nucleoside metabolic inhibitor that interferes with DNA and RNA synthesis, leading to a thymine deficiency that provokes unbalanced growth and death of the cell.

Route	Onset	Peak	Duration
IV, topical	Unknown	Unknown	Unknown

Half-life: 16 minutes (IV).

ADVERSE REACTIONS

CNS: malaise, acute cerebellar syndrome, headache, disorientation, confusion. **EENT:** visual changes, lacrimal duct stenosis, photophobia. **GI:** stomatitis, GI ulcer, nausea, vomiting, diarrhea, anorexia, *GI bleeding.* **Hematologic:** *leukopenia, thrombocytopenia, agranulocytosis,* anemia. **Skin:** dermatitis, erythema, scaling, pruritus, nail changes, pigmented palmar creases, erythematous contact dermatitis, desquamative rash of hands and feet, hand-foot syndrome with long-term use, photosensitivity reactions, reversible alopecia, pain, burning, soreness, suppuration, swelling, dryness, erosion with topical use. **Other:** *hypersensitivity reactions.*

INTERACTIONS

Drug-drug. *Leucovorin calcium:* May increase cytotoxicity and toxicity of fluorouracil. Monitor patient closely.
Live-virus vaccines: May increase risk of vaccine-induced adverse reactions. Concomitant use isn't recommended.
Warfarin: May prolong PT and increase INR. Monitor PT and INR closely; adjust warfarin dosage accordingly.

Drug-lifestyle. *Sun exposure:* May cause photosensitivity reactions. Advise patient to avoid excessive sunlight exposure.

EFFECTS ON LAB TEST RESULTS

- May increase alkaline phosphatase, AST, ALT, bilirubin, 5-hydroxyindoleacetic acid (in urine), and LDH levels. May decrease Hb and plasma albumin levels.
- May decrease granulocyte, platelet, RBC, and WBC counts.

CONTRAINDICATIONS & CAUTIONS

- Contraindicated in patients hypersensitive to drug. Some topical dosage forms contain peanut oil.

⚕ Patients with dihydropyrimidine dehydrogenase gene mutations have increased risk of acute early-onset of toxicity and severe, life-threatening, or fatal adverse reactions. Drug may need to be withheld or permanently discontinued based on clinical assessment of toxicities.

❸ *Alert:* Withhold IV drug for cardiotoxicity, hyperammonemic encephalopathy, neurologic toxicity, GI toxicity, hand-foot syndrome, and severe hematologic toxicity. Bone marrow suppression can be fatal.

- Use cautiously in patients who have received high-dose pelvic radiation or alkylating drugs and in those with impaired hepatic or renal function or widespread neoplastic infiltration of bone marrow.

Dialyzable drug: Yes.

⚠ *Overdose S&S:* Nausea, vomiting, diarrhea, GI ulceration and bleeding, bone marrow depression (thrombocytopenia, leukopenia, agranulocytosis).

PREGNANCY-LACTATION-REPRODUCTION

- There are no well-controlled studies in pregnant women. Drug may cause fetal harm. Use during pregnancy only if potential benefit justifies potential risk to the fetus. Inform patient about potential fetal hazard.
- Topical formulations contraindicated in women who are or may become pregnant during therapy.
- Women of childbearing potential and males with partners of childbearing potential should use effective contraception during therapy and for 3 months after final dose.
- Contraindicated in breastfeeding women.

Reactions in bold italics are *life-threatening*. Interactions may have a *rapid onset* or a *delayed onset*.

NURSING CONSIDERATIONS

⚠ *Alert:* IV drug should be administered under the supervision of a physician experienced in cancer chemotherapy. Patient should be hospitalized at least during the initial course of IV therapy.

• Ingestion and systemic absorption of topical form may cause leukopenia, thrombocytopenia, stomatitis, diarrhea, or GI ulceration, bleeding, and hemorrhage. Application to large ulcerated areas may cause systemic toxicity.

• Monitor patient and withhold drug and notify prescriber for signs and symptoms of cardiotoxicity (angina, MI, ischemia, arrhythmia, HF), neurologic toxicity (confusion, disorientation, ataxia, visual disturbances), GI toxicities (severe diarrhea, mucositis, stomatitis, or esophagopharyngitis with mucosal sloughing or ulceration), hyperammonemic encephalopathy (altered mental status, confusion, disorientation, coma, or ataxia, with elevated serum ammonia level), hand-foot syndrome (tingling pain, edema, erythema with tenderness, skin desquamation), and severe hematologic toxicity (neutropenia, thrombocytopenia, anemia).

• Encourage diligent oral hygiene to prevent superinfection of denuded mucosa.

• Monitor CBC with differential and platelet count before each treatment cycle and as clinically indicated.

• Watch for ecchymoses, petechiae, easy bruising, and anemia, especially in patients taking warfarin.

• Monitor fluid intake and output, LFT values, and renal function test results.

• Long-term use may cause erythematous, desquamative rash of the hands and feet (hand-foot syndrome). Syndrome gradually resolves over 5 to 7 days after therapy interruption.

• Dermatologic adverse effects are reversible when drug is stopped.

• To prevent bleeding, avoid IM injections when platelet count is below 50,000/mm^3.

• Anticipate blood transfusions because of cumulative anemia.

⚠ *Alert:* Toxicity may be delayed for 1 to 3 weeks.

• The WBC count nadir occurs 9 to 14 days after first dose; the platelet count nadir occurs in 7 to 14 days.

⚠ *Alert:* Drug may be ordered as "5-fluorouracil" or "5-FU." The numeral "5" is part of the drug name and shouldn't be confused with dosage units.

• *Look alike–sound alike:* Don't confuse fluorouracil with floxuridine, fludarabine, or flucytosine.

PATIENT TEACHING

• Advise patient to immediately report all adverse reactions, especially infection, bleeding, chest pain, palpitations, swelling, dyspnea, severe nausea, vomiting, diarrhea, dark urine, yellowing of skin or eyes, malaise, confusion, visual or gait disturbances, or redness of hands or feet.

• Advise patient to take temperature daily and to immediately report signs or symptoms of infection.

• Warn patient that hair loss may occur but usually is reversible after drug is stopped.

• Caution patient to avoid prolonged exposure to sunlight or ultraviolet light when topical form is used.

• Tell patient to use highly protective sunblock to avoid inflammatory skin irritation.

• Warn patient that topically treated area may be unsightly during therapy and for several weeks afterward. Complete healing may take 1 or 2 months.

• Advise female patient of childbearing potential and male patient with partner of childbearing potential to use effective contraception during therapy and for 3 months after final dose.

• Inform female patient not to breastfeed.

FLUoxetine hydrochloride

floo-OX-e-teen

Prozac◊, Sarafem

Therapeutic class: Antidepressants
Pharmacologic class: SSRIs

AVAILABLE FORMS

Capsules (delayed-release) ⓜ: 90 mg
Capsules (pulvules): 10 mg, 20 mg, 40 mg

Oral solution: 20 mg/5 mL
Tablets: 10 mg, 15 mg, 20 mg, 60 mg

INDICATIONS & DOSAGES
Adjust-a-dose (for all indications): For patients with renal or hepatic impairment and those taking several drugs at the same time, reduce dose or increase dosing interval.
➤ **Depression, OCD (excluding Sarafem)**
Adults: Initially, 20 mg PO in the morning; increase dosage after several weeks based on patient response. Doses over 20 mg/day can be given once daily in the morning or divided into b.i.d. dosing (morning and noon). Maximum daily dose is 80 mg.
Children ages 7 to 17 (OCD): 10 mg PO daily. After 2 weeks, increase to 20 mg daily. Dosage range is 20 to 60 mg daily.

In lower weight children, initially 10 mg/day. Consider additional dosage increases after several more weeks if insufficient clinical improvement is observed. Dosage range of 20 to 30 mg/day is recommended.
Children ages 8 to 18 (depression): 10 mg PO once daily for 1 week; then increase to 20 mg daily. Due to higher plasma levels in lower weight children, the starting and target dose in this group may be 10 mg/day. Consider a dosage increase to 20 mg/day after several weeks if insufficient clinical improvement is observed.
➤ **Maintenance therapy for depression in stabilized patients (not for newly diagnosed depression)**
Adults: 90 mg Prozac Weekly PO once weekly. Start once-weekly doses 7 days after the last daily dose of Prozac 20 mg.
➤ **Short-term and long-term treatment of bulimia nervosa (excluding Sarafem)**
Adults: 60 mg PO daily in the morning. For some patients, it may be advisable to titrate up to this target dose over several days.
➤ **Short-term treatment of panic disorder with or without agoraphobia (excluding Sarafem)**
Adults: 10 mg PO once daily for 1 week, then increase dose as needed to 20 mg daily. Maximum daily dose is 60 mg.
➤ **Depressive episodes associated with bipolar I disorder (with olanzapine)**
Adults: 20 mg PO with 5 mg PO olanzapine once daily in the evening. Dosage adjustments can be made based on efficacy and

tolerability within ranges of fluoxetine 20 to 50 mg and olanzapine 5 to 12.5 mg.
Children ages 10 to 17: Initially, 20 mg PO with 2.5 mg olanzapine PO once daily in evening. Dosage adjustments can be made based on efficacy and tolerability. Safety of doses above 12 mg olanzapine with 50 mg fluoxetine hasn't been evaluated in pediatric clinical studies.
➤ **Premenstrual dysphoric disorder**
Adults: 20 mg Sarafem PO daily continuously (every day of the menstrual cycle) or intermittently (20 mg daily starting 14 days before the anticipated onset of menstruation through first full day of menses and repeating with each new cycle). Maximum daily dose, 80 mg PO.
➤ **Treatment-resistant depression**
Adults: 20 mg PO with 5 mg PO olanzapine once daily in the evening. Dosage adjustments can be made based on efficacy and tolerability within ranges of fluoxetine 20 to 50 mg and olanzapine 5 to 20 mg.

ADMINISTRATION
PO
• Give drug without regard for food.
• Avoid giving drug in the afternoon, whenever possible, because doing so commonly causes nervousness and insomnia.
• Delayed-release capsules must be swallowed whole; don't crush or open.

ACTION
Thought to be linked to drug's inhibition of CNS neuronal uptake of serotonin.

Route	Onset	Peak	Duration
PO	Unknown	6–8 hr	Unknown

Half-life: Acute administration, 1 to 3 days; long-term administration, 4 to 6 days.

ADVERSE REACTIONS
CNS: nervousness, somnolence, anxiety, insomnia, headache, drowsiness, tremor, dizziness, asthenia, abnormal thinking, fatigue, fever, emotional lability. **CV:** palpitations, hot flashes, prolonged QT interval. **EENT:** nasal congestion, pharyngitis, sinusitis. **GI:** nausea, diarrhea, dry mouth, anorexia, dyspepsia, constipation, abdominal pain, vomiting, flatulence, increased appetite, taste perversion. **GU:** sexual

---

Reactions in bold italics are *life-threatening*. Interactions may have a *rapid onset* or a *delayed onset*.

dysfunction, decreased libido, micturition disorder. **Metabolic:** weight loss, hyponatremia. **Musculoskeletal:** muscle pain. **Respiratory:** URI, cough. **Skin:** rash, pruritus, diaphoresis. **Other:** flulike syndrome, chills.

INTERACTIONS
Drug-drug. *Amphetamines, antiemetics, antipsychotics, buspirone, dextromethorphan, dihydroergotamine, lithium salts, meperidine, opioids, other SSRIs or SSNRIs (duloxetine, venlafaxine), TCAs,* **tramadol,** *trazodone, tryptophan:* May increase the risk of serotonin syndrome. Avoid combinations of drugs that increase the availability of serotonin in the CNS; monitor patient closely if used together.
Antiplatelet agents, aspirin, NSAIDs: May increase risk of bleeding. Use together cautiously.
Benzodiazepines, lithium, TCAs: May increase levels of these drugs, resulting in additional CNS effects. Monitor patient closely.
Beta blockers, carbamazepine, flecainide, vinblastine: May increase levels of these drugs. Monitor drug levels and monitor patient for adverse reactions.
Cyclosporine: May increase renal toxicity of cyclosporine. Monitor patient carefully for cyclosporine toxicity.
Cyproheptadine: May reverse or decrease fluoxetine effect. Monitor patient closely.
Dextromethorphan: May cause unusual side effects such as visual hallucinations. Advise use of cough suppressant that doesn't contain dextromethorphan while taking fluoxetine.
Highly protein-bound drugs: May increase level of fluoxetine or other highly protein-bound drugs. Monitor patient closely.
Insulin, oral antidiabetics: May alter glucose level and antidiabetic requirements. Adjust dosage.
Linezolid, methylene blue: May cause serotonin syndrome. Use extreme caution and monitor closely.
MAO inhibitors (phenelzine, selegiline, tranylcypromine): May cause serotonin syndrome and signs and symptoms resembling NMS. Avoid using at the same time and for at least 5 weeks after stopping fluoxetine.

Phenytoin: May increase phenytoin level and risk of toxicity. Monitor phenytoin level and adjust dosage.
Pimozide, thioridazine: May increase levels of these drugs, increasing risk of serious ventricular arrhythmias and sudden death. Don't use together and don't use thioridazine for at least 5 weeks after stopping fluoxetine.
Tamoxifen: May decrease tamoxifen plasma level, leading to breast cancer recurrence. Monitor patient carefully.
Triptans: May cause weakness, hyperreflexia, incoordination, rapid changes in BP, nausea, and diarrhea. Monitor patient closely, especially at the start of treatment and when dosage increases.
Warfarin: May increase risk for bleeding. Monitor PT and INR.
Drug-herb. *Kava kava, St. John's wort, tryptophan, valerian:* May increase sedative and hypnotic effects; may cause serotonin syndrome. Discourage use together.
Drug-lifestyle. *Alcohol use:* May increase CNS depression. Discourage use together.

EFFECTS ON LAB TEST RESULTS
• May decrease sodium level.

CONTRAINDICATIONS & CAUTIONS
• Contraindicated in patients hypersensitive to drug, with pimozide, and within 14 days of stopping an MAO inhibitor intended to treat psychiatric disorders. MAO inhibitors shouldn't be started within 5 weeks of stopping fluoxetine. Avoid using thioridazine with fluoxetine or within 5 weeks after stopping fluoxetine.

Black Box Warning Drug may increase the risk of suicidal thinking and behavior in children, adolescents, and young adults with major depressive disorder or other psychiatric disorder. ∎

Black Box Warning Fluoxetine is approved for use in children with major depressive disorder and OCD. Fluoxetine isn't approved for use in children younger than age 7. Sarafem isn't approved for use in children. ∎

🜂 *Alert:* Concomitant use with linezolid or methylene blue can cause serotonin syndrome (fever, mental status changes, muscle twitching, excessive sweating, shivering or shaking, diarrhea, loss of coordination). Use drug with linezolid or methylene blue only for life-threatening or urgent conditions when the potential benefits outweigh the risks of toxicity.

• Use cautiously in patients at high risk for suicide and in those with history of diabetes mellitus, seizures, mania, or hepatic, renal, or CV disease.

Dialyzable drug: No.

⚠ *Overdose S&S:* Nausea, seizures, somnolence, tachycardia, vomiting, coma, delirium, ECG abnormalities, hypotension, mania, NMS-like reactions, pyrexia, stupor, syncope.

PREGNANCY-LACTATION-REPRODUCTION

• Use cautiously in pregnant women and only if benefit justifies possible risk to the fetus.

• Drug appears in human milk. Use in breastfeeding women isn't recommended.

NURSING CONSIDERATIONS

☙ *Alert:* If linezolid or methylene blue must be given, fluoxetine must be stopped and patient monitored for serotonin toxicity for 5 weeks or until 24 hours after final dose of linezolid or methylene blue, whichever comes first. Treatment with fluoxetine may be resumed 24 hours after final dose of linezolid or methylene blue.

• Use antihistamines or topical corticosteroids to treat rashes or pruritus.

• Watch for weight change during therapy, particularly in underweight or bulimic patients.

• Record mood changes. Watch for suicidal tendencies.

• Drug has a long half-life; monitor patient for adverse effects for up to 2 weeks after drug is stopped.

• Monitor patient for serotonin syndrome, particularly when drug is used in combination with other serotonergic agents.

☙ *Alert:* Combining triptans with an SSRI or an SSNRI may cause serotonin syndrome or NMS-like reactions. Serotonin syndrome may be more likely to occur when starting or increasing the dose of triptan, SSRI, or SSNRI.

• Monitor blood glucose level (in diabetic patients) and liver and renal function (baseline and as clinically indicated).

• Obtain ECG and monitor periodically in patients with risk factors for QT-interval prolongation and ventricular arrhythmia.

• Monitor mental status for depression, suicidal ideation (especially at beginning of therapy and with dosage changes), anxiety, social functioning, mania, or panic attacks.

• Observe for signs or symptoms of serotonin syndrome, akathisia, or sleep disturbances.

• When discontinuing drug, taper dosage over 2 weeks to 1 month to avoid withdrawal syndrome.

• *Look alike–sound alike:* Don't confuse fluoxetine with fluvoxamine or fluvastatin. Don't confuse Prozac with Proscar or Prilosec.

PATIENT TEACHING

Black Box Warning Advise family and caregivers to carefully observe patient for worsening suicidal thinking or behavior. ∎

☙ *Alert:* Teach patient to recognize and immediately report symptoms of serotonin toxicity (fever, mental status changes, muscle twitching, excessive sweating, shivering or shaking, diarrhea, loss of coordination).

• Tell patient to avoid taking drug in the afternoon whenever possible because doing so commonly causes nervousness and insomnia.

• Drug may cause dizziness or drowsiness. Warn patient to avoid driving and other hazardous activities that require alertness and good psychomotor coordination until effects of drug are known.

• Tell patient to consult prescriber before taking other prescription or OTC drugs.

• Advise patient that full therapeutic effect may not be seen for 4 weeks or longer.

---

fluPHENAZine decanoate
floo-FEN-a-zeen

fluPHENAZine hydrochloride

Therapeutic class: Antipsychotics
Pharmacologic class: Phenothiazines

AVAILABLE FORMS
fluphenazine decanoate
Depot injection: 25 mg/mL*

---

fluphenazine hydrochloride
Elixir: 2.5 mg/5 mL*
IM injection: 2.5 mg/mL
Oral concentrate: 5 mg/mL*
Tablets: 1 mg, 2.5 mg, 5 mg, 10 mg

INDICATIONS & DOSAGES
➤ **Psychotic disorders**
Adults: Initially, 2.5 to 10 mg fluphenazine hydrochloride PO daily in divided doses every 6 to 8 hours; may increase cautiously to 20 mg/day. Maintenance dose is 1 to 5 mg PO daily. IM doses are one-third to one-half of PO doses. Usual initial IM dose is 1.25 mg. Give more than 10 mg daily with caution.

Or, 12.5 to 25 mg of fluphenazine decanoate IM or subcut every 3 to 4 weeks (response may last up to 6 weeks in some patients); maintenance dose is 25 to 100 mg, as needed.
Elderly patients: 1 to 2.5 mg fluphenazine hydrochloride PO daily.

ADMINISTRATION
PO
• Oral liquid forms can cause contact dermatitis. Wear gloves when preparing solutions, and avoid contact with skin and clothing.
• Protect drug from light. Slight yellowing of concentrate is common and doesn't affect potency. Discard markedly discolored solutions.
• Use calibrated device to measure desired dose, and dilute liquid concentrate with 60 mL of tomato or fruit juice, uncaffeinated soft drinks, or milk just before administration. Don't dilute in beverages containing caffeine (coffee, cola), tannics (tea), or pectinates (apple juice).
IM
• Parenteral forms can cause contact dermatitis. Wear gloves when preparing solutions, and avoid contact with skin and clothing.
• Protect drug from light. Slight yellowing of injection is common and doesn't affect potency. Discard markedly discolored solutions.
• For long-acting form (decanoate), which is an oil preparation, use a dry needle of at least 21G.

Subcutaneous
• Long-acting form (decanoate) is indicated for subcut administration.
• Use a dry syringe and needle of at least 21G.
• Don't use if solution is cloudy or contains particulate matter.

ACTION
A piperazine phenothiazine that blocks postsynaptic dopamine receptors in the brain.

Route	Onset	Peak	Duration
PO	<1 hr	2.8 hr	6–8 hr
IM (decanoate)	24–72 hr	8–10 hr	4 wk
IM (hydrochloride)	<1 hr	90–120 min	6–8 hr
Subcut	Unknown	Unknown	Unknown

Half-life: Decanoate, 14 days; hydrochloride, 15 hours.

ADVERSE REACTIONS
CNS: extrapyramidal reactions, tardive dyskinesia, pseudoparkinsonism, *seizures, NMS,* sedation, EEG changes, drowsiness, dizziness. **CV:** orthostatic hypotension, tachycardia, ECG changes. **EENT:** blurred vision, ocular changes, nasal congestion. **GI:** dry mouth, constipation, increased appetite. **GU:** urine retention, dark urine, menstrual irregularities, inhibited ejaculation. **Hematologic:** *leukopenia, agranulocytosis, aplastic anemia, thrombocytopenia,* eosinophilia, hemolytic anemia. **Hepatic:** cholestatic jaundice. **Metabolic:** weight gain. **Skin:** mild photosensitivity reactions, allergic reactions. **Other:** gynecomastia, galactorrhea.

INTERACTIONS
Drug-drug. *Antacids:* May inhibit absorption of oral phenothiazines. Separate antacid and phenothiazine doses by at least 2 hours.
Anticholinergics: May increase anticholinergic effects. Use together cautiously.
Barbiturates, lithium: May decrease phenothiazine effect and increase neurologic adverse effects. Monitor patient.
Centrally acting antihypertensives: May decrease antihypertensive effect. Monitor BP.
CNS depressants: May increase CNS depression. Use together cautiously.

F

Black Box Warning *Opioid class warning:*
May cause slow or difficult breathing, sedation, and death. Avoid use together. If use together is necessary, limit dosage and duration of each drug to the minimum necessary for desired effect. ∎

Drug-herb. *St. John's wort:* May increase risk of photosensitivity reactions. Advise patient to avoid excessive sunlight exposure.

Drug-lifestyle. *Alcohol use:* May increase CNS depression, especially that involving psychomotor skills. Strongly discourage alcohol use.

Sun exposure: May increase risk of photosensitivity reactions. Advise patient to avoid excessive sunlight exposure.

EFFECTS ON LAB TEST RESULTS

• May increase LFT values. May decrease Hb level and hematocrit.

• May increase eosinophil count. May decrease granulocyte, platelet, and WBC counts.

• May cause false-positive results for urine pregnancy tests that use human chorionic gonadotropin.

CONTRAINDICATIONS & CAUTIONS

• Contraindicated in patients hypersensitive to drug and in those with coma, CNS depression, bone marrow suppression or other blood dyscrasia, subcortical damage, or liver damage.

Black Box Warning *Opioid class warning:*
Opioids should only be prescribed with benzodiazepines or other CNS depressants to patients for whom alternative treatment options are inadequate. ∎

• Use cautiously in elderly or debilitated patients and in those with pheochromocytoma, severe CV disease (may cause sudden drop in BP), peptic ulcer, respiratory disorder, hypocalcemia, seizure disorder (drug may lower seizure threshold), severe reactions to insulin or electroconvulsive therapy, mitral insufficiency, glaucoma, or prostatic hyperplasia.

• Use cautiously in patients exposed to extreme heat or cold (including antipyretic therapy) or phosphorus insecticides.

Dialyzable drug: Unknown.

⚠ *Overdose S&S:* Stupor, coma, seizures in children.

PREGNANCY-LACTATION-REPRODUCTION

• Safe use during pregnancy hasn't been established. Use if only clearly needed and if benefit justifies risk.

① *Alert:* Neonates exposed to antipsychotics during the third trimester are at risk for developing extrapyramidal signs and symptoms (repetitive muscle movements of the face and body) and withdrawal signs and symptoms (agitation, abnormally increased or decreased muscle tone, tremors, sleepiness, severe difficulty breathing, difficulty feeding) after delivery.

• Drug may appear in human milk. Use cautiously in breastfeeding women.

NURSING CONSIDERATIONS

• Monitor patient for tardive dyskinesia, which may occur after prolonged use. It may not appear until months or years later and may disappear spontaneously or persist for life, despite ending drug.

① *Alert:* Watch for signs and symptoms of NMS (extrapyramidal effects, hyperthermia, autonomic disturbance), which is rare but often fatal. It may not be related to length of drug use or type of neuroleptic.

• Withhold dose and notify prescriber if patient, especially child or pregnant woman, develops signs or symptoms of blood dyscrasia (fever, sore throat, infection, cellulitis, weakness) or extrapyramidal reactions persisting longer than a few hours.

Black Box Warning Elderly patients with dementia-related psychosis treated with atypical or conventional antipsychotics are at increased risk for death. Antipsychotics aren't approved for the treatment of dementia-related psychosis. ∎

• May increase the risk of falls due to somnolence, orthostatic hypotension, and motor or sensory instability. Complete fall risk assessments at baseline and periodically during treatment in patients with diseases or on medications that may also increase fall risk.

• Don't withdraw drug abruptly unless serious adverse reactions occur.

• Abrupt withdrawal of long-term therapy may cause gastritis, nausea, vomiting, dizziness, tremor, feeling of warmth or cold, diaphoresis, tachycardia, headache, or insomnia.

Reactions in bold italics are *life-threatening*. Interactions may have a *rapid onset* or a *delayed onset*.

PATIENT TEACHING

Black Box Warning *Opioid class warning:* Caution patient or caregiver of patient taking an opioid with a benzodiazepine, CNS depressant, or alcohol to seek immediate medical attention for dizziness, light-headedness, extreme sleepiness, slowed or difficult breathing, or unresponsiveness. ∎

• Warn patient to avoid activities that require alertness and good coordination until effects of drug are known. Drowsiness and dizziness usually subside after first few weeks.

• Warn patient to avoid alcohol while taking drug.

• Tell patient to relieve dry mouth with sugarless gum or hard candy.

• Have patient report signs of urine retention or constipation.

• Advise patient to use sunblock and wear protective clothing to avoid sensitivity to the sun.

• Tell patient that drug may discolor urine.

SAFETY ALERT!

flutamide
FLOO-ta-mide

Therapeutic class: Antineoplastics
Pharmacologic class: Nonsteroidal antiandrogens

AVAILABLE FORMS
Capsules: 125 mg, 250 mg✲

INDICATIONS & DOSAGES
➤ **Metastatic locally confined prostate cancer (stages B₂, C, D₂), combined with luteinizing hormone-releasing hormone analogues, such as leuprolide acetate or goserelin**
Men: 250 mg PO every 8 hours.

ADMINISTRATION
PO
• Drug is a hormonal agent and is considered a potential teratogen. Follow safe handling procedures.
• Give drug without regard for food.

ACTION
Inhibits androgen uptake or prevents binding of androgens in nucleus of cells in target tissues.

Route	Onset	Peak	Duration
PO	Unknown	2 hr	Unknown

Half-life: For steady-state metabolite, about 6 hours.

ADVERSE REACTIONS
CNS: drowsiness, confusion, depression, anxiety, nervousness, paresthesia. **CV:** peripheral edema, HTN, hot flashes. **GI:** diarrhea, nausea, vomiting, anorexia. **GU:** erectile dysfunction, urine discoloration, cystitis, decreased libido, impotence. **Hematologic:** anemia, *leukopenia, thrombocytopenia,* hemolytic anemia. **Skin:** injection-site reaction, rash, photosensitivity reactions. **Other:** gynecomastia.

INTERACTIONS
Drug-drug. *Warfarin:* May prolong PT. Monitor PT and INR.
Drug-lifestyle. *Sun exposure:* May cause photosensitivity reactions. Advise patient to avoid excessive sunlight exposure.

EFFECTS ON LAB TEST RESULTS
• May increase BUN, creatinine, Hb, and liver enzyme levels.
• May decrease platelet and WBC counts.
• May alter pituitary-gonadal system tests during therapy and for 12 weeks after.

CONTRAINDICATIONS & CAUTIONS
• Contraindicated in patients hypersensitive to drug, in those with severe liver dysfunction, and in women.
Dialyzable drug: Unlikely.
⚠ *Overdose S&S:* Gynecomastia, breast tenderness, increased AST level.

PREGNANCY-LACTATION-REPRODUCTION
• Not indicated for use in women. May cause fetal harm.

NURSING CONSIDERATIONS
Black Box Warning Drug may cause liver failure. Obtain LFTs before the start of therapy, monthly for the first 4 months of therapy, periodically thereafter, and at the first

signs and symptoms suggesting liver dysfunction (nausea, vomiting, anorexia, fatigue). Immediately stop drug if jaundice occurs or AST level rises above 2 × ULN. ∎

• Monitor CBC periodically.

• Monitor PSA.

• Patients with hemoglobin M disease or G6PD deficiency and smokers are at risk for methemoglobinemia, hemolytic anemia, and cholestatic jaundice. Monitor methemoglobin level.

• Flutamide must be taken continuously with drug used for medical castration (such as leuprolide) to allow full therapeutic benefit. Leuprolide suppresses testosterone production, whereas flutamide inhibits testosterone action at cellular level; together, they can impair growth of androgen-responsive tumors.

PATIENT TEACHING

• Advise patient not to stop drug without consulting prescriber.

• Tell patient drug may be taken without food, but if stomach irritation occurs, to take with food.

• Instruct patient to report adverse reactions promptly, especially dark yellow or brown urine, vomiting, or yellowing of the eyes or skin.

---

fluticasone furoate
floo-TIK-a-sone

Arnuity Ellipta, Flonase Sensimist Allergy Relief ◇

fluticasone propionate
Armonair RespiClick, Flonase Allergy Relief ◇, Flovent Diskus, Flovent HFA, Xhance

Therapeutic class: Corticosteroids
Pharmacologic class: Corticosteroids

AVAILABLE FORMS
Nasal spray (furoate): 27.5 mcg/spray
Nasal spray (propionate): 50 mcg/metered spray, 93 mcg/metered spray
Oral inhalation aerosol: 44 mcg, 110 mcg, 220 mcg

Oral inhalation powder: 50 mcg, 55 mcg, 100 mcg, 113 mcg, 200 mcg, 232 mcg, 250 mcg

INDICATIONS & DOSAGES
➤ **As preventive in maintenance of chronic asthma in patients requiring oral corticosteroid**
Armonair RespiClick
Adults and children age 12 and older: For patients not on inhaled corticosteroids, usual starting dose is 55 mcg b.i.d. After 2 weeks may increase dosage to provide additional asthma control.

For adults and children previously taking inhaled corticosteroids, base dosage on strength of the previously inhaled corticosteroid product and disease severity. Initially, 55 to 232 mcg b.i.d. Maximum benefit may not be achieved for 2 weeks after start of treatment.
Flovent Diskus
Adults and children age 12 and older not on an inhaled corticosteroid: Initially, inhaled dose of 100 mcg b.i.d. approximately 12 hours apart. For patients who don't respond adequately to starting dosage after 2 weeks of therapy, may increase dosage to maximum of 1,000 mcg b.i.d.
Adults and children age 12 and older previously taking inhaled corticosteroids: Base dosage on strength of previously inhaled corticosteroid product and disease severity, including consideration of patient's current control of asthma symptoms and risk of future exacerbation, to maximum of 1,000 mcg b.i.d.
Children ages 4 to 11: For patients not on an inhaled corticosteroid, recommended starting dosage is 50 mcg b.i.d. approximately 12 hours apart. For other patients, and for patients who don't respond adequately to starting dosage after 2 weeks of therapy, may increase dosage to maximum 100 mcg b.i.d.
Flovent HFA
Adults and children age 12 and older not on an inhaled corticosteroid: Initially, inhaled dose of 88 mcg b.i.d. approximately 12 hours apart. For patients who don't respond adequately to starting dosage after 2 weeks of therapy, may increase dosage to maximum of 880 mcg b.i.d.

Reactions in bold italics are *life-threatening*. Interactions may have a *rapid onset* or a *delayed onset*.

Adults and children age 12 and older previously taking inhaled corticosteroids: Base dosage on strength of previously inhaled corticosteroid product and disease severity, including consideration of patient's current control of asthma symptoms and risk of future exacerbation, to maximum of 880 mcg b.i.d.

Children ages 4 to 11: 88 mcg inhaled b.i.d. approximately 12 hours apart, regardless of prior therapy.

Arnuity Ellipta

Adults and children age 12 and older: Base starting dosage on patient's asthma severity. Usual recommended starting dose for patients not on an inhaled corticosteroid is 100 mcg given as 1 inhalation at the same time every day. For other patients, base starting dose on previous asthma drug therapy and disease severity. For patients who don't respond to 100 mcg after 2 weeks of therapy, replacement with 200-mcg formulation may provide additional control. Don't use more than once every 24 hours.

Children ages 5 to 11: 50 mcg given as 1 inhalation daily.

➤ **Nasal symptoms of seasonal and perennial allergic and nonallergic rhinitis**

Flonase

Adults: Initially, 2 sprays (100 mcg) in each nostril daily or 1 spray b.i.d. Once symptoms are controlled, decrease to 1 spray in each nostril daily. Or, for seasonal allergic rhinitis, 2 sprays in each nostril once daily, as needed, for symptom control.

Adolescents and children age 4 and older: Initially, 1 spray (50 mcg) in each nostril daily. If not responding, increase to 2 sprays in each nostril daily. Once symptoms are controlled, decrease to 1 spray in each nostril daily. Maximum dose is 2 sprays in each nostril daily.

Veramyst

Adults and children age 12 and older: 110 mcg once daily administered as 2 sprays (27.5 mcg/spray) in each nostril. When maximum benefit has been achieved and symptoms have been controlled, reduce dosage to 55 mcg (1 spray in each nostril) once daily.

Children ages 2 to 11: 55 mcg once daily administered as 1 spray (27.5 mcg/spray) in each nostril. May increase to 110 mcg (2 sprays in each nostril) once daily if

needed. Once symptoms have been controlled, reduce dosage to 55 mcg once daily.

➤ **Nasal polyps (*Xhance*)**

Adults: 1 spray (93 mcg/spray) in each nostril b.i.d. May increase to 2 sprays in each nostril b.i.d. (maximum dose).

ADMINISTRATION

Inhalational

• For best results, aerosol canister should be at room temperature.

• Prime and shake well before each use.

• Patients should rinse mouth after inhalation.

• Armonair RespiClick doesn't require priming. Never place inhaler in water; wipe mouthpiece clean if needed.

• Refer to specific manufacturer's guideline for discard date and storage.

Intranasal

• Prime and shake well before use.

ACTION

Anti-inflammatory and vasoconstrictor that may decrease inflammation by inhibiting mast cells, macrophages, and mediators such as leukotrienes.

Route	Onset	Peak	Duration
Inhalation (nasal)	12 hr	Several days	1–2 wk
Inhalation (oral)	24 hr	Several days	1–2 wk

Half-life: 3 hours.

ADVERSE REACTIONS

CNS: headache, dizziness, fever, migraine, nervousness. **EENT:** cataracts, conjunctivitis, dry eye, eye irritation, epistaxis, nasal burning or irritation, nasal discharge, blood in nasal mucus, rhinitis, sinusitis, pharyngitis, hoarseness, laryngitis. **GI:** oral candidiasis, abdominal discomfort, abdominal pain, diarrhea, mouth irritation, nausea, viral gastroenteritis, vomiting. **GU:** UTI. **Hematologic:** eosinophilia. **Metabolic:** cushingoid features, growth retardation in children, hyperglycemia, weight gain. **Musculoskeletal:** aches and pains, symptoms of neck sprain or strain, joint pain, muscular soreness, osteoporosis. **Respiratory:** URI, *bronchospasm,* asthma symptoms, bronchitis, chest congestion, cough, dyspnea.

F

Skin: dermatitis, urticaria. **Other:** *angioedema,* influenza, viral infections.

INTERACTIONS
Drug-drug. *Cobicistat:* May increase serum concentration of oral inhalation drug. Avoid use together.
Ketoconazole, other CYP3A4 inhibitors: May increase mean fluticasone level and systemic corticosteroid adverse effects. Use together cautiously.
Ritonavir: May cause systemic corticosteroid effects, such as Cushing syndrome and adrenal suppression. Avoid using together.

EFFECTS ON LAB TEST RESULTS
• Abnormal response to the 6-hour cosyntropin stimulation test may occur in patients taking high doses of fluticasone.

CONTRAINDICATIONS & CAUTIONS
• Contraindicated in patients hypersensitive to components in these preparations. Immediate hypersensitivity reactions, including anaphylaxis, can occur.
• Contraindicated as primary treatment of patients with status asthmaticus or other acute, intense episodes of asthma.
• Use cautiously in patients at risk for decreased bone mineralization.
• Drug can increase risk of infections, vasculitis, Kaposi sarcoma, psychiatric disturbances, HTN, fluid retention, GI perforation, and hyperglycemia.
Dialyzable drug: Unknown.
⚠ *Overdose S&S:* Hypercorticism.

PREGNANCY-LACTATION-REPRODUCTION
• Use during pregnancy only if potential benefit justifies potential risk to the fetus.
• Use cautiously in breastfeeding.

NURSING CONSIDERATIONS
• Because of risk of systemic absorption of inhaled corticosteroids, observe patient carefully for evidence of systemic corticosteroid effects.
🔆 *Alert:* Monitor patient, especially postoperatively, during periods of stress or severe asthma attack for evidence of inadequate adrenal response.

🔆 *Alert:* During withdrawal from oral corticosteroids, some patients may experience signs and symptoms of systemically active corticosteroid withdrawal, such as joint or muscle pain, lassitude, and depression, despite maintenance or even improvement of respiratory function. Deaths due to adrenal insufficiency have occurred with transfer from active corticosteroids to fluticasone propionate inhaler.
• For patients starting therapy who are currently receiving oral corticosteroid therapy, reduce dose of prednisone to no more than 2.5 mg/day on a weekly basis, beginning after at least 1 week of therapy with fluticasone.
🔆 *Alert:* As with other inhaled asthma drugs, bronchospasm may occur, with an immediate increase in wheezing after a dose. If bronchospasm occurs after a dose of inhalation aerosol, treat immediately with a fast-acting inhaled bronchodilator.
• Drug may increase risk of glaucoma and cataracts. Monitor patient.
• Inhaled corticosteroids can reduce growth trajectory in children. Monitor growth.
• If a dosage regimen fails to provide adequate control of asthma, reevaluate the therapeutic regimen and consider additional therapeutic options, such as replacing the current strength with a higher strength, initiating an inhaled corticosteroid and long-acting beta$_2$-agonist combination product, or initiating oral corticosteroids.
• After asthma stability has been achieved, titrate to the lowest effective dosage to reduce the possibility of adverse effects.

PATIENT TEACHING
• Advise patient to report all adverse reactions.
• Tell patient that inhalation drug isn't indicated for the relief of acute bronchospasm.
• Advise patient to use drug at regular intervals, as directed.
• Advise patient that maximum inhalation benefit may not be achieved for 1 to 2 weeks or longer after starting treatment.
• Instruct patient to contact prescriber if nasal spray doesn't improve condition after 4 days of treatment.
• Instruct patient to immediately contact prescriber if asthma episodes unresponsive

to bronchodilators occur during treatment with fluticasone. During such episodes, patient may need therapy with oral corticosteroids.
• Warn patient to avoid exposure to chickenpox or measles and, if exposed, to consult prescriber immediately.
• Tell patient to carry or wear medical identification indicating that patient may need supplementary corticosteroids during stress or a severe asthma attack.
⚠ *Alert:* During periods of stress or a severe asthma attack, instruct patient who has been withdrawn from systemic corticosteroids to resume prescribed oral corticosteroids immediately and to contact prescriber for further instruction.
• Teach patient how to prime and use (oral/nasal) inhaler if needed, according to manufacturer's instructions.
• Advise patient to avoid spraying inhalation aerosol into eyes.
• Advise patient to store fluticasone powder in a dry place.

fluticasone furoate–vilanterol trifenatate
floo-TIK-a-sone/vye-LAN-ter-ol

Breo Ellipta

Therapeutic class: Corticosteroids–bronchodilators
Pharmacologic class: Corticosteroids–beta$_2$-adrenergic agonists

AVAILABLE FORMS
Powder for inhalation: Inhaler containing two double-foil blister strips of powder formulation: One strip contains fluticasone furoate 100 mcg/blister or 200 mcg/blister; the other contains vilanterol 25 mcg/blister

INDICATIONS & DOSAGES
➤ **Asthma**
Adults: 1 inhalation of 100 mcg fluticasone furoate–25 mcg vilanterol trifenatate or 200 mcg fluticasone furoate–25 mcg vilanterol trifenatate once daily.
➤ **Maintenance treatment of COPD**
Adults: 1 inhalation of 100 mcg fluticasone furoate–25 mcg vilanterol trifenatate once daily.

ADMINISTRATION
Inhalational
• Patient shouldn't use more than 1 inhalation in 24 hours; may cause adverse effects.
• Have patient exhale fully before taking one long, steady, deep breath through the mouthpiece (patient shouldn't breathe through the nose), hold breath for 3 to 4 seconds, and exhale slowly and gently. After use, have patient rinse mouth with water without swallowing to help reduce the risk of oropharyngeal candidiasis.
• Give at the same time every day and not more than one time every 24 hours.
• Store at room temperature between 68° and 77° F (20° and 25° C) in a dry place away from heat and sunlight.
• Keep drug stored inside the unopened moisture-protective foil tray; remove from tray immediately before initial use.
• Discard drug 6 weeks after opening foil tray or when the counter reads "0" (after all blisters have been used).
• Inhaler isn't reusable.
• Don't attempt to take the inhaler apart.

ACTION
Fluticasone is an anti-inflammatory and vasoconstrictor that may decrease inflammation by inhibiting mast cells, macrophages, and mediators such as leukotrienes. Vilanterol trifenatate relaxes bronchial smooth muscle and inhibits inflammatory mediators, especially mast cells.

Route	Onset	Peak	Duration
Inhalation (fluticasone)	Unknown	30–60 min	Unknown
Inhalation (vilanterol)	Unknown	10 min	Unknown

Half-life: Fluticasone, 24 hours; vilanterol, 21 hours.

ADVERSE REACTIONS
CNS: headache, pyrexia. **CV:** HTN, peripheral edema, extrasystoles. **EENT:** nasopharyngitis, oropharyngeal candidiasis, oropharyngeal pain, pharyngitis, rhinitis, sinusitis. **GI:** diarrhea, upper abdominal pain. **Musculoskeletal:** back pain, arthralgia. **Respiratory:** URI, COPD, pneumonia, bronchitis, cough. **Other:** flulike symptoms.

INTERACTIONS

Drug-drug. *CYP3A4 inhibitors (clarithromycin, conivaptan, indinavir, itraconazole, ketoconazole, lopinavir, nefazodone, nelfinavir, ritonavir, saquinavir, telithromycin, troleandomycin, voriconazole):* May increase systemic effects of corticosteroids, and increased CV adverse effects may occur. Use together cautiously.

Loop or thiazide diuretics (furosemide, hydrochlorothiazide, torsemide): May increase risk of hypokalemia or ECG changes. Monitor patient closely with concurrent use.

MAO inhibitors, TCAs, other drugs known to prolong QTc interval: May increase adrenergic effects or risk of ventricular arrhythmias. Don't use together.

Nonselective beta blockers (carvedilol, propranolol, sotalol): May increase risk of bronchospasm. Use cardioselective agents only if absolutely needed.

Other long-acting beta-agonist drugs (arformoterol tartrate, formoterol fumarate, indacaterol, salmeterol): May increase risk of overdose. Don't use together.

EFFECTS ON LAB TEST RESULTS

• May increase glucose level. May decrease potassium level.

CONTRAINDICATIONS & CAUTIONS

• Contraindicated in patients with severe hypersensitivity to milk proteins and in those who have demonstrated hypersensitivity to fluticasone furoate, vilanterol, or their components.

• Use of long-acting beta$_2$-adrenergic agonists (LABAs) as monotherapy (without inhaled corticosteroids [ICS]) for asthma is associated with an increased risk of asthma-related death. Available data from controlled clinical trials also suggest that use of LABAs as monotherapy increases the risk of asthma-related hospitalization in children and adolescents. These findings are considered a class effect of LABA monotherapy. When LABAs are used in fixed-dose combination with ICS, data from large clinical trials don't show a significant increase in the risk of serious asthma-related events (hospitalizations, intubations, death) compared with ICS alone.

◑ **Alert:** Contraindicated as primary treatment of status asthmaticus or other acute episodes of COPD or asthma where other intensive measures are required.

◑ **Alert:** Don't exceed recommended dosage; serious adverse events, including fatalities, have been associated with excessive use of inhaled sympathomimetics.

• Use cautiously in patients with existing TB; fungal, bacterial, viral, or parasitic infections; or ocular herpes simplex. Drug may suppress the immune system and infection may worsen.

• Use cautiously in patients with thyrotoxicosis, diabetes mellitus, ketoacidosis, or CV disorders (coronary insufficiency, arrhythmias, HTN).

• Use cautiously in patients with increased IOP, cataracts, or glaucoma. Increased IOP, glaucoma, and cataracts have occurred with prolonged use.

• Use cautiously in patients with seizure disorders; beta agonists may cause CNS stimulation.

Dialyzable drug: Unknown.

PREGNANCY-LACTATION-REPRODUCTION

• Use cautiously in pregnant and breastfeeding women.

• Avoid use during labor as drug may interfere with uterine contractility.

NURSING CONSIDERATIONS

• If not already prescribed, initiate an inhaled, short-acting beta$_2$ agonist in patients taking this drug.

• Patients who have been taking oral or inhaled short-acting beta$_2$ agonists on a regular basis (q.i.d.) should discontinue regular use of these drugs and use them only for relief of acute respiratory symptoms.

• Determine if patient has an allergy or intolerance to lactose; anaphylactic reactions have occurred in patients with severe milk protein allergies.

• Monitor short-acting beta$_2$ agonist rescue use. Increased use signals disease deterioration.

• Slowly wean patients requiring oral corticosteroids from systemic corticosteroid use after switch to an inhaler. Reduce daily prednisone dosage by 2.5 mg on a weekly basis during therapy with inhaled drug.

Reactions in bold italics are *life-threatening*. Interactions may have a *rapid onset* or a *delayed onset*.

• Patients may require supplemental corticosteroid during times of stress when weaning from systemic corticosteroids.
• Monitor lung function and watch for COPD signs and symptoms and adrenal insufficiency (fatigue, lassitude, weakness, nausea, vomiting, hypotension).
• Discontinue drug slowly if hypercortisolism or adrenal suppression is suspected.
• Monitor patient periodically for candidal infections of the mouth. Have patient rinse mouth after inhalation without swallowing to help reduce the risk.
• Monitor patient for signs and symptoms of pneumonia.
• If paradoxical bronchospasm occurs, discontinue drug and institute alternative therapy.
• Monitor patient for increased IOP and for development or worsening of glaucoma or cataracts.
• Monitor patient for hypokalemia and hyperglycemia.
• Serious or even fatal courses of chickenpox or measles can occur in susceptible patients.
• Monitor patient for CV effects (tachycardia, HTN, supraventricular tachycardia, extrasystoles).
• Monitor patient for reduction in bone mineral density (BMD) initially and periodically with long-term use. Patients who use tobacco and those with prolonged immobilization, family history of osteoporosis, postmenopausal status, advanced age, poor nutrition, or long-term use of other drugs that can reduce BMD (anticonvulsants, oral corticosteroids) are at increased risk.
🛈 *Alert:* Orally inhaled corticosteroids may slow growth rate when given to children and adolescents.

PATIENT TEACHING
• Teach patient to rinse mouth without swallowing after inhalation to help reduce the risk of candidal infections.
• Caution patient not to use drug for acute symptoms or asthma.
• Warn patient not to use drug with other LABAs.
• Instruct patient to immediately notify health care provider if adverse reactions occur, symptoms worsen, more inhalations

than usual of rescue medication are needed, or a significant decrease in lung function occurs.
• Instruct patient not to discontinue drug without the guidance of health care provider.
• Advise patient to obtain regular eye examinations.
• Caution female patient to report pregnancy to health care provider as soon as possible.

fluticasone propionate (topical)
floo-TIK-a-sone

Cutivate

Therapeutic class: Corticosteroids
Pharmacologic class: Corticosteroids

AVAILABLE FORMS
Cream: 0.05%
Lotion: 0.05%
Ointment: 0.005%

INDICATIONS & DOSAGES
➤ **Inflammation and pruritus from dermatoses responsive to corticosteroids**
Adults: Apply a thin film of cream or ointment to affected area b.i.d.; rub in gently and completely.
Children age 3 months and older: Apply a thin film of cream to affected areas b.i.d. Rub in gently. Don't use for longer than 4 weeks.
➤ **Inflammation and pruritus from atopic dermatitis**
Adults and children age 3 months and older: Apply thin film of cream to affected areas once daily or b.i.d. Or, apply a thin film of lotion to affected areas once daily. Rub in gently. Don't use for longer than 4 weeks.

ADMINISTRATION
Topical
• Don't use drug with an occlusive dressing or in diaper area.

ACTION
Is diffused across cell membranes to form complexes with cytoplasmic receptors. Shows anti-inflammatory, antipruritic, vasoconstrictive, and antiproliferative activity.

Considered a medium-potency drug, according to vasoconstrictive properties.

Route	Onset	Peak	Duration
Topical	Rapid	Unknown	10 hr

Half-life: About 7½ hours.

ADVERSE REACTIONS
CNS: light-headedness. **GU:** glycosuria. **Metabolic:** hyperglycemia. **Skin:** urticaria, burning, hypertrichosis, pruritus, irritation, erythema, hives, dryness, telangiectasia. **Other:** *HPA axis suppression,* Cushing syndrome.

INTERACTIONS
None significant.

EFFECTS ON LAB TEST RESULTS
• May increase glucose level.

CONTRAINDICATIONS & CAUTIONS
• Contraindicated in patients hypersensitive to drug or its components.
• Don't use as monotherapy in primary bacterial, viral, fungal, herpetic, or tubercular skin infections or for treatment of rosacea, perioral dermatitis, or acne.
• Drug isn't for ophthalmic use.
Dialyzable drug: Unknown.
⚠ **Overdose S&S:** Systemic effects (including reversible HPA axis suppression, Cushing syndrome, hyperglycemia, glycosuria).

PREGNANCY-LACTATION-REPRODUCTION
• Use during pregnancy only if potential benefit justifies potential risk to the fetus.
• Use cautiously in breastfeeding women.

NURSING CONSIDERATIONS
• Don't mix drug with other bases or vehicles because doing so may affect potency.
• If adverse reactions occur, prescriber may order less potent drug.
• Stop drug if local irritation or systemic infection, absorption, or hypersensitivity occurs.
• May cause suppression of HPA axis in patients receiving high doses for prolonged periods, particularly in children.
• Absorption of corticosteroid is increased when drug is applied to inflamed or damaged skin, eyelids, or scrotal area; it's lowest when applied to intact normal skin, palms of hands, or soles of feet.
• *Look alike–sound alike:* Don't confuse fluticasone with fluconazole, fluocinolone, or fluocinonide.

PATIENT TEACHING
• Teach patient or family member how to apply drug using gloves, sterile applicator, or after careful hand washing.
• Tell patient to wash hands after application.
• Tell patient to avoid prolonged use and contact with eyes. Warn patient not to apply to face, in skin creases, or around eyes, genitals, underarms, or rectum.
• Instruct patient to notify prescriber of all adverse reactions, if condition persists or worsens, or if burning or irritation develops.

fluticasone propionate–salmeterol (inhalation)
floo-TIK-a-sone/sal-MEE-ter-ol

Advair Diskus 100/50, Advair Diskus 250/50, Advair Diskus 500/50, Advair HFA 45/21, Advair HFA 115/21, Advair HFA 230/21, Airduo RespiClick, Wixela Inhub

Therapeutic class: Antiasthmatics
Pharmacologic class: Corticosteroids–long-acting beta$_2$-adrenergic agonists

AVAILABLE FORMS
Inhalation powder: 55 mcg fluticasone propionate and 14 mcg salmeterol, 100 mcg fluticasone propionate and 50 mcg salmeterol, 113 mcg fluticasone propionate and 14 mcg salmeterol, 232 mcg fluticasone propionate and 14 mcg salmeterol, 250 mcg fluticasone propionate and 50 mcg salmeterol, 500 mcg fluticasone propionate and 50 mcg salmeterol
Aerosol spray: 45 mcg fluticasone propionate and 21 mcg salmeterol, 115 mcg fluticasone propionate and 21 mcg salmeterol, 230 mcg fluticasone propionate and 21 mcg salmeterol

INDICATIONS & DOSAGES
➤ **Treatment of asthma for patients not adequately controlled on a long-term**

asthma control medication such as inhaled corticosteroid (ICS) or whose disease warrants initiation of treatment with both ICS and long-acting beta₂-adrenergic agonist (LABA)

Adults and children age 12 and older: 1 inhalation of Advair Diskus b.i.d., at least 12 hours apart, or 2 inhalations of Advair HFA b.i.d., at least 12 hours apart. Starting doses are dependent on patient's disease severity, based on previous asthma therapy (including ICS dosage), current control of asthma symptoms, and risk of future exacerbation. May increase dose after 2 weeks in patients who aren't adequately controlled. Maximum dose of Advair Diskus is 1 inhalation of fluticasone 500 mcg and salmeterol 50 mcg b.i.d. Maximum dose of Advair HFA is 2 inhalations of fluticasone 230 mcg and salmeterol 21 mcg b.i.d.

Or, for patients not adequately controlled on a long-term asthma control medication such as ICS or whose disease warrants initiation of treatment with both ICS and LABA, base starting dose on patient's asthma severity; usual recommended starting dose for patients not on ICS is 55 mcg fluticasone/14 mcg salmeterol b.i.d. approximately 12 hours apart. For other patients, base starting dose on previous asthma drug therapy and disease severity.

For patients switching from another inhaled corticosteroid, base initial Airduo RespiClick dose strength on strength of previous ICS and disease severity. Highest recommended Airduo RespiClick dose is 232 mcg fluticasone/14 mcg salmeterol b.i.d.

Children ages 4 to 11 not controlled on ICS: 1 inhalation of Advair Diskus fluticasone 100 mcg and salmeterol 50 mcg b.i.d. about 12 hours apart.

➤ **Maintenance therapy for airflow obstruction in patients with COPD; to reduce exacerbations of COPD in patients with a history of exacerbations**

Adults: 1 inhalation of Advair Diskus 250/50 only b.i.d., about 12 hours apart.

ADMINISTRATION
Inhalational

• Prime Advair HFA before first use by releasing 4 test sprays into the air, away from the face, shaking well for 5 seconds before each spray. If inhaler hasn't been used for 4 weeks or has been dropped, prime inhaler again by shaking well before each spray and releasing 2 test sprays into the air.

• Discard Advair HFA canister when counter reads "000."

• Airduo RespiClick doesn't require priming. Never place inhaler in water; clean mouthpiece with dry cloth or tissue as needed.

• After administration, have patient rinse mouth without swallowing.

ACTION

Fluticasone is a synthetic corticosteroid with potent anti-inflammatory activity. Salmeterol xinafoate, a long-acting beta agonist, relaxes bronchial smooth muscle and inhibits release of mediators.

Route	Onset	Peak	Duration
Inhalation (fluticasone)	Unknown	1–2 hr	Unknown
Inhalation (salmeterol)	Unknown	5 min	Unknown

Half-life: Fluticasone, 8 hours; salmeterol, 5½ hours.

ADVERSE REACTIONS

CNS: headache, sleep disorders, tremors, pain. **CV:** palpitations. **EENT:** pharyngitis, blood in nasal mucosa, congestion, conjunctivitis, dental discomfort and pain, eye redness, hoarseness or dysphonia, keratitis, nasal irritation, rhinorrhea, rhinitis, sinusitis, sneezing, viral eye infections. **GI:** abdominal pain and discomfort, appendicitis, constipation, diarrhea, gastroenteritis, nausea, oral candidiasis, oral discomfort and pain, oral erythema and rashes, oral ulcerations, unusual taste, vomiting. **Musculoskeletal:** arthralgia, articular rheumatism, bone and cartilage disorders, muscle pain, muscle stiffness, rigidity, tightness. **Respiratory:** URI, bronchitis, cough, lower respiratory tract infection, pneumonia. **Skin:** disorders of sweat and sebum, infection, skin flakiness, sweating, urticaria. **Other:** allergic reactions, chest symptoms, fluid retention, viral or bacterial infections.

INTERACTIONS

Drug-drug. *Beta blockers:* Blocked pulmonary effect of salmeterol may produce severe bronchospasm in patients with asthma. Avoid using together. If necessary, use a cardioselective beta blocker cautiously.

Ketoconazole, other inhibitors of CYP450: May increase fluticasone level and adverse effects. Use together cautiously.

Loop diuretics, thiazide diuretics: Potassium-wasting diuretics may cause or worsen ECG changes or hypokalemia. Use together cautiously.

MAO inhibitors, TCAs: May potentiate the action of salmeterol on the vascular system. Separate doses by 2 weeks.

EFFECTS ON LAB TEST RESULTS
• May increase liver enzyme levels.

CONTRAINDICATIONS & CAUTIONS
• Contraindicated in patients hypersensitive to drug or its components, as primary treatment of status asthmaticus or other acute episodes of asthma or COPD in which intensive measures are required, and in those with severe hypersensitivity to milk proteins.
• Use of LABA as monotherapy (without ICS) for asthma is associated with an increased risk of asthma-related death. Available data from controlled clinical trials also suggest that use of LABA as monotherapy increases the risk of asthma-related hospitalization in children and adolescents. These findings are considered a class effect of LABA monotherapy. When LABAs are used in fixed-dose combination with ICS, data from large clinical trials don't show a significant increase in the risk of serious asthma-related events (hospitalizations, intubations, death) compared with ICS alone.
⚠ *Alert:* Don't use drug for transferring patients from systemic corticosteroid therapy. Deaths from adrenal insufficiency have occurred in patients with asthma during and after transfer from systemic corticosteroids to less systemically available inhaled corticosteroids.
• Use cautiously, if at all, in patients with active or quiescent respiratory TB infection; untreated systemic fungal, bacterial, viral, or parasitic infection; or ocular herpes simplex.
• Use cautiously in patients with CV disorders, seizure disorders, or thyrotoxicosis; in

patients unusually responsive to sympathomimetic amines; and in patients with hepatic impairment.

Dialyzable drug: Unknown.

⚠ *Overdose S&S:* Hypercorticism, angina, arrhythmias, dizziness, dry mouth, fatigue, headache, HTN, hypotension, insomnia, malaise, muscle cramps, nausea, nervousness, palpitations, seizures, tachycardia, prolonged QTc interval, hypokalemia, hyperglycemia, cardiac arrest, death.

PREGNANCY-LACTATION-REPRODUCTION
• Use during pregnancy only if potential benefit justifies potential risk to the fetus.
• Avoid use during labor as drug can interfere with uterine contractility.
• Use cautiously in breastfeeding women.

NURSING CONSIDERATIONS
⚠ *Alert:* Patient shouldn't be switched from systemic corticosteroids to Advair Diskus or Advair HFA because of HPA axis suppression. Death from adrenal insufficiency can occur. Several months are required for recovery of HPA function after withdrawal of systemic corticosteroids.
• Don't start therapy during rapidly deteriorating or potentially life-threatening episodes of asthma. Serious acute respiratory events, including fatality, can occur.
• The benefit of Advair 250/50 in treating patients with COPD for more than 6 months is unknown. If drug is used for longer than 6 months, periodically reevaluate patient to assess for benefits or risks of therapy.
• Monitor patient for urticaria, angioedema, rash, bronchospasm, or other signs of hypersensitivity.
• Don't use this drug to stop an asthma attack. Patients should carry an inhaled, short-acting beta$_2$ agonist (such as albuterol) for acute symptoms.
• If drug causes paradoxical bronchospasm, treat immediately with a short-acting inhaled bronchodilator (such as albuterol), and notify prescriber.
• Monitor patient for increased use of inhaled short-acting beta$_2$ agonist. The dose of Advair may need to be increased.
• Closely monitor children for growth suppression.

PATIENT TEACHING
• Instruct patient on proper use of the prescribed inhaler to provide effective treatment.
• Tell patient to avoid exhaling into the dry-powder multidose inhaler; to activate and use the dry-powder multidose inhaler in a level, horizontal position; and not to use Advair Diskus with a spacer device.
• Instruct patient to keep the dry-powder multidose inhaler in a dry place, away from direct heat or sunlight, and to avoid washing the mouthpiece or other parts of the device. Patient should discard device 1 month after removal from the moisture-protective overwrap pouch or after every blister has been used, whichever comes first. Warn patient not to attempt to take device apart.
• Instruct patient to rinse mouth after inhalation to prevent oral candidiasis.
• Instruct patient to discard Airduo RespiClick inhaler 30 days after opening the foil pouch or when the counter reads "0," whichever comes first (device isn't reusable).
• Advise patient, after removing Advair Diskus from the box and foil pouch, to write the "Pouch opened" and "Use by" dates on the label on top of the Diskus. The "Use by" date is 1 month from date of opening the pouch.
• Teach patient how to use the Diskus: Each time the lever is pushed back, a dose is ready to be inhaled. Don't close or tilt the Diskus after the lever is pushed back. Don't play with the lever or move the lever more than once. The dose indicator displays how many doses are left; when the numbers 5 to 0 appear in red, only a few doses remain.
• Advise patient to discard Diskus device 1 month after removing it from the foil pouch or when the dose counter reads "0" (whichever comes first).
• Inform patient that improvement may occur within 30 minutes after dose, but the full benefit may not occur for 1 week or more.
• Advise patient not to exceed recommended prescribing dose.
• Instruct patient not to relieve acute symptoms with Advair. Treat acute symptoms with an inhaled short-acting beta$_2$ agonist.

• Instruct patient to report decreasing effects or use of increasing doses of the inhaled short-acting beta$_2$ agonist.
• Tell patient to report all adverse reactions, especially palpitations, chest pain, rapid HR, tremor, or nervousness.
• Instruct patient to call prescriber immediately if exposed to chickenpox or measles.

fluvastatin sodium ▓
flue-va-STA-tin

Lescol XL

Therapeutic class: Antilipemics
Pharmacologic class: HMG-CoA reductase inhibitors

AVAILABLE FORMS
Capsules ⓞ: 20 mg, 40 mg
Tablets (extended-release) ⓞ: 80 mg

INDICATIONS & DOSAGES
➤ **To reduce LDL cholesterol (LDL-C) and total cholesterol levels in patients with primary hypercholesterolemia (types IIa and IIb); to slow progression of coronary atherosclerosis in patients with CAD; to reduce elevated triglyceride and apolipoprotein B (apo B) levels in patients with primary hypercholesterolemia and mixed dyslipidemia whose response to dietary restriction and other nonpharmacologic measures has been inadequate**
Adults: Initially, 20 to 40 mg PO at bedtime, increasing if needed to maximum of 80 mg daily in divided doses or 80 mg Lescol XL PO at bedtime for patients requiring LDL-C reduction to a goal of at least 25%, or 20 mg daily for patients requiring LDL-C reduction to a goal of less than 25%.
➤ **Adjunct to diet to reduce LDL-C, total cholesterol, and apo B levels in pediatric patients with heterozygous familial hypercholesterolemia whose response to dietary restriction hasn't been adequate and for whom the following findings are present: LDL-C remains at 190 mg/dL or more, or LDL-C remains at 160 mg/dL or more and there's a positive family history of premature CV disease or two or more other CV disease risk factors are present**

Adolescent boys and girls (who are at least 1 year postmenarche) ages 10 to 16: 20 mg PO once daily at bedtime. Dosage adjustments may be made at 6-week intervals up to maximum of 40 mg (capsule) PO b.i.d. or 80 mg extended-release tablet PO once daily.

➤ **To reduce risk of undergoing coronary revascularization procedures**
Adults: In patients who must reduce LDL-C level by at least 25%, initially 40 mg PO once daily or b.i.d.; or one 80-mg extended-release tablet as a single dose at any time of the day. In patients who must reduce LDL-C level by less than 25%, initially 20 mg PO daily. Dosages range from 20 to 80 mg daily.

ADMINISTRATION
PO
• Give drug without regard for meals.
• For once-daily dosage, give immediate-release capsules in the evening.
• Don't crush or break tablets; don't open or crush capsules.
• Administer extended-release tablet as a single dose at any time of the day.
• Don't give two 40-mg capsules at one time.

ACTION
Inhibits HMG-CoA reductase, an early (and rate-limiting) step in the cholesterol synthesis pathway.

Route	Onset	Peak	Duration
PO	Unknown	1 hr	Unknown

Half-life: About 3 hours.

ADVERSE REACTIONS
CNS: dizziness, fatigue, headache, insomnia. **EENT:** pharyngitis, rhinitis, sinusitis. **GI:** abdominal pain, constipation, diarrhea, dyspepsia, flatulence, nausea, vomiting. **GU:** UTI. **Hematologic:** *leukopenia, thrombocytopenia,* hemolytic anemia. **Musculoskeletal:** *rhabdomyolysis,* arthralgia, back pain, myalgia, arthropathy. **Respiratory:** URI, bronchitis, cough. **Other:** hypersensitivity reactions, accidental trauma, flulike illness.

INTERACTIONS
Drug-drug. *Cholestyramine, colestipol:* May bind with fluvastatin in the GI tract and

decrease absorption. Separate doses by at least 4 hours.
Cimetidine, omeprazole, ranitidine: May decrease fluvastatin metabolism. Monitor patient for enhanced effects.
Cyclosporine and other immunosuppressants, erythromycin, niacin: May increase risk of polymyositis and rhabdomyolysis. Avoid using together. Don't exceed 20 mg b.i.d. in patients taking cyclosporine.
Digoxin: May alter digoxin pharmacokinetics. Monitor digoxin level carefully.
Erythromycin, nicotinic acid: May increase risk of myopathy and rhabdomyolysis. Don't use together.
Fibric acids (fenofibrate, gemfibrozil): May cause severe myopathy or rhabdomyolysis. If coadministration can't be avoided, monitor CK closely.
Fluconazole, itraconazole, ketoconazole: May increase fluvastatin level and adverse effects. Use cautiously together or, if given together, reduce dose of fluvastatin. Don't exceed 20 mg b.i.d. in patients taking fluconazole.
Glyburide: May increase levels of both drugs. Monitor serum glucose and signs and symptoms of toxicity.
Phenytoin: May increase phenytoin levels. Monitor phenytoin levels.
Protease inhibitors (atazanavir, darunavir, fosamprenavir, indinavir, nelfinavir, ritonavir, saquinavir, tipranavir): May increase fluvastatin level and risk of myopathy and rhabdomyolysis. Use together cautiously.
Rifampin: May enhance fluvastatin metabolism and decrease levels. Monitor patient for lack of effect.
Warfarin: May increase anticoagulant effect with bleeding. Monitor PT and INR.
Drug-herb. *Eucalyptus, jin bu huan, kava:* May increase risk of hepatotoxicity. Discourage use together.
Red yeast rice: May increase risk of adverse reactions because herb contains compounds similar to those in drug. Discourage use together.
Drug-lifestyle. *Alcohol use:* May increase risk of hepatotoxicity. Discourage use together.

Reactions in bold italics are *life-threatening*. Interactions may have a *rapid onset* or a *delayed onset*.

EFFECTS ON LAB TEST RESULTS

- May increase ALT, AST, HbA$_{1c}$, fasting glucose, and CK levels. May decrease Hb level and hematocrit.
- May decrease platelet and WBC counts.

CONTRAINDICATIONS & CAUTIONS

- Contraindicated in patients hypersensitive to drug and in those with active liver disease or unexplained persistent elevations of transaminase levels; also contraindicated in women of childbearing potential.
- Drug may cause rhabdomyolysis in patients with renal function impairment.
- Use cautiously in patients with severe renal impairment or history of liver disease or heavy alcohol use, in those with inadequately treated hypothyroidism, and in patients age 65 or older.

Dialyzable drug: Unknown.

⚠ *Overdose S&S:* GI complaints, elevated AST and ALT levels.

PREGNANCY-LACTATION-REPRODUCTION

- Use contraindicated in pregnant and breastfeeding women.

NURSING CONSIDERATIONS

- Patient should follow a diet restricted in saturated fat and cholesterol during therapy.
- Exercise caution when giving to patients with a history of liver disease or heavy alcohol ingestion. Closely monitor these patients.
- Perform LFTs before initiating therapy and if signs and symptoms of liver injury occur.
- Monitor lipid levels before starting therapy, at 4 weeks, at times of dosage changes, and periodically thereafter.
- Watch for signs and symptoms of myopathy. Monitor patient for muscle pain or weakness with malaise and fever. Discontinue drug for markedly elevated CK levels or if myopathy is suspected or confirmed.
- *Look alike–sound alike:* Don't confuse fluvastatin with fluoxetine.

PATIENT TEACHING

- Tell patient that drug may be taken without regard for meals; if taken once daily, immediate-release capsules are taken in the evening.

- Advise patient who is also taking a bile acid sequestrant such as cholestyramine to take fluvastatin at bedtime, at least 4 hours after taking the sequestrant.
- Teach patient about proper dietary management, weight control, and exercise. Explain their importance in controlling elevated cholesterol and triglyceride levels.
- Warn patient to avoid alcohol.
- Tell patient to notify prescriber of adverse reactions, especially muscle aches and pains.
- Advise patient that it may take up to 4 weeks for the drug to be completely effective.

🔵 *Alert:* Tell female patient of childbearing potential to stop drug and notify prescriber immediately if she becomes pregnant.

---

fluvoxaMINE maleate
floo-VOX-a-meen

Therapeutic class: Antidepressants
Pharmacologic class: SSRIs

AVAILABLE FORMS

Capsules (extended-release) ⓞ: 100 mg, 150 mg
Tablets: 25 mg, 50 mg, 100 mg

INDICATIONS & DOSAGES

Adjust-a-dose (for all indications): In elderly patients and those with hepatic impairment, give lower first dose and adjust dose more slowly. When using extended-release capsules, titrate dosage more slowly after initial 100-mg dose.

➤ **OCD**
Adults: Initially, 50 mg (tablet) PO daily at bedtime; increase by 50 mg every 4 to 7 days. Maximum, 300 mg daily. Give total daily amounts above 100 mg in two divided doses. Or, 100-mg extended-release capsule PO once per day as a single daily dose at bedtime. Increase in 50-mg increments every week, as tolerated, until maximum therapeutic benefit is achieved. Maximum dose is 300 mg/day.
Children ages 8 to 17: Initially, 25 mg PO daily at bedtime; increase by 25 mg every 4 to 7 days. Maximum, 200 mg daily for children ages 8 to 11 and 300 mg daily

for children ages 12 to 17. Give total daily amounts over 50 mg in two divided doses.

ADMINISTRATION
PO
- Give drug without regard for food.
- Capsules shouldn't be crushed or chewed.
- Give extended-release capsules at bedtime.

ACTION
Unknown. Selectively inhibits the presynaptic neuronal uptake of serotonin, which may improve OCD.

Route	Onset	Peak	Duration
PO (capsules)	Unknown	Unknown	Unknown
PO (tablets)	Unknown	3–8 hr	Unknown

Half-life: 14 to 16 hours.

ADVERSE REACTIONS
CNS: agitation, headache, malaise, asthenia, somnolence, insomnia, nervousness, dizziness, tremor, anxiety, hypertonia, depression, CNS stimulation, hyperkinesia, manic reaction, myoclonus, syncope. **CV:** palpitations, vasodilation. **EENT:** amblyopia, rhinitis. **GI:** nausea, diarrhea, constipation, dyspepsia, vomiting, dry mouth, anorexia, flatulence, dysphagia, taste perversion, weight gain or loss. **GU:** abnormal ejaculation, urinary frequency, erectile dysfunction, anorgasmia, urine retention, dysmenorrhea, decreased libido. **Respiratory:** URI, dyspnea. **Skin:** rash, sweating. **Other:** tooth disorder, flulike syndrome, chills, yawning.

INTERACTIONS
Drug-drug. *Alosetron, pimozide, terfenadine, thioridazine, tizanidine:* May prolong QTc interval. Use together is contraindicated.

Antipsychotics, MAO inhibitors (phenelzine, selegiline, tranylcypromine): May cause serotonin syndrome (CNS irritability, shivering, altered consciousness) or NMS. Avoid using within 2 weeks of MAO inhibitor.

Benzodiazepines (alprazolam, diazepam, midazolam, triazolam): May reduce clearance of these drugs. Use together cautiously (except for diazepam, which shouldn't be used with fluvoxamine). Adjust dosage as needed. Initial alprazolam dosage should be

at least halved; titration to the lowest effective dosage is recommended.

Carbamazepine, clozapine, methadone, metoprolol, propranolol, TCAs, theophylline: May increase levels of these drugs. Use together cautiously, and monitor patient closely for adverse reactions. Dosage adjustments may be needed.

Diltiazem: May cause bradycardia. Monitor HR.

Linezolid, methylene blue: May cause serotonin syndrome. Don't start drug in patients receiving linezolid or methylene blue.

Lithium, tryptophan: May enhance effects of fluvoxamine. Use together cautiously.

Sumatriptan: May cause weakness, hyperreflexia, and incoordination. Monitor patient closely. May cause serotonin syndrome. Avoid using within 2 weeks of MAO inhibitor.

Tramadol: May cause serotonin syndrome. Monitor patient closely.

Warfarin, other drugs that interfere with hemostasis (aspirin, NSAIDs): May increase levels of these drugs and the risk of bleeding and prolong PT. Monitor INR and adjust anticoagulant dosage accordingly.

Drug-herb. *Alfalfa, anise, bilberry:* May increase antiplatelet activity. Avoid use together.

Kava kava, SAM-e, St. John's wort, tryptophan, valerian: May increase sedative-hypnotic effects and risk of serotonin syndrome. Avoid use together.

Melatonin: May increase melatonin bioavailability. Avoid use together.

Drug-lifestyle. *Alcohol use:* May increase CNS effects. Discourage use together.

Smoking: May decrease drug's effectiveness. Urge patient to stop smoking.

EFFECTS ON LAB TEST RESULTS
None reported.

CONTRAINDICATIONS & CAUTIONS
- Contraindicated in patients hypersensitive to drug or to other phenyl piperazine antidepressants; in those receiving pimozide, alosetron, tizanidine, or thioridazine therapy; and within 2 weeks of MAO inhibitor.
- **Alert:** Concomitant use with linezolid or methylene blue can cause serotonin syndrome (fever, mental status changes, muscle

twitching, excessive sweating, shivering or shaking, diarrhea, loss of coordination). Use drug with linezolid or methylene blue only for life-threatening or urgent conditions when the potential benefits outweigh the risks of toxicity.

• Use cautiously in patients with hepatic dysfunction, other conditions that may affect hemodynamic responses or metabolism, or history of mania or seizures.

Black Box Warning Fluvoxamine tablets aren't approved for use in children, except for those with OCD. Fluvoxamine extended-release capsules shouldn't be used in children. ∎

• Use cautiously in patients with CV disease. Fluvoxamine hasn't been systemically evaluated in patients with a recent history of MI or unstable heart disease.

• Bone fractures have been associated with antidepressant use. Consider the possibility of a fragility fracture if an antidepressant-treated patient presents with unexplained bone pain, point tenderness, swelling, or bruising.

Dialyzable drug: Unlikely.

⚠ *Overdose S&S:* Nausea, vomiting, diarrhea, coma, hypokalemia, hypotension, respiratory difficulties, somnolence, tachycardia, ECG abnormalities, seizures, dizziness, liver function disturbances, tremor, increased reflexes.

PREGNANCY-LACTATION-REPRODUCTION

• Neonates exposed to drug late in the third trimester have developed complications requiring prolonged hospitalization, respiratory support, and tube feeding. Neonates exposed to SSRIs in late pregnancy may have an increased risk of persistent pulmonary HTN of the newborn, which is associated with substantial neonatal morbidity and mortality. Risks and benefits of treatment should be carefully considered on a case-by-case basis.

• Drug appears in human milk. Patient should discontinue breastfeeding or discontinue drug.

NURSING CONSIDERATIONS

Black Box Warning Drug may increase the risk of suicidal thinking and behavior in young adults ages 18 to 24, especially during first few months of treatment. Monitor patient closely for clinical worsening. ∎

• Record mood changes. Monitor patient for suicidal tendencies.

⊕ *Alert:* Combining an SSRI with a triptan may cause serotonin syndrome or NMS-like reactions. Serotonin syndrome is more likely to occur when starting or increasing the dose of a triptan.

⊕ *Alert:* If linezolid or methylene blue must be given, fluvoxamine must be stopped and patient should be monitored for serotonin toxicity for 2 weeks or until 24 hours after final dose of linezolid or methylene blue, whichever comes first. Treatment with fluvoxamine may be resumed 24 hours after final dose of linezolid or methylene blue.

• Patients shouldn't stop drug without first consulting prescriber; abruptly stopping drug may cause withdrawal syndrome, including headache, muscle ache, and flulike symptoms.

• Consider age and gender differences when determining dosages in children and women; therapeutic effect in women may be achieved with lower doses.

• *Look alike–sound alike:* Don't confuse fluvoxamine with fluoxetine.

PATIENT TEACHING

Black Box Warning Advise families and caregivers to closely observe patient for increased suicidal thinking or behavior. ∎

⊕ *Alert:* Teach patient to recognize and immediately report symptoms of serotonin toxicity (fever, mental status changes, muscle twitching, excessive sweating, shivering or shaking, diarrhea, loss of coordination).

• Warn patient to avoid hazardous activities until CNS effects of drug are known.

• Tell women to notify prescriber about planned, suspected, or known pregnancy.

• Tell patient who develops a rash, hives, or a related allergic reaction to notify prescriber.

• Inform patient that several weeks of therapy may be needed to obtain full therapeutic effect. Once improvement occurs, advise patient not to stop drug until directed by prescriber.

• Suggest that patient keep a diary of changes in mood or behavior. Tell patient to report suicidal thoughts immediately.

• Advise patient to check with prescriber before taking OTC drugs; drug interactions can occur.
• Tell patient drug can be taken with or without food.

fondaparinux sodium
fon-da-PAR-i-nuks

Arixtra

Therapeutic class: Anticoagulants
Pharmacologic class: Activated factor X inhibitors

AVAILABLE FORMS
Injection: 2.5 mg/0.5 mL, 5 mg/0.4 mL, 7.5 mg/0.6 mL, 10 mg/0.8 mL in single-dose, prefilled syringe

INDICATIONS & DOSAGES
➤ **To prevent DVT, which may lead to PE, in patients undergoing surgery for hip fracture, hip replacement, knee replacement, or abdominal surgery**
Adults weighing 50 kg or more: 2.5 mg subcut once daily for 5 to 9 days. Give first dose after hemostasis is established, 6 to 8 hours after surgery. Giving the dose earlier than 6 hours after surgery increases the risk of major bleeding. Patients undergoing hip fracture surgery should receive an extended prophylaxis course of up to 24 additional days; a total of 32 days (perioperative and extended prophylaxis) has been tolerated.
➤ **Acute DVT (with warfarin); acute PE (with warfarin) when treatment is started in the hospital**
Adults weighing more than 100 kg: 10 mg subcut daily for 5 to 9 days (drug has been given for up to 26 days in clinical trials) and until INR is 2 to 3. Begin warfarin therapy as soon as possible, usually within 72 hours.
Adults weighing 50 to 100 kg: 7.5 mg subcut daily for 5 to 9 days (drug has been given for up to 26 days in clinical trials) and until INR is 2 to 3. Begin warfarin therapy as soon as possible, usually within 72 hours.
Adults weighing less than 50 kg: 5 mg subcut daily for 5 to 9 days (drug has been given for up to 26 days in clinical trials) and until

INR is 2 to 3. Begin warfarin therapy as soon as possible, usually within 72 hours.
➤ **Acute symptomatic superficial vein thrombosis (at least 5 cm in length) of the legs** ◆
Adults: 2.5 mg subcut once daily for 45 days.
➤ **ACS (non-ST-elevation ACS [NSTE-ACS] or ST-elevation MI [STEMI])** ◆
Adults: For NSTE-ACS, 2.5 mg subcut once daily for duration of hospitalization or until PCI is done. For STEMI, 2.5 mg IV once, then 2.5 mg subcut once daily starting the following day; treat for duration of hospitalization, up to 8 days, or until revascularization.

ADMINISTRATION
Subcutaneous
• Give subcut only, never IM. Inspect the single-dose, prefilled syringe for particulate matter and discoloration before giving.
🔵 *Alert:* To avoid loss of drug, don't expel air bubble from the syringe.
• Give drug in fatty tissue, rotating injection sites. If drug has been properly injected, the needle will pull back into the syringe security sleeve and the white safety indicator will appear above the blue upper body. A soft click may be heard or felt when the syringe plunger is fully released. After injection of the syringe contents, the plunger automatically rises while the needle withdraws from the skin and retracts into the security sleeve. Don't recap the needle.

ACTION
Binds to antithrombin III (AT-III) and potentiates the neutralization of factor Xa by AT-III, which interrupts coagulation and inhibits formation of thrombin and blood clots.

Route	Onset	Peak	Duration
Subcut	Unknown	2–3 hr	Unknown

Half-life: 17 to 21 hours.

ADVERSE REACTIONS
CNS: insomnia, dizziness, confusion. **CV:** hypotension. **EENT:** epistaxis. **Hematologic:** *hemorrhage,* anemia, hematoma, *postoperative hemorrhage, thrombocytopenia.* **Hepatic:** increased AST and ALT levels. **Metabolic:** hypokalemia. **Skin:** mild

local irritation (injection-site bleeding, rash, pruritus), bullous eruption, purpura, rash, increased wound drainage and infection.

INTERACTIONS

Drug-drug. *Drugs that increase risk of bleeding (anticoagulants, NSAIDs, platelet inhibitors):* May increase risk of hemorrhage. Stop these drugs before starting fondaparinux. If use together is unavoidable, monitor patient closely.

Drug-herb. *Angelica (dong quai), ginkgo, ginseng, willow:* May increase risk of bleeding. Discourage use together.

EFFECTS ON LAB TEST RESULTS

• May increase AST, ALT, and bilirubin levels. May decrease potassium and Hb levels and hematocrit.
• May decrease platelet count.

CONTRAINDICATIONS & CAUTIONS

• Contraindicated in patients with CrCl of less than 30 mL/minute and for venous thromboembolism prophylaxis in patients weighing less than 50 kg who are undergoing hip fracture, hip replacement, knee replacement, or abdominal surgery.
• Contraindicated in patients with history of serious hypersensitivity reaction (angioedema, anaphylactoid/anaphylactic reactions) to fondaparinux.
• Contraindicated in patients with active major bleeding, bacterial endocarditis, or thrombocytopenia with a positive test result for antiplatelet antibody after taking fondaparinux.
• Use cautiously in patients being treated with platelet inhibitors; in those at increased risk for bleeding, such as those with congenital or acquired bleeding disorders; in those with active ulcerative and angiodysplastic GI disease; in those with hemorrhagic stroke; and in patients shortly after brain, spinal, or ophthalmologic surgery.
• Use cautiously in elderly patients, in patients with CrCl of 30 to 50 mL/minute, and in those with a history of heparin-induced thrombocytopenia, a bleeding diathesis, uncontrolled arterial HTN, or a history of recent GI ulceration, diabetic retinopathy, or hemorrhage.

⊙ *Alert:* Use cautiously in latex-sensitive patients; the packaging (needle guard) contains dry natural rubber.
Dialyzable drug: Yes.
⚠ *Overdose S&S:* Hemorrhagic complications.

PREGNANCY-LACTATION-REPRODUCTION

• Use cautiously in pregnant women and only if benefit justifies risk to the fetus.
• It isn't known if drug appears in human milk. Use cautiously in breastfeeding women.

NURSING CONSIDERATIONS

• Don't use interchangeably with heparin, low–molecular-weight heparins, or heparinoids.

Black Box Warning Patients who receive epidural or spinal anesthesia, epidural catheters, or spinal puncture or have a history of spine deformity or surgery are at increased risk for developing an epidural or spinal hematoma, which may result in long-term or permanent paralysis. Other factors that increase risk include concurrent use of NSAIDs, platelet inhibitors, and other anticoagulants; use of indwelling epidural catheters; and history of traumatic or repeated epidural or spinal surgery. Monitor these patients closely for neurologic impairment, and treat urgently. Consider the risk before neuraxial intervention in patients anticoagulated or to be anticoagulated for thromboprophylaxis. ■

• Monitor renal function periodically, and stop drug in patients who develop unstable renal function or severe renal impairment while receiving therapy.
• Routinely assess patient for signs and symptoms of bleeding, and regularly monitor CBC, platelet count, creatinine level, and stool occult blood test results. Stop use if platelet count is less than $100,000/mm^3$.
• Anticoagulant effects may last for 2 to 4 days after stopping drug in patients with normal renal function.
• PT and aPTT aren't suitable monitoring tests to measure drug activity. If coagulation parameters change unexpectedly or patient develops major bleeding, stop drug.

- Refer to label and local protocol for additional details for transitioning between anticoagulants.

PATIENT TEACHING
- Tell patient to report all adverse reactions, especially signs and symptoms of bleeding or neurologic impairment.
- Instruct patient to avoid OTC products that contain aspirin or other salicylates.
- Advise patient to consult with prescriber before starting herbal therapy; many herbs have anticoagulant, antiplatelet, or fibrinolytic properties.
- Teach patient the correct technique for subcut use, if needed.

formoterol fumarate
for-MOH-te-rol

Perforomist

Therapeutic class: Bronchodilators
Pharmacologic class: Selective beta$_2$-adrenergic agonists

AVAILABLE FORMS
Inhalation solution: 20 mcg/2 mL vial

INDICATIONS & DOSAGES
➤ **Maintenance treatment of bronchoconstriction in patients with COPD (chronic bronchitis, emphysema)**
Adults: One 20 mcg/2 mL vial (Perforomist) by oral inhalation through a jet nebulizer every 12 hours. Maximum dose, 40 mcg/day.

ADMINISTRATION
Inhalational
- Give inhalational solution through a standard jet nebulizer connected to an air compressor.
- Store in foil pouch and remove immediately before use. Drug is colorless; discard drug if solution isn't colorless.

ACTION
Long-acting selective beta$_2$ agonist that causes bronchodilation. It ultimately increases cAMP, leading to relaxation of bronchial smooth muscle and inhibition of mediator release from mast cells.

Route	Onset	Peak	Duration
Inhalation solution	12 min	1–3 hr	12 hr

Half-life: 7 hours.

ADVERSE REACTIONS
CNS: tremor, dizziness, insomnia, nervousness, headache, fatigue, malaise, anxiety. **CV:** *arrhythmias,* chest pain, angina, HTN, hypotension, tachycardia, palpitations. **EENT:** dry mouth, tonsillitis, dysphonia, nasopharyngitis, sinusitis. **GI:** nausea, vomiting, diarrhea. **Metabolic:** *metabolic acidosis, hypokalemia,* hyperglycemia. **Musculoskeletal:** muscle cramps. **Respiratory:** bronchitis, chest infection, dyspnea. **Skin:** rash, pruritus. **Other:** viral infection.

INTERACTIONS
Drug-drug. *Adrenergics:* May potentiate sympathetic effects of formoterol. Use together cautiously.
Beta blockers: May antagonize effects of beta agonists, causing bronchospasm in asthmatic patients. Avoid use except when benefit outweighs risks. Use cardioselective beta blockers with caution to minimize risk of bronchospasm.
Diuretics, steroids, xanthine derivatives: May increase hypokalemic effect of formoterol. Use together cautiously.
MAO inhibitors, TCAs, other drugs that prolong QT interval: May increase risk of ventricular arrhythmias. Use together cautiously.
Non–potassium-sparing diuretics, such as loop or thiazide diuretics: May worsen ECG changes or hypokalemia. Use together cautiously, and monitor patient for toxicity.

EFFECTS ON LAB TEST RESULTS
- May increase glucose level. May decrease potassium level.

CONTRAINDICATIONS & CAUTIONS
- Contraindicated in patients hypersensitive to drug or its components, or with other long-acting beta$_2$ agonists (LABAs).
Black Box Warning LABAs increase risk of asthma-related death. Safety and effectiveness of drug in patients with asthma haven't been established. All LABAs,

including formoterol, are contraindicated in patients with asthma without use of a long-term asthma control medication. It isn't known if the rate of death in patients with COPD is increased by LABA use. ∎

• Don't begin drug in patients with acutely deteriorating COPD, which may be life-threatening.

• Don't use drug to relieve acute symptoms (such as rescue therapy for acute episodes of bronchospasm). Treat acute symptoms with an inhaled short-acting beta$_2$ agonist.

• Use cautiously in patients with CV disease, especially coronary insufficiency, cardiac arrhythmias, and HTN, and in those who are unusually responsive to sympathomimetic amines.

• Use cautiously in patients with diabetes mellitus because hyperglycemia and ketoacidosis have occurred rarely with the use of beta agonists.

• Use cautiously in patients with seizure disorders or thyrotoxicosis.

Dialyzable drug: Unknown.

⚠ *Overdose S&S:* Exaggeration of adverse reactions, hypotension, cardiac arrest.

PREGNANCY-LACTATION-REPRODUCTION

• Use cautiously in pregnant women and only if benefit outweighs risk to the fetus.

• Drug may interfere with uterine contractility if used during labor.

• Use cautiously in breastfeeding women.

NURSING CONSIDERATIONS

�𝕊 *Alert:* If maintenance regimen fails to provide usual response, contact prescriber immediately, as this indicates COPD destabilization.

�𝕊 *Alert:* As with all beta$_2$ agonists, drug may produce life-threatening paradoxical bronchospasm. If bronchospasm occurs, treat immediately and notify prescriber promptly.

�𝕊 *Alert:* If patient develops tachycardia, HTN, or other adverse CV effects, drug may need to be stopped.

• Watch for immediate hypersensitivity reactions, such as anaphylaxis, urticaria, angioedema, rash, and bronchospasm.

PATIENT TEACHING

• Tell patient not to increase dosage or frequency of use without medical advice and to only use drug with a nebulizer.

• Show patient how use nebulizer according to manufacturer's instructions.

• Advise patient who misses a dose to skip that dose and take the next dose at the usual time.

• Advise patient that drug isn't to be used for acute asthmatic episodes. Prescriber should give a short-acting beta$_2$ agonist for this use.

• Advise patient to immediately report worsening symptoms, treatment that becomes less effective, or increased use of short-acting beta$_2$ agonists.

• Tell patient to report nausea, vomiting, shakiness, headache, fast or irregular heartbeat, or sleeplessness.

• Advise female patient to notify prescriber if she becomes pregnant or is breastfeeding.

foscarnet sodium (PFA, phosphonoformic acid)
foss-CAR-net

Foscavir

Therapeutic class: Antivirals
Pharmacologic class: Pyrophosphate analogues

AVAILABLE FORMS
Injection: 24 mg/mL

INDICATIONS & DOSAGES
Adjust-a-dose (for all indications): Adjust dosage when CrCl is less than 1.4 mL/minute/kg. If CrCl falls below 0.4 mL/minute/kg, stop drug. Consult manufacturer's package insert for specific dosage adjustments.

Black Box Warning Drug is only indicated for use in immunocompromised patients with CMV retinitis and mucocutaneous acyclovir-resistant HSV infections. ∎

➤ **CMV retinitis in patients with AIDS**
Adults: Initially, for induction, 60 mg/kg IV over a minimum of 1 hour every 8 hours or 90 mg/kg IV over 1½ to 2 hours every 12 hours for 2 to 3 weeks, depending on

patient response. Follow with a maintenance infusion of 90 to 120 mg/kg over 2 hours daily. Maximum dosage, 180 mg/kg/day (initial dosage) and 120 mg/kg/day (maintenance dosage).

➤ **Acyclovir-resistant HSV infections**
Adults: 40 mg/kg IV over 1 hour every 8 to 12 hours for 2 to 3 weeks or until healed. Maximum dosage, 120 mg/kg/day.

ADMINISTRATION

IV

Black Box Warning To minimize renal toxicity, make sure patient is adequately hydrated before and during infusion. ▮
▾ Don't exceed the recommended dosage, rate, or frequency of infusion. Doses must be individualized according to patient's renal function.
▾ Drug may be infused via a central or peripheral vein with enough blood flow for rapid distribution and dilution. If infusing into a central vein, don't dilute the commercially available form (24 mg/mL). If infusing into a peripheral vein, dilute to 12 mg/mL with D_5W or NSS to decrease risk of local irritation. Use an infusion pump. Use diluted solutions within 24 hours.
▾ Give induction treatment over 1 to 2 hours, depending on dose, and maintenance infusions over 2 hours and at no more than 1 mg/kg/minute.
▾ **Incompatibilities:** Acyclovir, amphotericin B, dextrose 30%, diazepam, digoxin, ganciclovir, lactated Ringer solution, leucovorin, midazolam, pentamidine, phenytoin, prochlorperazine, promethazine, solutions containing calcium (such as total parenteral nutrition), trimetrexate, sulfamethoxazole–trimethoprim, vancomycin. Other drugs may also be incompatible. Consult a drug incompatibility reference for more information.

ACTION

Inhibits herpes virus replication in vitro by blocking the pyrophosphate-binding site on DNA polymerases and reverse transcriptases.

Route	Onset	Peak	Duration
IV	Unknown	Immediate	Unknown

Half-life: 3 to 4 hours.

ADVERSE REACTIONS

CNS: asthenia, dizziness, fatigue, fever, headache, hypoesthesia, malaise, neuropathy, paresthesia, *seizures,* abnormal coordination, agitation, aggression, amnesia, anxiety, aphasia, ataxia, cerebrovascular disorder, confusion, dementia, depression, EEG abnormalities, generalized spasms, hallucinations, insomnia, meningitis, nervousness, pain, sensory disturbances, somnolence, stupor, tremor. **CV:** ECG abnormalities, first-degree AV block, flushing, HTN, hypotension, palpitations, sinus tachycardia, chest pain, edema. **EENT:** conjunctivitis, eye pain, pharyngitis, rhinitis, sinusitis, visual disturbances. **GI:** abdominal pain, anorexia, diarrhea, nausea, vomiting, *pancreatitis,* constipation, dysphagia, dry mouth, dyspepsia, flatulence, melena, rectal hemorrhage, taste perversion, ulcerative stomatitis. **GU:** *acute renal failure,* abnormal renal function, albuminuria, candidiasis, dysuria, polyuria, urethral disorder, urine retention, UTI. **Hematologic:** anemia, *bone marrow suppression, granulocytopenia, leukopenia, thrombocytopenia,* thrombocytosis. **Hepatic:** abnormal hepatic function. **Metabolic:** hyperphosphatemia, hypocalcemia, hypokalemia, *hypomagnesemia,* hypophosphatemia, hyponatremia. **Musculoskeletal:** arthralgia, back pain, leg cramps, myalgia. **Respiratory:** *bronchospasm,* cough, dyspnea, hemoptysis, pneumonitis, *pneumothorax,* pulmonary infiltration, *respiratory insufficiency, stridor.* **Skin:** diaphoresis, rash, erythematous rash, facial edema, pruritus, seborrhea, skin discoloration, skin ulceration. **Other:** *sarcoma, sepsis,* abscess, bacterial or fungal infections, flulike symptoms, inflammation and pain at infusion site, lymphadenopathy, lymphoma-like disorder, rigors.

INTERACTIONS

Drug-drug. *Calcium:* May decrease serum level of ionized calcium. Avoid concurrent use.
Nephrotoxic drugs (acyclovir, aminoglycosides, amphotericin B, cyclosporine): May increase risk of nephrotoxicity. Avoid using together.
Pentamidine: May increase risk of nephrotoxicity; severe hypocalcemia also has been

---

Reactions in bold italics are *life-threatening*. Interactions may have a *rapid onset* or a *delayed onset*.

reported. Monitor renal function tests and electrolytes.

❸ Alert: *QT-interval prolonging drugs (amiodarone, dofetilide, fluoroquinolones, phenothiazines, procainamide, quinidine, some macrolides, sotalol, TCAs):* May increase risk of prolonged QT interval and torsades de pointes. Avoid use together.

EFFECTS ON LAB TEST RESULTS
• May increase alkaline phosphatase, ALT, AST, bilirubin, creatinine, and phosphate levels. May decrease calcium, Hb, magnesium, phosphate, potassium, and sodium levels.
• May increase platelet count. May decrease granulocyte, platelet, and WBC counts.

CONTRAINDICATIONS & CAUTIONS
• Contraindicated in patients hypersensitive to drug.

Black Box Warning In patients with abnormal renal function, use cautiously, maintain adequate hydration, and reduce dosage. Drug is nephrotoxic and can worsen renal impairment. Some degree of nephrotoxicity occurs in most patients. ∎
• Drug may cause QT-interval prolongation and increase risk of ventricular arrhythmias. Use cautiously in patients with a history of or at risk for QT-interval prolongation.
Dialyzable drug: Yes.
⚠ Overdose S&S: Seizures, renal impairment, paresthesia (limb or perioral), calcium and phosphate electrolyte disturbances.

PREGNANCY-LACTATION-REPRODUCTION
• Use cautiously in pregnant women and only if clearly needed. Monitoring of amniotic fluid volumes by ultrasound is recommended weekly after 20 weeks' gestation to detect oligohydramnios.
• Patient should discontinue breastfeeding or discontinue drug.

NURSING CONSIDERATIONS
❸ Alert: Because drug is highly toxic, which is probably dose-related, always use the lowest effective maintenance dose.
Black Box Warning Frequent monitoring of serum creatinine, with dosage adjustment for changes in renal function, is imperative. ∎

• Monitor CrCl frequently during therapy because of drug's adverse effects on renal function. Obtain a baseline 24-hour CrCl. Monitor level two to three times weekly during induction and at least once every 1 to 2 weeks during maintenance.
Black Box Warning Drug can cause seizures related to altered mineral and electrolyte levels; monitor levels using a schedule similar to that established for monitoring of CrCl. Assess patient for tetany and seizures, and treat with supplementation if necessary. ∎
• Monitor patient's Hb level and hematocrit. Anemia occurs in about one-third of patients and may be severe enough to require transfusions.
• Drug may cause a dose-related transient decrease in ionized calcium, which may not always show up in patient's laboratory values.

PATIENT TEACHING
• Explain the importance of adequate hydration throughout therapy.
• Advise patient to report all adverse reactions, including tingling around the mouth, numbness in the arms and legs, pins-and-needles sensations, chest pain, palpitations, dyspnea, and changes in urine volume or color.
• Tell patient to report discomfort at IV insertion site.

---

fosinopril sodium ✂
foe-SIN-oh-pril

Therapeutic class: Antihypertensives
Pharmacologic class: ACE inhibitors

AVAILABLE FORMS
Tablets: 10 mg, 20 mg, 40 mg

INDICATIONS & DOSAGES
➤ **HTN**
Adults: Initially, 10 mg PO daily; adjust dosage based on BP response at peak and trough levels. Usual dosage is 10 to 40 mg daily; maximum is 80 mg daily. Dosage may be divided.

Children age 6 and older weighing more than 50 kg: Initially, 5 to 10 mg PO once daily. Maximum dosage is 40 mg/day.

➤ **Adjunctive therapy for HF with diuretics or digoxin**

Adults: Initially, 10 mg PO once daily. Increase dosage over several weeks to a maximum of 40 mg PO daily, if needed.

ADMINISTRATION

PO

• Give drug without regard for meals.

ACTION

Inhibits ACE, preventing conversion of angiotensin I to angiotensin II, a potent vasoconstrictor. Less angiotensin II decreases peripheral arterial resistance, thus decreasing aldosterone secretion, which reduces sodium and water retention and lowers BP.

Route	Onset	Peak	Duration
PO	1 hr	3 hr	24 hr

Half-life: 11½ hours.

ADVERSE REACTIONS

CNS: dizziness, *stroke,* headache, fatigue, syncope, paresthesia, sleep disturbance, weakness. **CV:** *MI,* chest pain, angina pectoris, rhythm disturbances, palpitations, hypotension, orthostatic hypotension, flushing. **EENT:** tinnitus, sinusitis. **GI:** *pancreatitis,* nausea, vomiting, diarrhea, dry mouth, abdominal distention, abdominal pain, constipation. **GU:** sexual dysfunction, renal insufficiency, urinary frequency. **Hepatic:** *hepatitis.* **Metabolic:** *hyperkalemia.* **Musculoskeletal:** arthralgia, musculoskeletal pain, myalgia. **Respiratory:** dry, persistent, tickling, nonproductive cough; *bronchospasm.* **Skin:** urticaria, rash, photosensitivity reactions, pruritus. **Other:** *angioedema,* decreased libido, gout.

INTERACTIONS

Drug-drug. *Aliskiren:* Increases risk of hypotension, hyperkalemia, and renal dysfunction. Don't use together in patients with GFR less than 60 mL/minute. Contraindicated in patients with diabetes.

Antacids: May impair absorption. Separate dosage times by at least 2 hours.

ARBs: May increase toxic effects of ACE inhibitors. Avoid use together when possible.

Azathioprine: May increase risk of anemia or leukopenia. Monitor hematologic studies if used together.

Diuretics, other antihypertensives: May cause excessive hypotension. Stop diuretic or lower fosinopril dosage.

Everolimus: May increase risk of angioedema. Use extreme caution.

Lithium: May increase lithium level and lithium toxicity. Monitor lithium level.

Nesiritide: May increase hypotensive effects. Monitor BP.

NSAIDs: May decrease antihypertensive effects and increase potential for renal dysfunction. Monitor BP.

Potassium-sparing diuretics, potassium supplements: May cause hyperkalemia. Use cautiously and monitor patient closely.

Drug-herb. *Capsaicin:* May cause cough. Discourage use together.

Ma huang: May decrease antihypertensive effects. Discourage use together.

Drug-food. *Salt substitutes containing potassium:* May increase risk of hyperkalemia. Discourage use together.

EFFECTS ON LAB TEST RESULTS

• May increase BUN, creatinine, potassium, and Hb levels and hematocrit.

• May increase LFT values.

• May cause falsely low digoxin level with the Digi-Tab radioimmunoassay kit for digoxin.

CONTRAINDICATIONS & CAUTIONS

• Contraindicated in patients hypersensitive to drug or other ACE inhibitors.

• Use cautiously in patients with impaired renal or hepatic function.

Dialyzable drug: 2% to 7%.

⚠ *Overdose S&S:* Hypotension.

PREGNANCY-LACTATION-REPRODUCTION

• Use in pregnant and breastfeeding women isn't recommended.

Black Box Warning Use during pregnancy can cause injury and death to the developing fetus. When pregnancy is detected, stop drug as soon as possible. ∎

Reactions in bold italics are *life-threatening.* Interactions may have a *rapid onset* or a *delayed onset.*

NURSING CONSIDERATIONS

• Monitor BP for drug effect.

▓ Black patients who take ACE inhibitors as monotherapy for HTN have a smaller reduction in BP than non-Black patients. Black patients taking ACE inhibitors have a higher incidence of angioedema than non-Blacks.

• Drug can increase risk of angioedema, including intestinal angioedema. Monitor patient for facial swelling, airway obstruction, and abdominal pain.

• Monitor potassium intake and potassium level. Diabetic patients, those with impaired renal function, and those receiving drugs that can increase potassium level may develop hyperkalemia.

• Other ACE inhibitors may cause agranulocytosis and neutropenia. Monitor CBC with differential counts before therapy and periodically thereafter.

• Assess renal and hepatic function before and periodically throughout therapy.

• **Look alike–sound alike:** Don't confuse fosinopril with lisinopril. Don't confuse Monopril with Monurol.

PATIENT TEACHING

• Tell patient to avoid potassium-containing salt substitutes, which may increase risk of hyperkalemia when taken with fosinopril.

• Instruct patient to contact prescriber if light-headedness or fainting occurs.

• Advise patient to report evidence of infection, such as fever and sore throat.

• Instruct patient to report easy bruising or bleeding; swelling of tongue, lips, face, eyes, mucous membranes, arms, or legs; difficulty swallowing or breathing; cough; or hoarseness.

• Urge patient to use caution in hot weather and during exercise. Inadequate fluid intake, vomiting, diarrhea, and excessive perspiration can lead to light-headedness and fainting.

• Tell diabetic patient using oral antidiabetic agents or insulin who is starting an ACE inhibitor to closely watch for hypoglycemia, especially during first month of combined use.

• Tell female patient of childbearing potential to notify prescriber if pregnancy occurs. Drug will need to be stopped.

---

fosphenytoin sodium ▓
faws-FEN-i-toe-in

Cerebyx

Therapeutic class: Anticonvulsants
Pharmacologic class: Hydantoin derivatives

AVAILABLE FORMS

Injection: 100 mg phenytoin sodium equivalents/2 mL, 500 mg phenytoin sodium equivalents/10 mL vials

INDICATIONS & DOSAGES

Adjust-a-dose (for all indications): Phenytoin clearance is decreased slightly in elderly patients; lower or less frequent dosing may be required.

➤ **Status epilepticus**

Adults: Loading dose, 15 to 20 mg phenytoin sodium equivalent/kg IV at infusion rate of 100 to 150 mg phenytoin sodium equivalent/minute; then 4 to 6 mg phenytoin sodium equivalent/kg/day IV or IM in divided doses as maintenance dose.

Children from birth to younger than age 17: Loading dose, 15 to 20 mg phenytoin sodium equivalent/kg IV at 2 mg phenytoin sodium equivalent/minute or 150 mg phenytoin sodium equivalent/minute, whichever is slower; then 2 to 4 mg phenytoin sodium equivalent/kg IV given 12 hours after loading dose, then continued once every 12 hours at 1 to 2 mg phenytoin sodium equivalent/kg/minute or 100 mg/minute, whichever is slower.

➤ **To prevent and treat seizures during neurosurgery (nonemergent loading or maintenance dosing)**

Adults: Loading dose, 10 to 20 mg phenytoin sodium equivalent/kg IM or IV at infusion rate not exceeding 150 mg phenytoin sodium equivalent/minute. Maintenance dose is 4 to 6 mg phenytoin sodium equivalent/kg/day IV or IM in divided doses.

Children from birth to younger than age 17: Loading dose, 10 to 15 mg phenytoin sodium equivalent/kg IV at 1 to 2 mg phenytoin sodium equivalent/minute or 150 mg phenytoin sodium equivalent/minute, whichever is slower; then 2 to 4 mg phenytoin sodium equivalent/kg IV

---

given 12 hours after loading dose, then continued once every 12 hours at 1 to 2 mg phenytoin sodium equivalent/kg/minute or 100 mg/minute, whichever is slower.

ADMINISTRATION

IV

▼ If rapid phenytoin loading is a main goal, this form is preferred.

▼ For status epilepticus, give IV rather than IM because therapeutic phenytoin level occurs more rapidly.

▼ For infusion, dilute in D_5W or NSS for injection to yield 1.5 to 25 mg phenytoin sodium equivalent/mL.

Black Box Warning Don't give more than 150 mg phenytoin sodium equivalent/minute in adults and 2 mg phenytoin sodium equivalent/kg/minute (or 150 mg phenytoin sodium equivalent/minute) in children because of risk of severe hypotension and cardiac arrhythmias. Careful cardiac monitoring is needed during and after administering IV drug. Although risk of CV toxicity increases with infusion rates above the recommended infusion rate, these events have also been reported at or below the recommended infusion rate. Reducing rate of administration or discontinuing drug may be needed. ■

▼ Maintenance infusion rates in children shouldn't exceed 1 to 2 mg phenytoin sodium equivalent/kg/minute (or 100 mg phenytoin sodium equivalent/minute, whichever is slower).

▼ Patients receiving 20 mg phenytoin sodium equivalent/kg at 150 mg phenytoin sodium equivalent/minute typically feel discomfort, usually in the groin. To reduce discomfort, slow or temporarily stop infusion.

▼ Monitor patient's ECG, BP, and respirations continuously during maximum phenytoin level—about 10 to 20 minutes after end of fosphenytoin infusion. Severe CV complications are most common in elderly or gravely ill patients. If needed, decrease rate or stop infusion.

▼ Store drug under refrigeration. Don't store at room temperature longer than 48 hours. Discard vials that develop particulate matter.

▼ **Incompatibilities:** Other IV drugs.

IM

● Depending on dose ordered, may require two separate IM injections.

● IM administration generates systemic phenytoin levels similar enough to oral phenytoin sodium to allow essentially interchangeable use.

● Store drug under refrigeration. Don't store at room temperature longer than 48 hours. Discard vials that develop particulate matter.

ACTION

May stabilize neuronal membranes and limit seizure activity either by increasing efflux or decreasing influx of sodium ions across cell membranes in the motor cortex during generation of nerve impulses.

Route	Onset	Peak	Duration
IV	Unknown	End of infusion	Unknown
IM	Unknown	30 min	Unknown

Half-life: Fosphenytoin, 15 minutes; phenytoin, 12 to 29 hours.

ADVERSE REACTIONS

CNS: ataxia, dizziness, somnolence, ***brain edema, intracranial HTN,*** agitation, asthenia, dysarthria, extrapyramidal syndrome, fever, headache, hypesthesia, incoordination, increased or decreased reflexes, nervousness, paresthesia, speech disorders, stupor, thinking abnormalities, tremor, vertigo. **CV:** HTN, hypotension, tachycardia, vasodilation. **EENT:** nystagmus, amblyopia, deafness, diplopia, tinnitus. **GI:** constipation, dry mouth, taste perversion, tongue disorder, vomiting. **GU:** pelvic pain. **Metabolic:** *hypokalemia.* **Musculoskeletal:** back pain, myasthenia. **Respiratory:** pneumonia. **Skin:** pruritus, ecchymoses, injection-site reaction and pain, rash. **Other:** accidental injury, chills, facial edema, infection.

INTERACTIONS

Drug-drug. *Amiodarone, capecitabine, chloramphenicol, chlordiazepoxide, cimetidine, disulfiram, estrogens, ethosuximide, felbamate, 5-FU, fluconazole, fluoxetine, fluvastatin, fluvoxamine, H_2-receptor antagonists, isoniazid, itraconazole, ketoconazole, methylphenidate, miconazole, omeprazole, oxcarbazepine, phenothiazines, salicylates, sertraline, succinimides, sulfonamides,*

Reactions in bold italics are *life-threatening.* Interactions may have a *rapid onset* or a ***delayed onset.***

ticlopidine, tolbutamide, topiramate, tra-zodone, voriconazole, warfarin: May increase phenytoin level and effect. Use together cautiously.

Bleomycin, carbamazepine, carboplatin, cisplatin, diazepam, diazoxide, doxorubicin, folic acid, fosamprenavir, methotrexate, nelfinavir, reserpine, rifampin, ritonavir, theophylline, vigabatrin: May decrease phenytoin level. Monitor patient.

Cisatracurium, corticosteroids, delavirdine, doxycycline, estrogens, fluconazole, furosemide, hormonal contraceptives, irinotecan, itraconazole, ketoconazole, paclitaxel, pancuronium, paroxetine, posaconazole, quinidine, rifampin, rocuronium, sertraline, teniposide, theophylline, vecuronium, vitamin D, voriconazole, warfarin: May decrease effects of these drugs because of increased hepatic metabolism. Monitor patient closely.

Lithium: May increase lithium toxicity. Monitor patient's neurologic status closely. Marked neurologic symptoms have been reported despite normal lithium level.

Phenobarbital, valproate sodium, valproic acid: May increase or decrease phenytoin level. May increase or decrease levels of these drugs. Monitor patient.

TCAs: May lower seizure threshold and require adjustments in phenytoin dosage. Use together cautiously.

Drug-herb. *St. John's wort:* May decrease phenytoin level. Monitor patient.

Drug-lifestyle. *Alcohol use:* Acute intoxication may increase phenytoin level and effect. Discourage use together.

Long-term alcohol use: May decrease phenytoin level. Monitor patient and strongly discourage use together.

EFFECTS ON LAB TEST RESULTS
• May increase alkaline phosphatase, GGT, and glucose levels. May decrease folate, potassium, and T4 levels.
• May cause falsely low dexamethasone and metyrapone test results.

CONTRAINDICATIONS & CAUTIONS
• Contraindicated in patients hypersensitive to drug or its components, phenytoin, or other hydantoins.

• Contraindicated in patients with a history of prior acute hepatotoxicity attributable to fosphenytoin or phenytoin.
• Contraindicated in patients with sinus bradycardia, SA block, second- or third-degree AV block, or Adams-Stokes syndrome.
• Contraindicated in patients taking delavirdine because of potential loss of virologic response and possible resistance to delavirdine or to NNRTIs.

Black Box Warning There is an increased risk of severe hypotension and cardiac arrhythmia (bradycardia, heart block, QT-interval prolongation, ventricular tachycardia, ventricular fibrillation) with IV infusion rate of greater than 150 mg phenytoin sodium equivalent/minute. CV effects can also occur at lower infusion rates; therefore, cardiac monitoring is needed during and after infusion. Reduce rate or discontinue drug as clinically necessary. ∎

• Use cautiously in patients with porphyria and in those with history of hypersensitivity to similarly structured drugs, such as barbiturates, oxazolidinediones, and succinimide.

⊕ Alert: If patient develops acute hepatotoxicity, discontinue drug and don't readminister.

⊕ Alert: Serious and sometimes fatal toxic epidermal necrolysis and SJS have been reported; usually onset of symptoms occurs within 28 days but sometimes later. Discontinue drug at first sign of rash unless rash is clearly not drug related. If rash occurs, evaluate patient for signs and symptoms of DRESS syndrome.

Dialyzable drug: Unknown.

⚠ Overdose S&S: Asystole, bradycardia, cardiac arrest, hypocalcemia, hypotension, lethargy, metabolic acidosis, nausea, syncope, tachycardia, vomiting, death.

PREGNANCY-LACTATION-REPRODUCTION
• Drug is known to cause birth defects. Use with extreme caution in pregnant women after assessing maternal benefits and fetal risk.
• Prenatal exposure to phenytoin may increase the risk of congenital malformations and other adverse developmental outcomes.
• A potentially life-threatening bleeding disorder related to decreased levels of vitamin

K–dependent clotting factors may occur in newborns exposed to phenytoin in utero. This drug-induced condition can be prevented with vitamin K administration to the mother before delivery and to the neonate after birth.

• It isn't known if fosphenytoin appears in human milk but phenytoin does appear in human milk. Weigh benefits of breastfeeding along with the mother's need for drug and potential adverse effects on the breastfed infant.

NURSING CONSIDERATIONS

۞ Alert: Because of risk of cardiac and local toxicity with IV fosphenytoin administration, use oral phenytoin whenever possible.

• Most significant drug interactions are those commonly seen with phenytoin.

۞ Alert: Drug should always be prescribed and dispensed in phenytoin sodium equivalent units. Don't make adjustments in the recommended doses when substituting fosphenytoin for phenytoin, and vice versa.

• In status epilepticus, phenytoin may be used as maintenance instead of fosphenytoin, using the appropriate dose.

• Phosphate load provided by fosphenytoin (0.0037 millimole phosphate/mg phenytoin sodium equivalent) must be taken into consideration when treating patients who need phosphate restriction, such as those with severe renal impairment. Monitor laboratory values.

▓ Patients with Chinese ancestry who have tested positive for the allele HLA-B*1502 have a potentially increased risk of serious skin reactions, including SJS and toxic epidermal necrolysis. Monitor these patients carefully.

▓ Some patients treated with phenytoin have been shown to metabolize the drug slowly, which appears to be genetically determined. If early signs and symptoms of dose-related CNS toxicity develop, check serum levels immediately.

• If patient develops exfoliative, purpuric, or bullous rash or signs and symptoms of SLE, SJS, or toxic epidermal necrolysis, stop drug and notify prescriber. If rash is mild (measles-like or scarlatiniform), therapy may resume after rash disappears. If rash recurs when therapy is resumed, further

fosphenytoin or phenytoin administration is contraindicated. Document that patient is allergic to drug.

• Stop drug in patients with acute hepatotoxicity.

• Doses are usually selected to attain therapeutic serum total phenytoin concentrations of 10 to 20 mcg/mL (unbound phenytoin concentrations of 1 to 2 mcg/mL). Trough levels provide information about clinically effective serum level range and are obtained just before patient's next scheduled dose.

• After administration, phenytoin levels shouldn't be monitored until conversion to phenytoin is essentially complete—about 2 hours after the end of an IV infusion or 4 hours after IM administration.

• Interpret total phenytoin levels cautiously in patients with renal or hepatic disease or hypoalbuminemia caused by an increased fraction of unbound phenytoin. It may be more useful to monitor unbound phenytoin levels in these patients. When giving drug IV, monitor patients with renal and hepatic disease because they are at increased risk for more frequent and severe adverse reactions.

• Monitor glucose level closely in diabetic patients; drug may cause hyperglycemia.

۞ Alert: Abrupt withdrawal of drug may precipitate status epilepticus.

• **Look alike–sound alike:** Don't confuse Cerebyx with Cerezyme, Celexa, or Celebrex.

PATIENT TEACHING

• Warn patient that sensory disturbances may occur with IV administration.

• Instruct patient to immediately report adverse reactions, especially rash, palpitations, dyspnea, chest pain, and dizziness.

• Warn patient not to stop drug abruptly or adjust dosage without discussing with prescriber.

• Advise female patient of childbearing potential to discuss drug therapy with prescriber if considering pregnancy.

• Advise female patient of childbearing potential that the benefits of breastfeeding should be weighed along with her need for drug and potential adverse effects on the breastfed infant.

Reactions in bold italics are *life-threatening*. Interactions may have a *rapid onset* or a *delayed onset*.

• Recommend that pregnant patient taking drug enroll in the North American AED Pregnancy Registry (www.aedpregnancyregistry.org or 1-888-233-2334).

frovatriptan succinate
frow-vah-TRIP-tan

Frova*⊘*

Therapeutic class: Antimigraine drugs
Pharmacologic class: Serotonin 5-HT₁ receptor agonists

AVAILABLE FORMS
Tablets: 2.5 mg

INDICATIONS & DOSAGES
➤ **Acute treatment of migraine attacks with or without aura**
Adults: 2.5 mg PO taken at the first sign of migraine attack. If the headache recurs, a second tablet may be taken at least 2 hours after the first dose. The total daily dose (per 24 hours) shouldn't exceed 7.5 mg.

ADMINISTRATION
PO
• Give drug without regard for food.
• Give drug with fluids as soon as signs or symptoms appear.

ACTION
May cause vasoconstriction in response to excessive dilation of extracerebral and intracranial arteries during migraine headaches.

Route	Onset	Peak	Duration
PO	Unknown	2–4 hr	Unknown

Half-life: 26 hours.

ADVERSE REACTIONS
CNS: dizziness, headache, fatigue, paresthesia, insomnia, anxiety, somnolence, dysesthesia, hypoesthesia, hot or cold sensation, pain, drowsiness. **CV:** chest pain, palpitations, flushing. **EENT:** abnormal vision, tinnitus, sinusitis, rhinitis. **GI:** dry mouth, dyspepsia, vomiting, abdominal pain, diarrhea,

nausea. **Musculoskeletal:** skeletal pain. **Skin:** increased sweating.

INTERACTIONS
Drug-drug. *Ergotamine-containing or ergot-type drugs (dihydroergotamine or methysergide):* May cause prolonged vasospastic reactions. Separate doses by 24 hours.
5-HT₁ agonists (such as triptans): May cause additive effects. Separate doses by 24 hours.
MAO inhibitors, SSRIs (citalopram, fluoxetine, fluvoxamine, paroxetine, sertraline), TCAs: May cause serotonin syndrome. Discontinue drug if serotonin syndrome is suspected.

EFFECTS ON LAB TEST RESULTS
None reported.

CONTRAINDICATIONS & CAUTIONS
• Contraindicated in patients hypersensitive to drug or its components.
• Contraindicated in patients with history or symptoms of ischemic heart disease or coronary artery vasospasm, including Prinzmetal variant angina, Wolff-Parkinson-White syndrome, or other cardiac accessory conduction pathway disorders; in those with cerebrovascular disease or PVD, including ischemic bowel disease; in those with uncontrolled HTN; and in those with hemiplegic or basilar migraine.
• Contraindicated within 24 hours of another triptan, drug containing ergotamine, or ergot-type drug.
• Contraindicated in patients with risk factors for CAD, such as HTN, hypercholesterolemia, smoking, obesity, diabetes, strong family history of CAD, postmenopausal women, or men older than age 40, unless patient is free from cardiac disease. If drug is used in such a patient, monitor patient closely and consider obtaining an ECG after the first dose. Intermittent, long-term users of triptans or those with risk factors should undergo periodic cardiac evaluation while using drug.
• Safety of treating an average of more than four migraine headaches in a 30-day period hasn't been established.
Dialyzable drug: Unknown.

PREGNANCY-LACTATION-REPRODUCTION
• It isn't known if drug affects fetal development. Use during pregnancy only if potential benefit justifies potential risk to the fetus.
• It isn't known if drug appears in human milk. Patient should discontinue breastfeeding or discontinue drug.

NURSING CONSIDERATIONS
❸ **Alert:** Rare but serious cardiac events, including acute MI, life-threatening cardiac arrhythmias, and death, may occur within a few hours of a triptan dose.
• Use drug only when patient has a clear diagnosis of migraine. If patient has no response for the first migraine attack treated with frovatriptan, reconsider the diagnosis of migraine.
❸ **Alert:** Combining a triptan with an SSRI or SSNRI, a TCA, MAO inhibitors, or agents that reduce frovatriptan's metabolism may cause serotonin syndrome. Signs and symptoms may include restlessness, hallucinations, loss of coordination, fast heartbeat, rapid changes in BP, increased body temperature, hyperreflexia, nausea, vomiting, and diarrhea. Serotonin syndrome is more likely to occur when starting or increasing dosage of a serotonergic drug and usually occurs within minutes to hours.

PATIENT TEACHING
• Instruct patient to take dose at first sign of migraine headache. If headache comes back after first dose, patient may take a second dose after 2 hours. Tell patient not to take more than 3 tablets in 24 hours.
• Caution patient to take extra care or avoid driving and operating machinery if dizziness or fatigue develops after taking drug.
• Stress importance of reporting all adverse reactions. Advise patient to immediately report pain, tightness, heaviness, or pressure in chest, throat, neck, or jaw; or rash or itching after taking drug.
• Instruct patient not to take drug within 24 hours of taking another serotonin-receptor agonist or ergot-type drug.
• Tell patient dose may be taken with or without food, but to take with a full glass of fluid.

SAFETY ALERT!

fulvestrant ℞
full-VES-trant

Faslodex

Therapeutic class: Antineoplastics
Pharmacologic class: Estrogen antagonists

AVAILABLE FORMS
Injection: 50 mg/mL in 5-mL prefilled syringes*

INDICATIONS & DOSAGES
Adjust-a-dose (for all indications): For patients with moderate hepatic impairment (Child-Pugh class·B), give 250 mg IM slowly into buttocks over 1 to 2 minutes as one 5-mL injection on days 1, 15, and 29, then monthly thereafter.
➤ **Hormone receptor (HR)–positive metastatic breast cancer with disease progression after antiestrogen therapy**
Postmenopausal women: 500 mg IM slowly into buttocks (over 1 to 2 minutes per injection) as two 5-mL injections, one in each buttock on days 1, 15, and 29, then once monthly thereafter.
➤ **HR-positive, HER2-negative advanced or metastatic breast cancer in combination with palbociclib or abemaciclib in women with disease progression after endocrine therapy** ℞
Adults: 500 mg IM slowly into buttocks (1 to 2 minutes per injection) as two 5-mL injections, one in each buttock, on days 1, 15, 29, and then once monthly thereafter. Recommended palbociclib dose is a 125-mg capsule PO once daily for 21 consecutive days followed by 7 days off each 28-day cycle. Recommended abemaciclib dosage is one 150-mg tablet PO b.i.d. Premenopausal and perimenopausal women treated with this combination should be treated with luteinizing hormone-releasing hormone (LHRH) agonists according to current clinical practice standards.
Adjust-a-dose: Refer to palbociclib or abemaciclib prescribing information for dosage adjustments and management of toxicity, use with concomitant medications, and other

---

Reactions in bold italics are *life-threatening*. Interactions may have a *rapid onset* or a *delayed onset*.

relevant safety information related to palbociclib and abemaciclib.

➤ **HR-positive, HER2-negative advanced breast cancer in women not previously treated with endocrine therapy** ▧

Postmenopausal women: 500 mg IM slowly into buttocks (over 1 to 2 minutes per injection) as two 5-mL injections, one in each buttock on days 1, 15, and 29, then once monthly thereafter.

➤ **HR-positive, HER2-negative advanced or metastatic breast cancer in postmenopausal women in combination with ribociclib, as initial endocrine-based therapy or after disease progression on endocrine therapy** ▧

Adults: 500 mg IM slowly into buttocks (over 1 to 2 minutes per injection) as two 5-mL injections, one in each buttock on days 1, 15, and 29, then once monthly thereafter. Recommended ribociclib dose is 600 mg PO once daily for 21 consecutive days followed by 7 days off treatment for each 28-day cycle.

Adjust-a-dose: For patients with moderate hepatic impairment (Child-Pugh class B), give 250 mg IM slowly into buttocks over 1 to 2 minutes as one 5-mL injection on days 1, 15, 29, then monthly thereafter. Refer to ribociclib prescribing information for dosage adjustments and management of ribociclib-related toxicities.

ADMINISTRATION
IM
• Drug is a potential teratogen. Follow safe handling procedures.
• Drug may be warmed before use by storing at room temperature for 1 hour or rolling injection gently in hands.
• Expel gas bubble from syringe before giving.
• Give slowly into buttocks.

ACTION
Competitively binds estrogen receptors and downregulates estrogen-receptor protein in human breast cancer cells. It's effective in treating estrogen receptor–positive breast tumors.

Route	Onset	Peak	Duration
IM	Unknown	7 days	1 mo

Half-life: About 40 days.

ADVERSE REACTIONS
CNS: asthenia, headache, pain, dizziness, insomnia, fever, paresthesia, depression, anxiety, fatigue. **CV:** hot flashes, chest pain, peripheral edema, vasodilation. **EENT:** pharyngitis. **GI:** nausea, vomiting, constipation, abdominal pain, diarrhea, anorexia. **GU:** UTI. **Hematologic:** anemia. **Hepatic:** elevated AST and ALT levels. **Musculoskeletal:** bone pain, back pain, pelvic pain, arthritis. **Respiratory:** dyspnea, cough. **Skin:** injection-site pain, rash, sweating. **Other:** accidental injury, flulike syndrome.

INTERACTIONS
None reported.

EFFECTS ON LAB TEST RESULTS
• May increase ALT and AST levels.
• May decrease Hb level and hematocrit.
• May interfere with estradiol measurement by immunoassay, resulting in falsely elevated estradiol levels.

CONTRAINDICATIONS & CAUTIONS
• Contraindicated in patients allergic to drug or its components.
• Use cautiously in patients with moderate or severe hepatic impairment.
• When drug is used with palbociclib or abemaciclib, leukopenia, thrombocytopenia, neutropenia, and febrile neutropenia may occur.
Dialyzable drug: Unknown.

PREGNANCY-LACTATION-REPRODUCTION
• Drug can cause fetal harm. Women of childbearing potential should be advised not to become pregnant during therapy. If drug is used during pregnancy, or if patient becomes pregnant during therapy, apprise patient of potential hazard to the fetus. Women should use effective contraception during therapy and for 1 year after final dose.
• It isn't known if drug appears in human milk. Women shouldn't breastfeed during therapy and for 1 year after final dose.

NURSING CONSIDERATIONS
• Because drug is given IM, use cautiously in patients with bleeding diatheses or thrombocytopenia, and in those taking anticoagulants.
• Pregnancy testing is recommended within 7 days before initiating drug.

PATIENT TEACHING
• Caution female patient to avoid pregnancy and breastfeeding during therapy and for 1 year after final dose and to report suspected pregnancy immediately.
• Inform patient of the most common adverse effects, including pain at injection site, headache, GI symptoms, back pain, hot flashes, and sore throat. Advise patient to report all adverse reactions.

furosemide
fur-OH-se-mide

Lasix❧, Lasix Special✦

Therapeutic class: Antihypertensives
Pharmacologic class: Loop diuretics

AVAILABLE FORMS
Injection: 10 mg/mL
Oral solution: 10 mg/mL, 40 mg/5 mL
Tablets: 20 mg, 40 mg, 80 mg, 500 mg✦

INDICATIONS & DOSAGES
➤ **Acute pulmonary edema**
Adults: 40 mg IV injected slowly over 1 to 2 minutes; then 80 mg IV in 60 to 90 minutes if needed. Maximum is 200 mg/dose.
➤ **Edema**
Adults: 20 to 80 mg PO daily in the morning. If response is inadequate, give a second dose, and each succeeding dose, every 6 to 8 hours. Carefully increase dose in 20- to 40-mg increments up to 600 mg daily. Once effective dose is attained, may give once daily or b.i.d. Or, 20 to 40 mg IV or IM, increased by 20 mg 2 hours after previous dose until desired effect achieved.
Infants and children: 2 mg/kg PO daily, increased by 1 to 2 mg/kg in 6 to 8 hours if needed; carefully adjusted up to maximum of 6 mg/kg if needed. Or, 1 mg/kg slowly IV or IM. May increase dosage by 1 mg/kg

2 hours after previous dose if needed up to 6 mg/kg. Maximum dose is 1 mg/kg/day for premature infants.
➤ **HTN**
Adults: 20 to 40 mg PO b.i.d. Dosage adjusted based on response. Usual dose is 40 to 80 mg/day in two divided doses. May be used as adjunct to other antihypertensives if needed.

ADMINISTRATION
PO
• To prevent nocturia, give in the morning. Give second dose if ordered in early afternoon, 6 to 8 hours after morning dose.
• Store tablets in light-resistant container to prevent discoloration (doesn't affect potency). Refrigerate oral solution to ensure drug stability.
IV
▼ If discolored yellow, don't use.
▼ For direct injection, give over 1 to 2 minutes.
✪ *Alert:* For high-dose, intermittent infusion in adults, dilute with D_5W, NSS, or lactated Ringer solution. To avoid ototoxicity, infuse at a rate no greater than 4 mg/minute.
▼ Use prepared infusion solution within 24 hours.
▼ **Incompatibilities:** Acidic solutions, amrinone, ciprofloxacin, milrinone, and various others. Consult a drug incompatibility reference for more information.
IM
• To prevent nocturia, give in the morning. Give second dose if ordered in early afternoon, 6 to 8 hours after morning dose.
• Record administration site.

ACTION
Inhibits sodium and chloride reabsorption at the proximal and distal tubules and the ascending loop of Henle.

Route	Onset	Peak	Duration
PO	20–60 min	1–2 hr	6–8 hr
IV	Within 5 min	30 min	2 hr
IM	Unknown	30 min	2 hr

Half-life: 2 hours.

ADVERSE REACTIONS

CNS: vertigo, headache, dizziness, paresthesia, weakness, restlessness, fever. **CV:** orthostatic hypotension, thrombophlebitis with IV administration. **EENT:** blurred or yellowed vision, transient deafness, tinnitus. **GI:** abdominal discomfort and pain, diarrhea, anorexia, nausea, vomiting, constipation, *pancreatitis.* **GU:** azotemia, nocturia, polyuria, frequent urination, oliguria. **Hematologic:** *agranulocytosis, aplastic anemia, leukopenia, thrombocytopenia,* anemia. **Hepatic:** hepatic dysfunction, jaundice, increased liver enzyme levels. **Metabolic:** volume depletion and dehydration, asymptomatic hyperuricemia, impaired glucose tolerance, *hypokalemia,* hypochloremic alkalosis, hyperglycemia, dilutional hyponatremia, *hypocalcemia, hypomagnesemia.* **Musculoskeletal:** muscle spasm. **Skin:** dermatitis, purpura, photosensitivity reactions, transient pain at IM injection site, *toxic epidermal necrolysis, SJS, erythema multiforme.* **Other:** gout.

INTERACTIONS

Drug-drug. *Aminoglycoside antibiotics, cisplatin:* May increase ototoxicity. Use together cautiously.
Amphotericin B, corticosteroids, corticotropin, metolazone: May increase risk of hypokalemia. Monitor potassium level closely.
Antidiabetics: May decrease hypoglycemic effects. Monitor glucose level.
Antihypertensives: May increase risk of hypotension. Use together cautiously. Decrease antihypertensive dose if needed.
Cardiac glycosides, neuromuscular blockers: May increase toxicity of these drugs from furosemide-induced hypokalemia. Monitor potassium level.
Chlorothiazide, chlorthalidone, hydrochlorothiazide, indapamide, metolazone: May cause excessive diuretic response, causing serious electrolyte abnormalities or dehydration. Adjust doses carefully, and monitor patient closely for signs and symptoms of excessive diuretic response.
Ethacrynic acid: May increase risk of ototoxicity. Avoid using together.
Lithium: May decrease lithium excretion, resulting in lithium toxicity. Monitor lithium level.

NSAIDs: May inhibit diuretic response. Use together cautiously.
Phenytoin: May decrease diuretic effects of furosemide. Use together cautiously.
Propranolol: May increase propranolol level. Monitor patient closely.
Salicylates: May cause salicylate toxicity. Use together cautiously.
Sucralfate: May reduce diuretic and antihypertensive effect. Separate doses by 2 hours.
Drug-herb. *Aloe:* May increase drug effect. Discourage use together.
Bayberry, blue cohosh, cayenne, ephedra, ginger, ginseng (American), kola, licorice: May worsen HTN. Discourage use together.
Licorice: May cause unexpected rapid potassium loss. Discourage use together.
Drug-food. *Any food:* May decrease furosemide serum level. Don't give with food.
Drug-lifestyle. *Sun exposure:* May increase risk of photosensitivity reactions. Advise patient to avoid excessive sunlight exposure.

EFFECTS ON LAB TEST RESULTS

● May increase cholesterol, glucose, BUN, creatinine, liver enzyme, and uric acid levels. May decrease calcium, magnesium, potassium, and sodium levels.
● May decrease Hb level and granulocyte, platelet, and WBC counts.

CONTRAINDICATIONS & CAUTIONS

● Contraindicated in patients hypersensitive to drug and in those with anuria.
● Use cautiously in patients with hepatic cirrhosis and in those allergic to sulfonamides.
● **Alert:** Drug may cause tinnitus and reversible or irreversible hearing loss. Ototoxicity is associated with rapid injection, severe renal impairment, use of higher-than-recommended doses, hypoproteinemia, or use with other ototoxic drugs.
● Drug may exacerbate or activate SLE.
● Premature infants may be at increased risk for persistent patent ductus arteriosus with furosemide treatment during first weeks of life.
Dialyzable drug: No.
⚠ Overdose S&S: Dehydration, blood volume reduction, hypotension, electrolyte imbalance.

PREGNANCY-LACTATION-REPRODUCTION

• There are no well-controlled studies in pregnant women. Use during pregnancy only if potential benefit justifies potential risk to the fetus.

• Drug appears in human milk. Use cautiously in breastfeeding women.

NURSING CONSIDERATIONS

⚠ *Alert:* Monitor weight, BP, and pulse rate routinely with long-term use.

Black Box Warning Drug is potent diuretic and can cause severe diuresis with water and electrolyte depletion. Monitor patient closely and adjust dose carefully. ∎

• If oliguria or azotemia develops or increases, drug may need to be stopped.

• Monitor fluid intake and output and electrolyte, BUN, and carbon dioxide levels frequently.

• Watch for signs of hypokalemia, such as muscle weakness and cramps.

• Consult prescriber and dietitian about a high-potassium diet or potassium supplements.

• Monitor glucose level in diabetic patients.

• Drug may not be well absorbed orally in patient with severe HF. Drug may need to be given IV even if patient is taking other oral drugs.

• Monitor uric acid level, especially in patients with a history of gout.

• Monitor elderly patients, who are especially susceptible to excessive diuresis, because circulatory collapse and thromboembolic complications are possible.

• Monitor patients with severe symptoms of urine retention due to bladder emptying disorders, prostate enlargement, or urethral narrowing or worsening of symptoms, especially during initial treatment.

• Drug may increase fetal birth weight. Monitor fetal growth during pregnancy.

• Nephrocalcinosis and nephrolithiasis have occurred in premature infants and in children younger than age 4 on long-term furosemide therapy. Monitor renal function and renal ultrasounds.

• *Look alike–sound alike:* Don't confuse furosemide with torsemide. Don't confuse Lasix with Lonox, Lidex, or Luvox.

PATIENT TEACHING

• Advise patient to take drug in morning to prevent need to urinate at night. If a second dose is needed, tell patient to take it in early afternoon, 6 to 8 hours after morning dose.

• Inform patient of possible need for potassium or magnesium supplements.

• Instruct patient to stand slowly to prevent dizziness and to limit alcohol intake and strenuous exercise in hot weather to avoid worsening dizziness upon standing quickly.

• Advise patient to report all adverse reactions and to immediately report ringing in ears, severe abdominal pain, or sore throat and fever; these symptoms may indicate toxicity.

⚠ *Alert:* Discourage patient from storing different types of drugs in the same container, increasing risk of drug errors. (The most popular strengths of furosemide and digoxin are white tablets that are about equal in size.)

• Tell patient to consult prescriber or pharmacist before taking OTC drugs.

• Teach patient to avoid direct sunlight and to use protective clothing and sunblock because of risk of photosensitivity reactions.

gabapentin
gab-ah-PEN-tin

Gralise, Neurontin✦

gabapentin enacarbil
Horizant

Therapeutic class: Anticonvulsants
Pharmacologic class: GABA structural analogues

AVAILABLE FORMS

Capsules: 100 mg, 300 mg, 400 mg
Oral solution: 250 mg/5 mL
Tablets ⊖: 100 mg, 300 mg, 400 mg, 600 mg, 800 mg
Tablets (extended-release) ⊖: 300 mg, 600 mg

INDICATIONS & DOSAGES

Adjust-a-dose (for all indications): For immediate-release formulation in patients age 12 and older with CrCl of 30 to 59 mL/minute, give 400 to 1,400 mg daily divided into two doses. For CrCl of

15 to 29 mL/minute, give 200 to 700 mg daily in a single dose. For CrCl of less than 15 mL/minute, give 100 to 300 mg daily in a single dose. Reduce daily dosage in proportion to CrCl (patients with a CrCl of 7.5 mL/minute should receive half the daily dosage of those with a CrCl of 15 mL/minute). For patients receiving hemodialysis, maintenance dosage is based on estimates of CrCl. Give supplemental dose of 125 to 350 mg after each 4 hours of hemodialysis.

➤ **Adjunctive treatment of partial seizures with or without secondary generalization in patients with epilepsy (excluding Gralise and Horizant)**
Adults and children age 12 and older: Initially, 300 mg PO t.i.d. Increase dosage as needed and tolerated to 1,800 mg daily in three divided doses. Dosages up to 3,600 mg daily have been well tolerated.

➤ **Adjunctive treatment to control partial seizures in children (excluding Gralise and Horizant)**
Starting dosage, children ages 3 to 11: 10 to 15 mg/kg daily PO in three divided doses, adjusting over 3 days to reach effective dosage.
Effective dosage, children ages 5 to 11: 25 to 35 mg/kg daily PO in three divided doses.
Effective dosage, children ages 3 to 4: 40 mg/kg daily PO in three divided doses.

➤ **Moderate to severe primary restless legs syndrome (Horizant)**
Adults: 600 mg extended-release tablet PO daily at about 5 p.m. If dose isn't taken at the recommended time, the next dose should be taken the following day as prescribed.
Adjust-a-dose: If CrCl is 30 to 59 mL/minute, give 300 mg daily (may increase to 600 mg if needed). If CrCl is 15 to 29 mL/minute, give 300 mg daily in the morning; increase to 300 mg b.i.d. if needed. If CrCl is less than 15 mL/minute, give 300 mg every other day in the morning; increase to 300 mg once daily in the morning if needed. Don't give to patients receiving hemodialysis.

➤ **Postherpetic neuralgia (immediate-release)**
Adults: 300 mg PO once daily on first day, 300 mg b.i.d. on day 2, and 300 mg t.i.d. on day 3. Adjust as needed for pain to a

maximum daily dose of 1,800 mg in three divided doses.

➤ **Postherpetic neuralgia (Gralise)**
Adults: Titrate dosage to 1,800 mg PO once daily with the evening meal. On day 1, give 300 mg; on day 2, 600 mg; on days 3 to 6, 900 mg; on days 7 to 10, 1,200 mg; on days 11 to 14, 1,500 mg; and on day 15 and thereafter, 1,800 mg.
Adjust-a-dose: For patients with reduced renal function, initiate Gralise at a daily dose of 300 mg. For patients with CrCl of 30 to 60 mL/minute, titrate dosage to 600 to 1,800 mg daily as tolerated. Don't give Gralise to patients with CrCl of less than 30 mL/minute or to those receiving hemodialysis.

➤ **Postherpetic neuralgia (Horizant)**
Adults: 600 mg PO in morning for 3 days; increase to 600 mg b.i.d. on day 4. If dose isn't taken at recommended time, skip dose, and take next dose at time of next scheduled dose.
Adjust-a-dose: If CrCl is 30 to 59 mL/minute, give 300 mg in the morning for 3 days; then increase to 300 mg b.i.d. (may increase to 600 mg b.i.d. as needed). If CrCl is 15 to 29 mL/minute, give 300 mg in the morning on days 1 and 3, then 300 mg daily in the morning (increase to 300 mg b.i.d. if needed). If CrCl is less than 15 mL/minute, give 300 mg in the morning every other day (increase to 300 mg daily in the morning if needed). If CrCl is less than 15 mL/minute and patient is on hemodialysis, give 300 mg after each dialysis treatment (increase to 600 mg after every dialysis treatment if needed).

➤ **Neuropathic pain (immediate-release)** ♦
Adults: 1,200 to 3,600 mg/day in three divided doses. For critically ill patients, initially 100 mg t.i.d. in combination with IV opioids. Maintenance dose, 300 to 1,200 mg t.i.d.; maximum dose, 3,600 mg daily.

ADMINISTRATION
PO
• Give immediate-release forms without regard for food.
• Give extended-release tablets with food.
• Give Gralise tablets with the evening meal.

- When giving drug t.i.d., maximum interval between doses should be no more than 12 hours.
- Give drug 2 hours after an antacid.
- Refrigerate oral solution.
- Patient should swallow extended-release tablets whole and shouldn't cut, crush, or chew them.
- May divide scored 600- or 800-mg Neurontin tablets and give as a half-tablet. Use half-tablets within 28 days of dividing or discard.
- Gralise, Horizant, and other gabapentin products aren't interchangeable.

ACTION

Unknown. Structurally related to GABA but doesn't interact with GABA receptors, isn't converted into GABA or GABA agonist, doesn't inhibit GABA reuptake, and doesn't prevent degradation.

Route	Onset	Peak	Duration
PO (immediate-release)	Unknown	2–4 hr	Unknown
PO (extended-release)	Unknown	8 hr	Unknown
PO (enacarbil)	Unknown	5–7 hr	Unknown

Half-life: Gabapentin, 5 to 7 hours; gabapentin enacarbil, 5 to 6 hours.

ADVERSE REACTIONS

CNS: ataxia, dizziness, fatigue, somnolence, abnormal thinking, amnesia, depression, fever, dysarthria, incoordination, tremor, headache, drowsiness. **CV:** peripheral edema, vasodilation. **EENT:** amblyopia, diplopia, nystagmus, pharyngitis, dry throat, nasopharyngitis. **GI:** constipation, dry mouth, dyspepsia, increased appetite, flatulence, nausea, vomiting; diarrhea (Gralise). **GU:** erectile dysfunction; UTI (Gralise). **Hematologic:** *leukopenia.* **Metabolic:** weight gain. **Musculoskeletal:** back pain, fractures, myalgia, limb pain. **Respiratory:** coughing, bronchitis, URI. **Skin:** abrasion, pruritus. **Other:** dental abnormalities, viral infections.

INTERACTIONS

Drug-drug. *Antacids:* May decrease absorption of gabapentin. Separate dosage times by at least 2 hours.

CNS depressants: May increase risk of CNS depressant–related adverse effects. Monitor therapy.

Opioid analgesics (hydrocodone): May enhance CNS depressant effect of opioid analgesics. Consider therapy modification or limit dosages and duration of each drug.

Drug-herb. *Kava kava:* May enhance adverse/toxic CNS effects. Monitor therapy.

Drug-lifestyle. *Alcohol use:* May increase CNS effects. Avoid use.

EFFECTS ON LAB TEST RESULTS

- May decrease WBC count.
- May cause false-positive results with the Ames N-Multistix SG dipstick test for urine protein when used with other anticonvulsants.

CONTRAINDICATIONS & CAUTIONS

- Contraindicated in patients hypersensitive to drug.
- In elderly patients, adjust dosage based on CrCl values due to potentially decreased renal function.
- Gabapentin enacarbil isn't recommended for patients who must sleep during the day and remain awake at night.
- Anaphylaxis and angioedema can occur any time during therapy and require emergency treatment and discontinuation of drug.
- DRESS syndrome (with such symptoms as fever, rash, lymphadenopathy, and other organ system involvement), which can be life-threatening, can occur. Evaluate patient immediately if symptoms occur and discontinue drug.

Dialyzable drug: Yes.

⚠ Overdose S&S: Double vision, slurred speech, drowsiness, lethargy, diarrhea.

PREGNANCY-LACTATION-REPRODUCTION

- Use during pregnancy only if potential benefit justifies potential risk to the fetus.
- Use in breastfeeding women only if benefit to the mother outweighs potential risk to the infant.

NURSING CONSIDERATIONS

☉ Alert: Closely monitor all patients taking or starting AEDs for changes in behavior indicating worsening of suicidal thoughts or behavior or depression. Symptoms such

---

as anxiety, agitation, hostility, mania, and hypomania may be precursors to emerging suicidality.
• If drug is to be stopped or an alternative drug substituted, do so gradually over at least 1 week to minimize risk of precipitating seizures.
❸ Alert: Don't suddenly withdraw other anticonvulsants in patients starting gabapentin therapy.
• Routine monitoring of drug levels isn't necessary. Drug doesn't appear to alter levels of other anticonvulsants.

PATIENT TEACHING
• Advise patient that immediate-release form may be taken without regard for meals.
• Advise patient to take extended-release tablets with food.
• Instruct patient to take first dose at bedtime to minimize adverse reactions.
• Tell patient with seizures that the maximum time interval between doses shouldn't exceed 12 hours.
• Warn patient that extended-release formulas can cause significant dizziness and sleepiness.
• Warn patient to report all adverse reactions and to avoid driving and operating heavy machinery until drug's CNS effects are known.
• Advise patient not to take extended-release formulas with alcohol or other drugs that may cause sleepiness or dizziness.
• Advise patient not to stop drug abruptly.
• Advise female patient to discuss drug therapy with prescriber if considering pregnancy.
• Tell patient to keep oral solution refrigerated.

---

galantamine hydrobromide
gah-LAN-tah-meen

Razadyne, Razadyne ER

Therapeutic class: Anti-Alzheimer drugs
Pharmacologic class: Cholinesterase inhibitors

AVAILABLE FORMS
Capsules (extended-release): 8 mg, 16 mg, 24 mg

Oral solution: 4 mg/mL
Tablets: 4 mg, 8 mg, 12 mg

INDICATIONS & DOSAGES
➤ **Mild to moderate Alzheimer dementia**
Adults: Initially, 4 mg tablets or solution PO b.i.d., preferably with morning and evening meals. If dose is well tolerated after minimum of 4 weeks of therapy, increase dosage to 8 mg b.i.d. A further increase to 12 mg b.i.d. may be attempted, but only after at least 4 weeks of therapy at the previous dosage. Dosage range is 16 to 24 mg daily in two divided doses.
Or, 8 mg extended-release capsule PO once daily in the morning with food. Increase to 16 mg PO once daily after a minimum of 4 weeks. May further increase to 24 mg once daily after a minimum of 4 weeks, based on patient response and tolerability. Dosage range is 16 to 24 mg daily.
Adjust-a-dose: For patients with Child-Pugh score of 7 to 9, dosage usually shouldn't exceed 16 mg daily. Drug isn't recommended for patients with Child-Pugh score of 10 to 15. For patients with moderate renal impairment, dosage usually shouldn't exceed 16 mg daily. For patients with CrCl less than 9 mL/minute, drug isn't recommended.

ADMINISTRATION
PO
❸ Alert: Give Razadyne tablets b.i.d., preferably with morning and evening meals. Give Razadyne ER capsules once daily in the morning, preferably with food. To avoid dosing errors, verify any prescription that suggests a different dosing schedule.
• Give drug with food and antiemetics, and ensure adequate fluid intake to decrease the risk of nausea and vomiting.
• Use proper technique when dispensing the oral solution with the pipette provided by the manufacturer. Dilute dose in 100 mL of a nonalcoholic beverage and give to patient right away.

ACTION
Thought to enhance cholinergic function by increasing acetylcholine level in the brain by slowing the degradation of acetylcholine.

G

Route	Onset	Peak	Duration
PO	Unknown	1 hr	Unknown
PO (extended-release)	Unknown	4½ –5 hr	Unknown

Half-life: About 7 hours.

ADVERSE REACTIONS

CNS: asthenia, depression, dizziness, headache, tremor, somnolence, fatigue, syncope, lethargy, malaise. **CV: bradycardia, AV block. GI:** diarrhea, nausea, vomiting, abdominal pain, dyspepsia, anorexia, decreased appetite. **Hematologic:** anemia. **Metabolic:** weight loss. **Skin:** rash.

INTERACTIONS

Drug-drug. *Amitriptyline, fluoxetine, fluvoxamine, quinidine:* May decrease galantamine clearance. Monitor patient closely.
Anticholinergics: May antagonize anticholinergic activity. Monitor patient.
Antipsychotics: May enhance neurotoxic effects of antipsychotics; severe extrapyramidal symptoms have occurred. Monitor therapy.
Beta blockers: May enhance bradycardic effect of some beta blockers. Monitor therapy.
Cholinergics (bethanechol, succinylcholine): May have synergistic effect. Monitor patient closely. May need to avoid use before procedures using general anesthesia with succinylcholine-type neuromuscular blockers.
Cimetidine, clarithromycin, erythromycin, ketoconazole, paroxetine: May increase galantamine bioavailability. Monitor patient closely.
Corticosteroids: May enhance adverse/toxic effect of galantamine and increase muscle weakness. Monitor therapy.
Highest risk QTc-prolonging agents: May enhance QTc-prolonging effects. Monitor for QTc prolongation and arrhythmias; consider therapy modification.
NSAIDs: May increase risk of bleeding due to increased gastric acid secretion. Monitor patient for symptoms of active or occult GI bleeding.
Drug-lifestyle. *Alcohol use:* May increase CNS effects. Avoid use.

EFFECTS ON LAB TEST RESULTS

None reported.

CONTRAINDICATIONS & CAUTIONS

• Contraindicated in patients hypersensitive to drug or its components.
• Use cautiously in patients with supraventricular cardiac conduction disorders and in those taking other drugs that significantly slow HR.
• Use cautiously during or before procedures involving anesthesia using succinylcholine-type or similar neuromuscular blockers.
• Use cautiously in patients with history of peptic ulcer disease and in those taking NSAIDs. Because of the potential for cholinomimetic effects, use cautiously in patients with bladder outflow obstruction, seizures, asthma, or COPD.
Dialyzable drug: Unknown.
⚠ *Overdose S&S:* Muscle weakness, muscle fasciculations, nausea, vomiting, GI cramping, excessive salivation, excessive lacrimation, sweating, bradycardia, hypotension, respiratory depression, syncope, seizures, QT-interval prolongation, hallucinations.

PREGNANCY-LACTATION-REPRODUCTION

• There are no well-controlled studies in pregnant women. Use during pregnancy only if potential benefit justifies potential risk to the fetus.
• It isn't known if drug appears in human milk. Use cautiously in breastfeeding women.

NURSING CONSIDERATIONS

🕒 *Alert:* Drug may cause bradycardia and heart block. Consider all patients at risk for adverse effects on cardiac conduction.
• If drug is stopped for 3 days or longer, restart at the lowest dose and gradually increase, at 4-week or longer intervals, to the previous dosage level.
• Because of the risk of increased gastric acid secretion, monitor patients closely for symptoms of active or occult GI bleeding, especially those with an increased risk of developing ulcers.
• Monitor patient's weight during therapy.
• Monitor patients closely for seizures.

Reactions in bold italics are *life-threatening*. Interactions may have a *rapid onset* or a *delayed onset*.

• Serious skin reactions such as SJS have been reported. Monitor patient for serious rash and discontinue therapy if needed.

PATIENT TEACHING

• Advise caregiver to give drug with morning and evening meals (for the conventional form), or only in the morning (for the extended-release form) and with food.

• Inform patient that nausea and vomiting are common adverse effects.

• Teach caregiver the proper technique when measuring the oral solution with the pipette. Tell her to place measured amount in 100 mL of a nonalcoholic beverage and have patient drink right away.

• Urge patient or caregiver to report slow heartbeat immediately.

• Advise patient and caregiver that although drug may improve cognitive function, it doesn't alter the underlying disease process.

• Instruct patient to watch for serious skin reactions and to stop drug at first appearance of a rash.

ganciclovir (DHPG)
gan-SYE-kloe-vir

Cytovene, Zirgan

Therapeutic class: Antivirals
Pharmacologic class: Nucleosides–nucleotides

AVAILABLE FORMS
Injection: 500 mg/vial
Ophthalmic gel: 0.15%

INDICATIONS & DOSAGES
🔹 *Alert:* IV ganciclovir is indicated only for the treatment of CMV retinitis in immuno-compromised patients and for the prevention of CMV disease in transplant patients at risk for CMV disease.

Adjust-a-dose (for all indications): Adjust IV dosage in patient with renal impairment according to the table. If patient is receiving hemodialysis, give dose shortly after session is complete.

Initial IV therapy

CrCl (mL/min)	Dose (mg/kg)	Interval
50–69	2.5	12 hr
25–49	2.5	24 hr
10–24	1.25	24 hr
<10	1.25	3 times weekly after hemodialysis

Maintenance IV therapy

CrCl (mL/min)	Dose (mg/kg)	Interval
50–69	2.5	24 hr
25–49	1.25	24 hr
10–24	0.625	24 hr
<10	0.625	3 times weekly after hemodialysis

➤ **CMV retinitis in immunocompromised patients, including those with AIDS and normal renal function**
Adults: Induction treatment is 5 mg/kg IV (given at a constant rate over 1 hour) every 12 hours for 14 to 21 days. Maintenance treatment is 5 mg/kg IV daily 7 days per week or 6 mg/kg IV once daily five times weekly.

➤ **To prevent CMV disease in transplant recipients with normal renal function**
Adults: 5 mg/kg IV (given at a constant rate over 1 hour) every 12 hours for 7 to 14 days; then 5 mg/kg daily 7 days per week or 6 mg/kg once daily five times weekly. Duration of therapy depends on degree of immunosuppression.

➤ **Acute herpetic keratitis**
Adults and children age 2 and older: 1 drop in affected eye five times daily (approximately every 3 hours while awake) until the corneal ulcer heals; then 1 drop t.i.d. for 7 days.

ADMINISTRATION
IV
▼ Drug is hazardous. Use safe handling precautions. IV solutions are alkaline; avoid direct contact with skin or mucous membranes. If contact occurs, wash area thoroughly with soap and water; thoroughly rinse eyes with plain water.

▼ To reconstitute, add 10 mL sterile water for injection to 500-mg vial. Shake vial well to dissolve drug. Don't use bacteriostatic water containing parabens, as precipitation can result.

♣Canada   ◇OTC   ◆Off-label use   ✐Photoguide   ⊜Do not crush   *Liquid contains alcohol   ▨Genetic

▼ Further dilute in 50 to 250 mL (usually 100 mL) of compatible IV solution.

▼ If fluids are being restricted, dilute to no more than 10 mg/mL.

▼ Don't give as rapid or bolus injection.

▼ Use an infusion pump.

▼ Infuse slowly over at least 1 hour.

▼ Infusing drug too rapidly has toxic effects.

◑ **Alert:** Don't give subcut or IM.

▼ Discard vial if particulate matter or discoloration is observed.

▼ Reconstituted solution is stable at room temperature for 12 hours. Don't refrigerate. Use solution within 24 hours of dilution to reduce risk of bacterial contamination.

▼ **Incompatibilities:** None listed by manufacturer. Consult a drug incompatibility reference for more information.

Ophthalmic

• Store at 59° to 77° F (15° to 20° C). Don't freeze.

ACTION

Inhibits binding of deoxyguanosine triphosphate to DNA polymerase, resulting in inhibition of DNA synthesis.

Route	Onset	Peak	Duration
IV	Unknown	Immediate	Unknown
Ophthalmic	Unknown	Unknown	Unknown

Half-life: IV, about 3 to 5 hours; ophthalmic, unknown.

ADVERSE REACTIONS

CNS: fever, *coma, seizures,* abnormal thinking, agitation, altered dreams, amnesia, anxiety, asthenia, ataxia, confusion, dizziness, headache, somnolence, tremor, neuropathy, paresthesia. **EENT:** retinal detachment in CMV retinitis patients; blurred vision, eye irritation, punctate keratitis, conjunctival hyperemia (ophthalmic). **GI:** abdominal pain, anorexia, diarrhea, nausea, vomiting, dry mouth, dyspepsia, flatulence, decreased appetite. **GU:** increased serum creatinine level. **Hematologic:** anemia, *agranulocytosis, leukopenia, thrombocytopenia.* **Respiratory:** pneumonia. **Skin:** rash, sweating, inflammation, pruritus, pain and phlebitis at injection site. **Other:** *sepsis,* chills, infection.

INTERACTIONS

Drug-drug. *Amphotericin B, cyclosporine, other nephrotoxic drugs:* May increase risk of nephrotoxicity. Monitor renal function.

Cytotoxic drugs: May increase toxic effects, especially hematologic effects and stomatitis. Use together only if benefits outweigh risks; monitor patient closely.

Imipenem–cilastatin: May increase seizure activity. Use together only if potential benefits outweigh risks.

Immunosuppressants (azathioprine, corticosteroids, cyclosporine): May enhance immune and bone marrow suppression. Use together cautiously.

Probenecid: May increase ganciclovir level. Monitor patient closely.

Tenofovir products: May increase serum concentration of both drugs. Monitor therapy.

Zidovudine: May increase risk of agranulocytosis. Use together cautiously; monitor hematologic function closely.

EFFECTS ON LAB TEST RESULTS

• May increase alkaline phosphatase, ALT, AST, creatinine, and GGT levels. May decrease Hb level.

• May decrease granulocyte, neutrophil, platelet, and WBC counts.

CONTRAINDICATIONS & CAUTIONS

Black Box Warning Clinical toxicity of IV ganciclovir includes granulocytopenia, anemia, thrombocytopenia, and pancytopenia. Animal studies indicate that drug is carcinogenic and teratogenic. ▮

• Contraindicated in patients hypersensitive to drug or acyclovir and in those with an ANC below 500/mm^3 or a platelet count below 25,000/mm^3.

• Use cautiously and reduce dosage in patients with renal dysfunction. Monitor renal function tests.

Dialyzable drug: About 50%.

⚠ **Overdose S&S:** Persistent bone marrow suppression, reversible neutropenia or granulocytopenia, hepatitis, renal toxicity, seizures (all with IV form).

Reactions in bold italics are *life-threatening*. Interactions may have a *rapid onset* or a *delayed onset*.

PREGNANCY-LACTATION-REPRODUCTION

Black Box Warning Based on animal studies, IV ganciclovir may be teratogenic or embryotoxic at recommended doses. ■

• Use during pregnancy only if potential benefits justify risks to the fetus.

• Women of childbearing potential should use effective contraception during treatment and for 30 days after final dose. Men should practice barrier contraception during treatment and for at least 90 days after final dose.

• Women receiving IV ganciclovir shouldn't breastfeed. It isn't known when breastfeeding can be safely resumed after last dose.

Black Box Warning Based on animal data, IV drug at recommended doses may cause temporary or permanent aspermatogenesis in males, and may cause suppression of fertility in females. ■

NURSING CONSIDERATIONS

• Because of the frequency of agranulocytosis and thrombocytopenia, obtain neutrophil and platelet counts every 2 days during twice-daily dosing and at least weekly thereafter.

• Carefully monitor renal function, particularly in elderly patients and in patients taking other nephrotoxic drugs, at least weekly; adjust dosages in patients with renal impairment.

PATIENT TEACHING

• Explain importance of drinking plenty of fluids during therapy.

• Instruct patient to report adverse reactions promptly.

• Tell patient to report discomfort at IV insertion site.

Black Box Warning Advise patient that IV use may impair fertility. ■

• Advise female patient of childbearing potential to use effective contraception during IV treatment and for at least 30 days after final dose. Caution male patient to practice barrier contraception during and for at least 90 days after treatment.

• Advise patient to use soft toothbrush and electric razor because of increased bleeding risk with IV use.

• Emphasize importance of adhering to blood work as requested by prescriber.

• Advise patient using gel not to let dropper touch any surface because dropper is sterile.

• Advise patient not to wear contact lenses while undergoing ophthalmic treatment.

• Advise patient undergoing ophthalmic treatment to notify prescriber if eye pain, redness, itching, or inflammation becomes aggravated.

SAFETY ALERT!

gemcitabine hydrochloride
jem-SITE-ah-been

Gemzar, Infugem

Therapeutic class: Antineoplastics
Pharmacologic class: Pyrimidine analogues

AVAILABLE FORMS

Injection: 10 mg/mL
Powder for injection: 200-mg, 1-g vials
Solution for injection: 200-mg, 1-g, 2-g vials

INDICATIONS & DOSAGES

Adjust-a-dose (for all indications): If patient is on hemodialysis, begin hemodialysis 6 to 12 hours after drug infusion. If serum bilirubin level is greater than 1.6 mg/dL, use initial dose of 800 mg/m^2 and escalate if tolerated. Refer to manufacturer's instructions for toxicity-related dosage adjustments.

Permanently discontinue drug for any of the following nonhematologic adverse reactions: unexplained dyspnea or other evidence of severe pulmonary toxicity, severe hepatotoxicity, hemolytic-uremic syndrome, capillary leak syndrome, or posterior reversible encephalopathy syndrome. Withhold drug or reduce dosage by 50% for other severe (grade 3 or 4) nonhematologic toxicity until resolved.

➤ **Locally advanced (nonresectable stage II or III) or metastatic (stage IV) adenocarcinoma of pancreas in patients previously treated with 5-FU**
Adults: 1,000 mg/m^2 IV over 30 minutes once weekly for 7 weeks followed by 1 week rest, unless toxicity occurs. Subsequent cycles should consist of infusions once weekly for 3 consecutive weeks out of every 4 weeks. Monitor CBC with differential and platelet count before giving each dose.

➤ **With cisplatin, first-line treatment of inoperable, locally advanced (stage IIIA or IIIB), or metastatic (stage IV) NSCLC**
Adults: For 4-week schedule, 1,000 mg/m^2 IV over 30 minutes on days 1, 8, and 15 of each 28-day cycle. Administer cisplatin IV at 100 mg/m^2 on day 1 after gemcitabine infusion. For 3-week schedule, 1,250 mg/m^2 IV over 30 minutes on days 1 and 8 of each 21-day cycle. Administer cisplatin IV at 100 mg/m^2 on day 1 after gemcitabine infusion.

➤ **With carboplatin, for treatment of advanced ovarian cancer that relapsed at least 6 months after platinum-based therapy**
Adults: 1,000 mg/m^2 IV over 30 minutes on days 1 and 8 of each 21-day cycle. Check CBC with differential and platelet count before each dose.

➤ **With paclitaxel, metastatic breast cancer (first-line treatment after failure of adjuvant anthracycline chemotherapy)**
Adults: 1,250 mg/m^2 IV over 30 minutes on days 1 and 8 of each 21-day cycle. Adjust dosage based on total AGC and platelet counts taken on days 1 and 8 of the cycle. Check CBC with differential before each dose.

➤ **Pancreatic cancer (adjuvant therapy)** ◆
Adults: 1,000 mg/m^2 IV on days 1, 8, and 15 every 28 days (in combination with capecitabine) for six cycles beginning within 12 weeks of resection.

➤ **Bladder cancer (advanced or metastatic)** ◆
Adults: 1,000 mg/m^2 IV over 30 to 60 minutes days 1, 8, and 15; repeat cycle every 28 days (in combination with cisplatin), or 1,000 mg/m^2 IV over 30 minutes days 1 and 8; repeat cycle every 21 days (in combination with carboplatin) until disease progression or unacceptable toxicity.

➤ **Hepatobiliary cancer (advanced or metastatic)** ◆
1,000 mg/m^2 IV over 30 minutes days 1 and 8; repeat cycle every 21 days (in combination with cisplatin), or 1,000 mg/m^2 IV over 30 minutes days 1 and 8; repeat cycle every 21 days (in combination with capecitabine), or 1,000 mg/m^2 IV infused at 10 mg/m^2/minute every 2 weeks (in combination with oxaliplatin).

ADMINISTRATION

IV

▼ Preparing and giving parenteral drug may be mutagenic, teratogenic, or carcinogenic. Follow safe handling precautions and use gloves.

▼ To prepare solution, add 5 mL of unpreserved NSS for injection to 200-mg vial or 25 mL to 1-g vial. Shake to dissolve.

▼ Resulting concentration is 38 mg/mL (accounting for the volume displaced by the powder); reconstitution at concentrations higher than 40 mg/mL isn't recommended.

▼ If needed, dilute to as little as 0.1 mg/mL by adding NSS for injection.

▼ Make sure solution is clear to light straw-colored and free of particles.

▼ Don't extend infusion time beyond 60 minutes or give drug more often than once weekly; doing so may increase toxicity.

▼ Drug is stable for 24 hours at room temperature.

▼ Don't refrigerate reconstituted drug because it may crystallize.

▼ **Incompatibilities:** None listed by manufacturer. Consult a drug incompatibility reference for more information.

ACTION

Cytotoxic and specific to cell cycle; inhibits DNA synthesis and blocks progression of cells.

Route	Onset	Peak	Duration
IV	Unknown	30 min	Unknown

Half-life: About 2½ to 19 hours (influenced by length of the infusion, age, and gender).

ADVERSE REACTIONS

CNS: drowsiness, paresthesia, pain, fever. **CV:** edema, peripheral edema. **GI:** stomatitis, nausea, vomiting, diarrhea. **GU:** proteinuria, hematuria. **Hematologic:** anemia, *leukopenia, neutropenia, thrombocytopenia, hemorrhage.* **Hepatic:** *hepatotoxicity.* **Respiratory:** dyspnea, *bronchospasm, pneumonitis.* **Skin:** alopecia, rash, pain at

---

Reactions in bold italics are *life-threatening*. Interactions may have a *rapid onset* or a *delayed onset*.

injection site. **Other:** flulike syndrome, infection, injection-site reactions.

INTERACTIONS
Drug-drug. *Bleomycin:* May increase risk of pulmonary toxicity. Consider therapy modification.
Clozapine: May increase risk of neutropenia. Avoid combination.
Live-virus vaccines: May increase risk of vaccine-induced adverse reactions. Defer use of live-virus vaccines.
Warfarin: May increase the anticoagulant effect of warfarin. Monitor patient and INR.

EFFECTS ON LAB TEST RESULTS
• May increase ALT, AST, BUN, and creatinine levels. May decrease Hb level.
• May decrease neutrophil, platelet, and WBC counts.

CONTRAINDICATIONS & CAUTIONS
• Contraindicated in patients hypersensitive to drug.
• Use cautiously in patients with renal or hepatic impairment.
• Use cautiously when given within 7 days of radiation therapy.
• Prolonging infusion duration beyond 60 minutes or administering more frequently than weekly has resulted in an increased incidence of toxicities, including clinically significant hypotension, severe flulike symptoms, myelosuppression, and asthenia.
• Capillary leak syndrome with severe consequences has been reported when drug has been used alone or in combination with other chemotherapeutic agents. Discontinue if syndrome develops.
• Hemolytic-uremic syndrome that may lead to renal failure has been reported. Watch for evidence of anemia with microangiopathic hemolysis (elevated bilirubin or LDH level, reticulocytosis, severe thrombocytopenia, or renal failure), and monitor renal function at baseline and periodically during treatment. Permanently discontinue if hemolytic-uremic syndrome or severe renal impairment occurs; renal failure may not be reversible despite discontinuation.
• Myelosuppression, manifested by neutropenia, thrombocytopenia, and anemia,

occurs with gemcitabine used alone; risk increases when drug is combined with other cytotoxic drugs.
• Pulmonary toxicity, including interstitial pneumonitis, pulmonary fibrosis, pulmonary edema, and ARDS, has been reported; it may lead to respiratory failure (some fatal) despite discontinuation of therapy. Onset of pulmonary symptoms may occur up to 2 weeks after last dose of gemcitabine. Discontinue for unexplained dyspnea, with or without bronchospasm, or other evidence of pulmonary toxicity.
• Serious hepatotoxicity, including liver failure and death, has been reported with gemcitabine alone or in combination with other potentially hepatotoxic drugs. Administration in patients with concurrent liver metastases or preexisting medical history of hepatitis, alcoholism, or liver cirrhosis can lead to exacerbation of the underlying hepatic insufficiency. Assess hepatic function before initiating gemcitabine and periodically during treatment. Discontinue if severe liver injury develops.
• Posterior reversible encephalopathy syndrome (PRES) has been reported in patients receiving gemcitabine alone or in combination with other chemotherapeutic agents. PRES can present with headache, seizure, lethargy, HTN, confusion, blindness, and other visual and neurologic disturbances. Confirm PRES diagnosis with MRI; discontinue gemcitabine if PRES develops during therapy.
• Safety and effectiveness in children haven't been determined.
Dialyzable drug: Unknown.
⚠ *Overdose S&S:* Myelosuppression, paresthesia, severe rash.

PREGNANCY-LACTATION-REPRODUCTION
• There are no adequate studies in pregnant women. Based on drug's mechanism of action, its use is expected to result in adverse reproductive effects. If drug is used during pregnancy or if patient becomes pregnant during therapy, apprise her of potential fetal hazard.
• Patient should discontinue breastfeeding or discontinue drug.

NURSING CONSIDERATIONS
• Monitor patient closely. Expect dosage modification according to toxicity and degree of myelosuppression. Age, gender, and presence of renal impairment may predispose patient to toxicity.
• Monitor hematologic values carefully, especially neutrophil and platelet counts.
• Obtain baseline and periodic renal and hepatic laboratory tests.

PATIENT TEACHING
• Advise patient to report all adverse reactions and to immediately report evidence of infection (fever, sore throat, fatigue) and bleeding (easy bruising, nosebleeds, bleeding gums, tarry stools). Tell patient to take temperature daily.
• Advise patient to immediately report changes in color or volume of urine output.
• Advise patient to promptly report flulike symptoms, breathing problems, abdominal pain, or yellowing of skin.
• Tell patient that adverse effects may continue after treatment ends.

gemfibrozil
jem-FI-broe-zil

Lopid✱

Therapeutic class: Antilipemics
Pharmacologic class: Fibric acid derivatives

AVAILABLE FORMS
Tablets: 600 mg

INDICATIONS & DOSAGES
➤ **As adjunct to diet in adults with hypertriglyceridemia (types IV and V hyperlipidemia) unresponsive to diet and who are at risk for pancreatitis; to reduce risk of CAD in patients without CAD symptoms and with type IIb hyperlipidemia who are refractory to treatment with diet, exercise, and other drugs, and who have decreased HDL levels and increased LDL and triglyceride levels**
Adults: 1,200 mg PO daily in two divided doses, 30 minutes before morning and evening meals.

ADMINISTRATION
PO
• Give drug 30 minutes before breakfast and dinner.

ACTION
Inhibits peripheral lipolysis and reduces triglyceride synthesis in the liver; lowers triglyceride and VLDL levels and increases HDL levels.

Route	Onset	Peak	Duration
PO	2–5 days	1–2 hr	Unknown

Half-life: 1½ hours.

ADVERSE REACTIONS
CNS: fatigue, headache, vertigo. **GI:** abdominal and epigastric pain, dyspepsia, acute appendicitis, constipation, diarrhea, nausea, vomiting. **Hematologic:** *leukopenia, thrombocytopenia,* anemia, eosinophilia. **Hepatic:** bile duct obstruction. **Metabolic:** *hypokalemia.* **Skin:** dermatitis, eczema, pruritus, rash.

INTERACTIONS
Drug-drug. *Bile acid sequestrants:* May decrease absorption of fibric acid derivatives. Separate doses by at least 2 hours to minimize interaction; fenofibric acid labeling recommends giving drug 1 hour before or 4 to 6 hours after a bile acid sequestrant.
Colchicine: May increase risk of myopathy, especially in patients with renal dysfunction and in elderly patients. Use cautiously.
Colestipol: May decrease colestipol effects. Separate administration times by 2 hours.
Cyclosporine: May decrease cyclosporine level; may increase risk of nephrotoxicity. Monitor renal function and cyclosporine level, and adjust dose as needed.
CYP2C8, CYP2C9, CYP2C19 substrates: May increase levels of substrates metabolized through these enzymes. Consider therapy modification.
Dasabuvir: May prolong QT interval and increase risk of ventricular arrhythmias. Use together is contraindicated.
Ezetimibe: May enhance adverse/toxic effect of ezetimibe; may increase risk of myopathy and cholelithiasis. Avoid combination.

Reactions in bold italics are *life-threatening*. Interactions may have a *rapid onset* or a **delayed onset**.

Glyburide, pioglitazone: May increase hypoglycemic effects. Monitor glucose level, and watch for signs of hypoglycemia.

HMG-CoA reductase inhibitors: May cause myopathy with rhabdomyolysis. Avoid using together. Use with simvastatin is contraindicated.

Montelukast: May increase montelukast level and effects. Monitor clinical response and adjust montelukast dosage.

Repaglinide: May increase risk of severe hypoglycemia. Concurrent use is contraindicated.

Warfarin: May prolong PT and increase bleeding risk. Reduce warfarin dosage and monitor PT.

EFFECTS ON LAB TEST RESULTS
• May increase ALT, AST, bilirubin, and CK levels.
• May decrease potassium and Hb level and hematocrit.
• May decrease eosinophil, WBC, and platelet counts.

CONTRAINDICATIONS & CAUTIONS
• Contraindicated in patients hypersensitive to drug and in those with hepatic or severe renal dysfunction (including primary biliary cirrhosis) or gallbladder disease.
• Concomitant administration with simvastatin is contraindicated. The 2013 American College of Cardiology/American Heart Association guidelines on cholesterol recommend avoiding use of gemfibrozil with all statins.

Dialyzable drug: Unknown.

⚠ *Overdose S&S:* Abdominal cramps, abnormal LFT values, diarrhea, increased CK level, joint and muscle pain, nausea and vomiting.

PREGNANCY-LACTATION-REPRODUCTION
• Use in pregnancy only if potential benefit justifies potential risk to the fetus.
• Patient should discontinue breastfeeding or discontinue drug.

NURSING CONSIDERATIONS
• Check CBC and LFTs periodically during the first 12 months of therapy.
• If drug has no benefits after 3 months of therapy, stop drug.

PATIENT TEACHING
• Instruct patient to take drug 30 minutes before breakfast and dinner.
• Teach patient about proper dietary management of cholesterol and triglycerides. When appropriate, recommend weight control, exercise, and smoking cessation programs.
• Because of possible dizziness and blurred vision, advise patient to avoid driving and other hazardous activities until effects of drug are known.
• Tell patient to observe bowel movements and to report evidence of excess fat in feces or other signs of bile duct obstruction.
• Advise patient to report all adverse reactions and muscle pain to prescriber.

gemifloxacin mesylate
jem-ah-FLOX-a-sin

Factive

Therapeutic class: Antibiotics
Pharmacologic class: Fluoroquinolones

AVAILABLE FORMS
Tablets ⒪: 320 mg

INDICATIONS & DOSAGES
Adjust-a-dose (for all indications): If CrCl is 40 mL/minute or less, or if patient receives routine hemodialysis or continuous ambulatory peritoneal dialysis, reduce dosage to 160 mg PO once daily.

➤ **Acute bacterial worsening of chronic bronchitis caused by *Streptococcus pneumoniae, Haemophilus influenzae, H. parainfluenzae*, or *Moraxella catarrhalis***
Adults: 320 mg PO once daily for 5 days.

➤ **Mild to moderate community-acquired pneumonia caused by *S. pneumoniae* (including multidrug-resistant strains), *H. influenzae, M. catarrhalis, Mycoplasma pneumoniae, Chlamydia pneumoniae*, or *Klebsiella pneumoniae***
Adults: 320 mg PO once daily for 5 to 7 days.

ADMINISTRATION
PO
• Give drug with or without food; however, it must be given 2 hours before or 3 hours after an antacid or multivitamin.

• Don't give with dairy products, such as milk or yogurt, or calcium-fortified juices alone. May give with a meal that contains these products.
• Give plenty of fluids during treatment.

ACTION

Prevents cell growth by inhibiting DNA gyrase and topoisomerase IV, which interferes with DNA synthesis.

Route	Onset	Peak	Duration
PO	Unknown	½–2 hr	Unknown

Half-life: 4 to 12 hours.

ADVERSE REACTIONS

CNS: headache, dizziness. **GI:** diarrhea, nausea, abdominal pain, vomiting. **Hematologic:** *neutropenia,* neutrophilia. **Musculoskeletal:** ruptured tendons. **Skin:** rash.

INTERACTIONS

Drug-drug. *Antacids (magnesium or aluminum), didanosine (chewable tablets, buffered tablets, or pediatric powder for oral solution), ferrous sulfate or multivitamins containing metal cations (such as iron, magnesium or zinc), sucralfate:* May decrease gemifloxacin level. Give these drugs at least 3 hours before or 2 hours after gemifloxacin.
Antiarrhythmics of class IA (procainamide, quinidine) or class III (amiodarone, sotalol): May increase risk of prolonged QTc interval. Avoid using together.
Antipsychotics, erythromycin, ivabradine, mifepristone, TCAs: May increase risk of prolonged QTc interval. Use together cautiously.
Corticosteroids: May increase risk of tendinitis and tendon rupture. Monitor patient for tendon pain or inflammation.
Ivabradine: May prolong QTc interval and increase risk of ventricular arrhythmias. Monitor patient closely.
NSAIDs: May enhance neuroexcitatory or seizure-potentiating effect of quinolones. Monitor therapy.
Probenecid: May increase gemifloxacin level. May use with probenecid for this reason.
Sevelamer: May decrease gemifloxacin level. Give drug at least 2 hours before or

6 hours after sevelamer; consider therapy modification.
Sucralfate: May decrease gemifloxacin level. Use together cautiously.
Warfarin: May increase anticoagulation effect. Monitor PT and INR.
Drug-lifestyle. *Sun exposure:* May increase risk of photosensitivity. Advise patient to avoid excessive sunlight exposure.

EFFECTS ON LAB TEST RESULTS

• May increase alkaline phosphatase, ALT, AST, bilirubin, BUN, CK, creatinine, GGT, and potassium levels. May decrease albumin, protein, and sodium levels.
• May increase or decrease calcium and Hb levels and hematocrit.
• May increase or decrease neutrophil, platelet, and RBC counts.

CONTRAINDICATIONS & CAUTIONS

Black Box Warning Drug is associated with increased risk of tendinitis and tendon rupture, especially in patients older than age 60 and those with heart, kidney, or lung transplants. ■
Black Box Warning Drug may exacerbate muscle weakness in patients with myasthenia gravis. Avoid using fluoroquinolones in patients with a known history of myasthenia gravis. ■
Black Box Warning Fluoroquinolones have been associated with disabling and potentially irreversible serious adverse reactions that have occurred together, including tendinitis and tendon rupture, peripheral neuropathy, and CNS effects (seizures, toxic psychoses, increased ICP, pseudotumor cerebri, tremors, restlessness, anxiety, lightheadedness, confusion, hallucinations, paranoia, depression, nightmares, insomnia and, rarely, suicidal thoughts or acts). If any of these serious adverse reactions occur, discontinue drug immediately. ■
🕔 Alert: Drug may increase risk of aortic dissection or rupture when used systemically. Avoid use in patients with known aortic aneurysm and patients at risk for an aortic aneurysm, including those with peripheral atherosclerotic vascular diseases, HTN, certain genetic conditions (Marfan syndrome, Ehlers-Danlos syndrome), and elderly

---

Reactions in bold italics are *life-threatening*. Interactions may have a *rapid onset* or a *delayed onset*.

patients. Use drug in these patients only if no other treatment options are available.
• Contraindicated in patients hypersensitive to fluoroquinolones, gemifloxacin, or their components.
• Contraindicated in patients with a history of prolonged QTc interval, those with uncorrected electrolyte disorders (such as hypokalemia or hypomagnesemia), and those taking a drug that could prolong the QTc interval.
• Use cautiously in patients with a proarrhythmic condition, epilepsy, or a predisposition to seizures.
⚠ *Alert:* Patients receiving systemic drug have an increased risk of hypoglycemia, which can result in coma. Hypoglycemia has been reported more frequently in the elderly and in those with diabetes.
• Safety and effectiveness haven't been established in children younger than age 18.
Dialyzable drug: 20% to 30%.

PREGNANCY-LACTATION-REPRODUCTION
• Don't use in pregnant or breastfeeding women unless potential benefit justifies risk to the fetus or infant.

NURSING CONSIDERATIONS
• Use drug only for infections caused by susceptible bacteria.
⚠ *Alert:* Don't exceed recommended dosage because this increases the risk of prolonging the QTc interval.
Black Box Warning Monitor patient for symptoms of peripheral neuropathy (pain, burning, tingling, numbness, weakness, or a change in sensation to light touch, pain, temperature, or the sense of body position) and report them immediately to practitioner. ■
• Mild to moderate maculopapular rash may appear, usually 8 to 10 days after therapy starts. It's more likely in women younger than age 40 and postmenopausal women taking hormone therapy. Stop drug if rash appears.
⚠ *Alert:* Serious, occasionally fatal, hypersensitivity reactions may occur, even with first dose. Stop drug immediately if hypersensitivity reaction occurs, and treat severe reactions emergently.
Black Box Warning Fluoroquinolones may cause tendon rupture, arthropathy, or

osteochondrosis; stop drug if patient reports pain or inflammation or ruptures a tendon. ■
• Stop drug if patient has a photosensitivity reaction.
• Fluoroquinolones may cause CNS effects, such as tremors and anxiety. Monitor patient carefully.
⚠ *Alert:* Monitor patients receiving systemic drug for symptoms of hypoglycemia (confusion, pounding or rapid heartbeat, dizziness, pale skin, shakiness, sweating, unusual hunger, trembling, headache, weakness, irritability, unusual anxiety). Immediately discontinue drug for blood glucose disturbances, and switch to a nonfluoroquinolone antibiotic if possible.
⚠ *Alert:* Monitor patients receiving systemic drug for psychiatric adverse reactions (disturbances in attention, disorientation, agitation, nervousness, memory impairment, delirium). Discontinue drug for CNS side effects, including psychiatric adverse reactions.
• CDAD, ranging in severity from mild to fatal colitis, may occur, even up to months after therapy ends. Drug may need to be stopped.
• Keep patient adequately hydrated to avoid concentration of urine.

PATIENT TEACHING
Black Box Warning Warn patient to immediately report signs and symptoms of serious adverse reactions, including unusual joint or tendon pain, muscle weakness, "pins and needles" tingling or pricking sensation, numbness in the arms or legs, confusion, or hallucinations. ■
• Urge patient to finish full course of treatment, even if symptoms improve.
⚠ *Alert:* Caution patients that significantly low blood sugar levels can occur. Instruct patients how to manage symptoms and to immediately report any occurrence to their prescriber.
⚠ *Alert:* Advise patients with diabetes that they may need to monitor blood glucose levels more frequently during therapy.
⚠ *Alert:* Inform patients to immediately report psychiatric adverse reactions and that these can occur after just one dose.
• Tell patient that drug may be taken with or without food, but that it shouldn't be taken

within 3 hours before or 2 hours after an antacid or a multivitamin.

• Tell patient to stop drug and seek medical care if evidence of hypersensitivity reaction develops.

• Instruct patient to drink fluids liberally.

• Warn patient against taking OTC drugs or dietary supplements without consulting prescriber.

• Tell patient to avoid excessive exposure to sunlight or ultraviolet light.

• Urge patient to report all adverse reactions.

• Warn patient to avoid driving or other hazardous activities until effects of drug are known.

gentamicin sulfate (injection)
jen-ta-MYE-sin

Therapeutic class: Antibiotics
Pharmacologic class: Aminoglycosides

AVAILABLE FORMS
Injection: 40 mg/mL (adults), 10 mg/mL (children)
IV infusion (premixed): 80 mg, 100 mg, 120 mg, 160 mg, 200 mg in 100 mL NSS

INDICATIONS & DOSAGES
➤ **Serious infections caused by sensitive strains of** *Pseudomonas aeruginosa,* *Escherichia coli, Proteus, Klebsiella,* *Enterobacter, Serratia, Citrobacter,* **or** *Staphylococcus*
Adults: 3 mg/kg IM or IV infusion daily in three divided doses every 8 hours. For life-threatening infections, may give up to 5 mg/kg daily in divided doses every 8 hours; reduce dosage to 3 mg/kg daily as soon as patient improves.
Children: 2 to 2.5 mg/kg IM or IV infusion every 8 hours.
Neonates older than 1 week and infants: 2.5 mg/kg IM or IV infusion every 8 hours.
Neonates younger than 1 week and preterm infants: 2.5 mg/kg IM or IV infusion every 12 hours.
Adjust-a-dose: For adults with impaired renal function, dosages and frequency are determined by drug level and renal function.

Refer to manufacturer's instructions for renal function dosage adjustments. To maintain therapeutic levels, adults should receive 1 to 1.7 mg/kg IM or IV infusion after each dialysis session, and children should receive 2 to 2.5 mg/kg IM or IV infusion after each dialysis session.

ADMINISTRATION
IV
▼ Obtain specimen for culture and sensitivity tests before giving. Begin therapy while awaiting results.
▼ For intermittent infusion, dilute with 50 to 200 mL of D_5W or NSS for injection.
▼ Infuse over 30 minutes to 2 hours.
▼ After completing infusion, flush the line with NSS or D_5W.
▼ Premixed, single-dose, flexible containers should be administered IV only.
▼ **Incompatibilities:** Don't physically premix gentamicin with other drugs; administer separately according to the recommended route of administration and dosage schedule.
IM
• Obtain specimen for culture and sensitivity tests before giving. Begin therapy while awaiting results.
• Obtain blood for peak level 1 hour after IM injection or 30 minutes after IV infusion finishes; for trough levels, draw blood just before next dose. Don't collect blood in a heparinized tube; heparin is incompatible with aminoglycosides.

ACTION
Inhibits protein synthesis by binding directly to the 30S ribosomal subunit; bactericidal.

Route	Onset	Peak	Duration
IV	Immediate	30–60 min	Unknown
IM	Unknown	30–90 min	Unknown

Half-life: 2 to 3 hours; longer in patients with renal impairment and in infants.

ADVERSE REACTIONS
CNS: *encephalopathy, seizures,* fever, headache, lethargy, confusion, dizziness, numbness, depression, peripheral neuropathy, vertigo, ataxia, tingling. **CV:** hypotension. **EENT:** ototoxicity, blurred vision, tinnitus. **GI:** vomiting, nausea, weight loss.

GU: *nephrotoxicity,* possible increase in urinary excretion of casts. **Hematologic:** *agranulocytosis, leukopenia, thrombo-cytopenia,* anemia, eosinophilia. **Musculoskeletal:** muscle twitching, myasthenia gravis–like syndrome. **Respiratory:** *apnea.* **Skin:** rash, urticaria, pruritus, injection-site pain. **Other:** *anaphylaxis.*

INTERACTIONS
Drug-drug. Black Box Warning *Amikacin, carboplatin, cephaloridine, cidofovir, cisplatin, colistin, neomycin, paramycin, polymyxin B, streptomycin, tobramycin, vancomycin, viomycin, other aminoglycosides:* May increase ototoxicity and nephrotoxicity. Monitor hearing and renal function test results. Avoid concurrent or sequential use.∎

Atracurium, pancuronium, rocuronium, vecuronium: May increase effects of nondepolarizing muscle relaxants, including prolonged respiratory depression. Use together only when necessary, and expect to reduce dosage of nondepolarizing muscle relaxant.
Bisphosphonate derivatives: May enhance hypocalcemic effect of bisphosphonate derivatives. Monitor therapy.
General anesthetics: May increase neuromuscular blockade. Monitor patient closely.
Indomethacin: May increase peak and trough levels of gentamicin. Monitor gentamicin level.
Black Box Warning *IV loop diuretics (ethacrynic acid, furosemide):* May increase risk of ototoxicity. Avoid use together.∎
Parenteral penicillins (ampicillin, ticarcillin): May inactivate gentamicin in vitro. Don't mix together.

EFFECTS ON LAB TEST RESULTS
• May increase ALT, AST, bilirubin, BUN, creatinine, LDH, and nonprotein nitrogen levels.
• May decrease Hb and serum calcium, magnesium, sodium, and potassium levels.
• May increase eosinophil count. May decrease platelet and WBC counts.

CONTRAINDICATIONS & CAUTIONS
• Contraindicated in patients hypersensitive to drug or other aminoglycosides.

• Use cautiously in neonates, infants, elderly patients, and patients with impaired renal function or neuromuscular disorders.
• Use drug for short-term treatment if possible. Prolonged use may result in fungal or bacterial superinfection including CDAD.
Dialyzable drug: 50%.
⚠ *Overdose S&S:* Nephrotoxicity, neurotoxicity, ototoxicity.

PREGNANCY-LACTATION-REPRODUCTION
Black Box Warning Aminoglycosides can cause fetal harm when used during pregnancy.∎
• If drug is used during pregnancy or if patient becomes pregnant during therapy, apprise patient of potential hazard (deafness) to the fetus.
• Drug appears in human milk.

NURSING CONSIDERATIONS
Black Box Warning Evaluate patient's hearing before and during therapy. Notify prescriber if patient complains of tinnitus, vertigo, or hearing loss.∎
• Weigh patient and review renal function studies before therapy begins.
❸ *Alert:* Use preservative-free form when intrathecal or intraventricular route is used adjunctively for serious CNS infections, such as meningitis and ventriculitis.
Black Box Warning Maintain peak levels at 4 to 12 mcg/mL and trough levels at 1 to 2 mcg/mL. The maximum peak level is usually 8 mcg/mL, except in patients with cystic fibrosis, who need increased lung penetration. Prolonged peak levels of 10 to 12 mcg/mL or prolonged trough levels greater than 2 mcg/mL may increase risk of toxicity.∎
Black Box Warning Nephrotoxicity risk is greater in patients with renal impairment and in those who receive high-dosage or prolonged therapy. Monitor renal function: urine output, specific gravity, urinalysis, BUN and creatinine levels, and CrCl. Report to prescriber evidence of declining renal function.∎
Black Box Warning High-risk patients should have serial audiograms, especially if they show signs and symptoms of ototoxicity (dizziness, vertigo, ataxia, tinnitus, hearing loss).∎

G

• Watch for signs and symptoms of super-infection (especially of upper respiratory tract), such as continued fever, chills, and increased pulse rate.

• Therapy usually continues for 7 to 10 days. If no response occurs in 3 to 5 days, stop therapy and obtain new specimens for culture and sensitivity testing.

PATIENT TEACHING

• Instruct patient to promptly report adverse reactions, such as vision changes, dizziness, vertigo, unsteady gait, ringing in the ears, hearing loss, numbness, tingling, muscle twitching, seizures, changes in urine amount, edema.

• Encourage patient to drink plenty of fluids.

• Warn patient to avoid hazardous activities if adverse CNS reactions occur.

SAFETY ALERT!

glatiramer acetate
glah-TEER-ah-mer

Copaxone, Glatopa

Therapeutic class: MS drugs
Pharmacologic class: Biological response modifiers

AVAILABLE FORMS

Injection: 20 mg glatiramer acetate and 40 mg mannitol (20 mg/mL), USP, in a single-use prefilled syringe; 40 mg glatiramer acetate and 40 mg mannitol (40 mg/mL), USP, in a single-use prefilled syringe

INDICATIONS & DOSAGES

➤ **For first clinical episode and to reduce frequency of relapse in patients with relapsing-remitting MS**
Adults: 20 mg subcut daily, or 40 mg (Copaxone) subcut three times per week given at least 48 hours apart.

ADMINISTRATION
Subcutaneous

⊙ *Alert:* 20 mg/mL and 40 mg/mL formulations of glatiramer aren't interchangeable.

• Give drug only subcut in arms, abdomen, hips, or thighs; rotate injection sites to prevent lipoatrophy. Don't give IV.

• Administer 40-mg dose on same 3 days each week (e.g., Monday, Wednesday, Friday) at least 48 hours apart.

• Drug doesn't contain preservatives; discard if solution is cloudy or contains particulate matter.

• Don't try to expel the air bubble from the prefilled syringe. This may lead to loss of drug and an incorrect dose.

• Store drug in refrigerator (36° to 46° F [2° to 8° C]); allow drug to warm to room temperature for 20 minutes before use. If refrigeration isn't available, may store at room temperature for up to 1 month (refrigeration is preferred).

ACTION

May modify immune processes responsible for the pathogenesis of MS.

Route	Onset	Peak	Duration
Subcut	Unknown	Unknown	Unknown

Half-life: Unknown.

ADVERSE REACTIONS

CNS: anxiety, asthenia, abnormal dreams, agitation, confusion, emotional lability, fever, migraine, nervousness, pain, speech disorder, stupor, syncope, tremor, vertigo. **CV:** chest pain, palpitations, vasodilation, HTN, tachycardia, edema. **EENT:** eye disorder, diplopia, visual field deficit, ear pain, rhinitis, laryngismus, nasopharyngitis. **GI:** diarrhea, nausea, anorexia, bowel urgency, gastroenteritis, GI disorder, oral candidiasis, salivary gland enlargement, ulcerative stomatitis, vomiting. **GU:** urinary urgency, *vaginal hemorrhage,* abnormal Papanicolaou smear, amenorrhea, dysmenorrhea, hematuria, erectile dysfunction, menorrhagia, vaginal candidiasis. **Hematologic:** lymphadenopathy, ecchymosis. **Metabolic:** weight gain. **Musculoskeletal:** arthralgia, back pain, hypertonia, neck pain. **Respiratory:** dyspnea, cough, bronchitis, hyperventilation. **Skin:** diaphoresis, injection-site reaction, pruritus, rash, eczema, erythema or hemorrhage, residual mass at injection site, skin atrophy, urticaria, warts. **Other:** flulike syndrome, infection, bacterial infection, chills, cyst, herpes simplex and zoster, peripheral and facial edema.

Reactions in bold italics are *life-threatening*. Interactions may have a *rapid onset* or a *delayed onset*.

INTERACTIONS
Drug-drug. *Denosumab, natalizumab, roflumilast:* May increase risk of serious infection. Consider therapy modification.
Leflunomide: May increase risk of hematologic toxicity, such as pancytopenia, agranulocytosis, or thrombocytopenia. Consider therapy modification.
Live-virus vaccines: Immunosuppressants may enhance adverse or toxic effect of live-virus vaccines. Avoid use for at least 3 months after immunosuppressive therapy.
Pimecrolimus, tacrolimus (topical): May enhance adverse or toxic effect of immunosuppressants. Avoid this combination.
Tofacitinib: May enhance immunosuppressive effect of tofacitinib. Avoid combination.
Trastuzumab: May enhance neutropenic effect of immunosuppressants. Monitor therapy.
Drug-herb. *Echinacea:* May diminish therapeutic effect of immunosuppressants. Consider therapy modification.

EFFECTS ON LAB TEST RESULTS
• May diminish diagnostic effect of coccidioidin skin test.

CONTRAINDICATIONS & CAUTIONS
• Contraindicated in patients hypersensitive to drug or mannitol.
Dialyzable drug: Unknown.

PREGNANCY-LACTATION-REPRODUCTION
• There are no well-controlled studies in pregnant women. Use in pregnancy only if clearly needed.
• Use cautiously in breastfeeding women.

NURSING CONSIDERATIONS
• Immediate postinjection reactions may occur; symptoms include flushing, chest pain, palpitations, anxiety, dyspnea, constriction of the throat, and urticaria. They typically are transient and self-limiting and don't need specific treatment. Onset of postinjection reaction may occur several months after treatment starts, and patients may have more than one episode.
• Patient may experience at least one episode of transient chest pain, which usually begins at least 1 month after treatment starts; it isn't accompanied by other signs or symptoms.

PATIENT TEACHING
• Instruct patient how to self-inject drug. Supervise first injection. Injection sites include arms, abdomen, hips, and thighs.
• Tell patient to rotate injection sites daily.
• Explain need for aseptic self-injection techniques, and warn patient against reuse of needles and syringes. Periodically review proper disposal of needles, syringes, drug containers, and unused drug.
• Tell patient to notify prescriber about planned, suspected, or known pregnancy.
• Tell female patient to notify prescriber if she's breastfeeding.
• Advise patient not to change drug or dosage schedule or to stop drug without medical approval.
• Tell patient to notify prescriber of all adverse reactions and to immediately report if dizziness, flushing, fast heartbeat, anxiety, breathing problems or tightness in throat, swelling, rash, itching, hives, profuse sweating, chest pain, or severe pain occurs after drug injection.

glecaprevir–pibrentasvir ☒
glek-A-pre-vir/pi-BRENT-as-vir

Mavyret

Therapeutic class: Antivirals
Pharmacologic class: HCV NS3/4A protease inhibitors–HCV NS5A inhibitors

AVAILABLE FORMS
Tablets: 100 mg glecaprevir/40 mg pibrentasvir

INDICATIONS & DOSAGES
➤ **Treatment-naive patients with chronic HCV genotype 1, 2, 3, 4, 5, or 6 infection without cirrhosis** ☒
Adults: 3 tablets (total daily dose of 300 mg glecaprevir/120 mg pibrentasvir) PO once daily for 8 weeks.
➤ **Treatment-naive patients with chronic HCV genotype 1, 2, 3, 4, 5, or 6 infection with compensated cirrhosis (Child-Pugh class A)** ☒
Adults: 3 tablets (total daily dose of 300 mg glecaprevir/120 mg pibrentasvir) PO once daily for 12 weeks.

➤ **HCV genotype 1 infection with or without compensated cirrhosis (Child-Pugh class A) in patients previously treated with a regimen containing an HCV NS5A inhibitor but without an NS3/4A protease inhibitor (PI)** ⧖

Adults: 3 tablets (total daily dose of 300 mg glecaprevir/120 mg pibrentasvir) PO once daily for 16 weeks.

➤ **HCV genotype 1 infection with or without compensated cirrhosis (Child-Pugh class A) in patients who previously received an NS3/4A PI without prior treatment with an NS5A inhibitor** ⧖

Adults: 3 tablets (total daily dose of 300 mg glecaprevir/120 mg pibrentasvir) PO once daily for 12 weeks.

➤ **HCV genotype 1, 2, 4, 5, or 6 infection without cirrhosis in patients who previously received regimens containing interferon, pegylated interferon, ribavirin, or sofosbuvir but have no prior treatment experience with an HCV NS3/4A PI or NS5A inhibitor** ⧖

Adults: 3 tablets (total daily dose of 300 mg glecaprevir/120 mg pibrentasvir) PO once daily for 8 weeks.

➤ **HCV genotype 1, 2, 4, 5, or 6 infection and compensated cirrhosis (Child-Pugh class A) in patients who previously received regimens containing interferon, pegylated interferon, ribavirin, or sofosbuvir but have no prior treatment experience with an HCV NS3/4A PI or NS5A inhibitor** ⧖

Adults: 3 tablets (total daily dose of 300 mg glecaprevir/120 mg pibrentasvir) PO once daily for 12 weeks.

➤ **HCV genotype 3 infection with or without cirrhosis (Child-Pugh class A) in patients who previously received regimens containing interferon, pegylated interferon, ribavirin, or sofosbuvir but have no prior treatment experience with an HCV NS3/4A PI or NS5A inhibitor** ⧖

Adults: 3 tablets (total daily dose of 300 mg glecaprevir/120 mg pibrentasvir) PO once daily for 16 weeks.

ADMINISTRATION
PO
• Give with food.
• If a dose is missed and it's less than 18 hours from the scheduled time, give dose

as soon as possible, then resume normal schedule. If it has been more than 18 hours from the scheduled time, skip missed dose, then resume normal schedule.
• Store at or below 86° F (30° C).

ACTION
Glecaprevir is an HCV NS3/4A protease inhibitor, and pibrentasvir is an HCV NS5A inhibitor. They are both direct-acting antivirals that prevent viral replication of HCV.

Route	Onset	Peak	Duration
PO	Unknown	5 hr	Unknown

Half-life: Glecaprevir, 6 hours; pibrentasvir, 13 hours.

ADVERSE REACTIONS
CNS: headache, fatigue, asthenia. **GI:** nausea, diarrhea. **Skin:** pruritus.

INTERACTIONS
Drug-drug. *Atazanavir:* May increase glecaprevir and pibrentasvir levels and ALT level. Use together is contraindicated.
Atorvastatin, lovastatin, simvastatin: May increase statin level, increasing risk of myopathy and rhabdomyolysis. Use together isn't recommended.
Carbamazepine, efavirenz: May decrease glecaprevir and pibrentasvir levels. Use together isn't recommended.
Cyclosporine: May increase glecaprevir and pibrentasvir levels. Coadministration isn't recommended in patients requiring more than 100 mg cyclosporine/day.
Dabigatran: May increase dabigatran level. Refer to dabigatran prescribing information for dosage modifications in combination with P-gp inhibitors in patients with renal impairment.
Darunavir, lopinavir, ritonavir: May increase glecaprevir and pibrentasvir levels. Use together isn't recommended.
Digoxin: May increase digoxin level. Measure digoxin level before therapy with glecaprevir and pibrentasvir. Decrease digoxin dosage by 50% or by modifying dosing and frequency; continue monitoring.
Ethinyl estradiol: May increase ALT level. Use together isn't recommended.
Fluvastatin, pitavastatin: May increase fluvastatin and pitavastatin levels, increasing

---

risk of myopathy and rhabdomyolysis. Use lowest approved dosage of fluvastatin and pitavastatin. If higher doses are needed, use lowest dosage necessary based on risk and benefit analysis.

Pravastatin: May increase pravastatin level, increasing risk of myopathy and rhabdomyolysis. Reduce pravastatin dosage by 50%.

Rifampin: May decrease glecaprevir and pibrentasvir levels and their therapeutic effect. Use together is contraindicated.

Rosuvastatin: May increase rosuvastatin level, increasing risk of myopathy and rhabdomyolysis. Don't exceed 10 mg of rosuvastatin.

Drug-herb. *St. John's wort:* May decrease glecaprevir and pibrentasvir levels and reduce their therapeutic effect. Discourage use together.

EFFECTS ON LAB TEST RESULTS
• May increase total bilirubin level.

CONTRAINDICATIONS & CAUTIONS
• Contraindicated in patients with severe hepatic impairment (Child-Pugh class C) and in those taking atazanavir or rifampin.
• Drug isn't recommended in patients with moderate hepatic impairment (Child-Pugh class B).

Black Box Warning HBV reactivation may occur and can result in fulminant hepatitis, hepatic failure, and death. ∎
• Safety and effectiveness in children haven't been established.
Dialyzable drug: No.

PREGNANCY-LACTATION-REPRODUCTION
• There are no studies in pregnant women. Patients should postpone pregnancy until therapy is complete.
• It isn't known if drug appears in human milk. Consider benefit to the mother against possible risk to the infant.

NURSING CONSIDERATIONS
Black Box Warning Before initiating treatment, test all patients for evidence of current or prior HBV infection by measuring HBsAg and hepatitis B core antigen (anti-HBc). ∎
Black Box Warning Monitor HCV/HBV coinfected patients for hepatitis flare or

HBV reactivation during HCV treatment and posttreatment follow-up. Initiate appropriate management for HBV infection as clinically indicated. ∎
• Monitor LFT values at baseline and periodically when clinically indicated.
• *Look alike–sound alike:* Don't confuse Mavyret with Mavik.

PATIENT TEACHING
Black Box Warning Teach patient about risk of HBV reactivation in patients coinfected with HBV during or after treatment of HCV infection. Advise patient to tell prescriber about a history of HBV infection. ∎
• Advise patient to report all medications being taken, including OTC and herbal agents, because of the risk of drug interactions.
• Tell patient to report all adverse reactions and to immediately report signs and symptoms of hepatic impairment (fatigue, abdominal pain, nausea, vomiting, dark urine, light-colored stools, yellowing of the skin or eyes).
• Instruct patient not to skip doses and to take drug for entire treatment duration.

SAFETY ALERT!

glimepiride ⚕
glye-MEH-per-ide

Amaryl✔

Therapeutic class: Antidiabetics
Pharmacologic class: Sulfonylureas

AVAILABLE FORMS
Tablets: 1 mg, 2 mg, 3 mg, 4 mg, 6 mg, 8 mg

INDICATIONS & DOSAGES
➤ **Adjunct to diet and exercise to lower glucose level in patients with type 2 diabetes**
Adults: Initially, 1 or 2 mg PO once daily; usual maintenance dose is 1 to 4 mg PO once daily. After reaching 2 mg, dosage is increased in increments not exceeding 2 mg every 1 to 2 weeks, based on patient's glucose level response. Maximum dose is 8 mg daily.

Adjust-a-dose: For patients with renal impairment, those at risk for hypoglycemia, and elderly patients, initially, 1 mg PO once daily; then adjust cautiously to appropriate dosage, if needed.

ADMINISTRATION
PO
• Give drug with first main meal of the day.
• Patients on nothing-by-mouth status or those requiring decreased caloric intake may need doses withheld to avoid hypoglycemia.

ACTION
Lowers glucose level by stimulating release of insulin from functioning pancreatic beta cells, and may lead to increased sensitivity of peripheral tissues to insulin.

Route	Onset	Peak	Duration
PO	1 hr	2–3 hr	>24 hr

Half-life: 5 to 9 hours.

ADVERSE REACTIONS
CNS: dizziness, asthenia, headache. **GI:** nausea. **Metabolic:** *hypoglycemia,* dilutional hyponatremia. **Respiratory:** flulike symptoms.

INTERACTIONS
Many drugs may increase or decrease the glucose-lowering effect of glimepiride. Consult manufacturer's product information for additional information.
Drug-drug. *Beta blockers, clonidine, guanethidine, reserpine:* May mask symptoms of hypoglycemia. Monitor glucose level.
Colesevelam: May decrease glimepiride serum concentration. Give glimepiride at least 4 hours before colesevelam. Consider therapy modification.
CYP2C9 inducers (rifampin)/inhibitors (fluconazole): Inducers may increase glimepiride metabolism, leading to worsening glycemic control; inhibitors may decrease glimepiride metabolism, leading to hypoglycemia. Monitor therapy.
Drugs that tend to produce hyperglycemia (corticosteroids, estrogens, fosphenytoin, hormonal contraceptives, isoniazid, nicotinic acid, phenothiazines, phenytoin,

thyroid products): May lead to loss of glucose control. Adjust dosage.
Insulin: May increase risk of hypoglycemia. Use together cautiously.
Miconazole (oral): May increase serum concentration and enhance hypoglycemic effect of glimepiride. Monitor therapy.
NSAIDs, other drugs that are highly protein-bound (beta blockers, chloramphenicol, coumarin, MAO inhibitors, probenecid, sulfonamides): May increase hypoglycemic action of sulfonylureas such as glimepiride. Monitor glucose level carefully.
Rifamycins, thiazide diuretics: May increase risk of hyperglycemia. Monitor glucose level.
Salicylates: May increase hypoglycemic effects of sulfonylurea. Monitor glucose level.
Warfarin: Sulfonylureas may enhance anticoagulant effect of vitamin K antagonists; vitamin K antagonists may enhance hypoglycemic effect of sulfonylureas. Monitor therapy.
Drug-herb. *Herbs with hypoglycemic properties:* May enhance hypoglycemic effect of glimepiride. Monitor therapy.
Drug-lifestyle. *Alcohol use:* May alter glycemic control, most commonly causing hypoglycemia. May also cause disulfiram-like reaction. Discourage use together.

EFFECTS ON LAB TEST RESULTS
• May increase alkaline phosphatase, AST, BUN, and creatinine levels.
• May decrease glucose, Hb, and sodium levels.
• May decrease granulocyte, platelet, RBC, and WBC counts.

CONTRAINDICATIONS & CAUTIONS
• Contraindicated in patients hypersensitive to drug and in those with diabetic ketoacidosis, which should be treated with insulin.
• Contraindicated as sole therapy for type 1 diabetes.
• Contraindicated in patients with sulfonamide allergy.
• Use cautiously in debilitated or malnourished patients and in those with adrenal, pituitary, or renal insufficiency; these patients are more susceptible to the hypoglycemic action of glucose-lowering drugs.

• Use cautiously with drugs that can cause hypoglycemia.
• Use cautiously in elderly patients and in patients allergic to sulfonamides.
※ Patients with G6PD deficiency may be at increased risk for sulfonylurea-induced hemolytic anemia. Use cautiously and consider therapy modification.
• Safety and effectiveness in children haven't been established.
Dialyzable drug: Unknown.
⚠ *Overdose S&S:* Hypoglycemia.

PREGNANCY-LACTATION-REPRODUCTION
• Use drug in pregnancy only if potential benefit justifies potential risk to the fetus.
• Prolonged severe hypoglycemia (4 to 10 days) has been reported in neonates born to mothers receiving a sulfonylurea at the time of delivery.
• May cause hypoglycemia in breastfed infants. Patient should discontinue breastfeeding or discontinue drug.

NURSING CONSIDERATIONS
• Glimepiride and insulin may be used together in patients who lose glucose control after first responding to therapy.
• Monitor fasting glucose level periodically to determine therapeutic response. Also monitor HbA$_{1c}$ level, usually every 3 to 6 months, to precisely assess long-term glycemic control.
❸ *Alert:* Use of oral antidiabetics may carry higher risk of CV mortality than use of diet alone or of diet and insulin therapy.
• When changing patient from other sulfonylureas to glimepiride, a transition period isn't needed. Monitor patient carefully for 1 to 2 weeks when changing from longer half-life sulfonylureas, such as chlorpropamide.
• *Look alike–sound alike:* Don't confuse glimepiride with glyburide or glipizide. Don't confuse Amaryl with Altace.

PATIENT TEACHING
• Tell patient to take drug with first meal of the day.
• Make sure patient understands that therapy relieves symptoms but doesn't cure the disease. Patient should also understand

potential risks and advantages of taking drug and of other treatment methods.
• Stress importance of adhering to diet, weight reduction, exercise, and personal hygiene programs. Explain to patient and family how and when to monitor glucose level, and teach recognition of and intervention for signs and symptoms of high and low glucose levels.
• Advise patient to wear or carry medical identification at all times.
• Advise patient to consult prescriber before taking any OTC products or supplements.
• Teach patient to carry candy or other simple sugars to treat mild episodes of low glucose level. Patient experiencing severe episode may need hospital treatment.
• Advise patient to avoid alcohol, which lowers glucose level.

SAFETY ALERT!

glipiZIDE ※
GLIP-i-zide

Glucotrol✿, Glucotrol XL✿

Therapeutic class: Antidiabetics
Pharmacologic class: Sulfonylureas

AVAILABLE FORMS
Tablets (extended-release) ⓞⓣⓒ: 2.5 mg, 5 mg, 10 mg
Tablets (immediate-release): 5 mg, 10 mg

INDICATIONS & DOSAGES
➤ **Adjunct to diet and exercise to lower glucose level in patients with type 2 diabetes**
Immediate-release tablets
Adults: Initially, 5 mg PO daily 30 minutes before breakfast. Titrate by 2.5- to 5-mg increments no less than every few days based on blood glucose levels. Maximum once-daily dose is 15 mg. Divide doses of more than 15 mg. Maximum daily dose is 20 mg.
Adjust-a-dose: For patients with hepatic or renal insufficiency, patients older than age 65, or debilitated or malnourished patients, initially give 2.5 mg PO daily.
Extended-release tablets
Adults: Initially, 2.5 to 5 mg PO with breakfast daily. Increase by 5 mg every 3 months,

depending on level of glycemic control. Maximum daily dose is 20 mg.

➤ **To replace insulin therapy**
Adults: If insulin dosage is 20 units or less daily, insulin may be stopped when glipizide starts. If insulin dosage is more than 20 units daily, start patient at usual dosage in addition to 50% of insulin dose. In some cases, especially if insulin dose is more than 40 units daily, it may be advisable to transition to glipizide in a hospital setting.

ADMINISTRATION
PO
• Give immediate-release tablet about 30 minutes before meals.
• Give extended-release tablet with breakfast.
• Don't split or crush extended-release tablets.
• Patients on nothing-by-mouth status or those requiring decreased caloric intake may need doses withheld to avoid hypoglycemia.

ACTION
Stimulates insulin release from pancreatic beta cells, reduces glucose output by the liver, and increases peripheral sensitivity to insulin.

Route	Onset	Peak	Duration
PO (immediate-release)	15–30 min	1–3 hr	12–24 hr
PO (extended-release)	2–3 hr	6–12 hr	12–24 hr

Half-life: 2 to 5 hours.

ADVERSE REACTIONS
CNS: dizziness, headache, syncope, asthenia, nervousness, tremor, anxiety, depression, insomnia, pain. **EENT:** blurred vision. **GI:** nausea, dyspepsia, flatulence, constipation, diarrhea, vomiting. **GU:** polyuria. **Hematologic:** *leukopenia,* hemolytic anemia, *agranulocytosis, thrombocytopenia, aplastic anemia.* **Metabolic:** *hypoglycemia.* **Musculoskeletal:** arthralgia, leg cramps. **Respiratory:** rhinitis. **Skin:** pruritus, photosensitivity reactions.

INTERACTIONS
Many drugs may increase or decrease glucose-lowering effect of glipizide.

Consult manufacturer's product information for additional information.

Drug-drug. *Amantadine, anabolic steroids, antifungals, chloramphenicol, clofibrate, guanethidine, MAO inhibitors, NSAIDs, probenecid, quinolones, ranitidine,* **salicylates,** *sulfonamides:* May increase hypoglycemic activity. Monitor glucose level.
Beta blockers, clonidine, guanethidine, reserpine: May prolong hypoglycemic effect and mask symptoms of hypoglycemia. Use together cautiously.
Colesevelam: May decrease glipizide serum concentration. Give glipizide at least 4 hours before colesevelam. Consider therapy modification.
Corticosteroids, glucagon, phenytoin, **rifamycins, thiazide diuretics:** May decrease hypoglycemic response. Monitor glucose level.
Fluconazole: May increase glipizide serum concentration, leading to hypoglycemia. Monitor patient closely.
Miconazole (oral): May increase serum concentration and enhance hypoglycemic effect of glipizide. Monitor therapy.
Oral anticoagulants: May increase hypoglycemic activity or enhance anticoagulant effect. Monitor glucose level, PT, and INR.
Drug-herb. *Herbs with hypoglycemic properties:* May enhance hypoglycemic effect of glipizide. Monitor therapy.
Drug-lifestyle. *Alcohol use:* May alter glycemic control, most commonly causing hypoglycemia. May cause disulfiram-like reaction. Discourage use together.

EFFECTS ON LAB TEST RESULTS
• May increase alkaline phosphatase, AST, LDH, BUN, cholesterol, and creatinine levels.
• May decrease glucose and Hb levels.
• May decrease granulocyte, platelet, and WBC counts.

CONTRAINDICATIONS & CAUTIONS
• Contraindicated in patients hypersensitive to drug and in those with diabetic ketoacidosis with or without coma.
• Contraindicated in patients with sulfonamide allergy.
▓ Patients with G6PD deficiency may be at increased risk for sulfonylurea-induced

---

Reactions in bold italics are *life-threatening*. Interactions may have a *rapid onset* or a *delayed onset*.

hemolytic anemia. Use cautiously and consider therapy modification.
• Use cautiously in patients with severe GI disease or renal or hepatic disease, and in debilitated, malnourished, or elderly patients.
Dialyzable drug: Unknown.
⚠ *Overdose S&S:* Hypoglycemia.

PREGNANCY-LACTATION-REPRODUCTION
• Insulin is drug of choice to control diabetes during pregnancy. If used during pregnancy, discontinue at least 1 month before expected delivery date because prolonged severe hypoglycemia (4 to 10 days) has been reported in neonates born to mothers receiving a sulfonylurea at the time of delivery.
• Drug may cause hypoglycemia in breastfed infants. Patient should discontinue breastfeeding or discontinue drug.

NURSING CONSIDERATIONS
• Some patients may attain effective control on a once-daily regimen, whereas others respond better with divided dosing.
• Patient may switch from immediate-release to extended-release tablets at the nearest equivalent total daily dose.
• Glipizide is a second-generation sulfonylurea. The frequency of adverse reactions appears to be lower than with first-generation drugs such as chlorpropamide.
🔸 *Alert:* Use of oral antidiabetic drugs may carry a higher risk of CV mortality than use of diet alone or of diet and insulin therapy.
• During periods of increased stress, patient may need insulin therapy. Monitor patient closely for hyperglycemia in these situations.
• Patient switching from insulin therapy to an oral antidiabetic should check glucose level at least three times a day before meals. Patient may need hospitalization during transition.
• *Look alike–sound alike:* Don't confuse glipizide with glyburide or glimepiride.

PATIENT TEACHING
• Instruct patient about disease and importance of following therapeutic regimen, adhering to diet, losing weight, getting exercise, and avoiding infection. Explain how and when to monitor glucose level, and teach recognition of episodes of low and high glucose levels.

• Tell patient to carry candy or other simple sugars to treat mild low-glucose episodes. Patient experiencing severe episode may need hospital treatment.
• Instruct patient not to change drug dosage without prescriber's consent and to report abnormal blood or urine glucose test results.
• Tell patient not to take other drugs, including OTC drugs, without first checking with prescriber.
• Advise patient to wear or carry medical identification at all times.
• Advise patient to avoid alcohol, which lowers glucose level.
• Tell patient that something resembling a tablet may appear in the stool; assure patient that it's the nonabsorbable shell of the extended-release tablet.

SAFETY ALERT!

glyBURIDE (glibenclamide) ▨
GLYE-byoor-ide

Diabeta, Glynase

Therapeutic class: Antidiabetics
Pharmacologic class: Sulfonylureas

AVAILABLE FORMS
Tablets: 1.25 mg, 2.5 mg, 5 mg
Tablets (micronized): 1.5 mg, 3 mg, 6 mg

INDICATIONS & DOSAGES
➤ **Adjunct to diet to lower glucose level in patients with type 2 diabetes**
Nonmicronized form
Adults: Initially, 2.5 to 5 mg PO once daily with breakfast or first main meal. Adjust to maintenance dose at no more than 2.5-mg increments at weekly intervals. Usual daily maintenance dose is 1.25 to 20 mg, in single dose or divided doses. Maximum daily dose is 20 mg PO.
Micronized form
Adults: Initially, 1.5 to 3 mg PO daily with breakfast or first main meal. Adjust to maintenance dose at no more than 1.5-mg increments at weekly intervals. Usual daily maintenance dose is 0.75 to 12 mg. Dosages exceeding 6 mg daily may have better response with b.i.d. dosing. Maximum dose is 12 mg PO daily.

Adjust-a-dose: For elderly patients, patients who are more sensitive to antidiabetics, and for those with renal, hepatic, adrenal, or pituitary insufficiency, start with 1.25 mg (nonmicronized) or 0.75 mg (micronized) daily.

➤ **To replace insulin therapy**
Adults: If insulin dose is less than 40 units/day, patient may be switched directly to glyburide when insulin is stopped. If insulin dose is less than 20 units/day, initial dose is 2.5 to 5 mg (1.5 to 3 mg micronized) PO daily. If insulin dose is 20 to 40 units/day, initial dose is 5 mg (3 mg micronized) PO daily. If insulin dose is 40 or more units/day, initially, 5 mg (3 mg micronized) PO once daily in addition to 50% of insulin dose. Gradually taper off insulin as the glyburide dose is increased.

ADMINISTRATION
PO
- Give drug with breakfast or first main meal.
- Twice-daily dosing may be beneficial if conventional glyburide doses are greater than 10 mg or micronized glyburide doses are greater than 6 mg.
- Patients on nothing-by-mouth status or those requiring decreased caloric intake may need doses withheld to avoid hypoglycemia.

ACTION
Unknown. Probably stimulates insulin release from pancreatic beta cells, reduces glucose output by the liver, and increases peripheral sensitivity to insulin.

Route	Onset	Peak	Duration
PO (micronized)	1 hr	2–3 hr	<24 hr
PO (non-micronized)	2–4 hr	2–4 hr	<24 hr

Half-life: 4 to 10 hours.

ADVERSE REACTIONS
GI: nausea, epigastric fullness, heartburn. **Hematologic:** *leukopenia,* hemolytic anemia, *agranulocytosis, thrombocytopenia, aplastic anemia.* **Hepatic:** cholestatic jaundice, *hepatitis.* **Metabolic:** *hypoglycemia, hyponatremia.* **Musculoskeletal:** arthralgia, myalgia. **Skin:** rash, pruritus, other allergic reactions. **Other:** *angioedema.*

INTERACTIONS
Many drugs may increase or decrease glucose-lowering effect of glyburide. Consult manufacturer's product information for additional information.
Drug-drug. *Anabolic steroids, azole antifungals, chloramphenicol, clofibrate, fluoroquinolones, guanethidine, MAO inhibitors, NSAIDs, probenecid, phenylbutazone, ranitidine,* **salicylates,** *sulfonamides:* May increase hypoglycemic activity. Monitor glucose level.
Beta blockers: May prolong hypoglycemic effect and mask symptoms of hypoglycemia. Use together cautiously.
Bosentan: Increases risk of elevated LFT values. Use together is contraindicated.
Carbamazepine, corticosteroids, glucagon, **rifamycins, thiazide diuretics:** May decrease hypoglycemic response. Monitor glucose level.
Colesevelam: May decrease glyburide serum concentration. Give glyburide at least 4 hours before colesevelam.
Miconazole (oral): May increase serum concentration and enhance hypoglycemic effect of glyburide. Monitor therapy.
Oral anticoagulants: May increase hypoglycemic activity or enhance anticoagulant effect. Monitor glucose level, PT, and INR.
Drug-herb. *Herbs with hypoglycemic properties:* May enhance hypoglycemic effect of glimepiride. Monitor therapy.
Drug-lifestyle. *Alcohol use:* May alter glycemic control, most commonly causing hypoglycemia. May cause disulfiram-like reaction. Discourage use together.

EFFECTS ON LAB TEST RESULTS
- May increase alkaline phosphatase, AST, ALT, bilirubin, BUN, and cholesterol levels.
- May decrease glucose, sodium, and Hb levels.
- May decrease granulocyte, platelet, and WBC counts.

CONTRAINDICATIONS & CAUTIONS
- Contraindicated in patients hypersensitive to drug and in those with type 1 diabetes or diabetic ketoacidosis with or without coma.
- Use cautiously in patients with hepatic or renal impairment (eGFR less than 60 mL/minute); in debilitated, malnourished, or

---

elderly patients; and in patients allergic to sulfonamides.

☒ Patients with G6PD deficiency may be at increased risk for sulfonylurea-induced hemolytic anemia. Use cautiously and consider therapy modification.

Dialyzable drug: Unknown.

⚠ *Overdose S&S:* Hypoglycemia.

PREGNANCY-LACTATION-REPRODUCTION

• Insulin is drug of choice to control diabetes during pregnancy. If used during pregnancy, discontinue at least 2 weeks before expected delivery date.

• Prolonged severe hypoglycemia (4 to 10 days) has been reported in neonates born to mothers receiving a sulfonylurea at the time of delivery.

• Drug may cause hypoglycemia in breast-fed infants. Patient should discontinue breastfeeding or discontinue drug.

NURSING CONSIDERATIONS

❸ *Alert:* Micronized glyburide (Glynase) contains drug in a smaller particle size and isn't bioequivalent to regular glyburide tablets. In patients who have been taking nonmicronized form, adjust dosage.

• Although most patients may take drug once daily, those taking more than 10 mg conventional glyburide or 6 mg micronized glyburide daily may achieve better results with twice-daily dosage.

• Drug is a second-generation sulfonylurea. Adverse effects are less common with second-generation drugs than with first-generation drugs such as chlorpropamide.

❸ *Alert:* Use of oral antidiabetic drugs may carry a higher risk of CV mortality than use of diet alone or of diet and insulin therapy.

• During periods of increased stress, such as infection, fever, surgery, or trauma, patient may need insulin therapy. Monitor patient closely for hyperglycemia in these situations.

• Patient switching from insulin therapy to an oral antidiabetic should check glucose level at least three times a day before meals. Patient may need hospitalization during transition.

• *Look alike–sound alike:* Don't confuse glyburide with glimepiride or glipizide.

PATIENT TEACHING

• Teach patient about diabetes and the importance of following therapeutic regimen, adhering to specific diet, losing weight, getting exercise, following personal hygiene programs, and avoiding infection. Explain how and when to monitor glucose level, and teach recognition of and intervention for low and high glucose levels.

• Tell patient not to change drug dosage without prescriber's consent and to report abnormal blood or urine glucose test results.

• Teach patient to carry candy or other simple sugars for mild low glucose level. Patient experiencing severe episode may need hospital treatment.

• Advise patient not to take supplements or other drugs, including OTC drugs, without first checking with prescriber.

• Advise patient to wear or carry medical identification at all times.

❸ *Alert:* Instruct patient to report episodes of low glucose to prescriber immediately; a severely low glucose level is sometimes fatal in patients receiving as little as 2.5 to 5 mg daily.

• Advise patient to avoid alcohol, which may lower glucose level.

golimumab
go-LIM-myoo-mab

Simponi, Simponi Aria

Therapeutic class: Antiarthritics
Pharmacologic class: TNF blockers

AVAILABLE FORMS

Injection (IV): 50 mg/4 mL single-use vial
Injection (subcut): 50 mg/0.5 mL, 100 mg/mL prefilled syringe; 50 mg/ 0.5 mL, 100 mg/mL prefilled autoinjector

INDICATIONS & DOSAGES

➤ **Moderate to severe active RA in combination with methotrexate; active psoriatic arthritis or active ankylosing spondylitis alone or in combination with methotrexate or other nonbiologic DMARDs**

Adults: 50 mg subcut monthly. Or 2 mg/kg IV infusion over 30 minutes at weeks 0 and 4, then every 8 weeks thereafter.

➤ **Moderate to severe ulcerative colitis in patients who have demonstrated an inadequate response or intolerance to prior treatment or who require continuous steroid therapy**

Adults: Initially, 200 mg subcut, followed by 100 mg subcut at week 2, then 100 mg subcut every 4 weeks.

ADMINISTRATION

• The efficacy and safety of switching between IV and subcut formulations and routes of administration haven't been established.

IV

▼ Dilute with NSS or half NSS to a final volume of 100 mL.

▼ Administer over 30 minutes. Use a 0.22-micron low protein-binding filter.

▼ Don't infuse with other drugs in the same IV line.

▼ Solutions diluted for infusion may be stored at room temperature for 4 hours.

Subcutaneous

• Remove drug from refrigerator 30 minutes before administration and allow it to reach room temperature.

• Inspect solution before administration. Don't use solution if discolored or cloudy or if foreign particles are present. Drug is normally colorless to slightly opalescent to light yellow.

• Prefilled syringe and prefilled autoinjector contain latex. Don't handle if sensitive to latex.

• Don't use any leftover product remaining in prefilled syringe or prefilled autoinjector.

• Rotate injection sites. Don't inject drug into areas where skin is tender, bruised, red, or hard.

• If multiple injections are required, administer injections at different sites on the body.

ACTION

Binds to human TNF-alpha to neutralize its activity and inhibit its binding with receptors, thereby reducing the infiltration of inflammatory cells.

Route	Onset	Peak	Duration
IV	Unknown	12 weeks	Unknown
Subcut	Unknown	2–6 days	Unknown

Half-life: 2 weeks.

ADVERSE REACTIONS

CNS: dizziness, paresthesia, fever. **CV:** HTN. **EENT:** nasopharyngitis, oral herpes, pharyngitis, rhinitis, sinusitis. **Respiratory:** bronchitis, URI. **Skin:** injection-site reactions, superficial fungal infections, rash. **Other:** flulike syndrome, infection, antibody development.

INTERACTIONS

Drug-drug. *Abatacept, anakinra, other immunosuppressants:* May increase risk of serious infection. Avoid using together.

CYP450 substrates (cyclosporine, theophylline, warfarin): May alter levels of these drugs. Monitor patient closely and adjust dosages as needed.

Live-virus vaccines: May increase risk of infection. Postpone live-virus vaccine until 3 months after therapy has ended.

EFFECTS ON LAB TEST RESULTS

• May increase LFT values.

• May decrease platelet, WBC, and neutrophil counts.

• May diminish diagnostic effect of coccidioidin skin test.

• May cause positive ANA titer.

CONTRAINDICATIONS & CAUTIONS

• Use cautiously in patients with malignancies; invasive fungal infection; chronic infection (HBV, TB); history of recurrent infection, hematologic abnormalities, or HF; or preexisting or recent onset of CNS demyelination.

• Safe use in children hasn't been established.

Dialyzable drug: Unknown.

PREGNANCY-LACTATION-REPRODUCTION

• Use in pregnant women only if benefit justifies risk to the fetus and only if clearly needed.

• Administration of live-virus vaccines to infants exposed to golimumab in utero isn't recommended for 6 months after the mother's last dose during pregnancy.

• It isn't known if drug appears in human milk. Patient should discontinue breastfeeding or discontinue drug.

Reactions in bold italics are *life-threatening*. Interactions may have a *rapid onset* or a *delayed onset*.

NURSING CONSIDERATIONS

Black Box Warning Monitor patient closely for signs and symptoms of infection before and after treatment. TB, invasive fungal infection, and other bacterial and viral opportunistic infections, which are sometimes fatal, may occur in patients receiving golimumab. Stop drug if serious infection or sepsis develops during treatment. ■

Black Box Warning Evaluate patient for latent TB with tuberculin skin test before initiating treatment. Treat latent TB before therapy with golimumab. Monitor all patients for active TB during treatment even if initial latent TB test is negative. ■

• Drug increases risk of reactivation of HBV infection, which can be fatal, in patients who are HBV carriers. Before starting therapy, patient should be tested for HBV infection.

• Monitor patient for new or worsening HF; stop drug if signs and symptoms occur.

Black Box Warning Lymphoma and other malignancies, some fatal, have been reported in children and adolescents treated with TNF blockers, including golimumab. ■

• Monitor patient for lymphomas and other malignancies.

• Pancytopenia and other significant cytopenias, including aplastic anemia, can occur. Monitor CBC regularly during therapy. May discontinue drug if hematologic abnormalities develop.

PATIENT TEACHING

• Teach patient how to give subcut injection. First self-injection should be under supervision of qualified health care practitioner.

• Advise patient that prefilled syringes and prefilled autoinjectors contain latex or a latex derivative.

• Instruct patient to report all adverse reactions, especially signs and symptoms of infection, new or worsening HF, or liver or nervous system problems.

• Tell patient to avoid live-virus vaccines while taking drug.

granisetron
gran-IZ-e-tron

Sancuso, Sustol

granisetron hydrochloride

Therapeutic class: Antiemetics
Pharmacologic class: 5-HT$_3$ receptor antagonists

AVAILABLE FORMS

Injection: 0.1 mg/mL in 1-mL single-use vials; 1 mg/mL in 1-mL single-dose, preservative-free vials and 4-mL multidose vials containing benzyl alcohol
Injection (extended-release): 10 mg/0.4 mL single-dose syringe
Tablets: 1 mg
Transdermal patch: 3.1 mg per 24 hours

INDICATIONS & DOSAGES

➤ **Prevention of nausea and vomiting from emetogenic cancer chemotherapy**
Adults and children ages 2 to 16: 10 mcg/kg IV undiluted and given by direct injection over 30 seconds, or diluted and infused over 5 minutes. Start giving at least 30 minutes before chemotherapy. Or, for adults, 1 mg PO up to 1 hour before chemotherapy and repeated 12 hours later. Or, for adults, 2 mg PO daily given up to 1 hour before chemotherapy. Or, for adults, apply a single patch to the upper outer arm 24 to 48 hours before chemotherapy. Remove the patch a minimum of 24 hours after completion of chemotherapy or a maximum of 7 days.

Or, for adults, 10 mg extended-release form subcut with dexamethasone at least 30 minutes before chemotherapy on day 1. Don't give extended-release form more frequently than once every 7 days. Refer to manufacturer's instructions for dexamethasone dosages.
Adjust-a-dose: In patients with moderate renal impairment (CrCl of 30 to 59 mL/minute), don't give extended-release form more frequently than once every 14 days. Don't give extended-release form to patients with severe renal impairment (CrCl of less than 30 mL/minute).

➤ **Prevention of nausea and vomiting from radiation, including total body irradiation and fractionated abdominal radiation**

Adults: 2 mg PO once daily within 1 hour of radiation.

ADMINISTRATION
PO
• Store tablets between 68° and 77° F (20° and 25° C). Protect from light.

IV
▼ For direct injection, give drug undiluted over 30 seconds.

▼ For intermittent infusion, dilute with NSS for injection or D_5W to a volume of 20 to 50 mL.

▼ Infuse over 5 minutes, starting within 30 minutes before chemotherapy and only on days chemotherapy is given.

▼ Diluted solutions are stable for 24 hours at room temperature. Protect from light.

▼ Don't freeze vials.

▼ Once the multiuse vial is penetrated, use contents within 30 days.

▼ **Incompatibilities:** Other IV drugs.

Subcutaneous
• Extended-release form is for subcut injection only.

• Drug should only be administered by a health care provider.

• Remove extended-release form kit from refrigerator 1 hour before administration.

• Refer to manufacturer's syringe preparation instructions for warming syringe to body temperature using syringe warming pouches included in kit.

• Don't give drug if discoloration or particulate matter is noted in syringe; be aware that syringe is amber-colored glass.

• Give drug by subcut injection in the skin of the back of the upper arm or in the skin of the abdomen at least 1 inch (2.54 cm) from the umbilicus.

• Topical anesthetic may be used at injection site before giving drug.

• Avoid injecting into skin that's burned, hardened, inflamed, swollen, or otherwise compromised.

• Give drug as a slow, sustained subcut injection over 20 to 30 seconds.

• Store in refrigerator at 36° to 46° F (2° to 8° C). Protect from light; don't freeze.

• Once drug has been removed from refrigerator, it can remain at room temperature for up to 7 days.

Transdermal
• Apply patch to clean, intact, healthy skin on the upper outer arm.

• Each patch is packed in a pouch and should be applied directly after the pouch has been opened.

• Don't cut patch into pieces.

ACTION
May block $5\text{-}HT_3$ in the CNS in the chemoreceptor trigger zone and in the peripheral nervous system on nerve terminals of the vagus nerve.

Route	Onset	Peak	Duration
PO, IV	Unknown	Unknown	24 hr
Subcut (extended-release)	Unknown	11–12 hr	7 days
Transdermal	Unknown	48 hr	Unknown

Half-life: PO, IV, transdermal, 5 to 9 hours; extended-release, 24 hours.

ADVERSE REACTIONS
CNS: asthenia, headache, fever, agitation, anxiety, CNS stimulation, dizziness, insomnia, somnolence, pain, weakness, drowsiness, syncope. **CV:** HTN, hypotension, prolonged QT interval; atrial fibrillation (extended-release form). **GI:** constipation, nausea, vomiting, abdominal pain, decreased appetite, diarrhea, dyspepsia, flatulence, taste disorder, GERD. **Hematologic:** anemia, *leukocytosis, leukopenia, thrombocytopenia.* **Skin:** alopecia, rash, dermatitis, injection-site reactions, *hypersensitivity reactions.*

INTERACTIONS
Drug-drug. *Apomorphine:* May increase risk of profound hypotension and loss of consciousness. Avoid use together.

Drugs that prolong QT interval: May increase risk of life-threatening cardiac arrhythmias, including torsades de pointes. Use together cautiously and monitor patient.

Serotonin modulators (fentanyl, lithium, MAO inhibitors, methylene blue IV, mirtazapine, SSNRIs, SSRIs, tramadol): May increase risk of serotonin syndrome. Monitor therapy.

Reactions in bold italics are *life-threatening*. Interactions may have a *rapid onset* or a *delayed onset*.

EFFECTS ON LAB TEST RESULTS
• May increase ALT and AST levels. May decrease Hb level and hematocrit. May alter fluid and electrolyte levels with prolonged use.
• May decrease platelet and WBC counts.

CONTRAINDICATIONS & CAUTIONS
• Contraindicated in patients hypersensitive to drug or other 5-HT$_3$ receptor antagonists.
• Hypersensitivity reactions, including anaphylaxis, may occur up to 7 days or longer after administration of extended-release form.
☉ *Alert:* QT-interval prolongation has been reported, and drug may increase risk of ventricular arrhythmias. Use caution in patients with preexisting arrhythmias, cardiac conduction disorders, cardiac disease, or electrolyte abnormalities; in patients receiving cardiotoxic chemotherapy; and in those receiving medications that prolong QT interval.
• May increase risk of serotonin syndrome, which can be fatal, especially if drug is used with other serotonergic drugs.
• Use of extended-release form with successive emetogenic chemotherapy cycles for more than 6 months isn't recommended.
• Injection-site bruising and hematoma, which can be severe, may occur more than 5 days after administration of extended-release form. Patients receiving anticoagulants or antiplatelet drugs may be at greater risk.
Dialyzable drug: Unknown.
⚠ *Overdose S&S:* Headache.

PREGNANCY-LACTATION-REPRODUCTION
• Use in pregnancy only if clearly needed.
• Use cautiously in breastfeeding women.

NURSING CONSIDERATIONS
• Drug regimen is given only on days when chemotherapy is given. Treatment at other times isn't useful.
• Monitor patient for signs and symptoms of serotonin syndrome (mental status changes, neuromuscular signs and symptoms, autonomic instability, seizures, GI symptoms). If signs or symptoms of serotonin syndrome occur, discontinue drug and initiate treatment.

• Monitor patients receiving extended-release form for injection-site infections, bruising, and hematoma.
• Monitor patients receiving extended-release form for signs and symptoms of hypersensitivity reactions (dyspnea, wheezing, rash, hives, fever, swelling).
• Monitor patients for constipation and decreased bowel activity, especially patients at risk for GI obstruction.

PATIENT TEACHING
• Stress importance of taking second dose of oral drug 12 hours after the first for maximum effectiveness.
• Tell patient to report adverse reactions immediately.
• Teach patient receiving extended-release form that hypersensitivity reactions can occur up to 7 days or later after subcut administration and to immediately report signs and symptoms.
• Teach patient signs and symptoms of serotonin syndrome and advise patient to report them immediately.
• Tell patient to report injection-site reactions (infection, bruising, hematoma, pain, warmth, bleeding) to prescriber.
• Tell patient not to apply patch to red, irritated, or damaged skin and to cover patch with clothing to avoid natural or artificial sunlight. If patch loosens, advise patient to apply tape only to edges to secure. Caution patient not to apply heat (heating pad) over or in area of transdermal patch.

haloperidol
ha-loe-PER-i-dole

haloperidol decanoate
Haldol Decanoate, Haloperidol LA ✦

haloperidol lactate
Haldol

Therapeutic class: Antipsychotics
Pharmacologic class: Butyrophenone derivatives

AVAILABLE FORMS
haloperidol
Tablets: 0.5 mg, 1 mg, 2 mg, 5 mg, 10 mg, 20 mg

H

haloperidol decanoate
Injection: 50 mg/mL*, 100 mg/mL*
haloperidol lactate
Injection: 5 mg/mL
Oral solution (concentrate): 2 mg/mL

INDICATIONS & DOSAGES

Adjust-a-dose (for all indications): For indications with oral dosing and for oral dosing in elderly and debilitated patients, initially, 0.5 to 2 mg PO b.i.d. or t.i.d.; increase gradually, as needed.

➤ **Psychotic disorders**
Adults and children older than age 12:
Dosage varies for each patient. Initially, 0.5 to 5 mg PO b.i.d. or t.i.d. Maximum, 100 mg PO daily. Or, 2 to 5 mg lactate IM every 4 to 8 hours, although hourly administration may be needed until control is obtained.
Children ages 3 to 12 weighing 15 to 40 kg:
Initially, 0.5 mg PO in two or three divided doses daily. May increase dose by 0.5 mg at 5- to 7-day intervals, depending on therapeutic response and patient tolerance. Maintenance dose, 0.05 to 0.15 mg/kg PO daily given in two or three divided doses. Severely disturbed children may need higher doses.

➤ **Chronic psychosis requiring prolonged therapy**
Adults: 50 to 200 mg decanoate IM every 4 weeks.
Adjust-a-dose: For elderly or debilitated patients, lower initial dose and gradual adjustments are recommended. Recommended initial and maintenance dosage is 10 to 15 times the daily oral dose, administered IM every 4 weeks.

➤ **Nonpsychotic behavior disorders**
Children ages 3 to 12 weighing 15 to 40 kg: 0.05 to 0.075 mg/kg PO daily, in two or three divided doses. Maximum, 6 mg daily. Severely disturbed nonpsychotic or hyperactive children with conduct disorders may only require short-term use.

➤ **Tourette syndrome**
Adults: Initially, 0.5 to 5 mg PO b.i.d., t.i.d., or as needed. Up to about 100 mg/day may be needed.
Children ages 3 to 12 weighing 15 to 40 kg: 0.05 to 0.075 mg/kg PO daily, in two or three divided doses.

ADMINISTRATION
PO
🕒 *Alert:* Haloperidol isn't approved for IV use.
• Protect drug from light. Slight yellowing of concentrate is common and doesn't affect potency. Discard very discolored solutions.
IM
• Protect drug from light. Slight yellowing of solution is common and doesn't affect potency. Discard very discolored solutions.
• Use a 21G needle. Maximum volume per injection site shouldn't exceed 3 mL. Give in gluteal muscle by deep IM injection; Z-track techniques are recommended (haloperidol decanoate).
• When switching from tablets to IM decanoate injection, give 10 to 20 times the oral dose once a month (maximum, 100 mg). If initial dose conversion requires more than 100 mg, give in two injections (100 mg maximum) separated by 3 to 7 days. If patient is elderly or debilitated or if oral haloperidol dose is 10 mg/day or less, initiate dose at 10 to 15 times the daily oral dose. If patient is at high risk for relapse or oral haloperidol dose is greater than 10 mg/day, initiate dose at 20 times the oral daily dose.

ACTION

A butyrophenone that probably exerts antipsychotic effects by blocking postsynaptic dopamine receptors in the brain.

Route	Onset	Peak	Duration
PO	Unknown	2–6 hr	Unknown
IM (decanoate)	Unknown	6 days	Unknown
IM (lactate)	Unknown	10–20 min	Unknown

Half-life: PO, 14 to 37 hours; IM decanoate, 3 weeks; IM lactate, 20 hours.

ADVERSE REACTIONS

CNS: severe extrapyramidal reactions, dystonia, tardive dyskinesia, *NMS, seizures,* sedation, drowsiness, lethargy, headache, insomnia, confusion, vertigo, agitation, anxiety, depression, euphoria, restlessness, tonic-clonic seizures, hallucinations, parkinsonian-like syndrome. **CV:** tachycardia, hypotension, HTN, *prolonged QT interval* and other ECG changes, *torsades de pointes* with high doses. **EENT:** blurred vision, cataracts, retinopathy, oculogyric crisis. **GI:** dry mouth, anorexia, constipation, diarrhea, nausea, vomiting, dyspepsia. **GU:** urine retention, menstrual irregularities, priapism. **Hematologic:** *leukopenia,* leukocytosis. **Hepatic:** jaundice. **Metabolic:** hyperglycemia, hypoglycemia, hyponatremia. **Skin:** rash, other skin reactions, diaphoresis. **Other:** gynecomastia.

INTERACTIONS
Drug-drug. *Anticholinergics:* May increase anticholinergic effects and glaucoma. Use together cautiously.
Antiparkinsonian drugs (dopamine agonist): May diminish therapeutic effect of both haloperidol and antiparkinsonian drug (dopamine agonist). Avoid using together. If used together can't be avoided, monitor patient for decreased effects of both agents.
Azole antifungals, buspirone, macrolides: May increase haloperidol level. Monitor patient for increased adverse reactions; haloperidol dose may need to be adjusted.
Beta blockers: May cause an unexpected severe hypotensive reaction. If this occurs, provide supportive treatment.
Carbamazepine: May decrease haloperidol level. Monitor patient.
CNS depressants: May increase CNS depression. Use together cautiously.
Lithium: May cause lethargy and confusion after high doses. Monitor patient.
Black Box Warning *Opioid class warning:* May cause slow or difficult breathing, sedation, and death. Avoid use together. If use together is necessary, limit dosage and duration of each drug to minimum necessary for desired effect.
QT-interval-prolonging drugs: May prolong QT interval. Monitor ECG.
Rifampin: May decrease haloperidol level. Monitor patient for clinical effect.
Drug-lifestyle. *Alcohol use, cannabidiol:* May increase CNS depression. Discourage use together.
Smoking: May decrease haloperidol serum concentration. Monitor therapy.

EFFECTS ON LAB TEST RESULTS
• May increase LFT values. May decrease sodium level.
• May increase or decrease glucose level and WBC count.

CONTRAINDICATIONS & CAUTIONS
• Contraindicated in patients hypersensitive to drug and in those with dementia with Lewy bodies, Parkinson disease, coma, or CNS depression.
Black Box Warning *Opioid class warning:* Opioids should only be prescribed with benzodiazepines or other CNS depressants to patients for whom alternative treatment options are inadequate. ∎
• Use cautiously in elderly and debilitated patients; in patients with history of seizures or EEG abnormalities, prolonged QT interval and other severe CV disorders, allergies, glaucoma, or urine retention; and in those taking anticonvulsants, anticoagulants, antiparkinsonians, or lithium.
• Use cautiously in patients at risk for falls, including those with diseases or conditions or who are taking drugs that may cause somnolence, orthostatic hypotension, or motor or sensory instability.
• Decanoate form contains benzyl alcohol.
• Blood dyscrasias have been reported. Discontinue drug for ANC less than $1,000/mm^3$ or for leukopenia or agranulocytosis.
Dializable drug: Unknown.
⚠ Overdose S&S: Severe extrapyramidal reactions, hypotension, sedation, EEG abnormalities.

PREGNANCY-LACTATION-REPRODUCTION
☻ Alert: Antipsychotic use during the third trimester may result in abnormal muscle movements (extrapyramidal symptoms) and withdrawal symptoms in newborns. Use during pregnancy only if clearly needed. Use minimum effective maternal dose.
• Drug appears in human milk. Breastfeeding isn't recommended.

NURSING CONSIDERATIONS
• Monitor patient for tardive dyskinesia, which may occur after prolonged use. It may not appear until months or years later and may disappear spontaneously or persist for life, despite ending drug.
☻ Alert: Watch for signs and symptoms of NMS (extrapyramidal effects, hyperthermia, autonomic disturbance), which is rare but commonly fatal.
☻ Alert: Monitor ECG when drug is given in high doses or when patient is taking other

H

QT interval–prolonging drugs because of the increased risk of QT-interval prolongation and torsades de pointes.

Black Box Warning Elderly patients with dementia-related psychosis treated with atypical or conventional antipsychotics are at increased risk for death. Antipsychotics aren't approved for the treatment of dementia-related psychosis. ∎

• Don't withdraw drug abruptly unless required by severe adverse reactions.

• Complete fall risk assessments at start of antipsychotic treatment and recurrently for patients on long-term therapy, especially those at increased risk for falls.

• Esophageal dysmotility and aspiration can occur. Use cautiously in patients at risk for aspiration (those with pneumonia, Alzheimer disease).

• *Look alike–sound alike:* Don't confuse Haldol with Halcion or Halog.

PATIENT TEACHING

Black Box Warning *Opioid class warning:* Caution patient or caregiver of patient taking an opioid with a benzodiazepine, CNS depressant, or alcohol to seek immediate medical attention for dizziness, lightheadedness, extreme sleepiness, slowed or difficult breathing, or unresponsiveness. ∎

• Advise patient to report all adverse reactions.

• Although drug is the least sedating of the antipsychotics, warn patient to avoid activities that require alertness and good coordination until effects of drug are known. Drowsiness and dizziness usually subside after a few weeks.

• Advise patient that drug may cause somnolence, orthostatic hypotension, and motor and sensory instability, which may lead to falls.

• Warn patient to avoid alcohol during therapy.

• Tell patient to relieve dry mouth with sugarless gum or hard candy.

SAFETY ALERT!

heparin sodium
HEP-a-rin

Heparin Sodium Injection

Therapeutic class: Anticoagulants
Pharmacologic class: Anticoagulants

AVAILABLE FORMS
Products are derived from beef lung or pork intestinal mucosa.
heparin sodium
Carpuject: 5,000 units/mL
Premixed IV solutions: Units of heparin and type of solution vary by manufacturer.
Single-dose ampules and vials: 1,000 units/mL, 5,000 units/mL, 10,000 units/mL, 20,000 units/mL
Syringes: 1,000 units/mL, 5,000 units/mL, 10,000 units/mL, 20,000 units/mL
Unit-dose vials: 1,000 units/mL, 5,000 units/0.5 mL (2,500 units/mL), 5,000 units/mL, 7,500 units/mL, 10,000 units/mL, 20,000 units/mL
Vials (multidose): 1,000 units/mL, 5,000 units/mL, 10,000 units/mL, 20,000 units/mL

INDICATIONS & DOSAGES
➤ **Thromboprophylaxis**
Adults: 5,000 units subcut every 8 to 12 hours for a minimum of 7 days or for 10 to 14 days for patients undergoing total hip arthroplasty, total knee arthroplasty, or hip fracture surgery according to American College of Chest Physicians guidelines.
➤ **Full-dose continuous IV infusion therapy for DVT or PE**
Adults: Initially, 5,000 units (or 80 units/kg) by IV bolus; then 20,000 to 40,000 units/day (or 18 units/kg/hour) by IV infusion with pump. Titrate hourly rate based on aPTT results (every 4 to 6 hours in the early stages of treatment).
Children: Initially, 75 to 100 units/kg IV over 10 minutes; then, for infants, maintenance dose of 25 to 30 units/kg/hour IV. For children older than age 1 year, maintenance dose is 18 to 20 units/kg/hour IV. Titrate dosage based on aPTT.

Reactions in bold italics are *life-threatening*. Interactions may have a *rapid onset* or a *delayed onset*.

➤ **Full-dose subcut therapy for DVT or PE**
Adults: Initially, 5,000 units IV bolus and 10,000 to 20,000 units in a concentrated solution subcut; then 8,000 to 10,000 units subcut every 8 hours or 15,000 to 20,000 units in a concentrated solution subcut every 12 hours.

➤ **Full-dose intermittent anticoagulation IV therapy for DVT or PE**
Adults: Initially, 10,000 units by IV bolus; then 5,000 to 10,000 units (or 50 to 70 units/kg) IV every 4 to 6 hours titrated according to aPTT.

➤ **Fixed low-dose therapy for prevention of venous thrombosis, PE, embolism associated with atrial fibrillation, and postoperative DVT**
Adults: 5,000 units subcut every 12 hours. In surgical patients, give first dose 2 hours before procedure; then 5,000 units subcut every 8 to 12 hours for 5 to 7 days or until patient can walk.

ADMINISTRATION
IV
▼ Establish baseline coagulation parameters before therapy.
▼ Use an infusion pump to provide maximum safety. Check continuous infusions regularly, even when pumps are in good working order, to ensure correct dosing. Place notice above patient's bed to caution IV team or lab personnel to apply pressure dressings after taking blood.
▼ During intermittent infusion, always draw blood 30 minutes before next scheduled dose to avoid falsely prolonged aPTT. Blood for aPTT may be drawn 4 hours after continuous IV heparin therapy starts. Never draw blood for aPTT from the tubing of the heparin infusion or from the infused vein, because falsely prolonged aPTT will result. Always draw blood from the opposite arm.
▼ Don't skip a dose or try to "catch up" with a solution containing heparin. If solution runs out, restart it as soon as possible, and reschedule bolus dose immediately. Monitor aPTT.
▼ Concentrated heparin solutions (more than 100 units/mL) can irritate blood vessels.

▼ Never piggyback other drugs into an infusion line while heparin infusion is running. Never mix another drug and heparin in same syringe when giving a bolus.
▼ **Incompatibilities:** Alteplase, amiodarone, caspofungin, ciprofloxacin, doxorubicin, doxycycline hyclate, droperidol, ergotamine, filgrastim, haloperidol, idarubicin, levofloxacin, methotrimeprazine, mitoxantrone, nesiritide, phenytoin sodium, reteplase. For additional information, consult detailed drug reference.
Subcutaneous
• Give low-dose injections sequentially between iliac crests in lower abdomen deep into subcutaneous fat. Inject drug subcut slowly into fat pad.
• Don't massage injection site; watch for signs of bleeding there.
• Alternate sites. Record location.

ACTION
Accelerates formation of antithrombin III–thrombin complex and deactivates thrombin, preventing conversion of fibrinogen to fibrin.

Route	Onset	Peak	Duration
IV	Immediate	Immediate	Variable
Subcut	20–30 min	2–4 hr	Variable

Half-life: 1 to 2 hours. Half-life is dose-dependent and nonlinear and may be disproportionately prolonged at higher doses.

ADVERSE REACTIONS
CNS: fever. **EENT:** rhinitis. **Hematologic:** *hemorrhage, overly prolonged clotting time, thrombocytopenia, white clot syndrome.* **Metabolic:** *hyperkalemia,* hypoaldosteronism. **Musculoskeletal:** osteoporosis. **Skin:** irritation, mild pain, hematoma, ulceration, cutaneous or subcutaneous necrosis, pruritus, urticaria, transient alopecia. **Other:** hypersensitivity reactions, including chills; *anaphylactoid reactions*.

INTERACTIONS
Drug-drug. *Antihistamines, nitrates:* May decrease heparin effect. Monitor coagulation tests.
Antiplatelet drugs, salicylates: May increase anticoagulant effect. Use together cautiously. Monitor coagulation studies and patient closely.

H

Nitroglycerin: May decrease effects of heparin. Monitor patient closely.

Oral anticoagulants: May increase additive anticoagulation. Monitor PT, INR, and PTT. Avoid combination.

Oritavancin, telavancin: May diminish therapeutic effect of heparin; may artificially increase results of laboratory tests commonly used to monitor IV heparin. Avoid combination.

Thrombolytics: May increase risk of hemorrhage. Monitor patient closely.

Drug-herb. *Alfalfa, angelica (dong quai), anise, bilberry, feverfew, garlic, ginger, ginkgo, ginseng, licorice, red clover, white willow:* May increase risk of bleeding. Discourage herb use.

Drug-lifestyle. *Smoking:* May interfere with anticoagulant effect of heparin. Discourage smoking.

EFFECTS ON LAB TEST RESULTS

• May increase ALT, AST, and potassium levels.

• May increase INR and prolong PT and aPTT. May decrease platelet count.

• Drug may cause false elevations in some tests for thyroxine level.

CONTRAINDICATIONS & CAUTIONS

• Contraindicated in patients hypersensitive to drug or pork products. Conditionally contraindicated in patients with active bleeding, blood dyscrasia, or bleeding tendencies, such as hemophilia, thrombocytopenia, history of heparin-induced thrombocytopenia (HIT), or hepatic disease with hypoprothrombinemia; suspected intracranial hemorrhage; suppurative thrombophlebitis; inaccessible ulcerative lesions (especially of GI tract) and open ulcerative wounds; extensive denudation of skin; ascorbic acid deficiency; and other conditions that cause increased capillary permeability.

• Conditionally contraindicated during or after brain, eye, or spinal cord surgery; during spinal tap or spinal anesthesia; during continuous tube drainage of stomach or small intestine; and in subacute bacterial endocarditis, shock, advanced renal disease, threatened abortion, or severe HTN.

• Use cautiously in women during menses or after childbirth and in patients with mild hepatic or renal disease, alcoholism, occupations with high risk of physical injury, or history of allergies, asthma, or GI ulcerations.

• May reduce bone mineral density with prolonged use (longer than 6 months).

• Use cautiously in women older than age 60 because of an increased risk of bleeding.

Dialyzable drug: Unknown.

⚠ *Overdose S&S:* Bleeding, nosebleeds, hematuria, tarry stools, easy bruising, petechial formations.

PREGNANCY-LACTATION-REPRODUCTION

• Drug doesn't cross placental barrier. Use during pregnancy only if potential benefit justifies potential risk to the fetus.

• Use cautiously in breastfeeding women.

• Use preservative-free formulations (without benzyl alcohol) in pregnant and breastfeeding women and neonates.

NURSING CONSIDERATIONS

• Although heparin use is clearly hazardous in certain conditions, its risks and benefits must be evaluated.

🔔 *Alert:* Some commercially available heparin injections contain benzyl alcohol.

• Drug requirements are higher in early phases of thrombogenic diseases and febrile states; they are lower when patient's condition stabilizes.

• Elderly patients should usually start at lower dosage.

• Monitor patients for hyperkalemia during therapy.

🔔 *Alert:* Check order and vial carefully; heparin comes in various concentrations. It's now required that the label clearly state the strength of the entire container followed by how much medication is in 1 mL.

🔔 *Alert:* USP and international units aren't equivalent for heparin.

🔔 *Alert:* Heparin, low-molecular-weight heparins, and danaparoid aren't interchangeable.

🔔 *Alert:* Don't change concentrations of infusions unless absolutely necessary. This is a common source of dosage errors.

🔔 *Alert:* There is the potential for delayed onset of HIT, a serious antibody-mediated reaction resulting from irreversible aggregation of platelets. HIT may progress to the development of venous and arterial thromboses, a condition referred to as

---

heparin-induced thrombocytopenia and thrombosis (HITT). Thrombotic events may be the initial presentation for HITT, which can occur up to several weeks after stopping heparin therapy. Evaluate patients presenting with thrombocytopenia or thrombosis after stopping heparin for HIT and HITT.

• Draw blood for aPTT 4 to 6 hours after subcut dose.

• Avoid IM injections of other drugs to prevent or minimize hematoma.

• Measure aPTT carefully and regularly. Anticoagulation is present when aPTT values are 1½ to 2 × the control values.

• Monitor platelet count regularly. When new thrombosis accompanies thrombocytopenia (white clot syndrome), stop heparin.

• Regularly inspect patient for bleeding gums, bruises on arms or legs, petechiae, nosebleeds, melena, tarry stools, hematuria, and hematemesis.

• Monitor vital signs.

🖐 **Alert:** To treat severe overdose, use protamine sulfate (1% solution), a heparin antagonist. Dosage is based on the dose of heparin, its route of administration, and the time since it was given. Generally, 1 mg of protamine neutralizes 100 USP units of heparin. Don't give more than 50 mg protamine in a 10-minute period. Protamine can cause severe hypotension and anaphylactoid reactions. Ensure emergency treatment is available.

• Abrupt withdrawal may cause increased coagulability; warfarin therapy usually overlaps heparin therapy for continuation of prophylaxis or treatment.

• **Look alike–sound alike:** Don't confuse heparin with Hespan.

PATIENT TEACHING
• Instruct patient and family to report all adverse reactions.

• Advise patient and family to watch for signs and symptoms of bleeding or bruising and to notify prescriber immediately if any occur.

• Tell patient to avoid OTC drugs containing aspirin, other salicylates, or drugs that may interact with heparin unless ordered by prescriber.

• Advise patient to consult prescriber before starting herbal therapy; many herbs have

anticoagulant, antiplatelet, or fibrinolytic properties.

hydrALAZINE hydrochloride
hye-DRAL-a-zeen

Apresoline ❦

Therapeutic class: Antihypertensives
Pharmacologic class: Peripheral dilators

AVAILABLE FORMS
Injection: 20 mg/mL in 1-mL vial
Tablets: 10 mg, 25 mg, 50 mg, 100 mg

INDICATIONS & DOSAGES
➤ **Essential HTN**
Adults: Initially, 10 mg PO q.i.d. for the first 2 to 4 days, 25 mg q.i.d. for the balance of the first week; 50 mg q.i.d. from the second week on, based on patient tolerance and response.
Children age 1 and older: Initially, 0.75 mg/kg daily PO divided into four doses; gradually increase over 3 to 4 weeks to maximum of 7.5 mg/kg/day in four divided doses or 200 mg/day.
➤ **Severe essential HTN**
Adults: 20 to 40 mg IM or IV; repeat as needed. Switch to oral form as soon as possible.
Children: 1.7 to 3.5 mg/kg/day IM or IV divided into four to six doses.
➤ **HF with reduced ejection fraction ♦**
Adults: Initially, 25 to 50 mg PO t.i.d. or q.i.d. in combination with isosorbide dinitrate. Maximum dose is 300 mg daily in divided doses.

ADMINISTRATION
PO
• Give drug with food to increase absorption.
IV
▼ Give drug as a rapid bolus injection directly into the vein only when the drug can't be given orally. Repeat p.r.n., generally every 4 to 6 hours. It shouldn't be added to infusion solutions.
▼ Drug may discolor upon contact with metal; discolored solutions should be discarded. Use immediately after the vial is opened.

▼ **Incompatibilities:** Aminophylline, ampicillin sodium, chlorothiazide, D₅W, dextrose 10% in lactated Ringer solution, dextrose 10% in NSS, diazoxide, edetate calcium disodium, ethacrynate, fructose 10% in NSS, fructose 10% in water, furosemide, mephentermine, methohexital, nitroglycerin, phenobarbital sodium, verapamil.

IM
• Administer undiluted as IM injection.

ACTION
Not fully understood. A direct-acting peripheral vasodilator that relaxes arteriolar smooth muscle.

Route	Onset	Peak	Duration
PO	Unknown	1–2 hr	Unknown
IV, IM	10–80 min	Unknown	Up to 12 hr

Half-life: 3 to 7 hours.

ADVERSE REACTIONS
CNS: headache, dizziness, peripheral neuritis. **CV:** angina pectoris, palpitations, tachycardia, orthostatic hypotension, edema, flushing. **EENT:** conjunctivitis, nasal congestion. **GI:** nausea, vomiting, diarrhea, anorexia, constipation, paralytic ileus. **GU:** difficult urination. **Hematologic:** *neutropenia, leukopenia, agranulocytosis,* eosinophilia, *thrombocytopenia with or without purpura.* **Musculoskeletal:** muscle cramps, arthralgia. **Respiratory:** dyspnea. **Skin:** rash. **Other:** hypersensitivity reactions, chills.

INTERACTIONS
Drug-drug. *Diazoxide, MAO inhibitors:* May cause severe hypotension. Use together cautiously.
Diuretics, other hypotensive drugs: May cause excessive hypotension. Dosage adjustment may be needed.
NSAIDs: May decrease effects of hydralazine. Monitor BP.
Drug-food. *Any food:* Food may increase drug absorption. Encourage patient to take with food.

EFFECTS ON LAB TEST RESULTS
• May decrease Hb level.

• May decrease neutrophil, WBC, granulocyte, platelet, and RBC counts.
• May cause positive ANA titers.

CONTRAINDICATIONS & CAUTIONS
• Contraindicated in patients hypersensitive to drug.
• Drug may contain tartrazine and cause allergic reactions, especially in patients hypersensitive to aspirin.
• Contraindicated in those with CAD or mitral valvular rheumatic heart disease.
• Use cautiously in patients with suspected cardiac disease, stroke, or severe renal impairment and in those taking other antihypertensives.
• May cause blood dyscrasias. Discontinue drug if they occur.
Dialyzable drug: Unknown.
⚠ *Overdose S&S:* Hypotension, tachycardia, headache, flushing.

PREGNANCY-LACTATION-REPRODUCTION
• Drug crosses the placental barrier and is associated with fetal toxicity in the third trimester. Use during pregnancy only if expected benefit justifies potential risk to the fetus.
• Use cautiously in breastfeeding women.

NURSING CONSIDERATIONS
• Monitor patient's BP, pulse rate, and body weight frequently. Drug may be given with diuretics and beta blockers to decrease sodium retention and tachycardia and to prevent angina attacks.
• Elderly patients may be more sensitive to drug's hypotensive effects.
• Obtain CBC, lupus erythematosus cell preparation, and ANA titer determination before therapy and periodically during long-term therapy.
🔆 *Alert:* Monitor patient closely for signs and symptoms of lupuslike syndrome (sore throat, fever, muscle and joint aches, rash), and notify prescriber immediately if they develop. Long-term steroid therapy may be necessary.
• *Look alike–sound alike:* Don't confuse hydralazine with hydroxyzine.

Reactions in bold italics are *life-threatening*. Interactions may have a *rapid onset* or a *delayed onset*.

PATIENT TEACHING
• Instruct patient to take oral form with meals to increase absorption.
• Inform patient that low BP and dizziness upon standing can be minimized by rising slowly and avoiding sudden position changes.
• Tell patient to report all adverse reactions, including unexplained prolonged general tiredness or fever, muscle or joint aching, or chest pain.
• Tell female patient of childbearing potential to notify prescriber if she suspects pregnancy.

---

hydroCHLOROthiazide
hye-droe-klor-oh-THYE-a-zide

Microzide

Therapeutic class: Diuretics
Pharmacologic class: Thiazide diuretics

AVAILABLE FORMS
Capsules: 12.5 mg
Tablets: 12.5 mg, 25 mg, 50 mg

INDICATIONS & DOSAGES
Adjust-a-dose (for all indications): In patients older than age 65, 12.5 mg daily initially. Adjust in increments of 12.5 mg, if needed.
➤ **Edema**
Adults: 25 to 100 mg PO daily in one to two divided doses.
Children ages 6 months to 12 years: Initially, 1 to 2 mg/kg/day PO in a single dose or two divided doses. May increase to a maximum of 37.5 mg/day for children ages 6 months to 2 years and 100 mg/day for children ages 2 to 12 years.
Children younger than age 6 months: May give up to 3 mg/kg/day PO in two divided doses. Maximum dose, 37.5 mg/day.
➤ **HTN**
Adults: 12.5 to 50 mg PO daily in one to two divided doses. Increase or decrease daily dose based on BP.
Children ages 6 months to 12 years: Initially, 1 to 2 mg/kg/day PO in a single dose or two divided doses. May increase to a maximum of 37.5 mg/day for children ages 6 months to 2 years and 100 mg/day for children ages 2 to 12 years.

Children younger than age 6 months: May give up to 3 mg/kg/day PO in two divided doses. Maximum dose 37.5 mg/day.

ADMINISTRATION
PO
• Give with or without food.
• To prevent nocturia, give drug in morning. If second dose is needed, give in early afternoon, preferably not later than 6 p.m.
• Capsules aren't indicated for use in children.

ACTION
Increases sodium and water excretion by inhibiting sodium and chloride reabsorption in distal segment of the nephron.

Route	Onset	Peak	Duration
PO	2–6 hr	1–5 hr	6–12 hr

Half-life: About 6 to 15 hours.

ADVERSE REACTIONS
CNS: dizziness, vertigo, headache, paresthesia, weakness, restlessness. **CV:** hypotension, vasculitis. **GI:** *pancreatitis,* anorexia, nausea, epigastric distress, vomiting, abdominal pain, diarrhea, constipation. **GU:** *renal failure,* polyuria, frequent urination, interstitial nephritis, erectile dysfunction. **Hematologic:** *aplastic anemia, agranulocytosis, leukopenia, thrombocytopenia,* hemolytic anemia. **Hepatic:** jaundice. **Metabolic:** asymptomatic hyperuricemia; *hypokalemia*; hyperglycemia and impaired glucose tolerance; fluid and electrolyte imbalances, including dilutional hyponatremia and hypochloremia; metabolic alkalosis; hypercalcemia; volume depletion and dehydration. **Musculoskeletal:** muscle cramps. **Respiratory:** *respiratory distress,* pneumonitis. **Skin:** dermatitis, photosensitivity reactions, rash, purpura, alopecia, *erythema multiforme,* exfoliative dermatitis. **Other:** *anaphylactic reactions,* hypersensitivity reactions, gout.

INTERACTIONS
Drug-drug. *Allopurinol:* May increase allopurinol serum concentration and enhance potential for allergic or hypersensitivity reactions to allopurinol. Monitor allopurinol level.

Amphotericin B, corticosteroids, topiramate: May increase risk of hypokalemia. Monitor potassium level closely.

Antidiabetics: May decrease hypoglycemic effects. Adjust dosage if needed. Monitor glucose level.

Antihypertensives: May have additive antihypertensive effect. Use together cautiously.

Barbiturates, opioids: May increase orthostatic hypotensive effect. Monitor patient closely.

Bumetanide, ethacrynic acid, furosemide, torsemide: May cause excessive diuretic response, causing serious electrolyte abnormalities or dehydration. Adjust doses carefully, and monitor patient closely for signs and symptoms of excessive diuretic response.

Cardiac glycosides: May increase risk of digoxin toxicity from diuretic-induced hypokalemia. Monitor potassium and digoxin levels.

Cholestyramine, colestipol: May decrease intestinal absorption of thiazides. Separate doses by 2 hours.

Diazoxide: May increase antihypertensive, hyperglycemic, and hyperuricemic effects. Use together cautiously.

Lithium: May decrease lithium excretion, increasing risk of lithium toxicity. Consider therapy modification.

Multivitamins/minerals (with ADEK, folate, iron): May enhance hypercalcemic effect of these multivitamins/minerals. Monitor patient closely.

NSAIDs: May increase risk of renal failure. May decrease diuretic and antihypertensive effects. Monitor renal function and BP.

Drug-herb. *Licorice:* May cause unexpected rapid potassium loss. Discourage use together.

Drug-lifestyle. *Alcohol use:* May increase orthostatic hypotensive effect. Discourage use together.

EFFECTS ON LAB TEST RESULTS
• May increase glucose, cholesterol, triglyceride, calcium, and uric acid levels.
• May decrease potassium, sodium, chloride, serum protein-bound iodine, and Hb levels.
• May decrease granulocyte, WBC, and platelet counts.

CONTRAINDICATIONS & CAUTIONS
• Contraindicated in patients with anuria and patients hypersensitive to other thiazides or other sulfonamide derivatives.
• Drug can cause systemic lupus activation or exacerbation.
• Use cautiously in children and in patients with severe renal disease, gout, diabetes, hypercholesterolemia, impaired hepatic function, or progressive hepatic disease.

Dialyzable drug: Unknown.

⚠ *Overdose S&S:* Electrolyte imbalance, dehydration.

PREGNANCY-LACTATION-REPRODUCTION
• Drug crosses the placental barrier; maternal use may adversely affect fetus.
• Women using thiazide diuretics for treatment of HTN before pregnancy may continue their use.
• Patient should discontinue breastfeeding or discontinue drug.

NURSING CONSIDERATIONS
• Monitor fluid intake and output, weight, BP, and electrolyte levels; correct electrolyte disturbances before start of therapy.
• Watch for signs and symptoms of hypokalemia, such as muscle weakness and cramps.
• Drug may be used with potassium-sparing diuretic to prevent potassium loss.
• Consult prescriber and dietitian about a high-potassium diet or potassium supplement.
• Monitor creatinine and BUN levels regularly. Cumulative effects of drug may occur with impaired renal function.
• Monitor uric acid level, especially in patients with history of gout.
• Monitor glucose level, especially in diabetic patients.
• Monitor elderly patients, who are especially susceptible to excessive diuresis.
• Stop thiazides and thiazide-like diuretics before parathyroid function tests.
• In patients with HTN, therapeutic response may be delayed several weeks.

PATIENT TEACHING
• Instruct patient to take drug with food to minimize GI upset.

Reactions in bold italics are *life-threatening*. Interactions may have a *rapid onset* or a *delayed onset*.

- Advise patient to take drug in morning to avoid need to urinate at night; if patient needs second dose, tell patient to take it in early afternoon before 6 p.m.
- Advise patient to report all adverse reactions and to avoid sudden posture changes and to rise slowly to avoid dizziness upon standing quickly.
- Encourage sunblock use to prevent photosensitivity reactions.
- Tell patient to check with prescriber or pharmacist before using OTC drugs.
- Advise female patient to tell prescriber if she is pregnant or plans to become pregnant or is breastfeeding or plans to breastfeed.

SAFETY ALERT!

HYDROcodone bitartrate
hye-droe-KOE-done

Hysingla ER, Zohydro ER

Therapeutic class: Opioid analgesics
Pharmacologic class: Opioid analgesics
Controlled substance schedule: II

AVAILABLE FORMS
Capsules (extended-release) ⓓ: 10 mg, 15 mg, 20 mg, 30 mg, 40 mg, 50 mg

INDICATIONS & DOSAGES
➤ **Management of pain severe enough to require daily, around-the-clock, long-term opioid treatment and for which alternative treatment options are inadequate**
Adults who are opioid naive or who aren't opioid tolerant: Initially, 10 mg (Zohydro ER) PO every 12 hours. Gradually adjust dosage, preferably in increments of 10 mg every 12 hours every 3 to 7 days, until adequate pain relief and acceptable adverse reactions have been achieved.

Or, 20 mg (Hysingla ER) PO once daily. Increase dosage in increments of 10 to 20 mg once daily every 3 to 5 days as needed to achieve adequate analgesia. Patients who experience breakthrough pain may require a dosage increase or may need a rescue medication.
Adults who are opioid tolerant: Discontinue all other around-the-clock opioids before initiating therapy. Refer to manufacturer's instructions when converting from other oral opioids to Zohydro ER, Hysingla ER, doses aren't equianalgesic.
Adjust-a-dose: In patients with moderate renal impairment to ESRD, start with 50% of the Hysingla ER or initial dose or with low Zohydro ER dose, and monitor closely.

For severe hepatic impairment, start with 10 mg (Zohydro ER) PO every 12 hours or use 50% of initial dose of Hysingla ER. No dosage adjustments are recommended for Hysingla ER or Zohydro ER in patients with mild to moderate hepatic impairment.

Monitor patients closely for adverse events such as respiratory depression. Decrease initial dose in elderly patients, who may be more sensitive to adverse effects.

ADMINISTRATION
PO
Black Box Warning Give capsules whole. Don't crush, dissolve, or allow patient to chew capsules because of the risk of rapid release and absorption of a potentially fatal dose of hydrocodone. ∎
- Administer capsules one at a time with enough water to ensure complete swallowing immediately after placing in the mouth.
- Store at room temperature.

ACTION
Acts as a full agonist primarily at the mu opioid receptor, binding to and activating opioid receptors at various sites in the CNS to produce analgesia.

Route	Onset	Peak	Duration
PO (Hysingla ER)	Unknown	6–30 hr	Unknown
PO (Zohydro ER)	Unknown	5 hr	Unknown

Half-life: Hysingla ER, 7 to 9 hours; Zohydro ER, about 8 hours.

ADVERSE REACTIONS
CNS: somnolence, tremor, lethargy, anxiety, depression, insomnia, fatigue, dizziness, drowsiness, headache or migraine, pain, paresthesia, sedation. **CV:** peripheral edema, hot flashes, HTN. **EENT:** tinnitus, nasopharyngitis, nasal congestion, oropharyngeal pain, sinusitis, dry mouth. **GI:** constipation, nausea, vomiting, abdominal pain, GERD, decreased appetite, diarrhea, dyspepsia, viral gastroenteritis. **GU:** UTI.

Metabolic: dehydration, *hypokalemia.*
Musculoskeletal: muscle spasms, back pain, foot fracture, joint injury, joint sprain, muscle strain, arthralgia, musculoskeletal pain, myalgia, neck pain, extremity pain, noncardiac chest pain, osteoarthritis. **Respiratory:** URI, bronchitis, cough, dyspnea. **Skin:** pruritus, skin laceration, hyperhidrosis, night sweats, rash. **Other:** fall, flulike syndrome, chills.

INTERACTIONS

Drug-drug. *Anticholinergics:* May increase risk of urine retention, severe constipation, or paralytic ileus. Monitor patient for signs and symptoms of urine retention and constipation in addition to respiratory and CNS depression. Use together cautiously.

Black Box Warning *Benzodiazepines, CNS depressants:* May cause slow or difficult breathing, sedation, and death. Avoid use together. If use together is necessary, limit dosage and duration of each drug to the minimum necessary for desired effect. ∎

Black Box Warning *CYP3A4 inhibitors (amiodarone, erythromycin, ketoconazole, nefazodone, protease inhibitors, ritonavir, telithromycin):* May increase hydrocodone plasma concentration and prolong opioid effects, especially if use of CYP3A4 inhibitors is concomitant. Monitor patient for respiratory depression and sedation; consider dosage adjustments until drug effects are stable. ∎

Black Box Warning *CYP3A4 inducers (carbamazepine, phenytoin, rifampin):* May induce metabolism and decrease hydrocodone plasma concentration, decreasing efficacy and potentially causing withdrawal symptoms. Monitor patient for effectiveness of drug and for opioid withdrawal symptoms. Consider dosage adjustments until stable. If CYP3A4 inducer is stopped, monitor patient for increased therapeutic and adverse effects, especially respiratory depression. ∎

MAO inhibitors: May potentiate effects of opioid analgesics. Don't use in patients who have received MAO inhibitors within past 14 days.

Mixed agonist/antagonists (butorphanol, nalbuphine, pentazocine), partial agonists (buprenorphine): May reduce analgesic effect of hydrocodone or precipitate withdrawal symptoms. Avoid concurrent use.

⊘ *Alert: Serotonergic drugs (amoxapine, antimigraine drugs, buspirone, cyclobenzaprine, dextromethorphan, linezolid, lithium, MAO inhibitors, maprotiline, methylene blue, mirtazapine, nefazodone, SSNRIs, SSRIs, TCAs, trazodone, tryptophan, vilazodone):* May increase risk of serotonin syndrome; may enhance toxic effect of hydrocodone. Use together cautiously. Monitor patient for serotonin syndrome.

Drug-herb. ⊘ *Alert: St. John's wort:* May decrease hydrocodone serum concentration. Use together cautiously.

Drug-lifestyle. **Black Box Warning** *Alcohol use:* May increase hydrocodone plasma level and risk of fatal overdose. Patients shouldn't consume alcoholic beverages or use other drugs that contain alcohol. ∎

EFFECTS ON LAB TEST RESULTS

• May increase cholesterol and GGT levels.
• May decrease potassium level.

CONTRAINDICATIONS & CAUTIONS

Black Box Warning Drug exposes patient to risks of addiction, abuse, and misuse even at recommended doses, which can lead to overdose and death. Assess each patient's risk before prescribing, and monitor patients for these behaviors or conditions. ∎

Black Box Warning Accidental ingestion of even one dose of this drug, especially by children, can result in a fatal overdose of hydrocodone. ∎

Black Box Warning Opioids should only be prescribed with benzodiazepines or other CNS depressants to patients for whom alternative treatment options are inadequate. Limit dosages and durations to minimum required. ∎

Black Box Warning The FDA has required a REMS program for this drug. Drug companies with approved opioid analgesic products must make a REMS-compliant education program available to health care providers, who are strongly encouraged to complete the education program; discuss the safe use, serious risks, and proper storage and disposal of opioid analgesics with patients and their caregivers every time these medicines are prescribed; emphasize the

---

Reactions in bold italics are *life-threatening.* Interactions may have a *rapid onset* or a *delayed onset.*

importance of reading the Medication Guide every time an opioid analgesic is dispensed to them; and consider using other tools to improve patient, household, and community safety. Obtain additional information at www.opioidanalgesicrems.com or by calling 1-800-503-0784. ■

❸ **Alert:** Drug should only be prescribed by health care professionals knowledgeable in the use of potent opioids for pain management. Drug should only be used when alternative treatment options are ineffective, not tolerated, or otherwise inadequate to provide sufficient pain management.

❸ **Alert:** Drug may lead to rare but serious decrease in adrenal gland cortisol production.

❸ **Alert:** Drug may reduce sex hormone levels with long-term use.

• Contraindicated for use as an as-needed analgesic. Drug should be prescribed in the smallest appropriate quantity.

• Use cautiously in patients with hypersensitivity to morphine, oxycodone, and codeine because cross-reactivity may occur.

• Contraindicated in patients with significant respiratory depression, acute or severe bronchial asthma, known or suspected paralytic ileus, or hypersensitivity to drug or its components.

• Use cautiously in cachectic or debilitated patients; there is potential for crucial respiratory depression even at therapeutic dosages.

• Use cautiously in patients with a history of seizures and adrenal insufficiency.

❸ **Alert:** When giving first dose, it's preferable to underestimate patient's 24-hour oral hydrocodone requirements and provide rescue medication (immediate-release opioid) than to overestimate the 24-hour oral hydrocodone requirements, which could result in adverse reactions.

• Use cautiously in elderly patients and in those with chronic pulmonary disease, seizure disorder, hypotension or depleted blood volume, or hepatic or renal impairment.

❸ **Alert:** Avoid use in patients with head injuries, increased ICP, brain tumors, impaired consciousness, or coma. Drug reduces respiratory drive, increasing carbon dioxide retention and ICP.

• QTc interval may be prolonged when doses greater than 160 mg daily are used.

Use cautiously in patients with HF, bradyarrhythmias, or electrolyte abnormalities, and when patients are using other drugs known to prolong the QTc interval. Don't use in those with congenital long QT syndrome. If QTc-interval prolongation occurs, consider dosage reduction of 33% to 50% or change to another analgesic.

• Esophageal obstruction, dysphagia, and choking have occurred with Hysingla ER use. Patients with underlying GI disorders or with a small GI lumen are at greater risk. Consider another analgesic in these patients.

• Safety and effectiveness in children younger than age 18 haven't been established.

Dialyzable drug: Unknown.

⚠ **Overdose S&S:** Respiratory depression, somnolence (can lead to stupor or coma), skeletal muscle flaccidity, cold clammy skin, constricted pupils (although mydriasis rather than miosis may occur due to severe hypoxia in overdose situations), pulmonary edema, bradycardia, hypotension, death.

PREGNANCY-LACTATION-REPRODUCTION

• Use in pregnant women only if benefit outweighs risk to the fetus.

Black Box Warning Prolonged use during pregnancy can result in neonatal opioid withdrawal syndrome, which may be life-threatening if not recognized and treated according to protocols developed by neonatology experts. ■

Black Box Warning If opioid use is required for a prolonged period during pregnancy, advise patient of risk of neonatal opioid withdrawal syndrome (poor feeding, diarrhea, irritability, tremor, rigidity, seizures) and assure her that appropriate treatment will be available. ■

• Don't use during labor and delivery; neonatal respiratory depression may occur.

• Opioids may appear in human milk. Patient should discontinue breastfeeding or discontinue drug.

• Monitor infants exposed to drug through human milk for excess sedation and respiratory depression. Also watch for withdrawal symptoms in breastfeeding infants when maternal administration of an opioid analgesic is stopped, or when breastfeeding is stopped.

NURSING CONSIDERATIONS

• Drug may be targeted for theft, diversion, and misuse.

Black Box Warning Monitor patients for respiratory depression, especially within first 24 to 72 hours of drug initiation or after dosage increase. Serious, life-threatening, or fatal respiratory depression may occur. ■

Black Box Warning Monitor patients for abuse or misuse of drug, especially those with a personal or family history of substance abuse (drug or alcohol addiction or abuse, mental illness). Counsel patients about risks and proper use of drug. ■

◑ **Alert:** If patient is taking opioids with serotonergic drugs, watch for signs and symptoms of serotonin syndrome (agitation, hallucinations, rapid HR, fever, excessive sweating, shivering or shaking, muscle twitching or stiffness, trouble with coordination, nausea, vomiting, diarrhea), especially when starting treatment or increasing dosages. Signs and symptoms may occur within several hours of coadministration but may also occur later, especially after dosage increase. Discontinue the opioid, serotonergic drug, or both if serotonin syndrome is suspected.

◑ **Alert:** Monitor patient for signs and symptoms of adrenal insufficiency (nausea, vomiting, loss of appetite, fatigue, weakness, dizziness, low BP). Perform diagnostic testing if adrenal insufficiency is suspected. If adrenal insufficiency is confirmed, treat with corticosteroids and wean patient off opioids if appropriate. Discontinue corticosteroids when clinically appropriate.

◑ **Alert:** Monitor patient for signs and symptoms of decreased sex hormone levels (low libido, erectile dysfunction, amenorrhea, infertility). If signs and symptoms occur, evaluate patient and obtain laboratory testing.

◑ **Alert:** Don't stop drug abruptly; withdraw slowly and individualize the gradual tapering plan to prevent signs and symptoms of withdrawal, worsening pain, and psychological distress in physically dependent patients. Refer to manufacturer's label for specific tapering instructions.

◑ **Alert:** When tapering opioids, monitor patients closely for signs and symptoms of opioid withdrawal (restlessness, lacrimation, rhinorrhea, yawning, perspiration, chills, myalgia, mydriasis, irritability, anxiety, insomnia, backache, joint pain, weakness, abdominal cramps, anorexia, nausea, vomiting, diarrhea, increased BP or HR, increased respiratory rate). Such signs and symptoms may indicate a need to taper more slowly. Also monitor patients for suicidal thoughts, use of other substances, and mood changes.

• Patients considered opioid tolerant are those receiving, for 1 week or longer, at least 60 mg morphine per day, 25 mcg/hour transdermal fentanyl, 30 mg oral oxycodone per day, 8 mg oral hydromorphone per day or more, 25 mg oral oxymorphone per day or more, 60 mg oral hydrocodone, or an equianalgesic dose of another opioid.

• Closely monitor patients converting from methadone because methadone has a long half-life and can accumulate in plasma, resulting in significant respiratory depression.

• Closely monitor patients converting from fentanyl patches because of risk of additive effects.

• Elderly patients receiving drug may become confused and oversedated, especially those with impaired hepatic or renal function. Start with low doses of hydrocodone and observe closely for adverse events such as respiratory depression.

• Watch for decreased bowel motility in postoperative patients and for biliary spasm in patients with biliary tract disease or acute pancreatitis.

• Monitor patients with history of seizure disorder for worsening seizure control.

• Use lowest initial dose in patients with renal or hepatic impairment, and monitor patients closely for adverse events such as respiratory depression.

• Periodically reevaluate patient's need for therapy.

• **Look alike–sound alike:** Don't confuse hydrocodone ER with hydrocodone standard release. Don't confuse hydrocodone with oxycodone, oxymorphone, or hydromorphone.

PATIENT TEACHING

Black Box Warning Caution patient or caregiver of patient taking an opioid with a benzodiazepine, CNS depressant, or alcohol to seek immediate medical attention for dizziness, light-headedness, extreme

---

Reactions in bold italics are *life-threatening*. Interactions may have a *rapid onset* or a *delayed onset*.

sleepiness, slowed or difficult breathing, or unresponsiveness. ∎

Black Box Warning Instruct patient to avoid alcoholic beverages, prescription drugs, and OTC products that contain alcohol during treatment. ∎

Black Box Warning Instruct patient to swallow drug whole to avoid exposure to a potentially fatal dose of hydrocodone. Crushing, chewing, snorting, or injecting the dissolved product allows uncontrolled delivery of drug and may result in overdose and death. ∎

Black Box Warning Inform female patient that prolonged use of drug during pregnancy can result in neonatal opioid withdrawal syndrome, which may be life-threatening. ∎

⟳ *Alert:* Encourage patient to report all medications being taken, including prescription and OTC medications and supplements.

⟳ *Alert:* Caution patient to immediately report signs and symptoms of serotonin syndrome, adrenal insufficiency, and decreased sex hormone levels.

⟳ *Alert:* Counsel patient not to discontinue opioids without first discussing the need for a gradual tapering regimen with prescriber.

• Caution patient not to share drug and to protect it from theft or misuse.

• Inform patient that potentially serious additive effects may occur if drug is used with other CNS depressants and to avoid such drugs unless supervised by a health care provider.

• Advise patient to report signs and symptoms of respiratory depression (respiratory rate less than 12 breaths/minute, shortness of breath, confusion, excessive drowsiness, nausea, vomiting) and to seek immediate medical attention. Risk of respiratory depression is greatest at drug initiation and dosage increases.

• Warn patient that use of drug, even when taken as recommended, can result in addiction, abuse, and misuse, which can lead to overdose or death.

• Caution patient not to drive or operate dangerous machinery until drug's effects are known.

• Warn patient about potential for severe constipation; teach management instructions and when to seek medical attention.

• Inform patient that drug may cause orthostatic hypotension and fainting. Teach how to recognize signs and symptoms of low BP and how to reduce risk of serious consequences of hypotension (e.g., sit or lie down, carefully rise from a sitting or lying position).

• Caution patient to seek medical attention immediately if hypersensitivity reactions, including anaphylaxis, occur.

Black Box Warning Instruct patient to store drug securely and away from children, to dispose of drug properly when no longer needed, and not to throw in regular trash. Accidental ingestion, especially by children, may result in respiratory depression or death. ∎

• Inform patient to dispose of unused capsules through a drug take-back program. If such a program isn't available in patient's area, instruct patient to flush unused capsules down the toilet.

SAFETY ALERT!

HYDROcodone bitartrate–acetaminophen

hye-droe-KOE-done/a-seet-a-MIN-oh-fen

Norco

Therapeutic class: Opioid analgesics
Pharmacologic class: Opioid analgesics–para-aminophenol derivatives
Controlled substance schedule: II

AVAILABLE FORMS

Oral solution*: 7.5 mg hydrocodone/325 mg acetaminophen per 15 mL, 10 mg hydrocodone/300 mg acetaminophen per 15 mL
Tablets: 2.5 mg hydrocodone/325 mg acetaminophen, 5 mg hydrocodone/300 mg acetaminophen, 5 mg hydrocodone/325 mg acetaminophen, 7.5 mg hydrocodone/300 mg acetaminophen, 7.5 mg hydrocodone/325 mg acetaminophen, 10 mg hydrocodone/300 mg acetaminophen, 10 mg hydrocodone/325 mg acetaminophen

INDICATIONS & DOSAGES

➤ **Moderate to moderately severe pain**
Adults: Give 1 to 2 tablets (hydrocodone 2.5 to 5 mg/acetaminophen 300 to 325 mg)

PO every 4 to 6 hours or 1 tablet (hydrocodone 7.5 to 10 mg/acetaminophen 300 to 325 mg) PO every 4 to 6 hours. Or, for oral solution, give 15 mL (hydrocodone 7.5 mg/acetaminophen 325 mg) or 11.25 mL (hydrocodone 10 mg/acetaminophen 300 mg) PO every 4 to 6 hours as needed. Refer to manufacturer's instructions for maximum dosages.

Children age 2 and older (solution only):
Refer to manufacturer's instructions for specific weight- and age-based dosing. For hydrocodone 7.5 mg/acetaminophen 325 mg, give 0.27 mL/kg PO every 4 to 6 hours as needed. Or, for hydrocodone 10 mg/acetaminophen 300 mg, give 0.20 mL/kg PO every 4 to 6 hours as needed. Refer to manufacturer's instructions for maximum dosages.

Adjust-a-dose: Adjust dosage according to severity of pain and patient response. Use a low initial dose in elderly patients and in patients with hepatic or renal impairment; monitor closely for adverse events, such as respiratory depression and sedation. Total acetaminophen intake shouldn't exceed 4,000 mg/day in adults and in children age 14 and older.

ADMINISTRATION
PO
• Give drug with food or milk.
🔴 *Alert:* Ensure accuracy when prescribing, dispensing, and administering oral solution. Dosing errors due to confusion between mg and mL, and among other hydrocodone bitartrate–acetaminophen oral solutions of different concentrations, can result in accidental overdose and death.
• Administer oral solution by a calibrated device such as syringe or dropper.
• Only oral solution is approved for pediatric use.

ACTION
Inhibits synthesis of prostaglandins and binds to opiate receptors in CNS and peripherally blocks pain impulse generation; produces antipyresis by direct action on hypothalamic heat-regulating center; causes cough suppression by direct central action in medulla; may produce generalized CNS depression.

Route	Onset	Peak	Duration
PO (hydrocodone)	10–20 min	1–1.6 hr	4–8 hr
PO (acetaminophen)	Unknown	½–1 hr	4–6 hr

Half-life: Hydrocodone, 3.3 to 4.4 hours; acetaminophen, 2 to 3 hours.

ADVERSE REACTIONS
CNS: light-headedness, dizziness, sedation, drowsiness, mental clouding, lethargy, impairment of mental and physical performance, anxiety, fear, dysphoria, psychological dependence, mood changes, *stupor, coma.* **CV:** *bradycardia, cardiac arrest, circulatory collapse,* hypotension. **EENT:** hearing impairment, permanent hearing loss. **GI:** nausea, vomiting, constipation, abdominal pain, gastric distress, heartburn, peptic ulcer. **GU:** urethral spasms, spasm of vesical sphincters, urine retention, *renal tubular necrosis,* renal toxicity. **Hematologic:** *thrombocytopenia, agranulocytosis,* occult blood loss, hemolytic anemia, iron deficiency anemia, prolonged bleeding time. **Hepatic:** *hepatic necrosis, hepatitis,* increased LFT values. **Metabolic:** *hypoglycemia, hypoglycemic coma.* **Musculoskeletal:** muscle flaccidity. **Respiratory:** *respiratory depression, acute airway obstruction,* apnea, dyspnea. **Skin:** rash, pruritus, cold clammy skin, diaphoresis. **Other:** allergic reaction.

INTERACTIONS
Drug-drug. *Anticholinergics:* May increase risk of urine retention, severe constipation, or paralytic ileus. Avoid use together.
Black Box Warning *Antidepressants, antipsychotics, anxiolytics, barbiturates, benzodiazepines or other CNS depressants, other opioids:* May cause slow or difficult breathing, sedation, and death. Avoid use together. If use together is necessary, limit dosage and duration of each drug to minimum necessary for desired effect. ▮
Barbiturates, metyrapone, mipomersen: May increase risk of hepatotoxicity from acetaminophen. Monitor therapy.
Carbamazepine, dasatinib, hydantoins, isoniazid: May increase risk of hepatotoxicity from acetaminophen. Use cautiously together. Consider alternative therapy.

Reactions in bold italics are *life-threatening*. Interactions may have a *rapid onset* or a *delayed onset*.

Black Box Warning *CYP3A4 inhibitors (amiodarone, erythromycin, ketoconazole, nefazodone, protease inhibitors, ritonavir, telithromycin):* May increase hydrocodone plasma concentration and prolong opioid effects, especially if use of CYP3A4 inhibitors is concomitant. These effects may be more pronounced with concomitant use of both CYP3A4 and CYP2D6 inhibitors, particularly when an inhibitor is added after a stable dose is achieved. Monitor patient for respiratory depression and sedation; consider dosage adjustments until drug effects are stable. ∎

Black Box Warning *CYP3A4 inducers (carbamazepine, phenytoin, rifampin):* May induce metabolism and decrease hydrocodone plasma concentration, decreasing efficacy and potentially causing withdrawal symptoms. Monitor patient for effectiveness of drug and for opioid withdrawal symptoms. Consider dosage adjustments until stable. If CYP3A4 inducer is stopped, monitor patient for increased therapeutic and adverse effects, especially respiratory depression. ∎

MAO inhibitors: May potentiate effects of opioid analgesics. Don't use in patients who have received MAO inhibitors within past 14 days.

Mixed agonist/antagonists (butorphanol, nalbuphine, pentazocine), partial agonists (buprenorphine): May reduce analgesic effect of hydrocodone or precipitate withdrawal symptoms. Avoid concurrent use.

🐌 *Alert:* Serotonergic drugs (amoxapine, antimigraine drugs, buspirone, cyclobenzaprine, dextromethorphan, linezolid, lithium, MAO inhibitors, maprotiline, methylene blue, mirtazapine, nefazodone, SSNRIs, SSRIs, TCAs, trazodone, tryptophan, vilazodone): May increase risk of serotonin syndrome. Use together cautiously. Monitor patient for serotonin syndrome.

Sodium oxybate: May increase sleep duration and CNS depression. Consider therapy modification.

Drug-herb. *Kava kava, valerian:* May increase risk of excessive sedation. Avoid use together.

🐌 *Alert:* St. John's wort: May decrease hydrocodone serum concentration. Use together cautiously.

Drug-lifestyle. **Black Box Warning** *Alcohol use:* May increase hydrocodone plasma level and risk of fatal overdose. Patients shouldn't consume alcoholic beverages or use other drugs that contain alcohol. ∎

EFFECTS ON LAB TEST RESULTS
• May increase amylase and lipase levels.
• Acetaminophen may produce false-positive results on urinary 5-hydroxyindoleacetic acid test.

CONTRAINDICATIONS & CAUTIONS
Black Box Warning Acetaminophen has been associated with acute liver failure, at times resulting in liver transplant and death. Most liver injury has been associated with the use of acetaminophen at doses exceeding 4,000 mg/day, and often involves more than one acetaminophen-containing product. ∎

Black Box Warning Opioids should only be prescribed with benzodiazepines or other CNS depressants to patients for whom alternative treatment options are inadequate. Limit dosages and durations to minimum required. ∎

Black Box Warning Drug exposes patient to risks of addiction, abuse, and misuse, even at recommended doses, which can lead to overdose and death. Assess each patient's risk before prescribing; monitor patients for these behaviors or conditions. ∎

Black Box Warning The FDA has required a REMS program for this drug. Drug companies with approved opioid analgesic products must make a REMS-compliant education program available to health care providers, who are strongly encouraged to complete the education program; discuss the safe use, serious risks, and proper storage and disposal of opioid analgesics with patients and their caregivers every time these medicines are prescribed; emphasize the importance of reading the Medication Guide every time an opioid analgesic is dispensed to them; and consider using other tools to improve patient, household, and community safety. Obtain additional information at www.opioidanalgesicrems.com or by calling 1-800-503-0784. ∎

Black Box Warning Accidental ingestion of even one dose of this drug, especially by children, can result in a fatal hydrocodone overdose. ■

• Contraindicated in patients hypersensitive to hydrocodone or acetaminophen and in those with significant respiratory depression, acute or severe bronchial asthma in an unmonitored setting or in the absence of resuscitative equipment, or known or suspected GI obstruction, including paralytic ileus.

Black Box Warning Drug may cause serious, life-threatening, or fatal respiratory depression. ■

◑ *Alert:* May cause serious, potentially fatal skin reactions, including SJS, toxic epidermal necrolysis, and acute generalized exanthematous pustulosis. Reaction may occur with first or subsequent use when acetaminophen is used as monotherapy or when it's one component of combination drug therapy. Monitor patient for reddening of the skin, rash, blisters, and detachment of the upper surface of the skin. Stop drug immediately if skin reaction is suspected.

◑ *Alert:* Patients with any of the following conditions are at increased risk for oversedation and respiratory depression and require close monitoring: snoring or sleep apnea, first-time opioid use or previous (nonrecent) opioid use, opioid habituation or need for increased opioid doses, need for prolonged general anesthesia or other sedating drugs, preexisting pulmonary or cardiac disease, or thoracic or other surgical incisions that may impair breathing.

• Use cautiously in patients who are allergic to other opioids because cross-sensitivity may occur.

◑ *Alert:* Drug may lead to rare but serious decrease in adrenal gland cortisol production.

◑ *Alert:* Drug may reduce sex hormone levels with long-term use.

• Use cautiously in patients with a history of respiratory depression, drug abuse, head injury or increased ICP, seizures, acute abdominal conditions, liver disease, recent anesthesia, pulmonary disease, renal impairment, hypothyroidism, Addison disease, or BPH and urethral stricture, and in elderly or debilitated patients and those sensitive to CNS depressants.

Dialyzable drug: Unknown.

⚠ *Overdose S&S:* Hydrocodone: Loss of consciousness, pinpoint pupils, respiratory depression, stupor, coma, skeletal muscle flaccidity, cold clammy skin, bradycardia, hypotension, apnea, circulatory collapse, cardiac arrest, death. Acetaminophen: Fatal hepatic necrosis, renal tubular necrosis, hypoglycemic coma, thrombocytopenia, nausea, vomiting, diaphoresis, general malaise.

PREGNANCY-LACTATION-REPRODUCTION
• Use in pregnant women only if benefit outweighs risk to the fetus.

Black Box Warning Prolonged use during pregnancy can result in neonatal opioid withdrawal syndrome, which may be life-threatening if not recognized and treated according to protocols developed by neonatology experts. ■

Black Box Warning If opioid use is required for a prolonged period during pregnancy, advise patient of risk of neonatal opioid withdrawal syndrome (poor feeding, diarrhea, irritability, tremor, rigidity, seizures) and assure her that appropriate treatment will be available. ■

• Don't use during labor and delivery; neonatal respiratory depression may occur.

• Opioids may appear in human milk. A decision to breastfeed should take into account benefits to the mother and risks to the infant.

• Monitor infants exposed to drug through human milk for excess sedation and respiratory depression. Also watch for withdrawal symptoms in breastfed infants when mother stops an opioid analgesic, or when breastfeeding is stopped.

NURSING CONSIDERATIONS
• Monitor patients closely for an allergic reaction, particularly those who are allergic to other opioids.

• Drug may be targeted for theft, diversion, and misuse.

Black Box Warning Monitor patients for respiratory depression, especially within first 24 to 72 hours of drug initiation or after dosage increase. Serious, life-threatening, or fatal respiratory depression may occur. ■

Black Box Warning Monitor patients for abuse or misuse of drug, especially those with a personal or family history of substance abuse (drug or alcohol addiction or abuse, mental illness). Counsel patients about risks and proper use of drug. ■

Reactions in bold italics are *life-threatening*. Interactions may have a *rapid onset* or a *delayed onset*.

❸ Alert: Carefully monitor vital signs, pain level, respiratory status, and sedation level in all patients receiving opioids, especially those receiving IV drugs, even those given postoperatively.

❸ Alert: If patient is taking opioids with serotonergic drugs, watch for signs and symptoms of serotonin syndrome (agitation, hallucinations, rapid HR, fever, excessive sweating, shivering or shaking, muscle twitching or stiffness, trouble with coordination, nausea, vomiting, diarrhea), especially when starting treatment or increasing dosages. Signs and symptoms may occur within several hours of coadministration but may also occur later, especially after dosage increase. Discontinue the opioid, serotonergic drug, or both if serotonin syndrome is suspected.

❸ Alert: Monitor patient for signs and symptoms of adrenal insufficiency (nausea, vomiting, loss of appetite, fatigue, weakness, dizziness, low BP). Perform diagnostic testing if adrenal insufficiency is suspected. If adrenal insufficiency is confirmed, treat with corticosteroids and wean patient off opioids, if appropriate. Discontinue corticosteroids when clinically appropriate.

❸ Alert: Monitor patient for signs and symptoms of decreased sex hormone levels (low libido, erectile dysfunction, amenorrhea, infertility). If signs and symptoms occur, evaluate patient and obtain laboratory testing.

❸ Alert: Don't stop drug abruptly; withdraw slowly and individualize the gradual tapering plan to prevent signs and symptoms of withdrawal, worsening pain, and psychological distress in physically dependent patients. Refer to manufacturer's label for specific tapering instructions.

❸ Alert: When tapering opioids, monitor patients closely for signs and symptoms of opioid withdrawal (restlessness, lacrimation, rhinorrhea, yawning, perspiration, chills, myalgia, mydriasis, anxiety, insomnia, backache, joint pain, weakness, abdominal cramps, anorexia, nausea, vomiting, diarrhea, increased BP or HR, increased respiratory rate). Such signs and symptoms may indicate a need to taper more slowly. Also monitor patients for suicidal thoughts, use of other substances, and mood changes.

• Elderly patients receiving drug, especially those with impaired hepatic or renal function, may become confused or oversedated. Start with low doses of hydrocodone and observe closely for adverse events such as respiratory depression.

• Monitor patients who have had a head injury.

• Use of opioids in patients with acute abdominal disorders may mask symptoms.

• Constipation is a very common adverse effect. Treat constipation aggressively.

• Monitor patients with history of seizure disorder for worsening seizure control.

• Use lowest initial dose in patients with renal or hepatic impairment, and observe closely for adverse events such as respiratory depression.

• Monitor liver and kidney function. Acetaminophen elimination may be increased in patients with hepatic impairment.

• Monitor patient's ability to urinate; report urine retention.

• Monitor BP and pulse regularly.

• Periodically reevaluate patient's need for therapy.

PATIENT TEACHING

Black Box Warning Caution patient or caregiver of patient taking an opioid with a benzodiazepine, CNS depressant, or alcohol to seek immediate medical attention for dizziness, light-headedness, extreme sleepiness, slowed or difficult breathing, or unresponsiveness. ∎

Black Box Warning Instruct patient to avoid alcoholic beverages, prescription drugs, and OTC products that contain alcohol during treatment. ∎

Black Box Warning Inform female patient that prolonged use of drug during pregnancy can result in neonatal opioid withdrawal syndrome, which may be life-threatening. ∎

Black Box Warning Instruct patient to store drug securely and away from children, to dispose of drug properly when no longer needed, and not to throw in regular trash. Accidental ingestion, especially by children, may result in respiratory depression or death. ∎

❸ Alert: Counsel patient not to discontinue opioids without first discussing the need for a gradual tapering regimen with prescriber.

- Caution patient not to share drug and to protect it from theft or misuse.
- Warn patient that use of drug, even when taken as recommended, can result in addiction, abuse, and misuse, which can lead to overdose or death.
- Inform patient that drug may cause orthostatic hypotension and fainting. Teach patient how to recognize signs and symptoms of low BP and how to reduce risk of serious consequences of hypotension (e.g., by sitting or lying down or by carefully rising from a sitting or lying position).
- For best results, instruct patient to take drug before pain becomes severe.
- Explain the assessment and monitoring process to patient and family. Instruct them to immediately report difficulty breathing or other signs of a potential adverse opioid-related reaction.
- Advise patient that drug may impair judgment and not to operate heavy machinery or drive until drug's effects are known.
- Instruct patient to avoid alcohol while taking drug.

Black Box Warning Warn patient that drug contains acetaminophen (or Tylenol). Caution patient not to take more than 4,000 mg of acetaminophen on a daily basis (including from all medications being taken). Instruct patient to look for "acetaminophen" or "APAP" on package labels, not to use more than one product that contains acetaminophen, and to contact health care provider if patient has taken more than 4,000 mg in a day, even if feeling well. ■

◑ *Alert:* Encourage patient to report all medications being taken, including prescription and OTC medications and supplements.

◑ *Alert:* Caution patient to immediately report signs and symptoms of serotonin syndrome, adrenal insufficiency, and decreased sex hormone levels.

- Teach patient to eat a high-fiber diet, drink plenty of fluids, and use a stool softener or bulk laxative to prevent constipation.
- Tell patient to stop drug and immediately report blurred vision, rash, or yellowing of the skin.

◑ *Alert:* Warn patient to stop drug and seek medical attention immediately if rash or reaction occurs while using acetaminophen.

hydrocortisone (oral, injection, rectal)
hye-droe-KOR-ti-sone

Colocort, Cortef, Cortenema

hydrocortisone sodium succinate
Solu-Cortef

Therapeutic class: Corticosteroids
Pharmacologic class: Glucocorticoids

AVAILABLE FORMS
hydrocortisone
Enema: 100 mg/60 mL
Tablets: 5 mg, 10 mg, 20 mg
hydrocortisone sodium succinate
Injection*: 100-mg vial, 250-mg vial, 500-mg vial, 1,000-mg vial

INDICATIONS & DOSAGES
➤ **Rheumatic disorders (adjunctive therapy for short-term administration in psoriatic arthritis, RA, including juvenile RA, ankylosing spondylitis, acute and subacute bursitis, acute nonspecific tenosynovitis, acute gouty arthritis, posttraumatic osteoarthritis, synovitis of osteoarthritis, epicondylitis)**
Adults: 20 to 240 mg PO daily. Or, initially, 100 to 500 mg succinate IM or IV; repeat every 2, 4, or 6 hours.
➤ **Collagen diseases (SLE, acute rheumatic carditis, systemic dermatomyositis)**
Adults: 20 to 240 mg PO daily. Or, initially, 100 to 500 mg succinate IM or IV; repeat every 2, 4, or 6 hours as needed.
➤ **Dermatologic diseases (pemphigus, bullous dermatitis herpetiformis, severe erythema multiforme [SJS], exfoliative dermatitis, mycosis fungoides, severe psoriasis, severe seborrheic dermatitis)**
Adults: 20 to 240 mg PO daily. Or, initially, 100 to 500 mg succinate IM or IV; repeat every 2, 4, or 6 hours.
➤ **Severe or intractable allergic states (seasonal or perennial allergic rhinitis, bronchial asthma, contact dermatitis, atopic dermatitis, serum sickness, drug**

---

hypersensitivity reactions, transfusion reactions)
Adults: 20 to 240 mg PO daily. Or, initially, 100 to 500 mg succinate IM or IV; repeat every 2, 4, or 6 hours.
Children: 0.56 to 8 mg/kg/day IV or IM in three or four divided doses.

➤ **Severe acute and chronic allergic and inflammatory processes involving the eye and its adnexa (allergic conjunctivitis, keratitis, allergic corneal marginal ulcers, herpes zoster ophthalmicus, iritis and iridocyclitis, chorioretinitis, anterior segment inflammation, diffuse posterior uveitis and choroiditis, optic neuritis, sympathetic ophthalmia)**
Adults: 20 to 240 mg PO daily. Or, initially, 100 to 500 mg succinate IM or IV; repeat every 2, 4, or 6 hours.

➤ **Respiratory diseases (symptomatic sarcoidosis, Loeffler syndrome not manageable by other means, berylliosis, fulminating or disseminated pulmonary TB when used concurrently with appropriate antituberculous chemotherapy, aspiration pneumonitis)**
Adults: 20 to 240 mg PO daily. Or, initially, 100 to 500 mg succinate IM or IV; repeat every 2, 4, or 6 hours.

➤ **Hematologic disorders (ITP in adults [IM form is contraindicated], secondary thrombocytopenia in adults, acquired [autoimmune] hemolytic anemia, erythroblastopenia, congenital [erythroid] hypoplastic anemia)**
Adults: 20 to 240 mg PO daily. Or, initially, 100 to 500 mg succinate IM or IV; repeat every 2, 4, or 6 hours.

➤ **Neoplastic diseases (palliative management of leukemias and lymphomas in adults and acute leukemia of childhood)**
Adults: 20 to 240 mg PO daily. Or, initially, 100 to 500 mg succinate IM or IV; repeat every 2, 4, or 6 hours as needed.
Children older than age 1 month: 0.56 to 8 mg/kg/day IV or IM in three or four divided doses.

➤ **Edematous states (to induce diuresis or remission of proteinuria in nephrotic syndrome, without uremia, of the idiopathic type or that is due to SLE)**
Adults: 20 to 240 mg PO daily. Or, initially, 100 to 500 mg succinate IM or IV; repeat every 2, 4, or 6 hours.
Children older than age 2: 0.56 to 8 mg/kg/day IV or IM in three or four divided doses.

➤ **Ulcerative colitis, regional enteritis**
Adults: 20 to 240 mg PO daily. Or, initially, 100 to 500 mg succinate IM or IV; repeat every 2, 4, or 6 hours.

➤ **Nervous system disorders (cerebral edema associated with brain tumors or craniotomy [IV], tuberculous meningitis with subarachnoid block or impending block when used concurrently with appropriate antituberculotics, trichinosis with neurologic or myocardial involvement)**
Adults: 20 to 240 mg PO daily. Or, initially, 100 to 500 mg succinate IM or IV; repeat every 2, 4, or 6 hours.

➤ **Severe inflammation**
Adults: 20 to 240 mg PO daily. Or, initially, 100 to 500 mg succinate IM or IV; repeat every 2, 4, or 6 hours.

➤ **Endocrine disorders (adrenal insufficiency, congenital adrenal hyperplasia, nonsuppurative thyroiditis, hypercalcemia associated with cancer)**
Adults: 20 to 240 mg PO daily. Or, initially, 100 to 500 mg succinate IM or IV; repeat every 2, 4, or 6 hours.

➤ **Adjunctive treatment for ulcerative colitis and proctitis**
Adults: 1 enema (100 mg) PR nightly for 21 days. Or, 1 applicatorful (90-mg foam) PR daily or b.i.d. for 14 to 21 days.

➤ **Acute exacerbations of MS**
Adults: 800 mg IM or IV daily for 1 week, followed by 320 mg every other day for 1 month. Refer to manufacturer's instructions for oral dosing.

ADMINISTRATION
PO
● Give drug with milk or food when possible. Patient may need another drug to prevent GI irritation.

IV
▼ Reconstitute hydrocortisone sodium succinate with no more than 2 mL bacteriostatic water or bacteriostatic saline solution before adding to IV solutions. For doses of 500 mg or more, administer over 10 minutes. For direct injection, inject over

H

---

30 seconds to 10 minutes. For infusion, dilute with D_5W, NSS, or dextrose 5% in NSS to 1 mg/mL or less. Give intermittent IV infusion over 20 to 30 minutes.

▼ **Incompatibilities:** Solutions other than D_5W, NSS, or dextrose 5% in NSS, and other drugs.

IM
• Inject deep into gluteal muscle. Rotate injection sites to prevent muscle atrophy. Avoid subcut injection because atrophy and sterile abscesses may occur.
• Injectable forms aren't used for alternate-day therapy.

Rectal
• Have patient lie on the left side during administration and for 30 minutes afterward to allow fluid to distribute throughout the left colon. Have patient try to retain the enema for at least 1 hour but preferably all night.

ACTION

Not clearly defined. Decreases inflammation, mainly by stabilizing leukocyte lysosomal membranes; suppresses immune response; stimulates bone marrow; and influences protein, fat, and carbohydrate metabolism.

Route	Onset	Peak	Duration
PO	Variable	1 hr	Variable
IV, IM, PR	Variable	Variable	Variable

Half-life: Oral, 78 to 128 minutes; IV, 60 to 180 minutes.

ADVERSE REACTIONS

CNS: euphoria, insomnia, psychotic behavior, *pseudotumor cerebri,* vertigo, mood swings, headache, paresthesia, *seizures.* **CV:** *HF,* HTN, edema, *arrhythmias,* thrombophlebitis, *thromboembolism.* **EENT:** cataracts, glaucoma. **GI:** peptic ulceration, GI irritation, increased appetite, *pancreatitis,* nausea, vomiting. **GU:** menstrual irregularities, increased urine calcium levels. **Hematologic:** easy bruising. **Metabolic:** *hypokalemia,* hyperglycemia, carbohydrate intolerance, hypercholesterolemia, *hypocalcemia.* **Musculoskeletal:** growth suppression in children, muscle weakness, osteoporosis, tendon rupture. **Skin:** hirsutism, delayed wound healing, acne, skin eruptions, injection-site atrophy. **Other:** *anaphylaxis,*

angioedema, hypersensitivity reactions, cushingoid state, susceptibility to infections, *acute adrenal insufficiency after increased stress or abrupt withdrawal after long-term therapy.* **After abrupt withdrawal:** rebound inflammation, fatigue, weakness, arthralgia, fever, dizziness, lethargy, depression, fainting, orthostatic hypotension, dyspnea, anorexia, *hypoglycemia. After prolonged use, sudden withdrawal may be fatal.*

INTERACTIONS

Drug-drug. *Antacids:* May decrease bioavailability of corticosteroids. Separate doses by 2 hours.
Antidiabetic agents: May diminish antidiabetic therapeutic effects. Monitor therapy.
Aspirin, indomethacin, other NSAIDs: May increase risk of GI distress and bleeding. Use together cautiously.
Barbiturates, carbamazepine, fosphenytoin, phenytoin, rifampin: May decrease corticosteroid effect. Increase corticosteroid dosage.
Cyclosporine: May increase toxicity. Monitor patient closely.
CYP3A4 inducers (strong): May decrease serum concentration of hydrocortisone (systemic). Increase hydrocortisone dosage.
CYP3A4 inhibitors (strong): May increase serum concentration of corticosteroids (systemic). Decrease corticosteroid dosage.
Ketoconazole, troleandomycin: May decrease clearance of hydrocortisone. Titrate hydrocortisone dosage to avoid steroid toxicity.
Live attenuated virus vaccines, other toxoids and vaccines: May decrease antibody response and increase risk of neurologic complications. Avoid using together.
Oral anticoagulants: May alter dosage requirements. Monitor PT and INR closely.
Potassium-depleting drugs (thiazide diuretics): May enhance potassium-wasting effects of hydrocortisone. Monitor potassium level.
Skin-test antigens: May decrease response. Postpone skin testing until after therapy.
Tacrolimus (systemic): May decrease tacrolimus serum concentration. Conversely, when corticosteroid therapy is discontinued, tacrolimus concentration may increase. Monitor therapy.

Reactions in bold italics are *life-threatening*. Interactions may have a *rapid onset* or a *delayed onset*.

Tacrolimus (topical): May enhance adverse/toxic effect of immunosuppressants. Avoid combination.

Drug-herb. *Echinacea, ginseng:* May increase immune-stimulating effects. Discourage use together.

EFFECTS ON LAB TEST RESULTS

• May increase glucose and cholesterol levels. May decrease T_3, T_4, potassium, and calcium levels.

• May cause decreased ^{131}I uptake and protein-bound iodine levels in thyroid function tests. May cause false-negative results in nitroblue tetrazolium test for systemic bacterial infections. May alter reactions to coccidioidin skin tests.

CONTRAINDICATIONS & CAUTIONS

• Contraindicated in patients hypersensitive to drug or its ingredients, in those with systemic fungal infections, and in those receiving immunosuppressive doses together with live-virus vaccines.

• Use with caution in patients with recent MI.

• Use cautiously in patients with GI ulcer, renal disease, HTN, osteoporosis, diabetes mellitus, hypothyroidism, cirrhosis, diverticulitis, nonspecific ulcerative colitis, active hepatitis, recent intestinal anastomoses, thromboembolic disorders, seizures, myasthenia gravis, HF, TB, ocular herpes simplex, emotional instability, and psychotic tendencies.

• Drug can cause hypercorticism or suppression of the HPA axis, particularly in younger children or patients receiving high-dose therapy. Withdraw drug slowly.

• Kaposi sarcoma has been reported. Clinical remission is possible once corticosteroids are discontinued.

Dialyzable drug: Unknown.

PREGNANCY-LACTATION-REPRODUCTION

• Use cautiously in pregnant and breast-feeding women. When essential during pregnancy, use lowest possible dose for the shortest duration. Avoid high doses in first trimester.

• Steroids may alter the motility and number of sperm in some patients.

NURSING CONSIDERATIONS

• Determine whether patient is sensitive to other corticosteroids.

• Most adverse reactions to corticosteroids are dose- or duration-dependent.

• For better results and less toxicity, give a once-daily dose in morning.

❸ *Alert:* Salts aren't interchangeable.

❸ *Alert:* Only hydrocortisone sodium succinate can be given IV.

❸ *Alert:* Epidural corticosteroid injections to treat neck and back pain and radiating pain in the arms and legs may result in rare but serious adverse events (vision loss, stroke, paralysis, death). The use of epidural corticosteroid injections isn't approved by the FDA.

• Enema may produce same systemic effects as other forms of hydrocortisone. If enema therapy must exceed 21 days, taper off by giving every other night for 2 to 3 weeks.

• High-dose therapy usually isn't continued beyond 48 hours.

• Always adjust to lowest effective dose.

• Monitor patient's weight, BP, and electrolyte levels.

• Monitor patient for cushingoid effects, including moon face, buffalo hump, central obesity, thinning hair, HTN, and increased susceptibility to infection.

• Unless contraindicated, give a low-sodium diet that's high in potassium and protein. Give potassium supplements.

• Drug may mask or worsen infections, including latent amebiasis.

• Stress (fever, trauma, surgery, and emotional problems) may increase adrenal insufficiency. Increase dosage.

• Watch for depression or psychotic episodes, especially during high-dose therapy.

• Inspect patient's skin for petechiae.

• Diabetic patient may need increased insulin; monitor glucose level.

• Periodic measurement of growth and development may be needed during high-dose or prolonged therapy in children.

• Elderly patients may be more susceptible to osteoporosis with prolonged use.

• Gradually reduce dosage after long-term therapy.

• *Look alike–sound alike:* Don't confuse Solu-Cortef with Solu-Medrol. Don't confuse hydrocortisone with hydrocodone, hydroxychloroquine, or hydrochlorothiazide. Don't confuse Cortef with Coreg or Lortab.

PATIENT TEACHING
• Tell patient not to stop drug abruptly or without prescriber's consent.
• Instruct patient to take oral form of drug with milk or food.
• Warn patient on long-term therapy about cushingoid effects (moon face, buffalo hump) and the need to notify prescriber about sudden weight gain or swelling.
• Teach patient signs and symptoms of early adrenal insufficiency: fatigue, muscle weakness, joint pain, fever, anorexia, nausea, shortness of breath, dizziness, and fainting.
• Instruct patient to carry a card with prescriber's name and name and dosage of drug, indicating the need for supplemental systemic glucocorticoids during stress.
• Warn patient about easy bruising.
• Urge patient receiving long-term therapy to consider exercise or physical therapy. Also, tell patient to ask prescriber about vitamin D or calcium supplement.
• Advise patient receiving long-term therapy to have periodic eye exams.
• Caution patient to avoid exposure to infections (such as chickenpox or measles) and to notify prescriber if such exposure occurs.
• *Alert:* Counsel patient who receives epidural corticosteroid injections to seek immediate medical attention for vision loss or vision changes; tingling in the arms or legs; sudden weakness or numbness of the face, arm, or leg on one or both sides of the body; dizziness; severe headache; or seizures.
• *Alert:* Advise patient to discuss benefits and risks along with other possible treatments with health care provider before patient undergoes epidural corticosteroid injection.

hydrocortisone (topical)
hye-droe-KOR-ti-sone

Ala-Cort, Ala-Scalp, Anusol HC, Cortizone-10 ◇, Proctocort, Scalpicin ◇, Texacort

hydrocortisone acetate (topical, rectal)
Anusol HC ◇, Cortaid ◇, Corticaine ◇, Cortifoam, Gynecort 10 ◇, Micort-HC

hydrocortisone butyrate
Locoid, Locoid Lipocream

hydrocortisone probutate
Pandel

hydrocortisone valerate

Therapeutic class: Corticosteroids
Pharmacologic class: Corticosteroids

AVAILABLE FORMS
hydrocortisone
Cream: 0.5% ◇, 1% ◇, 1%, 2.5% ◇, 2.5%
Lotion: 1% ◇, 2%, 2.5% ◇
Ointment: 0.5% ◇, 1%, 2.5%
Rectal cream: 1%, 2.5% ◇
Rectal ointment: 1%
Topical solution: 1% ◇, 2.5%
hydrocortisone acetate
Cream: 1%, 2%, 2.5%, 2.5% ◇
Lotion: 2%
Rectal foam: 90 mg per application
Rectal suppositories: 25 mg
hydrocortisone butyrate
Cream: 0.1%
Ointment: 0.1%
Solution: 0.1%
hydrocortisone probutate
Cream: 0.1%
hydrocortisone valerate
Cream: 0.2%
Ointment: 0.2%

INDICATIONS & DOSAGES
➤ **Inflammation and pruritus from corticosteroid-responsive dermatoses, adjunctive topical management of seborrheic dermatitis of scalp**

Adults and children: Clean area; apply cream, lotion, ointment, or topical solution sparingly daily to q.i.d. as directed until acute phase is controlled; then reduce dosage to one to three times weekly as needed. Give children lowest dose that provides positive results.

➤ **Inflammation from proctitis; adjunctive treatment of chronic ulcerative colitis, cryptitis**

Adults: 1 applicatorful of rectal foam PR daily or b.i.d. for 2 to 3 weeks; then every other day as needed. Or, 1 suppository PR b.i.d. to t.i.d. or 2 suppositories PR b.i.d. for 2 weeks. In factitial proctitis, recommended duration of therapy is 6 to 8 weeks.

ADMINISTRATION
Rectal
- Refer to manufacturer's instructions to properly fill applicator barrel.
- Once applicator is properly filled, gently insert tip into anus. Once in place, push plunger to expel foam; then withdraw applicator.
- Thoroughly clean all applicator parts after each use.
- Avoid excessive handling of suppository, which is designed to melt at body temperature.
- Insert suppository, pointed end first, into rectum using gentle pressure.

Topical
- Gently wash skin before applying. To prevent skin damage, rub in gently, leaving a thin coat. When treating hairy sites, part hair and apply directly to lesions.
- Check individual products for frequency of administration.
- Avoid applying near eyes or mucous membranes or in ear canal; may be safely used on face, groin, armpits, and under breasts.
- Change dressing as prescribed. Stop drug and tell prescriber if skin infection, striae, or atrophy occurs.
- Continue treatment for a few days after lesions clear.

ACTION
Unclear. Diffuses across cell membranes to form complexes with cytoplasmic receptors, showing anti-inflammatory, antipruritic, vasoconstrictive, and antiproliferative activity. Considered a low-potency (hydrocortisone, hydrocortisone acetate) and a medium-potency (hydrocortisone butyrate, hydrocortisone probutate, hydrocortisone valerate) drug, according to vasoconstrictive properties.

Route	Onset	Peak	Duration
Topical, PR	Unknown	Unknown	Unknown

Half-life: Unknown.

ADVERSE REACTIONS
Topical
Skin: burning, pruritus, irritation, dryness, erythema, folliculitis, hypertrichosis, hypopigmentation, acneiform eruptions, allergic contact dermatitis, atrophy, maceration, secondary infection, striae, miliaria with occlusive dressings.

Rectal
CNS: *seizures, increased ICP,* vertigo, headache. **CV:** HTN. **EENT:** cataracts, glaucoma. **GI:** peptic ulcer, *pancreatitis,* abdominal distention. **GU:** menstrual irregularities, glycosuria. **Metabolic:** fluid or electrolyte disturbances, decreased carbohydrate tolerance, hyperglycemia. **Musculoskeletal:** muscle weakness, osteoporosis, necrosis and fractures in bone. **Skin:** impaired wound healing, fragile skin, petechiae, erythema, sweating. **Other:** *HPA axis suppression,* Cushing syndrome.

INTERACTIONS
None significant.

EFFECTS ON LAB TEST RESULTS
- May increase glucose level.

CONTRAINDICATIONS & CAUTIONS
- Contraindicated in patients hypersensitive to drug or its components. Rectal formulations are contraindicated in patients with some GI conditions and after surgery. Refer to individual product information.
- Drug can cause hypercorticism or suppression of the HPA axis, which can lead to adrenal crisis.
- Don't use as monotherapy in primary bacterial infections (impetigo, paronychia, erysipelas, cellulitis, angular cheilitis), treatment of rosacea, perioral dermatitis, or acne.

H

• Drug isn't for ophthalmic use.
Dialyzable drug: Unknown.
⚠ *Overdose S&S:* Systemic effects.

PREGNANCY-LACTATION-REPRODUCTION
• There are no well-controlled studies in pregnant women. Use during pregnancy only if potential benefit justifies potential risk to the fetus.
• Use cautiously in breastfeeding women.

NURSING CONSIDERATIONS
• If an occlusive dressing is applied and a fever develops, notify prescriber and remove dressing.
• If antifungal or antibiotic combined with corticosteroid fails to provide prompt improvement, stop corticosteroid until infection is controlled.
• Systemic absorption is likely with use of occlusive dressings, prolonged treatment, or extensive body surface treatment. Watch for symptoms, such as hyperglycemia, glycosuria, and HPA axis suppression.
• Avoid using plastic pants or tight-fitting diapers on treated areas in young children. Children may absorb larger amounts of drug and be more susceptible to systemic toxicity.
• Monitor patient for fluid or electrolyte disturbances (sodium and fluid retention, potassium loss, hypokalemic alkalosis, negative nitrogen balance from catabolism of protein).
• Drug may suppress skin reaction testing.
• *Look alike–sound alike:* Don't confuse hydrocortisone with hydrocodone, hydroxychloroquine, or hydrochlorothiazide.

PATIENT TEACHING
• Teach patient or family member how to apply drug.
• Tell patient to wash hands after application.
• If an occlusive dressing is ordered, advise patient to leave it in place for no longer than 12 hours each day and not to use the dressing on infected or weeping lesions.
• Teach patient how to use rectal foam applicator or suppository if needed.
• Tell patient to stop drug and report signs of systemic absorption, skin irritation or ulceration, hypersensitivity, infection, or lack of improvement.

• For perianal application, instruct patient to place small amount of drug on a tissue and gently rub in.
• Tell patient to disassemble applicator and clean with warm water after each use.
• Tell patient to stop using this product if condition worsens or if symptoms persist for more than 7 days.

SAFETY ALERT!

HYDROmorphone hydrochloride (dihydromorphinone hydrochloride)
hye-droe-MOR-fone

Dilaudid

Therapeutic class: Opioid analgesics
Pharmacologic class: Opioids
Controlled substance schedule: II

AVAILABLE FORMS
Injection (prefilled syringes): 1 mg/mL, 2 mg/mL, 4 mg/mL, 10 mg/mL
Oral liquid: 5 mg/5 mL
Tablets: 2 mg, 4 mg, 8 mg
Tablets (extended-release) ⓞⓝⓒ: 8 mg, 12 mg, 16 mg, 32 mg

INDICATIONS & DOSAGES
➤ **Management of pain severe enough to require opioid treatment and for which alternative treatment options are inadequate**
Adults: For opioid-naive patients, 2 to 4 mg immediate-release tablets PO every 4 to 6 hours p.r.n. Or, 1 to 2 mg IM or subcut every 2 to 3 hours. Or, 0.2 to 1 mg IV (slowly over at least 2 to 3 minutes) every 2 to 3 hours p.r.n. Or, 2.5 to 10 mg oral liquid every 3 to 6 hours p.r.n. Or, for opioid-tolerant adults currently on immediate-release hydromorphone who require continuous analgesia for an extended period, starting dose of extended-release form is equivalent to total daily dose of immediate-release form. May increase by 4 to 8 mg every 3 to 4 days as needed to achieve adequate analgesia.
Adjust-a-dose: For elderly patients, use cautiously and reduce initial oral starting dose. Initial IV starting dose for elderly or

---

debilitated patients should be 0.2 mg. For those with moderate renal impairment, reduce dose to 50% of usual starting dose. For those with renal or hepatic impairment, reduce dose to 25% to 50% of usual starting dose of immediate-acting forms. For extended-release forms, give patients with moderate hepatic impairment 25% of usual starting dose; give patients with moderate renal impairment 50%, and patients with severe renal impairment 25% of usual starting dose. Use an alternative analgesic for those with severe hepatic impairment.

ADMINISTRATION
PO

• Give drug with food if GI upset occurs.

Black Box Warning Patient should swallow extended-release tablets whole; don't break, chew, dissolve, crush, or inject them. ∎

Black Box Warning Don't give extended-release tablets with other extended-release opioids. ∎

Black Box Warning Ensure accuracy when prescribing, dispensing, and administering oral solution to avoid dosing errors due to confusion between mg and mL, which could result in accidental overdose and death. ∎

Black Box Warning For oral solution, use only a calibrated device that can measure and deliver prescribed dose accurately. ∎

IV

▼ Give by direct injection over no less than 2 minutes.

▼ Respiratory depression and hypotension can occur. Give slowly, and monitor patient constantly. Keep resuscitation equipment available.

▼ **Incompatibilities:** None listed by manufacturer. Consult a drug incompatibility reference for more information.

IM

• Document administration site.

Subcutaneous

• Rotate injection sites to avoid induration with subcut injection.

ACTION

Unknown. Binds with opioid receptors in the CNS, altering perception of and emotional response to pain. Also suppresses the cough reflex by direct action on the cough center in the medulla.

Route	Onset	Peak	Duration
PO	15–30 min	30–60 min	3–4 hr
PO (extended-release)	Gradually over 6–8 hr	12–16 hr	18–24 hr
IV	5 min	10–20 min	3–4 hr
IM	15 min	30–60 min	4–5 hr
Subcut	15 min	30–90 min	4 hr

Half-life: 2½ to 4 hours; PO (extended-release), 11 hours.

ADVERSE REACTIONS

CNS: sedation, somnolence, dizziness, euphoria, light-headedness, insomnia, drug withdrawal syndrome (extended-release form), headache, confusion, syncope. **CV:** *cardiac arrest,* hypotension, flushing, *bradycardia,* chest discomfort, edema, tachycardia. **EENT:** blurred vision, diplopia, nystagmus. **GI:** nausea, vomiting, constipation, anorexia, weight loss, diarrhea, ileus, dry mouth, abdominal pain, biliary colic. **GU:** urine retention, urinary frequency, urinary hesitancy, erectile dysfunction, sexual disorder, hypogonadism. **Musculoskeletal:** arthralgia, muscle contractions. **Respiratory:** *apnea, respiratory depression, bronchospasm.* **Skin:** diaphoresis, pruritus, hyperhidrosis. **Other:** induration with repeated subcut injections, physical dependence, pain.

INTERACTIONS

Drug-drug. *Anticholinergics:* May increase risk of urine retention or severe constipation. Use together cautiously.

Antipsychotics: May enhance opioid analgesic effects. Monitor therapy.

Black Box Warning *Benzodiazepines, CNS depressants:* May cause slow or difficult breathing, sedation, and death. Avoid use together. If use together is necessary, limit dosage and duration of each drug to the minimum necessary for desired effect. ∎

Droperidol, general anesthetics, minocycline, nabilone, neuromuscular blockers, other opioid analgesics, TCAs, tranquilizers: May cause additive effects. Monitor therapy carefully.

MAO inhibitors: May cause respiratory and CNS depression. Use together isn't recommended and use of extended-release tablets within 14 days of MAO inhibitors isn't

H

recommended. If coadministration of extended-release form and MAO inhibitors is unavoidable, monitor patient carefully for respiratory and CNS depression.

Opioids (mixed agonist/antagonist): May diminish analgesic effect of opioid analgesics or cause withdrawal signs and symptoms. Avoid using together.

◑ *Alert:* Serotonergic drugs (amoxapine, antimigraine drugs, buspirone, cyclobenzaprine, dextromethorphan, linezolid, lithium, MAO inhibitors, maprotiline, methylene blue, mirtazapine, nefazodone, SSNRIs, SSRIs, TCAs, trazodone, tryptophan, vilazodone):* May increase risk of serotonin syndrome. Use together cautiously and monitor patient for serotonin syndrome.

Drug-herb. *Kava kava, valerian:* May increase CNS depression. Avoid use together.

◑ *Alert: St. John's wort:* May increase risk of serotonin syndrome. Use together cautiously and monitor patient for serotonin syndrome.

Drug-lifestyle. Black Box Warning *Alcohol use:* May cause additive effects and risk of fatal overdose. Patients shouldn't consume alcoholic beverages or use other drugs that contain alcohol. ∎

EFFECTS ON LAB TEST RESULTS
• May decrease amylase level.
• May interfere with hepatobiliary imaging studies because delayed gastric emptying and contraction of sphincter of Oddi may increase biliary tract pressure.

CONTRAINDICATIONS & CAUTIONS
Black Box Warning Opioids should only be prescribed with benzodiazepines or other CNS depressants to patients for whom alternative treatment options are inadequate. ∎
• Contraindicated in patients hypersensitive to drug; in those with intracranial lesions that cause increased ICP; in those with paralytic ileus or narrowed or obstructed GI tract; for obstetric analgesia; and in those with depressed ventilation, such as in status asthmaticus, COPD, cor pulmonale, emphysema, and kyphoscoliosis.
Black Box Warning Extended-release form is contraindicated in opioid-naive patients. It isn't indicated for acute pain or postoperative pain or as a p.r.n. analgesic. Fatal respiratory depression may occur in patients

who aren't opioid-tolerant. Accidental intake, especially in children, can cause fatal hydromorphone overdose. ∎

Black Box Warning Hydromorphone is an opioid agonist with an abuse liability similar to other opioid agonists, legal or illicit. Risk of abuse is increased in patients with a personal or family history of substance abuse or mental illness. Use with ethanol, other opioids, and other CNS depressants can increase risk of adverse events, including death. ∎

Black Box Warning The FDA has required a REMS program for this drug. Drug companies with approved opioid analgesic products must make a REMS-compliant education program available to health care providers, who are strongly encouraged to complete the education program; discuss the safe use, serious risks, and proper storage and disposal of opioid analgesics with patients and their caregivers every time these medicines are prescribed; emphasize the importance of reading the Medication Guide every time an opioid analgesic is dispensed to them; and consider using other tools to improve patient, household, and community safety. Obtain additional information at www.opioidanalgesicrems.com or by calling 1-800-503-0784. ∎

◑ *Alert:* Patients with any of the following conditions are at increased risk for oversedation and respiratory depression and require close monitoring: sleep-disordered breathing; first-time opioid use or previous (nonrecent) opioid use; opioid habituation or need for increased opioid doses; need for prolonged general anesthesia or other sedating drugs; preexisting pulmonary or cardiac disease; or thoracic or other surgical incisions that may impair breathing.

◑ *Alert:* Drug may lead to rare but serious decrease in adrenal gland cortisol production.

◑ *Alert:* Drug may reduce sex hormone levels with long-term use.
• Drug may contain a sulfite that can cause allergic-type reactions, including anaphylactic symptoms and life-threatening or less severe asthmatic episodes in certain susceptible patients.
• Use cautiously in patients with a history of seizures and adrenal insufficiency.

⊘ *Alert:* Drug may cause severe hypotension, including orthostatic hypotension and syncope in ambulatory patients. Risk is increased in patients whose ability to maintain BP has already been compromised by a reduced blood volume or concurrent administration of certain CNS depressants (e.g., phenothiazines or general anesthetics).

• Use cautiously in elderly or debilitated patients and in those with hepatic or renal disease, hypothyroidism, Addison disease, prostatic hyperplasia, or urethral stricture.

Dialyzable drug: Unknown.

⚠ Overdose S&S: Constricted pupils, cold clammy skin, extreme somnolence progressing to stupor or coma, respiratory depression, skeletal muscle flaccidity, bradycardia, hypotension, apnea, cardiac arrest, circulatory collapse, death.

PREGNANCY-LACTATION-REPRODUCTION

⊘ *Alert:* Drug crosses placental barrier. Carefully weigh benefits and risks of using drug during pregnancy.

Black Box Warning Use in pregnancy can cause neonatal withdrawal syndrome, which can be life-threatening, and requires management by neonatology experts. Advise women of the risk, and ensure appropriate treatment is available. ∎

• Don't use during labor and delivery; neonatal respiratory depression may occur.

• Drug appears in human milk in low concentrations. Monitor breastfeeding infants exposed to opioids for excess sedation and respiratory depression. Also watch for withdrawal signs and symptoms in breastfeeding infants when maternal administration of an opioid analgesic is stopped, or when breastfeeding is stopped.

• Long-term use can cause hypogonadism and infertility.

NURSING CONSIDERATIONS

⊘ *Alert:* Vial stopper may contain latex.

• Reassess patient's level of pain at least 15 and 30 minutes after administration.

• For better analgesic effect, give drug on a regular schedule, before patient has intense pain.

Black Box Warning Routinely monitor all patients for signs and symptoms of misuse, abuse, and addiction during treatment. ∎

Black Box Warning Monitor patients for respiratory depression, especially within first 24 to 72 hours of drug initiation and after dosage increase. Serious, life-threatening, or fatal respiratory depression may occur. ∎

⊘ *Alert:* Carefully monitor vital signs, pain level, respiratory status, and sedation level in all patients receiving opioids, especially those receiving IV drugs, even those given postoperatively.

⊘ *Alert:* If patient is taking opioids with serotonergic drugs, watch for signs and symptoms of serotonin syndrome (agitation, hallucinations, rapid HR, fever, excessive sweating, shivering or shaking, muscle twitching or stiffness, trouble with coordination, nausea, vomiting, diarrhea), especially when starting treatment or increasing dosages. Signs and symptoms may occur within several hours of coadministration but may also occur later, especially after dosage increase. Discontinue the opioid, serotonergic drug, or both if serotonin syndrome is suspected.

⊘ *Alert:* Monitor patient for signs and symptoms of adrenal insufficiency (nausea, vomiting, loss of appetite, fatigue, weakness, dizziness, low BP). Perform diagnostic testing if adrenal insufficiency is suspected. If adrenal insufficiency is confirmed, treat with corticosteroids and wean patient off opioids, if appropriate. Discontinue corticosteroids when clinically appropriate.

⊘ *Alert:* Monitor patient for signs and symptoms of decreased sex hormone levels (low libido, erectile dysfunction, amenorrhea, infertility). If signs and symptoms occur, evaluate patient and obtain laboratory testing.

⊘ *Alert:* Don't stop drug abruptly; withdraw slowly and individualize the gradual tapering plan to prevent signs and symptoms of withdrawal, worsening pain, and psychological distress in physically dependent patients. Refer to manufacturer's label for specific tapering instructions.

⊘ *Alert:* When tapering opioids, monitor patients closely for signs and symptoms of opioid withdrawal (restlessness, lacrimation, rhinorrhea, yawning, perspiration, chills, myalgia, mydriasis, irritability, anxiety, insomnia, backache, joint pain, weakness, abdominal cramps, anorexia, nausea, vomiting, diarrhea, increased BP or HR, increased respiratory rate). Such signs and symptoms may indicate a need to taper more slowly. Also monitor patient for suicidal thoughts, use of other substances, and mood changes.

• Monitor patients with history of seizure disorder for worsening seizure control.

• Patients considered opioid tolerant are those receiving, for 1 week or longer, at least 60 mg morphine per day, 25 mcg/hour transdermal fentanyl, 30 mg oral oxycodone per day, 8 mg oral hydromorphone per day or more, 25 mg oral oxymorphone per day or more, or an equianalgesic dose of another opioid.

• Discontinue all other extended-release opioids before giving extended-release form of hydromorphone.

• Monitor respiratory and circulatory status and bowel function.

• Keep opioid antagonist (naloxone) available.

• Don't use extended-release form within 14 days of stopping MAO inhibitor.

• Discontinue use of extended-release form if stopped for more than 3 days.

• Drug may worsen or mask gallbladder pain.

• Drug is a commonly abused opioid.

• Drug may cause constipation. Assess bowel function and need for stool softeners and stimulant laxatives.

• *Look alike–sound alike:* Don't confuse hydromorphone with morphine or oxymorphone. Don't confuse Dilaudid with Dilantin.

PATIENT TEACHING

• Instruct patient to request or take drug before pain becomes intense and to report all adverse reactions.

Black Box Warning Caution patient or caregiver of patient taking an opioid with a benzodiazepine, CNS depressant, or alcohol to seek immediate medical attention for dizziness, light-headedness, extreme sleepiness, slowed or difficult breathing, or unresponsiveness. ∎

Black Box Warning Warn patient that extended-release tablets must be taken whole. Caution patient not to cut, chew, crush, dissolve, or inject them. ∎

🕓 *Alert:* Encourage patient to report all medications being taken, including prescription and OTC medications and supplements.

🕓 *Alert:* Caution patient to immediately report signs and symptoms of serotonin syndrome, adrenal insufficiency, and decreased sex hormone levels.

🕓 *Alert:* Counsel patient not to discontinue opioids without first discussing the need for a gradual tapering regimen with prescriber.

• Warn patient that use of drug, even when taken as recommended, can result in addiction, abuse, and misuse, which can lead to overdose or death. Instruct patient not to discontinue drug without first discussing the need for a tapering regimen with prescriber.

• Instruct patient to use only a calibrated device to measure and deliver prescribed dose of oral solution accurately to prevent accidental overdose.

• Explain the assessment and monitoring process to patient and family. Instruct them to immediately report if patient has any difficulty breathing or any other signs of a potential adverse opioid-related reaction.

• Advise patient to take drug with food if GI upset occurs.

• When drug is used after surgery, encourage patient to turn, cough, and breathe deeply to avoid lung problems.

• Teach patient how to recognize signs and symptoms of low BP and how to reduce risk of serious consequences of hypotension (e.g., by sitting or lying down or by carefully rising from a sitting or lying position).

Black Box Warning Instruct patient to store drug securely and away from children, to dispose of drug properly when no longer needed, and not to throw in regular trash. Accidental ingestion, especially by children, may result in respiratory depression or death. ∎

• Warn outpatient to avoid hazardous activities that require mental alertness until drug's CNS effects are known.

Black Box Warning Inform female patient that prolonged use of drug during pregnancy can result in neonatal opioid withdrawal syndrome, which may be life-threatening. ∎

Black Box Warning Instruct patient to avoid alcoholic beverages, prescription drugs, and OTC products that contain alcohol during treatment. ∎

Reactions in bold italics are *life-threatening*. Interactions may have a *rapid onset* or a *delayed onset*.

hydroxychloroquine sulfate ☒
hye-droks-ee-KLOR-oh-kwin

Plaquenil

Therapeutic class: Antimalarials
Pharmacologic class: Aminoquinolines

AVAILABLE FORMS
Tablets ⓄⓉⒸ: 200 mg (equivalent to 155 mg base)

INDICATIONS & DOSAGES
➤ **Suppressive prevention of malaria attacks caused by** *Plasmodium vivax, Plasmodium malariae, Plasmodium ovale,* **and susceptible strains of** *Plasmodium falciparum*
Adults: 400 mg PO weekly on the same day each week, beginning 2 weeks before entering malaria-endemic area and continuing for 4 weeks after leaving area.
Children: 6.5 mg/kg PO weekly on the same day each week, beginning 2 weeks before entering malaria-endemic area and continuing for 4 weeks after leaving area. Don't exceed adult dose.
➤ **Acute malarial attacks**
Adults: Initially, 800 mg PO, followed by 400 mg at 6 hours, 24 hours, and 48 hours after initial dose.
Children: Initially, 13 mg/kg (up to 800 mg) PO; then 6.5 mg/kg (up to 400 mg) at 6 hours, 24 hours, and 48 hours after first dose.
➤ **SLE**
Adults: 200 to 400 mg PO daily as a single dose or in two divided doses, continued for several weeks or months, depending on response.
➤ **RA**
Adults: Initially, 400 to 600 mg PO daily as a single dose or in two divided doses. When good response occurs, cut dosage in half and continue at 200 to 400 mg daily in one or two divided doses. Maximum dose is 600 mg or 6.5 mg/kg per day, whichever is lower.

ADMINISTRATION
PO
❸ *Alert:* Drug dosage may be discussed in "mg" or "mg base"; be aware of the difference.

• Give drug with food or milk to minimize GI upset.
• Don't crush or divide film-coated tablets.
• To improve compliance when drug is used for prevention, advise patient to take drug immediately before or after a meal on the same day each week.

ACTION
May bind to and alter the properties of DNA in susceptible organisms.

Route	Onset	Peak	Duration
PO	Unknown	3–4 hr	Unknown

Half-life: 40 to 50 days.

ADVERSE REACTIONS
CNS: *seizures,* irritability, nightmares, ataxia, psychosis, vertigo, dizziness, hypoactive deep tendon reflexes, lassitude, headache, fatigue, extrapyramidal disorders, pyrexia. **CV:** *cardiomyopathy, ventricular arrhythmias, torsades de pointes.* **EENT:** blurred vision, difficulty in focusing, reversible corneal changes, typically irreversible nystagmus, sometimes progressive or delayed retinal changes such as narrowing of arterioles, macular lesions, pallor of optic disk, optic atrophy, tinnitus, deafness. **GI:** decreased appetite, abdominal cramps, diarrhea, nausea, vomiting. ☒ **Hematologic:** *agranulocytosis, leukopenia, thrombocytopenia, hemolysis in patients with G6PD deficiency,* anemia, porphyria, *aplastic anemia, hyperleukocytosis.* **Hepatic:** acute hepatic failure, abnormal LFT values. **Metabolic:** weight loss, *hypoglycemia.* **Musculoskeletal:** skeletal muscle myopathy or neuromyopathy leading to progressive weakness and atrophy of proximal muscle groups, bone marrow failure. **Respiratory:** bronchospasm. **Skin:** pruritus, lichen planus eruptions, skin and mucosal pigmentary changes, pleomorphic skin eruptions, worsened psoriasis, alopecia, photosensitivity, bleaching of hair, urticaria. **Other:** *angioedema, suicidal behavior.*

INTERACTIONS
Drug-drug. *Aluminum salts (kaolin), magnesium:* May decrease GI absorption. Separate dose times by 4 hours.

Antidiabetics, insulin: May enhance effects of a hypoglycemic treatment. An insulin or antidiabetic dosage decrease may be required.

Artemether: May increase toxic effects of hydroxychloroquine. Avoid use together.

Beta blockers: May increase CV effects of certain beta blockers (metoprolol). Carefully monitor patient. Consider using alternative beta blocker (atenolol).

Digoxin: May increase digoxin level. Monitor drug levels; monitor patient for toxicity.

Mefloquine: May increase QTc-interval prolongation and seizure risk when used concurrently. Avoid use together.

Phenothiazines: May increase serum concentration of phenothiazines. Monitor therapy.

QTc-prolonging drugs: May enhance QTc-prolonging effect of highest-risk QTc-prolonging drugs. Avoid combination.

Tamoxifen: May increase risk of retinal toxicity. Monitor therapy.

EFFECTS ON LAB TEST RESULTS
• May decrease Hb level.
• May decrease granulocyte, WBC, and platelet counts.

CONTRAINDICATIONS & CAUTIONS
• Contraindicated in patients hypersensitive to drug, in those with retinal or visual field changes or porphyria, and for long-term treatment in children.
• Use cautiously in patients with severe GI, neurologic, or blood disorders.
• Use cautiously in patients with hepatic disease or alcoholism or when used with hepatotoxic drugs.
▓ Use with caution in those with G6PD deficiency or psoriasis because drug may worsen these conditions.
◑ **Alert:** Suicidal behavior has been reported in very rare cases.
Dialyzable drug: Unknown.
▲ **Overdose S&S:** Headache, drowsiness, visual disturbances, *CV collapse, seizures, sudden and early respiratory and cardiac arrest, atrial standstill, nodal rhythm, prolonged intraventricular conduction time, progressive bradycardia leading to ventricular fibrillation or arrest.*

PREGNANCY-LACTATION-REPRODUCTION
• Drug doesn't appear to pose a significant risk to the fetus, especially with lower doses.
• Pregnant women exposed to drug for the treatment of RA or SLE may be enrolled in the Organization of Teratology Information Specialists (OTIS) Autoimmune Diseases in Pregnancy Study (1-877-311-8972).
• Drug appears in human milk. Use cautiously in breastfeeding women; infants are extremely sensitive to toxic effects of 4-aminoquinolines such as hydroxychloroquine.

NURSING CONSIDERATIONS
• Before prescribing drug for treatment or prophylaxis of malaria, consult the CDC malaria website (www.cdc.org/parasites/malaria).
• Ensure that baseline and periodic ophthalmic exams are performed at baseline and annually. Check periodically for ocular muscle weakness after long-term use. Retinal toxicity is largely dose-related.
• Monitor CBC and LFTs periodically during long-term therapy; if severe blood disorder not caused by disease develops, drug may need to be stopped.
◑ **Alert:** Monitor patient for possible overdose, which can quickly lead to toxic signs or symptoms. Children are extremely susceptible to toxicity.

PATIENT TEACHING
• Advise patient taking drug for prevention to take immediately before or after a meal on the same day each week, to improve compliance.
• Instruct patient to report adverse reactions promptly.
• Tell patient that dizziness may occur and to use caution while driving or performing other tasks that require alertness, coordination, or physical dexterity.

Reactions in bold italics are *life-threatening*. Interactions may have a *rapid onset* or a *delayed onset*.

hydroxyurea
hye-droks-ee-yoor-EE-a

Droxia, Hydrea, Siklos

Therapeutic class: Antineoplastics
Pharmacologic class: Antimetabolites

AVAILABLE FORMS
Capsules: 200 mg, 300 mg, 400 mg, 500 mg
Tablets: 100 mg, 1,000 mg

INDICATIONS & DOSAGES
Adjust-a-dose (for all indications): Base
dosage on patient's actual or ideal weight,
whichever is less. Dosage adjustment is recommended in renal impairment. According to manufacturer, if CrCl is less than
60 mL/minute or in patients with ESRD,
give 50% of usual dose. If patient is on
hemodialysis, give 50% of usual dose after
dialysis on dialysis days. Prophylactic administration of folic acid is recommended.
➤ **Carcinoma of the head (excluding lip)
and neck, with radiation (Hydrea)**
Adults: 1,000 mg every 12 hours for 11 doses
per cycle, in combination with continuous
infusion 5-FU and radiation therapy.
➤ **Resistant chronic myelocytic leukemia
(Hydrea)**
Adults: Initially, 40 mg/kg/day (reduce initial dosage for thrombocytopenia); reduce
dosage to 20 mg/kg/day if WBC count is less
than 2,000/mm^3. Further individualize dose
based on WBC counts.
➤ **To reduce frequency of painful crises
and need for blood transfusions in adult
patients with sickle cell anemia with recurrent moderate to severe painful crises
(Droxia, Siklos)**
Adults (Droxia): 15 mg/kg PO once daily. If
blood counts are in acceptable range, dose
may be increased by 5 mg/kg daily every
12 weeks until maximum tolerated dose or
35 mg/kg daily has been reached. If blood
counts are considered toxic, withhold drug
until counts recover. Resume treatment after reducing dose by 2.5 mg/kg daily. Every
12 weeks, drug may then be adjusted up or
down in 2.5-mg/kg daily increments until

patient is at a stable, nontoxic dose for
24 weeks.
Adults and children age 2 and older (Siklos):
20 mg/kg PO once daily. If blood counts are
in acceptable range, may increase dosage by
5 mg/kg daily every 8 weeks or if a painful
crisis occurs until mild myelosuppression
(ANC 2,000 to 4,000/mm^3) is achieved, or
up to a maximum dose of 35 mg/kg/day. If
blood counts are considered toxic, withhold
drug until counts recover. Resume treatment
after reducing dosage by 5 mg/kg daily.
Every 8 weeks thereafter, may adjust dosage
up or down in 5-mg/kg daily increments until patient is at a stable, nontoxic dose for
24 weeks. Discontinue permanently if hematologic toxicity develops twice.
➤ **Thrombocythemia ◆**
Adults: 15 to 20 mg/kg PO daily. Titrate to
maintain platelet count of 400,000/mm^3
or less and ANC of greater than 1,000
cells/mm^3.
➤ **Polycythemia vera ◆**
Adults: 0.5 to 2.5 g PO daily or 10 to
15 mg/kg/day PO for up to 16 years. Give
with concurrent aspirin therapy, unless contraindicated due to high risk of bleeding.

ADMINISTRATION
PO
● Wear gloves when handling drug or its
container, and wash hands before and
after contact with bottle or capsule. If
powder from capsule is spilled, wipe up
immediately with a damp towel. Dispose
of towel in a closed container such as a
plastic bag.
● Patient must swallow capsules whole;
don't open.
● Patient should take tablets with a glass of
water.
● The 1,000-mg tablets have three score
lines and can be split into four parts (each
250 mg).
● Don't split the 100-mg tablets into smaller
parts.
● For patients who can't swallow tablets,
disperse them immediately before use in a
small quantity of water in a teaspoon.

ACTION
May inhibit DNA synthesis.

Route	Onset	Peak	Duration
PO	Unknown	1–4 hr	24 hr

Half-life: 2 to 4 hours.

ADVERSE REACTIONS
CNS: malaise, fever, drowsiness. **GI:** anorexia, nausea, vomiting, diarrhea, stomatitis, constipation. **Hematologic:** *leukopenia, thrombocytopenia,* anemia, macrocytosis, megaloblastosis, *bone marrow suppression.* **Metabolic:** hyperuricemia, weight gain. **Skin:** rash, itching, alopecia, cutaneous vasculitic toxicities (including vasculitic ulcerations and gangrene), nail discoloration. **Other:** chills.

INTERACTIONS
Drug-drug. ❸ *Alert: Antiretrovirals (didanosine, stavudine):* May cause hepatotoxicity and hepatic failure, resulting in death. When given with didanosine to HIV-infected patients, severe peripheral neuropathy or fatal pancreatitis may occur. Avoid using with didanosine and stavudine.
Cytotoxic drugs, radiation therapy: May enhance toxicity of hydroxyurea. Use together cautiously.
Interferon: May increase the risk of cutaneous vasculitic toxicities, including vasculitic ulcerations and gangrene. Stop drug.
Live-virus vaccines: May increase risk of vaccine-related adverse reactions, viral replication, and severe infection. Avoid vaccinations during and for 3 months after therapy ends.
Drug-herb. *Echinacea:* May diminish therapeutic effect of immunosuppressants. Consider therapy modification.

EFFECTS ON LAB TEST RESULTS
• May increase BUN, creatinine, hepatic enzyme, and uric acid levels. May decrease Hb level.
• May decrease WBC, RBC, and platelet counts.
• May interfere with lactic acid, urea, or uric acid assays, resulting in falsely elevated results.

CONTRAINDICATIONS & CAUTIONS
• Contraindicated in patients hypersensitive to drug or its components.

• Don't initiate treatment if bone marrow function is markedly depressed. Bone marrow suppression may occur, and leukopenia is generally its first and most common manifestation. Thrombocytopenia and anemia occur less often, and are seldom seen without a preceding leukopenia.
• Use cautiously in patients with renal dysfunction and in the elderly.
Dialyzable drug: 50% to 74%.
⚠ *Overdose S&S:* Acute mucocutaneous toxicity; soreness, violet erythema on palms and soles followed by scaling of hands and feet; severe generalized hyperpigmentation of the skin; stomatitis.

PREGNANCY-LACTATION-REPRODUCTION
• Drug can cause fetal harm; don't use during pregnancy. Advise women of childbearing potential who are taking drug to avoid pregnancy.
• Verify pregnancy status of women of childbearing potential before initiating therapy.
• Females of childbearing potential should use effective contraception during and for at least 6 months after therapy. Males with female sexual partners of childbearing potential should use effective contraception during and for at least 1 year after therapy ends.
• Patient should discontinue breastfeeding or discontinue drug.
• Azoospermia or oligospermia, sometimes reversible, has been observed.

NURSING CONSIDERATIONS
Black Box Warning Droxia may cause severe myelosuppression. Monitor blood counts at baseline and throughout therapy. Treatment interruption and dosage reductions may be needed. ∎
Black Box Warning Droxia is carcinogenic. Monitor patient for malignancies. ∎
• Routinely measure BUN, uric acid, liver enzyme, and creatinine levels; monitor blood counts every 2 weeks.
• Use fetal Hb (HbF) level to evaluate drug's efficacy in sickle cell anemia. Obtain HbF level every 3 to 4 months. Monitor patient for an increase in HbF level of at least twofold over baseline.

Reactions in bold italics are *life-threatening*. Interactions may have a *rapid onset* or a *delayed onset*.

• Acceptable blood counts during dosage adjustment for sickle cell anemia are neutrophil count of 2,500/mm^3 or more, platelet count of 95,000/mm^3 or more, Hb level more than 5.3 g/dL, and reticulocyte count (if Hb level is below 9 g/dL) at least 95,000/mm^3. Toxic levels are neutrophil count less than 2,000/mm^3, platelet count less than 80,000/mm^3, Hb level less than 4.5 g/dL, and reticulocyte count (if Hb level is below 9 g/dL) less than 80,000/mm^3.

• Hydroxyurea may dramatically lower WBC count in 24 to 48 hours.

🛈 **Alert:** Patients who have received or are currently receiving interferon may be at greater risk for developing cutaneous vasculitic toxicities. Monitor patients closely; discontinue drug if toxicities occur.

🛈 **Alert:** Patients with HIV infection who are also receiving didanosine may be at increased risk for severe peripheral neuropathy and fatal pancreatitis. Avoid this combination.

• Monitor patient for pancreatitis. If it occurs, discontinue drug permanently.

• Drug may increase risk of hyperuricemia. Monitor fluid intake and output; keep patient hydrated.

• To prevent bleeding, avoid all IM injections when platelet count is less than 50,000/mm^3.

• Blood transfusions may be necessary for cumulative anemia.

• Dosage change may be needed after chemotherapy or radiation therapy.

• Auditory and visual hallucinations and hematologic toxicity increase when renal function decreases.

• Drug crosses blood-brain barrier.

• Radiation therapy may increase risk or severity of GI distress or stomatitis.

PATIENT TEACHING

• Tell patient and caregiver to wear gloves when handling drug or its container and to wash their hands before and after contact with the bottle or capsule. If powder from capsule is spilled, they should wipe up immediately with a damp towel and dispose of the towel in a closed container such as a plastic bag.

• Advise patient to watch for signs and symptoms of infection (fever, sore throat, fatigue) and bleeding (easy bruising, nosebleeds, bleeding gums, tarry stools) and to take temperature daily.

• Advise female patient of childbearing potential to use effective contraception during and for at least 6 months after therapy.

• Counsel breastfeeding patient to discontinue breastfeeding.

• Advise male patient with female sexual partner of childbearing potential to use effective contraception during and for at least 1 year after therapy ends.

• Inform male patient about the possibility of sperm conservation before start of therapy because azoospermia or oligospermia, sometimes reversible, has occurred.

Black Box Warning Advise patient to use sun protection and inform patient that monitoring for development of secondary malignancies will be needed. ∎

---

hydrOXYzine hydrochloride
hye-DROKS-i-zeen

Atarax♣

hydrOXYzine pamoate
Vistaril

Therapeutic class: Antihistamines
Pharmacologic class: Piperazine derivatives

AVAILABLE FORMS
hydroxyzine hydrochloride
Injection: 25 mg/mL, 50 mg/mL
Syrup: 2 mg/mL♣, 10 mg/5 mL
Tablets: 10 mg, 25 mg, 50 mg
hydroxyzine pamoate
Capsules: 25 mg, 50 mg, 100 mg
Oral suspension: Equivalent to 25 mg hydroxyzine hydrochloride/5 mL

INDICATIONS & DOSAGES
Adjust-a-dose (for all indications): In elderly patients, initiate drug at the lower end of dosage range and observe closely.
➤ **Anxiety**
Adults: 50 to 100 mg PO q.i.d. Or, 50 to 100 mg IM t.i.d. or q.i.d.
Children age 6 and older: 50 to 100 mg PO daily in divided doses.
Children younger than age 6: 50 mg PO daily in divided doses.

➤ **Preoperative and postoperative adjunctive therapy for sedation**
Adults: 25 to 100 mg PO or IM.
Children: 0.6 mg/kg/dose PO or 1.1 mg/kg/dose IM.
➤ **Pruritus**
Adults: 25 mg PO or IM t.i.d. or q.i.d.
Children age 6 and older: 50 to 100 mg PO daily in divided doses.
Children younger than age 6: 50 mg PO daily in divided doses.
➤ **Nausea and vomiting**
Adults: 25 to 100 mg/dose IM.
Children: 1.1 mg/kg/dose IM.

ADMINISTRATION
PO
• Give drug without regard for meals.
• Shake suspension well before giving.
IM
• Parenteral form (hydroxyzine hydrochloride) is for IM use only, preferably by Z-track injection.
🕚 *Alert:* Never give drug IV, subcut, or intra-arterially.
• Aspirate IM injection carefully to prevent inadvertent IV injection. Inject deeply into a large muscle (don't inject into lower and mid-third of upper arm).

ACTION
Suppresses activity in certain essential regions of the subcortical area of the CNS.

Route	Onset	Peak	Duration
PO	15–30 min	2 hr	Varies
IM	Rapid	Unknown	Varies

Half-life: Children ages 1 to 14, 4 to 11 hours; adults, 20 hours; elderly patients, 29 hours.

ADVERSE REACTIONS
CNS: drowsiness, dizziness, fatigue, involuntary motor activity. **GI:** dry mouth. **Respiratory:** respiratory depression. **Skin:** pain at IM injection site.

INTERACTIONS
Drug-drug. *Anticholinergics:* May cause additive anticholinergic effects. Use together cautiously.
CNS depressants: May increase CNS depression. Use together cautiously; dosage adjustments may be needed.

Epinephrine: May inhibit and reverse vasopressor effect of epinephrine. Avoid using together.
Drug-lifestyle. *Alcohol, cannabidiol, cannabis use:* May increase CNS depression. Discourage use together.

EFFECTS ON LAB TEST RESULTS
• May cause false-negative skin allergen tests by reducing or inhibiting the cutaneous response to histamine.
• May cause false-positive serum TCA screen.

CONTRAINDICATIONS & CAUTIONS
• Contraindicated in patients hypersensitive to drug, in those with known hypersensitivity to cetirizine hydrochloride or levocetirizine hydrochloride, and in patients with prolonged QTc interval.
• Drug can prolong QTc interval. Use cautiously in patients with risk factors for QTc-interval prolongation and in patients with conditions that predispose to QTc-interval prolongation and ventricular arrhythmia, as well as in those with recent MI, uncompensated HF, and bradyarrhythmias. Use cautiously during concomitant use of drugs known to prolong QTc interval.
• Use cautiously in patients with glaucoma, BPH, urinary stricture, asthma, or COPD and in elderly patients.
Dialyzable drug: Unknown.
⚠ *Overdose S&S:* Hypersedation.

PREGNANCY-LACTATION-REPRODUCTION
• Contraindicated in early pregnancy and in breastfeeding women.

NURSING CONSIDERATIONS
• If patient takes other CNS drugs, watch for oversedation.
• Drug may rarely cause acute generalized exanthematous pustulosis (AGEP), a serious skin reaction involving fever, pustules, and large areas of edematous erythema. Discontinue at first sign of rash, worsening of preexisting skin reactions, or other signs or symptoms of hypersensitivity. If signs or symptoms suggest AGEP, don't resume therapy.

Reactions in bold italics are *life-threatening*. Interactions may have a *rapid onset* or a *delayed onset*.

• Elderly patients may be more sensitive to adverse anticholinergic effects; monitor these patients for dizziness, excessive sedation, confusion, hypotension, syncope, and dysuria.

• *Look alike–sound alike:* Don't confuse hydroxyzine with hydroxyurea, Hydrogesic, or hydralazine. Don't confuse Vistaril with Restoril.

PATIENT TEACHING

• Warn patient to avoid hazardous activities that require alertness and good coordination until effects of drug are known.

• Advise patient against simultaneous use of other CNS depressants, and to avoid use of alcohol during therapy because drug may increase alcohol's effect.

• Tell patient to report all adverse reactions, especially heart palpitations, dizziness, fainting, difficulty breathing, difficulty urinating, or vision changes.

---

ibandronate sodium
eh-BAN-drow-nate

Boniva✔

Therapeutic class: Antiosteoporotics
Pharmacologic class: Bisphosphonates

AVAILABLE FORMS
Injection: 3 mg/3 mL prefilled syringes
Tablets ⒹⓃⒸ: 150 mg

INDICATIONS & DOSAGES
Adjust-a-dose (for all indications): In patients with severe renal impairment (CrCl less than 30 mL/minute), drug isn't recommended.
➤ **To treat or prevent postmenopausal osteoporosis**
Women: 150 mg PO once monthly on the same day each month, with a large glass of plain water. Or, for treatment, 3 mg IV bolus once every 3 months.
➤ **Hypercalcemia of malignancy** ◆
Adults: 2 to 6 mg as a single IV infusion over 15 minutes to 4 hours every 4 weeks. May give additional infusions up to 6 mg (including initial dose) if the albumin-corrected serum calcium level hasn't normalized by day 4 after the initial infusion.

➤ **Metastatic bone disease due to breast cancer** ◆
Adults: 6 mg IV every 3 to 4 weeks.

ADMINISTRATION
PO
• Give drug 1 hour before first food or drink of the day and before any other drugs.
• Make sure patient doesn't lie down for at least 1 hour after receiving drug.
• Give drug with plain water only.
• Patient should swallow tablets whole only. Don't allow patient to chew or suck tablets as this may cause oropharyngeal ulceration.
IV
▼ Prefilled syringes are for single use only.
▼ Give undiluted using needle provided with the syringe.
▼ Give by IV bolus over 15 to 30 seconds.
▼ Don't use if drug is discolored or contains particulate matter.
▼ Store at room temperature.
▼ **Incompatibilities:** Calcium-containing solutions and other IV drugs.

ACTION
Inhibits bone breakdown and removal to reduce bone loss and increase bone mass.

Route	Onset	Peak	Duration
PO	Unknown	½–2 hr	Unknown
IV	Rapid	Unknown	Unknown

Half-life: PO, 37 to 157 hours for the 150-mg dose; IV, about 4½ to 25½ hours.

ADVERSE REACTIONS
CNS: asthenia, dizziness, depression, fatigue, headache, insomnia, vertigo. **CV:** HTN. **EENT:** nasopharyngitis, pharyngitis. **GI:** dyspepsia, abdominal pain, constipation, diarrhea, gastritis, nausea, vomiting. **GU:** cystitis, UTI. **Musculoskeletal:** back pain, arthralgia, arthritis, joint disorder, limb pain, localized osteoarthritis, muscle cramps, myalgia. **Respiratory:** bronchitis, URI, pneumonia. **Skin:** rash. **Other:** allergic reaction, infection, influenza, tooth disorder.

INTERACTIONS
Drug-drug. *Aspirin, NSAIDs:* May increase GI irritation. Use together cautiously.

Drugs that prolong QTc interval: May enhance QTc-prolonging effects. For high-risk QTc-prolonging agents, consider therapy modification. For moderate-risk QTc-prolonging drugs, monitor therapy.
PPIs: May decrease ibandronate therapeutic effects. Monitor therapy.
Products containing aluminum, calcium, magnesium, or iron: May decrease ibandronate absorption. Give oral ibandronate 1 hour before vitamins, minerals, or antacids.
Drug-food. *Food, milk, beverages (except water):* May decrease drug absorption. Give oral drug on an empty stomach with plain water.

EFFECTS ON LAB TEST RESULTS
• May decrease calcium and total alkaline phosphatase levels.
• May interfere with bone-imaging agents.

CONTRAINDICATIONS & CAUTIONS
• Contraindicated in patients hypersensitive to drug and in those with uncorrected hypocalcemia. Oral form is contraindicated in those who can't stand or sit upright for 60 minutes.
❸ *Alert:* There may be an increased risk of atypical fractures of the thigh in patients treated with bisphosphonates.
❸ *Alert:* Drug may cause osteonecrosis, mainly in the jaw. Avoid invasive dental procedures if possible.
• Drug may cause hypocalcemia, especially if dietary intake of calcium or vitamin D is inadequate.
• Don't give to patients with severe renal impairment (CrCl less than 30 mL/minute).
• Use cautiously in patients with a history of GI disorders.
Dialyzable drug: Yes.
⚠ *Overdose S&S:* Hypocalcemia, hypophosphatemia, hypomagnesemia, upset stomach, dyspepsia, esophagitis, gastritis, ulcer.

PREGNANCY-LACTATION-REPRODUCTION
• There are no adequate studies in pregnant women. Use during pregnancy only if potential benefit justifies potential risk to the fetus.
• It isn't known if drug appears in human milk. Use cautiously in breastfeeding women.

NURSING CONSIDERATIONS
• Correct hypocalcemia or other disturbances of bone and mineral metabolism before therapy.
• Make sure patient has adequate intake of calcium and vitamin D.
• Obtain serum creatinine level and perform an oral exam before each dose in patients receiving IV ibandronate.
• Watch for signs of esophageal irritation (dysphagia, painful swallowing, retrosternal pain, heartburn).
• Monitor patient for bone, joint, and muscle pain, which may be severe and incapacitating and may occur within days, months, or years of start of therapy. When drug is stopped, symptoms may resolve.
• Watch for signs of uveitis and scleritis.
• Use care to avoid intra-arterial or paravenous administration, which can lead to tissue damage; must only be administered IV.

PATIENT TEACHING
• Tell patient receiving IV form that if a dose is missed, to reschedule the missed dose as soon as possible. Subsequent injections should be rescheduled once every 3 months from that dose. Patient shouldn't receive more than one dose in a 3-month time frame.
• Tell patient taking monthly dose to take it on same date each month and to wait at least 7 days between doses if patient misses a scheduled dose.
• Instruct patient to take oral drug 1 hour before any food or fluids and before any other drugs, including OTC drugs.
• Advise patient to swallow drug whole with a full glass of plain water while standing or sitting and to remain upright for at least 1 hour after taking drug.
• Advise patient to take calcium and vitamin D supplements as prescribed.
• Tell patient to report any bone, joint, or muscle pain.
• Advise patient to stop drug and immediately report signs and symptoms of esophageal irritation.
• Advise patient to have periodic dental exams to monitor for osteonecrosis of jaw.

Reactions in bold italics are *life-threatening*. Interactions may have a *rapid onset* or a *delayed onset*.

SAFETY ALERT!

ibrutinib ⚥
eye-BROO-ti-nib

Imbruvica

Therapeutic class: Antineoplastics
Pharmacologic class: Kinase inhibitors

AVAILABLE FORMS
Capsules ⓄⓃⒸ: 70 mg, 140 mg
Tablets: 140 mg, 280 mg, 420 mg, 560 mg

INDICATIONS & DOSAGES
Adjust-a-dose (for all indications): Recommended dosage for patients with mild hepatic impairment is 140 mg daily; for those with moderate hepatic impairment, recommended dosage is 70 mg daily. Avoid use in patients with severe hepatic impairment. Refer to manufacturer's instructions for toxicity-related and drug interaction dosage adjustments.
➤ **Patients with mantle cell lymphoma who have received at least one prior therapy**
Adults: 560 mg PO once daily until disease progression or unacceptable toxicity.
➤ **Patients with chronic lymphocytic leukemia or small lymphocytic lymphoma; patients with chronic lymphocytic leukemia or small lymphocytic lymphoma with 17p deletion** ⚥
Adults: 420 mg PO once daily as a single agent or in combination with bendamustine and rituximab or with obinutuzumab until disease progression or unacceptable toxicity.
➤ **Patients with Waldenström macroglobulinemia**
Adults: 420 mg PO once daily as a single agent or in combination with rituximab until disease progression or unacceptable toxicity occurs.
➤ **Patients with marginal zone lymphoma who have received at least one prior anti-CD20-based therapy**
Adults: 560 mg PO once daily until disease progression or unacceptable toxicity.
➤ **Chronic GVHD**
Adults: 420 mg PO once daily until GVHD progresses, underlying malignancy recurs, unacceptable toxicity occurs, or patient no longer requires treatment.

ADMINISTRATION
PO
• Give capsules whole with water at approximately same time each day.
• Patient should swallow capsules whole. Don't break, open, or crush capsules.
• Consider giving ibrutinib before rituximab or obinutuzumab, if applicable, when given on the same day.
• If a dose is missed, administer as soon as missed dose is remembered on same day; return to normal scheduling the following day. Don't give extra capsules to make up for missed dose.
• Drug is hazardous; use safe handling precautions.
• Store at room temperature in original package.

ACTION
Inhibits Bruton tyrosine kinase activity, resulting in decreased malignant B-cell proliferation and survival.

Route	Onset	Peak	Duration
PO	Unknown	1–2 hr	Unknown

Half-life: 4 to 6 hours.

ADVERSE REACTIONS
CNS: dizziness, headache, fatigue, pyrexia, asthenia, subdural hematoma, insomnia, pain, anxiety. **CV:** atrial fibrillation, atrial flutter, HTN, peripheral edema, intracranial hemorrhage. **EENT:** blurred vision, decreased visual acuity, dry eye, increased lacrimation, epistaxis, sinusitis. **GI:** diarrhea, nausea, constipation, abdominal pain, vomiting, stomatitis, dyspepsia, decreased appetite, GERD, *GI bleeding.* **GU:** UTI, *renal failure,* hematuria. **Hematologic:** *neutropenia, thrombocytopenia,* anemia. **Metabolic:** dehydration, hyperuricemia, *hypokalemia,* hypoalbuminemia. **Musculoskeletal:** arthropathy, musculoskeletal pain, muscle spasms, arthralgia, weakness. **Respiratory:** URI, pneumonia, dyspnea, cough. **Skin:** skin infections, bruising, rash, petechiae, pruritus. **Other:** chills, other malignancies, infection.

INTERACTIONS

Drug-drug. *Anticoagulants, antiplatelet agents, omega-3 fatty acids, vitamin E (systemic):* May increase risk of bleeding. Monitor bleeding risk and patient closely.

Digoxin: May increase digoxin level. Monitor drug concentrations.

Moderate CYP3A inhibitors (amprenavir, aprepitant, atazanavir, ciprofloxacin, crizotinib, darunavir, diltiazem, erythromycin, fluconazole, fosamprenavir, imatinib, verapamil): May increase ibrutinib level. Avoid concurrent use. If ibrutinib must be used, refer to manufacturer's product information for dosage adjustments and monitor patient for toxicities.

Strong CYP3A inducers (carbamazepine, phenytoin, rifampin): May decrease ibrutinib level. Avoid concurrent use and consider agents with less CYP3A induction.

Strong CYP3A inhibitors (clarithromycin, indinavir, itraconazole, ketoconazole, nefazodone, nelfinavir, posaconazole, ritonavir, saquinavir, telithromycin, voriconazole): May increase ibrutinib level. Avoid concurrent use or withhold ibrutinib for antibiotic or antifungal regimens lasting less than 7 days. Monitor patient closely for toxicities.

Drug-herb. *Flaxseed oil:* May enhance antiplatelet effect. Monitor therapy.

St. John's wort: May decrease ibrutinib level. Avoid use together.

Drug-food. *Grapefruit products, Seville oranges:* May increase ibrutinib level. Avoid use together.

EFFECTS ON LAB TEST RESULTS

• May increase uric acid and creatinine levels. May decrease Hb level.

• May increase lymphocyte count. May decrease platelet and neutrophil counts.

CONTRAINDICATIONS & CAUTIONS

• Contraindicated in patients hypersensitive to drug or its components.

• Drug may increase risk of renal failure. Fatalities have been reported.

• Avoid use in patients with severe hepatic impairment (Child-Pugh class C).

• Drug may cause atrial fibrillation or atrial flutter, particularly in patients with cardiac risk factors, HTN, acute infections, or a previous history of atrial fibrillation.

• Use cautiously in elderly patients because of increased risk of adverse effects.

• Drug may increase risk of hemorrhage in patients receiving antiplatelet or anticoagulant therapy. Watch for signs and symptoms of bleeding.

Dialyzable drug: Unknown.

PREGNANCY-LACTATION-REPRODUCTION

• Drug may cause fetal harm; avoid use in pregnant women. Patient should avoid pregnancy for 1 month after therapy ends.

• Obtain pregnancy test in women of childbearing potential before starting drug.

• Men should avoid fathering a child during therapy and for 1 month after final dose.

• It isn't known if drug appears in human milk. Patient should discontinue breastfeeding or discontinue drug.

NURSING CONSIDERATIONS

• Monitor patients for signs and symptoms of hypersensitivity reactions (wheezing, chest tightness, fever, itching, heavy cough, blue-colored skin, seizures, or swelling of face, lips, tongue, or throat).

• Fatal bleeding events have occurred. Monitor patients for bleeding and evaluate risk-benefit of use in patients receiving anticoagulants or antiplatelet drugs.

• Consider interrupting therapy for 3 to 7 days before and after surgery, depending on procedure type and risk of bleeding.

• Monitor patients closely for fever and other signs of infection. Serious, sometimes fatal, infections have occurred.

• Monitor blood counts monthly, as indicated.

• Monitor for hyperuricemia and evaluate renal function; maintain hydration.

• Evaluate patients for new malignancy during treatment.

• Monitor patients for HTN or cardiac abnormalities.

• Assess patient's baseline risk of TLS (high tumor burden) and take appropriate precautions. Monitor patient closely and treat appropriately.

PATIENT TEACHING

• Caution patient to swallow capsules whole and not to open, break, or chew them.

• Caution patient to immediately report signs and symptoms of significant hypersensitivity reaction (wheezing, chest tightness, fever, itching, heavy cough, blue-colored skin, seizures, or swelling of face, lips, tongue, or throat).

• Instruct patient to contact prescriber if diarrhea, nausea, vomiting, abdominal pain, fever, infection, bleeding, or easy bruising occurs.

• Caution female patient to avoid becoming pregnant during therapy and for 1 month after therapy ends. Counsel patient to use effective birth control during treatment because drug may cause harm to the fetus.

• Advise male patient to avoid fathering a child during therapy and for 1 month after final dose.

• Teach patient appropriate precautions for safe handling and disposal of drug.

ibuprofen
eye-byoo-PROH-fen

Advil ◊, Advil Liqui-Gels ◊, Caldolor, Children's Advil ◊, Children's Motrin Jr Strength ◊, Ibuprofen ◊, Infants' Advil Concentrated Drops ◊, Junior Strength Advil ◊, Novo-Profen✹, pms-Ibuprofen✹

ibuprofen lysine
NeoProfen

Therapeutic class: NSAIDs
Pharmacologic class: NSAIDs

AVAILABLE FORMS
ibuprofen
Capsules: 200 mg ◊
Injection: 800 mg/8 mL (100 mg/mL) in single-dose vials
Oral drops: 40 mg/mL ◊, 50 mg/1.25 mL ◊
Oral suspension: 40 mg/mL ◊, 100 mg/ 5 mL ◊
Tablets: 100 mg ◊, 200 mg ◊, 400 mg, 600 mg, 800 mg
Tablets (chewable): 50 mg ◊, 100 mg ◊
ibuprofen lysine
Injection: EQ 20 mg base/2 mL (EQ 10 mg base/mL)

INDICATIONS & DOSAGES
➤ **RA, osteoarthritis, arthritis**
Adults: 300 to 800 mg PO t.i.d. or q.i.d. Maximum daily dose is 3.2 g.
➤ **Mild to moderate pain; moderate to severe pain as an adjunct to opioid analgesics; fever reduction in children**
Children ages 12 to 17: 400 mg IV every 4 to 6 hours p.r.n. Infusion time must be at least 10 minutes. Maximum daily dose is 2,400 mg.
Children ages 6 months to younger than 12 years: 10 mg/kg IV up to a maximum single dose of 400 mg every 4 to 6 hours p.r.n. Infusion time must be at least 10 minutes. Maximum daily dose is 40 mg/kg or 2,400 mg, whichever is less.
➤ **Mild to moderate pain, fever**
Adults: 200 to 400 mg PO every 4 to 6 hours p.r.n. Or, for pain, 400 to 800 mg IV every 6 hours p.r.n.; for fever, 400 mg IV followed by 400 mg IV every 4 to 6 hours or 100 to 200 mg IV every 4 hours p.r.n. Infuse over at least 30 minutes. Maximum dose, 3,200 mg/day. Use smallest effective dose.
Children age 12 and older: 200 to 400 mg PO every 4 to 6 hours. Maximum daily dose is 1.2 g. Use smallest effective dose.
Children age 11 weighing 33 to 43 kg: 300 mg chewable tablets or 15 mL (300 mg) oral suspension PO every 6 to 8 hours up to q.i.d.
Children ages 9 to 10 weighing 27 to 32 kg: 250 mg chewable tablets or 12.5 mL (250 mg) oral suspension PO every 6 to 8 hours up to q.i.d.
Children ages 6 to 8 weighing 22 to 27 kg: 200 mg chewable tablets or 10 mL (200 mg) oral suspension PO every 6 to 8 hours up to q.i.d.
Children ages 4 to 5 weighing 16 to 21 kg: 150 mg chewable tablets or 7.5 mL (150 mg) oral suspension PO every 6 to 8 hours up to q.i.d.
Children ages 2 to 3 weighing 11 to 16 kg: 100 mg (5 mL) oral suspension PO every 6 to 8 hours up to q.i.d.
Children ages 12 to 23 months weighing 8 to 10 kg: 75 mg (1.875 mL) oral drops PO every 6 to 8 hours up to q.i.d.
Children ages 6 to 11 months weighing 5 to 8 kg: 50 mg (1.25 mL) oral drops PO every 6 to 8 hours up to q.i.d.

Adjust-a-dose: For children ages 6 months to 11 years, use weight to determine dosage if possible; otherwise, use age. If needed, dose may be repeated every 6 to 8 hours but no more frequently than q.i.d. or a maximum of 30 mg/kg in 24 hours. Consult a health care provider before giving ibuprofen 100 mg chewable tablets to children younger than age 6 or those weighing less than 22 kg, 50 mg chewable tablets to children younger than age 4 or those weighing less than 16 kg, 50 mg oral suspension to children younger than age 2 or those weighing less than 11 kg, or 50 mg oral drops to infants younger than age 6 months or those weighing less than 5 kg. Ibuprofen oral drops should be dosed at 7.5 mg/kg of body weight.

➤ **Relief of signs and symptoms of juvenile arthritis**
Children: Recommended dose is 30 to 40 mg/kg/day of oral suspension PO divided into three or four doses; patients with milder disease may be adequately treated with 20 mg/kg/day. Doses above 50 mg/kg/day aren't recommended because they haven't been studied and may increase risk of serious adverse events. Lower dosage to the smallest dose needed to maintain adequate symptom control when clinical effect is obtained.

➤ **Migraine**
Adults: 400 mg (2 capsules) PO in 24 hours.
➤ **Clinically significant patent ductus arteriosus (PDA) (ibuprofen lysine)**
Premature infants weighing between 500 and 1,500 g who are no more than 32 weeks' gestational age: 10 mg/kg IV followed by 5 mg/kg IV 24 hours later followed by a third dose of 5 mg/kg IV 24 hours after second dose.
Adjust-a-dose: If anuria or marked oliguria (urine output less than 0.6 mL/kg/hour) is evident at the scheduled time of the second or third dose, don't give additional dose until renal function has returned to normal. If the ductus arteriosus closes or is significantly reduced in size after completion of the first course of ibuprofen lysine, no further doses are necessary.

ADMINISTRATION
PO
• Give drug with milk or meals.

• Shake oral suspension and drops well before using.
IV
▼ Dilute drug with NSS, 5% dextrose, or lactated Ringer solution. For 800-mg dose, use at least 200 mL of diluent. In adults, give over at least 30 minutes; in children, over at least 10 minutes; in neonates, over at least 15 minutes (lysine injection).
▼ For weight-based dosing at 10 mg/kg, ensure that drug concentration is 4 mg/mL or less.
▼ Diluted solutions are stable for 24 hours at room temperature.
▼ Correct dehydration before administering drug.
▼ **Incompatibilities:** TPN solutions.

ACTION
May inhibit prostaglandin synthesis, to produce anti-inflammatory, analgesic, and antipyretic effects.

Route	Onset	Peak	Duration
PO	Variable	1–2 hr	4–6 hr
IV	Unknown	Unknown	Unknown

Half-life: 2 to 4 hours.

ADVERSE REACTIONS
CNS: dizziness, headache, nervousness. **CV:** edema, fluid retention. **EENT:** tinnitus. **GI:** abdominal pain, bloating, constipation, decreased appetite, diarrhea, dyspepsia, epigastric distress, flatulence, heartburn, nausea, nonnecrotizing enterocolitis, vomiting. **GU:** *acute renal failure,* azotemia, cystitis, hematuria. **Hematologic:** *agranulocytosis, aplastic anemia, leukopenia, neutropenia, pancytopenia, thrombocytopenia,* anemia, prolonged bleeding time. **Metabolic:** *hypokalemia, hypoglycemia.* **Skin:** pruritus, rash, injection-site irritation.

INTERACTIONS
Drug-drug. *Anticoagulants (warfarin):* May increase risk of serious GI bleeding. Use with extreme caution if concomitant use can't be avoided. Monitor patient closely. *Antihypertensives, furosemide, thiazide diuretics:* May decrease the effectiveness of diuretics or antihypertensives. Monitor patient closely.

Reactions in bold italics are *life-threatening*. Interactions may have a *rapid onset* or a *delayed onset*.

Aspirin: May negate the antiplatelet effect of low-dose aspirin therapy. Advise patient on the appropriate spacing of doses.

Aspirin, corticosteroids: May cause adverse GI reactions. Avoid using together.

Bisphosphonates: May increase risk of gastric ulceration. Monitor patient for signs of gastric irritation or bleeding.

Cyclosporine: May increase nephrotoxicity of both drugs. Avoid using together.

Digoxin, lithium: May increase levels or effects of these drugs. Monitor patient for toxicity.

Direct thrombin inhibitors (apixaban, dabigatran, desirudin, edoxaban, rivaroxaban): May increase risk of bleeding. Coadminister with caution.

Methotrexate: May decrease methotrexate clearance and increase toxicity. Use together cautiously.

SSRIs (fluoxetine, venlafaxine): May increase risk of upper GI bleeding. If use together is unavoidable, closely watch for signs and symptoms of GI bleeding. Consider acid suppression therapy.

Triamterene: May increase risk of acute renal failure. Avoid using together; if unavoidable, closely monitor renal function.

Drug-herb. *Dong quai, feverfew, garlic, ginger, ginkgo biloba, horse chestnut, red clover:* May increase risk of bleeding, based on the known effects of components. Discourage use together.

White willow: Herb and drug contain similar components. Discourage use together.

Drug-lifestyle. *Alcohol use:* May cause adverse GI reactions. Discourage use together.

Sun exposure: May cause photosensitivity reactions. Advise patient to avoid excessive sunlight exposure.

EFFECTS ON LAB TEST RESULTS

• May increase BUN, creatinine, ALT, AST, and potassium levels.

• May decrease glucose and Hb levels and hematocrit.

• May decrease neutrophil, WBC, RBC, platelet, and granulocyte counts.

CONTRAINDICATIONS & CAUTIONS

• Contraindicated in patients hypersensitive to drug and in those with angioedema, syndrome of nasal polyps, or bronchospastic reaction to aspirin or other NSAIDs.

Black Box Warning Contraindicated for the treatment of perioperative pain after CABG surgery. ■

Black Box Warning NSAIDs can increase risk of heart attack or stroke in patients with or without heart disease or risk factors for heart disease. ■

Black Box Warning Risk of heart attack or stroke can occur as early as the first weeks of using an NSAID. Risk appears greater at higher doses. Use lowest effective dose for shortest duration possible. ■

Black Box Warning NSAIDs may increase risk of serious GI adverse events, including bleeding, ulceration, and perforation of the stomach or intestines, which can be fatal. These events can occur at any time during use and without warning symptoms. Elderly patients are at greater risk for serious GI events. ■

• Ibuprofen lysine injection is contraindicated in preterm infants with significant renal impairment, proven or suspected untreated infection or necrotizing enterocolitis, thrombocytopenia, coagulation defects, active bleeding, and congenital heart disease in whom patency of the ductus arteriosus is necessary for satisfactory pulmonary or systemic blood flow.

⊙ *Alert:* NSAIDs increase risk of HF.

• Use cautiously in elderly patients and in patients with GI disorders, history of peptic ulcer disease, hepatic or renal disease, cardiac decompensation, HTN, asthma, or intrinsic coagulation defects.

• Long-term NSAID use may result in renal papillary necrosis and other renal injury.

• May increase risk of aseptic meningitis, with fever and coma, particularly in patients with SLE and related connective tissue disease. If signs or symptoms of meningitis occur, consider whether they're related to ibuprofen therapy.

Dialyzable drug: Unknown.

⚠ *Overdose S&S:* Abdominal pain, nausea, vomiting, lethargy, drowsiness, headache, tinnitus, nystagmus, CNS depression, seizures, hypotension, bradycardia, tachycardia, atrial fibrillation, metabolic acidosis, coma, acute renal failure, hyperkalemia, respiratory depression and failure.

PREGNANCY-LACTATION-REPRODUCTION
• There are no adequate studies in pregnant women. Drug can cause fetal harm and is contraindicated in pregnant women starting at 30 weeks' gestation. Before 30 weeks' gestation, use during pregnancy only if potential benefit justifies potential risk to the fetus.
• Drug appears in human milk. Patient should discontinue breastfeeding or discontinue drug.

NURSING CONSIDERATIONS
• Check renal and hepatic function periodically in patients on long-term therapy. Stop drug if abnormalities occur and notify prescriber.
• Monitor BP because drug can lead to new-onset HTN or worsening of preexisting HTN, which may contribute to the increased incidence of CV events.
• Because of their antipyretic and anti-inflammatory actions, NSAIDs may mask signs and symptoms of infection.
• Blurred or diminished vision and changes in color vision may occur.
• Full anti-inflammatory effects may take 1 or 2 weeks to develop.
◐ **Alert:** Watch for and immediately evaluate signs and symptoms of heart attack (chest pain, shortness of breath or trouble breathing) or stroke (weakness in one part or side of the body, slurred speech).
▨ **Black Box Warning** NSAIDs cause an increased risk of serious GI adverse events, including bleeding, ulceration, and perforation of the stomach or intestines, which can be fatal. Elderly patients are at greater risk. ▪
• Monitor patients for signs and symptoms of GI ulceration and bleeding.
• Monitor patient for signs or symptoms of aseptic meningitis (fever, headache, sensitivity to light, vomiting) and report immediately if they occur.
▨ **Black Box Warning** NSAIDs may increase the risk of serious thrombotic events, MI, or stroke, which can be fatal. The risk may be greater with longer use or in patients with CV disease or risk factors for CV disease. ▪

• If patient consumes three or more alcoholic drinks per day, drug may cause stomach bleeding.

PATIENT TEACHING
• Tell patient to take with meals or milk to reduce adverse GI reactions.
◐ **Alert:** Drug is available OTC. Instruct patient not to exceed 3.2 g daily for adults and children age 12 and older or 30 mg/kg for children ages 6 months to 11 years, not to give to children younger than age 6 months, and not to take for extended periods (longer than 3 days for fever or longer than 10 days for pain) without consulting prescriber.
• Tell patient that full therapeutic effect for arthritis may be delayed for 2 to 4 weeks. Although pain relief occurs at low dosage levels, inflammation doesn't improve at dosages less than 400 mg q.i.d.
• Caution patient that use with aspirin, anticoagulants, alcohol, or corticosteroids may increase risk of GI adverse reactions.
• Teach patient to watch for and immediately report to prescriber signs and symptoms of GI bleeding, including blood in vomit, urine, or stool; coffee-ground vomit; and black, tarry stool.
◐ **Alert:** Advise patient to seek medical attention immediately if chest pain, shortness of breath or trouble breathing, weakness in one part or side of the body, or slurred speech occurs.
• Tell patient to contact prescriber before using this drug if fluid intake hasn't been adequate or if fluids have been lost as a result of vomiting or diarrhea.
• Warn patient to avoid hazardous activities that require mental alertness until effects on CNS are known.
• Tell patient taking ibuprofen not to take other OTC NSAIDs, such as naproxen or Aleve, as these are in the same class.
• Advise patient to wear sunscreen to avoid hypersensitivity to sunlight.

ibutilide fumarate
eye-BYOO-ti-lyed

Corvert

Therapeutic class: Antiarrhythmics
Pharmacologic class: Methanesulfonanilide derivatives

AVAILABLE FORMS
Injection: 0.1 mg/mL in 10-mL vials

INDICATIONS & DOSAGES
➤ **Rapid conversion of recent-onset atrial fibrillation or atrial flutter to sinus rhythm**
Adults weighing 60 kg or more: 1 mg IV infusion over 10 minutes. May repeat dose if arrhythmia doesn't respond within 10 minutes after completing first dose.
Adults weighing less than 60 kg: 0.01 mg/kg IV infusion over 10 minutes. May repeat dose if arrhythmia doesn't respond within 10 minutes after completing first dose.

ADMINISTRATION
IV
▼ Give drug undiluted or diluted in 50 mL of diluent and add to NSS for injection or D_5W before infusion. Add contents of 10-mL vial (0.1 mg/mL) to 50-mL infusion bag to form admixture of about 0.017 mg ibutilide/mL. Use drug with polyvinyl chloride plastic bags or polyolefin bags.
▼ Give drug over 10 minutes.
▼ Stop infusion if arrhythmia is terminated or patient develops ventricular tachycardia or marked prolongation of QT or QTc interval. If arrhythmia doesn't respond within 10 minutes after infusion ends, may repeat dose.
▼ Admixtures with approved diluents are stable for 24 hours at room temperature and for 48 hours if refrigerated.
▼ Don't infuse parenteral products that contain particulate matter or are discolored.
▼ **Incompatibilities:** None listed by manufacturer. Consult a drug incompatibility reference for more information.

ACTION
Prolongs action potential in isolated cardiac myocytes and increases atrial and ventricular refractoriness, namely class III electrophysiologic effects.

Route	Onset	Peak	Duration
IV	≤90 min	Unknown	Unknown

Half-life: Averages about 6 hours.

ADVERSE REACTIONS
CNS: headache. **CV:** *sustained polymorphic ventricular tachycardia, AV block, bradycardia, HF,* ventricular extrasystoles, *nonsustained ventricular tachycardia,* hypotension, bundle-branch block, HTN, *prolonged QT interval,* palpitations, tachycardia. **GI:** nausea.

INTERACTIONS
Drug-drug. *Class IA antiarrhythmics (disopyramide, procainamide, quinidine), other class III antiarrhythmics (amiodarone, sotalol):* May increase potential for prolonged refractoriness. Don't give these drugs for at least five half-lives before and 4 hours after ibutilide dose.
Digoxin: Supraventricular arrhythmias may mask cardiotoxicity from excessive digoxin level. Use with caution in patients who may have an increased digoxin therapeutic range.
H_1-*receptor antagonists, phenothiazines, TCAs, tetracyclic antidepressants, other drugs that prolong QT interval:* May increase risk for proarrhythmia. Monitor patient closely.

EFFECTS ON LAB TEST RESULTS
None reported.

CONTRAINDICATIONS & CAUTIONS
Black Box Warning Administer drug only when the benefits of maintaining sinus rhythm outweigh the immediate risks of ibutilide administration and the risks of maintenance therapy. ■
• Contraindicated in patients hypersensitive to drug or its components.
• Contraindicated in patients with history of polymorphic ventricular tachycardia.
• Use cautiously in patients with hepatic or renal dysfunction.

• Safety and effectiveness of drug haven't been established in children.

• Drug's effectiveness hasn't been determined in patients with arrhythmias of more than 90 days' duration.

Dialyzable drug: Unknown.

⚠ *Overdose S&S:* Ventricular ectopy, ventricular tachycardia, third-degree AV block.

PREGNANCY-LACTATION-REPRODUCTION

• Drug causes fetal harm in animals. Use during pregnancy only if clearly needed and potential benefit justifies potential risk to the fetus.

• It isn't known if drug appears in human milk. Use isn't recommended in breastfeeding women.

NURSING CONSIDERATIONS

Black Box Warning Drug can cause potentially fatal arrhythmias. Only skilled personnel trained in identification and treatment of acute ventricular arrhythmias, particularly polymorphic ventricular tachycardia, should give drug. ▮

• Before therapy, correct hypokalemia and hypomagnesemia to reduce risk of proarrhythmia.

Black Box Warning Patients with atrial fibrillation lasting longer than 2 to 3 days must be adequately anticoagulated, generally over at least 2 weeks. ▮

• Monitor ECG continuously during administration and for at least 4 hours afterward or until QTc interval returns to baseline; drug can induce or worsen ventricular arrhythmias. Longer monitoring is required if ECG shows arrhythmia or patient has hepatic insufficiency.

• Don't give class IA or other class III antiarrhythmics with infusion or for 4 hours afterward.

PATIENT TEACHING

• Tell patient to report adverse reactions promptly.

• Instruct patient to alert nurse of discomfort at injection site.

SAFETY ALERT!

IDArubicin hydrochloride
eye-duh-ROO-bi-sin

Idamycin PFS

Therapeutic class: Antineoplastics
Pharmacologic class: Semisynthetic anthracyclines

AVAILABLE FORMS

Injection: 1 mg/mL in 5-, 10-, and 20-mL single-dose vials

INDICATIONS & DOSAGES

Dosages vary. Check treatment protocol with prescriber.

Black Box Warning Reduce dosage in patients with hepatic or renal impairment. Don't give idarubicin if bilirubin level exceeds 5 mg/dL. ▮

➤ **Acute myeloid leukemia, including French-American-British classifications M1 through M7, with other approved antileukemic drugs**

Adults: 12 mg/m^2 daily for 3 days by slow IV injection (over 10 to 15 minutes) with 100 mg/m^2 daily of cytarabine for 7 days by continuous IV infusion. Or, cytarabine may be given as 25-mg/m^2 bolus; then 200 mg/m^2 daily for 5 days by continuous IV infusion. A second course may be given, if needed.

Adjust-a-dose: If patient experiences severe mucositis, delay second course of therapy until recovery is complete; reduce dosage by 25%. Consider dosage reduction if bilirubin or creatinine level is above normal range. If serum bilirubin level is 2.6 to 5 mg/dL, give 50% of usual dose.

➤ **Acute myeloid leukemia (newly diagnosed)** ◆

Infants, children, adolescents: Per clinical trial CCG-2961, for induction and consolidation, 5 mg/m^2/dose IV daily for 4 days on days 0 to 3 in combination with cytarabine, etoposide, thioguanine, and dexamethasone. Or, for consolidation only, 12 mg/m^2/dose IV daily for 3 days on days 0 to 2 in combination with fludarabine and cytarabine.

Adjust-a-dose: For patients with GFR of 50 mL/minute/1.73 m^2 or lower and those

---

Reactions in bold italics are *life-threatening*. Interactions may have a *rapid onset* or a *delayed onset*.

on intermittent hemodialysis, peritoneal dialysis, or continuous renal replacement therapy, give 75% of dose.

ADMINISTRATION

IV

▼ Preparing and giving parenteral drug may be mutagenic, teratogenic, or carcinogenic. Follow facility policy to reduce risks.

Black Box Warning Give drug over 10 to 15 minutes into a free-flowing IV infusion of NSS or D₅W. Don't give IM or subcut. Drug is a vesicant; tissue necrosis may occur. ■

▼ If extravasation occurs, stop infusion immediately and notify prescriber; infusion may be restarted in another vein. Treat with intermittent ice packs for ½ hour immediately and then for ½ hour q.i.d. for 3 days. Elevate affected extremity.

▼ Vials are sterile and for single use only; contain no preservative.

▼ Store refrigerated (36° to 46° F [2° to 8° C]); protect from light. Keep in carton until time of use.

▼ **Incompatibilities:** Many other drugs.

ACTION

Inhibits nucleic acid synthesis and interacts with the enzyme topoisomerase II. Drug is highly lipophilic, which increases rate of cellular uptake.

Route	Onset	Peak	Duration
IV	Unknown	Few min	Unknown

Half-life: 20 to 22 hours; primary active metabolite (idarubicinol), more than 45 hours.

ADVERSE REACTIONS

CNS: headache, changed mental status, peripheral neuropathy, *seizures,* fever. **CV:** *hemorrhage, HF, MI, myocardial insufficiency, arrhythmias, myocardial toxicity,* atrial fibrillation, chest pain, asymptomatic decline in LVEF. **GI:** nausea, vomiting, cramps, diarrhea, mucositis. **GU:** renal dysfunction, red urine. **Hematologic:** *myelosuppression.* **Hepatic:** changes in hepatic function. **Metabolic:** hyperuricemia. **Skin:** alopecia, rash, urticaria, bullous erythrodermatous rash on palms and soles, erythema at previously irradiated sites, tissue necrosis

if extravasation occurs. **Other:** *infection,* hypersensitivity reactions.

INTERACTIONS

Drug-drug. *Alkaline solutions, heparin:* These combinations are incompatible. Don't mix idarubicin with other drugs unless specific compatibility data are known.

Inactivated vaccines: May diminish therapeutic effect of inactivated vaccines. Complete all age-appropriate vaccinations at least 2 weeks before starting drug.

Live-virus vaccines: May increase risk of vaccine-induced adverse reactions. Avoid use together. Don't give live-attenuated vaccines for at least 3 months after final drug dose.

EFFECTS ON LAB TEST RESULTS

• May increase uric acid level. May decrease Hb level.

• May decrease WBC, neutrophil, and platelet counts.

CONTRAINDICATIONS & CAUTIONS

Black Box Warning Don't give idarubicin if serum bilirubin level exceeds 5 mg/dL. ■

• Don't use in patients with preexisting bone marrow suppression unless benefits outweigh risks.

• Use cautiously in patients with impaired hepatic or renal function, previous treatment with anthracyclines or cardiotoxic drugs, or a cardiac condition.

Dialyzable drug: Unlikely.

⚠ *Overdose S&S:* Severe and prolonged myelosuppression, increased severity of GI toxicity, severe arrhythmia, acute cardiac toxicity, increased incidence of delayed HF.

PREGNANCY-LACTATION-REPRODUCTION

• There are no adequate studies in pregnant women. If used during pregnancy, or if patient becomes pregnant during therapy, inform her of potential hazard to the fetus. Advise women of childbearing potential to avoid pregnancy.

• It isn't known if drug appears in human milk. Patient should stop breastfeeding before using drug.

NURSING CONSIDERATIONS

Black Box Warning Drug should be given only under the supervision of a physician experienced in the use of cancer chemotherapeutic agents. ■

Black Box Warning Cardiotoxicity is the dose-limiting toxicity of drug. It is more common in those who have received prior anthracyclines or who have preexisting cardiac disease. No maximum cumulative lifetime dose for cardiotoxicity has been determined. ■

• CV adverse effects occur with greater frequency in older patients.

• Make sure patient is adequately hydrated before treatment. Hyperuricemia may result from rapid lysis of leukemic cells. Allopurinol may be ordered.

• Assess patient for systemic infection and ensure that it's controlled before therapy begins.

• Give antiemetics to prevent or treat nausea and vomiting.

• Monitor LFTs and renal function tests and CBC frequently.

• To prevent bleeding, avoid all IM injections when platelet count is below 50,000/mm³.

Black Box Warning Severe myelosuppression may occur. ■

• Anticipate need for blood transfusions for anemia.

• Notify prescriber if signs or symptoms of HF occur.

• *Look alike–sound alike:* Don't confuse idarubicin with daunorubicin or doxorubicin.

PATIENT TEACHING

• Teach patient to recognize and report signs and symptoms of extravasation.

• Warn patient to watch for signs and symptoms of infection (fever, sore throat, fatigue) and bleeding (easy bruising, nosebleeds, bleeding gums, tarry stools).

• Advise patient that red urine for several days is normal and doesn't indicate presence of blood.

• Caution female patient of childbearing potential to avoid becoming pregnant during therapy. Recommend that she consult prescriber before becoming pregnant.

idaruCIZUmab ℞
EYE-da-roo-siz-ue-mab

Praxbind

Therapeutic class: Antidotes
Pharmacologic class: Humanized monoclonal antibody fragments

AVAILABLE FORMS
Injection: 2.5 g/50 mL in single-use vials

INDICATIONS & DOSAGES
➤ **To reverse anticoagulant effects of dabigatran etexilate mesylate (Pradaxa) for emergency surgery or urgent procedures; for life-threatening or uncontrolled bleeding**
Adults: 5 g (two 2.5-g vials) as two consecutive IV infusions by hanging the vials or as two bolus injections, injecting contents of both vials consecutively, one after the other, using syringes.

ADMINISTRATION
IV
▼ Inspect for discoloration and particulate matter before giving. Solution is colorless to slightly yellow and clear to slightly opalescent.

▼ Give drug within 1 hour of removal from vial.

▼ A preexisting IV line may be used for administration, but line must be flushed with NSS before infusion.

▼ Don't administer other infusions at the same time using the same IV access.

▼ Store vials in refrigerator at 36° to 46° F (2° to 8° C). Don't freeze or shake.

▼ Before use, unopened vial may be kept at room temperature (77° F [25° C]) for up to 48 hours if stored in the original package to protect from light, or up to 6 hours when exposed to light.

▼ **Incompatibilities:** Other IV drugs or infusions.

ACTION
A humanized monoclonal antibody fragment that binds specifically to dabigatran and its acylglucuronide metabolites with higher affinity than the binding affinity of

dabigatran to thrombin, neutralizing dabigatran's anticoagulant effects within minutes.

Route	Onset	Peak	Duration
IV	Rapid	Unknown	24 hr

Half-life: 10.3 hours.

ADVERSE REACTIONS
CNS: headache, delirium, pyrexia. **GI:** constipation. **Metabolic:** *hypokalemia.* **Respiratory:** pneumonia. **Other:** *hypersensitivity.*

INTERACTIONS
None reported.

EFFECTS ON LAB TEST RESULTS
• May decrease potassium level.
• May prolong aPTT and ecarin clotting time.

CONTRAINDICATIONS & CAUTIONS
• Hypersensitivity and anaphylactoid reactions, such as pyrexia, bronchospasm, hyperventilation, rash, and pruritus, may occur. If reactions occur, discontinue drug.
• Reversing dabigatran therapy exposes patients to the thrombotic risk of their underlying disease. To reduce this risk, consider resumption of anticoagulant therapy as soon as medically appropriate. Dabigatran therapy can be started 24 hours after idarucizumab is given.
▨ *Alert:* Drug contains sorbitol. Use cautiously in patients with hereditary fructose intolerance, as serious and even fatal reactions, including hypoglycemia, hypophosphatemia, metabolic acidosis, increased uric acid level, and acute liver failure, have been reported. The minimum amount of sorbitol at which serious adverse reactions may occur in these patients isn't known.
Dialyzable drug: Unknown.

PREGNANCY-LACTATION-REPRODUCTION
• There are no adequate studies in pregnant women. It isn't known if drug can cause fetal harm or affect reproductive capacity. Use during pregnancy only if clearly needed.
• It isn't known if drug appears in human milk. Use cautiously in breastfeeding women.

NURSING CONSIDERATIONS
• For patients with elevated coagulation parameters and reappearance of clinically relevant bleeding, or who require a second emergency surgery or urgent procedure, an additional 5 g of drug may be considered. Safety and effectiveness of repeat treatment haven't been established.
▨ Assess patient for history of hereditary fructose intolerance before giving drug.
• Drug hasn't been studied in patients with hepatic impairment.
• Safety and effectiveness in children haven't been established.

PATIENT TEACHING
• Warn patient to immediately report signs and symptoms of hypersensitivity and anaphylactoid reactions (fever, bronchospasm, dyspnea, rash, itching), as drug will need to be discontinued.
• Instruct patient to seek immediate medical attention for signs or symptoms of bleeding.
• Warn patient that reversing dabigatran therapy exposes patient to the thromboembolic risk of the underlying disease. Advise patient that anticoagulant therapy may be resumed as soon as possible to reduce this risk.
▨ Teach patient with hereditary fructose intolerance to report this condition before receiving drug because drug contains sorbitol and may cause serious and even fatal reactions.

SAFETY ALERT!

idelalisib
eye-DEL-a-lis-ib

Zydelig

Therapeutic class: Antineoplastics
Pharmacologic class: Kinase inhibitors

AVAILABLE FORMS
Tablets ⓪: 100 mg, 150 mg

INDICATIONS & DOSAGES
➤ **Relapsed chronic lymphocytic leukemia, in combination with rituximab, in patients for whom rituximab alone would be considered appropriate therapy due to other comorbidities; relapsed**

follicular B-cell non-Hodgkin lymphoma or relapsed small lymphocytic lymphoma in patients who have received at least two prior systemic therapies

Adults: 150 mg PO b.i.d. Continue treatment until disease progression or unacceptable toxicity.

Adjust-a-dose: Refer to manufacturer's instructions for toxicity-related dosage adjustments.

ADMINISTRATION
PO
• Drug is considered hazardous; use safe-handling precautions.
• Give without regard for food.
• Patients should swallow tablets whole. Don't crush or split tablets.
• If a dose is missed by less than 6 hours, give missed dose right away and give next dose as usual. If a dose is missed by more than 6 hours, wait to give the next dose at the usual time.

ACTION
Induces apoptosis and inhibits proliferation in cell lines derived from malignant B cells and in primary tumor cell. Also inhibits several cell-signaling pathways to halt movement of B cells to lymph nodes and bone marrow.

Route	Onset	Peak	Duration
PO	Unknown	1½ hr	Unknown

Half-life: About 8 hours.

ADVERSE REACTIONS
CNS: headache, pain, night sweats, pyrexia, fatigue, asthenia, insomnia. **CV:** peripheral edema. **EENT:** nasal congestion, sinusitis. **GI:** abdominal pain, nausea, vomiting, *diarrhea,* decreased appetite, GERD, stomatitis, *colitis.* **GU:** UTI. **Hematologic:** anemia, *neutropenia, leukopenia, lymphocytopenia, thrombocytopenia.* **Hepatic:** *hepatotoxicity.* **Metabolic:** dehydration. **Musculoskeletal:** arthralgia. **Respiratory:** pneumonia, cough, dyspnea, bronchitis, URI. **Skin:** rash. **Other:** chills, oral herpes, *sepsis.*

INTERACTIONS
Drug-drug. *CYP3A inducers (carbamazepine, phenytoin, rifampin):* May decrease idelalisib concentration. Avoid use together.
CYP3A inhibitors (ketoconazole, nefazodone, ritonavir, telithromycin): May increase idelalisib level. Monitor patient for toxicity; modify dosage if adverse reactions occur.
CYP3A substrates (alfentanil, cyclosporine, dihydroergotamine, ergotamine, fentanyl, pimozide, quinidine, sirolimus, tacrolimus): May increase substrate concentration. Avoid use together.
Hepatotoxic drugs: May increase risk of hepatotoxicity. Don't use together.
Other drugs that cause diarrhea: May increase risk of diarrhea and toxicity. Avoid use together.
Drug-herb. *St. John's wort:* May decrease idelalisib concentration. Don't use together.

EFFECTS ON LAB TEST RESULTS
• May increase ALT, AST, GGT, bilirubin, and triglyceride levels. May decrease sodium level.
• May increase or decrease glucose level.
• May decrease Hb level and neutrophil and platelet counts.
• May increase or decrease lymphocyte count.

CONTRAINDICATIONS & CAUTIONS
• Contraindicated in patients hypersensitive to drug or its components and in those with history of anaphylaxis or toxic epidermal necrolysis when exposed to drug.
• Drug isn't indicated and isn't recommended as first-line treatment.
• Severe or life-threatening cutaneous reactions can occur. Discontinue drug for any severe reaction.
Black Box Warning Drug may cause serious or fatal hepatotoxicity, severe diarrhea or colitis, pneumonitis, infections, or intestinal perforation. ▋
• Safety and effectiveness in children younger than age 18 haven't been established.
Dialyzable drug: Unknown.

Reactions in bold italics are *life-threatening*. Interactions may have a *rapid onset* or a *delayed onset*.

PREGNANCY-LACTATION-REPRODUCTION

• Women of childbearing potential should avoid becoming pregnant while taking drug. If drug is used during pregnancy, or if patient becomes pregnant while taking drug, she should be told of potential hazard to a fetus.

• Obtain pregnancy test in women of childbearing potential before starting drug.

• Women of childbearing potential should use effective contraception during treatment and for at least 1 month after last dose.

• Men with female partners of childbearing potential should use effective contraception during treatment and for 3 months after final dose.

• It isn't known if drug appears in human milk. Patient shouldn't breastfeed during therapy and for at least 1 month after final dose.

NURSING CONSIDERATIONS

Black Box Warning Monitor AST, ALT, and bilirubin levels because hepatotoxicity may occur; monitor patient carefully and discontinue drug if necessary. Obtain baseline LFTs every 2 weeks for first 3 months of treatment, every 4 weeks for next 3 months, then every 1 to 3 months thereafter. Obtain LFTs weekly to monitor for hepatotoxicity if ALT or AST level rises above $3 \times$ ULN; monitor levels until resolved. Withhold drug if ALT or AST level is greater than $5 \times$ ULN; continue to monitor AST, ALT, and total bilirubin levels weekly until the abnormality is resolved. ∎

Black Box Warning Monitor patient carefully for diarrhea, colitis, and intestinal perforation (new or worsening abdominal pain, chills, fever, nausea, or vomiting); discontinue drug if necessary. ∎

Black Box Warning Monitor patient for respiratory signs and symptoms (cough, dyspnea, hypoxia, bilateral interstitial infiltrates on X-ray, decrease in oxygen saturation level by more than 5%). If pneumonitis is suspected, interrupt therapy until cause of the pulmonary symptoms has been determined. If pneumonitis is secondary to drug, discontinue drug and treat with corticosteroids. ∎

Black Box Warning Serious infections (pneumonia, sepsis, febrile neutropenia), including fatal infections, have occurred.

Monitor for signs and symptoms of infection and interrupt drug for grade 3 or higher infection. ∎

⚠ Alert: Consider *Pneumocystis jiroveci* pneumonia (PJP) prophylaxis. Interrupt treatment in patient with suspected PJP infection of any grade and permanently discontinue drug if PJP infection is confirmed.

⚠ Alert: Interrupt treatment for positive CMV infection until infection has resolved. Monitor for CMV reactivation at least monthly if drug is resumed.

• Fatal cases of SJS and toxic epidermal necrolysis (TEN) have occurred. If SJS or TEN is suspected, interrupt therapy until cause of the reaction has been determined. If SJS or TEN is confirmed, permanently discontinue drug. Other severe or life-threatening (grade 3 or more) cutaneous reactions also have been reported. Monitor patients for development of severe cutaneous reactions and discontinue drug as appropriate.

• Monitor CBC, ANC, and platelet count at least every 2 weeks for first 3 months of therapy, and at least weekly in patients whose neutrophil count is less than $1,000$ cells/mm^3.

• Drug responds poorly to antimotility agents given for diarrhea.

• Monitor patient for rash.

• Older patients may have increased risk of adverse effects. Monitor these patients carefully.

• Monitor patients for anaphylaxis; discontinue drug if anaphylaxis occurs.

• **Look alike–sound alike:** Don't confuse Zydelig with Zykadia.

PATIENT TEACHING

• Advise patient to take drug exactly as prescribed. If a dose is missed by less than 6 hours, tell patient to take missed dose right away and to take next dose as usual. If a dose is missed by more than 6 hours, advise patient to wait and take next dose at usual time.

Black Box Warning Instruct patient to report jaundice, bruising, abdominal pain, or bleeding. ∎

Black Box Warning Caution patient to immediately notify prescriber if the number of bowel movements in a day increases by six or more. ∎

Black Box Warning Warn patient to immediately notify prescriber if severe abdominal pain, chills, fever, nausea, or vomiting occurs, because of risk of colitis and intestinal perforation. ■

• Advise patient to immediately notify prescriber if fever or signs or symptoms of infection occur.

Black Box Warning Advise patient to report new or worsening respiratory signs and symptoms, including cough or dyspnea. ■

• Instruct patient that blood tests will be needed periodically, as ordered, to minimize risk of adverse reactions.

• Caution patient that drug may cause severe cutaneous reactions and to notify prescriber immediately if a severe skin reaction develops.

• Counsel female patient to avoid pregnancy and to use adequate contraception during therapy and for at least 1 month after therapy ends.

• Counsel male patient with female partner of childbearing potential to use effective contraception during treatment and for 3 months after final dose.

• Advise female patient to contact prescriber if she becomes pregnant or suspects she is pregnant.

• Caution patient not to breastfeed during therapy and for 1 month after final dose.

SAFETY ALERT!

ifosfamide
eye-FOSS-fa-mide

Ifex

Therapeutic class: Antineoplastics
Pharmacologic class: Nitrogen mustards

AVAILABLE FORMS
Powder for injection: 1-g, 3-g vials

INDICATIONS & DOSAGES
➤ **Germ cell testicular cancer**
Adults: 1.2 g/m^2 IV daily for 5 consecutive days. Repeat treatment every 3 weeks or after patient recovers from hematologic toxicity. Don't repeat doses until WBC count exceeds 4,000/mm^3 and platelet count exceeds 100,000/mm^3.

ADMINISTRATION
IV
▼ Preparing and giving drug may be mutagenic, teratogenic, or carcinogenic. Follow facility policy to reduce risks.

▼ Give a protective drug such as mesna to prevent hemorrhagic cystitis. Ifosfamide and mesna are physically compatible and may be mixed in the same IV solution.

▼ Obtain urinalysis before each dose. If microscopic hematuria occurs, notify prescriber. Adjust dosage of mesna, if needed. Adequate fluid intake (at least 2 L daily, either PO or IV) is essential before, and 72 hours after, therapy.

▼ Reconstitute each gram of drug with 20 mL of diluent to yield a solution of 50 mg/mL. Use sterile water for injection or bacteriostatic water for injection. Solutions may then be further diluted with sterile water, dextrose 2.5% or 5% in water, half-NSS or NSS for injection, dextrose 5% and NSS for injection, or lactated Ringer injection.

▼ Infuse each dose over at least 30 minutes.

▼ Refrigerate constituted or constituted and further diluted solutions and use within 24 hours. Benzyl alcohol–containing solutions can reduce stability of ifosfamide.

▼ **Incompatibilities:** Cefepime, mesna with epirubicin, methotrexate sodium.

ACTION
Cross-links strands of cellular DNA and interferes with RNA transcription, causing an imbalance of growth that leads to cell death. Not specific to cell cycle.

Route	Onset	Peak	Duration
IV	Unknown	Unknown	Unknown

Half-life: Dose-dependent mean terminal, 7 to 15 hours.

ADVERSE REACTIONS
CNS: somnolence, confusion, hallucinations, depressive psychosis, fever, *seizures, coma.* **GI:** nausea, vomiting, anorexia. **GU:** hemorrhagic cystitis, hematuria, dysuria, urinary frequency. **Hematologic:** *leukopenia, thrombocytopenia, myelosuppression,* anemia. **Skin:** alopecia. **Other:** infection, phlebitis.

Reactions in bold italics are *life-threatening*. Interactions may have a *rapid onset* or a *delayed onset*.

INTERACTIONS

Drug-drug. *Anticoagulants, aspirin, NSAIDs:* May increase risk of bleeding. Avoid using together.

CYP3A4 inducers (carbamazepine, fosphenytoin, phenobarbital, phenytoin, rifampin): May increase metabolism of ifosfamide to its active alkylating metabolites; may increase formation of the neurotoxic/nephrotoxic metabolite chloroacetaldehyde. Closely monitor patient for toxicities; consider dosage adjustment.

CYP3A4 inhibitors (aprepitant, fluconazole, fosaprepitant, itraconazole, ketoconazole, sorafenib): May decrease metabolism of ifosfamide to its active alkylating metabolites, perhaps decreasing effectiveness of ifosfamide. Monitor therapy.

Live-virus vaccines: May increase risk of vaccine-induced adverse reactions. Avoid using together.

Myelosuppressive drugs: May enhance hematologic toxicity. Dosage adjustment may be needed.

Drug-herb. *St. John's wort:* May increase risk of toxicities. Closely monitor patient and consider dosage adjustment.

Drug-food. *Grapefruit, grapefruit juice:* May decrease effectiveness of ifosfamide treatment. Monitor therapy.

EFFECTS ON LAB TEST RESULTS

● May increase creatinine, BUN, and liver enzyme levels.
● May decrease WBC and platelet counts.

CONTRAINDICATIONS & CAUTIONS

● Contraindicated in patients hypersensitive to drug and in those with severe bone marrow suppression or urinary outflow obstruction.
● Unless clinically essential, avoid giving to patients with WBC less than 2,000/mm³ and platelet count less than 50,000/mm³.
● Use cautiously in patients with renal impairment or compromised bone marrow reserve, as indicated by leukopenia, granulocytopenia, extensive bone marrow metastases, previous radiation therapy, or previous therapy with cytotoxic drugs.
● Drug and its metabolites are excreted by the kidneys. Dosage reduction may be considered.

● Drug is extensively metabolized in the liver and forms both efficacious and toxic metabolites. Use cautiously.
● Drug may suppress immune response and increase risk of serious infection, sepsis, or septic shock. Use cautiously.
Dialyzable drug: 75% to 100%.

PREGNANCY-LACTATION-REPRODUCTION

● Drug can cause fetal harm. Women shouldn't become pregnant and men shouldn't father a child during therapy and for up to 6 months after therapy ends.
● Drug appears in human milk. Women mustn't breastfeed during therapy.
● Drug interferes with oogenesis and spermatogenesis. Amenorrhea, azoospermia, and sterility in both sexes have been reported and appear to depend on drug dosage, duration of therapy, and state of gonadal function at time of treatment. Sterility may be irreversible in some patients.

NURSING CONSIDERATIONS

Black Box Warning Urotoxic adverse effects, especially hemorrhagic cystitis, and CNS toxicities, such as confusion and coma, may require cessation of ifosfamide therapy. Hemorrhagic cystitis can be reduced by prophylactic use of mesna. ∎

Black Box Warning Myelosuppression can be severe and lead to fatal infections. Monitor blood counts before and at intervals after each treatment cycle. ∎

● Ensure that patient is adequately hydrated during therapy.
● Patients are at increased risk for hemorrhagic cystitis. Obtain urinalysis before each dose. Withhold drug for microscopic hematuria (greater than 10 RBCs per high power field) until completely resolved.
● If cystitis develops, stop drug and notify prescriber.
● Bladder irrigation with NSS may be done to treat cystitis.
● Monitor CBC, renal function, and LFT values.
● To prevent bleeding, avoid all IM injections when platelet count is less than 50,000/mm³.
● Anticipate blood transfusions because of cumulative anemia.

• Assess patient for CNS toxicity, which may be severe and cause death; dosage reduction may be needed. Discontinue drug if encephalopathy occurs.

• *Look alike–sound alike:* Don't confuse ifosfamide with cyclophosphamide.

PATIENT TEACHING

• Remind patient to urinate frequently to minimize contact of drug and its metabolites with the lining of the bladder.

• Advise patient to watch for signs and symptoms of infection (fever, sore throat, fatigue) and bleeding (easy bruising, nosebleeds, bleeding gums, tarry stools). Tell patient to take temperature daily.

• Instruct patient to avoid OTC products that contain aspirin.

• Advise female patient to stop breastfeeding during therapy because of possible risk of toxicity to infant.

• Advise male patient to avoid fathering a child during therapy and for up to 6 months after therapy ends.

• Caution female patient of childbearing potential to avoid becoming pregnant during therapy. Recommend that she consult prescriber before becoming pregnant.

iloperidone
ill-oh-PER-ih-done

Fanapt

Therapeutic class: Antipsychotics
Pharmacologic class: Dopamine–serotonin antagonists

AVAILABLE FORMS
Tablets: 1 mg, 2 mg, 4 mg, 6 mg, 8 mg, 10 mg, 12 mg

INDICATIONS & DOSAGES
➤ **Schizophrenia**
Adults: Initially, 1 mg PO b.i.d. Increase dosage daily as needed according to the following dosing schedule: 2 mg PO b.i.d. on day 2; 4 mg PO b.i.d. on day 3; 6 mg PO b.i.d. on day 4; 8 mg PO b.i.d. on day 5; 10 mg PO b.i.d. on day 6; 12 mg PO b.i.d. on day 7. Maximum dosage is 12 mg PO b.i.d.

Adjust-a-dose: For patients who are poor metabolizers of CYP2D6 and those taking CYP2D6 inhibitors (fluoxetine, paroxetine, quinidine) or CYP3A4 inhibitors (clarithromycin, ketoconazole), reduce dosage by 50%. Patients with moderate hepatic impairment may need dosage reduction if clinically indicated.

ADMINISTRATION
PO
• Give drug with or without food.
• When restarting drug after discontinuation (more than 3 days), follow initial titration schedule.

ACTION
May antagonize dopamine type 2 and serotonin type 2.

Route	Onset	Peak	Duration
PO	Unknown	2–4 hr	Unknown

Half-life: 18 to 37 hours.

ADVERSE REACTIONS
CNS: aggression, delusion, dizziness, extrapyramidal effects, fatigue, lethargy, restlessness, somnolence, tremor. **CV:** hypotension, orthostatic hypotension, palpitations, tachycardia. **EENT:** blurred vision, conjunctivitis, dry mouth, nasal congestion, nasopharyngitis. **GI:** abdominal discomfort, diarrhea, nausea. **GU:** ejaculation failure, erectile dysfunction, urinary incontinence. **Hematologic:** hyperprolactinemia. **Metabolic:** weight gain, weight loss. **Musculoskeletal:** arthralgia, muscle spasm, musculoskeletal stiffness, myalgia. **Respiratory:** dyspnea, URI. **Skin:** rash.

INTERACTIONS
Drug-drug. *Alpha₁ blockers:* May enhance antihypertensive effects. Use together cautiously.
CYP3A4 or CYP2D6 inhibitors (clarithromycin, fluoxetine, ketoconazole, paroxetine, quinidine): May increase iloperidone level. Reduce dosage by half.
Dextromethorphan: May increase dextromethorphan level. Avoid use together.
Drugs that prolong QT interval: May cause lethal arrhythmias. Avoid use together.

Reactions in bold italics are *life-threatening*. Interactions may have a *rapid onset* or a *delayed onset*.

Opioids: May cause slow or difficult breathing, sedation, and death. Avoid use together. If use together is necessary, limit dosage and duration of each drug to the minimum necessary for desired effect.

Drug-lifestyle. *Alcohol use:* May increase CNS effects. Discourage use together.

EFFECTS ON LAB TEST RESULTS
• May increase lipid and glucose levels.
• May decrease WBC count and hematocrit.

CONTRAINDICATIONS & CAUTIONS
• Contraindicated in patients hypersensitive to drug or its components; anaphylaxis, angioedema, and other hypersensitivity reactions have been reported.

Black Box Warning *Opioid class warning:* Opioids should only be prescribed with benzodiazepines or other CNS depressants to patients for whom alternative treatment options are inadequate. ∎

Black Box Warning Fatal CV events may occur in elderly patients with dementia. Drug isn't approved for use in patients with dementia-related psychosis. ∎

• Avoid use with other drugs known to prolong QT interval and in patients with history of cardiac arrhythmias.

• Use cautiously in patients with history of stroke, TIA, QT-interval prolongation, diabetes, seizures, orthostatic hypotension, NMS, tardive dyskinesia, leukopenia, neutropenia, agranulocytosis, suicidal ideation, or priapism.

• Use cautiously in patients at risk for falls, including those with diseases or conditions or who are taking drugs that may cause somnolence, orthostatic hypotension, or motor or sensory instability.

• Use cautiously in patients with moderate hepatic impairment. Use in patients with severe hepatic impairment isn't recommended.

Dialyzable drug: Unknown.

⚠ **Overdose S&S:** Prolonged QT interval, drowsiness, sedation, tachycardia, hypotension.

PREGNANCY-LACTATION-REPRODUCTION
• There are no adequate studies in pregnant women. Use during pregnancy only if potential benefit justifies potential risk to the fetus.

ⓘ **Alert:** Neonates exposed to antipsychotics during the third trimester are at risk for developing extrapyramidal symptoms (repetitive muscle movements of face and body) and withdrawal symptoms (agitation, abnormally increased or decreased muscle tone, tremors, sleepiness, severe difficulty breathing, difficulty feeding) after delivery.

• It isn't known if drug appears in human milk. Use in breastfeeding women isn't recommended.

NURSING CONSIDERATIONS
• Symptom control may be delayed during the first 1 to 2 weeks of treatment compared to other antipsychotics that don't require similar titration.

ⓘ **Alert:** Obtain baseline BP measurements before starting therapy, and monitor BP regularly. Watch for orthostatic hypotension, especially during first dosage adjustments.

ⓘ **Alert:** Watch for evidence of NMS (hyperthermia, muscle rigidity, altered mental status, and autonomic instability), which is rare but can be fatal.

ⓘ **Alert:** Life-threatening hyperglycemia may occur in patients taking atypical antipsychotics. Monitor patients with diabetes regularly. Monitor fasting blood glucose level at drug initiation and periodically during therapy in patients with risk factors for diabetes.

• Monitor patient for tardive dyskinesia, which may occur with prolonged use of drug. If tardive dyskinesia occurs, discontinue drug unless patient's condition warrants continued use.

• Monitor patient for suicidal thinking and behavior.

• Complete fall risk assessments when initiating drug and recurrently for patients on long-term therapy, especially for those with diseases or conditions that increase fall risk and in those who are taking other drugs that could increase fall risk.

• Dispense lowest appropriate quantity of drug to reduce the risk of overdose.

• Monitor patient for weight gain.

• Periodically reassess patient to determine continued need for therapy.

• Monitor CBC frequently during the first few months of therapy and discontinue drug

if WBC count drops with no other underlying cause.
• Monitor potassium and magnesium levels at baseline and periodically in patients at risk for electrolyte imbalance.
• Drug may lower seizure threshold in patients with a history of seizures; monitor these patients closely.

PATIENT TEACHING
Black Box Warning *Opioid class warning:* Caution patient or caregiver of patient taking an opioid with a benzodiazepine, CNS depressant, or alcohol to seek immediate medical attention for dizziness, lightheadedness, extreme sleepiness, slowed or difficult breathing, or unresponsiveness. ■
• Warn patient to avoid driving and other hazardous activities that require mental alertness until the drug's effects are known.
• Tell patient drug can be taken with or without food.
• Warn patient to rise slowly, avoid hot showers, and use other precautions to avoid fainting when starting therapy and to reduce risk of falls.
• Advise patient to avoid becoming overheated or dehydrated.
• Tell female patient of childbearing potential to notify prescriber about planned, suspected, or known pregnancy.
• Advise breastfeeding patient not to breastfeed during therapy.
• Instruct patient to report symptoms of dizziness, palpitations, or fainting to prescriber.
• Advise patient to avoid alcohol use while taking drug.
• Tell male patient to seek emergency medical care if an erection lasts more than 4 hours.
• Warn patient and caregiver about risk of NMS; advise them to seek emergency medical care if symptoms occur.
• Tell patient to notify prescriber about other prescription or OTC drugs that patient is taking or plans to take.

iloprost
EYE-loe-prost

Ventavis

Therapeutic class: Pulmonary vasodilators
Pharmacologic class: Prostacyclin analogues

AVAILABLE FORMS
Inhalation solution: 10 mcg/mL, 20 mcg/mL in single-dose ampules

INDICATIONS & DOSAGES
➤ **PAH in patients with NYHA Class III or IV symptoms**
Adults: Initially, 2.5 mcg inhaled using the I-neb Adaptive Aerosol Delivery (AAD) or Prodose AAD systems. As tolerated, increase to 5 mcg inhaled six to nine times daily while patient is awake, as needed, but to no more than every 2 hours. Maximum, 5 mcg nine times daily.
Adjust-a-dose: For patients with hepatic impairment (Child-Pugh class B or C), consider increasing dosing interval to every 3 to 4 hours depending on patient response.

ADMINISTRATION
Inhalational
• Use only I-neb AAD or Prodose AAD delivery devices, per manufacturer's instructions.

ACTION
Lowers pulmonary arterial pressure by dilating systemic and pulmonary arterial beds. Drug also affects platelet aggregation, although effect in PAH treatment isn't known.

Route	Onset	Peak	Duration
Inhalation	Unknown	Within 5 min	30–60 min

Half-life: 20 to 30 minutes.

ADVERSE REACTIONS
CNS: headache, insomnia, syncope. **CV:** hypotension, vasodilation, chest pain, *HF, supraventricular tachycardia,* palpitations, peripheral edema. **GI:** nausea, tongue pain, vomiting. **GU:** *renal failure.* **Musculoskeletal:** trismus, back pain, muscle cramps. **Respiratory:** cough, dyspnea,

hemoptysis, pneumonia. **Other:** flulike syndrome.

INTERACTIONS
Drug-drug. *Anticoagulants, antiplatelet drugs:* May increase risk of bleeding. Monitor patient closely.
Antihypertensives, vasodilators: May increase effects of these drugs. Monitor BP.

EFFECTS ON LAB TEST RESULTS
• May increase alkaline phosphatase and GGT levels.

CONTRAINDICATIONS & CAUTIONS
• No known contraindications. Avoid using in patients whose systolic BP is less than 85 mm Hg.
• Use cautiously in elderly patients, patients with hepatic or renal impairment, and patients with COPD, severe asthma, or acute pulmonary infection.
• PAH may worsen if drug is withdrawn abruptly or dosages are reduced.
Dialyzable drug: Unknown.
⚠ *Overdose S&S:* Diarrhea, flushing, headache, hypotension, nausea, vomiting.

PREGNANCY-LACTATION-REPRODUCTION
• There are no adequate studies in pregnant women. Use during pregnancy only if potential benefit justifies potential risk to the fetus.
• It isn't known if drug appears in human milk. Patient should discontinue breastfeeding or discontinue drug.

NURSING CONSIDERATIONS
• Keep drug away from skin and eyes.
• The 2-mL ampule must be used with the Prodose AAD and may be used with the I-neb AAD. The 1-mL ampule must be used only with the I-neb AAD.
• Monitor patient's vital signs carefully at start of treatment. Monitor patient for syncope.
• If patient develops evidence of pulmonary edema, stop treatment immediately.

PATIENT TEACHING
• Warn patient not to drink drug and that drug is for inhalation only.

• Advise patient to take drug exactly as prescribed.
• Advise patient to keep a backup Prodose AAD or I-neb AAD in case the original malfunctions.
• Tell patient to keep drug away from skin and eyes and to rinse the area immediately if contact occurs.
• Inform patient that drug may cause dizziness and fainting. Urge patient to stand up slowly from a sitting or lying position and to report to prescriber worsening of symptoms.
• Tell patient to take drug before physical exertion, no more than every 2 hours.
• Tell patient not to expose others, especially pregnant women and infants, to drug.
• Teach patient how to clean equipment and safely dispose of used ampules after each treatment. Caution patient not to save or use leftover solution.

SAFETY ALERT!

imatinib mesylate 🅖
eh-MAT-eh-nib

Gleevec

Therapeutic class: Antineoplastics
Pharmacologic class: Protein–tyrosine kinase inhibitors

AVAILABLE FORMS
Tablets 🅞🆃🅒: 100 mg, 400 mg

INDICATIONS & DOSAGES
Adjust-a-dose (for all indications): For patients with CrCl of 40 to 59 mL/minute, don't exceed 600 mg daily; if CrCl is 20 to 39 mL/minute, decrease starting dose by 50% and don't exceed 400 mg daily; if CrCl is less than 20 mL/minute, don't exceed 100 mg daily. For patients with severe hepatic impairment, reduce dosage by 25%. See manufacturer's package insert for full details on dosage adjustments for children; patients with neutropenia, thrombocytopenia, or hepatotoxicity; and those with adverse reactions.
➤ **Relapsed or refractory Philadelphia chromosome–positive (Ph+) acute lymphoblastic leukemia (ALL)** 🅖
Adults: 600 mg PO daily.

➤ **Newly diagnosed Ph+ ALL in pediatric patients in combination with chemotherapy** ⊠
Children age 1 and older: 340 mg/m^2 PO daily. Maximum dosage is 600 mg daily.
➤ **Aggressive systemic mastocytosis (ASM) without the D816V c-*Kit* mutation or with c-*Kit* mutational status unknown** ⊠
Adults: 400 mg PO daily.
Adjust-a-dose: For patients with ASM associated with eosinophilia, a clonal hematologic disease related to the fusion kinase FIP1L1-PDGFRα, initial dose is 100 mg/day. Increase dose from 100 mg to 400 mg/day if no adverse drug reactions occur and if there is insufficient response to therapy.
➤ **Hypereosinophilic syndrome (HES) or chronic eosinophilic leukemia (CEL), or both** ⊠
Adults: 400 mg PO daily.
Adjust-a-dose: In HES/CEL patients with demonstrated FIP1L1-PDGFRα fusion kinase, initial dose is 100 mg/day. Increase dose from 100 mg to 400 mg/day if no adverse drug reactions occur and if there is insufficient response to therapy.
➤ **Myelodysplastic syndrome (MDS) or myeloproliferative disease (MPD) with *PDGFR* gene rearrangements** ⊠
Adults: 400 mg PO daily.
➤ **Unresectable, recurrent, or metastatic dermatofibrosarcoma protuberans**
Adults: 400 mg PO b.i.d. (800 mg/day).
➤ **Chronic myeloid leukemia (CML) in blast crisis, in accelerated phase, or in chronic phase after failure of alfa interferon therapy; newly diagnosed Ph+ chronic-phase CML** ⊠
Adults: For chronic-phase CML, 400 mg PO daily as single dose. For accelerated-phase CML or blast crisis, 600 mg PO daily as single dose. Continue treatment as long as patient continues to benefit. May increase daily dose to 600 mg PO in chronic phase or to 800 mg PO (400 mg PO b.i.d.) in accelerated phase or blast crisis.
Children age 1 and older: For newly diagnosed Ph+ chronic-phase CML only, give 340 mg/m^2 daily PO. Don't exceed 600 mg/day.

➤ *Kit* **(CD117)-positive or GI stromal tumors (GISTs) after resection** ⊠
Adults: 400 mg PO daily.
➤ *Kit*-**positive unresectable or metastatic malignant GISTs** ⊠
Adults: 400 mg PO daily or b.i.d.

ADMINISTRATION
PO
• Give with a meal and large glass of water.
• Administer 400-mg or 600-mg dose once daily. Give 800-mg dose as 400 mg b.i.d.
• For daily dosing of 800 mg and above, use the 400-mg tablet to reduce exposure to iron.
• For patients unable to swallow tablets, disperse the tablets in water or apple juice (50 mL for 100-mg tablet and 200 mL for 400-mg tablet). Stir and have patient drink immediately.
• Drug is hazardous. Avoid exposure to crushed tablets. If necessary to manipulate tablets (e.g., to prepare an oral solution), double gloving, wearing a protective gown, and preparing in a controlled device is recommended.

ACTION
Inhibits the abnormal tyrosine kinase created by the Philadelphia chromosome abnormality in CML; it inhibits tumor growth of murine myeloid cells and leukemia lines from CML patients in blast crisis.

Route	Onset	Peak	Duration
PO	Unknown	2–4 hr	Unknown

Half-life: Adults, 18 hours (parent drug), 40 hours (active metabolite); children, 15 hours (parent drug).

ADVERSE REACTIONS
CNS: *cerebral hemorrhage,* fatigue, headache, pyrexia, weakness, depression, dizziness, insomnia, anxiety. **CV:** edema. **EENT:** epistaxis, nasopharyngitis. **GI:** *GI hemorrhage,* abdominal pain, anorexia, constipation, diarrhea, dyspepsia, nausea, vomiting. **Hematologic:** *hemorrhage, neutropenia, thrombocytopenia,* anemia. **Metabolic:** hypokalemia, weight increase. **Musculoskeletal:** arthralgia, myalgia, muscle cramps, musculoskeletal pain, growth suppression in children. **Respiratory:** cough, dyspnea, pneumonia.

Reactions in bold italics are *life-threatening.* Interactions may have a *rapid onset* or a *delayed onset.*

Skin: petechiae, rash, pruritus. **Other:** night sweats.

INTERACTIONS
Drug-drug. *CYP3A4 inducers (carbamazepine, dexamethasone, phenobarbital, phenytoin, rifampin):* May decrease imatinib level. Avoid concurrent use when possible. If combination must be used, increase imatinib dosage by at least 50%; monitor patient closely.

CYP3A4 inhibitors (clarithromycin, erythromycin, itraconazole, ketoconazole): May decrease metabolism and increase imatinib level. Monitor patient for toxicity.

Dihydropyridine–calcium channel blockers, certain HMG-CoA reductase inhibitors (simvastatin), cyclosporine, pimozide, triazolo-benzodiazepines: May increase levels of these drugs. Monitor patient for toxicity, and obtain drug levels, if appropriate.

Levothyroxine: May increase levothyroxine clearance, causing increased TSH levels and symptoms of hypothyroidism. Monitor thyroid function.

Warfarin: May alter metabolism of warfarin. Avoid using together; use standard heparin or a low–molecular-weight heparin.

Drug-herb. *Ginseng:* May increase risk of hepatotoxicity. Avoid use together.

St. John's wort: May decrease drug effects. Discourage use together.

Drug-food. *Grapefruit juice:* May increase imatinib level. Patient should avoid grapefruit juice.

EFFECTS ON LAB TEST RESULTS
• May increase creatinine, bilirubin, alkaline phosphatase, AST, and ALT levels. May decrease potassium and Hb levels.
• May decrease neutrophil and platelet counts.

CONTRAINDICATIONS & CAUTIONS
• Contraindicated in patients hypersensitive to drug or its components.
• Use cautiously in elderly patients and in those with hepatic or renal impairment.
• Severe HF and left ventricular dysfunction have occurred in patients taking imatinib. Use cautiously in patients with cardiac disease or risk factors for HF.

• Growth retardation has occurred in children and preadolescents receiving imatinib; long-term effects of prolonged treatment are unknown.
• Safety and effectiveness in children younger than age 1 haven't been established.
Dialyzable drug: Unknown.

⚠ **Overdose S&S:** Muscle cramps; ascites; creatinine, AST, ALT, and bilirubin levels.

PREGNANCY-LACTATION-REPRODUCTION
• Drug can harm fetus. Sexually active women should use highly effective contraception during therapy and for 14 days after final dose. A pregnancy test should be done before start of therapy.
• Drug appears in human milk. Patient shouldn't breastfeed during treatment and for 1 month after final dose.

NURSING CONSIDERATIONS
🧬 In adults with MDS/MPD or ASM, determine *PDGFRB* gene rearrangements status or D816V c-*Kit* mutational status, respectively, before starting therapy. For information on FDA-approved tests for detection of *PDGFRB* rearrangements and D816V c-*Kit* mutational status, go to www.fda.gov/medical-devices/vitro-diagnostics/companion-diagnostics.
• Monitor patient closely for possibly severe fluid retention. Elderly patients may have an increased risk of edema.
• There have been postmarketing reports of severe bullous skin reactions. Monitor patient for skin reactions. Drug may need to be withheld.
• Fatal TLS can occur. Correct dehydration and treat high uric acid levels before starting therapy.
• Monitor weight daily. Report unexpected, rapid weight gain.
• Monitor CBC weekly for first month, every other week for second month, and periodically thereafter.
• Monitor LFTs carefully because hepatotoxicity (occasionally severe) may occur; decrease dosage as needed.
• Monitor growth of children being treated with imatinib.
• May increase dosage if no severe adverse reactions or severe non–leukemia-related neutropenia or thrombocytopenia occur

in the following circumstances: disease progression, failure to achieve a satisfactory hematologic response after at least 3 months of treatment, or loss of a previously achieved hematologic response.

▓ In patients with HES and cardiac involvement, cases of cardiogenic shock/left ventricular dysfunction have been associated with the initiation of imatinib therapy. The condition is reversible with administration of systemic steroids and circulatory support measures, and by temporarily withholding imatinib. Monitor echocardiogram and serum troponin in patients with HES/CEL and in patients with MDS/MPD or ASM associated with high eosinophil levels.

▓ Grade 3/4 hemorrhage has been reported in patients with newly diagnosed CML and with GIST. GI tumor sites may be the source of GI bleeds in GIST.

• GI perforations, some fatal, have been reported.

PATIENT TEACHING

• Tell patient to take drug with food and a large glass of water.

• Advise patient unable to swallow tablets to mix them uncrushed in water or apple juice (50 mL for 100-mg tablet and 200 mL for 400-mg tablet) and to stir and drink immediately.

• Advise patient to report adverse effects, such as fluid retention and sudden weight gain.

• Advise patient that periodic laboratory tests will be needed to monitor therapy.

• Inform patient and caregivers that growth retardation has occurred in children and preadolescents receiving imatinib, and that long-term effects of prolonged treatment are unknown. Monitor growth closely.

• Advise patient of the risk of dizziness, blurred vision, or somnolence during treatment and to use caution when driving a car or operating machinery.

• Advise female patient that drug may cause fetal harm. Caution her to avoid pregnancy during therapy and for 14 days after therapy ends and to inform prescriber if she suspects pregnancy.

• Advise female patient not to breastfeed during therapy and for 1 month after final dose.

imipenem–cilastatin sodium
im-ih-PEN-em/sye-la-STAT-in

Primaxin 500✚, Primaxin IV

Therapeutic class: Antibiotics
Pharmacologic class: Carbapenems–beta-lactams

AVAILABLE FORMS
Powder for injection: 250 mg, 500 mg

INDICATIONS & DOSAGES
Adjust-a-dose (for all indications): If CrCl is less than 90 mL/minute, adjust dosage and monitor renal function test results. Consult manufacturer's package insert for specific dosage adjustments. For patients on hemodialysis, administer dose after hemodialysis and at intervals timed from the end of that dialysis session. Drug isn't recommended in children with renal impairment who weigh less than 30 kg.

➤ **Serious lower respiratory tract, bone, intra-abdominal, gynecologic, joint, skin, and soft-tissue infections; UTIs; endocarditis; and bacterial septicemia, caused by** *Acinetobacter, Enterococcus, Staphylococcus aureus, Streptococcus, Escherichia coli, Haemophilus, Klebsiella, Morganella, Proteus, Enterobacter, Pseudomonas aeruginosa,* **or** *Bacteroides,* **including** *B. fragilis*
Adults: For susceptible bacterial species, give 500 mg IV every 6 hours or 1,000 mg IV every 8 hours. For intermediate susceptibility bacterial species, give 1,000 mg IV every 6 hours. Refer to manufacturer's package insert for susceptibility test interpretive criteria. Maximum dosage is 4,000 mg/day.
Children age 3 months and older (except for CNS infections): 15 to 25 mg/kg IV every 6 hours. Maximum daily dose is 4 g.
Infants ages 4 weeks to 3 months weighing 1.5 kg or more (except for CNS infections): 25 mg/kg IV every 6 hours.
Neonates ages 1 to 4 weeks weighing 1.5 kg or more (except for CNS infections): 25 mg/kg IV every 8 hours.
Neonates younger than age 1 week weighing 1.5 kg or more (except for CNS infections): 25 mg/kg IV every 12 hours.

Reactions in bold italics are *life-threatening*. Interactions may have a *rapid onset* or a **delayed onset**.

➤ **Neutropenic fever ◆**
Adults: 500 mg IV every 6 hours.

ADMINISTRATION

IV

▼ Obtain specimens for culture and sensitivity testing before giving first dose. Begin therapy while awaiting results.

 Alert: Don't use diluents containing benzyl alcohol to reconstitute drug for administration to neonates; benzyl alcohol has been associated with toxicity in neonates. While toxicity hasn't been demonstrated in children older than age 3 months, small children in this age range may also be at risk for benzyl alcohol toxicity.

▼ Reconstitute powder by adding approximately 10 mL of appropriate diluent to vial; shake until solution is clear. Solution may be colorless to yellow; color variations within this range don't affect drug's potency.

▼ After reconstitution, transfer resulting suspension to 100 mL of an appropriate infusion solution. Repeat transfer of resulting suspension with an additional 10 mL of infusion solution to ensure complete transfer of vial contents to infusion solution. Agitate resulting mixture until clear before administering by IV infusion.

▼ After reconstitution, solution is stable for 4 hours at room temperature and for 24 hours when refrigerated.

▼ Refer to manufacturer's instructions for reconstitution, preparation, and storage instructions for ADD-Vantage vials.

▼ Don't give by direct IV bolus injection.

▼ For adults with normal renal function, give each 500-mg dose by IV infusion over 20 to 30 minutes. Infuse each 1-g dose over 40 to 60 minutes. For adults with renal impairment, refer to manufacturer's instructions for infusion rates.

▼ For children, infuse doses of 500 mg or less over 20 to 30 minutes. Infuse doses greater than 500 mg over 40 to 60 minutes. If nausea occurs, the infusion may be slowed.

▼ **Incompatibilities:** Allopurinol, antibiotics, amiodarone, azithromycin, fluconazole, gemcitabine, lorazepam, meperidine, midazolam, milrinone, sargramostim, sodium bicarbonate.

ACTION

Inhibits bacterial cell-wall synthesis. Cilastatin prevents metabolism of imipenem, resulting in increased urinary recovery and decreased renal toxicity.

Route	Onset	Peak	Duration
IV	Immediate	Immediate	Unknown

Half-life: 1 hour after IV dose.

ADVERSE REACTIONS

CNS: *seizures.* **CV:** thrombophlebitis, phlebitis, tachycardia. **GI:** diarrhea, nausea, vomiting, gastroenteritis, oral candidiasis. **GU:** urine discoloration, oliguria, anuria. **Skin:** injection-site irritation, rash.

INTERACTIONS

Drug-drug. *Cyclosporine:* May increase CNS adverse effects. Use together cautiously.
Ganciclovir: May cause seizures. Avoid using together.
Probenecid: May increase imipenem level. Don't give concurrently.
Valproic acid: May decrease valproic acid level and increase risk of seizures. Monitor patient and valproic acid level carefully. Adjust valproic acid level or consider alternative antibiotic.

EFFECTS ON LAB TEST RESULTS

● May increase BUN, creatinine, ALT, AST, alkaline phosphatase, bilirubin, chloride, and LDH levels. May increase or decrease sodium level.

● May increase eosinophil count. May decrease Hb level, hematocrit, and WBC and platelet counts.

● May interfere with glucose determination by Benedict solution, Fehling's solution, or Clinitest.

CONTRAINDICATIONS & CAUTIONS

● Contraindicated in patients hypersensitive to drug or its components and in those with CrCl of 5 mL/minute/1.73 m^2 or less unless hemodialysis is begun within 48 hours.

● Patients with CrCl of 15 to less than 30 mL/minute may have an increased risk of seizures.

● Use cautiously in patients allergic to penicillins or cephalosporins because drug has

similar chemical structure. Also use cautiously in patients with a history of sensitivity to multiple allergens. Serious anaphylactic reactions require immediate emergency measures.
- Use cautiously in patients with history of seizure disorders, especially if they also have compromised renal function.
- Drug may cause CDAD, ranging in severity from mild to fatal colitis and occurring even 2 months after drug administration.
- Prolonged use may result in superinfection.
- Repeated evaluation of patient's condition is essential.
- Use cautiously in children younger than age 3 months. Drug isn't recommended in children with impaired renal function who weigh less than 30 kg.
- Drug isn't indicated in patients with meningitis; safety and effectiveness haven't been established.
Dialyzable drug: Yes.

PREGNANCY-LACTATION-REPRODUCTION
- There are no adequate studies in pregnant women. Use during pregnancy only if potential benefit justifies potential hazards to the fetus.
- It isn't known if drug appears in human milk. Use cautiously in breastfeeding women.

NURSING CONSIDERATIONS
⚠ *Alert:* Don't use for CNS infections in children because of seizure risk.
⚠ *Alert:* If seizures develop and persist despite anticonvulsant therapy, stop drug.
- For patients receiving hemodialysis, drug is recommended only when benefits outweigh possible risk of seizures.
- Monitor patient for superinfections during and after therapy.
- Monitor organ system functions, including renal, hepatic, and hematopoietic, during prolonged therapy.

PATIENT TEACHING
- Instruct patient to report adverse reactions promptly.
- Tell patient to report discomfort at IV insertion site.

- Urge patient to notify prescriber as soon as possible about loose stools or diarrhea.
- Advise patient taking valproic acid or divalproex sodium that seizure therapy may need adjustment.

imipramine hydrochloride
im-IP-ra-meen

Tofranil

imipramine pamoate

Therapeutic class: Antidepressants
Pharmacologic class: TCAs

AVAILABLE FORMS
imipramine hydrochloride
Tablets: 10 mg, 25 mg, 50 mg
imipramine pamoate
Capsules: 75 mg, 100 mg, 125 mg, 150 mg

INDICATIONS & DOSAGES
➤ **Depression**
Adults: Initially, 75 mg (outpatients) to 100 mg (inpatients) PO daily in divided doses or (for outpatients) as a single bedtime dose. Maximum daily dose is 200 mg for outpatients and 300 mg for hospitalized patients.
Adolescents: 30 to 40 mg PO once daily, preferably at bedtime, or in divided doses if necessary. Dosage increases above 100 mg daily are generally unnecessary.
Elderly patients: Initially, 30 to 40 mg PO daily; maximum shouldn't exceed 100 mg daily.
➤ **Childhood enuresis**
Children age 6 and older: Initially, 25 mg imipramine hydrochloride PO 1 hour before bedtime. If patient doesn't improve within 1 week, increase dose to a maximum of 50 mg if child is younger than age 12; increase dose to a maximum of 75 mg for children age 12 and older. Don't exceed 2.5 mg/kg/day.

ADMINISTRATION
PO
- Give drug without regard for food.
- Give full dose at bedtime if possible.

Reactions in bold italics are *life-threatening*. Interactions may have a *rapid onset* or a *delayed onset*.

ACTION
Unknown. Increases norepinephrine, serotonin, or both in the CNS by blocking their reuptake by the presynaptic neurons.

Route	Onset	Peak	Duration
PO	Unknown	2–6 hr	Unknown

Half-life: 8 to 21 hours.

ADVERSE REACTIONS
CNS: drowsiness, dizziness, *seizures, stroke,* excitation, tremor, confusion, hallucinations, anxiety, ataxia, paresthesia, nervousness, EEG changes, extrapyramidal reactions, agitation, sleep disorders, tiredness. **CV:** orthostatic hypotension, tachycardia, ECG changes, *MI, arrhythmias, heart block,* HTN, *precipitation of HF,* palpitations. **EENT:** blurred vision, mydriasis, tinnitus. **GI:** dry mouth, constipation, nausea, vomiting, anorexia, paralytic ileus, abdominal cramps, black tongue, diarrhea. **GU:** urine retention, urinary frequency. **Hematologic:** *bone marrow depression, thrombocytopenia.* **Metabolic:** *hypoglycemia,* hyperglycemia. **Skin:** rash, urticaria, photosensitivity reactions, pruritus, diaphoresis, alopecia. **Other:** hypersensitivity reactions.

INTERACTIONS
Drug-drug. *Aclidinium:* May enhance anticholinergic effects. Avoid using together.
Barbiturates, CNS depressants: May enhance CNS depression. Avoid using together.
*Cimetidine, **fluoxetine, fluvoxamine, paroxetine, sertraline:** May increase imipramine level. Monitor drug levels and patient for signs of toxicity.
Clonidine: May cause life-threatening HTN. Avoid using together.
Epinephrine, norepinephrine: May increase hypertensive effect. Use together cautiously.
Linezolid, methylene blue: May cause serotonin syndrome. Use with extreme caution and monitor patient closely.
MAO inhibitors: May cause hyperpyretic crisis, severe seizures, and death. Don't use within 14 days of MAO inhibitor therapy.
QTc-prolonging drugs (quinidine, quinolones): May increase the risk of life-threatening arrhythmias. Avoid using together.

Drug-herb. *SAM-e, St. John's wort, yohimbe:* May cause serotonin syndrome. Discourage use together.
Drug-lifestyle. *Alcohol use:* May enhance CNS depression. Discourage use together.
Smoking: May lower level of drug. Monitor patient for lack of effect.
Sun exposure: May increase risk of photosensitivity reactions. Advise patient to avoid excessive sunlight exposure.

EFFECTS ON LAB TEST RESULTS
• May increase or decrease glucose level.
• May increase LFT values.

CONTRAINDICATIONS & CAUTIONS
Black Box Warning Antidepressants increase risk of suicidal thinking and behavior in children, adolescents, and young adults with major depressive disorder and other psychiatric disorders. Imipramine isn't approved for use in children except for those with nocturnal enuresis. ∎
• Contraindicated in patients hypersensitive to drug and in those receiving MAO inhibitors; also contraindicated during acute recovery phase of MI.
❸ *Alert:* Concomitant use with linezolid or methylene blue can cause serotonin syndrome (fever, mental status changes, muscle twitching, excessive sweating, shivering or shaking, diarrhea, and loss of coordination). Use imipramine with linezolid or methylene blue only for life-threatening or urgent conditions when the potential benefits outweigh the risks of toxicity.
• Use with extreme caution in patients at risk for suicide; in elderly patients and in patients with history of urine retention, angle-closure glaucoma, or seizure disorders; in patients with increased IOP, CV disease, impaired hepatic function, hyperthyroidism, or impaired renal function; and in patients receiving thyroid drugs.
❸ *Alert:* Imipramine pamoate shouldn't be used in children of any age because of increased risk of acute overdose.
Dialyzable drug: No.
▲ *Overdose S&S:* Cardiac arrhythmias, severe hypotension, seizures, CNS depression, coma, ECG changes, drowsiness, stupor, ataxia, restlessness, agitation, hyperactive reflexes, muscle rigidity, athetoid and

choreiform movements, tachycardia, HF, respiratory depression, cyanosis, shock, vomiting, hyperpyrexia, mydriasis, diaphoresis.

PREGNANCY-LACTATION-REPRODUCTION
• There are no adequate studies in pregnant women; however, fetal risk can't be excluded. Use during pregnancy only if potential benefit clearly justifies potential risk to the fetus.
• Drug appears in human milk. Use in breastfeeding women isn't recommended.

NURSING CONSIDERATIONS
❶ *Alert:* If linezolid or methylene blue must be given, discontinue imipramine and monitor patient for serotonin toxicity for 2 weeks (5 weeks if fluoxetine was taken) or until 24 hours after the last dose of methylene blue or linezolid, whichever comes first. May resume imipramine 24 hours after last dose of methylene blue or linezolid.
• Monitor WBC count during therapy, and monitor patient for fever and sore throat. Discontinue drug if pathologic neutrophil depression occurs.
• Monitor patient for nausea, headache, and malaise after abrupt withdrawal of long-term therapy; these symptoms don't indicate addiction.
• Safety of long-term use as adjunctive therapy for nocturnal enuresis in children age 6 or older hasn't been established. Consider a drug-free period after an adequate therapeutic trial with a favorable response.
• Don't withdraw drug abruptly.
• Because of hypertensive episodes during surgery in patients receiving TCAs, stop drug gradually several days before surgery.
• If signs or symptoms of psychosis occur or increase, expect prescriber to reduce dosage. Monitor mood changes. Monitor patient for suicidal tendencies, and allow only a minimum supply of drug.
• To prevent relapse in children receiving drug for enuresis, withdraw drug gradually.
• Recommend sugarless hard candy or gum to relieve dry mouth. Saliva substitutes may be useful.
❶ *Alert:* Tofranil may contain tartrazine.
• *Look alike–sound alike:* Don't confuse imipramine with desipramine.

PATIENT TEACHING
Black Box Warning Advise families and caregivers to closely observe patient for increased suicidal thinking and behavior. ∎
❶ *Alert:* Teach patient to recognize and immediately report symptoms of serotonin toxicity (fever, mental status changes, muscle twitching, excessive sweating, shivering or shaking, diarrhea, and loss of coordination).
• Tell patient to take full dose at bedtime whenever possible, but caution patient about possible morning dizziness upon standing up quickly.
• If child is an early-night bed-wetter, tell parents it may be more effective to divide dose and give the first dose earlier in day.
• Tell patient to avoid alcohol while taking this drug.
• Advise patient to consult prescriber before taking other prescription or OTC drugs.
• Warn patient to avoid hazardous activities that require alertness and good coordination until effects of the drug are known. Drowsiness and dizziness usually subside after a few weeks.
• Warn patient not to stop drug suddenly.
• To prevent oversensitivity to the sun, advise patient to use sunblock, wear protective clothing, and avoid prolonged exposure to strong sunlight.

indacaterol maleate
in-da-KA-ter-ol

Arcapta Neohaler, Onbrez Breezhaler✤

Therapeutic class: Bronchodilators
Pharmacologic class: Beta$_2$-adrenergic agonists

AVAILABLE FORMS
Capsules (powder for inhalation): 75 mcg

INDICATIONS & DOSAGES
➤ **Long-term maintenance therapy for COPD**
Adults: 75 mcg (1 capsule) daily by oral inhalation.

Reactions in bold italics are *life-threatening*. Interactions may have a *rapid onset* or a *delayed onset*.

ADMINISTRATION
Inhalational
• Patient shouldn't swallow capsules.
• Use inhalation capsules with the Neohaler device only. Always use the new Neohaler device that comes with each prescription. Administer inhaled capsules using the Neohaler device according to the package instructions.
• Don't wash the Neohaler device. The inhaler may be wiped between uses with a clean, dry, lint-free cloth or a clean, dry, soft brush.
• Don't use other inhaler devices from other inhaled medications to administer indacaterol capsules.
• Always store capsules in the blister packaging and remove just before using. Don't keep or store capsules in the Neohaler device. Protect capsules from light and moisture.
• Administer indacaterol at the same time each day; patient shouldn't use more than once in 24 hours.

ACTION
Binds to beta$_2$ receptors in the lung and increases cAMP levels, resulting in relaxation of bronchial smooth muscle.

Route	Onset	Peak	Duration
Inhalation	5 min	15 min	24 hr

Half-life: 46 to 126 hours.

ADVERSE REACTIONS
CNS: headache, dizziness. **CV:** peripheral edema, tachycardia, palpitations. **EENT:** nasopharyngitis, sinusitis, oropharyngeal pain. **GI:** nausea. **Metabolic:** hyperglycemia. **Musculoskeletal:** muscle spasm, musculoskeletal pain. **Respiratory:** cough, URI, dyspnea. **Skin:** pruritus, rash.

INTERACTIONS
Drug-drug. *Adrenergics (dobutamine, dopamine):* May increase risk of additive effects and adverse reactions. Use together cautiously.
Beta$_2$ agonists (formoterol): May result in overdose. Avoid use with other long-acting beta$_2$ agonists.
Beta blockers: May block therapeutic effects of beta-adrenergic agonists and cause

severe bronchospasm. If beta blocker use can't be avoided, administer indacaterol with extreme caution.
Drugs that prolong QTc interval, MAO inhibitors, TCAs: May increase risk of ventricular arrhythmias. Monitor carefully.
Xanthine derivatives (caffeine, theophylline), non-potassium-sparing diuretics, steroids: May cause hypokalemia. Monitor electrolyte levels closely.

EFFECTS ON LAB TEST RESULTS
• May increase glucose level. May decrease potassium level.

CONTRAINDICATIONS & CAUTIONS
Black Box Warning Long-acting beta$_2$-adrenergic agonists increase risk of asthma-related death. The safety and effectiveness of indacaterol in patients with asthma haven't been established. Inhaled indacaterol isn't indicated to treat asthma. ■
• Contraindicated in patients with acutely deteriorating COPD, when used more than once daily or at doses higher than prescribed, or in addition to drugs containing long-acting beta$_2$-adrenergic agonists.
• Use cautiously in patients with a history of CV disorders (coronary insufficiency, arrhythmias, HTN), seizures, thyrotoxicosis, diabetes, or abnormal electrolyte levels and in patients abnormally responsive to sympathomimetic amines.
Dialyzable drug: Unknown.
⚠ *Overdose S&S:* Angina, HTN or hypotension, tachycardia, cardiac arrest, arrhythmias, nervousness, headache, tremor, dry mouth, palpitations, muscle cramps, nausea, dizziness, fatigue, malaise, hypokalemia, hyperglycemia, metabolic acidosis, insomnia, death.

PREGNANCY-LACTATION-REPRODUCTION
• There are no adequate studies in pregnant women. Use during pregnancy only if potential benefit justifies potential risk to the fetus.
• Drug may interfere with uterine contractions. Use during labor only if benefit clearly outweighs risks.
• It isn't known if drug appears in human milk. Use cautiously in breastfeeding women.

NURSING CONSIDERATIONS

☻ *Alert:* Drug may produce paradoxical bronchospasm that may be life-threatening. If paradoxical bronchospasm occurs, discontinue drug immediately and institute alternative therapy.

• Discontinue routine use of short-acting beta$_2$-adrenergic agonists when indacaterol therapy is begun. Short-acting beta$_2$-adrenergic agonists should be used only for symptomatic relief of acute symptoms.

• As long as the capsule is empty after inhalation, the full dose of medication has been received even if patient coughs. Monitor patient for worsening of symptoms, decreased effectiveness, or increased need for short-acting rescue inhaler.

PATIENT TEACHING

Black Box Warning Inform patient that indacaterol isn't for use in asthma and can increase the risk of asthma-related death. ▪

• Instruct patient on the proper administration, use, and storage of the Neohaler device and capsules. Remind patient to use only the Neohaler device and no other inhaler to administer the medication.

• Warn patient that indacaterol isn't to be used for acute exacerbations of COPD and that acute symptoms should be treated with a short-acting inhaler such as albuterol.

• Advise patient not to use indacaterol with other long-acting beta-adrenergic agonists because of the risk of significant CV effects.

• Advise patient to notify prescriber of worsening symptoms, decreased effectiveness of drug, or the need for more frequent use of a short-acting inhaler.

• Warn patient not to stop therapy without first discussing with health care provider.

indapamide
in-DAP-a-mide

Lozide✦

Therapeutic class: Diuretics
Pharmacologic class: Thiazide-like diuretics

AVAILABLE FORMS
Tablets: 1.25 mg, 2.5 mg

INDICATIONS & DOSAGES
➤ **Edema of HF**
Adults: Initially, 2.5 mg PO daily in the morning, increased to 5 mg daily after 1 week, if needed.
➤ **HTN**
Adults: Initially, 1.25 mg PO daily in the morning, increased to 2.5 mg daily after 4 weeks, if needed. Increased to 5 mg daily after 4 more weeks, if needed. If response is inadequate, a second antihypertensive, given at 50% of the usual starting dose, may be needed.

ADMINISTRATION
PO
• Give drug with food or milk to minimize GI upset.
• To prevent nocturia, give drug in the morning.

ACTION
Enhances excretion of sodium chloride and water by interfering with sodium transport in the distal tubule.

Route	Onset	Peak	Duration
PO	Unknown	Within 2 hr	Unknown

Half-life: About 14 hours.

ADVERSE REACTIONS
CNS: headache, nervousness, dizziness, light-headedness, weakness, vertigo, restlessness, drowsiness, fatigue, anxiety, depression, numbness of limbs, irritability, agitation, lethargy, hypertonia. **CV:** orthostatic hypotension, palpitations, PVCs, arrhythmia, vasculitis, flushing, chest pain, edema. **EENT:** blurred vision, conjunctivitis, rhinorrhea, pharyngitis, sinusitis. **GI:** anorexia, nausea, epigastric distress, vomiting, abdominal pain or cramps, diarrhea, constipation, dyspepsia. **GU:** nocturia, polyuria, frequent urination, erectile dysfunction. **Metabolic:** asymptomatic hyperuricemia; fluid and electrolyte imbalances, including dilutional hyponatremia, hypochloremia, metabolic alkalosis, and *hypokalemia*; weight loss; volume depletion and dehydration; hyperglycemia. **Musculoskeletal:** muscle cramps and spasms. **Respiratory:** cough. **Skin:** rash, pruritus, urticaria. **Other:** gout, infection, flulike syndrome.

Reactions in bold italics are *life-threatening*. Interactions may have a *rapid onset* or a *delayed onset*.

INTERACTIONS
Drug-drug. *Amphotericin B, corticosteroids:* May increase risk of hypokalemia. Monitor potassium level closely.
Antidiabetics: May decrease hypoglycemic effect of sulfonylureas, causing elevated glucose levels. Adjust dosage, if needed. Monitor glucose level.
Barbiturates, opioids: May increase orthostasis. Monitor patient closely.
Bumetanide, ethacrynic acid, furosemide, torsemide: May cause excessive diuretic response, causing serious electrolyte abnormalities or dehydration. Adjust doses carefully, and monitor patient closely for signs and symptoms of excessive diuretic response.
Cardiac glycosides: May increase risk of digoxin toxicity from indapamide-induced hypokalemia. Monitor potassium and digoxin levels.
Cholestyramine, colestipol: May decrease absorption of thiazides. Separate doses by 2 hours.
Diazoxide: May increase antihypertensive, hyperglycemic, and hyperuricemic effects. Use together cautiously.
Lithium: May decrease lithium clearance, which may increase lithium toxicity. Avoid using together.
NSAIDs: May increase risk of NSAID-induced renal failure. Monitor patient for signs and symptoms of renal failure.
Drug-herb. *Licorice:* May cause unexpected rapid potassium loss and HTN. Discourage use together.
Drug-lifestyle. *Alcohol use:* May increase orthostatic hypotensive effect. Discourage use together.

EFFECTS ON LAB TEST RESULTS
• May increase BUN, creatinine, glucose, cholesterol, triglyceride, calcium, and uric acid levels.
• May decrease potassium, sodium, phosphate, and chloride levels.

CONTRAINDICATIONS & CAUTIONS
• Contraindicated in patients hypersensitive to other sulfonamide-derived drugs and in those with anuria.
• Use cautiously in patients age 65 and older and in patients with severe renal disease,

gout, impaired hepatic function, or progressive hepatic disease.
Dialyzable drug: Unknown.
⚠ ***Overdose S&S:*** Nausea, vomiting, GI disorders, weakness, electrolyte imbalance, hypotension, depressed respirations.

PREGNANCY-LACTATION-REPRODUCTION
• There are no adequate studies in pregnant women. Use during pregnancy only if clearly needed.
• It isn't known if drug appears in human milk. Patient should discontinue breastfeeding or discontinue drug.

NURSING CONSIDERATIONS
• Monitor fluid intake and output, weight, BP, and electrolyte levels.
• Watch for signs of hypokalemia, such as muscle weakness and cramps. Drug may be used with potassium-sparing diuretic to prevent potassium loss.
• Consult prescriber and dietitian about a high-potassium diet or potassium supplement.
• Monitor creatinine and BUN levels regularly. Cumulative effects of drug may occur in patients with renal impairment.
• Monitor uric acid level, especially in patients with history of gout.
• Monitor glucose level, especially in diabetic patients.
• Monitor elderly patients, who are especially susceptible to excessive diuresis.
• Stop thiazides and thiazide-like diuretics before parathyroid function tests.
• Therapeutic response may be delayed several weeks in hypertensive patients.

PATIENT TEACHING
• Instruct patient to take drug in morning to prevent need to urinate at night.
• Tell patient to take drug with food to minimize GI upset.
• Advise patient to avoid sudden posture changes and to rise slowly to avoid dizziness upon standing quickly.

indinavir sulfate

in-DIN-a-veer

Crixivan◆

Therapeutic class: Antiretrovirals
Pharmacologic class: Protease inhibitors

AVAILABLE FORMS
Capsules: 200 mg, 400 mg

INDICATIONS & DOSAGES
➤ **HIV infection, with other antiretrovirals, when antiretrovirals are warranted**
Adults: 800 mg PO every 8 hours. Consider reducing indinavir to 600 mg every 8 hours when patient is taking delavirdine 400 mg t.i.d. Reduce indinavir to 600 mg every 8 hours when patient is taking itraconazole 200 mg b.i.d. or ketoconazole. When patient is taking indinavir and rifabutin, decrease rifabutin to half the standard dosage and increase indinavir to 1,000 mg every 8 hours. If patient is taking indinavir and didanosine concomitantly, give at least 1 hour apart on an empty stomach.
Adjust-a-dose: For patients with mild to moderate hepatic insufficiency from cirrhosis, reduce dosage to 600 mg PO every 8 hours.

ADMINISTRATION
PO
• Give drug on an empty stomach with water 1 hour before or 2 hours after a meal. Or, give it with other liquids (such as skim milk, juice, coffee, or tea) or a light meal. A meal high in fat, calories, and protein reduces drug absorption.
• Store capsules in the original container and keep desiccant in the bottle; capsules are sensitive to moisture.

ACTION
Inhibits HIV protease by binding to the protease-active site and inhibiting activity of the enzyme, preventing cleavage of the viral polyproteins and forming immature noninfectious viral particles.

Route	Onset	Peak	Duration
PO	Rapid	<1 hr	Unknown

Half-life: 1½ to 2 hours.

ADVERSE REACTIONS
CNS: asthenia, dizziness, fatigue, headache, insomnia, malaise, somnolence, fever. **GI:** nausea, abdominal pain, acid regurgitation, anorexia, diarrhea, dry mouth, taste perversion, vomiting, dyspepsia. **GU:** hematuria, nephrolithiasis, dysuria, flank pain. **Hematologic:** *neutropenia, thrombocytopenia,* anemia. **Hepatic:** jaundice. **Metabolic:** hyperbilirubinemia, hyperglycemia. **Musculoskeletal:** back pain. **Respiratory:** cough. **Skin:** pruritus, rash. **Other:** flank pain.

INTERACTIONS
Drug-drug. *Alfuzosin, alprazolam, amiodarone, oral midazolam, pimozide, sildenafil (when used for PAH), triazolam:* May increase plasma concentrations of these drugs and cause life-threatening reactions. Use together is contraindicated.
Atorvastatin, pitavastatin, rosuvastatin: May increase level of statin and risk of myopathy and rhabdomyolysis. Use together cautiously and use the lowest appropriate statin dose.
Carbamazepine, phenobarbital, phenytoin: May decrease indinavir concentration and effectiveness. Use with caution.
Clarithromycin: May alter clarithromycin level. Dosage adjustments not needed.
Delavirdine, itraconazole, ketoconazole: May increase indinavir level. Consider reducing indinavir to 600 mg every 8 hours.
Didanosine: May alter absorption of indinavir. Separate doses by 1 hour and give on an empty stomach.
Direct factor Xa inhibitors (rivaroxaban): May increase plasma concentrations and effects of direct factor Xa inhibitors. Avoid use together.
Efavirenz, nevirapine: May decrease indinavir level. Closely monitor clinical response.
Ergot derivatives (dihydroergotamine, ergonovine, ergotamine, methylergonovine): May cause acute ergot toxicity, characterized by peripheral vasospasm and ischemia of the extremities and other tissues. Use together is contraindicated.
Lopinavir–ritonavir: May increase indinavir level. Adjust indinavir dosage to 600 mg b.i.d.

Reactions in bold italics are *life-threatening*. Interactions may have a *rapid onset* or a *delayed onset*.

Lovastatin, simvastatin: May increase levels of these drugs and increase risk of myopathy and rhabdomyolysis. Use together is contraindicated.

Nelfinavir: May increase indinavir level. Monitor patient closely.

PPIs: May reduce the antiviral activity of indinavir. Monitor clinical response and adjust indinavir dosage as needed.

Rifabutin: May increase rifabutin level and decrease indinavir level. Avoid using together or adjust dosages accordingly.

Rifampin: May decrease indinavir level. Avoid using together.

Ritonavir: May increase indinavir level twofold to fivefold. Monitor clinical response and adjust dosage if needed.

Sildenafil, tadalafil, vardenafil: May increase levels of these drugs and increase adverse effects (hypotension, visual changes, priapism). Tell patient not to exceed prescribed dosage. Sildenafil dosage shouldn't exceed 25 mg in a 48-hour period. Tadalafil dosage shouldn't exceed 10 mg in a 72-hour period. Vardenafil dosage shouldn't exceed 2.5 mg in a 24-hour period.

Drug-herb. *Garlic supplements:* May decrease indinavir level. Use together isn't recommended.

St. John's wort: May reduce drug level by more than half. Avoid use together.

Drug-food. *Grapefruit, grapefruit juice:* May decrease drug level and therapeutic effect. Discourage use together.

EFFECTS ON LAB TEST RESULTS
• May increase ALT, AST, bilirubin, amylase, and glucose levels.
• May decrease Hb and neutrophil and platelet counts.

CONTRAINDICATIONS & CAUTIONS
• Contraindicated in patients hypersensitive to drug or its components.
• Fatal cases of hemolytic anemia have occurred. If hemolytic anemia occurs, treat appropriately and discontinue drug.
• Immune reconstitution syndrome has been reported in patients treated with combination antiretroviral therapy, which may cause development of an inflammatory response to indolent or residual opportunistic infections or activation of autoimmune disorders.

• Use cautiously in patients with hepatic insufficiency from cirrhosis.
• Safety and effectiveness in children haven't been established.
Dialyzable drug: Unknown.

⚠ **Overdose S&S:** Nephrolithiasis/urolithiasis, flank pain, hematuria, nausea, vomiting, diarrhea.

PREGNANCY-LACTATION-REPRODUCTION
• There are no adequate studies in pregnant women. Use during pregnancy only if potential benefit justifies potential risk to the fetus.
• It isn't known if drug appears in human milk. HIV-infected mothers shouldn't breastfeed, to avoid postnatal transmission of HIV.

NURSING CONSIDERATIONS
• Drug must be taken at 8-hour intervals.
• Drug may cause nephrolithiasis. If signs and symptoms of nephrolithiasis occur, prescriber may stop drug for 1 to 3 days during acute phases.
• To prevent nephrolithiasis, patient should maintain adequate hydration (at least 48 oz or 1.5 L of fluids every 24 hours while taking indinavir).

PATIENT TEACHING
• Tell patient that drug doesn't cure HIV infection and that opportunistic infections and other complications of HIV infection may continue to develop. Drug hasn't been shown to reduce the risk of HIV transmission.
• Advise patient to use barrier protection during sexual intercourse.
• Caution patient not to adjust dosage or stop therapy without first consulting prescriber.
• Tell patient that drug may interact with many drugs and to report the use of other prescription or OTC drugs or supplements.
• Advise patient that if a dose is missed by less than 2 hours, to take dose immediately and resume regular dosing schedule. If dose is missed by more than 2 hours, tell patient to skip missed dose and resume at next regularly scheduled dose.
• Instruct patient to take drug on an empty stomach with water 1 hour before or 2 hours

after a meal. Or, patient may take it with other liquids (such as skim milk, juice, coffee, or tea) or a light meal.
• Instruct patient to store capsules in the original container and to keep desiccant in the bottle; capsules are sensitive to moisture.
• Tell patient to drink at least 48 oz (1.5 L) of fluid daily.
• Advise female patient to avoid breastfeeding because drug may appear in human milk. Advise HIV-positive patient not to breastfeed, to prevent transmitting virus to infant.

indomethacin
in-doe-METH-a-sin

Indocin, Tivorbex

indomethacin sodium trihydrate
Indocin IV

Therapeutic class: NSAIDs
Pharmacologic class: NSAIDs

AVAILABLE FORMS
indomethacin
Capsules: 20 mg, 25 mg, 40 mg, 50 mg
Capsules (extended-release): 75 mg
Injection: 1 mg base/vial
Oral suspension: 25 mg/5 mL
Suppositories: 50 mg, 100 mg✦
indomethacin sodium trihydrate
Injection: 1 mg base/vial

INDICATIONS & DOSAGES
➤ **Moderate to severe RA or osteoarthritis, ankylosing spondylitis (excluding Tivorbex)**
Adults and children age 15 and older: 25 mg PO b.i.d. or t.i.d. with food or antacids or 25 mg PR b.i.d. or t.i.d.; increase daily dose by 25 or 50 mg every 7 days until satisfactory response is obtained, up to total daily dose of 150 to 200 mg. Or, 75 mg extended-release capsules PO to start, in morning or at bedtime, followed by 75 mg extended-release capsules b.i.d. if needed.
➤ **Acute gouty arthritis (excluding Tivorbex)**
Adults and children age 15 and older: 50 mg PO or PR t.i.d. Reduce dose as soon as

possible; then stop therapy. Don't use extended-release form.
➤ **Acute painful shoulders (bursitis or tendinitis) (excluding Tivorbex)**
Adults and children age 15 and older: 75 to 150 mg PO or PR daily in divided doses t.i.d. or q.i.d. for 7 to 14 days. Or, 75 mg (extended-release) PO daily or b.i.d. for 7 to 14 days.
➤ **Mild to moderate acute pain (Tivorbex)**
Adults: 20 mg PO t.i.d. or 40 mg PO b.i.d. or t.i.d.
➤ **To close a hemodynamically significant patent ductus arteriosus in premature neonates**
Neonates older than age 7 days: 0.2 mg/kg IV; then two doses of 0.25 mg/kg at 12- to 24-hour intervals.
Neonates ages 2 to 7 days: 0.2 mg/kg IV; then two doses of 0.2 mg/kg at 12- to 24-hour intervals.
Neonates younger than 48 hours: 0.2 mg/kg IV; then two doses of 0.1 mg/kg IV at 12- to 24-hour intervals.

ADMINISTRATION
PO
• Give drug with food, milk, or antacid.
IV
▼ Reconstitute powder for injection with sterile water or NSS. For each 1-mg vial, add 1 or 2 mL of diluent for a solution containing 1 mg/mL or 0.5 mg/mL, respectively. Give over 20 to 30 minutes.
🌢 *Alert:* Use only preservative-free sterile saline solution or sterile water to prepare. Never use diluents containing benzyl alcohol because it has been linked to toxicity in newborns.
▼ Because injection contains no preservatives, reconstitute drug immediately before use and discard unused solution.
▼ If anuria or marked oliguria is evident, withhold administration of second or third scheduled IV dose and notify prescriber.
▼ Watch carefully for bleeding and for reduced urine output.
▼ **Incompatibilities:** None listed by manufacturer. Consult a drug incompatibility reference for more information.

Reactions in bold italics are *life-threatening*. Interactions may have a *rapid onset* or a ***delayed onset***.

Rectal
• If suppository is too soft, place in refrigerator for 15 minutes or run under cold water in wrapper.

ACTION

May inhibit prostaglandin synthesis, to produce anti-inflammatory, analgesic, and antipyretic effects.

Route	Onset	Peak	Duration
PO	30 min	2 hr	4–6 hr
IV	Immediate	Immediate	4–6 hr
PR	Unknown	Unknown	4–6 hr

Half-life: Adults (mean), 4½ hours; Tivorbex 7½ hours.

ADVERSE REACTIONS
PO and rectal
CNS: headache, dizziness, depression, fatigue, somnolence, syncope, vertigo. **CV:** edema, HTN. **EENT:** hearing loss, tinnitus. **GI:** *pancreatitis,* abdominal pain, constipation, diarrhea, dyspepsia, *GI bleeding,* nausea, peptic ulceration, vomiting. **Other:** hypersensitivity reactions.
IV
GU: hematuria, interstitial nephritis, proteinuria.

INTERACTIONS
Drug-drug. *ACE inhibitors (benazepril, enalaprilat), angiotensin II receptor blockers (candesartan, valsartan):* May reduce antihypertensive effects; may worsen renal function in those with impaired renal function. Monitor patient closely.
Aminoglycosides, cyclosporine, methotrexate: May enhance toxicity of these drugs. Avoid using together.
Anticoagulants: May cause bleeding. Monitor patient closely.
Antihypertensives: May decrease antihypertensive effect. Monitor patient closely.
Antihypertensives, furosemide, thiazide diuretics: May impair response to both drugs. Avoid using together, if possible.
Aspirin: May increase adverse reactions, including risk of GI toxicity. Avoid using together.
Bisphosphonates: May increase risk of gastric ulceration. Monitor patient for symptoms of gastric irritation or GI bleeding.

Corticosteroids: May increase risk of GI toxicity. Avoid using together.
Cyclosporine: May increase cyclosporine toxicity. Use cautiously and monitor renal function.
Diflunisal, probenecid: May decrease indomethacin excretion. Watch for increased indomethacin adverse effects.
Digoxin: May prolong half-life of digoxin. Use together cautiously.
Dipyridamole: May enhance fluid retention. Avoid using together.
Lithium: May increase lithium level. Monitor patient for toxicity.
Methotrexate: May increase methotrexate toxicity. Use together cautiously.
Penicillamine: May increase bioavailability of penicillamine. Monitor patient closely.
Phenytoin: May increase phenytoin level. Monitor patient closely.
SSRIs: May increase risk of GI bleeding. Adjust dosage as needed.
Triamterene: May cause nephrotoxicity. Avoid using together.
Drug-herb. *Alfalfa, anise, bilberry, dong quai, garlic:* May cause bleeding. Discourage use together.
Senna: May inhibit diarrheal effects. Discourage use together.
White willow: Herb and drug contain similar components. Don't use together.
Drug-lifestyle. *Alcohol use:* May cause GI toxicity. Discourage use together.

EFFECTS ON LAB TEST RESULTS
• May increase potassium level.
• May decrease Hb level and hematocrit.
• May increase LFT values.

CONTRAINDICATIONS & CAUTIONS
• Contraindicated in patients hypersensitive to drug and in those with a history of aspirin- or NSAID-induced asthma, rhinitis, or urticaria.
• Contraindicated in neonates with untreated infection, active bleeding, coagulation defects or thrombocytopenia, congenital heart disease needing patency of the ductus arteriosus, necrotizing enterocolitis, or significant renal impairment.
Black Box Warning NSAIDs can increase risk of heart attack or stroke in patients with

or without heart disease or risk factors for heart disease. ∎

Black Box Warning Risk of heart attack or stroke can occur as early as the first weeks of NSAID use. Risk appears greater at higher doses. Use lowest effective dose for shortest duration possible. ∎

Black Box Warning NSAIDs may increase risk of serious GI adverse events, including bleeding, ulceration, and perforation of the stomach or intestines, which can be fatal. These events can occur at any time during use and without warning symptoms. Elderly patients and patients with a prior history of peptic ulcer disease or GI bleeding are at greater risk for serious GI events. ∎

⊕ Alert: Avoid use in patients with severe HF unless benefits are expected to outweigh risk of worsening HF.

• Suppositories are contraindicated in patients with history of proctitis or recent rectal bleeding.

Black Box Warning Contraindicated for the treatment of perioperative pain after CABG surgery. ∎

• Use cautiously in elderly patients, those with history of GI disease, and those with epilepsy, parkinsonism, hepatic or renal disease, CV disease, infection, and mental illness or depression.

• Safety and effectiveness in children age 14 and younger (age 17 and younger for Tivorbex) haven't been established.

Dialyzable drug: Unknown.

⚠ Overdose S&S: Drowsiness, lethargy, confusion, nausea, vomiting, paresthesia, numbness, aggressive behavior, disorientation, seizures, headache, dizziness, GI bleeding.

PREGNANCY-LACTATION-REPRODUCTION

⊕ Alert: Drug can cause fetal harm starting at 30 weeks' gestation and cause premature closure of the ductus arteriosus; avoid use. Before 30 weeks' gestation, use during pregnancy only if potential benefit justifies potential risk to the fetus.

• Drug appears in human milk. Use in breastfeeding women isn't recommended by most manufacturers.

• Long-term use of NSAIDs in women of reproductive age may be associated with infertility that's reversible upon discontinuation of drug.

NURSING CONSIDERATIONS

• Because of the high risk of adverse effects from long-term use, drug shouldn't be used routinely as an analgesic or antipyretic.

⊕ Alert: Watch for and immediately evaluate signs and symptoms of heart attack (chest pain, shortness of breath or trouble breathing) or stroke (weakness in one part or side of the body, slurred speech).

• If ductus arteriosus reopens, a second course of one to three doses may be given. If ineffective, surgery may be needed.

• Watch for bleeding in patients receiving anticoagulants, patients with coagulation defects, and neonates.

• Because NSAIDs impair synthesis of renal prostaglandins, they can decrease renal blood flow and lead to reversible renal impairment, especially in patients with renal failure, HF, or hepatic dysfunction; in elderly patients; and in those taking diuretics. Monitor these patients closely.

• Drug causes sodium retention; watch for weight gain (especially in elderly patients) and increased BP in patients with HTN.

• Monitor patient for rash and respiratory distress, which may indicate a hypersensitivity reaction.

• Because of their antipyretic and antiinflammatory actions, NSAIDs may mask signs and symptoms of infection.

Black Box Warning NSAIDs cause an increased risk of serious GI adverse events, including bleeding, ulceration, and perforation of the stomach or intestines, which can be fatal. Elderly patients are at greater risk. ∎

Black Box Warning NSAIDs may increase the risk of serious thrombotic events, MI, or stroke, which can be fatal. The risk may be greater with longer use or in patients with CV disease or risk factors for CV disease. ∎

• Monitor patient on long-term oral therapy for toxicity by conducting regular eye exams, hearing tests, CBCs, and kidney function tests.

PATIENT TEACHING

• Tell patient to take oral dose with food, milk, or antacid to prevent GI upset.

⊕ Alert: Advise patient to seek medical attention immediately if chest pain, shortness of breath or trouble breathing, weakness

---

in one part or side of the body, or slurred speech occurs.
• Alert patient that using oral form with aspirin, alcohol, other NSAIDs, or corticosteroids may increase risk of adverse GI reactions.
• Teach patient signs and symptoms of GI bleeding (blood in vomit, urine, or stool; coffee-ground vomit; and black, tarry stools) and to notify prescriber immediately if any of these occurs.
• Tell patient to immediately report signs or symptoms of cardiac events, such as chest pain, shortness of breath, weakness, and slurred speech.
• Warn patient to avoid hazardous activities that require mental alertness until CNS effects are known.
• Tell patient to notify prescriber immediately if visual or hearing changes occur.
• Tell patient to notify prescriber if unexplained weight gain or edema occurs.

BIOSIMILAR DRUG

inFLIXimab
in-FLICKS-ih-mab

Remicade

inFLIXimab-abda
Renflexis

inFLIXimab-dyyb
Inflectra

inFLIXimab-qbtx
Ixifi

Therapeutic class: Anti-inflammatory drugs
Pharmacologic class: TNF blockers

AVAILABLE FORMS
Lyophilized powder for injection: 100-mg vials

INDICATIONS & DOSAGES
➤ **Moderately to severely active Crohn disease; reduction in the number of draining enterocutaneous and rectovaginal fistulas and maintenance of fistula closure in adults with fistulizing Crohn disease**

Adults: 5 mg/kg IV infusion over at least 2 hours. Repeat at 2 and 6 weeks, then every 8 weeks thereafter. For patients who respond and then lose their response, consider 10 mg/kg. Patients who don't respond by week 14 are unlikely to respond with continued therapy. In those patients, consider stopping drug.
Children ages 6 to 17: For Crohn disease, 5 mg/kg IV infusion over at least 2 hours. Repeat at 2 and 6 weeks, then every 8 weeks thereafter.
➤ **Moderately to severely active RA**
Adults: 3 mg/kg IV infusion over at least 2 hours. Repeat at 2 and 6 weeks after first infusion and every 8 weeks thereafter. Dose may be increased up to 10 mg/kg, or doses may be given every 4 weeks if response is inadequate. Use with methotrexate.
➤ **Moderate to severe ulcerative colitis**
Adults: Induction dose, 5 mg/kg IV over at least 2 hours. Repeat at 2 and 6 weeks, then every 8 weeks thereafter.
➤ **Moderate to severe ulcerative colitis in children who have had an inadequate response to conventional therapy (Remicade only)**
Children age 6 and older: Initially, 5 mg/kg IV infusion over at least 2 hours at 0, 2, and 6 weeks, followed by a maintenance regimen of 5 mg/kg IV infusion over at least 2 hours every 8 weeks.
➤ **Ankylosing spondylitis**
Adults: 5 mg/kg IV infusion over at least 2 hours. Repeat at 2 and 6 weeks, then every 6 weeks thereafter.
➤ **Psoriatic arthritis, with or without methotrexate**
Adults: 5 mg/kg IV infusion over at least 2 hours. Repeat at 2 and 6 weeks after first infusion, then every 8 weeks thereafter.
➤ **Chronic severe plaque psoriasis**
Adults: 5 mg/kg IV infusion over at least 2 hours. Repeat dose in 2 and 6 weeks, then give 5 mg/kg every 8 weeks thereafter.

ADMINISTRATION
IV
▼ Reconstitute with 10 mL sterile water for injection, using syringe with 21G or smaller needle. Don't shake; gently swirl to dissolve powder. Solution should be colorless to light yellow and opalescent. It may

also develop a few translucent particles; don't use if other types of particles develop or discoloration occurs.

▼ Dilute total volume of reconstituted drug to 250 mL with NSS for injection. Infusion concentration range is 0.4 to 4 mg/mL.

▼ Use an in-line, sterile, nonpyrogenic, low-protein-binding filter with a pore size smaller than 1.2 microns.

▼ Begin infusion within 3 hours of preparation and give over at least 2 hours.

▼ **Incompatibilities:** Other IV drugs. Don't infuse with other drugs.

ACTION

Binds to human TNF-alpha to neutralize its activity and inhibit its binding with receptors, thereby reducing the infiltration of inflammatory cells and TNF-alpha production in inflamed areas of the intestine.

Route	Onset	Peak	Duration
IV	Unknown	Unknown	Unknown

Half-life: 7½ to 9½ days.

ADVERSE REACTIONS

CNS: fatigue, fever, headache, depression, insomnia, malaise, pain, systemic and cutaneous vasculitis. **CV:** HTN, chest pain, flushing, hypotension, pericardial effusion, tachycardia, bradycardia. **EENT:** conjunctivitis, rhinitis, sinusitis, pharyngitis. **GI:** abdominal pain, diarrhea, dyspepsia, nausea. **GU:** UTI. **Hematologic:** *leukopenia, neutropenia,* anemia, hematoma. **Musculoskeletal:** arthralgia, back pain, arthritis, myalgia, bone fracture. **Respiratory:** cough, URI, bronchitis, dyspnea, pneumonia, respiratory tract allergic reaction. **Skin:** rash, pruritus, candidiasis, urticaria, cellulitis, skin ulceration, abscess. **Other:** hypersensitivity reactions, infusion reactions, serum sickness, development of antibodies, bacterial infection, *sepsis,* viral infections, candidiasis, *anaphylaxis,* chills, flulike syndrome.

INTERACTIONS

Drug-drug. *CYP450 substrates:* May normalize formation of CYP450 enzymes upon initiation or discontinuation of infliximab. Monitor effect or drug concentration; may adjust individual dose of drug product as needed.

Live-virus vaccines: May affect normal immune response. Postpone live-virus vaccine until therapy stops. Use live-virus vaccines cautiously in infants born to female patients treated with infliximab.
TNF blockers (abatacept, anakinra, golimumab, rilonacept): May increase risk of serious infections and neutropenia. Use together isn't recommended.
Tocilizumab: May increase risk of immunosuppression and infection. Avoid use together.
Drug-herb. *Echinacea:* May diminish therapeutic effect of immunosuppressants. Consider therapy modification.

EFFECTS ON LAB TEST RESULTS

• May increase liver enzyme levels. May decrease Hb level and hematocrit.
• May decrease RBC, WBC, and platelet counts.
• May produce false-negative TB test results.
• May cause false-positive ANA test result.

CONTRAINDICATIONS & CAUTIONS

• Contraindicated in patients hypersensitive to murine proteins or other components of drug. Doses greater than 5 mg/kg are contraindicated in patients with moderate to severe HF.

Black Box Warning Lymphoma and other malignancies, some fatal, have occurred in children and adolescents treated with TNF blockers, including infliximab. ▌

Black Box Warning Hepatosplenic T-cell lymphoma, a rare type of lymphoma that can be fatal, has occurred in adolescents and young adults with inflammatory bowel disease treated with TNF blockers, including infliximab. ▌

Black Box Warning Drug increases risk of serious infections, including TB, histoplasmosis, coccidioidomycosis, blastomycosis, bacterial sepsis, *Listeria, Legionella,* and other opportunistic infections. Patients with histoplasmosis or other invasive fungal infections may present with disseminated disease. Consider antifungal therapy in patients at risk for invasive fungal infections who develop severe systemic illness. ▌

Black Box Warning Carefully consider risks and benefits of treatment before

---

initiating inﬂiximab therapy in patients with long-term or recurrent infection. ∎

• Depending on the product, each vial contains between 50 and 500 mg of sucrose.

• Use cautiously in elderly patients; in patients with active infection, history of chronic or recurrent infections, a history of hematologic abnormalities, or preexisting or recent-onset CNS demyelinating or seizure disorders; or in those who have lived in regions where histoplasmosis is endemic.

• Rare cases of severe hepatic reactions (acute liver failure, jaundice, hepatitis, cholestasis) with or without elevations in aminotransferase levels have been reported in postmarketing data. Discontinue drug if signs and symptoms of liver injury occur.

• Use cautiously in patients with hematologic abnormalities. Serious and sometimes fatal cases of leukopenia, neutropenia, thrombocytopenia, and pancytopenia have been reported.

Dialyzable drug: Unknown.

PREGNANCY-LACTATION-REPRODUCTION

• Drug crosses placental barrier but it isn't known if drug can cause fetal harm or can affect reproductive capacity if used during pregnancy. Use in pregnant women only if clearly needed.

• Drug may be present in the serum of infants up to 6 months after birth. Exposed infants may be at increased risk for infection.

• It isn't known if drug appears in human milk. Patient should discontinue breastfeeding or discontinue drug.

NURSING CONSIDERATIONS

• Inﬂiximab-abda, inﬂiximab-dyyb, and inﬂiximab-qbtx are biosimilar to the FDA-approved reference product inﬂiximab (Remicade). There are no clinically meaningful differences between the biosimilar product and the reference product based on the conditions of their use. However, these drugs aren't considered to be interchangeable.

• Premedication with antihistamines, acetaminophen, and corticosteroids may be considered at prescriber's discretion to prevent infusion-related reactions.

• Monitor patients for signs and symptoms of hypersensitivity reactions (urticaria,

dyspnea, hypotension), which may occur during or within 2 hours of infusion and may be severe. Discontinue drug for severe reactions and treat appropriately.

⚠ **Alert:** Watch for infusion-related reactions, including fever, chills, pruritus, urticaria, dyspnea, hypotension, HTN, and chest pain during administration and for 2 hours afterward. If an infusion-related reaction occurs, stop drug, notify prescriber, and prepare to give acetaminophen, antihistamines, corticosteroids, and epinephrine.

• Don't give live-virus vaccines to infants exposed to drug in utero for at least 6 months after birth because of increased risk of infection, including disseminated infection, which can be fatal.

• Give for Crohn disease and ulcerative colitis only after patient has an inadequate response to conventional therapy.

• Consider stopping treatment in patient who develops significant hematologic abnormalities or CNS adverse reactions.

• Notify prescriber for symptoms of new or worsening HF.

Black Box Warning Patients with histoplasmosis or other invasive fungal infections may present with disseminated rather than localized disease. Antigen and antibody testing for histoplasmosis may be negative in some patients with active infection. Consider empirical antifungal therapy in patients at risk for invasive fungal infections who develop severe systemic illness. ∎

Black Box Warning Discontinue drug if serious infection or sepsis develops. ∎

Black Box Warning Watch for development of lymphoma and infection. Patient with chronic Crohn disease and long-term exposure to immunosuppressants is more likely to develop lymphoma and infection. ∎

• Drug may affect normal immune responses. Patient may develop autoimmune antibodies and lupuslike syndrome; stop drug if this happens. Symptoms should resolve.

Black Box Warning Drug may cause disseminated or extrapulmonary TB and fatal opportunistic infections. ∎

Black Box Warning Evaluate patient for latent TB infection with a tuberculin skin test. Treat latent TB infection before therapy. ∎

Black Box Warning Closely monitor patients for signs and symptoms of infection during and after infliximab treatment, including possible development of TB in patients who tested negative for latent TB infection before start of therapy. ∎

• TNF blockers may increase risk of reactivation of HBV in patients who are chronic carriers. Patients taking concomitant immunosuppressants are at increased risk. Test for HBV infection before therapy begins.

• Monitor patient for hepatotoxicity (jaundice, liver enzyme elevations 5 × ULN or more). Stop drug and closely evaluate patient if these signs or symptoms occur.

• *Look alike–sound alike:* Don't confuse Remicade with Renacidin. Don't confuse infliximab with rituximab. Don't confuse Inflectra with Renflexis, Entyvio, Enbrel, Infergen, or Injectafer.

PATIENT TEACHING
Black Box Warning Tell patient that testing for TB will be done before therapy and to immediately report signs and symptoms of infection. ∎

Black Box Warning Counsel patient about risk of lymphoma and other malignancies. ∎

• Tell patient about infusion-reaction symptoms and adverse effects and the need to report them promptly.

• Advise patient to report all adverse reactions and to seek immediate medical attention for signs and symptoms of infection (persistent fever, cough, shortness of breath, fatigue, unusual bleeding or bruising).

• Advise female patient to report if she is or plans to become pregnant before start of therapy. Tell patient not to breastfeed during therapy.

• Advise female patient who took drug during pregnancy that infant shouldn't receive live-virus vaccines for at least 6 months after birth.

• Tell patient to alert prescriber to therapy before receiving vaccines.

• Advise parent to make sure child is up-to-date for all vaccines before therapy.

ingenol mebutate
IN-je-nol

Picato

Therapeutic class: Immunomodulators
Pharmacologic class: Immune response modifiers

AVAILABLE FORMS
Topical gel: 0.015%, 0.05%

INDICATIONS & DOSAGES
➤ **Actinic keratosis on the face and scalp**
Adults: Apply 0.015% strength gel to affected area once daily for 3 days.
➤ **Actinic keratosis on the trunk and extremities**
Adults: Apply 0.05% strength gel to affected area once daily for 2 consecutive days.

ADMINISTRATION
Topical
• Store gel in refrigerator. Don't freeze.
• Spread evenly over treatment area using 1 unit-dose tube, and allow to dry.
• *Alert:* Don't apply to a treatment area of more than 25 cm².
• Wash hands after application to avoid transferring gel to other areas of the body, including periocular area, lips, and mouth.
• Avoid washing and touching treated area for 6 hours after application; after 6 hours, area may be washed with a mild soap.
• One unit-dose tube covers about a 2-inch × 2-inch (5 cm × 5 cm) area. Use each tube only once; throw away open tube after use even if it still contains gel.

ACTION
Unknown. Thought to induce cell death.

Route	Onset	Peak	Duration
Topical	Unknown	Unknown	Unknown

Half-life: Unknown.

ADVERSE REACTIONS
CNS: headache. **EENT:** periorbital edema, nasopharyngitis. **Skin:** erythema, flaking, scaling, crusting, swelling, vesiculation, pustulation, erosion, ulceration, pain, pruritus, infection at treatment site, irritation.

Reactions in bold italics are *life-threatening*. Interactions may have a *rapid onset* or a *delayed onset*.

INTERACTIONS
None reported.

EFFECTS ON LAB TEST RESULTS
None reported.

CONTRAINDICATIONS & CAUTIONS
۞ Alert: Allergic reactions, including anaphylaxis, allergic contact dermatitis, and
herpes zoster reactivation, have occurred in
patients using drug. For severe allergic reactions, stop drug immediately.
۞ Alert: Severe eye injury (severe pain,
chemical conjunctivitis, corneal burn, eyelid
edema, ptosis, periorbital edema) may occur
with eye exposure to drug.
• Drug can cause severe skin reactions in
treated area.
Dialyzable drug: Unknown.

PREGNANCY-LACTATION-REPRODUCTION
• There are no adequate studies in pregnant
women. Use during pregnancy only if potential benefit justifies potential risk to the
fetus.
• No data are available concerning breastfeeding.

NURSING CONSIDERATIONS
• Monitor skin for serious adverse effects.
• Gel is for external use only; don't use via
oral, ophthalmic, or intravaginal route.
• Don't use gel if skin hasn't healed from
previous drug therapy, sunburn, or surgical
treatment.
• Don't apply bandages or closed dressings
to the treated area.

PATIENT TEACHING
• Warn patient that gel is for external use
only and not to apply near mouth, eyes, or
vagina.
• Teach patient proper application technique
and to avoid drug transfer to nontreatment
areas such as the periocular area.
۞ Alert: Caution patient not to use on an area
of skin larger or for a period of time longer
than prescribed.
۞ Alert: Advise patient not to apply makeup
or insert contact lenses right after applying
gel.

• Advise patient to wash hands well after
applying drug to prevent transferring drug to
eye or mouth area.
۞ Alert: If accidental eye exposure occurs,
tell patient to flush eyes thoroughly with
water and seek medical care.
۞ Alert: Warn patient not to mix gel with
other topical drugs or lotions, or to cover
treatment area with a bandage, dressing, or
overlay.
• Instruct patient to keep drug out of the
reach of children.
• Tell patient to store gel in refrigerator and
not to freeze.
• Instruct patient to use gel only after skin
has healed from previous drug therapy, sunburn, or surgical treatment.
• Caution patient not to use gel immediately
after showering or less than 2 hours before
bedtime, and not to perform activities that
cause increased sweating for 6 hours after
applying gel. Advise patient to allow treated
area to dry for 15 minutes after application.
• Tell patient to report serious adverse skin
effects.
• Instruct patient to use each tube only once
and to throw away the open tube after use
even if there is still gel in it.

SAFETY ALERT!

insulin degludec–liraglutide
IN-su-lin de-GLOO-dek/LEER-ah-gloo-
tide

Xultophy 100/3.6

Therapeutic class: Antidiabetics
Pharmacologic class: Insulins–glucagon-
like peptide-1 receptor agonists

AVAILABLE FORMS
Injection (prefilled pen): 100 units insulin
degludec/3.6 mg liraglutide per mL in 3-mL
pens

INDICATIONS & DOSAGES
➤ **Adjunct to diet and exercise to improve
glycemic control in patients with type 2
diabetes mellitus**
Adults: In patients naive to basal insulin
or a glucagon-like peptide-1 (GLP-1) agonist, initially give 10 units (insulin degludec

10 units/liraglutide 0.36 mg) subcut once daily at same time each day. In patients currently on basal insulin or a GLP-1 agonist, initially give 16 units (insulin degludec 16 units/liraglutide 0.58 mg) subcut once daily at same time each day. Titrate dosage upwards or downwards by 2 units (insulin degludec 2 units/liraglutide 0.072 mg) every 3 to 4 days until desired fasting plasma glucose level is achieved. Maximum dose, 50 units (insulin degludec 50 units/liraglutide 1.8 mg)/day.

Adjust-a-dose: Titrate dosage to minimize risk of hypoglycemia or hyperglycemia; with changes in physical activity, meal patterns, or renal or hepatic function; during acute illness; or when drug is used with other drugs that affect glucose level.

ADMINISTRATION
Subcutaneous
• Discontinue other liraglutide products and basal insulins before start of therapy.
• **Alert:** Pens are for a single patient only; pens should never be shared.
• Dose counter displays numbers for the insulin units.
• Don't mix this product with other insulin products or solutions.
• May give drug with or without food.
• Visually inspect drug for particulate matter and discoloration before administration.
• Inject subcut into the thigh, upper arm, or abdomen; don't give IV or IM or use in an insulin infusion pump.
• Rotate injection sites within the same region from one injection to the next to reduce risk of lipodystrophy.
• Don't split the dose; give once daily.
• If a dose is missed, omit the missed dose and resume drug at next scheduled dose. Don't give an extra injection or increase dosage to make up for the missed dose.
• If more than 3 days have elapsed since the last dose, reinitiate drug at the starting dose to avoid GI symptoms associated with treatment reinitiation.
• Before first use, store pens between 36° and 46° F (2° and 8° C) until the expiration date printed on the label. Don't freeze.
• After first use, pens can be stored for 21 days at controlled room temperature

(59° to 86° F [15° to 30° C]) or in refrigerator (36° to 46° F [2° to 8° C]); keep all pens away from direct heat and light.

ACTION
Insulin degludec lowers blood glucose level by stimulating peripheral glucose uptake, especially by skeletal muscle and fat, and by inhibiting hepatic glucose production. Insulin also inhibits lipolysis and proteolysis while enhancing protein synthesis. Liraglutide is a GLP-1 receptor agonist that increases glucose-dependent insulin release, decreases glucagon secretion, and slows gastric emptying.

Route	Onset	Peak	Duration
Subcut	Unknown	Unknown	Unknown

Half-life: Insulin degludec, 25 hours; liraglutide, 13 hours.

ADVERSE REACTIONS
CNS: headache. **CV:** peripheral edema. **EENT:** nasopharyngitis. **GI:** nausea, diarrhea, vomiting, constipation, dyspepsia, gastritis, abdominal pain, flatulence, eructation, GERD, abdominal distention, decreased appetite, *pancreatitis.* **Metabolic:** *hypoglycemia,* weight gain. **Respiratory:** URI. **Skin:** injection-site reactions, lipodystrophy. **Other:** antibody formation.

INTERACTIONS
Drug-drug. *ACE inhibitors, antidiabetics, ARBs, disopyramide, fibrates, fluoxetine, MAO inhibitors, octreotide, pentoxifylline, pramlintide, salicylates, sulfonamide antibiotics:* May increase hypoglycemia risk. Monitor glucose level closely and adjust Xultophy dosage accordingly.

Atypical antipsychotics (olanzapine, clozapine), corticosteroids, danazol, diuretics, estrogens, glucagon, isoniazid, niacin, oral contraceptives, phenothiazines, progestogens in oral contraceptives, protease inhibitors, somatropin, sympathomimetic agents (albuterol, epinephrine, terbutaline), thyroid hormones: May decrease glucose-lowering effects. Monitor glucose level closely and adjust Xultophy dosage as needed.

Reactions in bold italics are *life-threatening*. Interactions may have a *rapid onset* or a *delayed onset*.

Beta blockers, clonidine, guanethidine, reserpine: May blunt or mask signs and symptoms of hypoglycemia. Monitor glucose level closely.

Beta blockers, clonidine, lithium salts, pentamidine: May increase risk of hypoglycemia or hyperglycemia. Monitor glucose level closely and adjust Xultophy dosage as needed.

Oral medications: May affect gastric absorption of other oral medications taken at the same time. Monitor effectiveness of oral medications.

Peroxisome proliferator-activated receptor (PPAR) gamma agonists (thiazolidinediones [pioglitazone, rosiglitazone]): May cause dose-related fluid retention, which can lead to or exacerbate HF. Discontinue or reduce dosage of PPAR gamma agonist as clinically indicated.

Potassium-lowering drugs (loop and thiazide diuretics, theophylline): May increase risk of hypokalemia. Monitor potassium level.

Drug-lifestyle. *Alcohol use:* May alter glucose level and insulin needs. Discourage use together.

EFFECTS ON LAB TEST RESULTS
• May increase bilirubin, calcitonin, lipase, and amylase levels.
• May decrease potassium level.

CONTRAINDICATIONS & CAUTIONS
Black Box Warning Liraglutide causes dose-dependent and treatment duration–dependent thyroid C-cell tumors at clinically relevant exposures in both genders of rats and mice. It isn't known if drug causes thyroid C-cell tumors, including medullary thyroid carcinoma (MTC), in humans, as the human relevance of liraglutide-induced rodent thyroid C-cell tumors hasn't been determined. ▪

Black Box Warning Contraindicated in patients with a personal or family history of MTC and in patients with multiple endocrine neoplasia syndrome type 2 (MEN 2). ▪
• Contraindicated during episodes of hypoglycemia and in patients with hypersensitivity to insulin degludec or liraglutide.

• Severe, life-threatening allergic reactions, including anaphylaxis, angioedema and bronchospasm, urticaria, rash, and pruritus, have been reported. If hypersensitivity reactions occur, discontinue drug. Use cautiously in patients with a history of angioedema resulting from use of another GLP-1 receptor agonist.
• Drug isn't recommended as first-line therapy for patients who have inadequate glycemic control with diet and exercise because of the uncertain relevance of the rodent C-cell tumor findings in humans.
• Use cautiously in patients at risk for pancreatitis. Pancreatitis has been observed in patients taking liraglutide. Drug hasn't been studied in patients with a history of pancreatitis; consider other antidiabetic therapies in these patients.
• Drug isn't indicated for use in patients with type 1 diabetes mellitus or diabetic ketoacidosis, or for use in combination with prandial insulin.
• Drug isn't recommended for use in combination with other products containing liraglutide or other GLP-1 receptor agonists.
• Postmarketing reports indicate incidences of acute renal failure and worsening of chronic renal failure, sometimes requiring hemodialysis, in patients treated with liraglutide. In most cases, these events occurred in patients who experienced nausea, vomiting, diarrhea, or dehydration.
• Drug can cause hypokalemia that, if untreated, can cause respiratory paralysis, ventricular arrhythmias, and death.
• Safety and effectiveness in children haven't been established.
• Use cautiously in elderly patients, as they may be more sensitive to drug's effects.
Dialyzable drug: No.
⚠ *Overdose S&S:* Hypoglycemia, hypokalemia, GI adverse reactions (severe nausea and vomiting).

PREGNANCY-LACTATION-REPRODUCTION
• Animal studies suggest drug may increase fetal adverse events. Use during pregnancy only if potential benefit justifies risk to the fetus.
• It isn't known if drug appears in human milk. Consider both the potential adverse effects to the breastfed infant and the

developmental and health benefits of breast-feeding.

NURSING CONSIDERATIONS
• Adjust dosages cautiously and only under medical supervision with frequent glucose monitoring.
• Monitor patients for dehydration. Drug can cause dehydration due to GI adverse reactions; take precautions to avoid fluid depletion.
• Monitor patients for signs and symptoms of pancreatitis (persistent severe abdominal pain that may radiate to the back, with or without vomiting). Discontinue drug if pancreatitis is confirmed.
• Monitor patients for URI.
• Monitor patients for hypersensitivity reactions (urticaria, rash, pruritus, anaphylactic reaction, angioedema).
• Evaluate patients with changes to the thyroid gland or significantly elevated serum calcitonin level.
• Monitor renal function and blood glucose, amylase, and lipase levels.
• Monitor serum potassium level in patients at risk for hypokalemia (patients taking potassium-lowering medication or medications sensitive to potassium levels).
• Monitor patients for development of lipodystrophy.
• *Look alike–sound alike:* Don't confuse Xultophy with Azulfidine or Xarelto.

PATIENT TEACHING
• Explain that dose counter on pen shows only the number of insulin units to be injected.
• Teach patient how to use dosage pen and how to administer drug, including rotating injection sites.
• Advise patient against sharing pens with other individuals because of the risk of contracting blood-borne pathogens.
• Instruct patient not to take more than 50 units of the pen per day and not to use with other GLP-1 receptor agonists.
• Advise patient not to split doses into two injections and not to mix other insulin or GLP-1 products in the same syringe.
• Emphasize to patient that glucose monitoring will need to be done regularly and that glucose level will need to be checked

more carefully with changes in amount of activity, meal patterns, and acute illness.
• Caution patient that dosage changes should only be made under medical supervision.
• Teach patient the signs and symptoms of hypoglycemia (confusion, dizziness, feeling shaky, rapid pulse) and how to manage it.
• Instruct patient to report all adverse effects and to immediately report edema, chest pain, or palpitations.
Black Box Warning Inform patient of risk of thyroid tumors, including cancer, and to immediately report neck lump or swelling, hoarseness, trouble swallowing, or shortness of breath. ∎
• Warn patient to immediately report severe pain in the abdomen that may or may not radiate to the back (with or without vomiting), as this type of pain may indicate pancreatitis.
• Counsel patient to avoid becoming dehydrated, as acute kidney injury may occur.

SAFETY ALERT!

insulin glargine–lixisenatide
IN-su-lin/lix-i-SEN-a-tide

Soliqua 100/33

Therapeutic class: Antidiabetics
Pharmacologic class: Insulins–glucagon-like peptide-1 receptor agonists

AVAILABLE FORMS
Injection: insulin glargine 100 units/mL and lixisenatide 33 mcg/mL in 3-mL pens

INDICATIONS & DOSAGES
➤ **Adjunct to diet and exercise to improve glycemic control in patients with type 2 diabetes mellitus**
Adults naive to basal insulin or to a glucagon-like peptide-1 (GLP-1) receptor agonist, currently on a GLP-1 receptor agonist, or currently on less than 30 units of basal insulin daily: Initially, 15 units (insulin glargine 15 units/lixisenatide 5 mcg) subcut once daily within the hour before first meal of the day.
Adults inadequately controlled on 30 to 60 units of basal insulin, with or without a GLP-1 receptor agonist: Initially, 30 units

(insulin glargine 30 units/lixisenatide 10 mcg) subcut once daily within the hour before the first meal of the day.

Adjust-a-dose: Titrate dosage up or down by 2 to 4 units every week based on patient's metabolic needs, blood glucose monitoring results, and glycemic goal until desired fasting glucose level is achieved. Dosage titration may also be needed with changes in activity, meal patterns, or renal or hepatic function; during acute illness; or when used with other medications that affect glucose level. Use alternative antidiabetic products if patients require a Soliqua 100/33 daily dosage below 15 units or above 60 units. Maximum dose, 60 units (insulin glargine 60 units/lixisenatide 20 mcg) daily.

ADMINISTRATION
Subcutaneous
• Discontinue therapy with a GLP-1 receptor agonist or basal insulin before starting Soliqua 100/33.
• Prefilled pen delivers doses from 15 to 60 units in a single injection.
• Refer to manufacturer's instructions and perform a safety test before each injection to check that pen and needle are working correctly and to ensure that correct dose will be delivered.
• Inspect pen before use. Solution should be clear and colorless to almost colorless.
• Inject into abdominal area, thigh, or upper arm, rotating injection sites within the same region to reduce risk of lipodystrophy.
• Don't administer IV, IM, or via an insulin pump.
• Don't dilute or mix with other insulins or solution.
• Don't administer drug in split doses.
• Remove needle after each injection and store pen without needle attached. Always use a new needle for each injection to prevent contamination.
• If a dose is missed, resume the once-daily regimen as prescribed with the next scheduled dose. Don't administer an extra dose or increase the dose to make up for the missed dose.
⚠ *Alert:* Pen is for single-patient use only because of risk of transmission of blood-borne pathogens even if needle is changed.

• Store drug in refrigerator at 36° to 46° F (2° to 8° C) before first use. Don't freeze. Discard drug if pen has been frozen. Protect from light.
• After first use, store pen at room temperature below 86° F (30° C). Replace pen cap after each use to protect from light. Discard pen 14 days after first use.

ACTION
Insulin glargine lowers blood glucose level by stimulating peripheral glucose uptake and by inhibiting hepatic glucose production. Lixisenatide increases glucose-dependent insulin release, decreases glucagon secretion, and slows gastric emptying.

Route	Onset	Peak	Duration
Subcut	Insulin glargine: 3–4 hr	Insulin glargine: no pronounced peak Lixisenatide: 2½–3 hr	Insulin glargine: about 24 hr

Half-life: 3 hours (lixisenatide).

ADVERSE REACTIONS
CNS: headache. **CV:** peripheral edema. **EENT:** nasopharyngitis. **GI:** diarrhea, nausea, *pancreatitis,* vomiting, constipation, dyspepsia, gastritis, abdominal pain, flatulence, GERD, abdominal distention, decreased appetite. **Metabolic:** *hypoglycemia, hypokalemia,* weight gain. **Respiratory:** URI. **Skin:** injection-site reactions, lipodystrophy. **Other:** antibody development, hypersensitivity reactions.

INTERACTIONS
Drug-drug. *ACE inhibitors, antidiabetics, ARBs, disopyramide, fibrates, fluoxetine, MAO inhibitors, pentoxifylline, pramlintide, salicylates, somatostatin analogues (octreotide), sulfonamide antibiotics:* May increase risk of hypoglycemia. Monitor glucose level closely and adjust dosage as necessary.
Acetaminophen, antibiotics and other oral medications dependent on threshold concentrations for efficacy: Lixisenatide may reduce rate of absorption of coadministered oral drugs. Give other drugs at least 1 hour before Soliqua 100/33.
Atypical antipsychotics (clozapine, olanzapine), corticosteroids, danazol, diuretics,

estrogens, glucagon, isoniazid, niacin, phenothiazines, protease inhibitors, somatropin, sympathomimetic agents (albuterol, epinephrine, terbutaline), thyroid hormones: May decrease blood glucose–lowering effect of Soliqua 100/33. Monitor glucose level closely and adjust Soliqua 100/33 dosage as needed.

Beta blockers, clonidine, guanethidine, reserpine: May mask signs and symptoms of hypoglycemia. Monitor glucose level closely and adjust Soliqua 100/33 dosage as needed.

Beta blockers, clonidine, lithium salts: May increase or decrease blood glucose–lowering effect of Soliqua 100/33. Monitor glucose level closely and adjust Soliqua 100/33 dosage as necessary.

Lixisenatide, other GLP-1 receptor agonists: May increase risk of overdose and hypoglycemia. Use together isn't recommended.

Oral contraceptives, progesterones: May delay rate of contraceptive absorption. Patient should take contraceptive at least 1 hour before or 11 hours after Soliqua 100/33.

Pentamidine: May cause hypoglycemia, which may be followed by hyperglycemia. Monitor glucose level closely and adjust Soliqua 100/33 dosage as needed.

Drug-lifestyle. *Alcohol use:* May increase or decrease blood glucose–lowering effect of Soliqua 100/33. Discourage use together.

Smoking: May decrease insulin absorption and increase insulin resistance. Discourage use together.

EFFECTS ON LAB TEST RESULTS

• May decrease glucose, HbA$_{1c}$, and potassium levels.

• May cause immunogenicity and antibody positivity.

CONTRAINDICATIONS & CAUTIONS

• Contraindicated during hypoglycemia episodes.

• Contraindicated in patients hypersensitive to either of the active drug substances or their components.

• Rarely, allergic reactions (urticaria, angioedema, anaphylaxis, bronchospasm, hypotension, shock) have been reported. Use cautiously in patients with a history of anaphylaxis or angioedema with use of another GLP-1 receptor agonist.

• Drug isn't indicated for use in patients with type 1 diabetes mellitus or for treatment of diabetic ketoacidosis.

• Acute pancreatitis has been reported with GLP-1 receptor agonists. Consider other antidiabetics in patients with a history of pancreatitis.

• Not recommended in patients with ESRD (eGFR <15 mL/minute/1.73 m^2) or in patients with severe gastroparesis. Consider other antidiabetics.

• Use with prandial insulin hasn't been studied.

• Use cautiously in patients with visual impairment who may rely on audible clicks to dial their dose.

• Safety and effectiveness in children haven't been established.

• Use cautiously in elderly patients. Initial dosing, dose increments, and maintenance dosing should be conservative to avoid hypoglycemia.

Dialyzable drug: Unknown.

⚠ **Overdose S&S:** Insulin glargine: hypoglycemia, hypokalemia. Lixisenatide: increased incidence of GI disorders.

PREGNANCY-LACTATION-REPRODUCTION

• Exposure to lixisenatide during pregnancy may cause fetal harm. Use in pregnant women only if potential benefits justify risk to the fetus.

• It isn't known if insulin glargine or lixisenatide appears in human milk. Effects on the breastfed infant or on milk production are unknown. Weigh benefits of breastfeeding and the mother's clinical need for drug against potential adverse effects on the breastfed infant.

NURSING CONSIDERATIONS

• Monitor patient for signs and symptoms of hypoglycemia; the long-acting effect of insulin glargine may delay recovery from hypoglycemia.

• Frequently monitor blood glucose level during dosage changes, which may predispose patient to hypoglycemia or hyperglycemia. Adjust concomitant oral antidiabetics as needed.

- Always check insulin label before giving drug, as accidental mix-ups among insulin products have been reported.
- Increase frequency of glucose monitoring with changes to meal pattern or physical activity and in patients with renal or hepatic impairment and hypoglycemia unawareness.
- Observe patients treated with insulin-containing products and a peroxisome proliferator-activated receptor (PPAR) (pioglitazone, rosiglitazone, fenofibrate, clofibrate) for signs and symptoms of HF. If HF develops, manage per standards of care; consider discontinuing drug or reducing dosage of the PPAR-gamma agonist.
- Monitor patient for signs and symptoms of pancreatitis (persistent severe abdominal pain, sometimes radiating to the back, with or without vomiting). If pancreatitis is suspected, discontinue drug and treat appropriately. If pancreatitis is confirmed, don't restart drug.
- Acute kidney injury and worsening of chronic renal failure have been reported. Monitor renal function and GI adverse effects when starting drug or increasing dosage in patients with renal impairment and in those reporting severe GI reactions. Assess fluid status closely.
- Monitor patient for worsening glycemic control or failure to achieve targeted glycemic control, significant injection-site reactions, or allergic reactions, as they may indicate antibody formation. Consider alternative antidiabetic therapy.
- Insulin-containing products may cause potassium to shift into the intracellular space, resulting in hypokalemia. Monitor potassium level in patients at risk for hypokalemia (patients using potassium-lowering drugs or drugs sensitive to serum potassium concentrations).
- **Look alike–sound alike:** Don't confuse insulin glargine with other insulin products.

PATIENT TEACHING

- Inform patient that serious hypersensitivity reactions, including anaphylaxis, have been reported. Instruct patient to stop drug and immediately seek medical attention for signs and symptoms of hypersensitivity reactions.
- Advise patient of risk of pancreatitis. Instruct patient to discontinue drug and report persistent abdominal pain, with or without vomiting.
- Teach patient to never share the pen with another person, even if the needle is changed, because of risk of transmission of blood-borne pathogens.
- Inform patient that hypoglycemia is the most common adverse reaction. Teach patient signs and symptoms of hypoglycemia and that regimen changes can predispose patient to hypoglycemia or hyperglycemia.
- Warn patient that hypoglycemia may impair mental alertness and to use caution while driving or operating machinery.
- Advise patient of risk of dehydration due to GI adverse reactions and to take precautions to avoid fluid depletion.
- Inform patient of risk of worsening renal function, which may require dialysis.
- Instruct patient to always check label before each injection to avoid medication errors due to confusion with other insulin products.
- Caution patient that administering more than 60 units of Soliqua 100/33 daily or concurrent use with other GLP-1 inhibitors can result in lixisenatide overdose.
- Instruct patient on self-management procedures, including glucose monitoring and management of hypoglycemia and hyperglycemia.
- Teach patient how to handle special situations, such as concurrent illness, stress, or emotional disturbances; inadequate or missed insulin dose; inadvertent administration of an increased insulin dose; inadequate food intake; and missed meals.
- Instruct patient on proper administration and handling. Caution patient not to dilute drug or mix drug with other insulin products or solutions.
- Advise female patient to tell physician if she is pregnant, intends to become pregnant, or is breastfeeding.

Insulins (fixed combinations)
IN-su-lins

insulin degludec–insulin aspart

insulin lispro protamine–insulin lispro
HumaLOG Mix 75/25, HumaLOG Mix 50/50

isophane insulin suspension–insulin injection combinations
HumuLIN 70/30 ◇, NovoLIN 70/30 ◇

insulin aspart (rDNA origin) protamine suspension–insulin aspart (rDNA origin) injection
NovoLOG Mix 70/30

Therapeutic class: Antidiabetics
Pharmacologic class: Insulins

AVAILABLE FORMS
Injection: Humalog Mix 75/25 (75% insulin lispro protamine suspension and 25% insulin lispro) and 50/50 (50% insulin lispro protamine suspension and 50% insulin lispro) 100 units/mL (U-100) in 10-mL vials, 3-mL prefilled KwikPen syringes
Injection: Humulin 70/30 (70% isophane insulin suspension and 30% regular insulin) 100 units/mL (U-100) in 3-mL and 10-mL vials, 3-mL prefilled pens, 3-mL KwikPen syringes
Injection: Novolog Mix 70/30 (70% insulin aspart protamine suspension and 30% insulin aspart) 100 units/mL (U-100) in 10-mL vials, 3-mL prefilled FlexPen syringes
Injection: Novolin 70/30 (70% isophane insulin suspension and 30% regular insulin) 100 units/mL (U-100) in 10-mL vials

INDICATIONS & DOSAGES
Adjust-a-dose (for all indications): Individualize dosage based on metabolic needs, blood glucose monitoring, and glycemic control goal. Insulin requirements may be altered during acute illness, emotional distress, or stress. Adjust as needed in patients who are elderly, have renal or hepatic dysfunction, or have changes in physical activity or meal patterns, and in patients concurrently taking drugs that lower blood glucose level. Refer to manufacturer's instructions for dosage adjustments when converting from other insulin regimens and formulations. Obese patients may need a maintenance dosage of up to 1.2 units/kg/day.

➤ **To improve glycemic control in patients with diabetes mellitus**
Adults: For Novolog Mix 70/30, usual dosage is 0.5 to 1 unit/kg/day subcut in divided doses within 15 minutes before a meal or, in type 2 diabetes, given up to 15 minutes after start of a meal. Drug isn't intended for initial treatment, but may be transitioned to after basal insulin requirements are determined. Generally, 50% to 75% daily insulin dose is given as an intermediate- or long-acting form of insulin in one to two daily subcut injections. The remaining portion of the 24-hour insulin requirement is divided and given as either regular insulin or a rapid-acting form of insulin at the same time before breakfast and dinner.
Adults: For Humalog Mix 50/50 and 75/25, dosage is individualized and given subcut within 15 minutes before a meal.
Adults and children: For Humulin 70/30 and Novolin 70/30, usual dosage is 0.5 to 1 unit/kg/day subcut divided into two doses given about 30 to 45 minutes before a meal. During puberty, insulin requirements may increase to 1.2 units/kg/day during growth spurts.

ADMINISTRATION
Subcutaneous
• Inspect vials and syringes. Drug should appear uniformly white and cloudy. Don't use if it looks clear or contains solid particles.
• Administer all insulin mixtures at room temperature.
• Don't freeze vials or pens; discard if frozen.
• Drug is a suspension; administer only subcut, never IV.
• Don't use in insulin infusion pumps.
• Don't mix with other insulins.
• Keep away from direct heat and sunlight.

Reactions in bold italics are *life-threatening*. Interactions may have a *rapid onset* or a *delayed onset*.

• Discard insulin exposed to temperatures above 98.6° F (37° C).

• Follow product-specific pen device directions for preparation and administration.

۞ Alert: Multidose pens are for single-patient use only. Pens should never be shared even if the needle is changed. Clearly label with patient identifying information where it won't obstruct dosing window, warning, or other product information.

Novolog Mix 70/30

• Keep all unopened Novolog Mix 70/30 refrigerated between 36° and 46° F (2° and 8° C) until expiration date.

• Once vial is opened or has been unopened but stored at room temperature, use within 28 days.

• Once a Novolog Mix 70/30 FlexPen has been punctured, it should be kept at temperatures below 86° F (30° C) for up to 14 days. Don't store a Novolog Mix 70/30 FlexPen that's in use in refrigerator.

Humulin 70/30

• Discard opened or unopened vials stored at room temperature after 31 days.

• Store unopened pen or KwikPen in refrigerator at 36° to 46° F (2° to 8° C). Discard unopened pens stored at room temperature after 10 days.

• Store opened pen or KwikPen at room temperature; discard after 10 days even if syringe contains insulin.

Novolin 70/30

• Store unopened vials in refrigerator at 36° to 46° F (2° to 8° C).

• If refrigeration isn't possible, may keep unopened vials at room temperature for up to 6 weeks (42 days), as long as temperature is at or below 77° F (25° C). Keep unopened vials in carton to protect from light.

• If unopened vials are stored in refrigerator, follow expiration date on label.

• Keep open vials at room temperature.

• Throw away open vial after 6 weeks (42 days) of use, even if insulin remains in vial.

Humalog Mix 75/25 and Humalog Mix 50/50

• Refrigerate vials and pens at 36° to 46° F (2° to 8° C) until ready to use.

• Unrefrigerated (below 86° F [30° C]) vials must be used within 28 days or discarded.

• Unrefrigerated (below 86° F [30° C]) KwikPen and pen must be used within 10 days and then discarded, even if syringe contains insulin.

ACTION

Regulates glucose metabolism by binding to insulin receptors on muscle, liver, and fat cells; facilitates cellular uptake of glucose; and promotes uptake and storage of glucose in the form of glycogen in the liver.

Route	Onset	Peak	Duration
Subcut (Novolog Mix 70/30)	10–20 min	1.8–3.6 hr	Up to 24 hr
Subcut (Humulin 70/30)	30–90 min	2.2 hr	Up to 24 hr
Subcut (Humalog Mix 75/25 and 50/50)	15 min	30–240 min	Up to 24 hr
Subcut (Novolin 70/30)	30 min	3.8–4.6 hr	Up to 24 hr

Half-life: Novolog Mix 70/30, 8 to 9 hours; Humulin 70/30 and Novolin 70/30, unknown; Humalog Mix 75/25 and 50/50, unknown.

ADVERSE REACTIONS

CNS: asthenia, headache, fever, pain. **CV:** peripheral edema. **EENT:** pharyngitis, rhinitis. **GI:** abdominal pain, diarrhea, nausea. **GU:** UTI, dysmenorrhea. **Metabolic:** *hypoglycemia, hypokalemia,* weight gain. **Musculoskeletal:** myalgia. **Respiratory:** bronchitis, cough. **Skin:** lipodystrophy, injection-site reactions, rash. **Other:** *allergic reactions,* insulin antibody production, flulike syndrome, infection.

INTERACTIONS

Drug-drug. *ACE inhibitors, antidiabetic agents (oral), ARBs, disopyramide, fibrates, fluoxetine,* **MAO inhibitors,** *octreotide, pentoxifylline, pramlintide, salicylates, sulfonamide antibiotics:* May increase risk of hypoglycemia. Monitor glucose level closely and adjust insulin dosage as needed.

Atypical antipsychotics, corticosteroids, danazol, diuretics, estrogens, glucagon, hormonal contraceptives, isoniazid, niacin, phenothiazines, protease inhibitors, sympathomimetics (albuterol, epinephrine, terbutaline), somatropin, thyroid hormones: May decrease blood glucose–lowering effects. Monitor glucose level closely and adjust insulin dosage as needed.

Beta blockers, clonidine, guanethidine, reserpine: May mask signs and symptoms of hypoglycemia. Avoid concurrent use, if possible, or monitor patient closely.

Beta blockers, clonidine, lithium salts, pentamidine: May cause hypoglycemia or hyperglycemia. Monitor glucose level closely.

Thiazolidinediones (TZDs; pioglitazone, rosiglitazone): May cause fluid retention that can lead to HF. Monitor patient closely and adjust or stop TZDs as clinically indicated.

Drug-herb. *Ginseng:* May increase drug's effects. Discourage use together.

Drug-lifestyle. *Alcohol use:* May cause hyperglycemia or hypoglycemia. Monitor glucose level closely and discourage concurrent use.

EFFECTS ON LAB TEST RESULTS
• May decrease blood glucose and potassium levels.

CONTRAINDICATIONS & CAUTIONS
• Contraindicated during episodes of hypoglycemia or ketoacidosis.
• Contraindicated in patients with a history of hypersensitivity to drug or its components. Severe, life-threatening, generalized allergy, including anaphylaxis, can occur with insulin products.
• Changes in insulin or oral antidiabetic dosages may affect glycemic control and should be made only under medical supervision.
• Use cautiously in patients susceptible to hypokalemia, such as patients who are fasting, are taking potassium-lowering drugs, or are concurrently taking drugs that may affect potassium levels, including IV insulin. Untreated hypokalemia can cause respiratory paralysis, ventricular arrhythmias, and death.
• Hypoglycemia is the most common adverse reaction. Severe hypoglycemia can cause seizures, and may be life-threatening or fatal. Hypoglycemia can occur suddenly, and signs and symptoms may differ. Risk increases with intensity of glycemic control

and changes in glycemic treatment, meal patterns, physical activity, or concomitant medications, and in patients with renal or hepatic impairment.
• Use cautiously in elderly patients, who may be at increased risk for adverse effects; signs and symptoms of hypoglycemia may be more difficult to recognize in these patients.

Dialyzable drug: Unknown.

⚠ *Overdose S&S:* Hypoglycemia, hypokalemia.

PREGNANCY-LACTATION-REPRODUCTION
• Use cautiously in pregnant women and only if clearly needed.
• Monitor blood glucose levels closely in pregnant patients, in women who have recently given birth, and in breastfeeding women; insulin requirements may change.
• It isn't known if insulin appears in human milk. Use cautiously in breastfeeding women.

NURSING CONSIDERATIONS
• Don't mix combination insulins with other insulins.
• Rotate injection sites to reduce risk of lipodystrophy.
• Subcut administration is usually made into thighs, arms, buttocks, or abdomen.
• The time course of the action of insulin mixtures may vary among patients and in the same patient depending on time of day, injection site, blood supply, temperature, and physical activity.
• Observe injection sites for reactions, such as redness, swelling, itching, or burning. These reactions should resolve within a few days or weeks.
• Assess patient and notify prescriber for signs and symptoms of hypoglycemia (sweating, shaking, trembling, confusion, headache, irritability, hunger, rapid, pulse, nausea) and hyperglycemia (drowsiness, fruity breath odor, frequent urination, thirst).
• Signs and symptoms of hypoglycemia may occur in patients with diabetes regardless of glucose value.
• Monitor blood glucose level and adjust insulin dosages as needed with medical supervision.

Reactions in bold italics are *life-threatening*. Interactions may have a *rapid onset* or a *delayed onset*.

• Closely monitor patients also taking other medications because other drugs can mask signs and symptoms of hypoglycemia or cause an increase or decrease in blood glucose level.

• Increase frequency of glucose monitoring in patients who are acutely ill or under emotional stress, or if changes in diet, exercise, or medication regimen occur. These situations may affect rate of insulin absorption.

• Increase frequency of glucose monitoring when initiating therapy or when changes in insulin strength, dosage, manufacturer, or type or method of administration are made. Such changes may affect glycemic control and increase risk of hypoglycemia.

• Monitor patient carefully for signs and symptoms of hypoglycemia. Symptom awareness may be decreased in patients with long-standing diabetes, diabetic nerve disease, renal disease, or hepatic impairment and in patients who have experienced recurrent hypoglycemia. Treat according to individual facility policy and procedure if necessary.

• Mild episodes of hypoglycemia may be treated with oral glucose. More severe episodes of hypoglycemia, such as coma, seizure, or neurologic impairment, may be treated with IM or subcut glucagon or concentrated IV glucose.

• Monitor potassium levels in patients at risk for hypokalemia (those receiving potassium-depleting drugs or IV insulin).

• Monitor patients for generalized allergic reactions, rash (including pruritus) over entire body, shortness of breath, wheezing, hypotension, rapid pulse, sweating, and anaphylaxis.

• Periodically measure HbA_{1c} levels.

• *Look alike–sound alike:* Don't confuse Novolog with Novolin; don't confuse Humalog with Humulin.

PATIENT TEACHING

• Caution patient not to mix insulin combination products with other insulins.

🔵 *Alert:* Warn patient not to share multidose pen with other people, even if the needle is changed, because of risk of bloodborne pathogen transmission, including HIV and hepatitis.

• Advise patient that hypoglycemic episodes can impair the ability to concentrate and react; advise patient to use caution while driving and operating machinery.

• Instruct patient to keep hard candy or glucose tablets on hand to treat mild cases of hypoglycemia.

• Advise patient to keep a log of glucose levels.

• Instruct patient on long-term sequelae of diabetes if not managed properly.

• Instruct patient to carry identification or wear jewelry indicating that patient has diabetes.

• Advise patient that allergic and hypersensitivity reactions can occur, including injection-site reactions (local pain, redness, or swelling), and to report symptoms to health care provider. Teach patient signs and symptoms of anaphylaxis and to seek emergency medical attention promptly if anaphylaxis occurs.

• Instruct patient on self-management procedures, including glucose monitoring, proper preparation and administration techniques, and management of hypoglycemia and hyperglycemia.

• Warn patient about special situations, such as concurrent conditions (illness, stress, or emotional disturbances), inadequate or skipped insulin dose, inadvertent administration of an increased insulin dose, inadequate food intake, and skipped meals.

• Advise female patient with diabetes to inform prescriber if she is pregnant or plans to become pregnant.

• Advise pregnant patient of the change in insulin requirements that may occur during pregnancy and after childbirth.

• Teach patient that alcohol and some other medications may increase or decrease glucose levels. Advise patient to inform prescriber of all medications and supplements being taken.

• Caution patient not to stop insulin abruptly or change amount taken without consulting prescriber.

• Advise patient that any insulin change should be made cautiously and only under medical supervision. Changes in insulin strength, manufacturer, type (regular, NPH, or insulin analogues), species (animal, human), or method of manufacture (rDNA versus animal-source insulin) may result in the need for a dosage change. Dosage of concomitant oral antidiabetic agents may need adjustment.

• Teach patient to give insulin at appropriate time around a meal, depending on product.
• Instruct patient to rotate injection sites and of the importance of avoiding lipodystrophy.
• Teach patient to store insulin products properly, depending on individual products.
• Explain importance of checking insulin label before each injection as accidental mix-ups among insulin types have been reported.

SAFETY ALERT!

Insulins (intermediate-acting)

IN-su-lins

isophane insulin suspension (NPH)
HumuLIN N ◊, HumuLIN N KwikPen ◊, NovoLIN N ◊

Therapeutic class: Antidiabetics
Pharmacologic class: Insulins

AVAILABLE FORMS
Injection: 100 units/mL in 3-mL and 10-mL vials, 3-mL pens (Humulin N)

INDICATIONS & DOSAGES
Adjust-a-dose (for all indications): Individualize dosage based on metabolic needs, blood glucose monitoring, and glycemic control goal. Adjust dosage to achieve premeal plasma glucose level of 90 to 130 mg/dL and peak postprandial plasma and bedtime glucose level of less than 180 mg/dL. Insulin requirements may be altered during acute illness, emotional distress, or stress. Adjust as needed in patients who are elderly, have renal or hepatic dysfunction, or have changes in physical activity or meal patterns, and in patients concurrently taking drugs that lower blood glucose level. Refer to manufacturer's instructions for dosage adjustments when converting from other insulin regimens and formulations.
➤ **Patients with type 1 diabetes mellitus; patients with type 2 diabetes mellitus that can't be properly controlled by diet, exercise, and weight control**
Adults and children age 12 and older: Usual dosage is 0.5 to 1 unit/kg/day, often given in two divided doses to provide a more constant level of basal insulin.

ADMINISTRATION
Subcutaneous
• Give by subcut injection only; not for IM, IV, or insulin pump administration.
• Give injection in abdominal region, buttocks, thigh, or upper arm. Subcut injection into abdominal wall is generally associated with faster absorption than other injection sites.
• Rotate injection sites within same region to reduce risk of lipodystrophy. A general rule is to not administer within 1 inch (2.5 cm) of same site for 1 month.
• Injection into a lifted skin fold minimizes risk of IM injection.
• Roll vial gently between the hands before each dose to uniformly disperse NPH insulin. Avoid vigorous shaking that may cause air bubbles or foam.
• NPH insulin should be uniformly cloudy or milky after gentle mixing and shouldn't contain particulate matter.
• When mixing NPH insulin with regular insulin, always draw clear regular insulin into syringe first; then administer immediately.
• NPH insulin is typically given within 60 minutes of a meal. However, time of administration depends on patient-specific variables; NPH insulin may be given with meal-time regular or Humalog insulin if indicated.
• *Alert:* Multidose pens are for single patient use only. Pens should never be shared even if the needle is changed. Clearly label with patient identifying information where it won't obstruct dosing window, warning, or other product information.
• Store Humulin N at room temperature, below 86° F (30° C), if not exposed to direct sunlight for 31 days (vial) or 14 days (pen). May store opened vials and unopened vials and pens in refrigerator at 36° to 46° F (2° to 8° C); don't refrigerate opened pens. Don't freeze vials or pens.
• Store opened or unopened Novolin N away from direct heat or light at room temperature,

---

below 77° F (25° C), for up to 42 days. Unopened Novolin N can be stored in refrigerator at 36° to 46° F (2° to 8° C) and used until expiration date on label. Don't freeze.

ACTION

Lowers blood glucose level by stimulating peripheral glucose uptake by binding to insulin receptors on skeletal muscle and in fat cells and by inhibiting hepatic glucose production; also inhibits lipolysis and proteolysis, and enhances protein synthesis. Intermediate-acting insulin suspensions of human insulin with protamine and zinc provide a slower onset and a longer duration of activity.

Route	Onset	Peak	Duration
Subcut	1–1½ hr	4–12 hr	Up to 24 hr

Half-life: About 4.4 hours.

ADVERSE REACTIONS

CV: peripheral edema. **Metabolic:** hypoglycemia, hypokalemia, weight gain. **Skin:** injection-site reaction, lipodystrophy, pruritus, rash. **Other:** allergic reactions, immunogenicity.

INTERACTIONS

Drug-drug. *ACE inhibitors, antidiabetic agents (oral), ARBs, disopyramide, fibrates, fluoxetine,* **MAO inhibitors,** *octreotide, pentoxifylline, pramlintide, salicylates, sulfonamide antibiotics:* May increase risk of hypoglycemia. Monitor glucose level closely and adjust insulin dosage as needed.
Atypical antipsychotics, corticosteroids, danazol, diuretics, estrogens, glucagon, hormonal contraceptives, isoniazid, niacin, phenothiazines, protease inhibitors, sympathomimetics (albuterol, epinephrine, terbutaline), somatropin, thyroid hormones: May decrease blood glucose–lowering effects. Monitor glucose level closely and adjust insulin dosage as needed.
Beta blockers, clonidine, guanethidine, reserpine: May mask signs and symptoms of hypoglycemia. Avoid concurrent use, if possible, and monitor patient closely.
Beta blockers, clonidine, lithium salts, pentamidine: May cause hypoglycemia or hyperglycemia. Monitor glucose level closely.

Thiazolidinediones (TZDs; pioglitazone, rosiglitazone): May cause fluid retention that can lead to HF. Monitor patient closely and adjust or stop TZDs as clinically indicated.
Drug-lifestyle. *Alcohol use:* May cause hyperglycemia or hypoglycemia. Monitor glucose level closely, and discourage concurrent use.

EFFECTS ON LAB TEST RESULTS

• May decrease blood glucose and potassium levels.
• May develop antibodies that react with human insulin.

CONTRAINDICATIONS & CAUTIONS

• Contraindicated during episodes of hypoglycemia or ketoacidosis.
• Contraindicated in patients with a history of hypersensitivity to drug or its components. Severe, life-threatening, generalized allergy, including anaphylaxis, can occur with insulin products.
• Use cautiously in patients susceptible to hypokalemia, such as patients who are fasting, are taking potassium-lowering drugs, or are concurrently taking drugs that may affect potassium level. Untreated hypokalemia can cause respiratory paralysis, ventricular arrhythmias, and death.
• Hypoglycemia is the most common adverse reaction. Severe hypoglycemia can cause seizures, and may be life-threatening or fatal. Hypoglycemia can occur suddenly and symptoms may differ. Risk increases with intensity of glycemic control and changes in glycemic treatment, meal patterns, physical activity, and concomitant medications and in patients with renal or hepatic impairment.
• Use cautiously in elderly patients, who may at increased risk for adverse effects; signs and symptoms of hypoglycemia may be more difficult to recognize in these patients.
Dialyzable drug: Unknown.
⚠ Overdose S&S: Hypoglycemia, hypokalemia.

PREGNANCY-LACTATION-REPRODUCTION

• Use cautiously in pregnant women and monitor patients closely.

• Monitor blood glucose levels closely in pregnant patients, in women who have recently given birth, and in breastfeeding women; insulin requirements may change.

• It isn't known if insulin appears in human milk. Use cautiously in breastfeeding women.

NURSING CONSIDERATIONS

• Monitor blood glucose levels and adjust insulin dosages as needed.

• Monitor patients taking other medications with insulin more closely because other drugs may mask signs and symptoms of hypoglycemia or may cause an increase or decrease in blood glucose level.

• Increase frequency of glucose monitoring in patients who are acutely ill or under emotional stress, or if changes in diet, exercise, or medication regimen occur, as these may affect rate of insulin absorption. Also closely monitor patients after changes to insulin dosage.

• Monitor patients carefully for signs and symptoms of hypoglycemia. Treat according to individual facility policy and procedure if necessary.

• Mild episodes of hypoglycemia may be treated with oral glucose. More severe episodes of hypoglycemia, such as coma, seizure, or neurologic impairment, may be treated with IM or subcut glucagon or concentrated IV glucose.

• Monitor potassium levels in patients at risk for hypokalemia, especially those taking potassium-depleting drugs.

• Assess patient for signs and symptoms of hypoglycemia (seizures, sweating, shaking, trembling, confusion) and hyperglycemia (drowsiness, fruity breath odor, frequent urination, thirst). Notify prescriber if any of these signs or symptoms occur.

• Periodically measure HbA_{1c} levels.

• Monitor patients for generalized allergic reactions, including anaphylaxis.

• *Look alike–sound alike:* Don't confuse Humulin with Humalog; don't confuse Novolin with Novolog.

PATIENT TEACHING

• Instruct patient in self-management, including glucose monitoring, injection preparation and technique, proper storage of insulin, and recognition and management of hypoglycemia and hyperglycemia.

• Explain to patient that insulin requirements may vary due to illness, stress or emotional disturbance, inadequate food intake, and skipped meals.

• Advise patient that hypoglycemic episodes can impair the ability to concentrate and react; advise patient to use caution while driving and operating machinery.

• Advise patient that allergic and hypersensitivity reactions can occur, including injection-site reactions (local pain, redness, or swelling), and to report signs and symptoms to health care provider. Teach patient signs and symptoms of anaphylaxis and to seek emergency medical attention promptly if anaphylaxis occurs.

• Instruct patient to rotate injection sites to avoid developing lipodystrophy.

⟲ *Alert:* Warn patient not to share multidose pen with other people, even if the needle is changed, because of risk of bloodborne pathogen transmission, including HIV and hepatitis.

• Explain importance of checking insulin label before each injection as accidental mix-ups among insulin types have been reported.

• Explain that intermediate-acting insulins can be mixed with regular insulin.

• Instruct patient to visually inspect insulin before use to ensure that there's no particulate matter in vial and that the medication appears uniformly cloudy.

• Teach patient that alcohol and some other medications may increase or decrease glucose levels. Advise patient to inform health care provider of all medications and supplements being taken.

• Instruct patient not to stop insulin abruptly or change amount injected without consulting prescriber.

• Advise patient that any insulin changes should be made cautiously and only under medical supervision. Changes in insulin strength, manufacturer, type (regular, NPH, or insulin analogues), species (animal, human), or method of manufacture (rDNA versus animal-source insulin) may result in the need for a dosage change. Dosage of concomitant oral antidiabetic agents may need adjustment.

Reactions in bold italics are *life-threatening*. Interactions may have a *rapid onset* or a *delayed onset*.

• Warn female patient to inform prescriber if she is pregnant or plans to become pregnant.
• Advise female patient of childbearing potential of importance of maintaining tight glucose control if she is pregnant or plans to become pregnant.
• Advise pregnant patient of the change in insulin requirements that may occur during pregnancy and after childbirth.
• Instruct patient not to use insulin after the printed expiration date; inform patient that vials are good for 31 days at room temperature and pens are good for 14 days at room temperature.

SAFETY ALERT!

Insulins (long-acting)

IN-su-lins

insulin degludec
Tresiba FlexTouch

insulin detemir (rDNA origin) injection
Levemir, Levemir FlexTouch

insulin glargine (rDNA origin) injection
Basaglar KwikPen, Lantus, Lantus SoloStar, Toujeo SoloStar

Therapeutic class: Antidiabetics
Pharmacologic class: Insulins

AVAILABLE FORMS
Injection: 100 units/mL in 10-mL vials and 3-mL pens, 200 units/mL in 3-mL pens, 300 units/mL in 1.5-mL pens

INDICATIONS & DOSAGES
Adjust-a-dose (for all indications): Individualize dosage based on metabolic needs, blood glucose monitoring, and glycemic control goal. Insulin requirements may be altered during acute illness, emotional distress, or stress. Adjust dosage as needed in patients who are elderly, in those who have renal or hepatic dysfunction or have changes in physical activity or meal patterns, and in patients who are concurrently taking drugs that lower blood glucose level. Refer to manufacturer's

instructions for dosage adjustments when converting from other insulin regimens and formulations.
➤ **To improve glycemic control in patients with type 1 diabetes mellitus**
Adults (degludec, detemir, glargine) and children age 2 and older (detemir) or age 6 and older (glargine [except Toujeo]) or age 1 and older requiring 5 units or more daily (degludec): In insulin-naive patients, initial dosage is approximately one-third (Basaglar, Levemir, Lantus) or one-third to one-half (Toujeo, Tresiba) of total daily insulin requirements subcut once daily at any time of day (Tresiba [adults]) or at any time of day but at same time every day (Tresiba [children], Basaglar, Lantus, Toujeo) or with evening meal or at bedtime. Satisfy the remainder of the daily insulin requirements with rapid- or short-acting premeal insulin. Or, in patients who require b.i.d. detemir dosing, give evening dose with evening meal, at bedtime, or 12 hours after morning dose.
➤ **To improve glycemic control in patients with type 2 diabetes mellitus**
Adults: Initial insulin degludec dosage is 10 units once daily subcut at any time of day. Initial insulin detemir dosage is 10 units (0.1 to 0.2 unit/kg) subcut once daily in evening or divided into two daily doses in patients inadequately controlled on oral antidiabetic agents, or once daily in the evening in patients inadequately controlled on a glucagon-like peptide 1 (GLP-1) receptor antagonist. Initial insulin glargine dosage is 0.2 unit/kg (up to 10 units) subcut once daily. Adjust dosage as needed.
Children age 1 and older (degludec only): Initial dosage in insulin-naive patients is 10 units subcut once daily at same time every day.

ADMINISTRATION
Subcutaneous
General
• Don't give long-acting insulins by insulin infusion pumps or by IM or IV injection.
• Administer by subcut injection only in the thigh, abdominal wall, or upper arm. Rotate sites within same region (abdomen, thigh, or deltoid) from one injection to the next to reduce risk of lipodystrophy.

• Don't mix or dilute long-acting insulins with other insulins or solutions because the pharmacokinetic and pharmacodynamic profile (onset of action, time to peak effect) of the insulin may be altered unpredictably.

• Inspect visually for particulate matter and discoloration before administration, whenever solution and container permit; use only if solution appears clear and colorless.

• Instructions for priming and using pens vary from one to another, are very detailed, and involve multiple steps. Refer to manufacturer's instructions for use.

◐ *Alert:* Multidose pens are for single patient use only. Pens should never be shared even if the needle is changed. Clearly label with patient identifying information where it won't obstruct dosing window, warning, or other product information.

Insulin degludec

• Give insulin degludec once daily at any time of day.

• Individualize and titrate dosage every 3 to 4 days based on patient's metabolic needs, blood glucose monitoring results, and glycemic control goal.

• Don't perform dose conversion when using FlexTouch pen. The dose window for both 100-unit and 200-unit pens shows the number of insulin units to be delivered and no conversion is needed.

• In adults with type 1 or type 2 diabetes mellitus already on insulin therapy, start insulin degludec at the same unit dose as the total daily long- or intermediate-acting insulin unit dose.

• In children age 1 and older already on insulin therapy, start at 80% of the total daily long- or intermediate-acting insulin unit dose to minimize risk of hypoglycemia. Not recommended for patients requiring less than 5 units of insulin degludec daily.

• Always use a new needle for each injection to help ensure sterility and prevent blocked needles.

• Store unused pens in refrigerator at 36° to 46° F (2° to 8° C); may be used until expiration date on label. Don't freeze or use if pens have been frozen.

• Store open pen away from heat or light at room temperature, below 86° F (30° C). Discard after 56 days, even if pen still

contains insulin and expiration date hasn't passed.

Insulin detemir

• Give insulin detemir once daily or b.i.d. For patients treated with insulin detemir once daily, give dose with evening meal or at bedtime. For patients who require b.i.d. dosing, administer evening dose with evening meal, at bedtime, or 12 hours after morning dose.

• When using insulin detemir with a GLP-1 receptor agonist, give as separate injections; never mix together. Insulin detemir and a GLP-1 receptor agonist may be injected in same body region, but the injections shouldn't be adjacent to each other.

• If converting from insulin glargine or NPH insulin to insulin detemir, maintain the same unit dose. Monitor glucose level closely during transition.

• Store unused (unopened) insulin detemir vials and pens between 36° and 46° F (2° and 8° C). Don't freeze and don't use if vials or pens have been frozen. Keep in carton so that vials or pens stay clean and protected from light.

• If refrigeration isn't possible, unused (unopened) insulin detemir can be kept unrefrigerated at room temperature, below 86° F (30° C), as long as it's kept as cool as possible and away from direct heat and light. Discard unrefrigerated insulin detemir 42 days after it's first kept out of the refrigerator, even if the pen or vial still contains insulin.

• After initial use, store vials in refrigerator; never freeze. If refrigeration isn't possible, the in-use vial can be kept unrefrigerated at room temperature, below 86° F (30° C), as long as it's kept as cool as possible and away from direct heat and light. Discard refrigerated insulin detemir vials 42 days after initial use.

• Pens (in use): After initial use, don't store insulin detemir pen in refrigerator and don't store with the needle in place; keep opened insulin detemir pen away from direct heat and light at room temperature, below 86° F (30° C). Discard unrefrigerated insulin detemir pens 42 days after they're first kept out of refrigerator.

Reactions in bold italics are *life-threatening*. Interactions may have a *rapid onset* or a ***delayed onset***.

Insulin glargine
- Give subcut once daily at same time every day, at any time during the day.
- If converting from insulin detemir to insulin glargine, maintain the same unit dose. Monitor glucose level closely during transition.
- If changing from once-daily Toujeo 300 units/mL to a different insulin glargine product, recommended initial dose is 80% of the Toujeo dose that's being discontinued.
- If changing from another insulin glargine product, 100 units/mL, to Basaglar, Basaglar dose should be the same as the other insulin glargine product, 100 units/mL, and prescriber should determine the time of day for administration.
- If changing from a treatment regimen with an intermediate- or long-acting insulin (other than an insulin glargine product, 100 units/mL) to a regimen with Basaglar, a change in the basal insulin dosage may be required and the amount and timing of shorter-acting insulins and dosages of any antidiabetic drugs may need adjustment.
- If switching from once-daily NPH insulin to once-daily Lantus, the recommended initial glargine dose is the same as the dose of NPH that is being discontinued.
- If switching from b.i.d. NPH insulin to once-daily Lantus or Basaglar, the recommended initial insulin glargine dose is 80% of the total NPH insulin dose that is being discontinued.
- Store unopened insulin glargine vials and pens at 36° to 46° F (2° to 8° C). Don't freeze; discard if frozen. If refrigeration isn't possible, the open vial in use can be kept unrefrigerated for up to 28 days away from direct heat and light, as long as the room temperature isn't above 86° F (30° C).
- Opened vials, whether or not refrigerated, must be used within a 28-day period or they must be discarded.
- Opened pens shouldn't be refrigerated but should be kept at room temperature, below 86° F (30° C), away from direct heat and light; discard opened pens kept at room temperature after 28 days.

ACTION

Lowers blood glucose level by stimulating peripheral glucose uptake by binding to insulin receptors on skeletal muscle and in fat cells, and by inhibiting hepatic glucose production; also inhibits lipolysis and proteolysis, and enhances protein synthesis.

Route	Onset	Peak	Duration
Subcut (degludec)	1 hr	9 hr	24+hr
Subcut (detemir)	Unknown	Constant	24 hr
Subcut (glargine)	3–6 hr	Constant	24 hr

Half-life: Degludec, 25 hours; detemir, 5 to 7 hours; glargine, unknown.

ADVERSE REACTIONS

CNS: headache, pyrexia. **CV:** peripheral edema, HTN. **EENT:** pharyngitis, rhinitis, cataract, retinopathy. **GI:** abdominal pain, gastroenteritis, nausea, vomiting, diarrhea. **GU:** UTI. **Metabolic:** *hypoglycemia,* sodium retention, weight gain. **Musculoskeletal:** back pain. **Respiratory:** URI, bronchitis, cough. **Skin:** injection-site reactions, lipodystrophy, pruritus, rash. **Other:** allergic reactions, flulike symptoms, infection.

INTERACTIONS

Drug-drug. *ACE inhibitors, antidiabetic agents (oral), ARBs, disopyramide, fibrates, fluoxetine, MAO inhibitors, octreotide, pentoxifylline, pramlintide, salicylates, sulfonamide antibiotics:* May increase blood glucose–lowering effect of insulin, increasing risk of hypoglycemia. Monitor glucose level and patient closely. Adjust insulin dosage as necessary.
Antiadrenergics (beta blockers, clonidine, guanethidine, reserpine): May mask signs and symptoms of hypoglycemia. Avoid concurrent use, if possible, and monitor patient closely.
Atypical antipsychotics, corticosteroids, danazol, diuretics, estrogens, glucagon, hormonal contraceptives, isoniazid, niacin, phenothiazines, protease inhibitors, somatropin, sympathomimetics (albuterol, epinephrine, terbutaline), thyroid hormones: May decrease blood glucose–lowering effect of insulin, increasing risk of hyperglycemia. Monitor glucose level and patient closely. Adjust insulin dosage as necessary.
Beta blockers, clonidine, lithium salts, pentamidine: May increase risk of either

hypoglycemia or hyperglycemia. Monitor glucose level closely.

GLP-1 receptor agonists (albiglutide, exenatide, liraglutide): May increase risk of hypoglycemia. Monitor glucose level closely and decrease insulin dosage if necessary.

Thiazolidinediones (TZDs; pioglitazone, rosiglitazone): May cause fluid retention that can lead to HF. Monitor patient closely, and adjust or stop TZD as clinically necessary.

Drug-lifestyle. *Alcohol use:* May cause hyperglycemia or hypoglycemia. Monitor glucose level and discourage concurrent use.

EFFECTS ON LAB TEST RESULTS
• May decrease blood glucose level.

CONTRAINDICATIONS & CAUTIONS
• Contraindicated during episodes of hypoglycemia or diabetic ketoacidosis.
• Contraindicated in patients hypersensitive to drug or its components. Severe, life-threatening, generalized allergy, including anaphylaxis, can occur with insulin products.
❸ **Alert:** Adjust insulin regimen only with appropriate glucose monitoring under medical supervision.
• Use cautiously in patients susceptible to hypokalemia, such as patients who are fasting, are taking potassium-lowering drugs, or are concurrently taking drugs that may affect potassium level. Untreated hypokalemia can cause respiratory paralysis, ventricular arrhythmias, and death.
• Hypoglycemia is the most common adverse reaction. Severe hypoglycemia can cause seizures, and may be life-threatening or fatal. Hypoglycemia can occur suddenly, and symptoms may differ. Risk increases with intensity of glycemic control and changes in glycemic treatment, meal patterns, physical activity, and concomitant medications and in patients with renal or hepatic impairment.
• Use cautiously in elderly patients, who may be at risk for increased sensitivity to drug's effects. Signs and symptoms of hypoglycemia may be more difficult to recognize in these patients.

• Use prefilled pens cautiously in patients with visual impairment who may rely on audible clicks to dial their dose.
Dialyzable drug: Unknown.
⚠ **Overdose S&S:** Hypoglycemia.

PREGNANCY-LACTATION-REPRODUCTION
• Insulin detemir: Use cautiously in pregnant women. Carefully monitor glucose level.
• Insulin degludec, glargine: There are no well-controlled studies in pregnant women. Use during pregnancy only if potential benefit justifies potential risk to the fetus.
• Closely monitor blood glucose levels in pregnant patients, in women who have recently given birth, and in breastfeeding women; insulin requirements may change.
• It isn't known if insulin appears in human milk. Use cautiously in breastfeeding women. Insulin doses may need adjustment.

NURSING CONSIDERATIONS
• Prolonged effect of long-acting insulin may delay recovery from hypoglycemia. Monitor patient carefully.
• Monitor patients taking other medications with insulin more closely because other drugs can mask signs and symptoms of hypoglycemia or cause an increase or a decrease in blood glucose level.
• Adjust dosages regularly, depending on patient-specific glucose measurements.
• Monitor patient carefully for signs and symptoms of hypoglycemia, especially in long-standing disease. Treat according to individual facility policy and procedure if necessary.
• Mild episodes of hypoglycemia may be treated with oral glucose. More severe episodes of hypoglycemia, such as coma, seizure, or neurologic impairment, may be treated with IM or subcut glucagon or concentrated IV glucose.
• Assess patient for signs and symptoms of hypoglycemia (sweating, shaking, trembling, confusion) and hyperglycemia (drowsiness, fruity breath odor, frequent urination, thirst). Notify prescriber if any of these signs or symptoms occur.
• Periodically measure HbA_{1c} levels.
• Increase frequency of glucose monitoring in patients who are acutely ill or under

---

emotional stress, or if changes in diet, exercise, or medication regimen occur, as these may affect the rate of insulin absorption. Also, closely monitor patient after changes to insulin dosage.

• *Look alike–sound alike:* Don't confuse insulin glargine with insulin glulisine.

PATIENT TEACHING

• Instruct patient in self-management, including glucose monitoring, injection technique, proper storage of insulin, and recognition and management of hypoglycemia and hyperglycemia.

• Explain to patient that insulin requirements may vary due to illness, stress or emotional disturbance, change in activity level, inadequate food intake, and skipped meals.

• Teach patient to watch for signs and symptoms of hypoglycemia (sweating, shaking, trembling, confusion) and hyperglycemia (drowsiness, frequent urination, thirst).

• Advise patient that hypoglycemic episodes may impair the ability to concentrate and react; advise patient to use caution while driving and operating machinery.

• Instruct patient to keep hard candy or glucose tablets on hand to treat mild cases of hypoglycemia.

• Advise patient that allergic and hypersensitivity reactions can occur, including injection-site reactions (local pain, redness, or swelling) and generalized reactions and to report signs or symptoms to health care provider. Teach patient signs and symptoms of anaphylaxis and to seek emergency medical attention promptly if anaphylaxis occurs.

• Instruct patient to rotate injection sites within same region to reduce risk of lipodystrophy.

• *Alert:* Warn patient not to share multidose pen with other people, even if the needle is changed, because of risk of bloodborne pathogen transmission, including HIV and hepatitis.

• Teach patient to store insulin products properly, depending on individual products, and to use only if solution appears clear and colorless.

• Explain importance of checking insulin label before each injection as accidental mix-ups among insulin types have been reported.

• Explain that long-acting insulins shouldn't be diluted or mixed with other insulins or drugs.

• Teach patient that alcohol may affect glucose levels and should be avoided.

• Inform patient that any insulin change should be made cautiously and only under medical supervision. Changes in insulin strength, manufacturer, type (regular, NPH, or insulin analogues), species (animal, human), or method of manufacture (rDNA versus animal-source insulin) may result in the need for a dosage change. Dosage of concomitant oral antidiabetic agents may need adjustment.

• Instruct patient not to stop insulin abruptly or change amount injected without consulting prescriber.

• Warn female patient to contact prescriber if she is pregnant or plans to become pregnant.

• Advise pregnant patient of the change in insulin requirements that may occur during pregnancy and after childbirth.

SAFETY ALERT!

Insulins (rapid-acting)

IN-su-lins

insulin aspart (rDNA origin) injection
NovoLOG, NovoRapid✤

insulin glulisine (rDNA origin) injection
Apidra, Apidra SoloStar

insulin (human)

insulin (lispro)
HumaLOG, Admelog

Therapeutic class: Antidiabetics
Pharmacologic class: Insulins

AVAILABLE FORMS
Inhalation powder (Afrezza): 4-unit, 8-unit, 12-unit single-use cartridges
Injection (aspart): 10-mL vials, 3-mL prefilled pens and cartridges
Injection (glulisine): 10-mL vials, 3-mL prefilled pens

Injection (lispro): 10-mL vials, 3-mL pre-filled pens and cartridges

INDICATIONS & DOSAGES

Adjust-a-dose (for all indications): Individualize dosage based on metabolic needs, blood glucose monitoring, and glycemic control goal. Insulin requirements may be altered during acute illness, emotional distress, or stress. Adjust as needed in patients who are elderly, have renal or hepatic dysfunction, or have changes in physical activity or meal patterns, and in those who are concurrently taking drugs that lower blood glucose level. Refer to manufacturer's instructions for dosage adjustments when converting from other insulin regimens or formulations. Obese patients and children during puberty may need increased maintenance doses.

➤ **To improve glycemic control in patients with diabetes mellitus (aspart, glulisine, lispro)**
Adults and children age 2 and older (aspart), age 3 and older (lispro), age 4 and older (glulisine): For insulin aspart, initially, 0.2 to 0.6 unit/kg/day in divided doses subcut immediately (5 to 10 minutes) before a meal. Usual maintenance dose is 0.5 to 1 unit/kg/day subcut in divided doses. When continuous subcut infusion pump is used, follow health care provider recommendations when setting basal and mealtime infusion rates. Usual IV concentration is 0.05 to 1 unit/mL in NSS infused under close medical supervision.

For insulin glulisine, usual maintenance dose is 0.5 to 1 unit/kg/day subcut in divided doses within 15 minutes before a meal or 20 minutes after starting a meal. When continuous subcut infusion pump is used, base initial dosing on total daily insulin dose of the previous regimen. Usual IV concentration is 0.05 to 1 unit/mL in NSS infused under close medical supervision.

For lispro, usual maintenance dose is 0.5 to 1 unit/kg/day subcut in divided doses within 15 minutes before a meal or immediately after a meal. When continuous subcut infusion pump is used, follow health care provider recommendations when setting basal and mealtime infusion rates. Usual IV concentration is 0.1 to 1 unit/mL in NSS infused under close medical supervision.

➤ **To improve glycemic control in patients with diabetes mellitus (inhalation)**
Adults: For insulin-naive patients, initially 4 units inhaled at beginning of each meal. To convert to inhaled insulin from subcut mealtime insulin, refer to manufacturer's instructions. For patients using subcut premixed insulin, estimate mealtime injected dose by dividing half of total daily injected premixed insulin dose equally among the three meals of the day; then convert each estimated injected mealtime dose to an appropriate inhaled dose according to manufacturer's instructions. Administer half of total daily injected premixed dose as an injected basal insulin dose.

ADMINISTRATION
General
• Rapid-acting insulins are usually given in a regimen that includes an intermediate-acting or a long-acting insulin.
• Don't use if solution is viscous or cloudy; use only if clear and colorless.
• Multidose pens are for single-patient use only. Pens should never be shared even if the needle is changed. Clearly label with patient identifying information where it won't obstruct dosing window, warning, or other product information.
• Store unopened insulin aspart vials, cartridges, and pens under refrigeration (36° to 46° F [2° to 8° C]) until expiration date or at room temperature of less than 86° F (30° C) for 28 days; don't freeze. Keep away from heat and sunlight. Once opened, may store vials under refrigeration or at room temperature of less than 86° F (30° C); use within 28 days. Store cartridges and pens that have been opened at temperatures less than 86° F (30° C) and use within 28 days; don't freeze or refrigerate.
• Store insulin glulisine under refrigeration at 36° to 46° F (2° to 8° C) and protect from light. Don't store in freezer. Don't allow insulin glulisine to freeze; discard if it has been frozen. Unopened vials and cartridge systems not stored in refrigerator must be used within 28 days. Opened vials, whether or not refrigerated, must be used within 28 days. If refrigeration isn't possible, can keep open vials at room temperature of less than 77° F (25° C) for up to 28 days away

from direct heat and light. Don't refrigerate opened cartridge system, but keep below 77° F (25° C) and away from direct heat and light. Discard opened cartridge systems after 28 days. Don't store pen, with or without cartridge system, in refrigerator at any time.
• Store lispro in refrigerator (36° to 46° F [2° to 8° C]), but not in freezer. Protect from direct heat and light. Don't use if frozen. Store unopened vials and pens in refrigerator until expiration date; if stored unopened at room temperature, discard after 28 days. May store opened vials for 28 days under refrigeration or at room temperature; may store opened pens and cartridges for 28 days at room temperature. Discard if exposed to temperatures greater than 98.6° F (37° C).
• **Incompatibilities:** Don't mix with any other insulin except NPH.

IV

▼ Rapid-acting insulin may be administered IV with close monitoring of blood glucose and serum potassium levels under appropriate medical supervision.
▼ Flush IV tubing with priming infusion of 20 mL from insulin infusion whenever new IV tubing set is added to insulin infusion container, to avoid adsorption to IV tubing.
▼ Use NSS and polyvinyl chloride or polypropylene infusion bags for IV infusions.
▼ Always administer IV infusions using an infusion pump.

Subcutaneous

• Administer by subcut injection in abdominal region, buttocks, thigh, or upper arm. Subcut injection into abdominal wall is generally associated with faster absorption than other injection sites.
• Rotate injection sites within same region to reduce risk of lipodystrophy.
• Injection into a lifted skin fold minimizes risk of IM injection.
• When used for continuous subcut insulin infusion, insulin aspart contained within an external insulin pump reservoir should be replaced at least every 6 days and infusion sets and insertion sites should be changed at least every 3 days. Discard if exposed to temperatures greater than 98.6° F (37° C).
• NovoLog may be diluted with Insulin Diluting Medium for NovoLog for subcut injection. Diluting one part NovoLog to nine

parts diluent will yield a concentration one-tenth that of NovoLog (equivalent to U-10). Diluting one part NovoLog to one part diluent will yield a concentration one-half that of NovoLog (equivalent to U-50).
• When using for continuous subcut insulin infusion, change insulin glulisine in reservoir and infusion set (reservoirs, tubing, and catheters) every 48 hours or after exposure to temperatures greater than 98.6° F (37° C).
• When using for continuous subcut insulin infusion, change lispro in reservoir every 7 days, and change infusion sets every 3 days.
• Don't use mixed insulins in external insulin pumps.

Inhalational

• Administer using a single inhalation per cartridge using Afrezza inhaler only. Inhaler can be used for the 4-unit, 8-unit, and 12-unit cartridges.
• Administer at beginning of a meal.
• Keep inhaler level, with white mouthpiece on top and purple base on bottom, after a cartridge has been inserted into inhaler.
• Loss of drug effect can occur if inhaler is turned upside down, held with mouthpiece pointing down, or shaken or dropped after the cartridge has been inserted but before dose has been administered. If any of these occur, replace cartridge before use.
• May mix and match between 4-unit (blue), 8-unit (green), and 12-unit (yellow) cartridges to obtain correct dose.
• Store unused foil packages of inhalation powder until expiration date under refrigeration (36° to 46° F [2° to 8° C]) or if at room temperature, use within 10 days. If in use, unopened blister cards and strips must be used within 10 days and opened strips must be used within 3 days.
• Inhaler can be refrigerated but should be at room temperature before use. Cartridges should be at room temperature for 10 minutes before use.
• Replace inhaler after 15 days of use.

ACTION

Lowers blood glucose level by stimulating peripheral glucose uptake by binding to insulin receptors on skeletal muscle and in fat cells and by inhibiting hepatic glucose production; also inhibits lipolysis and proteolysis, and enhances protein synthesis.

Route	Onset	Peak	Duration
Aspart (IV)	Immediate	Unknown	3–5 hr
Aspart (Subcut)	15 min	1–3 hr	3–5 hr
Glulisine (IV)	Immediate	Unknown	5 hr
Glulisine (Subcut)	5–15 min	1 hr	5 hr
Lispro (IV)	Immediate	Unknown	Unknown
Lispro (Subcut)	15–30 min	30–90 min	≤5 hr
Inhalation	Unknown	12–15 min	180 min

Half-life: Aspart IV, unknown; aspart subcut, 81 minutes; glulisine IV, 13 minutes; glulisine subcut, 42 minutes; lispro IV, 51 to 55 minutes; lispro subcut, 1 hour; inhalation, 28 to 39 minutes.

ADVERSE REACTIONS

CNS: headache, *seizures,* asthenia, fever, fatigue (inhalation), sensory disturbance. **CV:** HTN, peripheral edema. **EENT:** nasopharyngitis. **GI:** nausea, diarrhea. **GU:** UTI, dysmenorrhea. **Metabolic:** *hypoglycemia, hypokalemia,* weight gain. **Musculoskeletal:** myalgia. **Respiratory:** URI, cough; bronchospasm, throat pain or irritation, bronchitis, decreased pulmonary function (inhaled product). **Skin:** injection- or infusion-site reactions, lipodystrophy, pruritus, rash. **Other:** *allergic reactions, anaphylaxis,* insulin antibody production, flulike symptoms.

INTERACTIONS

Drug-drug. *ACE inhibitors, antidiabetic agents (oral), ARBs, disopyramide, fibrates, fluoxetine,* **MAO inhibitors***, octreotide, pentoxifylline, pramlintide, salicylates, sulfonamide antibiotics:* May increase risk of hypoglycemia. Monitor glucose level closely and adjust insulin dosage as needed.
Atypical antipsychotics, corticosteroids, danazol, diuretics, estrogens, glucagon, hormonal contraceptives, isoniazid, niacin, phenothiazines, protease inhibitors, somatropin, sympathomimetics (albuterol, epinephrine, terbutaline), thyroid hormones: May decrease blood glucose–lowering effects. Monitor glucose level closely and adjust insulin dosage as needed.
Beta blockers, clonidine, guanethidine, reserpine: May mask signs and symptoms of hypoglycemia. Avoid concurrent use, if possible, or monitor patient closely.
Beta blockers, clonidine, lithium salts, pentamidine: May cause hypoglycemia or hyperglycemia. Monitor glucose level closely.
Thiazolidinediones (TZDs; pioglitazone, rosiglitazone): May cause fluid retention that can lead to HF. Monitor patient closely and adjust or stop TZDs as clinically indicated.
Drug-lifestyle. *Alcohol use:* May cause hyperglycemia or hypoglycemia. Monitor glucose level closely and discourage concurrent use.

EFFECTS ON LAB TEST RESULTS
• May decrease glucose and potassium levels.

CONTRAINDICATIONS & CAUTIONS
Black Box Warning Inhaled insulin is contraindicated in patients with chronic lung disease, such as asthma or COPD, as acute bronchospasm has been observed in these patients. ∎
• Contraindicated during episodes of hypoglycemia.
• Contraindicated in patients with a history of hypersensitivity to drug or its components. Severe, life-threatening, generalized allergic reaction, including anaphylaxis, can occur with insulin products.
• Inhaled insulin may increase risk of diabetic ketoacidosis (DKA). Closely monitor patients at risk for DKA. Change to an alternative route of insulin delivery if needed.
• Inhaled insulin isn't recommended in patients who smoke or who have recently stopped smoking.
• Use cautiously in patients susceptible to hypokalemia, such as patients who are fasting, are taking potassium-lowering drugs, or are concurrently taking drugs that may affect potassium levels. Untreated hypokalemia can cause respiratory paralysis, ventricular arrhythmias, and death.
• Hypoglycemia is the most common adverse reaction. Severe hypoglycemia can cause seizures, and may be life-threatening or fatal. Hypoglycemia can occur suddenly, and symptoms may differ. Risk increases with intensity of glycemic control and changes in glycemic treatment, meal patterns, physical activity, and concomitant medications and in patients with renal or hepatic impairment.

Reactions in bold italics are *life-threatening*. Interactions may have a *rapid onset* or a *delayed onset*.

• Use cautiously in elderly patients, who may be at increased risk for adverse effects. Signs and symptoms of hypoglycemia may be more difficult to recognize in these patients.
• Use prefilled pens cautiously in patients with visual impairment who may rely on audible clicks to dial their dose.
Dialyzable drug: Unknown.
⚠ *Overdose S&S:* Hypoglycemia, hypokalemia.

PREGNANCY-LACTATION-REPRODUCTION
• There are no adequate studies in pregnant women. Don't use during pregnancy unless potential benefit justifies risk to the fetus.
• Monitor blood glucose levels closely in pregnant patients, in women who have recently given birth, and in breastfeeding women; insulin requirements may change.
• It isn't known if insulin appears in human milk. Refer to manufacturer's instructions for use in breastfeeding women.

NURSING CONSIDERATIONS
Black Box Warning Before initiating inhaled insulin, perform a detailed medical history, physical examination, and spirometry (forced expiratory volume in 1 second [FEV_1]) to identify potential lung disease in all patients. ▪
• Assess pulmonary function (spirometry) before initiating inhalation product, after 6 months of therapy, and annually, even in the absence of pulmonary symptoms.
• Increase frequency of pulmonary assessment in patients with such symptoms as wheezing, bronchospasm, breathing difficulties, or persistent or recurring cough. Switch to another form of drug for persistent symptoms or decline of 20% or more in FEV_1 from baseline.
• Monitor blood glucose level and adjust insulin dosage as needed.
• Closely monitor patients also taking other medications as other drugs can mask signs and symptoms of hypoglycemia or cause an increase or decrease in blood glucose level.
• Increase frequency of glucose monitoring in patients who are acutely ill or under emotional stress, or if changes in diet, exercise, or medication regimen occur, because these may affect rate of insulin absorption.

• Closely monitor patients at risk for DKA from acute illness or infection; consider changing from inhaled product to alternative route of insulin delivery.
• Increase frequency of glucose monitoring when initiating therapy or when changes in insulin strength, dosage, manufacturer, or type or method of administration are made. Changes may affect glycemic control and increase risk of hypoglycemia.
• Monitor patient carefully for signs and symptoms of hypoglycemia. Symptom awareness may be decreased in patients with long-standing diabetes, diabetic nerve disease, renal disease, or hepatic impairment and in patients who have experienced recurrent hypoglycemia. Treat according to individual facility policy if necessary.
• Mild episodes of hypoglycemia may be treated with oral glucose. More severe episodes of hypoglycemia, such as coma, seizure, or neurologic impairment, may be treated with IM or subcut glucagon or concentrated IV glucose.
• Monitor potassium levels in patients at risk for hypokalemia (those receiving potassium-depleting drugs or IV insulin).
• Monitor patients for generalized allergic reactions, including anaphylaxis.
• Assess patients and notify prescriber for signs or symptoms of hypoglycemia (sweating, shaking, trembling, confusion) and hyperglycemia (drowsiness, fruity breath odor, frequent urination, thirst).
• Periodically measure HbA_{1c} levels.
• Monitor external pump for malfunction as this may cause a rapid decline in blood glucose level.
• *Look alike–sound alike:* Don't confuse NovoLog with Novolog 70/30. Don't confuse Humalog with Humalog 50/50 or 75/25. Don't confuse insulin glulisine with insulin glargine.

PATIENT TEACHING
General
• Advise patient that hypoglycemic episodes can impair the ability to concentrate and react; advise patient to use caution while driving and operating machinery.
• Instruct patient to keep hard candy or glucose tablets on hand to treat mild cases of hypoglycemia.

- Advise patient to keep a log of glucose levels.
- Instruct patient on the long-term sequelae of diabetes if not managed properly.
- Instruct patient to carry identification or wear jewelry indicating that patient has diabetes.
- Advise patient that allergic and hypersensitivity reactions can occur, including injection-site reactions (local pain, redness or swelling), and to report symptoms to health care provider. Teach patient signs and symptoms of anaphylaxis and to seek emergency medical attention promptly if anaphylaxis occurs.
- Instruct patient on self-management procedures, including glucose monitoring, proper administration technique, and management of hypoglycemia and hyperglycemia.
- Warn patient that insulin requirements may vary due to illness, stress, emotional disturbances, inadequate or skipped insulin dose, inadvertent administration of an increased insulin dose, inadequate food intake, or skipped meals.
- ❸ *Alert:* Warn patient not to share multidose pen with other people, even if the needle is changed, because of risk of bloodborne pathogen transmission, including HIV and hepatitis.
- Advise female patient with diabetes to inform physician if she is pregnant or plans to become pregnant.
- Advise pregnant patient of change in insulin requirements that may occur during pregnancy and after childbirth.
- Teach patient that alcohol and some other medications may increase or decrease glucose levels. Advise patient to inform health care provider of all medications and supplements being taken.
- Caution patient not to stop insulin abruptly or change amount taken without consulting prescriber.
- Advise patient that any change of insulin should be made cautiously and only under medical supervision. Changes in insulin strength, manufacturer, type (regular, NPH, or insulin analogues), species (animal, human), or method of manufacture (rDNA versus animal-source insulin) may result in need for a dosage change. Dosage of con-

comitant oral antidiabetic agents may need adjustment.

Injection

- Teach patient to give insulin at appropriate time around a meal, depending on product.
- Instruct patient to rotate injection sites and of the importance of avoiding lipodystrophy.
- Instruct patient that when mixing two types of insulin, to always draw up the shorter-acting insulin first, followed by NPH insulin, and inject immediately.
- Teach patient how to use external insulin pumps properly, to use the appropriate insulin in the pump, not to dilute it or mix it with other insulin formulations, to change the infusion set every 3 days, to rotate infusion sites, and to follow instructions for patient's specific type of pump.
- Teach patient to store insulin products properly, depending on individual products.
- Explain importance of checking insulin label before each injection; accidental mix-ups among insulin types have been reported.
- Instruct patient not to share pens with others, even if needles are changed.

Inhalational

- Instruct patient to read inhaler's medication guide before starting inhalation therapy and to reread it each time the prescription is renewed.
- Caution patient not to open cartridges, place cartridges in mouth, or swallow cartridges.
- Inform patient that inhaled insulin can cause a decline in lung function and that lung function will be evaluated by spirometry before initiation of treatment and periodically during treatment.
- Instruct patient to promptly report respiratory difficulty or signs or symptoms of lung cancer (hemoptysis, cough).
- Inform patient that if inhaled product isn't being used, it should be stored in refrigerator. If inhaler is being used, tell patient to leave it at room temperature and use unopened strips within 10 days and opened strips within 3 days.
- Instruct patient never to wash inhaler but to wipe it with a clean, dry cloth.
- Advise patient that inhalers should be discarded and replaced every 15 days.

Reactions in bold italics are *life-threatening*. Interactions may have a *rapid onset* or a ***delayed onset***.

Insulins (short-acting)

IN-su-lins

insulin (regular)
HumuLIN R ◇, HumuLIN R U-500
(concentrated), HumuLIN R U-500
KwikPen, NovoLIN R ◇

Therapeutic class: Antidiabetics
Pharmacologic class: Insulins

AVAILABLE FORMS
Injection: 100 units/mL in 3-mL, 10-mL
vials; 500 units/mL in 3-mL pens and 20-mL
vials

INDICATIONS & DOSAGES
Adjust-a-dose (for all indications): Individualize dosage based on metabolic needs, blood
glucose monitoring, and glycemic control.
Insulin requirements may be altered during
acute illness, emotional distress, or stress.
Adjust dosage as needed in patients who are
elderly, have renal or hepatic dysfunction,
or have changes in physical activity or meal
patterns, and in those who are concurrently
taking drugs that lower blood glucose level.
Dosage may also need adjustment when
switching from another insulin formulation,
manufacturer, or strength. IV administration
of regular insulin is possible under medical
supervision with close monitoring of blood
glucose and potassium levels to avoid hypoglycemia and hypokalemia. IV administration of insulin is commonly used in the treatment of diabetic ketoacidosis, perioperative
management of diabetes, and maintenance
of glycemic control during labor in pregnant
women with diabetes.
➤ **As adjunct to diet and exercise to improve glycemic control in patients with
type 1 and type 2 diabetes mellitus**
Adults and children: Total daily insulin requirements vary and are usually between
0.5 and 1 unit/kg/day subcut in three or more
divided doses. Novolin R hasn't been studied in children with type 2 diabetes. Initial
doses may be lower, and maintenance doses
in obese patients and children during puberty may be higher. Give 30 minutes before
start of a meal. May give IV under medical

supervision with close monitoring of blood
glucose and potassium levels to avoid hypoglycemia and hypokalemia.
ⓘ *Alert:* U-500 concentrate is used for the
treatment of insulin-resistant patients with
diabetes who require daily doses of more
than 200 units because a large dose may be
given subcut in a reasonable volume. Don't
give U-500 concentrated insulin IV or IM.

ADMINISTRATION
General
• Store unopened vials and pens in refrigerator at 36° to 46° F (2° to 8° C). Don't freeze
and don't use if vial has been frozen.
ⓘ *Alert:* Multidose pens are for single patient
use only. Pens should never be shared even if
the needle is changed. Clearly label with patient identifying information where it won't
obstruct dosing window, warning, or other
product information.
• Novolin R vials can be kept at room temperature (not greater than 77° F [25° C]),
away from heat or light, for up to 42 days;
don't refrigerate after first use. Discard after
42 days even if vial is unopened or isn't
empty.
• Opened (in use) Humulin R vials can be
kept at room temperature (not greater than
86° F [30° C]), away from heat or light, for
up to 31 days. Discard after 31 days even if
vial is unopened or isn't empty.
• Opened and unopened Humulin R U-500
vials can be kept at room temperature, below 86° F (30° C); discard after 40 days.
Also discard opened refrigerated vials after
40 days.
• Opened and unopened Humulin R U-500
pens can be kept at room temperature, below
86° F (30° C); discard after 28 days. Don't
store opened pens in refrigerator.
IV
▼ Don't use if solution is viscous or cloudy;
use only if clear and colorless.
▼ IV administration requires close monitoring of blood glucose and serum potassium
levels. Appropriate medical supervision is
required.
▼ Onset of action when administered IV is
more rapid in comparison to subcut administration.

▼ Use of regular insulin in insulin pumps isn't recommended because of risk of precipitation.

▼ For IV use, Humulin R U-100 should be used at a concentration of 0.1 to 1 unit/mL in NSS using polyvinyl chloride infusion bags. Novolin R should be used at concentrations of 0.05 to 1 unit/mL in infusion systems using polypropylene infusion bags and one of the following infusion solutions: NSS, 5% dextrose, or 10% dextrose with potassium chloride 40 mmol/L.

▼ Always administer IV infusions using an infusion pump.

▼ Infusion bags prepared with Humulin R are stable when stored in refrigerator for 48 hours at 36° to 46° F (2° to 8° C) and may be used at room temperature for up to an additional 48 hours.

▼ Infusion bags prepared with Novolin R are stable at room temperature for 24 hours.

▼ **Incompatibilities:** Don't mix regular insulin with any other insulin except NPH; don't mix regular concentrated insulin with any other insulin.

Subcutaneous

● Regular insulin administered by subcut injection should generally be used in regimens that include an intermediate- or long-acting insulin. It may also be used in combination with oral antidiabetic agents.

● Subcut injection should be followed by a meal within 30 minutes of administration.

● Administer by subcut injection in abdominal region, buttocks, thigh, or upper arm. Subcut injection into abdominal wall is generally associated with faster absorption than other injection sites.

● Injection sites should be rotated within same region to reduce risk of lipodystrophy.

● Injection into a lifted skin fold minimizes risk of IM injection.

● Don't perform dose conversion when using the Humulin R U-500 KwikPen. The dose window of the pen shows the number of units of Humulin R U-500 to be injected, and no dose conversion is required.

● Don't transfer Humulin R U-500 from the pen into a syringe for administration because overdose and severe hypoglycemia can occur.

● Don't use if solution is viscous or cloudy; use only if clear and colorless.

ACTION

Lowers blood glucose level by stimulating peripheral glucose uptake by binding to insulin receptors on skeletal muscle and in fat cells and by inhibiting hepatic glucose production; also inhibits lipolysis and proteolysis, and enhances protein synthesis.

Route	Onset	Peak	Duration
IV	10–15 min	Unknown	4 hr
U-100 (Subcut)	30 min	1½–3½ hr	8 hr
U-500 (Subcut)	30 min	4–8 hr	13–24 hr

Half-life: IV, 30 to 60 minutes; subcut, 1½ hours.

ADVERSE REACTIONS

CV: peripheral edema. **Metabolic:** *hypoglycemia, hypokalemia,* weight gain. **Skin:** injection-site reactions, lipodystrophy, pruritus. **Other:** allergic reactions, *anaphylaxis,* insulin antibody production.

INTERACTIONS

Drug-drug. *ACE inhibitors, antidiabetic agents (oral), ARBs, disopyramide, fibrates, fluoxetine, MAO inhibitors, salicylates, sulfonamide antibiotics, octreotide, pentoxifylline, pramlintide:* May cause hypoglycemia. Monitor glucose level and adjust insulin dosage as needed.

Atypical antipsychotics, corticosteroids, danazol, diuretics, estrogens, glucagon, hormonal contraceptives, isoniazid, niacin, phenothiazines, protease inhibitors, somatropin, sympathomimetics (albuterol, epinephrine, terbutaline), thyroid hormones: May cause hyperglycemia. Monitor glucose level and adjust insulin dosage as needed.

Beta blockers, clonidine, guanethidine, reserpine: May mask signs and symptoms of hypoglycemia. Avoid concurrent use, if possible, or monitor patient closely.

Beta blockers, clonidine, lithium salts, pentamidine: May cause hypoglycemia or hyperglycemia. Monitor glucose level.

Thiazolidinediones (TZDs; pioglitazone, rosiglitazone): May cause fluid retention that can lead to HF. Monitor patient closely, and adjust or stop TZD as clinically necessary.

Drug-lifestyle. *Alcohol use:* May cause hyperglycemia or hypoglycemia. Monitor

---

Reactions in bold italics are *life-threatening*. Interactions may have a *rapid onset* or a *delayed onset*.

glucose level closely and discourage concurrent use.

EFFECTS ON LAB TEST RESULTS
• May decrease glucose and potassium levels.
• May develop antibodies that react with human insulin.

CONTRAINDICATIONS & CAUTIONS
• Contraindicated during episodes of hypoglycemia.
• Contraindicated in patients with a history of hypersensitivity to drug or its components. Severe, life-threatening, generalized allergic reactions, including anaphylaxis, can occur with insulin products.
• Use cautiously in patients susceptible to hypokalemia, such as patients who are fasting, are taking potassium-lowering drugs, or are concurrently taking drugs that may affect potassium level. Untreated hypokalemia can cause respiratory paralysis, ventricular arrhythmias, and death.
• Hypoglycemia is the most common adverse reaction. Severe hypoglycemia can cause seizures, and may be life-threatening or fatal. Hypoglycemia can occur suddenly, and symptoms may differ. Risk increases with intensity of glycemic control and changes in glycemic treatment, meal patterns, physical activity, and concomitant medications and in patients with renal or hepatic impairment.
• Use cautiously in elderly patients, who may be at increased risk for adverse effects. Signs and symptoms of hypoglycemia may be more difficult to recognize in these patients.
• Use Humulin R U-500 KwikPen cautiously in patients with visual impairment who may rely on audible clicks to dial their dose.
Dialyzable drug: Unknown.
⚠ *Overdose S&S:* Hypoglycemia, hypokalemia.

PREGNANCY-LACTATION-REPRODUCTION
• Use cautiously in pregnant women.
• Monitor blood glucose levels closely in pregnant women, in women who have recently given birth, and in breastfeeding women; insulin requirements may change.

• It isn't known if insulin appears in human milk. Use cautiously in breastfeeding women. Adjust insulin dose as needed.

NURSING CONSIDERATIONS
• Regular insulins are generally used in regimens that also include an intermediate- or long-acting insulin.
• Monitor blood glucose level and adjust insulin dosage as needed for patient-specific goals.
• Monitor patient carefully when initiating therapy. Time course of insulins varies with each patient.
• Monitor patient carefully for signs and symptoms of hypoglycemia, especially in long-standing disease. Treat according to individual facility policy if necessary.
• Mild episodes of hypoglycemia may be treated with oral glucose. More severe episodes of hypoglycemia, such as coma, seizure, or neurologic impairment, may be treated with IM or subcut glucagon or concentrated IV glucose.
• Assess patient and notify prescriber for signs and symptoms of hypoglycemia (sweating, shaking, trembling, confusion) and hyperglycemia (drowsiness, fruity breath odor, frequent urination, thirst).
• Periodically measure HbA_{1c} levels.
• Monitor potassium levels in patients at risk for hypokalemia, including those taking potassium-depleting drugs.
• Increase frequency of glucose monitoring in patients who are acutely ill or under emotional stress, or if changes in diet, exercise, or medication regimen occur because these may affect the rate of insulin absorption. Also monitor patient closely after changes to insulin dosage.
• Monitor patients for generalized allergic reactions, including anaphylaxis.
• *Look alike–sound alike:* Don't confuse Humulin with Humalog. Don't confuse Novolin with NovoLog.

PATIENT TEACHING
• Instruct patient in self-management, including glucose management, injection technique, proper storage of insulin, and recognition and management of hypoglycemia and hyperglycemia.

• Teach patient to eat within 30 minutes of injecting short-acting insulin.

• Instruct patient to only use syringes calibrated for their particular concentration of insulin.

⊙ *Alert:* Warn patient not to share multidose pen with other people, even if the needle is changed, because of risk of bloodborne pathogen transmission, including HIV and hepatitis.

• Teach patient to rotate injection sites and the importance of avoiding lipodystrophy.

• Instruct patient that when mixing two types of insulin, to always draw up the shorter-acting insulin first, followed by NPH, and inject immediately.

• Explain importance of checking insulin label before each injection; accidental mix-ups among insulin types have been reported.

• Instruct patient to keep hard candy or glucose tablets on hand to treat mild cases of hypoglycemia.

• Caution patient that hypoglycemic episodes can impair the ability to concentrate and react; advise patient to use caution while driving and operating machinery.

• Advise patient to track glucose levels.

• Instruct patient on long-term risks of diabetes if not managed properly.

• Instruct patient to carry identification or wear jewelry indicating that patient has diabetes.

• Advise patient that allergic reactions, including injection-site reactions (local pain, redness or swelling) and generalized allergic reaction and anaphylaxis (whole-body rash, shortness of breath, wheezing, reduced BP, fast pulse, sweating), can occur. Teach patient to immediately seek emergency medical attention for generalized reactions.

• Warn patient that insulin requirements may vary due to illness, stress, emotional disturbances, inadequate or skipped insulin dose, inadvertent administration of an increased insulin dose, inadequate food intake, skipped meals or pregnancy.

• Caution patient not to stop insulin abruptly or to change amount injected without consulting prescriber.

• Warn patient that any change in insulin should be made cautiously and only under medical supervision. Changes in insulin strength, manufacturer, type (regular, NPH,

or insulin analogues), species (animal, human), or method of manufacture (rDNA, animal-source insulin) may result in the need for a dosage change.

• Caution patient to discuss adjustments to the administration schedule if traveling across more than two time zones.

SAFETY ALERT!

interferon alfa-2b (recombinant) (IFN-alpha 2b)
in-ter-FEER-on

Intron A

Therapeutic class: Antivirals
Pharmacologic class: Biological response modifiers

AVAILABLE FORMS
Powder for injection: 10, 18, and 50 million international units/vial with diluent
Solution for injection: 18 and 25 million international units/vial (6 and 10 million international units/mL)

INDICATIONS & DOSAGES
Adjust-a-dose (for all indications): For all indications except condylomata acuminata, if adverse effects occur, stop drug until they abate; then resume drug at 50% of the previous dose. If intolerance persists, stop drug. See package insert for specific guidance.

➤ **Hairy cell leukemia**
Adults: 2 million international units/m^2 IM or subcut three times weekly for 6 months or more if patient is responding to treatment. Give subcut if platelet count is less than 50,000/mm^3.

➤ **AIDS-related Kaposi sarcoma**
Adults: 30 million international units/m^2 subcut or IM three times weekly. Maintain dose until disease progression or maximal response has been achieved after 16 weeks of treatment. Don't use solution for injection in vials for this indication.

➤ **Chronic HBV infection**
Adults: 30 to 35 million international units IM or subcut weekly, given as 5 million international units daily or 10 million international units three times weekly for 16 weeks.

Reactions in bold italics are *life-threatening*. Interactions may have a *rapid onset* or a *delayed onset*.

Children ages 1 to 17: 3 million international units/m² subcut three times weekly for first week; then increase to 6 million international units/m² subcut three times weekly (maximum is 10 million international units three times weekly) for total of 16 to 24 weeks.

Adjust-a-dose: If WBC count is less than 1.5×10^9/L, granulocyte count is less than 0.75×10^9/L, or platelet count is less than 50×10^9/L, reduce dose by 50%. Permanently discontinue drug if WBC count is less than 1×10^9/L, granulocyte count is less than 0.5×10^9/L, or platelet count is less than 25×10^9/L.

➤ **Chronic HCV infection**
Adults: 3 million international units IM or subcut three times weekly. In patients tolerating therapy with normalization of ALT at 16 weeks of therapy, continue for 18 to 24 months. In patients who haven't normalized the ALT, consider stopping therapy.

➤ **Adjunct to surgical treatment in patients with malignant melanoma who are asymptomatic after surgery but at high risk for systemic recurrence for up to 8 weeks after surgery**
Adults: Initially, 20 million international units/m² by IV infusion over 20 minutes 5 consecutive days weekly for 4 weeks; then maintenance dose of 10 million international units/m² subcut three times weekly for 48 weeks. Solution for injection in vials isn't recommended for IV administration and shouldn't be used for the induction phase.
Adjust-a-dose: Withhold dose if severe adverse reactions develop, including granulocyte count more than 250/mm³ but less than 500/mm³ or ALT/AST level of more than 5 to 10 × ULN, until adverse reactions abate. Restart at 50% of the previous dose.

➤ **First treatment of clinically aggressive follicular non-Hodgkin lymphoma with chemotherapy containing anthracycline**
Adults: 5 million international units subcut three times weekly for up to 18 months.
Adjust-a-dose: For neutrophil count of more than 1,000/mm³ but less than 1,500/mm³, decrease dosage by 50%. May resume starting dose if neutrophil count returns to more than 1,500/mm³. Withhold drug if neutrophil count is less than 1,000/mm³ or platelet count is less than 50,000/mm³.

➤ **Condylomata acuminata (genital or venereal warts)**
Adults: 1 million international units for each lesion (maximum five lesions in a single course) intralesionally three times weekly for 3 weeks. Additional course may be given at 12 to 16 weeks. Don't use the 18-million or 50-million international units powder for injection or the 18-million international units multidose solution for injection for this indication.

ADMINISTRATION
IV
▼ Prepare infusion solution immediately before use.
▼ Based on desired dose, reconstitute appropriate vial strength of drug with diluent provided. Withdraw dose and inject into a 100-mL bag of NSS. Final yield of drug shouldn't be less than 10 million international units/100 mL.
▼ Infuse over 20 minutes.
▼ Store solution in refrigerator. Store powder before and after reconstitution in refrigerator. Use within 24 hours.
▼ **Incompatibilities:** Dextrose solutions.
IM
• Carefully monitor injection sites in patient with thrombocytopenia. Avoid IM injections if possible.
• In patients whose platelet count is below 50,000/mm³, give subcutaneously.
• Give drug at bedtime to minimize daytime drowsiness.
Subcutaneous
• For condylomata acuminata intralesional injection, use only 10 million-international unit vial because dilution of other strengths for intralesional use results in a hypertonic solution.
• Don't reconstitute drug in 10 million-international unit vial with more than 1 mL of diluent.
• Use tuberculin or similar syringe and 25G to 30G needle.
• Don't inject too deep beneath lesion or too superficially. As many as five lesions can be treated at one time.
• To ease discomfort, give in evening with acetaminophen.

ACTION

Unknown. May inhibit tumor or viral cell replication and modulate host immune response by enhancing macrophage activity and improving specific lymphocytes' cytotoxicity for target cells.

Route	Onset	Peak	Duration
IV	Unknown	15–60 min	4 hr
IM, subcut	Unknown	3–12 hr	16 hr

Half-life: IV, 2 hours; IM, subcut, 2 to 3 hours.

ADVERSE REACTIONS

CNS: apathy, amnesia, asthenia, depression, difficulty in thinking or concentrating, dizziness, drowsiness, fatigue, insomnia, paresthesia, somnolence, anxiety, lethargy, nervousness, weakness, headache, rigors. **CV:** chest pain, *cyanosis,* edema, hypotension. **EENT:** conjunctivitis, earache, rhinorrhea, rhinitis, sinusitis, pharyngitis. **GI:** anorexia, diarrhea, dry mouth, dyspepsia, nausea, vomiting, abdominal pain, constipation, esophagitis, flatulence, stomatitis. **GU:** decreased libido, impotence, amenorrhea. **Hematologic:** *leukopenia, thrombocytopenia, anemia, neutropenia.* **Hepatic:** *hepatitis.* **Metabolic:** weight loss. **Respiratory:** coughing, dyspnea. **Skin:** alopecia, dryness, increased diaphoresis, pruritus, rash, dermatitis. **Other:** flulike syndrome, injection-site reaction.

INTERACTIONS

Drug-drug. *Aldesleukin, telbivudine:* May enhance adverse or toxic effects of these drugs. Avoid use together.
Aminophylline, theophylline: May reduce theophylline clearance. Monitor theophylline level.
CNS depressants: May increase CNS effects. Avoid using together.
Ribavirin: May enhance adverse effects, including hemolytic anemia. Monitor therapy.
Zidovudine: May cause synergistic adverse effects (higher risk of neutropenia). Carefully monitor WBC count.

EFFECTS ON LAB TEST RESULTS

• May increase calcium, phosphate, AST, ALT, LDH, alkaline phosphatase, triglyceride, and fasting glucose levels. May decrease Hb level.

• May increase INR and prolong PT and PTT.
• May decrease WBC and platelet counts.
• May increase or decrease TSH level.

CONTRAINDICATIONS & CAUTIONS

• Contraindicated in patients hypersensitive to drug or its components and in those with autoimmune hepatitis or decompensated liver disease.
• Combination therapy with ribavirin is additionally contraindicated in patients hypersensitive to ribavirin or other components of the product and in those with hemoglobinopathies or CrCl less than 50 mL/minute.
• Use cautiously in elderly patients and in those with history of CV disease, pulmonary disease, diabetes mellitus, coagulation disorders, renal impairment, and severe myelosuppression.
• Depression, psychosis, and suicidal behavior have been linked to drug use; patients with psychotic disorders, especially depression, shouldn't continue drug treatment.
❸ Alert: Neurotoxicity and cardiotoxicity are more common in elderly patients, especially those with underlying CNS or cardiac impairment.
Dialyzable drug: No.
⚠ Overdose S&S: Abnormal liver enzyme levels, renal failure, hemorrhage, MI.

PREGNANCY-LACTATION-REPRODUCTION

• There are no adequate studies in pregnant women. Use during pregnancy only if potential benefit justifies potential risk to the fetus.
❸ Alert: Combination therapy with ribavirin is contraindicated in pregnant women and in men whose female partners are pregnant.
❸ Alert: Because of fetal risk, warn women of childbearing potential and male patients with partners of childbearing potential who are receiving combination therapy with ribavirin to use two forms of contraception.
• It isn't known if drug appears in human milk. Patient should discontinue breastfeeding or discontinue drug.

NURSING CONSIDERATIONS

Black Box Warning Alpha interferons cause or aggravate fatal or life-threatening

---

Reactions in bold italics are *life-threatening*. Interactions may have a *rapid onset* or a *delayed onset*.

neuropsychiatric, autoimmune, ischemic, and infectious disorders. Monitor patients closely with periodic clinical and laboratory evaluations. Withdraw patients with persistently severe or worsening signs or symptoms of these conditions from therapy. ■

◆ *Alert:* Not all dosage forms are appropriate for all indications. Refer to manufacturer's instructions for approved indications before use.

• Powder for injection doesn't contain a preservative. Discard vial after reconstitution and withdrawal of a single dose; don't reenter vial.

• Ensure patient is well hydrated, especially at beginning of treatment.

• At start of treatment, monitor patient for flulike signs and symptoms, which tend to diminish with continued therapy. Premedicate patient with acetaminophen to minimize these symptoms.

• Periodically check for adverse CNS reactions, such as decreased mental status and dizziness, during therapy.

• Monitor CBC with differential, platelet count, and blood chemistry and electrolyte studies. Monitor ECG before and during treatment if patient has cardiac disorder or advanced stages of cancer.

• Monitor hepatic function (serum bilirubin, ALT, AST, alkaline phosphatase, and LDH) at 2, 8, and 12 weeks after start of therapy, then every 6 months during therapy. Permanently stop drug for evidence of severe (grade 3) hepatic injury or hepatic decompensation (Child-Pugh classes B and C).

• For patients who develop thrombocytopenia, exercise extreme care in performing invasive procedures; inspect injection site and skin frequently for signs and symptoms of bruising; limit frequency of IM injections; test urine, emesis fluid, stool, and secretions for occult blood.

• Severe adverse reactions may need dosage reduction to half or withholding of drug until reactions subside.

• Use with blood dyscrasia-causing drugs, bone marrow suppressants, or radiation therapy may increase bone marrow suppression. Dosage reduction may be needed.

• For condylomata acuminata, maximum response usually occurs in 4 to 8 weeks. If results are not satisfactory after 12 to 16 weeks, a second course may be started. Patients with 6 to 10 condylomata may receive a second course of treatment; patients with more than 10 condylomata may receive additional courses.

PATIENT TEACHING
• Advise patient to avoid contact with persons with viral illness; patient is at increased risk for infection during therapy.

• Advise patient that lab tests will be performed before and periodically during therapy.

• Teach patient proper oral hygiene during treatment because bone marrow suppressant effects of interferon may lead to microbial infection, delayed healing, and bleeding gums. Drug also may decrease saliva.

• Advise patient to check with prescriber for instructions after missing a dose.

• Stress need to follow prescriber's instructions about taking and recording temperature and how and when to take acetaminophen.

• Teach patient who will self-administer drug how to prepare injection and how to use disposable syringe. Provide information on drug stability.

• Tell patient that drug may cause temporary partial hair loss; hair should return after drug is stopped.

• Advise patient to report all adverse reactions and to immediately report neuropsychiatric symptoms (depression, mania, psychosis, suicidal ideation).

SAFETY ALERT!

interferon beta-1a
in-ter-FEER-on

Avonex, Rebif

Therapeutic class: Antivirals
Pharmacologic class: Biological response modifiers

AVAILABLE FORMS
Avonex (IM use only)
Lyophilized powder for injection: 30 mcg/single-use vials (6.6 million international units)
Prefilled syringe or autoinjector: 30 mcg (6 million international units)/0.5 mL

Rebif (subcut use only)
Parenteral: 8.8 mcg (2.4 million international units)/0.2 mL, 22 mcg (6 million international units)/0.5 mL, 44 mcg (12 million international units)/0.5 mL in prefilled syringes or autoinjectors

INDICATIONS & DOSAGES
Adjust-a-dose (for all indications): To decrease incidence and severity of flulike symptoms that may occur when initiating Avonex at a dose of 30 mcg, initiate once-weekly dosing with 7.5 mcg IM (week 1); then increase dose in increments of 7.5 mcg once weekly (weeks 2 to 4) up to recommended dose (30 mcg once weekly).
➤ **To slow accumulation of physical disability and decrease frequency of clinical worsening in patients with relapsing forms of MS**
Adults age 18 and older: 30 mcg Avonex IM once weekly. Or, initially, 4.4 or 8.8 mcg Rebif subcut three times weekly for 2 weeks; then increase dose to 11 or 22 mcg three times weekly for another 2 weeks. Then increase to a maintenance dose of 22 or 44 mcg subcut three times weekly.
Adjust-a-dose: For Rebif, in patients with leukopenia or elevated LFT values (ALT greater than 5 × ULN), reduce dosage until toxicity is resolved. Stop treatment if jaundice or other signs of hepatic injury occur.
➤ **First MS attack if brain MRI shows abnormalities consistent with MS**
Adults: 30 mcg Avonex IM once weekly.

ADMINISTRATION
Subcutaneous
• Visually inspect Rebif for particulate matter and discoloration before administration.
• Rotate sites of injection.
• Administer Rebif at same time on same 3 days at least 48 hours apart each week (late afternoon or evening on Monday, Wednesday, and Friday).
• Use only prefilled syringes for titration to 22 mcg prescribed dose of Rebif.
• Store Rebif in the refrigerator between 36° and 46° F (2° and 8° C). Don't freeze. Rebif may be stored at or below 77° F (25° C) for up to 30 days if away from heat and light.

IM
🜂 *Alert:* Syringe tip cap contains natural rubber latex, which may cause allergic reactions.
• To reconstitute lyophilized Avonex, inject 1.1 mL of supplied diluent (sterile water for injection) into vial and gently swirl to dissolve drug. Don't shake.
• Use drug as soon as possible; may be used up to 6 hours after being reconstituted if stored at 36° to 46° F.
• Rotate injection sites. Don't inject into areas where skin is red, bruised, or irritated.
• The Avonex and diluent vials are for single use only; discard unused portions.
• Store Avonex prefilled syringes and autoinjectors in the refrigerator at 36° to 46° F. If refrigeration is unavailable, may store at 77° F for up to 7 days. Once refrigerated, syringes and autoinjectors must not be stored above 77° F. Once removed from refrigerator, warm to room temperature (about 30 minutes). Don't use external heat sources, such as hot water, to warm syringe, or expose to high temperatures. Don't freeze. Protect from light.
• After giving each dose, discard any remaining product in the syringe or autoinjector.

ACTION
Unknown. Interacts with specific cell receptors found on the surface of cells. Binding of these receptors causes the expression of a number of interferon-induced gene products believed to mediate the biological actions of interferon beta-1a.

Route	Onset	Peak	Duration
Subcut	Unknown	16 hr	Unknown
IM	12 hr	6–36 hr	4 days

Half-life: Subcut, 69 hours; IM, 8 to 54 hours.

ADVERSE REACTIONS
CNS: asthenia, dizziness, fatigue, fever, headache, pain, sleep difficulty, depression, *seizures, suicidal ideation or attempt, suicidal tendency,* abnormal coordination, ataxia, hypertonia, malaise, speech disorder, syncope, rigors. **CV:** chest pain, vasodilation. **EENT:** abnormal vision, decreased hearing, otitis media, sinusitis. **GI:** abdominal pain, diarrhea, dyspepsia, nausea, anorexia, dry

---

Reactions in bold italics are *life-threatening*. Interactions may have a *rapid onset* or a *delayed onset*.

mouth. **GU:** increased urinary frequency, ovarian cyst, urinary incontinence, vaginitis, UTI. **Hematologic:** lymphadenopathy, *leukopenia, pancytopenia, thrombocytopenia,* anemia. **Hepatic:** abnormal hepatic function, *autoimmune hepatitis,* bilirubinemia, hepatic injury, *hepatitis.* **Metabolic:** hyperthyroidism, hypothyroidism. **Musculoskeletal:** back pain, muscle ache, skeletal pain, arthralgia, muscle spasm. **Respiratory:** URI, dyspnea, bronchitis. **Skin:** injection-site reaction, alopecia, ecchymosis at injection site, nevus, urticaria. **Other:** chills, flulike syndrome, infection, hypersensitivity reactions, herpes simplex, herpes zoster, neutralizing antibodies.

INTERACTIONS
Drug-drug. *Myelosuppressive drugs:* May cause added hematologic toxicities; use cautiously together. Monitor CBC.
Theophylline derivatives (except dyphylline): Interferon beta-1a may decrease metabolism of theophylline derivative. Monitor therapy.
Drug-lifestyle. *Sun exposure:* May cause photosensitivity reactions. Advise patient to take precautions against sun exposure.

EFFECTS ON LAB TEST RESULTS
• May increase liver enzyme levels. May decrease Hb level and hematocrit. May increase or decrease thyroid function test levels.
• May increase eosinophil count. May decrease WBC and platelet counts.

CONTRAINDICATIONS & CAUTIONS
• Contraindicated in patients hypersensitive to natural or recombinant interferon beta, human albumin, or other components of drug.
• Use cautiously in patients with depression, seizure disorders, or severe cardiac conditions.
• Thrombotic microangiopathy (TMA), including thrombotic thrombocytopenic purpura and hemolytic-uremic syndrome, sometimes fatal, has been reported with interferon beta products and may occur several weeks to years after start of therapy.

• Safety and effectiveness of drug in chronic progressive MS or in children younger than age 18 haven't been established.
Dialyzable drug: Unknown.

PREGNANCY-LACTATION-REPRODUCTION
• There are no adequate studies in pregnant women. Use during pregnancy only if potential benefit justifies potential risk to the fetus.
• It isn't known if drug appears in human milk. Use cautiously in breastfeeding women.

NURSING CONSIDERATIONS
• Monitor patient closely for depression and suicidal ideation. It isn't known if these symptoms are related to the underlying neurologic basis of MS or to the drug.
• Monitor thyroid function tests, WBC count, platelet count, and blood chemistries, including LFTs.
• Monitor patient for TMA and discontinue drug if clinical signs and symptoms and laboratory findings consistent with TMA occur; manage as clinically indicated.
• Give analgesics or antipyretics to decrease flulike symptoms.

PATIENT TEACHING
• Advise patient to read medication guide that comes with drug.
• Teach patient and family member how to reconstitute drug and give Avonex IM; explain that syringe tip cap contains natural rubber latex, which can cause allergic reactions.
• Advise patient not to inject where skin is irritated, red, bruised, scarred, or infected.
• Caution patient not to change dosage or schedule of administration. If a dose is missed, tell patient to take it as soon as remembered and then resume regular schedule. Tell patient not to take two injections within 48 hours of each other.
• Show patient how to store drug.
• Inform patient that flulike signs and symptoms (such as fever, fatigue, muscle aches, headache, chills, and joint pain) aren't uncommon at start of therapy and that analgesics/antipyretics may be prescribed on treatment days to lessen severity of flulike signs and symptoms.

- Advise patient to report depression, suicidal thoughts, or other adverse reactions.
- If pregnancy occurs, instruct patient to notify prescriber immediately.
- Instruct patient to keep syringes and needles away from children. Also, instruct patient not to reuse needles or syringes and to discard them in a syringe-disposal unit.
- Advise patient to use sunscreen and avoid sun exposure while taking drug because photosensitivity may occur.

SAFETY ALERT!

interferon beta-1b (recombinant)
in-ter-FEER-on

Betaseron, Extavia

Therapeutic class: Antivirals
Pharmacologic class: Biological response modifiers

AVAILABLE FORMS
Powder for injection: 9.6 million international units (0.3 mg)

INDICATIONS & DOSAGES
➤ **To reduce frequency of exacerbations in relapsing forms of MS, including patients who have experienced a first clinical episode and have MRI features consistent with MS**
Adults: 0.0625 mg subcut every other day for weeks 1 and 2; then 0.125 mg subcut every other day for weeks 3 and 4; then 0.1875 mg subcut every other day for weeks 5 and 6; then 0.25 mg subcut every other day thereafter.

ADMINISTRATION
Subcutaneous
🔴 *Alert:* The removable rubber cap of the Extavia diluent prefilled syringe contains natural rubber latex, which may cause allergic reactions and shouldn't be handled by latex-sensitive individuals.
- To reconstitute, inject 1.2 mL of supplied diluent (half-NSS for injection) into vial and gently swirl to dissolve drug.
- Reconstituted solution contains 8 million international units (0.25 mg)/mL.

- Don't shake. Discard vial that contains particulates or discolored solution.
- Inject immediately after preparation.
- Rotate injection sites to minimize local reactions and observe site for necrosis. Don't inject into red, sore, or infected skin.
- Store at room temperature. After reconstitution, if not used immediately, drug may be refrigerated for up to 3 hours.

ACTION
A naturally occurring antiviral and immunoregulatory drug derived from human fibroblasts. Drug attaches to membrane receptors and causes cellular changes, including increased protein synthesis.

Route	Onset	Peak	Duration
Subcut	Unknown	1–8 hr	Unknown

Half-life: 8 minutes to 4¼ hours.

ADVERSE REACTIONS
CNS: depression, anxiety, emotional lability, depersonalization, *suicidal tendencies,* confusion, hypertonia, asthenia, migraine, *seizures,* headache, pain, dizziness, malaise, fever, chills, insomnia, ataxia. **CV:** chest pain, peripheral edema, palpitations, HTN, tachycardia, peripheral vascular disorder. **EENT:** conjunctivitis, abnormal vision, sinusitis, laryngitis. **GI:** diarrhea, constipation, abdominal pain, vomiting, dyspepsia, nausea. **GU:** menstrual bleeding or spotting, early or delayed menses, fewer days of menstrual flow, menorrhagia, urgency, impotence, prostate disorder, frequency. **Hematologic:** *leukopenia,* lymphadenopathy. **Musculoskeletal:** myasthenia, arthralgia, myalgia, leg cramps. **Respiratory:** dyspnea. **Skin:** inflammation, pain, necrosis at injection site, diaphoresis, alopecia, rash, skin disorder. **Other:** breast pain, flulike syndrome, pelvic pain, generalized edema.

INTERACTIONS
None reported.

EFFECTS ON LAB TEST RESULTS
- May increase ALT and bilirubin levels.
- May decrease WBC and neutrophil counts.

CONTRAINDICATIONS & CAUTIONS

• Contraindicated in patients hypersensitive to interferon beta, human albumin, or components of drug.

• Drug-induced lupus erythematosus has been reported and has occurred with positive serologic testing (including positive antinuclear or anti-double-stranded DNA antibody testing).

• Thrombotic microangiopathy (TMA), including thrombotic thrombocytopenic purpura and hemolytic-uremic syndrome, sometimes fatal, has been reported with interferon beta products and may occur several weeks to years after start of therapy.

Dialyzable drug: Unknown.

PREGNANCY-LACTATION-REPRODUCTION

• There are no adequate studies in pregnant women; however, spontaneous abortions have been reported in clinical trials. Use during pregnancy only if potential benefit justifies potential risk to the fetus.

• It isn't known if drug appears in human milk. Patient should discontinue breastfeeding or discontinue drug.

NURSING CONSIDERATIONS

🟢 *Alert:* Serious liver damage, including hepatic failure requiring transplant, can occur. Monitor liver function at 1, 3, and 6 months after therapy starts and periodically thereafter.

• Drug is intended for use under the guidance and supervision of a physician. Administer first injection under the supervision of a health care provider. If patients or caregivers are to administer drug, train them in the proper technique for self-administering.

• Monitor patient for signs and symptoms of drug-induced lupus erythematosus (rash, serositis, polyarthritis, nephritis, Raynaud phenomenon); discontinue therapy if they occur.

• Monitor patient for TMA and discontinue drug if clinical signs and symptoms and laboratory findings consistent with TMA occur; manage as clinically indicated.

• Monitor patient for symptoms of depression and severe psychiatric effects (mania, suicidal behavior or ideation, psychosis).

• Monitor CBC at 1, 3, and 6 months after therapy starts and periodically thereafter.

• Monitor thyroid function tests every 6 months in patients being treated for thyroid disorder.

• Use of analgesics and antipyretics on treatment days may help ameliorate flulike symptoms associated with interferon beta-1b use.

PATIENT TEACHING

• Warn female patient about dangers to fetus. If pregnancy occurs during therapy, tell her to notify prescriber.

• Advise patient to read medication guide that comes with drug.

• Advise patient if a dose is missed to administer as soon as remembered but not to administer on 2 consecutive days. Tell patient to time subsequent doses every 48 hours.

• Advise patient to stay well hydrated.

• Teach patient how to perform subcut injections, including solution preparation, aseptic technique, injection-site rotation, and equipment disposal. Periodically reevaluate patient's technique.

• Tell patient to report sign and symptoms of drug-induced lupus erythematosus.

• Tell patient to take drug at bedtime to minimize mild flulike signs and symptoms that commonly occur.

• Advise patient to report suicidal thoughts or depression.

• Urge patient to immediately report signs or symptoms of tissue death at injection site.

• Advise patient of importance of obtaining routine blood tests.

SAFETY ALERT!

ipilimumab
IP-ih-LIM-yoo-mab

Yervoy

Therapeutic class: Antineoplastics
Pharmacologic class: Monoclonal antibodies

AVAILABLE FORMS

Injection: 50 mg/10 mL (5 mg/mL), 200 mg/40 mL (5 mg/mL)

INDICATIONS & DOSAGES
Adjust-a-dose (for all indications):
Black Box Warning For patients with severe immune-mediated reactions, initiate systemic high-dose corticosteroids and permanently discontinue ipilimumab. ■

Refer to manufacturer's instructions for other toxicity-related dosage adjustments.
➤ **Treatment of unresectable or metastatic melanoma**
Adults and children age 12 and older:
3 mg/kg IV infusion over 90 minutes every 3 weeks for a total of four doses. All treatment must be administered within 16 weeks of first dose.
➤ **Adjuvant treatment of cutaneous melanoma with pathologic involvement of regional lymph nodes of more than 1 mm after complete resection, including total lymphadenectomy**
Adults: 10 mg/kg IV over 90 minutes every 3 weeks for four doses, followed by 10 mg/kg every 12 weeks for up to 3 years or until documented disease recurrence or unacceptable toxicity. If toxicity occurs, omit, don't delay, doses.
➤ **Treatment of intermediate- or poor-risk, previously untreated advanced renal cell carcinoma in combination with nivolumab**
Adults: Nivolumab 3 mg/kg IV over 30 minutes followed by ipilimumab 1 mg/kg IV over 30 minutes on the same day every 3 weeks for a maximum of four doses, then nivolumab 240 mg IV over 30 minutes every 2 weeks or 480 mg IV over 30 minutes every 4 weeks.
➤ **Microsatellite instability-high (MSI-H) or mismatch repair-deficient (dMMR) metastatic colorectal cancer that has progressed following treatment with a fluoropyrimidine, oxaliplatin, and irinotecan, as a single agent or in combination with nivolumab**
Adults and children age 12 and older:
1 mg/kg IV over 30 minutes, immediately following nivolumab given on the same day, every 3 weeks for up to four doses or until intolerable toxicity or disease progression occurs. Review nivolumab prescribing information before administering ipilimumab.
➤ **First-line combination therapy for unresectable or metastatic melanoma ◆**

Adults: 3 mg/kg IV every 3 weeks with nivolumab for four combination doses. Continue nivolumab until disease progression or unacceptable toxicity.

ADMINISTRATION
IV
▼ Store vials in refrigerator at 36° to 46° F (2° to 8° C). Don't freeze or shake vials. Protect from light.
▼ Visually inspect solution. Solution may be clear to pale yellow. Discard if cloudy or discolored or if particles (other than translucent-to-white, amorphous particles) are present.
▼ Allow vials to come to room temperature for 5 minutes before preparing infusion.
▼ Withdraw required volume of drug and transfer into IV bag of NSS or D₅W. Final concentration should range from 1 to 2 mg/mL. Invert bag gently to mix.
▼ Store diluted solution up to 24 hours under refrigeration or at room temperature (68° to 77° F [20° to 25° C]).
▼ Administer diluted solution over 90 minutes through IV line containing a sterile, nonpyrogenic, low-protein-binding in-line filter.
▼ After each dose, flush IV line with NSS or D₅W.
▼ Discard unused portion of vial.
▼ **Incompatibilities:** Other IV drugs and solutions other than NSS or D₅W.

ACTION
Binds to the cytotoxic T-lymphocyte–associated antigen 4; this blockade has been shown to augment T-cell–mediated antitumor immune responses.

Route	Onset	Peak	Duration
IV	Rapid	Unknown	Unknown

Half-life: 15.4 days.

ADVERSE REACTIONS
CNS: fatigue, neuropathy, pyrexia, headache, insomnia. **GI:** diarrhea, colitis, enterocolitis, vomiting, decreased appetite. **GU:** nephritis. **Hepatic:** *hepatotoxicity.* **Metabolic:** endocrinopathy, hypopituitarism, weight loss. **Skin:** pruritus, rash, dermatitis, urticaria. **Other:** *adrenal insufficiency.*

Reactions in bold italics are *life-threatening.* Interactions may have a *rapid onset* or a *delayed onset.*

INTERACTIONS
None reported.

EFFECTS ON LAB TEST RESULTS
• May increase liver enzyme, alkaline phosphatase, bilirubin, amylase, lipase, and creatinine levels.
• May decrease Hb level.
• May increase eosinophil count.
• May increase or decrease thyroid hormone levels.

CONTRAINDICATIONS & CAUTIONS
• Contraindicated in patients hypersensitive to drug or its components.

Black Box Warning Ipilimumab can cause severe and fatal immune-mediated adverse reactions involving any organ system, especially such reactions as enterocolitis, hepatitis, dermatitis (including toxic epidermal necrolysis), neuropathy, and endocrinopathy. Reactions usually occur during treatment, but may present weeks to months after therapy ends. If severe immune-mediated reactions occur, permanently discontinue ipilimumab and initiate systemic high-dose corticosteroid therapy. Assess patient for these reactions. ■

• Permanently discontinue drug for any of the following: persistent moderate adverse reactions or inability to reduce corticosteroid dose to 7.5 mg of prednisone or equivalent daily; failure to complete full treatment course for unresectable or metastatic melanoma within 16 weeks from administration of first dose; severe or life-threatening adverse reactions, including colitis with abdominal pain, fever, ileus, or peritoneal signs and symptoms; diarrhea (seven or more loose stools over baseline); elevated transaminase or total bilirubin level; pneumonitis; elevated serum creatinine level; infusion reaction; hepatotoxicity; endocrinopathy; SJS; toxic epidermal necrolysis; rash complicated by full-thickness dermal ulceration or necrotic, bullous, or hemorrhagic manifestations; severe motor or sensory neuropathy; Guillain-Barré syndrome; myasthenia gravis; severe immune-mediated reactions involving any organ system (nephritis, pneumonitis, pancreatitis, noninfectious myocarditis); or

immune-mediated ocular disease unresponsive to topical immunosuppressive therapy.
Dialyzable drug: Unknown.

PREGNANCY-LACTATION-REPRODUCTION
• Based on its mechanism of action and data from animal studies, drug can cause fetal harm when given to pregnant women.
• Advise women of childbearing potential to use effective contraception during treatment and for 3 months after last dose.
• Drug may appear in human milk. Because of the risk of serious adverse reactions in breastfeeding infants, patient should discontinue breastfeeding or discontinue drug. Women shouldn't breastfeed for 3 months after final dose.

NURSING CONSIDERATIONS
Black Box Warning Assess patients for signs and symptoms of enterocolitis, dermatitis, neuropathy, and endocrinopathy, and evaluate clinical chemistry values, including ACTH level and LFT and thyroid function test results, at baseline and before each dose. ■

• Review LFT results and assess patient for signs and symptoms of hepatotoxicity (jaundice, dark urine, nausea, vomiting, right upper quadrant pain, abnormal bleeding or bruising) before each dose. For patients with hepatotoxicity (AST or ALT level more than 5 × ULN or total bilirubin level more than 3 × ULN), rule out infectious or malignant causes and increase frequency of LFT monitoring until resolution. When LFT results show sustained improvement or return to baseline, initiate corticosteroid tapering and continue to taper over 1 month. Withhold ipilimumab in patients with grade 2 hepatotoxicity.

• Monitor patients for signs and symptoms of enterocolitis and bowel perforation (abdominal pain, fever, ileus, or peritoneal signs and symptoms; increase in stool frequency to seven or more over patient's baseline; fecal incontinence; need for IV hydration for more than 24 hours; GI hemorrhage; GI perforation). Rule out infection and consider endoscopic evaluation for persistent or severe symptoms. With improvement to grade 1 or less, taper corticosteroid dosage over at least 1 month. If moderate symptoms occur, administer antidiarrheal and, if persistent for more than 1 week, start systemic corticosteroids (prednisone or equivalent) at 0.5 mg/kg/day. May consider adding anti-TNF or other immunosuppressive therapy for management of immune-mediated enterocolitis unresponsive to 3 to 5 days of systemic corticosteroids or recurring after symptomatic improvement.

• Monitor patients for signs and symptoms of motor or sensory neuropathy. Withhold ipilimumab in patients with moderate neuropathy. Permanently discontinue drug in patients with severe neuropathy that interferes with daily activities, such as Guillain-Barré–like syndromes (unilateral or bilateral weakness, sensory changes, paresthesia). Consider systemic corticosteroids (1 to 2 mg/kg/day prednisone or equivalent) for severe neuropathies.

• Monitor patients for signs and symptoms of dermatitis (rash, pruritus) and consider these symptoms immune-mediated unless an alternative cause is identified. Permanently discontinue ipilimumab in patients with SJS, toxic epidermal necrolysis, or rash complicated by full-thickness dermal ulceration or necrotic, bullous, or hemorrhagic manifestations. When dermatitis is controlled, taper corticosteroids over at least 1 month. For patients with mild to moderate dermatitis, treat symptomatically; give topical or systemic corticosteroids if there is no improvement within 1 week. Withhold ipilimumab in patients with moderate to severe signs and symptoms.

• Monitor patients for signs and symptoms of hypophysitis, adrenal insufficiency (including adrenal crisis), and hyperthyroidism or hypothyroidism (headaches, fatigue, feeling cold, weight gain, changes in mood or behavior, dizziness, or fainting). Endocrinopathies should be considered immune-mediated unless an alternative cause is identified. Withhold drug in symptomatic patients. Give corticosteroids and hormone replacement as appropriate.

• Monitor patients for ocular symptoms (vision changes, eye pain or redness). Administer corticosteroid eyedrops to patients who develop uveitis, iritis, or episcleritis. Permanently discontinue drug in patients with

immune-mediated ocular disease unresponsive to local immunosuppressive therapy.

PATIENT TEACHING
• Instruct patient to report history of immune system disorders, such as ulcerative colitis, Crohn disease, lupus, or sarcoidosis; organ transplant; or liver damage.
• Teach patient signs and symptoms of serious immune-mediated adverse reactions, and advise patient to immediately report them to prescriber.
• Advise patient that blood chemistry studies will be needed before start of therapy and before each dose.
• Instruct patient to read the Yervoy Medication Guide before taking each dose.
• Warn female patient that ipilimumab can cause fetal harm and to report pregnancy immediately.
• Advise female patient of childbearing potential to use effective contraception during treatment and for 3 months after last dose.
• Tell breastfeeding patient not to breastfeed during therapy and for 3 months after final dose.

ipratropium bromide
ih-pra-TROE-pee-um

Atrovent HFA, Ipravent✦

Therapeutic class: Bronchodilators
Pharmacologic class: Anticholinergics

AVAILABLE FORMS
Inhaler: 17 mcg/metered dose
Nasal spray: 0.03% (21 mcg/metered dose), 0.06% (42 mcg/metered dose)
Solution (for inhalation): 0.02% (500 mcg/vial)

INDICATIONS & DOSAGES
➤ **Bronchospasm in chronic bronchitis and emphysema**
Adults: Usually, 2 inhalations q.i.d.; patient may take additional inhalations as needed but shouldn't exceed 12 inhalations in 24 hours. Or, 500 mcg every 6 to 8 hours via oral nebulizer.
Children age 12 and older: 500 mcg every 6 to 8 hours (t.i.d. to q.i.d.) via oral nebulizer.

➤ **Rhinorrhea caused by allergic and nonallergic perennial rhinitis**
Adults and children age 6 and older: Two 0.03% nasal sprays (42 mcg) per nostril b.i.d. or t.i.d.

➤ **Rhinorrhea caused by the common cold**
Adults and children age 12 and older: Two 0.06% nasal sprays (84 mcg) per nostril t.i.d. or q.i.d.
Children ages 5 to 11: Two 0.06% nasal sprays (84 mcg) per nostril t.i.d.

➤ **Rhinorrhea caused by seasonal allergic rhinitis**
Adults and children age 5 and older: Two 0.06% nasal sprays (84 mcg) per nostril q.i.d. Total dose is 672 mcg/day.

➤ **Acute asthma exacerbations, in combination with a short-acting beta agonist ♦**
Adults and adolescents age 13 and older: 500 mcg via oral nebulizer every 20 minutes for three doses, then as needed; or 8 inhalations of inhalation aerosol every 20 minutes as needed for up to 3 hours.
Children ages 6 to 12: 250 to 500 mcg via oral nebulizer every 20 minutes for three doses, then as needed; or 4 to 8 inhalations of inhalation aerosol every 20 minutes as needed for up to 3 hours.
Children age 5 and younger: 250 mcg via oral nebulizer every 20 minutes for 1 hour; or 2 inhalations of inhalation aerosol every 20 minutes if needed for 1 hour.

ADMINISTRATION
Inhalational
• Prime inhaler before initial use by releasing 2 test sprays into the air. If inhaler not used for more than 3 days, reprime.
• If more than 1 inhalation is ordered, wait at least 2 minutes between inhalations.
• Use spacer device to improve drug delivery, if appropriate.
• Wash mouthpiece once a week for 30 seconds in warm water only and let air dry.
• Don't puncture inhaler, throw into a fire or incinerator, or use or store near heat or open flame.
• Inhalation solution is for use with oral nebulizer. Refer to manufacturer's instructions for use.
• Protect solution from light. Store unused vials in foil pouch.

• Store inhaler and solution between 59° and 86° F (15° and 30° C).
Intranasal
• Prime nasal spray with 7 sprays of pump before first use; prime with 2 sprays after pump hasn't been used for more than 24 hours.
• Tilt patient's head backward after dose to allow drug to spread to back of nose.
• Store between 59° and 77° F (15° and 25° C); avoid freezing.

ACTION
Inhibits vagally mediated reflexes by antagonizing acetylcholine at muscarinic receptors on bronchial smooth muscle.

Route	Onset	Peak	Duration
Inhalation	15 min	1–2 hr	2–8 hr
Intranasal	15 min	Unknown	Unknown

Half-life: Inhalation, about 2 hours; intranasal, 1.6 hours.

ADVERSE REACTIONS
CNS: dizziness, headache. **CV:** palpitations, chest pain, HTN. **EENT:** blurred vision, epistaxis, rhinitis, pharyngitis, sinusitis, nasal dryness. **GI:** nausea, dyspepsia, dry mouth, bitter taste, constipation. **GU:** UTI.
Musculoskeletal: back pain. **Respiratory:** URI, bronchitis, *bronchospasm*, cough, dyspnea, increased sputum. **Skin:** rash.
Other: flulike symptoms, hypersensitivity reactions.

INTERACTIONS
Drug-drug. *Anticholinergics:* May increase anticholinergic effects. Avoid using together.

EFFECTS ON LAB TEST RESULTS
None reported.

CONTRAINDICATIONS & CAUTIONS
• Contraindicated in patients hypersensitive to drug, atropine, or its derivatives.
• Use cautiously in patients with angle-closure glaucoma, prostatic hyperplasia, or bladder-neck obstruction.
• **Alert:** Drug isn't indicated for initial treatment of acute episodes of bronchospasm, for which rescue therapy is required for rapid response.

• Safety and effectiveness of nebulization or inhaler in children younger than age 12 haven't been established.
Dialyzable drug: Unknown.

PREGNANCY-LACTATION-REPRODUCTION
• There are no adequate studies in pregnant women. Use during pregnancy only if clearly needed and if potential benefit justifies potential risk to the fetus.
• It isn't known if drug appears in human milk. Use cautiously in breastfeeding women.

NURSING CONSIDERATIONS
• If patient uses a face mask for a nebulizer, take care to prevent leakage around the mask because eye pain or temporary blurring of vision may occur.
• Safety and effectiveness of intranasal use beyond 4 days in patients with a common cold haven't been established.

PATIENT TEACHING
• Warn patient that drug isn't effective for treating acute episodes of bronchospasm when rapid response is needed.
• Teach patient to use metered-dose inhaler (MDI) or oral nebulizer correctly. Refer to manufacturer's instructions for use.
• Tell patient to prime inhaler before initial use by releasing 2 test sprays into the air. If inhaler hasn't been used for more than 3 days, advise patient to reprime.
• Instruct patient to wash mouthpiece once a week for 30 seconds in warm water only and let air dry.
• Inform patient that use of a spacer device with an MDI may improve drug delivery to lungs.
• Warn patient to avoid accidentally spraying drug into eyes. Temporary blurring of vision may result.
• If more than 1 inhalation is prescribed, tell patient to wait at least 15 seconds before repeating procedure.
• Advise patient who is also using a corticosteroid inhaler to use ipratropium first and then to wait about 5 minutes before using the corticosteroid. This lets the bronchodilator open air passages for maximal effectiveness of the corticosteroid.

• Instruct patient to prime nasal spray by pumping seven times before first use or after it has not been used for 1 week. Prime with two pumps after it has not been used for 1 day.
• Instruct patient to sniff deeply after each spray and to breathe out through mouth. Tell patient to tilt head backward to allow drug to spread to back of nose.

irbesartan
er-bah-SAR-tan

Avapro◆

Therapeutic class: Antihypertensives
Pharmacologic class: Angiotensin II receptor antagonists

AVAILABLE FORMS
Tablets: 75 mg, 150 mg, 300 mg

INDICATIONS & DOSAGES
Adjust-a-dose (for all indications): For volume- and sodium-depleted patients, initially, 75 mg PO daily.
➤ **HTN**
Adults: Initially, 150 mg PO daily, increased to maximum of 300 mg daily, if needed.
➤ **Nephropathy in patients with type 2 diabetes**
Adults: Target maintenance dose is 300 mg PO once daily.

ADMINISTRATION
PO
• Give drug without regard for meals.

ACTION
Produces antihypertensive effect by competitive antagonist activity at the angiotensin II receptor.

Route	Onset	Peak	Duration
PO	1–2 hr	1½–2 hr	>24 hr

Half-life: 11 to 15 hours.

ADVERSE REACTIONS
CNS: fatigue, anxiety, dizziness, headache. **CV:** chest pain, edema, tachycardia. **EENT:** pharyngitis, rhinitis, sinus abnormality. **GI:** diarrhea, dyspepsia, abdominal pain,

---

Reactions in bold italics are *life-threatening*. Interactions may have a *rapid onset* or a *delayed onset*.

nausea, vomiting. **GU:** UTI. **Musculoskeletal:** musculoskeletal trauma or pain. **Respiratory:** URI, cough. **Skin:** rash. **Other:** flulike symptoms.

INTERACTIONS

Drug-drug. *ACE inhibitors:* May increase risk of hypotension, renal dysfunction, and hyperkalemia. Use together cautiously; closely monitor BP, renal function, and potassium level.

❸ Alert: *Aliskiren:* May increase risk of renal impairment, hypotension, and hyperkalemia in diabetic patients and those with moderate to severe renal impairment (GFR less than 60 mL/minute). Concomitant use is contraindicated in diabetic patients. Avoid concomitant use in those with moderate to severe renal impairment.

Lithium: May increase lithium concentration, possibly causing toxicity. Monitor lithium serum concentration, and observe patient's clinical response. Adjust lithium dosage as needed.

NSAIDs, selective cyclooxygenase-2 inhibitors (celecoxib): May result in deterioration of renal function, including possible acute renal failure, in patients who are elderly, volume-depleted (including those on diuretic therapy), or who have compromised renal function. May decrease antihypertensive effect of irbesartan. Periodically monitor renal function during coadministration.

Potassium-sparing diuretics, potassium supplements, trimethoprim: May increase risk of hyperkalemia. Closely monitor serum potassium concentration and adjust treatment as needed.

EFFECTS ON LAB TEST RESULTS

• May lead to false-negative aldosterone/renin ratio.

CONTRAINDICATIONS & CAUTIONS

• Contraindicated in patients hypersensitive to drug or its components.
• Use cautiously in patients with impaired renal function, HF, and renal artery stenosis.

Dialyzable drug: No.

⚠ Overdose S&S: Hypotension, tachycardia, bradycardia.

PREGNANCY-LACTATION-REPRODUCTION

Black Box Warning Use during pregnancy can cause injury and death to the developing fetus. When pregnancy is detected, stop drug as soon as possible. ■

• It isn't known if drug appears in human milk. Patient should discontinue breastfeeding or discontinue drug.

NURSING CONSIDERATIONS

• Drug may be given with a diuretic or other antihypertensive, if needed, for control of HTN.
• Symptomatic hypotension may occur in volume- or sodium-depleted patients (vigorous diuretic use or dialysis). Correct the cause of volume depletion before administration or before a lower dose is used.
• If hypotension occurs, place patient in a supine position and give an IV infusion of NSS, if needed. Once BP has stabilized after a transient hypotensive episode, drug may be continued.
• Dizziness and orthostatic hypotension may occur more frequently in patients with type 2 diabetes and renal disease.

PATIENT TEACHING

• Warn female patient of childbearing potential of consequences of drug exposure to fetus. Tell her to notify prescriber immediately if pregnancy is suspected.
• Tell patient that drug may be taken without regard for food.
• Tell patient to report all adverse reactions and to inform prescriber of other prescription and OTC drugs and supplements being taken.

SAFETY ALERT!

irinotecan hydrochloride ✂
eh-rin-OH-te-kan

Camptosar

Therapeutic class: Antineoplastics
Pharmacologic class: DNA topoisomerase inhibitors

AVAILABLE FORMS

Injection: 20 mg/mL in 2-, 5-, 15-, and 25-mL vials

INDICATIONS & DOSAGES

➤ **Metastatic carcinoma of the colon or rectum that has recurred or progressed after 5-FU therapy**

Adults: Initially, 125 mg/m^2 by IV infusion over 90 minutes on days 1, 8, 15, and 22; then 2-week rest period. Thereafter, additional courses of treatment may be repeated every 6 weeks with 4 weeks on and 2 weeks off. Subsequent doses may be adjusted to low of 50 mg/m^2 or maximum of 150 mg/m^2 in 25- to 50-mg/m^2 increments based on patient's tolerance. Or, 350 mg/m^2 by IV infusion over 90 minutes once every 3 weeks. Additional courses may continue indefinitely in patients who respond favorably and in those whose disease remains stable, provided intolerable toxicity doesn't occur.

Adjust-a-dose: Consider reducing starting dose in patients age 65 and older, in those who have received pelvic or abdominal radiation, or in those who have a performance status of 2 or increased bilirubin level. Give 300 mg/m^2 by IV infusion once every 3 weeks. Or, give 100 mg/m^2 by IV infusion once weekly. See manufacturer's instructions for details on dosage adjustments due to toxicities.

➤ **First-line therapy for metastatic colorectal cancer with 5-FU and leucovorin**
Regimen 1
Adults: 125 mg/m^2 IV infusion on days 1, 8, 15, and 22; then leucovorin 20 mg/m^2 IV bolus on days 1, 8, 15, and 22 and 5-FU 500 mg/m^2 IV bolus on days 1, 8, 15, and 22. Courses are repeated every 6 weeks.
Regimen 2
Adults: 180 mg/m^2 IV infusion on days 1, 15, and 29; then leucovorin 200 mg/m^2 IV over 2 hours on days 1, 2, 15, 16, 29, and 30; then 5-FU 400 mg/m^2 IV bolus on days 1, 2, 15, 16, 29, and 30 and 5-FU 600 mg/m^2 IV infusion over 22 hours on days 1, 2, 15, 16, 29, and 30.

Adjust-a-dose: Consider reducing starting dose by one dose level for patients with any of the following conditions: prior pelvic or abdominal radiotherapy, performance status of 2, or increased bilirubin level. See manufacturer's instructions for details on all dosage adjustments.

➤ **Esophageal cancer, metastatic or locally advanced ◆**

Adults: 65 mg/m^2 IV infusion on days 1, 8, 15, and 22 of a 6-week cycle (in combination with cisplatin), or 180 mg/m^2 IV infusion every 2 weeks (in combination with leucovorin and 5-FU), or 250 mg/m^2 IV every 3 weeks (in combination with capecitabine).

➤ **Gastric cancer, metastatic or locally advanced ◆**

Adults: 150 mg/m^2 IV infusion (as a single agent) on days 1 and 15 of a 4-week cycle, or 65 mg/m^2 IV infusion on days 1, 8, 15, and 22 of a 6-week cycle (in combination with cisplatin), or 70 mg/m^2 IV infusion on days 1 and 15 of a 4-week cycle (in combination with cisplatin) for up to six cycles, or 180 mg/m^2 IV infusion over 90 minutes every 2 weeks (in combination with leucovorin and 5-FU), or 250 mg/m^2 IV every 3 weeks (in combination with capecitabine).

➤ **NSCLC, advanced ◆**
Adults: 60 mg/m^2 IV infusion on days 1, 8, and 15 every 4 weeks (in combination with cisplatin).

➤ **Pancreatic cancer, advanced ◆**
Adults: 180 mg/m^2 IV infusion over 90 minutes every 2 weeks (in combination with oxaliplatin, leucovorin, and 5-FU).

➤ **Small-cell lung cancer, extensive stage ◆**

Adults: 60 mg/m^2 IV infusion on days 1, 8, and 15 every 4 weeks (in combination with cisplatin), or 65 mg/m^2 IV on days 1 and 8 every 3 weeks (in combination with cisplatin), or 175 mg/m^2 IV on day 1 every 3 weeks (in combination with carboplatin), or 50 mg/m^2 IV on days 1, 8, and 15 every 4 weeks (in combination with carboplatin).

➤ **Rhabdomyosarcoma (metastatic or relapsed/progressive) in children ◆**

Children: 50 mg/m^2 (maximum, 100 mg/dose) IV once daily for 5 days during protocol-specific weeks (in combination with ifosfamide, etoposide, vincristine, doxorubicin, cyclophosphamide, dactinomycin, and radiation; high-risk disease) or 50 mg/m^2 IV once daily for 5 days at weeks 1 and 4 (in combination with vincristine).

ADMINISTRATION

IV

▼ Drug packaged in plastic blister to protect against inadvertent breakage and leakage. Inspect vial for damage and signs of leakage before removing blister.

▼ Wear gloves while handling and preparing infusion solutions. If drug contacts skin, wash thoroughly with soap and water. If drug contacts mucous membranes, flush thoroughly with water.

▼ Dilute drug in D₅W injection (preferred) or NSS for injection before infusion to yield 0.12 to 2.8 mg/mL.

▼ Administer by IV infusion, usually over 90 minutes.

▼ Solution is stable for up to 24 hours at 77° F (25° C) in ambient fluorescent lighting. Solutions diluted in D₅W, stored at 36° to 46° F (2° to 8° C), and protected from light are stable for 48 hours. However, because microbial contamination may occur during dilution, use admixture within 24 hours if refrigerated or 4 to 12 hours if kept at room temperature. Refrigerating admixtures using NSS isn't recommended because of low and sporadic risk of visible particulate. Don't freeze admixture because drug may precipitate.

▼ Premedicate patient with antiemetic drugs on day of treatment starting at least 30 minutes before giving irinotecan.

▼ Watch for irritation and infiltration; extravasation can cause tissue damage. If extravasation occurs, flush site with sterile water and apply ice. Notify prescriber.

▼ Store vial at 59° to 86° F (15° to 30° C). Protect from light.

▼ **Incompatibilities:** Gemcitabine, pemetrexed.

ACTION
Interacts with topoisomerase I, inducing reversible single-strand DNA breaks. Drug binds to the topoisomerase I–DNA complex and prevents religation of these single-strand breaks.

Route	Onset	Peak	Duration
IV	Unknown	1 hr	Unknown

Half-life: About 6 to 12 hours; active metabolite, 10 to 20 hours.

ADVERSE REACTIONS
CNS: asthenia, dizziness, fever, headache, insomnia, pain, akathisia, confusion, somnolence. **CV:** edema, vasodilation,

orthostatic hypotension. **EENT:** rhinitis. **GI:** *diarrhea,* abdominal cramping, abdominal pain and enlargement, anorexia, constipation, dyspepsia, flatulence, nausea, stomatitis, vomiting. **Hematologic:** anemia, *leukopenia, neutropenia, thrombocytopenia.* **Metabolic:** dehydration, weight loss. **Musculoskeletal:** back pain. **Respiratory:** dyspnea, increased cough, pneumonia. **Skin:** alopecia, rash, sweating. **Other:** chills, infection.

INTERACTIONS
Drug-drug. *CYP3A4 enzyme-inducing anticonvulsants (carbamazepine, phenobarbital, phenytoin), rifampin, rifabutin:* May significantly decrease irinotecan levels. For patients requiring anticonvulsant treatment, consider substituting non–enzyme-inducing anticonvulsants at least 2 weeks before start of irinotecan therapy.

CYP3A4 inhibitors (clarithromycin, indinavir, itraconazole, lopinavir, nefazodone, nelfinavir, ritonavir, saquinavir, voriconazole), UGT1A1 inhibitors (atazanavir, gemfibrozil, indinavir): May increase systemic exposure to irinotecan. Discontinue strong CYP3A4 inhibitors at least 1 week before starting irinotecan. Don't give strong CYP3A4 or UGT1A1 inhibitors with irinotecan unless there are no therapeutic alternatives.

Diuretics: May increase risk of dehydration and electrolyte imbalance. Consider stopping diuretic during active periods of nausea and vomiting.

Ketoconazole: May increase irinotecan levels, leading to drug toxicity. Stop ketoconazole at least 1 week before starting irinotecan therapy. Ketoconazole is contraindicated during irinotecan therapy.

Laxatives: May increase risk of diarrhea. Avoid using together.

Live-virus vaccines: May cause serious or fatal infection. Don't give together.

Neuromuscular blockers: May prolong the neuromuscular-blocking effects of succinylcholine, and the neuromuscular blockade of nondepolarizing drugs may be antagonized. Monitor patient for prolonged effects of succinylcholine if given together.

Other antineoplastics: May cause additive adverse effects, such as myelosuppression and diarrhea. Monitor patient closely.
Prochlorperazine: May increase risk of akathisia. Monitor patient closely.
Vaccines (killed or inactivated virus): May diminish response to vaccine. Avoid use together.
Drug-herb. *St. John's wort:* May decrease drug levels. Use together is contraindicated.
Drug-food. *Grapefruit juice:* May increase irinotecan serum concentration. Avoid combination.

EFFECTS ON LAB TEST RESULTS
• May increase alkaline phosphatase, AST, and bilirubin levels.
• May decrease Hb level and platelet, WBC, and neutrophil counts.

CONTRAINDICATIONS & CAUTIONS
• Contraindicated in patients hypersensitive to drug.
▓ Patients with UGT1A1*28 allele or UGT1A1 7/7 genotype are at increased risk for neutropenia. Consider reducing starting dose by at least one level in patients known to be homozygous for the UGT1A1*28 allele; monitor patient closely.
• Fatal interstitial pulmonary disease (IPD) has been reported. Patients with preexisting lung disease, patients taking pulmonary toxic drugs or colony-stimulating factors, and patients receiving radiation therapy are at increased risk. If IPD is diagnosed, all chemotherapy will be discontinued.
• Rare cases of renal impairment and acute renal failure have been identified, usually in patients who became volume-depleted from severe vomiting or diarrhea.
• Safety and effectiveness in children haven't been established.
• Use cautiously in elderly patients.
Dialyzable drug: Unknown.
⚠ *Overdose S&S:* Severe neutropenia, severe diarrhea.

PREGNANCY-LACTATION-REPRODUCTION
• May cause fetal harm. Women of childbearing potential should avoid becoming pregnant during therapy.

• It isn't known if drug appears in human milk. Patient should discontinue breastfeeding or discontinue drug.

NURSING CONSIDERATIONS
• Administer drug under the supervision of a physician experienced with cancer chemotherapy.
Black Box Warning Drug may cause severe myelosuppression. ▪
Black Box Warning Drug can cause severe diarrhea. Treat diarrhea occurring within 24 hours of drug administration with 0.25 to 1 mg atropine IV, unless contraindicated. Treat late diarrhea (occurring more than 24 hours after irinotecan administration) promptly with loperamide. Monitor patient for dehydration, electrolyte imbalance, or sepsis; treat appropriately. Institute antibiotic therapy if ileus, fever, or severe neutropenia develops. Interrupt therapy and reduce subsequent doses if severe diarrhea occurs. ▪
• Delay subsequent doses until normal bowel function returns for at least 24 hours without an antidiarrheal.
• Pelvic or abdominal irradiation may increase risk of severe myelosuppression. Avoid use of drug in patients undergoing irradiation.
• If neutropenic fever occurs or if ANC drops below 500/mm^3, temporarily stop therapy. Reduce dosage, especially if WBC count is below 2,000/mm^3, neutrophil count is below 1,000/mm^3, Hb level is below 8 g/dL, or platelet count is below 100,000/mm^3.
• A colony-stimulating factor may be helpful in patients with significant neutropenia.
• Monitor WBC count with differential, Hb level, and platelet count before each dose.
• To decrease risk of dehydration, withhold diuretic during treatment and periods of active vomiting or diarrhea.
• Monitor patient for respiratory signs and symptoms (dyspnea, cough, fever) before and during treatment.
• *Look alike–sound alike:* Don't confuse irinotecan with topotecan.

PATIENT TEACHING
• Inform patient about risk of diarrhea and methods to treat it; tell patient to avoid laxatives.

Reactions in bold italics are *life-threatening*. Interactions may have a *rapid onset* or a ***delayed onset***.

• Instruct patient to report all adverse reactions and to immediately contact prescriber if any of the following occur: diarrhea for the first time during treatment; black or bloody stools; symptoms of dehydration such as light-headedness, dizziness, or faintness; inability to drink fluids due to nausea or vomiting; inability to control diarrhea within 24 hours; fever or infection; dyspnea or cough.

• Warn patient that hair loss may occur.

• Caution female patient to avoid pregnancy and breastfeeding during therapy.

iron dextran
DexIron✦, InFeD

Therapeutic class: Iron supplements
Pharmacologic class: Hematinics

AVAILABLE FORMS
1 mL iron dextran provides 50 mg elemental iron.
Injection: 50 mg elemental iron/mL in 2-mL single-dose vials

INDICATIONS & DOSAGES
➤ **Iron deficiency anemia**
Adults and children weighing more than 15 kg: IV or IM test dose is required. (See manufacturer's instructions.) Total dose may be calculated using dosage table in manufacturer's instructions or by using the following formula:

$$\text{Dose (mL)} = 0.0442 \text{ (desired Hb} - \text{observed Hb)} \times \text{LBW} + (0.26 \times \text{LWB})$$

Note: LBW = lean body weight in kg. For males, LBW = 50 kg + 2.3 kg for each inch of patient's height over 5 feet. For females, LBW = 45.5 kg + 2.3 kg for each inch of patient's height over 5 feet.
Children weighing 5 to 15 kg: Use dosage table in package insert or calculate dose as follows:

$$\text{Dose (mL)} = 0.0442 \text{ (desired Hb} - \text{observed Hb)} \times \text{weight in kg} + (0.26 \times \text{weight in kg})$$

IV
Adults and children: Inject 0.5-mL test dose over at least 5 minutes. If no reaction occurs in 1 hour, give remainder of therapeutic IV dose. Repeat therapeutic IV dose daily. Single daily dose shouldn't exceed 100 mg. Give slowly (1 mL/minute). Don't give drug in the first 4 months of life.

IM (by Z-track method)
Adults and children: Inject 0.5-mL test dose. If no reaction occurs in 1 hour, give remainder of dose. Daily dose ordinarily shouldn't exceed 0.5 mL (25 mg) for infants weighing less than 5 kg; 1 mL (50 mg) for those weighing less than 10 kg; and 2 mL (100 mg) for heavier children and adults. Don't give drug in the first 4 months of life.

➤ **Iron replacement for blood loss**
Adults and children older than age 4 months: Replacement iron (in mg) = blood loss (in mL) × hematocrit.
Note: This formula is based on the approximation that 1 mL of normocytic, normochromic red cells contains 1 mg of elemental iron.

ADMINISTRATION
IV
▼ Check facility policy before giving IV.
▼ Give at slow gradual rate not to exceed 50 mg (1 mL)/minute.
▼ After completing IV dose, flush the vein with 10 mL of NSS.
▼ Patient should rest for 15 to 30 minutes after IV administration.
▼ **Incompatibilities:** Other IV drugs, parenteral nutrition solutions for IV infusion.
IM
• Inject IM deep into upper outer quadrant of buttock—never into the arm or other exposed area—with a 2″ to 3″ 19G or 20G needle.
• Use Z-track method to avoid leakage into subcutaneous tissue and staining of skin.
• After drawing up drug, use a new sterile needle to give injection.

ACTION
Provides elemental iron, an essential component in the formation of Hb.

Route	Onset	Peak	Duration
IV	Unknown	7–9 days	Unknown
IM	72 hr	Unknown	3–4 wk

Half-life: 5 to 20 hours. Half-life values don't represent iron clearance from the body. Iron isn't easily eliminated, and the accumulation of iron can be toxic.

ADVERSE REACTIONS

CNS: headache, transitory paresthesia, dizziness, malaise, fever, chills, *seizures,* disorientation. **CV:** chest pain, tachycardia, *bradycardia,* hypotensive reaction, peripheral vascular flushing, arrhythmias, *cardiac arrest, shock,* HTN. **GI:** nausea, anorexia, abdominal pain, diarrhea, vomiting. **GU:** hematuria. **Hematologic:** leukocytosis, lymphadenopathy. **Musculoskeletal:** arthralgia, myalgia. **Respiratory:** *bronchospasm,* dyspnea, wheezing, *respiratory arrest.* **Skin:** rash, urticaria, soreness, inflammation, brown skin discoloration at IM injection site, local phlebitis at IV injection site, sterile abscess, necrosis, atrophy, cellulitis. **Other:** fibrosis, *anaphylaxis, delayed sensitivity reactions.*

INTERACTIONS

Drug-drug. *ACE inhibitors:* Increases risk of adverse systemic reactions. Stop one of the agents if interaction occurs.
Chloramphenicol: May increase iron level. Monitor patient closely.

EFFECTS ON LAB TEST RESULTS

• May cause false increase in bilirubin level and false decrease in calcium level. Use of more than 250 mg iron may color the serum brown. Drug may alter measurement of iron level and total iron-binding capacity for up to 3 weeks; IM injection may cause dense areas of activity for 1 to 6 days on bone scans using technetium-99m diphosphonate.

CONTRAINDICATIONS & CAUTIONS

Black Box Warning Fatal anaphylactic reactions have been reported. Fatal reactions have occurred when the test dose was tolerated. Patients with history of drug allergy may be at increased risk. Give only when indications have been clearly established. ∎
Black Box Warning IV or IM injections of iron are advisable only for patients in whom oral administration is impossible or ineffective. ∎

• Contraindicated in patients hypersensitive to drug, in those with acute infectious renal disease, and in those with any anemia except iron deficiency anemia.

• Use cautiously in patients who have serious hepatic impairment, RA, or other inflammatory diseases.

• Use cautiously in patients with history of significant allergies or asthma.

Dialyzable drug: No.

⚠ *Overdose S&S:* Hemosiderosis.

PREGNANCY-LACTATION-REPRODUCTION

• Use during pregnancy only if potential benefit justifies potential risk to the fetus.

• Traces of unmetabolized drug appear in human milk. Use caution in breastfeeding.

NURSING CONSIDERATIONS

Black Box Warning Administer test dose of iron dextran before first therapeutic dose. If no signs or symptoms of anaphylactic-type reactions follow test dose, administer full therapeutic iron dextran dose. Observe for signs and symptoms of anaphylactic-type reactions with every dose given. Have emergency equipment immediately available. ∎

• Don't give iron dextran with oral iron drug.

• Monitor Hb level, hematocrit, and reticulocyte count.

• Maximum daily dose should not exceed 2 mL undiluted iron dextran.

PATIENT TEACHING

• Teach patient signs and symptoms of hypersensitivity and iron toxicity; tell patient to report all adverse reactions to prescriber.

• Inform patient that drug may stain skin.

iron sucrose injection
Venofer

Therapeutic class: Iron supplements
Pharmacologic class: Hematinics

AVAILABLE FORMS

Injection: 20 mg/mL of elemental iron in 2.5-mL, 5-mL, and 10-mL single-dose vials

---

INDICATIONS & DOSAGES

➤ **Iron deficiency anemia in patients who are hemodialysis dependent**

Adults: 100 mg (5 mL) of elemental iron IV directly in the dialysis line by slow injection over 2 to 5 minutes or by infusion of 100 mg diluted in a maximum of 100 mL NSS over 15 minutes per consecutive hemodialysis session. Administer early during each dialysis session. Usual total treatment course is 1,000 mg; may repeat if iron deficiency recurs.

➤ **Iron deficiency anemia in chronic kidney disease patients not on dialysis**

Adults: 200 mg by undiluted slow IV injection over 2 to 5 minutes, or as an infusion of 200 mg in a maximum of 100 mL NSS over 15 minutes, on five separate occasions in a 14-day period to a total cumulative dose of 1,000 mg; may repeat if needed.

➤ **Iron deficiency anemia in peritoneal dialysis-dependent chronic kidney disease patients**

Adults: 300 mg IV infusion over 90 minutes on two separate occasions 14 days apart, followed by one 400-mg infusion over 2½ hours 14 days later. Dilute in a maximum of 250 mL NSS; may repeat if needed.

➤ **Maintenance treatment in pediatric patients with hemodialysis-dependent chronic kidney disease, nondialysis-dependent chronic kidney disease who are receiving erythropoietin, or peritoneal dialysis-dependent chronic kidney disease who are receiving erythropoietin**

Children ages 2 and older: 0.5 mg/kg IV every 4 weeks for 12 weeks. Give undiluted by slow IV injection over 5 minutes or diluted in 25 mL NSS and administered over 5 to 60 minutes. May repeat treatment if necessary. Don't give more than 100 mg per dose.

ADMINISTRATION

IV

▼ Inspect drug for particulate matter and discoloration before giving.

▼ For infusion, dilute 100 mg elemental iron in a maximum of 100 mL NSS immediately before infusion, and infuse over at least 15 minutes. Dilute dose 300 mg or greater in a maximum of 250 mL NSS.

▼ Store in original carton at 68° to 77° F (20° to 25° C). Excursions are permitted from 59° to 86° F (15° to 30° C). Don't freeze.

▼ Syringe is stable for 7 days at controlled room temperature or under refrigeration. IV admixture is stable for 7 days at controlled room temperature when added to an infusion bag containing NSS.

▼ **Incompatibilities:** Other IV drugs, parenteral nutrition solutions.

ACTION

Exogenous source of iron that replenishes depleted body iron stores and is essential for Hb synthesis.

Route	Onset	Peak	Duration
IV	Unknown	Unknown	Variable

Half-life: 6 hours.

ADVERSE REACTIONS

CNS: headache, asthenia, malaise, dizziness, fever. **CV:** *HF,* hypotension, chest pain, HTN, fluid retention, edema. **GI:** nausea, vomiting, diarrhea, abdominal pain, taste perversion. **Metabolic:** gout, *hypoglycemia,* hyperglycemia. **Musculoskeletal:** leg cramps, bone and muscle pain, arthralgia, back pain. **Respiratory:** dyspnea, wheezing, pneumonia, cough. **Skin:** rash, pruritus, injection-site reaction. **Other:** accidental injury, pain, *sepsis, hypersensitivity reactions.*

INTERACTIONS

Drug-drug. *Oral iron preparations:* May reduce absorption of oral iron preparations. Avoid using together.

EFFECTS ON LAB TEST RESULTS

None reported.

CONTRAINDICATIONS & CAUTIONS

• Contraindicated in patients with hypersensitivity to drug or its components, evidence of iron overload, or anemia not caused by iron deficiency.

Dialyzable drug: No.

⚠ *Overdose S&S:* Accumulation of iron in storage sites, potentially leading to hemosiderosis.

PREGNANCY-LACTATION-REPRODUCTION
• There are no adequate studies in pregnant women. Use during pregnancy only if clearly needed.
• It isn't known if drug appears in human milk. Use cautiously in breastfeeding women.

NURSING CONSIDERATIONS
🔴 *Alert:* Rare but fatal hypersensitivity reactions, characterized by anaphylactic shock, loss of consciousness, collapse, hypotension, dyspnea, or seizures, may occur, often within 30 minutes of completing infusion. Have emergency equipment and therapies readily available.
• Mild to moderate hypersensitivity reactions, with wheezing, dyspnea, hypotension, rash, or pruritus, may occur.
• Infusing drug may reduce hypotension risk.
• Transferrin saturation level increases rapidly after IV administration of drug. Obtain iron level 48 hours after IV use.
• Monitor ferritin level, transferrin saturation, Hb level, and hematocrit.
• Withhold dose in patient with signs and symptoms of iron overload.
• Keep dose selection in elderly patients conservative because of decreased hepatic, renal, or cardiac function; other disease; and other drug therapy.

PATIENT TEACHING
• Instruct patient to report all adverse reactions and notify prescriber immediately if symptoms of overdose or allergic reaction occur.

isavuconazonium sulfate
EYE-sa-vue-KOE-na-zoe-nee-um

Cresemba

Therapeutic class: Antifungals
Pharmacologic class: Triazole antifungals

AVAILABLE FORMS
Capsules ⓄⓉⒸ: 186 mg (equal to isavuconazole 100 mg)
Injection: 372 mg (equal to isavuconazole 200 mg)/vial

INDICATIONS & DOSAGES
➤ **Invasive aspergillosis; invasive mucormycosis fungal infection**
Adults: Give loading doses of 372 mg IV or PO every 8 hours for six doses (48 hours); then give maintenance dose of 372 mg IV or PO once daily. Initiate maintenance dose 12 to 24 hours after last loading dose. Switching between IV and PO formulations of isavuconazonium sulfate is acceptable for maintenance dosing. It isn't necessary to restart dosing with a loading dose when switching between formulations.

ADMINISTRATION
PO
• May give with or without food.
• Give capsules whole; capsules shouldn't be chewed, crushed, dissolved, or opened.
• Store capsules in original packaging at 68° to 77° F (20° to 25° C).

IV
▼ Reconstitute one vial of isavuconazonium with 5 mL sterile water for injection; shake gently to dissolve.
▼ Inspect for particulate matter and discoloration.
▼ Store intact vials at 36° to 46° F (2° to 8° C).
▼ Reconstituted solution may be stored below 77° F (25° C) for a maximum of 1 hour before preparation of the admixed solution.
▼ Remove 5 mL of reconstituted solution from vial and add it to an infusion bag containing 250 mL NSS or D_5W.
▼ Diluted solution may show visible translucent to white particulates of isavuconazole (which will be removed by the in-line filter). Use gentle mixing or roll bag to minimize formation of particulates. Avoid unnecessary vibration or vigorous shaking of solution. Don't use a pneumatic transport system.
▼ Infuse through an in-line filter with a microporous membrane pore size of 0.2 to 1.2 microns to remove particulates.
▼ Infuse over a minimum of 1 hour. Don't give as an IV bolus injection.
▼ Complete IV administration within 6 hours of dilution. If this isn't possible, immediately refrigerate admixed solution at 36° to 46° F (2° to 8° C) and complete infusion within 24 hours. Don't freeze.

Reactions in bold italics are *life-threatening*. Interactions may have a *rapid onset* or a ***delayed onset***.

▼ Flush IV line with NSS or D₅W before and after infusion.

▼ **Incompatibilities:** IV medications and IV solutions other than NSS or D₅W.

ACTION

Isavuconazonium, a prodrug of isavuconazole, inhibits synthesis of ergosterol, a key component of the fungal cell membrane, weakening the membrane structure and function.

Route	Onset	Peak	Duration
PO	Unknown	2–4 hr	Unknown
IV	Rapid	Within 1 hr	Unknown

Half-life: 130 hours (IV).

ADVERSE REACTIONS

CNS: anxiety, fatigue, headache, insomnia, delirium, confusion, hallucination, depression, drowsiness, *seizures,* encephalopathy, hypoesthesia, migraine, peripheral neuropathy, paresthesia, somnolence, stupor, syncope, tremor, malaise, chills, vertigo. **CV:** chest pain, hypotension, peripheral edema, thrombophlebitis, atrial fibrillation, atrial flutter, *bradycardia,* decreased QT interval, palpitations, supraventricular extrasystoles, supraventricular tachycardia, PVCs, *cardiac arrest,* catheter-site thrombosis. **EENT:** optic neuropathy, tinnitus, gingivitis, stomatitis. **GI:** abdominal pain, constipation, decreased appetite, diarrhea, nausea, vomiting, dyspepsia, dysgeusia, abdominal distention, gastritis, cholecystitis, cholelithiasis. **GU:** hematuria, proteinuria, *acute renal failure.* **Hematologic:** *agranulocytosis, leukopenia, pancytopenia.* **Hepatic:** increased bilirubin level, elevated LFT values, *hepatitis,* hepatomegaly, *hepatic failure.* **Metabolic:** hypoglycemia, *hypokalemia, hypomagnesemia,* hypoalbuminemia, hyponatremia. **Musculoskeletal:** back pain, myositis, bone pain, neck pain. **Respiratory:** cough, dyspnea, *bronchospasm,* tachypnea. **Skin:** pruritus, rash, alopecia, dermatitis, exfoliative dermatitis, erythema, petechiae, urticaria. **Other:** injection-site reactions, hypersensitivity reaction, falls.

INTERACTIONS

Drug-drug. *Atorvastatin:* May increase atorvastatin level. Monitor patient for atorvastatin-related adverse reactions.
Bupropion: May decrease bupropion level. Bupropion dosage increase may be needed but shouldn't exceed maximum recommended dose.
Cyclosporine, sirolimus, tacrolimus: May increase levels of concomitant drugs. Monitor concentrations of concomitant drugs; adjust their dosages as needed.
Digoxin: May increase digoxin level. Monitor digoxin level and titrate dose during concurrent use.
Lopinavir–ritonavir: May increase isavuconazonium level and decrease lopinavir and ritonavir levels, which may result in loss of antiviral efficacy. Use cautiously together, and monitor patient closely. Use with high-dose (400 mg) ritonavir is contraindicated.
Midazolam: May increase midazolam level. Consider midazolam dosage reduction.
Mycophenolate mofetil: May increase mycophenolate level. Monitor patient for mycophenolate–related toxicities.
Strong CYP3A4 inducers (carbamazepine, long-acting barbiturates, rifampin): May significantly decrease isavuconazonium level. Concomitant use is contraindicated.
Strong CYP3A4 inhibitors (ketoconazole, high-dose ritonavir): May significantly increase isavuconazonium level. Concomitant use is contraindicated.
Drug-herb. *St. John's wort:* May significantly decrease drug level. Concomitant use is contraindicated.

EFFECTS ON LAB TEST RESULTS

• May increase total bilirubin, AST, ALT, alkaline phosphatase, and GGT levels.
• May decrease potassium, magnesium, albumin, glucose, and sodium levels.
• May decrease WBC count.

CONTRAINDICATIONS & CAUTIONS

• Contraindicated in patients hypersensitive to drug or its components.
❸ **Alert:** Serious hypersensitivity reactions and severe skin reactions, such as anaphylaxis and SJS, have been reported with other azole antifungals. Discontinue drug for severe cutaneous reaction. Use cautiously

in patients with serious underlying medical conditions and in patients hypersensitive to other azole drugs.

• Contraindicated in patients with familial short QT syndrome; drug shortens QTc interval in a concentration-related manner.

• Use cautiously in patients with severe hepatic impairment and only when benefits outweigh risks.

• Safety and effectiveness in children younger than age 18 haven't been established.

Dialyzable drug: No.

⚠ *Overdose S&S:* Headache, dizziness, paresthesia, somnolence, disturbance in attention, dysgeusia, dry mouth, diarrhea, oral hypoesthesia, vomiting, hot flushes, anxiety, restlessness, palpitations, tachycardia, photophobia, arthralgia.

PREGNANCY-LACTATION-REPRODUCTION

• There are no adequate studies in pregnant women. Drug may cause fetal harm. Use during pregnancy only if potential benefit outweighs risk to the fetus.

• Women shouldn't breastfeed during therapy.

NURSING CONSIDERATIONS

• Obtain specimens for fungal culture to isolate and identify causative organism before initiating antifungal therapy. May start therapy before results are available; however, adjust therapy accordingly when results are known.

• Infusion-related reactions can occur; monitor patients for dyspnea, hypotension, chills, dizziness, paresthesia, and hypotension. Discontinue infusion if reaction occurs.

• Monitor patients for hypersensitivity reactions and severe skin reactions, including anaphylaxis and SJS. Discontinue drug for exfoliative cutaneous reaction.

• Assess LFT values before and periodically during treatment.

• Monitor patients who develop abnormal LFT values during therapy for development of more severe hepatic injury. Discontinue drug if liver disease develops that may be attributed to drug.

PATIENT TEACHING

• Advise patient that routine blood tests will be needed to evaluate liver function.

• Instruct patient to report any adverse reactions, including infusion-related and skin-related reactions, to prescriber.

• Counsel patient to swallow capsules whole.

• Instruct female patient to inform prescriber if she becomes pregnant during therapy. Inform her of risks to the fetus.

• Warn female patient not to breastfeed during therapy.

isoniazid (INH, isonicotinic acid hydrazide) 🔖
eye-soe-NYE-a-zid

PDP-Isoniazid ❖

Therapeutic class: Antituberculotics
Pharmacologic class: Isonicotinic acid hydrazines

AVAILABLE FORMS
Injection: 100 mg/mL
Oral solution: 50 mg/5 mL
Tablets: 100 mg, 300 mg

INDICATIONS & DOSAGES
Adjust-a-dose (for all indications): Give dose after hemodialysis.

➤ **Actively growing tubercle bacilli**
Adults and children age 15 and older: 5 mg/kg daily PO or IM in a single daily dose, up to 300 mg/day, with other drugs, continued for 6 months to 2 years. For intermittent multiple-drug regimen, 15 mg/kg (up to 900 mg) PO or IM up to 3 times/week.
Infants and children: 10 to 15 mg/kg PO or IM in a single daily dose, up to 300 mg/day, continued long enough to prevent relapse. Give with at least one other antituberculotic. For intermittent multidrug regimen, 20 to 40 mg/kg (up to 900 mg) PO or IM two or three times weekly.

➤ **Preventative therapy for TB**
Adults weighing more than 30 kg: 300 mg PO daily in a single dose, continued for 6 months to 1 year.
Infants and children: 10 mg/kg PO daily in a single dose, up to 300 mg/day, continued for up to 1 year. In situations in which adherence with daily preventive therapy can't be assured, 20 to 30 mg/kg (not to exceed

900 mg) twice weekly under the direct observation of a health care worker at the time of administration.

ADMINISTRATION

PO
- Always give drug with other antituberculotics to prevent development of resistant organisms.
- Don't give with food.

IM
- Solution may crystallize at a low temperature. Warm vial to room temperature before use to redissolve crystals.
- Inject deep IM into a large muscle mass.

ACTION

May inhibit cell-wall biosynthesis by interfering with lipid and DNA synthesis; bactericidal.

Route	Onset	Peak	Duration
PO, IM	Unknown	1–2 hr	Unknown

Half-life: ½ to 5 hours.

ADVERSE REACTIONS

CNS: peripheral neuropathy, *seizures, toxic encephalopathy,* memory impairment, toxic psychosis. **EENT:** optic neuritis and atrophy. **GI:** epigastric distress, nausea, vomiting. **Hematologic:** *agranulocytosis, aplastic anemia, thrombocytopenia,* eosinophilia, hemolytic anemia, sideroblastic anemia. **Hepatic:** *hepatitis,* bilirubinemia, jaundice. **Metabolic:** hyperglycemia, hypocalcemia, hypophosphatemia, *metabolic acidosis.* **Skin:** irritation at injection site. **Other:** gynecomastia, hypersensitivity reactions, pyridoxine deficiency, rheumatic and lupuslike syndromes.

INTERACTIONS

Drug-drug. *Acetaminophen:* May inhibit acetaminophen metabolism. Monitor patient closely for hepatotoxicity.
Antacids and laxatives containing aluminum: May decrease isoniazid absorption. Give isoniazid at least 1 hour before antacid or laxative.
Benzodiazepines (diazepam, triazolam): May inhibit metabolic clearance of benzodiazepines that undergo oxidative metabolism,

possibly increasing benzodiazepine activity. Monitor for adverse effects.
Carbamazepine: May increase carbamazepine levels. Monitor drug levels closely.
Cycloserine: May increase CNS adverse reactions. Use safety precautions.
Disulfiram: May cause neurologic symptoms, including changes in behavior and coordination. Avoid using together.
Enflurane: In rapid acetylators of isoniazid, may cause high-output renal failure because of nephrotoxic inorganic fluoride level. Monitor renal function.
Ketoconazole: May decrease ketoconazole level. Monitor for lack of effectiveness.
Meperidine: May increase CNS adverse reactions and hypotension. Use safety precautions.
Oral anticoagulants: May enhance anticoagulant activity. Monitor PT and INR.
Phenytoin: May inhibit phenytoin metabolism and increase phenytoin level. Monitor patient for phenytoin toxicity.
Rifampin: May increase risk of hepatotoxicity. Monitor LFT values closely.
Theophylline: May increase theophylline level and, in some instances, slightly decrease isoniazid elimination. Monitor theophylline level closely; adjust dosage as appropriate.
Valproate: May increase valproate plasma level. Monitor valproate plasma concentration; adjust dosage as necessary.
Drug-food. *Foods containing histamines (saury, skipjack tuna, other tropical fish):* May cause headache, sweating, palpitations, flushing, diarrhea, itching, wheezing, dyspnea, or hypotension. Patients should avoid these foods during therapy.
Foods containing tyramine (aged cheese, beer, chocolate): May cause hypertensive crisis. Patients should avoid such foods.
Drug-lifestyle. *Alcohol use:* May increase risk of drug-related hepatitis. Discourage use of alcohol.

EFFECTS ON LAB TEST RESULTS
- May increase transaminase, glucose, and bilirubin levels. May decrease calcium, phosphate, and Hb levels.
- May increase eosinophil count. May decrease granulocyte and platelet counts.

✤Canada ◇OTC ◆Off-label use ✐Photoguide ⊛Do not crush *Liquid contains alcohol ▨Genetic

• May alter result of urine glucose tests that use cupric sulfate method, such as Benedict reagent and Diastix.

CONTRAINDICATIONS & CAUTIONS

Black Box Warning Contraindicated in patients with acute hepatic disease or isoniazid-related liver damage. Severe and sometimes fatal hepatitis associated with drug may occur even after months of treatment but usually occurs during first 3 months of treatment. Risk of developing hepatitis is age-related (increases with age), increases with daily alcohol use, and may be more common in black and Hispanic women, particularly during the postpartum period. If signs or symptoms suggest hepatic damage, discontinue isoniazid because a more severe form of liver damage can occur. ■

• Use cautiously in the elderly, those with chronic non–isoniazid-related liver disease or chronic alcoholism, those with seizure disorders (especially if taking phenytoin), and those with severe renal impairment.

Dialyzable drug: Yes.

⚠ *Overdose S&S:* Nausea, vomiting, dizziness, slurring of speech, blurring of vision, visual hallucinations, respiratory distress, CNS depression progressing from stupor to coma, seizures, severe metabolic acidosis, acetonuria, hyperglycemia.

PREGNANCY-LACTATION-REPRODUCTION

• There are no adequate studies in pregnant women; however, drug should be used as a treatment for active TB during pregnancy because benefit justifies potential risk to the fetus.

• Weigh benefit of preventive therapy against possible risk to the fetus. Preventive therapy generally should be started after delivery to prevent putting fetus at risk for exposure.

• Small amounts of drug in human milk don't produce toxicity in breastfeeding infants. Breastfeeding shouldn't be discouraged.

NURSING CONSIDERATIONS

▩ Drug's pharmacokinetics vary among patients because drug is metabolized in the liver by genetically controlled acetylation.

Fast acetylators metabolize drug up to 5 times faster than slow acetylators. About 50% of Blacks and Whites are fast acetylators; more than 80% of Chinese, Japanese, and Inuits are fast acetylators. A report suggests the risk of fatal hepatitis increases in Black and Hispanic women and in the postpartum period. The risk of hepatitis increases with daily alcohol use and with age.

▩ Peripheral neuropathy is more common in patients who are slow acetylators, malnourished, alcoholic, or diabetic. Give pyridoxine to prevent peripheral neuropathy.

Black Box Warning Monitor and interview patients monthly. For those patients older than age 35, also measure hepatic enzyme levels before and periodically throughout treatment. Elevated LFT results occur in about 15% of patients; most abnormalities are mild and transient, but some may persist throughout treatment, and progressive liver dysfunction may occur. If LFT values exceed 3 to 5 × ULN, strongly consider discontinuing treatment. ■

PATIENT TEACHING

• Instruct patient to take drug exactly as prescribed; warn against stopping drug without prescriber's consent.

• Advise patient that drug shouldn't be taken with food.

Black Box Warning Tell patient to notify prescriber immediately if signs and symptoms of liver impairment occur, such as appetite loss, fatigue, malaise, yellowing of skin or eyes, dark urine, fever of more than 3 days' duration, and abdominal tenderness, particularly of the right upper quadrant. ■

• Advise patient to avoid alcoholic beverages while taking drug and to avoid certain foods: fish (such as skipjack tuna) and products containing tyramine (such as aged cheese, beer, and chocolate) because drug has some MAO inhibitor activity.

• Advise patient who is a slow acetylator, malnourished, alcoholic, or diabetic to take pyridoxine, as prescribed, to prevent peripheral neuropathy.

• Encourage patient to comply fully with treatment, which may take months or years.

Reactions in bold italics are *life-threatening*. Interactions may have a *rapid onset* or a *delayed onset*.

isosorbide dinitrate
eye-soe-SOR-bide

ISDN✥, Dilatrate-SR, Isordil Titradose

isosorbide mononitrate
Apo-ISMN✥, Imdur✥, Monoket, PMS-ISMN✥, PRO-ISMN✥

Therapeutic class: Antianginals
Pharmacologic class: Nitrates

AVAILABLE FORMS
isosorbide dinitrate
Capsules (sustained-release) ⓒ: 40 mg
Tablets: 5 mg, 10 mg, 20 mg, 30 mg, 40 mg
Tablets (extended-release) ⓒ: 40 mg
isosorbide mononitrate
Tablets: 10 mg, 20 mg
Tablets (extended-release) ⓒ: 30 mg, 60 mg, 120 mg

INDICATIONS & DOSAGES
➤ **Treatment (immediate-release isosorbide mononitrate only) and prevention of angina pectoris**
Adults (dinitrate): For immediate release, 5 to 20 mg PO b.i.d. to t.i.d., titrated to a maximum of 40 mg PO b.i.d. to t.i.d. For sustained release, usual dose is 40 to 160 mg PO daily. For Dilatrate-SR only, titrate to a maximum of 160 mg PO daily.
Adults (mononitrate): For immediate release, 5 to 20 mg PO b.i.d., with the two doses given 7 hours apart. For extended-release, 30 to 60 mg PO daily; titrate every 3 days to 120 mg PO daily. Rarely, 240 mg may be required.
➤ **HF (isosorbide dinitrate)** ◆
Adults: 20 to 30 mg immediate-release PO t.i.d. to q.i.d. (in combination with hydralazine) according to American College of Cardiology Foundation/American Heart Association HF guidelines. Maximum dosage is 120 mg daily in divided doses.

ADMINISTRATION
PO
• Tell patient taking isosorbide dinitrate to swallow oral tablet whole on an empty

stomach either 30 minutes before or 1 to 2 hours after meals.
• Store drug in a cool place, in a tightly closed container, and away from light.
• Don't crush or allow patient to chew extended- or sustained-release tablets or capsules.

ACTION
Thought to reduce cardiac oxygen demand by decreasing preload and afterload. Drug also may increase blood flow through the collateral coronary vessels.

Route	Onset	Peak	Duration
PO	30–45 min	Unknown	4–8 hr
PO (extended-release)	½–4 hr	Unknown	6–12 hr

Half-life: Dinitrate PO, 5 to 6 hours; mononitrate, about 5 hours.

ADVERSE REACTIONS
CNS: headache, dizziness, weakness. **CV:** orthostatic hypotension, tachycardia, palpitations, ankle edema, flushing, fainting. **EENT:** sublingual burning. **GI:** nausea, vomiting. **Skin:** cutaneous vasodilation, rash.

INTERACTIONS
Drug-drug. *Antihypertensives:* May increase hypotensive effects. Monitor patient closely during initial therapy.
PDE5 inhibitors (avanafil, sildenafil, tadalafil, vardenafil), riociguat: May cause life-threatening hypotension. Use of nitrates in any form with these drugs is contraindicated.
Drug-lifestyle. *Alcohol use:* May increase hypotension. Discourage use together.

EFFECTS ON LAB TEST RESULTS
• May falsely reduce value in cholesterol tests using the Zlatkis-Zak color reaction.

CONTRAINDICATIONS & CAUTIONS
• Contraindicated in patients with hypersensitivity or idiosyncrasy to nitrates and in those with severe hypotension, angle-closure glaucoma, increased ICP, shock, or acute MI with low left ventricular filling pressure.
• Use cautiously in patients with blood volume depletion (such as from diuretic

therapy), mild hypotension, or suspected right ventricular infarction.

Dialyzable drug: Mononitrate, yes; dinitrate, unknown.

⚠ *Overdose S&S:* Venous pooling, decreased cardiac output, hypotension, methemoglobinemia, headache, confusion, vertigo, fever, palpitations, nausea, vomiting (possibly with colic and bloody diarrhea), syncope, air hunger, dyspnea, slow breathing, diaphoresis, flushed skin, heart block, bradycardia, paralysis, coma.

PREGNANCY-LACTATION-REPRODUCTION

• There are no adequate studies in pregnant women. Use during pregnancy only if clearly needed.

• It isn't known if drug appears in human milk. Use cautiously in breastfeeding women.

NURSING CONSIDERATIONS

• To prevent tolerance, a nitrate-free interval of 10 to 14 hours per day is recommended. The regimen for isosorbide mononitrate (1 tablet on awakening with the second dose in 7 hours, or 1 extended-release tablet daily) is intended to minimize nitrate tolerance by providing a substantial nitrate-free interval.

• Monitor BP, HR, and intensity and duration of drug response.

• Drug may cause headaches, especially at beginning of therapy. Dosage may be reduced temporarily, but tolerance usually develops. Treat headache with aspirin or acetaminophen.

• Methemoglobinemia has been seen with nitrates. Symptoms are those of impaired oxygen delivery despite adequate cardiac output and adequate arterial partial pressure of oxygen.

• *Look alike–sound alike:* Don't confuse Isordil with Plendil, Isuprel, or Inderal.

PATIENT TEACHING

• Caution patient to take drug as prescribed and to keep it accessible at all times.

🚫 *Alert:* Advise patient that stopping drug abruptly may cause increased angina symptoms and risk of MI.

• Advise patient on isosorbide dinitrate to take oral tablet on an empty stomach either 30 minutes before or 1 to 2 hours after meals and to swallow oral tablets whole.

• Tell patient to change to an upright position slowly, to climb stairs carefully, and to lie down at first sign of dizziness.

• Caution patient to avoid alcohol because it may worsen low BP effects.

• Advise patient that use of sildenafil, tadalafil, vardenafil, or avanafil with any nitrate may cause severe low BP. Counsel patient to talk to prescriber before using these drugs together.

• Tell patient to store drug in a cool dark place, in a tightly closed container.

ISOtretinoin
eye-so-TRET-i-noyn

Absorica, Amnesteem, Claravis, Myorisan, Zenatane

Therapeutic class: Antiacne drugs
Pharmacologic class: Retinoic acid derivatives

AVAILABLE FORMS

Capsules: 10 mg, 20 mg, 25 mg, 30 mg, 35 mg, 40 mg

INDICATIONS & DOSAGES

➤ **Severe recalcitrant nodular acne that's unresponsive to conventional therapy**
Adults and adolescents age 12 and older: 0.5 to 1 mg/kg PO daily in two divided doses with food for 15 to 20 weeks. Or, 2 mg/kg/day for adults whose disease is very severe with scarring or whose disease is primarily on the trunk.

➤ **Moderate acne ◆**
Adults: 20 mg/day (approximately 0.3 to 0.4 mg/kg/day) for 6 months, or 0.25 to 0.4 mg/kg daily for 24 weeks.
Children and adolescents ages 12 to 17: 20 mg/day (approximately 0.3 to 0.4 mg/kg/day) for 6 months, or 0.3 to 0.5 mg/kg/day for 15 to 20 weeks.

➤ **Treatment of high-risk neuroblastoma in children, in combination with dinutuximab, sargramostim, and aldesleukin, when given after chemotherapy or hematopoietic stem cell transplantation ◆**

Children: 160 mg/m^2/day (in two divided doses) on days 15 through 28 of a 28-day cycle for six cycles, or 160 mg/m^2/day (in two divided doses) on days 1 through 14 every 28 days for six cycles, beginning after continuation chemotherapy or transplantation.

ADMINISTRATION
PO
• Hazardous agent; use safe handling and disposal precautions.
• Before use, have patient read patient information and sign consent form.
• Give drug with or shortly after meals to facilitate absorption, except Absorica, which may be given without regard to meals.
• Have patient swallow capsule whole with full glass of liquid.
• Absorica isn't substitutable with other forms of isotretinoin.

ACTION
May normalize keratinization, reversibly decrease size of sebaceous glands, and make sebum less viscous and less likely to plug follicles.

Route	Onset	Peak	Duration
PO	Unknown	3–5 hr	Unknown

Half-life: 21 to 24 hours.

ADVERSE REACTIONS
CNS: pseudotumor cerebri, depression, *psychosis, suicidal ideation or attempts, suicide, aggressive and violent behavior,* emotional instability, headache, fatigue, dizziness, drowsiness, insomnia, weakness. **CV:** palpitations, *stroke,* tachycardia. **EENT:** conjunctivitis, corneal deposits, dry eyes, decreased night vision, visual disturbances, hearing impairment (sometimes irreversible), epistaxis, drying of mucous membranes, dry nose. **GI:** nonspecific GI symptoms, nausea, vomiting, abdominal pain, dry mouth, anorexia, gum bleeding and inflammation, *acute pancreatitis,* inflammatory bowel disease. **GU:** abnormal menses, hematuria. **Hematologic:** increased erythrocyte sedimentation rate, anemia, *thrombocytosis.* **Hepatic:** *hepatitis.* **Metabolic:** hypertriglyceridemia, hyperglycemia. **Musculoskeletal:** *rhabdomyolysis,* skeletal

hyperostosis, tendon and ligament calcification, premature epiphyseal closure, decreased bone mineral density and other bone abnormalities, back pain, arthralgia, arthritis, tendinitis. **Respiratory:** *bronchospasm,* respiratory tract infections. **Skin:** cheilitis, cheilosis, fragility, rash, dry skin, facial skin desquamation, petechiae, pruritus, nail brittleness, thinning of hair, skin infection, peeling of palms and toes, photosensitivity reaction.

INTERACTIONS
Drug-drug. *Corticosteroids:* May increase risk of osteoporosis. Use together cautiously.
Fluoride, folate, iron, minerals, multivitamins: May enhance adverse or toxic effect of retinoic acid derivatives. Avoid combination.
Medicated soaps, cleansers, and cover-ups; preparations containing alcohol; topical resorcinol peeling agents (benzoyl peroxide): May have cumulative drying effect. Use together cautiously.
Micro-dose progesterone hormonal contraceptives ("minipills") that don't contain estrogen: May decrease effectiveness of contraceptive. Advise patient to use different contraceptive method.
Phenytoin: May increase risk of osteomalacia. Use together cautiously.
Products containing vitamin A: May increase toxic effects of isotretinoin. Avoid using together.
Tetracyclines: May increase risk of pseudotumor cerebri. Avoid using together.
Drug-herb. *St. John's wort:* May interact with hormonal contraceptives; pregnancies have been reported when used together. Avoid use together.
Drug-food. *Any high-fat food:* May increase absorption of drug. Advise patient to take drug with milk, a meal, or shortly after a meal.
Drug-lifestyle. *Alcohol use:* May increase risk of hypertriglyceridemia. Discourage use together.
Sun exposure: May increase photosensitivity reaction. Advise patient to avoid excessive sunlight exposure.

EFFECTS ON LAB TEST RESULTS
• May increase AST, ALT, alkaline phosphatase, triglyceride, glucose, and uric acid levels.

- May decrease serum HDL levels.
- May increase platelet count and erythrocyte sedimentation rate.

CONTRAINDICATIONS & CAUTIONS

- Contraindicated in patients hypersensitive to parabens (used as preservatives), vitamin A, or other retinoids.
- Use cautiously in patients with a history of mental illness or a family history of psychiatric disorders, asthma, liver disease, diabetes, heart disease, hearing impairment, hypertriglyceridemia, inflammatory bowel disease, osteoporosis, genetic predisposition for age-related osteoporosis, history of childhood osteoporosis, weak bones, anorexia nervosa, osteomalacia, or other disorders of bone metabolism.
- Drug may cause erythema multiforme and severe skin reactions (such as SJS or toxic epidermal necrolysis), which may be serious and result in hospitalization, disability, life-threatening events, or death.

Dialyzable drug: Unknown.

⚠ *Overdose S&S:* Vomiting, facial flushing, abdominal pain, headache, dizziness, ataxia.

PREGNANCY-LACTATION-REPRODUCTION

Black Box Warning Women and adolescents who are pregnant or who may become pregnant must not use drug. There is an extremely high risk of severe birth defects if pregnancy occurs while patient is taking isotretinoin in any amount, even for short periods. Potentially, any fetus exposed during pregnancy can be affected; there are no accurate means of determining whether an exposed fetus has been affected. There is an increased risk of spontaneous abortion, and premature births have been reported. Cases of IQ scores less than 85 with or without other abnormalities have been reported. Documented external abnormalities include skull abnormalities, ear abnormalities (anotia, micropinna, small or absent external auditory canals), eye abnormalities (microphthalmia), facial dysmorphia, and cleft palate. Documented internal abnormalities include CNS abnormalities (cerebral abnormalities, cerebellar malformation, hydrocephalus, microcephaly, cranial nerve deficit), CV abnormalities, thymus gland abnormality, and parathyroid hormone

deficiency. In some cases, these abnormalities have resulted in death. ▮

Black Box Warning To minimize risk of fetal exposure, drug is only available through a restricted FDA-approved distribution program called iPLEDGE. ▮

⟐ *Alert:* Patient must have negative results from two urine or serum pregnancy tests, one performed in the office when patient is qualified for therapy and the second performed during the first 5 days of the next normal menstrual period immediately preceding beginning of therapy. A pregnancy test must be repeated every month and must be negative before each course of therapy. For patients with amenorrhea, the second test should be done within 7 days after office visit and immediately preceding beginning of therapy. A pregnancy test must be repeated every month before patient receives the prescription. For patients with irregular cycles, or for those using a contraceptive method that precludes withdrawal bleeding, the second pregnancy test must be done within 7 days after office visit, immediately preceding beginning of therapy, and after patient has used two forms of contraception for 1 month.

Black Box Warning If pregnancy does occur during treatment, discontinue drug immediately and refer patient to an obstetrician-gynecologist experienced in reproductive toxicity. ▮

- It isn't known if drug appears in human milk. Patient should discontinue breastfeeding or discontinue drug.

NURSING CONSIDERATIONS

- If total nodule count has been reduced by more than 70% before patient has completed 15 to 20 weeks of treatment, drug may be discontinued.
- Monitor baseline lipid studies, LFTs, and pregnancy tests before therapy and at monthly intervals.
- Regularly monitor glucose level and CK levels in patients who participate in vigorous physical activity.
- Closely watch for and report severe skin reactions. Drug may need to be discontinued.
- Most adverse reactions occur at doses exceeding 1 mg/kg daily. Reactions are

---

Reactions in bold italics are *life-threatening*. Interactions may have a *rapid onset* or a *delayed onset*.

generally reversible when therapy is stopped or dosage is reduced.

⟐ *Alert:* If patient experiences headache, nausea and vomiting, or visual disturbances, screen for papilledema. Signs and symptoms of pseudotumor cerebri require stopping the drug immediately and beginning neurologic interventions promptly.

⟐ *Alert:* Monitor patient for mood disturbance, psychosis, aggressive behavior, or suicidal ideation. Drug may need to be discontinued and patient evaluated.

• A second course of therapy may begin 8 weeks after completion of the first course, if necessary. Improvements may continue after first course is complete.

• Patients may be at increased risk of bone fractures or injury when participating in sports with repetitive impact.

• Spontaneous reports of osteoporosis, osteopenia, bone fractures, and delayed healing of bone fractures have occurred in patients taking drug. To decrease this risk, don't exceed recommended doses and duration.

PATIENT TEACHING

⟐ *Alert:* Warn female patient of childbearing potential that if this drug is used during pregnancy, severe fetal abnormalities may occur. Advise her that she must commit to either abstain from sex or use two reliable forms of contraception simultaneously for 1 month before, during, and for 1 month after treatment. An isotretinoin medication guide must be given to patient each time isotretinoin is dispensed, as required by law.

• Advise patient to take drug with or shortly after meals to facilitate absorption, except Absorica, which can be taken without regard to meals.

• Tell patient to immediately report visual disturbances, tinnitus, and bone, muscle, or joint pain.

• Warn patient that contact lenses may feel uncomfortable during therapy.

• Advise patient not to drive at night until effect on vision is known. Drug may decrease night vision.

• Warn patient against using abrasives, medicated soaps and cleansers, acne preparations containing peeling drugs, and topical products containing alcohol (including cosmetics, aftershave, cologne) because they may cause cumulative irritation or excessive drying of skin.

• Tell patient to avoid prolonged sun exposure and to use sunblock. Drug may have additive effect if used with other drugs that cause photosensitivity reaction.

• Warn patient that transient exacerbations may occur during therapy.

• Warn patient not to donate blood during therapy and for 1 month after stopping drug because drug could harm fetus of a pregnant recipient.

• Advise patient to consult prescriber before taking OTC medications, vitamins, or herbal supplements.

• Tell patient to report adverse reactions immediately, especially depression, suicidal thoughts, persistent headaches, visual disturbances, severe skin reactions, and persistent GI pain.

⟐ *Alert:* Advise patient to read iPLEDGE carefully and to fully understand all information before signing it.

itraconazole
eye-tra-KON-a-zole

Onmel, Sporanox, Sporanox PulsePak

Therapeutic class: Antifungals
Pharmacologic class: Synthetic triazoles

AVAILABLE FORMS
Capsules ⓓ: 100 mg
Oral solution: 10 mg/mL
Tablets: 200 mg

INDICATIONS & DOSAGES
➤ **Pulmonary and extrapulmonary blastomycosis, nonmeningeal histoplasmosis (capsules)**
Adults: 200 mg PO daily; increase as needed and tolerated by 100 mg to maximum of 400 mg daily. Give dosages exceeding 200 mg PO daily in two divided doses. Continue treatment for at least 3 months. In life-threatening illness, give a loading dose of 200 mg PO t.i.d. for 3 days.
➤ **Aspergillosis (capsules)**
Adults: 200 to 400 mg PO daily for at least 3 months. In life-threatening illness, give

a loading dose of 200 mg PO t.i.d. for first 3 days of treatment.

➤ **Onychomycosis of the toenail (with or without fingernail involvement)**
Adults: 200 mg PO once daily for 12 consecutive weeks.

➤ **Onychomycosis of the fingernail**
Adults: 200 mg PO b.i.d. for 1 week, followed by 3 weeks drug-free. Repeat dosage.

➤ **Oropharyngeal candidiasis**
Adults: 200 mg oral solution swished in mouth vigorously and swallowed daily, for 1 to 2 weeks.

➤ **Oropharyngeal candidiasis in patients unresponsive to fluconazole tablets**
Adults: 100 mg oral solution swished in mouth vigorously and swallowed b.i.d., for 2 to 4 weeks.

➤ **Esophageal candidiasis**
Adults: 100 to 200 mg oral solution swished in mouth vigorously and swallowed daily, for at least 3 weeks. Treatment should continue for 2 weeks after symptoms resolve.

ADMINISTRATION
PO
• Before starting therapy, confirm diagnosis of onychomycosis by sending nail specimens for testing.
• Don't interchange capsules and tablets with oral solution.
• Give capsules and tablets with a full meal.
• Give oral solution on an empty stomach if possible.
• Have patient vigorously swish oral solution in mouth for several seconds and then swallow.
• Store oral solution at or below 77° F (25° C). Don't freeze. Protect from light and moisture.

ACTION
Interferes with fungal cell-wall synthesis by inhibiting ergosterol formation and increasing cell-wall permeability, leading to osmotic instability.

Route	Onset	Peak	Duration
PO	Unknown	2–5 hr	7–14 days

Half-life: Single dose, 16 to 28 hours; repeated dosing, 34 to 42 hours.

ADVERSE REACTIONS
CNS: headache, fever, dizziness, somnolence, fatigue, malaise, asthenia, pain, tremor, abnormal dreams, anxiety, depression. **CV:** *HF,* HTN, edema, orthostatic hypotension. **EENT:** rhinitis, sinusitis, pharyngitis. **GI:** nausea, vomiting, diarrhea, abdominal pain, anorexia, dyspepsia, flatulence, increased appetite, constipation, gastritis, gastroenteritis, ulcerative stomatitis, gingivitis. **GU:** albuminuria. **Hematologic:** *neutropenia.* **Hepatic:** *hepatotoxicity, liver failure,* impaired hepatic function. **Metabolic:** hypokalemia, hypertriglyceridemia. **Musculoskeletal:** myalgia. **Respiratory:** *pulmonary edema,* URI. **Skin:** rash, pruritus. **Other:** decreased libido, injury, herpes zoster, hypersensitivity reactions (urticaria, *angioedema, SJS*).

INTERACTIONS
Consult manufacturer's instructions for a full list of interactions.
Drug-drug. *Alprazolam:* May increase and prolong drug levels, CNS depression, and psychomotor impairment. Avoid using together.
Antacids, carbamazepine, H₂-receptor antagonists, isoniazid, phenobarbital, **phenytoin,** *rifabutin, rifampin:* May decrease itraconazole level. Avoid using together.
Chlordiazepoxide, clonazepam, clorazepate, diazepam, estazolam, flurazepam, quazepam: May increase and prolong drug levels, CNS depression, and psychomotor impairment. Avoid using together.
Clarithromycin, erythromycin: May increase itraconazole levels. Monitor patient for signs of itraconazole toxicity.
Cyclosporine, **digoxin,** *tacrolimus:* May increase levels of these drugs. Monitor drug levels.
Black Box Warning *Dofetilide, ergometrine, ergot alkaloids, ergotamine, felodipine, lovastatin, methadone, methylergotamine, midazolam (oral), nisoldipine, pimozide, quinidine, simvastatin, triazolam:* May increase levels of these drugs by CYP450 metabolism, causing serious CV events, including torsades de pointes, QT-interval prolongation, ventricular tachycardia, cardiac arrest, and sudden death. Use together is contraindicated. ▪

HMG-CoA reductase inhibitors (atorvastatin, fluvastatin, pravastatin): May increase levels and adverse effects of these drugs. Avoid using together, or reduce dose of HMG-CoA reductase inhibitor.

NNRTIs (nevirapine): May decrease itraconazole level. Use together isn't recommended.

Oral anticoagulants: May enhance anticoagulant effect. Monitor PT and INR.

Oral antidiabetics: May cause hypoglycemia, similar to effect of other antifungals. Monitor glucose level. Avoid using together.

PDE5 inhibitors (avanafil, sildenafil, tadalafil, vardenafil): May increase levels of these drugs, increasing adverse effects. Give PDE5 inhibitors with caution and in reduced doses.

Protease inhibitors (indinavir, ritonavir, saquinavir): May increase levels of these drugs; indinavir and ritonavir may increase itraconazole levels. Monitor patient for toxicity.

EFFECTS ON LAB TEST RESULTS
• May increase alkaline phosphatase, ALT, AST, bilirubin, triglyceride, and GGT levels.
• May decrease potassium, magnesium, calcium, and phosphate levels.

CONTRAINDICATIONS & CAUTIONS
Black Box Warning Contraindicated in patients hypersensitive to drug; in those receiving methadone, disopyramide, dofetilide, dronedarone, quinidine, isavuconazole, naloxegol, ergot alkaloids (dihydroergotamine, ergometrine [ergonovine], ergotamine, felodipine, methylergometrine [methylergonovine]), irinotecan, lurasidone, oral midazolam, pimozide, triazolam, nisoldipine, ivabradine, ranolazine, eplerenone, lomitapide, avanafil, lovastatin, simvastatin, or ticagrelor; colchicine, fesoterodine, and solifenacin in patients with varying degrees of renal or hepatic impairment; eliglustat in patients who are poor or intermediate metabolizers of CYP2D6; and in patients taking strong or moderate CYP2D6 inhibitors. Administration with itraconazole can cause elevated plasma concentrations and may increase or prolong pharmacologic effects and adverse reactions to these drugs. For example, increased plasma concentrations of some of these drugs can lead to QT-interval prolongation and ventricular tachyarrhythmias, including potentially fatal torsades de pointes. ▐
• Use cautiously in patients with hypochlorhydria; they may not absorb drug readily.

Black Box Warning Don't use drug to treat onychomycosis in patients with evidence of ventricular dysfunction, such as HF or history of HF. If signs or symptoms of HF occur while giving oral solution, reassess continued use. If signs or symptoms of HF occur while giving capsules or tablets, discontinue use. ▐
• Use cautiously in HIV-infected patients because hypochlorhydria can accompany HIV infection.
• Use cautiously in patients receiving other highly bound drugs.
• Drug may cause transient or permanent hearing loss, particularly in elderly patients.
Dialyzable drug: No.

PREGNANCY-LACTATION-REPRODUCTION
• Don't use to treat onychomycosis in pregnant women, those contemplating pregnancy, or women of childbearing potential unless they are using effective contraceptive measures and they begin therapy on the second or third day after onset of menses. Effective contraception should be continued throughout therapy and for 2 months after therapy ends.
• Drug may cause maternal or fetal harm. Use to treat systemic fungal infections in pregnant women only if benefit justifies potential risk.
• Drug appears in human milk. Weigh expected benefits for mother against potential risk to infant.

NURSING CONSIDERATIONS
• Perform baseline LFTs and monitor results periodically. In patients with baseline hepatic impairment, give drug only if patient's condition is life threatening. If liver dysfunction occurs during therapy, notify prescriber immediately.
• Monitor patient for hearing loss.

PATIENT TEACHING
• Teach patient to recognize and report signs and symptoms of liver disease (anorexia, dark urine, pale stools, unusual fatigue, and jaundice) or hearing loss.
• Instruct patient not to use oral solution interchangeably with capsules or tablets.
• For the oral solution, tell patient to take 10 mL at a time.
• Tell patient to take solution without food; capsules or tablets, with a full meal.
• Urge patient to list other drugs being taken, to avoid drug interactions.
• Advise female patient of childbearing potential that an effective form of contraception must be used during therapy and for two menstrual cycles after stopping therapy with capsules or tablets.

---

ivabradine
eye-VAB-ra-deen

Corlanor, Lancora✹

Therapeutic class: Antianginals
Pharmacologic class: Cyclic nucleotide-gated channel blockers

AVAILABLE FORMS
Tablets: 5 mg, 7.5 mg

INDICATIONS & DOSAGES
➤ **To reduce risk of hospitalization for worsening HF in patients with stable, symptomatic chronic HF with LVEF of 35% or less who are in sinus rhythm with resting HR of 70 beats/minute (bpm) or more and either are on maximally tolerated doses of beta blockers or have a contraindication to beta blocker use**
Adults: Initially, 5 mg PO b.i.d. with meals. After 2 weeks, adjust dosage to achieve resting HR of 50 to 60 bpm if necessary. Maximum dose is 7.5 mg b.i.d.
Adjust-a-dose: If HR is greater than 60 bpm, increase dosage by 2.5 mg b.i.d. up to a maximum of 7.5 mg b.i.d. If HR is less than 50 bpm or patient has signs and symptoms of bradycardia, decrease dosage by 2.5 mg b.i.d.; however, if current dosage is 2.5 mg b.i.d., discontinue therapy. In patients with a history of conduction defects and in those

whose bradycardia could lead to hemodynamic compromise, initiate therapy at 2.5 mg b.i.d. before increasing dosage based on HR.

ADMINISTRATION
PO
• Give with meals.
• Store tablets at room temperature.

ACTION
Reduces HR by blocking hyperpolarization-activated cyclic nucleotide-gated channel responsible for the cardiac pacemaker I_f current.

Route	Onset	Peak	Duration
PO	Rapid	1 – 2 hr	Unknown

Half-life: 6 hours.

ADVERSE REACTIONS
CV: *bradycardia, conduction disturbances,* HTN, atrial fibrillation. **EENT:** phosphenes, visual brightness.

INTERACTIONS
Drug-drug. *CYP3A4 inducers (barbiturates, phenytoin, rifampin):* May decrease ivabradine level. Avoid use together.
Drugs that decrease HR (amiodarone, beta blockers, digoxin): May increase risk of bradycardia. Monitor HR.
Moderate CYP3A4 inhibitors (diltiazem, verapamil): May increase ivabradine level, causing bradycardia and conduction disturbances. Avoid use together.
Strong CYP3A4 inhibitors (clarithromycin, HIV protease inhibitors [nelfinavir], itraconazole, nefazodone, telithromycin): May significantly increase ivabradine level, leading to bradycardia and conduction disturbances. Use together is contraindicated.
Drug-herb. *St. John's wort:* May decrease ivabradine level. Discourage use together.
Drug-food. *Grapefruit juice:* May increase ivabradine level, causing bradycardia and conduction disturbances. Discourage use together.

EFFECTS ON LAB TEST RESULTS
None reported.

CONTRAINDICATIONS & CAUTIONS
• Contraindicated in patients hypersensitive to drug or its components and in those with acute decompensated HF or BP less than 90/50 mm Hg; sick sinus syndrome, SA block, or third-degree AV block unless a functioning demand pacemaker is present; resting HR less than 60 bpm before treatment; severe hepatic impairment; pacemaker dependence (HR maintained exclusively by the pacemaker); or concomitant use of strong CYP3A4 inhibitors.
• Avoid use in patients with second-degree AV block unless a functioning demand pacemaker is present and in those taking diltiazem or verapamil concomitantly.
• Use cautiously in patients with sinus node dysfunction, conduction defects (first- or second-degree AV block, bundle-branch block), or ventricular dyssynchrony and in those taking other negative chronotropes (digoxin, amiodarone) concomitantly. Drug may increase risk of bradycardia, sinus arrest, and heart block.
• Not recommended in those with demand pacemakers set to rates of 60 bpm or greater.
• Safety and effectiveness in children haven't been established.
Dialyzable drug: Unknown.
⚠ ***Overdose S&S:*** Severe and prolonged bradycardia.

PREGNANCY-LACTATION-REPRODUCTION
• There are no adequate studies in pregnant women, but animal studies showed fetal harm. Avoid use during pregnancy because of risk of fetal harm; advise pregnant women of potential risk to the fetus. Women of childbearing potential should use effective contraception during treatment.
• If drug must be used during pregnancy, monitor patients, especially during first trimester, for destabilization of HF that could result from slowing HR. Monitor pregnant women with HF who are in the third trimester for signs and symptoms of preterm birth. Pregnant patients with LVEF less than 35% on maximally tolerated doses of beta blockers may be particularly HR-dependent for augmenting cardiac output.
• Drug may appear in human milk. Women shouldn't breastfeed during therapy.

NURSING CONSIDERATIONS
• Regularly monitor cardiac rhythm. Drug may increase risk of atrial fibrillation. Discontinue drug if atrial fibrillation develops.
• Monitor patient for bradycardia; drug may increase risk of QT-interval prolongation, which may lead to severe ventricular arrhythmias, including torsades de pointes, especially in patients with risk factors such as use of QT-prolonging drugs.
• Monitor patients for phosphenes (transient enhanced brightness in a limited area of the visual field, halos, image decomposition, colored bright lights, or multiple images), which may be triggered by sudden variations in light intensity. Onset is typically within first 2 months of treatment; phosphenes may resolve without discontinuing treatment.

PATIENT TEACHING
• Instruct patient to take tablets with meals.
• Warn female patient of childbearing potential that drug may cause fetal harm. Instruct her to use effective contraception during treatment and to notify prescriber if she is pregnant or suspects she is pregnant.
• Advise breastfeeding patient to avoid breastfeeding during therapy because of potential risk of fetal harm.
• Advise patient to immediately seek medical attention for significant decreases in HR or such signs and symptoms as dizziness, fatigue, or hypotension.
• Advise patient to report all adverse reactions and to immediately report signs and symptoms of atrial fibrillation (heart palpitations or racing, chest pressure, worsened shortness of breath).
• Warn patient about possibility of developing luminous phenomena (phosphenes), resulting in transient visual brightness. Advise patient to use caution while driving or operating machinery in situations in which sudden changes in light intensity may occur, especially at night. Inform patient that phosphenes may subside during treatment.
• Warn patient to avoid grapefruit juice and St. John's wort and to report all drugs and supplements being taken before starting drug.

ixazomib citrate
ix-AZ-oh-mib

Ninlaro

Therapeutic class: Antineoplastics
Pharmacologic class: Proteasome inhibitors

AVAILABLE FORMS
Capsules ⬤: 2.3 mg, 3 mg, 4 mg

INDICATIONS & DOSAGES
➤ **Multiple myeloma in combination with lenalidomide and dexamethasone in patients who have received at least one prior therapy**
Adults: 4 mg PO once a week on days 1, 8, and 15 of a 28-day treatment cycle, in combination with lenalidomide 25 mg on days 1 through 21 and dexamethasone 40 mg on days 1, 8, 15, and 22 of a 28-day treatment cycle. Before initiating a new cycle of therapy, ANC should be at least 1,000/mm³, platelet count should be at least 75,000/mm³, and nonhematologic toxicities should generally be recovered to patient's baseline or grade 1 or lower. Continue treatment until disease progression or unacceptable toxicity.
Adjust-a-dose: Reduce starting dose of drug to 3 mg in patients with moderate (total bilirubin level greater than 1.5 and less than 3 × ULN) or severe (total bilirubin level greater than 3 × ULN) hepatic impairment and in patients with severe renal impairment (CrCl of less than 30 mL/minute) or ESRD requiring dialysis. Refer to manufacturer's instructions for toxicity-related dosage adjustments. Refer to lenalidomide prescribing information for dosing recommendation in patients with renal impairment.

ADMINISTRATION
PO
• Hazardous drug: use safe handling and disposal precautions according to facility policy. Use gloves to administer intact capsules.
• Give drug once weekly on the same day, at approximately the same time.

• Give at least 1 hour before or at least 2 hours after food.
• Patient should swallow capsules whole with water and shouldn't chew them. Don't crush or open capsules.
• May give without regard to timing of dialysis.
• If dose is delayed or missed, give only if the next scheduled dose is 72 hours or more away; don't double-dose. Don't repeat dose if patient vomits after taking a dose; resume dosing at the time of the next scheduled dose.
• Store at room temperature. Don't store above 86° F (30° C). Don't freeze.
• Store capsules in original packaging until immediately before use.

ACTION
A reversible proteasome inhibitor that binds and inhibits the chymotrypsin-like activity of the beta 5 subunit of the 20S proteasome, thereby inducing death of multiple myeloma cell lines.

Route	Onset	Peak	Duration
PO	Unknown	1 hr	Unknown

Half-life: 9½ days.

ADVERSE REACTIONS
CNS: peripheral neuropathy. **CV:** peripheral edema. **EENT:** blurred vision, dry eyes, conjunctivitis. **GI:** diarrhea, constipation, nausea, vomiting. **Hematologic:** *thrombocytopenia, neutropenia.* **Hepatic:** hepatic impairment. **Musculoskeletal:** back pain. **Respiratory:** URI. **Skin:** rash.

INTERACTIONS
Drug-drug. *Strong CYP3A inducers (carbamazepine, phenytoin, rifampin):* May decrease ixazomib concentration. Avoid use together.
Drug-herb. *St. John's wort:* May decrease ixazomib concentration. Avoid use together.
Drug-food. *High-fat meals:* May decrease ixazomib concentration. Patient should take drug at least 1 hour before or at least 2 hours after food.

EFFECTS ON LAB TEST RESULTS
• May increase LFT values.
• May decrease platelet and neutrophil counts.

Reactions in bold italics are *life-threatening*. Interactions may have a *rapid onset* or a *delayed onset*.

CONTRAINDICATIONS & CAUTIONS
• Bone marrow suppression was commonly reported in clinical trials.
• Thrombocytopenia purpura and TLS can occur rarely.
• Drug isn't indicated for use in children.
Dialyzable drug: No.

PREGNANCY-LACTATION-REPRODUCTION
• Drug may cause fetal harm; advise women of risk. Lenalidomide is contraindicated during pregnancy.
• Males and females of reproductive potential must use effective contraception during treatment and for 90 days after final dose.
• It isn't known if drug appears in human milk. Breastfeeding isn't recommended.

NURSING CONSIDERATIONS
• Monitor patients for signs and symptoms of thrombocytopenia (bleeding, bruising). Platelet nadirs typically occur between days 14 and 21 of each 28-day cycle and recover to baseline by the start of the next cycle. Monitor platelet count at least monthly; consider more frequent monitoring during the first three cycles. Adjust dosage and consider platelet transfusions per standard medical guidelines if indicated.
• Monitor patients for GI adverse effects (severe diarrhea, constipation, nausea, vomiting); provide antidiarrheals, antiemetics, and supportive care as needed. Adjust dosage for grade 3 or 4 symptoms.
• Monitor patients for new or worsening peripheral neuropathy. Adjust dosage as clinically indicated.
• Monitor patients for rash; SJS can occur rarely. Provide supportive care or adjust dosage as clinically indicated.
• Monitor patients for peripheral edema. Evaluate for underlying causes and provide supportive care as clinically indicated. Adjust dexamethasone dosage per prescribing information or ixazomib dosage for grade 3 or 4 symptoms.
• Monitor liver enzyme levels regularly and adjust dosage for grade 3 or 4 symptoms.
• *Look alike–sound alike:* Don't confuse Ninlaro with Teflaro.

PATIENT TEACHING
• Advise patient to take drug once a week on the same day and at approximately the same time for the first 3 weeks of a 4-week cycle.
• Remind patient to take drug at least 1 hour before or at least 2 hours after food.
• Explain that capsules must be stored in original packaging until immediately before use.
• Warn patient not to open or crush capsules.
• Advise patient to avoid direct contact with the capsule contents: In case of capsule breakage, avoid direct contact of contents with the skin or eyes. If skin contact occurs, wash thoroughly with soap and water. If eye contact occurs, flush thoroughly with water.
• Teach patient to report all adverse reactions and to immediately report bleeding and easy bruising, diarrhea, constipation, nausea and vomiting, rash, abdominal pain, or yellowing of the skin.
• Advise patient to report new or worsening peripheral neuropathy signs and symptoms (tingling, numbness, pain, burning feeling in the feet or hands, weakness in the arms or legs).
• Instruct patient to report unusual extremity swelling or weight gain due to swelling.
• Remind male and female patient of reproductive potential that it's essential to use effective contraception during treatment and for 90 days after final dose.
• Inform female patient of risk to fetus with ixazomib use during pregnancy. Instruct her to immediately report suspected pregnancy.
• Caution female patient not to breastfeed during treatment.

ixekizumab
IX-e-kiz-ue-mab

Taltz

Therapeutic class: Immunomodulators
Pharmacologic class: Humanized interleukin-17A antagonists

AVAILABLE FORMS
Injection: 80 mg/mL autoinjector or pre-filled syringe

INDICATIONS & DOSAGES
➤ **Moderate to severe plaque psoriasis in patients who are candidates for systemic therapy or phototherapy**
Adults: Initially, 160 mg (two 80-mg injections) subcut followed by 80 mg subcut at weeks 2, 4, 6, 8, 10, and 12; then 80 mg every 4 weeks.
➤ **Active psoriatic arthritis**
Adults: Initially, 160 mg (two 80-mg injections) subcut followed by 80 mg subcut every 4 weeks. For patients with psoriatic arthritis who have coexistent moderate to severe plaque psoriasis, use the dosing regimen for plaque psoriasis. May be given alone or in combination with a conventional DMARD such as methotrexate.

ADMINISTRATION
Subcutaneous
• Allow medication to reach room temperature for 30 minutes before injection without removing needle cap.
• Inspect solution for particulate matter and discoloration before administration. Solution should be clear and colorless to slightly yellow. Don't use if solution contains particles or is discolored or cloudy. Don't shake.
• Inject the full 1 mL of medication in the autoinjector or prefilled syringe.
• Discard unused portion if any medication remains in the autoinjector or prefilled syringe after injection. Drug doesn't contain preservatives.
• Give each injection in a different location (upper arm, thigh, or abdomen) than previous injection.
• Don't inject into skin that is tender, bruised, erythematous, indurated, or affected by psoriasis.
• If a dose is missed, give as soon as possible; then resume dosing at the regularly scheduled time.
• Store in refrigerator at 36° to 46° F (2° to 8° C). Protect from light. Don't freeze.

ACTION
A humanized monoclonal IgG antibody that binds selectively to IL-17A receptors and inhibits release of proinflammatory cytokines and chemokines.

Route	Onset	Peak	Duration
Subcut	Unknown	4 days	Unknown

Half-life: 13 days.

ADVERSE REACTIONS
GI: nausea. **Hematologic:** *neutropenia, thrombocytopenia.* **Respiratory:** URI. **Skin:** injection-site reaction. **Other:** tinea infection, infection, development of neutralizing antibodies.

INTERACTIONS
Drug-drug. *CYP450 substrates (cyclosporine, warfarin):* May affect substrate levels, especially those with narrow therapeutic index. Monitor patient for effect and consider dosage modification of substrate.
Live-virus vaccines: May reduce effectiveness of live-virus vaccine. Immunocompromised patients may be at increased risk for vaccine-induced infection. Avoid use of live-virus vaccines.

EFFECTS ON LAB TEST RESULTS
• May decrease WBC and platelet counts.

CONTRAINDICATIONS & CAUTIONS
• Contraindicated in patients hypersensitive to drug or its components. Rarely, angioedema and urticaria were reported.
• Contraindicated in patients with active TB. Evaluate patients for TB before initiating treatment and consider providing TB treatment in patients with a history of latent or active TB in whom adequate treatment can't be confirmed.
• Use cautiously in patients at risk for serious infections and in those with Crohn disease or ulcerative colitis.
• Safety in children hasn't been established.
Dialyzable drug: Unknown.

PREGNANCY-LACTATION-REPRODUCTION
• No data exist on the use of drug during pregnancy. Human IgG is known to cross the placental barrier so it's possible that ixekizumab, a humanized IgG monoclonal antibody, may be transmitted from mother to fetus. Other agents are preferred for treatment of plaque psoriasis in pregnant women.

Reactions in bold italics are *life-threatening*. Interactions may have a *rapid onset* or a ***delayed onset***.

• It isn't known if drug appears in human milk. Weigh benefits to mother against potential risk to the infant.

NURSING CONSIDERATIONS

• Monitor patients for signs and symptoms of infection, including TB, during and after treatment.
• Monitor patients for hypersensitivity reactions (angioedema, urticaria). If serious reaction occurs, discontinue drug and initiate treatment.
• Monitor patients for onset or exacerbation of Crohn disease and ulcerative colitis.
• Before start of therapy, make sure all appropriate immunizations are up to date. Avoid live-virus vaccines.
• *Look alike–sound alike:* Don't confuse ixekizumab with infliximab, reslizumab, or rituximab.

PATIENT TEACHING

• Advise patient to report all adverse reactions and to promptly report signs or symptoms of infection (because drug may lower patient's ability to fight infection).
• Warn patient to seek immediate medical attention if signs or symptoms of severe hypersensitivity reaction occur.
• Teach patient and caregivers how to safely use autoinjectors or prefilled syringes.

ketoconazole (oral)
kee-toe-KOE-na-zole

Therapeutic class: Antifungals
Pharmacologic class: Imidazole derivatives

AVAILABLE FORMS
Tablets: 200 mg

INDICATIONS & DOSAGES
Black Box Warning Drug should only be used when other effective antifungal therapy isn't available or tolerated and potential benefits outweigh potential risks. ∎
➤ **Fungal infections (coccidioidomycosis, blastomycosis, histoplasmosis, chromomycosis, and paracoccidioidomycosis)**
Adults: Initially, 200 mg PO daily in a single dose. May increase dosage to 400 mg once daily in patients who don't respond.

Continue until fungal infection is resolved; usual duration of therapy for systemic infection is 6 months. Maximum dosage is 400 mg once daily.
Children age 2 and older: 3.3 to 6.6 mg/kg PO daily in a single dose. Continue until fungal infection is resolved; usual duration of therapy for systemic infection is 6 months. Maximum dosage is 400 mg once daily.
➤ **Prostate cancer, advanced ◆**
Adults: 400 mg PO t.i.d. (in combination with oral hydrocortisone) until disease progression.

ADMINISTRATION
PO
• Patient should wait at least 1 hour before or 2 hours after dose before taking antacids and H$_2$-receptor antagonists.

ACTION
Interferes with fungal cell-wall synthesis by inhibiting formation of ergosterol and increasing cell-wall permeability that makes the fungus susceptible to osmotic instability.

Route	Onset	Peak	Duration
PO	Unknown	1–2 hr	Unknown

Half-life: 8 hours.

ADVERSE REACTIONS
CNS: insomnia, nervousness, dizziness, asthenia, headache, fatigue, malaise, paresthesia, somnolence, fever, chills. **CV:** orthostatic hypotension, peripheral edema, prolonged QT interval. **EENT:** photophobia, epistaxis. **GI:** nausea, vomiting, upper abdominal pain, diarrhea, constipation, dry mouth, dysgeusia, dyspepsia, flatulence, increased appetite, anorexia, tongue discoloration. **GU:** menstrual disorder. **Hematologic:** hyperlipidemia, decreased platelet count. **Hepatic:** *hepatitis,* jaundice. **Musculoskeletal:** myalgia. **Skin:** pruritus, rash, *erythema multiforme,* dermatitis, erythema, alopecia, xeroderma. **Other:** *anaphylaxis,* gynecomastia, hot flush, adrenal insufficiency.

INTERACTIONS
Refer to manufacturer's instructions for complete list of drug-drug interactions.

K

Drug-drug. *Chlordiazepoxide, clonazepam, clorazepate, diazepam, estazolam, flurazepam, midazolam, quazepam, triazolam:* May increase and prolong levels of these drugs. May cause CNS depression and psychomotor impairment. Avoid using together.

Black Box Warning *Disopyramide, dofetilide, dronedarone, methadone, pimozide, quinidine, ranolazine:* There is risk of elevated plasma concentrations of these drugs and QT-interval prolongation. Use together is contraindicated. ∎

HMG-CoA reductase inhibitors (atorvastatin, fluvastatin, lovastatin, pravastatin, simvastatin): May increase levels and adverse effects of these drugs. Use together is contraindicated.

Drug-herb. *St. John's wort:* May decrease ketoconazole level. Consider therapy modification.

Drug-lifestyle. *Alcohol use:* May cause disulfiram-like reaction (flushing, rash, peripheral edema, nausea, headache). Don't use together.

EFFECTS ON LAB TEST RESULTS
• May increase lipid, alkaline phosphatase, ALT, and AST levels.
• May decrease Hb level and platelet count.

CONTRAINDICATIONS & CAUTIONS
• Contraindicated in patients hypersensitive to drug or its components.

Black Box Warning Drug can cause serious hepatotoxicity that may be fatal or require liver transplantation, even in patients with no obvious risk factors for liver disease. Drug is contraindicated in patients with acute or chronic liver disease. ∎

• Drug decreases adrenal corticosteroid secretions at doses of 400 mg. Don't exceed recommended dose of 400 mg.

Dialyzable drug: No.

PREGNANCY-LACTATION-REPRODUCTION
• There are no adequate studies in pregnant women. Use during pregnancy only if potential benefit justifies potential risk to the fetus.
• Drug has been shown to lower serum testosterone level, which returns to baseline when therapy is discontinued. Testosterone levels are impaired with doses of

800 mg daily and abolished by 1,600 mg daily. Clinical manifestations may include gynecomastia, impotence, and oligospermia.
• Drug appears in human milk. Women shouldn't breastfeed during therapy.

NURSING CONSIDERATIONS
◑ **Alert:** Because of risk of hepatotoxicity, drug shouldn't be used for less serious conditions, such as fungal infections of the skin or nails.

Black Box Warning Because of increased risk of hepatotoxicity, monitor patient for signs and symptoms of hepatotoxicity, including elevated liver enzyme levels, nausea that doesn't subside, unusual fatigue, jaundice, dark urine, or pale stool. ∎

◑ **Alert:** Drug is a potent inhibitor of the CYP450 enzyme system. Giving this drug with drugs metabolized by CYP3A4 may lead to increased drug levels, which could increase or prolong therapeutic and adverse effects.

• Monitor adrenal function in patients with adrenal insufficiency or borderline adrenal function and in those experiencing prolonged periods of stress (such as major surgery).
• Assess liver function status (AST, ALT, total bilirubin), alkaline phosphatase, PT, and INR before starting drug.
• Measure ALT level weekly for duration of treatment. If ALT levels increase above the ULN or 30% above baseline, or if patient develops signs and symptoms of hepatotoxicity, obtain a full set of LFTs. Repeat LFTs to ensure normalization of values. If drug is restarted, monitor patient frequently.
• Review all medications patient is receiving for potential drug interactions with ketoconazole.

PATIENT TEACHING
• Instruct patient to take antacids or H_2-receptor antagonists at least 1 hour before or 2 hours after taking ketoconazole.
• Make sure patient understands that treatment should continue until all tests indicate that active fungal infection has subsided. If drug is stopped too soon, infection will recur. Treatment for systemic fungal infections may last 6 months.

Reactions in bold italics are *life-threatening*. Interactions may have a *rapid onset* or a ***delayed onset***.

- Review signs and symptoms of hepatotoxicity with patient. Tell patient to stop drug and notify prescriber if they occur.
- Instruct patient to immediately report irregular heartbeats, palpitations, feeling faint, dizziness, or light-headedness.
- Advise patient to tell prescriber about any new drugs or herbal supplements being taken.
- Caution patient to avoid alcohol consumption during treatment.

ketoconazole (topical)
kee-toe-KOE-na-zole

Extina, Ketoderm✤, Nizoral, Nizoral A-D ◊, Xolegel

Therapeutic class: Antifungals
Pharmacologic class: Imidazoles

AVAILABLE FORMS
Cream: 2%
Foam: 2%
Gel: 2%
Shampoo: 1% ◊, 2%

INDICATIONS & DOSAGES
➤ **Seborrheic dermatitis in immunocompetent patients**
Adults and children age 12 and older: Apply foam to affected area b.i.d. for 4 weeks. Apply gel to affected area once daily for 2 weeks. Apply cream to affected area b.i.d. for 4 weeks or until clearing.
➤ **Tinea corporis, tinea cruris, tinea pedis, tinea versicolor from susceptible organisms; seborrheic dermatitis; cutaneous candidiasis**
Adults: Cover affected and immediate surrounding areas daily for at least 2 weeks. For seborrheic dermatitis, apply b.i.d. for 4 weeks. Patients with tinea pedis need 6 weeks of treatment. For tinea (pityriasis) versicolor, apply 2% shampoo to affected area of damp skin, lather, leave on for 5 minutes, and rinse (one application is usually sufficient).
➤ **Scaling caused by dandruff**
Adults and children age 12 and older: Using 1% OTC shampoo, wet hair, lather, and rinse thoroughly; repeat. Use every 3 to 4 days for

up to 8 weeks; then apply only as needed to control dandruff.

ADMINISTRATION
Topical
- For external use only. Don't let drug come in contact with eyes.
- When using foam, dispense into cap of can or other cool surface; don't spray directly onto affected skin or the hands. If fingers are warm, rinse them in cold water and dry well; then, using fingertips, gently massage foam into affected areas until it disappears.
- Don't wash areas where gel was applied for at least 3 hours. Have patient wait at least 20 minutes after application before applying makeup or sunscreen to the affected areas.

ACTION
Probably inhibits yeast growth by altering the permeability of the cell membrane.

Route	Onset	Peak	Duration
Topical	Unknown	Unknown	Unknown

Half-life: Unknown.

ADVERSE REACTIONS
Skin: pruritus, application-site reaction, oiliness or dryness of hair and scalp with shampoo use; application-site reaction, burning with foam or gel; severe irritation, pruritus, and stinging or burning with cream.

INTERACTIONS
None known.

EFFECTS ON LAB TEST RESULTS
None reported.

CONTRAINDICATIONS & CAUTIONS
- Product contains sodium sulfite anhydrous, which may cause severe or life-threatening allergic reactions, including anaphylaxis, in patients with asthma.
Dialyzable drug: No.

PREGNANCY-LACTATION-REPRODUCTION
- There are no adequate studies in pregnant women. Use during pregnancy only if potential benefit justifies potential risk to the fetus.
- It isn't known if drug appears in human milk. Use cautiously in breastfeeding

K

✤Canada   ◊OTC   ◆Off-label use   ✐Photoguide   ⊕Do not crush   *Liquid contains alcohol   ▩Genetic women only if benefits outweigh risk to infant.

NURSING CONSIDERATIONS
• Most patients show improvement soon after treatment begins.
• Treatment of tinea corporis or tinea cruris should continue for at least 2 weeks to reduce possibility of recurrence.

PATIENT TEACHING
• Tell patient to stop drug and notify prescriber if hypersensitivity reaction occurs.
• Advise patient to check with prescriber if condition worsens; drug may have to be stopped and diagnosis reevaluated.
• Tell patient to avoid using shampoo on scalp if skin is broken or inflamed.
• Advise patient that foam and gel are flammable and to avoid fire, flame, and smoking during and immediately after application.
• Instruct patient to dispense foam into cap of can or other cool surface and not to spray directly onto affected skin or the hands. If fingers are warm, tell patient to rinse them in cold water and dry well; then, using fingertips, to gently massage foam into affected areas until it disappears.
• Instruct patient to not wash areas where gel was applied for at least 3 hours and to wait at least 20 minutes after application before applying makeup or sunscreen to the affected areas.
• Instruct patient to wash hands before and after use, unless affected areas are on hands.
• Warn patient that shampoo applied to permanent-waved hair removes curl.
• Warn patient to avoid drug contact with eyes.
• Tell patient to continue drug for intended duration of therapy, even if signs and symptoms improve soon after starting treatment.
• Tell patient not to store drug above room temperature (77° F [25° C]) and to protect from light.

ketoprofen
kee-toe-PROE-fen

Therapeutic class: NSAIDs
Pharmacologic class: NSAIDs

AVAILABLE FORMS
Capsules: 50 mg, 75 mg
Capsules (extended-release) ⓞⓝⓒ: 200 mg

INDICATIONS & DOSAGES
Adjust-a-dose (for all indications): For patients age 75 and older, reduce dosage. For patients with mildly impaired renal function, maximum daily dose is 150 mg. For patients with GFR of less than 25 mL/minute/1.73 m^2, ESRD, or impaired liver function and serum albumin level less than 3.5 g/dL, maximum daily dose is 100 mg.
➤ **RA, osteoarthritis**
Adults: 75 mg PO t.i.d. or 50 mg PO q.i.d., or 200 mg as an extended-release capsule once daily. Maximum dose is 300 mg daily, or 200 mg daily for extended-release capsules.
➤ **Mild to moderate pain, dysmenorrhea**
Adults: 25 to 50 mg PO every 6 to 8 hours p.r.n. Maximum dose is 300 mg daily.
➤ **Ankylosing spondylitis** ♦
Adults: 100 mg PO b.i.d.

ADMINISTRATION
PO
• Tell patient to take drug with or without food and with a full glass of water.
• Don't open extended-release capsules.

ACTION
Unknown. Produces anti-inflammatory, analgesic, and antipyretic effects, possibly by inhibiting prostaglandin synthesis.

Route	Onset	Peak	Duration
PO	<30 min	30–120 min	6 hr
PO (extended-release)	2–3 hr	6–7 hr	Unknown

Half-life: Immediate-release capsules, 2 to 4 hours; extended-release capsules, 3 to 7½ hours.

ADVERSE REACTIONS
CNS: headache, dizziness, CNS excitation (insomnia, nervousness, and dreams) or

CNS depression (somnolence and malaise). **CV:** peripheral edema. **EENT:** visual disturbances, tinnitus. **GI:** dyspepsia, abdominal pain, anorexia, constipation, diarrhea, flatulence, nausea, stomatitis, vomiting. **GU:** *nephrotoxicity,* UTI signs and symptoms. **Skin:** rash.

INTERACTIONS
Drug-drug. *ACE inhibitors, ARBs:* May significantly decrease glomerular filtration and renal function. Monitor therapy.
Aspirin, corticosteroids: May increase risk of adverse GI reactions. Avoid using together.
Aspirin, probenecid: May increase ketoprofen level. Avoid using together.
Cyclosporine: May increase nephrotoxicity. Avoid using together.
Hydrochlorothiazide, other diuretics: May decrease diuretic effectiveness and increase nephrotoxicity. Monitor patient for adverse effects and lack of effect.
Lithium, methotrexate: May increase levels of these drugs, leading to toxicity. Monitor patient closely.
Probenecid: May increase ketoprofen serum concentration. Use together isn't recommended.
Warfarin: May increase risk of bleeding. Monitor patient closely.
Drug-herb. *Dong quai, feverfew, garlic, ginger, horse chestnut, red clover:* May cause bleeding based on the known effects of components. Discourage use together.
White willow: Herb and drug contain similar components. Discourage use together.
Drug-lifestyle. *Alcohol use:* May cause GI toxicity. Discourage use together.
Smoking: May increase risk of GI bleeding. Discourage use together.

EFFECTS ON LAB TEST RESULTS
• May increase creatinine, BUN, ALT, and AST levels.
• May increase bleeding time.
• May lead to false-positive aldosterone/renin ratio.

CONTRAINDICATIONS & CAUTIONS
• Contraindicated in patients hypersensitive to drug and in those with history of aspirin or NSAID-induced asthma, urticaria, or other allergic reactions.

Black Box Warning Contraindicated for the treatment of perioperative pain after CABG surgery. ■

Black Box Warning NSAIDs can increase risk of heart attack or stroke in patients with or without heart disease or risk factors for heart disease. Risk may increase with duration of use. ■

Black Box Warning NSAIDs may increase risk of serious GI adverse events, including bleeding, ulceration, and perforation of the stomach or intestines, which can be fatal. These events can occur at any time during use and without warning symptoms. Elderly patients and patients with a prior history of peptic ulcer disease or GI bleeding are at greater risk for serious GI events. ■

🕲 **Alert:** Risk of heart attack or stroke can occur as early as the first weeks of NSAID use. Risk appears greater at higher doses. Use lowest effective dose for shortest duration possible.
🕲 **Alert:** NSAIDs increase risk of HF.
• Drug isn't recommended for children.
• Use cautiously in patients with history of peptic ulcer disease, renal dysfunction, HTN, HF, or fluid retention.
Dialyzable drug: Unlikely.
⚠ **Overdose S&S:** Lethargy, drowsiness, nausea, vomiting, epigastric pain, respiratory depression, coma, seizures.

PREGNANCY-LACTATION-REPRODUCTION
🕲 **Alert:** Use during pregnancy only if potential benefit outweighs risk. Avoid use during last trimester because drug may cause premature closure of the ductus arteriosus.
• The drug appears in human milk. Women shouldn't breastfeed during therapy.

NURSING CONSIDERATIONS
• Don't use extended-release form for patients in acute pain.
• Because NSAIDs impair synthesis of renal prostaglandins, they can decrease renal blood flow and lead to reversible renal impairment, especially in patients with renal failure, HF, or liver dysfunction; in elderly patients; and in those taking diuretics. Monitor these patients closely.
• Check renal and hepatic function every 6 months or as indicated.

K

• Monitor BP at start of and throughout therapy.
❸ *Alert:* Watch for and immediately evaluate signs and symptoms of MI (chest pain, shortness of breath or trouble breathing) or stroke (weakness in one part or side of the body, slurred speech).
• Drug decreases platelet adhesion and aggregation, and can prolong bleeding time about 3 to 4 minutes from baseline.

Black Box Warning NSAIDs cause an increased risk of serious GI adverse events, including bleeding, ulceration, and perforation of the stomach or intestines, which can occur at any time during use and without warning signs and symptoms; it can be fatal. Elderly patients are at greater risk. ∎

Black Box Warning NSAIDs may increase the risk of serious thrombotic events, MI, or stroke, which can be fatal. The risk may be greater with longer use or in patients with CV disease or risk factors for CV disease. ∎

• NSAIDs may mask signs and symptoms of infection because of their antipyretic and anti-inflammatory actions.

PATIENT TEACHING

• Tell patient to take drug with or without food and with a full glass of water. If adverse GI reactions occur, patient may take drug with milk or meals.
• Tell patient not to open extended-release capsules.
❸ *Alert:* Advise patient to seek medical attention immediately if chest pain, shortness of breath or trouble breathing, weakness in one part or side of the body, or slurred speech occurs.
• Teach patient signs and symptoms of GI bleeding (blood in vomit, urine, or stool; coffee-ground vomit; and black, tarry stools) and to notify prescriber immediately if any of these occurs.
• Alert patient that using with aspirin, alcohol, other NSAIDs, or corticosteroids may increase risk of adverse GI reactions.
• Warn patient to avoid hazardous activities that require mental alertness until CNS effects are known.
• Because of possibility of sensitivity to the sun, advise patient to use a sunblock, wear protective clothing, and avoid prolonged exposure to sunlight.

• Instruct patient to report problems with vision or hearing immediately.
• Tell patient to protect drug from direct light and excessive heat and humidity.

ketorolac tromethamine (oral, nasal, injection)
KEE-toe-role-ak

Sprix, Toradol❧

Therapeutic class: NSAIDs
Pharmacologic class: NSAIDs

AVAILABLE FORMS
Injection*: 10 mg/mL in 1-mL ampules❧, 15 mg/mL in 1- and 2-mL vials and 1-mL Tubex syringes; 30 mg/mL in 1- and 2-mL single-dose vials, 1- and 2-mL Tubex syringes
Nasal spray: 15.75 mg/spray
Tablets: 10 mg

INDICATIONS & DOSAGES
➤ **Short-term management of moderately severe, acute pain for single-dose treatment**
Adults younger than age 65 and adolescents age 17 and older: 60 mg IM or 30 mg IV.
Adults age 65 and older: 30 mg IM or 15 mg IV.
Adjust-a-dose: For renally impaired patients or those who weigh less than 50 kg, 30 mg IM or 15 mg IV.
➤ **Short-term management of moderately severe, acute pain for multiple-dose treatment**
Adults younger than age 65 and adolescents age 17 and older: 30 mg IM or IV every 6 hours for maximum of 5 days. Maximum daily dose is 120 mg. Or, 31.5 mg (one 15.75-mg spray in each nostril) every 6 to 8 hours; maximum daily dose is 126 mg.
Adults age 65 and older: 15 mg IM or IV every 6 hours for maximum of 5 days. Maximum daily dose is 60 mg. Or, 15.75 mg (1 spray in only one nostril) every 6 to 8 hours; maximum daily dose is 63 mg.
Adjust-a-dose: For renally impaired patients or those who weigh less than 50 kg, 15 mg IM or IV every 6 hours. Maximum daily dose is 60 mg. Or, 15.75 mg (1 spray in only one nostril) every 6 to 8 hours; maximum daily dose is 63 mg.

➤ **Short-term management of moderately severe, acute pain when switching from parenteral to oral administration (oral therapy is indicated only as continuation of parenterally given drug and should never be given without patient first having received parenteral therapy)**

Adults younger than age 65 and adolescents age 17 and older: 20 mg PO as single dose; then 10 mg PO every 4 to 6 hours for maximum of 5 days (combined for both parenteral and oral). Maximum daily dose is 40 mg.

Adults age 65 and older: 10 mg PO as single dose; then 10 mg PO every 4 to 6 hours for maximum of 5 days (combined for both parenteral and oral). Maximum daily dose is 40 mg.

Adjust-a-dose: For renally impaired patients or those who weigh less than 50 kg, give 10 mg PO as single dose; then 10 mg PO every 4 to 6 hours. Maximum daily dose is 40 mg.

ADMINISTRATION
PO
• Give drug with food if GI upset occurs.

IV
▼ Dilute with NSS, D₅W, 5% dextrose and NSS, Ringer solution, lactated Ringer solution, or Plasma-Lyte A.
▼ Give injection over at least 15 seconds.
▼ Protect from light.
▼ **Incompatibilities:** Solutions that result in a relatively low pH, such as hydroxyzine, meperidine, morphine sulfate, and prochlorperazine.

IM
• When appropriate, give by deep IM injection.
• Patient may feel pain at injection site.
• Put pressure on site for 15 to 30 seconds after injection to minimize local effects.

Intranasal
• Discard nasal spray within 24 hours of first dose, even if bottle still contains medication.
• Each 1.7-g bottle contains eight sprays.
• Activate pump before first use by pumping five times.
• Have patient blow nose before use, sit upright or stand, and tilt head slightly forward.
• Insert tip into the nostril, point away from the septum, and spray once.

ACTION
May inhibit prostaglandin synthesis to produce anti-inflammatory, analgesic, and antipyretic effects.

Route	Onset	Peak	Duration
PO	30–60 min	2–3 hr	4–6 hr
IV, IM	About 30 min	≤2–3 hr	4–6 hr
Intranasal	20 min	¾ hr	Unknown

Half-life: PO, 2 to 9 hours; IV, 5 to 6 hours; IM, 5 to 6 hours; intranasal, 5 to 6 hours.

ADVERSE REACTIONS
CNS: headache, dizziness, drowsiness. **CV:** edema, HTN. **EENT:** tinnitus. Nasal spray only: increased lacrimation, nasal discomfort, rhinalgia, rhinitis, throat irritation. **GI:** dyspepsia, GI pain, nausea, constipation, diarrhea, flatulence, peptic ulceration, stomatitis, vomiting, *GI hemorrhage.* **GU:** renal impairment. **Hematologic:** anemia, decreased platelet adhesion, prolonged bleeding time, purpura. **Skin:** diaphoresis, pruritus, rash. **Other:** pain at injection site.

INTERACTIONS
Drug-drug. *ACE inhibitors, ARBs:* May cause renal impairment, particularly in volume-depleted patients. Avoid using together in volume-depleted patients.
Anticoagulants: May increase anticoagulant levels in the blood. Use together with extreme caution and monitor patient closely.
Antihypertensives, diuretics: May increase nephrotoxicity. May decrease effectiveness. Monitor patient closely.
Disulfiram: May cause severe alcohol intolerance because injection form contains alcohol. Don't use together.
Lithium: May increase lithium level. Monitor patient closely for lithium toxicity.
Methotrexate: May decrease methotrexate clearance and increase toxicity. Avoid using together.
Pentoxifylline: May increase risk of bleeding. Use together is contraindicated.
Probenecid: May increase level and toxicity of ketorolac. Use together is contraindicated.
Salicylates: May increase risk of bleeding. Use together is contraindicated.
SSRIs: May increase risk of GI bleeding. Use together cautiously.

K

Drug-herb. *Dong quai, feverfew, garlic, ginger, horse chestnut, red clover:* May cause bleeding. Discourage use together. *White willow:* Herb and drug contain similar components. Discourage use together.
Drug-lifestyle. *Alcohol use:* May increase risk of GI bleeding. Use with caution. *Smoking:* May increase risk of GI bleeding. Discourage use together.

EFFECTS ON LAB TEST RESULTS
• May increase ALT and AST levels.
• May decrease Hb level and hematocrit.
• May increase bleeding time.
• May lead to false-positive aldosterone/renin ratio.

CONTRAINDICATIONS & CAUTIONS
Black Box Warning Drug is contraindicated in patients who have previously demonstrated hypersensitivity to ketorolac or allergic manifestations to aspirin or other NSAIDs. Hypersensitivity reactions, ranging from bronchospasm to anaphylactic shock, have occurred and appropriate counteractive measures must be available when first dose of ketorolac injection is given. ■
Black Box Warning Contraindicated in children younger than age 17, as prophylactic analgesic before major surgery, and intraoperatively when hemostasis is critical; in patients with advanced renal impairment; and in those at risk for renal failure from volume depletion. ■
Black Box Warning Contraindicated in patients with suspected or confirmed cerebrovascular bleeding, hemorrhagic diathesis, or incomplete hemostasis, and in those at high risk for bleeding because drug inhibits platelet function. ■
Black Box Warning NSAIDs can cause peptic ulcers, GI bleeding, or perforation of the stomach or intestines, which can be fatal. These events can occur at any time during therapy and without warning. Contraindicated in patients with active peptic ulcer disease, recent GI bleeding or perforation, and a history of peptic ulcer disease or GI bleeding. Elderly patients are at greater risk for serious GI events. ■
Black Box Warning Contraindicated for treatment of perioperative pain in patients requiring CABG surgery. ■

Black Box Warning Contraindicated in patients currently receiving aspirin, probenecid, or other NSAIDs because of the cumulative risks of inducing serious NSAID-related adverse reactions. ■
Black Box Warning NSAIDs can increase risk of heart attack or stroke in patients with or without heart disease or risk factors for heart disease. Risk of heart attack or stroke can occur as early as the first weeks of NSAID use. Risk appears greater at higher doses. Use lowest effective dose for shortest duration possible. ■
❸ *Alert:* NSAIDs increase risk of HF.
• Use cautiously in patients who are elderly or have hepatic or renal impairment or cardiac decompensation.
Dialyzable drug: Unlikely.
⚠ *Overdose S&S:* Abdominal pain, nausea, vomiting, peptic ulcers, GI bleeding, renal dysfunction, HTN, lethargy, drowsiness, respiratory depression, coma, anaphylaxis.

PREGNANCY-LACTATION-REPRODUCTION
Black Box Warning Contraindicated in women during labor and delivery because drug may adversely affect fetal circulation and inhibit uterine contractions. ■
❸ *Alert:* Carefully weigh risks and benefits of use during pregnancy. Avoid use in late pregnancy due to effect on fetal CV system.
• Prolonged use of NSAIDs in women of childbearing potential may be associated with infertility that's reversible upon drug discontinuation.
• Low concentrations of drug appear in human milk. Use cautiously in breastfeeding women.

NURSING CONSIDERATIONS
• Correct hypovolemia before giving drug.
Black Box Warning Drug is indicated for short-term management (up to 5 days in adults) of moderately severe acute pain that requires analgesia at the opioid level and only as continuation treatment after IV or IM dosing, if necessary. Total combined duration of use of nasal spray, tablets, and injection shouldn't exceed 5 days because of increased risk of serious adverse events. Recommended total daily dose of ketorolac tablets (maximum, 40 mg) is significantly lower than for ketorolac injection (maximum, 120 mg). ■

Black Box Warning Contraindicated for epidural or intrathecal administration because of its alcohol content. ∎

Black Box Warning Drug isn't indicated for minor or long-term painful conditions. ∎

⚠ **Alert:** Watch for and immediately evaluate signs and symptoms of heart attack (chest pain, shortness of breath or trouble breathing) or stroke (weakness in one part or side of the body, slurred speech).

• Carefully observe patients with coagulopathies and those taking anticoagulants. Drug inhibits platelet aggregation and can prolong bleeding time.

Black Box Warning NSAIDs may increase the risk of serious thrombotic events, MI, or stroke, which can be fatal. The risk may be greater with longer use or in patients with CV disease or risk factors for CV disease. ∎

Black Box Warning Adjust dosage for patients age 65 and older, weighing less than 50 kg, and with moderately elevated serum creatinine level. Doses of ketorolac injection aren't to exceed 60 mg (total dose per day) in these patients. ∎

• NSAIDs may mask signs and symptoms of infection because of their antipyretic and anti-inflammatory actions.

• **Look alike–sound alike:** Don't confuse ketorolac with Ketalar.

PATIENT TEACHING

• Tell patient to discard nasal spray within 24 hours of the first dose, even if medication remains in the bottle.

• Warn patient using nasal spray that transient, mild to moderate nasal irritation may occur that lasts for a few minutes and won't worsen with next dose.

• Advise patient to take a sip of water after using nasal spray to decrease throat sensation.

• Teach patient to read package insert and full directions for use of nasal spray bottle.

• Warn patient not to take ketorolac with other NSAIDs.

⚠ **Alert:** Advise patient to seek medical attention immediately for chest pain, shortness of breath or trouble breathing, weakness in one part or side of the body, or slurred speech.

• Advise patient to maintain adequate fluid intake.

• Tell patient to promptly report edema and weight gain.

• Teach patient the warning signs and symptoms of hepatotoxicity (nausea, fatigue, lethargy, pruritus, jaundice, right upper quadrant abdominal tenderness, flulike symptoms). Advise patient to stop drug and seek medical help immediately if they occur.

• Instruct female patient to notify prescriber immediately if she is pregnant.

• Warn patient receiving drug IM that pain may occur at injection site.

• Teach patient signs and symptoms of GI bleeding (including blood in vomit, urine, or stool; coffee-ground vomit; and black, tarry stools) and to notify prescriber immediately if any of these occurs.

• Tell patient not to take drug for more than 5 days in a row.

SAFETY ALERT!

labetalol hydrochloride
la-BET-ah-loll

Trandate❖

Therapeutic class: Antihypertensives
Pharmacologic class: Alpha–beta blockers

AVAILABLE FORMS

Injection: 5 mg/mL in 20- and 40-mL multiple-dose vials and 4-mL syringes
Tablets: 100 mg, 200 mg, 300 mg

INDICATIONS & DOSAGES

➤ **HTN**

Adults (inpatients after IV therapy): Once supine diastolic BP has begun to rise, give 200 mg PO, followed by 200 to 400 mg PO in 6 to 12 hours depending on BP response. May increase by 200 mg PO b.i.d. at 1-day intervals. Usual dosage range is 100 to 300 mg PO b.i.d.

Adults (outpatients): 100 mg PO b.i.d. with or without a diuretic. If needed, dosage is increased to 200 mg b.i.d. after 2 to 3 days. Further increases may be made every 2 to 3 days until optimal response is reached. Usual maintenance dosage is 200 to 400 mg b.i.d. Maximum dose is 2.4 g daily in two divided doses given alone or with a diuretic.

▶ **Severe HTN, hypertensive emergencies**
Adults (inpatients): 200 mg diluted in 160 mL of a commonly used IV fluid infused at 2 mg/minute IV or 200 mg diluted in 250 mL of a commonly used IV fluid and administered at 3 mL/minute IV until satisfactory response is obtained; then infusion is stopped. Maximum dose is 300 mg.

Or, give by repeated IV injection; initially, 20 mg IV slowly over 2 minutes. Repeat injections of 40 to 80 mg every 10 minutes until maximum dose of 300 mg is reached, as needed.

ADMINISTRATION

PO
• If dizziness occurs, give dose at bedtime or in smaller doses t.i.d.
• Administer in a consistent manner with regard to meals.

IV
▼ Give by slow, direct IV injection over 2 minutes at 10-minute intervals.
▼ For IV infusion, prepare by diluting with D$_5$W, NSS, or other compatible IV solution (refer to manufacturer's instructions for other compatible solutions) to yield 1 mg/mL or 2 mg/3 mL. Infuse at 2 mg/minute.
▼ Give labetalol infusion with an infusion-control device.
▼ Monitor BP during and after completion of infusion or IV injections.
▼ Patient should remain supine for 3 hours after infusion. When given IV for hypertensive emergencies, drug produces a rapid, predictable fall in BP within 5 to 10 minutes.
▼ Store at room temperature. Protect from light.
▼ **Incompatibilities:** Alkali solutions, furosemide.

ACTION
May be related to reduced peripheral vascular resistance, as a result of alpha and beta blockade.

Route	Onset	Peak	Duration
PO	20–120 min	1–2 hr	8–12 hr
IV	2–5 min	5–15 min	16–18 hr

Half-life: IV, about 5½ hours; oral, 6 to 8 hours.

ADVERSE REACTIONS
CNS: dizziness, fatigue, headache, paresthesia, transient scalp tingling, syncope, vertigo, asthenia, somnolence. **CV:** edema, orthostatic hypotension, flushing, *ventricular arrhythmias.* **EENT:** nasal congestion. **GI:** nausea, vomiting, dyspepsia, taste distortion. **GU:** sexual dysfunction, urine retention. **Respiratory:** *bronchospasm,* dyspnea, wheezing. **Skin:** rash, increased sweating, pruritus.

INTERACTIONS
Drug-drug. *Beta agonists:* May blunt bronchodilator effect of these drugs in patients with bronchospasm. May need to increase dosages of these drugs.
Cardiac glycosides: May increase risk of bradycardia. Monitor therapy.
Cimetidine: May enhance labetalol's effect. Use together cautiously.
CV drugs, diuretics: May increase hypotensive effects. Monitor BP.
Halothane: May increase hypotensive effect. Monitor BP closely.
Insulin, oral antidiabetics: May alter dosage requirements in previously stabilized diabetic patient. Monitor patient closely.
Nitroglycerin: May blunt reflex tachycardia produced by nitroglycerin but not the hypotension. Monitor BP if used together.
NSAIDs: May decrease antihypertensive effects. Monitor BP.
TCAs: May increase incidence of tremor. Monitor patient for tremor.
Drug-herb. *Ma huang:* May decrease antihypertensive effects. Discourage use together.

EFFECTS ON LAB TEST RESULTS
• May increase transaminase, creatinine, and urea levels.
• May cause false-positive increase of urine free and total catecholamine levels when measured by a nonspecific trihydroxyindole fluorometric method. May cause false-positive test result for amphetamines when screening urine for drugs.

CONTRAINDICATIONS & CAUTIONS
• Contraindicated in patients hypersensitive to drug or its components and in those with bronchial asthma (history of obstructive

---

Reactions in bold italics are *life-threatening*. Interactions may have a *rapid onset* or a *delayed onset*.

airway disease), overt HF, greater than first-degree heart block (except in patients with a functioning pacemaker), cardiogenic shock, severe bradycardia, and other conditions that may cause severe and prolonged hypotension.
• Use cautiously in patients with HF, hepatic failure, chronic bronchitis, emphysema, PVD, and pheochromocytoma.
Dialyzable drug: No.
⚠ *Overdose S&S:* Orthostatic hypotension, bradycardia, HF, bronchospasm, seizures.

PREGNANCY-LACTATION-REPRODUCTION
• There are no adequate studies in pregnant women. Use during pregnancy only if potential benefit justifies potential risk to the fetus.
• Low amounts of drug appear in human milk and can be detected in the serum of breastfeeding infants. Use cautiously in breastfeeding women.

NURSING CONSIDERATIONS
• Monitor BP frequently. Drug masks common signs and symptoms of shock.
• Keep patient supine while patient is receiving IV therapy. Monitor BP closely before allowing patient to ambulate.
• In diabetic patients, monitor glucose level closely because beta blockers may mask certain signs and symptoms of hypoglycemia.
• Don't routinely withdraw long-term beta-blocker therapy before surgery.
• Rare occurrences of severe hepatic injury have been reported. Monitor LFTs.

PATIENT TEACHING
🔔 *Alert:* Tell patient that stopping drug abruptly can worsen chest pain and trigger a heart attack.
• Advise patient to take drug in a consistent manner with regard to meals.
• Advise patient that dizziness is the most common adverse reaction and tends to occur in the early stages of treatment, in patients taking diuretics, and with higher dosages. Inform patient that dizziness can be minimized by rising slowly and avoiding sudden position changes.
• Warn patient that occasional, harmless scalp tingling may occur, especially when therapy begins.

lacosamide
lah-COSS-ah-mide

Vimpat

Therapeutic class: Anticonvulsants
Pharmacologic class: Functionalized amino acids
Controlled substance schedule: V

AVAILABLE FORMS
Injection: 200 mg/20 mL vials
Oral solution: 10 mg/mL
Tablets: 50 mg, 100 mg, 150 mg, 200 mg

INDICATIONS & DOSAGES
Adjust-a-dose (for all indications): In patients with mild or moderate hepatic impairment, ESRD, or severe renal impairment (CrCl of 30 mL/minute or less), reduce maximum recommended daily dosage by 25%. Withhold drug in patients with severe hepatic impairment. Dosage supplementation of up to 50% should be considered following a 4-hour hemodialysis treatment. Reduce dosage as needed in patients with hepatic or renal impairment who are taking strong CYP3A4 and CYP2C9 inhibitors because of increased lacosamide exposure.
➤ **Adjunctive therapy for partial-onset seizures**
Adults and adolescents age 17 and older: Initially, 50 mg PO b.i.d.; increase by 50 mg b.i.d. at weekly intervals to recommended daily dosage of 100 to 200 mg PO b.i.d. Or, initially 200 mg PO as a single loading dose followed approximately 12 hours later by 100 mg PO b.i.d. for 1 week. Then, increase by 50 mg b.i.d. as needed based on patient response and tolerance up to recommended maintenance dose of 200 mg b.i.d. May administer IV at an equivalent daily dosage and frequency when oral administration is temporarily not feasible.
Children ages 4 to younger than 17: In patients weighing 50 kg or more, same dosing as adults; in those weighing 30 to less than 50 kg, initially, 1 mg/kg PO b.i.d.; increase as needed by 1 mg/kg b.i.d. at weekly intervals to recommended daily dosage of 2 to 4 mg/kg PO b.i.d.; in those weighing 11 to less than 30 kg, initially 1 mg/kg PO

b.i.d.; increase as needed by 1 mg/kg b.i.d. at weekly intervals to recommended daily dosage of 3 to 6 mg/kg PO b.i.d.

➤ **Monotherapy for partial-onset seizures**
Adults and adolescents age 17 and older:
Initially, 100 mg PO b.i.d.; increase at weekly intervals by 50 mg b.i.d. to recommended daily dosage of 150 to 200 mg PO b.i.d. Or, initially 200 mg PO as a single loading dose followed approximately 12 hours later by 100 mg PO b.i.d. for 1 week. Then, increase by 50 mg b.i.d. as needed based on patient response and tolerance up to recommended maintenance dose of 150 to 200 mg PO b.i.d. When converting from another single antiepileptic, titrate lacosamide to therapeutic dose of 150 to 200 mg PO b.i.d. and maintain for at least 3 days before initiating withdrawal of concomitant drug. Gradually withdraw concomitant drug over at least 6 weeks. May administer drug IV at an equivalent daily dosage and frequency when oral administration is temporarily not feasible.
Children ages 4 to younger than 17: In patients weighing 50 kg or more, same dosing as adults; in those weighing 30 to less than 50 kg, initially, 1 mg/kg PO b.i.d.; increase as needed by 1 mg/kg b.i.d. at weekly intervals to recommended daily dosage of 2 to 4 mg/kg PO b.i.d.; in those weighing 11 to less than 30 kg, initially, 1 mg/kg PO b.i.d.; increase as needed by 1 mg/kg b.i.d. at weekly intervals to recommended daily dosage of 3 to 6 mg/kg PO b.i.d.

ADMINISTRATION
PO
• Give drug with or without food.
• Use a calibrated measuring device to administer oral solution.
• May also give oral solution by NG or gastrostomy tube.
• Discard unused oral solution remaining after 7 weeks of first opening bottle.
IV
▼ Don't use injectable form in patients younger than age 17.
▼ Dilute with NSS, D₅W, or lactated Ringer solution. Discard solution if discolored or if particulate matter is present. Diluted solution is stable for 4 hours at room temperature. May administer without further dilution.
▼ Infuse over 15 to 60 minutes; 30 to 60 minutes is preferred.
▼ Discard unused solution in vial.
▼ Limit IV use to 5 days of consecutive treatment.
▼ **Incompatibilities:** None known.

ACTION
May selectively enhance slow inactivation of sodium channels, stabilizing hyperexcitable neuronal membranes and inhibiting repetitive neuronal firing.

Route	Onset	Peak	Duration
PO	Unknown	1–4 hr	Unknown
IV	Unknown	30–60 min	Unknown

Half-life: About 13 hours.

ADVERSE REACTIONS
CNS: asthenia, ataxia, balance disorder, depression, dizziness, fatigue, gait disturbance, headache, memory impairment, somnolence, oral paresthesia or hypoesthesia, tremor. **EENT:** blurred vision, diplopia, nystagmus, vertigo. **GI:** diarrhea, nausea, vomiting. **Skin:** pruritus, skin laceration. **Other:** contusion, injection-site pain or discomfort.

INTERACTIONS
Drug-drug. *Drugs that prolong PR interval (beta blockers, calcium channel blockers):* May increase risk of bradycardia or AV block. Monitor patient closely, especially with IV formulation.
Drug-lifestyle. *Alcohol use:* May cause additive drowsiness. Don't use together.

EFFECTS ON LAB TEST RESULTS
• May increase LFT values.

CONTRAINDICATIONS & CAUTIONS
• Not recommended for patients with severe hepatic impairment.
• Use cautiously in patients with known cardiac conduction problems, depression, myocardial ischemia, or HF and in those with a history of suicidal thoughts.
• Drug may predispose patients to atrial fibrillation or flutter, especially patients with diabetic neuropathy or CV disease.

• Use cautiously in patients with phenylke-tonuria because oral solution contains phenylalanine.

• Safety and effectiveness in children younger than age 17 haven't been estab-lished.

Dialyzable drug: 50%.

⚠ *Overdose S&S:* Coma.

PREGNANCY-LACTATION-REPRODUCTION

• There are no adequate studies in pregnant women. Use during pregnancy only if po-tential benefit justifies potential risk to the fetus.

• Encourage pregnant women taking drug to enroll in the Antiepileptic Drug (AED) Pregnancy Registry (1-888-233-2334 or www.aedpregnancyregistry.org).

• It isn't known if drug appears in human milk. Patient should discontinue breastfeed-ing or discontinue drug.

NURSING CONSIDERATIONS

❸ *Alert:* Give loading dose under medical su-pervision because of increased risk of CNS adverse reactions.

❸ *Alert:* Monitor patient for syncopal episodes; drug may increase risk of syncope, especially in patients with cardiac disease and in those receiving drugs that slow AV conduction.

❸ *Alert:* Obtain ECG before starting ther-apy and after titrating to maintenance dose in patients with known conduction problems (marked first-degree AV block, second- or third-degree AV block, or sick sinus syn-drome without pacemaker), sodium chan-nelopathies (Brugada syndrome), concomi-tant use of drugs that prolong PR interval, or severe cardiac disease (MI, HF, struc-tural heart disease). Also closely monitor this population when giving IV lacosamide.

• Monitor patient for signs and symptoms of DRESS syndrome, including fever, rash, eosinophilia, hepatitis, nephritis, lym-phadenopathy, and myocarditis. If reaction is suspected, discontinue drug and begin al-ternative treatment.

• Titrate dosage carefully in patients with renal or hepatic impairment.

❸ *Alert:* Withdraw drug gradually over 1 week to minimize potential for increased seizure activity.

❸ *Alert:* Drug may increase risk of suici-dal thinking and behavior. Monitor patient closely for worsening depression, suicidal thoughts or behavior, and unusual changes in mood or behavior.

PATIENT TEACHING

• Inform patient that drug may be taken without regard to meals.

• Tell patient to report mood changes or suicidal thoughts immediately.

• Warn patient to avoid driving and operat-ing heavy machinery until drug's CNS ef-fects are known; drug may cause dizziness and ataxia.

• Advise female patient to notify prescriber if she suspects or is considering pregnancy or plans to breastfeed.

• Warn patient not to stop drug abruptly.

• Tell patient to avoid alcohol while taking drug.

• Tell patient taking oral solution to use a calibrated measuring device and to discard unused oral solution remaining after 7 weeks of first opening bottle.

• Inform patient with phenylketonuria that a 200-mg dose of oral solution contains 0.32 mg of phenylalanine.

• Advise patient to report blurred vision, dizziness, double vision, nausea, uncoordi-nated movement, or vertigo.

lamiVUDine (3TC)
lam-ah-VEW-den

Epivir, Epivir-HBV, Heptovir✦

Therapeutic class: Antiretrovirals
Pharmacologic class: Nucleoside–nucleotide reverse transcriptase inhibitors

AVAILABLE FORMS
Epivir
Oral solution: 10 mg/mL
Tablets: 150 mg, 300 mg
Epivir-HBV
Oral solution: 5 mg/mL
Tablets: 100 mg

INDICATIONS & DOSAGES
Black Box Warning Lamivudine tablets and oral solution used to treat HIV-1

infection contain a higher dose of the active ingredient than do lamivudine tablets and oral solution used to treat chronic HBV infection. Patients with HIV-1 infection should receive only dosing forms appropriate for HIV-1 treatment. ■

➤ **HIV infection, with other antiretrovirals**
Adults: 300 mg Epivir PO once daily or 150 mg PO b.i.d.
Children ages 3 months and older: 5 mg/kg Epivir solution PO b.i.d. or 10 mg/kg PO once daily. Maximum dose is 300 mg daily.
Children weighing 14 kg or more who can reliably swallow tablets: For 14 to less than 20 kg, give 1 tablet (150 mg) PO once daily or ½ tablet (75 mg) PO b.i.d.; for 20 kg to less than 25 kg, give 1½ tablets (225 mg) PO once daily or ½ tablet (75 mg) PO in morning and 1 tablet (150 mg) PO in evening; for 25 kg or more, give 2 tablets (300 mg) PO once daily or 150 mg PO b.i.d.
Adjust-a-dose: For adults and adolescents weighing 25 kg or more with HIV infection and CrCl of 30 to 49 mL/minute, give 150 mg Epivir PO daily. If CrCl is 15 to 29 mL/minute, give 150 mg PO on day 1 and then 100 mg daily; if CrCl is 5 to 14 mL/minute, give 150 mg on day 1 and then 50 mg daily; if CrCl is less than 5 mL/minute, give 50 mg on day 1 and then 25 mg daily. Although there are insufficient data to recommend a specific dosage adjustment in children with renal impairment, consider a dosage reduction or an increase in the dosing interval.

➤ **Chronic HBV infection with evidence of HBV replication and active liver inflammation**
Adults: 100 mg Epivir-HBV PO once daily.
Children ages 2 to 17 years: 3 mg/kg Epivir-HBV PO once daily, up to a maximum dose of 100 mg daily. Use oral solution for doses less than 100 mg and in patients unable to swallow tablets. Optimum treatment duration isn't known.
Adjust-a-dose: For adults with chronic HBV infection and CrCl of 30 to 49 mL/minute, give first dose of 100 mg Epivir-HBV; then give 50 mg PO once daily. If CrCl is 15 to 29 mL/minute, give first dose of 100 mg; then give 25 mg PO once daily. If CrCl is 5 to 14 mL/minute, give first dose

of 35 mg; then give 15 mg PO once daily. If CrCl is less than 5 mL/minute, give first dose of 35 mg; then give 10 mg PO once daily. There are insufficient data to recommend a specific dosage in children with renal impairment.

ADMINISTRATION
PO
• Give without regard for food.

ACTION
A synthetic nucleoside analogue that inhibits HIV and HBV reverse transcription via viral DNA chain termination. Inhibits RNA- and DNA-dependent DNA polymerase activities.

Route	Onset	Peak	Duration
PO	Unknown	1–3 hr	Unknown

Half-life: Adults, 5 to 7 hours; children, 2 hours.

ADVERSE REACTIONS
Adverse reactions pertain to the combination therapy of lamivudine and zidovudine.
CNS: dizziness, fatigue, fever, headache, insomnia and other sleep disorders, malaise, neuropathy, depressive disorders, paresthesia. **EENT:** nasal symptoms. **GI:** anorexia, diarrhea, nausea, vomiting, abdominal cramps, abdominal pain, dyspepsia. **Hematologic:** *neutropenia, thrombocytopenia,* anemia. **Hepatic:** hepatomegaly (children), *hepatotoxicity.* **Metabolic:** *lactic acidosis.* **Musculoskeletal:** musculoskeletal pain, arthralgia, myalgia. **Respiratory:** cough. **Skin:** rash. **Other:** chills.

INTERACTIONS
Drug-drug. *Emtricitabine:* May increase adverse or toxic effects of emtricitabine. Avoid combination.
Orlistat: May decrease serum concentrations of antivirals. Use cautiously together.
Trimethoprim-containing drugs: May increase lamivudine level because of decreased clearance of drug. Monitor patient for toxicity.

EFFECTS ON LAB TEST RESULTS
• May increase ALT, bilirubin, and serum lipase and CK levels.
• May decrease Hb level and neutrophil and platelet counts.

Reactions in bold italics are *life-threatening*. Interactions may have a *rapid onset* or a *delayed onset*.

CONTRAINDICATIONS & CAUTIONS

◑ *Alert:* Lactic acidosis and severe hepatomegaly with steatosis, including fatal cases, have been reported.

• Contraindicated in patients hypersensitive to drug.

• Use cautiously in patients with renal impairment.

• Don't use with other combination drugs containing lamivudine or emtricitabine.

• Safety and effectiveness of lamivudine haven't been established for treatment of chronic HBV infection in patients dually infected with HIV-1 and HBV. Emergence of HBV variants associated with resistance to lamivudine has also been reported in HIV-1-infected patients who have received lamivudine-containing antiretroviral regimens in the presence of concurrent HBV infection.

• Use Epivir-HBV only when an alternative antiviral with a higher genetic barrier to resistance isn't available or appropriate. Drug hasn't been evaluated in patients with HBV/HIV-1 coinfection, HCV infection, or hepatitis delta virus; in patients with chronic HBV infection with decompensated liver disease; or in liver transplant recipients.

◑ *Alert:* Use drug cautiously, if at all, in children with history of pancreatitis or other significant risk factors for development of pancreatitis.

Dialyzable drug: Unknown.

PREGNANCY-LACTATION-REPRODUCTION

• There are no adequate studies of Epivir-HBV use in pregnant women. Use during pregnancy only if potential benefit justifies potential risk to the fetus.

• Epivir is one of the preferred drugs used for the treatment of HIV infection in pregnant women.

• The Antiretroviral Pregnancy Registry monitors maternal-fetal outcomes of pregnant women exposed to lamivudine. To register, call the registry at 1-800-258-4263.

• Because of the potential for HIV transmission, women taking Epivir shouldn't breastfeed.

• Epivir-HBV appears in human milk. Because of the potential for serious adverse reactions in breastfed infants, a decision should be made whether to discontinue breastfeeding, taking into consideration importance of continued HBV therapy to the mother and the benefits of breastfeeding.

NURSING CONSIDERATIONS

◑ *Alert:* Stop treatment immediately and notify prescriber if signs, symptoms, or laboratory abnormalities suggest pancreatitis. Monitor amylase level.

◑ *Alert:* Lactic acidosis and hepatotoxicity have been reported. Notify prescriber if signs of lactic acidosis or hepatotoxicity occur.

◑ *Alert:* Epivir scored tablet is the preferred formulation for HIV-1-infected children who weigh at least 14 kg and for whom a solid dosage form is appropriate because the oral solution has been shown to have lower rates of virologic suppression and lower plasma lamivudine exposure, and patients developed viral resistance more frequently. Monitor HIV-1 viral load more frequently when using Epivir oral solution.

Black Box Warning Severe acute exacerbations of hepatitis B have been reported in patients coinfected with HBV and HIV-1 and who have discontinued lamivudine or anti–hepatitis B therapy (including Epivir-HBV). Monitor hepatic function closely with both clinical and laboratory follow-up for at least several months in patients who discontinue lamivudine and are coinfected with HIV-1 and HBV or who discontinue anti–hepatitis B therapy. If appropriate, initiation of anti-HBV therapy may be warranted. ∎

Black Box Warning Provide HIV counseling and test patients for HIV before starting treatment and during therapy because form and dosage of lamivudine in Epivir-HBV aren't appropriate for those infected with both HBV and HIV. If lamivudine is given to patients with HBV and HIV, use the higher dosage indicated for HIV therapy as part of an appropriate combination regimen. ∎

• Monitor patient's CBC, platelet count, LFTs, and renal function studies. Report abnormalities.

• To reduce risk of resistance in patients receiving Epivir-HBV monotherapy, consider switching to an alternative regimen if serum HBV DNA remains detectable after

24 weeks of treatment. Guide optimal therapy by resistance testing.

PATIENT TEACHING

• Inform patient that long-term effects of drug aren't known.

• Stress importance of taking drug exactly as prescribed.

Black Box Warning Offer HIV counseling and testing to all patients before beginning treatment with Epivir-HBV and periodically during treatment because Epivir-HBV contains a lower dose of the same active ingredient as in lamivudine tablets and oral solution used to treat HIV. If treatment with Epivir-HBV is prescribed for chronic HBV infection in patient with unrecognized or untreated HIV infection, HIV resistance is likely because of the subtherapeutic dose and inappropriate monotherapy. ■

• Inform patient that drug doesn't cure HIV infection, that opportunistic infections and other complications of HIV infection may still occur, and that transmission of HIV to others through sexual contact or blood contamination is still possible.

• Teach parents or guardians signs and symptoms of pancreatitis. Advise them to report signs and symptoms immediately.

---

lamoTRIgine
la-MO-tri-geen

LaMICtal, LaMICtal CD, LaMICtal ODT, LaMICtal XR

Therapeutic class: Anticonvulsants
Pharmacologic class: Phenyltriazines

AVAILABLE FORMS

Tablets: 25 mg, 100 mg, 150 mg, 200 mg
Tablets (chewable dispersible): 2 mg, 5 mg, 25 mg
Tablets (extended-release) ⓞⓝⓒ: 25 mg, 50 mg, 100 mg, 200 mg, 250 mg, 300 mg
Tablets (ODTs): 25 mg, 50 mg, 100 mg, 200 mg

INDICATIONS & DOSAGES

🟢 *Alert:* Extended-release formula isn't for use as initial monotherapy or for conversion to monotherapy from two or more concomitant antiepileptic drugs (AEDs).

Adjust-a-dose (for all indications): No dosage adjustment is needed in patients with mild hepatic impairment. Generally, reduce initial, escalation, and maintenance doses by approximately 25% in patients with moderate and severe hepatic impairment without ascites and 50% in patients with severe hepatic impairment with ascites. May adjust escalation and maintenance doses according to clinical response. In patients with renal impairment, base initial doses on patients' concomitant medications; reduced maintenance doses may be effective for patients with significant renal impairment. Use cautiously in such patients.

➤ **Conversion to monotherapy using extended-release formula in patients with partial seizures who are receiving treatment with a single enzyme-inducing AED**
Adults and children age 13 and older: Add 50 mg extended-release tablet PO daily to current drug regimen for 2 weeks, followed by 100 mg PO daily for 2 weeks. Then, increase by 100 mg every week until a dosage of 500 mg PO daily is reached. The concomitant enzyme-inducing AED can then be gradually reduced by 20% decrements each week over a 4-week period. Two weeks after completing withdrawal of the enzyme-inducing AED, decrease lamotrigine (extended-release tablet) no faster than 100 mg/day each week to achieve the monotherapy maintenance dosage of 250 to 300 mg/day.

➤ **Conversion to monotherapy using extended-release formula in patients with partial seizures who are receiving adjunctive treatment with valproate**
Adults and children age 13 and older: Add 25 mg extended-release PO every other day for 2 weeks; then increase to 25 mg PO daily for weeks 3 and 4. Increase to 50 mg PO daily for week 5, 100 mg PO daily for week 6, and 150 mg PO daily for week 7. Maintain dosage at 150 mg PO daily while decreasing valproate dosage by no more than 500 mg/day each week until 500 mg/day is achieved; maintain for 1 week. Then, simultaneously increase extended-release tablet to 200 mg/day while decreasing valproate to 250 mg/day; maintain for 1 week. Increase to 250 or 300 mg PO daily as maintenance dosage and discontinue valproate.

Reactions in bold italics are *life-threatening*. Interactions may have a *rapid onset* or a *delayed onset*.

➤ **Conversion to monotherapy using extended-release formula in patients with partial seizures who are receiving treatment with a single drug other than an enzyme-inducing AED or valproate**
Adults and children age 13 and older: Add 25 mg extended-release PO daily for 2 weeks; then increase to 50 mg PO daily for weeks 3 and 4. Increase to 100 mg PO daily for week 5. Starting with week 6, continue increasing dosage each week by 50 mg PO daily until a dosage of 250 to 300 mg PO daily is achieved; then withdraw concomitant AED therapy by 20% decrements each week over a 4-week period. No additional lamotrigine (extended-release tablet) adjustment is needed.

➤ **Adjunctive treatment of partial seizures or primary generalized tonic-clonic seizures caused by epilepsy or generalized seizures of Lennox-Gastaut syndrome**
Adults and children older than age 12 taking valproate: 25 mg immediate-release PO every other day for 2 weeks; then 25 mg PO daily for 2 weeks. Continue to increase, as needed, by 25 to 50 mg daily every 1 to 2 weeks until an effective maintenance dosage of 100 to 400 mg daily given in one or two divided doses is reached. When added to valproate alone, the usual daily maintenance dose is 100 to 200 mg. Or, 25 mg extended-release PO every other day for 2 weeks; then 25 mg PO daily for 2 weeks; then 50 mg PO daily for 1 week; then 100 mg PO daily for 1 week; then 150 mg PO daily for 1 week. Daily maintenance dose is 200 to 250 mg.
Adults and children older than age 12 not taking carbamazepine, phenytoin, phenobarbital, primidone, or valproate: 25 mg extended-release PO daily for 2 weeks; then 50 mg PO daily for 2 weeks; then 100 mg PO daily for 1 week; then 150 mg PO daily for 1 week; then 200 mg PO daily for 1 week. Daily maintenance dose is 300 to 400 mg.
Adults and children older than age 12 taking anticonvulsant drugs but not carbamazepine, phenytoin, phenobarbital, primidone, or valproate: 25 mg immediate-release PO daily for 1 to 2 weeks; then 50 mg PO daily for another 2 weeks.

Continue to increase by 50 mg/day every 1 to 2 weeks until an effective maintenance dose is reached. Daily maintenance dose is 225 to 375 mg PO daily in two divided doses.
Adults and children older than age 12 taking carbamazepine, phenytoin, phenobarbital, or primidone but not valproate: 50 mg immediate-release PO daily for 2 weeks; then 100 mg PO daily in two divided doses for 2 weeks. Increase, as needed, by 100 mg daily every 1 to 2 weeks. Usual maintenance dosage is 300 to 500 mg PO daily in two divided doses. Or, 50 mg extended-release PO daily for 2 weeks; then 100 mg PO daily for 2 weeks; then 200 mg PO daily for 1 week; then 300 mg PO daily for 1 week; then 400 mg PO daily for 1 week. Daily maintenance dose is 400 to 600 mg.
Children ages 2 to 12 weighing 7 to 40 kg taking valproate: 0.15 mg/kg immediate-release PO daily in one or two divided doses (rounded down to nearest whole tablet) for 2 weeks. Increase to 0.3 mg/kg daily in one or two divided doses for 2 weeks, followed by increasing the daily dose every 1 or 2 weeks with an additional 0.3 mg/kg daily in one or two divided doses. Thereafter, usual maintenance dosage is 1 to 5 mg/kg daily (maximum, 200 mg daily in one to two divided doses). In patients weighing less than 30 kg, maintenance dosage may need to be increased by as much as 50% based on clinical response.
Children ages 2 to 12 weighing 7 to 40 kg taking anticonvulsant drugs but not carbamazepine, phenytoin, phenobarbital, primidone, or valproate: 0.3 mg/kg immediate-release PO daily in one or two divided doses (rounded down to the nearest whole tablet) for 2 weeks; then 0.6 mg/kg PO daily in two divided doses for another 2 weeks; then increase the daily dose every 1 to 2 weeks with an additional 0.6 mg/kg PO daily in two divided doses. Thereafter, usual maintenance dose is 4.5 to 7.5 mg/kg PO daily. Maximum dose is 300 mg daily in two divided doses. In patients weighing less than 30 kg, maintenance dosage may need to be increased by as much as 50% based on clinical response.
Children ages 2 to 12 weighing 7 to 40 kg taking carbamazepine, phenytoin, phenobarbital, or primidone but not

L

valproate: 0.6 mg/kg immediate-release PO daily in two divided doses (rounded down to nearest whole tablet) for 2 weeks. Increase to 1.2 mg/kg PO daily in two divided doses for 2 weeks; then increase the daily dose every 1 to 2 weeks with an additional 1.2 mg/kg daily in two divided doses. Usual maintenance dosage is 5 to 15 mg/kg PO daily (maximum 400 mg daily in two divided doses). In patients weighing less than 30 kg, maintenance dosage may need to be increased by as much as 50% based on clinical response.

➤ **To convert patients from therapy with a hepatic enzyme-inducing AED alone to lamotrigine therapy**
Adults and children age 16 and older: Add 50 mg immediate-release PO once daily to current drug regimen for 2 weeks, followed by 100 mg PO daily in two divided doses for 2 weeks. Then increase daily dosage by 100 mg every 1 to 2 weeks until maintenance dose of 500 mg daily in two divided doses is reached. The concomitant hepatic enzyme-inducing AED can then be gradually reduced by 20% decrements weekly for 4 weeks.

➤ **To convert patients with partial seizures from adjunctive therapy with valproate to therapy with lamotrigine alone**
Adults and children age 16 and older: Add immediate-release form until 200 mg daily is achieved; then gradually decrease valproate to 500 mg daily by decrements of no more than 500 mg daily per week. Maintain these dosages for 1 week, then increase lamotrigine to 300 mg daily while decreasing valproate to 250 mg daily. Maintain these dosages for 1 week, then stop valproate completely while increasing lamotrigine by 100 mg daily every week until a dose of 500 mg daily is reached.

➤ **Bipolar disorder for maintenance treatment to delay time to occurrence of mood episodes (depression, mania, hypomania, mixed episodes) in patients treated for acute mood episodes with standard therapy**
Adults: Initially, 25 mg immediate-release PO once daily for 2 weeks; then 50 mg PO once daily for 2 weeks. Dosage may then be doubled at weekly intervals, to maintenance dosage of 200 mg daily.

Adults taking carbamazepine or other hepatic enzyme-inducing drugs without valproate: Initially, 50 mg immediate-release PO once daily for 2 weeks; then 100 mg daily in two divided doses for 2 weeks. Dosage is then increased by 100 mg weekly to maintenance dosage of 400 mg daily, given in two divided doses.
Adults taking valproate: Initially, 25 mg immediate-release PO every other day for 2 weeks; then 25 mg PO once daily for 2 weeks. Dosage may then be doubled at weekly intervals to maintenance dosage of 100 mg daily.

ADMINISTRATION
PO
• Starter and titration kits are available to provide doses consistent with recommended titration schedule for the first 5 weeks of treatment.
• Chewable dispersible tablets may be swallowed whole, chewed, or dispersed in water or diluted fruit juice.
• If tablets are chewed, give a small amount of water or diluted fruit juice to aid in swallowing.
• ODTs should be placed on the tongue and moved around in the mouth.
• ODTs may be swallowed with or without water and without regard to food.
• Give extended-release tablets once daily with or without food. Patient must swallow tablets whole and must not chew, crush, or divide them.

ACTION
Inhibits release of glutamate (an excitatory neurotransmitter) in the brain via action at voltage-sensitive sodium channels. Is a weak inhibitor of the 5-HT$_3$ receptor.

Route	Onset	Peak	Duration
PO (immediate-release)	Unknown	1–5 hr	Unknown
PO (extended-release)	Unknown	4–11 hr	Unknown

Half-life: 7 to 148 hours, depending on age, dosage schedule, use of other anticonvulsants, and other medical conditions.

ADVERSE REACTIONS
CNS: ataxia, dizziness, drowsiness, headache, somnolence, fatigue, anxiety,

---

abnormal thinking, amnesia, depression, confusion, dysarthria, emotional lability, fever, incoordination, insomnia, irritability, malaise, *suicidal ideation.* **CV:** palpitations, chest pain, edema. **EENT:** blurred vision, diplopia, vision abnormality, nystagmus, rhinitis, epistaxis, pharyngitis, sinusitis. **GI:** nausea, vomiting, abdominal pain, anorexia, constipation, diarrhea, dry mouth, dyspepsia, flatulence, rectal hemorrhage, peptic ulcer. **GU:** amenorrhea, dysmenorrhea, urinary frequency, vaginitis, UTI. **Hematologic:** lymphadenopathy. **Metabolic:** weight loss. **Musculoskeletal:** arthralgia, back pain, muscle spasm, neck pain, weakness. **Respiratory:** cough, dyspnea, bronchitis, bronchospasm. **Skin:** rash, dermatitis, dry skin, sweating, photosensitivity. **Other:** infection, accidental injury, flulike syndrome.

INTERACTIONS
Drug-drug. *Acetaminophen:* May decrease therapeutic effects of lamotrigine. Monitor patient.

Atazanavir/ritonavir, ethosuximide, lopinavir/ritonavir, oxcarbazepine, phenobarbital, phenytoin, primidone: May decrease lamotrigine level. Monitor patient closely.

Carbamazepine: May decrease effects of lamotrigine while increasing toxicity of carbamazepine. Adjust doses and monitor patient.

Folate inhibitors (methotrexate, sulfamethoxazole–trimethoprim): May have additive effect because lamotrigine inhibits dihydrofolate reductase, an enzyme involved in folic acid synthesis. Monitor patient.

Hormonal contraceptives containing estrogen, rifampin: May decrease lamotrigine levels. Adjust dosage. By the end of the "pill-free" week, lamotrigine levels may double.

Organic cation transporter 2 substrates: May increase lamotrigine plasma level. Don't coadminister.

Valproate: May decrease clearance of lamotrigine, which increases lamotrigine level; also decreases valproate level. Monitor patient for toxicity.

Drug-lifestyle. *Sun exposure:* May cause photosensitivity reactions. Advise patient to avoid excessive sun exposure.

EFFECTS ON LAB TEST RESULTS
• May result in false-positive readings in rapid urine drug screens, particularly for phencyclidine.

CONTRAINDICATIONS & CAUTIONS
• Contraindicated in patients hypersensitive to drug or its components.
◑ *Alert:* Rare, multiorgan hypersensitivity reactions that can be fatal have occurred.
◑ *Alert:* Drug may cause hemophagocytic lymphohistiocytosis (HLH), a rare and life-threatening immune system reaction.
• Use cautiously in patients with renal, hepatic, or cardiac impairment.
• Drug isn't recommended for treatment of acute manic or mixed episodes of bipolar disorder because effectiveness hasn't been established.
Dialyzable drug: 20%.
⚠ *Overdose S&S:* Ataxia, nystagmus, increased seizures, decreased level of consciousness, coma, intraventricular conduction delay.

PREGNANCY-LACTATION-REPRODUCTION
• There are no adequate studies in pregnant women; in animal studies, lamotrigine was developmentally toxic. Use during pregnancy only if potential benefit justifies potential risk to the fetus.
• Pregnant patients are encouraged to register in the Antiepileptic Drug (AED) Pregnancy Registry (1-888-233-2334).
• Drug appears in human milk. Closely monitor breastfeeding infants for adverse events resulting from drug use. Women should discontinue breastfeeding if infants develop drug toxicity. Use cautiously in breastfeeding women.

NURSING CONSIDERATIONS
◑ *Alert:* Closely monitor all patients taking or starting AEDs for changes in behavior indicating worsening of suicidal thoughts or behavior or depression. Symptoms such as anxiety, agitation, hostility, mania, and hypomania may be precursors to emerging suicidality.

• Don't stop drug abruptly because this may increase seizure frequency. Instead, taper drug over at least 2 weeks.

Black Box Warning Serious rashes, including SJS, requiring hospitalization and discontinuation of treatment have been reported. Most life-threatening rashes have been documented between 2 and 8 weeks of treatment initiation, but isolated cases have been reported with prolonged treatment (e.g., 6 months). Rate of serious rash is greater in children than in adults. Don't exceed initial dose or recommended dosage escalation, or maintain coadministration with valproate. Stop drug at first sign of rash, unless rash is clearly not drug-related. ■

Black Box Warning Stopping treatment may not prevent a rash from becoming life-threatening or permanently disabling or disfiguring. ■

Black Box Warning Extended-release form isn't approved for children younger than age 13. ■

◑ *Alert:* Drug may cause aseptic meningitis. Monitor patient for symptoms such as headache, fever, neck stiffness, nausea, vomiting, rash, and photophobia. Discontinue drug if no other cause of meningitis is found.

• Reduce lamotrigine dose if drug is added to a multidrug regimen that includes valproic acid.

• Evaluate patients for changes in seizure activity. Check adjunct anticonvulsant level.

◑ *Alert:* Monitor patient for HLH (persistent fever, hepatosplenomegaly, rash, lymphadenopathy, neurologic symptoms, cytopenias, high serum ferritin level, and liver function and coagulation abnormalities). Evaluate patient with fever or rash promptly, and discontinue drug if HLH or another serious immune-related reaction is suspected or an alternative cause can't be identified.

• *Look alike–sound alike:* Don't confuse lamotrigine with lamivudine or levothyroxine. Don't confuse Lamictal with Lamisil, labetalol, or Lomotil.

PATIENT TEACHING

• Inform patient that drug may cause rash. Combination therapy of valproic acid and lamotrigine may cause a serious rash. Tell patient to report rash or signs or symptoms

of hypersensitivity promptly to prescriber; drug may need to be stopped.

• Strongly advise patient to visually inspect tablets with each prescription refill to verify the tablets are correct, to avoid medication errors.

• Warn patient not to engage in hazardous activity until drug's CNS effects are known.

• Warn patient to seek immediate medical attention if signs or symptoms of HLH occur, including fever; rash; abdominal pain, tenderness, or swelling; enlarged lymph nodes; yellowing of the skin or eyes; unusual bleeding; seizures; vision changes; or trouble walking.

• Teach patient or caregiver to immediately report headache, fever, mouth ulcers, bruising or petechiae, signs of infection (fever, cough, dyspnea), neck stiffness, nausea, vomiting, rash, drowsiness, confusion, or light sensitivity.

• Warn patient that the drug may trigger sensitivity to the sun and to take precautions until tolerance is determined.

• Warn patient not to stop drug abruptly.

◑ *Alert:* Advise female patient of childbearing potential to discuss drug therapy with prescriber if considering pregnancy. Infants exposed to drug during the first trimester have a greater risk of cleft lip or palate.

• Advise female patient of childbearing potential that breastfeeding isn't recommended during therapy.

lansoprazole
lanz-AH-pray-zol

Prevacid◈, Prevacid SoluTab, Prevacid 24 Hour ◇

Therapeutic class: Antiulcer drugs
Pharmacologic class: PPIs

AVAILABLE FORMS
Capsules (delayed-release) ⓞⓝⓒ*:* 15 mg, 30 mg
Tablets (ODT delayed-release): 15 mg, 30 mg

INDICATIONS & DOSAGES
Adjust-a-dose (for all indications): Recommended dosage in patients with severe

hepatic impairment (Child-Pugh class C) is 15 mg PO daily.

➤ **Short-term treatment of active duodenal ulcer**
Adults: 15 mg PO daily before eating for 4 weeks.

➤ **Maintenance of healed duodenal ulcers**
Adults: 15 mg PO daily.

➤ **Short-term treatment of active benign gastric ulcer**
Adults: 30 mg PO once daily for up to 8 weeks.

➤ **Short-term treatment of erosive esophagitis**
Adults: 30 mg PO daily before eating for up to 8 weeks. If healing doesn't occur, 8 more weeks of therapy may be given. Maintenance dosage for healing is 15 mg PO daily.
Children ages 12 to 17: 30 mg PO once daily for up to 8 weeks.
Children ages 1 to 11 weighing more than 30 kg: 30 mg PO once daily for up to 12 weeks.
Children ages 1 to 11 weighing 30 kg or less: 15 mg PO once daily for up to 12 weeks.

➤ **Long-term treatment of pathologic hypersecretory conditions, including Zollinger-Ellison syndrome**
Adults: Initially, 60 mg PO once daily. Increase dosage, as needed. Give daily amounts above 120 mg in evenly divided doses.

➤ *Helicobacter pylori* **eradication to reduce risk of duodenal ulcer recurrence**
Adults: For patients receiving dual therapy, 30 mg PO lansoprazole with 1 g PO amoxicillin, each given t.i.d. for 14 days. For patients receiving triple therapy, 30 mg PO lansoprazole with 1 g PO amoxicillin and 500 mg PO clarithromycin, all given b.i.d. for 10 to 14 days.

➤ **Short-term treatment of symptomatic GERD**
Adults: 15 mg PO once daily for up to 8 weeks.
Children ages 12 to 17: 15 mg PO once daily for up to 8 weeks.
Children ages 1 to 11 weighing more than 30 kg: 30 mg PO once daily for up to 12 weeks.
Children ages 1 to 11 weighing 30 kg or less: 15 mg PO once daily for up to 12 weeks.

➤ **NSAID-related ulcer in patients who continue NSAID use**
Adults: 30 mg PO daily for 8 weeks.

➤ **To reduce risk of NSAID-related ulcer in patients with history of gastric ulcer who need NSAIDs**
Adults: 15 mg PO daily for up to 12 weeks.

ADMINISTRATION
PO
• Give before a meal.
• Don't crush or allow patient to chew capsules.
• For patients who have difficulty swallowing capsules, the capsules can be opened and the intact granules sprinkled on 1 tablespoon of applesauce, Ensure pudding, cottage cheese, yogurt, or strained pears and swallowed immediately. Or, capsule contents may be emptied into a small volume (60 mL) of apple, orange, or tomato juice and swallowed.
• Contents of capsule can be mixed with 40 mL of apple juice in a syringe and given within 3 to 5 minutes via an NG or nasojejunal tube. Flush with additional apple juice to give entire dose and maintain patency of the tube.
• Place ODT on patient's tongue and allow it to disintegrate with or without water until the particles can be swallowed.
• To give ODTs using an oral syringe, dissolve a 15-mg tablet in 4 mL water or a 30-mg tablet in 10 mL water and give within 15 minutes. Refill syringe with about 2 mL (15-mg tablet) or 5 mL (30-mg tablet) of water, shake gently, and give any remaining contents.
• To give ODTs through an 8 French or larger NG tube, dissolve a 15-mg tablet in 4 mL water or a 30-mg tablet in 10 mL water and give within 15 minutes. Refill syringe with about 5 mL of water, shake gently, and flush the NG tube.
• ODTs contain 2.5 mg phenylalanine/ 15-mg tablet and 5.1 mg phenylalanine/ 30-mg tablet.

ACTION
Reduces acid secretion in gastric parietal cells through inhibition of (H^+, K^+)-ATPase enzyme system, inhibiting the final step in gastric acid production.

L

Route	Onset	Peak	Duration
PO	1–3 hr	1.7 hr	24 hr

Half-life: Less than 2 hours.

ADVERSE REACTIONS
GI: abdominal pain, constipation, diarrhea, nausea.

INTERACTIONS
Drug-drug. *Ampicillin esters, digoxin, erlotinib, iron salts, ketoconazole, mycophenolate mofetil:* May inhibit absorption of these drugs. Monitor patient closely.

Atazanavir, nelfinavir: May reduce GI absorption of atazanavir and nelfinavir, reducing antiviral activity. Don't use together.

Cefuroxime: May reduce cefuroxime absorption. Avoid combination.

Clarithromycin: May increase lansoprazole level and adverse effects. Monitor patient.

Digoxin: May cause hypomagnesemia. Monitor magnesium level before and during treatment.

Methotrexate: May increase methotrexate serum level. Monitor methotrexate concentration and adjust dosage as needed.

Rilpivirine: May decrease rilpivirine concentration. Use together is contraindicated.

Sucralfate: May cause delayed lansoprazole absorption. Give lansoprazole at least 30 minutes before sucralfate.

Tacrolimus: May increase whole blood levels of tacrolimus, especially in transplant patients who are intermediate or poor metabolizers of CYP2C19. Consider therapy modification.

Theophylline: May mildly increase theophylline clearance. Adjust theophylline dosage when lansoprazole is started or stopped. Use together cautiously.

Warfarin: May increase bleeding risk. Monitor INR and PT.

Drug-herb. *St. John's wort:* May increase risk of sun sensitivity. Advise patient to avoid excessive sunlight exposure.

Drug-food. *Any food:* May decrease rate and extent of GI absorption. Advise patient to take before meals.

EFFECTS ON LAB TEST RESULTS
• May increase LFT values and creatinine, serum potassium, and serum urea levels.

May increase gastrin, globulin, and LDH levels.

• May increase or decrease electrolyte levels.

• May cause abnormal CBC. May increase or decrease WBC and platelet counts.

• May cause false-positive results in diagnostic investigations for neuroendocrine tumors, urine screening tests for tetrahydrocannabinol, and gastrin secretion in response to secretin stimulation test.

CONTRAINDICATIONS & CAUTIONS
• Contraindicated in patients hypersensitive to drug or its components. Reactions may include anaphylaxis, anaphylactic shock, angioedema, bronchospasm, acute interstitial nephritis, and urticaria.

❸ **Alert:** Prolonged use of PPIs or use with medications such as digoxin or drugs that may cause hypomagnesemia (e.g., diuretics) may cause low magnesium levels that may require magnesium supplementation and possible discontinuation of drug. Monitor magnesium levels before starting treatment and periodically thereafter.

❸ **Alert:** There may be an increased risk of hip, wrist, and spine fractures associated with PPIs.

• Acute interstitial nephritis has been observed in patients taking PPIs, including lansoprazole. It may occur at any point during therapy, and is generally attributed to an idiopathic hypersensitivity reaction. Discontinue drug if condition develops.

• Prolonged treatment (2 years or more) may cause cyanocobalamin (vitamin B$_{12}$) malabsorption caused by hypochlorhydria or achlorhydria. Observe for clinical signs and symptoms consistent with cyanocobalamin deficiency.

• Prolonged PPI use (especially beyond 1 year) is associated with increased risk of fundic gland polyps. Use the shortest duration of PPI therapy appropriate to the condition being treated.

Dialyzable drug: No.

PREGNANCY-LACTATION-REPRODUCTION
• There are no adequate studies in pregnant women. Use during pregnancy only if clearly needed.

Reactions in bold italics are *life-threatening*. Interactions may have a *rapid onset* or a *delayed onset*.

• It isn't known if drug appears in human milk. Patient should discontinue breastfeeding or discontinue drug.

NURSING CONSIDERATIONS

⚠ *Alert:* Monitor patient for signs and symptoms of low magnesium level, such as abnormal HR or rhythm, palpitations, muscle spasms, tremor, or seizures. In children, abnormal HR may present as fatigue, upset stomach, dizziness, and light-headedness.

• New onset and exacerbation of existing cutaneous lupus erythematosus and SLE have been reported in patients taking PPIs, including lansoprazole. Avoid administering PPIs for longer than medically indicated. Discontinue drug and refer patient to appropriate specialist for evaluation if indicated.

⚠ *Alert:* May increase risk of CDAD. Evaluate for CDAD in patients who develop diarrhea that doesn't improve.

• Patients with severe liver disease may need dosage adjustment, but don't adjust dosage for elderly patients or those with renal insufficiency.

• Just because symptoms respond to therapy, gastric malignancy shouldn't be ruled out.

• *Look alike–sound alike:* Don't confuse Prevacid with Pepcid, Prilosec, or Prevpac.

PATIENT TEACHING

• For best effect, instruct patient to take drug before eating.

• Teach patient how to take drug and alternative methods if needed.

• Inform patient with phenylketonuria that ODTs contain 2.5 mg phenylalanine/15-mg tablet and 5.1 mg phenylalanine/30-mg tablet.

• Teach patient to recognize and report all adverse reactions, especially diarrhea that doesn't improve and signs and symptoms of low magnesium level or SLE.

ledipasvir–sofosbuvir ▧
LED-i-pas-vir/soe-FOS-bue-vir

Harvoni

Therapeutic class: Antivirals
Pharmacologic class: Antivirals

AVAILABLE FORMS
Tablets: 90 mg ledipasvir/400 mg sofosbuvir

INDICATIONS & DOSAGES

⚠ *Alert:* Sofosbuvir and its metabolite accumulate in patients with severe renal impairment (CrCl of less than 30 mL/minute) or ESRD. There are no dosing guidelines provided by the manufacturer.

➤ **Chronic HCV genotype 1 infection in treatment-naive patients without cirrhosis or with compensated cirrhosis or in treatment-experienced patients without cirrhosis** ▧

Adults and children age 12 and older or weighing at least 35 kg: One tablet PO once daily for 12 weeks. If pretreatment HCV-RNA is less than 6 million international units/mL in treatment-naive adults without cirrhosis, may consider treatment course of 8 weeks.

➤ **Chronic HCV genotype 1 infection in treatment-experienced patients with compensated cirrhosis** ▧

Adults and children age 12 and older or weighing at least 35 kg: One tablet PO once daily for 24 weeks.

➤ **Chronic HCV genotype 1 infection in treatment-naive and treatment-experienced patients with decompensated cirrhosis, in combination with ribavirin; chronic HCV genotype 1 or 4 infection in treatment-naive and treatment-experienced liver transplant patients without cirrhosis or with compensated cirrhosis, in combination with ribavirin** ▧

Adults: One tablet PO once daily with ribavirin for 12 weeks.

➤ **Chronic HCV genotype 4, 5, or 6 infection in treatment-naive and treatment-experienced patients without cirrhosis or with compensated cirrhosis** ▧

L

Adults and children age 12 and older or weighing at least 35 kg: One tablet PO once daily for 12 weeks.

ADMINISTRATION
PO
- May give without regard for food.
- Store at room temperature in original container.

ACTION
Ledipasvir and sofosbuvir are direct-acting antivirals against HCV. Ledipasvir inhibits the NS5A protein, and sofosbuvir inhibits the NS5B RNA polymerase, both of which are required for viral replication.

Route	Onset	Peak	Duration
PO (ledipasvir)	Unknown	4–4½ hr	Unknown
PO (sofosbuvir)	Unknown	0.8–1 hr	Unknown

Half-life: Ledipasvir, 47 hours; sofosbuvir, ½ hour.

ADVERSE REACTIONS
CNS: fatigue, asthenia, headache, insomnia, irritability, dizziness, depression. **GI:** nausea, diarrhea. **Hepatic:** increased bilirubin and lipase levels. **Musculoskeletal:** myalgia. **Respiratory:** cough, dyspnea.

INTERACTIONS
Drug-drug. ✪ *Alert: Amiodarone:* May increase risk of symptomatic bradycardia, requiring pacemaker intervention, and cardiac arrest. Avoid use together. If use together can't be avoided, advise patient of risk and monitor patient carefully.
Antacids (aluminum hydroxide, magnesium hydroxide): May decrease ledipasvir level. Separate administration of antacids and ledipasvir–sofosbuvir by 4 hours.
Anticonvulsants (carbamazepine, oxcarbazepine, phenobarbital, phenytoin), antimycobacterials (rifabutin, rifampin, rifapentine), P-gp inducers (rifampin): May decrease ledipasvir–sofosbuvir concentrations. Use together isn't recommended.
Atorvastatin: May increase atorvastatin level; may be associated with increased risk of myopathy. Monitor patient closely.
Digoxin: May increase digoxin concentration. Monitor digoxin level.

H₂-receptor antagonists (famotidine): May decrease ledipasvir level. Separate administration by 12 hours or administer simultaneously if H₂-receptor antagonist dose doesn't exceed equivalent of famotidine 40 mg b.i.d.
HIV antiretroviral regimen containing tenofovir disoproxil fumarate, an HIV protease inhibitor (atazanavir, darunavir, lopinavir), and ritonavir: May increase tenofovir-associated adverse reactions. Safety of use together hasn't been established. Consider alternative HCV or antiretroviral therapy or monitor patient closely for tenofovir-associated adverse reactions.
HIV antiretroviral regimen containing tenofovir disoproxil fumarate, cobicistat, elvitegravir, and emtricitabine: May increase tenofovir level. Safety of use together hasn't been established; use together isn't recommended.
HIV antiretroviral regimen containing tenofovir disoproxil fumarate, efavirenz, and emtricitabine: May increase tenofovir concentration and risk of toxicity. Monitor patient for tenofovir-associated adverse reactions.
HIV antiretroviral regimen containing tipranavir and ritonavir: May decrease ledipasvir–sofosbuvir concentrations and effectiveness. Use together isn't recommended.
HMG-CoA reductase inhibitors (rosuvastatin): May increase concentration of reductase inhibitor and increase risk of myopathy, including rhabdomyolysis. Use together isn't recommended.
Other products containing sofosbuvir: Duplicates therapy. Contraindicated for use together.
PPIs (omeprazole): May decrease ledipasvir level. May give PPI doses equivalent to 20 mg or less of omeprazole simultaneously with ledipasvir–sofosbuvir on an empty stomach.
Simeprevir: May increase ledipasvir–sofosbuvir concentrations. Use together isn't recommended.
Drug-herb. *St. John's wort:* May significantly decrease drug plasma level and reduce effectiveness. Discourage use together.

Reactions in bold italics are *life-threatening*. Interactions may have a *rapid onset* or a *delayed onset*.

EFFECTS ON LAB TEST RESULTS

• May increase bilirubin, lipase, and CK levels.

CONTRAINDICATIONS & CAUTIONS

• Contraindicated in patients hypersensitive to either drug or their components.

Black Box Warning Reactivation of hepatitis B virus (HBV) may occur in hepatitis C virus (HCV) co-infected patients, and result in fulminant hepatitis, hepatic failure, and death. Screen all patients for current or prior HBV infection before treatment; if positive for HBV infection, assess baseline HBV DNA. ■

• Use with other drugs containing sofosbuvir isn't recommended.

❸ Alert: Symptomatic bradycardia, including fatal cardiac arrest and cases requiring pacemaker intervention, have been reported when drug is given with amiodarone. Patients taking amiodarone who are also taking beta blockers or have underlying cardiac comorbidities or advanced liver disease may be at increased risk. Symptoms may occur within hours to up to 2 weeks after start of treatment of HCV infection.

• Safety and effectiveness haven't been established in children younger than age 12 or weighing less than 35 kg, in children with decompensated cirrhosis, or in children with liver transplants.

Dialyzable drug: Ledipasvir, unlikely; sofosbuvir, 18%.

PREGNANCY-LACTATION-REPRODUCTION

• Use in pregnant women hasn't been well studied. Use cautiously and only if benefits outweigh potential risk to the fetus.

• If drug is given with ribavirin, the combination regimen is contraindicated in pregnant women and in men whose female partners are pregnant.

• It isn't known if drug appears in human milk. Use cautiously in breastfeeding women and only if benefits outweigh potential risk to the fetus.

NURSING CONSIDERATIONS

Black Box Warning Monitor patient with current or prior HBV infection for hepatitis flare or HBV reactivation with laboratory testing, and watch for signs and symptoms of liver injury during active and post-treatment follow-up. ■

❸ Alert: Test all patients for evidence of current or prior HBV infection by measuring HBsAg and hepatitis B core antibody (anti-HBc) before initiating HCV treatment.

❸ Alert: Monitor patients taking amiodarone and those who must start amiodarone or who recently discontinued amiodarone for signs and symptoms of bradycardia (near-fainting or fainting, dizziness, light-headedness, malaise, weakness, excessive fatigue, shortness of breath, chest pain, confusion, or memory problems). Utilize inpatient cardiac monitoring for first 48 hours; continue outpatient or self-monitoring of HR for bradycardia daily through at least first 2 weeks of treatment. Discontinue HCV treatment if signs or symptoms of bradycardia occur.

• Monitor bilirubin, liver enzyme, and serum creatinine levels at baseline and periodically when clinically indicated.

• Monitor serum HCV-RNA level at baseline, during treatment, at end of treatment, during treatment follow-up, and when clinically indicated.

• Assess patient's concomitant medication use for potential drug interactions.

PATIENT TEACHING

Black Box Warning Warn patient to immediately report signs and symptoms of liver injury (fatigue, weakness, loss of appetite, nausea, vomiting, yellow skin or eyes, light-colored stool). ■

• Instruct patient to take only one tablet at same time each day, with or without food. If a dose is missed within the calendar day it's usually taken, patient should take dose as soon as possible. If the calendar day when dose is usually taken has passed, patient shouldn't take missed dose and should resume usual dosing schedule.

❸ Alert: Caution patient also taking amiodarone to seek immediate medical attention for signs and symptoms of bradycardia.

• Inform patient that the effect of treatment on HCV transmission isn't known and to follow precautions to prevent transmission.

• Advise patient to report to prescriber all other prescription drugs, OTC medications, vitamins, and herbal supplements being taken because drug interactions are possible.

• Caution patient not to stop drug without first discussing with prescriber.
• Tell patient to report signs and symptoms of adverse reactions (fatigue, nausea, and headache).
• Advise patient to immediately report signs and symptoms of hypersensitivity reactions (wheezing, chest tightness, fever, itching, or swelling of the face, lips, tongue, or throat).

leflunomide
leh-FLEW-no-mide

Arava

Therapeutic class: Antiarthritics
Pharmacologic class: Pyrimidine synthesis inhibitors

AVAILABLE FORMS
Tablets: 10 mg, 20 mg, 100 mg

INDICATIONS & DOSAGES
➤ Active RA
Adults: 100 mg PO loading dose every 24 hours for 3 days; then 20 mg (maximum daily dose) PO every 24 hours. Eliminating loading dose may decrease risk of adverse reactions, especially in patients at risk for hematologic or hepatic toxicity. Dose may be decreased to 10 mg daily if higher dose isn't well tolerated.

ADMINISTRATION
PO
• Give drug without regard for food.

ACTION
An immunomodulatory drug that inhibits dihydroorotate dehydrogenase, an enzyme involved in pyrimidine synthesis that has antiproliferative activity and anti-inflammatory effects.

Route	Onset	Peak	Duration
PO	Unknown	6–12 hr	Unknown

Half-life: Teriflunomide (active metabolite), 18 to 19 days.

ADVERSE REACTIONS
CNS: dizziness, headache, asthenia, somnolence, malaise. **CV:** HTN, chest pain, palpitations, varicose veins, thrombophlebitis.

EENT: blurred vision, eye disorder, papilledema, retinal disorder, retinal hemorrhage, rhinitis, sore throat. **GI:** diarrhea, abdominal pain, anorexia, dry mouth, enlarged salivary glands, flatulence, nausea, vomiting. **GU:** vaginal moniliasis. **Hematologic:** leukocytosis, thrombocytopenia. **Hepatic:** elevated liver enzyme levels, increased GGT and alkaline phosphatase levels, bilirubinemia, *hepatotoxicity.* **Musculoskeletal:** back pain, tenosynovitis. **Respiratory:** bronchitis, dyspnea. **Skin:** alopecia, rash, pruritus. **Other:** abscess, *anaphylaxis,* allergic reaction, flulike syndrome.

INTERACTIONS
Drug-drug. *Charcoal, cholestyramine:* May decrease leflunomide level. Sometimes used for this effect in leflunomide toxicity.
Methotrexate, other hepatotoxic drugs: May increase risk of hepatotoxicity. Monitor liver enzyme levels.
NSAIDs (diclofenac, ibuprofen): May increase NSAID level. Monitor patient.
Rifampin: May increase active leflunomide metabolite level. Use together cautiously.
Tacrolimus: May increase toxic effects of immunosuppressants. Avoid combination.
Tolbutamide: May increase tolbutamide level. Monitor patient.
Vaccines: May increase vaccine-related toxic effects. Modify therapy.
Vitamin K antagonists (warfarin): May enhance anticoagulant effect of these drugs. Monitor therapy.

EFFECTS ON LAB TEST RESULTS
• May increase AST, ALT, glucose, lipid, and CK levels.

CONTRAINDICATIONS & CAUTIONS
• Contraindicated in patients hypersensitive to drug or its components, in patients with severe hepatic impairment, and in those taking teriflunomide.
• Not recommended for patients with evidence of HBV or HBC infection, severe immunodeficiency, bone marrow dysplasia, or severe uncontrolled infections.
Black Box Warning Drug isn't recommended for patients with preexisting liver disease or ALT more than 2 × ULN. ∎

---

*Reactions in bold italics are **life-threatening**. Interactions may have a rapid onset or a **delayed onset**.*

Black Box Warning Use cautiously in patients taking other drugs that can cause liver damage. ∎

Black Box Warning If confirmed ALT elevations greater than 3 × ULN occur during treatment, stop drug and investigate cause. If ALT elevations are likely leflunomide-induced, start accelerated drug elimination procedure according to manufacturer's instructions; monitor LFTs weekly until normalized. ∎

• Use cautiously in patients with renal insufficiency.

• Severe infections including sepsis, which may be fatal, have been reported in patients receiving leflunomide, especially *Pneumocystis jiroveci* pneumonia, TB, and aspergillosis. Most reported cases were confounded by concomitant immunosuppressive therapy or comorbid illness that, in addition to RA, may predispose patients to infection.

• Drug isn't recommended in patients younger than age 18.

Dialyzable drug: No.

⚠ *Overdose S&S:* Diarrhea, abdominal pain, leukopenia, anemia, elevated LFT results.

PREGNANCY-LACTATION-REPRODUCTION

Black Box Warning Contraindicated in pregnant women and women of childbearing potential who aren't using reliable contraception because of the potential for fetal harm. Pregnancy must be excluded before start of therapy. ∎

• To monitor fetal outcomes of pregnant women exposed to leflunomide, patients should be registered with the Leflunomide Pregnancy Registry (1-877-311-8972).

• It isn't known if drug appears in human milk. Patient should discontinue breastfeeding or discontinue drug.

• Patients should avoid pregnancy after drug administration until undetectable serum concentrations (less than 0.02 mg/L) are verified, which may be accomplished by use of the recommended leflunomide removal protocol.

NURSING CONSIDERATIONS

• Before starting leflunomide, evaluate patient for active TB and screen for latent TB infection, check BP, and obtain blood for lab

tests, including serum ALT and Hb levels, hematocrit, and WBC and platelet counts.

• Vaccination with live-virus vaccines isn't recommended. Consider the long half-life of drug when contemplating giving a live-virus vaccine after stopping drug treatment.

• Risk of malignancy, particularly lymphoproliferative disorders, is increased with use of some immunosuppressants, including leflunomide.

Black Box Warning Monitor liver enzyme levels at least monthly for 6 months after beginning therapy and every 6 to 8 weeks thereafter. If ALT level rises to more than 3 × ULN, interrupt therapy. If drug is determined to be the cause, start cholestyramine washout (8 g PO t.i.d. for 11 days) or activated charcoal powder (50 g made into a suspension PO every 12 hours for 11 days) and monitor LFT values until normalized. ∎

• Without use of an accelerated drug elimination procedure, it may take up to 2 years to reach undetectable plasma concentrations of teriflunomide (active metabolite of leflunomide) after drug discontinuation.

◑ *Alert:* Monitor platelet and WBC counts and Hb level or hematocrit at baseline and monthly for 6 months after starting therapy and every 6 to 8 weeks thereafter.

◑ *Alert:* Continue monitoring AST, ALT, and serum albumin levels monthly if treatment includes methotrexate or other potential immunosuppressants.

• Monitor patient for peripheral neuropathy as drug may need to be stopped.

• Stop drug and start cholestyramine or charcoal therapy if bone marrow suppression occurs.

• Watch for overlapping hematologic toxicity when switching to another antirheumatic.

Black Box Warning Rare cases of severe liver injury, including cases with fatal outcome, have occurred during leflunomide therapy. Most cases occur within 6 months of therapy and in a setting of multiple risk factors for hepatotoxicity (liver disease, other hepatotoxins). ∎

• Carefully monitor patient after dose reduction. Because the active metabolite of leflunomide has a prolonged half-life, it may take several weeks for levels to decline.

• Rare cases of SJS, toxic epidermal necrolysis, and DRESS syndrome have been reported in patients receiving leflunomide. If patient develops any of these conditions, stop drug and perform an accelerated drug elimination procedure.

• ILD and worsening of preexisting ILD have been reported and can be fatal. Risk increases in patients with a history of ILD. If new-onset or worsening pulmonary symptoms (cough, dyspnea) with or without fever occur, drug may need to be discontinued and the etiology of symptoms investigated as appropriate.

PATIENT TEACHING
• Explain need for and frequency of required blood tests and monitoring.
Black Box Warning Instruct patient to use birth control during course of treatment and until it's been determined that drug is no longer active. ∎
• Warn patient to notify prescriber if signs or symptoms of pregnancy (such as late menstrual periods or breast tenderness) occur because of risk of fetal birth defects.
• Advise female patient to stop breastfeeding.
• Instruct patient to report all adverse reactions and to immediately report rash or mucous membrane lesions, unusual tiredness, abdominal pain, jaundice, easy bruising, bleeding, fever, recurrent infections, or pallor, which may be warnings of infrequent but serious adverse reactions.
• Inform patient that aspirin, other NSAIDs, and low-dose corticosteroids may continue to be taken during treatment.
• Inform patient that it may take 4 weeks to begin to see improvement from therapy.

lesinurad
le-SIN-ure-ad

Zurampic

Therapeutic class: Antigout drugs
Pharmacologic class: Uric acid transporter 1 inhibitors

AVAILABLE FORMS
Tablets: 200 mg

INDICATIONS & DOSAGES
Black Box Warning Don't use as monotherapy. Drug should only be used in combination with a xanthine oxidase inhibitor. ∎

➤ **Hyperuricemia associated with gout in combination with a xanthine oxidase inhibitor in patients who haven't achieved target serum uric acid levels with a xanthine oxidase inhibitor alone**
Adults: 200 mg PO once daily.
Adjust-a-dose: If creatinine level increases to more than 2 × baseline level, withhold drug. If lesinurad is found to be cause of creatinine elevation or when CrCl is persistently less than 45 mL/minute, discontinue drug. If treatment with xanthine oxidase inhibitor is interrupted, drug should also be withheld.

ADMINISTRATION
PO
• Give in the morning with food and water.
• Give at the same time as the morning dose of the xanthine oxidase inhibitor.
• Don't give a missed dose; give the next day.
• Store at room temperature. Protect from light.

ACTION
A uric acid transporter 1 and organic anion transporter 4 inhibitor that reduces serum uric acid levels by inhibiting the function of transporter proteins involved in renal uric acid reabsorption.

Route	Onset	Peak	Duration
PO	Rapid	1–4 hr	Unknown

Half-life: 5 hours.

ADVERSE REACTIONS
CNS: headache. **CV:** *major adverse CV event (MI, stroke, death).* **GI:** GERD. **GU:** elevated creatinine levels, *renal failure,* nephrolithiasis. **Other:** flulike symptoms.

INTERACTIONS
Drug-drug. *Aspirin:* May decrease effectiveness of lesinurad in combination with allopurinol. Avoid use together unless aspirin dose is 325 mg or less per day.

CYP2C9 inducers (carbamazepine, rifampin): May decrease lesinurad level. Monitor patient for decreased therapeutic effect.

CYP2C9 inhibitors (amiodarone, fluconazole): May increase lesinurad level. Use lesinurad cautiously in patients taking moderate CYP2C9 inhibitors and in CYP2C9 poor metabolizers.

CYP3A4 substrates (amlodipine, HMG-CoA reductase inhibitors, sildenafil): Lesinurad may decrease levels of CYP3A4 substrates. Monitor effectiveness of sensitive CYP3A4 substrates when used with lesinurad.

Epoxide hydrolase inhibitors (valproic acid): May interfere with lesinurad metabolism. Don't use together.

Hormonal contraceptives: Oral, injectable, transdermal, and implantable forms of hormonal contraceptives may not be reliable when used with lesinurad. Females should use additional methods of contraception.

EFFECTS ON LAB TEST RESULTS
• May increase creatinine level.

CONTRAINDICATIONS & CAUTIONS
• Contraindicated in patients with severe renal impairment (CrCl of less than 30 mL/minute) or ESRD, in kidney transplant recipients, and in patients on dialysis.
• Contraindicated in patients with TLS or Lesch-Nyhan syndrome.
Black Box Warning Use only in combination with a xanthine oxidase inhibitor. Acute renal failure has occurred with lesinurad use and was more common when drug was given alone. ∎
• Drug isn't recommended for treatment of asymptomatic hyperuricemia.
• Drug isn't recommended for patients taking daily doses of allopurinol less than 300 mg (or less than 200 mg in patients with CrCl of less than 60 mL/minute).
• Drug may increase risk of major adverse CV events (death, nonfatal MI, nonfatal strokes). Monitor patients as clinically appropriate.
• Safety and effectiveness in children younger than age 18 haven't been established.
Dialyzable drug: No.

PREGNANCY-LACTATION-REPRODUCTION
• Drug hasn't been studied in pregnant women. Use cautiously during pregnancy and only if benefit outweighs possible risk to the fetus.
• Hormonal contraceptives may not be reliable when used with drug. Women should use additional methods of contraception.
• It isn't known if drug appears in human milk. Use cautiously in breastfeeding women and only if benefit to the mother outweighs risk to the infant.

NURSING CONSIDERATIONS
• Don't start treatment in patients with CrCl of less than 45 mL/minute. Monitor renal function before start of therapy and periodically thereafter as clinically indicated. More frequent renal function monitoring is recommended in patients with CrCl of less than 60 mL/minute or serum creatinine level of 1.5 to 2 × baseline level.
• Monitor patients for signs and symptoms of acute uric acid nephropathy (flank pain, nausea, vomiting). Withhold drug and assess serum creatinine level if signs and symptoms occur.
• Monitor fluid intake. Patient should maintain adequate hydration of at least 68 oz (2 L) of liquid per day.
• Gout flares may occur after start of therapy and gout flare prophylaxis is recommended. Drug doesn't need to be stopped if a gout flare occurs.

PATIENT TEACHING
• Advise patient to take medication with food and water. Recommend that patient drink 68 oz (2 L) of fluid each day to stay hydrated.
Black Box Warning Warn patient not to take drug by itself. Drug should always be taken with a xanthine oxidase inhibitor, such as allopurinol or febuxostat. ∎
• Counsel patient that if a dose is missed in the morning, not to take the missed dose later in the day but to wait until the next day to take a dose. Advise patient not to double the dose.
• Inform patient that renal events, including increases in blood creatinine level and acute renal failure, may occur.

• Advise patient that periodic monitoring of blood creatinine levels is recommended.
• Teach patient that gout flares may occur after starting therapy and that gout flare prophylaxis medication is recommended to prevent gout flares. Advise patient not to discontinue drug if a gout flare occurs during treatment.
• Advise female patient to tell prescriber if she is pregnant, plans to become pregnant, or is breastfeeding.
• Caution female patient using hormonal contraceptives to use a back-up contraceptive method during treatment.

SAFETY ALERT!

letrozole
LE-tro-zol

Femara

Therapeutic class: Antineoplastics
Pharmacologic class: Aromatase inhibitors

AVAILABLE FORMS
Tablets: 2.5 mg

INDICATIONS & DOSAGES
Adjust-a-dose (for all indications): In patients with cirrhosis and severe hepatic impairment, give 2.5 mg every other day.
➤ **Metastatic breast cancer with disease progression after antiestrogen therapy (such as tamoxifen)**
Postmenopausal women: 2.5 mg PO as single daily dose until tumor progression is evident.
➤ **First-line treatment of hormone receptor–positive or hormone receptor–unknown, locally advanced, or metastatic breast cancer**
Postmenopausal women: 2.5 mg PO once daily until tumor progression is evident.
➤ **Adjuvant treatment of hormone-sensitive early breast cancer**
Postmenopausal women: 2.5 mg PO daily. Optimal duration of treatment is unknown.
➤ **Extended adjuvant treatment of early breast cancer following 5 years of adjuvant tamoxifen therapy**
Postmenopausal women: 2.5 mg PO once daily for 5 years.

ADMINISTRATION
PO
• Drug is a hormonal agent and considered a potential teratogen. Follow safe handling procedures.
• Give drug without regard for meals.

ACTION
Inhibits conversion of androgens to estrogens, which decreases tumor mass or delays progression of tumor growth in some women.

Route	Onset	Peak	Duration
PO	Unknown	2–6 wk (steady-state plasma)	Unknown

Half-life: About 2 days.

ADVERSE REACTIONS
CNS: *stroke,* headache, somnolence, insomnia, dizziness, fatigue, asthenia, mood changes, depression. **CV:** hot flashes or flushing, *MI, thromboembolism,* chest pain, edema, HTN. **EENT:** cataract. **GI:** nausea, vomiting, constipation, diarrhea, abdominal pain, anorexia, dyspepsia. **GU:** vaginal bleeding, vaginal irritation, vulvovaginal dryness, UTI. **Metabolic:** hypercholesterolemia, weight gain or loss. **Musculoskeletal:** bone pain, limb pain, back pain, arthralgia, fractures, osteopenia, osteoporosis, myalgia. **Respiratory:** dyspnea, cough, pleural effusion. **Skin:** rash, pruritus, alopecia, diaphoresis. **Other:** viral infections, breast pain, secondary malignancies.

INTERACTIONS
Drug-drug. *Estrogens:* May produce antagonistic effects with letrozole. Use together isn't recommended.
Methadone: May increase methadone serum concentration. Monitor therapy.
Tamoxifen: May reduce plasma letrozole levels. Monitor therapy.

EFFECTS ON LAB TEST RESULTS
• May increase cholesterol level.
• May decrease lymphocyte count.

CONTRAINDICATIONS & CAUTIONS
• Contraindicated in patients hypersensitive to drug or its components.

Reactions in bold italics are *life-threatening*. Interactions may have a *rapid onset* or a ***delayed onset***.

• Use cautiously in patients with severe liver impairment; dosage adjustment isn't needed in those with mild to moderate liver dysfunction.
Dialyzable drug: Unknown.

PREGNANCY-LACTATION-REPRODUCTION
• May cause fetal harm. Contraindicated in women who are or may become pregnant.
• Women of childbearing potential should use effective contraception during therapy and for at least 3 weeks after final dose.
• Rule out pregnancy before starting drug.
• It isn't known if drug appears in human milk. Patient shouldn't breastfeed during therapy and for 3 weeks after final dose.

NURSING CONSIDERATIONS
• Dosage adjustment isn't needed in patients with CrCl of 10 mL/minute or more.
• Use drug only in postmenopausal women.
• *Look alike–sound alike:* Don't confuse Femara with FemHRT.

PATIENT TEACHING
• Teach patient about safe handling of drug.
• Instruct patient to take drug exactly as prescribed.
• Tell patient to take drug with a small glass of water, with or without food.
• Inform patient about potential adverse effects and to report them.
• Advise patient to use caution performing tasks that require alertness, coordination, or dexterity, such as driving, until effects are known.
• Advise patient of childbearing potential to use adequate contraceptive methods during therapy and for 3 weeks after final dose.
• Advise patient not to breastfeed during therapy and for 3 weeks after final dose.
• Inform female patient who is recently menopausal of the need for adequate contraception until postmenopausal status is clinically well established.

SAFETY ALERT!

leuprolide acetate
loo-PROE-lide

Eligard, Lupron Depot, Lupron Depot-Ped

Therapeutic class: Antineoplastics
Pharmacologic class: Gonadotropin-releasing hormone analogues

AVAILABLE FORMS
Depot injection: 3.75 mg, 7.5 mg, 11.25 mg, 15 mg, 22.5 mg, 30 mg, 45 mg
Injection: 1 mg/0.2 mL, 5 mg/mL in 2.8-mL multiple-dose vials

INDICATIONS & DOSAGES
➤ **Advanced prostate cancer**
Adults: 1 mg subcut daily. Or, 7.5 mg IM depot injection monthly. Or, 7.5 mg subcut Eligard once monthly. Or, 22.5 mg IM depot injection every 3 months. Or, 22.5 mg subcut Eligard every 3 months. Or, 30 mg IM depot injection every 4 months. Or, 30 mg subcut Eligard every 4 months. Or, 45 mg subcut Eligard every 6 months. Or, 45 mg IM depot injection every 6 months.
➤ **Endometriosis (alone or in combination with norethindrone acetate)**
Adults: 3.75 mg IM depot injection as single injection once monthly for up to 6 months. Or, 11.25 mg IM every 3 months for up to 6 months.
➤ **Central precocious puberty**
Children: Initially, 50 mcg/kg/day subcut. Titrate dosage upward by 10 mcg/kg/day until no progression of condition is noted. Discontinue drug at the appropriate age of puberty onset.
Children age 2 and older (Lupron Depot-Ped): Initially, for child weighing more than 37.5 kg, 15 mg IM once monthly. For child weighing more than 25 to 37.5 kg, 11.25 mg IM once monthly. For child weighing 25 kg or less, 7.5 mg IM once monthly. Or, for 3-month formulation, usual dosage is 11.25 or 30 mg IM once every 3 months. If clinical suppression isn't achieved with starting dose, increase dose to next available higher dose. Discontinue drug at the appropriate age of puberty onset.

L

➤ **Anemia related to uterine fibroids (with iron therapy)**
Adults: 3.75 mg IM depot injection once monthly for up to 3 consecutive months. Or 11.25 mg IM depot injection for 1 dose.
➤ **Premenopausal ovarian suppression in breast cancer patients ◆**
Adults: 3.75 mg IM every 28 days for up to 24 months, or 11.25 mg IM every 3 months for up to 24 months.

ADMINISTRATION
• Products have specific mixing and administration instructions. Read manufacturer's directions closely.
• Hazardous drug; use safe-handling precautions.

IM
• Never give by IV injection.
• Give depot injections under medical supervision.
• Use supplied diluent to reconstitute drug (extra diluent is provided; discard remainder).
• Inject into vial; shake well. Suspension will appear milky. Use immediately.
• Draw appropriate amount into a syringe with a 22G needle.
• When using prefilled dual-chamber syringes, prepare for injection according to manufacturer's instructions.
• Gently shake syringe to form a uniform milky suspension. If particles adhere to stopper, tap syringe against your finger.
• Remove needle guard and advance plunger to expel air from syringe. Inject entire contents IM as with a normal injection.

Subcutaneous
• For the two-syringe mixing system, connect the syringes and inject the liquid contents according to manufacturer's instructions.
• Mix product by pushing contents back and forth between syringes for about 45 seconds; shaking the syringes won't mix the contents enough.
• Attach the needle provided in the kit and inject subcut.
• Suspension settles very quickly. Remix if settling occurs. Must be given within 30 minutes.
• Never give by IV injection.

ACTION
Stimulates and then inhibits release of FSH and luteinizing hormone, which suppresses testosterone and estrogen levels.

Route	Onset	Peak	Duration
IM, subcut	Variable	1–2 mo	60–90 days

Half-life: 3 hours.

ADVERSE REACTIONS
CNS: dizziness, depression, headache, pain, insomnia, paresthesia, asthenia, fatigue, lethargy, anxiety. **CV: *arrhythmias,*** angina, *MI,* peripheral edema, ECG changes, hypotension, HTN, murmur, hot flashes. **GI:** nausea, vomiting, anorexia, constipation. **GU:** impotence, vaginitis, urinary frequency, hematuria, UTI, amenorrhea. **Hematologic:** anemia. **Metabolic:** weight gain or loss. **Musculoskeletal:** transient bone pain during first week of treatment, joint disorder, myalgia, neuromuscular disorder, bone loss, back pain, arthralgia. **Respiratory:** dyspnea, sinus congestion, cough, *pulmonary fibrosis.* **Skin:** injection-site reactions, dermatitis, acne, injection-site pain, rash. **Other:** gynecomastia, androgen-like effects.

INTERACTIONS
None significant.

EFFECTS ON LAB TEST RESULTS
• May increase bilirubin, cholesterol, BUN, calcium, creatinine, glucose, LDH, phosphorus, AST, ALT, and uric acid levels.
• May decrease albumin, protein, and potassium levels.
• May increase WBC. May decrease Hb level and hematocrit.
• May prolong PT and PTT.
• May increase or decrease platelet count.
• May alter results of pituitary-gonadal system tests during therapy and for 12 weeks after.

CONTRAINDICATIONS & CAUTIONS
• Contraindicated in patients hypersensitive to drug or other gonadotropin-releasing hormone analogues and in women with undiagnosed vaginal bleeding.
• Androgen deprivation therapy may prolong QT/QTc interval. Consider if benefits

---

of therapy outweigh potential risks in patients with congenital long QT syndrome, HF, or frequent electrolyte abnormalities, and in patients taking drugs known to prolong QT interval.

• Seizures have been reported in patients taking leuprolide, including those with and without a history of seizures, epilepsy, cerebrovascular disorders, or CNS anomalies or tumors and in patients taking concomitant medications associated with seizures.

• The 30- and 45-mg depot injections are contraindicated in women and children.

• Use cautiously in patients hypersensitive to benzyl alcohol.

Dialyzable drug: Unknown.

PREGNANCY-LACTATION-REPRODUCTION

• May cause fetal harm; contraindicated in women who are or may become pregnant during therapy.

• It isn't known if drug appears in human milk. Use is contraindicated in breastfeeding women.

• May impair fertility in males of reproductive potential.

NURSING CONSIDERATIONS

• A fractional dose of drug formulated to give every 3, 4, or 6 months isn't equivalent to same dose of once-a-month formulation.

• Correct electrolyte abnormalities before starting drug; consider periodic monitoring of ECGs and electrolytes.

• After starting treatment for central precocious puberty, monitor patient response every 1 to 2 months with a gonadotropin-releasing hormone stimulation test and sex corticosteroid level determinations. Measure bone age for advancement every 6 to 12 months.

🔹 *Alert:* During first few weeks of treatment for prostate cancer, signs and symptoms of disease may temporarily worsen or additional signs and symptoms may occur.

• In patients treated with gonadotropin-releasing hormone analogues for prostate cancer, treatment is usually continued upon development of metastatic castration-resistant prostate cancer.

• May increase risk of diabetes and CV events. Monitor patient closely.

• *Look alike–sound alike:* Don't confuse Lupron Depot with Lupron Depot-Ped.

PATIENT TEACHING

• Before starting child on treatment for central precocious puberty, make sure parents understand importance of continuous therapy.

• Carefully instruct patient who will self-administer subcut injection about the proper technique. Advise patient to use only the syringes provided by manufacturer.

• Advise patient that, if another syringe must be substituted, a low-dose insulin syringe (U-100, 0.5 mL) may be an appropriate choice but that needle gauge should be no smaller than 22G.

• Instruct patient to store leuprolide acetate powder (depot) and diluent at room temperature, to refrigerate unopened vials of leuprolide acetate injection, and to protect leuprolide acetate injection from heat and light.

• Inform patient with history of undesirable effects from other endocrine therapies that leuprolide is easier to tolerate. Advise patient to report all adverse effects.

• Explain that symptoms may worsen at first.

• Advise female patient of childbearing potential to use a nonhormonal form of contraception during treatment.

---

levalbuterol hydrochloride
lev-al-BYOO-ter-ol

Xopenex

levalbuterol tartrate
Xopenex HFA

Therapeutic class: Bronchodilators
Pharmacologic class: Beta₂ agonists

AVAILABLE FORMS

Inhalation aerosol: 45 mcg per actuation
Solution for inhalation: 0.31 mg, 0.63 mg, or 1.25 mg in 3-mL vials; 1.25 mg/0.5 mL in vials (concentrate)

INDICATIONS & DOSAGES

➤ **To prevent or treat bronchospasm in patients with reversible obstructive airway disease**

Adults and adolescents age 12 and older: 0.63 mg by oral inhalation via nebulizer t.i.d. every 6 to 8 hours. Patients with more severe asthma who don't respond adequately to 0.63 mg t.i.d. may benefit from 1.25 mg t.i.d.

Children ages 6 to 11: 0.31 mg by oral inhalation via nebulizer t.i.d. Routine dosage shouldn't exceed 0.63 mg t.i.d.

Adults and children age 4 and older: 2 inhalations Xopenex HFA (90 mcg) every 4 to 6 hours. In some patients, 1 inhalation (45 mcg) every 4 hours is sufficient.

ADMINISTRATION
Inhalational
- Keep unopened vials of regular solution in foil pouch and use within 2 weeks of opening pouch. Use vials removed from pouch within 1 week and protect from light.
- Use vials of concentrated solution immediately after opening pouch.
- Discard vial if solution isn't colorless.
- Release four test sprays before first use of inhaler or after inhaler has not been used for more than 3 days.
- Shake canister well before use.
- Use a spacer device to improve inhalation, as appropriate.
- Wash actuator with warm water and air-dry thoroughly at least once a week.
- Dilute concentrated solution (1.25 mg/ 0.5 mL) with sterile NSS before administration by nebulization.

ACTION
Relaxes bronchial smooth muscle by stimulating beta$_2$ receptors; also inhibits release of mediators from mast cells in the airway.

Route	Onset	Peak	Duration
Inhalation	5–15 min	1 hr	3–4 hr

Half-life: 3¼ to 4 hours.

ADVERSE REACTIONS
CNS: dizziness, migraine, nervousness, pain, tremor, anxiety, asthenia, fever, headache, insomnia. **CV:** tachycardia. **EENT:** rhinitis, sinusitis, turbinate edema, pharyngitis. **GI:** dyspepsia, diarrhea, vomiting. **Musculoskeletal:** leg cramps. **Respiratory:** increased cough, asthma, bronchitis.

Other: viral infection, flulike syndrome, accidental injury, lymphadenopathy.

INTERACTIONS
Drug-drug. *Beta blockers:* May block pulmonary effect of the drug and cause severe bronchospasm. Avoid using together, if possible. If use together is unavoidable, consider a cardioselective beta blocker, but use cautiously.

Digoxin: May decrease digoxin levels up to 22%. Monitor digoxin level.

Loop or thiazide diuretics: May cause ECG changes and hypokalemia. Use together cautiously.

MAO inhibitors, TCAs: May potentiate action of levalbuterol on the vascular system. Avoid using within 2 weeks of MAO inhibitor or TCA therapy.

Other short-acting sympathomimetic aerosol bronchodilators, epinephrine: May increase adrenergic adverse effects. Use together cautiously.

EFFECTS ON LAB TEST RESULTS
None reported.

CONTRAINDICATIONS & CAUTIONS
- Contraindicated in patients hypersensitive to drug or to racemic albuterol.
- Use cautiously in patients with CV disorders (especially coronary insufficiency, HTN, and arrhythmias), seizure disorders, hyperthyroidism, or diabetes mellitus, and in those who are unusually responsive to sympathomimetic amines.

Dialyzable drug: Unknown.

⚠ **Overdose S&S:** Exaggeration of adverse reactions, hypokalemia, seizures, angina, HTN, hypotension, arrhythmias, muscle cramps, dry mouth, palpitations, nausea, insomnia, cardiac arrest, sudden death.

PREGNANCY-LACTATION-REPRODUCTION
- There are no adequate studies in pregnant women. Use during pregnancy only if potential benefit justifies potential risk to the fetus.
- Encourage enrollment in MotherToBaby Pregnancy Studies' Asthma & Pregnancy Study by calling 1-877-311-8972 or visiting www.mothertobaby.org/ongoing-study/asthma

---

Reactions in bold italics are *life-threatening*. Interactions may have a *rapid onset* or a *delayed onset*.

• It isn't known if drug appears in human milk. Patient should discontinue breastfeeding or discontinue drug.

NURSING CONSIDERATIONS

❸ **Alert:** As with other inhaled beta agonists, drug can produce paradoxical bronchospasm or life-threatening CV effects. If this occurs, stop drug immediately and notify prescriber.

• Drug may worsen diabetes mellitus and ketoacidosis.

• Monitor potassium level, as drug may temporarily decrease potassium level.

• The compatibility of levalbuterol mixed with other drugs in a nebulizer hasn't been established.

PATIENT TEACHING

• Tell patient not to increase dosage without consulting prescriber.

• Advise patient not to use more frequently than recommended.

• Urge patient to seek medical attention immediately if levalbuterol becomes less effective, if signs and symptoms worsen, or if patient is using drug more frequently than usual.

• Tell patient that the effects of levalbuterol may last up to 8 hours.

• Tell patient not to double the next dose if a dose is missed and to take doses at least 6 hours apart.

• Advise patient to use other inhalational drugs and antiasthmatics only as directed while taking levalbuterol.

• Inform patient that common adverse reactions include palpitations, rapid HR, headache, dizziness, tremor, and nervousness.

• Tell patient to keep unopened vials in foil pouch.

• After the foil pouch is opened, vials of regular solution must be used within 2 weeks. Inform patient that vials removed from the pouch, if not used immediately, should be protected from light and excessive heat and used within 1 week.

• Advise patient to use vials of concentrated solution immediately after opening pouch.

• Tell patient to discard vial if solution isn't colorless.

• Teach patient to use drug correctly when inhaling by nebulizer.

• Instruct patient to shake inhaler well before using and to breathe as calmly, deeply, and evenly as possible until no more mist is formed in the nebulizer reservoir (5 to 15 minutes).

• Tell patient using the inhaler to release four test sprays into the air away from the face before the first use or if it hasn't been used for more than 3 days.

• Instruct patient to thoroughly wash and dry plastic actuator of inhaler at least once a week to prevent medication build-up and blockage. If actuator becomes blocked, washing actuator will remove blockage.

• Tell patient to discard inhaler when dose indicator display window shows "0."

• Encourage female patient to contact prescriber if she becomes pregnant or is breastfeeding.

---

levETIRAcetam
lee-vah-tih-RACE-ah-tam

Keppra, Keppra XR, Roweepra, Spritam

Therapeutic class: Anticonvulsants
Pharmacologic class: Pyrrolidine derivatives

AVAILABLE FORMS

Injection: 500 mg/5 mL single-use vials
Injection (premixed in NSS): 500 mg/ 100 mL (5 mg/mL), 1,000 mg/100 mL (10 mg/mL), 1,500 mg/100 mL (15 mg/mL)
Oral solution: 100 mg/mL
Tablets ⬤: 250 mg, 500 mg, 750 mg, 1,000 mg
Tablets (extended-release) ⬤: 500 mg, 750 mg
Tablets for oral suspension: 250 mg, 500 mg, 750 mg, 1,000 mg

INDICATIONS & DOSAGES

Adjust-a-dose (for all indications): For immediate-release and oral solution, in adults with CrCl of 50 to 80 mL/minute, give 500 to 1,000 mg every 12 hours; if CrCl is 30 to 50 mL/minute, give 250 to 750 mg every 12 hours; if CrCl is less than 30 mL/minute, give 250 to 500 mg every 12 hours. For ESRD dialysis patients, give

500 to 1,000 mg every 24 hours. Give a 250- to 500-mg dose after dialysis.

For extended-release tablets, if CrCl is 50 to 80 mL/minute, give 1,000 to 2,000 mg every 24 hours. If CrCl is 30 to 50 mL/minute, give 500 to 1,500 mg every 24 hours. If CrCl is less than 30 mL/minute, give 500 to 1,000 mg every 24 hours.

➤ **Adjunctive therapy for myoclonic seizures of juvenile myoclonic epilepsy**
Adults and adolescents age 12 and older: Initially, 500 mg PO or IV b.i.d. Increase by 1,000 mg/day every 2 weeks to a dose of 1,500 mg PO or IV b.i.d. (3,000 mg/day).

➤ **Adjunctive therapy for primary generalized tonic-clonic seizures**
Adults and adolescents age 16 and older: Initially, 500 mg PO or IV b.i.d. Increase dose by 500 mg b.i.d. every 2 weeks to dose of 1,500 mg b.i.d.
Children ages 6 to younger than 16: Initially, 10 mg/kg PO or IV b.i.d. Increase dose by 10 mg/kg b.i.d. at 2-week intervals to dose of 30 mg/kg b.i.d. For children weighing more than 20 kg, use either tablets or oral solution. For children weighing 20 kg or less, use oral solution.

➤ **Adjunctive therapy for primary generalized tonic-clonic seizures (Spritam)**
Adults and children age 6 and older weighing more than 40 kg: 500 mg PO b.i.d.; increase as needed and tolerated by 500 mg PO b.i.d. every 2 weeks to a maximum recommended dose of 1,500 mg b.i.d.
Children age 6 and older weighing 20 to 40 kg: 250 mg PO b.i.d.; increase by 250 mg PO b.i.d. every 2 weeks to a maximum of 750 mg b.i.d.

➤ **Adjunctive treatment for partial-onset seizures in patients with epilepsy**
Adults and adolescents age 16 and older: Initially, 500 mg PO or IV b.i.d. Increase dosage by 500 mg b.i.d., as needed, for seizure control at 2-week intervals to maximum of 1,500 mg b.i.d.
Children ages 4 to younger than 16: Initially, 10 mg/kg PO or IV b.i.d. Increase dose by 10 mg/kg b.i.d. at 2-week intervals to recommended dose of 30 mg/kg b.i.d. If patient can't tolerate this dose, reduce it. For children who weigh 20 kg or less, use the oral solution.

Children ages 6 months to younger than 4 years: Initially, 10 mg/kg PO or IV b.i.d. Increase by 10 mg/kg b.i.d. at 2-week intervals to recommended dosage of 25 mg/kg b.i.d. Reduce dosage if patient can't tolerate total daily dose of 50 mg/kg.
Children ages 1 month to 6 months: Initially, 7 mg/kg PO or IV b.i.d. Increase by 7 mg/kg b.i.d. at 2-week intervals to recommended dosage of 21 mg/kg b.i.d.

➤ **Adjunctive treatment for partial-onset seizures in patients with epilepsy (Spritam)**
Adults and children age 4 and older weighing more than 40 kg: 500 mg PO b.i.d.; increase as needed and tolerated by 500 mg PO b.i.d. every 2 weeks to a maximum recommended dose of 1,500 mg b.i.d.
Children age 4 and older weighing 20 to 40 kg: 250 mg PO b.i.d.; increase by 250 mg PO b.i.d. every 2 weeks to a maximum of 750 mg b.i.d.

➤ **Adjunctive treatment for partial-onset seizures in patients with epilepsy (extended-release)**
Adults and children age 12 and older: Initially, 1,000 mg PO once daily. May adjust once-daily dosage in increments of 1,000 mg every 2 weeks to maximum recommended once-daily dose of 3,000 mg.

ADMINISTRATION
PO
• Give drug without regard for food.
• Oral and IV forms are bioequivalent.
• Tablets should be swallowed whole and shouldn't be chewed, broken, or crushed.
• Tablets for oral solution are intended to disintegrate in the mouth. Place tablet on tongue with a dry hand. Follow with a sip of liquid and have patient swallow only after tablet disintegrates; patient shouldn't swallow tablet intact. Or, add whole tablet to a small volume of liquid in a cup (1 tablespoon or enough to cover tablet); allow tablet to disperse, then have patient immediately consume entire contents. Don't give partial tablets.
• Don't push tablets for oral solution through the foil; peel foil from blister by bending up and lifting peel tab around the blister seal.

Reactions in bold italics are *life-threatening*. Interactions may have a *rapid onset* or a *delayed onset*.

• For children weighing more than 20 kg, use either tablets or oral solution. For children weighing 20 kg or less, use oral solution.

IV

▼ Dilute drug before giving.

▼ For adults and adolescents receiving adult dosages, dilute 500-mg, 1,000-mg, or 1,500-mg dose in 100 mL NSS, D$_5$W, or lactated Ringer injection to maximum levetiracetam concentration of 15 mg/mL of diluted solution, and infuse within 4 hours over 15 minutes.

▼ For children and patients requiring a smaller volume, calculate the amount of diluent to not exceed a maximum levetiracetam concentration of 15 mg/mL of diluted solution; infuse within 4 hours over 15 minutes.

▼ Drug is compatible with diazepam, lorazepam, and valproate sodium for 4 hours at a controlled room temperature.

▼ Store premixed solution for infusion at 68° to 77° F (20° to 25° C); don't dilute.

▼ Store vials for injection at 77° F (25° C); excursions permitted to 59° to 86° F (15° to 30° C).

▼ **Incompatibilities:** Unknown with other drugs or antiepileptics besides diazepam, lorazepam, and valproate sodium. Consult a drug incompatibility reference for more information.

ACTION

May act by inhibiting simultaneous neuronal firing that leads to seizure activity.

Route	Onset	Peak	Duration
PO (immediate-release), IV	1 hr	1 hr	12 hr
PO (extended-release)	Unknown	4 hr	Unknown

Half-life: About 6 to 8 hours in adult patients with normal renal function.

ADVERSE REACTIONS

CNS: asthenia, headache, somnolence, amnesia, anxiety, ataxia, depression, dizziness, emotional lability, hostility, nervousness, paresthesia, pain, vertigo, hypersomnia, irritability, insomnia, confusion, falls, sedation, abnormal gait, incoordination. **EENT:** diplopia, conjunctivitis, ear pain, rhinitis, sinusitis, nasal congestion, pharyngitis. **GI:** anorexia, vomiting, upper abdominal pain, diarrhea, constipation, gastroenteritis. **Hematologic:** *leukopenia, neutropenia.* **Musculoskeletal:** neck pain, joint sprain. **Respiratory:** cough. **Skin:** contusion. **Other:** infection, head injury, flulike symptoms.

INTERACTIONS

Drug-drug. *Antihistamines, benzodiazepines, opioids, other drugs that cause drowsiness, TCAs:* May lead to severe sedation. Avoid using together.

Drug-lifestyle. *Alcohol use:* May lead to severe sedation. Discourage use together.

EFFECTS ON LAB TEST RESULTS

• May alter LFT results. May decrease Hb and hematocrit.

• May decrease WBC, RBC, and neutrophil counts.

• May increase eosinophil count.

CONTRAINDICATIONS & CAUTIONS

• Contraindicated in patients hypersensitive to drug.

• Don't use extended-release form in patients with ESRD.

• Anaphylaxis and angioedema may occur after first dose or at any time during treatment.

• Use cautiously in patients with history of psychiatric symptoms, especially psychotic symptoms and behaviors.

• Serious skin reactions, including toxic epidermal necrolysis and SJS, have been reported. Recurrence following rechallenge is possible. Discontinue drug for hypersensitivity reaction or unspecified rash.

• Don't abruptly discontinue drug because withdrawal seizures may occur.

• Drug may cause hematologic abnormalities, including decreased RBC, WBC, and neutrophil counts, Hb level, and hematocrit, and increased eosinophil count. Cases of agranulocytosis have been reported in the postmarketing setting.

Dialyzable drug: 50%.

⚠ **Overdose S&S:** Drowsiness, aggression, agitation, coma, depressed level of consciousness, respiratory depression, somnolence.

L

PREGNANCY-LACTATION-REPRODUCTION

- There are no adequate studies in pregnant women. Use during pregnancy only if potential benefit justifies potential risk to the fetus.
- Pregnant patients taking drug should enroll themselves in the North American AED Pregnancy Registry (1-888-233-2334).
- Drug appears in human milk. Patient should discontinue breastfeeding or discontinue drug.

NURSING CONSIDERATIONS

- Use drug only with other anticonvulsants; it isn't recommended for monotherapy.
- Seizures can occur if drug is stopped abruptly. Tapering is recommended.
- Monitor patients for signs and symptoms of somnolence and fatigue. Somnolence and asthenia occurred most frequently within first 4 weeks of treatment.
- Monitor patients closely for such adverse reactions as dizziness, which may lead to falls.
- Discontinue drug and notify prescriber for signs and symptoms of anaphylaxis (hypotension, hives, rash, and respiratory distress) and of angioedema (swelling of face, lips, mouth, eyes, tongue, throat, and feet).
- Monitor renal function as acute kidney injury has been reported.
- Monitor patients ages 1 month to younger than 4 years for increases in diastolic BP.
- ⚠ **Alert:** Closely monitor all patients taking or starting antiepileptic drugs for changes in behavior indicating psychosis or worsening of suicidal thoughts or behavior or depression. Symptoms such as anxiety, agitation, hostility, mania, and hypomania may be precursors to emerging suicidality.
- **Look alike–sound alike:** Don't confuse levetiracetam with levofloxacin. Don't confuse Keppra with Kaletra or Keflex.

PATIENT TEACHING

- Tell patient to seek medical attention for emerging or worsening depression, suicidal thoughts or behavior, or unusual changes in mood or behavior and to report such symptoms as anxiety, agitation, hostility, mania, and hypomania, which may be precursors to emerging suicidality.
- Warn patient to use extra care when sitting or standing to avoid falling.
- Advise patient to seek immediate medical attention for signs and symptoms of anaphylaxis or angioedema.
- Advise patient to call prescriber and not to stop drug suddenly if adverse reactions occur.
- Tell patient to take with other prescribed seizure drugs.
- For the oral solution, tell patient or caregiver to use a calibrated measuring device, not a household spoon.
- Warn patient that drug may cause dizziness and somnolence and to avoid driving, operating heavy machinery, bike riding, or other hazardous activities until drug's effects are known.
- Inform patient that drug can be taken with or without food.
- Tell patient not to chew, crush, or break tablets.
- Teach patient how to use tablets for oral solution correctly.
- Advise patient not to stop drug abruptly because seizure activity may increase.

levocetirizine dihydrochloride

LEE-voe-se-TIR-a-zeen

Children's Xyzal Allergy 24HR ◇, Xyzal, Xyzal Allergy 24HR ◇

Therapeutic class: Antihistamines
Pharmacologic class: H_1-receptor antagonists

AVAILABLE FORMS

Oral solution: 2.5 mg/5 mL
Tablets: 5 mg

INDICATIONS & DOSAGES

➤ **Seasonal allergic rhinitis (OTC only)**
Adults and children age 12 and older: 5 mg PO once daily in the evening; 2.5 mg PO once daily in the evening may be adequate for some patients.
Children ages 6 to 11: 2.5 mg PO once daily in the evening.
Children ages 2 to 5: 1.25 mg (2.5 mL) PO once daily in the evening. Don't exceed this dose.

Reactions in bold italics are *life-threatening*. Interactions may have a *rapid onset* or a ***delayed onset***.

Adjust-a-dose: Use in the presence of renal impairment isn't recommended.

➤ **Chronic idiopathic urticaria**

Adults and children age 12 and older: 5 mg once daily in the evening; some patients with less severe symptoms may experience symptom relief with 2.5 mg once daily.

Children ages 6 to 11: 2.5 mg once daily in the evening. Maximum dosage, 2.5 mg/day.

Children ages 6 months to 5 years: 1.25 mg (2.5 mL) once daily in the evening. Maximum dosage, 1.25 mg/day.

Adjust-a-dose: For patients age 12 and older with CrCl of 50 to 80 mL/minute, give 2.5 mg PO once daily; with CrCl of 30 to 50 mL/minute, give 2.5 mg PO every other day; with CrCl of 10 to 30 mL/minute, give 2.5 mg PO twice weekly (once every 3 to 4 days). Use in patients with ESRD, those undergoing hemodialysis, and children younger than age 12 with any renal impairment is contraindicated.

➤ **Perennial allergic rhinitis**

Children ages 6 months to 5 years: 1.25 mg (2.5 mL) PO daily in the evening. Don't exceed this dose.

Adjust-a-dose: Use in the presence of renal impairment is contraindicated.

ADMINISTRATION

PO

• Give drug in the evening without regard for food.

ACTION

H_1-receptor inhibition creates antihistamine effect, relieving allergy symptoms.

Route	Onset	Peak	Duration
PO	1 hr	½–1 hr	24 hr

Half-life: Adults, 8 to 9 hours; children, 6 hours.

ADVERSE REACTIONS

CNS: asthenia, fatigue, pyrexia, somnolence. **EENT:** otitis media, epistaxis, nasopharyngitis, pharyngitis. **GI:** diarrhea, dry mouth, vomiting, constipation. **GU:** urine retention. **Respiratory:** cough.

INTERACTIONS

Drug-drug. *CNS depressants:* May have additive effects when taken together. Avoid using together.

Ritonavir: May increase serum concentration and increase half-life of levocetirizine. Use cautiously together.

Theophylline: May decrease the clearance of levocetirizine. Use cautiously together.

Drug-lifestyle. *Alcohol use:* May have additive effect when taken with levocetirizine. Discourage use together.

EFFECTS ON LAB TEST RESULTS

• May prevent, reduce, or mask positive result skin wheal in diagnostic skin test.

CONTRAINDICATIONS & CAUTIONS

• Contraindicated in patients hypersensitive to drug or to cetirizine.

• Contraindicated in patients with CrCl of less than 10 mL/minute or those undergoing hemodialysis.

• Contraindicated in patients younger than age 12 with impaired renal function, in those with ESRD, and in those undergoing dialysis.

• Use cautiously in elderly patients.

• Use cautiously in patients with predisposing factors for urine retention, such as spinal cord lesion or prostatic hyperplasia. Discontinue drug if urine retention occurs.

Dialyzable drug: Less than 10%.

⚠ **Overdose S&S:** Drowsiness; initial agitation and restlessness, then drowsiness (in children).

PREGNANCY-LACTATION-REPRODUCTION

• There are no adequate studies in pregnant women. Use only if clearly needed.

• Drug may appear in human milk. Use in breastfeeding women isn't recommended.

NURSING CONSIDERATIONS

• Monitor patient's renal function.

• Patient should avoid engaging in hazardous occupations requiring mental alertness and motor coordination, such as operating machinery or driving a motor vehicle.

• Safety and effectiveness in patients younger than age 6 months haven't been established.

PATIENT TEACHING

• Warn patient not to perform hazardous tasks or those requiring alertness and coordination until CNS effects are known.

L

• Advise patient to avoid use of alcohol and other CNS depressants while taking this drug.

• Advise patient not to take more than the recommended dose because of increased risk of somnolence at higher doses.

levodopa–carbidopa
lee-voe-DOE-pa/kar-bih-DOE-pa

Duopa, Rytary, Sinemet♦,
Sinemet CR♦

Therapeutic class: Antiparkinsonian drugs
Pharmacologic class: Decarboxylase inhibitors–dopamine precursors

AVAILABLE FORMS
Capsules (extended-release) ⓞ: 95 mg levodopa with 23.75 mg carbidopa, 145 mg levodopa with 36.25 mg carbidopa, 195 mg levodopa with 48.75 mg carbidopa, 245 mg levodopa with 61.25 mg carbidopa
Enteral suspension: levodopa 20 mg/mL with 4.63 mg/mL carbidopa in single-use cassettes
Tablets (extended-release) ⓞ: 200 mg levodopa with 50 mg carbidopa (Sinemet CR), 100 mg levodopa with 25 mg carbidopa (Sinemet CR)
Tablets (immediate-release): 100 mg levodopa with 10 mg carbidopa (Sinemet 10–100), 100 mg levodopa with 25 mg carbidopa (Sinemet 25–100), 250 mg levodopa with 25 mg carbidopa (Sinemet 25–250)
Tablets (ODTs): 100 mg levodopa with 10 mg carbidopa, 100 mg levodopa with 25 mg carbidopa, 250 mg levodopa with 25 mg carbidopa

INDICATIONS & DOSAGES
➤ **Idiopathic Parkinson disease, post-encephalitic parkinsonism, and symptomatic parkinsonism resulting from carbon monoxide or manganese intoxication**
Adults: 1 immediate-release tablet of 100 mg levodopa with 25 mg carbidopa PO t.i.d., increased by 1 tablet daily or every other day, as needed, to maximum daily dose of 8 tablets. May use 250 mg levodopa with 25 mg carbidopa or 100 mg levodopa with 10 mg carbidopa tablets, as directed, to

obtain maximal response. Optimum daily dose must be determined by careful adjustment for each patient. Or, 1 extended-release capsule of 95 mg levodopa with 23.75 mg carbidopa t.i.d. for 3 days; on day 4, increase to 145 mg levodopa with 36.25 mg carbidopa t.i.d. Adjust dose as needed; may increase dose up to 390 mg levodopa with 97.5 mg t.i.d. May increase frequency of dosing to maximum of five times daily if needed and tolerated. Maximum recommended daily dose is 2,450 mg levodopa with 612.5 mg carbidopa. Or, 1 extended-release tablet of 200 mg levodopa with 50 mg carbidopa b.i.d. at intervals of 6 hours or more. Increase or decrease doses and dosing intervals based on response. Most patients have been adequately treated with a dose that provides 400 to 1,600 mg of levodopa per day (divided doses) at intervals of 4 to 8 hours while awake. Allow at least a 3-day interval between dosage adjustments.

Refer to manufacturer's instructions to convert from immediate-release to extended-release formulations.

➤ **Motor fluctuations in patients with advanced Parkinson disease (Duopa)**
🛈 *Alert:* Before initiating enteral therapy, convert patient from all other forms of levodopa to oral immediate-release levodopa–carbidopa tablets (1:4 ratio).
Adults: Total daily dose (expressed in terms of levodopa) consists of a morning dose, a continuous dose, and extra doses, which can be used to manage acute "off" symptoms not controlled by the morning and continuous dose. Refer to manufacturer's labeling for morning dose and continuous dose calculations and titration instructions. Maximum dose of morning and continuous dose is 2,000 mg of the levodopa component over 16 hours. Maximum of extra doses is one extra dose every 2 hours. Give patient's routine nighttime dosage of oral immediate-release levodopa–carbidopa after discontinuation of daily infusion.
Adjust-a-dose: For dyskinesias or levodopa-related adverse reactions within 1 hour of morning dose on preceding day, decrease morning dose by 1 mL. For dyskinesias or adverse reactions lasting 1 hour or more on preceding day, decrease continuous dose by 0.3 mL/hour. For dyskinesias or adverse

reactions lasting for two or more periods of 1 hour or more on preceding day, decrease continuous dose by 0.6 mL/hour.

ADMINISTRATION
PO
• Give drug with food to decrease GI upset, but avoid giving with high-protein meals, which can impair absorption and reduce effectiveness.
• Don't crush or break extended-release form.
• Give ODT immediately after removing from bottle. Place tablet on patient's tongue, where it will dissolve in seconds and be swallowed with saliva. No additional fluid is needed.
• For patients who have difficulty swallowing, capsules may be opened and the entire contents sprinkled on a small amount of applesauce (1 to 2 tablespoons) and then consumed immediately (don't store for future use).
Enteral
• Before use, fully thaw in refrigerator. To ensure controlled thawing, take cartons containing the seven individual cassettes out of the transport box and separate cartons from each other.
• Assign a 12-week, use-by date based on the time the cartons are put into the refrigerator to thaw (may take up to 96 hours to thaw).
• Once thawed, individual cartons may be packed in a closer configuration within the refrigerator.
• Remove one cassette from refrigerator 20 minutes before administration (failure to use at room temperature may result in inaccurate dosage).
• Administer through either a nasojejunal tube (temporary administration) or a percutaneous endoscopic gastrostomy-jejunostomy tube (long-term administration) connected to the CADD-Legacy 1400 pump.
• Disconnect tube from the pump at end of infusion and flush tube with room temperature drinking water with a syringe.
• Cassettes are for single use only and should be discarded daily after infusion. Don't reuse opened cassettes.

ACTION
Levodopa, a dopamine precursor, relieves parkinsonian symptoms by being converted to dopamine in the brain. Carbidopa inhibits the decarboxylation of peripheral levodopa, which allows more intact levodopa to travel to the brain.

Route	Onset	Peak	Duration
PO	Unknown	30–120 min	Unknown
Enteral	Unknown	2½ hr	Unknown

Half-life: 1½ to 2 hours.

ADVERSE REACTIONS
CNS: syncope, agitation, bradykinetic episodes, confusion, dementia, *suicidal tendencies,* dizziness, dream abnormalities, headache, insomnia, *NMS,* paresthesia, psychotic episodes, somnolence. **CV:** cardiac irregularities, HTN, hypotension, orthostatic hypotension, palpitations, phlebitis, *MI.* **GI:** anorexia, constipation, dark saliva, duodenal ulcer, diarrhea, dry mouth, dyspepsia, *GI bleeding,* taste alterations, vomiting. **GU:** dark urine, urinary frequency, UTI. **Hematologic:** *agranulocytosis,* hemolytic and nonhemolytic anemia, *leukopenia, thrombocytopenia.* **Musculoskeletal:** back pain, muscle cramps, shoulder pain. **Respiratory:** dyspnea, URI. **Skin:** alopecia, rash, diaphoresis, dark sweat. **Other:** increased libido, hypersensitivity.

INTERACTIONS
Drug-drug. *Antihypertensives:* May cause additive hypotensive effects. Use together cautiously.
Antipsychotics (butyrophenones, phenothiazines, risperidone): May decrease levodopa activity and increase risk of NMS. Monitor patient closely.
Iron salts (oral): May reduce bioavailability of levodopa–carbidopa. Give iron 1 hour before or 2 hours after oral levodopa–carbidopa.
Isoniazid: May antagonize antiparkinsonian actions. Use together cautiously. Therapy modification may be necessary.
MAO inhibitors: May cause risk of severe HTN. Avoid using together.
Methylphenidate: May increase risk of adverse effects related to levodopa–carbidopa. Monitor patient carefully.

L

Metoclopramide: May decrease therapeutic effects of levodopa–carbidopa. Monitor therapeutic effects.

Papaverine, phenytoin: May antagonize antiparkinsonian actions. Avoid using together.

Sapropterin: May increase risk of levodopa-related adverse effects. Monitor patient carefully.

TCAs: May cause increase in BP and dyskinesia. Use together cautiously.

Drug-herb. *Kava:* May decrease action of drug. Discourage kava use altogether.

Drug-food. *Foods high in protein:* May decrease levodopa absorption. Don't give levodopa with high-protein foods.

EFFECTS ON LAB TEST RESULTS

• May increase BUN, creatinine, uric acid, ALT, AST, alkaline phosphatase, LDH, and bilirubin levels.

• May decrease Hb level and hematocrit and WBC, granulocyte, and platelet counts.

• May falsely increase urinary catecholamine level and serum and urinary uric acid levels in colorimetric tests. May falsely decrease urinary vanillylmandelic acid level. May cause false-positive results in urine ketone tests using sodium nitroprusside reagent and in urine glucose tests using cupric sulfate reagent. May cause false-negative urine glucose or false-positive urine acetone results in tests using glucose oxidase. May alter results of urine screening tests for phenylketonuria.

• May cause positive Coombs test.

CONTRAINDICATIONS & CAUTIONS

• Contraindicated in patients hypersensitive to drug and in those with angle-closure glaucoma, melanoma, or undiagnosed skin lesions.

• Contraindicated within 14 days of MAO inhibitor therapy.

• Use cautiously in patients with severe CV, renal, hepatic, endocrine, or pulmonary disorders; orthostatic hypotension; history of peptic ulcer; psychiatric illness; MI with residual arrhythmias; bronchial asthma; emphysema; or well-controlled, chronic open-angle glaucoma.

• Potentially fatal GI complications, including bezoar, ileus, implant-site erosion or ulcer, intestinal hemorrhage, intestinal ischemia, intestinal obstruction, intestinal perforation, pancreatitis, peritonitis, pneumoperitoneum, and postoperative wound infection, may occur in patients receiving enteral therapy.

• May increase risk of impulse-control disorders, dyskinesia, melanoma, orthostatic hypotension, and sudden somnolence.

Dialyzable drug: Unknown.

⚠ Overdose S&S: Muscle twitching, blepharospasm.

PREGNANCY-LACTATION-REPRODUCTION

• There are no adequate studies in pregnant women. Use during pregnancy only if potential benefit justifies potential risk to the fetus.

• Drug appears in human milk. Use cautiously in breastfeeding women.

NURSING CONSIDERATIONS

• Determine optimum daily dose by careful titration in each patient. Therapy should be individualized and adjusted according to the desired therapeutic response.

• Observe patient and monitor vital signs, especially changes in BP, when changing positions and while adjusting dosage. Report significant changes.

⟳ Alert: Because of risk of precipitating a symptom complex resembling NMS, observe patient closely if levodopa dosage is reduced abruptly or stopped.

• Hallucinations may require reduction or withdrawal of drug.

• Test patients receiving long-term therapy regularly for diabetes and acromegaly, and periodically for hepatic, renal, and hematopoietic function.

PATIENT TEACHING

• Tell patient to take drug with food to minimize GI upset; however, high-protein meals can impair absorption and reduce effectiveness.

• Tell patient not to chew or crush extended-release form.

• Advise patient to have skin checks.

• Warn patient and caregivers not to increase or decrease dosage without prescriber's orders.

• Caution patient about possible dizziness when standing up quickly, especially at start

---

Reactions in bold italics are *life-threatening*. Interactions may have a *rapid onset* or a *delayed onset*.

of therapy. Tell patient to change positions slowly and dangle legs before getting out of bed.
• Instruct patient to report adverse reactions (such as somnolence, loss of impulse control) and therapeutic effects.
• Advise patient receiving enteral therapy to immediately report abdominal pain, prolonged constipation, nausea, vomiting, fever, or melanotic stool.
• Inform patient that pyridoxine (vitamin B_6) doesn't reverse beneficial effects of levodopa–carbidopa. Multivitamins can be taken without reversing levodopa's effects.
• Teach patient to take ODT immediately after taking from bottle and to place on top of tongue. Tablet will dissolve in seconds and will be swallowed with saliva. No additional fluid is needed.

levodopa–carbidopa–entacapone
lee-voe-DOE-pa/kar-bih-DOE-pa/en-ta-KAP-own

Stalevo✐

Therapeutic class: Antiparkinsonian drugs
Pharmacologic class: Dopamine precursors–decarboxylase inhibitors–catecholamine-*O*-methyltransferase inhibitors

AVAILABLE FORMS
Tablets (film-coated) ⓞⓣⓒ: 50 mg levodopa, 12.5 mg carbidopa, and 200 mg entacapone; 75 mg levodopa, 18.75 mg carbidopa, and 200 mg entacapone; 100 mg levodopa, 25 mg carbidopa, and 200 mg entacapone; 125 mg levodopa, 31.25 mg carbidopa, and 200 mg entacapone; 150 mg levodopa, 37.5 mg carbidopa, and 200 mg entacapone; 200 mg levodopa, 50 mg carbidopa, and 200 mg entacapone

INDICATIONS & DOSAGES
➤ **Idiopathic Parkinson disease, to replace (with equivalent strengths) levodopa, carbidopa, and entacapone given individually or to replace immediate-release levodopa–carbidopa for patient who has end-of-dose "wearing off," who's** taking a total daily levodopa dose of 600 mg or less, and who has no dyskinesia
Adults: 1 tablet PO; determine dose and interval by therapeutic response. Maximum, 8 tablets/24 hours for all strengths except levodopa 200 mg, carbidopa 50 mg, and entacapone 200 mg; for these strengths, give maximum 6 tablets/24 hours.

ADMINISTRATION
PO
• Don't cut, crush, or allow patient to chew tablets.
• Give only 1 tablet at each dosing interval.
• Give drug with or without food, but avoid giving with a high-fat, high-calorie meal, which can decrease absorption.

ACTION
Levodopa, a dopamine precursor, relieves parkinsonian symptoms by converting to dopamine in the brain. Carbidopa inhibits the decarboxylation of peripheral levodopa, which allows more intact levodopa to travel to the brain. Entacapone is a reversible catecholamine-*O*-methyltransferase (COMT) inhibitor that increases levodopa level.

Route	Onset	Peak	Duration
PO	Unknown	1–3½ hr	Unknown

Half-life: Carbidopa, 1½ to 2 hours; levodopa, 1 to 3¼ hours; entacapone, ¾ to 1 hour.

ADVERSE REACTIONS
levodopa and carbidopa
CNS: syncope, agitation, bradykinetic episodes, confusion, dementia, *suicidal tendencies,* dizziness, dream abnormalities, headache, insomnia, *NMS,* paresthesia, psychotic episodes, somnolence, hallucinations. **CV:** cardiac irregularities, HTN, hypotension, orthostatic hypotension, palpitations, phlebitis, *MI.* **GI:** anorexia, constipation, dark saliva, duodenal ulcer, diarrhea, dry mouth, dyspepsia, *GI bleeding,* taste alterations, vomiting. **GU:** dark urine, urinary frequency, UTI. **Hematologic:** *agranulocytosis,* hemolytic and nonhemolytic anemia, *leukopenia, thrombocytopenia.* **Musculoskeletal:** back pain, muscle cramps, shoulder pain.

L

Respiratory: dyspnea, URI. **Skin:** alopecia, rash, diaphoresis, dark sweat. **Other:** increased libido, hypersensitivity.

entacapone

CNS: dyskinesia, hyperkinesia, agitation, anxiety, asthenia, dizziness, fatigue, hypokinesia, somnolence. **GI:** diarrhea, nausea, abdominal pain, constipation, dry mouth, dyspepsia, flatulence, gastritis, taste perversion, vomiting. **GU:** urine discoloration. **Musculoskeletal:** back pain. **Respiratory:** dyspnea. **Skin:** increased sweating, purpura. **Other:** bacterial infection.

INTERACTIONS

Drug-drug. *Ampicillin, chloramphenicol, cholestyramine, erythromycin, probenecid, rifampin:* May interfere with entacapone excretion. Use together cautiously.

Antihypertensives: May cause orthostatic hypotension. Adjust antihypertensive dosage as needed.

CNS depressants: Additive effects. Use together cautiously.

Dopamine (D2) receptor antagonists (butyrophenones, iron salts, isoniazid, metoclopramide, phenothiazines, phenytoin, risperidone): May decrease levodopa, carbidopa, and entacapone effects. Monitor patient for effectiveness.

Drugs metabolized by COMT (apomorphine, dobutamine, dopamine, epinephrine, isoetharine, isoproterenol, methyldopa, norepinephrine): May increase HR, arrhythmias, and excessive BP changes. Use together cautiously.

Iron salts (oral): May reduce bioavailability of levodopa–carbidopa–entacapone. Separate drugs by 2 or more hours; monitor therapy.

Metoclopramide: May increase availability of levodopa and carbidopa by increasing gastric emptying. Monitor patient for adverse effects.

Nonselective MAO inhibitors: May disrupt catecholamine metabolism. Use together is contraindicated.

Selegiline: May cause severe hypotension. Use together cautiously, and monitor BP.

TCAs: May increase risk of HTN and dyskinesia. Monitor patient closely.

Drug-food. *Foods high in protein:* May decrease levodopa absorption. Don't give drug with high-protein foods.

Drug-herb. *Kava kava:* May decrease action of drug. Discourage kava kava use altogether.

Drug-lifestyle. *Alcohol use:* May enhance CNS depressant effects. Monitor therapy.

EFFECTS ON LAB TEST RESULTS

• May increase alkaline phosphatase, AST, ALT, LDH, glucose, BUN, and bilirubin levels. May decrease Hb level and hematocrit.

• May decrease platelet and WBC counts.

• May cause false-positive reaction for urinary ketone bodies on a test tape. May cause false-negative result for glycosuria with glucose oxidase testing methods.

• May cause abnormal catecholamine and Coombs test.

CONTRAINDICATIONS & CAUTIONS

• Contraindicated in patients hypersensitive to drug or its components.

• Contraindicated in patients with angle-closure glaucoma, suspicious undiagnosed skin lesions, or a history of melanoma.

• Contraindicated within 2 weeks of MAO inhibitor therapy.

• Use cautiously in patients with past or current psychosis and in patients with severe pulmonary disease; bronchial asthma; biliary obstruction; peptic ulcer; or renal, hepatic, or endocrine disease.

• Use cautiously in patients with chronic open-angle glaucoma or hepatic impairment.

Dialyzable drug: Unlikely.

⚠ *Overdose S&S:* CNS disturbances, hypotension, tachycardia, rhabdomyolysis, transient renal insufficiency, abdominal pain, loose stools.

PREGNANCY-LACTATION-REPRODUCTION

• There are no adequate studies in pregnant women. Use only if potential benefit justifies potential risk to the fetus.

• It isn't known if drug appears in human milk. Use cautiously in breastfeeding women.

NURSING CONSIDERATIONS

• Certain CNS effects, such as dyskinesia, may occur at lower dosages and sooner with levodopa–carbidopa–entacapone than with levodopa alone. Dyskinesia may require a reduced dosage.

Reactions in bold italics are *life-threatening*. Interactions may have a *rapid onset* or a **delayed onset**.

• Monitor patients for orthostatic hypotension, especially during dosage escalation.
• NMS may develop when levodopa and carbidopa are reduced or stopped, especially in patients taking antipsychotic drugs. Watch patient carefully for fever, hyperthermia, muscle rigidity, involuntary movements, altered consciousness, mental status changes, and autonomic dysfunction.
• During extended therapy, periodically monitor hepatic, hematopoietic, CV, and renal function.
• Diarrhea is common; it usually develops 4 to 12 weeks after treatment starts but may appear as early as the first week or as late as many months after treatment starts.
۞ Alert: Monitor patient for hallucinations, depression, and suicidal tendencies.

PATIENT TEACHING
• Advise patient to take drug exactly as prescribed and not to split or crush tablets.
• Tell patient to report a "wearing-off" effect, which may occur at the end of the dosing interval.
• Tell patient that urine, sweat, and saliva may turn dark (red, brown, or black) during treatment.
• Advise patient to notify the prescriber if problems making voluntary movements increase.
• Tell patient that diarrhea is common with this treatment.
• Inform patient that hallucinations may occur.
• Urge patient to immediately report depression, suicidal thoughts, or loss of impulse control.
• Explain that patient may become dizzy if rising quickly. Urge patient to use caution when rising.
• Tell patient that excessive acidity, iron salts, or a high-fat, high-calorie, or high-protein diet may reduce drug's effectiveness.
• Urge patient to avoid hazardous activities until CNS effects of drug are known.
• Advise female patient to notify prescriber if she becomes pregnant.

levoFLOXacin
lee-voe-FLOX-a-sin

Levaquin✐

Therapeutic class: Antibiotics
Pharmacologic class: Fluoroquinolones

AVAILABLE FORMS
Infusion (premixed): 250 mg in 50 mL D₅W, 500 mg in 100 mL D₅W, 750 mg in 150 mL D₅W
Ophthalmic solution: 0.5%
Oral solution: 25 mg/mL
Single-use vials: 500 mg, 750 mg
Tablets: 250 mg, 500 mg, 750 mg

INDICATIONS & DOSAGES
Black Box Warning Use in patients with acute bacterial sinusitis, acute bacterial exacerbation of bronchitis, and uncomplicated UTI isn't recommended because of risk of serious adverse effects. Use in these patients only when they have no other treatment options. ∎
Adjust-a-dose (for all indications): For patients with CrCl of less than 50 mL/minute, adjust the oral or IV dosage regimen according to the manufacturer's instructions.
➤ **Acute bacterial sinusitis caused by susceptible strains of** *Streptococcus pneumoniae, Moraxella catarrhalis,* **or** *Haemophilus influenzae*
Adults: 500 mg PO or IV infusion over 60 minutes every 24 hours for 10 to 14 days or 750 mg PO or IV every 24 hours for 5 days.
➤ **Mild to moderate skin and skin-structure infections caused by** *Staphylococcus aureus* **or** *Streptococcus pyogenes*
Adults: 500 mg PO or IV infusion every 24 hours for 7 to 10 days.
➤ **Acute bacterial worsening of chronic bronchitis caused by** *S. aureus, S. pneumoniae, M. catarrhalis, H. influenzae,* **or** *Haemophilus parainfluenzae*
Adults: 500 mg PO or IV infusion every 24 hours for 7 days.
➤ **To prevent inhalation anthrax after confirmed or suspected exposure to** *Bacillus anthracis*

Adults: 500 mg IV infusion or PO every 24 hours for 60 days.

Children age 6 months and older weighing at least 50 kg: 500 mg PO or by slow IV infusion every 24 hours for 60 days.

Children age 6 months and older weighing less than 50 kg: 250 mg PO or 8 mg/kg (not to exceed 250 mg/dose) oral solution or by slow IV infusion every 12 hours for 60 days.

➤ **Chronic bacterial prostatitis caused by** *Escherichia coli, Enterococcus faecalis,* **or** *Staphylococcus epidermidis*
Adults: 500 mg PO or IV infusion every 24 hours for 28 days.

➤ **Community-acquired pneumonia from** *S. pneumoniae* **(excluding multidrug-resistant strains),** *H. influenzae, H. parainfluenzae, Mycoplasma pneumoniae,* **or** *Chlamydia pneumoniae*
Adults: 750 mg PO or IV infusion every 24 hours for 5 days.

➤ **Community-acquired pneumonia caused by methicillin-susceptible** *S. aureus, S. pneumoniae, H. influenzae, H. parainfluenzae, Klebsiella pneumoniae, M. catarrhalis, C. pneumoniae, Legionella pneumophila,* **or** *M. pneumoniae*
Adults: 500 mg PO or IV infusion every 24 hours for 7 to 14 days.

➤ **Complicated skin and skin-structure infections caused by methicillin-sensitive** *S. aureus, E. faecalis, S. pyogenes,* **or** *Proteus mirabilis*
Adults: 750 mg PO or IV infusion every 24 hours for 7 to 14 days.

➤ **Nosocomial pneumonia caused by methicillin-susceptible** *S. aureus, Pseudomonas aeruginosa, Serratia marcescens, E. coli, K. pneumoniae, H. influenzae,* **or** *S. pneumoniae*
Adults: 750 mg PO or IV infusion every 24 hours for 7 to 14 days.

➤ **Complicated UTI caused by** *E. faecalis, Enterobacter cloacae, E. coli, K. pneumoniae, P. mirabilis,* **or** *P. aeruginosa;* **acute pyelonephritis caused by** *E. coli*
Adults: 250 mg PO or IV infusion every 24 hours for 10 days.

➤ **Complicated UTI caused by** *E. coli, K. pneumoniae,* **or** *P. mirabilis;* **acute pyelonephritis caused by** *E. coli*
Adults: 750 mg PO or IV infusion daily for 5 days.

➤ **Mild to moderate uncomplicated UTI caused by** *E. coli, K. pneumoniae,* **or** *Staphylococcus saprophyticus*
Adults: 250 mg PO daily for 3 days.

➤ **Prophylaxis or treatment of pneumonic and septicemic plague** *(Yersinia pestis)*
Adults: 500 mg PO or IV infusion every 24 hours for 10 to 14 days.

Children age 6 months and older weighing 50 kg or more: 500 mg PO or by slow IV infusion every 24 hours for 10 to 14 days.

Children age 6 months and older weighing less than 50 kg: 250 mg PO or 8 mg/kg (not to exceed 250 mg/dose) oral solution or by slow IV infusion every 12 hours for 10 to 14 days.

➤ **Bacterial conjunctivitis**
Adults and children age 6 and older: On days 1 through 3, instill 1 to 2 drops in affected eye(s) every 30 minutes to 2 hours while patient is awake and approximately 4 and 6 hours after retiring. On days 4 through 7, instill 1 to 2 drops in affected eye(s) every 1 to 4 hours while patient is awake.

ADMINISTRATION
PO
• Obtain specimen for culture and sensitivity tests before therapy and as needed to determine if bacterial resistance has occurred.
• Give drug with plenty of fluids.
• Give 2 hours before or 2 hours after antacids, sucralfate, and products containing magnesium, aluminum, iron, or multivitamins with zinc.
• Give oral solution 1 hour before or 2 hours after a meal.

IV
▼ Obtain specimen for culture and sensitivity tests before therapy and as needed to determine if bacterial resistance has occurred.
▼ Give this form only by infusion.
▼ Dilute drug in single-use vials, according to manufacturer's instructions, with D_5W or NSS for injection to a final concentration of 5 mg/mL.
▼ Infuse doses of 500 mg or less over 60 minutes and doses of 750 mg over 90 minutes.
▼ Reconstituted solution should be clear, slightly yellow, and free of particulate matter.

▼ Reconstituted drug is stable for 72 hours at room temperature, for 14 days when refrigerated in plastic containers, and for 6 months when frozen.

▼ Thaw at room temperature or in refrigerator.

▼ **Incompatibilities:** The manufacturer recommends not mixing or infusing other drugs with levofloxacin.

Ophthalmic

• Avoid touching applicator tip to eye or other surfaces.

ACTION

Inhibits bacterial DNA gyrase and prevents DNA replication, transcription, repair, and recombination in susceptible bacteria.

Route	Onset	Peak	Duration
PO, IV	Unknown	1–2 hr	Unknown
Ophthalmic	Unknown	Unknown	Unknown

Half-life: About 6 to 8 hours.

ADVERSE REACTIONS

CNS: *encephalopathy, seizures,* dizziness, headache, insomnia; headache (ophthalmic). **CV:** edema, chest pain. **EENT:** foreign body or burning sensation in eye, eye pain, blurred vision, vision loss, photophobia (ophthalmic). **GI:** *pseudomembranous colitis,* abdominal pain, constipation, diarrhea, dyspepsia, nausea, vomiting. **GU:** vaginitis. **Hematologic:** *lymphopenia,* eosinophilia, hemolytic anemia. **Metabolic:** *hypoglycemia.* **Musculoskeletal:** back pain, tendon rupture. **Respiratory:** allergic pneumonitis, dyspnea. **Skin:** *erythema multiforme, SJS,* photosensitivity, pruritus, rash, injection-site reaction. **Other:** *anaphylaxis, multisystem organ failure, hypersensitivity reactions.*

INTERACTIONS

Drug-drug. *Aluminum hydroxide, aluminummagnesium hydroxide, calcium carbonate, didanosine, magnesium hydroxide, products containing zinc, sucralfate:* May interfere with GI absorption of levofloxacin. Give levofloxacin 2 hours before or 2 hours after these products.

Antiarrhythmics (Class IA [procainamide, quinidine] or Class III [amiodarone, dofetilide]), chlorpromazine, erythromycin,

fluconazole, haloperidol, imipramine, ondansetron, ziprasidone: May increase risk of life-threatening cardiac arrhythmias. Avoid use together.

Antidiabetics: May alter glucose level. Monitor glucose level closely.

Iron salts: May decrease absorption of levofloxacin, reducing anti-infective response. Separate doses by at least 2 hours.

NSAIDs: May increase CNS stimulation. Monitor patient for seizure activity.

Black Box Warning *Steroids:* May increase risk of tendinitis and tendon rupture. Monitor patient for tendon pain or inflammation. ∎

Theophylline: May decrease clearance of theophylline. Monitor theophylline level.

Warfarin and derivatives: May increase effect of oral anticoagulant. Monitor PT and INR.

Drug-lifestyle. *Sun exposure:* May cause photosensitivity reactions. Advise patient to avoid excessive sunlight exposure.

EFFECTS ON LAB TEST RESULTS

• May decrease glucose and Hb levels.

• May increase eosinophil count. May decrease WBC count.

• May produce false-positive opioid assay results.

CONTRAINDICATIONS & CAUTIONS

Black Box Warning Drug is associated with increased risk of tendinitis and tendon rupture, especially in patients older than age 60, in patients taking corticosteroids, and in those with heart, kidney, or lung transplants. ∎

Black Box Warning Drug may exacerbate muscle weakness in patients with myasthenia gravis. Avoid using fluoroquinolones in patients with a history of myasthenia gravis. ∎

Black Box Warning Reserve drug for patients who have no alternative treatment options for uncomplicated UTI, acute exacerbation of chronic bronchitis, and acute sinusitis. ∎

❸ *Alert:* Drug is associated with an increased incidence of musculoskeletal disorders (arthralgia, arthritis, tendinopathy, and gait abnormality) in pediatric patients. Testing of drug in immature animals has resulted in increased osteochondrosis, erosions in weight-bearing joints, and other signs and symptoms of arthropathy.

◑ *Alert:* Drug may increase risk of aortic dissection or rupture when used systemically. Avoid use in patients with known aortic aneurysm and in patients at risk for an aortic aneurysm, including those with peripheral atherosclerotic vascular diseases, HTN, certain genetic conditions (Marfan syndrome, Ehlers-Danlos syndrome), and elderly patients. Drug should only be used in these patients if no other treatment options are available.

• Contraindicated in patients hypersensitive to drug, its components, or other fluoroquinolones.

◑ *Alert:* Patients receiving systemic drug have an increased risk of hyperglycemia and hypoglycemia, which can result in coma. Hypoglycemia has been reported more frequently in the elderly and those with diabetes.

• Use cautiously in patients with history of seizure disorders or other CNS diseases, such as cerebral arteriosclerosis.

• Use cautiously and with dosage adjustment in patients with renal impairment.

• Drug is indicated in children (age 6 months and older) only for postexposure inhalational anthrax prevention and for plague.

Dialyzable drug: No.

PREGNANCY-LACTATION-REPRODUCTION
• There are no adequate studies in pregnant women. Use during pregnancy only if potential benefit justifies potential risk to the fetus.

• Drug probably appears in human milk. Patient should discontinue breastfeeding or discontinue drug.

NURSING CONSIDERATIONS
Black Box Warning Fluoroquinolones have been associated with disabling and potentially irreversible serious adverse reactions that have occurred together, including tendinitis and tendon rupture, peripheral neuropathy, and CNS effects (seizures, toxic psychoses, increased ICP, pseudotumor cerebri, tremors, restlessness, anxiety, light-headedness, confusion, hallucinations,

paranoia, depression, nightmares, insomnia and, rarely, suicidal thoughts or acts). If any of these serious adverse reactions occur, discontinue drug immediately. ■

◑ *Alert:* Monitor patients for signs and symptoms of aortic aneurysm, dissection, and rupture (sudden, severe, and constant pain in the stomach, chest, or back; throbbing in the stomach area, deep pain in the back or side of the stomach; steady, gnawing pain in the stomach that lasts for hours or days; pain in the jaw, neck, back, or chest; coughing or hoarseness; shortness of breath or trouble swallowing). Discontinue drug immediately if any of these aortic disorders are suspected.

• Patients with acute hypersensitivity reactions may need treatment with epinephrine, oxygen, IV fluids, antihistamines, corticosteroids, pressor amines, and airway management.

Black Box Warning Monitor patient for signs and symptoms of peripheral neuropathy (pain, burning, tingling, numbness, weakness, or a change in sensation to light touch, pain, temperature, or sense of body position), and report them immediately to health care provider. ■

• Most antibacterials can cause pseudomembranous colitis. If diarrhea occurs, notify prescriber; drug may be stopped.

• Drug may cause an abnormal ECG.

◑ *Alert:* Monitor patients receiving systemic drug for symptoms of hypoglycemia (confusion, pounding or rapid heartbeat, dizziness, pale skin, shakiness, sweating, unusual hunger, trembling, headache, weakness, irritability, unusual anxiety). Immediately discontinue drug for blood glucose disturbances, and switch to a nonfluoroquinolone antibiotic if possible.

◑ *Alert:* Monitor patients receiving systemic drug for psychiatric adverse reactions (disturbances in attention, disorientation, agitation, nervousness, memory impairment, delirium). Discontinue drug for CNS side effects, including psychiatric adverse reactions.

◑ *Alert:* If *P. aeruginosa* is a confirmed or suspected pathogen, use with a beta-lactam.

• Monitor glucose level and results of renal function tests, LFTs, and blood counts.

Reactions in bold italics are *life-threatening*. Interactions may have a *rapid onset* or a *delayed onset*.

• *Look alike–sound alike:* Don't confuse levofloxacin with levetiracetam.

PATIENT TEACHING
Black Box Warning Warn patient to immediately notify prescriber for signs and symptoms of serious adverse reactions, including unusual joint or tendon pain, muscle weakness, "pins and needles" tingling or prickling sensation, numbness in the arms or legs, confusion, or hallucinations. ∎

◑ *Alert:* Warn patient to seek immediate medical attention for signs and symptoms of aortic aneurysm, dissection, or rupture.

• Tell patient to take drug as prescribed, even if signs and symptoms disappear.

• Advise patient to take drug with plenty of fluids and to space antacids, sucralfate, and products containing iron or zinc.

• Tell patient to take oral solution 1 hour before or 2 hours after eating.

• Warn patient to avoid hazardous tasks until adverse effects of drug are known.

• Advise patient to avoid excessive sunlight exposure.

• Instruct patient to stop drug and notify prescriber if rash or other signs or symptoms of hypersensitivity develop.

• Instruct patient to notify prescriber of all adverse reactions, including loose stools or diarrhea.

• Tell patient not to take more than one dose in the same day, even if a dose is missed.

• Instruct patient not to use contact lenses during treatment for bacterial conjunctivitis.

◑ *Alert:* Caution patients that significantly low blood sugar level can occur. Instruct patients how to manage symptoms and to immediately report any occurrence to the prescriber.

◑ *Alert:* Advise patients with diabetes that they may need to monitor blood glucose levels more frequently during therapy.

◑ *Alert:* Inform patients to immediately report psychiatric adverse reactions and that these can occur after just one dose.

levomilnacipran hydrochloride
lee-voe-mil-NAY-sih-pran

Fetzima

Therapeutic class: Antidepressants
Pharmacologic class: SSNRIs

AVAILABLE FORMS
Capsules (extended-release) ⓓ: 20 mg, 40 mg, 80 mg, 120 mg

INDICATIONS & DOSAGES
➤ **Major depressive disorder**
Adults: Initially, 20 mg PO once daily for 2 days; then increase to 40 mg once daily. May increase in increments of 40 mg at intervals of 2 or more days. Maximum dosage is 120 mg once daily.
Adjust-a-dose: For patients with CrCl of 30 to 59 mL/minute, maximum maintenance dosage is 80 mg once daily. If CrCl is 15 to 29 mL/minute, maximum maintenance dosage is 40 mg once daily. Don't use for patients with ESRD.

ADMINISTRATION
PO
• Give drug with or without food.
• Make sure patient swallows extended-release capsules whole and doesn't chew, crush, or open them.
• Give drug at approximately the same time each day.

ACTION
A potent inhibitor of neuronal norepinephrine and serotonin reuptake.

Route	Onset	Peak	Duration
PO	Unknown	6–8 hr	Unknown

Half-life: 12 hours.

ADVERSE REACTIONS
CNS: syncope, agitation, extrapyramidal reaction, panic attack, migraine, paresthesia, tension, aggressive behavior, anger outburst, yawning. **CV:** orthostatic hypotension, HTN, angina, chest pain, flushing, palpitations, tachycardia, premature atrial contractions, PVCs. **EENT:** blurred vision, dry eye

syndrome, conjunctival hemorrhage. **GI:** abdominal pain, constipation, decreased appetite, dry mouth, flatulence, nausea, vomiting, thirst, teeth grinding. **GU:** hematuria, proteinuria, urinary frequency; in men—dysuria, ejaculation disorder, erectile dysfunction, libido decrease, prostatitis, scrotal pain, testicular pain, testicular swelling, urethral pain, urinary hesitation, urine retention, urine flow decrease. **Metabolic:** hypercholesterolemia. **Skin:** hyperhidrosis, pruritus, urticaria, rash, dry skin. **Other:** hot flashes.

INTERACTIONS
Drug-drug. *Antipsychotics (risperidone), cyclobenzaprine, dopamine antagonists (metoclopramide):* May increase risk of NMS and serotonin syndrome. If use together can't be avoided, closely monitor patient and if signs and symptoms occur, discontinue drug.
⊗ Alert: *Drugs that affect coagulation or bleeding (aspirin, NSAIDs, warfarin):* May increase risk of bleeding. Use together cautiously.
Lithium, other serotonergic drugs: May cause serotonin syndrome (diarrhea, dysreflexia, fever, hallucinations, loss of coordination, nausea, tachycardia). Avoid use together.
MAO inhibitors: May cause hyperthermia, rigidity, myoclonus, autonomic instability, rapid fluctuations of vital signs, agitation, delirium, and coma. Avoid using drug within 2 weeks after MAO inhibitor therapy; wait at least 7 days after stopping levomilnacipran before starting MAO inhibitor.
Methylene blue: May cause CNS toxicity and serotonin syndrome. Avoid use together.
Drug-herb. *Herbs with anticoagulant properties (alfalfa, anise, bilberry):* May increase bleeding risk. Discourage use together.
St. John's wort: Increases risk of serotonin syndrome. Don't use together.
Drug-lifestyle. *Alcohol use:* May cause more rapid release of levomilnacipran and enhance CNS depression.

EFFECTS ON LAB TEST RESULTS
• May increase LFT values.
• May decrease sodium level.

CONTRAINDICATIONS & CAUTIONS
• Contraindicated in patients hypersensitive to levomilnacipran, milnacipran hydrochloride, or components of the formulation.
• Contraindicated in patients being treated with MAO inhibitors (within 7 days of discontinuing drug or within 2 weeks of discontinuing MAO inhibitor), linezolid, or IV methylene blue.
• Drug isn't approved for treatment of fibromyalgia.
⊗ Alert: Pupillary dilation that occurs after drug use can lead to an angle-closure attack in patients with anatomically narrow angles who don't have a patent iridectomy.
⊗ Alert: Serotonin syndrome, a potentially life-threatening condition, may occur, particularly with concomitant use of serotonergic drugs (including triptans, TCAs, lithium, and tramadol) and drugs that impair serotonin metabolism (including MAO inhibitors). Discontinue drug for signs and symptoms of serotonin syndrome, including mental status changes (agitation, coma, hallucinations), autonomic instability (hyperthermia, labile BP, tachycardia), neuromuscular aberrations (hyperreflexia, incoordination), and diarrhea, nausea, and vomiting.
• Not recommended for use in patients with ESRD.
• Use cautiously in patients with a history of mania, seizures, HTN, tachyarrhythmias, CV disease, glaucoma, or dysuria.
• Avoid use in patients with bipolar disorder.
Dialyzable drug: Unlikely.

PREGNANCY-LACTATION-REPRODUCTION
• There are no adequate studies in pregnant women. Use during pregnancy only if potential benefit justifies potential risk to the fetus. Neonates exposed to SSRIs/SSNRIs late in the third trimester have developed complications requiring prolonged hospitalization, respiratory support, and tube feeding.
• It isn't known if drug appears in human milk. Patient should discontinue breastfeeding or discontinue drug, taking into account importance of drug to the mother.

NURSING CONSIDERATIONS
Black Box Warning Drug may increase the risk of suicidal thinking and behavior in children, adolescents, and young adults with

---

major depressive disorder or other psychiatric disorder. Drug isn't approved for use in children. ■

• At least 14 days should elapse between discontinuation of an MAO inhibitor and initiation of levomilnacipran. Allow at least 7 days after stopping levomilnacipran before starting an MAO inhibitor.

Black Box Warning Monitor patient closely for worsening depression or suicidal behavior, especially during first few months of therapy and with dosage adjustments. ■

• Screen patients with depressive symptoms for bipolar disorder.

• To prevent withdrawal signs and symptoms, decrease dosage gradually, and watch for signs and symptoms that may arise when drug is stopped, such as dysphoria, irritability, agitation, dizziness, sensory disturbances, anxiety, confusion, headache, lethargy, emotional lability, insomnia, hypomania, tinnitus, and seizures.

• Carefully monitor HR and BP.

• Monitor patient for signs of hyponatremia (headache, difficulty concentrating, memory impairment, confusion, weakness, unsteadiness, hallucination, syncope, seizures, coma, respiratory arrest). Volume depletion, diuretic use, and increased age increase risk.

• Monitor LFT values and sodium level before and during therapy.

PATIENT TEACHING

Black Box Warning Warn families and caregivers to immediately report signs and symptoms of worsening depression (such as agitation, irritability, insomnia, hostility, and impulsivity) and suicidal behavior. ■

• Tell patient to consult prescriber before taking other prescription or OTC drugs and to avoid taking NSAIDs and aspirin to reduce risk of bleeding.

• Tell patient to avoid alcohol while taking drug.

• Instruct patient that frequent HR and BP monitoring will be needed and to report dizziness, passing out, or palpitations.

• Tell patient to report urinary hesitation or urine retention.

• Instruct female patient of childbearing potential to notify prescriber if she becomes pregnant, is planning pregnancy during therapy, or is breastfeeding.

• Warn patient not to stop drug suddenly.

• Warn patient to avoid hazardous activities that require alertness and good coordination until drug's effects are known.

• Tell patient to take medication at the same time every day.

• Tell patient that drug may be taken with or without food but that food may increase tolerability.

• Instruct patient to swallow capsules whole and not to chew, crush, or open them.

levothyroxine sodium (T₄, ʟ-thyroxine sodium)
lee-voe-thye-ROX-een

Eltroxin✦, Euthyrox, Levo-T, Levoxyl𝒫, Synthroid𝒫, Tirosint, Unithroid

Therapeutic class: Thyroid hormone replacements
Pharmacologic class: Thyroid hormones

AVAILABLE FORMS

Capsules ⓓⓝⓒ: 13 mcg, 25 mcg, 50 mcg, 75 mcg, 88 mcg, 100 mcg, 112 mcg, 125 mcg, 137 mcg, 150 mcg
Powder for injection: 100 mcg, 200 mcg, 500 mcg
Tablets: 25 mcg, 50 mcg, 75 mcg, 88 mcg, 100 mcg, 112 mcg, 125 mcg, 137 mcg, 150 mcg, 175 mcg, 200 mcg, 300 mcg

INDICATIONS & DOSAGES

➤ **Thyroid hormone replacement**
Adults: In otherwise healthy, nonelderly individuals who have been hypothyroid for only a short time (such as a few months), initiate drug at approximately 1.6 mcg/kg PO once daily. (See individual manufacturer's instructions.) Monitor TSH level and adjust dosage every 4 to 6 weeks in 12.5- to 25-mcg increments until patient is euthyroid and TSH level normalizes.
Adults: For elderly patients or patients with underlying cardiac disease, initiate dose at 12.5 to 25 mcg PO daily. Adjust dosage every 6 to 8 weeks, if needed, until patient is euthyroid and TSH level normalizes.

Children in whom growth and puberty are complete: 1.6 mcg/kg PO once daily. (See individual manufacturer's instructions.)

Children older than age 12 in whom growth and puberty are incomplete: 2 to 3 mcg/kg PO daily.

Children ages 6 to 12: 4 to 5 mcg/kg PO daily.

Children ages 1 to 5: 5 to 6 mcg/kg PO daily.

Children ages 6 months to 1 year: 6 to 8 mcg/kg PO daily.

Children ages 3 to 6 months: 8 to 10 mcg/kg PO daily.

Infants and neonates birth to age 3 months: 10 to 15 mcg/kg PO daily. In neonates at risk for cardiac failure, consider a lower initial dose, and increase every 4 to 6 weeks as needed.

Children at risk for hyperactivity: Initiate at one-fourth the recommended full replacement dose, and increase weekly by one-fourth the full recommended replacement dose until the full recommended replacement dose is reached.

Adjust-a-dose: For children, adjust dosage based on clinical response and laboratory parameters.

➤ **Severe, long-standing hypothyroidism**

Adults and adolescents in whom growth and puberty are complete: 12.5 to 25 mcg PO daily. Increase in increments of 12.5 to 25 mcg every 2 to 4 weeks as needed.

➤ **Myxedema coma**

Adults: Initially, 300 to 500 mcg (0.3 to 0.5 mg) IV as solution followed by 50 to 100 mcg IV once daily until patient is able to tolerate oral administration. Consider smaller doses in patients with CV disease.

➤ **TSH suppression in well-differentiated thyroid cancer**

Adults: Dosage is highly individualized. Generally, TSH is suppressed to below 0.1 milliunits/L, which usually requires a dosage greater than 2 mcg/kg/day. However, in patients with high-risk tumors, target level for TSH suppression may be lower.

ADMINISTRATION

PO

• Synthroid may contain tartrazine.

• Don't crush, break, or allow patient to chew capsules.

• Give drug at same time each day on an empty stomach, preferably ½ to 1 hour before breakfast.

• Give drug at least 4 hours before or after drugs known to interfere with levothyroxine.

• Give tablets with a full glass of water to prevent difficulty swallowing.

• If necessary, crush tablet and suspend it in small amount of formula (except soy formula, which may decrease absorption), human milk, or water, and give by spoon or dropper. Crushed tablet can also be sprinkled over food, except foods containing large amounts of soybean, fiber, or iron.

IV

▼ Reconstitute by adding 5 mL NSS injection only.

▼ Shake vial.

▼ Use immediately after reconstitution.

▼ Discard any unused portion.

▼ **Incompatibilities:** Don't mix or give with anything other than NSS injection.

ACTION

Synthetic form of thyroxine that affects the growth of tissues, energy expenditure, and the turnover of all substrates.

Route	Onset	Peak	Duration
PO	3–5 days	2–4 hr	Unknown
IV	6–8 hr	Unknown	Unknown

Half-life: 6 to 8 days in euthyroidism; 3 to 4 days in hyperthyroidism; 9 to 10 days in hypothyroidism.

ADVERSE REACTIONS

CNS: insomnia, tremor, headache, fever, fatigue, anxiety, emotional lability. **CV:** tachycardia, palpitations, *arrhythmias,* angina pectoris, *cardiac arrest,* HTN, *HF, MI.* **GI:** diarrhea, vomiting, abdominal cramps. **GU:** menstrual irregularities. **Metabolic:** weight loss, increased appetite. **Musculoskeletal:** decreased bone density, muscle weakness, tremors. **Respiratory:** dyspnea. **Skin:** allergic skin reactions, diaphoresis, hair loss. **Other:** heat intolerance, impaired fertility.

INTERACTIONS

Drug-drug. *Amiodarone, iodide (including iodine-containing radiographic contrast agents), lithium:* May reduce thyroid hormone secretion. Monitor thyroid function studies if used together.

Reactions in bold italics are *life-threatening*. Interactions may have a *rapid onset* or a *delayed onset*.

Antacids, calcium carbonate, cholestyramine, colestipol, ferrous sulfate, orlistat, sucralfate: May impair levothyroxine absorption. Separate doses by 4 to 5 hours and monitor therapy.

Beta blockers: May reduce beta-blocker effects. Monitor patient.

Carbamazepine, hydantoins, phenobarbital, rifampin: May increase hepatic metabolism, resulting in hypothyroidism. Monitor patient.

Clofibrate, estrogens, 5-FU, methadone, mitotane, tamoxifen: May decrease thyroid levels. Monitor therapy.

Digoxin: May decrease cardiac glycoside effects. Monitor patient for clinical effect.

Fosphenytoin, phenytoin: May release free thyroid hormone. Monitor patient for tachycardia.

Insulin, oral antidiabetics: May alter glucose level. Monitor glucose level. Dosage adjustments may be needed.

Ketamine: May produce marked HTN and tachycardia. Use together cautiously.

SSRIs: May increase levothyroxine requirements. Adjust dosage as needed.

Sympathomimetics such as epinephrine: May increase risk of coronary insufficiency. Monitor patient closely.

TCAs, tetracyclic antidepressants: May increase therapeutic effects and toxicity of both drugs. Monitor patient closely.

Theophylline: May decrease theophylline clearance in hypothyroidism; clearance may return to normal when euthyroid state is achieved. Monitor theophylline level.

Warfarin: May increase anticoagulant effects. Monitor patient for bleeding, and check PT and INR closely. Warfarin dosage adjustment may be needed.

Drug-herb. *Horseradish:* May cause abnormal thyroid function. Discourage use in patients undergoing thyroid function tests.

Lemon balm: May have antithyroid effects; may inhibit TSH. Discourage use together.

Drug-food. *Cottonseed meal, dietary fiber, soybean flour, walnuts:* May decrease absorption of drug. Dosage adjustments may be needed.

Grapefruit juice: May delay absorption of drug. Avoid use.

EFFECTS ON LAB TEST RESULTS
• May decrease thyroid function test results. May alter results of liothyronine, protein-bound iodine, and radioactive[131]I uptake studies.

CONTRAINDICATIONS & CAUTIONS
• Contraindicated in patients hypersensitive to drug and in those with acute MI uncomplicated by hypothyroidism, untreated subclinical or overt thyrotoxicosis, or uncorrected adrenal insufficiency.

Black Box Warning Don't use either alone or with other therapeutic agents for treatment of obesity or for weight loss. ∎

Black Box Warning Doses beyond the range of daily hormonal requirements may produce serious or even life-threatening toxicities, especially if given with sympathomimetic amines. ∎

• Use cautiously in elderly patients and in those with angina pectoris, HTN, other CV disorders, renal insufficiency, or ischemia.

• Use cautiously in patients with diabetes mellitus, diabetes insipidus, or myxedema and during rapid replacement in those with arteriosclerosis.

Dialyzable drug: No.

⚠ *Overdose S&S:* Signs and symptoms of hyperthyroidism, confusion, disorientation, cerebral embolism, shock, coma, seizures, death.

PREGNANCY-LACTATION-REPRODUCTION
• Drug is safe to use in pregnancy and shouldn't be discontinued during pregnancy. If hypothyroidism is diagnosed during pregnancy, patient should be promptly treated.

• Dosage may need to be increased in pregnant women. Measure serum TSH and free T_4 levels as soon as pregnancy is confirmed and, at minimum, during each trimester of pregnancy. Reduce dosage to prepregnancy levels immediately after delivery and measure serum TSH level 4 to 8 weeks postpartum.

• For new-onset hypothyroidism during pregnancy, normalize thyroid function as rapidly as possible. In patients with moderate to severe signs and symptoms, start drug at 1.6 mcg/kg daily. In patients with mild hypothyroidism, start drug at 1 mcg/kg daily.

Evaluate serum TSH level every 4 weeks and adjust dosage as indicated.
• Drug appears minimally in human milk. Adequate replacement doses of levothyroxine are generally needed to maintain normal lactation and should be continued during breastfeeding.

NURSING CONSIDERATIONS
• Patients with diabetes mellitus may need increased antidiabetic doses when starting thyroid hormone replacement.
• Watch for angina, coronary occlusion, or stroke in patients with arteriosclerosis who are receiving rapid replacement.
• In patients with CAD who must receive thyroid hormone, observe carefully for possible coronary insufficiency.
• Patients with adult hypothyroidism are unusually sensitive to thyroid hormone. Start at lowest dosage, and adjust to higher dosages according to patient's symptoms and laboratory data until euthyroid state is reached.
• When changing from levothyroxine to liothyronine, stop levothyroxine and begin liothyronine. Increase dosage in small increments after residual effects of levothyroxine have disappeared. When changing from liothyronine to levothyroxine, start levothyroxine several days before withdrawing liothyronine to avoid relapse. Drugs aren't interchangeable.
• Long-term therapy causes bone loss in premenopausal and postmenopausal women. Consider a basal bone density measurement, and monitor patient closely for osteoporosis.
• Patients taking levothyroxine who need to have ^{131}I uptake studies performed must stop drug 4 weeks before test.
• Patients taking anticoagulants may need their dosage modified and require careful monitoring of coagulation status.
• Drug shouldn't be used for infertility (unless associated with hypothyroidism).
• *Look alike–sound alike:* Don't confuse levothyroxine with lamotrigine or Lanoxin.

PATIENT TEACHING
• Teach patient the importance of compliance, to take drug at same time each day (preferably ½ to 1 hour before breakfast), to maintain constant hormone levels, and help prevent insomnia.

• Make sure patient understands that replacement therapy is usually for life. The drug should never be stopped unless directed by prescriber.
• Warn patient (especially elderly patient) to notify prescriber immediately about chest pain, palpitations, sweating, nervousness, shortness of breath, or other signals of overdose or aggravated CV disease.
• Tell caregiver of infant or child who can't swallow tablets to crush tablet and suspend in small amount of water and give by spoon or dropper. Crushed tablet can be sprinkled over food, except foods containing large amounts of soybean, fiber, or iron.
• Tell patient using tablets to take them with plenty of water to avoid choking, gagging, or getting the pill stuck in throat.
• Advise patient who has achieved stable response not to change brands.
• Tell patient to report unusual bleeding and bruising or any other adverse reaction.
• Advise patient not to take herbal products or OTC or other prescription drugs without first consulting prescriber.
• Advise patient to tell prescriber about all medications, both OTC and prescription, and herbal products being taken.
• Tell patient who plans to have surgery to notify physician or dentist about taking levothyroxine.
• Advise patient to report pregnancy to prescriber because dosage may need adjustment.
• Advise patient to protect tablets from light and moisture.

SAFETY ALERT!

lidocaine hydrochloride (IV)
LYE-doe-kane

Xylocaine, Xylocard✦

Therapeutic class: Antiarrhythmics
Pharmacologic class: Amide derivatives

AVAILABLE FORMS
Infusion (premixed): 0.2% (2 mg/mL), 0.4% (4 mg/mL), 0.8% (8 mg/mL)
Injection (for direct IV use): 0.5% (5 mg/mL), 1% (10 mg/mL), 2% (20 mg/mL)
Injection (for IV admixtures): 4% (40 mg/mL), 10% (100 mg/mL), 20% (200 mg/mL)

INDICATIONS & DOSAGES

➤ **Ventricular arrhythmias caused by MI, cardiac manipulation, or cardiac glycosides**

Adults: 50 to 100 mg by IV bolus at 25 to 50 mg/minute. Bolus dose is repeated every 5 minutes until arrhythmias subside or adverse reactions develop. Don't exceed 300-mg total bolus during a 1-hour period. Simultaneously, constant infusion of 20 to 50 mcg/kg/minute (1 to 4 mg/minute) is begun. If single bolus has been given, smaller bolus dose may be repeated 15 to 20 minutes after start of infusion to maintain therapeutic level.

Elderly patients: Reduce dosage and rate of infusion.

➤ **Ventricular arrhythmias; shock-refractory ventricular fibrillation; pulseless ventricular tachycardia ◆**

Children: 1 mg/kg by IV or intraosseous bolus. Start infusion at 20 to 50 mcg/kg/minute.

Adjust-a-dose: For patients with HF, with renal or liver disease, or who weigh less than 50 kg, reduce dosage.

ADMINISTRATION

IV

▼ Injections (additive syringes and single-use vials) containing 40, 100, or 200 mg/mL are for the preparation of IV infusion solutions only and must be diluted before use.

▼ Prepare IV infusion by adding 1 g (using 25 mL of 4% or 5 mL of 20% injection) to 1 L of D₅W injection to provide a solution containing 1 mg/mL.

▼ Use a more concentrated solution of up to 8 mg/mL in fluid-restricted patient.

▼ Patients receiving infusions must be on a cardiac monitor and must be attended at all times. Use an infusion control device for giving infusion precisely. Don't exceed 4 mg/minute; faster rate greatly increases risk of toxicity.

▼ Avoid giving injections containing preservatives.

▼ **Incompatibilities:** None listed by manufacturer. Consult a drug incompatibility reference for more information.

ACTION

A class IB antiarrhythmic that decreases the depolarization, automaticity, and excitability in the ventricles during the diastolic phase by direct action on the tissues, especially the Purkinje network.

Route	Onset	Peak	Duration
IV	Rapid	Unknown	15–20 min

Half-life: 1½ to 2 hours (may be prolonged in patients with HF or hepatic disease).

ADVERSE REACTIONS

CNS: confusion, tremor, stupor, restlessness, light-headedness, *seizures,* lethargy, somnolence, anxiety, hallucinations, nervousness, paresthesia, muscle twitching.
CV: hypotension, *bradycardia, new or worsened arrhythmias, cardiac arrest.* **EENT:** blurred or double vision, tinnitus. **GI:** vomiting. **Respiratory:** *respiratory depression and arrest.* **Skin:** soreness at injection site.
Other: *anaphylaxis,* sensation of cold.

INTERACTIONS

Drug-drug. *Atenolol, metoprolol, nadolol, pindolol, propranolol:* May reduce hepatic metabolism of lidocaine, increasing the risk of toxicity. Give bolus doses of lidocaine at a slower rate, and monitor lidocaine level and patient closely.

Cimetidine: May decrease clearance of lidocaine, increasing the risk of toxicity. Consider a different H₂-receptor antagonist if possible. Monitor lidocaine level closely.

Ergot-type oxytocic drugs: May cause severe, persistent HTN or stroke. Avoid using together.

Mexiletine: May increase pharmacologic effects. Avoid using together.

Phenytoin, procainamide, propranolol, quinidine: May increase cardiac depressant effects. Monitor patient closely.

Succinylcholine: May prolong neuromuscular blockade. Monitor patient closely.

EFFECTS ON LAB TEST RESULTS

None reported.

CONTRAINDICATIONS & CAUTIONS

• Contraindicated in patients hypersensitive to amide-type local anesthetics.

• Contraindicated in those with Adams-Stokes syndrome, Wolff-Parkinson-White syndrome, and severe degrees of SA, AV, or intraventricular block in the absence of an artificial pacemaker.
• Use cautiously and at reduced dosages in patients with complete or second-degree heart block or sinus bradycardia, in elderly patients, in those with HF or renal or hepatic disease, and in those weighing less than 50 kg.
Dialyzable drug: No.
⚠ *Overdose S&S:* Circulatory depression, change in level of consciousness, seizures, hypoventilation.

PREGNANCY-LACTATION-REPRODUCTION
• There are no adequate studies with IV lidocaine in pregnant women. Use cautiously if clearly needed, especially during early pregnancy.
• Drug appears in human milk. Use cautiously in breastfeeding women.

NURSING CONSIDERATIONS
• Monitor drug level. Therapeutic levels are 1.5 to 5 mcg/mL.
⊙ *Alert:* Monitor patient for toxicity. In many severely ill patients, seizures may be the first sign of toxicity, but severe reactions are usually preceded by somnolence, confusion, tremors, and paresthesia. If signs of toxicity occur, stop drug at once and notify prescriber. Continuing could lead to seizures and coma. Give oxygen through a nasal cannula if not contraindicated. Keep oxygen and CPR equipment available.
• Monitor patient's response, especially BP and electrolytes, BUN, and creatinine levels. Notify prescriber if abnormalities occur.
• If arrhythmias worsen or ECG changes occur (for example, QRS complex widens or PR interval substantially prolongs), stop infusion and notify prescriber.

PATIENT TEACHING
• Tell patient to promptly report adverse reactions, such as palpitations, dyspnea, confusion, anxiety, vision changes, dizziness, tinnitus, nausea, and vomiting, because toxicity can occur.

SAFETY ALERT!

linagliptin
lin-a-GLIP-tin

Tradjenta

Therapeutic class: Antidiabetics
Pharmacologic class: DPP-4 inhibitors

AVAILABLE FORMS
Tablets: 5 mg

INDICATIONS & DOSAGES
➤ **Adjunct to diet and exercise to improve glycemic control in adults with type 2 diabetes as monotherapy or as combination therapy with an insulin secretagogue (such as a sulfonylurea) or insulin**
Adults: 5 mg PO daily.
Adjust-a-dose: When used in combination with an insulin secretagogue or insulin, use lower doses of those drugs to decrease the risk of hypoglycemia.

ADMINISTRATION
PO
• Give drug without regard for food.
• Store tablets at 77° F (25° C) with excursions permitted to between 59° and 86° F (15° and 30° C).
• Store tablets out of reach of children.

ACTION
Inhibits DPP-4, an enzyme that rapidly inactivates incretin hormones, which play a part in the body's regulation of glucose.

Route	Onset	Peak	Duration
PO	Rapid	1½ hr	Unknown

Half-life: About 12 hours (accumulation).

ADVERSE REACTIONS
CNS: headache. **EENT:** nasopharyngitis. **GI:** diarrhea, constipation. **Metabolic:** hyperlipidemia, weight gain, *hypoglycemia.* **Musculoskeletal:** arthralgia, back pain, myalgia. **Respiratory:** cough, URI.

INTERACTIONS
Drug-drug. *CYP3A4 or P-gp inducers (such as rifampin):* May decrease linagliptin level. Avoid use together.

Reactions in bold italics are *life-threatening*. Interactions may have a *rapid onset* or a *delayed onset*.

Ritonavir: May increase linagliptin effects and risk of adverse effects. Use with caution; monitor response, and adjust dosage as necessary.

Sulfonylureas (glyburide), insulin: May increase risk of hypoglycemia. Monitor glucose level carefully and adjust sulfonylurea or insulin dosage as necessary.

Drug-herb. *St. John's wort:* May decrease concentrations of CYP3A4 substrates. Avoid combination.

EFFECTS ON LAB TEST RESULTS
• May increase lipase and uric acid level.
• May decrease fasting glucose and HbA_{1c} levels.

CONTRAINDICATIONS & CAUTIONS
• Contraindicated in patients hypersensitive to drug (with such signs and symptoms as urticaria, angioedema, and bronchial hyperactivity).
• Drug not for use in patients with type 1 diabetes or for treatment of diabetic ketoacidosis.
• Acute pancreatitis, including fatal pancreatitis, has occurred in patients taking linagliptin. It's unknown whether patients with a history of pancreatitis are at increased risk for development of pancreatitis while using linagliptin.
❸ Alert: Drug may cause joint pain that can be severe and disabling. Report severe and persistent joint pain to prescriber; drug may need to be discontinued.
• Safety in children hasn't been established.
Dialyzable drug: Unlikely.

PREGNANCY-LACTATION-REPRODUCTION
• There are no adequate studies in pregnant women. Use during pregnancy only if clearly needed.
• It isn't known if drug appears in human milk. Use cautiously in breastfeeding women.

NURSING CONSIDERATIONS
• Monitor HbA_{1c} and fasting blood glucose levels periodically.
• Monitor patient for signs and symptoms of hypoglycemia (anxiety, confusion, diaphoresis, tachycardia, paresthesia) and hyperglycemia (excess thirst, urination).

• Monitor patient for signs and symptoms of pancreatitis (persistent, severe abdominal pain, which may radiate to the back, and vomiting). If pancreatitis is suspected, promptly discontinue linagliptin and initiate appropriate management.
• Postmarketing cases of bullous pemphigoid requiring hospitalization have been reported in patients taking DPP-4 inhibitors. Monitor patients for signs and symptoms, including blisters or erosions. If bullous pemphigoid is suspected, discontinue linagliptin and refer patient to dermatologist for diagnosis and appropriate treatment.

PATIENT TEACHING
• Inform patient of the potential risks and benefits of linagliptin and of alternative modes of therapy.
• Instruct patient to take drug only as prescribed. If a dose is missed, advise patient not to double the next dose.
• Explain the importance of proper diet, regular physical activity, and periodic blood glucose monitoring.
• Teach patient to recognize and manage hypoglycemia and hyperglycemia.
• Advise patient to notify the health care provider promptly during periods of stress (such as fever, trauma, infection, or surgery) because medication requirements may change.
• Teach patient signs and symptoms of pancreatitis and to immediately contact prescriber if they occur.
• Advise patient to contact prescriber if blisters or erosions develop.

L

linezolid
lih-NEH-zoe-lid

Zyvox

Therapeutic class: Antibiotics
Pharmacologic class: Oxazolidinones

AVAILABLE FORMS
Injection: 2 mg/mL
Powder for oral suspension: 100 mg/5 mL when reconstituted
Tablets: 600 mg

INDICATIONS & DOSAGES

Adjust-a-dose (for all indications): Administer after hemodialysis on dialysis days.

➤ **Vancomycin-resistant** *Enterococcus faecium* **infections, including those with concurrent bacteremia**

Adults and children age 12 and older:
600 mg IV or PO every 12 hours for 14 to 28 days.

Full-term neonates, infants, and children through age 11: 10 mg/kg IV or PO every 8 hours for 14 to 28 days.

Preterm neonates younger than age 7 days (gestational age less than 34 weeks):
10 mg/kg IV or PO every 12 hours for 14 to 28 days. Increase to 10 mg/kg every 8 hours when patient is 7 days old. Consider this dosage increase if neonate has inadequate response.

➤ **Hospital-acquired pneumonia caused by** *Staphylococcus aureus* **(methicillin-susceptible [MSSA] and MRSA strains) or** *Streptococcus pneumoniae* **(including multidrug-resistant strains [MDRSP]); complicated skin and skin-structure infections, including diabetic foot infections without osteomyelitis caused by** *S. aureus* **(MSSA and MRSA),** *Streptococcus pyogenes,* **or** *Streptococcus agalactiae;* **community-acquired pneumonia caused by** *S. pneumoniae* **(including MDRSP), including those with concurrent bacteremia, or** *S. aureus* **(MSSA only)**

Adults and children age 12 and older:
600 mg IV or PO every 12 hours for 10 to 14 days.

Full-term neonates, infants, and children through age 11: 10 mg/kg IV or PO every 8 hours for 10 to 14 days.

Preterm neonates younger than age 7 days (gestational age less than 34 weeks):
10 mg/kg IV or PO every 12 hours for 10 to 14 days. Increase to 10 mg/kg every 8 hours when patient is 7 days old. Consider this dosage increase if neonate has inadequate response.

➤ **Uncomplicated skin and skin-structure infections caused by** *S. aureus* **(MSSA only) or** *S. pyogenes*

Adults: 400 mg PO every 12 hours for 10 to 14 days.

Children ages 12 to 18: 600 mg PO every 12 hours for 10 to 14 days.

Children ages 5 to 11: 10 mg/kg PO every 12 hours for 10 to 14 days.

Full-term neonates, infants, and children younger than age 5: 10 mg/kg PO every 8 hours for 10 to 14 days.

Preterm neonates younger than age 7 days (gestational age less than 34 weeks):
10 mg/kg PO every 12 hours for 10 to 14 days. Increase to 10 mg/kg every 8 hours when patient is 7 days old. Consider this dosage increase if neonate has inadequate response.

ADMINISTRATION
PO
- Give tablets and suspension with or without meals.
- Reconstitute suspension according to manufacturer's instructions.
- Store reconstituted suspension at room temperature and use within 21 days.

IV
▼ Inspect solution for particulate matter and leaks.

▼ Drug is compatible with D_5W injection, NSS for injection, and lactated Ringer injection.

▼ Don't inject additives into infusion bag. Give other IV drugs separately or via a separate IV line to avoid incompatibilities. If single IV line is used, flush line before and after infusion with a compatible solution.

▼ Infuse over 30 minutes to 2 hours. Don't infuse drug in a series connection.

▼ Store drug at room temperature in its protective overwrap. Solution may turn yellow over time, but this doesn't affect drug's potency.

▼ **Incompatibilities:** Amphotericin B, ceftriaxone, chlorpromazine hydrochloride, diazepam, erythromycin lactobionate, pentamidine isethionate, phenytoin, trimethoprim–sulfamethoxazole.

ACTION
Prevents bacterial protein synthesis by interfering with DNA translation in the ribosomes. Also prevents formation of a functional 70S ribosomal subunit by binding to a site on the bacterial 50S ribosomal subunit.

Route	Onset	Peak	Duration
PO	Unknown	1–2 hr	Unknown
IV	Unknown	30 min	Unknown

Half-life: Adults, 4 to 5 hours; children age 1 week to 11 years, 1½ to 3 hours.

ADVERSE REACTIONS

CNS: headache, dizziness, fever, insomnia; vertigo (children). **GI:** diarrhea, nausea, altered taste, constipation, oral candidiasis, tongue discoloration, vomiting, abdominal pain. **GU:** vaginal candidiasis. **Hematologic:** *leukopenia, myelosuppression, neutropenia, thrombocytopenia,* anemia. **Skin:** rash. **Other:** fungal infection.

INTERACTIONS

Drug-drug. *Adrenergic drugs (dopamine, epinephrine, pseudoephedrine):* May cause HTN. Monitor BP and HR; start continuous infusions of dopamine and epinephrine at lower doses and titrate to response.
Insulin, oral antidiabetic agents: May cause symptomatic hypoglycemia. Monitor patient closely.
Serotonergic drugs: May cause serotonin syndrome, including confusion, delirium, restlessness, tremors, blushing, diaphoresis, and hyperpyrexia. Notify prescriber immediately of signs and symptoms of serotonin syndrome.
Drug-food. *Foods and beverages high in tyramine (aged cheeses, air-dried meats, red wines, sauerkraut, soy sauce, tap beers):* May increase BP. Provide a list of foods containing tyramine and advise patient that tyramine content of meals shouldn't exceed 100 mg.

EFFECTS ON LAB TEST RESULTS

• May increase ALT, AST, bilirubin, alkaline phosphatase, BUN, creatinine, amylase, lipase, LDH, and BUN levels. May decrease Hb level.
• May decrease glucose level and WBC, neutrophil, and platelet counts.

CONTRAINDICATIONS & CAUTIONS

• Contraindicated in patients hypersensitive to drug or its components.
🚫 *Alert:* Concomitant use with psychiatric drugs or within 2 weeks of taking

psychiatric drugs that work through the serotonin system of the brain (SSRIs, SSNRIs, TCAs, MAO inhibitors, and others) can cause serotonin syndrome (fever, mental status changes, muscle twitching, excessive sweating, shivering or shaking, diarrhea, and loss of coordination). Use linezolid with these drugs only for life-threatening or urgent conditions when the potential benefits outweigh the risks of toxicity.
Dialyzable drug: 30%.

PREGNANCY-LACTATION-REPRODUCTION

• There are no adequate studies in pregnant women. Use during pregnancy only if potential benefit justifies potential risk to the fetus.
• Drug may appear in human milk. Use cautiously in breastfeeding women.

NURSING CONSIDERATIONS

• No dosage adjustment is needed when switching from IV to oral forms.
🚫 *Alert:* Before giving linezolid, stop any serotonergic drug and monitor patient for serotonin toxicity for 2 weeks (5 weeks if fluoxetine was taken) or until 24 hours after the last dose of linezolid, whichever comes first. May resume serotonergic psychiatric drugs 24 hours after last dose of linezolid.
🚫 *Alert:* Nausea and vomiting may be symptoms of lactic acidosis. Monitor patient for unexplained acidosis or low bicarbonate level, and notify prescriber immediately if these occur.
🚫 *Alert:* Drug may cause thrombocytopenia. In patients at increased risk for bleeding, those with existing thrombocytopenia, those taking other drugs that may cause thrombocytopenia, and those receiving this drug for longer than 14 days, monitor platelet count.
🚫 *Alert:* Drug may lead to myelosuppression. Monitor CBC weekly.
🚫 *Alert:* Prolonged use can cause superinfection, including CDAD, which can occur more than 2 months after treatment ends. Consider these diagnoses and take appropriate measures in patients with persistent diarrhea or secondary infections.
🚫 *Alert:* Drug may cause symptomatic hypoglycemia in patients taking insulin or oral antidiabetic agents. Monitor patient closely.

L

• Inappropriate use of antibiotics may lead to development of resistant organisms; carefully consider other drugs before starting therapy, especially in outpatient setting.

• Peripheral and optic neuropathies can occur, especially in patients treated for a longer-than-recommended duration. If these neuropathies occur, drug may need to be discontinued. Patients with vision changes should receive prompt ophthalmic evaluation.

• Use cautiously in patients with seizure disorder.

• *Look alike–sound alike:* Don't confuse Zyvox with Zovirax. Both come in a 400-mg strength.

PATIENT TEACHING

• Tell patient that tablets and oral suspension may be taken with or without meals.

• Stress importance of completing entire course of therapy, even if patient feels better.

• Tell patient to report all adverse reactions promptly.

• Tell patient to alert prescriber if patient has high BP; is taking cough or cold preparations, insulin, or oral antidiabetic agents; or is being treated with SSRIs or other antidepressants.

❸ *Alert:* Teach patient to recognize and immediately report signs and symptoms of serotonin toxicity (fever, mental status changes, muscle twitching, excessive sweating, shivering or shaking, diarrhea, and loss of coordination).

• Advise patient taking prescribed psychiatric drugs that these drugs may need to be stopped during linezolid therapy but not to stop them without first speaking to prescriber.

• Teach patient to avoid eating large quantities of tyramine-containing foods (aged cheeses, soy sauce, tap beers, red wine) during therapy.

• Inform patient with phenylketonuria that each 5 mL of oral suspension contains 20 mg of phenylalanine. Tablets and injection don't contain phenylalanine.

SAFETY ALERT!

liraglutide
leer-ah-GLOO-tide

Saxenda, Victoza

Therapeutic class: Antidiabetics
Pharmacologic class: Glucagon-like peptide-1 receptor agonists

AVAILABLE FORMS
Injection: 0.6 mg, 1.2 mg, 1.8 mg, 2.4 mg, 3 mg in 6-mg/mL prefilled multidose pens

INDICATIONS & DOSAGES
➤ **As adjunct to diet and exercise to improve glycemic control in patients with type 2 diabetes mellitus (Victoza)**
Adults: Initially, 0.6 mg subcut daily; after 1 week, increase dosage to 1.2 mg subcut daily. May increase dosage to 1.8 mg subcut daily if needed to achieve glycemic control.

➤ **As adjunct to diet and exercise for long-term weight management in adults with initial BMI of 30 kg/m² or greater (obese) or 27 kg/m² or greater (overweight) in the presence of at least one weight-related comorbid condition (HTN, type 2 diabetes mellitus, or dyslipidemia) (Saxenda)**
Adults: Initially, 0.6 mg subcut once daily for 1 week. Increase by 0.6 mg/day subcut at weekly intervals to a target dose of 3 mg once daily. If patient can't tolerate an increased dose during titration period, consider delaying dose escalation for 1 week.

➤ **To reduce risk of major adverse CV events in patients with type 2 diabetes mellitus and established CV disease (Victoza)**
Adults: Initially, 0.6 mg subcut daily; after 1 week, increase dosage to 1.2 mg daily. May increase dosage to 1.8 mg subcut daily if needed to achieve glycemic control.

ADMINISTRATION
Subcutaneous
• Hazardous drug; use safe handling precautions.

• Give drug once daily at any time of day, independently of meals. Inject into abdomen,

---

thigh, or upper arm. Injection site and timing can be changed without dosage adjustment.
• Don't mix drug with insulin for injection or inject liraglutide and insulin in adjacent areas at the same time.
• If a dose is missed, don't double subsequent dose. Resume once-daily regimen. If more than 3 days have elapsed, initiate dose at 0.6 mg daily and, for Victoza, increase as directed by prescriber or, for Saxenda, increase weekly per titration schedule.
• Inspect solution before each injection. Use solution only if it is clear, colorless, and contains no particles.
🌢 *Alert:* Multidose pens are for single-patient use only. Pens should never be shared even if the needle is changed. Clearly label with patient identifying information where it won't obstruct dosing window, warning, or other product information.
• Before first use, store drug in refrigerator between 36° and 46° F (2° and 8° C). Discard if pen freezes.
• After initial use of liraglutide pen, pen can be stored for 30 days at room temperature (59° to 86° F [15° to 30° C]) or in refrigerator (36° to 46° F). Keep pen cap on when not in use. Discard pen after 30 days.

ACTION
Stimulates insulin secretion and reduces glucagon secretion; delays gastric emptying.

Route	Onset	Peak	Duration
Subcut	Unknown	8–12 hr	Unknown

Half-life: 13 hours.

ADVERSE REACTIONS
CNS: headache, dizziness, fatigue, insomnia, anxiety, weakness. **CV:** increased HR, tachycardia. **GI:** constipation, diarrhea, dyspepsia, nausea, vomiting, abdominal distention or pain, decreased appetite, flatulence, GERD, gastroenteritis, dry mouth. **GU:** UTI. **Hepatic:** cholelithiasis. **Metabolic:** *hypoglycemia.* **Respiratory:** URI. **Skin:** injection-site reactions. **Other:** flulike syndrome, *thyroid cancer,* anti-liraglutide antibody formation, infection.

INTERACTIONS
Drug-drug. *Insulin secretagogues (sulfonylureas):* May increase risk of hypoglycemia.

Reduce dosage of insulin secretagogue before beginning drug.
Oral medications: May impair absorption of oral drugs because of delayed gastric emptying. Use together cautiously.

EFFECTS ON LAB TEST RESULTS
• May increase serum bilirubin and lipase levels and serum calcitonin concentration.
• May decrease blood glucose level.

CONTRAINDICATIONS & CAUTIONS
Black Box Warning Drug causes dose-dependent and treatment duration–dependent thyroid C-cell tumors at clinically relevant exposures in both genders of rats and mice. It isn't known if drug causes thyroid C-cell tumors, including medullary thyroid carcinoma (MTC), in humans, as the human relevance of liraglutide-induced rodent thyroid C-cell tumors hasn't been determined. ▪
Black Box Warning Contraindicated in patients with personal or family history of MTC and in patients with multiple endocrine neoplasia syndrome type 2. ▪
• Contraindicated in patients with a prior serious hypersensitivity reaction to liraglutide or its components.
• Avoid use in patients with a history of suicidal attempts or active suicidal ideation.
• Use cautiously in patients with renal and hepatic impairment and in those with history of pancreatitis.
🌢 *Alert:* Acute pancreatitis, including fatal pancreatitis and nonfatal hemorrhagic or necrotizing pancreatitis, has occurred in patients taking liraglutide.
• Saxenda isn't indicated for treatment of type 2 diabetes mellitus.
• Saxenda and Victoza both contain the same active ingredient and shouldn't be used together.
• Saxenda shouldn't be used in combination with other GLP-1 receptor agonists.
• Saxenda hasn't been studied in patients taking insulin; don't use together.
• Safety and effectiveness of Saxenda in combination with other products intended for weight loss haven't been established.
• Elderly adults may be more sensitive to drug. Use cautiously.
Dialyzable drug: Unknown.

L

⚠ **Overdose S&S:** Nausea, vomiting, hypoglycemia.

PREGNANCY-LACTATION-REPRODUCTION
• There are no adequate studies of Victoza in pregnant women. Use during pregnancy only if potential benefit justifies potential risk to the fetus.
• Saxenda is contraindicated during pregnancy because weight loss offers no potential benefit to a pregnant patient and may result in fetal harm.
• It isn't known if drug appears in human milk. Patient should either discontinue breastfeeding or discontinue drug.

NURSING CONSIDERATIONS
Black Box Warning Drug may cause thyroid C-cell tumors, including MTC. Monitor patient closely. ■
• Discontinue Saxenda if dose of 3 mg once daily isn't tolerated because effectiveness hasn't been established at lower doses. Evaluate change in body weight 16 weeks after start of therapy; discontinue if body weight loss of at least 4% of baseline hasn't been achieved.
• Monitor patient closely for signs and symptoms of pancreatitis (persistent, severe abdominal pain, which may radiate to the back, and vomiting). Discontinue drug promptly if pancreatitis is suspected. Don't restart if pancreatitis is confirmed.
❸ **Alert:** Patients with thyroid nodules found on examination or neck imaging or with elevated serum calcitonin levels should be evaluated by an endocrinologist.
• Drug may increase risk of gallbladder and bile duct disease. If cholelithiasis is suspected, gallbladder studies and appropriate clinical follow-up are indicated.
• Monitor patients for emergence or worsening of depression, suicidal thoughts or behavior, and unusual changes in mood or behavior. Discontinue in patients who experience suicidal thoughts or behaviors.
• Drug isn't recommended for first-line therapy in patients who have inadequate glycemic control with diet and exercise.
• Victoza isn't a substitute for insulin; it shouldn't be used for treatment of diabetic ketoacidosis or type 1 diabetes mellitus.

• Victoza hasn't been studied in combination with prandial insulin.
• Monitor blood glucose and HbA$_{1c}$ levels. Consider decreasing insulin and insulin secretagogue (such as sulfonylurea) dosage when initiating liraglutide.
• Monitor patient for signs and symptoms of hypoglycemia (tachycardia, palpitations, anxiety, hunger, nausea, diaphoresis, tremors, pallor, restlessness, headache, and speech and motor dysfunction).
• Monitor GI status; drug slows gastric emptying.

PATIENT TEACHING
Black Box Warning Counsel patient regarding potential risk of MTC and describe signs and symptoms of thyroid tumors (neck mass, dysphagia, dyspnea, persistent hoarseness). Routine monitoring of serum calcitonin level or use of thyroid ultrasound is of uncertain value for early detection of MTC. ■
• Warn patient that drug may increase risk of thyroid tumor; tell patient to report such signs and symptoms as hoarseness, difficulty swallowing, difficulty breathing, or lump in the neck.
• Advise patient to report emergence or worsening of depression, suicidal thoughts or behavior, and unusual changes in mood or behavior.
• Advise patient to report signs and symptoms of acute gallbladder disease or cholelithiasis, including sudden and rapidly intensifying pain in the upper right portion of the abdomen or in the center of the abdomen, just below the breastbone; back pain between the shoulder blades; pain in the right shoulder; nausea; or vomiting.
• Advise patient to stop drug and report persistent, severe abdominal pain that may radiate to the back and may or may not be accompanied by vomiting.
❸ **Alert:** Warn patient not to share multidose pen with other people, even if needle is changed, because of risk of bloodborne pathogen transmission, including HIV and hepatitis.
• Tell patient that stress, such as fever, trauma, infection, or surgery, may change drug requirements and to seek medical advice promptly if these occur.

Reactions in bold italics are **life-threatening**. Interactions may have a *rapid onset* or a **delayed onset**.

• Emphasize to patient importance of adhering to a diet and exercise program and monitoring glucose and HbA$_{1c}$ levels.

• Advise patient of risk of dehydration; encourage hydration.

• Warn patient of risk of hypersensitivity reactions and advise patient to report reactions should they occur.

• Teach patient how to give subcut injection; instruct patient to rotate sites to prevent injection-site reactions.

• Instruct patient to discard pen after 30 days.

lisdexamfetamine dimesylate
lis-DEX-am-FET-a-meen

Vyvanse◆

Therapeutic class: CNS stimulants
Pharmacologic class: Amphetamines
Controlled substance schedule: II

AVAILABLE FORMS
Capsules ⓓⓝⓒ: 10 mg, 20 mg, 30 mg, 40 mg, 50 mg, 60 mg, 70 mg
Tablets (chewable): 10 mg, 20 mg, 30 mg, 40 mg, 50 mg, 60 mg

INDICATIONS & DOSAGES
Adjust-a-dose (for all indications): For patients with severe renal impairment (GFR of 15 mL to less than 30 mL/minute/1.73 m^2), maximum dose is 50 mg/day. For those with ESRD (GFR less than 15 mL/minute/1.73 m^2), maximum dose is 30 mg/day.
➤ **ADHD**
Adults and children ages 6 to 17: Initially, 30 mg PO once daily in the morning. Increase by 10 or 20 mg at weekly intervals to a maximum of 70 mg daily.
➤ **Moderate to severe binge eating disorder**
Adults: Initially, 30 mg PO once daily in the morning. Increase by 20 mg at weekly intervals to target dose of 50 to 70 mg/day. Maximum dose is 70 mg/day.

ADMINISTRATION
PO
• Give drug in the morning to prevent insomnia.

• Give drug without regard for meals.

• Have patient swallow capsules whole, or mix capsule contents in yogurt, water, or orange juice, dissolve completely, and have patient take immediately; don't store.

• For chewable tablets, make sure patient chews tablets thoroughly before swallowing.

• Capsules can be substituted with chewable tablets on a unit/mg basis.

• Don't divide the dose of a single capsule or chewable tablet or give less than one capsule or chewable tablet per day.

ACTION
Increases the release of norepinephrine and dopamine from nerve terminals and blocks their reuptake into the presynaptic neuron.

Route	Onset	Peak	Duration
PO	Rapid	1 hr	8–14 hr

Half-life: Lisdexamfetamine, less than 1 hour; dextroamphetamine, 10 to 13 hours.

ADVERSE REACTIONS
CNS: aggression, depression, dyskinesia, tics, *seizures.* **CV:** *cardiomyopathy,* chest pain. **EENT:** mydriasis, diplopia, blurred vision, impaired visual accommodation. **GI:** dysgeusia, bruxism, constipation. **GU:** frequent or prolonged erections, libido changes. **Hepatic:** eosinophilic hepatitis. **Musculoskeletal:** rhabdomyolysis. **Skin:** dermatillomania, urticaria, alopecia, *SJS.* **Other:** anaphylaxis, hypersensitivity, angioedema.

INTERACTIONS
Drug-drug. *Adrenergic blockers:* May inhibit adrenergic-blocking effects. Monitor BP and adjust adrenergic blocker dosage if necessary.
Antihistamines: May inhibit sedative effects of antihistamines. Monitor patient.
Antihypertensives, veratrum alkaloids: May inhibit antihypertensive effects of these drugs. If use together can't be avoided, closely monitor BP when lisdexamfetamine is started or stopped, and adjust antihypertensive dosage as needed.
Buspirone, fentanyl, lithium, SSNRIs, SSRIs, tramadol, triptans, tryptophan: May increase risk of serotonin syndrome. Start lisdexamfetamine treatment with lower

L

doses and monitor patients for signs and symptoms of serotonin syndrome, particularly during lisdexamfetamine initiation or dosage increases.

Chlorpromazine, haloperidol: May decrease effectiveness of amphetamines. Monitor patient closely.

CYP2D6 inhibitors (fluoxetine, paroxetine, quinidine, ritonavir): May increase exposure of dextroamphetamine and increase risk of serotonin syndrome. Start lisdexamfetamine treatment with lower doses and monitor patient during lisdexamfetamine initiation or dosage increases.

Ethosuximide: May delay absorption of this drug. Monitor patient closely.

Lithium: May inhibit anorectic and CNS stimulant effects of amphetamine. Monitor patient closely.

MAO inhibitors: May cause severe HTN or hypertensive crisis. Use is contraindicated within 14 days of MAO inhibitor therapy.

Meperidine: May increase the analgesic effect of meperidine. Use together cautiously.

Norepinephrine: May increase adrenergic effects of norepinephrine. Monitor patient closely.

Phenobarbital, phenytoin: May delay intestinal absorption of these drugs and enhance their anticonvulsant effects. Monitor patient closely.

TCAs: May cause adverse CV effects and increase risk of serotonin syndrome. Avoid use together.

Urine acidifiers (ammonium chloride, sodium acid phosphate), methenamine: May decrease serum level due to increased renal excretion of amphetamine. Monitor patient for decreased drug effects.

Urine alkalinizers (sodium bicarbonate): May increase lisdexamfetamine serum level because of decreased renal excretion of amphetamine. Monitor patient for increased drug effects and adjust dosage accordingly.

Drug-herb. *St. John's wort:* May increase risk of serotonin syndrome. Avoid use together.

Drug-food. *Caffeine:* May increase CNS stimulation. Discourage use together.

Drug-lifestyle. *Alcohol use:* May increase CNS depression. Don't use together.

EFFECTS ON LAB TEST RESULTS
• May increase corticosteroid level.
• May interfere with urinary steroid test.

CONTRAINDICATIONS & CAUTIONS
Black Box Warning Drug has a high potential for abuse and dependence. ∎
• Contraindicated in patients hypersensitive to sympathomimetic amines or in those with idiosyncratic reactions to them, in agitated patients, and in those with a history of drug abuse.
• Anaphylactic reactions, SJS, angioedema, and urticaria have been noted in postmarketing reports.
❸ Alert: Drug isn't indicated or recommended for weight loss.
• Contraindicated in patients with advanced arteriosclerosis, hyperthyroidism, symptomatic CV disease, structural cardiac abnormalities, cardiomyopathy, serious heart arrhythmia, moderate to severe HTN, or glaucoma, and those intolerant of changes in HR or BP.
• Use cautiously in patients with a history of arrhythmias, MI, stroke, or seizures.
• Use cautiously in patients with preexisting psychosis, bipolar disorder, aggressive behavior, or Tourette syndrome.
Dialyzable drug: No.
⚠ Overdose S&S: Assaultiveness, confusion, hallucinations, hyperpyrexia, hyperreflexia, panic states, rapid respiration, restlessness, rhabdomyolysis, tremor, fatigue, depression, arrhythmias, circulatory collapse, HTN, hypotension, abdominal cramps, diarrhea, nausea, vomiting, seizures, coma.

PREGNANCY-LACTATION-REPRODUCTION
• There are no adequate studies in pregnant women. Use during pregnancy only if potential benefit justifies potential risk to the fetus.
• Drug appears in human milk. Patient should discontinue breastfeeding or discontinue drug.

NURSING CONSIDERATIONS
• Diagnosis of ADHD must be based on complete history and evaluation of the child with consultation of psychological, educational, and social resources.

• Assess patient for cardiac disease, including a careful history, family history of sudden death or ventricular arrhythmia, and physical exam, before starting therapy.
• Evaluate for bipolar disorder before initiating therapy.
• Give the lowest effective dose in the morning. Afternoon doses may cause insomnia.
Black Box Warning Assess the risk of abuse before initiating therapy, and monitor patient for signs of drug dependence or abuse. Misuse may cause sudden death. ■
◑ Alert: Periodically monitor patients for changes in HR or BP.
• Abruptly stopping the drug can cause severe fatigue and depression.
• Monitor patient closely for adverse CV effects, new or worsening behavior (aggression, mania), vision problems, or seizures.
• Monitor BP and pulse routinely.
• Use cautiously in patients taking other drugs that increase risk of serotonin syndrome. Monitor these patients closely and consider an alternative nonserotonergic drug.
• Carefully observe patient for digital changes because stimulants used to treat ADHD are associated with peripheral vasculopathy, including Raynaud phenomenon.
• Effectiveness of this drug when taken longer than 4 weeks isn't known. Periodically interrupt therapy to determine whether continuation is necessary.
• Growth may be suppressed with long-term stimulant use. Monitor the child for growth and weight gain. Stop treatment if growth is suppressed or if weight gain is lower than expected.
• The drug may trigger Tourette syndrome. Monitor patient, especially at the start of therapy.
• Monitor patient for the appearance or worsening of aggressive behavior or hostility, especially when treatment is initiated.
• May cause psychotic or manic episodes in patients with no prior history or exacerbation of signs and symptoms in patients with preexisting psychosis.

PATIENT TEACHING
• Warn patient that the misuse of amphetamines can cause serious CV adverse events, including sudden death.

◑ Alert: Instruct patient to immediately report chest pain, shortness of breath, or fainting.
• Tell patient or caregiver that drug should be taken in the morning to prevent insomnia.
• Advise patient to swallow capsule whole but if patient can't, chewable tablets may be prescribed. Or, instruct patient to mix capsule's contents in yogurt, water, or orange juice, dissolve completely, and take immediately; tell patient not to store for later use.
• Tell patient using chewable tablets to chew them thoroughly before swallowing.
• Tell patient or caregiver that abruptly stopping drug can cause severe fatigue, depression, or general withdrawal reaction.
• Caution patient to avoid activities that require alertness or good psychomotor coordination until CNS effects of drug are known.
• Advise patient taking other drugs that increase risk of serotonin syndrome to immediately report signs and symptoms of serotonin syndrome (confusion, agitation, fever, rapid heartbeat, loss of muscle coordination, vomiting, sweating).
• Warn patient with seizure disorder that drug may decrease seizure threshold. Urge patient to notify prescriber if a seizure occurs.
• Instruct patient or caregiver to report palpitations or visual disturbances.
• Tell patient or caregiver to report worsening aggression, hallucinations, delusions, or mania.
• Advise patient or caregiver that drug may slow growth and cause weight loss.
• Instruct patient to immediately report unexplained wounds appearing on fingers or toes while taking drug.
• Advise patient to avoid caffeine and alcohol consumption while taking drug.

lisinopril 🎟
lye-SIN-oh-pril

Prinivil✔, Qbrelis, Zestril✔

Therapeutic class: Antihypertensives
Pharmacologic class: ACE inhibitors

AVAILABLE FORMS
Oral solution: 1 mg/mL

Tablets: 2.5 mg, 5 mg, 10 mg, 20 mg, 30 mg, 40 mg

INDICATIONS & DOSAGES
➤ **HTN**
Adults: Initially, 10 mg PO daily for patients not taking a diuretic. Most patients are well controlled on 20 to 40 mg daily as a single dose. For patients taking a diuretic, initially, 5 mg PO daily.
Children age 6 and older: Initially, 0.07 mg/kg (up to 5 mg) PO once daily. Increase dosage based on patient response and tolerance. Maximum dose, 0.61 mg/kg (don't exceed 40 mg). Don't use in children with a CrCl of less than 30 mL/minute.
Adjust-a-dose: In adults, if CrCl is 10 to 30 mL/minute, give 5 mg PO daily; if CrCl is less than 10 mL/minute, give 2.5 mg PO daily. May titrate dosage up to 40 mg/day.
➤ **Adjunctive treatment (with diuretics and cardiac glycosides) for HF**
Adults: Initially, 5 mg PO daily; increased as needed to maximum of 20 mg (40 mg for Zestril) PO daily.
Adjust-a-dose: If sodium level is less than 130 mEq/L, serum creatinine greater than 3 mg/dL, or CrCl less than 30 mL/minute, start treatment at 2.5 mg daily.
➤ **Hemodynamically stable patients within 24 hours of acute MI to improve survival**
Adults: Initially, 5 mg PO; then 5 mg after 24 hours, 10 mg after 48 hours, followed by 10 mg once daily for 6 weeks.
Adjust-a-dose: For patients with systolic BP 120 mm Hg or less when treatment is started or during first 3 days after an infarct, decrease dosage to 2.5 mg PO. If systolic BP drops to 100 mm Hg or less, reduce daily maintenance dose of 5 mg to 2.5 mg, if needed. If prolonged systolic BP stays under 90 mm Hg for longer than 1 hour, withdraw drug.
    If CrCl is 10 to 30 mL/minute, reduce initial dose to 2.5 mg PO daily and titrate as tolerated to a maximum of 40 mg daily. If patient is on hemodialysis or CrCl is less than 10 mL/minute, start treatment at 2.5 mg PO daily.

ADMINISTRATION
PO
• Give drug without regard for food.
• Oral solution is bioequivalent to lisinopril tablets.
• Store oral solution at room temperature in a tightly closed container. Protect from freezing and excessive heat.
• If tablets are made into a suspension by pharmacist, store at or below 77° F (25° C) for up to 4 weeks; shake before each use.

ACTION
Causes decreased production of angiotensin II and suppression of the RAAS.

Route	Onset	Peak	Duration
PO	1 hr	7 hr	24 hr

Half-life: 12 hours.

ADVERSE REACTIONS
CNS: dizziness, headache, fatigue, paresthesia, syncope. **CV:** orthostatic hypotension, hypotension, chest pain. **EENT:** nasal congestion. **GI:** diarrhea, nausea, dyspepsia. **GU:** impaired renal function, impotence. **Metabolic:** *hyperkalemia.* **Respiratory:** dyspnea; dry, persistent, tickling, nonproductive cough. **Skin:** rash. **Other:** *angioedema.*

INTERACTIONS
Drug-drug. *Aliskiren:* May increase risk of renal impairment, hypotension, and hyperkalemia in diabetic patients and those with moderate to severe renal impairment (GFR less than 60 mL/minute). Concomitant use is contraindicated in diabetic patients. Avoid concomitant use in those with moderate to severe renal impairment.
Allopurinol: May cause hypersensitivity reaction. Use together cautiously.
Azathioprine: May increase risk of anemia or leukopenia. Monitor hematologic studies if used together.
Diuretics, thiazide diuretics: May cause excessive hypotension with diuretics. Monitor BP closely.
Indomethacin, NSAIDs: May reduce hypotensive effects of drug. Adjust dose as needed.

Insulin, oral antidiabetics: May cause hypoglycemia, especially at start of lisinopril therapy. Monitor glucose level.

Lithium: May cause lithium toxicity. Monitor lithium levels.

Neprilysin inhibitors (sacubitril): May increase risk of angioedema. Use together is contraindicated. Don't give lisinopril within 36 hours of switching to or from sacubitril/valsartan.

Phenothiazines: May increase hypotensive effects. Monitor BP closely.

Potassium-sparing diuretics, potassium supplements: May cause hyperkalemia. Monitor laboratory values.

Tizanidine: May cause severe hypotension. Monitor patient.

Drug-herb. *Capsaicin:* May cause ACE inhibitor–induced cough. Discourage use together.

Ma huang: May decrease antihypertensive effects. Discourage use together.

Drug-food. *Potassium-containing salt substitutes:* May cause hyperkalemia. Monitor laboratory values.

EFFECTS ON LAB TEST RESULTS

• May increase BUN, creatinine, potassium, and bilirubin levels.

• May increase LFT values.

CONTRAINDICATIONS & CAUTIONS

• Contraindicated in patients hypersensitive to ACE inhibitors and in those with a history of angioedema related to previous treatment with ACE inhibitor.

• Use cautiously in patients with impaired renal function; adjust dosage.

• Use cautiously in patients at risk for hyperkalemia or hypotension and in those with aortic stenosis or hypertrophic cardiomyopathy. The safety and effectiveness of lisinopril on BP control in children younger than age 6 or in children with GFR less than 30 mL/minute hasn't been established.

▒ Although rare, angioedema, which can be fatal, may occur at any time during treatment, including after first dose; it may involve the head and neck (potentially compromising the airway) or the intestine (presenting with abdominal pain). Black patients and patients with idiopathic or hereditary angioedema may be at increased risk.

Patients concurrently receiving mammalian target of rapamycin (mTOR) inhibitor therapy (temsirolimus, sirolimus, everolimus) also may be at increased risk.

Dialyzable drug: Yes.

⚠ Overdose S&S: Hypotension.

PREGNANCY-LACTATION-REPRODUCTION

Black Box Warning Drug acts directly on the RAAS and can cause injury and death to a developing fetus. When pregnancy is detected, stop drug as soon as possible. ▮

• It isn't known if drug appears in human milk. Patient should discontinue breastfeeding or discontinue drug.

NURSING CONSIDERATIONS

• When using drug in acute MI, give patient the appropriate and standard recommended treatment, such as thrombolytics, aspirin, and beta blockers.

▒ Although ACE inhibitors reduce BP in all races, BP reduction is less in Blacks taking an ACE inhibitor alone. Black patients should take drug with a thiazide diuretic for a more favorable response.

• Monitor BP frequently. If drug doesn't adequately control BP, diuretics may be added.

• Monitor WBC with differential counts before therapy, every 2 weeks for first 3 months of therapy, and periodically thereafter.

• Monitor serum potassium level periodically.

• *Look alike–sound alike:* Don't confuse lisinopril with fosinopril or Lioresal. Don't confuse Zestril with Zostrix, Zetia, Zebeta, or Zyrtec. Don't confuse Prinivil with Proventil or Prilosec.

PATIENT TEACHING

🔴 *Alert:* Rarely, facial and throat swelling (including swelling of the larynx) or intestinal swelling may occur, especially after first dose. Advise patient to report abdominal pain, breathing problems, or swelling of face, eyes, lips, or tongue.

• Tell patient that light-headedness can occur, especially during first few days of therapy, to rise slowly to minimize this effect, and to report symptoms to prescriber. If fainting occurs, advise patient to stop drug and call prescriber immediately.

L

• If unpleasant adverse reactions occur, tell patient not to stop drug suddenly but to notify prescriber.

• Advise patient to report signs and symptoms of infection, such as fever and sore throat.

• Tell female patient of childbearing potential to notify prescriber if pregnancy occurs. Drug will need to be stopped.

• Advise patient to report signs and symptoms of hyperkalemia, such as muscle fatigue, weakness, nausea, or abnormal heart rhythm.

• Instruct patient not to use salt substitutes that contain potassium without first consulting prescriber.

• Inform patient that a dry, nonproductive cough may develop during therapy.

---

lisinopril–hydrochlorothiazide ℞

lye-SIN-oh-pril/hye-droe-klor-oh-THYE-a-zide

Zestoretic

Therapeutic class: Antihypertensives
Pharmacologic class: ACE inhibitors–thiazide diuretics

AVAILABLE FORMS

Tablets: 10 mg lisinopril and 12.5 mg hydrochlorothiazide, 20 mg lisinopril and 12.5 mg hydrochlorothiazide, 20 mg lisinopril and 25 mg hydrochlorothiazide

INDICATIONS & DOSAGES

➤ **HTN in patients not adequately controlled on lisinopril or hydrochlorothiazide monotherapy**

Adults: Initially, 10 mg lisinopril and 12.5 mg hydrochlorothiazide or 20 mg lisinopril and 12.5 mg hydrochlorothiazide PO once daily; titrate based on clinical response. Don't increase the hydrochlorothiazide component until 2 to 3 weeks have elapsed. In patients on adequate pressure control on single-agent hydrochlorothiazide 25 mg PO daily but with significant potassium loss, switch to 10 mg lisinopril and 12.5 mg hydrochlorothiazide tablets.

Maximum dosage is 80 mg lisinopril and 50 mg hydrochlorothiazide PO once daily.
Adjust-a-dose: Not for use in patients with CrCl of less than 30 mL/minute/1.73 m^2. Dosage selection for elderly patients should be cautious, usually starting at low end of dosing range.

ADMINISTRATION

PO

• Store at controlled room temperature; protect from excessive light and humidity.
• May give without regard for food.

ACTION

Lisinopril inhibits ACE, leading to decreased angiotensin II production, decreased aldosterone secretion, and increased potassium level. Hydrochlorothiazide inhibits sodium reabsorption in the distal tubules, causing increased excretion of sodium and water as well as potassium and hydrogen ions.

Route	Onset	Peak	Duration
PO (lisinopril)	1 hr	7 hr	24 hr
PO (hydrochloro-thiazide)	2 hr	4 hr	6–12 hr

Half-life: Lisinopril, 12 hours; hydrochlorothiazide, 5.6 to 14.8 hours.

ADVERSE REACTIONS

CNS: dizziness, headache, fatigue, asthenia, paresthesia. **CV:** orthostatic effects, hypotension. **GI:** diarrhea, nausea, vomiting, dyspepsia. **GU:** erectile dysfunction. **Metabolic:** *hypokalemia, hyperkalemia,* hyperglycemia. **Musculoskeletal:** muscle cramps. **Respiratory:** cough, URI. **Skin:** rash.

INTERACTIONS

Drug-drug. *Aliskiren:* May increase risk of renal impairment, hypotension, and hyperkalemia in diabetic patients and in those with moderate to severe renal impairment (GFR less than 60 mL/minute). Concomitant use is contraindicated in diabetic patients. Avoid concomitant use in patients with moderate to severe renal impairment.
Antidiabetic agents, insulin: May increase blood glucose level. Monitor patient carefully; adjust dosage of antidiabetic as needed.

Barbiturates, opioids: May increase risk of orthostatic hypotension. Avoid use together.

Colestipol resins, cholestyramine: May impair absorption of hydrochlorothiazide. Separate administration times by at least 4 hours.

Corticosteroids, corticotropin: May worsen electrolyte depletion, particularly hypokalemia. Monitor patient carefully.

Diuretics, other antihypertensives: May increase hypotensive effects. Monitor patient carefully.

Gold injections: May increase risk of nitritoid effects (flushing, nausea, vomiting, hypotension). Avoid use together.

Lithium: May increase lithium level. Monitor patient carefully.

Neprilysin inhibitors (sacubitril): May increase risk of angioedema. Use together is contraindicated. Don't give lisinopril within 36 hours of switching to or from sacubitril/valsartan.

Nondepolarizing skeletal muscle relaxants (tubocurarine): May increase response to muscle relaxant. Avoid use together.

NSAIDs: May diminish antihypertensive effects. Use cautiously together.

Potassium-sparing diuretics, potassium supplements: May increase risk of hyperkalemia. Avoid use together.

Pressor amines (norepinephrine): May decrease response to pressor amines. Use together cautiously.

Drug-food. *Potassium-containing salt substitutes:* May increase risk of hyperkalemia. Discourage use together.

Drug-lifestyle. *Alcohol use:* May increase risk of orthostatic hypotension. Discourage use together.

Sun exposure: May increase risk of photosensitivity. Discourage sun exposure.

EFFECTS ON LAB TEST RESULTS

• May increase glucose, cholesterol, triglyceride, BUN, creatinine, potassium, and bilirubin levels and LFT values.

• May decrease calcium, potassium, and magnesium levels and WBC count.

CONTRAINDICATIONS & CAUTIONS

• Contraindicated in patients hypersensitive to either drug or sulfonamides and in those with history of angioedema related to previous treatment with an ACE inhibitor, hereditary or idiopathic angioedema, or anuria.

• Use cautiously in patients with a history or risk of angioedema, anaphylactoid reactions, salt or volume depletion, collagen vascular disease, obstruction in the outflow tract of the left ventricle, HF, renal artery stenosis, renal disease, jaundice or hepatic disease, asthma, SLE, history of aortic stenosis, hypertrophic cardiomyopathy, existing hyperkalemia or other electrolyte imbalance, or hyperuricemia.

⬛ Although rare, angioedema, which can be fatal, may occur at any time during treatment, including after first dose; it may involve the head and neck (potentially compromising the airway) or the intestine (presenting with abdominal pain). Black patients and patients with idiopathic or hereditary angioedema may be at increased risk. Patients concurrently receiving mammalian target of rapamycin (mTOR) inhibitor therapy (temsirolimus, sirolimus, everolimus) also may be at increased risk.

Dialyzable drug: Yes (lisinopril); unknown (hydrochlorothiazide).

⚠ *Overdose S&S:* Hypotension, dehydration, electrolyte imbalance.

PREGNANCY-LACTATION-REPRODUCTION

Black Box Warning Drugs that act directly on the RAAS can cause injury and death to a developing fetus. When pregnancy is detected, discontinue drug as soon as possible. ∎

• It isn't known if lisinopril appears in human milk; hydrochlorothiazide does appear in human milk. Patient should discontinue breastfeeding or discontinue drug.

NURSING CONSIDERATIONS

• Drug isn't to be used for initial therapy. Begin combination therapy only after patient has failed to achieve desired effect with monotherapy.

• Consider ACE inhibitor–induced cough if patient develops cough of unknown etiology.

• Correct lisinopril-induced hypotension before major surgery and anesthesia.

• If hypotension occurs, place patient in supine position and give IV NSS if appropriate. May resume drug once BP has increased.

• Monitor glucose, electrolyte, and lipid levels during therapy.

• Monitor WBC count in patients with collagen vascular disease or renal disease.

• Monitor patient for jaundice and elevated liver enzyme levels. Discontinue drug and treat appropriately if these occur.

• Drug may cause intestinal angioedema. Monitor patient for abdominal pain.

• Monitor patient for angioedema of the face, extremities, lips, tongue, glottis, or larynx, which may occur at any time during treatment. If symptoms occur, discontinue drug, treat appropriately, and monitor patient until symptoms have resolved.

• If airway obstruction is likely, give subcut epinephrine solution 1:1,000 or other appropriate treatment as necessary to ensure patent airway.

▓ Black patients and patients with a history of angioedema unrelated to ACE inhibitors may be at increased risk for angioedema from ACE inhibitors.

▓ Black patients may have a more limited response to lisinopril than non-Black patients.

PATIENT TEACHING
Black Box Warning Counsel female patient to report possible pregnancy to prescriber as soon as possible. ■

• Instruct patient to stop drug and immediately report signs or symptoms suggesting angioedema (abdominal pain; swelling of the face, extremities, eyes, lips, or tongue; difficulty swallowing or breathing).

• Caution patient to report light-headedness, especially during first few days of therapy, and if syncope occurs, to discontinue drug and notify prescriber.

• Tell patient to consult prescriber if fluid losses occur (excessive perspiration, dehydration, vomiting, or diarrhea).

• Advise patient to immediately report signs and symptoms of fluid and electrolyte imbalance (dry mouth, thirst, weakness, lethargy, drowsiness, restlessness, confusion, seizures, muscle pains or cramps, muscle fatigue, decreased urination, rapid heartbeat, nausea, vomiting).

• Instruct patient to promptly report signs and symptoms of infection (sore throat, fever).

• Warn patient to avoid salt substitutes containing potassium.

• Inform patient that a dry, nonproductive cough may develop during therapy.

---

lithium carbonate
LITH-ee-um

Carbolith✦, Lithane✦, Lithobid

lithium citrate

Therapeutic class: Antimanics
Pharmacologic class: Alkali metals

AVAILABLE FORMS
lithium carbonate
Capsules: 150 mg, 300 mg, 600 mg
Tablets: 300 mg
Tablets (extended-release) ⓄⓃⒸ*:* 300 mg, 450 mg
lithium citrate
Syrup (sugarless): 8 mEq lithium/5 mL; 5 mL lithium citrate liquid contains 8 mEq lithium, equal to 300 mg lithium carbonate

INDICATIONS & DOSAGES
Adjust-a-dose (for all indications): In elderly patients and patients with CrCl of 30 to 89 mL/minute, start at lower doses. Immediate-release lithium isn't recommended in patients with CrCl of less than 30 mL/minute.

➤ **Acute mania in bipolar disorder**
Adults and children age 7 and older weighing more than 30 kg: Initially, 300 mg (immediate-release tablets or capsules) or 5 mL (8 mEq lithium) PO t.i.d. Increase by 300 mg or 5 mL every 3 days to a goal of 600 mg or 10 mL (16 mEq) PO b.i.d. or t.i.d. *Children age 7 and older weighing 20 to 30 kg:* 300 mg (immediate-release tablets or capsules) or 5 mL (8 mEq lithium) PO b.i.d. Increase by 300 mg or 5 mL weekly to a goal of 600 to 1,500 mg or 16 to 40 mEq (10 to 25 mL) PO in divided doses daily.

Reactions in bold italics are *life-threatening*. Interactions may have a *rapid onset* or a *delayed onset*.

Adults and children age 12 and older (extended-release tablets): 900 mg PO b.i.d. or 600 mg PO t.i.d.

Adjust-a-dose: Individualize dosage according to serum concentrations and clinical response. Titrate to serum lithium concentrations of 0.8 to 1.2 mEq/L (immediate-release forms) or 1 to 1.5 mEq/L (extended-release form).

➤ **Long-term control in bipolar disorder**
Adults and children age 7 and older weighing more than 30 kg: Usual dose, 300 to 600 mg (immediate-release tablets or capsules) or 5 to 10 mL (8 to 16 mEq lithium) PO b.i.d. or t.i.d.
Children age 7 and older weighing 20 to 30 kg: Usual dose, 600 to 1,200 mg (immediate-release tablets or capsules) or 10 to 20 mL (16 to 32 mEq lithium) PO in divided doses daily.
Adults and children age 12 and older (extended-release tablets): 900 to 1,200 mg/day in divided doses. Usual dose, 600 mg PO b.i.d.

Adjust-a-dose: Individualize dosage according to serum concentrations and clinical response. Titrate immediate-release formulations to serum lithium concentrations of 0.8 to 1 mEq/L. Desirable serum lithium concentrations for extended-release formulation is 0.6 to 1.2 mEq/L.

ADMINISTRATION
PO
• Give drug after meals with plenty of water to minimize GI upset.
• Don't crush extended-release tablets.

ACTION
Probably alters chemical transmitters in the CNS, possibly by interfering with ionic pump mechanisms in brain cells, and may compete with or replace sodium ions.

Route	Onset	Peak	Duration
PO (immediate-release)	Unknown	30 min–3 hr	Unknown
PO (extended-release)	Unknown	2–6 hr	Unknown
PO (syrup)	Unknown	¼–1 hr	Unknown

Half-life: 18 to 36 hours.

ADVERSE REACTIONS
CNS: fatigue, lethargy, *coma, seizures,* tremors, drowsiness, headache, confusion, restlessness, dizziness, psychomotor retardation, blackouts, EEG changes, worsened organic mental syndrome, impaired speech, ataxia, incoordination. **CV:** *arrhythmias, bradycardia,* reversible ECG changes, *severe bradycardia,* hypotension, Brugada syndrome. **EENT:** blurred vision, exophthalmos, nystagmus, tinnitus. **GI:** vomiting, anorexia, diarrhea, thirst, nausea, metallic taste, dry mouth, abdominal pain, flatulence, indigestion. **GU:** polyuria, *renal toxicity with long-term use,* glycosuria, decreased CrCl, albuminuria, urinary incontinence, erectile dysfunction. **Hematologic:** leukocytosis. **Metabolic:** transient hyperglycemia, goiter, hypothyroidism, hyponatremia. **Musculoskeletal:** muscle weakness. **Skin:** pruritus, rash, diminished or absent sensation, drying and thinning of hair, psoriasis, acne, alopecia. **Other:** ankle and wrist edema.

INTERACTIONS
Drug-drug. *ACE inhibitors:* May increase lithium level. Monitor lithium level; adjust lithium dosage, as needed.
Aminophylline, sodium bicarbonate, urine alkalinizers: May increase lithium excretion. Avoid excessive salt, and monitor lithium levels.
Antiarrhythmics and other drugs that prolong QT interval: May increase risk of life-threatening arrhythmias. Avoid use together.
Calcium channel blockers (verapamil): May decrease lithium levels and may increase risk of neurotoxicity. Use together cautiously.
Carbamazepine, fluoxetine, methyldopa, NSAIDs, probenecid: May increase effect of lithium. Monitor patient for lithium toxicity.
Neuromuscular blockers: May cause prolonged paralysis or weakness. Monitor patient closely.
Thiazide diuretics: May increase reabsorption of lithium by kidneys, with possible toxic effect. Use with caution, and monitor lithium and electrolyte levels (especially sodium).
Drug-food. *Caffeine:* May decrease lithium level and drug effect. Advise patient who ingests large amounts of caffeine to tell

L

prescriber before stopping caffeine. Adjust lithium dosage, as needed.

Sodium (salt): May change renal elimination of drug if sodium intake changes. Avoid major changes in sodium intake.

EFFECTS ON LAB TEST RESULTS

• May increase glucose and creatinine and TSH levels. May decrease sodium, T_3, T_4, and protein-bound iodine levels.
• May increase ^{131}I uptake and WBC and neutrophil counts.

CONTRAINDICATIONS & CAUTIONS

• Contraindicated if therapy can't be closely monitored.
• Use extreme caution in patients receiving neuromuscular blockers and diuretics; in elderly or debilitated patients; and in patients with thyroid disease, seizure disorder, infection, renal or CV disease, severe debilitation or dehydration, or sodium depletion.
• Patients with Brugada syndrome (abnormal ECG with increased risk of sudden death) or with risk factors for this condition shouldn't take lithium.

Dialyzable drug: Yes.

⚠ Overdose S&S: Diarrhea, vomiting, drowsiness, muscular weakness, lack of coordination, giddiness, ataxia, blurred vision, confusion, tinnitus, large output of dilute urine, slurred speech, loss of consciousness, myoclonic limb movements, agitation, urinary or fecal incontinence, seizures, arrhythmias, hypotension, peripheral vascular collapse, coma.

PREGNANCY-LACTATION-REPRODUCTION

• Drug may cause fetal harm if used during pregnancy; data from lithium birth registries suggest an increase in cardiac and other anomalies. If drug is used in women of childbearing potential or during pregnancy, or if patient becomes pregnant while taking drug, apprise patient of potential hazard to the fetus.
• If patient decides to continue lithium during pregnancy, monitor serum lithium concentration and adjust dosage if indicated. Two to three days before delivery, decrease lithium dosage or discontinue drug to reduce risk of maternal or neonatal toxicity. Monitor neonate and provide supportive care

until lithium is excreted and toxic signs and symptoms disappear, which may take up to 14 days. Consider fetal echocardiography between 16 and 20 weeks' gestation in a woman with first-trimester lithium exposure, because of the potential increased risk of cardiac malformations.
• Drug appears in human milk. Use in breastfeeding women isn't recommended.

NURSING CONSIDERATIONS

Black Box Warning Lithium toxicity is closely related to serum lithium levels and can occur at doses close to therapeutic levels. Facilities for prompt and accurate serum lithium determinations should be available before initiation of therapy. ■
• Monitor patient and discontinue drug for signs and symptoms of lithium toxicity (ataxia, drowsiness, weakness, tremor, vomiting).
• When drug level is less than 1.5 mEq/L, adverse reactions are usually mild.
• Monitor baseline ECG, thyroid studies, renal studies, and electrolyte levels.
• Check fluid intake and output, especially when surgery is scheduled.
• Weigh patient daily; check for edema or sudden weight gain.
• Adjust fluid and salt ingestion to compensate if excessive loss occurs from protracted diaphoresis or diarrhea. Under normal conditions, fluid intake should be 2½ to 3 L daily, and patient should follow a balanced diet with adequate salt intake.
• Check urine specific gravity and report level below 1.005, which may indicate diabetes insipidus.
• Drug alters glucose tolerance in diabetic patients. Monitor glucose level closely.
• Perform outpatient follow-up of thyroid and renal function every 2 to 3 months during 6 months of treatment, then as clinically indicated. Monitor CBC and ECG (patients older than age 40) before therapy and as needed. Monitor lithium level twice weekly, 12 hours after the last oral dose, until patient and levels are stable, then every 1 to 2 months or as needed.
• Palpate thyroid to check for enlargement. Monitor weight before and during therapy.

Reactions in bold italics are *life-threatening*. Interactions may have a *rapid onset* or a *delayed onset*.

• *Look alike–sound alike:* Don't confuse lithium carbonate with lanthanum carbonate.

PATIENT TEACHING

• Tell patient to take drug with plenty of water and after meals to minimize GI upset.
• Explain the importance of having regular blood tests to determine drug levels and to monitor therapy; even slightly high values can be dangerous.
• Warn patient and caregivers to expect transient nausea, large amounts of urine, thirst, and discomfort during first few days and to watch for evidence of toxicity.
• Instruct patient to withhold one dose and call prescriber immediately if signs and symptoms of toxicity appear, but not to stop drug abruptly.
• Warn patient to avoid hazardous activities that require alertness and good psychomotor coordination until CNS effects are known.
• Tell patient not to switch brands or take other prescription or OTC drugs without prescriber's guidance.
• Advise patient to immediately seek emergency assistance if fainting, light-headedness, abnormal heartbeat, or shortness of breath occurs because these signs and symptoms are associated with a potentially life-threatening heart disorder known as Brugada syndrome.
• Tell patient to wear or carry medical identification at all times.

SAFETY ALERT!

lixisenatide
lix-i-SEN-a-tide

Adlyxin

Therapeutic class: Antidiabetics
Pharmacologic class: Glucagon-like peptide-1 receptor antagonists

AVAILABLE FORMS
Injection: 10 mcg/dose in 3-mL prefilled pens (14 doses); 20 mcg/dose in 3-mL pre-filled pens (14 doses)

INDICATIONS & DOSAGES
➤ **Adjunct to diet and exercise to improve glycemic control in patients with type 2 diabetes**
Adults: Initially, 10 mcg subcut once daily for 14 days; then on day 15, increase to maintenance dose of 20 mcg subcut once daily.

ADMINISTRATION
Subcutaneous
• Inspect pen before each use; it should be clear and colorless. Don't use if there is particulate matter or discoloration.
• Administer subcut injection in abdomen, thigh, or upper arm once daily. Rotate injection site with every use.
• Give within 1 hour before first meal of the day, preferably the same meal every day. If a dose is missed, give dose 1 hour before next meal.
• Replace cap after each use. Don't store pen with needle attached.
• Store unused pen in refrigerator at 36° to 46° F (2° to 8° C) in original package; protect from light. After first dose, may store pen at room temperature, below 86° F (30° C). Discard pen after 14 days.
🛈 *Alert:* Use a new needle for each dose. Pens are for single patient use; don't share among patients even if needle is changed, because of risk of blood-borne pathogen transmission.

ACTION
Increases glucose-dependent insulin release, decreases glucagon secretion, and slows gastric emptying.

Route	Onset	Peak	Duration
Subcut	Unknown	1–3½ hr	Unknown

Half-life: 3 hours.

ADVERSE REACTIONS
CNS: headache, dizziness. **GI:** nausea, vomiting, diarrhea, dyspepsia, constipation, abdominal distention, abdominal pain. **Metabolic:** *hypoglycemia.* **Skin:** injection-site reactions. **Other:** immunogenicity.

INTERACTIONS
Drug-drug. *Basal insulin, sulfonylurea:* May increase risk of hypoglycemia. Reduce

L

basal insulin or sulfonylurea dosage as needed.

Oral contraceptives: May alter concentration of contraceptive. Patient should take contraceptive at least 1 hour before or at least 11 hours after lixisenatide injection.

Oral drugs dependent on threshold concentrations for efficacy (antibiotics) or for which a delay in effect is undesirable (acetaminophen): Lixisenatide causes delayed gastric emptying, which may affect concentrations of other drugs or cause delays in effects. Use together cautiously and give oral drugs 1 hour before lixisenatide injection.

EFFECTS ON LAB TEST RESULTS
• May decrease glucose level.

CONTRAINDICATIONS & CAUTIONS
• Contraindicated in patients hypersensitive to drug or its components. Hypersensitivity, including anaphylaxis, has occurred.
• Use cautiously in patients with a history of anaphylaxis or angioedema after receiving another GLP-1 receptor agonist.
• May increase risk of pancreatitis, especially in patients with history of cholelithiasis or alcohol abuse.
• Drug hasn't been studied in patients with chronic pancreatitis or a history of unexplained pancreatitis. Consider other antidiabetic therapies.
• May increase risk of acute kidney injury or worsening of renal impairment, especially in patients with nausea, vomiting, diarrhea, or dehydration. Use isn't recommended in patients with ESRD.
• Drug isn't indicated to treat type 1 diabetes or diabetic ketoacidosis.
• Use with short-acting insulin hasn't been studied. Use together isn't recommended.
• Drug hasn't been studied in patients with gastroparesis. Use isn't recommended.
• Antibodies to drug may develop, decreasing glycemic control and increasing risk of injection-site or allergic reactions. Consider alternative therapy if antibodies develop.
• Safety and effectiveness in children haven't been established.

Dialyzable drug: Unknown.

⚠ *Overdose S&S:* Increased GI disorders.

PREGNANCY-LACTATION-REPRODUCTION
• Data are limited concerning use in pregnant women. Use during pregnancy only if benefits outweigh risks.
• It isn't known if drug appears in human milk. Before use, consider clinical needs of the mother and potential adverse effects on the infant.

NURSING CONSIDERATIONS
• Monitor patient for hypersensitivity reactions, including anaphylaxis and angioedema. Discontinue drug and treat appropriately if reaction occurs.
• Monitor glucose level closely to evaluate effectiveness.
• Monitor renal function at beginning of therapy and at dosage escalations in patients with renal impairment or severe GI reactions.
• Monitor patient for signs and symptoms of pancreatitis. Discontinue drug and manage signs and symptoms clinically if pancreatitis is suspected. If pancreatitis is confirmed, don't restart drug.
• *Look alike–sound alike:* Don't confuse lixisenatide with liraglutide.

PATIENT TEACHING
• Tell patient to report all medications being taken before start of therapy.
• Teach patient how to prepare pen, to always use a new needle, and to administer drug according to manufacturer's instructions.
• Instruct patient to store pen in original container without the needle at room temperature, and to discard pen 14 days after first use.
• **Alert:** Teach patient not to share pens even if the needle is changed, because of risk of blood-borne pathogen transmission.
• Caution patient to report all adverse reactions, especially signs and symptoms of hypoglycemia (dizziness, confusion, weakness, feeling jittery, sweating), particularly if patient is taking a sulfonylurea or basal insulin, and pancreatitis (persistent, severe abdominal pain that may radiate to the back, with or without vomiting).
• Warn patient to watch for signs and symptoms of hypersensitivity reactions (fever, nausea, difficulty breathing, rash, swelling

---

Reactions in bold italics are *life-threatening*. Interactions may have a *rapid onset* or a *delayed onset*.

of the face, lips or tongue) and to stop drug and seek immediate medical attention if they occur.

• Teach patient to report nausea, vomiting, diarrhea, and dehydration promptly, because of risk of kidney injury.

• Advise female patient to inform prescriber if she is or plans to become pregnant or to breastfeed before start of therapy.

---

lofexidine hydrochloride ☒
loe-FEX-i-deen

Lucemyra

Therapeutic class: Opioid cessation drugs
Pharmacologic class: Alpha₂-adrenergic receptor agonists

AVAILABLE FORMS
Tablets: 0.18 mg

INDICATIONS & DOSAGES
➤ **Mitigation of opioid withdrawal symptoms to facilitate abrupt opioid discontinuation**
Adults: Initially, three 0.18-mg tablets PO q.i.d. during the peak withdrawal period (generally 5 to 7 days after last opioid dose). Allow 5 to 6 hours between doses and continue for up to 14 days, with dosing guided by symptoms. Maximum daily dose is 2.88 mg (16 tablets); maximum single dose is 0.72 mg (4 tablets). Discontinue treatment gradually over 2 to 4 days, reducing by 1 tablet per dose every 1 to 2 days.
Adjust-a-dose: For patients with mild hepatic impairment (Child-Pugh score 5 to 6), give 3 tablets q.i.d. (2.16 mg/day); for those with moderate hepatic impairment (Child-Pugh score 7 to 9), give 2 tablets q.i.d. (1.44 mg/day); for those with severe hepatic impairment (Child-Pugh score greater than 9), give 1 tablet q.i.d. (0.72 mg/day). For patients with mild to moderate renal impairment (eGFR of 30 to 89.9 mL/minute/1.73 m²), give 2 tablets q.i.d. (1.44 mg/day); for those with severe renal impairment, ESRD, or on dialysis (eGFR of less than 30 mL/minute/1.73 m²), give 1 tablet q.i.d. (0.72 mg/day).

ADMINISTRATION
PO
• May give with or without food.
• Store at controlled room temperature 77° F (25° C). Protect from excess moisture and heat. Don't remove desiccant pack from bottle.

ACTION
A central alpha₂-adrenergic agonist that binds to receptors on adrenergic neurons. It inhibits the release of norepinephrine in the central and peripheral nervous systems, reducing the signs and symptoms of opioid withdrawal.

Route	Onset	Peak	Duration
PO	Unknown	3–5 hr	Unknown

Half-life: 11 to 13 hours (first dose); 17 to 22 hours (at steady-state).

ADVERSE REACTIONS
CNS: insomnia, dizziness, somnolence, sedation, syncope. **CV:** orthostatic hypotension, *bradycardia,* hypotension. **EENT:** tinnitus, dry mouth.

INTERACTIONS
Drug-drug. *CNS depressants (barbiturates, benzodiazepines):* May enhance CNS depressant effects. Avoid use together.
CYP2D6 inhibitors (paroxetine): May increase lofexidine concentration. Use cautiously together. Monitor patient for orthostatic hypotension and bradycardia.
Drugs that decrease HR: May increase risk of excessive bradycardia. Avoid use together.
Drugs that increase QT interval (methadone): May further increase QT interval. Use together cautiously and monitor ECGs.
Drugs that lower BP: May increase hypotensive effects. Avoid use together.
Naltrexone: May decrease effectiveness of oral naltrexone if given within 2 hours of lofexidine. Monitor therapy and separate dosing times of drugs by 2 hours.
Drug-lifestyle. *Alcohol use:* May increase CNS depressive effects. Discourage use together.

EFFECTS ON LAB TEST RESULTS
None reported.

CONTRAINDICATIONS & CAUTIONS

• Avoid use in patients with severe coronary insufficiency, recent MI, cerebrovascular disease, chronic renal failure, and marked bradycardia. If drug must be used, monitor ECG, especially in patients with these conditions and electrolyte disturbances.

❸ *Alert:* Drug causes QT-interval prolongation, especially in patients with renal impairment; prolonged QT interval increases risk of ventricular arrhythmias. Avoid using in patients with congenital long QT syndrome.

• Use cautiously in patients with congestive HF, bradyarrhythmias, and hepatic or renal impairment.

• Use cautiously in outpatient setting. Patients should be capable of self-monitoring for adverse effects.

• Drug may decrease tolerance to opioids and increase the risk of fatal opioid overdose if patient resumes opioid use.

• Use drug for opioid use disorder only with a comprehensive treatment and management program.

❸ *Alert:* Drug may increase risk of discontinuation symptoms. Don't stop medication abruptly as it can cause a rise in BP, diarrhea, insomnia, chills, hyperhidrosis, and extremity pain.

▒ Use cautiously in patients who are CYP2D6 poor metabolizers. Monitor patients for orthostatic hypotension and bradycardia.

• Safety and effectiveness in children haven't been established.

• Use cautiously in elderly patients; consider utilizing dosage adjustments for renal impairment.

Dialyzable drug: Minimal.

⚠ *Overdose S&S:* Hypotension, bradycardia, sedation.

PREGNANCY-LACTATION-REPRODUCTION

• Safe use in pregnancy hasn't been established. Use only if benefits outweigh risks to fetus.

• It isn't known if drug appears in human milk or how drug affects breastfed infants or milk production. Use cautiously in breastfeeding women.

NURSING CONSIDERATIONS

• Monitor vital signs and watch for bradycardia and orthostatic hypotension before dosing. Reduce dosage or delay or skip next dose for clinically significant hypotension or bradycardia.

• Monitor ECG in patients with congestive HF, bradycardia, hepatic impairment, or renal impairment and in those taking medications that prolong QT interval, especially if electrolyte disturbances are present.

• Monitor electrolyte levels and correct abnormalities (hypokalemia, hypomagnesemia) before administering drug; monitor ECG when starting drug.

• Monitor patient for drug discontinuation signs and symptoms; manage by resuming previous dose, followed by gradual tapering if signs and symptoms occur.

PATIENT TEACHING

• Teach patient signs and symptoms of hypotension and to rise slowly from a seated or lying position.

• Caution patient to stay hydrated.

• Instruct patient to withhold dose and immediately contact prescriber if signs or symptoms of low BP or slow HR occur (dizziness, light-headedness, feeling faint at rest or when standing up).

• Instruct patient to avoid driving or operating heavy machinery until drug's effects are known.

• Instruct patient not to abruptly stop drug and to follow instructions for gradual drug discontinuation.

❸ *Alert:* Inform patient and caregivers of increased risk of overdose if opioids are resumed.

---

lomitapide mesylate ▒
lom-i-TA-pide

Juxtapid

Therapeutic class: Antilipemics
Pharmacologic class: Microsomal triglyceride transfer protein inhibitors

AVAILABLE FORMS
Capsules ⓄⒸ: 5 mg, 10 mg, 20 mg, 30 mg, 40 mg, 60 mg

INDICATIONS & DOSAGES
➤ **As an adjunct to low-fat diet and other lipid-lowering treatments, including LDL apheresis where available, to reduce LDL, total cholesterol, apolipoprotein B, and non-HDL cholesterol levels in patients with homozygous familial hypercholesterolemia (HoFH)** ▧

Adults: 5 mg PO once daily. May increase to 10 mg daily after at least 2 weeks; may increase at least 4 weeks later to 20 mg, then at least 4 weeks later to 40 mg, then at least 4 weeks later to 60 mg. Measure ALT and AST levels before any dosage increase. Maximum daily dosage is 60 mg.

Adjust-a-dose: In patients with ESRD receiving dialysis and in patients with mild hepatic impairment (Child-Pugh class A), don't exceed 40 mg PO daily. Refer to manufacturer's instructions for drug-interaction and toxicity-related dosage adjustments.

ADMINISTRATION
PO
• Give drug with a glass of water on an empty stomach at least 2 hours after evening meal.
• Don't crush or open capsules.
■Black Box Warning■ Check LFT values (ALT, AST, alkaline phosphatase, and total bilirubin) before starting and periodically during treatment. ▌
• To reduce risk of developing a fat-soluble nutrient deficiency, patients should take drug with concurrent daily doses of vitamin E, 400 international units; linoleic acid, 200 mg; alpha-linolenic acid, 210 mg; eicosapentaenoic acid, 110 mg; and docosahexaenoic acid, 80 mg.

ACTION
Inhibits microsomal triglyceride transfer protein, stopping synthesis of chylomicrons and VLDL, leading to reduced levels of plasma LDL cholesterol.

Route	Onset	Peak	Duration
PO	Unknown	6 hr	Unknown

Half-life: 39.7 hours.

ADVERSE REACTIONS
CNS: headache, dizziness, fever, fatigue.
CV: chest pain, angina pectoris, palpitations.

EENT: nasopharyngitis, pharyngolaryngeal pain, nasal congestion. **GI:** diarrhea, nausea, dyspepsia, vomiting, abdominal pain, abdominal discomfort, abdominal distention, constipation, flatulence, GERD, defecation urgency, rectal tenesmus, gastroenteritis. **Hepatic:** increased ALT level, hepatic steatosis, *hepatotoxicity.* **Metabolic:** weight loss. **Musculoskeletal:** back pain. **Other:** flulike symptoms.

INTERACTIONS
Drug-drug. *Bile acid sequestrants (cholestyramine, colesevelam, colesevelam hydrochloride, colestipol, colestipol hydrochloride):* May interfere with absorption of lomitapide. Separate doses by 4 hours.
Hepatotoxins (acetaminophen [more than 4 g/day for 3 days/week or more], amiodarone, isotretinoin, methotrexate, tamoxifen, tetracyclines): May accelerate liver injury. Use together cautiously and monitor LFTs frequently.
Lovastatin: May increase risk of myopathy. Use together cautiously; consider lower lovastatin dosage.
Moderate CYP3A4 inhibitors (amprenavir, aprepitant, atazanavir, ciprofloxacin, crizotinib, darunavir/ritonavir, diltiazem, erythromycin, fluconazole, fosamprenavir, imatinib, verapamil): May increase lomitapide concentration. Use together is contraindicated.
P-gp substrates (aliskiren, ambrisentan, colchicine, dabigatran, digoxin, everolimus, fexofenadine, imatinib, lapatinib, maraviroc, nilotinib, posaconazole, ranolazine, saxagliptin, sirolimus, sitagliptin, tolvaptan, topotecan): May increase level of substrate. Use together cautiously; consider substrate dosage reduction.
Simvastatin: May increase risk of myopathy. Decrease simvastatin dosage to 20 mg daily, or to 40 mg for patients previously taking 80 mg daily with no muscle toxicity in last year.
Strong CYP3A4 inhibitors (clarithromycin, conivaptan, indinavir, itraconazole, ketoconazole, lopinavir–ritonavir, nefazodone, nelfinavir, posaconazole, ritonavir, saquinavir, telithromycin, voriconazole): May increase lomitapide level. Use together is contraindicated.

L

Warfarin: May increase INR. Use together cautiously. Monitor INR carefully, especially after lomitapide dosage adjustments.

Weak CYP3A4 inhibitors (alprazolam, amiodarone, amlodipine, atorvastatin, bicalutamide, cilostazol, cimetidine, cyclosporine, fluoxetine, fluvoxamine, isoniazid, lapatinib, nilotinib, oral contraceptives, pazopanib, ranitidine, ranolazine, tipranavir/ritonavir, ticagrelor, zileuton): Use together cautiously, with maximum lomitapide dosage of 30 mg PO daily; maximum dosage is 40 mg PO daily with oral contraceptives.

Drug-herb. *Ginkgo biloba, goldenseal:* May increase lomitapide level. Use together cautiously, with maximum lomitapide dosage of 30 mg daily.

Drug-food. *Fat-soluble nutrients (alphalinolenic acid, docosahexaenoic acid, eicosapentaenoic acid, linoleic acid, vitamin E):* May decrease absorption of these nutrients. Supplements should be given.

Grapefruit juice: May adversely affect absorption. Discourage use together.

Drug-lifestyle. *Alcohol use:* May exacerbate liver injury and increase hepatic fat levels. Discourage consumption of more than one alcoholic drink per day.

EFFECTS ON LAB TEST RESULTS

• May increase INR and transaminase, bilirubin, and alkaline phosphatase levels.

CONTRAINDICATIONS & CAUTIONS

Black Box Warning Because of risk of hepatotoxicity, lomitapide is available only through a restricted program under a REMS called the Juxtapid REMS program. Safety and effectiveness haven't been established in patients with hypercholesterolemia who don't have HoFH. ■

• Contraindicated in patients hypersensitive to drug or its components and in those with moderate or severe hepatic impairment (Child-Pugh class B or C) or active liver disease, including unexplained persistent elevations of serum transaminases.

Black Box Warning Drug causes increased hepatic fat (steatosis), a risk factor for progressive liver disease, including steatohepatitis and cirrhosis. ■

• Drug hasn't been studied when given with other LDL-lowering agents that can also increase hepatic fat. Use together isn't recommended.

▨ Avoid use in patients with galactose intolerance, Lapp lactase deficiency, or glucose–galactose malabsorption; decreased absorption of concurrent drugs may result.

Dialyzable drug: Unlikely.

PREGNANCY-LACTATION-REPRODUCTION

⊕ *Alert:* Rule out pregnancy in women of childbearing potential before starting treatment.

• Drug may cause fetal harm and is contraindicated during pregnancy. Women of childbearing potential should use effective contraception during therapy.

• Women who become pregnant during therapy should stop drug immediately and notify their prescriber.

⊕ *Alert:* Discontinue drug immediately if pregnancy occurs during therapy and enroll patient in the Global Lomitapide Pregnancy Exposure Registry at 1-877-902-4099.

• It isn't known if drug appears in human milk. Patient should discontinue breastfeeding or discontinue drug.

NURSING CONSIDERATIONS

Black Box Warning Drug may cause hepatic steatosis or transaminase elevations. Measure AST, ALT, alkaline phosphatase, and total bilirubin levels before treatment; then obtain AST and ALT levels periodically and with dosage changes. Adjust dosage if AST or ALT level is greater than $3 \times$ ULN. Discontinue drug for clinically significant liver toxicity. ■

• Assess liver-related tests (ALT and AST, at a minimum) monthly or before each dosage increase, whichever occurs first during the first year; then assess at least every 3 months and before any dosage increase.

• If transaminase elevations are accompanied by clinical signs and symptoms of liver injury (nausea, vomiting, abdominal pain, fever, jaundice, lethargy, or flulike symptoms), increase in bilirubin level $2 \times$ ULN or more, or active liver disease, discontinue treatment and investigate probable cause.

• Monitor patient for GI adverse effects. Absorption of oral medications, including oral contraceptives, may be affected in patients with diarrhea and vomiting.

Reactions in bold italics are **life-threatening***. Interactions may have a* **rapid onset** *or a* **delayed onset***.*

• Monitor patients who are more susceptible to complications from diarrhea, such as older patients and patients taking drugs that can lead to volume depletion or hypotension, because of risk of severe diarrhea.

PATIENT TEACHING

• Inform patient about participation in drug's registry program. Information is available at www.juxtapid.com.
• Advise patient to limit alcohol to one drink daily.
• Instruct patient to report severe stomach upset or other GI signs and symptoms, fever, jaundice, lethargy, or flulike symptoms as these may be signs of liver injury.
• Instruct patient to stop drug and contact prescriber if severe diarrhea occurs or if patient experiences signs and symptoms of volume depletion, such as light-headedness, decreased urine output, or tiredness.
• Teach female patient that drug may harm a fetus and to use effective contraception during therapy and to discontinue drug and immediately notify prescriber if she becomes pregnant.
• Teach female patient of childbearing potential who is taking oral contraceptives to use additional contraceptive methods if vomiting and diarrhea occur.
• Remind patient to take vitamin E and other supplements as required.
• Caution patient to adhere to low-fat diet (less than 20% of calories from fat) and to take drug at least 2 hours after evening meal to minimize GI adverse effects.
• Warn patient to contact health care provider if drug has been stopped for more than a week.

lopinavir–ritonavir ▨
low-PIN-ah-ver/ri-TON-ah-veer

Kaletra*✐

Therapeutic class: Antiretrovirals
Pharmacologic class: Protease inhibitors

AVAILABLE FORMS
Solution: lopinavir 400 mg and ritonavir 100 mg/5 mL (80 mg/mL and 20 mg/mL)*

Tablets ⓓ*:* lopinavir 100 mg and ritonavir 25 mg; lopinavir 200 mg and ritonavir 50 mg

INDICATIONS & DOSAGES
➤ **HIV infection, with other antiretrovirals but not efavirenz, nevirapine, or nelfinavir** ▨
Adults: 800 mg lopinavir and 200 mg ritonavir PO once daily (only in patients with less than three lopinavir resistance–associated substitutions) or in two evenly divided doses.
Children older than 6 months to 18 years: 230 mg lopinavir and 57.5 mg/m^2 ritonavir (oral solution) PO b.i.d. with food. Or, if patient weighs more than 35 kg, give four tablets of lopinavir 100 mg and ritonavir 25 mg PO b.i.d. If patient weighs between 25 and 35 kg, give three tablets of lopinavir 100 mg and ritonavir 25 mg PO b.i.d. If patient weighs 15 to 25 kg, give two tablets of lopinavir 100 mg and ritonavir 25 mg PO b.i.d. Maximum dosage is lopinavir 400 mg and ritonavir 100 mg PO b.i.d.
Children ages 14 days to 6 months: 16 mg lopinavir and 4 mg ritonavir/kg oral solution PO b.i.d. Or, lopinavir 300 mg and ritonavir 75 mg/m^2 PO b.i.d.
Adjust-a-dose: In pregnant women with no documented lopinavir resistance–associated substitutions, give 400 mg lopinavir and 100 mg ritonavir tablets b.i.d.; avoid oral solution. Once-daily dosing isn't recommended. There are insufficient data to recommend dosing in pregnant women with documented lopinavir resistance–associated substitutions. No dosage adjustment is required during the postpartum period.
➤ **HIV infection, in combination with other antiretrovirals (efavirenz, nevirapine, or nelfinavir)**
Adults: 500 mg lopinavir and 125 mg ritonavir (tablets) PO b.i.d., or 520 mg lopinavir and 130 mg ritonavir (oral solution) PO b.i.d. with food.
Children older than 6 months to 18 years: 300 mg lopinavir and 75 mg/m^2 ritonavir (oral solution) PO b.i.d. with food. Maximum dosage is lopinavir 533 mg and ritonavir 133 mg (oral solution) PO b.i.d. with food. Or, if patient weighs more than 45 kg, give five tablets of lopinavir 100 mg and ritonavir 25 mg PO b.i.d. If patient weighs between 30 and 45 kg, give four tablets of

L

lopinavir 100 mg and ritonavir 25 mg PO b.i.d. If patient weighs 20 to 30 kg, give three tablets of lopinavir 100 mg and ritonavir 25 mg PO b.i.d. If patient weighs 15 to 20 kg, give two tablets of lopinavir 100 mg and ritonavir 25 mg PO b.i.d. Maximum dosage is lopinavir 500 mg and ritonavir 125 mg (tablets) PO b.i.d.

ADMINISTRATION
PO
❸ *Alert:* Many drug interactions are possible. Review all drugs patient is taking.
• Give oral solution with food. Give tablets without regard for food.
• Calculate children's doses based on either body weight or BSA.
• Tablets must be swallowed whole; don't crush or divide, and tell patient not to chew.
• Don't use oral solution with polyurethane feeding tubes because of potential incompatibility with ethanol and propylene glycol. Feeding tubes that are compatible with ethanol and propylene glycol, such as silicone and polyvinyl chloride feeding tubes, can be used.
• Refrigerated solution remains stable until expiration date on package. If stored at room temperature, use drug within 2 months.

ACTION
Lopinavir is an HIV protease inhibitor, which produces immature, noninfectious viral particles. Ritonavir, also an HIV protease inhibitor, slows lopinavir metabolism, thereby increasing lopinavir level.

Route	Onset	Peak	Duration
PO	Unknown	4 hr	Unknown

Half-life: About 5 to 6 hours.

ADVERSE REACTIONS
CNS: *encephalopathy,* abnormal dreams, abnormal thinking, agitation, amnesia, anxiety, asthenia, ataxia, confusion, depression, dizziness, dyskinesia, emotional lability, fever, headache, hypertonia, insomnia, malaise, nervousness, neuropathy, pain, paresthesia, peripheral neuritis, somnolence, tremors. **CV:** chest pain, *DVT,* edema, HTN, palpitations, thrombophlebitis, vasculitis. **EENT:** abnormal vision, eye disorder, otitis media, tinnitus, sinusitis. **GI:** *hemorrhagic*

colitis, pancreatitis, diarrhea, nausea, abdominal pain, abnormal stools, anorexia, cholecystitis, constipation, dry mouth, dyspepsia, dysphagia, enterocolitis, eructation, esophagitis, fecal incontinence, flatulence, gastritis, gastroenteritis, GI disorder, increased appetite, inflammation of the salivary glands, stomatitis, taste perversion, ulcerative stomatitis, vomiting. **GU:** abnormal ejaculation, hypogonadism, renal calculus, urine abnormality. **Hematologic:** *leukopenia, neutropenia, thrombocytopenia in children,* anemia. **Hepatic:** hyperbilirubinemia in children. **Metabolic:** Cushing syndrome, dehydration, decreased glucose tolerance, hypertriglyceridemia, hyperglycemia, hypercholesterolemia, hyperuricemia, hyponatremia in children, hypothyroidism, *lactic acidosis,* weight loss. **Musculoskeletal:** arthralgia, arthrosis, back pain, myalgia. **Respiratory:** bronchitis, dyspnea, lung edema. **Skin:** acne, alopecia, benign skin neoplasm, dry skin, exfoliative dermatitis, furunculosis, nail disorder, pruritus, rash, skin discoloration, sweating. **Other:** chills, decreased libido, facial edema, flu syndrome, gynecomastia, immune reconstitution syndrome, lymphadenopathy, viral infection.

INTERACTIONS
Drug-drug. *Alfuzosin:* Increases hypotension risk. Use together is contraindicated.
Amiodarone, bepridil, lidocaine, quinidine: May increase antiarrhythmic level. Use together cautiously. Monitor levels of these drugs, if possible.
Antiarrhythmics (dronedarone, flecainide, propafenone), pimozide: May increase risk of cardiac arrhythmias. Avoid using together. Dronedarone is contraindicated.
Aripiprazole: May enhance adverse effects of ritonavir. Modify therapy.
Atorvastatin: May increase level of this drug and risk of myopathy and rhabdomyolysis. Use lowest possible dose and monitor patient carefully.
Atovaquone, methadone: May decrease levels of these drugs. Consider increasing doses of these drugs.
Bosentan: May increase bosentan level. Withhold bosentan for at least 36 hours

---

Reactions in bold italics are *life-threatening*. Interactions may have a *rapid onset* or a ***delayed onset***.

before starting lopinavir–ritonavir, and decrease bosentan dosage and frequency.

Bupropion: May decrease bupropion level and antidepressant effect. Monitor patient for adequate clinical response and adjust bupropion dosage as needed.

Carbamazepine, phenobarbital, phenytoin: May decrease lopinavir level. Use together cautiously. Don't use once-daily lopinavir–ritonavir. Consider therapy modification.

Clarithromycin: May increase clarithromycin level in patients with renal impairment. Adjust clarithromycin dosage.

Cobicistat: May enhance therapeutic effects of ritonavir. Avoid use together.

Colchicine: May increase colchicine level. Contraindicated in patients with renal or hepatic impairment. Decrease colchicine dosage if used together in patient with normal renal and hepatic function.

Cyclosporine, rapamycin, tacrolimus: May increase levels of these drugs. Monitor therapeutic levels.

Dasatinib, nilotinib: May increase levels of these drugs and risk of adverse events. Adjust dasatinib and nilotinib dosages as needed.

Delavirdine: May increase lopinavir level. Avoid using together.

Didanosine: May decrease absorption of didanosine because lopinavir–ritonavir combination is taken with food. Give didanosine 1 hour before or 2 hours after lopinavir–ritonavir combination.

Disulfiram, metronidazole: May cause disulfiram-like reaction in patients using oral solution (contains alcohol). Avoid use together.

Drugs that prolong PR interval (atazanavir, beta blockers, calcium channel blockers, digoxin): May further prolong PR interval. Use cautiously together.

Drugs that prolong QT interval (amiodarone, flecainide, propafenone): May further prolong QT interval and increase risk of ventricular arrhythmias. Avoid use together.

Efavirenz, nelfinavir, nevirapine: May decrease lopinavir level. Consider increasing lopinavir–ritonavir combination dose. Don't use a once-daily regimen of lopinavir–ritonavir combination with these drugs.

Elvitegravir: May increase elvitegravir concentration. Reduce dosages of both drugs and consider modifying therapy.

Ergot derivatives (dihydroergotamine, ergonovine, ergotamine, methylergonovine): May increase risk of ergot toxicity characterized by peripheral vasospasm and ischemia. Use together is contraindicated.

Felodipine, nicardipine, nifedipine: May increase levels of these drugs. Use together cautiously.

Fentanyl, triazolam: May increase or prolong sedation or cause respiratory depression. Monitor patient carefully.

Fluticasone: May increase fluticasone plasma concentration, leading to decreased serum cortisol level, Cushing syndrome, and adrenal suppression. Use together isn't recommended unless benefits outweigh risks.

Fosamprenavir with ritonavir: May increase rate of adverse reactions. Appropriate doses of the combinations with respect to safety and effectiveness haven't been established.

Hormonal contraceptives (ethinyl estradiol): May decrease effectiveness of contraceptives. Recommend nonhormonal contraceptives.

Indinavir, saquinavir: May increase levels of these drugs. Avoid using together.

Itraconazole, ketoconazole: May increase levels of these drugs. Don't give more than 200 mg/day of these drugs.

Lovastatin, simvastatin: May increase risk of adverse reactions, such as myopathy and rhabdomyolysis. Use together is contraindicated.

Lurasidone, pimozide, ranolazine: Increases risk of life-threatening reactions. Use together is contraindicated.

Methadone: May decrease methadone level. Monitor clinical response and increase methadone dosage as needed.

Midazolam (oral), triazolam: May cause prolonged or increased sedation or respiratory depression. Use together is contraindicated.

Pitavastatin, pravastatin: May increase statin level and risk of myopathy and rhabdomyolysis. Use together cautiously.

Rifabutin: May increase rifabutin level. Decrease rifabutin dosage by at least 75% or a maximum of 150 mg every other day or

L

three times a week. Monitor patient carefully and adjust dosage as needed.

Rifampin: May decrease effectiveness of Kaletra. Avoid using together.

Rosuvastatin: May increase statin level and risk of myopathy and rhabdomyolysis. Rosuvastatin dosage shouldn't exceed 10 mg daily.

Salmeterol: May increase salmeterol level and risk of CV adverse reactions. Use together isn't recommended.

Sildenafil, tadalafil, vardenafil: May increase level of these drugs and adverse effects, such as hypotension and prolonged erection. Warn patient not to take more than 25 mg of sildenafil in 48 hours, more than 10 mg of tadalafil in 72 hours, or more than 2.5 mg vardenafil in 72 hours.

Trazodone: May increase trazodone level and risk of adverse reactions. Consider lower dosage of trazodone.

Vinblastine, vincristine: May increase levels of these drugs and risk of adverse reactions. Temporarily withhold antiretroviral regimen for hematologic or GI adverse reactions. If cancer treatment is prolonged, consider other antivirals.

Warfarin: May affect warfarin level. Monitor INR frequently.

Drug-herb. *Garlic supplements:* May decrease serum concentration of protease inhibitors. Concurrent use isn't recommended. If combination is used, monitor patient closely for signs or symptoms of therapeutic failure.

St. John's wort: May cause loss of virologic response and possible resistance to drug. Discourage use together.

Drug-food. *Any food:* May increase absorption of oral solution. Tell patient to take with food.

EFFECTS ON LAB TEST RESULTS

• May increase glucose, amylase, lipase, cholesterol, uric acid, and triglyceride levels and LFT values.
• May decrease Hb level and hematocrit.
• May decrease RBC, WBC, neutrophil, and platelet counts.

CONTRAINDICATIONS & CAUTIONS

• Contraindicated in patients hypersensitive to drug or its components.

• Concomitant use with certain other drugs may result in known or potentially significant drug interactions. Consult full prescribing information before and during treatment for potential drug interactions.
🧬 Genetic or phenotype testing and treatment history should guide use of drug. The number of baseline lopinavir resistance–associated substitutions affects drug's virologic response.
• Avoid use in patients with congenital long QT syndrome or hypokalemia and in those taking drugs that prolong QT interval. Correct potassium abnormalities before starting therapy.
• Use cautiously in patients with a history of pancreatitis, hepatic impairment, HBV or HCV infection, marked elevations in liver enzyme levels, or hemophilia.
• Use cautiously in patients with cardiac conduction abnormalities or underlying cardiac disease.
• Use cautiously in elderly patients.
• New-onset diabetes mellitus, exacerbation of preexisting diabetes mellitus, and hyperglycemia have been reported in HIV-1-infected patients receiving protease inhibitor therapy.
• Oral solution contains 42.4% (volume/volume) alcohol and 15.3% (weight/volume) propylene glycol; use with care, especially in infants and young children. Consider total amounts of alcohol and propylene glycol from all drugs given to children ages 14 days to 6 months to avoid toxicity.
◑ *Alert:* Safety and effectiveness in neonates younger than age 14 days haven't been established. Use only if benefit outweighs risk. Monitor neonates for toxicity, such as hyperosmolality with or without lactic acidosis, renal toxicity, CNS depression (stupor, coma, apnea), seizures, hypotonia, cardiac arrhythmias, ECG changes, and hemolysis. Toxicity in preterm neonates can be severe or fatal.
Dialyzable drug: Unlikely.
⚠ *Overdose S&S:* Alcohol-related toxicity.

PREGNANCY-LACTATION-REPRODUCTION

• Drug is recommended with dosage adjustments for pregnant women with HIV infection.

Reactions in bold italics are *life-threatening*. Interactions may have a *rapid onset* or a *delayed onset*.

• Avoid use of oral solution during pregnancy because it contains alcohol.

⚮ Once-daily dosing isn't recommended in pregnant women with any documented lopinavir resistance–associated amino acid substitutions.

• The Antiretroviral Pregnancy Registry monitors maternal-fetal outcomes of pregnant women taking Kaletra. Health care providers are encouraged to enroll patients by calling 1-800-258-4263.

• Patients with HIV-1 infection shouldn't breastfeed, to avoid risk of postnatal transmission of HIV-1.

NURSING CONSIDERATIONS

• Don't administer tablets or oral solution as a once-daily dosing regimen when combined with efavirenz, nevirapine, or nelfinavir.

• Avoid once-daily dosing in children younger than age 18.

• Calculate appropriate dose of drug for each individual pediatric patient based on body weight or BSA to avoid underdosing or exceeding the recommended adult dose.

• Assess children for ability to swallow intact tablets before drug is prescribed; use oral solution in a calibrated dosing syringe if a child is unable to reliably swallow a tablet.

• During initial phase of treatment, patients responding to antiretroviral therapy may develop an inflammatory response to indolent or residual opportunistic infections (CMV, *Mycobacterium avium* complex, *Pneumocystis jiroveci* pneumonia, TB), which may necessitate further evaluation and treatment. Autoimmune disorders (such as Graves disease, polymyositis, and Guillain-Barré syndrome) have also been reported in the setting of immune reconstitution; however, time to onset is more variable, and onset can occur many months after initiation of antiretroviral treatment.

• Monitor patient for signs of fat redistribution, including central obesity, buffalo hump, peripheral wasting, breast enlargement, and cushingoid appearance.

• Monitor glucose, total cholesterol, and triglyceride levels before starting therapy and periodically thereafter.

• Monitor patient for signs and symptoms of pancreatitis (nausea, vomiting, abdominal pain, or increased lipase and amylase values).

• Monitor patient for signs and symptoms of bleeding (hypotension, rapid HR) and for adverse reactions associated with concomitant drugs.

• Consider potential for drug interactions before and during therapy. Review concomitant medications and monitor patient for adverse reactions associated with the concomitant medications.

• *Look alike–sound alike:* Don't confuse Kaletra with Keppra.

PATIENT TEACHING

• Tell patient to take oral solution with food. Tablets may be taken without regard to food.

⚠ *Alert:* Tablets must be swallowed whole; don't crush or divide, and tell patient not to chew.

• Tell patient also taking didanosine to take it 1 hour before or 2 hours after lopinavir–ritonavir combination.

• Advise patient to report all side effects to prescriber.

• Teach patient signs and symptoms of acute pancreatitis and to seek emergency medical treatment if signs and symptoms occur.

• Tell patient to report all adverse reactions and to immediately report severe nausea, vomiting, or abdominal pain.

• Inform patient that drug doesn't cure HIV infection, that opportunistic infections and other complications of HIV infection may still occur, and that transmission of HIV to others through sexual contact or blood contamination remains possible.

• Advise patient taking an erectile dysfunction drug of the increased risk of adverse effects, including low BP, visual changes, and painful erections, and to promptly report any symptoms to prescriber. Tell patient not to take more often than directed.

• Warn patient to tell prescriber about other prescription or OTC drugs being taken, including herbal supplements.

SAFETY ALERT!

LORazepam
lor-AZ-e-pam

Ativan⬦, Lorazepam Intensol

Therapeutic class: Anxiolytics
Pharmacologic class: Benzodiazepines
Controlled substance schedule: IV

AVAILABLE FORMS
Injection: 2 mg/mL, 4 mg/mL
Oral solution: 2 mg/mL
Tablets: 0.5 mg, 1 mg, 2 mg

INDICATIONS & DOSAGES
➤ **Anxiety**
Adults: 2 to 6 mg PO daily in divided doses, with the largest dose taken before bedtime. Maximum, 10 mg daily.
Elderly patients: 1 to 2 mg PO daily in divided doses. Maximum, 10 mg daily.
➤ **Insomnia from anxiety or transient situational stress**
Adults: 2 to 4 mg PO at bedtime.
➤ **Preoperative sedation**
Adults: 2 mg IV total or 0.044 mg/kg IV, whichever is smaller, 15 to 20 minutes before the anticipated operative procedure. Larger doses up to 0.05 mg/kg IV, to total of 4 mg, may be needed. Or, 0.05 mg/kg IM 2 hours before procedure. Total dose shouldn't exceed 4 mg.
➤ **Status epilepticus**
Adults: 4 mg IV at a rate of 2 mg/minute. If seizures continue or recur after 10 to 15 minutes, an additional 4-mg dose may be given. Drug may be given IM if IV access isn't available.

ADMINISTRATION
PO
• Use only the calibrated dropper provided.
• Mix oral solution with liquid or semisolid food, such as water, juices, carbonated beverages, applesauce, or pudding. Gently stir liquid or food for a few seconds and have patient immediately consume entire mixture.
IV
▼ Keep emergency resuscitation equipment and oxygen available.

▼ Dilute with an equal volume of sterile water for injection, NSS for injection, or D_5W. Give slowly at no more than 2 mg/minute.
▼ Monitor respirations every 5 to 15 minutes and before each IV dose.
▼ Contains benzyl alcohol. Avoid use in neonates.
▼ Refrigerate intact vials and protect from light.
▼ **Incompatibilities:** None listed by manufacturer. Consult a drug incompatibility reference for more information.
IM
• For status epilepticus, drug may be given IM if IV access isn't available.
• For IM use, inject deeply into a muscle. Don't dilute.
• Refrigerate parenteral form to prolong shelf life.

ACTION
Potentiates the effects of GABA, depresses the CNS, and suppresses the spread of seizure activity.

Route	Onset	Peak	Duration
PO	1 hr	2 hr	12–24 hr
IV	5 min	60–90 min	6–8 hr
IM	15–30 min	60–90 min	6–8 hr

Half-life: 10 to 20 hours.

ADVERSE REACTIONS
CNS: drowsiness, sedation, amnesia, insomnia, agitation, dizziness, weakness, unsteadiness, disorientation, depression, headache, somnolence. **CV:** hypotension. **EENT:** visual disturbances, nasal congestion. **GI:** abdominal discomfort, nausea, change in appetite.
Respiratory: *respiratory failure, respiratory depression.*

INTERACTIONS
Drug-drug. *Clozapine:* May cause delirium, sedation, sialorrhea, and ataxia. Don't start simultaneously. Carefully monitor patient, especially during first 48 hours of coadministration.
Black Box Warning *Opioids:* May cause slow or difficult breathing, sedation, and death. Avoid use together. If use together is necessary, limit dosage and duration of each

---

Reactions in bold italics are *life-threatening*. Interactions may have a *rapid onset* or a *delayed onset*.

drug to the minimum necessary for desired effect. ∎

Oral hormonal contraceptives: May decrease lorazepam level. Monitor closely; lorazepam dosage may need to be increased.

Probenecid: May result in prolonged lorazepam half-life and a decrease in its total clearance. Reduce lorazepam dosage by 50% when coadministered.

Sodium oxybate: May result in additive effects, including increased sleep duration and CNS depression. Use together is contraindicated.

Valproate: May increase lorazepam plasma concentration. Reduce lorazepam dosage to 50% of normal adult dose when used together.

Drug-herb. *Kava kava:* May enhance adverse/toxic effects of CNS depressants. Monitor therapy.

Yohimbe: May diminish therapeutic effect of antianxiety agents. Monitor therapy.

Drug-lifestyle. *Alcohol use:* May cause additive CNS effects. Discourage use together.

Cannabis: May enhance CNS depressant effect of CNS depressants. Monitor therapy.

EFFECTS ON LAB TEST RESULTS

• May increase LDH and LFT values.

CONTRAINDICATIONS & CAUTIONS

• Contraindicated in patients hypersensitive to drug, other benzodiazepines, or the vehicle used in parenteral dosage form, and in patients with acute angle-closure glaucoma. IV administration is contraindicated in patients with sleep apnea and in patients with severe respiratory insufficiency, except those who are mechanically ventilated.

• Contraindicated for intra-arterial administration.

Black Box Warning *Opioid class warning:* Opioids should only be prescribed with benzodiazepines or other CNS depressants to patients for whom alternative treatment options are inadequate. ∎

🚱 *Alert:* Repeated or lengthy use of general anesthetic and sedation drugs during surgeries or procedures in children younger than age 3 or in pregnant women during the third trimester may affect brain development in children. Weigh benefits of appropriate anesthesia in young children and pregnant women against risks.

• Use cautiously in patients with pulmonary, renal, or hepatic impairment, or history of substance abuse.

• Use cautiously in elderly, acutely ill, or debilitated patients.

Dialyzable drug: Unknown.

⚠ *Overdose S&S:* Drowsiness, confusion lethargy, ataxia, hypotonia, hypotension, hypnotic state, stage 1 to 3 coma, death.

PREGNANCY-LACTATION-REPRODUCTION

• May cause fetal harm, including neonatal withdrawal symptoms. Avoid use during pregnancy except in life-threatening situations (status epilepticus) when safer drugs can't be used.

• Drug appears in human milk. Use in breastfeeding women isn't recommended.

NURSING CONSIDERATIONS

• Monitor hepatic, renal, and hematopoietic function periodically in patients receiving repeated or prolonged therapy.

🚱 *Alert:* Use of this drug may lead to abuse and addiction. Don't stop drug abruptly after long-term use because withdrawal symptoms may occur.

• *Look alike–sound alike:* Don't confuse lorazepam with alprazolam, clonazepam, or Lovaza. Don't confuse Ativan with Atgam.

PATIENT TEACHING

Black Box Warning *Opioid class warning:* Caution patient or caregiver of patient taking an opioid with a benzodiazepine, CNS depressant, or alcohol to seek immediate medical attention for dizziness, lightheadedness, extreme sleepiness, slowed or difficult breathing, or unresponsiveness. ∎

🚱 *Alert:* Discuss with pregnant women benefits, risks, and appropriate timing of surgery or procedures requiring anesthetic and sedation drugs.

• When used before surgery, drug causes substantial preoperative amnesia. Patient teaching requires extra care to ensure adequate recall. Provide written materials or inform a family member, if possible.

• Warn patient to avoid hazardous activities that require alertness or good coordination until effects of drug are known.

• Tell patient to avoid use of alcohol while taking drug.
• Notify patient that smoking may decrease drug's effectiveness.
• Warn patient not to stop drug abruptly because withdrawal symptoms may occur.
• Advise female patient to avoid pregnancy during therapy.

lorcaserin hydrochloride
lor-ca-SER-in

Belviq, Belviq XR

Therapeutic class: Appetite suppressants
Pharmacologic class: Serotonin 2C receptor agonists
Controlled substance schedule: IV

AVAILABLE FORMS
Tablets: 10 mg
Tablets (extended-release) (ORC): 20 mg

INDICATIONS & DOSAGES
➤ **Weight management in patients with initial BMI of 30 kg/m² or greater (obese) or 27 kg/m² or greater (overweight) in the presence of at least one weight-related comorbid condition as adjunct to reduced-calorie diet and increased physical activity**
Adults: 10 mg (immediate-release) PO b.i.d. or 20 mg (extended-release) PO once daily.
Adjust-a-dose: If patient hasn't lost at least 5% of baseline body weight by week 12, discontinue drug.

ADMINISTRATION
PO
• Store at room temperature.
• May give without regard for food.
• Make sure patient swallows extended-release tablets whole; don't crush, divide, or allow patient to chew them.

ACTION
Exact mechanism of action unknown. May decrease food consumption and promote satiety by selectively activating 5-HT$_{2C}$ receptors on anorexigenic proopiomelanocortin neurons located in the hypothalamus.

Route	Onset	Peak	Duration
PO (immediate-release)	Unknown	1½–2 hr	Unknown
PO (extended-release)	Unknown	10 hr	Unknown

Half-life: Immediate-release, 11 hours; extended-release, 12 hours.

ADVERSE REACTIONS
CNS: headache, dizziness, fatigue, anxiety, insomnia, stress, depression, impaired memory and attention, confusion. **CV:** HTN, *valvulopathy,* peripheral edema. **EENT:** eye disorder, nasopharyngitis, oropharyngeal pain, sinus congestion, toothache. **GI:** nausea, vomiting, diarrhea, constipation, gastroenteritis, dry mouth. **GU:** UTI. **Metabolic:** *hypoglycemia,* worsening of diabetes mellitus, decreased appetite. **Musculoskeletal:** back pain, musculoskeletal pain, muscle spasms. **Respiratory:** URI, cough. **Skin:** rash.

INTERACTIONS
Drug-drug. *Antipsychotics, bupropion, dextromethorphan, dopamine antagonists, linezolid, lithium, MAO inhibitors, SSNRIs, SSRIs, tramadol, TCAs, triptans:* May increase risk of serotonin syndrome or NMS-like reactions. Use together cautiously.
CYP2D6 substrates (antipsychotics, dextromethorphan, metoclopramide, SSNRIs, SSRIs, TCAs): May increase levels of CYP2D6 substrates. Use together cautiously.
Insulin, sulfonylureas: May increase risk of hypoglycemia in patients with type 2 diabetes. Monitor patient closely; adjust antidiabetic regimen as needed.
PDE5 inhibitors (sildenafil): May increase risk of priapism. Use together cautiously.
Potent 5-HT$_{2B}$ agonists (cabergoline): May increase risk of valvulopathy. Don't use together.
Drug-herb. *St. John's wort, tryptophan:* May increase risk of serotonin syndrome or NMS-like reactions. Discourage use together.

EFFECTS ON LAB TEST RESULTS
• May increase prolactin level. May decrease glucose level.
• May decrease Hb level and hematocrit and total WBC, lymphocyte, neutrophil, and total RBC counts.

Reactions in bold italics are *life-threatening*. Interactions may have a *rapid onset* or a *delayed onset*.

CONTRAINDICATIONS & CAUTIONS
• Contraindicated in patients hypersensitive to drug or its components. Drug isn't recommended in patients with severe renal impairment or ESRD.
• Use with extreme caution in combination with serotonergic and dopaminergic drugs that are potent 5-HT$_{2B}$ receptor agonists and are known to increase risk of heart valvulopathy.
• May increase risk of potentially life-threatening serotonin syndrome or NMS.
• Use cautiously in patients with moderate renal impairment, severe hepatic impairment, HF, hemodynamically significant valvular disease, bradycardia, or heart block greater than first degree.
• Use cautiously in patients with type 2 diabetes mellitus being treated with insulin or antidiabetic agents because weight loss may increase risk of hypoglycemia.
• Use cautiously in men who have conditions that might predispose them to priapism (sickle cell anemia, multiple myeloma, or leukemia) and in men with anatomic deformation of the penis (angulation, cavernosal fibrosis, or Peyronie disease).
Dialyzable drug: No.
⚠ **Overdose S&S:** Headache, nausea, abdominal discomfort, dizziness.

PREGNANCY-LACTATION-REPRODUCTION
• Contraindicated in pregnant women; drug may cause fetal harm. If used during pregnancy, or if patient becomes pregnant during therapy, apprise her of potential hazard to the fetus.
• It isn't known if drug appears in human milk. Patient should discontinue breastfeeding or discontinue drug.

NURSING CONSIDERATIONS
• Safety and effectiveness of using drug with other products intended for weight loss, including prescription drugs, OTC drugs, and herbal preparations, haven't been established.
• Measure blood glucose levels before and during treatment in patients with type 2 diabetes.
• Monitor patient for dyspnea, dependent edema, HF, or new murmur. Effect on CV

morbidity and mortality hasn't been established.
• Monitor CBC periodically.
• Measure prolactin level if gynecomastia or galactorrhea occurs.
• Monitor patient for serotonin syndrome (mental status changes, tachycardia, labile BP, hyperthermia, hyperreflexia, incoordination, nausea, vomiting, diarrhea).
• Monitor patient for confusion or impaired attention and memory.
• Monitor patient for new or worsening depression, suicidal thoughts or behaviors, or unusual changes in mood or behavior. Discontinue drug if symptoms occur.

PATIENT TEACHING
• Teach patient to use drug only in conjunction with a reduced-calorie diet and increased physical activity.
• Tell patient drug will be discontinued if 5% weight loss isn't achieved by 12 weeks of treatment.
• Warn patient to seek medical attention if signs or symptoms of valvular heart disease (dyspnea or dependent edema) occur.
• Advise patient to seek medical attention in the event of emerging or worsening depression, suicidal thoughts or behavior, or unusual changes in mood or behavior.
• Caution patient not to operate hazardous machinery, including automobiles, until drug's effects are known.
• Warn patient never to increase dosage.
• Advise male patient experiencing an erection lasting longer than 4 hours, whether painful or not, to immediately stop drug and seek emergency medical attention.
• Instruct patient to inform prescriber of all medications, nutritional supplements, and vitamins (including weight-loss products) being taken.
• Tell patient to swallow extended-release tablets whole and not to crush, chew, or divide them.
• Caution female patient to avoid pregnancy and not to breastfeed during therapy and to notify prescriber immediately if pregnancy occurs.

losartan potassium ℞
low-SAR-tan

Cozaar✍

Therapeutic class: Antihypertensives
Pharmacologic class: ARBs

AVAILABLE FORMS
Tablets: 25 mg, 50 mg, 100 mg

INDICATIONS & DOSAGES
Adjust-a-dose (for all indications): In adults
with mild to moderate hepatic impairment,
starting dose is 25 mg once daily.
➤ **HTN**
Adults: Initially, 50 mg PO daily. Maximum
daily dose is 100 mg.
Children age 6 and older: 0.7 mg/kg (up to
50 mg) PO daily, adjusted as needed up to
1.4 mg/kg/day (maximum 100 mg).
Adjust-a-dose: For adults with intravascular volume depletion (such as those taking diuretics), initially, 25 mg. Don't use
in children with eGFR less than 30 mL/
minute/1.73 m^2.
➤ **Nephropathy in patients with type 2
diabetes**
Adults: 50 mg PO once daily. Increase
dosage to 100 mg once daily based on BP
response.
➤ **To reduce risk of stroke in patients
with HTN and left ventricular hypertrophy**
Adults: Initially, 50 mg PO once daily. Adjust dosage based on BP response, adding
hydrochlorothiazide 12.5 mg once daily, increasing losartan to 100 mg daily, or both.
If further adjustments are required, may
increase the daily dosage of hydrochlorothiazide to 25 mg.

ADMINISTRATION
PO
• Give drug without regard for meals.
• If made into suspension by pharmacist,
store in refrigerator and shake well before
each use.

ACTION
Inhibits vasoconstrictive and aldosterone-
secreting action of angiotensin II by
blocking angiotensin II receptor on the surface of vascular smooth muscle and other
tissue cells.

Route	Onset	Peak	Duration
PO	6 hr	1–2 hr	Unknown

Half-life: Parent drug, about 1½ to 3 hours; active
metabolite, about 4½ to 10 hours.

ADVERSE REACTIONS
**Patients with HTN or left ventricular
hypertrophy**
CNS: dizziness, asthenia, fatigue, headache,
insomnia. **CV:** edema, chest pain. **EENT:**
nasal congestion, sinusitis, pharyngitis, sinus disorder. **GI:** abdominal pain, nausea, diarrhea, dyspepsia. **Musculoskeletal:** muscle cramps, myalgia, back or leg pain. **Respiratory:** cough, URI. **Other:** *angioedema.*
Patients with nephropathy
CNS: asthenia, fatigue, fever, hypoesthesia. **CV:** chest pain, hypotension, orthostatic
hypotension. **EENT:** cataract, sinusitis. **GI:**
diarrhea, dyspepsia, gastritis, nausea. **GU:**
UTI. **Hematologic:** anemia. **Metabolic:**
hyperkalemia, hypoglycemia, hyponatremia, weight gain. **Musculoskeletal:** back
pain, leg or knee pain, muscle weakness.
Respiratory: cough, bronchitis. **Skin:** cellulitis. **Other:** flulike syndrome, *diabetic
vascular disease, angioedema,* infection,
trauma, diabetic neuropathy.

INTERACTIONS
Drug-drug. *Aliskiren:* May increase risk of
renal impairment, hypotension, and hyperkalemia in diabetic patients and those with
moderate to severe renal impairment (GFR
less than 60 mL/minute). Concomitant use
is contraindicated in diabetic patients. Avoid
concomitant use in those with moderate to
severe renal impairment.
Amphetamines: May diminish antihypertensive effect. Monitor therapy.
Antifungals (azole derivatives, systemic):
May decrease losartan metabolism. Monitor
therapy.
Antipsychotics (atypical): May enhance hypotensive effect of these agents. Monitor
therapy.
Lithium: May increase lithium level. Monitor lithium level and patient for toxicity.

Reactions in bold italics are *life-threatening.* Interactions may have a *rapid onset* or a *delayed onset.*

NSAIDs: May decrease antihypertensive effects. Monitor BP and renal function.
Potassium-sparing diuretics, potassium supplements: May cause hyperkalemia. Monitor patient closely.
Drug-herb. *Ma huang:* May decrease antihypertensive effects. Discourage use together.
Drug-food. *Salt substitutes containing potassium:* May cause hyperkalemia. Monitor patient closely.

EFFECTS ON LAB TEST RESULTS
• May increase liver enzyme or bilirubin levels.

CONTRAINDICATIONS & CAUTIONS
• Contraindicated in patients hypersensitive to drug.
• Use cautiously in patients with impaired renal or hepatic function.
Dialyzable drug: No.
⚠ **Overdose S&S:** Hypotension, tachycardia, bradycardia.

PREGNANCY-LACTATION-REPRODUCTION
Black Box Warning Drugs that act directly on the RAAS can cause fetal injury and death. If pregnancy is suspected, notify prescriber because drug should be stopped as soon as possible. ∎
• It isn't known if drug appears in human milk. Patient should discontinue breastfeeding or discontinue drug, taking into account importance of drug to the mother.

NURSING CONSIDERATIONS
• Drug can be used alone or with other antihypertensives.
▨ Monitor patient's BP closely to evaluate effectiveness of therapy. When used alone, drug has less of an effect on BP in black patients than in patients of other races.
• Monitor patients who are also taking diuretics for symptomatic hypotension.
• Regularly assess patient's renal function (via creatinine and BUN levels).
• Patients with severe HF whose renal function depends on the angiotensin-aldosterone system may develop acute renal failure during therapy. Closely monitor patient's BP, renal function, and potassium levels,

especially during first few weeks of therapy and after dosage adjustments.
• **Look alike–sound alike:** Don't confuse Cozaar with Zocor or Colace.

PATIENT TEACHING
• Tell patient to avoid salt substitutes; these products may contain potassium, which can cause high potassium level in patients taking losartan.
• Inform female patient of childbearing potential about consequences of taking drug while pregnant. Advise her to notify prescriber immediately if she suspects she is pregnant.
• Advise patient not to breastfeed while taking drug.
• Advise patient to report all adverse reactions and to immediately report swelling of face, eyes, lips, or tongue or breathing difficulty.

lovastatin (mevinolin) ▨
loe-va-STA-tin

Altoprev

Therapeutic class: Antilipemics
Pharmacologic class: HMG-CoA reductase inhibitors

AVAILABLE FORMS
Tablets: 10 mg, 20 mg, 40 mg
Tablets (extended-release) ⓞ: 20 mg, 40 mg, 60 mg

INDICATIONS & DOSAGES
Adjust-a-dose (for all indications): Avoid use of lovastatin with fibrates or niacin at doses greater than 1 g daily. For patients also taking danazol, diltiazem, dronedarone, or verapamil, start lovastatin at 10 mg (immediate-release) and don't exceed 20 mg daily. For patients also taking amiodarone, lovastatin dosage shouldn't exceed 40 mg daily unless clinical benefit is likely to outweigh increased risk of myopathy or rhabdomyolysis. For elderly patients or patients with CrCl of less than 30 mL/minute, carefully consider dosage increase greater than 20 mg daily and implement cautiously if necessary. For patients requiring smaller reductions in

cholesterol levels, use immediate-release lovastatin.

➤ **To prevent and treat CAD; hyperlipidemia**

Adults: Initially, 20 mg (immediate-release) PO once daily with evening meal. Recommended range is 10 to 80 mg as a single dose or in two divided doses; maximum daily recommended dose is 80 mg. Or, 20 to 60 mg extended-release tablets PO at bedtime.

Make dosage adjustments at intervals of 4 weeks or more.

➤ **Heterozygous familial hypercholesterolemia in adolescents**

Adolescents ages 10 to 17: Give 10 to 40 mg (immediate-release) PO daily with evening meal. Patients requiring reductions in LDL cholesterol level of 20% or more should start with 20 mg daily. Make dosage adjustments at intervals of 4 weeks or more.

➤ **Primary prevention of CV disease**

Adults ages 40 to 75 with type 1 or type 2 diabetes (moderate-intensity therapy): 40 mg (immediate-release) PO once daily.

Adults ages 40 to 75 with an estimated 10-year atherosclerotic CV disease risk of 7.5% or more (moderate- to high-intensity therapy): 40 mg (immediate-release) PO once daily.

➤ **Secondary prevention of CV disease (moderate-intensity therapy)**

Adults older than age 75 or who aren't candidates for high-intensity therapy: 40 mg (immediate-release) PO once daily.

ADMINISTRATION
PO
- Give immediate-release drug with evening meal, which improves absorption and cholesterol biosynthesis. Give extended-release drug at bedtime.
- Don't crush, split, or allow patient to chew extended-release tablets.

ACTION
Inhibits HMG-CoA reductase, an early (and rate-limiting) step in cholesterol biosynthesis.

Route	Onset	Peak	Duration
PO	Unknown	2–4 hr	Unknown
PO (extended-release)	3 days	12–14 hr	Unknown

Half-life: 1.1 to 1.7 hours.

ADVERSE REACTIONS
CNS: headache, dizziness, insomnia, peripheral neuropathy. **EENT:** blurred vision. **GI:** abdominal pain or cramps, constipation, diarrhea, dyspepsia, flatulence, heartburn, nausea, vomiting. **GU:** UTI. **Musculoskeletal:** muscle cramps, myalgia, myositis, *rhabdomyolysis.* **Skin:** alopecia, rash, pruritus. **Other:** flulike syndrome, pain, infection.

INTERACTIONS
Drug-drug. *Amiodarone:* May decrease the metabolism of lovastatin. Avoid combining lovastatin at doses exceeding 40 mg daily with amiodarone unless clinical benefit is likely to outweigh increased risk of myopathy.

Azole antifungals: May cause myopathy and rhabdomyolysis. Avoid using together.

Colchicine: May increase risk of myopathy or rhabdomyolysis. If coadministration can't be avoided, monitor patient for unexplained muscle pain, tenderness, or weakness.

Cyclosporine, gemfibrozil: May cause severe myopathy and rhabdomyolysis. Avoid this combination.

Danazol, diltiazem, dronedarone, verapamil: May cause myopathy and rhabdomyolysis. Don't exceed 20 mg lovastatin daily.

Dronedarone: May increase lovastatin serum concentration. Limit lovastatin to maximum of 20 mg/day (in adults). Increase monitoring for signs and symptoms of lovastatin toxicity (such as myopathy and rhabdomyolysis). Consider therapy modification.

Erythromycin, protease inhibitors (atazanavir, darunavir, fosamprenavir, indinavir, nefazodone, nelfinavir, ritonavir, saquinavir, tipranavir), strong CYP3A inhibitors (clarithromycin, itraconazole, ketoconazole, posaconazole, telithromycin, voriconazole): Increase risk of myopathy and rhabdomyolysis. Use together is contraindicated.

Macrolides (azithromycin, clarithromycin, telithromycin), nefazodone: May decrease metabolism of HMG-CoA reductase inhibitor, increasing toxicity. Monitor patient for adverse effects and report unexplained muscle pain.

Mifepristone (CYP3A4 inhibitor): May increase lovastatin plasma level, increasing risk of toxicity. Use together is contraindicated.

Niacin, other fibrates: May increase the risk for adverse and toxic effects of lovastatin. Avoid use of lovastatin with fibrates or niacin at doses greater than 1 g daily.

Oral anticoagulants: May increase anticoagulant effect. Monitor patient closely.

Phenytoin: May decrease serum concentration of HMG-CoA reductase inhibitors. Consider therapy modification.

Ranolazine: May increase risk of myopathy and rhabdomyolysis. Consider lovastatin dosage adjustment.

Drug-herb. *Eucalyptus, kava:* May increase risk of hepatotoxicity. Discourage use together.

Red yeast rice: May increase risk of adverse reactions because herb contains compounds similar to those in drug. Discourage use together.

Drug-food. *Grapefruit juice:* May increase drug level, increasing risk of adverse effects. Discourage use together.

Drug-lifestyle. *Alcohol use:* May increase risk of hepatotoxicity. Discourage use together.

EFFECTS ON LAB TEST RESULTS
• May increase ALT, AST, and CK levels.
• May cause thyroid function test abnormalities.

CONTRAINDICATIONS & CAUTIONS
• Contraindicated in patients hypersensitive to drug and in those with active liver disease or unexplained persistently increased transaminase level.
• Use cautiously in patients who consume substantial quantities of alcohol or have a history of liver disease.
Dialyzable drug: Unknown.

PREGNANCY-LACTATION-REPRODUCTION
• Drug may cause fetal harm and is contraindicated in women who are pregnant or may become pregnant. Use in women of childbearing potential only when such patients are highly unlikely to conceive. If patient becomes pregnant during therapy, discontinue drug and apprise her of potential hazard to the fetus.

• It isn't known if drug appears in human milk. Use in breastfeeding women is contraindicated.

NURSING CONSIDERATIONS
• Have patient follow a diet restricted in saturated fat and cholesterol during therapy.
• Obtain LFT results at the start of therapy; then monitor results periodically.
▨ Heterozygous familial hypercholesterolemia can be diagnosed in adolescent boys and in girls who are at least 1 year postmenarche and are 10 to 17 years old; if after an adequate trial of diet therapy LDL cholesterol level remains over 189 mg/dL or LDL cholesterol over 160 mg/dL and patient has a positive family history of premature CV disease or two or more other CV disease risk factors.
• Obtain CK level in patients with unexplained muscle pain.
• Discontinue lovastatin immediately if markedly elevated CK levels occur or myopathy is diagnosed or suspected. Predisposing factors for skeletal muscle effects include advanced age (65 and older), female gender, uncontrolled hypothyroidism, and renal impairment.
• *Look alike–sound alike:* Don't confuse lovastatin with Lotensin.

PATIENT TEACHING
• Instruct patient to take immediate-release drug with the evening meal and extended-release drug at bedtime.
• *Alert:* Advise patient not to crush or chew extended-release tablets.
• Teach patient about proper dietary management of cholesterol and triglycerides. When appropriate, recommend weight control, exercise, and smoking cessation programs.
• Instruct patient to store tablets at room temperature in a light-resistant container.
• Advise patient of risk of myopathy and rhabdomyolysis and to promptly report unexplained muscle pain, tenderness, or weakness, particularly when accompanied by malaise or fever.
• Teach patient about substances that shouldn't be taken with lovastatin and to inform other health care providers about

taking lovastatin, especially if a new medication is being prescribed.

• Caution patient to avoid grapefruit juice while taking drug.

🕦 **Alert:** Tell female patient to stop drug and notify prescriber immediately if she is or may be pregnant or if she's breastfeeding.

lurasidone hydrochloride
loo-RAS-i-dohne

Latuda✏

Therapeutic class: Antipsychotics
Pharmacologic class: Dopamine–serotonin receptor antagonists

AVAILABLE FORMS
Tablets: 20 mg, 40 mg, 60 mg, 80 mg, 120 mg

INDICATIONS & DOSAGES
Adjust-a-dose (for all indications): For patients with moderate (CrCl of 30 to less than 50 mL/minute) or severe (CrCl of less than 30 mL/minute) renal impairment or those concomitantly taking a moderate CYP3A4 inhibitor (such as diltiazem), the recommended starting dose is 20 mg and the maximum recommended dose is 80 mg. For patients with moderate (Child-Pugh score 7 to 9) or severe (Child-Pugh score 10 to 15) hepatic impairment, the recommended starting dose is 20 mg. The maximum recommended dose is 80 mg for patients with moderate hepatic impairment and 40 mg for those with severe hepatic impairment.
➤ **Schizophrenia**
Adults: Initially, 40 mg PO once daily. May increase to maximum dose of 160 mg daily.
Adolescents ages 13 to 17: 40 mg PO once daily. May increase to maximum dose of 80 mg daily.
➤ **Depressive episodes associated with bipolar I disorder as monotherapy or as adjunctive therapy with lithium or valproate**
Adults: Initially, 20 mg PO once daily. May increase to maximum of 120 mg daily.
➤ **Depressive episodes associated with bipolar I disorder (monotherapy)**

Children ages 10 to 17: 20 mg PO once daily. May increase after 1 week to maximum dose of 80 mg daily.

ADMINISTRATION
PO
• Give with food (at least 350 calories).

ACTION
Exact mechanism is unknown. Drug's efficacy is mediated through antagonism at the dopamine type 2 and serotonin type 2 receptors.

Route	Onset	Peak	Duration
PO	Unknown	1–3 hr	Unknown

Half-life: 18 hours.

ADVERSE REACTIONS
CNS: somnolence, akathisia, parkinsonism (bradykinesia, cogwheel rigidity, drooling, extrapyramidal disorder, hypokinesia, muscle rigidity, psychomotor retardation, tremor), agitation, dystonia, dizziness, insomnia, anxiety, restlessness, seizures, fatigue. **CV:** tachycardia. **EENT:** blurred vision, nasopharyngitis. **GI:** nausea, vomiting, dyspepsia, abdominal pain, diarrhea, dysphagia, increased appetite. **GU:** UTI. **Metabolic:** dyslipidemia, hyperglycemia, weight gain. **Musculoskeletal:** back pain. **Skin:** rash, pruritus.

INTERACTIONS
Drug-drug. *Antihypertensives:* May increase risk of hypotension. Monitor orthostatic vital signs and adjust antihypertensive dosage as needed.
Centrally acting drugs: May increase risk of adverse effects (increased cognitive impairment). Avoid use together.
Epinephrine (systemic): May enhance hypotensive effect of lurasidone. Avoid combination.
Moderate inhibitors of CYP3A4 (atazanavir, diltiazem, erythromycin, fluconazole, verapamil): May increase lurasidone level. Use together cautiously and reduce lurasidone dosage by 50%. Initial recommended lurasidone dose is 20 mg daily, with maximum dose of 80 mg daily.
Black Box Warning *Opioid class warning:* May cause slow or difficult breathing,

sedation, and death. Avoid use together. If use together is necessary, limit dosage and duration of each drug to minimum necessary for desired effect. ■

Strong inducers of CYP3A4 (carbamazepine, phenytoin, rifampin): May significantly reduce lurasidone level. Don't use together.

Strong inhibitors of CYP3A4 (clarithromycin, ketoconazole, ritonavir, voriconazole): May significantly increase lurasidone level. Don't use together.

Drug-herb. *Kava kava:* May enhance adverse/toxic effect of CNS depressants. Monitor therapy.

St. John's wort: May significantly reduce lurasidone level. Don't use together.

Drug-food. *Grapefruit, grapefruit juice:* May increase lurasidone level. Patient should avoid grapefruit and grapefruit juice during therapy.

Drug-lifestyle. *Alcohol use, cannabidiol, cannabis:* May increase CNS depressant effect and risk of adverse effects (such as increased cognitive impairment). Discourage use together.

EFFECTS ON LAB TEST RESULTS

• May increase prolactin, total cholesterol, triglyceride, glucose, serum creatinine, AST, ALT, and CK levels.

• May decrease WBC, neutrophil, and granulocyte counts.

CONTRAINDICATIONS & CAUTIONS

• Contraindicated in patients hypersensitive to drug or its components.

• Contraindicated for concomitant use with strong CYP3A4 inhibitors or inducers. If used concomitantly with a moderate CYP3A4 inducer, it may be necessary to increase lurasidone dosage after long-term treatment (7 days or more) with the CYP3A4 inducer.

Black Box Warning *Opioid class warning:* Opioids should only be prescribed with benzodiazepines or other CNS depressants to patients for whom alternative treatment options are inadequate. ■

Black Box Warning Elderly patients with dementia-related psychosis treated with atypical or conventional antipsychotics are at increased risk for death. Antipsychotics

aren't approved for the treatment of dementia-related psychosis. ■

• Use cautiously in patients with hyperlipidemia, diabetes or risk factors for diabetes (family history, obesity), seizures or conditions that lower the seizure threshold (Alzheimer dementia), body temperature dysregulation, major depressive disorder, suicide attempts, dysphagia, or concomitant illness.

• Use cautiously in patients with known CV disease, cerebrovascular disease, and conditions that cause hypotension (dehydration, hypovolemia, antihypertensive use) and in antipsychotic-naive patients because of increased risk of dizziness, tachycardia or bradycardia, and syncope.

• Use cautiously in patients with preexisting low WBC count or a history of drug-induced neutropenia or leukopenia.

• Use cautiously in patients at risk for falls, including those with diseases or conditions or who are taking medications that may cause somnolence, orthostatic hypotension, or motor or sensory instability.

• Safety and effectiveness haven't been established in children with depression.

Dialyzable drug: Unknown.

PREGNANCY-LACTATION-REPRODUCTION

• There are no adequate studies in pregnant women. Use during pregnancy only if clearly needed and potential benefit justifies potential risk to the fetus. Drug may cause abnormal muscle movements (extrapyramidal symptoms) or withdrawal symptoms in newborns.

• Enroll women exposed to lurasidone during pregnancy in the National Pregnancy Registry for Atypical Antipsychotics (1-866-961-2388).

• It isn't known if drug appears in human milk. Patient should discontinue breastfeeding or discontinue drug.

NURSING CONSIDERATIONS

Black Box Warning Antidepressants increase risk of suicidal thinking and behavior in children, adolescents, and young adults. Monitor all patients for worsening of depression or emergence of suicidal thoughts and behaviors. ■

L

• Monitor patients for tardive dyskinesia. Risk increases in elderly patients and women and with long-term administration. Use the lowest dose for the shortest time possible to minimize risk. Discontinue drug if symptoms occur.

• Monitor patients for orthostatic hypotension, syncope, and excessive sedation.

• Monitor patients for signs and symptoms of NMS, such as fever, diaphoresis, muscle rigidity, altered mental status, irregular pulse or BP, cardiac arrhythmias, increased CK level, rhabdomyolysis, and acute renal failure. Discontinue drug immediately if NMS occurs.

• Monitor CBC, renal function, and prolactin level periodically; discontinue drug if severe neutropenia develops.

• Monitor patients for metabolic changes (such as weight gain and elevated blood glucose, triglyceride, or cholesterol levels), and treat appropriately.

• Complete fall risk assessments at start of therapy and recurrently for patients on long-term therapy, especially for patients with diseases or conditions or who are taking other medications that could exacerbate fall risk.

PATIENT TEACHING

Black Box Warning *Opioid class warning:* Caution patient or caregiver of patient taking an opioid with a benzodiazepine, CNS depressant, or alcohol to seek immediate medical attention for dizziness, lightheadedness, extreme sleepiness, slowed or difficult breathing, or unresponsiveness. ▉

Black Box Warning Advise family or caregivers to observe patient closely for worsening of depression or suicidal thoughts and behaviors. Encourage them to report such behaviors to health care provider immediately. ▉

• Advise patient to take drug on a regular basis and not to skip doses.

• Inform patient that periodic blood tests will be needed to monitor tolerance to the drug.

• Tell patient to avoid overheating and to maintain adequate hydration.

• Teach patient to monitor weight and maintain a healthy diet because drug may increase weight and blood glucose and cholesterol levels.

• Instruct patient to report all adverse reactions and to immediately report sudden changes in temperature or BP, irregular HR, or severe muscle rigidity.

• Counsel female patient to tell her prescriber if she is pregnant or breastfeeding before taking drug.

• Tell patient to avoid alcohol and grapefruit products during therapy.

• Warn patient to avoid driving or operating hazardous machinery until drug's effects are known.

SAFETY ALERT!

magnesium sulfate (injection)

Therapeutic class: Electrolyte replacements
Pharmacologic class: Minerals

AVAILABLE FORMS

Injectable: 4%, 8%, 50% in 2-, 10-, 20-, and 50-mL ampules, vials, and prefilled syringes
Injection solution: 1% in D_5W; 2% in D_5W or NSS; 4% in water for injection, D_5W, or NSS; 8% in water for injection, D_5W, or NSS

INDICATIONS & DOSAGES

Adjust-a-dose (for all indications): In severe renal impairment, reduce dosage and obtain frequent serum magnesium levels. *Note:* 1 g = 8.12 mEq of magnesium.

➤ **Mild hypomagnesemia**
Adults: 1 g IM every 6 hours for four doses, depending on magnesium level.

➤ **Symptomatic severe hypomagnesemia, with magnesium level of 0.8 mEq/L or less**
Adults: 5 g IV in 1 L of D_5W or NSS over 3 hours. Base subsequent doses on magnesium level.

➤ **Magnesium supplementation in total parenteral nutrition (TPN)**
Adults: 8 to 24 mEq IV daily added to TPN solution.
Infants: 2 to 10 mEq/day IV added to TPN solution.

➤ **Seizures in preeclampsia or eclampsia**
Adults: Total initial dose is 10 to 14 g IV. To accomplish this, give 4 to 5 g IV in 250 mL of solution and simultaneously give up to 10 g IM (5 g or 10 mL of the undiluted 50%

Reactions in bold italics are *life-threatening*. Interactions may have a *rapid onset* or a *delayed onset*.

solution in each buttock). After initial IV dose, some clinicians administer 1 to 2 g/hour by constant IV infusion. Base subsequent doses on magnesium level; serum magnesium level of 6 mg/100 mL is considered optimal for seizure control. Don't exceed 40 g in a 24-hour period. Maximum dose in patients with severe renal insufficiency is 20 g/48 hours.

ADMINISTRATION
IV/IM
• Store between 68° and 77° F (20° and 25° C). Protect from freezing.
• Discard unused portion.
IV
▼ Dilute concentration to concentrations of 20% or less.
▼ Inject bolus dose slowly at a rate of 150 mg/minute or less, or use infusion pump for continuous infusion to avoid respiratory or cardiac arrest. Maximum infusion rate is 150 mg/minute. Rapid drip causes feeling of heat.
▼ For severe hypomagnesemia, watch for respiratory depression and evidence of heart block. Respirations should be better than 16 breaths/minute before giving dose.
▼ **Incompatibilities:** Alcohol (in high concentrations); alkali carbonates, bicarbonates, and hydroxides; aminophylline; amiodarone; amphotericin B; barium; calcium chloride; calcium gluconate; cefuroxime; clindamycin; cyclosporine; dexamethasone sodium phosphate; diazepam; heavy metals; hydrocortisone sodium succinate; procaine; salicylates; soluble phosphates; strontium; tartrates.
IM
• Undiluted 50% solutions may be given by deep IM injection to adults. Dilute solutions to 20% or less for use in children.

ACTION
Replaces magnesium and maintains magnesium level; as an anticonvulsant, reduces muscle contractions by interfering with release of acetylcholine at myoneural junction.

Route	Onset	Peak	Duration
IV	Immediate	Unknown	30 min
IM	1 hr	Unknown	3–4 hr

Half-life: Unknown.

ADVERSE REACTIONS
CNS: toxicity, weak or absent deep tendon reflexes, paralysis, drowsiness, stupor. **CV:** slow, weak pulse; *arrhythmias*; hypotension; *circulatory collapse*; flushing. **GI:** diarrhea. **Metabolic:** hypocalcemia. **Respiratory:** *respiratory distress.* **Skin:** diaphoresis. **Other:** hypothermia.

INTERACTIONS
Drug-drug. *Calcium channel blockers:* May increase magnesium-related adverse effects. Monitor therapy.
Cardiac glycosides: May cause serious cardiac conduction changes. Use together with caution.
CNS depressants: May increase CNS depression. Use together cautiously.
Neuromuscular blockers: May cause increased neuromuscular blockage. Use together cautiously. Closely monitor clinical response.
Drug-lifestyle. *Alcohol use:* May decrease magnesium level. Discourage use together.

EFFECTS ON LAB TEST RESULTS
• May decrease calcium level.

CONTRAINDICATIONS & CAUTIONS
• Contraindicated in patients with myocardial damage, heart block, or coma.
• Use cautiously in patients with impaired renal function.
۞ Alert: Using magnesium sulfate to stop preterm labor isn't an FDA-approved use of drug; safety and effectiveness of drug for this indication haven't been established.
Dialyzable drug: Yes.
⚠ Overdose S&S: Hypotension, facial flushing, feeling of warmth, thirst, nausea, vomiting, lethargy, dysarthria, drowsiness, diminished deep tendon reflexes, shallow respirations, apnea, coma, cardiac arrest, respiratory paralysis, disappearance of patellar reflex.

PREGNANCY-LACTATION-REPRODUCTION
۞ Alert: Drug can cause fetal abnormalities (fetal hypocalcemia, bone abnormalities), especially when given beyond 5 to 7 days to pregnant women. Use during pregnancy only if clearly needed, and inform patient of potential fetal harm.

M

• When drug is administered by continuous IV infusion (especially for more than 24 hours preceding delivery) to control seizures in a toxemic woman, the neonate may show signs of magnesium toxicity, including neuromuscular or respiratory depression.

• Use cautiously and monitor closely in pregnant women in active labor, in pregnant women with preeclampsia or eclampsia who are at risk for seizures, and in pregnant women at risk for preterm delivery.

• Drug appears in human milk. Use cautiously in breastfeeding women.

NURSING CONSIDERATIONS

• Keep IV calcium available to reverse magnesium intoxication.

• Test knee-jerk and patellar reflexes before each additional dose. If absent, notify prescriber and give no more magnesium until reflexes return; otherwise, patient may develop temporary respiratory failure and need cardiopulmonary resuscitation or IV administration of calcium.

• Check magnesium level after repeated doses. Monitor levels hourly in patients with severe hypomagnesemia. Normal plasma magnesium level is 1.5 to 2.5 mEq/L.

• Monitor fluid intake and output. Output should be 100 mL or more during 4-hour period before dose.

• Monitor renal function.

• Drug may contain aluminum. Premature neonates are at higher risk for aluminum toxicity due to immature renal function. Aluminum exposure of more than 4 to 5 mcg/kg/day is associated with CNS and bone toxicity.

• Patients with prolonged exposure to magnesium sulfate who have impaired renal function are at risk for aluminum toxicity.

• *Look alike–sound alike:* Don't confuse magnesium sulfate with manganese sulfate.

PATIENT TEACHING

• Explain use and administration of drug to patient and family.

• Emphasize importance of keeping lab appointments.

• Tell patient about warning signs of high or low magnesium level. Encourage patient to report all adverse effects.

mannitol
MAN-i-tole

Osmitrol

Therapeutic class: Diuretics
Pharmacologic class: Osmotic diuretics

AVAILABLE FORMS
Injection: 5%, 10%, 15%, 20%, 25%
Solution for irrigation: 5 g/100 mL

INDICATIONS & DOSAGES
➤ **Oliguria**
Adults and children older than age 12: 50 to 100 g IV as a 20% solution over 90 minutes to several hours.
➤ **To prevent or treat oliguria or acute renal failure**
Adults and children older than age 12: 50 to 100 g IV of a 5% to 25% solution. Determine exact concentration by fluid requirements.
➤ **To reduce intraocular or intracranial pressure or cerebral edema**
Adults and children older than age 12: 1.5 to 2 g/kg as a 15%, 20%, or 25% IV solution over 30 to 60 minutes. For maximum IOP reduction before surgery, give 60 to 90 minutes preoperatively.
➤ **Diuresis in drug intoxication**
Adults and children older than age 12: 5% to 25% solution continuously up to 200 g IV, while maintaining 100 to 500 mL urine output/hour and a positive fluid balance.
➤ **Irrigating solution during transurethral surgical procedures**
Adults: Irrigate bladder with 2.5% to 5% solution.

ADMINISTRATION
IV
▼ Change IV administration apparatus every 24 hours.
▼ To redissolve crystallized solution (crystallization occurs at low temperatures or in concentrations higher than 15%), warm bottle or bag by appropriate means to approximately 140° F (60° C) with occasional shaking. Cool to body temperature before giving. Don't use solution with undissolved crystals.

Reactions in bold italics are *life-threatening*. Interactions may have a *rapid onset* or a *delayed onset*.

▼ Give as intermittent or continuous infusion at prescribed rate, using an inline filter and an infusion pump. Don't give as direct injection. Don't use plastic container in series connections.

▼ Check patency at infusion site before and during administration.

▼ Monitor patient for signs and symptoms of infiltration; if it occurs, watch for inflammation, edema, and necrosis.

▼ **Incompatibilities:** Blood products and other drugs.

ACTION

Increases osmotic pressure of glomerular filtrate, thus inhibiting tubular reabsorption of water and electrolytes. Drug elevates plasma osmolality and increases urine output.

Route	Onset	Peak	Duration
IV	½–3 hr	30–60 min	2–8 hr

Half-life: About 1½ hours.

ADVERSE REACTIONS

CNS: *seizures,* dizziness, headache, fever. **CV:** edema, thrombophlebitis, hypotension, HTN, *HF,* tachycardia, angina pectoris, vascular overload. **EENT:** blurred vision, rhinitis. **GI:** thirst, dry mouth, nausea, vomiting, diarrhea. **GU:** urine retention. **Metabolic:** dehydration, fluid and electrolyte imbalance. **Respiratory:** *pulmonary edema.* **Skin:** local pain, urticaria, injection-site reaction (infection, phlebitis, venous thrombosis). **Other:** chills, thirst.

INTERACTIONS

Drug-drug. *Lithium:* May increase urinary excretion of lithium. Monitor lithium level closely.

Nephrotoxic drugs (aminoglycosides, cyclosporine): May increase risk of toxicity and renal failure. Avoid use together.

Opioid analgesics: May increase diuretic-related adverse effects and diminish therapeutic effects of diuretics. Monitor therapy.

Sodium phosphates: May enhance nephrotoxic effect of sodium phosphates. Consider therapy modification.

Tobramycin: Mannitol (systemic) may enhance nephrotoxic effect of tobramycin (oral inhalation). Avoid combination.

EFFECTS ON LAB TEST RESULTS

• May increase or decrease electrolyte levels.

• May interfere with tests for inorganic phosphorus or ethylene glycol level.

CONTRAINDICATIONS & CAUTIONS

• Contraindicated in patients hypersensitive to drug.

• Contraindicated in patients with anuria; severe pulmonary congestion; frank pulmonary edema; active intracranial bleeding (except during craniotomy); severe dehydration; metabolic edema; previous progressive renal disease or dysfunction after starting drug, including increasing azotemia and oliguria; previous progressive HF or pulmonary congestion after treatment with drug; or failure to respond to test dose.

Dialyzable drug: Yes.

⚠ *Overdose S&S:* Increased electrolyte excretion, orthostatic tachycardia or hypotension, decreased central venous pressure, impaired neuromuscular function, intestinal dilation and ileus, HF, pulmonary edema or water intoxication if urine output is inadequate.

PREGNANCY-LACTATION-REPRODUCTION

• There are no adequate studies in pregnant women. Use during pregnancy only if clearly needed and potential benefit justifies potential risk to the fetus.

• It isn't known if drug appears in human milk. Use cautiously in breastfeeding women.

NURSING CONSIDERATIONS

• Monitor vital signs, including central venous pressure and fluid intake and output hourly. Report increasing oliguria. Check weight, renal function, fluid balance, and serum and urine sodium and potassium levels daily.

• In comatose or incontinent patient, use urinary catheter because therapy is based on strict evaluation of fluid intake and output. If patient has urinary catheter, use an hourly urometer collection bag to evaluate output accurately and easily.

• To relieve thirst, give frequent mouth care or fluids.

• Drug is commonly used in chemotherapy regimens to enhance diuresis of renally toxic drugs.

• Don't give electrolyte-free solutions with blood. If blood is given simultaneously, add at least 20 mEq of sodium chloride to each liter of drug solution to avoid pseudoagglutination.

PATIENT TEACHING

• Tell patient that thirstiness or dry mouth may occur; emphasize importance of drinking only the amount of fluids ordered.

• Instruct patient to promptly report adverse reactions and discomfort at IV site.

SAFETY ALERT!

maraviroc
mahr-AY-vih-rok

Celsentri✴, Selzentry

Therapeutic class: Antiretrovirals
Pharmacologic class: CCR5 co-receptor antagonists

AVAILABLE FORMS
Oral solution: 20 mg/mL
Tablets: 25 mg, 75 mg, 150 mg, 300 mg

INDICATIONS & DOSAGES
➤ **Combined with CYP3A4 inhibitors, including protease inhibitors (except tipranavir and ritonavir), delavirdine, elvitegravir–ritonavir, ketoconazole, itraconazole, clarithromycin, other potent CYP3A inhibitors (nefazodone, telithromycin), or boceprevir, to treat only CCR5-tropic HIV-1 infection**
Adults: 150 mg PO b.i.d.
Children age 2 and older weighing more than 40 kg: 150 mg PO b.i.d.
Children age 2 and older weighing 30 to less than 40 kg: 100 mg PO b.i.d.
Children age 2 and older weighing 20 to less than 30 kg: 75 mg (tablets) or 80 mg (oral solution) PO b.i.d.
Children age 2 and older weighing 10 to less than 20 kg: 50 mg PO b.i.d.
Adjust-a-dose: For adults with CrCl of 30 mL/minute or more, no adjustment is needed. Drug is contraindicated in patients

with CrCl of less than 30 mL/minute or in those with ESRD on regular hemodialysis.
➤ **Combined with noninteracting concomitant medications (all medications that aren't potent CYP3A inhibitors or inducers), including all NRTIs, tipranavir–ritonavir, nevirapine, raltegravir, or enfuvirtide to treat CCR5-tropic HIV-1 infection**
Adults and children age 2 and older weighing 30 kg or more: 300 mg PO b.i.d.
Adjust-a-dose: For adults with renal impairment, no dosage adjustment is needed. If patient with CrCl of less than 30 mL/minute or ESRD on hemodialysis experiences orthostatic hypotension, reduce dosage to 150 mg PO b.i.d.
➤ **Combined with potent CYP3A inducers (without a potent CYP3A inhibitor), including efavirenz, rifampin, etravirine, carbamazepine, phenobarbital, and phenytoin, to treat CCR5-tropic HIV-1 infection**
Adults: 600 mg PO b.i.d.
Adjust-a-dose: Use is contraindicated in patients with CrCl of less than 30 mL/minute or in those with ESRD on regular hemodialysis.

ADMINISTRATION
PO
• Give drug without regard for food.
• Use oral solution in children who are unable to reliably swallow tablets.
• Use oral dosing syringe for oral solution.

ACTION
Blocks viral entry into cells by binding to chemokine receptor type 5 co-receptor and preventing the initiation of HIV replication cycle.

Route	Onset	Peak	Duration
PO	Unknown	½–4 hr	Unknown

Half-life: 14 to 18 hours.

ADVERSE REACTIONS
CNS: anxiety, dizziness, paresthesia, sensory abnormalities, peripheral neuropathy, sleep disturbances, depressive disorders, pyrexia, pain, disturbances in consciousness, *stroke*. **CV:** unstable angina, *acute cardiac failure,* CAD, endocarditis, *MI,* myocardial

ischemia, vascular hypertensive disorders, edema. **EENT:** conjunctivitis, ocular infections, otitis media, nasal congestion, paranasal sinus disorders, sinusitis, rhinitis, esophageal candidiasis. **GI:** abdominal pain, constipation, dyspepsia, stomatitis, appetite disorders, diarrhea, flatulence, vomiting. **GU:** urinary tract signs and symptoms. **Hematologic:** anemia, *neutropenia*. **Hepatic:** *cirrhosis, hepatic failure*, cholestatic jaundice. **Metabolic:** lipodystrophies. **Musculoskeletal:** muscle pains, joint pain, myositis, osteonecrosis, *rhabdomyolysis*. **Respiratory:** URI, bronchitis, cough, pneumonia. **Skin:** rash, pruritus, dermatitis, eczema, folliculitis, condyloma acuminata. **Other:** herpes infection, immune reconstitution syndrome, influenza.

INTERACTIONS

Drug-drug. *Boceprevir, clarithromycin, CYP3A inhibitors (protease inhibitors except tipranavir–ritonavir), delavirdine, elvitegravir–ritonavir, itraconazole, ketoconazole, nefazodone, telithromycin:* May increase maraviroc level. May need to decrease maraviroc dosage.
CYP3A inducers (carbamazepine, efavirenz, etravirine, phenobarbital, phenytoin, rifampin): May decrease maraviroc level. May need to increase maraviroc dosage.
Drug-herb. *St. John's wort:* May decrease maraviroc level. Discourage use together.

EFFECTS ON LAB TEST RESULTS

• May increase AST, ALT, bilirubin, amylase, lipase, and CK levels.
• May decrease ANC.

CONTRAINDICATIONS & CAUTIONS

• Contraindicated in patients hypersensitive to drug or its components.
• Contraindicated in patients with severe renal impairment or ESRD (CrCl of less than 30 mL/minute) who are taking potent CYP3A inhibitors or inducers.
Black Box Warning Hepatotoxicity has been reported with maraviroc use. Severe rash or evidence of a systemic allergic reaction (fever, eosinophilia, or elevated IgE level) before the development of hepatotoxicity may occur. Immediately evaluate

patients with signs or symptoms of hepatitis or allergic reaction after drug use. ■
🜨 *Alert:* Before starting drug, test for CCR5 tropism. Outgrowth of preexisting low-level CXCR4- or dual/mixed-tropic HIV-1 not detected by tropism testing at screening has been associated with virologic failure.
• Severe and potentially life-threatening skin and hypersensitivity reactions, including SJS, toxic epidermal necrolysis, and DRESS syndrome, have been reported. Discontinue drug if signs or symptoms of hypersensitivity occur.
• Use cautiously in patients with preexisting liver dysfunction or patients who are infected with HBV or HCV.
• Use cautiously in patients at risk for CV events, with a history of postural hypotension, or taking another medication known to lower BP.
• During initial phase of treatment, patients treated with combination antiretroviral therapy may develop an inflammatory response to indolent or residual opportunistic infections (CMV, *Mycobacterium avium* complex, *Pneumocystis jiroveci* pneumonia, TB), which may necessitate further evaluation and treatment. Autoimmune disorders (such as Graves disease, polymyositis, and Guillain-Barré syndrome) have also been reported in the setting of immune reconstitution; however, time to onset is more variable, and onset can occur many months after initiation of antiretroviral treatment.
• Because of immune suppression, risk of malignancy may increase.
• Safety and effectiveness in children younger than age 2 haven't been established.
Dialyzable drug: No.

PREGNANCY-LACTATION-REPRODUCTION

• There are no adequate studies in pregnant women. Use during pregnancy only if potential benefit justifies potential risk to the fetus.
• Pregnant women exposed to drug should be registered in the Antiretroviral Pregnancy Registry (1-800-258-4263).
• Patient shouldn't breastfeed while taking drug because of potential for HIV transmission and serious adverse reactions in infants.

M

NURSING CONSIDERATIONS
• Effectiveness hasn't been established in patients with dual, mixed, or CXCR4-tropic HIV-1 infection.
• Monitor patient closely for signs and symptoms of infection, hepatic and renal impairment, and skin and hypersensitivity reactions.
• Monitor patient for malignancy with long-term use.

PATIENT TEACHING
• Instruct patient to immediately report signs or symptoms of hepatitis or allergic reaction (rash, yellow eyes or skin, dark urine, vomiting, and abdominal pain).
• Caution patient that drug doesn't cure HIV infection and that patient may still develop HIV-related illness, including opportunistic infections.
• Caution patient that drug doesn't reduce risk of transmission of HIV to others.
• If patient who feels dizzy while taking drug to avoid driving or operating machinery.
• Instruct female patient to tell prescriber if she's pregnant or planning to become pregnant while taking drug.
• Advise patient not to breastfeed during therapy.
• Advise patient to take drug every day as prescribed with other antiretrovirals. Tell patient not to change the dose or dosing schedule or stop any antiretroviral without consulting prescriber. If a dose is missed, tell patient to take it as soon as possible but not to double the next dose or take more than the prescribed dose.

---

medroxyPROGESTERone acetate
me-DROKS-ee-proe-JES-te-rone

Depo-Provera, Depo-subQ Provera 104, Meprogest❖, Provera♦

Therapeutic class: Estrogens
Pharmacologic class: Progestins

AVAILABLE FORMS
Injection (suspension): 104 mg/0.65 mL, 150 mg/mL, 400 mg/mL
Tablets: 2.5 mg, 5 mg, 10 mg

INDICATIONS & DOSAGES
➤ **Abnormal uterine bleeding caused by hormonal imbalance**
Women: 5 to 10 mg PO daily for 5 to 10 days beginning on day 16 or 21 of menstrual cycle. If patient also has received estrogen, give 10 mg PO daily for 10 days beginning on day 16 or 21 of cycle.
➤ **Secondary amenorrhea**
Women: 5 to 10 mg PO daily for 5 to 10 days. Start at any time during menstrual cycle (usually during latter half of cycle).
➤ **Endometrial hyperplasia**
Postmenopausal women (intact uterus) receiving conjugated estrogen 0.625 mg:
5 or 10 mg PO daily for 12 to 14 consecutive days per month, beginning day 1 or 16 of cycle.
➤ **Adjunctive therapy and palliative treatment of inoperable, recurrent, and metastatic endometrial or renal cancer**
Adults: 400 to 1,000 mg IM weekly. Dosage may be decreased to 400 mg/month when disease has stabilized.
➤ **Contraception**
Women: 150 mg (Depo-Provera) IM once every 3 months. Or, 104 mg Depo-subQ Provera subcut once every 3 months. Give first dose during first 5 days of normal menstrual period; only within first 5 days postpartum if patient isn't breastfeeding; and, if patient is exclusively breastfeeding, only at sixth postpartum week.
➤ **Endometriosis-associated pain**
Women: 104 mg subcut every 3 months (12 to 14 weeks).

ADMINISTRATION
• Hazardous drug; use safe handling and disposal precautions.
PO
• Giving drug immediately before or after a meal increases its bioavailability.
IM
• Shake vigorously before use.
• Give by deep IM injection in the gluteal or deltoid muscle.
• IM injection may be painful. Monitor sites for evidence of sterile abscess. Rotate injection sites to prevent muscle atrophy.
• For multidose vials, use a povidone-iodine solution or similar product to clean vial top before aspirating contents. Take special care

---

Reactions in bold italics are *life-threatening*. Interactions may have a *rapid onset* or a ***delayed onset***.

to prevent contamination of vial's contents, especially when multidose vial is used for endometrial or renal carcinoma.

Subcutaneous

• Shake vigorously for at least 1 minute before use.

• Give subcut injection over 5 to 7 seconds into the anterior thigh or abdomen.

ACTION

Suppresses ovulation, possibly by inhibiting pituitary gonadotropin secretion, thus preventing follicular maturation and causing endometrial thinning.

Route	Onset	Peak	Duration
PO	Rapid	2–4 hr	3–5 days
IM	Slow	3 wk	3–4 mo
Subcut	Unknown	1 wk	Unknown

Half-life: Oral, 12 to 17 hours; IM, 50 days; subcut, 43 days.

ADVERSE REACTIONS

CNS: anxiety, depression, fatigue, insomnia, somnolence, dementia, ***stroke,*** pain, dizziness, headache, nervousness. **CV:** thrombophlebitis, ***PE,*** edema, ***thromboembolism,*** syncope. **EENT:** exophthalmos, diplopia, optic neuritis, retinal vascular thrombosis. **GI:** bloating, abdominal pain, nausea, ***pancreatitis.*** **GU:** breakthrough bleeding, dysmenorrhea, amenorrhea, cervical erosion, abnormal secretions, decreased libido. **Hepatic:** cholestatic jaundice. **Metabolic:** weight changes. **Musculoskeletal:** osteoporosis. **Skin:** rash, induration, sterile abscesses, acne, pruritus, melasma, alopecia, hirsutism. **Other:** breast tenderness, enlargement, or secretion; hot flashes.

INTERACTIONS

Drug-drug. *Aminoglutethimide, carbamazepine, fosphenytoin, phenobarbital, phenytoin, rifampin, topiramate:* May decrease progestin effects. Monitor patient for diminished therapeutic response. Tell patient to use a nonhormonal contraceptive during therapy with these drugs.

Anticonvulsants, corticosteroids: These drugs can also reduce bone mass. Monitor patient.

Antidiabetics: May diminish antidiabetic therapeutic effects. Monitor therapy.

NNRTIs, protease inhibitors: May cause significant changes (increase or decrease) in plasma levels of progestins. Monitor patients for diminished progestin response and advise using nonhormonal contraception during therapy.

Strong CYP3A inducers (carbamazepine, phenobarbital, phenytoin, rifabutin, rifampin, rifapentine): May decrease progestin effects. Avoid use together.

Strong CYP3A inhibitors (clarithromycin, indinavir, itraconazole, ketoconazole, nefazodone, ritonavir, telithromycin, voriconazole): May increase progestin effects. Monitor therapy.

Drug-herb. *St. John's wort:* May decrease progestin effects. Avoid use together.

Drug-food. *Caffeine:* May increase caffeine level. Advise caution.

Grapefruit: May increase progestin effects. Monitor therapy.

Drug-lifestyle. *Smoking:* May increase risk of adverse CV effects. If smoking continues, may need alternative therapy.

EFFECTS ON LAB TEST RESULTS

• May increase LFT values, thyroid-binding globulin levels, HDL and triglyceride levels, coagulation tests, and prothrombin factors VII, VIII, IX, and X.

• May decrease plasma and urinary steroid levels, gonadotropin levels, and sex hormone–binding globulin concentrations.

• May reduce metyrapone test results. May alter glucose level.

CONTRAINDICATIONS & CAUTIONS

Black Box Warning Estrogens with progestins increase the risk of dementia in women age 65 and older. ■

• Contraindicated in patients hypersensitive to drug and in those with active thromboembolic disorders or history of thromboembolic disorders, cerebrovascular disease, stroke, breast cancer, history of breast cancer, known or suspected estrogen- or progesterone-dependent neoplasia, undiagnosed abnormal vaginal bleeding, missed abortion, or hepatic dysfunction. Tablets are contraindicated in patients with liver dysfunction.

Black Box Warning Injectable drug shouldn't be used for long-term birth control

M

(more than 2 years) unless other forms of birth control are inadequate. Loss of bone mineral density can occur and may not be reversible. ▪

• Use cautiously in patients with diabetes, seizures, migraine, cardiac or renal disease, strong family history of breast cancer, asthma, depression, or breast nodules.

Dialyzable drug: Unknown.

⚠ *Overdose S&S:* Nausea, vomiting, dizziness, breast tenderness, abdominal pain, drowsiness/fatigue, withdrawal bleeding.

PREGNANCY-LACTATION-REPRODUCTION

• Drug is contraindicated in women who are pregnant, suspected to be pregnant, or as a diagnostic test for pregnancy.

• Be alert to the possibility of an ectopic pregnancy in women using medroxyprogesterone contraceptive injection who become pregnant or complain of severe abdominal pain.

• Drug appears in human milk. Tablets aren't recommended for use in breastfeeding women. The manufacturer recommends that the injectable form be used with caution in breastfeeding women.

• High doses impair fertility.

NURSING CONSIDERATIONS

Black Box Warning Depo-Provera and Depo-subQ Provera may cause a significant loss of bone mineral density. Loss is greater with increasing duration of use and may not be reversible. In adolescents and young adults, drug may reduce peak bone mass and increase risk of osteoporotic fractures in later life. ▪

• Monitor patient for pain, swelling, warmth, or redness in calves; sudden, severe headaches; visual disturbances; numbness in extremities; signs of depression; and signs of liver dysfunction (abdominal pain, dark urine, jaundice).

PATIENT TEACHING

• According to FDA regulations, patient must read package insert explaining possible adverse effects of progestins before receiving first dose. Also, give patient verbal explanation.

Black Box Warning Teach patient that this product doesn't protect against HIV or other sexually transmitted diseases. ▪

• Advise patient to take medication with food if GI upset occurs.

🟢 *Alert:* Tell patient to report unusual symptoms immediately and to stop drug and notify prescriber about visual disturbances or migraine.

• Advise patient of the importance of an annual physical exam, including BP, breasts, abdomen, pelvic organs, and Papanicolaou test.

• Teach female patient how to perform routine breast self-exam.

• Advise patient to immediately report breast abnormalities, vaginal bleeding, swelling, yellowing of skin or eyes, dark urine, clay-colored stools, shortness of breath, chest pain, or pregnancy.

• Advise patient that injection must be given every 3 months to maintain adequate contraceptive effects.

• Tell patient that because this is a long-acting method of birth control, it may take some time for fertility to return after the last injection.

• Tell female patient to immediately report a suspected pregnancy.

• Advise patient that amenorrhea is possible with prolonged use.

• Encourage adequate intake of calcium and vitamin D.

mefloquine hydrochloride
ME-floe-kwin

Therapeutic class: Antimalarials
Pharmacologic class: Quinine derivatives

AVAILABLE FORMS
Tablets: 250 mg

INDICATIONS & DOSAGES

➤ **Acute malaria infections caused by mefloquine-sensitive strains of *Plasmodium falciparum* or *Plasmodium vivax***
Adults: 1,250 mg (five tablets) PO as a single dose with food and at least 8 oz of water. Patients with *P. vivax* infections should receive further therapy with primaquine or

other 8-aminoquinolines to avoid relapse after treatment of the initial infection.
Children age 6 months and older: 20 to 25 mg/kg PO as a single dose with food and at least 8 oz of water. Maximum dose, 1,250 mg. Dosage may be divided into two doses given 6 to 8 hours apart to reduce the incidence and severity of adverse effects. Patients with *P. vivax* infections should receive further therapy with primaquine or other 8-aminoquinolines to avoid relapse after treatment of the initial infection.

➤ **To prevent malaria**
Adults and children age 6 months and older weighing more than 45 kg: 250 mg PO once weekly. Preventive therapy should start 1 week before entering endemic area and continue for 4 weeks after returning. Give subsequent doses on same day of each week, preferably after main meal.
Children age 6 months and older weighing 30 to 45 kg: 187.5 mg (three-quarters of a 250-mg tablet) PO once weekly.
Children age 6 months and older weighing 20 to less than 30 kg: 125 mg (one-half of a 250-mg tablet) PO once weekly.

ADMINISTRATION
PO
• Patient should avoid taking drug on empty stomach and should always take with at least 240 mL of water.
• May crush tablets and suspend in a small amount of water, milk, or other beverage when giving to small children and other patients unable to swallow tablets whole.

ACTION
May be caused by drug's ability to form complexes with hemin and to raise intravesicular pH in parasite acid vesicles.

Route	Onset	Peak	Duration
PO	Unknown	6–24 hr	Unknown

Half-life: 2 to 4 weeks.

ADVERSE REACTIONS
CNS: *seizures, suicidal behavior,* fever, dizziness, syncope, headache, psychotic changes, hallucinations, confusion, anxiety, fatigue, vertigo, depression, abnormal dreams, insomnia, paresthesia, tremor, ataxia, mood changes, panic attacks, loss of balance, asthenia. **CV:** chest pain, edema, arrhythmia, conduction disorder. **EENT:** tinnitus, visual disturbances. **GI:** vomiting, nausea, loose stools, diarrhea, abdominal discomfort or pain, dyspepsia, loss of appetite. **Hematologic:** *leukopenia, thrombocytopenia.* **Musculoskeletal:** myalgia. **Skin:** rash, erythema, urticaria, hair loss, pruritus. **Other:** chills.

INTERACTIONS
Drug-drug. *Antiarrhythmics or beta blockers, antihistamines or H_1-blockers, calcium channel blockers, phenothiazines, TCAs:* May prolong QTc interval and increase risk of life-threatening cardiac arrhythmias. Coadminister with caution.
Carbamazepine, phenytoin, valproic acid: May decrease drug levels and loss of seizure control at start of mefloquine therapy. Monitor anticonvulsant level.
Chloroquine, quinidine, quinine: May increase risk of seizures and ECG abnormalities. Give mefloquine at least 12 hours after last dose.
CYP3A4 inducers: May decrease mefloquine plasma concentration and reduce drug's effect. Use together cautiously.
CYP3A4 inhibitors: May increase mefloquine plasma concentration and risk of adverse reactions. Use together cautiously.
Halofantrine: May cause fatal prolongation of QTc interval if given with or within 15 weeks of last mefloquine dose. Don't use together.
Ketoconazole: May increase mefloquine plasma concentration, leading to potentially fatal QT-interval prolongation. Don't use ketoconazole within 15 weeks of last dose of mefloquine.
Live-virus vaccines: May decrease immunization result. Complete vaccination at least 3 days before start of mefloquine.
Rifampin: May decrease mefloquine plasma concentration. Use together cautiously.

EFFECTS ON LAB TEST RESULTS
• May increase transaminase levels.
• May decrease hematocrit and platelet count.
• May increase or decrease WBC count.

M

CONTRAINDICATIONS & CAUTIONS

• Contraindicated in patients hypersensitive to mefloquine or related compounds, in those with a history of seizures, and in patients with active or recent history of depression, generalized anxiety disorder, psychosis, schizophrenia, or other major psychiatric disorders.

• Other IV antimalarials should be used to initially treat life-threatening or serious malarial infections. Mefloquine may be used after IV treatment is completed.

Black Box Warning Drug may cause neuropsychiatric adverse reactions that can persist after therapy ends. Drug shouldn't be prescribed for prophylaxis in patients with major psychiatric disorders. ■

• If psychiatric symptoms occur with prophylactic treatment, discontinue drug.

• Use cautiously when treating patients with cardiac disease or seizure disorders.

• Cases of agranulocytosis and aplastic anemia have been reported in patients taking mefloquine.

• Use cautiously in patients with hepatic impairment.

• In certain cases, such as when a traveler is taking other medications, it may be desirable to start prophylaxis 2 to 3 weeks before departure, to ensure that the combination of drugs is well tolerated.

Dialyzable drug: No.

⚠ *Overdose S&S:* Possibly more pronounced adverse reactions.

PREGNANCY-LACTATION-REPRODUCTION

• Studies in pregnant women have shown no increase in the risk of teratogenic effects after mefloquine use; however, risk to a developing fetus can't be ruled out. Use only if clearly needed.

• Drug appears in human milk in small amounts. Use cautiously in breastfeeding women.

NURSING CONSIDERATIONS

• Patients with *P. vivax* infections are at high risk for relapse because drug doesn't eliminate the hepatic-phase exoerythrocytic parasites. Give follow-up therapy with primaquine.

• Monitor LFT results periodically.

• If patient vomits within 30 minutes of receiving dose, repeat full dose; if within 30 to 60 minutes, give a half dose.

• If overdose is suspected, induce vomiting or perform gastric lavage because of risk of cardiotoxicity. Mefloquine has produced cardiac reactions similar to those caused by quinidine and quinine.

❸ *Alert:* Monitor patient for neurologic signs and symptoms (dizziness, vertigo, tinnitus, seizures, insomnia) or psychiatric signs and symptoms (anxiety, paranoia, hallucinations, depression, restlessness, confusion, behavior changes). Signs and symptoms may be more difficult to detect in children.

Black Box Warning During prophylactic use, if psychiatric or neurologic signs and symptoms occur, drug should be discontinued and an alternative drug prescribed. ■

PATIENT TEACHING

• Advise patient taking drug for prevention to take dose immediately before or after a meal on the same day each week, to improve compliance beginning 1 week before arrival at endemic area.

• Tell patient not to take drug on an empty stomach and always to take it with at least 8 oz of water.

• Instruct patient to read the medication guide and to always carry the information wallet card during therapy.

• Advise patient to use caution when performing activities that require alertness and coordination because dizziness, disturbed sense of balance, and neuropsychiatric reactions may occur.

❸ *Alert:* Inform patient that dizziness, vertigo, and tinnitus can occur during treatment, may continue for months or years after treatment, or may be permanent.

❸ *Alert:* Warn patient to immediately report neurologic or psychiatric signs or symptoms and not to stop drug until discussing with prescriber. Encourage patient to read the medication guide that comes with every prescription.

• Advise patient undergoing long-term therapy to have periodic ophthalmic exams because drug may cause ocular lesions.

• Advise patient that drug may cause insomnia.

• Advise female patient of childbearing potential to use reliable contraception during treatment.

SAFETY ALERT!

megestrol acetate
me-JES-trole

Megace ES, Apo-Megestrol ✤

Therapeutic class: Antineoplastics
Pharmacologic class: Progestins

AVAILABLE FORMS
Oral suspension: 40 mg/mL
Oral suspension (concentrated): 125 mg/mL
Tablets: 20 mg, 40 mg, 160 mg ✤

INDICATIONS & DOSAGES
➤ **Breast cancer (palliative treatment)**
Adults: 40 mg PO q.i.d. for at least 2 months. Use tablets only.
➤ **Endometrial cancer (palliative treatment)**
Adults: 40 to 320 mg PO daily in divided doses for at least 2 months. Use tablets only.
➤ **Anorexia, cachexia, or unexplained significant weight loss in patients with AIDS**
Adults: 400 to 800 mg PO (10 to 20 mL regular oral suspension) or 625 mg PO (5 mL concentrated oral suspension) once daily.
➤ **Hot flashes ◆**
Adults: 20 mg PO once daily.

ADMINISTRATION
PO
• Drug is a hormonal agent and is considered a teratogen. Follow safe handling procedures.
• Give drug without regard for meals.
• Shake suspension well before pouring.
• Protect tablets and oral suspension from heat; protect tablets from light.

ACTION
Inhibits hormone-dependent tumor growth by inhibiting pituitary and adrenal steroidogenesis. Drug may also have direct cytotoxicity; its appetite-stimulating mechanism is unknown.

Route	Onset	Peak	Duration
PO	Unknown	1–3 hr	Unknown

Half-life: Mean, 34.2 hours.

ADVERSE REACTIONS
CNS: confusion, seizures, depression, headache, neuropathy, insomnia, abnormal thinking, mood changes, fever, asthenia, malaise. **CV:** thrombophlebitis, *HF,* HTN, *thromboembolism, cardiomyopathy, PE,* palpitations, chest pain, edema. **EENT:** pharyngitis. **GI:** nausea, vomiting, diarrhea, flatulence, constipation, dry mouth, increased appetite, abdominal pain, dyspepsia. **GU:** breakthrough menstrual bleeding, erectile dysfunction, UTI, urinary incontinence, urinary frequency. **Hematologic:** *leukopenia.* **Hepatic:** hepatomegaly. **Metabolic:** hyperglycemia, weight gain. **Musculoskeletal:** carpal tunnel syndrome. **Respiratory:** dyspnea, pneumonia, cough. **Skin:** alopecia, rash, diaphoresis, pruritus. **Other:** gynecomastia, tumor flare, hot flushes.

INTERACTIONS
Drug-drug. *Anticoagulants:* May diminish therapeutic effect of anticoagulants. Weigh risks and benefits of therapy.
Antidiabetics: May diminish therapeutic effect of antidiabetics. Monitor therapy.
Dofetilide: May increase dofetilide plasma level, increasing risk of life-threatening cardiac arrhythmias, including torsades de pointes. Avoid use together.
Indinavir: May decrease exposure of indinavir. Consider increasing indinavir dosage when using together.
Rifamycins (rifampin): May increase megestrol metabolism due to induction of CYP3A4 pathway, reducing pharmacologic effects. Consider increasing megestrol dosage.
Drug-herb. *Bloodroot, yucca:* May enhance adverse/toxic effects of progestins. Monitor therapy.

EFFECTS ON LAB TEST RESULTS
• May increase glucose and LDH levels.

M

CONTRAINDICATIONS & CAUTIONS
• Contraindicated in patients hypersensitive to drug.
• Use cautiously in patients with history of thrombophlebitis or thromboembolism.
Dialyzable drug: Unlikely.

PREGNANCY-LACTATION-REPRODUCTION
• Drug may cause fetal harm. Oral solution is contraindicated in pregnancy. If tablets are used during pregnancy, or if patient becomes pregnant during therapy, apprise her of potential hazard to the fetus. Women of childbearing potential should avoid becoming pregnant.
• Drug appears in human milk. Women shouldn't breastfeed during therapy.

NURSING CONSIDERATIONS
• May increase glucose level in diabetic patients.
• Drug isn't intended for prophylactic use to avoid weight loss. Start treatment with megestrol acetate oral suspension only after treatable causes of weight loss are sought and addressed.
• Two months is an adequate trial period in patients with cancer.
• Drug may cause adrenal insufficiency, which can be fatal. Monitor patient for signs and symptoms, such as hypotension, nausea, vomiting, dizziness, or weakness. Glucocorticoid therapy may be needed.

PATIENT TEACHING
• Inform patient that therapeutic response isn't immediate. Drug must be taken for at least 2 months to determine effectiveness.
• Tell patient drug may be taken without regard for food.
◑ **Alert:** Tell patient that the ES oral suspension is more concentrated than the regular oral suspension, so a smaller amount is needed if prescription is changed.
• Advise female patient to stop breastfeeding during therapy because of risk of toxicity to infant.
• Advise female patient of childbearing potential to use an effective form of contraception while receiving drug.
• Tell patient to report all adverse reactions, especially signs and symptoms of adrenal insufficiency.

melphalan (L-PAM, phenylalanine mustard)
MEL-fa-lan

Alkeran✲

melphalan hydrochloride
Alkeran✲, Evomela

Therapeutic class: Antineoplastics
Pharmacologic class: Nitrogen mustards

AVAILABLE FORMS
Lyophilized powder for injection: 50 mg
Tablets: 2 mg

INDICATIONS & DOSAGES
➤ **Multiple myeloma (palliative treatment)**
Adults: Initially, 6 mg PO daily for 2 to 3 weeks; then stop drug for up to 4 weeks or until WBC and platelet counts stop dropping and begin to rise again; maintenance dose is 2 mg daily. Or, 10 mg/day for 7 to 10 days, followed by 2 mg/day when WBC is greater than 4,000 cells/mm^3 and platelet count is greater than 100,000 cells/mm^3; dosage is adjusted to between 1 and 3 mg/day depending on hematologic response. Or, 0.15 mg/kg PO daily for 7 days followed by a rest period of 2 to 6 weeks; maintenance dose is 0.05 mg/kg/day or less. Or 0.25 mg/kg/day for 4 consecutive days (or 0.2 mg/kg/day for 5 consecutive days) for a total dose of 1 mg/kg/course; repeat every 4 to 6 weeks.

Or, give IV to patients who can't tolerate oral therapy, 16 mg/m^2 given by infusion over 15 to 20 minutes at 2-week intervals for four doses. After patient has recovered from toxicity, give drug at 4-week intervals.
Adjust-a-dose: Withhold drug until recovery for WBC count less than 3,000/mm^3 or platelet count less than 100,000/mm^3. For moderate to severe renal impairment, consider a reduced PO dose initially. For patients with renal insufficiency (BUN level of 30 mg/dL or more), consider reducing IV dose 50%.

➤ **Nonresectable advanced epithelial ovarian cancer (palliative treatment)**

Reactions in bold italics are *life-threatening*. Interactions may have a *rapid onset* or a *delayed onset*.

Adults: 0.2 mg/kg PO daily for 5 days. Repeat every 4 to 5 weeks, depending on hematologic tolerance.

Adjust-a-dose: For moderate to severe renal impairment, consider a reduced dose initially.

➤ **Multiple myeloma (conditioning treatment before hematopoietic stem cell transplantation) (Evomela)**
Adults: 100 mg/m^2/day by IV infusion over 30 minutes for 2 consecutive days (day –3 and day –2) before autologous stem cell transplantation (day 0).

Adjust-a-dose: For patients weighing more than 130% of their ideal body weight, calculate BSA based on adjusted ideal body weight.

➤ **Amyloidosis, light chain ◆**
Adults: 0.22 mg/kg/day PO for 4 days every 28 days (in combination with oral dexamethasone), or 10 mg/m^2/day PO for 4 days every month (in combination with oral dexamethasone) for 12 to 18 treatment cycles.

ADMINISTRATION
PO
• Hazardous drug; use safe handling and disposal precautions.
• Give on an empty stomach; food decreases drug absorption.
• Store tablets in refrigerator. Protect from light.

IV
Black Box Warning Preparing and giving this form may be mutagenic, teratogenic, or carcinogenic. Follow facility safe handling policy to reduce risks. ∎

▼ IV drug is available in different formulations, with different indications and preparation and storage instructions.

▼ Because drug isn't stable in solution, reconstitute immediately before giving with the 10 mL of sterile diluent supplied by manufacturer, using 20G or larger needle. Shake vigorously until solution is clear. The resulting solution will contain 5 mg/mL of melphalan. Immediately dilute required dose in NSS for injection to no more than 0.45 mg/mL. Give infusion over at least 15 minutes.

▼ Monitor infusion carefully; drug is considered a vesicant and extravasation may cause local damage. If extravasation

occurs, stop infusion immediately, notify prescriber, and follow facility protocol for treatment.

▼ Reconstituted product begins to degrade within 30 minutes. After final dilution, nearly 1% of drug degrades every 10 minutes. Administration must be finished within 60 minutes of reconstitution.

▼ Don't refrigerate reconstituted product because precipitate will form.

Evomela
▼ Use 8.6 mL NSS as directed to reconstitute and make a 50-mg/10 mL (5-mg/mL) nominal concentration of melphalan. The NSS should appear to be pulled into vial by the negative pressure in vial. Discard any vial (and replace with another) if there is no vacuum present when reconstituting vial.

▼ Reconstituted drug is stable for 24 hours when refrigerated (41° F [5° C]) without any precipitation because of the high solubility, and is stable for 1 hour at room temperature.

▼ Withdraw required volume needed for dose from vial and add to the appropriate volume of NSS to a final concentration of 0.45 mg/mL.

▼ For conditioning treatment, infuse over 30 minutes via injection port or central venous catheter.

▼ For palliative treatment, administer as a single IV infusion over 15 to 20 minutes by injecting slowly into a fast-running IV infusion via a CVAD.

▼ Admixture solution is stable for 4 hours at room temperature in addition to the 1 hour after reconstitution.

▼ Don't mix Evomela with other melphalan hydrochloride for injection products.

▼ Extravasation may cause local tissue damage. Don't administer by direct injection into a peripheral vein.

▼ **Incompatibilities:** Amphotericin B, chlorpromazine, D_5W, lactated Ringer injection. Compatibility with NSS injection depends on the concentration; don't prepare solutions with a concentration exceeding 0.45 mg/mL.

ACTION
Cross-links strands of cellular DNA and interferes with RNA transcription, causing an

M

imbalance of growth that leads to cell death. Not specific to cell cycle.

Route	Onset	Peak	Duration
PO	Unknown	About 1–2 hr	Unknown
IV	Unknown	Unknown	Unknown

Half-life: Oral, about ½ to 2¼ hours; IV, about 75 minutes.

ADVERSE REACTIONS
CNS: fatigue. **CV:** vasculitis. **GI:** nausea, vomiting, diarrhea, oral ulceration, stomatitis, decreased appetite, constipation, abdominal pain. **GU:** amenorrhea, testicular suppression. **Hematologic:** *thrombocytopenia, leukopenia, bone marrow suppression,* hemolytic anemia. **Hepatic:** *hepatotoxicity.* **Metabolic:** *hypokalemia.* **Respiratory:** *pneumonitis, pulmonary fibrosis.* **Skin:** pruritus, alopecia, urticaria, ulceration at injection site. **Other:** *anaphylaxis,* hypersensitivity reactions.

INTERACTIONS
Drug-drug (IV melphalan only. There are no known drug interactions with oral form). *Anticoagulants, aspirin, NSAIDs:* May increase risk of bleeding. Avoid using together.
Carmustine: May decrease threshold for pulmonary toxicity. Use together cautiously.
Cimetidine: May decrease melphalan level. Monitor patient closely.
Cisplatin: May increase renal impairment, decreasing melphalan clearance. Monitor patient closely.
Clozapine: May increase risk of neutropenia. Monitor WBC count carefully.
Cyclosporine: May cause severe renal impairment. Monitor renal function closely.
Immunosuppressants (pimecrolimus): May increase risk of immunosuppression. Avoid concurrent use.
Live-virus vaccines: May increase risk of toxicity from live-virus vaccines. Postpone immunization with live-virus vaccines for at least 3 months after last dose of melphalan.
Nalidixic acid: May cause hemorrhagic ulcerative colitis or intestinal necrosis (children). Monitor therapy.
Drug-herb. *Echinacea:* May alter immune system activity. Consider therapy modification.

Drug-food. *Any food:* May decrease oral drug absorption. Advise patient to take drug on an empty stomach.

EFFECTS ON LAB TEST RESULTS
• May increase urine urea level. May decrease Hb level.
• May decrease RBC, WBC, and platelet counts.
• May cause a false-positive direct Coombs test.

CONTRAINDICATIONS & CAUTIONS
• Contraindicated in patients hypersensitive to drug and in those with disease resistant to drug.
• Contraindicated in patients with severe leukopenia, thrombocytopenia, or anemia and in those with chronic lymphocytic leukemia.
• Use cautiously in patients receiving radiation and chemotherapy.
• Drug is a vesicant and may cause local tissue damage if extravasation occurs. If signs or symptoms of extravasation develop, stop infusion immediately and notify prescriber.
Dialyzable drug: No.
⚠ **Overdose S&S:** Vomiting, ulceration of the mouth, diarrhea, GI hemorrhage, bone marrow suppression.

PREGNANCY-LACTATION-REPRODUCTION
• There are no adequate studies in pregnant women, but drug may cause fetal harm. Women of childbearing potential should avoid becoming pregnant by using an effective contraceptive.
• It isn't known if drug appears in human milk; however, excretion into human milk is likely. Don't give to breastfeeding women.
• Drug suppresses ovarian function in premenopausal women, resulting in amenorrhea in a significant number of patients.
• May damage spermatozoa and testicular tissue, resulting in possible genetic fetal abnormalities. Reversible and irreversible testicular suppression has also been reported.

NURSING CONSIDERATIONS
Black Box Warning Administer drug only under the supervision of a physician experienced in the use of cancer chemotherapeutic agents. ∎

Reactions in bold italics are *life-threatening*. Interactions may have a *rapid onset* or a *delayed onset*.

Black Box Warning Severe bone marrow suppression with resulting bleeding or infection may occur. ∎

Black Box Warning Drug is leukemogenic. It produces chromosomal aberrations in vitro and in vivo and should be considered potentially mutagenic in humans. ∎

Black Box Warning Controlled trials comparing IV to oral melphalan have shown more myelosuppression with the IV formulation. Hypersensitivity reactions, including anaphylaxis, have occurred in approximately 2% of patients who received the IV formulation. ∎

• Dosage may need to be reduced in patients with renal impairment.
• Monitor uric acid level and CBC.
• To prevent bleeding, avoid all IM injections when platelet count is less than 50,000/mm³.
• Blood transfusions may be needed for cumulative anemia.
• Drug is associated with moderate emetic potential.
• Anaphylaxis may occur. Keep antihistamines and steroids readily available to give if needed.
• *Look alike–sound alike:* Don't confuse melphalan with Mephyton.

PATIENT TEACHING

• Advise patient to take tablets on empty stomach.
• Advise patient to report pain or redness at IV site.
• Advise patient to report all adverse reactions and to watch for signs and symptoms of infection (fever, sore throat, fatigue) and bleeding (easy bruising, nosebleeds, bleeding gums, tarry stools). Tell patient to take temperature daily.
• Advise female patient to stop breastfeeding during therapy because of risk of toxicity to infant.
• Advise patient that drug can interfere with menstrual cycle and stop sperm production in men.
• Advise male patient with female sexual partners of childbearing potential to use effective contraception during and after treatment.
• Advise female patient of childbearing potential to avoid pregnancy (which may

include use of effective contraceptive methods) during and after treatment.
• Inform patient to report nausea, vomiting, and diarrhea. Antiemetics and antidiarrheals may be prescribed.

memantine hydrochloride
me-MAN-teen

Ebixa✤, Namenda✔, Namenda XR

Therapeutic class: Anti-Alzheimer drugs
Pharmacologic class: N-methyl-D-aspartate receptor antagonists

AVAILABLE FORMS
Capsules (extended-release) ⓓⓝⓒ: 7 mg, 14 mg, 21 mg, 28 mg
Oral solution: 2 mg/mL
Tablets: 5 mg, 10 mg

INDICATIONS & DOSAGES
➤ **Moderate to severe Alzheimer dementia**
Adults: Initially, 5 mg PO once daily. Increase by 5 mg/day every week until target dose is reached. Maximum, 10 mg PO b.i.d. Doses greater than 5 mg should be given in two divided doses.

Or, for extended-release capsules, initial dose is 7 mg PO once daily. Increase as tolerated by 7-mg increments each week to target dosage of 28 mg PO once daily.
To convert from immediate-release to extended-release form: Patients taking immediate-release 10 mg b.i.d. may switch to extended-release 28 mg once daily the day following the last immediate-release tablet. Patients with severe renal failure taking immediate-release 5 mg b.i.d. may switch to extended-release 14 mg once daily the day following the last immediate-release tablet.
Adjust-a-dose: For immediate-release form, no dosage adjustment is recommended for patients with mild to moderate renal impairment; target dosage of 5 mg b.i.d. is recommended for patients with severe renal impairment (CrCl of 5 to 29 mL/minute). For extended-release form, no dosage adjustment is recommended for patients with mild to moderate renal impairment; a target dosage of 14 mg/day is recommended for

M

patients with severe renal impairment (CrCl of 5 to 29 mL/minute).

ADMINISTRATION

PO

• Give drug without regard for food.

• Patients may take capsules intact or capsules may be opened, sprinkled on applesauce, then swallowed. Don't allow the patient to divide, chew, or crush capsules.

• Use dosing device provided with the oral solution to withdraw correct dose volume. Slowly squirt dose into the corner of patient's mouth.

• Don't mix oral solution with any other liquid.

ACTION

Antagonizes N-methyl-D-aspartate receptors, the persistent activation of which seems to increase Alzheimer symptoms.

Route	Onset	Peak	Duration
PO (tablets)	Unknown	3–7 hr	Unknown
PO (capsules)	Unknown	9–12 hr	Unknown

Half-life: 60 to 80 hours.

ADVERSE REACTIONS

CNS: aggressiveness, agitation, anxiety, ataxia, confusion, depression, dizziness, fatigue, hallucinations, headache, hypokinesia, insomnia, pain, somnolence, syncope, vertigo, drowsiness. **CV:** *HF,* edema, HTN, hypotension. **EENT:** cataracts, conjunctivitis. **GI:** anorexia, constipation, diarrhea, nausea, vomiting, abdominal pain. **GU:** incontinence, urinary frequency. **Hematologic:** anemia. **Metabolic:** weight loss or gain. **Musculoskeletal:** arthralgia, back pain. **Respiratory:** bronchitis, coughing, dyspnea, flulike symptoms, pneumonia, URI. **Skin:** rash. **Other:** abnormal gait, falls, injury, flulike symptoms.

INTERACTIONS

Drug-drug. *Cimetidine, hydrochlorothiazide, metformin, quinidine, ranitidine, triamterene:* May alter levels of both drugs. Monitor patient.

NMDA antagonists (amantadine, dextromethorphan, ketamine): Effects of combined use unknown. Use together cautiously.

Urine alkalinizers (carbonic anhydrase inhibitors, sodium bicarbonate): May decrease memantine clearance. Monitor patient for adverse effects.

Drug-food. *Foods that alkalinize urine:* May increase drug level and adverse effects. Use together cautiously.

Drug-lifestyle. *Alcohol use:* May alter drug adherence, decrease its effectiveness, or increase adverse effects. Discourage use together.

Nicotine: May alter levels of drug and nicotine. Discourage use together.

EFFECTS ON LAB TEST RESULTS

• May increase alkaline phosphatase level.

• May decrease Hb level and hematocrit.

CONTRAINDICATIONS & CAUTIONS

• Contraindicated in patients allergic to drug or its components.

• Use cautiously in patients with seizures, CV disease, or severe hepatic or renal impairment.

• Use cautiously in patients who may have an increased urine pH (from drugs, diet, renal tubular acidosis, or severe UTI).

Dialyzable drug: Unknown.

⚠ *Overdose S&S:* Restlessness, psychosis, visual hallucinations, somnolence, stupor, loss of consciousness, agitation, asthenia, bradycardia, confusion, coma, dizziness, ECG changes, HTN, lethargy, unsteady gait, vertigo, vomiting, weakness.

PREGNANCY-LACTATION-REPRODUCTION

• There are no adequate studies in pregnant women. Use during pregnancy only if potential benefit justifies potential risk to the fetus.

• It isn't known if drug appears in human milk. Use cautiously in breastfeeding women.

NURSING CONSIDERATIONS

• Monitor patient carefully for adverse reactions as patient may not be able to recognize changes or communicate effectively.

PATIENT TEACHING

• Explain that drug doesn't cure Alzheimer disease but may aid patient to maintain function for a longer period of time.

• Tell patient or caregiver to report adverse effects.

Reactions in bold italics are *life-threatening.* Interactions may have a *rapid onset* or a *delayed onset.*

• Urge patient to avoid alcohol during treatment.
• To avoid possible interactions, advise patient not to take herbal or OTC products without consulting prescriber.

SAFETY ALERT!

meperidine hydrochloride (pethidine hydrochloride)
me-PER-i-deen

Demerol◆

Therapeutic class: Opioid analgesics
Pharmacologic class: Opioids
Controlled substance schedule: II

AVAILABLE FORMS
Injection: 10 mg/mL, 25 mg/mL, 50 mg/mL, 75 mg/mL, 100 mg/mL
Solution: 50 mg/5 mL
Tablets: 50 mg, 100 mg

INDICATIONS & DOSAGES
Adjust-a-dose (for all indications): Reduce meperidine dosage by 25% to 50% when administered with phenothiazines or other tranquilizers because they potentiate the action of meperidine. Use cautiously and initiate at the lower end of the dosage range in elderly patients and in those with hepatic and renal impairment; if needed, titrate dosage slowly.
➤ **Moderate to severe pain that requires an opioid analgesic and for which alternative treatments are inadequate**
Adults: 50 to 150 mg PO, IM, or subcut every 3 to 4 hours p.r.n. Or, 10 mg IV slowly by patient-controlled analgesia device, with range of 1 to 5 mg per dose; lockout interval is 6 to 10 minutes. Or, continuous IV infusion of 15 to 35 mg/hour.
Children: 1.1 to 1.8 mg/kg PO, or 1.1 to 1.8 mg/kg IM or subcut every 3 to 4 hours. Maximum, 50 to 150 mg every 4 hours p.r.n.
➤ **Preoperative analgesia**
Adults: 50 to 100 mg IM or subcut 30 to 90 minutes before beginning of anesthesia.
Children: 1.1 to 2.2 mg/kg IM or subcut up to the adult dose 30 to 90 minutes before anesthesia.

➤ **Adjunct to anesthesia**
Adults: Repeated slow IV injections of fractional doses (10 mg/mL). Or, continuous IV infusion of a more dilute solution (1 mg/mL) titrated to patient's needs.
➤ **Obstetric analgesia**
Adults: 50 to 100 mg IM or subcut when pain becomes regular; may repeat at 1- to 3-hour intervals.

ADMINISTRATION
PO
• Solution has local anesthetic effect on mucous membranes if not diluted. Give with a half glass of water.
• Oral dose is less than half as effective as parenteral dose. Give IM if possible. When changing from parenteral to oral route, increase dosage.

IV
▼ Keep opioid antagonist (naloxone) available.
▼ Give drug slowly by direct injection.
▼ Drug may also be given by slow continuous infusion. Drug is compatible with most solutions, including D₅W, NSS, and Ringer or lactated Ringer solutions.
▼ Protect from light and store at room temperature.
▼ **Incompatibilities:** Aminophyllines, barbiturates, iodide, morphine, phenytoin, sodium bicarbonate, sulfadiazine.

IM
• Inject deep into large muscle mass, taking care to avoid nerve trunks.
Subcutaneous
• Subcut injection isn't recommended because it's very painful, but it may be suitable for occasional use. Monitor patient for pain at injection site, local tissue irritation, and induration after subcut injection.

ACTION
Unknown. Binds with opioid receptors in the CNS, altering perception of and emotional response to pain.

Route	Onset	Peak	Duration
PO	10–15 min	60–120 min	2–4 hr
IV	5 min	5–7 min	2–3 hr
IM, subcut	10–15 min	30–50 min	2–4 hr

Half-life: 2½ to 4 hours.

M

ADVERSE REACTIONS

CNS: agitation, incoordination, dizziness, euphoria, light-headedness, sedation, somnolence, *seizures,* hallucinations, headache, paradoxical anxiety, physical dependence, syncope, tremor, confusion, disorientation. **CV:** *bradycardia, cardiac arrest, shock,* hypotension, tachycardia, palpitations, flushing. **GI:** biliary tract spasms, constipation, dry mouth, ileus, nausea, vomiting. **GU:** urine retention. **Musculoskeletal:** muscle twitching, weakness. **Respiratory:** *respiratory arrest, respiratory depression.* **Skin:** diaphoresis, pruritus, urticaria. **Other:** induration, local tissue irritation, pain at injection site, phlebitis after IV delivery, *anaphylaxis.*

INTERACTIONS

Drug-drug. *Acyclovir:* Increases meperidine plasma concentration and risk of adverse reactions. Use together cautiously.
Aminophylline, barbiturates, heparin, methicillin, morphine sulfate, phenytoin, sodium bicarbonate, sulfonamides: Incompatible when mixed in same IV container. Avoid using together.

Black Box Warning *Benzodiazepines, CNS depressants:* May cause slow or difficult breathing, sedation, and death. Avoid use together. If use together is necessary, limit dosage and duration of each drug to the minimum necessary for desired effect. ∎

Chlorpromazine: May cause excessive sedation and hypotension. Avoid using together.
Cimetidine: May increase respiratory and CNS depression. Monitor patient closely.

Black Box Warning *CYP3A4 inducers (carbamazepine, phenytoin, rifampin):* May increase meperidine level and increase risk of toxicity if inducers are discontinued. Monitor patient closely when discontinuing an inducer. ∎

Black Box Warning *CYP3A4 inhibitors (erythromycin, ketoconazole, ritonavir):* May increase meperidine plasma concentration, which could increase or prolong adverse reactions; may cause fatal respiratory depression. Monitor patient closely. ∎

General anesthetics, phenothiazines, TCAs: May cause respiratory depression, hypotension, profound sedation, or coma. Use together with caution; reduce meperidine dosage.

Black Box Warning *MAO inhibitors:* May increase CNS and respiratory depression and hypotension that can be severe or fatal. Use of meperidine within 14 days of an MAO inhibitor is contraindicated. ∎

Phenytoin: May decrease meperidine level. Watch for decreased analgesia.
Protease inhibitors: May increase respiratory and CNS depression. Avoid using together.

◑ *Alert:* Serotonergic drugs (amoxapine, antiemetics [dolasetron, granisetron, ondansetron, palonosetron], antimigraine drugs, buspirone, cyclobenzaprine, dextromethorphan, linezolid, lithium, maprotiline, methylene blue, mirtazapine, nefazodone, SSNRIs, SSRIs, TCAs, trazodone, tryptophan, vilazodone):* May increase risk of serotonin syndrome. Use together cautiously and monitor patient for serotonin syndrome.
Sodium oxybate: May increase CNS depression and sleep duration. Use together is contraindicated.

Drug-herb. *Kava kava:* May enhance adverse effects of CNS depressants. Monitor therapy.

◑ *Alert:* *St. John's wort:* May increase risk of serotonin syndrome. Use together cautiously and monitor patient for serotonin syndrome.

Drug-lifestyle. **Black Box Warning** *Alcohol use:* May cause additive CNS and respiratory depressive effects. Don't use together. ∎

EFFECTS ON LAB TEST RESULTS

• May increase amylase, lipase, and CK levels.
• May increase bromsulphthalein retention.

CONTRAINDICATIONS & CAUTIONS

• Contraindicated in patients hypersensitive to drug and in those with significant respiratory depression, acute or severe bronchial asthma in an unmonitored setting or in the absence of resuscitative equipment, and with known or suspected GI obstruction, including paralytic ileus.

Black Box Warning Contraindicated in patients who have received MAO inhibitors within past 14 days. ∎

Reactions in bold italics are *life-threatening*. Interactions may have a *rapid onset* or a *delayed onset*.

Black Box Warning Opioids should only be prescribed with benzodiazepines or other CNS depressants to patients for whom alternative treatment options are inadequate. ∎

Black Box Warning Drug may increase risks of opioid addiction, abuse, and misuse, which can lead to overdose and death. Risks increase in patients with a personal or family history of substance abuse or mental illness. Assess risks before drug is prescribed. ∎

☙ *Alert:* Drug may lead to a rare but serious decrease in adrenal gland cortisol production.

☙ *Alert:* Drug may cause decreased sex hormone levels with long-term use.

☙ *Alert:* Patients are at increased risk for oversedation and respiratory depression if they snore or have a history of sleep apnea, haven't used opioids recently or are first-time opioid users, have increased opioid dosage requirements or opioid habituation, have received general anesthesia for longer lengths of time or received other sedating drugs, have preexisting pulmonary or cardiac disease, or have thoracic or other surgical incisions that may impair breathing. Monitor patients carefully.

• Use cautiously in elderly or debilitated patients and in those with increased ICP, head injury, asthma and other respiratory conditions, supraventricular tachycardias, seizures, abdominal conditions, decreased bowel motility conditions, hepatic or renal disease, hypothyroidism, Addison disease, urethral stricture, and prostatic hyperplasia.

• Meperidine can produce drug dependence of the morphine type and, therefore, has the potential for abuse. Psychic dependence, physical dependence, and tolerance may develop upon repeated administration.

Dialyzable drug: Unknown.

⚠ *Overdose S&S:* Respiratory depression, somnolence progressing to stupor, coma, bradycardia, hypotension, hypothermia, delirium, skeletal muscle flaccidity, circulatory collapse, death.

PREGNANCY-LACTATION-REPRODUCTION

Black Box Warning Prolonged use of drug during pregnancy can result in neonatal opioid withdrawal syndrome, which may be life-threatening and requires management according to protocols developed by neonatology experts. If prolonged use is needed,

advise patient of risks and ensure that appropriate treatment will be available. ∎

• Don't use in pregnant women before labor unless physician determines potential benefits outweigh possible risks; safe use in pregnancy before labor hasn't been established relative to possible adverse effects on fetal development.

• Drug appears in human milk. Patient should discontinue breastfeeding or discontinue drug.

NURSING CONSIDERATIONS

Black Box Warning Regularly monitor patients for development of opioid addiction, abuse, and misuse. ∎

Black Box Warning Serious, life-threatening, or fatal respiratory depression can occur. Monitor patient closely, especially within first 24 to 72 hours of starting drug and after a dosage increase. ∎

Black Box Warning Accidental ingestion of even one dose of drug, especially by children, can be fatal. ∎

• In elderly patients, patients using meperidine for longer than 48 hours, those with preexisting renal or CNS disease, and those taking more than 600 mg/day, the active metabolite may accumulate, causing increased adverse CNS reactions. Avoid prolonged use.

• Monitor patients with biliary tract disease, including acute pancreatitis, for worsening signs and symptoms.

☙ *Alert:* Carefully monitor vital signs, pain level, respiratory status, and sedation level in all patients receiving opioids, especially those receiving IV drugs, even those given postoperatively.

☙ *Alert:* If patient is taking opioids with serotonergic drugs, watch for signs and symptoms of serotonin syndrome (agitation, hallucinations, rapid HR, fever, excessive sweating, shivering or shaking, muscle twitching or stiffness, trouble with coordination, nausea, vomiting, diarrhea), especially when starting treatment or increasing dosages. Signs and symptoms may occur within several hours of coadministration but may also occur later, especially after dosage increase. Discontinue the opioid, serotonergic drug, or both if serotonin syndrome is suspected.

M

Alert: Monitor patient for signs and symptoms of adrenal insufficiency (nausea, vomiting, loss of appetite, fatigue, weakness, dizziness, low BP). Perform diagnostic testing if adrenal insufficiency is suspected. If adrenal insufficiency is confirmed, treat with corticosteroids and wean patient off opioids if appropriate. Discontinue corticosteroids when clinically appropriate.

Alert: Monitor patient for signs and symptoms of decreased sex hormone levels (low libido, erectile dysfunction, amenorrhea, infertility). If signs and symptoms occur, evaluate patient and obtain lab testing.

• When giving drug parenterally, make sure patient is lying down.

• Drug may be used in some patients who are allergic to morphine.

• Reassess patient's level of pain at least 15 and 30 minutes after administration.

• Because drug toxicity frequently appears after several days of treatment, drug isn't recommended for treatment of chronic pain.

• In neonates exposed to drug during labor, monitor respirations. Have resuscitation equipment and naloxone available.

• Monitor respiratory and CV status carefully. Don't give if respirations are below 12 breaths/minute, if respiratory rate or depth is decreased, or if change in pupils is noted.

• If drug is stopped abruptly after long-term use, monitor patient for withdrawal symptoms.

• In postoperative patients, monitor bladder function.

• Monitor bowel function. Patient may need a stimulant laxative and stool softener.

Alert: Don't stop drug abruptly; withdraw slowly and individualize gradual taper plan to prevent signs and symptoms of withdrawal, worsening pain, and psychological distress in physically dependent patients. Refer to manufacturer's label for specific tapering instructions.

Alert: When tapering opioids, monitor patient closely for signs and symptoms of opioid withdrawal (restlessness, lacrimation, rhinorrhea, yawning, perspiration, chills, myalgia, mydriasis, irritability, anxiety, insomnia, backache, joint pain, weakness, abdominal cramps, anorexia, nausea, vomiting, diarrhea, increased BP or HR, increased respiratory rate), which may indicate a need to taper more slowly. Also monitor patient for suicidal thoughts, use of other substances, and mood changes.

• **Look alike–sound alike:** Don't confuse Demerol with Demulen.

PATIENT TEACHING

Black Box Warning Caution patient or caregiver of patient taking an opioid with a benzodiazepine, CNS depressant, or alcohol to seek immediate medical attention for dizziness, light-headedness, extreme sleepiness, slowed or difficult breathing, or unresponsiveness. ■

Black Box Warning Advise patient that drug increases risk of opioid addiction, abuse, and misuse, which can lead to overdose and death. Teach patient proper use of drug. ■

Black Box Warning Warn patient to keep drug out of reach of children as accidental ingestion of even one dose can be fatal. ■

Alert: Explain assessment and monitoring process to patient and family. Instruct them to immediately report difficulty breathing or other signs or symptoms of an adverse opioid-related reaction.

Alert: Encourage patient to report all medications being taken, including prescription and OTC medications and supplements.

Alert: Caution patient to immediately report signs and symptoms of serotonin syndrome, adrenal insufficiency, and decreased sex hormone levels.

• Encourage postoperative patient to turn, cough, deep-breathe, and use an incentive spirometer to prevent lung problems.

• Caution ambulatory patient about getting out of bed or walking. Warn outpatient to avoid driving and other potentially hazardous activities that require mental alertness until drug's CNS effects are known.

• Advise patient to avoid alcohol and sleep aids during therapy.

• Caution patient that drug isn't intended for long-term use.

• Tell patient who has been taking drug regularly not to stop drug abruptly and that dosage must be tapered gradually.

Alert: Counsel patient not to discontinue opioids without first discussing with prescriber the need for a gradual tapering regimen.

Reactions in bold italics are *life-threatening*. Interactions may have a *rapid onset* or a *delayed onset*.

mercaptopurine
(6-mercaptopurine, 6-MP) ▨
mer-kap-toe-PURE-een

Purinethol✦, Purixan

Therapeutic class: Antineoplastics
Pharmacologic class: Purine antagonists

AVAILABLE FORMS
Oral suspension: 20 mg/mL
Tablets (scored): 50 mg

INDICATIONS & DOSAGES
➤ **Acute lymphoblastic leukemia as part of a combination regimen**
Adults and children: After remission is attained, usual maintenance dose for adults and children is 1.5 to 2.5 mg/kg once daily.
▨ *Adjust-a-dose:* Reduce initial dosage in patients known to have homozygous thiopurine S-methyltransferase (TPMT) or nucleotide diphosphatase (NUDT15) deficiency. Patients with heterozygous TPMT or NUDT15 deficiency may require dosage reduction based on toxicities. Patients who are heterozygous for both TPMT and NUDT15 may require more substantial dosage reductions.

For patients with impaired renal function, begin with lower dosages. Consider reducing dosage in patients with impaired hepatic function.
➤ **Acute promyelocytic leukemia, maintenance ◆**
Adults: 60 mg/m^2/day for 1 year (in combination with tretinoin and methotrexate).

ADMINISTRATION
PO
• Drug is a hazardous agent; follow safe handling and disposal procedures.
• Give total daily dosage at one time, calculated to the nearest multiple of 25 mg.
• Give on an empty stomach.
• Give in the evening to reduce risk of relapse.
• Shake oral suspension vigorously for at least 30 seconds to ensure it's well mixed.
• Once opened, use oral suspension within 8 weeks.

ACTION
Inhibits RNA and DNA synthesis.

Route	Onset	Peak	Duration
PO	Unknown	<2 hr	Unknown

Half-life: Adults, 47 minutes; children, 21 minutes.

ADVERSE REACTIONS
CNS: malaise. **GI:** nausea, vomiting, anorexia, painful oral ulcers, diarrhea, *pancreatitis*, GI ulceration. **Hematologic:** *leukopenia, thrombocytopenia,* anemia, myelosuppression. **Hepatic:** jaundice, *hepatotoxicity, hepatic necrosis.* **Metabolic:** hyperuricemia. **Skin:** rash, hyperpigmentation, alopecia, urticaria.

INTERACTIONS
Drug-drug. *Allopurinol:* May cause mercaptopurine toxicity (bone marrow suppression, nausea, vomiting). Purixan product information recommends avoiding concomitant use.
Aminosalicylate derivatives (mesalamine, olsalazine, sulfasalazine): May increase risk of myelosuppression. Use lowest possible dosages of each drug and monitor patient closely.
Azathioprine: Increased risk of severe myelosuppression. Avoid giving together.
Febuxostat: May increase risk of toxicity. Use together is contraindicated.
Hepatotoxic drugs: May enhance hepatotoxicity of mercaptopurine. Monitor patient for hepatotoxicity.
Live-virus vaccines: May increase risk of toxicity from vaccine and infection. Consider therapy modification.
Myelosuppressants: May increase bone marrow suppression when combined with other drugs whose primary or secondary toxicity is myelosuppression. Monitor CBC and adjust dosage if indicated.
Nondepolarizing neuromuscular blockers: May antagonize muscle relaxant effect. Notify anesthesiologist that patient is receiving mercaptopurine.
Sulfamethoxazole–trimethoprim: May enhance bone marrow suppression. Monitor CBC with differential carefully.
Warfarin: May decrease anticoagulant effect. Monitor PT and INR.

M

Drug-herb. *Echinacea:* May diminish therapeutic effect of immunosuppressants. Consider therapy modification.

EFFECTS ON LAB TEST RESULTS
• May increase uric acid, transaminase, alkaline phosphatase, and bilirubin levels.
• May decrease Hb level.
• May decrease WBC, RBC, and platelet counts.

CONTRAINDICATIONS & CAUTIONS
• Contraindicated in patients resistant or hypersensitive to drug.
▨ Patients with TPMT or NUDT15 deficiency are more sensitive to drug's myelosuppressive defects. Consider TPMT phenotype and genotype testing and NUDT15 genotype testing for severe toxicities and excessive myelosuppression. Homozygous patients may need up to a 90% dosage reduction. Heterozygous patients may need up to a 50% dosage reduction. Patients who are heterozygous for both TPMT and NUDT15 may require more substantial dosage reductions.
• Drug can cause myelosuppression and hepatotoxicity.
• Drug may increase risk of secondary neoplasia.
• Use cautiously in elderly patients.
Dialyzable drug: Unlikely.
⚠ *Overdose S&S:* Anorexia, nausea, vomiting, diarrhea, myelosuppression, hepatic dysfunction, gastroenteritis.

PREGNANCY-LACTATION-REPRODUCTION
• Drug may cause fetal harm. Women of childbearing potential should avoid becoming pregnant during therapy.
• Drug may appear in human milk. Patient should discontinue breastfeeding or discontinue drug.

NURSING CONSIDERATIONS
• Monitor CBC and transaminase, alkaline phosphatase, and bilirubin levels weekly during induction and monthly during maintenance to monitor ANC, platelet count, and hepatic function to ensure sufficient drug exposure and to adjust for excessive toxicity.
• Consider modifying dosage after chemotherapy or radiation therapy in patients who have depressed neutrophil or platelet counts or impaired hepatic or renal function.
🕓 *Alert:* Drug may be ordered as "6-mercaptopurine" or as "6-MP." The numeral 6 is part of drug name and doesn't refer to dosage.
• Leukopenia, thrombocytopenia, or anemia may persist for several days after drug is stopped.
• Watch for signs of bleeding and infection.
🕓 *Alert:* Watch for jaundice, clay-colored stools, and frothy, dark urine. Hepatic dysfunction is reversible when drug is stopped. If right-sided abdominal tenderness occurs, stop drug and notify prescriber.
• Anticipate need for blood transfusions because of cumulative anemia.

PATIENT TEACHING
• Educate patient or caregivers on proper handling, storage, administration, and disposal of drug and how to clean up accidental spillage of the solution.
• Instruct patient to watch for signs and symptoms of infection (fever, sore throat, fatigue) and bleeding (easy bruising, nosebleeds, bleeding gums, tarry stools). Tell patient to take temperature daily.
• Advise patient to avoid dental work until blood counts have returned to normal.
• Caution female patient of childbearing potential to consult prescriber before becoming pregnant.
• Advise female patient to stop breastfeeding during therapy because of risk of toxicity to infant.

meropenem
mare-oh-PEN-em

Merrem

Therapeutic class: Antibiotics
Pharmacologic class: Carbapenems

AVAILABLE FORMS
Powder for injection: 500 mg, 1 g

INDICATIONS & DOSAGES
Adjust-a-dose (for all indications): For adults with CrCl of 26 to 50 mL/minute, give usual

dose every 12 hours. If CrCl is 10 to 25 mL/minute, give half usual dose every 12 hours; if CrCl is less than 10 mL/minute, give half usual dose every 24 hours.

➤ **Complicated skin and skin-structure infections from *Staphylococcus aureus* (methicillin-susceptible isolates only), *Streptococcus pyogenes*, *Streptococcus agalactiae*, viridans group streptococci, *Enterococcus faecalis* (excluding vancomycin-resistant isolates), *Escherichia coli*, *Proteus mirabilis*, *Bacteroides fragilis*, or *Peptostreptococcus* species**

Adults and children weighing more than 50 kg: 500 mg IV every 8 hours.
Children age 3 months and older weighing 50 kg or less: 10 mg/kg IV every 8 hours; maximum dose is 500 mg IV every 8 hours.

➤ **Complicated skin and skin-structure infections caused by *Pseudomonas aeruginosa***

Adults and children weighing more than 50 kg: 1 g IV every 8 hours.
Children age 3 months and older weighing 50 kg or less: 20 mg/kg IV every 8 hours; maximum dose is 1 g IV every 8 hours.

➤ **Complicated intra-abdominal infections (including appendicitis and peritonitis) caused by viridans group streptococci, *E. coli*, *Klebsiella pneumoniae*, *P. aeruginosa*, *B. fragilis*, *Bacteroides thetaiotaomicron*, or *Peptostreptococcus* species**

Adults and children weighing more than 50 kg: 1 g IV every 8 hours.
Children age 3 months and older weighing 50 kg or less: 20 mg/kg IV every 8 hours; maximum dose is 1 g IV every 8 hours.
Children 32 weeks' or more gestational age (GA) and 14 days or more postnatal age (PNA): 30 mg/kg IV every 8 hours over 30 minutes.
Children 32 weeks' or more GA and less than 14 days PNA: 20 mg/kg IV every 8 hours.
Children less than 32 weeks' GA and 14 days or more PNA: 20 mg/kg IV every 8 hours.
Children less than 32 weeks' GA and less than 14 days PNA: 20 mg/kg IV every 12 hours.

➤ **Bacterial meningitis caused by *S. pneumoniae*, *Haemophilus influenzae*, or *Neisseria meningitidis***

Children weighing more than 50 kg: 2 g IV every 8 hours.
Children age 3 months and older weighing 50 kg or less: 40 mg/kg IV every 8 hours; maximum dose, 2 g IV every 8 hours.

ADMINISTRATION

IV

▼ Obtain specimen for culture and sensitivity tests before giving first dose. Begin therapy while awaiting results.

ⓘ *Alert:* Serious hypersensitivity reactions may occur in patients receiving beta-lactams. Before therapy begins, determine if patient has had previous hypersensitivity reactions to penicillins, cephalosporins, beta-lactams, or other allergens. If an allergic reaction occurs, stop drug and notify prescriber. Serious anaphylactic reactions require emergency treatment.

▼ Use freshly prepared solutions of drug immediately whenever possible. Stability of drug varies with form of drug used (injection vial, infusion vial, or ADD-Vantage container).

▼ For bolus, add 10 mL of sterile water for injection to 500-mg vial or 20 mL to 1-g vial. Shake to dissolve, and let stand until clear. Give over 3 to 5 minutes. May be stored for up to 3 hours at up to 77° F (25° C) or for 13 hours at up to 41° F (5° C).

▼ For infusion, an infusion vial (500 mg/100 mL or 1 g/100 mL) may be directly reconstituted with a compatible infusion fluid. Or, an injection vial may be reconstituted and the resulting solution added to an IV container and further diluted with an appropriate infusion fluid. Don't use ADD-Vantage vials for this purpose. Give over 15 to 30 minutes.

▼ Solutions prepared with NSS at 1 to 20 mg/mL may be stored for 1 hour at up to 77° F (25° C) or 15 hours at up to 41° F (5° C); use solutions prepared with D₅W immediately.

▼ For ADD-Vantage vials, constitute only with half-NSS for injection, NSS for injection, or D₅W in 50-, 100-, or 250-mL Abbott ADD-Vantage flexible diluent

M

containers. Follow manufacturer's guidelines closely when using ADD-Vantage vials.

▼ **Incompatibilities:** Compatibility with other drugs hasn't been established. Don't mix with or physically add to solutions containing other drugs.

ACTION

Inhibits cell-wall synthesis in bacteria. Readily penetrates cell wall of most grampositive and gram-negative bacteria to reach penicillin-binding protein targets.

Route	Onset	Peak	Duration
IV	Unknown	1 hr	Unknown

Half-life: 1 to 1½ hours.

ADVERSE REACTIONS

CNS: headache. **CV:** phlebitis, thrombophlebitis, peripheral vascular disorder. **EENT:** oral candidiasis, pharyngitis. **GI:** *CDAD,* constipation, diarrhea, glossitis, nausea, vomiting. **GU:** hematuria. **Hematologic:** anemia. **Hepatic:** hyperbilirubinemia. **Respiratory:** *apnea,* pneumonia. **Skin:** injection-site inflammation, pruritus, rash. **Other:** *anaphylaxis, sepsis,* hypersensitivity reactions, inflammation, pain.

INTERACTIONS

Drug-drug. *Probenecid:* May decrease renal excretion of meropenem; probenecid competes with meropenem for active tubular secretion, which significantly increases elimination half-life of meropenem and extent of systemic exposure. Avoid using together.

Valproic acid: May decrease valproic acid levels, increasing the risk of breakthrough seizures. Monitor levels frequently, and observe patient for seizure activity. Consider alternative antibiotic or supplemental anticonvulsant therapy.

EFFECTS ON LAB TEST RESULTS

• May increase ALT, AST, bilirubin, alkaline phosphatase, LDH, creatinine, and BUN levels.

• May decrease Hb level and hematocrit.

• May increase eosinophil count. May decrease WBC count. May increase or decrease INR and platelet count. May prolong or shorten PT and PTT.

• May produce a positive Coombs test.

CONTRAINDICATIONS & CAUTIONS

• Contraindicated in patients hypersensitive to components of drug or other drugs in same class and in patients who have had anaphylactic reactions to beta-lactams.

• Use cautiously in elderly patients and in those with a history of brain lesions, seizure disorders, or impaired renal function.

• Severe cutaneous adverse reactions, such as SJS, toxic epidermal necrolysis, DRESS syndrome, erythema multiforme, and acute generalized exanthematous pustulosis, have been reported with meropenem use.

Dialyzable drug: Yes.

⚠ *Overdose S&S:* Exaggerated adverse reactions.

PREGNANCY-LACTATION-REPRODUCTION

• There are no adequate studies in pregnant women. Use during pregnancy only if clearly needed.

• Drug appears in human milk. Use cautiously in breastfeeding women.

NURSING CONSIDERATIONS

• In patients with CNS disorders, bacterial meningitis, and compromised renal function, drug may cause seizures and other CNS adverse reactions.

• If seizures occur during therapy, stop infusion and notify prescriber. Dosage adjustment may be needed.

• Monitor patient for signs and symptoms of superinfection. Drug may cause overgrowth of nonsusceptible bacteria or fungi.

• Periodic assessment of organ system functions, including renal, hepatic, and hematopoietic function, is recommended during prolonged therapy.

• Monitor patient's fluid balance and weight carefully.

• If patient develops signs and symptoms suggestive of a severe cutaneous reaction, stop drug immediately and consider an alternative treatment.

• CDAD may occur up to months after last dose and range from mild diarrhea to fatal colitis. If CDAD occurs, drug will need to be stopped and appropriate treatment begun.

PATIENT TEACHING
- Instruct patient to report adverse reactions or signs and symptoms of superinfection.
- Advise patient to report loose stools to prescriber.
- ❸ **Alert:** Advise patient to stop drug and notify prescriber if rash, peeling skin, trouble swallowing or breathing, or other signs and symptoms of allergic reaction occur.
- Caution patient drug can interfere with mental alertness. Caution patient not to operate motorized vehicles or machinery until tolerance is known.

---

mesalamine
me-SAL-a-meen

Apriso, Asacol HD, Canasa, Delzicol, Lialda, Mezavant,✢, Pentasa, Rowasa, Salofalk✢, sfRowasa

Therapeutic class: Anti-inflammatory drugs
Pharmacologic class: Salicylates

AVAILABLE FORMS
Capsules (controlled-release) 🐶: 250 mg, 375 mg, 500 mg
Capsules (delayed-release) 🐶: 400 mg, 800 mg
Rectal suspension: 2 g/60 mL✢, 4 g/60 mL, 1 g/100 mL✢, 4 g/100 mL✢
Suppositories: 500 mg✢, 1,000 mg
Tablets (delayed-release) 🐶: 400 mg✢, 800 mg, 1.2 g

INDICATIONS & DOSAGES
➤ **Active mild to moderate distal ulcerative colitis, proctitis, or proctosigmoiditis**
Adults: Two 400-mg tablets (800 mg) PO t.i.d. for total dose of 2.4 g daily for 6 weeks. Or, 1 g capsules PO q.i.d. for total dose of 4 g up to 8 weeks. Or, 1,000 mg suppository PR, retained in the rectum for 1 to 3 hours or longer, once daily at bedtime for 3 to 6 weeks. Or, 4 g retention enema once daily (preferably at bedtime); retain approximately 8 hours for 3 to 6 weeks.
➤ **Remission-induction of active, mild to moderate ulcerative colitis**
Lialda
Adults: Two to four 1.2-g tablets (2.4 g) PO once daily with a meal for up to 8 weeks.

Pentasa
Adults: Four 250-mg capsules or two 500-mg capsules (1 g) PO q.i.d. for a total dose of 4 g for up to 8 weeks.
Delzicol
Adults: 1.6 g daily in two to four divided doses.
➤ **Maintenance of remission of ulcerative colitis**
Adults: 1.5 g Apriso PO once daily in the morning. Or, two 1.2-g Lialda tablets PO once daily. Or, 1 g Pentasa PO q.i.d. Or, 1.6 g Delzicol PO in two to four divided doses.
➤ **Treatment of ulcerative colitis (Delzicol)**
Children age 5 and older weighing 54 to 90 kg: 27 to 44 mg/kg/day PO in two divided doses daily for 6 weeks. Maximum dose is 2.4 g/day.
Children age 5 and older weighing 33 to less than 54 kg: 37 to 61 mg/kg/day PO in two divided doses daily for 6 weeks. Maximum dose is 2 g/day.
Children age 5 and older weighing 17 to less than 33 kg: 36 to 71 mg/kg/day PO in two divided doses daily for 6 weeks. Maximum dose 1.2 g/day.

ADMINISTRATION
PO
- Give Lialda with food.
- Give Apriso with or without food. Don't give with antacids.
- Don't crush or cut delayed-release or controlled-release forms.
- Intact or partially intact tablets may be seen in stool. Notify prescriber if this occurs repeatedly.
- Give Asacol HD on an empty stomach at least 1 hour before or 2 hours after a meal.
- Give Delzicol with or without food.
- If patient is unable to swallow Pentasa capsules whole, they may be opened and the contents sprinkled on applesauce or yogurt and consumed immediately.
Rectal
- Patient should retain rectal enema dosage form overnight (for about 8 hours). Usual course of therapy for rectal form is 3 to 6 weeks.
- Shake suspension well before each use and remove sheath before inserting into rectum.

M

• Patient should retain suppository for 1 to 3 hours or longer, if possible.

ACTION
An active metabolite of sulfasalazine, drug probably acts topically by inhibiting prostaglandin production in the colon.

Route	Onset	Peak	Duration
PO, PR	Unknown	3–12 hr	Unknown

Half-life: About 5 to 10 hours.

ADVERSE REACTIONS
CNS: headache, dizziness, fever, fatigue, malaise, asthenia, insomnia, pain, vertigo, syncope, anxiety. **CV:** chest pain, peripheral edema, HTN. **EENT:** nasopharyngitis, pharyngitis, rhinitis, sinusitis. **GI:** abdominal pain, cramps, discomfort, flatulence, diarrhea, rectal pain, bloating, nausea, vomiting, dyspepsia, constipation, eructation, *hemorrhage.* **GU:** interstitial nephritis, hematuria, urinary frequency, nephropathy, *nephrotoxicity.* **Musculoskeletal:** arthralgia, myalgia, back pain, hypertonia. **Respiratory:** bronchitis, cough, dyspnea. **Skin:** itching, rash, acne, urticaria, hair loss. **Other:** chills, pain, flulike symptoms.

INTERACTIONS
Drug-drug. *Antacids, H₂ antagonists, PPIs:* May cause premature release of delayed- or extended-release products. Avoid concurrent administration. Consider therapy modification.
Azathioprine, mercaptopurine: May cause blood disorders. Monitor blood cell counts and adjust therapy as needed.
NSAIDs, other nephrotoxic agents: May enhance nephrotoxic effect of 5-aminosalicylic acid derivatives. Monitor renal function and adverse reactions.
Vaccines (varicella virus): May enhance adverse effect of varicella virus–containing vaccines, causing Reye syndrome. Consider therapy modification.
Warfarin: May decrease anticoagulation effect. Monitor effectiveness of therapy closely.

EFFECTS ON LAB TEST RESULTS
• May increase bilirubin, BUN, creatinine, AST, ALT, alkaline phosphatase, LDH, amylase, triglyceride, and lipase levels.

• May decrease Hb level and hematocrit and RBC and WBC counts.

CONTRAINDICATIONS & CAUTIONS
• Contraindicated in children and in patients allergic to mesalamine, sulfites (including sulfasalazine), any salicylates, or any component of the preparation.
• Use cautiously in elderly patients, in patients with renal or hepatic impairment, and in those taking nephrotoxic drugs.
Dialyzable drug: Unknown.
⚠ *Overdose S&S:* Confusion, diarrhea, headache, hyperventilation, diaphoresis, tinnitus, vertigo, vomiting.

PREGNANCY-LACTATION-REPRODUCTION
• There are no adequate studies in pregnant women. Use during pregnancy only if clearly needed.
• Drug appears in human milk. Use cautiously in breastfeeding women.

NURSING CONSIDERATIONS
• Monitor periodic renal function studies and blood cell counts in patients on long-term therapy.
• Because the mesalamine rectal suspension contains potassium metabisulfite, it may cause hypersensitivity reactions in patients sensitive to sulfites.
• Absorption of drug may be nephrotoxic.
• Drug may be associated with an acute intolerance syndrome in which signs and symptoms (abdominal pain, cramping, bloody diarrhea, headache, fever, rash) may be similar to an ulcerative colitis exacerbation. If acute intolerance syndrome is suspected, discontinue drug.
• Apriso contains phenylalanine.
• *Look alike–sound alike:* Don't confuse Asacol with Os-Cal; mesalamine with mecamylamine, megestrol, memantine, metaxalone, or methenamine; or Apriso with Apri or Lialda with Aldara.

PATIENT TEACHING
• Instruct patient to carefully follow instructions supplied with drug and to swallow tablets whole without crushing or chewing.
• Tell patient not to take drug with antacids.
• Advise patient to report all adverse reactions and to stop drug if fever or rash occurs.

Reactions in bold italics are *life-threatening*. Interactions may have a *rapid onset* or a *delayed onset*.

Patient intolerant of sulfasalazine may also be hypersensitive to mesalamine.
• Tell patient to remove foil wrapper from suppositories before inserting into rectum.
• Teach patient about proper use of retention enema.

SAFETY ALERT!

metFORMIN hydrochloride
met-FOR-min

Glucophage*◊*, Glucophage XR*◊*, Glumetza, Riomet

Therapeutic class: Antidiabetics
Pharmacologic class: Biguanides

AVAILABLE FORMS
Oral solution: 500 mg/5 mL
Tablets: 500 mg, 850 mg, 1,000 mg
Tablets (extended-release) ⓓⓝⓒ: 500 mg, 750 mg, 1,000 mg

INDICATIONS & DOSAGES
Adjust-a-dose (for all indications): Obtain patient's eGFR before starting drug. Contraindicated in patients with eGFR below 30 mL/minute/1.73 m². Starting drug in patients with eGFR between 30 and 45 mL/minute/1.73 m² isn't recommended. If eGFR falls below 45 mL/minute/1.73 m² in patients taking drug, assess benefits and risks of continuing treatment. Discontinue if eGFR falls below 30 mL/minute/1.73 m². Obtain eGFR at least annually in all patients taking drug. In patients at increased risk for development of renal impairment such as the elderly, assess renal function more frequently.

For elderly or debilitated patients, use conservative initial and maintenance dosage because of potential decrease in renal function. Adjust dosage carefully. Don't adjust to maximum dosage.
➤ **Adjunct to diet to lower glucose level in patients with type 2 diabetes**
Adults: If using immediate-release tablets or oral solution, initially 500 mg PO b.i.d. given with morning and evening meals, or 850 mg PO once daily given with morning meal. Titrate immediate-release forms in increments of 500 mg weekly or 850 mg every

other week to maximum dose of 2,550 mg PO daily in divided doses. If using extended-release formulation, start therapy at 500 mg PO once daily with the evening meal. May increase dose as tolerated weekly (every 1 to 2 weeks for Glumetza) in increments of 500 mg daily, up to a maximum dose of 2,000 mg once daily. If higher doses are required, consider a trial of 1,000 mg b.i.d. or using the regular-release formulation up to its maximum dose.
Children ages 10 and older: 500 mg PO b.i.d. using the immediate-release formulation only. Increase dosage in increments of 500 mg weekly up to a maximum of 2,000 mg daily in divided doses.
➤ **Prevention of type 2 diabetes in patients with prediabetes (impaired glucose tolerance, impaired fasting glucose, or an HbA₁c of 5.7% to 6.4%), especially those with BMI of more than 35 kg/m², those younger than age 60, and women with prior history of gestational diabetes or polycystic ovary syndrome** ✦
Adults: 850 mg immediate-release tablets PO once daily for 1 month; then increase to 850 mg b.i.d., unless GI adverse effects warrant a longer titration period.

ADMINISTRATION
PO
• Give drug with meals. Maximum doses may be better tolerated if total dose is divided and given in three doses with meals (immediate-release tablets only).
• Don't cut or crush extended-release tablets.

ACTION
Decreases hepatic glucose production and intestinal absorption of glucose and improves insulin sensitivity (increases peripheral glucose uptake and use).

Route	Onset	Peak	Duration
PO (conventional)	Unknown	2–3 hr	Unknown
PO (extended-release)	Unknown	4–8 hr	Unknown
PO (solution)	Unknown	2½ hr	Unknown

Half-life: About 4 to 9 hours.

ADVERSE REACTIONS
CNS: asthenia, headache, dizziness, chills, light-headedness. **CV:** chest discomfort,

M

palpitations. **EENT:** rhinitis. **GI:** diarrhea, nausea, vomiting, abdominal bloating, flatulence, anorexia, taste disorder, abnormal stools, constipation, dyspepsia, weight loss. **Metabolic:** *hypoglycemia.* **Musculoskeletal:** myalgia, limb pain. **Respiratory:** URI. **Skin:** flushing, nail disorder, diaphoresis. **Other:** accidental injury, infection.

INTERACTIONS

Drug-drug. *Beta blockers:* Hypoglycemia may be difficult to recognize in patients using beta blockers. Monitor patient and blood glucose.

Calcium channel blockers, corticosteroids, estrogens, fosphenytoin, hormonal contraceptives, isoniazid, nicotinic acid, phenothiazines, phenytoin, sympathomimetics, thiazide and other diuretics, thyroid drugs: May produce hyperglycemia. Monitor patient's glycemic control. Metformin dosage may need to be increased.

Cationic drugs (amiloride, cimetidine, digoxin, morphine, procainamide, quinidine, quinine, ranitidine, triamterene, trimethoprim, vancomycin): May compete for common renal tubular transport systems, which may increase metformin level. Monitor glucose level.

Dolutegravir: Increases metformin exposure. Total daily dose of metformin shouldn't exceed 1,000 mg. Closely monitor response to metformin.

Nifedipine: May increase metformin level. Monitor patient closely. Metformin dosage may need to be decreased.

QT interval–prolonging drugs (such as antiarrhythmics, chlorpromazine, citalopram, dolasetron): May have an additive effect on QT-interval prolongation. Coadminister with caution.

Black Box Warning *Radiologic contrast dye:* May cause acute renal failure or lactic acidosis. Withhold metformin at the time of or prior to the procedure and 48 hours after the procedure. Restart drug only after renal function is evaluated and found to be normal. ∎

Drug-herb. *Guar gum:* May decrease hypoglycemic effect. Discourage use together.

Drug-lifestyle. **Black Box Warning** *Alcohol use:* May increase drug effects and potentiate metformin's effect on lactate metabolism. Discourage use together. ∎

EFFECTS ON LAB TEST RESULTS
• May decrease vitamin B_{12} and Hb levels.

CONTRAINDICATIONS & CAUTIONS
• Contraindicated in patients hypersensitive to drug and in those with hepatic disease or metabolic acidosis or lactic acidosis, including diabetic ketoacidosis with or without coma.
• Not indicated for use in patients with type 1 diabetes mellitus or diabetic ketoacidosis.
• Contraindicated in patients with eGFR below 30 mL/minute/1.73 m². Not recommended in patients with eGFR between 30 and 45 mL/minute/1.73 m².

Black Box Warning Metformin-associated lactic acidosis has resulted in death, hypothermia, hypotension, and resistant bradyarrhythmias. Onset is often subtle, accompanied only by nonspecific symptoms, such as malaise, myalgias, respiratory distress, somnolence, and abdominal pain. It's characterized by elevated blood lactate levels (>5 mmol/L), anion gap acidosis (without evidence of ketonuria or ketonemia), an increased lactate/pyruvate ratio, and metformin plasma levels generally above 5 mcg/mL. Metformin decreases liver uptake of lactate, increasing lactate blood levels, which may increase the risk of lactic acidosis, especially in patients at risk. ∎

Black Box Warning Risk factors for metformin-associated lactic acidosis include renal impairment, concomitant use of certain drugs, age 65 and older, having a radiologic study with contrast, surgery and other procedures, hypoxic states, excessive alcohol intake, and hepatic impairment. ∎

Black Box Warning Discontinue drug in the setting of acute CHF (particularly when accompanied by hypoperfusion and hypoxemia), CV collapse (shock), acute MI, sepsis, and other conditions associated with hypoxemia that have been associated with lactic acidosis and may cause prerenal azotemia. ∎

Black Box Warning Avoid using drug in patients with clinical or lab evidence of hepatic disease. ∎

Reactions in bold italics are *life-threatening*. Interactions may have a *rapid onset* or a ***delayed onset***.

• Administration of Glumetza with an insulin secretagogue (e.g., sulfonylurea) or insulin may require lower doses of the insulin secretagogue or insulin to reduce risk of hypoglycemia.

• Use cautiously in elderly, debilitated, or malnourished patients and in those with adrenal or pituitary insufficiency because of increased risk of hypoglycemia.

Dialyzable drug: Yes.

⚠ *Overdose S&S:* Hypoglycemia, lactic acidosis.

PREGNANCY-LACTATION-REPRODUCTION

• Abnormal blood glucose levels during pregnancy may cause fetal harm. Most experts recommend that insulin be used during pregnancy to maintain blood glucose levels as close to normal as possible. Use metformin during pregnancy only if clearly needed.

• Drug appears in human milk. Patient should discontinue breastfeeding or discontinue drug, taking into account importance of drug to the mother and risk of hypoglycemia in the infant. Consider insulin therapy.

NURSING CONSIDERATIONS

• Before therapy begins and at least annually thereafter, assess patient's renal function. Assess more frequently in patients at risk for renal impairment.

Black Box Warning If metformin-associated lactic acidosis is suspected, immediately discontinue drug and promptly institute general supportive measures in a hospital setting. Prompt hemodialysis is recommended, which has often resulted in reversal of symptoms and recovery. ∎

Black Box Warning Consider more frequent monitoring of patients taking drugs that may increase the risk of metformin-associated lactic acidosis, including drugs that impair renal function, result in significant hemodynamic change, interfere with acid-base balance, or increase metformin accumulation. ∎

• When switching patients from chlorpropamide to metformin, take care during the first 2 weeks of metformin therapy because the prolonged retention of chlorpropamide increases the risk of hypoglycemia during this time.

• Monitor patient's glucose level regularly to evaluate effectiveness of therapy. Notify prescriber if glucose level increases despite therapy.

• If patient hasn't responded to 4 weeks of therapy with maximum dosage, an oral sulfonylurea can be added while keeping metformin at maximum dosage. If patient still doesn't respond after several months of therapy with both drugs at maximum dosage, prescriber may stop both and start insulin therapy.

• Monitor patient closely during times of increased stress, such as infection, fever, surgery, or trauma. Insulin therapy may be needed in these situations.

Black Box Warning Stop drug at the time of, or before, an iodinated contrast imaging procedure in patients with an eGFR between 30 and 60 mL/minute/1.73 m^2; in patients with a history of hepatic impairment, alcoholism, or HF; or in patients who will be administered intra-arterial iodinated contrast. Reevaluate eGFR 48 hours after the imaging procedure; restart drug if renal function is stable. ∎

Black Box Warning Temporarily discontinue drug in patients with restricted food and fluid intake due to surgery or other procedures because of increased risk of volume depletion, hypotension, and renal impairment. ∎

• Monitor patient's hematologic status for evidence of megaloblastic anemia. Patients with inadequate vitamin B$_{12}$ or calcium intake or absorption appear to be predisposed to developing subnormal vitamin B$_{12}$ level. These patients should have routine vitamin B$_{12}$ level determinations every 2 to 3 years.

• *Look alike–sound alike:* Don't confuse Glucophage with Glucovance or Glucotrol; don't confuse metformin with metronidazole.

PATIENT TEACHING

• Instruct patient about nature of diabetes and importance of following therapeutic regimen, adhering to specific diet, losing weight, getting exercise, following personal hygiene programs, and avoiding infection. Explain how and when to monitor glucose level. Teach evidence of low and high glucose levels. Explain emergency measures.

Black Box Warning Instruct patient to stop drug and immediately notify prescriber about unexplained hyperventilation, muscle pain, malaise, dizziness, light-headedness, unusual sleepiness, unexplained stomach pain, feeling of coldness, slow or irregular HR, or other nonspecific symptoms of early lactic acidosis. ∎

Black Box Warning Warn patient against excessive alcohol intake while taking drug. ∎

• Tell patient not to change drug dosage without prescriber's knowledge. Encourage patient to report abnormal glucose level test results.

🌢 *Alert:* Advise patient not to cut, crush, or chew extended-release tablets; instruct patient to swallow them whole.

• Tell patient that inactive ingredients may be eliminated in the stool as a soft mass resembling the original tablet.

• Advise patient not to take other drugs, including OTC drugs, without first checking with prescriber.

• Instruct patient to carry medical identification at all times.

• Tell patient to report all adverse reactions and that diarrhea, nausea, and upset stomach generally subside over time.

SAFETY ALERT!

methadone hydrochloride⌀
METH-a-done

Dolophine, Metadol❋, Metadol-D❋, Methadose

Therapeutic class: Opioid analgesics
Pharmacologic class: Opioid agonists
Controlled substance schedule: II

AVAILABLE FORMS
Dispersible tablets and diskets (for methadone maintenance therapy): 40 mg
Injection: 10 mg/mL
Oral solution: 1 mg/mL❋, 5 mg/5 mL, 10 mg/5 mL, 10 mg/mL (concentrate)
Tablets: 1 mg❋, 5 mg, 10 mg, 25 mg❋

INDICATIONS & DOSAGES
Adjust-a-dose (for all indications): For elderly patients and those with renal or hepatic impairment, reduce initial dose.

➤ **Severe pain in opioid nontolerant patients**
Adults: Initiate dosing regimen for each patient individually, taking into account patient's prior analgesic treatment experience and risk factors for addiction, abuse, and misuse. Initially, 2.5 mg PO every 8 to 12 hours, or 2.5 to 10 mg IM, IV, or subcut every 8 to 12 hours. Titrate slowly, no more frequently than every 3 to 5 days, and increase dosage as needed or use rescue drug as needed to maintain analgesia.

➤ **Opioid detoxification; maintenance treatment of opioid addiction**
Adults: Initially, 20 to 30 mg PO daily to suppress withdrawal symptoms (highly individualized; some patients may require a higher dose). Initial dose shouldn't exceed 30 mg. Maintenance dose is 80 to 120 mg PO daily. Adjust dosage as needed.

ADMINISTRATION
PO
• Oral form legally required in maintenance programs. Completely dissolve dispersible tablets, disket, or oral solution in 4 oz (120 mL) of water, orange juice, or other acidic fruit beverage.
• Oral dose is half as potent as injected dose.

IV
▼ Store at controlled room temperature (59° to 86° F [15° to 30° C]).
▼ Protect from light.
▼ **Incompatibilities:** None listed by manufacturer. Consult a drug incompatibility reference for more information.

IM
• For parenteral use, IM injection is preferred. Rotate injection sites. Monitor site as local tissue reactions may occur.
• Store at controlled room temperature (59° to 86° F [15° to 30° C]).
• Protect from light.

Subcutaneous
• Monitor patient for pain at injection site, tissue irritation, and induration after injection.
• Store at controlled room temperature (59° to 86° F [15° to 30° C]).
• Protect from light.

Reactions in bold italics are *life-threatening*. Interactions may have a *rapid onset* or a *delayed onset*.

ACTION

Unknown. Binds with opioid receptors in the CNS, altering perception of and emotional response to pain.

Route	Onset	Peak	Duration
PO	30–60 min	1–7½ hr	4–8 hr
IV	Unknown	Unknown	4–8 hr
IM, subcut	10–20 min	1–2 hr	4–8 hr

Half-life: 8 to 59 hours.

ADVERSE REACTIONS

CNS: clouded sensorium, hallucinations, dizziness, light-headedness, sedation, somnolence, *seizures,* agitation, euphoria, headache, insomnia, syncope. **CV:** *arrhythmias, bradycardia, prolonged QT interval, cardiac arrest, shock, cardiomyopathy, HF,* flushing, phlebitis, edema, hypotension, palpitations. **EENT:** visual disturbances. **GI:** nausea, vomiting, abdominal pain, anorexia, biliary tract spasm, constipation, dry mouth, glossitis, ileus. **GU:** urine retention. **Metabolic:** hypokalemia, *hypomagnesemia,* weight gain. **Respiratory:** *respiratory arrest, respiratory depression, pulmonary edema.* **Skin:** diaphoresis, pruritus, urticaria. **Other:** decreased libido, induration, pain at injection site, physical dependence, tissue irritation.

INTERACTIONS

Drug-drug. *Ammonium chloride, other urine acidifiers:* May reduce methadone effect. Watch for decreased pain control.
Black Box Warning *Benzodiazepines, other CNS depressants (antipsychotics, anxiolytics, general anesthetics, hypnotics, MAO inhibitors, muscle relaxants, TCAs, tranquilizers):* May cause respiratory depression, hypotension, profound sedation, coma, or death. If alternative treatment options are inadequate, monitor patient closely and consider delaying or omitting daily methadone dosing for signs and symptoms of respiratory depression and sedation. ▮
Black Box Warning *CYP2B6, CYP2C9, CYP2C19, CYP2D6, or CYP3A4 inhibitors (all); CYP2B6, CYP2C9, CYP2C19, or CYP3A4 inducers:* Concomitant use of inhibitors and discontinuation of inducers may cause increased methadone plasma concentrations, resulting in potentially fatal

respiratory depression. Monitor patient closely and reduce methadone dosage if necessary. ▮
Black Box Warning *CYP2B6, CYP2C9, CYP2C19, or CYP3A4 inducers; CYP2B6, CYP2C9, CYP2C19, CYP2D6, or CYP3A4 inhibitors:* Adding inducers concomitantly with methadone or stopping inhibitors may decrease methadone effect and precipitate a withdrawal syndrome. Monitor patient closely. ▮
NNRTIs (delavirdine, efavirenz, nevirapine), protease inhibitors (lopinavir–ritonavir, nelfinavir, ritonavir), rifamycins: May increase methadone metabolism, causing opioid withdrawal symptoms. Monitor patient and adjust dose as needed.
Black Box Warning *Opioids:* May cause slow or difficult breathing, sedation, and death. Avoid use together. If use together is necessary, limit dosage and duration of each drug to the minimum necessary for desired effect. ▮
Protease inhibitors, cimetidine, fluvoxamine: May increase respiratory and CNS depression. Monitor patient closely.
☉ Alert: *Serotonergic drugs (amoxapine, antiemetics [dolasetron, granisetron, ondansetron, palonosetron], antimigraine drugs, buspirone, cyclobenzaprine, dextromethorphan, linezolid, lithium, MAO inhibitors, maprotiline, methylene blue, mirtazapine, nefazodone, SSNRIs, SSRIs, TCAs, trazodone, tryptophan, vilazodone):* May increase risk of serotonin syndrome. Use together cautiously and monitor patient for serotonin syndrome.
Black Box Warning *QT interval–prolonging drugs (such as antiarrhythmics, chlorpromazine, citalopram, dolasetron):* May increase risk of QT-interval prolongation and ventricular arrhythmias. Use with extreme caution. ▮
Drug-herb. ☉ Alert: *St. John's wort:* May reduce methadone effect and precipitate a withdrawal syndrome. May increase risk of serotonin syndrome. Use together cautiously and monitor patient closely.
Drug-lifestyle. **Black Box Warning** *Alcohol use:* May cause death. Use together is contraindicated. ▮

M

EFFECTS ON LAB TEST RESULTS
• May increase amylase level.

CONTRAINDICATIONS & CAUTIONS
• Contraindicated in patients hypersensitive to drug and in those with significant respiratory depression, acute or severe bronchial asthma in an unmonitored setting or in the absence of resuscitative equipment, or known or suspected GI obstruction, including paralytic ileus.

Black Box Warning Respiratory depression, including fatal cases, has been reported during initiation and conversion of patients to methadone, even when drug has been used as recommended and not misused or abused. Proper dosing and titration are essential and drug should only be prescribed by health care professionals knowledgeable in the use of methadone for detoxification and maintenance treatment of opioid addiction. Monitor patient for respiratory depression, especially during initiation or after a dosage increase. ∎

Black Box Warning Accidental ingestion of methadone, especially in children, can result in a fatal overdose of methadone. ∎

Black Box Warning Prolonged QT interval and serious arrhythmia (torsades de pointes) have occurred during methadone treatment. Most cases involve patients being treated for pain with large, multiple daily doses, although cases have been reported in patients receiving doses commonly used for maintenance treatment of opioid addiction. ∎

Black Box Warning Opioids should only be prescribed with benzodiazepines or other CNS depressants to patients for whom alternative treatment options are inadequate. ∎

❸ *Alert:* Drug may lead to a rare but serious decrease in adrenal gland cortisol production.

❸ *Alert:* The combined use of medication-assisted treatment (MAT) drugs methadone or buprenorphine with benzodiazepines or other CNS depressants increases the risk of serious adverse effects; however, the harm caused by untreated opioid addiction may outweigh these risks. Patients may require MAT for opioid addiction indefinitely and its use should continue for as long as patients are benefiting and the use of MAT contributes to the intended treatment goals.

❸ *Alert:* Drug may cause decreased sex hormone levels with long-term use.

• Use cautiously in elderly or debilitated patients and in those with severe hepatic or renal impairment, hypothyroidism, Addison disease, prostatic hyperplasia, urethral stricture, head injury, increased ICP, and respiratory conditions.

❸ *Alert:* Patients are at increased risk for oversedation and respiratory depression if they snore or have a history of sleep apnea, haven't used opioids recently or are first-time opioid users, have increased opioid dosage requirements or opioid habituation, have received general anesthesia for longer lengths of time or received other sedating drugs, have preexisting pulmonary or cardiac disease, or have thoracic or other surgical incisions that may impair breathing. Monitor patients carefully.

❸ *Alert:* Drug isn't indicated as a p.r.n. analgesic.

Dialyzable drug: No.

⚠ *Overdose S&S:* Miosis, respiratory depression, somnolence, coma, cool clammy skin, skeletal muscle flaccidity, hypotension, apnea, bradycardia, noncardiac pulmonary edema, death.

PREGNANCY-LACTATION-REPRODUCTION
• Use drug during pregnancy only if potential benefit justifies risk to the fetus. Methadone clearance may increase during pregnancy, particularly during second and third trimesters. Dosage may need to be increased or dosing interval decreased. Use lowest possible dosage.

Black Box Warning Prolonged use during pregnancy can cause neonatal opioid withdrawal syndrome, which can be life-threatening and requires management by neonatology experts. If use is required for a prolonged period during pregnancy, apprise patient of the risk and ensure that appropriate treatment will be available. ∎

• Drug appears in human milk. Sedation and respiratory depression in breastfeeding infants have been reported. Monitor infants for respiratory depression and sedation and slowly wean to prevent withdrawal symptoms.

• When methadone is used to treat opioid addiction in breastfeeding women, and if

---

additional illicit substances are being abused, patient should express and discard human milk until sobriety is established.

• Long-term opioid use may cause secondary hypogonadism, which may lead to sexual dysfunction or infertility.

• Advise patients who developed amenorrhea secondary to substance abuse that pregnancy may occur after initiation of methadone maintenance treatment. Provide contraception counseling to prevent unplanned pregnancies.

NURSING CONSIDERATIONS

Black Box Warning Methadone is an opioid agonist and Schedule II controlled substance with an abuse liability similar to that of other opioid agonists, legal or illicit. Assess each patient's risk of opioid abuse or addiction before prescribing methadone. Risk of opioid abuse increases in patients with personal or family history of substance abuse (including drug or alcohol abuse or addiction) or mental illness (such as major depressive disorder). Routinely monitor all patients receiving methadone for signs and symptoms of misuse, abuse, and addiction during treatment. ▮

Black Box Warning Oral methadone can only be dispensed by certified treatment programs or during inpatient care for conditions other than concurrent opioid addiction. ▮

Black Box Warning Respiratory depression that can be life-threatening or fatal, QT-interval prolongation, and torsades de pointes have been observed during treatment. Be vigilant during treatment initiation and dosage titration. ▮

Black Box Warning Carefully monitor vital signs, pain level, respiratory status, and sedation level in all patients receiving opioids, especially those receiving IV drugs, even when given postoperatively. ▮

Black Box Warning Caution patient or caregiver of patient taking an opioid with a benzodiazepine, CNS depressant, or alcohol to seek immediate medical attention for dizziness, light-headedness, extreme sleepiness, slowed or difficult breathing, or unresponsiveness. ▮

⊕ Alert: If patient is taking opioids with serotonergic drugs, watch for signs and symptoms of serotonin syndrome (agitation,

hallucinations, rapid HR, fever, excessive sweating, shivering or shaking, muscle twitching or stiffness, trouble with coordination, nausea, vomiting, diarrhea), especially when starting treatment or increasing dosages. Signs and symptoms may occur within several hours of coadministration but may also occur later, especially after dosage increase. Discontinue the opioid, serotonergic drug, or both if serotonin syndrome is suspected.

⊕ Alert: Work with patient to develop strategies to manage the use of prescribed or illicit benzodiazepines or other CNS depressants when starting MAT. Taper benzodiazepine or CNS depressant to discontinuation if possible.

⊕ Alert: If patient is receiving prescribed benzodiazepines or other CNS depressants for anxiety or insomnia, verify the diagnosis and consider other treatment options for these conditions if possible.

⊕ Alert: Coordinate care to ensure other prescribers are aware of patient's MAT.

⊕ Alert: Monitor patient for illicit drug use, including urine or blood screening.

⊕ Alert: Monitor patient for signs and symptoms of adrenal insufficiency (nausea, vomiting, loss of appetite, fatigue, weakness, dizziness, low BP). Perform diagnostic testing if adrenal insufficiency is suspected. If adrenal insufficiency is confirmed, treat with corticosteroids and wean patient off opioids if appropriate. Discontinue corticosteroids when clinically appropriate.

⊕ Alert: Monitor patient for signs and symptoms of decreased sex hormone levels (low libido, erectile dysfunction, amenorrhea, infertility). If signs and symptoms occur, evaluate patient and obtain lab testing.

• Reassess patient's level of pain at least 15 and 30 minutes after parenteral administration and 30 minutes after oral administration.

Black Box Warning When used for detoxification and maintenance of opioid dependence, treatment products in oral form shall be dispensed only by opioid treatment programs. Administer in accordance with treatment standards cited in 42 CFR (Code of Federal Regulations) Section 8, including limitations on unsupervised administration. Dispensing hospitals and pharmacies are

M

approved by the FDA and designated state authorities. ■

• An around-the-clock regimen is needed to manage severe, chronic pain.

• Patients treated in methadone maintenance program usually need an additional analgesic if pain control is needed.

• Monitor patient closely because drug has cumulative effect; marked sedation can occur after repeated doses.

• Monitor circulatory and respiratory status and bladder and bowel function. Patient may need a stool softener and stimulant laxative.

◐ *Alert:* Respiratory depressant effects may last longer than analgesic effects. Monitor patient's respiratory status closely.

• When used as an adjunct in the treatment of opioid addiction (maintenance), withdrawal is usually delayed and mild.

◐ *Alert:* Use caution when dosing. Confusion has occurred between milliliter and milligram doses.

◐ *Alert:* Don't stop drug abruptly; withdraw slowly and individualize gradual taper plan to prevent signs and symptoms of withdrawal, worsening pain, and psychological distress in physically dependent patients. Refer to manufacturer's label for specific tapering instructions.

◐ *Alert:* When tapering opioids, monitor patient closely for signs and symptoms of opioid withdrawal (restlessness, lacrimation, rhinorrhea, yawning, perspiration, chills, myalgia, mydriasis, irritability, anxiety, insomnia, backache, joint pain, weakness, abdominal cramps, anorexia, nausea, vomiting, diarrhea, increased BP or HR, increased respiratory rate), which may indicate a need to taper more slowly. Also monitor patient for suicidal thoughts, use of other substances, and mood changes.

• *Look alike–sound alike:* Don't confuse methadone with ketorolac, methylphenidate, dexmethylphenidate, and Mephyton.

PATIENT TEACHING

◐ *Alert:* Explain assessment and monitoring process to patient and family. Instruct them to immediately report difficulty breathing or other signs or symptoms of a potential adverse opioid-related reaction.

◐ *Alert:* Encourage patient to report all medications being taken, including prescription and OTC medications and supplements.

◐ *Alert:* Caution patient to immediately report signs and symptoms of serotonin syndrome, adrenal insufficiency, and decreased sex hormone levels.

◐ *Alert:* Teach patient not to take nonprescribed benzodiazepines, sedatives, or alcohol when taking MAT due to the increased risk of overdose and death.

◐ *Alert:* Advise patient to notify all prescribers of MAT and not to stop MAT or other prescribed drugs without first consulting prescriber.

• Caution ambulatory patient about getting out of bed or walking. Warn outpatient to avoid hazardous activities that require mental alertness until drug's CNS effects are known.

Black Box Warning Advise patient to keep drug out of reach of children. Accidental ingestion can result in fatal methadone overdose. ■

• Instruct patient to increase fluid and fiber in diet, if not contraindicated, to combat constipation.

• Advise patient to avoid alcohol during therapy.

• Instruct breastfeeding patient to monitor infant for respiratory depression and sedation; advise her when to contact health care provider for emergency care.

• Caution patients not to use CNS depressants during initiation of treatment with methadone.

◐ *Alert:* Counsel patient not to discontinue opioids without first discussing with prescriber the need for a gradual tapering regimen.

methIMAzole
meth-IM-a-zole

Tapazole

Therapeutic class: Antihyperthyroid drugs
Pharmacologic class: Thyroid hormone antagonists

AVAILABLE FORMS
Tablets: 5 mg, 10 mg

INDICATIONS & DOSAGES
➤ **Hyperthyroidism**
Adults: If mild, 15 mg PO daily in three divided doses given at 8-hour intervals. If moderately severe, 30 to 40 mg daily in three divided doses given at 8-hour intervals. If severe, 60 mg daily in three divided doses given at 8-hour intervals. Maintenance dosage is 5 to 15 mg daily.
Children: 0.4 mg/kg/day PO in three divided doses given at 8-hour intervals. Maintenance dosage is 0.2 mg/kg/day in three divided doses daily.

ADMINISTRATION
PO
• Hazardous drug; use gloves to administer intact tablets.

ACTION
Inhibits synthesis of thyroid hormones.

Route	Onset	Peak	Duration
PO	Rapid	1–2 hr	36–72 hr

Half-life: 4 to 6 hours.

ADVERSE REACTIONS
CNS: headache, drowsiness, vertigo, paresthesia, neuritis, CNS stimulation, fever.
CV: edema. **GI:** nausea, vomiting, salivary gland enlargement, loss of taste, epigastric distress. **Hematologic:** *agranulocytosis, leukopenia, thrombocytopenia, aplastic anemia.* **Hepatic:** jaundice, hepatic dysfunction, *hepatitis.* **Metabolic:** hypothyroidism, *hypoglycemic coma.* **Musculoskeletal:** arthralgia, myalgia. **Skin:** rash, urticaria, discoloration, pruritus, lupuslike syndrome, abnormal hair loss. **Other:** lymphadenopathy.

INTERACTIONS
Drug-drug. *Aminophylline, theophylline:* May decrease clearance of these drugs. Dosage may need adjustment.
Beta blockers: Beta-blocker clearance may be enhanced by hyperthyroidism. Dosage of beta blocker may need to be reduced when patient becomes euthyroid.
Cardiac glycosides: May increase cardiac glycoside level. Cardiac glycoside dosage may need to be reduced.

Potassium iodide: May decrease response to drug. Methimazole dosage may need to be increased.
Warfarin: May alter dosage requirements. Monitor PT and INR, and adjust warfarin dosage as needed.

EFFECTS ON LAB TEST RESULTS
• May increase LFT values and PT.
• May decrease Hb level and granulocyte, WBC, and platelet counts.
• May alter thyroid uptake of ^{123}I or ^{131}I.

CONTRAINDICATIONS & CAUTIONS
• Contraindicated in patients hypersensitive to drug.
• Drug may cause hypoprothrombinemia and bleeding. Monitor patient for bleeding.
Dialyzable drug: No.
⚠ **Overdose S&S:** Nausea, vomiting, epigastric distress, headache, fever, joint pain, pruritus, edema, aplastic anemia, agranulocytosis, hepatitis, nephrotic syndrome, exfoliative dermatitis, neuropathies, CNS stimulation or depression.

PREGNANCY-LACTATION-REPRODUCTION
• Drug may cause fetal harm, particularly in first trimester; consider other agents during this time. If used during pregnancy or if patient becomes pregnant during therapy, apprise her of potential hazard to the fetus.
• Pregnant women may need lower doses as pregnancy progresses, and drug may be stopped during last few weeks of pregnancy. Monitor thyroid function studies closely.
• Drug appears in human milk. Use cautiously and administer after breastfeeding and in divided doses.

NURSING CONSIDERATIONS
• Monitor CBC periodically to detect impending leukopenia, thrombocytopenia, aplastic anemia, and agranulocytosis; also monitor hepatic function. Stop drug if liver abnormality occurs.
🕓 **Alert:** Doses higher than 40 mg daily increase risk of agranulocytosis, which can be life-threatening. Monitor patient for sore throat, fever, and general malaise and report symptoms promptly.
• Watch for evidence of hypothyroidism (mental depression, cold intolerance, and

M

hard, nonpitting edema); notify prescriber because patient may need dosage adjustment.

⚠️ **Alert:** Stop drug and notify prescriber if severe rash or enlarged cervical lymph nodes develop.

• **Look alike–sound alike:** Don't confuse methimazole with mebendazole, methazolamide, metolazone, or metronidazole.

PATIENT TEACHING

• Warn patient to report fever, sore throat, mouth sores, skin eruptions, anorexia, itching, right upper quadrant pain, or yellow skin or eyes.

• Tell patient to ask prescriber about using iodized salt and eating shellfish because the iodine in these foods may make the drug less effective.

• Warn patient that drug may cause drowsiness; advise patient to use caution when operating machinery or a vehicle.

• Instruct patient to store drug in light-resistant container.

• Teach patient to watch for evidence of hypothyroidism (unexplained weight gain, fatigue, cold intolerance) and to notify prescriber if it arises.

SAFETY ALERT!

methotrexate (amethopterin)
meth-oh-TREKS-ate

Otrexup, Rasuvo, Xatmep

methotrexate sodium
Trexall, Metoject❖

Therapeutic class: Antineoplastics
Pharmacologic class: Folate antagonists

AVAILABLE FORMS

Autoinjector: 7.5 mg/0.15 mL, 7.5 mg/ 0.75 mL❖, 10 mg/mL❖, 10 mg/0.2 mL, 10 mg/0.4 mL, 12.5 mg/0.25 mL, 12.5 mg/ 0.4 mL, 15 mg/1.5 mL❖, 15 mg/0.3 mL, 15 mg/0.4 mL, 17.5 mg/0.35 mL, 17.5 mg/ 0.4 mL, 20 mg/0.4 mL, 22.5 mg/0.4 mL, 22.5 mg/0.45 mL, 25 mg/0.4 mL, 25 mg/ 0.5 mL, 30 mg/0.6 mL

Injection: 25 mg/mL preservative-free vials; 25 mg/mL in 2-mL and 10-mL vials containing benzyl alcohol
Lyophilized powder: 1,000-mg preservative-free vials
Oral solution: 2.5 mg/mL
Tablets: 2.5 mg, 5 mg, 7.5 mg, 10 mg, 15 mg

INDICATIONS & DOSAGES

Adjust-a-dose (for all indications): Reduce dosage in patients with impaired renal function.

➤ **Trophoblastic tumors (choriocarcinoma, hydatidiform mole) (except Otrexup, Rasuvo)**

Adults: 15 to 30 mg PO or IM daily for 5 days. Repeat after 1 or more weeks, based on response or toxicity. Number of courses is three to maximum of five.

➤ **Acute lymphocytic leukemia (except Otrexup, Rasuvo)**

Adults and children: 3.3 mg/m^2 daily PO (tablets), IV, or IM with 60 mg/m^2 prednisone daily for 4 to 6 weeks or until remission occurs; then 30 mg/m^2 PO or IM weekly in two divided doses or 2.5 mg/kg IV every 14 days. Or, for oral solution use in children, give 20 mg/m^2 once weekly.

➤ **Meningeal leukemia (except Otrexup, Rasuvo)**

Adults and children age 3 and older: 12 mg intrathecally every 2 to 5 days until CSF is normal.
Children ages 2 to younger than 3: 10 mg intrathecally every 2 to 5 days.
Children ages 1 to younger than 2: 8 mg intrathecally every 2 to 5 days.
Children younger than age 1: 6 mg intrathecally every 2 to 5 days.

➤ **Lymphoma (Burkitt tumor stage I, II) (except Otrexup, Rasuvo)**

Adults: 10 to 25 mg PO daily for 4 to 8 days, with 7- to 10-day rest intervals; commonly given with other agents.

➤ **Lymphosarcoma (stage III) (except Otrexup, Rasuvo)**

Adults: 0.625 to 2.5 mg/kg daily PO, IM, or IV; commonly given with other agents.

➤ **Osteosarcoma (except Otrexup, Rasuvo)**

Adults: Initially, 12 g/m^2 IV (maximum dose, 20 g) as 4-hour infusion. If dose isn't sufficient to produce peak serum

---

Reactions in bold italics are *life-threatening*. Interactions may have a *rapid onset* or a *delayed onset*.

methotrexate concentration of 1,000 mcM (10^{-3} mol/L), may increase subsequent doses to 15 g/m^2 IV, as 4-hour IV infusion at postoperative weeks 4, 5, 6, 7, 11, 12, 15, 16, 29, 30, 44, and 45. Give with leucovorin, 15 mg PO every 6 hours for 10 doses, beginning 24 hours after start of methotrexate infusion.

➤ **Mycosis fungoides (except Otrexup, Rasuvo)**
Adults: 5 to 50 mg PO or IM once weekly; if poor response, may increase to 15 to 37.5 mg IM twice weekly.

➤ **Psoriasis**
Adults: 10 to 25 mg PO, IM, IV, or subcut as single weekly dose; or 2.5 to 5 mg PO every 12 hours for three doses weekly. Dosage shouldn't exceed 30 mg/week.

➤ **RA**
Adults: Initially, 7.5 mg PO, IM, or subcut weekly, either in single dose or divided as 2.5 mg PO every 12 hours for three doses once weekly. Dosage may be gradually increased to maximum of 20 mg weekly.

➤ **Polyarticular course, juvenile RA**
Children and adolescents age 2 to 16: 10 mg/m^2 PO, IM, or subcut once weekly. Or, 20 to 30 mg/m^2/week IM or subcut.

➤ **Crohn disease ◆**
Adults: 25 mg IM or subcut once weekly; may reduce to 15 mg once weekly if steroid-free remission is maintained for 4 months.

ADMINISTRATION
PO
• Give drug on an empty stomach.
• Use an accurate measuring device to measure oral solution.
IV
▼ Preparing and giving parenteral drug may be mutagenic, teratogenic, or carcinogenic. Follow facility policy to reduce risks.
▼ Dilution of drug depends on product, and infusion guidelines vary, depending on dose.
▼ Reconstitute 20-mg vial to a concentration no greater than 25 mg/mL. Reconstitute 1-g vial with 19.4 mL of diluent to obtain a concentration of 50 mg/mL.
▼ If giving infusion, dilute total dose in D$_5$W.

▼ Reconstitute solutions without preservatives with NSS or D$_5$W immediately before use, and discard unused drug.
▼ For methotrexate therapy with leucovorin rescue, patients should be well hydrated. Administer 1 L/m^2 of IV fluids over 6 hours before initiation of methotrexate infusion. Continue hydration at 125 mL/m^2/hour during the methotrexate infusion and for 2 days after infusion has been completed.
▼ **Incompatibilities:** None listed by manufacturer. Consult a drug incompatibility reference for more information.
IM
• Preparing and giving parenteral drug may be mutagenic, teratogenic, or carcinogenic. Follow facility policy to reduce risks.
Subcutaneous
• Administer subcutaneously in the abdomen or thigh only.
• Otrexup and Rasuvo are single-dose autoinjectors for once-weekly subcut use only and are available in specific dosage strengths. Use another formulation for dosing by other routes, doses less than 7.5 mg/week, doses more than 30 mg/week, high-dose regimens, or dosage adjustments between the available doses.
Intrathecal
• Preparing and giving parenteral drug may be mutagenic, teratogenic, or carcinogenic. Follow facility policy to reduce risks.
Black Box Warning Use preservative-free form for intrathecal or high-dose administration. ∎

ACTION
Reversibly binds to dihydrofolate reductase, blocking reduction of folic acid to tetrahydrofolate, a cofactor necessary for purine, protein, and DNA synthesis.

Route	Onset	Peak	Duration
PO	Unknown	1–2 hr	Unknown
IV	Immediate	Immediate	Unknown
IM	Unknown	30 min–1 hr	Unknown
Subcut	Unknown	1–2 hr	Unknown
Intrathecal	Unknown	Unknown	Unknown

Half-life: For doses below 30 mg/m^2, about 3 to 10 hours; for doses of 30 mg/m^2 and above, 8 to 15 hours.

M

ADVERSE REACTIONS

CNS: *arachnoiditis within hours of intrathecal use,* subacute neurotoxicity possibly beginning a few weeks later, demyelination, malaise, fatigue, dizziness, aphasia, hemiparesis, fever. **CV:** thromboembolic events, chest pain, hypotension, pericardial effusion, pericarditis. **EENT:** pharyngitis, blurred vision. **GI:** gingivitis, stomatitis, diarrhea, GI ulceration, *GI bleeding,* enteritis, nausea, vomiting. **GU:** nephropathy, tubular necrosis, *renal failure,* menstrual dysfunction, abortion, cystitis. **Hematologic:** *leukopenia, thrombocytopenia.* **Hepatic:** *acute toxicity, chronic toxicity,* including cirrhosis, *hepatic fibrosis.* **Metabolic:** *diabetes,* hyperuricemia. **Musculoskeletal:** arthralgia, myalgia, osteoporosis in children on long-term therapy. **Respiratory:** *pulmonary interstitial infiltrates,* pneumonitis, *PE.* **Skin:** urticaria, pruritus, hyperpigmentation, erythematous rashes, ecchymoses, rash, photosensitivity reactions, alopecia, acne, psoriatic lesions aggravated by exposure to sun. **Other:** chills, reduced resistance to infection, *septicemia, sudden death.*

INTERACTIONS

Drug-drug. *Acitretin:* May increase the risk of hepatitis. Avoid using together.
Acyclovir: Use with intrathecal methotrexate may cause neurologic abnormalities. Monitor patient closely.
Digoxin: May decrease digoxin level. Monitor digoxin level closely.
Folic acid derivatives: Antagonizes methotrexate effect. Avoid using together, except for leucovorin rescue with high-dose methotrexate therapy.
Fosphenytoin, phenytoin: May decrease phenytoin and fosphenytoin levels. Monitor drug levels closely.
Hepatotoxic drugs: May increase risk of hepatotoxicity. Monitor patient closely.
NSAIDs, salicylates: May increase methotrexate toxicity. Avoid using together.
Oral antibiotics: May decrease absorption of methotrexate. Monitor patient closely.
Penicillins, sulfonamides, trimethoprim: May increase methotrexate level. Monitor patient for methotrexate toxicity.

Probenecid: May impair excretion of methotrexate, causing increased level, effect, and toxicity of methotrexate. Monitor methotrexate level closely and adjust dosage accordingly.
❸ *Alert: PPIs:* May cause methotrexate toxicity, especially when high doses of methotrexate are given. Use cautiously.
Procarbazine: May increase risk of nephrotoxicity. Monitor patient closely.
Theophylline: May increase theophylline level. Monitor theophylline level closely.
Thiopurines: May increase thiopurine level. Monitor patient closely.
Vaccines: May make immunizations ineffective; may cause risk of disseminated infection with live-virus vaccines. Postpone immunization, if possible.
Drug-food. *Any food:* May delay absorption and reduce peak level of methotrexate. Instruct patient to take drug on an empty stomach.
Drug-lifestyle. *Alcohol use:* May increase hepatotoxicity. Discourage use together.
Sun exposure: May cause photosensitivity reactions. Advise patient to avoid excessive sunlight exposure.

EFFECTS ON LAB TEST RESULTS

• May increase uric acid level.
• May decrease Hb level and WBC, RBC, and platelet counts.
• May alter results of lab assay for folate, which interferes with detection of folic acid deficiency.

CONTRAINDICATIONS & CAUTIONS

• Contraindicated in patients hypersensitive to drug and in those with psoriasis or RA who also have alcoholism, alcoholic liver, chronic liver disease, immunodeficiency syndromes, or blood dyscrasias.
Black Box Warning Use drug only in patients with life-threatening neoplastic diseases and in those with severe psoriasis or RA not adequately responsive to other therapy; deaths have occurred. Closely monitor patients for bone marrow, liver, lung, and kidney toxicities. ∎
Black Box Warning Methotrexate given with radiotherapy may increase the risk of soft-tissue necrosis and osteonecrosis. ∎

Reactions in bold italics are *life-threatening*. Interactions may have a *rapid onset* or a *delayed onset*.

Black Box Warning Unexpectedly severe (sometimes fatal) bone marrow suppression, aplastic anemia, and GI toxicity have been reported with concomitant administration of methotrexate (usually in high dosage) with some NSAIDs. ∎

Black Box Warning Use cautiously and at modified dosage in patients with impaired hepatic or renal function, bone marrow suppression, aplasia, leukopenia, thrombocytopenia, or anemia. ∎

• Use cautiously in very young, elderly, or debilitated patients and in those with infection, peptic ulceration, or ulcerative colitis.

Dialyzable drug: Yes (using a high-flux dialyzer).

⚠ *Overdose S&S:* Leukopenia, thrombocytopenia, anemia, pancytopenia, bone marrow suppression, mucositis, stomatitis, oral ulceration, nausea, vomiting, GI ulceration, GI bleeding, sepsis or septic shock, renal failure, aplastic anemia, headache, seizures, acute toxic encephalopathy, cerebellar herniation associated with increased ICP, death.

PREGNANCY-LACTATION-REPRODUCTION
Black Box Warning Contraindicated during pregnancy. Don't use in women of childbearing potential unless benefits outweigh risks. ∎

• Contraindicated in breastfeeding women.

• If either partner is receiving methotrexate, they should avoid conception during and for a minimum of 3 months after therapy for males, and during and for at least one ovulatory cycle after therapy for females.

• Drug has been reported to cause impaired fertility, oligospermia, and menstrual dysfunction during and for a short period after therapy ends.

NURSING CONSIDERATIONS
Black Box Warning Methotrexate should be used only by health care providers whose knowledge and experience include the use of antimetabolite therapy. ∎

Black Box Warning Drug can cause severe and fatal toxicities. Modify dosage or discontinue drug for bone marrow suppression, infection, and renal, GI, pulmonary, and dermatologic toxicities or hypersensitivity. ∎

Black Box Warning Methotrexate-induced lung disease, including acute or chronic interstitial pneumonitis, is a potentially dangerous lesion that may occur at any time during therapy. It isn't always fully reversible. Pulmonary symptoms (especially a dry, nonproductive cough) may require interruption of treatment and careful investigation. ∎

Black Box Warning Diarrhea and ulcerative stomatitis require interruption of therapy; hemorrhagic enteritis and death from intestinal perforation may occur. ∎

Black Box Warning Malignant lymphomas may occur in patients receiving low-dose methotrexate and may regress upon discontinuing drug. ∎

Black Box Warning Methotrexate may induce TLS in patients with rapidly growing tumors. ∎

Black Box Warning Severe, occasionally fatal skin reactions have been reported following single or multiple doses of methotrexate. Reactions have occurred within days of methotrexate administration. Recovery has been reported with discontinuation of therapy. ∎

Black Box Warning Potentially fatal opportunistic infections, especially *Pneumocystis jiroveci* pneumonia, may occur with methotrexate therapy. ∎

Black Box Warning The high-dose regimens for osteosarcoma require meticulous care. ∎

🕙 *Alert:* Drug may be given daily or once weekly, depending on the disease. To avoid administration errors, know patient's dosing schedule.

• Monitor pulmonary function tests periodically and fluid intake and output daily. Encourage fluid intake of 2 to 3 L daily.

• Monitor uric acid level.

• Drug distributes readily into pleural effusions and other third-space compartments, such as ascites, leading to prolonged systemic level and risk of toxicity. Use drug cautiously in these patients.

🕙 *Alert:* Alkalinize urine by giving sodium bicarbonate tablets or fluids to prevent precipitation of drug, especially at high doses. Maintain urine pH above 7. If BUN level is 20 to 30 mg/dL or creatinine level is 1.2 to 2 mg/dL, reduce dosage. If BUN level exceeds 30 mg/dL or creatinine level is higher

M

than 2 mg/dL, stop drug and notify prescriber.

Black Box Warning It's essential to monitor CBC with differential, platelet count, and liver and renal function periodically. Watch for increases in AST, ALT, and alkaline phosphatase levels, which may signal hepatic dysfunction. Periodic liver biopsies are recommended for psoriatic patients who are receiving long-term treatment. Monitor patients at risk for impaired drug elimination (renal dysfunction, pleural effusions, ascites) more frequently. ■

• Watch for signs and symptoms of bleeding (especially GI) and infection.

• To prevent bleeding, avoid all IM injections when platelet count is below 50,000/mm³.

• Give blood transfusions for cumulative anemia. Patient may receive injections of RBC colony-stimulating factors to promote RBC production and decrease need for blood transfusions.

• Leucovorin rescue is needed with doses of more than 100 mg and starts 24 hours after therapy starts. Leucovorin is continued until methotrexate level falls below 5×10^{-8} M. Consult specialized references for specific recommendations for leucovorin dosage. Monitor methotrexate level and adjust leucovorin dose.

• The WBC and platelet count nadirs usually occur on day 7.

PATIENT TEACHING

• Advise patient to watch for signs and symptoms of infection (fever, sore throat, fatigue) and bleeding (easy bruising, nosebleeds, bleeding gums, tarry stools). Tell patient to take temperature daily.

Black Box Warning Fully inform patient of the risks involved with methotrexate therapy. ■

• Teach and encourage diligent mouth care to reduce risk of superinfection in the mouth.

• Inform caregivers to always use an accurate measuring device when administering the oral solution.

• Instruct patient how to take leucovorin. Stress the importance of taking as prescribed until instructed by prescriber to stop.

• Tell patient to use highly protective sunblock when exposed to sunlight.

• Advise female patient to stop breastfeeding during therapy.

SAFETY ALERT!

methyldopa
meth-il-DOE-pa

Therapeutic class: Antihypertensives
Pharmacologic class: Centrally acting antiadrenergics

AVAILABLE FORMS
methyldopa
Tablets: 125 mg✿, 250 mg, 500 mg

INDICATIONS & DOSAGES
➤ **HTN, hypertensive crisis**
Adults: Initially, 250 mg PO b.i.d. to t.i.d. in first 48 hours. Increase if needed every 2 days. May give entire daily dose in evening or at bedtime. Adjust dosages if other antihypertensives are added to or deleted from therapy. Limit initial daily dose to 500 mg/day when drug is administered with other antihypertensives other than thiazide diuretics. Adjust dosage at 48-hour intervals. Maintenance dosage is 500 mg to 2 g daily in two to four divided doses. Maximum recommended PO daily dose is 3 g.
Children: Initially, 10 mg/kg/day PO daily in two to four divided doses. Maximum daily dose is 65 mg/kg or 3 g, whichever is less.

ADMINISTRATION
PO
• If unpleasant adverse reactions occur, patient shouldn't suddenly stop taking drug but should notify the prescriber.

ACTION
May inhibit the central vasomotor centers, decreasing sympathetic outflow to the heart, kidneys, and peripheral vasculature.

Route	Onset	Peak	Duration
PO	4–6 hr	Unknown	12–48 hr

Half-life: About 105 minutes.

ADVERSE REACTIONS
CNS: decreased mental acuity, sedation, headache, weakness, dizziness, paresthesia, parkinsonism, involuntary choreoathetoid

---

Reactions in bold italics are *life-threatening*. Interactions may have a *rapid onset* or a *delayed onset*.

movements, psychic disturbances, depression, nightmares. **CV:** orthostatic hypotension, edema, *bradycardia, HF, myocarditis,* aggravated angina. **EENT:** nasal congestion. **GI:** dry mouth, *pancreatitis,* nausea, vomiting, diarrhea, constipation, flatus, sore or "black" tongue, abdominal distention, colitis. **GU:** amenorrhea, breast enlargement, impotence. **Hematologic:** *thrombocytopenia, leukopenia, bone marrow depression,* hemolytic anemia. **Hepatic:** *hepatic necrosis, hepatitis,* jaundice. **Metabolic:** hyperprolactinemia, weight gain. **Musculoskeletal:** arthralgia, myalgia. **Skin:** rash. **Other:** drug-induced fever.

INTERACTIONS

Drug-drug. *Amphetamines, norepinephrine, pseudoephedrine, phenothiazines, TCAs:* May cause hypertensive effects. Monitor patient closely.
Anesthetics: May need lower doses of anesthetics. Use together cautiously.
Antihypertensives: May increase risk of hypotension. Use cautiously.
Barbiturates: May decrease actions of methyldopa. Monitor patient closely.
Ferrous sulfate: May decrease bioavailability of methyldopa. Separate doses.
Levodopa: May increase hypotensive effects, which may increase adverse CNS reactions. Monitor patient closely.
Lithium: May increase lithium level. Watch for increased lithium level and signs and symptoms of toxicity.
MAO inhibitors: May cause excessive sympathetic stimulation. Avoid using together.

EFFECTS ON LAB TEST RESULTS

• May increase creatinine level and LFT values.
• May decrease Hb level, hematocrit, and platelet and WBC counts.
• May interfere with results of urinary uric acid testing, serum creatinine test, and AST test. May cause positive Coombs test result. May falsely increase urine catecholamine level, interfering with the diagnosis of pheochromocytoma.

CONTRAINDICATIONS & CAUTIONS

• Contraindicated in patients hypersensitive to drug and in those with active hepatic disease (such as acute hepatitis) or active cirrhosis.
• Contraindicated in those whose previous methyldopa therapy caused liver problems and in those taking MAO inhibitors.
• Use cautiously in patients with history of impaired hepatic function or sulfite sensitivity.
Dialyzable drug: Yes.
⚠ *Overdose S&S:* Sedation, acute hypotension, weakness, bradycardia, dizziness, constipation, abdominal distention, flatus, diarrhea, nausea, vomiting, light-headedness.

PREGNANCY-LACTATION-REPRODUCTION

• There are no well-controlled studies in pregnant women in the first trimester. Use only if clearly needed. Available data show use during pregnancy doesn't cause fetal harm and may improve fetal outcomes.
• Drug appears in human milk. Use cautiously in breastfeeding women.

NURSING CONSIDERATIONS

• Monitor patient's BP regularly. Elderly patients are more likely to experience hypotension, syncope, and sedation.
• Occasionally, tolerance may occur, usually between the second and third months of therapy. Adding a diuretic or adjusting dosage may be needed. If patient's response changes significantly, notify prescriber.
• After dialysis, monitor patient for HTN and notify prescriber, if needed. Patient may need an extra dose of drug.
• Monitor CBC with differential counts before therapy and periodically thereafter.
• Patients who need blood transfusions should have direct and indirect Coombs tests to prevent cross-matching problems.
• Monitor patient's Coombs test results. In patients who have received drug for several months, positive reaction to direct Coombs test may indicate hemolytic anemia.
• Report involuntary choreoathetoid movements. Drug may be stopped.

PATIENT TEACHING

• If unpleasant adverse reactions occur, advise patient not to suddenly stop taking drug but to notify prescriber.

• Instruct patient to report signs and symptoms of infection, yellowing of the skin, flu-like symptoms, and muscle aches.

• Tell patient to check weight daily and to notify prescriber for a weight gain of 900 g in 1 day or 2.3 kg in 1 week. Sodium and water retention may occur but can be relieved with diuretics.

• Warn patient that, particularly at the start of therapy, drug may impair ability to perform tasks that require mental alertness. A once-daily dose at bedtime minimizes daytime drowsiness.

• Inform patient that low BP and dizziness upon rising can be minimized by rising slowly and avoiding sudden position changes and that dry mouth can be relieved by chewing gum or sucking on hard candy or ice chips.

• Tell patient that urine may turn dark if left sitting in toilet bowl or if toilet bowl has been treated with bleach.

---

methylnaltrexone bromide
meth-il-nal-TREKS-one

Relistor

Therapeutic class: GI drugs
Pharmacologic class: Peripherally acting mu-opioid receptor antagonists

AVAILABLE FORMS
Injection: 8 mg/0.4 mL, 12 mg/0.6 mL in single-use vials, 20 mg/mL✤
Tablets: 150 mg

INDICATIONS & DOSAGES
Adjust-a-dose (for all indications): If CrCl is less than 60 mL/minute, reduce dosage by half.

➤ **Opioid-induced constipation (OIC) in those receiving palliative care for advanced illness when response to laxatives is insufficient**
Adults weighing more than 114 kg: 0.15 mg/kg subcut every other day, as needed.
Adults weighing 62 to 114 kg: 12 mg subcut every other day, as needed.
Adults weighing 38 to less than 62 kg: 8 mg subcut every other day, as needed.

Adults weighing less than 38 kg: 0.15 mg/kg subcut every other day, as needed.
Adjust-a-dose: In patients with moderate or severe renal impairment, give subcut dose every other day. If patient weighs more than 114 kg, give 0.075 mg/kg; if weight is 62 to 114 kg, give 6 mg; if weight is 38 to less than 62 kg, give 4 mg; if weight is less than 38 kg, give 0.075 mg/kg.
➤ **OIC in patients with chronic non-cancer pain**
Adults: 450 mg PO or 12 mg subcut once daily. Discontinue maintenance laxative therapy before starting methylnaltrexone. May resume laxative after patient has taken methylnaltrexone for 3 days if OIC symptoms persist. Reevaluate need for drug when opioid regimen is changed.
Adjust-a-dose: For CrCl of less than 60 mL/minute, give 150 mg PO once daily or 6 mg subcut once daily. For moderate or severe hepatic impairment, give 150 mg PO once daily. Or, for moderate or severe hepatic impairment, if patient weighs more than 114 kg, give 0.075 mg/kg subcut; if weight is 62 to 114 kg, give 6 mg subcut; if weight is 38 to less than 62 kg, give 4 mg subcut; if weight is less than 38 kg, give 0.075 mg/kg subcut.

ADMINISTRATION
PO
• Give tablets with water on an empty stomach at least 30 minutes before first meal of the day.
Subcutaneous
• Administer no more than one dose within 24 hours.
• To determine injection volume for the 0.15 mg/kg dose, multiply patient's weight in pounds by 0.0034 and round up to the nearest 0.1 mL, or multiply patient's weight in kilograms by 0.0075 and round up to the nearest 0.1 mL.
• Store drug at room temperature, away from light.
• After drawn into a syringe as directed, drug is stable at room temperature for 24 hours. Vials are for single use only.
• Give injections subcutaneously into the abdomen, thighs, or upper arms; rotate injection sites. Don't inject into bruised, tender, red, or hard areas.

Reactions in bold italics are *life-threatening*. Interactions may have a *rapid onset* or a *delayed onset*.

ACTION
Antagonizes GI mu-opioid receptors, preventing opioid-induced slowing of GI motility and transit time.

Route	Onset	Peak	Duration
PO	Unknown	1½ hr	Unknown
Subcut	Unknown	30 min	Unknown

Half-life: PO, 15 hours.

ADVERSE REACTIONS
CNS: dizziness, tremor, headache, anxiety. **EENT:** rhinorrhea. **GI:** abdominal pain, abdominal distention, flatulence, nausea, diarrhea, vomiting. **Musculoskeletal:** muscle spasms. **Other:** chills, hot flushes, hyperhidrosis.

INTERACTIONS
Drug-drug. *Opioid antagonists:* May increase risk of opioid withdrawal. Avoid combination.

EFFECTS ON LAB TEST RESULTS
None reported.

CONTRAINDICATIONS & CAUTIONS
❸ *Alert:* Contraindicated in patients with known or suspected GI obstruction and in those at increased risk for recurrent obstruction because of increased risk of GI perforation.

❸ *Alert:* Use cautiously in patients with peptic ulcer disease, Ogilvie syndrome, diverticular disease, infiltrative GI tract malignancies, or peritoneal metastases because of increased risk of GI perforation.

• Contraindicated in patients hypersensitive to drug.

❸ *Alert:* GI perforation has occurred rarely in patients with reduced GI tract integrity. Use cautiously.

• Use cautiously in patients with peritoneal catheters.

• Patients with disruptions to the blood-brain barrier may be at increased risk for opioid withdrawal or reduced analgesia. Consider overall risk-benefit profile.

• Drug hasn't been studied in patients with ESRD requiring dialysis.

• Safety and effectiveness in children haven't been established.

Dialyzable drug: Unknown.

⚠ *Overdose S&S:* Orthostatic hypotension, signs and symptoms of opioid withdrawal.

PREGNANCY-LACTATION-REPRODUCTION
• Don't use in pregnant women unless benefits outweigh risks to the fetus. Use in pregnancy may cause opioid withdrawal in a fetus.

• It isn't known if drug appears in human milk. Patient should discontinue breastfeeding or discontinue drug.

NURSING CONSIDERATIONS
❸ *Alert:* Watch for symptoms of perforation (severe, persistent, or worsening abdominal pain). If symptoms occur, stop drug and evaluate patient.

• Discontinue drug if treatment with the opioid pain medication is also discontinued.

PATIENT TEACHING
• Inform patient that drug may be effective within a few minutes to a few hours after administration.

• Instruct patient to discontinue drug and notify prescriber if severe, persistent, or worsening abdominal pain or diarrhea or rash occurs.

• Tell patient to take tablets once daily with water at least 30 minutes before first meal of the day.

• Inform patient that vial is for single-use only; remaining drug should be discarded.

• Advise patient to avoid injecting the drug into areas where the skin is tender, bruised, red, or hard, to avoid areas with scars or stretch marks, and to rotate injection sites.

• Warn patient that no more than one dose should be taken within a 24-hour period.

• Advise patient to report loss of analgesia or signs and symptoms of opioid withdrawal (hyperhidrosis, chills, diarrhea, abdominal pain, anxiety, yawning).

• Warn patient to report all adverse reactions, to immediately report severe, worsening, or persistent abdominal pain, and to discontinue drug for severe or persistent diarrhea.

M

methylphenidate hydrochloride
meth-il-FEN-i-date

Aptensio XR, Biphentin✤,
Concerta✞, Cotempla XR-ODT,
Methylin, QuilliChew ER, Quillivant
XR, Ritalin✞, Ritalin LA, Ritalin-SR✞

methylphenidate transdermal system
Daytrana

Therapeutic class: CNS stimulants
Pharmacologic class: Piperidine derivatives
Controlled substance schedule: II

AVAILABLE FORMS
Oral solution (Methylin): 5 mg/5 mL,
10 mg/5 mL
Tablets (chewable): 2.5 mg, 5 mg, 10 mg
Tablets (Ritalin): 5 mg, 10 mg, 20 mg
Extended-release
Capsules (Aptensio XR, Biphentin) **ⓄⓃⒸ***:*
10 mg, 15 mg, 20 mg, 30 mg, 40 mg, 50 mg,
60 mg, 80 mg✤
Capsules (Ritalin LA) **ⓄⓃⒸ***:* 10 mg, 20 mg,
30 mg, 40 mg
Oral suspension: 25 mg/5 mL
Tablets (chewable; QuilliChew ER) **ⓄⓃⒸ***:*
20 mg, 30 mg, 40 mg
Tablets (Concerta) **ⓄⓃⒸ***:* 18 mg, 27 mg,
36 mg, 54 mg
Tablets (ODTs; Cotempla XR-ODT) **ⓄⓃⒸ***:*
8.6 mg, 17.3 mg, 25.9 mg
Sustained-release
Tablets (Ritalin-SR) **ⓄⓃⒸ***:* 20 mg
Transdermal system
Patch: 10 mg, 15 mg, 20 mg, 30 mg

INDICATIONS & DOSAGES
➤ **ADHD**
Adults: 20 to 30 mg (immediate-release)
PO b.i.d. or t.i.d. Dosage varies; maximum
dosage is 60 mg daily.
Children age 6 and older: Initially, 5 mg PO
b.i.d. immediate-release form before breakfast and lunch, increasing by 5 to 10 mg at
weekly intervals, as needed, until an optimum daily dose of 2 mg/kg is reached, not to
exceed 60 mg/day.

To use Ritalin-SR tablets in place of
immediate-release methylphenidate tablets,
calculate methylphenidate dosage in 8-hour
intervals.
Concerta
*Adults ages 18 to 65 not taking methyl-
phenidate, or for patients taking other stimulants:* Initially, 18 or 36 mg PO daily. May
increase dosage in 18-mg increments at weekly
intervals to maximum of 72 mg daily.
*Adolescents ages 13 to 17 not currently tak-
ing methylphenidate, or for patients taking other stimulants:* 18 mg PO extended-
release Concerta once daily in the morning.
Adjust dosage by 18 mg at weekly intervals
to a maximum of 72 mg PO once daily in the
morning.
*Children ages 6 to 12 not currently taking
methylphenidate, or for patients taking other
stimulants:* 18 mg extended-release PO
once daily every morning. Adjust dosage by
18 mg at weekly intervals to a maximum of
54 mg daily every morning.
Adult currently taking methylphenidate: If
previous methylphenidate dosage was 5 mg
b.i.d. or t.i.d., give 18 mg PO every morning. If previous dosage was 10 mg b.i.d. or
t.i.d., give 36 mg PO every morning. If previous dosage was 15 mg b.i.d. or t.i.d., give
54 mg PO every morning. If previous dosage
was 20 mg b.i.d. or t.i.d., give 72 mg every
morning.
*Adolescents and children age 6 and older
currently taking methylphenidate:* If previous methylphenidate dosage was 5 mg b.i.d.
or t.i.d., give 18 mg PO every morning. If
previous dosage was 10 mg b.i.d. or t.i.d.,
give 36 mg PO every morning. If previous
dosage was 15 mg b.i.d. or t.i.d., give 54 mg
PO every morning. Maximum conversion
daily dose is 54 mg. Once conversion is
complete, adjust maximum dose in adolescents ages 13 to 17 to 72 mg once daily.
Aptensio XR
Adults and children age 6 and older: Initially, 10 mg PO daily in the morning. Increase dosage weekly in increments of
10 mg to maximum of 60 mg daily.
Ritalin LA
Adults and children age 6 and older: Initially, 20 mg PO once daily. Increase by
10 mg at weekly intervals to a maximum
of 60 mg daily. If previous methylphenidate

Reactions in bold italics are *life-threatening*. Interactions may have a *rapid onset* or a *delayed onset*.

dosage was 5 mg PO b.i.d., give 10 mg PO once daily. If previous methylphenidate dosage was 10 mg b.i.d., give 20 mg PO once daily. If previous methylphenidate dosage was 15 mg b.i.d., give 30 mg PO once daily. If previous methylphenidate dosage was 20 mg b.i.d., give 40 mg PO once daily. If previous methylphenidate dosage was 30 mg b.i.d., give 60 mg PO once daily.

Daytrana
Adults and children ages 6 to 17: Initially, apply one 10-mg patch to clean, dry, nonirritated skin on the hip, alternating sites daily. Apply 2 hours before desired effect and remove 9 hours later. Increase dose weekly as needed to a maximum of 30 mg daily. Base final dose and wear time on patient response.

Quillivant XR
Children age 6 and older: Initially, 10 to 20 mg PO once daily in a.m. May titrate weekly in dosages of 10 to 20 mg. Maximum dosage is 60 mg daily.

QuilliChew ER
Children age 6 and older: Initially, 20 mg PO once daily in the morning. Titrate dose up or down weekly in increments of 10 mg, 15 mg, or 20 mg. Maximum dosage is 60 mg daily.

Cotempla XR-ODT
Children age 6 and older: Initially, 17.3 mg PO daily in the morning. May increase dosage weekly in increments of 8.6 to 17.3 mg per day. Don't exceed a daily dosage of 51.8 mg.
➤ **Narcolepsy (except Aptensio XR, Concerta, Cotempla XR-ODT, Ritalin LA, QuilliChew ER, and Quillivant XR)**
Adults: 10 mg immediate-release PO b.i.d. or t.i.d. 30 to 45 minutes before meals. Dosage varies; maximum dose is 60 mg/day.
Children age 6 and older: Initially, 5 mg immediate-release PO b.i.d. (before breakfast and lunch). Increase dosage, if needed, by 5 to 10 mg weekly. Maximum dose is 60 mg. To use Ritalin-SR tablets in place of immediate-release methylphenidate tablets, calculate the dose of methylphenidate in 8-hour intervals.

ADMINISTRATION
PO
• Give chewable tablet with at least 240 mL of water or other liquid.
• Give immediate-release tablets, chewable tablets, and oral solution in divided doses

b.i.d. or t.i.d., preferably 30 to 45 minutes before meals. Give last daily dose before 6 p.m. to prevent insomnia.
• Aptensio XR or Ritalin LA may be swallowed whole, or the contents of the capsule may be sprinkled onto a small amount of cool applesauce and taken immediately. Administer with or without food.
• Extended-release and sustained-release tablets (Ritalin-SR) must be swallowed whole and never crushed, chewed, or divided.
• Concerta may be taken with or without food and must be swallowed whole. Don't crush, divide, or allow patient to chew Concerta tablets.
• Vigorously shake oral suspension bottle for 10 seconds before administering dose. Use oral dosing dispenser to measure dose. May give with or without food.
• For ODT, remove tablet with dry hands from blister pack and immediately place on patient's tongue. Allow it to disintegrate and be swallowed without chewing or crushing; no liquid is needed.

Transdermal
• Avoid placing the patch on the waistline or where tight clothing may rub it off. If possible, alternate sides of the body daily.

ACTION
Releases nerve terminal stores of norepinephrine, promoting nerve impulse transmission. At high doses, effects are mediated by dopamine.

Route	Onset	Peak	Duration
PO (Methylin, Ritalin)	Unknown	2 hr	Unknown
PO (Ritalin-SR)	Unknown	5 hr	8 hr
PO (Aptensio XR)	Unknown	2 hr; 8 hr	Unknown
PO (Ritalin LA)	Unknown	1–3 hr; 4–7 hr	Unknown
PO (Concerta)	Unknown	6–10 hr	Unknown
PO (QuilliChew XR, Quillivant XR)	Unknown	5 hr	Unknown
PO (Cotempla XR-ODT)	Unknown	4½–5 hr	Unknown
Transdermal	2 hr	8–10 hr	Unknown

Half-life: Conventional, 3 to 6 hours; extended-release (Ritalin-SR), 3 to 8 hours; (Concerta, Ritalin LA), 3.5 hours; (Aptensio XR), 5 hours; (Quillivant XR), 6 hours; (QuilliChew XR), 5 hours; (Cotempla XR-ODT), 3½ to 5½ hours; transdermal, 3 to 4 hours.

M

ADVERSE REACTIONS

CNS: nervousness, headache, insomnia, *seizures,* tics, dizziness, akathisia, dyskinesia, drowsiness, mood swings, anxiety, irritability, depression, tremor, vertigo, confusion. **CV:** palpitations, tachycardia, *arrhythmias,* HTN. **EENT:** blurred vision, pharyngitis, sinusitis, bruxism. **GI:** nausea, abdominal pain, anorexia, decreased appetite, vomiting, constipation, dyspepsia. **Hematologic:** *thrombocytopenia, thrombocytopenic purpura, leukopenia,* anemia. **Metabolic:** weight loss. **Respiratory:** cough, URI. **Skin:** exfoliative dermatitis, *erythema multiforme,* rash, urticaria, application-site irritation (redness, swelling, papules). **Other:** viral infection, hyperhidrosis.

INTERACTIONS

Drug-drug. *Antacids, H₂ antagonists, PPIs:* May interfere with normal release of Ritalin LA extended-release tablets. Monitor therapy.

Anticonvulsants (such as phenobarbital, phenytoin, primidone), SSRIs, TCAs (clomipramine, desipramine, imipramine), warfarin: May increase levels of these drugs. Monitor patient for adverse reactions, and decrease dose of these drugs as needed. Monitor drug levels (or coagulation times if patient is also taking warfarin).

Antihypertensives: May decrease antihypertensive effect. Monitor BP.

Centrally acting alpha₂ agonists, clonidine: May cause serious adverse events. Avoid using together.

MAO inhibitors: May cause severe HTN or hypertensive crisis. Avoid using within 14 days of MAO inhibitor therapy.

Drug-food. *Caffeine:* May increase amphetamine and related amine effects. Discourage use together.

Drug-lifestyle. *Alcohol use:* May increase methylphenidate concentration, causing toxicity. Patient should avoid alcohol during therapy.

EFFECTS ON LAB TEST RESULTS

• May decrease Hb level and hematocrit.
• May decrease platelet and WBC counts.

CONTRAINDICATIONS & CAUTIONS

• Contraindicated in patients hypersensitive to drug and within 14 days of MAO inhibitor therapy. Some formulations are contraindicated in patients with glaucoma, motor tics, family history or diagnosis of Tourette syndrome, or history of marked anxiety, tension, or agitation. Refer to individual manufacturer's instructions.

• Avoid use in patients with structural cardiac abnormalities.

🔴 *Alert:* Drug may increase risk of prolonged, painful erection (priapism) in males of any age, with or without sexual stimulation. Incidence is rare, but if not treated immediately, priapism may lead to permanent damage to the penis.

• Because it doesn't dissolve, Concerta isn't recommended in patients with a history of peritonitis or with severe GI narrowing (such as small-bowel inflammatory disease, short-gut syndrome caused by adhesions or decreased transit time, cystic fibrosis, chronic intestinal pseudo-obstruction, or Meckel diverticulum).

• Use cautiously in patients with a history of emotional disorder, preexisting psychosis or bipolar disorder, seizures, EEG abnormalities, or HTN, and in patients whose underlying medical conditions might be compromised by increases in BP or HR, such as those with preexisting HTN, HF, recent MI, or hyperthyroidism.

Black Box Warning Drug has a high potential for abuse and dependence. Use cautiously in patients with a history of drug dependence or alcoholism. Long-term abusive use can lead to tolerance and psychological dependence. Psychotic episodes can occur. Monitor patient for severe depression and the effects of chronic overactivity during drug withdrawal. ■

🔴 *Alert:* Chewable tablets contain phenylalanine.

🔴 *Alert:* The transdermal patch may cause irreversible chemical leukoderma (loss of skin color) at patch application site and other areas of the body. Although not harmful, if hypopigmentation occurs, consider alternative treatments.

Dializable drug: Unknown.

⚠ *Overdose S&S:* Agitation, cardiac arrhythmias, confusion, seizures, coma, delirium,

---

Reactions in bold italics are *life-threatening*. Interactions may have a *rapid onset* or a *delayed onset*.

dryness of mucous membranes, euphoria, flushing, hallucinations, headache, hyperpyrexia, hyperreflexia, HTN, muscle twitching, mydriasis, palpitations, sweating, tachycardia, tremors, vomiting.

PREGNANCY-LACTATION-REPRODUCTION
• There are no adequate studies in pregnant women. Use during pregnancy only if potential benefit justifies potential risk to the fetus.
• Drug appears in human milk. Use cautiously in breastfeeding women. ∎

NURSING CONSIDERATIONS
• Don't use drug to prevent fatigue or treat severe depression.
• Before starting drug, assess for the presence of cardiac disease by performing a careful history, family history of sudden death or ventricular arrhythmia, and physical exam.

Black Box Warning Assess risk of abuse before prescribing; monitor patients for signs and symptoms of abuse and dependence during therapy. Maintain careful prescription records; educate patients about abuse; monitor patients for signs and symptoms of abuse and overdose; and periodically reevaluate the need for use. ∎

• Drug may trigger Tourette syndrome in children. Monitor patient, especially at start of therapy.
• Observe patient for signs of excessive stimulation. Monitor BP.
• Check CBC, differential, and platelet counts with long-term use, particularly if patient shows signs or symptoms of hematologic toxicity (fever, sore throat, easy bruising).
• Monitor height and weight in children on long-term therapy. Drug may delay growth spurt, but children will attain normal height when drug is stopped.
• Monitor patient for tolerance or psychological dependence.
• Carefully observe patient for digital changes because stimulants used to treat ADHD are associated with peripheral vasculopathy, including Raynaud phenomenon.
• If ADHD hasn't improved after a 1-month period at the appropriate dose, prescriber may discontinue drug.

❸ **Alert:** Monitor patients using patch for chemical leukoderma. Report skin changes to prescriber.
• **Look alike–sound alike:** Don't confuse methylphenidate with methadone. Don't confuse Ritalin with ritodrine or Rifadin. Don't confuse Ritalin-SR with Ritalin LA.

PATIENT TEACHING
• Tell patient or caregiver to give drug 30 to 45 minutes before meals and to give last daily dose at 6 p.m. to prevent insomnia.
• Advise patient to avoid alcohol during therapy.
❸ **Alert:** Advise patient with phenylketonuria that the chewable tablets contain phenylalanine.
❸ **Alert:** Inform male patient of any age and caregivers of the rare but possible risk of priapism. Caution patient to seek medical attention if priapism or an erection lasting longer than 4 hours occurs.
• Warn patient against chewing sustained-release tablets.
• Advise patient that Ritalin LA may be swallowed whole, or the contents of the capsule may be sprinkled onto a small amount of cool applesauce and taken immediately.
❸ **Alert:** Warn patient to take chewable tablet with at least 240 mL of water. Not using enough liquid to swallow tablet may cause the tablet to swell and block the throat, causing choking.
• Advise patient using ODT to remove tablet with dry hands from blister pack, immediately place on tongue and allow it to disintegrate and be swallowed without chewing or crushing; no liquid is needed.
❸ **Alert:** Advise patient and caregiver to watch for signs of chemical leukoderma, especially under skin patch site, and to report any skin changes to prescriber. Caution patient not to stop treatment without first consulting prescriber.
• Caution patient to avoid activities that require alertness or good psychomotor coordination until CNS effects of drug are known.
• Warn patient with seizure disorder that drug may decrease seizure threshold and to notify prescriber if seizure occurs.
• Advise patient to avoid beverages containing caffeine while taking drug.

M

- Teach parent to always use oral dosing dispenser to measure oral suspension dose.
- Tell parent to apply patch in morning immediately after opening and not to use the pouch if the seal is broken. Provide caregivers with these instructions: Don't cut or trim patch. Press patch firmly in place for about 30 seconds using the palm of your hand, being sure there is good contact with the skin, especially around the edges. Once the patch has been applied correctly, the child may shower, bathe, or swim as usual.
- Inform parent that, if patch comes off, a new one may be applied on a different site, but the total wear time for that day should be 9 hours. Upon removal, fold patch in half so the sticky sides adhere to each other, then flush down toilet or dispose of in a lidded container.
- If the applied patch is missing, have parent ask the child when or how the patch came off. Teach child that patch shouldn't be shared or removed except by parent or health care provider.
- Encourage parent to use the application chart provided with patch carton to keep track of application and removal.
- Tell parent to remove patch sooner than 9 hours if the child has decreased evening appetite or has difficulty sleeping.
- Tell parent the effects of the patch last for several hours after its removal.
- Warn parent and patient to avoid exposing patch to direct external heat sources, such as heating pads, electric blankets, and heated water beds.
- Tell parent to notify prescriber if the child develops bumps, swelling, or blistering at the patch application site or is experiencing blurred vision or other serious side effects.

methylPREDNISolone
meth-il-pred-NIS-oh-lone

Medrol

methylPREDNISolone acetate
Depo-Medrol

methylPREDNISolone sodium succinate
Solu-Medrol

Therapeutic class: Corticosteroids
Pharmacologic class: Glucocorticoids

AVAILABLE FORMS
methylprednisolone
Tablets: 2 mg, 4 mg, 8 mg, 16 mg, 32 mg
methylprednisolone acetate
Injection (suspension): 20 mg/mL, 40 mg/mL, 80 mg/mL
methylprednisolone sodium succinate
Injection: 40-mg vial, 125-mg vial, 500-mg vial, 1,000-mg vial, 2,000-mg vial

INDICATIONS & DOSAGES
➤ **Severe inflammation or immunosuppression**
Adults and children: 4 to 48 mg PO daily depending on the disease treated. After favorable response is noted, determine maintenance dosage by decreasing until lowest dosage that will maintain adequate clinical response is achieved. Or, 4 to 120 mg acetate IM daily, or 10 to 40 mg succinate IM or IV, with subsequent doses dictated by patient's clinical response and condition. Or, 4 to 10 mg acetate into small joints, 10 to 40 mg acetate into medium joints, or 20 to 80 mg acetate into larger joints. Intralesional use is usually 20 to 60 mg acetate. Repeat intralesional and intra-articular injections every 1 to 5 weeks.
Children: 0.11 to 1.6 mg/kg/day PO, IM, or IV in three to four divided doses (sodium succinate).

ADMINISTRATION
PO
- Give drug with milk or food when possible. Critically ill patients may need to take

drug with an antacid or H₂-receptor antagonist.

IV

▼ Use only methylprednisolone sodium succinate, never the acetate form.

▼ Reconstitute according to manufacturer's directions using supplied diluent, or use bacteriostatic water for injection with benzyl alcohol.

⊘ *Alert:* Don't use formulations containing benzyl alcohol in neonates, which can cause potentially fatal toxicity.

▼ Compatible solutions include D_5W, NSS, and dextrose 5% in NSS.

▼ For direct injection, inject diluted drug into vein or free-flowing compatible IV solution over at least 1 minute.

▼ For IV infusion, dilute solution according to manufacturer's instructions and give over prescribed duration.

▼ For doses greater than 0.5 g, give IV over at least 30 to 60 minutes to prevent arrhythmias and circulatory collapse. Recommended infusion rate is giving over at least 30 minutes.

▼ Discard reconstituted solution after 48 hours.

▼ **Incompatibilities:** None listed by manufacturer. Consult a drug incompatibility reference for more information.

IM

● Give injection deeply into gluteal muscle. Avoid injection into the deltoid muscle. Avoid subcut injection because atrophy and sterile abscesses may occur.

● Dermal atrophy may occur with large doses of acetate form. Use several small injections rather than a single large dose, and rotate injection sites.

ACTION

Not clearly defined. Decreases inflammation, mainly by stabilizing leukocyte lysosomal membranes; suppresses immune response; stimulates bone marrow; and influences protein, fat, and carbohydrate metabolism.

Route	Onset	Peak	Duration
PO	Rapid	2–3 hr	30–36 hr
IV	1 hr	Immediate	12 hr
IM	6–48 hr	4–8 days	4–8 days
Intra-articular	Rapid	7 days	1–5 wk

Half-life: 2 to 36 hours.

ADVERSE REACTIONS

CNS: euphoria, insomnia, psychotic behavior, pseudotumor cerebri, vertigo, headache, depression, personality changes, paresthesia, *seizures,* malaise, emotional lability, insomnia. **CV:** *arrhythmias, HF, cardiomyopathy,* HTN, bradycardia, tachycardia, syncope, myocardial rupture after MI, edema, thrombophlebitis, *thromboembolism, cardiac arrest, CV collapse.* **EENT:** cataracts, glaucoma, IOP, exophthalmoses, rhinitis. **GI:** peptic ulceration, GI irritation, increased appetite, *pancreatitis,* nausea, vomiting. **GU:** menstrual irregularities. **Metabolic:** hypokalemia, hyperglycemia, sodium and water retention, carbohydrate intolerance, hypercholesterolemia, hypocalcemia. **Musculoskeletal:** growth suppression in children, muscle weakness, osteoporosis, tendon rupture, aseptic necrosis. **Respiratory:** *pulmonary edema.* **Skin:** hirsutism, delayed wound healing, acne, skin eruptions, cutaneous and subcutaneous atrophy. **Other:** cushingoid state, susceptibility to infections, *acute adrenal insufficiency after increased stress or abrupt withdrawal after long-term therapy, hypersensitivity reactions.*

INTERACTIONS

Drug-drug. *Aspirin, indomethacin, other NSAIDs:* May increase risk of GI distress and bleeding. Use together cautiously.

Barbiturates, carbamazepine, phenytoin, rifampin: May decrease corticosteroid effect. Increase corticosteroid dosage.

Cyclosporine: May increase toxicity. Monitor patient closely.

Ketoconazole and macrolide antibiotics: May decrease methylprednisolone clearance. Decreased dose may be required.

Mifepristone: May diminish methylprednisolone's therapeutic effects. Avoid combination.

Oral anticoagulants: May alter dosage requirements. Monitor PT and INR closely.

Potassium-depleting drugs (thiazide diuretics): May enhance potassium-wasting effects of methylprednisolone. Monitor potassium level.

Salicylates: May decrease salicylate levels. Monitor patient for lack of salicylate effectiveness.

M

Skin-test antigens: May decrease response. Postpone skin testing until after therapy.

Toxoids, vaccines: May decrease antibody response and may increase risk of neurologic complications. Avoid using together.

Drug-herb. *Echinacea:* May decrease therapeutic effects of immunosuppressants. Discourage use together.

Ginseng: May increase immune-regulating response. Discourage use together.

EFFECTS ON LAB TEST RESULTS

• May increase glucose and cholesterol levels and ALT, AST, alkaline phosphatase, and urine calcium levels.

• May decrease T_3, T_4, potassium, and calcium levels.

• May decrease ^{131}I uptake and protein-bound iodine levels in thyroid function tests. May cause false-negative results in nitroblue tetrazolium test for systemic bacterial infections. May alter reactions to skin tests.

CONTRAINDICATIONS & CAUTIONS

• Contraindicated in patients hypersensitive to drug or its ingredients, in those with systemic fungal infections, in premature infants (acetate and succinate), and in patients receiving immunosuppressive doses together with live-virus vaccines.

• IM injections are contraindicated in patients with idiopathic thrombocytopenia purpura.

• Use cautiously in patients with GI ulceration or renal disease, HTN, osteoporosis, diabetes mellitus, hypothyroidism, cirrhosis, diverticulitis, nonspecific ulcerative colitis, recent intestinal anastomoses, thromboembolic disorders, seizures, active hepatitis, myasthenia gravis, HF, TB, ocular herpes simplex, emotional instability, and psychotic tendencies.

• Prolonged use may increase risk of infection, mask signs of infection, and activate latent infections.

Dialyzable drug: Unknown.

PREGNANCY-LACTATION-REPRODUCTION

• There are no adequate studies in pregnant women. Use during pregnancy only if potential benefit justifies potential risk to the fetus. Use lowest effective dose for shortest duration.

• Monitor infants born to mothers who received corticosteroids during pregnancy for hypoadrenalism.

• Drug appears in human milk. Patient should discontinue breastfeeding or discontinue drug.

NURSING CONSIDERATIONS

۞ Alert: Epidural corticosteroid injections to treat neck and back pain and radiating pain in the arms and legs may result in rare but serious adverse events (loss of vision, stroke, paralysis, death). The use of epidural corticosteroid injections isn't approved by the FDA.

۞ Alert: Counsel patients who receive epidural corticosteroid injections to seek immediate medical attention if they experience loss of vision or vision changes; tingling in the arms or legs; sudden weakness or numbness of the face, arm, or leg on one or both sides of the body; dizziness; severe headache; or seizures.

۞ Alert: Drug may cause suppression of the HPA axis, which can lead to adrenal crisis. Younger children and patients receiving high doses are at increased risk. Withdrawal from corticosteroids should be done slowly and with careful patient monitoring.

• Medrol may contain tartrazine. Watch for allergic reaction to tartrazine in patients with sensitivity to aspirin.

• Drug may be used for alternate-day therapy.

• Most adverse reactions to corticosteroids are dose- or duration-dependent. For better results and less toxicity, give a once-daily dose in the morning.

۞ Alert: Different salts aren't interchangeable.

۞ Alert: Don't give Solu-Medrol intrathecally because severe adverse reactions may occur.

• If immediate onset of action is needed, don't use acetate form.

• Always adjust to lowest effective dose.

• Monitor patient's weight, BP, electrolyte level, and sleep patterns. Euphoria may initially interfere with sleep, but patients typically adjust to therapy in 1 to 3 weeks.

• Monitor patient for cushingoid effects, including moon facies, supraclavicular fat pad, central obesity, thinning hair, HTN, and increased susceptibility to infection.

• Measure growth and development periodically in children during high-dose or prolonged treatment.

• Watch for depression or psychotic episodes, especially in high-dose therapy.

• Diabetic patient may need increased insulin; monitor glucose level.

• Watch for an enhanced response to drug in patients with hypothyroidism or cirrhosis.

• Unless contraindicated, give low-sodium diet that's high in potassium and protein. Give potassium supplements as needed.

• Elderly patients may be more susceptible to osteoporosis with prolonged use.

• Taper off dosage after long-term therapy.

• **Look alike–sound alike:** Don't confuse Solu-Medrol with Solu-Cortef. Don't confuse methylprednisolone with medroxyprogesterone or methyltestosterone.

PATIENT TEACHING

☉ **Alert:** Counsel patient to discuss benefits and risks and other possible treatments with health care provider before undergoing epidural corticosteroid injection.

• Tell patient not to stop drug abruptly or without prescriber's consent.

• Instruct patient to take oral form of drug with milk or food.

• Teach patient signs and symptoms of early adrenal insufficiency: fatigue, muscle weakness, joint pain, fever, anorexia, nausea, shortness of breath, dizziness, and fainting.

• Instruct patient to carry or wear medical identification indicating the need for supplemental systemic glucocorticoids during stress. This card should contain prescriber's name, name of drug, and dosage taken.

• Warn patient on long-term therapy about cushingoid effects (moon facies, supraclavicular fat pad) and the need to notify prescriber about sudden weight gain or swelling.

• Advise patient receiving long-term therapy to consider exercise or physical therapy. Also, tell patient to ask prescriber about vitamin D or calcium supplement.

• Instruct patient to avoid exposure to infections (such as chickenpox or measles) and to contact prescriber if such exposure occurs.

methylTESTOSTERone
meth-il-tes-TOS-te-rone

Android 25, Testred

Therapeutic class: Androgens
Pharmacologic class: Androgens
Controlled substance schedule: III

AVAILABLE FORMS
Capsules: 10 mg
Tablets: 10 mg, 25 mg

INDICATIONS & DOSAGES
➤ **Metastatic breast cancer**
Women 1 to 5 years after menopause: 50 to 200 mg PO daily.
➤ **Hypogonadism; delayed puberty in carefully selected males**
Men and adolescents: 10 to 50 mg PO daily.

ADMINISTRATION
PO
• Drug is hazardous; use safe handling and disposal precautions.
• Give without regard for food.

ACTION
Stimulates target tissues to develop normally in androgen-deficient men. May have some antiestrogen properties, making it useful in treating certain estrogen-dependent breast cancers.

Route	Onset	Peak	Duration
PO	Unknown	Unknown	Unknown

Half-life: Varies from 10 to 100 minutes.

ADVERSE REACTIONS
CNS: headache, anxiety, depression, paresthesia, *stroke.* **CV:** edema, *HF,* venous thromboembolism, *MI.* **GI:** irritation of oral mucosa with buccal administration, nausea. **GU:** oligospermia, decreased ejaculatory volume, priapism, amenorrhea. **Hematologic:** *suppression of clotting factors,* polycythemia. **Hepatic:** reversible jaundice, *cholestatic hepatitis.* **Metabolic:** hypernatremia, *hyperkalemia,* hyperphosphatemia, hypercholesterolemia, hypercalcemia. **Skin:** hypersensitivity reactions, acne. **Other:** androgenic effects in women, altered libido,

M

gynecomastia, hypoestrogenic effects in women, excessive hormonal effects in men, male-pattern baldness.

INTERACTIONS

Drug-drug. *Cyclosporine (systemic):* May increase cyclosporine-associated hepatotoxicity. Consider therapy modification.
Hepatotoxic drugs: May increase risk of hepatotoxicity. Monitor liver function closely.
Insulin, oral antidiabetics: May decrease glucose level; may alter dosage requirements. Monitor glucose level in diabetic patients.
Oral anticoagulants: May increase sensitivity to oral anticoagulants; may alter dosage requirements. Monitor PT and INR.
Drug-herb. *Saw palmetto:* May cause hormone-like effects. Don't use together.

EFFECTS ON LAB TEST RESULTS

• May increase sodium, potassium, phosphate, liver enzyme, lipid, and calcium levels. May decrease thyroxine-binding globulin and total T_4 levels.
• May increase RBC count and resin uptake of T_3 and T_4.

CONTRAINDICATIONS & CAUTIONS

• Contraindicated in men with breast or prostate cancer.
• Use cautiously in elderly patients; patients with cardiac, renal, or hepatic disease or diabetes; and healthy males with delayed puberty.
Dialyzable drug: Unknown.
⚠ *Overdose S&S:* Nausea, edema.

PREGNANCY-LACTATION-REPRODUCTION

• Contraindicated in women who are or may become pregnant. Use during pregnancy may cause virilization of the female fetus. If patient becomes pregnant during therapy, apprise her of potential hazard to the fetus.
• It isn't known if drug appears in human milk. Patient should discontinue breastfeeding or discontinue drug.

NURSING CONSIDERATIONS

• In children, obtain X-rays of wrist bones before therapy begins to establish bone maturation level. During treatment, bones

may mature more rapidly than they grow in length. Review X-rays every 6 months to monitor bone maturation.
• Drug is typically used only for intermittent therapy. Because of potential hepatotoxicity, watch closely for jaundice.
• Promptly report evidence of virilization in women, such as deepening of the voice, increased hair growth, acne, or baldness.
• Watch for hypoestrogenic effects in women (flushing, diaphoresis, vaginal bleeding, nervousness, emotional lability, menstrual irregularities, and vaginitis, including itching, dryness, and burning).
• Watch for excessive hormonal effects in men. If patient is prepubertal, watch for premature epiphyseal closure, acne, priapism, growth of body and facial hair, and phallic enlargement. If patient is postpubertal, watch for testicular atrophy, oligospermia, decreased ejaculatory volume, impotence, gynecomastia, and epididymitis.
• Unless contraindicated, use with high-calorie, high-protein diet. Give small, frequent meals.
• Periodically check cholesterol, calcium, and Hb levels, hematocrit, and cardiac and LFT results.
• Check weight regularly. Control edema with sodium restriction or diuretics.
🕓 *Alert:* In breast cancer, therapeutic response usually occurs within 3 months. If disease appears to progress, stop drug.
• Report signs of hypercalcemia. In metastatic breast cancer, hypercalcemia may indicate progression of bone metastases.
• Evaluate semen every 3 to 4 months, especially in adolescent boys.
🕓 *Alert:* Don't use to enhance athletic performance or physique.
• *Look alike–sound alike:* Testosterone and methyltestosterone aren't interchangeable. Don't confuse methyltestosterone with medroxyprogesterone.

PATIENT TEACHING

• Ensure patient understands importance of using effective contraception during therapy.
• Teach patient about potential adverse reactions and to report them.
• Tell female patient of childbearing potential to report menstrual irregularities and to stop drug while awaiting exam.

Reactions in bold italics are *life-threatening*. Interactions may have a *rapid onset* or a *delayed onset*.

• Instruct patient to stop drug immediately and notify prescriber if pregnancy is suspected.
• Tell female patient to immediately report evidence of virilization, such as acne, swelling, weight gain, increased hair growth, hoarseness, clitoral enlargement, decreased breast size, deepening of voice, changes in libido, male pattern baldness, and oily skin or hair.
• Teach patient signs and symptoms of low glucose level (hypoglycemia) and method for checking glucose level; drug enhances hypoglycemia. Instruct patient to report signs or symptoms of hypoglycemia immediately.
• Advise adolescent and parents about the potential adverse effect on bone maturation before start of therapy.

metoclopramide hydrochloride ▓
met-oh-KLOE-pra-mide

Metonia✦, Reglan

Therapeutic class: GI stimulants
Pharmacologic class: Dopamine antagonists

AVAILABLE FORMS
Injection: 5 mg/mL
Oral solution: 5 mg/5 mL
Tablets: 5 mg, 10 mg
Tablets (ODTs): 5 mg, 10 mg

INDICATIONS & DOSAGES
▓ *Adjust-a-dose (for all indications):* Refer to manufacturer's product information for dosage adjustments, if indicated, for elderly patients, for patients with hepatic or renal impairment or ESRD, in CYP2D6 poor metabolizers, and with concomitant use with strong CYP2D6 inhibitors.
➤ **To prevent or reduce nausea and vomiting from emetogenic cancer chemotherapy**
Adults: 1 to 2 mg/kg IV 30 minutes before chemotherapy; repeat every 2 hours for two doses, then every 3 hours for three doses.
➤ **To prevent or reduce postoperative nausea and vomiting**

Adults: 10 to 20 mg IM near end of surgical procedure.
➤ **To facilitate small-bowel intubation**
Adults and children older than age 14: 10 mg IV as a single dose over 1 to 2 minutes.
Children ages 6 to 14: 2.5 to 5 mg IV as a single dose slowly over 1 to 2 minutes.
Children younger than age 6: 0.1 mg/kg IV as a single dose slowly over 1 to 2 minutes.
➤ **To aid in radiologic exam**
Adults: 10 mg IV as a single dose over 1 to 2 minutes.
➤ **Delayed gastric emptying secondary to diabetic gastroparesis**
Adults: 10 mg PO 30 minutes before each meal and at bedtime for mild symptoms. Maximum daily dosage is 40 mg. Or, give 10 mg IM or by slow IV push over 1 to 2 minutes 30 minutes before each meal and at bedtime for up to 10 days for severe symptoms; then PO dose may be started and continued for 2 to 8 weeks.
➤ **GERD**
Adults: 10 to 15 mg PO q.i.d., as needed, 30 minutes before meals and at bedtime.

ADMINISTRATION
PO
• Give drug 30 minutes before each meal and at bedtime when used for gastroparesis and GERD.
PO (ODT)
• Give drug at least 30 minutes before eating and at bedtime.
• Give immediately after opening sealed blister. If the tablet breaks or crumbles, throw it away and obtain a new one.
• Place tablet on patient's tongue. Tell patient to let it melt for approximately 1 minute and then swallow.
IV
▼ Drug is compatible with D_5W, NSS for injection, dextrose 5% in half-NSS, Ringer injection, and lactated Ringer injection. NSS is the preferred diluent; drug is most stable in this solution.
▼ Give doses of 10 mg or less by direct injection over 1 to 2 minutes. Dilute doses larger than 10 mg in 50 mL of compatible diluent, and infuse over at least 15 minutes. Monitor BP closely.

M

▼ There is no need to protect drug from light if infusion mixture is given within 24 hours. If protected from light and refrigerated, it's stable for 48 hours.

▼ **Incompatibilities:** Cephalothin, chloramphenicol, sodium bicarbonate.

IM

• Inspect for particulate matter and discoloration. If either is present, don't use.
• Inject into a large muscle.

ACTION

Stimulates motility of upper GI tract, increases lower esophageal sphincter tone, and blocks dopamine receptors at the chemoreceptor trigger zone.

Route	Onset	Peak	Duration
PO	30–60 min	1–2 hr	1–2 hr
IV	1–3 min	Unknown	1–2 hr
IM	10–15 min	Unknown	1–2 hr

Half-life: 4 to 6 hours.

ADVERSE REACTIONS

CNS: anxiety, drowsiness, dystonic reactions, fatigue, lassitude, restlessness, *seizures, suicidal ideation,* akathisia, confusion, depression, dizziness, extrapyramidal symptoms, fever, hallucinations, headache, insomnia, tardive dyskinesia. **CV:** *bradycardia, supraventricular tachycardia,* hypotension, transient HTN, *HF.* **GI:** bowel disorders, diarrhea, nausea. **GU:** incontinence, urinary frequency, erectile dysfunction. **Hematologic:** *agranulocytosis, neutropenia.* **Skin:** rash, urticaria. **Other:** loss of libido, prolactin secretion, gynecomastia, amenorrhea.

INTERACTIONS

Drug-drug. *Anticholinergics, opioid analgesics:* May antagonize GI motility effects of metoclopramide. Use together cautiously.
Antiparkinsonians (dopamine agonists): May decrease therapeutic effects of antiparkinsonians. Monitor therapy.
Antipsychotics: May increase toxic effects of antipsychotics. Don't use together.
CNS depressants: May cause additive CNS effects. Avoid using together.
Cyclosporine: May increase cyclosporine absorption. Monitor therapy.

CYP2D6 inhibitors (bupropion, fluoxetine, paroxetine, quinidine): May increase metoclopramide level. Adjust metoclopramide dosage as indicated.
Digoxin: May diminish digoxin absorption. Monitor therapy.
MAO inhibitors: May increase release of catecholamines in patients with HTN. Use together cautiously.
Phenothiazines: May increase risk of extrapyramidal effects. Monitor patient closely.
Drug-lifestyle. *Alcohol use:* May cause additive CNS effects. Discourage use together.

EFFECTS ON LAB TEST RESULTS

• May increase LFT values, aldosterone levels, and prolactin levels.
• May decrease neutrophil and granulocyte counts.

CONTRAINDICATIONS & CAUTIONS

• Contraindicated in patients hypersensitive to drug and in those with pheochromocytoma or other catecholamine-releasing paragangliomas, tardive dyskinesia, or seizure disorders.
• Contraindicated in patients for whom stimulation of GI motility might be dangerous (those with hemorrhage, obstruction, or perforation).

Black Box Warning Drug can cause irreversible tardive dyskinesia, even after drug is stopped. Risk increases with duration of therapy and total cumulative dose; there is no treatment. Discontinue drug if signs and symptoms occur. Except in rare cases, avoid treatment for longer than 12 weeks. ■

• In addition to tardive dyskinesia, drug may cause other extrapyramidal signs and symptoms, parkinsonian symptoms, and motor restlessness.
• Metoclopramide isn't recommended for use in children due to the risk of tardive dyskinesia and other extrapyramidal signs and symptoms as well as the risk of methemoglobinemia in neonates.
• Galactorrhea, amenorrhea, gynecomastia, and impotence have been reported with prolactin-elevating drugs, including metoclopramide.
① Alert: NMS has occurred rarely and may be fatal. If signs and symptoms develop

---

Reactions in bold italics are *life-threatening*. Interactions may have a *rapid onset* or a *delayed onset*.

(fever, CNS symptoms, irregular pulse, cardiac arrhythmias, or abnormal BP), discontinue drug.
• Use cautiously in patients with history of depression, Parkinson disease, or HTN.
Dialyzable drug: No.
⚠ *Overdose S&S:* Drowsiness, disorientation, extrapyramidal reactions; seizures, lethargy (in infants and children).

PREGNANCY-LACTATION-REPRODUCTION
• There are no adequate studies in pregnant women. Use during pregnancy only if clearly needed.
• Drug appears in human milk. Use cautiously in breastfeeding women.

NURSING CONSIDERATIONS
• Monitor bowel sounds.
• Safety and effectiveness of drug haven't been established for therapy lasting longer than 12 weeks.
• Drug may cause tardive dyskinesia, parkinsonian symptoms, and motor restlessness. Monitor patient for involuntary movements of face, tongue, and extremities, which may indicate tardive dyskinesia or other extrapyramidal adverse effects.
• Monitor patient for fever, CNS symptoms, irregular pulse, cardiac arrhythmias, or abnormal BP, which may indicate NMS.
• Monitor patient for dizziness, headache, or nervousness after metoclopramide is stopped; these may indicate withdrawal.
• Diphenhydramine or benztropine may be used to counteract extrapyramidal adverse effects from high doses.

PATIENT TEACHING
• Instruct patient to take ODTs 30 minutes before food and at bedtime and not to repeat dose if inadvertently taken with food.
• Tell patient taking ODTs to open blister pack with dry hands and immediately place tablet on tongue, let it melt completely, and then swallow. (Taking it with water isn't necessary.) If tablet breaks or crumbles, advise patient to throw it away and take a new tablet out of the blister pack.
• Tell patient to avoid activities that require alertness for 2 hours after doses.
• Urge patient to report persistent or serious adverse reactions promptly.

• Teach patient signs and symptoms of tardive dyskinesia, other extrapyramidal signs and symptoms, and NMS. Advise patient to discontinue drug and to seek immediate medical attention if such signs and symptoms occur.
• Advise patient not to drink alcohol during therapy.

metOLazone
me-TOLE-a-zone

Zaroxolyn

Therapeutic class: Diuretics
Pharmacologic class: Thiazide-like diuretics

AVAILABLE FORMS
Tablets: 2.5 mg, 5 mg, 10 mg

INDICATIONS & DOSAGES
➤ **Edema in HF or renal disease**
Adults: 5 to 20 mg PO once daily.
➤ **HTN**
Adults: 2.5 to 5 mg PO once daily. Base maintenance dosage on BP.

ADMINISTRATION
PO
• Give drug in the morning without regard for meals.

ACTION
Increases sodium and water excretion by inhibiting sodium reabsorption in ascending loop of Henle.

Route	Onset	Peak	Duration
PO	1 hr	8 hr	≥24 hr

Half-life: 6 to 20 hours.

ADVERSE REACTIONS
CNS: dizziness, headache, fatigue, vertigo, paresthesia, weakness, restlessness, drowsiness, anxiety, depression, nervousness, blurred vision. **CV:** orthostatic hypotension, palpitations, chest pain, venous thrombosis. **GI:** *pancreatitis,* anorexia, nausea, epigastric pain, vomiting, abdominal pain, diarrhea, constipation, dry mouth. **GU:** nocturia, polyuria, impotence. **Hematologic:** *aplastic anemia, agranulocytosis, leukopenia.*

M

Hepatic: jaundice, *hepatitis.* **Metabolic:** hyperglycemia, *hypokalemia, hypomagnesemia,* hyponatremia, hypochloremia, metabolic alkalosis, hypercalcemia, volume depletion and dehydration. **Musculoskeletal:** muscle cramps. **Skin:** dermatitis, photosensitivity reactions, rash, pruritus, urticaria, skin necrosis, purpura, *SJS, toxic epidermal necrolysis,* necrotizing angiitis.

INTERACTIONS

Drug-drug. *Amphotericin B, corticosteroids:* May increase risk of hypokalemia. Monitor potassium level closely.

Anticoagulants: May decrease anticoagulant response. Monitor PT and INR.

Antidiabetics: May alter glucose level and require dosage adjustment of antidiabetics. Monitor glucose level.

Barbiturates, opioids: May increase orthostatic hypotensive effect. Monitor patient closely.

Bumetanide, ethacrynic acid, furosemide, torsemide: May cause excessive diuretic response, causing serious electrolyte abnormalities or dehydration. Adjust doses carefully, and monitor patient closely for signs and symptoms of excessive diuretic response.

Calcium salts: May decrease calcium excretion. Monitor therapy.

Carbamazepine: May increase risk of hyponatremia. Monitor therapy.

Cholestyramine, colestipol: May decrease intestinal absorption of thiazides. Separate doses.

Diazoxide: May increase antihypertensive, hyperglycemic, and hyperuricemic effects. Use together cautiously.

Levodopa–carbidopa: May increase risk of hypotension. Monitor therapy.

Lithium: May decrease lithium clearance, increasing risk of lithium toxicity. Monitor lithium level.

NSAIDs: May increase risk of renal failure. May decrease diuretic and antihypertensive effects. Monitor renal function and BP.

Other antihypertensives: May have additive effects. Use together cautiously.

QT-interval-prolonging drugs: May increase risk of QT-interval prolongation and ventricular arrhythmias. Avoid use together.

Drug-herb. *Licorice:* May cause hypokalemia. Discourage use together.

Drug-lifestyle. *Alcohol use:* May increase orthostatic hypotensive effect. Discourage use together.

Sun exposure: May cause photosensitivity reaction. Advise patient to avoid excessive sunlight exposure.

EFFECTS ON LAB TEST RESULTS

● May increase glucose, calcium, cholesterol, BUN, and triglyceride levels. May decrease potassium, sodium, magnesium, and chloride levels.

● May decrease Hb level and granulocyte and WBC counts.

CONTRAINDICATIONS & CAUTIONS

● Contraindicated in patients hypersensitive to thiazides, other sulfonamide-derived drugs, or metolazone and in those with anuria, hepatic coma, or precoma.

● Use cautiously in patients with impaired renal or hepatic function, electrolyte imbalances, hyperuricemia, SLE, diabetes, or gout.

Dialyzable drug: Unlikely.

⚠ *Overdose S&S:* Orthostatic hypotension, dizziness, drowsiness, lethargy, syncope, CNS depression, electrolyte abnormalities, hemoconcentration, depressed respirations, GI irritation and hypermotility.

PREGNANCY-LACTATION-REPRODUCTION

● There are no adequate studies in pregnant women. Use during pregnancy only if clearly needed.

● Drug appears in human milk. Patient should discontinue breastfeeding or discontinue drug.

NURSING CONSIDERATIONS

● Monitor fluid intake and output, weight, BP, and electrolyte levels.

● Watch for signs and symptoms of hypokalemia, such as muscle weakness and cramps. Drug may be used with potassium-sparing diuretic to prevent potassium loss.

● Consult dietitian about a high-potassium diet.

● Monitor glucose level, especially in diabetic patients.

Reactions in bold italics are *life-threatening*. Interactions may have a *rapid onset* or a *delayed onset*.

- Monitor uric acid level, especially in patients with history of gout.
- Monitor elderly patients, who are especially susceptible to excessive diuresis.
- In hypertensive patients, therapeutic response may be delayed several weeks.
- Monitor BP. If response is inadequate, another antihypertensive may be added.
- Metolazone and furosemide may be used together to enhance diuretic effect.
- Unlike thiazide diuretics, metolazone is effective in patients with decreased renal function.
- Stop thiazides and thiazide-like diuretics before parathyroid function tests.
- *Look alike–sound alike:* Don't confuse metolazone with methadone or methimazole.

PATIENT TEACHING
- Tell patient to take drug in morning to prevent need to urinate at night.
- Advise patient to avoid sudden posture changes and to rise slowly to avoid dizziness upon standing quickly.
- Instruct patient to use a sunblock to prevent photosensitivity reactions.
- Instruct patient to increase dietary intake of potassium-containing foods.
- Teach patient about adverse reactions and to report them promptly.

metoprolol succinate
me-toe-PROE-lole

Toprol-XL⌀

metoprolol tartrate
Lopresor✤, Lopresor SR✤, Lopressor⌀

Therapeutic class: Antihypertensives
Pharmacologic class: Selective beta-adrenergic blockers

AVAILABLE FORMS
metoprolol succinate
Tablets (extended-release) ⓞⓝⓒ: 25 mg, 50 mg, 100 mg, 200 mg
metoprolol tartrate
Injection: 1 mg/mL in 5-mL ampules
Tablets: 25 mg, 37.5 mg, 50 mg, 75 mg, 100 mg

Tablets (extended-release) ⓞⓝⓒ: 100 mg✤, 200 mg✤

INDICATIONS & DOSAGES
➤ **HTN**
Adults: Initially, 50 mg PO b.i.d. or 100 mg PO once daily; then up to 100 to 400 mg daily in two or three divided doses. Or, 25 to 100 mg extended-release tablets (tartrate equivalent) PO once daily. Adjust dosage as needed and tolerated at intervals of not less than 1 week to maximum of 400 mg (extended-release) daily or 450 mg (immediate-release) daily.
Children older than age 6 (metoprolol succinate): Initially, 1 mg/kg PO once daily, not to exceed 50 mg PO daily. Adjust dosage based on BP response. Doses greater than 2 mg/kg or in excess of 200 mg/day haven't been studied.
➤ **Early intervention in acute MI**
Adults: 5 mg metoprolol tartrate IV bolus every 2 minutes for three doses. Then, starting 15 minutes after the last IV dose, 25 to 50 mg PO every 6 hours for 48 hours. Maintenance dosage is 100 mg PO b.i.d.
➤ **Angina pectoris**
Adults: Initially, 100 mg PO daily as a single dose or in two equally divided doses; increased at weekly intervals until an adequate response or a pronounced decrease in HR is seen. Effects of daily dose beyond 400 mg aren't known. Or, 100 mg extended-release tablets (tartrate equivalent) once daily. Adjust dosage as needed and tolerated at intervals of not less than 1 week to maximum of 400 mg daily.
➤ **Stable symptomatic HF (NYHA Class II) resulting from ischemia, HTN, or cardiomyopathy**
Adults: 25 mg Toprol-XL PO once daily for 2 weeks. Double the dose every 2 weeks, as tolerated, to a maximum of 200 mg daily.
Adjust-a-dose: In patients with more severe HF, start with 12.5 mg Toprol-XL PO once daily for 2 weeks.

ADMINISTRATION
PO
- Give drug with or immediately after meal.
- Extended-release tablets may be cut in half on scored line, but never crushed or chewed.

M

✤Canada   ◇OTC   ◆Off-label use   ⌀Photoguide   ⓞⓝⓒDo not crush   *Liquid contains alcohol   ᛒGenetic

IV

▼ Give drug undiluted by direct injection in an intensive care setting.

▼ Store drug at room temperature and protect from light. Discard solution if it's discolored or contains particles.

▼ **Incompatibilities:** None listed by manufacturer. Consult a drug incompatibility reference for more information.

ACTION

Unknown. A selective beta blocker that selectively blocks beta₁ receptors; decreases cardiac output, peripheral resistance, and cardiac oxygen consumption; and depresses renin secretion.

Route	Onset	Peak	Duration
PO	15 min	1 hr	6–12 hr
PO (extended-release)	15 min	6–12 hr	24 hr
IV	5 min	20 min	5–8 hr

Half-life: 3 to 10 hours.

ADVERSE REACTIONS

CNS: fatigue, dizziness, depression, headache, insomnia, mental confusion, nightmares, short-term memory loss, hallucinations, vertigo. **CV:** hypotension, *brady-cardia, HF,* edema, palpitations, *stroke.* **EENT:** blurred vision, tinnitus, rhinitis. **GI:** nausea, diarrhea, constipation, heartburn, dry mouth, flatulence, gastric pain, vomiting. **GU:** decreased libido, erectile dysfunction. **Musculoskeletal:** pain. **Respiratory:** dyspnea, wheezing, *bronchospasm.* **Skin:** rash, pruritus.

INTERACTIONS

Drug-drug. *Amiodarone:* May increase bradycardic effects. Monitor therapy.
Barbiturates: May reduce metoprolol effect. Monitor therapy.
Calcium channel blockers: May increase hypotensive effects. Monitor therapy.
Cardiac glycosides: May cause excessive bradycardia and increased depressant effect on myocardium. Use together cautiously.
Catecholamine-depleting drugs (MAO inhibitors): May have additive effect. Monitor patient for hypotension and bradycardia.
Clonidine: May increase risk of bradycardia. If clonidine and a beta blocker are

coadministered, withdraw the beta blocker several days before the gradual withdrawal of clonidine.
CYP2D6 inhibitors (fluoxetine, paroxetine, propafenone, quinidine): May increase metoprolol level. Monitor vital signs carefully. Metoprolol dosage reduction may be needed.
Hydralazine: May increase levels and effects of both drugs. Monitor patient closely. May need to adjust dosage.
Indomethacin, NSAIDs: May decrease antihypertensive effect. Monitor BP and adjust dosage.
Insulin, oral antidiabetics: May alter dosage requirements in previously stabilized diabetic patients. Monitor patient closely.
IV lidocaine: May reduce hepatic metabolism of lidocaine, increasing risk of toxicity. Give bolus doses of lidocaine at a slower rate, and monitor lidocaine level closely.
Terbutaline: May antagonize bronchodilatory effects of terbutaline. Monitor patient.
Verapamil: May increase effects of both drugs. Monitor cardiac function closely, and decrease dosages as needed.
Drug-herb. *Ma huang:* May decrease antihypertensive effects. Discourage use together.
Drug-food. *Any food:* May increase absorption. Encourage patient to take drug with food.

EFFECTS ON LAB TEST RESULTS

• May increase transaminase, alkaline phosphatase, LDH, and uric acid levels.

CONTRAINDICATIONS & CAUTIONS

• Contraindicated in patients hypersensitive to drug or other beta blockers.
• Contraindicated in patients with sinus bradycardia, greater than first-degree heart block, cardiogenic shock, sick sinus syndrome (unless a permanent pacemaker is in place), or overt cardiac failure when used to treat HTN or angina. When used to treat MI, drug is contraindicated in patients with HR less than 45 beats/minute, greater than first-degree heart block, PR interval of 0.24 second or longer with first-degree heart block, systolic BP less than 100 mm Hg, or moderate to severe cardiac failure.

• Use cautiously in patients with HF, diabetes, or respiratory or hepatic disease.
• Avoid initiating high-dose, extended-release drug in patients undergoing noncardiac surgery because drug has been associated with bradycardia, hypotension, stroke, and death.
• Don't routinely withdraw long-term beta-blocker therapy before surgery.
Dialyzable drug: Yes.
⚠ *Overdose S&S:* Bradycardia, hypotension, bronchospasm, cardiac failure, cardiac arrest, coma, AV block, nausea, vomiting.

PREGNANCY-LACTATION-REPRODUCTION
• There are no adequate studies in pregnant women. Use during pregnancy only if clearly needed.
• Drug appears in human milk in very small quantities; an infant consuming 1 L of human milk daily would receive a metoprolol dose of less than 1 mg. Consider possible infant exposure when giving to breastfeeding women.

NURSING CONSIDERATIONS
• Always check patient's apical pulse rate before giving drug. If it's slower than 60 beats/minute, withhold drug and call prescriber immediately.
• In diabetic patients, monitor glucose level closely because drug masks common signs and symptoms of hypoglycemia.
• Monitor BP frequently; drug masks common signs and symptoms of shock.
• Beta blockers may mask tachycardia caused by hyperthyroidism. In patients with suspected thyrotoxicosis, taper off beta blocker to avoid thyroid storm.
Black Box Warning When stopping therapy, taper dosage over 1 to 2 weeks. Abrupt discontinuation may cause exacerbations of angina or MI. Don't discontinue therapy abruptly even in patients treated only for HTN. ∎
• Beta selectivity is lost at higher doses. Watch for peripheral side effects.
• *Look alike–sound alike:* Don't confuse metoprolol succinate with metoprolol tartrate. Don't confuse metoprolol with metaproterenol, misoprostol, or metolazone. Don't confuse Toprol-XL with Topamax, Tegretol, or Tegretol-XR.

PATIENT TEACHING
• Instruct patient to take drug exactly as prescribed and with meals.
• Caution patient to avoid driving and other tasks requiring mental alertness until response to therapy has been established.
• Advise patient to inform dentist or prescriber about use of this drug before procedures or surgery.
• Tell patient to report all adverse reactions, especially shortness of breath.
Black Box Warning Instruct patient not to stop drug suddenly but to notify prescriber about unpleasant adverse reactions. Inform patient that drug must be withdrawn gradually over 1 or 2 weeks. ∎

---

metroNIDAZOLE (oral, injection)
met-roe-NYE-da-zole

Flagyl R

metroNIDAZOLE hydrochloride
Flagyl IV RTU, Metro IV in Plastic Container

Therapeutic class: Antiprotozoals
Pharmacologic class: Nitroimidazoles

AVAILABLE FORMS
Capsules: 375 mg, 500 mg✤
Injection: 500 mg/100 mL in ready-to-use (RTU) minibags
Tablets: 250 mg, 500 mg

INDICATIONS & DOSAGES
Black Box Warning Use metronidazole only for the conditions for which it's indicated because it may be carcinogenic. Avoid unnecessary use. ∎
Adjust-a-dose (for all indications): For severe hepatic impairment (Child-Pugh class C), reduce dose of immediate-release tablets and IV infusion by 50%.
➤ **Amebic liver abscess**
Adults: 500 to 750 mg PO t.i.d. for 5 to 10 days; or, 500 mg IV every 6 hours for 10 days if patient can't tolerate oral route.
Children: 35 to 50 mg/kg PO daily in three divided doses for 7 to 10 days.

M

➤ **Intestinal amebiasis (immediate-release)**
Adults: 750 mg PO t.i.d. for 7 to 10 days.
Children: 35 to 50 mg/kg PO daily in three divided doses for 7 to 10 days. IV form may be necessary for severe infection or extraintestinal disease.
Adjust-a-dose: For severe hepatic impairment (Child-Pugh class C), reduce dose to 375 mg PO every 8 hours.

➤ **Trichomoniasis (immediate-release)**
Adults: One 250-mg tablet PO t.i.d. for 7 days, or 2 g PO in single dose (may give the 2-g dose in two 1-g doses, both on the same day); wait 4 to 6 weeks before repeating course. Or, one 375-mg capsule PO b.i.d. for 7 days.
Adjust-a-dose: For severe hepatic impairment (Child-Pugh class C), reduce dose to 375 mg PO once daily.

➤ **Bacterial infections caused by anaerobic microorganisms**
Adults: Loading dose is 15 mg/kg IV infused over 1 hour. Maintenance dose is 7.5 mg/kg IV or 500 mg PO every 6 hours. Give first maintenance dose 6 hours after loading dose. Maximum dose shouldn't exceed 4 g daily.

➤ **To prevent postoperative infection in contaminated or potentially contaminated colorectal surgery**
Adults: Infuse 15 mg/kg IV over 30 to 60 minutes and complete about 1 hour before surgery. Then, infuse 7.5 mg/kg IV over 30 to 60 minutes at 6 and 12 hours after first dose.

➤ **Bacterial vaginosis (nonpregnant women)**
Adults: 500 mg PO b.i.d. for 7 days.

➤ **Giardiasis ◆**
Adults: 250 to 500 mg t.i.d. or 500 mg b.i.d. for 5 to 7 days.

➤ **Pouchitis ◆**
Adults: (Acute) 500 mg to 1 g every 12 hours for 14 days. (Chronic) 500 mg every 12 hours in combination with ciprofloxacin for at least 28 days.

ADMINISTRATION
PO
• Give tablets and capsules with food if GI upset occurs.

IV
▼ Flagyl IV RTU minibags need no preparation.
▼ Don't use aluminum needles or hubs to reconstitute the drug or to transfer reconstituted drug. Equipment that contains aluminum will turn the solution orange; the potency isn't affected.
▼ To reconstitute lyophilized vials, add 4.4 mL of sterile water for injection, bacteriostatic water for injection, sterile NSS for injection, or bacteriostatic NSS for injection. Reconstituted drug contains 100 mg/mL. Add contents of vial to 100 mL of D_5W, lactated Ringer injection, or NSS to yield 5 mg/mL. Neutralize this highly acidic solution by carefully adding 5 mEq sodium bicarbonate to each 500 mg; the carbon dioxide gas that forms may need to be vented.
▼ Don't give by IV push. Infuse over 30 to 60 minutes.
▼ Don't refrigerate the neutralized diluted solution; precipitation may occur. Refrigerated Flagyl IV RTU may form crystals, which disappear after the solution warms to room temperature.
▼ **Incompatibilities:** Other IV drugs. Avoid contact of drug solution with equipment containing aluminum.

ACTION
Direct-acting trichomonacide and amebicide that works inside and outside the intestines. It's thought to enter the cells of microorganisms that contain nitroreductase, forming unstable compounds that bind to DNA and inhibit synthesis, causing cell death.

Route	Onset	Peak	Duration
PO	Unknown	1–2 hr	Unknown
IV	Immediate	1 hr	Unknown

Half-life: 6 to 8 hours.

ADVERSE REACTIONS
CNS: headache, *seizures,* fever, vertigo, ataxia, dizziness, syncope, incoordination, confusion, irritability, depression, weakness, insomnia, peripheral neuropathy. **CV:** flattened T wave, edema, flushing, thrombophlebitis after IV infusion. **EENT:** rhinitis, sinusitis, pharyngitis. **GI:** nausea, abdominal pain, stomatitis, epigastric distress,

---

Reactions in bold italics are *life-threatening*. Interactions may have a *rapid onset* or a *delayed onset*.

vomiting, anorexia, diarrhea, constipation, proctitis, dry mouth, metallic taste. **GU:** vaginitis, darkened urine, polyuria, dysuria, cystitis, dyspareunia, dryness of vagina and vulva, vaginal candidiasis, genital pruritus, *UTI,* dysmenorrhea. **Hematologic:** *transient leukopenia, neutropenia.* **Musculoskeletal:** transient joint pains. **Respiratory:** URI. **Skin:** rash. **Other:** decreased libido; overgrowth of nonsusceptible organisms, *candidiasis;* flulike symptoms.

INTERACTIONS

Drug-drug. *Busulfan:* May increase busulfan toxicity. Avoid using together.

Cimetidine: May increase risk of metronidazole toxicity because of inhibited hepatic metabolism. Monitor for toxicity.

CYP3A4 substrates: May increase concentration of aripiprazole, dofetilide, lomitapide, and pimozide. Monitor therapy.

Disulfiram: May cause acute psychosis and confusion. Avoid giving metronidazole within 2 weeks of disulfiram.

Lithium: May increase lithium level, which may cause toxicity. Monitor lithium level.

Mebendazole: May increase risk of SJS or toxic epidermal necrolysis. Consider therapy modification.

Phenobarbital, phenytoin: May decrease metronidazole effectiveness; may reduce total phenytoin clearance. Monitor patient.

QT-interval-prolonging drugs: May increase risk of QT-interval prolongation and ventricular arrhythmias. Avoid use together.

Warfarin: May increase anticoagulant effects and risk of bleeding. Reduce warfarin as needed.

Drug-lifestyle. *Alcohol use:* May cause disulfiram-like reaction, including nausea, vomiting, headache, cramps, and flushing. Warn patient to avoid alcohol during and for 3 days after completing drug therapy.

EFFECTS ON LAB TEST RESULTS

• May decrease WBC and neutrophil counts.
• May falsely decrease triglyceride and aminotransferase levels.
• May interfere with ALT, AST, glucose, and LDH testing.

CONTRAINDICATIONS & CAUTIONS

• Contraindicated in patients hypersensitive to drug or other nitroimidazole derivatives. The use of disulfiram within 2 weeks of metronidazole therapy and the use of alcohol or propylene glycol products during treatment and for 3 days after treatment ends are contraindicated.

• Use cautiously in patients with history of blood dyscrasia, CNS disorder, or retinal or visual field changes.

• Use cautiously in patients who take hepatotoxic drugs or have hepatic disease, alcoholism, or renal impairment.

Dialyzable drug: Yes.

⚠ *Overdose S&S:* Nausea, vomiting, ataxia, neurotoxicity.

PREGNANCY-LACTATION-REPRODUCTION

• Contraindicated during first trimester. Consult current guidelines for appropriate use in pregnant women.

• Drug appears in human milk. Patient should discontinue breastfeeding or discontinue drug.

NURSING CONSIDERATIONS

• Monitor LFT results carefully in elderly patients.

• Observe patient for edema, especially if patient is receiving corticosteroids; Flagyl IV RTU may cause sodium retention.

• Record number and character of stools when drug is used to treat amebiasis. Give drug only after *Trichomonas vaginalis* infection is confirmed by wet smear or culture or *Entamoeba histolytica* is identified.

• Sexual partners of patients being treated for *T. vaginalis* infection, even if asymptomatic, must also be treated to avoid reinfection.

• *Look alike–sound alike:* Don't confuse metronidazole with metformin.

PATIENT TEACHING

• Inform patient with trichomoniasis of need for sexual partners to be treated simultaneously to avoid reinfection.

• Tell patient to avoid alcohol and alcohol-containing drugs during and for at least 3 days after treatment course.

• Tell patient that a metallic taste and dark or red-brown urine may occur.

M

• Tell patient to report signs and symptoms of candidal overgrowth.

• Tell patient to report all adverse reactions immediately, especially neurologic symptoms (seizures, peripheral neuropathy).

metroNIDAZOLE (topical, vaginal)
me-troe-NI-da-zole

MetroCream, MetroGel, MetroGel Vaginal, MetroLotion, Noritate, Nuvessa, Vandazole

Therapeutic class: Antibacterials (topical)
Pharmacologic class: Nitroimidazoles

AVAILABLE FORMS
Topical cream: 0.75%, 1%
Topical gel: 0.75%, 1%
Topical lotion: 0.75%
Vaginal gel: 0.75%, 1.3%

INDICATIONS & DOSAGES
➤ **Inflammatory papules and pustules of acne rosacea**
Adults: If using a 0.75% preparation, apply thin film to affected area b.i.d., morning and evening. If using a 1% preparation, apply thin film to affected area once daily. After response is seen (usually within 3 weeks), adjust frequency and duration of therapy.
➤ **Bacterial vaginosis**
Adults: One applicatorful of 0.75% (approximately 37.5 mg) vaginally daily or b.i.d. for 5 days. For once-daily use, give at bedtime. Or, one applicatorful (approximately 65 mg) of 1.3% vaginal gel intravaginally once as a single dose at bedtime.

ADMINISTRATION
Topical
• Clean area thoroughly before use; then wait 15 to 20 minutes before applying drug to minimize risk of local irritation. Avoid contact with eyes.
• Patient should wait at least 5 minutes after using lotion before applying cosmetics.
Vaginal
• Screw the end of the applicator onto the tube and squeeze slowly. The plunger will stop when the applicator is full.

• Wash plunger and barrel in warm, soapy water and rinse thoroughly. Dry before reassembling.

ACTION
Unknown. May cause bactericidal effect by interacting with bacterial DNA. Drug is active against many anaerobic gram-negative bacilli, anaerobic gram-positive cocci, *Gardnerella vaginalis*, and *Campylobacter fetus*.

Route	Onset	Peak	Duration
Topical	Unknown	8–12 hr	Unknown
Vaginal	Unknown	6–12 hr	Unknown

Half-life: Unknown.

ADVERSE REACTIONS
Topical form
CNS: headache. **CV:** HTN. **GU:** UTI. **Skin:** transient redness, dryness, mild burning, stinging, contact dermatitis, pruritus, rash.
Vaginal form
CNS: headache, dizziness, depression. **GI:** cramps, nausea, loose stools, metallic or bad taste in mouth, pain, vomiting, diarrhea. **GU:** cervicitis, vaginitis, perineal and vulvovaginal itching, vaginal burning, vaginal discharge, pelvic discomfort. **Skin:** transient redness, dryness, mild burning, stinging. **Other:** overgrowth of nonsusceptible organisms.

INTERACTIONS
Drug-drug. *Disulfiram:* May cause disulfiram-like reaction when used with vaginal form of metronidazole. Don't use together, and wait 2 weeks after stopping disulfiram before starting metronidazole vaginal therapy.
Lopinavir: May enhance adverse/toxic effect of lopinavir and result in a disulfiram-like reaction. Monitor therapy.
Oral anticoagulants: May increase anticoagulant effect. Monitor patient for adverse reactions.
Tipranavir: May enhance adverse/toxic effect of tipranavir. Monitor therapy.
Drug-lifestyle. *Alcohol use:* May cause disulfiram-like reaction when used with vaginal form. Don't use together.

EFFECTS ON LAB TEST RESULTS
• May interfere with AST, ALT, LDH, triglyceride, and glucose levels.
• May increase or decrease WBC count.

CONTRAINDICATIONS & CAUTIONS
• Contraindicated in patients hypersensitive to drug or its ingredients, such as parabens, and other nitroimidazole derivatives.
• Use cautiously in patients with history or evidence of blood dyscrasia and in those with hepatic impairment.
• Use vaginal gel cautiously in patients with history of CNS diseases. Oral form may cause seizures and peripheral neuropathy.
• Prolonged use of vaginal form can lead to fungal or bacterial superinfection.
Dialyzable drug: Unknown.

PREGNANCY-LACTATION-REPRODUCTION
• There are no adequate studies in pregnant women. Use during pregnancy only if clearly needed and benefit justifies potential risk to the fetus.
• Drug may appear in human milk after vaginal or topical use because some of drug is absorbed systemically. Patient should discontinue breastfeeding or discontinue drug.

NURSING CONSIDERATIONS
• Topical therapy hasn't been linked to the adverse effects observed with parenteral or oral therapy, but some drug may be absorbed after topical use.
• Don't use vaginal gel in patients who have taken disulfiram within past 2 weeks.
• Monitor patient for worsening symptoms.

PATIENT TEACHING
• Instruct patient to avoid use of topical gel around eyes.
• Advise patient to clean area thoroughly before use and to wait 15 to 20 minutes after cleaning skin before applying drug to minimize risk of local irritation. Cosmetics may be used 5 minutes after medication has dried.
• If local reactions occur, advise patient to apply drug less frequently or stop using it and notify prescriber.
• Advise patient to avoid sexual intercourse while using vaginal preparation.

• Caution patient to avoid alcohol while being treated with vaginal preparation.

micafungin sodium
mi-ka-FUN-gin

Mycamine

Therapeutic class: Antifungals
Pharmacologic class: Echinocandins

AVAILABLE FORMS
Lyophilized powder for injection: 50 mg, 100 mg in single-use vials

INDICATIONS & DOSAGES
➤ **Candidemia, acute disseminated candidiasis, and** *Candida* **peritonitis and abscesses**
Adults: 100 mg IV daily for 10 to 47 days (mean duration, 15 days).
Children age 4 months and older: 2 mg/kg IV once daily. Maximum dosage is 100 mg daily.
➤ **Esophageal candidiasis**
Adults: 150 mg IV daily for 10 to 30 days (mean duration, 15 days).
Children age 4 months and older weighing more than 30 kg: 2.5 mg/kg IV once daily. Maximum dosage is 150 mg daily.
Children age 4 months and older weighing 30 kg or less: 3 mg/kg IV once daily.
➤ **To prevent candidal infection in hematopoietic stem cell transplant recipients**
Adults: 50 mg IV daily for 6 to 51 days (mean duration, 19 days).
Children age 4 months and older: 1 mg/kg IV once daily. Maximum dosage is 50 mg daily.

ADMINISTRATION
IV
▼ Use aseptic technique when preparing drug.
▼ Reconstitute each 50-mg or 100-mg vial with 5 mL of NSS without a bacteriostatic agent or D_5W for injection. To minimize foaming, dissolve powder by swirling the vial; don't shake it.
▼ For adult, dilute dose in 100 mL of NSS or D_5W for injection.

M

▼ For children's doses: Add reconstituted drug to NSS or D₅W IV infusion bag or syringe. Ensure that final concentration of solution is between 0.5 and 4 mg/mL. To minimize risk of infusion reactions, administer concentrations of greater than 1.5 mg/mL via central catheter.

▼ Flush line with NSS for injection before infusing drug.

▼ Infuse drug over 1 hour.

▼ Reconstituted product and diluted infusion may be stored for up to 24 hours at room temperature.

▼ Protect diluted solution from light.

▼ **Incompatibilities:** Don't mix or confuse with other medications. Drug may precipitate when mixed with commonly used drugs.

ACTION

Inhibits synthesis of an essential component of fungal cell walls. Drug is active against *Candida albicans, C. glabrata, C. krusei, C. parapsilosis,* and *C. tropicalis.*

Route	Onset	Peak	Duration
IV	Unknown	Unknown	Unknown

Half-life: 11 to 21 hours.

ADVERSE REACTIONS

CNS: headache, insomnia, anxiety, dizziness, *seizures, intracranial hemorrhage.* **CV:** atrial fibrillation, bradycardia, cardiac disorders, HTN, hypotension, tachycardia, vascular disorders, edema, *cardiac arrest, MI, pericardial effusion.* **GI:** abdominal pain, diarrhea, nausea, vomiting, anorexia, dyspepsia, mucositis, constipation. **Hematologic:** *leukopenia, neutropenia, thrombocytopenia,* anemia. **Hepatic:** elevated LFT values, hepatic injury, hepatomegaly, hyperbilirubinemia. **Metabolic:** hypocalcemia, hypokalemia, *hypomagnesemia,* hypophosphatemia, *hyperglycemia, hypoglycemia, hyperkalemia,* hypernatremia, *hypocalcemia.* **Respiratory:** cough, dyspnea. **Skin:** infusion-site inflammation, phlebitis, pruritus, rash. **Other:** pyrexia, rigors.

INTERACTIONS

Drug-drug. *CYP3A4 substrates:* May increase concentration of aripiprazole, dofetilide, lomitapide, and pimozide. Monitor therapy.

Itraconazole: May increase itraconazole level. Monitor for itraconazole toxicity, and reduce itraconazole dose if needed.

Nifedipine: May increase nifedipine level. Monitor BP, and decrease nifedipine dose if needed.

Sirolimus: May increase sirolimus level. Monitor patient for evidence of toxicity, and decrease sirolimus dose if needed.

EFFECTS ON LAB TEST RESULTS

• May increase alkaline phosphatase, ALT, AST, bilirubin, BUN, creatinine, and LDH levels.

• May decrease calcium, magnesium, phosphorus, potassium, and Hb levels and hematocrit.

• May decrease neutrophil and platelet counts.

CONTRAINDICATIONS & CAUTIONS

• Contraindicated in patients hypersensitive to drug.

• Effects of micafungin are unknown in patients with severe hepatic disease.

Dialyzable drug: No.

PREGNANCY-LACTATION-REPRODUCTION

• There are no adequate studies in pregnant women. Use during pregnancy only if potential benefit justifies potential risk to the fetus.

• It isn't known if drug appears in human milk. Use cautiously in breastfeeding women.

NURSING CONSIDERATIONS

• Injection-site reactions occur more often in patients receiving drug by peripheral IV.

• To reduce the risk of histamine-mediated reactions, infuse drug over at least 1 hour.

❸ *Alert:* If patient develops signs of serious hypersensitivity reaction, including shock, stop infusion and notify prescriber immediately.

• Monitor hepatic and renal function during therapy.

• Monitor patient for hemolysis and hemolytic anemia.

PATIENT TEACHING
• Advise patient to report pain or redness at infusion site.
• Teach patient about adverse reactions and to report them immediately.
• Tell patient lab tests will most likely be needed to monitor hematologic, renal, and hepatic function.

miconazole
my-KON-a-zole

Oravig

miconazole nitrate
Fungoid Tincture ◇, Lotrimin AF ◇, Lotrimin AF Liquid Spray ◇, Lotrimin AF Powder ◇, Lotrimin AF Powder Spray ◇, Micaderm, Micatin ◇, Micozole✤ ◇, Monistat 1 ◇, M-Zole 3 ◇, Tetterine ◇, Vagistat-3 ◇, Zeasorb-AF ◇

Therapeutic class: Antifungals
Pharmacologic class: Imidazoles

AVAILABLE FORMS
Aerosol powder: 2% ◇
Aerosol spray: 2% ◇
Buccal tablets ⓞⓣⓒ: 50 mg
Lotion: 2% ◇
Powder: 2% ◇
Topical cream: 2% ◇
Topical ointment: 2% ◇
Topical solution: 2% ◇
Vaginal cream: 2% ◇, 4% ◇
Vaginal suppositories: 100 mg ◇, 200 mg ◇, 1,200 mg ◇

INDICATIONS & DOSAGES
➤ **Tinea corporis, tinea cruris, tinea pedis, cutaneous candidiasis, common dermatophyte infections**
Adults and children older than age 2: Apply sparingly b.i.d. for 2 weeks (tinea cruris) to 4 weeks (tinea pedis and corporis). Powder or spray can be used liberally over affected area. In children younger than age 2, use only under the direction and supervision of a physician.
➤ **Vulvovaginal candidiasis**
Adults and children age 12 and older: One applicatorful 2% or 100-mg suppository

vaginally at bedtime for 7 days; repeat course, if needed. Or, one applicatorful 4% or 200-mg suppository vaginally at bedtime for 3 days. Or, one 1,200-mg Monistat 1 suppository vaginally at bedtime for 1 day. May apply topical cream sparingly to affected area b.i.d. for 7 days or as needed for external symptoms.
➤ **Oropharyngeal candidiasis**
Adults and children age 16 and older: One 50-mg buccal tablet to the upper gum region once daily for 14 consecutive days.

ADMINISTRATION
PO
• Apply buccal tablet to the gum in the morning with dry hands after patient has brushed teeth.
• Place the rounded surface of the tablet against the gum just above the incisor. Apply slight pressure over the upper lip for 30 seconds to ensure adhesion.
• Alternate sides of the mouth for each dose.
• Instruct patient not to crush, chew, or swallow buccal tablets.
Topical
• Don't use occlusive dressings.
• Lotion is preferred in skin folds.
Vaginal
• Suppository is inserted high into vagina with applicator provided.
• Store between 59° and 86° F (15° and 30° C).

ACTION
Fungicidal; disrupts fungal cell membrane permeability.

Route	Onset	Peak	Duration
PO	Unknown	7 hr	15 hr
Topical, vaginal	Unknown	Unknown	Unknown

Half-life: Unknown.

ADVERSE REACTIONS
CNS: headache, fatigue, pain. **GI:** diarrhea, nausea, dysgeusia, upper abdominal pain, vomiting (buccal tablets), oral discomfort, dry mouth, gastroenteritis. **GU:** pelvic cramps, pruritus, and irritation with vaginal cream; vulvovaginal burning. **Hematologic:** anemia, *lymphopenia, neutropenia.* **Respiratory:** URI. **Skin:** allergic contact dermatitis, burning, irritation, maceration, pain, edema.

INTERACTIONS

Drug-drug. *Progesterone:* Vaginal form of drug may diminish progesterone effects. Avoid use together.

Warfarin: Buccal form of drug may enhance anticoagulant effect. Monitor PT and INR, and observe patient for bleeding. Oral form of drug may increase warfarin concentration. Monitor therapy.

Drug-herb. *Saccharomyces boulardii:* Antifungals may decrease therapeutic effect. Consider alternative therapy.

EFFECTS ON LAB TEST RESULTS

None.

CONTRAINDICATIONS & CAUTIONS

• Contraindicated in patients hypersensitive to drug or its components. Cross-sensitivity to imidazole antifungals may occur.

• Safety and effectiveness of Oravig haven't been established for children younger than age 16.

• Don't use in younger children because of risk of choking.

Dialyzable drug: Unknown.

PREGNANCY-LACTATION-REPRODUCTION

• There are no adequate studies in pregnant women. Use oral form during pregnancy only if potential benefit justifies potential risk to the fetus.

◑ *Alert:* Vaginal preparation shouldn't be used during first trimester and should be used during pregnancy only if recommended by prescriber.

• It isn't known if drug appears in human milk. Topical and vaginal administration should result in low systemic absorption. Use cautiously in breastfeeding women.

• Vaginal form can weaken latex condoms and diaphragms.

NURSING CONSIDERATIONS

• Carefully monitor patients with hepatic impairment who are taking oral form.

PATIENT TEACHING

• Advise patient that vaginal form of drug is for perineal or vaginal use only and to keep drug out of eyes.

• Caution patient that frequent or persistent yeast infections may suggest a more serious medical problem.

• Tell patient to cautiously insert vaginal form high into the vagina with applicator provided.

• Tell patient that drug may stain clothing.

• Warn patient to stop drug if sensitivity or chemical irritation occurs.

• Tell patient to use drug for full treatment period prescribed and to notify prescriber if symptoms persist or worsen despite therapy.

• Advise patient to avoid tampons and sexual intercourse during vaginal treatment.

• Instruct patient to apply sparingly in skin folds and rub in well to prevent skin breakdown.

• Tell patient to store vaginal product between 59° and 86° F (15° and 30° C).

• Tell patient not to crush, chew, or swallow buccal tablets.

• Emphasize that patient can eat and drink with the buccal tablet in place but to avoid chewing gum.

• Instruct patient how to use buccal tablet.

• Tell patient that if the tablet falls off or is swallowed after being in place for at least 6 hours, not to apply a new tablet until the next regularly scheduled dose.

SAFETY ALERT!

midazolam hydrochloride
MID-aye-zoe-lam

Therapeutic class: Anxiolytics
Pharmacologic class: Benzodiazepines
Controlled substance schedule: IV

AVAILABLE FORMS

Injection: 1 mg/mL, 5 mg/mL
Injection (preservative-free): 1 mg/mL, 5 mg/mL
Syrup: 2 mg/mL

INDICATIONS & DOSAGES

➤ **Preoperative sedation (to induce sleepiness or drowsiness and relieve apprehension)**
Adults: 0.07 to 0.08 mg/kg IM 30 to 60 minutes before surgery. Usual dose is 5 mg.

➤ **Moderate sedation before short diagnostic or endoscopic procedures**

Adults younger than age 60: Initially, small dose not to exceed 2.5 mg IV given slowly over at least 2 minutes; wait at least 2 minutes to evaluate sedative effect. Then repeat in 2 minutes p.r.n., in small increments of first dose over at least 2 minutes each to achieve desired effect. Total dose of up to 5 mg may be used. Additional doses to maintain desired level of sedation may be given by slow titration in increments of 25% of dose used to first reach the sedative end point.

Patients age 60 or older and debilitated patients: 0.5 to 1.5 mg IV over at least 2 minutes. Incremental doses shouldn't exceed 1 mg. A total dose of up to 3.5 mg is usually sufficient.

➤ **To induce sleepiness and amnesia and to relieve apprehension before anesthesia or before and during procedures**
PO
Children ages 6 to 16 who are cooperative: 0.25 to 0.5 mg/kg PO as a single dose, up to 20 mg.

Infants and children ages 6 months to 5 years or less cooperative, older children: 0.25 to 1 mg/kg PO as a single dose, up to 20 mg.
IV
Children ages 12 to 16: Initially, no more than 2.5 mg IV given slowly; repeat in 2 minutes, if needed, in small increments of first dose over at least 2 minutes to achieve desired effect. Total dose of up to 10 mg may be used. Additional doses to maintain desired level of sedation may be given by slow titration in increments of 25% of dose used to first reach the sedative end point.

Children ages 6 to 12: 0.025 to 0.05 mg/kg IV over 2 or 3 minutes. Additional doses may be given in small increments after 2 to 3 minutes. Total dose of up to 0.4 mg/kg, not to exceed 10 mg, may be used.

Children ages 6 months to 5 years: 0.05 to 0.1 mg/kg IV over 2 to 3 minutes. Additional doses may be given in small increments after 2 to 3 minutes. Total dose of up to 0.6 mg/kg, not to exceed 6 mg, may be used.
IM
Children: 0.1 to 0.15 mg/kg IM. Use up to 0.5 mg/kg in more anxious patients.

Adjust-a-dose: For obese children, base dose on ideal body weight; high-risk or

debilitated children and children receiving other sedatives need lower doses.

➤ **To induce general anesthesia**
Adults older than age 55: 0.3 mg/kg IV infusion over 20 to 30 seconds if patient hasn't received premedication, or 0.2 mg/kg IV infusion over 20 to 30 seconds if patient has received a sedative or opioid premedication. Allow 2 minutes for effect. Additional increments of 25% of first dose may be needed to complete induction.

Adults younger than age 55: 0.3 to 0.35 mg/kg IV infusion over 20 to 30 seconds if patient hasn't received premedication, or 0.25 mg/kg IV infusion over 20 to 30 seconds if patient has received a sedative or opioid premedication. Allow 2 minutes for effect. Additional increments of 25% of first dose may be needed to complete induction.

Adjust-a-dose: For debilitated patients, initially, 0.2 to 0.25 mg/kg. As little as 0.15 mg/kg may be needed. Reduce doses in elderly patients.

➤ **As continuous infusion to sedate intubated patients in critical care unit**
Adults: Initially, 0.01 to 0.05 mg/kg may be given IV over several minutes, repeated at 10- to 15-minute intervals until adequate sedation is achieved. To maintain sedation, usual initial infusion rate is 0.02 to 0.1 mg/kg/hour. Higher loading dose or infusion rates may be needed in some patients. Use the lowest effective rate.

Children: Initially, 0.05 to 0.2 mg/kg may be given IV over 2 to 3 minutes or longer; then continuous infusion at rate of 0.06 to 0.12 mg/kg/hour. Increase or decrease infusion to maintain desired effect.

Neonates more than 32 weeks' gestational age: Initially, 0.06 mg/kg/hour IV. Adjust rate, as needed, using lowest possible rate.

Neonates less than 32 weeks' gestational age: Initially, 0.03 mg/kg/hour IV. Adjust rate, as needed, using lowest possible rate.

Black Box Warning Avoid rapid injection (less than 2 minutes) in neonates because rapid injection has been associated with severe hypotension, particularly when neonate has also received fentanyl. Severe hypotension has also been observed in neonates receiving a continuous infusion of midazolam who then receive a rapid IV injection of

M

---

fentanyl. Seizures have been reported in several neonates after rapid IV administration. ■

➤ **Status epilepticus (seizures lasting longer than 5 minutes or occurring after patient has had intermittent seizures without regaining consciousness for longer than 5 minutes)** ◆

Children age 1 and older: For patients weighing more than 40 kg, give 10 mg IM once; for those weighing 13 to 40 kg, give 5 mg IM once.

ADMINISTRATION
PO

Black Box Warning Midazolam syrup has been associated with respiratory depression and respiratory arrest, especially when used in noncritical-care settings. Midazolam syrup should only be used in hospital or ambulatory care settings that can provide continuous respiratory and cardiac function monitoring. Availability of appropriate resuscitative drugs and equipment and personnel trained in their use and skilled in airway management should be ensured. ■

• Give drug without regard for food. Dispense syrup directly into the mouth and don't mix with any liquid (such as grapefruit juice) before dispensing.
• Refer to manufacturer's instructions for use of oral dispenser and press-in bottle dispenser.

IV

Black Box Warning IV midazolam has been associated with respiratory depression and respiratory arrest, especially when used in noncritical-care settings. It should only be used in hospital or ambulatory care settings, including physicians' and dental offices that can provide continuous monitoring of cardiac and respiratory function. Availability of appropriate resuscitative drugs and equipment and personnel trained in their use and skilled in airway management should be ensured. ■

▼ Drug may be mixed in the same syringe with morphine sulfate, meperidine, atropine, or scopolamine.
▼ When mixing infusion, use 5-mg/mL vial and dilute to 0.5 mg/mL with D_5W or NSS.

Black Box Warning Give slowly over at least 2 minutes, and wait at least 2 minutes when initiating or titrating doses to fully evaluate therapeutic effect. Initial adult dose shouldn't exceed 2.5 mg. Lower initial doses are necessary for adults age 60 and older, for debilitated patients, and for those receiving concomitant opioids or other CNS depressants. ■

Black Box Warning Don't administer by rapid injection in the neonatal population. ■

▼ **Incompatibilities:** None listed by manufacturer. Consult a drug incompatibility reference for more information.

IM
• Inject deeply into a large muscle.

ACTION

May potentiate the effects of GABA, depress the CNS, and suppress the spread of seizure activity.

Route	Onset	Peak	Duration
PO	10–20 min	45–60 min	2–6 hr
IV	90 sec–5 min	Rapid	2–6 hr
IM	15 min	15–60 min	2–6 hr

Half-life: 2 to 6 hours.

ADVERSE REACTIONS

CNS: oversedation, drowsiness, amnesia, headache, seizures, involuntary movements, nystagmus, hiccups, paradoxical behavior or excitement. **CV:** variations in BP and pulse rate. **EENT:** nystagmus. **GI:** nausea, vomiting. **Respiratory:** *apnea,* decreased respiratory rate, oxygen desaturation, coughing. **Other:** pain at injection site, redness.

INTERACTIONS

Drug-drug. *Cimetidine:* May increase and prolong sedation. Avoid use together.
CNS depressants: May cause apnea. Use together cautiously. Adjust dosage of midazolam if used with opiates or other CNS depressants.
CYP3A4 inducers (carbamazepine, phenytoin, rifampin): May decrease midazolam level. Use cautiously and adjust dosage as needed.
CYP3A4 inhibitors (calcium channel blockers, fluconazole, itraconazole, ketoconazole, macrolide antibiotics [erythromycin]): May increase and prolong midazolam level, CNS depression, and psychomotor impairment. Avoid using together. If must be given together, monitor patient closely.

Reactions in bold italics are *life-threatening*. Interactions may have a *rapid onset* or a *delayed onset*.

Hormonal contraceptives: May prolong half-life of midazolam. Use together cautiously.

Black Box Warning *Opioids:* May cause slow or difficult breathing, sedation, and death. Avoid use together. If use together is necessary, limit dosage and duration of each drug to minimum necessary for desired effect. ■

Protease inhibitors (ritonavir, saquinavir): May increase midazolam level and prolong sedation. Use together cautiously.

Theophylline: May antagonize sedative effect of midazolam. Use together cautiously.

Drug-herb. *Ginkgo biloba, St. John's wort:* May decrease drug level. Discourage use together.

Drug-food. *Grapefruit juice:* May increase bioavailability of oral drug. Don't use together.

Drug-lifestyle. *Alcohol use:* May cause additive CNS effects. Don't use together.

EFFECTS ON LAB TEST RESULTS
None reported.

CONTRAINDICATIONS & CAUTIONS
• Contraindicated in patients hypersensitive to drug or its components and in those with acute angle-closure glaucoma, shock, coma, or acute alcohol intoxication.

• Intrathecal or epidural injection of parenteral forms containing benzyl alcohol is contraindicated.

❸ *Alert:* Drug should only be used with individualization of the dosage.

• Use cautiously in elderly or debilitated patients; in patients with uncompensated acute illness, HF, impaired gag reflex, or respiratory, renal, or hepatic disease; and in patients at risk for falls.

• Benzodiazepines are associated with paradoxical reactions (agitation, aggressive behavior, involuntary movements) and anterograde amnesia.

Black Box Warning Pediatric dosages must be calculated on a mg/kg basis, and all dosages should be titrated slowly. ■

Black Box Warning Midazolam should only be administered by persons specifically trained in the use of anesthetics and the management of respiratory effects of anesthetics, including resuscitation of patients in the age-group being treated. The appropriate

emergency equipment must always be immediately available. ■

Black Box Warning Opioids should only be prescribed with benzodiazepines or other CNS depressants to patients for whom alternative treatment options are inadequate. ■

• When overdose is suspected, flumazenil may be used as a reversal agent. It's used as an adjunct to proper benzodiazepine overdose management.

• Abrupt discontinuation of midazolam after prolonged use can result in withdrawal symptoms.

❸ *Alert:* Repeated or lengthy use of general anesthetics and sedation drugs during surgeries or procedures in children younger than age 3 and in pregnant women during the third trimester may affect the development of children's brains. Weigh benefits of appropriate anesthesia in young children and pregnant women against risks.

Dialyzable drug: Unknown.

⚠ *Overdose S&S:* Excessive sedation, somnolence, confusion, impaired coordination, diminished reflexes, coma, altered vital signs.

PREGNANCY-LACTATION-REPRODUCTION
• Several studies suggest an increased risk of congenital malformations associated with benzodiazepine use. Use in pregnancy isn't recommended.

• Drug appears in human milk. Use cautiously in breastfeeding women.

NURSING CONSIDERATIONS
Black Box Warning A qualified individual, other than the practitioner performing the procedure, should monitor patient throughout procedure. Have oxygen and resuscitation equipment available in case of severe respiratory depression. Excessive amounts and rapid infusion have been linked to respiratory arrest. Continuously monitor patient, including children taking syrup form, for life-threatening respiratory depression. ■

• Monitor BP, HR and rhythm, respirations, airway integrity, and pulse oximetry during procedure.

PATIENT TEACHING
• Teach patient about drug's use and potential adverse reactions; advise patient to immediately report difficulty breathing.

Black Box Warning Caution patient or caregivers of patient taking an opioid with a benzodiazepine, CNS depressant, or alcohol to seek immediate medical attention for dizziness, light-headedness, extreme sleepiness, slowed or difficult breathing, or unresponsiveness. ■

• Because drug diminishes patient's recall of events around the time of surgery, provide written information, family member instructions, and follow-up contact.

🔵 *Alert:* Discuss with parents or caregivers of child younger than age 3 and with female patient who is pregnant the benefits, risks, and appropriate timing of surgery or procedures requiring anesthetics and sedation drugs.

• Warn patient to avoid hazardous activities that require alertness or good coordination until effects of drug are known.

SAFETY ALERT!

miglitol
MIG-li-tol

Glyset

Therapeutic class: Antidiabetics
Pharmacologic class: Alpha-glucosidase inhibitors

AVAILABLE FORMS
Tablets: 25 mg, 50 mg, 100 mg

INDICATIONS & DOSAGES
➤ **Adjunct to diet in patients with type 2 diabetes, alone or with a sulfonylurea**
Adults: 25 mg PO t.i.d. May start with 25 mg PO daily and increase gradually to t.i.d. to minimize GI upset; dosage may be increased after 4 to 8 weeks to 50 mg PO t.i.d. Dosage may then be further increased after 3 months, based on HbA$_{1c}$ level, to maximum of 100 mg PO t.i.d.

ADMINISTRATION
PO
• Give drug with first bite of each main meal.

ACTION
Lowers glucose level by inhibiting enzymes in the small intestine, which delays the digestion of carbohydrates after a meal, resulting in a smaller increase in postprandial glucose level.

Route	Onset	Peak	Duration
PO	Unknown	2–3 hr	Unknown

Half-life: About 2 hours.

ADVERSE REACTIONS
GI: abdominal pain, diarrhea, flatulence.
Skin: rash.

INTERACTIONS
Drug-drug. *Digoxin, propranolol, ranitidine:* May decrease bioavailability of these drugs. Monitor clinical response and adjust dosage.
Insulin, sulfonylureas: May increase risk of hypoglycemia. Consider decreasing dosages of miglitol, insulin, and sulfonylureas.
Intestinal adsorbents (charcoal), digestive enzyme preparations (amylase, pancreatin): May reduce effect of miglitol. Avoid using together.

EFFECTS ON LAB TEST RESULTS
• May decrease iron level.

CONTRAINDICATIONS & CAUTIONS
• Contraindicated in patients hypersensitive to drug or its components and in those with diabetic ketoacidosis, inflammatory bowel disease, colonic ulceration, partial intestinal obstruction, chronic intestinal diseases with marked disorders of digestion or absorption, or conditions that may deteriorate because of increased gas formation in the intestine.
• Contraindicated in patients predisposed to intestinal obstruction.
• Drug isn't recommended in patients with CrCl of less than 25 mL/minute or if serum creatinine level is more than 2 mg/dL.
• Fever, trauma, infection, or surgery can cause a temporary loss of blood glucose control; temporary insulin therapy may be needed.
Dializable drug: Unknown.
⚠ *Overdose S&S:* Transient increases in flatulence, diarrhea, and abdominal discomfort.

Reactions in bold italics are *life-threatening*. Interactions may have a *rapid onset* or a *delayed onset*.

PREGNANCY-LACTATION-REPRODUCTION

• Safe use in pregnancy hasn't been established. Abnormal blood glucose levels during pregnancy may cause harm to the fetus. Most experts recommend insulin be used during pregnancy to maintain blood glucose levels. Don't use miglitol during pregnancy unless clearly needed.
• Drug appears in human milk. Use in breastfeeding women isn't recommended.

NURSING CONSIDERATIONS

• In patients also taking insulin or a sulfonylurea, dosage adjustment of these drugs may be needed. Monitor patient for hypoglycemia.
• Diabetes management should include diet control, an exercise program, and regular testing of urine and glucose level.
• Monitor glucose level regularly, especially during situations of increased stress, such as infection, fever, surgery, or trauma.
• Monitor HbA_{1c} level every 3 months to evaluate long-term glycemic control.
• Treat mild to moderate hypoglycemia with a ready form of sugar, such as glucose tablets or gel. Severe hypoglycemia may necessitate IV glucose or glucagon.
• Monitor patient for adverse GI effects.

PATIENT TEACHING

• Stress importance of adhering to diet, weight reduction, and exercise instructions. Urge patient to have glucose and HbA_{1c} levels tested regularly.
• Inform patient that drug treatment relieves symptoms but doesn't cure diabetes.
• Teach patient how to recognize high and low glucose levels.
• Instruct patient to have a source of glucose readily available to treat hypoglycemia.
• Advise patient that sucrose (table sugar, cane sugar) or fruit juices shouldn't be used to treat low-glucose reactions with this drug. Oral glucose (dextrose) or glucagon is necessary to increase glucose.
• Advise patient to seek medical advice promptly during periods of stress, such as fever, trauma, infection, or surgery, because dosage may have to be adjusted.
• Instruct patient to take drug three times daily with first bite of each main meal.

• Show patient how and when to monitor glucose level.
• Advise patient that adverse GI effects are most common during first few weeks of therapy and should improve over time.
• Urge patient to carry medical identification at all times.

milnacipran hydrochloride
mil-NAY-ci-pran

Savella𝒫

Therapeutic class: Antifibromyalgia drugs
Pharmacologic class: SSNRIs

AVAILABLE FORMS
Tablets: 12.5 mg, 25 mg, 50 mg, 100 mg

INDICATIONS & DOSAGES
➤ **Fibromyalgia**
Adults: Initially, 12.5 mg PO once daily; increase dosage to 12.5 mg b.i.d. on days 2 and 3, followed by 25 mg b.i.d. on days 4 to 7. Increase to 50 mg b.i.d. after day 7. May increase to 100 mg PO b.i.d. based on individual response; recommended dosage is 50 mg b.i.d.
Adjust-a-dose: For patients with CrCl of 5 to 29 mL/minute, give 25 mg b.i.d. May increase to 50 mg b.i.d. based on individual tolerance.

ADMINISTRATION
PO
• Give drug with or without food, but giving with food may improve tolerability.

ACTION
Unclear. Milnacipran is a potent inhibitor of neuronal norepinephrine and serotonin reuptake; however, it doesn't affect the uptake of dopamine or other transmitters.

Route	Onset	Peak	Duration
PO	Unknown	2–4 hr	36–48 hr

Half-life: 6 to 8 hours; active metabolite, 8 to 10 hours.

ADVERSE REACTIONS
CNS: anxiety, depression, dizziness, falls, fatigue, fever, hypesthesia, irritability,

M

insomnia, migraine, paresthesia, *seizures,* stress, somnolence, headache, tremors. **CV:** chest discomfort, chest pain, flushing, HTN, palpitations, peripheral edema, tachycardia, fever. **EENT:** blurred vision. **GI:** abdominal distention, abdominal pain, constipation, decreased appetite, diarrhea, dry mouth, flatulence, GERD, dyspepsia, dysgeusia, nausea, vomiting. **GU:** cystitis, UTI; in men—dysuria, ejaculation disorder, ejaculation failure, erectile dysfunction, libido decrease, prostatitis, scrotal pain, testicular pain, testicular swelling, urethral pain, urinary hesitation, urine retention, urine flow decrease. **Metabolic:** hypercholesterolemia, weight loss or gain. **Respiratory:** dyspnea, URI. **Skin:** hyperhidrosis, pruritus, rash. **Other:** chills, contusion, hot flush, night sweats.

INTERACTIONS
Drug-drug. *Amphetamines, antipsychotics (risperidone), buspirone, cyclobenzaprine, dopamine antagonists (metoclopramide):* May cause serotonin syndrome (diarrhea, dysreflexia, fever, hallucinations, loss of coordination, nausea, tachycardia). If use together can't be avoided, closely monitor patient for signs and symptoms of serotonin syndrome.
◑ *Alert: Aspirin, NSAIDs, platelet inhibitors, warfarin:* May increase risk of bleeding. Use together cautiously.
Clomipramine: May cause euphoria and orthostatic hypotension when switching from clomipramine to milnacipran. Use together may also increase risk of serotonin syndrome. Monitor patient closely.
Clonidine: May decrease antihypertensive effect of clonidine. Monitor therapy.
Digoxin: May cause orthostatic hypotension and tachycardia and digoxin-related adverse effects. Avoid use of digoxin IV; when using oral digoxin and drug together, monitor patient closely.
Lithium, other serotonergic drugs (SSNRIs, SSRIs, TCAs, tramadol, triptans): May cause serotonin syndrome. Avoid use together.
MAO inhibitors: May cause serotonin syndrome. Avoid using drug within 2 weeks after MAO inhibitor therapy; wait at least 5 days after stopping milnacipran or before starting MAO inhibitor.

Methylene blue: May cause CNS toxicity and serotonin syndrome. Avoid use together.
Drug-herb. *Herbs with anticoagulant properties (alfalfa, anise, bilberry):* May increase risk of bleeding. Use together cautiously.
St. John's wort: May increase risk of serotonin syndrome. Avoid using together.
Drug-lifestyle. *Alcohol use:* May enhance psychomotor impairment and aggravate preexisting liver disease. Don't administer to patients using alcohol or with chronic liver disease.

EFFECTS ON LAB TEST RESULTS
• May increase LFT values.
• May decrease sodium level.

CONTRAINDICATIONS & CAUTIONS
• Contraindicated in patients hypersensitive to drug or its components.
• Contraindicated in patients being treated with MAO inhibitors, such as linezolid or IV methylene blue.
◑ *Alert:* Pupillary dilation that occurs after drug use may trigger an angle-closure attack in patients with anatomically narrow angles who don't have a patent iridectomy.
◑ *Alert:* Serotonin syndrome, a potentially life-threatening condition, may occur, particularly with concomitant use of serotonergic drugs (including triptans and tramadol) and drugs that impair serotonin metabolism (including MAO inhibitors). Signs and symptoms of serotonin syndrome include mental status changes (agitation, coma, hallucinations), autonomic instability (hyperthermia, labile BP, tachycardia), neuromuscular aberrations (hyperreflexia, incoordination), and diarrhea, nausea, and vomiting.
• Use cautiously in patients with a history of mania, seizures, severe hepatic impairment, or dysuria; in patients who consume substantial amounts of alcohol; and in those with HTN or controlled angle-closure glaucoma.
• Drug isn't approved for use in children.
Dialyzable drug: Unlikely.
⚠ *Overdose S&S:* HTN, cardiac arrest, decreased level of consciousness, confusion, dizziness, elevated LFT results.

Reactions in bold italics are *life-threatening*. Interactions may have a *rapid onset* or a *delayed onset*.

PREGNANCY-LACTATION-REPRODUCTION
• There are no adequate studies in pregnant women. Use during pregnancy only if potential benefit justifies potential risk to the fetus. Neonates exposed to SSRIs/SSNRIs late in the third trimester have developed complications requiring prolonged hospitalization, respiratory support, and tube feeding.
• Manufacturer advises pregnant patients to enroll in the Savella Pregnancy Registry (1-844-726-3512).
• Drug appears in human milk. Use cautiously in breastfeeding women.

NURSING CONSIDERATIONS
Black Box Warning Drug may increase risk of suicidal thinking and behavior in children, adolescents, and young adults with major depressive disorder or other psychiatric disorder. Drug isn't approved for use in children. ∎
• At least 14 days should elapse between discontinuation of an MAO inhibitor and initiation of milnacipran. Allow at least 5 days after stopping milnacipran before starting an MAO inhibitor.
• Monitor patient closely for worsening depression or suicidal behavior, especially during the first few months of therapy and with dosage adjustments.
• To prevent withdrawal signs and symptoms, decrease dosage gradually, and watch for signs and symptoms that may arise when drug is stopped, such as dysphoria, irritability, agitation, dizziness, sensory disturbances, anxiety, confusion, headache, lethargy, emotional lability, insomnia, hypomania, tinnitus, and seizures.
• Carefully monitor HR and BP.
• Monitor patient for signs and symptoms of hyponatremia (headache, difficulty concentrating, memory impairment, confusion, weakness, unsteadiness, hallucination, syncope, seizures, coma, respiratory arrest).
• Monitor LFT values and sodium level before and during therapy.

PATIENT TEACHING
Black Box Warning Warn families and caregivers to immediately report signs and symptoms of worsening depression (such as agitation, irritability, insomnia, hostility, and impulsivity) and suicidal behavior. ∎

• Advise patient to avoid taking NSAIDs and aspirin while taking drug to reduce risk of bleeding.
• Tell patient to avoid alcohol while taking drug.
• Instruct patient to have frequent HR and BP monitoring.
• Tell patient to report urinary hesitation or urine retention.
• Instruct female patient of childbearing potential to notify prescriber if she becomes pregnant, is planning pregnancy during therapy, or is breastfeeding.
• Warn patient not to stop drug suddenly.
• Tell patient to consult prescriber before taking other prescription or OTC drugs or herbal supplements.
• Warn patient to avoid hazardous activities that require alertness and good coordination until drug's effects are known.
• Tell patient that drug may be taken with or without food but that food may increase tolerability.

SAFETY ALERT!

milrinone lactate
MIL-ri-none

Therapeutic class: Inotropes
Pharmacologic class: Bipyridine phosphodiesterase inhibitors

AVAILABLE FORMS
Injection: 1 mg/mL
Injection (premixed): 200 mcg/mL in D_5W

INDICATIONS & DOSAGES
➤ **Short-term treatment of acutely decompensated HF**
Adults: Give first loading dose of 50 mcg/kg IV slowly over 10 minutes; then give continuous IV infusion of 0.375 to 0.75 mcg/kg/minute. Titrate infusion dose based on clinical and hemodynamic responses. Don't exceed 1.13 mg/kg/day.
Adjust-a-dose: If CrCl is 50 mL/minute, infusion rate is 0.43 mcg/kg/minute; if 40 mL/minute, infusion rate is 0.38 mcg/kg/minute; if 30 mL/minute, infusion rate is 0.33 mcg/kg/minute; if 20 mL/minute, infusion rate is 0.28 mcg/kg/minute; if 10 mL/minute, infusion rate is 0.23 mcg/kg/minute;

M

and if 5 mL/minute, infusion rate is
0.2 mcg/kg/minute.

ADMINISTRATION

IV

▼ Give loading dose undiluted as a direct
injection over 10 minutes.

▼ For continuous IV infusion, dilute vials
labeled as containing 10, 20, or 50 mg of
milrinone with 40, 80, or 200 mL, respectively, of ½ NSS, NSS, or D5W to provide solutions containing approximately
200 mcg/mL of milrinone. Don't dilute
200-mcg/mL commercially available bags.

▼ **Incompatibilities:** None listed by manufacturer. Consult a drug incompatibility
reference for more information.

ACTION

Produces inotropic action by increasing cellular levels of cAMP and vasodilation by
relaxing vascular smooth muscle.

Route	Onset	Peak	Duration
IV	5–15 min	1–2 hr	3–6 hr

Half-life: 2.4 hours.

ADVERSE REACTIONS

CNS: headache. **CV:** *ventricular arrhythmias,* ventricular ectopic activity, *ventricular tachycardia,* hypotension, nonsustained
ventricular tachycardia, chest pain.

INTERACTIONS

None significant.

EFFECTS ON LAB TEST RESULTS

● May cause abnormal LFT results.
● May cause electrolyte changes.

CONTRAINDICATIONS & CAUTIONS

● Contraindicated in patients hypersensitive
to drug. Solutions containing dextrose may
be contraindicated in patients with known
allergy to corn or corn products.

❸ *Alert:* Use of milrinone for more than
48 hours in patients with HF hasn't been
shown to be safe or effective.

❸ *Alert:* Drug has been associated with increased frequency of ventricular arrhythmias, including nonsustained ventricular tachycardia and supraventricular and

ventricular arrhythmias in the high-risk population. Closely monitor patient.

● Drug isn't recommended for use in patients with severe aortic or pulmonic valvular disease in place of surgery and during
acute phase after an MI.

● Use cautiously in patients with atrial flutter or fibrillation because drug may increase
ventricular response rate.

Dialyzable drug: Unknown.

⚠ *Overdose S&S:* Hypotension.

PREGNANCY-LACTATION-REPRODUCTION

● There are no adequate studies in pregnant
women. Use during pregnancy only if potential benefit justifies potential risk to the
fetus.

● It isn't known if drug appears in human
milk. Use cautiously in breastfeeding
women.

NURSING CONSIDERATIONS

● In patients with atrial flutter or fibrillation,
drug is typically given with digoxin and diuretics.

● Improved cardiac output may increase
urine output. Reduce diuretic dosage when
HF improves. Potassium loss may cause
digitalis toxicity.

● Monitor fluid and electrolyte status, BP,
HR, and renal function during therapy. Excessive decrease in BP requires stopping or
slowing rate of infusion.

● Correct hypoxemia and electrolyte imbalances, especially hypokalemia and hypomagnesemia, before use and throughout
therapy.

PATIENT TEACHING

● Instruct patient to report adverse reactions
promptly, especially angina or palpitations.

● Tell patient that drug may cause headache,
which can be treated with analgesics.

● Tell patient to report discomfort at IV
insertion site.

---

minocycline hydrochloride
mi-noe-SYE-kleen

Dynacin, Minocin, Minolira, Solodyn, Ximino

Therapeutic class: Antibiotics
Pharmacologic class: Tetracyclines

AVAILABLE FORMS
Capsules ⓞⓝⓒ: 50 mg, 75 mg, 100 mg
Injection: 100 mg
Tablets: 50 mg, 75 mg, 100 mg
Tablets (extended-release) ⓞⓝⓒ: 45 mg, 55 mg, 65 mg, 80 mg, 90 mg, 105 mg, 115 mg, 135 mg

INDICATIONS & DOSAGES
Adjust-a-dose (for all indications): Decrease dosage or increase dosing interval in patients with renal impairment. Don't exceed 200 mg (immediate-release) in 24 hours.
➤ **Infections caused by susceptible gram-negative and gram-positive organisms (including** *Haemophilus ducreyi, Yersinia pestis,* **and** *Campylobacter fetus),* *Rickettsiae* **species,** *Mycoplasma pneumoniae,* **or** *Chlamydia trachomatis;* **psittacosis; granuloma inguinale**
Adults: 200 mg PO or IV initially; then 100 mg PO or IV every 12 hours. May use 100 or 200 mg PO initially; then 50 mg q.i.d.
Children older than age 8: Initially, 4 mg/kg PO or IV; then, 2 mg/kg PO or IV every 12 hours. Maximum dose is 100 mg/dose or 200 mg/dose for the loading dose.
➤ **Gonorrhea in patients allergic to penicillin**
Adults: Initially, 200 mg PO or IV; then 100 mg PO or IV every 12 hours for at least 4 days. Obtain samples for follow-up cultures within 2 to 3 days after treatment.
➤ **Syphilis in patients allergic to penicillin**
Adults: Initially, 200 mg PO or IV; then 100 mg PO or IV every 12 hours for 10 to 15 days.
➤ **Meningococcal carrier state**
Adults: 100 mg PO every 12 hours for 5 days.

➤ **Uncomplicated urethral, endocervical, or rectal infection caused by** *C. trachomatis* **or** *Ureaplasma urealyticum*
Adults: 100 mg PO every 12 hours for at least 7 days. Or, 200 mg IV initially; then 100 mg IV every 12 hours, not to exceed 400 mg in 24 hours.
➤ **Uncomplicated gonococcal urethritis**
Men: 100 mg PO every 12 hours for 5 days.
➤ **Treatment of inflammatory lesions of nonnodular moderate to severe acne vulgaris**
Adults and children age 12 and older: 1 mg/kg extended-release tablets PO once daily for 12 weeks.
➤ **Acne vulgaris**
Adults: Initially, 200 mg (immediate-release) PO; then 100 mg PO every 12 hours. Or, initially 100 to 200 mg (immediate-release) PO followed by 50 mg PO every 6 hours.
Children age 8 and older: Initially, 4 mg/kg (immediate-release) PO followed by 2 mg/kg PO every 12 hours. Maximum is 200 mg for the loading dose and 100 mg/dose for additional doses.

ADMINISTRATION
PO
• Obtain specimen for culture and sensitivity tests before first dose. Begin therapy while awaiting results.
• Give drug with a full glass of water. Patient may take with food to help decrease esophageal irritation.
• Drug shouldn't be given within 1 hour of bedtime, to avoid esophageal irritation or ulceration.
• Give capsules and extended-release tablets at the same time each day, with or without food.
• Capsules and extended-release tablets must be swallowed whole and not crushed, chewed, or split.

IV
▼ Reconstitute powder with 5 mL sterile water for injection; further dilute to 100 to 1,000 mL with sodium chloride injection, dextrose injection, or dextrose and sodium chloride injection, or to 250 to 1,000 mL with Ringer injection or lactated Ringer injection. (Don't use solutions containing

M

calcium except for lactated Ringer, because a precipitate may form.)

▼ Infuse over 60 minutes, avoid rapid administration, and don't administer with other drugs.

▼ Parenteral therapy is indicated only when oral therapy is inadequate or isn't tolerated. Institute oral therapy as soon as possible.

▼ **Incompatibilities:** Other drugs.

ACTION

May be bacteriostatic by binding to microorganism's ribosomal subunits, inhibiting protein synthesis; may also alter the cytoplasmic membrane of susceptible microorganisms.

Route	Onset	Peak	Duration
PO	Unknown	1–4 hr	Unknown
PO (extended-release)	Unknown	3½–4 hr	Unknown
IV	Unknown	Unknown	Unknown

Half-life: PO, 11 to 17 hours; IV, 15 to 23 hours.

ADVERSE REACTIONS

CNS: *intracranial HTN,* headache, lightheadedness, dizziness, vertigo, fatigue, mood alterations, somnolence, malaise, drowsiness, fever, paresthesia, hypesthesia, sedation. **CV:** thrombophlebitis, pericarditis. **EENT:** tooth disorder, tinnitus. **GI:** anorexia, diarrhea, nausea, dysphagia, glossitis, oral candidiasis, vomiting, dyspepsia, pancreatitis, dry mouth, stomatitis, *pseudomembranous colitis.* **GU:** *acute renal failure,* vaginitis. **Hematologic:** *neutropenia, thrombocytopenia,* eosinophilia, hemolytic anemia. **Hepatic:** *hepatotoxicity.* **Musculoskeletal:** arthralgia, myalgia, joint swelling. **Respiratory:** *bronchospasm,* cough, dyspnea, asthma exacerbation, pneumonitis. **Skin:** increased pigmentation, maculopapular and erythematous rashes, photosensitivity reactions, pruritus, urticaria, alopecia, *erythema multiforme, SJS.* **Other:** *anaphylaxis,* enamel defects, hypersensitivity reactions, superinfection, pain at injection site, lupuslike syndrome, serum sickness–like syndrome.

INTERACTIONS

Drug-drug. *Antacids (including sodium bicarbonate) and laxatives containing aluminum, magnesium, or calcium; antidiarrheals:* May decrease antibiotic absorption. Give antibiotic 1 hour before or 2 hours after these drugs.

Ferrous sulfate and other iron products, zinc: May decrease antibiotic absorption. Give drug 2 hours before or 3 hours after iron.

Hormonal contraceptives: May decrease contraceptive effectiveness and increase risk of breakthrough bleeding. Advise patient to use nonhormonal contraceptive.

Isotretinoin: May increase ICP. Don't use together.

Live-virus vaccines: May decrease vaccine effectiveness. Avoid administering together.

Oral anticoagulants: May increase anticoagulant effect. Monitor PT and INR, and adjust dosage.

Penicillins: May disrupt bactericidal action of penicillins. Avoid using together.

Retinoids: May increase risk of pseudotumor cerebri. Avoid administering together.

Drug-lifestyle. *Sun exposure:* May cause photosensitivity reactions. Advise patient to avoid excessive sunlight exposure.

EFFECTS ON LAB TEST RESULTS

● May increase BUN and liver enzyme levels. May decrease Hb level.

● May increase eosinophil count. May decrease platelet and neutrophil counts.

● May falsely elevate fluorometric test results for urine catecholamines. Parenteral form may cause false-positive results on copper sulfate test (Clinitest). May cause false-negative results on urine glucose tests using glucose oxidase reagent (Diastix or Chemstrip uG).

CONTRAINDICATIONS & CAUTIONS

● Contraindicated in patients hypersensitive to drug or other tetracyclines.

🚫 *Alert:* Severe cases of anaphylaxis, serious skin reactions (SJS, erythema multiforme, DRESS syndrome), and death have been reported.

🚫 *Alert:* Some products may contain tartrazine, which can cause allergy-type reactions (including bronchial asthma).

Reactions in bold italics are *life-threatening.* Interactions may have a *rapid onset* or a ***delayed onset.***

Although incidence of this sensitivity is low, these reactions are frequently seen in patients who are also sensitive to aspirin.
• Use cautiously in patients with impaired renal or hepatic function. Use of these drugs during last half of pregnancy and in children younger than age 8 may cause permanent discoloration of teeth, enamel defects, and bone growth retardation.
• Drug may cause superinfection. If overgrowth of nonsusceptible organisms occurs, discontinue drug and begin appropriate therapy.
• Increases in ICP and pseudotumor cerebri have been reported. If visual disturbances occur, a prompt ophthalmologic exam is needed.
Dialyzable drug: No.
⚠ *Overdose S&S:* Dizziness, nausea, vomiting.

PREGNANCY-LACTATION-REPRODUCTION
• There are no adequate studies in pregnant women. Drug may cause fetal harm. Avoid use in pregnancy.
• If patient becomes pregnant during therapy, stop drug immediately and apprise her of potential hazard to the fetus.
• Drug appears in human milk. Patient should discontinue breastfeeding or discontinue drug.
• Drug shouldn't be used to treat acne in males or females attempting to conceive a child.

NURSING CONSIDERATIONS
• Monitor renal function and LFT results.
🔔 *Alert:* Check expiration date. Outdated or deteriorated drug may cause reversible nephrotoxicity (Fanconi syndrome).
• Don't expose drug to light or heat. Keep cap tightly closed.
• If large doses are given, therapy is prolonged, or patient is at high risk, monitor patient for signs and symptoms of superinfection.
• Drug may cause mild to severe CDAD, which can occur up to 2 months after therapy ends. If diarrhea occurs, evaluate patient for CDAD. Drug may need to be discontinued and appropriate therapy begun.
• Check patient's tongue for signs of candidal infection. Stress good oral hygiene.

• Drug may discolor teeth in older children and young adults, more commonly when used as long-term treatment. Watch for brown pigmentation, and notify prescriber if it occurs.
• Photosensitivity reactions may occur within a few minutes to several hours after exposure. Photosensitivity lasts after therapy ends.
• Monitor patient for DRESS syndrome. Discontinue drug immediately if syndrome occurs.
• *Look alike–sound alike:* Don't confuse Minocin with niacin or minoxidil.

PATIENT TEACHING
• Tell patient to take entire amount of drug exactly as prescribed, even if feeling better.
• Instruct patient to take drug with a full glass of water. Drug may be taken with food. Tell patient not to take within 1 hour of bedtime to avoid esophageal irritation or ulceration.
• Teach patient about potential adverse reactions and to report them promptly.
• Warn patient to avoid driving or other hazardous tasks because of possible adverse CNS effects.
• Caution patient to avoid direct sunlight and ultraviolet light, wear protective clothing, and use sunscreen.
• Tell patient to take extended-release tablets at the same time each day.
• Tell patient to swallow extended-release tablet whole and not to crush, chew, or split tablet.
• Warn patient not to take more than one extended-release tablet each day.
• Warn patient that diarrhea may occur up to 2 months after last dose. Tell patient to report diarrhea to prescriber.
• Tell female patient not to take drug if pregnant or trying to become pregnant because of potential fetal hazard.
• Warn patient that drug can decrease hormonal contraceptive effectiveness. Advise the use of a nonhormonal method.

M

mipomersen sodium ℞
mi-poe-MER-sen

Therapeutic class: Antilipemics
Pharmacologic class: Oligonucleotides

AVAILABLE FORMS
Injection: 200 mg/mL single-use vials or prefilled syringes

INDICATIONS & DOSAGES
➤ **Adjunctive treatment for homozygous familial hypercholesterolemia (HoFH) with lipid-lowering medications and diet to reduce LDL cholesterol, apolipoprotein B, total cholesterol, and non-HDL cholesterol** ℞
Adults: 200 mg subcut once weekly on same day each week.
Adjust-a-dose: Refer to manufacturer's instructions for toxicity-related dosage adjustments.

ADMINISTRATION
Subcutaneous
Black Box Warning Before beginning treatment, obtain ALT, AST, alkaline phosphatase, and total bilirubin levels. ∎
• Store refrigerated at 36° to 46° F (2° to 8° C). Protect from light and keep in original carton until time of use. If refrigeration isn't possible, store at or below 86° F (30° C), away from heat sources, for up to 14 days.
• Remove from refrigeration at least 30 minutes before use.
• Inspect solution for clarity or particulate matter; if solution is cloudy or contains particles, return product to pharmacy.
• Administer first dose under supervision of health care provider.
• Administration sites include the abdomen, thigh region, and outer area of the upper arm. Alternate sites.
• Don't inject in areas of active skin disease or injury (such as sunburn, rash, inflammation, skin infection, or active areas of psoriasis). Avoid tattooed and scarred skin.
• Vials and syringes are for single use only. Discard excess solution; product contains no preservatives.
• Don't give IV or IM.

• Don't mix or administer this drug with other products.
• If a dose is missed, give missed dose at least 3 days from the next scheduled weekly dose.

ACTION
Inhibits synthesis of apolipoprotein B-100, a primary component of LDL cholesterol and its metabolic precursor, VLDL.

Route	Onset	Peak	Duration
Subcut	Unknown	3–4 hr	Unknown

Half-life: 1 to 2 months.

ADVERSE REACTIONS
CNS: fatigue, headache, fever, chills, insomnia. **CV:** angina pectoris, palpitations, peripheral edema, HTN. **GI:** nausea, vomiting, abdominal pain. **GU:** proteinuria. **Hepatic:** *hepatotoxicity,* hepatic steatosis, hepatic enzyme increase. **Musculoskeletal:** extremity pain, musculoskeletal pain. **Skin:** injection-site reactions (pain, hematoma, erythema, pruritus, swelling, discoloration). **Other:** flulike symptoms, benign neoplasms, *malignant neoplasms.*

INTERACTIONS
Drug-drug. *Hepatotoxic drugs (acetaminophen, amiodarone, isotretinoin, methotrexate, tamoxifen, tetracyclines):* May increase risk of liver injury. Monitor LFTs frequently.
Drug-lifestyle. *Alcohol use:* May increase risk of hepatotoxicity. Limit alcohol intake to one drink per day.

EFFECTS ON LAB TEST RESULTS
• May increase AST, ALT, and urine protein levels.

CONTRAINDICATIONS & CAUTIONS
Black Box Warning Drug may cause elevated transaminase levels and may increase hepatic fat, with or without concomitant increases in transaminase levels. Hepatic steatosis is a risk factor for advanced liver disease, including steatohepatitis and cirrhosis. Measure ALT, AST, alkaline phosphatase, and total bilirubin levels before initiating treatment, and monitor ALT and AST levels regularly as recommended.

Reactions in bold italics are *life-threatening*. Interactions may have a *rapid onset* or a *delayed onset*.

During treatment, withhold dose if ALT or AST level is 3 × ULN or more. Discontinue drug for clinically significant liver toxicity. ∎
• Contraindicated in patients with known hypersensitivity to drug or its components and in those with moderate or severe hepatic impairment (Child-Pugh class B or C) or active liver disease, including unexplained, persistent serum transaminase elevations.
Black Box Warning Only patients with a clinical or lab diagnosis of HoFH should use drug. Safety and effectiveness haven't been established in patients with hypercholesterolemia who don't have HoFH. ∎
• Drug isn't recommended in patients with severe renal impairment or clinically significant proteinuria, or in patients on renal dialysis.
• Using drug as an adjunct to LDL apheresis isn't recommended.
Dialyzable drug: Unlikely.

PREGNANCY-LACTATION-REPRODUCTION
• Drug may cause fetal harm. Women of childbearing potential should use effective contraception during therapy. Use drug only if clearly needed.
• It isn't known if drug appears in human milk. Patient should discontinue breastfeeding or discontinue drug.

NURSING CONSIDERATIONS
• If baseline LFT values are abnormal, consider treatment only after appropriate evaluation and resolution or explanation of any abnormalities.
• Obtain LFT values monthly for first year, then at least every 3 months thereafter. Discontinue drug if persistent or clinically significant increases occur.
• If transaminase elevations are accompanied by clinical signs and symptoms of liver injury (nausea, vomiting, abdominal pain, fever, jaundice, lethargy, flulike symptoms), increases in bilirubin to 2 × ULN or more, or active liver disease, discontinue drug and identify probable cause.
• Measure lipid levels at least every 3 months for first year. Assess LDL levels after 6 months, since maximum LDL reduction occurs at that time. Assess whether drug is effective, taking into account possible hepatotoxicity.

Black Box Warning Because of hepatotoxicity, only providers and pharmacies certified through the Kynamro REMS program may prescribe and administer this medication. For more information, call 1-877-KYNAMRO (1-877-596-2676) or go to www.kynamrorems.com. ∎
• Drug's effect on CV morbidity and mortality hasn't been determined.
• Proper injection technique may help decrease risk of injection-site reactions, which occur in the majority of patients and typically consist of one or more of the following: erythema, pain, tenderness, pruritus, and local swelling.
• Flulike symptoms, which typically develop within 2 days after an injection, may occur and include one or more of the following: flulike illness, pyrexia, chills, myalgia, arthralgia, malaise, and fatigue.

PATIENT TEACHING
• Caution patient that there must be at least 3 days between a missed dose and the next regularly scheduled weekly dose.
• Instruct patient or caregiver on the proper technique for administering this drug, including use of aseptic technique. Needles or syringes may only be used once, and should be properly disposed of in a suitable puncture-resistant container. Proper administration technique may decrease risk of injection-site reactions.
• Advise patient to avoid or limit alcohol to one drink per day because of additive liver toxicity.
• Tell patient to report signs and symptoms of liver damage, including nausea, vomiting, fever, anorexia, fatigue, jaundice, dark urine, pruritus, and abdominal pain. Encourage compliance with follow-up blood tests to monitor safe use of drug.
• Advise patient that injection-site reactions (erythema, pain, tenderness, pruritus, or local swelling) may occur.
• Advise patient that flulike symptoms, typically appearing within 2 days after an injection, may occur and include flulike illness, pyrexia, chills, myalgia, arthralgia, malaise, and fatigue.

M

mirabegron
mir-a-BEG-ron

Myrbetriq

Therapeutic class: Bladder antispasmodics
Pharmacologic class: Beta-3 adrenergic agonists

AVAILABLE FORMS
Tablets (extended-release) ⓄⓉⒸ: 25 mg, 50 mg

INDICATIONS & DOSAGES
Adjust-a-dose (for all indications): For patients with severe renal impairment (CrCl of 15 to 29 mL/minute) or moderate hepatic impairment (Child-Pugh class B), give no more than 25 mg daily. Drug isn't recommended for patients with ESRD (CrCl of less than 15 mL/minute) or for patients with severe hepatic impairment (Child-Pugh class C).

➤ **Overactive bladder with symptoms of urge incontinence, urgency, and frequency**
Adults: Initially, 25 mg PO once daily. Drug is effective within 8 weeks. Based on individual patient effectiveness and tolerability, may increase dosage to 50 mg once daily.

➤ **Overactive bladder with symptoms of urge incontinence, urgency, and frequency in combination with solifenacin succinate**
Adults: Initially, mirabegron 25 mg PO once daily with solifenacin 5 mg PO once daily. May increase mirabegron to 50 mg PO once daily with solifenacin 5 mg PO once daily after 4 to 8 weeks if necessary.

ADMINISTRATION
PO
• May give without regard to food.
• Patient should swallow tablets whole with water; don't crush or divide tablets.

ACTION
Relaxes the detrusor smooth muscle during storage phase of the urinary bladder fill-void cycle, increasing bladder capacity.

Route	Onset	Peak	Duration
PO	Unknown	3½ hr	Unknown

Half-life: 50 hours.

ADVERSE REACTIONS
CNS: headache, fatigue, dizziness. **CV:** HTN, tachycardia. **EENT:** nasopharyngitis, dry mouth, sinusitis. **GI:** constipation, diarrhea, abdominal pain. **GU:** UTI, cystitis, urine retention. **Musculoskeletal:** arthralgia, back pain. **Respiratory:** URI. **Other:** flulike symptoms.

INTERACTIONS
Drug-drug. *Digoxin:* May increase digoxin level. Monitor digoxin level and titrate mirabegron to lowest effective dosage.
Drugs metabolized by CYP2D6 (desipramine, flecainide, metoprolol, propafenone, thioridazine): May increase levels of these drugs. Monitor patient for adverse events; adjust dosage as needed.
Ketoconazole: May increase mirabegron concentration. Monitor patient response.
Metoprolol: May alter metoprolol concentration. Monitor BP closely.
Rifampin: May decrease mirabegron concentration. Monitor patient response.
Warfarin: May increase warfarin level. Monitor INR; adjust warfarin dosage as necessary.

EFFECTS ON LAB TEST RESULTS
• May increase ALT, AST, GGT, LDH, and digoxin levels.
• May increase INR.

CONTRAINDICATIONS & CAUTIONS
• Contraindicated in patients hypersensitive to drug or its components.
• Drug isn't recommended for use in patients with severe, uncontrolled HTN (systolic BP 180 mm Hg or higher or diastolic BP 110 mm Hg or higher).
• Use cautiously in patients with HTN, QT-interval prolongation, or bladder outlet obstruction, as the risk of urine retention may be increased.
• Safety and effectiveness in children haven't been established.
Dialyzable drug: Unknown.

Reactions in bold italics are *life-threatening*. Interactions may have a *rapid onset* or a *delayed onset*.

⚠ *Overdose S&S:* Palpitations, increased HR, increased BP.

PREGNANCY-LACTATION-REPRODUCTION
• There are no adequate studies in pregnant women. Use during pregnancy only if potential benefit justifies potential risk to the fetus.
• It isn't known if drug appears in human milk. Patient should discontinue breastfeeding or discontinue drug.

NURSING CONSIDERATIONS
• Monitor BP and pulse regularly, especially in patients with HTN or atrial fibrillation.
• Monitor patient for angioedema of the face, lips, tongue, or larynx, which may be life threatening and can occur after first dose. Promptly discontinue drug if involvement of the tongue, hypopharynx, or larynx occurs, and ensure a patent airway.
• Monitor patient closely for urine retention and bladder obstruction, especially in those already taking bladder antispasmodics.
• Monitor LFT values periodically.
• Monitor patients for rash or pruritus.

PATIENT TEACHING
• Tell patient not to crush, chew, or cut tablets; inform patient that drug may be taken without regard to food.
• Warn patient that drug may cause an increase in BP or pulse. Teach patient to monitor BP and pulse at home and to report increases to the health care provider.
• Advise patient that difficulty in emptying the bladder and infrequent bladder infections may occur and to report concerns to health care provider.
• Tell patient to report rash or itching, which may indicate an allergy or a serious adverse reaction.
• Advise patient to immediately report signs and symptoms of a significant reaction (fast heartbeat, palpitations, back pain, bloody urine, chills, severe dizziness, passing out, severe headache, wheezing, chest tightness, fever, bad cough, blue skin, seizures, or swelling of face, lips, tongue, or throat).
• Teach female patient to report pregnancy to her health care provider as soon as possible.

mirtazapine
mir-TAZ-a-peen

Remeron, Remeron SolTab

Therapeutic class: Antidepressants
Pharmacologic class: Tetracyclic antidepressants

AVAILABLE FORMS
Tablets: 7.5 mg, 15 mg, 30 mg, 45 mg
Tablets (ODTs) ⓓⓝⓖ: 15 mg, 30 mg, 45 mg

INDICATIONS & DOSAGES
➤ **Major depressive disorder**
Adults: Initially, 15 mg PO at bedtime. Maintenance dose is 15 to 45 mg daily. Adjust dosage at intervals of at least 1 week.

ADMINISTRATION
PO
• Give drug without regard for food.
• Remove ODT from blister pack and immediately place on patient's tongue.
• ODT may be given with or without water.
• Don't split or crush ODT.

ACTION
Thought to enhance central noradrenergic and serotonergic activity.

Route	Onset	Peak	Duration
PO	Unknown	2 hr	Unknown

Half-life: About 20 to 40 hours.

ADVERSE REACTIONS
CNS: somnolence, dizziness, asthenia, abnormal dreams, abnormal thinking, tremors, confusion, drowsiness, agitation, amnesia, anxiety, apathy, depression, hypoesthesia, malaise, myasthenia, paresthesia, twitching, vertigo. **CV:** edema, peripheral edema, HTN, vasodilation. **EENT:** dry mouth. **GI:** increased appetite, dry mouth, constipation, abdominal pain, anorexia, vomiting, nausea. **GU:** urinary frequency, UTI. **Metabolic:** weight gain. **Musculoskeletal:** myalgia, weakness, back pain. **Respiratory:** dyspnea, cough. **Skin:** pruritus, rash. **Other:** flulike syndrome.

INTERACTIONS

Drug-drug. *CYP2D6, CYP3A4 inhibitors:* May increase mirtazapine level. Consider therapy modification.

CYP3A4 inducers: May decrease mirtazapine level. Consider therapy modification.

Diazepam, other CNS depressants: May cause additive CNS effects. Avoid using together.

❸ Alert: *Linezolid, methylene blue:* May cause serotonin syndrome. Use together is contraindicated.

❸ Alert: *MAO inhibitors:* May sometimes cause fatal reactions. Avoid using within 14 days of MAO inhibitor therapy.

QT interval–prolonging agents (antiarrhythmics, fluoroquinolones, macrolides): May cause additive QT interval–prolonging effects. Coadminister with caution.

Serotonergic drugs (antidepressants, antiemetics [5-HT₃ antagonists], buspirone, fentanyl, lithium, TCAs, tramadol, triptans, tryptophan): May increase risk of serotonin syndrome. Monitor therapy.

Warfarin: May increase anticoagulant effect. Closely monitor INR when mirtazapine is started or stopped, and adjust warfarin dosage as needed.

Drug-herb. *St. John's wort:* May increase risk of serotonin syndrome. Use together cautiously and monitor patient closely for adverse reactions.

Drug-lifestyle. *Alcohol use:* May cause additive CNS effects. Discourage use together.

EFFECTS ON LAB TEST RESULTS

• May increase cholesterol and triglyceride levels and LFT values.

CONTRAINDICATIONS & CAUTIONS

• Contraindicated in patients hypersensitive to drug and within 14 days of MAO inhibitor therapy.

❸ Alert: Concomitant use with linezolid or methylene blue can cause serotonin syndrome (fever, mental status changes, muscle twitching, excessive sweating, shivering or shaking, diarrhea, or loss of coordination). Use together is contraindicated.

Black Box Warning Drug may increase risk of suicidal thinking and behavior in children, adolescents, and young adults with major depressive or other psychiatric disorders. Drug isn't approved for use in children. ∎

• Use cautiously in patients with CV or cerebrovascular disease, seizure disorders, suicidal thoughts, hepatic or renal impairment, or history of mania or hypomania.

• Use cautiously in patients with conditions that predispose them to hypotension, such as dehydration, hypovolemia, or antihypertensive therapy.

• Give drug cautiously to elderly patients; decreased clearance has occurred in this age group.

Dialyzable drug: Unknown.

⚠ Overdose S&S: Disorientation, drowsiness, impaired memory, tachycardia.

PREGNANCY-LACTATION-REPRODUCTION

• There are no adequate studies in pregnant women. Use during pregnancy only if clearly needed.

• Drug may appear in human milk. Use cautiously in breastfeeding women.

NURSING CONSIDERATIONS

❸ Alert: If linezolid or methylene blue must be given, mirtazapine must be stopped and patient should be monitored for serotonin toxicity for 2 weeks, or until 24 hours after the last dose of methylene blue or linezolid, whichever comes first. Treatment with mirtazapine may be resumed 24 hours after last dose of methylene blue or linezolid.

• Don't use within 14 days of MAO inhibitor therapy.

Black Box Warning Appropriately monitor and closely observe patients of all ages who are started on antidepressants for clinical worsening, mood changes, suicidality, or unusual changes in behavior. ∎

• Monitor patient for distressing restlessness and need to move, which is most likely to occur within first few weeks of treatment.

• Although agranulocytosis occurs rarely, stop drug and monitor patient closely if a sore throat, fever, stomatitis, or other signs and symptoms of infection with a low WBC count develop.

• Lower dosages tend to be more sedating than higher dosages.

PATIENT TEACHING

Black Box Warning Advise families and caregivers to closely observe patient for increasing suicidal thinking and behavior. ■

🕕 **Alert:** Teach patient to recognize and immediately report signs and symptoms of serotonin toxicity.

• Instruct patient to take drug at bedtime. Caution patient to avoid hazardous activities if feeling too sleepy.

• Tell patient to report signs and symptoms of infection, such as fever, chills, sore throat, mucous membrane irritation, or flulike syndrome.

• Instruct patient not to use alcohol or other CNS depressants while taking drug.

• Instruct patient not to take other drugs or stop drug abruptly without prescriber's approval.

• Tell female patient of childbearing potential to report suspected pregnancy immediately and to notify prescriber if breastfeeding.

• Instruct patient to remove ODTs from blister pack and place immediately on tongue. Tell patient to be sure hands are clean and dry when touching the tablet.

• Advise patient not to break or split tablet.

SAFETY ALERT!

mitoMYcin (mitomycin-C)
mye-toe-MYE-sin

Therapeutic class: Antineoplastics
Pharmacologic class: Antineoplastic antibiotics

AVAILABLE FORMS
Powder for injection: 5-mg, 20-mg, 40-mg vials

INDICATIONS & DOSAGES
Dosage and indications vary. Check treatment protocol with prescriber.

➤ **Disseminated adenocarcinoma of stomach or pancreas in combination with other chemotherapeutic agents**
Adults: 20 mg/m^2 IV as a single dose at 6- to 8-week intervals if patient has full hematologic recovery. Fully evaluate patient after each cycle and reduce dosage

if toxicities occur. Discontinue drug if disease progresses after two courses of therapy.
Adjust-a-dose: Refer to manufacturer's instructions for toxicity-related dosage instructions.

➤ **Anal cancer ♦**
Adults: 10 mg/m^2 IV on days 1 and 29 (maximum dose, 20 mg/dose) in combination with 5-FU and radiation therapy. Or, 10 mg/m^2 IV on day 1 (maximum dose, 15 mg/dose) in combination with capecitabine and radiation therapy. Or, 12 mg/m^2 IV on day 1 (maximum dose, 20 mg/dose) in combination with capecitabine and radiation therapy. Or, 12 mg/m^2 or 15 mg/m^2 on day 1 in combination with 5-FU and radiation therapy.

➤ **Bladder cancer (muscle invasive) ♦**
Adults: 12 mg/m^2 IV on day 1 in combination with 5-FU and radiation therapy.

ADMINISTRATION

IV

🕕 **Alert:** Don't give to patients with serum creatinine level greater than 1.7 mg/dL.

▼ Preparing and giving drug may be mutagenic, teratogenic, or carcinogenic. Use safe handling and disposal precautions.

▼ Drug is a vesicant. Never give drug IM or subcut. Consider using a CVAD.

▼ Using sterile water for injection, reconstitute drug in 5-mg vials with 10 mL, 20-mg vials with 40 mL, and 40-mg vials with 80 mL. Solution will appear clear to pale blue. Protect from light.

▼ Give drug by slow IV push or slow IV infusion into the side arm of a free-flowing IV line.

▼ When reconstituted with sterile water, solution is stable for 14 days under refrigeration and for 7 days at room temperature, if protected from light. When further diluted, drug is stable in D$_5$W for no more than 3 hours, in NSS for no more than 12 hours, and in sodium lactate for no more than 24 hours.

▼ The combination of mitomycin (5 to 15 mg) and heparin (1,000 to 10,000 units) in 30 mL NSS is stable for 48 hours at room temperature.

▼ Stop infusion immediately and notify prescriber if extravasation occurs because

M

of potential for severe ulceration and necrosis.

▼ **Incompatibilities:** None listed by manufacturer. Consult a drug incompatibility reference for more information.

ACTION
Similar to an alkylating drug, cross-linking strands of DNA and causing an imbalance of cell growth, leading to cell death.

Route	Onset	Peak	Duration
IV	Unknown	Unknown	Unknown

Half-life: About 50 minutes.

ADVERSE REACTIONS
CNS: headache, neurologic abnormalities, confusion, drowsiness, fatigue, fever, pain. **EENT:** blurred vision. **GI:** mucositis, nausea, vomiting, anorexia, diarrhea, stomatitis. **GU:** *renal toxicity, hemolytic-uremic syndrome.* **Hematologic:** *thrombocytopenia, leukopenia, microangiopathic hemolytic anemia.* **Respiratory:** *interstitial pneumonitis, pulmonary edema,* dyspnea, nonproductive cough. **Skin:** cellulitis, induration, desquamation, pruritus, pain at injection site, reversible alopecia, purple bands on nails, rash, sloughing with extravasation, alopecia. **Other:** *septicemia,* ulceration.

INTERACTIONS
None reported in prescribing information.

EFFECTS ON LAB TEST RESULTS
• May increase BUN and creatinine levels. May decrease Hb level.
• May decrease WBC and platelet counts.

CONTRAINDICATIONS & CAUTIONS
• Contraindicated in patients hypersensitive to drug and in those with thrombocytopenia, coagulation disorders, or an increased bleeding tendency from other causes.
• Don't give to patients with serum creatinine level greater than 1.7 mg/dL.
Dialyzable drug: Unknown.

PREGNANCY-LACTATION-REPRODUCTION
• Drug can cause fetal harm. If used during pregnancy, or if patient becomes pregnant during therapy, apprise her of potential hazard to the fetus and potential risk of loss of the pregnancy.
• It isn't known if drug appears in human milk. Patient should discontinue breastfeeding or discontinue drug.

NURSING CONSIDERATIONS
Black Box Warning Administer drug under the supervision of a physician experienced with cancer chemotherapeutic agents. ∎
Black Box Warning Bone marrow suppression (thrombocytopenia and leukopenia), which may contribute to overwhelming infections in an already compromised patient, is the most common and severe toxic effect. ∎
• Reevaluate patient fully after each course of mitomycin, and reduce dosage if patient has experienced toxicities.
🚹 *Alert:* Pulmonary toxicity, which may be severe and life-threatening, has been reported infrequently. Signs and symptoms may include dyspnea with a nonproductive cough and pulmonary infiltrates on X-ray. Drug may need to be discontinued.
🚹 *Alert:* Extravasation may occur, causing cellulitis, ulceration, and tissue slough. If signs or symptoms of these conditions occur, stop infusion immediately and notify prescriber. Withdraw 3 to 5 mL of blood; then remove infusion needle. If skin necrosis develops, skin grafting may be necessary.
• Continue CBC and blood studies at least 8 weeks after therapy stops. Leukopenia and thrombocytopenia are cumulative. If WBC count falls below 2,000/mm³ or granulocyte count falls below 1,000/mm³, follow institutional policy for infection control in immunocompromised patients.
• If disease progresses after two courses of mitomycin, chances of response are minimal and drug should be discontinued.
• Anticipate need for blood transfusions to combat anemia.
• Monitor patient for dyspnea with nonproductive cough; chest X-ray may show infiltrates.
• Monitor renal function tests.
• Leukopenia may occur up to 8 weeks after therapy and may be cumulative with successive doses.
Black Box Warning Drug can cause hemolytic-uremic syndrome, which is

---

Reactions in bold italics are *life-threatening*. Interactions may have a *rapid onset* or a *delayed onset*.

characterized by microangiopathic hemolytic anemia, thrombocytopenia, and irreversible renal failure. The syndrome may occur at any time during systemic therapy with mitomycin as a single agent or in combination with other cytotoxic drugs; however, most cases occur at doses of 60 mg or more. Blood product transfusion may exacerbate symptoms associated with this syndrome. ∎

PATIENT TEACHING

• Advise patient to report all adverse reactions and to immediately report pain or burning at injection site during or after administration.
• Warn patient to watch for signs and symptoms of infection (fever, sore throat, fatigue), bleeding (easy bruising, nosebleeds, bleeding gums, tarry stools), and pulmonary toxicity (dyspnea with nonproductive cough). Tell patient to take temperature daily.
• Inform patient that hair loss may occur but that it's usually reversible.
• Inform patient of the potential for fetal harm if drug is used during pregnancy or if patient becomes pregnant during therapy.

SAFETY ALERT!

mitoXANTRONE hydrochloride
mye-toe-ZAN-trone

Therapeutic class: Antineoplastics
Pharmacologic class: DNA-reactive drugs–anthracenediones

AVAILABLE FORMS
Injection: 2 mg/mL

INDICATIONS & DOSAGES
➤ **Combination initial therapy for acute nonlymphocytic leukemia (ANLL)**
Adults: Induction begins with 12 mg/m² IV daily on days 1 to 3, with 100 mg/m² daily of cytarabine on days 1 to 7 as a continuous 24-hour infusion. A second induction with mitoxantrone for 2 days and cytarabine for 5 days may be given if response isn't adequate. Consolidation therapy: 12 mg/m² IV infusion daily on days 1 and 2 and cytarabine 100 mg/m² for 5 days given as a continuous 24-hour infusion on days 1 through 5. The first course is given approximately 6 weeks

after the final induction course; the second is generally given 4 weeks after the first. Severe myelosuppression has occurred with this regimen.
➤ **To reduce neurologic disability and frequency of relapse in chronic progressive, progressive relapsing, or worsening relapsing-remitting MS**
Adults: 12 mg/m² IV over 5 to 15 minutes every 3 months. Maximum cumulative lifetime dose is 140 mg/m². Dosage adjustments based on package insert.
➤ **Advanced hormone-refractory prostate cancer**
Men: 12 to 14 mg/m² as a short IV infusion every 21 days. Drug is given as an adjunct to corticosteroid therapy.

ADMINISTRATION
IV
▼ Preparing and giving drug may be mutagenic, teratogenic, or carcinogenic. Follow facility policy to reduce risks.
▼ Dilute dose in at least 50 mL of NSS for injection or D₅W injection. Don't mix with other drugs. Can further dilute in D₅W, NSS, or D₅NSS; use immediately if further diluted.
Black Box Warning Give slowly into a free-flowing IV infusion of NSS or D₅W injection over at least 3 minutes. ∎
Black Box Warning Never give subcutaneously, intra-arterially, intramuscularly, or intrathecally. ∎
Black Box Warning Severe local tissue damage may result if extravasation occurs. ∎
▼ If extravasation occurs, stop infusion immediately and notify prescriber. Place ice packs over the area intermittently.
▼ Once vial is penetrated, undiluted solution may be stored for 7 days at room temperature or 14 days in refrigerator. Don't freeze.
▼ **Incompatibilities:** Other drugs.

ACTION
Reacts with DNA, producing cytotoxic effect. Probably not specific to cell cycle.

Route	Onset	Peak	Duration
IV	Unknown	Unknown	Unknown

Half-life: Terminal half-life, 23 to 215 hours.

ADVERSE REACTIONS

CNS: fever, headache, *seizures,* asthenia.
CV: *arrhythmias,* ECG abnormalities, *HF,*
tachycardia, edema, *hemorrhage.* **EENT:**
conjunctivitis, sinusitis, pharyngitis, rhinitis.
GI: abdominal pain, bleeding, constipation,
diarrhea, mucositis, nausea, stomatitis, vomiting. **GU:** amenorrhea, menstrual disorder,
UTI, *renal failure.* **Hematologic:** *myelosuppression,* anemia. **Hepatic:** jaundice.
Metabolic: hyperuricemia, *hypocalcemia,*
hyponatremia. **Musculoskeletal:** back
pain. **Respiratory:** cough, dyspnea, URI,
pneumonia. **Skin:** alopecia, ecchymoses, local irritation or phlebitis, petechiae, *sepsis.*
Other: fungal infections, *sepsis.*

INTERACTIONS

Drug-drug. *Clozapine:* May increase risk of
neutropenia. Monitor patient closely.
Cyclosporine: May increase effects of mitoxantrone. Monitor patient closely.
Live-virus vaccines: May increase risk of
vaccine-induced adverse reactions. Defer
vaccination until mitoxantrone therapy has
been completed.
Natalizumab: May increase risk of concurrent infection. Avoid use together.
Palifermin: May increase severity of oral
mucositis. Don't give palifermin within
24 hours before or after mitoxantrone dose.
Pimecrolimus, tacrolimus (topical): May enhance adverse/toxic effect of mitoxantrone.
Avoid use together.
Tofacitinib: May increase immunosuppressive effect of tofacitinib. Avoid use together.
Trastuzumab: May increase risk of
trastuzumab-induced cardiac dysfunction.
Monitor patient closely for signs and symptoms of cardiac dysfunction.

EFFECTS ON LAB TEST RESULTS

• May increase ALT, AST, bilirubin, GGT,
and uric acid levels.
• May decrease calcium and sodium levels.
• May decrease WBC and granulocyte
counts, Hb level, and hematocrit.

CONTRAINDICATIONS & CAUTIONS

• Contraindicated in patients hypersensitive
to drug.
Black Box Warning Present or history of
CV disease, radiotherapy to mediastinal/

pericardial area, previous therapy with other
anthracyclines or anthracenediones, or use
of other cardiotoxic drugs may increase risk
of cardiotoxicity. ■
• Significantly myelosuppressed patients
shouldn't receive drug unless benefits outweigh risks.
• Use cautiously in patients with hepatic impairment.
Dialyzable drug: No.
⚠ *Overdose S&S:* Severe leukopenia.

PREGNANCY-LACTATION-REPRODUCTION

• Drug may cause fetal harm. Women of
childbearing potential should avoid becoming pregnant during therapy. If used during
pregnancy or if patient becomes pregnant
during therapy, apprise her of potential risk
to the fetus.
• There are no adequate studies in pregnant
women. Women with MS who are biologi-
cally capable of becoming pregnant should
have a pregnancy test before each dose, and
results should be known before drug administration.
• Drug appears in human milk. Patient
should discontinue breastfeeding before
starting drug.

NURSING CONSIDERATIONS

Black Box Warning Administer under the
supervision of a physician experienced with
cytotoxic chemotherapy. ■
Black Box Warning Except when used to
treat ANLL, mitoxantrone should generally
not be given to patients with baseline neutrophil counts less than 1,500 cells/mm^3.
Frequently monitor peripheral blood cell
counts for all patients using drug. ■
Black Box Warning Assess all patients
for cardiac signs and symptoms by history,
physical exam, and ECG before start of therapy. Assess patients with MS for cardiac
signs and symptoms by history, physical
exam, and ECG before each dose. ■
Black Box Warning Patients with MS
shouldn't receive a cumulative mitoxantrone
dose greater than 140 mg/m^2. ■
• Closely monitor hematologic and lab
chemistry parameters, including LFTs. Obtain CBC and platelet count before each
course of treatment. Patient may require

Reactions in bold italics are *life-threatening*. Interactions may have a *rapid onset* or a *delayed onset*.

blood transfusion or RBC or WBC colony-stimulating factors.
• Avoid all IM injections in patients with thrombocytopenia.

Black Box Warning Drug can cause potentially fatal HF during therapy or months to years after therapy. All patients should have baseline quantitative evaluation of LVEF. In patients with MS, evaluate LVEF before initiating treatment and before administering each dose of mitoxantrone. Patients with MS with a baseline LVEF below the lower limit of normal shouldn't be treated with mitoxantrone. All patients with MS who have finished treatment should receive yearly, quantitative LVEF evaluation to detect late-occurring cardiotoxicity. Additional doses of mitoxantrone shouldn't be given to patients with MS who have experienced either a drop in LVEF to below the lower limit of normal or a clinically significant reduction in LVEF during mitoxantrone therapy. ■

Black Box Warning Use of drug has been associated with cardiotoxicity; risk of cardiotoxicity increases with cumulative dose of 140 mg/m^2, although toxicities may occur at any dose. Continue ongoing cardiac monitoring to detect late occurring cardiotoxicity. ■
• If severe nonhematologic toxicity occurs during first course, delay second course until patient recovers.

Black Box Warning Secondary acute myelocytic leukemia has been reported with mitoxantrone therapy. ■

⚫ Alert: Women of childbearing potential with MS should have a pregnancy test even if they are using contraception. Results should be known before administration of each dose.

PATIENT TEACHING
• Advise patient to immediately report injection-site discomfort.
• Tell patient that urine may appear blue-green within 24 hours after receiving drug and that the whites of the eyes may turn blue. These effects are not harmful but may persist during therapy.
• Teach patient about potential adverse reactions and tell patient to report them. Advise patient to watch for signs and symptoms of bleeding and infection.

• Advise female patient to use appropriate contraceptive method to avoid pregnancy while receiving drug.

modafinil
moe-DAF-i-nil

Alertec✲, Provigil✐

Therapeutic class: CNS stimulants
Pharmacologic class: Analeptics
Controlled substance schedule: IV

AVAILABLE FORMS
Tablets: 100 mg, 200 mg

INDICATIONS & DOSAGES
➤ **To improve wakefulness in patients with excessive daytime sleepiness caused by narcolepsy, obstructive sleep apnea-hypopnea syndrome, and shift-work sleep disorder**
Adults: 200 mg PO daily, as a single dose in the morning. Patients with shift-work sleep disorder should take dose about 1 hour before the start of their shift. Maximum dose is 400 mg PO daily as a single dose.
Adjust-a-dose: In patients with severe hepatic impairment, give 100 mg PO daily as a single dose in the morning. Consider lower doses and close monitoring in elderly patients.

ADMINISTRATION
PO
• Give drug without regard for food; however, food may delay effect of drug.

ACTION
Unknown. Similar to action of sympathomimetics, including amphetamines, but drug is structurally distinct from amphetamines and doesn't alter release of dopamine or norepinephrine.

Route	Onset	Peak	Duration
PO	Unknown	2–4 hr	Unknown

Half-life: 15 hours.

ADVERSE REACTIONS
CNS: headache, nervousness, dizziness, drowsiness, insomnia, depression, anxiety,

paresthesia, hypertonia, confusion, emotional lability, vertigo, tremor, dyskinesia, agitation. **CV:** HTN, vasodilation, chest pain, palpitations, tachycardia, edema. **EENT:** abnormal vision, epistaxis, rhinitis, dry mouth, mouth ulcer, pharyngitis. **GI:** nausea, diarrhea, anorexia, gingivitis, thirst, dyspepsia, constipation, flatulence, taste perversion, decreased appetite, abdominal pain. **GU:** abnormal urine. **Hematologic:** eosinophilia. **Metabolic:** weight loss. **Musculoskeletal:** back or neck pain. **Respiratory:** *asthma.* **Skin:** sweating. **Other:** chills.

INTERACTIONS

Drug-drug. *Carbamazepine, phenobarbital, rifampin, other inducers of CYP3A4:* May alter modafinil level. Monitor patient closely.

Cyclosporine, theophylline: May reduce levels of these drugs. Use together cautiously.

CYP3A4/5 substrates (cyclosporine, midazolam, steroidal contraceptives, triazolam): May decrease level of the substrate. Adjust substrate dosage as needed.

Dextroamphetamine, methylphenidate: May cause 1-hour delay in modafinil absorption. Separate dosing times.

Diazepam, phenytoin, propranolol, other drugs metabolized by CYP2C19: May inhibit CYP2C19 and lead to higher levels of drugs metabolized by this enzyme. Use together cautiously; adjust dosage as needed.

Hormonal contraceptives: May reduce contraceptive effectiveness. Advise patient to use alternative or additional method of contraception during modafinil therapy and for 1 month after drug is stopped.

Itraconazole, ketoconazole, other CYP3A4 inhibitors: May alter modafinil level. Monitor patient closely.

Phenytoin, warfarin: May inhibit CYP2C9 and increase phenytoin and warfarin levels. Monitor patient closely for toxicity.

TCAs: May increase TCA level. Reduce dosage of these drugs.

Drug-lifestyle. *Alcohol use:* Coadministration hasn't been studied. Avoid using together.

EFFECTS ON LAB TEST RESULTS
• May increase glucose, GGT, and AST levels.
• May increase eosinophil count.

CONTRAINDICATIONS & CAUTIONS
• Contraindicated in patients hypersensitive to modafinil or armodafinil or its inactive ingredients.
• Drug isn't recommended in patients with a history of left ventricular hypertrophy or ischemic ECG changes, chest pain, arrhythmias, or other evidence of mitral valve prolapse linked to CNS stimulant use.
• Use cautiously in patients with recent MI or unstable angina and in those with history of psychosis or mania.
• Use cautiously and give reduced dosage to patients with severe hepatic impairment, with or without cirrhosis.
• Use cautiously in patients taking MAO inhibitors.
• Safety and effectiveness in patients with severe renal impairment haven't been determined.
• Modafinil isn't approved for use in children.

Dialyzable drug: Unknown.

⚠ **Overdose S&S:** Agitation or excitation, insomnia, slight or moderate elevations in hemodynamic parameters, aggressiveness, anxiety, confusion, shortened PT, diarrhea, irritability, nausea, nervousness, palpitations, sleep disturbances, tremor, bradycardia, chest pain, HTN, tachycardia, hallucination, restlessness.

PREGNANCY-LACTATION-REPRODUCTION
• There are no adequate studies in pregnant women. Use during pregnancy only if potential benefit justifies potential risk to the fetus.
• A pregnancy registry has been established to collect information on pregnancy outcomes of women exposed to modafinil. Prescribers are encouraged to register pregnant patients, or pregnant women may self-enroll in the Provigil Pregnancy Registry, by calling 1-866-404-4106.
• Caution patient that use of hormonal contraceptives (including depot or implantable contraceptives) with modafinil may reduce contraceptive effectiveness. Recommend an alternative method of contraception during therapy and for 1 month after therapy ends.
• It isn't known if drug appears in human milk. Use cautiously in breastfeeding women.

Reactions in bold italics are *life-threatening*. Interactions may have a *rapid onset* or a ***delayed onset***.

NURSING CONSIDERATIONS

• Life-threatening angioedema, SJS, and DRESS syndrome can occur. Monitor patient for rash, dysphagia, bronchospasm, fever, and organ dysfunction. Stop drug and begin appropriate treatment.

• Monitor patient for emergence or exacerbation of psychiatric signs and symptoms and HTN.

• *Look alike–sound alike:* Don't confuse Provigil with Nuvigil; don't confuse Alertec with Arthrotec.

PATIENT TEACHING

❸ *Alert:* Advise patient to stop drug and notify prescriber if rash, peeling skin, trouble swallowing or breathing, or other symptoms of allergic reaction occur. Rare cases of serious rash, including SJS, toxic epidermal necrolysis, and DRESS syndrome, have been reported.

• Advise female patient to notify prescriber about planned, suspected, or known pregnancy, or if she's breastfeeding.

• Tell patient to avoid alcohol while taking drug.

• Warn patient to avoid activities that require alertness or good coordination until CNS effects of drug are known.

---

mometasone furoate
moe-MET-a-sone

Asmanex HFA, Asmanex Twisthaler, Elocon

mometasone furoate monohydrate
Nasonex

Therapeutic class: Anti-inflammatory drugs
Pharmacologic class: Glucocorticoids

AVAILABLE FORMS

Cream: 0.1%
Inhalation aerosol: 100 mcg/actuation, 200 mcg/actuation
Inhalation powder: 110 mcg/inhalation, 220 mcg/inhalation
Lotion: 0.1%
Nasal spray: 50 mcg/spray
Ointment: 0.1%

INDICATIONS & DOSAGES

➤ **Maintenance therapy for asthma; asthma in patients who take an oral corticosteroid**
Asmanex Twisthaler
Adults and children age 12 and older who previously used a bronchodilator or inhaled corticosteroid: Initially, 220 mcg by oral inhalation every day in the evening. Maximum, 440 mcg/day.
Adults and children age 12 and older who previously received an oral corticosteroid: 440 mcg by oral inhalation b.i.d. Maximum, 880 mcg/day.
Adjust-a-dose: For patients on long-term oral corticosteroid therapy, reduce oral prednisone dosage by no more than 2.5 mg/day at weekly intervals, beginning at least 1 week after starting mometasone. After stopping oral corticosteroid, reduce mometasone dosage to lowest effective amount. Carefully monitor patient for signs and symptoms of asthma instability and adrenal insufficiency.
Children ages 4 to 11 regardless of prior therapy: 110 mcg by oral inhalation once daily in the evening.
Asmanex HFA
Adults and children age 12 and older who previously used a medium-dose inhaled corticosteroid: Using a 100-mcg inhaler, 2 inhalations b.i.d. (morning and evening). Maximum, 800 mcg/day.
Adults and children age 12 and older who previously used a high-dose inhaled corticosteroid: Using a 200-mcg inhaler, 2 inhalations b.i.d. (morning and evening). Maximum, 800 mcg/day.
Adults and children age 12 and older who previously received an oral corticosteroid: 200 mcg by oral inhalation b.i.d. (morning and evening). Maximum, 800 mcg/day.
Adjust-a-dose: For patients currently receiving long-term oral corticosteroid therapy, wean prednisone slowly, beginning after at least 1 week of Asmanex HFA therapy. Carefully monitor patient for signs and symptoms of asthma instability and adrenal insufficiency. If a dosage regimen fails to provide adequate asthma control, reevaluate the therapeutic regimen and consider additional therapeutic options, such as replacing the current strength of inhaler with a higher strength, initiating an inhaled corticosteroid

M

---

and long-acting beta₂-agonist combination product, or initiating oral corticosteroids.

➤ **Allergic rhinitis; nasal congestion associated with seasonal allergic rhinitis**
Adults and children age 12 and older:
2 sprays (50 mcg/spray) in each nostril once daily.
Children ages 2 to 11: 1 spray (50 mcg/ spray) in each nostril once daily.

➤ **Prophylaxis of seasonal allergic rhinitis**
Adults and children age 12 and older:
2 sprays (50 mcg/spray) in each nostril once daily 2 to 4 weeks before anticipated start of pollen season.

➤ **Nasal polyps**
Adults: 2 sprays (50 mcg/spray) in each nostril once daily to b.i.d.

➤ **Dermatoses**
Adults: Apply thin film of cream or ointment to affected areas once daily. Or, apply a few drops of lotion to affected areas and massage lightly. Discontinue when control is achieved. If no improvement is seen within 2 weeks, reassess diagnosis.
Children age 12 and older: Apply a few drops of lotion to affected areas once daily and massage lightly. Discontinue when control is achieved. If no improvement is seen within 2 weeks, reassess diagnosis.
Children age 2 and older: Apply thin film of cream or ointment to affected areas once daily. Discontinue when control is achieved. If no improvement is seen within 2 weeks, reassess diagnosis.

ADMINISTRATION
Inhalational aerosol
• Shake well before each inhalation.
• Prime before first use by releasing four test sprays into the air, away from the face, shaking well before each spray.
• If the inhaler hasn't been used for more than 5 days, prime inhaler again with four test sprays.
• Have patient rinse mouth with water without swallowing after administration.
Inhalational powder
• Have patient exhale fully before bringing Twisthaler up to the mouth, placing between lips, and inhaling quickly and deeply.
• Patient shouldn't breathe out through inhaler but should remove inhaler and hold breath for 10 seconds if possible.

• Have patient rinse mouth after administration.
• Discard 45 days after opening foil pouch or when dose counter reads "00."
Intranasal
• Before initial use, prime nasal spray pump 10 times or until fine spray appears.
• Pump may be stored for 1 week without repriming. If unused for more than 1 week, reprime two times or until a fine spray appears.
• Shake well before each use.
Topical
• Drug is for topical use only; not for oral, ophthalmic, or intravaginal use. Avoid use on axillae, groin, or face.
• Don't use with occlusive dressings or in diaper area if child still requires diapers or plastic pants unless directed by prescriber.

ACTION
Unknown, although corticosteroids inhibit many cells and mediators involved in inflammation and the asthmatic response.

Route	Onset	Peak	Duration
Inhalation	Unknown	1–2½ hr	Unknown
Intranasal	Unknown	Unknown	Unknown
Topical	8 hr	Unknown	Unknown

Half-life: Oral, 5 hours; nasal and topical, unknown.

ADVERSE REACTIONS
CNS: headache, depression, fatigue, insomnia, pain, paresthesia. **EENT:** allergic rhinitis, pharyngitis, dry throat, dysphonia, earache, epistaxis, nasal irritation, sinus congestion, sinusitis, oral candidiasis. **GI:** abdominal pain, anorexia, dyspepsia, flatulence, gastroenteritis, nausea, vomiting, thrush. **GU:** dysmenorrhea, menstrual disorder, UTI. **Metabolic:** decreased glucocorticoid levels. **Musculoskeletal:** arthralgia, back pain, myalgia. **Respiratory:** URI, respiratory disorder. **Skin:** burning, pruritus, skin atrophy, furunculosis, folliculitis, skin depigmentation, candidiasis, bacterial infection. **Other:** flulike symptoms, infection, fever.

INTERACTIONS
Drug-drug. *Strong CYP3A4 inhibitors (atazanavir, clarithromycin, cobicistat-containing products, indinavir, itraconazole,*

Reactions in bold italics are *life-threatening*. Interactions may have a *rapid onset* or a ***delayed onset***.

ketoconazole, nefazodone, nelfinavir, riton-avir, saquinavir): May increase systemic exposure to mometasone and increase risk of systemic adverse effects, especially with long-term use. Use together cautiously.

EFFECTS ON LAB TEST RESULTS
None reported.

CONTRAINDICATIONS & CAUTIONS
• Contraindicated in patients hypersensitive to drug or its components, in those hypersensitive to milk proteins (Asmanex Twisthaler only), and in those with status asthmaticus or other acute forms of asthma or bronchospasm (as primary treatment).
• Use cautiously in patients at high risk for decreased bone mineral content (those with a family history of osteoporosis, prolonged immobilization, long-term use of drugs that reduce bone mass), patients switching from a systemic to an inhaled corticosteroid, and patients with active or dormant TB, untreated systemic infections, cataracts, glaucoma, ocular herpes simplex, diabetes, myasthenia, MI, thyroid disease, psychiatric disturbances, or immunosuppression.
• Drug may cause HPA axis suppression with potential for glucocorticosteroid insufficiency during treatment or after treatment withdrawal. Evaluate patient periodically for HPA suppression.
🔴 *Alert:* Children treated with topical corticosteroids are at greater risk than adults for HPA axis suppression and Cushing syndrome. Don't use in treatment of diaper dermatitis.
• If patient develops allergic contact dermatitis, usually diagnosed by a failure to heal, drug should be discontinued.
• If skin infections are present or develop, topical drug may need to be discontinued until infection is controlled.
Dialyzable drug: Unknown.
⚠ *Overdose S&S:* Hypercorticism with long-term overdose.

PREGNANCY-LACTATION-REPRODUCTION
• There are no adequate studies in pregnant women. Use during pregnancy only if clearly needed and potential benefit justifies potential risk to the fetus.

• Systemically administered corticosteroids appear in human milk and could suppress growth, interfere with endogenous corticosteroid production, or cause other untoward effects. Use cautiously in breastfeeding women.

NURSING CONSIDERATIONS
🔴 *Alert:* Don't use inhalation form for acute bronchospasm. Life-threatening paradoxical bronchospasm can occur after inhalation. Stop drug and use a fast-acting bronchodilator.
• Wean patients slowly from a systemic corticosteroid after they switch to mometasone. Monitor pulmonary function tests, beta-agonist use, and asthma symptoms.
🔴 *Alert:* If patient is switching from an oral corticosteroid to an inhaled form, watch closely for evidence of adrenal insufficiency, such as fatigue, lethargy, weakness, nausea, vomiting, and hypotension.
• After an oral corticosteroid is withdrawn, HPA function may not recover for months. Patient experiencing trauma, stress, infection, or surgery during this HPA recovery period is particularly vulnerable to adrenal insufficiency or adrenal crisis.
• Because inhaled and topical corticosteroids can be systemically absorbed, watch for cushingoid effects.
• Assess patient for bone loss during long-term use.
• Watch for evidence of localized mouth infections, vision changes, loss of glucose control, and immunosuppression.
• If female patient has taken a corticosteroid during pregnancy, monitor neonate for hypoadrenalism.
• Monitor elderly patients for increased sensitivity to drug effects.

PATIENT TEACHING
• Instruct patient on proper use and routine care of the inhaler or nasal spray pump.
• Tell patient to use drug regularly and at the same time each day. Advise patient who uses drug only once daily to do so in the evening.
• Caution patient not to use drug for immediate relief of an asthma attack or bronchospasm. Verify patient has a rescue inhaler prescribed.

• Inform patient that maximal benefits might not occur for 1 to 2 weeks or longer after therapy starts. Instruct patient to notify prescriber if condition fails to improve or worsens.

• Tell patient that if bronchospasm occurs after taking drug, to immediately use a fast-acting bronchodilator. Urge patient to contact prescriber immediately if bronchospasm doesn't respond to the fast-acting bronchodilator.

⏲ *Alert:* Urge patient who has been weaned from an oral corticosteroid to contact prescriber immediately if an asthma attack occurs or if patient is experiencing a period of stress. The oral corticosteroid may need to be resumed.

• Warn patient to avoid exposure to chickenpox or measles and to notify prescriber if such contact occurs.

• Long-term use of an inhaled corticosteroid may increase risk of cataracts or glaucoma; tell patient to report vision changes.

• Advise patient to write the date on a new inhaler on the day inhaler is opened and to discard the inhaler after 45 days or when the dose counter reads "00."

• Instruct patient not to use topical form with occlusive dressings or diapers unless instructed by prescriber.

montelukast sodium
mon-te-LOO-kast

Singulair⬦

Therapeutic class: Antiasthmatics
Pharmacologic class: Leukotriene-receptor antagonists

AVAILABLE FORMS
Oral granules: 4-mg packet
Tablets (chewable): 4 mg, 5 mg
Tablets (film-coated): 10 mg

INDICATIONS & DOSAGES
➤ **Asthma, seasonal allergic rhinitis, perennial allergic rhinitis**
Adults and children age 15 and older: 10 mg PO once daily in evening.
Children ages 6 to 14: 5 mg chewable tablet PO once daily in evening.

Children ages 2 to 5: 4 mg chewable tablet or 1 packet of 4-mg oral granules PO once daily in the evening.
Children ages 12 to 23 months (asthma only): 1 packet of 4-mg oral granules PO once daily in the evening.
Children ages 6 to 23 months (perennial allergic rhinitis only): 1 packet of 4-mg oral granules PO once daily in the evening.
➤ **Prevention of exercise-induced bronchoconstriction**
Adults and children age 15 and older: 10 mg PO at least 2 hours before exercise. Patients already taking a daily dose shouldn't take an additional dose. Also, an additional dose shouldn't be taken within 24 hours of a previous dose.
Children ages 6 to 14: 5 mg PO at least 2 hours before exercise (1 chewable tablet). An additional dose shouldn't be taken within 24 hours of a previous dose.

ADMINISTRATION
PO
• Give oral granules directly in the mouth, dissolved in 5 mL of cold or room-temperature baby formula or human milk, or mixed with a spoonful of cold or room-temperature soft foods (use only applesauce, carrots, rice, or ice cream). Use within 15 minutes of opening the packet.
• May be taken without regard to food.

ACTION
Reduces early and late-phase bronchoconstriction from antigen challenge.

Route	Onset	Peak	Duration
PO (chewable, granules)	Unknown	2–2½ hr	24 hr
PO (film-coated)	Unknown	3–4 hr	24 hr

Half-life: 2¾ to 5½ hours.

ADVERSE REACTIONS
CNS: headache, asthenia, dizziness, fatigue, fever, somnolence, weakness. **EENT:** conjunctivitis, otitis media, nasal congestion, nosebleed, laryngitis, sinusitis, pharyngitis, rhinitis, tonsillitis, dental pain. **GI:** abdominal pain, dyspepsia, gastroenteritis, nausea, diarrhea. **GU:** pyuria. **Hematologic:** systemic eosinophilia. **Respiratory:** URI, cough, wheezing, pneumonia, bronchitis.

Reactions in bold italics are *life-threatening*. Interactions may have a *rapid onset* or a *delayed onset*.

Skin: rash, dermatitis, urticaria, eczema.
Other: flulike symptoms, trauma, varicella, viral infection.

INTERACTIONS

Drug-drug. *Gemfibrozil:* May increase montelukast plasma concentration. Adjust montelukast dosage as needed.
Phenobarbital, rifampin: May decrease bioavailability of montelukast because of hepatic metabolism induction. Monitor patient for effectiveness.

EFFECTS ON LAB TEST RESULTS

• May increase ALT and AST levels.

CONTRAINDICATIONS & CAUTIONS

• Contraindicated in patients hypersensitive to drug or its ingredients.
• Avoid use with aspirin and other NSAIDs in patients with known aspirin sensitivity because drug hasn't been shown to affect the bronchoconstrictor response to aspirin and other NSAIDs in aspirin-sensitive asthmatic patients.
• Patients with asthma may present with systemic eosinophilia that may manifest as clinical features of vasculitis consistent with Churg-Strauss syndrome. Churg-Strauss syndrome is often treated with systemic corticosteroid therapy. These reactions have sometimes been associated with reduction of oral corticosteroid dosage. Be alert to development of eosinophilia, vasculitic rash, worsening pulmonary symptoms, cardiac complications, or neuropathy.
• Use cautiously and with appropriate monitoring in patients whose dosages of systemic corticosteroids are reduced.
🛈 **Alert:** Neuropsychiatric events have been reported in adults, adolescents, and children taking montelukast. Postmarketing reports include agitation, aggressive behavior or hostility, anxiousness, depression, disorientation, disturbance in attention, dream abnormalities, hallucinations, insomnia, irritability, memory impairment, restlessness, somnambulism, suicidal thinking and behavior (including suicide), and tremor.
• Use caution when using drug in patients with hepatic disease, jaundice, or hepatitis.
Dialyzable drug: Unknown.

⚠ *Overdose S&S:* Headache, vomiting, psychomotor hyperactivity, thirst, somnolence, hyperkinesia, abdominal pain.

PREGNANCY-LACTATION-REPRODUCTION

• There are no adequate studies in pregnant women. Use during pregnancy only if clearly needed.
• It isn't known if drug appears in human milk. Use cautiously in breastfeeding women.

NURSING CONSIDERATIONS

• Assess patient's underlying condition; monitor patient for effectiveness.
🛈 **Alert:** Don't abruptly substitute drug for inhaled or oral corticosteroids. Dose of inhaled corticosteroids may be reduced gradually.
🛈 **Alert:** Drug isn't indicated for use in patients with acute asthmatic attacks, status asthmaticus, or as monotherapy for management of exercise-induced bronchospasm. Continue appropriate rescue drug for acute worsening.
• Drug may cause behavior and mood changes. Monitor patient and consider discontinuing drug if neuropsychiatric symptoms develop.

PATIENT TEACHING

• Inform caregiver that the oral granules may be given directly into the child's mouth, dissolved in 1 teaspoon of cold or room-temperature baby formula or human milk, or mixed in a spoonful of applesauce, carrots, rice, or ice cream.
• Tell caregiver not to open packet until ready to use and, after opening, to give the full dose within 15 minutes. If drug is mixed with food, tell caregiver not to store excess for future use and to discard the unused portion.
• Advise patient to take drug daily, even if asymptomatic, and to contact prescriber if asthma isn't well controlled.
• Warn patient not to reduce or stop taking other prescribed antiasthmatics without prescriber's approval.
• Advise patient to seek medical attention if short-acting inhaled bronchodilators are needed more often than usual during drug therapy.

M

• Warn patient that drug isn't beneficial in acute asthma attacks or in acute exercise-induced bronchospasm. Advise patient to keep appropriate rescue drugs available.

• Warn patient that drug may cause behavior and mood changes, and to report development of these symptoms to prescriber.

• Advise patient with known aspirin sensitivity to continue to avoid using aspirin and NSAIDs during drug therapy.

🚫 **Alert:** Advise patient with phenylketonuria that chewable tablet contains phenylalanine.

SAFETY ALERT!

morphine hydrochloride
MOR-feen

Doloral✦

morphine sulfate
Arymo ER, Duramorph PF, Infumorph, Kadian, M-Ediat✦, M-Eslon✦, MorphaBond, Morphine LP Epidural✦, MS Contin, MS.IR✦, Statex✦, Statex DPS✦

Therapeutic class: Opioid analgesics
Pharmacologic class: Opioids
Controlled substance schedule: II

AVAILABLE FORMS
morphine hydrochloride
Syrup: 1 mg/mL*✦, 5 mg/mL*✦
morphine sulfate
Capsules (extended-release microgranules [M-Eslon]) ⓒ: 10 mg✦, 15 mg✦, 30 mg✦, 60 mg✦, 100 mg✦, 200 mg✦
Capsules (extended-release pellets) ⓒ: 30 mg, 45 mg, 60 mg, 75 mg, 90 mg, 120 mg
Capsules (extended-release pellets [Kadian]) ⓒ: 10 mg, 20 mg, 30 mg, 40 mg, 50 mg, 60 mg, 70 mg, 80 mg, 100 mg, 130 mg, 150 mg, 200 mg
Capsules (immediate-release [M-Ediat]): 5 mg✦, 10 mg✦, 20 mg✦, 30 mg✦
Drops (Statex): 20 mg/mL✦, 50 mg/mL✦
Injection with preservative: 0.5 mg/mL, 1 mg/mL, 2 mg/mL, 5 mg/mL, 10 mg/mL, 15 mg/mL, 50 mg/mL
Injection without preservative (Duramorph, Infumorph): 0.5 mg/mL, 1 mg/mL, 10 mg/mL, 25 mg/mL ampules

Injection without preservative (Carpuject and prefilled syringes and vials): 2 mg/mL, 4 mg/mL, 8 mg/mL, 10 mg/mL, 15 mg/mL
Oral solution: 10 mg/5 mL, 20 mg/5 mL, 20 mg/mL (concentrate), 100 mg/5 mL (concentrate)
Suppositories: 5 mg, 10 mg, 20 mg, 30 mg
Syrup (Statex): 1 mg/mL✦, 5 mg/mL✦, 10 mg/mL
Tablets: 5 mg✦, 10 mg✦, 15 mg, 20 mg✦, 25 mg✦, 30 mg✦, 50 mg✦
Tablets (extended-release) ⓒ: 15 mg, 30 mg, 60 mg, 100 mg, 200 mg
Tablets (extended-release, abuse deterrent) ⓒ: 15 mg, 30 mg, 60 mg, 100 mg

INDICATIONS & DOSAGES
🚫 **Alert:** Initiate dosing for each patient individually and use the lowest effective dosage for the shortest duration consistent with individual treatment goals.

➤ **Moderate to severe pain**
Adults: Initially, 10 mg (based on 70 kg individual) IM or 0.1 to 0.2 mg/kg IV every 4 hours p.r.n. Or, 15 to 30 mg (immediate-release tablets) PO, or 10 to 20 mg (oral solution) PO, or 10 to 20 mg PR every 4 hours p.r.n.

For extended-release tablet, give 15 or 30 mg PO every 8 to 12 hours.

For epidural injection, give 5 mg by epidural catheter; then, if pain isn't relieved adequately in 1 hour, give supplementary doses of 1 to 2 mg at intervals sufficient to assess effectiveness. Maximum total epidural dose shouldn't exceed 10 mg/24 hours.

For intrathecal injection, a single dose of 0.2 to 1 mg may provide pain relief for 24 hours (only in the lumbar area). Don't repeat injections.

➤ **Moderate to severe pain requiring continuous, around-the-clock oral opioid**
Adults: For patients receiving other oral morphine formulations, may convert to extended-release capsules by administering patient's total daily oral morphine dose as extended-release capsules once daily (Kadian) or by administering one-half of patient's total daily oral morphine dose b.i.d. (Kadian capsules, MS Contin tablets, Arymo ER tablets). Patients 24-hour morphine requirement may also be divided every 8 hours and given as MS Contin tablets or Arymo

---

Reactions in bold italics are *life-threatening*. Interactions may have a *rapid onset* or a *delayed onset*.

ER tablets. Initial dosage in opioid-naive or opioid-nontolerant patients is 15 mg (Arymo ER tablets) PO every 8 or 12 hours. Don't give Kadian more frequently than every 12 hours. MS Contin shouldn't be used more frequently than every 8 hours.

ADMINISTRATION
PO
Black Box Warning Take care when administering morphine oral solution to avoid dosing errors because of confusion among different concentrations and between milligrams and milliliters, which could result in accidental overdose and death. Take care to ensure the proper dose is communicated and dispensed. ■

Black Box Warning Oral solutions of various concentrations and an intensified oral solution (20 mg/mL) are available. Carefully note strength given. The 20-mg/mL concentration is indicated for use only in opioid-tolerant patients because of the risk of fatal respiratory depression in opioid-naive patients. It's packaged with a calibrated oral syringe for accurate dosing. ■

Black Box Warning Instruct patient to swallow extended-release or long-acting morphine sulfate oral formulations whole, without crushing, chewing, or dissolving, which may cause rapid, uncontrolled release and absorption of a potentially fatal dose of morphine. If necessary, capsules (Kadian) may be carefully opened and entire contents poured into cool, soft foods such as applesauce and swallowed immediately without chewing. ■

• Give morphine sulfate without regard to food.

• May give Kadian capsules through a gastrostomy tube; flush tube with water, sprinkle contents of capsules in 10 mL of water, and flush through tube.

IV
▼ For direct injection, dilute 2.5 to 15 mg in 4 or 5 mL of sterile water for injection and give slowly over 4 to 5 minutes.

▼ For continuous infusion, mix drug with D_5W to yield 0.1 to 1 mg/mL, and give by a continuous infusion device.

▼ In adults with severe, chronic pain, maintenance IV infusion is 0.8 to 80 mg/hour; sometimes higher doses are needed.

▼ Make sure an opioid antagonist is immediately available before administering IV.

Black Box Warning Infumorph and Duramorph are supplied in sealed ampules. Treat accidental dermal exposure to these drugs by removing contaminated clothing and rinsing affected area with water. ■

Black Box Warning Inspect parenteral drug products for particulate matter before opening the amber ampule and again for color after removing contents from ampule. Don't use if solution in the unopened ampule contains a precipitate that doesn't disappear upon shaking. After removal, don't use unless solution is colorless or pale yellow. ■

▼ **Incompatibilities:** None listed by manufacturer. Consult a drug incompatibility reference for more information.

IM
• Document injection site.
• Store injection solution at room temperature and protect from light.

Black Box Warning Solution may darken with age. Don't use if injection is darker than pale yellow, discolored, or contains precipitate. ■

Epidural/intrathecal
• Document injection site; limit to lumbar area.

🕒 *Alert:* Intrathecal dosage is usually one-tenth that of epidural dosage.

• Verify proper placement of needle or catheter in the intrathecal or epidural space before injecting drug.

Black Box Warning Inspect for particulate matter and discoloration before administration. Don't use if it's darker than pale yellow, discolored in any other way, or contains a precipitate. ■

• Store injection solution at room temperature until ready to use; discard unused portion.

• Protect from light; don't freeze or heat sterilize.

Rectal
• Refrigeration of rectal suppository isn't needed.

ACTION
Unknown. Binds with opioid receptors in the CNS, altering perception of and emotional response to pain.

M

Route	Onset	Peak	Duration
PO	30 min	1–2 hr	3–5 hr
PO (extended-release)	1–2 hr	3–4 hr	8–24 hr
IV	5–10 min	20 min	4–5 hr
IM	10–30 min	30–60 min	4–5 hr
PR	20–60 min	20–60 min	3–7 hr
Epidural	15–60 min	15–60 min	24 hr
Intrathecal	15–60 min	30–60 min	24 hr

Half-life: Immediate release, 2 to 4 hours; extended release, 11 to 24 hours.

ADVERSE REACTIONS

CNS: dizziness, drowsiness, headache, euphoria, light-headedness, nightmares, sedation, somnolence, *seizures,* depression, hallucinations, nervousness, physical dependence, syncope, anxiety. **CV:** *bradycardia, cardiac arrest, shock,* HTN, hypotension, tachycardia, palpitations, peripheral circulatory collapse, peripheral edema, chest pain, syncope. **EENT:** miosis, blurred vision. **GI:** constipation, nausea, vomiting, anorexia, biliary tract spasms, dry mouth, ileus, flatulence, abdominal pain. **GU:** urine retention. **Hematologic:** *thrombocytopenia, anemia, leukopenia.* **Respiratory:** *apnea, respiratory arrest, respiratory depression.* **Skin:** diaphoresis, edema, pruritus, skin flushing, pain at injection site. **Other:** decreased libido.

INTERACTIONS

Drug-drug. *Alvimopan:* May enhance adverse/toxic effects of alvimopan. Alvimopan is contraindicated in patients receiving therapeutic doses of opioids for more than 7 consecutive days immediately before alvimopan initiation. Consider therapy modification.

Black Box Warning *Benzodiazepines, CNS depressants:* May cause slow or difficult breathing, sedation, and death. Avoid use together. If use together is necessary, limit dosage and duration of each drug to the minimum necessary for desired effect. ∎

Cimetidine: May increase respiratory and CNS depression when given with morphine sulfate. Monitor patient closely.

General anesthetics, hypnotics, MAO inhibitors, other opioid analgesics, TCAs: May cause respiratory depression, hypotension, profound sedation, or coma. Use together with caution, reduce morphine dose, and monitor patient response.

❸ *Alert: Serotonergic drugs (amoxapine, antiemetics [dolasetron, granisetron, ondansetron, palonosetron], antimigraine drugs, buspirone, cyclobenzaprine, dextromethorphan, linezolid, lithium, MAO inhibitors, maprotiline, methylene blue, mirtazapine, nefazodone, SSNRIs, SSRIs, TCAs, trazodone, tryptophan, vilazodone):* May increase risk of serotonin syndrome. Use together cautiously and monitor patient for serotonin syndrome.

Drug-herb. ❸ *Alert: St. John's wort:* May increase risk of serotonin syndrome. Use together cautiously and monitor patient for serotonin syndrome.

Drug-lifestyle. **Black Box Warning** *Alcohol use:* May cause additive CNS effects and fatal overdose. Warn patient to avoid alcohol and products containing alcohol. ∎

EFFECTS ON LAB TEST RESULTS

- May increase amylase level. May decrease Hb level (morphine sulfate).
- May decrease platelet count.
- May cause abnormal LFT values (morphine sulfate).

CONTRAINDICATIONS & CAUTIONS

- Contraindicated in patients hypersensitive to drug and in those with conditions that would preclude IV administration of opioids (acute bronchial asthma or upper airway obstruction).

Black Box Warning Opioids should only be prescribed with benzodiazepines or other CNS depressants to patients for whom alternative treatment options are inadequate. ∎

Black Box Warning Use of extended-release or long-acting morphine sulfate forms may increase the risk of addiction, abuse, and misuse, even at recommended doses, and has a greater risk of overdose and death. Reserve their use for patients for whom alternative treatment options are ineffective, not tolerated, or are otherwise insufficient to provide adequate pain management. ∎

Black Box Warning Accidental ingestion of even one dose of extended-release or long-acting forms of morphine sulfate, especially by children, can result in a fatal overdose. Keep out of reach of children. ▪

🖲 *Alert:* Drug may lead to a rare but serious decrease in adrenal gland cortisol production.

🖲 *Alert:* Drug may cause decreased sex hormone levels with long-term use.

🖲 *Alert:* Patients are at increased risk for oversedation and respiratory depression if they snore or have a history of sleep apnea, haven't used opioids recently or are first-time opioid users, have increased opioid dosage requirements or opioid habituation, have received general anesthesia for longer lengths of time or received other sedating drugs, have preexisting pulmonary or cardiac disease, or have thoracic or other surgical incisions that may impair breathing. Monitor patients carefully.

• Contraindicated in patients with GI obstruction.

• Use with caution in elderly or debilitated patients and in those with head injury, increased ICP, seizures, chronic pulmonary disease, prostatic hyperplasia, severe hepatic or renal disease, acute abdominal conditions, hypothyroidism, Addison disease, and urethral stricture.

• Use with caution in patients with circulatory shock, biliary tract disease, CNS depression, toxic psychosis, acute alcoholism, delirium tremens, and seizure disorders.

Dialyzable drug: Yes.

⚠ *Overdose S&S:* Miosis, CNS depression, respiratory depression, apnea, flaccid skeletal muscles, bradycardia, hypotension, circulatory collapse, cardiac arrest, respiratory arrest, death.

PREGNANCY-LACTATION-REPRODUCTION

🖲 *Alert:* Carefully weigh risks and benefits of using drug in pregnant women. Drug should be used in pregnancy only if need for opioid analgesia clearly outweighs potential risks to the fetus.

Black Box Warning Prolonged use of opioids during pregnancy can result in neonatal opioid withdrawal syndrome, which may be life-threatening if not recognized and treated, and requires management according to protocols developed by neonatology experts. If opioid use is required for a prolonged period, apprise pregnant patient of

risk to the neonate and ensure appropriate treatment will be available. ▪

• Because of the potential for serious adverse reactions in breastfeeding infants, including respiratory depression, sedation, and possibly withdrawal symptoms upon cessation of morphine to the mother, patient should discontinue breastfeeding or discontinue drug, taking into account importance of drug to the mother.

• If morphine use is necessary in a breastfeeding patient, use cautiously. Limit use and supplement with nonopioid agents. Monitor infant for increased sleepiness, difficulty feeding or breathing, and limpness.

NURSING CONSIDERATIONS

Black Box Warning Assess each patient's risk of addiction, abuse, or misuse before prescribing extended-release or long-acting forms of morphine sulfate, and monitor all patients regularly for development of these behaviors. ▪

Black Box Warning Monitor patients for respiratory depression, especially during initiation of extended-release or long-acting morphine sulfate or after a dosage increase. Serious, life-threatening, or fatal respiratory depression may occur. ▪

🖲 *Alert:* If patient is taking opioids with serotonergic drugs, watch for signs and symptoms of serotonin syndrome (agitation, hallucinations, rapid HR, fever, excessive sweating, shivering or shaking, muscle twitching or stiffness, trouble with coordination, nausea, vomiting, diarrhea), especially at start of treatment and at dosage increases. Signs and symptoms may occur within several hours of coadministration but may also occur later, especially after dosage increase. Discontinue the opioid, serotonergic drug, or both if serotonin syndrome is suspected.

🖲 *Alert:* Monitor patient for signs and symptoms of adrenal insufficiency (nausea, vomiting, loss of appetite, fatigue, weakness, dizziness, low BP). Perform diagnostic testing if adrenal insufficiency is suspected. If adrenal insufficiency is confirmed, treat with corticosteroids and wean patient off opioids if appropriate. Discontinue corticosteroids when clinically appropriate.

🖲 *Alert:* Monitor patient for signs and symptoms of decreased sex hormone levels (low

M

libido, erectile dysfunction, amenorrhea, infertility). If signs and symptoms occur, evaluate patient and obtain lab testing.

❸ Alert: Carefully monitor vital signs, pain level, respiratory status, and sedation level in all patients receiving opioids, especially those receiving IV drugs, even those given postoperatively.

• Reassess patient's level of pain at least 15 and 30 minutes after giving parenterally and 30 minutes after giving orally.

❸ Alert: Extended-release capsules aren't for use on an as-needed basis.

Black Box Warning Keep opioid antagonist (naloxone) and resuscitation equipment available. ∎

• Monitor circulatory, respiratory, bladder, and bowel functions carefully. Drug may cause hypotension, urine retention, nausea, vomiting, ileus, or altered level of consciousness regardless of the route.

❸ Alert: Intrathecal dosage is usually one-tenth of epidural dosage.

Black Box Warning Life-threatening respiratory depression may occur with morphine use, even when drug has been used as recommended and not misused or abused. Proper dosing and titration are essential, and morphine should only be prescribed by health care providers knowledgeable in the use of potent opioids for management of long-term pain. Monitor patients for respiratory depression, especially during initiation of morphine or after a dosage increase. Instruct patients to swallow morphine capsule whole; Kadian capsule can be opened and contents sprinkled on applesauce and swallowed without chewing. Crushing, dissolving, or chewing pellets within the capsule can cause rapid release and absorption of a potentially fatal dose of morphine. ∎

• If respirations drop below 12 breaths/minute, withhold dose and notify prescriber.

Black Box Warning Morphine has an abuse liability similar to other opioid analgesics and may be misused, abused, or diverted. ∎

❸ Alert: Extended-release tablets and capsules aren't for use on an as-needed basis for mild or acute pain or for postoperative pain, unless patient has already been receiving long-term opioid therapy before surgery or if postoperative pain is expected to be

moderate to severe and persist for an extended period.

• Preservative-free preparations are available for epidural and intrathecal use.

• Epidural administration has been associated with less potential for immediate or late adverse effects than intrathecal administration; use epidural route whenever possible.

• A constant IV infusion of naloxone, 0.6 mg/hour, for 24 hours after intrathecal injection may be used to reduce potential adverse effects.

Black Box Warning When the epidural or intrathecal route is used, observe patients in a fully equipped and staffed environment for at least 24 hours after the initial dose. ∎

Black Box Warning Infumorph isn't recommended for single-dose IV, IM, or subcut administration. ∎

Black Box Warning Improper or erroneous substitution of Infumorph 200 or 500 (10 or 25 mg/mL, respectively) for regular Duramorph (0.5 or 1 mg/mL) is likely to result in serious overdose, leading to seizures, respiratory depression, and possibly fatal outcome. ∎

• When drug is given epidurally, monitor patient closely for respiratory depression up to 24 hours after the injection. Check respiratory rate and depth every 30 to 60 minutes for 24 hours. Watch for pruritus and skin flushing.

• Morphine is drug of choice in relieving MI pain; may cause transient decrease in BP.

• An around-the-clock regimen best manages severe, chronic pain. Verify patient has a breakthrough pain medication prescribed in addition to the around-the-clock medication.

• Morphine may worsen or mask gallbladder pain.

• Constipation is commonly severe with maintenance dose. Ensure that stool softener or stimulant laxative is ordered.

• Taper morphine sulfate therapy gradually when stopping therapy.

Black Box Warning Each ampule of Infumorph and Duramorph contains a large amount of a potent opioid that has been associated with abuse and dependence among health care providers. Due to the limited indications for this product, risk of overdose, and risk of its diversion and abuse,

---

Reactions in bold italics are *life-threatening*. Interactions may have a *rapid onset* or a *delayed onset*.

special measures should be taken to control this product within the hospital or clinic. Infumorph and Duramorph should be subject to rigid accounting, rigorous control of wastage, and restricted access. ■

Black Box Warning Accidental consumption of morphine, especially by children, can result in a fatal overdose of morphine. ■

🕙 *Alert:* Don't stop drug abruptly; withdraw slowly and individualize gradual taper plan to prevent signs and symptoms of withdrawal, worsening pain, and psychological distress in physically dependent patients. Refer to manufacturer's label for specific tapering instructions.

🕙 *Alert:* When tapering opioids, monitor patient closely for signs and symptoms of opioid withdrawal (restlessness, lacrimation, rhinorrhea, yawning, perspiration, chills, myalgia, mydriasis, irritability, anxiety, insomnia, backache, joint pain, weakness, abdominal cramps, anorexia, nausea, vomiting, diarrhea, increased BP or HR, increased respiratory rate), which may indicate a need to taper more slowly. Also monitor patient for suicidal thoughts, use of other substances, and mood changes.

• *Look alike–sound alike:* Don't confuse morphine with hydromorphone. Don't confuse MS Contin with Oxycontin.

PATIENT TEACHING
Black Box Warning Caution patient or caregiver of patient taking an opioid with a benzodiazepine, CNS depressant, or alcohol to seek immediate medical attention for dizziness, light-headedness, extreme sleepiness, slowed or difficult breathing, or unresponsiveness. ■

🕙 *Alert:* Explain assessment and monitoring process to patient and family. Instruct them to immediately report difficulty breathing or other signs or symptoms of a potential adverse opioid-related reaction.

🕙 *Alert:* Encourage patient to report all medications being taken, including prescription and OTC medications and supplements.

• Warn patient that morphine can cause constipation.

🕙 *Alert:* Caution patient to immediately report signs and symptoms of serotonin syndrome, adrenal insufficiency, and decreased sex hormone levels.

• When drug is used after surgery, encourage patient to turn, cough, deep-breathe, and use incentive spirometer to prevent lung problems.

• Caution ambulatory patient about getting out of bed or walking. Warn outpatient to avoid driving and other potentially hazardous activities that require mental alertness until drug's adverse CNS effects are known.

Black Box Warning Drinking alcohol or taking drugs containing alcohol while taking extended-release capsules may cause additive CNS effects and potentially fatal overdose. Warn patient to read labels on OTC drugs carefully for alcohol content and not to use alcohol in any form. ■

• Tell patient to swallow morphine sulfate whole or to open capsule and sprinkle beads or pellets on a small amount of applesauce immediately before taking.

Black Box Warning Tell patient to keep morphine oral preparations out of the reach of children. In case of accidental ingestion, advise patient to seek emergency medical help immediately. ■

🕙 *Alert:* Counsel patient not to discontinue opioids without first discussing with prescriber the need for a gradual tapering regimen.

🕙 *Alert:* Warn patient not to crush, break, or chew extended-release forms.

SAFETY ALERT!

morphine sulfate–naltrexone hydrochloride
MOR-feen/nal-TREKS-own

Embeda

Therapeutic class: Opioid analgesics
Pharmacologic class: Opioid agonist–antagonists
Controlled substance schedule: II

AVAILABLE FORMS
Capsules 🔵: 20 mg morphine/0.8 mg naltrexone, 30 mg morphine/1.2 mg naltrexone, 50 mg morphine/2 mg naltrexone, 60 mg morphine/2.4 mg naltrexone, 80 mg morphine/3.2 mg naltrexone, 100 mg morphine/4 mg naltrexone

M

INDICATIONS & DOSAGES

➤ **Moderate to severe pain when a continuous, around-the-clock opioid analgesic is needed for an extended period of time**

Adults: Individualize dosage according to patient's previous analgesic treatment, general condition, concurrent medication, type and severity of pain, and degree of opioid tolerance. Initially, give lowest dose possible; titrate no more frequently than every other day to allow for stabilization before escalating dosage. If pain relief is inadequate, administer every 12 hours.

Initial treatment with Embeda as patient's first opioid analgesic or in patients who aren't opioid tolerant is one 20-mg morphine/0.8-mg naltrexone capsule PO every 24 hours. Use of higher starting doses in patients who aren't opioid tolerant may cause fatal respiratory depression. The 100-mg morphine/4-mg naltrexone capsules are for use only in opioid-tolerant patients. First dose of Embeda may be taken with last dose of any immediate-release (short-acting) opioid medication because of extended-release characteristics of Embeda.

Adjust-a-dose: For patients receiving other morphine preparations, convert by administering half of patient's daily morphine dose as Embeda every 12 hours or by administering total morphine dose as Embeda every 24 hours.

ADMINISTRATION
PO

Black Box Warning If patient has difficulty swallowing whole capsule, open capsule, sprinkle pellets onto small amount of applesauce, and administer immediately. Caution patient not to chew pellets. Have patient rinse mouth to make sure all pellets are swallowed. ∎

Black Box Warning Crushing, chewing, cutting, or dissolving morphine–naltrexone capsules can cause rapid release and absorption of a potentially fatal dose of morphine. ∎

• Don't administer pellets through an NG or gastric tube.

ACTION

Morphine is a selective mu agonist that produces analgesia and sedation by binding with the mu opioid receptor. Naltrexone is a centrally acting mu antagonist that reverses subjective and analgesic effects of morphine by competing for mu receptor sites.

Route	Onset	Peak	Duration
PO	Unknown	7½ hr	Days

Half-life: 29 hours.

ADVERSE REACTIONS

CNS: anxiety, depression, dizziness, fatigue, headache, insomnia, irritability, lethargy, restlessness, sedation, somnolence, tremor. **CV:** *cardiac arrest,* flushing, hypotension, peripheral edema, *shock.* **EENT:** miosis. **GI:** abdominal pain, anorexia, constipation, decreased appetite, diarrhea, dyspepsia, flatulence, nausea, stomach discomfort, vomiting, dry mouth. **Musculoskeletal:** arthralgia, muscle spasms. **Respiratory:** *apnea, respiratory arrest, respiratory depression.* **Skin:** hyperhidrosis, pruritus. **Other:** hot flush, chills.

INTERACTIONS

Drug-drug. *Anticholinergics:* May cause urine retention, severe constipation, or paralytic ileus. Use together cautiously and monitor patient closely.

Black Box Warning *Benzodiazepines, CNS depressants:* May cause slow or difficult breathing, sedation, and death. Avoid use together. If use together is necessary, limit dosage and duration of each drug to the minimum necessary for desired effect. ∎

Cimetidine: May cause confusion and severe respiratory depression. Avoid use together.

General anesthetics: May cause respiratory depression, hypotension, profound sedation, or coma. Use together cautiously; reduce initial dosage of one or both agents by at least 50% and monitor patient closely.

Diuretics: May cause antidiuretic hormone release, rendering diuretics ineffective, and urine retention due to bladder sphincter spasm. Use together cautiously.

MAO inhibitors: May cause anxiety, confusion, significant respiratory depression, or coma. Use together and within 14 days of treatment with MAO inhibitors is contraindicated.

Mixed agonist–antagonist opioid analgesics (butorphanol, nalbuphine, pentazocine):

Reactions in bold italics are *life-threatening*. Interactions may have a *rapid onset* or a *delayed onset*.

May reduce analgesic effects and precipitate withdrawal symptoms. Consider therapy modification.

Muscle relaxants: May enhance neuromuscular blocking action of skeletal muscle relaxants, causing respiratory depression. Use together cautiously.

P-gp inhibitors (such as quinidine): May increase morphine level and risk of adverse effects. Use together cautiously.

Rifamycins (rifampin): May reduce morphine level and analgesic effects. Monitor response and increase morphine–naltrexone dosage if necessary.

❸ *Alert:* Serotonergic drugs (amoxapine, antiemetics [dolasetron, granisetron, ondansetron, palonosetron], antimigraine drugs, buspirone, cyclobenzaprine, dextromethorphan, linezolid, lithium, MAO inhibitors, maprotiline, methylene blue, mirtazapine, nefazodone, SSNRIs, SSRIs, TCAs, trazodone, tryptophan, vilazodone): May increase risk of serotonin syndrome. Use together cautiously and monitor patient for serotonin syndrome.

Drug-herb. ❸ *Alert:* St. John's wort: May increase risk of serotonin syndrome. Use together cautiously and monitor patient for serotonin syndrome.

Drug-lifestyle. Black Box Warning *Alcohol use:* May cause additive CNS effects and fatal overdose. Warn patient to avoid alcohol. ∎

EFFECTS ON LAB TEST RESULTS
• May interfere with tests that use enzymes to detect opioids.

CONTRAINDICATIONS & CAUTIONS
• Contraindicated in patients hypersensitive to drug or its components and in those with significant respiratory depression, known or suspected paralytic ileus, acute or severe bronchial asthma, or hypercapnia in unmonitored settings without resuscitative equipment.

Black Box Warning Opioids should only be prescribed with benzodiazepines or other CNS depressants to patients for whom alternative treatment options are inadequate. ∎

• Drug should be prescribed only by health care professionals knowledgeable in the use of potent opioids for management of chronic pain.

❸ *Alert:* Drug may lead to a rare but serious decrease in adrenal gland cortisol production.

❸ *Alert:* Drug may cause decreased sex hormone levels with long-term use.

❸ *Alert:* Patients are at increased risk for oversedation and respiratory depression if they snore or have a history of sleep apnea, haven't used opioids recently or are first-time opioid users, have increased opioid dosage requirements or opioid habituation, have received general anesthesia for longer lengths of time or received other sedating drugs, have preexisting pulmonary or cardiac disease, or have thoracic or other surgical incisions that may impair breathing. Monitor patients carefully.

• Use cautiously in patients with mental health conditions, COPD, cor pulmonale, decreased respiratory reserve, hypoxia, hypercapnia, head injury, increased ICP, shock, seizures, biliary tract disease including pancreatitis, CNS depression, toxic psychosis, acute alcoholism, or delirium tremens.

• Use cautiously in elderly and debilitated patients and in those with severe renal or hepatic insufficiency, Addison disease, myxedema, hypothyroidism, prostatic hypertrophy, and urethral stricture.

• Individualize dosing regimen for each patient.

Dialyzable drug: Morphine, yes; naltrexone, no.

⚠ *Overdose S&S:* Respiratory depression, somnolence progressing to stupor or coma, skeletal muscle flaccidity, cold and clammy skin, constricted pupils, pulmonary edema, bradycardia, hypotension, death.

PREGNANCY-LACTATION-REPRODUCTION
• There are no adequate studies in pregnant women. Use during pregnancy only if clearly needed and potential benefit justifies potential risk to the fetus.

Black Box Warning Prolonged use during pregnancy can result in neonatal opioid withdrawal syndrome, which may be life-threatening if not recognized and treated, and requires management according to protocols developed by neonatology experts. If opioid use is required for a prolonged period,

M

advise pregnant patient of risk to neonate and ensure that appropriate treatment will be available. ∎

• Morphine appears in human milk. Because of potential for adverse reactions in breastfed infants, patient should discontinue breastfeeding or discontinue drug, taking into account importance of drug to the mother.

• Closely monitor infants of breastfeeding women receiving drug. Withdrawal symptoms can occur in breastfed infants when maternal administration of morphine is stopped.

• Long-term opioid use may cause secondary hypogonadism, which may lead to sexual dysfunction or infertility.

NURSING CONSIDERATIONS

Black Box Warning Capsules contain pellets of morphine sulfate. The pellets shouldn't be crushed, dissolved, or chewed because drug will be released and absorbed rapidly; resulting dose may be fatal, especially in opioid-naive patients. ∎

Black Box Warning Drug has an abuse liability similar to that of other opioid agonists, legal or illicit. Assess each patient's risk of opioid abuse or addiction before prescribing. Risk of opioid abuse increases in patients with personal or family history of substance abuse (including drug or alcohol abuse or addiction) or mental illness (such as major depressive disorder). Routinely monitor all patients receiving drug for signs and symptoms of misuse, abuse, and addiction during treatment. ∎

◑ **Alert:** If patient is taking opioids with serotonergic drugs, watch for signs and symptoms of serotonin syndrome (agitation, hallucinations, rapid HR, fever, excessive sweating, shivering or shaking, muscle twitching or stiffness, trouble with coordination, nausea, vomiting, diarrhea), especially when at start of treatment or at dosage increases. Signs and symptoms may occur within several hours of coadministration but may also occur later, especially after dosage increase. Discontinue the opioid, serotonergic drug, or both if serotonin syndrome is suspected.

◑ **Alert:** Monitor patient for signs and symptoms of adrenal insufficiency (nausea,

vomiting, loss of appetite, fatigue, weakness, dizziness, low BP). Perform diagnostic testing if adrenal insufficiency is suspected. If adrenal insufficiency is confirmed, treat with corticosteroids and wean patient off opioids if appropriate. Discontinue corticosteroids when clinically appropriate.

◑ **Alert:** Monitor patient for signs and symptoms of decreased sex hormone levels (low libido, erectile dysfunction, amenorrhea, infertility). If signs and symptoms occur, evaluate patient and obtain lab testing.

• If patient is currently taking a CNS depressant and the decision is made to begin this drug, start with 33% to 50% of the recommended starting dosage; monitor patient for signs and symptoms of sedation, respiratory depression, and hypotension; and consider using a lower dosage of the concomitant CNS depressant.

• Monitor patients closely for respiratory depression, especially within first 24 to 72 hours of start of therapy.

◑ **Alert:** Don't use for mild or acute pain, on an as-needed basis, or for postoperative pain, unless patient has already been receiving long-term opioid therapy before surgery or if postoperative pain is expected to be moderate to severe and persist for an extended period.

• Morphine 100 mg/naltrexone 4 mg is for use in opioid-tolerant patients only.

Black Box Warning Respiratory depression, including fatal cases, may occur with morphine–naltrexone, even when drug has been used as recommended and not misused or abused. Proper dosing and titration are essential, and drug should only be prescribed by health care professionals knowledgeable in the use of potent opioids for management of chronic pain. Monitor patient for respiratory depression, especially during initiation of drug or after a dosage increase. ∎

◑ **Alert:** Carefully monitor vital signs, pain level, respiratory status, and sedation level in all patients receiving opioids, especially those receiving IV drugs, even those given postoperatively.

• Monitor circulatory, respiratory, bladder, and bowel functions carefully. Drug may cause hypotension, urine retention, nausea, vomiting, constipation, ileus, or altered level of consciousness.

Reactions in bold italics are *life-threatening*. Interactions may have a *rapid onset* or a *delayed onset*.

• Taper drug gradually when stopping therapy to avoid withdrawal symptoms.

Black Box Warning Accidental ingestion of even one dose of drug can result in fatal overdose of morphine, especially in children. ∎

• Keep opioid antagonist (naloxone) and resuscitation equipment available.

⊙ Alert: Don't stop drug abruptly; withdraw slowly and individualize the gradual tapering plan to prevent signs and symptoms of withdrawal, worsening pain, and psychological distress in physically dependent patients. Refer to manufacturer's label for specific tapering instructions.

⊙ Alert: When tapering opioids, monitor patient closely for signs and symptoms of opioid withdrawal (restlessness, lacrimation, rhinorrhea, yawning, perspiration, chills, myalgia, mydriasis, irritability, anxiety, insomnia, backache, joint pain, weakness, abdominal cramps, anorexia, nausea, vomiting, diarrhea, increased BP or HR, increased respiratory rate), which may indicate a need to taper more slowly. Also monitor patient for suicidal thoughts, use of other substances, and mood changes.

PATIENT TEACHING

Black Box Warning Caution patient or caregiver of patient taking an opioid with a benzodiazepine, CNS depressant, or alcohol to seek immediate medical attention for dizziness, light-headedness, extreme sleepiness, slowed or difficult breathing, or unresponsiveness. ∎

• Explain assessment and monitoring process to patient and family. Instruct them to immediately report difficulty breathing or other signs or symptoms of a potential adverse opioid-related reaction.

• Tell patient that drug must be tapered gradually when stopping therapy.

Black Box Warning Warn patient taking drug that consuming alcoholic beverages or prescription or OTC drugs containing alcohol may cause dose to be fatal. ∎

Black Box Warning Tell patient to swallow capsules whole or open capsule and sprinkle pellets on small amount of applesauce immediately before taking; instruct patient that capsules shouldn't be crushed, cut, dissolved, or chewed. ∎

⊙ Alert: Encourage patient to report all medications being taken, including prescription and OTC medications and supplements.

⊙ Alert: Caution patient to immediately report breakthrough pain and signs and symptoms of serotonin syndrome, adrenal insufficiency, and decreased sex hormone levels.

• Caution patient that drug has potential for abuse and should be protected from theft.

Black Box Warning Tell patient to keep morphine oral preparations out of the reach of children. In case of accidental ingestion, advise patient to seek emergency medical help immediately. ∎

• Warn patient to avoid driving and other potentially hazardous activities that require mental alertness until drug's effects are known.

• Caution ambulatory patient about getting out of bed or walking because drug may cause a drop in BP with position change.

• Tell patient the importance of dietary changes, stool softeners, and laxatives to prevent constipation, a common adverse effect of drug.

⊙ Alert: Counsel patient not to discontinue opioids without first discussing with prescriber the need for a gradual tapering regimen.

moxifloxacin hydrochloride
mox-i-FLOKS-a-sin

Avelox⌀, Moxeza, Vigamox

Therapeutic class: Antibiotics
Pharmacologic class: Fluoroquinolones

AVAILABLE FORMS
Injection: 400 mg/250 mL
Ophthalmic solution: 0.5%
Tablets (film-coated): 400 mg

INDICATIONS & DOSAGES
Black Box Warning Use in patients with acute bacterial sinusitis or acute bacterial exacerbation of bronchitis isn't recommended due to risk of serious adverse effects. Use drug in these patients only when they have no other treatment options. ∎

M

➤ **Acute bacterial sinusitis caused by** *Streptococcus pneumoniae, Haemophilus influenzae,* **or** *Moraxella catarrhalis*
Adults: 400 mg PO or IV every 24 hours for 10 days.

➤ **Complicated skin and skin-structure infections caused by methicillin-susceptible** *Staphylococcus aureus, Escherichia coli, Klebsiella pneumoniae,* **or** *Enterobacter cloacae*
Adults: 400 mg PO or IV every 24 hours for 7 to 21 days.

➤ **Complicated intra-abdominal infection caused by** *E. coli, Bacteroides fragilis, Streptococcus anginosus, Streptococcus constellatus, Enterococcus faecalis, Proteus mirabilis, Clostridium perfringens, Bacteroides thetaiotaomicron,* **or** *Peptostreptococcus* **species**
Adults: 400 mg PO or IV every 24 hours for 5 to 14 days. Start with the IV form; switch to PO when appropriate.

➤ **Community-acquired pneumonia from multidrug-resistant** *S. pneumoniae* **(resistance to two or more of the following antibiotics: penicillin, second-generation cephalosporins, macrolides, sulfamethoxazole–trimethoprim, tetracyclines),** *S. aureus, M. catarrhalis, H. influenzae, Haemophilus parainfluenzae, K. pneumoniae, Chlamydia pneumoniae, Legionella pneumophila,* **or** *Mycoplasma pneumoniae*
Adults: 400 mg PO or IV every 24 hours for 7 to 14 days.

➤ **Acute bacterial exacerbation of chronic bronchitis caused by** *S. pneumoniae, H. influenzae, H. parainfluenzae, K. pneumoniae, S. aureus,* **or** *M. catarrhalis*
Adults: 400 mg PO or IV every 24 hours for 5 days.

➤ **Uncomplicated skin-structure or skin infection caused by** *S. aureus* **or** *Streptococcus pyogenes*
Adults: 400 mg PO or IV every 24 hours for 7 days.

➤ **Plague (pneumonic and septicemic) caused by susceptible isolates of** *Yersinia pestis*
Adults: For prophylaxis and treatment, 400 mg PO or IV every 24 hours for 10 to 14 days.

➤ **Bacterial conjunctivitis caused by susceptible strains of aerobic gram-positive and gram-negative organisms and** *Chlamydia trachomatis*
Adults and children age 1 and older (Vigamox): 1 drop into affected eye(s) t.i.d. for 7 days.
Adults and children age 4 months and older (Moxeza): 1 drop into affected eye(s) b.i.d. for 7 days.

ADMINISTRATION
PO
• Give drug without regard for food. Give at same time each day.
• Give dose 4 hours before or 8 hours after antacids, sucralfate, multivitamins, didanosine buffered tablets for oral suspension or pediatric powder for oral solution, and other products containing aluminum, magnesium, iron, and zinc, to avoid decreasing drug's therapeutic effects.
• Store drug at controlled room temperature.
IV
▼ Don't refrigerate. Product precipitates if refrigerated.
▼ Don't use if particulate matter is visible.
▼ Flush IV line with a compatible solution such as D_5W, NSS, or lactated Ringer solution before and after use.
▼ Give only by infusion over 1 hour. Avoid rapid or bolus infusion.
▼ **Incompatibilities:** Other IV drugs.
Ophthalmic
• Place gentle pressure on lacrimal duct for 1 to 2 minutes after instilling drop.
• Solution isn't for injection subconjunctivally or into anterior chamber of the eye.

ACTION
Interferes with action of enzymes needed for bacterial replication. Inhibits topoisomerases I (DNA gyrase) and IV, impairing bacterial DNA replication, transcription, repair, and recombination.

Route	Onset	Peak	Duration
PO, IV	Unknown	1–3 hr	Unknown
Ophthalmic	Unknown	Unknown	Unknown

Half-life: PO, IV, about 12 hours; ophthalmic, 13 hours.

Reactions in bold italics are *life-threatening*. Interactions may have a *rapid onset* or a ***delayed onset***.

ADVERSE REACTIONS
CNS: dizziness, headache, insomnia, fever. **EENT:** with ophthalmic use: conjunctivitis; dry eyes; increased lacrimation; keratitis; ocular discomfort, pain, or pruritus; reduced visual acuity; subconjunctival hemorrhage; otitis media; pharyngitis; rhinitis. **GI:** abdominal pain, anorexia, constipation, diarrhea, dyspepsia, nausea, vomiting. **Hematologic:** anemia. **Hepatic:** abnormal liver function. **Metabolic:** hypokalemia. **Respiratory:** *hypoxia.*

INTERACTIONS
Drug-drug. *Aluminum hydroxide, aluminum–magnesium hydroxide, calcium carbonate, didanosine, magnesium hydroxide, multivitamins, products containing zinc:* May interfere with GI absorption of moxifloxacin. Give moxifloxacin 4 hours before or 8 hours after these products.
Antidiabetics: May cause hyperglycemia and hypoglycemia. Monitor blood glucose control.
Class IA antiarrhythmics (procainamide, quinidine), class III antiarrhythmics (amiodarone, sotalol): May increase risk of cardiac arrhythmias. Avoid using together.
Drugs that prolong QT interval (antipsychotics, erythromycin, TCAs): May have additive effect. Avoid using together.
Live-virus vaccines: May decrease effectiveness of live-virus vaccines. Don't give live-virus vaccines during therapy.
NSAIDs: May increase risk of CNS stimulation and seizures. Monitor patient and adjust treatment as needed.
Black Box Warning *Steroids:* May increase risk of tendinitis and tendon rupture. Monitor patient for tendon pain or inflammation. ∎
Sucralfate: May decrease absorption of moxifloxacin, reducing anti-infective response. If use together can't be avoided, take oral form 4 hours before or 8 hours after sucralfate.
Warfarin: May increase anticoagulant effects. Monitor PT and INR closely.
Drug-lifestyle. *Sun exposure:* May cause moderate to severe photosensitivity reactions. Advise patient to avoid excessive sunlight exposure.

EFFECTS ON LAB TEST RESULTS
• May increase ALT; ionized calcium, chloride, globulin, and albumin levels; and PT and INR.
• May decrease potassium, glucose, and amylase levels and oxygen partial pressure.
• May increase or decrease bilirubin and glucose levels.
• May increase WBC count. May decrease RBC, eosinophil, and basophil counts and Hb level and hematocrit. May increase or decrease neutrophil count.

CONTRAINDICATIONS & CAUTIONS
Black Box Warning Drug is associated with increased risk of tendinitis and tendon rupture, especially in patients older than age 60, patients taking corticosteroids, and those with heart, kidney, or lung transplants. ∎
❸ *Alert:* Drug may increase risk of aortic dissection or rupture when used systemically. Avoid use in patients with known aortic aneurysm and patients at risk for an aortic aneurysm, including those with peripheral atherosclerotic vascular diseases, HTN, or certain genetic conditions (Marfan syndrome, Ehlers-Danlos syndrome), and elderly patients. Drug should only be used in these patients if no other treatment options are available.
❸ *Alert:* Patients receiving systemic drug have an increased risk of hypoglycemia, which can result in coma. Hypoglycemia has been reported more frequently in elderly patients and in those with diabetes.
• Contraindicated in patients hypersensitive to drug or other fluoroquinolones, in those with prolonged QT interval or uncorrected hypokalemia, and in those taking class IA (procainamide) or class III (amiodarone) antiarrhythmics.
❸ *Alert:* Drug can prolong QT interval in some patients. Use cautiously in patients with ongoing proarrhythmic conditions, such as clinically significant bradycardia or acute myocardial ischemia.
• Discontinue drug at first sign of rash, jaundice, or other signs or symptoms of hypersensitivity.
• Seizures, increased ICP, and pseudotumor cerebri have been reported in patients taking fluoroquinolones. Drug may cause CNS events (including agitation, anxiety,

M

confusion, depression, insomnia and, rarely, suicidal ideation), which may occur after first dose. Use cautiously in patients who may have CNS disorders or risk factors for seizures. Drug may need to be discontinued.

Black Box Warning Drug may exacerbate muscle weakness in patients with myasthenia gravis. Avoid use of fluoroquinolones in patients with known history of myasthenia gravis. ∎

• Drug may cause CDAD, ranging in severity from mild diarrhea to fatal colitis, which can occur more than 2 months after therapy. If CDAD is suspected or confirmed, drug may need to be discontinued and appropriate therapy initiated.

• Safety and effectiveness in children and adolescents younger than age 18 haven't been established.

Dialyzable drug: No.

PREGNANCY-LACTATION-REPRODUCTION

• There are no adequate studies in pregnant women. Use during pregnancy only if potential benefit justifies potential risk to the fetus.

• Drug may appear in human milk. Patient should discontinue breastfeeding or discontinue drug.

NURSING CONSIDERATIONS

Black Box Warning Fluoroquinolones have been associated with disabling and potentially irreversible serious adverse reactions that have occurred together, including tendinitis and tendon rupture, peripheral neuropathy, and CNS effects (seizures, toxic psychoses, increased ICP, pseudotumor cerebri, tremors, restlessness, anxiety, lightheadedness, confusion, hallucinations, paranoia, depression, nightmares, insomnia and, rarely, suicidal thoughts or acts). If any of these serious adverse reactions occur, discontinue drug immediately. ∎

Black Box Warning Monitor patient for signs and symptoms of peripheral neuropathy (pain, burning, tingling, numbness, weakness, or change in sensation to light touch, pain or temperature, or sense of body position) and immediately report them. ∎

• Monitor patient for hypersensitivity reactions, including anaphylaxis.

• If diarrhea develops during therapy, send stool specimen for *Clostridium difficile* test.

• Rupture of the Achilles and other tendons is linked to fluoroquinolone use. If pain, inflammation, or tendon rupture occurs, stop drug and notify prescriber.

⊙ *Alert:* Monitor patient for signs and symptoms of aortic aneurysm, dissection, and rupture (sudden, severe, constant pain in the stomach, chest, or back; throbbing in the stomach area; deep pain in the back or side of the stomach; steady, gnawing pain in the stomach that lasts for hours or days; pain in the jaw, neck , back, or chest; coughing or hoarseness; shortness of breath; trouble swallowing). Discontinue drug immediately if any of these aortic disorders are suspected.

⊙ *Alert:* Monitor patients receiving systemic drug for symptoms of hypoglycemia (confusion, pounding or rapid heartbeat, dizziness, pale skin, shakiness, sweating, unusual hunger, trembling, headache, weakness, irritability, unusual anxiety). Immediately discontinue drug for blood glucose disturbances and switch to a nonfluoroquinolone antibiotic if possible.

⊙ *Alert:* Monitor patients receiving systemic drug for psychiatric adverse reactions (disturbances in attention, disorientation, agitation, nervousness, memory impairment, delirium). Discontinue drug for CNS adverse effects, including psychiatric adverse reactions.

• ***Look alike–sound alike:*** Don't confuse Avelox with Avonex; don't confuse Vigamox with Amoxil.

PATIENT TEACHING

Black Box Warning Warn patient to immediately report signs and symptoms of serious adverse reactions, including unusual joint or tendon pain, muscle weakness, "pins and needles" tingling or prickling sensation, numbness in the arms or legs, confusion, or hallucinations. ∎

⊙ *Alert:* Warn patient to seek immediate medical attention for signs and symptoms of aortic aneurysm.

• Instruct patient to take drug once daily, at the same time each day, without regard to meals.

• Tell patient to finish entire course of therapy, even if symptoms are relieved.

- Advise patient to drink plenty of fluids.
- Tell patient to space antacids, sucralfate, multivitamins, and products containing aluminum, magnesium, iron, and zinc to avoid decreasing drug's therapeutic effects.

☉ Alert: Caution patient that significantly low blood glucose levels can occur. Instruct patient how to manage signs and symptoms of low glucose level and to immediately report signs and symptoms to prescriber.

☉ Alert: Advise patient with diabetes that more frequent blood glucose monitoring may be needed during therapy.

☉ Alert: Inform patient to immediately report psychiatric adverse reactions, which can occur after just one dose.

- Instruct patient to contact prescriber and stop drug if allergic reaction, rash, heart palpitations, fainting, or persistent diarrhea occurs.
- Direct patient to contact prescriber, stop drug, rest, and refrain from exercise if pain, inflammation, or tendon rupture occurs.
- Warn patient that drug may cause dizziness and light-headedness. Tell patient to avoid hazardous activities, such as driving or operating machinery, until effects of drug are known.
- Instruct patient to avoid excessive sunlight exposure and ultraviolet light and to report photosensitivity reactions to prescriber.
- Tell patient not to wear contact lenses during ophthalmic treatment.
- Instruct patient not to touch ophthalmic dropper tip to anything, including eyes and fingers.

---

mupirocin
myoo-PEER-oh-sin

Centany

Therapeutic class: Antibacterials (topical)
Pharmacologic class: Antibiotics

AVAILABLE FORMS
Topical cream: 2%
Topical ointment: 2%

INDICATIONS & DOSAGES
➤ **Impetigo (topical ointment)**
Adults and children age 2 months and older:
Apply to affected areas t.i.d. Reevaluate

patient in 3 to 5 days; may cover affected area with dressing.
➤ **Traumatic skin lesions infected with *Staphylococcus aureus* or *Streptococcus pyogenes* (cream)**
Adults and children age 3 months and older:
Apply thin film with cotton swab or gauze pad t.i.d. for 10 days; may cover with gauze dressing, if needed. Reevaluate patient if improvement doesn't occur in 3 to 5 days.
➤ **To eradicate nasal colonization by MRSA in adult patients and health care workers (intranasal ointment)**
Adults and children age 12 and older: Divide ointment in single-use tube between nostrils (half tube per nostril) b.i.d. for 5 days. After application, close nostrils by pressing together and releasing sides of nose repeatedly for 1 minute to spread ointment throughout nares.

ADMINISTRATION
Topical
- Apply topical ointment and cream with gauze pad or cotton swab to avoid contamination.
- Don't apply topical ointment to the eye or in the nose.
- Patient should not use cosmetics and other skin products on treated area.

Intranasal
- Patient shouldn't use other nasal products with intranasal ointment.
- Don't apply to the eyes.

ACTION
Inhibits bacterial protein synthesis by reversibly and specifically binding to bacterial isoleucyl transfer-RNA synthetase.

Route	Onset	Peak	Duration
Topical, intranasal	Unknown	Unknown	Unknown

Half-life: Unknown.

ADVERSE REACTIONS
CNS: headache. **EENT:** rhinitis, pharyngitis, burning or stinging with intranasal use.
GI: taste perversion, nausea. **Respiratory:** respiratory tract congestion, cough with intranasal use. **Skin:** burning, erythema with topical use, pain, pruritus, rash, stinging.

M

INTERACTIONS
Drug-drug. *Bacillus Calmette-Guérin (BCG):* May diminish therapeutic effect of BCG. Avoid combination.
Other nasal products: May interfere with absorption of other nasal drugs. Don't use together.
Sodium picosulfate, typhoid vaccine: May diminish therapeutic effect of sodium picosulfate and typhoid vaccine. Consider therapy modification.

EFFECTS ON LAB TEST RESULTS
None reported.

CONTRAINDICATIONS & CAUTIONS
• Contraindicated in patients hypersensitive to drug or its components.
• Use cautiously in patients with burns or large open wounds and in those with impaired renal function because serious renal toxicity may occur.
Dialyzable drug: Unknown.

PREGNANCY-LACTATION-REPRODUCTION
• There are no adequate studies in pregnant women. Use during pregnancy only if clearly needed.
• It isn't known if drug appears in human milk. Use cautiously in breastfeeding women.

NURSING CONSIDERATIONS
• Drug isn't for ophthalmic or internal use.
• Prolonged use may cause CDAD, ranging in severity from mild diarrhea to fatal colitis, which can occur more than 2 months after therapy ends. If CDAD is suspected or confirmed, drug may need to be discontinued and appropriate therapy initiated.
• Discontinue drug if sensitization or severe local irritation occurs.
• Prolonged use may cause overgrowth of nonsusceptible bacteria and fungi.

PATIENT TEACHING
• Tell patient to notify prescriber immediately if condition doesn't improve or gets worse in 3 to 5 days.
• Advise patient to avoid contact with eyes and if accidental contact occurs, to rinse well with water.

• Urge patient to immediately report diarrhea.
• Tell patient not to use other nasal products with intranasal ointment.
• Warn patient about local adverse reactions related to drug use.
• Caution patient not to use cosmetics or other skin products on treated area.

mycophenolate mofetil
my-koe-FIN-oh-late

CellCept

mycophenolate mofetil hydrochloride
CellCept, CellCept Intravenous

mycophenolic acid (mycophenolate sodium)
Myfortic

Therapeutic class: Immunosuppressants
Pharmacologic class: Mycophenolic acid derivatives

AVAILABLE FORMS
mycophenolate mofetil
Capsules 🔴*:* 250 mg
Powder for oral suspension: 200 mg/mL
Tablets: 500 mg
mycophenolate mofetil hydrochloride
Injection: 500 mg/vial
mycophenolic acid
Tablets (extended-release) 🔴*:* 180 mg, 360 mg

INDICATIONS & DOSAGES
➤ **To prevent organ rejection in patients receiving allogeneic renal transplants**
Adults: 1 g IV or PO (regular-release) b.i.d. with corticosteroids and cyclosporine. Or, 720 mg extended-release tablets PO b.i.d. 1 hour before or 2 hours after food.
Children ages 5 to 16 (extended-release): 400 mg/m^2 PO b.i.d. Maximum dose, 720 mg PO b.i.d. Or, for patients with body surface area (BSA) of 1.19 to 1.58 m^2, give 540 mg PO b.i.d. If BSA is greater than 1.58 m^2, give 720 mg PO b.i.d. Extended-release formulation isn't recommended for BSA of less than 1.19 m^2.

Reactions in bold italics are *life-threatening*. Interactions may have a *rapid onset* or a *delayed onset*.

Children ages 3 months to 18 years: For oral suspension, give 600 mg/m^2 PO b.i.d.; maximum dose is 1 g b.i.d. Or, for patients with BSA of 1.25 to 1.5 m^2, give 750 mg (capsules) PO b.i.d. If BSA is greater than 1.5 m^2, give 1 g (tablets or capsules) PO b.i.d.

Adjust-a-dose: For patients with severe chronic renal impairment (GFR less than 25 mL/minute/1.73 m^2) outside of immediate posttransplant period, avoid doses above 1 g b.i.d. If neutropenia develops, interrupt or reduce dosage.

➤ **To prevent organ rejection in patients receiving allogeneic cardiac transplant**
Adults: 1.5 g PO or IV b.i.d. with cyclosporine and corticosteroids.

➤ **To prevent organ rejection in patients receiving allogeneic hepatic transplants**
Adults: 1 g IV b.i.d. over no less than 2 hours or 1.5 g PO b.i.d. with cyclosporine and corticosteroids.

Adjust-a-dose: If neutropenia develops, stop or reduce dosage.

ADMINISTRATION
PO
🕙 *Alert:* Drug is considered a potential mutagen and teratogen. Follow safe-handling procedures when preparing, administering, or dispensing.
• Don't crush tablets; don't open or crush capsules.
• Give on an empty stomach (1 hour before or 2 hours after a meal). In stable renal transplant patients, may give with food if necessary.
• Avoid inhaling powder in capsule or having it contact skin or mucous membranes. If contact occurs, wash skin thoroughly with soap and water, and rinse eyes with water.
• The extended-release tablets are not interchangeable with other forms.
• Suspension may be administered via NG tube with a minimum size 8 French catheter (at least 1.7-mm interior diameter).
IV
▼ Reconstitute using 14 mL of D$_5$W. Further dilute to 6 mg/1 mL: 1-g doses in 140 mL of D$_5$W and 1.5-g doses in 210 mL of D$_5$W.
▼ Never give by rapid or bolus IV injection. Infuse drug over at least 2 hours.

▼ Use within 4 hours of reconstitution and dilution.
▼ **Incompatibilities:** Other IV drugs or solutions.

ACTION
Inhibits proliferative response of T and B lymphocytes, suppresses antibody formation by B lymphocytes, and may inhibit recruitment of leukocytes into sites of inflammation and graft rejection.

Route	Onset	Peak	Duration
PO	Unknown	1–1½ hr	7–18 hr
PO (extended-release)	Unknown	1½–2¾ hr	8–17 hr
IV	Unknown	Unknown	10–17 hr

Half-life: Oral, 8 to 18 hours; IV, 17 hours.

ADVERSE REACTIONS
CNS: asthenia, fever, headache, pain, tremor, dizziness, insomnia, depression, psychosis, anxiety. **CV:** chest pain, edema, HTN, hypotension, tachycardia, *hemorrhage.* **EENT:** conjunctivitis, visual disturbance, ear pain, deafness, pharyngitis. **GI:** abdominal pain, constipation, diarrhea, dyspepsia, nausea, anorexia, oral candidiasis, vomiting, *hemorrhage.* **GU:** hematuria, UTI, *renal tubular necrosis, acute renal failure.* **Hematologic:** anemia, *leukopenia, thrombocytopenia,* hypochromic anemia, leukocytosis. **Metabolic:** hypercholesterolemia, hyperglycemia, *hyperkalemia,* hypokalemia, hypophosphatemia. **Musculoskeletal:** back pain. **Respiratory:** cough, dyspnea, infection, bronchitis, pneumonia. **Skin:** acne, rash, alopecia, skin carcinoma. **Other:** infection, *sepsis.*

INTERACTIONS
Drug-drug. *Acyclovir, ganciclovir, other drugs that undergo renal tubular secretion:* May increase risk of toxicity for both drugs. Monitor patient closely.
Antacids with magnesium and aluminum hydroxides: May decrease mycophenolate absorption. Separate dosing times.
Azathioprine: May increase risk of bone marrow suppression. Don't use together.
Bile acid sequestrants, cholestyramine, oral activated charcoal, other drugs that

M

interfere with enterohepatic recirculation:
May interfere with enterohepatic recirculation, reducing mycophenolate bioavailability. Avoid using together.

*Cyclosporine, drugs that alter normal GI
flora, rifamycins (rifampin):* May decrease
mycophenolate level. Monitor response to
therapy and increase dosage if necessary.

Hormonal contraceptives: May decrease effectiveness of contraceptive. Recommend
addition of barrier form of contraception
during treatment and for 6 weeks after treatment ends.

*Immunosuppressants (sirolimus, tacro-
limus):* May increase mycophenolate level.
Monitor patient closely.

Live-virus vaccines: May decrease vaccine
effectiveness. Avoid using together.

Probenecid, salicylates: May increase mycophenolate level. Monitor patient closely.

*Sevelamer, other calcium-free phosphate
binders:* May decrease mycophenolate level.
Avoid using together. If concomitant use is
unavoidable, give 2 hours after mycophenolate to minimize impact on absorption.

Drug-herb. *Cat's claw, echinacea:* May increase immunostimulation. Discourage use
together.

Drug-food. *Any food:* May delay absorption
of extended-release form. Advise patient to
take on an empty stomach 1 hour before or
2 hours after a meal.

EFFECTS ON LAB TEST RESULTS

• May increase cholesterol and glucose levels. May decrease phosphorus level. May
increase or decrease potassium level.

• May decrease Hb level and platelet count.
May increase or decrease WBC count.

CONTRAINDICATIONS & CAUTIONS

• Contraindicated in patients hypersensitive to drug, its ingredients, or mycophenolic
acid and in patients sensitive to polysorbate
80.

• Use cautiously in patients with GI disorders. Bleeding and perforation may occur.

• Oral suspension contains aspartame; use
cautiously in patients with phenylketonuria.

• Use cautiously in patients with severe renal impairment, diabetes, or liver disease.

• Immunosuppression can lead to increased
risk of other infection.

• Drug concentrations should be determined
before changes to immunosuppressive
therapy are made.

Dialyzable drug: No.

⚠ *Overdose S&S:* Nausea, vomiting, diarrhea, neutropenia.

PREGNANCY-LACTATION-REPRODUCTION

Black Box Warning Use during pregnancy
is associated with increased risk of first-
trimester pregnancy loss and congenital malformations. Women of childbearing potential must be counseled regarding pregnancy
prevention and planning and to use acceptable contraception during therapy and for
6 weeks after final dose. ■

• For women using drug at any time during
pregnancy and those becoming pregnant
within 6 weeks of discontinuing therapy,
prescriber should report pregnancy to the
Mycophenolate Pregnancy Registry (1-800-
617-8191).

• It isn't known if drug appears in human
milk. Breastfeeding isn't recommended during therapy and for 6 weeks after therapy
ends.

NURSING CONSIDERATIONS

Black Box Warning Increased risk of infection and lymphoma may result from
immunosuppression. ■

Black Box Warning Drug should only be
used by health care providers experienced
in immunosuppressive therapy and management of renal, cardiac, or hepatic transplant patients and in facilities equipped and
staffed with adequate lab and supportive
medical resources. ■

• Start drug therapy within 24 hours after
transplantation. Use IV form in patients unable to take oral forms.

• IV form can be given for up to 14 days;
switch patient to capsules or tablets as soon
as oral drugs can be tolerated.

🔆 *Alert:* Polyomavirus-associated nephropathy, progressive multifocal leukoencephalopathy, CMV infections, and reactivation of HBV or HCV infection have been
reported in patients treated with immunosuppressants. Consider reducing immunosuppressant dosage in patients who develop
evidence of new or reactivated viral infections.

Reactions in bold italics are *life-threatening*. Interactions may have a *rapid onset* or a *delayed onset*.

◐ *Alert:* Drugs causing immunosuppression increase the risk of opportunistic infections, including activation of latent viral infections such as BK virus-associated neuropathy, which may lead to serious outcomes, including kidney graft loss.

◐ *Alert:* Pure red cell aplasia (PRCA) has occurred in patients treated with this drug in combination with other immunosuppressants. Patients may experience fatigue, lethargy, or pallor. PRCA may be reversible with dose reduction or stopping drug. However, this may put graft at risk.

PATIENT TEACHING

• Warn patient not to open or crush capsules nor to cut, crush, or chew extended-release tablets, but to swallow them whole on an empty stomach 1 hour before or 2 hours after a meal.

• Stress importance of following treatment as prescribed.

• Inform patient of the importance of follow-up visits and ongoing lab tests during therapy.

• Tell female patient to have a pregnancy test 1 week before therapy begins and then again 8 to 10 days later. Inform her that repeat tests should be performed during routine follow-up visits.

• Instruct female patient to use two forms of contraception during therapy and for 6 weeks afterward, even if she has a history of infertility. Tell her to notify prescriber immediately if she suspects pregnancy.

• Instruct breastfeeding patient that she shouldn't breastfeed during therapy and for 6 weeks after final dose.

Black Box Warning Warn patient of the increased risk of infection and lymphoma and other malignancies. ∎

• Caution patient to promptly report signs and symptoms of infection (fever, cough, malaise, erythema, wound drainage, pain).

• Caution patient not to drive or operate heavy machinery if somnolence, confusion, dizziness, tremor, or hypotension occurs.

nadolol
nay-DOE-lol

Corgard

Therapeutic class: Antihypertensives, antianginals
Pharmacologic class: Nonselective beta blockers

AVAILABLE FORMS
Tablets: 20 mg, 40 mg, 80 mg, 160 mg ✹

INDICATIONS & DOSAGES
Adjust-a-dose (for all indications): If CrCl is 31 to 50 mL/minute, change dosing interval to every 24 to 36 hours; if CrCl is 10 to 30 mL/minute, every 24 to 48 hours; and if CrCl is less than 10 mL/minute, every 40 to 60 hours.

➤ **Angina pectoris**
Adults: 40 mg PO once daily. Increase in 40- to 80-mg increments at 3- to 7-day intervals until optimal response occurs. Usual maintenance dose is 40 to 80 mg once daily; up to 240 mg once daily may be needed.

➤ **HTN**
Adults: 40 mg PO once daily. Increase in 40- to 80-mg increments until optimal response occurs. Usual maintenance dose is 40 to 80 mg once daily. Doses up to 320 mg daily may be needed.

ADMINISTRATION
PO

• Give drug without regard for food.

• Store at room temperature and avoid heat. Protect from light.

• Check apical pulse before giving drug. If slower than 60 beats/minute, withhold drug and call prescriber.

Black Box Warning Abruptly stopping drug may worsen angina and cause an MI. Reduce dosage gradually over 1 to 2 weeks. ∎

ACTION
Reduces cardiac oxygen demand by blocking catecholamine-induced increases in HR, BP, and force of myocardial contraction. Depresses renin secretion.

N

Route	Onset	Peak	Duration
PO	Unknown	3–4 hr	17–24 hr

Half-life: About 20 to 24 hours.

ADVERSE REACTIONS

CNS: fatigue, dizziness, drowsiness, insomnia, depression, sedation, fever. **CV:** *bradycardia, HF,* hypotension, PVD, rhythm and conduction disturbances, edema, palpitations, Raynaud phenomenon.

INTERACTIONS

Drug-drug. *Acetylcholinesterase inhibitors, amiodarone, dipyridamole, ivabradine, midodrine:* May enhance bradycardic effect. Monitor HR.

Amphetamine, methylphenidate: May decrease antihypertensive effect. Monitor BP.

Anilidopiperidine opioids: May increase bradycardic and hypotensive effects. Monitor HR and BP.

Antihypertensives: May increase antihypertensive effect. Monitor BP closely.

Antipsychotics (second-generation atypicals): May enhance hypotensive effect. Monitor BP.

Barbiturates, calcium channel blockers, diazoxide, duloxetine, levodopa, methoxyflurane, pentoxifylline, PDE5 inhibitors, prostacyclin analogues, quinagolide: May enhance hypotensive effect. Monitor BP.

Beta₂ agonists: May diminish bronchodilatory effect. Avoid combination.

Bretylium: May increase bradycardic and AV blockade effects. Monitor HR and BP.

Cardiac glycosides: May cause excessive bradycardia and additive effects on AV conduction. Use together cautiously.

Ceritinib: May increase bradycardic effect. Avoid use together. If use together is necessary, monitor BP and HR.

Cholinergic agonists: May increase potential for cardiac conduction abnormalities and bronchoconstriction. Administer with caution; monitor patient for conduction disturbances.

Disopyramide: May increase bradycardic and negative inotropic effects. Monitor HR and BP.

Dronedarone: May enhance bradycardic effect and increase nadolol serum

concentration. Use lower initial nadolol dosage and monitor therapy.

Epinephrine: May decrease patient response to epinephrine for treatment of an allergic reaction. Monitor patient closely for decreased clinical effect.

Ergot derivatives: May increase vasoconstricting effect. Consider other therapies.

Fingolimod: May enhance bradycardic effect. Avoid concomitant use. If not possible, patient should have overnight continuous ECG monitoring after first fingolimod dose. Monitor HR.

Floctafenine, methacholine: May enhance adverse/toxic effect. Avoid combination.

General anesthetics: May increase hypotensive effects. Consider stopping nadolol before surgery.

Insulin, oral antidiabetic agents: May mask symptoms of hypoglycemia (such as tachycardia), as a result of beta blockade. May also alter dosage requirements in previously stabilized patients with diabetes. Monitor glucose level closely and use with caution in patients with diabetes.

IV lidocaine: May reduce hepatic metabolism of lidocaine, increasing the risk of toxicity. Give bolus doses of lidocaine at a slower rate and monitor lidocaine level closely.

Lacosamide: May enhance AV blockade effect. Monitor patient.

MAO inhibitors: May enhance orthostatic hypotensive effect. Monitor patient.

NSAIDs: May decrease antihypertensive effect. Monitor BP and adjust dosage.

Obinutuzumab: May enhance hypotensive effect. Consider withholding nadolol for 12 hours before to 1 hour after infusion of obinutuzumab.

Phenothiazines: May increase hypotensive effects. Monitor BP.

Prazosin: May increase risk of orthostatic hypotension in the early phases of use together. Assist patient to stand slowly until effects are known.

Reserpine: May increase hypotension or bradycardia. Monitor patient for adverse effects, such as dizziness, syncope, and postural hypotension.

Verapamil: May increase effects of both drugs. Monitor cardiac function closely and decrease dosages as necessary.

Reactions in bold italics are ***life-threatening***. Interactions may have a *rapid onset* or a ***delayed onset***.

Drug-herb. *Dong quai, ephedra, garlic, ginseng, licorice, yohimbe:* May worsen HTN or affect fluid and electrolytes. Avoid use.
Drug-food. *Green tea:* May decrease nadolol serum concentration. Patient should minimize green tea consumption while using nadolol.

EFFECTS ON LAB TEST RESULTS
• May lead to false-positive aldosterone/renin ratio.

CONTRAINDICATIONS & CAUTIONS
• Contraindicated in patients with bronchial asthma, sinus bradycardia and greater than first-degree heart block (except in patients with functional pacemaker), cardiogenic shock, and overt (uncompensated) HF.
• Use cautiously in patients with HF, chronic bronchitis, emphysema, renal or hepatic impairment, myasthenia gravis, PVD, psoriasis, or psychiatric disease and in patients undergoing major surgery involving general anesthesia. Drug shouldn't be routinely withdrawn before major surgery.
• Generally, patients with bronchospastic disease shouldn't receive beta blockers because they may block bronchodilation.
• Use cautiously in diabetic patients because beta blockers may mask certain signs and symptoms of hypoglycemia.
Black Box Warning Exacerbation of ischemic heart disease may occur following abrupt withdrawal of drug. Exacerbation of angina and, in some cases, MI have occurred after abrupt discontinuation of therapy. ∎
Dialyzable drug: Yes.
⚠ *Overdose S&S:* Bradycardia, cardiac failure, hypotension, bronchospasm.

PREGNANCY-LACTATION-REPRODUCTION
• Use cautiously in pregnant women and only if benefit justifies possible risk to the fetus.
• Drug appears in human milk. Patient should discontinue breastfeeding or discontinue drug.

NURSING CONSIDERATIONS
• Monitor BP and HR frequently. If patient develops severe hypotension, give vasopressors, as prescribed.

• Drug masks signs and symptoms of shock, hypoglycemia, and hyperthyroidism.
Black Box Warning If nadolol is to be discontinued after long-term administration, particularly in patients with ischemic heart disease, dosage should be gradually reduced over a period of 1 to 2 weeks and patient carefully monitored. If angina markedly worsens or acute coronary insufficiency develops after drug cessation, nadolol should be temporarily restarted and other measures taken to appropriately manage unstable angina. Because CAD is common and may be unrecognized, don't discontinue nadolol therapy abruptly, even in patients treated only for HTN. ∎
• *Look alike–sound alike:* Don't confuse Corgard with Coreg.

PATIENT TEACHING
• Explain importance of taking drug as prescribed, with or without regard to food, even when patient feels well.
• Teach patient how to check pulse rate and to check it before each dose. If pulse rate is below 60 beats/minute, tell patient to notify prescriber.
Black Box Warning Warn patient not to stop drug suddenly. ∎

nafcillin sodium
naf-SIL-in

Therapeutic class: Antibiotics
Pharmacologic class: Penicillinase-resistant penicillins

AVAILABLE FORMS
Infusion: 1-g, 2-g, 10-g premixed or Add-Vantage vials

INDICATIONS & DOSAGES
Adjust-a-dose (for all indications): In patients with concomitant renal failure and hepatic insufficiency, measure nafcillin serum levels and adjust dosage accordingly. Duration of therapy depends on type and severity of the infection and overall condition of patient. In severe infection, continue for at least 14 days. Continue for at least 48 hours after patient is afebrile and asymptomatic and cultures are negative. Treatment of endocarditis

N

and osteomyelitis may require a longer duration of therapy.

➤ **Systemic infection caused by susceptible organisms (methicillin-sensitive *Staphylococcus aureus*)**
Adults: 500 mg IV every 4 hours, or 500 mg IM every 4 to 6 hours. For severe infections, 1 g IV or IM every 4 hours.
Infants and children weighing less than 40 kg: 25 mg/kg IM b.i.d.
Neonates: 10 mg/kg IM b.i.d.

ADMINISTRATION
IV

▼ Before giving drug, ask patient about allergic reactions to penicillin.

▼ Obtain specimen for culture and sensitivity tests before giving. Begin therapy while awaiting results.

▼ Check container for leaks, cloudiness, or precipitate before use. Discard if present.

▼ Give drug over 30 to 60 minutes.

▼ Change site every 48 hours to prevent vein irritation.

▼ Vials may be reconstituted with sterile water for injection or NSS.

▼ Reconstituted vials of 10 to 40 mg/mL are stable for 24 hours at room temperature.

▼ **Incompatibilities:** Other drugs.

IM

● Reconstitute with sterile water for injection, NSS for injection, or bacteriostatic water for injection. Add 6.6 mL to 2-g vial. Reconstituted vials contain 250 mg/mL.

● Administer clear solution by deep intragluteal IM injection immediately after reconstitution.

ACTION
Inhibits cell-wall synthesis during bacterial multiplication.

Route	Onset	Peak	Duration
IV	Immediate	Immediate	Unknown
IM	Unknown	30–60 min	Unknown

Half-life: About 33 to 61 minutes.

ADVERSE REACTIONS
CNS: *neurotoxicity.* **CV:** thrombophlebitis, vein irritation. **GI:** nausea, *pseudomembranous colitis,* diarrhea, vomiting, CDAD. **GU:** renal tubular damage, interstitial nephritis. **Hematologic:** *agranulocytosis,* *leukopenia, neutropenia, thrombocytopenia,* anemia, eosinophilia. **Hepatic:** cholestasis. **Skin:** severe tissue necrosis (with subcutaneous extravasation), injection-site pain and reactions. **Other:** *anaphylaxis,* hypersensitivity reactions.

INTERACTIONS
Drug-drug. *Aminoglycosides:* May have synergistic effect; drugs are chemically and physically incompatible. Don't combine in same IV solution.
Antivirals: May decrease serum concentration of antivirals. Avoid combination.
Bedaquiline: May decrease bedaquiline serum concentration. Avoid combination.
Clarithromycin: May decrease clarithromycin serum concentration. Consider alternative antimicrobial therapy.
Clozapine: May decrease clozapine serum concentration. Monitor therapy.
Cyclosporine: May cause subtherapeutic cyclosporine levels. Monitor cyclosporine levels.
CYP3A4 substrates: May decrease serum concentration of the substrates. Use with caution.
Deflazacort: May decrease serum concentration of active metabolite(s) of deflazacort. Avoid combination.
Fentanyl: May decrease fentanyl serum concentration. Monitor pain level.
Guanfacine: May decrease guanfacine serum concentration. Increase guanfacine dosage by up to double when initiating concomitant therapy. Increase guanfacine dosage gradually over 1 to 2 weeks if nafcillin therapy is just starting.
Hormonal contraceptives: May decrease contraceptive effectiveness. Advise use of additional form of contraception during therapy.
Hydrocodone: May decrease hydrocodone serum concentration. Monitor pain level.
Live-virus vaccines: May reduce effectiveness of live-virus vaccine. Don't use concurrently.
Lurasidone: May decrease lurasidone serum concentration. Monitor patient for decreased lurasidone effects.
Methotrexate: May cause methotrexate toxicity. Monitor patient closely.

Mycophenolate: May decrease serum concentration of active metabolites of mycophenolate. Monitor patient.

Probenecid: May increase nafcillin level. Probenecid may be used for this purpose.

Ranolazine: May decrease ranolazine serum concentration. Avoid combination.

Rifampin: May cause dose-dependent antagonism. Monitor patient closely.

Tetracycline: May decrease nafcillin's effectiveness. Avoid concurrent use.

Warfarin: May decrease effects of warfarin. Monitor PT and INR closely.

Zolpidem: May decrease zolpidem serum concentration. Monitor patient.

EFFECTS ON LAB TEST RESULTS

• May increase liver transaminase levels.
• May decrease Hb level and hematocrit and neutrophil, WBC, eosinophil, granulocyte, and platelet counts.
• May cause false-positive Coombs test and false-positive urinary and serum protein levels.

CONTRAINDICATIONS & CAUTIONS

• Contraindicated in patients hypersensitive to drug or other penicillins.
• Use cautiously in patients with asthma, GI distress, or hepatic impairment and in those with other drug allergies (especially to cephalosporins) because of possible cross-sensitivity.
• Superinfection and CDAD can occur during therapy and up to 2 months after therapy ends. Drug may need to be discontinued and appropriate treatment initiated.
• Drug may infrequently cause renal tubular damage and interstitial nephritis, especially with large IV doses.
• Skin sloughing from subcutaneous extravasation has been reported.
Dialyzable drug: No.
⚠ *Overdose S&S:* Neurotoxic reactions.

PREGNANCY-LACTATION-REPRODUCTION

• Use during pregnancy only if clearly needed.
• Penicillins appear in human milk. Use cautiously in breastfeeding women.

NURSING CONSIDERATIONS

• If large doses are given or if therapy is prolonged, bacterial or fungal superinfection may occur, especially in elderly, debilitated, or immunosuppressed patients.
• Serious and fatal hypersensitivity reactions can occur, including anaphylactic reactions requiring treatment with epinephrine. Monitor patient during and after drug administration and obtain complete drug allergy history.
• Monitor sodium level because each gram of drug contains 2.9 mEq of sodium.
• Monitor WBC counts twice weekly in patients receiving drug for longer than 2 weeks. Neutropenia commonly occurs in the third week.
• Monitor patient for signs and symptoms of interstitial nephritis (abnormal urinalysis results, rash, fever, eosinophilia, hematuria, proteinuria, renal insufficiency).

PATIENT TEACHING

• Tell patient to report burning or irritation at the IV site.
• Advise patient to notify prescriber of all adverse reactions, especially rash or signs and symptoms of superinfection (recurring fever, chills, malaise) or CDAD (unexplained diarrhea).

SAFETY ALERT!

nalbuphine hydrochloride
NAL-byoo-feen

Nubain✶

Therapeutic class: Opioid analgesics
Pharmacologic class: Opioid agonist-antagonists–opioid partial agonists

AVAILABLE FORMS

Injection: 10 mg/mL, 20 mg/mL

INDICATIONS & DOSAGES

Adjust-a-dose (for all indications): In patients with renal or hepatic impairment, decrease dosage.
➤ **Moderate to severe pain (non-opioid-tolerant patients)**
Adults: For patient weighing about 70 kg, 10 to 20 mg subcut, IM, or IV every 3 to

N

6 hours p.r.n. Maximum, 160 mg daily. Adjust dosage according to the severity of pain, physical status, and other drugs patient is receiving.

➤ **Adjunct to balanced anesthesia; preoperative and postoperative analgesia; obstetric analgesia during labor and delivery**

Adults: 0.3 to 3 mg/kg IV over 10 to 15 minutes; then maintenance dose of 0.25 to 0.5 mg/kg in single IV dose p.r.n.

ADMINISTRATION
IV
▼ Inject slowly over at least 2 to 3 minutes into a vein or into an IV line containing a compatible, free-flowing IV solution, such as D5W, NSS, or lactated Ringer solution.

▼ Respiratory depression can be reversed with naloxone. Keep resuscitation equipment available, particularly when giving IV.

▼ **Incompatibilities:** None listed by manufacturer. Consult a drug incompatibility reference for more information.

IM
• Document injection site.
• Store vial in carton to protect from light.

Subcutaneous
• Document injection site.
• Store vial in carton to protect from light.

ACTION
Unknown. Binds with opioid receptors in the CNS, altering perception of and emotional response to pain.

Route	Onset	Peak	Duration
IV	2–3 min	2–3 min	3–6 hr
IM, subcut	<15 min	<15 min	3–6 hr

Half-life: 5 hours.

ADVERSE REACTIONS
CNS: dizziness, headache, sedation, vertigo. **CV:** *bradycardia,* hypotension. **EENT:** dry mouth. **GI:** nausea, vomiting. **Respiratory:** *respiratory depression.* **Skin:** clamminess, diaphoresis.

INTERACTIONS
Drug-drug. *CNS depressants, general anesthetics, hypnotics, MAO inhibitors, sedatives, tranquilizers, TCAs:* May cause respiratory depression, HTN, profound sedation, or coma. Use together with caution, and monitor patient response.

Naltrexone: May result in opioid withdrawal signs and symptoms and decreased opioid effectiveness. Avoid combination.

Black Box Warning *Opioids, CNS depressants:* May cause respiratory depression, profound sedation, coma, and death. Avoid use together. If use together is necessary, limit dosage and duration of each drug to minimum necessary for desired effect. Monitor patient response closely. ∎

⊗ Alert: *Serotonergic drugs (amoxapine, antiemetics [dolasetron, granisetron, ondansetron, palonosetron], antimigraine drugs, buspirone, cyclobenzaprine, dextromethorphan, linezolid, lithium, MAO inhibitors, maprotiline, methylene blue, mirtazapine, nefazodone, SSNRIs, SSRIs, TCAs, trazodone, tryptophan, vilazodone):* May increase risk of serotonin syndrome. Use together cautiously. Monitor patient for serotonin syndrome. Avoid using MAO inhibitors during treatment and don't use drug within 14 days of MAO inhibitor therapy.

Drug-lifestyle. *Alcohol use:* May cause additive effects. Discourage use together.

⊗ Alert: *St. John's wort:* May increase risk of serotonin syndrome. Use together cautiously. Monitor patient for serotonin syndrome.

EFFECTS ON LAB TEST RESULTS
• May interfere with enzymatic methods for detection of opioids.

CONTRAINDICATIONS & CAUTIONS
• Contraindicated in patients hypersensitive to drug or its components and in those with significant respiratory depression, known or suspected GI obstruction (including paralytic ileus), and acute or severe asthma in an unmonitored setting or in the absence of resuscitative equipment.

• Use cautiously and at low doses in patients with preexisting respiratory compromise.

⊗ Alert: Drug should only be administered as a supplement to general anesthesia by those specifically trained in the use of IV anesthetics and management of respiratory effects of potent opioids. Naloxone hydrochloride and emergency resuscitative equipment should be readily available.

Reactions in bold italics are *life-threatening*. Interactions may have a *rapid onset* or a *delayed onset*.

◐ *Alert:* Patients are at increased risk for oversedation and respiratory depression if they snore or have a history of sleep apnea, haven't used opioids recently or are first-time opioid users, have increased opioid dosage requirements or opioid habituation, have received general anesthesia for longer lengths of time or received other sedating drugs, have preexisting pulmonary or cardiac disease, or have thoracic or other surgical incisions that may impair breathing. Monitor patients carefully.

◐ *Alert:* Drug may lead to a rare but serious decrease in adrenal gland cortisol production.

◐ *Alert:* Drug may cause decreased sex hormone levels with long-term use.

• Use cautiously in patients with history of drug abuse and in those with emotional instability, head injury, increased ICP, impaired ventilation, MI accompanied by nausea and vomiting, upcoming biliary surgery, or hepatic, renal, or adrenal insufficiency.

• Drug may cause mood disorders and osteoporosis.

◐ *Alert:* Certain commercial preparations contain sodium metabisulfite.

Dialyzable drug: Unknown.

⚠ *Overdose S&S:* Sleepiness, mild dysphoria.

PREGNANCY-LACTATION-REPRODUCTION

• There are no adequate studies in pregnant women. Use only if clearly needed.

◐ *Alert:* When used for pain relief during labor, fetal bradycardia can occur. Monitor fetuses and newborns for bradycardia.

• Prolonged use of drug during pregnancy can result in neonatal withdrawal syndrome, which may be life-threatening and which requires management according to neonatology expert protocols.

• Use cautiously in breastfeeding women.

• Long-term opioid use can cause secondary hypogonadism, infertility, and sexual dysfunction.

NURSING CONSIDERATIONS

• Reassess patient's level of pain at least 15 and 30 minutes after parenteral administration.

◐ *Alert:* Carefully monitor vital signs, pain level, respiratory status, and sedation level

in all patients receiving opioids, especially those receiving IV drugs, even those given postoperatively.

Black Box Warning Drug can cause life-threatening or fatal respiratory depression. Monitor patient for respiratory depression, especially within first 24 to 72 hours of the start of therapy and after dosage increase. ▌

Black Box Warning Before starting drug, assess patient's risk of opioid abuse, misuse, and addiction. Regularly monitor patients for development of these behaviors or conditions. ▌

◐ *Alert:* If patient is taking opioids with serotonergic drugs, watch for signs and symptoms of serotonin syndrome (agitation, hallucinations, rapid HR, fever, excessive sweating, shivering or shaking, muscle twitching or stiffness, trouble with coordination, nausea, vomiting, diarrhea), especially at start of therapy and after dosage increase. Signs and symptoms may occur within several hours of coadministration but may also occur later, especially after dosage increase. Discontinue opioid, serotonergic drug, or both if serotonin syndrome is suspected.

◐ *Alert:* Monitor patient for signs and symptoms of adrenal insufficiency (nausea, vomiting, loss of appetite, fatigue, weakness, dizziness, low BP). Perform diagnostic testing if adrenal insufficiency is suspected. If adrenal insufficiency is confirmed, treat with corticosteroids and wean patient off opioids if appropriate. Discontinue corticosteroids when clinically appropriate.

◐ *Alert:* Monitor patient for signs and symptoms of decreased sex hormone levels (low libido, erectile dysfunction, amenorrhea, infertility). If signs and symptoms occur, evaluate patient and obtain lab testing.

◐ *Alert:* Don't stop drug abruptly; withdraw slowly and individualize the gradual tapering plan to prevent signs and symptoms of withdrawal, worsening pain, and psychological distress in physically dependent patients. Refer to manufacturer's label for specific tapering instructions.

◐ *Alert:* When tapering opioids, monitor patient closely for signs and symptoms of opioid withdrawal (restlessness, lacrimation, rhinorrhea, yawning, perspiration, chills, myalgia, mydriasis, irritability, anxiety, insomnia, backache, joint pain, weakness,

N

abdominal cramps, anorexia, nausea, vomiting, diarrhea, increased BP or HR, increased respiratory rate), which may indicate a need to taper more slowly. Also monitor patient for suicidal thoughts, use of other substances, and mood changes.

• Drug acts as an opioid antagonist and may cause withdrawal syndrome. For patients who have received long-term opioids, give 25% of the usual dose initially. Watch for signs of withdrawal.

❸ Alert: Drug causes respiratory depression, which at 10 mg is equal to respiratory depression produced by 10 mg of morphine.

• Monitor circulatory and respiratory status and bladder and bowel function. If respirations are shallow or rate is below 12 breaths/minute, withhold dose and notify prescriber.

• Constipation is commonly severe with maintenance therapy. Make sure stool softener or other stimulant laxative is ordered.

• Psychological and physical dependence may occur with prolonged use.

• **Look alike–sound alike:** Don't confuse Nubain with Navane or Nebcin. Don't confuse nalbuphine with naloxone.

PATIENT TEACHING

❸ Alert: Encourage patient to report all medications being taken, including prescription and OTC medications and supplements.

❸ Alert: Counsel patient not to discontinue opioids without first discussing with prescriber the need for a gradual tapering regimen.

Black Box Warning Caution patient or caregiver of patient taking an opioid with a benzodiazepine, CNS depressant, or alcohol to seek immediate medical attention for dizziness, light-headedness, extreme sleepiness, slowed or difficult breathing, or unresponsiveness. ■

❸ Alert: Caution patient to immediately report signs and symptoms of serotonin syndrome, adrenal insufficiency, and decreased sex hormone levels.

• Explain assessment and monitoring process to patient and family. Instruct them to immediately report difficulty breathing or other signs and symptoms of a potential adverse opioid-related reaction.

• Caution ambulatory patient about getting out of bed or walking. Warn outpatient to avoid driving and other hazardous activities that require mental alertness until drug's CNS effects are known.

• Teach patient how to manage troublesome adverse effects such as constipation.

• Caution patient to avoid taking drug with alcohol.

naloxone hydrochloride
nal-OX-one

Evzio, Narcan

Therapeutic class: Antidotes
Pharmacologic class: Opioid antagonists

AVAILABLE FORMS
Injection: 0.4 mg/mL, 1 mg/mL
Injection (prefilled autoinjector): 2 mg/ 0.4 mL
Nasal spray: 4 mg/0.1 mL

INDICATIONS & DOSAGES
➤ **Known or suspected opioid-induced respiratory depression, including that caused by pentazocine, methadone, nalbuphine, and butorphanol**
Adults: 0.4 to 2 mg IV, IM, or subcut. Repeat dose every 2 to 3 minutes, p.r.n. If patient doesn't respond after 10 mg have been given, question diagnosis of opioid-induced toxicity. After reversal, additional dose(s) may be needed at a later interval (e.g., 20 to 60 minutes) depending on type and duration of opioid. May also give via ET tube at 2 to 2.5 × initial IV dose (e.g., 0.8 to 5 mg).
Children age 1 month and older: 0.01 mg/kg IV; then, second dose of 0.1 mg/kg IV, if needed. If IV route isn't available, drug may be given IM or subcut in divided doses.
Neonates: 0.01 mg/kg IV, IM, or subcut. Repeat dose every 2 to 3 minutes, p.r.n.
➤ **Postoperative opioid depression**
Adults: 0.1 to 0.2 mg IV every 2 to 3 minutes, p.r.n. Repeat doses may be required within 1- or 2-hour intervals depending on amount, type (short- or long-acting), and time interval since last administration. Supplemental IM doses have produced a longer-lasting effect.

Reactions in bold italics are *life-threatening*. Interactions may have a *rapid onset* or a *delayed onset*.

Children: 0.005 to 0.01 mg IV repeated every 2 to 3 minutes, p.r.n.

➤ **Emergency treatment of known or suspected opioid overdose**

Adults and children: 0.4 to 2 mg IM or subcut. If desired response isn't obtained after 2 or 3 minutes, may give another dose. If there is still no response and additional doses are available, every 2 or 3 minutes until emergency medical assistance arrives. Or, contents of 1 nasal spray (2 mg or 4 mg) intranasally as a single dose; may repeat dose every 2 to 3 minutes in alternating nostrils until emergency medical assistance arrives. In neonates with known or suspected exposure to maternal opioid use, consider using another form to allow dosing according to weight and titration to effect.

Adjust-a-dose: Restrict prescription of naloxone 2-mg nasal spray to opioid-dependent patients expected to be at risk for severe opioid withdrawal in situations in which there is low risk of accidental or intentional opioid exposure by household contacts.

➤ **Opioid-induced pruritus** ◆

Adults: 0.25 mcg/kg/hour IV. Monitor pain control; verify that drug isn't reversing analgesia.

ADMINISTRATION

IV

▼ Give continuous infusion to control adverse effects of epidural morphine.

▼ Dilute 2 mg of drug in 500 mL D_5W or NSS to yield a concentration of 0.004 mg/mL; use within 24 hours.

▼ Titrate rate to patient's response.

▼ **Incompatibilities:** Alkaline solutions, amphotericin B cholesteryl sulfate, preparations containing bisulfite, sulfite, long-chain or high-molecular-weight anions.

IM

• Use mixtures within 24 hours. After 24 hours, discard.

• May give autoinjector doses IM or subcut into the anterolateral thigh through clothing.

🕭 *Alert:* When autoinjector is used, seek emergency medical assistance as soon as possible.

• For children younger than age 1, the caregiver should pinch the thigh muscle while administering the autoinjector dose.

• Each autoinjector can only be used once.

• Each autoinjector has a speaker that provides voice instructions to guide patients and caregivers through each step of the instructions. If the voice instructions don't work, the autoinjector will still work. Follow the instructions on the label.

• To use the autoinjector, remove it from the outer case, pull off the red safety guard, place the black end against the outer thigh, press firmly, and hold in place for 5 seconds. The needle will inject and then retract back into the autoinjector. After use, the viewing window will contain a red indicator.

• Store autoinjector at room temperature in the case provided.

Intranasal

• Don't prime or test the device before administration.

• Each container contains a single intranasal spray; don't reuse.

• To administer nasal spray, place patient in the supine position and support the back of the neck to allow the head to tilt back. After administration, turn patient on side.

• If repeat administration is necessary, use a new container and alternate nostrils.

Subcutaneous

• Use mixtures within 24 hours. After 24 hours, discard.

ACTION

May displace opioid analgesics from their receptors (competitive antagonism); drug has no pharmacologic activity of its own.

Route	Onset	Peak	Duration
IV	1–2 min	5–15 min	Variable
IM, subcut	2–5 min	5–15 min	Variable
Intranasal	8–13 min	20–30 min	Variable

Half-life: IV, IM, or subcut, 30 to 81 minutes in adults, 3 hours in neonates; intranasal, about 2 hours.

ADVERSE REACTIONS

CNS: *seizures,* tremors, headache. **CV:** *ventricular fibrillation, ventricular tachycardia,* HTN with higher-than-recommended doses, hypotension. **EENT:** nasal dryness, edema, congestion, inflammation. **GI:** nausea, vomiting. **Musculoskeletal:** pain. **Respiratory:** *pulmonary edema.* **Skin:** diaphoresis, injection-site pain and erythema. **Other:** withdrawal symptoms in

N

opioid-dependent patients with higher-than-recommended doses.

INTERACTIONS

Drug-drug. *Methylnaltrexone, naldemedine, naloxegol:* May enhance risk of opioid withdrawal. Avoid combination.

EFFECTS ON LAB TEST RESULTS

None reported.

CONTRAINDICATIONS & CAUTIONS

• Contraindicated in patients hypersensitive to drug.

۞ Alert: Use cautiously in patients with cardiac irritability or opioid addiction. Abrupt reversal of opioid-induced CNS depression may result in sudden opioid withdrawal signs and symptoms (such as nausea, vomiting, diaphoresis, tachycardia, CNS excitement, and increased BP).

۞ Alert: In infants younger than age 4 weeks, sudden opioid withdrawal can be life-threatening. Signs and symptoms include excessive crying, increased reflexes, and seizures.

Dialyzable drug: Unknown.

PREGNANCY-LACTATION-REPRODUCTION

• Pregnant women should receive drug if there is a clear indication for its use. Drug shouldn't be withheld because of fears of teratogenicity.

• Drug crosses the placental barrier and may precipitate withdrawal in the fetus and the opioid-dependent mother. Monitor fetus for distress.

• It isn't known if drug appears in human milk. Use cautiously; however, because drug is used for opioid reversal, consider the opioid concentration in the milk of a breastfeeding mother and potential transfer of the opioid to the infant.

NURSING CONSIDERATIONS

• Duration of action of the opioid may exceed that of naloxone, and patients may relapse into respiratory depression. Monitor patients closely and repeat dose if needed.

• Respiratory rate increases within 1 to 2 minutes.

• Abrupt postoperative reversal of opioid depression may result in adverse CV effects; monitor patients closely.

• Large doses of naloxone are required to antagonize buprenorphine; reversal effects have a gradual onset.

• Methohexital may block the acute onset of withdrawal symptoms induced by naloxone in opioid-addicted patients.

۞ Alert: Drug is only effective for reversing respiratory depression caused by opioids and not for other drug-induced respiratory depression, including that caused by benzodiazepines.

• Monitor patients, especially infants younger than age 4 weeks, for opioid withdrawal signs and symptoms.

• Patients who receive drug to reverse opioid-induced respiratory depression may exhibit tachypnea.

• Monitor respiratory depth and rate. Provide oxygen, ventilation, and other resuscitation measures.

• *Look alike–sound alike:* Don't confuse naloxone with naltrexone.

PATIENT TEACHING

• Reassure family that patient will be monitored closely until effects of opioid resolve.

• Instruct patient and family about signs and symptoms of opioid toxicity emergency (unusual sleepiness or inability to awaken the person, breathing problems, pinpoint pupils).

• Instruct patient and caregivers on the use of autoinjector and to seek emergency care as soon as possible when it's used. Advise patient to refer to manufacturer's instructions.

• Instruct person who will be administering intranasal drug to read instructions carefully before use. Remind the person that the spray is single-use only; if signs and symptoms of an opioid emergency return and more drug is needed, a second container must be used.

• Instruct person who will be administering intranasal drug to seek emergency help immediately after giving first dose of drug.

• Instruct patient and caregivers that naloxone administration can precipitate acute opioid withdrawal symptoms, which can be fatal in neonates.

---

naltrexone
nal-TREX-one

Vivitrol

naltrexone hydrochloride
Revia

Therapeutic class: Opioid cessation drugs
Pharmacologic class: Opioid antagonists, antidotes

AVAILABLE FORMS
naltrexone
Injection: 380-mg vial dose kit
naltrexone hydrochloride
Tablets: 25 mg, 50 mg, 100 mg

INDICATIONS & DOSAGES
➤ **Adjunct for maintaining opioid-free state in detoxified patients**
Adults: Initially, 25 mg PO. If no withdrawal signs or symptoms occur after initiation, may start patient on 50 mg every 24 hours the following day. Or, 50 mg PO every weekday with a 100-mg dose on Saturday, 100 mg every other day, or 150 mg every third day. Or, 380 mg IM in gluteal muscle every 4 weeks or once a month.
➤ **Alcohol dependence**
Adults: 50 mg PO once daily for up to 12 weeks, or 380 mg IM in gluteal muscle every 4 weeks or once monthly.

ADMINISTRATION
• Don't give to patients who haven't been opioid free for at least 7 to 10 days. May consider a naloxone challenge test.
PO
• Keep container tightly closed and protect from light.
• Give without regard to meals; give with food if GI upset occurs.
IM
• Use only the diluent, needles, and other components supplied with the dose kit. Don't substitute.
• Allow drug to reach room temperature before administering.
• Administer IM into gluteal muscle, alternating buttocks for each subsequent administration. Avoid giving IV, subcut, or inadvertently into fatty tissue. Monitor injection site.
• Store in refrigerator or up to 7 days at controlled room temperature. Don't freeze.

ACTION
Probably reversibly blocks the effects of exogenous opioids by competitively occupying opiate receptors in the brain. Mechanism of action in alcohol dependence is unknown; however, may be related to the endogenous system.

Route	Onset	Peak	Duration
PO	15–30 min	1 hr	24–72 hr
IM	Unknown	2 hr	>30 days

Half-life: PO, about 4 hours; IM, 5 to 10 days.

ADVERSE REACTIONS
CNS: insomnia, anxiety, nervousness, headache, depression, dizziness, fatigue, somnolence, syncope, low energy, irritability, nervousness, suicidal ideation, depression. **CV:** HTN. **EENT:** nasopharyngitis. **GI:** nausea, diarrhea, vomiting, abdominal pain, anorexia, constipation, dry mouth, toothache, increased thirst, decreased appetite. **GU:** delayed ejaculation, decreased potency. **Musculoskeletal:** muscle and joint pain, muscle cramps, back pain. **Skin:** injection-site reaction, rash. **Other:** chills, flulike symptoms.

INTERACTIONS
Drug-drug. *Methylnaltrexone, naloxegol:* May enhance adverse/toxic effect; increases risk of opioid withdrawal. Avoid use together.
Products that contain opioids: May decrease effect of opioid. Avoid using together.

EFFECTS ON LAB TEST RESULTS
• May increase AST, ALT, and LDH levels.
• May increase lymphocyte count.
• May be cross-reactive with certain immunoassay methods for detection of opioids in urine.

CONTRAINDICATIONS & CAUTIONS
• Contraindicated in patients hypersensitive to drug or components of the diluent, those currently dependent on opioids, those receiving opioid analgesics, those who fail

N

the naloxone challenge test or who have a positive urine screen for opioids, or those in acute opioid withdrawal.

• Drug may precipitate opioid withdrawal.

• Fatal overdose may occur if patient uses opioids at the end of a dosing interval, after missing a dose, or after discontinuing treatment. Attempts by patient to overcome blockade may also lead to fatal overdose.

• Dose-related hepatic injury is possible. Use cautiously in patients with mild hepatic disease or history of recent hepatic disease.

• Suicidal ideation and depression have been noted in postmarketing reports.

• Drug should be part of a comprehensive treatment plan that includes psychosocial support.

• Safety and effectiveness is children haven't been evaluated.

Dialyzable drug: Unknown.

⚠ *Overdose S&S:* Injection-site reaction, nausea, abdominal pain, somnolence, dizziness.

PREGNANCY-LACTATION-REPRODUCTION

• Use during pregnancy only if potential benefit justifies potential risk to the fetus.

• Drug appears in human milk. Use cautiously in breastfeeding women.

NURSING CONSIDERATIONS

❸ *Alert:* Patient must be completely free from opioids before taking naltrexone or severe withdrawal symptoms may occur. Patients who have been addicted to short-acting opioids, such as heroin and meperidine, must wait at least 7 days after last opioid dose before starting drug. Patients who have been addicted to longer-acting opioids such as methadone should wait at least 10 days.

❸ *Alert:* Discontinue drug if patient develops signs or symptoms of acute hepatitis.

• Monitor patient for the development of depression or suicidal thinking.

• Don't begin treatment for opioid dependence until patient receives naloxone challenge, a test of opioid dependence. If signs and symptoms of opioid withdrawal persist after naloxone challenge, don't give drug.

• In an emergency, patient may be given an opioid analgesic, but dose must be higher than usual to overcome naltrexone's effect.

Watch for respiratory depression from the opioid; it may be longer and deeper.

• For patients expected to be noncompliant because of history of opioid dependence, use a flexible maintenance-dose regimen of 100 mg on Monday and Wednesday and 150 mg on Friday.

• Monitor patient for an injection-site reaction, including pain, tenderness, swelling, erythema, bruising, or pruritus. In some cases, an injection-site reaction may be very severe, with induration, cellulitis, hematoma, abscess, sterile abscess, and necrosis.

• Use drug only as part of a comprehensive rehabilitation program.

• *Look alike–sound alike:* Don't confuse naltrexone with naloxone or methylnaltrexone.

PATIENT TEACHING

• Advise patient to carry medical identification and to inform medical personnel about taking naltrexone.

• Tell patient that drug can block the effects of opioids and opioid-like drugs, including heroin, pain medicine, antidiarrheals, or cough medicine.

❸ *Alert:* Warn patient that using large doses of heroin or any other opioid can cause serious injury, coma, or death.

• Advise patient who previously used opioids that patient may be more sensitive to lower doses of opioids once naltrexone therapy is stopped.

• Warn patient of risk of hepatic injury and to seek medical attention if signs or symptoms of acute hepatitis occur.

❸ *Alert:* Tell caregiver of alcohol-dependent patient to monitor patient closely for signs of depression or suicidal ideation and to report this immediately to prescriber.

• Provides names of nonopioid drugs that patient can continue to take for pain, diarrhea, or cough.

• Tell patient to report pain, swelling, tenderness, induration, bruising, pruritus, or redness at the injection site.

• Advise patient that drug may cause an allergic pneumonia and to immediately notify prescriber if signs and symptoms of pneumonia, including dyspnea, coughing, or wheezing, develop.

Reactions in bold italics are *life-threatening*. Interactions may have a *rapid onset* or a *delayed onset*.

naproxen
na-PROX-en

EC-Naprosyn, Naprosyn✒

naproxen sodium
Aleve ◇, Anaprox DS, Flanax Pain
Relief ◇, Maxidol✤ ◇, Mediproxen ◇,
Motrimax ◇

Therapeutic class: NSAIDs
Pharmacologic class: NSAIDs

AVAILABLE FORMS
naproxen
Oral suspension: 125 mg/5 mL
Tablets: 250 mg, 375 mg, 500 mg
Tablets (delayed-release) ⓝⓒ: 375 mg,
500 mg, 750 mg
naproxen sodium
Capsules: 105 mg✤ ◇, 200 mg ◇,
220 mg✤ ◇
Tablets (extended-release) ⓝⓒ: 375 mg,
500 mg, 750 mg
Tablets (film-coated) ⓝⓒ: 220 mg ◇, 275 mg,
550 mg
Note: 275 mg of naproxen sodium contains
250 mg of naproxen

INDICATIONS & DOSAGES
Adjust-a-dose (for all indications): Consider
lower dosage in elderly patients and patients
with renal or hepatic impairment. Not recommended for patients with moderate or
severe renal impairment (CrCl less than
30 mL/minute).
➤ **Acute gout**
Adults: 750 mg naproxen PO; then 250 mg
every 8 hours until attack subsides. Or,
825 mg naproxen sodium PO; then 275
mg every 8 hours until attack subsides. Or,
1,000 to 1,500 mg extended-release tablets
PO on day 1, followed by 1,000 mg daily
until attack subsides.
➤ **Acute tendinitis, bursitis, pain, primary dysmenorrhea**
Adults: 550 mg naproxen sodium PO, then
550 mg PO every 12 hours or 275 mg every
6 to 8 hours. Initial total daily dose shouldn't
exceed 1,375 mg; thereafter, total daily dose
shouldn't exceed 1,100 mg. Or, 500 mg
naproxen PO followed by 500 mg PO every

12 hours or 250 mg PO every 6 to 8 hours.
Or, 1,000 mg extended-release tablets PO
once daily for a limited time.
➤ **Ankylosing spondylitis, osteoarthritis,
RA**
Adults: 275 to 550 mg naproxen sodium
PO b.i.d. Or, 250 to 500 mg naproxen tablet
or suspension PO b.i.d. Or, 375 or 500 mg
naproxen delayed-release tablet PO b.i.d. Or,
750 to 1,000 mg extended-release tablets
PO once daily. During long-term administration, the dose of naproxen may be adjusted up or down depending on patient's
clinical response. In patients who tolerate
lower doses well, the dose may be increased
to 1,500 mg/day when a higher level of anti-
inflammatory/analgesic activity is required.
➤ **Juvenile arthritis**
Children age 2 and older: 10 mg/kg
naproxen suspension PO daily in two divided doses. Don't exceed 15 mg/kg/day.

ADMINISTRATION
PO
• Give drug with food or milk to minimize
GI upset. Have patient drink a full glass of
water or other liquid with each dose.
• Shake suspension well.
• Make sure patient swallows delayed-
release, extended-release, and film-coated
tablets whole and doesn't break, crush, or
chew them.

ACTION
May inhibit prostaglandin synthesis to produce anti-inflammatory, analgesic, and antipyretic effects.

Route	Onset	Peak	Duration
PO (immediate-release)	30–60 min	2–4 hr	<12 hr
PO (delayed-release)	30–60 min	4–24 hr	<12 hr
PO (suspension)	60 min	1–4 hr	<12 hr

Half-life: 8 to 21 hours.

ADVERSE REACTIONS
CNS: dizziness, drowsiness, headache, vertigo. **CV:** edema, palpitations. **EENT:** tinnitus, auditory disturbances, visual disturbances. **GI:** abdominal pain, constipation, diarrhea, dyspepsia, epigastric pain,
heartburn, nausea, occult blood loss, peptic

N

ulceration, stomatitis, thirst. **Hematologic:** ecchymoses, increased bleeding time. **Respiratory:** dyspnea. **Skin:** diaphoresis, pruritus, purpura.

INTERACTIONS

Drug-drug. *ACE inhibitors, tacrolimus:* May cause renal impairment. Use together cautiously.

Anticoagulants, antiplatelets, corticosteroids, other NSAIDs, salicylates, TCAs: May cause adverse GI reactions and bleeding. Avoid use together.

Antihypertensives, diuretics: May decrease effect of these drugs. Monitor patient closely.

Cyclosporine: May increase risk of nephrotoxicity. Monitor renal function; consider therapy modification.

Digoxin: May increase serum digoxin level. Monitor levels.

Lithium: May increase lithium level. Observe patient for toxicity and monitor level. Adjustment of lithium dosage may be required.

Loop diuretics, thiazide diuretics: May reduce diuretic effects. Monitor patient and consider therapy modification.

Methotrexate: May cause toxicity. Monitor patient closely.

Oral anticoagulants, NSAIDs, SSRIs, other sulfonylureas, highly protein-bound drugs: May cause toxicity. Monitor patient closely.

Pemetrexed: May result in pemetrexed toxicity (myelosuppression, renal toxicity, and GI toxicity). Consider therapy modification.

Potassium-sparing diuretics: May reduce antihypertensive effects and enhance hyperkalemic effects. Monitor patient closely.

Probenecid: May decrease elimination of naproxen. Monitor patient for toxicity.

Drug-herb. *Alfalfa, anise, bilberry, dong quai, feverfew, garlic, ginger, ginkgo, horse chestnut, licorice, red clover:* May cause bleeding, based on the known effects of components. Discourage use together.

White willow: Herb and drug contain similar components. Discourage use together.

Drug-lifestyle. *Alcohol use:* May cause GI irritation and bleeding. Avoid use together.

EFFECTS ON LAB TEST RESULTS

• May increase BUN, creatinine, ALT, AST, and potassium levels.
• May increase bleeding time.
• May interfere with urinary 5-hydroxy-indoleacetic acid and 17-hydroxycorticosteroid determinations.

CONTRAINDICATIONS & CAUTIONS

• Contraindicated in patients hypersensitive to drug and in those with the syndrome of aspirin-sensitive asthma, rhinitis, and nasal polyps.
• Drug can cause serious skin reactions (SJS, toxic epidermal necrolysis). Stop drug at first sign of rash or hypersensitivity.

Black Box Warning Naproxen is contraindicated for the treatment of perioperative pain after CABG surgery. ▌

• Use cautiously in elderly patients and in patients with HTN, hyperkalemia, renal disease, CV disease, GI disorders, hepatic disease, or history of peptic ulcer disease.
• Drug may increase risk of aseptic meningitis, especially in patients with lupus and mixed connective tissue disorders.

Dialyzable drug: No.

⚠ *Overdose S&S:* Drowsiness, heartburn, indigestion, nausea, vomiting, seizures.

PREGNANCY-LACTATION-REPRODUCTION

• Drug shouldn't be used in pregnant women, especially during last trimester, as closure of the ductus arteriosus can occur.
• Avoid use in breastfeeding women.

NURSING CONSIDERATIONS

• Because NSAIDs impair synthesis of renal prostaglandins, they can decrease renal blood flow and lead to reversible renal impairment, especially in patients with renal failure, HF, or liver dysfunction; in elderly patients; and in those taking diuretics. Monitor these patients closely.
• Monitor CBC and renal and hepatic function every 4 to 6 months during long-term therapy.
• Monitor patient for neurologic effects (drowsiness, dizziness, blurred vision), which may impair physical or mental abilities.

🕙 *Alert:* Watch for and immediately evaluate signs and symptoms of heart attack (chest

---

pain, shortness of breath or trouble breathing), or stroke (weakness in one part or side of the body, slurred speech).

Black Box Warning NSAIDs cause an increased risk of serious GI adverse events, including bleeding, ulceration, and perforation of the stomach or intestines, which can be fatal. Elderly patients are at greater risk. These events may occur at any time during therapy and without warning. ■

Black Box Warning NSAIDs may increase the risk of serious thrombotic events, MI, or stroke, which can be fatal. The risk may be greater with longer use or in patients with CV disease or risk factors for CV disease. ■

• Because of their antipyretic and anti-inflammatory actions, NSAIDs may mask signs and symptoms of infection.
• Drug may prolong bleeding time and anemias can occur.

PATIENT TEACHING

◑ *Alert:* Drug is available without prescription (naproxen sodium, 220 mg). Instruct adult not to take more than 440 mg of naproxen sodium in any 8- to 12-hour period or 660 mg of naproxen sodium in a 24-hour period.
• Advise patient to take drug with food or milk to minimize GI upset and to drink a full glass of water or other liquid with each dose.
• Tell patient taking prescription doses for arthritis that full therapeutic effect may be delayed 2 to 4 weeks.
• Warn patient against taking naproxen and naproxen sodium at the same time.
◑ *Alert:* Advise patient to seek medical attention immediately if chest pain, shortness of breath or trouble breathing, weakness in one part or side of the body, or slurred speech occurs.
• Teach patient signs and symptoms of GI bleeding (including blood in vomit, urine, or stool; coffee-ground vomit; and black, tarry stools) and to notify prescriber immediately if any of these occurs.
• Caution patient that use with aspirin, alcohol, other NSAIDs, or corticosteroids may increase risk of adverse GI reactions.
• Warn patient against hazardous activities that require mental alertness until CNS effects are known.

naratriptan hydrochloride
nar-ah-TRIP-tan

Amerge, Apo-Naratriptan✦,
Sandoz Naratriptan✦

Therapeutic class: Antimigraine drugs
Pharmacologic class: Serotonin 5-HT₁ receptor agonists

AVAILABLE FORMS
Tablets: 1 mg, 2.5 mg

INDICATIONS & DOSAGES
➤ **Acute migraine attacks with or without aura**
Adults: 1 or 2.5 mg PO as a single dose as soon as symptoms appear. If headache returns or responds only partially, may repeat dose after 4 hours. Maximum, 5 mg in 24 hours.
Adjust-a-dose: For patients with mild to moderate renal or hepatic impairment, reduce dosage. Maximum, 2.5 mg in 24 hours; a 1-mg starting dose is recommended.

ADMINISTRATION
PO
• Give drug with fluid without regard for food.

ACTION
May act as an agonist at serotonin receptors on extracerebral intracranial blood vessels, which constricts the affected vessels, inhibits neuropeptide release, and reduces pain transmission in the trigeminal pathways.

Route	Onset	Peak	Duration
PO	1–2 hr	2–3 hr	Unknown

Half-life: 6 hours.

ADVERSE REACTIONS
CNS: paresthesia, dizziness, drowsiness, malaise, fatigue, vertigo, pain. **CV:** *tachyarrhythmias,* abnormal ECG changes, palpitations, HTN. **EENT:** photophobia; ear, nose, and throat infections; throat pain. **GI:** nausea, hyposalivation, vomiting. **Musculoskeletal:** neck pain. **Other:** sensations of warmth, cold, pressure, tightness, or heaviness.

N

INTERACTIONS

Drug-drug. *Antiemetics (5-HT₃ antagonists), antipsychotics, bromocriptine, linezolid, MAO inhibitors, methylene blue, methylphenidate, opioids, SSNRIs, SSRIs, TCAs, tedizolid:* May increase risk of serotonin syndrome. Monitor therapy.

Drugs that prolong QT interval (antiarrhythmics, arsenic trioxide, chlorpromazine, dolasetron, droperidol, mefloquine, mesoridazine, moxifloxacin, pentamidine, pimozide, tacrolimus, thioridazine, ziprasidone): May cause an additive effect and prolong QT interval. Monitor patient closely.

Ergot-containing or ergot-type drugs (dihydroergotamine, methysergide), other 5-HT₁ agonists: May prolong vasospastic reactions. Avoid using within 24 hours of naratriptan.

Hormonal contraceptives: May slightly increase naratriptan level. Monitor patient.

Tramadol: May increase risk of serotonin syndrome and seizures. Monitor therapy. Monitor patient.

Drug-herb. *St. John's wort:* May increase serotonergic effect. Discourage use together.

Drug-lifestyle. *Smoking:* May increase naratriptan clearance. Discourage smoking.

EFFECTS ON LAB TEST RESULTS
None reported.

CONTRAINDICATIONS & CAUTIONS
• Contraindicated in patients hypersensitive to drug or its components and in those with prior or current cardiac ischemia, Wolff-Parkinson-White syndrome, vasospastic CAD, arrhythmias associated with accessory conduction pathways, cerebrovascular (stroke, TIA) or peripheral vascular syndromes, hemiplegic or basilar migraines, ischemic bowel disease, or uncontrolled HTN.

• Contraindicated in elderly patients, patients with severe renal impairment (CrCl less than 15 mL/minute), patients with severe hepatic impairment (Child-Pugh class C), and patients who have used ergot-containing, ergot-type, or other 5-HT₁ agonists within 24 hours.

◑ **Alert:** Coronary artery spasm, transient ischemia, MI, ventricular tachycardia, and ventricular fibrillation and death have been reported within a few hours of administration. Discontinue drug if these occur. If signs or symptoms of angina occur after dose, evaluate patient for CAD or Prinzmetal angina before additional doses are given and monitor ECG.

• Use cautiously in patients with risk factors for CAD, such as HTN, hypercholesterolemia, obesity, diabetes, smoking, strong family history of CAD, and postmenopausal women, and men older than age 40, unless patient is free from cardiac disease. Monitor patient closely after first dose.

• Use cautiously in patients with renal or hepatic impairment.

• Safety and effectiveness when treating cluster headaches or more than four headaches in a 30-day period haven't been established.

Dialyzable drug: Unknown.

⚠ **Overdose S&S:** Chest pain, ischemic ECG changes, increased BP resulting in lightheadedness, neck tension, tiredness, loss of coordination.

PREGNANCY-LACTATION-REPRODUCTION
• There are no adequate studies in pregnant women. Use only if potential benefit justifies potential risk to the fetus.

• It isn't known if drug appears in breast milk. Patient should discontinue breastfeeding or discontinue drug.

NURSING CONSIDERATIONS
• Assess cardiac status in patients who develop risk factors for CAD.

◑ **Alert:** Drug can cause coronary artery vasospasm and increased risk of cerebrovascular events.

• Drug isn't intended to prevent migraines or manage hemiplegic or basilar migraine.

• Drug can cause significant BP elevations, including in patients with no history of HTN. Monitor BP.

• Use drug only when patient has a clear diagnosis of migraine.

◑ **Alert:** Combining drug with other serotonin-modulating drugs may cause serotonin syndrome. Symptoms include restlessness, hallucinations, loss of coordination, fast heartbeat, rapid changes in BP, increased body temperature, hyperreflexia, nausea, vomiting, and diarrhea. Serotonin syndrome is more likely to occur when

---

Reactions in bold italics are *life-threatening*. Interactions may have a *rapid onset* or a *delayed onset*.

starting or increasing the dose of naratriptan, the SSRI, or the SSNRI.
• *Look alike–sound alike:* Don't confuse Amerge with Altace or Amaryl.

PATIENT TEACHING
• Instruct patient to take drug only as prescribed and to read the accompanying patient instruction leaflet before using drug.
• Tell patient to seek immediate medical care for chest pain, difficulty breathing, irregular heartbeat, weakness, swelling of the face, rash or hives, or slurring of speech.
• Tell patient not to take other prescription or OTC drugs or herbal preparations without first consulting prescriber.
• Inform patient that somnolence and dizziness can occur with naratriptan use. Instruct patient to evaluate ability to perform complex tasks while taking drug.
• Tell patient that drug is intended to relieve, not prevent, migraines.
• Instruct patient to take dose soon after headache starts. If no response occurs with first tablet, tell patient to seek medical approval before taking second tablet. Tell patient that if more relief is needed after first tablet (if a partial response occurs or headache returns), and prescriber has approved a second dose, patient may take a second tablet (but not sooner than 4 hours after first tablet). Tell patient not to exceed 2 tablets within 24 hours.
• Advise patient to increase fluid intake.
• Advise patient not to use drug if she suspects or knows that she's pregnant.
• Advise female patient to notify prescriber if she is breastfeeding or plans to breastfeed.
• Tell patient to alert prescriber about bothersome adverse effects.
• Encourage patient to keep a headache diary record of headache frequency and medication use.

natalizumab
nah-tah-LIZ-yoo-mab

Tysabri

Therapeutic class: Immunomodulators
Pharmacologic class: Monoclonal antibodies

AVAILABLE FORMS
Injection: 300 mg/15 mL single-use vials

INDICATIONS & DOSAGES
➤ **As monotherapy for the treatment of patients with relapsing forms of MS; to induce and maintain clinical response and remission in patients with moderately to severely active Crohn disease with evidence of inflammation who have had an inadequate response to, or are unable to tolerate, conventional therapies and inhibitors of TNF-α**
Adults: 300 mg IV over 1 hour every 4 weeks.

ADMINISTRATION
IV
▼ Dilute 300 mg in 100 mL NSS to final concentration of 2.6 mg/mL.
▼ Invert IV bag gently to mix solution; don't shake.
▼ Infuse over 1 hour; don't give by IV push or bolus.
▼ Flush IV line with NSS after infusion is complete.
▼ Refrigerate solution and use within 8 hours if not used immediately.
▼ Refrigerate single-dose vials between 36° and 46° F (2° and 8° C). Don't shake or freeze; protect from light.
▼ **Incompatibilities:** Don't mix or infuse with other drugs. Don't use any diluent other than NSS.

ACTION
May block interaction between adhesion molecules on inflammatory cells and receptors on endothelial cells of vessel walls.

Route	Onset	Peak	Duration
IV	Unknown	Unknown	Unknown

Half-life: 3 to 17 days.

N

ADVERSE REACTIONS

CNS: depression, dysesthesia, fatigue, headache, vertigo, syncope. **CV:** chest discomfort, peripheral edema. **EENT:** tonsillitis. **GI:** abdominal discomfort, diarrhea, gastroenteritis, nausea, dyspepsia, constipation. **GU:** UTI, vaginitis, amenorrhea, dysmenorrhea, irregular menstruation, urinary frequency, urinary urgency, ovarian cyst. **Hepatic:** cholelithiasis. **Metabolic:** weight increase or decrease. **Musculoskeletal:** arthralgia, extremity pain, muscle cramps, swollen joints, back pain. **Respiratory:** upper and lower respiratory tract infection. **Skin:** rash, dermatitis, pruritus, urticaria, night sweats, thermal injury, skin laceration. **Other:** hypersensitivity reaction, infusion-related reaction, tooth infections, herpes infection, rigors, seasonal allergy, flulike symptoms.

INTERACTIONS

Drug-drug. *Corticosteroids, immunosuppressants, TNF inhibitors:* May increase risk of infection. Avoid using together.
Live-virus vaccines: May cause reduced effectiveness of the vaccine. Defer vaccine administration until immune function has returned.
Drug-herb. *Echinacea:* May decrease effectiveness of natalizumab. Consider therapy modification.

EFFECTS ON LAB TEST RESULTS

• May increase LFT values and lymphocyte, monocyte, eosinophil, basophil, and nucleated RBC counts.
• May cause transient decrease in Hb level.

CONTRAINDICATIONS & CAUTIONS

• Contraindicated in patients hypersensitive to drug or its components or in those with current or history of PML. Use with other immunosuppressants or TNF-α inhibitors isn't recommended.
Black Box Warning Patients who test positively for anti-JC virus antibodies are at increased risk for developing PML. Consider testing for anti-JC virus antibodies before or during treatment if antibody status is unknown. Use drug cautiously in patients who are anti-JC virus antibody-positive and

especially in those with one or more additional PML risk factors. ∎
• Safety and effectiveness in patients with chronic progressive MS haven't been established.
Dialyzable drug: Unknown.

PREGNANCY-LACTATION-REPRODUCTION

• Use in pregnancy only if benefit justifies potential risk to the fetus.
• Drug appears in human milk. Effects on infants are unknown.

NURSING CONSIDERATIONS

Black Box Warning Only prescribers registered in the TOUCH Prescribing Program may prescribe drug. Contact the TOUCH Prescribing Program at 1-800-456-2255. ∎
• Report serious opportunistic and atypical infections to Biogen Idec at 1-800-456-2255 and to the FDA's MedWatch Program at 1-800-FDA-1088.
• Safety and effectiveness of natalizumab treatment beyond 2 years are unknown. When used for Crohn disease, discontinue drug after 12 weeks if patient hasn't experienced therapeutic benefit.
Black Box Warning Drug may cause PML. Withhold drug immediately at the first signs or symptoms suggestive of PML. Symptoms include clumsiness; progressive weakness; and visual, speech, and sometimes personality changes. Gadolinium-enhanced MRI and CSF analysis for JC viral DNA are recommended for diagnosis. ∎
Black Box Warning Risk of PML increases with duration of therapy, number of infusions, prior use of immunosuppressants, and presence of anti–JC virus antibodies. Consider these factors in the context of expected benefit when initiating and continuing treatment. ∎
• Obtain a brain MRI scan before starting therapy.
☉ Alert: Watch for evidence of hypersensitivity reaction during and for 1 hour after infusion, which may include dizziness, urticaria, fever, rash, rigors, pruritus, nausea, flushing, hypotension, dyspnea, and chest pain.
• If hypersensitivity reaction occurs, stop drug and notify prescriber.

Reactions in bold italics are *life-threatening*. Interactions may have a *rapid onset* or a *delayed onset*.

⊙ Alert: Drug increases risk of developing encephalitis, acute retinal necrosis, and meningitis caused by herpes simplex and varicella zoster viruses. Monitor patient for signs and symptoms of these conditions. Discontinue drug if any of these signs and symptoms occur and initiate appropriate treatment.

• Other serious infections, including opportunistic infections, have occurred. Concurrent use of antineoplastics, immunosuppressants, or immunomodulating agents may increase the risk. Discontinue therapy until successful resolution of the infection.

• For patients who start therapy while on long-term corticosteroids, begin steroid taper as soon as a therapeutic benefit has occurred. If corticosteroids can't be tapered within 6 months, discontinue drug.

• Patients who develop antibodies to drug have an increased risk of infusion-related reaction.

• Discontinue drug in patients with jaundice or other evidence of significant liver injury. Elevated serum hepatic enzymes and elevated total bilirubin levels may occur as early as 6 days after the first dose.

PATIENT TEACHING
• Inform patient that enrollment in and compliance with the TOUCH program is required.

• Tell patient to read the "Medication Guide for Tysabri" before each infusion.

• Urge patient to immediately report progressively worsening symptoms persisting over several days, including changes in eyesight, balance, strength, and thinking, memory, and orientation leading to confusion and personality changes.

• Advise patient to inform all health care providers about receiving this drug.

• Tell patient to schedule follow-up appointments with prescriber at 3 and 6 months after the first infusion, then at least every 6 months thereafter.

• Urge patient to immediately report rash, hives, dizziness, fever, shaking chills, or itching while drug is infusing or up to 1 hour afterward.

• Tell patient about the potential for liver injury.

nateglinide ⚶
na-te-GLYE-nide

Starlix

Therapeutic class: Antidiabetics
Pharmacologic class: Meglitinide derivatives

AVAILABLE FORMS
Tablets: 60 mg, 120 mg

INDICATIONS & DOSAGES
➤ **Type 2 diabetes as an adjunct to diet and exercise to improve glycemic control**
Adults: 120 mg PO t.i.d. taken 1 to 30 minutes before meals. Patients near goal HbA_{1c} level when treatment is started may receive 60 mg PO t.i.d.

ADMINISTRATION
PO
• Give drug 1 to 30 minutes before a meal.
• If a meal is skipped, dose should be skipped to reduce risk of hypoglycemia.

ACTION
Lowers glucose level by stimulating insulin secretion from pancreatic beta cells.

Route	Onset	Peak	Duration
PO	20 min	1 hr	4 hr

Half-life: About 1½ hours.

ADVERSE REACTIONS
CNS: dizziness. **GI:** diarrhea. **Metabolic:** *hypoglycemia,* hyperuricemia, weight gain. **Musculoskeletal:** back pain, arthropathy. **Respiratory:** URI. **Other:** flulike symptoms, accidental trauma.

INTERACTIONS
Drug-drug. *Androgens, antidiabetic agents, glucomannan, guanethidine, MAO inhibitors, nonselective beta blockers, NSAIDs, pegvisomant, quinolones, salicylates, SSRIs, thioacetic acid:* May increase hypoglycemic action of nateglinide. Monitor glucose level closely. Consider dosage reduction.

N

Beta blockers, clonidine, guanethidine: May mask signs and symptoms of hypoglycemia. Increase frequency of glucose monitoring.
Ceritinib, eltrombopag: May increase nateglinide serum concentration. Monitor glucose level closely.
Corticosteroids, rifamycins, somatostatin analogues, somatropin, sympathomimetics, thiazides, thyroid products: May decrease hypoglycemic action of nateglinide. Monitor glucose level closely. Consider dosage increase.
CYP2C9 inducers (phenytoin, rifampin): May decrease hypoglycemic action of nateglinide. Monitor glucose level closely. Consider dosage increase.
CYP2C9 inhibitors (amiodarone, fluconazole, sulfinpyrazone, voriconazole): May increase hypoglycemic action of nateglinide. Monitor glucose level closely. Consider dosage reduction.
Dabrafenib, enzalutamide: May decrease nateglinide serum concentration. Consider alternative therapy.
Mifepristone: May increase nateglinide serum concentration. Use lowest recommended dosage of nateglinide. Monitor patient closely for adverse effects during and for 2 weeks after mifepristone treatment.
Drug-herb. *Gymnema sylvestre:* May increase hypoglycemic action of nateglinide. Monitor glucose level closely.
St. John's wort: May decrease hypoglycemic action of nateglinide. Monitor glucose level closely.
Drug-lifestyle. *Alcohol use:* May increase hypoglycemic action of nateglinide. Monitor glucose level closely.

EFFECTS ON LAB TEST RESULTS
• May increase uric acid level.

CONTRAINDICATIONS & CAUTIONS
• Contraindicated in patients hypersensitive to drug and in those with type 1 diabetes or diabetic ketoacidosis.
• Use cautiously in patients with moderate to severe liver dysfunction or adrenal or pituitary insufficiency, and in elderly and malnourished patients.
⚖ Patients known to be poor metabolizers of CYP2C9 substrates may need dosage reductions and increased glucose monitoring.

• Safety and effectiveness in children haven't been established.
Dialyzable drug: Yes.
⚠ **Overdose S&S:** Hypoglycemic symptoms.

PREGNANCY-LACTATION-REPRODUCTION
• It isn't known if drug can cause fetal harm when administered to a pregnant woman. Use during pregnancy only if the potential benefit justifies the potential risk to the fetus.
• It isn't known if drug appears in human milk. Patient should discontinue breastfeeding or discontinue drug.

NURSING CONSIDERATIONS
• Don't use with glyburide or other oral antidiabetics; may use with metformin or a thiazolidinedione.
• Monitor glucose level regularly to evaluate drug's effectiveness.
• Observe patient for signs and symptoms of hypoglycemia. To minimize risk of hypoglycemia, make sure patient has a meal immediately after dose. If hypoglycemia occurs and patient remains conscious, give patient an oral form of glucose. If patient is unconscious, treat with IV glucose.
• Risk of hypoglycemia increases with strenuous exercise, alcohol ingestion, or insufficient caloric intake.
• Symptoms of hypoglycemia may be masked in patients with autonomic neuropathy and in those who use beta blockers, clonidine, or guanethidine.
• Insulin therapy may be needed for glycemic control in patients with fever, infection, or trauma and in those undergoing surgery.
• Monitor glucose level closely when other drugs are started or stopped, to detect possible drug interactions.
• Periodically monitor HbA$_{1c}$ level.
• Drug's effectiveness may decrease over time.
• Usually, no special dosage adjustments are necessary in elderly patients, but some elderly patients may have greater sensitivity to glucose-lowering effect.

PATIENT TEACHING
• Tell patient to take drug 1 to 30 minutes before a meal.

Reactions in bold italics are *life-threatening*. Interactions may have a *rapid onset* or a *delayed onset*.

- Advise patient who misses a meal to skip the scheduled dose to reduce risk of hypoglycemia.
- Instruct patient on risk of hypoglycemia, its signs and symptoms (sweating, rapid pulse, trembling, confusion, headache, irritability, and nausea), and ways to treat these symptoms by eating or drinking something containing sugar.
- Teach patient how to monitor and log glucose levels to evaluate diabetes control.
- Advise patient to notify prescriber for persistent low or high glucose level.
- Instruct patient to adhere to prescribed diet and exercise regimen.
- Explain possible long-term complications of diabetes and importance of regular preventive therapy.
- Encourage patient to wear a medical identification bracelet.
- Inform patient of potential drug-drug interactions with nateglinide.

---

nebivolol hydrochloride
neh-BIH-voh-lawl

Bystolic✐

Therapeutic class: Antihypertensives
Pharmacologic class: Beta blockers

AVAILABLE FORMS
Tablets: 2.5 mg, 5 mg, 10 mg, 20 mg

INDICATIONS & DOSAGES
➤ **HTN**
Adults: Initially, 5 mg PO once daily. Increase at 2-week intervals to a maximum dose of 40 mg, if needed.
Adjust-a-dose: For patients with severe renal impairment (CrCl less than 30 mL/minute) or moderate hepatic impairment, start with 2.5 mg PO once daily. Increase dose cautiously, if needed.

ADMINISTRATION
PO
- May give drug without regard to food.

ACTION
Selectively blocks beta$_1$-adrenergic receptors, reducing HR, myocardial contractility,

and sympathetic tone. Nebivolol also reduces BP by suppressing renin activity and decreasing peripheral vascular resistance.

Route	Onset	Peak	Duration
PO	Unknown	1½–4 hr	Unknown

Half-life: 12 to 19 hours.

ADVERSE REACTIONS
CNS: dizziness, fatigue, headache, insomnia. **CV:** *bradycardia,* chest pain, peripheral edema. **GI:** diarrhea, nausea. **Metabolic:** hyperuricemia. **Respiratory:** dyspnea. **Skin:** rash.

INTERACTIONS
Drug-drug. *Acetylcholinesterase inhibitors, dipyridamole, midodrine, regorafenib, ruxolitinib:* May enhance bradycardic effect. Monitor HR.
Alpha$_1$ blockers: May enhance severity and duration of hypotension. A smaller starting dose of alpha$_1$ blocker may be necessary.
Amifostine: May enhance hypotensive effect of amifostine. Withhold BP medication for 24 hours before amifostine administration.
Amiodarone, calcium channel blockers (nonhydropyridine), digoxin, disopyramide: May increase risk of bradycardia. Monitor ECG and vital signs.
Amphetamines, methylphenidate: May decrease antihypertensive effect of nebivolol. Monitor BP.
Antidiabetic agents (insulin, sulfonylureas): May mask signs of hypoglycemia. Monitor blood glucose level.
Antipsychotics (second-generation atypicals), diazoxide, duloxetine, levodopa, methoxyflurane, nitroprusside, PDE5 inhibitors, pentoxifylline, prostacyclin analogues, quinagolide: May enhance hypotensive effect. Monitor BP.
Barbiturates: May decrease serum concentration and enhance hypotensive effect of nebivolol. Monitor BP and HR.
Beta agonists (dobutamine, isoproterenol): May reverse nebivolol effects or cause protracted, severe hypotension. Avoid concomitant use.
Beta blockers (atenolol, nadolol): May increase synergistic activity and bradycardia. Don't use together.

N

♣Canada   ◇OTC   ◆Off-label use   ✐Photoguide   ⊜Do not crush   *Liquid contains alcohol   ▨Genetic

Bretylium, lacosamide: May enhance brady-cardic effect and AV blockade. Monitor HR.

Catecholamine-depleting drugs (guanethi-dine, reserpine): May cause bradycardia or severe hypotension. Monitor patient closely.

Ceritinib, rivastigmine: May increase brady-cardic effect. Avoid combination if possible.

Clonidine: May cause further decrease in BP. Simultaneous withdrawal may cause life-threatening rebound HTN. Discontinue nebivolol for several days before gradual tapering of clonidine.

CYP2D6 inhibitors (fluoxetine, paroxetine, propafenone, quinidine), dronedarone: May increase nebivolol level. Monitor BP closely, and adjust nebivolol dose as needed.

Ergot derivatives: May enhance vasocon-stricting effect. Consider therapy modifica-tion.

Fingolimod, ivabradine: May increase risk of bradycardia. Monitor patient closely.

Mefloquine: May cause CV toxicity. Con-sider an alternative drug.

NSAIDs: May decrease antihypertensive ef-fect. Monitor BP; adjust nebivolol dosage as needed.

Obinutuzumab: May enhance hypoten-sive effect. Consider withholding nebivolol for 12 hours before to 1 hour after obinu-tuzumab infusion.

Rifamycin derivatives (except rifabutin): May decrease nebivolol serum concentra-tion. Monitor BP.

SSRIs: May increase nebivolol serum con-centration. Monitor BP and HR.

EFFECTS ON LAB TEST RESULTS
• May increase BUN, uric acid, and triglyc-eride levels. May decrease HDL and choles-terol levels.
• May decrease platelet count.

CONTRAINDICATIONS & CAUTIONS
• Contraindicated in patients hypersensitive to drug and in those with decompensated HF, severe bradycardia, second- or third-degree AV block, sick sinus syndrome (unless a per-manent pacemaker is in place), cardiogenic shock, or severe hepatic impairment (greater than Child-Pugh class B).
• In general, patients with bronchial asthma or related bronchospastic diseases shouldn't receive beta blockers.

• Use cautiously in patients with compen-sated HF, in perioperative patients receiving anesthetics that depress myocardial function (such as cyclopropane and trichloroethy-lene), in diabetic patients receiving insulin or oral antidiabetics or who are subject to spontaneous hypoglycemia, in patients with moderate hepatic impairment or severe re-nal impairment, and in patients with thyroid disease (use may mask hyperthyroidism and withdrawal may worsen it), pheochromocy-toma, or PVD (may cause or worsen symp-toms of arterial insufficiency).
• Don't stop drug abruptly in patients with CAD, angina, or MI as severe exacerbations and ventricular arrhythmias can occur.
• Don't withdraw drug routinely before ma-jor surgery; continue drug throughout peri-operative period if possible.
• Safety and effectiveness in children haven't been established.
Dialyzable drug: Unknown.
⚠ *Overdose S&S:* Bradycardia, hypotension, cardiac failure, fatigue, dizziness, hypo-glycemia, vomiting, bronchospasm, heart block.

PREGNANCY-LACTATION-REPRODUCTION
• Use drug during pregnancy only if benefit justifies potential risk to the fetus.
• Don't use drug in breastfeeding women.

NURSING CONSIDERATIONS
🔵 *Alert:* Patients with a history of severe anaphylactic reaction to several allergens may be more reactive to repeated expo-sure to nebivolol (accidental, diagnostic, or therapeutic), and they may not respond to amounts of epinephrine typically used to treat allergic reactions.
• Check patient's BP and HR often.
• Monitor LFTs and renal function test results.
• If nebivolol must be stopped, do so gradu-ally over 1 to 2 weeks. If angina worsens or ACS occurs, restart drug promptly.
• Because beta blockers may mask tachy-cardia caused by hyperthyroidism, be sure to withdraw nebivolol gradually in patients with suspected thyrotoxicosis to avoid thy-roid storm.
• Observe a diabetic patient closely because drug may mask evidence of hypoglycemia.

Reactions in bold italics are *life-threatening*. Interactions may have a *rapid onset* or a *delayed onset*.

• If patient has a history of HF, watch for worsening symptoms, renal dysfunction, or fluid retention. Patient's diuretic dosage may need to be increased.

• In patients with known or suspected pheochromocytoma, initiate an alpha blocker before use of a beta blocker.

• Store drug at room temperature in a light-resistant container.

PATIENT TEACHING

• Instruct patient not to stop drug suddenly but to notify prescriber about unpleasant adverse reactions. Explain that drug must be withdrawn gradually over 1 or 2 weeks.

• Caution patient to avoid driving and other tasks requiring alertness until response to therapy is known.

• Tell patient to alert prescriber if shortness of breath occurs.

• Caution patient with diabetes or spontaneous hypoglycemia that drug may mask symptoms of low blood glucose level, especially increased HR.

• Urge female patient not to breastfeed.

SAFETY ALERT!

necitumumab
ne-si-TOOM-oo-mab

Portrazza

Therapeutic class: Antineoplastics
Pharmacologic class: Epidermal growth factor receptor antagonists

AVAILABLE FORMS

Injection: 800 mg/50 mL in single-dose vials

INDICATIONS & DOSAGES

➤ **First-line treatment of metastatic squamous cell NSCLC in combination with gemcitabine and cisplatin**

Adults: 800 mg IV infusion on days 1 and 8 of each 3-week cycle given before gemcitabine and cisplatin infusions. Continue until disease progression or unacceptable toxicity occurs.

Adjust-a-dose: **Black Box Warning** For grade 3 or 4 electrolyte abnormalities (such as hypomagnesemia, hypocalcemia, or

hypokalemia), withhold drug and replace electrolytes as medically indicated. Resume subsequent cycles after electrolyte abnormalities improve to grade 2 or less. ∎

Refer to manufacturer's instructions for other toxicity-related dosage adjustments and premedication instructions.

ADMINISTRATION

IV

▼ Inspect solution for particulate matter and discoloration. If present, discard solution.

▼ Dilute to a final volume of 250 mL in NSS. Don't use solutions containing dextrose.

▼ Gently invert to ensure mixing; don't shake.

▼ Store diluted infusions up to 24 hours at 36° to 46° F (2° to 8° C) or up to 4 hours at room temperature (up to 77° F [25° C]).

▼ Discard vial with any unused portion.

▼ Administer via infusion pump over 60 minutes through a separate infusion line. Flush line with NSS at end of infusion.

▼ Give drug before gemcitabine and cisplatin.

▼ Refrigerate vials at 36° to 46° F (2° to 8° C); don't freeze. Protect from light.

▼ **Incompatibilities:** Dextrose, electrolytes, other drugs.

ACTION

A recombinant human IgG1 monoclonal antibody that binds to human epidermal growth factor receptor (EGFR) and blocks binding of EGFR to ligands, inhibiting angiogenesis and malignant progression, and allowing apoptosis.

Route	Onset	Peak	Duration
IV	Unknown	Unknown	Unknown

Half-life: 14 days.

ADVERSE REACTIONS

CNS: headache, *stroke, cerebral ischemia.* **CV:** *cardiopulmonary arrest, sudden death, MI, arterial thromboembolism, PE, venous thromboembolism.* **EENT:** conjunctivitis, oropharyngeal pain. **GI:** vomiting, diarrhea, stomatitis, dysphagia. **Metabolic:** weight loss, *hypomagnesemia, hypokalemia,*

N

hypocalcemia, hypophosphatemia. **Musculoskeletal:** muscle spasms. **Respiratory:** hemoptysis. **Skin:** rash, dermatitis, acneiform rash, acne, pruritus, dry skin, skin fissures, erythema, skin toxicity. **Other:** paronychia, infusion reaction.

INTERACTIONS
Drug-lifestyle. *Sun exposure:* May increase photosensitivity. Patient should avoid sun exposure.

EFFECTS ON LAB TEST RESULTS
• May decrease magnesium, potassium, calcium, and phosphorus levels.

CONTRAINDICATIONS & CAUTIONS
Black Box Warning Drug may increase risk of cardiopulmonary arrest and sudden death when used in combination with gemcitabine and cisplatin. Closely monitor electrolyte levels, including magnesium, potassium, and calcium. ■

Black Box Warning May increase risk of hypomagnesemia. Monitor electrolyte levels and replace electrolytes as needed. ■

• Drug isn't indicated for nonsquamous NSCLC.

• Drug increases risk of venous thromboembolism (VTE) and arterial thromboembolism (ATE), which can be fatal. Discontinue drug for serious or life-threatening VTE or ATE.

• Safety and effectiveness in children haven't been established.

• Use cautiously in elderly patients, because they may have increased risk of adverse reactions.

Dialyzable drug: Unknown.

PREGNANCY-LACTATION-REPRODUCTION
• Contraindicated for use in pregnancy; drug may cause fetal harm. Advise women to use effective contraception during therapy and for 3 months after therapy ends.

• There are no data about breastfeeding. Women shouldn't breastfeed during treatment and for 3 months after last dose.

NURSING CONSIDERATIONS
Black Box Warning Closely monitor electrolyte levels, including magnesium,

potassium, and calcium, before each dose and for at least 8 weeks after last dose. ■

Black Box Warning Aggressively replace electrolytes as indicated. ■

• Monitor patients for infusion reaction.

• Monitor patients for skin reactions, which may be severe and usually develop within first 2 weeks of treatment; drug may need to be withheld or discontinued, or dosage reduced.

• Monitor patients for signs and symptoms of ATE (pain, pallor, pulselessness, loss of function, coldness) and VTE (pain, swelling, erythema, dyspnea, hypotension, tachycardia).

PATIENT TEACHING
• Teach patient about adverse reactions and to immediately report them.

• Explain that drug may reduce blood levels of magnesium, calcium, and potassium and that these levels must be carefully monitored. Advise patient to take any supplements prescribed.

• Advise patient that lab monitoring will be needed to monitor for adverse reactions to treatment.

• Teach patient signs and symptoms of infusion reactions (fever, chills, difficulty breathing) and to report them immediately.

• Warn female patient of childbearing potential to use contraception during therapy and for 3 months after final dose.

• Instruct female patient not to breastfeed during therapy and for 3 months after final dose.

• Caution patient to minimize sun exposure, wear protective clothing, and use sunscreen.

nelfinavir mesylate
nell-FIN-ah-veer

Viracept

Therapeutic class: Antiretrovirals
Pharmacologic class: Protease inhibitors

AVAILABLE FORMS
Tablets: 250 mg, 625 mg

Reactions in bold italics are *life-threatening*. Interactions may have a *rapid onset* or a *delayed onset*.

INDICATIONS & DOSAGES
➤ **HIV infection, in combination with other antiretrovirals**
Adults and children age 13 and older:
1,250 mg PO b.i.d. or 750 mg PO t.i.d. Maximum dosage is 2,500 mg/day.
Children ages 2 to 12: 45 to 55 mg/kg PO b.i.d. or 25 to 35 mg/kg PO t.i.d.; don't exceed 2,500 mg/day (b.i.d. dosing) or 2,250 mg/day (t.i.d. dosing).

ADMINISTRATION
PO
- Give tablets with a meal.
- May dissolve tablets in a small amount of water. Give the cloudy liquid immediately, rinse the glass, and give the rinse to patient to ensure entire dose is consumed.

ACTION
An HIV-1 protease inhibitor, which prevents cleavage of the viral polyprotein, resulting in the production of immature, noninfectious virus.

Route	Onset	Peak	Duration
PO	Unknown	2–4 hr	Unknown

Half-life: 3½ to 5 hours.

ADVERSE REACTIONS
CNS: *seizures, suicidal ideation,* anxiety, asthenia, depression, dizziness, emotional lability, headache, hyperkinesia, insomnia, malaise, migraine, paresthesia, sleep disorder, somnolence, fever. **CV:** *QTc prolongation, torsades de pointes.* **EENT:** acute iritis, eye disease, pharyngitis, rhinitis, sinusitis. **GI:** diarrhea, *pancreatitis,* flatulence, nausea, abdominal pain, anorexia, dyspepsia, epigastric pain, GI bleeding, mouth ulceration, pancreatitis, vomiting. **GU:** sexual dysfunction, urine abnormality. **Hematologic:** *leukopenia, thrombocytopenia, anemia.* **Hepatic:** *hepatitis,* abnormal LFT values. **Metabolic:** *hypoglycemia,* hyperglycemia, dehydration, *diabetes mellitus,* hyperlipidemia, hyperuricemia. **Musculoskeletal:** arthralgia, arthritis, back pain, cramps, myasthenia, myopathy. **Respiratory:** dyspnea. **Skin:** rash, dermatitis, folliculitis, fungal dermatitis, pruritus, sweating, urticaria. **Other:** redistribution or accumulation of body fat, allergic reaction, accidental injury.

INTERACTIONS
⊕ Alert: Consult full prescribing information for potential drug interactions before and during treatment.
Drug-drug. *Alfuzosin, amiodarone, ergot derivatives, oral midazolam, pimozide, quinidine, triazolam:* May increase levels of these drugs, causing increased risk of life-threatening adverse events. Use together is contraindicated.
⊕ Alert: *Atorvastatin:* May increase statin level and risk of myopathy and rhabdomyolysis. Atorvastatin dosage shouldn't exceed 40 mg/day.
Azithromycin: May increase azithromycin level. Monitor patient for liver impairment.
Carbamazepine, phenobarbital: May reduce the effectiveness of nelfinavir. Use together cautiously.
Colchicine: May cause increased colchicine plasma concentration and increased risk of toxicity. Avoid combination.
Cyclosporine, sirolimus, tacrolimus: May increase levels of these immunosuppressants. Use together cautiously.
Delavirdine, HIV protease inhibitors (indinavir, saquinavir): May increase levels of protease inhibitors. Use together cautiously.
Didanosine: May decrease didanosine absorption. Take nelfinavir with food at least 2 hours before or 1 hour after didanosine.
Drugs that prolong QT interval: May increase risk of life-threatening cardiac arrhythmias such as torsades de pointes. Monitor patient and ECG closely.
Ethinyl estradiol: May decrease contraceptive level and effectiveness. Advise patient to use alternative contraceptive measures during therapy.
⊕ Alert: *Lovastatin, simvastatin:* May increase statin level and risk of myopathy and rhabdomyolysis. Use together is contraindicated.
Methadone, phenytoin: May decrease levels of these drugs. Adjust dosage of these drugs accordingly.
Rifabutin: May increase rifabutin level and decrease nelfinavir level. Reduce dosage of rifabutin to half the usual dose and increase nelfinavir to 1,250 mg b.i.d.

N

Rifampin: May decrease nelfinavir level. Use together is contraindicated.

Sildenafil: May increase adverse effects of sildenafil. Caution patient not to exceed 25 mg of sildenafil in a 48-hour period. Contraindicated when used for treatment of PAH.

Drug-herb. *St. John's wort:* May decrease drug level. Use together is contraindicated.

EFFECTS ON LAB TEST RESULTS

• May increase ALT, AST, alkaline phosphatase, bilirubin, GGT, amylase, CK, uric acid, and lipid levels.
• May increase or decrease glucose level.
• May decrease Hb level, WBC count, and platelet count.

CONTRAINDICATIONS & CAUTIONS

• Contraindicated in patients hypersensitive to drug or its components and in those with moderate or severe hepatic impairment.
• Contraindicated with drugs that are highly dependent on CYP3A for clearance (alfuzosin, amiodarone, ergot derivatives, rifampin, lovastatin, simvastatin, pimozide, quinidine, sildenafil used for pulmonary HTN, oral midazolam, triazolam).
• Use cautiously in patients with mild hepatic dysfunction or hemophilia types A or B. Monitor LFT results.
• Hyperglycemia requiring treatment with insulin or oral antidiabetics has been reported in postmarketing reports. A causal relationship hasn't been established.
• Immune reconstitution syndrome has been reported in patients treated with combination antiretroviral therapy. During the initial phase of treatment, patients whose immune system responds may develop inflammatory response to indolent or residual opportunistic infections, which may require further evaluation and treatment. Autoimmune disorders have also been reported in the setting of immune reconstitution; however, the time to onset is more variable, and can occur many months after initiation of treatment.
Dialyzable drug: Unlikely.

PREGNANCY-LACTATION-REPRODUCTION

• Use in pregnant women only if potential benefit justifies potential risk to the fetus.

• Enroll pregnant women taking nelfinavir in the Antiretroviral Pregnancy Registry (1-800-258-4263).
• Minimal amounts of drug appear in human milk. Women shouldn't breastfeed during therapy because of risk of transmitting HIV to infant.

NURSING CONSIDERATIONS

• Drug may increase bleeding risk in patients with hemophilia. Monitor closely.
• Drug may cause hyperglycemia. Monitor glucose levels carefully.
• *Look alike–sound alike:* Don't confuse nelfinavir with nevirapine. Don't confuse Viracept with Viramune or Viramune XR.

PATIENT TEACHING

• Advise patient to take drug with food.
• Inform patient that drug doesn't cure HIV infection.
• Tell patient that long-term effects of drug are unknown and that there are no data stating that nelfinavir reduces risk of HIV transmission.
• Advise patient to take drug daily as prescribed and not to alter dose or stop drug without medical approval.
• Tell patient who misses a dose to take it as soon as possible and then return to the normal schedule. Advise patient not to double the dose.
• Tell patient that diarrhea is the most common adverse effect and that it can be controlled with loperamide, if needed.
• Instruct patient taking hormonal contraceptives to use alternative or additional contraceptive measures while taking nelfinavir.
• ❸ *Alert:* Advise patient taking sildenafil for erectile dysfunction about an increased risk of sildenafil-related adverse events, including low BP, visual changes, and painful erections. Tell patient to promptly report any symptoms and not to exceed 25 mg of sildenafil in a 48-hour period.
• Advise patient to report use of other prescribed or OTC drugs or herbal products because of possible drug interactions.

neomycin sulfate
nee-o-MYE-sin

Therapeutic class: Antibiotics
Pharmacologic class: Aminoglycosides

AVAILABLE FORMS
Tablets: 500 mg

INDICATIONS & DOSAGES
➤ **To suppress intestinal bacteria before surgery**
Adults: After saline cathartic, 1 g neomycin with 1 g erythromycin base PO at 1 p.m., 2 p.m., and 11 p.m. on day before 8 a.m. surgery.
➤ **Adjunctive treatment for hepatic coma**
Adults: 4 to 12 g PO daily in divided doses for 5 to 6 days.
➤ **Chronic hepatic insufficiency**
Adults: 4 g PO daily for an indefinite period. Treatment for longer than 2 weeks isn't recommended.

ADMINISTRATION
PO
• For preoperative disinfection, provide a low-residue diet and a cathartic immediately before therapy.

ACTION
Inhibits protein synthesis by binding directly to the 30S ribosomal subunit; bactericidal.

Route	Onset	Peak	Duration
PO	Unknown	1–4 hr	48–72 hr

Half-life: 2 to 3 hours.

ADVERSE REACTIONS
CNS: *neuromuscular blockade.* **EENT:** ototoxicity. **GI:** nausea, vomiting, diarrhea, malabsorption syndrome, CDAD. **GU:** *nephrotoxicity,* possible increase in urinary excretion of casts.

INTERACTIONS
Drug-drug. **Black Box Warning** *Acyclovir, amphotericin B, cephalosporins, cidofovir, cisplatin, methoxyflurane, vancomycin, other aminoglycosides:* May increase nephrotoxicity. Monitor renal function test results. ∎

Black Box Warning *Anesthetics, neuromuscular blockers (decamethonium, succinylcholine, tubocurarine):* May increase effects of nondepolarizing muscle relaxants, including prolonged respiratory depression and respiratory paralysis. Use together only when necessary, and expect to reduce dosage of nondepolarizing muscle relaxants. Mechanical ventilation may be needed. ∎
Digoxin: May decrease digoxin absorption. Monitor digoxin level.
Black Box Warning *IV loop diuretics (furosemide):* May increase ototoxicity. Monitor patient's hearing. ∎
Oral anticoagulants: May inhibit vitamin K–producing bacteria; may increase anticoagulant effect. Monitor PT and INR.

EFFECTS ON LAB TEST RESULTS
• May increase BUN, creatinine, and nonprotein nitrogen levels.

CONTRAINDICATIONS & CAUTIONS
• Contraindicated in patients hypersensitive to neomycin or other aminoglycosides and in those with intestinal obstruction or inflammatory or ulcerative GI disease.
• Use cautiously in elderly patients and in those with impaired renal function or neuromuscular disorders.
• Prolonged use can cause superinfection including CDAD, which can occur 2 months after therapy ends.
• Safety and effectiveness of oral neomycin sulfate in patients younger than age 18 haven't been established.
Dialyzable drug: Yes.
⚠ *Overdose S&S:* Neurotoxicity, ototoxicity, nephrotoxicity.

PREGNANCY-LACTATION-REPRODUCTION
• Drug may cause fetal harm. Use during pregnancy only if clearly needed.
• Patient should discontinue breastfeeding or discontinue drug.

NURSING CONSIDERATIONS
Black Box Warning Due to increased risk of nephrotoxicity, monitor renal function: urine output, specific gravity, urinalysis, BUN and creatinine levels, and creatinine clearance. Report evidence of declining renal function to prescriber. ∎

Black Box Warning Due to increased risk of neurotoxicity and ototoxicity, evaluate patient's hearing before and during prolonged therapy. Notify prescriber if patient has tinnitus, vertigo, or hearing loss. Deafness may start several weeks after drug is stopped. ∎

Black Box Warning Don't use with other aminoglycosides or neurotoxic or nephrotoxic drugs; risk of toxicities increase. ∎

• Watch for signs and symptoms of superinfection (chills, fever, diarrhea), including CDAD, which can occur more than 2 months after therapy ends.

Black Box Warning Neuromuscular blockade and respiratory paralysis have been reported after administration of aminoglycosides. Monitor patient closely. ∎

• For adjunctive treatment for hepatic coma, decrease patient's dietary protein and assess neurologic status frequently during therapy.

• The ototoxic and nephrotoxic properties of drug limit its usefulness.

PATIENT TEACHING
• Instruct patient to report all adverse reactions promptly, especially fever, chills, diarrhea, changes in hearing, changes in urine amount, or dark urine.

• Encourage patient to maintain adequate fluid intake.

SAFETY ALERT!

neratinib ☒
ner-A-ti-nib

Nerlynx

Therapeutic class: Antineoplastics
Pharmacologic class: Tyrosine kinase inhibitors

AVAILABLE FORMS
Tablets ⓞⓝⓒ: 40 mg

INDICATIONS & DOSAGES
➤ **Extended adjuvant treatment of early-stage HER2-overexpressed/amplified breast cancer, after adjuvant trastuzumab-based therapy** ☒
Adults: 240 mg (6 tablets) PO once daily with food for 1 year. Prophylaxis with an antidiarrheal is recommended, starting with

first dose of neratinib and continuing for at least the first 56 days of treatment.
Adjust-a-dose: For severe hepatic impairment (Child-Pugh class C), reduce dosage to 80 mg once daily. Refer to manufacturer's instructions for toxicity-related adjustments.

ADMINISTRATION
PO
• Give with food at the same time each day.
• Patient must swallow tablets whole and not crush, chew, or split them.
• If a dose is missed, skip the missed dose and resume normal schedule.
• Store at room temperature (68° to 77° F [20° to 25° C]).

ACTION
A kinase inhibitor that irreversibly binds to epidermal growth factor receptor, HER2, and HER4, inhibiting their activity and causing antitumor activity.

Route	Onset	Peak	Duration
PO	Unknown	2–8 hr	Unknown

Half-life: 7 to 17 hours.

ADVERSE REACTIONS
CNS: fatigue. **CV:** *dehydration.* **EENT:** epistaxis. **GI:** diarrhea, nausea, abdominal pain, vomiting, stomatitis, decreased appetite, tongue burning, mucosal inflammation, dyspepsia, abdominal distention, dry mouth. **GU:** UTI. **Metabolic:** weight loss. **Musculoskeletal:** muscle spasms. **Skin:** rash, dermatitis, dry skin, nail disorders, skin fissures.

INTERACTIONS
Drug-drug. *Antacids:* May decrease neratinib level. Give neratinib 3 hours after antacids.
H₂-receptor antagonists: May decrease neratinib level. Give neratinib at least 2 hours before or 10 hours after H$_2$-receptor antagonists.
Moderate and strong CYP3A4 inducers (bosentan, carbamazepine, efavirenz, phenytoin, rifampin): May decrease neratinib level. Avoid use together.
Moderate and strong CYP3A4 inhibitors (aprepitant, clarithromycin, ciprofloxacin,

---

diltiazem, ketoconazole, ritonavir): May increase neratinib level. Avoid use together.

P-gp substrates (dabigatran, digoxin, fexofenadine): May increase P-gp substrate level and increase risk of substrate-related adverse reactions. Adjust P-gp substrate dosage, if clinically indicated.

PPIs: May decrease neratinib level. Avoid use together.

Drug-herb. *St. John's wort:* May decrease neratinib level. Discourage use together.

Drug-food. *Grapefruit juice:* May increase neratinib level. Discourage use together.

EFFECTS ON LAB TEST RESULTS
• May increase AST and ALT levels.

CONTRAINDICATIONS & CAUTIONS
• Use cautiously in patients with severe hepatic impairment (Child-Pugh class C).
• Safety and effectiveness in children haven't been established.
• Use cautiously in elderly patients because of increased severity of adverse reactions.
Dialyzable drug: Unknown.
⚠ *Overdose S&S:* Diarrhea, nausea, vomiting, dehydration.

PREGNANCY-LACTATION-REPRODUCTION
• Drug may cause fetal harm. Women of childbearing potential should have a pregnancy test before treatment.
• Women of childbearing potential should use effective contraception during treatment and for at least 1 month after last dose.
• Male patients with female partners of childbearing potential should use effective contraception during treatment and for 3 months after last dose.
• Serious adverse reactions may occur in a breastfed infant. Women shouldn't breastfeed during treatment and for at least 1 month after final dose.

NURSING CONSIDERATIONS
• Measure total bilirubin, AST, ALT, and alkaline phosphatase levels at baseline, monthly for the first 3 months, then every 3 months during treatment and as clinically indicated.
• Monitor patients for sign and symptoms of hepatotoxicity (worsening fatigue, nausea, vomiting, right upper quadrant tenderness,

fever, rash, eosinophilia). Therapy may need to be interrupted, dosage reduced, or drug permanently discontinued.
• Prophylaxis with an antidiarrheal is recommended during the first two cycles starting with first dose of neratinib and titrating to one to two bowel movements per day. See manufacturer's instructions for suggested loperamide prophylaxis dosages. Additional antidiarrheals, dosing interruptions, and dosage reductions may be necessary to manage diarrhea.
• Monitor patients for diarrhea, vomiting, and dehydration, especially elderly patients. For severe diarrhea, administer fluid and electrolytes as needed, interrupt treatment, and reduce subsequent doses. Perform stool cultures as clinically indicated to exclude infectious causes of grade 3 or 4 diarrhea or diarrhea of any grade with complicating features (dehydration, fever, neutropenia).
• *Look alike–sound alike:* Don't confuse neratinib with nesiritide.

PATIENT TEACHING
• Caution female patient of childbearing potential that drug can cause fetal harm and that a pregnancy test will be performed before therapy begins.
• Advise female patient of childbearing potential to use effective contraception during treatment and for at least 1 month after last dose. Male patient with female partner of childbearing potential should use effective contraception during treatment and for at least 3 months after final dose.
• Advise female patient not to breastfeed during therapy and for at least 1 month after last dose.
• Tell patient that lab testing will be needed during therapy.
• Stress importance of antidiarrheal prophylaxis with loperamide. Remind patient to immediately report severe episodes of diarrhea.
• Caution patient to report all adverse reactions, especially signs and symptoms of liver toxicity, such as worsening fatigue, nausea, vomiting, right upper quadrant tenderness, fever, or rash.

N

nesiritide
neh-SIR-ih-tide

Natrecor

Therapeutic class: Vasodilators
Pharmacologic class: Human B-type natri-uretic peptides

AVAILABLE FORMS
Injection: Single-dose vials of 1.5 mg ster-ile, lyophilized powder

INDICATIONS & DOSAGES
➤ **Acutely decompensated HF in patients with dyspnea at rest or with minimal activity**
Adults: 2 mcg/kg by IV bolus over 60 sec-onds, followed by continuous infusion of 0.01 mcg/kg/minute. Don't titrate up more frequently than every 3 hours. Maximum dosage is 0.03 mcg/kg/minute. Loading dose may not be appropriate for patients with sys-tolic BP less than 110 mm Hg or those re-cently treated with afterload reducers.
Adjust-a-dose: If hypotension develops dur-ing administration, reduce dosage or stop drug. Restart drug at dosage reduced by 30% with no bolus doses.

ADMINISTRATION
IV
▼ Reconstitute one 1.5-mg vial with 5 mL of diluent (such as D_5W, NSS, 5% dextrose and 0.2% saline solution injection, or 5% dextrose and half-NSS) from a prefilled 250-mL IV bag.
▼ Gently rock (don't shake) vial until solu-tion becomes clear and colorless.
▼ Withdraw contents of vial and add back to the 250-mL IV bag to yield 6 mcg/mL. Invert the bag several times to ensure com-plete mixing, and use the solution within 24 hours.
▼ Use the formulas below to calculate bo-lus volume (2 mcg/kg) and infusion flow rate (0.01 mcg/kg/minute):

Bolus volume = patient weight ÷ 3
    (mL)   (kg)

Infusion flow rate = 0.1 × patient weight
    (mL/hr)   (kg)

▼ Before giving bolus dose, prime the IV tubing with 5 mL of solution. Withdraw the bolus and give over 60 seconds through an IV port in the tubing.
⑤ *Alert:* Drug binds to heparin, including the heparin lining of a coated catheter, de-creasing the amount of nesiritide deliv-ered. Don't give nesiritide through a central heparin-coated catheter.
▼ Immediately after giving bolus, in-fuse drug at 0.1 mL/kg/hour to deliver 0.01 mcg/kg/minute.
▼ Use central hemodynamic monitoring.
▼ Store drug at 68° to 77° F (20° to 25° C). Protect from light. May store re-constituted vials at 36° to 77° F (2° to 25° C) for up to 24 hours.
▼ **Incompatibilities:** Bumetanide, enalaprilat, ethacrynate sodium, furosemide, heparin, hydralazine, insulin, sodium metabisulfite.

ACTION
Increases cyclic guanosine monophosphate level, relaxes smooth muscle, and dilates veins and arteries. Drug reduces pulmonary capillary wedge pressure and systemic arte-rial pressure in patients with HF.

Route	Onset	Peak	Duration
IV	15 min	1 hr	3 hr

Half-life: 18 minutes.

ADVERSE REACTIONS
CNS: dizziness, headache, light-headedness. **CV:** hypotension. **GI:** nausea. **GU:** renal insufficiency. **Hematologic:** anemia. **Metabolic:** *hypoglycemia.* **Musculoskele-tal:** back pain. **Skin:** injection-site reactions, rash, pruritus.

INTERACTIONS
Drug-drug. *ACE inhibitors, ARBs:* May in-crease hypotension symptoms. Monitor BP closely.

EFFECTS ON LAB TEST RESULTS
• May increase creatinine level more than 0.5 mg/dL above baseline.
• May decrease glucose level, Hb level, and hematocrit.

Reactions in bold italics are *life-threatening*. Interactions may have a *rapid onset* or a *delayed onset*.

CONTRAINDICATIONS & CAUTIONS

• Contraindicated in patients hypersensitive to drug or its components.
• Contraindicated in patients with cardiogenic shock or systolic BP below 100 mm Hg.
• Use cautiously in patients with low cardiac filling pressures, conditions in which cardiac output depends on venous return, or conditions that make vasodilators inappropriate (valvular stenosis, restrictive or obstructive cardiomyopathy, constrictive pericarditis, pericardial tamponade).
• Use cautiously with prolonged infusions.
• Safety and effectiveness in children haven't been established.
Dialyzable drug: Unknown.
⚠ Overdose S&S: Excessive hypotension.

PREGNANCY-LACTATION-REPRODUCTION

• Use during pregnancy only if potential benefit justifies possible risk to the fetus.
• It isn't known if drug appears in human milk. Use cautiously if breastfeeding.

NURSING CONSIDERATIONS

• Don't start drug at higher-than-recommended dosage; this may cause hypotension and increase creatinine level.
❸ Alert: This drug may cause hypotension. Monitor patient's BP closely, particularly if patient is also taking an ACE inhibitor or ARB.
• Drug may affect renal function. In patients with severe HF whose renal function depends on the RAAS, use may lead to azotemia; monitor serum creatinine level.
• There is limited experience with giving this drug for longer than 96 hours.

PATIENT TEACHING

• Tell patient to report IV site discomfort.
• Urge patient to report to prescriber symptoms of hypotension, such as dizziness, light-headedness, blurred vision, or sweating.
• Tell patient to report other adverse effects to prescriber promptly.

---

nevirapine
neh-VEER-ah-pine

Viramune, Viramune XR

Therapeutic class: Antiretrovirals
Pharmacologic class: NRTIs

AVAILABLE FORMS

Oral suspension: 50 mg/5 mL
Tablets: 200 mg
Tablets (extended-release) ⊙: 100 mg, 400 mg

INDICATIONS & DOSAGES

➤ **Treatment of HIV-1, in combination with other antiretrovirals**
Black Box Warning Adhere strictly to 14-day lead-in period with nevirapine 200-mg daily dosing. ▪
Adults: 200 mg (immediate-release) PO daily for the first 14 days; then 200 mg PO b.i.d. Or, 400 mg (extended-release) PO once daily after 14-day lead-in period with 200-mg daily dosing.
Children and adolescents, infants 15 days and older (immediate-release): 150 mg/m^2/dose (maximum dose, 200 mg/dose) PO once daily for first 14 days; then increase to 150 mg/m^2/dose (maximum, 200 mg/dose) PO b.i.d.
Children age 6 and older with BSA of 1.17 m^2 or greater (extended-release): Initially, 150 mg/m^2 (immediate-release) PO once daily for 14 days. If patient has already completed the lead-in period and is on a b.i.d. regimen of immediate-release formulation, another lead-in period isn't required. Then increase to 400 mg (extended-release) PO once daily. Maximum dose, 400 mg/day.
Adjust-a-dose: Don't increase immediate-release lead-in dose if patient experiences mild to moderate rash without constitutional symptoms during 14-day lead-in period of 200 mg/day (150 mg/m^2/day in children) until rash has resolved. For patients on dialysis, give an additional 200-mg (immediate-release) dose after each dialysis treatment. Patients with a CrCl equal to or greater than 20 mL/minute don't require dosage adjustment. Extended-release formula hasn't been studied in patients with renal impairment.

N

ADMINISTRATION
PO
• Use drug with at least one other antiretroviral.
• Administer with or without food, antacid, or didanosine.
• Extended-release tablets must be swallowed whole and shouldn't be crushed, chewed, or divided.
• Shake suspension gently before administering. An oral dosing syringe is recommended. If using a dosing cup, rinse the cup and administer the rinse also.

ACTION
Binds directly to reverse transcriptase and blocks RNA-dependent and DNA-dependent DNA polymerase activities by disrupting the enzyme's catalytic site.

Route	Onset	Peak	Duration
PO (immediate-release)	Unknown	4 hr	Unknown
PO (extended-release)	Unknown	24 hr	Unknown

Half-life: 25 to 30 hours.

ADVERSE REACTIONS
CNS: fever, headache, fatigue. **GI:** nausea, abdominal pain, diarrhea. **Hematologic:** *neutropenia.* **Hepatic:** *hepatitis.* **Musculoskeletal:** myalgia, arthralgia. **Skin:** blistering, rash, *S.JS.*

INTERACTIONS
Drug-drug. *Artemether, calcium channel blockers, cyclophosphamide, fentanyl, immunosuppressants:* May decrease exposure of these drugs. Monitor therapy effectiveness.
Atazanavir: May increase risk of virologic failure due to decreased atazanavir exposure; may increase risk of nevirapine toxicity. Avoid combination.
Boceprevir, telaprevir: May decrease boceprevir or telaprevir level. Don't use together.
Delavirdine, etravirine, rilpivirine: May alter nevirapine concentration. Don't use together, as combination hasn't proved beneficial.
Drugs extensively metabolized by CYP450: May lower levels of these drugs. Dosage adjustment of these drugs may be needed.

Efavirenz: May decrease efavirenz concentration and increase adverse reactions. Concurrent use isn't recommended.
Fluconazole, voriconazole: May increase nevirapine exposure. Monitor patient for increased adverse effects; consider therapy modification.
Fosamprenavir, saquinavir: May decrease plasma concentrations of these drugs and increase adverse events. Monitor patient.
Ketoconazole: May decrease ketoconazole level. Avoid using together.
Protease inhibitors, hormonal contraceptives: May decrease levels of these drugs. Use together cautiously.
Rifabutin, rifampin: May decrease levels of these drugs. Dosage adjustment may be needed. Monitor patient closely. Avoid concomitant use of rifampin if possible.
Warfarin: May increase anticoagulant effect of warfarin. Monitor INR and adjust warfarin dose as needed.
Drug-herb. *St. John's wort:* May decrease drug level. Don't use together.

EFFECTS ON LAB TEST RESULTS
• May increase ALT, AST, GGT, bilirubin, LDL, amylase, and serum cholesterol levels.
• May decrease serum phosphate and Hb levels and neutrophil count.

CONTRAINDICATIONS & CAUTIONS
• Contraindicated in patients hypersensitive to drug.
Black Box Warning Use in patients with moderate or severe hepatic impairment or as part of occupational or nonoccupational postexposure prophylaxis regimens is contraindicated because of increased risk of hepatic failure. ■
Black Box Warning Severe, life-threatening and, in some cases, fatal hepatotoxicity, particularly in the first 18 weeks, has been reported in patients treated with nevirapine. In some cases, patients presented with nonspecific prodromal signs or symptoms of hepatitis and progressed to hepatic failure. These events are often associated with rash and fever. ■
Black Box Warning Women and patients with higher CD4$^+$ cell counts at start of therapy are at increased risk for life-threatening hepatotoxicity. Women with

---

Reactions in bold italics are *life-threatening*. Interactions may have a *rapid onset* or a *delayed onset*.

CD4$^+$ cell counts higher than 250/mm^3, including pregnant women receiving drug in combination with other antiretrovirals for treatment of HIV-1 infection, are at greatest risk. However, hepatotoxicity associated with nevirapine use can occur in both genders, at all CD4$^+$ cell counts, and at any time during treatment. ∎

Black Box Warning Severe, life-threatening, sometimes fatal skin reactions have occurred, including SJS, toxic epidermal necrolysis, and hypersensitivity reactions characterized by rash, constitutional findings, and organ dysfunction. ∎

• Use cautiously in patients with mild hepatic impairment; pharmacokinetics haven't been evaluated in these patients.

• Unless the benefit outweighs the risk, drug isn't indicated in adult females with CD4$^+$ cell counts greater than 250 cells/mm^3 or adult males with CD4$^+$ cell counts greater than 400 cells/mm^3.

• Immune reconstitution syndrome has been reported in patients treated with combination antiretroviral therapy. During the initial phase of treatment, patients whose immune system responds may develop inflammatory response to indolent or residual opportunistic infections, which may require further evaluation and treatment. Autoimmune disorders have also been reported in the setting of immune reconstitution; however, the time to onset is more variable, and can occur many months after initiation of treatment.

Dialyzable drug: Yes.

⚠ *Overdose S&S:* Edema, erythema nodosum, fatigue, fever, headache, insomnia, nausea, pulmonary infiltrates, rash, vertigo, vomiting, weight decrease.

PREGNANCY-LACTATION-REPRODUCTION

• Use cautiously in pregnant women. Advise women who are pregnant or may become pregnant to enroll in the Antiretroviral Pregnancy Registry (1-800-258-4263).

• Women with HIV infection shouldn't breastfeed.

• Drug may reduce fertility in women of childbearing potential, based on animal studies.

NURSING CONSIDERATIONS

• Perform lab tests, including renal function tests, before therapy and regularly throughout.

Black Box Warning Monitor patient intensively during first 18 weeks of therapy to detect potentially life-threatening hepatotoxicity or skin reactions. Extra vigilance is warranted during first 6 weeks of therapy, which is the period of greatest risk of these reactions. ∎

⊕ *Alert:* Monitor patient for blistering, oral lesions, conjunctivitis, muscle or joint aches, or general malaise. Especially look for severe rash or rash accompanied by fever. Immediately report these signs and symptoms to prescriber.

⊕ *Alert:* Be vigilant for signs or symptoms of hepatitis, such as fatigue, malaise, anorexia, nausea, jaundice, bilirubinuria, acholic stools, liver tenderness, or hepatomegaly. Consider diagnosis of hepatotoxicity in this setting, even if transaminase levels are initially normal or alternative diagnoses are possible.

Black Box Warning Check AST and ALT levels immediately if patient has signs or symptoms suggestive of hepatitis or hypersensitivity reaction. Check these levels for all patients who develop a rash in first 18 weeks of treatment. ∎

Black Box Warning Patients with signs or symptoms of hepatitis or with increased ALT or AST levels combined with rash or other systemic symptoms, including hypersensitivity reactions, must stop drug and immediately seek medical evaluation. ∎

Black Box Warning Don't restart drug after clinical hepatitis, elevated transaminase levels combined with rash or other systemic symptoms, or after severe rash or hypersensitivity reactions. In some cases, hepatic injury has progressed despite discontinuation of treatment. ∎

⊕ *Alert:* If mild to moderate rash occurs during 14-day lead-in period with immediate-release nevirapine, don't increase dosage until the rash has resolved. Total duration of the once-daily lead-in dosing shouldn't exceed 28 days, at which point an alternative regimen should be sought.

⊕ *Alert:* If rash is present beyond 14-day lead-in period with immediate-release

N

formulation, don't begin extended-release drug. The lead-in period before switching to extended-release formula isn't required if patient is already taking twice-daily immediate-release formulation in combination with other antiretrovirals.

🕩 *Alert:* Patients who have stopped therapy for more than 7 days should restart therapy with lead-in dosing as if receiving drug for the first time.

• Antiretroviral therapy may be changed if disease progresses during nevirapine therapy. Drug shouldn't be used as monotherapy for HIV infection because of the rapid emergence of resistance.

• Drug may cause body-fat redistribution.

• *Look alike–sound alike:* Don't confuse nevirapine with nelfinavir. Don't confuse Viramune with Viracept.

PATIENT TEACHING

• Inform patient that drug doesn't cure HIV and that illnesses from advanced HIV infection still may occur. Explain that drug doesn't reduce risk of HIV transmission.

• Instruct patient to report rash immediately and to stop drug until told to resume.

• Tell patient with signs or symptoms of hepatitis (such as fatigue, malaise, anorexia, nausea, jaundice, liver tenderness or hepatomegaly, with or without initially abnormal transaminase levels) to stop drug and seek medical evaluation immediately.

• Instruct patient that clinical and lab monitoring is essential, especially during the first 18 weeks of therapy, to detect potentially life-threatening hepatotoxicity and skin reactions.

• Stress importance of taking drug exactly as prescribed. If a dose is missed, tell patient to take the next dose as soon as possible and not to double next dose.

• Advise patient that if therapy is interrupted for more than 7 days, the 14-day lead-in dosages will be needed.

• Tell patient not to use other drugs or herbal products unless approved by prescriber.

• Advise female patient of childbearing potential not to use hormonal contraceptives and other hormonal methods of birth control while taking nevirapine.

niCARdipine hydrochloride
nye-KAR-de-peen

Cardene IV

Therapeutic class: Antihypertensives, antianginals
Pharmacologic class: Calcium channel blockers

AVAILABLE FORMS
Capsules: 20 mg, 30 mg
Injection: 2.5 mg/mL vials; 20 mg/200 mL, 40 mg/200 mL in premixed bags

INDICATIONS & DOSAGES
➤ **Chronic stable angina (used alone or with other antianginals)**
Adults: Initially, 20-mg capsule PO t.i.d. Adjust dosage no sooner than every 3 days based on patient response. Usual range, 20 to 40 mg t.i.d.
➤ **HTN**
Adults: Initially, 20 mg capsule PO t.i.d.; range, 20 to 40 mg t.i.d. Adjust dosage every 3 days based on patient response. Or, for a drug-free patient who is starting on nicardipine and can't take oral form, 5 mg/hour IV infusion initially; then, increase by 2.5 mg/hour every 5 minutes for rapid control or every 15 minutes for gradual control to maximum of 15 mg/hour. After achieving BP goal, decrease infusion rate to 3 mg/hour. Or, as a substitute for oral nicardipine therapy, if patient is taking 20 mg PO every 8 hours, give 0.5 mg/hour IV infusion; if patient is taking 30 mg PO every 8 hours, give 1.2 mg/hour IV infusion; if patient is taking 40 mg PO every 8 hours, give 2.2 mg/hour IV infusion.
Adjust-a-dose: For patients with renal impairment, use starting dose of 20 mg PO t.i.d. with slow titration. For patients with hepatic impairment, use starting dose of 20 mg b.i.d. with slow titration.

ADMINISTRATION
PO
• Give drug with or without food, but avoid giving with high-fat meal.
• Patient should avoid grapefruit juice during therapy.

IV

▼ Dilute 25-mg vial with 240 mL D$_5$W, dextrose 5% in NSS or half-NSS, or NSS or half-NSS to a concentration of 0.1 mg/mL.

▼ Check premixed bags for leaks, solution clarity, and intact seal. Don't add other drugs to bag.

▼ Give by slow infusion.

▼ Closely monitor BP during and after completion of infusion.

▼ If hypotension or tachycardia occurs, titrate infusion rate.

▼ Administer via central line or through a large peripheral vein. To minimize risk of peripheral venous irritation, change infusion site every 12 hours.

▼ Don't combine premixed or injection with any product in the same IV line or premixed container.

▼ When switching to oral form, give first dose of t.i.d. regimen 1 hour before stopping infusion. If using a different oral drug, start it when infusion ends.

▼ If solution is kept at room temperature, use within 24 hours.

▼ **Incompatibilities:** Sodium bicarbonate (5%) injection, lactated Ringer injection. Consult a drug incompatibility reference for other possible incompatibilities.

ACTION

Inhibits calcium ion influx across cardiac and smooth muscle cells but is more selective to vascular smooth muscle than cardiac muscle. Drug also dilates coronary arteries and arterioles.

Route	Onset	Peak	Duration
PO	½–2 hr	1–2 hr	8 hr
IV	Immediate	45 min	<8 hr

Half-life: 2 to 4 hours (PO); 3 minutes to 14 hours (IV).

ADVERSE REACTIONS

CNS: headache, dizziness, light-headedness, asthenia, drowsiness, paresthesia, somnolence. **CV:** angina, peripheral edema, palpitations, flushing, hypotension, tachycardia. **GI:** nausea, vomiting, abdominal discomfort, dry mouth, dyspepsia. **Musculoskeletal:** myalgia and weakness (IV form). **Skin:** rash, diaphoresis, injection-site reaction.

INTERACTIONS

Drug-drug. *Antihypertensives, protease inhibitors:* May increase antihypertensive effect. Monitor BP closely.

Cimetidine: May decrease metabolism of calcium channel blockers. Monitor patient for increased pharmacologic effect.

Cyclosporine, tacrolimus: May increase plasma levels of these drugs. Monitor patient for toxicity.

Digoxin: May increase digoxin level. Monitor digoxin level.

Drugs that prolong QT interval: May have an additive effect. Monitor patient and ECG.

Fentanyl: May cause severe hypotension. Closely monitor BP.

Fluconazole: May increase nicardipine serum concentration and toxicity. Monitor therapy.

Drug-food. *Grapefruit and grapefruit juice:* May increase bioavailability of nicardipine. Discourage use together.

High-fat foods: May decrease absorption of nicardipine. Discourage use together.

EFFECTS ON LAB TEST RESULTS

None reported.

CONTRAINDICATIONS & CAUTIONS

• Contraindicated in patients hypersensitive to drug and in those with advanced aortic stenosis.

• Use cautiously in patients with hypotension or impaired hepatic or renal function and in elderly patients.

• Avoid systemic hypotension when administering drug to patients who have sustained an acute cerebral infarction or hemorrhage.

• Consider lower dosages and closely monitor responses in patients with hepatic impairment or reduced hepatic blood flow.

• Titrate gradually in patients with renal impairment.

• MI and increased angina have been noted when calcium channel blockers have been started or doses titrated. Abrupt withdrawal can cause rebound angina in patients with CAD.

• Avoid use of drug, a calcium channel blocker, in patients with HF due to increased risk of worse outcomes.

N

• Safety and effectiveness in patients younger than age 18 haven't been established.

Dialyzable drug: No.

⚠ ***Overdose S&S:*** Hypotension, bradycardia, palpitations, flushing, drowsiness, confusion, slurred speech.

PREGNANCY-LACTATION-REPRODUCTION

• There are no adequate studies in pregnant women. Use during pregnancy only if potential benefits outweigh risk to the fetus.

• Use cautiously in breastfeeding women, and monitor infant for adverse effects. Some manufacturers recommend that patient should avoid breastfeeding during therapy.

NURSING CONSIDERATIONS

• Closely monitor BP and HR. Drug can cause symptomatic hypotension or tachycardia. Measure BP frequently during initial therapy. Maximal response occurs in about 1 hour. Check for orthostatic hypotension. Because large swings in BP may occur based on drug level, assess antihypertensive effect 8 hours after dosing.

❸ ***Alert:*** Only immediate-release form is approved for treatment of angina.

• To reduce risk of venous thrombosis, phlebitis, and vascular impairment, don't use small veins, such as those on the dorsum of the hand or wrist. Use extreme care to avoid intra-arterial administration or extravasation.

• ***Look alike–sound alike:*** Don't confuse nicardipine with niacinamide, nifedipine, or nimodipine. Don't confuse Cardene with Cardura, Cardizem, or codeine.

PATIENT TEACHING

• Tell patient to take oral form exactly as prescribed.

• Tell patient to report injection-site pain.

• Advise patient to report chest pain immediately. Some patients may experience increased frequency, severity, or duration of chest pain at beginning of therapy or during dosage adjustments.

• Tell patient to get up from a sitting or lying position slowly to avoid dizziness caused by a decrease in BP.

• Tell patient drug may be taken with or without food but shouldn't be taken with high-fat foods or grapefruit products.

nicotine
NIK-oh-teen

Habitrol ◇, Nicoderm CQ ◇, Nicotine Transdermal System Patch Kit ◇, Nicotrol, Nicotrol NS

nicotine polacrilex
Commit ◇, Habitrol ◇, Nicorelief ◇, Nicorette ◇, Nicorette Mini ◇, Thrive ◇

Therapeutic class: Smoking cessation aids
Pharmacologic class: Nicotinic agonists

AVAILABLE FORMS
Gum: 2 mg, 4 mg per piece
Lozenges: 2 mg, 4 mg
Nasal spray: 10 mg/mL (0.5 mg/actuation)
Oral inhaler: 10-mg cartridge (4 mg delivered)
Transdermal patch: 7 mg, 14 mg, 21 mg

INDICATIONS & DOSAGES
➤ **As an aid to smoking cessation for the relief of nicotine withdrawal signs and symptoms as part of a comprehensive behavioral smoking cessation program**
Adults: For gum, initially patient should slowly chew 1 piece every 1 to 2 hours weeks 1 to 6, then 1 piece every 2 to 4 hours weeks 7 to 9, then 1 piece every 4 to 8 hours weeks 10 to 12. Maximum dosage is 24 pieces/day. Patient who smokes first cigarette more than 30 minutes after waking up should use 2-mg pieces; patient who smokes first cigarette within 30 minutes of waking up should use 4-mg pieces. For best results, at least 9 pieces should be chewed per day for first 6 weeks.

For oral inhaler, patient should use 6 to 16 cartridges per day weeks 1 to 12; adjust dosage based on signs or symptoms of nicotine withdrawal or excess. After 12 weeks, taper dosage over 6 to 12 additional weeks. Use beyond 6 months isn't recommended.

For nasal spray, initially one or two doses per hour (one dose is 1 spray in each nostril); may increase to a maximum recommended dose of 40 mg (80 sprays)/day. For best results, at least eight doses per day are recommended. Don't exceed five doses per hour or 40 doses per day. Treat for 3 months. Use beyond 6 months isn't recommended.

For transdermal patch (Habitrol) in patients who smoke more than 10 cigarettes a day, apply one 21-mg patch daily during weeks 1 to 4; during weeks 5 to 6, decrease patch strength to 14 mg; during weeks 7 to 8, decrease patch strength to 7 mg, then discontinue. If patient smokes 10 or fewer cigarettes per day, start with 14-mg patch daily for 6 weeks, then 7-mg patch for 2 weeks, then discontinue. Patch may be worn for 16 or 24 hours.

For transdermal patch (Nicoderm CQ) in patients who smoke more than 10 cigarettes a day, apply one 21-mg patch daily during weeks 1 to 6; during weeks 7 to 8, decrease patch strength to 14 mg; during weeks 9 to 10, decrease patch strength to 7 mg, then discontinue. If patient smokes 10 or fewer cigarettes per day, start with 14-mg patch daily for 6 weeks, then 7-mg patch for 2 weeks, then discontinue. Patch may be worn for 16 or 24 hours.

ADMINISTRATION

• Hazardous drug; use safe handling and disposal precautions.

Buccal (gum)

• Patient shouldn't eat or drink for 15 minutes before chewing or while chewing a piece of nicotine gum.

• Patient should chew the gum slowly until it tingles, then place it between cheek and gum. When the tingle is gone, patient should begin chewing again until the tingle returns. This process should be repeated until most of the tingle is gone (about 30 minutes).

• Store at room temperature.

Buccal (lozenge)

• Patient shouldn't eat or drink 15 minutes before using lozenge or while lozenge is in mouth.

• Patient should place lozenge in mouth and allow lozenge to slowly dissolve (about 20 to 30 minutes); there may be a warm or tingling sensation. Patient should minimize swallowing and not chew or swallow lozenge.

• Occasionally patient should move lozenge from one side of mouth to the other until it's completely dissolved (about 20 to 30 minutes).

• Patient shouldn't use more than one lozenge at a time or continuously use one lozenge after another because GI adverse effects may occur.

• Patient who slips and has a cigarette should continue use.

• Store at room temperature; protect from light.

Inhalational

• Follow manufacturer's directions for assembling inhaler.

• Each cartridge may be used multiple times to provide a total of about 20 minutes of active puffing time. When not in use, keep mouthpiece in locked position out of reach of children and pets.

• Store mouthpiece in plastic storage case. Clean regularly with soap and water.

• Store and use at room temperature; protect from light.

Intranasal (spray)

• See manufacturer's instructions for use of device.

• Give with patient's head tilted back slightly; patient shouldn't sniff, swallow, or inhale through the nose during actuation.

• Patient shouldn't blow nose for 2 to 3 minutes after administration.

• Avoid contact with solution. If skin, lips, mouth, eyes, or ears come in contact with nicotine solution, immediately rinse with water.

Transdermal (patch)

• Apply one new patch every 24 hours on dry, clean, and hairless skin on upper body or outer arm. Save pouch for patch disposal after use.

• Remove backing from patch and immediately press onto skin for 10 seconds. After handling patch, wash hands with water only.

• Don't cut patch or use a patch that's damaged on opening protective pouch.

• Don't apply patch to skin that is oily, burned, broken out, cut, or irritated. Avoid using soaps, lotions, oils, or creams that contain aloe, lanolin, or glycerin moisturizers on skin where the patch will be applied.

• Apply patch at the same time each day and rotate application sites. Allow at least 1 week before applying to previously used skin.

• Patient shouldn't wear more than one patch at a time and patches shouldn't be left

N

---

on for more than 24 hours; patches lose potency after 24 hours and increased skin irritation may occur.
• Throw away the patch by folding sticky ends together. Replace in pouch and discard.

ACTION

Binds to nicotinic-cholinergic receptors in the adrenal medulla, neuromuscular junctions, and in the brain, causing stimulation and reward effects. Replaces endogenous nicotine effects obtained from smoking or other forms of tobacco. When appropriate doses are used, reduces withdrawal symptoms, including nicotine craving associated with quitting smoking.

Route	Onset	Peak	Duration
Buccal (gum, lozenge)	Unknown	Unknown	Unknown
Inhalation	Unknown	Within 15 min	Unknown
Intranasal	Rapid	10–20 min	Unknown
Transdermal	Unknown	2–8 hr	Unknown

Half-life: Inhaler and nasal spray, 1 to 2 hours; transdermal patch, 4 hours.

ADVERSE REACTIONS

CNS: impaired concentration, confusion, fever, headache, nervousness, pain, tremor, incoordination, increased dreaming, apathy, withdrawal signs and symptoms (dizziness, anxiety, restlessness, cravings, sleep disorder, depression, drug dependence, fatigue), paresthesia. **CV:** tachycardia, HTN, palpitations, chest discomfort/tightness, facial flushing (nasal spray). **EENT:** Gum: gum problems, tooth disorder, stomatitis, glossitis. Inhaler: mouth and throat irritation, taste disturbance, rhinitis, sinusitis, tooth disorder. Nasal spray: transient epistaxis, transient changes in sense of smell and taste, earache, numbness of nose or mouth, burning of nose or eyes, hoarseness, watery eyes, sneezing or runny nose, nasal mucosa irritation, ulcer, or blister. **GI:** dyspepsia, flatulence, hiccups, nausea, constipation, diarrhea, gingival bleeding, increased salivation, xerostomia, increased appetite. **GU:** menstrual disorder. **Metabolic:** weight gain. **Musculoskeletal:** back pain, arthralgia, jaw/neck pain (inhaler, gum), myalgia. **Respiratory:** cough (inhaler), bronchitis, dyspnea. **Skin:** rash, acne, application-site reaction, diaphoresis, pruritus. **Other:** allergic reaction, flulike symptoms.

INTERACTIONS

Drug-drug. *Acetaminophen, adrenergic antagonists (labetalol, prazosin), beta blockers (propranolol and others), imipramine, oxazepam, pentazocine, theophylline:* May cause a deinduction of hepatic enzymes on smoking cessation with or without nicotine replacement. A decrease in dosage of these drugs after smoking cessation may be needed. Monitor patient closely.
Adenosine: May enhance AV-blocking and tachycardic effects of adenosine. Monitor therapy.
Adrenergic agonists (isoproterenol, phenylephrine): May decrease circulating catecholamines with smoking cessation with or without nicotine replacement. An increase in dosage of these drugs after cessation of smoking may be needed. Monitor patient.
Cimetidine: May increase nicotine concentration. Monitor therapy.
Insulin: May increase subcutaneous absorption of insulin. A decrease in insulin dosage after cessation of smoking may be needed. Monitor patient closely.
Nasal vasoconstrictors (xylometazoline): May delay time to onset and peak nicotine concentration of nasal formulation. Advise patient of delay in nicotine effect.
Niacin: May increase flushing and dizziness. Use cautiously together.
TCAs: May affect pharmacokinetics of TCAs with smoking cessation with or without nicotine replacement. Monitor patient and adjust TCA dosage as necessary.
Drug-herb. *Lobelia:* May result in additive nicotine effects. Discourage use together.
Drug-food. *Acidic foods and beverages:* May decrease absorption of lozenge. Discourage use together.
Caffeine: May increase caffeine's effects after smoking cessation. Monitor patient.
Drug-lifestyle. *Smoking:* May have additive nicotine effect and increase risk of toxicity. Discourage smoking.

EFFECTS ON LAB TEST RESULTS
None reported.

Reactions in bold italics are *life-threatening*. Interactions may have a *rapid onset* or a *delayed onset*.

CONTRAINDICATIONS & CAUTIONS
• Contraindicated in patients with known hypersensitivity or allergy to nicotine or components of the products, including menthol (inhaler) or soy (lozenges).
• Nicotine from any source can be toxic and addictive; dependence on nicotine replacements has occurred.
• Use cautiously in patients with recent MI, serious arrhythmias, CAD, severe or worsening angina, HTN, vasospastic diseases, or PVD.
• Use oral inhaler cautiously in patients with bronchospastic disease because of potential for airway irritation. Other forms of nicotine replacement may be preferred.
• Nasal spray isn't recommended in patients with chronic allergy, rhinitis, nasal polyps, sinusitis, or severe reactive airway disease.
• Use patch cautiously in patients with skin problems and in those allergic to adhesive tape.
• Use cautiously in patients with insulin-dependent diabetes, hyperthyroidism, pheochromocytoma, or severe renal or hepatic impairment.
• Use cautiously in patients with oropharyngeal inflammation, history of esophagitis, or peptic ulcer disease because healing of GI disorders may be delayed.
• Nicotine gum may cause severe occlusal stress due to its heavier viscosity compared to ordinary chewing gum. The gum may loosen inlays or fillings, damage oral mucosa and natural teeth, and stick to dentures.
⚠ **Alert:** Nicotine exposure by children and pets may cause poisoning and is potentially fatal.
• Use in children hasn't been studied.
• Use cautiously in patients older than age 65.
Dialyzable drug: Unknown.
⚠ **Overdose S&S:** Lethargy, pallor, cold sweat, nausea, salivation, vomiting, abdominal pain, diarrhea, headache, dizziness, disturbed hearing and vision, tremor, mental confusion, and weakness, ataxia, hypotension, seizures, arrhythmias, vascular collapse, central respiratory paralysis, coma.

PREGNANCY-LACTATION-REPRODUCTION
• Nicotine may cause fetal harm, including spontaneous abortion. Encourage

pregnant women to attempt smoking cessation through nonpharmacologic means. Use during pregnancy only if the likelihood of smoking cessation justifies the potential risk of using nicotine by the pregnant patient who might continue to smoke.
• Nicotine appears in human milk; however, the amount of nicotine from nicotine replacement products in human milk isn't known. Encourage breastfeeding patients not to smoke. Weigh risk of exposure of the infant to nicotine from nicotine replacement therapy against risks associated with the mother's use of replacement therapy and continued smoking.

NURSING CONSIDERATIONS
• Connect patients who smoke with programs to assist with smoking cessation, such as government-based quit lines.
• Successful smoking cessation programs are individualized and include frequent supportive care.
• For patients older than age 65, consider initiating treatment at the low end of the dosage range.
• Monitor patients for withdrawal signs and symptoms (craving, nervousness, restlessness, irritability, mood lability, anxiety, drowsiness, sleep disturbances, impaired concentration, increased appetite, headache, myalgia, constipation, fatigue, weight gain).
• Monitor patients for tachycardia and other arrhythmias. Discontinue drug if CV signs and symptoms occur.
• Monitor patients for signs and symptoms of toxicity and overuse (nausea, abdominal pain, vomiting, diarrhea, diaphoresis, flushing, dizziness, disturbed hearing and vision, confusion, weakness, palpitations, altered respiration, hypotension); ensure that drug is used only as directed.
• Monitor patients for temporomandibular joint dysfunction and pain due to excessive chewing of gum.
• Strategies for discontinuing nasal spray include using only half a dose (1 spray) at a time, using spray less frequently, tallying daily usage, setting a steadily reducing usage target, skipping a dose by not medicating every hour, and setting a planned "quit date" for stopping spray.

• Discontinue patch if skin redness caused by the patch doesn't resolve after 4 days or if inflammation or rash occurs.

• OTC products aren't for sale to individuals younger than age 18.

• *Look alike–sound alike:* Don't confuse nicotine brand names.

PATIENT TEACHING

• Emphasize that patient should stop smoking completely while on nicotine replacement therapy to avoid additive nicotine levels higher than smoking alone.

• Teach patient how to properly apply or use products.

• Warn patient to adhere to maximum dosage ranges for these products.

• Advise patient to read all patient education material that comes with each product being used.

• Inform patient using nasal spray that nasal irritation is likely to occur but may lessen with continued use.

• Tell patient that onset of nasal spray's effect may be delayed if patient has a cold or rhinitis.

• Advise patient using gum to report jaw or tooth pain.

• Alert patient using gum that gum can stick to and damage dentures and dental work.

• Instruct patient to use hard, sugarless candy between doses of gum to help provide oral stimulation.

• Advise patient that participating in a comprehensive smoking cessation program improves success.

• Discuss benefits and risks of nicotine replacement versus smoking with female patient who is or plans to become pregnant or breastfeed.

• Caution patient that dosages of other drugs patient may be taking may need adjustment because of the impact smoking cessation may have on the drugs' pharmacokinetics.

• **Alert:** Advise patient to keep all nicotine products, including used inhaler cartridges, nasal spray bottles, and patches, out of reach of children and pets.

NIFEdipine
nye-FED-i-peen

Adalat CC, Adalat XL✚, Procardia, Procardia XL◆

Therapeutic class: Antihypertensives, antianginals
Pharmacologic class: Calcium channel blockers

AVAILABLE FORMS
Capsules: 5 mg✚, 10 mg, 20 mg
Tablets (extended-release) ⒪: 20 mg✚, 30 mg, 60 mg, 90 mg

INDICATIONS & DOSAGES
Adjust-a-dose (for all indications): For elderly patients and patients with renal and hepatic impairment, initiate drug at the low end of the dosing range.

➤ **Vasospastic angina (Prinzmetal or variant angina), classic chronic stable angina pectoris**
Adults: Initially, 10 mg short-acting capsule PO t.i.d. Usual effective dosage range is 10 to 20 mg t.i.d. Some patients may require up to 30 mg q.i.d. Maximum daily dose is 180 mg/day. Adjust dosage over 7 to 14 days to evaluate response. Or, 30 to 60 mg (extended-release tablets, except Adalat CC) PO once daily. Maximum daily dose is 120 mg. Adjust dosage over 7 to 14 days to evaluate response. Use doses of more than 90 mg cautiously and only when clinically warranted.

➤ **HTN**
Adults: Initially, 30 mg extended-release tablet (Adalat CC) or 30 or 60 mg extended-release tablet (Procardia XL) PO once daily, adjusted over 7 to 14 days. Maximum dose is 90 mg (Adalat CC) or 120 mg/day (Procardia XL).

➤ **Ureteral calculi (distal)** ◆
Adults: 10 to 30 mg PO t.i.d. for up to 4 weeks or until expulsion of lower stones.

ADMINISTRATION
PO
• May give immediate-release form with or without food. If flushing occurs, may give with a low-fat meal.

Reactions in bold italics are *life-threatening*. Interactions may have a *rapid onset* or a *delayed onset*.

• Give extended-release form (Adalat CC)
on an empty stomach.

◑ Alert: Don't use capsules SL to rapidly reduce severe high BP because the result may
be fatal.

• Give extended-release tablets whole; don't
break or crush tablet.

• Don't give drug with grapefruit juice.

• Protect capsules from direct light and
moisture and store at room temperature.

ACTION

Thought to inhibit calcium ion influx across
cardiac and smooth muscle cells, decreasing
contractility and oxygen demand. Drug may
also dilate coronary arteries and arterioles.

Route	Onset	Peak	Duration
PO	20 min	30–60 min	4–8 hr
PO (extended-release)	20 min	2½–5 hr	24 hr

Half-life: 2 to 7 hours.

ADVERSE REACTIONS

CNS: dizziness, light-headedness, giddiness,
headache, weakness, nervousness, mood
changes, shakiness, sleep disturbances,
fever. **CV:** flushing, heat sensation, peripheral edema, palpitations, transient hypotension. **EENT:** nasal congestion, sore throat,
blurred vision. **GI:** nausea, heartburn, diarrhea, constipation, cramps, flatulence. **Musculoskeletal:** muscle cramps, tremor, inflammation, joint stiffness. **Respiratory:**
dyspnea, cough, wheezing, chest congestion,
shortness of breath. **Skin:** dermatitis, pruritus, urticaria, sweating. **Other:** difficulties
in balance, chills, sexual difficulties.

INTERACTIONS

Drug-drug. *ACE inhibitors (benazepril):*
May increase hypotensive effects. Monitor
BP and adjust nifedipine dosage as needed.
Alpha₁ blockers (doxazosin): May increase
nifedipine plasma concentration. Monitor
BP and adjust nifedipine dosage as needed.
Antiretrovirals, cimetidine, verapamil: May
decrease nifedipine metabolism. Monitor BP
closely; adjust nifedipine dose as needed.
*Azole antifungals, erythromycin, nefaz-
odone, quinupristin–dalfopristin, valproic
acid:* May increase the effects of nifedipine.

Monitor BP closely and decrease nifedipine
dosage as needed.
Clopidogrel: May decease antiplatelet effect
and increase thrombotic events. Monitor
patient.
Cyclosporine, tacrolimus: May increase
serum levels of these drugs and increase risk
of toxicity. Monitor serum levels and adjust
dosage as needed.
Digoxin: May cause elevated digoxin level.
Monitor digoxin level.
Diltiazem: May increase the effects of
nifedipine. Monitor patient closely.
Diuretics, fentanyl: May increase hypotensive effects. Monitor BP.
PDE5 inhibitors (sildenafil): Increases
risk of hypotension. Monitor BP and adjust
nifedipine dosage if needed.
Propranolol, other beta blockers: May cause
hypotension and HF. Use together cautiously.
Quinidine: May decrease levels and effects
of quinidine while increasing effects of
nifedipine. Monitor HR and adjust nifedipine dose as needed.
*Strong CYP3A4 inducers (carbamazepine,
dexamethasone, phenytoin, rifabutin, rifampin):* May decrease nifedipine level. Use
together is contraindicated.
Vincristine: May increase risk of vincristine
toxicity. Monitor therapy.
Warfarin: May increase PT. Monitor coagulation parameters and adjust warfarin dosage
as needed.
Drug-herb. *Melatonin, St. John's wort:* May
interfere with antihypertensive effect. Discourage use together.
Drug-food. *Grapefruit juice:* May increase
bioavailability of drug. Discourage use
together.

EFFECTS ON LAB TEST RESULTS

• May increase ALT, AST, alkaline phosphatase, and LDH levels.

CONTRAINDICATIONS & CAUTIONS

• Contraindicated in patients hypersensitive to drug, in those taking strong CYP450
inducers (rifampin), and in patients with cardiogenic shock or ST-segment elevation MI.

• Increased angina and MI have occurred at
start of therapy or with dosage titration of
dihydropyridine calcium channel blockers.

N

Reflex tachycardia may occur, resulting in angina or MI in patients with obstructive coronary disease, especially in the absence of concurrent beta blockade.

• BP must be lowered at a rate appropriate for patient's clinical condition to avoid symptomatic hypotension with or without syncope. The use of immediate-release nifedipine in hypertensive emergencies and urgencies is neither safe nor effective. Serious adverse events (death, cerebrovascular ischemia, syncope, stroke, acute MI, fetal distress) have been reported. Don't use immediate-release nifedipine for acute BP reduction or to manage primary HTN.

• Avoid use in patients with HF; drug may worsen symptoms.

• Use with extreme caution in patients with severe aortic stenosis. Drug may reduce coronary perfusion, resulting in ischemia.

• Use cautiously in patients with hypertrophic cardiomyopathy and outflow tract obstruction because reduction in afterload may worsen symptoms.

• Use cautiously before major surgery. Cardiopulmonary bypass, intraoperative blood loss, or vasodilating anesthesia may result in severe hypotension or increased fluid requirements. Consider withdrawing nifedipine more than 36 hours before surgery if possible.

• Rare reversible elevations in BUN and serum creatinine levels have been reported in patients with preexisting chronic renal insufficiency.

• Use cautiously in patients with hepatic impairment. Clearance of nifedipine is reduced in cirrhotic patients, leading to increased systemic exposure and possibly increasing toxicities; monitor patient and consider dosage adjustments.

⊙ *Alert:* Immediate-release drug is considered a high-risk drug for elderly patients because of the potential for hypotension and increased risk of precipitating myocardial ischemia in this population. Avoid use.

⊙ *Alert:* Use extended-release form cautiously because of an increased risk of serious GI obstruction in patients both with and without risk factors. (Risk factors for GI obstruction include altered GI anatomy, GI hypomotility related to GERD, colon cancer, ileus, obesity, hypothyroidism,

diabetes, and concomitant use of H_2 blockers, NSAIDs, laxatives, anticholinergic agents, and levothyroxine.)

• Safety and effectiveness in children haven't been established.

Dialyzable drug: Unlikely.

⚠ *Overdose S&S:* Hypotension, dizziness, palpitations, flushing, nervousness.

PREGNANCY-LACTATION-REPRODUCTION

• There are no adequate studies in pregnant women. Use only when potential benefit justifies possible risk to the fetus.

• Drug appears in human milk. Use cautiously in breastfeeding women. Monitor breastfed infants for adverse effects.

NURSING CONSIDERATIONS

• Monitor BP and HR regularly, especially in patients who take beta blockers or antihypertensives.

• Watch for symptoms of HF.

• The most common adverse effect is peripheral edema, which occurs within 2 to 3 weeks of start of therapy.

• Don't give immediate-release capsules within 1 week of acute MI or in ACS.

• *Look alike–sound alike:* Don't confuse nifedipine with nimodipine, nisoldipine, or nicardipine. Don't confuse Procardia XL with Cartia XT.

PATIENT TEACHING

• If patient is kept on nitrate therapy while nifedipine dosage is being adjusted, urge continued compliance. Patient may take SL nitroglycerin, as needed, for acute chest pain.

• Tell patient that chest pain may worsen briefly as therapy starts or dosage increases.

• Instruct patient to swallow extended-release tablets without breaking, crushing, or chewing them.

• Advise patient to avoid taking drug with grapefruit juice.

• Tell patient not to abruptly stop drug unless directed by prescriber. Abrupt withdrawal may cause rebound angina in patients with CAD.

• Advise patient that Adalat CC tablets contain lactose and shouldn't be used by patients with galactose intolerance, Lapp

---

lactase deficiency, or glucose-galactose malabsorption.
• Reassure patient taking the extended-release tablet that the wax mold may be passed in the stools. Assure patient that drug has already been completely absorbed.
• Tell patient to protect capsules from direct light and moisture and to store at room temperature.

SAFETY ALERT!

niraparib
nye-RAP-a-rib

Zejula

Therapeutic class: Antineoplastics
Pharmacologic class: Poly (ADP-ribose) polymerase inhibitors

AVAILABLE FORMS
Capsules ⊙: 100 mg

INDICATIONS & DOSAGES
➤ **Maintenance treatment of recurrent epithelial ovarian, fallopian tube, or primary peritoneal cancer in patients who are in complete or partial response to platinum-based chemotherapy**
Adults: 300 mg (3 capsules) PO once daily beginning no later than 8 weeks after most recent platinum-containing regimen. Continue treatment until disease progression or unacceptable toxicity occurs.
Adjust-a-dose: For toxicity-related dosage adjustments, consider treatment interruption, dosage reduction, or drug discontinuation according to manufacturer's instructions.

ADMINISTRATION
PO
• Hazardous drug; use safe handling and disposal precautions.
• May give with or without food.
• Give at approximately the same time each day; bedtime administration may help diminish nausea.
• Patients should swallow capsules whole.
• If dose is missed or vomited, don't make up dose; resume at next scheduled time.

ACTION
An inhibitor of poly (ADP-ribose) polymerase (PARP) enzymes PARP-1 and PARP-2, which have a role in DNA repair. Inhibition of PARP enzymatic activity and increased formation of PARP–DNA complexes result in DNA damage, apoptosis, and cell death.

Route	Onset	Peak	Duration
PO	Unknown	3 hr	Unknown

Half-life: 36 hours.

ADVERSE REACTIONS
CNS: fatigue, headache, dizziness, insomnia, anxiety, depression, asthenia. **CV:** palpitations, HTN, *hypertensive crisis,* tachycardia, peripheral edema. **EENT:** conjunctivitis, epistaxis, nasopharyngitis. **GI:** nausea, constipation, vomiting, abdominal pain/distention, mucositis, stomatitis, diarrhea, dyspepsia, dysgeusia, decreased appetite, dry mouth. **GU:** UTI. **Hematologic:** anemia, *neutropenia, leukopenia, thrombocytopenia.* **Hepatic:** increased liver enzyme levels. **Metabolic:** weight loss, *hypokalemia.* **Musculoskeletal:** myalgia, arthralgia, back pain. **Respiratory:** dyspnea, cough, bronchitis. **Skin:** rash.

INTERACTIONS
None reported. Formal drug interaction studies haven't been performed.

EFFECTS ON LAB TEST RESULTS
• May increase LFT values and creatinine level.
• May decrease potassium level.
• May decrease Hb level, platelet and WBC counts, and ANC.

CONTRAINDICATIONS & CAUTIONS
• Contraindicated in patients hypersensitive to drug or its components.
• Drug may increase risk of bone marrow suppression, myelodysplastic syndrome (MDS), or acute myeloid leukemia (AML). Discontinue drug if MDS or AML is confirmed.
• HTN and hypertensive crisis have occurred in patients treated with drug. Closely monitor patients with CV disorders.

N

• Use in severe renal disease, ESRD, and in moderate to severe hepatic impairment hasn't been studied.
• Safety and effectiveness in children haven't been established.
Dializable drug: Unknown.

PREGNANCY-LACTATION-REPRODUCTION
• Drug may cause fetal harm. Advise women of childbearing potential to use appropriate contraception during and for at least 6 months after final dose.
• It isn't known if drug appears in human milk. Advise women not to breastfeed during treatment and for 1 month after final dose.
• Drug may impair male fertility.

NURSING CONSIDERATIONS
• Assess CBC before treatment; don't give drug until hematologic toxicity from previous chemotherapy has resolved.
• Monitor CBC weekly for first month, then monthly for 11 months, then periodically.
• Monitor BP and HR monthly for 1 year and periodically thereafter. Manage HTN with medication and dosage adjustments as clinically indicated. Closely monitor patients with cardiac disorders.
• Obtain pregnancy test before start of treatment.

PATIENT TEACHING
• Explain that lab testing will be needed to monitor treatment.
• Advise patient to report all adverse reactions.
• Warn patient of risk of blood disorders and to report weakness, fatigue, fever, weight loss, frequent infections, bruising, bleeding easily, blood in urine or stool, and breathlessness.
• Inform patient that BP and HR will be monitored during therapy.
• Advise female patient that a pregnancy test will be needed before therapy begins and that drug can cause fetal harm. Advise patient to use contraception during treatment and for 6 months after final dose.
• Inform male patient that drug may impair fertility.

• Caution female patient not to breastfeed during therapy and for 1 month after final dose.

---

nitrofurantoin macrocrystals ▨
nye-troh-fyoo-RAN-toyn

Macrobid, Macrodantin⬦

nitrofurantoin microcrystals ▨
Furadantin

Therapeutic class: Antibiotics
Pharmacologic class: Nitrofurans

AVAILABLE FORMS
nitrofurantoin macrocrystals
Capsules: 25 mg, 50 mg, 100 mg
nitrofurantoin microcrystals
Oral suspension: 25 mg/5 mL

INDICATIONS & DOSAGES
➤ **UTIs caused by susceptible *Escherichia coli*, *Staphylococcus aureus*, enterococci, or certain strains of *Klebsiella* and *Enterobacter* species**
Adults and children older than age 12: 50 to 100 mg PO q.i.d. with meals and at bedtime. Continue for 1 week or for at least 3 days after sterility of urine is obtained. Or, 100 mg Macrobid PO every 12 hours for 7 days.
Children ages 1 month to 12 years: 5 to 7 mg/kg PO daily in four divided doses. Continue for 1 week or for at least 3 days after sterility of urine is obtained.
➤ **UTI prophylaxis**
Adults: 50 to 100 mg PO daily at bedtime.
Children: 1 to 2 mg/kg PO daily in a single dose at bedtime or divided into two doses given every 12 hours.

ADMINISTRATION
PO
• Obtain urine specimen for culture and sensitivity tests before giving. Repeat as needed. Begin therapy while awaiting results.
• Shake suspension well before use.
• Give with food or milk to minimize GI distress and improve absorption.
• Protect from light.

Reactions in bold italics are *life-threatening*. Interactions may have a *rapid onset* or a **delayed onset**.

ACTION
May interfere with bacterial enzyme systems and bacterial cell-wall formation.

Route	Onset	Peak	Duration
PO	Unknown	Unknown	Unknown

Half-life: 20 minutes to 1 hour.

ADVERSE REACTIONS
CNS: *ascending polyneuropathy with high doses or renal impairment,* dizziness, drowsiness, headache, peripheral neuropathy, vertigo, confusion, depression, asthenia. **CV:** ECG changes. **EENT:** nystagmus. **GI:** anorexia, diarrhea, nausea, vomiting, abdominal pain. **GU:** overgrowth of nonsusceptible organisms in urinary tract. **Hematologic:** *agranulocytosis, hemolysis in patients with G6PD deficiency, thrombocytopenia.* **Hepatic:** *hepatic necrosis, hepatitis.* **Respiratory:** *asthmatic attacks,* pulmonary sensitivity reactions, cough, cyanosis, dyspnea, pneumonitis, pulmonary fibrosis. **Skin:** *SJS*; exfoliative dermatitis; maculopapular, erythematous, or eczematous eruption; pruritus; transient alopecia; urticaria. **Other:** *anaphylaxis,* drug fever, hypersensitivity reactions.

INTERACTIONS
Drug-drug. *Antacids containing magnesium:* May decrease nitrofurantoin absorption. Separate dosage times by 1 hour.
Dapsone (topical), nitric oxide, prilocaine, sodium nitrite, tetracaine (topical): May enhance nitrofurantoin adverse/toxic effects. Monitor therapy.
Eplerenone, spironolactone: May enhance hyperkalemic effect. Monitor potassium level.
Live vaccines (BCG, cholera, typhoid): May diminish therapeutic effect of live vaccines. Avoid combination.
Magnesium trisilicate: May decrease nitrofurantoin concentration. Avoid combination.
Probenecid, sulfinpyrazone: May inhibit excretion of nitrofurantoin, increasing drug levels and risk of toxicity. The resulting decreased urinary levels could lessen antibacterial effects. Avoid using together.
Drug-food. *Any food:* May increase absorption. Advise patient to take drug with food or milk.

EFFECTS ON LAB TEST RESULTS
• May increase AST, ALT, bilirubin, and alkaline phosphatase levels.
• May increase eosinophil count.
• May decrease Hb level and WBC, granulocyte, and platelet counts.
• May cause false-positive results in urine glucose tests using cupric sulfate (such as Benedict reagent, Fehling solution, or Chemstrip uG).

CONTRAINDICATIONS & CAUTIONS
• Contraindicated in infants age 1 month and younger; in patients with anuria, oliguria, or CrCl less than 60 mL/minute; in patients with a history of cholestatic jaundice or hepatic dysfunction associated with nitrofurantoin use; and in patients with a known hypersensitivity to drug.
• Use cautiously in patients with renal impairment, asthma, anemia, diabetes mellitus, electrolyte abnormalities, vitamin B deficiency, debilitating disease, and G6PD deficiency.
• Peripheral neuropathy, which may become severe or irreversible, has occurred.
• Optic neuritis has been reported rarely in postmarketing experience with nitrofurantoin formulations.
▧ Patients with G6PD deficiency have an increased risk of developing hemolytic anemia. This deficiency is found in 10% of Blacks and a small percentage of ethnic groups of Mediterranean and Near-Eastern origin. If hemolytic anemia occurs, discontinue drug. Hemolysis ceases when drug is stopped.
Dialyzable drug: Yes.
⚠ *Overdose S&S:* Vomiting.

PREGNANCY-LACTATION-REPRODUCTION
• Contraindicated in pregnant women at 38 to 42 weeks' gestation, during labor and delivery, and when onset of labor is imminent due to possible hemolytic anemia in the neonate.
• Because of possible serious adverse reactions in infants younger than age 1 month, patient should discontinue breastfeeding or discontinue drug.

N

NURSING CONSIDERATIONS

• Drug may cause an asthma attack in patients with a history of asthma.

• Monitor fluid intake and output carefully. Treatment may turn urine brown or dark yellow.

• Monitor LFT values, because of risk of fatal hepatic reactions. Stop drug immediately if hepatitis occurs, and treat appropriately.

• Monitor CBC, renal function, and pulmonary status regularly.

❸ *Alert:* Monitor patient for signs and symptoms of superinfection, which can occur up to 2 months after therapy ends. Use of nitrofurantoin may result in growth of nonsusceptible organisms, especially *Pseudomonas* species, or cause fungal or bacterial superinfection, such as CDAD and pseudomembranous colitis.

• Monitor patient for pulmonary sensitivity reactions, including cough, chest pain, fever, chills, dyspnea, and pulmonary infiltration with consolidation or effusions.

❸ *Alert:* Hypersensitivity may develop when drug is used for long-term therapy.

• Some patients may experience fewer adverse GI effects with nitrofurantoin macrocrystals.

• Dual-release capsules (25 mg nitrofurantoin macrocrystals combined with 75 mg nitrofurantoin monohydrate) enable patients to take drug only twice daily.

• Continue treatment for 3 days after sterile urine specimens have been obtained.

• Store drug in amber container. Don't store in metals other than stainless steel or aluminum to avoid precipitation.

PATIENT TEACHING

• Instruct patient to take drug for as long as prescribed, exactly as directed, even after feeling better.

• Tell patient to take drug with food or milk to minimize stomach upset.

• Instruct patient to report adverse reactions, especially peripheral neuropathy, which can become severe or irreversible.

• Alert patient that drug may turn urine dark yellow or brown.

• Warn patient not to store drug in metals other than stainless steel or aluminum.

• Advise patient not to use antacid preparations containing magnesium trisilicate.

---

nitroglycerin (glyceryl trinitrate)
nye-troe-GLIH-ser-in

GoNitro, Minitran, Nitro-Dur, Nitrolingual, NitroMist, Nitrostat,◆, Rectiv, Trinipatch✤

Therapeutic class: Vasodilators, antianginals
Pharmacologic class: Nitrates

AVAILABLE FORMS

Aerosol (translingual): 0.4 mg/metered spray
Injection: 5 mg/mL, 100 mcg/mL, 200 mcg/mL, 400 mcg/mL
Ointment: 0.4%, 2%
Powder (SL): 400 mcg
Tablets (SL): 0.3 mg (½₀₀ grain), 0.4 mg (⅒₅₀ grain), 0.6 mg (⅒₀₀ grain)
Transdermal patch: 0.1 mg/hour, 0.2 mg/hour, 0.3 mg/hour, 0.4 mg/hour, 0.6 mg/hour, 0.8 mg/hour release rate

INDICATIONS & DOSAGES

➤ **To prevent chronic anginal attacks**
Adults: For 2% ointment: Start dosage with ½ inch ointment, increasing by ½-inch increments until desired results are achieved. Range of dosage with ointment is ½ inch to 5 inches (1.25 to 12.7 cm). Usual dose is 1 to 2 inches (2.5 to 5.08 cm) every 6 to 8 hours. Transdermal patch: Starting dose is 0.2 to 0.4 mg/hour once daily applied for 12 to 14 hours a day (with a patch-off period of 10 to 12 hours).

➤ **Acute angina pectoris; to prevent or minimize anginal attacks before stressful events**
Adults: 1 SL tablet (½₀₀ grain, ⅒₅₀ grain, or ⅒₀₀ grain) dissolved under the tongue or in the buccal pouch as soon as angina begins. Repeat every 5 minutes, if needed, to a maximum of three doses within a 15-minute period. May be used prophylactically 5 to 10 minutes before activities that might precipitate an acute angina attack. Or, 1 or 2 metered-dose sprays Nitrolingual into mouth, preferably onto or under the tongue. Repeat every 3 to 5 minutes, if

---

needed, to a maximum of three doses within a 15-minute period. Or, 1 or 2 packets of SL powder dissolved under the tongue at onset of angina or 5 to 10 minutes before activities that might precipitate an acute angina attack. Give 1 additional packet every 5 minutes as needed but not more than 3 total packets (1,200 mcg) within a 15-minute period.

➤ **HTN from surgery, HF after MI, angina pectoris in acute situations; to produce controlled hypotension during surgery (by IV infusion)**
Adults: Initially, infuse at 5 mcg/minute, increasing as needed by 5 mcg/minute every 3 to 5 minutes until response occurs. If a 20-mcg/minute rate doesn't produce a response, increase dosage by as much as 20 mcg/minute every 3 to 5 minutes. Up to 100 mcg/minute may be needed.

➤ **Moderate to severe pain from chronic anal fissure**
Adults: 1 inch (2.5 cm) of ointment PR every 12 hours for up to 3 weeks.

ADMINISTRATION

IV
▼ Dilute with D₅W or NSS for injection. Concentration shouldn't exceed 400 mcg/mL.
▼ Always give with an infusion control device and titrate to desired response.
▼ Regular polyvinyl chloride tubing can bind up to 80% of drug, making it necessary to infuse higher dosages. A special nonabsorbent polyvinyl chloride tubing is available from the manufacturer. Always mix in glass bottles and avoid using a filter.
▼ Use the same type of infusion set when changing lines.
▼ When changing the concentration of infusion, flush the administration set with 15 to 20 mL of the new concentration before use. This will clear the line of the old drug solution.
▼ **Incompatibilities:** Other drugs.

Topical
• To apply ointment, measure the prescribed amount on the application paper; then place the paper on any nonhairy area. Don't rub in. Cover with plastic film to aid absorption and to protect clothing. Remove all excess ointment from previous site before applying the next dose. Avoid getting ointment on fingers.

Rectal
• Cover a finger with plastic wrap, disposable surgical glove, or a finger cot.
• Apply 1 inch of ointment onto the covered finger.
• Gently insert the ointment into the anal canal using the covered finger no further than the first finger joint. Wash hands after use.

Transdermal
• Apply patch to any nonhairy part of the skin except distal parts of the arms or legs. (Absorption won't be maximal at distal sites.) Patch may cause contact dermatitis.
• Remove patch after 12 to 14 hours. Rotate patch sites.
• A cardioverter-defibrillator shouldn't be discharged through a paddle electrode that overlies a nitroglycerin patch.
• Remove patch before defibrillation. Because of the aluminum backing on the patch, the electric current may cause arcing that can damage the paddles and burn patient.
• When stopping transdermal treatment of angina, gradually reduce the dosage and frequency of application over 4 to 6 weeks.

Sublingual
• Give tablet at first sign of attack. Patient should wet the tablet with saliva and place it under tongue until absorbed. Dose may be repeated every 5 minutes for a maximum of three doses. If drug doesn't provide relief, obtain prompt medical attention. Tablet shouldn't be crushed, chewed, or swallowed.
• Give dose of 1 or 2 packets of SL powder as prescribed. Hold packet close to patient's mouth, tear packet at red line, and pour all of the powder under the tongue. Patient shouldn't swallow until all of the powder has dissolved. Patient shouldn't rinse or spit for 5 minutes after dose.

Buccal
• The tablet should be placed between the lip and gum above the incisors or between the cheek and gum. Tablets shouldn't be swallowed or chewed.

Translingual
• Patient using translingual aerosol form shouldn't inhale the spray but should release it onto or under the tongue, then wait about 10 seconds or so before swallowing. Patient shouldn't rinse or spit for 5 to 10 minutes after a dose.

N

ACTION

Reduces cardiac oxygen demand by decreasing left ventricular end-diastolic pressure (preload) and, to a lesser extent, systemic vascular resistance (afterload). Also increases blood flow through the collateral coronary vessels.

Route	Onset	Peak	Duration
IV	Immediate	Immediate	3–5 min
Topical	15–30 min	1 hr	7 hr
Transdermal	30 min	2 hr	10–12 hr
SL	1–3 min	5–7 min	25 min
Buccal	3 min	Unknown	3–5 hr
Translingual	1–3 min	4–15 min	25 min
PR	Immediate	Unknown	Unknown

Half-life: About 1 to 4 minutes.

ADVERSE REACTIONS

CNS: headache, dizziness, syncope, weakness. **CV:** orthostatic hypotension, bradycardia, flushing, palpitations, peripheral edema. **EENT:** pharyngitis, rhinitis, SL burning. **GI:** nausea, vomiting, abdominal pain. **Respiratory:** dyspnea. **Skin:** contact dermatitis, rash. **Other:** hypersensitivity reactions.

INTERACTIONS

Drug-drug. *Alteplase:* May decrease tissue plasminogen activator antigen level. Avoid using together; if unavoidable, use lowest effective dose of nitroglycerin.
Antihypertensives: May increase hypotensive effect. Monitor BP closely.
Ergotamine, ergot derivatives: May diminish vasodilatory effect of nitroglycerin. Avoid combination.
Heparin: IV nitroglycerin may interfere with anticoagulant effect of heparin. Monitor PTT.
Nitric oxide: May increase risk of methemoglobinemia. Monitor therapy.
Riociguat: May cause hypotension. Use together is contraindicated.
Sildenafil, tadalafil, vardenafil: May cause severe hypotension. Use of nitrates in any form with these drugs is contraindicated.
Drug-lifestyle. *Alcohol use:* May increase hypotension. Discourage use together.

EFFECTS ON LAB TEST RESULTS

• May falsely decrease values in cholesterol determination tests using the Zlatkis-Zak color reaction.

CONTRAINDICATIONS & CAUTIONS

• Contraindicated in patients hypersensitive to drug.
• Contraindicated in patients with early MI (oral and sublingual), severe anemia, increased ICP, angle-closure glaucoma, orthostatic hypotension, allergy to adhesives (transdermal), or hypersensitivity to nitrates.
• IV nitroglycerin is contraindicated in patients hypersensitive to IV form and in those with cardiac tamponade, restrictive cardiomyopathy, or constrictive pericarditis.
• Use cautiously in patients with hypotension or volume depletion.
Dialyzable drug: Unknown.
⚠ *Overdose S&S:* Vasodilation, decreased cardiac output, venous pooling, severe hypotension, methemoglobinemia.

PREGNANCY-LACTATION-REPRODUCTION

• There are no adequate studies in pregnant women. Use only if clearly needed.
• It isn't known if drug appears in human milk. Use cautiously in breastfeeding women.

NURSING CONSIDERATIONS

• Closely monitor vital signs, particularly BP, during infusion, especially in patient with an MI. Excessive hypotension can worsen ischemia.
• Monitor BP and intensity and duration of drug response.
• Drug may cause headaches, especially at beginning of therapy. Dosage may be reduced temporarily, but tolerance usually develops. Treat headache with aspirin or acetaminophen.
• Tolerance to drug can be minimized with a 10- to 12-hour nitrate-free interval. To achieve this, remove the transdermal system in the early evening and apply a new system the next morning or omit the last daily dose of a buccal, sustained-release, or ointment form. Check with the prescriber for alterations in dosage regimen if tolerance is suspected.
• Wipe off nitroglycerin paste or remove patch before defibrillation to avoid patient burns.
• *Look alike–sound alike:* Don't confuse nitroglycerin with nitroprusside or

---

Reactions in bold italics are *life-threatening*. Interactions may have a *rapid onset* or a *delayed onset*.

nitrofurantoin. Don't confuse Nitroderm with Nicoderm.

PATIENT TEACHING

• Caution patient to take nitroglycerin regularly, as prescribed, and to have it accessible at all times.

⊙ Alert: Advise patient that stopping drug abruptly may cause coronary artery spasm.

• Teach patient how to give the prescribed form of nitroglycerin.

• Tell patient to take SL tablet at first sign of attack. Patient should wet the tablet with saliva, place it under the tongue until absorbed, and then sit down and rest. Patient may repeat dose every 5 minutes for a maximum of three doses. If drug doesn't provide relief, patient should obtain medical help promptly.

• Advise patient who complains of a tingling sensation with SL drug to try holding tablet in cheek.

• Tell patient not to use more than 3 packets of SL powder in a 15-minute period and to obtain medical help promptly if drug doesn't provide relief. Advise patient not to swallow or spit for 5 minutes after taking each packet.

• Tell patient to take oral tablets on an empty stomach either 30 minutes before or 1 to 2 hours after meals, to swallow oral tablets whole, and not to chew tablets.

• Remind patient using translingual aerosol form not to inhale the spray but to release it onto or under the tongue, and to wait about 10 seconds or so before swallowing.

• Tell patient to place the buccal tablet between the lip and gum above the incisors or between the cheek and gum. Tablets shouldn't be swallowed or chewed.

• Tell patient to take an additional dose before anticipated stress or at bedtime if chest pain occurs at night.

• Urge patient using skin patches to dispose of them carefully because enough medication remains after normal use to be hazardous to children and pets.

• If patients using skin patches are scheduled for an MRI scan, advise them to notify the facility that they are wearing a patch.

• Advise patient to avoid alcohol.

• To minimize dizziness when standing up, advise patient to rise slowly, to go up and down stairs carefully, and to lie down at the first sign of dizziness.

⊙ Alert: Advise patient that use of sildenafil, tadalafil, or vardenafil with any nitrate may cause life-threatening low BP. Use together is contraindicated.

• Tell patient to store drug in cool, dark place in a tightly closed container and to remove cotton from container because it absorbs drug.

• Tell patient to store SL tablets in original container or other container specifically approved for this use and to carry the container in a jacket pocket or purse, not in a pocket close to the body.

SAFETY ALERT!

nitroprusside sodium
nye-troe-PRUSS-ide

Nipride❋, Nitropress, Nipride RTU

Therapeutic class: Antihypertensives
Pharmacologic class: Vasodilators

AVAILABLE FORMS

Injection: 25 mg/mL, 10 mg/50 mL, 20 mg/100 mL, 50 mg/100 mL

INDICATIONS & DOSAGES

➤ **To lower BP quickly in hypertensive emergencies; to produce controlled hypotension to reduce bleeding during surgery; treatment of acute HF**

Adults and children: Begin infusion at 0.3 mcg/kg/minute IV and gradually titrate every few minutes (no less than 5 minutes) until desired effect is achieved or until the maximum dose of 10 mcg/kg/minute.

Adjust-a-dose: Patients also taking other antihypertensives are extremely sensitive to nitroprusside. Titrate dosage accordingly. Use with caution in patients with severe renal impairment or hepatic insufficiency; use minimum effective dose.

ADMINISTRATION

IV

▼ Prepare solution by dissolving 50 mg in 2 to 3 mL of D₅W injection or according to manufacturer's instructions.

Black Box Warning Drug isn't for direct injection and must be further diluted before infusion. Further dilute concentration in 250, 500, or 1,000 mL of D₅W to provide solutions with 200, 100, or 50 mcg/mL, respectively. ∎

Black Box Warning Immediately discontinue infusion if adequate BP reduction isn't obtained within 10 minutes at maximum dose. ∎

▼ Reconstitute ADD-Vantage vials labeled as containing 50 mg of drug according to manufacturer's directions.

▼ Because drug is sensitive to light, wrap solution in foil or other opaque material; it's not necessary to wrap the tubing. Fresh solution has a faint brownish tint. Discard if solution is discolored, particulate matter is visible, or if it's been 24 hours since dilution.

◑ *Alert:* Use an infusion pump. Drug is best given via piggyback through a peripheral line with no other drug. Don't titrate rate of main IV line while drug is being infused. Even a small bolus can cause severe hypotension.

Black Box Warning Use drug only when available equipment and personnel allow BP to be continuously monitored using either a continually reinflated sphygmomanometer or (preferably) an intra-arterial pressure sensor. ∎

▼ When drug is used to treat HF, titration of infusion rate must be guided by results of invasive hemodynamic monitoring with simultaneous monitoring of urine output.

▼ Confirm drug's effect at any infusion rate after an additional 5 minutes before titrating to a higher dose to achieve desired BP.

▼ If severe hypotension occurs, stop infusion; effects of drug quickly reverse. Notify prescriber.

▼ **Incompatibilities:** Other drugs.

ACTION
Relaxes arteriolar and venous smooth muscle.

Route	Onset	Peak	Duration
IV	Immediate	1–2 min	10 min

Half-life: 2 minutes.

ADVERSE REACTIONS
CNS: headache, dizziness, *increased ICP,* loss of consciousness, apprehension, restlessness. **CV:** *bradycardia,* hypotension, tachycardia, palpitations, ECG changes, flushing. **GI:** nausea, abdominal pain, ileus. **Hematologic:** *methemoglobinemia,* decreased platelet aggregation. **Metabolic:** acidosis, hypothyroidism. **Musculoskeletal:** muscle twitching. **Skin:** diaphoresis, pink color, rash. **Other:** *thiocyanate toxicity, cyanide toxicity,* venous streaking, irritation at IV site.

INTERACTIONS
Drug-drug. *Amphetamines, methylphenidate:* May decrease antihypertensive effect. Monitor BP.
Antipsychotics (second-generation, atypical), barbiturates, brimonidine (topical), diazoxide, duloxetine, ganglionic blockers, general anesthetics, levodopa, lormetazepam, negative inotropic drugs, pentoxifylline, prostacyclin analogues, other antihypertensives: May cause additive effects. Monitor BP closely.
Dapsone (topical), nitric oxide, prilocaine, sodium nitrite, tetracaine (topical): May enhance adverse/toxic effects. Monitor patient closely for hypoxia and cyanosis.
Riociguat, sildenafil, vardenafil: May increase hypotensive effects. Use together is contraindicated.

EFFECTS ON LAB TEST RESULTS
• May increase serum cyanide and creatinine levels.
• May decrease RBC and WBC counts.

CONTRAINDICATIONS & CAUTIONS
• Contraindicated in patients hypersensitive to drug.
• Contraindicated in patients with compensatory HTN (such as in arteriovenous shunt or coarctation of the aorta), inadequate cerebral circulation, acute HF with reduced peripheral vascular resistance (e.g., high-output HF in endotoxic sepsis), congenital optic atrophy, or tobacco-induced amblyopia, and in moribund patients coming to emergency surgery.
• Use with extreme caution in patients with increased ICP.

- Use cautiously in patients with hypothyroidism, hepatic or renal disease, hyponatremia, or low vitamin B level and in those who are poor surgical risks.

Dialyzable drug: Yes.

⚠ *Overdose S&S:* Hypotension, acidosis, cyanide or thiocyanate toxicity.

PREGNANCY-LACTATION-REPRODUCTION
- There are no adequate studies in pregnant women. Use only if clearly needed.
- It isn't known if drug appears in human milk. Patient should discontinue breastfeeding or discontinue drug.

NURSING CONSIDERATIONS

Black Box Warning Drug can cause severe hypotension, which can lead to ischemic injuries or death. Use drug only when available equipment and personnel allow BP to be continuously monitored. ∎

- Obtain baseline vital signs before giving drug; ascertain parameters prescriber wants to achieve. Monitor BP continuously. Patients receiving other antihypertensives may be more sensitive to drug.
- Keep patient in supine position when starting therapy or titrating drug.

Black Box Warning Giving excessive doses of 500 mcg/kg delivered faster than 2 mcg/kg/minute or using maximum infusion rate of 10 mcg/kg/minute for more than 10 minutes can cause cyanide toxicity. ∎

Black Box Warning Although acid-base balance and venous oxygen concentration should be monitored and may indicate cyanide toxicity, these lab tests provide imperfect guidance. ∎

☝ *Alert:* If patient is at risk, check thiocyanate level every 72 hours. Level higher than 100 mcg/mL may be toxic. If profound hypotension, metabolic acidosis, dyspnea, headache, confusion, loss of consciousness, ataxia, or vomiting occurs, stop drug immediately and notify prescriber.

- *Look alike–sound alike:* Don't confuse nitroprusside with nitroglycerin.

PATIENT TEACHING
- Instruct patient to report all adverse reactions promptly, especially signs and symptoms of hypotension and cyanide toxicity.

- Tell patient to alert nurse if discomfort occurs at IV insertion site.

SAFETY ALERT!

nivolumab ☒
neh-VOL-you-mab

Opdivo

Therapeutic class: Antineoplastics
Pharmacologic class: Monoclonal antibodies

AVAILABLE FORMS
Injection: 40 mg/4 mL, 100 mg/10 mL

INDICATIONS & DOSAGES

Adjust-a-dose (for all indications): Refer to manufacturer's instructions for dosage adjustments for adverse reactions and treatment-related toxicities.

➤ **Unresectable or metastatic melanoma; adjuvant treatment of melanoma with lymph node involvement or metastatic disease in patients who have undergone complete resection**

Adults: 240 mg IV infusion every 2 weeks or 480 mg every 4 weeks until disease progression or unacceptable toxicity occurs.

➤ **Metastatic NSCLC with progression on or after platinum-based chemotherapy; patients with epidermal growth factor receptor (*EGFR*) or *ALK* genomic tumor aberrations should have disease progression on FDA-approved therapy for these aberrations before nivolumab ☒**

Adults: 240 mg IV infusion every 2 weeks or 480 mg every 4 weeks until disease progression or unacceptable toxicity occurs.

➤ **Unresectable or metastatic melanoma, in combination with ipilimumab**

Adults: 1 mg/kg IV infusion over 30 minutes followed by ipilimumab 3 mg/kg IV infusion over 90 minutes on the same day, every 3 weeks for a maximum of four doses or until unacceptable toxicity; then nivolumab 240 mg IV infusion every 2 weeks or 480 mg every 4 weeks until disease progression or unacceptable toxicity.

➤ **Advanced renal carcinoma in patients who have received prior anti-angiogenic therapy**

N

Adults: 240 mg IV infusion once every 2 weeks or 480 mg every 4 weeks until disease progression or unacceptable toxicity occurs.

➤ **Intermediate or poor risk, previously untreated advanced renal cell carcinoma, in combination with ipilimumab**
Adults: 3 mg/kg IV infusion over 30 minutes followed by ipilimumab 1 mg/kg IV infusion over 30 minutes on the same day every 3 weeks for four doses; then nivolumab 240 mg as a single-agent IV infusion every 2 weeks or 480 mg every 4 weeks over 30 minutes until disease progression or unacceptable toxicity.

➤ **Classical Hodgkin lymphoma that has relapsed or progressed after autologous hematopoietic stem cell transplantation (HSCT) and posttransplantation brentuximab vedotin; after three or more lines of systemic therapy that includes autologous HSCT; recurrent or metastatic squamous cell carcinoma of the head and neck with disease progression on or after platinum-based therapy**
Adults: 240 mg IV infusion every 2 weeks or 480 mg every 4 weeks until disease progression or unacceptable toxicity.

➤ **Locally advanced or metastatic urothelial carcinoma in patients with disease progression during or after platinum-containing chemotherapy, or who have disease progression within 12 months of neoadjuvant or adjuvant treatment with a platinum-containing chemotherapy**
Adults: 240 mg IV infusion every 2 weeks or 480 mg every 4 weeks until disease progression or unacceptable toxicity occurs.

➤ **Microsatellite instability-high (MSI-H) or mismatch repair deficient (dMMR) metastatic colorectal cancer that has progressed following treatment with a fluoropyrimidine, oxaliplatin, and irinotecan**
Adults and children age 12 and older: 240 mg IV infusion every 2 weeks until disease progression or unacceptable toxicity occurs.

➤ **MSI-H or dMMR metastatic colorectal cancer that has progressed after treatment with a fluoropyrimidine, oxaliplatin, and irinotecan in combination with ipilimumab**
Adults and children age 12 and older: 3 mg/kg IV infusion over 30 minutes, followed by ipilimumab 1 mg/kg IV infusion over 30 minutes on the same day, every 3 weeks for four doses, then nivolumab 240 mg as a single-agent IV infusion over 30 minutes every 2 weeks until disease progression or unacceptable toxicity occurs.

➤ **Hepatocellular carcinoma in patients previously treated with sorafenib**
Adults: 240 mg IV infusion every 2 weeks or 480 mg every 4 weeks until disease progression or unacceptable toxicity occurs.

➤ **Metastatic small-cell lung cancer with progression after platinum-based chemotherapy and at least one other line of therapy**
Adults: 240 mg IV infusion over 30 minutes every 2 weeks until disease progression or unacceptable toxicity.

ADMINISTRATION
IV
▼ When administering with ipilimumab, infuse nivolumab first followed by ipilimumab on the same day. Use separate infusion bags and filters for each infusion.
▼ Visually inspect for particulate matter and discoloration (solution should be clear to opalescent, colorless to pale yellow).
▼ Store vial refrigerated at 36° to 46° F (2° to 8° C). Don't freeze.
▼ Protect from light by storing in original package until time of use.
▼ To prepare: Withdraw required volume of nivolumab and dilute with NSS or 5% dextrose injection to yield a final concentration of 1 to 10 mg/mL. Don't exceed total volume of 160 mL. For patients weighing less than 40 kg, the total volume mustn't exceed 4 mL/kg of body weight. Mix by gentle inversion; don't shake.
▼ Discard all partially used or empty vials.
▼ Diluted solution is stable at room temperature for no more than 8 hours, including room temperature storage of infusion in the IV container and time for administration of infusion.
▼ Diluted solution is stable under refrigeration (36° to 46° F [2° to 8° C]) for no more than 24 hours from time of infusion preparation. Don't freeze.

▼ Give through IV line containing a sterile, nonpyrogenic, low-protein-binding in-line filter (pore size, 0.2 to 1.2 microns) over 30 minutes.

▼ Flush IV line at end of infusion.

▼ **Incompatibilities:** Don't administer with other drugs through same IV line.

ACTION

A humanized monoclonal antibody that binds to the PD1 receptor found on the surface of T cells, reversing T-cell suppression and resulting in decreased tumor growth.

Route	Onset	Peak	Duration
IV	Unknown	Unknown	Unknown

Half-life: About 25 days.

ADVERSE REACTIONS

CNS: dizziness, peripheral and sensory neuropathy, fatigue, headache, neuritis, asthenia. **CV:** peripheral edema, *ventricular arrhythmia,* chest pain. **EENT:** iridocyclitis, stomatitis. **GI:** abdominal pain, colitis, nausea, vomiting, constipation, diarrhea, stomatitis. **GU:** renal dysfunction, nephritis, renal insufficiency. **Hematologic:** anemia, lymphopenia, thrombocytopenia, *neutropenia.* **Hepatic:** increased AST, ALT, and alkaline phosphatase levels; *hepatitis.* **Metabolic:** hyponatremia, *hyperkalemia, hypokalemia,* hyperglycemia, hypercalcemia, *hypocalcemia, hypomagnesemia,* weight loss, decreased appetite. **Respiratory:** cough, URI, dyspnea, pneumonitis, *ILD,* pleural effusion. **Skin:** rash, pruritus, exfoliative dermatitis, *erythema multiforme,* psoriasis, skin depigmentation. **Musculoskeletal:** pain. **Other:** infusion-related reactions, thyroiditis, fever.

INTERACTIONS

Drug-drug. *Immunosuppressants:* May diminish therapeutic effect of nivolumab. Consider therapy modification.

EFFECTS ON LAB TEST RESULTS

• May increase creatinine, total bilirubin, potassium, amylase, lipase, ALT, AST, alkaline phosphatase, glucose, triglyceride, cholesterol, and thyroid function levels.

• May decrease sodium, thyroid, and magnesium level.

• May increase or decrease potassium and calcium levels.

• May decrease RBC, lymphocyte, neutrophil, and platelet counts.

CONTRAINDICATIONS & CAUTIONS

• Contraindicated in patients hypersensitive to drug or its components.

🛈 *Alert:* If nivolumab is withheld for an adverse reaction, also withhold ipilimumab.

🛈 *Alert:* Drug can cause severe immune-mediated pneumonitis or ILD, which can be fatal.

• Drug can cause the following immune-mediated conditions: colitis, hepatitis, nephritis, and renal dysfunction, hypothyroidism and hyperthyroidism, life-threatening rash, encephalitis, and other serious adverse reactions.

• Drug can cause hypophysitis and adrenal insufficiency.

• Nivolumab shouldn't be used for the treatment of multiple myeloma. The use of nivolumab in combination with a thalidomide analogue plus dexamethasone showed an increased risk of mortality in clinical trials. This combination isn't recommended outside the setting of a clinical trial.

• Drug hasn't been studied in patients with moderate or severe hepatic impairment.

• Safety and effectiveness in children haven't been established.

Dialyzable drug: Unknown.

PREGNANCY-LACTATION-REPRODUCTION

🛈 *Alert:* Use cautiously in pregnant women. Drug may cause fetal harm and increase risk of abortion and premature infant death.

• Women of childbearing potential should use effective contraception during treatment and for at least 5 months after last dose.

• It isn't known if drug appears in human milk. Patient should discontinue breastfeeding during treatment because of possible serious adverse effects in breastfeeding infants.

NURSING CONSIDERATIONS

• Infusion-related reactions, which can be severe or life-threatening, can occur. Discontinue drug for severe or life-threatening reactions. For mild to moderate reactions,

N

either interrupt infusion or decrease infusion rate.

• Drug can cause type 1 diabetes mellitus. Monitor glucose levels and withhold drug for severe hyperglycemia until metabolic control is achieved; permanently discontinue for life-threatening hyperglycemia.

• Monitor patients for acute GVHD and hepatic veno-occlusive disease. Transplant-related mortality has occurred.

• Monitor patient for signs and symptoms of immune-mediated severe pneumonitis or ILD (fever, cough, dyspnea, chest pain) or colitis (fever, abdominal pain, diarrhea, bloody stools). Adjust dosage or discontinue drug as needed. Refer to manufacturer's instructions for corticosteroid treatment if indicated.

• Obtain LFT values at baseline and monitor periodically during treatment because of risk of immune-mediated hepatitis. Adjust dosages or discontinue drug as needed. Refer to manufacturer's instructions for corticosteroid treatment if indicated.

• Obtain serum creatinine level at baseline and monitor periodically during treatment because of risk of immune-mediated nephritis and renal dysfunction. Adjust dosages or discontinue drug as needed. Refer to manufacturer's instructions for corticosteroid treatment if indicated.

• Monitor thyroid function at baseline and periodically during treatment because of risk of immune-mediated hypothyroidism and hyperthyroidism. Administer hormone replacement therapy for hypothyroidism, or initiate medical management for control of hyperthyroidism. There are no recommended nivolumab dosage adjustments for hypothyroidism or hyperthyroidism.

• Monitor patient for other immune-mediated adverse reactions, which may occur during or after nivolumab has been discontinued. Rule out other causes of reactions first. Based on severity of reaction, withhold drug, administer corticosteroids, or initiate hormone-replacement therapy, if appropriate.

• *Look alike–sound alike:* Don't confuse Opdivo with Optivite or Osphena. Don't confuse nivolumab with Nabilone, natalizumab, nebivolol, nepafenac, NephPlex, or nofetumomab.

PATIENT TEACHING

• Instruct patient to inform prescriber if patient has known disease that affects the immune system, lungs, liver, or kidney or has had an organ transplant.

• Educate patient and family to recognize and immediately report signs and symptoms of pneumonitis (new or worsening cough, chest pain, shortness of breath), colitis (diarrhea, bloody stools, dark tarry stools, severe abdominal pain or tenderness), hepatic dysfunction (dark urine, yellowing of eyes, nausea, vomiting, right-sided abdominal pain, lethargy, easy bruising or bleeding), renal dysfunction (decreased urine output, blood in urine, edema, loss of appetite), hormone gland problems (weight gain or loss, feeling hot or cold, constipation, persistent or unusual headaches, extreme fatigue, changes in mood or behavior, dizziness, hair loss, deepening voice), rash, vision changes, severe or persistent muscle or joint pains, or severe muscle weakness.

◑ *Alert:* Warn pregnant patient of the possibility of fetal harm. Advise female patient of childbearing potential to use effective contraception during and for at least 5 months after last dose.

• Advise female patient to report known or suspected pregnancy to prescriber.

• Caution female patient not to breastfeed while taking drug.

• Reinforce importance of lab tests and instruct patient to keep follow-up appointments to monitor drug's safety and effectiveness.

norelgestromin–ethinyl estradiol transdermal system
nor-el-JES-troe-min/ETH-i-nill ess-tra-DYE-ole

Xulane

Therapeutic class: Contraceptives
Pharmacologic class: Estrogen–progestin combinations

AVAILABLE FORMS
Transdermal patch: norelgestromin 4.86 mg and ethinyl estradiol 0. 53 mg per patch, delivering 150 mcg norelgestromin and 35 mcg ethinyl estradiol daily

---

INDICATIONS & DOSAGES
➤ Contraception
Women of childbearing potential: Apply
1 patch weekly for 3 weeks (21 total days).
Apply each new patch on the same day of the
week. Week 4 is patch-free, and withdrawal
bleeding is expected. On the day after week
4 ends, apply a new patch to start a new
4-week cycle. The patch-free interval between cycles should never be longer than
7 days.

ADMINISTRATION
Transdermal
• Apply patch to a clean, dry area of the skin
on the buttocks, abdomen, upper outer arm,
or upper torso. Don't apply to the breasts or
to skin that is red, irritated, or cut, or on the
same location as the previous patch.
• Don't cut, damage, or alter the size of the
patch, as contraception may be impaired.

ACTION
Combination hormonal contraceptives act
by suppressing gonadotropins. The primary
mechanism of this action is ovulation inhibition. However, changes in cervical mucus
increase the difficulty of sperm entry into the
uterus, and changes in the endometrium decrease the likelihood of implantation.

Route	Onset	Peak	Duration
Transdermal	Rapid	2 days	Unknown

Half-life: Norelgestromin, 28 hours; ethinyl
estradiol, about 17 hours.

ADVERSE REACTIONS
CNS: headache, emotional lability, dizziness, fatigue, migraine, anxiety. **CV:** increased BP, *PE.* **EENT:** contact lens intolerance, changes in corneal curvature. **GI:**
nausea, diarrhea, abdominal pain, vomiting,
abdominal distention, cholestatic jaundice.
GU: dysmenorrhea, changes in menstrual
flow, vulvovaginal candidiasis, genital discharge, uterine spasm, vaginal dryness, vulvar dryness, premenstrual syndrome, libido
changes. **Metabolic:** weight changes, fluid
retention. **Skin:** application-site reaction,
melasma, pruritus, acne, dermatitis, erythema. **Other:** breast tenderness, enlargement, or secretion.

INTERACTIONS
Drug-drug. *Acetaminophen, clofibric acid,
morphine, salicylic acid, temazepam:* May
decrease levels or increase clearance of these
drugs. Monitor for lack of effect.
*Ampicillin, barbiturates, carbamazepine,
felbamate, griseofulvin, nevirapine, oxcarbazepine, phenylbutazone, phenytoin, rifampin, tetracyclines, topiramate:* May reduce contraceptive effectiveness, resulting
in unintended pregnancy or breakthrough
bleeding. Encourage backup method of contraception if used together.
Anticoagulants: May increase or decrease
effect of anticoagulant. Monitor patient and
lab values.
*Ascorbic acid, atorvastatin, etravirine, itra-
conazole, ketoconazole:* May increase hormone levels. Use together cautiously.
*Cyclosporine, prednisolone, theophylline,
tizanidine:* May increase levels of these
drugs. Monitor patient for adverse reactions.
HIV protease inhibitors: May affect contraceptive effectiveness and safety. Use together cautiously.
Ombitasvir, paritaprevir, ritonavir: May
cause elevated ALT level. Use is contraindicated.
Sugammadex: May decrease contraceptive
effectiveness. Patient should use backup
contraception while using sugammadex and
for 7 days after.
Drug-herb. *St. John's wort:* May reduce
effectiveness of drug. Don't use together.
Drug-lifestyle. Black Box Warning *Smoking:* May increase risk of CV adverse effects,
related to age and smoking 15 or more
cigarettes daily. Urge patient not to smoke. ∎

EFFECTS ON LAB TEST RESULTS
• May increase circulating total thyroid hormone, triglyceride, other binding protein,
sex hormone–binding globulin, total circulating endogenous sex steroid, corticoid, and
factor VII, VIII, IX, and X levels. May decrease antithrombin III and folate levels.
• May decrease free T_3 resin uptake and glucose tolerance.

CONTRAINDICATIONS & CAUTIONS
Black Box Warning Cigarette smoking
increases the risk of serious adverse cardiac effects from hormonal contraceptive

use. Risk increases with age, especially in women older than age 35, and with the number of cigarettes smoked. Hormonal contraceptives are contraindicated in women older than age 35 who smoke. ■

Black Box Warning There is an increased risk of venous thromboembolism in women ages 15 to 44 using the norelgestromin–ethinyl estradiol transdermal system compared to women using oral contraceptives containing 30 to 35 mcg of ethinyl estradiol and either levonorgestrel or norgestimate. ■

Black Box Warning The contraceptive patch has higher steady-state concentrations and lower peak concentrations than oral contraceptives. It's unknown whether there are changes in the risk of serious adverse events based on the differences in pharmacokinetic profiles of ethinyl estradiol in women using the contraceptive patch compared with women using oral contraceptives containing ethinyl estradiol 30 to 35 mcg. Increased estrogen exposure may increase the risk of adverse events, including venous thromboembolism. ■

• Contraindicated in patients hypersensitive to components of drug; in those with history of DVT or related disorder; in patients at high risk for arterial or venous thrombotic diseases or with current or past history of cerebrovascular disease or CAD; in those with uncontrolled HTN and inherited or acquired hypercoagulopathies; and in patients with headaches with focal neurologic conditions, migraine headaches with aura, or migraine headaches if older than age 35.

• Contraindicated in patients with past or current known or suspected breast cancer or other known or suspected estrogen- or progestin-sensitive neoplasia and in those with hepatic adenoma or cancer.

• Contraindicated in patients with thrombophlebitis, thromboembolic disorders, valvular heart disease with complications, diabetes with vascular involvement, major surgery with prolonged immobilization, undiagnosed abnormal genital bleeding, cholestatic jaundice of pregnancy or jaundice with previous hormonal contraceptive use, benign or malignant liver tumors or liver disease, or acute or chronic hepatocellular disease with abnormal hepatic function.

• Contraindicated with hepatitis C drug combinations containing ombitasvir/paritaprevir/ritonavir, with or without dasabuvir, due to potential for ALT elevations.

• Use cautiously in patients with CV disease risk factors, conditions that might be aggravated by fluid retention, or history of depression.

Dialyzable drug: Unknown.

⚠ *Overdose S&S:* Nausea, vomiting, withdrawal uterine bleeding.

PREGNANCY-LACTATION-REPRODUCTION

• Contraindicated in women who are or may be pregnant. Studies haven't shown an increased risk of birth defects when drug was inadvertently taken during early pregnancy.

• Breastfeeding women should use alternative forms of contraception until infant is completely weaned.

• In women who choose not to breastfeed, don't begin drug until 4 weeks after childbirth.

NURSING CONSIDERATIONS

🕓 *Alert:* Patients taking combination hormonal contraceptives may be at increased risk for thrombophlebitis, venous thrombosis with or without embolism, PE, MI, cerebral hemorrhage, cerebral thrombosis, HTN, gallbladder disease, hepatic adenomas, benign liver tumors, mesenteric thrombosis, and retinal thrombosis.

• Increased risk of MI occurs primarily in smokers and women with HTN, hypercholesterolemia, morbid obesity, and diabetes.

• Encourage women with a history of HTN or renal disease to use a different contraceptive. If this drug is used, monitor BP closely and stop use if HTN occurs.

• Drug may be less effective in women who weigh 90 kg or more.

• The risk of thromboembolic disease increases if therapy is used postpartum or postabortion.

• Rule out pregnancy if withdrawal bleeding fails to occur for two consecutive cycles.

• If skin becomes irritated, the patch may be removed and a new patch applied at a different site.

• Stop drug and notify prescriber at least 4 weeks before and for 2 weeks after an elective surgery that increases the risk of thromboembolism, and during and after prolonged immobilization. Teach patient about alternative methods of contraception during this time.

• Stop drug and notify prescriber if patient has headaches, vision loss, proptosis, diplopia, papilledema, retinal vascular lesions, jaundice, or depression.

PATIENT TEACHING
• Emphasize the importance of having regular annual physical exams to check for adverse effects or developing contraindications.

• Tell patient that drug doesn't protect against HIV and other sexually transmitted diseases.

• Advise patient to initiate and apply patch on the first day of menstrual cycle and then on the same day each week.

• Advise patient to use a backup method of contraception for the first 7 days.

• Tell patient switching from estrogen–progestin oral contraceptives to apply first patch on the first day of withdrawal bleeding. If no bleeding occurs within 5 days of last hormonally active pill, advise patient to obtain a pregnancy test.

• Advise patient to immediately apply a new patch once the used patch is removed, on the same day of the week every 7 days for 3 weeks. Week 4 is patch-free. Withdrawal bleeding is expected to occur during this time.

• Tell patient to apply each patch to a clean, dry area of the skin on the buttocks, abdomen, upper outer arm, or upper torso. Tell patient not to apply to the breasts or to skin that's red, irritated, or cut, or on the same location as the previous patch.

• Tell patient to carefully fold the used patch in half so that it sticks to itself before discarding.

• Tell female patient to immediately stop use if pregnancy is confirmed.

• Tell patient who wears contact lenses to report visual changes or changes in lens tolerance.

• Advise patient not to smoke while using the patch.

• Tell patient that if a patch becomes detached for less than 1 day, to reapply it or replace it immediately and continue the schedule. If the patch is detached for more than 1 day, a new cycle should be started and back-up contraception should be used for the first week.

• Stress that if patient isn't sure what to do about mistakes with patch use, she should use a backup method of birth control and contact her health care provider.

• Tell patient undergoing an MRI scan to alert facility that she's using a transdermal patch.

• Advise patient to report all drugs and supplements she is taking as some can decrease contraceptive effectiveness; a backup contraceptive method may be needed.

• Advise female patient on thyroid hormone replacement therapy that she may require increased doses of thyroid hormone medication.

SAFETY ALERT!

norepinephrine bitartrate (levarterenol bitartrate, noradrenaline acid tartrate)
nor-ep-i-NEF-rin

Levophed

Therapeutic class: Vasopressors
Pharmacologic class: Alpha/beta agonists

AVAILABLE FORMS
Injection: 1 mg/mL

INDICATIONS & DOSAGES
➤ **To restore BP in acute hypotension; severe hypotension during cardiac arrest**
Adults: Initially, 8 to 12 mcg/minute by IV infusion; then titrate to maintain systolic BP at 80 to 100 mm Hg in previously normotensive patients and 40 mm Hg below preexisting systolic BP in previously hypertensive patients. Average maintenance dose is 2 to 4 mcg/minute.

ADMINISTRATION
IV
▼ Use a central venous catheter (preferred) or large vein, such as the antecubital fossa,

to minimize risk of extravasation. Give in D₅W alone or D₅W in NSS for injection. Use continuous infusion pump to regulate infusion flow rate and a piggyback setup so IV line stays open if norepinephrine is stopped.

▼ Never leave patient unattended during infusion. Check BP every 2 minutes until stabilized; then check every 5 minutes.

▼ During infusion, frequently monitor ECG, cardiac output, central venous pressure, pulmonary artery wedge pressure, pulse rate, urine output, and color and temperature of limbs. Titrate infusion rate based on findings and prescriber guidelines.

Black Box Warning Check site frequently for signs and symptoms of extravasation. If they appear, stop infusion immediately and call prescriber. To prevent sloughing and necrosis, use a fine hypodermic needle to infiltrate area with 5 to 10 mg phentolamine in 10 to 15 mL of NSS as soon as possible. Immediate local hyperemic changes will occur if area is infiltrated within 12 hours. Also, check for blanching along course of infused vein, which may progress to superficial sloughing. ■

▼ Protect drug from light. Discard discolored solution or solution that contains precipitate. Solution will deteriorate after 24 hours.

▼ If prolonged therapy is needed, change injection site frequently.

▼ Avoid mixing with alkaline solutions, oxidizing drugs, or iron salts. The use of NSS alone isn't recommended because of the lack of oxidation protection.

▼ **Incompatibilities:** Alkalis, drotrecogin alfa, iron salts, oxidizers, regular insulin, thiopental.

ACTION

Stimulates alpha and beta₁ receptors in the sympathetic nervous system, causing vasoconstriction and cardiac stimulation.

Route	Onset	Peak	Duration
IV	Immediate	Immediate	1–2 min after infusion

Half-life: About 1 minute.

ADVERSE REACTIONS

CNS: headache, anxiety. **CV:** *bradycardia, severe HTN, arrhythmias, ischemic injury.* **Respiratory:** respiratory difficulties. **Skin:** irritation with extravasation, necrosis and gangrene secondary to extravasation. **Other:** *anaphylaxis.*

INTERACTIONS

Drug-drug. *Alpha blockers:* May antagonize drug effects. Monitor perfusion and BP. *Antihistamines, atropine, ergot alkaloids, guanethidine, imipramine, linezolid, MAO inhibitors, methyldopa, oxytocics, TCAs:* May cause severe HTN. Use together with extreme caution.
Atomoxetine: May enhance hypertensive and tachycardic effects. Monitor BP and HR.
Inhaled anesthetics: May increase risk of arrhythmias. Don't use together.
TCAs: May potentiate the pressor response and cause arrhythmias. Use together cautiously.

EFFECTS ON LAB TEST RESULTS
None reported.

CONTRAINDICATIONS & CAUTIONS
● Contraindicated in patients with mesenteric or peripheral vascular thrombosis (unless drug is deemed necessary as a life-saving procedure), profound hypoxia, hypercarbia, or hypotension resulting from blood volume deficit (except as an emergency measure).
● Contraindicated during cyclopropane and halothane anesthesia due to risk of ventricular arrhythmias.
● Use cautiously in patients with sulfite sensitivity.
Dialyzable drug: Unknown.
⚠ *Overdose S&S:* Headache, severe HTN, reflex bradycardia, increased peripheral resistance, decreased cardiac output.

PREGNANCY-LACTATION-REPRODUCTION
● Safe use in pregnancy hasn't been established. Use in pregnant women only if clearly needed.
● It isn't known if drug appears in human milk. Use cautiously in breastfeeding women.

Reactions in bold italics are *life-threatening*. Interactions may have a *rapid onset* or a *delayed onset*.

NURSING CONSIDERATIONS

• Drug isn't a substitute for blood or fluid replacement therapy. If patient has volume deficit, replace fluids before giving vasopressors.

• Keep emergency drugs on hand to reverse effects of drug: atropine for reflex bradycardia, phentolamine to decrease vasopressor effects, and propranolol for arrhythmias.

• Notify prescriber immediately of decreased urine output.

• When stopping drug, gradually slow infusion rate. Continue monitoring vital signs, watching for possible severe drop in BP.

↻ Alert: Monitor infusion site carefully as extravasation can cause tissue necrosis.

• **Look alike–sound alike:** Don't confuse norepinephrine with epinephrine.

PATIENT TEACHING

• Tell patient to report adverse reactions promptly.

• Advise patient that vital signs will be monitored frequently and to immediately report discomfort at IV insertion site.

---

norethindrone
nor-ETH-in-drone

Camila, Errin, Heather, Incassia, Jencycla, Movisse✤, Nor-QD

norethindrone acetate
Aygestin, Norlutate✤

Therapeutic class: Contraceptives
Pharmacologic class: Progestins

AVAILABLE FORMS
norethindrone
Tablets: 0.35 mg
norethindrone acetate
Tablets: 5 mg

INDICATIONS & DOSAGES

➤ **Amenorrhea, abnormal uterine bleeding**
Women: 2.5 to 10 mg norethindrone acetate PO daily for 5 to 10 days, beginning in the assumed latter half of the menstrual cycle.

➤ **Endometriosis**
Women: 5 mg norethindrone acetate PO daily for 14 days; then increased by

2.5 mg/day every 2 weeks, up to 15 mg daily. Therapy may continue for 6 to 9 months or until breakthrough bleeding warrants temporary termination.

➤ **Contraception**
Women of childbearing potential and menarchal girls: Initially, 0.35 mg norethindrone PO on first day of menstruation; then 0.35 mg daily.

ADMINISTRATION
PO
• When used for contraception, give drug at same time every day, continuously, with no interruption between pill packs.

• Give norethindrone acetate without regard to meals. May give with food if GI upset occurs.

ACTION

Suppresses ovulation, possibly by inhibiting pituitary gonadotropin secretion, and forms thick cervical mucus.

Route	Onset	Peak	Duration
PO	Unknown	2 hr	Unknown

Half-life: 8 to 10 hours.

ADVERSE REACTIONS

CNS: depression, *stroke,* headache, mood swings, dizziness, fatigue, insomnia, migraine, nervousness. **CV:** thrombophlebitis, *PE,* edema, *thromboembolism.* **GI:** bloating, abdominal pain or cramping nausea, vomiting. **GU:** breakthrough bleeding, dysmenorrhea, amenorrhea, cervical erosion, abnormal secretions. **Hepatic:** cholestatic jaundice. **Metabolic:** weight changes. **Skin:** melasma, rash, acne, pruritus, alopecia, hirsutism, hemorrhagic skin eruptions. **Other:** breast tenderness, enlargement, or secretion; premenstrual-like syndrome, *anaphylactic reactions.*

INTERACTIONS

Drug-drug. *Barbiturates, carbamazepine, fosphenytoin, phenytoin, rifampin:* May decrease progestin effects. Monitor patient for diminished therapeutic response.
Ulipristal: May decrease effectiveness of both drugs. Avoid norethindrone within 5 days of stopping ulipristal.

N

Drug-lifestyle. *Smoking:* May increase risk of adverse CV effects. If smoking continues, may need alternative therapy.

EFFECTS ON LAB TEST RESULTS
• May increase LFT values. May alter thyroid function tests.
• May decrease metyrapone test results and HDL levels. May increase LDL/HDL ratio.

CONTRAINDICATIONS & CAUTIONS
• Contraindicated in patients hypersensitive to drug and in those with breast cancer, undiagnosed abnormal vaginal bleeding, impaired liver function or hepatic disease, benign or malignant liver tumors, current or recent thromboembolic disorders (stroke, MI), or active DVT, PE, or history of these conditions.
• Use cautiously in patients with diabetes, seizures, migraines, cardiac or renal disease, asthma, and depression.
◆ *Alert:* Norethindrone acetate may cause papilledema or retinal vascular lesions. If these occur, discontinue drug.
Dialyzable drug: Unknown.

PREGNANCY-LACTATION-REPRODUCTION
• Contraindicated in pregnant women or as a diagnostic test for pregnancy; may cause fetal harm.
• Use cautiously in breastfeeding women.

NURSING CONSIDERATIONS
• If switching from combined oral contraceptives to progestin-only pills (POPs), take the first POP the day after the last active combined pill.
• If switching from POPs to combined pills, take the first active combined pill on the first day of menstruation, even if the POP pack isn't finished.
◆ *Alert:* Norethindrone acetate is twice as potent as norethindrone. Norethindrone acetate shouldn't be used for contraception.
• Patients with menstrual disorders usually need preliminary estrogen treatment.
• Watch patient closely for signs of edema.
• Monitor BP.

PATIENT TEACHING
• According to FDA regulations, patient must read package insert explaining possible adverse effects before receiving first dose. Also, give patient verbal explanation.
• Tell patient to take drug at the same time every day when used as a contraceptive. If she's more than 3 hours late taking the pill or if she has missed a pill, she should take the pill as soon as she remembers, and then continue the normal schedule. Also tell her to use a backup method of contraception for the next 48 hours.
◆ *Alert:* Tell patient to report unusual symptoms immediately and to stop drug and notify prescriber about visual disturbances or migraine, or pain or numbness in her arms or legs.
• Teach patient how to perform routine breast self-exam.
• Tell patient to report suspected pregnancy to prescriber.
• Encourage patient to stop or reduce smoking because of the risk of CV complications.
• Tell patient with diabetes that glucose levels may be affected and to closely monitor her levels.
• Advise patient to immediately report sudden partial or complete loss of vision, diplopia, migraine, or bulging of the eye.
• Tell patient that drug does not protect against HIV or other sexually transmitted diseases.
• Tell patient that if she vomits soon after taking a pill to use a back-up method of birth control for 48 hours.

---

nortriptyline hydrochloride ◙
nor-TRIP-ti-leen

Aventyl✣, Pamelor✑

Therapeutic class: Antidepressants
Pharmacologic class: TCAs

AVAILABLE FORMS
Capsules: 10 mg, 25 mg, 50 mg, 75 mg
Oral solution: 10 mg/5 mL*

INDICATIONS & DOSAGES
➤ **Depression**
Adults: 25 mg PO t.i.d. or q.i.d., gradually increased to maximum of 150 mg daily. Or, give total daily dose at bedtime.

Elderly patients and adolescents: 30 to 50 mg PO daily given once or in divided doses.

ADMINISTRATION
PO
• Give drug without regard for food.
• Whenever possible, give full dose at bedtime.

ACTION
Unknown. Increases the amount of norepinephrine, serotonin, or both in the CNS by blocking reuptake by the presynaptic neurons.

Route	Onset	Peak	Duration
PO	Unknown	4–9 hr	Unknown

Half-life: 14 to 51 hours.

ADVERSE REACTIONS
CNS: *stroke,* numbness, tingling, paresthesia of extremities, incoordination, ataxia, tremors, peripheral neuropathy, extrapyramidal symptoms, *seizures,* alteration in EEG, confusional states with hallucinations, delusions, disorientation, panic, anxiety, restlessness, agitation, insomnia, nightmares, hypomania, exacerbation of psychosis, drowsiness, dizziness, weakness, fatigue, headache. **CV:** edema, hypotension, HTN, tachycardia, palpitations, *MI,* arrhythmias, *heart block,* flushing. **EENT:** blurred vision, disturbance of accommodation, mydriasis, tinnitus. **GI:** dry mouth, constipation, paralytic ileus, nausea and vomiting, anorexia, epigastric distress, diarrhea, peculiar taste, stomatitis, abdominal cramps, black tongue. **GU:** urine retention, delayed micturition, dilation of the urinary tract, erectile dysfunction, testicular swelling, urinary frequency, nocturia, increased or decreased libido. **Hematologic:** bone marrow depression, eosinophilia, purpura, *thrombocytopenia.* **Hepatic:** jaundice, altered liver function. **Metabolic:** weight gain or loss, SIADH. **Skin:** rash, petechiae, urticaria, itching, photosensitivity, alopecia, diaphoresis. **Other:** drug fever, gynecomastia, breast enlargement and galactorrhea in women, *suicidal ideation.*

INTERACTIONS
Drug-drug. *Barbiturates, CNS depressants:* May enhance CNS depression. Avoid using together.
Cimetidine, **fluoxetine, fluvoxamine, paroxetine, sertraline:** May increase nortriptyline level. Monitor drug levels and patient for signs of toxicity.
Clonidine: May cause life-threatening HTN. Avoid using together.
Drugs that prolong QT interval: May increase risk of life-threatening cardiac arrhythmias, including torsades de pointes. Monitor patient and ECG.
Epinephrine, norepinephrine: May increase hypertensive effect. Use together cautiously.
Linezolid, methylene blue: May cause serotonin syndrome. Use extreme caution and monitor patient closely.
MAO inhibitors: May cause severe excitation, hyperpyrexia, or seizures, usually with high doses. Avoid using within 14 days of MAO inhibitor therapy.
Quinolones: May increase the risk of life-threatening arrhythmias. Avoid using together.
Drug-herb. *Evening primrose oil:* May cause additive or synergistic effect, lowering seizure threshold and increasing the risk of seizure. Discourage use together.
St. John's wort, SAM-e, yohimbe: May cause serotonin syndrome and reduced drug level. Discourage use together.
Drug-lifestyle. *Alcohol use:* May enhance CNS depression. Discourage use together.
Smoking: May decrease drug level. Monitor patient for lack of effect.
Sun exposure: May increase risk of photosensitivity reactions. Advise patient to avoid excessive sunlight exposure.

EFFECTS ON LAB TEST RESULTS
• May increase or decrease glucose level.
• May increase eosinophil count and LFT values.
• May decrease WBC, RBC, granulocyte, and platelet counts.

CONTRAINDICATIONS & CAUTIONS
• Contraindicated in patients hypersensitive to drug and during acute recovery phase of MI; also contraindicated within 14 days of MAO inhibitor therapy.

Black Box Warning Nortriptyline isn't approved for use in children. ■

◑ *Alert:* Concomitant use with linezolid or methylene blue can cause serotonin syndrome (fever, mental status changes, muscle twitching, excessive sweating, shivering or shaking, diarrhea, loss of coordination). Use drug with linezolid or methylene blue only for life-threatening or urgent conditions when the potential benefits outweigh the risks of toxicity.

▨ Patients who are poor metabolizers of CYP2D6 have higher plasma concentration when given usual doses. Approximately 7% to 10% of Whites are poor metabolizers.

• Drug isn't approved for use in patients with bipolar depression. Screen for bipolar depression before starting drug.

• Use with extreme caution in patients with glaucoma, suicidal tendency, history of urine retention or seizures, CV disease, or hyperthyroidism and in those receiving thyroid drugs.

Dialyzable drug: No.

⚠ *Overdose S&S:* Cardiac arrhythmias, severe hypotension, shock, HF, pulmonary edema, seizures, CNS depression, coma, ECG changes, confusion, restlessness, disturbed concentration, transient visual hallucinations, dilated pupils, agitation, hyperactive reflexes, stupor, drowsiness, muscle rigidity, vomiting, hypothermia, hyperpyrexia.

PREGNANCY-LACTATION-REPRODUCTION

• Safe use during pregnancy and breastfeeding hasn't been established. Weigh potential benefits against possible hazards.

• Monitor pregnant women and breastfeeding infants for adverse reactions.

NURSING CONSIDERATIONS

◑ *Alert:* If linezolid or methylene blue must be given, stop nortriptyline and monitor patient for serotonin toxicity for 2 weeks or until 24 hours after the last dose of methylene blue or linezolid, whichever comes first. Treatment with nortriptyline may resume 24 hours after the last dose of methylene blue or linezolid.

• To withdraw drug, gradually taper dosage and monitor patient for reemerging symptoms.

• Because patients using TCAs may suffer hypertensive episodes during surgery, stop drug gradually several days before surgery.

• If signs or symptoms of psychosis occur or increase, expect to reduce dosage. Record mood changes. Monitor patient for suicidal tendencies; allow patient only a minimum supply of drug.

Black Box Warning Drug may increase the risk of suicidal thinking and behavior in children, adolescents, and young adults with major depressive disorder or other psychiatric disorder. ■

• *Look alike–sound alike:* Don't confuse nortriptyline with amitriptyline. Don't confuse Pamelor with Tambocor.

PATIENT TEACHING

Black Box Warning Advise families and caregivers to closely observe patient for increased suicidal thinking or behavior. ■

• Teach patient to recognize and immediately report signs and symptoms of serotonin syndrome (fever, mental status changes, muscle twitching, excessive sweating, shivering or shaking, diarrhea, loss of coordination).

• Advise patient to take full dose at bedtime whenever possible to reduce risk of dizziness upon standing quickly.

• Warn patient to avoid activities that require alertness and good coordination until effects of drug are known. Drowsiness and dizziness usually subside after a few weeks.

• Recommend use of sugarless hard candy or gum to relieve dry mouth. Saliva substitutes may be needed.

• Tell patient to consult prescriber before taking other prescription or OTC drugs.

• Warn patient not to stop drug suddenly.

• To prevent oversensitivity to the sun, advise patient to use sun block, wear protective clothing, and avoid prolonged exposure to strong sunlight.

Reactions in bold italics are *life-threatening*. Interactions may have a *rapid onset* or a *delayed onset*.

nystatin
nye-STAT-in

Nystop, Nyaderm✤

Therapeutic class: Antifungals
Pharmacologic class: Polyene macrolides

AVAILABLE FORMS
Cream: 25,000 units/g✤, 100,000 units/g
Ointment: 100,000 units/g
Oral suspension: 100,000 units/mL
Powder: 100,000 units/g
Tablets: 500,000 units

INDICATIONS & DOSAGES
➤ **Intestinal candidiasis**
Adults: 500,000 to 1 million units PO as
tablets t.i.d.
➤ **Mycotic infections**
Adults and children: Apply cream or ointment liberally to affected areas b.i.d. Or,
apply powder to lesions b.i.d. to t.i.d. until
lesions have healed.
➤ **Oral candidiasis (thrush)**
Adults and children: 400,000 to 600,000
units PO as oral suspension q.i.d. for up to
14 days.
Infants: 200,000 units PO as oral suspension
q.i.d.

ADMINISTRATION
PO
• To treat oral candidiasis, after patient's
mouth is clean of food debris, have patient
hold suspension in mouth for several minutes before swallowing. When treating infants, swab medication on oral mucosa.
• Shake suspension well before use.
• Suspension made with bulk powder contains no preservatives. Use immediately.
Don't store.
Topical
• Store at room temperature.
• For fungal infection of the feet, apply the
powder to feet and all footwear.

ACTION
Probably binds to sterols in fungal cell membrane, altering cell permeability and allowing leakage of intracellular components.

Route	Onset	Peak	Duration
PO, topical	24–72 hr	Unknown	Unknown

Half-life: Unknown.

ADVERSE REACTIONS
GI: transient nausea, vomiting, diarrhea,
GI upset. **GU:** irritation, sensitization, vulvovaginal burning (vaginal form). **Skin:**
rash.

INTERACTIONS
Drug-drug. *Progesterone:* May diminish
therapeutic effect of progesterone. Avoid
combination with vaginal use.

EFFECTS ON LAB TEST RESULTS
None reported.

CONTRAINDICATIONS & CAUTIONS
• Contraindicated in patients hypersensitive
to drug.
• Rarely, SJS has been reported.
• Don't use topical powder for the treatment
of systemic, oral, intravaginal, or ophthalmic
infections.
Dialyzable drug: Unknown.
⚠ **Overdose S&S:** Nausea, GI upset.
• **Look alike–sound alike:** Don't confuse ny-
statin with atorvastatin, fluvastatin, or any
other statins. Don't confuse nystatin with
Nitrostat.

PREGNANCY-LACTATION-REPRODUCTION
• Use cautiously in pregnant and breastfeeding women and only when clearly
needed.

NURSING CONSIDERATIONS
• Drug isn't effective against systemic infec-
tions.
• Monitor patient for rash.
• Avoid skin contact when applying.

PATIENT TEACHING
• Advise patient to continue taking drug for
at least 2 days after signs and symptoms resolve.
• Instruct patient to continue therapy during
menstruation.
• Advise patient to report redness, swelling,
or irritation.

N

- Tell patient that overusing mouthwash or wearing poorly fitting dentures may promote infection.
- For fungal foot infections, teach patient to dust powder freely on the feet and footwear.

SAFETY ALERT!

obinutuzumab
OH-bi-nue-TOOZ-ue-mab

Gazyva

Therapeutic class: Antineoplastics
Pharmacologic class: Monoclonal antibodies

AVAILABLE FORMS
Solution: 25 mg/mL (1,000 mg/40 mL)

INDICATIONS & DOSAGES
Adjust-a-dose (for all indications): Refer to manufacturer's instructions for toxicity-related dosage adjustments.
➤ **Chronic lymphocytic leukemia previously untreated, in combination with chlorambucil**
Adults: Each cycle lasts 28 days. Cycle 1, day 1: 100 mg IV at 25 mg/hour over 4 hours; don't increase infusion rate. Cycle 1, day 2: 900 mg IV at 50 mg/hour; may increase infusion rate in increments of 50 mg/hour every 30 minutes to maximum rate of 400 mg/hour. Cycle 1, days 8 and 15: If no infusion reaction occurred during previous infusion and final infusion rate was 100 mg/hour or faster, give 1,000 mg IV weekly at 100 mg/hour; may increase infusion rate by 100 mg/hour every 30 minutes to maximum rate of 400 mg/hour. For cycles 2 to 6 on day 1 only, give every 28 days for five doses: If no infusion reaction occurred during previous infusion and final infusion rate was 100 mg/hour or faster, give 1,000 mg IV at 100 mg/hour; may increase infusion rate in increments of 100 mg/hour every 30 minutes to maximum of 400 mg/hour.
If a dose is missed, administer dose as soon as possible and adjust future doses accordingly to maintain the time interval between chemotherapy cycles. If appropriate, patients who don't complete the day-1,

cycle-1 dose may proceed to the day-2, cycle-1 dose.
➤ **Follicular lymphoma, in combination with bendamustine followed by obinutuzumab monotherapy in patients who relapsed after, or are refractory to, a rituximab-containing regimen**
Adults: Each cycle lasts 28 days. Cycle 1, day 1: 1,000 mg IV at 50 mg/hour; may increase infusion rate in increments of 50 mg/hour every 30 minutes to maximum rate of 400 mg/hour. Cycle 1, days 8 and 15: If no infusion reaction occurred during previous infusion and final infusion rate was 100 mg/hour or faster, give 1,000 mg IV at 100 mg/hour; may increase infusion rate by 100 mg/hour every 30 minutes to maximum rate of 400 mg/hour. For cycles 2 to 6 on day 1 only: If no infusion reaction occurred during previous infusion and final infusion rate was 100 mg/hour or faster, give 1,000 mg IV at 100 mg/hour; may increase infusion rate in increments of 100 mg/hour every 30 minutes to maximum rate of 400 mg/hour. Give dose on day 1 every 28 days for five doses.

Give missed dose as soon as possible and adjust future doses accordingly to maintain the time interval between chemotherapy cycles. During monotherapy, maintain the original dosing schedule for subsequent doses.

Patients who achieve stable disease, complete response, or partial response to the initial 6 cycles of obinutuzumab in combination with bendamustine should continue on obinutuzumab 1,000 mg as monotherapy once every 2 months for 2 years, beginning approximately 2 months after last dose during the induction phase.
➤ **Previously untreated stage II bulky, III, or IV follicular lymphoma in combination with chemotherapy, followed by obinutuzumab monotherapy in patients achieving at least a partial remission**
Adults: Cycle 1, day 1: 1,000 mg IV at 50 mg/hour; may increase infusion rate in increments of 50 mg/hour every 30 minutes to maximum rate of 400 mg/hour. Cycle 1, days 8 and 15: If no infusion reaction occurred during previous infusion and final infusion rate was 100 mg/hour or faster, give 1,000 mg IV at 100 mg/hour; may increase infusion rate by 100 mg/hour every 30 minutes to maximum rate of 400 mg/hour.

For cycles 2 to 6 or 2 to 8, on day 1 only: If no infusion reaction occurred during previous infusion and final infusion rate was 100 mg/hour or faster, give 1,000 mg IV at 100 mg/hour; may increase infusion rate in increments of 100 mg/hour every 30 minutes to maximum rate of 400 mg/hour.

Treat concurrently with one of the following chemotherapy regimens: six 28-day cycles in combination with bendamustine; or six 21-day cycles in combination with cyclophosphamide, doxorubicin, vincristine, and prednisone, followed by two additional 21-day cycles of obinutuzumab alone; or eight 21-day cycles in combination with cyclophosphamide, vincristine, and prednisone.

Patients who achieve a complete response or partial response to the initial six or eight cycles of obinutuzumab should continue on obinutuzumab 1,000 mg as monotherapy once every 2 months, maintaining the original dosing schedule for up to 2 years.

Give missed dose as soon as possible and adjust future doses accordingly to maintain the time interval between chemotherapy cycles.

ADMINISTRATION

IV

🖐 **Alert:** Premedicate all patients with acetaminophen and an antihistamine (such as diphenhydramine) at least 30 minutes before infusion and a glucocorticoid (dexamethasone or methylprednisolone) at least 1 hour before each infusion to reduce infusion-related reactions. Refer to manufacturer's instructions for premedication dosage instructions.

▼ Store vials in refrigerator at 36° to 46° F (2° to 8° C).

▼ Protect vials from light; don't freeze or shake vials.

▼ Administer through a dedicated IV line; don't administer as an IV push or bolus.

▼ Solution should be used immediately but is stable in refrigerator for up to 24 hours followed by 48 hours (including infusion time) at room temperature.

▼ **Incompatibilities:** Don't mix with other drugs or solutions, other than NSS.

ACTION

Binds to CD20 antigen, mediating lysis of both normal and malignant B cells.

Route	Onset	Peak	Duration
IV	Rapid	Unknown	Unknown

Half-life: 25.5 to 35.3 days.

ADVERSE REACTIONS

CNS: pyrexia, asthenia, fatigue. **CV:** *worsening of cardiac conditions, causing death.* **EENT:** sinusitis, nasopharyngitis, nasal congestion. **GI:** nausea, vomiting, dyspepsia, diarrhea, constipation. **GU:** UTI. **Hematologic:** *neutropenia, lymphopenia, leukopenia, thrombocytopenia,* anemia. **Hepatic:** elevated ALT, AST, and alkaline phosphatase levels; *reactivation of HBV.* **Metabolic:** *hypocalcemia, hypokalemia, hyperkalemia,* hyponatremia, hypoalbuminemia. **Musculoskeletal:** bone and muscle pain, arthralgia, extremity pain, weakness. **Respiratory:** cough, URI. **Skin:** pruritus. **Other:** *infusion-related reaction, TLS, sepsis.*

INTERACTIONS

Drug-drug. *Alfuzosin, amifostine, antipsychotics (second generation [atypical]), barbiturates, brimonidine (topical), diazoxide, duloxetine, nicorandil, PDE5 inhibitors, pentoxifylline, prostacyclin analogues:* May increase risk of hypotension. Monitor therapy closely.

Anticoagulants, antiplatelet drugs (aspirin, NSAIDs): May increase risk of bleeding. Consider withholding anticoagulants, platelet inhibitors, or other medications that may increase bleeding risk, especially during first cycle. Monitor therapy closely.

Antihypertensives: May increase risk of hypotension. Consider withholding antihypertensives for 12 hours before, during, and for first hour after giving obinutuzumab.

Belimumab: May enhance adverse effects of belimumab. Avoid use together.

Deferiprone: May increase risk of neutropenia. Avoid use together.

Denosumab, natalizumab: May increase risk of serious infections. Monitor patient closely.

Fingolimod: May increase risk of immuno-suppression. Avoid use together if possible or consider therapy modification.

Inactivated vaccines: May diminish therapeutic effect of inactivated vaccines. Complete all appropriate vaccinations at least 2 weeks before starting drug. If patient is vaccinated during obinutuzumab therapy, revaccinate at least 3 months after drug is discontinued.

Leflunomide: May increase risk of hematologic toxicity. Monitor patient for bone marrow suppression at least monthly. Consider modifying leflunomide dosage.

Live-virus vaccines: May increase risk of infection. Live-virus vaccination isn't recommended during treatment and until B-cell recovery. Avoid use together.

Nivolumab: May diminish effect of nivolumab. Consider therapy modification.

Pimecrolimus, tacrolimus (topical): May enhance adverse effects of obinutuzumab. Avoid use together.

Roflumilast: May enhance immunosuppressive effect. Consider therapy modification.

Sipuleucel-T: May diminish effect of Sipuleucel-T. Monitor therapy closely.

Tofacitinib: May enhance immunosuppressive effect of tofacitinib. Avoid use together.

Trastuzumab: May enhance neutropenic effect of obinutuzumab. Monitor patient closely.

Drug-herb. *Echinacea:* May diminish therapeutic effect of obinutuzumab. Avoid use together.

EFFECTS ON LAB TEST RESULTS
• May increase creatinine, alkaline phosphatase, AST, and ALT levels.
• May decrease calcium, sodium, phosphate, and albumin levels.
• May increase or decrease potassium level.
• May decrease creatinine clearance.
• May decrease Hb level and WBC, lymphocyte, and platelet counts.
• May diminish diagnostic effect of coccidioidin skin test.

CONTRAINDICATIONS & CAUTIONS
• Contraindicated in patients hypersensitive to drug or its components and in those who experienced serum sickness with prior obinutuzumab use.

Black Box Warning HBV reactivation, including fulminant hepatitis, hepatic failure, and death, may occur. Screen all patients for HBV infection before starting therapy and monitor carriers for active HBV infection during and for several months after therapy is complete. Discontinue therapy and any concomitant chemotherapy if HBV reactivates and treat appropriately. The decision to restart therapy should be discussed with physician experienced in treating HBV infection. ■

Black Box Warning JC virus infection, resulting in progressive multifocal leukoencephalopathy (PML), has been reported. Monitor patients for new-onset neurologic symptoms or change in existing neurologic symptoms. Discontinue therapy and reduce or stop concomitant chemotherapy or immunosuppressive therapy in patients who develop PML. ■

• Use cautiously in patients with history of recurring or chronic infections.
• Patients with severe and long-lasting neutropenia (lasting more than 1 week) should receive antimicrobial prophylaxis throughout treatment. Also consider antiviral and antifungal prophylaxis and G-CSFs.
• Consider withholding other drugs that may increase bleeding risk.
• May cause severe infusion reactions, including bronchospasm, shortness of breath, tachycardia, hypotension, HTN, nausea, vomiting, diarrhea, headache, and chills. Delayed reactions (up to 24 hours) may occur. Premedicate appropriately and consider infusion rate reduction, interruption of therapy, or discontinuation if reactions persist.
• Give in a facility with access to resuscitative emergency equipment.
• Use cautiously in patients with cardiac or pulmonary conditions; these patients may be at increased risk for serious infusion reactions.
• Consider temporarily withholding antihypertensives for 12 hours before, during, and for 1 hour after administration due to risk of hypotension.

Dialyzable drug: Unknown.

Reactions in bold italics are *life-threatening*. Interactions may have a *rapid onset* or a *delayed onset*.

PREGNANCY-LACTATION-REPRODUCTION
• There are no adequate studies in pregnant women. Use only if potential benefit justifies potential risk to the fetus.
• Adverse effects were observed in animal reproduction studies. Monoclonal antibodies are known to cross the placental barrier.
• It isn't known if drug appears in human milk. Patient should discontinue breastfeeding or discontinue drug.

NURSING CONSIDERATIONS
❸ *Alert:* Monitor patient for infusion reactions (hypotension, tachycardia, dyspnea, respiratory symptoms, nausea, vomiting, diarrhea, HTN, flushing headache, pyrexia, chills), which can be fatal. Symptoms may occur up to 24 hours after infusion.
• Premedicate patient with acetaminophen, antihistamine, and IV glucocorticoid to reduce risk of infusion reactions.
• Cases of TLS with fatalities have been reported. Acute renal failure, hyperkalemia, hypocalcemia, hyperuricemia, or hyperphosphatemia may occur. Administer prophylaxis (antihyperuricemic therapy [e.g., allopurinol] and hydration) in patients at high risk or with high tumor burden or renal impairment before therapy. Correct electrolyte abnormalities and monitor renal function and hydration.
• Patient may develop detectable antibodies to obinutuzumab.
• Regularly monitor blood counts. If neutropenia occurs, consider prophylaxis with antiviral and antifungal agents. Neutropenia may occur 28 days or more after end of treatment and last for more than 28 days.
• Regularly monitor renal function and electrolyte and uric acid levels.
• Monitor patient for clinical and lab signs and symptoms of hepatitis or HBV reactivation during and for several months after treatment.
• Monitor patient for bleeding and thrombocytopenia. Transfuse blood products if appropriate.
• Monitor BP before, during, and after infusion. Consider withholding antihypertensives for 12 hours before, during, and for 1 hour after infusion if appropriate.
• *Look alike–sound alike:* Don't confuse obinutuzumab with blinatumomab,

dinutuximab, obiltoxaximab, ocrelizumab, ofatumumab, olaratumab, omalizumab, or rituximab.

PATIENT TEACHING
• Advise patient to seek immediate medical attention for infusion-related reactions, such as dizziness, nausea, chills, fever, vomiting, diarrhea, breathing problems, or chest pain.
• Advise patient to seek immediate medical attention for signs and symptoms of TLS, such as nausea, vomiting, diarrhea, and lethargy.
• Tell patient to report signs and symptoms of infection, including fever and cough.
■ Black Box Warning ■ Advise patient to report signs and symptoms of hepatitis, such as worsening fatigue or yellowing of skin or eyes and that patient will be monitored for hepatitis reactivation and treated appropriately. ■
■ Black Box Warning ■ Advise patient to immediately report new or changed neurologic signs and symptoms, such as confusion, dizziness or loss of balance, difficulty talking or walking, or vision problems. ■

ocrelizumab
oh-kre-LIZ-oo-mab

Ocrevus

Therapeutic class: MS drugs
Pharmacologic class: Monoclonal antibodies

AVAILABLE FORMS
Injection: 30 mg/mL (300 mg/10 mL) in single-dose, preservative-free vials

INDICATIONS & DOSAGES
➤ **Relapsing or primary progressive MS**
Adults: Initially, 300 mg IV infusion on day 1 followed by 300 mg IV infusion 2 weeks later. Then, 600 mg IV infusion every 6 months beginning 6 months after first 300-mg dose. Before each infusion, premedicate with 100 mg IV methylprednisolone (or equivalent corticosteroid) 30 minutes before infusion and an antihistamine such as diphenhydramine 30 to 60 minutes before infusion. May also add an antipyretic such as acetaminophen.

Adjust-a-dose: For life-threatening or disabling infusion reactions, immediately stop infusion, provide supportive treatment, and permanently discontinue drug. For mild, moderate, and severe infusion reactions, refer to manufacturer's instructions for interrupting therapy and IV infusion rates.

ADMINISTRATION

IV

▼ For 300-mg dose, withdraw 10 mL of drug and dilute into an infusion bag containing 250 mL NSS. For 600-mg dose, withdraw 20 mL of drug and dilute into 500 mL NSS.

▼ Use infusion solution immediately or store up to 24 hours in refrigerator at 36° to 46° F (2° to 8° C) or up to 8 hours at room temperature (up to 77° F [25° C]), including infusion time. Discard any excess solution that's not used the same day.

▼ Inspect for particulate matter or discoloration before use.

▼ Administer diluted solution through a dedicated line using an infusion set with an 0.2- or 0.22-micron in-line filter. No incompatibilities with polyvinyl chloride or polyolefin bags and IV administration sets have been observed.

▼ Administer infusion when solution is at room temperature.

▼ Begin 300-mg dose infusion at 30 mL/hour and increase by 30 mL/hour every 30 minutes to a maximum rate of 180 mL/hour. Duration of infusion is 2½ hours or longer.

▼ Begin 600-mg dose infusion at 40 mL/hour and increase by 40 mL/hour every 30 minutes to a maximum rate of 200 mL/hour. Duration of infusion is 3½ hours or longer.

▼ If a dose is missed, administer as soon as possible and reset the dose schedule to give the next dose 6 months later. Doses must be separated by at least 5 months.

▼ Keep vials in the carton to protect from light and store in refrigerator at 36° to 46° F (2° to 8° C). Don't freeze or shake vials.

▼ **Incompatibilities:** Don't give with solutions other than NSS.

ACTION

A recombinant humanized monoclonal antibody directed against CD20-expressing B cells, which causes antibody-dependent cellular cytolysis and complement-mediated lysis.

Route	Onset	Peak	Duration
IV	14 days	Unknown	72 wk

Half-life: 26 days.

ADVERSE REACTIONS

CNS: depression. **CV:** peripheral edema. **GI:** diarrhea. **Musculoskeletal:** back pain, extremity pain. **Respiratory:** URI, lower respiratory tract infections, cough. **Skin:** skin infections. **Other:** *infusion reactions,* herpes infections.

INTERACTIONS

Drug-drug. *Coccidioides immitis skin test:* Immunosuppressants may decrease diagnostic effect of *C. immitis* skin test. Monitor patient closely.

Immunosuppressants and immune-modulating therapies (corticosteroids, daclizumab, fingolimod, mitoxantrone, natalizumab, teriflunomide): May increase risk of immunosuppression when used in combination or when switching from listed drugs to ocrelizumab. Use cautiously together.

Other MS drugs: Use of ocrelizumab with other MS drugs hasn't been studied. Consider the potential for increased immunosuppressive effects.

Tacrolimus (topical): May enhance adverse effects of immunosuppressants. Avoid combination.

Vaccines (live-attenuated or live-virus): May decrease vaccine's effects or increase infection risk. These vaccines aren't recommended during or after discontinuation of treatment until B-cell repletion occurs. Give all necessary immunizations according to immunization guidelines at least 6 weeks before initiation of ocrelizumab.

Drug-herb. *Echinacea:* May decrease therapeutic effect of immunosuppressants. Avoid combination.

EFFECTS ON LAB TEST RESULTS
• May decrease total Ig level.
• May decrease neutrophil count.

Reactions in bold italics are *life-threatening*. Interactions may have a *rapid onset* or a *delayed onset*.

CONTRAINDICATIONS & CAUTIONS

• Contraindicated in patients with active HBV infection; screen patients for HBV infection before therapy begins. For patients who are negative for HBsAg and positive for HB core antibody (HBcAb+) or are carriers of HBV (HBsAg+), consult a liver disease specialist before therapy begins and during treatment.

• Contraindicated in patients with a history of a life-threatening infusion reaction to ocrelizumab.

• Drug may increase frequency of herpes and other infections.

• Drug may cause an increase in malignancy, including breast cancer. Follow standard cancer screening guidelines.

• Safety and effectiveness in children haven't been established.

Dialyzable drug: Unknown.

PREGNANCY-LACTATION-REPRODUCTION

• Drug hasn't been studied in pregnant women. Immunoglobulins cross the placental barrier. Infants born to mothers exposed to other anti-CD20 antibodies experienced transient peripheral B-cell depletion and lymphocytopenia.

• Women of childbearing potential should use contraception during therapy and for 6 months after final infusion.

• Drug may appear in human milk. Risk of infant harm during breastfeeding is unknown. Before patient starts breastfeeding, consider mother's clinical need for drug along with the potential adverse reactions in the infant.

NURSING CONSIDERATIONS

• Administer drug under supervision of an experienced health care provider with access to supportive measures to manage severe reactions.

• Before every infusion, monitor patient for signs and symptoms of infection (fever, chills, persistent cough, herpes [cold sores, shingles, genital sores]). Delay infusion until an active infection resolves.

• Monitor patient for infusion reactions during and for at least 1 hour after completion of the infusion. Reactions include pruritus, rash, urticaria, erythema, bronchospasm, throat irritation, oropharyngeal pain, dyspnea, pharyngeal or laryngeal edema, flushing, hypotension, pyrexia, fatigue, headache, dizziness, nausea, and tachycardia. Infusion reactions can occur up to 24 hours after the infusion. If infusion reaction occurs, interrupt or discontinue infusion or decrease rate depending on severity of reaction.

• Progressive multifocal leukoencephalopathy (PML) caused by the John Cunningham virus has occurred in patients treated with other MS drugs and can lead to severe disability or death. Monitor patient for new or worsening signs or symptoms of neurologic function changes (problems with thinking, clumsiness, vision changes, personality changes, weakness on one side of the body). At first sign or symptom, withhold drug and obtain an appropriate diagnostic evaluation, including an MRI.

• *Look alike–sound alike:* Don't confuse ocrelizumab with eculizumab, obiltoxaximab, obinutuzumab, ofatumumab, omalizumab, or rituximab.

PATIENT TEACHING

• Advise patient to undergo standard cancer screenings because drug may increase the risk of malignancy.

• Advise patient to immediately report signs and symptoms of an infusion reaction; teach patient that signs and symptoms can occur 24 hours after the infusion ends.

• Instruct patient to immediately report signs and symptoms of infection (fever, chills, cough, herpes [including cold sores, shingles, or genital sores]).

• Teach patient to immediately report signs and symptoms associated with PML, such as new or worsening neurologic function changes.

• Remind female patient of childbearing potential to use contraception during therapy and for 6 months after final infusion.

• Caution female patient to tell prescriber if she is pregnant or breastfeeding before therapy begins.

• Inform patient that drug can cause reactivation of HBV infection, that testing for HBV will be performed before therapy begins, and that monitoring is required if patient is at risk.

• Advise patient that all necessary vaccinations will be completed at least 6 weeks before therapy begins.

octreotide acetate
ok-TREE-oh-tide

Octreotide Acetate Omega✦,
Sandostatin, Sandostatin LAR
Depot

Therapeutic class: Endocrine-metabolic agents
Pharmacologic class: Somatostatin analogues

AVAILABLE FORMS
Injection (ampules): 50 mcg/mL, 100 mcg/mL, 500 mcg/mL
Injection (single-dose vials): 50 mcg/mL, 100 mcg/mL, 500 mcg/mL
Injection (multidose vials): 200 mcg/mL, 1,000 mcg/mL
Injection for LAR (powder for suspension): 10 mg/5 mL, 20 mg/5 mL, 30 mg/5 mL

INDICATIONS & DOSAGES
➤ **Flushing and diarrhea from carcinoid tumors**
Adults: 100 to 600 mcg subcut or IV daily in two to four divided doses for first 2 weeks of therapy. Usual daily dosage is 450 mcg but can range from 50 to 1,500 mcg/day. Base subsequent dosage on individual response. If Sandostatin LAR Depot is used, give 20 mg IM (intragluteally) at 4-week intervals for 2 months. Patients should continue to receive octreotide solution subcut for 2 weeks at same dosage they were taking before the switch. After 2 months, adjust dosage based on symptoms.
➤ **Watery diarrhea from vasoactive intestinal polypeptide–secreting tumors (VIPomas)**
Adults: 200 to 300 mcg subcut or IV daily in two to four divided doses for first 2 weeks of therapy. Base subsequent dosage on individual response. Range is 150 to 750 mcg/day, but usually shouldn't exceed 450 mcg daily. If Sandostatin LAR Depot is used, give 20 mg IM (intragluteally) at 4-week intervals for 2 months. Patients should continue

to receive octreotide solution subcut for 2 weeks at same dosage they were taking before the switch. After 2 months, adjust dosage based on symptoms.
➤ **Acromegaly**
Adults: Initially, 50 mcg subcut or IV t.i.d.; then adjust based on IGF-1 (somatomedin C) levels every 2 weeks. Or, may obtain multiple growth hormone levels at 0 to 8 hours after octreotide administration to permit more rapid dose titration.
Usual dosage is 100 mcg subcut or IV t.i.d.; some patients require up to 500 mcg t.i.d. If Sandostatin LAR Depot is used, give 20 mg IM (intragluteally) at 4-week intervals for 3 months; then adjust dosage based on growth hormone and somatomedin C levels and symptoms. See manufacturer's instructions for a detailed dosing schedule. For depot injection, drug should be withdrawn yearly for 4-week interval in patients who have received irradiation.
Adjust-a-dose: In patients with cirrhosis of the liver or renal failure requiring dialysis, starting dose of Sandostatin LAR Depot is 10 mg IM every 4 weeks.
➤ **Dumping syndrome ◆**
Adults: 50 to 100 mcg subcut once daily to t.i.d. before meals (range, 25 to 600 mcg/day), or Sandostatin LAR Depot 10 to 20 mg per month. Octreotide therapy has been documented for as long as 17 years' duration.
➤ **Gastroesophageal variceal hemorrhage ◆**
Adults: 25 to 100 mcg as an IV bolus, followed by a continuous IV infusion of 25 to 50 mcg/hour for 2 to 5 days. May repeat a bolus within the first hour of treatment if hemorrhage isn't controlled.
➤ **Gastroenteropancreatic neuroendocrine tumors (metastatic) ◆**
Adults: 30 mg IM every 4 weeks until tumor progression or death. Ensure tolerability by initiating with the subcut formulation for 3 to 7 days (and continue with subcut formulation for approximately the first 14 days after the initial IM depot dose). Then initiate 20 to 30 mg IM every 28 days (subcut doses of 200 to 600 mcg/day should receive 20 mg IM and subcut doses of 750 to 1,500 mcg/day should receive 30 mg IM); IM range is 20 to 60 mg every 28 days.

Reactions in bold italics are *life-threatening*. Interactions may have a *rapid onset* or a *delayed onset*.

ADMINISTRATION

IV
▼ Dilute in 50 to 200 mL D$_5$W or NSS and infuse over 15 to 30 minutes.

▼ May be given by IV push over 3 minutes.

▼ Store solution in refrigerator between 36° and 46° F (2° and 8° C). May store at room temperature of 70° to 86° F (20° to 30° C) for up to 14 days. Discard multidose vials within 14 days after initial entry.

▼ Solution is stable for 24 hours as a parenteral admixture.

▼ Protect from light.

▼ **Incompatibilities:** Total parenteral nutrition.

IM
• Don't use if particulates or discoloration are observed.

• Follow the mixing instructions included in the packaging and give immediately after mixing.

• For LAR depot suspension: Before dilution, store refrigerated between 36° and 46° F (2° and 8° C). May store at room temperature of 68° to 77° F (20° to 25° C) for up to 10 days. Depot kit may be at room temperature for 30 to 60 minutes before use.

• Rotate injection sites.

• Avoid deltoid muscle injections. May cause significant discomfort.

⭘ *Alert:* Never give the injectable suspension by IV or subcut routes.

Subcutaneous
• Don't use if particulates or discoloration is observed.

ACTION

Mimics action of naturally occurring somatostatin.

Route	Onset	Peak	Duration
IV	Rapid	Unknown	Unknown
IM	Unknown	1 hr	Unknown
Subcut	30 min	30 min	6–12 hr

Half-life: 1.7 to 1.9 hours, increased in elderly patients and patients with cirrhosis and renal impairment; long-acting, unknown.

ADVERSE REACTIONS

CNS: confusion, dizziness, fatigue, headache, light-headedness, depression, weakness, pain. **CV:** *arrhythmias, bradycardia,* conduction abnormalities, peripheral edema, HTN. **EENT:** blurred vision, hearing loss. **GI:** abdominal pain or discomfort, diarrhea, gallbladder abnormalities, loose stools, nausea, *pancreatitis,* constipation, fat malabsorption, flatulence, vomiting. **GU:** urinary frequency, UTI. **Metabolic:** *hypoglycemia,* hyperglycemia, hypothyroidism, suppressed secretion of growth hormone and gastroenterohepatic peptides (gastrin, VIP, insulin, glucagon, secretin, motilin, and pancreatic polypeptide). **Musculoskeletal:** backache, joint pain. **Skin:** alopecia, erythema or pain at injection site, flushing, wheal, bruising, hair loss, pruritus. **Other:** cold symptoms, flulike symptoms, pain or burning at subcut injection site.

INTERACTIONS

Drug-drug. *Androgens, MAO inhibitors, quinolone antibiotics, salicylates, SSRIs:* May increase risk of hypoglycemia. Monitor patient closely.

Beta blockers (propranolol) and other drugs that may cause bradycardia, ivabradine: May have additive effect and further lower HR. Decrease beta blocker dosage as needed.

Bromocriptine: May increase bromocriptine availability. Monitor therapy.

Codeine: May decrease codeine metabolism and decrease morphine formation. Monitor therapy.

Cyclosporine: May decrease cyclosporine level. Consider therapy modification; monitor patient closely.

Drugs that prolong QT interval (antiarrhythmics, SSRIs, TCAs): May increase risk of life-threatening cardiac arrhythmias, including torsades de pointes. Monitor patient and ECG.

Insulin, oral antidiabetics: May inhibit secretion of insulin and glucagon. Monitor patient and adjust dosage of antidiabetics as needed.

Lacosamide: May increase risk of AV-blocking effect of lacosamide. Monitor patient closely.

Quinidine, rifampin: May decrease excretion of these drugs. Use with caution and reduce dosage as needed.

Drug-food. *Any food:* May alter absorption of dietary fats. Administer injections between meals.

O

EFFECTS ON LAB TEST RESULTS
• May decrease vitamin B_{12} level. May increase or decrease glucose level.
• May alter LFT and TSH values.

CONTRAINDICATIONS & CAUTIONS
• Contraindicated in patients hypersensitive to drug or its components.
• Use cautiously in elderly patients, who may be more sensitive to drug.
• Use cautiously in patients with pancreatitis, gallbladder or bile disorders, cardiac abnormalities, diabetes, or nutritional disorders; octreotide may cause or exacerbate these conditions.
• Use cautiously in patients with renal impairment requiring dialysis or hepatic cirrhosis. Dosage adjustment may be needed.
Dialyzable drug: Unknown.
⚠ *Overdose S&S:* Hypoglycemia, flushing, dizziness, nausea.

PREGNANCY-LACTATION-REPRODUCTION
• Use cautiously in pregnant women and only if clearly needed and benefit justifies possible risks to the fetus.
• Drug appears in human milk. Use cautiously in breastfeeding women.

NURSING CONSIDERATIONS
• Monitor baseline thyroid function tests.
• Monitor somatomedin C levels every 2 weeks. Dosage adjustments are based on this level.
• Periodically monitor lab tests, such as thyroid function, glucose, urine 5-hydroxyindoleacetic acid, plasma serotonin, vitamin B_{12} level, and plasma substance P (for carcinoid tumors).
• Monitor patient regularly for gallbladder disease. Therapy may be related to the development of cholelithiasis because of its effect on gallbladder motility or fat absorption.
• Monitor patient closely for signs and symptoms of glucose imbalance. Patients with type 1 diabetes mellitus and those receiving oral antidiabetics or oral diazoxide may need dosage adjustments during therapy. Monitor glucose level.
• Monitor patient closely for bradycardia, arrhythmias, conduction abnormalities, and other ECG changes (e.g., prolonged QT interval).

• Drug may alter fluid and electrolyte balance; other therapies may need adjusting.
• Half-life may be altered in patients with ESRD who are receiving dialysis.
• *Look alike–sound alike:* To avoid giving drug by the wrong route, don't confuse octreotide acetate injection with injectable depot suspension product.
• *Look alike–sound alike:* Don't confuse Sandostatin with Sandimmune, Sandoglobulin, Sandostatin LAR, sargramostim, or simvastatin.

PATIENT TEACHING
• Urge patient to report signs and symptoms of abdominal discomfort immediately.
• Stress importance of the need for periodic lab testing during octreotide therapy.
• Advise patient that drug may restore fertility in some women with acromegaly and that patient should use effective birth control if pregnancy isn't desired.
• Counsel patient to discontinue long-acting formulation approximately 2 months before planned pregnancy; short-acting formulation may be used until conception.
• Tell patient that drug may cause dizziness, drowsiness, wheezing, chest tightness, bad cough, fever, blue skin, vision changes, or swelling of face, lips, tongue, or throat and that these symptoms may increase with alcohol use or certain other medications. Advise patient not to drive or perform hazardous tasks until drug's effects are known.
• Warn diabetic patient to monitor blood glucose level closely and to discuss results with prescriber before making dosage changes.

ofloxacin (oral)
oh-FLOKS-a-sin

Therapeutic class: Antibiotics
Pharmacologic class: Fluoroquinolones

AVAILABLE FORMS
Tablets: 200 mg, 300 mg, 400 mg

INDICATIONS & DOSAGES
Black Box Warning Use in patients with acute bacterial exacerbation of bronchitis and uncomplicated UTIs isn't recommended

because of risk of serious adverse effects. Use drug in these patients only when they have no other treatment options. ■

Adjust-a-dose (for all indications): For patients with CrCl of 20 to 50 mL/minute, give first dose as recommended; then give usual maintenance dose every 24 hours. For patients with CrCl less than 20 mL/minute, give 50% of recommended dose every 24 hours. For patients with severe hepatic impairment, don't exceed 400 mg/day.

➤ **Acute bacterial worsening of chronic bronchitis, uncomplicated skin and skin-structure infections, and community-acquired pneumonia**
Adults: 400 mg PO every 12 hours for 10 days.

➤ **Acute, uncomplicated urethral and cervical gonorrhea**
Adults: 400 mg PO as a single dose.

➤ **Mixed infection of the urethra and cervix due to *Chlamydia trachomatis* and *Neisseria gonorrhoeae*; nongonococcal cervicitis/urethritis due to *C. trachomatis***
Adults: 300 mg PO every 12 hours for 7 days.

➤ **Uncomplicated cystitis caused by *Escherichia coli*, *Klebsiella pneumoniae*, or other organisms**
Adults: 200 mg PO every 12 hours for 3 days *(E. coli* or *K. pneumoniae)* or 200 mg PO every 12 hours for 7 days (other organisms).

➤ **Complicated UTI**
Adults: 200 mg PO every 12 hours for 10 days.

➤ **Prostatitis from *E. coli***
Adults: 300 mg PO every 12 hours for 6 weeks.

➤ **Acute pelvic inflammatory disease**
Adults: 400 mg PO every 12 hours with metronidazole for 10 to 14 days.

➤ **Spontaneous bacterial peritonitis ◆**
Adults: 400 mg PO b.i.d.

ADMINISTRATION
PO
• Give drug with or without food but not at the same time as antacids and vitamins.
• Give drug with plenty of fluids.

ACTION
Interferes with DNA gyrase, which is needed for synthesis of bacterial DNA. Spectrum of action includes many gram-positive and gram-negative aerobic bacteria, including *Enterobacteriaceae* and *Pseudomonas aeruginosa.*

Route	Onset	Peak	Duration
PO	Unknown	60–120 min	Unknown

Half-life: 4 to 7½ hours.

ADVERSE REACTIONS
CNS: dizziness, fatigue, fever, headache, insomnia, lethargy, nervousness, sleep disorders. **CV:** chest pain, phlebitis. **EENT:** visual disturbances, pharyngitis. **GI:** nausea, *pseudomembranous colitis,* abdominal pain or discomfort, anorexia, constipation, diarrhea, dry mouth, dysgeusia, flatulence, vomiting, decreased appetite. **GU:** external genital pruritus in women, glycosuria, hematuria, proteinuria, vaginal discharge, vaginitis. **Hematologic:** *leukopenia, neutropenia,* anemia, eosinophilia, leukocytosis. **Musculoskeletal:** body pain, tendon rupture, myalgia. **Skin:** pruritus, rash. **Other:** *anaphylactoid reaction,* hypersensitivity reactions.

INTERACTIONS
Drug-drug. *Aluminum hydroxide, aluminum-magnesium hydroxide, calcium carbonate, magnesium hydroxide:* May decrease effects of ofloxacin. Give antacid at least 2 hours before or 2 hours after ofloxacin.
Antidiabetics: May affect glucose level, causing hypoglycemia or hyperglycemia. Monitor patient closely.
Didanosine (chewable or buffered tablets or pediatric powder for oral solution): May interfere with GI absorption of ofloxacin. Separate doses by 2 hours.
Drugs that prolong QT interval (antiarrhythmics, pimozide, ziprasidone): May increase risk of life-threatening ventricular arrhythmias. Avoid use together.
Iron salts: May decrease absorption of ofloxacin, reducing anti-infective response. Separate doses by at least 2 hours.
NSAIDs: May enhance seizure-potentiating effect of ofloxacin. Monitor therapy closely.
Black Box Warning *Steroids:* May increase risk of tendinitis and tendon

O

rupture. Monitor patient for tendon pain or inflammation. ∎

Sucralfate: May decrease absorption of ofloxacin, reducing anti-infective response. If use together can't be avoided, give ofloxacin 2 hours before or 6 hours after sucralfate.

Theophylline: May increase theophylline level. Monitor patient closely and adjust theophylline dosage as needed.

Warfarin: May prolong PT and INR. Monitor PT and INR.

Drug-lifestyle. *Sun exposure:* May cause photosensitivity reactions. Advise patient to avoid excessive sunlight exposure.

EFFECTS ON LAB TEST RESULTS

• May increase BUN, creatinine, and liver enzyme levels. May increase or decrease glucose level.

• May increase erythrocyte sedimentation rate and eosinophil count.

• May decrease Hb level, hematocrit, and neutrophil count. May increase or decrease WBC count.

• May produce false-positive urine screen results for opiates.

CONTRAINDICATIONS & CAUTIONS

Black Box Warning Drug is associated with increased risk of tendinitis and tendon rupture, especially in patients older than age 60, patients taking corticosteroids, and those with heart, kidney, or lung transplants. ∎

Black Box Warning Drug may exacerbate muscle weakness in patients with myasthenia gravis. Avoid use in patients with a known history of myasthenia gravis. ∎

• Contraindicated in patients hypersensitive to drug or other fluoroquinolones.

۞ Alert: Serious, even fatal, hypersensitivity reactions can occur, even after first dose. Discontinue drug at first sign of rash or hypersensitivity. Emergency treatment with epinephrine and resuscitative measures may be needed.

Black Box Warning Oral or parenteral fluoroquinolones may increase the risk of peripheral neuropathy of the arms or legs. Symptoms can occur at any time during treatment and can last for months or years or be permanent. Stop drug immediately if

patient develops symptoms, and switch to a nonfluoroquinolone antibacterial drug. ∎

• Use cautiously in patients with seizure disorders, CNS diseases such as cerebral arteriosclerosis, hepatic disorders, or renal impairment.

۞ Alert: Patients receiving systemic drug have an increased risk of hypoglycemia, which can result in coma. Hypoglycemia has been reported more frequently in elderly patients and those with diabetes.

• Mild to life-threatening CDAD can occur during therapy and up to 2 months after therapy ends. Monitor patient for diarrhea as drug may need to be discontinued and other therapy begun.

• Safety and effectiveness in children younger than age 18 haven't been established.

۞ Alert: Drug may increase risk of aortic dissection or rupture when used systemically. Avoid use in patients with known aortic aneurysm and patients at risk for an aortic aneurysm, including those with peripheral atherosclerotic vascular diseases, HTN, certain genetic conditions (Marfan syndrome, Ehlers-Danlos syndrome), and elderly patients. Drug should only be used in these patients if no other treatment options are available.

Dialyzable drug: No.

⚠ Overdose S&S: Nausea, vomiting, seizures, vertigo, dysgeusia, psychosis, dizziness, drowsiness, hot and cold flushes, facial swelling and numbness, slurred speech, mild to moderate disorientation.

PREGNANCY-LACTATION-REPRODUCTION

• There are no adequate studies in pregnant women. Drug does cross the placental barrier. Use only if potential benefit justifies risks to the fetus.

• Drug appears in human milk in levels similar to those found in plasma. Patient should discontinue breastfeeding or discontinue drug.

NURSING CONSIDERATIONS

Black Box Warning Fluoroquinolones have been associated with disabling and potentially irreversible serious adverse reactions that have occurred together, including tendinitis and tendon rupture, peripheral

---

neuropathy, and CNS effects (seizures, toxic psychoses, increased ICP, pseudotumor cerebri, tremors, restlessness, anxiety, light-headedness, confusion, hallucinations, paranoia, depression, nightmares, insomnia and, rarely, suicidal thoughts or acts). If any of these serious adverse reactions occur, discontinue drug immediately. ■

Black Box Warning Monitor patient for symptoms of peripheral neuropathy (pain, burning, tingling, numbness, weakness, or a change in sensation to light touch, pain, temperature, or the sense of body position) and report them immediately. ■

❸ Alert: Patients treated for gonorrhea should be tested for syphilis. Drug isn't effective against syphilis, and treating gonorrhea may mask or delay syphilis symptoms.

• Periodically assess organ system functions during prolonged therapy.

• Monitor patient for overgrowth of nonsusceptible organisms.

• Monitor renal and hepatic studies and CBC in prolonged therapy.

• Test for *Clostridium difficile* if patient develops diarrhea.

❸ Alert: Monitor patients receiving systemic drug for signs and symptoms of hypoglycemia (confusion, pounding or rapid heartbeat, dizziness, pale skin, shakiness, sweating, unusual hunger, trembling, headache, weakness, irritability, unusual anxiety). Immediately discontinue drug for blood glucose disturbances and switch to a nonfluoroquinolone antibiotic, if possible.

❸ Alert: Monitor patients receiving systemic drug for psychiatric adverse reactions (disturbances in attention, disorientation, agitation, nervousness, memory impairment, delirium). Discontinue drug for CNS adverse effects, including psychiatric adverse reactions.

• Monitor patient for adverse CNS effects, including dizziness, headache, seizures, or depression. Stop drug and notify prescriber if these effects occur.

• Monitor patient for hypersensitivity reactions. Stop drug and initiate supportive therapy, as indicated.

❸ Alert: Monitor patient for signs and symptoms of aortic aneurysm, dissection, and rupture (sudden, severe, and constant pain in the stomach, chest, or back; throbbing in

the stomach area; deep pain in the back or side of the stomach; steady, gnawing pain in the stomach that lasts for hours or days; pain in the jaw, neck, back, or chest; coughing or hoarseness; shortness of breath or trouble swallowing). Discontinue drug immediately if any of these aortic disorders are suspected.

PATIENT TEACHING
Black Box Warning Warn patient to immediately report signs and symptoms of serious adverse reactions, including unusual joint or tendon pain, muscle weakness, "pins and needles" tingling or prickling sensation, numbness in the arms or legs, confusion, or hallucinations. ■

• Tell patient to drink plenty of fluids during drug therapy and to finish the entire prescription, even after starting to feel better.

• Tell patient drug may be taken with or without food, but not to take antacids and vitamins at the same time as ofloxacin.

❸ Alert: Caution patient that significantly low blood glucose level can occur. Show patient how to manage signs and symptoms of low blood glucose level and to immediately report such occurrences to prescriber.

❸ Alert: Advise patient with diabetes that more frequent monitoring of blood glucose levels may be needed during therapy.

❸ Alert: Inform patient to immediately report psychiatric adverse reactions and warn that these can occur after just one dose.

• Warn patient that dizziness and light-headedness may occur. Advise caution when driving or operating hazardous machinery until effects of drug are known.

• Warn patient that hypersensitivity reactions may follow first dose. Advise patient to stop drug at first sign of rash or other allergic reaction and call prescriber immediately.

• Advise patient to avoid prolonged exposure to direct sunlight and to use a sunscreen when outdoors.

• Advise patient to report severe bloody diarrhea.

❸ Alert: Warn patient to seek immediate medical attention for signs and symptoms of aortic aneurysm.

OLANZapine
oh-LAN-za-peen

Zyprexa✔, Zyprexa Zydis

OLANZapine pamoate
Zyprexa Relprevv

Therapeutic class: Antipsychotics
Pharmacologic class:
Thienobenzodiazepines

AVAILABLE FORMS
Injection: 10 mg
Injection (extended-release): 210-mg base/vial, 300-mg base/vial, 405-mg base/vial
Tablets: 2.5 mg, 5 mg, 7.5 mg, 10 mg, 15 mg, 20 mg
Tablets (ODTs): 5 mg, 10 mg, 15 mg, 20 mg

INDICATIONS & DOSAGES
➤ **Schizophrenia**
Adults: Initially, 5 to 10 mg PO once daily with the goal to be at 10 mg daily within several days of starting therapy. Adjust dose in 5-mg increments at intervals of 1 week or more. Most patients respond to 10 to 15 mg daily. Safety of dosages greater than 20 mg daily hasn't been established. Or, for maintenance dosing, 150 mg (extended-release) IM every 2 weeks, or 300 mg (extended-release) IM every 2 or 4 weeks, or 210 mg (extended-release) IM every 2 weeks, or 405 mg (extended-release) IM every 4 weeks.
Children age 13 and older: 2.5 or 5 mg PO once daily. Adjust dose as needed in increments of 2.5 or 5 mg. Maintenance dose is 10 mg/day.
➤ **Short-term treatment of acute manic episodes linked to bipolar I disorder**
Adults: Initially, 10 to 15 mg PO daily. Adjust dosage as needed in 5-mg daily increments at intervals of 24 hours or more. Maximum, 20 mg PO daily. Duration of treatment is usually 2 weeks.
Children age 13 and older: 2.5 or 5 mg PO once daily. Adjust dose as needed in increments of 2.5 or 5 mg. Maintenance dose is 10 mg/day. Maximum dose is 20 mg/day.

➤ **Short-term treatment, with lithium or valproate, of acute mixed or manic episodes linked to bipolar I disorder**
Adults: 10 mg PO once daily. Dosage range is 5 to 20 mg daily. Duration of treatment is 6 weeks.
➤ **Long-term treatment of bipolar I disorder**
Adults: 5 to 20 mg PO daily.
Adjust-a-dose: In elderly or debilitated patients, those predisposed to hypotensive reactions, patients who may metabolize olanzapine more slowly than usual (nonsmoking women older than age 65) or may be more pharmacodynamically sensitive to olanzapine, initially, 5 mg PO. Increase dose cautiously.
➤ **Agitation caused by schizophrenia and bipolar I mania**
Adults: 10 mg IM (short-acting) (range, 2.5 to 10 mg). Subsequent doses of up to 10 mg may be given 2 hours after the first dose or 4 hours after the second dose, up to 30 mg IM daily. If maintenance therapy is required, convert patient to 5 to 20 mg PO daily.
Adjust-a-dose: In elderly patients, give 5 mg IM. In debilitated patients, in those predisposed to hypotension, and in patients sensitive to effects of drug, give 2.5 mg IM.
➤ **Depressive episodes associated with bipolar I disorder**
Adults: 5 mg PO with fluoxetine 20 mg PO once daily in the evening. Dosage adjustments can be made based on effectiveness and tolerability within ranges of olanzapine 5 to 12.5 mg and fluoxetine 20 to 50 mg.
Children age 10 and older: 2.5 mg PO with 20 mg fluoxetine PO once daily in the evening. Adjust dosage based on effectiveness and tolerability. Doses above 12 mg (olanzapine) with fluoxetine doses above 50 mg haven't been evaluated.
➤ **Treatment-resistant depression**
Adults: 5 mg PO with 20 mg fluoxetine PO once daily in the evening. Dosage adjustments can be made based on effectiveness and tolerability within ranges of olanzapine 5 to 20 mg and fluoxetine 20 to 50 mg.
➤ **Preventing chemotherapy-associated acute and delayed nausea or vomiting ◆**
Adults: 10 mg PO on day of chemotherapy (day 1) followed by 10 mg once daily on

---

Reactions in bold italics are *life-threatening*. Interactions may have a *rapid onset* or a ***delayed onset***.

days 2 to 4 (in combination with dexamethasone and palonosetron on day 1 only).
➤ **Chemotherapy-associated breakthrough nausea or vomiting ♦**
Adults: 10 mg PO once daily for 3 days.
Infants, children, and adolescents: 0.1 mg/kg/dose PO once daily. Maximum dose is 10 mg/day.

ADMINISTRATION

PO
• Give drug without regard for food.
• Don't push tablet through foil backing; remove foil from package, then remove tablet.
• Place ODT on patient's tongue immediately after opening package.
• ODT may be given without water.

IM
• Inspect IM solution for particulate matter and discoloration before administration.
• To reconstitute IM injection, dissolve contents of one vial with 2.1 mL of sterile water for injection to yield a clear yellow 5 mg/mL solution. Store at room temperature and give within 1 hour of reconstitution. Discard any unused solution.
• For Zyprexa Relprevv extended-release injection, follow specific manufacturer's instructions for the appropriate diluent to add for each dosage.
• Olanzapine extended-release formula is intended for deep gluteal IM injection only.

ACTION

May block dopamine and 5-HT$_2$ receptors.

Route	Onset	Peak	Duration
PO	1–6 wk	6 hr	Unknown
IM	Rapid	15–45 min	Unknown
IM (extended-release)	Unknown	1 wk	Months

Half-life: 21 to 54 hours; extended release, 30 days.

ADVERSE REACTIONS

CNS: somnolence, insomnia, parkinsonism, dizziness, *NMS, suicide attempt,* abnormal gait, asthenia, personality disorder, akathisia, headache, tremor, articulation impairment, tardive dyskinesia, fever, extrapyramidal events (IM). **CV:** orthostatic hypotension, tachycardia, chest pain, HTN, ecchymosis, peripheral edema, hypotension (IM). **EENT:** amblyopia, rhinitis, pharyngitis, conjunctivitis. **GI:** constipation, dry mouth, dyspepsia, increased appetite, increased salivation, vomiting, thirst. **GU:** hematuria, metrorrhagia, urinary incontinence, UTI, amenorrhea, vaginitis. **Hematologic:** *leukopenia.* **Metabolic:** hyperglycemia, weight gain. **Musculoskeletal:** joint pain, extremity pain, back pain, neck rigidity, twitching, hypertonia. **Respiratory:** increased cough, dyspnea. **Skin:** sweating, ecchymosis, injection-site pain (IM). **Other:** flulike syndrome, injury.

INTERACTIONS

Drug-drug. *Amphetamines:* May decrease stimulatory effect of amphetamines. Monitor therapy.
Anticholinergic agents: May increase adverse effects of anticholinergic agents. Monitor therapy.
Antihypertensives: May potentiate hypotensive effects. Monitor BP closely.
Carbamazepine, omeprazole, rifampin: May increase clearance of olanzapine. Monitor patient.
Ciprofloxacin: May increase olanzapine level. Monitor patient for increased adverse effects.
Diazepam: May increase CNS effects. Monitor patient.
Dopamine agonists, levodopa: May antagonize activity of these drugs. Monitor patient.
Fluoxetine: May increase olanzapine level. Use together cautiously.
Fluvoxamine: May increase olanzapine level. May need to reduce olanzapine dose.
Lamotrigine: May increase sedative effect of olanzapine. Monitor patient.
Opioid agonists: May cause slow or difficult breathing, sedation, and death. Avoid use together. If use together is necessary, limit dosage and duration of each drug to minimum necessary for desired effect.
QT-prolonging agents: May enhance QTc-prolonging effect of QT-prolonging agents. Consider therapy modification.
Drug-herb. *Kava kava:* May increase adverse/toxic effect of olanzapine. Monitor patient.
St. John's wort: May decrease drug level. Discourage use together.
Drug-lifestyle. *Alcohol use:* May increase CNS effects. Don't use together.

Smoking: May increase drug clearance. Urge patient to quit smoking.

EFFECTS ON LAB TEST RESULTS
• May increase AST, ALT, GGT, CK, glucose, triglyceride, uric acid, and prolactin levels.
• May decrease bilirubin level.
• May increase eosinophil count. May decrease WBC count.

CONTRAINDICATIONS & CAUTIONS
• Contraindicated in patients hypersensitive to drug.
Black Box Warning Sedation (including coma) or delirium have been reported following injections of olanzapine extended-release formula. This drug must be administered in a registered health care facility with ready access to emergency response services. After each injection, patient must be observed at the health care facility by a health care provider for at least 3 hours. Olanzapine extended-release is available only through the restricted Zyprexa Relprevv Patient Care Program (1-877-772-9390). ▮
Black Box Warning Drug may increase risk of CV or infection-related death in elderly patients with dementia. Olanzapine isn't approved to treat patients with dementia-related psychosis. ▮
• Opioids should only be prescribed with benzodiazepines or other CNS depressants to patients for whom alternative treatment options are inadequate.
• Use cautiously in patients with heart disease, cerebrovascular disease, conditions that predispose patient to hypotension, history of seizures or conditions that might lower the seizure threshold, and hepatic impairment.
• Use cautiously in elderly patients, those with a history of paralytic ileus, and those at risk for aspiration pneumonia, prostatic hyperplasia, or angle-closure glaucoma.
• Use cautiously during initiation of therapy in patients at high-risk for suicide.
• Impaired core body temperature regulation may occur. Patient should use caution with strenuous exercise, heat exposure, and dehydration.
Dialyzable drug: No.

⚠ *Overdose S&S:* Agitation, aggressiveness, dysarthria, tachycardia, extrapyramidal symptoms, reduced level of consciousness, aspiration, cardiopulmonary arrest, cardiac arrhythmias, delirium, NMS, respiratory depression or arrest, seizures, HTN, hypotension.

PREGNANCY-LACTATION-REPRODUCTION
• There are no adequate studies in pregnant women. Use only if potential benefit justifies potential risk to the fetus. Use during pregnancy should be individualized.
❸ *Alert:* Neonates exposed to antipsychotics during the third trimester are at risk for developing extrapyramidal signs and symptoms (repetitive muscle movements of the face and body) and withdrawal signs and symptoms (agitation, abnormally increased or decreased muscle tone, tremors, sleepiness, severe difficulty breathing, difficulty feeding) after delivery and may require intensive care support.
• Prescribers should enroll women exposed to drug during pregnancy in the National Pregnancy Registry for Atypical Antipsychotics (1-866-961-2388).
• Drug appears in human milk. Breastfeeding isn't recommended.

NURSING CONSIDERATIONS
❸ *Alert:* Watch for evidence of NMS (hyperpyrexia, muscle rigidity, altered mental status, autonomic instability), which is rare but commonly fatal. Stop drug immediately; monitor and treat patient as needed.
❸ *Alert:* Drug may cause hyperglycemia. Monitor patients with diabetes regularly. In patients with risk factors for diabetes, obtain fasting blood glucose test results at baseline and periodically.
❸ *Alert:* Monitor patient for symptoms of metabolic syndrome (significant weight gain and increased BMI, HTN, hyperglycemia, hypercholesterolemia, and hypertriglyceridemia).
❸ *Alert:* Monitor patient for DRESS syndrome, which can be fatal. DRESS syndrome consists of three or more of the following signs and symptoms: cutaneous reaction, eosinophilia, fever, and lymphadenopathy, plus one or more of the following systemic complications: hepatitis, myocarditis,

pericarditis, nephritis, and pneumonia. Discontinue drug immediately if DRESS syndrome is suspected and provide supportive care.

Black Box Warning When using olanzapine and fluoxetine in combination, also refer to the Boxed Warning section of the package insert for Symbyax. ∎

• ODTs contain phenylalanine.

• Monitor patient for abnormal body temperature regulation, especially if patient exercises, is exposed to extreme heat, takes anticholinergics, or is dehydrated.

• Obtain baseline and periodic LFT results.

• Monitor patient for weight gain.

• Monitor patient for mental status changes, sedation, coma, or delirium.

• Monitor patient for tardive dyskinesia, which may occur after prolonged use. It may not appear until months or years later and may disappear spontaneously or persist for life, despite stopping drug.

• Periodically reevaluate the long-term usefulness of olanzapine.

• Patient who feels dizzy or drowsy after an IM injection should remain recumbent until assessment for orthostatic hypotension and bradycardia can be done. Patient should rest until the feeling passes.

• Taper dosage slowly when discontinuing.

🌑 *Alert:* Drug may increase risk of suicidal thinking and behavior in young adults ages 18 to 24 during first 2 months of treatment.

Black Box Warning Monitor patient receiving extended-release injection for postinjection delirium sedation syndrome (PDSS). Signs and symptoms that may be consistent with overdose and PDSS include sedation, coma, delirium, confusion, disorientation, agitation, anxiety, and other cognitive impairment. Other possible signs and symptoms of PDSS include dysarthria, ataxia, aggression, dizziness, weakness, HTN, and seizures. ∎

Black Box Warning After receiving extended-release injection and after postinjection observation period, patients must be alert, oriented, and absent of signs or symptoms of PDSS before release. Patients must be accompanied to their destination upon leaving the facility. If PDSS is suspected, patients must remain under medical supervision. ∎

• *Look alike–sound alike:* Don't confuse olanzapine with olsalazine or quetiapine. Don't confuse Zyprexa with Zyrtec, Zestril, Reprexain, or Celexa. Don't confuse Zyprexa Zydis with Zelapar or zolpidem.

PATIENT TEACHING

• Caution patient or caregiver of patient taking an opioid with a benzodiazepine, CNS depressant, or alcohol to seek immediate medical attention for dizziness, lightheadedness, extreme sleepiness, slowed or difficult breathing, or unresponsiveness.

🌑 *Alert:* Inform patient of risk of DRESS syndrome and importance of reporting symptoms immediately.

• Warn patient to avoid hazardous tasks until full effects of drug are known.

• Warn patient against exposure to extreme heat; drug may impair body's ability to reduce temperature.

• Inform patient of potential for weight gain.

• Advise patient to avoid alcohol.

• Tell patient to rise slowly to avoid dizziness upon standing up quickly.

• Inform patient that ODTs contain phenylalanine.

• Tell patient to peel foil away from ODT, not to push tablet through. Have patient take tablet immediately, allowing tablet to dissolve on tongue and be swallowed with saliva; no additional fluid is needed.

• Tell patient to take drug with or without food.

• Instruct patient with diabetes to closely monitor blood glucose level. Drug may cause hyperglycemia.

• Urge female patient of childbearing potential to notify prescriber if she becomes pregnant or plans or suspects pregnancy. Tell her not to breastfeed during therapy.

Black Box Warning Warn patient not to drive or operate heavy machinery for rest of day after receiving extended-release injection and to seek medical attention if signs and symptoms of PDSS occur. ∎

O

olmesartan medoxomil ⊠
ol-ma-SAR-tan

Benicar◈, Olmetec✦

Therapeutic class: Antihypertensives
Pharmacologic class: Angiotensin II
receptor antagonists

AVAILABLE FORMS
Tablets: 5 mg, 20 mg, 40 mg

INDICATIONS & DOSAGES
➤ **HTN**
Adults: 20 mg PO once daily if patient has
no volume depletion. May increase dosage
to 40 mg PO once daily if BP isn't reduced
after 2 weeks of therapy.
Children ages 6 to 16: For children weighing
35 kg or more, initially, 20 mg PO daily, with
maintenance dosage of 20 to 40 mg daily.
For children weighing 20 to less than 35 kg,
initially, 10 mg PO daily, with maintenance
dosage of 10 to 20 mg daily.
Adjust-a-dose: In patients with possible depletion of intravascular volume (those with
impaired renal function who are taking diuretics), consider a lower starting dose. Use
cautiously in patients with CrCl less than
20 mL/minute.

ADMINISTRATION
PO
• Give drug without regard for food.
• Drug may be made into suspension by
pharmacist if patient is unable to swallow
pills.
• Refrigerate suspension, which may be
stored for up to 28 days.
• Shake suspension well before use.

ACTION
Blocks vasoconstrictor and aldosterone-
secreting effects of angiotensin II by selectively blocking the binding of angiotensin II
to the angiotensin I, or AT_1, receptor in the
vascular smooth muscle.

Route	Onset	Peak	Duration
PO	Rapid	1–2 hr	24 hr

Half-life: 13 hours.

ADVERSE REACTIONS
CNS: headache, dizziness. **EENT:** pharyngitis, rhinitis, sinusitis. **GI:** diarrhea. **GU:**
hematuria. **Metabolic:** hyperglycemia, hypertriglyceridemia. **Musculoskeletal:** back
pain. **Respiratory:** bronchitis, URI. **Other:**
flulike symptoms.

INTERACTIONS
Drug-drug. *ACE inhibitors:* May increase
risk of hyperkalemia and decrease renal
function. Consider monotherapy; if coadministration can't be avoided, monitor renal
function and serum potassium level.
❸ *Alert: Aliskiren:* May increase risk of renal impairment, hypotension, and hyperkalemia in diabetic patients and those with
moderate to severe renal impairment (GFR
less than 60 mL/minute). Concomitant use
is contraindicated in diabetic patients. Avoid
concomitant use in those with moderate to
severe renal impairment.
Colesevelam: Reduces olmesartan level.
Give olmesartan at least 4 hours before colesevelam.
Cyclo-oxygenase-2 inhibitors, NSAIDs:
May decrease antihypertensive effects of
olmesartan. Coadministration in elderly or
volume-depleted patients or in those with
compromised renal function may result in
deterioration of renal function, including
possible acute renal failure. Monitor BP and
renal function periodically.
Lithium: May increase serum lithium level
and risk of toxicity. Closely monitor serum
lithium level and adjust dosage as needed.
Potassium: May increase risk of hyperkalemia, possibly with cardiac arrhythmias
or arrest. Closely monitor serum potassium
level and renal function; adjust therapy as
needed.
Potassium-sparing diuretics: May increase
risk of hyperkalemia. Closely monitor serum
potassium level.
NSAIDs: May increase risk of renal impairment and decrease antihypertensive effect.
Monitor therapy.
Trimethoprim: May increase risk of hyperkalemia, especially in elderly patients. If use
together can't be avoided, closely monitor
potassium level.

Reactions in bold italics are *life-threatening*. Interactions may have a *rapid onset* or a *delayed onset*.

Drug-herb. *Yohimbe:* May decrease antihypertensive effect of olmesartan. Closely monitor patient.

EFFECTS ON LAB TEST RESULTS
• May increase glucose, triglyceride, uric acid, liver enzyme, bilirubin, and CK levels.
• May decrease Hb level and hematocrit.

CONTRAINDICATIONS & CAUTIONS
• Contraindicated in patients hypersensitive to drug or its components and in patients with diabetes who are also taking aliskiren.
• Avoid use in patients who experienced angioedema with other ARBs and in those with renal impairment who are also taking aliskiren.
• Use cautiously in patients who are volume- or sodium-depleted, those whose renal function depends on the RAAS (such as patients with severe HF), and those with unilateral or bilateral renal artery stenosis.
◑ *Alert:* Drug can cause spruelike enteropathy (severe chronic diarrhea with substantial weight loss).
Dializable drug: Unknown.
⚠ *Overdose S&S:* Hypotension, tachycardia, bradycardia.

PREGNANCY-LACTATION-REPRODUCTION
Black Box Warning Drug may cause fetal and neonatal complications and death. If patient becomes pregnant, stop drug immediately. ∎
• It isn't known if drug appears in human milk. Patient should discontinue breastfeeding or discontinue drug.

NURSING CONSIDERATIONS
• Symptomatic hypotension may occur in patients who are volume- or sodium-depleted, especially those being treated with high doses of a diuretic. If hypotension occurs, place patient supine and treat supportively. Treatment may continue once BP is stabilized.
• If BP isn't adequately controlled, a diuretic or other antihypertensive drugs also may be prescribed.
• Closely monitor patients with HF for oliguria, azotemia, and acute renal failure.
• Watch for signs and symptoms of angioedema.

• Monitor BUN and creatinine level in patients with unilateral or bilateral renal artery stenosis.
▩ The antihypertensive effects of ACE inhibitors and ARBs are reduced in Black patients; use of these drugs as initial antihypertensive therapy in these patients isn't recommended.
• *Look alike–sound alike:* Don't confuse Benicar with Mevacor.

PATIENT TEACHING
• Tell patient to take drug exactly as prescribed and not to stop taking it, even if feeling better.
• Tell patient to take drug without regard to meals.
• Tell patient to promptly report all adverse reactions, especially light-headedness and fainting.
• Teach patient signs and symptoms of angioedema (wheezing, swelling of face, lips, tongue, or throat).
◑ *Alert:* Tell patient to contact prescriber if severe chronic diarrhea with substantial weight loss develops, even if months to years have elapsed before symptoms occur.
• Advise female patient of childbearing potential that drug can cause fetal harm and to immediately report pregnancy to health care provider.
• Inform diabetic patient that glucose readings may rise and that dosage of diabetes drugs may need adjustment.
• Warn patient that inadequate fluid intake, excessive perspiration, diarrhea, or vomiting may lead to an excessive drop in BP, light-headedness, and possibly fainting.
• Instruct patient that other antihypertensives can have additive effects. Patient should inform prescriber of all medications being taken, including OTC drugs and herbal products.

olodaterol
OH-loe-DA-ter-ol

Striverdi Respimat

Therapeutic class: Bronchodilators
Pharmacologic class: Long-acting selective beta₂-adrenergic agonists

AVAILABLE FORMS
Inhalation aerosol: 2.5 mcg/actuation

INDICATIONS & DOSAGES
➤ **Long-term maintenance treatment of airway obstruction in patients with COPD, including chronic bronchitis and emphysema**
Adults: 2 inhalations once daily. Maximum dose is 2 inhalations in 24 hours.

ADMINISTRATION
Inhalational
• Prime inhaler by spraying toward ground until aerosol cloud is seen; then repeat spray three more times before first use or if inhaler hasn't been used for more than 21 days. If not used for more than 3 days, spray once toward ground to prime.
• To administer dose, have patient breathe in slowly through the mouth and press the dose release button. Patient should then continue to breathe in slowly as long as possible and then hold breath for 10 seconds if possible. Repeat for the second inhalation.
• While patient is inhaling dose, have patient hold inhaler flat; make sure patient doesn't cover air vents on the mouthpiece.
• Give at same time each day.
• Store at 77° F (25° C); avoid freezing. Discard 3 months after cartridge has been inserted into inhaler.

ACTION
Binds and activates beta₂ adrenoceptors in the lungs, resulting in relaxation of smooth muscle cells and bronchodilation.

Route	Onset	Peak	Duration
Inhalation	5 min	10–20 min	24 hr

Half-life: 7½ hours.

ADVERSE REACTIONS
CNS: pyrexia. **EENT:** nasopharyngitis. **GI:** constipation. **GU:** UTI. **Musculoskeletal:** back pain, arthralgia. **Respiratory:** URI, bronchitis, pneumonia. **Skin:** rash.

INTERACTIONS
Drug-drug. *Atomoxetine, linezolid, tedizolid:* May have additive tachycardic effect. Monitor patient carefully.
Beta blockers: May diminish effect of both drugs and increase risk of bronchospasm. Avoid combination if possible.
Cannabinoid-containing products: May increase tachycardic effect of olodaterol. Monitor therapy closely.
Corticosteroids, non-potassium-sparing diuretics, xanthine derivatives (caffeine, theophylline): May increase risk of hypokalemia. Monitor potassium level.
Drugs that prolong QT interval (antiarrhythmics, droperidol, haloperidol, mifepristone, TCAs, thioridazine): May increase risk of life-threatening cardiac arrhythmias. Use together cautiously.
Linezolid: May cause additive hypertensive effect. Consider therapy modification.
Loop diuretics, thiazide and thiazide-like diuretics: May increase hypokalemic effect of diuretics. Monitor potassium level.
MAO inhibitors, TCAs: May increase CV effects. Use together cautiously.
Other beta₂ agonists (long-acting): May have additive risk of toxic adverse effects. Use together is contraindicated.
Tedizolid: May increase hypertensive and tachycardic effects of olodaterol. Monitor therapy closely.
Drug-food. *Caffeine:* May increase risk of hypokalemia. Discourage use together.

EFFECTS ON LAB TEST RESULTS
• May increase glucose level. May decrease potassium level.

CONTRAINDICATIONS & CAUTIONS
Black Box Warning Long-acting beta agonists such as olodaterol have been associated with increased risk of asthma-related death. Safety and effectiveness in patients with asthma haven't been established. Drug isn't indicated for use in asthma. ∎

Reactions in bold italics are *life-threatening*. Interactions may have a *rapid onset* or a *delayed onset*.

❸ *Alert:* Rare, paradoxical, life-threatening bronchospasm has been reported. Discontinue drug immediately and treat emergently.
• Discontinue drug if hypersensitivity reactions such as angioedema occur.
• Don't initiate drug in patients with acute deterioration of COPD.
• Contraindicated as rescue therapy for acute symptoms.
• Use cautiously in patients with extreme sensitivity to other sympathomimetics, CV conditions (coronary insufficiency, cardiac arrhythmias, hypertrophic obstructive cardiomyopathy, HTN), seizure disorders, diabetes, or thyrotoxicosis.
• Use cautiously in patients with known or suspected prolongation of QT interval.
• Safety and effectiveness in children haven't been established.
Dialyzable drug: Unknown.
⚠ *Overdose S&S:* CV toxicity, HTN or hypotension, tachycardia, arrhythmias, palpitations, dizziness, nervousness, insomnia, anxiety, headache, tremor, dry mouth, muscle spasms, nausea, fatigue, malaise, hypokalemia, hyperglycemia, metabolic acidosis.

PREGNANCY-LACTATION-REPRODUCTION
• There are no adequate studies in pregnant women. Use during pregnancy only if potential benefit justifies potential risks to the fetus.
• It isn't known if drug appears in human milk but it's likely. Use cautiously in breastfeeding women.

NURSING CONSIDERATIONS
• Patient must also be prescribed a short-acting inhaled beta$_2$ agonist to provide symptomatic relief.
• Monitor patient for increased use of inhaled beta$_2$ agonist and decreased control of symptoms of bronchospasm. Evaluate for deterioration of disease.
• Monitor FEV$_1$, FVC, and other pulmonary function tests; serum potassium and serum glucose levels; and BP and HR.
❸ *Alert:* Excessive use of drug by using more frequently, increasing the number of inhalations, or using in combination with other medications containing long-acting beta$_2$ agonists may cause CV effects and death.

• Monitor patient for hypokalemia (which may increase risk of cardiac arrhythmias) and hyperglycemia.
• *Look alike–sound alike:* Don't confuse olodaterol with olopatadine. Don't confuse Striverdi Respimat with Combivent Respimat.

PATIENT TEACHING
Black Box Warning Warn patient that drug isn't approved for treatment of asthma. People with asthma who take long-acting beta$_2$ agonists have an increased risk of death from asthma complications. ∎
• Teach patient how to use the Respimat device; then ask patient to demonstrate its use.
• Advise patient to take medication at same time each day.
• Explain that drug has a long-acting effect and should never be used as a "rescue medication" to relieve acute symptoms. Advise patient to always carry a rescue inhaler.
• Advise patient to report worsening signs or symptoms of COPD, increased frequency of rescue medication use, and decrease in effectiveness of rescue medication.
• Warn patient not to use drug with other long-acting beta$_2$ agonists and not to regularly use short-acting beta$_2$ agonists. Short-acting beta$_2$ agonists should only be used for acute symptoms.
• Instruct patient to report palpitations, chest pain, rapid heartbeat, muscle spasms, weakness, tremor or nervousness, URI, confusion, flushed dry skin, excessive thirst, urination, or hunger.
• Teach patient to seek emergency medical care for serious allergic reactions (breathing problems, rash, hives, or swelling of the face, mouth, or tongue).
• Caution patient not to stop drug without first discussing with prescriber.
• Instruct patient to consult prescriber before starting new prescription or OTC medications or herbal or nutritional supplements.
• Advise female patient to inform prescriber if she becomes pregnant, intends to become pregnant, or is breastfeeding.

olsalazine sodium

ol-SAL-uh-zeen

Dipentum

Therapeutic class: Anti-inflammatory drugs
Pharmacologic class: Salicylates

AVAILABLE FORMS
Capsules: 250 mg

INDICATIONS & DOSAGES
➤ **Maintenance of remission of ulcerative colitis in patients intolerant of sulfasalazine**
Adults: 500 mg PO b.i.d.

ADMINISTRATION
PO
• Give drug with food.

ACTION
Unknown. After oral use, converts to 5-aminosalicylic acid (5-ASA, or mesalamine) in the colon, where it has local anti-inflammatory effect.

Route	Onset	Peak	Duration
PO	Unknown	1 hr	Unknown

Half-life: About 1 hour.

ADVERSE REACTIONS
CNS: headache, depression, vertigo, dizziness, fatigue. **GI:** diarrhea, nausea, abdominal pain/cramps, dyspepsia, bloating, anorexia, stomatitis, vomiting. **Musculoskeletal:** arthralgia. **Respiratory:** URI. **Skin:** rash, itching.

INTERACTIONS
Drug-drug. *Anticoagulants:* May prolong PT and increase INR and bleeding risk. If concurrent use is necessary, monitor patient and therapy closely.
Cardiac glycosides: May decrease serum concentration of cardiac glycosides. Monitor therapy.
NSAIDs: May enhance nephrotoxic effect of 5-aminosalicylic acid derivatives. Monitor therapy.

Thiopurine analogues: May decrease metabolism of thiopurine analogues. Monitor therapy.
Varicella virus–containing vaccines: May increase risk of Reye syndrome. Avoid salicylate use for 6 weeks after patient has received a varicella vaccine.
Drug-food. *Any food:* May decrease GI irritation. Advise patient to take drug with food.

EFFECTS ON LAB TEST RESULTS
• May increase ALT and AST levels.
• May decrease WBC and platelet counts.

CONTRAINDICATIONS & CAUTIONS
• Contraindicated in patients hypersensitive to olsalazine, other salicylates, or any of the excipients.
• Use cautiously in patients with severe allergies, asthma, hepatic impairment, and renal disease.
• Safety and effectiveness in children haven't been established.
Dialyzable drug: Unknown.

PREGNANCY-LACTATION-REPRODUCTION
• There are no adequate studies in pregnant women. Use only if potential benefit justifies risks to the fetus.
• Drug appears in human milk. Use in breastfeeding women only if benefits outweigh risks.

NURSING CONSIDERATIONS
• Regularly monitor BUN and creatinine levels and urinalysis in patients with renal disease.
• Monitor liver enzyme levels in patients with hepatic impairment.
• Absorption of drug or its metabolites may cause renal tubular damage.
• Diarrhea sometimes occurs during therapy. Although diarrhea appears to be dose-related, it's difficult to distinguish from worsening of disease symptoms.
• Similar drugs have caused worsening of disease.
• *Look alike–sound alike:* Don't confuse olsalazine with olanzapine or sulfasalazine.
• Don't confuse Dipentum with Dilantin.

Reactions in bold italics are *life-threatening*. Interactions may have a *rapid onset* or a *delayed onset*.

PATIENT TEACHING
• Teach patient to take drug in evenly divided doses and with food to minimize adverse GI reactions.
• Instruct patient to report persistent or severe adverse reactions promptly.

omalizumab
oh-mah-lye-ZOO-mab

Xolair

Therapeutic class: Antiasthmatics
Pharmacologic class: Monoclonal antibodies

AVAILABLE FORMS
Powder for injection: 150 mg in 5-mL vials
Prefilled syringe: 75 mg/0.5 mL (0.5 mL), 150 mg/mL (1 mL)

INDICATIONS & DOSAGES
➤ **Moderate to severe persistent asthma in patients with positive skin test or in vitro reactivity to a perennial aeroallergen and whose symptoms aren't adequately controlled by inhaled corticosteroids**
Adults and children age 6 and older: 75 to 375 mg subcut every 2 or 4 weeks. Dose and frequency vary with pretreatment IgE level (international units/mL) and patient weight. (Refer to manufacturer's instructions.) Divide doses larger than 150 mg among more than one injection site.
➤ **Chronic idiopathic urticaria in patients who are symptomatic despite antihistamine treatment**
Adults and adolescents age 12 and older: 150 to 300 mg subcut every 4 weeks. Dosing isn't dependent on serum IgE level or body weight. Periodically reassess need for continued therapy; treatment duration hasn't been evaluated.

ADMINISTRATION
Subcutaneous
• Reconstitute with 1.4 mL of sterile water for injection only. Swirl gently, don't shake. Continue to swirl for 5 to 10 seconds approximately every 5 minutes until there are no visible gel-like particles in the solution.

• The lyophilized product takes 15 to 20 minutes to dissolve completely. Don't use if vial's contents don't dissolve completely by 40 minutes.
• The fully reconstituted product will appear clear or slightly opalescent and may have a few small bubbles or foam around edge of vial.
• Use 18G needle to draw medication into syringe, then replace with a 25G needle for administration.
• Because the solution is slightly viscous, it may take 5 to 10 seconds to administer.
• Use reconstituted solution within 4 hours if at room temperature or within 8 hours if refrigerated. Protect from sunlight.
• Store vials before reconstitution and prefilled syringes under refrigeration at 36° to 46° F (2° to 8° C).

ACTION
Inhibits binding of IgE to high-affinity receptor on surface of mast cells and basophils, which limits release of allergic response mediators.

Route	Onset	Peak	Duration
Subcut	Slow	7–8 days	Unknown

Half-life: About 24 to 26 days.

ADVERSE REACTIONS
CNS: anxiety, headache, dizziness, fatigue, pain, migraine, fever. **CV:** *MI, PE, thrombosis,* angina pectoris, peripheral edema. **EENT:** pharyngitis, sinusitis, earache. **GI:** abdominal pain, gastroenteritis, toothache. **GU:** UTI. **Musculoskeletal:** arm pain, arthralgia, fracture, leg pain. **Respiratory:** URI, cough, asthma. **Skin:** injection-site reaction, dermatitis, pruritus, bleeding, bruising, burning, redness, pain, inflammation, stinging, swelling, warmth. **Other:** viral and fungal infections, alopecia.

INTERACTIONS
Drug-drug. *Belimumab:* May enhance adverse/toxic effect of belimumab. Avoid combination.
Loxapine (inhalation only): May enhance adverse/toxic effect of loxapine. Avoid combination.

EFFECTS ON LAB TEST RESULTS
• May increase IgE level, which may remain elevated for up to 1 year after treatment ends.
• May increase eosinophil count.

CONTRAINDICATIONS & CAUTIONS
• Contraindicated in patients severely hypersensitive to drug.

Black Box Warning Anaphylaxis presenting as bronchospasm, hypotension, syncope, urticaria, or angioedema of the throat or tongue has been reported after administration as early as the first dose and even after a year of treatment. ∎
• Drug should be given only in a health care setting under direct medical supervision because of the risk of anaphylaxis.
۞ Alert: Drug isn't indicated for other allergic conditions or other forms of urticaria.
• Safety and effectiveness in children younger than age 6 haven't been established.
Dialyzable drug: Unknown.

PREGNANCY-LACTATION-REPRODUCTION
• There are no adequate studies in pregnant women. Use only if clearly needed.
• Encourage patients exposed to drug during pregnancy to call the manufacturer (Genentech) at 888-835-2555. The EXPECT Xolair Pregnancy Registry has closed; preliminary data have been published.
• It isn't known if drug appears in human milk. Use cautiously in breastfeeding women.

NURSING CONSIDERATIONS
۞ Alert: Don't use this drug to treat acute bronchospasm or status asthmaticus.
• Don't abruptly stop systemic or inhaled corticosteroid when omalizumab therapy starts; taper the dose gradually and under supervision.
• Recommended injection sites are upper arm, stomach, or front and middle of the thighs for lyophilized powder, or upper arm and the front and middle of the thighs for prefilled syringe.
• Don't inject into moles, scars, bruises, tender areas, or broken skin.
• Injection-site reactions, such as bruising, redness, warmth, burning, stinging, itching, hives, pain, induration, and inflammation,

may occur, usually within 1 hour after the injection. These reactions last fewer than 8 days and decrease in frequency with subsequent injections.

Black Box Warning Observe patient for an appropriate time period after the injection, and keep drugs available to respond to anaphylactic reactions (such as bronchospasm, hypotension, syncope, urticaria, or angioedema of the throat or tongue). These reactions usually occur within 2 hours of subcut injection; however, delayed reactions may occur up to 24 hours after administration. Anaphylaxis has also occurred beyond 1 year after beginning regularly administered treatment. If patient has a severe hypersensitivity reaction, stop treatment. ∎
۞ Alert: Drug may slightly increase risk of CV and cerebrovascular events (TIA, MI, chest pain, pulmonary HTN, DVT, PE). Periodically reassess the need for continued therapy based on disease severity and asthma control.
• Drug increases IgE level, so it can't be used to determine appropriate dosage during therapy or for 1 year after therapy ends.
• Monitor pulmonary function test results for signs and symptoms of infection.
• Patient medication guide must be given with each dose.
• **Look alike–sound alike:** Don't confuse omalizumab with obinutuzumab or ofatumumab.

PATIENT TEACHING
• Tell patients not to stop or reduce the dosage of any other asthma drugs unless directed by the prescriber. Patient medication guide must be given with each dose.
• Explain that patient may not notice an immediate improvement in asthma after therapy starts.

Black Box Warning Teach patient signs and symptoms of anaphylaxis and to seek immediate medical care if symptoms occur. ∎

ombitasvir–paritaprevir–ritonavir–dasabuvir

om-BIT-as-vir/par-i-TA-pre-vir/
ri-TOE-na-vir/da-SA-bue-vir

Viekira Pak, Viekira XR

Therapeutic class: Antivirals
Pharmacologic class: Antivirals

AVAILABLE FORMS
Copackaged 28-day supply
Tablets: 12.5 mg ombitasvir/75 mg pari-
taprevir/50 mg ritonavir
Tablets: dasabuvir 250 mg
Tablets (24-hour extended-release) �MC:
8.33 mg ombitasvir/50 mg paritaprevir/
33.33 mg ritonavir/200 mg dasabuvir

INDICATIONS & DOSAGES
➤ **Chronic HCV genotype 1 infection,
including patients with compensated
cirrhosis, with or without ribavirin**
Adults: For Viekira Pak, give two
ombitasvir–paritaprevir–ritonavir tablets PO
once daily (in morning) and one dasabuvir
tablet PO b.i.d. (morning and evening), with
a meal, or 3 tablets (Viekira XR) PO once
daily with a meal.
Adjust-a-dose: For patients with HCV genotype 1a infection or unknown genotype without cirrhosis, give Viekira Pak or Viekira
XR plus ribavirin for 12 weeks. For patients
with genotype 1a infection or unknown
genotype with compensated cirrhosis, give
Viekira Pak or Viekira XR plus ribavirin
for 24 weeks. For patients with genotype
1b infection with or without compensated
cirrhosis, give Viekira Pak or Viekira XR
for 12 weeks. For liver transplant patients
with normal hepatic function and mild fibrosis, regardless of genotype 1 subtype, give
Viekira Pak or Viekira XR plus ribavirin for
24 weeks. For ALT level greater than 10 ×
ULN, consider discontinuing antiviral therapy. If ALT level is elevated and associated
with liver inflammation, increasing bilirubin
or alkaline phosphatase level or INR, discontinue treatment.
    Use in patients with Child-Pugh class B
or C is contraindicated.

ADMINISTRATION
PO
● Must give with a meal but without regard
to fat or calorie content.
● Patient should swallow extended-release
tablets whole and not split, crush, or chew
them.
● Store at room temperature.

ACTION
Ombitasvir inhibits HCV NS5A, an enzyme
needed for viral RNA replication and assembly of virions. Paritaprevir inhibits HCV
NS3/4A protease, an enzyme essential for
viral replication and responsible for HCV
protein cleavage. Ritonavir doesn't have activity against HCV but acts as a potent inhibitor of CYP3A, thereby significantly increasing paritaprevir exposure. Dasabuvir
inhibits NS5B polymerase, an enzyme essential for replication of the viral genome.

Route	Onset	Peak	Duration
PO (ombitasvir)	Unknown	4–5 hr	Unknown
PO (paritaprevir)	Unknown	4–5 hr	Unknown
PO (ritonavir)	Unknown	4–5 hr	Unknown
PO (dasabuvir)	Unknown	4–8 hr	Unknown

Half-life: Ombitasvir, 21 to 25 hours; paritaprevir,
5½ hours; ritonavir, 4 hours; dasabuvir, 5½ to
6 hours.

ADVERSE REACTIONS
CNS: insomnia, fatigue, asthenia, headache.
EENT: scleral icterus. **GI:** nausea, diarrhea.
Hematologic: anemia. **Hepatic:** ALT and
serum bilirubin elevations. **Musculoskeletal:** muscle spasms. **Respiratory:** cough,
dyspnea. **Skin:** pruritus, rash, erythema,
eczema, dermatitis, exfoliation, psoriasis,
ulcer, urticaria, photosensitivity.

INTERACTIONS
Drug-drug. *Alpha$_1$-adrenergic antagonists
(alfuzosin):* May increase risk of hypotension. Use together is contraindicated.
Alprazolam: May increase alprazolam level.
Monitor patient closely for clinical effects of
alprazolam and decrease dosage if indicated.
*Antiarrhythmics (amiodarone, bepridil,
disopyramide, flecainide, lidocaine
[systemic], mexiletine, propafenone,
quinidine):* May increase antiarrhythmic

concentration. Use together cautiously and monitor drug levels, if available.

Antidiabetic agents: May enhance hypoglycemic effect. Use together cautiously.

Atazanavir/ritonavir: May increase paritaprevir concentration. Give atazanavir 300 mg without ritonavir in morning.

Calcium channel blockers (amlodipine): May increase amlodipine level. Consider amlodipine dosage reduction and monitor patient closely.

Cannabidiol and cannabis: May increase serum concentration of these agents. Monitor therapy closely.

Corticosteroids, fluticasone (inhaled/nasal): May increase fluticasone level and decrease cortisol concentration. Consider alternative corticosteroids, especially if using long term.

Darunavir/ritonavir: May decrease darunavir trough level. Use together isn't recommended.

Dihydroergotamine, ergonovine, ergotamine, methylergonovine: May increase risk of acute ergot toxicity (vasospasm, tissue ischemia) when given with ritonavir. Use together is contraindicated.

Diuretics (furosemide): May increase furosemide maximum concentration. Monitor patient and adjust furosemide dosage as clinically indicated.

Drugs highly dependent on CYP3A for clearance (oral midazolam, triazolam): May increase risk of high plasma levels of drugs dependent on CYP3A for clearance and serious or life-threatening adverse effects. Use together is contraindicated.

Efavirenz: Caused liver enzyme elevations in clinical trials. Use together is contraindicated.

Estrogen (conjugated estrogens for hormone replacement therapy, estradiol): May increase ALT level. Use cautiously together and monitor liver enzyme levels.

◑ *Alert:* *Ethinyl estradiol (combined oral contraceptives):* May significantly increase ALT level. Use together is contraindicated. Discontinue ethinyl estradiol–containing medication before starting antiviral treatment. Alternative methods of contraception (progestin only or nonhormonal) are recommended. Ethinyl estradiol may be restarted

2 weeks after completion of antiviral treatment.

Immunosuppressants (cyclosporine, tacrolimus): May increase cyclosporine and tacrolimus levels. Reduce cyclosporine dosage to one-fifth of patient's dose and closely monitor cyclosporine blood concentration. Reduce tacrolimus dosage to 0.5 mg every 7 days, monitor tacrolimus level frequently, and adjust dosage as needed. May resume higher doses after completion of antiviral therapy based on cyclosporine or tacrolimus level.

Ketoconazole: May increase ketoconazole level. Limit daily dose of ketoconazole to 200 mg.

Long-acting beta agonists (salmeterol): May increase salmeterol concentration and risk of QT-interval prolongation. Coadministration isn't recommended.

Lopinavir–ritonavir: May increase paritaprevir level. Use together isn't recommended.

Lovastatin, simvastatin: May significantly increase risk of myopathy, including rhabdomyolysis. Use together is contraindicated.

Metformin: May increase risk of lactic acidosis. Monitor therapy closely.

Opioid analgesics (buprenorphine/naloxone, hydrocodone): May increase concentrations of opioids. Monitor patient closely for sedative and cognitive effects and reduce hydrocodone dosage by 50%.

Pimozide: May increase risk of cardiac arrhythmias. Use together is contraindicated.

PPIs (omeprazole): May decrease omeprazole concentration. Monitor patient closely for omeprazole effectiveness and consider increasing omeprazole dosage if symptoms aren't well controlled; avoid using more than 40 mg/day of omeprazole.

Pravastatin, rosuvastatin: May increase pravastatin and rosuvastatin levels. Limit pravastatin to 40 mg/day and rosuvastatin to 10 mg/day.

Rilpivirine: May increase rilpivirine level and risk of QT-interval prolongation. Use together isn't recommended.

Sildenafil (at doses for treatment of PAH): May increase risk of sildenafil-associated adverse effects (visual disturbances,

---

Reactions in bold italics are *life-threatening*. Interactions may have a *rapid onset* or a **delayed onset**.

hypotension, priapism, syncope). Use together is contraindicated.

Strong CYP2C8 and CYP3A inducers (carbamazepine, phenobarbital, phenytoin, rifampin): May reduce effectiveness of ombitasvir, paritaprevir, ritonavir, and dasabuvir, and increase risk of resistance. Use together is contraindicated.

Strong CYP2C8 inhibitors (gemfibrozil): May increase dasabuvir level and risk of QT-interval prolongation. Use together is contraindicated.

Voriconazole: May decrease voriconazole level. Use together isn't recommended unless benefit outweighs risks.

Drug-herb. *St. John's wort:* May decrease ombitasvir, paritaprevir, ritonavir, and dasabuvir levels. Use together is contraindicated.

Drug-lifestyle. *Alcohol use:* May alter release of extended-release tablets. Avoid use 4 hours before or after taking drug.

EFFECTS ON LAB TEST RESULTS
• May increase ALT and bilirubin levels.

CONTRAINDICATIONS & CAUTIONS
• If ombitasvir–paritaprevir–ritonavir and dasabuvir are administered with ribavirin, the contraindications for ribavirin also apply.
• Contraindicated in patients hypersensitive to any of the drugs or their components. Contraindicated in patients with known hypersensitivity (toxic epidermal necrolysis or SJS) to ritonavir.
• Contraindicated with drugs that are extensively metabolized by CYP3A, are strong inducers of CYP3A and CYP2C8, or are strong inhibitors of CYP2C8.
◐ **Alert:** Contraindicated in patients with moderate or severe hepatic impairment (Child-Pugh class B or C) because of potential toxicity.
◐ **Alert:** Patients with cirrhosis are at risk for hepatic decompensation and hepatic failure, including liver transplantation and death, during therapy.
Black Box Warning Reactivation of HBV may occur in patients coinfected with HCV, and result in fulminant hepatitis, hepatic failure, and death. Screen all patients for current or prior HBV infection before

treatment and if positive for HBV infection, assess baseline HBV DNA. ∎
• Use cautiously in patients with HIV infection. HIV-positive patients should also be on suppressive antiretroviral regimen to reduce risk of HIV-1 protease inhibitor drug resistance.
• Safety and effectiveness in children haven't been established.
Dialyzable drug: Unknown.

PREGNANCY-LACTATION-REPRODUCTION
• Use in pregnant women, without concomitant ribavirin, only if clearly needed.
• It isn't known if drug combination causes fetal harm. Drug combination, when taken with concomitant ribavirin, is contraindicated in pregnant women and in men whose female partners are pregnant.
• Encourage pregnant women with HCV/HIV-1 coinfection who are taking concomitant antiretrovirals to register with the Antiretroviral Pregnancy Registry (1-800-258-4263).
• It isn't known if ombitasvir, paritaprevir, dasabuvir, or their metabolites appear in human milk. Ritonavir appears in breast milk. Use cautiously in breastfeeding women. HIV-infected women shouldn't breastfeed.

NURSING CONSIDERATIONS
Black Box Warning Use lab testing to monitor patient with current or prior HBV infection for hepatitis flare or HBV reactivation and watch for signs and symptoms of hepatic injury during active and posttreatment follow-up. ∎
◐ **Alert:** Perform LFTs at baseline, during first 4 weeks of therapy, then as clinically indicated. If ALT level, bilirubin level, or both are elevated above baseline, repeat tests and monitor patient closely. Drug may need to be discontinued if ALT level remains persistently greater than 10 × ULN.
◐ **Alert:** Monitor patient for hepatic decompensation (elevated bilirubin level, ascites, hepatic encephalopathy, variceal hemorrhage). Discontinue drug if hepatic decompensation occurs.
• Monitor INR, CBC, and serum creatinine level at baseline and periodically. In patients with diabetes, monitor blood glucose level

and watch for signs or symptoms of hypoglycemia.

• Monitor serum HCV-RNA level at baseline, end of treatment, during treatment follow-up, and when clinically indicated.

• Review patient's medication profile carefully before and periodically during therapy; many drug interactions are possible.

• Monitor patient for hepatotoxicity (fatigue, weakness, lack of appetite, nausea, vomiting, jaundice, discolored feces).

PATIENT TEACHING

• Explain to patient that this combination therapy is supplied as a monthly carton for a total of 28 days of treatment.

• Teach patient to take medication with a meal and not to crush, chew, or split extended-release tablets.

• Tell patient not to drink alcohol within 4 hours of taking extended-release form of drug.

❸ Alert: Inform patient with cirrhosis of the increased risk of hepatic decompensation and failure with therapy, and the need for close monitoring.

Black Box Warning Warn patient to immediately report signs and symptoms of hepatic injury (fatigue, weakness, appetite loss, nausea, vomiting, yellowing of the skin or eyes, light-colored stool). ▮

• Advise female patient to avoid becoming pregnant during therapy, especially if using drug combination concomitantly with ribavirin. Counsel her to notify prescriber immediately if she becomes pregnant.

• Inform female patient that contraceptives containing ethinyl estradiol are contraindicated during treatment and for 2 weeks after therapy ends; tell her to use alternative contraceptive methods.

• Instruct patient to report all current or new medications to prescriber because of possible drug-drug interactions.

• Inform patient to take medication as prescribed, without missing any doses. If a dose of ombitasvir–paritaprevir–ritonavir is missed, it can be taken within 12 hours of missed dose. If a dose of dasabuvir is missed, it can be taken within 6 hours of missed dose. If more than 12 hours have passed since ombitasvir–paritaprevir–ritonavir is typically taken or more than

6 hours have passed since dasabuvir is typically taken, patient shouldn't take the missed dose but should take the next scheduled dose per the usual schedule.

• Caution patient to take medication as prescribed for full treatment period, to avoid virologic treatment failure and resistance.

• Explain to patient importance of obtaining lab tests as ordered.

• Advise patient to continue precautions to prevent HCV transmission during treatment.

omega-3–fatty acids
oh-MEG-a-three/FAT-tee-AS-ids

Lovaza✎, Vascepa

Therapeutic class: Antilipemics
Pharmacologic class: Fatty acids

AVAILABLE FORMS
Capsules ⓞⓝⓒ: 0.5 g, 1 g

INDICATIONS & DOSAGES
➤ **Adjunct to diet to reduce triglyceride levels 500 mg/dL or higher**
Adults: 2 or 4 g PO once daily. Or, 4 g (Lovaza) PO once daily or divided as 2 g PO b.i.d. Or, 2 g (Vascepa) PO b.i.d.

ADMINISTRATION
PO
• May give Lovaza with or without meals. Give Vascepa with meals.

• Make sure patient swallows capsules whole and doesn't chew, crush, dissolve, or extract contents of capsule.

ACTION
May reduce hepatic formation of triglycerides because two components of drug are poor substrates for the necessary enzymes. These components also block formation of other fatty acids.

Route	Onset	Peak	Duration
PO	Unknown	5–9 hr	Unknown

Half-life: Eicosapentaenoic acid, about 37 to 89 hours; docosahexaenoic acid, about 46 hours.

ADVERSE REACTIONS
GI: altered taste, abdominal pain, belching, dyspepsia, diarrhea, nausea. **Musculoskeletal:** arthralgia, back pain. **Skin:** rash.

INTERACTIONS
Drug-drug. *Anticoagulants, antiplatelet drugs:* May prolong bleeding time. Monitor patient.
Ibrutinib: May enhance antiplatelet effect of ibrutinib. Monitor therapy.

EFFECTS ON LAB TEST RESULTS
• May increase bleeding time and ALT, AST, and LDL cholesterol levels.

CONTRAINDICATIONS & CAUTIONS
• Contraindicated in patients hypersensitive to drug or its components.
• Use cautiously in patients sensitive to fish.
• Use cautiously in patients with coagulopathy and in those receiving therapeutic anticoagulation or antiplatelet therapy because of risk of prolonged bleeding time.
• Effect of drug on risk of pancreatitis and on CV mortality and morbidity hasn't been determined.
• Safety and effectiveness in children haven't been established.
Dialyzable drug: Unknown.

PREGNANCY-LACTATION-REPRODUCTION
• There are no adequate studies in pregnant women. Use cautiously and only if benefit justifies possible risks to the fetus.
• Drug may appear in human milk. Use cautiously in breastfeeding women.

NURSING CONSIDERATIONS
• Assess patient for conditions that contribute to increased triglycerides, such as diabetes and hypothyroidism, before treatment.
• Monitor patient for changes in INR after drug initiation and after omega-3 fatty acid dosage changes in patients receiving warfarin.
• Evaluate patient's current drug regimen for any drugs known to sharply increase triglyceride levels, including estrogen therapy, thiazide diuretics, and beta blockers. Stopping

these drugs, if appropriate, may negate the need for drug.
• Continue diet and lifestyle modifications during treatment.
• Obtain baseline triglyceride levels to confirm that they're consistently abnormal before therapy; then recheck periodically during treatment. If patient has an inadequate response after 2 months, stop drug.
• Monitor LDL level to make sure it doesn't increase excessively during treatment.
• *Look alike–sound alike:* Don't confuse Lovaza with lorazepam or lovastatin.

PATIENT TEACHING
• Explain that taking drug doesn't reduce the importance of following the recommended diet and exercise plan.
• Remind patient of the need for follow-up blood work to evaluate progress.
• Advise patient to swallow capsules whole and not to chew, crush, dissolve, or extract contents of capsule.
• Advise patient to notify prescriber about bothersome side effects.
• Tell patient to report planned or suspected pregnancy.

---

omeprazole ☒
oh-MEP-ra-zole

Losec ✦

omeprazole magnesium
Prilosec OTC ◇, Prilosec Packets

Therapeutic class: Antiulcer drugs
Pharmacologic class: PPIs

AVAILABLE FORMS
Capsules (delayed-release) ⓞ: 10 mg, 20 mg, 40 mg
Powder (for delayed-release oral suspension): 2.5 mg/packet, 10 mg/packet
Suspension: 2 mg/mL
Tablets (delayed-release) ⓞ: 20 mg ◇

INDICATIONS & DOSAGES
➤ **Symptomatic GERD without esophageal lesions**
Adults: 20 mg PO, as delayed-release form or oral suspension, daily for 8 weeks for

patients who respond poorly to customary medical treatment, usually including an adequate course of H_2-receptor antagonists.
Children ages 1 to 16 weighing 20 kg or more: 20 mg PO daily for up to 4 weeks.
Children ages 1 to 16 weighing 10 to less than 20 kg: 10 mg PO daily for up to 4 weeks.
Children ages 1 to 16 weighing 5 to less than 10 kg: 5 mg PO daily for up to 4 weeks.
➤ **Erosive esophagitis (EE)** ▨
Adults: 20 mg PO daily. For recurrent EE or GERD signs and symptoms, treat for up to 12 months.
Adjust-a-dose: When drug is used for maintenance of healing of EE, dosage reduction to 10 mg once daily is recommended for patients with hepatic impairment (Child-Pugh class A, B, or C) and Asian patients.
Children ages 1 to 16 weighing 20 kg or more: 20 mg PO daily for 4 to 8 weeks.
Children ages 1 to 16 weighing 10 to less than 20 kg: 10 mg PO daily for 4 to 8 weeks.
Children ages 1 to 16 weighing 5 to less than 10 kg: 5 mg PO daily for 4 to 8 weeks.
Infants weighing 3 to less than 5 kg: 2.5 mg once daily for up to 6 weeks.
➤ **Pathologic hypersecretory conditions (such as Zollinger-Ellison syndrome)**
Adults: Initially, 60 mg PO daily; adjust dosage based on patient response. If daily dose exceeds 80 mg, give in divided doses. Doses up to 120 mg t.i.d. have been given. Continue therapy as long as clinically indicated.
➤ **Duodenal ulcer (short-term treatment)**
Adults: 20 mg PO, as delayed-release form or oral suspension, daily for 4 weeks.
➤ *Helicobacter pylori* **infection and duodenal ulcer disease, to eradicate** *H. pylori* **with clarithromycin (dual therapy)**
Adults: 40 mg PO every morning with clarithromycin 500 mg PO t.i.d. for 14 days. For patients with an ulcer at start of therapy, give another 14 days of omeprazole 20 mg PO once daily.
➤ *H. pylori* **infection and duodenal ulcer disease, to eradicate** *H. pylori* **with clarithromycin and amoxicillin (triple therapy)**
Adults: 20 mg PO with clarithromycin 500 mg PO and amoxicillin 1,000 mg PO, each given b.i.d. for 10 days. For patients

with an ulcer at start of therapy, give another 18 days of omeprazole 20 mg PO once daily.
➤ **Short-term treatment of active benign gastric ulcer**
Adults: 40 mg PO once daily for 4 to 8 weeks.
➤ **Frequent heartburn (2 or more days a week)**
Adults: 20 mg Prilosec OTC PO once daily before breakfast for 14 days. May repeat the 14-day course every 4 months.
➤ **Dyspepsia** ◆
Adults: 20 mg once daily for up to 4 weeks.

ADMINISTRATION
PO
• Don't crush tablets or capsules. For patients who have difficulty swallowing, capsules may be opened and contents mixed with 15 mL of applesauce. Follow with water to ensure complete swallowing of pellets.
• Give drug at least 30 to 60 minutes before meals; best if taken before breakfast. If administering twice daily, give first dose before breakfast and the second dose before dinner.
• For oral suspension, empty contents of 2.5-mg packet into container containing 5 mL water; empty contents of 10-mg packet into container containing 15 mL water. Stir and leave for 2 to 3 minutes to thicken. Stir and administer within 30 minutes. If material remains after drinking, add more water, stir, and give immediately.
• For patients with an NG or gastric tube in place, add 5 mL water to catheter-tipped syringe; then add contents of 2.5-mg packet (or 15 mL water for 10-mg packet). Immediately shake syringe and leave for 2 to 3 minutes to thicken. Shake syringe and inject through NG or gastric tube, #6 French or larger, into stomach within 30 minutes. Refill syringe with an equal amount of water. Shake and flush any remaining contents from NG or gastric tube into stomach.

ACTION
Inhibits proton pump activity by binding to hydrogen–potassium adenosine triphosphatase, located at secretory surface of gastric parietal cells, to suppress gastric acid secretion.

Route	Onset	Peak	Duration
PO	1 hr	30 min–2 hr	<3 days

Half-life: 30 to 60 minutes.

ADVERSE REACTIONS
CNS: asthenia, dizziness, headache. **GI:** abdominal pain, constipation, diarrhea, flatulence, nausea, vomiting, acid regurgitation. **Musculoskeletal:** back pain, weakness. **Respiratory:** cough, URI. **Skin:** rash.

INTERACTIONS
Drug-drug. *Ampicillin esters, azole antifungals (such as ketoconazole), erlotinib, iron derivatives, nilotinib:* May cause poor bioavailability of these drugs because they need a low gastric pH for optimal absorption. Avoid using together.
Atazanavir, nelfinavir: May decrease plasma concentrations of these drugs, possibly resulting in loss of therapeutic effect. Avoid use together.
Benzodiazepines (metabolized by hepatic oxidation), fosphenytoin, phenytoin, warfarin: May decrease hepatic clearance, possibly leading to increased levels of these drugs. Monitor drug levels.
Bisphosphonates: May decrease therapeutic effect of bisphosphonates. Monitor therapy.
Calcium salts: May decrease GI absorption of calcium salts. Closely monitor clinical response and increase calcium dosage if needed.
Cilostazol: May increase cilostazol level. Reduce cilostazol dosage.
Clopidogrel: May decrease antiplatelet activity. Avoid use together.
Cyclosporine: May increase cyclosporine serum concentration. Monitor cyclosporine level closely.
Digoxin: May increase digoxin level, causing toxicity. Monitor digoxin level.
Fluvoxamine: May increase omeprazole level. Monitor patient for increased adverse reactions.
Fosphenytoin: May increase fosphenytoin serum concentration; fosphenytoin may decrease omeprazole serum concentration. Monitor therapy closely.
Iron salts: May interfere with iron absorption. Omeprazole may need to be temporar-

ily stopped, or parenteral iron may be given as an alternative.
Mycophenolate: May decrease mycophenolate serum concentration; may reduce formation of active metabolite for mycophenolate. Monitor therapy.
Methotrexate: May increase methotrexate level, causing toxicity. Monitor patient closely.
Rifampin: May substantially decrease omeprazole concentration. Avoid concomitant use.
Salicylates: Enteric-coated forms may dissolve faster, increasing risk of gastric adverse effects. Use together cautiously.
Saquinavir: May increase saquinavir serum concentration, resulting in increased toxicity. Monitor therapy.
Tacrolimus: May increase tacrolimus level and risk of toxicity. Monitor tacrolimus trough concentration when omeprazole is started and stopped.
Voriconazole: May increase serum concentrations of both drugs. Consider reducing omeprazole dosage by 50%; monitor therapy.
Drug-herb. *St. John's wort:* May substantially decrease omeprazole concentration. Avoid concomitant use.
Drug-food. *Vitamin B_{12}:* Prolonged treatment with omeprazole (2 years or longer) may lead to malabsorption of dietary vitamin B_{12}. Avoid concomitant use.

EFFECTS ON LAB TEST RESULTS
● May increase LFT values and falsely elevate serum chromogranin A (CgA) level.
● May decrease magnesium, sodium, glucose, and vitamin B_{12} levels.

CONTRAINDICATIONS & CAUTIONS
● Contraindicated in patients hypersensitive to drug or its components and in patients receiving rilpivirine-containing products.
◑ **Alert:** High-dose, long-term PPI therapy may be associated with an increased risk of hip, wrist, and spine fractures.
▧ Bioavailability is increased in patients of Asian descent, and reduced dosages are recommended when used for healing EE.
● Use cautiously in patients with hypokalemia and respiratory alkalosis and in patients on a low-sodium diet.

• Risk of fundic gland polyps increases with long-term use, especially beyond 1 year.

• Long-term administration of bicarbonate with calcium or milk can cause milk-alkali syndrome.

Dialyzable drug: Unlikely.

⚠ *Overdose S&S:* Confusion, drowsiness, blurred vision, tachycardia, nausea, vomiting, diaphoresis, flushing, headache, dry mouth.

PREGNANCY-LACTATION-REPRODUCTION

• Use during pregnancy only if potential benefit justifies risks to the fetus. When treating GERD in pregnant women, PPIs may be used when necessary; however, lifestyle modification is the initial treatment.

• Drug appears in human milk. Use cautiously in breastfeeding women.

NURSING CONSIDERATIONS

⊙ *Alert:* May increase risk of CDAD. Evaluate for CDAD in patients who develop diarrhea that doesn't improve.

• False-positive results in diagnostic investigations for neuroendocrine tumors may occur due to increased CgA level. Temporarily stop omeprazole treatment at least 14 days before assessing CgA level and consider repeating the test if initial CgA level is high. If serial tests are performed (e.g., for monitoring), the same commercial lab should be used for testing, as reference ranges between tests may vary.

• Long-term therapy may cause vitamin B_{12} absorption problems. Assess patient for signs and symptoms of cyanocobalamin deficiency (weakness, heart palpitations, dyspnea, paresthesia, pale skin, smooth tongue, CNS changes, loss of appetite).

• Because risk of fundic gland polyps increases with long-term use, especially beyond 1 year, use drug for shortest duration appropriate to the condition being treated.

⚖ Dosage adjustments may be necessary in Asians and patients with hepatic impairment.

• Periodically assess patient for osteoporosis.

• Monitor patient for signs and symptoms of acute interstitial nephritis.

• Discontinue drug if signs or symptoms of cutaneous lupus erythematosus or SLE de-

velop; refer patient to the appropriate specialist for evaluation.

• Drug increases its own bioavailability with repeated doses. Drug is unstable in gastric acid; less drug is lost to hydrolysis because drug increases gastric pH.

• Gastrin level rises in most patients during the first 2 weeks of therapy.

⊙ *Alert:* Prolonged use of PPIs may cause low magnesium levels. Monitor magnesium levels before starting treatment and periodically thereafter.

⊙ *Alert:* Monitor patients for signs and symptoms of low magnesium level, such as abnormal HR or rhythm, palpitations, muscle spasms, tremors, or seizures. In children, an abnormal HR may present as fatigue, upset stomach, dizziness, and lightheadedness. Magnesium supplementation or drug discontinuation may be required.

• *Look alike–sound alike:* Don't confuse Prilosec OTC with Plendil, Prevacid, prednisone, Pristiq, Prozac, prilocaine, or Prinivil. Don't confuse omeprazole with aripiprazole, esomeprazole, or fomepizole.

PATIENT TEACHING

• Tell patient to swallow tablets whole and not to open, crush, or chew them.

• Give patient instructions on how to take oral suspension.

• Instruct patient to take drug at least 30 to 60 minutes before meals.

• Caution patient to avoid hazardous activities if dizziness occurs.

• Advise patient that Prilosec OTC isn't intended to treat infrequent heartburn (one episode of heartburn a week or less), or for those who want immediate relief of heartburn.

• Inform patient that Prilosec OTC may take 1 to 4 days for full effect, although some patients may get complete relief of symptoms within 24 hours.

• Teach patient to recognize and report signs and symptoms of low magnesium levels.

---

onabotulinumtoxinA
oh-nuh-BOT-yoo-lin-num-TOKS-in aye

Botox

onabotulinumtoxinA (cosmetic)
Botox Cosmetic

Therapeutic class: Neuromuscular transmission blockers
Pharmacologic class: Acetylcholine release inhibitors

AVAILABLE FORMS
onabotulinumtoxinA
Injection: 50 units/vial, 100 units/vial, 200 units/vial
onabotulinumtoxinA (cosmetic)
Injection: 50 units/vial, 100 units/vial

INDICATIONS & DOSAGES
Adjust-a-dose (for all indications): When adults are being treated for one or more indications, maximum cumulative dose generally shouldn't exceed 400 units in a 3-month interval (Botox) or 360 units in a 3-month interval (Botox Cosmetic).

➤ **Overactive bladder signs and symptoms (urge urinary incontinence, urgency, and frequency) in patients with inadequate response to or intolerant of anticholinergic medication (Botox)**
Adults: Recommended total dose is 100 units, given as 0.5 mL (5 units) IM across 20 sites into the detrusor muscle. Give prophylactic antibiotics (except aminoglycosides) 1 to 3 days before treatment, on treatment day, and 1 to 3 days after treatment to reduce likelihood of procedure-related UTI. Discontinue antiplatelet therapy at least 3 days before administration. Consider retreatment no sooner than 12 weeks from prior injection.

➤ **Urinary incontinence due to detrusor overactivity associated with a neurologic condition, such as spinal cord injury or MS, after inadequate response to or intolerance of anticholinergic medication (Botox)**
Adults: Recommended total dose is 200 units, given as 30 injections of 1 mL (6.7 units) each (total volume of 30 mL) IM across 30 sites into the detrusor muscle. For the final injection, inject approximately 1 mL of sterile NSS to ensure that the remaining medication in the needle is delivered to the bladder. Give prophylactic antibiotics (except aminoglycosides) 1 to 3 days before treatment, on treatment day, and 1 to 3 days after treatment to reduce likelihood of procedure-related UTI. Consider retreatment no sooner than 12 weeks from prior injection. Discontinue antiplatelet therapy at least 3 days before administration.

➤ **Prophylaxis of headaches in patients with chronic migraine (15 days per month or more, with headache lasting 4 hours a day or longer) (Botox)**
Adults: Recommended total dose is 155 units, given as 0.1 mL (5 units), IM divided across seven head/neck muscles every 12 weeks. Injections should be equally divided and administered bilaterally into 31 total sites. Refer to manufacturer's instructions for injection-site diagrams.

➤ **Upper limb spasticity (Botox)**
Adults: 12.5 to 50 units per site IM. Up to 200 units divided into four sites for biceps brachii. The lowest recommended starting dose should be used. Tailor dosing in initial and sequential treatment sessions to the individual based on the size, number, and location of muscles involved; severity of spasticity; presence of local muscle weakness; and patient's response to previous treatment or adverse event history with onabotulinumtoxinA. Administer no more than 50 units per site. Refer to manufacturer's instructions for specific sites and dosages. Consider retreatment no sooner than 12 weeks from prior injection.

➤ **Lower limb spasticity (Botox)**
Adults: 300 to 400 units IM divided among five muscles (gastrocnemius, soleus, tibialis posterior, flexor hallucis longus, and flexor digitorum longus). Use lowest recommended starting dose and administer no more than 50 units per site. Individualize dosing in initial and sequential treatment sessions based on size, number, and location of muscles involved; severity of spasticity; presence of local muscle weakness; and patient's response to previous treatment or adverse event history with

O

onabotulinumtoxinA. Refer to manufacturer's instructions for specific sites and dosages. May repeat therapy no sooner than 12 weeks, with appropriate dosage based on clinical condition of patient at time of retreatment.

➤ **Cervical dystonia to reduce severity of abnormal head position and neck pain (Botox)**

Adults and children age 16 and older: Adjust initial and subsequent dosing based on patient's head and neck position, localization of pain, muscle hypertrophy, patient response, and adverse event history. Use lower initial dose in botulinum toxin–naive patients. Administer no more than 50 units per site. See prescribing information for mean doses and ranges used in studies.

➤ **Severe axillary hyperhidrosis inadequately managed by topical agents (Botox)**

Adults: 50 units (2 mL) injected intradermally in 0.1- to 0.2-mL aliquots to each axilla, evenly distributed in 10 to 15 sites approximately 1 to 2 cm apart. May administer repeat injections when clinical effect of a previous injection diminishes.

➤ **Blepharospasm associated with dystonia (Botox)**

Adults and children age 12 and older: 1.25 to 2.5 units (0.05 to 0.1 mL volume at each site) IM into medial and lateral pretarsal orbicularis oculi of upper lid and into lateral pretarsal orbicularis oculi of lower lid. Cumulative dose in a 30-day period shouldn't exceed 200 units.

➤ **Strabismus (Botox)**

Adults and children age 12 and older: It's recommended that several drops of local anesthetic and an ocular decongestant be given several minutes before injection.

For vertical muscles, and for horizontal strabismus of less than 20 prism diopters: 1.25 to 2.5 units in any one muscle. For horizontal strabismus of 20 to 50 prism diopters: 2.5 to 5 units in any one muscle. Maximum dose is 25 units for any one muscle. For reexamination and subsequent dosing, see prescribing information.

➤ **Persistent cranial nerve VI palsy lasting 1 month or longer**

Adults: 1.25 to 2.5 units IM in medial rectus muscle.

➤ **Temporary improvement in appearance of moderate to severe glabellar lines associated with corrugator or procerus muscle activity (Botox Cosmetic)**

Adults: Inject 4 units (0.1 mL) IM into each of five sites, two in each corrugator muscle and one in the procerus muscle for a total dose of 20 units; administer no more frequently than every 3 to 4 months. An effective dose for facial lines is determined by gross observation of patient's ability to activate the superficial muscles injected.

➤ **Temporary improvement in appearance of moderate to severe lateral canthal lines associated with orbicularis oculi activity (Botox Cosmetic)**

Adults: Inject 4 units (0.1 mL) IM into each of three sites per side (six total injection points) in the lateral orbicularis oculi muscle for a total of 24 units (0.6 mL) (12 units per side); administer no more frequently than every 3 months. For simultaneous treatment with glabellar lines, dose is 24 units for lateral canthal lines and 20 units for glabellar lines, with total dose of 44 units.

➤ **Temporary improvement in appearance of moderate to severe forehead lines associated with frontalis muscle activity (Botox Cosmetic)**

Adults: 0.1 mL (4 units) IM into each of five forehead line sites (20 units) with 0.1 mL (4 units) IM into each of five glabellar line sites (20 units). Recommended total dose for forehead lines and glabellar lines together is 40 units. Administer no more frequently than every 3 months.

➤ **Spasticity of cerebral palsy**

Children and adolescents: 1 to 30 units/kg per session. Total dose per muscle is 0.5 to 6 units/kg.

ADMINISTRATION
IM, intradermal

🕭 *Alert:* Don't use Botox and contact Allergan (1-800-890-4345) if carton labeling doesn't contain an intact seal with a translucent silver Allergan logo (on both ends of carton) or the seal has a black circle with a diagonal line through it (i.e., prohibition sign), if vial label doesn't contain a holographic film containing the name "Allergan" within rainbow-colored horizontal lines, or if the U.S. license number 1145 isn't present on the vial label and carton labeling.

• Store unopened vials refrigerated at 36° to 46° F (2° to 8° C) for up to 36 months or until expiration date.

• Reconstitute each vial with sterile, non-preserved NSS for injection by drawing up proper amount of diluent (see manufacturer's instructions) in appropriate-sized syringe (see manufacturer's instructions) and slowly injecting diluent into vial.

• Gently mix drug with the NSS by rotating vial.

• Administer within 24 hours after reconstitution; store in refrigerator until administration.

ACTION
Blocks neuromuscular transmission by inhibiting release of acetylcholine. IM doses chemically denervate muscle, reducing muscular activity either temporarily or permanently. Intradermal administration causes temporary chemical denervation of sweat glands, resulting in local reduction in sweating. Intradetrusor injection affects detrusor muscle activity via inhibition of acetylcholine release.

Route	Onset	Peak	Duration
IM, intradermal	Varies by site	Varies by site	Varies by site

Half-life: Unknown.

ADVERSE REACTIONS
Overactive bladder symptoms
GU: UTI, dysuria, urine retention, bacteriuria, residual urine volume, hematuria. **Other:** injection-site soreness or *hemorrhage*.
Urinary incontinence due to detrusor overactivity associated with a neurologic condition
GI: constipation. **GU:** UTI, dysuria, urine retention, hematuria. **Musculoskeletal:** weakness, muscle spasm, gait disturbance, falls. **Other:** injection-site soreness or *hemorrhage*.
Chronic migraine headache prophylaxis
CNS: headache, worsening migraine. **CV:** HTN. **EENT:** ptosis, facial paresis. **Musculoskeletal:** neck pain, weakness, stiffness, myalgia, muscle spasm. **Respiratory:**

bronchitis. **Other:** injection-site pain.
Upper and lower limb spasticity
CNS: fatigue. **GI:** nausea. **Musculoskeletal:** extremity pain, weakness. **Respiratory:** bronchitis, URI. **Other:** injection-site soreness or *hemorrhage*.
Cervical dystonia
CNS: headache, dizziness, fever, speech disorder, numbness, asthenia, drowsiness. **EENT:** ptosis, diplopia, blepharoptosis. rhinitis, oral dryness. **GI:** nausea, dysphagia. **Musculoskeletal:** neck pain, back pain, stiffness, hypertonia. **Respiratory:** URI, increased cough, dyspnea. **Other:** flulike syndrome, injection-site soreness, antibody formation.
Severe axillary hyperhidrosis
CNS: headache, fever, anxiety, dizziness. **EENT:** pharyngitis. **GI:** nausea. **Metabolic:** nonaxillary sweating. **Musculoskeletal:** neck or back pain. **Skin:** pruritus. **Other:** flulike syndrome, injection-site pain or *hemorrhage*, infection.
Blepharospasm associated with dystonia
EENT: ptosis, superficial punctate keratitis, eye dryness, irritation, tearing, lagophthalmos, photophobia, ectropion, keratitis, diplopia, entropion, local swelling of eyelid skin. **Skin:** diffuse rash. **Other:** injection-site soreness or *hemorrhage*.
Strabismus
EENT: vertical deviation due to effect on adjacent extraocular muscles, ptosis. **Other:** injection-site soreness or *hemorrhage*.
Persistent cranial nerve VI palsy
Other: injection-site soreness or *hemorrhage*.
Glabellar lines
CNS: facial paresis. **EENT:** eyelid ptosis. **Musculoskeletal:** muscular weakness. **Other:** facial pain.
Lateral canthal lines
EENT: eyelid edema.
Forehead lines
CNS: headache. **EENT:** eyelid ptosis. **Skin:** brow ptosis, skin tightness.

INTERACTIONS
Drug-drug. *Aminoglycosides, neuromuscular blockers (curare or curare-like compounds):* May increase effect of toxin and risk of respiratory depression. Don't use together.

O

Anticholinergics: May increase systemic anticholinergic effects. Avoid use together.

Anticoagulants, antiplatelet drugs: May increase risk of bleeding. Discontinue antiplatelet therapy at least 3 days before injection procedure; monitor patients on anticoagulant therapy carefully.

Muscle relaxants, other botulinum neurotoxin products: May cause excessive neuromuscular weakness. Avoid use together.

EFFECTS ON LAB TEST RESULTS
None reported.

CONTRAINDICATIONS & CAUTIONS
Black Box Warning The effects of onabotulinumtoxinA and all botulinum toxin products may spread from the injection area to produce signs and symptoms consistent with botulinum toxin effects. These may include asthenia, generalized muscle weakness, diplopia, ptosis, dysphagia, dysphonia, dysarthria, urinary incontinence, and breathing difficulties, which have reportedly occurred hours to weeks after injection. Swallowing and breathing difficulties can be life-threatening; deaths have been reported. Risk of symptoms developing is probably greatest in children treated for spasticity, but symptoms can also occur in adults treated for spasticity and other conditions, particularly in those with an underlying condition predisposing them to these symptoms. In unapproved uses (including spasticity in children) and in approved indications, cases of spread of effect have been reported at doses comparable to those used to treat cervical dystonia and at lower doses. ∎

☉ *Alert:* In the event of overdose, antitoxin against botulinum toxin is available from the CDC. However, the antitoxin will not reverse botulinum toxin-induced effects already apparent by the time of antitoxin administration. In the event of suspected or actual cases of botulinum toxin poisoning, contact your local or state health department to process a request for antitoxin through the CDC. If you don't receive a response within 30 minutes, contact the CDC directly at 1-800-232-4636.

• Contraindicated in known hypersensitivity to botulinum toxin and in patient with infection at injection sites.

• Contraindicated in patients being treated for overactive bladder with UTIs and in patients with overactive bladder or detrusor overactivity associated with a neurologic condition who have postvoid residual urine volume greater than 200 mL but don't catheterize routinely (patients with MS or diabetes mellitus).

• Use cautiously in patients with bleeding disorders and in those receiving anticoagulation therapy.

• Use cautiously in patients with inflammation at the proposed injection site or when excessive weakness or atrophy is present in the target muscle.

• Use cautiously in patients with preexisting neuromuscular disorders, compromised respiratory function, or corneal exposure and ulceration due to reduced blinking.

Dialyzable drug: Unknown.

⚠ *Overdose S&S:* Neuromuscular weakness, aspiration pneumonia, respiratory muscle paralysis, respiratory failure, death.

PREGNANCY-LACTATION-REPRODUCTION
• There are no adequate studies in pregnant women. Use only if benefit justifies risks to the fetus.

• It isn't known if drug appears in human milk. Use cautiously in breastfeeding women.

NURSING CONSIDERATIONS
☉ *Alert:* Signs and symptoms of overdose usually don't occur immediately after injection. Should accidental injection or oral ingestion occur or overdose be suspected, patient should be medically supervised for several weeks for signs and symptoms of systemic muscular weakness, which could be local or distant from the injection.

Black Box Warning Monitor patient for swallowing and breathing difficulties, which can lead to death. ∎

• Prescribers administering the drug must understand the relevant neuromuscular or orbital anatomy and any alterations to that anatomy due to prior surgical procedures.

• Understanding of standard electromyographic techniques is required for treatment of strabismus and upper limb spasticity, and may be useful for the treatment of cervical dystonia.

- Botox and Botox Cosmetic contain the same active ingredient in the same formulation but aren't interchangeable.
- Drug isn't interchangeable with other preparations of botulinum toxin products and can't be converted into units of other botulinum toxin products.
- Start treatment at lowest recommended dosage.
- Watch for bronchitis and URI in patients being treated for upper limb spasticity.
- Discontinue antiplatelet therapy at least 3 days before the injection procedure; patients on anticoagulant therapy need to be managed appropriately to decrease bleeding risk.
- Repeat treatment may be administered when effect of previous injection has diminished, but generally no sooner than 12 weeks after previous injection.
- Degree or pattern of muscle spasticity at the time of reinjection may necessitate alterations in dosage and of muscles to be injected.
- To prepare eye for injection, several drops of a local anesthetic and an ocular decongestant are instilled several minutes before injection.
- Monitor patient for retrobulbar hemorrhages and compromised retinal circulation after eye injections.

PATIENT TEACHING

Black Box Warning Caution patient to seek immediate medical attention if serious side effects occur, such as difficulty swallowing, speaking, or breathing. These side effects can occur hours, days, or even weeks after injection and can be fatal. ■

- Teach patient to report signs and symptoms of botulism toxicity, such as loss of strength or muscle weakness, double vision, blurred vision, drooping eyelids, hoarseness, change in or loss of voice, trouble speaking clearly, or loss of bladder control. Inform patient that, if these side effects occur, patient shouldn't drive a car, operate machinery, or perform other dangerous activities.
- Advise patient that onabotulinumtoxinA injections may cause reduced blinking or reduced effectiveness of blinking, and to seek immediate medical attention if eye pain or irritation occurs after treatment.

- Instruct patient to report voiding difficulties after bladder injections for urinary incontinence.

ondansetron
on-DAN-sah-tron

Zuplenz

ondansetron hydrochloride
Zofran, Zofran ODT

Therapeutic class: Antiemetics
Pharmacologic class: Selective serotonin (5-HT$_3$) receptor antagonists

AVAILABLE FORMS
Injection: 2 mg/mL, 4 mg/2 mL
Oral soluble film: 4 mg, 8 mg
Oral solution: 4 mg/5 mL
Tablets: 4 mg, 8 mg, 24 mg
Tablets (ODTs): 4 mg, 8 mg

INDICATIONS & DOSAGES
Adjust-a-dose (for all indications): For patients with severe hepatic impairment (Child-Pugh class C), total daily dose shouldn't exceed 8 mg.
➤ **To prevent nausea and vomiting from highly emetogenic chemotherapy**
Adults: Administer in combination with neurokinin 1 receptor antagonist and dexamethasone, with or without olanzapine. Give 24 mg PO as a single dose or 8 mg PO b.i.d. for two doses 30 minutes before chemotherapy. Or, three successive 8-mg PO doses (ODT, film) 30 minutes before start of single-day highly emetogenic chemotherapy.

If patient can't take oral form, give 0.15 mg/kg IV over 15 minutes beginning 30 minutes before chemotherapy. Give a second 0.15-mg/kg IV dose 4 hours later, then a third 0.15-mg/kg IV dose 8 hours after first dose. Don't exceed 16 mg/dose.
Children ages 6 months to 18 years: 0.15 mg/kg IV over 15 minutes beginning 30 minutes before chemotherapy. Give second dose of 0.15 mg/kg IV over 15 minutes 4 hours after first dose. Give third 0.15-mg/kg IV dose 8 hours after first dose. No single IV dose should exceed 16 mg.

O

➤ **To prevent nausea and vomiting from moderately emetogenic chemotherapy**
Adults: Administer in combination with neurokinin 1 receptor antagonist and dexamethasone for carboplatin-based regimens or in combination with dexamethasone for non-carboplatin-based regimens. Give 8 mg PO 30 minutes before chemotherapy. Then, 8 mg PO 8 hours after first dose. Then, 8 mg PO every 12 hours for 1 to 2 days after completion of chemotherapy. Or, one dose of 0.15 mg/kg IV. No single IV dose should exceed 16 mg. Or, 8 mg PO (film) 30 minutes before chemotherapy, followed by 8 mg PO (film) 8 hours after first dose. Then give 8 mg PO (film) every 12 hours for 1 to 2 days after completing chemotherapy.
Children ages 12 and older: 8 mg PO (ODT, tablet, solution) 30 minutes before chemotherapy, then 8 mg PO 4 hours and 8 hours after first dose. Then, 8 mg every 8 hours for 1 to 2 days after completion of chemotherapy. Or, for soluble film, 8 mg PO 30 minutes before start of emetogenic chemotherapy, then a subsequent dose 8 hours after first dose, then 8 mg every 12 hours for 1 to 2 days after completion of chemotherapy.
Children ages 4 to 11: 4 mg PO 30 minutes before chemotherapy. Then, 4 mg PO 4 and 8 hours after first dose. Then, 4 mg PO every 8 hours for 1 to 2 days after completion of chemotherapy.
Infants and children ages 6 months to 18 years: Three doses of 0.15 mg/kg IV. Give first dose 30 minutes before chemotherapy; give subsequent doses 4 and 8 hours after first dose. Infuse drug over 15 minutes. No single IV dose should exceed 16 mg.
➤ **To prevent postoperative nausea and vomiting**
Adults: 4 mg undiluted solution for injection IM or IV over 2 to 5 minutes at end of surgery. Or, 8 mg ODT or oral soluble film PO as a single dose 30 to 60 minutes before surgery.
Children ages 1 month to 12 years weighing more than 40 kg: 4 mg IV as a single dose over 2 to 5 minutes.
Children ages 1 month to 12 years weighing 40 kg or less: 0.1 mg/kg IV as a single

dose over 2 to 5 minutes. Maximum dose is 4 mg/dose.
➤ **To prevent nausea and vomiting from radiation therapy in patients receiving total body irradiation, single high-dose fraction radiation therapy to abdomen, or daily fractionated radiation therapy to abdomen**
Adults: For patients receiving total body irradiation, give 8 mg PO ODT or oral soluble film 1 to 2 hours before each fraction of radiation therapy each day. May administer b.i.d. Give in combination with dexamethasone. For patients receiving single high-dose fraction radiation therapy to the abdomen, give 8 mg PO ODT or oral soluble film 1 to 2 hours before therapy, then every 8 hours for 1 to 2 days after completion of therapy. For patients receiving daily fractionated radiation therapy, give 8 mg PO ODT or oral soluble film 1 to 2 hours before therapy, then every 8 hours for each day therapy is given.

ADMINISTRATION
PO
• Open blister of ODT just before use by peeling backing off. Don't push ODT through foil blister.
• For Zuplenz, open film pouch with dry hands and immediately place film on top of the tongue, where it will dissolve in 4 to 20 seconds. Then have patient swallow with or without liquid. Wash hands after giving Zuplenz. If using more than one film, allow each film to dissolve completely before administering the next film.
• Protect 4-mg tablets and oral solution from light.
IV
⚠ Alert: No single IV dose should exceed 16 mg due to the risk of QT-interval prolongation.
▼ If precipitate is noted in vial, shake vigorously until dissolved.
▼ Dilute drug in 50 mL of D_5W injection or NSS for injection.
▼ Drug is stable for up to 48 hours after dilution in NSS, D_5W, 5% dextrose in half-NSS for injection, 5% dextrose in NSS.
▼ Infuse over 15 minutes.
▼ **Incompatibilities:** Alkaline solutions.

IM
• Document injection site.
• If precipitate is noted in vial, shake vigorously until dissolved.
• Give IM injection undiluted.

ACTION
May block 5-HT$_3$ in the CNS in the chemoreceptor trigger zone and in the peripheral nervous system on nerve terminals of the vagus nerve.

Route	Onset	Peak	Duration
PO	30 min	1–2 hr	Unknown
IV	Immediate	Unknown	Unknown
IM	Unknown	Unknown	Unknown

Half-life: About 3 to 6 hours.

ADVERSE REACTIONS
CNS: dizziness, fatigue, headache, malaise, sedation, extrapyramidal syndrome, fever, agitation, anxiety, pain. **CV:** *arrhythmias,* chest pain. **GI:** constipation, diarrhea. **GU:** gynecologic disorders, urine retention. **Respiratory:** *hypoxia.* **Skin:** pruritus, rash. **Other:** chills, injection-site reaction.

INTERACTIONS
Drug-drug. ❸ *Alert: Apomorphine:* May cause profound hypotension and loss of consciousness. Use together is contraindicated.
Drugs (such as cimetidine) that alter hepatic drug-metabolizing enzymes, phenobarbital, rifampin: May change pharmacokinetics of ondansetron, but there is no need to adjust dosage based on clinical data.
Drugs that prolong QTc interval (antiarrhythmics, antipsychotics, antidepressants): May result in ventricular arrhythmias. Use cautiously and avoid combination with drugs at highest risk for QTc-interval prolongation.
SSNRIs, SSRIs: May result in serotonin syndrome. Use cautiously and monitor patient for mental status changes, tachycardia, sweating, flushing, nausea, vomiting, tremors, and muscle rigidity.
Drug-herb. *Horehound:* May enhance serotonergic effects. Discourage use together.
St. John's wort: May decrease ondansetron serum concentration. Consider therapy modification.

EFFECTS ON LAB TEST RESULTS
• May increase ALT and AST levels.

CONTRAINDICATIONS & CAUTIONS
• Contraindicated in patients hypersensitive to drug.
• ECG changes, including prolonged QT interval and torsades de pointes, have been reported. Avoid use in patients with congenital long QT syndrome. Monitor patient carefully.
• Use cautiously in patients with hepatic impairment.
Dialyzable drug: Unlikely.
⚠ *Overdose S&S:* Sudden transient blindness, severe constipation, hypotension.

PREGNANCY-LACTATION-REPRODUCTION
• There are no adequate studies in pregnant women. Drug crosses placental barrier during first trimester. Use only if clearly needed.
• It isn't known if drug appears in human milk. Use cautiously in breastfeeding women.

NURSING CONSIDERATIONS
❸ *Alert:* Drug may increase the risk of prolonged QT interval and torsades de pointes (a potentially fatal heart rhythm). Monitor ECG in patients with congenital long QT syndrome, in those with HF or bradyarrhythmias, and in those taking other medications that can prolong the QT interval.
❸ *Alert:* Correct electrolyte abnormalities (hypokalemia or hypomagnesemia) before infusing drug.
• Monitor LFT results. Don't exceed 8 mg in patients with hepatic impairment.
• Monitor patient for signs and symptoms of serotonin syndrome.
• *Look alike–sound alike:* Don't confuse Zofran with Zosyn, Zantac, or Zoloft. Don't confuse ondansetron with dolasetron, granisetron, or palonosetron.

PATIENT TEACHING
❸ *Alert:* Caution patient to contact health care provider immediately for signs and symptoms of abnormal HR or rhythm, such as palpitations, dyspnea, or dizziness.
• Tell patient that an ECG may be necessary to monitor HR and rhythm.

- Instruct patient to immediately report difficulty breathing after drug administration.
- Tell patient receiving drug IV to report discomfort at insertion site.
- Tell patient taking ODTs to open blister just before use by peeling backing off and not by pushing through foil blister and that taking ODT with liquid isn't required.
- Teach patient to place ODTs or film on tongue, allow to dissolve, then swallow with saliva.

oritavancin diphosphate
or-it-a-VAN-sin

Orbactiv

Therapeutic class: Antibiotics
Pharmacologic class: Lipoglycopeptides

AVAILABLE FORMS
Powder for injection: 400-mg vial

INDICATIONS & DOSAGES
➤ **Acute bacterial skin and skin-structure infections caused or suspected to be caused by susceptible gram-positive bacteria, including *Staphylococcus aureus* (methicillin-sensitive and methicillin-resistant); *Streptococcus* species, including *S. pyogenes, S. agalactiae, S. dysgalactiae, S. anginosus, S. intermedius,* and *S. constellatus*; and vancomycin-susceptible *Enterococcus faecalis***
Adults: A single dose of 1,200 mg IV.

ADMINISTRATION
IV
▼ Obtain specimen for culture and sensitivity testing before giving.
▼ Prepare three 400-mg vials for a single 1,200-mg IV dose.
▼ Reconstitute each vial with 40 mL of sterile water for injection to provide a solution containing 10 mg/mL/vial. Inspect for particulate matter. Solution should be clear and colorless to pale yellow.
▼ For infusion, further dilute in 1,000 mL D₅W; withdraw 120 mL from 1,000-mL D₅W bag and add oritavancin reconstituted solution.

▼ Infuse drug over 3 hours. If IV line is also used to infuse other drugs, flush it with D₅W before and after each infusion.
▼ Refrigerate solution after reconstitution and use within 12 hours or within 6 hours when stored at room temperature, including 3-hour infusion time.
▼ **Incompatibilities:** NSS.

ACTION
Disrupts bacterial cell-wall synthesis and bacterial membrane integrity.

Route	Onset	Peak	Duration
IV	Unknown	Unknown	Unknown

Half-life: 245 hours.

ADVERSE REACTIONS
CNS: headache, dizziness. **CV:** tachycardia, peripheral edema, injection-site phlebitis, *leukocytoclastic vasculitis.* **GI:** nausea, vomiting, diarrhea. **Hematologic:** anemia, eosinophilia. **Hepatic:** elevated ALT, AST, and bilirubin levels. **Metabolic:** *hypoglycemia,* hyperuricemia. **Musculoskeletal:** tenosynovitis, myalgia, osteomyelitis. **Respiratory:** *bronchospasm,* wheezing. **Skin:** limb and subcutaneous abscesses, rash, urticaria, *erythema multiforme,* cellulitis. **Other:** infusion reaction, infusion-site erythema, extravasation, induration, pruritus, hypersensitivity, *angioedema.*

INTERACTIONS
Drug-drug. *Dextromethorphan, midazolam:* May decrease concentrations of these drugs. Monitor patient for effectiveness.
Omeprazole: May increase omeprazole level. Monitor patient for omeprazole toxicity.
Unfractionated heparin sodium (IV): May falsely elevate aPTT test results for up to 120 hours (5 days). Heparin use is contraindicated for 120 hours after oritavancin administration.
Warfarin: May increase warfarin level and risk of bleeding. Monitor INR and patient for bleeding.

EFFECTS ON LAB TEST RESULTS
- May artificially prolong aPTT for up to 120 hours, prolong PT and increase INR for up to 12 hours, and prolong activated

---

clotting time for up to 24 hours after dose is given.
• May increase AST, ALT, uric acid, and total bilirubin levels. May decrease glucose level.

CONTRAINDICATIONS & CAUTIONS
• Contraindicated in patients hypersensitive to drug or its components.
• Use of unfractionated heparin IV is contraindicated for 120 hours after oritavancin administration.
• Use cautiously in patients with history of hypersensitivity to glycopeptides (vancomycin, telavancin, dalbavancin); serious hypersensitivity reactions have been reported. If acute reaction occurs, discontinue drug and treat immediately.
• Drug can cause superinfection, including CDAD and pseudomembranous colitis, which can occur more than 2 months after therapy ends.
• Drug may increase risk of osteomyelitis; an alternative antibacterial therapy may be needed.
• Drug hasn't been studied in patients with severe renal or hepatic impairment.
Dialyzable drug: No.

PREGNANCY-LACTATION-REPRODUCTION
• There are no adequate studies in pregnant women. Use only if potential benefit justifies potential risks to the fetus.
• It isn't known if drug appears in human milk. Use cautiously in breastfeeding women.

NURSING CONSIDERATIONS
• Monitor patient for signs and symptoms of superinfection (frequent, watery stools) and osteomyelitis (fever, erythema, edema, pain).
• Infusion-related reactions (pruritus, urticaria, flushing) have been reported. Slow rate or interrupt infusion if reaction develops.
• If anticoagulation is needed, consider using anticoagulants that don't require PTT or INR monitoring.
• *Look alike–sound alike:* Don't confuse Orbactiv with Activase, Vibativ, or Factive. Don't confuse oritavancin with telavancin or dalbavancin.

PATIENT TEACHING
• Explain that antibiotics can change normal intestinal flora and that patient should report severe watery or bloody diarrhea as this may indicate a more serious intestinal infection.
• Instruct patient to report discomfort at IV insertion site.
• Warn patient that allergic reactions, including serious allergic reactions, can occur and require immediate treatment.

oseltamivir phosphate
oh-sel-TAM-i-ver

Tamiflu✍

Therapeutic class: Antivirals
Pharmacologic class: Selective neuraminidase inhibitors

AVAILABLE FORMS
Capsules: 30 mg, 45 mg, 75 mg
Oral suspension: 6 mg/mL after reconstitution

INDICATIONS & DOSAGES
➤ **To prevent influenza during a community outbreak or within 2 days after close contact with an infected person**
Adults and adolescents age 13 and older: 75 mg PO (capsule or 12.5 mL suspension) once daily for 1 week after last exposure if vaccinated or 2 weeks if unvaccinated. For a community outbreak, safety and effectiveness have been demonstrated for up to 6 weeks in immunocompetent patients.
Children ages 1 to 12 weighing 40.1 kg or more: 75 mg (12.5 mL suspension) PO once daily for 10 days.
Children ages 1 to 12 weighing 23.1 to 40 kg: 60 mg (10 mL suspension) PO once daily for 10 days.
Children ages 1 to 12 weighing 15.1 to 23 kg: 45 mg (7.5 mL suspension) PO once daily for 10 days.
Children ages 1 to 12 weighing 15 kg or less: 30 mg (5 mL suspension) PO once daily for 10 days.
Children age 3 months or older: 3 mg/kg PO once daily. Duration is variable.
Adjust-a-dose: For adults and adolescents with CrCl of 30 to 60 mL/minute, reduce

dosage to 30 mg PO once daily. For CrCl of 10 to 30 mL/minute, reduce dosage to 30 mg every other day. For patients on hemodialysis (CrCl <10 mL/minute), give 30 mg PO immediately, then 30 mg after every hemodialysis session for 5 days. For patients on continuous ambulatory peritoneal dialysis (CrCl <10 mL/minute), give 30 mg PO immediately and 30 mg once weekly.

➤ **To treat influenza**
Adults and adolescents age 13 and older: 75 mg PO b.i.d. (capsule or 12.5 mL suspension) for 5 days. Begin treatment within 2 days of onset of influenza symptoms.
Children ages 1 to 12 weighing 40.1 kg or more: 75 mg (12.5 mL suspension) PO b.i.d. for 5 days.
Children ages 1 to 12 weighing 23.1 to 40 kg: 60 mg (10 mL) PO b.i.d. for 5 days.
Children ages 1 to 12 weighing 15.1 to 23 kg: 45 mg (7.5 mL) PO b.i.d. for 5 days.
Children ages 1 to 12 weighing 15 kg or less: 30 mg (5 mL) PO b.i.d. for 5 days.
Children ages 2 weeks to younger than 1 year: 3 mg/kg PO b.i.d. for 5 days. Begin treatment within 2 days of influenza onset.
Adjust-a-dose: For adults and adolescents with CrCl of 30 to 60 mL/minute, reduce dosage to 30 mg PO b.i.d. for 5 days. For CrCl of 10 to 30 mL/minute, reduce dosage to 30 mg PO once daily for 5 days. For patients on hemodialysis (CrCl <10 mL/minute), give 30 mg PO immediately after hemodialysis, then 30 mg after each hemodialysis cycle. Don't exceed treatment duration of longer than 5 days. For patients on continuous ambulatory peritoneal dialysis (CrCl <10 mL/minute), give a single dose of 30 mg PO immediately after dialysis exchange.

ADMINISTRATION
PO
• Give drug with meals to decrease GI adverse effects.
• Store at controlled room temperature (59° to 86° F [15° to 30° C]).
• May open capsules and mix contents with sweetened liquids, such as regular or sugar-free chocolate syrup, corn syrup, caramel topping, or light brown sugar (dissolved in water).

• Oral suspension is preferred for patients who can't swallow capsules.
• Shake oral suspension well before use.
• For emergency (e.g., shortage), pharmacists can compound an oral suspension (6 mg/mL) from capsules.
• May give via NG or orogastric tube. Dissolve powder from capsule in 20 mL sterile water and inject in tube; follow with 10-mL sterile water flush.
• Once reconstituted, store oral suspension in refrigerator at 36° to 46° F (2° to 8° C) or at room temperature. Use within 10 days of preparation if stored at room temperature or within 17 days of preparation if stored under refrigeration.

ACTION
Inhibits influenza A and B virus enzyme neuraminidase, which is thought to play a role in viral particle aggregation and release from the host cell and appears to interfere with viral replication.

Route	Onset	Peak	Duration
PO	Unknown	Unknown	Unknown

Half-life: 1 to 10 hours.

ADVERSE REACTIONS
CNS: headache, pain. **GI:** nausea, vomiting.

INTERACTIONS
Drug-drug. *Live/attenuated influenza virus vaccine:* May decrease effect of live/attenuated influenza virus vaccine. Avoid oseltamivir 48 hours before vaccination and 2 weeks after.
Probenecid: May increase active metabolite of oseltamivir. Consider alternative to probenecid, or reduced oseltamivir dosage may be needed.

EFFECTS ON LAB TEST RESULTS
None reported.

CONTRAINDICATIONS & CAUTIONS
• Contraindicated in patients hypersensitive to drug or its components.
• Use cautiously in patients with renal failure, chronic cardiac or respiratory diseases, or any medical condition that may require imminent hospitalization.

• Don't administer live/attenuated influenza vaccine within 2 weeks before or 48 hours after oseltamivir administration unless medically indicated.

Dialyzable drug: Yes.

⚠ *Overdose S&S:* Nausea, vomiting.

PREGNANCY-LACTATION-REPRODUCTION
• Drug is recommended for treatment or prophylaxis of influenza in pregnant women and in women up to 2 weeks postpartum. It shouldn't be used as a substitute for vaccination in pregnant women.
• Drug appears in human milk in small amounts. According to the CDC, patient may continue oseltamivir while breastfeeding.

NURSING CONSIDERATIONS
• Drug must be given within 2 days of onset of symptoms.
• Safety and effectiveness of repeated treatment courses haven't been established.
❸ *Alert:* Closely monitor patients with influenza for neuropsychiatric symptoms, such as hallucinations, delirium, and abnormal behavior. Risks and benefits of continuing drug should be evaluated.
• *Look alike–sound alike:* Don't confuse Tamiflu with Tambocor or Thera-Flu.

PATIENT TEACHING
• Instruct patient to begin treatment as soon as possible after appearance of flu symptoms.
• Inform patient that drug may be taken with or without meals. If nausea or vomiting occurs, patient can take drug with food or milk.
• Tell patient to take a missed dose as soon as possible. However, if next dose is due within 2 hours, tell patient to skip the missed dose and take the next dose on schedule.
• Advise patient to complete the full course of treatment, even if symptoms resolve.
• Alert patient that drug isn't a replacement for the annual influenza vaccination. Patients for whom vaccine is indicated should continue to receive the vaccine each fall.

SAFETY ALERT!

osimertinib mesylate ▨
oh-sim-ER-ti-nib

Tagrisso

Therapeutic class: Antineoplastics
Pharmacologic class: Tyrosine kinase inhibitors

AVAILABLE FORMS
Tablets ⓓⓒ: 40 mg, 80 mg

INDICATIONS & DOSAGES
Adjust-a-dose (for all indications): Refer to manufacturer's instructions for toxicity-related dosage adjustments. If drug must be given with a strong CYP3A4 inducer, increase osimertinib dosage to 160 mg daily. Resume osimertinib at 80 mg daily 3 weeks after discontinuing the strong CYP3A4 inducer.

➤ **Metastatic epidermal growth factor receptor *(EGFR)* T790M mutation-positive NSCLC in patients who have progressed on or after EGFR tyrosine kinase inhibitor therapy**
Adults: 80 mg PO once daily until disease progression or unacceptable toxicity.

➤ **First-line treatment of metastatic NSCLC in patients whose tumors have *EGFR* exon 19 deletions or exon 21 L858R mutations, as detected by an FDA-approved test** ▨
Adults: 80 mg PO once daily until disease progression or unacceptable toxicity occurs.

ADMINISTRATION
PO
• Hazardous drug; use safe handling and disposal precautions. Use single gloves to administer intact tablets. Avoid exposure to crushed tablets.
• May give with or without food.
• Don't make up for a missed dose. Resume dosing at next scheduled dose.
• If patient is unable to swallow solids, disperse tablet in approximately 60 mL of non-carbonated water. Stir until tablet is completely dispersed into small pieces and have patient swallow immediately. Rinse

O

---

container with 120 to 240 mL of water and give to patient immediately.

• To give through an NG tube, disperse tablet in 15 mL noncarbonated water and use an additional 15 mL of water to transfer any residual to the syringe. Give through the NG tube followed by a 30 mL water flush.

• Prepare oral liquid in a controlled device using double gloves and protective gown. Don't crush, heat, or ultrasonicate during preparation.

• Store at room temperature (68° to 77° F [20° to 25° C]).

ACTION

A kinase inhibitor of EGFR that binds irreversibly to select mutant forms of EGFR, including T790M, L858R, and exon 19 deletion. In vitro, drug also inhibited the activity of HER2, HER3, HER4, ACK1, and BLK at clinically relevant concentrations.

Route	Onset	Peak	Duration
PO	Unknown	6 hr	Unknown

Half-life: 48 hours.

ADVERSE REACTIONS

CNS: headache, fever, fatigue, *stroke.* **CV: *venous thromboembolism, QTc-interval prolongation,*** reduced LVEF, *cardiomyopathy.* **EENT:** eye disorders. **GI:** diarrhea, nausea, decreased appetite, constipation, stomatitis, vomiting. **Hematologic:** *lymphopenia, thrombocytopenia,* anemia, *neutropenia.* **Metabolic:** hypermagnesemia, hyponatremia, hypokalemia, hyperglycemia. **Hepatic:** increased AST, ALT, and bilirubin levels. **Musculoskeletal:** back pain. **Respiratory:** cough, pneumonia, URI, interstitial pneumonitis, *PE.* **Skin:** rash, dry skin, pruritus, nail toxicity.

INTERACTIONS

Drug-drug. *Breast cancer resistance protein (BCRP) substrate (rosuvastatin, sulfasalazine, topotecan):* Use together may increase exposure to the BCRP substrate and risk of exposure-related toxicity. Monitor patient for BCRP substrate–related adverse reactions.
CYP1A2 drugs with narrow therapeutic indices (carbamazepine, phenytoin), sensitive substrates of CYP3A (cyclosporine, ergot

alkaloids, fentanyl, quinidine): May decrease plasma concentrations of these drugs. Avoid use together.
Drugs that prolong QT interval (amiodarone, chlorpromazine, disopyramide, gatifloxacin, moxifloxacin, procainamide, quinidine, sotalol, thioridazine, ziprasidone): May cause additive QT-interval prolongation and increased risk of cardiac arrhythmia. Avoid use together.
Strong CYP3A inducers (carbamazepine, phenytoin, rifampin): May decrease osimertinib plasma concentration. Avoid use together.
Strong CYP3A inhibitors (antifungals [itraconazole], antivirals [ritonavir], macrolide antibiotics [telithromycin], nefazodone): May increase osimertinib level. Avoid concomitant administration. If no alternative exists, monitor patient closely for adverse reactions.
Drug-herb. *Echinacea:* May decrease effect of osimertinib. Use together isn't recommended.
St. John's wort: May decrease osimertinib plasma concentration. Discourage use together.

EFFECTS ON LAB TEST RESULTS

• May increase AST, ALT, bilirubin, magnesium, and blood glucose levels.

• May decrease sodium and potassium levels.

• May decrease Hb level and lymphocyte, platelet, and neutrophil counts.

CONTRAINDICATIONS & CAUTIONS

• Use cautiously in patients with congenital long QTc syndrome, HF, or electrolyte abnormalities and in those taking medications known to prolong QTc interval.

• ILD and cardiomyopathy (cardiac failure, pulmonary edema, decreased ejection fraction, stress cardiomyopathy) may occur with treatment.

• Safety and effectiveness in children haven't been established.

Dialyzable drug: Unknown.

PREGNANCY-LACTATION-REPRODUCTION

• Based on animal study data, drug may cause fetal harm. Advise women of childbearing potential of potential risk to the

---

Reactions in bold italics are *life-threatening.* Interactions may have a *rapid onset* or a *delayed onset.*

fetus and to use effective contraception during therapy and for up to 6 weeks after last dose.

• Men should use contraception during therapy and for up to 4 months after last dose.

• It isn't known if drug appears in human milk. Because of potential for adverse effects in the infant, women shouldn't breastfeed during therapy and for 2 weeks after last dose.

• Drug may impair fertility in men and women of reproductive potential. It isn't known if the effects are reversible.

NURSING CONSIDERATIONS

• Wear single gloves during receiving, unpacking, placing drug in storage, and administering intact tablets. If preparing drug for oral suspension, double gloving, a protective gown, and preparation in a controlled device is recommended.

▧ Confirm T790M, exon 19 deletions, or exon 21 L858R *EGFR* mutations in tumor or plasma specimens, as appropriate, before initiation of treatment.

• Verify pregnancy status of women of childbearing potential before starting drug.

• Assess LVEF by echocardiogram or MUGA before therapy begins and every 3 months during therapy.

• Monitor ECG and electrolyte levels in patients with congenital long QTc syndrome, HF, or electrolyte abnormalities and in those taking medications known to prolong QTc interval.

• Monitor patient for signs and symptoms of ILD (dyspnea, cough, fever, worsening respiratory symptoms). Interrupt treatment and promptly evaluate for ILD. Discontinue drug if ILD is confirmed.

• Monitor patient for signs and symptoms of keratitis (eye inflammation, light sensitivity, lacrimation, vision changes, pain); if they occur, refer patient to an ophthalmologist for evaluation.

• Monitor patient for skin toxicity (rash, nail changes, dry skin, itching).

• *Look alike–sound alike:* Don't confuse osimertinib with olaparib or ospemifene. Don't confuse Tagrisso with Targretin or Tasigna.

PATIENT TEACHING

• Instruct patient to swallow tablets whole and not to crush or chew them. Tell patient to report difficulty swallowing tablets.

• Tell patient if a dose is missed, not to make up the missed dose, but to take the next dose at the scheduled time.

• Teach patient to promptly report all adverse reactions, especially new or worsening cough, trouble breathing, shortness of breath, fever or symptoms of keratitis.

• Teach patient to seek medical attention for rapid heartbeat or heart pounding, swollen feet or ankles, dizziness, light-headedness, or faintness.

• Advise female patient not to breastfeed during therapy and for up to 2 weeks after therapy ends.

• Warn female patient of risk to the fetus, and to use contraception during therapy and for 6 weeks after therapy ends. Teach men to use contraception during therapy and for 4 months after therapy ends.

• Caution female patient to contact prescriber if she becomes pregnant or suspects she is pregnant during treatment.

---

ospemifene
os-PEM-i-feen

Osphena

Therapeutic class: Selective estrogen receptor modulators
Pharmacologic class: Selective estrogen agonists–antagonists

AVAILABLE FORMS
Tablets: 60 mg

INDICATIONS & DOSAGES
➤ **Moderate to severe dyspareunia due to vulvar and vaginal atrophy of menopause**
Adults: 60 mg PO once daily.
✷ *NEW INDICATION:* **Moderate to severe vaginal dryness, a symptom of vulvar and vaginal atrophy, due to menopause**
Adults: 60 mg PO once daily.

ADMINISTRATION
PO
- Hazardous drug; use safe handling and disposal precautions, including single gloving for administration.
- Give with food.
- Store medication at room temperature.

ACTION
Binds to estrogen receptors, activating estrogenic pathways in some tissues (agonism) and blocking estrogenic pathways in others (antagonism).

Route	Onset	Peak	Duration
PO	12 wk	2 hr	Unknown

Half-life: 26 hours.

ADVERSE REACTIONS
CNS: headache. **CV:** hot flash. **GU:** vaginal or genital discharge, proliferative endometrium, endometrial hyperplasia. **Musculoskeletal:** muscle spasms. **Skin:** hyperhidrosis.

INTERACTIONS
Drug-drug. *CYP2C9, CYP2C19, CYP3A4 inducers (rifampin):* May decrease ospemifene level, decreasing therapeutic effect. Avoid use together.
CYP2C9, CYP2C19, CYP3A4 inhibitors (fluconazole, ketoconazole, omeprazole): May increase ospemifene level, increasing risk of ospemifene-related adverse effects. Avoid use together.
Estrogen agonists–antagonists, estrogens: Safety of concomitant use hasn't been established. Don't use together.
Highly protein-bound drugs (phenytoin, tolbutamide): May increase exposure of ospemifene or highly protein-bound drug, increasing adverse reactions. Monitor clinical response when either drug is started or stopped.
Drug-herb. *St. John's wort:* May decrease drug level and therapeutic effect. Avoid use together.

EFFECTS ON LAB TEST RESULTS
None reported.

CONTRAINDICATIONS & CAUTIONS
- Contraindicated in women hypersensitive to drug or its components; in women with undiagnosed abnormal genital bleeding or known or suspected estrogen-dependent neoplasm; and in those with active or previous DVT or PE or active or previous arterial thromboembolic disease (stroke, MI).
- Don't use in women with known or suspected breast cancer or in those with a history of breast cancer. Drug hasn't been studied in this population.
- Don't use in women with severe hepatic impairment.
- Use cautiously in women with an increased risk of CV disorders, arterial vascular disease, or venous thromboembolism (obesity, SLE, family history, personal history).
Dialyzable drug: Unknown.

PREGNANCY-LACTATION-REPRODUCTION
- Drug may cause fetal harm and is contraindicated in women who are or may become pregnant.
- It isn't known if drug appears in human milk.

NURSING CONSIDERATIONS
■ Black Box Warning ■ Risk of endometrial cancer is increased in women with a uterus who use unopposed estrogens; consider adding a progestin in these women. Women without a uterus don't need a progestin. Evaluate patient for uterine cancer if patient experiences persistent or recurrent abnormal genital bleeding. ∎
■ Black Box Warning ■ Postmenopausal women who received daily oral conjugated estrogens as part of the Women's Health Initiative experienced an increased risk of stroke and DVT. To reduce these risks, this drug should be used for the shortest period of time necessary. Periodically reevaluate the need to continue therapy. ∎
- Discontinue drug immediately if a venous thromboembolism or thromboembolic or hemorrhagic stroke is suspected or occurs.
- Discontinue drug at least 4 to 6 weeks before surgery that's associated with an increased risk of thromboembolism or during periods of extended immobilization.

• Monitor patient for signs and symptoms of PE or cardiac event (sudden onset of shortness of breath and chest pain).
• *Look alike–sound alike:* Don't confuse ospemifene with osimertinib, raloxifene, or toremifene.

PATIENT TEACHING
• Instruct patient to take drug with food for better absorption.
• Inform patient that drug may initiate or worsen hot flashes.
• Advise patient to immediately report all adverse reactions, especially unusual vaginal discharge or bleeding.

SAFETY ALERT!

oxaliplatin
ox-AL-i-pla-tin

Eloxatin

Therapeutic class: Antineoplastics
Pharmacologic class: Platinum-containing compounds

AVAILABLE FORMS
Solution for injection: 5 mg/mL

INDICATIONS & DOSAGES
Adjust-a-dose (for all indications): For patients with severe renal impairment (CrCl <30 mL/minute), initial recommended dose is 65 mg/m^2. Refer to manufacturer's instructions for toxicity-related dosage adjustments.

➤ **First-line treatment of advanced colorectal cancer with 5-FU and leucovorin (5-FU/LV)**
Adults: On day 1, give 85 mg/m^2 oxaliplatin IV in 250 to 500 mL D$_5$W and leucovorin 200 mg/m^2 IV in D$_5$W simultaneously over 120 minutes, in separate bags using a Y-line, followed by 5-FU 400 mg/m^2 IV bolus over 2 to 4 minutes, followed by 600 mg/m^2 5-FU IV infusion in 500 mL D$_5$W over 22 hours.

On day 2, give 200 mg/m^2 leucovorin IV infusion over 120 minutes, followed by 400 mg/m^2 5-FU IV bolus over 2 to 4 minutes, followed by 600 mg/m^2 5-FU IV infusion in 500 mL D$_5$W over 22 hours.

Repeat cycle every 2 weeks until disease progression or unacceptable toxicity occurs.
➤ **With 5-FU/LV for the adjuvant treatment of stage III colon cancer in patients who have had complete resection of the primary tumor**
Adults: On day 1, give oxaliplatin, 85 mg/m^2 IV in 250 to 500 mL D$_5$W and 200 mg/m^2 leucovorin IV infusion in D$_5$W, both over 120 minutes at the same time, in separate bags, using a Y-line. Follow with 400 mg/m^2 5-FU IV bolus over 2 to 4 minutes, then 600 mg/m^2 5-FU in 500 mL D$_5$W as a 22-hour continuous infusion.

On day 2, give leucovorin, 200 mg/m^2 IV infused over 120 minutes, followed by 400 mg/m^2 5-FU as an IV bolus over 2 to 4 minutes, then 600 mg/m^2 5-FU in 500 mL D$_5$W as a 22-hour infusion.

Repeat cycle every 2 weeks for a total of 6 months.
➤ **Esophageal cancer** ◆
Adults: 130 mg/m^2 IV on day 1 every 3 weeks (in combination with epirubicin and either capecitabine or 5-FU) for up to eight cycles, or 85 mg/m^2 IV on day 1 every 2 weeks (in combination with docetaxel, leucovorin, and 5-FU) for up to eight cycles, or 85 mg/m^2 IV on day 1 every 2 weeks (in combination with leucovorin and 5-FU; FOLFOX4) for six cycles.
➤ **Gastric cancer** ◆
Adults: 130 mg/m^2 IV on day 1 every 3 weeks (in combination with capecitabine) for eight cycles.
➤ **Pancreatic cancer, adjuvant therapy** ◆
Adults: 85 mg/m^2 IV every 2 weeks (in combination with 5-FU, leucovorin, and irinotecan; modified FOLFIRINOX regimen) for 24 weeks.
➤ **Pancreatic cancer, advanced or metastatic** ◆
Adults: 85 mg/m^2 IV every 2 weeks (in combination with 5-FU, leucovorin, and irinotecan; FOLFIRINOX regimen) for up to 6 months, or 110 to 130 mg/m^2 IV on day 1 every 3 weeks (in combination with capecitabine) until disease progression or unacceptable toxicity.

ADMINISTRATION

IV

▼ Preparing and giving drug may be mutagenic, teratogenic, or carcinogenic. Follow facility policy to reduce risks.

▼ Wear single glove during receiving, unpacking, and placing in storage. Double gloving and gown are required during administration.

▼ Reconstitute powder using sterile water for injection or D_5W. Add 10 mL to a 50-mg vial or 20 mL to a 100-mg vial, for a yield of 5 mg/mL. Never reconstitute with sodium chloride solution or other solution containing chloride.

▼ Reconstituted solutions must be further diluted in an infusion solution of 250 to 500 mL of D_5W.

▼ Inspect bag for particulate matter and discoloration before giving, and discard if present.

▼ Don't use needles or IV administration sets that contain aluminum because it displaces the platinum, causing it to lose potency and form a black precipitate.

▼ Premedicate with antiemetics, with or without dexamethasone.

▼ Give oxaliplatin and leucovorin over 2 hours at the same time in separate bags, using a Y-line. Extend the infusion time to 6 hours to decrease acute toxicities.

▼ When used in combination with 5-FU, infuse oxaliplatin first.

▼ Store unopened vials at room temperature. Reconstituted solutions are stable if refrigerated (36° to 46° F [2° to 8° C]) for up to 24 hours. After final dilution, solutions are stable for 6 hours at room temperature and up to 24 hours under refrigeration.

▼ **Incompatibilities:** Alkaline solutions or drugs such as 5-FU. Flush infusion line with D_5W before giving any other drugs simultaneously.

ACTION

Inhibits cell replication and transcription by forming platinum complexes that cross-link with DNA molecules. Not specific to cell cycle.

Route	Onset	Peak	Duration
IV	Unknown	Unknown	Unknown

Half-life: 391 hours (long, terminal phase).

ADVERSE REACTIONS

CNS: pain, peripheral neuropathy, fatigue, headache, dizziness, insomnia, fever, anxiety, depression. **CV:** chest pain, *thromboembolism,* edema, flushing, peripheral edema, hypotension. **EENT:** rhinitis, pharyngolaryngeal dysesthesias, pharyngitis, epistaxis, abnormal lacrimation. **GI:** nausea, vomiting, diarrhea, stomatitis, abdominal pain, anorexia, constipation, dyspepsia, taste perversion, gastroesophageal reflux, flatulence, mucositis, dysphagia. **GU:** dysuria, hematuria, increased serum creatinine level. **Hematologic:** *febrile neutropenia,* anemia, *leukopenia, thrombocytopenia.* **Hepatic:** veno-occlusive disease, increased AST, ALT, and bilirubin levels. **Metabolic:** *hypokalemia,* hypocalcemia, dehydration. **Musculoskeletal:** back pain, arthralgia, myalgia. **Respiratory:** dyspnea, cough, URI, hiccups, *pulmonary toxicity.* **Skin:** injection-site reaction, rash, alopecia, dry skin, pruritus, sweating. **Other:** *anaphylaxis,* hand-foot syndrome, allergic reaction, rigors.

INTERACTIONS

Drug-drug. *Anticoagulants:* May increase risk of hemorrhage. Monitor patient closely.
Bacille Calmette-Guérin vaccine (BCG): May diminish therapeutic effect of BCG (intravesical). Avoid combination.
Clozapine: May increase risk of agranulocytosis. Avoid use together.
Deferiprone: May increase risk of neutropenia. Avoid combination.
Denosumab: May increase risk of serious infections. Monitor therapy.
Fosphenytoin, phenytoin: May decrease serum concentration of fosphenytoin and phenytoin. Monitor therapy.
Leflunomide: May increase risk of pancytopenia, agranulocytosis, or thrombocytopenia. Consider not using a leflunomide loading dose in patients receiving other immunosuppressants. Monitor patient for bone marrow suppression at least monthly. Consider therapy modification.

Reactions in bold italics are *life-threatening*. Interactions may have a *rapid onset* or a *delayed onset*.

Live-virus vaccines, pimecrolimus, tacro-limus (topical): May enhance adverse or toxic effects of these drugs. Avoid combination.

Natalizumab: May enhance adverse or toxic effect of natalizumab; specifically, may increase risk of concurrent infection. Avoid combination.

Nephrotoxic drugs (such as gentamicin): May decrease elimination of these drugs and increase gentamicin level. Monitor patient for toxicity.

Roflumilast: May enhance immunosuppressive effect of roflumilast. Consider therapy modification.

Sipuleucel-T: May diminish sipuleucel-T therapeutic effect. Monitor therapy.

Taxane derivatives: May enhance myelosuppressive effect of taxane derivatives. Administer taxane derivative before platinum derivative when given as sequential infusions to limit toxicity. Consider therapy modification.

Tofacitinib: May enhance immunosuppressive effect of tofacitinib. Avoid combination.

Topotecan: May enhance adverse or toxic effect of topotecan. Consider therapy modification.

Trastuzumab: May increase neutropenia. Monitor therapy.

Vaccines (inactivated): May diminish therapeutic effect of inactivated vaccines. Monitor therapy.

EFFECTS ON LAB TEST RESULTS
• May increase glucose, creatinine, bilirubin, AST, and ALT levels. May decrease potassium, albumin, calcium, sodium, and Hb levels.
• May decrease neutrophil, WBC, and platelet counts.

CONTRAINDICATIONS & CAUTIONS
• Contraindicated in patients allergic to drug or other platinum-containing compounds.
• Oxaliplatin may cause early-onset (occurs within hours or 1 to 2 days) or persistent (greater than 14 days) peripheral sensory neuropathy.
• Oxaliplatin has been associated with rare, sometimes fatal, pulmonary fibrosis.
• Extravasation of oxaliplatin can cause tissue necrosis. If extravasation occurs, stop

infusion and notify health care provider immediately.
• Use cautiously in patients with renal impairment or peripheral sensory neuropathy.
• Use cautiously in patients with CV disease. May cause QT-interval prolongation and ventricular arrhythmias.
Dialyzable drug: Unknown.
⚠ **Overdose S&S:** Thrombocytopenia, dyspnea, wheezing, paresthesia, vomiting, chest pain, respiratory failure, bradycardia, dysesthesia, laryngospasm, myelosuppression, nausea, diarrhea, neurotoxicity.

PREGNANCY-LACTATION-REPRODUCTION
• Drug may cause fetal harm. If used during pregnancy or if patient becomes pregnant while using oxaliplatin, drug may cause harm to the fetus. Female patients of childbearing potential should use effective contraception during therapy.
• It isn't known if drug appears in human milk. Patient should discontinue breastfeeding or discontinue drug.

NURSING CONSIDERATIONS
• Administer drug under the supervision of a physician experienced in the use of cancer chemotherapeutic agents.
Black Box Warning Monitor patient for anaphylactic reactions, which may occur within minutes of administration. Keep epinephrine, corticosteroids, and antihistamines available. ■
• Premedication with antiemetics, including 5-HT$_3$ receptor antagonists with or without dexamethasone, is recommended.
• Drug doesn't require patient prehydration.
• Drug clearance is reduced in patients with renal impairment.
• Monitor CBC, platelet count, LFTs, and kidney function tests before each chemotherapy cycle.
• Monitor patient for injection-site reaction; extravasation with necrosis may occur. If extravasation occurs, stop infusion immediately and disconnect; gently aspirate extravasated solution; remove needle; and elevate extremity.
• Monitor patient for neuropathy and pulmonary toxicity. Peripheral neuropathy may be acute or persistent. Acute neuropathy is reversible; it occurs within 2 days of dosing

and resolves within 14 days. Persistent peripheral neuropathy occurs more than 14 days after dosing and causes paresthesia, dysesthesia, hypoesthesia, and other neurologic impairments that can interfere with daily activities (such as walking or swallowing).
• Avoid ice and cold exposure during infusion of drug because cold temperatures can worsen acute neurologic symptoms. Cover patient with a blanket during infusion.
• Diarrhea, dehydration, hypokalemia, and fatigue may occur more frequently in elderly patients.
• *Look alike–sound alike:* Don't confuse oxaliplatin with Aloxi, carboplatin, or cisplatin.

PATIENT TEACHING
• Inform patient of potential serious adverse reactions and of need to report them promptly.
• Tell patient to avoid exposure to cold or cold objects (such as cold drinks or ice cubes), which can bring on or worsen acute symptoms of peripheral neuropathy. Advise patient to drink warm drinks, wear warm clothing, and cover any exposed skin (hands, face, and head).
• Tell patient to immediately report trouble breathing or signs and symptoms of an allergic reaction, such as rash, hives, swelling of lips or tongue, or sudden cough.
• Tell patient to report fever, signs and symptoms of infection, persistent vomiting, diarrhea, or signs and symptoms of dehydration (thirst, dry mouth, light-headedness, and decreased urination).
• Warn female patient of childbearing potential of the risk of harm to the fetus if oxaliplatin is used during pregnancy. Advise use of effective contraception.
• Advise male and female patient of reproductive potential desiring children to consider fertility preservation before therapy.

SAFETY ALERT!

oxazepam
oks-A-ze–pam

Therapeutic class: Anxiolytics
Pharmacologic class: Benzodiazepines
Controlled substance schedule: IV

AVAILABLE FORMS
Capsules: 10 mg, 15 mg, 30 mg

INDICATIONS & DOSAGES
➤ **Alcohol withdrawal, severe anxiety**
Adults: 15 to 30 mg PO t.i.d. or q.i.d.
➤ **Mild to moderate anxiety**
Adults and children older than age 12: 10 to 15 mg PO t.i.d. or q.i.d.
Elderly patients: Initially, 10 mg PO t.i.d.; cautiously increase to 15 mg t.i.d. to q.i.d.
➤ **Severe anxiety syndromes; agitation; anxiety associated with depression**
Adults and children older than age 12: 15 to 30 mg PO t.i.d. or q.i.d.
➤ **Anxiety, tension, irritability, agitation**
Elderly patients: 10 mg PO t.i.d. May increase cautiously to 15 mg t.i.d. or q.i.d.

ADMINISTRATION
PO
• Give drug without regard for meals.

ACTION
May stimulate GABA receptors in the ascending reticular activating system.

Route	Onset	Peak	Duration
PO	Unknown	3 hr	Unknown

Half-life: About 8 hours.

ADVERSE REACTIONS
CNS: drowsiness, lethargy, dizziness, vertigo, headache, syncope, tremor, slurred speech, changes in EEG patterns. **CV:** edema. **GI:** nausea. **Hepatic:** *hepatic dysfunction.* **Skin:** rash. **Other:** altered libido.

INTERACTIONS
Drug-drug. *CNS depressants:* May increase CNS depression. Use together cautiously.
Melatonin: May enhance sedative effect of benzodiazepines. Use with caution.

Reactions in bold italics are *life-threatening*. Interactions may have a *rapid onset* or a *delayed onset*.

Black Box Warning *Opioids:* May cause slow or difficult breathing, sedation, and death. Avoid use together. If use together is necessary, limit dosage and duration of each drug to minimum necessary for desired effect. ■

Drug-herb. *Kava kava:* May increase sedation. Discourage use together.

Yohimbe: May decrease effect of oxazepam. Discourage use together.

Drug-lifestyle. *Alcohol use:* May cause additive CNS effects. Don't use together.

EFFECTS ON LAB TEST RESULTS
• May increase LFT values.

CONTRAINDICATIONS & CAUTIONS
• Contraindicated in patients hypersensitive to drug and in those with psychoses.

Black Box Warning Opioids should only be prescribed with benzodiazepines or other CNS depressants to patients for whom alternative treatment options are inadequate. ■

• Use cautiously in elderly patients and in those with history of substance abuse or in whom a decrease in BP might lead to cardiac problems.

• Safety and effectiveness in children younger than age 6 haven't been established. Absolute dosage for children ages 6 to 12 isn't established.

Dialyzable drug: No.

⚠ Overdose S&S: Drowsiness, confusion, lethargy, ataxia, hypotonia, hypotension, hypnotic state, stage 1 to 3 coma, death.

PREGNANCY-LACTATION-REPRODUCTION
• Drug crosses placental barrier and may adversely affect the fetus (premature birth, low birth weight, hypoglycemia, respiratory problems), especially in first and third trimesters. Use during pregnancy should almost always be avoided.

• Drug appears in human milk. Drowsiness, lethargy, or weight loss may occur in breastfed infants. Breastfeeding isn't recommended.

NURSING CONSIDERATIONS
• Monitor hepatic, renal, and hematopoietic function periodically in patients receiving repeated or prolonged therapy.

❸ Alert: Use of this drug may lead to abuse and addiction. Don't stop drug abruptly because withdrawal symptoms may occur.

• *Look alike–sound alike:* Don't confuse oxazepam with oxaprozin, oxcarbazepine, or quazepam.

PATIENT TEACHING
Black Box Warning Caution patient or caregiver of patient taking an opioid with a benzodiazepine, CNS depressant, or alcohol to seek immediate medical attention if patient experiences dizziness, lightheadedness, extreme sleepiness, slowed or difficult breathing, or unresponsiveness. ■

• Warn patient to avoid hazardous activities that require alertness or good coordination until effects of drug are known.

• Tell patient to avoid use of alcohol.

• Notify patient that smoking may decrease drug's effectiveness.

• Warn patient not to stop drug abruptly because withdrawal symptoms may occur.

• Warn female patient of childbearing potential to avoid use during pregnancy.

OXcarbazepine ⚡
ox-car-BAZ-e-peen

Oxtellar XR, Trileptal

Therapeutic class: Anticonvulsants
Pharmacologic class: Carboxamide derivatives

AVAILABLE FORMS
Oral suspension: 300 mg/5 mL (60 mg/mL)
Tablets (extended-release) ⓓ: 150 mg, 300 mg, 600 mg
Tablets (film-coated): 150 mg, 300 mg, 600 mg

INDICATIONS & DOSAGES
Adjust-a-dose (for all indications): If CrCl is less than 30 mL/minute, start therapy at 150 mg PO b.i.d. (one-half usual starting dose) and increase slowly to achieve desired response. In patients with ESRD on dialysis, use immediate-release formulation instead of extended-release formulation.

➤ **Adjunctive treatment of partial seizures in patients with epilepsy**

Adults: Initially, 300 mg immediate-release tablets or suspension PO b.i.d. Increase by a maximum of 600 mg daily (300 mg PO b.i.d.) at weekly intervals. Maximum recommended daily dose is 1,200 mg PO in two divided doses. Or, 600 mg extended-release tablets PO daily. May increase at weekly intervals in 600-mg/day increments. Usual dosage is 1,200 to 2,400 mg daily.

Children ages 4 to 16 (immediate-release): Initially, 8 to 10 mg/kg PO daily in two divided doses, not to exceed 600 mg daily. The target maintenance dose depends on patient's weight and should be divided in to two doses. If patient weighs between 20 and 29 kg, target maintenance dose is 900 mg daily in two divided doses. If patient weighs between 29.1 and 39 kg, target maintenance dose is 1,200 mg daily in two divided doses. If patient weighs more than 39 kg, target maintenance dose is 1,800 mg daily in two divided doses. Target doses should be achieved over 2 weeks.

Children ages 2 to younger than 4 (immediate-release): Initially, 8 to 10 mg/kg PO daily in two divided doses, not to exceed 600 mg daily. If patient weighs less than 20 kg, a starting dose of 16 to 20 mg/kg may be considered. Maximum maintenance dosage should be achieved over 2 to 4 weeks and shouldn't exceed 60 mg/kg/day in a two-dose divided regimen.

Children ages 6 to 17 (extended-release): 8 to 10 mg/kg PO once daily, not to exceed 600 mg daily in first week. May increase at weekly intervals in 8- to 10-mg/kg increments once daily, not to exceed 600 mg. Target daily dose in patients weighing more than 39 kg is 1,800 mg/day; from 29.1 to 39 kg, 1,200 mg/day; and from 20 to 29 kg, 900 mg/day.

Elderly patients: When using extended-release tablets, consider a lower starting dose (300 or 450 mg/day). Dosage increases can be made at weekly intervals in increments of 300 to 450 mg/day.

Adjust-a-dose: Dosage adjustment is recommended with concomitant use of strong CYP3A4 enzyme inducers or UGT inducers, which include certain antiepileptic drugs. Consider initiating dosage of extended-release formulation at 900 mg once daily.

Refer to Interactions section and product insert for more information.

➤ **To change from multidrug to single-drug treatment of partial seizures in patients with epilepsy**
Adults: Initially, 300 mg immediate-release tablets or suspension PO b.i.d., while reducing dose of concomitant anticonvulsant. Increase oxcarbazepine by a maximum of 600 mg daily at weekly intervals over 2 to 4 weeks. Recommended daily dose is 2,400 mg PO in two divided doses. Withdraw other anticonvulsant completely over 3 to 6 weeks.

Children ages 4 to 16: Initially, 8 to 10 mg/kg immediate-release tablets or suspension PO daily in two divided doses, while reducing dose of concomitant anticonvulsant. Increase oxcarbazepine by a maximum of 10 mg/kg daily at weekly intervals to achieve the recommended daily dose by weight listed in the manufacturer's instructions. Withdraw other anticonvulsant completely over 3 to 6 weeks. See manufacturer's instructions for weight-based maintenance dosing with oxcarbazepine monotherapy.

➤ **To start single-drug treatment of partial seizures in patients with epilepsy**
Adults: Initially, 300 mg immediate-release tablets or suspension PO b.i.d. Increase dosage by 300 mg daily every third day to a daily dose of 1,200 mg in two divided doses. Or, 600 mg extended-release tablets PO daily. May increase at weekly intervals in 600-mg/day increments. Usual dosage is 1,200 to 2,400 mg once daily.

Children ages 4 to 16: Initially, 8 to 10 mg/kg immediate-release tablets or suspension PO daily in two divided doses, increasing dosage by 5 mg/kg daily every third day to the recommended daily dose range by weight in the manufacturer's instructions.

✳ *NEW INDICATION:* **Monotherapy for partial-onset seizures**
Adults: Initially, 600 mg extended-release tablets PO daily. May increase at weekly intervals in 600-mg/day increments. Usual dosage is 1,200 to 2,400 mg daily.

Children ages 6 to 17: Initially, 8 to 10 mg/kg extended-release tablets PO daily, not to exceed 600 mg daily in first week. May increase at weekly intervals in increments of 8 to 10 mg/kg once daily, not to exceed

600 mg. Target daily dose in patients weighing more than 39 kg is 1,800 mg/day; from 29.1 to 39 kg, 1,200 mg /day; and from 20 to 29 kg, 900 mg/day.

ADMINISTRATION

PO

• Shake suspension well.

• Mix suspension with water or give directly from syringe.

• Use suspension within 7 weeks of first opening container.

• Give immediate-release tablets without regard for food.

• Give extended-release tablets on an empty stomach (at least 1 hour before or 2 hours after a meal). Don't cut, crush, or allow patient to chew tablets. For ease of swallowing, use multiple lower-strength tablets for appropriate dose.

• When converting from immediate-release to extended-release form, higher doses may be needed.

• Oral tablets and suspension may be interchanged at equal doses.

ACTION

Thought to prevent seizure spread in the brain by blocking voltage-sensitive sodium channels and to produce anticonvulsant effects by increasing potassium conduction and modulating high-voltage activated calcium channels.

Route	Onset	Peak	Duration
PO	Unknown	Immediate: 3–13 hr; extended-release: 7 hr	Unknown

Half-life: Immediate-release: About 2 hours for the drug; about 9 hours for the active metabolite. Children younger than age 8 have a 30% to 40% increase in clearance. Extended-release: 7 to 11 hours.

ADVERSE REACTIONS

CNS: abnormal gait, ataxia, dizziness, drowsiness, fatigue, headache, tremor, vertigo, *seizures,* abnormal coordination, agitation, amnesia, anxiety, asthenia, confusion, emotional lability, feeling abnormal, fever, hypoesthesia, impaired concentration, insomnia, nervousness, speech disorder, falls. **CV:** chest pain, edema, hypotension. **EENT:** abnormal vision, diplopia, nystagmus, abnormal accommodation, ear pain, epistaxis, pharyngitis, rhinitis, sinusitis. **GI:** abdominal pain, nausea, vomiting, rectal hemorrhage, anorexia, constipation, diarrhea, dry mouth, dyspepsia, gastritis, taste perversion, thirst. **GU:** urinary frequency, UTI, vaginitis. **Hematologic:** lymphadenopathy. **Metabolic:** hyponatremia, weight gain. **Musculoskeletal:** back pain, muscular weakness. **Respiratory:** URI, bronchitis, pulmonary infection, coughing, pneumonia. **Skin:** acne, bruising, hot flashes, increased sweating, purpura, rash. **Other:** allergic reaction, infection, toothache.

INTERACTIONS

Drug-drug. *Carbamazepine, valproic acid, verapamil:* May decrease level of active metabolite of oxcarbazepine. Monitor patient and level closely.

CYP3A4 substrates (cyclosporine, itraconazole, rivaroxaban): May decrease serum concentrations of substrates. Substrate dosage modifications may be needed.

Dolutegravir, elvitegravir, ledipasvir, rilpivirine, simeprevir, sofosbuvir, tenofovir, ulipristal: May decrease serum concentration of these drugs. Avoid combination.

Hormonal contraceptives: May decrease levels of ethinyl estradiol and levonorgestrel, reducing hormonal contraceptive effectiveness. Caution women of childbearing potential to use alternative forms of contraception.

Phenobarbital: May decrease level of active metabolite of oxcarbazepine; may increase phenobarbital level. Monitor patient closely.

Phenytoin: May decrease level of active metabolite of oxcarbazepine; may increase phenytoin level in adults receiving high doses of oxcarbazepine. Monitor phenytoin level closely when starting therapy in these patients.

Rifampin: May decrease serum concentrations of active metabolite(s) of oxcarbazepine. Monitor therapy.

Selegiline: May enhance serotonergic effect of selegiline. Avoid combination.

Thiazide and thiazide-like diuretics: May enhance oxcarbazepine adverse effects, specifically hyponatremia. Monitor therapy.

Drug-lifestyle. *Alcohol use:* May increase CNS depression. Discourage use together.

0

EFFECTS ON LAB TEST RESULTS
• May decrease sodium and thyroxine levels.

CONTRAINDICATIONS & CAUTIONS
• Contraindicated in patients hypersensitive to drug or its components or to eslicarbazepine acetate.

❸ *Alert:* Serious dermatologic reactions, including SJS and toxic epidermal necrolysis, have been reported in both children and adults in association with oxcarbazepine use. Such serious skin reactions may be life-threatening, and some patients have required hospitalization, with very rare reports of fatal outcome. The median time of onset for reported cases was 19 days after treatment initiation. Recurrence of serious skin reactions after rechallenge with oxcarbazepine has also been reported.

❧ Screen patients of Asian ancestry for the human leukocyte antigen allele (HLA-B*1502) before therapy; these patients may be at increased risk for SJS or toxic epidermal necrolysis with oxcarbazepine therapy.

• Fatal or life-threatening DRESS syndrome has been reported. This disorder varies in expression and frequently first presents with fever and lymphadenopathy.

Dialyzable drug: Unknown.

PREGNANCY-LACTATION-REPRODUCTION
• There are no adequate studies in pregnant women; drug may cause fetal harm. Use cautiously in pregnant women and only if benefit justifies possible risk to the fetus.

• Patients exposed to drug during pregnancy are encouraged to enroll themselves in the North American AED Pregnancy Registry (1-888-233-2334).

• Drug and its active metabolite appear in human milk in small amounts. Patient should discontinue breastfeeding or discontinue drug.

NURSING CONSIDERATIONS
❸ *Alert:* Between 25% and 30% of patients with history of hypersensitivity reaction to carbamazepine may develop hypersensitivities to oxcarbazepine. Ask patient about carbamazepine hypersensitivity and stop drug immediately if signs or symptoms of hypersensitivity occur.

❸ *Alert:* Closely monitor all patients taking or starting antiepileptic drugs for changes in behavior indicating worsening of suicidal thoughts or behavior or depression. Symptoms such as anxiety, agitation, hostility, mania, and hypomania may be precursors to emerging suicidality.

❸ *Alert:* Withdraw drug gradually to minimize potential for increased seizure frequency.

❸ *Alert:* Rare serious and sometimes fatal dermatologic reactions can occur. If skin reactions occur, discontinue drug.

• Watch for signs and symptoms of hyponatremia, including nausea, malaise, headache, lethargy, confusion, and decreased sensation.

• Monitor sodium level in patients receiving oxcarbazepine for maintenance treatment, especially patients receiving other therapies that may decrease sodium levels.

• Oxcarbazepine use has been linked to several nervous system-related adverse reactions, including psychomotor slowing, difficulty with concentration, speech or language problems, somnolence, fatigue, and coordination abnormalities, such as ataxia and gait disturbances.

• *Look alike–sound alike:* Don't confuse oxcarbazepine with carbamazepine, oxazepam, or oxaprozin.

PATIENT TEACHING
• Tell patient to take drug with or without food. For extended-release, tell patient to take on an empty stomach and not to cut, crush, or chew tablets.

• Tell patient to contact prescriber before interrupting or stopping drug.

• Advise patient not to discontinue drug abruptly because of the risk of increasing seizure frequency.

• Advise patient to report signs and symptoms of low sodium in the blood, such as nausea, malaise, headache, lethargy, and confusion.

❸ *Alert:* DRESS syndrome hypersensitivity reactions may occur. Tell patient to report fever and swollen lymph nodes to prescriber.

❸ *Alert:* Serious skin reactions, including SJS and toxic epidermal necrolysis, can occur. Advise patient to immediately report rashes to prescriber.

• Caution patient to avoid driving and other potentially hazardous activities that require

mental alertness until effects of drug are known.
• Instruct female patient using hormonal contraceptives to use alternative form of contraception while taking drug.
• Tell patient to avoid alcohol while taking drug.
• Advise patient to inform prescriber if patient has ever experienced hypersensitivity reaction to carbamazepine.

oxybutynin
oks-i-BYOO-ti-nin

Oxytrol, Oxytrol for Women ◇

oxybutynin chloride
Ditropan XL, Gelnique

Therapeutic class: Urinary antispasmodics
Pharmacologic class: Antimuscarinics

AVAILABLE FORMS
oxybutynin
Transdermal patch: 36-mg patch delivering 3.9 mg/day ◇
oxybutynin chloride
Syrup: 5 mg/5 mL
Tablets: 5 mg
Tablets (extended-release) ⓞⓝⓖ: 5 mg, 10 mg, 15 mg
Topical gel: 10%

INDICATIONS & DOSAGES
➤ **Bladder instability associated with voiding**
Adults: 5 mg (immediate-release) PO b.i.d. to t.i.d., to maximum of 5 mg q.i.d.
Children age 5 and older: 5 mg (immediate-release) PO b.i.d., to maximum of 5 mg t.i.d.
Elderly patients: A lower initial starting dose of 2.5 mg (immediate-release) PO b.i.d. or t.i.d. is recommended.
➤ **Overactive bladder**
Adults: 5 mg (immediate-release tablet) PO b.i.d. to t.i.d.; maximum, 5 mg q.i.d. Or, 5 to 10 mg (extended-release tablet) PO once daily. Dosage adjustments may be made weekly in 5-mg increments, as needed, to maximum of 30 mg PO daily. Or, apply one patch twice weekly (every 3 to 4 days) to dry, intact skin on the abdomen, hip, or buttock. Or, 1 g topical gel (10%) once daily

applied to dry, intact skin on the abdomen, upper arms or shoulders, or thighs.
Elderly patients: A lower initial starting dose of 2.5 mg (immediate-release) PO b.i.d. or t.i.d. is recommended.
➤ **Symptoms of detrusor overactivity associated with a neurologic condition (e.g., spina bifida)**
Children age 5 and older (immediate-release): 5 mg PO b.i.d. or t.i.d.
Children age 6 and older (extended-release): 5 mg once daily; adjust in 5-mg increments at weekly intervals. Maximum daily dose, 20 mg/day.

ADMINISTRATION
PO
• Don't crush extended-release tablets.
• Give extended-release tablets without regard for food.
Topical (gel)
• Use immediately after sachets are opened.
• Apply to dry, intact skin on the abdomen, upper arms or shoulders, or thighs.
• Don't apply to recently shaved skin.
• Rotate application sites.
• Patient shouldn't bathe, shower, or swim for 1 hour after gel application.
Transdermal
• Apply immediately after removing from protective pouch.
• Apply to dry, intact skin on the abdomen, hip, or buttock.
• Don't apply to areas with cuts, scrapes, or irritation.
• Avoid reapplication to the same site within 7 days.
• Don't expose patch to sunlight.

ACTION
Relaxes smooth muscle of bladder by antagonizing muscarinic receptors, relieving symptoms of overactive bladder.

Route	Onset	Peak	Duration
PO	30–60 min	60 min	6–10 hr
PO (extended-release)	Unknown	4–6 hr	24 hr
Topical (gel)	Unknown	Unknown	Unknown
Transdermal	Unknown	24–48 hr	96 hr

Half-life: Tablets or oral solution, 2 to 3 hours; extended-release tablets, 12 to 13 hours; patch, 7 to 8 hours; transdermal gel, 64 hours.

0

ADVERSE REACTIONS
PO
CNS: dizziness, insomnia, nervousness, drowsiness, restlessness, hallucinations, asthenia, fever, headache, somnolence, confusion. **CV:** palpitations, tachycardia, vasodilation, peripheral edema. **EENT:** mydriasis, cycloplegia, decreased lacrimation, amblyopia, blurred vision, dry eyes. **GI:** constipation, dry mouth, nausea, vomiting, dyspepsia, decreased GI motility, abdominal pain. **GU:** urinary hesitancy, urine retention, impotence, UTI. **Skin:** rash, decreased diaphoresis. **Other:** suppression of lactation.
Topical (gel)
CNS: dizziness, fatigue. **EENT:** dry mouth. **GI:** viral gastroenteritis. **GU:** UTI. **Metabolic:** increased serum glucose level. **Respiratory:** URI. **Skin:** application-site reaction.
Transdermal patch
CNS: fatigue, somnolence, headache. **CV:** flushing. **EENT:** abnormal vision. **GI:** dry mouth, diarrhea, abdominal pain, nausea, flatulence, constipation. **GU:** dysuria. **Musculoskeletal:** back pain. **Skin:** pruritus, erythema, vesicles, macules, rash, burning at application site.

INTERACTIONS
Drug-drug. *Amantadine, anticholinergics:* May increase anticholinergic effects. Use together cautiously.
Cannabinoid-containing products: May enhance tachycardic effect of oxybutynin. Monitor therapy closely.
CNS depressants: May increase CNS effects. Use together cautiously.
CYP3A4 inhibitors (ketoconazole): May alter oxybutynin concentration. Use together cautiously.
Opioid agonists: May increase risk of constipation and urine retention. Monitor therapy closely.
Drug-lifestyle. *Alcohol use:* May increase CNS effects. Discourage use together.
Exercise, hot weather: May cause heatstroke. Advise patient to use with caution in hot weather.

EFFECTS ON LAB TEST RESULTS
• May suppress the wheal and flare reactions to skin test antigens.

CONTRAINDICATIONS & CAUTIONS
• Contraindicated in patients hypersensitive to drug or its components and in those with GI obstruction and conditions that decrease GI motility, uncontrolled narrow-angle glaucoma, urine or gastric retention, or obstructive uropathy.
• Angioedema may occur after a single dose.
• Use cautiously in elderly patients and in those with autonomic neuropathy, reflux esophagitis, myasthenia gravis, Parkinson disease, or hepatic or renal disease.
• Extended-release form isn't recommended for children who can't swallow the tablet whole without chewing, dividing, or crushing or for children younger than age 6.
• Use extended-release form cautiously in patients with bladder outflow obstruction, gastric obstruction, ulcerative colitis, intestinal atony, myasthenia gravis, or gastroesophageal reflux and in those taking drugs that worsen esophagitis (bisphosphonates).
Dialyzable drug: Unknown.
⚠ Overdose S&S: Restlessness, tremors, irritability, seizures, delirium, hallucinations, flushing, fever, dehydration, cardiac arrhythmias, vomiting, urine retention, hypotension or HTN, respiratory failure, paralysis, coma.

PREGNANCY-LACTATION-REPRODUCTION
• Use cautiously in pregnant women and only if benefit justifies risk to the fetus.
• It isn't known if drug appears in human milk. Use cautiously in breastfeeding women.
• Lactation suppression has been reported.

NURSING CONSIDERATIONS
• Drug may aggravate symptoms of hyperthyroidism, CAD, HF, arrhythmias, tachycardia, HTN, or prostatic hyperplasia.
• Oxytrol for Women has been FDA-approved as an OTC product. The 3.9-mg/day patch should be applied to the skin every 3 to 4 days.
• ***Look alike–sound alike:*** Don't confuse Ditropan with Detrol, diazepam, Diprivan, or dithranol. Don't confuse oxybutynin with Oxycontin.

Reactions in bold italics are *life-threatening*. Interactions may have a *rapid onset* or a ***delayed onset***.

PATIENT TEACHING

• Warn patient to avoid hazardous activities, such as operating machinery or driving, until CNS effects of drug are known.

• Caution patient that using drug during very hot weather may cause fever or heatstroke because it suppresses sweating.

• Tell patient to swallow extended-release tablet whole and not to chew or crush it.

• Instruct patient to measure syrup with a teaspoon.

• Instruct patient using transdermal patch to change patch twice a week (every 3 to 4 days) and to choose a new application site with each new patch to avoid the same site within 7 days. Warn patient to only wear one patch at a time. Tell patient to dispose of old patches carefully in the trash in a manner that prevents accidental application or ingestion by children and pets.

• Tell patient using transdermal patch to keep patch in sealed pouch until immediately before application, not to expose patch to sunlight, and to wear patch under clothing.

• Tell patient to remove patch before undergoing an MRI scan.

• Advise patient using topical gel to rotate application sites.

• Advise patient to avoid alcohol while taking drug.

• Tell patient that drug may cause dry mouth.

SAFETY ALERT!

oxyCODONE
oks-i-KOE-done

Xtampza ER

oxyCODONE hydrochloride
Oxaydo, OxyCONTIN♂, Oxy.IR♣, OxyNEO♣, Roxicodone, Supeudol♣

Therapeutic class: Opioid analgesics
Pharmacologic class: Opioids
Controlled substance schedule: II

AVAILABLE FORMS
oxycodone
Capsules (extended-release, 12-hour abuse deterrent): 9-mg base, 13.5-mg base, 18-mg base, 27-mg base, 36-mg base

oxycodone hydrochloride
Capsules: 5 mg
Oral solution: 5 mg/5 mL
Oral solution (concentrate): 20 mg/mL
Tablets (extended-release, 12-hour abuse deterrent) ⬤: 10 mg, 15 mg, 20 mg, 30 mg, 40 mg, 60 mg, 80 mg
Tablets (immediate-release): 5 mg, 10 mg, 15 mg, 20 mg, 30 mg
Tablets (immediate-release, abuse deterrent): 5 mg, 7.5 mg

INDICATIONS & DOSAGES
➤ **Moderate to severe pain**
Adults: 5 to 15 mg immediate-release form or oral solution PO every 4 to 6 hours. Titrate dosage based on response. For control of severe, chronic pain, give on a regularly scheduled basis every 4 to 6 hours.
➤ **Moderate to severe pain in patients not currently receiving opioids, who need a continuous, around-the-clock analgesic for an extended period of time**
Adults: 10 mg extended-release tablets or 9 mg extended-release capsules PO every 12 hours. May increase dose every 1 to 2 days until desired pain control is achieved. For pediatric dosing, refer to manufacturer's recommendations.
Adjust-a-dose: For elderly or debilitated patients and those with hepatic or renal impairment, or if patient is receiving CNS depressants, decrease initial starting dose by one-third to one-half.

ADMINISTRATION
PO
• To minimize GI upset, give drug after meals or with milk.
Black Box Warning Patient must swallow extended-release tablets whole. ∎
⊕ *Alert:* The 60- and 80-mg extended-release tablets, or a single 40-mg dose, or a total daily dose of more than 80 mg is limited to opioid-tolerant patients.
Black Box Warning Oxycodone concentrated oral solution, available as a 20-mg/mL concentration, is indicated for use in opioid-tolerant patients only. ∎
⊕ *Alert:* Oxycodone extended-release capsules aren't bioequivalent to oxycodone hydrochloride extended-release tablets.

O

- Don't crush or dissolve extended-release tablets.

ACTION
Unknown. Binds with opioid receptors in the CNS, altering perception of and emotional response to pain.

Route	Onset	Peak	Duration
PO (immediate-release)	10–15 min	½–1 hr	3–6 hr
PO (extended-release)	Unknown	4–5 hr	12 hr

Half-life: 3 to 4 hours. Extended-release tablets, 4.5 hours; extended-release capsules, 5.6 hours.

ADVERSE REACTIONS
CNS: clouded sensorium, dizziness, euphoria, light-headedness, physical dependence, sedation, somnolence, headache, asthenia, fever, abnormal dreams, confusion. **CV:** *bradycardia,* hypotension, edema, flushing, HTN, tachycardia. **EENT:** blurred vision, pharyngitis, rhinitis, sinusitis. **GI:** constipation, nausea, vomiting, ileus, diarrhea, anorexia, gastritis. **GU:** urine retention. **Hematologic:** anemia; decreased Hb level, platelet count, RBC count. **Hepatic:** increased ALT level. **Metabolic:** hypochloremia, hyponatremia, hyperglycemia. **Musculoskeletal:** weakness, arthralgia, back pain, tremor. **Respiratory:** *respiratory depression,* cough, dyspnea. **Skin:** diaphoresis, pruritus.

INTERACTIONS
Drug-drug. *Alvimopan:* May enhance alvimopan-related toxicity. Alvimopan is contraindicated in patients receiving opioids for more than 7 consecutive days before starting alvimopan.
Anticholinergic agents: May increase risk of constipation and urine retention. Monitor therapy closely.
Anticoagulants: Oxycodone hydrochloride products containing aspirin may increase anticoagulant effect. Monitor clotting times. Use together cautiously.
Black Box Warning *Benzodiazepines, CNS depressants:* May cause slow or difficult breathing, sedation, and death. Avoid use together. If use together is necessary, limit dosage and duration of each drug to minimum necessary for desired effect. ∎

Black Box Warning *CYP3A4 inducers (such as carbamazepine, phenytoin, rifampin):* May increase oxycodone level and cause oxycodone-related adverse reactions if inducer is discontinued. Taper inducers cautiously and adjust oxycodone dosage as needed. ∎
Black Box Warning *CYP3A4 inhibitors such as azole antifungals (ketoconazole), macrolide antibiotics (erythromycin), protease inhibitors (ritonavir):* May increase oxycodone level, increase or prolong adverse effects, and cause fatal respiratory depression. Carefully monitor patient over extended period of time and adjust oxycodone dosage as needed. ∎
General anesthetics, hypnotics, MAO inhibitors, TCAs: May cause additive adverse effects (e.g., CNS or respiratory depression). Use together with caution. Reduce oxycodone dose and monitor patient response.
❸ *Alert: Serotonergic drugs (amoxapine, antiemetics [dolasetron, granisetron, ondansetron, palonosetron], antimigraine drugs, buspirone, cyclobenzaprine, dextromethorphan, linezolid, lithium, MAO inhibitors, maprotiline, methylene blue, mirtazapine, nefazodone, SSNRIs, SSRIs, TCAs, trazodone, tryptophan, vilazodone):* May increase risk of serotonin syndrome. Use together cautiously and monitor patient for serotonin syndrome.
Drug-herb. *Kava kava:* May enhance adverse effects of CNS depressants. Monitor therapy carefully.
❸ *Alert: St. John's wort:* May increase risk of serotonin syndrome. May decrease oxycodone serum concentration. Use together cautiously.
Drug-lifestyle. **Black Box Warning** *Alcohol use:* May increase risk of profound sedation, respiratory depression, coma, and death. Don't use together. ∎

EFFECTS ON LAB TEST RESULTS
- May increase blood glucose and ALT levels.
- May decrease serum chloride and sodium levels.
- Decrease hemoglobin level and RBC and platelet count.

• Quinolones (levofloxacin, ofloxacin) may cause a false-positive urine screen result for opioids.

CONTRAINDICATIONS & CAUTIONS
• Drug should be prescribed only by health care professionals knowledgeable in the use of potent opioids for the management of chronic pain.

Black Box Warning Opioids should only be prescribed with benzodiazepines or other CNS depressants to patients for whom alternative treatment options are inadequate. ■

☻ *Alert:* Patients are at increased risk for oversedation and respiratory depression if they snore or have a history of sleep apnea, haven't used opioids recently or are first-time opioid users, have increased opioid dosage requirements or opioid habituation, have received general anesthesia for longer lengths of time or received other sedating drugs, have preexisting pulmonary or cardiac disease, or have thoracic or other surgical incisions that may impair breathing. Monitor patients carefully.

☻ *Alert:* Drug may lead to rare but serious decrease in adrenal gland cortisol production.

☻ *Alert:* Drug may cause decreased sex hormone levels with long-term use.

• Contraindicated in patients hypersensitive to drug.

• Contraindicated in known or suspected paralytic ileus, significant respiratory depression, and acute or severe bronchial asthma.

• Use with caution in elderly and debilitated patients and in those with head injury, increased ICP, seizures, asthma, COPD, prostatic hyperplasia, severe hepatic or renal disease, acute abdominal conditions, urethral stricture, hypothyroidism, Addison disease, and arrhythmias.

Black Box Warning Serious, life-threatening, or fatal respiratory depression may occur with use of extended-release oxycodone. Monitor patient for respiratory depression, especially during initiation of therapy and after a dosage increase. Instruct patient to swallow extended-release oxycodone tablets whole; crushing, dissolving, or chewing the tablets can cause rapid release and absorption of a potentially fatal dose of oxycodone. ■

Black Box Warning Accidental ingestion of even one dose of drug, especially by children, can result in a fatal oxycodone overdose. ■

Black Box Warning Patients must be screened for increased risk of opioid abuse (personal or family history of substance abuse or mental illness) before being prescribed opioids. ■

Black Box Warning Oxycodone extended-release tablets are indicated for the management of moderate to severe pain, when a continuous, around-the-clock opioid analgesic is needed for an extended period of time. They aren't intended for use as as-needed analgesics. ■

Dialyzable drug: Unknown.

⚠ *Overdose S&S:* CNS depression, respiratory depression, apnea, flaccid skeletal muscles, bradycardia, hypotension, circulatory collapse, cardiac arrest, respiratory arrest, death.

PREGNANCY-LACTATION-REPRODUCTION
☻ *Alert:* Carefully weigh risks and benefits of using drug during pregnancy.

Black Box Warning Prolonged use of extended-release oxycodone during pregnancy can result in neonatal opioid withdrawal syndrome, which may be life-threatening if not recognized and treated and requires management according to protocols developed by neonatology experts. If prolonged use is required, advise patient of risks and ensure appropriate treatment is available. ■

• There are no adequate studies in pregnant women. Use only if potential benefit justifies potential risks to the fetus.

• Drug isn't recommended for use during or immediately before labor as uterine contractions may be adversely affected.

• Prolonged opioid use during pregnancy may cause respiratory depression or withdrawal signs and symptoms in the neonate. Naloxone should be available to reverse opioid-induced respiratory depression in the neonate.

• Drug appears in human milk. Breastfeeding isn't recommended.

O

• Long-term opioid use may cause secondary hypogonadism, which may lead to sexual dysfunction or infertility.

NURSING CONSIDERATIONS

Black Box Warning Use care when prescribing and administering oxycodone concentrated oral solution, to avoid dosing errors due to confusion between milligram and milliliter and among other oxycodone solutions with different concentrations, which could result in accidental overdose and death. Take care to ensure the proper dose is communicated and dispensed. ▮

Black Box Warning Serious, life-threatening or fatal respiratory depression can occur. Monitor patient closely, especially within first 24 to 72 hours of starting drug and after a dosage increase. ▮

Black Box Warning Routinely monitor all patients on opioids for signs and symptoms of misuse, abuse, and addiction. ▮

Black Box Warning Accidental ingestion of even one dose of drug, especially by children, can be fatal. ▮

❸ Alert: Carefully monitor vital signs, pain level, respiratory status, and sedation level in all patients receiving opioids, especially those receiving IV drugs, even when given postoperatively.

• Reassess patient's level of pain at least 15 and 30 minutes after administration.

• For full analgesic effect, give drug before patient has intense pain.

• Keep opioid antagonist (naloxone) and resuscitation equipment available.

❸ Alert: If patient is taking opioids with serotonergic drugs, watch for signs and symptoms of serotonin syndrome (agitation, hallucinations, rapid HR, fever, excessive sweating, shivering or shaking, muscle twitching or stiffness, trouble with coordination, nausea, vomiting, diarrhea), especially at start of treatment or with dosages increases. Signs and symptoms may occur within several hours of coadministration but may also occur later, especially after dosage increase. Discontinue opioid, serotonergic drug, or both if serotonin syndrome is suspected.

❸ Alert: Monitor patient for signs and symptoms of adrenal insufficiency (nausea, vomiting, loss of appetite, fatigue, weakness,

dizziness, low BP). Perform diagnostic testing if adrenal insufficiency is suspected. If adrenal insufficiency is confirmed, treat with corticosteroids and wean patient off opioids if appropriate. Discontinue corticosteroids when clinically appropriate.

❸ Alert: Monitor patient for signs and symptoms of decreased sex hormone levels (low libido, erectile dysfunction, amenorrhea, infertility). If signs and symptoms occur, evaluate patient and obtain lab testing.

• Patients taking extended-release form around-the-clock may need to take immediate-release form for worsening of pain or prevention of incident pain (e.g., breakthrough pain).

• Single-drug oxycodone solution or tablets are especially useful for patients who shouldn't take aspirin or acetaminophen.

• Monitor circulatory and respiratory status closely, especially within the first 24 to 72 hours of initiation of therapy. Withhold dose and notify prescriber if respirations are shallow or if respiratory rate falls below 12 breaths/minute.

• Monitor patient's bladder and bowel patterns. Patient may need a stimulant laxative because drug has a constipating effect.

• For patients who are taking more than 60 mg daily, stop drug gradually to prevent withdrawal symptoms.

• Extended-release formula isn't intended for as-needed use or for immediate postoperative pain. Drug is indicated only for postoperative use if patient was receiving it before surgery or if pain is expected to persist for an extended time.

❸ Alert: Drug is potentially addictive, even at recommended doses, and if drug is misused. Chewing, crushing, snorting, or injecting it can lead to overdose and death.

• OxyContin has been formulated to prevent immediate access to full-dose oxycodone by cutting, chewing, or breaking the tablet. Attempts to dissolve tablets will result in a gummy substance that can't be drawn up into a syringe or injected.

❸ Alert: Don't stop drug abruptly; withdraw slowly and individualize gradual taper plan to prevent signs and symptoms of withdrawal, worsening of pain, and psychological distress in physically dependent patients.

Reactions in bold italics are *life-threatening*. Interactions may have a *rapid onset* or a ***delayed onset***.

Refer to manufacturer's label for specific tapering instructions.

❸ *Alert:* When tapering opioids, monitor patients closely for signs and symptoms of opioid withdrawal (restlessness, lacrimation, rhinorrhea, yawning, perspiration, chills, myalgia, mydriasis, irritability, anxiety, insomnia, backache, joint pain, weakness, abdominal cramps, anorexia, nausea, vomiting, diarrhea; increased BP or HR and increased respiratory rate), which may indicate a need to taper more slowly. Also monitor patients for suicidal thoughts, use of other substances, or changes in mood.

• *Look alike–sound alike:* Don't confuse oxycodone with hydrocodone, Oxycontin, or oxymorphone. Don't confuse Oxycontin with MS Contin or oxybutynin, or Roxicodone with Roxanol.

PATIENT TEACHING

Black Box Warning Caution patient or caregiver of patient taking an opioid with a benzodiazepine, CNS depressant, or alcohol to seek immediate medical attention if patient experiences dizziness, lightheadedness, extreme sleepiness, slowed or difficult breathing, or unresponsiveness. ∎

Black Box Warning Advise patient that drug increases risk of opioid addiction, abuse, and misuse, which can lead to overdose and death. Teach patient proper use of drug. ∎

• Instruct patient to take drug before pain is intense.

• Explain assessment and monitoring process to patient and family. Instruct them to immediately report difficulty breathing or other signs or symptoms of a potential adverse opioid-related reaction.

• Tell patient to take drug with milk or after eating.

Black Box Warning Instruct patient or caregiver to keep drug out of the reach of children because accidental ingestion can result in a fatal oxycodone overdose. Advise patient or caregiver that if accidental ingestion occurs, to seek emergency medical help immediately. ∎

Black Box Warning Tell patient to swallow extended-release tablets whole. ∎

❸ *Alert:* Encourage patient to report all medications being taken, including prescription and OTC medications and supplements.

❸ *Alert:* Caution patient to immediately report symptoms of serotonin syndrome, adrenal insufficiency, and decreased sex hormone levels.

• Caution ambulatory patient about getting out of bed or walking. Warn outpatient to avoid driving and other hazardous activities that require mental alertness until drug's CNS effects are known.

• Advise patient to avoid alcohol use during therapy.

• Tell patient not to stop drug abruptly.

• Inform patient that urine drug testing and review of state prescription drug monitoring program will be done periodically.

❸ *Alert:* Counsel patient not to discontinue opioids without first discussing with prescriber the need for a gradual tapering regimen.

SAFETY ALERT!

oxyCODONE hydrochloride–acetaminophen
oks-i-KOE-done/a-seet-a-MIN-oh-fen

Percocet, Primlev, Roxicet

Therapeutic class: Opioid analgesics
Pharmacologic class: Opioid agonists–para-aminophenol derivatives
Controlled substance schedule: II

AVAILABLE FORMS

Oral solution: 5 mg oxycodone hydrochloride/325 mg acetaminophen per 5 mL (5 mL, 500 mL)
Tablets: 2.5 mg oxycodone hydrochloride/300 mg acetaminophen, 5 mg oxycodone hydrochloride/300 mg acetaminophen, 7.5 mg oxycodone hydrochloride/300 mg acetaminophen, 10 mg oxycodone hydrochloride/300 mg acetaminophen, 2.5 mg oxycodone hydrochloride/325 mg acetaminophen, 5 mg oxycodone hydrochloride/325 mg acetaminophen, 7.5 mg oxycodone hydrochloride/325 mg acetaminophen, 10 mg oxycodone hydrochloride/325 mg acetaminophen

INDICATIONS & DOSAGES

❸ Alert: Use in patients for whom alternative treatments are ineffective, not tolerated, or are inadequate.

➤ **Moderate to moderately severe pain (immediate-release)** Initial dose based on oxycodone content; maximum daily dose based on acetaminophen content.

Adults: Oxycodone 2.5 to 10 mg and acetaminophen 325 mg PO every 6 hours as needed for pain. Adjust dosage based on pain severity and patient response. Maximum daily doses shouldn't exceed 60 mg oxycodone or 4 g acetaminophen.

Adjust-a-dose: Consider decreased dosage in patients with renal or hepatic impairment, chronic alcoholics, elderly patients, and patients overly sensitive to effects of opioids. Gradually taper dosage if therapy lasts for more than a few weeks.

➤ **Acute pain (extended-release)**
Adults: 2 tablets PO every 12 hours. May give second dose early (8 hours after first dose) if needed, with subsequent doses of 2 tablets every 12 hours. Maximum daily doses shouldn't exceed 4 g acetaminophen.

Adjust-a-dose: For patients with renal or hepatic impairment, consider an initial dose of 1 tablet PO every 12 hours and adjust as needed.

ADMINISTRATION
PO

• Administer without regard to food.
• Store drug at room temperature.
• Don't crush, split, dissolve, break, or allow patient to chew extended-release tablets.

ACTION

Oxycodone binds with opioid receptors in the CNS, altering perception of and emotional response to pain. Acetaminophen is thought to produce analgesia by inhibiting prostaglandin and other substances that sensitize pain receptors. The combination reduces pain more effectively than acetaminophen alone.

Route	Onset	Peak	Duration
PO (acetaminophen)	<1 hr	10–60 min	4–6 hr
PO (oxycodone)	10–15 min	30 min–1 hr	3–6 hr

Half-life: Acetaminophen, 2 to 3 hours; oxycodone, 3½ to 4 hours.

ADVERSE REACTIONS

CNS: paresthesia, hypoesthesia, dizziness, drowsiness, fatigue, headache, dysphoria, insomnia. **CV:** peripheral edema, circulatory depression, hypotension, *shock.* **EENT:** dry mouth. **GI:** constipation, dyspepsia, nausea, vomiting, diarrhea. **GU:** dysuria. **Hematologic:** *hemolytic anemia, neutropenia, pancytopenia, thrombocytopenia.* **Hepatic:** increased liver enzyme levels. **Respiratory:** cough, *apnea, respiratory arrest,* respiratory depression. **Skin:** pruritus, erythema, erythematous dermatitis, excoriation, rash, flushing. **Other:** *anaphylactoid reaction.*

INTERACTIONS

Drug-drug. *Anticholinergics (atropine, dicyclomine, scopolamine):* May increase risk of paralytic ileus. Monitor patient closely.

Black Box Warning *Benzodiazepines, CNS depressants:* May cause slow or difficult breathing, sedation, and death. Avoid use together. If use together is necessary, limit dosage and duration of each drug to minimum necessary for desired effect. ∎

Beta blockers (propranolol): May inhibit acetaminophen metabolism. Use together carefully.

Black Box Warning *CYP3A4 inducers (carbamazepine, phenytoin, rifampin):* May increase oxycodone level and cause oxycodone-related adverse reactions if inducer is discontinued. Taper inducers cautiously and adjust oxycodone dosage as needed. ∎

Black Box Warning *CYP3A4 inhibitors (such as azole antifungals [ketoconazole]):* May increase oxycodone level, increase or prolong adverse effects, and cause fatal respiratory depression. Carefully monitor patient over extended period and adjust oxycodone dosage as needed. ∎

Desmopressin: May increase desmopressin-related toxicity. Monitor therapy.

Reactions in bold italics are *life-threatening*. Interactions may have a *rapid onset* or a *delayed onset*.

General anesthetics, neuromuscular blockers: May increase CNS depression. Use together cautiously, decreasing dosage of one or both agents.

Lamotrigine, loop diuretics, zidovudine: May decrease effects of these drugs when used with acetaminophen. Use together cautiously.

Mixed opioid agonist–antagonist combinations: May decrease effects of oxycodone and precipitate withdrawal. Use together carefully.

Oral contraceptives: May decrease acetaminophen half-life. Use together cautiously.

Probenecid: May increase effectiveness of acetaminophen. Use together cautiously.

❸ *Alert: Serotonergic drugs (amoxapine, antiemetics [dolasetron, granisetron, ondansetron, palonosetron], antimigraine drugs, buspirone, cyclobenzaprine, dextromethorphan, linezolid, lithium, MAO inhibitors, maprotiline, methylene blue, mirtazapine, nefazodone, SSNRIs, SSRIs, TCAs, trazodone, tryptophan, vilazodone):* May increase risk of serotonin syndrome. Use together cautiously and monitor patient for serotonin syndrome.

Drug-herb. *Kava kava:* May enhance adverse effects of CNS depressants. Monitor therapy carefully.

❸ *Alert: St. John's wort:* May increase risk of serotonin syndrome. May decrease oxycodone serum concentration. Use together cautiously.

Drug-lifestyle. Black Box Warning *Alcohol use:* May increase risk of profound sedation, respiratory depression, coma, and death. Don't use together. ∎

EFFECTS ON LAB TEST RESULTS
• May increase potassium, amylase, bilirubin, or liver enzyme levels. May increase or decrease blood glucose level.
• May decrease platelet count.
• Oxycodone may cause cross-reactivity with urinary assays used to detect cocaine and marijuana.
• Quinolones (levofloxacin, ofloxacin) may cause a false-positive urine screen result for opioids.

• Acetaminophen may cause false-positive result for urinary 5-hydroxyindoleacetic acid.

CONTRAINDICATIONS & CAUTIONS
• Contraindicated in patients hypersensitive to components of drug and in those with significant respiratory depression, acute or severe bronchial asthma, hypercarbia, or suspected or known paralytic ileus.

Black Box Warning Acetaminophen may increase risk of acute liver failure, liver transplant, and death. Liver injury is generally associated with use of acetaminophen at doses exceeding 4,000 mg/day and the use of more than one acetaminophen-containing product. ∎

Black Box Warning Serious, life-threatening, or fatal respiratory depression may occur with use of oxycodone–acetaminophen extended-release form. Monitor patient for respiratory depression, especially during initiation of therapy and after a dosage increase. Instruct patients to swallow oxycodone–acetaminophen extended-release tablets whole; crushing, dissolving, or chewing tablets can cause rapid release and absorption of a potentially fatal dose of oxycodone. ∎

Black Box Warning Accidental ingestion of even one dose of extended-release oxycodone–acetaminophen, especially by children, can result in a fatal overdose of oxycodone. ∎

Black Box Warning Patients must be screened for increased risk of opioid abuse (personal or family history of substance abuse or mental illness) before being prescribed opioids. ∎

Black Box Warning Opioids should only be prescribed with benzodiazepines or other CNS depressants to patients for whom alternative treatment options are inadequate. ∎

❸ *Alert:* Patients are at increased risk for oversedation and respiratory depression if they snore or have a history of sleep apnea, haven't used opioids recently or are first-time opioid users, have increased opioid dosage requirements or opioid habituation, have received general anesthesia for longer lengths of time or received other sedating drugs, have preexisting pulmonary or cardiac disease, or have thoracic or other surgical incisions that may impair breathing. Monitor patients carefully.

🜂 *Alert:* May cause serious, potentially fatal skin reactions, including SJS, toxic epidermal necrolysis, and acute generalized exanthematous pustulosis. Reaction may occur with first or subsequent use when acetaminophen is used as monotherapy or when it is one component of combination drug therapy. Monitor for reddening of the skin, rash, blisters, and detachment of the upper surface of the skin. Stop drug immediately if skin reaction is suspected.

🜂 *Alert:* Drug may lead to rare but serious decrease in adrenal gland cortisol production.

🜂 *Alert:* Drug may cause decreased sex hormone levels with long-term use.

• Use cautiously in patients with increased sensitivity to codeine, head injury, increased ICP, intracranial lesions, seizures, alcoholism, delirium tremens, biliary disease including pancreatitis, liver disease, COPD, preexisting respiratory impairment, or cor pulmonale.

• Use cautiously in acute abdominal conditions because this drug may obscure diagnostic signs or markedly increase respiratory depression or CSF pressure.

• Use cautiously in hypotensive patients, elderly or debilitated patients, and in those with severe renal or hepatic impairment, hypothyroidism, urethral stricture, or Addison disease.

Dialyzable drug: Oxycodone, unknown; acetaminophen, unknown.

⚠ *Overdose S&S:* Oxycodone: Pinpoint pupils, respiratory depression, loss of consciousness, somnolence, stupor, coma, skeletal muscle flaccidity, cold and clammy skin, bradycardia, hypotension, apnea, circulatory collapse, cardiac arrest, death. Acetaminophen: Nausea, vomiting, diaphoresis, general malaise, hepatic necrosis, renal tubular necrosis, hypoglycemic coma, coagulation defects.

PREGNANCY-LACTATION-REPRODUCTION

🜂 *Alert:* Carefully weigh risks and benefits of using drug during pregnancy.

Black Box Warning Prolonged use of extended-release oxycodone–acetaminophen during pregnancy can result in neonatal opioid withdrawal syndrome, which may be life-threatening if not recognized and treated and requires management according to protocols developed by neonatology experts. If prolonged use is required, advise patient of risks and ensure appropriate treatment is available. ∎

• Don't use immediately before labor. Prolonged use of opioids during pregnancy can result in neonatal withdrawal syndrome. Use only if benefits outweigh risks to the fetus.

• Use during breastfeeding isn't recommended.

NURSING CONSIDERATIONS

• Monitor circulatory and respiratory status closely, especially within the first 24 to 72 hours of initiating therapy. Withhold dose and notify prescriber if respirations are shallow or if respiratory rate falls below 12 breaths/minute.

🜂 *Alert:* Carefully monitor vital signs, pain level, respiratory status, and sedation level in all patients receiving opioids, especially those receiving IV drugs, even those given postoperatively.

• Keep opioid antagonist (naloxone) and resuscitation equipment available.

• The lowest effective dosage should be prescribed for the shortest period of time. Inform patients of risks and signs and symptoms of morphine toxicity.

Black Box Warning Assess patients identified as potential abusers; drug should be prescribed with extreme care. Drug may cause physical dependence and tolerance with long-term therapy. ∎

Black Box Warning Drug is potentially addictive. Chewing, crushing, dissolving, or injecting it can lead to overdose and death. ∎

Black Box Warning All patients using opioids should be routinely monitored for signs and symptoms of misuse, abuse, and addiction. ∎

Black Box Warning Serious, life-threatening or fatal respiratory depression can occur. Monitor patient closely, especially within first 24 to 72 hours of starting drug and after a dosage increase. ∎

Black Box Warning Accidental ingestion of even one dose of drug, especially by children, can be fatal. ∎

Reactions in bold italics are *life-threatening*. Interactions may have a *rapid onset* or a *delayed onset*.

❷ *Alert:* If patient is taking opioids with serotonergic drugs, watch for signs and symptoms of serotonin syndrome (agitation, hallucinations, rapid HR, fever, excessive sweating, shivering or shaking, muscle twitching or stiffness, trouble with coordination, nausea, vomiting, diarrhea), especially at start of treatment and at dosage increases. Signs and symptoms may occur within several hours of coadministration but may also occur later, especially after dosage increase. Discontinue opioid, serotonergic drug, or both if serotonin syndrome is suspected.

❷ *Alert:* Monitor patient for signs and symptoms of adrenal insufficiency (nausea, vomiting, loss of appetite, fatigue, weakness, dizziness, low BP). Perform diagnostic testing if adrenal insufficiency is suspected. If adrenal insufficiency is confirmed, treat with corticosteroids and wean patient off opioids if appropriate. Discontinue corticosteroids when clinically appropriate.

❷ *Alert:* Monitor patient for signs and symptoms of decreased sex hormone levels (low libido, erectile dysfunction, amenorrhea, infertility). If signs and symptoms occur, evaluate patient and obtain lab testing.

• Monitor patients for orthostatic hypotension.

• Monitor patients with head injury carefully. Oxycodone's effects on pupillary response and consciousness may mask worsening of neurologic status.

• Monitor patients with acute abdominal conditions closely. Drug may mask signs and symptoms in these patients.

• Observe for seizures in patients with convulsive disorders.

• Monitor bowel motility postoperatively, especially after intra-abdominal surgery.

❷ *Alert:* Don't stop drug abruptly; withdraw slowly and individualize gradual taper plan to prevent signs and symptoms of withdrawal, worsening of pain, and psychological distress in physically dependent patients. Refer to manufacturer's label for specific tapering instructions.

❷ *Alert:* When tapering opioids, monitor patients closely for signs and symptoms of opioid withdrawal (such as restlessness, lacrimation, rhinorrhea, yawning, perspiration, chills, myalgia, mydriasis, irritability, anxiety, insomnia, backache, joint pain,

weakness, abdominal cramps, anorexia, nausea, vomiting, diarrhea; increased BP or HR and increased respiratory rate), which may indicate a need to taper more slowly. Also monitor patients for suicidal thoughts, use of other substances, or changes in mood.

• *Look alike–sound alike:* Don't confuse oxycodone and acetaminophen with hydrocodone and acetaminophen. Don't confuse Endocet with Indocid, Percocet with Fioricet, Percodan, or Procet-30, or Roxicet with Roxanol.

PATIENT TEACHING

Black Box Warning Caution patient or caregiver of patient taking an opioid with a benzodiazepine, CNS depressant, or alcohol to seek immediate medical attention if patient experiences dizziness, lightheadedness, extreme sleepiness, slowed or difficult breathing, or unresponsiveness. ∎

Black Box Warning Teach patient to look for acetaminophen on labels of all prescriptions and OTC medications being taken and to not use more than one product containing acetaminophen. Warn patient to seek medical attention if acetaminophen intake exceeds 4,000 mg/day even if feeling well. ∎

Black Box Warning Advise patient that drug increases risk of opioid addiction, abuse, and misuse which can lead to overdose and death. Teach patient proper use of drug. ∎

• Explain assessment and monitoring process to patient and family. Instruct them to immediately report difficulty breathing or other signs or symptoms of a potential adverse opioid-related reaction.

Black Box Warning Instruct patient or caregiver to keep drug out of the reach of children because accidental ingestion can result in a fatal overdose of oxycodone. Advise patient or caregiver that if accidental ingestion occurs, to seek emergency medical help immediately. ∎

Black Box Warning Tell patient to swallow oxycodone–acetaminophen extended-release tablets whole. ∎

❷ *Alert:* Encourage patient to report all medications being taken, including prescription and OTC medications and supplements.

❷ *Alert:* Caution patient to immediately report signs and symptoms of serotonin syndrome, adrenal insufficiency, and decreased sex hormone levels.

🌢 **Alert:** Warn patient to stop drug and seek medical attention immediately if rash or reaction occurs while using acetaminophen.

• Inform patient with severe hepatic or renal disease that serial blood tests will be needed.

• Advise patient not to drive a car or operate heavy machinery while taking this drug.

• Warn patient to avoid alcohol and other CNS depressants.

Black Box Warning Caution patient that oxycodone may be habit-forming and to take drug only as long as prescribed in the amounts prescribed. Advise patient that if drug is taken for more than a few weeks, it should be tapered off gradually. ■

• Caution breastfeeding patient not to use drug because it can cause morphine toxicity (sleepiness, difficulty breastfeeding, breathing difficulties, limpness) in infants.

• Inform patient that urine drug testing and review of state prescription drug monitoring program will be done periodically.

🌢 **Alert:** Counsel patient not to discontinue opioids without first discussing with prescriber the need for a gradual tapering regimen.

SAFETY ALERT!

oxyMORphone hydrochloride
oks-i-MOR-fone

Opana

Therapeutic class: Opioid analgesics
Pharmacologic class: Opioids
Controlled substance schedule: II

AVAILABLE FORMS
Tablets (extended-release): 5 mg, 7.5 mg, 10 mg, 15 mg, 20 mg, 30 mg, 40 mg
Tablets (immediate-release): 5 mg, 10 mg

INDICATIONS & DOSAGES
Adjust-a-dose (for all indications): For elderly patients or those with mild hepatic impairment or CrCl less than 50 mL/minute, start with the lowest possible dose and slowly increase as tolerated. For patients receiving CNS depressants, begin at one third to one half of usual dose.

Adjust-a-dose: Refer to manufacturer's product information for instructions about converting to immediate-release tablets from other opioids and extended-release formulation.

➤ **Acute pain severe enough to require an opioid analgesic and for which alternative treatments are inadequate**
Adults: In opioid-naive patients, 5 to 10 mg immediate-release PO every 4 to 6 hours. Adjust dosage based on patient response.

➤ **Chronic pain**
Adults: 5 mg extended-release PO every 12 hours. Adjust dosage based on patient response.

ADMINISTRATION
PO
🌢 **Alert:** Starting doses of more than 20 mg aren't recommended because of potential serious adverse reactions.

• Give tablets 1 hour before or 2 hours after a meal.

Black Box Warning Patient should swallow extended-release tablets whole. Don't break, crush, dissolve, or allow patient to chew tablets, which can cause rapid release and can be fatal. ■

ACTION
May bind with opioid receptors in the CNS, altering perception of and emotional response to pain.

Route	Onset	Peak	Duration
PO	Varies	Varies	Varies

Half-life: Immediate-release, 7 to 9 hours; extended-release, 9 to 11 hours.

ADVERSE REACTIONS
CNS: clouded sensorium, dizziness, euphoria, headache, sedation, drowsiness, somnolence, *seizures,* dysphoria, light-headedness, hallucinations, physical dependence, fever, confusion, anxiety. **CV:** hypotension, HTN, *bradycardia,* palpitations, tachycardia, flushing. **EENT:** blurred vision, diplopia, miosis. **GI:** constipation, nausea, vomiting, ileus, dry mouth, abdominal pain, dyspepsia, flatulence. **GU:** urine retention. **Respiratory:** *respiratory depression, laryngeal edema, bronchospasm.* **Skin:** increased sweating, pruritus.

Reactions in bold italics are *life-threatening*. Interactions may have a *rapid onset* or a *delayed onset*.

INTERACTIONS

Drug-drug. *Agonist or antagonist analgesics (mixed or partial):* May reduce analgesic effect or precipitate withdrawal symptoms. Don't use together.

Anticholinergics: May increase risk of urine retention or severe constipation, leading to paralytic ileus. Monitor patient for abdominal pain or distention.

Black Box Warning *Benzodiazepines, CNS depressants:* May cause slow or difficult breathing, sedation, and death. Avoid use together. If use together is necessary, limit dosage and duration of each drug to minimum necessary for desired effect. ■

Cimetidine: May increase CNS reactions. Monitor patient closely.

CNS depressants, general anesthetics, phenothiazines, sedative-hypnotics, TCAs: May cause additive effects. Use together with caution and reduce opioid dosage.

Eluxadoline: May increase constipation. Avoid combination.

MAO inhibitors: May cause severe opioid potentiation. Don't use opioids if patient has received MAO inhibitors within 14 days. Avoid combination.

Propofol: May increase bradycardia risk. Monitor ECG closely.

☷ Alert: *Serotonergic drugs (amoxapine, antiemetics [dolasetron, granisetron, ondansetron, palonosetron], antimigraine drugs, buspirone, cyclobenzaprine, dextromethorphan, linezolid, lithium, MAO inhibitors, maprotiline, methylene blue, mirtazapine, nefazodone, SSNRIs, SSRIs, TCAs, trazodone, tryptophan, vilazodone):* May increase risk of serotonin syndrome. Use together cautiously and monitor patient for serotonin syndrome.

Drug-lifestyle. **Black Box Warning** *Alcohol use:* Alcoholic beverages or medications containing alcohol may cause additive effects and result in a potentially fatal overdose of oxymorphone. Don't use together. ■

Drug-herb. *Kava kava:* May enhance adverse effects of CNS depressants. Monitor therapy closely.

☷ Alert: *St. John's wort:* May increase risk of serotonin syndrome. Use together cautiously and monitor patient for serotonin syndrome.

EFFECTS ON LAB TEST RESULTS

• May increase amylase and lipase levels.
• Some quinolones (most consistently levofloxacin and ofloxacin) may produce false-positive urine screening results for opioids using commercially available immunoassay kits.

CONTRAINDICATIONS & CAUTIONS

• Contraindicated in patients hypersensitive to drug; in those with acute or severe bronchial asthma in an unmonitored setting or in the absence of resuscitative equipment, severe respiratory depression, upper airway obstruction, or GI obstruction, including paralytic ileus; and in those with moderate to severe hepatic impairment.

Black Box Warning Opioids should only be prescribed with benzodiazepines or other CNS depressants to patients for whom alternative treatment options are inadequate. ■

Black Box Warning Accidental ingestion of even one dose of oxymorphone, especially by children, can result in a fatal oxymorphone overdose. ■

Black Box Warning Patients must be screened for increased risk of opioid abuse (personal or family history of substance abuse or mental illness) before being prescribed opioids. ■

☷ Alert: Drug may lead to rare but serious decrease in adrenal gland cortisol production.

☷ Alert: Drug may cause decreased sex hormone levels with long-term use.

☷ Alert: Patients are at increased risk for oversedation and respiratory depression if they snore or have a history of sleep apnea, haven't used opioids recently or are first-time opioid users, have increased opioid dosage requirements or opioid habituation, have received general anesthesia for longer lengths of time or received other sedating drugs, have preexisting pulmonary or cardiac disease, or have thoracic or other surgical incisions that may impair breathing. Monitor patients carefully.

• Use with caution in elderly or debilitated patients and in those with head injury, increased ICP, seizures, asthma, COPD, acute abdominal conditions, biliary tract disease (including pancreatitis), acute alcoholism, delirium tremens, prostatic hyperplasia,

O

renal or mild hepatic impairment, urethral stricture, respiratory depression, hypothyroidism, Addison disease, and arrhythmias.
Dialyzable drug: Unknown.

⚠ *Overdose S&S:* Miosis, CNS depression, respiratory depression, apnea, flaccid skeletal muscles, bradycardia, hypotension, circulatory collapse, cardiac arrest, respiratory arrest, death.

PREGNANCY-LACTATION-REPRODUCTION
• Opioids cross placental barrier. During pregnancy, use minimum effective dose and only if benefit justifies risks to the fetus.
• Use cautiously during labor as uterine contractions and fetal HR may be affected.

Black Box Warning Prolonged use of oxymorphone during pregnancy can result in neonatal opioid withdrawal syndrome, which may be life-threatening if not recognized and treated and requires management according to protocols developed by neonatology experts. If drug is used for a prolonged period during pregnancy, advise patient of risk of withdrawal and ensure appropriate treatment will be available. ∎

⚙ *Alert:* Use cautiously in breastfeeding women. Use the lowest dose for the shortest duration of time, and only if drug is needed. Monitor infants for apnea and sedation.

NURSING CONSIDERATIONS
• Keep opioid antagonist (naloxone) and resuscitation equipment available.

Black Box Warning Monitor circulatory and respiratory status closely, especially within the first 24 to 72 hours of initiation of therapy or after a dosage increase. Withhold dose and notify prescriber for signs or symptoms of respiratory depression. ∎

Black Box Warning Assess patients identified as potential abusers; drug should be prescribed with extreme care. Drug may cause physical dependence and tolerance with long-term use. ∎

Black Box Warning Drug is potentially addictive. Chewing, crushing, snorting, or injecting it can lead to overdose and death. ∎

Black Box Warning All patients using opioids should be routinely monitored for signs and symptoms of misuse, abuse, and addiction. ∎

⚙ *Alert:* Carefully monitor vital signs, pain level, respiratory status, and sedation level in all patients receiving opioids.

⚙ *Alert:* If patient is taking opioids with serotonergic drugs, watch for signs and symptoms of serotonin syndrome (agitation, hallucinations, rapid HR, fever, excessive sweating, shivering or shaking, muscle twitching or stiffness, trouble with coordination, nausea, vomiting, diarrhea), especially at start of treatment or dosage increases. Signs and symptoms may occur within several hours of coadministration but may also occur later, especially after dosage increase. Discontinue opioid, serotonergic drug, or both if serotonin syndrome is suspected.

⚙ *Alert:* Monitor patient for signs and symptoms of adrenal insufficiency (nausea, vomiting, loss of appetite, fatigue, weakness, dizziness, low BP). Perform diagnostic testing if adrenal insufficiency is suspected. If adrenal insufficiency is confirmed, treat with corticosteroids and wean patient off opioids if appropriate. Discontinue corticosteroids when clinically appropriate.

⚙ *Alert:* Monitor patient for signs and symptoms of decreased sex hormone levels (low libido, erectile dysfunction, amenorrhea, infertility). If signs and symptoms occur, evaluate patient and obtain lab testing.

• Use of this drug may worsen gallbladder pain.
• Drug isn't for mild pain. For better effect, give drug before patient has intense pain.
• Monitor bladder and bowel function. Patient may need a stimulant laxative.

⚙ *Alert:* Closely monitor neonate whose mother received opioid analgesics during labor for signs and symptoms of respiratory depression. A specific opioid antagonist, such as naloxone or nalmefene, should be available for reversal of opioid-induced respiratory depression in a neonate.

⚙ *Alert:* Don't stop drug abruptly; withdraw slowly and individualize gradual taper plan to prevent signs and symptoms of withdrawal, worsening of pain, and psychological distress in physically dependent patients. Refer to manufacturer's label for specific tapering instructions.

⚙ *Alert:* When tapering opioids, monitor patients closely for signs and symptoms of opioid withdrawal (such as restlessness,

---

Reactions in bold italics are *life-threatening*. Interactions may have a *rapid onset* or a *delayed onset*.

lacrimation, rhinorrhea, yawning, perspiration, chills, myalgia, mydriasis, irritability, anxiety, insomnia, backache, joint pain, weakness, abdominal cramps, anorexia, nausea, vomiting, diarrhea; increased BP or HR and increased respiratory rate), which may indicate a need to taper more slowly. Also monitor patients for suicidal thoughts, use of other substances, or changes in mood.

• *Look alike–sound alike:* Don't confuse oxymorphone with hydromorphone, oxymetholone, or oxycodone.

PATIENT TEACHING

◐ *Alert:* Encourage patient to report all medications being taken, including prescription and OTC medications and supplements.

◐ *Alert:* Caution patient to immediately report signs and symptoms of serotonin syndrome, adrenal insufficiency, and decreased sex hormone levels.

• Instruct patient to ask for drug before pain is intense.

• Explain the assessment and monitoring process to patient and family. Instruct them to immediately report difficulty breathing or other signs of a potential adverse opioid-related reaction.

Black Box Warning Caution patient or caregiver of patient taking an opioid with a benzodiazepine, CNS depressant, or alcohol to seek immediate medical attention if patient experiences dizziness, lightheadedness, extreme sleepiness, slowed or difficult breathing, or unresponsiveness. ∎

Black Box Warning Inform patient that the use of oxymorphone, even when taken as recommended, can result in addiction, abuse, and misuse, which can lead to overdose or death. ∎

• Instruct patient not to share oxymorphone with others and to take steps to protect oxymorphone from theft or misuse.

• Caution ambulatory patient about getting out of bed or walking. Warn outpatient to avoid driving and other hazardous activities that require mental alertness until drug's CNS effects are known.

Black Box Warning Caution patient not to consume alcohol or take any prescription or OTC drug containing alcohol with oral form as this can lead to an overdose. ∎

• Tell patient to take tablets 1 hour before or 2 hours after a meal. Advise patient to swallow ER tablets whole and not to break, crush, dissolve, or chew them.

Black Box Warning Instruct patient to keep tablets in a child-resistant container and in a safe place out of the reach of children. Accidental ingestion by a child can result in death. In case of accidental ingestion, seek emergency medical help immediately. ∎

◐ *Alert:* Counsel patient not to discontinue opioids without first discussing with prescriber the need for a gradual tapering regimen.

SAFETY ALERT!

oxytocin (synthetic injection)
oks-i-TOE-sin

Pitocin

Therapeutic class: Oxytocics
Pharmacologic class: Exogenous hormones

AVAILABLE FORMS
Injection: 10 units/mL

INDICATIONS & DOSAGES
➤ **To induce or stimulate labor**
Adults: Initially, 0.5 to 1 milliunit/minute IV infusion. Increase rate by 1 to 2 milliunits/minute at 30- to 60-minute intervals until normal contraction pattern is established. Decrease rate when labor is firmly established. Rates exceeding 9 to 10 milliunits/minute are rarely required.

➤ **To reduce postpartum bleeding after expulsion of placenta**
Adults: 10 to 40 units in 1,000 mL of lactated Ringer solution, or NSS IV infused at rate needed to sustain uterine contraction and control uterine atony. Also, may give 10 units IM after delivery of placenta.

➤ **Incomplete, inevitable, or elective abortion**
Adults: 10 units IV infusion at 10 to 20 milliunits (20 to 40 drops)/minute. Don't exceed 30 units in 12 hours.

ADMINISTRATION
IV
▼ Never give drug simultaneously by more than one route.

▼ To induce or stimulate labor, dilute drug by adding 10 units to 1 L of NSS or lactated Ringer solution.

▼ To produce intense uterine contractions and reduce postpartum bleeding, dilute drug by adding 10 units to 1,000 mL of NSS or lactated Ringer solution.

▼ To treat abortion, add 10 units to 500 mL NSS.

▼ Don't give bolus injection; use an infusion pump. Give drug only by piggyback infusion so that it may be stopped without interrupting IV line.

▼ **Incompatibilities:** None listed by manufacturer. Consult a drug incompatibility reference for more information.

IM
• Drug isn't recommended for routine IM use, but 10 units may be given IM after delivery of placenta to control postpartum uterine bleeding.

• Never give drug simultaneously by more than one route.

ACTION
Causes potent and selective stimulation of uterine and mammary gland smooth muscle.

Route	Onset	Peak	Duration
IV	1 min	Unknown	1 hr
IM	3–5 min	Unknown	2–3 hr

Half-life: 1 to 6 minutes.

ADVERSE REACTIONS
Maternal
CNS: *subarachnoid hemorrhage, seizures, coma.* **CV:** *arrhythmias,* HTN, PVCs, hypotension, tachycardia. **GI:** nausea, vomiting. **GU:** *abruptio placentae,* tetanic uterine contractions, *postpartum hemorrhage, uterine rupture,* impaired uterine blood flow, pelvic hematoma, increased uterine motility. **Hematologic:** *afibrinogenemia, possibly related to postpartum bleeding, pelvic hematoma.* **Other:** *anaphylaxis, death from oxytocin-induced water intoxication,* hypersensitivity reactions.

Fetal
CNS: *infant brain damage, seizures.* **CV:** *bradycardia, arrhythmias,* PVCs. **EENT:** neonatal retinal hemorrhage. **Hepatic:** neonatal jaundice. **Other:** *low Apgar scores at 5 minutes, death.*

INTERACTIONS
Drug-drug. *Carboprost tromethamine:* May enhance adverse/toxic effect of oxytocin. Avoid combination.

Cyclopropane anesthetics: May cause less pronounced bradycardia and hypotension. Use together cautiously.

Dinoprostone: May enhance oxytocic effects of oxytocin. Concomitant use isn't recommended. If used sequentially, monitor uterine activity closely. Administer oxytocin 30 minutes after removing dinoprostone vaginal insert and 6 to 12 hours after application of dinoprostone gel.

Drugs that prolong QT interval: May increase risk of life-threatening cardiac arrhythmias, including torsades de pointes. Use together cautiously.

Misoprostol: May increase oxytocin adverse effects. Don't use together.

Vasoconstrictors: May cause severe HTN if oxytocin is given within 3 to 4 hours of vasoconstrictor in patient receiving caudal block anesthetic. Avoid using together.

EFFECTS ON LAB TEST RESULTS
None reported.

CONTRAINDICATIONS & CAUTIONS
• Contraindicated in patients hypersensitive to drug.

• Contraindicated when vaginal delivery isn't advised (placenta previa, vasa previa, invasive cervical carcinoma, genital herpes), when cephalopelvic disproportion is present, or when delivery requires conversion, as in transverse lie.

• Contraindicated in fetal distress when delivery isn't imminent, in prematurity, in other obstetric emergencies, and in patients with severe toxemia or hypertonic uterine patterns.

• Use cautiously, if at all, in patients with invasive cervical cancer and in those with previous cervical or uterine surgery (including cesarean section), grand multiparity, uterine sepsis, traumatic delivery, or overdistended uterus.

❸ Alert: May cause antidiuretic effect and risk of severe water intoxication, seizures, or death.

Dialyzable drug: Unknown.

⚠ Overdose S&S: Uterine hypersensitivity, tumultuous labor, uterine rupture, cervical and vaginal lacerations, postpartum hemorrhage, uteroplacental hypoperfusion, variable deceleration of fetal HR, fetal hypoxia, hypercapnia, perinatal hepatic necrosis, water intoxication, seizures, death.

PREGNANCY-LACTATION-REPRODUCTION
Black Box Warning Drug is only indicated for the medical, rather than the elective, induction of labor. ■
• Use cautiously during first and second stages of labor because uterine hypertonicity, tetanic contraction, cervical laceration, uterine rupture, and maternal and fetal death have been reported.
• Use cautiously in pregnant or breastfeeding women. May disrupt breastfeeding initiation.

NURSING CONSIDERATIONS
❸ Alert: All patients receiving oxytocin IV must be under continuous observation by trained personnel who have a thorough knowledge of the drug.
❸ Alert: Discontinue oxytocin infusion immediately if uterine hyperactivity or fetal distress occurs. Administer oxygen to the mother. Mother and fetus must be evaluated by the responsible practitioner.
• Drug is used to induce or reinforce labor only when pelvis is known to be adequate, when vaginal delivery is indicated, when fetal maturity is assured, and when fetal position is favorable. Use drug only in hospital where critical care facilities and prescriber are immediately available.
• Monitor fluid intake and output. Antidiuretic effect may lead to fluid overload, seizures, and coma from water intoxication.
• Monitor and record uterine contractions, HR, BP, intrauterine pressure, fetal HR, and blood loss at least every 15 minutes.

PATIENT TEACHING
• Explain use and administration of drug to patient and family.

• Instruct patient to promptly report adverse reactions.

SAFETY ALERT!

PACLitaxel (conventional)
pac-li-TAKS-el

Therapeutic class: Antineoplastics
Pharmacologic class: Taxoids

AVAILABLE FORMS
Injection: 6 mg/mL in 5-mL, 16.7-mL, 25-mL, 50-mL vials

INDICATIONS & DOSAGES
➤ **AIDS-related Kaposi sarcoma**
Adults: 135 mg/m^2 IV over 3 hours every 3 weeks, or 100 mg/m^2 IV over 3 hours every 2 weeks.
Adjust-a-dose: For patients with hepatic impairment, reduce first 135 mg/m^2 3-hour infusion based on transaminase and bilirubin levels. If transaminase levels are less than $10 \times$ ULN and bilirubin levels are $1.25 \times$ ULN or less, give 175 mg/m^2. If transaminase levels are less than $10 \times$ ULN and bilirubin levels are 1.26 to $2 \times$ ULN, give 135 mg/m^2. Refer to manufacturer's instructions for toxicity-related dosage adjustments and management.
➤ **First-line and subsequent therapy for advanced ovarian cancer**
Adults (previously untreated): 175 mg/m^2 IV over 3 hours every 3 weeks, followed by cisplatin 75 mg/m^2; or 135 mg/m^2 IV over 24 hours every 3 weeks, followed by cisplatin 75 mg/m^2 every 3 weeks.
Adults (previously treated): 135 or 175 mg/m^2 IV over 3 hours every 3 weeks.
Adjust-a-dose: For patients with hepatic impairment, reduce first 3-hour dose based on transaminase and bilirubin levels. If transaminase levels are less than $10 \times$ ULN and bilirubin levels are $1.25 \times$ ULN or less, give 175 mg/m^2. If transaminase levels are less than $10 \times$ ULN and bilirubin levels are 1.26 to $2 \times$ ULN, give 135 mg/m^2. If transaminase levels are less than $10 \times$ ULN and bilirubin levels are 2.01 to $5 \times$ ULN, give 90 mg/m^2. Refer to manufacturer's instructions for toxicity-related dosage adjustments and management.

P

➤ Breast cancer after failure of combination chemotherapy for metastatic disease or relapse within 6 months of adjuvant chemotherapy (previous therapy should have included an anthracycline unless contraindicated); adjuvant therapy for node-positive breast cancer given sequentially to standard doxorubicin-containing combination chemotherapy

Adults: 175 mg/m^2 IV over 3 hours every 3 weeks for four cycles.

Adjust-a-dose: For patients with hepatic impairment, reduce first 3-hour dose based on transaminase and bilirubin levels. If transaminase levels are less than $10 \times$ ULN and bilirubin levels are $1.25 \times$ ULN or less, give 175 mg/m^2. If transaminase levels are less than $10 \times$ ULN and bilirubin levels are 1.26 to $2 \times$ ULN, give 135 mg/m^2. If transaminase levels are less than $10 \times$ ULN and bilirubin levels are 2.01 to $5 \times$ ULN, give 90 mg/m^2. Refer to manufacturer's instructions for toxicity-related dosage adjustments and management.

➤ First treatment of advanced NSCLC in patients who aren't candidates for curative surgery or radiation

Adults: 135 mg/m^2 IV infusion over 24 hours, followed by cisplatin 75 mg/m^2. Repeat cycle every 3 weeks.

Adjust-a-dose: For patients with hepatic impairment, adjust doses for the first courses of therapy as follows: For first 24-hour infusion if transaminase levels are less than $2 \times$ ULN and bilirubin levels are 1.5 mg/dL or less, give 135 mg/m^2. If transaminase levels are 2 to less than $10 \times$ ULN and bilirubin levels are 1.5 mg/dL or less, give 100 mg/m^2. If transaminase levels are less than $10 \times$ ULN and bilirubin levels are 1.6 to 7.5 mg/dL, give 50 mg/m^2. Refer to manufacturer's instructions for toxicity-related dosage adjustments and management.

ADMINISTRATION

IV

⊕ *Alert:* Preparing and giving drug may be mutagenic, teratogenic, or carcinogenic. Follow institutional safe handling and disposal policies to reduce risks. Mark all waste materials with CHEMOTHERAPY HAZARD labels.

Black Box Warning To reduce risk or severity of hypersensitivity, patients must receive pretreatment with antihistamines and corticosteroids. Both H$_1$-receptor antagonists such as diphenhydramine and H$_2$-receptor antagonists, such as cimetidine or ranitidine, may be used. Fatal reactions have occurred despite premedication. ▌

▼ Prepare and store infusion solutions in glass containers or polypropylene bottles, or use polypropylene or polyolefin bags. Undiluted concentrate shouldn't contact polyvinyl chloride IV bags or tubing.

▼ Dilute concentrate before infusion. Compatible solutions include NSS for injection, D$_5$W, 5% dextrose in NSS for injection, and 5% dextrose in lactated Ringer injection. Dilute to yield 0.3 to 1.2 mg/mL. Diluted solutions are stable for 27 hours at room temperature. Prepared solution may appear hazy.

▼ Give through polyethylene-lined administration sets, and use an in-line 0.22-micron filter.

⊕ *Alert:* Watch for irritation and infiltration; extravasation can cause tissue damage and necrosis. Administration of hyaluronidase may be needed.

▼ Closely monitor patient and vital signs during infusion, especially during the first hour.

▼ Store diluted solution in glass or polypropylene bottles, or use polypropylene or polyolefin bags.

▼ **Incompatibilities:** Y-site incompatibilities: amiodarone, amphotericin B cholesteryl sulfate, amphotericin conventional, amphotericin B liposomal, chlorpromazine, diazepam, digoxin, gemtuzumab ozogamicin, hydroxyzine, idarubicin, indomethacin, labetalol, methylprednisolone sodium succinate, phenytoin, propranolol.

ACTION

Prevents depolymerization of cellular microtubules, inhibiting normal reorganization of microtubule network needed for mitosis and other vital cellular functions.

Route	Onset	Peak	Duration
IV	Unknown	Unknown	Unknown

Half-life: 13 to 53 hours.

ADVERSE REACTIONS
CNS: peripheral neuropathy, asthenia, fever. **CV:** *bradycardia,* hypotension, abnormal ECG. **GI:** nausea, vomiting, diarrhea, mucositis. **Hematologic:** *neutropenia, leukopenia, thrombocytopenia,* anemia, *bleeding.* **Hepatic:** elevated LFT values, elevated bilirubin level. **Musculoskeletal:** myalgia, arthralgia. **Skin:** alopecia, cellulitis and phlebitis at injection site. **Other:** hypersensitivity reactions, *anaphylaxis,* infections.

INTERACTIONS
Drug-drug. *Cisplatin:* May cause additive myelosuppressive effects. Give paclitaxel before cisplatin.
CYP450 inducers (carbamazepine, phenobarbital): May decrease serum concentration of CYP3A4 substrates (high risk with inducers). Monitor therapy.
*CYP450 inhibitors (clarithromycin, cyclosporine, dexamethasone, diazepam, etoposide, felodipine, **ketoconazole**, quinidine, retinoic acid, teniposide, testosterone, verapamil, vincristine):* May increase paclitaxel level. Monitor patient for toxicity.
Doxorubicin: May increase plasma levels of doxorubicin and its active metabolite, doxorubicinol. Use together cautiously.
Live-virus vaccines: May increase risk of vaccine-induced adverse reactions. Use together isn't recommended. Patients with malignancies who are in remission can receive live-virus vaccines 3 months after completion of chemotherapy.

EFFECTS ON LAB TEST RESULTS
• May increase alkaline phosphatase, ALT/AST, bilirubin, and triglyceride levels.
• May decrease Hb level and neutrophil, WBC, and platelet counts.

CONTRAINDICATIONS & CAUTIONS
• Contraindicated in patients hypersensitive to drug or polyoxyethylated castor oil.
Black Box Warning Patients who experience hypersensitivity reactions shouldn't be rechallenged with drug. ∎
Black Box Warning Contraindicated in those with baseline neutrophil counts below 1,500/mm^3 and platelet counts below 100,000/mm^3, or in those with AIDS-related Kaposi sarcoma with baseline neutrophil counts below 1,000/mm^3. ∎
• Use cautiously in patients with hepatic impairment.
Dialyzable drug: No.
⚠ *Overdose S&S:* Bone marrow suppression, sensory neurotoxicity, mucositis, acute ethanol toxicity (in children), CNS toxicity (in children).

PREGNANCY-LACTATION-REPRODUCTION
• Women of childbearing potential should avoid becoming pregnant during therapy. Men shouldn't father a child during therapy.
• Drug may appear in human milk. Patient should discontinue breastfeeding or discontinue drug.

NURSING CONSIDERATIONS
Black Box Warning Administer drug under the supervision of a prescriber experienced with cancer chemotherapeutic agents and only when adequate diagnostic and treatment facilities are readily available to manage complications. ∎
• Patient may experience peripheral neuropathies, which may be cumulative and dose related. Patients with severe symptoms may need dosage reduction.
Black Box Warning Monitor blood counts before and during therapy. Bone marrow toxicity is the most common and dose-limiting toxicity. Institute bleeding precautions, as indicated. ∎
• Premedicate with dexamethasone 20 mg PO or IV approximately 12 and 6 hours before paclitaxel; diphenhydramine 50 mg IV 30 to 60 minutes before paclitaxel; and cimetidine 300 mg, ranitidine 50 mg, or famotidine 20 mg IV 30 to 60 minutes before paclitaxel. Premedication for patients with advanced HIV disease: Reduce dexamethasone to 10 mg.
• If patient develops significant cardiac conduction abnormalities, use indicated therapy and continuous cardiac monitoring during therapy and subsequent infusions.
🌢 *Alert:* When indicated, cisplatin dose should follow dose of paclitaxel.
• *Look alike–sound alike:* Don't confuse paclitaxel with paroxetine or with paclitaxel protein-bound particles.

P

PATIENT TEACHING

- Advise patient to report any pain or burning at site of injection.
- Urge patient to report fever, sore throat, fatigue, easy bruising, nosebleeds, bleeding gums, or tarry stools. Tell patient to take temperature daily.
- Teach patient to report tingling or burning sensation or numbness in limbs immediately.
- Warn patient that reversible hair loss will probably occur.
- Caution female patient of childbearing potential to avoid becoming pregnant or breastfeeding during therapy. Recommend that she consult prescriber before becoming pregnant.

SAFETY ALERT!

PACLitaxel protein-bound particles
pac-li-TAKS-el

Abraxane

Therapeutic class: Antineoplastics
Pharmacologic class: Taxoids

AVAILABLE FORMS
Lyophilized powder for injection: 100 mg in single-use vials

INDICATIONS & DOSAGES
➤ **Metastatic breast cancer after failure of combination chemotherapy or relapse within 6 months of adjuvant chemotherapy (previous therapy should have included an anthracycline unless clinically contraindicated at the time)**
Adults: 260 mg/m^2 IV over 30 minutes every 3 weeks.
Adjust-a-dose: For patients with moderate hepatic impairment (serum bilirubin level greater than 1.5 to 3 × ULN and AST level 1 to 10 × ULN) and patients with severe hepatic impairment (serum bilirubin level greater than 3 to 5 × ULN and AST level 1 to 10 × ULN), recommended dosage is 200 mg/m^2/dose initially; may increase dosage to 260 mg/m^2/dose in subsequent courses if patient tolerates reduced dosage for two cycles. Don't give to patients with very severe hepatic impairment (serum

bilirubin level more than 5 × ULN or AST level more than 10 × ULN).
Refer to manufacturer's instructions for toxicity-related dosage adjustments.
➤ **NSCLC as first-line treatment in combination with carboplatin in patients who aren't candidates for surgery or radiation therapy**
Adults: 100 mg/m^2 IV over 30 minutes on days 1, 8, and 15 of each 21-day cycle. Give carboplatin immediately after paclitaxel protein-bound particles dose on day 1 of each 21-day cycle. Refer to manufacturer's instructions for carboplatin dosage.
Adjust-a-dose: For patients with moderate hepatic impairment (serum bilirubin level greater than 1.5 to 3 × ULN and AST level 1 to 10 × ULN) and severe hepatic impairment (serum bilirubin level greater than 3 to 5 × ULN and AST level 1 to 10 × ULN), recommended dosage is 80 mg/m^2/dose; may increase dosage to 100 mg/m^2/dose in subsequent courses if patient tolerates reduced dosage for two cycles. Don't give to patients with very severe hepatic impairment (serum bilirubin level more than 5 × ULN or AST level more than 10 × ULN).
Don't administer paclitaxel on day 1 of a cycle until ANC is at least 1,500/mm^3 and platelet count is at least 100,000/mm^3.
Refer to manufacturer's instructions for toxicity-related dosage adjustments.
➤ **Metastatic pancreatic adenocarcinoma as first-line treatment in combination with gemcitabine**
Adults: 125 mg/m^2 IV over 30 to 40 minutes on days 1, 8, and 15 of each 28-day cycle. Give gemcitabine 1,000 mg/m^2 IV immediately after each paclitaxel dose.
Adjust-a-dose: For patients with mild hepatic impairment (bilirubin level greater than ULN to 1.5 × ULN and AST less than 10 × ULN), no dosage adjustment is needed. Drug isn't recommended for patients with moderate to severe hepatic impairment.
Refer to manufacturer's instructions for toxicity-related dosage adjustments.

ADMINISTRATION
IV
▼ Because of drug's cytotoxicity, handle it cautiously and wear gloves. If drug

---

contacts skin, wash area thoroughly with soap and water. If drug contacts mucous membranes, flush thoroughly with water.

▼ Reconstitute the vial with 20 mL of NSS to yield 5 mg/mL of drug. Direct the stream slowly, over at least 1 minute, onto the inside wall of the vial to avoid foaming. Let the vial sit for 5 minutes to ensure proper wetting of the powder. Gently swirl or turn the vial for at least 2 minutes until completely dissolved. If foaming occurs, let the solution stand for 15 minutes for the foam to subside. If particles are visible, gently invert the vial again to ensure complete resuspension. The solution should appear milky and uniform. Inject the correct dose into an empty polyvinyl chloride-type IV bag and use immediately.

▼ Give drug over 30 minutes (breast cancer and NSCLC) or over 30 to 40 minutes (pancreatic adenocarcinoma).

▼ The suspension for infusion, when prepared in an infusion bag, can be stored at 36° to 46° F (2° to 8° C), protected from bright light, for up to 24 hours.

▼ Store unopened vials at room temperature in the original package. Store reconstituted vials at 36° to 46° F (2° to 8° C) for up to 24 hours, protected from light.

▼ The total combined refrigerated storage time of reconstituted solution in vial and infusion bag is 24 hours. This may be followed by storage in infusion bag at ambient temperature and lighting conditions for a maximum of 4 hours.

▼ **Incompatibilities:** None listed by manufacturer.

ACTION

Prevents depolymerization of cellular microtubules, inhibiting reorganization of the microtubule network and disrupting mitosis and other vital cell functions.

Route	Onset	Peak	Duration
IV	Unknown	Unknown	Unknown

Half-life: 13 to 27 hours.

ADVERSE REACTIONS

CNS: asthenia, depression, peripheral neuropathy, headache, fatigue, sensory neuropathy, fever. **CV:** abnormal ECG, edema, HTN, hypotension. **EENT:** visual distur-

bances, epistaxis. **GI:** anorexia, diarrhea, nausea, oral candidiasis, vomiting, intestinal obstruction, *ischemic colitis, pancreatitis, perforation,* mucositis. **GU:** *renal failure, UTI.* **Hematologic:** anemia, *neutropenia, thrombocytopenia, bleeding, myelosuppression.* **Hepatic:** *hepatic encephalopathy, hepatic necrosis.* **Musculoskeletal:** arthralgia, myalgia. **Respiratory:** *PE,* cough, dyspnea, pneumonia, respiratory tract infection. **Skin:** alopecia, rash, injection-site reactions. **Other:** infections, hypersensitivity reactions, dehydration, *sepsis.*

INTERACTIONS

Drug-drug. *Clozapine:* May increase risk of agranulocytosis. Avoid use together.
CYP450 inhibitors: May decrease paclitaxel metabolism. Use together cautiously.
Live-virus vaccines: May increase vaccine-related adverse effects. Avoid use together. Don't give vaccines for at least 3 months after immunosuppressants.
Vaccines (inactivated): May diminish vaccine therapeutic effects. Monitor therapy.

EFFECTS ON LAB TEST RESULTS

● May increase alkaline phosphatase, AST, bilirubin, creatinine, and GGT levels. May decrease Hb level.

● May decrease neutrophil and platelet counts.

CONTRAINDICATIONS & CAUTIONS

Black Box Warning Contraindicated in patients with baseline neutrophil count of less than 1,500/mm³. ■

● Contraindicated in patients hypersensitive to drug or its components; severe and sometimes fatal hypersensitivity reactions can occur. Don't rechallenge patients who experience a hypersensitivity reaction.

● Don't repeat dose until neutrophil counts recover to more than 1,500/mm³ and platelet count recovers to more than 100,000/mm³.

● Use hasn't been studied in patients with creatinine level less than 30 mL/minute.
Dialyzable drug: Unknown.

⚠ *Overdose S&S:* Bone marrow suppression, sensory neurotoxicity, acute ethanol toxicity (in children), CNS toxicity (in children).

PREGNANCY-LACTATION-REPRODUCTION

• Women of childbearing potential should avoid becoming pregnant during therapy. Males shouldn't father a child during therapy.

• Drug appears in human milk. Patient shouldn't breastfeed during therapy and for 2 weeks after final dose.

NURSING CONSIDERATIONS

⚠ *Alert:* Give only under supervision of practitioner experienced in using chemotherapy in a facility that can manage complications of therapy.

Black Box Warning Don't substitute Abraxane for other forms of paclitaxel. ▮

Black Box Warning Monitor CBC frequently to evaluate for neutropenia, which may be severe and may result in infection. ▮

⚠ *Alert:* Obtain CBC before dosing on day 1 for metastatic breast cancer and before days 1, 8, and 15 for NSCLC or pancreatic cancer.

⚠ *Alert:* If patient becomes febrile (regardless of ANC), initiate treatment with broad-spectrum antibiotics.

⚠ *Alert:* Watch for pneumonitis in patients receiving drug in combination with gemcitabine. If pneumonitis is suspected, interrupt treatment. If pneumonitis is diagnosed, permanently discontinue treatment with paclitaxel and gemcitabine.

• Dosage reductions or drug discontinuation may be needed based on severe hematologic, neurologic, cutaneous, or GI toxicities.

• Because drug contains human albumin, a remote risk exists of transmitting viruses and Creutzfeldt-Jakob disease.

• Assess patient for symptoms of sensory neuropathy and severe neutropenia.

• Monitor LFT and renal function test results.

• Monitor infusion site closely.

PATIENT TEACHING

• Warn patient that alopecia commonly occurs but is reversible after therapy.

• Teach patient to recognize signs of neuropathy, such as tingling, burning, and numbness in arms and legs.

• Tell patient to report signs of infection, severe abdominal pain, or severe diarrhea.

• Advise patient to contact prescriber if nausea and vomiting persist or interfere with

adequate nutrition. Reassure patient that an antiemetic can be prescribed.

• Explain that many patients experience weakness and fatigue, so it's important to rest.

• To reduce or prevent mouth sores, remind patient to perform proper oral hygiene.

• Tell female patient to avoid pregnancy and not to breastfeed. Advise male patient to avoid fathering a child during therapy.

SAFETY ALERT!

palbociclib ☒
pal-boe-SYE-klib

Ibrance

Therapeutic class: Antineoplastics
Pharmacologic class: Kinase inhibitors

AVAILABLE FORMS
Capsules ⊙*:* 75 mg, 100 mg, 125 mg

INDICATIONS & DOSAGES

➤ **Hormone receptor (HR)–positive, HER2-negative advanced or metastatic breast cancer, as initial endocrine-based therapy in postmenopausal women in combination with an aromatase inhibitor or in combination with fulvestrant in women with disease progression after endocrine therapy** ☒

Adults: 125 mg PO daily for 21 consecutive days followed by 7 days off to complete a cycle of 28 days. When given with an aromatase inhibitor, refer to prescribing information for the inhibitor being used. When given with fulvestrant, recommended dosage of fulvestrant is 500 mg PO on days 1, 15, and 29, and once monthly thereafter; refer to full prescribing information for fulvestrant.

Premenopausal and perimenopausal women treated with the combination of palbociclib and fulvestrant should be treated with luteinizing hormone-releasing hormone agonists according to current standards.

Adjust-a-dose: Refer to manufacturer's instructions for toxicity-related dosage adjustments.

Reactions in bold italics are *life-threatening*. Interactions may have a *rapid onset* or a *delayed onset*.

ADMINISTRATION
PO
• Drug is hazardous; use appropriate safe handling and disposal precautions.
• Give capsule whole with food. Don't crush.
• If patient vomits after taking a dose or misses a dose, patient should take next prescribed dose at the usual time.

ACTION
Inhibits cyclin-dependent kinase 4 and 6. Reduces cellular proliferation of ER-positive breast cancer cell line by blocking progression of cell from G_1 to S phase of the cell cycle, resulting in decreased phosphorylation and decreased tumor growth.

Route	Onset	Peak	Duration
PO	N/A	6–12 hr	N/A

Half-life: 24 to 34 hours.

ADVERSE REACTIONS
CNS: peripheral neuropathy, asthenia, fatigue, fever. **EENT:** blurred vision, dry eyes, epistaxis. **GI:** decreased appetite, stomatitis, nausea, diarrhea, vomiting. **Hematologic:** *neutropenia, febrile neutropenia, leukopenia,* anemia, *thrombocytopenia.* **Skin:** alopecia, rash, infections.

INTERACTIONS
Drug-drug. *Alfentanil, cyclosporine, dihydroergotamine, ergotamine, everolimus, fentanyl, midazolam, pimozide, quinidine, sirolimus, tacrolimus:* May increase concentrations of these drugs. Dosages of these drugs may need to be decreased.
Strong or moderate CYP3A inducers: May decrease palbociclib concentration. Avoid concurrent use.
Strong CYP3A inhibitors: May increase palbociclib concentration. Avoid use together; if unavoidable, decrease palbociclib dosage to 75 mg daily. If strong inhibitor is discontinued, increase palbociclib dosage after three to five half-lives have passed from CYP3A dose.
Drug-herb. *St. John's wort:* May decrease palbociclib concentration. Discourage use together.
Drug-food. *Grapefruit, grapefruit juice:* May increase palbociclib concentration. Discourage use together.

EFFECTS ON LAB TEST RESULTS
• May decrease Hb level and WBC, neutrophil, lymphocyte, and platelet counts.

CONTRAINDICATIONS & CAUTIONS
• Contraindicated in patients hypersensitive to drug or its components.
⊘ *Alert:* May cause severe or fatal interstitial lung disease (ILD) and pneumonitis.
• May cause neutropenia and risk of infection.
• Drug hasn't been studied in children.
• Use cautiously in elderly patients, who may experience a greater sensitivity to drug's effects.
• There is no antidote for overdose. Use general supportive measures.
Dialyzable drug: Unknown.

PREGNANCY-LACTATION-REPRODUCTION
• Contraindicated in pregnant women. Women of childbearing potential should use effective contraception during treatment and for at least 3 weeks after last dose.
• Advise women not to breastfeed during treatment and for 3 weeks after final dose.
• Advise male patients with female partners of childbearing potential to use effective contraception during treatment and for 3 months after final dose.

NURSING CONSIDERATIONS
• Monitor CBC before start of therapy, at beginning of each cycle, on day 15 of first two cycles, and as clinically indicated. Interrupt therapy and adjust dosage as necessary.
⊘ *Alert:* Monitor patients for new or worsening pulmonary symptoms; if they occur, interrupt therapy immediately and evaluate the patient. If infection, neoplasm and other causes are excluded, permanently discontinue treatment in patients with severe ILD or pneumonitis.
• Monitor patient for myelosuppression or infection; treat appropriately.

PATIENT TEACHING
⊘ *Alert:* Warn patients to immediately report difficulty or discomfort with breathing or shortness of breath while at rest or with low activity; these may be symptoms of ILD or pneumonitis.

P

- Instruct patient to take with food and to swallow capsules whole.
- Advise patient that if vomiting occurs after taking a dose or if patient misses a dose not to make it up but to take the next prescribed dose at the usual time.
- Teach patient to report signs and symptoms of decreased bone marrow function and infection.
- Tell patient to report chest pain or rapid heartbeat.
- Instruct patient to tell prescriber of all medications being taken, including prescription and OTC drugs and herbal products.
- Caution patient to avoid grapefruit and grapefruit juice.

---

paliperidone
pal-ee-PER-i-done

Invega

paliperidone palmitate
Invega Sustenna, Invega Trinza

Therapeutic class: Antipsychotics
Pharmacologic class: Benzisoxazole derivatives

AVAILABLE FORMS
Injection: 39 mg/0.25 mL, 78 mg/0.5 mL, 117 mg/0.75 mL, 156 mg/mL, 234 mg/ 1.5 mL, 273 mg/0.875 mL, 410 mg/ 1.315 mL, 546 mg/1.75 mL, 819 mg/ 2.625 mL
Tablets (extended-release) Ⓓ: 1.5 mg, 3 mg, 6 mg, 9 mg

INDICATIONS & DOSAGES
Adjust-a-dose (for all indications): In patients with CrCl of 50 to 80 mL/minute, initial dosage is 3 mg PO once daily and maximum dosage is 6 mg once daily; in patients with CrCl of 10 to 49 mL/minute, initial dosage is 1.5 mg PO once daily and maximum dosage is 3 mg once daily; in patients with CrCl less than 10 mL/minute, use isn't recommended. If using injectable form (Invega Sustenna) and CrCl is 50 to 80 mL/minute, give 156 mg IM on day 1 and 117 mg IM 1 week later, followed by monthly injections of 78 mg IM. If using injectable 3-month form

(Invega Trinza) and CrCl is 50 to less than 80 mL/minute, adjust dosage and stabilize patient using the monthly IM injection, then transition to the 3-month IM injection.

➤ **Schizophrenia and schizoaffective disorder**
Adults: 6 mg PO once daily in the morning; may increase or decrease dose in 3-mg increments not sooner than every 4 days to a range of 3 to 12 mg daily; maximum dose is 12 mg/day. Or, 234 mg IM on treatment day 1 and 156 mg IM 1 week later, both administered in deltoid muscle. Recommended maintenance dosage is 117 mg IM monthly (range, 39 to 234 mg based on tolerability and efficacy). Adjustments may be made monthly. Maximum recommended monthly dose is 234 mg. See manufacturer's instructions for missed dosage schedules.

Use 3-month IM paliperidone (Invega Trinza) only after monthly IM paliperidone (Invega Sustenna) has been established as adequate treatment for at least 4 months. The last two doses of monthly IM paliperidone should be the same dosage strength before starting 3-month IM paliperidone. Initiate 3-month IM paliperidone when next monthly IM paliperidone dose is scheduled. Base 3-month dose on the previous monthly dose, using the equivalent 3.5 times higher dose. May adjust dosage of 3-month paliperidone every 3 months in increments ranging from 273 to 819 mg based on response and tolerability. Because of long-acting nature of Invega Trinza, patient's response to an adjusted dose may not be apparent for several months.

➤ **Schizophrenia**
Adolescents ages 12 to 17: Initially, 3 mg PO daily. May increase dosage by 3 mg/day every 5 days based on clinical response. Maximum dose is 12 mg/day for patients weighing 51 kg or more and 6 mg/day for patients weighing less than 51 kg.

ADMINISTRATION
PO
- Give tablet whole with or without food; don't crush or break.
IM
- Inspect for particulate matter and discoloration.
- Don't give IV or subcut.

• Inject slowly and deeply into deltoid or gluteal muscle.

• Injection is for single use only. Don't administer dose in divided injections.

• For Invega Sustenna, shake syringe vigorously for at least 10 seconds to ensure a homogenous suspension before administration.

• Administer first two doses of Invega Sustenna into deltoid muscle. After second dose, can give monthly maintenance doses in deltoid or gluteal muscle.

• For Invega Trinza, shake syringe vigorously for at least 15 seconds within 5 minutes before administration.

• For Invega Trinza, use the thin-wall needles provided. DON'T use needles from the 1-month pack or other commercially available needles, to reduce the risk of blockage.

• If incomplete administration occurs, don't reinject the dose remaining in the syringe. Don't administer another dose.

• For Invega Trinza, alternate injection sites at each administration.

• Injection is for single use only. Don't administer dose in divided injections.

• May give monthly or 3-month IM paliperidone maintenance doses within 7 days before or after next monthly dose date.

ACTION

May antagonize both central dopamine (D_2) and serotonin type 2 receptors, as well as alpha$_1$, alpha$_2$, and H$_1$ receptors. Drug is a major active metabolite of risperidone.

Route	Onset	Peak	Duration
PO	Unknown	24 hr	Unknown
IM	24 hr	13 days	126 days

Half-life: 23 hours (oral); 25 to 49 days (IM).

ADVERSE REACTIONS

CNS: akathisia, headache, parkinsonism, somnolence, anxiety, asthenia, dizziness, dystonia, extrapyramidal disorder, fatigue, hypertonia, pyrexia, tremor, dyskinesia, hyperkinesia, insomnia, *suicidal ideation.* **CV:** HTN, orthostatic hypotension, edema, palpitations, sinus arrhythmia, bradycardia, tachycardia, *AV block,* bundle-branch block. **EENT:** blurred vision, nasopharyngitis, rhinitis, epistaxis. **GI:** abdominal pain, dry mouth, dyspepsia, nausea, salivary hypersecretion, vomiting, diarrhea, constipation, dry mouth. **GU:** amenorrhea, galactorrhea, decreased male libido, erectile dysfunction. **Metabolic:** blood insulin increases, hyperprolactinemia, weight gain or loss. **Musculoskeletal:** back pain, extremity pain, musculoskeletal stiffness, myalgia. **Respiratory:** cough, URI. **Skin:** pruritus, rash, injection-site reaction.

INTERACTIONS

Drug-drug. *Anticholinergics:* May worsen side effects. Use cautiously together.
Antihypertensives: May worsen orthostatic hypotension. Avoid using together.
Centrally acting drugs: May worsen CNS side effects. Use cautiously together.
Divalproex sodium: Increases paliperidone concentration. Consider dosage reduction.
Drugs that prolong QTc interval, such as antiarrhythmics (amiodarone, procainamide, quinidine, sotalol), antipsychotics (chlorpromazine, thioridazine), quinolone antibiotics (moxifloxacin): May further prolong QTc interval. Avoid using together.
Levodopa, other dopamine agonists: May antagonize effects of these drugs. Use cautiously together.
Opioid agonists: Opioids may cause slow or difficult breathing, sedation, and death. Avoid use together. If use together is necessary, limit dosage and duration of each drug to minimum necessary for desired effect.
Risperidone: May increase toxic effects of paliperidone. Use alternative combination if possible.
Serotonin modulators: May increase risk of NMS and serotonin syndrome. Monitor therapy.
Strong CYP3A and P-gp inducers: May decrease paliperidone concentration. Dosage may need to be increased or decreased depending on use. Avoid use of Invega Trinza during 3-month dosing interval, if possible.
Drug-herb. *St. John's wort:* May increase serum concentration of paliperidone. Consider therapy modification.
Drug-lifestyle. *Alcohol use:* May worsen CNS side effects. Discourage use together.

EFFECTS ON LAB TEST RESULTS

• May increase blood glucose, lipid, and prolactin levels.

• May decrease WBC count.

P

CONTRAINDICATIONS & CAUTIONS

• Contraindicated in patients hypersensitive to paliperidone or risperidone.

• Elderly patients with dementia-related psychosis treated with atypical or conventional antipsychotics are at increased risk for death. Antipsychotics aren't approved for the treatment of dementia-related psychosis.

• Contraindicated in patients with congenital long QT syndrome or history of cardiac arrhythmias.

• Contraindicated in patients with preexisting severe GI narrowing.

• Use cautiously in patients with a history of seizures, diabetes, or Parkinson disease; in those at risk for aspiration pneumonia or impaired temperature regulation; and in those with bradycardia, hypokalemia, hypomagnesemia, CV disease, cerebrovascular disease, dehydration, or hypovolemia.

• Use cautiously in patients taking antihypertensives and drugs that lower the seizure threshold.

• Use cautiously in patients with history of suicide attempts.

• Somnolence, orthostatic hypotension, and motor and sensory instability may lead to falls and fall-related injuries.

• Drug may inhibit reproductive function owing to hyperprolactinemia.

• Rare cases of priapism (requiring surgery) have been reported.

Dialyzable drug: Unknown.

⚠ *Overdose S&S:* Extrapyramidal symptoms, unsteady gait, drowsiness, sedation, tachycardia, hypotension, prolonged QT interval.

PREGNANCY-LACTATION-REPRODUCTION

• Use in pregnancy only if potential benefit justifies risk to the fetus.

• Pregnant women exposed to drug should enroll in the National Pregnancy Registry for Atypical Antipsychotics (1-866-961-2388).

🜂 *Alert:* Neonates exposed to antipsychotics during the third trimester are at increased risk for developing extrapyramidal signs and symptoms and withdrawal signs and symptoms after delivery.

• Drug appears in human milk. The known benefits of breastfeeding should outweigh the unknown risks of infant's exposure to paliperidone.

NURSING CONSIDERATIONS

• Establish tolerability with oral paliperidone or oral risperidone before initiating treatment with paliperidone injection.

🜂 *Alert:* Monitor patient for atypical ventricular tachycardia, such as torsades de pointes, and ECG changes, particularly lengthening of the QT interval.

• Obtain baseline BP before starting therapy, and monitor BP regularly. Watch for orthostatic hypotension.

🜂 *Alert:* Watch for evidence of NMS, which is rare but deadly.

• Monitor patient for tardive dyskinesia; it may disappear spontaneously or persist for life despite discontinuing drug. Seek smallest dosage and shortest duration of treatment that produce a satisfactory clinical response.

🜂 *Alert:* Drug may cause hyperglycemia. Monitor patient with diabetes regularly. In patient with risk factors for diabetes, obtain fasting blood glucose test results at baseline and periodically.

• Monitor patient for seizure activity.

• Monitor patient for dysphagia.

• Monitor patient for abnormal body temperature regulation, especially if patient exercises, is exposed to extreme heat, takes anticholinergics, or is dehydrated.

• Monitor patient for somnolence and sedation. Antipsychotics, including paliperidone, have the potential to impair judgment, thinking, or motor skills.

• Complete fall risk assessments at start of treatment and recurrently for patients on long-term therapy.

• Dispense lowest appropriate quantity of drug, to reduce risk of overdose.

PATIENT TEACHING

• Caution patient or caregiver of patient taking an opioid with a benzodiazepine, CNS depressant, or alcohol to seek immediate medical attention if patient experiences dizziness, light-headedness, extreme sleepiness, slowed or difficult breathing, or unresponsiveness.

• Tell patient that remains of the tablet may appear in feces.

• Tell patient to swallow whole with liquids and not to chew, crush, or break tablets.

• Instruct patient not to perform activities that require mental alertness until effects of drug are known.

• Advise patient that drug may cause somnolence, orthostatic hypotension, and motor and sensory instability, which may lead to falls and fall-related injuries.

• Warn patient to use caution in performing excessively strenuous activities because body temperature may be disrupted.

• Advise patient that drug may lower BP and to change positions slowly.

• Advise patient to seek medical attention for an erection lasting more than 4 hours.

• Instruct patient to contact prescriber before taking any other drugs to avoid potential interactions.

• Advise patient to avoid alcohol while taking this medication.

• Advise patient to contact prescriber if she becomes pregnant or wants to breastfeed.

palonosetron hydrochloride
pal-oh-NOE-se-tron

Aloxi

Therapeutic class: Antiemetics
Pharmacologic class: Selective serotonin (5-HT₃) receptor antagonists

AVAILABLE FORMS
Injection: 0.075 mg in 1.5-mL, 0.25 mg in 5-mL single-use vials

INDICATIONS & DOSAGES
➤ **To prevent acute nausea and vomiting from moderately or highly emetogenic chemotherapy or delayed nausea and vomiting from moderately emetogenic chemotherapy**
Adults: 0.25 mg given IV over 30 seconds, 30 minutes before chemotherapy starts.
➤ **To prevent acute nausea and vomiting associated with initial and repeat courses of emetogenic, including highly emetogenic, cancer chemotherapy**
Children age 1 month to younger than 17 years: Infuse 20 mcg/kg IV over 15 minutes beginning approximately 30 minutes before chemotherapy starts. Maximum dose is 1.5 mg.

➤ **To prevent postoperative nausea and vomiting for up to 24 hours following surgery**
Adults: 0.075 mg IV over 10 seconds immediately before anesthesia induction.

ADMINISTRATION
IV
▼ Flush with NSS before and after injection.
▼ Give by rapid IV injection through a peripheral or central IV line.
▼ Protect from light. Don't freeze.
▼ **Incompatibilities:** Don't mix with other drugs.

ACTION
Antagonizes 5-HT₃ receptors in the GI tract and brain, which inhibits emesis caused by chemotherapy.

Route	Onset	Peak	Duration
IV	30 min	Unknown	5 days

Half-life: 40 hours (adults); 20 to 30 hours (children).

ADVERSE REACTIONS
CNS: anxiety, dizziness, headache, weakness. **CV:** *bradycardia, nonsustained ventricular tachycardia,* hypotension, *QT-interval prolongation.* **GI:** constipation, diarrhea. **GU:** urine retention. **Metabolic:** *hyperkalemia.* **Skin:** pruritus.

INTERACTIONS
Drug-drug. *Antiarrhythmics or other drugs that prolong the QTc interval, diuretics that induce electrolyte abnormalities, high-dose anthracycline:* May increase risk of prolonged QTc interval. Use together cautiously.
Apomorphine: May cause profound hypotension and loss of consciousness. Use together is contraindicated.
Fentanyl, 5-HT₃ receptor antagonists, IV methylene blue, lithium, MAO inhibitors, mirtazapine, SSNRIs, SSRIs, tramadol: May increase risk of serotonin syndrome. Avoid use together.

EFFECTS ON LAB TEST RESULTS
• May increase potassium level.
• May increase serum ALT or AST level.

CONTRAINDICATIONS & CAUTIONS

• Contraindicated in patients hypersensitive to palonosetron or its ingredients.
• Use cautiously in patients hypersensitive to other 5-HT$_3$ antagonists, in those taking drugs that affect cardiac conduction, and in those with cardiac conduction abnormalities, hypokalemia, or hypomagnesemia.
• There is no antidote for overdose. Use supportive care; monitor patient for adverse events.
Dialyzable drug: Unlikely.

PREGNANCY-LACTATION-REPRODUCTION

• Use in pregnancy only if clearly needed.
• It isn't known if drug appears in human milk. Patient should discontinue breastfeeding or discontinue drug.

NURSING CONSIDERATIONS

• Before giving this drug, check patient's potassium level.
• Consider adding corticosteroids to the antiemetic regimen, particularly for patients receiving highly emetogenic chemotherapy.
• Make sure patient has additional antiemetics for breakthrough nausea or vomiting.
• If patient has cardiac conduction abnormalities, check the ECG before giving drug.

PATIENT TEACHING

• Advise patient to take a different antiemetic for breakthrough nausea or vomiting at the first sign of nausea rather than waiting until symptoms are severe.
• Urge patient with a history of cardiac conduction abnormalities to report any changes in drug regimen, such as adding or stopping an antiarrhythmic.

pamidronate disodium
pa-mi-DROE-nate

Therapeutic class: Antiosteoporotics
Pharmacologic class: Bisphosphonates

AVAILABLE FORMS

Powder for injection: 30 mg/vial, 90 mg/vial
Solution for injection: 3 mg/mL, 6 mg/mL, 9 mg/mL in 10-mL vials

INDICATIONS & DOSAGES

➤ **Moderate to severe hypercalcemia from cancer (with or without bone metastases)**
Adults: Dosage depends on severity of hypercalcemia. Correct calcium level for albumin. Corrected calcium (CCa) level is calculated using this formula:

$$\text{CCa (mg/dL)} = \text{serum calcium (mg/dL)} + 0.8(4 - \text{serum albumin)(g/dL)}$$

Give patients with CCa levels of 12 to 13.5 mg/dL 60 to 90 mg by IV infusion as a single dose over 2 to 24 hours. Give patients with CCa levels greater than 13.5 mg/dL 90 mg by IV infusion over 2 to 24 hours. Allow at least 7 days before retreatment to permit full response to first dose.
➤ **Moderate to severe Paget disease**
Adults: 30 mg IV as a 4-hour infusion on 3 consecutive days for total dose of 90 mg. Repeat cycle as needed.
➤ **Osteolytic bone metastases of breast cancer with standard antineoplastic therapy**
Adults: 90 mg IV infusion over 2 hours every 3 to 4 weeks.
➤ **Osteolytic bone lesions of multiple myeloma**
Adults: 90 mg IV over 4 hours once monthly.

ADMINISTRATION

IV

▼ Hazardous drug; use safe handling and disposal precautions.
▼ Reconstitute drug with 10 mL of sterile water for injection. After drug is completely dissolved, add to 250 mL (2-hour infusion), 500 mL (4-hour infusion), or 1,000 mL (up to 24-hour infusion) of half-NSS or NSS for injection or D$_5$W.
▼ Inspect solution for precipitate before use.
▼ Give drug only by IV infusion. Injecting a bolus may cause nephropathy.
▼ Infusions longer than 2 hours may reduce the risk of renal toxicity, particularly in patients with preexisting renal insufficiency.
▼ Solution is stable for 24 hours at room temperature.
▼ Store reconstituted drug at 36° to 46° F (2° to 8° C) for up to 24 hours.

Reactions in bold italics are *life-threatening*. Interactions may have a *rapid onset* or a *delayed onset*.

▼ **Incompatibilities:** Calcium-containing infusion solutions, such as Ringer injection. Give in a line separate from all other drugs.

ACTION
An antihypercalcemic that inhibits resorption of bone but apparently not bone formation. Adsorbs to hydroxyapatite crystals in bone and may directly block calcium phosphate dissolution and mature osteoclast formation.

Route	Onset	Peak	Duration
IV	Unknown	Unknown	Unknown

Half-life: 21 to 35 hours.

ADVERSE REACTIONS
CNS: *seizures,* fatigue, somnolence, fever, headache, psychosis, anxiety, drowsiness. **CV:** atrial fibrillation/flutter, tachycardia, HTN, fluid overload, syncope. **EENT:** sinusitis, rhinitis. **GI:** abdominal pain, anorexia, dyspepsia, constipation, diarrhea, nausea, vomiting, *GI hemorrhage.* **GU:** renal dysfunction, UTI, *renal failure.* **Hematologic:** *leukopenia, thrombocytopenia,* anemia. **Hepatic:** elevated live enzyme levels. **Metabolic:** hypophosphatemia, *hypokalemia, hypomagnesemia, hypocalcemia.* **Musculoskeletal:** arthralgia, back pain, myalgia, weakness, osteonecrosis of the jaw. **Respiratory:** cough, dyspnea, pleural effusions, URI, crackles. **Skin:** infusion-site reaction, pain at infusion site. **Other:** metastases.

INTERACTIONS
Nephrotoxic drugs: Increases risk of renal dysfunction. Use with caution.

EFFECTS ON LAB TEST RESULTS
• May increase creatinine level.
• May decrease phosphate, potassium, magnesium, calcium, and Hb levels.
• May decrease WBC and platelet counts.
• May interfere with technetium-99m diphosphonate imaging agents.

CONTRAINDICATIONS & CAUTIONS
• Contraindicated in patients hypersensitive to drug or other bisphosphonates.

🚯 *Alert:* There may be an increased risk of atypical fractures of the thigh in patients treated with bisphosphonates.
• Use with caution, considering risks versus benefits, in patients with renal impairment.
Dialyzable drug: Yes.
⚠ *Overdose S&S:* High fever, hypotension, taste perversion, hypocalcemia.

PREGNANCY-LACTATION-REPRODUCTION
• Contraindicated in pregnant women.
• It isn't known if drug appears in human milk. Patient should discontinue breastfeeding or discontinue drug.

NURSING CONSIDERATIONS
• Assess hydration before treatment. Use drug only after patient has been vigorously hydrated with NSS. In patients with mild to moderate hypercalcemia, hydration alone may be sufficient.
• Because drug can cause electrolyte disturbances, carefully monitor electrolyte levels, especially calcium, phosphate, and magnesium. Short-term use of calcium may be needed in patients with severe hypocalcemia. Also monitor CBC and differential count, creatinine and Hb levels, and hematocrit.
• Carefully monitor patients with preexisting anemia, leukopenia, or thrombocytopenia during first 2 weeks of therapy.
• Monitor patient's temperature. Patient may experience a slight elevation for 24 to 48 hours after therapy.
🚯 *Alert:* Because renal dysfunction may lead to renal failure, single doses shouldn't exceed 90 mg.
• Monitor creatinine level before each treatment.
• In patients treated for bone metastases who have renal dysfunction, withhold dose until renal function returns to baseline. Treating bone metastases in patients with severe renal impairment isn't recommended. For other indications, determine whether the potential benefit outweighs the potential risk.
• Severe musculoskeletal pain has been associated with bisphosphonate use and may occur within days, months, or years of start of therapy. When drug is stopped, symptoms may resolve partially or completely.

P

• Bisphosphonates can interfere with bone-imaging agents.

⚠ **Alert:** Patients should have a dental exam with appropriate preventive dentistry before taking drug, especially those with risk factors, including cancer, chemotherapy, corticosteroid therapy, and poor oral hygiene. These patients should avoid dental procedures, if possible, during therapy.

PATIENT TEACHING

• Explain use and administration of drug to patient and family.
• Instruct patient to report adverse reactions promptly.
• Tell patient to immediately report groin or thigh pain.
• Advise female patient to tell prescriber if she is pregnant or breastfeeding.

---

pancrelipase
pan-kre-LYE-pase

Creon, Pancreaze, Pertzye, Ultresa, Viokace, Zenpep

Therapeutic class: Digestive enzymes
Pharmacologic class: Pancreatic enzymes

AVAILABLE FORMS
Creon
Capsules (delayed-release) 🔴: 3,000 units lipase, 9,500 units protease, 15,000 units amylase; 6,000 units lipase, 19,000 units protease, 30,000 units amylase; 12,000 units lipase, 38,000 units protease, 60,000 units amylase; 24,000 units lipase, 76,000 units protease, 120,000 units amylase; 36,000 units lipase, 114,000 units protease, 180,000 units amylase
Pancreaze
Capsules (delayed-release) 🔴: 2,600 units lipase, 6,200 units protease, 10,850 units amylase; 4,200 units lipase, 10,000 units protease, 17,500 units amylase; 10,500 units lipase, 25,000 units protease, 43,750 units amylase; 16,800 units lipase, 40,000 units protease, 70,000 units amylase; 21,000 units lipase, 37,000 units protease, 61,000 units amylase

Pertzye
Capsules (delayed-release) 🔴: 4,000 units lipase, 14,375 units protease, 15,125 units amylase; 8,000 units lipase, 28,750 units protease, 30,250 units amylase; 16,000 units lipase, 57,500 units protease, 60,500 units amylase; 24,000 units lipase, 86,250 units protease, 90,750 units amylase
Ultresa
Capsules (delayed-release) 🔴: 13,800 units lipase, 27,600 units protease, 27,600 units amylase; 20,700 units lipase, 41,400 units protease, 41,400 units amylase; 23,000 units lipase, 46,000 units protease, 46,000 units amylase
Viokace
Tablets 🔴: 10,440 units lipase, 39,150 units protease, 39,150 units amylase; 20,880 units lipase, 78,300 units protease, 78,300 units amylase
Zenpep
Capsules (enteric-coated beads) 🔴: 3,000 units lipase, 10,000 units protease, 14,000 units amylase; 5,000 units lipase, 17,000 units protease, 24,000 units amylase; 10,000 units lipase, 32,000 units protease, 42,000 units amylase; 15,000 units lipase, 47,000 units protease, 63,000 units amylase; 20,000 units lipase, 63,000 units protease, 84,000 units amylase; 25,000 units lipase, 79,000 units protease, 105,000 units amylase; 40,000 units lipase, 126,000 units protease, 168,000 units amylase

INDICATIONS & DOSAGES
➤ **Exocrine pancreatic secretion insufficiency; cystic fibrosis in adults and children; steatorrhea and other disorders of fat metabolism caused by insufficient pancreatic enzymes**
Adults and children older than age 4: 500 lipase units/kg PO per meal to a maximum of 2,500 lipase units/kg per meal (or 10,000 lipase units/kg per day) or less than 4,000 lipase units/g fat ingested per day.
Children older than age 12 months to 4 years: 1,000 lipase units/kg PO per meal up to maximum dose of 2,500 lipase units/kg per meal, 10,000 lipase units/kg daily, or 4,000 lipase units/g of fat ingested daily.

Reactions in bold italics are *life-threatening*. Interactions may have a *rapid onset* or a *delayed onset*.

Infants up to age 12 months: 2,000 to 4,000 lipase units PO per 120 mL of formula or per breastfeeding.

➤ **Exocrine pancreatic insufficiency due to chronic pancreatitis or pancreatectomy (Creon)**
Adults: 72,000 lipase units PO per meal while consuming at least 100 g of fat per day. Or, 500 lipase units/kg per meal. Adjust dosage to patient's response.

➤ **Exocrine pancreatic insufficiency due to chronic pancreatitis or pancreatectomy, with a PPI (Viokace)**
Adults: 500 lipase units/kg PO per meal to a maximum of 2,500 lipase units/kg per meal (or 10,000 lipase units/kg/day) or less than 4,000 lipase units/g fat ingested per day. Adjust dosage to patient's response.

➤ **Exocrine pancreatic insufficiency due to cystic fibrosis or other conditions**
Adults and children age 4 and older weighing 16 kg or more: Pertzye: 500 lipase units/kg PO per meal to a maximum of 2,500 lipase units/kg per meal (or 10,000 lipase units/kg or less per day), or less than 4,000 lipase units/g fat ingested per day.
Adults and children age 4 and older: Ultresa: 500 lipase units/kg PO per meal to a maximum of 2,500 lipase units/kg per meal (or 10,000 lipase units/kg or less per day) or less than 4,000 lipase units/g fat ingested per day.
Children age 12 months to 4 years weighing 8 kg or more: Pertzye: 1,000 lipase units/kg PO per meal to a maximum of 2,500 lipase units/kg per meal (or 10,000 lipase units/kg or less per day), or less than 4,000 lipase units/g fat ingested per day.
Children older than age 12 months to younger than 4 years: Ultresa: 1,000 lipase units/kg per meal to a maximum of 2,500 lipase units/kg per meal (or 10,000 lipase units/kg or less per day), or less than 4,000 lipase units/g fat per day.

ADMINISTRATION
PO
• Give drug before or with meals and snacks.
• Don't crush or allow patient to chew capsules. Capsules containing enteric-coated microspheres may be opened and sprinkled on a small quantity of soft food at room temperature. Have patient swallow immediately,

without chewing, and follow dose with glass of water or juice.
• For infants, mix capsule contents with applesauce and give within 15 minutes of each feeding. Follow with 120 mL of formula or human milk. Don't mix directly with formula or human milk. Capsule contents may be administered directly into infant's mouth before feeding. Avoid contact with or inhalation of powder because it may be highly irritating. Older children may swallow capsules with food.
• Viokace tablets aren't enteric-coated; patient should take with a PPI.

ACTION
Replaces endogenous exocrine pancreatic enzymes and aids digestion of starches, fats, and proteins.

Route	Onset	Peak	Duration
PO	Variable	Variable	Variable

Half-life: Unknown.

ADVERSE REACTIONS
CNS: headache, dizziness. **EENT:** nasopharyngitis, pharyngolaryngeal pain, epistaxis. **GI:** abdominal pain, nausea, cramping, diarrhea with high doses, dyspepsia, vomiting, weight loss, flatulence. **Metabolic:** hyperglycemia, *hypoglycemia.* **Respiratory:** cough. **Other:** biliary tract stones, anal pruritus.

INTERACTIONS
Drug-drug. *Antacids:* May destroy enteric coating and enhance degradation of pancrelipase. Avoid using together.
Oral iron supplement: May decrease iron response. Monitor patient for decreased effectiveness.

EFFECTS ON LAB TEST RESULTS
• May increase uric acid level.

CONTRAINDICATIONS & CAUTIONS
• Use cautiously in patients with a known allergy to proteins of porcine origin.
• Use cautiously in patients with gout, renal impairment, or hyperuricemia.
Dialyzable drug: Unknown.
⚠ *Overdose S&S:* Transient intestinal upset, diarrhea.

P

PREGNANCY-LACTATION-REPRODUCTION
• Use cautiously in pregnant women and only if clearly needed. Nutrition should be optimized during pregnancy.
• It isn't known if drug appears in human milk. Use cautiously in breastfeeding women.

NURSING CONSIDERATIONS
❸ *Alert:* Use drug only for confirmed exocrine pancreatic insufficiency. It isn't effective in GI disorders unrelated to enzyme deficiency.
❸ *Alert:* Fibrosing colonopathy is associated with high-dose use of pancreatic enzymes. Use cautiously when doses exceed 2,500 lipase units/kg per meal (or are greater than 10,000 lipase units/kg per day).
• Lipase activity is greater than with other pancreatic enzymes.
• Monitor patient's stools. Adequate replacement decreases number of bowel movements and improves stool consistency.
• Individual products aren't bioequivalent and shouldn't be interchanged without prescriber supervision.
• Dosage varies with degree of maldigestion and malabsorption, amount of fat in diet, and enzyme activity of individual preparations.
• Enteric coating on some products may reduce available enzyme in upper portion of jejunum.
• Viokace tablets aren't enteric-coated and should be taken with a PPI.

PATIENT TEACHING
• Instruct patient to take drug before or with meals and snacks, but always with food and generous amounts of liquid.
• Advise patient not to crush or chew capsules; retention of a capsule in the mouth before swallowing may cause mucosal irritation and stomatitis.
• Capsules containing enteric-coated microspheres may be opened and sprinkled on a small quantity of soft food at room temperature. Stress importance of swallowing immediately, without chewing, and following with glass of water or juice.
• Warn patient not to inhale powder form or powder from capsules; it may irritate skin or mucous membranes.

• Tell patient to store drug in airtight container at room temperature.
• Instruct patient not to change brands without consulting prescriber.
• Advise patient to report unusual or severe stomach area pain, bloating, trouble passing stool, nausea, vomiting, or diarrhea, which may indicate fibrosing colonopathy.

SAFETY ALERT!

pancuronium bromide
pan-kyoo-ROE-nee-um

Therapeutic class: Skeletal muscle relaxants
Pharmacologic class: Nondepolarizing neuromuscular blockers

AVAILABLE FORMS
Injection: 1 mg/mL, 2 mg/mL

INDICATIONS & DOSAGES
➤ **Adjunct to anesthesia to relax skeletal muscle, facilitate intubation, and assist with mechanical ventilation**
Adults and children age 1 month and older: Initially, 0.04 to 0.1 mg/kg IV; then 0.01 mg/kg IV every 25 to 60 minutes. For ET intubation, a bolus dose of 0.06 to 0.1 mg/kg IV is recommended. Conditions satisfactory for intubation are usually present within 2 to 3 minutes.
Neonates: Individualize dosage. It's recommended that a test dose of 0.02 mg/kg IV be given first to measure responsiveness.

ADMINISTRATION
IV
Black Box Warning This drug should be administered by adequately trained individuals familiar with its actions, characteristics, and hazards. ∎
▼ Only staff skilled in airway management should use drug.
▼ Drug has no known effect on consciousness, pain threshold, or cerebration. To avoid patient distress, don't induce neuromuscular blockade before unconsciousness.
▼ Keep ET equipment, ventilator, oxygen, atropine, edrophonium, epinephrine, and neostigmine immediately available.

Reactions in bold italics are *life-threatening*. Interactions may have a *rapid onset* or a *delayed onset*.

▼ Store in refrigerator. The 10-mL vial will maintain full clinical potency for up to 6 months at room temperature.

▼ Compatible in solution with NSS, dextrose 5%, dextrose 5% and sodium chloride, and lactated Ringer solution.

▼ When mixed with approved solutions in glass or plastic containers, drug will remain stable in solution for 48 hours with no alteration in potency or pH.

▼ **Incompatibilities:** Alkaline solutions, barbiturates, diazepam, thiopental sodium.

ACTION
Prevents acetylcholine from binding to receptors on the motor end plate, blocking neuromuscular transmission.

Route	Onset	Peak	Duration
IV	30–45 sec	3–4½ min	35–65 min

Half-life: 89 to 161 minutes.

ADVERSE REACTIONS
CV: tachycardia, increased BP, flushing. **EENT:** excessive salivation. **Musculoskeletal:** residual muscle weakness. **Respiratory:** *prolonged respiratory insufficiency or apnea.* **Skin:** transient rashes. **Other:** allergic or idiosyncratic hypersensitivity reactions.

INTERACTIONS
Drug-drug. *Aminoglycosides (amikacin, gentamicin, neomycin, streptomycin, tobramycin), magnesium salts:* May increase the effects of pancuronium, including prolonged respiratory depression. Use together only when necessary. Dose of pancuronium may need to be reduced.

Azathioprine: May reverse neuromuscular blockade induced by pancuronium. Monitor patient.

Beta blockers, clindamycin, general anesthetics (enflurane, halothane, isoflurane), ketamine, lincomycin, magnesium sulfate, polymyxin antibiotics (colistin, polymyxin B sulfate), quinidine, quinine, verapamil: May enhance neuromuscular blockade, increasing skeletal muscle relaxation and prolonging effect of pancuronium. Use together cautiously during and after surgery.

Carbamazepine, phenytoin: May decrease effects of pancuronium. May need to increase pancuronium dose.

Diuretics: May cause electrolyte imbalance or alter neuromuscular blockade. Monitor electrolytes before giving drug.

Lithium, opioid analgesics: May enhance neuromuscular blockade, increasing skeletal muscle relaxation and possibly causing respiratory paralysis. Use cautiously, and reduce dose of pancuronium.

Succinylcholine: May increase intensity and duration of neuromuscular blockade. Allow effects of succinylcholine to subside before giving pancuronium.

TCAs: May increase risk of ventricular arrhythmias in patients anesthetized with both halothane and pancuronium. Monitor ECG closely in patients taking TCAs before surgery.

Theophylline: May produce a dose-dependent reversal of neuromuscular blocking effects. Monitor patient for clinical effect.

EFFECTS ON LAB TEST RESULTS
None reported.

CONTRAINDICATIONS & CAUTIONS
• Contraindicated in patients hypersensitive to bromides, those with tachycardia, and those for whom even a minor increase in HR is undesirable.

• Use cautiously in elderly or debilitated patients; in patients with renal, hepatic, or pulmonary impairment; and in those with respiratory depression, myasthenia gravis, myasthenic syndrome related to lung cancer, dehydration, thyroid disorders, CV disease, collagen diseases, porphyria, electrolyte disturbances, hyperthermia, severe obesity, and toxemic states. Also, use large doses cautiously in patients undergoing cesarean section.

Dialyzable drug: Unknown.

⚠ **Overdose S&S:** Residual neuromuscular blockade (skeletal muscle weakness, decreased respiratory reserve, low tidal volume, apnea).

PREGNANCY-LACTATION-REPRODUCTION
• It isn't known if drug can cause fetal harm. Use during pregnancy only if benefit justifies risk to the fetus.

• There is no information on the use of drug in breastfeeding women.

NURSING CONSIDERATIONS
• Dosage depends on anesthetic used, individual needs, and response. Dosages are representative and must be adjusted.
• Allow succinylcholine effects to subside before giving this drug.
• Monitor baseline electrolyte determinations (electrolyte imbalance can potentiate neuromuscular effects) and vital signs, especially respirations and HR.
• Measure fluid intake and output; renal dysfunction may prolong duration of action because 25% of drug is excreted unchanged in the urine.
• A nerve stimulator and train-of-four monitoring are recommended to confirm antagonism of neuromuscular blockade and recovery of muscle strength. Make sure there's some evidence of spontaneous recovery before attempting pharmacologic reversal with neostigmine.
• Monitor respirations closely until patient recovers fully from neuromuscular blockade, as indicated by tests of muscle strength (hand grip, head lift, and ability to cough).
• After spontaneous recovery starts, neuromuscular blockade may be reversed with an anticholinesterase (such as neostigmine or edrophonium), which is usually given with an anticholinergic (such as atropine).
• Drug doesn't cause histamine release or hypotension, but it may raise HR and BP.
• Give analgesics for pain.
⊙ **Alert:** Careful dosage calculation is essential. Always verify dosage with another health care professional.

PATIENT TEACHING
• Explain all events and procedures to patient because patient can still hear.

pantoprazole sodium
pan-TOE-pray-zol

Pantoloc❦, Protonix◊, Protonix IV

Therapeutic class: Antiulcer drugs
Pharmacologic class: PPIs

AVAILABLE FORMS
Injection: 40 mg/vial
Suspension (delayed-release) ⓄⓃⒸ: 40 mg
Tablets (delayed-release) ⓄⓃⒸ: 20 mg, 40 mg
Tablets (enteric-coated) ⓄⓃⒸ: 20 mg❦, 40 mg❦

INDICATIONS & DOSAGES
➤ **Maintenance of healing of erosive esophagitis**
Adults: 40 mg PO once daily.
➤ **Short-term treatment of erosive esophagitis associated with GERD**
Adults: 40 mg PO once daily for up to 8 weeks. For patients who haven't healed after 8 weeks of treatment, another 8-week course may be considered. Or, 40 mg IV once daily for 7 to 10 days. Switch to PO form as soon as patient is able to take orally.
Children age 5 and older weighing 40 kg or more: 40 mg PO once daily for up to 8 weeks.
Children age 5 and older weighing 15 to less than 40 kg: 20 mg PO once daily for up to 8 weeks.
Adjust-a-dose: Consider dosage reduction in children who are poor CYP2C19 metabolizers.
➤ **Long-term maintenance of healing erosive esophagitis and reduction in relapse rates of daytime and nighttime heartburn symptoms in patients with GERD**
Adults: 40 mg PO once daily.
➤ **Treatment of pathologic hypersecretion caused by Zollinger-Ellison syndrome**
Adults: Individualize dosage. Usual dosage is 40 mg PO b.i.d. Usual IV dose is 80 mg IV every 12 hours for no more than 6 days. For those needing a higher dose, 80 mg every 8 hours is expected to maintain acid output below 10 mEq/hour. Maximum daily dose is 240 mg/day. When converting from IV to PO form, ensure continuity of suppression of acid secretion.

Reactions in bold italics are *life-threatening*. Interactions may have a *rapid onset* or a *delayed onset*.

➤ **Dyspepsia**
Adults: 20 to 40 mg once daily for 4 weeks.

ADMINISTRATION
PO
• Give tablets without regard for food and make sure patient swallows them whole.
• May give with antacids.
• Don't crush or split tablets. Don't allow patient to chew granules (delayed-release oral suspension).
• Give delayed-release oral suspension in 1 tsp applesauce or 1 tsp apple juice 30 minutes before a meal. Don't give in water or other liquids or foods.
• Delayed-release packets can't be divided to make a smaller dose.
IV
▼ Safety and effectiveness of the IV form to start therapy for GERD are unknown.
▼ Reconstitute each vial with 10 mL of NSS.
▼ Compatible diluents for infusion include NSS, D_5W, and lactated Ringer solution for injection.
▼ For patients with GERD, further dilute with 100 mL of diluent to yield 0.4 mg/mL.
▼ For patients with hypersecretion, combine two reconstituted vials and further dilute with 80 mL of diluent to a total volume of 100 mL, to yield 0.8 mg/mL.
▼ Infuse diluted solutions over 15 minutes at a rate of about 7 mL/minute.
▼ For a 2-minute infusion, give the reconstituted vials (final yield of about 4 mg/mL) over at least 2 minutes.
▼ Reconstituted 15-minute infusion (0.4 mg/mL) may be stored for up to 6 hours and the diluted solutions for up to 24 hours at room temperature.
▼ Reconstituted 2-minute solution (4 mg/mL) may be stored for up to 24 hours at room temperature before infusion.
▼ **Incompatibilities:** Midazolam, zinc-containing products or solutions. Don't give another infusion simultaneously through the same line.

ACTION
Inhibits proton pump activity by binding to hydrogen-potassium adenosine triphosphatase, located at secretory surface of gastric parietal cells, to suppress gastric acid secretion.

Route	Onset	Peak	Duration
PO	Unknown	2½ hr	>24 hr
IV	15–30 min	Unknown	24 hr

Half-life: 1 hour.

ADVERSE REACTIONS
CNS: anxiety, asthenia, dizziness, headache, insomnia, migraine, pain, depression, vertigo. **CV:** chest pain, edema, thrombophlebitis. **EENT:** blurred vision, pharyngitis, rhinitis, sinusitis. **GI:** abdominal pain, constipation, diarrhea, dyspepsia, eructation, flatulence, gastroenteritis, GI disorder, nausea, rectal disorder, vomiting. **GU:** urinary frequency, UTI. **Hematologic:** *leukopenia, thrombocytopenia.* **Hepatic:** elevated liver enzyme levels. **Metabolic:** hyperglycemia, hyperlipidemia. **Musculoskeletal:** arthralgia, back pain, hypertonia, neck pain. **Respiratory:** bronchitis, dyspnea, increased cough, URI. **Skin:** rash, pruritus, urticaria. **Other:** flulike syndrome, infection, injection-site reaction, photosensitivity reactions.

INTERACTIONS
Drug-drug. *Ampicillin esters, iron salts, ketoconazole, mycophenolate:* May decrease absorption of these drugs. Monitor patient closely and separate doses.
Azole antifungals (itraconazole, ketoconazole): May decrease plasma levels of these drugs. Avoid this combination if possible.
Methotrexate: May increase methotrexate concentration and risk of toxicity. Closely monitor methotrexate concentration, and watch for signs and symptoms of methotrexate toxicity.
Protease inhibitors (atazanavir, indinavir, nelfinavir): May reduce antiviral activity of these drugs. Adjust dosage as needed; administration of atazanavir or nelfinavir with pantoprazole isn't recommended.
Salicylates: Enteric-coated salicylates may dissolve more rapidly, increasing gastric adverse reactions. Monitor patient.
Warfarin: May increase INR and prolong PT. Monitor patient and lab values.
Drug-herb. *St. John's wort:* May increase risk of sunburn. Advise patient to avoid excessive sunlight exposure.

P

Drug-lifestyle. *Sun exposure:* May increase risk of sunburn. Advise patient to avoid excessive sunlight exposure.

EFFECTS ON LAB TEST RESULTS
• May increase glucose and lipid levels.
• May increase LFT result values.
• May cause false-positive urine screen test for tetrahydrocannabinol.
• May increase serum chromogranin A level, causing a false-positive result in diagnostic investigation for neuroendocrine tumors.

CONTRAINDICATIONS & CAUTIONS
• Contraindicated in patients hypersensitive to any component of the formulation.
• PPI therapy may be associated with an increased risk of osteoporosis-related fractures. Patients should use lowest dose and shortest duration of therapy appropriate to condition being treated.
• Cutaneous lupus erythematosus (CLE) and SLE have been reported, occurring as both new onset and an exacerbation of existing autoimmune disease in patients of all ages within weeks to years after continuous drug therapy.
Dialyzable drug: No.

PREGNANCY-LACTATION-REPRODUCTION
• There are no adequate studies in pregnant women. Use cautiously and only if clearly needed.
• Drug appears in human milk. Patient should discontinue breastfeeding or discontinue drug.

NURSING CONSIDERATIONS
• Symptomatic response to therapy doesn't preclude the presence of gastric malignancy.
❸ *Alert:* Prolonged use of PPIs may cause low magnesium levels. Monitor magnesium levels before start of treatment and periodically thereafter.
❸ *Alert:* Monitor patient for signs and symptoms of low magnesium level, such as abnormal HR or rhythm, palpitations, muscle spasms, tremor, or seizures. In children, abnormal HR may present as fatigue, upset stomach, dizziness, and light-headedness. Magnesium supplementation or drug discontinuation may be required.

❸ *Alert:* May increase risk of CDAD. Evaluate for CDAD in patients who develop diarrhea that doesn't improve.
• If signs or symptoms consistent with CLE or SLE are noted, discontinue drug and refer patient to the appropriate specialist for evaluation. Most patients improve with discontinuation of the PPI alone in 4 to 12 weeks.
• *Look alike–sound alike:* Don't confuse Protonix with Prilosec, Prozac, or Prevacid. Don't confuse pantoprazole with aripiprazole.

PATIENT TEACHING
• Instruct patient to take exactly as prescribed and at about the same time every day.
• Advise patient that drug can be taken without regard to meals.
• Tell patient to swallow tablet whole and not to crush, split, or chew it.
• Tell patient that antacids don't affect drug absorption.
• Teach patient to report all adverse reactions and to recognize and report signs and symptoms of low magnesium levels.

PARoxetine hydrochloride
pa-ROKS-e-teen

Paxil, Paxil CR

PARoxetine mesylate
Brisdelle, Pexeva

Therapeutic class: Antidepressants
Pharmacologic class: SSRIs

AVAILABLE FORMS
paroxetine hydrochloride
Suspension: 10 mg/5 mL
Tablets ⓞ: 10 mg, 20 mg, 30 mg, 40 mg
Tablets (controlled-release) ⓞ: 12.5 mg, 25 mg, 37.5 mg
paroxetine mesylate
Capsules: 7.5 mg
Tablets ⓞ: 10 mg, 20 mg, 30 mg, 40 mg

INDICATIONS & DOSAGES
Adjust-a-dose (for all indications): For elderly and debilitated patients and those with renal or hepatic impairment taking immediate-release form, initially, 10 mg

PO daily, preferably in morning. If patient doesn't respond after full antidepressant effect has occurred, increase dose in 10-mg/day increments at intervals of at least 1 week to a maximum of 40 mg daily. If using controlled-release form, start therapy at 12.5 mg daily. Don't exceed 50 mg daily.

➤ **Depression (excluding Brisdelle)**
Adults: Initially, 20 mg PO daily, preferably in morning, as indicated. If patient doesn't improve, increase dose by 10 mg daily at intervals of at least 1 week to a maximum of 50 mg daily. If using controlled-release form, initially, 25 mg PO daily. Increase dose in 12.5-mg/day increments at intervals of at least 1 week to a maximum of 62.5 mg daily.

➤ **OCD (Paxil and Pexeva only)**
Adults: Initially, 20 mg PO daily, preferably in morning. Increase dose in 10-mg day increments at intervals of at least 1 week. Recommended daily dose is 40 mg. Maximum daily dose is 60 mg.

➤ **Panic disorder (excluding Brisdelle)**
Adults: Initially, 10 mg PO daily. Increase dose in 10-mg/day increments at intervals of at least 1 week, up to a maximum of 60 mg daily. Or, 12.5 mg Paxil CR PO as a single daily dose. Increase dose in 12.5-mg/day increments at intervals of at least 1 week, up to a maximum of 75 mg daily.

➤ **Social anxiety disorder (Paxil and Paxil CR only)**
Adults: Initially, 20 mg PO daily. Dosage range is 20 to 60 mg daily. Adjust dosage to maintain patient on lowest effective dose. Or, 12.5 mg Paxil CR PO as a single daily dose. Increase dose in 12.5-mg/day increments at intervals of at least 1 week, up to a maximum of 37.5 mg daily.

➤ **Generalized anxiety disorder (Paxil and Pexeva only)**
Adults: 20 mg PO daily initially. Increase dose in 10-mg/day increments at intervals of at least 1 week, up to a maximum of 50 mg daily. Doses greater than 20 mg/day don't appear to have an added benefit.

➤ **Posttraumatic stress disorder (Paxil only)**
Adults: Initially, 20 mg PO daily. Increase dose in 10-mg/day increments at intervals of at least 1 week. Maximum daily dose is 50 mg PO.

➤ **Premenstrual dysphoric disorder (PMDD) (Paxil CR only)**
Adults: Initially, 12.5 mg Paxil CR PO as a single daily dose. May be given daily throughout menstrual cycle or daily during the luteal phase of menstrual cycle. Dose changes should occur at intervals of at least 1 week. Maximum dose is 25 mg PO daily.

➤ **Moderate to severe vasomotor symptoms associated with menopause (Brisdelle only)**
Adults: 7.5 mg PO daily at bedtime.

ADMINISTRATION
PO
• Give drug in the morning without regard for food.
• Don't split or crush controlled-release tablets.
• Shake oral suspension well before each use. Measure with oral syringe or calibrated measuring device.

ACTION
Thought to be linked to drug's inhibition of CNS neuronal uptake of serotonin.

Route	Onset	Peak	Duration
PO	Unknown	2–8 hr	Unknown
PO (controlled-release)	Unknown	6–10 hr	Unknown

Half-life: Paroxetine, 21 hours; controlled-release, 15 to 20 hours; paroxetine mesylate, 33.2 hours.

P

ADVERSE REACTIONS
CNS: asthenia, dizziness, headache, insomnia, somnolence, tremor, nervousness, *suicidal behavior,* anxiety, paresthesia, confusion, agitation. **CV:** palpitations, vasodilation, HTN, tachycardia, chest pain. **EENT:** blurred vision, tinnitus, lump or tightness in throat, pharyngitis, rhinitis, sinusitis. **GI:** dry mouth, nausea, constipation, diarrhea, flatulence, vomiting, dyspepsia, dysgeusia, increased or decreased appetite, abdominal pain. **GU:** ejaculatory disturbances, sexual dysfunction, urinary frequency, other urinary disorders, dysmenorrhea, female genital tract disease. **Musculoskeletal:** myopathy, myalgia, myasthenia, back pain. **Skin:** diaphoresis, rash, pruritus. **Respiratory:** dyspnea. **Other:** decreased libido, yawning.

INTERACTIONS
Drug-drug. *Amphetamines, metoclopramide, serotonergics, sibutramine,* L-*tryptophan, sympathomimetics:* May increase risk of serotonin syndrome. Monitor patient closely.

Anticoagulants, platelet inhibitors: May impair platelet aggregation and increase risk of bleeding. Monitor patient for signs and symptoms of bleeding.

Atomoxetine: May alter atomoxetine level. Initiate atomoxetine at a reduced dosage.

Barbiturates (phenobarbital), phenytoin: May alter pharmacokinetics of both drugs. Dosage adjustments may be needed.

Cimetidine: May decrease hepatic metabolism of paroxetine, leading to risk of adverse reactions. Dosage adjustments may be needed.

Cyclosporine: May increase cyclosporine level and toxicity. Monitor cyclosporine level when adding or discontinuing paroxetine; adjust cyclosporine dosage as needed.

Digoxin: May decrease digoxin level. Use together cautiously.

Drugs that prolong QT interval (antiarrhythmics [amiodarone, bretylium, disopyramide, dofetilide, procainamide, quinidine, sotalol], arsenic trioxide, chlorpromazine, cisapride, dolasetron, droperidol, mefloquine, mesoridazine, moxifloxacin, pentamidine, pimozide, tacrolimus, thioridazine, ziprasidone): May increase risk of life-threatening cardiac arrhythmias, including torsades de pointes. Monitor patient closely.

Fosamprenavir, ritonavir: May decrease paroxetine plasma level. Adjust dosage as needed.

Galantamine: May alter oral bioavailability of galantamine. Use together cautiously.

IV methylene blue, linezolid: May cause serotonin syndrome. Allow at least 2 weeks after stopping linezolid before giving paroxetine.

Lithium: May enhance serotonergic effects of paroxetine. Use with caution.

MAO inhibitors (phenelzine, selegiline, tranylcypromine): May cause serotonin syndrome and signs and symptoms resembling NMS. Avoid using within 14 days of MAO inhibitor therapy.

NSAIDs: May increase risk of GI bleeding. If possible, avoid concurrent use. If coadministration can't be avoided, consider shortening NSAID treatment duration, decreasing dosage, or switching to acetaminophen or a TCA.

Phenothiazines (thioridazine): May increase phenothiazine plasma level, increasing pharmacologic and adverse reactions of phenothiazine. Use together is contraindicated.

Pimozide: May increase pimozide level. Use together is contraindicated.

Procyclidine: May increase procyclidine level. Reduce procyclidine dosage if anticholinergic effects occur.

Risperidone: May increase risperidone level, increasing risk of adverse reactions; serotonin syndrome may occur. Use together cautiously.

Sympathomimetics: May increase sensitivity to the effect of sympathomimetics and increase risk of serotonin syndrome. Monitor patient.

Tamoxifen: May reduce plasma concentration of active tamoxifen metabolite. Avoid combination.

TCAs: May increase plasma concentration and elimination half-life of TCAs. TCA dosage reduction may be needed.

Theophylline: May increase theophylline plasma concentration. Theophylline dosage reduction may be needed.

Drug-herb. *SAM-e:* May increase risk of serotonin syndrome. Avoid use together.

St. John's wort: May increase sedative-hypnotic effects and risk of serotonin syndrome. Discourage use together.

Drug-lifestyle. *Alcohol use:* May alter psychomotor function. Discourage use together.

EFFECTS ON LAB TEST RESULTS
None reported.

CONTRAINDICATIONS & CAUTIONS
• Contraindicated in patients hypersensitive to drug, within 14 days of MAO inhibitor therapy, and in those taking thioridazine or pimozide.

Black Box Warning Antidepressants increase the risk of suicidal thinking and behavior in children, adolescents, and young adults with depression and other psychiatric disorders. Health professionals considering the use of paroxetine in a child, adolescent, or young adult must balance this risk with the clinical need. Paroxetine isn't approved for use in children. ■

◑ *Alert:* Use with linezolid or methylene blue can cause serotonin syndrome (fever, mental status changes, muscle twitching, excessive sweating, shivering or shaking, diarrhea, loss of coordination). Use drug with linezolid or methylene blue only for life-threatening or urgent conditions when the potential benefits outweigh the risks of toxicity.

• Use cautiously in patients with history of seizure disorders or mania and in those with other severe, systemic illness.

• Use cautiously in patients at risk for volume depletion and monitor them appropriately.

• Don't discontinue an SSRI abruptly, to avoid withdrawal signs and symptoms.

Dialyzable drug: Unlikely.

⚠ *Overdose S&S:* Coma, confusion, dizziness, nausea, somnolence, tachycardia, tremor, vomiting, acute renal failure, aggressive reactions, bradycardia, dystonia, hepatic necrosis, HTN, hypotension, jaundice, manic reactions, mydriasis, myoclonus, rhabdomyolysis, seizures, serotonin syndrome, stupor, hepatic impairment, syncope, urine retention, ventricular arrhythmias.

PREGNANCY-LACTATION-REPRODUCTION
• Drug can cause fetal harm, especially if taken in the first trimester. Manufacturer suggests discontinuing drug or switching to another antidepressant unless benefits justify continuing treatment. Consider other treatment options for women who are planning to become pregnant.

• Contraindicated for treatment of vasomotor symptoms in pregnant women.

• Drug appears in human milk. Use in breastfeeding women only if benefit of treating postpartum depression with this drug outweighs risk. Monitor infants for growth.

NURSING CONSIDERATIONS
• Patients taking Paxil CR for PMDD should be periodically reassessed to determine the need for continued treatment.

• If signs or symptoms of psychosis occur or increase, expect prescriber to reduce dosage. Record mood changes. Monitor patient for suicidal tendencies, and allow only a minimum supply of drug.

Black Box Warning Drug may increase the risk of suicidal thinking and behavior in children, adolescents, and young adults ages 18 to 24 during the first 2 months of treatment, especially in those with major depressive disorder or other psychiatric disorder. ■

Black Box Warning Monitor patients of all ages who are started on antidepressant therapy and observe closely for clinical worsening, suicidality, or unusual changes in behavior. ■

◑ *Alert:* If linezolid or methylene blue must be given, stop paroxetine and monitor patient for serotonin toxicity for 2 weeks or until 24 hours after the last dose of methylene blue or linezolid, whichever comes first. Treatment with paroxetine may be resumed 24 hours after the last dose of methylene blue or linezolid.

• Monitor patient for complaints of sexual dysfunction. In men, they include anorgasmia, erectile difficulties, and delayed ejaculation or orgasm; in women, they include anorgasmia or difficulty with orgasm.

◑ *Alert:* Don't stop drug abruptly. Withdrawal or discontinuation syndrome may occur if drug is stopped abruptly. Symptoms include headache, myalgia, lethargy, and general flulike symptoms. Taper drug slowly over 1 to 2 weeks.

◑ *Alert:* Combining triptans with an SSRI or an SSNRI may cause serotonin syndrome or NMS-like reactions. Signs and symptoms of serotonin syndrome may include restlessness, hallucinations, loss of coordination, fast heartbeat, rapid changes in BP, increased body temperature, overactive reflexes, nausea, vomiting, and diarrhea. Serotonin syndrome may be more likely to occur when starting or increasing the dose of triptan, SSRI, or SSNRI.

• *Look alike–sound alike:* Don't confuse paroxetine with fluoxetine or paclitaxel. Don't confuse Paxil with Doxil, paclitaxel, Plavix, or Taxol.

PATIENT TEACHING
Black Box Warning Advise families and caregivers to closely observe patient for increased suicidal thinking and behavior. ■

◑ *Alert:* Teach patient to recognize and immediately report signs and symptoms of serotonin toxicity.

- Tell patient that drug may be taken with or without food, usually in morning.
- Tell patient not to break, crush, or chew controlled-release tablets.
- Warn patient to avoid activities that require alertness and good coordination until effects of drug are known.
- Advise female patient of childbearing potential to contact prescriber if she becomes pregnant or plans to become pregnant during therapy or if she's currently breastfeeding.
- Tell patient to avoid alcohol and to consult prescriber before taking other prescription or OTC drugs or herbal medicines.
- Instruct patient not to stop taking drug abruptly.

SAFETY ALERT!

pegaspargase
(PEG-L-asparaginase)
peg-AHS-per-jays

Oncaspar

Therapeutic class: Antineoplastics
Pharmacologic class: Modified L-asparaginases

AVAILABLE FORMS
Injection: 3,750 international units/5-mL solution in single-use vial (750 international units/mL)

INDICATIONS & DOSAGES
➤ **As part of a multidrug chemotherapy regimen in the treatment of acute lymphoblastic leukemia, and acute lymphoblastic leukemia with hypersensitivity to native forms of L-asparaginase**
Adults and children older than age 1:
2,500 international units/m² IV or IM every 14 days.

ADMINISTRATION
IV
▼ Give IV only if IM route is contraindicated. Don't administer by IV push.
▼ Give IV over 1 to 2 hours in 100 mL of NSS or D₅W injection through an infusion that's already running.
▼ Drug may be a contact irritant, and solution must be handled and given with care.

Wear gloves. Avoid inhalation of vapors and contact with skin or mucous membranes, especially in the eyes. If contact occurs, wash with generous amounts of water for at least 15 minutes.
▼ Don't use if cloudy or contains precipitate. Avoid excessive agitation of drug; don't shake.
▼ Don't freeze or use drug that has been frozen because freezing destroys drug's effectiveness.
▼ Discard unused portions. Use only one dose per vial; don't reenter vial.
▼ Don't use if stored at room temperature for longer than 48 hours. Keep refrigerated at 36° to 46° F (2° to 8° C). Protect infusion bags from light.
▼ **Incompatibilities:** None listed by manufacturer. Consult a drug incompatibility reference for more information.

IM
- IM is the preferred route and is associated with lower incidence of adverse effects.
- When giving IM, limit volume given at a single injection site to 2 mL. If volume to be given exceeds 2 mL, use multiple injection sites.
- Administer as deep IM injection into a large muscle.

ACTION
A modified version of the enzyme L-asparaginase that exerts cytotoxic effects by inactivating the amino acid asparagine, which tumor cells need to synthesize proteins.

Route	Onset	Peak	Duration
IV	Unknown	Unknown	2–4 wk
IM	Unknown	Unknown	21 days

Half-life: IV, about 7 days; IM, about 6 days.

ADVERSE REACTIONS
CNS: *stroke.* **GI:** *pancreatitis.* **Hematologic:** *coagulopathy.* **Hepatic:** abnormal LFT values, hyperbilirubinemia. **Metabolic:** hyperglycemia. **Other:** hypersensitivity reactions.

INTERACTIONS
Drug-drug. *Aspirin, dipyridamole, heparin, NSAIDs, warfarin:* May cause imbalances in coagulation factors, predisposing patient

---

Reactions in bold italics are *life-threatening*. Interactions may have a *rapid onset* or a ***delayed onset***.

to bleeding or thrombosis. Use together cautiously.

Immunosuppressants: May enhance adverse/toxic effect of immunosuppressants; specifically, may increase risk of serious infections. Use together cautiously.

Live-virus vaccines: May increase adverse or toxic effects of vaccines; may diminish vaccines' therapeutic effects. Avoid use together. Don't give live-virus vaccines for at least 3 months after drug.

Vaccines (inactivated): May diminish therapeutic effect of vaccines. Monitor therapy.

EFFECTS ON LAB TEST RESULTS

• May increase BUN, creatinine, amylase, lipase, bilirubin, ALT, AST, uric acid, and ammonia levels. May decrease sodium and protein levels. May increase or decrease glucose level.

• May prolong PT and aPTT, and increase INR and PTT.

• May decrease Hb level and antithrombin III, WBC, RBC, platelet, and granulocyte counts.

CONTRAINDICATIONS & CAUTIONS

• Contraindicated in patients with pancreatitis or history of pancreatitis with prior L-asparaginase therapy, in those who have had significant thrombosis or hemorrhagic events related to previous treatment with L-asparaginase, and in those with history of serious allergic reactions to drug, such as generalized urticaria, bronchospasm, laryngeal edema, hypotension, or other unacceptable adverse reactions.

• Discontinue drug in patients with serious thrombotic events.

• Use cautiously in patients with hepatic impairment.

• Use cautiously in patients with a history of diabetes.

Dialyzable drug: Unknown.

⚠ *Overdose S&S:* Elevated liver enzyme levels, rash.

PREGNANCY-LACTATION-REPRODUCTION

• It isn't known if drug causes fetal harm. Use only if clearly needed.

• It isn't known if drug appears in human milk. Patient should discontinue breastfeeding or discontinue drug.

NURSING CONSIDERATIONS

• Take preventive measures (including adequate hydration) before starting treatment. Hyperuricemia may result from rapid lysis of leukemic cells.

🔸 *Alert:* Monitor patients closely for hypersensitivity (including life-threatening anaphylaxis), especially those hypersensitive to other forms of L-asparaginase. Observe patient for 1 hour after giving drug and have emergency equipment and other drugs needed to treat anaphylaxis readily available. Moderate to life-threatening hypersensitivity requires stopping L-asparaginase.

• To assess effects of therapy, monitor patient's peripheral blood count and bone marrow. A drop in circulating lymphoblasts is often noted after therapy starts, sometimes accompanied by a marked rise in uric acid level.

• Obtain frequent amylase and lipase determinations to detect pancreatitis. Monitor patient's glucose level during therapy to detect hyperglycemia.

• Monitor patient for liver dysfunction when drug is used with hepatotoxic chemotherapeutic drugs.

• Drug may affect several plasma proteins; monitor fibrinogen, PT, INR, and PTT at baseline and periodically during and after treatment.

• *Look alike–sound alike:* Don't confuse pegaspargase with asparaginase.

PATIENT TEACHING

• Inform patient of risk of hypersensitivity reactions and importance of reporting them immediately.

• Tell patient not to take other drugs, including OTC preparations, until approved by prescriber because risk of bleeding is higher when pegaspargase is given with drugs such as aspirin. Drug may also increase toxicity of other drugs.

• Advise patient to use an electric razor and soft toothbrush to minimize bleeding.

• Urge patient to report all adverse reactions and signs and symptoms of infection (fever, chills, and malaise); drug may suppress the immune system. Advise patient to avoid crowds, if possible, and people who are sick.

P

- Advise patient to report signs and symptoms of thrombosis (severe headache, arm or leg swelling, acute shortness of breath, and chest pain).
- Tell patient to report severe abdominal pain, which may indicate pancreatitis.
- Teach patient to report excessive thirst or an increase in the volume or frequency of urination.
- Encourage patient to drink plenty of fluids every 24 hours (unless instructed not to).
- Caution female patient of childbearing potential to avoid pregnancy and breastfeeding during therapy.

SAFETY ALERT!

pegfilgrastim
peg-fil-GRA-stim

Lapelga, Neulasta, Neulasta Onpro Kit

pegfilgrastim-jmdb
Fulphila

pegfilgrastim-cbqv
Udenyca

Therapeutic class: Colony-stimulating factors
Pharmacologic class: Hematopoietics

AVAILABLE FORMS
Injection: 6 mg/0.6 mL syringe; 6 mg/0.6 mL single-dose prefilled syringe packaged with On-body injector

INDICATIONS & DOSAGES
➤ **To reduce frequency of infection in patients with nonmyeloid malignancies receiving myelosuppressive chemotherapy that may cause febrile neutropenia**
Adults weighing more than 45 kg: 6 mg subcut once per chemotherapy cycle. Don't give in period between 14 days before and 24 hours after administration of cytotoxic chemotherapy.
Children: Give once per chemotherapy cycle, beginning 24 hours after completion of chemotherapy. If weight is 31 to 44 kg, give 4 mg subcut. If weight is 21 to 30 kg, give 2.5 mg subcut. If weight is 10 to 20 kg, give 1.5 mg subcut. If weight is less than 10 kg, give 0.1 mg/kg subcut.

➤ **To increase survival in patients acutely exposed to myelosuppressive doses of radiation (Neulasta, Neulasta Onpro Kit)**
Adults and children weighing 45 kg or more: 6 mg subcut as soon as possible after suspected or confirmed exposure. Repeat 1 week after first dose.
Children weighing 31 to 44 kg: 4 mg (0.4 mL) subcut as soon as possible after suspected or confirmed exposure. Repeat 1 week after first dose.
Children weighing 21 to 30 kg: 2.5 mg (0.25 mL) subcut as soon as possible after suspected or confirmed exposure. Repeat 1 week after first dose.
Children weighing 10 to 20 kg: 1.5 mg (0.15 mL) subcut as soon as possible after suspected or confirmed exposure. Repeat 1 week after first dose.
Children weighing less than 10 kg: 0.1 mg/kg (0.01 mL/kg) subcut as soon as possible after suspected or confirmed exposure. Repeat 1 week after first dose.

ADMINISTRATION
Subcutaneous
ⓘ *Alert:* Don't use prefilled syringe for patients requiring less than 6 mg (0.6 mL), as syringe doesn't have graduated markings for smaller doses. Transfer drug to appropriately marked syringe to measure dose of less than 0.6 mL.
- Allow drug to come to room temperature before giving; protect from light.
- Don't shake.
- Don't use if discoloration or particulate matter is seen.
- Refrigerate Neulasta; don't freeze.
- Discard Fulphila if frozen more than once. If frozen, thaw in refrigerator before administration.
- Refer to manufacturer's instructions for administering drug using the On-body injector and for its removal and disposal.
- Discard drug if left at room temperature for more than 48 hours.

ACTION
Binds cell receptors to stimulate proliferation, differentiation, commitment, and end-cell function of neutrophils.

Reactions in bold italics are *life-threatening*. Interactions may have a *rapid onset* or a ***delayed onset***.

Route	Onset	Peak	Duration
Subcut	Unknown	Unknown	Unknown

Half-life: 15 to 80 hours.

ADVERSE REACTIONS

CNS: dizziness, fatigue, fever, headache, insomnia, asthenia. **CV:** peripheral edema. **GI:** abdominal pain, anorexia, constipation, diarrhea, dyspepsia, mucositis, nausea, stomatitis, taste perversion, vomiting. **Hematologic:** *granulocytopenia, neutropenic fever.* **Musculoskeletal:** arthralgia, bone pain, generalized weakness, myalgia, skeletal pain. **Skin:** alopecia.

INTERACTIONS
None.

EFFECTS ON LAB TEST RESULTS
• May increase LDH, alkaline phosphatase, and uric acid levels.
• May decrease granulocyte, platelet, and RBC counts.

CONTRAINDICATIONS & CAUTIONS
• Contraindicated in patients hypersensitive to *Escherichia coli*–derived proteins, filgrastim, or any component of the drug. Don't use for peripheral blood progenitor cell mobilization.
• Use cautiously in patients with sickle cell disease, those receiving chemotherapy causing delayed myelosuppression, those receiving radiation therapy, and during breastfeeding.
• Infants, children, and adolescents who weigh less than 45 kg shouldn't receive the 6-mg single-use syringe dose.
Dialyzable drug: Unknown.
⚠ Overdose S&S: Leukocytosis, bone pain, edema, dyspnea, pleural effusions.

PREGNANCY-LACTATION-REPRODUCTION
• There are no adequate studies in pregnant women. Use only if potential benefit justifies potential risk to the fetus.
• Women who become pregnant during treatment should enroll in Amgen's Pregnancy Surveillance Program (1-800-772-6436).
• It isn't known if drug appears in human milk. Use cautiously in breastfeeding women.

NURSING CONSIDERATIONS
❸ Alert: Splenic rupture may occur rarely. Assess patient who experiences signs or symptoms of left upper abdominal or shoulder pain for an enlarged spleen or splenic rupture.
• Obtain CBC and platelet count before therapy.
• Monitor patient's Hb level, hematocrit, CBC, and platelet count, as well as LDH, alkaline phosphatase, and uric acid levels during therapy.
• Monitor patient for allergic-type reactions, including anaphylaxis, skin rash, and urticaria, which can occur with first or subsequent treatment.
• Evaluate patient with fever, lung infiltrates, or respiratory distress for adult respiratory distress syndrome. Notify prescriber if respiratory status worsens.
• Keep patient with sickle cell disease well hydrated, and monitor for symptoms of sickle cell crisis.
• Monitor patient for capillary leak syndrome (hypotension, hypoalbuminemia, edema, hemoconcentration) and manage with symptomatic treatment, if necessary.
• Pegfilgrastim may act as a growth factor for tumors.
❸ Alert: After acute radiation exposure, obtain a baseline CBC but don't delay drug administration if a CBC isn't readily available. Estimate patient's absorbed radiation dose (level of radiation exposure) based on information from public health authorities, biodosimetry if available, or clinical findings, such as time to onset of vomiting or lymphocyte depletion kinetics.
• *Look alike–sound alike:* Don't confuse Neulasta with Neumega, Neupogen, or Lunesta.

PATIENT TEACHING
• Advise patient to report all adverse reactions.
• Tell patient to report signs and symptoms of allergic reactions, fever, or breathing problems.
❸ Alert: Rarely, splenic rupture may occur. Advise patient to immediately report upper left abdominal or shoulder tip pain.
• Tell patient with sickle cell disease to keep drinking fluids and report signs or symptoms of sickle cell crisis.

P

♣Canada   ◇OTC   ♦Off-label use   *Photoguide   ⊕Do not crush   *Liquid contains alcohol   ▨Genetic

• Instruct patient or caregiver how to give drug if it's to be given at home.

• Instruct patient using On-body injector not to expose injector to oxygen-rich environments (e.g., hyperbaric chamber), MRI, X-ray (including airport X-ray), CT scan, or ultrasound (may damage injector system).

• Instruct patient to keep On-body injector at least 4 inches (10 cm) away from electrical equipment, including cell phones, cordless phones, microwaves, and other common appliances (injector may not work properly).

• Advise patient to avoid activities, such as traveling, driving, or operating machinery, for 26 to 29 hours after using On-body injector.

• Advise patient not to reuse syringes.

SAFETY ALERT!

peginterferon alfa-2a
peg-in-ter-FEER-on

Pegasys, Pegasys ProClick

Therapeutic class: Antivirals
Pharmacologic class: Interferons

AVAILABLE FORMS
Injection: 180 mcg/1 mL single-dose vials; 180 mcg/0.5 mL prefilled syringe; 135 mcg/0.5 mL, 180 mcg/0.5 mL autoinjector

INDICATIONS & DOSAGES
Adjust-a-dose (for all indications): Refer to manufacturer's instructions for toxicity-related dosage adjustments.

➤ **Chronic HCV infection with compensated hepatic disease in patients not previously treated with interferon alfa, in combination with other HCV antiviral drugs**
Adults with HCV genotype 1 or 4: 180 mcg subcut in abdomen or thigh once weekly as monotherapy or combination therapy with ribavirin for 48 weeks. Refer to prescribing information of the other HCV antiviral for duration of entire treatment regimen. If used with ribavirin with or without other HCV antivirals, treatment duration is 48 weeks.
Adults with HCV genotype 2 or 3: 180 mcg subcut in abdomen or thigh once weekly. Refer to prescribing information of the other

HCV antiviral for duration of entire treatment regimen. If used with ribavirin with or without other HCV antivirals, treatment duration is 24 weeks.
Children age 5 and older: 180 mcg/1.73 m² × BSA subcut once weekly in combination with ribavirin. Treat patients with genotype 2 or 3 for 24 weeks, other genotypes for 48 weeks. Maximum dose is 180 mcg once weekly.
➤ **Chronic HCV infection (regardless of genotype) in HIV-infected patients who haven't previously been treated with interferon alfa**
Adults: 180 mcg subcut in abdomen or thigh once weekly. When used with ribavirin, treatment duration is 48 weeks. When used with other HCV antivirals, refer to prescribing information of the other HCV antiviral for treatment duration.
➤ **Chronic HBV infection in patients with compensated liver disease and evidence of viral replication and liver inflammation**
Adults: 180 mcg subcut in abdomen or thigh once weekly for 48 weeks.
➤ **Hepatitis B e-antigen (HbeAg)-positive chronic HBV infection in noncirrhotic children who have evidence of viral replication and elevation in serum ALT level**
Children age 3 and older: 180 mcg/1.73 m² × BSA subcut once weekly in combination with ribavirin. Maximum recommended dosage is 180 mcg weekly; recommended duration of therapy is 48 weeks. Patients who turn age 18 during therapy should maintain the recommended pediatric dosage through completion of therapy.

ADMINISTRATION
Subcutaneous
• Vials and prefilled syringes are for single use only. Discard unused portion.
• Don't shake. Allow to reach room temperature before use, but don't leave out of refrigerator for more than 24 hours. Don't freeze.
• Protect from light.
• Visually inspect drug for particulate matter and discoloration before administration; don't use if particulate matter is visible or product is discolored.

ACTION
Causes reversible decreases in leukocyte and platelet counts, partially through stimulation of production of effector proteins in vitro. Inhibits HCV RNA replication.

Route	Onset	Peak	Duration
Subcut	Unknown	3–4 days	<1 wk

Half-life: 160 hours (range, 84 to 353 hours).

ADVERSE REACTIONS
CNS: depression, dizziness, fatigue, headache, insomnia, irritability, pain, pyrexia, anxiety, asthenia, concentration impairment, memory impairment, mood alteration, nervousness. **EENT:** blurred vision. **GI:** abdominal pain, anorexia, diarrhea, nausea, dry mouth, vomiting, weight loss. **Hematologic:** *neutropenia, thrombocytopenia,* anemia, *lymphopenia.* **Musculoskeletal:** arthralgia, myalgia, back pain. **Respiratory:** cough, dyspnea. **Skin:** alopecia, pruritus, dermatitis, increased sweating, rash, dry skin, eczema. **Other:** injection-site reaction, rigors.

INTERACTIONS
Drug-drug. *Methadone:* May increase methadone level. Monitor patient closely and decrease methadone dosage as needed.
NRTIs: May cause severe and potentially fatal hepatic decompensation. If used together in patients coinfected with HIV who are taking NRTIs, monitor for toxicities.
Ribavirin: May cause additive hematologic toxicity. Monitor hematologic function.
Telbivudine: May increase risk of peripheral neuropathy. Avoid use together.
Theophylline, other drugs metabolized by CYP1A2: May increase theophylline level and may interact with other drugs metabolized by this enzyme system. Monitor theophylline level and adjust dosage as needed.
Zidovudine: May enhance adverse/toxic effect of zidovudine; may decrease zidovudine metabolism. Monitor therapy.

EFFECTS ON LAB TEST RESULTS
• May increase triglyceride and ALT levels. May decrease Hb level and hematocrit.
• May decrease ANC, WBC, and platelet counts. May increase or decrease thyroid function test values.

CONTRAINDICATIONS & CAUTIONS
• Contraindicated in patients hypersensitive to interferon alfa-2a or any components of formulation.
• Contraindicated in patients with autoimmune hepatitis or decompensated liver disease (with monoinfection or coinfection with HIV) before or during treatment with drug and in neonates and infants.
• Use cautiously in patients with a history of depression.
• Use cautiously in patients with baseline neutrophil counts less than 1,500/mm^3, baseline platelet counts less than 90,000/mm^3, or baseline Hb level less than 10 g/dL.
• Use cautiously in patients with CrCl less than 50 mL/minute.
• Use cautiously in patients with cardiac disease or HTN, thyroid disease, autoimmune disorders, pulmonary disorders, colitis, pancreatitis, and ophthalmologic disorders.
• Use cautiously in elderly patients because they may be at increased risk for adverse reactions.
❸ *Alert:* Use cautiously in patients also taking ribavirin. Ribavirin is also known to cause hemolytic anemia, which may worsen cardiac disease.
• Safety and effectiveness haven't been established in patients who have failed to respond to other interferon alfa treatments, in solid organ transplant recipients, and in patients also infected with HBV.
Dialyzable drug: No.
⚠ *Overdose S&S:* Fatigue, elevated liver enzyme levels, neutropenia, thrombocytopenia.

PREGNANCY-LACTATION-REPRODUCTION
• There are no adequate studies of drug used as monotherapy in pregnant women. Manufacturer advises using drug as monotherapy only if potential benefit justifies potential risk to the fetus and only in women of childbearing potential when they are using effective contraception. Some professional guidelines recommend that drug not be used during pregnancy.
• Combination therapy with ribavirin may cause fetal birth defects or death; combination therapy with ribavirin in pregnant women is contraindicated. Patient must have a confirmed negative pregnancy test

P

immediately before start of combination treatment. Monthly pregnancy tests must be performed. Women of childbearing potential and men must use two forms of effective contraception during therapy and for at least 6 months after therapy ends.

• It isn't known if drug appears in human milk. Patient should discontinue breastfeeding or discontinue drug.

NURSING CONSIDERATIONS

Black Box Warning Alpha interferons may cause or aggravate *fatal or life-threatening neuropsychiatric, autoimmune, ischemic, and infectious disorders.* Monitor patients closely with periodic clinical and lab evaluations. Withdraw patients with persistently severe or worsening signs or symptoms of these conditions from therapy. ∎

• Obtain CBC before treatment and monitor counts routinely during therapy. Stop drug in patients who develop severe decrease in neutrophil or platelet counts.

• Stop drug if uncontrollable thyroid disease, hyperglycemia, hypoglycemia, or diabetes mellitus occurs during treatment.

• If persistent or unexplained pulmonary infiltrates or pulmonary dysfunction occur, stop drug.

• Stop drug if signs and symptoms of colitis occur, such as abdominal pain, bloody diarrhea, and fever. Symptoms should resolve within 1 to 3 weeks.

• Stop drug if signs and symptoms of pancreatitis occur, including fever, malaise, and abdominal pain.

• Obtain baseline eye exam and periodically monitor eye exams during treatment. Stop drug if new or worsening eye disorders occur.

• Monitor patient with impaired renal function for interferon toxicity.

• Use in women of childbearing potential only when effective contraception is being used.

• *Look alike–sound alike:* Don't confuse peginterferon alfa-2a with interferon alfa-2a, interferon alfa-2b, interferon alfa-n3, or peginterferon alfa-2b.

PATIENT TEACHING

• Advise patient to read medication guide that comes with drug.

• Teach patient proper way to give drug and dispose of needles and syringes.

• Tell patient to immediately report depression or suicidal ideation.

• Tell patient to report signs and symptoms of pancreatitis, colitis, eye disorders, or respiratory disorders.

• Advise patient who feels dizzy, tired, confused, or sleepy to avoid driving or operating machinery.

• Advise patient not to switch to another brand of interferon without consulting health care provider.

• Advise female patient that drug may alter menstrual cycles and impaired fertility is possible.

🖐 *Alert:* When drug is used with ribavirin, tell male and female patients and their partners to take extreme care to avoid pregnancy during treatment with ribavirin and for 6 months after treatment ends.

SAFETY ALERT!

peginterferon alfa-2b
peg-in-ter-FEER-on

PegIntron, PegIntron Redipen, Sylatron

Therapeutic class: Antivirals
Pharmacologic class: Interferons

AVAILABLE FORMS

Injection: 50 mcg/0.5 mL, 80 mcg/0.5 mL, 120 mcg/0.5 mL, 150 mcg/0.5 mL
Powder for injection: 200-mcg, 300-mcg, 600-mcg single-use vials

INDICATIONS & DOSAGES

Adjust-a-dose (for all indications): Refer to manufacturer's instructions for toxicity-related dosage adjustments.

➤ **Chronic HCV infection, as monotherapy in patients with compensated liver disease not previously treated with interferon alfa (PegIntron, PegIntron Redipen)**
Adults: 1 mcg/kg subcut once weekly for up to 1 year on same day each week. Volume to be injected depends on the strength of drug and patient's body weight. Refer to manufacturer's instructions for weight-based tables.

➤ **Chronic HCV infection in patients with compensated liver disease, combined with ribavirin (PegIntron, PegIntron Redipen)**
Adults: 1.5 mcg/kg subcut once weekly for 12 to 48 weeks depending on combination regimen chosen. See guidelines for specific treatment lengths. Treatment duration depends on genotype and treatment status (naive versus prior treatment failures). For interferon alfa–naive patients with HCV genotype 1, treatment duration is 48 weeks; for patients with HCV genotypes 2 and 3, treatment duration is 24 weeks. Treatment duration for patients who previously failed therapy is 48 weeks, regardless of HCV genotype. For patients with HCV genotype 1 who previously failed therapy, PegIntron and ribavirin without an HCV NS3/4A protease inhibitor should only be used if there are contraindications, significant intolerance, or other clinical factors that wouldn't warrant use of an HCV NS3/4A protease inhibitor. Volume to be injected depends on the strength of PegIntron and patient's body weight. Refer to manufacturer's instructions for weight-based tables and for ribavirin dosages.
Children ages 3 to 17: 60 mcg/m^2 subcut on same day every week. Treatment duration for patients with HCV genotype 1 is 48 weeks; patients with HCV genotypes 2 and 3 should be treated for 24 weeks. Refer to manufacturer's instructions for ribavirin weight-based dosage tables. Patients who reach age 18 while receiving combination therapy should remain on the pediatric dosing regimen.
Adjust-a-dose: Refer to manufacturer's instructions for toxicity-related dosage adjustments.

➤ **For adjuvant treatment of melanoma with microscopic or gross nodal involvement within 84 days of definitive surgical resection including complete lymphadenectomy (Sylatron only)**
Adults: 6 mcg/kg/week subcut for eight doses, followed by 3 mcg/kg/week subcut for up to 5 years. Premedicate with acetaminophen 500 to 1,000 mg PO 30 minutes before the first dose and as needed for subsequent doses.

Adjust-a-dose: Refer to manufacturer's instructions for toxicity-related dosage adjustments.

ADMINISTRATION
Subcutaneous
• To reconstitute the lyophilized peginterferon alfa-2b in the Redipen, hold the Redipen upright (dose button down), and press the two halves of the pen together until there is an audible click.
• Gently invert the pen to mix the solution. Don't shake.
• Keeping the pen upright, attach the supplied needle, and select the appropriate peginterferon alfa-2b dose by pulling back on the dosing button until the dark bands are visible and turning the button until the dark band is aligned with the correct dose.
• The Redipen is for single use only.
• Reconstitute the peginterferon alfa-2b lyophilized product with only 0.7 mL of supplied diluent (sterile water for injection). Discard the remaining diluent.
• Swirl gently to dissolve completely. Don't shake.
• Before mixing, store PegIntron Redipen in refrigerator between 36° and 46° F (2° and 8° C) and store vials at room temperature between 68° and 77° F (20° and 25° C).
• Administer subcut. Rotate injection sites.
• **Incompatibilities:** Don't add any other medication to solutions containing peginterferon alfa-2b.

ACTION
Binds to specific membrane receptors on the cell surface, inducing certain enzymes, suppressing cell proliferation and immunomodulating activities, and inhibiting virus replication in virus-infected cells. Increases levels of effector proteins and body temperature, and decreases leukocyte and platelet counts.

Route	Onset	Peak	Duration
Subcut	Unknown	15–44 hr	Unknown

Half-life: PegIntron, 40 hours (range, 22 to 60 hours); Sylatron, 43 to 51 hours.

ADVERSE REACTIONS
CNS: anxiety, depression, dizziness, emotional lability, fatigue, fever, headache,

insomnia, irritability, *suicidal behavior,* hypertonia, malaise, agitation, nervousness. **CV:** flushing, chest pain, *bundle-branch block, ventricular tachycardia, MI.* **EENT:** conjunctivitis, blurred vision, pharyngitis, sinusitis, rhinitis, dry mouth, taste perversion. **GI:** abdominal pain, anorexia, diarrhea, nausea, dyspepsia, right upper quadrant pain, vomiting. **GU:** menstrual disorder. **Hematologic:** *neutropenia, thrombocytopenia,* anemia. **Hepatic:** hepatomegaly. **Metabolic:** weight loss, hypothyroidism, hyperthyroidism. **Musculoskeletal:** musculoskeletal pain, myalgia, arthralgia. **Respiratory:** cough, dyspnea. **Skin:** alopecia, dry skin, increased sweating, injection-site inflammation or reaction, pruritus, rash, injection-site pain. **Other:** flulike symptoms, rigors, viral infection.

INTERACTIONS

Drug-drug. *Drugs metabolized by CYP2C8, CYP2C9 (phenytoin, warfarin), or CYP2D6 (flecainide):* May decrease serum levels of these drugs. Monitor patient response and drug levels; adjust dosage as needed.
Fluoxetine: May decrease fluoxetine serum concentration. Monitor patient closely and adjust dosage as needed.
Methadone: May increase methadone level. Monitor patient closely and decrease methadone dosage as needed.
NRTIs: May cause severe and potentially fatal hepatic decompensation. If used together in patient coinfected with HIV, monitor patient for toxicities.
Ribavirin: May cause additive hematologic toxicity. Monitor therapy.
Telbivudine: May increase risk of peripheral neuropathy. Avoid use together.

EFFECTS ON LAB TEST RESULTS

• May increase serum bilirubin, uric acid, triglyceride, and ALT levels. May increase or decrease TSH level.
• May decrease Hb level.
• May decrease neutrophil and platelet counts.

CONTRAINDICATIONS & CAUTIONS

• Contraindicated in patients hypersensitive to drug or any of its components, in patients with autoimmune hepatitis or decompensated liver disease, in those with diabetes or thyroid disorders that can't be controlled with medication, in patients who have failed to respond to other alpha interferon treatment or have had an organ transplant, and in those with HIV or HBV.
• Use cautiously in patients with psychiatric disorders, diabetes mellitus, CV disease, CrCl less than 50 mL/minute, pulmonary infiltrates, pulmonary function impairment, or autoimmune, ischemic, or infectious disorders.
• If overdose occurs, use symptomatic treatment and close observation.
Dialyzable drug: No.
⚠ *Overdose S&S:* Fatigue, headache, myalgia, neutropenia, thrombocytopenia.

PREGNANCY-LACTATION-REPRODUCTION

Black Box Warning Use of drug with ribavirin may cause birth defects and fetal death. Combination use is contraindicated in women who are pregnant and in male partners of women who are pregnant. ∎
• Combination therapy with ribavirin should begin only after obtaining a negative pregnancy test immediately before start of therapy. Obtain pregnancy tests monthly during therapy and for 6 months after therapy ends. Patients should use two effective forms of contraception.
• There are no adequate studies of drug used as monotherapy in pregnancy. Manufacturer recommends that drug be used in pregnancy only if potential benefit justifies potential risks to the fetus and that women of childbearing potential use effective contraception during treatment. Some professional guidelines recommend that drug not be used in pregnant women.
• It isn't known if drug appears in human milk. Patient should discontinue breastfeeding or discontinue drug.

NURSING CONSIDERATIONS

• Obtain eye exam in patient with diabetes or HTN before starting drug. Retinal hemorrhages, cotton-wool spots, and retinal artery or vein obstruction may occur.
Black Box Warning Drug may cause or aggravate fatal or life-threatening neuropsychiatric, autoimmune, ischemic, and infectious disorders. Monitor patients closely with periodic clinical and lab evaluations. In

---

Reactions in bold italics are *life-threatening*. Interactions may have a *rapid onset* or a *delayed onset*.

patient with persistently severe or worsening signs or symptoms of these conditions from therapy, withhold drug. In many but not all cases, these disorders resolve after stopping PegIntron therapy. ■

Black Box Warning The risk of serious depression with suicidal ideation, completed suicides, and other neuropsychiatric disorders increases with use of alpha interferons, including Sylatron. Permanently discontinue Sylatron in patients with persistently severe or worsening signs or symptoms of depression, psychosis, or encephalopathy. These disorders may not resolve after stopping Sylatron. ■

• Combination therapy with ribavirin for HCV infection is preferred over monotherapy because of better response rates, unless contraindication or intolerance exists. Monotherapy is only indicated for previously untreated adults.

Black Box Warning If used in combination therapy with ribavirin, monitor patient for worsening cardiac disease secondary to hemolytic anemia. ■

• Drug may cause or aggravate hypothyroidism, hyperthyroidism, or diabetes.

• Perform ECG on patient with history of MI or arrhythmias before starting drug.

• Start treatment in patient who is well hydrated.

• Monitor patient with history of MI or arrhythmias closely for hypotension, arrhythmias, tachycardia, cardiomyopathy, and signs and symptoms of MI.

• Monitor patient for depression and other mental health disorders. If symptoms are severe, stop drug and refer patient for psychiatric care.

• Monitor patient for signs and symptoms of colitis, such as abdominal pain, bloody diarrhea, and fever. Stop drug if colitis occurs. Symptoms should resolve 1 to 3 weeks after stopping drug.

• Monitor patient for signs and symptoms of pancreatitis (due to elevated triglyceride levels) or hypersensitivity reactions, and stop drug if these occur.

• Monitor patient with pulmonary disease for dyspnea, pulmonary infiltrates, pneumonitis, and pneumonia.

• Monitor patient with renal disease for signs and symptoms of toxicity.

• Monitor CBC count, platelet count, and AST, ALT, bilirubin, and TSH levels before starting drug and periodically during treatment.

• Notify prescriber if severe neutropenia or thrombocytopenia occurs.

• Children may experience growth delays in height and weight.

• Monitor patient for effectiveness of treatment. If HCV viral levels remain elevated after 6 months of therapy, discontinue treatment.

• **Look alike–sound alike:** Don't confuse peginterferon alfa-2b with interferon alfa-2a, interferon alfa-2b, interferon alfa-n3, or peginterferon alfa-2a. Don't confuse Peg Intron with Intron A.

PATIENT TEACHING

• Teach patient the appropriate use of the drug and the benefits and risks of treatment. Tell patient that adverse reactions may continue for several months after treatment is stopped.

• Tell patient to immediately report symptoms of depression or suicidal thoughts.

• Instruct patient on importance of proper disposal of needles and syringes. Caution patient against reuse of old needles and syringes.

• Tell patient that drug won't prevent transmission of HCV to others and may not cure HCV infection or prevent cirrhosis, liver failure, or liver cancer that may result from HCV infection.

• Advise patient that lab tests are needed before starting therapy and periodically thereafter.

• Tell patient to take drug at bedtime and to use fever-reducing drugs to decrease risk of flulike signs and symptoms.

• Inform breastfeeding patient of the potential for adverse reactions in infants. Tell her to either stop using drug or stop breastfeeding.

• Advise patient to brush teeth thoroughly at least twice a day, have regular dental exams, and rinse mouth thoroughly after emesis.

Black Box Warning Tell patient using combination therapy to avoid pregnancy. ■

P

pembrolizumab ▨
pem-broe-LIZ-ue-mab

Keytruda

Therapeutic class: Antineoplastics
Pharmacologic class: Monoclonal antibodies

AVAILABLE FORMS
Injection: 50 mg lyophilized powder in single-use vial; 25 mg/mL (4 mL) solution in single-use vial

INDICATIONS & DOSAGES
Adjust-a-dose (for all indications): Refer to manufacturer's instructions for toxicity-related dosage adjustments.

➤ **Unresectable or metastatic melanoma**
Adults: 200 mg IV infusion over 30 minutes every 3 weeks until disease progression or unacceptable toxicity occurs.

➤ **Recurrent or metastatic head and neck squamous cell carcinoma (HNSCC) in patients with disease progression on or after platinum-containing chemotherapy; first-line treatment for metastatic NSCLC in patients whose tumors have high PD-L1 expression and don't have EGFR or ALK genomic tumor aberrations; metastatic NSCLC in patients whose tumors express PD-L1 as determined by an FDA-approved test and who have disease progression on or after platinum-containing chemotherapy** ▨
Adults: 200 mg IV infusion every 3 weeks until disease progression or unacceptable toxicity occurs, or up to 24 months in patients without disease progression on drug.

➤ **Treatment of patients with refractory classical Hodgkin lymphoma or who have relapsed after three or more prior lines of therapy; unresectable or metastatic, microsatellite instability-high or mismatch repair deficient solid tumors that have progressed after prior treatment in patients who have no satisfactory alternative treatment options; colorectal cancer that has progressed after treatment with a fluoropyrimidine, oxaliplatin, and irinotecan** ▨
Adults: 200 mg IV infusion every 3 weeks until disease progression or unacceptable toxicity occurs, or up to 24 months in patients without disease progression.
Children age 2 and older: 2 mg/kg (up to a maximum of 200 mg/dose) IV infusion every 3 weeks until disease progression or unacceptable toxicity occurs, or up to 24 months in patients without disease progression.

➤ **First-line treatment in patients with metastatic nonsquamous NSCLC in combination with pemetrexed and carboplatin; locally advanced or metastatic urothelial carcinoma in patients who aren't eligible for cisplatin-containing chemotherapy or who have disease progression during or after platinum-containing chemotherapy or within 12 months of neoadjuvant or adjuvant treatment with platinum-containing chemotherapy**
Adults: 200 mg IV infusion every 3 weeks until disease progression or unacceptable toxicity occurs, or up to 24 months in patients without disease progression.

➤ **Gastric cancer**
Adults: 200 mg IV infusion every 3 weeks until disease progression or unacceptable toxicity occurs, or up to 24 months in patients without disease progression.

➤ **Urothelial carcinoma**
Adults: 200 mg IV infusion every 3 weeks until disease progression or unacceptable toxicity occurs, or up to 24 months in patients without disease progression.

➤ **Microsatellite instability-high cancer**
Adults: 200 mg IV infusion every 3 weeks until disease progression or unacceptable toxicity occurs, or up to 24 months in patients without disease progression.

➤ **Recurrent or metastatic cervical cancer with disease progression on or after chemotherapy in patients whose tumors express PD-L1 as determined by an FDA-approved test**
Adults: 200 mg IV infusion every 3 weeks until disease progresses or unacceptable toxicity occurs, or up to 24 months in patients without disease progression.

➤ **Primary mediastinal large B-cell lymphoma (PMBCL) in patients with refractory PMBCL, or who have relapsed after** two or more prior lines of therapy and who don't require urgent cytoreductive therapy

Adults: 200 mg IV infusion every 3 weeks until disease progression or unacceptable toxicity occurs, or up to 24 months in patients without disease progression.

Children age 2 and older: 2 mg/kg (up to a maximum of 200 mg/dose) IV infusion every 3 weeks until disease progression or unacceptable toxicity occurs, or up to 24 months in patients without disease progression.

➤ **First-line treatment of patients with metastatic nonsquamous NSCLC with no EGFR or ALK genomic tumor aberrations, in combination with pemetrexed and platinum chemotherapy** ⚹

Adults: 200 mg IV infusion every 3 weeks prior to other chemotherapy when given the same day. Continue until disease progression, unacceptable toxicity or up to 24 months in patients without disease progression.

✳ *NEW INDICATION:* **First-line treatment of patients with metastatic or unresectable recurrent HNSCC, in combination with platinum and 5-FU chemotherapy**

Adults: 200 mg IV infusion every 3 weeks until disease progression or unacceptable toxicity occurs, or up to 24 months in patients without disease progression. Give pembrolizumab before chemotherapy when given the same day.

✳ *NEW INDICATION:* **First-line treatment of HNSCC in patients with metastatic or unresectable recurrent tumors that express PD-L1 (combined positive score of ≥1) as determined by an FDA-approved test**

Adults: 200 mg IV infusion every 3 weeks until disease progression or unacceptable toxicity occurs, or up to 24 months in patients without disease progression.

✳ *NEW INDICATION:* **Metastatic small-cell lung cancer (SCLC) in patients with disease progression on or after platinum-based chemotherapy and at least one other prior line of therapy**

Adults: 200 mg IV infusion every 3 weeks until disease progression or unacceptable toxicity occurs, or up to 24 months in patients without disease progression.

✳ *NEW INDICATION:* **Hepatocellular carcinoma in patients previously treated with sorafenib**

Adults: 200 mg IV infusion over 30 minutes every 3 weeks until disease progression or unacceptable toxicity occurs, or up to 24 months in patients without disease progression.

✳ *NEW INDICATION:* **Recurrent locally advanced or metastatic Merkel cell carcinoma**

Adults: 200 mg IV infusion over 30 minutes every 3 weeks until disease progression or unacceptable toxicity occurs, or up to 24 months in patients without disease progression.

Children: 2 mg/kg (up to maximum of 200 mg) IV infusion over 30 minutes every 3 weeks until disease progression or unacceptable toxicity occurs, or up to 24 months in patients without disease progression.

✳ *NEW INDICATION:* **Adjuvant treatment of melanoma with lymph node involvement after complete resection**

Adults: 200 mg IV over 30 minutes every 3 weeks until disease recurrence or unacceptable toxicity, or up to 12 months in patients without disease recurrence.

✳ *NEW INDICATION:* **First-line treatment of stage III NSCLC in patients who aren't candidates for surgical resection or definitive chemoradiation, or metastatic NSCLC, and whose tumors have no EGFR or ALK genomic aberrations and express PD-L1 (tumor proportion score ≥1%) as determined by an FDA-approved test**

Adults: 200 mg IV infusion every 3 weeks until disease progression or unacceptable toxicity occurs, or up to 24 months in patients without disease progression.

✳ *NEW INDICATION:* **First-line treatment of patients with advanced renal cell carcinoma in combination with axitinib**

Adults: 200 mg IV infusion every 3 weeks in combination with 5 mg axitinib PO b.i.d. until disease progression or unacceptable toxicity occurs, or up to 24 months in patients without disease progression. May consider axitinib dosage escalation above initial 5-mg dose at intervals of 6 weeks or longer. Refer to manufacturer's instructions for axitinib dosing recommendations.

P

✦Canada   ◇OTC   ◆Off-label use   ✐Photoguide   ⊛Do not crush   *Liquid contains alcohol   ✄Genetic

✳ *NEW INDICATION:* **Recurrent locally advanced or metastatic squamous cell carcinoma of the esophagus in patients whose tumors express PD-L1 as determined by an FDA-approved test, with disease progression after one or more prior lines of systemic therapy** ▧

Adults: 200-mg IV infusion every 3 weeks until disease progression or unacceptable toxicity occurs, or up to 24 months in patients without disease progression.

✳ *NEW INDICATION:* **Recurrent locally advanced or metastatic Merkel cell carcinoma**

Adults: 200 mg IV infusion over 30 minutes every 3 weeks until disease progression or unacceptable toxicity occurs, or up to 24 months in patients without disease progression.

Children: 2 mg/kg (up to a maximum of 200 mg) IV infusion over 30 minutes every 3 weeks until disease progression or unacceptable toxicity occurs, or up to 24 months in patients without disease progression.

✳ *NEW INDICATION:* **Adjuvant treatment of melanoma with lymph node involvement following complete resection**

Adults: 200 mg IV over 30 minutes every 3 weeks until disease recurrence or unacceptable toxicity occurs, or up to 12 months in patients without disease recurrence.

✳ *NEW INDICATION:* **First-line treatment of stage III NSCLC in patients who aren't candidates for surgical resection or definitive chemoradiation or metastatic NSCLC, and whose tumors have no EGFR or ALK genomic aberrations and express PD-L1 (tumor proportion score [TPS] ≥1%) as determined by an FDA-approved test**

Adults: 200 mg IV infusion every 3 weeks until disease progression or unacceptable toxicity occurs, or up to 24 months in patients without disease progression.

✳ *NEW INDICATION:* **First-line treatment of patients with advanced renal cell carcinoma in combination with axitinib**

Adults: 200-mg IV infusion every 3 weeks in combination with 5 mg axitinib PO b.i.d. until disease progression or unacceptable toxicity occurs, or up to 24 months in patients without disease progression. Dose escalation of axitinib above the initial 5-mg dose

may be considered at intervals of 6 weeks or longer.

✳ *NEW INDICATION:* **Advanced endometrial carcinoma that's not microsatellite instability-high or mismatch repair deficient in patients who have disease progression following prior systemic therapy and are not candidates for curative surgery or radiation in combination with lenvatinib**

Adults: 200 mg IV infusion every 3 weeks in combination with lenvatinib 20 mg PO once daily until disease progression or unacceptable toxicity occurs, or (for pembrolizumab), up to 24 months in patients without disease progression. Refer to the lenvatinib prescribing information for recommended dosing information.

ADMINISTRATION

IV

▼ Don't give as IV push or bolus.

▼ Reconstitute lyophilized powder with 2.3 mL of sterile water to yield vial concentration of 25 mg/mL.

▼ After reconstitution, slowly swirl vial; don't shake. Allow up to 5 minutes for bubbles to clear. Inspect for particulate matter and discoloration.

▼ Dilute to yield 1 to 10 mg/mL in bag of NSS or D₅W. Gently invert bag to mix solution.

▼ Discard unused portion left in vial.

▼ Administer infusion over 30 minutes using an IV line with a nonpyrogenic, low-protein-binding 0.2- to 5-micron filter.

▼ Diluted solution is stable for 24 hours if refrigerated and for 6 hours at room temperature. Don't freeze.

▼ **Incompatibilities:** Other drugs.

ACTION

A humanized monoclonal antibody that binds to the PD1 receptor found on the surface of T cells, reversing T-cell suppression and resulting in decreased tumor growth.

Route	Onset	Peak	Duration
IV	Unknown	Unknown	Unknown

Half-life: 22 days.

ADVERSE REACTIONS

CNS: fatigue, fever, confusion, peripheral neuropathy, weakness, headache, dizziness, insomnia. **CV:** peripheral edema. **EENT:** uveitis. **GI:** nausea, constipation, diarrhea, vomiting, abdominal pain, colitis. **GU:** *renal failure,* nephritis, UTI. **Hematologic:** anemia, lymphocytopenia, *thrombocytopenia.* **Hepatic:** *hepatitis.* **Metabolic:** decreased appetite; hypophysitis; immune-mediated hyperthyroidism; immune-mediated hypothyroidism; hyperglycemia; hyponatremia; hypoalbuminemia; hypertriglyceridemia; increased AST, ALT, and alkaline phosphatase levels; hypocalcemia. **Musculoskeletal:** arthralgia, musculoskeletal pain, myalgia, myositis, immune-mediated arthritis. **Respiratory:** cough, dyspnea, URI, pneumonitis, pneumonia, pleural effusion, *respiratory failure.* **Skin:** pruritus, rash, immune-mediated rash, vitiligo. **Other:** antibody development, chills, *sepsis.*

INTERACTIONS

Drug-drug. *Thalidomide:* May increase mortality in patients with multiple myeloma when used with pembrolizumab and dexamethasone. This combination isn't recommended.

EFFECTS ON LAB TEST RESULTS

• May increase glucose, triglyceride, cholesterol, creatinine, alkaline phosphatase, ALT, and AST levels.
• May decrease sodium, calcium, WBC, and albumin levels.
• May decrease Hb level and lymphocyte and platelet counts.

CONTRAINDICATIONS & CAUTIONS

• Contraindicated in patients hypersensitive to drug or its components.
▧ ◐ *Alert:* Patients with EGFR or ALK genomic tumor aberrations should have disease progression on FDA-approved therapy for these aberrations before receiving pembrolizumab.
◐ *Alert:* Drug can cause immune-mediated reactions (such as pneumonitis, hepatitis, endocrinopathies, colitis, nephritis, and renal dysfunction); drug may need to be withheld or permanently discontinued.

• Severe, life-threatening infusion-related reactions have occurred in patients receiving drug. Stop infusion immediately and administer supportive care.
• Use hasn't been studied in patients with moderate or severe hepatic impairment.
• Safety and effectiveness in children younger than age 18 haven't been established.
Dialyzable drug: Unknown.

PREGNANCY-LACTATION-REPRODUCTION

• Drug may cause fetal harm. Don't use in pregnant women. Women of childbearing potential should use highly effective contraception during therapy and for 4 months after final dose.
• It isn't known if drug appears in human milk. Patient shouldn't breastfeed during therapy and for 4 months after final dose.

NURSING CONSIDERATIONS

• Must be administered with 0.2- to 5-micron filter.
• Monitor patient closely for signs and symptoms of hypersensitivity or infusion reactions. Stop infusion and have drugs, such as epinephrine, antihistamines, and corticosteroids, available for immediate treatment of such a reaction.
• Assess for signs and symptoms of immune-mediated reactions. Thyroid disorders, liver toxicity, and hypophysitis typically occur early in treatment. Pulmonary, renal, and GI toxicity may develop after 6 months of treatment.
• Monitor patient for immune-mediated pneumonitis (shortness of breath, chest pain, new or worsening cough). Evaluate radiographically, give corticosteroids if clinically indicated, and withhold or discontinue drug based on grade.
• Monitor patient for signs and symptoms of immune-mediated colitis (increased frequency of bowel movements or diarrhea; abdominal pain or tenderness; melena; black, tarry stools). Give corticosteroids as clinically indicated and withhold or discontinue drug based on toxicity grade.
• Monitor patient for signs and symptoms of immune-mediated hepatitis (elevated liver

P

enzyme levels, jaundice, tea-colored urine, nausea, vomiting, anorexia, right upper quadrant abdominal pain, abnormal bleeding or bruising). Give corticosteroids as clinically indicated and withhold or discontinue drug based on toxicity grade.

• Monitor patient for signs and symptoms of hypophysitis, the immune-mediated inflammation of the pituitary gland (persistent or unusual headaches, extreme weakness, dizziness, fainting, vision changes). Give corticosteroids and hormone replacement as clinically indicated and withhold or discontinue drug based on toxicity grade.

• Monitor patient for signs and symptoms of immune-mediated endocrine disorders (hypothyroidism, hyperthyroidism, adrenal insufficiency), which may include tachycardia, weight loss or gain, edema, and hair loss. Assess hormone levels at baseline, periodically during treatment, and as clinically indicated. Give corticosteroids and hormone replacement as clinically indicated and withhold or discontinue drug based on toxicity grade.

• Be aware of potential for less common immune-mediated adverse reactions, such as exfoliative dermatitis, uveitis, arthritis, myositis, pancreatitis, hemolytic anemia, and partial seizures in patients with inflammatory foci in the brain. Based on severity of adverse reaction, withhold drug and administer corticosteroids. Upon improvement to grade 1 or less, initiate corticosteroid tapering and continue to taper over at least 1 month. Restart drug if adverse reaction remains at grade 1 or less. Permanently discontinue drug for any severe or grade 3 immune-mediated adverse reaction that recurs and for any life-threatening immune-mediated adverse reaction.

PATIENT TEACHING

• Caution patient about the risk of immune-mediated adverse effects that may require corticosteroid treatment and interruption of therapy or discontinuation of drug.

• Teach patient signs and symptoms of lung problems (dyspnea, chest pain, cough), colitis (diarrhea; black, tarry stools; abdominal pain), liver problems (yellowing of the skin

or eyes, dark urine, nausea or vomiting, decreased appetite, abdominal pain, bleeding or bruising), hormone gland problems (rapid heartbeat, weight loss, increased sweating, weight gain, hair loss, feeling cold), renal problems (changes in the amount or color of urine), and other problems (rash, vision changes, muscle or joint pain, muscle weakness) and to report them to prescriber.

• Advise female patient to inform prescriber if she becomes pregnant, plans to become pregnant, or is breastfeeding.

• Inform patient of potential hazard to the fetus and advise female patient to use contraception during therapy and for 4 months after final dose.

• Advise breastfeeding patient to stop breastfeeding during therapy and for 4 months after final dose.

• Instruct patient to keep lab test appointments as requested by prescriber to monitor drug's safety and effectiveness.

SAFETY ALERT!

PEMEtrexed disodium
pem-e-TREKS-ed

Alimta

Therapeutic class: Antineoplastics
Pharmacologic class: Folate antagonists

AVAILABLE FORMS
Injection: 100 mg, 500 mg in single-use vials

INDICATIONS & DOSAGES
Adjust-a-dose (for all indications): Refer to manufacturer's instructions for toxicity-related dosage adjustments.

➤ **Malignant pleural mesothelioma in patients whose disease is unresectable or who aren't candidates for curative surgery, in combination with cisplatin; locally advanced or metastatic NSCLC (nonsquamous) as initial treatment, in combination with cisplatin**
Adults: 500 mg/m^2 IV infusion over 10 minutes on day 1 of each 21-day cycle. Starting 30 minutes after pemetrexed infusion ends.

➤ **Locally advanced or metastatic NSCLC after prior chemotherapy; as maintenance therapy for patients whose disease hasn't progressed after four cycles of platinum-based first-line chemotherapy, as single-agent therapy**
Adults: 500 mg/m^2 IV infusion on day 1 of each 21-day cycle.

➤ **Initial treatment of metastatic, non-squamous NSCLC in combination with platinum chemotherapy and pembrolizumab**
Adults: 500 mg/m^2 IV infusion administered before carboplatin on day 1 of each 21-day cycle for four cycles. After completion of platinum-based therapy, may give pemetrexed as maintenance therapy, alone or with pembrolizumab, until disease progression or unacceptable toxicity occurs. Give pembrolizumab before pemetrexed when both drugs are administered on the same day. Refer to the full prescribing information for pembrolizumab and carboplatin.

✳ *NEW INDICATION:* **In combination with cisplatin for initial treatment of patients with locally advanced or metastatic, non-squamous NSCLC**
Adults: 500 mg/m^2 IV infusion over 10 minutes administered before cisplatin on day 1 of each 21-day cycle for up to six cycles in the absence of disease progression or unacceptable toxicity.

✳ *NEW INDICATION:* **Initial treatment of metastatic nonsquamous NSCLC with no EGFR or ALK genomic tumor aberrations, in combination with pembrolizumab and platinum chemotherapy**
Adults: 500 mg/m^2 IV infusion over 10 minutes administered after pembrolizumab and before carboplatin or cisplatin on day 1 of each 21-day cycle for four cycles. After completion of platinum-based therapy, may give pemetrexed as maintenance therapy, alone or with pembrolizumab, until disease progression or unacceptable toxicity occurs. Refer to the full prescribing information for pembrolizumab and carboplatin or cisplatin.

ADMINISTRATION

IV

▼ Hazardous drug; use safe handling and disposal precautions.

▼ Premedicate with folic acid 400 to 1,000 mcg PO once daily beginning 7 days before first dose of drug and continued during therapy and for 21 days after last dose. Administer vitamin B$_{12}$ 1 mg IM 1 week before first dose of pemetrexed and every three cycles thereafter. Administer dexamethasone 4 mg PO b.i.d. the day before, the day of, and the day after pemetrexed administration.

▼ Reconstitute 100-mg vial with 4.2 mL or 500-mg vial with 20 mL of preservative-free NSS to yield 25 mg/mL.

▼ Swirl vial gently until powder is completely dissolved. Solution should be clear and colorless to yellow or yellow-green.

▼ Calculate appropriate dose, and further dilute with NSS so total volume of solution is 100 mL.

▼ Give over 10 minutes.

▼ Reconstituted solution and dilution are stable for 24 hours refrigerated.

▼ **Incompatibilities:** Calcium-containing diluents, including Ringer or lactated Ringer for injection; other drugs or diluents.

ACTION

Disturbs cell replication by inhibiting several folate-dependent enzymes involved in nucleotide synthesis. When given with other antineoplastics, drug inhibits growth of mesothelioma cell lines.

Route	Onset	Peak	Duration
IV	Unknown	Unknown	Unknown

Half-life: 3½ hours.

ADVERSE REACTIONS

CNS: depression, fatigue, fever, neuropathy. **CV:** *cardiac ischemia*, edema, thrombosis. **EENT:** pharyngitis, conjunctivitis. **GI:** anorexia, constipation, diarrhea, nausea, stomatitis, vomiting, esophagitis, painful, difficult swallowing, taste disturbance. **GU:** *renal failure.* **Hematologic:** anemia, *leukopenia, neutropenia, febrile neutropenia, thrombocytopenia.* **Metabolic:** dehydration, elevated creatinine level,

P

hyperglycemia, hypoalbuminemia, hyponatremia, hypophosphatemia, increased alkaline phosphatase level, hypocalcemia, hyperkalemia, hypokalemia. **Musculoskeletal:** arthralgia, myalgia. **Respiratory:** dyspnea. **Skin:** alopecia, rash. **Other:** allergic reaction, infection.

INTERACTIONS
Drug-drug. *Nephrotoxic drugs, probenecid:* May delay pemetrexed clearance. Monitor patient.
NSAIDs: May decrease pemetrexed clearance in patients with mild to moderate renal insufficiency. For NSAIDs with short half-lives, avoid use for 2 days before, during, and 2 days after pemetrexed therapy. For NSAIDs with long half-lives, avoid use for 5 days before, during, and 2 days after pemetrexed therapy.

EFFECTS ON LAB TEST RESULTS
• May increase ALT, AST, and creatinine levels. May decrease Hb level and hematocrit.
• May decrease absolute neutrophil, platelet, and WBC counts.

CONTRAINDICATIONS & CAUTIONS
• Contraindicated in patients with a history of severe hypersensitivity reaction to drug.
• Don't use in patients with CrCl of less than 45 mL/minute.
• There is increased risk of renal impairment in patients taking ibuprofen. In patients with CrCl between 45 and 79 mL/minute, avoid ibuprofen 2 days before, the day of, and 2 days after pemetrexed administration.
Dialyzable drug: Unknown.
⚠ *Overdose S&S:* Neutropenia, anemia, thrombocytopenia, mucositis, rash, infection with or without fever, diarrhea.

PREGNANCY-LACTATION-REPRODUCTION
• There are no adequate studies in pregnant women. Drug can cause fetal harm. Women should avoid becoming pregnant and use effective contraception during therapy and for 6 months after final dose. Male partners should use contraception during treatment and for 3 months after final dose.

• If drug is used during pregnancy or if patient becomes pregnant during therapy, apprise her of potential for harm to the fetus.
• It isn't known if drug appears in human milk. Patient should discontinue breastfeeding or discontinue drug.

NURSING CONSIDERATIONS
• Patient shouldn't start a new cycle of treatment unless ANC is 1,500/mm³ or more, platelet count is 100,000/mm³ or more, and CrCl is 45 mL/minute or more.
• Patients with pleural effusion and ascites may need to have effusion drained before therapy.
• Monitor renal function, CBC, platelet count, Hb level, hematocrit, and LFT values.
• Assess patient for neurotoxicity, mucositis, and diarrhea. Severe symptoms may warrant dosage adjustment.
🛈 *Alert:* To reduce the occurrence and severity of cutaneous reactions, give a corticosteroid, such as dexamethasone 4 mg PO b.i.d., the day before, the day of, and the day after giving this drug.
🛈 *Alert:* To reduce toxicity, patient should take 400 to 1,000 mcg of folic acid daily, 5 days before therapy until 21 days after therapy.
🛈 *Alert:* Give vitamin B₁₂ 1,000 mcg IM once during the week before the first dose and every three cycles thereafter. After the first cycle, vitamin injections may be given on the first day of the cycle.
• *Look alike–sound alike:* Don't confuse pemetrexed with methotrexate or pralatrexate.

PATIENT TEACHING
• Inform patient that corticosteroids and vitamins will be given before pemetrexed to help minimize its adverse effects.
• Tell patient to avoid NSAIDs for several days before, during, and after treatment.
• Urge patient to report adverse effects, especially fever, sore throat, infection, diarrhea, fatigue, bleeding, cough, shortness of breath, and limb pain.

penicillin G benzathine (benzathine benzylpenicillin)
pen-i-SILL-in

Bicillin L-A

Therapeutic class: Antibiotics
Pharmacologic class: Natural penicillins

AVAILABLE FORMS
Injection: 600,000 units/mL per syringe (1 mL); 1,200,000 units per syringe (2 mL); 2,400,000 units per syringe (4 mL)

INDICATIONS & DOSAGES
➤ **Congenital syphilis**
Children ages 2 to 12: Adjust dosage based on adult dosage schedule.
Children younger than age 2: 50,000 units/kg (up to 2.4 million units) IM as a single dose.
➤ **Group A streptococcal URIs**
Adults: 1.2 million units IM as a single injection.
Children weighing 27 kg or more: 900,000 units IM as a single injection.
Infants and children weighing less than 27 kg: 300,000 to 600,000 units IM as a single injection.
➤ **To prevent poststreptococcal rheumatic fever and glomerulonephritis**
Adults and children: 1.2 million units IM once monthly or 600,000 units IM every 2 weeks.
➤ **Syphilis (primary, secondary, and latent)**
Adults: 2.4 million units IM as a single dose.
➤ **Syphilis (tertiary and neurosyphilis)**
Adults: 2.4 million units IM once every 7 days for 3 weeks.
➤ **Yaws, bejel, and pinta**
Adults: 1.2 million units IM as a single injection.

ADMINISTRATION
IM
Black Box Warning Inadvertent IV use may cause cardiac arrest and death. ■
• Before giving drug, ask patient about allergic reactions to penicillin.

• Obtain specimen for culture and sensitivity tests before giving first dose. Begin therapy while awaiting results.
• Shake well before injecting.
• Inject deep into upper outer quadrant of buttocks in adults and in midlateral thigh in infants and small children. Rotate injection sites. Avoid injection into or near major nerves or blood vessels to prevent permanent neurovascular damage.
• Injection may be painful, but ice applied to the site may ease discomfort.
• Store in refrigerator at 36° to 46° F (2° to 8° C); don't freeze.

ACTION
Inhibits cell-wall synthesis during bacterial multiplication.

Route	Onset	Peak	Duration
IM	Unknown	13–24 hr	1–4 wk

Half-life: Unknown.

ADVERSE REACTIONS
CNS: neuropathy. **GI:** *pseudomembranous colitis,* enterocolitis, nausea, vomiting. **GU:** nephropathy. **Hematologic:** *agranulocytosis, leukopenia, thrombocytopenia,* eosinophilia, hemolytic anemia. **Skin:** exfoliative dermatitis, maculopapular rash. **Other:** *anaphylaxis,* hypersensitivity reactions, sterile abscess at injection site.

INTERACTIONS
Drug-drug. *Aminoglycosides:* Physical and chemical incompatibility. Give separately.
Live-virus vaccines: May decrease effectiveness of live-virus vaccines. Avoid concurrent use.
Methotrexate: May increase risk of methotrexate toxicity. Monitor patient closely.
Probenecid: May increase penicillin level. Probenecid may be used for this purpose.
Tetracycline: May antagonize penicillin G benzathine effects. Avoid using together.
Warfarin: May increase anticoagulant effects. Monitor therapy.

EFFECTS ON LAB TEST RESULTS
• May increase BUN, creatinine, and AST levels.

P

• May decrease Hb level.
• May increase eosinophil count. May decrease platelet, WBC, and granulocyte counts. May cause positive Coombs test results.
• May falsely decrease aminoglycoside level. May cause false-positive CSF protein test results. May alter urine glucose testing using cupric sulfate (Benedict reagent).

CONTRAINDICATIONS & CAUTIONS
• Contraindicated in patients hypersensitive to drug or other penicillins.
Black Box Warning Not for IV use or to be mixed with other IV solutions. Risk of cardiorespiratory arrest and death. ∎
• Inadvertent intravascular administration, including inadvertent direct intra-arterial injection or injection immediately adjacent to arteries, has resulted in severe neurovascular damage, including transverse myelitis with permanent paralysis, gangrene requiring amputation of digits and more proximal portions of extremities, and necrosis and sloughing at and surrounding the injection site.
• Use cautiously in patients allergic to other drugs, especially to cephalosporins, because of possible cross-sensitivity.
• Use cautiously in patients with a history of significant allergies or asthma.
• Drug may cause CDAD ranging in severity from mild diarrhea to fatal colitis. If CDAD is suspected or confirmed, drug may need to be discontinued and treatment initiated.
Dialyzable drug: Yes.
⚠ *Overdose S&S:* Neuromuscular hyperexcitability, seizures.

PREGNANCY-LACTATION-REPRODUCTION
• There are no adequate studies in pregnant women and there is no evidence of adverse effects on fetus; neither have animal studies shown adverse fetal effects. Use during pregnancy only if clearly needed.
• Drug appears in human milk. Use cautiously in breastfeeding women.

NURSING CONSIDERATIONS
◉ *Alert:* Bicillin L-A is the only penicillin G benzathine product indicated for sexually

transmitted infections. Don't substitute Bicillin C-R because it may not be effective.
• Monitor patient for diarrhea. Drug may need to be stopped.
• Drug's extremely slow absorption time makes allergic reactions difficult to treat.
• If large doses are given or if therapy is prolonged, bacterial or fungal superinfection may occur, especially in elderly, debilitated or immunosuppressed patients.
• *Look alike–sound alike:* Don't confuse penicillin G benzathine with Polycillin, penicillamine, or the various other types of penicillin.

PATIENT TEACHING
• Tell patient to report adverse reactions promptly.
• Inform patient that fever and increased WBC count are the most common reactions.
• Warn patient that IM injection may be painful but that ice applied to the site may ease discomfort.

penicillin G potassium (benzylpenicillin potassium)
pen-i-SILL-in

Pfizerpen

Therapeutic class: Antibiotics
Pharmacologic class: Natural penicillins

AVAILABLE FORMS
Injection: 1 million units, 5 million units, 20 million units
Premixed injection: 1 million units/50 mL, 2 million units/50 mL, 3 million units/50 mL

INDICATIONS & DOSAGES
Adjust-a-dose (for all indications): For uremic patients with a CrCl greater than 10 mL/minute/1.73 m^2, give full loading dose followed by one-half of loading dose every 4 to 5 hours. If CrCl is less than 10 mL/minute/1.73 m^2, give full loading dose followed by one-half of loading dose every 8 to 10 hours. Make additional dosage modification in patients with hepatic disease and renal impairment.

➤ **Actinomycosis**
Adults: For cervicofacial infections, 1 to 6 million units/day in divided doses IM or IV every 4 to 6 hours. For thoracic or abdominal infections, 10 to 20 million units/day in divided doses IM or IV every 4 to 6 hours or by continuous IV infusion.

➤ **Anthrax**
Adults: 8 million units/day in divided doses IM or IV every 6 hours; higher doses may be required depending on susceptibility of the organism.

➤ **Clostridial infections**
Adults: 20 million units/day in divided doses IM or IV every 4 to 6 hours.

➤ **Diphtheria**
Adults: 2 to 3 million units/day in divided doses IM or IV every 4 to 6 hours for 10 to 12 days.
Children: 150,000 to 250,000 units/kg/day in equal doses IM or IV every 6 hours for 7 to 10 days.

➤ **Disseminated gonococcal infections**
Adults: 10 million units/day in divided doses IM or IV every 4 to 6 hours. Duration depends on type of infection.
Children weighing 45 kg or more with arthritis, endocarditis, or meningitis: 10 million units/day in four equally divided doses IM or IV, with duration of therapy depending on type of infection.
Children weighing less than 45 kg with arthritis: 100,000 units/kg/day in four equally divided doses IM or IV for 7 to 10 days.
Children weighing less than 45 kg with endocarditis: 250,000 units/kg/day in equal doses IM or IV every 4 hours for 4 weeks.
Children weighing less than 45 kg with meningitis: 250,000 units/kg/day in equal doses IM or IV every 4 hours for 10 to 14 days.

➤ *Erysipelothrix* **endocarditis**
Adults: 12 to 20 million units/day in divided doses IM or IV every 4 to 6 hours for 4 to 6 weeks.

➤ **Fusospirochetosis**
Adults: 5 to 10 million units/day in divided doses IM or IV every 4 to 6 hours.

➤ **Haverhill fever; rat bite fever**
Adults: 12 to 20 million units/day in divided doses IM or IV every 4 to 6 hours for 3 to 4 weeks.

➤ **Haverhill fever (with endocarditis caused by** *Streptobacillus moniliformis***); rat bite fever**
Children: 150,000 to 250,000 units/kg/day in equal doses every 4 hours for 4 weeks.

➤ *Listeria monocytogenes* **endocarditis or meningitis**
Adults: 15 to 20 million units/day in divided doses IM or IV every 4 to 6 hours. Treat for 2 weeks for meningitis and 4 weeks for endocarditis.

➤ **Meningococcal meningitis or septicemia**
Adults: 24 million units/day as 2 million units IM or IV every 2 hours.

➤ **Neurosyphilis**
Adults: 12 to 24 million units/day (2 to 4 million units every 4 hours) IM or IV for 10 to 14 days. Many experts recommend penicillin G benzathine 2.4 million units IM weekly for 3 weeks following completion of this regimen.

➤ *Pasteurella multocida* **bacteremia or meningitis**
Adults: 4 to 6 million units/day in divided doses IM or IV every 4 to 6 hours for 2 weeks.

➤ **Serious staphylococcal infections**
Adults: 5 to 24 million units/day in equally divided doses IM or IV every 4 to 6 hours.

➤ **Serious streptococcal infections**
Adults: 12 to 24 million units/day in equally divided doses IM or IV every 4 to 6 hours.

➤ **Meningitis caused by susceptible strains of pneumococcus and meningococcus**
Children: 250,000 units/kg/day in equal doses IM or IV every 4 hours for 7 to 14 days, depending on infecting organism. Maximum dosage is 12 to 20 million units/day.

➤ **Serious streptococcal infections, such as pneumonia and endocarditis (***Streptococcus pneumoniae***), and meningococcal infections**
Children: 150,000 to 300,000 units/kg/day in equal doses IM or IV every 4 to 6 hours. Duration of therapy depends on infecting organism and type of infection.

➤ **Syphilis (congenital and neurosyphilis) after newborn period**

P

Children: 200,000 to 300,000 units/kg/day (administered as 50,000 units/kg IV every 4 to 6 hours) for 10 to 14 days.

➤ **Leptospirosis**
Adults: 1.5 million units IV every 6 hours for 7 days.

ADMINISTRATION

• May give IM or by continuous IV infusion for dosages of 500,000, 1 million, or 5 million units. Drug is also suitable for intrapleural, intra-articular, intrathecal, and other local instillations.

• Administer 20 million unit dosage form by IV infusion only.

❸ *Alert:* Don't use in children requiring less than 1 million units/dose.

IV

▼ Before giving drug, ask patient about allergic reactions to penicillin.

▼ Obtain specimen for culture and sensitivity tests before giving first dose. Begin therapy while awaiting results.

▼ Reconstitute drug with sterile water for injection or NSS for injection. Volume of diluent varies with manufacturer.

▼ Reconstituted solution may be stored in refrigerator for up to 7 days.

▼ For continuous infusion, add reconstituted drug to 1 to 2 L of compatible solution. Determine how much fluid is needed and what the rate should be for a 24-hour period; then, add the drug to this fluid.

▼ Don't administer premixed solutions to patients requiring less than 1 million units per dose.

▼ Intermittent IV infusions have been administered over 15 to 30 minutes for infants and children and over 1 to 2 hours for adults.

▼ Thaw frozen bags at room temperature. May keep at room temperature for 24 hours or under refrigeration for 14 days. Don't refreeze thawed antibiotics.

▼ **Incompatibilities:** None listed by manufacturer. Consult a drug incompatibility reference for more information.

IM

• Vials containing more than 5 million units aren't intended for IM use.

• Before giving drug, ask patient about allergic reactions to penicillin.

• Obtain specimen for culture and sensitivity tests before giving first dose. Begin therapy while awaiting results.

• IM is the preferred route. Keep total volume of injection small.

• Give deep into large muscle; injection may be extremely painful.

• IM injection may be painful, but ice applied to the site may help alleviate discomfort.

ACTION

Inhibits cell-wall synthesis during bacterial multiplication.

Route	Onset	Peak	Duration
IV	Immediate	Immediate	Unknown
IM	Unknown	15–30 min	Unknown

Half-life: 30 to 60 minutes.

ADVERSE REACTIONS

CNS: *seizures,* agitation, anxiety, confusion, depression, dizziness, fatigue, hallucinations, lethargy, hyperreflexia, myoclonic twitches, neuropathy. **CV:** thrombophlebitis, *cardiac arrest, arrhythmias.* **GI:** *pseudomembranous colitis,* enterocolitis, nausea, vomiting. **GU:** interstitial nephritis, nephropathy. **Hematologic:** *agranulocytosis, leukopenia, thrombocytopenia,* anemia, eosinophilia, hemolytic anemia. **Metabolic:** *hyperkalemia.* **Musculoskeletal:** arthralgia, myalgia. **Skin:** exfoliative dermatitis, maculopapular eruptions, pain at injection site. **Other:** *anaphylaxis,* hypersensitivity reactions, overgrowth of nonsusceptible organisms.

INTERACTIONS

Drug-drug. *Aminoglycosides:* Physically and chemically incompatible. Administer separately.

Aspirin, furosemide, indomethacin, sulfonamides, thiazide diuretics: May compete with penicillin for renal tubular secretion, prolonging penicillin half-life. Monitor patient.

Bacteriostatic antibacterial agents (chloramphenicol, macrolide antibiotics, sulfonamides, tetracyclines): Physically and chemically incompatible. Give separately.

Reactions in bold italics are *life-threatening*. Interactions may have a *rapid onset* or a *delayed onset*.

Heparin: May increase risk of bleeding. Closely monitor patient and adjust heparin dosage as needed.

Hormonal contraceptives: May decrease hormonal contraceptive effectiveness. Advise use of additional form of contraception during therapy.

Live-virus vaccines: May decrease effectiveness of live-virus vaccines. Don't use together.

Methotrexate: May increase risk of methotrexate toxicity. Monitor patient closely.

Oral anticoagulants: May increase or decrease anticoagulant effects. Monitor PT and INR.

Potassium-sparing diuretics: May increase risk of hyperkalemia. Avoid using together.

Probenecid: May increase penicillin level. Probenecid may be used for this purpose.

EFFECTS ON LAB TEST RESULTS
• May increase potassium level. May decrease Hb level.
• May increase eosinophil count. May decrease platelet, WBC, and granulocyte counts.
• May cause positive Coombs test result.
• May falsely decrease aminoglycoside levels. May cause false-positive CSF protein test result. May alter urine glucose testing using cupric sulfate (Benedict reagent).

CONTRAINDICATIONS & CAUTIONS
• Contraindicated in patients hypersensitive to drug or other penicillins.
• Use cautiously in patients with other drug allergies, especially to cephalosporins, because of possible cross-sensitivity.
• Use cautiously in patients with renal impairment or asthma.
• Drug may cause CDAD ranging in severity from mild diarrhea to fatal colitis. If CDAD is suspected or confirmed, drug may need to be discontinued and treatment initiated.
Dialyzable drug: Yes.
⚠ *Overdose S&S:* Agitation, confusion, asterixis, hallucinations, stupor, coma, multifocal myoclonus, seizures, encephalopathy, hyperkalemia.

PREGNANCY-LACTATION-REPRODUCTION
• There are no adequate studies in pregnant women. Animal studies reveal no evidence of fetal harm. Use during pregnancy only if clearly needed.
• Use cautiously in breastfeeding women.

NURSING CONSIDERATIONS
• Before starting drug, obtain culture and susceptibility tests to identify organisms causing infection.
• Monitor renal function closely. Patients with poor renal function may have increased levels of penicillin and are at increased risk for adverse effects.
• Due to increased risk of electrolyte imbalances, monitor potassium and sodium levels closely in patients receiving more than 10 million units IV daily.
• Observe patient closely. With large doses and prolonged therapy, bacterial or fungal superinfection may occur, especially in elderly, debilitated, or immunosuppressed patients.
• For most acute infections, continue treatment for at least 48 to 72 hours after patient becomes asymptomatic. For group A betahemolytic streptococcal infections, maintain treatment for at least 10 days to reduce risk of rheumatic fever.
• *Look alike–sound alike:* Don't confuse penicillin G potassium with Polycillin, penicillamine, or the various other types of penicillin.

PATIENT TEACHING
• Tell patient to notify prescriber if rash, fever, or chills develop. A rash is the most common allergic reaction.
• Warn patient that IM injection may be painful but that ice applied to the site may help alleviate discomfort.

P

penicillin G procaine
(benzylpenicillin procaine)
pen-i-SILL-in

Therapeutic class: Antibiotics
Pharmacologic class: Natural penicillins

AVAILABLE FORMS
Injection: 600,000 units/mL

INDICATIONS & DOSAGES
➤ **Cutaneous anthrax**
Adults: 600,000 to 1 million units/day IM.
➤ **Inhalational anthrax (postexposure)**
Adults: 1.2 million units IM every 12 hours. Available safety data for penicillin G procaine at this dose would best support a duration of therapy of 2 weeks or less.
Children: 25,000 units/kg (maximum, 1.2 million units) IM every 12 hours.
Note: Treatment of inhalational anthrax (postexposure) must be continued for a total of 60 days. Consider risks and benefits of continuing administration of penicillin G procaine for more than 2 weeks or switching to an effective alternative treatment.
➤ **Bacterial endocarditis (group A streptococci), only in extremely sensitive infections**
Adults: 600,000 to 1 million units/day IM.
➤ **Adjunctive therapy for diphtheria with antitoxin**
Adults: 300,000 to 600,000 units/day IM for 14 days.
➤ **Diphtheria carrier state**
Adults: 300,000 units/day IM for 10 days.
➤ **Erysipeloid**
Adults: 600,000 to 1 million units/day IM.
➤ **Fusospirochetosis (Vincent infection)**
Adults: 600,000 to 1 million units/day IM.
➤ **Pneumonia (pneumococcal), moderately severe (uncomplicated)**
Adults and children weighing 27.3 kg or more: 600,000 to 1 million units/day IM for a minimum of 10 days.
➤ **Rat bite fever (*Streptobacillus moniliformis* and *Spirillum minus*)**
Adults: 600,000 to 1 million units/day IM.
➤ **Staphylococcal infections, moderately severe to severe**
Adults and children weighing 27.3 kg or more: 600,000 to 1 million units/day IM for a minimum of 10 days.
Children weighing less than 27.3 kg: 300,000 units/day IM.
➤ **Streptococcal infections (group A), including moderately severe to severe tonsillitis, erysipelas, scarlet fever, URI, and skin and soft-tissue infections**
Adults: 600,000 to 1 million units/day IM for minimum of 10 days.
Children weighing less than 27.3 kg: 300,000 units/day IM.

➤ **Syphilis (primary, secondary, and latent syphilis with negative spinal fluid)**
Adults and children older than age 12: 600,000 units/day IM for 8 days; total, 4.8 million units.
➤ **Late syphilis (tertiary syphilis, neurosyphilis, and latent syphilis with positive spinal fluid exam or no spinal fluid exam)**
Adults: 600,000 units/day IM for 10 to 15 days; total, 6 to 9 million units.
➤ **Yaws, bejel, pinta**
Adults: Treatment as for syphilis in the corresponding stage of disease.

ADMINISTRATION
IM
• Before giving drug, ask patient about allergic reactions to penicillin.
• Obtain specimen for culture and sensitivity tests before giving first dose. Begin therapy while awaiting results.
• Give deep in upper outer quadrant of buttocks in adults and in midlateral thigh in small children. Rotate injection sites. Don't give subcut. Don't massage injection site. Avoid injection near major nerves or blood vessels.
• Inject at a slow, steady rate to avoid needle blockage caused by high concentration of suspended material in product.
❸ *Alert:* Inadvertent IV, intravascular, or intra-arterial administration may cause severe or permanent neurovascular damage.
• IM injection may be painful, but ice applied to the site may help alleviate discomfort.

ACTION
Inhibits cell-wall synthesis during bacterial multiplication.

Route	Onset	Peak	Duration
IM	Unknown	1–4 hr	15–20 hr

Half-life: 30 to 60 minutes.

ADVERSE REACTIONS
CNS: *seizures,* agitation, anxiety, confusion, depression, dizziness, fatigue, hallucinations, lethargy, chills, fever. **GI:** *pseudomembranous colitis,* enterocolitis, nausea, vomiting. **GU:** interstitial nephritis, nephropathy. **Musculoskeletal:** arthralgia.

Reactions in bold italics are *life-threatening*. Interactions may have a *rapid onset* or a *delayed onset*.

Skin: rash. **Other:** *anaphylaxis,* hypersensitivity reactions, overgrowth of nonsusceptible organisms.

INTERACTIONS
Drug-drug. *Aminoglycosides:* Physically and chemically incompatible. Give separately.
Hormonal contraceptives: May decrease hormonal contraceptive effectiveness. Advise use of additional form of contraception during therapy.
Live-virus vaccines: May decrease vaccine effectiveness. Avoid concurrent use.
Methotrexate: May increase risk of methotrexate toxicity. Monitor patient closely.
Oral anticoagulants (warfarin): May increase or decrease effects of warfarin. Monitor coagulation status and adjust warfarin dosage as needed.
Probenecid: May increase penicillin level. Probenecid may be used for this purpose.
Tetracycline: May antagonize bactericidal effect of penicillin. Avoid concurrent use of these drugs.

EFFECTS ON LAB TEST RESULTS
• May decrease Hb level.
• May increase eosinophil count. May decrease platelet, WBC, and granulocyte counts.

CONTRAINDICATIONS & CAUTIONS
• Contraindicated in patients hypersensitive to drug or other penicillins.
• Use cautiously in patients with other drug allergies, especially to cephalosporins, because of possible cross-sensitivity. Some formulations contain sulfites, which may cause allergic reactions in sensitive people.
• In patients with a history of hypersensitivity to procaine, administer intradermal test with 0.1 mL of 1% or 2% procaine solution and observe for wheal, flare, or eruption. If these occur, don't use drug and treat sensitivity supportively.
• Use cautiously in patients with a history of seizure disorders and renal impairment.
• Drug may cause CDAD ranging in severity from mild diarrhea to fatal colitis. If CDAD is suspected or confirmed, drug may need to be discontinued and treatment initiated.

Dializable drug: Yes.
⚠ *Overdose S&S:* Neuromuscular hyperexcitability, seizures.

PREGNANCY-LACTATION-REPRODUCTION
• There are no adequate studies in pregnant women and there is no human evidence of adverse effects on the fetus if drug is used during pregnancy. Use during pregnancy only when clearly needed.
• Drug appears in human milk. Use cautiously in breastfeeding women.

NURSING CONSIDERATIONS
❸ *Alert:* Continue postexposure treatment for inhalation anthrax for 60 days. Prescriber should consider the risk-benefit ratio of continuing penicillin longer than 2 weeks, compared with switching to another drug.
• Monitor patient for diarrhea and initiate therapeutic measures as needed. Drug may need to be stopped.
• Allergic reactions are hard to treat because of drug's slow absorption rate.
• Monitor renal and hematopoietic function periodically.
• If large doses are given or if therapy is prolonged, bacterial or fungal superinfection may occur, especially in elderly, debilitated, or immunosuppressed patients.
• Treatment duration depends on site and cause of infection.
• *Look alike–sound alike:* Don't confuse penicillin G procaine with Polycillin, penicillamine, or the various other types of penicillin.

PATIENT TEACHING
• Tell patient to report adverse reactions promptly. A rash is the most common allergic reaction.
• Warn patient that IM injection may be painful but that ice applied to the site may help alleviate discomfort.

P

penicillin G sodium (benzylpenicillin sodium)
pen-i-SILL-in

Therapeutic class: Antibiotics
Pharmacologic class: Natural penicillins

AVAILABLE FORMS
Injection: 5 million-unit vial

INDICATIONS & DOSAGES
Adjust-a-dose (for all indications): If CrCl is less than 10 mL/minute, give the full loading dose followed by 50% of the loading dose every 8 to 10 hours. If patient is uremic and CrCl is more than 10 mL/minute, give full loading dose; then give half the loading dose every 4 to 5 hours for additional doses. Make additional dosage adjustments in patients with hepatic disease and renal impairment.

➤ **Actinomycosis**
Adults: For cervicofacial infections, 1 to 6 million units/day in divided doses IM or IV every 4 to 6 hours. For thoracic or abdominal infections, 10 to 20 million units/day in divided doses every 4 to 6 hours.

➤ **Anthrax**
Adults: 8 million units/day in divided doses IM or IV every 6 hours; higher dosages may be required depending on susceptibility of the organism.
Infants, children, and adolescents: 400,000 units/kg/day IV in divided doses every 4 hours; maximum, 4 million units/dose. Use in combination with clindamycin, linezolid, doxycycline, or rifampin for 14 days or more until clinical stability is achieved.

➤ **Clostridial infections**
Adults: 20 million units/day in divided doses IM or IV every 4 to 6 hours.

➤ **Diphtheria**
Adults: 2 to 3 million units/day in divided doses IM or IV every 4 to 6 hours for 10 to 12 days.

➤ **Endocarditis or pericarditis due to penicillin-susceptible viridans streptococci and *Streptococcus bovis***
Adults: 12 to 18 million units/day IV, either as a continuous infusion or in four to six equally divided doses for 4 weeks for native valve. Or 24 million units/day for 6 weeks

with or without gentamicin for prosthetic valve/material endocarditis.

➤ ***Erysipelothrix* endocarditis**
Adults: 12 to 20 million units/day in divided doses IM or IV every 4 to 6 hours for 4 to 6 weeks.

➤ **Fusospirochetosis**
Adults: 5 to 10 million units/day in divided doses IM or IV every 4 to 6 hours.

➤ **Haverhill fever; rat bite fever**
Adults: 12 to 20 million units/day in divided doses IM or IV every 4 to 6 hours for 3 to 4 weeks.
Infants, children, and adolescents: 20,000 to 50,000 units/kg/day IM or IV divided every 6 hours for 7 to 10 days or 5 to 7 days; then oral penicillin V for 7 days.

➤ **Haverhill fever with endocarditis caused by *Streptobacillus moniliformis*; rat bite fever**
Children: 150,000 to 250,000 units/kg/day IM or IV in equal doses every 4 hours for 4 weeks.

➤ ***Listeria monocytogenes* endocarditis or meningitis**
Adults: 15 to 20 million units/day in divided doses IM or IV every 4 to 6 hours. Treat for 2 weeks for meningitis and 4 weeks for endocarditis.

➤ **Meningococcal meningitis or septicemia**
Adults: 24 million units/day as 2 million units IM or IV every 2 hours.

➤ **Neurosyphilis**
Adults: 12 to 24 million units/day (2 to 4 million units IM or IV every 4 hours) for 10 to 14 days. Many experts recommend benzathine penicillin G 2.4 million units IM weekly for 3 weeks following completion of this regimen.

➤ ***Pasteurella multocida* bacteremia or meningitis**
Adults: 4 to 6 million units/day in divided doses IM or IV every 4 to 6 hours for 2 weeks.

➤ **Serious staphylococcal and streptococcal infections**
Adults: 5 to 24 million units/day in equally divided doses IM or IV every 4 to 6 hours.

➤ **Diphtheria (adjunctive therapy to antitoxin and for prevention of carrier state)**
Children: 150,000 to 250,000 units/kg/day in equal doses IM or IV every 6 hours for 7 to 10 days.

Reactions in bold italics are *life-threatening*. Interactions may have a *rapid onset* or a **delayed onset**.

➤ **Meningitis caused by susceptible strains of pneumococcus and meningococcus**

Children: 250,000 units/kg/day in equal doses IM or IV every 4 hours for 7 to 14 days, depending on infecting organism. Maximum dosage is 12 to 20 million units/day.

➤ **Serious streptococcal infections, such as pneumonia and endocarditis (***Streptococcus pneumoniae***), and meningococcal infections**

Children: 150,000 units/kg/day in equal doses IM or IV every 4 to 6 hours. Duration of therapy depends on infecting organism and type of infection.

➤ **Syphilis (congenital and neurosyphilis) after newborn period**

Children: 200,000 to 300,000 units/kg/day (administered as 50,000 units/kg IM or IV every 4 to 6 hours) for 10 to 14 days.

ADMINISTRATION

ℹ *Alert:* Don't use in children requiring less than 1 million units/dose.

IV

▼ Before giving drug, ask patient about allergic reactions to penicillin.

▼ Obtain specimen for culture and sensitivity tests before giving first dose. Begin therapy while awaiting results.

▼ Reconstitute drug with sterile water for injection, NSS for injection, or D₅W. Check manufacturer's instructions for volume of diluent necessary to produce desired drug level.

▼ Give by intermittent infusion: Dilute drug in 50 to 100 mL, and give over 30 minutes to 2 hours every 4 to 6 hours.

▼ In infants and children, give divided doses over 15 to 30 minutes.

▼ Sterile reconstituted solution may be kept in refrigerator for up to 3 days.

▼ **Incompatibilities:** None listed by manufacturer. Consult a drug incompatibility reference for more information.

IM

ℹ *Alert:* Before giving drug, ask patient about allergic reactions to penicillin and cephalosporin.

● IM is the preferred route.

● Obtain specimen for culture and sensitivity tests before giving first dose. Begin therapy while awaiting results.

● Injection may be painful, but ice applied to site may help alleviate discomfort.

● Give deep in upper outer quadrant of buttocks in adults and in midlateral thigh in small children. Rotate injection sites. Don't give subcut.

ACTION

Inhibits cell-wall synthesis during bacterial multiplication.

Route	Onset	Peak	Duration
IV	Immediate	Immediate	Unknown
IM	Unknown	15–30 min	Unknown

Half-life: 30 to 60 minutes.

ADVERSE REACTIONS

CNS: neuropathy, *seizures,* agitation, anxiety, confusion, depression, dizziness, fatigue, hallucinations, lethargy. **CV:** *HF,* thrombophlebitis. **GI:** enterocolitis, ischemic colitis, nausea, vomiting, *pseudomembranous colitis.* **GU:** nephropathy, interstitial nephritis. **Hematologic:** hemolytic anemia, *agranulocytosis, leukopenia, thrombocytopenia,* anemia, eosinophilia. **Musculoskeletal:** arthralgia. **Other:** hypersensitivity reactions, *anaphylaxis,* overgrowth of nonsusceptible organisms, injection-site pain, vein irritation.

INTERACTIONS

Drug-drug. *Aminoglycosides:* Physically and chemically incompatible. Give separately.

Aspirin, furosemide, indomethacin, sulfonamides, thiazide diuretics: May compete with penicillin for renal tubular secretion, prolonging the half-life of penicillin. Monitor patient.

Bacteriostatic antibacterial agents (chloramphenicol, macrolide antibiotics, sulfonamides, tetracyclines): May antagonize bactericidal effect of penicillin. Avoid concomitant use.

Heparin: May increase risk of bleeding. Closely monitor coagulation status. Adjust heparin dosage as needed.

Hormonal contraceptives: May decrease hormonal contraceptive effectiveness.

P

Advise use of additional form of contraception during penicillin therapy.

Live-virus vaccines: May decrease effectiveness of live-virus vaccines. Avoid concurrent use.

Methotrexate: May increase risk of methotrexate toxicity. Monitor patient closely.

Oral anticoagulants: May increase or decrease anticoagulant effects. Monitor PT and INR.

Probenecid: May increase penicillin level. Probenecid may be used for this purpose.

Tetracyclines: May interfere with bactericidal action of penicillins. Avoid coadministration.

EFFECTS ON LAB TEST RESULTS

• May decrease Hb level.
• May cause positive Coombs test result. May increase eosinophil count. May decrease platelet, WBC, granulocyte, and RBC counts.
• May cause false-positive CSF protein test result. May falsely decrease aminoglycoside level. May alter urine glucose testing using cupric sulfate (Benedict reagent).

CONTRAINDICATIONS & CAUTIONS

• Contraindicated in patients hypersensitive to drug or other penicillins and in those on sodium-restricted diets.
• Drug may cause CDAD ranging in severity from mild diarrhea to fatal colitis. If CDAD is suspected or confirmed, drug may need to be discontinued and treatment initiated.
• Use cautiously in patients with other drug allergies, especially to cephalosporins, because of possible cross-sensitivity.
Dialyzable drug: Yes.
⚠ *Overdose S&S:* Neuromuscular hyperexcitability, seizures.

PREGNANCY-LACTATION-REPRODUCTION

• There are no adequate studies in pregnant women but experience hasn't shown evidence of adverse fetal effects. Use during pregnancy only if clearly needed.
• Drug appears in human milk. Use cautiously in breastfeeding women.

NURSING CONSIDERATIONS

• Drug may alter normal colon flora. Monitor patient for diarrhea, and initiate therapeutic measures as needed. Drug may need to be stopped.
• Observe patient closely. With large doses and prolonged therapy, bacterial or fungal superinfection may occur, especially in elderly, debilitated, or immunosuppressed patients.
• Antibiotic use can cause overgrowth of nonsusceptible organisms (superinfection). Monitor patient for infection.
• For most acute infections, continue treatment for at least 48 to 72 hours after patient becomes asymptomatic. Maintain antibiotic therapy for group A beta-hemolytic streptococcal infections for at least 10 days to reduce risk of rheumatic fever.
• Give high doses (above 10 million units) by IV slowly because of the potential adverse effects of electrolyte imbalance from the sodium content, which is 1.68 mEq of sodium per million units.
• *Look alike–sound alike:* Don't confuse penicillin G sodium with Polycillin, penicillamine, or the various other types of penicillin.

PATIENT TEACHING

• Tell patient to report adverse reactions promptly, especially hypersensitivity reactions and diarrhea.
• Instruct patient to report discomfort at IV site.
• Warn patient receiving IM injection that the injection may be painful but that ice applied to site may help alleviate discomfort.

penicillin V potassium (phenoxymethyl penicillin potassium)
pen-i-SIL-in

Penicillin-VK

Therapeutic class: Antibiotics
Pharmacologic class: Natural penicillins

AVAILABLE FORMS

Oral suspension: 125 mg/5 mL, 250 mg/ 5 mL (after reconstitution)
Tablets: 250 mg, 500 mg

INDICATIONS & DOSAGES

➤ **Fusospirochetosis (Vincent infection) and staphylococcal infections**
Adults and children age 12 and older: 250 to 500 mg PO every 6 to 8 hours.

➤ **Pneumococcal infections**
Adults and children age 12 and older: 250 to 500 mg PO every 6 hours until patient has been afebrile for at least 2 days.

➤ **Streptococcal infections**
Adults and children age 12 and older: 125 to 250 mg PO every 6 to 8 hours for 10 days.

➤ **Group A beta-hemolytic streptococcal pharyngitis**
Adults and children age 12 and older: 500 mg PO b.i.d. to t.i.d., or 250 mg PO q.i.d. for 10 days.

➤ **To prevent recurrent rheumatic fever or chorea**
Adults and children age 12 and older: 125 to 250 mg PO b.i.d.

ADMINISTRATION
PO
• Before giving drug, ask patient about allergic reactions to penicillins.
• Obtain specimen for culture and sensitivity tests before giving first dose. Begin therapy while awaiting results.
• Give drug with food if patient has stomach upset.
• Store oral solution in refrigerator. Discard any portion after 14 days.

ACTION
Inhibits cell-wall synthesis during bacterial multiplication.

Route	Onset	Peak	Duration
PO	Unknown	30–60 min	Unknown

Half-life: 30 minutes.

ADVERSE REACTIONS
GI: epigastric distress, nausea, diarrhea, black hairy tongue, vomiting, fever. **Hematologic:** *leukopenia, thrombocytopenia,* eosinophilia, hemolytic anemia.
Other: *anaphylaxis,* hypersensitivity reactions, overgrowth of nonsusceptible organisms.

INTERACTIONS
Drug-drug. *Methotrexate:* May increase risk of methotrexate toxicity. Monitor patient closely.
Probenecid: May increase penicillin level. Probenecid may be used for this purpose.
Tetracyclines: May impair bactericidal effects of penicillin V. Avoid use together.
Warfarin: May increase anticoagulant effects. Monitor therapy.

EFFECTS ON LAB TEST RESULTS
• May decrease Hb level.
• May increase eosinophil count. May decrease platelet, WBC, and granulocyte counts.
• May alter results of turbidimetric test methods using sulfosalicylic acid, acetic acid, trichloroacetic acid, and nitric acid.

CONTRAINDICATIONS & CAUTIONS
• Contraindicated in patients hypersensitive to drug or other penicillins.
• Drug may cause CDAD ranging in severity from mild diarrhea to fatal colitis. If CDAD is suspected or confirmed, drug may need to be discontinued and treatment initiated.
• Use cautiously in patients with GI disturbances, seizure disorders, or renal impairment and in those with other drug allergies, especially to cephalosporins, because of possible cross-sensitivity.
Dialyzable drug: Unknown.
⚠ *Overdose S&S:* Neuromuscular hyperexcitability, seizures.

PREGNANCY-LACTATION-REPRODUCTION
• May use cautiously in pregnant and breastfeeding women.

NURSING CONSIDERATIONS
• Drug may alter normal colon flora. Monitor patient for diarrhea, and initiate therapeutic measures as needed. Drug may need to be stopped.
• Periodically assess renal and hematopoietic function in patients receiving long-term therapy.
• If large doses are given or if therapy is prolonged, bacterial or fungal superinfection may occur, especially in elderly, debilitated, or immunosuppressed patients.

P

• After treatment for streptococcal infections, reculture patient to determine whether streptococci have been eradicated.

• Amoxicillin is the preferred drug to prevent endocarditis because GI absorption is better and drug levels are sustained longer. Penicillin V is considered an alternative drug.

• *Look alike–sound alike:* Don't confuse penicillin V potassium with Polycillin, penicillamine, or the various other types of penicillin.

PATIENT TEACHING

• Instruct patient to take entire quantity of drug exactly as prescribed, even after feeling better.

• Tell patient to take drug with food if stomach upset occurs.

• Advise patient to discard any unused reconstituted suspension after 14 days.

• Advise patient to notify prescriber if rash, fever, or chills develop. A rash is the most common allergic reaction.

---

pentamidine isethionate
pen-TAM-i-deen

NebuPent, Pentam

Therapeutic class: Antiprotozoals
Pharmacologic class: Diamidine derivatives

AVAILABLE FORMS
Aerosol, injection, powder for injection: 300-mg vial

INDICATIONS & DOSAGES

➤ *Pneumocystis jiroveci* **pneumonia**
Adults and children age 4 months and older: 4 mg/kg IV over 1 to 2 hours or IM once daily for 14 to 21 days.

➤ **To prevent** *P. jiroveci* **pneumonia in high-risk patients**
Adults: 300 mg by inhalation using a Respirgard II nebulizer once every 4 weeks.

ADMINISTRATION
IV
▼ Reconstitute drug with 3 to 5 mL sterile water for injection or D_5W.

▼ Dilute reconstituted drug in 50 to 250 mL D_5W.

▼ Infuse over 60 to 120 minutes.

▼ IV infusion solutions prepared in D_5W are stable at room temperature for up to 24 hours.

▼ To minimize risk of hypotension, infuse drug slowly with patient lying down. Closely monitor BP.

◑ *Alert:* Closely monitor infusion. Extravasation may cause ulceration, tissue necrosis, or sloughing and may require surgical debridement and skin grafting. If extravasation occurs, discontinue infusion immediately and manage symptoms.

▼ **Incompatibilities:** None listed by manufacturer. Consult a drug incompatibility reference for more information.

IM
• Reconstitute drug with 3 mL sterile water for a solution containing 100 mg/mL.

• Give deep into muscle.

• Patient may have pain and induration at injection site.

• Rotate injection sites.

Inhalational
• Drug is considered a biohazardous agent. Follow safe-handling procedures.

• Give aerosol form only by Respirgard II nebulizer. Dosage recommendations are based on particle size and delivery rate of this device. Deliver dose until nebulizer chamber is empty (about 30 to 45 minutes).

• To give aerosol, mix contents of one vial in 6 mL sterile water for injection. Don't use NSS. Don't mix with other drugs.

• Don't use the Respirgard II to administer a bronchodilator because there may be an incompatibility between pentamidine and the bronchodilator.

• Don't use low-pressure (less than 20 pounds per square inch [psi]) compressors. The flow rate should be 5 to 7 L/minute from 40- to 50-psi air or oxygen source.

ACTION
May interfere with biosynthesis of DNA, RNA, phospholipids, and proteins in susceptible organisms.

Reactions in bold italics are *life-threatening*. Interactions may have a *rapid onset* or a *delayed onset*.

Route	Onset	Peak	Duration
IV	Unknown	1 hr	Unknown
IM	Unknown	30 min	Unknown
Inhalation	Unknown	Unknown	Unknown

Half-life: IV, about 5 to 8 hours; IM, 7 to 11 hours; inhalation, unknown.

ADVERSE REACTIONS

CNS: confusion, hallucinations, headache. **CV:** chest pain, hypotension. **GI:** nausea, metallic taste, diarrhea, anorexia. **Hematologic:** *leukopenia, thrombocytopenia,* anemia. **Metabolic:** *hypoglycemia.* **Respiratory:** cough, wheezing. **Skin:** rash; sterile abscess or necrosis, pain, or induration at site of IM injection. **Other:** night sweats, infection.

INTERACTIONS

Drug-drug. *Aminoglycosides, amphotericin B, capreomycin, cisplatin, methoxyflurane, polymyxin B, vancomycin:* May increase risk of nephrotoxicity. Monitor renal function test results closely.
Antidiabetic agents: May initially cause hypoglycemia, then hyperglycemia, because pentamidine may harm pancreatic cells. Monitor blood glucose levels and adjust dosages when needed.
Antineoplastics: May cause additive bone marrow suppression. Use together cautiously; monitor hematologic study results.
Drugs that prolong the QT interval (antipsychotics; antiarrhythmics, such as amiodarone, disopyramide, procainamide, quinidine, sotalol; fluoroquinolones; macrolides; TCAs): May cause additive effect. Use together cautiously; monitor patient for adverse cardiac effects.

EFFECTS ON LAB TEST RESULTS

• May increase BUN, creatinine, and potassium levels and LFT values. May decrease Hb level and hematocrit. May increase or decrease glucose level.
• May decrease WBC and platelet counts.

CONTRAINDICATIONS & CAUTIONS

• Contraindicated in patients with history of anaphylactic reaction to drug.
• Use cautiously in patients with HTN, hypotension, hypoglycemia, hypocalcemia,

leukopenia, thrombocytopenia, anemia, diabetes, pancreatitis, SJS, or hepatic or renal dysfunction.
🛈 *Alert:* Severe hypotension may occur after a single IV or IM dose. Monitor patients closely.
Dialyzable drug: No.
⚠ *Overdose S&S:* Renal and hepatic impairment, hypotension, cardiopulmonary arrest.

PREGNANCY-LACTATION-REPRODUCTION

• It isn't known if drug causes fetal harm. Use in pregnant women only if potential benefits justify unknown risks and only if clearly needed.
• It isn't known if drug appears in human milk. Use cautiously in breastfeeding women and only if potential benefits justify unknown risks.

NURSING CONSIDERATIONS

🛈 *Alert:* Monitor glucose, creatinine, and BUN levels daily. After parenteral administration, glucose level may decrease initially; hypoglycemia may be severe in 5% to 10% of patients. After several months of therapy, this may be followed by hyperglycemia and type 1 diabetes mellitus, which may be permanent.
• Monitor CBC, platelet count, LFT, calcium level, and ECG before, during, and after therapy.
🛈 *Alert:* Monitor BP during and after infusion because of increased risk of severe hypotension with IV or IM administration.
• Extravasation can lead to ulceration, tissue necrosis, or sloughing at injection site. Monitor IV site closely.
• Inhalation drug may cause bronchospasm or cough, especially in patients with a history of asthma or smoking. Use of an inhaled bronchodilator before each inhaled pentamidine dose may minimize symptom recurrence.
• Use of aerosolized drug has been associated with acute pancreatitis. Discontinue drug if signs or symptoms of acute pancreatitis occur.
• Obtain the following tests before, during, and after therapy: BUN and creatinine levels, CBC, platelet count, LFT, serum calcium level, and ECG.

P

- In patients with AIDS, drug may produce less severe adverse reactions than sulfamethoxazole–trimethoprim.

PATIENT TEACHING
- Instruct patient to use the aerosol device until the chamber is empty, which may take up to 45 minutes.
- Warn patient that IM injection is painful.
- Instruct patient to complete the full course, even if feeling better.
- Tell patient to report signs and symptoms of pulmonary infection, such as shortness of breath, fever, or cough.

SAFETY ALERT!

pertuzumab ⚕
per-TU-zoo-mab

Perjeta

Therapeutic class: Antineoplastics
Pharmacologic class: Monoclonal antibodies

AVAILABLE FORMS
Injection: 420 mg/14 mL (30 mg/mL) in single-use vials

INDICATIONS & DOSAGES
Adjust-a-dose (for all indications): If a dose is missed or delayed and the time between infusions is less than 6 weeks, give 420-mg dose when possible; don't wait until the next planned dose. If the time between the two infusions is 6 weeks or more, give 840 mg loading dose followed by maintenance dose 3 weeks later. Withhold drug for at least 3 weeks if LVEF is less than 40% or is 40% to 45% with a 10% or more decrease below pretreatment values. Repeat LVEF assessment in 3 weeks. Discontinue both pertuzumab and trastuzumab if LVEF isn't improved or is worse, unless benefit outweighs risk. Dosage reductions aren't recommended for pertuzumab.

➤ **HER2-positive metastatic breast cancer with trastuzumab and docetaxel in patients who haven't received prior anti-HER2 therapy or chemotherapy for metastatic disease** ⚕

Adults: Initial loading dose of 840 mg IV as a 60-minute infusion in combination with trastuzumab 8 mg/kg and docetaxel 75 mg/m². Administer a maintenance regimen every 3 weeks with pertuzumab 420 mg IV as a 30- to 60-minute infusion in combination with trastuzumab 6 mg/kg and docetaxel (may increase docetaxel dose to 100 mg/m² if initial dose is tolerated).

➤ **Neoadjuvant treatment of HER2-positive, locally advanced, inflammatory, or early-stage breast cancer (either greater than 2 cm in diameter or node positive) in combination with other drugs** ⚕

Adults: Initial loading dose of 840 mg IV as a 60-minute infusion, then a maintenance regimen every 3 weeks with pertuzumab 420 mg IV as a 30- to 60-minute infusion in combination with either four preoperative cycles with trastuzumab and docetaxel followed by three or four postoperative cycles of 5-FU, epirubicin, and cyclophosphamide (FEC); or three preoperative cycles of FEC alone followed by three or four postoperative cycles of pertuzumab in combination with docetaxel and trastuzumab; or six preoperative cycles of pertuzumab in combination with docetaxel, carboplatin, and trastuzumab (TCH). Following surgery, continue trastuzumab to complete 1 year of treatment regardless of regimen used.

➤ **Adjuvant treatment of patients with HER2-positive early breast cancer at high risk for recurrence as part of a complete regimen for breast cancer, including anthracycline or taxane-based chemotherapy**

Adults: Initial loading dose, 840 mg IV as a 60-minute infusion in combination with trastuzumab 8 mg/kg starting day 1 of first taxane-containing cycle. Administer a maintenance regimen every 3 weeks with pertuzumab 420 mg IV as a 30- to 60-minute infusion in combination with trastuzumab 6 mg/kg. Continue maintenance regimen for a total of 1 year (up to 18 cycles) or until disease recurrence or unmanageable toxicity, whichever occurs first. Don't give pertuzumab without trastuzumab; withhold or discontinue pertuzumab if trastuzumab is withheld or discontinued.

Reactions in bold italics are *life-threatening*. Interactions may have a *rapid onset* or a *delayed onset*.

ADMINISTRATION
IV
▼ Hazardous drug; use safe handling and disposal precautions.
▼ Don't administer as IV push or bolus.
▼ Refrigerate vials. Store in outer carton to protect from light.
▼ Inspect solution for particulates and discoloration. Solution should be clear to slightly opalescent and colorless to pale brown.
▼ Withdraw appropriate amount of pertuzumab and dilute in 250 mL NSS in a PVC or non-PVC polyolefin infusion bag.
▼ Invert bag gently to mix solution; don't shake. Administer immediately.
▼ May store diluted solution, refrigerated, for up to 24 hours.
▼ Administer pertuzumab sequentially. Pertuzumab and trastuzumab can be given in any order. Give docetaxel after pertuzumab and trastuzumab. Wait 30 to 60 minutes after infusing pertuzumab before administering the other drugs.
▼ **Incompatibilities:** Other drugs. Only mix with NSS.

ACTION
Binds to HER2 protein receptor, causing inhibition of signaling pathways, which results in cell growth arrest and apoptosis. The combination of pertuzumab and trastuzumab synergistically increases their antitumor activity.

Route	Onset	Peak	Duration
IV	Unknown	Unknown	Unknown

Half-life: 18 days.

ADVERSE REACTIONS
CNS: fatigue, asthenia, pyrexia, peripheral neuropathy, headache, dizziness, insomnia. **CV:** peripheral edema, *left ventricular dysfunction.* **EENT:** nasopharyngitis, increased tearing. **GI:** diarrhea, nausea, vomiting, constipation, stomatitis, dysgeusia, decreased appetite, abdominal pain. **Hematologic:** *neutropenia,* anemia, *leukopenia, febrile neutropenia.* **Hepatic:** elevated liver enzyme levels. **Metabolic:** *hypokalemia,* hyperuricemia, hyperphosphatemia. **Musculoskeletal:** myalgia, arthralgia. **Respiratory:** URI, dyspnea, pleural effusion. **Skin:**

alopecia, rash, pruritus, dry skin, paronychia, nail disorder. **Other:** mucosal inflammation, infusion-related hypersensitivity, immunogenicity.

INTERACTIONS
Drug-drug. *Belimumab:* Monoclonal antibodies may enhance adverse or toxic effect of belimumab. Avoid combination.
Clozapine: Increases risk or severity of clozapine-induced neutropenia. Monitor patient for neutropenia.

EFFECTS ON LAB TEST RESULTS
• May decrease WBC and RBC counts.

CONTRAINDICATIONS & CAUTIONS
Black Box Warning Pertuzumab can cause subclinical and clinical cardiac failure. Evaluate LVEF in all patients before and during treatment. Discontinue drug treatment for a confirmed clinically significant decrease in left ventricular function. ■
Alert: The safe use of pertuzumab with a doxorubicin-containing regimen or administration of more than 6 cycles for early breast cancer has not been established.
• Contraindicated in patients hypersensitive to drug or its components.
• Use cautiously in patients with a history of HF or reduced LVEF and in those with severe renal impairment. Prior exposure to radiotherapy may increase risk of left ventricular dysfunction.
Dialyzable drug: Unknown.

PREGNANCY-LACTATION-REPRODUCTION
Black Box Warning Exposure to drug during pregnancy can result in embryo or fetal death, delayed renal development, and other birth defects. Verify pregnancy status before starting drug. Advise patients of risks and the need for effective contraception during therapy and for 7 months after therapy ends. ■
• Women exposed to drug during pregnancy or within 7 months before conception should be enrolled in the MotHER Pregnancy Registry (1-800-690-6720) and the exposure reported to the Genentech Adverse Event Line (1-888-835-2555).
• If patient becomes pregnant during therapy, monitor closely. If oligohydramnios occurs, perform fetal testing.

• It isn't known if drug appears in human milk. Patient should discontinue breastfeeding or discontinue drug. Consider drug's extended half-life when making breastfeeding decisions after therapy ends.

NURSING CONSIDERATIONS

☒ Verify HER2 status with reputable lab. Drug is only useful in patients with HER2 protein overexpression.

Black Box Warning Assess LVEF before starting treatment and every 3 months during treatment for metastatic disease or every 6 weeks during neoadjuvant treatment. ∎

• Withhold or discontinue pertuzumab if trastuzumab is withheld or discontinued. If docetaxel is discontinued, treatment with pertuzumab and trastuzumab may continue.

• Monitor patient for hypersensitivity or infusion reactions for 60 minutes after first infusion and for 30 minutes after subsequent infusions. For significant infusion-related reactions, slow or interrupt infusion and treat symptoms. If severe reactions occur, consider permanently discontinuing drug.

• Monitor CBC regularly.

• Monitor patients for fever or infection.

• An increased incidence of febrile neutropenia has occurred in Asian patients.

• Assess LVEF before starting treatment and every 3 months during treatment.

PATIENT TEACHING

Black Box Warning Inform female patient of childbearing potential that drug may cause fetal harm. Counsel patient to use reliable birth control methods while taking this drug and for 7 months after therapy ends. ∎

• Teach patient that hair loss (alopecia) and skin and nail adverse reactions are common during treatment.

• Instruct patient to immediately report fever or other signs and symptoms of infection.

• Caution patient to immediately report shortness of breath, unusual edema, weight gain, or excessive fatigue.

• Tell patient that lab monitoring of cardiac function will be needed.

phentermine hydrochloride
FEN-ter-meen

Adipex-P, Lomaira

Therapeutic class: Anorexiants
Pharmacologic class: Sympathomimetic amines
Controlled substance schedule: IV

AVAILABLE FORMS

Capsules: 15 mg, 30 mg, 37.5 mg
Tablets: 8 mg, 37.5 mg

INDICATIONS & DOSAGES

➤ **Short-term adjunct in exogenous obesity for patients with an initial BMI of 30 kg/m² or more, or of 27 kg/m² or more in the presence of other risk factors (e.g., controlled HTN, diabetes, hyperlipidemia)**

Adults and children age 17 and older: 15 to 37.5 mg PO daily as a single dose before breakfast or 1 to 2 hours after breakfast. Or, 8 mg (Lomaira) PO t.i.d. 30 minutes before meals. Individualize dose to obtain an adequate response with the lowest effective dose.

Adjust-a-dose: Maximum dose of Adipex-P is 15 mg daily for patients with severe renal impairment (eGFR 15 to 29 mL/minute/ 1.73 m²). Avoid use in patients with eGFR less than 15 mL/minute/1.73 m² or ESRD requiring dialysis. Use caution when administering Lomaira to patients with renal impairment.

ADMINISTRATION
PO

• Adipex-P tablets may be split and given in two divided doses if desired.

• Avoid giving drug in the late evening, to prevent insomnia.

ACTION

Unknown. Phentermine is a sympathomimetic amine with pharmacologic properties similar to amphetamines. The mechanism of action in reducing appetite may be secondary to CNS effects, including stimulation of the hypothalamus to release norepinephrine.

Reactions in bold italics are *life-threatening*. Interactions may have a *rapid onset* or a ***delayed onset***.

Route	Onset	Peak	Duration
PO	Unknown	3–4.4 hr	Unknown

Half-life: About 20 hours.

ADVERSE REACTIONS
CNS: insomnia, overstimulation, headache, restlessness, euphoria, dysphoria, dizziness, tremor, psychosis. **CV:** palpitations, tachycardia, ischemic events, increased BP, *primary pulmonary HTN*. **GI:** dry mouth, dysgeusia, constipation, diarrhea, unpleasant taste, other GI disturbances. **GU:** erectile dysfunction. **Skin:** urticaria. **Other:** altered libido.

INTERACTIONS
Drug-drug. *Acetazolamide, antacids, sodium bicarbonate:* May increase renal reabsorption. Monitor patient for enhanced effects.
Adrenergic neuron blockers: May reduce hypotensive effect. Monitor patient for cardiac changes.
Ammonium chloride, ascorbic acid: May decrease level and increase renal excretion of phentermine. Monitor patient for decreased phentermine effects.
Hormonal contraceptives: May reduce effectiveness of hormonal contraceptives. Advise patient to use alternative methods of contraception during treatment and for 1 month after discontinuation of therapy.
Insulin, oral antidiabetics: May alter antidiabetic requirements. Monitor glucose level.
MAO inhibitors: May cause severe HTN or hypertensive crisis. Contraindicated within 14 days of MAO inhibitor therapy.
Serotonin uptake inhibitors (fluoxetine, fluvoxamine, paroxetine, sertraline): May increase risk of serotonin syndrome. Use together isn't recommended.
Drug-food. *Alcohol use:* May increase risk of adverse drug reactions. Monitor patient.
Caffeine: May increase CNS stimulation. Discourage use together.

EFFECTS ON LAB TEST RESULTS
None reported.

CONTRAINDICATIONS & CAUTIONS
• Contraindicated in patients hypersensitive to sympathomimetic amines, in those with idiosyncratic reactions to them, in agitated patients, and within 14 days after taking an MAO inhibitor.
• Contraindicated in patients with history of drug abuse, hyperthyroidism, moderate to severe or uncontrolled HTN, advanced arteriosclerosis, symptomatic CV disease, or glaucoma.
• Contraindicated in patients with history of heart disease, stroke, CAD, CHF, and arrhythmias.
• Rare cases of valvular heart disease have been reported in patients who have taken phentermine alone.
• Use cautiously in patients with mild HTN or seizure disorders.
Dialyzable drug: Unknown.
⚠ *Overdose S&S:* Restlessness, tremor, hyperreflexia, rapid respiration, confusion, assaultiveness, hallucinations, panic states, fatigue, depression, arrhythmias, HTN, hypotension, circulatory collapse, nausea, vomiting, diarrhea, abdominal cramps, seizures, coma.

PREGNANCY-LACTATION-REPRODUCTION
• Contraindicated in pregnant and breastfeeding women.

NURSING CONSIDERATIONS
• Use drug with a weight-reduction program.
• Monitor patient for tolerance, dependence, or potential abuse. Drug is chemically related to amphetamines, which carry a high abuse potential.
• Don't stop drug abruptly; taper dosage.
• *Look alike–sound alike:* Don't confuse phentermine with phentolamine or phenytoin.

PATIENT TEACHING
• Counsel patient in use of effective contraception. Advise her to inform prescriber immediately if pregnancy occurs.
• Instruct patient to immediately report shortness of breath or dyspnea, which could be an early sign of a serious adverse effect such as primary pulmonary HTN.
• Advise patient to avoid products that contain caffeine and to report evidence of excessive stimulation.

P

♣Canada ◇OTC ◆Off-label use ✐Photoguide ⊜Do not crush *Liquid contains alcohol ▒Genetic

• Warn patient that fatigue may result as drug effects wear off and that patient will need more rest.
• Warn patient that drug may lose its effectiveness over time.
• Advise patient not to stop drug abruptly. Remind patient that drug is for short-term use (usually a few weeks).
• Stress importance of eating healthy and other healthy lifestyle choices.

phentermine hydrochloride–topiramate
FEN-ter-meen/toe-PIE-rah-mate

Qsymia

Therapeutic class: Anorexiants–anticonvulsants
Pharmacologic class: Sympathomimetic amines–sulfamate-substituted monosaccharides
Controlled substance schedule: IV

AVAILABLE FORMS
Capsules ⒹⓂⒸ: 3.75 mg phentermine/23 mg topiramate extended-release, 7.5 mg phentermine/46 mg topiramate extended-release, 11.25 mg phentermine/69 mg topiramate extended-release, 15 mg phentermine/92 mg topiramate extended-release

INDICATIONS & DOSAGES
➤ **Chronic weight management, as an adjunct to diet and increased physical activity in patients with initial BMI of 30 kg/m² or greater (obese) or 27 kg/m² or greater (overweight) and at least one weight-related comorbidity, such as HTN, type 2 diabetes mellitus, or dyslipidemia**
Adults: Initially, 3.75 mg phentermine/23 mg topiramate extended-release PO every morning for 14 days; then increase to 7.5 mg phentermine/46 mg topiramate extended-release every morning. Evaluate weight loss after 12 weeks of treatment. If patient hasn't lost at least 3% of baseline body weight, discontinue drug or escalate dosage to 11.25 mg phentermine/69 mg topiramate extended-release every morning for 14 days, followed by 15 mg phentermine/92 mg topiramate extended-release every

morning. Evaluate weight loss 12 weeks after dosage escalation. If patient hasn't lost at least 5% of baseline body weight, discontinue drug by decreasing dosage to every other day for at least 1 week before stopping treatment altogether.
Adjust-a-dose: For patients with moderate renal impairment (CrCl of 30 to less than 50 mL/minute), severe renal impairment (CrCl less than 30 mL/minute), or moderate hepatic impairment (Child-Pugh class B), don't exceed 7.5 mg phentermine/46 mg topiramate once daily. Drug isn't for use in patients with ESRD on dialysis or those with severe hepatic impairment.

ADMINISTRATION
PO
• Give drug in morning with or without food. Don't give in evening due to risk of insomnia.
• Don't open, cut, or crush capsules.

ACTION
Phentermine: Unknown. Drug is a sympathomimetic amine with pharmacologic properties similar to amphetamines. The mechanism of action in reducing appetite may be secondary to CNS effects, including stimulation of the hypothalamus to release norepinephrine.
   Topiramate: Unknown in weight management. May involve appetite suppression and satiety enhancement via a variety of neurotransmitter or enzymatic effects.

Route	Onset	Peak	Duration
PO	Unknown	6 hr (phentermine); 9 hr (topiramate)	Unknown

Half-life: Phentermine, 20 hours; topiramate, 65 hours.

ADVERSE REACTIONS
CNS: paresthesia, headache, dizziness, dysgeusia, hypoesthesia, disturbance in attention or memory, cognitive disorder, insomnia, depression, anxiety, fatigue, irritability, *suicidal behavior.* **CV:** palpitations, chest discomfort, palpitations. **EENT:** blurred vision, eye pain, dry eye, dry mouth, nasopharyngitis, sinusitis, sinus congestion, pharyngolaryngeal pain, nasal congestion. **GI:** constipation, nausea, diarrhea, dyspepsia,

---

Reactions in bold italics are *life-threatening*. Interactions may have a *rapid onset* or a *delayed onset*.

GERD, oral paresthesia, gastroenteritis, decreased appetite, thirst. **GU:** UTI, kidney stones, dysmenorrhea. **Metabolic:** elevated creatinine level, *hypokalemia, metabolic acidosis, hypoglycemia.* **Musculoskeletal:** back pain, extremity pain, muscle spasms, musculoskeletal pain, neck pain. **Respiratory:** cough, bronchitis, URI. **Skin:** alopecia, rash. **Other:** procedural pain, flulike symptoms.

INTERACTIONS
Drug-drug. *Amitriptyline:* May increase amitriptyline level. Monitor therapy.
Anticholinergics (atropine, benztropine): May increase risk of heat-related disorders, such as decreased sweating and increased body temperature. Use together cautiously.
Carbamazepine, phenytoin: May decrease topiramate plasma concentration. Use together cautiously.
Carbonic anhydrase inhibitors (acetazolamide, methazolamide, zonisamide): May increase risk of metabolic acidosis and kidney stones. May also increase risk of heat-related disorders, such as decreased sweating and increased body temperature. Avoid concurrent use.
CNS depressants (barbiturates, benzodiazepines, sleep medications): May increase CNS depressant effects. Avoid use together.
Diltiazem: May decrease diltiazem level and increase topiramate level. Use together cautiously.
Lithium: High topiramate dosage may increase lithium level. Monitor lithium level.
MAO inhibitors: May increase risk of hypertensive crisis. Use is contraindicated during or within 14 days of MAO inhibitor administration.
Non-potassium-sparing diuretics (loop and thiazide diuretics): May increase risk of hypokalemia. Monitor potassium level.
Oral antidiabetics, insulin: May increase risk of hypoglycemia. Monitor glucose level closely.
Oral contraceptives (progestins): May decrease contraceptive effectiveness. Consider therapy modification and adding an additional, nonhormonal contraceptive method.
Other weight-loss drugs: Use with other weight-loss drugs hasn't been studied. Avoid use together.

Serotonin uptake inhibitors (fluoxetine, fluvoxamine, paroxetine, sertraline): May increase risk of serotonin syndrome. Use together isn't recommended.
Valproic acid: May increase risk of hyperammonemia and encephalopathy. Monitor patient and measure blood ammonia level if symptoms develop.
Drug-herb. *Weight-loss supplements:* Use with other weight-loss products hasn't been studied. Avoid use together.
Drug-food. *Ketogenic diet (high-protein, low-carbohydrate):* May increase risk of kidney stones. Use together cautiously.
Drug-lifestyle. *Alcohol use:* May increase CNS depressant effects. Discourage use together.

EFFECTS ON LAB TEST RESULTS
• May increase creatinine level. May decrease sodium bicarbonate, potassium, and glucose levels.

CONTRAINDICATIONS & CAUTIONS
• Contraindicated in patients hypersensitive to drug or its components or with idiosyncrasy to the sympathomimetic amines; in those with glaucoma or hyperthyroidism; and during or within 14 days after administration of MAO inhibitors.
• Avoid use in patients with severe hepatic impairment or ESRD and in those with a history of or active suicidal ideation or attempts.
• Use cautiously in patients with increased resting HR, especially those with cardiac or cerebrovascular disease (history of MI or stroke in the past 6 months, life-threatening arrhythmias, HF); in patients with depression or suicidal thoughts; in elderly patients; and in those at risk for development of metabolic acidosis or kidney stones.
• Use cautiously in patients with a history of depression.
❸ *Alert:* Drug is a controlled substance because it can be abused, leading to drug dependence.
• The safety and effectiveness of this drug in combination with other products intended for weight loss, including prescription and OTC drugs and herbal preparations, haven't been established.

P

• Drug is only available through certified pharmacies that are enrolled in the Qsymia certified pharmacy network; see www. qsymiarems.com or call 1-888-998-4887.

Dialyzable drug: Unknown.

⚠ *Overdose S&S:* Phentermine: Restlessness, tremor, rapid respiration, confusion, hallucinations, arrhythmias, changes in BP, nausea, vomiting, diarrhea. Topiramate: Metabolic acidosis, seizures, drowsiness, speech disturbance, blurred vision, hypotension, abdominal pain, agitation, dizziness, depression.

PREGNANCY-LACTATION-REPRODUCTION

• Contraindicated in pregnant and breastfeeding women.

• Assess for pregnancy before and monthly during treatment. Women of childbearing potential should use effective contraception during therapy.

• Prescribers and patients should report pregnancies that occur during therapy to the Qsymia Pregnancy Surveillance Program (1-888-998-4887).

NURSING CONSIDERATIONS

• Gradually decrease dosage when discontinuing drug to lower risk of seizures. If it's necessary to stop drug immediately, monitor patient closely.

• Monitor patient for mood disorders and insomnia; if present, decrease dosage or discontinue drug.

• Monitor patient for emergence or worsening of depression, suicidal thoughts or behavior, or unusual changes in mood or behavior. Discontinue drug in patients who experience suicidal thoughts or behaviors.

• Monitor resting HR. If sustained tachycardia occurs, decrease dosage or stop drug.

• Assess electrolyte, glucose, and bicarbonate levels before and periodically during treatment.

• Drug causes decreased sweating, which can predispose patients to heat-related disorders. Monitor fluid loss, especially in hot weather.

• Monitor BP regularly, especially in patients with history of HTN.

• Monitor patient for ocular changes (acute myopia, severe and persistent eye pain, vision changes, anterior chamber shallowing,

redness, increased IOP, mydriasis). Discontinue drug immediately if any of these symptoms occur.

• Monitor patient for potential abuse of drug. Phentermine has a known potential for abuse.

• Phentermine is related chemically and pharmacologically to amphetamines.

PATIENT TEACHING

• Advise patient to take drug once daily in the morning and to avoid nighttime dosing because of insomnia.

• Inform patient that drug is only available through certified pharmacies that are enrolled in the Qsymia certified pharmacy network. Pharmacies can be found at www.qsymiarems.com or by calling 1-888-998-4887.

ℹ *Alert:* Tell patient to keep drug in a safe place and protect it from theft. Advise patient never to give drug to anyone else because it can cause harm or death and is against the law.

• Warn patient not to increase dosage without first discussing with prescriber.

• Advise female patient of childbearing potential that pregnancy testing will be done before start of therapy and monthly during therapy.

• Counsel patient to use effective contraception. Advise her to inform prescriber immediately if pregnancy occurs.

• Instruct patient to tell all health care providers about all medications, nutritional supplements, and vitamins (including weight-loss products) that are being taken or may be taken during therapy.

• Caution patient to report sustained periods of heart pounding or racing while at rest; mood changes, depression, or suicidal ideation; prolonged diarrhea; scheduled surgery; occurrence or history of seizures; or use of a high-protein, low-carbohydrate diet.

• Teach patient to immediately report severe and persistent eye pain or significant vision changes.

• Instruct patient to report changes in attention, concentration, memory, or difficulty finding words.

• Tell patient to avoid operating hazardous machinery, including automobiles, until effects of drug are known.

Reactions in bold italics are *life-threatening*. Interactions may have a *rapid onset* or a *delayed onset*.

• Advise diabetic patient to monitor glucose level closely and to report episodes of hypoglycemia. Medication regimen may need adjustment.

• Caution patient to watch for decreased sweating or increased body temperature during physical activity, especially during hot weather.

• Warn patient not to stop drug abruptly as seizures may result.

• Advise patient to increase fluid intake to avoid kidney stones and to report severe side or back pain or blood in urine.

---

phenytoin (diphenylhydantoin) 🎗
FEN-i-toe-in

Dilantin-125, Dilantin Infatabs

phenytoin sodium
Dilantin, Phenytek

Therapeutic class: Anticonvulsants
Pharmacologic class: Hydantoin derivatives

AVAILABLE FORMS
phenytoin
Oral suspension: 125 mg/5 mL*
Tablets (chewable): 50 mg
phenytoin sodium
Injection: 50 mg/mL (46 mg base)
phenytoin sodium (extended)
Capsules (extended-release): 30 mg (27.6 mg base), 100 mg (92 mg base), 200 mg (184 mg base), 300 mg (276 mg base)

INDICATIONS & DOSAGES
➤ **To control tonic-clonic (grand mal) and complex partial (temporal lobe) seizures**
Adults: Highly individualized. Initially, 100 mg (immediate-release, extended-release) PO t.i.d. Adjust dosage at no less than 7- to 10-day intervals until desired response is obtained. Usual range is 300 to 600 mg daily. If patient is stabilized on 100-mg extended-release capsules t.i.d., once-daily dosing with 300-mg extended-release capsules is possible as an alternative. Or, 125 mg oral solution t.i.d. in patients

without previous treatment. May increase to 625 mg daily.
Children: 5 mg/kg/day in two to three equally divided doses. Adjust dosage at no less than 7- to 10-day intervals. Usual maintenance dose range is 4 to 8 mg/kg daily. Maximum dose is 300 mg/day.
➤ **To control tonic-clonic (grand mal) and complex partial (temporal lobe) seizures in patients requiring a loading dose**
Adults: Initially, 1 g (extended-release) PO divided into three doses, which are given at 2-hour intervals with careful monitoring. Begin maintenance dosage of 100 mg (extended-release) PO t.i.d. to q.i.d. 24 hours after loading dose.
➤ **To prevent and treat seizures occurring during neurosurgery**
Adults: 100 to 200 mg IM every 4 hours during and after surgery.
➤ **Status epilepticus**
Adults: Loading dose of 10 to 15 mg/kg IV (1 to 1.5 g may be needed) at a rate not exceeding 50 mg/minute; then maintenance dosage of 100 mg PO or IV every 6 to 8 hours.
Children: Loading dose of 15 to 20 mg/kg IV, at a rate not exceeding 1 to 3 mg/kg/minute or 50 mg/minute, whichever is slower; then highly individualized maintenance dosages.
Elderly patients: May need lower dosages.

ADMINISTRATION
PO
• Give divided doses with or after meals to decrease adverse GI reactions.
• For chewable tablets, patient may chew thoroughly before swallowing or may swallow whole.
• Shake suspension well before use. Administer dose using a calibrated oral dosing syringe.
• Different oral forms aren't interchangeable.
• Don't crush or allow patient to chew extended-release capsules.
• For oral suspension, withhold enteral feedings for 1 hour before and 1 hour after giving drug.
IV
▼ Clear tubing with NSS. Use only clear solution for injection. A slight yellow color is acceptable.

P

▼ To give as an infusion, dilute in NSS to a final concentration of phenytoin sodium in the solution of no less than 5 mg/mL. Begin infusion immediately after mixture has been prepared. Infusion must be completed within 1 to 4 hours.

▼ Infusion must begin within 1 hour after preparation and should run through an in-line filter.

▼ Check patency of catheter before giving. Monitor site for extravasation because it can cause severe tissue damage.

Black Box Warning Drug must be administered slowly. In adults, don't exceed 50 mg/minute IV. In children, administer drug at a rate not exceeding 1 to 3 mg/kg/minute or 50 mg/minute, whichever is slower because of the risk of severe hypotension and cardiac arrhythmias. ▪

▼ Follow each injection with injection of sterile NSS through the same needle or catheter.

▼ If possible, don't give by IV push into veins on back of hand to avoid purple glove syndrome. Inject into larger veins or central venous catheter, if available.

▼ Continuous monitoring of BP and ECG during IV administration is essential.

▼ Discard 4 hours after preparation. Don't refrigerate.

▼ **Incompatibilities:** Amikacin, aminophylline, amphotericin B, bretylium, cephapirin, ciprofloxacin, D_5W, diltiazem, dobutamine, enalaprilat, fat emulsions, hydromorphone, insulin (regular), levorphanol, lidocaine, lincomycin, meperidine, morphine sulfate, nitroglycerin, norepinephrine, other IV drugs or infusion solutions, pentobarbital sodium, potassium chloride, procaine, propofol, streptomycin, sufentanil citrate, theophylline, vitamin B complex with C. If giving as an infusion, don't mix drug with D_5W because it will precipitate.

IM

• Give IM only if dosage adjustments are made; IM dose is 50% greater than oral dose.

• Be aware that drug may precipitate at injection site, cause pain, and be absorbed erratically.

• Don't give by IM route for treatment of status epilepticus as peak plasma levels may not be attained for up to 24 hours.

ACTION

May stabilize neuronal membranes and limit seizure activity either by increasing efflux or decreasing influx of sodium ions across cell membranes in the motor cortex during generation of nerve impulses.

Route	Onset	Peak	Duration
PO	Unknown	1½– 3 hr	Unknown
PO (extended-release)	Unknown	4–12 hr	Unknown
IV	Immediate	1–2 hr	Unknown
IM	Unknown	Unknown	Unknown

Half-life: Varies with dose and concentration changes.

ADVERSE REACTIONS

CNS: ataxia, decreased coordination, mental confusion, slurred speech, dizziness, headache, insomnia, nervousness, twitching, peripheral neuropathy, vertigo. **CV:** *bradycardia,* periarteritis nodosa, hypotension, *CV shock.* **EENT:** diplopia, nystagmus, blurred vision, thickening of facial features. **GI:** gingival hyperplasia, nausea, vomiting, constipation. **Hematologic:** *agranulocytosis, leukopenia, pancytopenia, thrombocytopenia,* macrocythemia, megaloblastic anemia. **Hepatic:** *toxic hepatitis.* **Metabolic:** hyperglycemia. **Musculoskeletal:** osteomalacia. **Skin:** *SJS, toxic epidermal necrolysis,* bullous or purpuric dermatitis, discoloration of skin if given by IV push in back of hand, exfoliative dermatitis, hypertrichosis, inflammation at injection site, necrosis, pain, photosensitivity reactions, scarlatiniform or morbilliform rash. **Other:** lymphadenopathy, SLE.

INTERACTIONS

Drug-drug. *Acetaminophen:* May decrease the therapeutic effects of acetaminophen and increase the incidence of hepatotoxicity. Monitor for toxicity.

Amiodarone, antihistamines, chloramphenicol, **cimetidine,** *cycloserine, diazepam,* **fluconazole, isoniazid,** *metronidazole, omeprazole, phenylbutazone, salicylates,* **sulfonamides, ticlopidine,** *valproate:* May increase

---

Reactions in bold italics are *life-threatening*. Interactions may have a *rapid onset* or a *delayed onset*.

phenytoin activity and toxicity. Monitor patient for toxicity and adjust dosage as needed.

Atracurium, cisatracurium, pancuronium, rocuronium, vecuronium: May decrease the effects of nondepolarizing muscle relaxant. May need to increase the nondepolarizing muscle relaxant dose.

Barbiturates, carbamazepine, dexamethasone, diazoxide, folic acid, rifampin: May decrease phenytoin activity. Monitor phenytoin level.

Carbamazepine, cardiac glycosides, doxycycline, quinidine, theophylline, valproic acid: May decrease effects of these drugs. Monitor patient.

Colesevelam: May impair phenytoin absorption. Administer phenytoin 4 hours prior to colesevelam.

Corticosteroids: May decrease phenytoin level and corticosteroid effects. Measure phenytoin level and adjust phenytoin and corticosteroid dosages as needed.

Cyclosporine: May decrease cyclosporine levels, risking organ rejection. Monitor cyclosporine levels closely and adjust dosage as needed.

Delavirdine: May cause loss of virologic response. Use together is contraindicated.

Disulfiram: May increase toxic effects of phenytoin. Monitor phenytoin level closely and adjust dosage as needed.

Efavirenz: May increase phenytoin level and decrease efavirenz level. Monitor patient and adjust dosages of either or both drugs if needed.

Erlotinib: May increase phenytoin level and decrease erlotinib level. Monitor patient response.

Hormonal contraceptives: May increase phenytoin level and decrease contraceptive effectiveness. Monitor phenytoin level and adjust dosage if needed. Alternative form of contraception is recommended during therapy.

Isoniazid: May increase phenytoin level. Monitor phenytoin level and patient for toxicity.

Lithium: May increase toxicity of lithium, despite normal lithium levels. Monitor patient for adverse effects.

Methylphenidate: May increase phenytoin level. Monitor phenytoin level and adjust phenytoin dosage as needed.

Protease inhibitors (fosamprenavir, lopinavir–ritonavir): May decrease levels of both drugs. Measure phenytoin level and adjust dosage of phenytoin or protease inhibitor as needed.

Warfarin: May increase effects of warfarin. Monitor patient for bleeding.

Drug-herb. *St. John's wort:* May decrease phenytoin level. Monitor phenytoin level.

Drug-food. *Enteral tube feedings:* May interfere with absorption of oral drug. Stop enteral feedings for 2 hours before and 2 hours after drug use. Monitor serum drug level more frequently.

Drug-lifestyle. *Alcohol use (long-term):* May decrease drug's activity. Strongly discourage use together.

EFFECTS ON LAB TEST RESULTS
• May increase alkaline phosphatase, GGT, and glucose levels. May decrease urinary 17-hydroxysteroid, 17-ketosteroid, and Hb levels and hematocrit.
• May decrease platelet, WBC, RBC, and granulocyte counts.
• May increase urine 6-hydroxycortisol excretion. May decrease dexamethasone suppression and metyrapone test results.
• May decrease T_3 and T_4 levels.
• May falsely reduce protein-bound iodine or free T_4 level test results.

CONTRAINDICATIONS & CAUTIONS
• Contraindicated in patients hypersensitive to hydantoin, in those taking delavirdine, and in those with a history of prior acute hepatotoxicity attributable to phenytoin. Parenteral phenytoin is also contraindicated in patients with sinus bradycardia, SA block, second- or third-degree AV block, or Adams-Stokes syndrome.
• Use cautiously in patients with hepatic dysfunction, hypotension, myocardial insufficiency, diabetes, or respiratory depression; in elderly or debilitated patients; and in those receiving other hydantoin derivatives.
• Elderly patients tend to metabolize drug slowly and may need reduced dosages.
Dialyzable drug: Yes.

P

⚠ *Overdose S&S:* Ataxia, dysarthria, nystagmus, hyperreflexia, lethargy, nausea, slurred speech, tremor, vomiting, coma, hypotension, circulatory and respiratory depression.

PREGNANCY-LACTATION-REPRODUCTION
• Drug may cause fetal harm. Prenatal exposure may increase the risk of congenital malformations and other adverse outcomes. Avoid use during pregnancy when possible and monotherapy is recommended.
• If drug is necessary, pregnant women may need dosage adjustments to maintain clinical response. Therapeutic dose needs usually increase during pregnancy.
• A potentially life-threatening bleeding disorder related to decreased levels of vitamin K–dependent clotting factors that may occur in neonates exposed to phenytoin in utero can be prevented with vitamin K administration to the mother before delivery and to the neonate after birth.
• Drug may interact with hormone-containing contraceptives; use of nonhormonal contraceptives is recommended.
• Women exposed to drug during pregnancy should enroll in the North American AED Pregnancy Registry (1-888-233-2334).
• Drug appears in human milk. Breastfeeding isn't recommended.

NURSING CONSIDERATIONS
Black Box Warning Carefully monitor cardiac status during and after IV administration. CV toxicity may increase with infusion rates above those recommended. Toxicity has also been reported at or below the recommended infusion rate. Reduction in administration rate or discontinuation of dosing may be needed. ■
🦺 Asian patients who have tested positive for the allele HLA-B*1502 have a potentially increased risk of serious skin reactions, including SJS and toxic epidermal necrolysis. Monitor these patients carefully.
• If rash appears, stop drug. If rash is scarlatiniform or morbilliform, resume drug after rash clears. If rash reappears, stop therapy. If rash is exfoliative, purpuric, or bullous, don't resume drug.
• Don't stop drug suddenly because this may worsen seizures. Call prescriber immediately if adverse reactions develop.

• Monitor drug level. Therapeutic level of total phenytoin is 10 to 20 mcg/mL in adults and children and 8 to 15 mcg/mL in neonates. Therapeutic range of free phenytoin is 1 to 2 mcg/mL.
• Long-term use may decrease bone mineral density. Vitamin D and calcium supplements may be needed.
• Because of the risks of cardiac and local toxicity with parenteral phenytoin, use oral form when possible.
• Monitor CBC and calcium level every 6 months, and periodically monitor hepatic function. If megaloblastic anemia is evident, prescriber may order folic acid and vitamin B$_{12}$.
• Maintain seizure precautions, as needed.
🛈 *Alert:* Closely monitor all patients for changes in behavior that may indicate worsening of suicidal thoughts or behavior or depression.
• Watch for gingival hyperplasia, especially in children.
🛈 *Alert:* Doubling the dose doesn't double the level but may cause toxicity. Consult pharmacist for specific dosing recommendations.
• If seizure control is established with divided doses, once-daily dosing may be considered.
• *Look alike–sound alike:* Don't confuse phenytoin with mephenytoin, fosphenytoin, phenelzine, phentermine, or phenobarbital. Don't confuse Dilantin with Dilaudid, diltiazem, or Dipentum.

PATIENT TEACHING
• Tell patient to report all adverse reactions and to notify prescriber if rash develops.
• Advise patient and caregivers to immediately report changes in behavior that may indicate worsening of suicidal thoughts or behavior or depression.
• Advise patient to avoid driving and other potentially hazardous activities that require mental alertness until drug's CNS effects are known.
• Advise patient not to change brands or dosage forms once stabilized on therapy.
• Dilantin capsules are the only oral form that can be given once daily. Toxic levels may result if any other brand or form is

---

Reactions in bold italics are *life-threatening*. Interactions may have a *rapid onset* or a *delayed onset*.

given once daily. Dilantin tablets and oral suspension should never be taken once daily.
• Tell patient not to use capsules that are discolored.
• Advise patient to avoid alcohol.
• Warn patient and parents not to stop drug abruptly.
• Stress importance of good oral hygiene and regular dental exams. Surgical removal of excess gum tissue may be needed periodically if dental hygiene is poor.
• Advise female patient of childbearing potential who isn't planning a pregnancy to use effective contraception; warn her that there's a potential for decreased hormonal contraceptive efficacy.
• Instruct female patient to notify prescriber if she becomes pregnant or intends to become pregnant during therapy, and if she's breastfeeding or intends to breastfeed during therapy.
• Advise patient that drug may cause an increase in blood glucose levels.

pilocarpine hydrochloride (oral)
pye-loe-KAR-peen

Salagen

Therapeutic class: Cholinergic agonists
Pharmacologic class: Cholinergic agonists

AVAILABLE FORMS
Tablets: 5 mg, 7.5 mg

INDICATIONS & DOSAGES
Adjust-a-dose (for all indications): For patients with moderate hepatic impairment, initial dose is 5 mg PO b.i.d. Adjust dosage based on tolerance.
➤ **Xerostomia from salivary gland hypofunction caused by radiotherapy for cancer of head and neck**
Adults: 5 mg PO t.i.d.; may increase to 10 mg PO t.i.d., as needed.
➤ **Dry mouth in patients with Sjögren syndrome**
Adults: 5 mg PO q.i.d.

ADMINISTRATION
PO
• Don't give drug with a high-fat meal.
• Give with full glass of water.

ACTION
Cholinergic parasympathomimetic that increases secretion of salivary glands, eliminating dryness.

Route	Onset	Peak	Duration
PO	20 min	1 hr	3–5 hr

Half-life: 45 minutes to 1½ hours.

ADVERSE REACTIONS
CNS: asthenia, dizziness, headache, tremor. **CV:** flushing, HTN, tachycardia, edema. **EENT:** abnormal vision, rhinitis, sinusitis, lacrimation, amblyopia, pharyngitis, voice alteration, conjunctivitis, epistaxis. **GI:** nausea, dyspepsia, diarrhea, abdominal pain, vomiting, dysphagia, taste perversion. **GU:** urinary frequency. **Musculoskeletal:** myalgia. **Skin:** sweating, rash, pruritus. **Other:** chills.

INTERACTIONS
Drug-drug. *Beta blockers:* May increase risk of conduction disturbances. Use together cautiously.
Drugs with anticholinergic effects: May antagonize anticholinergic effects. Use together cautiously.
Drugs with parasympathomimetic effects: May result in additive pharmacologic effects. Monitor patient closely.
Drug-food. *High-fat meals:* May reduce drug absorption. Discourage patient from eating high-fat meals.

EFFECTS ON LAB TEST RESULTS
None reported.

CONTRAINDICATIONS & CAUTIONS
• Contraindicated in patients hypersensitive to pilocarpine, in those with uncontrolled asthma, and in those for whom miosis is undesirable, as in acute iritis or angle-closure glaucoma.
• Use in severe hepatic impairment isn't recommended.
• Use cautiously in patients with CV disease, uncontrolled asthma, chronic

P

bronchitis, COPD, cholelithiasis, biliary tract disease, nephrolithiasis, or cognitive or psychiatric disturbances.

• Safety and effectiveness in children haven't been established.

Dialyzable drug: Unknown.

⚠ *Overdose S&S:* Exaggerated parasympathetic effects, CV depression, bronchoconstriction, death.

PREGNANCY-LACTATION-REPRODUCTION

• There are no adequate studies in pregnant women. Use only if potential benefit justifies potential risk to the fetus.

• It isn't known if drug appears in human milk. Patient should discontinue breastfeeding or discontinue drug.

NURSING CONSIDERATIONS

• Examine patient's fundus carefully before beginning therapy because retinal detachment may occur in patients with retinal disease.

• Monitor patient for signs and symptoms of toxicity: headache, visual disturbance, lacrimation, sweating, respiratory distress, GI spasm, nausea, vomiting, diarrhea, AV block, tachycardia, bradycardia, hypotension, HTN, shock, mental confusion, arrhythmia, and tremors. Immediately notify prescriber of suspected toxicity.

• *Look alike–sound alike:* Don't confuse Salagen with selegiline.

PATIENT TEACHING

• Warn patient that driving ability may be impaired, especially at night, by drug-induced visual disturbances.

• Advise patient to drink plenty of fluids to prevent dehydration.

• Tell elderly patient with Sjögren syndrome that this age-group may be especially prone to urinary frequency, diarrhea, and dizziness.

• Advise patient not to take drug with a high-fat meal.

pimavanserin tartrate
pim-a-VAN-ser-in

Nuplazid

Therapeutic class: Antipsychotics
Pharmacologic class: 5-HT receptor inverse agonist and antagonists

AVAILABLE FORMS
Capsules: 34 mg
Tablets: 10 mg

INDICATIONS & DOSAGES
➤ **Hallucinations and delusions associated with Parkinson disease psychosis**
Adults: 3 mg PO once daily.
Adjust-a-dose: If drug is used with strong CYP3A4 inhibitors, reduce pimavanserin dosage to 10 mg once daily.

ADMINISTRATION
PO
• May give with or without food.
• Store at 68° to 77° F (20° to 25° C).

ACTION
Unknown. Effects may be mediated through inverse agonist and antagonist activity at serotonin (5-HT$_{2A}$ and 5-HT$_{2C}$) receptors.

Route	Onset	Peak	Duration
PO	Unknown	6 hr (mean)	Unknown

Half-life: Pimavanserin, 57 hours; N-desmethylated metabolite, 200 hours.

ADVERSE REACTIONS
CNS: confusion, hallucinations, fatigue, gait disturbance. **CV:** peripheral edema, *QT-interval prolongation.* **GI:** nausea, constipation. **GU:** UTI.

INTERACTIONS
Drug-drug. *Drugs that prolong QT interval (amiodarone, chlorpromazine, disopyramide, gatifloxacin, moxifloxacin, procainamide, quinidine, sotalol, thioridazine, ziprasidone):* May cause additive QT-interval prolongation and increased risk of cardiac arrhythmia. Avoid use together.
Opioid class warning: May cause slow or difficult breathing, sedation, and death.

Reactions in bold italics are *life-threatening*. Interactions may have a *rapid onset* or a **delayed onset**.

Avoid use together. If use together is necessary, limit dosage and duration of each drug to minimum necessary for desired effect.
Strong CYP3A4 inducers (carbamazepine, phenytoin, rifampin): May decrease pimavanserin level and therapeutic effects. Monitor patient for reduced response and increase pimavanserin dosage as appropriate.
Strong CYP3A4 inhibitors (clarithromycin, indinavir, itraconazole, ketoconazole): May increase pimavanserin level. If used together, reduce pimavanserin dosage to 10 mg once daily.
Drug-herb. *St. John's wort:* May decrease pimavanserin level and therapeutic response. Monitor patient and increase pimavanserin dosage if needed.

EFFECTS ON LAB TEST RESULTS
None reported.

CONTRAINDICATIONS & CAUTIONS
• Contraindicated in patients hypersensitive (rash, urticaria, tongue swelling, circumoral edema, throat tightness, dyspnea) to drug or its components.

Black Box Warning Elderly patients with dementia-related psychosis treated with antipsychotics are at an increased risk for death. Pimavanserin isn't approved for the treatment of patients with dementia-related psychosis unrelated to hallucinations and delusions associated with Parkinson disease psychosis. ∎

• Drug prolongs QT interval. Avoid use with drugs that prolong QT interval, in patients with a history of cardiac arrhythmias, and in those with other conditions that increase risk of torsades de pointes ventricular arrhythmia or sudden death, including symptomatic bradycardia, hypokalemia or hypomagnesemia, and the presence of congenital prolongation of QT interval.
• Drug may cause orthostatic hypotension. Use cautiously in patients at risk for hypotension and in patients who wouldn't tolerate transient hypotension.
• Safety and effectiveness in children haven't been established.
Dialyzable drug: Unknown.
⚠ *Overdose S&S:* Nausea and vomiting, QT-interval prolongation.

PREGNANCY-LACTATION-REPRODUCTION
• There are no well-controlled studies in pregnant women. Use during pregnancy only if clearly needed.
• Drug hasn't been evaluated in breastfeeding women. Effects of exposure to drug on the breastfed infant are unknown.

NURSING CONSIDERATIONS
• Monitor patient for QT-interval prolongation.
• Monitor patient for orthostatic hypotension.
• *Look alike–sound alike:* Don't confuse pimavanserin with palivizumab, pamidronate, or pitavastatin.

PATIENT TEACHING
• Counsel patient to report changes in medications or supplements, because of potential for drug interactions.
• Warn patient to immediately report signs and symptoms of ventricular arrhythmia (dizziness or fainting, rapid or irregular heartbeat) or hypotension (dizziness, weakness).
• Advise patient to report swelling in the arms or legs.
• Instruct patient to report confusion or hallucinations that are new or worse after start of therapy.

pimecrolimus
py-meck-roh-LY-mus

Elidel

Therapeutic class: Immunosuppressants (topical)
Pharmacologic class: Topical immunomodulators

AVAILABLE FORMS
Cream: 1%*

INDICATIONS & DOSAGES
➤ **Second-line therapy for short and noncontinuous prolonged treatment of mild to moderate atopic dermatitis in nonimmunocompromised patients in whom use of other conventional therapies is deemed inadvisable, or in patients with**

inadequate response to or intolerance of conventional therapies
Adults and children age 2 and older: Apply a thin layer to the affected skin b.i.d. and rub in gently and completely. Discontinue therapy when signs and symptoms (itch, rash, redness) resolve. If signs and symptoms persist beyond 6 weeks, reevaluate patient.

ADMINISTRATION
Topical
• Drug may be used on all skin surfaces, including the head, neck, and intertriginous areas.
• Clear infections at treatment sites before using.
• Don't use with occlusive dressing.

ACTION
Unknown. Inhibits T-cell activation and prevents the release of inflammatory cytokines and mediators from mast cells.

Route	Onset	Peak	Duration
Topical	Unknown	Unknown	Unknown

Half-life: Unknown.

ADVERSE REACTIONS
CNS: headache, fever. **EENT:** nasopharyngitis, otitis media, sinusitis, pharyngitis, tonsillitis, eye infection, nasal congestion, rhinorrhea, sinus congestion, rhinitis, epistaxis, conjunctivitis, earache. **GI:** gastroenteritis, abdominal pain, vomiting, diarrhea, nausea, constipation, loose stools. **GU:** dysmenorrhea. **Musculoskeletal:** back pain, arthralgias. **Respiratory:** URI, bronchitis, cough, *asthma,* pneumonia, wheezing, dyspnea. **Skin:** application-site reaction (burning, irritation, erythema, pruritus), skin infections, impetigo, folliculitis, molluscum contagiosum, herpes simplex, varicella, papilloma, urticaria, acne. **Other:** flulike illness, hypersensitivity, toothache, bacterial infection, staphylococcal infection, viral infection.

INTERACTIONS
Drug-drug. *CYP3A4 inhibitors (calcium channel blockers, erythromycin, fluconazole, itraconazole, ketoconazole):* May affect metabolism of pimecrolimus. Use together cautiously.

Immunosuppressants (except cytarabine [liposomal]): May enhance adverse or toxic effect of immunosuppressants. Avoid use together.
Drug-lifestyle. *Natural or artificial sun exposure:* May worsen atopic dermatitis. Advise patient to avoid or minimize sunlight exposure.

EFFECTS ON LAB TEST RESULTS
None reported.

CONTRAINDICATIONS & CAUTIONS
• Contraindicated in patients hypersensitive to drug or its components, in patients with Netherton syndrome, and in immunocompromised patients.
Black Box Warning Long-term safety of topical calcineurin inhibitors hasn't been established. ∎
Black Box Warning Although a causal relationship hasn't been established, rare cases of malignancy (e.g., skin malignancy, lymphoma) have been reported in patients treated with topical calcineurin inhibitors, including pimecrolimus. ∎
• Contraindicated in patients with active cutaneous viral infections or infected atopic dermatitis.
• Contraindicated in patients with malignant or premalignant skin conditions.
• Use cautiously in patients with varicella zoster virus infection, HSV infection, or eczema herpeticum.
Black Box Warning Not indicated for use in children younger than age 2. ∎
Dialyzable drug: Unknown.

PREGNANCY-LACTATION-REPRODUCTION
• There are no adequate studies in pregnant women. Use only if potential benefit justifies potential risk to the fetus.
• It's unknown if drug appears in human milk. Serious adverse reactions may occur in breastfeeding infants exposed to drug. Patient should discontinue breastfeeding or discontinue drug.

NURSING CONSIDERATIONS
◑ *Alert:* Use drug only after other therapies have failed because of the risk of cancer.
Black Box Warning Long-term safety hasn't been established. Avoid continuous

---

Reactions in bold italics are *life-threatening*. Interactions may have a *rapid onset* or a *delayed onset*.

long-term use of drug and limit application to areas of involvement of atopic dermatitis. ■
• If symptoms persist longer than 6 weeks, reevaluate patient.
• May cause local symptoms such as skin burning. Most local reactions start within 1 to 5 days after treatment, are mild to moderately severe, and last no longer than 5 days.
• Monitor patient for lymphadenopathy. If lymphadenopathy occurs and its cause is unknown, or if patient develops acute infectious mononucleosis, consider stopping drug.
• Drug use may cause papillomas or warts. Consider stopping drug if papillomas worsen or don't respond to conventional treatment.
• **Look alike–sound alike:** Don't confuse pimecrolimus with tacrolimus.

PATIENT TEACHING
• Inform patient that drug is for external use only and to use it as directed.
• Tell patient to report adverse reactions.
• Tell patient not to use with an occlusive dressing.
• Instruct patient to wash hands before and after application if hands aren't treated and that skin should be dry before applying cream.
• Caregivers should wash their hands with soap and water after applying cream.
• Tell patient to stop therapy after signs and symptoms have resolved. If signs and symptoms persist longer than 6 weeks, advise patient to contact prescriber.
• Tell patient to resume treatment at first signs of recurrence.
• Stress that patient should minimize or avoid exposure to natural or artificial sunlight (including tanning beds and UVA-UVB treatment) while using this drug.
• Tell patient to expect application-site reactions but to notify prescriber if reaction is severe or persists for longer than 1 week.

pioglitazone hydrochloride
pye-oh-GLI-ta-zone

Actos✔

Therapeutic class: Antidiabetics
Pharmacologic class: Thiazolidinediones

AVAILABLE FORMS
Tablets: 15 mg, 30 mg, 45 mg

INDICATIONS & DOSAGES
➤ **Type 2 diabetes mellitus, alone or with a sulfonylurea, metformin, or insulin as an adjunct to diet and exercise to improve glycemic control**
Adults: Initially, 15 or 30 mg PO once daily. Maximum daily dose, if used alone or in combination therapy, is 45 mg.
Adjust-a-dose: For patients taking pioglitazone with insulin, reduce insulin by 10% to 25% if patient reports hypoglycemia. Maximum recommended dose of pioglitazone is 15 mg when used with gemfibrozil or other strong CYP2C8 inhibitors. Start with 15 mg in patients with NYHA Class I or II HF.

ADMINISTRATION
PO
• Give drug without regard for meals.

ACTION
Lowers glucose level by decreasing insulin resistance and hepatic glucose production. Improves sensitivity of insulin in muscle and adipose tissue.

Route	Onset	Peak	Duration
PO	30 min	≤2 hr	Unknown

Half-life: 3 to 7 hours.

ADVERSE REACTIONS
CNS: headache, dizziness. **CV:** edema, *HF, HTN,* chest pain. **EENT:** sinusitis, pharyngitis, macular edema. **GI:** diarrhea, flatulence. **Hematologic:** anemia. **Metabolic:** *hypoglycemia,* weight gain. **Musculoskeletal:** myalgia, fractures. **Respiratory:** URI. **Other:** tooth disorder.

INTERACTIONS

Drug-drug. *Atorvastatin:* May decrease atorvastatin and pioglitazone levels. Monitor patient and glucose level.

CYP2C8 inducers (rifampin): May decrease pioglitazone concentration. Don't exceed maximum recommended pioglitazone dose.

Hormonal contraceptives: May decrease level of hormonal contraceptives, reducing contraceptive effectiveness. Advise patient taking drug and hormonal contraceptives to consider additional birth control measures.

Insulin: May increase incidence of edema and HF and may cause additive or synergistic pharmacologic effects. If hypoglycemia occurs, decrease insulin dosage.

Ketoconazole: May inhibit pioglitazone metabolism. Monitor glucose level more frequently.

Strong CYP2C8 inhibitors (gemfibrozil): May increase pioglitazone level. Monitor patient and glucose level. Maximum pioglitazone dose is 15 mg.

Sulfonylureas: May increase risk of hypoglycemia. If hypoglycemia occurs, reduce sulfonylurea dosage.

Drug-herb. *Eucalyptus:* May increase hypoglycemic effects. Discourage use together.

Drug-lifestyle. *Alcohol use:* May alter glycemic control and increase risk of hypoglycemia. Discourage use together.

EFFECTS ON LAB TEST RESULTS

• May increase CK, ALT, HDL, LDL, and total cholesterol levels.

• May decrease glucose, triglyceride, and Hb levels and hematocrit.

CONTRAINDICATIONS & CAUTIONS

Black Box Warning Contraindicated in patients with NYHA Class III or IV HF; not recommended in those with symptomatic HF. ∎

• Contraindicated in patients hypersensitive to drug or its components and in those with active bladder cancer.

• Don't use in patients with type 1 diabetes mellitus and diabetic ketoacidosis; use cautiously in those with active liver disease.

Black Box Warning Use cautiously in patients with edema or HF or patients at risk for HF. ∎

• Safety and effectiveness in children haven't been established.

Dialyzable drug: Unknown.

PREGNANCY-LACTATION-REPRODUCTION

• Use during pregnancy only if benefit justifies risk to the fetus. Insulin is preferred antidiabetic during pregnancy.

• It isn't known if drug appears in human milk. Patient should discontinue breastfeeding or discontinue drug.

NURSING CONSIDERATIONS

❸ Alert: Measure liver enzyme levels at start of therapy, every 2 months for first year of therapy, and periodically thereafter. Obtain LFT results in patients who develop signs and symptoms of liver dysfunction, such as nausea, vomiting, abdominal pain, fatigue, anorexia, or dark urine. Stop drug if patient develops jaundice or if LFT results show ALT level greater than 3 × ULN.

Black Box Warning Drug can cause fluid retention, leading to or worsening HF. Observe patients carefully for signs and symptoms of HF (including excessive, rapid weight gain; dyspnea; and edema). If these signs and symptoms develop, the HF should be managed according to the current standards of care. Also, stopping or reducing dose of pioglitazone must be considered. ∎

• Hb level and hematocrit may drop, usually during first 4 to 12 weeks of therapy.

• Management of type 2 diabetes should include diet control. Because caloric restrictions, weight loss, and exercise help improve insulin sensitivity and help make drug therapy effective, these measures are essential for proper diabetes management.

❸ Alert: Watch for hypoglycemia, especially in patients receiving combination therapy. Dosage adjustments of these drugs may be needed.

• Monitor glucose level regularly, especially during situations of increased stress, such as infection, fever, surgery, and trauma.

❸ Alert: Drug may be associated with an increased risk of bladder cancer when used for more than 1 year. Monitor patients for signs and symptoms of bladder cancer (such as blood in urine or abdominal pain). If considering use in patients with a history of bladder cancer, weigh benefits of blood glucose

---

control with drug against unknown risks of cancer recurrence.

• Risk of fractures (forearm, hand, wrist, foot, ankle, fibula, and tibia) in female patients receiving long-term treatment is increased. Give only if risk outweighs benefits.

• *Look alike–sound alike:* Don't confuse pioglitazone with rosiglitazone. Don't confuse Actos with Actidose or Actonel.

PATIENT TEACHING

• Instruct patient to adhere to dietary instructions and to have glucose and HbA$_{1c}$ levels tested regularly.

• Teach patient taking pioglitazone with insulin or oral antidiabetics the signs and symptoms of hypoglycemia.

• Advise patient to notify prescriber during periods of stress, such as fever, trauma, infection, or surgery, because dosage may need adjustment.

• Instruct patient how and when to monitor glucose level.

• Notify patient that blood tests of liver function will be performed before therapy starts, every 2 months for the first year, and periodically thereafter.

• Tell patient to immediately report all adverse reactions, especially unexplained nausea, vomiting, abdominal pain, fatigue, anorexia, and dark urine, because these symptoms may indicate liver problems.

• Warn patient to contact health care provider for signs or symptoms of HF (unusually rapid increase in weight, swelling, or shortness of breath).

• Advise anovulatory, premenopausal female patient with insulin resistance that therapy may cause resumption of ovulation; recommend using contraception.

• Tell patient to have regular eye exams and to report any visual changes immediately.

• Advise patient to report blood in the urine, red-colored urine, new or worsening urge to urinate, or pain when urinating; these symptoms may indicate bladder cancer.

---

piperacillin sodium–tazobactam sodium
pi-PER-a-sil-in/ta-zoe-BAK-tam

Zosyn

Therapeutic class: Antibiotics
Pharmacologic class: Extended-spectrum penicillins–beta-lactamase inhibitors

AVAILABLE FORMS
Powder for injection: 2 g piperacillin and 0.25 g tazobactam per vial, 3 g piperacillin and 0.375 g tazobactam per vial, 4 g piperacillin and 0.5 g tazobactam per vial
Premixed, frozen solution for injection: 2 g piperacillin and 0.25 g tazobactam per 50-mL container, 3 g piperacillin and 0.375 g tazobactam per 50-mL container, 4 g piperacillin and 0.5 g tazobactam per 100-mL container

INDICATIONS & DOSAGES
➤ **Moderate to severe infections from piperacillin-resistant, piperacillin-tazobactam–susceptible, beta-lactamase–producing strains of microorganisms in appendicitis (complicated by rupture or abscess) and peritonitis caused by *Escherichia coli, Bacteroides fragilis, B. ovatus, B. thetaiotaomicron,* or *B. vulgatus;* skin and skin-structure infections caused by *Staphylococcus aureus;* postpartum endometritis or pelvic inflammatory disease caused by *E. coli;* moderately severe community-acquired pneumonia caused by *Haemophilus influenzae***
Adults: 3.375 g (3 g piperacillin/0.375 g tazobactam) every 6 hours by IV infusion for 7 to 10 days.
Adjust-a-dose: If CrCl is 20 to 40 mL/minute, give 2.25 g (2 g piperacillin/0.25 g tazobactam) every 6 hours; if CrCl is less than 20 mL/minute, give 2.25 g (2 g piperacillin/0.25 g tazobactam) every 8 hours. In continuous ambulatory peritoneal dialysis (CAPD) patients, give 2.25 g (2 g piperacillin/0.25 g tazobactam) every 12 hours. In hemodialysis patients, give 2.25 g (2 g piperacillin/0.25 g tazobactam) every 12 hours with a supplemental

P

dose of 0.75 g (0.67 g piperacillin/0.08 g tazobactam) after each dialysis period.

➤ **Appendicitis, peritonitis**

Children weighing more than 40 kg with normal renal function: 3.375 g (3 g piperacillin/0.375 g tazobactam) every 6 hours by IV infusion for 7 to 10 days.

Children age 9 months and older weighing 40 kg or less with normal renal function: 100 mg piperacillin/12.5 mg tazobactam per kg of body weight every 8 hours by IV infusion for 7 to 10 days.

Children age 2 to 9 months: 80 mg piperacillin/10 mg tazobactam per kg of body weight every 8 hours by IV infusion for 7 to 10 days.

➤ **Moderate to severe nosocomial pneumonia caused by piperacillin-resistant, beta-lactamase–producing strains of *S. aureus* or by piperacillin-tazobactam–susceptible *Acinetobacter baumannii*, *H. influenzae*, *Klebsiella pneumoniae*, and *Pseudomonas aeruginosa***

Adults: 4.5 g (4 g piperacillin/0.5 g tazobactam) IV every 6 hours with aminoglycoside. Patients with *P. aeruginosa* should continue aminoglycoside or antipseudomonal fluoroquinolone treatment; if *P. aeruginosa* isn't isolated, aminoglycoside or fluoroquinolone treatment may be stopped. Duration of treatment is usually 7 to 14 days.

Adjust-a-dose: If CrCl is 20 to 40 mL/minute, give 3.375 g (3 g piperacillin/0.375 g tazobactam) every 6 hours; if CrCl is less than 20 mL/minute, give 2.25 g (2 g piperacillin/0.25 g tazobactam) every 6 hours. In patients with CAPD, give 2.25 g (2 g piperacillin/0.25 g tazobactam) every 8 hours. In hemodialysis patients, give 2.25 g (2 g piperacillin/0.25 g tazobactam) every 8 hours with a supplemental dose of 0.75 g (0.67 g piperacillin/0.08 g tazobactam) after each dialysis period.

ADMINISTRATION

IV

▼ Before giving drug, ask patient about allergic reactions to penicillins, cephalosporins, or beta-lactamase inhibitors.

▼ Obtain specimen for culture and sensitivity tests before giving first dose. Therapy may begin while awaiting results.

▼ Reconstitute each gram with 5 mL of diluent, such as sterile or bacteriostatic water for injection, NSS for injection, bacteriostatic NSS for injection, D_5W, dextrose 5% in NSS for injection, or dextran 6% in NSS for injection.

▼ Shake until dissolved.

▼ Further dilute to 50 to 150 mL before infusion.

▼ Use drug immediately after reconstitution.

▼ Stop any primary infusion during administration, if possible.

▼ Infuse over at least 30 minutes.

▼ Discard unused drug in single-dose vials after 24 hours if stored at room temperature or 48 hours if refrigerated.

▼ Diluted drug is stable in IV bags for 24 hours at room temperature or for 1 week refrigerated.

▼ Store premixed, frozen solution containers at or below –4° F (–20° C).

▼ Thaw frozen container at room temperature (68° to 77° F [20° to 25° C]) or under refrigeration (36° to 46° F [2° to 8° C]). Don't force-thaw by immersion in water baths or by microwave irradiation.

▼ Check for minute leaks by squeezing container firmly. If leaks are detected, discard solution as sterility may be impaired.

▼ Visually inspect solution, which may precipitate while frozen but will dissolve upon reaching room temperature with little or no agitation. If, after visual inspection, solution remains cloudy, an insoluble precipitate is noted, or if any seals or outlet ports aren't intact, discard container.

▼ Don't use plastic containers in series connections.

▼ **Incompatibilities:** Other drugs.

ACTION

Inhibits cell-wall synthesis during bacterial multiplication.

Route	Onset	Peak	Duration
IV	Immediate	Immediate	Unknown

Half-life: About 0.7 to 1.5 hours.

ADVERSE REACTIONS

CNS: headache, insomnia, fever, *seizures,* agitation, anxiety, dizziness, pain. **CV:** *arrhythmia,* chest pain, edema, HTN,

---

tachycardia. **EENT:** rhinitis. **GI:** diarrhea, constipation, nausea, *pseudomembranous colitis,* abdominal pain, dyspepsia, stool changes, vomiting, oral candidiasis. **GU:** candidiasis, interstitial nephritis. **Hematologic:** *leukopenia, neutropenia, thrombocytopenia,* anemia, eosinophilia. **Respiratory:** dyspnea. **Skin:** pruritus, rash. **Other:** *anaphylaxis,* hypersensitivity reactions, inflammation, phlebitis at IV site.

INTERACTIONS
Drug-drug. *Aminoglycosides:* Penicillins may decrease serum concentration of aminoglycosides. Consider therapy modification.
Anticoagulants, heparin: May prolong effectiveness and increase risk of bleeding. Monitor PT and INR closely.
Hormonal contraceptives: May decrease contraceptive effectiveness. Advise using another form of contraception.
Live-virus vaccines: May decrease vaccine effectiveness. Don't use together.
Methotrexate: May increase risk of methotrexate toxicity. Monitor closely.
Probenecid: May increase piperacillin level. Probenecid may be used for this purpose.
Vancomycin: May increase nephrotoxicity. Monitor therapy.
Vecuronium: May prolong neuromuscular blockade. Monitor patient closely.

EFFECTS ON LAB TEST RESULTS
• May increase serum sodium level because of increased sodium in drug.
• May decrease Hb level.
• May increase eosinophil count. May decrease neutrophil, platelet, and WBC counts.
• May cause false-positive result for urine glucose tests using copper reduction method such as Clinitest. May cause false-positive test for *Aspergillus.*

CONTRAINDICATIONS & CAUTIONS
• Contraindicated in patients hypersensitive to drug, other penicillins, cephalosporins, or beta-lactamase inhibitors.
• Drug can cause CDAD. Consider possibility of CDAD in all patients who present with diarrhea after antibiotic use.
• Use cautiously in patients with bleeding tendencies, uremia, hypokalemia, and allergies to other drugs.

Dialyzable drug: Yes.
⚠ *Overdose S&S:* Neuromuscular hyperexcitability, seizures.

PREGNANCY-LACTATION-REPRODUCTION
• There are no adequate studies in pregnant women. Use only if clearly needed.
• Drug appears in low concentrations in human milk. Use cautiously if breastfeeding.

NURSING CONSIDERATIONS
• Drug may cause CDAD ranging in severity from mild diarrhea to fatal colitis. Monitor patient for diarrhea and initiate therapeutic measures as needed. Drug may need to be stopped.
• Studies have shown that drug is an independent risk factor for renal failure and delayed renal function recovery in critically ill patients. Alternative treatments should be considered; if alternative treatment options are inadequate or unavailable, monitor renal function during therapy.
• Serious skin reactions can occur. If rash develops, monitor patient closely and discontinue if lesion progresses.
• Hemodialysis removes 30% to 40% of a dose in 4 hours. Additional doses may be needed after each dialysis period.
• If large doses are given or if therapy is prolonged, bacterial or fungal superinfection may occur, especially in elderly, debilitated, or immunosuppressed patients.
• Drug contains 2.84 mEq (65 mg) sodium per gram of piperacillin. Monitor patient's sodium intake and electrolyte levels.
• Monitor hematologic and coagulation parameters.
• Patients with cystic fibrosis may have a higher rate of fever and rash. Monitor these patients closely.
• *Look alike–sound alike:* Don't confuse Zosyn with Zofran or Zyvox.

PATIENT TEACHING
• Tell patient to report adverse reactions promptly.
• Tell patient to report discomfort at the IV site.

P

pitavastatin
pih-tav-a-STAT-in

Livalo, Zypitamag

Therapeutic class: Antilipemics
Pharmacologic class: HMG-CoA reductase inhibitors

AVAILABLE FORMS
Tablets: 1 mg, 2 mg, 4 mg

INDICATIONS & DOSAGES
Adjust-a-dose (for all indications): For patients with GFR of 15 to 59 mL/minute/1.73 m² who aren't receiving hemodialysis and for those with ESRD who are receiving hemodialysis, start with 1 mg PO daily; maximum dosage is 2 mg daily.

➤ **Adjunctive therapy with diet to decrease total cholesterol (TC), LDL cholesterol (LDL-C), and apolipoprotein B (apo B) triglyceride levels, and to increase HDL cholesterol level in patients with primary hyperlipidemia and mixed dyslipidemia**
Adults: Initially, 2 mg PO daily. May increase dosage as needed, to maximum of 4 mg PO daily.

✳ *NEW INDICATION:* **Heterozygous familial hypercholesterolemia in children to reduce elevated TC, LDL-C, and apo B levels**
Children age 8 and older: Initially, 2 mg PO daily. May increase as needed, to maximum of 4 mg daily.

ADMINISTRATION
PO
• May give without regard to food at any time of the day.

ACTION
Inhibits HMG-CoA reductase, a hepatic enzyme that's needed for cholesterol biosynthesis.

Route	Onset	Peak	Duration
PO	Unknown	1 hr	Unknown

Half-life: 12 hours.

ADVERSE REACTIONS
CNS: headache. **EENT:** nasopharyngitis. **GI:** constipation, diarrhea. **Musculoskeletal:** back pain, myalgia, extremity pain, *rhabdomyolysis*. **Other:** flulike symptoms.

INTERACTIONS
Drug-drug. ❸ *Alert: Atazanavir, atazanavir and ritonavir, darunavir and ritonavir, lopinavir–ritonavir:* May increase statin level and risk of myopathy and rhabdomyolysis. Avoid concurrent use with lopinavir–ritonavir combination; use together cautiously with other agents.
Colchicine: May cause myopathy, including rhabdomyolysis. Use cautiously together.
Cyclosporine: May increase pitavastatin level. Use together is contraindicated.
Erythromycin: May increase pitavastatin levels. Don't exceed 1 mg pitavastatin daily.
Fibrates (gemfibrozil, niacin): May increase risk of myopathy. Use together cautiously; consider reducing pitavastatin dosage when combined with niacin.
Rifampin: May increase pitavastatin levels. Don't exceed 2 mg pitavastatin daily.
Vitamin K antagonists (warfarin): May enhance anticoagulant effect. Monitor therapy.
Drug-herb. *Herbal cholesterol-lowering products:* May increase pitavastatin levels. Discourage using together.
Drug-food. *Grapefruit juice:* May increase pitavastatin levels and increase risk of adverse effects, including rhabdomyolysis and myopathy. Avoid using together.

EFFECTS ON LAB TEST RESULTS
• May increase AST, ALT, CK, bilirubin, HbA₁c, and glucose levels.

CONTRAINDICATIONS & CAUTIONS
• Contraindicated in patients hypersensitive to drug or its components and in those with active liver disease, which may include unexplained persistent elevations of hepatic transaminase levels.
• Use cautiously in elderly patients and in those with renal impairment, inadequately treated hypothyroidism, or a history of myopathy or rhabdomyolysis.
• Statin therapy should be interrupted if patient shows signs of serious liver injury, hyperbilirubinemia, or jaundice. The drug

shouldn't be restarted if another cause can't be found.

• Drug hasn't been studied in Fredrickson Type I, III, and V dyslipidemias.

• Safety and effectiveness in children haven't been established.

Dialyzable drug: Unlikely.

PREGNANCY-LACTATION-REPRODUCTION

• Drug may cause fetal harm. Contraindicated in women who are or may become pregnant.

• Drug is contraindicated during breastfeeding.

NURSING CONSIDERATIONS

• Start pitavastatin only after diet and other nondrug therapies have proved ineffective.

• Monitor PT and INR in patients taking warfarin when pitavastatin is added.

• Monitor LFT results and CK levels before therapy is started, 12 weeks after therapy is initiated, after a dosage change, and periodically thereafter.

• Monitor lipid levels at baseline, 4 weeks after start of therapy, and at titration; adjust dosage accordingly.

• Discontinue drug if myopathy develops or if CK level markedly increases. Doses greater than 4 mg once daily were associated with an increased risk of severe myopathy in premarketing clinical studies. Don't exceed 4 mg once daily.

• Temporarily withhold drug if patient develops sepsis; hypotension; dehydration; severe metabolic, endocrine, or electrolyte disorders; uncontrolled seizures; or trauma or if patient requires major surgery. These conditions may predispose patient to myopathy or rhabdomyolysis.

• **Look alike–sound alike:** Don't confuse pitavastatin with atorvastatin, fluvastatin, lovastatin, nystatin, pravastatin, rosuvastatin, or simvastatin.

PATIENT TEACHING

• Tell patient that drug may be taken without regard to meals.

• Explain the importance of controlling serum lipid levels. Teach appropriate dietary management (restricting saturated fat and cholesterol intake), weight control, and exercise.

• Advise female patient of childbearing potential to use contraception during therapy and to discuss future pregnancy and breastfeeding plans with health care provider.

• Advise patient to report unexplained muscle pain, tenderness, or weakness, especially if accompanied by fever or malaise.

• Advise patient that blood tests to check liver enzyme levels will be needed at 12 weeks after the start of therapy, after a dosage increase, and periodically thereafter.

• Tell patient that drug may increase blood glucose level; however, the CV benefits are thought to outweigh blood glucose level increase.

plecanatide
ple-KAN-a-tide

Trulance

Therapeutic class: Laxatives
Pharmacologic class: Guanylate cyclase-C agonists

AVAILABLE FORMS
Tablets: 3 mg

INDICATIONS & DOSAGES
➤ **Chronic idiopathic constipation or IBS with constipation**
Adults: 3 mg (1 tablet) PO daily.

ADMINISTRATION
PO
• May give with or without food.
• Patient should swallow tablets whole, if possible.
• For patients with swallowing difficulties, may crush tablet and mix with 1 tsp of room temperature applesauce; give immediately.
• May dissolve tablet by placing whole tablet in a cup and adding 30 mL of room temperature water; swirl for at least 10 seconds. Give mixture immediately. To give any portion left in cup, add an additional 30 mL of water and swirl for at least 10 seconds. Give immediately; don't store mixture.
• If giving dissolved tablet by NG or gastric feeding tube, place tablet in 30 mL of water and swirl for at least 15 seconds. Draw up mixture using an appropriate syringe and

P

administer. Flush tube with 30 mL of water before and at least 10 mL of water after administration.

• Skip a missed dose and give next dose at regularly scheduled time. Don't double dose.

• Store in dry place at room temperature. Keep drug in its original bottle with supplied desiccant.

ACTION
Plecanatide and its active metabolite bind to guanylate cyclase-C and act locally on the luminal surface of the intestinal epithelium, resulting in increased secretion of chloride and bicarbonate into the intestinal lumen, mainly through activation of the cystic fibrosis transmembrane conductance regulator ion channel, resulting in increased intestinal fluid and accelerated transit.

Route	Onset	Peak	Duration
PO	Unknown	Unknown	Unknown

Half-life: Unknown.

ADVERSE REACTIONS
CNS: dizziness. **EENT:** sinusitis, nasopharyngitis. **GI:** diarrhea, abdominal distention, flatulence, abdominal tenderness, nausea. **GU:** UTI. **Hepatic:** elevated liver enzyme levels. **Respiratory:** URI.

INTERACTIONS
None reported.

EFFECTS ON LAB TEST RESULTS
• May increase AST and ALT levels.

CONTRAINDICATIONS & CAUTIONS
Black Box Warning Contraindicated in patients younger than age 6 because of risk of serious dehydration. ∎
Black Box Warning Safety and effectiveness in patients younger than age 18 haven't been established. Avoid use in patients age 6 to younger than age 18. ∎
• Contraindicated in patients with known or suspected mechanical GI obstruction.
• Don't administered to patients with severe diarrhea. Diarrhea is the most common adverse effect of plecanatide.
• Use cautiously in elderly patients.
Dialyzable drug: Unlikely.

PREGNANCY-LACTATION-REPRODUCTION
• Drug isn't absorbed systemically; therefore, use in pregnant women isn't expected to result in fetal exposure.
• It isn't known if drug appears in human milk. Use only if benefits to mother outweigh risks to infant.

NURSING CONSIDERATIONS
• Monitor patient for diarrhea. If severe diarrhea occurs, withhold drug and rehydrate patient.
• *Look alike–sound alike:* Don't confuse Trulance with Trulicity.

PATIENT TEACHING
• Instruct patient to stop taking drug if severe diarrhea occurs and to contact prescriber.
• Instruct patient to swallow tablets whole. Show patient with swallowing difficulties how to dissolve tablet in water or take with applesauce.
• Advise patient not to make up a missed dose.
🔆 *Alert:* Warn patient to securely store drug away from children. Accidental ingestion may cause severe diarrhea and dehydration.

---

posaconazole
poe-sa-KON-a-zole

Noxafil, Posanol❈

Therapeutic class: Antifungals
Pharmacologic class: Triazole antifungals

AVAILABLE FORMS
Injection: 18 mg/mL
Oral suspension: 40 mg/mL
Tablets (delayed-release) ⊙: 100 mg

INDICATIONS & DOSAGES
➤ **Prevention of invasive** *Aspergillus* **and** *Candida* **infections in high-risk immunocompromised patients**
Adults: 200 mg (5 mL) oral suspension PO t.i.d. with a full meal or a liquid nutritional supplement. Or, 300 mg delayed-release tablet PO with food b.i.d. on first day, then 300 mg once daily. Or, 300 mg IV b.i.d. on first day, then 300 mg once daily. Duration of

---

therapy is based on recovery from neutropenia or immunosuppression.

Children ages 13 to 17: 200 mg (5 mL) oral suspension PO t.i.d. with a full meal or a liquid nutritional supplement. Or, 300 mg delayed-release tablet PO b.i.d. with food on first day, then 300 mg once daily. Duration of therapy is based on recovery from neutropenia or immunosuppression.

➤ **Oropharyngeal candidiasis**
Adults and children age 13 and older:
100 mg (2.5 mL) PO b.i.d. on first day, then 100 mg (2.5 mL) once daily for 13 days with a full meal or a liquid nutritional supplement.

➤ **Oropharyngeal candidiasis resistant to itraconazole or fluconazole treatment**
Adults and children age 13 and older:
400 mg (10 mL) PO b.i.d. with a full meal or a liquid nutritional supplement; duration of treatment is based on severity of underlying disease and patient response.

ADMINISTRATION
PO
• Delayed-release tablets and oral suspension aren't to be used interchangeably because of differences in the dosing of each formulation.
PO (suspension)
• Give with a full meal, liquid nutritional supplement, or an acidic carbonated beverage (e.g., ginger ale).
• Shake well before giving it.
• Measure doses using calibrated spoon provided with the drug, which has two markings, one for 2.5 mL and one for 5 mL. After patient takes dose, fill spoon with water and have patient drink it to ensure a full dose.
• Store at room temperature.
PO (delayed-release tablets)
• Patient should swallow tablets whole; don't divide, crush, or allow patient to chew tablets.
• Administer with food.
• Delayed-release oral formulation is preferred for prophylaxis due to higher plasma drug exposures.
IV
▼ Bring refrigerated vial to room temperature.
▼ To prepare, transfer one vial of drug to IV bag or bottle of half-NSS, NSS, D₅W,

D₅W half-NSS, D₅W NSS, or D₅W with 20 mEq potassium chloride to achieve a final concentration that's between 1 and 2 mg/mL. Solution may be colorless to yellow.
▼ Use mixture immediately after preparation, or it can be stored up to 24 hours refrigerated (36° to 46° F [2° to 8° C]).
❸ *Alert:* Infuse over 90 minutes via central venous line. When multiple dosing is required, administer via central venous line. Don't give by IV push or bolus.
▼ If a central venous line isn't available, administer only once through peripheral venous catheter over 30 minutes in advance of central venous line placement or to bridge period during which central venous line is replaced or is in use for other IV treatment; multiple peripheral infusions given through the same vein have resulted in infusion-site reactions.
▼ An in-line filter (0.22-micron polyethersulfone or polyvinylidene difluoride) must be used during infusion.
▼ **Incompatibilities:** Diluents, including lactated Ringer solution, 5% dextrose with lactated Ringer solution, 4.2% sodium bicarbonate. Consult a drug incompatibility reference for more information.

ACTION
Blocks the synthesis of ergosterol, a vital component of the fungal cell membrane.

Route	Onset	Peak	Duration
PO (suspension)	Unknown	3–5 hr	Unknown
PO (tablets)	Unknown	4–5 hr	Unknown
IV	Unknown	Unknown	Unknown

Half-life: Suspension, 20 to 66 hours; tablets, 26 to 31 hours; injection, 27 hours.

ADVERSE REACTIONS
CNS: anxiety, dizziness, fatigue, fever, headache, insomnia, weakness. **CV:** edema, HTN, hypotension, tachycardia. **EENT:** epistaxis, pharyngitis, altered taste, blurred vision. **GI:** abdominal pain, constipation, diarrhea, dyspepsia, mucositis, nausea, vomiting. **GU:** *vaginal hemorrhage.* **Hematologic:** anemia, petechiae, *febrile neutropenia, neutropenia, thrombocytopenia.* **Hepatic:** bilirubinemia. **Metabolic:** anorexia, hyperglycemia, *hypokalemia,*

hypomagnesemia, hypocalcemia. **Musculoskeletal:** arthralgia, back pain, musculoskeletal pain. **Respiratory:** cough, dyspnea, URI. **Skin:** pruritus, rash, diaphoresis. **Other:** bacteremia, CMV infection, herpes simplex, rigors, chills.

INTERACTIONS

Drug-drug. *Atazanavir, ritonavir:* May increase plasma concentrations of these drugs. Frequently monitor for adverse effects and toxicity during coadministration.

Calcium channel blockers, cyclosporine, phenytoin, tacrolimus: May increase levels of these drugs. Reduce dosages, increase monitoring of levels, and observe patient for adverse effects.

Cimetidine, phenytoin: May decrease level and effectiveness of posaconazole. Avoid using together.

CYP3A4 substrates (astemizole, cisapride, halofantrine, pimozide, quinidine, terfenadine): May lead to QT-interval prolongation and torsades de pointes. Use together is contraindicated.

Digoxin: May increase digoxin level. Monitor digoxin level.

Efavirenz: May significantly decrease posaconazole plasma concentration. Avoid use together unless benefit outweighs risks.

Ergot alkaloids (dihydroergotamine, ergotamine): May increase ergot level. Use together is contraindicated.

Fosamprenavir: May decrease posaconazole level. Monitor patient closely for breakthrough fungal infection.

HMG-CoA reductase inhibitors metabolized through CYP3A4, sirolimus: May increase levels of these drugs. Use with posaconazole is contraindicated.

Metoclopramide: May decrease posaconazole level when used with posaconazole suspension. (No such effect when used with posaconazole tablets.) Monitor patient for breakthrough fungal infections.

Midazolam: May significantly increase midazolam concentration and potentiate or prolong sedative or hypnotic effects. Reversal agents should be readily available.

PPIs: May decrease posaconazole level. Consider therapy modification.

QTc interval–prolonging drugs: May enhance prolongation of QTc interval.

When used with moderate QTc interval–prolonging drugs, monitor therapy. Avoid use with high-risk QTc interval–prolonging drugs; if use together is unavoidable, monitor QTc interval and cardiac rhythm closely.

Rifabutin: May decrease level and effectiveness of posaconazole while increasing rifabutin level and risk of toxicity. Avoid using together. If unavoidable, monitor patient for uveitis, leukopenia, and other adverse effects.

Sirolimus: May increase sirolimus blood concentration, resulting in sirolimus toxicity. Use together is contraindicated.

Vinca alkaloids (vincristine, vinblastine): May increase plasma concentrations of vinca alkaloids, leading to neurotoxicity and other serious adverse reactions. Don't use together unless there are no alternative antifungal treatment options.

Drug-food. *Any food, liquid nutritional supplements:* May greatly enhance absorption of drug. Always give drug with liquid supplement or food.

EFFECTS ON LAB TEST RESULTS

- May increase AST, ALT, bilirubin, creatinine, alkaline phosphatase, and glucose levels.
- May decrease potassium, magnesium, and calcium levels.
- May decrease WBC, RBC, and platelet counts.

CONTRAINDICATIONS & CAUTIONS

- Contraindicated in patients hypersensitive to drug or its components and in patients taking sirolimus, HMG-CoA reductase inhibitors that are primarily metabolized through CYP3A4 (atorvastatin, lovastatin, simvastatin), CYP3A4 substrates that prolong the QT interval (pimozide, quinidine), other antifungal agents, or ergot derivatives.
- Use cautiously in patients hypersensitive to other azole antifungals, patients with potentially proarrhythmic conditions, and patients with hepatic or renal insufficiency.
- Safety in children younger than age 13 hasn't been established.

⟳ Alert: Drug may prolong QT interval and increase risk of torsades de pointes.

Dialyzable drug: No.

Reactions in bold italics are *life-threatening*. Interactions may have a *rapid onset* or a **delayed onset**.

PREGNANCY-LACTATION-REPRODUCTION

• There are no adequate studies in pregnant women. Drug may cause fetal harm. Use during pregnancy only if potential benefit outweighs potential risk to the fetus.

• It isn't known if drug appears in human milk. Patient should discontinue breastfeeding or discontinue drug.

NURSING CONSIDERATIONS

• Use IV route only when oral administration isn't possible.

• Avoid IV route in patients with moderate or severe renal impairment (eGFR <50 mL/minute), unless benefit vs. risk to patient justifies its use. Closely monitor serum creatinine level; if increases occur, consider changing to oral therapy.

• Don't use delayed-release tablets and oral suspension interchangeably.

• Correct electrolyte imbalances, especially potassium, magnesium, and calcium imbalances, before therapy.

• Monitor patient for signs and symptoms of electrolyte imbalance, including a slow, weak, or irregular pulse; ECG change; nausea; neuromuscular irritability; and tetany.

• Obtain baseline LFTs, including bilirubin level, before therapy and periodically during treatment. Notify prescriber if patient develops signs or symptoms of hepatic dysfunction.

• Monitor patient weighing more than 120 kg closely for breakthrough fungal infections because of lower plasma drug exposure.

• Monitor patient who has severe vomiting or diarrhea for breakthrough fungal infection.

• *Look alike–sound alike:* Don't confuse posaconazole with fluconazole, ketoconazole, itraconazole, or voriconazole. Don't confuse Noxafil with minoxidil.

PATIENT TEACHING

• Instruct patient who can't take a liquid supplement or eat a full meal to notify prescriber. A different anti-infective may be needed, or monitoring may need to be increased.

• Tell patient to notify prescriber about an irregular heartbeat, fainting, or severe diarrhea or vomiting.

• Explain the signs and symptoms of liver dysfunction, including abdominal pain, yellowing skin or eyes, pale stools, and dark urine.

• Urge patient to contact the prescriber or pharmacist before taking other prescription or OTC drugs, herbal supplements, or dietary supplements.

• Tell patient to shake the suspension well before taking it.

• Instruct patient to measure doses using the spoon provided with the drug. Household spoons vary in size and may yield an incorrect dose.

• Point out that the calibrated spoon has two markings: one for 2.5 mL and one for 5 mL. Make sure patient understands which mark to use for the prescribed dose.

• After patient takes dose, tell patient to fill the spoon with water and drink it, to ensure a full dose, and to clean the spoon with water before putting it away.

• Tell patient not to break, crush, or chew delayed-release tablets.

potassium acetate

Therapeutic class: Potassium supplements
Pharmacologic class: Potassium salts

AVAILABLE FORMS

Injection: 2 mEq/mL in 20-mL, 50-mL, and 100-mL vials

INDICATIONS & DOSAGES

➤ **Hypokalemia**

Adults age 19 and older: Individualize dosage and give by IV infusion; normal daily requirements are 40 to 80 mEq/24 hours.

Children: Individualize dosage and give by IV infusion; normal daily requirements are 2 to 3 mEq/kg/24 hours. For newborns, normal daily requirement is 2 to 6 mEq/kg/24 hours.

ADMINISTRATION

IV

▼ Use only in life-threatening hypokalemia or when oral replacement isn't feasible.

▼ Don't give undiluted potassium. Maximum infusion rate is 1 mEq/kg/hour.

P

▼ Don't add potassium to a hanging bag. Mix well to avoid layering.

▼ To prevent pain, use largest peripheral vein and a well-placed small-bore needle.

▼ Give only by infusion, never IV push or IM. Watch for pain and redness at infusion site.

▼ Give slowly as diluted solution; rapid infusion may cause fatal hyperkalemia.

▼ **Incompatibilities:** None listed by manufacturer. Consult a drug incompatibility reference for more information.

ACTION
Replaces potassium and maintains potassium level.

Route	Onset	Peak	Duration
IV	Immediate	Immediate	Unknown

Half-life: Unknown.

ADVERSE REACTIONS
CNS: paresthesia of limbs, listlessness, mental confusion, weakness or heaviness of legs, flaccid paralysis, pain, fever. **CV:** *arrhythmias, cardiac arrest, heart block,* ECG changes, hypotension. **GI:** nausea, vomiting, abdominal pain, diarrhea. **Metabolic:** *hyperkalemia.* **Respiratory:** *respiratory paralysis.* **Skin:** redness at infusion site.

INTERACTIONS
Drug-drug. *ACE inhibitors, aldosterone blockers, ARBs, potassium-sparing diuretics:* May increase risk of hyperkalemia. Use together with caution.
Digoxin: May cause digoxin toxicity from hypokalemia if drug is stopped. Stop potassium cautiously if patient is taking digoxin.
Eplerenone: May increase hyperkalemia risk. Use together is contraindicated when eplerenone is used to treat HTN.
Heparin: May enhance hyperkalemic effects of potassium salts. Monitor therapy.
Drug-food. *Potassium-containing salt substitutes:* May increase risk of hyperkalemia. Use together cautiously.

EFFECTS ON LAB TEST RESULTS
• May increase potassium level.

CONTRAINDICATIONS & CAUTIONS
• Contraindicated in patients with severe renal impairment with oliguria, anuria, or azotemia.

• Contraindicated in patients with adrenal insufficiency and in those with diseases in which high potassium levels are encountered.

• Use cautiously in patients with cardiac disease or renal impairment.
Dialyzable drug: Unknown.

⚠ *Overdose S&S:* Paresthesia, flaccid paralysis, listlessness, confusion, weakness and heaviness of legs, hypotension, cardiac arrhythmias, heart block, ECG changes, cardiac arrest.

PREGNANCY-LACTATION-REPRODUCTION
• Safe use in pregnant women hasn't been established. Use only if benefit justifies potential risk to the fetus.

• It isn't known if drug appears in human milk. Use cautiously in breastfeeding women.

NURSING CONSIDERATIONS
• During therapy, monitor ECG, renal function, fluid intake and output, and potassium, creatinine, and BUN levels. Never give potassium postoperatively until urine flow is established.

• Many adverse reactions may reflect hyperkalemia, muscle weakness or paralysis, and cardiac conduction abnormalities (heart block, ventricular arrhythmias, asystole).

⚠ *Alert:* Consider a separate storage area for concentrated IV potassium. Fatal outcomes are possible if concentrated potassium is administered by IV push.

• Use great care when giving solutions containing acetate ions to patients with metabolic or respiratory alkalosis and to those with conditions such as hepatic impairment in which the acetate levels may be increased or the utilization of the ion may be impaired.

⚠ *Alert:* Product contains aluminum and may reach toxic levels with prolonged parenteral administration in patients with renal impairment. Premature neonates are particularly at risk.

• *Look alike–sound alike:* Potassium preparations aren't interchangeable; verify preparation before use.

PATIENT TEACHING
• Explain use and administration to patient and family.
• Tell patient to report adverse effects, especially pain at insertion site.
• Advise patient to immediately report signs and symptoms of hyperkalemia (arrhythmia, bradycardia, weakness).

SAFETY ALERT!

potassium chloride
Klor-Con, Klor-Con 10, Klor-Con M10, Klor-Con M15, Klor-Con M20, Klor-Con Sprinkle, K-Tab

Therapeutic class: Potassium supplements
Pharmacologic class: Potassium salts

AVAILABLE FORMS
Capsules (extended-release) ⊕*:* 8 mEq, 10 mEq
Injection concentrate: 2 mEq/mL
Injection for IV infusion: 0.1 mEq/mL, 0.2 mEq/mL, 0.4 mEq/mL
Oral liquid: 20 mEq/15 mL, 40 mEq/15 mL
Powder for oral administration: 20 mEq/packet
Tablets (extended-release) ⊕*:* 8 mEq, 10 mEq, 15 mEq, 20 mEq

INDICATIONS & DOSAGES
➤ **To prevent hypokalemia**
Adults: Initially, 16 to 24 mEq of potassium supplement PO daily, in divided doses. Adjust dosage, as needed, based on potassium levels. Patient should take no more than 20 or 25 mEq at a single dose.
➤ **Hypokalemia**
Adults: 40 to 100 mEq PO in two to five divided doses daily. Patient should take no more than 20 or 25 mEq at a single dose. Maximum dose of diluted IV potassium chloride is 40 mEq/L at 10 mEq/hour. Don't exceed 200 mEq daily. Further doses are based on potassium levels and blood pH. Give IV potassium replacement only with monitoring of ECG and potassium level.

➤ **Severe hypokalemia**
Adults: Dilute potassium chloride in a suitable IV solution of less than 80 mEq/L, and give at no more than 40 mEq/hour.
Further doses are based on potassium level. Don't exceed 400 mEq IV daily. Give IV potassium replacement only with monitoring of ECG and potassium level.

ADMINISTRATION
PO
• Make sure powders are completely dissolved before giving.
• Enteric-coated tablets are not recommended because of increased risk of GI bleeding and small-bowel ulcerations.
• Patient should take with meals and a full glass of water or other liquid to minimize risk of GI irritation.
• Tablets in wax matrix may lodge in the esophagus and cause ulceration in cardiac patients with esophageal compression from an enlarged left atrium. Use sugar-free liquid form in these patients and in those with esophageal stasis or obstruction. Have patient sip slowly to minimize GI irritation.
• Don't crush extended-release forms.
IV
▼ Use only when oral replacement isn't feasible or when hypokalemia is life-threatening.
▼ Give by infusion only, never IV push or IM. Give slowly as dilute solution; rapid infusion may cause fatal hyperkalemia.
▼ Administer high concentrations (300 and 400 mEq/L) exclusively via a central route and infusion pump.
▼ If burning occurs during infusion, decrease rate.
▼ Drug is a vesicant/irritant (at concentrations greater than 0.1 mEq/mL); ensure proper needle or catheter placement before and during infusion. Avoid extravasation.
▼ **Incompatibilities:** None listed by manufacturer. Consult a drug incompatibility reference for more information.

ACTION
Replaces potassium and maintains potassium level.

Route	Onset	Peak	Duration
PO	Unknown	Unknown	Unknown
IV	Immediate	Immediate	Unknown

Half-life: Unknown.

ADVERSE REACTIONS
CNS: paresthesia of limbs, listlessness, confusion, weakness or heaviness of limbs, flaccid paralysis. **CV:** postinfusion phlebitis, *arrhythmias, heart block, cardiac arrest,* ECG changes, hypotension. **GI:** nausea, vomiting, abdominal pain, diarrhea. **Metabolic:** *hyperkalemia.* **Respiratory:** *respiratory paralysis.* **Skin:** injection-site reactions.

INTERACTIONS
Drug-drug. *ACE inhibitors, ARBs, digoxin, heparins, potassium-sparing diuretics:* May cause hyperkalemia. Use together with extreme caution. Monitor potassium level. *Eplerenone:* May increase hyperkalemia risk. Use together is contraindicated when eplerenone is used to treat HTN.

EFFECTS ON LAB TEST RESULTS
• May increase potassium level.

CONTRAINDICATIONS & CAUTIONS
• Contraindicated in patients hypersensitive to potassium chloride or components of the formulation, in patients with renal failure, and in those with conditions in which potassium retention is present.
• Use cautiously in patients with cardiac disease, renal impairment, and acid-base disorders.
Dialyzable drug: Yes.
⚠ *Overdose S&S:* ECG changes, weakness, flaccidity, respiratory paralysis, cardiac arrhythmias, death.

PREGNANCY-LACTATION-REPRODUCTION
• It isn't known if drug causes fetal harm. Use only if clearly needed.
• It isn't known if drug appears in human milk. Use cautiously in breastfeeding women.

NURSING CONSIDERATIONS
• Patients at increased risk for GI lesions when taking oral potassium include those with scleroderma, diabetes, mitral valve replacement, cardiomegaly, or esophageal strictures, and elderly or immobile patients.
• Drug is commonly used orally with potassium-wasting diuretics to maintain potassium levels.
• Monitor continuous ECG and electrolyte levels during therapy.
• Monitor renal function. After surgery, don't give drug until urine flow is established.
• Many adverse reactions may reflect hyperkalemia.
• Patient may be sensitive to tartrazine in some of these products.
❸ *Alert:* Consider a separate storage area for concentrated IV potassium. Fatal outcomes are possible if concentrated potassium is administered by IV push.
• *Look alike–sound alike:* Potassium preparations aren't interchangeable; verify preparation before use and don't switch products. Don't confuse Kaon-Cl-10 with Kaolin, KCl with HCl, KlorCon with Klaron, or Micro-K with Macrobid or Micronase.

PATIENT TEACHING
• Teach patient how to prepare powders and how to take drug. Tell patient to take with or after meals with full glass of water or fruit juice to lessen GI distress.
• Teach patient signs and symptoms of hyperkalemia, and tell patient to notify prescriber if they occur.
• Tell patient to report discomfort at IV insertion site.
• Warn patient not to use salt substitutes concurrently, except with prescriber's permission.
• Tell patient not to be concerned if wax matrix appears in stool because the drug has already been absorbed.

pramipexole dihydrochloride
pram-ah-PEX-ole

Mirapex, Mirapex ER

Therapeutic class: Antiparkinsonians
Pharmacologic class: Nonergot dopamine agonists

AVAILABLE FORMS
Tablets: 0.125 mg, 0.25 mg, 0.5 mg, 0.75 mg, 1 mg, 1.5 mg

Tablets (extended-release) ⓓⓝⓒ*:* 0.375 mg, 0.75 mg, 1.5 mg, 2.25 mg, 3 mg, 3.75 mg, 4.5 mg

INDICATIONS & DOSAGES
➤ **Signs and symptoms of idiopathic Parkinson disease**
Adults: Initially, 0.375 mg PO daily in three divided doses. Adjust doses slowly (not more often than every 5 to 7 days) over several weeks until desired therapeutic effect is achieved. Maintenance dosage is 1.5 to 4.5 mg daily in three divided doses. Or, 0.375 mg (extended-release form) PO once daily. May titrate dosage gradually (not more often than every 5 to 7 days), first to 0.75 mg PO daily, then by 0.75-mg increments to maximum recommended dosage of 4.5 mg/day.
Adjust-a-dose: For patients with CrCl over 50 mL/minute, first dosage of immediate-release tablets is 0.125 mg PO t.i.d., up to 1.5 mg t.i.d. For those with CrCl of 30 to 50 mL/minute, first dosage is 0.125 mg PO b.i.d., up to 0.75 mg t.i.d. For those with CrCl of 15 mL/minute to less than 30 mL/minute, first dosage is 0.125 mg PO daily, up to 1.5 mg daily. If using extended-release tablets, in patients with CrCl of 30 to 50 mL/minute, initially give dose every other day. Use caution and assess response and tolerability before increasing to daily dosing after 1 week and before titration. Titrate dosage in 0.375-mg increments up to 2.25 mg/day, no more frequently than at weekly intervals. Don't use extended-release tablets in patients with CrCl of less than 30 mL/minute or in hemodialysis patients.
➤ **Moderate to severe primary restless leg syndrome (immediate-release only)**
Adults: 0.125 mg PO daily, 2 to 3 hours before bedtime. May increase after 4 to 7 days to 0.25 mg PO daily, as needed. May increase again after 4 to 7 days to 0.5 mg PO daily, if needed.
Adjust-a-dose: For patients with CrCl of 20 to 60 mL/minute, increase the duration between titration steps to 14 days.

ADMINISTRATION
PO
• Give drug with or without food; giving with food may reduce nausea.

• Patient must swallow extended-release tablets whole; tablets shouldn't be chewed, crushed, or divided.
• If a significant interruption in therapy occurs, retitration of therapy may be warranted.

ACTION
Thought to stimulate dopamine receptors.

Route	Onset	Peak	Duration
PO	Rapid	2–6 hr	8–12 hr

Half-life: About 8½ hours.

ADVERSE REACTIONS
CNS: asthenia, confusion, dizziness, dream abnormalities, dyskinesia, extrapyramidal syndrome, hallucinations, insomnia, somnolence, amnesia, akathisia, drowsiness, delusions, dystonia, gait abnormalities, hypoesthesia, hypertonia, myoclonus, paranoid reaction, malaise, sleep disorders, thought abnormalities, fever. **CV:** orthostatic hypotension, chest pain, peripheral edema. **EENT:** accommodation abnormalities, diplopia, rhinitis, vision abnormalities. **GI:** constipation, nausea, dry mouth, anorexia, dysphagia, vomiting. **GU:** erectile dysfunction, urinary frequency, UTI, urinary incontinence. **Metabolic:** weight loss. **Musculoskeletal:** arthritis, bursitis, myasthenia, twitching. **Respiratory:** dyspnea, cough, pneumonia. **Skin:** skin disorders. **Other:** accidental injury, decreased libido, general edema, impulse control disorders.

INTERACTIONS
Drug-drug. *Antipsychotics (typical):* May diminish therapeutic effects of pramipexole. Avoid use together if possible; if use together is unavoidable, monitor therapy carefully.
Cimetidine, diltiazem, quinidine, quinine, ranitidine, triamterene, verapamil: May decrease pramipexole clearance. Adjust dosage as needed.
Dopamine antagonists: May reduce pramipexole effectiveness. Monitor patient closely.
Drug-lifestyle. *Alcohol use:* May increase sedative effects. Avoid use together.

EFFECTS ON LAB TEST RESULTS
• May increase CK level.

CONTRAINDICATIONS & CAUTIONS
• Contraindicated in patients hypersensitive to drug or its components.
• Use cautiously in patients with renal impairment.
• Use cautiously in patients with a known major psychotic disorder due to risk of exacerbating psychosis.
• Use cautiously in patients with hypotension.
• Drug may cause somnolence, and patients may fall asleep without warning.
Dialyzable drug: Unknown.

PREGNANCY-LACTATION-REPRODUCTION
• There are no studies in pregnant women. Animal studies suggest drug may cause fetal harm. Use only if benefit clearly justifies potential risk to the fetus.
• It isn't known if drug appears in human milk. Drug inhibits prolactin secretion and may inhibit lactation. Patient should discontinue breastfeeding or discontinue drug.

NURSING CONSIDERATIONS
• Drug should be tapered off at a rate of 0.75 mg/day until daily dose has been reduced to 0.75 mg. Thereafter, dose may be reduced by 0.375 mg/day.
• Drug may cause orthostatic hypotension, especially during dosage increases. Monitor patient carefully.
• Drug may cause intense impulse control and compulsive behaviors. Monitor patient for problems with impulse control (such as gambling urges, intense sexual urges, binge eating).
• Adjust dosage gradually to achieve maximal therapeutic effect, balanced against the main adverse effects of dyskinesia, hallucinations, somnolence, and dry mouth.
• Assess patients for preexisting sleep disorder and monitor for daytime sleepiness and for episodes of falling asleep without warning. Drug may need to be discontinued.
• *Look alike–sound alike:* Don't confuse Mirapex with Hiprex, Mifeprex, or MiraLax.

PATIENT TEACHING
• Instruct patient not to rise rapidly after sitting or lying down because of risk of dizziness.

• Tell patient about potential for daytime sleepiness and falling asleep without warning and to report episodes to prescriber. Caution patient to avoid hazardous activities until CNS response to drug is known.
• Tell patient to use caution before taking drug with other CNS depressants.
• Tell patient (especially elderly patient) to immediately report hallucinations and changes in impulse control behaviors.
• Advise patient to take drug with food if nausea develops.
• Tell female patient to notify prescriber if she is or will be breastfeeding.
• Advise patient that it may take 4 weeks for effects of drug to be noticed because of slow adjustment schedule.
• Instruct patient that drug should be tapered gradually and not stopped abruptly.
• Instruct patient to report problems with muscle control (dyskinesias).

SAFETY ALERT!

pramlintide acetate
PRAM-lin-tide

SymlinPen 60, SymlinPen 120

Therapeutic class: Antidiabetics
Pharmacologic class: Human amylin analogues

AVAILABLE FORMS
Injection: 1 mg/mL in 1.5-mL and 2.7-mL multidose pen injectors

INDICATIONS & DOSAGES
➤ **Adjunct to insulin in patients with type 1 diabetes mellitus**
Adults: Initially, 15 mcg subcut before major meals (more than 250 calories or 30 g of carbohydrates). Reduce prandial rapid-acting or short-acting insulin dose, including fixed-mix insulin such as 70/30, by 50%. Increase pramlintide dose by 15-mcg increments every 3 days if no nausea occurs, to a maintenance dose of 30 to 60 mcg. Adjust insulin dose as needed.
Adjust-a-dose: If significant nausea at 45 or 60 mcg persists, decrease to 30 mcg. If nausea persists at 30 mcg, consider stopping.

Reactions in bold italics are *life-threatening*. Interactions may have a *rapid onset* or a *delayed onset*.

➤ **Adjunct to insulin in patients with type 2 diabetes mellitus, with or without a sulfonylurea or metformin**

Adults: Initially, 60 mcg subcut immediately before major meals. Reduce preprandial rapid-acting or short-acting insulin dose, including fixed-mix insulin, by 50%. Increase pramlintide dose to 120 mcg if no significant nausea occurs for at least 3 days. Adjust insulin dose as needed.

Adjust-a-dose: If significant nausea persists at 120 mcg, decrease to 60 mcg.

ADMINISTRATION
Subcutaneous

• Before starting drug, review patient's HbA_{1c} level, recent blood glucose monitoring data, hypoglycemic episodes, current insulin regimen, and body weight. Reduce preprandial, rapid-acting or short-acting insulin dosages, including fixed-mix insulins, by 50%.
• Allow medication to reach room temperature before injecting.
• Give each dose subcut into abdomen or thigh. Rotate injection sites.
• Administer immediately before each major meal consisting of 250 kcal or more or containing 30 g or more of carbohydrates.
• Always administer pramlintide and insulin as separate injections. The injection site for pramlintide should be distinct from the site for concomitant insulin injection.
• Don't transfer drug to syringe for administration. Don't mix with any type of insulin.
🜂 **Alert:** Multidose pens are for single-patient use only. Pens should never be shared, even if the needle is changed. Clearly label with patient identifying information where it won't obstruct the dosing window, warning, or other product information.
• After initial use, may keep refrigerated or at room temperature (86° F [30° C]).
• Discard after 30 days; protect from light.

ACTION

Slows rate at which food leaves the stomach, reducing the initial postprandial increase in glucose level. Decreases hyperglycemia by reducing postprandial glucagon level and reduces total caloric intake by reducing appetite.

Route	Onset	Peak	Duration
Subcut	Unknown	19–21 min	3 hr

Half-life: Parent drug and metabolite, about 48 minutes each.

ADVERSE REACTIONS
CNS: dizziness, fatigue, headache. **EENT:** pharyngitis. **GI:** abdominal pain, anorexia, nausea, vomiting. **Metabolic:** *hypoglycemia.* **Musculoskeletal:** arthralgia. **Respiratory:** cough. **Skin:** injection-site reaction. **Other:** allergic reaction, accidental injury.

INTERACTIONS
Drug-drug. *ACE inhibitors, disopyramide, fibrates, fluoxetine, MAO inhibitors, oral antidiabetics, pentoxifylline, propoxyphene, salicylates, sulfonamide antibiotics:* May increase risk of hypoglycemia. Monitor glucose level closely.
Alpha-glucosidase inhibitors (acarbose), anticholinergics (atropine, benztropine, TCAs): May alter GI motility and slow intestinal absorption. Avoid using together.
Beta blockers, clonidine, guanethidine, reserpine: May mask signs of hypoglycemia. Monitor glucose level closely.
Oral drugs dependent on rapid onset of action (such as analgesics, antibiotics, oral contraceptives): May delay absorption because of slowed gastric emptying. If rapid effect is needed, give oral drug 1 hour before or 2 hours after pramlintide.

EFFECTS ON LAB TEST RESULTS
None reported.

CONTRAINDICATIONS & CAUTIONS
• Contraindicated in patients hypersensitive to drug or its components, including metacresol, and in patients with gastroparesis or hypoglycemia unawareness.
• Don't use in patients nonadherent with current insulin and glucose monitoring regimen, patients with an HbA_{1c} level greater than 9%, patients with severe hypoglycemia during the previous 6 months, and patients who take drugs that stimulate GI motility.
• Safe use in children hasn't been established.
• Use cautiously in elderly patients.

P

Dialyzable drug: Unknown.

⚠ *Overdose S&S:* Severe nausea, vomiting, diarrhea, vasodilation, dizziness.

PREGNANCY-LACTATION-REPRODUCTION

• There are no adequate studies in pregnant women. Use only if potential benefit justifies potential risk to the fetus. Other agents are currently recommended to treat diabetes in pregnant women.

• It isn't known if drug appears in human milk. Use in breastfeeding women only if benefit clearly outweighs risk to infant.

NURSING CONSIDERATIONS

Black Box Warning When used with insulin, drug may increase risk of insulin-induced severe hypoglycemia, particularly in patients with type 1 diabetes. Risk of severe hypoglycemia is highest within first 3 hours after an injection. Serious injuries may occur if severe hypoglycemia develops while patient is operating a motor vehicle or heavy machinery or engaging in other high-risk activities. ∎

Black Box Warning Appropriate patient selection, careful patient instruction, and insulin dosage adjustments are critical elements for reducing risk of hypoglycemia. ∎

• Symptoms of hypoglycemia may be masked in patients with a long history of diabetes, diabetic nerve disease, or intensified diabetes control.

• Notify prescriber of severe nausea and vomiting. A reduced dose may be needed.

• If patient has persistent nausea or recurrent, unexplained hypoglycemia that requires medical assistance, stop drug.

• If patient doesn't comply with glucose monitoring or drug dosage adjustments, drug will need to be stopped.

PATIENT TEACHING

• Teach patient how to take drug exactly as prescribed, at mealtimes. Explain that it doesn't replace daily insulin but may lower the amount of insulin needed.

• Explain that a meal is considered more than 250 calories or 30 g of carbohydrates.

• Caution patient not to mix drug with insulin. Instruct patient to give the injections at separate sites.

• Instruct patient not to change doses of pramlintide or insulin without consulting prescriber.

• Instruct patient not to transfer drug from pen injector to syringe.

🔔 *Alert:* Warn patient not to share the multidose pen with other people, even if the needle is changed, because of the risk of bloodborne pathogen transmission, including HIV and hepatitis virus.

Black Box Warning Tell patient to refrain from driving, operating heavy machinery, or performing other risky activities that may cause harm to patient or others until drug's effects on glucose level are known. ∎

Black Box Warning Caution patient about possibility of severe hypoglycemia, particularly within 3 hours after injection. ∎

• Teach patient and family members the signs and symptoms of hypoglycemia, including hunger, headache, sweating, tremor, irritability, and difficulty concentrating.

• Instruct patient and family members what to do if patient develops hypoglycemia.

• Tell patient to report severe nausea and vomiting to prescriber.

• Advise female patient of childbearing potential to tell prescriber if she is, could be, or is planning to become pregnant.

• Teach patient how to handle unplanned situations, such as illness or stress, low or forgotten insulin dose, accidental use of too much insulin or drug, not enough food, or missed meals.

• Tell patient to keep unopened injector pens refrigerated and protected from light; in-use pens can be refrigerated or kept at room temperature. Patient should discard after 30 days.

SAFETY ALERT!

prasugrel hydrochloride
PRA-soo-grel

Effient♦

Therapeutic class: Antiplatelet drugs
Pharmacologic class: Adenosine diphosphate–induced platelet aggregation inhibitors

AVAILABLE FORMS
Tablets: 5 mg, 10 mg

INDICATIONS & DOSAGES

➤ To reduce thrombotic events in patients with ACS (unstable angina and non-ST-elevation MI) managed with PCI; to reduce thrombotic events in patients with ACS (ST-elevation MI) managed with primary or delayed PCI

Adults: Initially, single 60-mg loading dose; then 10 mg PO once daily. Patient should also take aspirin 75 to 325 mg PO daily.

Adjust-a-dose: For adults weighing less than 60 kg, consider reducing dosage to 5 mg PO once daily.

ADMINISTRATION

PO

• May give drug with or without food.
• Don't break tablets. In an emergent primary PCI setting, crushing tablets (using a commercially available syringe crusher) and mixing with 25 mL water led to faster absorption and a quicker, more potent antiplatelet effect (seen as early as 30 minutes). Also, tablets may be chewed and swallowed (bitter to taste) or crushed and mixed in food or liquid (applesauce, juice, water) and immediately given by mouth or gastric tube.
• Administration via an enteral tube that bypasses the acidic environment of the stomach may result in reduced bioavailability of prasugrel.

ACTION

Inhibits platelet activation and aggregation through irreversible binding of its active metabolite to the P2Y12 class of ADP receptors on platelets.

Route	Onset	Peak	Duration
PO	Rapid	30 min	5–9 days

Half-life: 7 hours (range, 2 to 15 hours).

ADVERSE REACTIONS

CNS: dizziness, fatigue, headache, fever. **CV:** atrial fibrillation, bradycardia, HTN or hypotension, peripheral edema. **GI:** *GI bleeding,* nausea, diarrhea. **EENT:** epistaxis. **Hematologic:** *bleeding,* leukopenia, *thrombotic thrombocytopenic purpura.* **Metabolic:** hypercholesterolemia, hyperlipidemia. **Musculoskeletal:** back pain, extremity pain. **Respiratory:** cough, dyspnea. **Skin:** rash. **Other:** noncardiac chest pain.

INTERACTIONS

Drug-drug. *Direct factor Xa inhibitors (rivaroxaban), direct thrombin inhibitors (dabigatran, desirudin), fibrinolytics (tenecteplase), heparin, low-molecular-weight heparin, NSAIDs (long-term use), platelet inhibitors, warfarin:* May increase the risk of bleeding. Use together cautiously.
Opioids: Delay absorption of prasugrel due to slowed gastric emptying. Consider therapy modification.
Vitamin E (systemic): May enhance antiplatelet effect of agents with antiplatelet properties. Monitor therapy.
Drug-herb. *Fish oil, garlic, ginger, ginkgo, omega-3 fatty acids:* Inhibit platelet aggregation. Use cautiously together; monitor patient for signs and symptoms of bleeding.

EFFECTS ON LAB TEST RESULTS

• May increase cholesterol and lipid levels.
• May decrease WBC and platelet counts.

CONTRAINDICATIONS & CAUTIONS

Black Box Warning Contraindicated in patients with pathologic bleeding (such as peptic ulcer or intracranial hemorrhage) and in those with a history of TIA or stroke. ■
Black Box Warning Prasugrel is generally not recommended in patients age 75 and older because of the increased risk of intracranial and fatal bleeding and uncertain benefit, except in high-risk situations (patients with diabetes or a history of prior MI). In these situations, drug's effect appears to be greater and its use may be considered. ■
Black Box Warning Use cautiously in patients who weigh less than 60 kg and in those with a propensity to bleed or who are using drugs that increase bleeding risk (warfarin, heparin, fibrinolytic therapy, long-term NSAID use) because of increased risk of bleeding. ■
• Contraindicated in patients with hypersensitivity to prasugrel or its components. Angioedema can occur.
• Use cautiously in patients at risk for increased bleeding from trauma, surgery, or other pathologic conditions and in those with severe hepatic impairment.
Dialyzable drug: Unlikely.
⚠ *Overdose S&S:* Bleeding due to impaired clotting ability.

P

PREGNANCY-LACTATION-REPRODUCTION
• There are no adequate studies in pregnant women. Use during pregnancy and breast-feeding only if potential maternal benefit justifies potential risk to the fetus.

NURSING CONSIDERATIONS
Black Box Warning Drug may cause significant, sometimes fatal, bleeding. Suspect bleeding in patient who is hypotensive and has recently undergone PCI, CABG, or other surgical procedure. Manage bleeding without stopping drug, if possible. Stopping drug within first few weeks after ACS occurrence increases the risk of further CV events. ■
• Monitor patient for unusual bleeding or bruising.
• Drug should be taken with aspirin (75 to 325 mg daily).
Black Box Warning Discontinue drug 7 days before CABG or any surgery. Don't start drug if patient is likely to undergo urgent CABG. ■
• Bleeding associated with CABG may be treated with transfusion of blood products, such as RBCs and platelets; however, platelets may be ineffective if given within 6 hours of loading dose or within 4 hours of maintenance dose.
🕓 *Alert:* Drug may cause fatal thrombotic thrombocytopenic purpura (thrombocytopenia, hemolytic anemia, neurologic signs and symptoms, renal dysfunction, and fever) that requires urgent treatment, including plasmapheresis.
• *Look alike–sound alike:* Don't confuse prasugrel with pravastatin or propranolol.

PATIENT TEACHING
• Advise patient that drug can be taken without regard to food and not to break tablets.
• Inform patient that bruising will occur more easily and that it may take longer than usual to stop bleeding.
• Instruct patient to report prolonged or excessive bleeding, bruising, blood in the stool or urine, or fever, fatigue, low urine output, or neurologic signs and symptoms.
• Advise patient to inform health care providers of prasugrel use before scheduling surgery or taking new drugs.
• Advise patient that duration of therapy may be determined by the type of stent used

and not to discontinue drug without first consulting prescriber.

---

pravastatin sodium (eptastatin) ⚗
prah-va-STA-tin

Pravachol⬧

Therapeutic class: Antilipemics
Pharmacologic class: HMG-CoA reductase inhibitors

AVAILABLE FORMS
Tablets: 20 mg, 40 mg, 80 mg

INDICATIONS & DOSAGES
Adjust-a-dose (for all indications): In patients with renal dysfunction, start with 10 mg PO daily. In patients taking immunosuppressants, begin with 10 mg PO at bedtime and adjust to higher dosages with caution. Most patients treated with the combination of immunosuppressants and pravastatin receive up to 20 mg pravastatin daily. In patients taking clarithromycin, limit dose to 40 mg once daily.

➤ **Primary and secondary prevention of coronary events; hyperlipidemia**
Adults: Initially, 40 mg PO once daily at the same time each day, with or without food. Adjust dosage every 4 weeks, based on patient tolerance and response; maximum daily dose is 80 mg. Dosage range is 10 to 80 mg/day.

➤ **Heterozygous familial hypercholesterolemia** ⚗
Adolescents ages 14 to 18: Give 40 mg PO once daily. Maximum dose is 40 mg daily.
Children ages 8 to 13: Give 20 mg PO once daily. Maximum dose is 20 mg daily.

ADMINISTRATION
PO
• Give drug without regard for meals.
• If patient is also taking a bile acid resin (cholestyramine), administer pravastatin 1 hour before or 4 hours after the resin.

ACTION
Inhibits HMG-CoA reductase, an early (and rate-limiting) step in cholesterol biosynthesis.

Reactions in bold italics are *life-threatening*. Interactions may have a *rapid onset* or a *delayed onset*.

Route	Onset	Peak	Duration
PO	Unknown	60–90 min	Unknown

Half-life: 1¼ to 2¼ hours.

ADVERSE REACTIONS
CNS: dizziness, fatigue, headache. **CV:** chest pain. **EENT:** rhinitis. **GI:** nausea, abdominal pain, constipation, diarrhea, flatulence, heartburn, vomiting. **GU:** *renal failure caused by myoglobinuria,* urinary abnormality. **Hepatic:** elevated liver enzyme levels. **Musculoskeletal:** localized muscle pain, *rhabdomyolysis,* myalgia, myopathy, myositis. **Respiratory:** common cold, cough. **Skin:** rash. **Other:** flulike symptoms, influenza.

INTERACTIONS
Drug-drug. *Azole antifungals (fluconazole, ketoconazole), erythromycin, fibric acid derivatives (gemfibrozil), niacin:* May increase risk of severe myopathy or rhabdomyolysis. Avoid using together.
Cholestyramine, colestipol: May decrease pravastatin level. Give pravastatin 1 hour before or 4 hours after these drugs.
Clarithromycin: May increase pravastatin level. Limit pravastatin to 40 mg once daily.
Colchicine: May increase risk of myopathy/rhabdomyolysis. Consider therapy modification.
Cyclosporine: May increase pravastatin level and pravastatin-related adverse reactions. If concomitant use can't be avoided, begin therapy with pravastatin 10 mg once daily at bedtime and titrate to higher doses with caution. Most patients received a maximum dose of pravastatin 20 mg daily.
🕐 *Alert: Darunavir and ritonavir, lopinavir–ritonavir:* May increase pravastatin level and risk of myopathy and rhabdomyolysis. Use together cautiously.
Fenofibrate: May increase risk of muscle pain and weakness. Avoid combination unless there are no other options.
Hepatotoxic drugs: May increase risk of hepatotoxicity. Avoid using together.
Protease inhibitors (ritonavir, saquinavir): May reduce pravastatin level. Monitor clinical response.

Rifamycins: May increase or decrease pravastatin levels. Carefully monitor clinical response.
Drug-herb. *Kava kava:* May increase risk of hepatotoxicity. Discourage use together.
Red yeast rice: May increase risk of adverse reactions because herb contains compounds similar to those in drug. Discourage use together.
Drug-food. *Oat bran:* May decrease effectiveness of pravastatin. Separate administration times as much as possible.
Drug-lifestyle. *Alcohol use:* May increase risk of hepatotoxicity. Discourage use together.

EFFECTS ON LAB TEST RESULTS
• May increase ALT, AST, CK, alkaline phosphatase, HbA$_{1c}$, fasting glucose, and bilirubin levels.
• May alter thyroid function test values.

CONTRAINDICATIONS & CAUTIONS
• Contraindicated in patients hypersensitive to drug and in those with active liver disease or conditions that cause unexplained, persistent elevations of transaminase levels.
• Use cautiously in patients who consume large quantities of alcohol or have history of liver disease.
• Statin therapy should be interrupted if patient shows signs of serious liver injury, hyperbilirubinemia, or jaundice. The drug shouldn't be restarted if another cause can't be found.
• Safety and effectiveness in children younger than age 8 haven't been established.
Dialyzable drug: Unknown.

PREGNANCY-LACTATION-REPRODUCTION
• Contraindicated in pregnant and breast-feeding women and in women of childbearing potential.

NURSING CONSIDERATIONS
• Patient should follow a diet restricted in saturated fat and cholesterol during therapy.
🧬 Use in children with heterozygous familial hypercholesterolemia if LDL cholesterol level is at least 190 mg/dL, or if LDL cholesterol is at least 160 mg/dL and patient has either a positive family history of premature

P

CV disease or two or more other CV disease risk factors.

• Obtain LFT results at start of therapy and then periodically. A liver biopsy may be performed if elevated liver enzyme levels persist.

• Monitor patient for fatigue and severe signs or symptoms affecting muscles. Evaluate patient for conditions that increase risk of muscle problems and obtain CK and creatinine levels and urinalysis for myoglobinuria. Drug may need to be withheld or discontinued.

• *Look alike–sound alike:* Don't confuse Pravachol with Prevacid, Prinivil, or propranolol. Don't confuse pravastatin with nystatin, pitavastatin, or prasugrel.

PATIENT TEACHING
• Advise patient who is also taking a bile acid resin such as cholestyramine to take pravastatin at least 1 hour before or 4 hours after taking resin.

• Tell patient to notify prescriber of adverse reactions, particularly muscle aches and pains.

• Inform patient that LFTs will be performed before and periodically throughout treatment.

• Tell patient to promptly report signs and symptoms of liver injury, including fatigue, anorexia, right upper quadrant discomfort, dark urine, or jaundice.

• Tell patient to promptly report any unexplained muscle pain, tenderness, or weakness, especially if accompanied by malaise or fever or if symptoms persist after discontinuing drug.

• Tell patient that the drug may increase blood sugar levels; however, the CV benefits are thought to outweigh the slight increase in risk.

• Teach patient about proper dietary management of cholesterol and triglycerides. When appropriate, recommend weight control, exercise, and smoking cessation programs.

• Inform patient that it will take up to 4 weeks to achieve full therapeutic effect.

۞ Alert: Tell female patient of childbearing potential to stop drug and notify prescriber immediately if she is or may be pregnant or if she's breastfeeding.

prazosin hydrochloride
PRA-zoh-sin

Minipress

Therapeutic class: Antihypertensives
Pharmacologic class: Alpha blockers

AVAILABLE FORMS
Capsules: 1 mg, 2 mg, 5 mg

INDICATIONS & DOSAGES
➤ **Mild to moderate HTN**
Adults: Initially, 1 mg PO b.i.d. or t.i.d. Dosage may be increased slowly. Maximum daily dose is 20 mg. Maintenance dosage is 6 to 15 mg daily in divided doses. Some patients need larger dosages (up to 40 mg daily in divided doses).

If other antihypertensives or diuretics are added to therapy, decrease prazosin dosage to 1 to 2 mg t.i.d. and retitrate to maintenance dosage.

ADMINISTRATION
PO
• Give drug without regard for meals.

ACTION
Unknown. Thought to act by blocking alpha-adrenergic receptors.

Route	Onset	Peak	Duration
PO	30–90 min	2–4 hr	10–24 hr

Half-life: 2 to 3 hours.

ADVERSE REACTIONS
CNS: dizziness, **first-dose syncope,** headache, drowsiness, nervousness, paresthesia, weakness, depression, vertigo, lack of energy. **CV:** orthostatic hypotension, palpitations, edema. **EENT:** blurred vision, conjunctivitis, epistaxis, nasal congestion. **GI:** vomiting, diarrhea, abdominal cramps, nausea, constipation. **GU:** urinary frequency. **Musculoskeletal:** arthralgia, myalgia. **Respiratory:** dyspnea. **Skin:** rash.

INTERACTIONS
Drug-drug. *Acebutolol, atenolol, betaxolol, carteolol, esmolol, metoprolol, nadolol, pindolol, propranolol, sotalol, timolol; calcium channel blockers:* May increase the risk of

orthostatic hypotension in the early phases of use together. Monitor therapy and help patient stand slowly until effects are known.

Antihypertensives, diuretics: May increase hypotension. Reduce prazosin dosage to 1 or 2 mg t.i.d. and retitrate as needed.

PDE5 inhibitors: May increase frequency of hypotensive effect or syncope with loss of consciousness. Initiate PDE5 inhibitor at the lowest dose.

Verapamil: May increase prazosin level. Monitor patient closely.

Drug-herb. *Ma huang:* May decrease antihypertensive effects. Discourage use together.

Yohimbe: May reduce prazosin effect. Discourage use together.

EFFECTS ON LAB TEST RESULTS
• May increase levels of BUN, uric acid, and urinary metabolite of norepinephrine and vanillylmandelic acid.
• May increase LFT values. May alter results of screening tests for pheochromocytoma.
• May cause positive ANA titer.

CONTRAINDICATIONS & CAUTIONS
• Contraindicated in patients hypersensitive to drug or its components, quinazolines, or other alpha blockers.
• Use cautiously in patients receiving other antihypertensives.
• Not approved for use in children.
Dialyzable drug: No.
⚠ **Overdose S&S:** Profound drowsiness, depressed reflexes, hypotension.

PREGNANCY-LACTATION-REPRODUCTION
• There are no adequate studies in pregnant women. Use during pregnancy only if maternal benefits justify potential maternal and fetal risk.
• Drug appears in human milk. Use cautiously in breastfeeding women.

NURSING CONSIDERATIONS
• Monitor patient's BP and pulse rate frequently.
• Elderly patients may be more sensitive to drug's hypotensive effects.
• Adherence might be improved with twice-daily dosing. Discuss dosing change with

prescriber if compliance problems are suspected.
◑ *Alert:* If first dose is more than 1 mg, first-dose syncope may occur.
• *Look alike–sound alike:* Don't confuse prazosin with prednisone.

PATIENT TEACHING
• Warn patient that dizziness may occur with first dose. If dizziness occurs, tell patient to sit or lie down. Reassure patient that this effect disappears with continued dosing.
• Caution patient to avoid driving or performing hazardous tasks for the first 24 hours after starting this drug or increasing the dose.
• Tell patient not to suddenly stop taking drug, but to notify prescriber if unpleasant adverse reactions occur.
• Advise patient to minimize low BP and dizziness upon standing by rising slowly and avoiding sudden position changes.
• Priapism may occur. Advise patient to seek emergency treatment for erections lasting longer than 4 hours.

prednisoLONE
pred-NISS-oh-lone

Millipred

prednisoLONE sodium phosphate
Millipred, Orapred ODT, Pediapred, Veripred 20

Therapeutic class: Corticosteroids
Pharmacologic class: Glucocorticoids–mineralocorticoids

AVAILABLE FORMS
prednisolone
Syrup: 15 mg/5 mL
Tablets: 5 mg
prednisolone sodium phosphate
Oral solution: 5 mg/5 mL, 10 mg/5 mL, 15 mg/5 mL, 20 mg/5 mL, 25 mg/5 mL
Tablets (ODTs) ⬛: 10 mg, 15 mg, 30 mg

INDICATIONS & DOSAGES
➤ **Severe inflammation, immunosuppression**
Adults: 5 to 60 mg PO daily.

Children: 0.1 to 2 mg/kg/day PO in three or four divided doses (4 to 60 mg/m^2/day).
➤ **Uncontrolled asthma in those taking inhaled corticosteroids and long-acting bronchodilators**
Children: 1 to 2 mg/kg/day prednisolone sodium phosphate in single or divided doses. Continue short course (or "burst" therapy) until child achieves a peak expiratory flow rate of 80% of personal best, or until symptoms resolve. This usually requires 3 to 10 days of treatment but can take longer. Tapering the dose after improvement doesn't necessarily prevent relapse.
➤ **Acute exacerbations of MS**
Adults and children: 200 mg/day prednisolone sodium phosphate PO as single or divided dose for 7 days; then 80 mg every other day for 1 month.
➤ **Nephrotic syndrome**
Children: 60 mg/m^2 prednisolone sodium phosphate PO in three divided doses daily for 4 weeks, followed by 4 weeks of single-dose alternate-day therapy at 40 mg/m^2/day.

ADMINISTRATION
PO
• Give drug with food or milk to reduce GI irritation. Patient may need another drug to prevent GI irritation.
• Don't cut or crush ODTs.
• Don't remove ODTs from blister pack until right before dosing.
• Patient may swallow ODT whole or allow to dissolve in mouth with or without water.

ACTION
Not clearly defined. Decreases inflammation, mainly by stabilizing leukocyte lysosomal membranes; suppresses immune response; stimulates bone marrow; and influences protein, fat, and carbohydrate metabolism.

Route	Onset	Peak	Duration
PO	Rapid	1–2 hr	18–36 hr

Half-life: 2 to 4 hours.

ADVERSE REACTIONS
CNS: euphoria, insomnia, *pseudotumor cerebri, seizures,* psychotic behavior, vertigo, headache, paresthesia. **CV:** *arrhythmias, HF, thromboembolism,* HTN, edema, thrombophlebitis. **EENT:** cataracts, glaucoma. **GI:** peptic ulceration, *pancreatitis,* GI irritation, increased appetite, nausea, vomiting. **GU:** menstrual irregularities, increased urine calcium levels. **Metabolic:** *hypokalemia,* hyperglycemia, carbohydrate intolerance, hypercholesterolemia, *hypocalcemia.* **Musculoskeletal:** growth suppression in children, muscle weakness, osteoporosis. **Skin:** hirsutism, delayed wound healing, acne, various skin eruptions. **Other:** after increased stress— *acute adrenal insufficiency,* susceptibility to infections, cushingoid state; after abrupt withdrawal—rebound inflammation, fatigue, weakness, arthralgia, fever, dizziness, lethargy, depression, fainting, orthostatic hypotension, dyspnea, anorexia, *hypoglycemia*; after prolonged use followed by sudden withdrawal—*possible death.*

INTERACTIONS
Drug-drug. *Aspirin, indomethacin, other NSAIDs:* May increase risk of GI distress and bleeding. Use together cautiously.
Azole antifungals (fluconazole, ketoconazole): May increase antifungal toxicity. Reduce steroid dosage as needed.
Barbiturates, carbamazepine, fosphenytoin, phenytoin, rifampin: May decrease corticosteroid effect. Increase corticosteroid dosage.
Cyclosporine: May increase toxicity and risk of seizures. Monitor patient closely.
Drugs that deplete potassium (thiazide diuretics, amphotericin B): May enhance potassium-wasting effects of prednisolone. Monitor potassium level.
Estrogens: May increase pharmacologic and toxic effects of prednisolone. Monitor patient closely.
Oral anticoagulants (warfarin): May alter anticoagulant dosage requirements. Monitor PT and INR closely.
Salicylates: May decrease salicylate level. Monitor patient for lack of salicylate effectiveness.
Skin-test antigens: May decrease response. Postpone skin testing until therapy is completed.
Toxoids, vaccines: May decrease antibody response and may increase risk of neurologic complications. Avoid using together.

Reactions in bold italics are *life-threatening*. Interactions may have a *rapid onset* or a *delayed onset*.

EFFECTS ON LAB TEST RESULTS

• May increase glucose and cholesterol levels. May decrease T_3, T_4, potassium, and calcium levels.

• May decrease ^{131}I uptake and protein-bound iodine levels in thyroid function tests. May alter skin-test results. May cause false-negative results in nitroblue tetrazolium test for systemic bacterial infections.

CONTRAINDICATIONS & CAUTIONS

• Contraindicated in patients hypersensitive to drug or its ingredients, in those with systemic fungal infections, and in those receiving immunosuppressive doses together with live-virus vaccines.

• Use cautiously in patients with recent MI, GI ulcer, renal disease, HTN, osteoporosis, diabetes mellitus, hypothyroidism, cirrhosis, active hepatitis, diverticulitis, nonspecific ulcerative colitis, recent intestinal anastomoses, thromboembolic disorders, seizures, myasthenia gravis, HF, TB, ocular herpes simplex, emotional instability, and psychotic tendencies.

◑ *Alert:* Prolonged use can increase incidence of secondary infection, activate latent infections, prolong viral infections, and mask infections.

• Drug can suppress HPA axis, which can lead to adrenal crisis. Always withdraw drug slowly and carefully.

Dialyzable drug: Unknown.

⚠ *Overdose S&S:* Abnormal fat deposits, accentuated menopausal symptoms, acne, adrenal insufficiency, decreased glucose tolerance, decreased resistance to infection, dry scaly skin, ecchymosis, excessive appetite, fluid retention, fractures, headache, hypertrichosis, hypokalemia, increased BP, increased sweating, menstrual disorder, mental symptoms, moon face, negative nitrogen balance with delayed bone and wound healing, neuropathy, osteoporosis, peptic ulcer, pigmentation, striae, tachycardia, thinning scalp hair, thrombophlebitis, weakness, weight gain; hepatomegaly, abdominal distention (in children).

PREGNANCY-LACTATION-REPRODUCTION

• There are no adequate and well-controlled studies in pregnant women. Use during pregnancy only if potential benefit justifies potential risk to the fetus. Refer to individual manufacturer's instructions for each product.

• Infants born to mothers who have received corticosteroids during pregnancy should be carefully observed for signs and symptoms of hypoadrenalism.

• Drug appears in human milk and could suppress growth, interfere with endogenous corticosteroid production, or cause other untoward effects in the breastfed child. Use cautiously in breastfeeding women. Refer to individual manufacturer's instructions for each product.

NURSING CONSIDERATIONS

• Determine whether patient is sensitive to other corticosteroids.

• Always adjust to lowest effective dose.

• Drug may be used for alternate-day therapy.

• Most adverse reactions to corticosteroids are dose- or duration-dependent.

• Monitor patient's weight, BP, and electrolyte level.

• Monitor patient for cushingoid effects, including moon face, buffalo hump, central obesity, thinning hair, HTN, and increased susceptibility to infection.

• Watch for depression or psychotic episodes, especially during high-dose therapy.

• Patients with diabetes may need increased insulin; monitor glucose level.

• Give patient low-sodium diet that's high in potassium and protein. Give potassium supplements as needed.

• Elderly patients may be more susceptible to osteoporosis with long-term use.

• Gradually reduce dosage after long-term therapy.

• *Look alike–sound alike:* Don't confuse prednisolone with prednisone.

PATIENT TEACHING

• Tell patient not to stop drug abruptly or without prescriber's consent.

• Instruct patient to take oral form of drug with food or milk.

• Teach patient signs and symptoms of early adrenal insufficiency: fatigue, muscle weakness, joint pain, fever, anorexia, nausea, shortness of breath, dizziness, and fainting.

- Instruct patient to carry medical identification that includes prescriber's name and name, dosage of drug, and the need for supplemental systemic glucocorticoids during stress.
- Warn patient on long-term therapy about cushingoid effects and the need to notify prescriber about sudden weight gain or swelling.
- Tell patient to report slow healing.
- Advise patient receiving long-term therapy to consider exercise or physical therapy and to ask prescriber about vitamin D or calcium supplement.
- Instruct patient to avoid exposure to infections and to notify prescriber if exposure occurs.
- Tell patient to avoid immunizations while taking drug.
- **ⓘ Alert:** Tell patient not to cut, crush, or chew ODTs.
- Instruct patient not to remove the ODT from the blister pack until ready to take it. The tablet can be swallowed whole or allowed to dissolve on the tongue with or without water.

prednisoLONE acetate (ophthalmic suspension)
pred-NISS-oh-lone

Omnipred, Pred Forte, Pred Mild

prednisoLONE sodium phosphate (solution)

Therapeutic class: Anti-inflammatory drugs (ophthalmic)
Pharmacologic class: Corticosteroids

AVAILABLE FORMS
prednisolone acetate
Ophthalmic suspension: 0.12%, 1%
prednisolone sodium phosphate
Ophthalmic solution: 1%

INDICATIONS & DOSAGES
➤ **Inflammation of palpebral and bulbar conjunctiva, cornea, and anterior segment of globe**
Prednisolone acetate
Adults: 1 or 2 drops into affected eye b.i.d. to q.i.d. In severe conditions, may increase dosing frequency if needed. If signs and symptoms fail to improve after 2 days, reevaluate. In chronic conditions, taper doses gradually.
Prednisolone sodium phosphate
Adults: 1 or 2 drops into conjunctival sac hourly during the day and every 2 hours at night until response is observed. May reduce to 1 drop every 4 hours, then 1 drop t.i.d. to q.i.d. as needed for adequate response. In chronic conditions, taper doses gradually.

ADMINISTRATION
Ophthalmic
- Shake suspension and check dosage before giving to ensure correct strength. Store in tightly covered container.
- Apply light finger pressure on lacrimal sac for 1 to 2 minutes after instillation.
- Don't touch dropper tip to eyelids or other surfaces when placing drops in eyes.
- May contain benzalkonium chloride, which may be absorbed by soft contact lenses. Have patient remove contacts before using drops and wait 15 minutes before reinserting.

ACTION
Suppresses edema, fibrin deposition, capillary dilation, leukocyte migration, capillary proliferation, and collagen deposition.

Route	Onset	Peak	Duration
Ophthalmic	Unknown	Unknown	Unknown

Half-life: Unknown.

ADVERSE REACTIONS
EENT: cataracts, corneal ulceration, discharge, discomfort, foreign body sensation, glaucoma worsening, increased IOP, increased susceptibility to viral or fungal corneal infection, interference with corneal wound healing, optic nerve damage with excessive or long-term use, visual acuity and visual field defects. **Other:** adrenal suppression with excessive or long-term use, systemic effects.

INTERACTIONS
None significant.

EFFECTS ON LAB TEST RESULTS
None reported.

Reactions in bold italics are *life-threatening*. Interactions may have a *rapid onset* or a *delayed onset*.

CONTRAINDICATIONS & CAUTIONS
• Contraindicated in patients hypersensitive to prednisolone or components of the formulation, after uncomplicated removal of a superficial corneal foreign body (prednisolone sodium phosphate), and in patients with acute, untreated, purulent ocular infections; acute superficial herpes simplex (dendritic keratitis); vaccinia, varicella, or other viral or fungal eye diseases; or ocular TB.
• Use cautiously in patients with corneal thinning or corneal abrasions that may be contaminated (especially with herpes).
• Use after cataract surgery may delay healing and increase the incidence of bleb formation.
• Use in the presence of thin corneal or thin scleral tissue may lead to perforation.
• Withdraw drug by gradually tapering dosage in patients with chronic conditions.
• Prolonged use may result in glaucoma and cataracts.
Dialyzable drug: Unknown.

PREGNANCY-LACTATION-REPRODUCTION
• There are no adequate studies in pregnant women. The amount of drug that crosses placental barrier through ophthalmic drops isn't known. Use during pregnancy only if potential benefit justifies potential risks to the fetus.
• It isn't known if drug appears in human milk. Patient should discontinue breastfeeding or discontinue drug.

NURSING CONSIDERATIONS
• IOP can increase with prolonged use. Use cautiously in patients with glaucoma. Monitor IOP and visual acuity in patients receiving treatment for 10 days or longer.
• *Look alike–sound alike:* Don't confuse prednisolone with prednisone.

PATIENT TEACHING
• Teach patient how to instill drops and to wash hands before and after instillation. Warn patient not to touch tip of dropper to eye or surrounding area.
• Advise patient to remove contact lenses before administration and wait 15 minutes before reinserting.

• Advise patient to apply light finger pressure on lacrimal sac for 1 minute after instillation.
• Tell patient on long-term therapy to have IOP tested frequently.
• Tell patient not to share drug, washcloths, or towels with family members and to notify prescriber if anyone develops the same signs or symptoms.
• Stress importance of compliance with recommended therapy.
• Tell patient to notify prescriber if improvement doesn't occur within several days or if pain, itching, or swelling of eye occurs.
• Warn patient not to use leftover drug for new eye inflammation because serious problems may occur.

---

predniSONE
PRED-ni-sone

Prednisone Intensol*, Rayos, Winpred✦

Therapeutic class: Corticosteroids
Pharmacologic class: Adrenocorticoids

AVAILABLE FORMS
Oral solution: 5 mg/5 mL*, 5 mg/mL (concentrate)*
Tablets: 1 mg, 2.5 mg, 5 mg, 10 mg, 20 mg, 50 mg
Tablets (delayed-release) ⓓⓝⓒ: 1 mg, 2 mg, 5 mg

INDICATIONS & DOSAGES
➤ **Severe inflammation, immunosuppression, endocrine disorders (immediate-release, delayed-release)**
Adults and children: Initially, 5 to 60 mg PO daily in single dose or as two to four divided doses. Maintenance dosage given daily or every other day (immediate-release only). Use lowest dose that will maintain adequate clinical response. Dosage must be individualized, and constant monitoring is needed.
➤ **Acute exacerbations of MS (immediate-release)**
Adults: 200 mg PO daily for 7 days; then 80 mg PO every other day for 1 month.

➤ **Treatment of metastatic castration-resistant prostate cancer (with abiraterone); hormone-refractory metastatic prostate cancer (with docetaxel); metastatic castration-resistant prostate cancer that has progressed during or after docetaxel-based therapy (with cabazitaxel)** ◆

Adults: 5 mg b.i.d. (in combination with abiraterone) until disease progression or unacceptable toxicity occurs, or 10 mg once daily (in combination with cabazitaxel) for up to 10 cycles, or 5 mg b.i.d. (in combination with docetaxel) for up to 10 cycles.

➤ **Multiple myeloma (previously untreated; transplant-ineligible)** ◆

Adults age 65 and older or younger than age 65 and transplant-ineligible: 60 mg/m^2/day for 4 days (days 1 to 4) every 6 weeks for nine cycles (dexamethasone 20 mg was substituted for prednisone on day 1 of each cycle), in combination with daratumumab, bortezomib, and melphalan. After cycle 9, daratumumab is continued as a single agent. Or, 60 mg/m^2/day for 4 days (days 1 to 4) every 6 weeks (in combination with bortezomib and melphalan) for nine cycles, or 2 mg/kg/day for 4 days (days 1 to 4) every 6 weeks (in combination with melphalan and thalidomide) for 12 cycles.

Adults age 65 or older: 2 mg/kg/day for 4 days (days 1 to 4) every 6 weeks (in combination with melphalan) for 12 cycles.

ADMINISTRATION
PO
• Unless contraindicated, give drug with food to reduce GI irritation. Patient may need another drug to prevent GI irritation.
• Solution may be diluted in juice or other flavored diluent or semisolid food such as applesauce before using.
• Make sure patient swallows delayed-release tablets whole and doesn't break, chew, or divide them.
• Discard opened bottle of solution after 90 days. Administer only using the provided calibrated dropper.

ACTION
Not clearly defined. Decreases inflammation, mainly by stabilizing leukocyte lysosomal membranes; suppresses immune response; stimulates bone marrow; and influences protein, fat, and carbohydrate metabolism.

Route	Onset	Peak	Duration
PO (immediate-release)	Variable	2 hr	Variable
PO (delayed-release)	4 hr	6–6½ hr	Unknown

Half-life: 2 to 3 hours.

ADVERSE REACTIONS
CNS: euphoria, insomnia, psychotic behavior, *pseudotumor cerebri,* vertigo, headache, paresthesia, *seizures.* **CV:** *HF,* HTN, edema, *arrhythmias,* thrombophlebitis, *thromboembolism.* **EENT:** cataracts, glaucoma. **GI:** peptic ulceration, *pancreatitis,* GI irritation, increased appetite, nausea, vomiting, abdominal distention. **GU:** menstrual irregularities, increased urine calcium level. **Metabolic:** *hypokalemia,* hyperglycemia, carbohydrate intolerance, hypercholesterolemia, *hypocalcemia,* weight gain. **Musculoskeletal:** growth suppression in children, muscle weakness, osteoporosis. **Skin:** hirsutism, delayed wound healing, acne, various skin eruptions. **Other:** cushingoid state, susceptibility to infections, *acute adrenal insufficiency* after increased stress or abrupt withdrawal after long-term therapy. **After abrupt withdrawal:** rebound inflammation, fatigue, weakness, arthralgia, fever, dizziness, lethargy, depression, fainting, orthostatic hypotension, dyspnea, anorexia, *hypoglycemia. After prolonged use, sudden withdrawal may be fatal.*

INTERACTIONS
Drug-drug. *Aspirin, indomethacin, other NSAIDs:* May increase risk of GI distress and bleeding. Use together cautiously.
Barbiturates, carbamazepine, fosphenytoin, phenobarbital, phenytoin, rifampin: May decrease corticosteroid effect. Increase corticosteroid dosage.
Cyclosporine: May increase toxicity and cause seizures. Monitor patient closely.
Ketoconazole, troleandomycin: May inhibit the metabolism of corticosteroids and decrease their clearance. Titrate the dose of corticosteroid to avoid toxicity.
Oral anticoagulants: May alter dosage requirements. Monitor PT and INR closely.

Potassium-depleting drugs (thiazide diuretics, amphotericin B): May enhance potassium-wasting effects of prednisone. Monitor potassium level.

Salicylates: May decrease salicylate level. Monitor patient for lack of salicylate effectiveness.

Skin-test antigens: May decrease response. Postpone skin testing until therapy is completed.

Toxoids, vaccines: May decrease antibody response and may increase risk of neurologic complications. Avoid using together.

EFFECTS ON LAB TEST RESULTS

• May increase glucose and cholesterol levels. May decrease T_3, T_4, potassium, and calcium levels.

• May decrease ^{131}I uptake and protein-bound iodine values in thyroid function tests. May cause false-negative results in nitroblue tetrazolium test for systemic bacterial infections. May alter reactions to skin tests.

CONTRAINDICATIONS & CAUTIONS

• Contraindicated in patients hypersensitive to drug or its components; in those with systemic fungal infections (immediate-release only), cerebral malaria, or active ocular herpes simplex; and in those receiving immunosuppressive doses together with live-virus vaccines.

• Use cautiously in patients with recent MI, GI ulcer, renal disease, HTN, osteoporosis, diabetes mellitus, seizures, hypothyroidism, cirrhosis, active hepatitis, diverticulitis, nonspecific ulcerative colitis, recent intestinal anastomoses, thromboembolic disorders, myasthenia gravis, HF, TB, ocular herpes simplex, and psychiatric disturbances.

🔵 *Alert:* Patients are more susceptible to infections (from mild to fatal) during therapy. Drug can also mask signs and symptoms of infection.

• Drug can cause cataracts or glaucoma.

🔵 *Alert:* High-dose therapy is associated with acute myopathy that most often occurs in patients receiving neuromuscular drugs or in those with diseases such as myasthenia gravis.

Dialyzable drug: Unknown.

PREGNANCY-LACTATION-REPRODUCTION

• Some studies have shown that corticosteroids are teratogenic in many species when given in doses equivalent to human doses. Use only if potential benefits justify potential risks to the fetus.

• Monitor infants born to mothers who received substantial amounts of drug during pregnancy for signs and symptoms of hypoadrenalism.

• Drug appears in human milk. Patient should discontinue breastfeeding or discontinue drug.

• Drug may increase or decrease motility and number of sperm.

NURSING CONSIDERATIONS

• Determine if patient is sensitive to other corticosteroids.

• Immediate-release drug may be used for alternate-day therapy.

• Always adjust to lowest effective dose.

• Most adverse reactions to corticosteroids are dose- or duration-dependent.

• For better results and less toxicity, give a once-daily dose in the morning.

• Monitor patient's BP, sleep patterns, and potassium level.

• If therapy lasts 6 weeks, monitor IOP.

• Weigh patient daily; report sudden weight gain to prescriber.

• Drug can cause HPA axis suppression and result in corticosteroid insufficiency if withdrawn. Reduce dosage gradually and reinstitute corticosteroid therapy if needed.

• Monitor patient for HPA axis suppression and cushingoid effects, including moon face, buffalo hump, central obesity, thinning hair, HTN, and increased susceptibility to infection.

• Watch for depression or psychotic episodes, especially during high-dose therapy.

• Patient with diabetes may need increased insulin; monitor glucose level.

• Elderly patients may be more susceptible to osteoporosis with long-term use.

• Patients with thyroid status changes may need dosage adjustment.

• Drug can cause osteoporosis at any age. Monitor bone density in patients on long-term therapy and bone growth in children.

P

Institute bone-loss prevention measures if therapy is expected to last 3 months or more.

• Monitor patient for signs and symptoms of infection. Drug may mask or worsen infections, including latent amebiasis.

• Unless contraindicated, give low-sodium diet that's high in potassium and protein. Give potassium supplements as needed.

• Gradually reduce dosage after long-term therapy.

• *Look alike–sound alike:* Don't confuse prednisone with prednisolone or primidone.

PATIENT TEACHING

• Tell patient not to stop drug abruptly or without prescriber's consent.

• Advise patient to report all adverse reactions.

• Instruct patient to take drug with food or milk and to swallow delayed-release tablets whole.

• Teach patient signs and symptoms of early adrenal insufficiency: fatigue, muscle weakness, joint pain, fever, anorexia, nausea, shortness of breath, dizziness, and fainting.

• Instruct patient to carry or wear medical identification indicating the need for supplemental systemic glucocorticoids during stress. It should include prescriber's name and name and dosage of drug.

• Warn patient on long-term therapy about cushingoid effects (moon face, buffalo hump) and the need to notify prescriber about sudden weight gain or swelling.

• Advise patient receiving long-term therapy to consider exercise or physical therapy. Also, tell patient to ask prescriber about vitamin D or calcium supplement.

• Tell patient to report slow healing.

• Advise patient receiving long-term therapy to have periodic eye exams.

• Instruct patient to report infection, to avoid exposure to infections, and to contact prescriber if exposure occurs.

pregabalin
pre-GAB-a-lin

Lyrica◆, Lyrica CR

Therapeutic class: Anticonvulsants
Pharmacologic class: CNS drugs
Controlled substance schedule: V

AVAILABLE FORMS

Capsules: 25 mg, 50 mg, 75 mg, 100 mg, 150 mg, 200 mg, 225 mg, 300 mg
Oral solution: 20 mg/mL
Tablets (extended-release) ⊕: 82.5 mg, 165 mg, 330 mg

INDICATIONS & DOSAGES

Adjust-a-dose (for all indications): Refer to specific product information for guidelines regarding dosing in patients with renal impairment.

➤ **Fibromyalgia**
Adults: (immediate-release and oral solution): 75 mg PO b.i.d. (150 mg/day). May increase to 150 mg b.i.d. (300 mg/day) within 1 week, based on patient response. If pain relief insufficient with 300 mg/day, increase to 225 mg b.i.d. (450 mg/day).

➤ **Diabetic peripheral neuropathy**
Adults: Initially, 50 mg PO t.i.d. May increase to 100 mg PO t.i.d. within 1 week based on patient response. Maximum dose is 300 mg/day. Or, initially 165 mg (extended-release) PO once daily after an evening meal. Increase to 330 mg within 1 week, based on patient response. Maximum dose is 330 mg once daily.

➤ **Neuropathic pain associated with spinal cord injury**
Adults: Initially, 75 mg PO b.i.d. (150 mg/ day). May increase to 150 mg b.i.d. (300 mg/ day) within 1 week based on patient response. If pain relief is insufficient after 2 to 3 weeks, increase to 300 mg b.i.d. Maximum dose is 600 mg/day.

➤ **Postherpetic neuralgia**
Adults: Initially, 75 mg PO b.i.d. or 50 mg PO t.i.d. May increase to 300 mg/day in two or three equally divided doses within 1 week based on patient response. If pain relief insufficient after 2 to 3 weeks, may increase to 300 mg b.i.d. or 200 mg t.i.d. Or, initially

165 mg (extended-release) PO once daily after an evening meal. Increase to 330 mg within 1 week, based on patient response. If pain relief is insufficient after 2 to 4 weeks and patient tolerates drug, may increase up to 660 mg. Maximum dose is 660 mg once daily.

➤ **Partial onset seizures (adjunctive therapy)**
Adults: Initially, 75 mg PO b.i.d. or 50 mg PO t.i.d. Range, 150 to 600 mg/day. Dosage may be increased to maximum 600 mg/day.
Children ages 4 to 16 weighing 30 kg or more: 2.5 mg/kg/day PO in two or three divided doses. May increase weekly up to 10 mg/kg/day (maximum, 600 mg/day).
Children ages 4 to 16 weighing 11 to 29 kg: 3.5 mg/kg/day PO in two or three divided doses. May increase to 14 mg/kg/day.

ADMINISTRATION
PO
• Give immediate-release form without regard for food.
• Give extended-release form after an evening meal. Don't crush, split, or allow patient to chew extended-release tablets.
• Don't stop drug abruptly. Instead, taper gradually over at least 1 week.
• Follow manufacturer's instructions when switching from immediate-release to extended-release.
• Store Lyrica CR in original container.

ACTION
May contribute to analgesic and anticonvulsant effects by binding to sites in CNS.

Route	Onset	Peak	Duration
PO (immediate-release)	Unknown	1½–3 hr	Unknown
PO (extended-release)	Unknown	8 hr	Unknown

Half-life: 6 hours.

ADVERSE REACTIONS
CNS: ataxia, dizziness, somnolence, tremor, abnormal gait, abnormal thinking, amnesia, anxiety, asthenia, confusion, fatigue, depersonalization, euphoria, headache, hypesthesia, hypertonia, incoordination, myoclonus, nervousness, nystagmus, pain, paresthesia, stupor, twitching, vertigo. **CV:** edema, PR-interval prolongation. **EENT:** blurred or abnormal vision, conjunctivitis, diplopia, eye disorder, otitis media, tinnitus. **GI:** dry mouth, abdominal pain, constipation, flatulence, gastroenteritis, vomiting, nausea. **GU:** anorgasmia, impotence, urinary incontinence, urinary frequency. **Metabolic:** *hypoglycemia,* weight gain, increased or decreased appetite. **Musculoskeletal:** arthralgia, back and chest pain, leg cramps, myalgia, myasthenia, neuropathy, tremor. **Respiratory:** bronchitis, dyspnea. **Skin:** ecchymosis, pruritus. **Other:** accidental injury, infection, allergic reaction, decreased libido, flu syndrome.

INTERACTIONS
Drug-drug. *ACE inhibitors:* May increase risk of angioedema with concomitant use. Monitor patient.
CNS depressants: May have additive effects on cognitive and gross motor function. Monitor patient for increased dizziness and somnolence.
Pioglitazone, rosiglitazone: May cause additive fluid retention and weight gain. Monitor patient closely.
Drug-lifestyle. *Alcohol use:* May have additive depressant effects on cognitive and gross motor function. Discourage alcohol use.

EFFECTS ON LAB TEST RESULTS
• May increase CK level.
• May decrease platelet count.

CONTRAINDICATIONS & CAUTIONS
• Contraindicated in patients hypersensitive to drug or its components.
• Use cautiously in patients with NYHA Class III or IV HF.
✪ *Alert:* Use cautiously in patients with depression. Drug may increase risk of suicidal thoughts or behavior.
✪ *Alert:* Use cautiously in patients with history of substance abuse. Drug may cause physical and psychological dependence.
Dialyzable drug: Yes.
⚠ *Overdose S&S:* Exaggerated adverse effects.

PREGNANCY-LACTATION-REPRODUCTION
• There are no adequate studies in pregnant women. Drug may cause fetal harm. Use in

pregnancy only if potential benefit clearly justifies risk to the fetus.

• Patients exposed to drug during pregnancy should enroll in the North American AED Pregnancy Registry (1-888-233-2334).

• Drug appears in human milk. Patient should discontinue breastfeeding or discontinue drug.

NURSING CONSIDERATIONS

❸ *Alert:* Monitor patient for signs and symptoms of angioedema (including swelling of face, mouth, and neck), which may compromise breathing. Discontinue drug immediately if angioedema occurs.

❸ *Alert:* Monitor patient for worsening depression, suicidal thoughts or behavior, or unusual mood or behavior changes.

• Monitor patient's weight and fluid status, especially if patient has HF.

• Check for changes in vision.

• Withdraw drug gradually over 1 week, especially in patients with seizure disorder.

❸ *Alert:* Watch for signs of rhabdomyolysis, such as dark, red, or cola-colored urine; muscle tenderness; generalized weakness; or muscle stiffness or aching.

• *Look alike–sound alike:* Don't confuse Lyrica with Lopressor or Hydrea.

PATIENT TEACHING

• Explain that immediate-release form of drug may be taken without regard to food.

• Advise patient to take extended-release form of drug after an evening meal.

• Warn patient not to stop drug abruptly and that it should be tapered over at least 1 week.

• Advise patient that drug may cause angioedema, with swelling of the face, mouth (lip, gum, and tongue), and neck (larynx and pharynx) that can lead to life-threatening respiratory compromise. Instruct patient to discontinue drug and immediately seek medical care if these symptoms occur.

• Tell patient to seek immediate medical care for a hypersensitivity reaction, such as blisters, dyspnea, hives, rash, or wheezing.

❸ *Alert:* Counsel patient, caregiver, and family about risk of suicidal thoughts and behaviors. Advise them of the need to be alert for the emergence or worsening of symptoms of depression, unusual changes in mood or behavior, or the emergence of suicidal

thoughts, behavior, or thoughts about self-harm and to immediately report behaviors of concern to health care provider.

• Caution patient to avoid hazardous activities until drug's effects are known.

• Instruct patient to watch for weight changes and water retention.

• Advise patient to report vision changes and malaise or fever accompanied by muscle pain, tenderness, or weakness.

• Tell male patient taking pregabalin who plans to father a child to consult prescriber about potential risk to a fetus because of male-mediated teratogenicity.

• Urge patient with diabetes to inspect skin closely for ulcer formation.

• Advise patient to avoid alcohol.

primaquine phosphate ▧
PRIM-a-kwin

Therapeutic class: Antimalarials
Pharmacologic class: Aminoquinolines

AVAILABLE FORMS
Tablets: 26.3 mg (equivalent to 15-mg base)

INDICATIONS & DOSAGES
➤ **Relapsing *Plasmodium vivax* malaria, eliminating symptoms and infection completely; to prevent relapse**
Adults: 15 mg base PO daily for 14 days. Begin therapy during the last 2 weeks of, or after, a course of suppression with chloroquine or comparable drug.

ADMINISTRATION
PO

❸ *Alert:* Drug dosage may be discussed in "mg" or "mg base"; be aware of the difference.

• Give drug with or without food. Give with a meal if stomach irritation occurs.

ACTION
May bind to and alter the properties of DNA in susceptible parasites.

Route	Onset	Peak	Duration
PO	Unknown	1–3 hr	Unknown

Half-life: 3.7 to 9.6 hours.

ADVERSE REACTIONS

CNS: dizziness. **CV:** *arrhythmias, prolonged QT interval.* **GI:** nausea, vomiting, epigastric distress, abdominal cramps. **Hematologic:** *hemolytic anemia (in patients with G6PD deficiency), leukopenia, methemoglobinemia.* **Skin:** rash, pruritus.

INTERACTIONS

Drug-drug. *QTc interval–prolonging drugs:* May increase QTc interval and risk of ventricular arrhythmias. Monitor therapy.
Quinacrine: May increase risk of toxicity. Concomitant use is contraindicated.
Vaccine (rabies): May decrease antibody response to rabies vaccine. International travelers should complete a three-dose rabies vaccination series before starting primaquine. If this isn't possible, the rabies vaccine should be given intramuscularly and not intradermally.
Drug-food. *Grapefruit juice:* May increase drug plasma concentration and toxic effects. Advise patient to avoid grapefruit products.

EFFECTS ON LAB TEST RESULTS

• May decrease Hb level.
• May decrease RBC count. May increase or decrease WBC count.

CONTRAINDICATIONS & CAUTIONS

▓ Contraindicated in patients with systemic diseases in which agranulocytosis may develop, such as lupus erythematosus or RA, and in those with severe G6PD deficiency or who are taking a bone marrow suppressant, quinacrine, or hemolytic drugs.
▓ Use cautiously in patients with previous idiosyncratic reaction involving hemolytic anemia, methemoglobinemia, or leukopenia; in those with a family or personal history of favism; and in those with mild to moderate G6PD or nicotinamide-adenine-dinucleotide (NADH) methemoglobin reductase deficiency.
▓ Testing for G6PD deficiency must be performed before therapy begins. Moderate to severe hemolytic reactions may occur in patients with G6PD deficiency. Areas of high prevalence of G6PD deficiency are Africa, Southern Europe, Mediterranean region, Middle East, Southeast Asia, and Oceania.

• May prolong QTc interval. Monitor ECG in patients with risk factors for QTc-interval prolongation.
Dialyzable drug: Unknown.
⚠ **Overdose S&S:** Abdominal cramps, anemia, burning epigastric distress, CNS and CV disturbances, cyanosis, methemoglobinemia, moderate leukocytosis or leukopenia, vomiting, granulocytopenia, acute hemolytic anemia, acute hemolysis.

PREGNANCY-LACTATION-REPRODUCTION

• Contraindicated in pregnant women. Pregnancy testing should be performed before therapy begins.
• Females of childbearing potential should use effective contraception (methods with less than 1% pregnancy rates) during therapy and after therapy ends until completion of an ongoing ovulatory cycle (up to the next menses). Males undergoing treatment whose partners may become pregnant should use a condom during treatment and for 3 months after therapy ends.
▓ It isn't known if drug appears in human milk. If drug is needed, test mother and infant for G6PD deficiency; may use drug in breastfeeding patients and infants with normal G6PD levels.

NURSING CONSIDERATIONS

• Use drug with a fast-acting antimalarial such as chloroquine to reduce possibility of drug-resistant strains.
▓ Monitor CBC and glucose and electrolyte levels. Patients with G6PD deficiency will need more frequent monitoring.
• Monitor patient for markedly darkened urine and for suddenly reduced Hb level or RBC or WBC count, which suggest impending hemolytic reactions. Stop drug immediately and notify prescriber.
• **Look alike–sound alike:** Don't confuse primaquine with primidone.

PATIENT TEACHING

• Instruct patient to take drug with meals to minimize stomach upset. If nausea, vomiting, or stomach pain persists, tell patient to notify prescriber.
• Tell patient to report to prescriber chills, fever, chest pain, and bluish skin

P

discoloration; these signs and symptoms may suggest a hemolytic reaction.
• Tell patient to stop drug and notify prescriber immediately if urine darkens markedly.
• Stress importance of completing full course of therapy.

SAFETY ALERT!

procainamide hydrochloride
proe-KANE-a-myed

Therapeutic class: Antiarrhythmics
Pharmacologic class: Procaine derivatives

AVAILABLE FORMS
Injection: 100 mg/mL, 500 mg/mL

INDICATIONS & DOSAGES
➤ **Life-threatening ventricular arrhythmias**
Adults: Loading dose: 100 mg every 5 minutes by slow IV push, no faster than 25 to 50 mg/minute, until arrhythmias disappear, adverse effects develop, or 500 mg has been given. Or, give a loading dose of 500 to 600 mg IV infusion over 25 to 30 minutes. Maximum total dose given by repeated bolus injections or loading infusion is 1 g. Maintenance infusion: To maintain therapeutic levels, give continuous infusion of 2 to 6 mg/minute based on clinical response and patient condition; monitor closely.

For patients with less-threatening arrhythmias but who are nauseated, vomiting, or are ordered to receive nothing by mouth, give 50 mg/kg IM divided into fractional doses of one eighth to one fourth every 3 to 6 hours. If more than three injections are given, prescriber may wish to assess patient factors, such as age and renal function, clinical response and, if available, blood levels of procainamide and *N*-acetylprocainamide (NAPA) in adjusting further dosages for that patient. For arrhythmias occurring during surgery, give 100 to 500 mg IM.
Adjust-a-dose: For patients with renal or hepatic dysfunction, decrease dosage or increase dosing interval, as needed.

ADMINISTRATION
IV
▼ Vials for IV injection contain 1 g of drug: 100 mg/mL (10 mL) or 500 mg/mL (2 mL).
▼ Direct injection into a vein or into tubing of an established IV line should be done slowly at a rate not to exceed 50 mg/minute.
▼ For loading dose infusion, dilute with compatible IV solution, such as D_5W injection (1 g diluted to 50 mL), and give with patient supine at a rate not exceeding 25 to 50 mg/minute. Keep patient supine during IV administration.
▼ For IV infusion to maintain therapeutic levels, dilute 1 g procainamide in 500 or 250 mL D_5W and administer at 2 to 6 mg/minute based on patient response and clinical condition.
▼ Attend patient receiving infusion at all times. Use an infusion-control device to give infusion precisely.
❸ *Alert:* Monitor BP and ECG continuously during IV administration. Watch for prolonged QTc intervals and widening of the QRS complexes, heart block, or increased arrhythmias. If such reactions occur, withhold drug, obtain rhythm strip, and notify prescriber immediately. If drug is given too rapidly, hypotension can occur. Watch closely for adverse reactions during infusion, and notify prescriber if they occur.
▼ Solution may turn slightly yellow upon standing. Discard solutions that are slightly darker than yellow or discolored in any other way.
▼ **Incompatibilities:** Bretylium, 5% dextrose in normal saline, esmolol, ethacrynate, milrinone, phenytoin sodium.
IM
• Use IM route only if IV route isn't feasible. IM injection may be painful and can increase CK level.

ACTION
Decreases excitability, conduction velocity, automaticity, and membrane responsiveness with prolonged refractory period. Larger than usual doses may induce AV block.

Reactions in bold italics are *life-threatening*. Interactions may have a *rapid onset* or a *delayed onset*.

Route	Onset	Peak	Duration
IV	Immediate	Immediate	Unknown
IM	10–30 min	15–60 min	Unknown

Half-life: About 2½ to 4¾ hours.

ADVERSE REACTIONS

CNS: fever, *seizures,* hallucinations, psychosis, giddiness, confusion, depression, dizziness. **CV:** hypotension, *bradycardia, AV block, ventricular fibrillation, ventricular asystole.* **GI:** abdominal pain, nausea, vomiting, anorexia, diarrhea, bitter taste. **Skin:** maculopapular rash, urticaria, pruritus, flushing. **Other:** lupuslike syndrome, *angioneurotic edema.*

INTERACTIONS

Drug-drug. *Amiodarone:* May increase procainamide level and toxicity and have additive effects on QTc interval and QRS complex. Avoid using together.
Antiarrhythmics: May enhance antiarrhythmic and hypotensive effects. Avoid using together.
Anticholinergics: May increase antivagal effects. Monitor patient closely.
Beta blockers, ranitidine, trimethoprim: May increase procainamide level. Watch for toxicity.
Cimetidine, ranitidine: May increase procainamide level. Avoid using together if possible. Monitor procainamide level closely and adjust the dosage as necessary.
Macrolides and related antibiotics (azithromycin, clarithromycin, erythromycin, telithromycin): May prolong the QT interval. Use with caution. Avoid use with telithromycin.
Neuromuscular blockers: May increase skeletal muscle relaxant effect. May need to decrease dosage of neuromuscular blocker.
Quinolones: Life-threatening arrhythmias, including torsades de pointes, can occur. Avoid using together; sparfloxacin is contraindicated.
Thioridazine, ziprasidone: May prolong QTc interval. Avoid using together.
Drug-herb. *Licorice:* May prolong QTc interval. Urge caution.
Drug-lifestyle. *Alcohol use:* May reduce drug level. Discourage use together.

EFFECTS ON LAB TEST RESULTS

• May increase ALT, AST, alkaline phosphatase, LDH, and bilirubin levels.
• May decrease Hb level, hematocrit, and WBC and platelet counts.
• May cause positive ANA titers and positive direct antiglobulin (Coombs) tests.

CONTRAINDICATIONS & CAUTIONS

• Contraindicated in patients hypersensitive to this drug and related drugs.
• Drug contains sulfite, which can cause allergic-type reactions, including anaphylaxis. Sensitivity to sulfites may be more frequent in patients with asthma.
• Contraindicated in those with complete second- or third-degree heart block in the absence of an artificial pacemaker. Also contraindicated in those with SLE or atypical ventricular tachycardia (torsades de pointes).
• Use with extreme caution in patients with ventricular tachycardia during coronary occlusion and in patients with myasthenia gravis.
• Use cautiously in patients with HF or other conduction disturbances, such as bundle-branch heart block, sinus bradycardia, or digoxin intoxication, and in those with hepatic or renal insufficiency.
Black Box Warning Use cautiously in patients with blood dyscrasias or bone marrow suppression. ▪
Dialyzable drug: Procainamide, 20 to 50%; metabolite NAPA, less than 5%.
⚠ *Overdose S&S:* Progressive widening of QRS complex, prolonged QT and PR intervals, lowered R and T waves, increasing AV block, ventricular ectopy, ventricular tachycardia, hypotension, CNS depression, tremor, respiratory depression.

PREGNANCY-LACTATION-REPRODUCTION

• Use during pregnancy only if clearly needed. It isn't known if drug can harm the fetus.
• Procainamide and metabolite NAPA appear in human milk. Patient should discontinue breastfeeding or discontinue drug.

NURSING CONSIDERATIONS

Black Box Warning Because of its proarrhythmic effects, procainamide should be

P

reserved for patients with life-threatening ventricular arrhythmias. ∎

• Digitalize or cardiovert patients with atrial flutter or fibrillation before therapy with procainamide to prevent ventricular rate acceleration in patient.

• Monitor level of drug and its active metabolite NAPA.

• Monitor ECG closely. If QRS widens more than 25% or marked prolongation of the QTc interval occurs, check for overdosage.

• Hypokalemia predisposes patient to arrhythmias. Monitor electrolytes, especially potassium level.

• Elderly patients may be more likely to develop hypotension. Monitor BP carefully.

Black Box Warning Agranulocytosis, bone marrow depression, neutropenia, hypoplastic anemia, and thrombocytopenia have been noted in patients during the first 12 weeks of therapy. It is recommended that CBCs be performed at weekly intervals for the first 3 months of therapy and periodically thereafter. ∎

Black Box Warning Perform CBCs promptly if patient develops signs of infection, bruising, or bleeding. If hematologic disorder is identified, discontinue drug. Blood counts usually return to normal within 1 month of discontinuation. ∎

Black Box Warning Positive ANA titer is common in about 60% of patients who don't have symptoms of lupuslike syndrome. This response seems to be related to prolonged use, not dosage. If positive ANA titer develops, assess the benefits and risks of continued therapy. ∎

• Discontinue IV therapy if persistent conduction disturbances or hypotension develops. As soon as cardiac rhythm is stabilized, start oral antiarrhythmic maintenance therapy 3 to 4 hours after last IV dose.

PATIENT TEACHING

• Instruct patient to report all adverse reactions and to immediately report fever, rash, muscle pain, diarrhea, bleeding, bruises, pleuritic chest pain, or signs and symptoms of infection.

• Instruct patient to report sulfite sensitivity before receiving drug.

SAFETY ALERT!

procarbazine hydrochloride
pro-KAR-ba-zeen

Matulane

Therapeutic class: Antineoplastics
Pharmacologic class: Methylhydrazine derivatives

AVAILABLE FORMS
Capsules: 50 mg

INDICATIONS & DOSAGES

➤ **Single-agent therapy or adjunctive treatment of Hodgkin lymphoma (stages III and IV) and other cancers using nitrogen mustard, vincristine, procarbazine, prednisone (MOPP) regimen**

Adults: For single-agent therapy, give 2 to 4 mg/kg/day PO in single dose or divided doses for first week. Then, 4 to 6 mg/kg/day until WBC count falls below 4,000/mm^3, platelet count falls below 100,000/mm^3, or maximum response is obtained. Maintenance dose is 1 to 2 mg/kg/day after bone marrow recovery. For MOPP regimen, 100 mg/m^2 daily PO for first 14 days of 28-day cycle.

Children: The prescribing information provides this dosage schedule as a guideline only: For single-agent therapy, give 50 mg/m^2/day PO for first week; then 100 mg/m^2/day until response or toxicity occurs. Maintenance dose is 50 mg/m^2/day PO after bone marrow recovery. In combination with other agents, procarbazine 100 mg/m^2/day (maximum, 150 mg) PO on days 1 to 15 has been used.

➤ **CNS tumors, anaplastic oligodendroglioma/oligoastrocytoma ♦ *PCV regimen***

Adults: 60 mg/m^2 PO on days 8 to 21 every 6 weeks (in combination with lomustine and vincristine beginning within 4 weeks after radiotherapy) for six cycles, or 75 mg/m^2 PO on days 8 to 21 every 6 weeks (in combination with lomustine and vincristine, followed by radiotherapy) for up to four cycles.

➤ **CNS tumors (low-grade gliomas)** ♦
PCV regimen
Adults: 60 mg/m^2 PO on days 8 to 21 every
8 weeks (after radiotherapy; in combination
with lomustine and vincristine) for six
cycles.
TPCV regimen
Children younger than age 10: 50 mg/m^2
PO every 6 hours for four doses (at hours
60, 66, 72, and 78) during a 42-day cycle (in
combination with thioguanine, vincristine,
and lomustine) for a total of eight cycles.
Adjust-a-dose: Base dose on actual weight.
If patient is obese or exhibits weight gain
due to fluid retention, use ideal body weight.

ADMINISTRATION
PO
• Give drug with or after meals. May give
once daily or in two to three divided doses.

ACTION
Unknown. Thought to inhibit DNA, RNA,
and protein synthesis.

Route	Onset	Peak	Duration
PO	Unknown	Unknown	Unknown

Half-life: About 1 hour.

ADVERSE REACTIONS
CNS: ataxia, hallucinations, *coma,* confusion, depression, dizziness, headache, insomnia, nervousness, neuropathy, nightmares, paresthesia, syncope, *seizures.* **CV:**
flushing, hypotension, tachycardia. **EENT:**
nystagmus, photophobia, retinal hemorrhage, diplopia, hearing loss. **GI:** nausea,
vomiting, abdominal pain, anorexia, constipation, diarrhea, dry mouth, dysphagia,
hematemesis, melena, stomatitis. **GU:**
hematuria, nocturia, urinary frequency.
Hematologic: *anemia, bleeding tendency, leukopenia, thrombocytopenia,*
eosinophilia, hemolytic anemia. **Hepatic:**
hepatotoxicity, jaundice. **Musculoskeletal:** myalgia, arthralgia, tremors. **Respiratory:** pleural effusion, cough, pneumonitis. **Skin:** dermatitis, hyperpigmentation,
pruritus, rash, reversible alopecia. **Other:**
secondary malignancies, allergic reaction,
gynecomastia, herpes outbreak.

INTERACTIONS
Drug-drug. *Anticoagulants (warfarin):*
May increase anticoagulant effect. Monitor
coagulation status (PT and INR) and adjust
dosage as needed.
CNS depressants: May cause additive depressant effects. Avoid using together.
Digoxin: May decrease digoxin level. Monitor digoxin level closely.
*Drugs high in tyramine, local anesthet-
ics, MAO inhibitors, sympathomimetics,
TCAs:* May cause tremor, palpitations, and
increased BP. Monitor patient closely.
Methotrexate: The nephrotoxicity of
methotrexate may be increased. Wait
72 hours or longer between giving the final
dose of procarbazine and starting a high-
dose methotrexate infusion.
Drug-food. *Caffeine:* May result in arrhythmias and severe HTN. Discourage caffeine
intake.
Foods high in tyramine (cheese, Chianti):
May cause tremor, palpitations, and increased BP. Monitor patient closely; advise
patient to avoid or limit intake.
Drug-lifestyle. ❶ *Alert:Alcohol use:* Mild
disulfiram-like reaction may cause flushing,
headache, nausea, and hypotension. Warn
patient to avoid alcoholic beverages.

EFFECTS ON LAB TEST RESULTS
• May decrease Hb level.
• May increase eosinophil count. May de-
crease platelet, RBC, and WBC counts.

CONTRAINDICATIONS & CAUTIONS
• Contraindicated in patients hypersensitive
to drug and in those with inadequate bone
marrow reserve as shown by bone marrow
aspiration.
• Consider hospitalization for the initial
course of treatment when appropriate for patients with renal or hepatic impairment, as
toxicity can occur.
Dialyzable drug: 25% to 49%.
⚠ *Overdose S&S:* Nausea, vomiting,
diarrhea, enteritis, hypotension, tremors,
seizures, coma.

PREGNANCY-LACTATION-REPRODUCTION
• Drug can cause fetal harm. Women should
avoid becoming pregnant during therapy.
• Women shouldn't breastfeed during therapy.

NURSING CONSIDERATIONS

Black Box Warning Give drug only under the supervision of a physician experienced with potent antineoplastic drugs. Adequate clinical and lab facilities should be available. ■

• Obtain baseline lab data before starting therapy. Monitor hematologic status at least every 3 or 4 days, including Hb level, hematocrit, and WBC, differential, reticulocyte, and platelet counts.

❺ *Alert:* Prompt discontinuation of therapy is recommended if patient develops CNS signs or symptoms, such as paresthesia, neuropathies, or confusion; leukopenia (WBC count less than 4,000 cell/mm^3); thrombocytopenia (platelet count less than 100,000/mm^3); hypersensitivity reaction; stomatitis; diarrhea; or hemorrhage or bleeding tendencies.

• Bone marrow depression begins 2 to 8 weeks after the start of treatment.

• Avoid all IM injections when platelet count is below 50,000/mm^3.

• Evaluate hepatic and renal function before starting therapy. Monitor urinalysis, ALT, AST, alkaline phosphatase, and BUN levels at least weekly.

• Drug has high emetic potential; give antiemetics to prevent nausea and vomiting.

• The manufacturer recommends that if radiation or chemotherapeutic agents with bone marrow depressant activity have been used, give patient a 1-month interval without such therapy before beginning procarbazine therapy.

• *Look alike–sound alike:* Don't confuse procarbazine with dacarbazine.

PATIENT TEACHING

• To decrease nausea and vomiting, advise patient to take drug at bedtime and in divided doses and to take antiemetics as prescribed.

• Tell patient to watch for fever, sore throat, fatigue, easy bruising, nosebleeds, bleeding gums, or tarry stools. Tell patient to take temperature daily.

• Tell patient not to consume alcohol or alcohol-containing products during therapy, and to discontinue tobacco use.

• Instruct patient to avoid OTC medications that contain antihistamines and

sympathomimetics and to avoid foods and drinks high in tyramine, such as wine, tea, coffee, cola, cheese, and bananas.

• Warn patient to avoid hazardous activities that require alertness and good motor coordination until CNS effects of drug are known.

• Caution female patient of childbearing potential to avoid becoming pregnant during therapy and to consult prescriber before becoming pregnant.

---

prochlorperazine
proe-klor-PER-a-zeen

Compro

prochlorperazine edisylate

prochlorperazine maleate
Prochlorazine✤

Therapeutic class: Antiemetics
Pharmacologic class: Dopamine antagonists

AVAILABLE FORMS
prochlorperazine
Suppositories: 10 mg✤, 25 mg
prochlorperazine edisylate
Injection: 5 mg/mL
prochlorperazine maleate
Tablets: 5 mg, 10 mg

INDICATIONS & DOSAGES
➤ **To control preoperative nausea**
Adults: 5 to 10 mg IM 1 to 2 hours before induction of anesthesia; repeat once in 30 minutes, if needed. Or, 5 to 10 mg IV at no more than 5 mg/minute 15 to 30 minutes before induction of anesthesia; repeat once, if needed. Maximum IM and IV dose is 40 mg/day.
➤ **Severe nausea and vomiting**
Adults: 5 to 10 mg PO t.i.d. or q.i.d.; 25 mg PR b.i.d.; or 5 to 10 mg IM, repeated every 3 to 4 hours, as needed. Maximum IM dose is 40 mg daily. Or, 2.5 to 10 mg IV at no more than 5 mg/minute. Maximum IV dose is 40 mg daily.
Children weighing 18 to 39 kg: 2.5 mg PO t.i.d.; or 5 mg PO b.i.d. or 2.5 mg PR t.i.d. Maximum, 15 mg daily. Or, 0.132 mg/kg

---

by deep IM injection t.i.d. to q.i.d. Control is usually achieved with one dose.

Children weighing 14 to 17 kg: 2.5 mg PO b.i.d. or t.i.d. or 2.5 mg PR b.i.d. to t.i.d. Maximum, 10 mg daily. Or, 0.132 mg/kg by deep IM injection t.i.d. to q.i.d. Control is usually achieved with one dose.

Children weighing 9 to 13 kg: 2.5 mg PO once daily or b.i.d. or 2.5 mg PR daily to b.i.d. Maximum, 7.5 mg daily. Or, 0.132 mg/kg by deep IM injection t.i.d. to q.i.d. Control is usually achieved with one dose.

➤ **Schizophrenia**

Adults: Treatment guidelines may not include drug as recommended therapy for this indication. According to prescribing information, for mild conditions, 5 or 10 mg PO t.i.d. or q.i.d. For moderate to severe conditions, start with 10 mg PO t.i.d. or q.i.d.; increase by small increments every 2 or 3 days until symptoms are controlled or adverse reactions become bothersome. Patients may respond on 50 to 75 mg/day in divided doses. For severe conditions, 100 to 150 mg PO daily. Or, for severe symptoms, 10 to 20 mg by deep IM injection. Repeat the initial IM dose every 2 to 4 hours (or, in resistant cases, every hour) to gain control of patient, as necessary. More than three or four IM doses are seldom necessary. If, in rare cases, parenteral therapy is needed for a prolonged period, give 10 to 20 mg IM every 4 to 6 hours. After control is achieved, switch patient to an oral form of drug at same dosage level or higher.

Children ages 2 to 12: Initially, 2.5 mg PO b.i.d. or t.i.d., not to exceed 10 mg on the first day. Increase dosage according to patient's response. Maximum dose is 20 mg/day (ages 2 to 5) or 25 mg/day (ages 6 to 12). Or, 0.132 mg/kg IM as a single dose. Don't exceed 10 mg/day on first day of therapy.

➤ **Nonpsychotic anxiety**

Adults: Treatment guidelines may not include drug as recommended therapy for this indication. According to prescribing information, give 5 mg PO t.i.d. or q.i.d. Maximum dose is 20 mg/day for no longer than 12 weeks.

ADMINISTRATION

PO

• Administer without regard to meals.

IV

▼ Give undiluted or diluted in isotonic solution by slow IV injection or infusion at a rate not to exceed 5 mg/minute. Don't exceed 10 mg in a single dose or total IV dose of 40 mg/day.

▼ Don't give by bolus injection.

▼ To prevent contact dermatitis, avoid getting injection solution on hands or clothing.

▼ Protect from light.

▼ **Incompatibilities:** Other IV drugs.

IM

• For IM use, inject deeply into upper outer quadrant of gluteal region.

• Don't give by subcut route or mix in syringe with another drug.

• To prevent contact dermatitis, avoid getting injection solution on hands or clothing.

• Store in light-resistant container. Slight yellowing doesn't affect potency; discard extremely discolored solutions.

Rectal

• Don't remove from wrapper until ready to use.

• Moisten suppository with water before insertion.

• If suppository is too soft because of warm storage, chill in refrigerator for 30 minutes or run cold water over it before removing wrapper.

ACTION

Acts on the chemoreceptor trigger zone to inhibit nausea and vomiting; in larger doses, it partially depresses vomiting center.

Route	Onset	Peak	Duration
PO	30–60 min	Unknown	3–12 hr
IV	Unknown	Unknown	Unknown
IM	30–60 min	Unknown	3–4 hr
PR	1 hr	Unknown	4–6 hr

Half-life: Unknown.

ADVERSE REACTIONS

CNS: extrapyramidal reactions, dizziness, EEG changes, pseudoparkinsonism, sedation, drowsiness, motor restlessness, dystonia, tardive dyskinesia. **CV:** orthostatic hypotension, ECG changes, tachycardia. **EENT:** blurred vision, ocular changes.

GI: constipation, dry mouth, increased appetite. **GU:** urine retention, dark urine, inhibited ejaculation, menstrual irregularities. **Hematologic:** *agranulocytosis, transient leukopenia.* **Hepatic:** cholestatic jaundice. **Metabolic:** weight gain. **Skin:** mild photosensitivity reactions, allergic reactions, exfoliative dermatitis. **Other:** gynecomastia, hyperprolactinemia.

INTERACTIONS
Drug-drug. *Antacids:* May inhibit absorption of oral phenothiazines. Separate antacid and phenothiazine doses by at least 2 hours.
Anticholinergics, including antidepressants and antiparkinsonians: May increase anticholinergic activity and may aggravate parkinsonian symptoms. Use together cautiously.
Anticoagulants: May decrease anticoagulant effects. Monitor PT and INR, and adjust dosage as needed.
Anticonvulsants: May lower seizure threshold; dosage adjustments of anticonvulsants may be needed.
Barbiturates: May decrease phenothiazine effect. Monitor patient for decreased antiemetic effect.
CNS depressants (anesthetics, opioids): May intensify or prolong action of these drugs. Monitor patient.
Loop diuretics, thiazides: May add to orthostatic hypotension caused by prochlorperazine. Monitor BP.
Propranolol: May increase plasma levels of both drugs. Observe for increased adverse effects.
Drug-herb. *Dong quai, St. John's wort:* May increase risk of photosensitivity. Advise patient to avoid excessive sun exposure.
Kava: May increase risk of dystonic reactions. Discourage use together.
Drug-lifestyle. *Alcohol use:* May increase CNS depression, particularly psychomotor skills. Strongly discourage use together.

EFFECTS ON LAB TEST RESULTS
• May decrease WBC and granulocyte counts.
• May cause false-positive results for phenylketonuria and pregnancy tests. May cause abnormal LFT results.

CONTRAINDICATIONS & CAUTIONS
• Contraindicated in patients hypersensitive to phenothiazines and in patients with CNS depression, including those in a coma.
• Contraindicated during pediatric surgery, when using spinal or epidural anesthetic or adrenergic blockers, and in children younger than age 2 or weighing less than 9 kg.
Black Box Warning Drug isn't approved for the treatment of elderly patients with dementia-related psychosis due to an increased risk of death. ■
• Use cautiously in patients with impaired CV function, glaucoma, seizure disorders, and Parkinson disease; in those who have been exposed to extreme heat; and in children with acute illness.
⚠ Alert: Potentially irreversible tardive dyskinesia and potentially fatal NMS have been reported with antipsychotic use.
Dialyzable drug: No.
⚠ Overdose S&S: Dystonic reactions, CNS depression, agitation, restlessness, seizures, ECG changes, cardiac arrhythmias, fever, hypotension, dry mouth, ileus.

PREGNANCY-LACTATION-REPRODUCTION
• Safe use in pregnant women hasn't been established. Use during pregnancy only if potential benefit justifies potential risks to the fetus.
⚠ Alert: Neonates exposed to antipsychotics in the third trimester are at risk for extrapyramidal or withdrawal symptoms after delivery that may range in severity from mild to severe and may require intensive care support.
• Drug may appear in human milk. Use cautiously in breastfeeding women.

NURSING CONSIDERATIONS
Black Box Warning Elderly patients with dementia-related psychosis treated with antipsychotics are at an increased risk for death. ■
• Watch for orthostatic hypotension, especially when giving drug IV.
• To reduce hypotension risk, patients receiving IV drug must remain supine and be observed for at least 30 minutes after administration.
• Monitor CBC and LFTs during long-term therapy.

⊕ Alert: Use drug only when vomiting can't be controlled by other measures or when only a few doses are needed. If more than four doses are needed in 24 hours, notify prescriber.
• Immediately report signs and symptoms of tardive dyskinesia (involuntary rhythmic movements of the face, tongue, or jaw) as drug may need to be discontinued.
• Immediately report signs and symptoms of NMS (high fever, confusion, muscle rigidity, unstable vital signs) as drug should be discontinued and supportive therapy begun.
• *Look alike–sound alike:* Don't confuse prochlorperazine with chlorpromazine.

PATIENT TEACHING
• Advise patient to report all adverse reactions and to immediately report signs and symptoms of tardive dyskinesia and NMS.
• Tell patient to avoid extreme heat because drug may interfere with the body's thermoregulatory mechanisms.
• Advise patient to avoid alcohol while taking drug because of increased CNS depression.
• Tell patient to call prescriber if more than four doses are needed within 24 hours.

SAFETY ALERT!

promethazine hydrochloride
proe-METH-a-zeen

Histantil, Promethazine Plain, Promethegan

Therapeutic class: Antiemetics
Pharmacologic class: Phenothiazines

AVAILABLE FORMS
Injection: 25 mg/mL, 50 mg/mL
Suppositories: 12.5 mg, 25 mg, 50 mg
Syrup: 6.25 mg/5 mL*
Tablets: 12.5 mg, 25 mg, 50 mg

INDICATIONS & DOSAGES
➤ **Motion sickness**
Adults: 25 mg PO or PR taken 30 minutes to 1 hour before departure. May repeat dose 8 to 12 hours later p.r.n. Then, 25 mg PO b.i.d. on successive travel days on rising and again before the evening meal.

Children older than age 2: 12.5 to 25 mg PO or PR 30 minutes to 1 hour before departure. May repeat dose 8 to 12 hours later p.r.n.
➤ **Nausea and vomiting**
Adults: 12.5 to 25 mg PO, IM, IV, or PR every 4 to 6 hours p.r.n.
Children older than age 2 weighing at least 9.1 kg: 0.25 to 1 mg/kg PO or PR every 4 to 6 hours p.r.n. Or, 0.132 mg/kg IM.
➤ **Rhinitis, allergy symptoms**
Adults: 25 mg PO or PR at bedtime; or, 12.5 mg PO or PR t.i.d. and at bedtime. Or, 25 mg deep IM or IV. May repeat dose within 2 hours if needed. Use oral dosing as soon as possible.
Children older than age 2: Maximum dose is 25 mg PO or PR at bedtime; or, 6.25 to 12.5 mg PO or PR t.i.d. Use lowest effective dose and avoid other respiratory depressants.
➤ **Nighttime sedation**
Adults: 25 to 50 mg PO, IM, or PR at bedtime. Or, 25 mg IV at bedtime.
Children older than age 2: 1.1 mg/kg/dose (maximum, 25 mg) PO or PR at bedtime. Manufacturer doesn't provide exact dosage of parenteral promethazine. Use lowest possible effective dose.
➤ **Adjunct to analgesics for routine preoperative or postoperative sedation**
Adults: 25 to 50 mg IM, PO, or PR. Or, 25 mg IV in combination with an appropriately reduced dose of opioid or barbiturate and the required amount of a belladonna alkaloid.
Children older than age 2: 0.25 to 1.1 mg/kg PO, IM, or PR in combination with an appropriately reduced dose of opioid or barbiturate and the appropriate dose of an atropine-like drug.
➤ **Obstetric sedation**
Adults: 25 to 50 mg deep IM or IV in the early stages of labor. When labor is definitely established, may give 25 to 75 mg IM or IV with an appropriately reduced dose of desired opioid. If necessary, may repeat once or twice at 4-hour intervals. Maximum dose is 100 mg/24 hours.

ADMINISTRATION
PO
• Reduce GI distress by giving drug with food or milk.

IV

▼ If solution is discolored or contains a precipitate, discard.

▼ Give injection through a free-flowing IV line; consider giving over 10 to 15 minutes to minimize risk of phlebitis.

Black Box Warning Be alert for extravasation. Severe chemical irritation and damage can result. ∎

🕙 *Alert:* Don't give at a concentration above 25 mg/mL or a rate above 25 mg/minute.

Black Box Warning Don't give IV solution subcutaneously or intra-arterially. ∎

▼ **Incompatibilities:** None listed by manufacturer. Consult a drug incompatibility reference for more information.

IM

Black Box Warning IM injection is the preferred parenteral route. Inject deep IM into large muscle mass. ∎

• Rotate injection sites.

Rectal

• If suppository is too soft, place wrapped in refrigerator for 15 minutes or run under cold water.

• Store in refrigerator between 36° and 46° F (2° and 8° C).

ACTION

Phenothiazine derivative that competes with histamine at H_1-receptor sites on effector cells. Prevents, but doesn't reverse, histamine-mediated responses. At high doses, drug also has local anesthetic effects.

Route	Onset	Peak	Duration
PO	15–60 min	Unknown	<12 hr
IV	3–5 min	Unknown	<12 hr
IM, PR	20 min	Unknown	<12 hr

Half-life: 10-14 hours.

ADVERSE REACTIONS

CNS: drowsiness, sedation, confusion, sleepiness, dizziness, disorientation, extrapyramidal symptoms, insomnia. **CV:** hypotension, HTN. **EENT:** dry mouth, blurred vision. **GI:** nausea, vomiting. **GU:** urine retention. **Hematologic:** *leukopenia, agranulocytosis, thrombocytopenia.* **Metabolic:** hyperglycemia. **Respiratory:** *respiratory depression, apnea.* **Skin:** photosensitivity, rash, injection-site reaction.

INTERACTIONS

Drug-drug. *Anticholinergics, TCAs:* May increase anticholinergic effects. Avoid using together.

Antipsychotics: May increase risk of NMS. Monitor patient; discontinue promethazine if interaction is suspected.

CNS depressants: May increase sedation. Use together cautiously. If used together, reduce CNS depressant dosage.

Epinephrine: May block or reverse effects of epinephrine. Use other pressor drugs instead.

Levodopa: May decrease antiparkinsonian action of levodopa. Avoid using together.

Lithium: May reduce GI absorption or enhance renal elimination of lithium. Avoid using together.

MAO inhibitors: May increase extrapyramidal effects. Avoid using together.

Drug-lifestyle. *Alcohol use:* May increase sedation. Discourage use together.

Sun exposure: May cause photosensitivity reactions. Advise patient to avoid extensive sunlight exposure and to use sun block.

EFFECTS ON LAB TEST RESULTS

• May increase Hb level and hematocrit and blood glucose level.

• May decrease WBC, platelet, and granulocyte counts.

• May prevent, reduce, or mask positive result in diagnostic skin test. May cause false-positive or false-negative pregnancy test result. May interfere with blood grouping in the ABO system.

• May cause false-positive or false-negative with urine detection of amphetamine/methamphetamine.

CONTRAINDICATIONS & CAUTIONS

• Contraindicated in patients hypersensitive to drug, in those who have experienced adverse reactions to phenothiazines, in comatose patients, and in the treatment of lower respiratory tract signs and symptoms, including asthma.

Black Box Warning Contraindicated in children younger than age 2 because of the potential for fatal respiratory depression. Use the lowest effective dose in children older than age 2 and avoid

---

Reactions in bold italics are *life-threatening*. Interactions may have a *rapid onset* or a *delayed onset*.

administering with drugs that can cause respiratory depression. ▮

• Use cautiously in patients with a history of seizures and in those taking drugs that affect the seizure threshold as drug can lower the seizure threshold.

• Use cautiously in patients with pulmonary, hepatic, or CV disease; acutely ill or dehydrated children; and in those with intestinal obstruction, prostatic hyperplasia, bladder-neck obstruction, angle-closure glaucoma, seizure disorders, CNS depression, or stenosing or peptic ulcerations.

Dialyzable drug: No.

⚠ *Overdose S&S:* Hypotension, respiratory depression, ataxia, athetosis, positive Babinski reflex, unconsciousness, hyperreflexia, hypertonia, dry mouth, fixed dilated pupils, flushing, GI symptoms, seizures, sudden death; hyperexcitability, nightmares (in children).

PREGNANCY-LACTATION-REPRODUCTION

• There are no adequate studies in pregnant women. Use only if potential benefit justifies risks to the fetus.

• Use of drug within 2 weeks of delivery may inhibit platelet aggregation in the newborn.

• It isn't known if drug appears in human milk. Patient should discontinue breastfeeding or discontinue drug.

NURSING CONSIDERATIONS

Black Box Warning Perivascular extravasation, unintentional intra-arterial injection, or intraneuronal or perineuronal infiltration of the drug may result in irritation and tissue damage. Adverse reactions include burning, pain, thrombophlebitis, tissue necrosis, and gangrene. ▮

• Monitor patient for NMS: altered mental status, autonomic instability, muscle rigidity, and hyperpyrexia.

• Stop drug 4 days before diagnostic skin testing because antihistamines can prevent, reduce, or mask positive skin test response.

• Drug is used as an adjunct to analgesics, usually to increase sedation; it has no analgesic activity.

• *Look alike–sound alike:* Don't confuse promethazine with chlorpromazine or prednisone.

PATIENT TEACHING

• Tell patient to take oral form with food or milk.

• When treating motion sickness, tell patient to take first dose 30 to 60 minutes before travel; dose may be repeated in 8 to 12 hours, if necessary. On succeeding days of travel, patient should take dose upon arising and with evening meal.

• Warn patient to avoid alcohol and hazardous activities that require alertness until CNS effects of drug are known.

• Tell patient to report all adverse reactions promptly.

• Warn patient about possible photosensitivity reactions. Advise use of a sun block.

• Advise patient to report discomfort at IV site immediately.

• Instruct patient to report involuntary muscle movements.

propafenone hydrochloride
proe-PAF-a-non

Rythmol SR

Therapeutic class: Antiarrhythmics
Pharmacologic class: Sodium channel antagonists

AVAILABLE FORMS

Capsules (extended-release) ⓞ*:* 225 mg, 325 mg, 425 mg
Tablets (immediate-release): 150 mg, 225 mg, 300 mg

INDICATIONS & DOSAGES

Adjust-a-dose (for all indications): Consider reducing dosage in patients with hepatic impairment, significant widening of the QRS complex, or second- or third-degree AV block. Reduce dosage in elderly patients.

➤ **To treat life-threatening ventricular arrhythmias such as sustained ventricular tachycardia; to prolong time to recurrence of paroxysmal supraventricular tachycardia (PSVT) and paroxysmal atrial fibrillation or flutter in patients without structural heart disease**

Adults: Initially, 150 mg immediate-release tablet PO every 8 hours. May increase dosage every 3 or 4 days to 225 mg every

8 hours. If needed, may increase dosage to 300 mg every 8 hours. Maximum daily dose, 900 mg.

➤ **To prolong time until recurrence of symptomatic atrial fibrillation (AF) in patients with episodic AF who don't have structural heart disease**

Adults: Initially, 150-mg immediate-release tablet PO every 8 hours. May increase dosage after 3 to 4 days to 225- to 300-mg immediate-release tablet PO every 8 hours. Maximum dosage is 900 mg/day. Or, 225 mg extended-release capsule PO every 12 hours. May increase dose after 5 days to 325 mg PO every 12 hours. May increase dose to 425 mg every 12 hours.

ADMINISTRATION

PO
- Give without regard to food.
- Don't crush or open the extended-release capsules.

ACTION

Reduces inward sodium current in cardiac cells, prolongs refractory period in AV node, and decreases excitability, conduction velocity, and automaticity in cardiac tissue.

Route	Onset	Peak	Duration
PO (immediate-release)	Unknown	3½ hr	Unknown
PO (extended-release)	Unknown	3–8 hr	Unknown

Half-life: Estimated at 10 to 32 hours.

ADVERSE REACTIONS

CNS: dizziness, anxiety, ataxia, drowsiness, fatigue, headache, insomnia, syncope, tremor, weakness. **CV:** *HF, bradycardia, arrhythmias, ventricular tachycardia, PVCs, ventricular fibrillation,* AF, bundle-branch block, angina, chest pain, edema, first-degree AV block, hypotension, prolonged QRS complex, intraventricular conduction delay, palpitations. **EENT:** blurred vision. **GI:** nausea, vomiting, abdominal pain or cramps, constipation, diarrhea, dyspepsia, anorexia, flatulence, dry mouth, unusual taste. **Musculoskeletal:** arthralgia. **Respiratory:** dyspnea. **Skin:** rash, diaphoresis.

INTERACTIONS

Drug-drug. *Antiarrhythmics, fluoxetine, paroxetine, sertraline:* May increase risk of prolonged QTc interval and arrhythmias. Avoid use together.

Beta blockers (metoprolol, propranolol): May decrease metabolism of these drugs. Adjust dosage of beta blocker as needed and monitor therapy.

Cimetidine: May increase propafenone levels. Monitor patient for adverse effects and toxicity.

Cyclosporine, **digoxin:** May increase levels of these drugs, causing toxicity. Monitor patient closely; dosage adjustment may be necessary.

CYP2D6 inhibitors (paroxetine, ritonavir, sertraline), CYP3A4 inhibitors (erythromycin, ketoconazole, saquinavir): May increase propafenone level. Avoid use together.

Desipramine, haloperidol, imipramine, venlafaxine: May decrease metabolism of these drugs. Monitor patient closely.

Lidocaine: May decrease lidocaine metabolism. Monitor patient for increased CNS adverse effects and lidocaine toxicity.

Local anesthetics: May increase risk of CNS toxicity. Monitor patient closely.

Mexiletine: May decrease mexiletine metabolism, increasing level and adverse reactions. Monitor mexiletine level and patient closely.

Orlistat: May reduce fraction of propafenone available for absorption. Abrupt discontinuation of orlistat can result in severe adverse events. Use together with caution.

Phenobarbital, rifampin: May increase propafenone clearance. Watch for decreased antiarrhythmic effect.

QTc interval–prolonging drugs: Use together may enhance QTc-interval prolongation and risk of ventricular arrhythmias. Monitor patient closely and consider therapy modification.

Quinidine: May decrease propafenone metabolism. Avoid use together.

Ritonavir: May increase propafenone level, causing life-threatening arrhythmias. Avoid using together.

SSRIs, TCAs: May increase risk of cardiac arrhythmias. Avoid use together.

Reactions in bold italics are *life-threatening.* Interactions may have a *rapid onset* or a *delayed onset.*

Theophylline: May decrease theophylline metabolism. Monitor theophylline level and ECG closely.

Warfarin: May increase warfarin level. Monitor PT and INR closely, and adjust warfarin dose as needed.

Drug-food. *Grapefruit, grapefruit juice:* May increase drug level. Discourage use together.

Drug-lifestyle. *Smoking:* May increase propafenone level and risk of cardiac arrhythmias.

EFFECTS ON LAB TEST RESULTS
• May increase alkaline phosphatase, ALT, and AST levels.
• May cause positive ANA titers.

CONTRAINDICATIONS & CAUTIONS
• Contraindicated in patients hypersensitive to drug and in those with severe or uncontrolled HF; cardiogenic shock; SA, AV, or intraventricular disorders of impulse conduction without a pacemaker; bradycardia; Brugada syndrome; marked hypotension; bronchospastic disorders and severe obstructive pulmonary disease; or electrolyte imbalances.
• Drug has caused new or worsened arrhythmias. ECG monitoring is essential before and during therapy.
• Use cautiously in patients with a history of HF because drug may weaken the contraction of the heart.
• Use cautiously in patients taking other cardiac depressants and in those with hepatic or renal impairment.
• Use cautiously in patients with myasthenia gravis; may cause exacerbation.
Dialyzable drug: Unlikely.
⚠ Overdose S&S: Hypotension, somnolence, bradycardia, intra-atrial and intraventricular conduction disturbance.

PREGNANCY-LACTATION-REPRODUCTION
• There are no adequate studies in pregnant women. Use only if potential benefit justifies potential risk to the fetus.
• Drug appears in human milk. Patient should discontinue breastfeeding or discontinue drug.

NURSING CONSIDERATIONS
Black Box Warning Because of its proarrhythmic effects, propafenone should be reserved for patients with life-threatening ventricular arrhythmias. ■
☉ Alert: Perform continuous cardiac monitoring at start of therapy and during dosage adjustments. If PR interval or QRS complex increases by more than 25%, reduce dosage.
• If using with digoxin, frequently monitor ECG and digoxin level.
• Pacing and sensing thresholds of artificial pacemakers may change; monitor pacemaker function.
• Agranulocytosis may develop during first 2 to 3 months of therapy. If patient has an unexplained fever, monitor leukocyte count. WBC count usually normalizes 14 days after drug is discontinued.

PATIENT TEACHING
• Stress importance of taking drug exactly as prescribed.
• Tell patient that if a dose is missed, not to double the dose but to take the next dose at the usual time.
• Tell patient to report all adverse reactions promptly, including fever, sore throat, chills, and other signs and symptoms of infection.
• Tell patient to report palpitations, dizziness, passing out, swelling in arms or legs, trouble breathing, or sudden weight gain.
• Instruct patient to notify prescriber if prolonged diarrhea, sweating, vomiting, or loss of appetite or thirst occurs; these may cause an electrolyte imbalance.
• Tell patient not to crush, chew, or open the extended-release capsules.
• Tell patient to avoid grapefruit juice.

SAFETY ALERT!

propofol
PROE-po-fole

Diprivan

Therapeutic class: Hypnotics
Pharmacologic class: Phenol derivatives

AVAILABLE FORMS
Injection*: 10 mg/mL

INDICATIONS & DOSAGES

➤ **To induce general anesthesia**

Adults younger than age 55 classified as American Society of Anesthesiologists (ASA) Physical Status (PS) category I or II: 2 to 2.5 mg/kg IV. Give in 40-mg boluses every 10 seconds until desired response is achieved.

Children ages 3 to 16 classified as ASA PS I or II: 2.5 to 3.5 mg/kg IV over 20 to 30 seconds.

Adjust-a-dose: In geriatric, debilitated, hypovolemic, or ASA PS III or IV patients, give half the usual induction dose, in 20-mg boluses, every 10 seconds. For cardiac anesthesia, give 20 mg (0.5 to 1.5 mg/kg) every 10 seconds until desired response is achieved. For neurosurgical patients, give 20 mg (1 to 2 mg/kg) every 10 seconds until desired response is achieved.

➤ **To maintain anesthesia**

Healthy adults younger than age 55: 0.1 to 0.2 mg/kg/minute (6 to 12 mg/kg/hour) IV. Or, 25- to 50-mg intermittent boluses, p.r.n.

Healthy children ages 2 months to 16 years: Initially, 200 to 300 mcg/kg/minute for 30 minutes, then 125 to 150 mcg/kg/minute (7.5 to 9 mg/kg/hour) IV titrated to achieve desired clinical effect. Younger children may require higher maintenance infusion rates than older children.

Adjust-a-dose: In elderly, debilitated, hypovolemic, or ASA PS III or IV patients, give half the usual maintenance dose (0.05 to 0.1 mg/kg/minute or 3 to 6 mg/kg/hour). For cardiac anesthesia with secondary opioid, 100 to 150 mcg/kg/minute; low dose with primary opioid, 50 to 100 mcg/kg/minute. For neurosurgical patients, 100 to 200 mcg/kg/minute (6 to 12 mg/kg/hour).

➤ **Monitored anesthesia care**

Healthy adults younger than age 55: Initially, 100 to 150 mcg/kg/minute (6 to 9 mg/kg/hour) IV for 3 to 5 minutes or a slow injection of 0.5 mg/kg over 3 to 5 minutes. For maintenance dose, give infusion of 25 to 75 mcg/kg/minute (1.5 to 4.5 mg/kg/hour) for first 10 to 15 minutes, then reduce dosage to 25 to 50 mcg/kg/minute or incremental 10- or 20-mg boluses.

Adjust-a-dose: In elderly, debilitated, or ASA PS III or IV patients, give 80% of usual adult maintenance dose. Don't use rapid bolus.

➤ **To sedate intubated ICU patients**

Adults: Initially, 5 mcg/kg/minute (0.3 mg/kg/hour) IV for 5 minutes. Increments of 5 to 10 mcg/kg/minute (0.3 to 0.6 mg/kg/hour) over 5 to 10 minutes may be used until desired sedation is achieved. Maintenance rate, 5 to 50 mcg/kg/minute (0.3 to 3 mg/kg/hour).

ADMINISTRATION

IV

⊖ Alert: Maintain strict aseptic technique when handling solution. Drug can support growth of microorganisms; don't use if solution might be contaminated. Don't access vial more than once or use on multiple patients.

▼ Shake well.

▼ Dilute only with D₅W. Don't dilute to less than 2 mg/mL.

▼ Don't use if emulsion shows evidence of separation.

▼ Don't infuse through a filter with a pore size smaller than 5 microns. Give via larger veins in arms to decrease injection-site pain.

▼ Titrate drug daily to maintain minimum effective level. Allow 3 to 5 minutes between dosage adjustments to assess effects.

▼ Discard tubing and unused portions of drug after 12 hours.

▼ Store between 40° and 77° F (4° and 25° C); don't freeze. Protect from light.

▼ **Incompatibilities:** Other IV drugs, blood and plasma.

ACTION

Unknown. Rapid-acting IV sedative-hypnotic.

Route	Onset	Peak	Duration
IV	<40 sec	Unknown	10–15 min

Half-life: Initial (distribution) phase, about 2 to 10 minutes; second (redistribution) phase, 21 to 70 minutes; terminal (elimination) phase, 1½ to 31 hours.

ADVERSE REACTIONS

CNS: dystonic or choreiform movement.
CV: *bradycardia,* hypotension, HTN,

---

decreased cardiac output. **Metabolic:** hyperlipidemia. **Respiratory:** *apnea, respiratory acidosis.* **Skin:** rash, pruritus. **Other:** burning or stinging at injection site.

INTERACTIONS

Drug-drug. *Inhaled anesthetics (enflurane, halothane, isoflurane), opioids (alfentanil, fentanyl, meperidine, morphine), sedatives (barbiturates, benzodiazepines, chloral hydrate, droperidol):* May increase anesthetic and sedative effects and further decrease BP and cardiac output. Monitor patient closely.
Drug-lifestyle. *Alcohol use:* May enhance CNS depressant effect of alcohol. Monitor therapy.

EFFECTS ON LAB TEST RESULTS

• May increase serum triglyceride levels.

CONTRAINDICATIONS & CAUTIONS

• Contraindicated in patients hypersensitive to drug or its components (soybean oil, glycerol, egg lecithin, disodium edetate, sodium hydroxide); in patients with allergies to eggs, egg products, soybeans, or soy products; and in those unable to undergo general anesthesia or sedation.
❸ Alert: Repeated or lengthy use of general anesthetic and sedation drugs during surgeries or procedures in children younger than age 3 or in pregnant women during the third trimester may affect the development of children's brains. Weigh benefits of appropriate anesthesia in young children and pregnant women against risks.
• Drug isn't recommended for obstetric surgery, including cesarean deliveries, because of potential neonatal depression.
• Use cautiously in patients who are hemodynamically unstable or who have seizures, disorders of lipid metabolism, or increased ICP.
Dialyzable drug: Unknown.
⚠ Overdose S&S: Cardiorespiratory depression.

PREGNANCY-LACTATION-REPRODUCTION

• There are no adequate studies in pregnant women. Use only if clearly needed.
• Drug isn't recommended for obstetric uses as it may cause neonatal CNS and respiratory depression.

• Drug appears in human milk. Avoid use in breastfeeding women.

NURSING CONSIDERATIONS

• If drug is used for prolonged sedation in ICU, urine may turn green.
• For general anesthesia or monitored anesthesia care sedation, trained staff not involved in the surgical or diagnostic procedure should give drug. For ICU sedation, persons skilled in managing critically ill patients and trained in cardiopulmonary resuscitation and airway management should give drug.
• Continuously monitor vital signs.
❸ Alert: The FDA issued an alert after receiving reports of chills, fever, and body aches in several clusters of patients shortly after patients received propofol for sedation or general anesthesia. Various lots of the drug were tested, but no toxins, bacteria, or other signs of contamination were found. The FDA advises all health care providers to carefully follow the handling and use sections of the prescribing information for this drug. They recommend that all patients be evaluated for possible reactions following use of the drug, and that anyone experiencing signs of acute febrile reactions be evaluated for possible bacterial sepsis. They ask that any adverse events following the use of propofol be reported to MedWatch.
• Monitor patient at risk for hyperlipidemia for elevated triglyceride levels.
• Drug contains 0.1 g of fat (1.1 kcal)/mL. Reduce other lipid products if given together.
• Some formulations contain ethylenediaminetetraacetic acid, a strong metal chelator. Consider supplemental zinc during prolonged therapy and in patients predisposed to zinc deficiency (those with burns, sepsis, or diarrhea).
• Some formulations contain sodium metabisulfite, a sulfite, which may cause allergic-type reactions, including anaphylactic signs and symptoms and life-threatening or less severe asthmatic episodes, in certain susceptible people.
• When giving drug in the ICU, assess patient's CNS function daily to determine minimum dose needed.

P

• Stop drug gradually to prevent abrupt awakening and increased agitation.

• Drug may be misused. Manage drug to prevent risk of diversion.

• *Look alike–sound alike:* Don't confuse Diprivan with Ditropan or Diflucan.

PATIENT TEACHING

• Advise patient that performance of activities requiring mental alertness may be impaired for some time after drug use.

• Tell patient that abnormal dreams or anesthesia awareness may occur.

🌢 *Alert:* Discuss with parents or caregivers of child younger than age 3 and with pregnant patients the benefits, risks, and appropriate timing of surgery or procedures requiring anesthetic and sedation drugs.

SAFETY ALERT!

propranolol hydrochloride ⚠
proe-PRAN-oh-lol

Hemangeol, Inderal LA✿, Inderal XL, InnoPran XL

Therapeutic class: Antihypertensives
Pharmacologic class: Nonselective beta blockers

AVAILABLE FORMS

Capsules (extended-release) ⒹⓃⒼ*:* 60 mg, 80 mg, 120 mg, 160 mg
Injection: 1 mg/mL
Oral solution: 4 mg/mL, 4.28 mg/mL, 8 mg/mL
Tablets: 10 mg, 20 mg, 40 mg, 60 mg, 80 mg

INDICATIONS & DOSAGES
➤ **Angina pectoris**
Adults: Total doses of 80 to 320 mg/day (immediate-release) PO in two to four divided doses. Or, one 80-mg extended-release capsule daily. Increase dosage at 3- to 7-day intervals until optimal response is obtained or a maximum of 320 mg PO daily has been given.
➤ **To decrease risk of death after MI**
Adults: Initially, 40 mg PO t.i.d. After 1 month, titrate to 60 to 80 mg t.i.d. as tolerated. Maintenance dose is 180 to 240 mg/day in divided doses b.i.d., t.i.d., or q.i.d.

➤ **Supraventricular, ventricular, and atrial arrhythmias; tachyarrhythmias caused by excessive catecholamine action during anesthesia, hyperthyroidism, or pheochromocytoma**
Adults: 1 to 3 mg by slow IV push, not to exceed 1 mg/minute. After 3 mg have been given, another dose may be given in 2 minutes; subsequent doses, no sooner than every 4 hours. Transfer to oral therapy as soon as possible. Usual maintenance dose is 10 to 30 mg PO t.i.d. or q.i.d.
➤ **HTN**
Adults: Initially, 80 mg PO daily in two divided doses or extended-release form once daily. Increase at 3- to 7-day intervals to maximum daily dose of 640 mg. Usual maintenance dose is 120 to 240 mg daily or 120 to 160 mg daily as extended-release. For InnoPran XL, dose is 80 mg PO once daily at bedtime. Give consistently with or without food. Adjust to maximum of 120 mg daily if needed. Full effects are seen in about 2 to 3 weeks.
➤ **Essential tremor**
Adults: 40 mg (tablets or oral solution) PO b.i.d. Usual maintenance dose is 120 to 320 mg daily in three divided doses.
➤ **Hypertrophic subaortic stenosis**
Adults: 20 to 40 mg PO t.i.d. or q.i.d., or 80 to 160 mg extended-release capsules once daily.
➤ **Adjunctive therapy in pheochromocytoma**
Adults: 60 mg PO daily in divided doses with an alpha blocker 3 days before surgery.
➤ **Prevention of migraine**
Adults: Initially, 80 mg PO daily in divided doses. May increase to 160 to 240 mg/day.
➤ **Proliferating infantile hemangioma requiring systemic therapy (Hemangeol)**
Infants ages 5 weeks to 5 months: Initially, 0.6 mg/kg PO b.i.d. for 1 week. Increase to 1.1 mg/kg PO b.i.d. after 1 week. Increase to maintenance dose of 1.7 mg/kg PO b.i.d. after 2 weeks of treatment and maintain for 6 months. Administer doses at least 9 hours apart during or after feeding.
Adjust-a-dose: Readjust dosage periodically for changes in child's weight.
➤ **Gastroesophageal varices** ◆
Adults: Initially, 20 mg PO b.i.d. Titrate to maximum tolerable dose.

ADMINISTRATION
PO
• Give immediate-release tablets on an empty stomach. Give extended-release capsules with or without food, but patient should always take consistently (with or without food). Food may increase absorption of propranolol.
• Adherence may be improved by giving drug twice daily or as extended-release capsules. Check with prescriber.
• Check BP and apical pulse before giving drug. If hypotension or extremes in pulse rate occur, withhold drug and notify prescriber.
• Monitor HR and BP for 2 hours after first dose and when increasing Hemangeol dosage.
• Give Hemangeol during or right after a feeding. Skip dose if child isn't eating or is vomiting. Don't shake before use.
• Give Hemangeol directly into child's mouth using the oral dosing syringe. If needed, may dilute with a small quantity of milk or fruit juice and give in baby's bottle.
• Don't substitute extended-release form for immediate-release on a milligram-for-milligram basis. Retitration may be necessary.

IV
▼ For direct injection, give into a large vessel or into the tubing of a free-flowing, compatible IV solution; don't give by continuous IV infusion.
▼ Drug is compatible with D_5W, half-NSS, NSS, and lactated Ringer solution.
▼ Infusion rate shouldn't exceed 1 mg/minute.
▼ Double-check dose and route. IV doses are much smaller than oral doses.
▼ Monitor BP, ECG, central venous pressure, and HR and rhythm frequently, especially during IV administration. If patient develops severe hypotension, notify prescriber; a vasopressor may be prescribed.
▼ For overdose, give IV isoproterenol, IV atropine, or glucagon; refractory cases may require a pacemaker.
▼ **Incompatibilities:** Amphotericin B, diazoxide.

ACTION
Reduces cardiac oxygen demand by blocking catecholamine-induced increases in HR, BP, and force of myocardial contraction. Drug depresses renin secretion and prevents vasodilation of cerebral arteries.

Route	Onset	Peak	Duration
PO	30 min	1–4 hr	12 hr
PO (Hemangeol)	Rapid	≤2 hr	Unknown
PO (extended-release)	Unknown	6–14 hr	24 hr
IV	Immediate	1 min	5 min

Half-life: About 3 to 6 hours; 8 hours for InnoPran XL; 3½ hours for Hemangeol.

ADVERSE REACTIONS
CNS: fatigue, lethargy, fever, vivid dreams, hallucinations, mental depression, light-headedness, dizziness, insomnia. **CV:** hypotension, *bradycardia, HF, intensification of AV block,* intermittent claudication. **GI:** abdominal cramping, constipation, diarrhea, nausea, vomiting. **Hematologic:** *agranulocytosis.* **Respiratory:** *bronchospasm.* **Skin:** rash.

INTERACTIONS
Drug-drug. *Aminophylline:* May antagonize beta-blocking effects of propranolol. Use together cautiously.
Amiodarone, diltiazem, verapamil: May cause hypotension, bradycardia, and increased depressant effect on myocardium. Use together cautiously.
Cardiac glycosides: May reduce the positive inotrope effect of the glycoside. Monitor patient for clinical effect.
Cimetidine, ciprofloxacin, fluconazole, fluoxetine, paroxetine: May inhibit metabolism of propranolol. Watch for increased beta-blocking effect.
Epinephrine: May cause severe vasoconstriction. Monitor BP and observe patient carefully.
Glucagon, isoproterenol: May antagonize propranolol effect. May be used therapeutically and in emergencies.
Haloperidol: May cause cardiac arrest. Avoid using together.
Insulin, oral antidiabetics: May alter requirements for these drugs in previously stabilized diabetics. Monitor patient for hypoglycemia.
Lidocaine: May reduce clearance of lidocaine. Monitor lidocaine level closely.

P

♣Canada ◇OTC ♦Off-label use ✐Photoguide ⓓDo not crush *Liquid contains alcohol ⚕Genetic

Phenothiazines (chlorpromazine, thiori-dazine): May increase risk of serious adverse reactions to either drug. Use with thioridazine is contraindicated. If chlorpromazine must be used, monitor patient's pulse and BP; decrease propranolol dose as needed.

Propafenone, quinidine: May increase propranolol level. Monitor cardiac function, and adjust propranolol dose as needed.

Theophylline derivatives: May decrease theophylline clearance by 30% to 52% and diminish their bronchodilatory effect. Consider therapy modification.

Drug-herb. *Ma huang:* May decrease antihypertensive effects. Discourage use together.

Drug-lifestyle. *Alcohol use:* May increase or decrease propranolol level. Discourage alcohol use.

Smoking: May decrease propranolol level. Monitor clinical response and adjust dosage as needed. Discourage smoking.

EFFECTS ON LAB TEST RESULTS

• May increase T_4, BUN, transaminase, alkaline phosphatase, potassium, and LDH levels. May decrease T_3 level.

• May decrease granulocyte count.

CONTRAINDICATIONS & CAUTIONS

Black Box Warning Abrupt withdrawal of drug may cause exacerbation of angina or MI. To discontinue drug, gradually reduce dosage over 1 to 2 weeks. If angina worsens or acute coronary insufficiency develops, resume therapy at least temporarily. Because CAD may be unrecognized, don't discontinue drug abruptly, even when taken for other indications. ∎

• Contraindicated in patients with known hypersensitivity to drug, bronchial asthma, sinus bradycardia and heart block greater than first-degree, cardiogenic shock, and overt and decompensated HF (unless failure is secondary to a tachyarrhythmia that can be treated with propranolol).

• Hemangeol is contraindicated in infants weighing less than 2 kg, premature infants with corrected age younger than 5 weeks, infants with an HR less than 80 beats/minute or BP lower than 50/30 mm Hg, and in infants with greater than first-degree heart block, decompensated HF, asthma,

pheochromocytoma, or history of bronchospasm.

• Use cautiously in patients with hepatic or renal impairment, Wolff-Parkinson-White syndrome, nonallergic bronchospastic diseases, or hepatic disease and in those taking other antihypertensives.

• Use cautiously in patients who have diabetes mellitus because drug masks some symptoms of hypoglycemia.

• In patients with thyrotoxicosis, use drug cautiously because it may mask the signs and symptoms. Abrupt withdrawal may exacerbate symptoms of hyperthyroidism, including thyroid storm.

• Elderly patients may experience enhanced adverse reactions and may need dosage adjustment.

Dialyzable drug: No.

⚠ *Overdose S&S:* Bradycardia, hypotension.

PREGNANCY-LACTATION-REPRODUCTION

• There are no adequate studies in pregnant women. Use only if potential benefit justifies potential risk to the fetus.

• Drug is associated with fetal intrauterine growth retardation and neonatal bradycardia, hypoglycemia, and respiratory depression. If drug is used during pregnancy, ensure adequate monitoring of infants is available at birth.

• Drug appears in human milk, with peak concentrations occurring 2 to 3 hours after oral doses. Use cautiously in breastfeeding women. Monitor infants for signs and symptoms of beta blockade and hypoglycemia.

NURSING CONSIDERATIONS

• Drug masks common signs and symptoms of shock and hypoglycemia.

▨ Some antihypertensives are less effective in lowering BP when used as monotherapy in black patients. Monitor black patients for expected therapeutic effects; dosage and therapy adjustments may be necessary.

❸ *Alert:* Don't stop drug before surgery for pheochromocytoma. Before any surgical procedure, tell anesthesiologist that patient is receiving propranolol.

• *Look alike–sound alike:* Don't confuse propranolol with prasugrel or Pravachol. Don't confuse Inderal with Isordil, Adderall, or Imuran.

PATIENT TEACHING

• Caution patient to continue taking drug as prescribed, even if feeling well, and to promptly report adverse reactions.

• Instruct patient to take immediate-release product without food and extended-release product consistently with or without food.

• Advise patient that propranolol may interfere with glaucoma screening because it can reduce IOP.

• Teach caregiver to skip Hemangeol dose if child isn't eating or is vomiting.

Black Box Warning Caution patient not to stop drug without advice from prescriber because abruptly stopping drug can worsen chest pain or cause an MI. ∎

• Advise patient to avoid smoking and alcohol.

pyridostigmine bromide
peer-id-oh-STIG-meen

Mestinon*, Mestinon-SR✽, Regonol*

Therapeutic class: Muscle stimulants
Pharmacologic class: Cholinesterase inhibitors

AVAILABLE FORMS
Injection: 5 mg/mL
Syrup: 60 mg/5 mL*
Tablets: 60 mg
Tablets (extended-release) ⓝ: 180 mg

INDICATIONS & DOSAGES
Adjust-a-dose (for all indications): Smaller doses may be required in patients with renal disease. Adjust dosage to achieve desired effect.

➤ **Antidote for nondepolarizing neuromuscular blockers**
Adults: 0.1 to 0.25 mg/kg IV. Immediately before or with dose, also give atropine sulfate 0.6 to 1.2 mg IV or an equipotent dose of glycopyrrolate.

➤ **Myasthenia gravis**
Adults: 60 to 120 mg immediate-release PO every 3 or 4 hours. Average dosage is 600 mg daily, but dosages up to 1,500 mg daily may be needed. Dosage must be adjusted for each patient, based on response and tolerance. Or, 180 to 540 mg

extended-release tablets PO daily or b.i.d., with at least 6 hours between doses.

ADMINISTRATION
PO
• Don't crush extended-release tablets.

• If patient has trouble swallowing, give syrup form. If patient can't tolerate sweet flavor, give over ice chips.

IV
🔸 *Alert:* Drug should only be administered by individuals familiar with its actions, characteristics, and hazards.

▼ Don't use solution if it contains particulate matter or is discolored.

▼ Position patient to ease breathing. Keep atropine injection available, and be prepared to give it immediately.

▼ Monitor vital signs frequently, especially respirations. Provide respiratory support as needed.

▼ Give injection no faster than 1 mg/minute. Rapid infusion may cause bradycardia and seizures.

▼ **Incompatibilities:** Alkaline solutions.

ACTION
Inhibits acetylcholinesterase, blocking destruction of acetylcholine from the parasympathetic and somatic efferent nerves. Acetylcholine accumulates, promoting increased stimulation of the receptors.

Route	Onset	Peak	Duration
PO	20–30 min	2 hr	3–6 hr
PO (extended-release)	30–60 min	1–2 hr	6–12 hr
IV	2–5 min	Unknown	2–4 hr

Half-life: 1 to 3 hours, depending on route.

ADVERSE REACTIONS
CNS: headache with high doses, weakness, syncope. **CV:** *bradycardia, cardiac arrest,* hypotension, thrombophlebitis. **EENT:** miosis, rhinorrhea. **GI:** nausea, vomiting, abdominal cramps, diarrhea, excessive salivation, increased peristalsis. **GU:** urinary frequency, urinary urgency. **Musculoskeletal:** muscle cramps, muscle fasciculations, muscle weakness, tingling in extremities. **Respiratory:** *bronchospasm, bronchoconstriction,* increased bronchial secretions. **Skin:** rash, diaphoresis.

INTERACTIONS

Drug-drug. *Anticholinergics, atropine, corticosteroids, general or local anesthetics, magnesium, procainamide, quinidine:* May antagonize cholinergic effects. Observe patient for lack of drug effect.

Beta blockers: May increase bradycardia risk. Monitor therapy.

Ganglionic blockers: May increase risk of hypotension. Monitor patient closely.

Succinylcholine: May prolong the phase I block of the depolarizing muscle relaxant. Avoid using together.

EFFECTS ON LAB TEST RESULTS

None reported.

CONTRAINDICATIONS & CAUTIONS

• Contraindicated in patients hypersensitive to anticholinesterases or bromides and in those with mechanical obstruction of the intestinal or urinary tract.

• Use cautiously in patients with bronchial asthma, bradycardia, arrhythmias, epilepsy, recent coronary occlusion, vagotonia, renal impairment, hyperthyroidism, glaucoma, or peptic ulcer.

• Use cautiously in patients taking beta blockers for HTN or glaucoma.

• Safety and effectiveness in children haven't been established.

Dialyzable drug: Unknown.

PREGNANCY-LACTATION-REPRODUCTION

• Drug may cross placental barrier. Use during pregnancy only if potential benefits justify potential maternal and fetal hazards.

• Drug appears in human milk. Use cautiously in breastfeeding women.

NURSING CONSIDERATIONS

• Stop all other cholinergics before giving this drug.

• Monitor and document patient's response after each dose. Optimum dosage is difficult to judge.

• ❸ **Alert:** Regonol contains benzyl alcohol preservative, which may cause toxicity in neonates if given in high doses.

• Mestinon syrup contains 5% alcohol.

• ***Look alike–sound alike:*** Don't confuse pyridostigmine with physostigmine. Don't confuse Regonol with Reglan or Renagel.

PATIENT TEACHING

• Advise patient to report all adverse reactions.

• When giving drug for myasthenia gravis, stress importance of taking exactly as prescribed, on time, in evenly spaced doses. For extended-release tablets, tell patient to take at same time each day, at least 6 hours apart.

• Advise patient not to crush or chew extended-release tablets.

• Explain that patient may have to take drug for life.

• Advise patient to wear or carry medical identification that indicates patient has myasthenia gravis.

QUEtiapine fumarate

kwe-TYE-a-peen

Seroquel✐, Seroquel XR

Therapeutic class: Antipsychotics
Pharmacologic class: Dibenzothiazepine derivatives

AVAILABLE FORMS

Tablets: 25 mg, 50 mg, 100 mg, 150 mg, 200 mg, 300 mg, 400 mg
Tablets (extended-release) ⓞⓝⓒ*:* 50 mg, 150 mg, 200 mg, 300 mg, 400 mg

INDICATIONS & DOSAGES

Adjust-a-dose (for all indications): Use slower titration rates and lower target doses in patients who are elderly or debilitated or who are predisposed to hypotension. Begin elderly patients on 50 mg/day (immediate-release or extended-release) and increase by 50 mg/day as needed depending on clinical response and tolerability. Patients with hepatic impairment should begin with 25 mg/day (immediate-release or extended-release) and increase by 25 mg/day to 50 mg/day to an effective dose, depending on clinical response and tolerability.

Adjust dosage when drug is used in combination with CYP3A4 inducers and inhibitors.

➤ **Schizophrenia**
Adults: Initially, 25 mg (immediate-release) PO b.i.d., with increases in increments of 25 to 50 mg b.i.d. or t.i.d. on days 2 and 3,

as tolerated. Target range is 300 to 400 mg daily divided into two or three doses by day 4. Further dosage adjustments, if indicated, should occur at intervals of not less than 2 days. Dosage can be increased or decreased by 25 to 50 mg b.i.d. Effect generally occurs at 150 to 750 mg daily. Maximum dosage is 750 mg/day for acute therapy, or 800 mg/day for maintenance treatment.

Or, initially, 300 mg/day extended-release tablets PO once daily, preferably in the evening. Titrate within a dose range of 400 to 800 mg/day, depending on the response and tolerance of the individual. Increase at intervals as short as 1 day and in increments of up to 300 mg/day. Maximum dose is 800 mg/day (extended-release).

Adolescents ages 13 to 17: For immediate-release tablets, usual dosage is 400 to 800 mg/day, which may be divided into three doses per day depending on response and tolerability; maximum dosage, 800 mg/day. Initially, 25 mg PO b.i.d. on day 1; 50 mg b.i.d. on day 2; 100 mg b.i.d. on day 3; 150 mg b.i.d. on day 4; and 200 mg b.i.d. on day 5. Adjust dosage by no more than 100 mg/day. For extended-release tablets, usual dosage is 400 to 800 mg/day; maximum dosage, 800 mg/day. Initially, 50 mg/day PO on day 1; 100 mg/day on day 2; 200 mg/day on day 3; 300 mg/day on day 4; and 400 mg/day on day 5. Make adjustments in increments of no greater than 100 mg/day.

➤ **Monotherapy and adjunctive therapy with lithium or divalproex for the short-term treatment of acute manic episodes associated with bipolar I disorder; adjunctive maintenance therapy with lithium or divalproex**

Adults: Initially, 50 mg (immediate-release) PO b.i.d. on day 1; 100 mg b.i.d. on day 2; 150 mg b.i.d. on day 3; and 200 mg b.i.d. on day 4. Further dosage adjustments after day 4 should be no greater than 200 mg daily to a maximum daily dose of 800 mg. Usual dose is 400 to 800 mg daily. For maintenance therapy with lithium or divalproex, continue treatment at the dosage required to maintain symptom remission.

Or, start with 300 mg (extended-release) PO on day 1 and 600 mg PO on day 2 once daily in the evening. Dosage may be ad-justed based on response and tolerability to maximum dosage of 800 mg/day.

➤ **Bipolar I disorder, acute manic episodes**

Children and adolescents ages 10 to 17: Total daily dosage for initial 5 days of therapy is 50 mg PO on day 1, then 100 mg on day 2, then 200 mg on day 3, then 300 mg on day 4, and 400 mg on day 5, usually given in divided doses b.i.d. (immediate-release) or daily (extended-release). After day 5, adjust dosage in increments of no more than 100 mg/day within the recommended range of 400 to 600 mg/day. Maximum dosage is 600 mg/day.

➤ **Bipolar depression**

Adults: Initially, 50 mg PO once daily at bedtime; increase on day 2 to 100 mg; increase on day 3 to 200 mg; increase on day 4 to maintenance dose of 300 mg/day. Maximum dose is 300 mg/day.

➤ **Major depressive disorder, adjunctive therapy with antidepressants**

Adults: 50 mg PO (extended-release) once daily in the evening on days 1 and 2. On day 3, may increase dosage to 150 mg PO once daily in the evening. Dosages ranging from 150 to 300 mg/day have proved effective.

ADMINISTRATION

PO

- Don't crush or allow patient to chew extended-release tablets.
- Give immediate-release tablets without regard for food; give extended-release tablets without food or with a light meal (about 300 calories), preferably in the evening.
- Patients who are currently being treated with divided doses of the immediate-release form may be switched to extended-release tablets at the equivalent total daily dose taken once daily. Individual dosage adjustments may be necessary.

ACTION

Blocks dopamine type 2 (D_2) and serotonin type 2A ($5\text{-}HT_{2a}$) receptors. Its action may be mediated through this antagonism.

Route	Onset	Peak	Duration
PO	Unknown	1½ hr	Unknown
PO (extended-release)	Unknown	6 hr	Unknown

Half-life: 6 hours; extended-release, 7 to 12 hours.

Q

ADVERSE REACTIONS

CNS: dizziness, headache, drowsiness, somnolence, *NMS, seizures,* hypertonia, dysarthria, asthenia, agitation, extrapyramidal reaction, fatigue, lethargy, pain, change in dreams, anxiety, paresthesia, restlessness, migraine, ataxia, confusion, disorientation, fever, depression. **CV:** orthostatic hypotension, tachycardia, palpitations, peripheral edema, hypotension, HTN, syncope. **EENT:** blurred vision, amblyopia, ear pain, epistaxis, nasal congestion, pharyngitis, rhinitis, sinusitis, toothache. **GI:** dry mouth, dyspepsia, abdominal pain, constipation, nausea, anorexia, vomiting, increased appetite, increased thirst, diarrhea, gastroenteritis, dysphagia, gastroesophageal reflux. **GU:** UTI. **Hematologic:** *leukopenia, neutropenia, agranulocytosis.* **Metabolic:** weight gain, hyperglycemia. **Musculoskeletal:** back pain, arthralgia, myalgia, weakness, tremor, dyskinesia. **Respiratory:** increased cough, dyspnea. **Skin:** rash, diaphoresis, pallor, acne. **Other:** flulike syndrome.

INTERACTIONS

Drug-drug. *Antihypertensives:* May increase effects of antihypertensives. Monitor BP.

CNS depressants: May increase CNS effects. Use together cautiously.

Dopamine agonists, levodopa: May antagonize the effects of these drugs. Monitor patient.

Lorazepam: May decrease lorazepam clearance and increase CNS depression. Monitor patient for increased CNS effects.

Opioids: May cause slow or difficult breathing, sedation, and death. Avoid use together if possible. If use together is necessary, limit dosage and duration of each drug to minimum necessary for desired effect. Consider therapy modification.

QTc interval–prolonging drugs: May enhance QTc-interval prolongation and risk of ventricular arrhythmias. Avoid use in highest risk patients; monitor therapy for those at lower risk.

Strong CYP3A4 inducers (carbamazepine, phenobarbital, phenytoin, rifampin, thioridazine): May decrease quetiapine serum concentration. Increase quetiapine dosage up to fivefold of the original dose when used

in combination with prolonged treatment (greater than 7 to 14 days); titrate based on clinical response and tolerability. When the CYP3A4 inducer is discontinued, reduce quetiapine dosage to the original level within 7 to 14 days.

Strong CYP3A4 inhibitors (erythromycin, fluconazole, indinavir, itraconazole, ketoconazole, nefazodone, ritonavir): May increase quetiapine serum concentration. Reduce quetiapine dosage to one-sixth of original dose when used together. When the CYP3A4 inhibitor is discontinued, increase quetiapine dosage by sixfold.

Voriconazole: May decrease quetiapine metabolism. Consider therapy modification.

Drug-herb. *St. John's wort:* May increase risk of serotonin syndrome and decrease quetiapine serum concentration. Consider therapy modification.

Drug-lifestyle. *Alcohol use, cannabis/cannabidiol:* May increase CNS effects. Discourage use together.

EFFECTS ON LAB TEST RESULTS

• May increase liver enzyme, prolactin, cholesterol, triglyceride, and glucose levels. May decrease T_4 and TSH levels.

• May decrease WBC count.

• May cause false-positive results in urine enzyme immunoassays for methadone and TCAs.

CONTRAINDICATIONS & CAUTIONS

• Contraindicated in patients hypersensitive to drug or its ingredients.

Black Box Warning The risk of death is increased in elderly patients with dementia-related psychosis. Quetiapine isn't approved for the treatment of patients with dementia-related psychosis. ∎

Black Box Warning Suicidal thoughts and behavior may occur in children, adolescents, and young adults (younger than age 24) who are taking quetiapine. In patients of all ages who are started on antidepressant therapy, monitor closely for clinical worsening and for emergence of suicidal thoughts and behavior. Advise families and caregivers of the need for close observation and communication with prescriber. Quetiapine isn't approved for use in children younger than age 10. ∎

Reactions in bold italics are *life-threatening*. Interactions may have a *rapid onset* or a ***delayed onset***.

• Avoid use when risk of torsades de pointes or sudden death may be increased, including in patients with a history of cardiac arrhythmias such as bradycardia, hypokalemia, or hypomagnesemia. Also avoid use with other drugs that prolong the QTc interval and in patients with congenital prolongation of the QT interval.

• Use cautiously in patients with increased risk of QT-interval prolongation, such as those with CV disease, family history of QT-interval prolongation, HF, or heart hypertrophy, and in elderly patients.

• Use cautiously in patients at risk for falls, including those with diseases, conditions, or who are taking medications that may cause somnolence, orthostatic hypotension, or motor or sensory instability.

• Use cautiously in patients with CV disease, cerebrovascular disease, conditions that predispose to hypotension, a history of seizures or conditions that lower the seizure threshold, and conditions in which core body temperature may be elevated.

• Rare cases of NMS have been reported. Monitor patients for mental status changes, fever, muscle rigidity, or autonomic instability. Other blood dyscrasias (leukopenia, neutropenia, and agranulocytosis) have also been reported.

• Drug may cause extrapyramidal signs and symptoms. Consider stopping drug for signs or symptoms of tardive dyskinesia.

• Use cautiously in patients with renal disease; experience is limited.

• Use cautiously in patients at risk for aspiration pneumonia.

Dialyzable drug: Unknown.

⚠ Overdose S&S: Drowsiness, hypotension, sedation, tachycardia, hypokalemia, QTc-interval prolongation, first-degree heart block.

PREGNANCY-LACTATION-REPRODUCTION

�উ Alert: Neonates exposed to antipsychotics during the third trimester are at risk for developing extrapyramidal signs and symptoms (repetitive muscle movements of the face and body) and withdrawal signs and symptoms (agitation, abnormally increased or decreased muscle tone, tremors, sleepiness, severe difficulty breathing, difficulty feeding) after delivery. Use in pregnancy

only if potential benefit justifies risk to the fetus.

• Women exposed to drug during pregnancy should be enrolled in the National Pregnancy Registry for Atypical Antipsychotics (1-866-961-2388 or www.womensmentalhealth.org/research/pregnancy registry).

• Drug appears in human milk. Breastfeeding isn't recommended.

NURSING CONSIDERATIONS

• Dispense lowest appropriate quantity of drug to reduce risk of overdose.

Black Box Warning Drug isn't indicated for use in elderly patients with dementia-related psychosis because of increased risk of death from CV disease or infection. ∎

�উ Alert: Watch for evidence of NMS (extrapyramidal effects, hyperthermia, autonomic disturbance), which is rare but deadly.

• Complete fall risk assessments when initiating antipsychotic treatment and recurrently for patients on long-term therapy, especially for patients with diseases, conditions, or who are taking other drugs that could exacerbate fall risk.

• Monitor patient for tardive dyskinesia, which may occur after prolonged use. It may not appear until months or years later and may disappear spontaneously or persist for life, despite ending drug. Consider discontinuing therapy if signs or symptoms of tardive dyskinesia occur.

• Hyperglycemia may occur in patients taking drug. Monitor patients with diabetes regularly. All patients should be monitored for signs and symptoms of hyperglycemia and undergo a fasting blood glucose test if signs or symptoms develop during treatment.

• Monitor patient for weight gain by checking waist circumference and BMI.

�উ Alert: Monitor patient for symptoms of metabolic syndrome (significant weight gain and increased BMI, HTN, hyperglycemia, hypercholesterolemia, and hypertriglyceridemia).

• Drug use may cause cataract formation.

• Obtain baseline ophthalmologic examination and reassess every 6 months.

• *Look alike–sound alike:* Don't confuse Seroquel with Serzone.

PATIENT TEACHING
• Advise patient and caregiver to use caution when quetiapine is being taken with other centrally acting drugs because of the risk of increased CNS effects.
• Advise patient to avoid alcohol and cannabis/cannabidiol while taking drug.
• Warn patient about risk of dizziness when standing up quickly. The risk is greatest during the 3- to 5-day period of first dosage adjustment, when resuming treatment, and when increasing dosages.
• Tell patient to avoid becoming overheated or dehydrated.
• Advise patient to report signs and symptoms of hyperglycemia (excessive thirst, excessive urination, excessive hunger or weakness).
• Warn patient to avoid activities that require mental alertness until effects of drug are known, especially during first dosage adjustment or dosage increases.
• Remind patient to have an eye examination at start of therapy and every 6 months during therapy to check for cataracts.
• Tell patient to notify prescriber about other prescription or OTC drugs being taken.
• Tell female patient of childbearing potential to notify prescriber about planned, suspected, or known pregnancy.
• Advise female patient not to breastfeed during therapy.
• Tell patient to take immediate-release drug with or without food.
• Tell patient not to crush, chew, or break extended-release tablets.
• Tell patient to take extended-release tablets once daily without food or with a light meal, preferably in the evening.
• Tell patient and caregivers to report all adverse reactions and to be alert for fever, muscle rigidity, repetitive muscle movements of the face, anxiety, agitation, panic attacks, insomnia, irritability, hostility, aggressiveness, impulsivity, motor restlessness, hypomania, mania, other unusual changes in behavior, worsening of depression, and suicidal thoughts.
• Advise patient that drug may cause somnolence, orthostatic hypotension, and motor and sensory instability, which may lead to falls, fractures, or other injuries.

• Tell patient not to stop medication abruptly.

quinapril hydrochloride ▧
KWIN-a-pril

Accupril✦

Therapeutic class: Antihypertensives
Pharmacologic class: ACE inhibitors

AVAILABLE FORMS
Tablets: 5 mg, 10 mg, 20 mg, 40 mg

INDICATIONS & DOSAGES
➤ **HTN**
Adults: Initially, 10 to 20 mg PO daily. May adjust dosage based on patient response at intervals of at least 2 weeks. Most patients are controlled at 10 to 80 mg daily as a single dose or in two divided doses. If patient is taking a diuretic, start therapy with 5 mg daily.
Elderly patients: For patients age 65 and older, start therapy at 10 mg PO daily and titrate to optimal response.
Adjust-a-dose: For adults with CrCl over 60 mL/minute, give 10 mg once daily initially; for CrCl of 30 to 60 mL/minute, 5 mg PO daily initially; for CrCl of 10 to 30 mL/minute, 2.5 mg PO daily initially.
➤ **HF**
Adults: 5 mg PO b.i.d. initially. Dosage may be increased at weekly intervals. Usual effective dose is 20 to 40 mg daily in two equally divided doses.
Adjust-a-dose: For patients with CrCl over 30 mL/minute, first dose is 5 mg PO daily. If tolerated, increase to b.i.d. dosing the next day. Adjust dosage at weekly intervals thereafter. If CrCl is 10 to 30 mL/minute, first dose is 2.5 mg PO daily. If tolerated, increase to b.i.d. dosing the next day. Adjust dosage at weekly intervals thereafter.

ADMINISTRATION
PO
• Don't give drug with a high-fat meal because this may decrease absorption of drug.

ACTION
Prevents conversion of angiotensin I to angiotensin II, a potent vasoconstrictor. Less

angiotensin II decreases peripheral arterial resistance, decreasing aldosterone secretion, which reduces sodium and water retention and lowers BP.

Route	Onset	Peak	Duration
PO	1 hr	1–4 hr	24 hr

Half-life: Quinapril, 0.8 hour; quinaprilat, 3 hours.

ADVERSE REACTIONS

CNS: headache, dizziness, fatigue. **CV:** *hypertensive crisis,* hypotension, chest pain. **GI:** abdominal pain, vomiting, nausea, diarrhea. **GU:** erectile dysfunction, UTI, *acute renal failure.* **Metabolic:** elevated creatinine and BUN levels, *hyperkalemia.* **Musculoskeletal:** back pain. **Respiratory:** cough, dyspnea.

INTERACTIONS

Drug-drug. ❸ *Alert: Aliskiren:* May increase risk of renal impairment, hypotension, and hyperkalemia in diabetic patients and those with moderate to severe renal impairment (GFR less than 60 mL/minute). Concomitant use is contraindicated in diabetic patients. Avoid concomitant use in those with moderate to severe renal impairment.
Diuretics, other antihypertensives: May cause excessive hypotension. Stop diuretic or reduce dose of quinapril, as needed.
Lithium: May increase lithium level and lithium toxicity. Monitor lithium level.
Neprilysin inhibitors (sacubitril, sacubitril–valsartan): May increase risk of angioedema. Use together is contraindicated.
NSAIDs: May decrease antihypertensive effects. Monitor BP. Combination may result in a significant decrease in renal function. Monitor renal function.
Potassium-sparing diuretics, potassium supplements: May cause hyperkalemia. Monitor patient closely.
Tetracycline: May decrease absorption if taken with quinapril. Separate dosing times by at least 2 hours if used together. Consider therapy modification.
Drug-herb. *Yohimbe:* May decrease antihypertensive effects. Monitor therapy.
Drug-food. *Salt substitutes containing potassium:* May cause hyperkalemia. Discourage use together.

EFFECTS ON LAB TEST RESULTS

• May increase potassium, BUN, and creatinine levels, and LFT values.
• May lead to false-negative aldosterone/renin ratio.

CONTRAINDICATIONS & CAUTIONS

• Contraindicated in patients hypersensitive to ACE inhibitors and in those with a history of angioedema related to treatment with an ACE inhibitor.
• Contraindicated when used within 36 hours of switching to or from a neprilysin inhibitor, such as sacubitril or the combination drug sacubitril–valsartan.
• Use cautiously in patients with impaired renal function.
• Acute renal failure and hypertensive crisis have been reported.
Dialyzable drug: No.
⚠ **Overdose S&S:** Severe hypotension.

PREGNANCY-LACTATION-REPRODUCTION

Black Box Warning Use of drugs that act directly on the RAAS during pregnancy can cause injury and death to the developing fetus. When pregnancy is detected, stop drug as soon as possible. ▮
• Drug appears in human milk. Use cautiously in breastfeeding women.

NURSING CONSIDERATIONS

• Assess renal and hepatic function before and periodically throughout therapy.
• Monitor BP for effectiveness of therapy. When adjusting dosage, measure BP before giving dose (trough) and 2 to 6 hours after dosing (peak).
• Monitor potassium level. Risk factors for the development of hyperkalemia include renal insufficiency, diabetes, and concomitant use of drugs that raise potassium level.
❧ Although ACE inhibitors reduce BP in all races, they reduce it less in blacks taking an ACE inhibitor alone. Black patients should take drug with a thiazide diuretic for a better response.
❧ ACE inhibitors appear to increase risk of angioedema in black patients.
• Other ACE inhibitors have caused agranulocytosis and neutropenia. Monitor CBC with differential counts before therapy and periodically thereafter.

Q

PATIENT TEACHING
• Advise patient to report signs of infection, such as fever and sore throat.
🕄 *Alert:* Facial and throat swelling (including swelling of the tongue and larynx) may occur, especially after first dose. Advise patient to report signs or symptoms of breathing difficulty or swelling of face, eyes, lips, or tongue.
• Light-headedness can occur, especially during first few days of therapy. Tell patient to rise slowly to minimize effect and to report signs and symptoms to prescriber. If fainting occurs, patient should stop taking drug and call prescriber immediately.
• Inform patient that inadequate fluid intake, vomiting, diarrhea, and excessive perspiration can lead to light-headedness and fainting. Tell patient to use caution in hot weather and during exercise.
• Tell patient to avoid salt substitutes. These products may contain potassium, which can cause high potassium level in patients taking quinapril.
• Advise female patient of childbearing potential about potential fetal hazards and to notify prescriber at once if pregnancy occurs. Drug will need to be stopped.
• Tell patient to avoid taking with a high-fat meal because this may decrease absorption of drug.

SAFETY ALERT!

quiNIDine gluconate
KWIN-i-deen

quiNIDine sulfate
Therapeutic class: Antiarrhythmics–antimalarials
Pharmacologic class: Cinchona alkaloids

AVAILABLE FORMS
quinidine gluconate (62% quinidine base)
Tablets (extended-release) 🔴: 324 mg
quinidine sulfate (83% quinidine base)
Tablets: 200 mg, 300 mg

INDICATIONS & DOSAGES
Adjust-a-dose (for all indications): In patients with hepatic impairment or HF, reduce dosage.

Discontinue drug if QRS complex widens to 130% of pretreatment duration, QTc interval widens to 130% of pretreatment duration and is longer than 500 msec, P waves disappear, or patient develops significant tachycardia, symptomatic bradycardia, or hypotension.
➤ **Atrial flutter or fibrillation (pharmacologic conversion)**
Adults: 400 mg quinidine sulfate or equivalent base PO every 6 hours. If no cardioversion after three or four doses, may increase cautiously to desired effect. Or, quinidine gluconate 648 mg (two 324-mg tablets) PO every 8 hours if no cardioversion after three or four doses, may increase cautiously to desired effect.
➤ **Paroxysmal atrial fibrillation/flutter, maintenance of sinus rhythm**
Adults: For quinidine gluconate, initially 324 mg (extended-release) every 8 to 12 hours. May increase dosage cautiously to desired effect to usual dosage range of 324 to 648 mg every 8 hours. For quinidine sulfate, initially 200 mg (immediate-release) every 6 hours. May increase dosage cautiously to desired effect.
➤ **Ventricular arrhythmias**
Note: Dosing regimens for suppression of life-threatening ventricular arrhythmias haven't been adequately studied. For patients with structural heart disease or other risk factors for toxicity, initiate or adjust dosage in a setting where continuous monitoring and resuscitation are available. Monitor patients for 2 to 3 days once the appropriate dosage has been achieved.
Adults: For quinidine gluconate, 324 mg (extended-release) every 8 to 12 hours. May increase dosage cautiously up to 648 mg every 8 to 12 hours. For quinidine sulfate, initially 200 mg (immediate-release) every 6 hours. May increase dosage cautiously up to 600 mg every 6 to 12 hours.

ADMINISTRATION
PO
• Give drug with food to avoid adverse GI reactions.
• Don't crush extended-release tablets. If necessary, scored tablets may be broken in half to adjust quinidine dose.

Reactions in bold italics are *life-threatening*. Interactions may have a *rapid onset* or a *delayed onset*.

- Avoid changes in dietary salt intake
- Don't give drug with grapefruit juice.

ACTION

A class IA antiarrhythmic with direct and indirect (anticholinergic) effects on cardiac tissue. Decreases automaticity, conduction velocity, and membrane responsiveness; prolongs effective refractory period; and reduces vagal tone.

Route	Onset	Peak	Duration
PO	1–3 hr	2–5 hr	6–8 hr

Half-life: Adults, 6 to 8 hours.

ADVERSE REACTIONS

CNS: ataxia, syncope, headache, fatigue, sleep disturbance, tremor, weakness, nervousness, dizziness, fever. **CV:** ECG changes, tachycardia, angina pectoris, palpitations. **EENT:** abnormal vision. **GI:** diarrhea, nausea, vomiting, esophagitis, abdominal pain. **Skin:** rash.

INTERACTIONS

Drug-drug. *Amiloride:* May increase the risk of arrhythmias. If use together can't be avoided, monitor ECG closely.

Amiodarone: May increase quinidine level, producing life-threatening cardiac arrhythmias. Monitor quinidine level closely if use together can't be avoided. Adjust quinidine as needed.

Antacids, sodium bicarbonate: May increase quinidine level. Monitor patient for increased effect.

Azole antifungals: May increase quinidine plasma concentration and enhance QTc-prolonging effect of quinidine. Use together is contraindicated.

Barbiturates, phenytoin, rifampin: May accelerate quinidine elimination and decrease quinidine level. Monitor patient for decreased effect.

Cimetidine: May increase quinidine level. Monitor patient for increased arrhythmias and toxicity. Consider therapy modification.

Digoxin: May increase digoxin level after starting quinidine therapy. Monitor digoxin level.

Drugs that prolong QT interval (amisulpride, antipsychotics, ceritinib, chloroquine, citalopram, disopyramide, nilotinib, *procainamide, sotalol, TCAs):* May have additive effect with quinidine and cause life-threatening cardiac arrhythmias. Avoid using together when possible.

Fluvoxamine, nefazodone, TCAs: May increase antidepressant level, thus increasing its effect. Monitor patient for adverse reactions.

Macrolides and related antibiotics (azithromycin, clarithromycin, erythromycin): May cause additive effects or prolongation of the QT interval. Use with caution (azithromycin); avoid combination with clarithromycin and erythromycin.

Neuromuscular blockers: May potentiate effects of these drugs. Avoid use of quinidine immediately after surgery.

Other antiarrhythmics (lidocaine, procainamide, propranolol): May increase risk of toxicity. Use together cautiously.

Protease inhibitors (lopinavir, nelfinavir, ritonavir): May significantly increase quinidine levels and toxicity. Use together is contraindicated.

Quinolones: May cause life-threatening arrhythmias, including torsades de pointes. Avoid using together.

Verapamil: May decrease quinidine clearance and cause hypotension, bradycardia, AV block, or pulmonary edema. Avoid use together.

Warfarin: May increase anticoagulant effect. Monitor patient closely.

Drug-herb. Licorice: May decrease potassium level and increase risk for arrhythmias. Don't use together.

Drug-food. Grapefruit: May increase quinidine level. Avoid combination.

EFFECTS ON LAB TEST RESULTS

- May decrease Hb level.
- May decrease platelet and granulocyte counts.

CONTRAINDICATIONS & CAUTIONS

- Contraindicated in patients with idiosyncrasy or hypersensitivity to quinidine or related cinchona derivatives.
- Contraindicated in patients affected by anticholinergic activity (e.g., myasthenia gravis, complete AV block, patients whose cardiac rhythm depends on a junctional or idioventricular pacemaker).

Q

- Contraindicated in patients with a history of immune thrombocytopenia (quinidine gluconate only) or who developed thrombocytopenia after exposure to quinidine or quinine.

Black Box Warning In many trials of antiarrhythmic therapy for non-life-threatening arrhythmias, active antiarrhythmic therapy has resulted in increased mortality. Risk of active therapy is probably greatest in patients with structural heart disease. ∎

- Use cautiously in patients with HF; drug may exacerbate HF.
- Use may cause QT-interval prolongation and subsequent torsades de pointes. Monitor patient and adjust dosage to prevent QTc-interval prolongation. Use extreme care in patients with a history of torsades de pointes (from any cause) or who have experienced marked QTc lengthening while using quinapril in the past.
- Use cautiously in patients with hepatic or renal impairment because systemic accumulation may occur.
- Use cautiously in patients at risk for heart block; drug can unmask sick sinus syndrome.
- Thrombocytopenia (including severe) may occur.

Dialyzable drug: No.

⚠ *Overdose S&S:* Depressed mental function, headache, nausea, vomiting, diarrhea, abdominal pain, tachyarrhythmias, depressed cardiac automaticity and conduction, hypotension, HF, hypokalemia, acidosis, high-frequency hearing loss, vertigo, blurred vision, diplopia, photophobia.

PREGNANCY-LACTATION-REPRODUCTION

- There are no adequate studies in pregnant women. Use only if clearly needed.
- Drug appears in human milk. Avoid use in breastfeeding women.

NURSING CONSIDERATIONS

- Check apical pulse rate and BP before therapy. If extremes in pulse rate are detected, withhold drug and notify prescriber at once.
- Anticoagulant therapy is commonly advised before quinidine therapy in long-standing atrial fibrillation because restoration of normal sinus rhythm may result in

thromboembolism caused by dislodgment of thrombi from atrial wall.

- Monitor patient for atypical ventricular tachycardia, such as torsades de pointes and ECG changes, particularly widening of QRS complex, widened QT and PR intervals, and disappearance of P waves.

⟁ *Alert:* When changing route of administration or oral salt form, prescriber should alter dosage to compensate for variations in quinidine base content.

⟁ *Alert:* Hospitalize patients with severe malaria in an intensive care setting, with continuous monitoring. Decrease infusion rate if quinidine level exceeds 6 mcg/mL, uncorrected QT interval exceeds 0.6 second, or QRS complex widening exceeds 25% of baseline.

- Monitor CBC, LFT values, and renal function test results during long-term administration.
- Monitor quinidine level. Therapeutic levels for antiarrhythmic effects are 2 to 6 mcg/mL.
- Correct electrolyte imbalances before and during therapy.
- Monitor patient response carefully. If adverse GI reactions occur, especially diarrhea, notify prescriber as these may be symptoms of quinidine toxicity.
- *Look alike–sound alike:* Don't confuse quinidine with quinine or clonidine.

PATIENT TEACHING

- Stress importance of taking drug exactly as prescribed and taking it with food if adverse GI reactions occur.

⟁ *Alert:* Instruct patient not to crush or chew extended-release tablets. If necessary, patient may break scored tablets in half to adjust quinidine dose.

- Tell patient to avoid grapefruit juice because it may delay drug absorption and inhibit drug metabolism.
- Instruct patient to avoid changes in dietary salt intake.
- Advise patient to report all adverse reactions promptly, especially signs and symptoms of quinidine toxicity (ringing in the ears, visual disturbances, dizziness, headache, nausea), palpitations, chest pain, and slow or fast heartbeat.

Reactions in bold italics are *life-threatening*. Interactions may have a *rapid onset* or a *delayed onset*.

RABEprazole sodium
ra-BEP-ra-zole

Aciphex✔, Aciphex Sprinkle

Therapeutic class: Antiulcer drugs
Pharmacologic class: PPIs

AVAILABLE FORMS
Capsules (delayed-release) ⓄⓃⒸ*:* 5 mg, 10 mg
Tablets (delayed-release) ⓄⓃⒸ*:* 20 mg

INDICATIONS & DOSAGES
➤ **Healing of erosive or ulcerative GERD**
Adults: 20 mg PO daily for 4 to 8 weeks.
Additional 8-week course may be considered, if needed.
➤ **Maintenance of healing of erosive or ulcerative GERD**
Adults: 20 mg PO daily for up to 12 months.
➤ **Healing of duodenal ulcers**
Adults: 20 mg PO daily after morning meal for up to 4 weeks.
➤ **Pathologic hypersecretory conditions, including Zollinger-Ellison syndrome**
Adults: Initially, 60 mg PO daily; may increase, as needed, to 100 mg PO daily or 60 mg PO b.i.d.
➤ **Symptomatic GERD, including daytime and nighttime heartburn**
Adults: 20 mg PO daily for 4 weeks. May consider additional 4-week course, if needed.
Children age 12 and older: 20 mg PO daily for up to 8 weeks.
➤ **GERD (Aciphex Sprinkle)**
Children ages 1 to 11 weighing 15 kg or more: 10 mg PO once daily for up to 12 weeks.
Children ages 1 to 11 weighing less than 15 kg: 5 mg PO once daily for up to 12 weeks. May increase to 10 mg once daily if inadequate response.
➤ *Helicobacter pylori* **eradication, to reduce risk of duodenal ulcer recurrence**
Adults: 20 mg PO b.i.d., combined with amoxicillin 1,000 mg PO b.i.d. and clarithromycin 500 mg PO b.i.d., for 7 days with morning and evening meals.

ADMINISTRATION
PO
• Don't crush, split, or allow patient to chew tablets.
• Give tablets without regard for food but if used for treatment of duodenal ulcers, give after a meal; when used for *H. pylori* eradication, give with food.
• Open Aciphex Sprinkle delayed-release capsules and empty onto a spoonful of soft food (applesauce) or liquid that's at or below room temperature.
• Give whole dose within 15 minutes of sprinkling and 30 minutes before a meal. Don't store for future use.
• Sprinkle granules shouldn't be chewed or crushed.

ACTION
Blocks proton pump activity and gastric acid secretion by inhibiting gastric hydrogen–potassium adenosine triphosphatase (an enzyme) at secretory surface of gastric parietal cells.

Route	Onset	Peak	Duration
PO	<1 hr	1–6½ hr	24 hr

Half-life: 1 to 2 hours.

ADVERSE REACTIONS
CNS: headache, pain, dizziness. **CV:** peripheral edema. **EENT:** pharyngitis. **GI:** abdominal pain, constipation, diarrhea, flatulence, nausea, vomiting, dry mouth, taste perversion. **Hepatic:** elevated liver enzyme levels, *hepatitis, hepatic encephalopathy.* **Musculoskeletal:** arthralgia, myalgia. **Other:** infection.

INTERACTIONS
Drug-drug. *Clarithromycin:* May increase rabeprazole level. Monitor patient closely.
Cyclosporine: May inhibit cyclosporine metabolism. Use together cautiously.
Dabigatran: May decrease dabigatran serum concentration. Monitor therapy.
Digoxin, diuretics: May augment hypomagnesemia; may also increase digoxin level. Monitor magnesium and digoxin levels.
Ketoconazole, other gastric pH-dependent drugs: May reduce absorption of these drugs because of rabeprazole's effect on reducing intragastric acidity. Monitor patient closely.

R

Methotrexate: May increase methotrexate concentration and risk of toxicity. Closely monitor methotrexate concentration, and watch for signs and symptoms of methotrexate toxicity. Rabeprazole may need to be suspended or stopped in patients taking high-dose methotrexate.

Protease inhibitors (atazanavir, indinavir, nelfinavir, saquinavir): May decrease levels of these drugs. Monitor clinical response. Contraindicated with atazanavir.

Rilpivirine-containing products: May reduce antiviral effect and promote drug resistance. Use together is contraindicated.

Salicylates (aspirin): May increase release of salicylate from enteric coating, increasing gastric side effects. Use together cautiously.

Warfarin: May inhibit warfarin metabolism. Monitor PT and INR.

EFFECTS ON LAB TEST RESULTS

• May decrease magnesium level.
• Can cause false-positive in the diagnosis of neuroendocrine tumors and gastrinoma.
• Can cause false-positive for tetrahydrocannabinol urine screening tests.

CONTRAINDICATIONS & CAUTIONS

• Contraindicated in patients hypersensitive to drug, other benzimidazoles (lansoprazole, omeprazole), or components of these formulations and with rilpivirine-containing products.
• In *H. pylori* eradication, clarithromycin is contraindicated in patients hypersensitive to macrolides and in those taking pimozide; amoxicillin is contraindicated in patients hypersensitive to penicillin or cephalosporins.
• Avoid use in patients with severe hepatic impairment. If necessary, monitor for adverse reactions.
• Long-term (1 year or more) and multiple daily-dose rabeprazole therapy may be associated with an increased risk of osteoporosis-related fractures of the hip, wrist, or spine. Use lowest dosage and shortest duration of therapy appropriate to condition being treated. May consider vitamin D and calcium supplementation and following appropriate guidelines to reduce risk of fractures in patients at risk.
• Acute interstitial nephritis has been observed in patients taking rabeprazole and

may occur at any point during therapy. Discontinue drug if this condition develops.
• Vitamin B$_{12}$ malabsorption and deficiency have been reported in patients receiving prolonged daily treatment (longer than 3 years) with acid suppressants.
• Cutaneous lupus erythematosus (CLE) and SLE have been reported, occurring as both new onset and an exacerbation of existing autoimmune disease in patients of all ages within weeks to years after continuous drug therapy.
• Long-term use (1 year or more) may increase risk of fundic gland polyps. Use lowest dosage and shortest duration of therapy appropriate to condition being treated.
Dialyzable drug: No.

PREGNANCY-LACTATION-REPRODUCTION

• There are no adequate studies in pregnant women. Use during pregnancy only if potential benefit justifies potential risk to the fetus.
• In *H. pylori* eradication, clarithromycin is contraindicated in pregnant women.
• It isn't known if drug appears in human milk. Use cautiously in breastfeeding women.

NURSING CONSIDERATIONS

• Consider additional courses of therapy if duodenal ulcer or GERD isn't healed after first course of therapy.
• If *H. pylori* eradication is unsuccessful, do susceptibility testing. If patient is resistant to clarithromycin or susceptibility testing isn't possible, expect to start therapy using a different antimicrobial.
⊕ *Alert:* Prolonged use of PPIs (longer than 3 months) may cause low magnesium levels, especially if patient is on concurrent magnesium-lowering drugs, such as digoxin and diuretics. Monitor magnesium levels before starting treatment and periodically thereafter.
⊕ *Alert:* Monitor patients for signs and symptoms of low magnesium level, such as abnormal HR or rhythm, palpitations, muscle spasms, tremor, or seizures. In children, abnormal HR may present as fatigue, upset stomach, dizziness, and light-headedness. Magnesium supplementation or drug discontinuation may be needed.

Reactions in bold italics are *life-threatening*. Interactions may have a *rapid onset* or a *delayed onset*.

- Symptomatic response to therapy doesn't preclude presence of gastric malignancy.
- **Alert:** Patients treated for *H. pylori* eradication have developed pseudomembranous colitis with nearly all antibiotics, including clarithromycin and amoxicillin. Monitor patient closely.
- **Alert:** May increase CDAD. Evaluate for CDAD in patients who develop diarrhea that doesn't improve. Use lowest dosage and shortest duration appropriate to condition being treated.
- If signs or symptoms consistent with CLE or SLE are noted, discontinue drug and refer patient to the appropriate specialist for evaluation. Most patients improve with discontinuation of the PPI alone in 4 to 12 weeks.
- Drug may cause false-positive in the diagnosis of neuroendocrine tumors and gastrinoma. Temporarily stop treatment at least 14 days before testing.
- **Look alike–sound alike:** Don't confuse Aciphex with Accupril or Aricept. Don't confuse rabeprazole with aripiprazole.

PATIENT TEACHING
- Explain importance of taking drug exactly as prescribed.
- Advise patient to swallow delayed-release tablet whole and not to crush, chew, or split the tablet.
- Inform patient that delayed-release tablet may be taken without regard to meals.
- Tell patient or caregiver to open Aciphex Sprinkle delayed-release capsules and empty onto a spoonful of soft food (applesauce) or liquid that's at or below room temperature, and to take the whole dose within 15 minutes of sprinkling and 30 minutes before a meal.
- Advise patient or caregiver that Aciphex Sprinkle granules shouldn't be chewed or crushed.
- Inform patient that drug may increase the risk of osteoporosis-related fractures of the hip, wrist, or spine with multiple daily doses that are continued for longer than 1 year.
- Teach patient to recognize and report signs and symptoms of low magnesium levels.

raloxifene hydrochloride
ral-OKS-i-feen

Evista*⌀*

Therapeutic class: Antiosteoporotics
Pharmacologic class: Selective estrogen receptor modulators

AVAILABLE FORMS
Tablets: 60 mg

INDICATIONS & DOSAGES
➤ **To prevent or treat osteoporosis; to reduce risk of invasive breast cancer in postmenopausal women with osteoporosis and postmenopausal women at high risk for invasive breast cancer**
Postmenopausal women: 60 mg PO once daily.

ADMINISTRATION
PO
- Give drug without regard for food.
- Stop drug at least 72 hours before prolonged immobilization and resume only after patient is fully mobilized.

ACTION
Reduces resorption of bone and decreases overall bone turnover. These effects on bone are manifested as reductions in serum and urine levels of bone turnover markers and increases in bone mineral density, which decrease fracture incidence.

Route	Onset	Peak	Duration
PO	Unknown	Unknown	Unknown

Half-life: 27½ to 32½ hours.

ADVERSE REACTIONS
CNS: depression, insomnia, fever, migraine. **CV:** chest pain, peripheral edema, varicose veins, syncope, *thromboembolism.* **EENT:** sinusitis, pharyngitis, laryngitis. **GI:** nausea, diarrhea, dyspepsia, vomiting, flatulence, gastroenteritis, abdominal pain. **GU:** vaginitis, UTI, cystitis, leukorrhea, endometrial disorder, vaginal bleeding. **Metabolic:** weight gain. **Musculoskeletal:** arthralgia, myalgia, arthritis, leg cramps, muscle spasms. **Respiratory:** increased cough,

R

pneumonia, bronchitis. **Skin:** rash, diaphoresis. **Other:** infection, flulike syndrome, hot flashes.

INTERACTIONS
Drug-drug. *Bile acid sequestrants (cholestyramine):* May cause significant reduction in absorption of raloxifene. Avoid using together.
Highly protein-bound drugs (clofibrate, diazepam, diazoxide, ibuprofen, indomethacin, naproxen): May interfere with binding sites. Use together cautiously.
Levothyroxine: May decrease levothyroxine absorption. Consider therapy modification.
Ospemifene: May increase adverse toxic effects of raloxifene. Avoid combination.
Systemic estrogens: Safety of concomitant use hasn't been established. Use together isn't recommended.
Warfarin: May cause a decrease in PT. Monitor PT and INR closely.

EFFECTS ON LAB TEST RESULTS
• May increase triglyceride level.

CONTRAINDICATIONS & CAUTIONS
Black Box Warning Increased risk of venous thromboembolism and death from stroke. Contraindicated in women with a history of, or active, venous thromboembolism, including DVT, PE, and retinal vein thrombosis. Consider risk-benefit balance in women at risk for stroke, including those with documented CAD or who are at increased risk for major coronary events. ■
• Raloxifene shouldn't be used for primary or secondary prevention of CV disease.
• Use cautiously in patients with moderate or severe hepatic or renal impairment.
• Safety and effectiveness of drug in men haven't been evaluated.
• Safety of use with systemic estrogens and use in premenopausal women haven't been established. Use isn't recommended.
Dialyzable drug: Unknown.
⚠ **Overdose S&S:** Leg cramps, dizziness, ataxia, flushing, rash, tremors, vomiting, elevated alkaline phosphatase level.

PREGNANCY-LACTATION-REPRODUCTION
• Contraindicated during pregnancy and in women who may become pregnant; drug

may cause fetal harm. If drug is used during pregnancy or if patient becomes pregnant during therapy, apprise her of potential hazard to the fetus.
• Contraindicated in breastfeeding women.

NURSING CONSIDERATIONS
• Watch for signs of blood clots. Greatest risk of thromboembolic events occurs during first 4 months of treatment.
• Watch for breast abnormalities; drug doesn't eliminate risk of breast cancer.
• Conduct breast examinations and mammograms before starting, and regularly during, therapy.
• Effect on bone mineral density beyond 2 years of drug treatment isn't known.
• For osteoporosis treatment, add supplemental calcium (average of 1,500 mg daily) and vitamin D (400 to 800 units daily) to the diet if daily intake is inadequate.
• Monitor triglyceride level if previous treatment with estrogen caused elevation.

PATIENT TEACHING
• Advise patient to avoid long periods of restricted movement (such as during traveling) because of increased risk of venous thromboembolic events.
• Inform patient that hot flashes or flushing may occur and that drug doesn't aid in reducing them.
• Instruct patient to practice other bone loss-prevention measures, including taking supplemental calcium and vitamin D if dietary intake is inadequate, performing weight-bearing exercises, and stopping alcohol consumption and smoking.
• Tell patient that drug may be taken without regard for food.
• Advise patient to report unexplained uterine bleeding or breast abnormalities during therapy.
• Explain adverse reactions and instruct patient to read patient information insert before starting therapy and each time prescription is renewed.

Reactions in bold italics are *life-threatening*. Interactions may have a *rapid onset* or a **delayed onset**.

raltegravir potassium

ral-TEG-ra-vir

Isentress, Isentress HD

Therapeutic class: Antiretrovirals
Pharmacologic class: HIV integrase strand transfer inhibitors

AVAILABLE FORMS
Powder for oral suspension: 100-mg packets
Tablets (chewable): 25 mg, 100 mg
Tablets (film-coated) ⓞ: 400 mg, 600 mg

INDICATIONS & DOSAGES
➤ **HIV-1 infection, with other antiretrovirals, in patients age 4 weeks and older weighing at least 3 kg**
Adults and children weighing 40 kg or more who are treatment-naive or virologically suppressed on an initial regimen of raltegravir 400-mg tablet b.i.d.: 1,200 mg (two 600-mg tablets) PO once daily or 400-mg tablet PO b.i.d. or 300 mg chewable tablets b.i.d. if child is unable to swallow a tablet.
Adults who are treatment-experienced: 400-mg tablet PO b.i.d.
Adults and children age 18 and older: When administered concomitantly with rifampin, give 800 mg (two 400-mg tablets) PO b.i.d.
Children weighing 28 to less than 40 kg: 400-mg tablet b.i.d. or 200 mg chewable tablets PO b.i.d. if child is unable to swallow a tablet.
Children weighing 25 to less than 28 kg: 400-mg tablet b.i.d. or 150 mg chewable tablets PO b.i.d. if child is unable to swallow a tablet.
Children at least age 4 weeks weighing 20 to less than 25 kg: 150 mg chewable tablets PO b.i.d.
Children at least age 4 weeks weighing 14 to less than 20 kg: 100 mg chewable tablets or 100 mg oral suspension (10 mL) PO b.i.d.
Children at least age 4 weeks weighing 11 to less than 14 kg: 75 mg chewable tablets or 80 mg oral suspension (8 mL) PO b.i.d.
Children at least age 4 weeks weighing 8 to less than 11 kg: 60 mg oral suspension (6 mL) PO b.i.d.

Children at least age 4 weeks weighing 6 to less than 8 kg: 40 mg oral suspension (4 mL) PO b.i.d.
Children at least age 4 weeks weighing 4 to less than 6 kg: 30 mg oral suspension (3 mL) PO b.i.d.
Children at least age 4 weeks weighing 3 to less than 4 kg: 25 mg oral suspension (2.5 mL) PO b.i.d.

ADMINISTRATION
PO
• Don't substitute chewable tablets or oral suspension for film-coated tablets.
• Give drug without regard for meals.
Tablets and chewable tablets
• Maximum dosage of chewable tablets is 300 mg b.i.d.
• Patient must swallow film-coated tablets whole.
• The 100-mg chewable tablet can be broken into two equal halves.
• Chewable tablets can be chewed or swallowed whole.
Oral suspension
• Maximum dosage of oral suspension is 100 mg b.i.d.
• Patients can remain on oral suspension as long as weight is below 20 kg.
• To administer, open foil packet of drug (100 mg). Measure 10 mL of water in provided mixing cup. Pour packet contents into the water, close lid, and swirl for 45 seconds. Don't shake or turn mixing cup upside down. Final concentration, 10 mg/mL.
• When mixed, measure recommended suspension dose into the oral syringe provided.
• Give within 30 minutes of mixing with water. Discard any remaining suspension in the trash.
• See detailed "Instructions for Use" that come with the oral suspension.

ACTION
Inhibits HIV-1 integrase, an enzyme required for HIV-1 replication.

Route	Onset	Peak	Duration
PO	Rapid	3 hr	Unknown

Half-life: About 9 hours.

ADVERSE REACTIONS

CNS: headache, fatigue, dizziness, insomnia, asthenia, abnormal dreams, depression, nightmares. **GI:** nausea, abdominal pain, vomiting, diarrhea, flatulence, decreased appetite. **Hematologic:** anemia, *neutropenia, thrombocytopenia.* **Metabolic:** hyperglycemia. **Musculoskeletal:** myopathy, *rhabdomyolysis.* **Skin:** rash.

INTERACTIONS

Drug-drug. *Antacids containing aluminum, magnesium, or calcium carbonate:* Ingestion with raltegravir at any time may significantly decrease raltegravir plasma level. Coadministration or staggered administration isn't recommended.

Fibric acid derivatives, HMG-CoA reductase inhibitors: May increase risk of rhabdomyolysis. Monitor therapy.

Strong inducers of drug-metabolizing enzymes (carbamazepine, phenobarbital, phenytoin): May affect raltegravir metabolism. Coadministration isn't recommended.

UGT1A1 inducers (rifampin): May decrease raltegravir level. Adjust raltegravir dosage to 800 mg b.i.d. when administering with rifampin.

EFFECTS ON LAB TEST RESULTS

• May increase bilirubin, AST, ALT, alkaline phosphatase, amylase, lipase, glucose, and CK levels. May decrease Hb level.
• May decrease neutrophil and platelet counts.

CONTRAINDICATIONS & CAUTIONS

❸ *Alert:* Severe, potentially life-threatening and fatal skin reactions have been reported, including SJS and toxic epidermal necrolysis. Hypersensitivity reactions, including rash; organ dysfunction, including hepatic failure; and general malaise, muscle or joint aches, edema, conjunctivitis, facial edema, angioedema, oral blisters, and eosinophilia have also been reported. Discontinue drug immediately if signs or symptoms of severe skin reactions or hypersensitivity reactions occur.
• Use cautiously in elderly patients, especially those with hepatic, renal, and cardiac insufficiency.

• Safety and effectiveness haven't been established in children younger than age 4 weeks.
Dialyzable drug: Unknown.

PREGNANCY-LACTATION-REPRODUCTION

• There are no adequate studies in pregnant women. Use during pregnancy only if potential benefit justifies potential risk to the fetus.
• Enroll pregnant women exposed to drug in the Antiretroviral Pregnancy Registry (1-800-258-4263).
• Mothers with HIV-1 infection shouldn't breastfeed to avoid risking postnatal HIV-1 transmission.

NURSING CONSIDERATIONS

• Perform laboratory tests, including viral load, CD4 count, CBC, platelet count, and LFTs, before therapy and regularly throughout therapy.
• Use drug with at least one other antiretroviral.
• Watch for signs and symptoms of myopathy or rash.
• Monitor patient for signs and symptoms of depression and suicidal ideation.
• Monitor patient for immune reconstitution syndrome. During initial phase of treatment, patients responding to antiretroviral therapy may develop an inflammatory response to indolent or residual opportunistic infections (CMV, *Mycobacterium avium* complex, *Pneumocystis jiroveci* pneumonia, TB), which may necessitate further evaluation and treatment. Autoimmune disorders (such as Graves disease, polymyositis, and Guillain-Barré syndrome) have also been reported in the setting of immune reconstitution; however, time to onset is more variable, and can occur many months after initiation of antiretroviral treatment.
• Avoid dosing before a dialysis session because the extent to which drug may be dialyzable is unknown.

PATIENT TEACHING

• Inform patient that drug doesn't cure HIV infection, that patient may continue to develop opportunistic infections and other complications of HIV infection, and transmission of HIV to others through

---

Reactions in bold italics are *life-threatening*. Interactions may have a *rapid onset* or a *delayed onset*.

sexual contact or blood contamination is still possible.
• Advise patient to use barrier protection during sexual intercourse.
• Tell female patient that breastfeeding isn't recommended.
• Advise patient to immediately report worsening symptoms or unexplained muscle pain, tenderness, or weakness while taking the drug.
• Instruct patient to avoid missing any doses to decrease the risk of developing HIV resistance.
• Inform patient that severe and potentially life-threatening rash has been reported and to immediately contact the health care provider if a rash develops. Instruct patient to immediately stop taking raltegravir and seek medical attention if the rash is associated with any of the following signs or symptoms: fever; generally ill feeling; extreme tiredness; muscle or joint aches; blisters; oral lesions; eye inflammation; facial swelling; swelling of the eyes, lips, or mouth; breathing difficulty; or signs and symptoms of liver problems (such as yellowing of the skin or whites of the eyes, dark or tea-colored urine, pale-colored stools or bowel movements, nausea, vomiting, loss of appetite, pain, aching or sensitivity on the right side below the ribs).
• Advise patient with phenylketonuria that the 25-mg and 100-mg chewable tablets contain phenylalanine.
• Tell patient if a dose is missed to take the next dose as soon as possible and not to double the next dose.
• Advise patient to report use of other drugs, including OTC drugs; this drug interacts with other drugs.
• Tell patient that drug may be taken without regard for meals.
• Tell patient or caregiver to carefully follow directions in manufacturer's "Instructions for Use" when preparing and administering oral solution. Use calibrated syringe to administer dose.
• Tell patient or caregiver to administer oral solution within 30 minutes of mixing.
• Instruct patient to swallow film-coated tablets whole.

• Inform patient that chewable tablets or oral suspension can't be substituted for film-coated tablets.

ramelteon
ra-MEL-tee-on

Rozerem

Therapeutic class: Hypnotics
Pharmacologic class: Melatonin receptor agonists

AVAILABLE FORMS
Tablets ⓞⓝⓒ: 8 mg

INDICATIONS & DOSAGES
➤ **Insomnia characterized by trouble falling asleep**
Adults: 8 mg PO within 30 minutes of bedtime. Maximum dose is 8 mg daily.

ADMINISTRATION
PO
• Don't give drug with or immediately after a high-fat meal.
• Give drug within 30 minutes of bedtime.
• Don't break, crush, or allow patient to chew tablets. Patient should swallow tablets whole.

ACTION
Acts on receptors believed to maintain the circadian rhythm underlying the normal sleep-wake cycle.

Route	Onset	Peak	Duration
PO	Rapid	½–1½ hr	Unknown

Half-life: Parent compound, 1 to 2½ hours; metabolite M-II, 2 to 5 hours.

ADVERSE REACTIONS
CNS: complex sleep-related behaviors, depression, dizziness, fatigue, headache, somnolence, worsened insomnia. **GI:** nausea.

INTERACTIONS
Drug-drug. *CNS depressants:* May cause excessive CNS depression. Use together cautiously.
Donepezil, doxepin: May increase ramelteon level. Monitor patient closely.

Opioids: May cause slow or difficult breathing, sedation, and death. Avoid use together. If use together is necessary, limit dosage and duration of each drug to minimum necessary for desired effect.

Strong CYP enzyme inducer (rifampin): May decrease ramelteon level. Monitor patient for lack of effect.

Strong CYP1A2 inhibitor (fluvoxamine): May increase ramelteon level. Don't use together.

Strong CYP2C9 inhibitor (fluconazole), strong CYP3A4 inhibitor (ketoconazole), weak CYP1A2 inhibitors: May increase ramelteon level. Use together cautiously.

Drug-food. *Food (especially high-fat meals):* May delay time to peak drug effect. Tell patient to take drug on an empty stomach.

Drug-lifestyle. *Alcohol use:* May cause excessive CNS depression. Discourage alcohol use.

EFFECTS ON LAB TEST RESULTS
- May increase prolactin level.
- May decrease testosterone level.

CONTRAINDICATIONS & CAUTIONS
- Contraindicated in patients hypersensitive to drug or its components. Don't use in patients taking fluvoxamine or in those with severe hepatic impairment, severe sleep apnea, or severe COPD.
- Opioids should only be prescribed with benzodiazepines or other CNS depressants to patients for whom alternative treatment options are inadequate.
- Use cautiously in patients with depression or moderate hepatic impairment.
- Drug is associated with abnormal thinking and behavior changes, including hallucinations, aggression, bizarre behavior, agitation, mania, amnesia, anxiety, and other neuropsychiatric symptoms, which may occur unpredictably.

Dialyzable drug: No.

PREGNANCY-LACTATION-REPRODUCTION
- There are no adequate studies in pregnant women. Drug may cause fetal harm. Use during pregnancy only if clearly needed and potential benefit justifies potential risk to the fetus.

- It isn't known if drug appears in human milk. Use cautiously in breastfeeding women.
- Drug has been associated with decreased testosterone levels and increased prolactin levels. Effects on reproduction are unknown.

NURSING CONSIDERATIONS
- ☻ *Alert:* Anaphylaxis and angioedema may occur as early as the first dose. Monitor patient closely. Emergency treatment may be needed.
- Thoroughly evaluate the cause of insomnia before starting drug.
- Assess patient for behavioral or cognitive disorders.
- Failure of insomnia to resolve after 7 to 10 days of treatment may indicate the presence of a primary psychiatric or medical illness that should be evaluated.
- ☻ *Alert:* Monitor patient for signs and symptoms of depression, worsening of depression, and suicidal ideation or behaviors.
- Drug doesn't cause physical dependence.
- *Look alike–sound alike:* Don't confuse Rozerem with Razadyne. Don't confuse ramelteon with Remeron.

PATIENT TEACHING
- Caution patient or caregiver of patient taking an opioid with a benzodiazepine, CNS depressant, or alcohol to seek immediate medical attention for dizziness, lightheadedness, extreme sleepiness, slowed or difficult breathing, or unresponsiveness.
- ☻ *Alert:* Warn patient that drug may cause allergic reactions, facial swelling, and complex sleep-related behaviors, such as driving, eating, and making phone calls while asleep. Advise patient to report these and all adverse effects.
- Advise patient and caregiver to report signs and symptoms of depression, worsening of depression, suicidal thoughts or behavior changes, nightmares, or hallucinations.
- Instruct patient to take dose within 30 minutes of bedtime and to only perform activities needed to get ready for bed.
- Tell patient not to take drug with or after a heavy meal.
- Tell patient not to break, chew, or crush tablets. Tablets must be swallowed whole.

Reactions in bold italics are *life-threatening*. Interactions may have a *rapid onset* or a ***delayed onset***.

• Caution against performing activities that require mental alertness or physical coordination after taking drug.
• Caution patient to avoid alcohol while taking drug.
• Tell patient to consult prescriber if insomnia worsens or behavior changes.
• Urge female patient to consult prescriber if menses stops or, for both genders, if libido decreases or galactorrhea or fertility problems develop.

ramipril ℞
RA-mi-pril

Altace

Therapeutic class: Antihypertensives
Pharmacologic class: ACE inhibitors

AVAILABLE FORMS
Capsules 🚫: 1.25 mg, 2.5 mg, 5 mg, 10 mg

INDICATIONS & DOSAGES
➤ **HTN**
Adults: Initially, 2.5 mg PO once daily for patients not taking a diuretic, and 1.25 mg PO once daily for patients taking a diuretic. Increase dosage, if needed, based on patient response. Maintenance dose is 2.5 to 20 mg daily as a single dose or in divided doses.
Adjust-a-dose: For patients with CrCl less than 40 mL/minute, give 1.25 mg PO daily. Adjust dosage gradually based on response. Maximum daily dose is 5 mg.
➤ **HF after MI**
Adults: Initially, 2.5 mg PO b.i.d. If hypotension occurs, decrease dosage to 1.25 mg PO b.i.d. Adjust as tolerated, with dosage increase (as tolerated) at 1 week and subsequent increases about 3 weeks apart, to target dosage of 5 mg PO b.i.d.
Adjust-a-dose: For patients with CrCl less than 40 mL/minute, give 1.25 mg PO daily. Adjust dosage gradually based on response. Maximum dosage is 2.5 mg b.i.d.
➤ **To reduce risk of MI, stroke, and death from CV causes**
Adults age 55 and older: 2.5 mg PO once daily for 1 week, then 5 mg PO once daily for 3 weeks. Increase as tolerated to a maintenance dose of 10 mg PO once daily.

Adjust-a-dose: In patients who are hypertensive or who have recently had an MI, daily dose may be divided.

ADMINISTRATION
PO
• Give drug without regard for meals.
• Patient should swallow capsules whole.
• If patient can't swallow capsules, open capsule and sprinkle contents on a small amount of applesauce (4 oz) or mix with 120 mL of water or apple juice. May store for up to 24 hours at room temperature or up to 48 hours under refrigeration if not given immediately.

ACTION
Prevents conversion of angiotensin I to angiotensin II, a potent vasoconstrictor. Less angiotensin II decreases peripheral arterial resistance, decreasing aldosterone secretion, which reduces sodium and water retention and lowers BP.

Route	Onset	Peak	Duration
PO	1–2 hr	2–4 hr	24 hr

Half-life: 13 to 17 hours.

ADVERSE REACTIONS
CNS: headache, dizziness, fatigue, asthenia, vertigo, syncope. **CV:** *HF,* MI, hypotension, angina pectoris, chest pain, edema. **GI:** nausea, vomiting, diarrhea. **Metabolic:** *hyperkalemia.* **Respiratory:** dyspnea; dry, persistent, tickling, nonproductive cough.

INTERACTIONS
Drug-drug. ❶ *Alert: Aliskiren:* May increase risk of renal impairment, hypotension, and hyperkalemia in diabetic patients and those with moderate to severe renal impairment (GFR less than 60 mL/minute). Concomitant use is contraindicated in diabetic patients. Avoid concomitant use in those with moderate to severe renal impairment.
Diuretics: May cause excessive hypotension, especially at start of therapy. Stop diuretic at least 3 days before therapy begins, increase sodium intake, or reduce starting dose of ramipril.
Insulin, oral antidiabetics: May cause hypoglycemia, especially at start of ramipril therapy. Monitor glucose level closely.

Iron dextran: May increase risk of anaphylactic-type reaction. If drugs must be given concurrently, have resuscitation equipment and trained personnel on hand before iron dextran administration and the use of a test dose before first therapeutic dose.

Lanthanum: May decrease ramipril serum concentration. Give ramipril at least 2 hours before or after lanthanum.

Lithium: May increase lithium level. Use together cautiously and monitor lithium level.

Neprilysin inhibitors (sacubitril, sacubitril–valsartan): May increase risk of angioedema. Use together is contraindicated.

NSAIDs: May decrease antihypertensive effects. Monitor BP.

Potassium-sparing diuretics, potassium supplements: May cause hyperkalemia; ramipril attenuates potassium loss. Monitor potassium level closely.

Salicylates (aspirin): May decrease antihypertensive effects of ramipril. Ramipril dosage increase or aspirin dosage decrease may be needed.

Telmisartan: May increase risk of renal dysfunction. Avoid use together.

Tizanidine: May cause severe hypotension. Use cautiously and monitor BP closely.

Drug-herb. *Capsaicin:* May cause cough. Discourage use together.

Grass pollen allergen extract (5 grass extract): May increase risk of severe allergic reaction to 5 grass extract. Don't use together.

Ma huang: May decrease antihypertensive effects. Discourage use together.

Drug-food. *Salt substitutes containing potassium:* May cause hyperkalemia; ramipril attenuates potassium loss. Discourage use of salt substitutes during therapy.

EFFECTS ON LAB TEST RESULTS
• May increase BUN, creatinine, bilirubin, liver enzyme, glucose, and potassium levels.
• May decrease Hb level and hematocrit.
• May decrease RBC and platelet counts.

CONTRAINDICATIONS & CAUTIONS
• Contraindicated in patients hypersensitive to ACE inhibitors and in those with a history of angioedema related to treatment with an ACE inhibitor.

• Use cautiously in patients with renal impairment.
• Anaphylactoid reactions have been reported in patients dialyzed with high-flux membranes and also treated with ACE inhibitors and in those undergoing LDL apheresis with dextran sulfate absorption.
Dialyzable drug: Unknown.
⚠ **Overdose S&S:** Hypotension.

PREGNANCY-LACTATION-REPRODUCTION
Black Box Warning Use during pregnancy can cause injury and death to the developing fetus. When pregnancy is detected, stop drug as soon as possible. ∎
• Drug may appear in human milk. Use in breastfeeding women isn't recommended.

NURSING CONSIDERATIONS
• Monitor BP regularly for drug effectiveness.
• Correct fluid and electrolyte imbalances before starting therapy.
• Closely assess renal function in patients during first few weeks of therapy. Regular assessment of renal function is advisable. Patients with severe HF whose renal function depends on the RAAS have experienced acute renal failure during ACE inhibitor therapy. Hypertensive patients with unilateral or bilateral renal artery stenosis also may show signs of worsening renal function during first few days of therapy. Dose reduction or drug stoppage may be necessary.
⚕ Although ACE inhibitors reduce BP in all races, they reduce it less in blacks taking the ACE inhibitor alone. Black patients should use drug in combination therapy for a more favorable response.
⚕ ACE inhibitors appear to increase risk of angioedema in black patients.
• Discontinue drug if patient develops jaundice or significant hepatic enzyme elevation (rare).
• Monitor CBC with differential counts before therapy and periodically thereafter.
• Drug may reduce Hb and WBC, RBC, and platelet counts, especially in patients with impaired renal function or collagen vascular diseases (SLE or scleroderma).
• Monitor potassium level. Risk factors for the development of hyperkalemia include

---

renal insufficiency, diabetes, and concomitant use of drugs that raise potassium level.

PATIENT TEACHING

• Tell patient to report adverse reactions. Dosage adjustment or stoppage of drug may be needed.

❸ *Alert:* Rarely, swelling of the face and throat (including swelling of the larynx) may occur, especially after first dose. Advise patient to report breathing difficulty or swelling of face, eyes, lips, or tongue.

• Inform patient that light-headedness can occur, especially during first few days of therapy. Tell patient to rise slowly to minimize this effect and to report light-headedness to prescriber. If fainting occurs, advise patient to stop drug and call prescriber immediately.

• Tell patient who has difficulty swallowing capsules to open capsules and sprinkle contents on a small amount of applesauce (about 4 oz [120 mL]) or mix in 120 mL of water or apple juice.

• Advise patient to report signs and symptoms of infection, such as fever and sore throat.

• Tell patient to avoid salt substitutes. These products may contain potassium, which can cause high potassium level in patients taking ramipril.

Black Box Warning Tell female patient of childbearing potential to notify prescriber if pregnancy occurs. Drug will need to be stopped. ∎

SAFETY ALERT!

ramucirumab 🗒
ra-mue-SIR-ue-mab

Cyramza

Therapeutic class: Antineoplastics
Pharmacologic class: Monoclonal antibodies

AVAILABLE FORMS
Injection: 10-mg/mL single-dose vial

INDICATIONS & DOSAGES
Adjust-a-dose (for all indications): Refer to manufacturer's instructions for toxicity-related dosage adjustments and infusion

rates. If severe HTN can't be controlled, permanently discontinue drug. For urine protein level of 3 g/24 hours or more, confirmed diagnosis of reversible posterior leukoencephalopathy syndrome (RPLS), severe HTN that can't be controlled, arterial thromboembolic event (ATE), or nephrotic syndrome, permanently discontinue drug. There are no manufacturer dosage adjustment recommendations for hepatic impairment.

If GI perforation or severe bleeding occurs, permanently discontinue drug.

Withhold drug before surgery and discontinue if patient develops wound-healing complications.

➤ **Advanced gastric cancer or gastroesophageal junction adenocarcinoma, as a single agent or in combination with paclitaxel, after prior fluoropyrimidine- or platinum-containing chemotherapy**
Adults: 8 mg/kg IV over 60 minutes every 2 weeks. Continue until disease progression or unacceptable toxicity. When given in combination, administer ramucirumab before paclitaxel.

➤ **Metastatic NSCLC in combination with docetaxel in patients with disease progression on or after platinum-based chemotherapy. (Patients with *EGFR* or *ALK* genomic tumor aberrations should have shown disease progression on FDA-approved therapy for these before treatment with ramucirumab.)** 🗒
Adults: 10 mg/kg IV over 60 minutes on day 1 of a 21-day cycle before docetaxel infusion. Continue until disease progression or unacceptable toxicity.

➤ **Colorectal cancer in combination with FOLFIRI (irinotecan, folinic acid, and 5-FU) in patients with disease progression on or after therapy with bevacizumab, oxaliplatin, and a fluoropyrimidine**
Adults: 8 mg/kg IV over 60 minutes every 2 weeks before FOLFIRI administration. Continue until disease progression or unacceptable toxicity.

✱ *NEW INDICATION:* **Treatment of patients with hepatocellular carcinoma who have an alpha-fetoprotein of at least 400 ng/mL and have been treated with sorafenib**
Adults: 8 mg/kg IV infusion over 60 minutes every 2 weeks. Continue until disease progression or unacceptable toxicity.

R

ADMINISTRATION

IV

▼ Administer as IV infusion only, not as IV push or bolus.

▼ For each infusion, premedicate with IV histamine (H₁) antagonist (diphenhydramine). For patients with prior grade 1 or 2 infusion-related reaction (IRR), also premedicate with dexamethasone or equivalent and acetaminophen before each infusion.

▼ Dilute drug with NSS to final volume of 250 mL. Diluted solution is stable for 24 hours if refrigerated or 4 hours at room temperature. Gently invert container; don't shake.

▼ Inspect solution for particles and discoloration before administration.

▼ Give infusion through separate infusion line using a protein-sparing 0.22-micron filter. Flush line with NSS at end of infusion.

▼ Store vials in refrigerator at 36° to 46° F (2° to 8° C) until ready to use. Keep vial in outer carton to protect from light. Don't freeze or shake vial.

▼ Drug is a hazardous agent; use appropriate handling and disposal precautions.

▼ **Incompatibilities:** Dextrose solutions, electrolytes, other medications.

ACTION

A vascular endothelial growth factor receptor 2 antagonist that inhibits proliferation and migration of human endothelial cells, angiogenesis, and tumor growth.

Route	Onset	Peak	Duration
IV	Unknown	Unknown	Unknown

Half-life: 14 days.

ADVERSE REACTIONS

CNS: headache, fatigue, asthenia. **CV:** HTN, peripheral edema, *arterial thromboembolic events, hemorrhage.* **EENT:** epistaxis. **GI:** diarrhea, intestinal obstruction, decreased appetite, abdominal pain. **GU:** proteinuria. **Hematologic:** anemia, hyponatremia, *neutropenia.* **Skin:** rash. **Other:** antibody development, hypothyroidism.

INTERACTIONS

None reported.

EFFECTS ON LAB TEST RESULTS

• May increase urine protein level and decrease serum sodium level.

• May decrease RBC count.

CONTRAINDICATIONS & CAUTIONS

• Drug increases risk of hemorrhage and GI hemorrhage, including severe and sometimes fatal hemorrhagic events. Permanently discontinue drug in patients who experience severe bleeding.

• Withhold drug before surgery. Resume after the surgical intervention based on clinical judgment of adequate wound healing. If patient develops wound-healing complications during therapy, discontinue drug until wound is fully healed.

• Permanently discontinue drug in patients who experience GI perforation, a potentially fatal event.

• Use cautiously in patients with cirrhosis (Child-Pugh class B or C). Use in patients with hepatic impairment (Child-Pugh class B or C) only if potential benefits outweigh potential risks.

❸ *Alert:* Rare and sometimes fatal RPLS has been reported.

• Safety and effectiveness in children haven't been established.

Dialyzable drug: Unknown.

PREGNANCY-LACTATION-REPRODUCTION

• Drug may cause fetal harm. Women of childbearing potential should use effective contraception during and for at least 3 months after last ramucirumab dose.

• It isn't known if drug appears in human milk. Because of the potential risk of serious adverse reactions in breastfeeding infants, breastfeeding isn't recommended during treatment.

• Based on animal data, drug may impair fertility in women.

NURSING CONSIDERATIONS

❸ *Alert:* Serious, sometimes fatal, ATEs, including MI, cardiac arrest, stroke, and cerebral ischemia, have occurred. Monitor patient closely, and permanently discontinue drug in patients who experience a severe ATE.

• Assess BP every 2 weeks or more frequently as clinically indicated. Control HTN

Reactions in bold italics are *life-threatening*. Interactions may have a *rapid onset* or a *delayed onset*.

before start of therapy. If severe HTN occurs, withhold drug until controlled. Discontinue drug permanently if HTN can't be controlled, in hypertensive crisis, or in hypertensive encephalopathy.
• Premedicate patient before each infusion, and monitor patient for IRR.
❸ *Alert:* Assess patient for signs and symptoms of GI perforation (severe abdominal pain, nausea, vomiting, fever).
❸ *Alert:* Monitor recent wounds for complications during therapy. For wound healing complications, withhold drug until wound is fully healed.
• Monitor patients with cirrhosis (Child-Pugh class B or C) for new-onset or worsening encephalopathy, ascites, or hepatorenal syndrome.
• Monitor patient for signs and symptoms of RPLS (HTN, headache, visual disturbances, altered consciousness, seizures). Confirm diagnosis with MRI; discontinue drug and provide supportive care.
• Monitor thyroid function because of risk of hypothyroidism.

PATIENT TEACHING
❸ *Alert:* Inform patient that drug can cause severe bleeding. Advise patient to contact prescriber for bleeding or symptoms of bleeding, including light-headedness.
• Warn patient of increased risk of ATE.
• Advise patient to undergo routine BP monitoring and to contact health care provider if BP is elevated or if signs and symptoms of HTN (severe headache, light-headedness, or neurologic symptoms) occur.
❸ *Alert:* Caution patient to notify health care provider for severe diarrhea, vomiting, or severe abdominal pain.
❸ *Alert:* Warn patient that drug may impair wound healing. Instruct patient not to undergo surgery without first discussing potential risk with health care provider.
• Teach patient about potential risk of maintaining pregnancy, risk to fetus, and risk to postnatal infant development during and after treatment with ramucirumab. Discuss the need to avoid pregnancy, including use of adequate contraception, for at least 3 months after last dose.
• Advise female patient of childbearing potential that drug may impair fertility.

• Counsel patient on the need to discontinue breastfeeding during treatment.

ranibizumab
RA-ni-BIZ-oo-mab

Lucentis

Therapeutic class: Vascular endothelial growth factor A inhibitors
Pharmacologic class: Monoclonal antibodies

AVAILABLE FORMS
Intravitreal injection: 6 mg/mL, 10 mg/mL in single-use glass vials; 6 mg/mL, 10 mg/mL in single-use prefilled syringe

INDICATIONS & DOSAGES
➤ **Neovascular (wet) age-related macular degeneration or macular edema after retinal vein occlusion**
Adults: 0.5 mg (0.05 mL of 10-mg/mL solution) by intravitreal injection once a month (approximately 28 days between doses).
➤ **Diabetic macular edema; diabetic retinopathy**
Adults: 0.3 mg (0.05 mL of 6-mg/mL solution) by intravitreal injection once a month (approximately 28 days between doses).
➤ **Myopic choroidal neovascularization**
Adults: 0.5 mg (0.05 mL of 10-mg/mL solution) by intravitreal injection once a month (approximately 28 days between doses) for up to 3 months. May retreat if needed.

ADMINISTRATION
Ophthalmic intravitreal injection
• Store vials in original carton under refrigeration until use. Don't freeze.
• Protect from light.
• Withdraw vial contents through a 5-micron, 19G filter needle attached to a 1-mL tuberculin syringe; discard filter needle after withdrawal of vial contents.
• Replace filter needle with a sterile 30G × ½-inch needle for the intravitreal injection. Expel contents until 0.05 mL remains in syringe.
• Follow manufacturer's instructions for use of the prefilled syringe.

R

• Carry out intravitreal injection procedure under aseptic conditions with adequate anesthesia and a broad-spectrum microbicide given before injection.

ACTION

Binds to the receptor-binding site of active forms of vascular endothelial growth factor A, reducing endothelial cell proliferation, vascular leakage, and new blood vessel formation.

Route	Onset	Peak	Duration
Intravitreal injection	Unknown	1 day	Unknown

Half-life: 9 days.

ADVERSE REACTIONS

CNS: headache, peripheral neuropathy. **CV:** atrial fibrillation, peripheral edema, *arterial thromboembolic events.* **EENT:** conjunctival hemorrhage, eye pain, vitreous floaters, increased IOP, vitreous detachment, intraocular inflammation, cataract, foreign body sensation in eyes, eye irritation, increased lacrimation, blepharitis, dry eye, visual disturbance or blurred vision, eye pruritus, ocular hyperemia, retinal disorder, maculopathy, retinal degeneration, ocular discomfort, conjunctival hyperemia, posterior capsule opacification, injection-site hemorrhage, nasopharyngitis, sinusitis. **GI:** nausea, constipation, GERD. **GU:** renal failure, chronic renal failure. **Hematologic:** anemia. **Metabolic:** hypercholesterolemia. **Musculoskeletal:** arthralgia. **Respiratory:** URI, bronchitis, COPD, cough. **Skin:** wound healing complications. **Other:** seasonal allergy, flulike symptoms, antibody formation.

INTERACTIONS

None reported.

EFFECTS ON LAB TEST RESULTS

None reported.

CONTRAINDICATIONS & CAUTIONS

• Contraindicated in patients with known hypersensitivity to drug or its components and in patients with ocular or periocular infections.
• May increase risk of arterial thromboembolic events (nonfatal stroke, nonfatal MI, vascular death, or death of unknown cause), especially in diabetic patients.
• May cause serious intraocular inflammation if drug is given within 9 days after verteporfin photodynamic therapy.
Dialyzable drug: Unknown.

PREGNANCY-LACTATION-REPRODUCTION

• There are no studies in pregnant women, and it isn't known if drug can cause fetal harm. Based on its mechanism of action, drug may pose a risk to embryo-fetal development (including teratogenicity) and reproductive capacity. Use during pregnancy only if clearly needed.
• It isn't known if drug appears in human milk. Use cautiously in breastfeeding women.

NURSING CONSIDERATIONS

• Before and 30 minutes after intravitreal injection, monitor patient for elevated IOP using tonometry.
• Check for perfusion of the optic nerve head immediately after injection.
• Use one vial per treatment of a single eye. If second eye treatment is necessary, use new vial and reestablish sterile field.
• Monitor patient for hypersensitivity reactions, which may present as severe intraocular inflammation.
• Monitor patient for signs and symptoms suggestive of endophthalmitis (eye redness, sensitivity to light, eye pain, vision changes).
• Monitor patient for arterial thromboembolic events.

PATIENT TEACHING

• Instruct patient to seek immediate care from the ophthalmologist for eye redness, sensitivity to light, eye pain, or vision changes.

Reactions in bold italics are *life-threatening*. Interactions may have a *rapid onset* or a *delayed onset*.

raNITIdine hydrochloride
ra-NYE-te-deen

Acid Reducer✸ ◇, Zantac℘,
Zantac 75 ◇, Zantac 150 ◇,
Zantac 300

Therapeutic class: Antiulcer drugs
Pharmacologic class: H_2-receptor
antagonists

AVAILABLE FORMS
Capsules: 150 mg, 300 mg
Injection: 25 mg/mL
Syrup: 15 mg/mL*
Tablets: 75 mg ◇, 150 mg ◇, 300 mg

INDICATIONS & DOSAGES
Adjust-a-dose (for all indications): For patients with CrCl below 50 mL/minute,
150 mg PO every 24 hours or 50 mg IV every 18 to 24 hours. Refer to specific product
information for guidelines regarding renal
dosing for children.
➤ **Active duodenal and gastric ulcer**
Adults: 150 mg PO b.i.d. or 300 mg daily
after evening meal or at bedtime. Or, 50 mg
IV or IM every 6 to 8 hours. Maximum daily
IV dose, 400 mg. Or, 150 mg by continuous
infusion at 6.25 mg/hour over 24 hours.
Children ages 1 month to 16 years: For
duodenal and gastric ulcers only, 2 to
4 mg/kg PO b.i.d., up to 300 mg/day. Or,
2 to 4 mg/kg/day IV, divided every 6 to
8 hours, up to a maximum of 50 mg every
6 to 8 hours.
➤ **Maintenance therapy for duodenal or
gastric ulcer**
Adults: 150 mg PO at bedtime.
Children ages 1 month to 16 years: 2 to
4 mg/kg PO daily, up to 150 mg daily.
➤ **Pathologic hypersecretory conditions,
such as Zollinger-Ellison syndrome**
Adults: 150 mg PO b.i.d.; doses up to 6 g or
more frequent intervals may be needed in
patients with severe disease. Or, infuse continuously at 1 mg/kg/hour. After 4 hours,
if patient remains symptomatic or gastric
acid output is greater than 10 mEq/hour, increase dose in increments of 0.5 mg/kg/hour
and recheck gastric acid output. Doses up

to 2.5 mg/kg/hour and infusion rates up to
220 mg/hour have been used.
➤ **GERD**
Adults: 150 mg PO b.i.d.
Children ages 1 month to 16 years: 5 to
10 mg/kg PO daily given as two divided
doses.
➤ **Erosive esophagitis**
Adults: 150 mg PO q.i.d. Maintenance
dosage is 150 mg PO b.i.d.
Children ages 1 month to 16 years: 5 to
10 mg/kg PO daily given as two divided
doses.
➤ **Heartburn**
Adults and children age 12 and older: 75 to
150 mg (OTC only) PO 30 to 60 minutes before food or beverages that cause heartburn
or as symptoms occur, up to 300 mg daily.
Don't use more than twice daily or exceed
2 weeks of continuous treatment.

ADMINISTRATION
PO
● Give once-daily dose after evening meal or
at bedtime.
IM
● Administer undiluted.
IV
▼ To prepare IV injection, dilute 2 mL
(50 mg) ranitidine with compatible IV solution to a total volume of 20 mL, and inject over at least 5 minutes. Compatible
solutions include sterile water for injection, NSS for injection, D_5W, and lactated
Ringer injection.
▼ To give drug by intermittent IV infusion,
dilute 50 mg (2 mL) in 100 mL compatible
solution and infuse at a rate of 5 to 7 mL/
minute. Infuse over 15 to 20 minutes.
▼ For continuous infusion to treat active
duodenal or gastric ulcer, dilute 150 mg in
250 mL of D_5W. For hypersecretory conditions such as Zollinger-Ellison syndrome,
dilute with D_5W or other compatible solution to no more than 2.5 mg/mL.
▼ Administer continuous IV infusion at
6.25 mg/hour. For patients with Zollinger-
Ellison syndrome, administer at 1 mg/kg/
hour. Rapid IV administration has been
associated with bradycardia (rarely), particularly in patients predisposed to cardiac
rhythm disturbances. Don't exceed recommended infusion rates.

R

▼ After dilution, solution is stable for 48 hours at room temperature.

▼ Store IV injection at 39° to 86° F (4° to 30° C).

▼ **Incompatibilities:** None listed by manufacturer. Consult a drug incompatibility reference for more information.

ACTION

Competitively inhibits action of histamine at H_2-receptor sites of parietal cells, decreasing gastric acid secretion.

Route	Onset	Peak	Duration
PO	1 hr	2–3 hr	13 hr
IV	Unknown	Unknown	Unknown

Half-life: 2 to 3 hours.

ADVERSE REACTIONS

CNS: headache, malaise, vertigo. **EENT:** blurred vision. **Hepatic:** jaundice. **Other:** *anaphylaxis, angioedema,* burning and itching at injection site.

INTERACTIONS

Drug-drug. *Atazanavir:* May impair atazanavir absorption. Use cautiously.
Delavirdine: May impair delavirdine absorption. Prolonged use isn't recommended.
Glipizide: May increase hypoglycemic effect. Adjust glipizide dosage, as directed.
Iron salts: May reduce absorption of iron salts. Monitor therapy.
Ketoconazole: May decrease ketoconazole serum concentration. Give at least 2 hours before ranitidine.
Methylphenidate: May decrease absorption and interfere with normal release of extended-release formulations of methylphenidate. Monitor therapy.
Midazolam, triazolam: May prolong sedation. Monitor patient for excessive sedation.
Procainamide: May decrease renal clearance of procainamide. Monitor patient closely for toxicity.
Warfarin: May interfere with warfarin clearance. Monitor patient closely.

EFFECTS ON LAB TEST RESULTS

• May increase creatinine and ALT levels.
• May cause false-positive results in urine protein tests using Multistix.

CONTRAINDICATIONS & CAUTIONS

• Contraindicated in patients hypersensitive to drug and in those with acute porphyria.
• Use cautiously in patients with hepatic dysfunction. Adjust dosage in patients with impaired renal function.
• Rarely, drug may cause confusion; risk is greater in elderly or severely ill patients and in those with renal or hepatic impairment.
• Prolonged treatment (at least 2 years) may lead to vitamin B_{12} malabsorption and deficiency. The magnitude of deficiency is dose-related and association is stronger in women and those younger than age 30.
Dialyzable drug: Yes.
⚠ *Overdose S&S:* Exaggeration of adverse reactions, abnormal gait, hypotension.

PREGNANCY-LACTATION-REPRODUCTION

• There are no adequate studies in pregnant women. Use during pregnancy only if clearly needed.
• Drug appears in human milk. Use cautiously in breastfeeding women.

NURSING CONSIDERATIONS

• Assess patient for abdominal pain. Note presence of blood in emesis, stool, or gastric aspirate.
• Drug may be added to total parenteral nutrition solutions.
• High doses (100 mg or more) or prolonged IV therapy (5 days or longer) may increase ALT level. Monitor ALT level daily for remainder of treatment.
• Don't use OTC forms in children younger than age 12 unless directed by health care provider.
• *Look alike–sound alike:* Don't confuse ranitidine with rimantadine. Don't confuse Zantac with Xanax or Zyrtec.

PATIENT TEACHING

• Instruct patient on proper use of OTC preparation, as indicated.
• Remind patient to take once-daily prescription drug at bedtime for best results.
• Instruct patient to take without regard to meals because absorption isn't affected by food.
• Urge patient to avoid cigarette smoking because this may increase gastric acid secretion and worsen disease.

Reactions in bold italics are *life-threatening*. Interactions may have a *rapid onset* or a *delayed onset*.

• Advise patient to report all adverse reactions, especially abdominal pain, blood in stool or emesis, coffee-ground emesis, or black, tarry stools.

ranolazine
ra-NOE-la-zeen

Ranexa✔

Therapeutic class: Antianginals
Pharmacologic class: CV drugs

AVAILABLE FORMS
Tablets (extended-release) ⓓⓝⓒ: 500 mg, 1,000 mg

INDICATIONS & DOSAGES
➤ **Chronic angina**
Adults: Initially, 500 mg PO b.i.d. Increase, if needed, to maximum of 1,000 mg b.i.d.
Adjust-a-dose: Limit maximum dose to 500 mg b.i.d. in patients on moderate CYP3A inhibitors, such as diltiazem, fluconazole, verapamil, and erythromycin. Avoid use with strong CYP3A inhibitors or any CYP3A inducer.

ADMINISTRATION
PO
• Give drug without regard for meals.
• Give drug whole; don't crush or cut tablets.
• Don't give drug with grapefruit juice.
• If a dose is missed, give at next scheduled time; don't double a dose.

ACTION
May result from increased efficiency of myocardial oxygen use when myocardial metabolism is shifted away from fatty acid oxidation toward glucose oxidation. Antianginal and anti-ischemic properties don't decrease HR or BP and don't increase myocardial work.

Route	Onset	Peak	Duration
PO	Rapid	2–5 hr	Unknown

Half-life: 7 hours.

ADVERSE REACTIONS
CNS: dizziness, headache, confusion, weakness, vertigo. **CV:** palpitations, peripheral edema, syncope, hypotension. **EENT:** tinnitus. **GI:** abdominal pain, constipation, dry mouth, nausea, vomiting. **Respiratory:** dyspnea.

INTERACTIONS
Drug-drug. *Antipsychotics or TCAs metabolized by CYP2D6:* May increase levels of these drugs. Dosage reduction may be needed.
Clarithromycin, nefazodone, protease inhibitors: May cause QTc prolongation. Use together is contraindicated.
Cyclosporine, paroxetine, ritonavir: May increase ranolazine level. Use cautiously together, and monitor patient for increased adverse effects.
Digoxin: May increase digoxin level. Monitor digoxin level periodically; digoxin dosage may need to be reduced.
Diltiazem, ketoconazole and other azole antifungals, macrolide antibiotics (azithromycin, erythromycin), verapamil, other CYP3A inhibitors: May increase ranolazine level and prolong QT interval. Avoid using together.
Drugs that prolong the QT interval (antiarrhythmics [dofetilide, quinidine, sotalol], antipsychotics [chlorpromazine, ziprasidone]): May increase risk of prolonged QT interval and ventricular arrhythmia. Use cautiously together.
Metformin: May increase metformin level when given with ranolazine 1,000 mg b.i.d. Limit metformin dosage to 1,700 mg/day and monitor blood glucose level.
Rifabutin, rifampin, rifapentine, other CYP3A inducers (carbamazepine, phenobarbital, phenytoin): May reduce plasma concentration of ranolazine to subtherapeutic levels. Don't use together.
Simvastatin: May increase simvastatin level. Limit simvastatin dosage to 20 mg once daily, and monitor patient for adverse effects.
Drug-herb. *St. John's wort:* May reduce plasma concentration of ranolazine to subtherapeutic levels. Don't use together.
Drug-food. *Grapefruit products:* May increase drug level and prolong QT interval. Discourage use together.

R

EFFECTS ON LAB TEST RESULTS
• May increase creatinine and BUN levels. May decrease Hb and HbA$_{1c}$ levels and hematocrit.
• May increase eosinophil count.

CONTRAINDICATIONS & CAUTIONS
• Contraindicated in patients taking QT interval–prolonging drugs, CYP3A inducers (rifampin, phenobarbital, St. John's wort), or strong CYP3A inhibitors (clarithromycin, ketoconazole, nelfinavir), and in patients with ventricular tachycardia, hepatic impairment, or prolonged QT interval.
• Use cautiously in patients with renal impairment. Discontinue drug if patient develops acute renal failure.
Dialyzable drug: Unlikely.

PREGNANCY-LACTATION-REPRODUCTION
• There are no adequate studies in pregnant women. Use during pregnancy only if potential benefit justifies potential risk to the fetus.
• It isn't known if drug appears human milk. Patient should discontinue breastfeeding or discontinue drug.

NURSING CONSIDERATIONS
🚯 **Alert:** Drug prolongs the QT interval according to the dose. If drug is given with other drugs that prolong the QTc interval, torsades de pointes or sudden death may occur. Don't exceed maximum dosage.
• Obtain baseline ECG and monitor subsequent ECG for prolonged QT interval. Measure the QTc interval regularly.
• If patient has renal insufficiency, monitor BP closely.

PATIENT TEACHING
• Teach patient about this drug's potential to affect the heart's rhythm. Advise patient to immediately report palpitations or fainting.
• Urge patient to tell prescriber about all other prescription or OTC drugs or herbal supplements being taken.
• Tell patient to keep taking other drugs prescribed for angina.
• Tell patient that drug may be taken with or without food.
• Advise patient to avoid grapefruit products while taking drug.

• Advise patient that if a dose is missed, to take it at the next scheduled time and not to double the dose.
🚯 **Alert:** Warn patient that tablets must be swallowed whole and not crushed, broken, or chewed.
• Explain that drug won't stop a sudden anginal attack. Advise patient to keep other treatments, such as S.L. nitroglycerin, readily available.
• Tell patient to avoid activities that require mental alertness until effects of the drug are known.

rasagiline mesylate
ra-SA-ji-leen

Azilect⬦

Therapeutic class: Antiparkinsonians
Pharmacologic class: Irreversible, selective MAO inhibitors type B

AVAILABLE FORMS
Tablets: 0.5 mg, 1 mg

INDICATIONS & DOSAGES
➤ **Idiopathic Parkinson disease, as monotherapy or with levodopa**
Adults: As monotherapy, 1 mg PO once daily. As adjunctive therapy, initial dose is 0.5 mg PO once daily. May increase to 1 mg PO once daily.
Adjust-a-dose: If patient has mild hepatic impairment or takes a CYP1A2 inhibitor such as ciprofloxacin, give 0.5 mg once daily.

ADMINISTRATION
PO
• Give drug without regard to meals.

ACTION
Unknown. May increase extracellular dopamine level in the CNS, improving neurotransmission and relieving signs and symptoms of Parkinson disease.

Route	Onset	Peak	Duration
PO	Variable	1 hr	1 wk

Half-life: 3 hours.

Reactions in bold italics are *life-threatening*. Interactions may have a *rapid onset* or a ***delayed onset***.

ADVERSE REACTIONS
Monotherapy
CNS: dizziness, falls, headache, depression, fever, hallucinations, malaise, paresthesia, syncope, vertigo. **CV:** chest pain, angina pectoris, orthostatic hypotension, peripheral edema. **EENT:** conjunctivitis, gingivitis. **GI:** anorexia, diarrhea, dyspepsia, gastroenteritis, vomiting, nausea. **GU:** albuminuria, impotence. **Hematologic:** *leukopenia.* **Musculoskeletal:** arthralgia, arthritis, neck pain. **Respiratory:** asthma, flu syndrome, rhinitis. **Skin:** alopecia, *carcinoma,* ecchymosis, vesiculobullous rash. **Other:** allergic reaction, decreased libido.

Combined with levodopa
CNS: confusion, falls, headache, abnormal dreams, amnesia, ataxia, dyskinesia, dystonia, hallucinations, paresthesia, somnolence, sweating, abnormal gait, anxiety, asthenia, hyperkinesia, hypertonia, neuropathy, tremor. **CV:** bundle-branch block, orthostatic hypotension. **EENT:** epistaxis, gingivitis. **GI:** nausea, abdominal pain, anorexia, constipation, diarrhea, dry mouth, dyspepsia, dysphagia, vomiting, weight loss, *GI hemorrhage.* **GU:** albuminuria, hematuria, urinary incontinence. **Hematologic:** *hemorrhage,* anemia. **Musculoskeletal:** arthralgia, arthritis, bursitis, hernia, leg cramps, myasthenia, neck pain, tenosynovitis. **Respiratory:** dyspnea, increased cough. **Skin:** *carcinoma,* ecchymosis, pruritus, rash, ulcer. **Other:** infection.

INTERACTIONS
Drug-drug. *Ciprofloxacin and other CYP1A2 inhibitors:* May double rasagiline level. Decrease rasagiline dosage to 0.5 mg daily.
Cyclobenzaprine: May enhance serotonergic effects. Concomitant use is contraindicated.
Dextromethorphan: May cause episodes of psychosis or bizarre behavior. Concomitant use is contraindicated.
Levodopa: May increase rasagiline level. Watch for dyskinesia, dystonia, hallucinations, and hypotension, and reduce levodopa dosage if needed.
MAO inhibitors: May cause hypertensive crisis. Contraindicated with other MAO inhibitors.

Opiate agonists (fentanyl, meperidine, methadone, tramadol): May cause severe, sometimes fatal, serotonin syndrome. Concomitant use is contraindicated.
SSNRIs, SSRIs, TCAs: May cause severe or fatal CNS toxicity. Stop rasagiline for at least 14 days before starting an antidepressant. Stop fluoxetine for 5 weeks before starting rasagiline.
Drug-herb. *St. John's wort:* May cause severe reaction. Use together is contraindicated.
Drug-food. *Foods with very high levels of tyramine (more than 150 mg), such as aged cheeses, cured meats, fava beans:* May cause hypertensive reaction. Urge patient to avoid foods high in tyramine.

EFFECTS ON LAB TEST RESULTS
• May increase liver enzyme levels.
• May decrease WBC count.

CONTRAINDICATIONS & CAUTIONS
• Contraindicated in patients with pheochromocytoma or moderate to severe hepatic impairment and with concomitant use of cyclobenzaprine, St. John's wort, or dextromethorphan.
• Contraindicated for use with or within 14 days of an MAO inhibitor (including selective MAO-B inhibitors), meperidine, methadone, or tramadol.
• Exacerbation of HTN may occur during treatment, which may require medication adjustment if sustained.
• Potentially life-threatening serotonin syndrome has been reported in patients treated with antidepressants concomitantly with rasagiline. Use together isn't recommended.
• Somnolence and falling asleep without prior warning while engaged in ADLs (including operating motor vehicles) have been reported in some patients. Evaluate patient for factors that may increase these risks.
• Use cautiously in patients with mild hepatic impairment. Dosage reduction may be needed.
Dialyzable drug: Unknown.
⚠ **Overdose S&S:** Drowsiness, dizziness, faintness, irritability, hyperactivity, agitation, severe headache, hallucinations, trismus, opisthotonos, seizures, coma, rapid and irregular pulse, HTN, hypotension and

R

vascular collapse, precordial pain, respiratory depression and failure, hyperpyrexia, diaphoresis, cool and clammy skin.

PREGNANCY-LACTATION-REPRODUCTION
• There are no adequate studies in pregnant women. Use during pregnancy only if potential benefit justifies potential risk to the fetus.
• It isn't known if drug appears in human milk. Use cautiously in breastfeeding women.

NURSING CONSIDERATIONS
• Orthostatic hypotension occurs most frequently during first 2 months of therapy; help patient to rise from a reclining position.
• Monitor patient for new-onset HTN or HTN that isn't adequately controlled after starting drug.
• Monitor patient taking antidepressants and rasagiline concomitantly for serotonin syndrome.
• Monitor patient for drowsiness, significant daytime sleepiness, or episodes of falling asleep during activities that require active participation. Discontinue drug if these symptoms occur.
• Ask patient or caregiver about development or worsening of impulsive or compulsive behaviors, such as new or increased gambling urges, sexual urges, uncontrolled spending, or other urges; patient may not recognize these behaviors as abnormal.
• Notify prescriber if patient experiences adverse effects; levodopa dose may need to be reduced.
• Examine patient's skin periodically for possible melanoma because patients with Parkinson disease have a higher risk of skin cancer.
• Notify prescriber if patient is having elective surgery; drug should be stopped at least 2 weeks before.
• **Look alike–sound alike:** Don't confuse Azilect with Aricept.

PATIENT TEACHING
• Explain the risk of hypertensive crisis if patient ingests foods containing very high levels of tyramine while taking rasagiline. Give patient a list of these foods and products.

• Advise patient to rise slowly after prolonged sitting or lying down.
• Advise patient taking antidepressants concomitantly with rasagiline to immediately report confusion, hallucinations, agitation, delirium, syncope, shivering, sweating, high fever, tachycardia, nausea, diarrhea, muscle rigidity or twitching, or tremors.
• Advise patient that drug may cause patient to fall asleep during activities that require active participation and to report if drowsiness, significant daytime sleepiness, or episodes of falling asleep during such activities occur.
• Tell patient to report difficulty controlling impulsive or compulsive behaviors, such as new or increased gambling urges, sexual urges, uncontrolled spending, or other urges.
• Urge patient to watch for skin changes that could suggest melanoma and to have periodic skin examinations.
• Instruct patient to maintain usual dosage schedule if a dose is missed and not to double the next dose.
• Tell female patient to inform prescriber if she plans to become pregnant or breastfeed.
• Advise patient to contact prescriber before discontinuing rasagiline.

SAFETY ALERT!

repaglinide
re-PAG-li-nide

Therapeutic class: Antidiabetics
Pharmacologic class: Meglitinides

AVAILABLE FORMS
Tablets: 0.5 mg, 1 mg, 2 mg

INDICATIONS & DOSAGES
➤ **Type 2 diabetes, as adjunct to diet and exercise**
Adults: For patients not previously treated or whose HbA$_{1c}$ level is below 8%, starting dose is 0.5 mg PO within 30 minutes before each meal. For patients previously treated with glucose-lowering drugs and whose HbA$_{1c}$ is 8% or more, first dose is 1 to 2 mg PO within 30 minutes before each meal. Recommended dosage range is 0.5 to 4 mg before meals b.i.d., t.i.d., or q.i.d. Maximum daily dose is 16 mg.

Reactions in bold italics are *life-threatening*. Interactions may have a *rapid onset* or a *delayed onset*.

Determine dosage by glucose response. May double dosage up to 4 mg before each meal until satisfactory glucose response is achieved. At least 1 week should elapse between dosage adjustments to assess response to each dose.

A thiazolidinedione may be added if repaglinide monotherapy is inadequate; no initial repaglinide dosage adjustment is necessary; however, dosage adjustment may be needed if patient experiences hypoglycemic episodes.

Adjust-a-dose: In patients with severe renal impairment (CrCl of 20 to 40 mL/minute), starting dosage is 0.5 mg PO within 30 minutes before meals. Gradually titrate dosage, if needed, to achieve glycemic control. Use cautiously in patients with impaired liver function and allow longer intervals between dosage adjustments to allow full assessment of response.

ADMINISTRATION
PO
• Give drug within 30 minutes before meals.
• If patient skips a meal, skip the scheduled dose to reduce the risk of hypoglycemia.

ACTION
Stimulates insulin release from beta cells in the pancreas by closing adenosine triphosphate (ATP)-dependent potassium channels in beta cell membranes, which causes calcium channels to open. Increased calcium influx induces insulin secretion; the overall effect is to lower glucose level.

Route	Onset	Peak	Duration
PO	15–60 min	1 hr	6 hr

Half-life: 1 hour.

ADVERSE REACTIONS
CNS: headache, paresthesia. **CV:** angina. **EENT:** rhinitis, sinusitis. **GI:** constipation, diarrhea, dyspepsia, nausea, vomiting. **GU:** UTI. **Metabolic:** *hypoglycemia,* hyperglycemia. **Musculoskeletal:** arthralgia, back pain. **Respiratory:** bronchitis, URI. **Other:** tooth disorder.

INTERACTIONS
Drug-drug. *Barbiturates, carbamazepine, rifampin:* May increase repaglinide metabolism. Monitor glucose level.
Beta blockers, chloramphenicol, coumarin derivatives, MAO inhibitors, NSAIDs, other drugs that are highly protein bound, probenecid, salicylates, sulfonamides: May increase hypoglycemic action of repaglinide. Monitor glucose level.
Calcium channel blockers, corticosteroids, estrogens, fosphenytoin, hormonal contraceptives, isoniazid, nicotinic acid, phenothiazines, phenytoin, sympathomimetics, thiazides and other diuretics, thyroid products: May produce hyperglycemia, resulting in a loss of glycemic control. Monitor glucose level.
Clarithromycin: May increase repaglinide levels. Adjust repaglinide dosage.
Clopidogrel: May increase repaglinide level. Start repaglinide at 0.5 mg before each meal. Maximum dosage is 4 mg/day. Avoid use together if possible.
Cyclosporine: May increase repaglinide serum concentration. Don't exceed repaglinide dosage of 6 mg/day.
Erythromycin, itraconazole, ketoconazole, miconazole, similar inhibitors of CYP3A4: May inhibit repaglinide metabolism. Monitor glucose level.
Gemfibrozil: Significantly increases repaglinide level. Use together is contraindicated.
Drug-herb. *Burdock:* May increase hypoglycemic effects. Discourage use together.
St. John's wort: May decrease repaglinide level and its therapeutic effect. Don't use together.
Drug-food. *Grapefruit juice:* May inhibit metabolism of drug. Discourage use together.
Drug-lifestyle. *Alcohol use:* May alter glycemic control, most commonly causing hypoglycemia. Discourage use together.

EFFECTS ON LAB TEST RESULTS
• May increase or decrease glucose level.

CONTRAINDICATIONS & CAUTIONS
• Contraindicated in patients hypersensitive to drug or its inactive ingredients, in those

R

with type 1 diabetes or diabetic ketoacidosis with or without coma, and with gemfibrozil.
• Drug isn't indicated for use in combination with NPH insulin.
• Use with caution in elderly, debilitated, or malnourished patients and in those with hepatic, adrenal, or pituitary insufficiency.
Dialyzable drug: Unknown.
⚠ *Overdose S&S:* Hypoglycemia, severe hypoglycemic reactions (coma, seizures, neurologic impairment).

PREGNANCY-LACTATION-REPRODUCTION
• Safety in pregnant women hasn't been established. Use during pregnancy only if clearly needed.
• Abnormal blood glucose levels during pregnancy may cause fetal harm. Most experts recommend that insulin be used during pregnancy to maintain blood glucose levels as close to normal as possible.
• It isn't known if drug appears in human milk. Patient should discontinue breastfeeding or discontinue drug.

NURSING CONSIDERATIONS
• Increase dosage carefully in patients with impaired renal function or renal failure requiring dialysis.
• Metformin may be added if repaglinide alone is inadequate.
• Monitor glucose and HbA$_{1c}$ levels for loss of glycemic control, especially during stress, such as fever, trauma, infection, or surgery.
• Hypoglycemia may be difficult to recognize in patients with longstanding diabetes or diabetic nerve disease, in elderly patients, and in patients taking beta blockers.
• When switching to a different oral antidiabetic, begin new drug on day after last dose of repaglinide.
• *Look alike–sound alike:* Don't confuse Prandin with Avandia.

PATIENT TEACHING
• Stress importance of diet and exercise with drug therapy.
• Discuss symptoms of hypoglycemia with patient and family.
• Encourage patient to keep regular appointments and have HbA$_{1c}$ level checked every 3 months to determine long-term glucose control.

• Tell patient to take drug within 30 minutes before meals; time can vary from immediately preceding meal to up to 30 minutes before meal.
• Tell patient that if a meal is skipped or added, to skip dose or add an extra dose of drug for that meal, respectively.
• Instruct patient to monitor glucose level carefully. Teach patient what to do when ill, undergoing surgery, or under added stress.
• Advise female patient planning pregnancy to first consult prescriber. Insulin may be needed during pregnancy and breastfeeding.
• Teach patient to carry candy or other simple sugars to treat mild hypoglycemia episodes. Patient experiencing severe episode may need emergency treatment.
• Advise patient to avoid alcohol, which lowers glucose level.

reslizumab
res-LIZ-ue-mab

Cinqair

Therapeutic class: Immunomodulators
Pharmacologic class: Interleukin-5 antagonist monoclonal antibodies

AVAILABLE FORMS
Injection: 100 mg/10 mL single-use vial

INDICATIONS & DOSAGES
➤ **Add-on maintenance treatment of patients with severe asthma with an eosinophilic phenotype**
Adults: 3 mg/kg IV every 4 weeks.

ADMINISTRATION
IV
▼ Don't give as IV push or bolus.
▼ Visually inspect for particulate matter and discoloration. Solution should be clear to slightly hazy/opalescent, colorless to slightly yellow. Particles that appear as translucent-to-white amorphous particulates may be present. Discard if solution is discolored or if other foreign particulates are present.
▼ To minimize foaming, don't shake.
▼ Discard any unused portion. Drug doesn't contain preservative.

▼ Slowly inject required volume into a 50-mL NSS infusion bag of polyvinyl chloride or polyolefin. Gently invert bag. Don't shake. Don't mix or dilute with other drugs.

▼ Time between preparation and administration shouldn't exceed 16 hours. If not used immediately, store diluted reslizumab solution in refrigerator at 36° to 46° F (2° to 8° C) or at room temperature (up to 77° F [25° C]), protected from light, for up to 16 hours.

▼ If refrigerated before administration, allow diluted solution to warm to room temperature.

▼ Use an infusion set with an in-line, low-protein-binding, 0.2-micron polyethersulfone, polyvinylidene fluoride nylon, or cellulose acetate in-line infusion filter.

▼ Infuse over 20 to 50 minutes (depending on the volume to be infused based on patient weight); then flush IV administration set with NSS to ensure that all reslizumab has been administered.

▼ **Incompatibilities:** Physical and biochemical compatibility studies haven't been conducted. Don't infuse with other drugs or solutions other than NSS.

ACTION
Binds to interleukin-5, reducing production and survival of eosinophils, which limits inflammation, a component of the pathogenesis of asthma; however, its exact mechanism in asthma hasn't been established.

Route	Onset	Peak	Duration
IV	Unknown	Unknown	Unknown

Half-life: 24 days.

ADVERSE REACTIONS
EENT: oropharyngeal pain. **Musculoskeletal:** myalgia, musculoskeletal chest pain, neck pain, muscle spasm, extremity pain, muscle fatigue, musculoskeletal pain. **Other:** antibody development.

INTERACTIONS
None reported.

EFFECTS ON LAB TEST RESULTS
• May increase CK level.
• May decrease blood eosinophil count.

CONTRAINDICATIONS & CAUTIONS
Black Box Warning Anaphylaxis has occurred in patients receiving reslizumab and was reported as early as the second dose. Give only in a health care setting prepared to manage anaphylactic reactions. ∎
• Contraindicated in patients hypersensitive to drug or its components.
• Drug isn't indicated for status asthmaticus, acute bronchospasm, or acute asthma exacerbations.
• Drug isn't indicated for eosinophilic conditions other than severe asthma with an eosinophilic phenotype.
• Safety and effectiveness in children haven't been established.
Dialyzable drug: Unlikely.

PREGNANCY-LACTATION-REPRODUCTION
• Use in pregnancy hasn't been studied. Weigh risks to the developing fetus against risks of the mother's poorly controlled asthma.
• Monoclonal antibodies such as reslizumab are known to cross the placental barrier, so drug may affect a fetus. The possibility is likely to be greater during the second and third trimesters.
• It isn't known if reslizumab appears in human milk; however, human IgG is known to appear in human milk. Closely monitor the level of asthma control in pregnant women and adjust reslizumab dosage as necessary to maintain optimal control. Weigh risks to the breastfed infant against the mother's need for the drug.

NURSING CONSIDERATIONS
◆ *Alert:* Monitor patient for signs and symptoms of anaphylaxis (dyspnea, decreased oxygen saturation, wheezing, vomiting, urticaria) during infusion and for an appropriate amount of time after infusion has been completed. Discontinue drug immediately if severe systemic reaction occurs.
• If patient has preexisting parasitic infection, treat infection before initiating reslizumab. If patient becomes infected with parasites while receiving drug and doesn't respond to antiparasitic treatment, discontinue reslizumab until infection resolves.
• Don't abruptly discontinue systemic or inhaled corticosteroids upon initiation of

reslizumab. If appropriate, decrease corticosteroid dosage gradually.
• *Look alike–sound alike:* Don't confuse reslizumab with infliximab, ixekizumab, or rituximab.

PATIENT TEACHING
Black Box Warning Teach patient signs and symptoms of anaphylaxis (mucosal swelling, airway compromise, reduced BP, rash, hives, itching). Instruct patient to immediately report signs and symptoms of an allergic reaction that occur during or after receiving a reslizumab infusion. ■
• Explain to patient that reslizumab doesn't treat acute asthma symptoms or exacerbations. Advise patient to seek medical attention if asthma remains uncontrolled or worsens after initiation of reslizumab.
• Inform patient that there is a small risk of malignancy associated with reslizumab therapy.
• Warn patient not to discontinue systemic or inhaled corticosteroids except under medical supervision. Inform patient that reducing corticosteroid dosage may be associated with signs and symptoms of systemic withdrawal or may unmask conditions previously suppressed by corticosteroid therapy.
• Tell patient to notify health care provider for an existing or developing parasitic infection.
• Teach patient to report all adverse reactions to prescriber.

ribavirin
rye-ba-VYE-rin

Ibavyr♣, Rebetol, Ribasphere, Ribasphere RibaPak, Virazole

Therapeutic class: Antivirals
Pharmacologic class: Nucleosides–nucleotides

AVAILABLE FORMS
Capsules ⓄⓉⒸ: 200 mg
Oral solution: 40 mg/mL
Powder to be reconstituted for inhalation: 6 g in 100-mL glass vial
Tablets: 200 mg, 400 mg, 500 mg, 600 mg

INDICATIONS & DOSAGES
Adjust-a-dose (for all indications): Refer to manufacturer's instructions for each formulation for dosage adjustments in patients with impaired renal function or hematologic toxicities. Some formulations are contraindicated in patients with CrCl of less than 50 mL/minute or in patients with hepatic decompensation (Child-Pugh classes B and C).
Black Box Warning Ribavirin alone isn't effective for treatment of chronic HCV infection. ■
➤ **Hospitalized infants and young children infected by RSV**
Infants and young children: Solution in concentration of 20 mg/mL delivered via the Viratek Small Particle Aerosol Generator (SPAG-2) and mechanical ventilator, oxygen hood, oxygen tent, or face mask. Treatment is given for 12 to 18 hours/day for at least 3 days, and no longer than 7 days.
➤ **Chronic HCV infection (monoinfection), in combination with peginterferon alfa-2b (capsules, oral solution)**
Adults weighing more than 105 kg: 1,400 mg PO daily in two divided doses, 600 mg in the morning and 800 mg in the evening.
Adults weighing 81 to 105 kg: 1,200 mg PO daily in two divided doses, 600 mg in the morning and 600 mg in the evening.
Adults weighing 66 to 80 kg: 1,000 mg PO daily in two divided doses, 400 mg in the morning and 600 mg in the evening.
Adults weighing less than 66 kg: 800 mg PO daily in two divided doses, 400 mg in the morning and 400 mg in the evening.
    For HCV genotype 1, treatment duration is 48 weeks; for HCV genotypes 2 and 3, treatment duration is 24 weeks. Recommended treatment duration for patients of any genotype who previously failed therapy is 48 weeks.
➤ **Chronic HCV infection (monoinfection), in combination with interferon alfa-2b (capsules)**
Adults weighing more than 75 kg: 1,200 mg PO daily in two divided doses, 600 mg in the morning and 600 mg in the evening. Individualize therapy duration (24 to 48 weeks).
Adults weighing 75 kg or less: 1,000 mg PO daily in two divided doses, 400 mg in the

---

morning and 600 mg in the evening. Individualize therapy duration (24 to 48 weeks).

➤ **Chronic HCV infection (monoinfection) in children, in combination with peginterferon alfa-2b or interferon alfa-2b (capsules, oral solution)**

Children age 3 and older weighing more than 73 kg: 1,200 mg PO daily in two divided doses, 600 mg in the morning and 600 mg in the evening.

Children age 3 and older weighing 60 to 73 kg: 1,000 mg PO daily in two divided doses, 400 mg in the morning and 600 mg in the evening.

Children age 3 and older weighing 47 to 59 kg: 800 mg PO daily in two divided doses, 400 mg in the morning and 400 mg in the evening.

Children age 3 and older weighing less than 47 kg: 15 mg/kg/day (oral solution) PO in two divided doses, in the morning and evening.

For children with HCV genotypes 2 or 3, recommended therapy duration is 24 weeks; for all other genotypes, therapy duration is 48 weeks.

➤ **Chronic HCV infection (monoinfection), in combination with peginterferon alfa-2a (tablets)**

Adults with genotype 1 or 4 weighing 75 kg or more: 1,200 mg PO daily in two divided doses for 48 weeks.

Adults with genotype 1 or 4 weighing less than 75 kg: 1,000 mg daily in two divided doses for 48 weeks.

Adults with genotype 2 or 3: 800 mg PO daily in two divided doses for 24 weeks.

Adolescents and children age 5 and older weighing 75 kg or more: 1,200 mg PO daily in two divided doses, 600 mg in the morning and 600 mg in the evening.

Adolescents and children age 5 and older weighing 60 to 74 kg: 1,000 mg PO daily in two divided doses, 400 mg in the morning and 600 mg in the evening.

Adolescents and children age 5 and older weighing 47 to 59 kg: 800 mg PO daily in two divided doses, 400 mg in the morning and 400 mg in the evening.

Adolescents and children age 5 and older weighing 34 to 46 kg: 600 mg PO daily in two divided doses, 200 mg in the morning and 400 mg in the evening.

Adolescents and children age 5 and older who weigh 23 to 33 kg: 400 mg PO daily in two divided doses, 200 mg in the morning and 200 mg in the evening.

Treatment duration for children and adolescents with genotype 2 or 3 is 24 weeks and for all other genotypes is 48 weeks.

➤ **Chronic HCV infection (regardless of genotype) in HIV-infected patients, in combination with peginterferon alfa-2a**

Adults: 800 mg (tablets) PO daily in two divided doses for 48 weeks.

ADMINISTRATION

⊘ *Alert:* Drug is a hazardous agent. Use appropriate precautions for handling and disposal.

Inhalational
• Give by the Viratek SPAG-2 only. Don't use any other aerosol-generating device.
• Use sterile USP water for injection, not bacteriostatic water. Water used to reconstitute this drug must not contain any antimicrobial product. Follow manufacturer's instructions for preparation.
• Discard solutions placed in the SPAG-2 unit at least every 24 hours before adding newly reconstituted solution.
• Store reconstituted solutions at room temperature for 24 hours.

PO
• Give drug with food and at the same time every day.
⊘ *Alert:* Capsules should never be opened, crushed, or broken.

ACTION

Inhibits viral activity by an unknown mechanism, possibly by inhibiting RNA and DNA synthesis by depleting intracellular nucleotide pools.

Route	Onset	Peak	Duration
Inhalation	Unknown	Unknown	Unknown
PO	Unknown	2 hr	Unknown

Half-life: First phase, 9¼ hours; second phase, 40 hours.

ADVERSE REACTIONS

CNS: fatigue, anxiety, depression, dizziness, headache, insomnia, agitation, rigors, irritability, nervousness, fever. **CV:** *bradycardia, cardiac arrest.* **EENT:** blurred vision, conjunctivitis, rhinitis, sinusitis, taste perversion. **GI:** anorexia, diarrhea, nausea, vomiting, weight loss, abdominal pain. **Hematologic:** anemia, *hemolytic anemia, leukopenia, neutropenia, thrombocytopenia,* reticulocytosis. **Musculoskeletal:** myalgia, arthralgia. **Respiratory:** *apnea, bronchospasm,* bacterial pneumonia, *pneumothorax, pulmonary edema,* worsening respiratory state, cough. **Skin:** flushing, alopecia, pruritus, rash, dry skin, diaphoresis, injection-site reaction. **Other:** chills, flulike illness, pain, homicidal ideation, *suicidal ideation.*

INTERACTIONS
Drug-drug. *Azathioprine:* May induce severe pancytopenia and increase risk of myelotoxicity (neutropenia, thrombocytopenia, anemia). Monitor closely for signs of myelosuppression. Consider an alternative agent if possible.
Didanosine: May increase toxicity. Coadministration is contraindicated.
Lamivudine, stavudine, zidovudine: May decrease antiretroviral activity and enhance hepatotoxic effects. Use together cautiously; consider therapy modification.

EFFECTS ON LAB TEST RESULTS
• May increase ALT, AST, and bilirubin levels. May decrease Hb level.
• May increase reticulocyte count. May decrease WBC and platelet counts.

CONTRAINDICATIONS & CAUTIONS
Black Box Warning Monotherapy is ineffective for treatment of chronic HCV infection; drug shouldn't be used alone for this indication. ▪
Black Box Warning Aerosol form isn't indicated for use in adults. ▪
Black Box Warning Ribavirin may cause hemolytic anemia and worsen cardiac disease, leading to potentially fatal MI. Patients with a history of significant or unstable cardiac disease shouldn't be treated with ribavirin. ▪
Black Box Warning Ribavirin has been shown to be teratogenic in all animal species in which adequate studies have been conducted (rodents and rabbits). ▪

• Aerosol form is contraindicated in patients hypersensitive to drug.
• Oral form is contraindicated in patients with known hypersensitivity reactions to ribavirin or its components; in patients with autoimmune hepatitis, hemoglobinopathies, or CrCl of less than 50 mL/minute; and when administered with didanosine.
• Ribavirin tablets and peginterferon alfa-2a combination therapy is contraindicated in hepatic decompensation (Child-Pugh score greater than 6; class B and C) in cirrhotic chronic HCV monoinfected patients before treatment and in hepatic decompensation (Child-Pugh score of 6 or greater) in cirrhotic chronic HCV patients coinfected with HIV before treatment.
Black Box Warning In infants, aerosolized ribavirin has been associated with sudden deterioration of respiratory function. Monitor respiratory function carefully and stop treatment if sudden respiratory deterioration occurs. Reinstitute only with extreme caution, continuous monitoring, and consideration of concomitant administration of bronchodilators. ▪
• Use cautiously in elderly patients and patients with hepatic or renal insufficiency.
• Patients who initiate oral treatment before their 18th birthday should maintain pediatric dosing through completion of therapy.
Dialyzable drug: 50%.
⚠ **Overdose S&S:** Increased severity of adverse reactions.

PREGNANCY-LACTATION-REPRODUCTION
Black Box Warning Contraindicated in pregnant women and in men whose partners are pregnant; significant teratogenic and embryocidal effects have occurred in all animal species exposed to ribavirin. ▪
Black Box Warning Women receiving ribavirin and female partners of men receiving ribavirin should use extreme care to avoid pregnancy during therapy and for 6 months after therapy ends and should use at least two reliable forms of effective contraception during therapy and during 6-month post-treatment follow-up. ▪
• If pregnancy occurs during therapy or during 6 months after therapy ends, patient must be advised of teratogenic fetal risk.

Reactions in bold italics are *life-threatening*. Interactions may have a *rapid onset* or a *delayed onset*.

• Women of childbearing potential must have a negative pregnancy test immediately before start of therapy. Pregnancy tests must be performed monthly during therapy and for 6 months after therapy ends.

• Advise pregnant health care workers to avoid unnecessary exposure to aerosol form.

• Report pregnancies that occur during therapy to the Ribavirin Pregnancy Registry (1-800-593-2214).

• It isn't known if drug appears in human milk. Patient should discontinue breastfeeding or discontinue drug, taking into account importance of drug to the mother.

NURSING CONSIDERATIONS
Aerosol form

◑ Alert: The long-term and cumulative effects in health care personnel exposed to this form aren't known. Eye irritation and headache may occur.

Black Box Warning Use in mechanically ventilated patients should only be undertaken by health care providers and staff familiar with this mode of administration and the specific ventilator used. Experienced providers and staff should use procedures that minimize accumulation of drug precipitate, which can result in ventilator dysfunction and increases in pulmonary pressures. ▪

• This form is indicated only for severe lower respiratory tract infection caused by RSV. Although you should begin treatment while awaiting test results, an RSV infection must be documented eventually.

• Most infants and children with RSV infection don't require treatment with antivirals because the disease is commonly mild and self-limiting. Premature infants or those with cardiopulmonary disease experience RSV in its most severe form and benefit most from treatment with ribavirin aerosol.

Oral form

• Don't start therapy until a negative pregnancy test is confirmed in patient or partner of patient; they should take a pregnancy test every month during therapy and for 6 months afterward.

• Monitor hematologic status, liver and renal function, and TSH level at baseline and throughout therapy.

• Combination therapy has been observed to inhibit growth in children ages 5 to 17.

Monitor child's height and weight during therapy.

◑ Alert: Monitor patient for suicidal ideation, severe depression, hemolytic anemia, bone marrow suppression, autoimmune and infective disorders, ophthalmic disorders, CV disorders, pulmonary dysfunction, pancreatitis, and diabetes.

• Stop drug if pulmonary infiltrates or severe pulmonary impairment or pancreatitis occurs.

• In patients receiving azathioprine with ribavirin, monitor CBC, including platelet counts, weekly for first month, twice monthly for second and third months of treatment, then monthly or more frequently if dosage or other therapy changes are necessary.

PATIENT TEACHING

• Inform parents of need for drug, and answer any questions.

• Tell patient not to crush, chew, or open capsules.

• Encourage parents to immediately report any subtle change in child.

• Inform patient that oral form may be taken without regard to meals but should be taken in a consistent manner.

• Warn female patient of childbearing potential that drug is a teratogen, and provide contraception counseling. Advise patient that extreme care must be taken to avoid pregnancy during therapy and for 6 months after completion of treatment.

• Advise female patient to immediately report a pregnancy.

SAFETY ALERT!

ribociclib ⚇
RYE-boe-sye-klib

Kisqali

Therapeutic class: Antineoplastics
Pharmacologic class: Cyclin-dependent kinase inhibitors

AVAILABLE FORMS
Tablets ⓞⓣⓒ: 200 mg

INDICATIONS & DOSAGES

➤ **Initial endocrine-based therapy for treatment of hormone receptor–positive, HER2–negative advanced or metastatic breast cancer in combination with aromatase inhibitor** ⚕

Postmenopausal women: 600 mg (three 200-mg tablets) PO once daily for 21 consecutive days followed by 7 days off therapy. Letrozole 2.5 mg once daily is given throughout the 28-day cycle. For dosing and administration with other aromatase inhibitors, refer to the respective prescribing information.

Adjust-a-dose: Refer to manufacturer's instructions for toxicity-related dosage adjustment. For patients with moderate (Child-Pugh class B) or severe (Child-Pugh class C) hepatic impairment, decrease starting dose to 400 mg once daily.

ADMINISTRATION

PO

- Hazardous drug; use safe handling and disposal precautions.
- May give with or without food.
- Patients should swallow tablets whole and not chew, crush, or split them before swallowing. Don't use cracked, broken, or damaged tablets.
- Give medication at the same time each day, preferably in the morning.
- Skip a missed dose or a dose lost due to vomiting after intake. Give the next dose at its usual time.

ACTION

A cyclin-dependent kinase inhibitor that prevents progression through the cell cycle, resulting in arrest in the G1 phase. The combination of ribociclib and an aromatase inhibitor causes increased inhibition of tumor growth compared to each agent alone.

Route	Onset	Peak	Duration
PO	Unknown	1–4 hr	Unknown

Half-life: 30 to 55 hours.

ADVERSE REACTIONS

CNS: headache, insomnia, fatigue, dizziness, vertigo, pyrexia. **CV:** peripheral edema, *prolonged QT interval,* syncope. **GI:** nausea, diarrhea, vomiting, constipation, stomatitis, abdominal pain, decreased appetite. **GU:** UTI. **Hematologic:** *neutropenia, leukopenia, lymphopenia,* anemia. **Hepatic:** abnormal LFT values. **Musculoskeletal:** back pain, arthralgia. **Respiratory:** dyspnea. **Skin:** alopecia, rash, pruritus.

INTERACTIONS

Drug-drug. *CYP3A substrates with narrow therapeutic index (alfentanil, cyclosporine, dihydroergotamine, ergotamine, everolimus, fentanyl, midazolam, pimozide, quinidine, sirolimus, tacrolimus):* May increase exposure to these drugs. Decrease substrate dosage when concomitant use with ribociclib is necessary.

Drugs that prolong QT interval (amiodarone, bepridil, chloroquine, clarithromycin, disopyramide, haloperidol, methadone, moxifloxacin, ondansetron, pimozide, procainamide, quinidine, sotalol): May increase risk of prolonged QT interval and ventricular arrhythmias. Avoid use together.

Strong CYP3A4 inducers (carbamazepine, phenytoin, rifampin): May decrease ribociclib level. Avoid use together.

Strong CYP3A4 inhibitors (clarithromycin, conivaptan, indinavir, itraconazole, ketoconazole, lopinavir/ritonavir, nefazodone, nelfinavir, posaconazole, ritonavir, saquinavir, voriconazole): May increase ribociclib level. Avoid use together. If coadministration is unavoidable, decrease ribociclib dosage to 400 mg daily. If strong inhibitor is discontinued, resume prior ribociclib dosage after at least five half-lives of the CYP3A inhibitor.

Drug-herb. *St. John's wort:* May decrease ribociclib level. Don't use together.

Drug-food. *Grapefruit or grapefruit juice, pomegranates or pomegranate juice:* May increase ribociclib plasma concentration. Don't use together.

EFFECTS ON LAB TEST RESULTS

- May increase ALT, AST, and serum creatinine levels. May decrease phosphorus and potassium levels.
- May decrease Hb level and leukocyte, neutrophil, lymphocyte, and platelet counts.

CONTRAINDICATIONS & CAUTIONS

⚡ Alert: Cyclin-dependent kinase 4/6 (CDK4/6) inhibitors may cause rare but severe or fatal interstitial lung disease (ILD) and pneumonitis.

• Drug may prolong QT interval. Avoid use in patients with long QT syndrome, uncontrolled or significant cardiac disease (recent MI, HF, unstable angina, bradyarrhythmias), or electrolyte abnormalities and in those taking strong CYP3A inhibitors or drugs known to prolong the QTc interval.

• Drug may increase risk of hepatobiliary toxicity and neutropenia.

Dialyzable drug: Unknown.

PREGNANCY-LACTATION-REPRODUCTION

• Based on mechanism of action, drug may cause fetal harm; avoid use in pregnant women. Obtain a pregnancy test before start of therapy. Females of childbearing potential should use effective contraception during therapy and for at least 3 weeks after final dose.

• It isn't known if drug appears in human milk. Women shouldn't breastfeed during therapy and for at least 3 weeks after final dose.

• Drug may impair fertility in males.

NURSING CONSIDERATIONS

⚡ Alert: Monitor patients for new or worsening pulmonary symptoms (hypoxia, cough, dyspnea, interstitial infiltrates on radiologic images); if they occur, interrupt therapy immediately and evaluate the patient. If infection, neoplasm and other causes are excluded, permanently discontinue treatment in patients with severe ILD or pneumonitis.

• Monitor LFTs before start of therapy, every 2 weeks for the first two cycles, then at the beginning of each subsequent four cycles, and as clinically indicated because of the risk of hepatobiliary toxicity. Interrupt therapy, reduce dosage, or discontinue drug based on LFT values as directed in manufacturer's instructions.

• Monitor electrolyte levels (potassium, calcium, phosphorus, magnesium) before start of therapy, at the beginning of the first six cycles, and as clinically indicated. Correct electrolyte abnormalities before therapy begins.

• Assess ECG before treatment. Initiate treatment only in patients with a baseline

QTcF (QT interval corrected for HR via Fridericia's method) of less than 450 msec. Repeat ECG on day 14 of the first cycle, at the beginning of the second cycle, and as clinically indicated. Interrupt therapy, reduce dosage, or discontinue drug based on QT-interval prolongation as directed in manufacturer's instructions.

• Assess CBC before start of therapy, every 2 weeks for the first two cycles, at the beginning of each subsequent four cycles, then as clinically indicated. Interrupt therapy, reduce dosage, or discontinue drug based on CBC results as directed in manufacturer's instructions.

• Monitor patient closely for hepatobiliary toxicity and neutropenia.

PATIENT TEACHING

⚡ Alert: Warn patients to immediately report difficulty or discomfort with breathing or shortness of breath while at rest or with low activity; these may be symptoms of ILD or pneumonitis.

• Teach patient to immediately report signs and symptoms related to QT-interval prolongation (fast or irregular heartbeat, dizziness, syncope).

• Advise patient to immediately report signs and symptoms of liver dysfunction (jaundice, dark or brown urine, fatigue, loss of appetite, upper abdominal pain, bleeding or bruising more easily than usual) and infection (fever, chills, pain, malaise).

---

rifAMPin (rifampicin)

rif-AM-pin

Rifadin, Rimactane, Rofact✚

Therapeutic class: Antituberculotics
Pharmacologic class: Semisynthetic rifamycins

AVAILABLE FORMS

Capsules: 150 mg, 300 mg
Powder for injection: 600 mg/vial

INDICATIONS & DOSAGES

➤ **Pulmonary TB, with other antituberculotics**
Adults: 10 mg/kg PO or IV daily in single dose. Give oral doses 1 hour before or

2 hours after meals with a full glass of water. Maximum daily dose is 600 mg.
Children: 10 to 20 mg/kg PO or IV daily in single dose. Give oral doses 1 hour before or 2 hours after meals with a full glass of water. Maximum daily dose is 600 mg.

➤ **Meningococcal carriers**
Adults: 600 mg PO or IV every 12 hours for 2 days.
Children ages 1 month to 12 years: 10 mg/kg PO or IV every 12 hours for 2 days, not to exceed 600 mg/day.
Neonates: 5 mg/kg PO or IV every 12 hours for 2 days.

➤ **Cholestatic pruritus**
Adults: 150 mg/day PO if bilirubin level is less than 3 mg/dL or 150 mg PO b.i.d. if bilirubin level is 3 mg/dL or higher.

ADMINISTRATION
PO
• For pulmonary TB, give drug with other antituberculotics.
• For best absorption, give capsules 1 hour before or 2 hours after a meal with a full glass of water.
• For patients who can't tolerate capsules on an empty stomach or those who have difficulty swallowing capsules or when lower doses are needed, consult pharmacist for preparation of an oral suspension.

IV
▼ Reconstitute drug with 10 mL of sterile water for injection to yield 60 mg/mL.
▼ Add to 100 mL of D$_5$W and infuse over 30 minutes, or add to 500 mL of D$_5$W and infuse over 3 hours.
▼ When dextrose is contraindicated, dilute with NSS for injection. Once prepared, dilutions in D$_5$W are stable for up to 4 hours and dilutions in NSS are stable for up to 24 hours at room temperature.
▼ **Incompatibilities:** Diltiazem, other IV solutions.

ACTION
Inhibits DNA-dependent RNA polymerase, which impairs RNA synthesis; bactericidal.

Route	Onset	Peak	Duration
PO	Unknown	2–4 hr	<24 hr
IV	Unknown	Unknown	<24 hr

Half-life: 1¼ to 5 hours.

ADVERSE REACTIONS
CNS: headache, fatigue, drowsiness, behavioral changes, dizziness, mental confusion, generalized numbness, ataxia, fever. **CV:** *shock.* **EENT:** visual disturbances, exudative conjunctivitis, tooth discoloration. **GI:** *pancreatitis, pseudomembranous colitis,* epigastric distress, anorexia, nausea, vomiting, abdominal pain, diarrhea, flatulence, sore mouth and tongue. **GU:** *acute renal failure,* hemoglobinuria, hematuria, menstrual disturbances. **Hematologic:** *thrombocytopenia, transient leukopenia,* eosinophilia, hemolytic anemia. **Hepatic:** *hepatotoxicity.* **Metabolic:** hyperuricemia. **Musculoskeletal:** muscular weakness, pain in extremities. **Respiratory:** shortness of breath, wheezing. **Skin:** pruritus, urticaria, rash. **Other:** flulike syndrome, discoloration of body fluids, porphyria exacerbation.

INTERACTIONS
Drug-drug. *Amiodarone, analgesics, anticonvulsants, barbiturates, bazedoxifene, beta blockers, bosentan, cardiac glycosides, chloramphenicol, citalopram, clofibrate,* **corticosteroids, cyclosporine,** *dapsone, delavirdine, diazepam, digoxin, disopyramide, doxycycline, enalapril, fluoroquinolones, hormonal contraceptives, hydantoins, losartan, methadone, mexiletine, midazolam, nifedipine, ondansetron, opioids, progestins, propafenone, quinidine,* **ritonavir,** *sulfonylureas,* **tacrolimus,** *TCAs, theophylline, tocainide, triazolam, verapamil, zidovudine, zolpidem:* May decrease effectiveness of these drugs. Monitor effectiveness.
Anticoagulants: May increase requirements for anticoagulant. Monitor PT and INR closely, and adjust dosage of anticoagulants.
Atazanavir, boceprevir, darunavir, fosamprenavir, tipranavir: May decrease plasma concentrations of antivirals, resulting in loss of antiviral efficacy or development of viral resistance. Use together is contraindicated.
Halothane: May increase risk of hepatotoxicity. Monitor LFT results.
Isoniazid: May increase risk of hepatotoxicity. Monitor LFT results.
Ketoconazole, para-aminosalicylate sodium: May interfere with absorption of rifampin. Separate doses by 8 to 12 hours.

Reactions in bold italics are *life-threatening*. Interactions may have a *rapid onset* or a *delayed onset*.

Macrolide antibiotics, protease inhibitors: May inhibit rifampin metabolism but increase metabolism of other drug. Monitor patient for clinical and adverse effects.

Probenecid: May increase rifampin levels. Use together cautiously.

Saquinavir: May increase risk of severe hepatocellular toxicity. Use together is contraindicated.

Voriconazole: May decrease voriconazole's therapeutic effects while increasing the risk of rifampin adverse effects. Use together is contraindicated.

Drug-lifestyle. *Alcohol use:* May increase risk of hepatotoxicity. Discourage use together.

EFFECTS ON LAB TEST RESULTS
• May increase ALT, AST, alkaline phosphatase, bilirubin, and uric acid levels. May decrease Hb level.
• May increase eosinophil counts. May decrease platelet and WBC counts.
• May alter standard folate and vitamin B_{12} assay results.

CONTRAINDICATIONS & CAUTIONS
• Contraindicated in patients hypersensitive to rifampin or related drugs.
• Use cautiously in patients with liver disease or diabetes.
Dialyzable drug: Poorly.
⚠ Overdose S&S: Nausea; vomiting; abdominal pain; pruritus; headache; increasing lethargy; unconsciousness; transient increases in liver enzyme or bilirubin levels; brownish red or orange discoloration of skin, urine, sweat, saliva, tears, and feces; facial or periorbital edema; hypotension; tachycardia; ventricular arrhythmias; seizures; cardiac arrest; liver enlargement; jaundice.

PREGNANCY-LACTATION-REPRODUCTION
• There are no adequate studies in pregnant women. Use during pregnancy only if clearly needed and potential benefit justifies potential risk to the fetus.
• Reportedly, drug can cause postnatal hemorrhages in the mother and infant when given during last few weeks of pregnancy; treatment with vitamin K may be indicated.

• Drug appears in human milk. Patient should discontinue breastfeeding or discontinue drug.

NURSING CONSIDERATIONS
• Monitor hepatic function, hematopoietic studies, and uric acid level. Drug's systemic effects may asymptomatically raise LFT values and uric acid level. In patients with existing impaired hepatic function, monitor LFT values, especially AST and ALT, before therapy, then every 2 to 4 weeks during therapy.
• Watch for and report to prescriber signs and symptoms of hepatic impairment.
• For TB, a three-drug regimen of rifampin, isoniazid (INH), and pyrazinamide is recommended in the initial phase of short-course therapy, which is usually continued for 2 months. Guidelines also recommend that either streptomycin or ethambutol be added as a fourth drug if community rates of INH resistance are 4% or greater. After the initial phase, continue treatment for at least 4 months or longer if patient is still sputum or culture positive, if resistant organisms are present, or if patient is HIV-positive.
• *Look alike–sound alike:* Don't confuse rifampin with rifabutin, rifaximin, rifapentine, or Rifamate.

PATIENT TEACHING
• Advise patient who is unable to swallow capsules whole or can't tolerate capsules on an empty stomach that an oral suspension can be prepared by the pharmacist.
• Warn patient that drowsiness may occur and that drug can turn body fluids red-orange and permanently stain contact lenses.
• Advise female patient using hormonal contraceptives to consider another form of contraception.
• Advise patient to report fever, loss of appetite, malaise, nausea, vomiting, dark urine, or yellowing of eyes or skin.
• Advise patient to avoid alcohol during drug therapy.
• Instruct patient on importance of not missing any doses and completing full course of therapy.

rifapentine
rif-a-PEN-teen

Priftin

Therapeutic class: Antituberculotics
Pharmacologic class: Synthetic rifamycins

AVAILABLE FORMS
Tablets (film-coated): 150 mg

INDICATIONS & DOSAGES
◔ *Alert:* Give drug as directly observed therapy for all indications.
➤ **Pulmonary TB, with at least one other antituberculotic to which the isolate is susceptible**
Adults and children age 12 and older: During intensive phase of short-course therapy, 600 mg PO twice weekly for 2 months, with an interval between doses of at least 3 days (72 hours). During continuation phase of short-course therapy, 600 mg PO once weekly for 4 months, combined with isoniazid or another drug to which the isolate is susceptible.
Elderly patients: Begin therapy at low end of dosing range.
➤ **Latent TB infection caused by *Mycobacterium tuberculosis*, in combination with isoniazid, in patients at high risk for progression to TB disease**
Adults and children age 12 and older: Rifapentine dosage is based on patient's weight and administered PO once weekly. If patient weighs more than 50 kg, give 900 mg; if weight is 32.1 to 50 kg, give 750 mg; if weight is 25.1 to 32 kg, give 600 mg; if weight is 14.1 to 25 kg, give 450 mg; if weight is 10 to 14 kg, give 300 mg. Maximum dose is 900 mg once weekly. Recommended isoniazid dose is 15 mg/kg (rounded to nearest 50 or 100 mg) up to maximum of 900 mg once weekly for 12 weeks.
Children ages 2 to 11: Rifapentine dosage is based on patient's weight and is administered PO once weekly. If patient weighs more than 50 kg, give 900 mg; if weight is 32.1 to 50 kg, give 750 mg; if weight is 25.1 to 32 kg, give 600 mg; if weight is 14.1 to 25 kg, give 450 mg; if weight is 10 to 14 kg, give 300 mg. Maximum dose is 900 mg once

weekly. Recommended isoniazid dose is 25 mg/kg (rounded to nearest 50 or 100 mg) up to maximum of 900 mg once weekly for 12 weeks.

ADMINISTRATION
PO
• Give drug with meals to increase oral bioavailability and possibly reduce the incidence of GI upset, nausea, and vomiting.
• For patients who can't swallow tablets, tablets may be crushed and added to small amount of semisolid food and consumed immediately.
◔ *Alert:* Give drug with appropriate daily companion drugs. Compliance with all drug regimens, especially with daily companion drugs on the days when rifapentine isn't given, is crucial for early sputum conversion and protection from relapse of TB.

ACTION
Inhibits DNA-dependent RNA polymerase in susceptible strains of *M. tuberculosis.* Demonstrates bactericidal activity against the organism both intracellularly and extracellularly.

Route	Onset	Peak	Duration
PO	Unknown	3–10 hr	Unknown

Half-life: 17 hours.

ADVERSE REACTIONS
CNS: headache, dizziness, pain. **CV:** chest pain. **EENT:** conjunctivitis, epistaxis. **GI:** anorexia, nausea, vomiting, dyspepsia, diarrhea. **GU:** hyperuricemia, pyuria, proteinuria, hematuria, urinary casts. **Hematologic:** *leukopenia, neutropenia,* anemia, *thrombocytosis.* **Metabolic:** hyperuricemia. **Musculoskeletal:** arthralgia. **Respiratory:** hemoptysis, cough. **Skin:** rash, pruritus, acne, maculopapular rash.

INTERACTIONS
Drug-drug. *Antiarrhythmics (disopyramide, mexiletine, quinidine, tocainide), antibiotics (chloramphenicol, clarithromycin, dapsone, doxycycline, fluoroquinolones), anticonvulsants (phenytoin), antifungals (fluconazole, itraconazole, ketoconazole), barbiturates, benzodiazepines (diazepam), beta blockers, calcium channel blockers*

Reactions in bold italics are **life-threatening**. Interactions may have a *rapid onset* or a **delayed onset**.

*(diltiazem, nifedipine, verapamil), cardiac glycosides, clofibrate, **corticosteroids**, haloperidol, HIV protease inhibitors (indinavir, nelfinavir, ritonavir, saquinavir), hormonal contraceptives, **immunosuppressants (cyclosporine, tacrolimus)**, levothyroxine, opioid analgesics (methadone), oral anticoagulants (warfarin), oral antidiabetics (sulfonylureas), progestins, quinine, reverse transcriptase inhibitors (delavirdine, zidovudine), sildenafil, TCAs (amitriptyline, nortriptyline), theophylline:* May decrease activity of these drugs because of cytochrome P-450 enzyme metabolism. May need to adjust dosage.

Ritonavir: May decrease ritonavir levels. Carefully monitor patient's response.

EFFECTS ON LAB TEST RESULTS
• May increase uric acid, ALT, and AST levels.
• May decrease blood glucose level.
• May increase platelet count.
• May decrease Hb level and neutrophil and WBC counts.
• May alter folate and vitamin B_{12} assay results.

CONTRAINDICATIONS & CAUTIONS
• Contraindicated in patients hypersensitive to rifamycins (rifapentine, rifampin, or rifabutin).
• May cause hypersensitivity reactions, including anaphylaxis (flulike illness, hypotension, urticaria, angioedema, bronchospasm, conjunctivitis, thrombocytopenia, neutropenia). If signs or symptoms occur, stop drug and notify prescriber.
• Patients with abnormal LFT values or liver disease and those initiating treatment for active pulmonary TB should receive rifapentine only in cases of necessity and under strict medical supervision.
• For HIV-infected patients with active pulmonary TB, don't use drug once weekly in the continuation phase regimen in combination with isoniazid because of a higher rate of failure or relapse with rifampin-resistant organisms. Rifapentine hasn't been studied as part of the initial phase treatment regimen in HIV-infected patients with active pulmonary TB.

• Rule out active TB disease before starting treatment for latent TB infection.
• Patients considered at high risk for progression to TB disease include those in close contact with patients with active TB or recent conversion to a positive result on tuberculin skin test, patients with pulmonary fibrosis on X-ray, and HIV-infected patients.
• Rifapentine in combination with isoniazid isn't recommended for patients presumed to be exposed to rifamycin- or isoniazid-resistant *M. tuberculosis*.
• Use cautiously in patients with cavitary pulmonary lesions or positive sputum cultures after initial treatment phase and in patients with bilateral pulmonary disease; higher relapse rates may occur in these patients.
• CDAD has been reported, ranging from mild diarrhea to fatal colitis, and can occur more than 2 months after therapy ends. Drug may need to be discontinued and appropriate measures initiated.
• Avoid using drug in patients with porphyria.
Dialyzable drug: Unlikely.
⚠ *Overdose S&S:* Hematuria, neutropenia, hyperglycemia, hyperuricemia, arthritis, increased ALT level, pruritus.

PREGNANCY-LACTATION-REPRODUCTION
• There are no adequate studies in pregnant women. Use during pregnancy only if potential benefit justifies potential risk to the fetus.
• Reportedly, postnatal hemorrhages in the mother and infant have occurred when another rifamycin (rifampin) was given during last few weeks of pregnancy. Monitor PT of pregnant women and neonates exposed to rifapentine during last few weeks of pregnancy. Treatment with vitamin K may be indicated.
• It isn't known if drug appears in human milk. Patient should discontinue breastfeeding or discontinue drug.

NURSING CONSIDERATIONS
• Monitor patient for signs and symptoms of hypersensitivity reaction; if they occur, use supportive measures and discontinue drug.
• Rifamycin antibiotics may cause hepatotoxicity. In patients with abnormal LFT

R

values or liver disease and patients starting treatment for active pulmonary TB, obtain serum transaminase levels before start of therapy and every 2 to 4 weeks during therapy. Discontinue drug if evidence of liver injury occurs.

• *Look alike–sound alike:* Don't confuse rifapentine with rifabutin or rifampin.

PATIENT TEACHING

• Stress importance of strict compliance with this drug regimen and that of daily companion drugs, as well as needed follow-up visits and laboratory tests.

• Advise female patient to use nonhormonal contraceptive methods.

• Tell patient to take drug with meals to increase oral bioavailability and possibly reduce the incidence of GI upset, nausea, and vomiting.

• Instruct patient to report all adverse reactions, especially fever, appetite loss, malaise, nausea, vomiting, darkened urine, yellowish skin and eyes, joint pain or swelling, or excessive loose stools or diarrhea.

• Instruct patient to protect pills from excessive heat.

• Tell patient that drug may turn body fluids red-orange and permanently stain contact lenses. Instruct patient to remove soft contact lenses during therapy. Advise patient with dentures that permanent staining of dentures may occur.

rifAXIMin
rif-AX-i-min

Xifaxan

Therapeutic class: Antibiotics
Pharmacologic class: Rifamycin antibacterials

AVAILABLE FORMS
Tablets: 200 mg, 550 mg

INDICATIONS & DOSAGES

➤ **Traveler's diarrhea from noninvasive strains of** *Escherichia coli*
Adults and children age 12 and older: 200 mg PO t.i.d. for 3 days.

➤ **Hepatic encephalopathy**
Adults: 550 mg PO b.i.d.
➤ **IBS with diarrhea**
Adults: 550 mg PO t.i.d. for 14 days. May repeat regimen twice if symptoms recur.

ADMINISTRATION
PO
• Give drug without regard for food.

ACTION
Binds to the beta-subunit of bacterial DNA-dependent RNA polymerase, which inhibits bacterial RNA synthesis and kills *E. coli.*

Route	Onset	Peak	Duration
PO	Unknown	1 hr	Unknown

Half-life: 1.8 to 6 hours.

ADVERSE REACTIONS
CNS: depression, dizziness, fatigue, fever, headache, insomnia. **CV:** peripheral edema. **EENT:** nasopharyngitis. **GI:** ascites, abdominal pain, constipation, defecation urgency, flatulence, nausea, rectal tenesmus, vomiting. **Hematologic:** anemia. **Musculoskeletal:** arthralgia, muscle spasms, myalgia. **Respiratory:** dyspnea. **Skin:** rash, pruritus.

INTERACTIONS
Drug-drug. *BCG (intravesical):* May diminish therapeutic effect of BCG. Avoid combination.
Cyclosporine: May increase systemic exposure of rifaximin. Monitor therapy.

EFFECTS ON LAB TEST RESULTS
• May increase CK and ALT levels.

CONTRAINDICATIONS & CAUTIONS
• Contraindicated in patients hypersensitive to rifaximin or its components, rifamycin, or other antimicrobial agents.
• Use with caution in patients with severe hepatic impairment.
Dialyzable drug: Unknown.

PREGNANCY-LACTATION-REPRODUCTION
• Safety in pregnant women hasn't been established; some animal studies have demonstrated adverse events. Because of limited absorption of rifaximin in patients with

normal hepatic function, fetal exposure to drug is expected to be low.
• It isn't known if drug appears in human milk. Patient should discontinue breastfeeding or discontinue drug.

NURSING CONSIDERATIONS
• Don't use drug in patients whose illness may be caused by *Campylobacter jejuni, Shigella*, or *Salmonella*.
🜂 **Alert:** Don't use drug in patients with blood in the stool, diarrhea with fever, or diarrhea from pathogens other than *E. coli*.
• Stop drug if diarrhea worsens or lasts longer than 24 to 48 hours. Patient may need a different antibiotic.
• Patients who have diarrhea after antibiotic therapy may have CDAD, which may range from mild to life-threatening.
• Monitor patient for overgrowth of nonsusceptible organisms.

PATIENT TEACHING
• Explain that drug may be taken with or without food.
• Tell patient to take all the prescribed drug, even if feeling better before drug is finished.
• Advise patient to notify prescriber if diarrhea worsens or lasts longer than 1 or 2 days after starting treatment. A different treatment may be needed.
• Tell patient to report fever or bloody stool.
• Explain that this drug is only for treating diarrhea caused by contaminated foods or beverages while traveling and not for any other type of infection.
• Caution patient not to share drug with others.

rilpivirine hydrochloride
ril-pi-VIR-een

Edurant

Therapeutic class: Antiretrovirals
Pharmacologic class: NNRTIs

AVAILABLE FORMS
Tablets: 25 mg

INDICATIONS & DOSAGES
➤ **Treatment of HIV-1 infection in antiretroviral-naive patients with HIV-1**

RNA 100,000 copies/mL or less at start of therapy, in combination with other antiretrovirals
Adults and children age 12 and older weighing at least 35 kg: 25 mg PO once daily.
Adjust-a-dose: For patients concomitantly receiving rifabutin, increase rilpivirine dosage to 50 mg once daily. When rifabutin is stopped, decrease rilpivirine to 25 mg once daily.
For pregnant patients who were already on a stable regimen before pregnancy and who are virologically suppressed (HIV-1 RNA less than 50 copies per mL), recommended dosage is 25 mg once daily.

ADMINISTRATION
PO
• Give drug with a normal to high-calorie meal.
• Patient should swallow tablets whole with water.
• Store tablets at room temperature and in the original bottle to protect from light.

ACTION
Inhibits HIV-1 replication by noncompetitive inhibition of HIV-1 reverse transcriptase but doesn't inhibit the human cellular DNA polymerases alpha, beta, and gamma.

Route	Onset	Peak	Duration
PO	Rapid	4–5 hr	Unknown

Half-life: 50 hours.

ADVERSE REACTIONS
CNS: abnormal dreams, dizziness, fatigue, headache, insomnia, depression. **GI:** nausea, vomiting, abdominal pain. **Skin:** rash.

INTERACTIONS
Drug-drug. *Antacids (aluminum or magnesium hydroxide, calcium carbonate):* May significantly decrease rilpivirine level. Give antacids either 2 hours before or at least 4 hours after rilpivirine.
Anticonvulsants (carbamazepine, oxcarbazepine, phenobarbital, phenytoin): May decrease rilpivirine level, decrease response, and increase risk of resistance to NNRTIs. Use together is contraindicated.
Azole antifungals (fluconazole, itraconazole, ketoconazole, posaconazole, voriconazole):

R

May increase rilpivirine level and decrease antifungal level. Monitor effectiveness of antifungal.

Delavirdine: May increase rilpivirine level. Don't use together.

Dexamethasone (more than a single dose): May decrease rilpivirine level and virologic response, and increase risk of resistance to NNRTIs. Use together is contraindicated.

Didanosine (buffered): May decrease rilpivirine level. Administer didanosine at least 2 hours before or 4 hours after rilpivirine.

Drugs that prolong QT interval: May increase risk of torsades de pointes. Use together cautiously.

H2-receptor antagonists (cimetidine, famotidine, nizatidine, ranitidine): May significantly decrease rilpivirine level. Give H2-receptor antagonists at least 12 hours before or 4 hours after rilpivirine.

Macrolide antibiotics (clarithromycin, erythromycin, troleandomycin): May increase rilpivirine level. When possible, consider an alternative such as azithromycin.

Methadone: May decrease levels of both drugs. Monitor effectiveness of methadone and adjust methadone dosage as needed.

Other NNRTIs (efavirenz, etravirine, nevirapine): May decrease rilpivirine level. Don't use together.

PPIs (esomeprazole, lansoprazole, pantoprazole, rabeprazole): May decrease rilpivirine level, decrease virologic response, and increase risk of resistance to NNRTIs. Use together is contraindicated.

Rifamycins (rifampin, rifapentine): May decrease rilpivirine level, decrease virologic response, and increase risk of resistance to NNRTIs. Use together is contraindicated.

Systemic glucocorticoids (dexamethasone): May decrease rilpivirine level if more than one dose of dexamethasone is administered. Use together is contraindicated.

Drug-herb. *St. John's wort:* May decrease rilpivirine level, decrease virologic response, and increase risk of resistance to NNRTIs. Use together is contraindicated.

Drug-food. *Grapefruit products:* May inhibit metabolism of rilpivirine. Avoid use during therapy.

EFFECTS ON LAB TEST RESULTS
• May increase AST, ALT, bilirubin, creatinine, total cholesterol, and LDL and triglyceride levels.

CONTRAINDICATIONS & CAUTIONS
• Contraindicated in patients hypersensitive to drug or its components.
• Use cautiously when administering with drugs known to prolong QT interval, in elderly patients, and in those with severe renal impairment, ESRD, or severe hepatic impairment.
• Redistribution or accumulation of body fat, including central obesity, dorsocervical fat enlargement (buffalo hump), peripheral wasting, facial wasting, breast enlargement, and "cushingoid appearance," has occurred in patients receiving antiretroviral therapy. The mechanism and long-term consequences of these events are currently unknown. A causal relationship hasn't been established.
• Hepatic adverse events have been reported. Patients with underlying HBV or HCV infection or marked elevations in transaminase levels before treatment may be at increased risk for worsening or development of transaminase elevations. A few cases of hepatotoxicity have been reported in patients who had no preexisting hepatic disease or other identifiable risk factors.
• Severe skin and hypersensitivity reactions have been reported, including severe rash or rash accompanied by fever, blisters, mucosal involvement, conjunctivitis, facial edema, angioedema, hepatitis, eosinophilia, or DRESS syndrome. Most rashes occurred within first 4 to 6 weeks of therapy. Discontinue drug if hypersensitivity reaction or rash develops.

Dialyzable drug: Unlikely.

PREGNANCY-LACTATION-REPRODUCTION
• Enroll pregnant women exposed to drug in the Antiretroviral Pregnancy Registry (1-800-258-4263).
• It isn't known if drug appears in human milk. Patients shouldn't breastfeed during therapy.
• The CDC recommends that an HIV-infected mother not breastfeed to avoid postnatal transmission of HIV.

Reactions in bold italics are *life-threatening*. Interactions may have a *rapid onset* or a *delayed onset*.

NURSING CONSIDERATIONS

- Patients should take drug with a regular meal and not with a protein drink; taking drug with a protein-rich nutritional drink alone may lower the exposure of rilpivirine by 50%.
- Always use rilpivirine in combination with other antiretrovirals.
- Drug isn't a cure for HIV infection. Patients must stay on continuous antiretroviral therapy to control HIV infection and decrease HIV-related illnesses.
- Monitor patient for severe rash or rash accompanied by fever, blisters, mucosal involvement, conjunctivitis, facial edema, angioedema, hepatitis, eosinophilia, or DRESS syndrome. Discontinue drug if hypersensitivity reaction or rash develops; initiate appropriate therapy.
- Assess patient for redistribution or accumulation of body fat.
- Monitor patients for reemergence of infections, such as *Mycobacterium avium*, cytomegalovirus, *Pneumocystis jiroveci* pneumonia, and TB, during initial phase of combination treatment. Treat infections appropriately.
- Monitor patients for depressive disorders (depressed mood, dysphoria, negative thoughts, suicidal ideation or attempt). Weigh risks of continued therapy against benefits of treatment.
- Monitor liver enzyme levels before and during treatment for patients with underlying hepatic disease, including HBV or HCV infection, and for patients with marked transaminase elevations. Consider monitoring liver enzyme levels for patients without preexisting hepatic dysfunction or other risk factors. Monitor patients with severe renal impairment or ESRD for adverse reactions during treatment.

PATIENT TEACHING

- Advise patient that rilpivirine isn't a cure for HIV infection or AIDS and that patient must stay on continuous antiretroviral therapy so that the HIV infection can be controlled.
- Tell patient to report all medications and supplements being taken because many of them may interact with rilpivirine.

- Instruct patient to take rilpivirine once daily with a full meal and to keep tablets in the original container to protect them from light.
- Inform patient that if a dose is missed, not to take the missed dose if the next scheduled dose is within 12 hours.
- Warn patient that rilpivirine may cause depressed or altered mood and to report mood changes or symptoms of depression immediately.
- Advise patient to immediately report hypersensitivity reaction or rash.
- Tell female patient to report pregnancy immediately. Also advise patient not to breastfeed.

---

risedronate sodium
ris-ED-roe-nate

Actonel✐, Atelvia

Therapeutic class: Antiosteoporotics
Pharmacologic class: Bisphosphonates

AVAILABLE FORMS
Tablets ⓓⓝⓒ: 5 mg, 30 mg, 35 mg, 150 mg
Tablets (delayed-release) ⓓⓝⓒ: 35 mg

INDICATIONS & DOSAGES
Adjust-a-dose (for all indications): Don't use if CrCl is less than 30 mL/minute.
➤ **To prevent and treat postmenopausal osteoporosis**
Women: 5-mg immediate-release tablet PO once daily, or 35-mg immediate-release tablet PO once weekly.
➤ **To treat postmenopausal osteoporosis**
Women: 35-mg delayed-release tablet PO once weekly.
➤ **To prevent or treat postmenopausal osteoporosis when fewer dosing days are desirable**
Women: 75 mg PO on 2 consecutive days for a total of 150 mg each month. Or, one 150-mg immediate-release tablet PO once each month.
➤ **To increase bone mass in men with osteoporosis**
Men: One 35-mg immediate-release tablet PO once weekly.

➤ **To prevent or treat glucocorticoid-induced osteoporosis in patients taking 7.5 mg or more of prednisone or equivalent glucocorticoid daily**
Adults: 5 mg immediate-release tablet PO daily.

➤ **Paget disease (immediate-release)**
Adults: 30 mg PO daily for 2 months. If relapse occurs or alkaline phosphatase level doesn't normalize, may repeat treatment course 2 months or more after completing first treatment course.

ADMINISTRATION
PO
• Give immediate-release tablets at least 30 minutes before the first food, drink, or medication of the day, other than water. Give with 8 oz of plain water while patient is sitting or standing.
• Patient shouldn't eat or drink anything except plain water or take other medications for at least 30 minutes after taking immediate-release risedronate.
• Give delayed-release tablet in the morning immediately after breakfast and not under fasting conditions because of a higher risk of abdominal pain if taken when fasting. Give with 8 oz of plain water while patient is sitting or standing.
• Warn patient against lying down for 30 minutes after taking drug.
• Make sure patient doesn't chew, crush, cut, or suck tablets.

ACTION
Reverses the loss of bone mineral density by reducing bone turnover and bone resorption. In patients with Paget disease, drug causes bone turnover to return to normal.

Route	Onset	Peak	Duration
PO	1 hr	1 hr	Unknown
PO (delayed-release)	Unknown	3 hr	Unknown

Half-life: Immediate-release, 23 hours; delayed-release, 561 hours.

ADVERSE REACTIONS
CNS: asthenia, headache, depression, dizziness, insomnia, anxiety, neuralgia, vertigo, hypertonia, paresthesia, pain. **CV:** HTN, CV disorder, angina pectoris, chest pain, peripheral edema. **EENT:** pharyngitis, rhinitis, sinusitis, cataract, conjunctivitis, otitis media, amblyopia, tinnitus. **GI:** nausea, diarrhea, abdominal pain, flatulence, gastritis, rectal disorder, constipation. **GU:** UTI, cystitis. **Hematologic:** ecchymosis, anemia. **Musculoskeletal:** arthralgia, neck pain, back pain, myalgia, bone pain, leg cramps, bursitis. **Respiratory:** URI, bronchitis. **Skin:** rash, pruritus. **Other:** infection, tooth disorder.

INTERACTIONS
Drug-drug. *Aspirin, NSAIDs:* May increase risk of gastric ulcers. Use cautiously together.
Calcium supplements; antacids that contain calcium, magnesium, or aluminum: May interfere with risedronate absorption. Advise patient to separate dosing times.
H₂ antagonists, PPIs: May affect enteric coating on delayed-release tablets, decreasing bioavailability. Use together isn't recommended.
Drug-food. *Any food:* May interfere with absorption of drug. Advise patient to take immediate-release tablets at least 30 minutes before first food or drink of the day (other than water).

EFFECTS ON LAB TEST RESULTS
• May decrease calcium and phosphorus levels.

CONTRAINDICATIONS & CAUTIONS
• Contraindicated in patients hypersensitive to any component of the product, in hypocalcemic patients, in patients with conditions that delay esophageal emptying, and in those who can't stand or sit upright for 30 minutes after administration.
• Drug isn't recommended for use in patients with CrCl less than 30 mL/minute.
• Hypersensitivity and skin reactions have been reported, including angioedema, generalized rash, bullous skin reactions, SJS, and toxic epidermal necrolysis.
⚠ Alert: There may be an increased risk of fractures of the thigh in patients treated with bisphosphonates.
• Drug increases risk of osteonecrosis of the jaw, which can occur spontaneously. For patients requiring invasive dental procedures, discontinuing bisphosphonate treatment may reduce risk.

Reactions in bold italics are *life-threatening*. Interactions may have a *rapid onset* or a *delayed onset*.

- Use cautiously in patients with upper GI disorders, such as dysphagia, esophagitis, and esophageal or gastric ulcers.
- Treat hypocalcemia and other disturbances of bone and mineral metabolism before starting treatment.
- Immediate-release and delayed-release formulations contain the same active ingredient and must not be given together.
Dialyzable drug: Unknown.
⚠ *Overdose S&S:* Hypocalcemia, hypophosphatemia.

PREGNANCY-LACTATION-REPRODUCTION
- There are no adequate studies in pregnant women. Use during pregnancy only if potential benefit justifies potential risk to the fetus.
- It isn't known if drug appears in human milk. Patient should discontinue breastfeeding or discontinue drug.

NURSING CONSIDERATIONS
- Monitor patient for osteonecrosis of the jaw. Associated risk factors include invasive dental procedures, cancer diagnosis, concomitant treatment such as chemotherapy and steroids, poor oral hygiene, and preexisting dental disease. If signs or symptoms occur, stop drug and refer patient to oral surgeon.
- ⚠ *Alert:* Drug may cause dysphagia, esophagitis, and esophageal or gastric ulcers. Monitor patient for symptoms of esophageal disease.
- Severe musculoskeletal pain has been associated with bisphosphonate use and may occur within days, months, or years of start of therapy. When drug is stopped, symptoms may resolve partially or completely.
- Give supplemental calcium and vitamin D if dietary intake is inadequate. Because calcium supplements and drugs containing calcium, aluminum, or magnesium may interfere with risedronate absorption, separate dosing times.
- Periodically evaluate need for continued therapy in all patients. Consider discontinuation of therapy in patients at low risk for fracture after 3 to 5 years of use. Periodically evaluate risk of fracture in patients who discontinue therapy.

- Bisphosphonates can interfere with bone-imaging agents.
- *Look alike–sound alike:* Don't confuse Actonel with Actos.

PATIENT TEACHING
- Explain that drug may reverse bone loss by stopping more bone loss and increasing bone strength.
- Caution patient about the importance of adhering to special dosing instructions, including staying in an upright position for 30 minutes after taking drug with plain water.
- Tell patient not to chew, cut, crush, or suck the tablet because doing so may irritate the mouth.
- Advise patient to immediately report GI discomfort (such as difficulty or pain when swallowing, retrosternal pain, or severe heartburn).
- Tell patient that Actonel and Atelvia contain the same active ingredient and must not be taken together.
- Advise patient to take calcium and vitamin D if dietary intake is inadequate, but to take them at a different time than risedronate.
- Instruct patient to avoid taking other medications for at least 30 minutes after a risedronate dose.
- Advise patient to stop smoking and drinking alcohol, as appropriate. Also, advise patient to perform weight-bearing exercise.
- Tell patient to store drug in a cool, dry place, at room temperature, and away from children.
- Tell patient that if a dose of the immediate-release or delayed-release tablet is missed, to follow the manufacturer's instructions.

R

risperiDONE
ris-PEER-i-dohn

Perseris, Risperdal✔, Risperdal Consta

Therapeutic class: Antipsychotics
Pharmacologic class: Benzisoxazole derivatives

AVAILABLE FORMS
Injection: 12.5 mg, 25 mg, 37.5 mg, 50 mg, 90 mg, 120 mg

Oral solution: 1 mg/mL
Tablets: 0.25 mg, 0.5 mg, 1 mg, 2 mg, 3 mg, 4 mg
Tablets (ODTs): 0.25 mg, 0.5 mg, 1 mg, 2 mg, 3 mg, 4 mg

INDICATIONS & DOSAGES

Adjust-a-dose (for all indications): When oral formulations are administered with an enzyme inducer, such as carbamazepine, phenytoin, rifampin, or phenobarbital, increase risperidone dosage up to double patient's usual dosage; decrease dosage when the enzyme inducer is discontinued. When administered with an enzyme inhibitor, such as fluoxetine or paroxetine, reduce risperidone dosage; titrate slowly and don't exceed 8 mg/day in adults. It may be necessary to increase risperidone dosage when the enzyme inhibitor is discontinued.

➤ **Schizophrenia**

Adults: Drug may be given once daily or b.i.d. Initial dosing is generally 2 mg PO daily. Increase dosage at intervals not less than 24 hours, in increments of 1 to 2 mg/day, as tolerated, to a recommended dose of 4 to 8 mg/day. Periodically reassess to determine the need for maintenance treatment with an appropriate dose. Maximum dose is 16 mg/day.

Adjust-a-dose: In elderly or hypotensive patients and in those with CrCl of less than 30 mL/minute or severe hepatic impairment, use lower starting dosage of 0.5 mg PO b.i.d. May increase in increments of 0.5 mg or less b.i.d. Increase to dosages above 1.5 mg b.i.d. at intervals of at least 1 week.

Adolescents ages 13 to 17: Start treatment with 0.5 mg PO once daily, given as a single daily dose in either the morning or evening. Adjust dose, if indicated, at intervals of not less than 24 hours, in increments of 0.5 or 1 mg/day, as tolerated, to a recommended dose of 3 mg/day. Reassess periodically to determine need for maintenance treatment with an appropriate dose. Maximum dose is 6 mg/day.

➤ **Parenteral maintenance therapy for schizophrenia or bipolar I disorder (as monotherapy or as combination therapy with lithium or valproate)**

Adults: Establish tolerance to oral risperidone before giving IM. Give 25 mg deep IM into the buttock every 2 weeks, alternating injections between the two buttocks.

Adjust dose no sooner than every 4 weeks. Maximum, 50 mg IM every 2 weeks. Continue oral antipsychotic for 3 weeks after first IM injection, then stop oral therapy. Continue therapy at lowest dose needed. Periodically reevaluate long-term risks and benefits of drug for the individual patient.

For subcut dosing, inject 90 or 120 mg once monthly where 90 mg corresponds to 3 mg/day oral risperidone and Perseris 120 mg corresponds to 4 mg/day oral risperidone.

Adjust-a-dose: In patients with hepatic or renal impairment, titrate slowly to 2 mg PO daily for 1 week. If tolerated, give 25 mg IM every 2 weeks, or may consider initial dose of 12.5 mg IM. Continue oral form of risperidone (or another antipsychotic) with the first injection and for 3 subsequent weeks to maintain therapeutic drug levels.

At initiation of therapy with carbamazepine or other known CYP3A4 hepatic enzyme inducers, closely monitor patient during first 4 to 8 weeks. A dosage increase or additional oral risperidone may need to be considered. On discontinuation of carbamazepine or other CYP3A4 hepatic enzyme inducers, reevaluate risperidone injection dosage and, if necessary, decrease dosage. Patients may be placed on a lower risperidone injection dosage between 2 and 4 weeks before the planned discontinuation of carbamazepine or other CYP3A4 inducers to adjust for the expected increase in risperidone plasma concentration.

➤ **Monotherapy or combination therapy with lithium or valproate for 3-week treatment of acute manic or mixed episodes from bipolar I disorder**

Adults: Initially, 2 to 3 mg PO once daily. Adjust dose by 1 mg daily. Dosage range is 1 to 6 mg daily. Or, 25 mg IM every 2 weeks. Some patients may benefit from a higher dose of 37.5 or 50 mg.

Adjust-a-dose: In elderly or hypotensive patients, or those with severe renal or hepatic impairment, start with 0.5 mg PO b.i.d. Increase dosage by 0.5 mg b.i.d. Increase in dosages above 1.5 mg b.i.d. should occur at least 1 week apart. Subsequent switches to once-daily dosing may be made after patient is on a twice-daily regimen for 2 to 3 days at the target dose.

Children and adolescents ages 10 to 17: 0.5 mg PO as a single daily dose in either the morning or evening. Adjust dose, if indicated, at intervals not less than 24 hours, in increments of 0.5 or 1 mg/day, as tolerated, to a recommended dose of 2.5 mg/day.

➤ **Irritability, including aggression, self-injury, and temper tantrums, associated with an autistic disorder**

Adolescents and children ages 5 to 17 weighing 20 kg or more: Initially, 0.5 mg PO once daily or in two divided doses. After 4 days, increase dose to 1 mg. Increase dosage further in 0.5-mg increments at intervals of at least 2 weeks.

Children ages 5 to 17 weighing more than 15 and less than 20 kg: Initially, 0.25 mg PO once daily or in two divided doses. After 4 days, increase dose to 0.5 mg. Increase dosage further in 0.25-mg increments at intervals of at least 2 weeks.

ADMINISTRATION

PO

• Give drug without regard for meals.

• Oral solution isn't compatible with cola or tea.

• Open package for ODTs immediately before giving by peeling off foil backing with dry hands. Don't push tablets through the foil. ODTs can be swallowed with or without liquid.

IM

• Continue oral therapy for the first 3 weeks of IM injection therapy until injections take effect, then stop oral therapy.

• Bring injection to room temperature for at least 30 minutes before reconstitution (don't warm any other way).

• To reconstitute IM injection, inject pre-measured diluent into vial and shake vigorously for at least 10 seconds. Suspension appears uniform, thick, and milky; particles are visible, but no dry particles remain. Use drug immediately after reconstitution. If more than 2 minutes pass before injection, shake vigorously again. See manufacturer's package insert for more detailed instructions.

• Refrigerate IM injection kit and protect it from light. Drug can be stored at

temperature less than 77° F (25° C) for no more than 7 days before administration.

Subcutaneous

• For abdominal subcut injection only. Don't give by any other route.

• Only a health care professional should administer drug.

• Allow package to come to room temperature for at least 15 minutes before preparation.

• Prepare medication immediately before administration.

ACTION

Blocks dopamine, 5-HT$_2$, alpha$_1$ and alpha$_2$ adrenergic, and H$_1$ histaminergic receptors in the brain.

Route	Onset	Peak	Duration
PO	Unknown	1 hr	Unknown
IM	3 wk	4–6 wk	7 wk
Subcut	Unknown	4–6 hr	4 wk

Half-life: PO, 3 to 20 hours; IM, 3 to 6 days; subcut, 9 to 11 days.

ADVERSE REACTIONS

CNS: akathisia, somnolence, dystonia, headache, insomnia, agitation, anxiety, pain, parkinsonism, *NMS,* dizziness, fever, hallucination, mania, impaired concentration, abnormal thinking and dreaming, tremor, hypoesthesia, fatigue, depression, nervousness, parkinsonism. **CV:** tachycardia, chest pain, orthostatic hypotension, peripheral edema, syncope, HTN. **EENT:** rhinitis, sinusitis, pharyngitis, abnormal vision, ear disorder (IM). **GI:** constipation, nausea, vomiting, dyspepsia, abdominal pain, anorexia, dry mouth, increased saliva, diarrhea. **GU:** urinary incontinence, increased urination, abnormal orgasm, decreased libido, vaginal dryness, amenorrhea. **Metabolic:** weight gain or loss, hyperglycemia, gynecomastia. **Musculoskeletal:** arthralgia, back pain, leg pain, myalgia. **Respiratory:** coughing, dyspnea, URI. **Skin:** rash, dry skin, photosensitivity reactions, acne, injection-site pain (IM). **Other:** toothache, injury.

INTERACTIONS

Drug-drug. *Antihypertensives:* May enhance hypotensive effects. Monitor BP.

R

Carbamazepine, phenobarbital, phenytoin, rifampin: May increase risperidone clearance and decrease effectiveness. Monitor patient closely.

Clozapine: May decrease risperidone clearance, increasing toxicity. Monitor patient closely.

CNS depressants: May cause additive CNS depression. Use together cautiously.

Dopamine agonists, levodopa: May antagonize effects of these drugs. Use together cautiously and monitor patient.

Fluoxetine, paroxetine: May increase the risk of risperidone's adverse effects, including serotonin syndrome. Monitor patient closely and decrease risperidone dose as needed.

Black Box Warning *Opioids:* May cause slow or difficult breathing, sedation, and death. Avoid use together. If use together is necessary, limit dosage and duration of each drug to minimum necessary for desired effect. ∎

QTc interval–prolonging drugs: May increase risk of QTc-interval prolongation and risk of life-threatening ventricular arrhythmias. Use together cautiously unless contraindicated.

Drug-lifestyle. *Alcohol use:* May cause additive CNS depression. Discourage use together.

EFFECTS ON LAB TEST RESULTS
• May increase AST, ALT, blood glucose, and prolactin levels.
• May decrease Hb level, hematocrit, and WBC count.

CONTRAINDICATIONS & CAUTIONS
• Contraindicated in patients hypersensitive to drug.
• Opioids should only be prescribed with benzodiazepines or other CNS depressants to patients for whom alternative treatment options are inadequate.

Black Box Warning Elderly patients with dementia-related psychosis treated with antipsychotics are at increased risk for death. Drug isn't approved to treat elderly patients with dementia-related psychosis. ∎

• Use cautiously in patients with prolonged QT interval, CV disease, cerebrovascular disease, dehydration, hypovolemia, history

of seizures, or conditions that could affect metabolism or hemodynamic responses.
• Use cautiously in patients exposed to extreme heat.
• Use caution in patients at risk for aspiration pneumonia.
• Use IM injection cautiously in those with hepatic or renal impairment.
• Somnolence, orthostatic hypotension, and motor and sensory instability have been reported, which may lead to falls and fall-related injuries.

Dialyzable drug: Unknown.

⚠ **Overdose S&S:** Drowsiness, sedation, tachycardia, hypotension, extrapyramidal symptoms, QT-interval prolongation, seizures, torsades de pointes.

PREGNANCY-LACTATION-REPRODUCTION
⊕ **Alert:** Neonates exposed to antipsychotics during the third trimester are at risk for developing extrapyramidal signs and symptoms (repetitive muscle movements of the face and body) and withdrawal signs and symptoms (agitation, abnormally increased or decreased muscle tone, tremors, sleepiness, severe difficulty breathing, difficulty feeding) after delivery. Use in pregnant women only if potential benefit justifies risk to the fetus.
• Enroll women exposed to drug during pregnancy in the National Pregnancy Registry for Atypical Antipsychotics (1-866-961-2388).
• Drug appears in human milk. Patient should discontinue breastfeeding or discontinue drug.
• Breastfeeding is contraindicated for 12 weeks after last IM injection.
• Drug may cause hyperprolactinemia, which may decrease reproductive function in both men and women.

NURSING CONSIDERATIONS
⊕ **Alert:** Obtain baseline BP measurements before starting therapy, and monitor BP regularly. Watch for orthostatic hypotension, especially during first dosage adjustment.

Black Box Warning Elderly patients with dementia-related psychosis treated with antipsychotics are at increased risk for death. Drug isn't approved to treat elderly patients with dementia-related psychosis. ∎

Reactions in bold italics are *life-threatening*. Interactions may have a *rapid onset* or a *delayed onset*.

• Monitor patient for tardive dyskinesia, which may occur after prolonged use. It may not appear until months or years later and may disappear spontaneously or persist for life, despite stopping drug.

🚫 **Alert:** Watch for evidence of NMS (extrapyramidal effects, hyperthermia, autonomic disturbance), which is rare but can be fatal.

• Life-threatening hyperglycemia may occur in patients taking atypical antipsychotics. Monitor patients with diabetes regularly.

🚫 **Alert:** Monitor patient for symptoms of metabolic syndrome (significant weight gain and increased BMI, HTN, hyperglycemia, hypercholesterolemia, and hypertriglyceridemia).

• Periodically reevaluate drug's risks and benefits, especially during prolonged use.

• Patients experiencing persistent somnolence may benefit from administering half the daily PO dose b.i.d.

• Monitor patient for weight gain.

• Complete fall risk assessments when initiating treatment and recurrently for patients on long-term therapy, especially for elderly patients and patients with diseases, conditions, or who are taking other drugs that could increase fall risk.

• **Look alike–sound alike:** Don't confuse risperidone with reserpine or ropinirole. Don't confuse Risperdal with Restoril.

PATIENT TEACHING

• Warn patient to avoid activities that require alertness until effects of drug are known.

• Caution patient or caregiver of patient taking an opioid with a benzodiazepine, CNS depressant, or alcohol to seek immediate medical attention for dizziness, lightheadedness, extreme sleepiness, slowed or difficult breathing, or unresponsiveness.

• Warn patient to rise slowly, and use other precautions to avoid fainting when starting therapy.

• Advise patient that drug may increase fall risk due to somnolence, orthostatic hypotension, and motor and sensory instability.

• Advise patient to use caution in hot weather to prevent heatstroke.

• Tell patient to take drug with or without food.

• Instruct patient to keep the ODT in the blister pack until just before taking it. After opening the pack, patient should dissolve the tablet on the tongue without cutting or chewing. Tell patient to use dry hands to peel apart the foil to expose the tablet. Patient shouldn't attempt to push tablet through the foil.

• Advise female patient not to become pregnant or to breastfeed for 12 weeks after final IM injection.

• Advise patient to avoid alcohol during therapy.

ritonavir
ri-TOE-na-veer

Norvir

Therapeutic class: Antiretrovirals
Pharmacologic class: Protease inhibitors

AVAILABLE FORMS
Oral powder: 100 mg
Oral solution: 80 mg/mL*
Tablets 🚫: 100 mg

INDICATIONS & DOSAGES
➤ **HIV infection, with other antiretrovirals**
Adults: 600 mg PO b.i.d. with meals. To reduce adverse GI effects, begin with 300 mg PO b.i.d. and increase by 100 mg b.i.d. at 2- to 3-day intervals.
Children older than age 1 month: 350 to 400 mg/m^2 PO b.i.d.; don't exceed 600 mg PO b.i.d. Initially, start with 250 mg/m^2 b.i.d. and increase by 50 mg/m^2 PO every 12 hours at 2- to 3-day intervals. If children can't reach b.i.d. doses of 400 mg/m^2 because of adverse effects, consider alternative therapy.
Adjust-a-dose: Dosage reduction is necessary when drug is used with other protease inhibitors: atazanavir, darunavir, fosamprenavir, saquinavir, and tipranavir. Consult full prescribing information for dosage modification.

ADMINISTRATION
PO
• Give drug with meals.

R

- Don't administer ritonavir oral solution to neonates before a postmenstrual age (first day of the mother's last menstrual period to birth plus the time elapsed after birth) of 44 weeks has been attained.
- Oral solution may be mixed with chocolate milk or enteral nutrition therapy liquids, such as Ensure or Advera, within 1 hour of dosing. Shake well.
- When giving oral solution to children, use a calibrated dosing syringe, if possible.
- Don't use oral powder for doses less than 100 mg or for incremental doses between 100-mg intervals; use oral solution instead.
- Mix oral powder with soft food, such as applesauce or vanilla pudding, or with liquid, such as water, chocolate milk, or infant formula, to lessen bitter aftertaste of oral powder. Give within 2 hours of preparation; discard and prepare new dose if more than 2 hours have elapsed since preparation.
- Make sure patient swallows tablets whole and doesn't break, crush, or chew them.

ACTION

An HIV-1 and HIV-2 protease inhibitor. Drug binds to the protease-active site and inhibits activity of the enzyme, preventing cleavage of the viral polyproteins and causing formation of immature, noninfectious viral particles.

Route	Onset	Peak	Duration
PO	Unknown	2–4 hr	Unknown

Half-life: 3 to 5 hours.

ADVERSE REACTIONS

CNS: asthenia, *seizure,* anxiety, circumoral paresthesia, confusion, depression, dizziness, fever, headache, insomnia, malaise, pain, paresthesia, peripheral paresthesia, somnolence, thinking abnormality. **CV:** syncope, vasodilation. **EENT:** blurred vision, pharyngitis. **GI:** diarrhea, nausea, taste perversion, vomiting, *pancreatitis, pseudomembranous colitis,* abdominal pain, anorexia, constipation, dyspepsia, flatulence. **Hematologic:** anemia, *leukopenia, thrombocytopenia.* **Hepatic:** *hepatitis.* **Metabolic:** *diabetes mellitus,* weight loss, lipid disorders. **Musculoskeletal:** arthralgia, myalgia. **Skin:** sweating, flushing. **Other:** hypersensitivity reactions, fat redistribution or accumulation, immune reconstitution syndrome.

INTERACTIONS

Drug-drug. Black Box Warning *Alfuzosin, bepridil, ergot derivatives, flecainide, lurasidone, methylergonovine, oral midazolam, pimozide, propafenone, quinidine, sildenafil (Revatio when used to treat PAH), simvastatin, triazolam:* May cause life-threatening adverse reactions due to possible effects of ritonavir on the hepatic metabolism of these drugs. Use together is contraindicated. ∎

Amiodarone, dronedarone, flecainide, propafenone, quinidine: May cause cardiac arrhythmias. Use together is contraindicated.

Apixaban: May increase apixaban concentration. Refer to manufacturer's instructions for possible dosage reductions.

Atazanavir, darunavir, fosamprenavir, saquinavir, tipranavir: Protease inhibitors may increase the serum concentration of other protease inhibitors. Ritonavir dosage reduction is necessary when ritonavir is used with other protease inhibitors. Consult full prescribing information and clinical study information of these protease inhibitors if they are administered with a reduced ritonavir dosage.

◑ *Alert: Atorvastatin, pitavastatin, pravastatin, rosuvastatin:* May increase statin level and risk of myopathy and rhabdomyolysis. Use together cautiously at the recommended dosage for the statin given in combination with ritonavir. Refer to prescribing information for statin drug dosage limitations.

Atovaquone, divalproex, lamotrigine, phenytoin: May decrease levels of these drugs. Use together cautiously and monitor drug levels closely.

Beta blockers, disopyramide, fluoxetine, mexiletine, nefazodone: May increase levels of these drugs, causing cardiac and neurologic events. Use together cautiously.

Bupropion, buspirone, calcium channel blockers, carbamazepine, clonazepam, clorazepate, cyclosporine, desipramine, dexamethasone, diazepam, **digoxin***, dronabinol, estazolam, ethosuximide, flurazepam, lidocaine, methamphetamine, metoprolol, perphenazine, prednisone, quinine, risperidone, sirolimus, SSRIs, tacrolimus, TCAs,*

Reactions in bold italics are *life-threatening.* Interactions may have a *rapid onset* or a *delayed onset.*

thioridazine, timolol, tramadol, zolpidem: May increase levels of these drugs. Use cautiously together and consider decreasing the dosage of these drugs by almost 50%. Monitor therapeutic levels.

Clarithromycin: May increase clarithromycin level. If CrCl is 30 to 60 mL/minute, reduce clarithromycin dosage by 50%. If CrCl is less than 30 mL/minute, reduce clarithromycin dosage by 75%.

Clozapine, piroxicam: May increase levels and toxicity of these drugs. Avoid using together.

Colchicine: May increase risk of serious or life-threatening reactions in patients with renal or hepatic impairment. Use together is contraindicated.

Delavirdine: May increase ritonavir level. Adjusted dose recommendations aren't established. Use together cautiously.

Didanosine: May decrease didanosine absorption. Separate doses by 2½ hours.

Disulfiram, metronidazole: May increase risk of disulfiram-like reactions because ritonavir formulations contain alcohol. Monitor patient.

Edoxaban: May increase edoxaban serum concentration. Consider dosage adjustment if using for venous thromboembolism. (Dosage adjustment isn't needed for atrial fibrillation.)

Ethinyl estradiol: May decrease ethinyl estradiol level. Use an alternative or additional method of birth control.

Fluticasone: May significantly increase fluticasone exposure, significantly decreasing cortisol concentrations and causing systemic corticosteroid effects (including Cushing syndrome). Don't use together, if possible.

HMG-CoA reductase inhibitors: May cause large increase in statin levels, resulting in myopathy. Use cautiously with atorvastatin and rosuvastatin, using lowest doses possible; monitor patient carefully. Consider using fluvastatin or pravastatin.

Indinavir: May increase indinavir levels. Use together cautiously.

Itraconazole, ketoconazole: May increase levels of these drugs. Don't exceed 200 mg/day of these drugs.

🔴 *Alert: Lovastatin, simvastatin:* May increase statin level and risk of myopathy and rhabdomyolysis. Use together is contraindicated.

Meperidine: May decrease meperidine level and increase level of its metabolite. Dosage increases and long-term use together aren't recommended because of CNS effects. Use cautiously together.

Methadone: May decrease methadone levels. Consider increasing methadone dosage.

PDE5 inhibitors (sildenafil, tadalafil, vardenafil): May increase levels of PDE5 inhibitor, causing hypotension, syncope, visual changes, or prolonged erection. Use together cautiously and increase monitoring for adverse reactions. Tell patient not to exceed 25 mg of sildenafil in a 48-hour period, 10 mg of tadalafil in a 72-hour period, or 2.5 mg of vardenafil in a 72-hour period.

Quinine: May increase quinine level. Consider decreased quinine dosage when used together.

Rifabutin: May increase rifabutin levels. Monitor patient and reduce rifabutin daily dosage by at least 75% of usual dose.

Rifampin, rifapentine: May decrease ritonavir levels. Consider using rifabutin.

Rivaroxaban: May lead to risk of increased bleeding. Avoid use together.

Saquinavir: May increase saquinavir plasma levels. Adjust dosage by taking saquinavir 400 mg b.i.d. and ritonavir 400 mg b.i.d.

Saquinavir: May prolong QT and PR intervals. Avoid concomitant use in patients with history of prolonged QT interval and in those already receiving drugs known to prolong QT interval (class I or class III antiarrhythmics).

Theophylline: May decrease theophylline levels. Increase dose based on blood levels.

Trazodone: May increase trazodone level, causing nausea, dizziness, hypotension, and syncope. Avoid using together. If unavoidable, use cautiously and lower trazodone dose.

Voriconazole: Decreases voriconazole level and reduces antifungal response. Voriconazole is contraindicated with ritonavir doses of 400 mg every 12 hours or greater.

Warfarin: May affect INR. Monitor patient frequently after initiating coadministration and adjust warfarin dosage as needed.

Drug-herb. *St. John's wort:* May substantially reduce drug levels. Use together is contraindicated.

Drug-lifestyle. *Smoking:* May decrease drug levels. Discourage smoking.

EFFECTS ON LAB TEST RESULTS
• May increase ALT, AST, GGT, glucose, triglyceride, lipid, CK, and uric acid levels. May decrease Hb level and hematocrit.
• May decrease WBC, RBC, platelet, and neutrophil counts.

CONTRAINDICATIONS & CAUTIONS
Black Box Warning Administration with sedative-hypnotics, antiarrhythmics, or ergot alkaloid preparations may result in potentially serious or life-threatening adverse events because of possible effects on the hepatic metabolism of certain drugs. Review medications taken by patients before administering ritonavir or when administering other medications to patients already taking ritonavir. ■
• Contraindicated in patients hypersensitive to drug or its components.
🔵 *Alert:* Consult full prescribing information before and during treatment for potential drug interactions.
• Use cautiously in patients with hepatic disease, liver enzyme abnormalities, or hepatitis.
🔵 *Alert:* Patients with advanced HIV infection may have increased risk of elevated triglyceride levels and in some cases fatal pancreatitis.
• In postmarketing surveillance, hyperglycemia requiring treatment has been reported. A causal relationship with ritonavir hasn't been established.
• Safety and effectiveness in children younger than age 1 month haven't been established.
• May cause toxicity in preterm neonates. Don't use oral solution in preterm neonates in the immediate postnatal period. A safe and effective dose in this patient population hasn't been established.
Dialyzable drug: Unlikely.
⚠ *Overdose S&S:* Paresthesia, renal failure with eosinophilia, alcohol-related toxicity with oral solution.

PREGNANCY-LACTATION-REPRODUCTION
• There are no adequate studies in pregnant women. Use only if potential benefit justifies potential risk to the fetus.
• Enroll pregnant women exposed to drug in the Antiretroviral Pregnancy Registry (1-800-258-4263).
• Once-daily dosing isn't recommended during pregnancy. Avoid using oral solution during pregnancy because it contains alcohol.
• Breastfeeding is contraindicated because of the potential for postnatal HIV-1 transmission.

NURSING CONSIDERATIONS
• When ritonavir is used with other protease inhibitors, consult full prescribing information and clinical study information of the other drugs.
• Monitor patient for immune reconstitution syndrome. During initial phase of treatment, patients responding to antiretroviral therapy may develop an inflammatory response to indolent or residual opportunistic infections (CMV, *Mycobacterium avium* complex, *Pneumocystis jiroveci* pneumonia, TB), which may necessitate further evaluation and treatment. Autoimmune disorders (such as Graves disease, polymyositis, and Guillain-Barré syndrome) have also been reported in the setting of immune reconstitution; however, time to onset is more variable, and can occur many months after initiation of antiretroviral treatment.
• Patients beginning regimens with ritonavir and nucleosides may improve GI tolerance by starting ritonavir alone and then adding nucleosides before completing 2 weeks of ritonavir.
• Patients who switch from soft gel capsule to tablet formulation may experience increased GI adverse reactions because of greater maximum plasma concentration achieved with the tablet formulation relative to the capsule.
• In patients with liver disease, monitor liver enzyme and triglyceride levels frequently, especially during the first 3 months of treatment.
• Monitor patient for redistribution or accumulation of body fat, which has been observed with antiretroviral therapy.
• Monitor total amounts of alcohol and propylene glycol from all drugs given to children ages 1 to 6 months, to avoid alcohol-related toxicity.

Reactions in bold italics are *life-threatening*. Interactions may have a *rapid onset* or a *delayed onset*.

• **Look alike–sound alike:** Don't confuse Norvir with Norvasc.

PATIENT TEACHING
• Explain that drug doesn't cure HIV infection and that opportunistic infections and other complications of HIV infection may continue to develop. Drug hasn't been shown to reduce the risk of transmitting HIV to others through sexual contact or blood contamination.
• Caution patient to take drug as prescribed and not to adjust dosage or stop therapy without first consulting prescriber.
• Advise patient who is experiencing increased GI adverse effects, such as nausea, vomiting, abdominal pain, or diarrhea, after switching from soft gel capsule to tablet formulation that these effects may diminish as therapy continues.
• Tell patient that taste of oral solution may be improved by mixing it with chocolate milk, Ensure, or Advera within 1 hour of the scheduled dose.
• Advise patient not to chew, crush, or break tablets.
• Instruct patient to take drug with a meal.
• Tell patient that if a dose is missed, to take the next dose as soon as possible. Advise patient not to double the next dose.
• Advise patient taking a PDE5 inhibitor for erectile dysfunction to promptly report hypotension, dizziness, visual changes, and prolonged erection to prescriber. Caution against exceeding the recommended reduced dosage.
• Advise patient using estrogen-based contraceptives to use an alternative contraceptive method during therapy.
• Caution patient to report signs and symptoms of pancreatitis (nausea, vomiting, and abdominal pain) immediately.
• Counsel patient that ritonavir must always be taken in combination with other antiretrovirals.
• Advise patient to report use of other drugs, including OTC drugs; this drug interacts with many drugs.

SAFETY ALERT!
BIOSIMILAR DRUG

riTUXimab
ri-TUK-si-mab

Rituxan

riTUXimab-pvvr
Ruxience

Therapeutic class: Antineoplastics
Pharmacologic class: Monoclonal antibodies

AVAILABLE FORMS
Injection: 10 mg/mL in 10-mL and 50-mL single-use, sterile vials

INDICATIONS & DOSAGES
➤ **Maintenance therapy for patients with previously untreated follicular, CD20-positive, B-cell non-Hodgkin lymphoma (NHL) who achieve response to rituximab in combination with chemotherapy**
Adults: 375 mg/m^2 IV as single agent every 8 weeks for 12 doses beginning 8 weeks after completion of combination therapy.
➤ **Wegener granulomatosis (WG); microscopic polyangiitis (MPA) in combination with glucocorticoids**
Adults: 375 mg/m^2 IV once weekly for 4 weeks. Give methylprednisolone 1,000 mg/day IV for 1 to 3 days followed by oral prednisone 1 mg/kg/day (not to exceed 80 mg/day and tapered per clinical need) to treat severe vasculitis symptoms. This regimen should begin within 14 days before or with the initiation of rituximab and may continue during and after the 4-week course of rituximab treatment.
Children ages 2 to 17: 375 mg/m^2 IV once weekly for 4 weeks. Give IV methylprednisolone 30 mg/kg (not to exceed 1 g/day) once daily for 3 days. Refer to manufacturer's instructions for follow-up treatment dosing for adults and children.
➤ **Previously untreated, follicular CD20-positive, B-cell NHL with cyclophosphamide-vincristine-prednisolone (CVP) chemotherapy regimen**
Adults: 375 mg/m^2 IV given on day 1 of each CVP cycle, for up to eight doses.

R

➤ **Previously untreated low-grade, CD20-positive, B-cell NHL following first-line treatment with CVP chemotherapy**
Adults: For patients who fail to progress after six to eight cycles of CVP chemotherapy, give 375 mg/m^2 IV once weekly for 4 doses every 6 months for up to 16 doses.

➤ **CD20-positive chronic lymphocytic leukemia (CLL) in combination with fludarabine and cyclophosphamide**
Adults: 375 mg/m^2 IV given day before combination treatment. Then give 500 mg/m^2 IV on day 1 of cycles two through six in combination with fludarabine and cyclophosphamide (every 28 days).

➤ **Relapsed or refractory low-grade or follicular, CD20-positive, B-cell NHL**
Adults: Initially, 375 mg/m^2 IV once weekly for four or eight doses. Retreatment for patients with progressive disease, 375 mg/m^2 IV infusion once weekly for four doses.

➤ **With ibritumomab tiuxetan (Zevalin) for relapsed or refractory low-grade, follicular or transformed B-cell NHL**
Adults: 250 mg/m^2 IV 4 hours before indium-111 Zevalin infusion. Repeat in 7 to 9 days, 4 hours before yttrium-90 Zevalin infusion.

➤ **With methotrexate to reduce the signs and symptoms of moderate to severely active RA in patients who have had an inadequate response to one or more TNF antagonists**
Adults: Two 1,000-mg IV infusions 2 weeks apart. To reduce the incidence and severity of infusion reactions, give methylprednisolone 100 mg IV, or its equivalent, 30 minutes before each infusion.

➤ **Diffuse large B-cell, CD20-positive NHL, given with cyclophosphamide-Adriamycin (doxorubicin)-Oncovin (vincristine)-prednisone (CHOP) chemotherapy regimen or other anthracycline-based chemotherapy regimens**
Adults: 375 mg/m^2 IV on day 1 of each chemotherapy cycle for up to eight infusions.

➤ **Moderate to severe pemphigus vulgaris**
Adults: Initially, give two 1,000-mg IV infusions separated by 2 weeks in combination with a tapering course of glucocorticoids; then use a maintenance schedule of rituximab 500-mg IV infusion at month 12 and every 6 months thereafter or based on clinical evaluation. If patient relapses, give rituximab 1,000-mg IV infusion with consideration to resuming or increasing the dosage of the glucocorticoid based on clinical evaluation. Allow at least 16 weeks between rituximab infusions. Methylprednisolone 100 mg IV or equivalent glucocorticoid is recommended 30 minutes before each rituximab infusion.

➤ **Burkitt lymphoma ◆**
Adults: 375 mg/m^2 IV on days 1 and 11 of cycles one and three and days 2 and 8 of cycles two and four. Or, 375 mg/m^2 IV at start of each chemotherapy cycle, followed by two additional doses 3 and 6 weeks after completion of chemotherapy. Or, 50 mg/m^2 IV on day 8 and 375 mg/m^2 IV on days 10 and 12 of cycle two, followed by 375 mg/m^2 IV on day 8 of cycles three to seven.

ADMINISTRATION

IV
▼ Protect vials from direct sunlight.
▼ Give as an infusion; don't give as IV push or bolus.
▼ Begin infusion at rate of 50 mg/hour. If no hypersensitivity or infusion-related events occur, increase rate by 50 mg/hour every 30 minutes, to maximum of 400 mg/hour. Start subsequent infusions at 100 mg/hour and increase by 100 mg/hour every 30 minutes, to maximum of 400 mg/hour as tolerated.
▼ For previously untreated follicular NHL and diffuse large B-cell NHL, patients may receive a 90-minute infusion in cycle 2 with a glucocorticoid-containing chemotherapy regimen if they didn't experience a grade 3 or 4 infusion-related adverse event during cycle 1. Refer to manufacturer's instructions.
▼ Dilute to yield 1 to 4 mg/mL in bag of D$_5$W or NSS. Gently invert bag to mix solution.
▼ Discard unused portion left in vial.
▼ Store diluted solutions in refrigerator at 36° to 46° F (2° to 8° C) because they don't contain a preservative.
▼ **Incompatibilities:** Other IV drugs.

Reactions in bold italics are *life-threatening*. Interactions may have a *rapid onset* or a *delayed onset*.

ACTION
A murine and human monoclonal antibody directed against CD20 antigen found on the surface of normal and malignant B lymphocytes. Binding to this antigen mediates the lysis of the B cells.

Route	Onset	Peak	Duration
IV	Variable	Variable	6–12 mo

Half-life: Varies widely, possibly because of differences in tumor burden among patients and changes in CD-positive B-cell populations on repeated therapy.

ADVERSE REACTIONS
CNS: asthenia, fever, headache, agitation, dizziness, fatigue, hypesthesia, hypertonia, insomnia, malaise, nervousness, pain, paresthesia, somnolence, vertigo. **CV:** hypotension, *arrhythmias, bradycardia,* chest pain, edema, flushing, HTN, peripheral edema, tachycardia, *HF.* **EENT:** conjunctivitis, rhinitis, sinusitis, sore throat. **GI:** nausea, abdominal pain or enlargement, anorexia, diarrhea, dyspepsia, taste perversion, vomiting. **GU:** *acute renal failure.* **Hematologic:** *leukopenia, neutropenia, thrombocytopenia, lymphopenia,* anemia. **Metabolic:** hyperglycemia, hypocalcemia, weight gain. **Musculoskeletal:** back pain, myalgia. **Respiratory:** *bronchospasm,* bronchitis, cough increase, dyspnea. **Skin:** pruritus, rash, *severe mucocutaneous reactions,* pain at injection site, urticaria. **Other:** chills, rigors, *angioedema, infusion reaction,* infection, *serious infection, TLS,* tumor pain.

INTERACTIONS
Drug-drug. *Certolizumab, denosumab, tocilizumab:* May increase risk of serious infection. Avoid use together.
Cisplatin: May cause renal toxicity. Monitor renal function tests.
Leflunomide: May increase risk of hematologic toxicity. Monitor patient for bone marrow suppression at least monthly if both medications are needed.
🟥 *Alert: Live-virus vaccines:* Virus replication may occur. Avoid vaccination with live-virus vaccines.

EFFECTS ON LAB TEST RESULTS
• May increase glucose and LDH levels. May decrease calcium and phosphate levels.

• May decrease Hb level and WBC, platelet, and neutrophil counts.

CONTRAINDICATIONS & CAUTIONS
Black Box Warning HBV reactivation, including fulminant hepatitis, hepatic failure, and death, may occur in patients treated with rituximab. ■
🟥 *Alert:* Consult hepatitis expert when screening identifies patients at risk for HBV reactivation due to prior HBV infection.
Dialyzable drug: Unknown.

PREGNANCY-LACTATION-REPRODUCTION
• Based on human data, drug can cause adverse developmental outcomes, including B-cell lymphocytopenia, in infants exposed to drug in utero. Advise pregnant women of the risk to a fetus.
• Women of childbearing potential should use effective contraception during therapy and for 12 months after therapy ends.
• It isn't known if drug appears in human milk. Patient should discontinue breastfeeding or discontinue drug, taking into account importance of drug to the mother.

NURSING CONSIDERATIONS
Black Box Warning Deaths from infusion reactions have occurred; 80% of fatal reactions are associated with the first infusion. Monitor patient for infusion reaction complex, including hypoxia, pulmonary infiltrates, ARDS, MI, or cardiogenic shock. Interrupt infusion or slow infusion rate until symptoms improve; then continue infusion at no more than one-half the previous rate. Closely monitor patient. Discontinue rituximab infusion for severe reactions and administer medical treatment for grade 3 or 4 infusion reactions. ■
• Monitor patient's BP closely during infusion. If hypotension, bronchospasm, or angioedema occurs, stop infusion and restart at half the rate when symptoms resolve.
• If serious or life-threatening arrhythmias occur, stop infusion. If patient develops significant arrhythmias, monitor cardiac function during and after subsequent infusions.
• *Pneumocystis jiroveci* pneumonia and antiherpetic viral prophylaxis is recommended for patients with CLL during and for up to 12 months after treatment ends.

Black Box Warning Screen all patients for HBV infection before treatment by measuring HbsAg and hepatitis B core antibody. Monitor patients with evidence of current or prior HBV infection during and for several months after therapy. If HBV reactivation occurs, discontinue rituximab and concomitant chemotherapy and begin appropriate treatment. ■

• Monitor patients with WG and MPA carefully for signs and symptoms of infection (fever, pain, cold or flu symptoms, erythema) if biological agents or DMARDs are used concomitantly.

❶ *Alert:* Prophylaxis for *P. jiroveci* pneumonia is recommended for patients with WG and MPA during treatment with rituximab and for at least 6 months after the last infusion.

Black Box Warning Severe mucocutaneous reactions (including toxic epidermal necrolysis, SJS, paraneoplastic pemphigus, and lichenoid or vesiculobullous dermatitis) may occur, with variable onset. Avoid further infusions and promptly start treatment of the skin reaction. ■

• Infusion-related reactions are most severe with the first infusion. Subsequent infusions are generally well tolerated.

❶ *Alert:* Acute renal failure requiring dialysis has been reported in the setting of TLS after treatment of patients with NHL.

• Patients at high risk for TLS may receive prophylactic allopurinol and hydration to correct hyperuricemia. Monitor renal function and fluid balance, and correct electrolyte abnormalities.

Black Box Warning JC virus infection resulting in progressive multifocal leukoencephalopathy has been reported in patients within 12 months of their last rituximab infusion. Monitor patient for new-onset neurologic manifestations. ■

• Obtain CBC at regular intervals and more frequently in patients in whom cytopenias develop.

• Monitor patients at risk for HBV infection closely. Discontinue drug at first sign of HBV infection.

• Monitor patient for abdominal pain. Bowel obstruction and perforation have occurred with chemotherapy.

PATIENT TEACHING

• Provide patient with medication guide to read before each treatment session.

• Tell patient to report signs and symptoms of hypersensitivity, such as itching, rash, chills, or rigor, during and after infusion.

• Urge patient to report all adverse reactions, especially fever, sore throat, fatigue, easy bruising, nosebleeds, bleeding gums, abdominal pain, or tarry stools and to take temperature daily.

• Advise breastfeeding patient to stop breastfeeding until drug levels are undetectable.

SAFETY ALERT!

rivaroxaban ⚠
riv-a-ROX-a-ban

Xarelto⌀

Therapeutic class: Anticoagulants
Pharmacologic class: Factor Xa inhibitors

AVAILABLE FORMS
Tablets: 2.5 mg, 10 mg, 15 mg, 20 mg

INDICATIONS & DOSAGES

➤ **Prophylaxis of DVT that may lead to PE in patients undergoing knee or hip replacement surgery**
Adults: 10 mg PO once daily, 6 to 10 hours after surgery once hemostasis has been established. Treat for 35 days after hip replacement surgery and 12 days after knee replacement surgery.

Adjust-a-dose: If CrCl is less than 30 mL/minute, avoid use. Use cautiously in patients with moderate renal impairment (CrCl ranging from 30 to less than 50 mL/minute).

➤ **Treatment of DVT or PE**
Adults: 15 mg PO b.i.d. with food for 21 days; then 20 mg PO once daily for remainder of treatment.

Adjust-a-dose: If CrCl is less than 30 mL/minute, avoid use.

➤ **To decrease risk of recurrent DVT or PE after initial 6 months of treatment**
Adults: 20 mg PO once daily with food.

Adjust-a-dose: If CrCl is less than 30 mL/minute, avoid use.

Reactions in bold italics are *life-threatening*. Interactions may have a *rapid onset* or a *delayed onset*.

➤ **Stroke and systemic embolism risk reduction in patients with nonvalvular atrial fibrillation**

Adults: 20 mg once daily with evening meal.
Adjust-a-dose: In patients with CrCl of 15 to 50 mL/minute, reduce dosage to 15 mg once daily with evening meal. Avoid use in patients with CrCl less than 15 mL/minute.

➤ **To reduce risk of major cardiovascular events in patients with chronic coronary artery disease or peripheral artery disease, in combination with aspirin**

Adults: 2.5 mg PO b.i.d., with or without food, in combination with aspirin (75–100 mg) once daily.

ADMINISTRATION
PO

• Give 2.5- or 10-mg tablets without regard for food. Give 15- and 20-mg tablets with food. For nonvalvular atrial fibrillation, give with evening meal.

• For patients unable to swallow tablets whole, crush tablet and mix with applesauce immediately before use; administer orally. Immediately follow administration of a crushed 15- or 20-mg tablet with food.

• For administration via NG or gastric feeding tube, crush tablet and suspend in 50 mL of water; confirm gastric placement and administer within 4 hours. Delivery of drug into the small intestine will result in reduced absorption. Immediately follow administration of a crushed 15- or 20-mg tablet with an enteral feeding.

ACTION

Selectively blocks the active site of factor Xa, which is necessary for coagulation.

Route	Onset	Peak	Duration
PO	Unknown	2–4 hr	Unknown

Half-life: 5 to 9 hours.

ADVERSE REACTIONS

CNS: syncope, fatigue, dizziness, anxiety, depression. **EENT:** oropharyngeal pain, sinusitis. **GI:** abdominal pain, dyspepsia, *GI hemorrhage.* **GU:** UTI. **Hematologic:** *bleeding events (including hemorrhage).* **Musculoskeletal:** extremity pain, muscle spasm, back pain. **Skin:** wound secretion, pruritus, blister.

INTERACTIONS

Drug-drug. *Anticoagulants (warfarin), antithrombotic agents, aspirin, fibrinolytics, NSAIDs, P2Y12 platelet aggregation inhibitors, thienopyridines, SSNRIs, SSRIs:* May increase bleeding risk. Avoid use together. Monitor patient carefully for bleeding if drugs must be given together.
Combined P-gp and strong CYP3A4 inducers (carbamazepine, phenytoin, rifampin): May significantly decrease rivaroxaban level. Avoid use together.
Combined P-gp and strong CYP3A4 inhibitors (conivaptan, indinavir/ritonavir, itraconazole, ketoconazole, lopinavir–ritonavir, ritonavir): May significantly increase rivaroxaban level. Avoid use together.
Combined P-gp and weak or moderate CYP3A4 inhibitors (amiodarone, azithromycin, diltiazem, dronedarone, erythromycin, felodipine, quinidine, ranolazine, verapamil): May increase rivaroxaban level. Use together only if benefit outweighs risk.
Mifepristone: May increase risk of bleeding. Avoid use together.
Drug-herb. *St. John's wort:* May significantly decrease rivaroxaban level. Avoid use together.

EFFECTS ON LAB TEST RESULTS

• May increase AST, ALT, total bilirubin, and GGT levels.

CONTRAINDICATIONS & CAUTIONS

Black Box Warning There is an increased risk of epidural or spinal hematomas, possibly resulting in long-term or permanent paralysis, in patients who have received anticoagulants and are receiving neuraxial anesthesia or undergoing spinal puncture. Factors that can increase the risk of epidural or spinal hematomas in these patients include use of indwelling epidural catheters; concomitant use of other drugs that affect hemostasis, such as NSAIDs, platelet inhibitors, and other anticoagulants; history of traumatic or repeated epidural or spinal punctures; and history of spinal deformity or spinal surgery. Monitor patients frequently for neurologic impairment. If neurologic compromise is noted, urgent treatment is necessary. Consider risks and benefits before neuraxial procedures in

R

patients who have received anticoagulants for thromboprophylaxis. ∎

Black Box Warning Discontinuing rivaroxaban places patients at increased risk for thrombotic events. If anticoagulation with rivaroxaban must be discontinued for a reason other than pathological bleeding or completion of a course of therapy, consider coverage with another anticoagulant. ∎

• Contraindicated in patients hypersensitive to drug and in those with active major bleeding.

• Use isn't recommended in patients with prosthetic heart valves.

• Use cautiously in conditions associated with increased risk of hemorrhage, with concurrent use of drugs affecting hemostasis (platelet aggregation inhibitors, other antithrombotic agents, fibrinolytics, thienopyridines, long-term NSAIDs, SSNRIs, SSRIs), and in elderly patients.

• Avoid use in patients with CrCl of less than 30 mL/minute who are taking drug for PE or DVT treatment or recurrence prophylaxis or prophylaxis of DVT after hip or knee replacement surgery.

• In patients with nonvalvular atrial fibrillation, assess renal function more frequently in situations in which renal function may decline and adjust therapy accordingly. Consider dosage adjustment or drug discontinuation in patients who develop acute renal failure.

• Avoid use in patients with moderate or severe hepatic impairment (Child-Pugh class B or C) and in those with hepatic disease associated with coagulopathy.

• Avoid use in patients receiving drugs that are concurrent P-gp and strong CYP3A4 inhibitors or inducers.

※ Use cautiously in Japanese patients because drug exposure in these patients may be increased up to 40% when compared to other ethnicities, but differences are reduced when values are corrected for body weight.

• Safety and effectiveness in children haven't been established.

Dialyzable drug: No.

⚠ ***Overdose S&S:*** Hemorrhage.

PREGNANCY-LACTATION-REPRODUCTION

• There are no adequate studies in pregnant women. Use cautiously and only if potential benefit justifies potential risk to the fetus because of the potential for pregnancy-related hemorrhage or emergent delivery with use of an anticoagulant that isn't readily reversible.

• It isn't known if drug appears in human milk. Patient should discontinue breastfeeding or discontinue drug.

NURSING CONSIDERATIONS

Black Box Warning Monitor patient frequently for signs and symptoms of neurologic impairment. If neurologic compromise is noted, urgent treatment is necessary. ∎

Black Box Warning Consider the benefits and risks before neuraxial intervention in patients anticoagulated or to be anticoagulated for thromboprophylaxis. Optimal timing between rivaroxaban administration and neuraxial procedures isn't known. ∎

• Don't remove an epidural catheter earlier than 18 hours after last administration of drug, and don't give next dose until 6 hours after catheter removal unless traumatic puncture occurred; if puncture has occurred, wait 24 hours before giving next dose.

• Monitor patient carefully for bleeding, which can occur at any site during therapy.

• If an anticoagulant must be discontinued to reduce risk of bleeding with surgical or other procedures, stop drug at least 24 hours before procedure. When deciding whether to delay a procedure until 24 hours after last dose, weigh the increased risk of bleeding against the urgency of intervention. Restart drug after procedure when adequate hemostasis has been established, as the time to onset of therapeutic effect is short.

❶ ***Alert:*** Watch for signs and symptoms of blood loss. Search for a bleeding site if an unexplained fall in hematocrit or BP occurs. Patients with moderate renal failure (CrCl ranging from 30 to less than 50 mL/minute) are at increased risk.

PATIENT TEACHING

• Instruct patient to take drug only as directed and not to discontinue drug without consulting prescriber.

• Tell patient on once-daily dosing that if a dose is missed, to take dose as soon as patient remembers and to resume normal regimen the following day.

● Alert: If patient has had neuraxial anesthesia or spinal puncture, especially if taking concomitant NSAIDs or platelet inhibitors, advise patient to watch for signs and symptoms of spinal or epidural hematoma (midline back pain, tingling, numbness of the limbs, muscular weakness, bowel or bladder dysfunction). If any of these signs and symptoms occur, advise patient to contact prescriber immediately.

• Advise patient to watch for bleeding risks, especially if patient had a spinal catheter or is currently taking drugs or supplements that increase bleeding risk.

• Instruct female patient to consult prescriber if she is pregnant, plans to become pregnant, or intends to breastfeed.

• Caution patient to report changes in medications or herbal supplements or unusual bleeding or bruising.

• Advise patient who can't swallow the tablet whole to crush tablet and combine with a small amount of applesauce followed by food.

• Instruct patient with an NG or gastric feeding tube to crush the tablet and mix it with 50 mL of water before administering via the tube and to follow administration of 15- or 20-mg tablet with an enteral feeding.

• Instruct patient to inform all health care providers that patient is taking rivaroxaban before any invasive procedure (including dental procedures) is scheduled.

---

rivastigmine
ri-va-STIG-meen

Exelon Patch

rivastigmine tartrateℇ
Exelon

Therapeutic class: Anti-Alzheimer drugs
Pharmacologic class: Cholinesterase inhibitors

AVAILABLE FORMS
Capsules ⎒: 1.5 mg, 3 mg, 4.5 mg, 6 mg
Transdermal patch: 4.6 mg/24 hours, 9.5 mg/24 hours, 13.3 mg/24 hours

INDICATIONS & DOSAGES
Adjust-a-dose (for all indications): Patients with moderate to severe renal impairment (GFR less than 50 mL/minute) or mild to moderate hepatic impairment (Child-Pugh score of 5 to 9) may be able to only tolerate lower doses of oral drug. For patients with mild to moderate hepatic impairment, consider using 4.6 mg/24 hours transdermal patch for both initial and maintenance dose. For patients weighing less than 50 kg, watch for toxicities (nausea, vomiting) and if they occur, consider reducing maintenance dose; reduce dose of transdermal patch to 4.6 mg/24 hours.

➚ **Mild to moderate Alzheimer dementia**
Adults: Initially, 1.5 mg PO b.i.d. with food. If tolerated, may increase to 3 mg b.i.d. after 2 weeks. After 2 weeks at this dose, may increase to 4.5 mg b.i.d. and to 6 mg b.i.d., as tolerated. Effective dosage range is 6 to 12 mg daily; maximum, 12 mg daily. Or, 4.6 mg/24 hours transdermal patch. After 4 weeks, if tolerated, increase to 9.5 mg/ 24 hours transdermal patch for as long as therapeutic benefit persists; if needed after at least 4 weeks, increase to 13.3 mg/24 hours transdermal patch. Maximum dose is 13.3 mg/24 hours.

➚ **Severe Alzheimer dementia (transdermal patch only)**
Adults: Initially, 4.6 mg/24 hours transdermal patch once daily. After 4 weeks, if tolerated, increase to 9.5 mg/24 hours transdermal patch; then, if tolerated after an additional 4 weeks, increase to 13.3 mg/24 hours transdermal patch.

➚ **Mild to moderate dementia associated with Parkinson disease**
Adults: Initially, 1.5 mg PO b.i.d. May increase, as tolerated, to 3 mg b.i.d., then to 4.5 mg b.i.d., and finally to 6 mg b.i.d. after a minimum of 4 weeks at each dose; maximum dose is 12 mg daily.

Or, 4.6 mg/24 hours transdermal patch. After 4 weeks, if tolerated, increase to 9.5 mg/24 hours transdermal patch for as long as therapeutic benefit persists; if needed after at least 4 weeks, increase to 13.3 mg/ 24 hours transdermal patch. Maximum dose is 13.3 mg/24 hours.

R

➤ **Treatment of neuropsychiatric symptoms associated with Lewy body dementia** ◆

Adults: Initially, 1.5 mg PO b.i.d.; increase as tolerated by 1.5 mg b.i.d. every 2 weeks to a maximum of 6 mg b.i.d. Ongoing therapy is required.

ADMINISTRATION

PO
- Give drug with food in the morning and evening.
- Patient should swallow capsule whole.

Transdermal
- Apply patch once daily to clean, dry, hairless skin on the upper or lower back, upper arm, or chest, in a place not rubbed by tight clothing.
- Change the site daily, and don't use the same site within 14 days. Avoid exposing patch to external heat sources (sauna, excess sunlight).
- Press patch firmly into place until the edges stick well.
- Avoid eye contact; wash hands with soap and water after removing patch. In case of contact with eyes or if eyes become red after handling patch, rinse immediately with plenty of water. Seek medical advice if symptoms don't resolve.

ACTION

Thought to increase acetylcholine level by inhibiting cholinesterase enzyme, which causes acetylcholine hydrolysis.

Route	Onset	Peak	Duration
PO	Unknown	1 hr	8–10 hr
Transdermal	Unknown	8–16 hr	24 hr

Half-life: Oral, 1½ hours; transdermal, 3 hours.

ADVERSE REACTIONS

CNS: headache, dizziness, syncope, fatigue, asthenia, malaise, somnolence, tremor, insomnia, confusion, depression, anxiety, hallucinations, aggressive reaction, vertigo, agitation, nervousness, delusion, paranoid reaction, pain. **CV:** HTN, chest pain, peripheral edema. **EENT:** rhinitis, pharyngitis. **GI:** nausea, vomiting, diarrhea, anorexia, abdominal pain, dyspepsia, constipation, flatulence, eructation, *GI bleeding.* **GU:** UTI, incontinence. **Metabolic:** weight loss.

Musculoskeletal: bradykinesia, dyskinesia, hypokinesia, weakness, cogwheel rigidity. **Respiratory:** URI, cough, bronchitis. **Skin:** increased sweating, rash. **Other:** flu-like symptoms.

INTERACTIONS

Drug-drug. *Anticholinergics:* May decrease effectiveness of anticholinergic. Monitor patient for expected therapeutic effects.
Beta blockers, bradycardia-inducing drugs: May worsen bradycardia. Use together isn't recommended.
Bethanechol, succinylcholine, other neuromuscular-blocking drugs or cholinergic antagonists: May have synergistic effect. Monitor patient closely.
Metoclopramide: May enhance risk of extrapyramidal reactions. Concomitant use isn't recommended.
NSAIDs: May increase gastric acid secretions. Monitor patient for symptoms of active or occult GI bleeding.
Drug-lifestyle. *Smoking:* May increase drug clearance. Discourage smoking.

EFFECTS ON LAB TEST RESULTS

None reported.

CONTRAINDICATIONS & CAUTIONS

- Contraindicated in patients hypersensitive to drug, other carbamate derivatives, or other components of drug.
- Isolated cases of disseminated allergic dermatitis, irrespective of administration route (oral or transdermal), have been noted in postmarketing reports. Discontinue drug if disseminated allergic dermatitis occurs.
- Contraindicated in patients with history of transdermal patch application-site reaction suggestive of allergic contact dermatitis.
- Use cautiously in patients with history of CV disease, GI bleeding, seizure disorder, GU conditions, asthma, or obstructive pulmonary disease.

Dialyzable drug: No.

⚠ **Overdose S&S:** Nausea, vomiting, excessive salivation, sweating, bradycardia, hypotension, respiratory depression, syncope, seizures, muscle weakness.

Reactions in bold italics are *life-threatening*. Interactions may have a *rapid onset* or a *delayed onset*.

PREGNANCY-LACTATION-REPRODUCTION

• There are no adequate studies in pregnant women. Use during pregnancy only if clearly needed.

• It isn't known if drug appears in human milk. Patient should discontinue breastfeeding or discontinue drug.

NURSING CONSIDERATIONS

• Expect significant GI adverse effects (such as nausea, vomiting, anorexia, and weight loss). These effects are less common during maintenance doses.

• Monitor patient for evidence of active or occult GI bleeding.

• Dramatic memory improvement is unlikely. As disease progresses, the benefits of drug may decline.

• Monitor patient for severe nausea, vomiting, and diarrhea, which may lead to dehydration and weight loss.

• Carefully monitor patient with a history of GI bleeding, NSAID use, arrhythmias, seizures, or pulmonary conditions for adverse effects.

• If adverse reactions, such as diarrhea, loss of appetite, nausea, or vomiting, occur with transdermal patch, stop use for several days, then restart at the same or lower dose. If treatment is interrupted for more than several days, restart patch at the lowest dose and retitrate.

• Patients weighing less than 50 kg may experience more adverse reactions when using the transdermal patch.

• Application-site reactions may occur with the transdermal patch. Discontinue treatment if application-site reaction spreads beyond the patch size, if there's evidence of a more intense local reaction (increasing erythema, edema, papules, vesicles), and if symptoms don't significantly improve within 48 hours after patch removal.

• When switching from oral form to the transdermal patch, patients on a total daily dose of less than 6 mg can be switched to 4.6 mg/24 hours. Patients taking 6 to 12 mg PO can switch to the 9.5 mg/24 hour patch. The patch should be applied on the day after the last oral dose.

PATIENT TEACHING

• Tell caregiver to give drug with food in the morning and evening.

• Advise patient that memory improvement may be subtle and that drug more likely slows future memory loss.

• Tell patient to report nausea, vomiting, or diarrhea.

• Tell patient to consult prescriber before using OTC drugs.

• Tell patient to apply patch once daily to clean, dry, hairless skin in a place not rubbed by tight clothing and to retain pouch for disposal.

• Teach patient that the recommended sites for patch placement include the upper or lower back, upper arm, or chest.

• Tell patient to change the site daily and not to use the same site within 14 days.

• Tell patient to press the patch firmly into place until the edges stick well.

• Advise patient to remove used patch, place in previously saved pouch and discard in trash (away from pets or children), and then wash hands with soap and water. In case of contact with eyes or if eyes become red after handling patch, tell patient to rinse immediately with plenty of water and seek medical advice if symptoms don't resolve.

roflumilast
roe-FLUE-mi-last

Daliresp

Therapeutic class: Miscellaneous respiratory drugs
Pharmacologic class: Selective phosphodiesterase inhibitors

R

AVAILABLE FORMS
Tablets: 250 mcg, 500 mcg

INDICATIONS & DOSAGES
➤ **To reduce risk of COPD exacerbations in patients with severe COPD associated with chronic bronchitis and a history of exacerbations**
Adults: 250 mcg once daily for 4 weeks and increasing to 500 mcg PO daily (maintenance dose).

ADMINISTRATION

PO

- Give drug without regard to food.

ACTION

Selectively inhibits phosphodiesterase-4 (PDE₄), which is a cAMP-metabolizing enzyme in the lung tissue. Inhibition of PDE₄ leads to accumulation of intracellular cAMP. Effects of drug are thought to be related to the increased intracellular cAMP in lung cells.

Route	Onset	Peak	Duration
PO	Unknown	1–2 hr	Unknown

Half-life: 17 hours; N-oxide metabolite, 30 hours.

ADVERSE REACTIONS

CNS: headache, insomnia, dizziness.
GI: diarrhea, nausea, decreased appetite.
Metabolic: weight loss. **Musculoskeletal:** back pain. **Other:** flulike symptoms.

INTERACTIONS

Drug-drug. *Ciprofloxacin (systemic):* May increase roflumilast serum concentration. Monitor therapy.
CYP450 inducers (carbamazepine, phenobarbital, phenytoin, rifampin): May decrease the effectiveness of roflumilast. Avoid use together.
CYP450 inhibitors (cimetidine, erythromycin, fluvoxamine, ketoconazole): May increase roflumilast concentration and risk of adverse reactions. Use together cautiously.
Immunosuppressants (except for beclomethasone [oral inhalation], cytarabine [liposomal], fluticasone [oral inhalation]): May enhance immunosuppressive effect. Consider therapy modification.

EFFECTS ON LAB TEST RESULTS

None reported.

CONTRAINDICATIONS & CAUTIONS

- Contraindicated in patients hypersensitive to drug or its components and in those with moderate to severe hepatic impairment (Child-Pugh class B or C).
- Use cautiously in patients with history of depression or suicidal thoughts and behaviors.

Dialyzable drug: Unlikely.

PREGNANCY-LACTATION-REPRODUCTION

- There are no adequate studies in pregnant women. Use only if potential benefit justifies potential risk to the fetus.
- Don't use during labor and delivery.
- Drug may appear in human milk. Patient should discontinue breastfeeding or discontinue drug.

NURSING CONSIDERATIONS

- Drug isn't a bronchodilator and isn't indicated for the relief of acute bronchospasm.
- Monitor patients for signs and symptoms of psychiatric adverse events, including insomnia, anxiety, depression, suicidal ideation, and suicide attempts. If events occur, evaluate the risks versus benefits of continuing drug.
- Monitor weight regularly; if unexplained or significant weight loss occurs, evaluate cause and consider stopping drug.

PATIENT TEACHING

- Educate patient that drug isn't a bronchodilator and isn't to be used for the relief of acute bronchospasm.
- Advise patient, family, and caregivers to watch for signs and symptoms of psychiatric adverse events, including insomnia, anxiety, depression, suicidal ideation, and suicide attempts, and to report any occurrences to the health care provider.
- Tell patient to report unexplained or significant weight loss.

rolapitant hydrochloride
roe-LA-pi-tant

Varubi

Therapeutic class: Antiemetics
Pharmacologic class: Substance P and neurokinin-1 receptor antagonists

AVAILABLE FORMS

Injectable emulsion: 166.5 mg/92.5 mL
Tablets: 90 mg

INDICATIONS & DOSAGES

➤ **Prevention of delayed nausea and vomiting associated with emetogenic chemotherapy, including but not limited**

Reactions in bold italics are *life-threatening*. Interactions may have a *rapid onset* or a ***delayed onset***.

to highly emetogenic chemotherapy (in combination with other antiemetics)
Adults: 180 mg PO or 166.5 mg IV infusion over 30 minutes. Administer within 2 hours of chemotherapy on day 1. Give dexamethasone 20 mg on day 1, 30 minutes before chemotherapy and then 8 mg PO b.i.d. on days 2, 3, and 4. Also give a 5-HT₃ receptor antagonist on day 1. Refer to manufacturer's instructions for appropriate dosing information.

➤ **Prevention of delayed nausea and vomiting associated with anthracycline and cyclophosphamide–based or moderately emetogenic chemotherapy, in combination with other antiemetics**
Adults: 180 mg PO or 166.5 mg IV infusion over 30 minutes. Administer within 2 hours of chemotherapy on day 1. Give dexamethasone 20 mg PO 30 minutes before chemotherapy on day 1. Also give a 5-HT₃ receptor antagonist on day 1. Refer to manufacturer's instructions for appropriate dosing information.

ADMINISTRATION
PO
- Give drug before each scheduled chemotherapy cycle, but at no less than 2-week intervals.
- Give without regard to meals.
- Store at room temperature.

IV
▼ Inspect injectable emulsion for particulate matter and discoloration before administration; discard if particulates or discoloration is present. Don't use if contamination is suspected.

▼ Use and maintain aseptic technique while handling injectable emulsion.

▼ Don't add diluents or other medications directly to vial.

▼ Administer dose by inserting a vented IV set through the septum of the vial. Once the stopper is punctured, use immediately. Don't dilute injectable emulsion.

▼ Infuse 92.5 mL from vial over 30 minutes.

▼ **Incompatibilities:** None listed by manufacturer. Consult a drug incompatibility reference for more information.

ACTION
A selective and competitive antagonist of human substance P/neurokinin-1 receptors in the brain. Appears to be synergistic with 5-HT₃ antagonists and corticosteroids.

Route	Onset	Peak	Duration
PO	30 min	4 hr	Unknown
IV	Rapid	30 min	Unknown

Half-life: About 7 days.

ADVERSE REACTIONS
CNS: dizziness. **GI:** abdominal pain, decreased appetite, dyspepsia, stomatitis. **GU:** UTI. **Hematologic:** *neutropenia,* anemia. **Respiratory:** hiccups. **Other:** infusion-related reactions.

INTERACTIONS
Drug-drug. *Breast cancer resistance protein (BCRP) substrates with a narrow therapeutic index (irinotecan, methotrexate, rosuvastatin, topotecan):* May increase plasma concentrations of BCRP substrates and risk of BCRP-related adverse reactions. Monitor patient for increased adverse effects. Use lowest effective rosuvastatin dose.
CYP2D6 substrates (dextromethorphan, TCAs): May increase plasma concentrations of CYP2D6 substrates. Monitor patient closely for increased adverse effects.
CYP2D6 substrates with a narrow therapeutic index (pimozide, thioridazine): May increase pimozide and thioridazine level and risk of QT-interval prolongation. Use is contraindicated.
Dabigatran, edoxaban: May increase serum concentration of anticoagulant. Consider therapy modification.
P-gp substrates with a narrow therapeutic index (digoxin): May increase plasma concentrations of P-gp substrates and risk of P-gp–related adverse reactions. Monitor drug levels and watch for increased adverse reactions if concomitant use can't be avoided.
Strong CYP3A4 inducers (rifampin): May decrease plasma concentration and therapeutic effect of rolapitant. Avoid concomitant use, if possible.
Warfarin: May increase warfarin level. Monitor INR and PTT; adjust doses as needed to maintain target INR.

R

EFFECTS ON LAB TEST RESULTS

• May decrease Hb level and neutrophil count.

CONTRAINDICATIONS & CAUTIONS

• Contraindicated in patients hypersensitive to drug or its components (including soybean oil). Because cross reactions to other allergens are possible, closely monitor patients with known allergies to legumes or other related allergens.

• Contraindicated in patients receiving thioridazine and pimozide because of risk of QT-interval prolongation and torsades de pointes.

• Use cautiously in patients receiving drugs that affect the CYP2D6 enzyme system. Inhibitory effects of rolapitant on CYP2D6 may last for 7 days or longer.

• Drug hasn't been studied in patients with severe hepatic impairment (Child-Pugh class C); avoid use. Monitor closely for adverse reactions if use can't be avoided.

• Safety and effectiveness in children haven't been established.

Dialyzable drug: Unlikely.

PREGNANCY-LACTATION-REPRODUCTION

• There are no data regarding use of rolapitant in pregnant women. Use only if benefits outweigh potential risks to the fetus.

• It isn't known if drug appears in human milk. Give only if benefits outweigh potential risks to breastfed infant.

NURSING CONSIDERATIONS

🔴 *Alert:* Before giving drug, assess patient's current drug list for potential drug-drug interactions.

• Drug is used to prevent, not treat, nausea and vomiting.

• Always use drug in combination with a corticosteroid and a 5-HT₃ inhibitor.

• If anaphylaxis or other serious hypersensitivity or infusion reactions occur in patients receiving injectable emulsion, immediately stop injectable emulsion and begin appropriate emergency interventions.

• *Look alike–sound alike:* Don't confuse rolapitant with aprepitant or fosaprepitant.

PATIENT TEACHING

• Remind patient that rolapitant is taken in combination with a corticosteroid and a 5-HT₃ inhibitor.

• Instruct patient to take breakthrough antiemetics rather than taking more rolapitant if nausea or vomiting isn't controlled.

• Remind patient to take drug 1 to 2 hours before scheduled chemotherapy.

• Inform patient that rolapitant is associated with drug-drug interactions and that it's important to report all medications being taken, including OTC drugs and supplements, before starting therapy.

• Advise patient to inform prescriber and pharmacist of dosage changes or new prescription drug therapy because drug interactions can be delayed after rolapitant is discontinued.

• Advise female patient to inform prescriber if she is or plans to become pregnant or is breastfeeding.

rOPINIRole hydrochloride
roe-PIN-i-role

Requip, Requip XL

Therapeutic class: Antiparkinsonians
Pharmacologic class: Nonergot dopamine agonists

AVAILABLE FORMS

Tablets: 0.25 mg, 0.5 mg, 1 mg, 2 mg, 3 mg, 4 mg, 5 mg
Tablets (extended-release) 🔴*:* 2 mg, 4 mg, 6 mg, 8 mg, 12 mg

INDICATIONS & DOSAGES

Adjust-a-dose (for all indications): For patients with ESRD on hemodialysis using immediate-release formula, give 0.25 mg PO t.i.d. for Parkinson disease and 0.25 mg PO daily for restless legs syndrome. Base further dosage escalations on tolerability and need for efficacy. Recommended maximum total daily dose in patients receiving regular dialysis is 18 mg/day for Parkinson disease and 3 mg daily for restless legs syndrome. Supplemental doses after dialysis aren't required. No dosage adjustment is necessary in patients with moderate renal impairment (CrCl of 30 to 50 mL/ minute).

For patients with ESRD on hemodialysis using extended-release formula, give 2 mg once daily initially. May titrate dosage upward for a maximum dose of 18 mg/day if needed. Supplemental doses after dialysis aren't required.

➤ **Idiopathic Parkinson disease**
Adults: Initially, 0.25 mg PO t.i.d. Increase dose by 0.25 mg t.i.d. at weekly intervals for 4 weeks. After week 4, daily dosage may be increased by 1.5 mg/day on a weekly basis up to a dose of 9 mg/day, and then by up to 3 mg/day weekly to a total dose of 24 mg/day (8 mg t.i.d.). For extended-release form, starting dosage is 2 mg PO once daily for 1 to 2 weeks. May increase by 2 mg/day at 1-week or longer intervals. Although the maximum dosage is 24 mg/day, patients with advanced Parkinson disease should generally be maintained at 8 mg or lower daily and patients with early Parkinson disease should generally be maintained at 12 mg or lower daily. To switch from immediate-release to extended-release tablets, refer to manufacturer's instructions.
Elderly patients: Adjust dosages individually, according to patient response; clearance may be reduced in these patients.

➤ **Moderate to severe restless legs syndrome (immediate-release)**
Adults: Initially, 0.25 mg PO 1 to 3 hours before bedtime. May increase dose as needed and tolerated after 2 days to 0.5 mg, then to 1 mg by the end of the first week. May further increase dose as needed and tolerated as follows: Week 2, give 1 mg once daily. Week 3, give 1.5 mg once daily. Week 4, give 2 mg once daily. Week 5, give 2.5 mg once daily. Week 6, give 3 mg once daily. Week 7, give 4 mg once daily. Maximum dosage is 4 mg/day. Patient should take all doses 1 to 3 hours before bedtime.

ADMINISTRATION
PO
• Give drug with food if nausea occurs.
• Patient must swallow extended-release tablets whole; they mustn't be chewed, crushed, or divided.

ACTION
Thought to stimulate dopamine (D2) receptors.

Route	Onset	Peak	Duration
PO (immediate-release)	Unknown	1–2 hr	6 hr
PO (extended-release)	Unknown	6–10 hr	Unknown

Half-life: 6 hours.

ADVERSE REACTIONS
Early Parkinson disease (without levodopa)
CNS: dizziness, fatigue, somnolence, syncope, hallucinations, aggravated Parkinson disease, headache, confusion, hyperkinesia, hypoesthesia, vertigo, amnesia, impaired concentration, malaise, asthenia, pain. **CV:** orthostatic hypotension, orthostatic symptoms, HTN, edema, chest pain, extrasystoles, atrial fibrillation, palpitations, tachycardia, flushing. **EENT:** pharyngitis, abnormal vision, eye abnormality, xerophthalmia, rhinitis, sinusitis. **GI:** nausea, vomiting, dyspepsia, dry mouth, flatulence, abdominal pain, anorexia, constipation. **GU:** UTI, erectile dysfunction. **Musculoskeletal:** back pain. **Respiratory:** bronchitis, dyspnea, yawning. **Other:** viral infection, increased sweating, peripheral ischemia.
Advanced Parkinson disease (with levodopa)
CNS: dizziness, somnolence, headache, hallucinations, aggravated parkinsonism, insomnia, abnormal dreaming, confusion, tremor, anxiety, nervousness, amnesia, paresis, paresthesia, syncope, pain. **CV:** hypotension, HTN. **EENT:** diplopia. **GI:** nausea, abdominal pain, dry mouth, vomiting, constipation, diarrhea, dysphagia, flatulence, increased saliva. **GU:** UTI, pyuria, urinary incontinence. **Hematologic:** anemia. **Metabolic:** weight decrease, suppressed prolactin. **Musculoskeletal:** dyskinesia, arthralgia, arthritis, hypokinesia, back pain. **Respiratory:** URI, dyspnea. **Skin:** increased sweating. **Other:** falls, injury, viral infection.
Restless legs syndrome
CNS: fatigue, somnolence, dizziness, vertigo, paresthesia. **CV:** peripheral edema. **EENT:** nasopharyngitis, nasal congestion. **GI:** nausea, vomiting, diarrhea, dyspepsia,

R

dry mouth. **Musculoskeletal:** arthralgia, muscle cramps, extremity pain, back pain. **Respiratory:** cough. **Skin:** increased sweating. **Other:** influenza.

INTERACTIONS
Drug-drug. *BP-lowering agents:* May enhance hypotensive effect. Monitor BP carefully.
Cimetidine, ciprofloxacin, fluvoxamine, inhibitors or substrates of CYP1A2, ritonavir: May alter ropinirole clearance. Adjust ropinirole dosage if other drugs are started or stopped during treatment.
CNS depressants: May increase CNS effects. Use together cautiously.
Dopamine antagonists (neuroleptics), metoclopramide: May decrease ropinirole effects. Avoid using together.
Estrogens: May decrease ropinirole clearance. Adjust ropinirole dosage if estrogen therapy is started or stopped during treatment.
Drug-lifestyle. *Alcohol use:* May increase sedative effect. Discourage use together.
Smoking: May increase drug clearance. Discourage use together.

EFFECTS ON LAB TEST RESULTS
• May increase BUN and alkaline phosphatase levels. May decrease Hb level.

CONTRAINDICATIONS & CAUTIONS
• Contraindicated in patients hypersensitive to drug.
• Use cautiously in patients with severe hepatic or renal impairment.
Dialyzable drug: 30%.
⚠ **Overdose S&S:** Nausea, dizziness, visual hallucinations, hyperhidrosis, claustrophobia, chorea, palpitations, asthenia, nightmares, vomiting, increased coughing, fatigue, syncope, vasovagal syncope, dyskinesia, agitation, chest pain, orthostatic hypotension, somnolence, confusion.

PREGNANCY-LACTATION-REPRODUCTION
• There are no adequate studies in pregnant women. Use only if potential benefit justifies potential risk to the fetus.
• Drug inhibits prolactin secretion and could potentially inhibit lactation. It isn't known if drug appears in human milk. Use cautiously in breastfeeding women.

NURSING CONSIDERATIONS
🔔 *Alert:* Monitor patient carefully for orthostatic hypotension, especially during dosage increases.
• Drug may potentiate the adverse effects of levodopa and may cause or worsen dyskinesia. Dosage may be decreased.
• Although not reported with ropinirole, other adverse reactions reported with dopaminergic therapy include hyperpyrexia, fibrotic complications, and confusion, which may occur with rapid dosage reduction or withdrawal of drug.
• Patient may have syncope, with or without bradycardia. Monitor patient carefully, especially for 4 weeks after start of therapy and with dosage increases.
• Rapid dosage reduction or withdrawal of drug can cause signs and symptoms resembling NMS (elevated temperature, muscular rigidity, altered consciousness, autonomic instability). When used for Parkinson disease, withdraw drug gradually over 7 days. For immediate-release form, reduce frequency from t.i.d. to b.i.d. for 4 days; then, for next 3 days, reduce frequency to once daily before complete withdrawal.
• Withdraw extended-release form gradually over 7 days.
• When used for restless legs syndrome, gradual reduction of the daily dose is recommended.
• Drug can cause somnolence and sudden episodes of falling asleep. Continually reassess patient for drowsiness or sleepiness and for factors that could contribute to sleepiness.
• Avoid use in patients with major psychotic disorders. Drug may cause changes in or worsening of mental status, abnormal thinking, and behavioral changes, which may be severe and include paranoid ideation, delusions, hallucinations, confusion, psychotic-like behavior, disorientation, aggressive behavior, agitation, and delirium.
• Augmentation (an increase in symptoms or earlier onset of symptoms in the evening or even the afternoon, or spread of symptoms to other extremities) and early-morning rebound symptoms (onset of symptoms in

---

the early morning) have been observed in a postmarketing trial in restless legs syndrome. Review use of drug, adjust dosage, or discontinue treatment if augmentation or early-morning rebound symptoms occur.

• Ask patient about development or worsening of impulsive or compulsive behaviors, such as new or increased gambling urges, sexual urges, uncontrolled spending, or other urges, because patient may not recognize these behaviors as abnormal.

• Patients with Parkinson disease have an increased risk of melanoma. Monitor patient for melanoma development during periodic dermatologic screenings.

• *Look alike–sound alike:* Don't confuse ropinirole with risperidone.

PATIENT TEACHING

• Advise patient to take drug with food if nausea occurs.

• Tell patient not to crush, chew, or divide extended-release tablets.

• Advise patient to inform prescriber if starting or stopping medications, OTC drugs or herbs, or smoking.

• Tell patient (especially elderly patient) to contact prescriber if paranoid ideation, delusions, hallucinations, confusion, psychotic-like behavior, disorientation, aggressive behavior, agitation, or delirium occurs.

• Instruct patient not to rise rapidly after sitting or lying down because of risk of dizziness, which may occur more frequently early in therapy or when dosage increases.

• Sleepiness and sudden episodes of falling asleep can occur, sometimes without warning. Warn patient to minimize hazardous activities until CNS effects of drug are known.

• Tell patient to contact prescriber if experiencing difficulty controlling impulsive or compulsive behaviors, such as new or increased gambling urges, sexual urges, uncontrolled spending, or other urges.

• Teach patient about melanoma and to report skin changes to prescriber.

• Advise patient to avoid alcohol.

• Tell female patient to notify prescriber about planned, suspected, or known pregnancy; also tell her to inform prescriber if she's breastfeeding.

SAFETY ALERT!

rosiglitazone maleate
roh-si-GLI-ta-zone

Avandia⏀

Therapeutic class: Antidiabetics
Pharmacologic class: Thiazolidinediones

AVAILABLE FORMS
Tablets: 2 mg, 4 mg, 8 mg

INDICATIONS & DOSAGES
➤ **Type 2 diabetes mellitus, alone or with a sulfonylurea or metformin, in patients currently benefiting from therapy or in patients unable to achieve glucose control with other medications**
Adults: Initially, 4 mg PO daily in the morning or in two divided doses (morning and evening). Increase to 8 mg PO daily or in two divided doses if fasting glucose level doesn't improve after 8 to 12 weeks of treatment. Maximum dose is 8 mg/day.

ADMINISTRATION
PO
• Give drug without regard for food.

ACTION
Lowers glucose level by improving insulin sensitivity.

Route	Onset	Peak	Duration
PO	Unknown	1 hr	Unknown

Half-life: 3 to 4 hours.

ADVERSE REACTIONS
CNS: headache, fatigue. **CV:** edema, *worsening HF.* **EENT:** sinusitis. **GI:** diarrhea. **Hematologic:** anemia. **Metabolic:** hyperglycemia, weight gain. **Musculoskeletal:** back pain, fractures. **Respiratory:** URI. **Other:** accidental injury.

INTERACTIONS
Drug-drug. *Atazanavir, fluvoxamine, gemfibrozil, ketoconazole, trimethoprim:* May increase rosiglitazone levels, increasing hypoglycemic effects and adverse reactions. Monitor glucose; dosage adjustment may be necessary.

R

Insulin: May increase incidence of edema and risk of MI. Use together isn't recommended.

MAO inhibitors, salicylates, SSRIs, sulfonylureas: May enhance hypoglycemic effects. Monitor therapy.

Quinolone antibiotics: May enhance hypoglycemic effect or diminish therapeutic blood glucose–lowering effect of rosiglitazone. Carefully monitor therapy and glucose level.

Rifampin: May decrease rosiglitazone levels. Monitor glucose; dosage adjustment may be necessary.

EFFECTS ON LAB TEST RESULTS
• May increase glucose, HDL, LDL, total cholesterol, and ALT levels.
• May decrease Hb level and hematocrit.
• May decrease free fatty acid levels.

CONTRAINDICATIONS & CAUTIONS
• Don't use for treatment of diabetic ketoacidosis or type 1 diabetes mellitus.
• Administration with insulin isn't recommended.
• Contraindicated in patients hypersensitive to drug or its components.
Black Box Warning Drug isn't recommended in patients with symptomatic HF. Initiating drug in patients with established NYHA Class III or IV HF is contraindicated. ∎
• Contraindicated in patients with active liver disease, increased baseline liver enzyme levels (ALT level greater than 2½ × ULN), type 1 diabetes, or diabetic ketoacidosis and in those who experienced jaundice while taking troglitazone.
• Stop drug if ALT level remains 3 × ULN or if patient develops jaundice.
• Don't start drug in patients experiencing acute coronary syndrome.
• Use cautiously in patients with edema or HF.
Dialyzable drug: No.

PREGNANCY-LACTATION-REPRODUCTION
• There are no adequate studies in pregnant women. Use only if potential benefit justifies potential risk to the fetus.
• Careful monitoring of glucose control is essential during pregnancy. Insulin monotherapy is recommended to maintain blood glucose levels as close to normal as possible.
• Drug can cause ovulation in some premenopausal anovulatory women and increase risk of pregnancy. Premenopausal women should use adequate contraception.
• It isn't known if drug appears in human milk. Patient should discontinue breastfeeding or discontinue drug.

NURSING CONSIDERATIONS
⊘ *Alert:* Monitor liver enzyme levels every 2 months for first 12 months and periodically thereafter. If ALT level becomes elevated, recheck as soon as possible. Stop drug if levels remain elevated.
Black Box Warning Drug may cause or exacerbate CHF in some patients. After drug initiation and after dosage increases, observe patient carefully for signs and symptoms of HF (excessive, rapid weight gain, dyspnea, edema). If these develop, manage HF according to current standards of care. Consider discontinuing drug or reducing dosage. ∎
• Management of type 2 diabetes should include diet control. Because caloric restriction, weight loss, and exercise help improve insulin sensitivity and effectiveness of drug therapy, these measures are essential to proper diabetes treatment.
• Check glucose and HbA$_{1c}$ levels periodically to monitor therapeutic response to drug.
• Hb level and hematocrit may drop during therapy, usually during first 4 to 8 weeks. Increases in total cholesterol, LDL, and HDL levels and decreases in free fatty acid level also may occur.
• For patients inadequately controlled with a maximum dose of a sulfonylurea or metformin, add rosiglitazone to, rather than substituting it for, the sulfonylurea or metformin.
• Drug may increase the incidence of bone fractures (most common in the arm, hand, and foot) in women.
• *Look alike–sound alike:* Don't confuse rosiglitazone with pioglitazone. Don't confuse Avandia with Prandin.

PATIENT TEACHING

• Advise patient that drug can be taken with or without food.

• Notify patient that blood will be tested to check liver function before therapy starts, every 2 months for first 12 months, and then periodically thereafter.

• Tell patient to immediately notify prescriber about unexplained signs and symptoms, such as nausea, vomiting, abdominal pain, fatigue, anorexia, or dark urine; these may indicate liver problems.

• Tell patient to immediately notify prescriber of changes in vision as this may indicate macular edema.

• Warn patient to report signs or symptoms of HF (unusually rapid increase in weight or swelling, shortness of breath) or MI (chest pain or pressure, dyspnea).

• Recommend use of contraceptives to premenopausal, anovulatory female patient with insulin resistance because ovulation may resume with therapy.

• Advise patient that management of diabetes includes diet control, calorie restriction, weight loss, and exercise, and that these measures improve effectiveness of drug therapy.

• Instruct patient to monitor glucose level carefully. Tell patient what to do if ill, undergoing surgery, or under added stress.

rosuvastatin calcium 🎗

roe-SOO-va-staT-tin

Crestor⌀

Therapeutic class: Antilipemics
Pharmacologic class: HMG-CoA reductase inhibitors

AVAILABLE FORMS

Tablets: 5 mg, 10 mg, 20 mg, 40 mg

INDICATIONS & DOSAGES

🎗 *Adjust-a-dose (for all indications):* If CrCl is less than 30 mL/minute/1.73 m² initially, give 5 mg once daily; don't exceed 10 mg once daily. For Asian patients, initial dose is 5 mg. For patients also taking cyclosporine, limit rosuvastatin dose to 5 mg once daily. For patients taking atazanavir and ritonavir,

lopinavir and ritonavir, or simeprevir, initially, 5 mg once daily; don't exceed 10 mg once daily. Avoid concomitant use with gemfibrozil. If concomitant use can't be avoided, initially give 5 mg once daily; don't exceed 10 mg once daily.

➤ **Risk reduction in patients without clinical evidence of CAD but with multiple risk factors**

Adults: Initially, 10 mg PO once daily; 5 mg PO once daily in patients needing less aggressive LDL cholesterol reduction. For aggressive lipid reduction (LDL greater than 190 mg/dL) initially, 20 mg PO once daily. Increase as needed to maximum of 40 mg PO daily. Dosage may be titrated every 2 to 4 weeks, based on lipid levels.

➤ **Children with heterozygous familial hypercholesterolemia to reduce total cholesterol, LDL cholesterol, and apolipoprotein B levels after failing an adequate trial of diet therapy when LDL cholesterol is more than 190 mg/dL, or more than 160 mg/dL and there is a positive family history of premature CV disease or two or more other CV disease risk factors** 🎗

Children ages 10 to 17: 5 to 20 mg PO daily.
Children ages 8 to younger than 10: 5 to 10 mg PO daily.

Adjust-a-dose: May titrate dosage every 4 weeks or more, based on lipid levels.

➤ **Children with homozygous familial hypercholesterolemia to reduce LDL cholesterol, total cholesterol, non-HDL cholesterol, and apolipoprotein B levels after failing an adequate trial of diet therapy** 🎗

Children ages 7 to 17: 20 mg PO once daily either alone or with other lipid-lowering treatments.

➤ **Adjunct to diet to reduce LDL cholesterol, total cholesterol, apolipoprotein B, non-HDL cholesterol, and triglyceride (TG) levels and to increase HDL cholesterol level in patients with primary hypercholesterolemia (heterozygous familial and nonfamilial) and mixed dyslipidemia (Fredrickson types IIa and IIb); adjunct to diet to treat elevated TG level (Fredrickson type IV); adjunct to diet to treat primary dysbetalipoproteinemia** 🎗

R

Adults: Initially, 10 mg PO once daily; 5 mg PO once daily in patients needing less aggressive LDL cholesterol reduction or those predisposed to myopathy. For aggressive lipid lowering when LDL is greater than 190 mg/dL, initially, 20 mg PO once daily. Increase as needed to maximum of 40 mg PO daily. Dosage may be titrated every 2 to 4 weeks, based on lipid levels.

➤ **Adjunct to diet to slow atherosclerosis progression in patients with elevated cholesterol**

Adults: Initially, 10 mg PO daily. Increase as needed every 2 to 4 weeks based on lipid levels, to maximum of 40 mg daily.

➤ **Adjunct to lipid-lowering therapies; to reduce LDL cholesterol, apolipoprotein B, and total cholesterol levels in homozygous familial hypercholesterolemia** ▩

Adults: Initially, 20 mg PO once daily. Maximum, 40 mg once daily.

ADMINISTRATION
PO
• Give drug without regard for meals.
• Wait 2 hours after giving dose to give aluminum- or magnesium-containing antacid.

ACTION
Inhibits HMG-CoA reductase, increases LDL receptors on liver cells, and inhibits hepatic synthesis of very–low-density lipoprotein.

Route	Onset	Peak	Duration
PO	1 wk	3–5 hr	Unknown

Half-life: About 19 hours.

ADVERSE REACTIONS
CNS: asthenia, dizziness, headache. **GI:** abdominal pain, constipation, diarrhea, dyspepsia, nausea, vomiting. **GU:** cystitis. **Hematologic:** anemia, ecchymosis. **Metabolic:** diabetes mellitus. **Musculoskeletal:** arthralgia, myalgia, neck pain.

INTERACTIONS
Drug-drug. *Antacids:* May decrease rosuvastatin level. Give antacids at least 2 hours after rosuvastatin.
Atazanavir, atazanavir–ritonavir, lopinavir–ritonavir, simeprevir: May increase rosuvastatin level and risk of myopathy and rhabdomyolysis. Rosuvastatin dosage shouldn't exceed 10 mg daily.
Colchicine: May increase risk of myopathy and rhabdomyolysis. Avoid use together. If use together is necessary, monitor patient for signs and symptoms of myopathy and elevated CK level during use and after dosage increases.
Cyclosporine: May increase rosuvastatin level and risk of myopathy or rhabdomyolysis. Don't exceed 5 mg of rosuvastatin daily. Watch for evidence of toxicity.
Daptomycin: May increase risk of rhabdomyolysis. Withhold rosuvastatin temporarily or monitor patient and CK level closely during coadministration.
Eltrombopag: May increase rosuvastatin level and risk of toxicity. Consider reducing rosuvastatin dosage.
Fenofibrate: May increase rosuvastatin level and risk of myopathy or rhabdomyolysis. Use together cautiously.
Gemfibrozil: May significantly increase rosuvastatin level and risk of myopathy or rhabdomyolysis. Avoid use together. If used together, don't exceed 10 mg/day of rosuvastatin.
Hormonal contraceptives: May increase ethinyl estradiol and norgestrel levels. Watch for adverse effects.
Niacin: May increase risk of myopathy or rhabdomyolysis. Monitor patient closely.
Warfarin: May increase INR and risk of bleeding. Monitor INR, and watch for evidence of increased bleeding.
Drug-lifestyle. *Alcohol use:* May increase risk of hepatotoxicity. Discourage use together.

EFFECTS ON LAB TEST RESULTS
• May increase HbA_{1c}, fasting blood sugar, CK, ALT, AST, glucose, glutamyl transpeptidase, alkaline phosphatase, and bilirubin levels.
• May cause thyroid function abnormalities, dipstick-positive proteinuria, and microscopic hematuria.

CONTRAINDICATIONS & CAUTIONS
• Contraindicated in patients hypersensitive to rosuvastatin or its components, patients with active liver disease, and those with

unexplained persistently increased transaminase levels.

• Use cautiously in patients who drink substantial amounts of alcohol or have a history of liver disease and in those at increased risk for myopathies, such as those with renal impairment, advanced age, or hypothyroidism.

🧬 Use cautiously in Asian patients because they have a greater risk of elevated drug levels.

• Rare postmarketing reports of cognitive impairment (memory loss, forgetfulness, amnesia, memory impairment, confusion) have been associated with statin use. These reported symptoms are generally not serious and are reversible upon statin discontinuation, with variable times to symptom onset (1 day to years) and symptom resolution (median of 3 weeks).

Dialyzable drug: No.

⚠ *Overdose S&S:* Unexplained muscle pain, tenderness, or weakness, especially with malaise or fever.

PREGNANCY-LACTATION-REPRODUCTION

• May cause fetal harm when given to pregnant women. Use during pregnancy is contraindicated. Discontinue drug before conception. If patient becomes pregnant during therapy, apprise her of potential fetal risks and the lack of known clinical benefit with continued use during pregnancy.

• Drug may appear in human milk. Use while breastfeeding is contraindicated.

NURSING CONSIDERATIONS

• Before therapy starts, assess patient for underlying causes of hypercholesterolemia, including poorly controlled diabetes, hypothyroidism, nephrotic syndrome, dyslipoproteinemias, obstructive liver disease, drug interaction, and alcoholism.

• Before therapy starts, advise patient to control hypercholesterolemia with diet, exercise, and weight reduction.

• Interrupt statin therapy if patient shows signs or symptoms of serious liver injury, hyperbilirubinemia, or jaundice. Don't restart drug if another cause can't be found.

• Monitor LFTs at baseline and with any indication of hepatotoxicity.

🔔 *Alert:* Rarely, rhabdomyolysis with acute renal failure has developed in patients taking drugs in this class, including rosuvastatin.

• Monitor lipid panel at baseline and a fasting lipid profile within 4 to 12 weeks after initiation or dosage adjustment and every 3 to 12 months thereafter.

• Patients who are age 65 or older, have hypothyroidism, or have renal insufficiency may be at a greater risk for developing myopathy while receiving a statin.

• Notify prescriber if CK level becomes markedly elevated or myopathy is suspected, or if routine urinalysis shows persistent proteinuria and patient is taking 40 mg daily.

• Withhold drug temporarily if patient becomes predisposed to myopathy or rhabdomyolysis because of sepsis, hypotension, major surgery, trauma, uncontrolled seizures, or severe metabolic, endocrine, or electrolyte disorders.

• Rare cases of immune-mediated necrotizing myopathy have been reported.

PATIENT TEACHING

• Instruct patient to take drug exactly as prescribed.

• Teach patient about diet, exercise, and weight control.

• Inform patient that rare instances of memory loss and confusion have occurred with statin use. These reported events were generally not serious and resolved when drug was discontinued.

• Tell patient that drug may increase blood glucose level but that the CV benefits are thought to outweigh the slight increase in risk.

• Tell patient to immediately report unexplained muscle pain, tenderness, or weakness (especially if accompanied by malaise or fever) and loss of appetite, upper abdominal pain, dark-colored urine, or yellowing of skin or eyes.

• Instruct patient to take drug at least 2 hours before taking aluminum- or magnesium-containing antacids.

🔔 *Alert:* Tell female patient to stop drug and notify prescriber immediately if she is or may be pregnant or if she's breastfeeding.

R

rucaparib camsylate ⚠
roo-KAP-a-rib

Rubraca

Therapeutic class: Antineoplastics
Pharmacologic class: Poly (ADP-ribose)
polymerase (PARP) inhibitors

AVAILABLE FORMS
Tablets: 200 mg, 250 mg, 300 mg

INDICATIONS & DOSAGES
Adjust-a-dose (for all indications): To manage any adverse reaction, interrupt therapy
or consider dosage reduction. First dosage
reduction is to 500 mg b.i.d.; second dosage
reduction is to 400 mg b.i.d.; third dosage
reduction is to 300 mg b.i.d. For prolonged
hematologic toxicities, interrupt therapy and
monitor blood counts weekly until recovery. If levels haven't recovered to grade 1 or
less after 4 weeks, refer patient to hematol-
ogist for further investigation. If myelodysplastic syndrome/acute myeloid leukemia
(MDS/AML) is confirmed, discontinue drug.
➤ **Epithelial ovarian, fallopian tube, or**
primary peritoneal cancer in patients
with deleterious *BRCA* mutation (germline
or somatic) and who have been treated
with two or more chemotherapies ⚠
Adults: 600 mg PO b.i.d. Continue treatment
until disease progression or unacceptable
toxicity occurs.
➤ **Maintenance treatment of patients**
with recurrent epithelial ovarian, fallop-
ian tube, or primary peritoneal cancer
who are in a complete or partial response
to platinum-based chemotherapy
Adults: 600 mg PO b.i.d. Continue treatment
until disease progression or unacceptable
toxicity occurs.

ADMINISTRATION
PO
• May give without regard for food.
• Omit a missed dose and give next dose at its
scheduled time. Don't replace vomited doses.
• Store at 68° to 77° F (20° to 25° C);
excursions permitted to 59° to 86° F
(15° to 30° C).

ACTION
Induces cytotoxicity by inhibiting PARP enzyme activity and increased formation of
PARP–DNA complexes, resulting in DNA
damage, apoptosis, and cell death.

Route	Onset	Peak	Duration
PO	Unknown	1.9 hr	Unknown

Half-life: 17 to 19 hours.

ADVERSE REACTIONS
CNS: asthenia, fatigue, dizziness, pyrexia,
depression. **CV:** peripheral edema. **EENT:**
nasopharyngitis. **GI:** nausea, vomiting, constipation, decreased appetite, diarrhea, abdominal pain, dysgeusia, dyspepsia. **Hema-**
tologic: anemia, *thrombocytopenia, neu-*
tropenia, febrile neutropenia. **Respira-**
tory: dyspnea, URI. **Skin:** rash, photosensitivity reaction, pruritus, hand-foot
syndrome.

INTERACTIONS
Drug-lifestyle. *Sun exposure:* May cause
photosensitivity. Patient should use appropriate sun protection to avoid sunburn.

EFFECTS ON LAB TEST RESULTS
• May increase creatinine, ALT, AST, alkaline phosphatase, and cholesterol levels.
• May decrease Hb level, ANC, and lymphocyte and platelet counts.

CONTRAINDICATIONS & CAUTIONS
• Use cautiously in patients with renal or
liver impairment; starting dosage adjustments haven't been established for patients
with CrCl of less than 30 mL/minute, for
those on dialysis, or for patients with moderate to severe hepatic impairment (bilirubin
level greater than 1.5 × ULN).
• Drug may increase risk of MDS/AML.
Discontinue drug if MDS/AML is confirmed.
• Safety and effectiveness in children
haven't been established.
• Use cautiously in elderly patients.
Dialyzable drug: Unknown.

PREGNANCY-LACTATION-REPRODUCTION
• Drug can cause fetal harm. Advise women
of childbearing potential to use effective contraception during therapy and for

6 months after final dose. Pregnancy testing is recommended before therapy begins.
• Advise women not to breastfeed during therapy and for 2 weeks after final dose.

NURSING CONSIDERATIONS

🧬 Patients should be tested for *BRCA* mutation (germline or somatic) using an FDA-approved test before treatment. Information on tests may be found at https://www.fda.gov/medical-devices/vitro-diagnostics/list-cleared-or-approved-companion-diagnostic-devices-vitro-and-imaging-tools.
• Monitor CBC at baseline and monthly thereafter. Don't start therapy until patient has recovered from hematologic toxicity caused by prior chemotherapy (grade 1 or less).

PATIENT TEACHING

• Instruct patient to take drug twice daily with or without food 12 hours apart. If a dose is missed, instruct patient to skip missed dose and resume normal schedule.
• Advise patient of childbearing potential to use effective contraception during treatment and for 6 months after final dose. Tell patient that pregnancy testing will be performed before treatment begins.
• Advise patient not to breastfeed during treatment and for 2 weeks after final dose.
• Warn patient that drug may cause photosensitivity and to use appropriate sun protection.
• Advise patient to report all adverse reactions, especially weakness, fatigue, fever, weight loss, frequent infections, bruising, easy bleeding, dyspnea, blood in urine or stool, nausea, and vomiting.

SAFETY ALERT!

ruxolitinib phosphate
rux-oh-LI-ti-nib

Jakafi

Therapeutic class: Antineoplastics
Pharmacologic class: Janus-associated kinase inhibitors

AVAILABLE FORMS
Tablets: 5 mg, 10 mg, 15 mg, 20 mg, 25 mg

INDICATIONS & DOSAGES

➤ **Treatment of patients with intermediate or high-risk myelofibrosis, including primary myelofibrosis, post–polycythemia vera myelofibrosis, and post–essential thrombocythemia myelofibrosis**
Adults: Initially, 20 mg PO b.i.d. if platelet count is greater than 200×10^9/L, 15 mg PO b.i.d. if platelet count is 100 to 200×10^9/L, or 5 mg PO b.i.d. if platelet count is 50 to less than 100×10^9/L. May increase in 5-mg increments b.i.d. to a maximum of 25 mg b.i.d. Don't increase during the first 4 weeks of therapy and not more frequently than every 2 weeks. Consider dosage increases in patients who meet all of the following conditions: failure to achieve either a 50% reduction from pretreatment baseline in palpable spleen length or a 35% reduction in spleen volume as measured by CT scan or MRI; platelet count greater than 125×10^9/L at 4 weeks and never below 100×10^9/L; and ANC greater than 0.75×10^9/L. Long-term maintenance at a 5-mg b.i.d. dosage hasn't shown response; limit continued use at this dosage to patients in whom benefits outweigh risks. Discontinue drug after 6 months if there is no spleen reduction or symptom improvement. If drug needs to be stopped for any reason except thrombocytopenia, taper gradually by 5 mg b.i.d. each week.
Adjust-a-dose: For moderate to severe renal impairment (CrCl of 15 to 59 mL/minute) and platelet count between 100 and 150×10^9/L, initial dose is 10 mg b.i.d. For moderate to severe renal impairment (CrCl of 15 to 59 mL/minute) and platelet count between 50 and less than 100×10^9/L, initial dose is 5 mg daily For patients with ESRD on dialysis and with platelet count between 100 and 200×10^9/L, initial dose is 15 mg once after dialysis. For patients with hepatic impairment and platelet count between 100 and 150×10^9/L, initial dose is 10 mg b.i.d. and for patients with platelet count between 50 and less than 100×10^9/L, initial dose is 5 mg daily.

Modify dosage when giving concomitantly with strong CYP3A4 inhibitors and fluconazole. Avoid use with fluconazole doses greater than 200 mg daily.

R

Refer to manufacturer's instructions for toxicity-related dosage adjustments.

➤ **Polycythemia vera in patients with an inadequate response to or who are intolerant of hydroxyurea**

Adults: Initially, 10 mg PO b.i.d. If response is inadequate and platelet count is 140×10^9 or greater, Hb level is 12 g/dL or greater, and ANC is 1.5×10^9/L or greater, may increase dose by 5 mg b.i.d. to a maximum of 25 mg b.i.d. (Maximum is 50 mg/day.) Doses shouldn't be increased during first 4 weeks of therapy and not more frequently than every 2 weeks. Inadequate response is defined as one of the following: continued need for phlebotomy, WBC count higher than ULN, platelet count greater than ULN, or palpable spleen that's reduced by less than 25% from baseline.

Adjust-a-dose: Recommended starting dose in patients with any degree of hepatic impairment or moderate to severe renal impairment (CrCl of 15 to 59 mL/minute) is 5 mg b.i.d. Recommended starting dose in patients with ESRD on dialysis is 10 mg. Avoid use in those with ESRD not requiring dialysis.

Modify dosage when giving concomitantly with strong CYP3A4 inhibitors and fluconazole. Avoid use with fluconazole doses greater than 200 mg daily.

Refer to manufacturer's instructions for toxicity-related dosage adjustments.

✳ *NEW INDICATION:* **Treatment of steroid-refractory acute GVHD**

Adults and children age 12 and older: Initially 5 mg PO b.i.d. May increase to 10 mg b.i.d after at least 3 days of treatment if ANC and platelet counts aren't decreased by 50% or more from first day of dosing.

Adjust-a-dose: Recommended starting dose in patients with Stage 3 or 4 liver GVHD, moderate to severe renal impairment (CrCl of 15 to 59 mL/minute), or ESRD on dialysis is 5 mg once daily. Modify dosage when giving concomitantly with fluconazole. After 6 months of treatment in patients who have discontinued corticosteroids, taper drug by one dose level every 8 weeks (10 mg b.i.d. to 5 mg b.i.d. to 5 mg once daily). Consider retreatment if acute GVHD recurs during or after taper. Refer to manufacturer's instructions for toxicity-related dosage adjustments.

ADMINISTRATION
PO
- May give without regard to food.
- To give through an NG tube (8 French or greater), place one tablet in approximately 40 mL water and stir for 10 minutes to dissolve. Give within 6 hours of preparing the suspension, using an appropriate syringe. Rinse NG tube with 75 mL water.
- Drug is a hazardous agent; use safe handling precautions.

ACTION
Inhibits signaling of cytokines and growth factors important for hematopoiesis and immune functions. Prevents splenomegaly by decreasing circulating inflammatory cytokines.

Route	Onset	Peak	Duration
PO	Rapid	1–2 hr	10 hr

Half-life: 3 hours.

ADVERSE REACTIONS
CNS: dizziness, headache, insomnia, fatigue. **EENT:** nasopharyngitis, epistaxis. **GI:** flatulence, abdominal pain, diarrhea, constipation. **GU:** UTI. **Hematologic:** *neutropenia, thrombocytopenia,* anemia. **Hepatic:** increased AST/ALT levels. **Metabolic:** hypercholesterolemia, hypertriglyceridemia, weight gain. **Musculoskeletal:** muscle spasm, weakness. **Respiratory:** dyspnea, cough. **Skin:** bruising, pruritus. **Other:** serious bacterial, mycobacterial, fungal, or viral infections.

INTERACTIONS
Drug-drug. *CYP3A4 inducers (rifampin):* May decrease ruxolitinib level. No initial dosage adjustment is necessary. Monitor patients closely and titrate dosage if necessary. *Fluconazole (doses of 200 mg or less):* May increase ruxolitinib level. Avoid using fluconazole doses greater than 200 mg daily concomitantly with ruxolitinib. If patient with myelofibrosis is taking fluconazole 200 mg or less daily and platelet count is 100×10^9/L or more, start ruxolitinib at 10 mg b.i.d. If patient is taking fluconazole 200 mg or less daily and platelet count is 50 to less than 100×10^9/L, start ruxolitinib at 5 mg once daily. If patient is taking

fluconazole 200 mg or less daily and is on stable ruxolitinib dose of 10 mg or more b.i.d., reduce ruxolitinib dosage by 50% (rounded up to closest available tablet strength). If patient is taking fluconazole 200 mg or less and is on stable ruxolitinib dose of 5 mg b.i.d., reduce ruxolitinib dosage to 5 mg once daily. If patient is on stable ruxolitinib dose of 5 mg once daily, avoid use of fluconazole or interrupt ruxolitinib treatment for duration of fluconazole use. For concomitant administration during polycythemia vera treatment, decrease ruxolitinib dose by 50%; if dose is 5 mg daily, avoid concomitant administration. Make additional dosage modifications with careful monitoring of safety and effectiveness.

Strong CYP3A4 inhibitors (clarithromycin, conivaptan, indinavir, itraconazole, ketoconazole, lopinavir–ritonavir, mibefradil, nefazodone, nelfinavir, posaconazole, ritonavir, saquinavir, voriconazole): May increase ruxolitinib level. If patient with myelofibrosis is taking a strong CYP3A4 inhibitor and platelet count is 100×10^9/L or more, start ruxolitinib at 10 mg b.i.d. If patient is taking a strong CYP3A4 inhibitor and platelet count is 50 to less than 100×10^9/L, start ruxolitinib at 5 mg once daily. If patient is taking a strong CYP3A4 inhibitor and is on stable ruxolitinib dose of 10 mg or more b.i.d., reduce ruxolitinib dosage by 50% (rounded up to closest available tablet strength). If patient is taking a strong CYP3A4 inhibitor and is on stable ruxolitinib dose of 5 mg b.i.d., reduce ruxolitinib dosage to 5 mg once daily. If patient is on stable ruxolitinib dose of 5 mg once daily, avoid use of strong CYP3A4 inhibitor or interrupt ruxolitinib treatment for duration of strong CYP3A4 inhibitor use. For concomitant administration during polycythemia vera treatment, decrease ruxolitinib dose by 50%; if dose is 5 mg daily, avoid concomitant administration. Make additional dosage modifications with careful monitoring of safety and effectiveness.

Drug-food. *Grapefruit juice:* May increase ruxolitinib level. Don't use together.

EFFECTS ON LAB TEST RESULTS
• May increase total cholesterol, LDL cholesterol, triglyceride, AST, and ALT levels.
• May decrease platelet and neutrophil counts.
• May decrease Hb level.

CONTRAINDICATIONS & CAUTIONS
• Contraindicated in patients hypersensitive to drug and in those with ESRD not requiring dialysis, moderate to severe renal failure and platelet count less than 100×10^9/L, or hepatic impairment with platelet count less than 100×10^9/L.
• Use cautiously in patients with thrombocytopenia, anemia, or neutropenia.
• Serious bacterial, mycobacterial (including TB), fungal, or viral infections (such as herpes zoster) have occurred. Evaluate patient for TB before treatment. Serious infections should be resolved before start of treatment. Progressive multifocal leukoencephalopathy (PML) has been reported; discontinue drug and evaluate patient if suspected.
• Acute relapse of myelofibrosis signs and symptoms have been reported about 1 week after ruxolitinib is discontinued, with some patients experiencing one or more adverse effects, including fever, respiratory distress, hypotension, DIC, and multiorgan failure. Evaluate and treat any illness, and consider restarting or increasing ruxolitinib dosage.
• Drug may increase risk of nonmelanoma skin cancer.
Dialyzable drug: Unlikely.

PREGNANCY-LACTATION-REPRODUCTION
• There are no adequate studies in pregnant women. Use during pregnancy only if potential benefit justifies potential risk to the fetus.
• It isn't known if drug appears in human milk. Patient should discontinue breastfeeding or discontinue drug.

NURSING CONSIDERATIONS
• Obtain platelet, RBC, and WBC counts before starting drug, every 2 to 4 weeks until dosage is stabilized, then as needed.

R

- Resolve active infections before starting therapy.
- Blood transfusions may be necessary to manage anemia.
- Monitor patient for signs and symptoms of serious bacterial, mycobacterial, fungal, or viral infections (such as herpes zoster) during therapy; begin treatment for infection, if necessary, as soon as possible.
- Monitor patient for skin cancer.
- Monitor lipid levels 8 to 12 weeks after start of therapy and treat according to clinical guidelines for management of hyperlipidemia.
- To discontinue drug, consider tapering dosage gradually rather than stopping drug abruptly unless drug is being discontinued because of thrombocytopenia or neutropenia.

PATIENT TEACHING
- Inform patient that drug must be taken daily and not to change dosage or stop drug without consulting prescriber. Myelofibrosis and related signs and symptoms will return if drug is discontinued.
- Instruct patient not to drink grapefruit juice.
- Instruct patient that if a dose is missed, not to take an additional dose but to take the next usual prescribed dose.
- Inform patient on dialysis to not take a dose before dialysis, but to wait and take it after dialysis.
- Inform patient that blood tests will be needed to monitor for adverse effects and possible dosage adjustment.
- Inform patient of increased risk of infection. Advise patient to immediately report signs and symptoms of illness (fever, cough, malaise, skin eruptions).
- Tell patient that drug can cause low blood cell counts and to report bleeding, bruising, fatigue, or shortness of breath.
- Warn patient that skin cancers have occurred in those taking drug and to report new or changing skin lesions.

sacubitril–valsartan ⚕
sak-UE-bi-tril/val-SAR-tan

Entresto

Therapeutic class: Antihypertensives
Pharmacologic class: Neprilysin inhibitors–ARBs

AVAILABLE FORMS
Tablets: 24 mg sacubitril/26 mg valsartan, 49 mg sacubitril/51 mg valsartan, 97 mg sacubitril/103 mg valsartan

INDICATIONS & DOSAGES
➤ **To reduce risk of CV death and hospitalization for HF in patients with chronic HF (NYHA Class II to IV) and reduced ejection fraction, usually in conjunction with other HF therapies, in place of an ACE inhibitor or other ARB**
Adults: Initially, 49 mg sacubitril/51 mg valsartan PO b.i.d. Increase after 2 to 4 weeks to target maintenance dose of 97 mg sacubitril/103 mg valsartan, as tolerated.

Adjust-a-dose: In patients not currently taking an ACE inhibitor or ARB or previously taking a low dose of these agents and in patients with severe renal impairment (estimated GFR less than 30 mL/minute/1.73 m^2) or moderate hepatic impairment (Child-Pugh class B), reduce starting dose to 24 mg sacubitril/26 mg valsartan b.i.d. Double the dose every 2 to 4 weeks to target maintenance dose of 97 mg sacubitril/103 mg valsartan, as tolerated.

✱ *NEW INDICATION:* **Symptomatic heart failure in pediatric patients with systemic left ventricular systolic dysfunction**
Children age 1 year and older weighing at least 50 kg: Initially, 49 mg sacubitril/51 mg valsartan PO twice daily. If tolerated, may increase to 72 mg sacubitril/78 mg valsartan after 2 weeks, then increase to 97 mg sacubitril/103 mg valsartan after 2 additional weeks.
Children age 1 year and older weighing at least 40 kg to less than 50 kg: Initially, 24 mg sacubitril/26 mg valsartan PO twice daily. If tolerated, may increase to 49 mg sacubitril/51 mg valsartan after 2 weeks, then increase to 72 mg sacubitril/78 mg valsartan after 2 additional weeks.

Children age 1 year and older weighing less than 40 kg: Use oral suspension and the recommended mg/kg doses of the combined amount of both sacubitril and valsartan. Initially, 1.6 mg/kg PO twice daily. If tolerated, may increase to 2.3 mg/kg after 2 weeks, then increase to 3.1 mg/kg after 2 additional weeks.

ADMINISTRATION
PO
● If patient is switching to or from an ACE inhibitor, allow a washout period of 36 hours between giving the two drugs.
● May give with or without food.
● If a dose is missed, give as soon as possible on the same day, then resume twice-daily dosing. If missed dose is close to the scheduled next dose, omit it.

ACTION
Inhibits neprilysin and angiotensin II, enhancing the protective neurohormonal systems of the heart (natriuretic peptide system) while suppressing the harmful RAAS.

Route	Onset	Peak	Duration
PO	Unknown	½–2 hr	Unknown

Half-life: Sacubitril, 1.4 hours; valsartan, 9.9 hours.

ADVERSE REACTIONS
CNS: dizziness. **CV:** *hypotension.* **GU:** *renal failure.* **Hematologic:** anemia. **Metabolic:** *hyperkalemia.* **Respiratory:** cough. **Other:** *angioedema (black patients),* falls.

INTERACTIONS
Drug-drug. *ACE inhibitors:* May increase risk of angioedema. Use together is contraindicated. Don't give sacubitril–valsartan within 36 hours of switching from or to an ACE inhibitor.
Aliskiren: May increase risk of renal failure. Contraindicated for use together in patients with diabetes. Avoid use in patients with renal impairment (GFR less than 60 mL/minute/1.73 m^2).
ARBs: Will cause dual blockade of the RAAS. Avoid concurrent use as product contains valsartan.
Canagliflozin: May enhance hyperkalemic and hypotensive effects. Monitor potassium level and BP carefully.

Cyclooxygenase-2 inhibitors, NSAIDs: May increase risk of renal failure, especially in patients who are elderly, volume-depleted, or with prior impaired renal function. Monitor renal function closely.
Lithium: May increase lithium level and risk of lithium toxicity. Monitor serum lithium level.
Potassium-sparing diuretics (amiloride, spironolactone, triamterene), potassium supplements: May increase serum potassium level. Use cautiously and monitor patient closely.
Sodium phosphates: May enhance risk of acute phosphate nephropathy. Seek alternatives to oral sodium phosphate bowel preparations.

EFFECTS ON LAB TEST RESULTS
● May increase serum creatinine and potassium levels.
● May decrease Hb level and hematocrit.

CONTRAINDICATIONS & CAUTIONS
● Contraindicated in patients with a history of angioedema related to previous ACE or ARB therapy, in patients currently receiving ACE inhibitors or within 36 hours of using an ACE inhibitor, and in patients with diabetes who are using aliskiren.
● Use in patients with severe hepatic impairment (Child-Pugh class C) isn't recommended.
▧ Drug may cause angioedema requiring emergency treatment and which can be fatal. Risk is greater in black than in non-black patients.
● Drug lowers BP and may cause symptomatic hypotension.
● ACE inhibitors and ARBs have been associated with oliguria, progressive azotemia, acute renal failure, hyperkalemia, and death. Monitor patient closely.
● Safety and effectiveness in children haven't been established.
Dialyzable drug: Unlikely.
⚠ *Overdose S&S:* Hypotension.

PREGNANCY-LACTATION-REPRODUCTION
Black Box Warning Use during pregnancy can cause injury and death to the developing fetus from effects on the RAAS. Stop drug as soon as pregnancy is detected. ∎

S

• Use during pregnancy only if there is no appropriate alternative therapy and if drug is considered lifesaving for the mother. Advise pregnant women of potential risk to the fetus.
• It isn't known if drug appears in human milk. Because of the potential for serious reactions in breastfed infants, breastfeeding isn't recommended during therapy.

NURSING CONSIDERATIONS
• Drug is usually given with other HF therapies, in place of an ACE inhibitor or other ARB.
• Don't give with or within 36 hours of an ACE inhibitor.
• To help prevent hypotension, correct volume or salt depletion before start of therapy.
• Monitor patients for hypotension. Patients who are volume- or salt-depleted, such as those on high-dose diuretics, may be at increased risk. Consider dosage adjustment of diuretics and concomitant antihypertensives and treat other cause of hypotension such as hypovolemia. Reduce dosage or temporarily discontinue sacubitril–valsartan for persistent hypotension.
▧ Monitor all patients, especially black patients, for angioedema (swelling of the face, tongue, throat, and lips; airway compromise; dyspnea). Discontinue drug and treat emergently.
• Monitor renal function and reduce dosage or temporarily interrupt therapy in patients who develop clinically significant decreased renal function.
• Monitor serum potassium level periodically and treat appropriately. Patients with severe renal impairment, diabetes, hypoaldosteronism, or a high-potassium diet may be at increased risk for hyperkalemia. Reduce dosage or interrupt therapy as clinically indicated.

PATIENT TEACHING
• Explain to patient that drug is usually used with other HF therapies, in place of an ACE inhibitor or other ARB therapy.
• Advise patient to report all adverse reactions, especially signs and symptoms of angioedema and allergic reaction (swelling of the face, lips, tongue, or throat; trouble breathing). Advise patient to seek immediate emergency medical help if they occur.

• Instruct patient to take drug exactly as prescribed and not to take within 36 hours of an ACE inhibitor.
• Tell female patient to notify prescriber if she becomes pregnant. Drug will need to be stopped. Caution patient not to breastfeed during therapy.
• Caution patient to contact prescriber if dizziness, light-headedness, or extreme fatigue occurs.

safinamide mesylate
sa-FIN-a-mide

Xadago

Therapeutic class: Antiparkinsonians
Pharmacologic class: MAO-B inhibitors

AVAILABLE FORMS
Tablets: 50 mg, 100 mg

INDICATIONS & DOSAGES
➤ **Parkinson disease in patients experiencing "off" episodes as adjunctive treatment to levodopa–carbidopa**
Adults: 50 mg PO once daily. After 2 weeks, may increase to 100 mg daily based on individual need and tolerability.
Adjust-a-dose: For patients with moderate hepatic impairment (Child-Pugh class B), maximum recommended dosage is 50 mg once daily. If patient progresses to severe hepatic impairment, discontinue drug. When discontinuing drug, taper 100-mg dose before stopping drug by decreasing dosage to 50 mg for 1 week.

ADMINISTRATION
PO
• May give with or without food.
• Give at the same time each day. Always administer with levodopa–carbidopa.
• If a dose is missed, patient should take the next dose at same time the next day.
• Store at room temperature.

ACTION
An inhibitor of MAO-B. Blockade of MAO-B is thought to result in an increase in dopamine levels by blocking the catabolism of dopamine, which then increases dopaminergic activity in the brain.

Route	Onset	Peak	Duration
PO	Unknown	2–3 hr	Unknown

Half-life: 20 to 26 hours.

ADVERSE REACTIONS
CNS: dyskinesia, insomnia, anxiety. **CV:** orthostatic hypotension, HTN. **GI:** nausea, dyspepsia. **Respiratory:** cough. **Other:** fall.

INTERACTIONS
Drug-drug. *Cold remedies; nasal, oral, and ophthalmic decongestants; sympathomimetic medications (amphetamine, methylphenidate):* May increase risk of hypertensive crisis. Use together is contraindicated.

Cyclobenzaprine, MAO inhibitor class drugs or other drugs that are potent inhibitors of MAO (e.g., linezolid, MAO-B inhibitors), opioids (meperidine and derivatives, methadone, propoxyphene, tramadol), SSNRIs, TCAs, tetracyclic antidepressants, triazolopyridine: May increase risk of serotonin syndrome. Use together is contraindicated. Allow at least 14 days to lapse after discontinuing safinamide and starting these drugs.

Dextromethorphan: May cause episodes of psychosis or bizarre behavior. Use together is contraindicated.

Dopamine antagonists (antipsychotics, metoclopramide): May decrease effectiveness of safinamide and exacerbate Parkinson symptoms. Monitor therapy.

Isoniazid: Isoniazid has some MAO-inhibiting activity. Watch for HTN and reaction to dietary tyramine in patients taking both drugs.

SSRIs: May cause serotonin syndrome. Monitor patient for signs and symptoms of serotonin syndrome; use lowest effective dosage of SSRI with safinamide.

Substrates of breast cancer resistance protein (BCRP) (imatinib, irinotecan, lapatinib, methotrexate, mitoxantrone, rosuvastatin, sulfasalazine, topotecan): May increase plasma concentrations of BRCP substrate. Monitor patient for increased adverse effects of BRCP substrate.

Drug-herb. *St John's wort:* May increase risk of serotonin syndrome. Discourage use together. Allow 14 days to lapse between discontinuing safinamide and starting St. John's wort.

Drug-food. *Tyramine-containing foods (aged, fermented, cured, pickled, or smoked food):* May increase risk of HTN. Avoid these types of food. Monitor patient closely.

Drug-lifestyle. *Alcohol use:* May increase sedative effects. Don't use together.

EFFECTS ON LAB TEST RESULTS
• May increase ALT and AST levels.

CONTRAINDICATIONS & CAUTIONS
• Contraindicated in patients hypersensitive to drug or its components and in patients with severe hepatic impairment (Child-Pugh class C).

• Concomitant use of other drugs in the MAO inhibitor class or other drugs that are potent inhibitors of MAO, including linezolid, may result in increased BP or hypertensive crisis.

• Concomitant use of opioids (e.g., meperidine and its derivatives, methadone, propoxyphene, or tramadol); SSNRIs; tricyclic, tetracyclic, or triazolopyridine antidepressants; cyclobenzaprine; methylphenidate, amphetamine, and their derivatives; or St. John's wort could result in life-threatening serotonin syndrome.

• Concomitant use of dextromethorphan may cause episodes of psychosis or abnormal behavior.

• Use cautiously in patients with moderate hepatic impairment (Child-Pugh class B).

• Use cautiously in patients with major psychotic disorder; drug may exacerbate psychosis. Consider dosage reduction or drug discontinuation if patient develops hallucinations or psychotic-like behaviors.

• Safinamide isn't effective alone for the treatment of Parkinson disease. Patients should take levodopa–carbidopa with this drug.

• Safety and effectiveness in children haven't been studied.

Dialyzable drug: Unknown.

PREGNANCY-LACTATION-REPRODUCTION
• There are no adequate or well-controlled studies in pregnant women. Developmental toxicity and teratogenic effects were observed in animal studies. Use only if benefits outweigh risks to the fetus.

S

• It isn't known if drug appears in human milk. Patient should discontinue breastfeeding or discontinue drug.

NURSING CONSIDERATIONS
• Monitor patients for hypersensitivity reactions, including dyspnea and swelling of the tongue and oral mucosa.
• Monitor patients for new-onset HTN or uncontrolled HTN.
• Monitor patients for serotonin syndrome (mental status changes [including agitation, hallucinations, delirium, coma], tachycardia, labile BP, dizziness, diaphoresis, flushing, hyperthermia, rigidity, monoclonus, hyperreflexia, incoordination, seizures, nausea, vomiting, diarrhea).
• Monitor LFT values.
• Patients may experience excessive drowsiness and fall asleep suddenly without warning. Monitor patients for daytime sleepiness or falling asleep during activities (driving, talking, eating). Drug may need to be discontinued.
• Monitor patients for new-onset or exacerbated dyskinesia. Reducing levodopa or other dopaminergic drug dosage may be needed.
• A withdrawal syndrome (elevated temperature, muscular rigidity, confusion, altered consciousness, autonomic instability) resembling NMS may occur with rapid dosage reduction, drug withdrawal, or changes in drug regimen that increase central dopaminergic tone. Adjust dosage carefully and taper dosage before discontinuation.
• Drug may exacerbate psychotic behaviors and cause hallucinations or psychotic-like behaviors. If signs and symptoms occur, dosage reduction or drug discontinuation may be needed.
• Drug may cause impulse control or compulsive behaviors. Monitor patients for new or increased gambling urges, sexual urges, uncontrolled spending, binge eating, or other intense urges and the inability to control these urges. If signs or symptoms occur, dosage reduction or drug discontinuation may be needed.
• Periodically monitor for visual changes in patients with a history of retinal or macular degeneration, uveitis, personal or family history of retinal disease, albinism, retinitis pigmentosa, diabetic retinopathy, or other retinopathy.

PATIENT TEACHING
• Tell patient to report all adverse reactions to prescriber.
• Inform patient that drug may elevate BP. Advise patient to monitor BP and report elevations.
• Teach patient signs and symptoms of serotonin syndrome and to report them should they occur.
• Explain that drug can cause sleepiness and patient can fall asleep suddenly during daily activities. Caution patient not to drive, operate heavy machinery, work in high places, or engage in other dangerous activities until drug's effects are known.
• Advise patient to avoid foods that contain large amounts of tyramine (aged, fermented, cured, smoked, or pickled foods) because of the potential for substantial increases in BP.
• Warn patient not to discontinue drug rapidly; drug should be tapered to avoid withdrawal.
• Explain that drug may cause retinal changes. Tell patient to notify prescriber if visual changes occur.
• Advise patient to immediately report hallucinations, psychotic behavior, compulsive behaviors, or problems with impulse control (gambling, spending money, sexual urges, binge eating).
• Advise female patient not to become pregnant or breastfeed during therapy.

salmeterol xinafoate
sal-ME-te-role

Serevent Diskus

Therapeutic class: Bronchodilators
Pharmacologic class: Long-acting selective beta$_2$ agonists

AVAILABLE FORMS
Inhalation powder: 50 mcg/dose

INDICATIONS & DOSAGES
➤ **Long-term maintenance of asthma; to prevent bronchospasm only as concomitant therapy with an inhaled corticosteroid**

---

in patients with nocturnal asthma or reversible obstructive airway
Adults and children age 4 and older: 1 inhalation (50 mcg) b.i.d. in the morning and evening, about 12 hours apart.
➤ **To prevent exercise-induced bronchospasm**
Adults and children age 4 and older: 1 inhalation (50 mcg) at least 30 minutes before exercise. Additional doses shouldn't be taken for at least 12 hours.
➤ **COPD, emphysema, or chronic bronchitis**
Adults: 1 inhalation (50 mcg) b.i.d. in the morning and evening, about 12 hours apart.

ADMINISTRATION
Inhalational
• Give drug 30 minutes before exercise to prevent exercise-induced bronchospasm.
• Don't use a spacer device with this drug.

ACTION
Unclear. Selectively activates beta$_2$ receptors, which results in bronchodilation; also, blocks the release of allergic mediators from mast cells lining the respiratory tract.

Route	Onset	Peak	Duration
Inhalation	30–120 min	20 min	12 hr

Half-life: 5½ hours.

ADVERSE REACTIONS
CNS: anxiety, headache, dizziness, tremor, nervousness, paresthesia, sleep disturbance, fever. **CV:** tachycardia, palpitations, HTN. **EENT:** conjunctivitis, keratitis, nasopharyngitis, pharyngitis, hoarseness, nasal cavity or sinus disorder, candidiasis of mouth/throat, hyposalivation, sinusitis, rhinitis. **GI:** nausea, vomiting, diarrhea, heartburn. **Musculoskeletal:** joint and back pain, myalgia. **Respiratory:** URI, cough, lower respiratory tract infection, *asthma.* **Other:** hypersensitivity reactions, rash, urticaria, flulike symptoms, photodermatitis.

INTERACTIONS
Drug-drug. *Antiarrhythmics (amiodarone, disopyramide, sotalol), chlorpromazine, dolasetron, droperidol, moxifloxacin, pentamidine, pimozide, tacrolimus, thioridazine, ziprasidone:* May prolong QT interval and increase risk of life-threatening cardiac arrhythmias. Monitor QT interval closely.
Beta agonists, other methylxanthines, theophylline: May cause adverse cardiac effects with excessive use. Monitor patient.
Beta blockers (nonselective): May diminish bronchodilatory effects. Use cardioselective beta blockers if therapy is indicated.
CYP3A4 inhibitors (atazanavir, clarithromycin, itraconazole, ketoconazole, ritonavir): May increase cardiac effects. Avoid use together.
Diuretics (non-potassium-sparing): May worsen hypokalemia and ECG changes. Use cautiously together.
MAO inhibitors: May cause risk of severe adverse CV effects. Avoid use within 14 days of MAO inhibitor therapy.
TCAs: May cause risk of moderate to severe adverse CV effects. Avoid use together within 14 days.

EFFECTS ON LAB TEST RESULTS
None reported.

CONTRAINDICATIONS & CAUTIONS
• Contraindicated in patients hypersensitive to drug or its ingredients.
Black Box Warning Contraindicated for treatment of asthma without a concomitant long-term asthma control medication such as an inhaled corticosteroid. Using without a long-term asthma control medication may increase the risk of asthma-related death. ∎
• Paradoxical bronchospasm that may be life-threatening may occur; distinguish from inadequate response.
🟢 *Alert:* Don't use drug with other medications containing long-acting beta$_2$ agonists.
🟢 *Alert:* Don't use as the primary treatment for acute episodes of asthma or COPD.
• Use cautiously in patients unusually responsive to sympathomimetics and those with coronary insufficiency, arrhythmias, HTN, other CV disorders, thyrotoxicosis, hepatic impairment, diabetes, or seizure disorders.
Dialyzable drug: Unknown.
⚠ *Overdose S&S:* Exaggeration of adverse reactions, hypokalemia, seizures, angina, HTN, hypotension, dry mouth, muscle cramps, dizziness, fatigue, insomnia,

S

tachycardia, ventricular arrhythmias, cardiac arrest, sudden death.

PREGNANCY-LACTATION-REPRODUCTION

• There are no adequate studies in pregnant women, but drug may be teratogenic. Use during pregnancy only if potential benefit justifies potential risk to the fetus.
• It isn't known if drug appears in human milk. Use cautiously in breastfeeding women.

NURSING CONSIDERATIONS

Black Box Warning Drug may increase the risk of asthma-related death. Only use salmeterol as additional therapy for patients whose condition is not adequately controlled on other medications or patients whose disease severity warrants initiation of treatment with two maintenance therapies. ■

Black Box Warning Once asthma control is achieved and maintained, assess patient at regular intervals; step down therapy (e.g., discontinue salmeterol) if possible without loss of asthma control and maintain patient on a long-term asthma control medication such as an inhaled corticosteroid. Don't use salmeterol for patients whose asthma is adequately controlled on low- or medium-dose inhaled corticosteroids. ■

Black Box Warning Long-acting beta$_2$ agonists may increase risk of asthma-related hospitalization in children and adolescents. For children and adolescents with asthma who require addition of a long-acting beta$_2$ agonist to an inhaled corticosteroid, a fixed-dose combination product containing both an inhaled corticosteroid and a long-acting beta$_2$ agonist should ordinarily be used to ensure adherence with both drugs. In cases in which use of a separate long-term asthma-control medication (such as an inhaled corticosteroid) and a long-acting beta$_2$ agonist is clinically indicated, appropriate steps must be taken to ensure adherence with both treatment components. If adherence can't be ensured, a fixed-dose combination product containing both an inhaled corticosteroid and a long-acting beta$_2$ agonist is recommended. ■

• Drug isn't indicated for acute bronchospasm.

❸ *Alert:* Monitor patient for rash and urticaria, which may signal a hypersensitivity reaction.
• Rarely, potentially life-threatening paradoxical bronchospasm can occur. Distinguish this symptom from inadequate response.

PATIENT TEACHING

Black Box Warning Teach parents of child or adolescent who requires the use of a separate long-term asthma-control medication (such as an inhaled corticosteroid) and a long-acting beta$_2$ agonist that appropriate steps must be taken to ensure adherence with both treatment components, because of the increased risk of asthma-related death. If adherence can't be ensured, a fixed-dose combination product containing both an inhaled corticosteroid and a long-acting beta$_2$ agonist is recommended. ■

• Remind patient to take drug at about 12-hour intervals for optimal effect and to take drug even when feeling better.
• Advise patient that immediate hypersensitivity reactions (such as urticaria, angioedema, rash, bronchospasm, and hypotension, including anaphylaxis) may occur after administration of this drug and to seek immediate medical attention if such reactions occur.
• If patient is taking drug to prevent exercise-induced bronchospasm, tell patient to take it 30 minutes before exercise.
❸ *Alert:* Tell patient drug shouldn't be used to treat acute bronchospasm. Patient must use a short-acting beta$_2$ agonist, such as albuterol, to treat worsening symptoms.
❸ *Alert:* Rare serious asthma episodes or asthma-related deaths may occur in patients using salmeterol. Black patients may be at greater risk.
• Tell patient to contact prescriber if the short-acting agonist no longer provides sufficient relief or if patient needs more than 4 inhalations daily. This may be a sign that the asthma symptoms are worsening. Tell patient not to increase the dosage of salmeterol.
• If patient takes an inhaled corticosteroid, patient should continue to use it regularly. Warn patient not to take other drugs without prescriber's consent.

• If patient takes the inhalation powder (in a multidose inhaler), instruct patient not to exhale into the device. Patient should activate and use it only in a level, horizontal position.
• Tell patient not to use dry-powder multidose inhaler with a spacer.
• Instruct patient never to wash mouthpiece or any part of dry-powder multidose inhaler; it must be kept dry.
• Advise female patient to contact physician if she becomes pregnant during therapy.

SAFETY ALERT!

sargramostim (GM-CSF; granulocyte-macrophage colony-stimulating factor)
sar-GRAM-oh-stim

Leukine

Therapeutic class: Hematopoietics
Pharmacologic class: Colony-stimulating factors

AVAILABLE FORMS
Powder for injection: 250 mcg
Solution for injection: 500 mcg/mL*

INDICATIONS & DOSAGES
➤ **To accelerate hematopoietic reconstitution after autologous or allogeneic bone marrow transplantation in patients with malignant lymphoma or acute lymphoblastic leukemia or in patients with Hodgkin lymphoma**
Adults: 250 mcg/m^2 daily given as 2-hour IV infusion beginning 2 to 4 hours after bone marrow transplantation and not less than 24 hours after last dose of chemotherapy or radiotherapy. Don't give until post–marrow infusion ANC is less than 500 cells/mm^3. Continue until ANC is more than 1,500/mm^3 for 3 consecutive days.
Adjust-a-dose: Discontinue immediately if blast cells appear or disease progression occurs. Temporarily discontinue or reduce dosage by 50% if a severe adverse reaction occurs. Interrupt therapy or reduce dosage by 50% if ANC exceeds 20,000 cells/mm^3 or WBC count is more than 50,000 cells/mm^3.

➤ **Neutrophil recovery following chemotherapy in acute myelogenous leukemia**
Adults age 55 and older: Initially, 250 mcg/m^2 IV once daily over 4 hours beginning day 11 or 4 days after completion of induction therapy; initiate only if bone marrow is hypoplastic with less than 5% blasts on day 10. If a second induction cycle is needed, begin sargramostim 4 days after completing chemotherapy and only if bone marrow is hypoplastic with less than 5% blasts. Continue until the ANC is more than 1,500/mm^3 for 3 consecutive days or for a maximum of 42 days.
Adjust-a-dose: Discontinue immediately if leukemic regrowth occurs. Reduce dosage by 50% or temporarily discontinue if a severe adverse reaction occurs. Interrupt therapy or reduce dosage by 50% if ANC exceeds 20,000 cells/mm^3.

➤ **Mobilization of peripheral blood progenitor cells (PBPCs)**
Adults: 250 mcg/m^2 by continuous IV infusion over 24 hours or by subcut injection once daily. Continue through PBPC collection.
Adjust-a-dose: If WBC count is more than 50,000/mm^3, reduce dosage by 50%. If adequate numbers of cells aren't collected, consider other mobilization therapy.

➤ **Post-PBPC transplantation**
Adults: 250 mcg/m^2 by continuous IV infusion over 24 hours or by subcut injection once daily beginning immediately after PBPC infusion; continue until ANC is more than 1,500/mm^3 for 3 consecutive days.

➤ **Bone marrow transplantation failure or engraftment delay**
Adults: 250 mcg/m^2 as a 2-hour IV infusion daily for 14 days. This course of therapy may be repeated after 7 days of no therapy. If engraftment still hasn't occurred, a third course of 500 mcg/m^2 daily IV for 14 days may be attempted after another therapy-free 7 days.
Adjust-a-dose: Stimulation of marrow precursors may result in rapid rise of WBC count. If blast cells appear or increase to 10% or more of WBC count or if the underlying disease progresses, stop therapy. If WBC count is more than 50,000 cells/mm^3 or ANC is above 20,000/mm^3, temporarily stop drug or reduce dose by 50%.

S

➤ **To increase survival in patients acutely exposed to myelosuppressive doses of radiation (hematopoietic syndrome of acute radiation syndrome) given as soon as possible after suspected or confirmed exposure to radiation doses greater than 2 gray**
Adults and children weighing more than 40 kg: 7 mcg/kg subcut once daily. Continue until ANC remains more than 1,000/mm³ for three consecutive CBCs obtained every third day, or exceeds 10,000/mm³ after a radiation-induced nadir.
Children weighing 15 to 40 kg: 10 mcg/kg subcut once daily. Continue until ANC remains more than 1,000/mm³ for three consecutive CBCs obtained every third day, or exceeds 10,000/mm³ after a radiation-induced nadir.
Children weighing less than 15 kg: 12 mcg/kg subcut once daily. Continue until ANC remains more than 1,000/mm³ for three consecutive CBCs obtained every third day, or exceeds 10,000/mm³ after a radiation-induced nadir.
➤ **Neuroblastoma in high-risk children ♦**
Children and adolescents: 250 mcg/m² subcut or IV once daily for 14 days, beginning 3 days before administration of dinutuximab (each cycle is 28 days); sargramostim is administered during cycles 1, 3, and 5 (regimen also includes dinutuximab, isotretinoin, and aldesleukin).

ADMINISTRATION
IV
▼ Reconstitute powder for injection with 1 mL of sterile or bacteriostatic water for injection. Direct stream of sterile water against side of vial and gently swirl contents to minimize foaming. Avoid excessive or vigorous agitation or shaking.
▼ Dilute in NSS. If drug yield is below 10 mcg/mL, add human albumin at final concentration of 0.1% to NSS before adding sargramostim to prevent adsorption to components of the delivery system. To yield 0.1% human albumin, add 1 mg human albumin to each milliliter of NSS (dilute 1 mL of 5% human albumin in 50 mL of NSS).
▼ Don't use in-line filter.
▼ Give as soon as possible after mixing and no later than 6 hours after reconstituting.

▼ **Incompatibilities:** Other IV drugs, unless specific compatibility data are available.
Subcutaneous
• Further dilution of injection or reconstituted solution isn't needed.

ACTION
Induces cellular responses by binding to specific receptors on surfaces of target cells.

Route	Onset	Peak	Duration
IV	15 min	Immediate	Unknown
Subcut	15 min	2–3 hr	Unknown

Half-life: IV, about 1 hour; subcut, about 3 hours.

ADVERSE REACTIONS
CNS: asthenia, CNS disorders, fever, headache, malaise, anxiety, insomnia. **CV:** *hemorrhage,* edema, peripheral edema, HTN, supraventricular arrhythmias, pericardial effusion, tachycardia. **EENT:** pharyngitis, rhinitis, epistaxis. **GI:** anorexia, diarrhea, abdominal pain, GI disorders, nausea, stomatitis, vomiting, *GI hemorrhage.* **GU:** urinary tract disorder, abnormal kidney function. **Hematologic:** blood dyscrasias. **Hepatic:** liver damage, bilirubinemia. **Musculoskeletal:** arthralgias, bone pain. **Respiratory:** dyspnea, lung disorders, pleural effusion. **Skin:** alopecia, pruritus, rash. **Other:** mucous membrane disorder, chills.

INTERACTIONS
Drug-drug. *Bleomycin, cyclophosphamide:* May enhance risk of pulmonary toxicity. Monitor patient closely.
Corticosteroids, lithium: May increase myeloproliferative effects of sargramostim. Use cautiously together.

EFFECTS ON LAB TEST RESULTS
• May increase BUN, creatinine, AST, ALT, alkaline phosphatase, bilirubin, glucose, and cholesterol levels.
• May decrease calcium and albumin levels.

CONTRAINDICATIONS & CAUTIONS
• Contraindicated in patients hypersensitive to drug or its components or to yeast-derived products and in those with excessive leukemic myeloid blasts in bone marrow or peripheral blood.

Reactions in bold italics are *life-threatening.* Interactions may have a *rapid onset* or a *delayed onset.*

• Infusion-related reactions (respiratory distress, hypoxia, flushing, hypotension, syncope, and tachycardia) may occur after administration of the first dose.

• Concomitant use within 24 hours of chemotherapy or radiation is contraindicated.

• Use cautiously in patients with cardiac disease, hypoxia, fluid retention, pulmonary infiltrates, HF, or impaired renal or hepatic function because these conditions may be worsened.

• Drug may interfere with bone imaging studies; increased hematopoietic activity of the bone marrow may appear as transient positive bone imaging changes.

• Safety and effectiveness haven't been established in children.

Dialyzable drug: Unknown.

⚠ **Overdose S&S:** Dyspnea, malaise, nausea, fever, rash, sinus tachycardia, headache, chills.

PREGNANCY-LACTATION-REPRODUCTION

• There are no adequate studies in pregnant women. Use during pregnancy only if clearly needed.

• It isn't known if drug appears in human milk. Use in breastfeeding women only if clearly needed.

NURSING CONSIDERATIONS

• If severe adverse reactions occur, reduce dose by 50% or temporarily stop drug and notify prescriber. Resume therapy when reactions decrease. Transient rash and local reactions at injection site may occur.

• Monitor patient for infusion-related reactions (respiratory distress, hypoxia, flushing, hypotension, syncope, and tachycardia), which may occur after administration of the first dose. If patient exhibits signs of dyspnea, reduce rate of infusion by 50%; if symptoms persist or worsen, discontinue infusion.

• Solution for injection contains benzyl alcohol, which has been associated with fatal "gasping syndrome" in neonates. Don't administer to neonates.

• Rapidly dividing progenitor cells may be sensitive to cytotoxic therapies, making the drug ineffective; don't give within 24 hours of last dose of chemotherapy or radiotherapy.

• Monitor CBC with differential, including examination for presence of blast cells, biweekly.

• Drug accelerates myeloid recovery in patients receiving bone marrow that is either unpurged or purged by anti-B cell monoclonal antibodies more than in those who receive bone marrow that is chemically purged.

• Drug may produce a limited response in transplant patients who have received extensive radiotherapy or who have received other myelotoxic drugs.

• Drug can act as a growth factor for any tumor type, particularly myeloid malignant disease.

PATIENT TEACHING

• Review administration schedule with patient and caregivers, and address their concerns.

• Urge patient to report all adverse reactions promptly.

---

sarilumab
sar-IL-ue-mab

Kevzara

Therapeutic class: Antirheumatics
Pharmacologic class: Monoclonal antibodies

AVAILABLE FORMS
Injection: 150 mg/1.14 mL, 200 mg/1.14 mL single-dose prefilled syringes and pens

INDICATIONS & DOSAGES
➤ **Treatment of moderately to severely active RA in patients who have had an inadequate response or intolerance to one or more DMARDs, as monotherapy or in combination with methotrexate or other conventional DMARDs**
Adults: 200 mg subcut once every 2 weeks.
Adjust-a-dose: Reduce dosage to 150 mg every 2 weeks for management of neutropenia, thrombocytopenia, and elevated liver enzyme levels. Refer to manufacturer's instructions for specific toxicity-related dosage adjustments.

ADMINISTRATION
Subcutaneous
• Allow prefilled syringe to sit at room temperature for 30 minutes or prefilled pen to sit at room temperature for 60 minutes before subcut injection; don't warm in any other way.
• Inspect solution before use. Don't use if solution is cloudy, discolored, or contains particles, or if any part of prefilled syringe appears to be damaged.
• Inject the full amount in the syringe or pen (1.14 mL).
• Rotate injection sites with each injection. Don't inject into skin that is tender, damaged, or has bruises or scars.
• Keep unused syringes or pens in original carton to protect from light and store in refrigerator between 36° and 46° F (2° and 8° C); don't freeze or heat.
• May store drug at room temperature up to 77° F (25° C) for up to 14 days in carton. Use syringe or pen within 14 days after removing from refrigerator.

ACTION
An interleukin 6 (IL-6) receptor antagonist that binds to both soluble and membrane-bound IL-6 receptors causing an anti-inflammatory effect that leads to a reduction in C-reactive protein levels.

Route	Onset	Peak	Duration
Subcut	Unknown	2–4 days	28 days (150-mg dose), 43 days (200-mg dose)

Half-life: 150-mg dose, 8 days; 200-mg dose, 10 days.

ADVERSE REACTIONS
EENT: nasopharyngitis. **GU:** UTI. **Hematologic:** *neutropenia, leukopenia, thrombocytopenia.* **Hepatic:** increased ALT and AST levels. **Metabolic:** hypertriglyceridemia. **Respiratory:** URI. **Skin:** injection-site erythema, injection-site pruritus. **Other:** infection, immunosuppression, hypersensitivity reactions.

INTERACTIONS
Drug-drug. *Biological DMARDs (anti-CD20 monoclonal antibodies, IL-1R antagonists, selective costimulation modulators,*

TNF antagonists): May increase risk of immunosuppression and infection. Avoid use together.
Corticosteroids: May increase risk of immunosuppression and infection. Monitor patient closely.
Corticosteroids, NSAIDs: May increase risk of GI perforation. Avoid concurrent use.
CYP450 substrates (atorvastatin, lovastatin, oral contraceptives, theophylline, warfarin): May alter substrate concentrations. Use cautiously together. Monitor substrate levels if possible and adjust substrate dosage as needed.
Live-virus vaccines: May increase risk of infection. Avoid use together.

EFFECTS ON LAB TEST RESULTS
• May increase AST, ALT, LDL, HDL, and triglyceride levels.
• May decrease neutrophil and platelet counts.

CONTRAINDICATIONS & CAUTIONS
• Contraindicated in patients with hypersensitivity to drug or its components.
Black Box Warning Serious infections leading to hospitalization or death, including bacterial, viral, invasive fungal, TB, and other opportunistic infections, can occur. Avoid use in patients with an active infection. ■
• Consider risks and benefits of use in patients with chronic or recurrent infection, a history of serious or opportunistic infections, underlying conditions in addition to RA that may predispose them to infections, exposure to TB, or a history of living or traveling to areas of endemic TB or mycoses.
• Risk of GI perforation may increase in patients with concurrent diverticulitis or use of NSAIDs or corticosteroids.
• Drug isn't recommended in patients with active hepatic disease or hepatic impairment (ALT or AST level more than 1.5 × ULN).
• Drug may increase risk of viral reactivation, including herpes zoster.
• Drug may increase risk of malignancies.
• Drug use hasn't been studied in patients with hepatic impairment or severe renal impairment.
• Safety and effectiveness in children haven't been established.

Reactions in bold italics are *life-threatening.* Interactions may have a *rapid onset* or a ***delayed onset.***

• Use cautiously in elderly patients (age 65 and older) because of increased risk of infections.
Dialyzable drug: Unknown.

PREGNANCY-LACTATION-REPRODUCTION
• Effect of drug on a fetus is unknown; however, monoclonal antibodies cross the placental barrier in the third trimester and drug may affect immune response in infants exposed in utero. Use in pregnancy only if potential benefit justifies potential risk to the fetus.
• It isn't known if drug appears in human milk. Consider benefits and risks of drug before patient starts breastfeeding.
• Enroll patients exposed to drug during pregnancy in a pregnancy registry to monitor outcomes by calling 1-877-311-8972.

NURSING CONSIDERATIONS
Black Box Warning Monitor patients for infection during treatment. Interrupt treatment if serious or opportunistic infection occurs; don't restart drug until infection is controlled. ∎
• Perform prompt and complete testing to evaluate a new infection during treatment and initiate appropriate antimicrobial therapy while closely monitoring patient.
Black Box Warning Assess patient for TB risk factors and test for latent TB before drug initiation. If positive, start treatment for TB before beginning therapy. Consider anti-TB therapy for patients with a history of TB in whom an adequate course of treatment can't be confirmed and in patients who test negatively for latent TB but have risk factors for TB. ∎
• Monitor neutrophil and platelet counts before therapy, 4 to 8 weeks after start of therapy, and every 3 months thereafter.
• Monitor ALT and AST levels before therapy, 4 to 8 weeks after start of therapy, and every 3 months thereafter. Assess bilirubin level or other LFT values as clinically indicated.
• Monitor patients for hypersensitivity reactions (injection-site rash, generalized rash, urticaria). If anaphylaxis or other severe hypersensitivity reaction occurs, stop drug immediately.

• Monitor patients with concurrent diverticulitis and those who are taking corticosteroids or NSAIDs for GI perforation. Promptly evaluate acute abdominal signs and symptoms.
• *Look alike–sound alike:* Don't confuse sarilumab with sirolimus. Don't confuse Kevzara with Keppra.

PATIENT TEACHING
Black Box Warning Warn patient that drug may lower resistance to infection and to contact prescriber immediately if signs and symptoms of infection appear, to ensure rapid evaluation and appropriate treatment. ∎
• Assess patient for the ability to self-administer drug. Instruct patient or caregivers in injection technique and syringe disposal.
• Advise patient to seek immediate medical attention for signs or symptoms of serious allergic reactions (shortness of breath, chest pain, dizziness, moderate or severe stomach pain or vomiting, or swelling of the lips, tongue, or face).
• Caution patient (especially if taking NSAIDs or steroids or with a history of tears of the stomach or intestines) of increased risk of GI perforation. Instruct patient to seek medical attention immediately for severe, persistent abdominal pain.
• Tell patient to discuss plans for surgery or a medical procedure with prescriber.
• Instruct patient to keep carton in an insulated bag with an ice pack when traveling.
• Caution female patient to immediately report pregnancy that occurs during treatment.

SAFETY ALERT!

sAXagliptin
sax-a-GLIP-tin

Onglyza⟡

Therapeutic class: Antidiabetics
Pharmacologic class: DPP-4 enzyme inhibitors

AVAILABLE FORMS
Tablets: 2.5 mg, 5 mg

INDICATIONS & DOSAGES

➤ **Adjunct to diet and exercise to improve glycemic control in type 2 diabetes**

Adults: 2.5 or 5 mg PO once daily.

Adjust-a-dose: For patients with eGFR of 45 mL/minute/1.73 m^2 or less or ESRD requiring hemodialysis, give 2.5 mg PO once daily. If patient requires hemodialysis or patient is taking strong CYP3A4/5 inhibitors, give 2.5 mg once daily after treatment.

ADMINISTRATION

PO

- Give drug with or without food.
- Don't split or cut tablets.

ACTION

Inhibits DPP-4, an enzyme that rapidly inactivates incretin hormones, which play a part in the body's regulation of glucose. By increasing active incretin levels, drug helps to increase insulin release and decrease circulating glucose.

Route	Onset	Peak	Duration
PO	Unknown	2 hr	24 hr

Half-life: 2½ hours.

ADVERSE REACTIONS

CNS: headache. **CV:** facial edema, peripheral edema. **EENT:** sinusitis. **GI:** abdominal pain, gastroenteritis, vomiting. **GU:** UTI. **Metabolic:** *hypoglycemia.* **Respiratory:** URI. **Skin:** urticaria.

INTERACTIONS

Drug-drug. *Strong CYP3A4/5 inhibitors (atazanavir, clarithromycin, indinavir, itraconazole, ketoconazole, nefazodone, nelfinavir, ritonavir, saquinavir):* May increase saxagliptin level. Reduce dosage to 2.5 mg PO daily.

EFFECTS ON LAB TEST RESULTS

- May decrease lymphocyte count.

CONTRAINDICATIONS & CAUTIONS

- Contraindicated in patients hypersensitive to drug or its components.
- Hypersensitivity reactions, including anaphylaxis, angioedema, and exfoliative skin conditions such as bullous pemphigoid, have occurred within first 3 months of therapy

initiation. Discontinue drug if hypersensitivity is suspected.

❶ *Alert:* Use cautiously in patients with a history of HF or renal disease. Drug may increase risk of HF in these patients.

- Use cautiously in patients taking secretagogues (such as sulfonylureas) because of increased risk of hypoglycemia.
- Discontinue drug if pancreatitis is suspected. Drug isn't indicated to treat type 1 diabetes or diabetic ketoacidosis.
- Safety and effectiveness in children haven't been established.

Dialyzable drug: 23%.

PREGNANCY-LACTATION-REPRODUCTION

- There are no adequate studies in pregnant women. Use during pregnancy only if clearly needed.
- It isn't known if drug appears in human milk. Use cautiously in breastfeeding women.

NURSING CONSIDERATIONS

❶ *Alert:* Drug may cause joint pain that can be severe and disabling. Report severe and persistent joint pain to prescriber as drug may need to be discontinued.

❶ *Alert:* Monitor patient for signs and symptoms of HF (dyspnea, orthopnea, tiredness, weakness, fatigue, weight gain, peripheral or abdominal edema). Drug may need to be discontinued and other antidiabetic drugs may be required.

- Monitor blood glucose level and watch for signs and symptoms of hypoglycemia.
- Monitor HbA$_{1c}$ level periodically to assess long-term glycemic control.
- Monitor patient for signs and symptoms of pancreatitis. If pancreatitis is suspected, discontinue drug and initiate appropriate management.
- Assess renal function before starting drug and periodically thereafter.
- Monitor patient for skin blistering or erosions. Discontinue drug if bullous pemphigoid is suspected and consider referral to a dermatologist.
- Management of type 2 diabetes should also include diet control and exercise. Because calorie restriction, weight loss, and exercise help improve insulin sensitivity and help make drug therapy effective, these

---

Reactions in bold italics are *life-threatening.* Interactions may have a *rapid onset* or a *delayed onset.*

measures are essential for proper diabetes management.
• *Look alike–sound alike:* Don't confuse saxagliptin with sitagliptin.

PATIENT TEACHING
• Tell patient drug may be taken with or without food.
• Instruct patient not to split or cut tablets.
• Tell patient to stop drug and seek immediate medical attention for signs and symptoms of hypersensitivity, including rash, flaking or peeling skin, itching, or swelling of the skin, face, lips, tongue, or throat.
◑ *Alert:* Instruct patient to immediately report signs and symptoms of HF to prescriber. Patient should not stop drug without first discussing with prescriber.
◑ *Alert:* Instruct patient to report severe and persistent joint pain to prescriber as drug may need to be discontinued.
• Advise patient that drug isn't a substitute for diet and exercise and that it's important to follow a prescribed dietary and physical activity routine and to monitor glucose levels.
• Inform patient and family members of the signs and symptoms of hypoglycemia and hyperglycemia and the steps to take should these occur, including notifying the prescriber.
• Tell patient to notify prescriber during periods of stress, such as fever, infection, or surgery, because dosage may need adjustment.
• Tell patient to stop drug if signs and symptoms of pancreatitis (persistent severe abdominal pain, sometimes radiating to the back; vomiting) occur.
• Advise patient to immediately report skin blisters or erosions.

selegiline
se-LE-ji-leen

Emsam

selegiline hydrochloride (L-deprenyl hydrochloride)
Eldepryl, Zelapar

Therapeutic class: Antiparkinsonians
Pharmacologic class: MAO inhibitors

AVAILABLE FORMS
selegiline
Transdermal system: 6 mg/24 hours, 9 mg/24 hours, 12 mg/24 hours
selegiline hydrochloride
Capsules: 5 mg
Tablets: 5 mg
Tablets (ODTs): 1.25 mg

INDICATIONS & DOSAGES
➤ **Adjunctive treatment with levodopa–carbidopa in managing signs and symptoms of Parkinson disease**
Adults: For capsules and tablets, 10 mg PO daily divided as 5 mg at breakfast and 5 mg at lunch. After 2 or 3 days, gradual decrease of levodopa–carbidopa dosage may be needed. Or, if using ODTs, start with 1.25 mg PO once daily before breakfast and without liquid. Increase to 2.5 mg daily after at least 6 weeks, if tolerated and needed. Maximum dose is 10 mg/day for tablets and capsules and 2.5 mg once daily for ODTs.
➤ **Major depressive disorder**
Adults: Apply one patch daily to dry intact skin on the upper torso, upper thigh, or upper arm. Initially, use 6 mg/day. Increase, if needed, in increments of 3 mg/day at intervals of 2 or more weeks. Maximum daily dose, 12 mg.
Elderly patients: 6 mg transdermal patch daily.

ADMINISTRATION
PO
• Don't give food or liquids for 5 minutes before and after giving ODTs.

- Don't push ODTs through the foil backing; peel the backing off and gently remove the tablet.
- Place tablet on top of tongue.

Transdermal
- Apply patch to dry, intact skin on the upper torso, upper thigh, or outer surface of the upper arm once every 24 hours.
- Apply at the same time each day and rotate application sites.
- Don't cut the transdermal patch into smaller pieces.

ACTION
May inhibit MAO type B (mainly found in the brain) and dopamine metabolism. At higher-than-recommended doses, drug non-selectively inhibits MAO, including MAO type A (mainly found in the intestine). May also directly increase dopaminergic activity by decreasing the reuptake of dopamine into nerve cells.

Route	Onset	Peak	Duration
PO (tablet, capsule)	Unknown	40–90 min	Unknown
PO (ODT)	5 min	10–15 min	Unknown
Transdermal	Unknown	Unknown	24 hr

Half-life: Selegiline, 2 to 10 hours; N-desmethyl-deprenyl, 2 hours; L-amphetamine, 17¾ hours; L-methamphetamine, 20½ hours.

ADVERSE REACTIONS
Oral form
CNS: dizziness, agitation, delusions, loss of balance, depression, increased bradykinesia, involuntary movements, headache, confusion, hallucinations, vivid dreams, insomnia, syncope, pain. **CV:** *arrhythmias,* orthostatic hypotension, HTN, new or increased angina. **EENT:** pharyngitis, rhinitis. **GI:** nausea, dry mouth, abdominal pain, diarrhea. **Musculoskeletal:** leg cramps, myalgia, back pain. **Respiratory:** dyspnea. **Skin:** rash, ecchymosis.

Transdermal form
CNS: headache, insomnia. **CV:** chest pain, hypotension, orthostatic BP. **GI:** diarrhea, dry mouth, dyspepsia. **Metabolic:** weight gain, weight loss. **Respiratory:** pharyngitis, sinusitis. **Skin:** application-site reaction, rash.

INTERACTIONS
Drug-drug. *Bupropion, cyclobenzaprine, dextromethorphan, meperidine, methadone, mirtazapine, MAO inhibitors, sympathomimetic amines (including amphetamines, cold products, and weight-loss preparations containing vasoconstrictors), TCAs, tramadol:* May cause hypertensive crisis. Separate use by at least 2 weeks.
Carbamazepine, oxcarbazepine: May increase selegiline levels. Use together is contraindicated.
Citalopram, duloxetine, fluoxetine, fluvoxamine, nefazodone, paroxetine, sertraline, venlafaxine: May cause serotonin syndrome (CNS irritability, shivering, and altered consciousness). Separate use by at least 2 weeks (5 weeks if switching to or from fluoxetine).
Hormonal contraceptives: May increase plasma selegiline level and increase adverse reactions. Monitor patient closely.
Linezolid, methylene blue: May cause serotonin syndrome. Don't administer within 14 days of each other.
Drug-herb. *St. John's wort:* May cause increased serotonergic effects. Warn against using together.
Drug-food. ✪ *Alert: Foods high in tyramine:* May cause hypertensive crisis, especially at increased doses. Provide patient with a list of foods to avoid.

EFFECTS ON LAB TEST RESULTS
- May cause positive result for amphetamine on urine drug screen.

CONTRAINDICATIONS & CAUTIONS
- Contraindicated in patients hypersensitive to drug, in patients with pheochromocytoma, and in those taking bupropion, carbamazepine, cyclobenzaprine, dextromethorphan, duloxetine, methadone, meperidine, mirtazapine, MAO inhibitors, oxcarbazepine, SSRIs, sympathomimetics, tramadol, TCAs, or venlafaxine.
- ✪ *Alert:* Concomitant use with linezolid or methylene blue can cause serotonin syndrome (fever, mental status changes, muscle twitching, excessive sweating, shivering or shaking, diarrhea, loss of coordination). Use drug with linezolid or methylene blue only for life-threatening or urgent conditions

---

Reactions in bold italics are *life-threatening.* Interactions may have a *rapid onset* or a *delayed onset.*

when the potential benefits outweigh the risks of toxicity.

• Don't use oral drug with the transdermal system.

• Don't use ODTs at daily doses exceeding 2.5 mg/day.

• Orthostatic hypotension may occur during first 2 months of therapy or after dosage increases, especially in older patients.

• Potentially life-threatening serotonin syndrome and hyperpyrexia have been reported in patients taking antidepressants concomitantly with selegiline. Use together isn't recommended.

• Somnolence and falling asleep without prior warning while engaged in ADLs (including operating motor vehicles) have been reported in some patients. Evaluate patients for factors that may increase these risks, such as elderly patients with sleep disorders and those taking sedatives.

• Avoid use in patients with major psychotic disorders. Drug may cause changes in or worsening of mental status, abnormal thinking, and behavioral changes, which may be severe and include paranoid ideation, delusions, hallucinations, confusion, psychotic-like behavior, disorientation, aggressive behavior, agitation, and delirium. Drug isn't approved for bipolar depression.

• Hypertensive reactions have been reported in patients who ingested tyramine-containing foods while receiving oral selegiline.

Dialyzable drug: Unknown.

⚠ ***Overdose S&S:*** Drowsiness, dizziness, faintness, irritability, hyperactivity, agitation, severe headache, hallucinations, trismus, opisthotonos, seizures, coma, rapid and irregular pulse, HTN, hypotension and vascular collapse, precordial pain, respiratory depression and failure, hyperpyrexia, diaphoresis, cool and clammy skin.

PREGNANCY-LACTATION-REPRODUCTION

• There are no adequate studies in pregnant women. Use during pregnancy only if potential benefit justifies potential risk to the fetus.

• It isn't known if drug appears in human milk. Use cautiously in breastfeeding women.

NURSING CONSIDERATIONS

🛈 ***Alert:*** Some patients experience new or increased adverse reactions to levodopa, such as dyskinesia, when it's used with selegiline. These patients need a 10% to 30% reduction of levodopa–carbidopa dosage.

▐ Black Box Warning ▌ Transdermal system used to treat depression may increase risk of suicidal thinking and behavior in children, adolescents, and young adults ages 18 to 24, especially during the first few months of treatment, especially in those with major depressive or other psychiatric disorder. Contraindicated in patients younger than age 12 because of risk of hypertensive crisis. ▪

🛈 ***Alert:*** If linezolid or methylene blue must be given, stop selegiline and monitor patient for serotonin toxicity for 2 weeks, or until 24 hours after the last dose of methylene blue or linezolid, whichever comes first. May resume selegiline 24 hours after last dose of methylene blue or linezolid.

• Monitor patients with major depressive disorder for worsening of symptoms and of suicidal behavior, especially during the first few weeks of treatment and during dosage changes.

🛈 ***Alert:*** Monitor patient carefully for orthostatic hypotension, especially during first 2 months of treatment and after dosage increases. Help patient rise from a reclining position.

• Monitor patient for new-onset HTN or HTN that isn't adequately controlled after starting drug.

• Monitor patient taking antidepressants and selegiline concomitantly for serotonin syndrome and hyperpyrexia.

• Monitor patient for drowsiness, significant daytime sleepiness, or episodes of falling asleep during activities that require active participation. Discontinue drug if present.

• Monitor patient for psychotic-like behavior, changes in or worsening of mental status, abnormal thinking, and behavioral changes.

• Ask patient about the development or worsening of impulsive or compulsive behaviors, such as new or increased gambling urges, sexual urges, binge eating, uncontrolled spending, or other urges, because patient may not recognize these behaviors as abnormal.

S

• Examine patient's skin periodically for possible melanoma, because of risk of skin cancer associated with drug and with Parkinson disease.

• Examine patient's mouth for irritation or ulceration; be aware of patient complaints of swallowing or mouth pain when taking ODTs.

• *Look alike–sound alike:* Don't confuse Eldepryl with enalapril.

PATIENT TEACHING

❶ *Alert:* Teach patient to recognize and immediately report signs and symptoms of serotonin toxicity (fever, mental status changes, muscle twitching, excessive sweating, shivering or shaking, diarrhea, loss of coordination).

• Advise patient not to take drug in the evening because doing so may cause insomnia.

• Explain risk of hypertensive crisis if patient ingests foods or beverages containing tyramine during therapy; if using a 9-mg/day or higher transdermal system, patient should avoid these products altogether. Give patient a list of tyramine-containing foods and products.

• Advise patient to avoid liquids for 5 minutes before and after taking ODTs.

❶ *Alert:* Warn patient about the many drugs, including OTC drugs, that may interact with this drug and about the need to consult a pharmacist or prescriber before using them.

• Teach patient and family the signs and symptoms of hypertensive crisis, including severe headache, sore or stiff neck, nausea, vomiting, sweating, rapid heartbeat, dilated pupils, and photophobia.

• Instruct patient not to rise rapidly after sitting or lying down because of risk of dizziness, which may occur more frequently early in therapy or after dosage increases.

• Advise patient taking antidepressants concomitantly with selegiline to immediately report such signs and symptoms as confusion, hallucinations, agitation, delirium, syncope, shivering, sweating, high fever, tachycardia, nausea, diarrhea, muscle rigidity or twitching, or tremors.

• Explain that drug may cause patient to fall asleep during activities that require active participation. Advise patient to contact

prescriber if drowsiness, significant daytime sleepiness, or episodes of falling asleep during such activities occur.

• Tell patient to report paranoid ideation, delusions, hallucinations, confusion, psychotic-like behavior, disorientation, aggressive behavior, agitation, or delirium.

• Tell patient to contact prescriber if experiencing difficulty controlling impulsive or compulsive behaviors, such as new or increased gambling urges, sexual urges, binge eating, uncontrolled spending, or other urges.

• Urge patient to watch for skin changes that could suggest melanoma and to have periodic skin examinations by a health professional.

• Advise patient taking ODTs to report mouth pain, pain when swallowing, or ulcerations.

• Advise patient to contact prescriber before discontinuing selegiline.

• Tell patient that each ODT contains 1.25 mg phenylalanine.

Black Box Warning Advise family members of patient using transdermal system to watch for anxiety, agitation, insomnia, irritability, hostility, and aggressiveness and to report these immediately to prescriber. ∎

• Tell patient to apply transdermal system to dry, intact skin on the upper torso (below the neck and above the waist), upper thigh, or the outer surface of the upper arm at the same time each day. Advise patient to choose a new site each day.

• Tell patient to avoid exposing transdermal system to direct external heat sources, such as heating pads, electric blankets, hot tubs, heated water beds, and prolonged sunlight.

• Tell patient to stop using the transdermal system 10 days before having surgery requiring general anesthesia.

• Tell patient not to cut the transdermal system into smaller pieces.

• Advise female patient planning pregnancy or breastfeeding to first contact prescriber.

Reactions in bold italics are *life-threatening*. Interactions may have a *rapid onset* or a *delayed onset*.

semaglutide
sem-a-GLOO-tide

Ozempic, Rybelsus

Therapeutic class: Antidiabetic agents
Pharmacologic class: Human glucagon-like peptide-1 receptor agonists

AVAILABLE FORMS
Injection: 2 mg/1.5 mL prefilled pen injector, delivering 0.25 mg, 0.5 mg, or 1 mg per injection

INDICATIONS & DOSAGES
➤ **Adjunct to diet and exercise to improve glycemic control in patients with type 2 diabetes mellitus**
Adults: Initially, 0.25 mg subcut once weekly for 4 weeks; then increase to 0.5 mg once weekly. After 4 weeks, if needed, may increase to 1 mg once weekly. Maximum dosage is 1 mg once weekly.

ADMINISTRATION
Subcutaneous
• Drug may be considered hazardous; refer to facility policy for administration precautions.
• Semaglutide is a clear and colorless solution. Don't use if particulate matter or coloration is seen.
• Use 0.25-mg dose for initiating treatment. It isn't effective for glycemic control.
• Give drug once weekly on the same day each week at any time of day, without regard to meals.
• Administer subcut in the abdomen, thigh, or upper arm. Rotate injection sites.
• Administer insulin as a separate injection; never mix the products. May inject semaglutide and insulin in the same body region but don't inject in sites adjacent to one another.
• May change the day of weekly administration as long as the time between two doses is at least 48 hours.
• Give a missed dose as soon as possible within 5 days after the missed dose. If more than 5 days have passed, skip the missed dose and give the next dose on the regularly scheduled day.

❸ *Alert:* Device is for single patient use. Never share this device with others, even if the needle has been changed, since it could transmit blood-borne pathogens.
• Store pen capped without a needle attached. Always use a new needle for each use. After each use, always remove and safely discard needle.
• Before first use, refrigerate pen between 36° and 46° F (2° and 8° C). Don't store in freezer or directly adjacent to the refrigerator cooling element.
• After first use, store pen for up to 56 days at controlled room temperature (59° to 86° F [15° to 30° C]) or refrigerated (36° to 46° F [2° to 8° C]); don't freeze. Protect from excessive heat and sunlight.

ACTION
Stimulates the release of insulin and lowers glucagon secretion in the presence of elevated glucose levels. It also causes a minor delay in gastric emptying in the early postprandial phase.

Route	Onset	Peak	Duration
Subcut	Unknown	1–3 days	Unknown

Half-life: About 1 week.

ADVERSE REACTIONS
EENT: diabetic retinopathy complications.
GI: nausea, vomiting, diarrhea, abdominal pain, constipation, dyspepsia, eructation, flatulence, GERD, gastritis, cholelithiasis.
Hematologic: *hypoglycemia.* **Other:** immunogenicity.

INTERACTIONS
Drug-drug. *Insulin, insulin secretagogues (glipizide, repaglinide):* May increase risk of hypoglycemia. A reduced insulin or insulin secretagogue dosage may be required.
Oral medications: May change therapeutic effect of oral drugs because semaglutide delays gastric emptying. Monitor patient closely.

EFFECTS ON LAB TEST RESULTS
• May increase amylase and lipase levels.

CONTRAINDICATIONS & CAUTIONS
• Contraindicated in patients hypersensitive to drug or its components.

S

- Drug isn't indicated for type 1 diabetes mellitus or the treatment of diabetic ketoacidosis, or as a substitute for insulin.

Black Box Warning Semaglutide caused thyroid adenomas and carcinomas after lifetime exposure in rodents. It isn't known whether drug causes thyroid C-cell tumors, including medullary thyroid carcinoma (MTC). ■

Black Box Warning Contraindicated in patients with a personal or family history of MTC and in patients with multiple endocrine neoplasia syndrome type 2 (MEN 2). ■

- Drug isn't recommended as first-line therapy due to the uncertain relevance of rodent tumor findings to humans.
- Use cautiously in patients with a history of diabetic retinopathy. Rapid improvement in glucose control has been associated with temporary worsening of diabetic retinopathy. The effect of long-term improved glucose control using this drug and diabetic retinopathy hasn't been studied.
- Use cautiously in patients with a history of chronic renal failure; worsening of renal function has been reported, particularly in patients who experienced nausea, vomiting, and diarrhea.
- Cases of pancreatitis have occurred. If pancreatitis is suspected, discontinue drug and treat appropriately. If pancreatitis is confirmed, don't restart drug.
- Use in patients with a history of pancreatitis hasn't been studied. Consider use of other antidiabetic drugs.
- There are no studies establishing conclusive evidence of macrovascular risk reduction when this drug is used.
- Safety and effectiveness in children haven't been determined.

Dialyzable drug: Unknown.

PREGNANCY-LACTATION-REPRODUCTION
- Based on animal studies, drug may adversely affect a fetus. Poorly controlled diabetes, especially in pregnant women, carries many risks. Use during pregnancy only if the benefits outweigh risks to the fetus.
- It isn't known if drug appears in human milk or how it affects a breastfed infant or milk production. Use in pregnancy only if benefits outweigh risks to infant.

- Women who are planning pregnancy should discontinue drug at least 2 months before pregnancy.

NURSING CONSIDERATIONS
Black Box Warning Monitor patients for MTC or MEN 2. It isn't known if routine monitoring of serum calcitonin level or thyroid ultrasound can detect these cancers early. Further evaluate patients with elevated serum calcitonin level or thyroid nodules on physical examination or neck imaging. ■

⊙ *Alert:* Monitor patients for hypersensitivity reactions, including anaphylaxis and angioedema. Discontinue drug and treat appropriately if reaction occurs. Use cautiously in patients with a history of hypersensitivity to another glucagon-like peptide-1 agonist.
- Monitor patients for pancreatitis (persistent severe abdominal pain that may radiate to the back or be accompanied by vomiting). If pancreatitis is suspected, discontinue drug.
- Monitor patients with a history of diabetic retinopathy for disease progression.
- Monitor patients for acute kidney injury. Assess renal function at baseline and during dosage adjustments. Assess for nausea, vomiting, diarrhea, or dehydration, which are associated with worsening of renal function.
- Monitor glucose level and HbA$_{1c}$.
- Monitor patients for signs and symptoms of hypoglycemia (confusion, irritability, shakiness, sweating, hunger, palpitations, pallor, speech and motor dysfunction).
- *Look alike–sound alike:* Don't confuse semaglutide with sitagliptin.

PATIENT TEACHING
- Instruct patient to report all adverse reactions.
- Teach patient proper drug administration and storage.
- Tell patient how to manage missed doses.

⊙ *Alert:* Caution patient never to share injection pen with another person, even if the needle is changed, due to risk of blood-borne pathogen transmission.

Black Box Warning Counsel patient on the potential risk of MTC and MEN 2 and to report signs and symptoms of thyroid tumors

---

(neck mass, dysphagia, dyspnea, persistent hoarseness). ■

• Caution patient to discontinue drug and seek immediate medical attention for hypersensitivity reactions (difficulty breathing, throat or tongue swelling).

• Advise patient to immediately report signs and symptoms of pancreatitis and to discontinue drug.

• Instruct patient to report vision changes.

• Inform patient of the risk of kidney injury. Risk increases with risk of dehydration due to GI adverse effects. Instruct patient to take precautions to avoid fluid depletion and to report nausea, vomiting, diarrhea, or dehydration to prescriber. Advise patient that worsening renal impairment may require dialysis.

• Caution female patient about the use of drug during pregnancy and while breastfeeding. Encourage patient to discuss drug with prescriber before a planned pregnancy.

• Stress importance of adhering to proper diet and regular physical activity and that glucose and HbA$_{1c}$ levels and other laboratory tests will be monitored during therapy.

• Teach patient to recognize and manage hypoglycemia. Caution patient who is also taking insulin or insulin secretagogues about the increased risk of hypoglycemia.

• Tell patient to immediately report stresses to the body (fever, surgery, trauma, infection) because drug requirements may change.

• Tell patient that nausea, vomiting, and diarrhea are common at start of therapy but decrease over time for most patients.

sertraline hydrochloride
SIR-trah-leen

Apo-Sertraline✤, Zoloft⟋

Therapeutic class: Antidepressants
Pharmacologic class: SSRIs

AVAILABLE FORMS
Oral concentrate:* 20 mg/mL
Tablets: 25 mg, 50 mg, 100 mg

INDICATIONS & DOSAGES
Adjust-a-dose (for all indications): If dosage changes are needed, increase by 25 to 50 mg (except when used for premenstrual dysmorphic disorder) at intervals of no less than 1 week. For patients with mild hepatic impairment (Child-Pugh score 5 or 6), both the recommended starting dosage and therapeutic range are half the recommended daily dosage.

➤ **Depression**
Adults: 50 mg PO daily. Adjust dosage as needed and tolerated; dosage range is 50 to 200 mg daily.

➤ **OCD**
Adults: 50 mg PO once daily. If patient doesn't improve, increase dosage, up to 200 mg daily.
Children ages 6 to 17: Initially, 25 mg PO daily in children ages 6 to 12, or 50 mg PO daily in adolescents ages 13 to 17. Increase dosage, as needed, up to 200 mg daily.

➤ **Panic disorder**
Adults: Initially, 25 mg PO daily for 3 to 7 days; then increase to 50 mg PO daily. If patient doesn't improve, increase dose to maximum of 200 mg daily.

➤ **Posttraumatic stress disorder**
Adults: Initially, 25 mg PO once daily. Increase to 50 mg PO once daily after 1 week. Increase as needed at weekly intervals to a maximum of 200 mg daily. Maintain patient on lowest effective dose.

➤ **Premenstrual dysphoric disorder**
Adults: Initially, 25 mg PO daily either continuously or only during the luteal phase of the menstrual cycle. If patient doesn't respond, may increase dose 50 mg per menstrual cycle, up to 150 mg daily for use throughout the menstrual cycle or up to 150 mg daily for luteal-phase doses. If a 100-mg daily dose has been established with luteal-phase dosing, give 50 mg daily for 2 to 3 days at the beginning of each luteal phase before increasing to 150 mg.

➤ **Social anxiety disorder**
Adults: Initially, 25 mg PO once daily. Increase dosage to 50 mg PO once daily after 1 week of therapy. Dose range is 50 to 200 mg daily. Adjust to the lowest effective dosage and periodically reassess patient to determine the need for long-term treatment.

➤ **Generalized anxiety disorder ◆**
Adults: Initially, 25 mg once daily. May increase based on response and tolerability in increments of 25 to 50 mg at intervals

of 1 to 2 weeks or more. Usual dose, 50 to 150 mg/day. Maximum dose, 200 mg/day.

ADMINISTRATION
PO
- Give drug without regard for food.
- Don't use oral concentrate dropper, which is made of rubber, for patient with latex allergy.
- Mix oral concentrate with 4 oz (118 mL) of water, ginger ale, lemon-lime soda, lemonade, or orange juice only, and give immediately.

ACTION
Thought to be linked to drug's inhibition of CNS neuronal reuptake of serotonin.

Route	Onset	Peak	Duration
PO	1 wk	4–8 hr	Unknown

Half-life: 62 to 104 hours.

ADVERSE REACTIONS
CNS: fatigue, headache, tremor, dizziness, insomnia, somnolence, ***suicidal behavior,*** paresthesia, hypesthesia, nervousness, anxiety, malaise, agitation, ataxia, coma, confusion, hallucinations, irritability, ***seizure,*** hypertonia, pain. **CV:** palpitations, chest pain, hot flashes. edema, HTN, syncope, tachycardia, vasodilation. **EENT:** visual disturbances, blurred vision, mydriasis. **GI:** dry mouth, nausea, diarrhea, loose stools, dyspepsia, vomiting, constipation, thirst, flatulence, anorexia, abdominal pain, decreased appetite. **GU:** male sexual dysfunction, decreased libido (both genders). **Musculoskeletal:** myalgia. **Skin:** rash, pruritus, diaphoresis, alopecia.

INTERACTIONS
Drug-drug. *Agents with antiplatelet properties (NSAIDs, P2Y12 inhibitors, SSRIs), aspirin, clopidogrel, heparin:* May enhance antiplatelet effect and bleeding risk. Monitor therapy.
Amphetamines, buspirone, dextromethorphan, dihydroergotamine, lithium salts, meperidine, other SSRIs or SSNRIs (duloxetine, venlafaxine), sumatriptan, TCAs, ***tramadol,*** *trazodone, tryptophan:* May increase the risk of serotonin syndrome. Avoid combinations of drugs that increase the availabil-ity of serotonin in the CNS; monitor patient closely if used together.
Apixaban, dabigatran, edoxaban, rivaroxaban: May increase bleeding risk. Monitor patient carefully.
Cimetidine: May decrease clearance of sertraline. Monitor patient closely.
CYP2D6 substrates (atomoxetine, desipramine, dextromethorphan, flecainide, metoprolol, nebivolol, perphenazine, propafenone, thioridazine, tolterodine, venlafaxine): May increase exposure of the substrate. If concurrent use is needed, decrease the substrate dosage. If sertraline is discontinued, an increased substrate dosage may be needed.
Disulfiram: Oral concentrate contains alcohol, which may react with drug. Use together is contraindicated.
Fosphenytoin, phenytoin: May increase phenytoin concentration. Monitor phenytoin level and reduce phenytoin dosage if needed.
Linezolid, methylene blue: May cause serotonin syndrome. Use extreme caution and monitor patient closely.
MAO inhibitors (phenelzine, selegiline, tranylcypromine): May cause serotonin syndrome or signs and symptoms resembling NMS. Avoid using within 14 days of MAO inhibitor therapy.
Pimozide: May increase risk of QT-interval prolongation and ventricular arrhythmias. Use together is contraindicated.
Triptans: May cause serotonin syndrome (restlessness, hallucinations, loss of coordination, fast heartbeat, rapid changes in BP, increased body temperature, hyperreflexia, nausea, vomiting, and diarrhea) or NMS-like reactions. Use cautiously, with close monitoring, especially at the start of treatment and during dosage adjustments.
Warfarin, other highly protein-bound drugs: May increase level of sertraline or other highly protein-bound drug. May prolong PT, or INR may increase by 8%. Monitor patient closely; monitor PT and INR.
Drug-herb. *Alfalfa, anise, bilberry:* May increase risk of bleeding. Consider alternative agents.
St. John's wort: May cause additive effects and serotonin syndrome. Discourage use together.

Reactions in bold italics are *life-threatening*. Interactions may have a *rapid onset* or a ***delayed onset***.

EFFECTS ON LAB TEST RESULTS

• May increase ALT and AST levels.
• May decrease sodium level.
• May show false-positive urine immunoassay screening tests for benzodiazepines.

CONTRAINDICATIONS & CAUTIONS

• Contraindicated in patients hypersensitive to drug or its components.
ⓘ **Alert:** Concomitant use with other serotonergic agents, such as SSRIs, SSNRIs, triptans, linezolid, or methylene blue, can cause serotonin syndrome (fever, mental status changes, muscle twitching, excessive sweating, shivering or shaking, diarrhea, loss of coordination). Use drug with linezolid or methylene blue only for life-threatening or urgent conditions when the potential benefits outweigh the risks of toxicity.
• Contraindicated in patients taking pimozide or MAO inhibitors or within 14 days of MAO inhibitor therapy.
ⓘ **Alert:** Oral concentrate is contraindicated with disulfiram because it contains alcohol.
• Use cautiously in patients at risk for suicide and in those with seizure disorders, major affective disorder, or diseases or conditions that affect metabolism or hemodynamic responses.
• Avoid use in patients with angle-closure glaucoma.
• Use with caution in patients with risk factors for QT-interval prolongation.
• Screen patients for bipolar disorder, as drug may activate manic or hypomanic states.
ⓘ **Alert:** Sertraline isn't approved for use in children except those with OCD.
ⓘ **Alert:** Drug may increase risk of bleeding, especially with concomitant use of aspirin, NSAIDs, other antiplatelet drugs, warfarin, and other anticoagulants.
Dialyzable drug: Unknown.
⚠ *Overdose S&S:* Somnolence, vomiting, tachycardia, nausea, dizziness, agitation, tremor, bradycardia, bundle-branch block, coma, seizures, delirium, hallucinations, HTN, hypotension, manic reactions, pancreatitis, prolonged QT interval, serotonin syndrome, stupor, syncope.

PREGNANCY-LACTATION-REPRODUCTION

• There are no adequate studies in pregnant women. Use only if potential benefit justifies potential risk to the fetus.
• Neonates exposed to sertraline and other SSRIs or SSNRIs late in the third trimester have developed complications requiring prolonged hospitalization, respiratory support, and tube feeding.
• Neonates exposed to SSRIs during pregnancy may be at increased risk for persistent pulmonary HTN of the newborn.
• It isn't known if drug appears in human milk. Use cautiously in breastfeeding women.

NURSING CONSIDERATIONS

• Give sertraline once daily, either in morning or evening, with or without food.
• Make dosage adjustments at intervals of no less than 1 week.
• Record mood changes. Monitor patient for suicidal tendencies, and allow only a minimum supply of drug.
‖ Black Box Warning ‖ Drug may increase the risk of suicidal thinking and behavior in children, adolescents, and young adults with major depressive disorder or other psychiatric disorder. ∎
‖ Black Box Warning ‖ Closely monitor all patients being treated with antidepressants for clinical worsening, suicidal thoughts, and unusual changes in behavior, especially during initial few months of treatment or at times of dosage increases or decreases. ∎
ⓘ **Alert:** If linezolid or methylene blue must be given, stop sertraline and monitor patient for serotonin toxicity for 2 weeks, or until 24 hours after the last dose of methylene blue or linezolid, whichever comes first. May resume sertraline 24 hours after last dose of methylene blue or linezolid.
• Don't use the oral concentrate dropper, which is made of rubber, for patient with latex allergy.
ⓘ **Alert:** Combining triptans with an SSRI or an SSNRI may cause serotonin syndrome or NMS-like reactions. Signs and symptoms of serotonin syndrome may include restlessness, hallucinations, loss of coordination, fast heartbeat, rapid changes in BP, increased body temperature, overactive reflexes, nausea, vomiting, and diarrhea.

S

Serotonin syndrome may be more likely to occur when starting or increasing the dose of triptan, SSRI, or SSNRI.

• *Look alike–sound alike:* Don't confuse sertraline with cetirizine or Soriatane.

PATIENT TEACHING
Black Box Warning Advise families and caregivers to closely observe patient for increased suicidal thinking and behavior. ∎

◆ *Alert:* Teach patient to recognize and immediately report signs and symptoms of serotonin toxicity (fever, mental status changes, muscle twitching, excessive sweating, shivering or shaking, diarrhea, loss of coordination).

• Advise patient to use caution when performing hazardous tasks that require alertness.

• Tell patient to avoid alcohol and to consult prescriber before taking OTC drugs.

• Advise patient to mix the oral concentrate with 4 oz (½ cup; 120 mL) of water, ginger ale, lemon-lime soda, lemonade, or orange juice only, and to take the dose right away.

• Instruct patient to avoid stopping drug abruptly.

---

sevelamer carbonate
se-VEL-a-mer

Renvela

sevelamer hydrochloride
Renagel

Therapeutic class: Hypophosphatemics
Pharmacologic class: Polymeric phosphate binders

AVAILABLE FORMS
sevelamer carbonate
Oral suspension: 0.8-g, 2.4-g packets
Tablets (film-coated) ⓞⓉⓒ*:* 800 mg
sevelamer hydrochloride
Tablets (film-coated) ⓞⓉⓒ*:* 400 mg, 800 mg

INDICATIONS & DOSAGES
➤ **To control phosphorus level in chronic kidney disease patients on dialysis**
Adults not taking a phosphate binder: Initially, 800 to 1,600 mg (one to two 800-mg

tablets, or two to four 400-mg tablets, or one to two 0.8-g packets) PO with each meal, based on phosphorus level. If phosphorus level is greater than 5.5 mg/dL and less than 7.5 mg/dL, start with 800 mg t.i.d. with meals. If phosphorus level is greater than or equal to 7.5 mg/dL and less than 9 mg/dL, start with two 800-mg tablets t.i.d., or three 400-mg tablets t.i.d. with meals. If phosphorus level is 9 mg/dL or more, start with 1,600 mg t.i.d. (two 800-mg tablets, or four 400-mg tablets, or two 0.8-g packets) with meals.

Adults switching from calcium acetate: Initially, if taking one 667-mg calcium acetate tablet per meal, start with 800 mg PO per meal. If taking two 667-mg calcium acetate tablets per meal, start with two 800-mg tablets, or three 400-mg tablets, or two 0.8-g packets per meal. If taking three 667-mg calcium acetate tablets per meal, start with three 800-mg tablets, or five 400-mg tablets, or one 2.4-g packet per meal.

Adjust-a-dose: If phosphorus level is greater than 5.5 mg/dL, increase by one tablet per meal at 2-week intervals. If phosphorus level is 3.5 to 5.5 mg/dL, maintain current dose. If phosphorus level is less than 3.5 mg/dL, decrease dose by one tablet per meal.

Children age 6 and older not taking a phosphate binder (Renvela only): Initially, 800 to 1,600 mg PO t.i.d. with meals, based on BSA. For BSA of 0.75 m^2 to less than 1.2 m^2, give 800 mg per meal or snack. Increase or decrease by 400 mg/dose at 2-week intervals as needed to achieve target levels. For BSA of 1.2 m^2 or greater, give 1,600 mg per meal or snack. Increase or decrease by 800 mg/dose at 2-week intervals as needed to achieve target levels.

ADMINISTRATION
PO
• Don't cut, crush, or allow patient to chew tablets.

• Mix powder packets with appropriate amount of water as directed. Stir mixture vigorously (it doesn't dissolve) and have patient drink entire preparation within 30 minutes.

• Give drug with meals.

Reactions in bold italics are *life-threatening*. Interactions may have a *rapid onset* or a *delayed onset*.

• Drug may bind to other drugs and decrease their bioavailability. Give other drugs 1 hour before or 3 hours after this drug.
• Take special precautions when using antiarrhythmics or anticonvulsants with this drug.

ACTION

Inhibits intestinal phosphate absorption and decreases phosphorus levels.

Route	Onset	Peak	Duration
PO	Unknown	Unknown	Unknown

Half-life: Unknown.

ADVERSE REACTIONS

GI: diarrhea, dyspepsia, vomiting, nausea, constipation, flatulence, abdominal pain.
Metabolic: hypercalcemia.

INTERACTIONS

Drug-drug. *Ciprofloxacin, other quinolones:* May decrease effectiveness of ciprofloxacin or other quinolones. Give quinolones either 2 hours before or 6 hours after sevelamer.
Mycophenolate: May decrease mycophenolic acid plasma concentration, decreasing effectiveness. Administer sevelamer 2 hours after mycophenolate.
Thyroid hormones (levothyroxine): May decrease effectiveness of hormones. Separate administration times by at least several hours. Consider therapy modification.

EFFECTS ON LAB TEST RESULTS

None reported.

CONTRAINDICATIONS & CAUTIONS

• Contraindicated in patients hypersensitive to drug or its components and in those with hypophosphatemia or bowel obstruction.
• Use cautiously in patient with dysphagia, swallowing disorders, severe GI motility disorders, or major GI tract surgery.
• May reduce absorption of vitamins D, E, and K and folic acid.
Dialyzable drug: Unknown.

PREGNANCY-LACTATION-REPRODUCTION

• There are no adequate studies in pregnant women. Use only if potential benefit justifies potential risk to the fetus.

• No information is available regarding use in breastfeeding women.

NURSING CONSIDERATIONS

• Monitor calcium, bicarbonate, and chloride levels.
• *Look alike–sound alike:* Don't confuse Renvela with Renagel.

PATIENT TEACHING

• Instruct patient to take with meals and to adhere to prescribed diet.
🜊 *Alert:* Inform patient that tablets must be taken whole because contents expand in water. Warn patient not to cut, crush, or chew tablets.
• Advise patient to take reconstituted oral suspension immediately or within 30 minutes.
• Tell patient to check with pharmacist before taking other drugs at the same time as sevelamer.
• Inform patient about common adverse reactions, including constipation that, if left untreated, may lead to severe complications.

sildenafil citrate
sil-DEN-a-fill

Revatio, Viagra🖋

Therapeutic class: Erectile dysfunction drugs–pulmonary vasodilators
Pharmacologic class: PDE5 inhibitors

AVAILABLE FORMS

Injection: 10 mg/12.5 mL single-use vials
Oral suspension (Revatio): 10 mg/mL
Tablets (Revatio): 20 mg
Tablets (Viagra): 25 mg, 50 mg, 100 mg

INDICATIONS & DOSAGES

➤ **Erectile dysfunction (Viagra only)**
Adult men younger than age 65: About 1 hour before sexual activity, 50 mg PO, as needed. Dosage range is 25 to 100 mg based on effectiveness and tolerance. Maximum is 100 mg daily.
Elderly male patients (age 65 and older): 25 mg PO, as needed, about 1 hour before sexual activity. Dosage may be adjusted based on patient response.

S

Adjust-a-dose: For adults with hepatic or severe renal impairment (CrCl less than 30 mL/minute), 25 mg PO about 1 hour before sexual activity. May adjust dosage based on patient response.

➤ **To improve exercise ability and delay clinical worsening in patients with WHO Group 1 PAH (Revatio only)**
Adults: 5 or 20 mg PO t.i.d., 4 to 6 hours apart. Or, 2.5 or 10 mg IV bolus t.i.d.

ADMINISTRATION

🌢 *Alert:* Don't substitute Viagra for Revatio because there isn't an equivalent dose.

PO
• Give without regard for food.
• Don't give to patients taking nitrates.
• Follow manufacturer's directions for reconstitution of powder for oral suspension.
• Label Revatio suspension with expiration date, which is 60 days from date of reconstitution.

IV
▼ Inspect solution visually for particulate matter and discoloration before administering.
▼ Don't give to patients taking nitrates.
▼ Ten-mg IV dose is equivalent to 20-mg oral dose (Revatio).
▼ **Incompatibilities:** None listed by manufacturer. Consult a drug incompatibility reference for more information.

ACTION

When used for erectile dysfunction, drug increases effect of nitric oxide by inhibiting PDE5, which is responsible for degradation of cyclic guanosine monophosphate (cGMP) in the corpus cavernosum. When sexual stimulation causes local release of nitric oxide, inhibition of PDE5 by sildenafil causes increased levels of cGMP in the corpus cavernosum, resulting in smooth muscle relaxation and inflow of blood to the corpus cavernosum. In PAH, drug increases cGMP level by preventing its breakdown by phosphodiesterase, prolonging smooth muscle relaxation of the pulmonary vasculature, which leads to vasodilation.

Route	Onset	Peak	Duration
PO	15–30 min	30–120 min	4 hr
IV	Unknown	Unknown	Unknown

Half-life: 4 hours.

ADVERSE REACTIONS

CNS: headache, *seizures,* anxiety, dizziness, insomnia, somnolence, vertigo, paresthesia, fever. **CV:** flushing. **EENT:** diplopia, temporary vision loss, photophobia, altered color perception, blurred vision, nasal congestion, epistaxis, rhinitis, sinusitis. **GI:** dyspepsia, diarrhea, gastritis, nausea. **GU:** UTI. **Musculoskeletal:** back pain, myalgia. **Respiratory:** dyspnea. **Skin:** erythema, rash.

INTERACTIONS

Drug-drug. *Alpha blockers:* May cause symptomatic hypotension. Consider dosage reduction.
Amyl nitrate: May increase vasodilatory effects. Don't use together.
Antihypertensives: May increase hypotension. Use cautiously.
Bosentan: May decrease sildenafil level and increase bosentan level. Monitor patient closely for bosentan adverse reactions.
CYP3A inhibitors (erythromycin, itraconazole, ketoconazole, protease inhibitors, ritonavir, saquinavir): May increase sildenafil level, increasing risk of adverse events, including hypotension, visual changes, and priapism. Reduce Viagra starting dose to 25 mg when used with itraconazole, ketoconazole, erythromycin, or protease inhibitors. When used with ritonavir, atazanavir, or darunavir, maximum Viagra dose is 25 mg in a 48-hour period. Use with Revatio isn't recommended.
CYP450 inducers, rifampin: May reduce sildenafil level. Monitor effect.
Guanylate cyclase (GC) stimulators (riociguat): May potentiate hypotensive effects of GC stimulators. Use together is contraindicated.
Hepatic isoenzyme inhibitors (cimetidine, erythromycin, itraconazole, ketoconazole): May reduce sildenafil clearance. Avoid using together.
Isosorbide, nitroglycerin: May cause severe hypotension. Use of nitrates in any form with sildenafil is contraindicated.

Reactions in bold italics are *life-threatening*. Interactions may have a *rapid onset* or a *delayed onset*.

Other PDE5 inhibitors: May increase risk of hypotension. Don't use together.

Vitamin K antagonists: May increase risk of bleeding (primarily epistaxis). Monitor patient.

Drug-herb. *St. John's wort:* May decrease sildenafil level. Don't use together.

Drug-food. *Grapefruit:* May increase drug level, while delaying absorption. Advise patient to avoid using together.

Drug-lifestyle. *Alcohol use:* Excessive alcohol intake may increase risk of hypotension. Advise patient to avoid or limit alcohol consumption.

EFFECTS ON LAB TEST RESULTS
• May increase liver enzyme levels.

CONTRAINDICATIONS & CAUTIONS
• Contraindicated in patients hypersensitive to drug or its components and in those taking organic nitrates or GC stimulators.

• Use cautiously in patients age 65 and older; in patients with hepatic or severe renal impairment, retinitis pigmentosa, bleeding disorders, or active peptic ulcer disease; in those who have suffered an MI, stroke, or life-threatening arrhythmia within past 6 months; in those with history of cardiac failure, CAD, uncontrolled high or low BP, or anatomic deformation of the penis (such as angulation, cavernosal fibrosis, or Peyronie disease); and in those with conditions that may predispose them to priapism (such as sickle cell anemia, multiple myeloma, or leukemia).

• Vision loss, including permanent loss of vision, has been reported in patients taking drug for erectile dysfunction and may be a sign of nonarteritic anterior ischemic optic neuropathy (NAION). Risk may increase with history of vision loss. Other risk factors for NAION include low cup-to-disk ratio ("crowded disk"), CAD, diabetes, HTN, hyperlipidemia, smoking, and age older than 50.

• Pulmonary vasodilators used to treat PAH can worsen the CV status of patients with pulmonary veno-occlusive disease (PVOD). Use in patients with PVOD isn't recommended. If pulmonary edema occurs after drug is administered for PAH, consider the possibility of PVOD.

• Safe and effective use of drug to treat PAH in patients with sickle cell anemia hasn't been established.

• Safe use of drug to treat PAH in children hasn't been established.

• Decreased hearing and hearing loss have been reported. Obtain prompt medical attention for hearing loss.

Dialyzable drug: Unlikely.

PREGNANCY-LACTATION-REPRODUCTION
• Viagra isn't indicated for use in women. There are no adequate studies of use in pregnant or breastfeeding women.

• Information regarding use of drug to treat PAH in pregnant women is limited. Current guidelines recommend that women with PAH use effective contraception and avoid pregnancy.

• It isn't known if Revatio appears in human milk. Use cautiously in breastfeeding women.

NURSING CONSIDERATIONS
🔔 *Alert:* Systemic vasodilatory properties cause transient decreases in supine BP and cardiac output (about 2 hours after ingestion).

• The serious CV events linked to this drug's use in erectile dysfunction mainly involve patients with underlying CV disease who are at increased risk for cardiac effects related to sexual activity.

• Patients with PAH caused by connective tissue disease are more prone to epistaxis during therapy than those with primary pulmonary HTN.

• Oral Revatio and IV Revatio doses aren't equivalent: A 10-mg IV dose is predicted to provide pharmacologic effect equivalent to that of a 20-mg oral dose.

• IV use is for patients with PAH currently unable to take oral medications.

• *Look alike–sound alike:* Don't confuse Viagra with Allegra.

PATIENT TEACHING
• Advise patient that drug shouldn't be used with nitrates or GC stimulators under any circumstances. Revatio and Viagra or other PDE5 inhibitors used for erectile dysfunction shouldn't be used together.

S

• Advise patient of potential cardiac risk of sexual activity, especially in presence of CV risk factors. Instruct patient to notify prescriber and refrain from further activity if such symptoms as chest pain, dizziness, or nausea occur when starting sexual activity.

• Warn patient that erections lasting longer than 4 hours and priapism (painful erections lasting longer than 6 hours) may occur; tell patient to seek immediate medical attention if either of these occurs. Penile tissue damage and permanent loss of potency may result if priapism isn't treated immediately.

• Inform patient that drug used for erectile dysfunction doesn't protect against sexually transmitted diseases; advise patient to use protective measures such as condoms.

• Advise patient receiving HIV medications of the increased risk of sildenafil adverse events, including low BP, visual changes, and priapism, and to promptly report such symptoms to prescriber. Tell patient not to exceed 25 mg of sildenafil.

• Instruct patient to take drug for erectile dysfunction 30 minutes to 4 hours before sexual activity; maximum benefit can be expected less than 2 hours after ingestion.

• Advise patient that drug can be taken without regard for food.

• Inform patient that impairment of color discrimination (blue, green) may occur and to avoid hazardous activities that rely on color discrimination.

• Instruct patient to immediately notify prescriber of vision or hearing changes.

• Caution patient to take drug only as prescribed.

silodosin
SI-lo-doe-sin

Rapaflo

Therapeutic class: BPH drugs
Pharmacologic class: Alpha₁ blockers

AVAILABLE FORMS
Capsules ⓄⓃⒼ: 4 mg, 8 mg

INDICATIONS & DOSAGES
➤ **To improve symptoms of BPH**
Men: 8 mg PO once daily.

Adjust-a-dose: For patients with CrCl of 30 to 50 mL/minute, give 4 mg once daily.

ADMINISTRATION
PO
• Give drug once daily with a meal.
• For patients who can't swallow capsules, contents of capsule may be sprinkled on a tablespoonful of applesauce (not hot), swallowed within 5 minutes without chewing, and followed with 8 oz of cool water to ensure complete swallowing of the powder. Don't store for future use.

ACTION
Causes relaxation of smooth muscles in the prostate and bladder tissues by antagonizing postsynaptic alpha₁ adrenoreceptors, thereby improving urine flow and reducing signs and symptoms of BPH.

Route	Onset	Peak	Duration
PO	Unknown	3 hr	Unknown

Half-life: About 13 hours.

ADVERSE REACTIONS
CNS: asthenia, dizziness, headache, insomnia. **CV:** orthostatic hypotension. **EENT:** nasal congestion, nasopharyngitis, rhinorrhea, sinusitis. **GI:** abdominal pain, diarrhea. **GU:** retrograde ejaculation.

INTERACTIONS
Drug-drug. *Alpha blockers:* May cause interactions. Avoid use together.
Antihypertensives: May cause dizziness and orthostatic hypotension. Use together cautiously and monitor patient for adverse reactions.
Moderate CYP3A4 inhibitors (diltiazem, erythromycin, verapamil): May increase silodosin level. Use together cautiously.
PDE5 inhibitors: May cause symptomatic hypotension. Monitor patient closely.
Strong CYP3A4 inhibitors (clarithromycin, itraconazole, ketoconazole, ritonavir): May increase silodosin level. Use together is contraindicated.
Strong P-gp/ABCB1 inhibitors (cyclosporine, ketoconazole, ritonavir, verapamil): May increase silodosin levels. Don't use together.

Reactions in bold italics are *life-threatening*. Interactions may have a *rapid onset* or a *delayed onset*.

Drug-herb. *St. John's wort:* May decrease silodosin level and its effects. Consider modifying therapy.

EFFECTS ON LAB TEST RESULTS
None reported.

CONTRAINDICATIONS & CAUTIONS
• Contraindicated in patients hypersensitive to drug or its components, in those with severe renal or hepatic impairment, and in those taking strong CYP3A4 inhibitors.
Dialyzable drug: Unlikely.
⚠ *Overdose S&S:* Orthostatic hypotension.

PREGNANCY-LACTATION-REPRODUCTION
• Drug isn't approved for use in women.

NURSING CONSIDERATIONS
• Because BPH and prostate cancer cause similar signs and symptoms, prostate cancer should be ruled out before the start of silodosin therapy.
• Monitor patient for orthostatic hypotension. Carefully monitor older patients for hypotension because risk of orthostatic hypotension increases with age.
• Don't use drug to treat HTN.
• Current or previous use of an alpha blocker may predispose patient to floppy-iris syndrome during cataract surgery.

PATIENT TEACHING
• Tell patient to take silodosin with the same meal each day.
• Advise patient who can't swallow capsules to sprinkle contents of capsule on a tablespoonful of applesauce (not hot), swallow within 5 minutes without chewing, and follow with 8 oz (240 mL) of cool water to ensure complete swallowing of the powder. Tell patient not to store for future use.
• Warn patient about possible hypotension, and explain that it may cause dizziness.
• Caution patient against driving or operating hazardous machinery until drug's effects are known.
• Advise patient who needs cataract surgery to inform ophthalmologist about taking silodosin.
• Advise patient about the possibility of retrograde ejaculation, which is reversible

upon drug discontinuation and doesn't pose a safety concern.

simvastatin ⚥
sim-va-STAT-in

Zocor⚖

Therapeutic class: Antilipemics
Pharmacologic class: HMG-CoA reductase inhibitors

AVAILABLE FORMS
Tablets: 5 mg, 10 mg, 20 mg, 40 mg, 80 mg

INDICATIONS & DOSAGES
Adjust-a-dose (for all indications): In patients taking fibrates, maximum is 10 mg PO daily. In patients taking dronedarone, diltiazem, or verapamil, maximum is 10 mg PO daily. In patients taking amiodarone, amlodipine, lomitapide, or ranolazine, maximum is 20 mg PO daily. In patients with severe renal insufficiency, start with 5 mg PO daily.
➤ **To reduce risk of death from CV disease and CV events in patients at high risk for coronary events; to reduce total and LDL cholesterol, apolipoprotein B, and triglyceride levels and increase HDL cholesterol level in patients with primary hyperlipidemia and mixed dyslipidemia; to reduce triglyceride levels; to reduce triglyceride levels and VLDL cholesterol level in patients with dysbetalipoproteinemia**
Adults: Initially, 10 to 20 mg PO daily in evening. In patients at high risk for a CAD event due to existing CAD, diabetes, PVD, or history of stroke, the recommended initial dose is 40 mg PO daily. Adjust dosage every 4 weeks based on patient tolerance and response. Patients unable to achieve their LDL-cholesterol goals utilizing simvastatin 40 mg shouldn't be titrated to 80-mg dose but should be placed on alternative LDL-cholesterol lowering treatment.
➤ **To reduce total and LDL cholesterol levels in patients with homozygous familial hypercholesterolemia ⚥**
Adults: 40 mg PO daily in evening.

S

➤ **Heterozygous familial hypercholes-terolemia in boys and postmenarchal girls** ⊠
Children ages 10 to 17: Give 10 mg PO once daily in the evening. Maximum, 40 mg daily.

ADMINISTRATION
PO
• Give drug in the evening.

ACTION
Inhibits HMG-CoA reductase, an early (and rate-limiting) step in cholesterol biosynthesis.

Route	Onset	Peak	Duration
PO	Unknown	1–2 hr	Unknown

Half-life: Unknown.

ADVERSE REACTIONS
CNS: asthenia, headache, vertigo. **CV:** edema, atrial fibrillation. **EENT:** sinusitis. **GI:** abdominal pain, constipation, nausea. **GU:** UTI. **Musculoskeletal:** myalgia. **Respiratory:** URI, bronchitis. **Skin:** eczema.

INTERACTIONS
Drug-drug. *Amiodarone, amlodipine, ranolazine:* May increase risk of myopathy and rhabdomyolysis. Don't exceed 20 mg simvastatin daily.
Azole antifungals (fluconazole, itraconazole, ketoconazole), **macrolides (azithromycin, clarithromycin, erythromycin):** May increase simvastatin level and adverse effects. Avoid using together or, if it can't be avoided, suspend simvastatin therapy for course of treatment.
Bile acid sequestrants (cholestyramine, colestipol): May decrease GI absorption of simvastatin. Separate administration times by at least 4 hours.
Cyclosporine, *danazol, gemfibrozil:* May increase risk of myopathy and rhabdomyolysis. Use together is contraindicated.
Digoxin: May slightly increase digoxin level. Closely monitor digoxin levels at the start of simvastatin therapy.
Dronedarone, diltiazem, **verapamil:** May increase risk of myopathy and rhabdomyolysis. Don't exceed 10 mg simvastatin daily.
Efavirenz, rifampin: May decrease simvastatin level. Monitor effectiveness.

Fibrates (other than gemfibrozil): Increase risk of myopathy. Use cautiously together.
Hepatotoxic drugs: May increase risk for hepatotoxicity. Avoid using together.
Lomitapide: May increase risk of myopathy or rhabdomyolysis. Reduce simvastatin dosage by 50% when starting lomitapide; don't exceed simvastatin 20 mg/day (or 40 mg/day for patients who previously tolerated simvastatin 80 mg/day for 1 year or more without muscle toxicity).
Nefazodone, protease inhibitors (amprenavir, atazanavir, darunavir, fosamprenavir, indinavir, lopinavir–ritonavir, nelfinavir, ritonavir, saquinavir): May inhibit metabolism of simvastatin and increase the risk of adverse effects, including rhabdomyolysis. Use together is contraindicated.
⊠ *Niacin:* May increase risk of myopathy and rhabdomyolysis with niacin dose of 1 g/day or more. Use cautiously in Chinese patients when administering with simvastatin doses exceeding 20 mg/day. Chinese patients and possibly others of Asian descent shouldn't receive simvastatin 80 mg with lipid-modifying dose of niacin-containing products.
Warfarin: May slightly enhance anticoagulant effect. Monitor PT and INR when therapy starts or dose is adjusted.
Drug-herb. *Eucalyptus, kava kava:* May increase risk of hepatotoxicity. Discourage use together.
Red yeast rice: May increase risk of rhabdomyolysis. Discourage use together.
St. John's wort: May decrease simvastatin level. Discourage use together.
Drug-food. *Grapefruit juice:* Large amounts (greater than 1 quart/day [1 L/day]) may increase drug levels, increasing risk of adverse effects, including myopathy and rhabdomyolysis. Discourage use together.
Drug-lifestyle. *Alcohol use:* May increase risk of hepatotoxicity. Discourage use together.

EFFECTS ON LAB TEST RESULTS
• May increase HbA_{1c}, fasting blood glucose, ALT, AST, alkaline phosphatase, GGT, and CK levels.

Reactions in bold italics are *life-threatening*. Interactions may have a *rapid onset* or a *delayed onset*.

CONTRAINDICATIONS & CAUTIONS

• Simvastatin occasionally causes myopathy manifested as muscle pain, tenderness, or weakness, with CK level more than 10 × ULN. Myopathy sometimes takes the form of rhabdomyolysis with or without acute renal failure secondary to myoglobinuria, and rare fatalities have occurred. The risk of myopathy, including rhabdomyolysis, is dose related. Predisposing factors for myopathy include advanced age (age 65 and older), female gender, uncontrolled hypothyroidism, and renal impairment.

• Contraindicated in patients hypersensitive to drug and in those with active liver disease or conditions that cause unexplained persistent elevations of transaminase levels.

• Contraindicated for use at its highest dosage (80 mg/day) in patients not previously prescribed simvastatin or in patients who have had prior muscle toxicity. Patients who can't reach their goal LDL cholesterol level on 40-mg dose should be switched to an alternative agent. Only patients who have tolerated the 80-mg dose without muscle toxicity for more than 12 months should continue taking 80 mg daily.

• Use cautiously in patients who consume large amounts of alcohol or have a history of liver disease.

• Rare reports of cognitive impairment (memory loss, forgetfulness, amnesia, memory impairment, confusion) have been associated with statin use. These reported symptoms are generally not serious and are reversible upon statin discontinuation, with variable times to symptom onset (1 day to years) and symptom resolution (median of 3 weeks).

🗟 Use cautiously when treating Chinese patients with simvastatin dosages exceeding 20 mg/day administered with lipid-modifying doses of niacin-containing products (niacin 1 g/day or more) because of the increased risk of myopathy. Don't give Chinese patients simvastatin 80 mg with lipid-modifying doses of niacin-containing products. It's unknown whether this increased risk of myopathy also applies to other Asian patients.

Dialyzable drug: Unknown.

PREGNANCY-LACTATION-REPRODUCTION

• Contraindicated in women who are pregnant or may become pregnant; drug may cause fetal harm. Use in women of childbearing potential only when they are highly unlikely to conceive.

• Discontinue drug immediately if pregnancy occurs. Apprise patient of potential hazard to the fetus.

• Contraindicated in breastfeeding women.

NURSING CONSIDERATIONS

• Obtain LFT results before initiation of treatment and thereafter when clinically indicated. Obtain lipid determinations after 4 weeks of therapy and periodically thereafter.

• Monitor all patients for myopathy (unexplained muscle pain, weakness, or tenderness). Periodic CK determinations may be considered in patients starting therapy or in patients whose dosage is being increased, but there's no assurance that such monitoring will prevent myopathy.

• Patient should follow a diet restricted in saturated fat and cholesterol during therapy.

• Interrupt statin therapy if patient shows signs or symptoms of serious liver injury, hyperbilirubinemia, or jaundice. Don't restart drug if another cause can't be found.

• A daily dose of 40 mg significantly reduces risk of death from CAD, nonfatal MI, stroke, and revascularization procedures.

• *Look alike–sound alike:* Don't confuse Zocor with Cozaar.

PATIENT TEACHING

• Instruct patient to take drug in the evening.

• Teach patient about proper dietary management of cholesterol and triglycerides. When appropriate, recommend weight control, exercise, and smoking cessation programs.

• Inform patient that rare instances of memory loss and confusion have occurred with statin use. These reported events were generally not serious and resolved when drug was discontinued.

• Tell patient that drug may increase blood glucose level, but the CV benefits are thought to outweigh the slight increase in risk.

S

• Tell patient to immediately report unexplained muscle pain, tenderness, or weakness (especially if accompanied by malaise or fever) and loss of appetite, upper abdominal pain, dark-colored urine, or yellowing of skin or eyes.

◑ **Alert:** Tell female patient to stop drug and notify prescriber immediately if she is or may be pregnant or if she is breastfeeding.

SAFETY ALERT!

sirolimus
sir-OH-li-mus

Rapamune

Therapeutic class: Immunosuppressants
Pharmacologic class: Immunosuppressants

AVAILABLE FORMS
Oral solution: 1 mg/mL
Tablets ⓄⓃⒼ: 0.5 mg, 1 mg, 2 mg

INDICATIONS & DOSAGES
➤ **With cyclosporine and corticosteroids, to prevent organ rejection in patients receiving renal transplants**
Adults and adolescents: Initially, 6 mg PO for patients with low to moderate immunologic risk weighing 40 kg or more or 3 mg/m^2 for patients weighing less than 40 kg as one-time dose as soon as possible after transplantation but 4 hours after administration of cyclosporine; then maintenance dose of 2 mg PO once daily for patients weighing 40 kg or more or 1 mg/m^2 PO once daily for patients weighing less than 40 kg. For patients with high immunologic risk, may give up to 15 mg PO on day 1 after transplantation, then 5 mg/day PO beginning on day 2 after transplantation. Obtain trough concentration between days 5 and 7 and adjust dosage as needed.

Maximum daily dose shouldn't exceed 40 mg. If a daily dose exceeds 40 mg due to a loading dose, give the loading dose over 2 days. Monitor trough concentrations at least 3 to 4 days after a loading dose.
Children age 13 and older weighing less than 40 kg: First dose is 3 mg/m^2 PO as one-time dose after transplantation; then 1 mg/m^2 PO once daily.

Adjust-a-dose: When maintenance dosage is adjusted, continue on the new maintenance dosage for at least 7 to 14 days before further dosage adjustments with concentration monitoring because drug has a long half-life.

For patients with mild to moderate hepatic impairment, reduce maintenance dose by about one-third, and by about one-half in patients with severe hepatic impairment. It isn't necessary to reduce loading dose. Two to 4 months after transplant in patients with low to moderate risk of graft rejection, taper off cyclosporine over 4 to 8 weeks. While tapering cyclosporine, adjust sirolimus dose every 1 to 2 weeks to obtain levels between 16 and 24 nanograms/mL. Base dosage adjustments on clinical status, tissue biopsies, and laboratory findings.
➤ **Lymphangioleiomyomatosis**
Adults: Initially, 2 mg PO daily consistently with or without food at same time each day. Measure trough concentration in 10 to 20 days and adjust dosage to achieve sirolimus trough level of between 5 and 15 nanograms/mL, allowing at least 7 to 14 days on new dose before further dosage adjustment. Once a stable dosage is achieved, perform therapeutic drug monitoring at least every 3 months.

ADMINISTRATION
PO
• Follow safe-handling procedures when preparing, administering, and dispensing drug.
• Give drug consistently either with or without food.
• Patients should swallow tablets whole. Don't crush or split tablets.
• Dilute oral solution before use. After dilution, use immediately and discard oral solution syringe.
• When diluting oral solution, empty correct amount into glass or plastic (not Styrofoam) container holding at least ¼ cup (60 mL) of either water or orange juice. Don't use grapefruit juice or any other liquid. Stir vigorously and have patient drink immediately. Refill container with at least ½ cup (120 mL) of water or orange juice, stir again, and have patient drink all contents.
• A slight haze may develop during refrigeration, which doesn't affect potency of drug.

If haze develops, bring to room temperature and shake until haze disappears.

• Store away from light, and refrigerate at 36° to 46° F (2° to 8° C). After opening bottle, use contents within 1 month. If needed, store bottles and pouches at room temperature (up to 77° F [25° C]) for several days. Drug may be kept in oral amber syringe for 24 hours at room temperature.

• Store tablets between 68° and 77° F (20° and 25° C).

ACTION

Inhibits T-cell activation and proliferation that occurs in response to antigenic and cytokine stimulation. Also inhibits antibody formation.

Route	Onset	Peak	Duration
PO	Unknown	1–3 hr (solution) 1–6 hr (tablet)	Unknown

Half-life: Adults, about 46 to 78 hours; children, 13.7 ± 6.2 hours.

ADVERSE REACTIONS

CNS: fever, headache, dizziness. **CV:** chest pain, edema, HTN, peripheral edema, tachycardia, *thrombosis.* **EENT:** epistaxis, nasopharyngitis. **GI:** abdominal pain, constipation, diarrhea, nausea, ascites, stomatitis. **GU:** UTI, *toxic nephropathy,* dysuria, glycosuria, hematuria, hemolytic-uremic syndrome, polynephritis. **Hematologic:** anemia, *thrombocytopenia, leukopenia, thrombotic thrombocytopenic purpura,* ecchymosis. **Hepatic:** *hepatic artery thrombosis, hepatotoxicity.* **Metabolic:** hypercholesteremia, *hyperkalemia,* hyperlipidemia, hypokalemia, hypophosphatemia, hypertriglyceridemia, *hypoglycemia, acidosis, diabetes mellitus,* dehydration, hypercalcemia, hyperglycemia. **Musculoskeletal:** arthralgia, back pain, bone necrosis, myalgia. **Respiratory:** atelectasis, cough, dyspnea, URI, *ILD, asthma,* bronchitis, *hypoxia,* lung edema, pleural effusion, pneumonia. **Skin:** acne, rash, fungal dermatitis, pruritus, *melanoma, squamous cell carcinoma, basal cell carcinoma.* **Other:** *sepsis;* abnormal healing, including fascial dehiscence and anastomotic disruption (wound, vascular, airway, ureteral, biliary); abscess; flu syndrome; infection; lymphadenopathy; lymphocele; hypersensitivity reactions; *angioedema;* herpes simplex; herpes zoster.

INTERACTIONS

Drug-drug. *Aminoglycosides, amphotericin B, other nephrotoxic drugs:* May increase risk of nephrotoxicity. Use with caution.
Amiodarone, bromocriptine, cimetidine, clarithromycin, clotrimazole, danazol, erythromycin, fluconazole, indinavir, itraconazole, metoclopramide, nicardipine, posaconazole, ritonavir, verapamil, voriconazole, other drugs that inhibit CYP3A4: May increase blood levels of sirolimus. Monitor sirolimus levels closely.
Carbamazepine, phenobarbital, phenytoin, rifabutin, rifapentine, other drugs that induce CYP3A4: May decrease blood levels of sirolimus. Monitor patient closely.
Cyclosporine: May increase sirolimus level and toxicity. Give sirolimus 4 hours after cyclosporine; monitor levels and adjust dosage as needed.
Diltiazem: May increase sirolimus levels. Monitor sirolimus level, as needed.
HMG-CoA reductase inhibitors or fibrates: May increase risk of rhabdomyolysis with the combination of sirolimus and cyclosporine. Monitor patient closely.
Ketoconazole: May increase rate and extent of sirolimus absorption. Avoid using together.
Live-virus vaccines: May reduce vaccine effectiveness. Avoid using together.
Rifampin: May decrease sirolimus level. Alternative therapy to rifampin may be prescribed.
Drug-herb. *St. John's wort:* May decrease sirolimus levels. Discourage use together.
Drug-food. *Grapefruit juice:* May decrease drug metabolism. Discourage use together.
Drug-lifestyle. *Sun exposure:* May increase risk of skin cancer. Advise patient to avoid sunlight exposure.

EFFECTS ON LAB TEST RESULTS

• May increase creatinine, liver enzyme, cholesterol, and lipid levels. May increase or decrease phosphate, potassium, and glucose levels.

• May increase RBC count. May decrease platelet count. May increase or decrease WBC count.

S

CONTRAINDICATIONS & CAUTIONS

• Contraindicated in patients hypersensitive to active drug, its derivatives, or components of product.

• Use cautiously in patients with hyperlipidemia and impaired liver or renal function.

• Cases of ILD, including pneumonitis, bronchiolitis obliterans organizing pneumonia, and pulmonary fibrosis (some fatal), have occurred. ILD may be associated with pulmonary HTN and risk may increase with higher trough levels. ILD may resolve with reduced doses or with drug discontinuation.

Black Box Warning Fatal bronchial anastomotic dehiscence has been reported in lung transplant patients when sirolimus has been used as part of an immunosuppressive regimen. Safety and effectiveness of sirolimus as immunosuppressive therapy haven't been established in liver or lung transplant patients. Use in these patients isn't recommended. ∎

Dialyzable drug: No.

⚠ *Overdose S&S:* Exaggerated adverse effects.

PREGNANCY-LACTATION-REPRODUCTION

• There are no adequate studies in pregnant women; drug may cause fetal harm. Patient must use effective contraception before and during therapy and for 12 weeks after therapy ends. Use during pregnancy only if potential benefit outweighs potential risk to the fetus.

• It isn't known if drug appears in human milk. Patient should discontinue breastfeeding or discontinue drug.

NURSING CONSIDERATIONS

Black Box Warning Using this drug with tacrolimus or cyclosporine may cause hepatic artery thrombosis, leading to graft loss and death in liver transplant patients. ∎

Black Box Warning Only those experienced in immunosuppressive therapy and management of kidney transplant patients should prescribe drug. Manage patients receiving drug in facilities equipped and staffed with adequate laboratory and supportive medical resources. ∎

Black Box Warning Patients taking drug are more susceptible to infection and lymphoma and other malignancies. ∎

🌙 *Alert:* Drugs causing immunosuppression increase the risk of opportunistic infections, including activation of latent viral infections such as BK virus-associated neuropathy, which may lead to serious outcomes, including kidney graft loss.

🌙 *Alert:* This drug has been associated with angioedema; using it with ACE inhibitors increases the risk. Monitor patient closely.

• Use drug in regimen with cyclosporine and corticosteroids; have patient take drug 4 hours after cyclosporine dose. After 2 to 4 months of combined therapy, wean off cyclosporine as cyclosporine inhibits the metabolism and transport of sirolimus. Sirolimus concentration may decrease when cyclosporine is discontinued unless the sirolimus dosage is increased.

• Cyclosporine withdrawal in patients with high risk of graft rejection isn't recommended. This includes patients with Banff grade III acute rejection or vascular rejection before cyclosporine withdrawal, those who are dialysis dependent, those with serum creatinine level greater than 4.5 mg/dL, black patients, patients with retransplants or multiorgan transplants, and patients with high panel of reactive antibodies.

• After transplantation, give antimicrobial prophylaxis for *Pneumocystis jiroveci* for 1 year and for cytomegalovirus for 3 months.

• Monitor renal function tests because use with cyclosporine may cause creatinine level to increase. Adjustment of immunosuppressive regimen may be needed.

• Monitor cholesterol and triglyceride levels. Treatment with lipid-lowering drugs during therapy isn't uncommon. If hyperlipidemia is detected, additional interventions, such as diet and exercise, should begin.

• Check for rhabdomyolysis.

• Monitor drug levels in patients age 13 and older who weigh less than 40 kg, patients with hepatic impairment, those also receiving drugs that induce or inhibit CYP3A4, and patients in whom cyclosporine dosing is markedly reduced or stopped.

• Monitor patient for impaired or delayed wound healing, including wound dehiscence, and fluid accumulation, including edema, lymphedema, pleural effusion, ascites, and pericardial effusion.

Reactions in bold italics are *life-threatening*. Interactions may have a *rapid onset* or a *delayed onset*.

PATIENT TEACHING
• Teach patient how to properly store, dilute, and give drug.
• Advise female patient about risks during pregnancy. Tell her to use effective contraception before and during therapy and for 12 weeks after stopping therapy.
• Tell patient to take drug consistently with or without food to minimize absorption variability.
• Tell patient to take drug 4 hours after cyclosporine to avoid drug interactions.
• Advise patient to wash area with soap and water if drug solution touches skin or mucous membranes.
• Advise patient to limit ultraviolet light and sun exposure because of the increased risk of skin cancer.

SAFETY ALERT!

SITagliptin phosphate
sit-a-GLIP-tin

Januvia✐

Therapeutic class: Antidiabetics
Pharmacologic class: DPP-4 enzyme inhibitors

AVAILABLE FORMS
Tablets: 25 mg, 50 mg, 100 mg

INDICATIONS & DOSAGES
➤ **To improve glycemic control in addition to diet and exercise in patients with type 2 diabetes, alone or in combination therapy**
Adults: 100 mg PO once daily.
Adjust-a-dose: For patients with eGFR of 30 to less than 45 mL/minute/1.73 m^2, give 50 mg once daily; for patients with eGFR less than 30 mL/minute/1.73 m^2 or ESRD with hemodialysis or peritoneal dialysis, give 25 mg once daily. Give without regard to timing of dialysis session.

ADMINISTRATION
PO
• Give drug without regard for food.

ACTION
Inhibits DPP-4, an enzyme that rapidly inactivates incretin hormones, which play a part in the body's regulation of glucose. By increasing and prolonging active incretin levels, the drug helps to increase insulin release and decrease circulating glucose.

Route	Onset	Peak	Duration
PO	Rapid	1–4 hr	Unknown

Half-life: About 12½ hours.

ADVERSE REACTIONS
CNS: headache. **EENT:** nasopharyngitis. **GI:** abdominal pain, nausea, diarrhea. **Metabolic:** *hypoglycemia.* **Respiratory:** URI.

INTERACTIONS
Drug-drug. *Digoxin:* Causes a slight increase in digoxin peak. Monitor patient when used together.
Insulin, insulin secretagogues: May produce hypoglycemia. Dosage adjustment may be required.

EFFECTS ON LAB TEST RESULTS
• May increase creatinine level.
• May increase WBC count.

CONTRAINDICATIONS & CAUTIONS
• Contraindicated in patients with type 1 diabetes or diabetic ketoacidosis.
• Consider risk and benefits before initiating drug in patients at risk for HF.
• Contraindicated in patients with a history of hypersensitivity to sitagliptin. Angioedema, anaphylaxis, and exfoliative skin conditions such as SJS have been reported, some after first dose or up to 3 months after drug initiation.
• Bullous pemphigoid has been reported in patients taking DPP-4 inhibitors.
• Use cautiously in patients with moderate to severe renal insufficiency or a history of pancreatitis and in those taking other antidiabetics.
• Safety and effectiveness in children haven't been evaluated.
• Drug used alone or in combination with other hypoglycemics can cause hypoglycemia.
Dialyzable drug: 13.5%.

S

PREGNANCY-LACTATION-REPRODUCTION
• There are no adequate studies in pregnant women. Use only if clearly needed.
• Report prenatal exposure to the Januvia Pregnancy Registry (1-800-986-8999).
• It isn't known if drug appears in human milk. Use cautiously in breastfeeding women.

NURSING CONSIDERATIONS
• In elderly patients and those at risk for renal insufficiency, periodically assess renal function.
• Assess renal function before start of therapy and periodically thereafter.
• Monitor HbA_{1c} level periodically to assess long-term glycemic control.
• Management of type 2 diabetes should include diet control. Because caloric restrictions, weight loss, and exercise help improve insulin sensitivity and help make drug therapy effective, these measures are essential for proper diabetes management.
• Watch for hypoglycemia, especially in patients receiving combination therapy.
• Monitor patient for pancreatitis (persistent abdominal pain with or without vomiting). Discontinue drug if pancreatitis is suspected.
• Monitor patient for skin blistering or erosions. Discontinue drug if bullous pemphigoid is suspected and consider referral to a dermatologist.
◑ *Alert:* Drug may cause joint pain that can be severe and disabling. Report severe and persistent joint pain to prescriber; drug may need to be discontinued.
• *Look alike–sound alike:* Don't confuse sitagliptin with saxagliptin.

PATIENT TEACHING
• Tell patient that drug isn't a substitute for diet and exercise and that it's important to follow a prescribed dietary and physical activity routine and to monitor glucose level.
• Instruct patient to immediately report persistent, severe abdominal pain that may radiate to the back, with or without vomiting.
• Inform patient and family members of the signs and symptoms of hyperglycemia and hypoglycemia and the steps to take if these symptoms occur.
• Advise patient to report all adverse reactions, and to immediately report signs and

symptoms of hypersensitivity (rash, swelling of the face).
• Instruct patient that during periods of stress (such as fever, trauma, infection, or surgery), medication requirements may change. Advise patient to seek medical advice promptly.
◑ *Alert:* Instruct patient to immediately report new or worsening joint pain that's severe and persistent because drug may need to be discontinued.
• Provide patient with information on complications associated with diabetes and ways to assess for them.
• Tell patient to notify prescriber during periods of stress, such as fever, infection, or surgery; dosage may need adjustment.
• Tell patient drug may be taken without regard for food.

sodium ferric gluconate complex
Ferrlecit

Therapeutic class: Iron supplements
Pharmacologic class: Macromolecular iron complexes–hematinics

AVAILABLE FORMS
Injection: 62.5 mg elemental iron (12.5 mg/mL) in 5-mL ampules

INDICATIONS & DOSAGES
➤ **Iron deficiency anemia in patients receiving long-term hemodialysis and supplemental erythropoietin**
Adults and children older than age 15: 10 mL (125 mg elemental iron) IV over 1 hour per dialysis session. Most patients need minimum cumulative dose of 1 g elemental iron given over more than eight sequential dialysis treatments to achieve a favorable Hb or hematocrit response.
Children ages 6 to 15: 1.5 mg/kg (maximum 125 mg/dose) IV over 1 hour per dialysis session. Maximum dosage is 125 mg per dose.

ADMINISTRATION
IV
▼ Drug contains benzyl alcohol. Don't use in neonates.

Reactions in bold italics are *life-threatening*. Interactions may have a *rapid onset* or a *delayed onset*.

▼ For adults, dilute in 100 mL NSS; for children, dilute in 25 mL NSS. Give immediately over 1 hour.

▼ Alternatively, give to adults undiluted at a rate not to exceed 1 mL/minute (12.5 mg/minute) per dialysis session.

▼ Life-threatening hypersensitivity reactions, such as CV collapse, cardiac arrest, bronchospasm, oral or pharyngeal edema, dyspnea, angioedema, urticaria, and pruritus—sometimes linked to pain and muscle spasm of chest or back—may occur during infusion. Have adequate supportive measures readily available. Monitor patient closely during infusion and for at least 30 minutes after infusion until clinically stable.

▼ During or after administration, profound hypotension with flushing, lightheadedness, malaise, fatigue, weakness, or severe chest, back, flank, or groin pain may occur; these symptoms may not be hypersensitivity reactions. Monitor patient closely.

▼ **Incompatibilities:** Other IV drugs. Don't add drug to parenteral nutrition solutions for infusion.

ACTION

Restores total body iron content, which is critical for normal Hb synthesis and oxygen transport.

Route	Onset	Peak	Duration
IV	Unknown	Varies	Unknown

Half-life: 1 hour in healthy, iron-deficient adults.

ADVERSE REACTIONS

CNS: asthenia, headache, fatigue, malaise, dizziness, paresthesia, agitation, insomnia, somnolence, syncope, pain, chills, fever. **CV:** hypotension, HTN, tachycardia, *bradycardia,* angina, chest pain, *MI,* edema, flushing. **EENT:** conjunctivitis, abnormal vision, rhinitis. **GI:** nausea, vomiting, diarrhea, rectal disorder, dyspepsia, eructation, flatulence, melena, abdominal pain. **GU:** UTI. **Hematologic:** anemia. **Metabolic:** *hyperkalemia, hypoglycemia, hypokalemia,* hypervolemia. **Musculoskeletal:** myalgia, arthralgia, back pain, arm pain, cramps. **Respiratory:** dyspnea, coughing, URI, pneumonia, pulmonary edema. **Skin:**

pruritus, increased sweating, rash, injection-site reaction. **Other:** infection, rigors, flu syndrome, *sepsis, carcinoma,* hypersensitivity reactions, lymphadenopathy.

INTERACTIONS

Drug-drug. *ACE inhibitors:* May cause sensitivity reactions. Stop IV iron if sensitivity reactions occur.

Oral iron preparations: May reduce absorption of oral iron preparations. Avoid using together.

EFFECTS ON LAB TEST RESULTS

• May increase hematologic and iron parameters (Hb, hematocrit, serum ferritin, and transferrin saturation).

CONTRAINDICATIONS & CAUTIONS

• Contraindicated in patients hypersensitive to drug or its components (such as benzyl alcohol) and in those with iron overload or anemias not related to iron deficiency.

• Don't use in patients with elevated ferritin levels.

• Use cautiously in elderly patients.

Dialyzable drug: No.

⚠ *Overdose S&S:* Abdominal pain, diarrhea, vomiting, pallor or cyanosis, lassitude, drowsiness, hyperventilation, CV collapse.

PREGNANCY-LACTATION-REPRODUCTION

• There are no adequate studies in pregnant women. Use only if clearly needed.

• It isn't known if drug appears in human milk and drug contains benzyl alcohol. Use cautiously in breastfeeding women.

NURSING CONSIDERATIONS

⚕ *Alert:* Dosage is expressed in milligrams of elemental iron.

⚕ *Alert:* Before administering, assess patients for prior history of reactions to iron products.

⚕ *Alert:* Closely monitor patients for life-threatening hypersensitivity reactions during infusion and for at least 30 minutes after infusion until clinically stable. Ensure that emergency measures to treat anaphylaxis are immediately available.

⚕ *Alert:* Closely monitor patients during and after drug administration for profound hypotension with flushing, light-headedness,

S

malaise, fatigue, weakness, or severe chest, back, flank, or groin pain.

☻ Alert: Drug contains benzyl alcohol, which is associated with adverse events and death in children. The minimum amount of benzyl alcohol that may cause toxicity isn't known.

• Drug shouldn't be used in patients with iron overload, which often occurs in hemoglobinopathies and other refractory anemias.

• Monitor ferritin level, iron saturation, Hb level, and hematocrit.

• In hemodialysis patients, adverse reactions may be related to dialysis itself or to chronic renal failure.

• Check with patient about other potential sources of iron, such as OTC iron preparations and iron-containing multiple vitamins with minerals.

PATIENT TEACHING

• Teach patient to immediately report all adverse reactions, especially those occurring during and after the infusion.

• Abdominal pain, diarrhea, vomiting, drowsiness, and rapid breathing may indicate iron poisoning. Urge patient to notify prescriber immediately.

sodium zirconium cyclosilicate
SOE-dee-um zir-KOE-nee-um
SYE-kloe-sil-i-kate

Lokelma

Therapeutic class: Antidotes
Pharmacologic class: Potassium binders

AVAILABLE FORMS

Powder for oral suspension: 5-g, 10-g packets

INDICATIONS & DOSAGES

➤ **Treatment of hyperkalemia**

Adults: Initially, 10 g PO t.i.d. for up to 48 hours. For continued treatment after 48 hours, give 10 g PO once daily. Maintenance dosage range is 5 g PO every other day to 15 g PO once daily.

Adjust-a-dose: Monitor serum potassium level and adjust dosage based on target potassium level range. During maintenance

treatment, up-titrate dosage based on potassium level at intervals of 1 week or longer and in increments of 5 g. Decrease dosage or stop drug if potassium level is below desired target range.

ADMINISTRATION
PO

• Empty entire contents of packet(s) into a glass containing at least 3 tablespoons of water or more if desired, stir well, and have patient drink immediately. If powder remains in the glass, add water, stir, and have patient drink immediately. Repeat until no powder remains.

• Give other oral medications 2 hours before or 2 hours after giving Lokelma.

• Store at 59° to 86° F (15° to 30° C).

ACTION

A potassium binder that preferentially exchanges potassium for hydrogen and sodium. Increases fecal potassium excretion through the binding of potassium in the lumen of the GI tract; reduces concentration of free potassium in the GI lumen and lowers serum potassium levels.

Route	Onset	Peak	Duration
PO	Unknown	Unknown	Unknown

Half-life: Unknown.

ADVERSE REACTIONS
CV: edema. **Metabolic:** *hypokalemia.*

INTERACTIONS

Drug-drug. *Drugs with pH-dependent solubility (atorvastatin, clopidogrel, dabigatran, furosemide):* May increase or decrease efficacy of coadministered drugs that have pH-dependent solubility. Separate drug administration from other oral medications by at least 2 hours.

EFFECTS ON LAB TEST RESULTS

• May decrease potassium and bicarbonate levels.

CONTRAINDICATIONS & CAUTIONS

☻ Alert: Drug shouldn't be used as an emergency treatment for life-threatening hyperkalemia because of its delayed onset of action.

Reactions in bold italics are *life-threatening*. Interactions may have a *rapid onset* or a **delayed onset**.

• Drug hasn't been studied in patients with motility disorders (severe constipation, bowel obstruction or impaction, postoperative bowel motility disorders). Avoid use in these patients as drug may be ineffective and may worsen GI conditions.
• Safety and effectiveness in children haven't been established.
Dialyzable drug: No.
⚠ *Overdose S&S:* Hypokalemia.

PREGNANCY-LACTATION-REPRODUCTION
• Drug isn't absorbed systemically and isn't expected to result in fetal exposure.
• Breastfeeding isn't expected to result in exposure of infant to drug.

NURSING CONSIDERATIONS
• Monitor potassium level and adjust dosage based on serum potassium level and desired target range.
• Monitor patient for signs and symptoms of edema, especially in patients who should restrict sodium intake or are prone to fluid overload (HF, renal disease). Each 5-g dose contains 400 mg of sodium. Adjust dietary sodium, if appropriate, and increase diuretic dosage as needed.

PATIENT TEACHING
• Teach patient to report all adverse reactions.
• Stress importance of drinking the entire dose.
• Advise patient taking other oral medications to separate dosing of drug by at least 2 hours (before or after).
• Instruct patient to adjust dietary sodium, if appropriate.

---

sofosbuvir 🧬
soe-FOS-bue-vir

Sovaldi

Therapeutic class: Antivirals
Pharmacologic class: Nucleotide analogue NS5B polymerase inhibitors

AVAILABLE FORMS
Tablets: 400 mg

INDICATIONS & DOSAGES
Adjust-a-dose (for all indications): Sofosbuvir dosage reduction isn't recommended. Discontinue sofosbuvir if concomitant antivirals are stopped. Adjust concomitant ribavirin or peginterferon alfa dosage if GFR is less than 50 mL/minute or hepatic decompensation or adverse reactions occur. Refer to manufacturer's instructions for ribavirin or peginterferon alfa dosage adjustments.
➤ **Chronic HCV infection (genotype 1 or 4) with or without HIV coinfection, as component of combination antiviral regimen in treatment-naive patients without cirrhosis or with compensated cirrhosis (Child-Pugh class A)** 🧬
Adults: 400 mg PO daily with peginterferon alfa and ribavirin for 12 weeks. For patients with HCV genotype 1 who can't receive interferon, give 400 mg PO daily with ribavirin for 24 weeks.
➤ **Chronic HCV infection (genotype 2) with or without HIV coinfection, as part of combination antiviral regimen in treatment-naive and treatment-experienced patients without cirrhosis or with compensated cirrhosis (Child-Pugh class A)** 🧬
Adults and children age 12 and older weighing at least 35 kg: 400 mg PO daily with ribavirin for 12 weeks.
➤ **Chronic HCV infection (genotype 3) with or without HIV coinfection, as part of combination antiviral regimen in treatment-naive and treatment-experienced patients without cirrhosis or with compensated cirrhosis (Child-Pugh class A)** 🧬
Adults and children age 12 and older weighing at least 35 kg: 400 mg PO daily with ribavirin for 24 weeks.
➤ **Chronic HCV infection with hepatocellular carcinoma in patients awaiting liver transplant**
Adults: 400 mg PO daily with ribavirin for 48 weeks or until liver transplant.

ADMINISTRATION
PO
• Give without regard for food.

S

ACTION

Inhibits HCV NS5B RNA polymerase, inhibiting viral replication.

Route	Onset	Peak	Duration
PO	Unknown	½–2 hr	Unknown

Half-life: 0.4 hour.

ADVERSE REACTIONS

CNS: headache, insomnia, asthenia, pyrexia, fatigue, irritability. **GI:** nausea, diarrhea. **Hematologic:** anemia, *neutropenia.* **Metabolic:** decreased appetite, chills. **Musculoskeletal:** myalgia. **Skin:** pruritus, rash. **Other:** flulike illness.

INTERACTIONS

Drug-drug. ❸ *Alert: Amiodarone:* May increase risk of symptomatic bradycardia, including cardiac arrest and cases requiring pacemaker intervention. Avoid use together. If use together can't be avoided, advise patient of risk and monitor carefully.
Anticonvulsants (carbamazepine, oxcarbazepine, phenobarbital, phenytoin, primidone), antimycobacterials (rifabutin, rifampin, rifapentine), HIV protease inhibitors (tipranavir, ritonavir): May decrease sofosbuvir level. Avoid use together.
Drug-herb. *St. John's wort:* May decrease sofosbuvir plasma concentration. Don't use together.

EFFECTS ON LAB TEST RESULTS

• May increase CK, bilirubin, and lipase levels.
• May decrease Hb level and neutrophil and platelet counts.

CONTRAINDICATIONS & CAUTIONS

• Contraindicated in patients hypersensitive to drug or its components. When used in combination with other drugs, the contraindications applicable to those agents also apply to combination therapies.
Black Box Warning Reactivation of HBV may occur in HCV coinfected patients and result in fulminant hepatitis, hepatic failure, and death. Screen all patients for current or prior HBV infection before treatment by measuring HBsAg and anti-HBc; if patient is positive for HBV infection, assess baseline HBV DNA. ■

❸ *Alert:* Symptomatic bradycardia, including fatal cardiac arrest and cases requiring pacemaker intervention, has been reported when sofosbuvir is administered with amiodarone. Patients taking amiodarone who are also taking beta blockers or who have underlying cardiac comorbidities or advanced liver disease may be at increased risk. Signs and symptoms may occur within hours to up to 2 weeks after start of HCV therapy.
• Safety and effectiveness of drug haven't been studied in patients with estimated GFR of less than 30 mL/minute, ESRD, or decompensated cirrhosis.
• Using Sovaldi with other products containing sofosbuvir isn't recommended.
• Refer to prescribing information for peginterferon alfa and ribavirin for contraindications when drug is given in these combination regimens.
Dialyzable drug: 18%.

PREGNANCY-LACTATION-REPRODUCTION

• Contraindicated in pregnant women and in men whose female partners are pregnant. Obtain baseline negative pregnancy test before start of therapy.
• Women of childbearing potential and their male partners must use two forms of effective nonhormonal contraception while receiving treatment regimens that include ribavirin and for 6 months after therapy ends.
• Men whose partners are exposed to ribavirin through sexual intercourse while pregnant and pregnant women who are themselves exposed to ribavirin should enroll in the Ribavirin Pregnancy Registry (1-800-593-2214).
• Pregnant patients coinfected with HCV/HIV-1 who are taking concomitant antiretrovirals should enroll in the Antiretroviral Pregnancy Registry (1-800-258-4263).
• Contraindicated in breastfeeding women. Patients must discontinue breastfeeding or discontinue drug.

NURSING CONSIDERATIONS

• Sofosbuvir isn't recommended as monotherapy. Always use as part of combination regimen.
Black Box Warning Monitor patient with current or prior HBV infection for hepatitis flare or HBV reactivation with laboratory

---

Reactions in bold italics are *life-threatening.* Interactions may have a *rapid onset* or a *delayed onset.*

testing; watch for signs and symptoms of liver injury during active and posttreatment follow-up. ■

❸ *Alert:* Monitor patients who must take amiodarone and those who must start amiodarone or who recently discontinued amiodarone for signs and symptoms of bradycardia (near-fainting or fainting, dizziness, light-headedness, malaise, weakness, excessive fatigue, shortness of breath, chest pain, confusion or memory problems). Inpatient cardiac monitoring should be utilized for first 48 hours, then outpatient monitoring or self-monitoring of HR for bradycardia should continue daily through at least first 2 weeks of treatment. Discontinue HCV treatment if signs or symptoms occur.

• Refer to ribavirin or peginterferon alfa prescribing information for complete guidance on their concomitant use.

• Refer to sofosbuvir prescribing information for ribavirin dosage in children.

• Monitor blood counts and bilirubin, liver enzyme, and serum creatinine levels at baseline and periodically when clinically indicated.

• Monitor serum HCV-RNA level at baseline, during treatment, at end of treatment, during treatment follow-up, and when clinically indicated.

• Obtain baseline negative pregnancy test before initiation of therapy and monthly thereafter until 6 months after treatment is discontinued.

• Treatment response varies based on patient and viral factors. Monitor patient carefully.

PATIENT TEACHING

• Advise patient that using drug as single agent isn't recommended. Sofosbuvir must always be used as part of combination regimen with ribavirin or peginterferon and ribavirin.

Black Box Warning Warn patient to immediately report signs and symptoms of liver injury (fatigue, weakness, loss of appetite, nausea, vomiting, yellowing of skin or eyes, light-colored stool). ■

• Teach patient to immediately report signs and symptoms of hypersensitivity reaction (wheezing, chest tightness, fever, itching, heavy cough, blue-colored skin, seizures, or swelling of face, lips, tongue, or throat) and to seek medical attention.

❸ *Alert:* Caution patient to seek immediate medical attention for signs and symptoms of bradycardia.

• Explain to patient and partner the risk of birth defects, contraception requirements, and pregnancy testing related to therapy.

• Teach patient to report all signs and symptoms of adverse reactions, such as headache, dyspepsia, and insomnia.

• Caution patient not to use other medications while taking this drug without first notifying prescriber.

• Teach patient to keep drug in original container.

• Advise patient to report liver problems (other than HCV infection), history of liver transplant, severe kidney problems or dialysis, positive HIV status, or other medical conditions.

• Warn female patient not to breastfeed while taking drug.

• Instruct patient not to discontinue drug without first discussing with prescriber.

sofosbuvir–velpatasvir ▨
soe-FOS-bue-vir/vel-PAT-as-vir

Epclusa

Therapeutic class: Antivirals
Pharmacologic class: Nucleotide analogue NS5B polymerase inhibitors/HCV NS5A inhibitors

AVAILABLE FORMS

Tablets: 400 mg sofosbuvir and 100 mg velpatasvir

INDICATIONS & DOSAGES

➤ **Chronic HCV genotype 1, 2, 3, 4, 5, or 6 infection without cirrhosis or with compensated cirrhosis (Child-Pugh class A) or with decompensated cirrhosis (Child-Pugh class B or C) in combination with ribavirin ▨**

Adults: One tablet PO once daily for 12 weeks.

S

ADMINISTRATION
PO
- Keep drug in original container.
- May give with or without food.
- Store below 86° F (30° C).

ACTION
Sofosbuvir and velpatasvir are direct-acting antivirals that inhibit viral replication of HCV.

Route	Onset	Peak	Duration
PO (sofosbuvir)	Unknown	½–1 hr	Unknown
PO (velpatasvir)	Unknown	3 hr	Unknown

Half-life: Sofosbuvir, ½ hour; velpatasvir, 15 hours.

ADVERSE REACTIONS
CNS: headache, fatigue, asthenia, insomnia, irritability, depression. **GI:** nausea, diarrhea, lipase elevations. **Hematologic:** anemia. **Metabolic:** CK elevations. **Skin:** rash.

INTERACTIONS
Drug-drug. *Antacids (aluminum hydroxide, magnesium hydroxide):* May decrease velpatasvir level. Separate antacid and drug administration by 4 hours.
❸ Alert: *Amiodarone:* May result in serious symptomatic bradycardia. Use together isn't recommended but if coadministration is necessary, cardiac monitoring is recommended.
Anticonvulsants (carbamazepine, oxcarbazepine, phenobarbital, phenytoin), antimycobacterial drugs (rifabutin, rifampin, rifapentine): May decrease levels of both antivirals. Avoid use together.
Atorvastatin, rosuvastatin: May significantly increase statin level and increase risk of rhabdomyolysis. Use together cautiously and monitor patient closely.
Digoxin: May increase digoxin level. Monitor digoxin level and adjust digoxin dosage as needed.
Efavirenz: May decrease velpatasvir level. Use together isn't recommended.
H_2 antagonists (famotidine): May decrease velpatasvir level. Give H_2 antagonist simultaneously or 12 hours apart from drug at a dose that doesn't exceed an equivalent of famotidine 40 mg b.i.d.
Moderate to potent CYP2B6, CYP2C8, or CYP3A4 inducers (carbamazepine, rifampin), P-gp inducers: May significantly decrease sofosbuvir or velpatasvir level, reducing therapeutic effect. Use together isn't recommended.
PPIs (omeprazole): May decrease velpatasvir level. Avoid use together, but if coadministration is necessary, give drug 4 hours before omeprazole 20 mg.
Tenofovir: May increase tenofovir level. Monitor patient for tenofovir-associated adverse reactions.
Tipranavir/ritonavir: May decrease levels of both antivirals. Avoid use together.
Topotecan: May increase topotecan level. Avoid use together.
Drug-herb. *St. John's wort:* May decrease antiviral levels and therapeutic effects. Use together isn't recommended.

EFFECTS ON LAB TEST RESULTS
- May increase lipase, CK, and indirect bilirubin levels.
- May decrease Hb level.

CONTRAINDICATIONS & CAUTIONS
- Combination regimen with ribavirin is contraindicated in patients for whom ribavirin is contraindicated. Refer to ribavirin manufacturer's instructions for contraindications.
- Warnings and precautions for ribavirin apply when used in combination with Epclusa. Refer to ribavirin prescribing information.

Black Box Warning Reactivation of HBV infection may occur in HCV coinfected patients and result in fulminant hepatitis, hepatic failure, and death. Screen all patients for current or prior HBV infection by measuring HBsAg and anti-hepatitis B core antibody (anti-HBc) before treatment and if positive for HBV infection, assess baseline HBV DNA level. ∎

❸ Alert: Serious symptomatic bradycardia may occur in patients taking amiodarone, particularly in patients also taking beta blockers, in those with underlying cardiac comorbidities, and in patients with advanced liver disease.
- Safety and effectiveness in children haven't been established.

Dialyzable drug: Sofosbuvir active metabolite, 53%; velpatasvir, unlikely.

PREGNANCY-LACTATION-REPRODUCTION

• Use of sofosbuvir and velpatasvir in pregnancy hasn't been studied.

• Combination regimen with ribavirin is contraindicated in pregnant women and in men whose female partners are pregnant.

• Advise patients using combination treatment with ribavirin to use two effective forms of contraception during treatment and for 6 months after therapy ends. Refer to ribavirin manufacturer's instructions for pregnancy testing before, during, and after therapy and for information about breastfeeding.

• It isn't known if sofosbuvir and velpatasvir and their metabolites appear in human milk, affect human milk production, or have effects on the breastfed infant. Use cautiously, weighing benefits for the mother and risk of breastfeeding for the infant.

NURSING CONSIDERATIONS

Black Box Warning Monitor patient with current or prior HBV infection for hepatitis flare or HBV reactivation with laboratory testing. Watch for signs and symptoms of liver injury during active therapy and post-treatment follow-up. ∎

🛈 **Alert:** For patients taking amiodarone (with or without beta blockers) who have no other treatment options and must begin Epclusa, cardiac monitoring in an inpatient setting for first 48 hours of coadministration is recommended, followed by outpatient or self-monitoring of HR daily for at least 2 weeks. Patients who discontinue amiodarone just before starting Epclusa and those who must begin amiodarone while taking Epclusa should also undergo similar cardiac monitoring.

• Monitor patient for bradycardia (near fainting, syncope, dizziness, lightheadedness, malaise, weakness, excessive fatigue, shortness of breath, chest pain, confusion, memory problems) and report it immediately.

• Clinical and hepatic laboratory monitoring, including direct bilirubin, is recommended for patients with decompensated cirrhosis taking Epclusa plus ribavirin.

• Monitor patient for anemia.

PATIENT TEACHING

Black Box Warning Warn patient to immediately report signs and symptoms of liver injury (fatigue, weakness, loss of appetite, nausea, vomiting, yellowing of skin or eyes, and light-colored stool). ∎

• Advise patient to report other prescription or OTC medications or herbal products being taken, including St. John's wort.

• Inform patient that it's important not to miss or skip doses and to take this medication for as long as recommended by prescriber.

• Advise patient to avoid pregnancy during combination treatment with ribavirin and to contact prescriber immediately if pregnancy occurs.

🛈 **Alert:** Counsel patient who is also taking amiodarone about the risk of symptomatic bradycardia. Teach patient to self-monitor HR.

• Caution patient to seek medical attention for signs and symptoms of bradycardia.

---

sofosbuvir–velpatasvir–voxilaprevir ▒

soe-FOS-bue-vir/vel-PAT-as-vir/vox-i-LA-pre-vir

Vosevi

Therapeutic class: Antivirals
Pharmacologic class: Nucleotide analogue HCV NS5B polymerase inhibitors—NS5A inhibitors—NS3/4A protease inhibitors

AVAILABLE FORMS

Tablets: 400 mg sofosbuvir/100 mg velpatasvir/100 mg voxilaprevir

INDICATIONS & DOSAGES

➤ **Chronic HCV infection without cirrhosis or with compensated cirrhosis (Child-Pugh class A) in patients who have genotype 1, 2, 3, 4, 5, or 6 infection and have previously been treated with an HCV regimen containing an NS5A inhibitor or in patients who have genotype 1a or 3 infection who have previously been treated with an HCV regimen containing sofosbuvir without an NS5A inhibitor** ▒
Adults: 1 tablet PO daily for 12 weeks.

S

ADMINISTRATION
PO
- Give with food to increase drug absorption.
- Store below 86° F (30° C) in original container.

ACTION
Sofosbuvir inhibits HCV NS5B RNA-dependent RNA polymerase; velpatasvir inhibits HCV NS5A protein; and voxilaprevir is a protease inhibitor. All three work together to halt HCV viral replication.

Route	Onset	Peak	Duration
PO	Unknown	2 hr (sofosbuvir); 4 hr (velpatasvir, voxilaprevir)	Unknown

Half-life: Sofosbuvir, ½ hour; velpatasvir, 17 hours; voxilaprevir, 33 hours.

ADVERSE REACTIONS
CNS: headache, insomnia, asthenia, depression, fatigue. **CV:** *symptomatic bradycardia.* **GI:** diarrhea, nausea. **Skin:** rash.

INTERACTIONS
Drug-drug. ◑ Alert: *Amiodarone:* May increase risk of symptomatic bradycardia, including cardiac arrest and cases requiring pacemaker intervention. Avoid use together. If administration can't be avoided, advise patient of risk and monitor carefully.
Antacids: May decrease velpatasvir concentration. Separate antacids and drug by 4 hours.
Atazanavir, cyclosporine, lopinavir: May increase voxilaprevir level. Use together isn't recommended.
Atorvastatin, fluvastatin, lovastatin, simvastatin: May increase statin concentration. Avoid use together. If necessary, give lowest necessary statin dose based on risks and benefits.
Dabigatran: May increase dabigatran concentration, especially in patient with moderate renal impairment. Use cautiously together, monitor patient closely, and refer to dabigatran prescribing information for dosage adjustments.
Digoxin: May increase digoxin concentration. Use cautiously together and monitor digoxin level.

Efavirenz: May decrease velpatasvir and voxilaprevir plasma concentrations. Use together isn't recommended.
H_2-receptor antagonists (famotidine): May decrease velpatasvir concentration. Limit concurrent H_2 antagonist to equivalent of famotidine 40 mg b.i.d.
Moderate to potent inducers of CYP2B6, CYP2C8, or CYP3A4 (carbamazepine, oxcarbazepine, phenobarbital, phenytoin, rifabutin, rifapentine), P-gp inducers: May significantly decrease sofosbuvir–velpatasvir–voxilaprevir plasma concentration. Use together isn't recommended.
Pitavastatin, rosuvastatin: May increase rosuvastatin and pitavastatin levels and risk of myopathy and rhabdomyolysis. Use together isn't recommended.
PPIs (omeprazole and others): May decrease velpatasvir concentration. Limit omeprazole to a dose of 20 mg. Other PPIs haven't been studied.
Pravastatin: May increase pravastatin level and risk of myopathy and rhabdomyolysis. Limit pravastatin dose to 40 mg.
Rifabutin, rifapentine: May decrease sofosbuvir–velpatasvir–voxilaprevir concentration. Use together isn't recommended.
Rifampin: May significantly alter sofosbuvir–velpatasvir–voxilaprevir plasma concentration. Use together is contraindicated.
Substrates of BCRP, OATP1B1, OATP1B3, OATP2B1, P-gp (imatinib, irinotecan, lapatinib, methotrexate, mitoxantrone, rosuvastatin, sulfasalazine, topotecan): May decrease concentrations of these substrates. Use together isn't recommended.
Tenofovir disoproxil fumarate: May increase tenofovir concentration, especially in patients with renal impairment. Monitor patient for tenofovir-associated adverse reactions; refer to tenofovir prescribing information for dosage adjustments.
Tipranavir/ritonavir: May decrease sofosbuvir and velpatasvir plasma concentrations. Use together isn't recommended.
Drug-herb. *St. John's wort:* May significantly decrease sofosbuvir, velpatasvir, or voxilaprevir plasma concentration. Discourage use together.
Drug-food. *Any food:* Increases drug concentrations. Give concurrently with food.

Reactions in bold italics are *life-threatening*. Interactions may have a *rapid onset* or a *delayed onset*.

EFFECTS ON LAB TEST RESULTS
• May increase lipase, creatine kinase, and total bilirubin levels.

CONTRAINDICATIONS & CAUTIONS
Black Box Warning HBV reactivation has been reported, in some cases resulting in fulminant hepatitis, hepatic failure, and death. Test all patients for evidence of current or prior HBV infection before initiation of HCV treatment. ∎

❸ *Alert:* Use cautiously in patients with risk factors for liver failure (hepatocellular carcinoma, alcohol abuse).

❸ *Alert:* Symptomatic bradycardia, including fatal cardiac arrest and cases requiring pacemaker intervention, has been reported when amiodarone has been administered with a sofosbuvir-containing regimen. Patients taking amiodarone who are also taking beta blockers, or who have underlying cardiac comorbidities or advanced liver disease, may be at increased risk. Signs and symptoms may occur within hours to up to 2 weeks after start of HCV therapy.

• Drug isn't recommended in patients with moderate or severe hepatic impairment (Child-Pugh class B or C).

• Use cautiously in patients with severe renal impairment (eGFR less than 30 mL/minute/1.73 m²) or ESRD, as sofosbuvir metabolite accumulates with renal impairment.

• Safety and effectiveness in children haven't been established.

Dialyzable drug: Sofosbuvir metabolite, yes; velpatasvir and voxilaprevir, unlikely.

PREGNANCY-LACTATION-REPRODUCTION
• Drug hasn't been studied in pregnant women and the safety of using drug during pregnancy hasn't been established.

• It isn't known if drug or its metabolites appear in human milk, affect milk production, or affect a breastfed infant. Consider benefits and risks before use in breastfeeding women.

NURSING CONSIDERATIONS
Black Box Warning Before initiating HCV treatment, test all patients for current or prior HBV infection by measuring HBsAg and hepatitis B core antibody (anti-HBc). ∎

Black Box Warning Monitor HCV/HBV coinfected patients for HBV reactivation and hepatitis flare during HCV treatment and posttreatment follow-up. Begin appropriate management for HBV infection as clinically indicated. ∎

❸ *Alert:* Monitor closely for liver failure, and discontinue drug in patients who develop signs and symptoms of decompensation or as clinically indicated.

❸ *Alert:* Coadministration with amiodarone isn't recommended. If these drugs must be used together or if amiodarone has been discontinued just before beginning HCV therapy, monitor patient for signs and symptoms of bradycardia (near-fainting, fainting, dizziness, light-headedness, malaise, weakness, excessive fatigue, shortness of breath, chest pain, confusion, or memory problems). Utilize inpatient cardiac monitoring for first 48 hours; then outpatient monitoring or self-monitoring of HR for bradycardia should continue daily for at least first 2 weeks of treatment. Discontinue drug if signs or symptoms of bradycardia occur.

• *Look alike–sound alike:* Don't confuse sofosbuvir–velpatasvir combination with sofosbuvir–velpatasvir–voxilaprevir combination.

PATIENT TEACHING
• Advise patient to report a history of HBV infection before therapy begins.

• Warn patient that therapy can increase risk of HBV reactivation and that laboratory testing for HBV exposure will be needed before therapy begins. Explain that for therapy to be effective, patient needs to take drug exactly as prescribed for the entire duration.

❸ *Alert:* Caution patient to seek immediate medical attention for signs and symptoms of bradycardia.

❸ *Alert:* Warn patient to immediately report signs and symptoms of liver injury (fatigue, weakness, loss of appetite, nausea, vomiting, yellowing of skin or eyes, light-colored stool).

• Caution patient not to stop treatment without first discussing with prescriber.

solifenacin succinate
sole-ah-FEN-ah-sin

VESIcare✦

Therapeutic class: Urinary antispasmodics
Pharmacologic class: Antimuscarinics

AVAILABLE FORMS
Tablets (film-coated) ⒪ⓃⒸ: 5 mg, 10 mg

INDICATIONS & DOSAGES
➤ **Overactive bladder with urinary urgency, frequency, and urge incontinence**
Adults: 5 mg PO once daily. May increase to 10 mg once daily if 5-mg dose is well tolerated.
Adjust-a-dose: If CrCl is less than 30 mL/minute or patient has moderate liver impairment (Child-Pugh class B), or if drug is taken concurrently with CYP3A4 inhibitors, maximum dose is 5 mg.

ADMINISTRATION
PO
• Give drug without regard for food.
• Patient should swallow tablet whole with water.

ACTION
Relaxes smooth muscle of bladder by antagonizing muscarinic receptors, relieving symptoms of overactive bladder.

Route	Onset	Peak	Duration
PO	Unknown	3–8 hr	Unknown

Half-life: About 45 to 68 hours.

ADVERSE REACTIONS
CNS: depression, dizziness, fatigue. **CV:** HTN, leg swelling. **EENT:** blurred vision, dry eyes, pharyngitis. **GI:** constipation, dry mouth, dyspepsia, nausea, upper abdominal pain, vomiting. **GU:** urine retention, UTI. **Respiratory:** cough. **Other:** influenza.

INTERACTIONS
Drug-drug. *Drugs that prolong QT interval:* May increase risk of serious cardiac arrhythmias. Monitor patient and ECG closely.
Potent CYP3A4 inducers (carbamazepine, phenobarbital, phenytoin, rifampin): May decrease solifenacin concentration. Monitor effectiveness. Some drugs may be contraindicated.
Potassium chloride (solid oral dosage forms only): May increase ulcer risk. Avoid using any solid oral dosage form of potassium chloride.
Potent CYP3A4 inhibitors (ketoconazole): May increase solifenacin level. Don't exceed solifenacin dose of 5 mg daily when used together.

EFFECTS ON LAB TEST RESULTS
None reported.

CONTRAINDICATIONS & CAUTIONS
• Contraindicated in patients hypersensitive to drug or its components and in patients with urine or gastric retention or uncontrolled narrow-angle glaucoma. Don't use in patients with severe hepatic impairment (Child-Pugh class C). Angioedema has been reported after first dose.
• Use cautiously in elderly patients and in patients with a history of prolonged QT interval, those being treated for angle-closure glaucoma, and those with bladder outflow obstruction, decreased GI motility, renal insufficiency, or moderate liver impairment.
• CNS anticholinergic effects can occur, including headache, confusion, hallucinations, and somnolence.
Dialyzable drug: Unknown.
⚠ *Overdose S&S:* Anticholinergic effects (fixed and dilated pupils, blurred vision, failure of heel-to-toe examination, tremors, dry skin).

PREGNANCY-LACTATION-REPRODUCTION
• There are no adequate studies in pregnant women. Use only if potential benefit justifies potential risk to the fetus.
• It isn't known if drug appears in human milk. Patient should discontinue breastfeeding or discontinue drug.

NURSING CONSIDERATIONS
• Assess bladder function, and monitor drug effects.
• If patient has bladder outlet obstruction, watch for urine retention.
• Monitor patient for decreased gastric motility and constipation.

• Monitor patient for signs and symptoms of anticholinergic CNS effects (including headache, confusion, hallucinations, and somnolence), particularly after beginning treatment or increasing dosage. If patient experiences anticholinergic CNS effects, consider dosage reduction or drug discontinuation.

• Safety and effectiveness are similar in older and younger adults, but levels and half-life may be increased in the elderly.

• *Look alike–sound alike:* Don't confuse VESIcare with Vesanoid.

PATIENT TEACHING

• Explain that drug may cause blurred vision. Tell patient to use caution when performing hazardous activities or tasks that require clear vision until effects of the drug are known.

• Discourage use of other drugs that may cause dry mouth, constipation, urine retention, or blurred vision.

• Urge patient to report all adverse reactions, especially swelling in the face, lips, or tongue or abdominal pain or constipation that lasts 3 days or longer.

• Tell patient that drug decreases the ability to sweat normally, and advise cautious use in hot environments or during strenuous activity.

• Tell patient to swallow tablet whole with water.

• Inform patient that drug may be taken with or without food.

• Advise patient not to drive or operate heavy machinery until drug's effects are known.

---

somatropin ᛟ
soe-ma-TROE-pin

Genotropin, Genotropin MiniQuick, Humatrope, Norditropin FlexPro, Nutropin AQ NuSpin, Omnitrope, Saizen, Serostim, Zomacton, Zorbtive

Therapeutic class: Growth hormones
Pharmacologic class: Anterior pituitary hormones

AVAILABLE FORMS

Genotropin injection: 5 mg and 12 mg in two-chamber cartridges

Genotropin MiniQuick injection: 0.2 mg/vial, 0.4 mg/vial, 0.6 mg/vial, 0.8 mg/vial, 1 mg/vial, 1.2 mg/vial, 1.4 mg/vial, 1.6 mg/vial, 1.8 mg/vial, 2 mg/vial

Humatrope injection: 5 mg (about 15 international units/vial), 6 mg (18 international units/cartridge), 12 mg (36 international units/cartridge), 24 mg (72 international units/cartridge)

Norditropin injection: 5 mg/1.5 mL, 10 mg/1.5 mL, 15 mg/1.5 mL, 30 mg/3 mL cartridges

Nutropin AQ injection: 5 mg (about 15 international units)/2-mL device, 10 mg (about 30 international units)/2-mL device or pen, 20 mg (about 60 international units)/2-mL device or pen

Omnitrope injection: 5.8 mg/vial, 5 mg/1.5 mL injection cartridge, 10 mg/1.5 mL injection cartridge

Saizen injection: 5 mg (about 15 international units/vial), 8.8 mg (about 26.4 international units/vial)

Serostim injection: 4 mg (about 12 international units/vial), 5 mg (about 15 international units/vial), 6 mg (about 18 international units/vial)

Zomacton* injection: 5-mg and 10-mg vials
Zorbtive injection: 8.8 mg (approximately 26.4 international units)/vial

INDICATIONS & DOSAGES

➤ **Long-term treatment of growth failure in children with inadequate secretion of endogenous growth hormone (GH)**
Children: 0.18 to 0.3 mg/kg/week Humatrope subcut, divided equally and given six times weekly or once daily. Or, up to 0.3 mg/kg Nutropin AQ subcut weekly in daily divided doses; in pubertal patients, a weekly dosage of up to 0.7 mg/kg (Nutropin AQ) in daily divided doses may be used. Or, Saizen 0.18 mg/kg/week subcut divided into equal doses given on 3 alternate days, 6 times per week, or daily. Or, Norditropin 0.024 to 0.034 mg/kg/day subcut, given on six or seven days cach week. Or, 0.16 to 0.24 mg/kg Genotropin or Omnitrope subcut weekly, divided into six or seven doses. Or, up to 0.1 mg/kg Zomacton subcut three times per week (up to 0.3 mg/kg/week total).

S

➤ **Growth failure from chronic renal insufficiency up to time of renal transplantation**
Children: Up to 0.35 mg/kg/week Nutropin AQ subcut divided into daily doses.

➤ **Long-term treatment of short stature from Turner syndrome**
Children: Up to 0.375 mg/kg/week Humatrope or Nutropin AQ subcut, divided into equal doses given three to seven times weekly. Or, up to 0.067 mg/kg/day Norditropin subcut. Or, 0.33 mg/kg/week Genotropin or Omnitrope divided into six or seven once-daily subcut injections per week.

➤ **Short stature in children with Noonan syndrome**
Children: Up to 0.46 mg/kg Norditropin subcut weekly, divided into six or seven equal daily doses.

➤ **Long-term treatment of growth failure in children with Prader-Willi syndrome diagnosed by genetic testing**
Children: 0.24 mg/kg Genotropin, Norditropin, or Omnitrope subcut weekly, divided into six or seven doses. Individualize dosage based on growth response.

➤ **Replacement of endogenous GH in adult patients with GH deficiency**
Adults: Initially, not more than 0.006 mg/kg Humatrope or Nutropin AQ subcut daily. May increase to maximum of 0.0125 mg/kg Humatrope daily. Or, initially 0.004 mg/kg Norditropin subcut daily. May increase to a maximum of 0.16 mg/kg/day. May increase Norditropin to maximum of 0.016 mg/kg daily after about 6 weeks; or increase by 0.1 to 0.2 mg/day every 1 to 2 months based on clinical response and insulin-like growth factor-1 concentration.

Nutropin AQ dosages may be increased to maximum of 0.025 mg/kg daily in patients younger than age 35 or 0.0125 mg/kg daily in patients older than age 35. Or, starting dosages not exceeding 0.04 mg/kg Genotropin or Omnitrope subcut weekly, divided into six or seven doses, may be increased at 4- to 8-week intervals to a maximum dose of 0.08 mg/kg subcut weekly, divided into six or seven doses. Or, initially, not more than 0.005 mg/kg Saizen daily. May increase after 4 weeks to a maximum dose of 0.01 mg/kg daily based on patient tolerance and clinical response.

➤ **HIV wasting or cachexia**
Adults and children weighing more than 55 kg: 6 mg Serostim subcut at bedtime.
Adults and children weighing 45 to 55 kg: 5 mg Serostim subcut at bedtime.
Adults and children weighing 35 to 45 kg: 4 mg Serostim subcut at bedtime.
Adults and children weighing less than 35 kg: 0.1 mg/kg/day Serostim subcut at bedtime.

➤ **Long-term treatment of growth failure in children born small for gestational age (SGA) who don't catch up by age 2**
Children: 0.48 mg/kg Genotropin or Omnitrope subcut weekly, divided into six or seven doses.

➤ **Short stature in children born SGA who don't catch up by age 2 to 4**
Children: Up to 0.067 mg/kg/day Norditropin or Humatrope subcut.

➤ **Idiopathic short stature**
Children: Up to 0.37 mg/kg Humatrope subcut weekly, divided into six or seven equal doses. Or, up to 0.47 mg/kg/week Genotropin, Omnitrope, or Norditropin subcut, divided into six or seven equal doses. Or, up to 0.3 mg/kg/week Nutropin AQ subcut divided into equal daily doses.

➤ **Short bowel syndrome**
Adults: 0.1 mg/kg/day Zorbtive subcut daily for 4 weeks. Maximum dosage, 8 mg/day.

➤ **Treatment of short stature or growth failure in children with short stature homeobox-containing (*SHOX*) gene deficiency** 🖹
Children: Humatrope 0.35 mg/kg subcut weekly divided into equal doses 6 or 7 days/week.

ADMINISTRATION
• Refer to product insert for brand-specific reconstitution instructions.

IM
• To prepare solution, inject supplied diluent into vial containing drug by aiming stream of liquid against wall of glass vial. Then swirl vial gently until contents are completely dissolved. Don't shake vial.
• After reconstitution, make sure solution is clear. Don't inject solution if it's cloudy or contains particles.
• For patients on hemodialysis, give drug before bedtime or 3 to 4 hours after dialysis.

Reactions in bold italics are *life-threatening*. Interactions may have a *rapid onset* or a ***delayed onset***.

For long-term cycling peritoneal dialysis, give drug in the morning after completion of dialysis. For long-term ambulatory peritoneal dialysis, give drug in the evening at the time of the overnight exchange.

• Store reconstituted drug in refrigerator; use within manufacturer's recommended time frame for each drug.

• If patient develops sensitivity to diluent, reconstitute drug with sterile water for injection. When drug is reconstituted in this way, use only one reconstituted dose per vial, refrigerate solution if it isn't used immediately after reconstitution, use reconstituted dose within 24 hours, and discard unused portion.

🔔 **Alert:** When administering to newborn, reconstitute with sterile water for injection.

Subcutaneous

• To prepare solution, inject supplied diluent into vial containing drug by aiming stream of liquid against wall of glass vial. Then swirl vial gently until contents are completely dissolved. Don't shake vial.

🔔 **Alert:** Don't use Zomacton 5-mg vials in neonates or if patient has a known benzyl alcohol sensitivity.

• After reconstitution, make sure solution is clear. Don't inject solution if it's cloudy or contains particles.

• For patients on hemodialysis, give drug before bedtime or 3 to 4 hours after dialysis. For long-term cycling peritoneal dialysis, give drug in the morning after completion of dialysis. For long-term ambulatory peritoneal dialysis, give drug in the evening at the time of the overnight exchange.

• Rotate injection sites to avoid tissue atrophy.

• Store reconstituted drug in refrigerator; use within manufacturer's recommended time frame for each drug.

• If patient develops sensitivity to diluent, reconstitute drug with sterile water for injection. When drug is reconstituted in this way, use only one reconstituted dose per vial, refrigerate solution if it isn't used immediately after reconstitution, use reconstituted dose within 24 hours, and discard unused portion.

🔔 **Alert:** When administering to newborn, reconstitute with sterile water for injection.

ACTION

Purified GH of recombinant DNA origin that stimulates skeletal, linear, muscle, and organ growth.

Route	Onset	Peak	Duration
IM, subcut	Unknown	Varies by route and brand	18–20 hr

Half-life: Varies by route and brand. Refer to manufacturer's drug label.

ADVERSE REACTIONS

CNS: headache, weakness, paresthesia, fatigue. **CV:** mild, transient edema; peripheral edema. **EENT:** otitis media. **Hematologic:** *leukemia.* **Metabolic:** mild hyperglycemia, hypothyroidism. **Musculoskeletal:** localized muscle pain, arthralgia, stiffness of extremities. **Respiratory:** URI. **Skin:** injection-site pain. **Other:** antibodies to GH.

INTERACTIONS

Drug-drug. *Corticotropin, corticosteroids:* Long-term use may inhibit growth response to GH. Monitor patient for lack of effect.
Estrogen replacement: May decrease somatropin level in adult women. Increase somatropin dosage as necessary.
Insulin, oral antidiabetic agents: Somatropin may decrease insulin sensitivity. Antidiabetic agent dosage may need adjustment.

EFFECTS ON LAB TEST RESULTS

• May increase glucose, serum phosphorus, alkaline phosphatase, and parathyroid hormone levels.

CONTRAINDICATIONS & CAUTIONS

• Contraindicated in patients with hypersensitivity to somatropin or its excipients.

• Contraindicated in patients with closed epiphyses, active proliferative or severe nonproliferative diabetic retinopathy, or an active underlying intracranial lesion.

• Contraindicated in patients with active malignancy. An increased risk of second neoplasm has been reported in childhood cancer survivors treated with somatropin. Patients with HIV and children with short stature (genetic cause) have increased baseline risk of developing malignancies.

S

Consider risk and benefits before initiating therapy; monitor these patients carefully.
• Contraindicated in patients with Prader-Willi syndrome who are severely obese, have a history of upper airway obstruction or sleep apnea, or have severe respiratory impairment.
• For patients hypersensitive to either metacresol or glycerin, don't use supplied diluent to reconstitute Humatrope.
• Contraindicated in patients with acute critical illness due to complications following open heart or abdominal surgery, trauma, or acute respiratory failure. Safety of continuing somatropin treatment in patients receiving replacement doses for approved indications who concurrently develop acute critical illnesses hasn't been established. Weigh potential benefit of treatment continuation against potential risks.
• Serious systemic hypersensitivity reactions, including anaphylactic reactions and angioedema, have been reported.
• Use cautiously in children with hypothyroidism and in those with GH deficiency caused by intracranial lesion.
• Use cautiously in patients with diabetes.
• May increase risk of pancreatitis. Monitor patient for persistent abdominal pain with or without vomiting.
• Patients receiving somatropin who have or are at risk for pituitary hormone deficiency may be at risk for reduced serum cortisol levels or unmasking of central (secondary) hypoadrenalism. Also, patients treated with glucocorticoid replacement for previously diagnosed hypoadrenalism may require an increase in maintenance or stress doses once somatropin therapy begins.
Dialyzable drug: Unknown.
⚠ *Overdose S&S:* Fluid retention, hypoglycemia followed by hyperglycemia, glucose intolerance, gigantism, acromegaly.

PREGNANCY-LACTATION-REPRODUCTION
• There are no adequate studies in pregnant women. Use only if clearly needed.
• It isn't known if drug appears in human milk. Use cautiously in breastfeeding women.

NURSING CONSIDERATIONS
• Frequently examine children with hypothyroidism and those whose GH deficiency is caused by an intracranial lesion for progression or recurrence of underlying disease.
• Obtain hip X-rays to check for slipped capital femoral epiphysis or femoral avascular necrosis before starting somatropin in patients with growth failure secondary to chronic kidney disease.
⚠ *Alert:* In patients with Prader-Willi syndrome who are morbidly obese and in those with a history of respiratory impairment, sleep apnea, or unidentified respiratory infection, therapy may be life-threatening. Assess patients with Prader-Willi syndrome for sleep apnea and upper airway obstruction before treatment. Interrupt treatment if signs of upper airway obstruction occur.
• Monitor patient with Prader-Willi syndrome for signs of respiratory infection.
• Monitor child's height regularly. Regular checkups, including monitoring of blood and radiologic studies, are also needed.
• Monitor patient's glucose level regularly because GH may induce a state of insulin resistance or new-onset diabetes mellitus.
• Excessive glucocorticoid therapy inhibits somatropin's growth-promoting effect. Patients with coexisting corticotropin deficiency should have their glucocorticoid replacement dosage carefully adjusted to avoid growth inhibition.
• Watch for slipped capital femoral epiphysis or progression of scoliosis in patients with rapid growth.
• Monitor results of periodic thyroid function tests for hypothyroidism; condition may need thyroid hormone treatment.
• Patient should have ophthalmic examinations to monitor for intracranial HTN before therapy (to establish baseline) and periodically thereafter.
• Monitor patients with preexisting tumors or growth failure secondary to an intracranial lesion for recurrence or progression of underlying disease; discontinue therapy with evidence of recurrence.
• Monitor all patients for increased growth, or potential malignant changes, of skin lesions.

- Monitor patients for signs and symptoms of serious systemic hypersensitivity reactions.
- Only adults with GH deficiency alone or together with multiple hormone deficiencies from pituitary or hypothalamic disease, surgery, radiation, or trauma or those who were GH deficient as children and have been confirmed GH deficient as adults can take Saizen.
- **Look alike–sound alike:** Don't confuse somatropin with somatrem or sumatriptan or Humatrope with homatropine.

PATIENT TEACHING
- Inform parents that child with endocrine disorders (including GH deficiency) may have an increased risk of slipped capital epiphyses. Tell parents to notify prescriber if they notice their child limping.
- Advise parents to be alert for limping or complaints of hip or knee pain in children being treated with Nutropin AQ for growth failure secondary to chronic kidney disease.
- Instruct patient with diabetes to monitor glucose level closely and report changes to prescriber.
- Instruct patient or parents in appropriate injection technique and needle disposal. Tell them to rotate injection sites.
- Advise patient or parents that serious systemic hypersensitivity reactions, including anaphylaxis and angioedema, can occur and to seek immediate medical attention if an allergic reaction occurs.
- Stress importance of close follow-up care and of reporting all adverse reactions.

sotalol hydrochloride
SOE-ta-lole

Betapace, Betapace AF, Sorine, Sotylize

Therapeutic class: Antiarrhythmics
Pharmacologic class: Nonselective beta blockers

AVAILABLE FORMS
Solution for injection: 15 mg/mL
Betapace
Tablets: 80 mg, 120 mg, 160 mg, 240 mg

Betapace AF
Tablets: 80 mg, 120 mg, 160 mg
Sorine
Tablets: 80 mg, 120 mg, 160 mg, 240 mg
Sotylize
Oral solution: 5 mg/mL

INDICATIONS & DOSAGES
Black Box Warning Calculate CrCl before dosing; adjust dosing interval based on CrCl. Don't initiate therapy with IV sotalol or oral solution if baseline QTc is longer than 450 msec.

Black Box Warning Don't substitute sotalol for sotalol AF.

➤ **Documented, life-threatening ventricular arrhythmias (Betapace, Betapace AF, Sorine, Sotylize)**
Adults: Initially, 80 mg PO b.i.d. Increase dosage gradually (increments of 80 mg/day for Sotylize) every 3 days as needed and tolerated. Most patients respond to 160 to 320 mg/day, although some patients with refractory arrhythmias need up to 640 mg/day. Or, 75 mg IV once daily or b.i.d. based on CrCl. After 3 days, dosage may be increased to 75 to 150 mg IV once daily or every 12 hours based on CrCl. For refractory life-threatening arrhythmias, dosage may be increased to 225 to 300 mg IV once daily or every 12 hours.
Children age 2 and older with normal renal function: Initially, 30 mg/m^2 PO t.i.d. Titrate dosage to a maximum of 60 mg/m^2 (equivalent to 320 mg total daily dose for adults). Guide titration by clinical response, HR, and QTc interval. Allow at least 36 hours between dose increments.
Children younger than age 2 with normal renal function: The reduced dosage is calculated based on an age factor plotted on a logarithmic scale found in manufacturer's instructions.
Adjust-a-dose: Adults: For oral route, if CrCl is 30 to 60 mL/minute, increase dosage interval to every 24 hours; if CrCl is 10 to 29 mL/minute, increase interval to every 36 to 48 hours; and if CrCl is less than 10 mL/minute, individualize dosage. For IV route, if CrCl is 40 to 59 mL/minute, give IV drug once daily; don't give if CrCl is less than 40 mL/minute.

S

Children: Use in any age-group with decreased renal function should be at lower dosages or at increased intervals between doses. Use of sotalol in children with renal impairment hasn't been investigated. Use with particular caution in children if QTc interval is greater than 500 msec on therapy; seriously consider reducing dosage or discontinuing therapy when QTc interval exceeds 550 msec.

➤ **To maintain normal sinus rhythm or to delay recurrence of atrial fibrillation or atrial flutter in patients with symptomatic atrial fibrillation or flutter who are currently in sinus rhythm (Betapace, Betapace AF, Sotylize, sotalol IV)**
Adults: 80 mg PO b.i.d. (Don't use if baseline QT interval is greater than 450 msec.) Increase dosage as needed to 120 mg PO b.i.d. after 3 days if the QTc interval is less than 500 msec. Maximum dosage is 160 mg PO b.i.d. Or, 75 mg IV once daily or every 12 hours based on CrCl. After 3 days, dosage may be increased to 112.5 to 150 mg IV once daily or every 12 hours based on clearance.
Children age 2 and older with normal renal function: Initially, 30 mg/m² PO t.i.d. Titrate dosage to a maximum of 60 mg/m² (equivalent to 320 mg total daily dose for adults). Guide titration by clinical response, HR, and QTc interval. Allow at least 36 hours between dose increments.
Children younger than age 2 with normal renal function: Initially, 30 mg/m² PO t.i.d. multiplied by age factor plotted on a logarithmic scale found in manufacturer's instructions.
Adjust-a-dose: Adults: For oral route, if CrCl is 40 to 60 mL/minute, increase dosage interval to every 24 hours; if CrCl is less than 40 mL/minute, use is contraindicated. For IV route, if CrCl is 40 to 59 mL/minute, give IV drug once daily; don't give if CrCl is less than 40 mL/minute.
Children: Use in any age-group with decreased renal function should be at lower dosages or at increased intervals between doses. Use of sotalol in children with renal impairment hasn't been investigated. Use with particular caution in children if QTc interval is greater than 500 msec on therapy; seriously consider reducing dosage or dis-

continuing therapy when QTc interval exceeds 550 msec.

ADMINISTRATION
PO
• Give 1 hour before or 2 hours after antacids.
• May give without regard for food, but patient should take the same way each time.
IV
▼ Dilute drug with NSS, D_5W, or lactated Ringer solution in a volume of 120 to 250 mL to compensate for dead space in the infusion set.
▼ Use an infusion pump to administer drug at a constant rate over 5 hours.
▼ **Incompatibilities:** None listed by manufacturer. Consult a drug incompatibility reference for more information.

ACTION
Depresses sinus HR, slows AV conduction, decreases cardiac output, and lowers systolic and diastolic BP. Drug also has class III antiarrhythmic properties and can prolong duration of the cardiac action potential.

Route	Onset	Peak	Duration
PO	1–2 hr	2–4 hr	Unknown
IV	5–10 min	Unknown	Unknown

Half-life: Adults, 12 hours; children, 9½ hours.

ADVERSE REACTIONS
CNS: asthenia, headache, dizziness, weakness, fatigue, light-headedness, sleep problems, anxiety, confusion, paresthesia, mood changes, fever. **CV:** chest pain, palpitations, *bradycardia, arrhythmias, HF, AV block, proarrhythmic events (including polymorphic ventricular tachycardia, PVCs, ventricular fibrillation),* edema, ECG abnormalities, hypotension. **EENT:** visual disturbance. **GI:** nausea, vomiting, diarrhea, dyspepsia, abdominal pain. **Metabolic:** hyperglycemia, decreased appetite. **Musculoskeletal:** pain. **Respiratory:** dyspnea, URI, *bronchospasm.* **Skin:** hyperhidrosis, rash. **Other:** infection, influenza.

INTERACTIONS
Drug-drug. *Antacids containing aluminum oxide and magnesium hydroxide:* May reduce bradycardic effect. Avoid sotalol administration within 2 hours of antacid.

Reactions in bold italics are *life-threatening*. Interactions may have a *rapid onset* or a *delayed onset*.

Antiarrhythmics: May increase drug effects. Avoid using together.

Antihypertensives, catecholamine-depleting drugs (guanethidine, reserpine): May increase hypotensive effects or cause marked bradycardia. Monitor BP and pulse closely.

Beta₂-agonists (albuterol, isoproterenol, terbutaline, isoproterenol): May diminish the bronchodilatory effect. Dosage increase may be needed.

Calcium channel blockers: May increase myocardial depression. Avoid using together.

Clonidine: May enhance rebound effect after withdrawal of clonidine. Stop sotalol several days before withdrawing clonidine.

Drugs that prolong the QT interval (class I and III antiarrhythmics, bepridil, phenothiazines, TCAs): May cause excessive QT prolongation. Monitor QT interval.

General anesthetics: May increase myocardial depression. Monitor patient closely.

Insulin, oral antidiabetics: May cause hyperglycemia and may mask signs and symptoms of hypoglycemia. Adjust dosage accordingly.

Macrolides and related antibiotics (azithromycin, clarithromycin, erythromycin), quinolones, TCAs: May cause additive effects or prolong the QT interval. Use with caution.

Prazosin: May increase the risk of orthostatic hypotension. Assist patient to stand slowly until effects are known.

Theophylline: May decrease bronchodilating effects. Avoid using together.

EFFECTS ON LAB TEST RESULTS
• May increase glucose level.
• May cause false-positive catecholamine level.

CONTRAINDICATIONS & CAUTIONS
• Contraindicated in patients hypersensitive to drug.
• Contraindicated in those with severe sinus node dysfunction, sinus bradycardia, second- and third-degree AV block unless patient has a pacemaker, congenital or acquired long QT-interval syndrome, cardiogenic shock, uncontrolled HF, CrCl of less than 40 mL/minute, serum potassium level of less than 4 mEq/L, and bronchial asthma.

• Contraindicated in patients with hypomagnesemia before correction of imbalance.

Black Box Warning Sotalol can cause life-threatening ventricular tachycardia associated with QT-interval prolongation. ∎

• Use cautiously in patients with renal impairment or diabetes mellitus (beta blockers may mask signs and symptoms of hypoglycemia).

Dialyzable drug: Yes.

⚠ *Overdose S&S:* Bradycardia, bronchospasm, HF, hypoglycemia, hypotension, asystole, QT-interval prolongation, torsades de pointes, ventricular tachycardia, death.

PREGNANCY-LACTATION-REPRODUCTION
• There are no adequate studies in pregnant women. Use only if potential benefit justifies potential risk to the fetus. Drug crosses placental barrier and appears in amniotic fluid.
• Drug appears in human milk. Patient should discontinue breastfeeding or discontinue drug.

NURSING CONSIDERATIONS
Black Box Warning Because proarrhythmic events may occur at the start of therapy and during dosage adjustments, patients should be hospitalized for a minimum of 3 days in a facility that can provide calculations of CrCl, continuous ECG monitoring, and cardiac resuscitation. Calculate CrCl before dosing; adjust the dosing interval based on CrCl. ∎

Black Box Warning The baseline QTc interval must be less than or equal to 450 msec before starting sotalol IV or oral suspension. If QT interval is 500 msec or more, dosage or frequency must be decreased or drug discontinued. ∎

• Assess patient for new or worsened symptoms of HF.

• Although patients receiving IV lidocaine may start sotalol therapy without ill effects, withdraw other antiarrhythmics before therapy begins. Sotalol therapy typically is delayed until two or three half-lives of the withdrawn drug have elapsed. After withdrawing amiodarone, give sotalol only after QT interval normalizes.

• Adjust dosage slowly, allowing 3 days between dosage increments for adequate

S

monitoring of QT intervals and for drug levels to reach a steady-state level.
• Monitor electrolytes regularly, especially if patient is receiving diuretics. Electrolyte imbalances, such as hypokalemia or hypomagnesemia, may enhance QT-interval prolongation and increase the risk of serious arrhythmias such as torsades de pointes.
• *Look alike–sound alike:* Don't confuse sotalol with Sudafed.

PATIENT TEACHING
• Explain that patient will need to be hospitalized for initiation of drug therapy.
• Warn patient to report all adverse reactions and to immediately report fast, irregular heartbeat; light-headedness; or fainting.
• Stress need to take drug as prescribed, even when feeling well. Caution patient against stopping drug suddenly.
• Caution patient against using OTC drugs and decongestants while taking drug.
• Advise patient to take drug consistently with or without food.
• Because antacids can interfere with absorption, tell patient to take drug 2 hours before or after antacids.
• Warn patient not to double the next dose if a dose is missed.

spironolactone
speer-on-oh-LAK-tone

Aldactone✦, CaroSpir

Therapeutic class: Diuretics
Pharmacologic class: Potassium-sparing diuretics–aldosterone receptor antagonists

AVAILABLE FORMS
Oral suspension: 25 mg/5 mL
Tablets: 25 mg, 50 mg, 100 mg

INDICATIONS & DOSAGES
➤ **Edema due to HF, hepatic cirrhosis, or nephrotic syndrome (except CaroSpir)**
Adults: Initially, 100 mg PO (tablets) daily given as a single dose or in divided doses. Usual range is 25 to 200 mg PO daily.
➤ **HTN**
Adults: 50 to 100 mg (tablets) PO daily or in divided doses. Some practitioners use

a lower dosage range of 25 to 50 mg daily and add another antihypertensive to the regimen, rather than continually increasing this drug. Or, 20 to 75 mg suspension PO daily in single or divided doses. May titrate dosage at 2-week intervals. Dosages higher than 75 mg/day generally don't provide additional BP reductions.
➤ **Diuretic-induced hypokalemia (except CaroSpir)**
Adults: 25 to 100 mg (tablets) PO daily.
➤ **To detect primary hyperaldosteronism (except CaroSpir)**
Adults: 400 mg (tablets) PO daily for 4 days (short test) or 3 to 4 weeks (long test). If hypokalemia and HTN are corrected, a presumptive diagnosis of primary hyperaldosteronism is made.
➤ **To manage primary hyperaldosteronism (except CaroSpir)**
Adults: 100 to 400 mg (tablets) PO daily. Use lowest effective dose.
➤ **Severe HF (class III or IV), as adjunct to ACE inhibitor or loop diuretic, with or without cardiac glycoside (except CaroSpir)**
Adults: 25 mg (tablets) PO daily if serum potassium level is 5 mEq/L or eGFR is 50 mL/minute. May increase to 50 mg (tablets) PO daily as clinically indicated.
Adjust-a-dose: Patients who don't tolerate 25 mg daily may have dosage decreased to every other day.
➤ **NYHA HF (Class III or IV) with other HF therapies (CaroSpir)**
Adults: Initially, 20 mg suspension PO once daily in patients with serum potassium level of 5.0 mEq/L or less and eGFR greater than 50 mL/minute/1.73 m^2. May increase dosage to 37.5 mg if 20-mg dose is tolerated.
Adjust-a-dose: In patients with eGFR between 30 and 50 mL/minute/1.73 m^2, consider initial dose of 10 mg, because of risk of hyperkalemia. If patient develops hyperkalemia on 20-mg once-daily therapy, may reduce dosage to 20 mg every other day.
➤ **Edema from hepatic cirrhosis (CaroSpir)**
Adults: Initially, 75 mg suspension PO daily in either single or divided doses. Initiate therapy in a hospital setting and slowly titrate. When used as the sole agent for diuresis, give for at least 5 days before

---

Reactions in bold italics are *life-threatening*. Interactions may have a *rapid onset* or a *delayed onset*.

increasing dosage. If patient requires more than 100 mg, use another formulation.

ADMINISTRATION
PO
• CaroSpir suspension isn't therapeutically equivalent to Aldactone tablets.
• To enhance absorption, give tablets with meals.
• May give suspension with or without food but give consistently with respect to food.

ACTION
Antagonizes aldosterone in the distal tubules, increasing sodium and water excretion.

Route	Onset	Peak	Duration
PO (tablets)	Unknown	3–4 hr	2–3 days
PO (suspension)	Unknown	2½–5 hr	Unknown

Half-life: Tablets, 1¼ hours; suspension, 1 to 2 hours.

ADVERSE REACTIONS
CNS: headache, drowsiness, lethargy, confusion, ataxia. **GI:** diarrhea, *gastric bleeding,* ulceration, cramping, gastritis, vomiting. **GU:** *renal failure,* inability to maintain erection, menstrual disturbances, postmenopausal bleeding. **Hematologic:** *agranulocytosis.* **Metabolic:** *hyperkalemia,* dehydration, hyponatremia, mild acidosis. **Skin:** urticaria, hirsutism, maculopapular eruptions. **Other:** *anaphylaxis,* gynecomastia, breast soreness, drug fever.

INTERACTIONS
Drug-drug. *ACE inhibitors, ARBs:* May increase risk of severe hyperkalemia. Use together with caution and monitor potassium levels.
Acetylsalicylic acid: May reduce therapeutic effects of spironolactone. Monitor spironolactone effects and increase maintenance dose as needed.
Anticoagulants: May decrease anticoagulant effects. Monitor PT and INR.
Aspirin and other salicylates: May block diuretic effect of spironolactone. Watch for diminished spironolactone response.

Cholestyramine: May increase risk of metabolic acidosis and hyperkalemia. Monitor therapy.
Digoxin: May alter digoxin clearance, increasing risk of toxicity. Monitor digoxin level.
🚫 *Alert: Eplerenone:* May increase risk of severe hyperkalemia. Use together is contraindicated.
Heparin, low–molecular-weight heparins: May increase risk of hyperkalemia. Use cautiously and monitor potassium level.
Lithium: May reduce lithium renal clearance and increase risk of lithium toxicity. Monitor patient closely.
NSAIDs, potassium-sparing diuretics, potassium supplements: May result in hyperkalemia. Don't use together.
Drug-herb. *Licorice:* May block ulcer-healing and aldosterone-like effects of herb; may increase risk of hypokalemia. Discourage use together.
Drug-food. *Potassium-rich foods, such as citrus fruits and tomatoes, salt substitutes containing potassium:* May increase risk of hyperkalemia. Urge caution.

EFFECTS ON LAB TEST RESULTS
• May increase glucose, uric acid, BUN, and potassium levels.
• May decrease sodium, magnesium, and calcium levels.
• May decrease granulocyte count.
• May cause hypochloremic alkalosis.
• May alter fluorometric determinations of plasma and urinary 17-hydroxycorticosteroid levels.

CONTRAINDICATIONS & CAUTIONS
• Use spironolactone only for those conditions for which it's indicated. Drug has been shown to be tumorigenic in long-term toxicity studies in rats. Avoid unnecessary use.
• Contraindicated in patients hypersensitive to drug and in those with anuria, acute or progressive renal insufficiency, Addison disease, or hyperkalemia.
• Use cautiously in patients with fluid or electrolyte imbalances and in those with impaired renal or hepatic function.
• CaroSpir should be initiated in a hospital setting for patients with hepatic disease with cirrhosis and ascites. Drug can cause

fluid and electrolyte disturbances, impair neurologic function, and worsen hepatic encephalopathy and coma.

• Safety and effectiveness in children haven't been established.

⚠ *Overdose S&S:* Drowsiness, confusion, rash, nausea, vomiting, dizziness, diarrhea, hyperkalemia.

PREGNANCY-LACTATION-REPRODUCTION

• Use of diuretics to treat edema during normal pregnancies isn't appropriate. Drug may cause fetal harm because of its antiandrogenic activity; avoid use in the first trimester. Use during pregnancy only if clearly needed and potential benefit justifies potential risk to the fetus.

• A major metabolite of drug appears in human milk. Patient should discontinue breastfeeding or discontinue drug, taking into account importance of drug to the mother.

NURSING CONSIDERATIONS

• Monitor electrolyte levels, fluid intake and output, weight, and BP closely.

• Monitor elderly patients closely, who are more susceptible to excessive diuresis.

• Inform laboratory that patient is taking spironolactone because drug may interfere with tests that measure digoxin level.

• Drug is less potent than thiazide and loop diuretics and is useful as an adjunct to other diuretic therapy. Diuretic effect is delayed 2 to 3 days when used alone.

• Maximum antihypertensive response may be delayed for up to 2 weeks.

• Watch for hyperchloremic metabolic acidosis, especially in patients with hepatic cirrhosis.

• *Look alike–sound alike:* Don't confuse Aldactone with Aldactazide.

PATIENT TEACHING

• Instruct patient to take oral suspension consistently either with or without food.

• Tell patient to report all adverse reactions.

❸ *Alert:* To prevent serious hyperkalemia, warn patient to avoid excessive ingestion of potassium-rich foods (such as citrus fruits, tomatoes, bananas, dates, and apricots), salt substitutes containing potassium, and potassium supplements.

• Caution patient not to perform hazardous activities if adverse CNS reactions occur.

• Advise patient about possible breast tenderness or enlargement.

stavudine (2′ 3′-didehydro-3-deoxythymidine, d4T)
STAV-yoo-deen

Zerit

Therapeutic class: Antiretrovirals
Pharmacologic class: Nucleosides–nucleotide reverse transcriptase inhibitors

AVAILABLE FORMS
Capsules: 15 mg, 20 mg, 30 mg, 40 mg

INDICATIONS & DOSAGES
➤ **HIV infection, with other antiretrovirals**
Adults weighing 60 kg or more: 40 mg PO every 12 hours.
Adults weighing less than 60 kg: 30 mg PO every 12 hours.
Children weighing 30 kg or more: Use the recommended adult dosage every 12 hours. Current clinical guidelines recommended 30 mg PO every 12 hours for patients weighing 60 kg or less to decrease risk of toxicity.
Neonates age 14 days and older and children weighing less than 30 kg: 1 mg/kg PO every 12 hours.
Neonates age 13 days and younger: 0.5 mg/kg PO every 12 hours.
Adjust-a-dose: For patients experiencing peripheral neuropathy, stop therapy and consider permanent discontinuation. For adults with CrCl of 26 to 50 mL/minute, adjust dosage to 20 mg (if weight exceeds 60 kg) or 15 mg (if weight is less than 60 kg) PO every 12 hours; if CrCl is 10 to 25 mL/minute or in adults undergoing dialysis, 20 mg (if weight exceeds 60 kg) or 15 mg (if weight is less than 60 kg) PO every 24 hours. There are insufficient data to recommend a specific dosage adjustment in children.

ADMINISTRATION
PO
• Give drug without regard for meals.
• May open capsule and disperse in a small amount of water; administer immediately.

- Reconstitute oral solution with 202 mL of purified water. Shake solution well before giving.
- Give drug after hemodialysis on hemodialysis treatment days.
- Discard unused solution after 30 days.

ACTION

A thymidine nucleoside analogue that prevents replication of retroviruses, including HIV, by inhibiting the enzyme reverse transcriptase and causing termination of DNA chain growth.

Route	Onset	Peak	Duration
PO	Unknown	1 hr	Unknown

Half-life: 1 to 2 hours.

ADVERSE REACTIONS

CNS: asthenia, fever, anxiety, headache, insomnia, malaise, motor weakness, nervousness, peripheral neuropathy. **GI:** abdominal pain, anorexia, diarrhea, nausea, vomiting, *pancreatitis.* **Hematologic:** *neutropenia, thrombocytopenia,* anemia. **Hepatic:** *hepatotoxicity,* severe hepatomegaly with steatosis. **Metabolic:** *lactic acidosis,* lipodystrophy, lipoatrophy, weight loss, diabetes mellitus, hyperglycemia. **Musculoskeletal:** myalgia. **Respiratory:** dyspnea. **Skin:** pruritus, rash. **Other:** chills.

INTERACTIONS

Drug-drug. *Didanosine, hydroxyurea:* Coadministration may increase risk for lactic acidosis, hepatotoxicity, pancreatitis, or peripheral neuropathy. Consider therapy modification.
Doxorubicin, ribavirin: May decrease effectiveness of stavudine. Use together cautiously.
Zidovudine: May inhibit phosphorylation of stavudine. Avoid using together.

EFFECTS ON LAB TEST RESULTS

- May increase amylase, lipase, bilirubin, ALT, and AST levels. May decrease Hb level.
- May decrease neutrophil and platelet count.

CONTRAINDICATIONS & CAUTIONS

- Contraindicated in patients hypersensitive to drug.

Black Box Warning Lactic acidosis and severe hepatomegaly with steatosis, including fatal cases, have been reported. Administration with didanosine is contraindicated. ∎
Black Box Warning Fatal and nonfatal cases of pancreatitis have occurred in combination therapy with didanosine. ∎
- Use cautiously in patients with renal impairment, liver dysfunction, or history of peripheral neuropathy. Adjust dosage for CrCl of less than 50 mL/minute; stop drug in patients with peripheral neuropathy.
- Safe use in patients with underlying hepatic impairment hasn't been established.
Dialyzable drug: Yes.
⚠ *Overdose S&S:* Peripheral neuropathy, hepatotoxicity.

PREGNANCY-LACTATION-REPRODUCTION

Black Box Warning Use cautiously in pregnant women and only if potential benefit clearly outweighs potential risk; fatal lactic acidosis may occur in pregnant women who receive stavudine and didanosine with other antiretrovirals. ∎
- Register patients in the Antiretroviral Pregnancy Registry (1-800-258-4263).
- The CDC recommends that mothers infected with HIV-1 not breastfeed, to avoid risking postnatal transmission of HIV-1.

NURSING CONSIDERATIONS

Black Box Warning Due to increased risk of pancreatic toxicity, monitor patient for signs and symptoms of pancreatitis, especially if stavudine is taken with didanosine. ∎
☉ *Alert:* Hepatotoxicity and fatal hepatic failure have been reported in patients treated with hydroxyurea and other antiretrovirals. Fatal hepatic events were most often reported in patients treated with combination of hydroxyurea, didanosine, and stavudine. Avoid using together and monitor LFTs.
☉ *Alert:* Motor weakness mimicking the signs and symptoms of Guillain-Barré syndrome (including respiratory failure) in HIV patients taking stavudine with other antiretrovirals may occur, especially in patients with lactic acidosis. Monitor patient for characteristics of lactic acidosis, including generalized fatigue, GI problems, tachypnea, and dyspnea. Patients with these symptoms should promptly interrupt antiretroviral

S

therapy and rapidly receive a full medical workup. Consider permanently stopping drug. Symptoms may continue or worsen when drug is stopped.

• Monitor patient for lipoatrophy and lipodystrophy, and consider the risk and benefit of treatment.

❸ Alert: Peripheral neuropathy may be the major dose-limiting adverse effect; it may or may not resolve after drug is stopped.

• Monitor CBC results and creatinine.

PATIENT TEACHING

• Tell patient that drug may be taken without regard to meals.

• Warn patient not to take other drugs for HIV or AIDS unless prescriber has approved them.

• Inform patient that drug doesn't cure HIV infection, that opportunistic infections and other complications of HIV infection may still occur, and that transmission of HIV to others through sexual contact or blood contamination is still possible.

• Teach patient signs and symptoms of peripheral neuropathy (pain, burning, aching, weakness, or pins and needles in the limbs). Advise patient to report these immediately.

• Tell patient to report symptoms of lactic acidosis, including fatigue, GI problems, dyspnea, or tachypnea.

• Tell patient to report symptoms of pancreatitis, including abdominal pain, nausea, vomiting, weight loss, or fatty stools.

• Tell patient to monitor weight patterns and report weight loss or gain.

SAFETY ALERT!

succinylcholine chloride (suxamethonium chloride) ⬜
suks-in-il-KOE-leen

Anectine, Quelicin

Therapeutic class: Skeletal muscle relaxants
Pharmacologic class: Depolarizing neuromuscular blockers

AVAILABLE FORMS
Injection: 20 mg/mL

INDICATIONS & DOSAGES

➤ **Adjunct to anesthesia to facilitate tracheal intubation; to provide skeletal muscle relaxation during surgery or mechanical ventilation**

Adults: 0.6 mg/kg IV given over 10 to 30 seconds. Dosage range is 0.3 to 1.1 mg/kg. For longer response, give 1 mg/mL solution as a continuous infusion at 0.5 to 10 mg/minute, or give an initial IV injection of 0.3 to 1.1 mg/kg followed by further injections of 0.04 to 0.07 mg/kg, as needed, to maintain relaxation. Or, 3 to 4 mg/kg IM. Maximum IM dose is 150 mg.
Children: 1 to 2 mg/kg IV or 3 to 4 mg/kg IM. Maximum IM dose is 150 mg.

ADMINISTRATION

IV

▼ Only staff skilled in airway management should use drug.

▼ Give test dose of 5 to 10 mg after patient has been anesthetized. If no respiratory depression occurs or transient depression lasts for up to 5 minutes, then patient can metabolize drug, and it is safe to continue. Don't give if patient develops respiratory paralysis sufficient to need ET intubation. (Recovery should occur within 30 to 60 minutes.)

▼ Use within 24 hours after reconstitution.

▼ Store injectable form in refrigerator.

▼ **Incompatibilities:** Alkaline solutions, barbiturates, nafcillin, sodium bicarbonate, solutions with pH above 8.5, thiopental sodium.

IM

• Inject deeply, preferably high into deltoid muscle. Use IM route only when IV access isn't available.

• Store injectable form in refrigerator.

ACTION

Binds with a high affinity to cholinergic receptors, prolonging depolarization of the motor end plate and ultimately producing muscle paralysis.

Route	Onset	Peak	Duration
IV	30–60 sec	1–2 min	4–6 min
IM	2–3 min	Unknown	10–30 min

Half-life: Unknown.

ADVERSE REACTIONS

CV: *arrhythmias, bradycardia, cardiac arrest,* tachycardia, HTN, hypotension, flushing. **EENT:** increased IOP. **GI:** excessive salivation. **Metabolic:** *hyperkalemia.* **Musculoskeletal:** postoperative muscle pain, muscle fasciculation, jaw rigidity, *rhabdomyolysis with acute renal failure.* **Respiratory:** *apnea, bronchoconstriction, prolonged respiratory depression.* **Skin:** rash. **Other:** allergic or idiosyncratic hypersensitivity reactions, *anaphylaxis, malignant hyperthermia.*

INTERACTIONS

Drug-drug. *Aminoglycosides, anticholinesterases (echothiophate, edrophonium, neostigmine, physostigmine, pyridostigmine), aprotinin, general anesthetics (enflurane, halothane, isoflurane), glucocorticoids, hormonal contraceptives, lidocaine, lithium, magnesium, metoclopramide, oxytocin, polymyxin antibiotics (colistin, polymyxin B sulfate), procainamide, quinine:* May enhance neuromuscular blockade, increasing skeletal muscle relaxation and potentiating effect. Use together cautiously during and after surgery.
Cardiac glycosides: May cause arrhythmias. Use together cautiously.
Cyclophosphamide, lithium, MAO inhibitors: May enhance neuromuscular blockade and prolong apnea. Use together cautiously.
Opioid analgesics: May enhance neuromuscular blockade, increasing skeletal muscle relaxation and possibly causing respiratory paralysis. Use together cautiously.
Parenteral magnesium sulfate: May enhance neuromuscular blockade, may increase skeletal muscle relaxation, and may cause respiratory paralysis. Use together cautiously, preferably at reduced doses.

EFFECTS ON LAB TEST RESULTS

• May increase myoglobin and potassium levels.

CONTRAINDICATIONS & CAUTIONS

▨ Contraindicated in patients hypersensitive to drug and in those with personal or family history of malignant hyperthermia.

• Contraindicated in patients with skeletal muscle myopathies and after the acute phase of injury following acute major burns, multiple trauma, skeletal muscle denervation, or upper motor neuron injury.
• Drug increases IOP. Use only when potential benefit outweighs potential risk when an increase in IOP is undesirable, such as in narrow-angle glaucoma or penetrating eye injury.
▨ Use carefully in patients with reduced plasma cholinesterase activity due to risk of prolonged neuromuscular block. Plasma cholinesterase activity may be diminished in the presence of genetic abnormalities of plasma cholinesterase, pregnancy, severe liver or kidney disease, malignant tumors, infections, burns, anemia, decompensated heart disease, peptic ulcer, myxedema, and certain drugs and chemicals.
• Use cautiously in elderly or debilitated patients; in patients receiving quinidine or cardiac glycoside therapy; in patients with hepatic, renal, or pulmonary impairment; and in those with respiratory depression, severe burns or trauma, electrolyte imbalances, hyperkalemia, paraplegia, spinal CNS injury, stroke, degenerative or dystrophic neuromuscular disease, myasthenia gravis, myasthenic syndrome related to lung cancer, dehydration, thyroid disorders, collagen diseases, porphyria, fractures, muscle spasms, dislocations, eye surgery, and pheochromocytoma.
Dialyzable drug: Unknown.
⚠ Overdose S&S: Prolonged neuromuscular blockade.

PREGNANCY-LACTATION-REPRODUCTION

• There are no adequate studies in pregnant women. Use during pregnancy only if clearly needed.
• Use large doses cautiously in patients undergoing cesarean section.
• It isn't known if drug appears in human milk. Use cautiously in breastfeeding women.

NURSING CONSIDERATIONS

• Drug has no known effect on consciousness, pain threshold, or cerebration. To avoid patient distress, don't induce neuromuscular blockade before unconsciousness.

• Dosage depends on anesthetic used, individual needs, and response. Recommended dosages must be individually adjusted. Drug should only be administered by experienced personnel trained in its use.

Black Box Warning Drug may cause acute rhabdomyolysis with hyperkalemia followed by ventricular arrhythmias, cardiac arrest, and death after administration to apparently healthy children who have undiagnosed skeletal muscle myopathy, most frequently Duchenne muscular dystrophy. Institute treatment for hyperkalemia when a healthy-appearing infant or child develops cardiac arrest soon after administration of succinylcholine. In children, drug should be reserved for use in emergency intubation, for instances when securing the airway is necessary, or for IM use when a suitable vein is inaccessible. ■

⌘ Assess patients for personal or family history of malignant hyperthermia as drug is contraindicated in these patients.

• Children may be less sensitive to drug than adults.

• May cause a transient increase in ICP, and may increase intragastric pressure, which could result in regurgitation and possible aspiration of stomach contents.

• Monitor baseline electrolyte determinations and vital signs. Check respirations every 5 to 10 minutes during infusion.

• Monitor respirations closely until tests of muscle strength (hand grip, head lift, and ability to cough) indicate full recovery from neuromuscular blockade.

○ *Alert:* Don't use reversing drugs. Unlike nondepolarizing drugs, neostigmine or edrophonium may worsen neuromuscular blockade if given before succinylcholine is metabolized by cholinesterase.

• Repeated or continuous infusions aren't advisable; they may cause reduced response or prolonged muscle relaxation and apnea.

• Give analgesics for pain.

• Keep airway clear. Have emergency respiratory support equipment (ET equipment, ventilator, oxygen, atropine, and epinephrine) immediately available.

○ *Alert:* Careful dosage calculation is essential. Always verify dosage with another health care professional.

PATIENT TEACHING
• Explain all events and procedures to patient because patient can still hear.

• Reassure patient that postoperative stiffness is normal and will soon subside.

sucralfate
soo-KRAL-fayt

Carafate⊘

Therapeutic class: Antiulcer drugs
Pharmacologic class: GI protectants

AVAILABLE FORMS
Suspension: 1 g/10 mL
Tablets: 1 g

INDICATIONS & DOSAGES
Adjust-a-dose (for all indications): Dosage selection for elderly patients should be cautious, usually starting at the low end of the dosing range; monitor renal function.

➤ **Short-term (up to 8 weeks) treatment of duodenal ulcer**
Adults: 1 g PO q.i.d. 1 hour before meals and at bedtime for 4 to 8 weeks unless healing has been demonstrated by X-ray or endoscopic examination.

➤ **Maintenance therapy for duodenal ulcer**
Adults: 1 g PO b.i.d.

ADMINISTRATION
PO
• Shake suspension well before pouring.

• After administration, flush NG tube with water to ensure passage into stomach.

• Give drug on an empty stomach 1 hour before meals.

ACTION
Selectively forms a coating that acts locally to protect the gastric lining against peptic acid, pepsin, and bile salts.

Route	Onset	Peak	Duration
PO	Unknown	Unknown	6 hr

Half-life: Unknown.

ADVERSE REACTIONS
GI: constipation.

INTERACTIONS
Drug-drug. *Antacids:* May decrease binding of drug to gastroduodenal mucosa, impairing effectiveness. Separate doses by 30 minutes.

Cimetidine, digoxin, fosphenytoin, ketoconazole, phenytoin, quinidine, ranitidine, tetracycline, theophylline: May decrease absorption. Separate doses by at least 2 hours.

Ciprofloxacin, levofloxacin, moxifloxacin, ofloxacin: May decrease absorption of these drugs, reducing anti-infective response. If use together can't be avoided, give at least 6 hours apart.

Diclofenac: May decrease effectiveness of diclofenac. Monitor patient response.

Warfarin: May decrease anticoagulant effect. Monitor effectiveness and adjust dosage as necessary.

EFFECTS ON LAB TEST RESULTS
None reported.

CONTRAINDICATIONS & CAUTIONS
• Contraindicated in patients with known hypersensitivity reactions to the active substance or to the components.

• Use cautiously in patients with chronic renal failure; toxic reactions may be greater in patients with impaired renal function.

• Safety and effectiveness in children haven't been established.

Dialyzable drug: Unknown.

⚠ *Overdose S&S:* Dyspepsia, abdominal pain, nausea, vomiting.

PREGNANCY-LACTATION-REPRODUCTION
• There are no adequate studies in pregnant women. Use during pregnancy only if clearly needed.

• It isn't known if drug appears in human milk. Use cautiously in breastfeeding women.

NURSING CONSIDERATIONS
• Drug is minimally absorbed and causes few adverse reactions.

• Monitor patient for severe, persistent constipation.

• Drug is as effective as cimetidine in healing duodenal ulcer.

• Drug contains aluminum but isn't classified as an antacid. Monitor patient with renal insufficiency for aluminum toxicity.

• Hyperglycemia has been reported in patients with diabetes who are taking suspension. Closely monitor blood glucose level and adjust dosage of antidiabetic drugs if indicated.

PATIENT TEACHING
• Tell patient to take sucralfate on an empty stomach, 1 hour before each meal and at bedtime.

• Instruct patient to continue prescribed regimen to ensure complete healing. Pain and other ulcer signs and symptoms may subside within first few weeks of therapy.

• Urge patient to avoid cigarette smoking, which may increase gastric acid secretion and worsen disease.

• Antacids may be used while taking drug, but separate doses by 30 minutes.

SAFETY ALERT!

SUFentanil
soo-FEN-ta-nil

Dsuvia

Therapeutic class: Opioid analgesics
Pharmacologic class: Opioid agonists
Controlled substance schedule: II

AVAILABLE FORMS
Tablets (SL): 30 mcg

INDICATIONS & DOSAGES
➤ **Management of acute pain severe enough to require an opioid analgesic and for which alternative treatments are inadequate**

Adults: 30 mcg SL as needed with a minimum of 1 hour between doses. Maximum cumulative dose is 360 mcg/day (12 tablets). Don't use for more than 72 hours.

ADMINISTRATION
Sublingual

Black Box Warning Drug is only to be administered by a health care professional in a medically certified health care setting. ∎

• Drug is packaged as a single-use product. Don't reuse. Don't use if pouch is broken or single-dose applicator (SDA) is damaged.

S

• Wear gloves when administering drug and dispose of SDA in biohazard waste.
• Follow manufacturer's instructions for use of delivery applicator.
• If patient has excessively dry mouth, provide ice chips before giving drug.
• Patient should allow drug to dissolve under the tongue and not chew or swallow the tablet.
• Patient should minimize talking and not eat or drink for 10 minutes after each dose.
• Visually confirm SL tablet placement.
• Store at 68° to 77° F (20° to 25° C) in a secure, limited-access location in accordance with institutional procedures for Schedule II products.

ACTION

An opioid agonist that is relatively selective for the mu-opioid receptor, although it can bind to other opioid receptors at higher doses. The analgesia and sedation effects are thought to be mediated through opioid-specific receptors throughout the CNS, with no ceiling effect to analgesia.

Route	Onset	Peak	Duration
SL	Unknown	1 hr	Unknown

Half-life: 13.4 hours.

ADVERSE REACTIONS

CNS: dizziness, hemiparesis, somnolence, syncope, headache. **CV:** hypotension. **GI:** nausea, vomiting. **Respiratory:** *respiratory depression,* decreased oxygen saturation.

INTERACTIONS

Drug-drug. *Anticholinergics:* May increase risk of urine retention or severe constipation, which may lead to paralytic ileus. Monitor patient for signs and symptoms of urine retention or reduced gastric motility.

Black Box Warning *Benzodiazepines, CNS depressants:* May increase risk of hypotension, respiratory depression, sedation, coma, and death. Use together only in patients with no alternative treatment options, and limit dosages and durations to the minimum required. Monitor patients closely for signs or symptoms of respiratory depression and sedation. ■

Black Box Warning *CYP3A4 inducers (carbamazepine, phenytoin, rifampin):* May decrease sufentanil level and lead to decreased efficacy or withdrawal symptoms in patients who have developed physical dependence. If use together is necessary, consider an alternative medication that permits dosage titration. Monitor patient for opioid withdrawal. If the CYP3A4 inducer is discontinued, consider decreasing sufentanil dosage and monitor patient for signs and symptoms of respiratory depression. ■

Black Box Warning *CYP3A4 inhibitors (erythromycin, ketoconazole, ritonavir):* May increase sufentanil level, leading to increased or prolonged opioid effects. Monitor patient for respiratory depression and sedation. If use together is necessary, consider an alternative medication that permits dosage titration. If the CYP3A4 inhibitor is discontinued, consider increasing sufentanil dosage until stable drug effects are achieved and monitor patient for opioid withdrawal symptoms. ■

Diuretics: May decrease the effects of diuretics by inducing the release of ADH. Monitor patients for signs and symptoms of diminished diuresis or effects on BP and increase the diuretic dosage as needed.

MAO inhibitors (linezolid, phenelzine, tranylcypromine): May increase risk of serotonin syndrome or opioid toxicity. Use of sufentanil isn't recommended for patients taking MAO inhibitors or within 14 days of stopping MAO inhibitor treatment.

Mixed agonist/antagonist and partial opioid analgesics (buprenorphine, butorphanol, nalbuphine, pentazocine): May reduce analgesic effect of sufentanil or precipitate withdrawal symptoms. Avoid use together.

Muscle relaxants: May enhance neuromuscular blocking action of skeletal muscle relaxants and produce increased respiratory depression. Monitor patient for signs and symptoms of respiratory depression, decrease dosage of the skeletal muscle relaxant, or consider discontinuing sufentanil.

Serotonergic drugs (mirtazapine, SSNRIs, SSRIs, TCAs, tramadol, trazodone, triptans): May increase risk of serotonin syndrome. If use together is necessary, monitor patient closely, especially during treatment initiation and dosage adjustment. Discontinue sufentanil if serotonin syndrome is suspected.

Reactions in bold italics are *life-threatening.* Interactions may have a *rapid onset* or a *delayed onset.*

Drug-lifestyle. Black Box Warning *Alcohol use:* May increase risk of hypotension, respiratory depression, sedation, coma, and death. Don't use together. ■

EFFECTS ON LAB TEST RESULTS
• May increase amylase level.

CONTRAINDICATIONS & CAUTIONS
• Contraindicated in patients with significant respiratory depression, acute or severe bronchial asthma in an unmonitored setting or in the absence of resuscitative equipment, known or suspected GI obstruction (including paralytic ileus), or known hypersensitivity to sufentanil or its components.
Black Box Warning Accidental exposure to or ingestion of sufentanil, even a single dose, can result in respiratory depression and death, especially in children. ■
Black Box Warning Because of the potential for life-threatening respiratory depression due to accidental exposure, sufentanil is only available through a REMS program. Drug may only be dispensed in a certified medically supervised health care setting and drug must be discontinued before discharge or transfer from that setting. ■
Black Box Warning Serious, life-threatening, or fatal respiratory depression has been reported with the use of opioids, even when used as recommended. Unrecognized respiratory depression may lead to respiratory arrest and death. Risk is greatest during the initiation of therapy but can occur at any time. ■
Black Box Warning Sufentanil is a Schedule II controlled substance and exposes users to the risks of addiction, abuse, and misuse, including overdose and death. ■
• Use cautiously in patients with chronic pulmonary disease and in elderly, cachectic, or debilitated patients, as they are at increased risk for respiratory depression, even at recommended doses. Consider nonopioid analgesics whenever possible.
• Drug may cause severe hypotension, including orthostatic hypotension and syncope in ambulatory patients. Use cautiously in patients with hypovolemia or CV disease and in those taking drugs that may exaggerate hypotensive effects. Avoid use in patients with circulatory shock.

• Avoid use in patients with impaired consciousness or coma. Sufentanil isn't suitable for use in patients who aren't alert and unable to follow directions.
• Drug may mask clinical changes in patients with head injury.
• Drug may increase the frequency of seizures in patients with seizure disorders and may increase the risk of seizures occurring in other clinical settings associated with seizures.
• Use cautiously in patients with brady-arrhythmias; drug may lower HR.
• Drug isn't approved for use in children, or for long-term or home use.
Dialyzable drug: Unknown.
⚠ *Overdose S&S:* Respiratory depression, somnolence, stupor, coma, skeletal muscle flaccidity, cold and clammy skin, constricted pupils, pulmonary edema, bradycardia, hypotension, partial or complete airway obstruction, atypical snoring, marked hypoxia-related mydriasis, death.

PREGNANCY-LACTATION-REPRODUCTION
⚠ *Alert:* Prolonged use of opioids during pregnancy can cause neonatal opioid withdrawal syndrome, which may be life-threatening. If prolonged opioid therapy is required in a pregnant woman, ensure protocols for management by neonatology experts are available and warn mother of risk to the neonate.
• Opioids cross the placental barrier and may produce respiratory depression and psycho-physiologic effects in neonates. Sufentanil shouldn't be used in pregnant women during or immediately before labor when other analgesics are more appropriate.
• Infants exposed to sufentanil through human milk should be monitored for excess sedation and respiratory depression. Withdrawal symptoms can occur in breastfed infants when maternal administration of an opioid analgesic is stopped or when breast-feeding is stopped.
• Long-term use of opioids may reduce fertility in females and males of reproductive potential. It isn't known if these effects on fertility are reversible.

S

NURSING CONSIDERATIONS

Black Box Warning Monitor patients closely for respiratory depression, sedation, and hypotension, especially during initiation of therapy. Ensure opioid antagonist (naloxone) and emergency equipment are readily available. ■

Black Box Warning Assess patients' risk of addiction, abuse, and misuse before prescribing sufentanil, and monitor patients regularly for these behaviors and conditions. Risk increases in patients with a personal or family history of substance abuse or mental illness. ■

Black Box Warning Watch for serotonin syndrome in patient who is taking concomitant serotonergic drugs. Assess for mental status changes (agitation, hallucinations, coma), autonomic instability (tachycardia, labile BP, hyperthermia), neuromuscular abnormalities (hyperreflexia, loss of coordination, rigidity), and GI signs and symptoms (nausea, vomiting, diarrhea). If serotonin syndrome is suspected, discontinue sufentanil. ■

• Use cautiously in patients with hepatic and severe renal impairment and monitor patients closely for respiratory depression, sedation, and hypotension.

• Monitor patients with a history of seizure disorders for worsened seizure control.

• Monitor patients for adrenal insufficiency (nausea, vomiting, anorexia, fatigue, weakness, dizziness, hypotension). If adrenal insufficiency is diagnosed, treat with physiologic replacement of corticosteroids, and wean patient off of the opioid.

• Monitor patients for hypotension, especially for changes in HR, particularly when initiating therapy.

• Monitor patients with biliary tract disease (acute pancreatitis) for worsening symptoms.

• Use cautiously in patients susceptible to the intracranial effects of carbon dioxide retention, such as those with brain tumors or increased ICP. Drug may decrease respiratory drive. Monitor patients for sedation and respiratory depression.

• Monitor neonates exposed to opioids during labor for excess sedation and respiratory depression. Monitor neonates with prolonged exposure in utero for opioid withdrawal syndrome (irritability, hyperactivity, abnormal sleep pattern, high-pitched cry, tremor, vomiting, diarrhea, failure to gain weight).

Black Box Warning Drug must be discontinued before patient leaves the certified medically supervised setting. Don't use for more than 72 hours. ■

• *Look alike–sound alike:* Don't confuse Dsuvia with Duavee.

PATIENT TEACHING

Black Box Warning Inform patient that accidental exposure may result in respiratory depression or death, especially in children, and that the risk is greatest at start of therapy but can occur at any time. ■

Black Box Warning Inform patient that the use of sufentanil can result in addiction, abuse, and misuse, even when taken as recommended. ■

Black Box Warning Teach patient that drug can only be administered by a health care professional in a certified medically supervised setting and that drug must be discontinued before patient is discharged or transferred. ■

• Teach patient to report all adverse reactions.

• Warn patient that hypersensitivity reactions, including anaphylaxis, have been reported. Advise patient to immediately report signs and symptoms of hypersensitivity reactions.

• Teach patient to allow sufentanil to dissolve under the tongue and not to chew or swallow the tablet. Advise patient not to eat or drink and to minimize talking for 10 minutes after each dose.

• Caution patient that sufentanil may cause orthostatic hypotension and syncope. Teach patient how to recognize signs and symptoms of low BP and how to reduce the risk of serious consequences should hypotension occur.

• Inform patient that opioids can cause adrenal insufficiency, and to report signs and symptoms of adrenal insufficiency if they occur.

• Warn patient with a history of seizure disorder that drug can increase risk of seizures.

• Inform female patient of childbearing potential that sufentanil can cause fetal harm and to tell prescriber if she is pregnant or suspects she is pregnant.

Reactions in bold italics are *life-threatening*. Interactions may have a *rapid onset* or a *delayed onset*.

- Advise breastfeeding patient to monitor infant for increased sleepiness (more than usual), breathing difficulties, or limpness. Instruct her to seek immediate medical care if any of these signs or symptoms occur.

sulfamethoxazole–trimethoprim ⚕

sul-fa-meth-OX-a-zole/tri-meth-O-prim

Bactrim, Bactrim DS✐, Septra, Septra Injection✤, Septra DS, Sulfatrim*

Therapeutic class: Antibiotics
Pharmacologic class: Sulfonamides–folate antagonists

AVAILABLE FORMS

Injection: sulfamethoxazole 80 mg/mL and trimethoprim 16 mg/mL in 5-mL vials*
Oral suspension: sulfamethoxazole 200 mg and trimethoprim 40 mg/5 mL*, sulfamethoxazole 80 mg and trimethoprim 16 mg/mL*✤
Tablets (double-strength): sulfamethoxazole 800 mg and trimethoprim 160 mg
Tablets (single-strength): sulfamethoxazole 400 mg and trimethoprim 80 mg, sulfamethoxazole 100 mg and trimethoprim 20 mg✤

INDICATIONS & DOSAGES

Adjust-a-dose (for all indications): For patients with CrCl of 15 to 30 mL/minute, reduce daily dose by 50%. Don't give to those with CrCl less than 15 mL/minute.
➤ **Shigellosis or UTIs caused by susceptible strains of *Escherichia coli, Proteus:* (indole positive or negative), *Klebsiella, Morganella morganii,* or *Enterobacter* species**
Adults: 800 mg sulfamethoxazole/160 mg trimethoprim PO every 12 hours for 10 to 14 days in UTIs and for 5 days in shigellosis. If indicated, give 8 to 10 mg/kg/day IV, based on trimethoprim component, in two to four divided doses every 6, 8, or 12 hours for 5 days for shigellosis or up to 14 days for severe UTIs. Maximum daily dose is 60 mL trimethoprim.

Children age 2 months and older: 8 mg/kg/day PO, based on trimethoprim component, in two divided doses every 12 hours for 10 days for UTIs and 5 days for shigellosis. If indicated, give 8 to 10 mg/kg/day IV, based on trimethoprim component, in two to four divided doses every 6, 8, or 12 hours for up to 14 days for severe UTIs and 5 days for shigellosis. Don't exceed adult dose.
➤ **Otitis media in patients with penicillin allergy or penicillin-resistant infection**
Children age 2 months and older: 8 mg/kg/day PO, based on trimethoprim component, in two divided doses every 12 hours for 10 days.
➤ **Chronic bronchitis, URIs**
Adults: 800 mg sulfamethoxazole/160 mg trimethoprim PO every 12 hours for 14 days.
➤ **Traveler's diarrhea**
Adults: 800 mg sulfamethoxazole/160 mg trimethoprim PO b.i.d. for 5 days.
➤ ***Pneumocystis jiroveci* pneumonia treatment**
Adults and children older than age 2 months: 15 to 20 mg/kg/day IV or PO, based on trimethoprim component, in equally divided doses every 6 hours (PO) or in divided doses every 6 to 8 hours (IV) for 14 days. Some guidelines recommend treatment duration of 21 days.
➤ ***P. jiroveci* pneumonia prophylaxis**
Adults: 800 mg sulfamethoxazole/160 mg trimethoprim every 24 hours.
Children older than age 2 months: 750 mg/m^2 sulfamethoxazole with trimethoprim 150 mg/m^2 daily in equally divided doses b.i.d., on 3 consecutive days per week.

ADMINISTRATION
PO
- Before giving drug, ask if patient is allergic to sulfa drugs.
- Obtain specimen for culture and sensitivity tests before giving. Begin therapy while awaiting results.
- Shake suspension well before using.
- Give drug with 8 oz (240 mL) of water.
IV
▼ Before giving drug, ask patient if patient is allergic to sulfa drugs.
▼ Obtain specimen for culture and sensitivity tests before giving. Begin therapy while awaiting results.

S

▼ Don't give by rapid infusion or bolus injection.

▼ Dilute each 5 mL of concentrate in 75 to 125 mL of D₅W. Don't mix with other drugs or solutions.

▼ Infuse slowly over 60 to 90 minutes.

▼ Don't refrigerate; use within 6 hours if diluted in 125 mL, within 4 hours if diluted in 100 mL, and within 2 hours if diluted in 75 mL.

▼ Discard solution if it's cloudy or crystallized.

▼ Never give drug IM.

▼ **Incompatibilities:** None listed by manufacturer. Consult a drug incompatibility reference for more information.

ACTION

Sulfamethoxazole inhibits formation of dihydrofolic acid from PABA; trimethoprim inhibits dihydrofolate reductase formation. Both decrease bacterial folic acid synthesis and are bactericidal.

Route	Onset	Peak	Duration
PO	Unknown	1–4 hr	Unknown
IV	Immediate	Unknown	Unknown

Half-life: Sulfamethoxazole, 9 to 12 hours; trimethoprim, 6 to 11 hours.

ADVERSE REACTIONS

CNS: *seizures,* apathy, aseptic meningitis, ataxia, depression, fatigue, hallucinations, headache, insomnia, nervousness, tinnitus, vertigo. **CV:** thrombophlebitis. **GI:** *pancreatitis, pseudomembranous colitis,* diarrhea, nausea, vomiting, abdominal pain, anorexia, stomatitis. **GU:** *toxic nephrosis with oliguria and anuria,* crystalluria, hematuria, interstitial nephritis, *renal failure.* **Hematologic:** *agranulocytosis, aplastic anemia, leukopenia, neutropenia, thrombocytopenia,* hemolytic anemia, megaloblastic anemia. **Hepatic:** *hepatic necrosis,* jaundice. **Metabolic:** *hyperkalemia, hypoglycemia,* hyponatremia. **Musculoskeletal:** arthralgia, muscle weakness, myalgia. **Respiratory:** pulmonary infiltrates, cough, shortness of breath. **Skin:** generalized skin eruption, *erythema multiforme, SJS, toxic epidermal necrolysis,* exfoliative dermatitis, photosensitivity reactions, pruritus, urticaria, rash. **Other:** *anaphylaxis,* drug fever, hypersensitivity reactions, serum sickness.

INTERACTIONS

Drug-drug. *Cyclosporine:* May decrease cyclosporine level and increase nephrotoxicity risk. Avoid using together.
Digoxin: May increase digoxin level. Monitor digoxin level.
Diuretics: May increase incidence of thrombocytopenia with purpura in elderly patients receiving certain diuretics, mainly thiazides. Avoid concomitant use.
Dofetilide: May increase dofetilide level and effects. May increase risk of prolonged QT-interval syndrome and fatal ventricular arrhythmias. Avoid using together.
Indomethacin: May increase sulfamethoxazole blood level. Avoid concomitant use.
Methotrexate: May increase methotrexate level. Monitor methotrexate level.
Oral antidiabetics: May increase hypoglycemic effect. Monitor glucose level.
Phenytoin: May inhibit hepatic metabolism of phenytoin. Monitor phenytoin level.
Procainamide: May prolong QT interval. Closely monitor patient for clinical and ECG signs of toxicity.
TCAs: May decrease efficacy of TCAs. Monitor therapeutic response to TCAs and adjust dosage accordingly.
Warfarin: May increase anticoagulant effect. Monitor patient for bleeding; monitor PT and INR.
Drug-herb. *St. John's wort:* May decrease drug level. Consider therapy modification.
Drug-lifestyle. *Sun exposure:* May cause photosensitivity reactions. Advise patient to avoid excessive sunlight exposure.

EFFECTS ON LAB TEST RESULTS

• May increase aminotransferase, bilirubin, potassium, BUN, and creatinine levels.
• May decrease sodium level.
• May decrease Hb level and granulocyte, platelet, and WBC counts.

CONTRAINDICATIONS & CAUTIONS

• Contraindicated in patients hypersensitive to trimethoprim or sulfonamides and in patients with a history of trimethoprim or sulfonamide drug-induced immune thrombocytopenia.

Reactions in bold italics are *life-threatening*. Interactions may have a *rapid onset* or a *delayed onset*.

• Severe, life-threatening, and fatal cases of thrombocytopenia have been reported and may be immune-mediated. Once drug is discontinued, thrombocytopenia usually resolves within 1 week.

• Contraindicated in those with CrCl less than 15 mL/minute, porphyria, megaloblastic anemia from folate deficiency, or marked hepatic damage.

• Contraindicated in infants younger than age 2 months.

• Some forms may contain benzyl alcohol, which, in newborn infants, has been associated with an increased incidence of neurologic and other complications that are sometimes fatal. Avoid use in neonates.

• Use cautiously and in reduced dosages in patients with CrCl of 15 to 30 mL/minute, severe allergy or bronchial asthma, or blood dyscrasia.

🜲 Use cautiously in patients with G6PD deficiency as hemolytic anemia can result.

• May cause CDAD ranging from mild diarrhea to fatal colitis.

• Using sulfamethoxazole–trimethoprim with antiarrhythmics (amiodarone, bretylium, disopyramide, dofetilide, procainamide, quinidine, sotalol), arsenic trioxide, chlorpromazine, dolasetron, droperidol, mefloquine, mesoridazine, moxifloxacin, pentamidine, pimozide, tacrolimus, thioridazine, and ziprasidone may prolong QT interval and increase the risk of life-threatening cardiac arrhythmias, including torsades de pointes.

Dialyzable drug: Moderately.

⚠ *Overdose S&S:* Headache, drowsiness, unconsciousness, pyrexia, depression, confusion, anorexia, colic, nausea, vomiting, diarrhea, hematuria, crystalluria; blood dyscrasias and jaundice (late signs).

PREGNANCY-LACTATION-REPRODUCTION
• There are no well-controlled studies in pregnant women; drug may cause fetal harm. Use only if potential benefit justifies potential risk to the fetus.

• Contraindicated in breastfeeding women because of potential risk of bilirubin displacement and kernicterus.

NURSING CONSIDERATIONS
🛈 *Alert:* Double-check dosage, which may be written as trimethoprim component.

🛈 *Alert:* "DS" product means "double strength."

• Monitor renal function test, CBC, and LFT results.

• Promptly report rash, sore throat, fever, cough, mouth sores, or iris lesions— early signs and symptoms of erythema multiforme, which may progress to life-threatening SJS, or blood dyscrasias.

• Watch for signs and symptoms of superinfection, such as fever, chills, and increased pulse.

🛈 *Alert:* Adverse reactions, especially hypersensitivity reactions, rash, and fever, occur much more frequently in patients with AIDS.

PATIENT TEACHING
• Tell patient to take drug as prescribed, even if feeling better.

• Encourage patient to drink plenty of fluids to prevent crystalluria and kidney stone formation.

• Tell patient to report adverse reactions promptly, especially fever, rash, bruising, bleeding, and throat or other pain.

• Instruct patient receiving drug IV to report discomfort at IV insertion site.

• Advise patient to avoid prolonged sun exposure, wear protective clothing, and use sunscreen.

• Instruct patient to take oral form with 8 oz (240 mL) of water.

S

sulfaSALAzine (salazosulfapyridine, sulphasalazine) 🜲
sul-fuh-SAL-uh-zeen

Azulfidine, Azulfidine EN-tabs, Salazopyrin✤, Salazopyrin EN-Tabs✤

Therapeutic class: Anti-inflammatory drugs
Pharmacologic class: Sulfonamide salicylates

AVAILABLE FORMS
Tablets: 500 mg
Tablets (delayed-release) 🔵: 500 mg

INDICATIONS & DOSAGES

➤ **Mild to moderate ulcerative colitis, adjunctive therapy in severe ulcerative colitis, prolongation of remission period between acute ulcerative colitis attacks**
Adults: Initially, 3 to 4 g PO daily in evenly divided doses not exceeding 8 hours apart; may start with 1 to 2 g, with gradual increase to minimize adverse effects. Usual maintenance dose is 2 g PO daily.
Children age 6 and older: Initially, 40 to 60 mg/kg PO daily, divided into three to six doses; may start at lower dose if GI intolerance occurs. Maintenance dose is 30 mg/kg in each 24-hour period, divided into four doses.

➤ **RA in patients who have responded inadequately to salicylates or NSAIDs**
Adults (delayed-release tablets): 2 g PO daily in two evenly divided doses. To reduce possible GI intolerance, start at 0.5 to 1 g daily.

➤ **Polyarticular-course juvenile RA in patients who have responded inadequately to salicylates or other NSAIDs**
Children age 6 and older (delayed-release tablets): 30 to 50 mg/kg PO daily in two evenly divided doses. Maximum dose is 2 g daily. To reduce possible GI intolerance, start with one-quarter to one-third of planned maintenance dose and increase weekly until reaching maintenance dose at 1 month.

ADMINISTRATION
PO
• Give drug with food to decrease GI irritation.
• Patient must swallow delayed-release tablets whole and mustn't crush, chew, or split them.

ACTION
May be related to observed anti-inflammatory or immunomodulatory properties.

Route	Onset	Peak	Duration
PO	Unknown	3–12 hr	Unknown

Half-life: 4 to 11 hours.

ADVERSE REACTIONS
CNS: *seizures,* dizziness, headache, depression, hallucinations. **GI:** nausea, vomiting, diarrhea, abdominal pain, gastric distress, anorexia, stomatitis, dyspepsia. **GU:** oligospermia, infertility. **Hematologic:** *agranulocytosis, leukopenia, thrombocytopenia, aplastic anemia,* megaloblastic anemia, *hemolytic anemia.* **Hepatic:** *hepatotoxicity,* urticaria, pruritus. **Other:** drug fever.

INTERACTIONS
Drug-drug. *Digoxin:* May reduce absorption of digoxin. Monitor patient closely.
Folic acid: May decrease absorption of folic acid. Monitor patient.
Heparin, oral anticoagulants: May increase anticoagulant effect. Watch for bleeding.
Methotrexate: May enhance hepatotoxic effect of methotrexate. Monitor patient for hematologic toxicity and adverse GI events, especially nausea.
Prilocaine: May increase risk of significant methemoglobinemia. Monitor patient. Avoid lidocaine and prilocaine in infants receiving such agents.
Thiopurines (azathioprine, mercaptopurine): May increase leukopenia. Monitor WBC count closely.
Drug-herb. *Dong quai, St. John's wort:* May also cause photosensitization. Avoid use together.

EFFECTS ON LAB TEST RESULTS
• May increase ALT and AST levels. May decrease Hb level.
• May decrease granulocyte, platelet, and WBC counts.
• May interfere with measurements, by liquid chromatography, of urinary normetanephrine and cause false-positive test results in patients exposed to sulfasalazine or its metabolite.

CONTRAINDICATIONS & CAUTIONS
• Contraindicated in patients hypersensitive to drug, its metabolites, sulfonamides, or salicylates and in those with porphyria or intestinal and urinary obstruction.
• Use cautiously and in reduced doses in patients with impaired hepatic or renal function, severe allergy, or bronchial asthma.
⚲ Use cautiously in patients with G6PD deficiency as hemolytic anemia can result.

Reactions in bold italics are *life-threatening*. Interactions may have a *rapid onset* or a *delayed onset*.

- Serious skin reactions, some fatal, including exfoliative dermatitis, SJS, and toxic epidermal necrolysis, have been reported. Patients are at highest risk for these events early in therapy, with most events occurring within the first month of treatment. Discontinue drug at the first appearance of rash or mucosal lesions.
- Serious CNS reactions can occur, including seizures, meningitis, spinal cord disorders, peripheral neuropathy, hearing loss, ataxia, and hallucinations.

Dialyzable drug: Yes.

⚠ *Overdose S&S:* Nausea, gastric distress, abdominal pain, drowsiness, seizures.

PREGNANCY-LACTATION-REPRODUCTION

- There are no adequate studies in pregnant women. Use only if clearly needed.
- Drug and its active metabolite appear in human milk. Use cautiously in breastfeeding women; monitor infant for kernicterus and diarrhea or bloody stools.
- Oligospermia and infertility have been observed in men treated with drug; stopping drug may reverse these effects.

NURSING CONSIDERATIONS

- Therapeutic response in patients with RA may occur as soon as 4 weeks after starting therapy, but it may take up to 12 weeks in others.
- Drug may cause urine discoloration.
- **✆ Alert:** Stop drug immediately and notify prescriber if patient shows signs and symptoms of hypersensitivity.
- Maintain adequate fluid intake to prevent crystalluria and stone formation.
- Obtain CBCs, including differential WBC count and LFTs, before start of treatment and every second week during first 3 months of therapy. During second 3 months, do the same tests once monthly and thereafter once every 3 months and as clinically indicated. Obtain a urinalysis with careful microscopic examination and an assessment of renal function periodically during treatment.
- Serum sulfapyridine levels greater than 50 mcg/mL appear to be associated with an increased incidence of adverse reactions.
- 🅖 Observe patients with G6PD deficiency closely for signs and symptoms of hemolytic anemia.

- *Look alike–sound alike:* Don't confuse sulfasalazine with sulfisoxazole, salsalate, or sulfadiazine.

PATIENT TEACHING

- Instruct patient to take drug after eating and to space doses evenly.
- Warn patient to avoid ultraviolet light; drug may increase risk of sunburn. Advise patient to use sunscreen and wear protective clothing and to avoid sunlamps and tanning booths.
- Advise patient that drug may produce an orange-yellow discoloration of skin and urine and may cause contact lenses to turn yellow.
- Teach patient about adverse reactions and to report them. Advise patient of the need for careful medical supervision. A sore throat, fever, pallor, purpura, or jaundice may indicate a serious blood disorder.
- Tell patient to drink plenty of water and to swallow tablets whole without crushing or chewing.
- Advise patient that blood and urine tests will be needed to monitor treatment and that it's important to keep laboratory and physician appointments.

SUMAtriptan succinate
sue-mah-TRIP-tan

Imitrex✐, Imitrex STATdose, Onzetra Xsail, Zembrace SymTouch

Therapeutic class: Antimigraine drugs
Pharmacologic class: Serotonin 5-HT$_1$ receptor agonists

AVAILABLE FORMS

Injection: 4 mg/0.5 mL, 6 mg/0.5 mL prefilled syringes; 6 mg/0.5 mL vials; 3 mg/0.5 mL, 6 mg/0.5 mL single-dose autoinjector, prefilled-syringe
Injection (needle-free): 4 mg/0.5 mL, 6 mg/0.5 mL jet-injector
Nasal powder: 11 mg (base)/disposable nosepiece
Nasal solution: 5 mg/0.1 mL, 20 mg/0.1 mL
Tablets ⊚: 25 mg, 50 mg, 100 mg (base)

INDICATIONS & DOSAGES
➤ **Acute migraine attacks (with or without aura)**
Adults: 1 to 6 mg subcut depending on product; maximum dose is 12 mg in 24 hours, separated by at least 1 hour. Or 25 to 100 mg PO, initially. If desired response isn't achieved in 2 hours, may give second dose of 25 to 100 mg. Additional doses may be used in at least 2-hour intervals. Maximum daily oral dose, 200 mg.

For nasal spray, give 5 mg, 10 mg, or 20 mg once in one nostril; may repeat once after 2 hours, for maximum daily dose of 40 mg.

For nasal powder, one 11 mg nosepiece in each nostril (22 mg total), using the Xsail breath-powered delivery device. If desired response isn't achieved in 2 hours, or migraine returns after a transient improvement, may give second dose of 22 mg. Maximum recommended dose within 24 hours is two doses (44 mg/4 nosepieces) or one dose of 22 mg and one dose of another sumatriptan product, separated by at least 2 hours.
Adjust-a-dose: In patients with mild to moderate hepatic impairment, the maximum single oral dose shouldn't exceed 50 mg.
➤ **Cluster headache (except Zembrace)**
Adults: 6 mg subcut. Maximum recommended dose is two 6-mg injections in 24 hours, separated by at least 1 hour.

ADMINISTRATION
PO
• Give drug without regard for food.
• Give drug whole; don't crush or break tablet.
Subcutaneous
• Redness or pain at injection site should subside within 1 hour after injection.
• Use injection site with adequate skin and subcutaneous tissue thickness to accommodate length of needle.
• Use only the abdomen or thigh for needle-free injection system.
Intranasal spray
• Have patient blow nose before use.
• Give medication on inhalation in one nostril, while blocking the other nostril.
Intranasal powder
• Use with the Xsail device only; insert disposable nosepiece into the device body.

• Pierce capsule inside nosepiece by pressing and releasing the white piercing button one time on the device body.
• Insert nosepiece into one nostril, ensuring a tight seal; rotate device, place mouthpiece into mouth, and blow forcefully through mouthpiece for 2 to 3 seconds to deliver powder into the nasal cavity.
• Remove and discard nosepiece; repeat in other nostril, using a second nosepiece.

ACTION
May act as an agonist at serotonin receptors on extracerebral intracranial blood vessels, which constricts the affected vessels, inhibits neuropeptide release, and reduces pain transmission in the trigeminal pathways.

Route	Onset	Peak	Duration
PO	30 min	2–2½ hr	Unknown
Subcut	10 min	12 min	Unknown
Intranasal spray	15–30 min	5–23 min	Unknown
Intranasal powder	Unknown	45 min	Unknown

Half-life: About 2 hours; intranasal, about 3 hours.

ADVERSE REACTIONS
CNS: dizziness, vertigo, drowsiness, headache, anxiety, malaise, fatigue. **CV:** *atrial fibrillation, ventricular fibrillation, ventricular tachycardia, coronary artery vasospasm, transient myocardial ischemia, MI,* pressure or tightness in chest. **EENT:** discomfort of throat, nasal cavity or sinus, mouth, jaw, or tongue; altered vision. **GI:** abdominal discomfort, dysphagia, diarrhea, nausea, vomiting, unusual or bad taste (nasal spray). **Musculoskeletal:** myalgia, muscle cramps, neck pain. **Respiratory:** upper respiratory tract inflammation and dyspnea (PO). **Skin:** injection-site or application-site reaction, tingling, diaphoresis, flushing. **Other:** warm or hot sensation, burning sensation, heaviness, pressure or tightness, tight feeling in head, cold sensation, numbness.

INTERACTIONS
Drug-drug. *Antipsychotics, metoclopramide, serotonin modulators:* May enhance adverse or toxic effect of other serotonin modulators, increasing risk of serotonin syndrome. Monitor therapy.

Reactions in bold italics are *life-threatening*. Interactions may have a *rapid onset* or a *delayed onset*.

Ergot and ergot derivatives, other 5-HT$_1$ agonists: May prolong vasospastic effects. Don't use within 24 hours of sumatriptan therapy.

MAO inhibitors: May reduce sumatriptan clearance. Use with or within 2 weeks of MAO inhibitor is contraindicated.

Methylene blue, SSRIs: May cause serotonin syndrome. Monitor patient closely for weakness, hyperreflexia, and incoordination if use together can't be avoided.

Drug-herb. *St. John's wort:* May increase serotonin levels. Use together cautiously.

EFFECTS ON LAB TEST RESULTS
• May increase liver enzyme levels.

CONTRAINDICATIONS & CAUTIONS
• Contraindicated in patients with hypersensitivity to drug or its components and in those with history, symptoms, or signs of ischemic cardiac, cerebrovascular (such as stroke or TIA), or peripheral vascular syndromes (such as ischemic bowel disease); hemiplegic or basilar migraine; significant underlying CV diseases, including angina pectoris, MI, and silent myocardial ischemia; Wolff-Parkinson-White syndrome or arrhythmias associated with other cardiac accessory conduction pathway disorders; uncontrolled HTN; or severe hepatic impairment.
• Contraindicated within 24 hours of another 5-HT agonist or drug containing ergotamine and within 2 weeks of MAO inhibitor.
• Use cautiously in patient with risk factors for CAD, such as postmenopausal women, men older than age 40, or patients with HTN, hypercholesterolemia, obesity, diabetes, smoking, or family history of CAD.
Dialyzable drug: Unknown.

PREGNANCY-LACTATION-REPRODUCTION
• There are no adequate studies in pregnant women. Use only if potential benefit justifies potential risk to the fetus.
• Drug appears in human milk after subcut administration. Refer to individual manufacturer's instructions regarding breastfeeding. Some manufacturers don't recommend breastfeeding and other sources note that

patient doesn't have to discontinue breast-feeding.

NURSING CONSIDERATIONS
🛈 *Alert:* When giving drug to patient at risk for CAD, give first dose in presence of other medical personnel. Rarely, serious adverse cardiac effects can follow administration.
🛈 *Alert:* Combining drug with an SSRI or an SSNRI may cause serotonin syndrome. Symptoms include restlessness, hallucinations, loss of coordination, fast heartbeat, rapid changes in BP, increased body temperature, hyperreflexia, nausea, vomiting, and diarrhea. Serotonin syndrome may occur when starting or increasing the dose of drug, SSRI, or SSNRI.
• Monitor patient for seizures. Seizures have been reported in patients with and without a history of seizures.
• After subcut injection, most patients experience relief in 1 to 2 hours.
• *Look alike–sound alike:* Don't confuse sumatriptan with somatropin.

PATIENT TEACHING
• Inform patient that drug is intended only to treat migraine attacks, not to prevent them or reduce their occurrence.
• If patient is pregnant or may become pregnant, tell her not to use drug but to discuss with prescriber the risks and benefits of using drug during pregnancy.
• Tell patient that drug may be taken at any time during a migraine attack, as soon as signs or symptoms appear.
• Review information about drug's injectable form, which is available in a spring-loaded injector system for easier patient use. Make sure patient understands how to load the injector, give the injection, and dispose of used syringes.
• Teach patient to select subcut administration sites with adequate subcutaneous tissue thickness.
• Teach patient using intranasal powder how to use Xsail device correctly.
• Teach patient to blow nose before using nasal spray. Patient should block other nostril while inhaling gently during administration and should keep head upright and breathe gently for 10 to 20 seconds after dose is given.

⚠ *Alert:* Tell patient to report all adverse reactions and to immediately report persistent or severe chest pain. Warn patient to stop using drug and to call prescriber if pain or tightness in the throat, wheezing, heart throbbing, rash, lumps, hives, or swollen eyelids, face, or lips develop.

SAFETY ALERT!

SUNItinib malate
su-NIT-e-nib

Sutent⬦

Therapeutic class: Antineoplastics
Pharmacologic class: Protein-tyrosine kinase inhibitors

AVAILABLE FORMS
Capsules: 12.5 mg, 25 mg, 37.5 mg, 50 mg

INDICATIONS & DOSAGES
➤ **GI stromal tumor that's progressing despite imatinib therapy or because patient is intolerant of imatinib; advanced renal cell carcinoma**
Adults: 50 mg PO once daily for 4 weeks, followed by 2 weeks off the drug. Repeat cycle.
Adjust-a-dose: Increase or decrease dosage in 12.5-mg increments based on individual safety and tolerability. If drug must be administered with a strong CYP3A4 inhibitor such as ketoconazole, reduce dosage to a minimum of 37.5 mg/day. If drug must be administered with a CYP3A4 inducer such as rifampin, consider increasing dosage to 87.5 mg daily; carefully monitor patient for toxicity. Refer to package insert for dosage adjustments for toxicities.
➤ **Progressive, well-differentiated pancreatic neuroendocrine tumors in patients with unresectable, locally advanced, or metastatic disease**
Adults: 37.5 mg PO once daily given continuously without a scheduled off-treatment period. Maximum recommended dosage is 50 mg daily.
Adjust-a-dose: Increase or decrease in 12.5-mg increments based on patient tolerance and safety. If drug must be administered with a strong CYP3A4 inhibitor such

as ketoconazole, consider decreasing dosage to 25 mg daily. If drug must be administered with a CYP3A4 inducer such as rifampin, consider increasing dosage to 62.5 mg daily and carefully monitor patient for toxicity. Refer to manufacturer's instructions for dosage adjustments for toxicities.
➤ **Adjuvant treatment of patients at high risk for recurrent renal cell carcinoma after nephrectomy**
Adults: 50 mg PO once daily, on a schedule of 4 weeks on treatment followed by 2 weeks off treatment for nine 6-week cycles.
Adjust-a-dose: Refer to manufacturer's instructions for toxicity-related dosage adjustments.

ADMINISTRATION
PO
• Hazardous agent; use safe handling and disposal precautions according to facility policy. Avoid contact with broken capsules.
• Give drug without regard for meals.

ACTION
A multi-kinase inhibitor targeting several receptor tyrosine kinases, which are involved in tumor growth, pathologic angiogenesis, and metastatic progression of cancer.

Route	Onset	Peak	Duration
PO	Unknown	6–12 hr	Unknown

Half-life: 40 to 60 hours; primary metabolite, 80 to 110 hours.

ADVERSE REACTIONS
CNS: asthenia, dizziness, fatigue, fever, headache, peripheral neuropathy. **CV:** *decreased LVEF, thromboembolic events,* HTN, peripheral edema, chest pain. **EENT:** increased lacrimation, periorbital edema.
GI: *GI perforation, pancreatitis,* abdominal pain, altered taste, anorexia, appetite disturbance, burning sensation in mouth, constipation, diarrhea, dyspepsia, flatulence, mucositis, nausea, oral pain, stomatitis, vomiting.
Hematologic: *bleeding, leukopenia, lymphopenia, neutropenia, thrombocytopenia,* anemia. **Metabolic:** dehydration, hypernatremia, hyperuricemia, hypokalemia, *hyperkalemia,* hyponatremia, hypophosphatemia, hypothyroidism. **Musculoskeletal:** arthralgia, back pain, limb pain, myalgia.

Reactions in bold italics are *life-threatening*. Interactions may have a *rapid onset* or a *delayed onset*.

Respiratory: cough, dyspnea. **Skin:** alopecia, dry skin, hair color changes, hand-foot syndrome, rash, skin discoloration, skin blistering. **Other:** *adrenal insufficiency.*

INTERACTIONS

Drug-drug. *Azole antifungals, CYP3A4 inducers (carbamazepine, dexamethasone, phenobarbital, phenytoin, rifabutin, rifampin, rifapentine):* May decrease sunitinib level and effects. If use together can't be avoided, increase sunitinib dosage.
Bevacizumab: May enhance hypertensive effect of sunitinib and increase risk of microangiopathic hemolytic anemia. Avoid use together.
QTc interval–prolonging drugs: May increase risk of QTc interval prolongation and ventricular arrhythmias. Carefully monitor ECG and QT interval. Consider therapy modification.
Strong CYP3A4 inhibitors (atazanavir, clarithromycin, indinavir, itraconazole, ketoconazole, nefazodone, nelfinavir, ritonavir, saquinavir, voriconazole): May increase sunitinib level and toxicity. If use together can't be avoided, decrease sunitinib dosage.
Drug-herb. *Echinacea, St. John's wort:* May cause an unpredictable decrease in drug level. Discourage use together.
Drug-food. *Grapefruit:* May increase drug level. Discourage use together.

EFFECTS ON LAB TEST RESULTS

• May increase AST, ALT, alkaline phosphatase, total and indirect bilirubin, amylase, lipase, creatinine, uric acid, and TSH levels.
• May decrease phosphorus and Hb levels and hematocrit.
• May increase or decrease potassium and sodium levels.
• May decrease RBC, neutrophil, lymphocyte, WBC, and platelet counts.

CONTRAINDICATIONS & CAUTIONS

• Contraindicated in patients hypersensitive to drug or its components.
• Use cautiously in patients with electrolyte imbalance or a history of HTN, QT-interval prolongation, concurrent antiarrhythmic use, bradycardia, MI, angina, CABG, symptomatic HF, stroke, TIA, or PE.

• Thrombotic microangiopathy (TMA), including thrombotic thrombocytopenic purpura and hemolytic-uremic syndrome, sometimes leading to renal failure or a fatal outcome, has been reported. Discontinue if TMA develops.
• Proteinuria and nephrotic syndrome have been reported, and some cases have resulted in renal failure and fatal outcomes. Monitor patient for development or worsening of proteinuria. Obtain urinalysis at baseline and periodically during treatment, with follow-up measurement of 24-hour urine protein as clinically indicated.
• Severe cutaneous reactions have been reported, including erythema multiforme, SJS, and toxic epidermal necrolysis (TEN), some of which were fatal. If patient develops signs or symptoms of a progressive rash, often with blisters or mucosal lesions, discontinue drug. If a diagnosis of SJS or TEN is suspected, don't restart drug.
• Necrotizing fasciitis, including of the perineum and secondary to fistula formation, sometimes fatal, has been reported. Discontinue drug if necrotizing fasciitis develops.
• Drug has been associated with symptomatic hypoglycemia, which may result in loss of consciousness or require hospitalization. Blood glucose level reductions may be worse in patients with diabetes. Check blood glucose levels regularly during and after discontinuation of treatment. Assess if antidiabetic drug dosage needs adjustment to minimize risk of hypoglycemia.
• Using sunitinib malate with antiarrhythmics (amiodarone, bretylium, disopyramide, dofetilide, procainamide, quinidine, sotalol), arsenic trioxide, chlorpromazine, cisapride, dolasetron, droperidol, mefloquine, mesoridazine, moxifloxacin, pentamidine, pimozide, tacrolimus, thioridazine, and ziprasidone may prolong QT interval and increase the risk of life-threatening cardiac arrhythmias, including torsades de pointes.
Dialyzable drug: No.

PREGNANCY-LACTATION-REPRODUCTION

• Drug can cause fetal harm when used in pregnant women. Women of childbearing potential should avoid becoming pregnant during therapy. If drug is used during pregnancy, or if patient becomes pregnant while

S

taking drug, apprise her of potential hazard to the fetus.

• It isn't known if drug appears in human milk. Patient should discontinue breastfeeding or discontinue drug.

NURSING CONSIDERATIONS

Black Box Warning Drug may cause severe, sometimes fatal, hepatotoxicity. Monitor liver function before and during each cycle of therapy. ■

❸ Alert: Drug may cause CV events, including HF, myocardial disorders, and cardiomyopathy, which may be fatal. Monitor CV status closely.

• Obtain CBC with platelet count and serum chemistries, including phosphate level, before each treatment cycle.

• Obtain LFTs at baseline, before each treatment cycle, and when clinically indicated.

• Obtain baseline evaluation of LVEF in all patients before treatment. If patient had a cardiac event in the year before treatment, check LVEF periodically.

• Interrupt therapy or decrease dosage in patients with LVEF less than 50% and more than 20% below baseline.

• Monitor patient's BP closely. If severe HTN occurs, notify prescriber. Drug may need to be withheld until BP is controlled.

• Monitor patient for signs and symptoms of HF, especially if there is a history of heart disease.

• Patient who has seizures may have reversible posterior leukoencephalopathy syndrome. Signs and symptoms include HTN, headache, decreased alertness, altered mental functioning, and vision loss. Stop treatment temporarily.

• Impaired wound healing has been reported during therapy. Temporarily interrupt therapy in patients undergoing major surgical procedures. May resume drug when health care provider determines patient has recovered.

• If patient will be undergoing surgery or suffers trauma or severe infection, assess for adrenal insufficiency (muscle weakness, weight loss, depression, salt craving, low BP).

• Provide antiemetics or antidiarrheals as needed for adverse GI effects.

• Monitor patient with renal cell carcinoma or GI stromal tumor with high tumor burden closely and treat as clinically indicated because of the risk of TLS. Correct dehydration and high uric acid levels before treatment.

• Osteonecrosis of the jaw has been reported. Consider preventive dentistry before treatment with sunitinib. If possible, avoid invasive dental procedures, particularly in patients receiving IV bisphosphonate therapy.

❸ Alert: Drug may cause bleeding in GI tract, urinary tract, respiratory tract, and brain, which may be fatal. Monitor patient and CBC closely.

PATIENT TEACHING

• Advise patient to keep appointments for blood tests and periodic heart function evaluations.

• Tell patient about common adverse effects, such as diarrhea, nausea, vomiting, fatigue, mouth pain, and taste disturbance, and to report all adverse reactions.

• Advise patient that severe hypoglycemia can occur. Inform patient of the signs, symptoms, and risks associated with hypoglycemia.

• Inform patient about changes that may occur in skin and hair, including color changes and dry, red, blistering skin of the hands and feet.

• Urge patient to tell prescriber about all prescribed and OTC drugs or herbal supplements.

• Warn patient not to consume grapefruit products during therapy.

• Tell patient to notify prescriber about unusual bleeding, trouble breathing, fainting, light-headedness, and heart palpitations, wheezing, severe or prolonged diarrhea or vomiting, or swelling of the hands or lower legs.

• Advise female patient of childbearing potential to avoid becoming pregnant during therapy.

Reactions in bold italics are *life-threatening*. Interactions may have a *rapid onset* or a ***delayed onset***.

suvorexant
soo-voe-REX-ant

Belsomra

Therapeutic class: Hypnotics
Pharmacologic class: Orexin receptor antagonists
Controlled substance schedule: IV

AVAILABLE FORMS
Tablets: 5 mg, 10 mg, 15 mg, 20 mg

INDICATIONS & DOSAGES
➤ **Insomnia characterized by difficulties with sleep onset or sleep maintenance**
Adults: 10 mg PO daily within 30 minutes of going to bed. If 10-mg dose is tolerated but not effective, increase to a maximum of 20 mg PO daily. Don't exceed more than one dose per night.
Adjust-a-dose: For patients taking concomitant moderate CYP3A4 inhibitors, give 5 mg PO daily at night. Maximum dose is 10 mg daily.

ADMINISTRATION
PO
• Give drug within 30 minutes of bedtime and ensure at least 7 hours remain before planned time of awakening.
• May give with or without food; however, the time to drug's effect is delayed if drug is taken with or soon after a meal.

ACTION
Blocks orexin receptors, suppressing the system responsible for promoting wakefulness.

Route	Onset	Peak	Duration
PO	30 min	2 hr	Unknown

Half-life: 12 hours.

ADVERSE REACTIONS
CNS: somnolence, behavioral changes, headache, dizziness, abnormal dreams. **EENT:** dry mouth. **GI:** diarrhea. **Respiratory:** cough, URI.

INTERACTIONS
Drug-drug. *CNS depressants, including other drugs that treat insomnia:* May cause excessive CNS depression. Use together isn't recommended.
Digoxin: May decrease digoxin metabolism. Monitor digoxin level.
Moderate CYP3A4 inhibitors (amprenavir, aprepitant, atazanavir, ciprofloxacin, diltiazem, erythromycin, fluconazole, fosamprenavir, imatinib, verapamil): May decrease suvorexant metabolism. Decrease initial suvorexant daily dose to 5 mg; don't exceed a dose of 10 mg.
Opioids: May cause slow or difficult breathing, sedation, and death. Avoid use together. If use together is necessary, limit dosage and duration of each drug to minimum necessary for desired effect.
Strong CYP3A4 inducers (carbamazepine, phenytoin, rifampin): May decrease clinical effect of suvorexant. Monitor patient for reduced therapeutic effect.
Strong CYP3A4 inhibitors (clarithromycin, conivaptan, indinavir, itraconazole, ketoconazole, nefazodone, nelfinavir, posaconazole, ritonavir, saquinavir, telaprevir): May increase risk of additive toxicity. Avoid use together.
Drug-food. *Grapefruit juice:* May decrease drug metabolism and increase drug level. Decrease suvorexant dosage.
Drug-lifestyle. *Alcohol use:* May cause excessive CNS depression. Discourage use together.

EFFECTS ON LAB TEST RESULTS
• May increase cholesterol level.

CONTRAINDICATIONS & CAUTIONS
• Contraindicated in patients hypersensitive to drug or its components and in those with narcolepsy.
• Opioids should only be prescribed with benzodiazepines or other CNS depressants to patients for whom alternative treatment options are inadequate.
• Not recommended for use in patients with severe hepatic impairment.
• **Alert:** Drug may increase risk of suicidal ideation. Immediately evaluate patients who report suicidal ideation or exhibit new behavioral signs or symptoms.

S

- Use cautiously in patients with compromised respiratory status (obstructive sleep apnea, COPD) or a history of drug abuse or dependence.
- Safety and effectiveness in children haven't been studied.

Dialyzable drug: Unknown.

⚠ *Overdose S&S:* Increased frequency and duration of somnolence.

PREGNANCY-LACTATION-REPRODUCTION

- Drug hasn't been studied in pregnant women. Use cautiously during pregnancy and only if benefits outweigh risk to the fetus.
- It isn't known if drug appears in human milk. Use cautiously in breastfeeding women.

NURSING CONSIDERATIONS

- Use the smallest effective dosage in all patients. Lower dosages may be necessary in obese or female patients because a higher incidence of adverse effects have been observed.
- Complex behaviors, such as "sleep driving" (driving while not fully awake), preparing and eating food, making phone calls, or having sex with subsequent amnesia of the event, have been reported with therapeutic doses; use of alcohol and other CNS depressants increases the risk. Discontinue drug for complex sleep behavior.
- Monitor patient for daytime somnolence. Decrease dosage or discontinue drug if daytime somnolence develops in patients who drive.
- Carefully evaluate patient for physical or psychiatric causes of sleep disturbances before drug is prescribed. If insomnia persists for more than 7 to 10 days, reevaluate patient.
- Monitor patients for sleep paralysis (inability to move or speak during sleep-wake transitions), hallucinations, and mild cataplexy signs and symptoms (periods of leg weakness).

🔹 *Alert:* Worsening of depression or suicidal thinking may occur. Be alert for signs and symptoms of depression or behavioral changes.

- *Look alike–sound alike:* Don't confuse suvorexant with Serevent.

PATIENT TEACHING

- Caution patient or caregiver of patient taking an opioid with a benzodiazepine, CNS depressant, or alcohol to seek immediate medical attention for dizziness, lightheadedness, extreme sleepiness, slowed or difficult breathing, or unresponsiveness.
- Teach patient to take drug immediately before going to bed and to allow at least 7 hours for sleep before planned awakening.
- Inform patient that drug may be taken with or without food but, for more rapid sleep onset, to avoid taking drug with or after meals.
- Advise patient to avoid alcohol and other drugs that cause sleepiness while taking suvorexant.
- Tell patient to notify prescriber if abnormal thoughts and behavior, symptoms of depression (changes in mood, excessive tiredness), or insomnia that persists for more than 7 to 10 days occurs.

🔹 *Alert:* Caution patient to immediately report suicidal ideation or new behavioral signs or symptoms.

- Inform patient that sleep paralysis (inability to move or speak during sleep-wake transitions), vivid and disturbing perceptions, and temporary leg weakness can occur.
- Warn patient that daytime somnolence can occur and to avoid performing activities that require mental alertness or physical coordination (such as driving) until fully awake.
- Warn patient of the risk of performing complex behaviors, such as driving, eating, and making phone calls, while asleep and to report if these symptoms occur.
- Instruct patient not to increase dosage without first consulting prescriber.
- Advise female patient to inform prescriber if she's pregnant, intends to become pregnant, or is breastfeeding.

Reactions in bold italics are *life-threatening*. Interactions may have a *rapid onset* or a *delayed onset*.

tacrolimus (topical)
tack-ROW-lim-us

Protopic

Therapeutic class: Immunosuppressants
Pharmacologic class: Calcineurin inhibitors

AVAILABLE FORMS
Ointment: 0.03%, 0.1%

INDICATIONS & DOSAGES
➤ **Moderate to severe atopic dermatitis in patients unresponsive to other therapies or unable to use other therapies because of potential risks**
Adults and children age 16 and older: Thin layer of 0.03% or 0.1% strength applied to affected areas b.i.d. and rubbed in completely.
Children ages 2 to 15: Thin layer of 0.03% strength applied to affected areas b.i.d. and rubbed in completely.

ADMINISTRATION
Topical
• In patients with infected atopic dermatitis, clear infections at treatment site before using drug.
• Don't use with occlusive dressings.
• Stop drug when signs and symptoms resolve.

ACTION
Unknown. Probably acts as an immune system modulator in the skin by inhibiting T-lymphocyte activation, which causes immunosuppression. Drug also inhibits the release of mediators from mast cells and basophils in skin.

Route	Onset	Peak	Duration
Topical	Unknown	Unknown	Unknown

Half-life: Unknown.

ADVERSE REACTIONS
CNS: headache, hyperesthesia, asthenia, insomnia, fever, pain. **CV:** peripheral edema, HTN, facial edema. **EENT:** otitis media, pharyngitis, rhinitis, sinusitis, conjunctivitis. **GI:** diarrhea, vomiting, nausea, abdominal pain, gastroenteritis, dyspepsia. **GU:** dysmenorrhea. **Musculoskeletal:** back pain,

myalgia. **Respiratory:** increased cough, *asthma,* pneumonia, bronchitis. **Skin:** burning, pruritus, erythema, infection, herpes simplex, eczema herpeticum, pustular rash, folliculitis, urticaria, maculopapular rash, fungal dermatitis, acne, sunburn, tingling, benign skin neoplasm, vesiculobullous rash, dry skin, varicella zoster, herpes zoster, eczema, exfoliative dermatitis, contact dermatitis. **Other:** flulike symptoms, accidental injury, infection, alcohol intolerance, periodontal abscess, cyst, allergic reaction.

INTERACTIONS
Drug-drug. *Calcium channel blockers, cimetidine, CYP3A4 inhibitors (erythromycin, itraconazole, ketoconazole, fluconazole, protease inhibitors):* May increase tacrolimus level if systemic absorption occurs. Use together cautiously.
Immunosuppressants: May enhance adverse effects of other immunosuppressants. Use together cautiously.
Tacrolimus (systemic): May increase toxicity. Use together cautiously and decrease dosage as needed.
Drug-food. *Grapefruit juice:* May increase tacrolimus level if absorbed systemically. Monitor therapy.
Drug-lifestyle. *Alcohol use:* May cause flushing. Discourage use together.
Sun exposure: May cause phototoxicity. Advise patient to avoid excessive sunlight or artificial ultraviolet light exposure.

EFFECTS ON LAB TEST RESULTS
None reported.

CONTRAINDICATIONS & CAUTIONS
• Contraindicated in patients hypersensitive to drug.
Black Box Warning Long-term safety of topical calcineurin inhibitors such as tacrolimus hasn't been established. ∎
Black Box Warning Don't use in children younger than age 2. Only 0.03% ointment is indicated for children ages 2 to 15. ∎
• Don't use in immunocompromised patients or in patients with skin conditions with a skin barrier defect in which there is a potential for increased systemic absorption, such as Netherton syndrome or generalized erythroderma.

T

- Effects on the developing immune system and safe use with long-term therapy are unknown. Safety hasn't been established beyond 1 year of noncontinuous use.
- **❸ Alert:** Use only after other therapies have failed or aren't advisable.
- **Dialyzable drug:** Unknown.

PREGNANCY-LACTATION-REPRODUCTION
- There are no adequate studies of topical tacrolimus use in pregnant women, and experience is too limited for assessment of its safe use during pregnancy. Use only if potential benefit justifies potential risk to the fetus.
- Drug appears in human milk. Patient should discontinue breastfeeding or discontinue drug.

NURSING CONSIDERATIONS
Black Box Warning Use drug only for short-term or intermittent long-term therapy. Limit application to areas of involvement with atopic dermatitis. Rare cases of malignancy have been reported without confirmation of causal relationship. ▪
- If signs and symptoms of atopic dermatitis don't improve within 6 weeks, reevaluate patient to confirm the diagnosis.
- Use of this drug may increase the risk of varicella zoster, HSV, and eczema herpeticum.
- Consider stopping drug in patients with lymphadenopathy if cause is unknown or acute mononucleosis is diagnosed.
- Monitor all cases of lymphadenopathy until resolution.
- Local adverse effects are most common during the first few days of treatment.
- Avoid use on areas of skin affected by premalignant and malignant skin conditions.

PATIENT TEACHING
- Tell patient to wash hands before and after applying drug and to avoid applying drug to wet skin.
- Tell patient to apply a thin layer only to affected area.
- Urge patient not to use bandages or other occlusive dressings.
- Tell patient not to bathe, shower, or swim immediately after application because doing so could wash the ointment off.

- Tell patient that a moisturizer can be applied after topical tacrolimus.
- Tell patient to stop treatment when the signs and symptoms resolve.
- Advise patient to avoid or minimize exposure to natural or artificial sunlight.
- Caution patient not to use drug for any disorder other than that for which it was prescribed.
- Encourage patient to report adverse reactions.
- Tell patient to store the ointment at room temperature.

tadalafil ☒
tah-DAL-ah-fill

Adcirca, Alyq, Cialis⦸

Therapeutic class: Erectile dysfunction drugs
Pharmacologic class: PDE5 inhibitors

AVAILABLE FORMS
Tablets (film-coated): 2.5 mg, 5 mg, 10 mg, 20 mg

INDICATIONS & DOSAGES
➤ **Erectile dysfunction (Cialis)**
Adults: 10 mg PO as a single dose, as needed, at least 30 minutes before sexual activity. Range is 5 to 20 mg, based on effectiveness and tolerance. Maximum is one dose daily. Or 2.5 mg PO once daily without regard to timing of sexual activity. May increase to 5 mg PO daily.
Adjust-a-dose: If CrCl is 30 to 50 mL/minute, starting dosage is 5 mg once daily and maximum is 10 mg once every 48 hours. If CrCl is less than 30 mL/minute or in patients with ESRD on hemodialysis, maximum is 5 mg once every 72 hours as needed; daily use isn't recommended. Use cautiously in patients with mild or moderate hepatic impairment (Child-Pugh class A or B); don't exceed 10 mg daily. Patients taking potent CYP3A4 inhibitors (erythromycin, itraconazole, ketoconazole, ritonavir) shouldn't exceed one 10-mg dose every 72 hours if taken as needed; the once-daily dose shouldn't exceed 2.5 mg.

➤ **PAH (Adcirca, Alyq)**
Adults: 40 mg (two 20-mg tablets) PO once daily. Dividing dose over course of the day isn't recommended.
Adjust-a-dose: For patients with CrCl of 31 to 80 mL/minute, start with 20 mg PO once daily. Increase to 40 mg once daily if tolerated. Avoid use in patients with CrCl of 30 mL/minute or less and in those on hemodialysis. Consider starting dose of 20 mg PO once daily in patients with Child-Pugh class A or B. In patients receiving ritonavir for at least 1 week, start at 20 mg PO once daily and increase to 40 mg as tolerated. Don't use Adcirca when starting ritonavir; stop Adcirca at least 24 hours before starting ritonavir. After at least 1 week, may give 20 mg PO once daily and increase to 40 mg as tolerated.
➤ **BPH (Cialis)**
Adults: 5 mg PO once daily taken at approximately the same time every day. When used with finasteride, recommended dose of Cialis is 5 mg once daily taken at approximately the same time every day for up to 26 weeks.
Adjust-a-dose: In patients with CrCl of 30 to 50 mL/minute, starting dose is 2.5 mg PO daily. May increase to 5 mg PO daily based on individual response. Not recommended for patients with CrCl less than 30 mL/minute or in patients on hemodialysis.
➤ **BPH and erectile dysfunction (Cialis)**
Adults: 5 mg PO once daily taken at approximately the same time every day, without regard to the timing of sexual activity.
Adjust-a-dose: In patients with CrCl of 30 to 50 mL/minute, starting dose is 2.5 mg PO daily. May increase to 5 mg PO daily based on individual response. Not recommended for patients with CrCl less than 30 mL/minute or in patients on hemodialysis.

ADMINISTRATION
PO
• Give drug without regard for food.

ACTION
Inhibits PDE5 enzyme, which leads to increased cyclic guanosine monophosphate levels, prolonged smooth muscle relaxation, and increased blood flow into the corpus cavernosum and pulmonary arteries. Effect is also seen in the smooth muscle of the prostate and bladder and their vascular supply.

Route	Onset	Peak	Duration
PO	Within 1 hr	½–6 hr	Up to 36 hr

Half-life: 15 to 17½ hours; PAH (in patients not receiving bosentan), 35 hours.

ADVERSE REACTIONS
CNS: dizziness, headache. **CV:** flushing, HTN. **EENT:** decrease in or loss of hearing, nasal congestion, tinnitus, nasopharyngitis. **GI:** dyspepsia, abdominal pain, diarrhea, GERD, gastroenteritis, nausea. **GU:** UTI. **Musculoskeletal:** back pain, limb pain, myalgia. **Respiratory:** bronchitis, cough, URI.

INTERACTIONS
Drug-drug. *Alpha blockers:* May increase risk of hypotension. For erectile dysfunction, patient should be on stable dose before starting tadalafil at lowest recommended dosage. Use with tadalafil for BPH treatment isn't recommended. Stop alpha blocker at least 1 day before starting tadalafil.
Guanylate cyclase (GC) stimulators (riociguat): May increase hypotension. Use together is contraindicated.
Nitrates: May enhance hypotensive effects. Use together is contraindicated.
Potent CYP3A4 inhibitors (ketoconazole, protease inhibitors, ritonavir): May increase tadalafil level. For erectile dysfunction, don't exceed a 10-mg dose of Cialis every 72 hours if taken as needed or 2.5 mg as the once-daily dose.
Rifampin, other CYP450 inducers: May decrease tadalafil level. Monitor patient closely.
Drug-food. *Grapefruit:* May increase drug level. Discourage use together.
Drug-lifestyle. *Alcohol use:* May increase risk of headache, dizziness, orthostatic hypotension, and increased HR. Discourage use together.

EFFECTS ON LAB TEST RESULTS
None reported.

CONTRAINDICATIONS & CAUTIONS
• Contraindicated in patients hypersensitive to drug or its components and in those taking nitrates or GC stimulators.

- Use cautiously in patients with mild or moderate hepatic impairment (Child-Pugh class A or B).
- Drug isn't recommended for patients with severe hepatic impairment (Child-Pugh class C), unstable angina, angina that occurs during sexual intercourse, NYHA Class II or greater HF within past 6 months, uncontrolled arrhythmias, hypotension (lower than 90/50 mm Hg), uncontrolled HTN (higher than 170/100 mm Hg), stroke within past 6 months, or an MI within past 90 days.
- Use cautiously in patients with left ventricular outflow obstruction. Use in patients with pulmonary veno-occlusive disease isn't recommended.
- ⚕ Drug isn't recommended for patients whose cardiac status makes sexual activity inadvisable or for those with known hereditary degenerative retinal disorders.
- Nonarteritic anterior ischemic optic neuropathy (NAION), a rare cause of decreased vision, including permanent vision loss, has been reported with all PDE5 inhibitors; a causal relationship hasn't been established. Most, but not all, of these patients had underlying risk factors for NAION.
- Use cautiously in patients with bleeding disorders, significant peptic ulceration, or renal impairment.
- Use cautiously in patients with conditions predisposing them to priapism (sickle cell anemia, multiple myeloma, and leukemia) and in those with anatomic penis abnormalities.
- Use cautiously in elderly patients.
Dialyzable drug: No.

PREGNANCY-LACTATION-REPRODUCTION
- There are no adequate studies in pregnant women. Drug isn't indicated for use in women.
- It isn't known if drug appears in human milk. Drug isn't indicated for use in women.

NURSING CONSIDERATIONS
- ❸ *Alert:* Sexual activity may increase cardiac risk. Evaluate patient's cardiac risk before starting drug.
- Before drug initiation, assess patient for underlying causes of erectile dysfunction.
- Transient decreases in supine BP may occur. Monitor patient for orthostatic hypotension.

- Prolonged erections and priapism may occur.
- Monitor patients for (rare) vision or hearing loss and report immediately.
- *Look alike–sound alike:* Don't confuse tadalafil with sildenafil or vardenafil. Don't confuse Adcirca with Advair Discus, Advair HFA, or Advicor.

PATIENT TEACHING
- Warn patient that taking drug with nitrates could cause a serious drop in BP, which increases the risk of heart attack or stroke.
- Tell patient to seek immediate medical attention if chest pain develops after taking the drug.
- Tell patient that drug doesn't protect against sexually transmitted diseases and to use protective measures.
- Urge patient to seek emergency medical care for an erection lasting more than 4 hours.
- Tell patient to take drug about 30 to 60 minutes before anticipated sexual activity if using as needed. Explain that drug has no effect without sexual stimulation.
- Warn patient not to change dosage unless directed by prescriber.
- Caution patient against drinking large amounts of alcohol while taking drug.
- Advise patient to avoid grapefruit juice.
- Instruct patient to notify prescriber of vision or hearing changes, especially sudden loss of vision in one or both eyes.

SAFETY ALERT!

tamoxifen citrate
ta-MOX-i-fen

Nolvadex-D✚, Soltamox

Therapeutic class: Antineoplastics
Pharmacologic class: Nonsteroidal antiestrogens

AVAILABLE FORMS
Oral solution: 10 mg/5 mL*
Tablets: 10 mg, 20 mg

INDICATIONS & DOSAGES
➤ **Estrogen receptor–positive metastatic breast cancer in adults**

Reactions in bold italics are *life-threatening*. Interactions may have a *rapid onset* or a *delayed onset*.

Adults: 20 to 40 mg PO daily; divide doses of more than 20 mg/day into two doses.
➤ **Adjuvant treatment of early-stage estrogen–receptor-positive breast cancer; to reduce occurrence of contralateral breast cancer**
Adults: 20 mg PO daily for 5 to 10 years.
➤ **To reduce breast cancer occurrence**
High-risk women: 20 mg PO daily for 5 years.
➤ **Ductal carcinoma in situ (DCIS) after breast surgery and radiation**
Adults: 20 mg PO daily for 5 years.
➤ **Gynecomastia ◆**
Adults: 20 mg PO daily for 1 to 12 months.

ADMINISTRATION
PO
• Drug is a hormonal agent and is considered a potential teratogen. Follow safe-handling procedures.
• Give drug without regard to food.
• Store between 68° and 77° F (20° and 25° C). Protect from light.
• Don't freeze or refrigerate oral solution; use within 3 months of opening.

ACTION
Competes with estrogen for estrogen receptor–positive breast cancer cells, thereby preventing their growth.

Route	Onset	Peak	Duration
PO	1 mo–several mo	5 hr	Several wk

Half-life: Terminal phase, 5 to 7 days for tamoxifen and 14 days for the metabolite.

ADVERSE REACTIONS
CNS: *stroke,* confusion, weakness, sleepiness, headache, fatigue, depression. **CV:** fluid retention, chest pain, HTN, flushing, *thromboembolism.* **EENT:** corneal changes, cataracts, retinopathy. **GI:** nausea, vomiting, diarrhea, constipation. **GU:** amenorrhea, irregular menses, vaginal discharge, *endometrial cancer, uterine sarcoma,* vaginal bleeding. **Hematologic:** *leukopenia, thrombocytopenia.* **Hepatic:** elevated liver enzyme levels. **Metabolic:** hypercalcemia, weight gain or loss, hypercholesterolemia. **Musculoskeletal:** brief worsening of pain from osseous metastases, arthralgia. **Respiratory:** *PE,* cough. **Skin:** skin changes,

rash, alopecia. **Other:** temporary bone or tumor pain, hot flashes.

INTERACTIONS
Drug-drug. *Coumarin-type anticoagulants:* May significantly increase anticoagulant effect. Monitor patient, PT, and INR closely. Use is contraindicated when tamoxifen is used to reduce risk of breast cancer in high-risk women and women with DCIS.
CYP3A4 inducers (such as rifampin): May increase tamoxifen metabolism and may lower drug levels. Monitor patient for clinical effects.
CYP3A4 inhibitors: May increase tamoxifen serum concentration. Consider therapy modification.
Cytotoxic drugs: May increase risk of thromboembolic events. Monitor patient.
Drugs that prolong QTc interval: May increase risk of life-threatening cardiac arrhythmias. Use together cautiously.
Letrozole: May decrease letrozole serum concentration. Monitor therapy.
Strong CYP2D6 inhibitors (fluoxetine, paroxetine, sertraline): May decrease serum concentration of highly potent active metabolite(s) of tamoxifen and decrease tamoxifen's therapeutic effects. Avoid use together.
Drug-herb. *St. John's wort:* May decrease tamoxifen serum concentration. Avoid use together.
Drug-food. *Grapefruit, grapefruit juice:* May decrease tamoxifen metabolism. Avoid use together.

EFFECTS ON LAB TEST RESULTS
• May increase serum creatinine, calcium, T_4, cholesterol, bilirubin, lipid, and liver enzyme levels.
• May decrease WBC and platelet counts.

CONTRAINDICATIONS & CAUTIONS
• Contraindicated in patients hypersensitive to drug.
• Contraindicated as therapy to reduce risk of breast cancer in high-risk women and women with DCIS who concurrently are taking coumarin-type anticoagulants or in women with history of DVT or PE.
Black Box Warning Serious and life-threatening events associated with tamoxifen

have occurred in the risk-reduction setting (women at high risk for cancer and women with DCIS) and include uterine malignancies, stroke, and PE. ∎

• Use cautiously in patients with leukopenia, thrombocytopenia, or bone marrow suppression.

• Drug increases risk of endometrial changes, including hyperplasia, polyps, endometrial cancer, and uterine cancer.

Dialyzable drug: No.

⚠ *Overdose S&S:* Tremors, hyperreflexia, unsteady gait, dizziness, seizures, prolonged QT interval.

PREGNANCY-LACTATION-REPRODUCTION

• May cause fetal harm when used in pregnant women. Advise women not to become pregnant during therapy or within 2 months of stopping drug and to use barrier or non-hormonal contraceptive measures if sexually active.

• Rule out pregnancy before therapy.

• Breastfeeding is contraindicated during therapy and for 3 months after final dose.

NURSING CONSIDERATIONS

• Monitor lipid levels during long-term therapy in patients with hyperlipidemia.

• Monitor calcium level. At start of therapy, drug may compound hypercalcemia related to bone metastases.

• Monitor patient for signs and symptoms of venous thromboembolism.

• Monitor bone mineral density in premenopausal women.

• Women should have baseline and periodic gynecologic exams because of a slight increased risk of endometrial cancer.

• Women should have periodic eye exams because of increased risk of cataracts, retinal vein thrombosis, and retinopathy.

• Monitor CBC closely in patients with leukopenia or thrombocytopenia.

• Patient may initially experience worsening symptoms.

• In postmenopausal women, karyopyknotic index of vaginal smears and various degrees of estrogen effect of Papanicolaou smears may vary.

Black Box Warning Discuss potential benefits versus potential risks with women at high risk for breast cancer and women with

DCIS who are considering tamoxifen to reduce their risks of developing breast cancer. Benefits of drug outweigh its risks in women already diagnosed with breast cancer. ∎

• *Look alike–sound alike:* Don't confuse tamoxifen with tamsulosin.

PATIENT TEACHING

• Reassure patient that acute worsening of bone pain during therapy usually indicates drug will produce good response. Give analgesics to relieve pain.

• Strongly encourage women who are taking or have taken drug to have regular gynecologic exams because drug may increase risk of uterine cancer.

• Encourage women to have mammograms and breast exams as recommended.

• Advise patient to use a barrier form of contraception because short-term therapy induces ovulation in premenopausal women.

• Instruct patient to report vaginal bleeding or changes in menstrual cycle.

• Caution women to avoid becoming pregnant during therapy and for first 2 months after stopping drug. Advise consulting prescriber before becoming pregnant.

• Tell patient to report all adverse reactions, especially signs and symptoms of stroke (headache, vision changes, confusion, difficulty speaking, weakness of face, arm, or leg, especially on one side of the body), PE (chest pain, difficulty breathing, rapid breathing, sweating, fainting), and DVT (leg swelling, tenderness).

• Advise patient to report vision changes.

• Tell patient not to freeze or refrigerate oral solution, to protect solution from light, and to use it within 3 months of opening.

tamsulosin hydrochloride
tam-soo-LOE-sin

Flomax✧, Flomax CR✦

Therapeutic class: BPH drugs
Pharmacologic class: Alpha blockers

AVAILABLE FORMS
Capsules ⓄⓉⒸ: 0.4 mg

INDICATIONS & DOSAGES
➤ **BPH**
Adults: 0.4 mg PO once daily, given 30 minutes after same meal each day. If no response after 2 to 4 weeks, increase dosage to 0.8 mg PO once daily.
➤ **Adjunctive treatment of ureteral stones ◆**
Adults: 0.4 mg PO daily at bedtime for up to 6 weeks or until expulsion of stones.

ADMINISTRATION
PO
• Don't crush, open, or allow patient to chew capsules.

ACTION
Selectively blocks alpha receptors in the prostate, leading to relaxation of smooth muscles in the bladder neck and prostate, improving urine flow and reducing symptoms of BPH.

Route	Onset	Peak	Duration
PO	Unknown	4–7 hr	9–15 hr

Half-life: 9 to 13 hours.

ADVERSE REACTIONS
CNS: dizziness, headache, asthenia, insomnia, somnolence, syncope, vertigo. **CV:** chest pain, orthostatic hypotension. **EENT:** rhinitis, amblyopia, pharyngitis, sinusitis. **GI:** diarrhea, nausea. **GU:** decreased libido, abnormal ejaculation. **Musculoskeletal:** back pain. **Respiratory:** increased cough. **Other:** infection, tooth disorder.

INTERACTIONS
Drug-drug. *Alpha blockers:* May interact with tamsulosin. Avoid using together.
Cimetidine: May decrease tamsulosin clearance. Use together cautiously.
CYP3A4 inducers (strong): May increase tamsulosin metabolism. Consider therapy modification. Some combinations may be specifically contraindicated. Consult appropriate manufacturer labeling.
CYP3A4 inhibitors (moderate): May decrease tamsulosin metabolism. Use cautiously and monitor therapy.
CYP3A4 inhibitors (strong): May increase tamsulosin serum concentration. Avoid combination.

PDE5 inhibitors: May cause symptomatic hypotension. Use together cautiously.
Warfarin: Limited studies are inconclusive. Use together cautiously.
Drug-herb. *St. John's wort:* May decrease tamsulosin serum concentration. Consider therapy modification.

EFFECTS ON LAB TEST RESULTS
None reported.

CONTRAINDICATIONS & CAUTIONS
• Contraindicated in patients hypersensitive to drug or its components.
• Use cautiously in patients with serious or life-threatening sulfa allergy.
• Intraoperative floppy iris syndrome has been observed during cataract and glaucoma surgery in some patients who are taking or had previously taken alpha$_1$ blockers, including tamsulosin, which may increase risk of eye complications during and after surgery. Initiation of drug in patients for whom cataract or glaucoma surgery is scheduled isn't recommended.
• Drug may cause orthostatic hypotension and syncope, especially with first dose.
Dialyzable drug: Unlikely.
⚠ *Overdose S&S:* Severe headache, hypotension.

PREGNANCY-LACTATION-REPRODUCTION
• Drug isn't indicated for use in women.
• Don't use drug for off-label indication in pregnant or breastfeeding women.

NURSING CONSIDERATIONS
• Monitor patient for decreases in BP.
• Symptoms of BPH and prostate cancer are similar; rule out prostate cancer before starting therapy.
• If treatment is interrupted for several days or more, restart therapy at the 0.4-mg PO once-daily dose.
• Rare but serious priapism can occur and must be treated urgently.
• *Look alike–sound alike:* Don't confuse Flomax with Fosamax, Flonase, or Flovent.

PATIENT TEACHING
• Instruct patient not to crush, chew, or open capsules.

T

• Advise patient that drug may cause sudden drop in BP, especially after first dose or when changing doses. Tell patient to rise slowly from a chair or bed when starting therapy and to avoid situations in which injury could occur as a result of fainting.

• Warn patient that rarely, priapism can occur and to report it immediately.

• Instruct patient not to drive or perform hazardous tasks for 12 hours after first dose or changes in dose until response can be monitored.

• Tell patient to take drug about 30 minutes after same meal each day.

• Advise patient considering cataract or glaucoma surgery to inform the ophthalmologist about taking drug.

telavancin
tell-uh-VAN-sin

Vibativ

Therapeutic class: Antibiotics
Pharmacologic class: Lipoglycopeptides

AVAILABLE FORMS
Lyophilized powder for injection: 750-mg single-use vials

INDICATIONS & DOSAGES
☉ *Alert:* Drug should be used to prevent or treat bacterial infections only. Reserve use for when alternative treatments aren't suitable.

Adjust-a-dose (for all indications): For patients with CrCl of 30 to 50 mL/minute, give 7.5 mg/kg every 24 hours; if CrCl is 10 to 29 mL/minute, give 10 mg/kg every 48 hours.

➤ **Complicated skin and skin-structure infections caused by susceptible gram-positive organisms, such as *Staphylococcus aureus*, MRSA, *Streptococcus pyogenes*, *Streptococcus agalactiae*, *Streptococcus anginosus* group, or *Enterococcus faecalis* (vancomycin-susceptible isolates only)**
Adults: 10 mg/kg IV infusion once every 24 hours for 7 to 14 days.

➤ **Hospital-acquired and ventilator-associated bacterial pneumonia caused by susceptible isolates of *S. aureus* (including methicillin-susceptible and methicillin-resistant isolates)**
Adults: 10 mg/kg IV once every 24 hours for 7 to 21 days.

ADMINISTRATION
IV

▼ Reconstitute 750-mg vial with 45 mL sterile water for injection. Solutions of D₅W and NSS for injection also may be used. Mix thoroughly but don't shake; reconstitution may take up to 20 minutes. Resultant solution has a concentration of 15 mg/mL.

▼ Further dilute doses of 150 to 800 mg in 100 to 250 mL of D₅W, NSS, or lactated Ringer solution before infusion. Further dilute doses less than 150 mg or greater than 800 mg to a final concentration of 0.6 to 8 mg/mL.

▼ Inspect for particulate matter before infusion.

▼ Infuse drug over 60 minutes.

▼ Reconstituted solution is stable for 12 hours at room temperature or 7 days if refrigerated.

▼ Diluted IV solution is stable for 12 hours at room temperature, 7 days if refrigerated, or 32 days if frozen (includes reconstituted time).

▼ **Incompatibilities:** Other IV drugs. If line is used for other IV drugs, flush with D₅W, NSS, or lactated Ringer solution before and after infusion.

ACTION
Inhibits bacterial cell-wall synthesis by binding to the bacterial cell membrane and disrupting its function.

Route	Onset	Peak	Duration
IV	Unknown	Unknown	Unknown

Half-life: About 6½ to 9½ hours.

ADVERSE REACTIONS
CNS: dizziness. **CV:** QTc-interval prolongation. **GI:** abdominal pain, decreased appetite, diarrhea, nausea, taste disturbance, vomiting, CDAD. **GU:** foamy urine, new-onset or worsening renal impairment, *acute renal failure.* **Skin:** generalized pruritus,

---

Reactions in bold italics are *life-threatening*. Interactions may have a *rapid onset* or a *delayed onset*.

infusion-site pain, infusion-site erythema, rash. **Other:** rigors.

INTERACTIONS
Drug-drug. *Drugs that prolong QTc interval:* May enhance QTc-prolonging effect of highest-risk QTc-prolonging drugs. Avoid combination. May enhance QTc-prolonging effect of other moderate-risk QTc-prolonging drugs. Avoid such combinations when possible. Use should be accompanied by close monitoring for evidence of QT prolongation or other cardiac rhythm alterations.
Heparin: May artificially prolong PTT, which could lead to incorrect decrease of heparin dosage. Concomitant use with IV unfractionated heparin is contraindicated.
Vaccines (cholera, live attenuated Ty21a strain of typhoid): May diminish vaccine's effect. Avoid cholera vaccine within 14 days of oral or parenteral antibiotics; don't give typhoid vaccine until at least 3 days after stopping antibiotic.

EFFECTS ON LAB TEST RESULTS
• May falsely prolong PT, PTT, and activated clotting time, and may increase factor Xa and INR.
• May falsely affect urine qualitative dipstick protein assays and quantitative dye methods, such as pyrogallol red-molybdate.

CONTRAINDICATIONS & CAUTIONS
⊙ *Alert:* Serious and potentially fatal hypersensitivity reactions, including anaphylactic reactions, may occur after first or subsequent doses. Use cautiously in patients with known hypersensitivity to vancomycin.
⊙ *Alert:* Concomitant use of IV unfractionated heparin sodium is contraindicated because aPTT test results are expected to be artificially prolonged for 0 to 18 hours after administration.
• Avoid use in patients with prolonged QTc interval, uncompensated HF, or severe left ventricular hypertrophy.
Black Box Warning Drug may cause nephrotoxicity. Monitor renal function in all patients. Use drug in patients with preexisting moderate to severe renal impairment (CrCl of 50 mL/minute or less) only

when anticipated benefit outweighs potential risk. ∎

Black Box Warning Decreased effectiveness has occurred among patients with moderate to severe preexisting renal impairment being treated for skin and skin-structure infections. Consider alternative drug when selecting antibacterial therapy for patients with baseline CrCl of 50 mL/minute or less. ∎
• Safety and effectiveness in children haven't been established.
Dialyzable drug: 5.9%.

PREGNANCY-LACTATION-REPRODUCTION
Black Box Warning Women of childbearing potential should have a pregnancy test before therapy. Avoid use during pregnancy unless benefits outweigh potential risks to the fetus. ∎

Black Box Warning Adverse developmental outcomes observed in three animal species at clinically relevant doses raise concerns about potential adverse developmental outcomes in humans. ∎
• Register pregnant women exposed to drug in the Vibativ Pregnancy Registry (1-855-633-8479).
• It isn't known if drug appears in human milk. Use cautiously in breastfeeding women.

NURSING CONSIDERATIONS
Black Box Warning Monitor renal function before and during therapy. ∎
⊙ *Alert:* Rapid IV infusion may cause "redman syndrome" (flushing of the upper body, urticaria, pruritus, or rash on the face, neck, trunk, or upper extremities). Infuse over at least 60 minutes.
• If diarrhea develops, test patient for CDAD, which can be fatal and can occur up to 2 months after last dose.
• Watch for signs and symptoms of superinfection, such as continued fever, chills, and increased pulse rate.
• Reduce dosage in elderly who have diminished renal function.
• *Look alike–sound alike:* Don't confuse Vibativ with Viactiv.

PATIENT TEACHING
• Advise women of childbearing potential to use an effective method of contraception during therapy.

T

• Tell patient to report a history of kidney problems, heart problems (including QTc-interval prolongation), or diabetes before starting drug.
• Tell patient not to skip doses or to stop treatment without notifying prescriber.
• Tell patient to notify prescriber of all adverse reactions, especially if diarrhea develops during treatment or within 2 months of completing treatment.

---

telmisartan
tell-mah-SAR-tan

Micardis✍

Therapeutic class: Antihypertensives
Pharmacologic class: ARBs

AVAILABLE FORMS
Tablets: 20 mg, 40 mg, 80 mg

INDICATIONS & DOSAGES
Adjust-a-dose (for all indications): In patients with biliary obstructive disorders or hepatic insufficiency, initiate at low doses and up titrate slowly.
➤ **HTN (used alone or with other antihypertensives)**
Adults: 40 mg PO once daily. BP response is dose-related over a range of 20 to 80 mg once daily.
➤ **CV risk reduction in patients at high risk and unable to take ACE inhibitors**
Adults age 55 and older: 80 mg PO once daily.

ADMINISTRATION
PO
• Give drug without regard to meals.

ACTION
Blocks vasoconstricting and aldosterone-secreting effects of angiotensin II by preventing angiotensin II from binding to the angiotensin I receptor.

Route	Onset	Peak	Duration
PO	3 hr	30–60 min	24 hr

Half-life: 24 hours.

ADVERSE REACTIONS
CNS: dizziness, pain, fatigue, headache. **CV:** chest pain, HTN, peripheral edema, intermittent claudication. **EENT:** pharyngitis, sinusitis. **GI:** nausea, abdominal pain, diarrhea, dyspepsia. **GU:** UTI. **Musculoskeletal:** back pain, myalgia. **Respiratory:** cough, URI. **Other:** flulike symptoms.

INTERACTIONS
Drug-drug. *ACE inhibitors:* May affect renal function and cause acute renal failure. Consider therapy modification.
Aliskiren: Increases risk of renal impairment, hypotension, and hyperkalemia in diabetic patients. Use together is contraindicated. Also avoid coadministration in patients with moderate to severe renal impairment (GFR less than 60 mL/minute).
COX-2 inhibitors, NSAIDs: May result in worsening renal function. Monitor renal function periodically.
Digoxin: May increase digoxin level. Monitor digoxin level closely.
Lithium: May cause reversible increase in lithium level and toxicity. Monitor lithium level, and adjust lithium dose as needed.
Ramipril, ramiprilat: May increase levels of these drugs and decrease telmisartan level. Avoid use together.
Drug-food. *Salt substitutes containing potassium:* May cause hyperkalemia. Discourage use together.

EFFECTS ON LAB TEST RESULTS
• May increase BUN and potassium, serum creatinine, and liver enzyme levels.
• May decrease Hb level.

CONTRAINDICATIONS & CAUTIONS
• Contraindicated in patients hypersensitive to drug or its components and in patients with diabetes or renal impairment (GFR less than 60 mL/minute) also taking aliskiren.
• Use cautiously in patients with hypotension, biliary obstruction disorders, or renal and hepatic insufficiency and in those with an activated RAAS, such as volume- or sodium-depleted patients (for example, those being treated with high doses of diuretics).
Dialyzable drug: No.

Reactions in bold italics are *life-threatening*. Interactions may have a *rapid onset* or a *delayed onset*.

⚠ **Overdose S&S:** Hypotension, dizziness, tachycardia, bradycardia.

PREGNANCY-LACTATION-REPRODUCTION

Black Box Warning Use during pregnancy can cause injury and death to a developing fetus because drug acts directly on the RAAS. When pregnancy is detected, stop drug as soon as possible. ∎

• It isn't known if drug appears in human milk. Patient should discontinue breastfeeding or discontinue drug.

NURSING CONSIDERATIONS

• Monitor patient for hypotension after starting drug. Place patient supine if hypotension occurs, and give IV NSS, if needed.

• If possible, correct volume and sodium depletion before first dose. Use cautiously in patients with hyperkalemia.

• Most of the antihypertensive effect occurs within 2 weeks. Maximal BP reduction is usually reached after 4 weeks. Diuretic may be added if BP isn't controlled by drug alone.

❂ Alert: In patients whose renal function may depend on the activity of the RAAS (such as those with severe HF), drug may cause oliguria or progressive azotemia and (rarely) acute renal failure or death.

• Drug isn't removed by hemodialysis. Patients undergoing dialysis may develop orthostatic hypotension. Closely monitor BP.

• Monitor patients with impaired hepatic function or biliary obstruction carefully.

• Angioedema has been reported rarely. Monitor patient for signs of angioedema (swelling of head and neck). Discontinue drug immediately.

• Rhabdomyolysis has been reported rarely. Monitor patient for myalgia, stiffness, and muscle weakness.

PATIENT TEACHING

• Inform female patient of childbearing potential of the consequences of second- and third-trimester exposure to drug and to immediately report pregnancy.

• Advise breastfeeding patient that she will need to stop breastfeeding or stop drug.

• Tell patient that if dizziness or low BP occurs on standing, to lie down, rise slowly

from a lying to standing position, and climb stairs slowly.

• Tell patient that drug may be taken without regard to meals.

• Tell patient not to remove drug from blister-sealed packet until just before use.

• Tell patient to report all OTC drugs being taken before starting drug and to report all adverse reactions.

• Tell patient not to use salt substitutes containing potassium.

telotristat ethyl
tel-OH-tri-stat

Xermelo

Therapeutic class: Antidiarrheals
Pharmacologic class: Tryptophan hydroxylase inhibitors

AVAILABLE FORMS
Tablets: 250 mg

INDICATIONS & DOSAGES

➤ **Treatment of carcinoid syndrome diarrhea in combination with somatostatin analogue (SSA) therapy in patients inadequately controlled by SSA therapy**
Adults: 250 mg PO t.i.d.

ADMINISTRATION
PO

• Give with food to improve systemic drug exposure.

• Skip a missed dose and give next dose at the regular time. Don't give two doses at the same time.

• Store at controlled room temperature of 59° to 86° F (15° to 30° C).

ACTION

Patients with carcinoid syndrome experience an overproduction of serotonin, which mediates the secretion, motility, inflammation, and sensation of the GI tract. Telotristat ethyl reduces the production of serotonin, thus reducing the frequency of carcinoid syndrome diarrhea.

T

Route	Onset	Peak	Duration
PO	Unknown	½–2 hr	Unknown

Half-life: 0.6 hour; active metabolite, 5 hours.

ADVERSE REACTIONS

CNS: headache, depression, fever. **CV:** peripheral edema. **GI:** nausea, flatulence, decreased appetite, abdominal pain and distention, constipation.

INTERACTIONS

Drug-drug. *CYP3A4 substrates (midazolam):* May decrease effectiveness of CYP3A4 substrates. Monitor patient for suboptimal effects and consider increasing substrate dosage if necessary.
Octreotide (short-acting): May decrease levels of telotristat ethyl and its active metabolite. Administer short-acting octreotide at least 30 minutes after administering telotristat ethyl.

EFFECTS ON LAB TEST RESULTS

• May increase GGT, alkaline phosphatase, AST, and ALT levels.

CONTRAINDICATIONS & CAUTIONS

• Avoid use in patients with constipation.
• Safety and effectiveness in children haven't been established.
Dialyzable drug: Unknown.

PREGNANCY-LACTATION-REPRODUCTION

• Drug hasn't been studied in pregnant women. Adverse effects were observed in some animal studies.
• It isn't known if drug appears in human milk. Before patient starts breastfeeding, consider maternal benefits and potential adverse effects on the infant. If patient breastfeeds, monitor infant for constipation.

NURSING CONSIDERATIONS

• Monitor patient for constipation and severe, persistent, or worsening abdominal pain. Discontinue drug if these symptoms develop.
• *Look alike–sound alike:* Don't confuse Xermelo with Xarelto.

PATIENT TEACHING

• Advise patient to take drug with food.
• Instruct patient that if a dose is missed, to skip the missed dose and take the next dose at the regular time. Caution patient not to take two doses at the same time.
• Warn patient to discontinue drug and contact prescriber if constipation or severe, persistent, or worsening abdominal pain occurs.
• Caution female patient to notify prescriber if she is pregnant or plans to breastfeed.

SAFETY ALERT!

temazepam
te-MAZ-e-pam

Restoril◆

Therapeutic class: Hypnotics
Pharmacologic class: Benzodiazepines
Controlled substance schedule: IV

AVAILABLE FORMS

Capsules: 7.5 mg, 15 mg, 22.5 mg, 30 mg

INDICATIONS & DOSAGES

➤ **Short-term treatment (7 to 10 days) of insomnia**
Adults: 7.5 to 30 mg PO at bedtime.
Elderly or debilitated patients: Initially, 7.5 mg PO at bedtime until individualized response is determined.

ADMINISTRATION

PO
• Give drug 15 to 30 minutes before bedtime.
• Give drug without regard for food.

ACTION

Potentiates GABA neuronal inhibition in the CNS.

Route	Onset	Peak	Duration
PO	10–20 min	1½ hr	Unknown

Half-life: Terminal, 3½ to 18 hours.

ADVERSE REACTIONS

CNS: complex sleep-related behaviors, drowsiness, dizziness, hangover effect, lethargy, disturbed coordination, daytime sedation, confusion, nightmares, vertigo, euphoria, weakness, headache, fatigue, nervousness, anxiety, depression, minor changes in EEG patterns (usually low-voltage fast activity). **EENT:** blurred vision. **GI:** abdominal discomfort, diarrhea, nausea, dry mouth. **GU:** decreased libido. **Skin:** rash, diaphoresis.

INTERACTIONS

Drug-drug. *Antacids (aluminum hydroxide–containing):* May decrease or delay sedative effects. Monitor patient closely.

Clozapine: May cause delirium, sedation, sialorrhea, and ataxia. Don't start drugs simultaneously, and monitor patient carefully.

CNS depressants: May increase CNS depression. Use together cautiously.

Digoxin: May increase digoxin level. Monitor patient carefully for digoxin toxicity.

Diphenhydramine: May increase effects of both drugs. Use together cautiously.

Hormonal contraceptives: May increase temazepam clearance. Monitor patient closely.

Black Box Warning *Opioids:* May cause slow or difficult breathing, sedation, and death. Avoid use together. If use together is necessary, limit dosage and duration of each drug to minimum necessary for desired effect. ∎

Probenecid: May cause rapid or prolonged temazepam effects. Monitor patient for increased sedation or lethargy with concurrent use.

Theophylline: May decrease sedative effects. Monitor patient closely.

Drug-herb. *Calendula, kava kava, lemon balm, passion flower, skullcap, valerian:* May enhance sedation. Don't use together.

Drug-lifestyle. *Alcohol use:* May cause additive CNS depressant effects. Discourage use together.

EFFECTS ON LAB TEST RESULTS

• May increase LFT values.

CONTRAINDICATIONS & CAUTIONS

• Contraindicated in patients hypersensitive to drug or other benzodiazepines.

Black Box Warning Opioids should only be prescribed with benzodiazepines or other CNS depressants to patients for whom alternative treatment options are inadequate. ∎

• Use cautiously in patients with chronic pulmonary insufficiency, impaired hepatic or renal function, severe or latent depression, suicidal tendencies, and history of drug abuse. Abrupt discontinuation can result in withdrawal symptoms.

• Use cautiously in debilitated patients, those age 65 and older, and others at increased risk for oversedation, dizziness, confusion, ataxia, and falls.

⚠ *Alert:* Drug may cause rare but serious injury, including death, due to complex sleep behaviors, such as sleepwalking, sleep driving, and engaging in other activities while not fully awake. These behaviors can occur even at the lowest recommended doses and after just one dose.

Dialyzable drug: Unknown.

⚠ *Overdose S&S:* Somnolence, impaired coordination, slurred speech, confusion, coma, decreased reflexes, hypotension, seizures, respiratory depression, apnea.

PREGNANCY-LACTATION-REPRODUCTION

• Contraindicated in women who are or may become pregnant; may cause fetal harm. If used during pregnancy, or if patient becomes pregnant during therapy, apprise her of potential hazard to the fetus.

• It isn't known if drug appears in human milk. Use cautiously in breastfeeding women; monitor infants for possible drowsiness, lethargy, or weight loss.

NURSING CONSIDERATIONS

⚠ *Alert:* Monitor patient closely. Anaphylaxis and angioedema may occur as early as the first dose (rare).

• Assess mental status before starting therapy and reduce doses in elderly patients; these patients may be more sensitive to drug's adverse CNS effects.

• Take precautions to prevent drug hoarding by patients who are depressed, suicidal, or drug-dependent or who have a history of drug abuse.

• Don't stop drug abruptly as this may cause withdrawal symptoms (cramps, seizures, tremor, and sweating). To discontinue drug, follow a gradual dosage-tapering schedule.

• *Look alike–sound alike:* Don't confuse Restoril with Risperdal or Vistaril. Don't confuse temazepam with flurazepam.

T

PATIENT TEACHING

🜲 *Alert:* Warn patient that drug may cause allergic reactions (rare), facial swelling (rare), and complex sleep-related behaviors, such as driving, eating, and making phone calls while asleep. Advise patient to report these adverse effects.

Black Box Warning Caution patient or caregiver of patient taking an opioid with a benzodiazepine, CNS depressant, or alcohol to seek immediate medical attention if patient experiences dizziness, lightheadedness, extreme sleepiness, slowed or difficult breathing, or unresponsiveness. ∎

• Tell patient to avoid alcohol.

• Caution patient that drug increases risk of falls and to avoid performing activities that require mental alertness or physical coordination.

🜲 *Alert:* Warn patient of risk of injury or death related to complex sleep behaviors. Direct patient to stop drug and immediately report an episode of complex sleep behavior or not remembering activities performed while taking drug.

• Instruct patient to stop drug before becoming pregnant.

• Warn patient not to stop drug abruptly.

• Warn patient that psychological and physical dependence may occur with prolonged use.

• Tell patient to not take drug unless patient can stay in bed a full night (7 to 8 hours) before becoming active again.

SAFETY ALERT!

tenecteplase
teh-NEK-ti-plaze

TNKase

Therapeutic class: Thrombolytics
Pharmacologic class: Recombinant tissue plasminogen activators

AVAILABLE FORMS

Injection: 50 mg/vial

INDICATIONS & DOSAGES

➤ **To reduce risk of death from an acute MI**
Adults weighing 90 kg or more: 50 mg (10 mL) by IV bolus over 5 seconds.

Adults weighing 80 to less than 90 kg: 45 mg (9 mL) by IV bolus over 5 seconds.
Adults weighing 70 to just under 80 kg: 40 mg (8 mL) by IV bolus over 5 seconds.
Adults weighing 60 to just under 70 kg: 35 mg (7 mL) by IV bolus over 5 seconds.
Adults weighing less than 60 kg: 30 mg (6 mL) by IV bolus over 5 seconds. Maximum dose is 50 mg.

ADMINISTRATION

IV

▼ Give IV only. Don't give IM or subcut.

▼ Use syringe prefilled with 10 mL sterile water for injection (don't use bacteriostatic water for injection), and inject the entire contents into drug vial. Gently swirl solution once mixed. Don't shake. Visually inspect product for particulate matter before administration.

▼ Draw up the appropriate dose needed from the reconstituted vial with the syringe and discard any unused portion. Give drug immediately, or refrigerate and use within 8 hours.

▼ Give drug in a designated line. Flush dextrose-containing lines with NSS before administration.

▼ Give the drug rapidly over 5 seconds.

▼ Store vial in refrigerator at 36° to 46° F (2° to 8° C).

▼ **Incompatibilities:** Solutions containing dextrose, other IV drugs.

ACTION

Promotes fibrinolysis by binding to fibrin and converting plasminogen to plasmin.

Route	Onset	Peak	Duration
IV	Immediate	Immediate	Unknown

Half-life: 90 to 130 minutes.

ADVERSE REACTIONS

CNS: *stroke, intracranial hemorrhage.*
EENT: pharyngeal bleeding, epistaxis.
GI: *GI bleeding.* **GU:** hematuria. **Skin:** hematoma. **Other:** bleeding at puncture site.

INTERACTIONS

Drug-drug. Anticoagulants *(direct thrombin inhibitors, heparin, vitamin K antagonists), drugs that alter platelet function*

(aspirin, dipyridamole, glycoprotein IIb/IIIa inhibitors, NSAIDs): May increase risk of bleeding when used before, during, or after tenecteplase use. Use together cautiously.

Drug-herb. *Alfalfa, anise, bilberry:* May increase bleeding risk. Consider therapy modification.

EFFECTS ON LAB TEST RESULTS
• May prolong PT and PTT, and increase INR.

CONTRAINDICATIONS & CAUTIONS
• Contraindicated in patients with hypersensitivity to drug; active internal bleeding; history of stroke; intracranial or intraspinal surgery or trauma during previous 2 months; intracranial neoplasm, aneurysm, or arteriovenous malformation; severe uncontrolled HTN; or bleeding diathesis.
• Use cautiously in patients who have had recent major surgery (such as CABG), organ biopsy, obstetric delivery, or previous puncture of noncompressible vessels.
• Use cautiously in patients age 75 and older and patients with recent trauma, recent GI or GU bleeding, high risk of left ventricular thrombus, acute pericarditis, systolic BP 180 mm Hg or higher or diastolic BP 110 mm Hg or higher, severe hepatic dysfunction, hemostatic defects, subacute bacterial endocarditis, septic thrombophlebitis, diabetic hemorrhagic retinopathy, or cerebrovascular disease.
Dialyzable drug: Unknown.

PREGNANCY-LACTATION-REPRODUCTION
• There are no adequate studies in pregnant women. Use only if potential benefit justifies potential risk to the fetus.
• It isn't known if drug appears in human milk. Use cautiously in breastfeeding women.

NURSING CONSIDERATIONS
• Begin therapy as soon as possible after onset of MI symptoms.
• Avoid noncompressible arterial punctures and internal jugular and subclavian venous punctures. Minimize all arterial and venous punctures during treatment.
• Avoid IM injections and nonessential patient handling for first few hours after treatment.

• Give heparin as prescribed but not in the same IV line.
• Monitor patient for bleeding. If serious bleeding occurs, stop heparin and antiplatelet drugs immediately.
⚠ *Alert:* Use exact patient weight for dosage. An overestimation in patient weight can lead to significant increase in bleeding or intracerebral hemorrhage.
• Monitor ECG for reperfusion arrhythmias.
• Life-threatening cholesterol embolism has been rarely reported in patients treated with thrombolytics. Signs and symptoms may include livedo reticularis (blue toe syndrome), acute renal failure, gangrenous digits, HTN, pancreatitis, MI, cerebral infarction, spinal cord infarction, retinal artery occlusion, bowel infarction, and rhabdomyolysis.

PATIENT TEACHING
• Tell patient to immediately report all adverse reactions, including bleeding.
• Explain use of drug to patient and family.

---

tenofovir disoproxil fumarate
te-NOE-fo-veer

Viread℗

Therapeutic class: Antiretrovirals
Pharmacologic class: Nucleoside–nucleotide reverse transcriptase inhibitors

AVAILABLE FORMS
Oral powder: 40 mg. One level scoop delivers 1 g of powder containing tenofovir 40 mg
Tablets: 150 mg, 200 mg, 250 mg, 300 mg

INDICATIONS & DOSAGES
Adjust-a-dose (for all indications): For adults with CrCl of 30 to 49 mL/minute, 300 mg PO every 48 hours. For CrCl of 10 to 29 mL/minute, 300 mg PO every 72 to 96 hours. For patients receiving hemodialysis, 300 mg PO every 7 days or after a total of about 12 hours of hemodialysis. Give dose after session. There are no recommendations for patients with CrCl of less than 10 mL/minute not receiving hemodialysis or for children with renal impairment.
➤ **HIV-1 infection, with other antiretrovirals; chronic HBV infection**

Tablets

Adults and children age 2 and older weighing 35 kg or more: 300 mg PO once daily.

Adults and children age 2 and older weighing 17 to less than 35 kg and able to swallow intact tablet: 8 mg/kg PO once daily up to maximum of 300 mg. Refer to product insert for specific weight-based dosing.

Powder

Adults and children age 2 and older weighing at least 10 kg and unable to swallow tablet: 8 mg/kg PO once daily. Maximum dosage is 300 mg/day. See product insert for weight-based dosing.

ADMINISTRATION
PO

• Give without regard to food.

• Monitor weight periodically and adjust dosage accordingly.

• For patients receiving tenofovir and didanosine (enteric-coated form), give under fasting conditions or with a light meal (less than 400 kcal, 20% fat). Buffered form of didanosine taken with tenofovir should be given under fasting conditions.

• For patients receiving tenofovir powder, measure only with supplied dosing scoop. Mix in container with 2 to 4 oz of soft food not requiring chewing (such as applesauce, baby food, or yogurt). Patient should ingest entire mixture immediately to avoid bitter taste. Don't administer tenofovir in a liquid because the powder may float on top of the liquid, even after stirring.

ACTION
Hydrolyzed to produce tenofovir, a nucleoside analogue of adenosine monophosphate that yields tenofovir diphosphate. Tenofovir diphosphate inhibits HIV replication by inhibiting viral RNA-dependent DNA polymerase. Tenofovir inhibits replication of HBV by inhibiting HBV polymerase.

Route	Onset	Peak	Duration
PO	Unknown	36–144 min	Unknown

Half-life: 17 hours.

ADVERSE REACTIONS
CNS: asthenia, headache, pain, fever, peripheral neuropathy, insomnia, dizziness, depression, anxiety, fatigue, weakness. **CV:** chest pain. **EENT:** sinusitis, nasopharyngitis. **GI:** nausea, abdominal pain, dyspepsia, diarrhea, vomiting, anorexia, flatulence. **GU:** hematuria, *renal failure.* **Hematologic:** *neutropenia.* **Hepatic:** hepatomegaly, *hepatitis.* **Metabolic:** hyperglycemia, *lactic acidosis,* weight loss. **Musculoskeletal:** arthralgia, back pain, myalgia, decreased bone mineral density. **Respiratory:** URI, pneumonia. **Skin:** rash, pruritus, diaphoresis. **Other:** lipodystrophy.

INTERACTIONS
Drug-drug. *Adefovir:* May diminish therapeutic effect of tenofovir; may increase serum concentration of both drugs, resulting in additive nephrotoxicity. Avoid combination.

Atazanavir: May decrease atazanavir level, causing resistance. Give both drugs with ritonavir.

Atazanavir with ritonavir, darunavir with ritonavir, lopinavir–ritonavir: May increase tenofovir-associated adverse reactions. Monitor patient carefully.

Didanosine (buffered or enteric-coated form): May increase didanosine bioavailability. For adults weighing more than 60 kg, reduce didanosine dose to 250 mg PO once daily; for those weighing less than 60 kg, reduce didanosine dose to 200 mg PO once daily. Use together cautiously and monitor patient closely for didanosine-associated adverse reactions.

Drugs that reduce renal function or compete for renal tubular secretion (acyclovir, aminoglycosides, cidofovir, ganciclovir, NSAIDs, valacyclovir, valganciclovir): May increase levels of tenofovir or other renally eliminated drugs. Monitor patient for adverse effects.

Ledipasvir/sofosbuvir: May increase tenofovir exposure. When given with tenofovir without an HIV-1 protease inhibitor/ritonavir or an HIV-1 protease inhibitor/cobicistat combination, monitor patient for adverse reactions associated with tenofovir. When given with tenofovir and an HIV-1 protease inhibitor/ritonavir or an HIV-1 protease inhibitor/cobicistat combination, consider modifying therapy. If use together is necessary, monitor patient for tenofovir-associated adverse effects.

Reactions in bold italics are *life-threatening*. Interactions may have a *rapid onset* or a *delayed onset*.

Sofosbuvir/velpatasvir: May increase tenofovir exposure. Monitor patient for tenofovir-associated adverse effects.
Drug-food. *Fatty meals:* May increase tenofovir bioavailability. Monitor patient for adverse effects.

EFFECTS ON LAB TEST RESULTS
• May increase amylase, AST, ALT, alkaline phosphatase, CK, serum and urine glucose, creatinine, phosphate, cholesterol, and triglyceride levels.
• May decrease neutrophil count.

CONTRAINDICATIONS & CAUTIONS
• Contraindicated in patients hypersensitive to components of drug.
• Use very cautiously in patients with risk factors for liver disease or with hepatic impairment.
• Use cautiously in patients with renal impairment; avoid use with concurrent or recent nephrotoxic therapy.
• Use cautiously in patients at higher risk for decreased renal function, including elderly patients and patients with recent or concurrent use of nephrotoxic drugs.
• Don't use tenofovir for the treatment of HIV-1 infection in combination with the fixed-dose combination products that also contain tenofovir, such as Atripla, Complera, Descovy, Genvoya, Odefsey, Stribild, Truvada, or Vemlidy. Don't administer tenofovir with adefovir.
Dialyzable drug: Yes.

PREGNANCY-LACTATION-REPRODUCTION
• There are no adequate studies in pregnant women. Use only if clearly needed.
• Register pregnant women exposed to drug in the Antiretroviral Pregnancy Registry (1-800-258-4263).
• The CDC recommends that mothers with HIV-1 infection not breastfeed to avoid risking postnatal transmission of HIV-1. Advise women not to breastfeed.

NURSING CONSIDERATIONS
• Before starting drug, test patient for HBV infection and HIV-1 infection. Don't use tenofovir alone in patients with HIV-1 infection.

◑ *Alert:* Drug may cause lactic acidosis and hepatomegaly with steatosis, even fatal cases. These effects may occur without elevated transaminase levels. Risk factors include long-term antiretroviral use, obesity, and being female. Monitor all patients closely.
• Assess estimated CrCl and serum creatinine, urine glucose, and urine protein levels at baseline and during therapy as clinically appropriate in all patients. In patients with chronic kidney disease, also assess serum phosphorus level.
Black Box Warning Severe acute exacerbations of hepatitis have been reported in HBV-infected patients after anti-HBV therapy has stopped. Monitor hepatic function closely for at least several months. Resumption of therapy may be warranted. ∎
• Drug may be linked to osteomalacia and decreased bone mineral density, increased creatinine and BUN levels, and phosphaturia. Monitor patient carefully.
• Drug may lead to decreased HIV-RNA level and CD4$^+$ cell counts.
• Monitor patient for immune reconstitution syndrome, an inflammatory response to indolent or residual opportunistic infections, which may require further evaluation and treatment. Autoimmune disorders have also been reported.

PATIENT TEACHING
• Instruct patient to take drug with or without food.
• Inform patient that drug doesn't cure HIV infection, that opportunistic infections and other complications of HIV infection may still occur, and that transmission of HIV to others through sexual contact or blood contamination is still possible.
• Instruct patient taking tenofovir and didanosine (buffered or enteric-coated form) to take these drugs on an empty stomach or with a light meal (less than 400 kcal, 20% fat).
• Tell patient to report adverse effects, including nausea, vomiting, diarrhea, flatulence, and headache.
• Advise patient to consult prescriber before taking OTC or other prescription medications or supplements, vitamins, or herbal supplements.
• Advise female patient not to breastfeed.

terazosin hydrochloride
ter-AY-zoe-sin

Therapeutic class: Antihypertensives
Pharmacologic class: Alpha blockers

AVAILABLE FORMS
Capsules: 1 mg, 2 mg, 5 mg, 10 mg

INDICATIONS & DOSAGES
➤ **HTN**
Adults: Initially, 1 mg PO at bedtime. May increase dosage gradually based on response. Usual dosage range is 1 to 5 mg daily. Maximum recommended dosage is 20 mg daily. If response is substantially diminished at 24 hours, consider a dosage increase or use of a twice-daily regimen.
➤ **Symptomatic BPH**
Adults: Initially, 1 mg PO at bedtime. Dosage may be titrated to 2, 5, or 10 mg once daily to achieve optimal response. Most patients need 10 mg daily for optimal response. Maximum recommended dosage is 20 mg/day.

ADMINISTRATION
PO
• Give drug without regard for meals.
• If drug is discontinued for several days or longer, restart drug with the initial dosing regimen.

ACTION
Improves urine flow in patients with BPH by blocking alpha-adrenergic receptors in the bladder neck and prostate, relieving urethral pressure. Drug also reduces peripheral vascular resistance and BP via arterial and venous dilation.

Route	Onset	Peak	Duration
PO	15 min	1 hr	24 hr

Half-life: About 12 hours.

ADVERSE REACTIONS
CNS: headache, dizziness, asthenia, first-dose syncope, nervousness, paresthesia, drowsiness, somnolence. **CV:** peripheral edema, palpitations, orthostatic hypotension, tachycardia. **EENT:** conjunctivitis, blurred vision, tinnitus, nasal congestion, sinusitis.

GI: nausea, constipation, dyspepsia, vomiting. **GU:** erectile dysfunction. **Hematologic:** *thrombocytopenia.* **Musculoskeletal:** back pain, muscle pain. **Respiratory:** dyspnea, flulike symptoms, cough. **Skin:** pruritus, rash, sweating.

INTERACTIONS
Drug-drug. *Antihypertensives, antipsychotics, calcium channel blockers (verapamil), PDE5 inhibitors (tadalafil, vardenafil):* May cause excessive hypotension. Use together cautiously.
Drug-herb. *Yohimbe:* May diminish antihypertensive effect of drug. Monitor therapy.

EFFECTS ON LAB TEST RESULTS
• May decrease total protein, albumin, total cholesterol, and combined LDL and VLDL levels. May decrease Hb level and hematocrit.
• May decrease WBC and platelet counts.

CONTRAINDICATIONS & CAUTIONS
• Contraindicated in patients hypersensitive to drug.
• May cause marked lowering of BP, especially orthostatic hypotension, and syncope in association with first dose or first few days of therapy. A similar effect can be expected if therapy is interrupted for several days, then restarted.
• Intraoperative floppy iris syndrome has been observed during cataract and glaucoma surgery in some patients who are taking or had previously taken alpha$_1$ blockers, which may increase risk of eye complications during and after surgery. Initiation of drug in patients for whom cataract or glaucoma surgery is scheduled isn't recommended.
• May cause CNS depression and impair mental alertness.
• Rare cases of priapism have been reported.
Dialyzable drug: 10%.
⚠ *Overdose S&S:* Hypotension.

PREGNANCY-LACTATION-REPRODUCTION
• There are no adequate studies in pregnant women, and safety in pregnancy hasn't been established. Use only if potential benefit justifies potential risk to the fetus.

Reactions in bold italics are *life-threatening*. Interactions may have a *rapid onset* or a ***delayed onset***.

• It isn't known if drug appears in human milk. Use cautiously in breastfeeding women.

NURSING CONSIDERATIONS
• Monitor BP frequently.
• Symptoms of BPH and prostate cancer are similar. Rule out prostate cancer before start of therapy.

PATIENT TEACHING
• Tell patient not to stop drug suddenly but to notify prescriber if adverse reactions occur.
• Inform patient about the rare but serious possibility of priapism and to report it immediately.
• Warn patient to avoid hazardous activities that require mental alertness, such as driving or operating heavy machinery, for 12 hours after first dose.
• Tell patient that light-headedness from hypotension can occur. Advise patient to rise slowly and to report signs and symptoms to prescriber.
• Advise patient considering cataract or glaucoma surgery to inform ophthalmologist about taking terazosin.

terbinafine hydrochloride (oral)
ter-BIN-ah-fin

Lamisil

Therapeutic class: Antifungals
Pharmacologic class: Synthetic allylamine derivatives

AVAILABLE FORMS
Tablets: 250 mg

INDICATIONS & DOSAGES
➤ **Fingernail and toenail onychomycosis caused by dermatophytes (tinea unguium)**
Adults: 250 mg PO once daily for 6 weeks for fingernail infection and 12 weeks for toenail infection.

ADMINISTRATION
PO
• Obtain pretreatment transaminase levels for all patients taking drug to evaluate for chronic or active liver disease.

• Give tablets without regard for food.
• Store tablets below 77° F (25° C); protect from light.

ACTION
Prevents biosynthesis of ergosterol, causing a deficiency of this essential component of fungal cell membranes.

Route	Onset	Peak	Duration
PO	Unknown	≤2 hr	Unknown

Half-life: Adults, 36 hours; children, 27 to 31 hours.

ADVERSE REACTIONS
CNS: headache, pyrexia. **EENT:** vision disturbances, smell disturbances, nasopharyngitis. **GI:** taste disturbances, diarrhea, dyspepsia, abdominal pain, flatulence. **Hematologic:** *neutropenia, thrombocytopenia.* **Hepatic:** liver enzyme elevations. **Skin:** rash, pruritus, urticaria.

INTERACTIONS
Drug-drug. *Antiarrhythmics class 1C (flecainide) and beta blockers:* Inhibits drugs metabolized by CYP2D6 isozyme. Monitor patient carefully and decrease dosage as necessary.
Caffeine: May decrease caffeine clearance. Use cautiously together.
Cimetidine: May decrease clearance of terbinafine by a third. Avoid using together.
Codeine: May decrease serum concentration of codeine's active metabolite. Monitor therapy.
Cyclosporine: May increase cyclosporine clearance. Monitor cyclosporine level.
CYP2C9, CYP3A4 enzyme inhibitors (amiodarone, fluconazole): May substantially increase systemic exposure of terbinafine. Use together cautiously.
CYP2D6 substrates: May inhibit substrate metabolism. Dosage adjustment may be needed. Monitor therapy.
Rifampin: Increases terbinafine clearance by 100%. Avoid use together.
SSRIs (paroxetine, venlafaxine): May increase SSRI levels. Monitor patient carefully and adjust SSRI dosage as necessary.
Tamoxifen: May decrease serum concentration of tamoxifen's active metabolite. Consider alternative to terbinafine.

T

Tramadol: May decrease serum concentration of tramadol's active metabolite. Monitor patient closely.

EFFECTS ON LAB TEST RESULTS
• May increase AST and ALT levels.
• May decrease neutrophil and lymphocyte counts.

CONTRAINDICATIONS & CAUTIONS
• Contraindicated in patients hypersensitive to drug or its components.
❸ Alert: Contraindicated in patients with chronic or active liver disease.
• Cases of liver failure, some leading to liver transplant or death, have occurred in patients with and without preexisting liver disease.
• Serious skin reactions (SJS, toxic epidermal necrolysis, and others) and hypersensitivity reactions have occurred. If these occur, discontinue drug.
• Thrombotic microangiopathy (TMA), including thrombotic thrombocytopenic purpura and hemolytic-uremic syndrome, can occur and fatalities have been reported.
• There have been postmarketing reports of new and worsened cases of cutaneous lupus erythematosus and SLE. Discontinue drug in patients with signs and symptoms suggestive of SLE.
Dialyzable drug: Unknown.
⚠ Overdose S&S: Abdominal pain, dizziness, frequent urination, headache, nausea, rash, vomiting.

PREGNANCY-LACTATION-REPRODUCTION
• There are no adequate studies in pregnant women. Because treatment can be postponed until after pregnancy is completed, it's recommended that terbinafine not be initiated during pregnancy.
• Drug appears in human milk. Use in breastfeeding women isn't recommended.

NURSING CONSIDERATIONS
❸ Alert: Rarely, patients may suffer life-threatening liver failure.
• Monitor CBC and hepatic enzyme levels in patients taking drug for longer than 6 weeks, especially those with known or suspected immunodeficiency. Stop drug if hepatobiliary dysfunction or cholestatic hepatitis develops.

• Monitor and evaluate patients who develop unexplained thrombocytopenia and anemia for TMA. Discontinue drug if clinical signs and symptoms and lab findings consistent with TMA occur.
• **Look alike–sound alike:** Don't confuse terbinafine with terbutaline.

PATIENT TEACHING
• Inform patient that successful treatment may take 12 weeks for toenail infections and 6 weeks for fingernail infections.
• Tell patient to immediately report depression; smell, taste, or vision disturbances (changes in the ocular lens and retina may occur); and persistent nausea, anorexia, fatigue, vomiting, right upper quadrant pain, jaundice, dark urine, or pale stools.

terbutaline sulfate
ter-BYOO-ta-leen

Therapeutic class: Bronchodilators
Pharmacologic class: Beta₂ agonists

AVAILABLE FORMS
Injection: 1 mg/mL
Tablets: 2.5 mg, 5 mg

INDICATIONS & DOSAGES
➤ **Prevention and reversal of bronchospasm in patients with asthma and reversible bronchospasm associated with bronchitis and emphysema**
Adults and children age 12 and older:
0.25 mg subcut. If needed, repeat in 15 to 30 minutes. Maximum, 0.5 mg in 4 hours. If patient fails to respond to second dose, consider other measures.
Adults and adolescents older than age 15:
2.5 to 5 mg PO t.i.d. every 6 hours while awake. Maximum, 15 mg daily.
Children ages 12 to 15: 2.5 mg PO t.i.d. every 6 hours while awake. Maximum, 7.5 mg daily.

ADMINISTRATION
PO
• Give drug without regard for food.
Subcutaneous
• Give subcut injections into the side of the deltoid.

• Protect drug from light. Don't use if discolored.

ACTION
Relaxes bronchial smooth muscle by stimulating beta$_2$ receptors.

Route	Onset	Peak	Duration
PO	30 min	½–3 hr	4–8 hr
Subcut	6–15 min	30 min	1½–4 hr

Half-life: Oral, 3.4 hours; subcut, 2.9 to 14 hours.

ADVERSE REACTIONS
CNS: nervousness, tremor, drowsiness, dizziness, headache, weakness, anxiety, somnolence, insomnia. **CV:** palpitations, *arrhythmias,* tachycardia, flushing. **GI:** vomiting, nausea, dry mouth. **Metabolic:** hypokalemia, transient hyperglycemia. **Respiratory:** dyspnea. **Skin:** diaphoresis, pain at injection site.

INTERACTIONS
Drug-drug. *Cardiac glycosides, cyclopropane, halogenated inhaled anesthetics, levodopa:* May increase risk of arrhythmias. Monitor patient closely, and avoid using together with levodopa.
CNS stimulants: May increase CNS stimulation. Avoid using together.
Diuretics (loop, thiazide): May increase risk of hypokalemia. Use together cautiously.
Drugs that prolong QTc interval: May increase risk of QTc-interval prolongation. Monitor therapy closely.
MAO inhibitors (including linezolid and tedizolid), TCAs: When given with sympathomimetics, may cause severe HTN (hypertensive crisis). Avoid using together or within 2 weeks.
Propranolol, other beta blockers: May block bronchodilating effects of terbutaline. Avoid using together.
Sympathomimetics (ephedrine): May result in additive CV effects. Monitor HR and rhythm.

EFFECTS ON LAB TEST RESULTS
• May increase glucose level.
• May decrease potassium level.

CONTRAINDICATIONS & CAUTIONS
• Contraindicated in patients hypersensitive to drug or sympathomimetic amines.
• Use cautiously in patient with CV disorders, hyperthyroidism, diabetes, or seizure disorders.
Dialyzable drug: Unknown.
⚠ Overdose S&S: Seizures, angina, HTN, hypotension, tachycardia, arrhythmias, nervousness, headache, tremors, dry mouth, palpitations, nausea, dizziness, fatigue, insomnia, hypokalemia.

PREGNANCY-LACTATION-REPRODUCTION
• There are no adequate studies in pregnant women. Use only if potential benefit justifies potential risk to the fetus.
Black Box Warning Injectable form is contraindicated in pregnant women for prevention or prolonged treatment (beyond 48 to 72 hours) of preterm labor in either the hospital or outpatient setting because of the potential for serious maternal heart problems and death. Oral terbutaline is contraindicated for prevention or for any treatment of preterm labor. ∎
• It isn't known if drug appears in human milk. Use during breastfeeding only if potential benefit justifies potential risk to the infant.

NURSING CONSIDERATIONS
• Monitor glucose and potassium levels, pulmonary function, and CV effects (HR, BP, ECG, QTc-interval prolongation) in pregnant patients.
• *Look alike–sound alike:* Don't confuse terbutaline with tolbutamide or terbinafine.

PATIENT TEACHING
• Ensure patient and caregivers understand drug's use.
• Instruct patient to immediately report changes in heart rate or rhythm, which patient may experience as feeling anxious, palpitations, or a racing heart.
• Advise patient to immediately report wheezing, chest tightness, bad cough, blue skin color, or difficulty breathing.

T

terconazole
ter-CONE-uh-zole

Therapeutic class: Antifungals
Pharmacologic class: Triazole derivatives

AVAILABLE FORMS
Vaginal cream: 0.4%*, 0.8%*
Vaginal suppositories: 80 mg

INDICATIONS & DOSAGES
➤ **Vulvovaginal candidiasis**
Adults: One applicatorful of cream or 1 suppository inserted into vagina at bedtime; 0.4% cream used for 7 consecutive days; 0.8% cream or 80-mg suppository for 3 consecutive days. Repeat course, if needed, after reconfirmation by smear or culture.

ADMINISTRATION
Vaginal
• Insert drug high in vagina (unless patient is pregnant).
• Wash applicator after each use and allow it to dry thoroughly.
• Store drug at room temperature.

ACTION
May increase *Candida* cell membrane permeability.

Route	Onset	Peak	Duration
Vaginal	Unknown	5–10 hr	Unknown

Half-life: 6.4 to 8.5 hours.

ADVERSE REACTIONS
CNS: headache, fever. **GI:** abdominal pain. **GU:** dysmenorrhea, genital pain, vulvovaginal burning. **Skin:** pruritus, irritation. **Other:** body aches, chills.

INTERACTIONS
None significant.

EFFECTS ON LAB TEST RESULTS
None reported.

CONTRAINDICATIONS & CAUTIONS
• Contraindicated in patients hypersensitive to drug or its inactive ingredients.
Dialyzable drug: Unknown.

PREGNANCY-LACTATION-REPRODUCTION
• Because drug is absorbed from the vagina, it shouldn't be used in the first trimester unless prescriber considers it essential to patient's welfare.
• May use during the second and third trimesters if potential benefit outweighs potential risks to the fetus.
• It isn't known if drug appears in human milk. Patient should discontinue breastfeeding or discontinue drug.

NURSING CONSIDERATIONS
• Therapeutic effect of drug is unaffected by menstruation or hormonal contraceptive use.
• Assess patient's ability to self-administer. Self-administration may be difficult in patients with arthritis or limited range of motion.
• *Look alike–sound alike:* Don't confuse terconazole with tioconazole.

PATIENT TEACHING
• Advise patient to administer drug at bedtime.
• Advise patient to continue treatment during menstrual period. However, tell her not to use tampons.
• Instruct patient on self-administration of drug; remind her to insert drug high in vagina (except during pregnancy).
• Tell patient to use drug for full treatment period prescribed. Explain how to prevent reinfection.
• Instruct patient to notify prescriber and stop drug if fever, chills, other flulike signs and symptoms, or sensitivity develops.
• Caution patient to refrain from sexual intercourse during treatment.
• Tell patient that drug base may react with latex or rubber, causing decreased effectiveness of condoms and diaphragms (for up to 72 hours after treatment is completed).
• Advise patient that her partner also may need treatment if he has symptoms.
• Instruct patient to wash applicator after each use and to allow it to dry thoroughly.

Reactions in bold italics are *life-threatening*. Interactions may have a *rapid onset* or a ***delayed onset***.

teriparatide (rDNA origin)
tehr-ih-PAHR-uh-tide

Forteo

Therapeutic class: Antiosteoporotics
Pharmacologic class: Recombinant human
parathyroid hormones

AVAILABLE FORMS
Injection: 20 mcg/dose in multidose prefilled pen

INDICATIONS & DOSAGES
➤ **Osteoporosis in postmenopausal
women at high risk for fracture; primary
or hypogonadal osteoporosis in men at
high risk for fracture; glucocorticoid-
induced osteoporosis in men and women**
Adults: 20 mcg subcut in thigh or abdominal
wall once daily for up to 2 years.

ADMINISTRATION
Subcutaneous
• Give drug without regard to meals or time
of day.
• Keep refrigerated at all times; minimize
time out of refrigerator during use.
• After each use, safely remove the needle,
recap the delivery device, and put it back in
the refrigerator right away.
• Inspect solution before giving.
• Drug is a colorless, clear liquid. Don't use
if solid particles are present or if solution is
cloudy or colored.
• Give while patient is sitting or lying down
to avoid orthostatic hypotension.
• Rotate administration sites.
• Discard pen after 28-day use, even if some
unused solution still remains.

ACTION
Promotes new bone formation, skeletal bone
mass, and bone strength by regulating calcium and phosphorus metabolism in bones
and kidneys.

Route	Onset	Peak	Duration
Subcut	Rapid	30 min	3 hr

Half-life: 1 hour.

ADVERSE REACTIONS
CNS: asthenia, depression, dizziness,
headache, insomnia, pain, syncope, vertigo. **CV:** angina pectoris, HTN, orthostatic
hypotension. **EENT:** pharyngitis, rhinitis. **GI:** constipation, diarrhea, dyspepsia,
gastritis, nausea, tooth disorder, vomiting.
Metabolic: hypercalcemia, hyperuricemia.
Musculoskeletal: arthralgia, leg cramps,
neck pain. **Respiratory:** dyspnea, increased
cough, pneumonia. **Skin:** rash, sweating.
Other: herpes zoster.

INTERACTIONS
Drug-drug. *Calcium supplements:* May increase urinary calcium excretion. Dosage
may need adjustment.
Digoxin: May predispose hypercalcemic patient to digitalis toxicity. Use together cautiously.

EFFECTS ON LAB TEST RESULTS
• May increase calcium and uric acid levels.
May decrease phosphorus level.
• May increase urinary calcium and phos-
phorus excretion.

CONTRAINDICATIONS & CAUTIONS
• Contraindicated in patients hypersensitive
to drug or its components.
Black Box Warning Drug increases risk
of osteosarcoma and is contraindicated in
patients at increased risk for osteosarcoma,
such as those with Paget disease or unexplained alkaline phosphatase elevations,
children and young adults with open epiphyses, and patients who have had skeletal
radiation. ■
• Contraindicated in patients with bone
metastases; a history of skeletal malignancies, hypercalcemia, or metabolic bone diseases other than osteoporosis; and in patients
with hypercalcemia.
• Use cautiously in patients with active or
recent urolithiasis; hepatic, renal, or cardiac
disease; or hypotension.
Dialyzable drug: Unknown.
⚠ *Overdose S&S:* Hypercalcemia, orthostatic
hypotension, nausea, vomiting, dizziness,
headache.

T

PREGNANCY-LACTATION-REPRODUCTION
• There are no adequate studies in pregnant women. Use only if potential benefit justifies potential risk to the fetus.
• There are no indications for use in pregnant or premenopausal women.
• It isn't known if drug appears in human milk. Patient should discontinue breastfeeding or discontinue drug.

NURSING CONSIDERATIONS
• Treatment shouldn't exceed 2 years.
• If patient may have urolithiasis or hypercalciuria, measure urinary calcium excretion before treatment.
• Monitor patient for orthostatic hypotension.
• Monitor calcium level. If persistent hypercalcemia develops, stop drug and evaluate possible cause.
• *Look alike–sound alike:* Don't confuse Forteo with Forfivo XL.

PATIENT TEACHING
• Instruct patient on proper use and disposal of prefilled pen.
• Tell patient not to share pen with others.
• Advise patient to remain in a sitting position while taking drug to prevent orthostatic hypotension.
• Advise patient to sit or lie down if drug causes a fast heartbeat, light-headedness, or dizziness. Tell patient to report persistent or worsening symptoms.
• Urge patient to report persistent symptoms of hypercalcemia, which include nausea, vomiting, constipation, lethargy, and muscle weakness.
• Tell patient to discard pen after 28-day use period, even if some unused solution remains.
• Encourage adequate calcium and vitamin D intake in the diet or by supplementation.
• Encourage patient to enroll in the Forteo Patient Registry (1-866-382-6813 or www.forteoregistry.rti.org) to monitor potential risk of osteosarcoma.

testosterone
tes-TOS-te-rone

Natesto, Striant, Testopel

testosterone cypionate
Depo-Testosterone

testosterone enanthate
Xyosted

testosterone undecanoate
Aveed, Jatenzo

Therapeutic class: Androgens
Pharmacologic class: Androgens
Controlled substance schedule: III

AVAILABLE FORMS
testosterone
Blister packs (buccal; extended-release) ⒪ⒷⒸ:
30 mg
Nasal gel (metered): 5.5 mg/actuation
Pellets (subcut implant): 75 mg
testosterone cypionate
Injection (in oil): 100 mg/mL*,
200 mg/mL*
testosterone enanthate
Autoinjector: 50 mg/0.5 mL, 75 mg/0.5 mL,
100 mg/0.5 mL
Injection (in oil): 200 mg/mL
testosterone undecanoate
Capsules: 158 mg, 198 mg, 237 mg
Injection (in oil): 250 mg/mL

INDICATIONS & DOSAGES
➤ **Hypogonadism**
Men: 50 to 400 mg cypionate or enanthate in oil IM every 2 to 4 weeks. Or, 75 mg enanthate autoinjector subcut in abdominal region once a week. Or, 750 mg undecanoate in oil IM, followed by 750 mg IM 4 weeks later, then 750 mg IM every 10 weeks thereafter. Or, initially, 237 mg undecanoate capsules PO b.i.d. (morning and evening). Or, 150 to 450 mg (2 to 6 pellets) implanted subcut every 3 to 6 months. Or, apply 1 buccal system (30 mg) to the gum region just above the incisor tooth on either side of the mouth b.i.d. (morning and evening) about 12 hours apart. Alternate sides of the mouth with each application. Or, 11 mg (2 pump actuations;

1 actuation per nostril) intranasally t.i.d., once in the morning, once in the afternoon, and once in the evening (6 to 8 hours apart), preferably at same time each day for a total daily dose of 33 mg.

Adjust-a-dose: When total testosterone concentration consistently exceeds 1,050 ng/dL, discontinue therapy. If total testosterone concentration is consistently below 300 ng/dL, consider alternative treatment. Adjust dosage as indicated in product inserts and periodic measurement of serum testosterone concentration.

➤ **Delayed puberty**
Men and boys: 50 to 200 mg enanthate IM every 2 to 4 weeks for 4 to 6 months. Or, 150 to 450 mg (2 to 6 pellets) implanted subcut every 3 to 6 months for a limited duration (e.g., 4 to 6 months).

➤ **Metastatic breast cancer**
Women 1 to 5 years after menopause: 200 to 400 mg enanthate IM every 2 to 4 weeks.

ADMINISTRATION

• Hazardous drug; use safe handling and disposal precautions according to facility policy.

PO
• Give with food.

IM
• Store IM preparations at room temperature. If crystals appear, warm and shake bottle to disperse them.
• Inject deep into upper outer quadrant of gluteal muscle. Rotate injection sites; report soreness at site.

Subcutaneous
• In most men, the pellets are implanted in an area on the anterior abdominal wall.
• Enanthate autoinjector isn't for IM or IV administration.
• Don't use autoinjector if liquid is cloudy, if visible particles are present, or if the seal is broken.
• Don't use autoinjector within 2 inches of the navel; where skin is tender, bruised, red, scaly, or hard; and in areas with scars, tattoos, or stretch marks.

Buccal
• The buccal system should be placed with the curved side against the upper gum region just above the incisor tooth on either side of the mouth.

• Have patient rotate sides of the mouth with each administration.
• Make sure patient doesn't chew or swallow the buccal system.
• The buccal system should remain in place until the next dosing. Check placement after toothbrushing, mouthwash use, eating, and drinking.
• To remove the system, gently slide it downward from the gum toward the tooth.

Intranasal
• Prime pump before first use by inverting then depressing pump 10 times (discard this portion of product into sink).
• Have patient blow nose before application.
• To administer, insert actuator into nostril until pump reaches base of nose; tilt so tip is in contact with lateral wall of nostril. Depress slowly until pump stops, then remove from nose while wiping tip to transfer gel to lateral side of nostril.
• After administration, press on nostrils just below bridge of nose and lightly massage.
• Make sure patient refrains from blowing nose or sniffing for 1 hour after administration.
• If gel gets on hands, wash with warm soap and water.

ACTION

Stimulates target tissues to develop normally in androgen-deficient men. May have some antiestrogen properties, making it useful in treating certain estrogen-dependent breast cancers.

Route	Onset	Peak	Duration
PO	Unknown	2–4 hr	Unknown
IM	Unknown	4–42 days	2–10 wk
Subcut (implant)	Unknown	Unknown	3–6 mo
Subcut (enanthate)	Unknown	6–168 hr	Unknown
Buccal	Unknown	10–12 hr	2–4 hr
Intranasal	Unknown	40 min	Unknown

Half-life: 10 to 100 minutes; cypionate, about 8 days.

ADVERSE REACTIONS

Refer to manufacturer's prescribing information for each product for additional adverse reactions not listed here.

CNS: headache, anxiety, depression, paresthesia, sleep apnea, mood swings, aggressive

T

behavior, irritability. **CV:** edema, HTN.
EENT: nasal discomfort, nasopharyngitis,
rhinorrhea, epistaxis, parosmia, nasal dryness or congestion, nasal scabbing. **GI:** nausea; gum or mouth irritation; bitter taste;
gum pain, tenderness, or edema; taste perversion (with buccal application); diarrhea.
GU: amenorrhea, oligospermia, decreased
ejaculatory disorder, priapism, prostatitis.
Hematologic: polycythemia, *suppression
of clotting factors.* **Hepatic:** reversible jaundice, *cholestatic hepatitis.* **Metabolic:** hypernatremia, *hyperkalemia,* hypercalcemia,
hyperphosphatemia, hypercholesterolemia,
weight gain. **Musculoskeletal:** back pain,
arthralgia. **Respiratory:** URI. **Skin:** pain,
application-site reaction, induration at injection site, local edema, acne, hyperhidrosis. **Other:** androgenic effects in women,
gynecomastia, hypersensitivity reactions,
hypoestrogenic effects in women, excessive
hormonal effects in men, male pattern baldness.

INTERACTIONS
Drug-drug. *Corticosteroids:* May increase
risk of edema. Use together cautiously, especially in patients with cardiac, hepatic, or
renal disease.
Cyclosporine: Androgens may enhance hepatotoxic effects. Consider therapy modification.
Hepatotoxic drugs: May increase risk of
hepatotoxicity. Monitor liver function
closely.
Insulin, oral antidiabetics: May decrease
glucose level; may alter dosage requirements. Monitor glucose level in diabetic patients.
Oral anticoagulants (warfarin): May increase sensitivity; may alter dosage requirements. Monitor PT and INR; decrease anticoagulant dose if necessary.
Oxyphenbutazone: May increase
oxyphenbutazone level. Monitor patient.
Drug-food. *Licorice:* May decrease testosterone level. Avoid use.

EFFECTS ON LAB TEST RESULTS
• May increase LFT values and sodium,
potassium, phosphate, cholesterol, calcium,
creatinine, and serum PSA levels.

• May increase Hb level, hematocrit, and
RBC count. May decrease leukocyte count.
• May increase resin uptake of T_3 and T_4.
• May decrease thyroxine-binding globulin,
total T_4 levels, and 17-ketosteroid level.
• May cause abnormal glucose tolerance test
results.

CONTRAINDICATIONS & CAUTIONS
• Contraindicated in patients hypersensitive
to drug or its components and in those with
hypercalcemia or cardiac, hepatic, or renal
decompensation.
• Contraindicated in men with breast or
known or suspected prostate cancer.
• Venous thromboembolic events (VTEs),
including DVT and PE, have been reported
in patients using testosterone products.
Black Box Warning Serious pulmonary oil
microembolism reactions, involving urge
to cough, dyspnea, throat tightening, chest
pain, dizziness, and syncope, and episodes
of anaphylaxis, including life-threatening
reactions, have been reported to occur during or immediately after administration of
testosterone undecanoate injection. These
reactions can occur after any injection of
testosterone undecanoate during the course
of therapy, including after first dose. Observe patients for 30 minutes after each dose.
Drug is available only through a restricted
program under a REMS called the Aveed
REMS Program. ∎
♦ *Alert:* Drug has potential for abuse, usually at doses higher than those prescribed
and usually in conjunction with other anabolic androgenic steroids (AASs). Abuse
is associated with serious safety risks, such
as MI, HF, stroke, depression, hostility, aggression, liver toxicity, and male infertility.
Withdrawal signs and symptoms (depression, fatigue, irritability, loss of appetite, decreased libido, and insomnia) can occur in
patients abusing high testosterone doses.
♦ *Alert:* Contraindicated in men with age-related low testosterone signs and symptoms
only. Testosterone replacement therapy is
only approved for men with primary or secondary hypogonadism resulting from certain medical conditions and with low testosterone levels confirmed by lab testing.
♦ *Alert:* Drug may increase risk of heart
attack and stroke.

• Prolonged use of high doses of androgens has been associated with the development of peliosis hepatis and hepatic neoplasms, including hepatocellular carcinoma.

• Use cautiously in elderly patients.

• Intranasal form isn't recommended for use with nasally administered drugs other than sympathomimetic decongestants or for use in patients with mucosal inflammatory disorders, sinus disease or history of nasal disorders, nasal or sinus surgery, nasal fracture within previous 6 months, or nasal fracture that caused a deviated anterior nasal septum.

• Use cautiously in patients with sleep apnea or those with risk factors for sleep apnea (obesity, chronic lung disease).

Dialyzable drug: Unknown.

⚠ *Overdose S&S:* Stroke (with enanthate injection).

PREGNANCY-LACTATION-REPRODUCTION

• Drug is teratogenic and may cause fetal harm. Use is contraindicated in pregnant women and women who may become pregnant. If a woman becomes pregnant during therapy, apprise her of potential hazard to the fetus.

• Contraindicated in breastfeeding women because of potential for virilization in breastfed infants.

NURSING CONSIDERATIONS

• Don't give to women of childbearing potential until pregnancy is ruled out.

• Cypionate, enanthate, and undecanoate are long-acting solutions.

🖑 *Alert:* If testosterone abuse is suspected, check serum testosterone concentrations to ensure they are within therapeutic range. Consider possibility of testosterone and AAS abuse in suspected patients who present with serious CV or psychiatric adverse events.

• If patient experiences severe rhinitis, temporarily discontinue intranasal therapy until signs and symptoms resolve. If signs and symptoms persist, an alternative testosterone replacement therapy is recommended.

• Monitor patient's liver function, and check PSA, cholesterol, and HDL levels periodically.

• Check Hb and hematocrit levels periodically.

🖑 *Alert:* Confirm low testosterone levels on at least two mornings before initiating therapy. Avoid measuring testosterone level later in the day when levels can be low, even in men who don't have hypogonadism.

• Monitor testosterone levels after initial dosage titration, and periodically as described in prescribing information for each product.

• Evaluate patients who report pain, edema, or warmth and erythema in lower extremity for DVT; evaluate those who present with acute shortness of breath for PE. If a VTE is suspected, discontinue drug and initiate appropriate workup and management.

• In patients with metastatic breast cancer, hypercalcemia usually indicates progression of bone metastases. Report signs and symptoms of hypercalcemia.

• Report evidence of virilization in women. Androgenic effects include acne, edema, weight gain, increased hair growth, hoarseness, clitoral enlargement, decreased breast size, changes in libido, male pattern baldness, and oily skin or hair.

• Watch for hypoestrogenic effects in women (flushing; diaphoresis; vaginitis, including itching, drying, and burning; vaginal bleeding; menstrual irregularities).

• Watch for excessive hormonal effects in men and boys. In prepubertal boy, watch for premature epiphyseal closure, acne, priapism, growth of body and facial hair, and phallic enlargement. In postpubertal men, watch for testicular atrophy, oligospermia, decreased ejaculatory volume, impotence, gynecomastia, and epididymitis.

• Drug may increase risk of depression and suicidal ideation. Evaluate patients with new-onset or worsening depression, anxiety, mood changes, or suicidal ideation or behavior.

• Monitor patient's weight and BP routinely.

• Monitor prepubertal boys by X-ray for rate of bone maturation.

• The treatment of hypogonadal men with testosterone esters may potentiate sleep apnea. Monitor patients with risk factors such as obesity or chronic lung diseases.

🖑 *Alert:* Therapeutic response in breast cancer is usually apparent within 3 months. If disease progresses, stop drug.

T

• Androgens may alter results of lab studies during therapy and for 2 to 3 weeks after therapy ends.

🚯 *Alert:* Testosterone salts aren't interchangeable.

• *Look alike–sound alike:* Don't confuse testosterone with testolactone.

PATIENT TEACHING

• Make sure patient understands importance of using an effective nonhormonal contraceptive during therapy.

🚯 *Alert:* Warn patient to seek immediate medical attention for signs and symptoms of heart attack (chest pain, shortness of breath, trouble breathing) or stroke (weakness in one part or side of the body, slurred speech).

• Instruct patient to stop drug immediately and notify prescriber if pregnancy is suspected.

• Advise patient and caregiver to seek medical attention for manifestations of new-onset or worsening depression, suicidal ideation or behavior, anxiety, or other mood changes.

• Review signs and symptoms of virilization with female patient, and instruct her to notify prescriber if they occur.

• Advise female patient to wear cotton underwear and to wash after intercourse to decrease risk of vaginitis.

• Instruct male patient to report priapism, reduced ejaculatory volume, or gynecomastia.

• Warn diabetic patient to be alert for hypoglycemia and to notify prescriber if it occurs.

• Instruct boys using testosterone for delayed puberty to have X-rays of hand and wrist obtained every 6 months during treatment.

• Tell patient to report sudden weight gain.

• Warn patient that drug shouldn't be used to enhance athletic performance.

• Instruct patient how to use the buccal system.

• Advise patient to avoid dislodging buccal system and ensure that the system is in place after toothbrushing, use of mouthwash, and eating or drinking.

• Tell male patient not to chew or swallow buccal system.

• Show patient how to administer drug intranasally.

testosterone transdermal
tes-TOS-te-rone

Androderm, AndroGel, Fortesta, Testim, Vogelxo

Therapeutic class: Androgens
Pharmacologic class: Androgens

AVAILABLE FORMS
1% gel* : 25 mg, 50 mg per unit dose; 12.5 mg per pump actuation
1.62% gel* : 20.25 mg, 40.5 mg per unit dose; 20.25 mg per pump actuation
2% gel: 10 mg per pump actuation
Transdermal solution* : 30 mg per metered-dose pump
Transdermal system: 2 mg/day, 4 mg/day

INDICATIONS & DOSAGES
➤ **Primary or hypogonadotropic hypogonadism**
Men: One Androderm 4 mg/day system (don't use two 2-mg/day patches) applied to back, abdomen, arm, or thigh nightly for total dosage of 4 mg daily. Dose may be increased to 6 mg once daily or decreased to 2 mg once daily, depending on morning serum testosterone levels.

Or, initially, 50 mg of AndroGel 1% (two 25-mg packets or one 50-mg packet) applied every morning to shoulders, upper arms, or abdomen. Check testosterone level after about 2 weeks. If response is inadequate, may increase AndroGel to 75 mg daily. Then, adjust to 100 mg if needed.

Or, 50 mg of Testim applied once daily in the morning to shoulders and upper arms. Don't apply to genitals or abdomen. May increase dosage to a maximum 100 mg/day, if needed, based on testosterone levels.

Or, initially, 40.5 mg (2 pumps) of AndroGel 1.62% applied once daily in the morning to upper arms or shoulders. May adjust dosage between a minimum of 20.25 mg (1 pump) and a maximum of 81 mg (4 pumps) titrated based on the predose morning serum testosterone concentration at about 14 days and 28 days after starting treatment or the last dosage adjustment.

Or, initially 40 mg (4 pumps) of Fortesta once daily to the thighs in the morning. May adjust dosage between 10 mg and maximum of 70 mg based on testosterone concentration drawn 2 hours after application approximately 14 days and 35 days after start of treatment and the last dosage adjustment.

Or, initially 60 mg (2 pumps) of solution, one actuation to each axilla, once daily. May adjust dosage between 30 mg (1 actuation) and a maximum of 120 mg (4 actuations) based on serum testosterone concentration drawn 2 to 8 hours after application and at least 14 days after starting treatment or the last dosage adjustment. For doses of more than 60 mg daily, alternate axillae, allowing them to dry completely before applying next actuation.

Or, 50 mg of Vogelxo once daily to shoulders or upper arms. If serum testosterone concentration is below normal range, increase dose to 100 mg of testosterone.

ADMINISTRATION
• Hazardous drug; use safe handling and disposal precautions according to facility policy.
Transdermal
• Wear gloves when handling patches. Fold used patches with adhesive sides together to discard.
• Apply patch nightly to clean, dry, intact skin of the back, abdomen, upper arms, or thighs only and not to the genitals or bony prominences. Rotate sites; don't reuse a site for 7 days.
Topical
• AndroGel 1.62% and AndroGel 1% and topical solution aren't interchangeable.
• Fully prime the pumps by pumping three times before first use (except Fortesta). Discard this portion of the product.
• Prime the twist-actuated metered-dose pump by twisting the dose dial three times before first use. Discard this portion of the product.
• Before first dose of Fortesta, prime the pump by depressing it eight times; discard this portion of the product.
• Wear gloves to apply gel to clean, dry, intact skin as directed for each product. Don't apply to the genitals or bony prominences.
• Application in the morning is preferable. Allow application sites to dry before dressing. Cover the application sites with clothing.

• Patient should avoid swimming or washing the administration site for 2 to 5 hours after application, depending on product.
• Gel contains alcohol and is flammable. Patient should avoid fire, flames, or smoking until gel has dried.
• Apply topical solution, using the applicator provided, to clean, dry, intact skin of the axilla as directed. Don't use the fingers or hand to rub the solution into the skin.
• Patient should apply deodorant at least 2 minutes before applying the solution.

ACTION
Releases testosterone, which stimulates target tissues to develop normally in androgen-deficient men.

Route	Onset	Peak	Duration
Transdermal, topical	Unknown	4–24 hr	24 hr– 10 days

Half-life: 10 to 100 minutes.

ADVERSE REACTIONS
CNS: *stroke,* asthenia, depression, headache, sleep apnea, aggressive behavior, mood swings, fatigue, insomnia, irritability. **CV:** HTN. **GI:** *GI bleeding,* diarrhea. **GU:** prostatitis, prostate abnormalities, UTI, ejaculation disorder, polyuria. **Hepatic:** *cholestatic hepatitis,* reversible jaundice. **Metabolic:** hypernatremia, hyperkalemia, hypercalcemia, hyperphosphatemia, hypercholesterolemia, weight gain. **Skin:** pruritus, blister under patch, acne irritation, allergic contact dermatitis, burning, hyperhidrosis. **Other:** gynecomastia, breast tenderness, flulike syndrome.

INTERACTIONS
Drug-drug. *Corticosteroids:* May increase risk of edema. Use together cautiously, especially in patients with renal, cardiac, or hepatic disease.
Cyclosporine: Androgens may enhance hepatotoxic effect. Consider therapy modification.
Hepatotoxic drugs: May increase risk of hepatotoxicity. Monitor liver function closely.
Insulin, oral antidiabetics: May enhance hypoglycemic effect and alter dosage

requirements of listed drugs. Monitor glucose level in patients with diabetes.

Oral anticoagulants (warfarin): May alter anticoagulant dosage requirements. Monitor PT and INR.

Oxyphenbutazone: May increase oxyphenbutazone level. Monitor patient.

EFFECTS ON LAB TEST RESULTS

• May increase PSA, sodium, potassium, phosphate, cholesterol, liver enzyme, calcium, and creatinine levels, and resin uptake of T_3 and T_4.

• May decrease glucose and total T_4 levels.

• May increase Hb level and hematocrit and RBC count.

CONTRAINDICATIONS & CAUTIONS

• Contraindicated in patients hypersensitive to drug, in women, in men with known or suspected breast or prostate cancer, and in patients with CV, renal, or hepatic disease.

❸ *Alert:* Contraindicated in men with age-related low testosterone symptoms only. Testosterone replacement therapy is only approved for men with primary or secondary hypogonadism resulting from certain medical conditions and with low testosterone levels confirmed by lab testing.

• Use cautiously in cancer patients at risk for hypercalcemia (and associated hypercalciuria).

❸ *Alert:* Drug has potential for abuse, usually at doses higher than those prescribed and usually in conjunction with other anabolic androgenic steroids (AASs). Abuse is associated with serious safety risks, such as MI, HF, stroke, depression, hostility, aggression, liver toxicity, and male infertility. Withdrawal signs and symptoms (depression, fatigue, irritability, loss of appetite, decreased libido, and insomnia) can occur in patients abusing high testosterone doses.

❸ *Alert:* Drug may increase risk of heart attack and stroke.

• Venous thromboembolic events (VTEs), including DVT and PE, have been reported in patients using testosterone products.

• Prolonged use of high doses of androgens has been associated with development of peliosis hepatis and hepatic neoplasms, including hepatocellular carcinoma.

• Use cautiously in elderly men.

Dialyzable drug: Unknown.

PREGNANCY-LACTATION-REPRODUCTION

• Drug is teratogenic; may cause fetal harm. Use is contraindicated in pregnant women and women who may become pregnant. If a woman becomes pregnant during therapy, apprise her of potential hazard to the fetus.

• Contraindicated in women who are breastfeeding because of potential for virilization in breastfed infants.

NURSING CONSIDERATIONS

Black Box Warning Virilization in children and women can occur after secondary exposure to transdermal application sites on men. Women and children should avoid contact with application sites. ∎

• Monitor serum calcium concentrations in cancer patients at risk for hypercalcemia (and associated hypercalciuria).

❸ *Alert:* If testosterone abuse is suspected, check serum testosterone concentrations to ensure they are within therapeutic range. Consider possibility of testosterone and AAS abuse in suspected patients who present with serious CV or psychiatric adverse events.

• Treatment of hypogonadal men with testosterone esters may potentiate sleep apnea. Monitor patients with risk factors, such as obesity or chronic lung diseases.

• Periodically assess LFT results, lipid profiles, Hb level, hematocrit (with long-term use), and levels of prostatic acid phosphatase and PSA.

❸ *Alert:* Confirm low testosterone levels on at least two mornings before initiating therapy. Avoid measuring testosterone level later in the day when levels can be low, even in men who don't have hypogonadism.

• Watch for excessive hormonal effects.

• Evaluate patients who report pain, edema, or warmth and erythema in lower extremity for DVT; evaluate those who present with acute shortness of breath for PE. If a VTE is suspected, discontinue treatment and initiate appropriate workup and management.

• Remove topical patch before an MRI because patch contains aluminum.

Reactions in bold italics are *life-threatening*. Interactions may have a *rapid onset* or a *delayed onset*.

PATIENT TEACHING

• Teach patient how to prime pumps and self-administer drug according to individual manufacturer's instructions.

• Tell patient to apply patch to skin immediately after removing from pouch; to rotate patch sites, allowing 7 days between applications to the same site; not to apply to bony areas or parts of the body that are subject to prolonged pressure while sleeping or sitting; and not to apply to oily, damaged, or irritated skin.

Black Box Warning Instruct patient to strictly adhere to recommended instructions for use. ■

• Instruct patient to thoroughly wash the application site with soap and water before situations in which direct skin-to-skin contact is anticipated.

• Tell patient using patch to apply it at night.

• Tell patient using gel to apply in the morning.

Black Box Warning Tell patient to wash hands thoroughly after using product and to cover treated area with clothing. ■

• Instruct patient that patch must be changed every 24 hours.

• For best results, advise patient not to swim or shower for 2 to 5 hours after applying gel, depending on product.

• Tell patient that if the patch falls off, it may be reapplied. If patch falls off and can't be reapplied, and it has been worn at least 12 hours, a new patch may be applied at the next application time.

• Warn diabetic patient that drug may decrease glucose level and to be alert for hypoglycemia.

🕒 **Alert:** Warn patient to seek immediate medical attention for signs and symptoms of heart attack (chest pain, shortness of breath, trouble breathing) or stroke (weakness in one part or side of the body, slurred speech).

• Advise patient to report persistent erections, nausea, vomiting, changes in skin color, ankle swelling, or sudden weight gain to prescriber.

Black Box Warning Tell patient that women and children should avoid contact with application sites. ■

• Tell patient that Androderm doesn't have to be removed during sexual intercourse or while showering.

• Tell patient undergoing an MRI to alert the facility about using a transdermal patch.

tetracycline hydrochloride
tet-ra-SYE-kleen

Therapeutic class: Antibiotics
Pharmacologic class: Tetracyclines

AVAILABLE FORMS
Capsules: 250 mg, 500 mg

INDICATIONS & DOSAGES
Adjust-a-dose (for all indications): Decrease recommended dosages or extend dosing intervals in patients with renal impairment.
➤ **Infections caused by susceptible gram-negative and gram-positive organisms, such as** *Haemophilus ducreyi, Yersinia pestis, Campylobacter fetus, Rickettsiae* **species,** *Mycoplasma pneumoniae, Chlamydia trachomatis, Entamoeba histolytica, Actinomyces* **species,** *Bacillus anthracis, Vibrio cholerae, Listeria monocytogenes, Fusobacterium fusiforme,* **and** *Treponema* **species;** *Francisella tularensis; Clostridium* **species;** *Escherichia coli; Enterobacter aerogenes; Shigella* **species;** *Klebsiella* **species;** *Borrelia* **species;** *Streptococcus pneumoniae; Streptococcus pyogenes; Staphylococcus aureus; Staphylococcus pyogenes;* **psittacosis; granuloma inguinale**
Adults: 1 to 2 g/day PO in two or four divided doses depending on the severity of infection.
Children older than age 8: 25 to 50 mg/kg PO daily, in divided doses every 6 hours.
➤ **Uncomplicated urethral, endocervical, or rectal infections caused by** *C. trachomatis*
Adults: 500 mg PO q.i.d. for at least 7 days.
➤ **Brucellosis**
Adults: 500 mg PO every 6 hours for 3 weeks in combination with streptomycin.
➤ **Uncomplicated gonorrhea in patients allergic to penicillin**
Adults: 500 mg PO every 6 hours for 7 days.
➤ **Syphilis in patients allergic to penicillin**
Adults and adolescents: 500 mg PO q.i.d. for 15 days. If infection has lasted 1 year or longer, treat for 30 days.

T

➤ **Acne (severe; long-term therapy)**
Adults and adolescents: Initially, 1 g PO daily in divided doses. For maintenance, 125 to 500 mg daily. (Alternate-day or intermittent therapy may be adequate in some patients.)

ADMINISTRATION
PO
• Obtain specimen for culture and sensitivity tests before giving first dose. Begin therapy while awaiting results.
• For streptococcal infections, continue therapy for 10 days.
• Effectiveness is reduced when drug is given with milk or other dairy products, antacids, or iron products. For best drug absorption, give drug with a full glass of water on an empty stomach, at least 1 hour before or 2 hours after meals.
• Give drug with adequate amount of fluid at least 1 hour before bedtime to prevent esophageal irritation or ulceration.
⚠ *Alert:* Be careful not to administer outdated drug because of the highly increased risk of nephrotoxicity and Fanconi syndrome.

ACTION
May exert bacteriostatic effect by binding to the 30S and possibly 50S ribosomal subunits of microorganisms, thus inhibiting protein synthesis. May also alter the cytoplasmic membrane of susceptible microorganisms.

Route	Onset	Peak	Duration
PO	Unknown	2–4 hr	Unknown

Half-life: 6 to 11 hours.

ADVERSE REACTIONS
CNS: *intracranial HTN,* dizziness, headache. **EENT:** sore throat. **GI:** diarrhea, epigastric distress, nausea, anorexia, dysphagia, enterocolitis, esophagitis, glossitis, oral candidiasis, stomatitis, vomiting. **GU:** inflammatory lesions in anogenital region. **Hematologic:** *neutropenia, thrombocytopenia,* eosinophilia. **Hepatic:** hepatotoxicity. **Musculoskeletal:** bone growth retardation in children younger than age 8. **Skin:** candidal superinfection, increased pigmentation, maculopapular and erythematous rash, photosensitivity reactions, urticaria.

Other: enamel defects, hypersensitivity reactions, permanent discoloration of teeth.

INTERACTIONS
Drug-drug. *Antacids, laxatives, and multivitamins containing aluminum, magnesium, or calcium;* *antidiarrheals containing kaolin, pectin, or bismuth subsalicylate:* May decrease antibiotic absorption. Give antibiotic 1 hour before or 2 hours after these drugs.
CYP3A4 inducers: May decrease tetracycline serum concentration. Some combinations may be contraindicated. Refer to manufacturer's instructions. Consult appropriate manufacturer labeling. Consider therapy modification.
Digoxin: May increase digoxin absorption. Monitor digoxin levels and monitor patient for signs of toxicity.
Ferrous sulfate and other iron products, zinc: May decrease antibiotic absorption. Give tetracycline 2 hours before or 3 hours after these products.
Hormonal contraceptives: May decrease contraceptive effectiveness and increase risk of breakthrough bleeding. Advise patient to use nonhormonal contraceptive.
Isotretinoin: May increase risk of pseudotumor cerebri. Avoid use together.
⚠ *Alert: Methoxyflurane:* May cause fatal nephrotoxicity. Avoid using together.
Oral anticoagulants: May increase anticoagulant effects. Monitor PT and INR, and adjust anticoagulant dosage.
Penicillins: May interfere with bactericidal action of penicillins. Avoid using together.
Drug-herb. *St. John's wort:* May decrease tetracycline serum concentration. Consider an alternative for one of the agents.
Drug-food. *Dairy products;* May decrease antibiotic absorption. Give antibiotic 1 hour before or 2 hours after eating or drinking dairy products.
Drug-lifestyle. *Sun exposure:* May cause photosensitivity reactions. Advise patient to avoid excessive sunlight exposure.

EFFECTS ON LAB TEST RESULTS
• May increase BUN and liver enzyme levels.
• May increase eosinophil count. May decrease platelet and neutrophil counts.

Reactions in bold italics are *life-threatening.* Interactions may have a *rapid onset* or a ***delayed onset.***

CONTRAINDICATIONS & CAUTIONS
• Contraindicated in patients hypersensitive to drug or other tetracyclines.
• Some tetracyclines may contain sulfites and are contraindicated in patients with sulfite hypersensitivity.
• CDAD, ranging in severity from mild diarrhea to fatal colitis, has been reported with use of nearly all antibacterial drugs, including tetracyclines.
• Use cautiously in patients with renal or hepatic impairment. Avoid using or use cautiously in children younger than age 8 because drug may cause permanent discoloration of teeth, enamel defects, and bone growth retardation.
Dialyzable drug: No.
⚠ *Overdose S&S:* Dizziness, nausea, vomiting.

PREGNANCY-LACTATION-REPRODUCTION
• Don't use during pregnancy unless absolutely necessary. May have toxic effects on the developing fetus (often related to retardation of skeletal development) and teeth. If used during pregnancy or if patient becomes pregnant during therapy, apprise her of potential hazard to the fetus.
• Pregnant women with renal disease may be more prone to developing tetracycline-associated liver failure.
• Drug appears in human milk. Patient should discontinue breastfeeding or discontinue drug.

NURSING CONSIDERATIONS
🖐 *Alert:* Check expiration date. Using outdated or deteriorated drug has been linked to severe reversible nephrotoxicity (Fanconi syndrome).
• Don't expose drug to light or heat.
• If CDAD is suspected or confirmed, discontinue ongoing use of antibacterial drugs not directed at *Clostridium difficile.* Institute appropriate fluid and electrolyte management, protein supplementation, and antibacterial treatment of *C. difficile.*
• If large doses are given, therapy is prolonged, or patient is at high risk, monitor patient for signs and symptoms of superinfection.
• Pseudotumor cerebri (benign intracranial HTN) in adults has been associated with tetracycline use. Monitor patient for clinical manifestations, including headache, blurred vision, diplopia, and vision loss; papilledema can be found on funduscopy.
• In patients with renal or hepatic impairment, monitor renal function tests and LFT values.
• Check patient's tongue for signs of candidal infection. Emphasize good oral hygiene.
• Drug isn't indicated for treatment of neurosyphilis.
• Photosensitivity reactions may occur within a few minutes to several hours after sun exposure. Photosensitivity lasts after therapy ends.

PATIENT TEACHING
• Tell patient to take drug exactly as prescribed, even after feeling better, and to take entire amount prescribed.
• Tell patient to check drug's expiration date and not to use if outdated.
• Advise patient to promptly report all adverse reactions and to immediately report headache, blurred vision, diplopia, vision loss, watery diarrhea, abdominal cramping and pain, fever, or blood or pus in the stool.
• Warn patient that use of tetracyclines with oral contraceptives may make contraceptives less effective.
• Explain that effectiveness is reduced when drug is taken within 2 hours before or after ingestion of milk or other dairy products, antacids, laxatives, multivitamins, or iron products. For best drug absorption, tell patient to take each dose with a full glass of water on an empty stomach, at least 1 hour before or 2 hours after meals. Also tell patient to take it at least 1 hour before bedtime to prevent esophageal irritation or ulceration.
• Warn patient to avoid direct sunlight and ultraviolet light and to use sun protection.

T

tetrahydrozoline hydrochloride (intranasal)
tet-rah-hi-DRAZ-oh-leen

Tyzine

Therapeutic class: Decongestants
Pharmacologic class: Sympathomimetics

AVAILABLE FORMS
Nasal solution: 0.05%, 0.1%
Nasal spray: 0.1%

INDICATIONS & DOSAGES
➤ **Nasal congestion**
Adults and children age 6 and older: 2 to 4 drops or 3 to 4 sprays of 0.1% solution in each nostril no more often than every 3 hours, p.r.n.
Children ages 2 to 5: Give 2 to 3 drops of 0.05% solution in each nostril no more often than every 3 hours, p.r.n.

ADMINISTRATION
Intranasal
• Instill nose drops with patient in lateral head-low position.
• Give nasal spray with patient's head tilted back slightly. Wait 1 to 2 minutes between sprays.
• Rinse spray tip in hot water and dry with a clean tissue.

ACTION
Thought to cause local vasoconstriction of dilated arterioles, reducing blood flow and nasal congestion.

Route	Onset	Peak	Duration
Intranasal	Few min	Unknown	4–8 hr

Half-life: Unknown.

ADVERSE REACTIONS
CNS: headache, drowsiness, weakness, tremors, light-headedness, insomnia. **CV:** palpitations. **EENT:** rebound nasal congestion, sneezing, transient burning or stinging, mucosal dryness.

INTERACTIONS
Drug-drug. *MAO inhibitors:* May cause headache, HTN, and hyperpyrexia. Use together or within 14 days of stopping an MAO inhibitor is contraindicated.

EFFECTS ON LAB TEST RESULTS
None reported.

CONTRAINDICATIONS & CAUTIONS
• Contraindicated in patients hypersensitive to drug and in children younger than age 2. The 0.1% solution is contraindicated in children younger than age 6.
• Use cautiously in patients with hyperthyroidism, HTN, CAD, or diabetes mellitus.
Dialyzable drug: Unknown.

⚠ *Overdose S&S:* HTN, bradycardia, drowsiness, rebound hypotension, shock, profuse sweating.

PREGNANCY-LACTATION-REPRODUCTION
• It isn't known if drug can cause fetal harm when used in pregnant women or if it can affect reproduction capacity. Use during pregnancy only if clearly needed.
• It isn't known if drug appears in human milk. Use cautiously in breastfeeding women.

NURSING CONSIDERATIONS
• Monitor BP and HR.
• Drug should be used for only 3 to 5 days.
• Overdose in young children may cause oversedation, coma, bradycardia, or respiratory depression.

PATIENT TEACHING
• Teach patient how to use drug.
• Advise patient to keep drug out of reach of small children. Accidental ingestion of even a small amount (1 to 2 mL) may result in bradycardia, respiratory depression, sedation, or coma. Tell patient to contact a poison control center and immediately seek emergency medical care for accidental ingestion.
• Caution patient not to share drug because this could spread infection.
• Tell patient not to exceed recommended dosage and to use only as needed for 3 to 5 days.

SAFETY ALERT!

thiotepa (TESPA, triethyl-enethiophosphoramide, TSPA) ▨
thye-oh-TEE-pa

Tepadina

Therapeutic class: Antineoplastics
Pharmacologic class: Alkylating drugs

AVAILABLE FORMS
Injection: 15 mg, 100 mg per vial

INDICATIONS & DOSAGES
➤ **Breast and ovarian cancers**
Adults: 0.3 to 0.4 mg/kg IV every 1 to 4 weeks. Adjust maintenance dose weekly

---

based on blood counts; don't give more often than weekly.

> **Superficial papillary bladder carcinoma**

Adults: 60 mg in 30 to 60 mL of NSS instilled in bladder for 2 hours once weekly for 4 weeks.

> **Neoplastic effusions**

Adults: 0.6 to 0.8 mg/kg intracavitarily every 1 to 4 weeks. Adjust maintenance dose weekly based on blood counts; don't give more often than weekly.

> **To reduce risk of graft rejection when used in conjunction with high-dose busulfan and cyclophosphamide as a preparative regimen for allogeneic hematopoietic progenitor (stem) cell transplantation (HSCT) for children with class 3 beta-thalassemia** ☒

Children older than age 1 month: Two doses of 5 mg/kg IV approximately 12 hours apart on the 6th day before allogeneic HSCT (in combination with high-dose busulfan and cyclophosphamide).

ADMINISTRATION

● Preparing and giving drug may be mutagenic, teratogenic, or carcinogenic. Follow facility policy to reduce risks.

IV

▼ Reconstitute with 1.5 mL of sterile water for injection in 15-mg vial to yield 10 mg/mL; or, with 10 mL of sterile water for injection in 100-mg vial to yield 10 mg/mL. Don't reconstitute with other solutions. Mix manually by repeated inversions.

▼ Reconstituted solution is stable for 8 hours when stored under refrigeration.

▼ Further dilute reconstituted solution in 500 mL NSS if dose is 250 to 500 mg, or in 1,000 mL if dose is greater than 500 mg. If dose is less than 250 mg, dilute with NSS to a final concentration of 0.5 to 1 mg/mL.

▼ After dilution, Tepadina is stable for 24 hours when refrigerated or for 4 hours at room temperature. Generic product should be used immediately. Microbiologically, the product should be used immediately.

▼ If solution appears grossly opaque or has a precipitate, discard it. Make sure solution is clear to slightly opaque.

▼ Infuse via a central venous catheter over 3 hours using an infusion set equipped with a 0.2-micron in-line filter. Before and after infusion, flush catheter with approximately 5 mL NSS.

▼ If pain occurs at insertion site, dilute drug further or use a local anesthetic to reduce pain. Make sure drug doesn't infiltrate.

▼ Refrigerate and protect dry powder from direct sunlight to avoid possible drug breakdown.

▼ **Incompatibilities:** None listed by manufacturer. Consult a drug incompatibility reference for more information.

Intravesical

● Recommended dose is 60 mg in 30 to 60 mL of NSS instilled into bladder by catheter; ask patient to retain solution for 2 hours. If discomfort is too great with 60 mL, reduce volume to 30 mL. Reposition patient every 15 minutes for maximum area contact.

Intracavitary

● For intracavitary instillation, drug may be given through the same tubing used to remove the fluid from the cavity involved.

ACTION

Cross-links strands of cellular DNA and interferes with RNA transcription, causing an imbalance of growth that leads to cell death. Not specific to cell cycle.

Route	Onset	Peak	Duration
IV	Unknown	Unknown	Unknown

Half-life: Adults, 1.4 to 3.7 hours; active metabolite, 4.9 to 17.6 hours. Children, 1.7 hours; active metabolite, 4 hours.

ADVERSE REACTIONS

CNS: headache, dizziness, fatigue, weakness, fever, *seizure, encephalopathy, intracranial hemorrhage.* **EENT:** blurred vision, conjunctivitis. **GI:** diarrhea, nausea, vomiting, abdominal pain, anorexia, mucositis, stomatitis, *hemorrhage.* **GU:** amenorrhea, hematuria, decreased spermatogenesis, dysuria, increased urine levels of uric acid, urine retention, hemorrhagic cystitis (with intravesical administration). **Hematologic:** *leukopenia, thrombocytopenia, neutropenia,* anemia. **Hepatic:** elevated

T

liver enzyme levels, hyperbilirubinemia, veno-occlusive disease. **Respiratory:** *laryngeal edema,* pneumonia. **Skin:** dermatitis, alopecia, injection-site pain, urticaria, rash. **Other:** GVHD, infection, hypersensitivity reactions, including *anaphylaxis.*

INTERACTIONS
Drug-drug. *Anticoagulants, aspirin, NSAIDs:* May increase risk of bleeding. Avoid using together.
Live-virus or attenuated virus vaccines: May increase risk of infection. Use together is contraindicated.
Myelosuppressive agents: May increase myelosuppression. Monitor patient.
Neuromuscular blockers: May prolong muscular paralysis. Monitor patient.
Other alkylating drugs, irradiation therapy: May intensify toxicity rather than enhance therapeutic response. Avoid using together.
Strong CYP3A4 inducers (phenytoin, rifampin): May increase serum concentrations of active metabolite(s) of thiotepa and decrease thiotepa serum concentration. Avoid using together; if use together is unavoidable, monitor patient for adverse effects.
Strong CYP3A4 inhibitors (clarithromycin, itraconazole, ritonavir): May decrease serum concentrations of active metabolite(s) of thiotepa and increase thiotepa serum concentration. Avoid using together; if use together is unavoidable, monitor patient for adverse effects and decreased efficacy.
Drug-herb. *Echinacea:* May decrease therapeutic effect of drug. Avoid using together.

EFFECTS ON LAB TEST RESULTS
• May increase uric acid, AST, ALT, and bilirubin levels.
• May decrease pseudocholinesterase level.
• May decrease Hb level and lymphocyte, platelet, WBC, RBC, and neutrophil counts.

CONTRAINDICATIONS & CAUTIONS
• Contraindicated in patients hypersensitive to drug.
• Generally contraindicated in patients with existing hepatic or renal dysfunction or bone marrow suppression or damage. However, if need outweighs risk in such patients, may use drug cautiously in low

dosage, and accompanied by hepatic, renal, and hematopoietic function tests.
Black Box Warning May cause severe bone marrow suppression, and high doses may cause marrow ablation with resulting infection or bleeding. Monitor hematologic lab parameters. HSCT is required to prevent potentially fatal complications of the prolonged myelosuppression after high doses of drug. ■
Black Box Warning Drug is potentially carcinogenic in humans. ■
• Myelodysplastic syndromes and acute nonlymphocytic leukemia have been reported in patients treated with thiotepa.
• Death has occurred after intravesical administration, caused by bone marrow depression from systemically absorbed drug, and from septicemia and hemorrhage as a direct result of hematopoietic depression.
Dialyzable drug: Yes.
⚠ *Overdose S&S:* Hematopoietic toxicity, bleeding.

PREGNANCY-LACTATION-REPRODUCTION
• Drug can cause fetal harm when used in pregnant women. If used during pregnancy, or if pregnancy occurs during therapy, apprise patient and patient's partner of potential hazard to the fetus.
• Verify pregnancy status of women of childbearing potential before starting drug.
• Women of childbearing potential should use highly effective contraception during treatment and for at least 6 months after therapy ends. Males with partners of childbearing potential should use effective contraception during treatment and for at least 1 year after therapy ends.
• It isn't known if drug appears in human milk. Patient should discontinue breastfeeding or discontinue drug.
• May interfere with spermatogenesis.

NURSING CONSIDERATIONS
• Monitor CBC weekly for at least 3 weeks after last dose.
• Drug is excreted through the skin of patients receiving high-dose therapy and may cause skin discoloration and reactions. Take precautions to prevent skin toxicity.
• Hepatic veno-occlusive disease may occur in patients who have received high-dose

---

therapy in conjunction with busulfan and cyclophosphamide. Monitor patient by physical exam and by observing serum transaminase and bilirubin levels daily through bone marrow transplant day +28.

• If WBC count drops below 3,000/mm^3 or if platelet count falls below 150,000/mm^3, stop drug and notify prescriber.

• Therapeutic effects are commonly accompanied by toxicity.

• Give blood transfusions for cumulative anemia.

• Doses of 300 mg/m^2 or greater are associated with high emetic potential in children. Antiemetics are recommended to prevent nausea and vomiting.

• *Look alike–sound alike:* Don't confuse thiotepa with thioguanine.

PATIENT TEACHING
• Instruct patient to shower or bathe with water, change the occlusive dressing, and clean the covered skin at least twice daily through 48 hours after the drug has been administered to prevent skin toxicities.

• Instruct patient to change bed sheets daily during therapy.

• Advise patient to watch for signs and symptoms of infection (fever, sore throat, fatigue) and bleeding (easy bruising, nosebleeds, bleeding gums, tarry stools). Tell patient to take temperature daily and to report even mild infections.

• Instruct patient to avoid OTC products containing aspirin or NSAIDs.

• Advise female patient to stop breastfeeding during therapy because of risk of toxicity to infant.

• Advise female patient of childbearing potential to use highly effective contraception during treatment and for at least 6 months after therapy ends. Advise male patient with partner of childbearing potential to use effective contraception during treatment and for at least 1 year after therapy ends.

tiaGABine hydrochloride
tye-AG-ah-been

Gabitril Filmtabs

Therapeutic class: Anticonvulsants
Pharmacologic class: GABA enhancers

AVAILABLE FORMS
Tablets: 2 mg, 4 mg, 12 mg, 16 mg

INDICATIONS & DOSAGES
➤ **Adjunctive treatment of partial seizures in patients taking enzyme-inducing anticonvulsants**
Adults: Initially, 4 mg PO once daily. Total daily dose may be increased by 4 to 8 mg at weekly intervals until clinical response or up to 56 mg daily. Give total daily dose in two to four divided doses.
Children ages 12 to 18: Initially, 4 mg PO once daily. Total daily dose may be increased by 4 mg at beginning of week 2 and thereafter by 4 to 8 mg per week until clinical response or up to 32 mg daily. Give total daily dose in two to four divided doses.
Adjust-a-dose: For patients with hepatic impairment, reduce first and maintenance doses or increase dosing intervals.

ADMINISTRATION
PO
• Give drug with food.
• If patient doesn't take a dose at the scheduled time, don't attempt to make up for the missed dose by increasing the next dose. If more than one dose has been missed, drug may need to be retitrated.

ACTION
Unknown. May act by facilitating the effects of the inhibitory neurotransmitter GABA. By binding to recognition sites linked to GABA uptake carrier, drug may make more GABA available.

Route	Onset	Peak	Duration
PO	Rapid	45 min (fasting)	Unknown

Half-life: 2 to 5 hours when given with enzyme inducers; 7 to 9 hours when given without enzyme inducers.

ADVERSE REACTIONS
CNS: asthenia, dizziness, nervousness, somnolence, abnormal gait, agitation, ataxia, confusion, depression, difficulty with concentration and attention, difficulty with memory, emotional lability, hostility, insomnia, language problems, paresthesia, speech disorder, tremor, pain, malaise, syncope, paranoia, migraine, hallucination. **CV:** vasodilation, chest pain, HTN, palpitations, tachycardia, edema. **EENT:** amblyopia, nystagmus, abnormal vision, ear pain, otitis media, tinnitus, epistaxis, pharyngitis. **GI:** nausea, abdominal pain, diarrhea, increased appetite, mouth ulceration, vomiting, gingivitis, stomatitis. **GU:** UTI, dysmenorrhea, dysuria, metrorrhagia, urinary incontinence, vaginitis. **Hematologic:** lymphadenopathy. **Metabolic:** weight gain or loss. **Musculoskeletal:** generalized weakness, myasthenia, neck pain, arthralgia, myalgia, hyperkinesia, hypokinesia. **Respiratory:** increased cough, bronchitis, dyspnea, pneumonia. **Skin:** pruritus, rash, ecchymoses, alopecia, dry skin, sweating. **Other:** accidental injury, flulike syndrome, infection.

INTERACTIONS
Drug-drug. *Cannabidiol, cannabis:* May enhance CNS depressant effect of tiagabine. Monitor therapy.
Carbamazepine, phenobarbital, phenytoin, other CYP3A4 inducers: May increase tiagabine clearance. Monitor patient closely.
CNS depressants (benzodiazepines, muscle relaxants, opioids, SSRIs): May enhance CNS effects. Avoid use together if possible.
CYP3A4 inhibitors (including conivaptan): May decrease tiagabine metabolism. Monitor therapy.
Drug-herb. *Kava kava:* May enhance adverse CNS effects of tiagabine. Monitor patient closely.
St. John's wort: May enhance tiagabine metabolism. Monitor patient closely.
Drug-lifestyle. *Alcohol use:* May enhance CNS effects. Use together cautiously and monitor therapy.

EFFECTS ON LAB TEST RESULTS
None reported.

CONTRAINDICATIONS & CAUTIONS
• Contraindicated in patients hypersensitive to drug or its components.
🔴 *Alert:* Drug may cause new-onset seizures and status epilepticus in patients without a history of epilepsy. In these patients, stop drug and evaluate for underlying seizure disorder. Drug shouldn't be used for off-label uses.
• Use cautiously in patients with psychiatric symptoms.
• Safety and effectiveness haven't been established for any indication other than as adjunctive therapy for partial seizures in adults and children age 12 and older.
Dialyzable drug: Unlikely.
⚠ *Overdose S&S:* Somnolence, impaired consciousness, agitation, confusion, speech difficulty, hostility, depression, weakness, seizures.

PREGNANCY-LACTATION-REPRODUCTION
• Drug may cause fetal harm, but there are no adequate studies in pregnant women. Use during pregnancy only if clearly needed.
• Pregnant women taking drug should enroll in the North American AED (Antiepileptic Drug) Pregnancy Registry (1-888-233-2334 or www.aedpregnancyregistry.org).
• It isn't known if drug or its metabolites appear in human milk. Use in breastfeeding women only if benefit clearly outweighs risks.

NURSING CONSIDERATIONS
🔴 *Alert:* Closely monitor all patients taking or starting antiepileptic drugs for changes in behavior indicating worsening of suicidal thoughts or behavior or depression. Symptoms such as anxiety, agitation, hostility, mania, and hypomania may be precursors to emerging suicidality.
• Withdraw drug gradually unless safety concerns require a more rapid withdrawal because sudden withdrawal may cause more frequent seizures.
🔴 *Alert:* Use of anticonvulsants, including tiagabine, may cause status epilepticus and sudden unexpected death in patients with and without epilepsy.
• Patients who aren't receiving at least one enzyme-inducing anticonvulsant when

---

Reactions in bold italics are *life-threatening*. Interactions may have a *rapid onset* or a *delayed onset*.

starting tiagabine may need lower doses or slower dosage adjustment.

• Monitor patient for cognitive and neuropsychiatric symptoms, including impaired concentration, speech or language problems, confusion, somnolence, and fatigue.

• Drug may cause moderately severe to incapacitating generalized weakness, which resolves after dosage is reduced or drug stopped.

• Monitor LFT values periodically, especially in patients with moderate hepatic impairment.

• *Look alike–sound alike:* Don't confuse tiagabine with tizanidine; both have 4-mg starting doses.

PATIENT TEACHING

❸ *Alert:* Advise patient, caregivers, and family to immediately report new-onset or worsening depression, emergence of suicidal thoughts or behavior, thoughts of self-harm, or other unusual changes in mood or behavior.

• Advise patient to take drug only as prescribed.

• Tell patient to take drug with food.

• Warn patient that drug may cause dizziness, somnolence, and other signs and symptoms of CNS depression. Advise patient to avoid driving and other potentially hazardous activities that require mental alertness until drug's CNS effects are known.

• Tell female patient of childbearing potential to call prescriber if she becomes pregnant or plans to become pregnant during therapy.

• Instruct female patient of childbearing potential to notify prescriber if she's planning to breastfeed because it isn't known if drug appears in human milk.

• Advise patient not to discontinue drug abruptly because of risk of seizures.

• Advise patient not to drink alcohol while taking drug.

ticagrelor
TYE-ka-GREL-or

Brilinta

Therapeutic class: Antiplatelet drugs
Pharmacologic class: P2Y$_{12}$ platelet inhibitors

AVAILABLE FORMS
Tablets: 60 mg, 90 mg

INDICATIONS & DOSAGES

➤ **ACS or a history of MI to reduce rate of CV death, MI, and stroke; after stent placement for treatment of ACS to reduce rate of thrombosis**

Adults: Initially, 180 mg PO as a loading dose; then, a maintenance dose of 90 mg PO b.i.d. during first year after an ACS event. After 1 year, give 60 mg b.i.d. Give daily maintenance dose with 75 to 100 mg of aspirin daily.

ADMINISTRATION
PO
• Give drug without regard to food.

• For patients unable to swallow tablets whole, tablets can be crushed, mixed with water, and drunk. The mixture can also be given via an NG tube.

• Store at room temperature in the original container. Keep away from moisture and humidity.

ACTION
Inhibits platelet aggregation by reversibly interacting with the P2Y$_{12}$ ADP receptor.

Route	Onset	Peak	Duration
PO	Rapid	1–5 hr	8 hr

Half-life: 7 hours (ticagrelor), 9 hours (active metabolite).

ADVERSE REACTIONS
CNS: headache, dizziness, fatigue, syncope, loss of consciousness. **CV:** *bleeding,* atrial fibrillation, HTN, hypotension, chest pain, bradyarrhythmias, abnormal ECG. **GI:** nausea, diarrhea. **Musculoskeletal:** back pain, noncardiac chest pain. **Respiratory:** cough, dyspnea.

T

INTERACTIONS

Drug-drug. *Anticoagulants, fibrinolytics, long-term NSAIDs, omega-3 fatty acids, vitamin E:* May increase risk of bleeding. Use cautiously together.

Black Box Warning *Aspirin:* Maintenance doses of aspirin greater than 100 mg/day may decrease ticagrelor effectiveness and increase risk of bleeding. Maintenance doses of aspirin shouldn't exceed 100 mg/day. ∎

CYP3A4 strong inducers (carbamazepine, dexamethasone, phenobarbital, phenytoin, rifampin): May significantly decrease ticagrelor and active metabolite levels and therapeutic effect. Avoid use together.

CYP3A4 strong inhibitors (atazanavir, clarithromycin, indinavir, itraconazole, ketoconazole, nefazodone, nelfinavir, ritonavir, saquinavir, telithromycin, voriconazole): May significantly increase ticagrelor level and risk of adverse reactions. Avoid use together.

Digoxin: May increase digoxin level. Monitor digoxin level at start of treatment and with any changes to treatment.

Other P2Y$_{12}$ platelet inhibitors: Increases risk of bleeding. Use together is contraindicated.

Statins: May increase levels of these drugs. Don't exceed 40 mg of simvastatin or lovastatin with concurrent ticagrelor use.

Drug-herb. *Alfalfa, anise, bilberry:* May increase risk of bleeding. Avoid using together.

St. John's wort: May increase metabolism of ticagrelor and decrease drug's effectiveness. Avoid using together.

Drug-food. *Grapefruit juice:* May increase ticagrelor level. Monitor therapy closely.

EFFECTS ON LAB TEST RESULTS

• May increase uric acid and creatinine levels.

CONTRAINDICATIONS & CAUTIONS

Black Box Warning Drug can cause serious, sometimes fatal bleeding. Contraindicated in patients with history of intracranial hemorrhage or active pathologic bleeding (including peptic ulcer). ∎

Black Box Warning Don't start ticagrelor in patients who will undergo planned urgent CABG. If possible, discontinue ticagrelor at least 5 days before any surgery. ∎

• Don't give drug with another oral P2Y$_{12}$ platelet inhibitor.

• Contraindicated in patients hypersensitive to drug. Avoid use in those with severe hepatic impairment.

• Use cautiously in patients with moderate hepatic failure, elderly patients, patients with history of a bleeding disorder, and patients who have had percutaneous invasive procedures.

⚕ Alert: Drug can cause ventricular pauses. Bradyarrhythmias, including AV block, have been reported. Patients with a history of sick sinus syndrome, second- or third-degree AV block, or bradycardia-related syncope (without pacemakers) weren't studied.

Dialyzable drug: No.

⚠ Overdose S&S: Bleeding, nausea, vomiting, diarrhea, ventricular pauses.

PREGNANCY-LACTATION-REPRODUCTION

• There are no adequate studies in pregnant women. Use only if potential benefit justifies potential risk to the fetus.

• It isn't known if drug or its active metabolites appear in human milk. Patient should discontinue breastfeeding or discontinue drug.

NURSING CONSIDERATIONS

Black Box Warning If possible, manage bleeding without discontinuing ticagrelor; premature discontinuation of treatment increases risk of MI, stent thrombosis, or death. If drug must be temporarily stopped, restart as soon as possible. ∎

• Monitor patient for bleeding.

• Monitor patient for dyspnea and rule out underlying conditions that require treatment in patients with new, prolonged, or worsened difficulty breathing. Dyspnea secondary to ticagrelor therapy is usually mild to moderate, and often self-limiting with continued treatment. If ticagrelor is discontinued for intolerable dyspnea, consider another antiplatelet agent.

• Ticagrelor can be given to patients with ACS who have already been given a loading dose of clopidogrel.

• **Look alike–sound alike:** Don't confuse Brilinta with Brintellix.

PATIENT TEACHING

Black Box Warning Tell patient not to take more than 100 mg of aspirin per day. Warn that other OTC products may also contain aspirin. ∎

Reactions in bold italics are *life-threatening*. Interactions may have a *rapid onset* or a **delayed onset**.

• Inform patient that bleeding or bruising may occur more easily and it will take longer for the bleeding to stop. Tell patient to immediately report unexpected, prolonged, or excessive bleeding, or blood in the urine or stool.

• Warn patient not to stop drug without consulting prescriber.

• Instruct patient to notify all health care providers about taking ticagrelor before any scheduled surgery or dental appointment. Advise patient to discuss with original prescriber recommendations by other providers to stop taking ticagrelor.

• Tell patient that ticagrelor may cause mild to moderate shortness of breath and to report unexpected shortness of breath, especially if it's severe.

• Advise patient that if a dose is missed to take the next dose at its scheduled time and not to take extra medication to make up for the missed dose.

• Tell female patient who is pregnant or planning to become pregnant to consult her primary health care provider before using this medication.

• Warn female patient taking drug not to breastfeed.

SAFETY ALERT!

tinidazole
teh-NID-ah-zol

Therapeutic class: Antiprotozoals
Pharmacologic class: Antiprotozoals

AVAILABLE FORMS
Tablets: 250 mg, 500 mg

INDICATIONS & DOSAGES
Black Box Warning Use tinidazole only for the conditions for which it's indicated. ∎
Adjust-a-dose (for all indications): For patients receiving hemodialysis, give an additional dose equal to half the recommended dose after the hemodialysis session.
➤ **Bacterial vaginosis in adult women**
Adults: 2 g PO once daily for 2 days, or 1 g PO once daily for 5 days.
➤ **Trichomoniasis caused by *Trichomonas vaginalis***

Adults: 2 g PO as a single dose. Sexual partners should be treated at the same time with the same dose.
➤ **Giardiasis caused by *Giardia lamblia* (*G. duodenalis*)**
Adults: 2 g PO as a single dose.
Children age 3 and older: Give 50 mg/kg (up to 2 g) PO as a single dose.
➤ **Intestinal amebiasis caused by *Entamoeba histolytica***
Adults: 2 g PO daily for 3 days.
Children age 3 and older: Give 50 mg/kg (up to 2 g) PO daily for 3 days.
➤ **Amebic liver abscess (amebiasis)**
Adults: 2 g PO daily for 3 to 5 days.
Children age 3 and older: Give 50 mg/kg (up to 2 g) PO daily for 3 to 5 days.

ADMINISTRATION
PO
• Give drug with food to minimize adverse GI effects.
• For children who can't swallow pills, drug can be compounded by the pharmacy by crushing tablets into fine powder and mixing with 10 mL of artificial cherry syrup. Suspension is stable at room temperature for 7 days. Shake well before administration.

ACTION
For *Trichomonas*, cell extracts of *Trichomonas* reduce the compound's nitro group into a free nitro radical that may be responsible for the antiprotozoal activity. Mechanism of action against *Giardia* and *Entamoeba* is unknown.

Route	Onset	Peak	Duration
PO	Unknown	1–2 hr	Unknown

Half-life: 12 to 15 hours.

ADVERSE REACTIONS
CNS: *seizures,* dizziness, fatigue, headache, malaise, weakness. **GI:** anorexia, constipation, cramps, diarrhea, abdominal pain, dyspepsia, metallic taste, nausea, vomiting, decreased appetite, flatulence. **GU:** UTI, painful urination, urine abnormality, pelvic pain, vulvovaginal discomfort, vaginal odor, menorrhagia. **Respiratory:** URI.

INTERACTIONS

Drug-drug. *Cholestyramine:* May decrease oral bioavailability of tinidazole. Separate dosing times.

Cyclosporine, tacrolimus: May increase cyclosporine or tacrolimus level. Monitor closely for toxicity, including headache, nausea, vomiting, nephrotoxicity, and electrolyte abnormalities.

CYP450 inducers (fosphenytoin, phenobarbital, phenytoin, rifampin): May increase tinidazole elimination. Monitor patient.

CYP450 inhibitors (cimetidine, ketoconazole): May prolong tinidazole half-life and decrease clearance. Monitor patient.

Disulfiram: May cause psychotic reactions and may increase abdominal cramping, nausea, vomiting, headaches, and flushing. Separate doses by 2 weeks.

5-FU: May decrease 5-FU clearance, increasing adverse effects without added benefit. Monitor patient for rash, nausea, vomiting, stomatitis, and leukopenia.

Fosphenytoin, phenytoin: May prolong phenytoin half-life and decrease clearance of IV drug. Monitor patient for toxicity.

Lactobacillus: May decrease therapeutic effect of lactobacillus. Monitor therapy.

Lithium: May increase lithium level. Monitor patient; monitor lithium and creatinine levels.

Warfarin, other oral anticoagulants: May increase anticoagulant effect. Anticoagulant dosage may need adjustment during and for up to 8 days after tinidazole therapy.

Drug-herb. *St. John's wort:* May increase or decrease drug level. Discourage use together.

Drug-lifestyle. *Use of alcohol and alcohol-containing products:* May increase abdominal cramps, nausea, vomiting, headaches, and flushing. Avoid using together and for 3 days after stopping drug.

EFFECTS ON LAB TEST RESULTS

• May increase AST, ALT, glucose, LDH, and triglyceride levels.
• May decrease WBC count.

CONTRAINDICATIONS & CAUTIONS

• Contraindicated in patients hypersensitive to drug, its component, or other nitroimidazole derivatives.

Black Box Warning Carcinogenicity has been seen in mice and rats treated long-term

with metronidazole, another nitroimidazole agent. Although such data haven't been reported for tinidazole, both drugs are structurally related and have similar biologic effects. ■

• Use cautiously in patients with CNS disorders, the elderly, and in those with blood dyscrasias or hepatic dysfunction.

Dialyzable drug: 43% in 6 hours.

PREGNANCY-LACTATION-REPRODUCTION

• Available data of use during pregnancy are insufficient to identify risk of major birth defects, miscarriage, or adverse maternal or fetal outcomes. Weigh potential benefits against potential risks to both mother and fetus.

• Drug appears in human milk for up to 72 hours after administration. Patient shouldn't breastfeed during therapy and for 3 days after final dose.

• Based on animal studies, drug may impair fertility in males of reproductive potential.

NURSING CONSIDERATIONS

• If therapy exceeds 3 days, monitor children closely.

🔹 *Alert:* If abnormal neurologic signs, such as seizures or paresthesia of the arms or legs, occur, stop drug immediately.

• Superinfection and CDAD can occur up to 2 months after therapy ends. Monitor patient for diarrhea.

• If candidiasis develops during therapy, patient may need an antifungal.

• Use cautiously in elderly patients, who may have decreased liver or kidney function.

• Monitor CBC.

PATIENT TEACHING

• Tell patient to take drug with food.

🔹 *Alert:* Tell patient to report to prescriber seizures and numbness in arms or legs.

• Warn patient not to drink alcohol or use alcohol-containing products while taking drug and for 3 days afterward.

• Advise female patient to notify prescriber if she becomes pregnant.

• Tell female patient to stop breastfeeding during therapy and for 3 days after final dose.

• If patient is being treated for a sexually transmitted infection, explain that patient's sexual partners should be treated at the same time.

Reactions in bold italics are *life-threatening*. Interactions may have a *rapid onset* or a ***delayed onset***.

tiotropium bromide
tye-oh-TROH-pee-um

Spiriva HandiHaler, Spiriva Respimat

Therapeutic class: Bronchodilators
Pharmacologic class: Anticholinergics

AVAILABLE FORMS
Capsules (powder for inhalation): 18 mcg
Spray inhaler (Respimat): 1.25 mcg/actuation, 2.5 mcg/actuation

INDICATIONS & DOSAGES
Adjust-a-dose (for all indications): Closely monitor patients with moderate to severe renal impairment for anticholinergic effects.
➤ **To reduce COPD exacerbations; maintenance treatment of bronchospasm in COPD, including chronic bronchitis and emphysema**
Adults: 2 oral inhalations of 1 capsule (18 mcg) once daily using HandiHaler inhalation device. Or, 2 inhalations (2.5 mcg each) of spray once daily.
➤ **Long-term maintenance treatment of asthma (Spiriva Respimat)**
Adults and children age 6 and older: 2 inhalations of 1.25 mcg/actuation spray once daily; total dose equals 2.5 mcg of tiotropium. Maximum benefits in lung function may take up to 4 to 8 weeks of dosing.

ADMINISTRATION
Inhalational
Capsules
• Give capsules only by oral inhalation with the HandiHaler device; don't store in device.
• Open capsule blister immediately before use.
• Capsules aren't for oral ingestion.
Respimat spray inhaler
• Before first use, insert cartridge into the inhaler.
• Prime the unit before using it for the first time by actuating the inhaler toward the ground until an aerosol cloud is visible; then repeat the process three more times.
• If not used for more than 3 days, the inhaler should be actuated once to prepare it for use. If not used for more than 21 days,

the inhaler should be actuated until an aerosol cloud is visible; then repeat the process three more times.

ACTION
Competitive, reversible inhibition of muscarinic receptors in smooth muscle leads to bronchodilation.

Route	Onset	Peak	Duration
Inhalation	Unknown	5–7 min	>24 hr

Half-life: COPD, 25 hours; asthma, 44 hours.

ADVERSE REACTIONS
CNS: depression, paresthesia, headache, dizziness, fever, insomnia. **CV:** *angina pectoris,* chest pain, edema, palpitations, HTN. **EENT:** cataract, glaucoma, epistaxis, sinusitis, laryngitis, dysphonia, pharyngitis, rhinitis, oropharyngeal candidiasis. **GI:** dry mouth, abdominal pain, constipation, dyspepsia, GERD, stomatitis, vomiting, diarrhea. **GU:** UTI. **Metabolic:** hypercholesterolemia, hyperglycemia. **Musculoskeletal:** arthritis, leg pain, myalgia, skeletal pain. **Respiratory:** URI, cough, bronchitis. **Skin:** rash, pruritus. **Other:** accidental injury, allergic reaction, candidiasis, flulike syndrome, herpes zoster, infections, candidiasis.

INTERACTIONS
Drug-drug. *Anticholinergics:* May increase the risk of adverse reactions. Avoid using together.
Glucagon: May increase risk of GI adverse effects. Avoid combination.
Opioids: May increase risk of constipation and urine retention. Monitor patient closely.
Potassium chloride: May increase ulcer risk. Avoid combination.

EFFECTS ON LAB TEST RESULTS
• May increase cholesterol and glucose levels.

CONTRAINDICATIONS & CAUTIONS
• Contraindicated in patients hypersensitive to atropine, its derivatives, ipratropium, or components of the product.
• Immediate hypersensitivity reactions can occur, including urticaria, angioedema, rash, itching, and anaphylaxis.

T

• Use cautiously in patients with CrCl of less than 60 mL/minute, and in patients with angle-closure glaucoma, prostatic hyperplasia, or bladder neck obstruction.
• Use capsule cautiously in patients with severe hypersensitivity to milk protein.
Dialyzable drug: Unknown.
⚠ *Overdose S&S:* Change in mental status, tremors, abdominal pain, severe constipation.

PREGNANCY-LACTATION-REPRODUCTION
• There are no adequate studies in pregnant women. Use only if potential benefit justifies potential risk to the fetus.
• It isn't known if drug appears in human milk. Use cautiously in breastfeeding women.

NURSING CONSIDERATIONS
🌓 *Alert:* Use drug for maintenance treatment of COPD or asthma, not for acute bronchospasm.
• Watch for evidence of hypersensitivity (especially angioedema) and paradoxical bronchospasm. Discontinue drug immediately.
• Monitor patients for signs and symptoms of narrow-angle glaucoma and urine retention. In patients with renal impairment, watch for anticholinergic adverse reactions.
• *Look alike–sound alike:* Don't confuse Spiriva with Inspra.

PATIENT TEACHING
• Inform patient that drug is for maintenance treatment of COPD or asthma and not for immediate relief of breathing problems.
🌓 *Alert:* Explain that capsules are for inhalation and shouldn't be swallowed.
• Provide full instructions for the HandiHaler device or the Respimat spray inhaler. Demonstrate use and observe return demonstration from patient.
• Tell patient not to get powder or spray in eyes.
• Tell patient not to take more than one dose (2 inhalations) in 24 hours.
• Review signs and symptoms of hypersensitivity (especially angioedema) and paradoxical bronchospasm. Tell patient to stop the drug and contact prescriber if they occur.

• Advise patient to report eye pain, blurred vision, visual halos, colored images, or red eyes immediately.
• Tell patient to keep capsules in sealed blisters and to remove each capsule just before use. Caution against storing capsules in the HandiHaler device.
• Instruct patient to store capsules and cartridges at 77° F (25° C) and not to expose them to extreme temperatures or moisture.
• Advise patient that when the labeled number of actuations (28 or 60) has been dispensed from the Respimat inhaler, a locking mechanism will be engaged and no more actuations can be dispensed.

tipranavir
tih-PRAN-uh-veer

Aptivus

Therapeutic class: Antiretrovirals
Pharmacologic class: Protease inhibitors

AVAILABLE FORMS
Capsules ⓄⒷⒸ: 250 mg*
Oral solution: 100 mg/mL

INDICATIONS & DOSAGES
➤ **HIV-1 in patients with viral replication who are highly treatment-experienced or have HIV-1 strains resistant to multiple protease inhibitors, in combination with ritonavir and other antiretrovirals**
Adults: 500 mg PO b.i.d. with 200 mg of ritonavir b.i.d.
Children ages 2 to 18: 14 mg/kg with ritonavir 6 mg/kg (or tipranavir 375 mg/m^2 with ritonavir 150 mg/m^2) b.i.d., not to exceed dosage of tipranavir 500 mg with ritonavir 200 mg b.i.d. For children who develop intolerance or toxicity, may consider decreasing dosage to tipranavir 12 mg/kg with ritonavir 5 mg/kg (or tipranavir 290 mg/m^2 with ritonavir 115 mg/m^2) b.i.d. provided the virus isn't resistant to multiple protease inhibitors.
Adjust-a-dose: Discontinue if asymptomatic AST or ALT elevations greater than 10 × ULN occur. Also discontinue if AST or ALT elevations greater than 5 to 10 × ULN occur concurrently with total bilirubin level greater than 2.5 × ULN.

ADMINISTRATION
PO
• Give with ritonavir and other antiretrovirals.
• Make sure patient swallows capsules whole and doesn't break, crush, or chew them.
• When given with ritonavir tablets, drug must only be taken with meals; when given with ritonavir capsules or solution, drug can be taken with or without meals.
• Don't freeze or refrigerate oral solution.
• Store unopened capsule bottle in refrigerator; after bottle is opened, store at room temperature.
• Use within 60 days of opening capsule or oral solution bottle.

ACTION
Inhibits virus-specific processing of polyproteins in HIV-1 infected cells, preventing formation of mature virions.

Route	Onset	Peak	Duration
PO	Unknown	3 hr	Unknown

Half-life: Adults, 6 hours; children age 2 to younger than age 6, 8 hours; children age 6 to younger than age 12, 7 hours; children ages 12 to 18, 5 hours.

ADVERSE REACTIONS
CNS: dizziness, fatigue, headache, insomnia, malaise, peripheral neuropathy, pyrexia, sleep disorder, somnolence, *intracranial hemorrhage.* **GI:** diarrhea, *pancreatitis,* abdominal distention, abdominal pain, dyspepsia, flatulence, GERD, nausea, vomiting. **GU:** renal insufficiency. **Hematologic:** *neutropenia, thrombocytopenia,* anemia. **Hepatic:** *hepatic failure, hepatitis.* **Metabolic:** anorexia, decreased appetite, dehydration, diabetes mellitus, facial wasting, hyperglycemia, hyperlipidemia, hypertriglyceridemia, weight loss. **Musculoskeletal:** muscle cramps, myalgia. **Respiratory:** cough, dyspnea. **Skin:** rash, acquired lipodystrophy, exanthem, lipoatrophy, lipohypertrophy, pruritus. **Other:** flulike illness, hypersensitivity, reactivation of herpes simplex and varicella zoster.

INTERACTIONS
Refer to manufacturer's prescribing information for complete list of drug interactions.

Drug-drug. *Alfuzosin:* May increase alfuzosin serum concentration. Avoid combination.

Amiodarone, bepridil, flecainide, propafenone, quinidine: May increase levels of these drugs and risk of life-threatening arrhythmias. Use together is contraindicated.

Anticoagulants: May increase anticoagulant effect. Monitor patient closely.

🚯 *Alert: Atorvastatin:* May increase levels of both drugs and risk of myopathy and rhabdomyolysis. Avoid use together.

Bosentan: May decrease tipranavir serum concentration; may increase bosentan serum concentration. Use bosentan 62.5 mg/day or every other day in adults taking tipranavir/ritonavir for at least 10 days. Temporarily stop bosentan (for at least 36 hours) before starting tipranavir/ritonavir; wait at least 10 days before restarting bosentan. Consider therapy modification.

Clarithromycin: May increase levels of both drugs. If CrCl is 30 to 60 mL/minute, decrease clarithromycin dose by 50%. If CrCl is less than 30 mL/minute, decrease clarithromycin dose by 75%.

Clozapine: May increase clozapine serum concentration. Monitor patient closely.

Codeine: May decrease effectiveness of codeine. Consider therapy modification.

Colchicine: May increase risk of life-threatening and fatal colchicine toxicity. Use together is contraindicated in patients with renal or hepatic impairment. In patients with healthy renal and hepatic function, reduce colchicine dosage according to manufacturer's instructions.

Contraceptives (progestins and estrogens): May decrease contraceptive effectiveness. Patient should use alternative or additional contraceptive method.

Cyclosporine, sirolimus, tacrolimus: May cause unpredictable interaction. Monitor drug levels closely until they've stabilized.

CYP3A4 inducers: May increase metabolism of protease inhibitors. Consider therapy modification.

Desipramine: May increase desipramine level. Decrease dose and monitor desipramine level.

Didanosine: May decrease didanosine level. Separate dosing by at least 2 hours.

T

Diltiazem, felodipine, nicardipine, nisoldipine, verapamil: May cause unpredictable interaction. Use together cautiously, and monitor patient closely.

Disulfiram, metronidazole: May cause disulfiram-like reaction when used with capsules. Use together cautiously.

Ergot derivatives (dihydroergotamine, ergonovine, ergotamine, methylergonovine): May cause acute ergot toxicity, including peripheral vasospasm and ischemia of extremities. Use together is contraindicated.

Estrogen-based hormone therapy: May decrease estrogen level, and rash may occur. Monitor patient carefully. Advise using nonhormonal contraception.

Fluoxetine, paroxetine, sertraline: May increase levels of these drugs. Adjust dosages as needed.

Glimepiride, glipizide, glyburide, pioglitazone, repaglinide, tolbutamide: May affect glucose levels. Monitor glucose level carefully.

❸ *Alert:* *Lovastatin, simvastatin:* May increase risk of myopathy and rhabdomyolysis. Use together is contraindicated.

Meperidine: May increase normeperidine metabolite. Avoid using together.

Methadone: May decrease methadone level by 50%. Consider increasing methadone dosage.

Midazolam, triazolam: May cause prolonged or increased sedation or respiratory depression. Use together is contraindicated.

Pimozide: May cause life-threatening arrhythmias. Use together is contraindicated.

Rifabutin: May increase rifabutin level. Decrease rifabutin dose by 75%.

Rifampin: May lead to loss of virologic response and resistance to tipranavir and other protease inhibitors. Use together is contraindicated.

Sildenafil, tadalafil, vardenafil: May increase levels of these drugs. Use together cautiously. Tell patient not to exceed 25 mg sildenafil in 48 hours, 10 mg tadalafil every 72 hours, or 2.5 mg vardenafil every 72 hours. Use of sildenafil (Revatio) for treatment of PAH is contraindicated.

Tamoxifen: May decrease serum concentration of active metabolite of tamoxifen. Avoid combination.

Trazodone: May increase trazodone serum concentration. Use together cautiously and consider a lower trazodone dose.

Valproic acid: May reduce valproic acid plasma level. Use with caution.

Warfarin: May cause unpredictable reaction. Check INR often.

Drug-herb. *Garlic:* May decrease serum concentration of protease inhibitors. Use together isn't recommended.

St. John's wort: May lead to loss of virologic response and resistance to tipranavir and other antiretrovirals. Don't use together.

EFFECTS ON LAB TEST RESULTS

• May increase total cholesterol, triglyceride, blood glucose, amylase, lipase, GGT, CK, ALT, and AST levels.

• May decrease Hb level and hematocrit and WBC, neutrophil, and platelet counts.

CONTRAINDICATIONS & CAUTIONS

Black Box Warning Administration of tipranavir has been associated with fatal and nonfatal intracranial hemorrhage, clinical hepatitis, and hepatic decompensation. ∎

• Contraindicated in patients hypersensitive to ingredients of the product, patients with moderate or severe (Child-Pugh class B or C) hepatic insufficiency, and patients taking drugs that are potent CYP3A inducers or that depend on CYP3A for clearance plus ritonavir.

• Use cautiously in patients with bleeding risk, sulfonamide allergy, diabetes, liver disease, HBV or HCV infection, or hemophilia A or B.

Dialyzable drug: No.

PREGNANCY-LACTATION-REPRODUCTION

• There are no adequate studies in pregnant women. Use only if potential benefit justifies potential risk to the fetus.

• To monitor maternal-fetal outcomes, register patients exposed to drug in the Antiretroviral Pregnancy Registry (1-800-258-4263).

• The CDC recommends that mothers with HIV-1 infection not breastfeed to avoid risking postnatal transmission of HIV-1.

NURSING CONSIDERATIONS

Black Box Warning Patients with chronic HBV or HCV infection are at increased risk for hepatotoxicity; fatalities have been reported. ■

• Assess for evidence of hepatitis, such as fatigue, malaise, anorexia, nausea, jaundice, bilirubinemia, acholic stools, liver tenderness, and hepatomegaly. If patient develops signs or symptoms of hepatitis, notify prescriber.

❸ **Alert:** Don't give drug to treatment-naive patients.

• To be effective, drug must be given with ritonavir and with other antiretrovirals.

❸ **Alert:** Monitor patient for signs and symptoms of intracranial hemorrhage, including headache, nausea and vomiting, change in mental status, speech or balance difficulties, and seizures.

❸ **Alert:** Obtain thorough patient drug history. Many drugs may interact with tipranavir. Consider potential for drug interactions before and during therapy; review concomitant medications during therapy; and monitor patient for adverse reactions associated with concomitant medications.

• Monitor LFTs at start of treatment and often during treatment.

• In diabetic patients, monitor glucose level closely; hyperglycemia may occur.

• Obtain baseline cholesterol and triglyceride levels at start of and periodically during therapy.

• Monitor patient for cushingoid symptoms, such as central obesity, buffalo hump, peripheral wasting, facial wasting, and breast enlargement.

• Use cautiously in elderly patients because they are more likely to have decreased organ function, multidrug therapy, and other illnesses.

PATIENT TEACHING

• Explain that drug doesn't cure HIV infection and doesn't reduce the risk of transmitting the virus to others.

❸ **Alert:** Many drugs may interfere with this drug. Urge patient to report all prescription and OTC drugs and herbal products being taken.

• Tell patient that drug is effective only when taken with ritonavir and other antiretrovirals.

• Instruct patient taking ritonavir tablets to take them with meals; patient taking ritonavir capsules or solution can take them with or without meals.

• Tell patient to store unopened capsule bottle in refrigerator, to store at room temperature after bottle is opened, and to use within 60 days of opening. Advise patient not to freeze or refrigerate oral solution.

• Tell patient to swallow capsules whole and to not break, crush, or chew them.

• Instruct patient taking oral solution not to take supplemental vitamin E in an amount greater than a standard multivitamin.

• Urge patient to report all adverse reactions and to stop drug and contact prescriber if signs and symptoms of hepatitis or intracranial hemorrhage occur.

• If female patient uses hormonal contraceptives, advise use of barrier contraception.

• Tell patient that redistribution or accumulation of body fat may occur.

• Advise female patient that breastfeeding isn't recommended during therapy.

SAFETY ALERT!

tirofiban hydrochloride
tye-row-FYE-ban

Aggrastat

Therapeutic class: Antiplatelet drugs
Pharmacologic class: Glycoprotein IIb/IIIa receptor antagonists

AVAILABLE FORMS

Injection (premixed bag): 50 mcg/mL in 250 mL
Injection (vials): 50 mcg/mL in 100 mL, 250 mcg/mL in 15 mL (bolus)

INDICATIONS & DOSAGES

➤ **In patients with non-ST elevation ACS to reduce the rate of thrombotic CV events (combined endpoint of death, MI, or refractory ischemia/repeat cardiac procedure)**
Adults: IV loading dose of 25 mcg/kg administered within 5 minutes, followed by 0.15 mcg/kg/minute for up to 18 hours.
Adjust-a-dose: If CrCl is 60 mL/minute or less, use an IV loading dose of 25 mcg/kg

T

administered within 5 minutes, followed by 0.075 mcg/kg/minute for up to 18 hours.

➤ **To support PCI (administered at the time of PCI) for ST-elevation MI ◆**
Adults: Loading dose of 25 mcg/kg IV administered over 5 minutes or less at the time of PCI, followed by maintenance infusion of 0.15 mcg/kg/minute in combination with heparin or bivalirudin in selected patients; was continued for 18 to 24 hours in clinical trials.

ADMINISTRATION

IV

▼ Inspect solution for particulate matter before giving, and check for leaks by squeezing the inner bag firmly. If bag leaks or particles are visible, discard solution.

▼ Avoid use of noncompressible sites (such as subclavian or jugular veins).

▼ Don't use plastic containers in series connections; may result in air embolism by drawing air from the first bag if it's empty of solution.

▼ May give tirofiban through same IV line as heparin, atropine sulfate, dobutamine, epinephrine hydrochloride, furosemide, midazolam hydrochloride, morphine sulfate, nitroglycerin, propranolol hydrochloride, dopamine, lidocaine, potassium chloride, and famotidine.

▼ Discard unused solution 24 hours after the start of infusion.

▼ Store drug at room temperature. Protect from light.

▼ **Incompatibilities:** Amphotericin B, dantrolene, diazepam, lansoprazole, phenytoin.

ACTION

Reversibly binds to the glycoprotein IIb/IIIa receptor on human platelets and inhibits platelet aggregation.

Route	Onset	Peak	Duration
IV	10 min	Immediate	4–8 hr

Half-life: About 2 hours.

ADVERSE REACTIONS

CNS: dizziness, headache, fever. **CV:** *brady-cardia, coronary artery dissection, hemor-rhage,* edema, vasovagal reaction. **GI:** occult bleeding, nausea. **Hematologic:** bleeding

at arterial access site, *thrombocytopenia.*
Musculoskeletal: leg pain. **Skin:** sweating.
Other: pelvic pain.

INTERACTIONS

Drug-drug. ❸ *Alert: Anticoagulants and antiplatelet agents, such as aspirin, apixaban, clopidogrel, dabigatran, dipyridamole, edoxaban, fibrinolytics, heparin, NSAIDs, rivaroxaban, ticlopidine, and warfarin; glucosamine, omega-3 fatty acids, vitamin E:* May increase risk of bleeding. Monitor patient closely.
Levothyroxine, omeprazole: May increase tirofiban renal clearance. Monitor patient.
Tipranavir: May increase antiplatelet effect of tirofiban. Monitor patient closely.
Drug-herb. *Alfalfa, anise, bilberry:* May increase risk of bleeding. Urge patient to avoid herbal supplements.

EFFECTS ON LAB TEST RESULTS

• May decrease Hb level and hematocrit.
• May decrease platelet count.

CONTRAINDICATIONS & CAUTIONS

• Contraindicated in patients hypersensitive to drug or its components.
• Contraindicated in patients with active internal bleeding or history of bleeding diathesis within previous 30 days, major surgical procedure or physical trauma within previous month, thrombocytopenia after previous exposure to drug, and severe HTN.
• Use cautiously in patients with renal impairment and those with increased risk of bleeding, including patients with hemorrhagic retinopathy or platelet count less than 150,000/mm³.
• Safety and effectiveness haven't been studied in patients younger than age 18.
Dialyzable drug: Yes.
⚠ *Overdose S&S:* Bleeding.

PREGNANCY-LACTATION-REPRODUCTION

• There are no adequate studies in pregnant women; adverse events haven't been observed in animal reproduction studies.
• It isn't known if drug appears in human milk. Patient should discontinue breastfeeding or discontinue drug.

Reactions in bold italics are *life-threatening*. Interactions may have a *rapid onset* or a *delayed onset*.

NURSING CONSIDERATIONS
• Monitor Hb level, hematocrit, and platelet count before starting therapy, 6 hours after loading dose, and at least daily during therapy. If thrombocytopenia occurs, notify prescriber.
• Monitor aPTT before treatment and 6 hours after the start of heparin infusion.
• Monitor patient for bleeding.
☻ **Alert:** The most common adverse effect is bleeding at the arterial access site for cardiac catheterization.
• Minimize use of arterial and venous punctures, IM injections, urinary catheters, and nasotracheal and NG tubes.
• Elderly patients have a higher risk of bleeding complications.
• Discontinue drug at least 2 to 4 hours before CABG surgery.
• **Look alike–sound alike:** Don't confuse Aggrastat with argatroban or Aggrenox.

PATIENT TEACHING
• Explain that drug is used to prevent chest pain and heart attack.
• Explain that the benefits of the drug far outweigh the risk of serious bleeding.
• Instruct patient to report chest discomfort or other adverse effects immediately.
• Tell patient that frequent blood sampling may be needed to evaluate therapy.

tiZANidine hydrochloride
tis-AN-i-deen

Zanaflex

Therapeutic class: Skeletal muscle relaxants
Pharmacologic class: Centrally acting alpha$_2$-adrenergic agonists

AVAILABLE FORMS
Capsules: 2 mg, 4 mg, 6 mg
Tablets: 2 mg, 4 mg

INDICATIONS & DOSAGES
➤ **Acute and intermittent management of increased muscle tone with spasticity**
Adults: Initially, 2 mg PO every 6 to 8 hours, as needed, to maximum of three doses in 24 hours. Dosage can be increased gradually in 2- to 4-mg increments, with 1 to 4 days between increases. Maximum, 36 mg daily.
Adjust-a-dose: Use cautiously and reduce dosage during titration in patients with hepatic impairment or renal insufficiency (CrCl of less than 25 mL/minute). If higher dosages are needed, increase individual doses rather than frequency.

ADMINISTRATION
PO
• Give drug consistently as either tablets or capsules and with or without food for same absorption rate and effect.

ACTION
Central alpha$_2$ agonist that may reduce spasticity by increasing presynaptic inhibition of motor neurons at the level of the spinal cord.

Route	Onset	Peak	Duration
PO	Unknown	1–2 hr	3–6 hr

Half-life: 2½ hours; metabolites, 20 to 40 hours.

ADVERSE REACTIONS
CNS: somnolence, sedation, asthenia, weakness, tiredness, dizziness, speech disorder, dyskinesia, nervousness, hallucinations, delusions, increased spasms, paresthesia. **CV:** hypotension, arrhythmia, *bradycardia.* **EENT:** amblyopia, visual field defect, pharyngitis, rhinitis, sinusitis. **GI:** dry mouth, constipation, vomiting, dyspepsia. **GU:** UTI, urinary frequency, vaginitis. **Hepatic:** hepatic injury. **Metabolic:** weight loss. **Musculoskeletal:** myasthenia, pathologic fracture. **Skin:** sweating, urticaria. **Other:** infection, *sepsis,* flulike syndrome.

INTERACTIONS
Drug-drug. *Acetaminophen:* May delay acetaminophen absorption time. Monitor patient for clinical effect.
Antihypertensives, other alpha agonists (such as clonidine): May cause hypotension; monitor patient closely. Avoid using together.
Baclofen, benzodiazepines, cannabis, dronabinol, magnesium sulfate, other CNS depressants: May have additive CNS depressant effects. Avoid using together.
CYP1A2 inhibitors (amiodarone, acyclovir, cimetidine, ciprofloxacin, famotidine,

T

fluoroquinolones, fluvoxamine, mexiletine, propafenone, ticlopidine, verapamil, zileuton): May cause significant increases in tizanidine levels. Use together should be avoided; use of ciprofloxacin or fluvoxamine with tizanidine is contraindicated.

Drugs that prolong QTc interval: May increase QTc interval and risk of ventricular arrhythmias. Monitor therapy.

Black Box Warning *Opioids:* May cause slow or difficult breathing, sedation, and death. Avoid use together. If use together is necessary, limit dosage and duration of each drug to minimum necessary for desired effect. ∎

Oral contraceptives: May decrease tizanidine clearance. Reduce tizanidine dosage.

Drug-herb. *Kava kava:* May enhance adverse CNS effects. Monitor patient closely.

Drug-lifestyle. *Alcohol use:* May increase CNS depression. Discourage use together.

EFFECTS ON LAB TEST RESULTS
• May increase AST and ALT levels.

CONTRAINDICATIONS & CAUTIONS
• Contraindicated in patients hypersensitive to drug and in patients taking potent CYP1A2 inhibitors, such as fluvoxamine or ciprofloxacin.

Black Box Warning *Opioid class warning:* Opioids should only be prescribed with benzodiazepines or other CNS depressants to patients for whom alternative treatment options are inadequate. ∎

• Use cautiously in patients who are taking antihypertensives, in those with renal or hepatic impairment or psychiatric disorders, and in elderly patients.

• Safety and effectiveness in children haven't been established.

Dialyzable drug: Unlikely.

⚠ *Overdose S&S:* Lethargy, somnolence, confusion, coma, bradycardia, hypotension, respiratory depression, depressed cardiac function.

PREGNANCY-LACTATION-REPRODUCTION
• Drug hasn't been studied in pregnant women. Use only if potential benefit justifies potential risk to the fetus.

• It isn't known if drug appears in human milk. Use cautiously in breastfeeding women.

NURSING CONSIDERATIONS
❸ *Alert:* The capsules and tablets are bioequivalent only if taken on an empty stomach.

• Obtain LFT results before treatment; during treatment at 1, 3, and 6 months; and then periodically thereafter.

• Monitor renal function, especially in elderly patients and those with renal insufficiency.

• May prolong QT interval and cause bradycardia and hypotension. Closely monitor vital signs, especially in patients receiving maximum recommended dosage and those taking other drugs that prolong QT interval.

• Monitor patient for signs and symptoms of excess sedation if patient is taking drug along with another CNS depressant.

• Consider discontinuing drug in patients who develop hallucinations.

❸ *Alert:* Stop drug gradually, especially in patients taking high doses for a prolonged period. Decrease dose slowly to minimize the potential for rebound HTN, tachycardia, and hypertonia.

• *Look alike–sound alike:* Don't confuse tizanidine with tiagabine; both have 4-mg starting doses. Don't confuse Zanaflex with Xiaflex.

PATIENT TEACHING
Black Box Warning *Opioid class warning:* Caution patient or caregiver of patient taking an opioid with a benzodiazepine, CNS depressant, or alcohol to seek immediate medical attention for dizziness, lightheadedness, extreme sleepiness, slowed or difficult breathing, or unresponsiveness. ∎

• Caution patient to avoid alcohol and activities that require alertness, such as driving or operating machinery, until drug's effects are known. Drug may cause drowsiness.

• Inform patient that dizziness upon standing quickly can be minimized by rising slowly.

❸ *Alert:* Advise patient that tizanidine absorption varies depending on whether drug is taken with or without food and that it should always be taken the same way to

---

reduce risk of changes in efficacy and adverse reactions.
• Instruct patient to inform the health care provider and pharmacist when medications are added or removed from patient's regimen.
• Advise patient not to suddenly stop taking medication.

tobramycin
toe-bra-MYE-sin

Tobrex

tobramycin sulfate
Bethkis, Kitabis Pak, TOBI, TOBI Podhaler

Therapeutic class: Antibiotics
Pharmacologic class: Aminoglycosides

AVAILABLE FORMS
Capsules (for inhalation): 28 mg
Multidose vials (pediatric): 10 mg/mL, 40 mg/mL
Nebulizer solution (for inhalation): 300 mg/4 mL, 300 mg/5 mL
Ophthalmic ointment: 0.3%
Ophthalmic solution: 0.3%
Premixed parenteral injection for infusion: 80 mg in 100 mL NSS

INDICATIONS & DOSAGES
➤ **Serious infection caused by sensitive strains of *Escherichia coli, Proteus, Klebsiella, Enterobacter, Serratia, Morganella morganii, Staphylococcus aureus, Citrobacter, Pseudomonas*, or *Providencia***
Adults: 3 mg/kg/day IM or IV in three equal doses every 8 hours. For life-threatening infections, give up to 5 mg/kg/day in divided doses every 6 to 8 hours; reduce to 3 mg/kg daily as soon as clinically indicated.
Children older than age 1 week: 6 to 7.5 mg/kg/day IM or IV, in three or four divided doses.
Neonates younger than age 1 week or preterm infants: Up to 4 mg/kg/day IV or IM in two equal doses every 12 hours.
Adjust-a-dose: For patients with renal impairment, give loading dose of 1 mg/kg; then give decreased doses at 8-hour intervals

or same dose at prolonged intervals. For hemodialysis patients, give 50% of the normal dose after dialysis and adjust according to serum concentrations. For patients with severe cystic fibrosis, initial dose is 10 mg/kg/day IV or IM, in four divided doses.
➤ **To manage cystic fibrosis patients with *Pseudomonas aeruginosa* infection**
Adults and children age 6 and older: 300 mg via nebulizer every 12 hours for 28 days. Continue cycle of 28 days on drug and 28 days off. Or, using TOBI Podhaler device, have patient inhale contents of four 28-mg capsules every 12 hours for 28 days, stop therapy for 28 days, then repeat and continue cycles of 28 days on drug and 28 days off.
➤ **External ocular infections by susceptible bacteria**
Adults and children age 2 months and older: In mild to moderate infections, instill 1 or 2 drops into affected eye every 4 hours, or apply ½-inch (1.27-cm) ribbon of ointment every 8 to 12 hours. In severe infections, instill 2 drops into infected eye every 60 minutes until condition improves; then reduce frequency. Or, apply ½-inch ribbon of ointment every 3 to 4 hours until condition improves; then reduce frequency to b.i.d. to t.i.d.

ADMINISTRATION
• For IV, IM, and inhalational use, obtain specimen for culture and sensitivity tests before giving. Begin therapy while awaiting results.

IV
▼ For adults, dilute in 50 to 100 mL of NSS or D₅W; use a smaller volume for children.
▼ Keep reconstituted solution in refrigerator and use within 96 hours or keep at room temperature for 24 hours.
▼ Infuse over 20 to 60 minutes.
▼ After infusion, flush line with NSS or D₅W.
▼ Obtain blood for peak level 30 minutes after infusion stops; draw blood for trough level just before next dose. Don't collect blood in a heparinized tube because of incompatibility.
▼ **Incompatibilities:** Don't mix with other drugs; administer separately.

T

IM

- Obtain blood for peak level 1 hour after IM injection; draw blood for trough level just before next dose. Don't collect blood in a heparinized tube because of incompatibility.
- Withdraw appropriate dose directly from vial.

Inhalational

- Capsules aren't for oral ingestion.
- Give nebulizer solution over 10 to 15 minutes using handheld Pari LC Plus reusable nebulizer with DeVilbiss Pulmo-Aide compressor.
- Give capsules only by oral inhalation using Podhaler device. A new Podhaler device is supplied with each weekly pack of capsules. Use only for 7 days; then discard.
- Store capsules in blister packs at room temperature and remove immediately before use.
- Give doses as close to 12 hours apart as possible. Doses shouldn't be taken less than 6 hours apart.
- Store solution in refrigerator until expiration date or at room temperature for up to 28 days. Protect from light.

Ophthalmic

- When two different ophthalmic solutions are used, allow at least 10 minutes between instillations.
- Apply light finger pressure on lacrimal sac for 1 minute after drops are instilled.
- Apply ointment to conjunctiva. Don't let tube touch eye.

ACTION

Generally bactericidal. Inhibits protein synthesis by binding directly to the 30S ribosomal subunit.

Route	Onset	Peak	Duration
IV	Immediate	30 min	8 hr
IM	Unknown	30–60 min	8 hr
Inhalation	Unknown	60 min	Unknown
Ophthalmic	Unknown	Unknown	Unknown

Half-life: Adults: IV, 2 to 3 hours; inhalation, 3 to 4 hours. Adults with impaired renal function, 5 to 70 hours. Neonates weighing 1,200 g or less, 11 hours; neonates weighing more than 1,200 g, 2 to 9 hours. Infants, 3 to 5 hours. Children and adolescents, ½ to 3 hours.

ADVERSE REACTIONS

CNS: *seizures,* headache, lethargy, confusion, disorientation, fever, dizziness, vertigo. **EENT:** blurred vision (ophthalmic); hearing loss, tinnitus, ototoxicity, dysphonia, pharyngitis. **GI:** vomiting, nausea, diarrhea. **GU:** *nephrotoxicity,* possible increase in urinary excretion of casts. **Hematologic:** anemia, eosinophilia, *leukopenia, thrombocytopenia, agranulocytosis.* **Metabolic:** electrolyte imbalances. **Musculoskeletal:** muscle twitching, chest pain. **Respiratory:** cough, dyspnea, hemoptysis, *bronchospasm.* **Skin:** rash, urticaria, pruritus, dermatitis, pain at injection site.

INTERACTIONS

Drug-drug. **Black Box Warning** *Acyclovir, amphotericin B, cephalosporins, cidofovir, cisplatin, colistin, methoxyflurane, polymyxin B, vancomycin, other aminoglycosides:* May increase nephrotoxicity when used with injectable tobramycin formulation. Monitor renal function. ∎

Atracurium, pancuronium, rocuronium, vecuronium: May increase effects of nondepolarizing muscle relaxants, including prolonged respiratory depression. Use together only when necessary, and expect to reduce dosage of nondepolarizing muscle relaxant.

Cyclosporine, foscarnet, NSAIDs: May increase risk of nephrotoxicity. Avoid combination.

General anesthetics: May increase neuromuscular blockade. Monitor patient for increased clinical effects.

Black Box Warning *IV loop diuretics (ethacrynic acid, furosemide):* May increase ototoxicity when used with injectable tobramycin. Monitor patient's hearing. ∎

Parenteral penicillins: May inactivate tobramycin in vitro. Don't mix together.

EFFECTS ON LAB TEST RESULTS

- May increase AST, ALT, LDH, bilirubin, BUN, creatinine, nonprotein nitrogen, and urine urea levels.
- May decrease calcium, magnesium, sodium, and potassium levels.
- May increase eosinophil count. May decrease Hb level and hematocrit and platelet count.
- May increase or decrease WBC count.

CONTRAINDICATIONS & CAUTIONS
• Contraindicated in patients hypersensitive to drug or other aminoglycosides.

Black Box Warning Use tobramycin injection cautiously in premature infants and neonates because of their renal immaturity and resulting prolongation of drug's serum half-life. ■

Black Box Warning For injectable tobramycin, neurotoxicity manifested as both auditory and vestibular ototoxicity can occur. Auditory changes are irreversible, are usually bilateral, and may be partial or total. Other manifestations of neurotoxicity may include numbness, skin tingling, muscle twitching, and seizures. Risk of hearing loss increases with degree of exposure to either high peak or high trough serum concentrations; other factors that may increase patient risk are advanced age and dehydration. Patients who develop cochlear damage may not have symptoms during therapy to warn them of eighth-nerve toxicity, and partial or total irreversible bilateral deafness may continue to develop after drug discontinuation. ■

۞ Alert: Avoid concurrent or sequential use with other drugs with neurotoxic, nephrotoxic, or ototoxic potential.
• Use cautiously in patients with impaired renal function or neuromuscular disorders and in elderly patients.
• Wheezing and bronchospasm have been reported with tobramycin inhalation. Treat as medically appropriate.

Dialyzable drug: Yes.

⚠ Overdose S&S: Nephrotoxicity, dizziness, tinnitus, vertigo, loss of high-tone hearing acuity, neuromuscular blockade, respiratory failure, respiratory paralysis (systemic); punctate keratitis, erythema, tearing, edema, eyelid itching (ophthalmic).

PREGNANCY-LACTATION-REPRODUCTION
Black Box Warning Aminoglycosides can cause fetal harm when given to pregnant women. ■
• There are no adequate studies in pregnant women. If used during pregnancy, or if patient becomes pregnant during therapy, apprise her of potential hazard to the fetus.
• Amount of drug that appears in human milk isn't known. Because of the potential for adverse effects in breastfed infants, patient should discontinue breastfeeding or discontinue drug.

NURSING CONSIDERATIONS
• It's recommended that dosage be determined by appropriate pharmacokinetic methods and patient-specific parameters.

۞ Alert: Tobramycin ophthalmic solution isn't for injection.
• If topical ocular tobramycin is given with systemic tobramycin, carefully monitor levels.
• Weigh patient and review renal function studies before therapy.

۞ Alert: If patient complains of tinnitus, vertigo, or hearing loss, notify prescriber.

Black Box Warning If possible, obtain serial audiograms in patients old enough to be tested, particularly high-risk patients. Evidence of impairment of renal, vestibular, or auditory function requires drug discontinuation or dosage adjustment. ■
• Don't dilute or mix with other drugs, including dornase alfa, in a nebulizer. If giving multiple inhaled therapies, administer this drug last.
• Unrefrigerated inhalation solution, which is normally slightly yellow, may darken with age. This doesn't affect product quality.
• Avoid exposing ampules to intense light.
• Follow facility policy for when to obtain serum samples for peak and trough levels. As a guide, obtain serum for peak levels 30 minutes after IV infusion or 1 hour after IM injection. Obtain serum for trough levels at 8 hours or just before next dose.

Black Box Warning Peak levels over 12 mcg/mL and trough levels over 2 mcg/mL may increase risk of toxicity. Periodically monitor peak and trough serum concentrations during therapy to ensure adequate levels and to avoid potentially toxic levels. ■

Black Box Warning Due to increased risk of nephrotoxicity, monitor renal function: urine output, specific gravity, urinalysis, serum creatinine, CrCl, and BUN. Notify prescriber about signs and symptoms of decreasing renal function. ■

Black Box Warning Closely monitor patient treated with tobramycin injection because of the inherent potential for ototoxicity and nephrotoxicity. ■

T

♣Canada   ◇OTC   ◆Off-label use   ✐ Photoguide   ⓓ Do not crush   *Liquid contains alcohol   ✠ Genetic

Black Box Warning Monitor patient for manifestations of neurotoxicity, including numbness, skin tingling, muscle twitching, and seizures. ■

• Carefully monitor peak and trough levels in order to determine appropriate dosage in patients with burns or cystic fibrosis as altered pharmacokinetics may cause reduced drug serum concentrations. Reserve higher peak levels for patients with cystic fibrosis, who need a greater lung penetration.

• Monitor tobramycin serum concentration only through venipuncture and not through fingerstick blood sampling. Skin contamination with tobramycin may lead to falsely increased serum levels.

• Watch for signs and symptoms of superinfection, such as continued fever, chills, and increased pulse rate.

• Monitor electrolyte levels.

• If no response occurs in 3 to 5 days, therapy may be stopped and new specimens obtained for culture and sensitivity testing.

• *Look alike–sound alike:* Don't confuse Tobrex with TobraDex.

PATIENT TEACHING

🛈 *Alert:* Explain that capsules are for inhalation only and shouldn't be swallowed.

• Provide full instructions for the Podhaler device and tell patient to always use the new Podhaler device provided with each weekly pack.

• Advise patient not to get powder in eyes.

• Tell patient to keep capsules in sealed blisters and to remove each capsule immediately before use.

• Instruct patient to store capsules at room temperature.

• Instruct patient to report all adverse reactions promptly.

• Caution patient not to perform hazardous activities if adverse CNS reactions occur.

• Encourage patient to maintain adequate fluid intake.

• Teach patient how to use and maintain nebulizer.

• Warn patient not to dilute or mix other drugs in the nebulizer with tobramycin.

• Tell patient using multiple inhaled therapies to use this drug last.

• Instruct patient not to use if the inhalation solution is cloudy or contains particles or if

it has been stored at room temperature for longer than 28 days.

• Tell patient to clean excessive discharge from eye area before applying ocular tobramycin.

• Tell patient to remove contact lenses before using ocular tobramycin and not to wear contact lenses when signs or symptoms of ocular infection are present.

• Teach patient how to instill drops or apply ointment. Advise patient to wash hands before and after applying and to avoid touching tip of dropper to eye or surrounding tissue.

• Instruct patient to apply light finger pressure on lacrimal sac for 1 minute after drops are instilled.

• Tell patient to wait at least 10 minutes before instilling other eyedrops.

---

tocilizumab ⌧
toe-sih-LIZ-oo-mab

Actemra

Therapeutic class: Antiarthritics
Pharmacologic class: Interleukin-6 receptor inhibitors

AVAILABLE FORMS

Injection (for IV use): 80 mg/4 mL, 200 mg/10 mL, 400 mg/20 mL in single-use vials
Injection (for subcut use): 162 mg/0.9 mL in prefilled syringe or autoinjector

INDICATIONS & DOSAGES

Adjust-a-dose (for all indications): Refer to manufacturer's instructions for toxicity-related dosage adjustments.

➤ **Systemic juvenile idiopathic arthritis (SJIA) alone or in combination with methotrexate** ⌧

Children age 2 and older weighing 30 kg or more: 8 mg/kg IV infusion over 60 minutes once every 2 weeks. Or, 162 mg subcut once each week.

Children age 2 and older weighing less than 30 kg: 12 mg/kg IV infusion over 60 minutes once every 2 weeks. Or, 162 mg subcut once every 2 weeks.

Adjust-a-dose: If appropriate, concomitant methotrexate or other medications should be

---

dose-modified or stopped and tocilizumab dosage adjusted until the clinical situation has been evaluated. In SJIA, the decision to discontinue tocilizumab for a lab abnormality should be based on medical assessment of the individual patient.

➤ **As monotherapy or with methotrexate or other nonbiologic DMARDs for moderately to severely active RA when response to one or more DMARDs is inadequate**
Adults: Initially, 4 mg/kg IV infusion over 60 minutes every 4 weeks. May increase dosage to 8 mg/kg every 4 weeks based on clinical response. Maximum dose is 800 mg per infusion. Or, for patients weighing 100 kg or more, 162 mg subcut once each week. Or, for patients weighing less than 100 kg, 162 mg subcut every other week, followed by an increase to every week based on clinical response.

➤ **Polyarticular juvenile idiopathic arthritis (PJIA) alone or in combination with methotrexate** 🧬
Children age 2 and older weighing 30 kg or more: 8 mg/kg IV infusion over 60 minutes once every 4 weeks. Or, 162 mg subcut once every 2 weeks.
Children age 2 and older weighing less than 30 kg: 10 mg/kg IV infusion once every 4 weeks. Or, 162 mg subcut once every 3 weeks.
Adjust-a-dose: If appropriate, concomitant methotrexate or other medications should be dose-modified or stopped and tocilizumab dosage adjusted until the clinical situation has been evaluated. In PJIA, the decision to discontinue tocilizumab for a lab abnormality should be based on medical assessment of the individual patient.

➤ **Treatment of giant cell arteritis (GCA)** 🧬
Adults: 162 mg subcut once each week in combination with a tapering course of glucocorticoids. Or, 162 mg subcut once every other week in combination with a tapering course of glucocorticoids as clinically indicated. May continue tocilizumab after glucocorticoids are stopped. Don't give IV.

➤ **Chimeric antigen receptor (CAR) T cell–induced severe or life-threatening cytokine release syndrome (CRS), alone or in combination with corticosteroids**

Adults and children age 2 and older weighing 30 kg or more: 8 mg/kg IV infusion over 60 minutes. May repeat infusion up to three more doses at least 8 hours apart if no clinical improvement in signs and symptoms of CRS. Maximum dose is 800 mg per infusion.
Adults and children age 2 and older weighing less than 30 kg: 12 mg/kg IV infusion over 60 minutes. May repeat infusion up to three more doses at least 8 hours apart if no clinical improvement in signs and symptoms of CRS.

ADMINISTRATION
IV
▼ Check body weight before calculating each dose. For adults and PJIA and SJIA patients at or above 30 kg, dilute to 100 mL in NSS or half-NSS for IV infusion following manufacturer's instructions. For adults and PJIA and SJIA patients less than 30 kg, dilute to 50 mL in NSS or half-NSS for IV infusion following manufacturer's instructions. Allow diluted solutions to reach room temperature before infusing.
▼ Don't use solution if it's discolored or contains particulate matter.
▼ Store NSS infusion solutions at 36° to 46° F (2° to 8° C) or at room temperature for up to 24 hours, or half-NSS infusion solutions at 36° to 46° F for up to 24 hours or at room temperature for up to 4 hours. Protect all solutions from light.
▼ Administer infusion over 60 minutes; infusion must be administered with infusion set. Don't administer as IV push or bolus.
▼ **Incompatibilities:** Don't infuse in same line with other IV drugs.
Subcutaneous
● When transitioning from IV therapy to subcut administration, administer the first subcut dose instead of the next scheduled IV dose.
● Interruption of dose or reduction in frequency of administration of subcut dose from every week to every other week dosing is recommended for management of certain dose-related lab changes, including elevated liver enzymes, neutropenia, and thrombocytopenia.
● Remove prefilled syringe from refrigerator 30 minutes before use or autoinjector

T

45 minutes before use. Don't warm in any other way.

• Don't use if product contains particulate matter or is cloudy or discolored, or if any part of syringe or autoinjector is damaged.

• Inject full amount in the syringe or autoinjector (0.9 mL).

• Rotate injection sites with each injection; never give into moles, scars, or areas where skin is tender, bruised, red, hard, or not intact. Don't rub injection site.

ACTION

Inhibits interleukin-6–mediated inflammatory processes by decreasing inflammatory markers such as C-reactive protein, rheumatoid factor, and erythrocyte sedimentation rate.

Route	Onset	Peak	Duration
IV	Unknown	Unknown	Unknown
Subcut	Unknown	3–4½ days	Unknown

Half-life: IV, 11 to 13 days; subcut, 5 to 13 days.

ADVERSE REACTIONS

CNS: dizziness, headache. **CV:** HTN, peripheral edema. **EENT:** nasopharyngitis. **GI:** gastritis, stomatitis, upper abdominal pain, gastric ulcer, diarrhea. **Hematologic:** *thrombocytopenia, neutropenia.* **Hepatic:** elevated liver enzyme levels. **Metabolic:** elevated lipid levels. **Respiratory:** bronchitis, URI. **Skin:** pruritus, rash, urticaria, injection-site reactions. **Other:** *antibody development, malignancy,* infection, infusion-related reactions.

INTERACTIONS

Drug-drug. *Biological DMARDs (anti-CD20 monoclonal antibodies, interleukin-1 receptor antagonists, TNF antagonists):* May increase risk of serious infection. Don't use together.

Cyclosporine, theophylline, warfarin: May decrease drug levels. Monitor levels closely and adjust dosage as needed.

CYP3A4 substrates (atorvastatin, lovastatin, omeprazole, simvastatin): May affect levels of these drugs. Avoid use together.

Hormonal contraceptives: May decrease effects of contraceptives. Consider nonhormonal alternatives for contraception.

Live-virus vaccines: No data are available on secondary transmission of infection from live-virus vaccine. Avoid using together.
Drug-herb. *Echinacea:* May decrease effect of immunosuppressants. Avoid combination.

EFFECTS ON LAB TEST RESULTS

• May increase bilirubin, ALT, AST, and lipid levels.

• May decrease leukocyte, platelet, and neutrophil counts.

CONTRAINDICATIONS & CAUTIONS

Black Box Warning Risks and benefits of treatment with tocilizumab should be carefully considered before start of therapy in patients with chronic or recurrent infection. ∎

Black Box Warning Patients treated with tocilizumab are at increased risk for developing serious infections (active pulmonary or extrapulmonary TB; invasive fungal infections [candidiasis, aspergillosis, pneumocystis]; or bacterial, viral, and other infections caused by opportunistic pathogens) that may lead to hospitalization or death. Most patients who developed these infections were taking concomitant immunosuppressants, such as methotrexate or corticosteroids. ∎

• Months to years after treatment, serious cases of hepatic injury have been observed in patients taking drug IV or subcut, some cases resulting in liver transplant or death.

• Don't initiate drug in patients with ANC less than 2,000/mm³ or platelet count less than 100,000/mm³, or in those with ALT or AST level more than 1.5 × ULN.

• Contraindicated in patients hypersensitive to drug or its components. Avoid use in those with active infection, active hepatic disease, or hepatic impairment.

◐ *Alert:* Use cautiously in patients who have been exposed to TB, in those with history of chronic or recurrent infection, serious or opportunistic infection, or underlying conditions that increase risk of infection. Use cautiously in those who have resided or traveled in areas with endemic TB or mycosis.

◐ *Alert:* Patients with severe or life-threatening CRS frequently have cytopenias or elevated ALT or AST level due to chemotherapy or CRS. Before start of

---

Reactions in bold italics are *life-threatening*. Interactions may have a *rapid onset* or a *delayed onset*.

therapy, consider the potential benefit of treating the CRS versus the risks of short-term treatment with tocilizumab.

• Use cautiously in patients at risk for GI perforation.

• Use cautiously in patients with preexisting CNS demyelinating disorders such as MS.

• For patients older than age 65 being treated with tocilizumab, give drug cautiously because serious infections are more common in this population.

Dialyzable drug: Unknown.

PREGNANCY-LACTATION-REPRODUCTION

• Based on animal data, there may be a risk to the fetus. Use in pregnant women only if benefit outweighs risk to the fetus.

• Encourage pregnant patients taking drug to register with the OTIS Autoimmune Diseases in Pregnancy Study (1-877-311-8972).

• It isn't known if drug appears in human milk. Patient should discontinue breastfeeding or discontinue drug.

NURSING CONSIDERATIONS

Black Box Warning Sepsis or serious infections, including TB and bacterial, invasive fungal, viral, and other opportunistic infections, may occur. Monitor patient closely for signs and symptoms of infection during and after treatment. Drug may need to be discontinued if infection occurs during treatment. ▌

Black Box Warning Patient should be evaluated and treated, if necessary, for latent TB before start of therapy. Monitor patient for possible TB development during therapy, even if patient tested negative before therapy. ▌

• Before starting drug, screen patient for prior HBV infection due to risk of viral reactivation.

• Suspect GI perforation in patient with new-onset abdominal symptoms.

• Monitor lipid levels and neutrophil and platelet counts at baseline and every 4 to 8 weeks during therapy.

• For RA and GCA patients, obtain LFTs before starting drug, every 4 to 8 weeks after start of therapy for first 6 months of treatment, and every 3 months thereafter.

• For PJIA and SJIA patients, monitor LFTs at the time of second administration and

thereafter every 4 to 8 weeks for PJIA patients and every 2 to 4 weeks for SJIA patients.

• Measure LFT values promptly in patients with signs and symptoms that may indicate liver injury, such as fatigue, anorexia, right upper abdominal discomfort, dark urine, or jaundice.

• Ensure availability of appropriate supportive measures to treat possible hypersensitivity reaction.

• Drug may increase risk of malignancy.

• Monitor patient closely for signs and symptoms of demyelinating disorders.

• Recommended immunizations (except live-virus vaccines) should be brought up-to-date before beginning therapy.

• Subcut injection is intended for use under the guidance of a health care practitioner. After proper training, patient may self-inject drug or patient's caregiver may administer drug if a health care practitioner determines that it's appropriate. Assess suitability of patient for subcut home use.

PATIENT TEACHING

❸ *Alert:* Warn patient to seek immediate medical attention if abdominal pain, fatigue, anorexia, dark urine, jaundice, or signs and symptoms of infection occur.

• Teach patient or caregiver proper subcut injection technique and to follow directions in manufacturer's instructions. Caution patient to inform prescriber before administering next dose if signs or symptoms of allergic reaction occur.

• Instruct patient that TB and hepatitis B screening will be needed before therapy begins.

• Advise female patient to consult prescriber if she becomes pregnant or plans to breastfeed.

• Tell patient to avoid exposure to infections.

• Remind patient to contact prescriber before scheduling surgery.

• Advise patient to avoid live-virus vaccines during therapy.

• Recommend that patient use nonhormonal contraception during therapy.

T

tofacitinib citrate ⌦
TOE-fa-SYE-ti-nib

Xeljanz, Xeljanz XR

Therapeutic class: Antirheumatics
Pharmacologic class: Janus kinase inhibitors

AVAILABLE FORMS
Tablets: 5 mg, 10 mg
Tablets (extended-release) ⓞⓝⓒ: 11 mg

INDICATIONS & DOSAGES
Adjust-a-dose (for all indications): Refer to manufacturer's instructions for toxicity-related dosage adjustments.

➤ **Moderately to severely active RA in patients who have had an inadequate response or intolerance to methotrexate, as monotherapy or in combination with methotrexate or other nonbiologic DMARDs**
Adults: 5 mg (immediate-release) PO b.i.d. Or, 11 mg (extended-release) once daily.
Adjust-a-dose: Reduce dosage to 5 mg (immediate-release) once daily in patients with moderate or severe renal insufficiency or moderate hepatic impairment, in those receiving concurrent potent CYP3A4 inhibitors (such as ketoconazole), and in those receiving a drug that moderates inhibition of CYP3A4 and acts as a potent inhibitor of CYP2C19 (such as fluconazole).

➤ **Active psoriatic arthritis in patients who have had an inadequate response or are intolerant to methotrexate or other DMARDs, in combination with nonbiologic DMARDs**
Adults: 5 mg (immediate-release) PO b.i.d. Or, 11 mg (extended-release) once daily.
Adjust-a-dose: Reduce dosage to 5 mg (immediate-release) once daily in patients with moderate or severe renal insufficiency or moderate hepatic impairment, in those receiving concurrent potent CYP3A4 inhibitors (such as ketoconazole), and in those receiving a drug that moderates inhibition of CYP3A4 and acts as a potent inhibitor of CYP2C19 (such as fluconazole).

➤ **Moderately to severely active ulcerative colitis in patients who have an inadequate response or are intolerant to TNF blockers**
Adults: 10 mg PO b.i.d. for at least 8 weeks followed by 5 or 10 mg b.i.d., depending on therapeutic response. Use lowest effective dose to maintain response. Discontinue after 16 weeks of treatment with 10 mg b.i.d. if adequate therapeutic benefit isn't achieved.
Adjust-a-dose: In patients with moderate or severe renal insufficiency or moderate hepatic impairment, in those receiving concurrent potent CYP3A4 inhibitors (such as ketoconazole), and in those receiving a drug that moderates inhibition of CYP3A4 and acts as a potent inhibitor of CYP2C19 (such as fluconazole): If patient is taking 10 mg b.i.d., reduce dosage to 5 mg b.i.d. or, if patient is taking 5 mg b.i.d., reduce dosage to 5 mg once daily.

ADMINISTRATION
PO
• May give with or without food.
• Make sure patient swallows extended-release tablets whole and intact. Don't crush, split, or allow patient to chew tablets.
• Store at room temperature.

ACTION
Inhibits activity of Janus kinases, preventing activation of certain intracellular activities that influence immune cell function.

Route	Onset	Peak	Duration
PO (immediate-release)	Unknown	½–1 hr	Unknown
PO (extended-release)	Unknown	4 hr	Unknown

Half-life: Immediate-release, 3 hours; extended-release, 6 hours.

ADVERSE REACTIONS
CNS: headache, paresthesia, insomnia, fever, fatigue. **CV:** HTN, peripheral edema. **EENT:** nasopharyngitis, sinus congestion. **GI:** diarrhea, abdominal pain, dyspepsia, vomiting, gastritis, nausea. **GU:** UTI. **Hematologic:** anemia. **Metabolic:** dehydration. **Musculoskeletal:** muscle and bone pain, arthralgia, tendon disorder, joint swelling. **Respiratory:** URI, dyspnea, cough. **Skin:** rash, erythema, pruritus, cancer, acne. **Other:** infection.

INTERACTIONS

Drug-drug. *Conivaptan:* May increase tofacitinib serum concentration. Avoid combination.

Black Box Warning *Immunosuppressants (corticosteroids, methotrexate):* May increase risk of serious infection. If infection occurs, discontinue tofacitinib until infection is controlled. ∎

Live-virus vaccines: May increase adverse effects of vaccines. Avoid using together; don't give live-attenuated vaccines for at least 3 months after immunosuppressants.

Moderate CYP3A4 inhibitors plus potent CYP2C19 inhibitors (fluconazole), potent CYP3A4 inhibitors (ketoconazole): May increase tofacitinib plasma level. Decrease tofacitinib dosage per manufacturer's instructions.

Potent immunosuppressants (abatacept, adalimumab, anakinra, azathioprine, certolizumab, cyclosporine, etanercept, golimumab, infliximab, rituximab, tacrolimus, tocilizumab): May significantly increase risk of immunosuppression and infection. Don't use together.

Potent CYP3A4 inducers (rifampin): May decrease tofacitinib plasma level. Use together isn't recommended.

Drug-herb. *Echinacea:* May diminish therapeutic effect of immunosuppressants. Avoid combination.

St. John's wort: May decrease serum concentration of CYP3A4 substrates. Consider therapy modification.

EFFECTS ON LAB TEST RESULTS

• May increase creatinine, liver enzyme, and lipid levels.
• May decrease Hb level.
• May decrease lymphocyte and neutrophil counts.

CONTRAINDICATIONS & CAUTIONS

• Contraindicated in patients hypersensitive to drug or its components.
• Use in patients with severe hepatic impairment isn't recommended.
• **Alert:** Use cautiously in patients at risk for serious infection (including those who have resided or traveled in areas of endemic TB or mycoses), those at risk for GI perforation (history of diverticulitis), and those with known malignancy.

Black Box Warning Serious infections leading to hospitalization or death, including TB and bacterial, invasive fungal, viral, and other opportunistic infections, have occurred in patients receiving tofacitinib, especially patients on concomitant immunosuppressants, such as methotrexate or corticosteroids. Weigh risk before starting therapy in patients with chronic or recurrent infection. If a serious infection develops, interrupt therapy until infection is controlled. ∎

Black Box Warning Lymphoma and other malignancies have been observed in patients treated with tofacitinib. ∎

Black Box Warning Epstein-Barr virus–associated post-transplant lymphoproliferative disorder has been increasingly observed in renal transplant patients treated with tofacitinib and concomitant immunosuppressants. ∎

Black Box Warning Patients age 50 and older with RA and at least one CV risk factor have increased risk of thrombosis, including serious events and death. Avoid drug in patients at risk. Dosage of 10 mg immediate-release b.i.d. or 22 mg extended-release once daily isn't recommended for patients with RA or psoriatic arthritis. ∎

• Patients shouldn't receive live-virus vaccines during therapy. Update immunizations according to current guidelines before starting drug.
• Use in combination with biologic DMARDs or with potent immunosuppressants, such as azathioprine, tacrolimus, and cyclosporine, isn't recommended.
• Use cautiously when giving extended-release formulation to patients with preexisting severe GI narrowing (pathologic or iatrogenic). There have been rare reports of obstructive signs and symptoms in patients with known strictures in association with ingestion of other drugs utilizing a nondeformable extended-release formulation.
• Consider risks and benefits of treatment before initiating therapy in patients with a known malignancy other than a successfully treated nonmelanoma skin cancer or when considering continuing tofacitinib in patients who develop a malignancy.

• Safety and effectiveness in children haven't been established.

• Effectiveness of tofacitinib as monotherapy hasn't been studied in patients with psoriatic arthritis.

• Use cautiously in patients with a history of chronic lung disease or in those who develop ILD, patients with diabetes, and patients older than age 65 because of increased risk of serious infection.

Dialyzable drug: Unknown.

PREGNANCY-LACTATION-REPRODUCTION

• There are no adequate studies in pregnant women, but drug may cause fetal harm. Use only if clearly needed and potential benefit justifies potential risk to the fetus.

• Encourage pregnant patients taking drug to register with the OTIS Autoimmune Diseases in Pregnancy Study (1-877-311-8972).

• It isn't known if drug appears in human milk. Patient shouldn't breastfeed while taking drug and for at least 18 hours after final dose of immediate-release form or 36 hours after final dose of extended-release form.

NURSING CONSIDERATIONS

Black Box Warning Before therapy, patients should be tested for latent TB. If test is positive, treatment for TB should begin before start of tofacitinib therapy. Monitor all patients for active TB during treatment, even if initial latent TB test is negative. ▪

Black Box Warning Monitor patients for thrombosis, including PE, DVT, and arterial thrombosis. Promptly evaluate patients if signs or symptoms occur and discontinue drug. ▪

⚕ Drug may reactivate viral infections such as herpes zoster. Risk of reactivation of herpes zoster appears to be higher in patients treated in Japan and Korea.

• The impact of drug on chronic viral hepatitis reactivation is unknown. Screen for viral hepatitis in accordance with clinical guidelines before starting therapy.

• Patients treated with Xeljanz 5 mg twice daily may be switched to Xeljanz XR 11 mg once daily the day after last dose of Xeljanz 5 mg.

• Interrupt treatment if serious infection occurs; don't restart until infection is resolved.

• Monitor lymphocyte count at baseline and every 3 months thereafter.

• Monitor neutrophil count, platelet, and Hb level at baseline, after 4 to 8 weeks of treatment, and every 3 months thereafter.

• Don't initiate therapy if lymphocyte count is less than 500/mm^3, ANC is less than 1,000/mm^3, or Hb level is less than 9 g/dL.

• Monitor LFT results regularly, especially in patients with history of taking DMARDs such as methotrexate. If drug-induced liver injury is suspected, stop drug until drug cause is ruled out.

• Assess lipid levels 4 to 8 weeks after drug initiation and then periodically; manage appropriately as needed.

• Monitor patients for GI perforation. Promptly evaluate patients with sudden new-onset abdominal pain or other GI signs and symptoms, especially those also taking NSAIDs.

• Perform periodic skin exam of patients who are at increased risk for skin cancer.

• May cause HTN; monitor BP.

PATIENT TEACHING

Black Box Warning Warn patient to stop drug and immediately report signs and symptoms of thrombosis (sudden shortness of breath, chest pain that worsens with breathing, swelling of the leg or arm, leg pain or tenderness, red or discolored skin in an affected extremity). ▪

• Advise patient to inform prescriber of all adverse reactions, especially signs and symptoms of infection, abdominal pain, or illness.

• Caution patient to obtain lab tests (CBC, liver enzymes, lipids) regularly as directed.

• Instruct female patient to contact prescriber if she becomes pregnant or plans to become pregnant.

• Warn patient to avoid live-virus vaccines.

---

tolcapone
TOLE-ka-pone

Tasmar

Therapeutic class: Antiparkinsonians
Pharmacologic class: Catechol-O-methyltransferase inhibitors

AVAILABLE FORMS
Tablets: 100 mg

INDICATIONS & DOSAGES
➤ **Adjunct to levodopa–carbidopa for signs and symptoms of idiopathic Parkinson disease in patients who have symptom fluctuation or haven't responded to other adjunctive treatment**
Adults: Initially, 100 mg PO t.i.d. with levodopa–carbidopa. May increase dosage to 200 mg PO t.i.d. if clinical benefit is justified, as this dosage is associated with increased frequency of ALT elevation. Recommended daily dosage is 100 mg PO t.i.d. Levodopa dosage may need to be reduced by about 30% to minimize risk of dyskinesias, especially when levodopa dose is over 600 mg daily. Stop drug if patient shows no benefit within 3 weeks.

ADMINISTRATION
PO
• Give drug without regard for food.
• Give first dose of the day with first daily dose of levodopa–carbidopa. Give subsequent doses 6 and 12 hours later.

ACTION
May reversibly inhibit catechol-O-methyltransferase when given with levodopa–carbidopa, increasing levodopa bioavailability. This causes a more constant dopaminergic stimulation in the brain.

Route	Onset	Peak	Duration
PO	Unknown	2 hr	Unknown

Half-life: 2 to 3 hours.

ADVERSE REACTIONS
CNS: dyskinesia, sleep disorder, dystonia, excessive dreaming, somnolence, confusion, headache, hallucinations, dizziness, fever, hyperkinesia, hypertonia, fatigue, falling, syncope, balance loss, depression, tremor, speech disorder, paresthesia, agitation, irritability, mental deficiency, hyperactivity, hypokinesia, euphoria. **CV:** orthostatic complaints, chest pain, chest discomfort, palpitations, hypotension. **EENT:** cataract, tinnitus, pharyngitis, sinus congestion. **GI:** nausea, anorexia, diarrhea, vomiting, flatulence, constipation, abdominal pain, dyspepsia, dry mouth. **GU:** UTI, urine discoloration, hematuria, micturition disorder, urinary incontinence, impotence. **Hepatic:** *hepatotoxicity.* **Musculoskeletal:** muscle cramps, stiffness, arthritis, neck pain, myalgia. **Respiratory:** bronchitis, dyspnea, URI. **Skin:** increased sweating, rash, alopecia. **Other:** flulike syndrome, infection, accidental injury.

INTERACTIONS
Drug-drug. *Antihypertensives, PDE5 inhibitors:* May enhance hypotensive effect of tolcapone. Use together cautiously.
CNS depressants: May cause additive effects. Monitor patient closely.
Nonselective MAO inhibitors (phenelzine, tranylcypromine): May cause hypertensive crisis. Avoid using together.
Phenytoin, tolbutamide: May increase serum concentrations of these drugs. Monitor patient closely.
SSRIs, TCAs: May increase risk of adverse effects. Use together cautiously.
Warfarin: May cause increased warfarin level. Monitor INR and adjust warfarin dosage as needed.
Drug-herb. *Herbs with hypotensive properties (black cohosh, garlic, hawthorn):* May enhance hypotensive effect of tolcapone. Use together cautiously.
Kava kava: May enhance CNS depressant effect of tolcapone. Monitor therapy.
Drug-lifestyle. *Alcohol use:* May increase CNS depressant effect of alcohol. Avoid use together.

EFFECTS ON LAB TEST RESULTS
• May increase LFT values.

CONTRAINDICATIONS & CAUTIONS
• Contraindicated in patients with liver disease, in those who were withdrawn from tolcapone because of evidence of drug-induced

hepatocellular injury, in those who have demonstrated hypersensitivity to drug or its components, and in those with history of drug-related confusion and hyperpyrexia or nontraumatic rhabdomyolysis.

Black Box Warning Don't initiate tolcapone therapy if patient exhibits clinical evidence of liver disease or two ALT or AST values greater than ULN. ∎

Black Box Warning Use cautiously in patients with severe dyskinesia or dystonia. ∎

Black Box Warning Cases of severe hepatocellular injury, including fulminant liver failure resulting in death, have been reported. ∎

• Use cautiously in patients with severe renal impairment.

• May cause new or worsening mental status and behavioral changes, which may be severe and include psychotic-like behavior, hallucinations, paranoid ideation, delusions, confusion, disorientation, aggressive behavior, agitation, and delirium.

• Reports suggest that patients may experience an intense urge to gamble, increased sexual urges, intense urge to spend money, binge eating, or other intense urges, and the inability to control these urges.

Dialyzable drug: Unlikely.

⚠ *Overdose S&S:* Nausea, vomiting, dizziness.

PREGNANCY-LACTATION-REPRODUCTION

• There are no adequate studies in pregnant women. Use only if potential benefit justifies potential risk to the fetus.

• It isn't known if drug appears in human milk. Use cautiously in breastfeeding women.

NURSING CONSIDERATIONS

Black Box Warning Because of risk of hepatotoxicity, stop treatment if patient shows no benefit within 3 weeks. ∎

Black Box Warning Because of risk of fatal hepatic failure, use drug only in patients taking levodopa–carbidopa who don't respond to or who aren't appropriate candidates for other adjunctive therapies. If drug is discontinued because of hepatocellular injury, don't reintroduce. ∎

• Drug shouldn't be used by patient until there has been a complete discussion of the risks; make sure patient provides written informed consent before taking drug.

Black Box Warning Prescribers who elect to use drug in the face of the increased risk of liver injury are strongly advised to monitor patients for evidence of emergent liver injury. ∎

Black Box Warning Monitor LFT results before starting drug, every 2 to 4 weeks for first 6 months of therapy, then periodically at intervals deemed clinically relevant. If dosage is increased to 200 mg t.i.d., obtain liver enzyme levels before increasing dosage, then every 2 to 4 weeks for 6 months, then periodically. Also, discontinue treatment if ALT or AST level exceeds 2 × ULN or if clinical signs and symptoms suggest onset of hepatic failure. Frequent lab monitoring may not prevent fulminant liver failure. Early detection of hepatic injury along with immediate withdrawal of the suspect drug may enhance likelihood for recovery. ∎

• Monitor patient for orthostatic hypotension and syncope.

• Monitor patient closely and adjust other dopaminergic treatments as needed if drug is discontinued. Syndrome resembling NMS may occur.

• *Look alike–sound alike:* Don't confuse tolcapone with tolazamide, tolbutamide, or tolterodine.

PATIENT TEACHING

• Advise patient to take drug exactly as prescribed and not to stop drug abruptly.

Black Box Warning Teach patient to immediately report signs and symptoms of liver injury (clay-colored stools, yellow eyes or skin, fatigue, loss of appetite, persistent nausea, itching, dark urine, right upper abdominal tenderness, lethargy). ∎

• Inform patient that routine lab monitoring is required during therapy.

• Warn patient that dizziness may occur upon standing up quickly; advise patient to stand up cautiously.

• Advise patient to avoid hazardous activities until CNS effects of drug are known.

• Tell patient that nausea may occur early in therapy.

• Inform patient that diarrhea is common, sometimes occurring 2 to 12 weeks after

---

Reactions in bold italics are *life-threatening*. Interactions may have a *rapid onset* or a *delayed onset*.

therapy begins, and usually resolves when therapy stops.
• Advise patient about risk of increased problems making voluntary movements or impaired muscle tone.
• Inform patient and caregivers that drug may cause new or worsening mental status and behavioral changes, which may be severe and include psychotic-like behavior, hallucinations, paranoid ideation, delusions, confusion, disorientation, aggressive behavior, agitation, and delirium.
• Instruct patient and caregivers to report intense urges to gamble, increased sexual urges, increased urge to spend money, binge eating, and other intense urges as well as the inability to control these urges.
• Tell female patient to notify prescriber about planned, suspected, or known pregnancy.
• Inform patient that drug may be taken without regard to meals.

tolterodine tartrate
toll-TEAR-oh-deen

Detrol✏, Detrol LA

Therapeutic class: Urinary antispasmodics
Pharmacologic class: Antimuscarinics

AVAILABLE FORMS
Capsules (extended-release) ⓄⓃⒸ: 2 mg, 4 mg
Tablets: 1 mg, 2 mg

INDICATIONS & DOSAGES
➤ **Overactive bladder in patients with symptoms of urinary frequency, urgency, or urge incontinence**
Adults: 2-mg tablet PO b.i.d. or 4-mg extended-release capsule PO once daily. Dose may be reduced to 1-mg tablet PO b.i.d. or 2-mg extended-release capsule PO once daily, based on patient response and tolerance.
Adjust-a-dose: For patients with mild to moderate hepatic impairment (Child-Pugh class A or B) or significantly reduced renal function (CrCl of 10 to 30 mL/minute) or those taking a potent CYP3A4 inhibitor, such as ketoconazole, clarithromycin, or

ritonavir, give 1-mg tablet PO b.i.d. or 2-mg extended-release capsule PO daily.

ADMINISTRATION
PO
• Give extended-release capsules with liquid because they must be swallowed whole. Don't crush or allow patient to chew capsules.
• Give without regard to meals.

ACTION
Relaxes smooth muscle of bladder by antagonizing muscarinic receptors, relieving symptoms of overactive bladder.

Route	Onset	Peak	Duration
PO	Unknown	1–2 hr	Unknown
PO (extended-release)	Unknown	2–6 hr	Unknown

Half-life: Immediate-release tablet, 2 to 11 hours; extended-release capsule, about 18 hours.

ADVERSE REACTIONS
CNS: headache, fatigue, paresthesia, vertigo, dizziness, nervousness, somnolence, drowsiness, anxiety. **CV:** chest pain. **EENT:** abnormal vision, xerophthalmia, sinusitis. **GI:** dry mouth, abdominal pain, constipation, diarrhea, dyspepsia. **GU:** dysuria, urine retention. **Metabolic:** weight gain. **Musculoskeletal:** arthralgia. **Respiratory:** bronchitis. **Skin:** dry skin. **Other:** flulike syndrome, infection.

INTERACTIONS
Drug-drug. *Anticholinergics (ipratropium, tiotropium):* Coadministration may increase frequency or severity of anticholinergic adverse reactions (such as blurred vision, constipation, dry mouth, or somnolence). Monitor patient closely.
Antifungals (itraconazole, ketoconazole, miconazole), CYP3A4 inhibitors (clarithromycin, erythromycin): May increase tolterodine level. Don't give more than 1-mg tablet b.i.d. or 2-mg extended-release capsule once daily of tolterodine if used together.
Cannabinoid-containing products: May increase risk of tachycardia. Monitor patient closely.

T

♣Canada   ◇OTC   ◆Off-label use   ✏Photoguide   ⓄⓃⒸDo not crush   *Liquid contains alcohol   ▓Genetic

Conivaptan: May increase tolterodine serum concentration. Avoid combination.

CYP3A4 inducers: May decrease tolterodine serum concentration. Monitor patient closely.

Fluoxetine: May increase tolterodine level. Monitor patient. No dosage adjustment is needed.

Opioid analgesics: May increase risk of constipation and urine retention. Monitor therapy closely.

Drug-food. *Grapefruit juice:* May increase drug level. Don't use together.

EFFECTS ON LAB TEST RESULTS

None reported.

CONTRAINDICATIONS & CAUTIONS

• Contraindicated in patients hypersensitive to drug or its components or to fesoterodine fumarate and in those with uncontrolled angle-closure glaucoma or urine or gastric retention.

• Use cautiously in patients with significant bladder outflow obstruction, GI obstructive disorders (such as pyloric stenosis), controlled angle-closure glaucoma, myasthenia gravis, and hepatic or renal impairment.

⚠ *Alert:* Anaphylaxis and angioedema requiring hospitalization and emergency medical treatment have occurred with the first or subsequent doses of tolterodine. Discontinue drug and promptly initiate appropriate therapy if difficulty breathing, upper airway obstruction, or fall in BP occurs.

• An additive effect of tolterodine with other drugs that prolong the QT interval cannot be excluded, which increases risk of life-threatening cardiac arrhythmias. Consider this when tolterodine is prescribed to patients with known history of QT-interval prolongation or those who are taking other drugs that prolong the QT interval, such as Class IA (procainamide, quinidine) or Class III (amiodarone, sotalol) antiarrhythmics.

• Extended-release capsules aren't recommended for use in patients with severe hepatic impairment (Child-Pugh class C) or those with CrCl of less than 10 mL/minute.

• Effectiveness in children hasn't been established.

Dialyzable drug: Unknown.

⚠ *Overdose S&S:* Dry mouth, severe central anticholinergic effects, QT-interval prolongation.

PREGNANCY-LACTATION-REPRODUCTION

• There are no adequate studies in pregnant women. Use only if potential benefit justifies potential risk to the fetus.

• It isn't known if drug appears in human milk. Patient should discontinue breastfeeding or discontinue drug.

NURSING CONSIDERATIONS

• Assess baseline bladder function and monitor therapeutic effects.

• Monitor patient for residual urine after voiding.

• Monitor relevant lab values in patients with hepatic or renal impairment.

• *Look alike–sound alike:* Don't confuse tolterodine with fesoterodine or Detrol with Ditropan.

PATIENT TEACHING

• Advise patient to avoid driving or other potentially hazardous activities until effects of drug are known.

• Instruct patient to immediately report all adverse reactions and signs and symptoms of infection, urine retention, GI problems, or difficulty breathing.

• Tell patient taking extended-release form to swallow capsule whole and to take with liquids.

• Advise female patient to stop breastfeeding during therapy.

• Advise patient not to consume grapefruit or grapefruit juice during therapy.

---

tolvaptan ⊠
tol-VAP-tan

Jinarc✿, Jynarque, Samsca

Therapeutic class: Vasopressin antagonists
Pharmacologic class: Selective vasopressin receptor antagonists

AVAILABLE FORMS

Tablets: 15 mg, 30 mg, 45 mg, 60 mg, 90 mg

INDICATIONS & DOSAGES

➤ **Hypervolemic and euvolemic hyponatremia (serum sodium level less than 125 mEq/L and symptomatic hyponatremia) in hospitalized patients, including those with HF or SIADH (Samsca only)**
Adults: Initially, 15 mg PO once daily. After 24 hours, may increase to 30 mg PO once daily, to maximum dosage of 60 mg PO once daily for no more than 30 days. Titrate dosage at 24-hour intervals to desired serum sodium concentration.

➤ **To slow kidney function decline in patients at risk for rapidly progressing autosomal dominant polycystic kidney disease (ADPKD) (Jynarque only)** ⬚
Adults: Initially, 60 mg PO daily as 45 mg taken on waking and 15 mg taken 8 hours later. Titrate to 60 mg plus 30 mg, then to 90 mg plus 30 mg per day if tolerated, with at least weekly intervals between titrations. May be down-titrated based on tolerability.
Adjust-a-dose: When administered with a moderate CYP3A inhibitor, reduce Jynarque dosage per manufacturer's instructions. Use with strong CYP3A inhibitors is contraindicated.

ADMINISTRATION
PO

⬚ **Black Box Warning** Samsca isn't for use for ADPKD. Tolvaptan can cause serious and potentially fatal liver injury and shouldn't be prescribed or used outside of the FDA-approved REMS for ADPKD patients. Jynarque is available only through the Jynarque REM Program. Further information is available by calling 1-866-244-9446 or at www.jynarquerems.com. ■

• Give drug with or without food.
• For patients with hyponatremia, avoid restricting fluids during the first 24 hours of therapy.
• Make sure patient drinks water when thirsty, and throughout the day and night if awake.
• Patient should avoid grapefruit and grapefruit juice during therapy.

ACTION

Antagonizes the effect of vasopressin, causing an increase in urine excretion, which results in an increase in free water clearance, a decrease in urine osmolality, and ultimately an increase in serum sodium level.

Route	Onset	Peak	Duration
PO	2–4 hr	2–4 hr	Unknown

Half-life: Dose-dependent, 3 to 12 hours.

ADVERSE REACTIONS

CNS: asthenia, fatigue, dizziness, fever, *stroke.* **CV:** *intracardiac thrombus, PE, ventricular fibrillation, DVT,* palpitations. **GI:** anorexia, constipation, nausea, GI bleeding, abdominal distention, decreased appetite, diarrhea, dyspepsia, dry mouth, thirst. **GU:** polyuria, urinary frequency or urgency, urethral hemorrhage, vaginal hemorrhage, nocturia. **Hematologic:** *DIC.* **Metabolic:** fluid imbalance, hyperglycemia, hyperuricemia, *diabetic ketoacidosis.* **Musculoskeletal:** *rhabdomyolysis.* **Respiratory:** *respiratory failure.* **Skin:** dry skin, rash.

INTERACTIONS

Drug-drug. *ACE inhibitors, ARBs, potassium-sparing diuretics:* May increase hyperkalemic effect of these drugs. Monitor therapy closely.
BCRP substrates (rosuvastatin): May inhibit BCRP substrates. Avoid using together.
CYP3A inducers (barbiturates, carbamazepine, phenytoin, rifabutin, rifampin, rifapentine): May decrease tolvaptan level. Avoid concomitant use with strong inducers if possible; monitor patient response and adjust dosage as needed.
Hypertonic sodium chloride solution: May increase risk of a too-rapid increase in serum sodium concentrations. Avoid using together.
Moderate CYP3A inhibitors (aprepitant, conivaptan, diltiazem, erythromycin, fluconazole, verapamil): May increase tolvaptan level. Avoid using together or adjust tolvaptan dosage as needed.
OATP1B1/B3 and OAT3 substrates (bosentan, furosemide, glyburide, methotrexate, nateglinide, repaglinide, statins): May increase plasma concentrations of these substrates. Avoid using together.
P-gp inhibitors (such as cyclosporine): May increase tolvaptan level. Reduce tolvaptan dosage.

P-gp substrates (digoxin): May increase digoxin level. Monitor patient, and adjust digoxin dosage as needed.

V₂-agonists (desmopressin): May decrease therapeutic effect of desmopressin. Avoid using with a V₂-agonist.

Drug-herb. *St John's wort:* May decrease drug level. Don't use together.

Drug-food. *Grapefruit juice:* May increase drug level. Don't use together.

EFFECTS ON LAB TEST RESULTS

• May increase glucose, potassium, ALT, AST, and bilirubin levels.
• May prolong PT.

CONTRAINDICATIONS & CAUTIONS

Black Box Warning Tolvaptan can cause serious and potentially fatal liver injury. Acute liver failure requiring liver transplantation has been reported. ■

• Contraindicated in patients hypersensitive to drug or its components.

• Contraindicated in patients with hypovolemic hyponatremia and in those who require urgent rise in serum sodium level, are anuric, or are unable to sense or appropriately respond to thirst.

• Contraindicated in patients receiving strong CYP3A inhibitors.

• Jynarque is also contraindicated in patients with a history or signs or symptoms of significant liver impairment or injury (doesn't apply to uncomplicated polycystic liver disease), uncorrected abnormal blood sodium concentrations, or uncorrected urinary outflow obstruction.

• Limit duration of therapy for hyponatremia to 30 days.

• Use cautiously in patients with dehydration; avoid use in those receiving hypertonic saline solution.

• Avoid use in patients with underlying liver disease, including cirrhosis, because the ability to recover from liver injury may be impaired; use not recommended in patients with CrCl of less than 10 mL/minute.

Dialyzable drug: Unlikely.

⚠ Overdose S&S: Polyuria, thirst, dehydration, hypovolemia.

PREGNANCY-LACTATION-REPRODUCTION

• There are no adequate studies in pregnant women. Use only if potential benefit justifies potential risk to the fetus.
• It isn't known if drug appears in human milk. Patient shouldn't breastfeed during therapy.

NURSING CONSIDERATIONS

Black Box Warning Initiate and reinitiate Samsca in hospital setting where serum sodium level can be monitored closely. ■

Black Box Warning Don't correct hyponatremia (for example, more than 12 mEq/L/ 24 hours) too rapidly; doing so may cause osmotic demyelination resulting in dysarthria, mutism, dysphagia, lethargy, affective changes, spastic quadriparesis, seizures, coma, and death. Slower correction may be necessary in patients with severe malnutrition, alcoholism, or advanced liver disease. ■

Black Box Warning To reduce risk of significant or irreversible liver injury, perform ALT, AST, and bilirubin blood testing before start of ADPKD treatment, at 2 and 4 weeks after initiation, monthly for 18 months, and every 3 months thereafter. Monitor patient for concurrent signs and symptoms that may indicate liver injury. Prompt action in response to lab abnormalities or signs and symptoms indicative of hepatic injury can mitigate, but not eliminate, risk of serious hepatotoxicity. ■

• Immediately discontinue Jynarque for signs or symptoms consistent with hepatic injury or if ALT, AST, or bilirubin level increases to greater than 2 × ULN. Obtain repeat tests within 48 to 72 hours, and continue testing as appropriate. If lab abnormalities stabilize or resolve, restart drug with more frequent monitoring as long as ALT and AST levels remain below 3 × ULN. Don't restart drug in patients who experience signs or symptoms consistent with hepatic injury or whose ALT or AST level exceeds 3 × ULN at any time during treatment, unless there's another explanation for liver injury and the injury has resolved.

• In patients taking Jynarque who have a stable, low baseline AST or ALT level, an increase above 2 × baseline, even if less than 2 × ULN, may indicate early liver injury.

Reactions in bold italics are *life-threatening*. Interactions may have a *rapid onset* or a *delayed onset*.

Such elevations may warrant treatment suspension and prompt (48 to 72 hours) reevaluation of LFT trends before reinitiation of therapy with more frequent monitoring.

• During Jynarque therapy, if serum sodium level increases above normal range or patient becomes hypovolemic or dehydrated and fluid intake can't be increased, suspend drug until serum sodium level, hydration status, and volume status are within normal range.

◑ *Alert:* Drug may increase risk of irreversible and potentially fatal liver injury. Monitor LFT values and assess liver function promptly in patients reporting fatigue, anorexia, right upper abdominal discomfort, dark urine, or jaundice. If liver injury is suspected, stop drug immediately, initiate treatment, and investigate cause. Don't reinitiate drug unless cause for the observed liver injury is definitively established to be unrelated to tolvaptan treatment.

• Monitor serum electrolyte levels, volume status, and neurologic status when therapy is begun, during dosage titration, and regularly during therapy.

• Monitor potassium level in patients with potassium level greater than 5 mEq/L and in those who are taking drugs known to increase potassium level.

• After treatment for hyponatremia has ended, patients should resume fluid restriction. Monitor patients for changes in serum sodium level and volume status.

• Monitor patients for weight loss, tachycardia, and hypotension, which may signal dehydration.

PATIENT TEACHING

• Advise patient to promptly report all adverse reactions, especially difficulty speaking or swallowing, drowsiness, mood changes, trouble controlling body movement, seizures, fatigue, anorexia, right upper abdominal discomfort, dark urine, or jaundice.

• Advise patient to inform prescriber of all drugs, herbs, and supplements being taken because of the potential for interactions.

• Advise patient to continue ingestion of fluid in response to thirst during therapy and to resume previous fluid restriction after tolvaptan is discontinued.

• Tell patient who misses a dose to take next dose at its scheduled time.

• Advise patient to prevent dehydration.

• Tell patient not to stop or restart drug without first consulting prescriber; Samsca should only be restarted in the hospital where sodium level can be monitored closely.

• Advise female patient not to breastfeed.

• Inform patient that drug can be taken without regard to food but to avoid grapefruit products during therapy.

---

topiramate
toe-PIE-rah-mate

Qudexy XR, Topamax✐, Trokendi XR

Therapeutic class: Anticonvulsants
Pharmacologic class: Sulfamate-substituted monosaccharides

AVAILABLE FORMS
Capsules, sprinkles: 15 mg, 25 mg
Capsules (extended-release) ⓞⓝⓖ: 25 mg, 50 mg, 100 mg, 150 mg, 200 mg
Tablets ⓞⓝⓖ: 25 mg, 50 mg, 100 mg, 200 mg

INDICATIONS & DOSAGES
Adjust-a-dose (for all indications): For adults, if CrCl is less than 70 mL/minute/1.73 m^2, reduce dosage by 50%. For patients at high risk for renal insufficiency, obtain an estimated CrCl before dosing. For hemodialysis patients, supplemental doses may be needed to avoid rapid drops in drug level during prolonged dialysis treatment.

➤ **Initial monotherapy for partial-onset or primary generalized tonic-clonic seizures**
Adults and children age 10 or older: Recommended daily dose is 400 mg (immediate-release) PO in two divided doses (morning and evening). To achieve this dosage, adjust as follows: first week, 25 mg PO b.i.d.; second week, 50 mg PO b.i.d.; third week, 75 mg PO b.i.d.; fourth week, 100 mg PO b.i.d.; fifth week, 150 mg PO b.i.d.; and sixth week, 200 mg PO b.i.d. Or, using extended-release capsules, initially 50 mg PO once daily. Increase dosage weekly by increments

T

of 50 mg for first 4 weeks, then 100 mg for weeks 5 and 6 to recommended 400 mg once daily.

Children ages 2 to younger than 10 (immediate-release and Qudexy XR extended-release) or children ages 6 to younger than 10 (Trokendi XR extended-release): During titration period, initially 25 mg/day (immediate-release or extended-release) PO nightly for first week. Based on tolerability, can increase to 50 mg/day (once daily for extended-release or 25 mg PO b.i.d. for immediate-release) in the second week. Can increase by 25 to 50 mg/day each subsequent week as tolerated. Attempt titration to the minimum maintenance dosage over 5 to 7 weeks of the total titration period. Based on tolerability and seizure control, can attempt additional titration to a higher dosage (up to the maximum maintenance dosage) at 25 to 50 mg/day in weekly increments. Total daily dosage shouldn't exceed the maximum maintenance dosage for each range of body weight.

Give maintenance doses of extended-release form once daily; give maintenance doses of immediate-release form in two equally divided PO doses daily. If patient weighs up to 11 kg, maintenance dosage range is 150 mg/day to a maximum of 250 mg/day. If patient weighs 12 to 22 kg, maintenance dosage range is 200 mg/day to a maximum of 300 mg/day. If patient weighs 23 to 31 kg, maintenance dosage range is 200 mg/day to a maximum of 350 mg/day. If patient weighs 32 to 38 kg, maintenance dosage range is 250 mg/day to a maximum of 350 mg/day. If patient weighs more than 38 kg, maintenance dosage range is 250 mg/day to a maximum of 400 mg/day.

➤ **Adjunctive treatment for partial-onset or primary generalized tonic-clonic seizures or Lennox-Gastaut syndrome**
Adults and children age 17 and older: Initially, 25 to 50 mg PO daily; increase gradually by 25 to 50 mg/week until an effective daily dose is reached. Adjust to recommended daily dose of 200 to 400 mg PO in two divided doses of immediate-release or once daily of extended-release for adults with partial-onset seizures or Lennox-Gastaut syndrome, or 400 mg PO in two divided doses of immediate-release or once daily of extended-release for adults with primary generalized tonic-clonic seizures.

Children ages 6 to 16 (Trokendi) or ages 2 to 16 (Qudexy XR): Initially, 25 mg PO daily at bedtime (based on range of 1 to 3 mg/kg once daily) for first week. Increase dosage at 1- or 2-week intervals by increments of 1 to 3 mg/kg daily. Guide dosage titration by clinical outcome. Recommended daily dose is 5 to 9 mg/kg once daily.

Children ages 2 to 16 (immediate-release): Initially, 25 mg/day (or less, based on a range of 1 to 3 mg/kg/day) PO given at bedtime for 1 week. Increase at 1- or 2-week intervals by 1 to 3 mg/kg daily (given in two divided doses) to achieve optimal response. Guide titration by clinical outcome. Recommended daily dose is 5 to 9 mg/kg, in two divided doses. Maximum, 400 mg/day.

➤ **To prevent migraine headache**
Adults and adolescents age 12 and older: For immediate-release, initially, 25 mg PO daily in evening for first week. Then, 25 mg PO b.i.d. in morning and evening for second week. For third week, 25 mg PO in morning and 50 mg PO in evening. For fourth week, 50 mg PO b.i.d. in morning and evening. Recommended total daily dose is 100 mg.

For extended-release, initially, 25 mg PO once daily. After 1 week, increase by 25 mg daily, then weekly by 25 mg daily until recommended daily dose of 100 mg is reached. Guide dosage and titration rate according to clinical outcome. Can use longer intervals between dosage adjustments if needed.

ADMINISTRATION
PO
● Give drug without regard for food.
● Immediate-release and Qudexy XR capsules may be opened and contents sprinkled on a teaspoon of soft food. Patient should swallow immediately without chewing.
● Patient should swallow Trokendi XR capsules whole and intact. Don't sprinkle capsule contents on food or allow patient to chew or crush capsules; doing so may disrupt the triphasic release properties.
● Don't break tablets, due to bitter taste.

ACTION
Unknown. May block a sodium channel, potentiate the activity of GABA, and inhibit

kainate's ability to activate an amino acid receptor, and inhibit carbonic anhydrase.

Route	Onset	Peak	Duration
PO (immediate-release)	Unknown	1–4 hr	Unknown
PO (extended-release)	Unknown	About 20 hr (Qudexy XR); 24 hr (Trokendi XR)	Unknown

Half-life: Immediate-release, 21 hours; extended-release, 31 to 56 hours.

ADVERSE REACTIONS

CNS: anxiety, asthenia, ataxia, confusion, difficulty with memory, dizziness, fatigue, nervousness, paresthesia, psychomotor slowing, somnolence, speech disorders, tremor, *generalized tonic-clonic seizures, suicide attempts,* abnormal coordination, aggressive reaction, agitation, apathy, depression, depersonalization, emotional lability, euphoria, fever, hallucination, hyperkinesia, hypertonia, hypoesthesia, hypokinesia, insomnia, malaise, mood problems, personality disorder, psychosis, stupor, vertigo; difficulty with concentration, attention, or language. **CV:** chest pain, edema, palpitations, vasodilation, flushing. **EENT:** abnormal vision, diplopia, nystagmus, conjunctivitis, eye pain, hearing problems, tinnitus, epistaxis, pharyngitis, sinusitis, rhinitis. **GI:** anorexia, nausea, abdominal pain, constipation, diarrhea, dry mouth, dyspepsia, flatulence, gastroenteritis, gingivitis, taste perversion, vomiting, GERD. **GU:** amenorrhea, dysuria, dysmenorrhea, hematuria, impotence, intermenstrual bleeding, leukorrhea, menstrual disorder, menorrhagia, urinary frequency, renal calculi, urinary incontinence, UTI, vaginitis, vaginal hemorrhage, cystitis. **Hematologic:** *leukopenia,* anemia. **Metabolic:** decreased weight, increased weight. **Musculoskeletal:** arthralgia, back or leg pain, muscle weakness, myalgia, rigors. **Respiratory:** URI, bronchitis, coughing, dyspnea, pneumonia. **Skin:** acne, alopecia, increased sweating, pruritus, rash. **Other:** body odor, breast pain, decreased libido, flulike syndrome, hot flashes, lymphadenopathy, infection.

INTERACTIONS
Drug-drug. *Cannabidiol, cannabis:* May enhance CNS depressant effect of topiramate. Monitor therapy.
Carbamazepine: May decrease topiramate level. Monitor patient.
Carbonic anhydrase inhibitors (acetazolamide, dichlorphenamide): May cause renal calculus formation. Avoid using together.
CNS depressants (including opioids), magnesium sulfate: May cause CNS depression and other adverse cognitive and neuropsychiatric events. Use together cautiously.
Fosphenytoin, phenytoin: May decrease topiramate level and increase phenytoin level. Monitor levels.
Hormonal contraceptives: May decrease effectiveness. Report changes in menstrual patterns. Advise patient to use another contraceptive method.
Lithium: May increase serum lithium level. Monitor patient closely.
Salicylates: May enhance toxicity of both agents. Avoid using together.
Valproic acid: May decrease valproic acid and topiramate level. Monitor patient.
Drug-herb. *Kava kava:* May increase CNS depressant effects. Avoid using together.
Drug-food. *Ketogenic diet:* May increase possibility of acidosis or kidney stones. Monitor patient for adverse effects.
Drug-lifestyle. *Alcohol use:* May cause CNS depression and other adverse cognitive and neuropsychiatric events. Discourage use together.

EFFECTS ON LAB TEST RESULTS
• May increase liver enzyme and ammonia levels. May decrease bicarbonate and Hb levels and hematocrit.
• May decrease WBC count.

CONTRAINDICATIONS & CAUTIONS
• Contraindicated in patients hypersensitive to drug or its components.
• Use cautiously in patients with hepatic and renal impairment.
• **Alert:** Alcohol use is contraindicated within 6 hours before and 6 hours after taking Trokendi XR.
• Bioequivalence hasn't been demonstrated between Trokendi XR and Qudexy XR.

T

• Acute myopia associated with secondary angle-closure glaucoma has been reported in adults and children receiving topiramate. Such symptoms as acute-onset decreased visual acuity or ocular pain typically occur within 1 month of therapy initiation. Discontinue drug as rapidly as possible, according to judgment of health care provider.

• Use cautiously with other drugs that predispose patients to heat-related disorders, including other carbonic anhydrase inhibitors and anticholinergics.

Dialyzable drug: Yes.

⚠ **Overdose S&S:** Abdominal pain, abnormal coordination, agitation, blurred vision, seizures, depression, diplopia, dizziness, drowsiness, hypotension, lethargy, impaired mentation, speech disturbance, stupor, severe metabolic acidosis.

PREGNANCY-LACTATION-REPRODUCTION

🜂 **Alert:** Drug is associated with increased risk of oral clefts (cleft lip or palate) and small-for-gestational-age infants born to women treated with topiramate during pregnancy. Use in pregnant women only if potential benefit outweighs risk to the fetus. Consider alternative medications with a lower risk of adverse outcomes for these patients.

🜂 **Alert:** Women who become pregnant during therapy should register with the North American Antiepileptic Drug (AED) Pregnancy Registry (1-888-233-2334).

• Although drug's effect on labor and delivery hasn't been established, development of topiramate-induced metabolic acidosis in the mother or fetus may result in adverse effects and fetal death.

• Tell women of childbearing potential that drug may decrease effectiveness of hormonal contraceptives. Advise women using hormonal contraceptives to report change in menstrual patterns.

• Drug appears in human milk, but effect of exposure in infants isn't known. Use cautiously in breastfeeding women.

NURSING CONSIDERATIONS

🜂 **Alert:** Closely monitor all patients taking or starting antiepileptic drugs for changes in behavior indicating worsening of suicidal thoughts or behavior or depression. Symptoms such as anxiety, agitation, hostility,

mania, and hypomania may be precursors to emerging suicidality.

• If needed, withdraw anticonvulsant (including topiramate) gradually to minimize risk of increased seizure activity.

• Monitoring topiramate level isn't necessary.

• Drug may infrequently cause oligohidrosis and hyperthermia, mainly in children. Monitor patient closely, especially in hot weather.

• Drug may cause hyperchloremic, nonanion gap metabolic acidosis from renal bicarbonate loss. Factors that may predispose patients to acidosis, such as renal disease, severe respiratory disorders, status epilepticus, diarrhea, surgery, ketogenic diet, or drugs, may add to topiramate's bicarbonate-lowering effects.

• Measure baseline and periodic bicarbonate levels. If metabolic acidosis develops and persists, consider reducing the dose, gradually stopping the drug, or offering alkali treatment.

• Monitor renal function, electrolyte and ammonia levels, and weight.

• Drug is rapidly cleared by dialysis. A prolonged period of dialysis may cause low drug level and seizures. A supplemental dose may be needed.

• Stop drug if patient experiences acute myopia and secondary angle-closure glaucoma.

• **Look alike–sound alike:** Don't confuse Topamax with Toprol-XL, Tegretol, or Tegretol-XR.

PATIENT TEACHING

• Tell patient not to consume alcohol within 6 hours before to 6 hours after taking Trokendi XR form.

• Instruct patient to report all adverse reactions and to immediately seek medical attention if blurred vision, visual disturbances, or eye pain occurs, to reduce risk of permanent vision loss.

• Advise patient to immediately report high or persistent fever or decreased sweating.

• Tell patient to use appropriate caution when engaging in activities in which loss of consciousness could result in serious danger to patient or others nearby. Some patients with epilepsy will continue to have unpredictable seizures and may need to avoid such activities entirely.

Reactions in bold italics are *life-threatening*. Interactions may have a *rapid onset* or a *delayed onset*.

• Tell patient to drink plenty of fluids during therapy to minimize risk of forming kidney stones.

• Advise patient that a ketogenic diet may increase kidney stone or acidosis risk.

• Advise patient not to drive or operate hazardous machinery until CNS effects of drug are known. Drug can cause sleepiness, dizziness, confusion, and concentration problems.

🛈 *Alert:* Teach female patient of childbearing potential to use effective contraceptive while taking topiramate, and explain about the drug's effect on fetal development. Tell her to contact prescriber if she becomes pregnant or plans to become pregnant during therapy.

• Inform patient that drug can be taken without regard to food.

• Tell patient taking Trokendi XR to swallow capsules whole and intact and not to chew or crush capsules or sprinkle capsule contents on food.

• Tell patient taking Qudexy XR that capsules may be swallowed whole or opened and the contents sprinkled on a spoonful of soft food; patient should swallow immediately and not chew.

• Tell patient that immediate-release capsules may either be swallowed whole or carefully opened and contents sprinkled on a teaspoonful of soft food. Tell patient to swallow immediately without chewing.

• Instruct patient not to stop drug abruptly, to prevent onset of seizures.

SAFETY ALERT!

topotecan hydrochloride
toh-poh-TEE-ken

Hycamtin

Therapeutic class: Antineoplastics
Pharmacologic class: DNA topoisomerase inhibitors

AVAILABLE FORMS
Capsules 🔘: 0.25 mg, 1 mg
Injection: 4-mg single-dose vial (preservative-free)

INDICATIONS & DOSAGES
🛈 *Alert:* Verify dosage using BSA before dispensing. Recommended IV dosage should generally not exceed 4 mg. For obese patients, use actual body weight to calculate BSA or weight-based dosing.

Adjust-a-dose (for all indications): Refer to manufacturer's instructions for toxicity-related dosage adjustments.

➤ **Relapsed small-cell lung cancer (SCLC) in patients with a prior complete or partial response who are at least 45 days from the end of first-line chemotherapy**
Adults: 2.3 mg/m^2/day PO once daily for 5 consecutive days, starting on day 1 of a 21-day cycle. Repeat cycle every 21 days. Round the calculated dose to the nearest 0.25 mg.

Adjust-a-dose: For patients with moderate renal impairment (CrCl 30 to 49 mL/minute), give 1.5 mg/m^2/day. For patients with severe renal impairment (CrCl less than 30 mL/minute), give 0.6 mg/m^2/day. For all patients with dosage adjustment due to renal impairment, dosage can be increased after the first course by 0.4 mg/m^2/day if no severe hematologic or GI toxicities occur.

➤ **With cisplatin, stage IVB recurrent or persistent cervical cancer unresponsive to surgery or radiation**
Adults: 0.75 mg/m^2 by IV infusion on days 1, 2, and 3, followed by 50 mg/m^2 cisplatin by IV infusion on day 1. Repeat cycle every 21 days. Adjust subsequent doses of drug based on hematologic toxicities.

➤ **Metastatic carcinoma of the ovary after failure of first or subsequent chemotherapy; SCLC in patients with platinum-sensitive disease who progressed at least 60 days after initiation of first-line chemotherapy**
Adults: 1.5 mg/m^2 IV infusion daily for 5 consecutive days, starting on day 1 of a 21-day cycle. For ovarian cancer, continue until disease progression or unacceptable toxicity.

Adjust-a-dose: For patients with CrCl of 20 to 39 mL/minute, decrease dosage to 0.75 mg/m^2.

T

ADMINISTRATION
PO
- Hazardous drug; avoid direct contact with capsule contents.
- Give drug without regard to food.
- Don't crush or divide capsules.
- If patient vomits after taking dose, don't give a replacement dose.

IV
▼ Hazardous drug; use safe handling and disposal precautions according to facility policy.
▼ Reconstitute each 4-mg vial with 4 mL sterile water for injection. Further dilute appropriate volume of reconstituted solution in either NSS or D$_5$W before giving.
▼ Lyophilized form contains no antibacterial preservative; use reconstituted product immediately.
▼ Infuse over 30 minutes and monitor insertion site during infusion. Extravasation injuries have been reported, some severe. If extravasation occurs, immediately discontinue infusion and notify prescriber.
▼ When giving topotecan with cisplatin, always give topotecan first.
▼ If stored at 68° to 77° F (20° to 25° C) and exposed to normal lighting, reconstituted drug is stable for 24 hours. Protect unopened vials from light.
▼ **Incompatibilities:** Many drugs are incompatible with topotecan. Consult a drug incompatibility reference for information.

ACTION
Interacts with topoisomerase I, inducing reversible single-strand DNA breaks. Drug binds to the topoisomerase I–DNA complex and prevents repair of these single-strand breaks.

Route	Onset	Peak	Duration
PO	Unknown	1–2 hr	Unknown
IV	Unknown	Unknown	Unknown

Half-life: Oral, 3 to 6 hours; IV, 2 to 3 hours.

ADVERSE REACTIONS
CNS: asthenia, fatigue, fever, headache.
GI: abdominal pain, anorexia, constipation, *severe diarrhea,* nausea, stomatitis, vomiting. **Hematologic:** anemia, *leukopenia, neutropenia, thrombocytopenia.*
Hepatic: elevated liver enzyme levels,

hyperbilirubinemia, *hepatotoxicity.* **Musculoskeletal:** weakness, back and skeletal pain. **Respiratory:** coughing, dyspnea, pneumonia. **Skin:** alopecia, rash. **Other:** infection, *sepsis.*

INTERACTIONS
Drug-drug. *Breast cancer resistance protein inhibitors (cyclosporine, eltrombopag), P-gp inhibitors (cyclosporine, ketoconazole, ritonavir):* May increase systemic exposure to oral topotecan. Avoid concomitant use.
Cisplatin, cytotoxic agents: May increase severity of myelosuppression. Use together with extreme caution. Dosage reductions may be needed.
Fosphenytoin, phenytoin: May decrease topotecan serum concentration. Consider using alternative agent to phenytoin.
G-CSF: May prolong duration of neutropenia. If G-CSF is to be used, don't start it until day 6 of the course, 24 hours after completion of IV topotecan treatment.
Vaccines: May increase adverse effects of vaccines. Patient should avoid vaccines for at least 3 months after using topotecan.
Drug-herb. *Echinacea:* May diminish therapeutic effect of topotecan. Avoid use together.

EFFECTS ON LAB TEST RESULTS
- May increase ALT, AST, and bilirubin levels. May decrease Hb level.
- May decrease WBC, platelet, and neutrophil counts.

CONTRAINDICATIONS & CAUTIONS
❸ *Alert:* Administer drug under the supervision of a health care provider experienced in the use of chemotherapeutic agents. Ensure that appropriate diagnostic and treatment facilities are readily available.
- Contraindicated in patients hypersensitive to drug or its components.
- Use cautiously in patients with renal impairment and in patients with a history of ILD.
- Safety and effectiveness of drug in children haven't been established.
Dialyzable drug: Unknown.
⚠ *Overdose S&S:* Bone marrow suppression.

PREGNANCY-LACTATION-REPRODUCTION

• Drug can cause fetal harm. If used during pregnancy, or if patient becomes pregnant during therapy, apprise her of potential hazard to a fetus.

• Women should use highly effective contraception during treatment and for at least 6 months after therapy ends.

• Drug may damage spermatozoa, possibly resulting in genetic and fetal abnormalities. Advise males with a female partner of childbearing potential to use effective contraception during and for 3 months after therapy ends.

• It isn't known if drug appears in human milk. Patient should discontinue breastfeeding or discontinue drug.

• Drug may have both acute and long-term adverse effects on male and female fertility. Patient should seek counseling on fertility and family planning options before starting treatment.

NURSING CONSIDERATIONS

Black Box Warning Before first course of therapy is started, patient must have baseline neutrophil count of 1,500/mm³ or more and platelet count of 100,000/mm³ or more. Perform peripheral blood counts frequently to monitor patient for bone marrow suppression, primarily neutropenia, which may be severe and result in infection and death. ∎

• Don't give subsequent courses until neutrophil count recovers to more than 1,000/mm³, platelet count recovers to more than 100,000/mm³, and Hb level recovers to 9 g/dL (with transfusion, if needed).

• Bone marrow suppression indicates toxic levels of topotecan. The nadir occurs at about 11 days. Neutropenia isn't cumulative over time.

• Duration of thrombocytopenia is about 5 days, with nadir at 15 days. The nadir for anemia is 15 days. Blood or platelet transfusions may be needed.

• WBC colony-stimulating factors may promote cell growth and decrease risk for infection.

• **Alert:** Fatalities due to neutropenic colitis have been reported. Consider possibility of neutropenic colitis in patients presenting with fever, neutropenia, and a compatible pattern of abdominal pain.

• **Alert:** Drug may cause ILD, which may be fatal. Monitor patient for cough, fever, dyspnea, and hypoxia; stop drug if they occur.

• Monitor CBC with differential and platelet count, renal function tests, and bilirubin level before each infusion and regularly during therapy.

• If extravasation occurs, discontinue infusion immediately and manage appropriately. Ensure proper needle and catheter placement before and during infusion.

• **Look alike–sound alike:** Don't confuse topotecan with irinotecan. Don't confuse Hycamtin with Mycamine.

PATIENT TEACHING

• Urge patient to promptly report all adverse reactions, especially sore throat, fever, chills, or unusual bleeding or bruising.

• Advise patient that although diarrhea is common, it may become severe and should be reported to health care provider.

• Caution patient to avoid contact with people with infections.

• Inform patient of potential hazard to the fetus if drug is used during pregnancy, or if patient becomes pregnant while taking drug.

• Advise female patient to use highly effective contraception during treatment and for at least 6 months after last dose and to contact health care provider if she becomes pregnant or suspects she is pregnant during therapy.

• Advise male patient with a female partner of childbearing potential to use effective contraception during and for 3 months after therapy ends.

• Caution female patient to avoid breastfeeding during therapy.

• Teach patient and family about drug's adverse reactions and need for frequent monitoring of blood counts.

• Advise patient that capsules can be taken without regard to food.

• Tell patient not to chew, crush, or divide capsules; they should be swallowed whole.

torsemide ⚱
TOR-seh-mide

Demadex⬧

Therapeutic class: Diuretics
Pharmacologic class: Loop diuretics

AVAILABLE FORMS
Tablets: 5 mg, 10 mg, 20 mg, 100 mg

INDICATIONS & DOSAGES
➤ **Diuresis in patients with HF**
Adults: Initially, 10 to 20 mg PO once daily.
If response is inadequate, double dose until
desired effect is achieved. Maximum,
200 mg daily.
➤ **Diuresis in patients with chronic renal
failure**
Adults: Initially, 20 mg PO once daily. If
response is inadequate, double dose until
response is obtained. Maximum, 200 mg
daily.
➤ **Diuresis in patients with hepatic cirrhosis**
Adults: Initially, 5 to 10 mg PO once
daily with an aldosterone antagonist or a
potassium-sparing diuretic. If response is
inadequate, double dose until desired effect
is achieved. Maximum, 40 mg daily.
➤ **HTN**
Adults: Initially, 5 mg PO daily. Increase
to 10 mg if needed and tolerated after 4 to
6 weeks. Add another antihypertensive if
response is still inadequate.

ADMINISTRATION
PO
• May give with or without food.
• To prevent nocturia, give drug in the
morning.

ACTION
Enhances excretion of sodium, chloride,
and water by acting on the ascending loop
of Henle.

Route	Onset	Peak	Duration
PO	1 hr	1–2 hr	6–8 hr

Half-life: 3½ hours.

ADVERSE REACTIONS
CNS: asthenia, dizziness, headache, nervousness, insomnia, weakness. **CV:** ECG
abnormalities, chest pain, edema, orthostatic
hypotension. **EENT:** rhinitis, sore throat. **GI:**
excessive thirst, diarrhea, constipation, nausea, dyspepsia. **GU:** excessive urination, impotence. **Metabolic:** electrolyte imbalances,
including *hypokalemia* and *hypomagnesemia; dehydration;* hypochloremic alkalosis; hyperuricemia. **Musculoskeletal:**
arthralgia, myalgia. **Respiratory:** cough.

INTERACTIONS
Drug-drug. *Aminoglycoside antibiotics,
cisplatin:* May increase ototoxicity. Use
together cautiously.
*Amphotericin B, corticosteroids, metola-
zone:* May increase risk of hypokalemia.
Monitor potassium level.
Antidiabetics: May decrease hypoglycemic
effect, resulting in higher glucose level.
Monitor glucose level.
*Chlorothiazide, chlorthalidone, hydrochloro-
thiazide, indapamide, metolazone:* May cause
excessive diuretic response, resulting in serious electrolyte abnormalities or dehydration.
Adjust doses carefully, and monitor patient
closely for signs and symptoms of excessive
diuretic response.
Cholestyramine: May decrease absorption
of torsemide. Give torsemide at least 1 hour
before or 4 to 6 hours after cholestyramine.
CYP2C9 inducers (rifampin): May increase
torsemide clearance and decrease plasma
concentrations. Monitor patient closely and
adjust torsemide dosage if indicated.
*CYP2C9 inhibitors (amiodarone, flucona-
zole, miconazole, oxandrolone):* May decrease torsemide clearance and increase
plasma concentrations. Monitor patient
closely and adjust torsemide dosage if
indicated.
*CYP2C9 substrates (sensitive ones such as
celecoxib and those with a narrow therapeutic range, such as warfarin or phenytoin):*
May affect efficacy and safety of substrate.
Monitor patient and adjust dosages if necessary.
Digoxin: Electrolyte imbalance caused by
diuretic may lead to digoxin-induced arrhythmia. Use together cautiously.

Reactions in bold italics are *life-threatening*. Interactions may have a *rapid onset* or a **delayed onset**.

Lithium: May increase lithium level and cause toxicity. Use together cautiously and monitor lithium level.

Methotrexate: May increase methotrexate serum concentration; may diminish therapeutic effects of torsemide. Consider therapy modification.

NSAIDs: May decrease effects of loop diuretics. Use together cautiously.

Probenecid: May decrease diuretic effect. Avoid using together.

Salicylates: May decrease excretion, possibly leading to salicylate toxicity. Avoid using together.

Drug-herb. *Licorice:* May cause unexpected rapid potassium loss. Discourage use together.

Yohimbe: May decrease antihypertensive effect of torsemide. Monitor therapy closely.

EFFECTS ON LAB TEST RESULTS
• May increase BUN, creatinine, cholesterol, glucose, and uric acid levels.
• May decrease calcium, sodium, potassium, and magnesium levels.
• Can cause false-negative aldosterone/renin ratios.

CONTRAINDICATIONS & CAUTIONS
• Contraindicated in patients hypersensitive to drug, other sulfonamide derivatives, or povidone and in those with anuria or hepatic coma.
• Use cautiously in patients with hepatic disease and related cirrhosis and ascites; sudden changes in fluid and electrolyte balance may precipitate hepatic coma in these patients.
• Serious skin reactions, including SJS and toxic epidermal necrolysis, leukopenia, thrombocytopenia, pancreatitis, and ototoxicity have been reported in association with torsemide use.
⚖ The antihypertensive effects of torsemide are, on average, greater in black patients than in nonblack patients.
Dialyzable drug: No.
⚠ **Overdose S&S:** Dehydration, hypovolemia, hypotension, hypokalemia, hypochloremic alkalosis, hemoconcentration.

PREGNANCY-LACTATION-REPRODUCTION
• There are no adequate studies in pregnant women. Use only if clearly needed.

• It isn't known if drug appears in human milk. Diuretics can suppress lactation. Use cautiously in breastfeeding women.

NURSING CONSIDERATIONS
• Monitor fluid intake and output, renal function, electrolyte levels, BP, weight, and pulse rate during rapid diuresis and routinely with long-term use. Drug can cause profound diuresis and water and electrolyte depletion.
• Watch for signs of hypokalemia, such as muscle weakness and cramps.
• Consult prescriber and dietitian about providing a high-potassium diet or potassium supplement. Foods rich in potassium include citrus fruits, bananas, and dates.
• Monitor elderly patients, who are especially susceptible to excessive diuresis with potential for circulatory collapse and thromboembolic complications.
• *Look alike–sound alike:* Don't confuse torsemide with furosemide. Don't confuse Demadex with Denorex.

PATIENT TEACHING
• Tell patient to take drug in morning to prevent the need to urinate at night.
• Advise patient to change positions slowly to prevent dizziness and to limit alcohol intake and strenuous exercise in hot weather to prevent dizziness.
• Advise patient to immediately report ringing in ears because it may indicate toxicity.
• Tell patient to report weakness, cramping, nausea, and dizziness.
• Tell patient to check with prescriber or pharmacist before taking OTC drugs.

---

traMADol hydrochloride
TRAM-uh-dohl

ConZip, Durela✣, Ralivia✣, Tridural✣, Ultram, Zytram XL✣

Therapeutic class: Analgesics
Pharmacologic class: Synthetic centrally active analgesics
Controlled substance schedule: IV

AVAILABLE FORMS
Capsules (extended-release) ⓝⓒ: 100 mg, 150 mg, 200 mg, 300 mg

T

Tablets: 50 mg
Tablets (extended-release) ◉: 75 mg✹,
100 mg, 150 mg✹, 200 mg, 300 mg,
400 mg✹

INDICATIONS & DOSAGES
❶ Alert: Initiate dosing regimen for each patient individually, taking into account patient's severity of pain, response, prior analgesic treatment experience, and risk factors
for addiction, abuse, and misuse. Use lowest
effective dosage for shortest duration consistent with individual patient treatment goals.
➤ **Moderate to moderately severe chronic
pain**
Adults age 17 and older: Initially, 25 mg
(immediate-release) PO in the morning. Adjust by 25 mg every 3 days to 100 mg/day
(25 mg q.i.d.). Thereafter, adjust by 50 mg
every 3 days to reach 200 mg/day (50 mg
q.i.d.). Thereafter, give 50 to 100 mg PO
every 4 to 6 hours p.r.n. Maximum, 400 mg
daily.
*Adults age 18 and older not taking
immediate-release tablets:* 100 mg
extended-release form PO once daily. Titrate
by 100 mg every 5 days to relieve pain. Do
not exceed 300 mg/day.
*Adults age 18 and older currently taking
immediate-release tablets:* Calculate the
24-hour tramadol immediate-release dose
and initiate a total daily dose of extended-
release product rounded down to the next
lowest 100-mg increment. Subsequently, individualize according to patient need. Maximum dose is 300 mg daily.
Adjust-a-dose: For immediate-release form,
if CrCl is less than 30 mL/minute, increase
dose interval to every 12 hours; maximum
is 200 mg daily. For patients with cirrhosis, give 50 mg (immediate-release) every
12 hours. For patients older than age 75,
maximum is 300 mg (immediate-release)
daily in divided doses. Don't use extended-
release form in patients with severe hepatic
or renal impairment.

ADMINISTRATION
PO
Black Box Warning To ensure that the
benefits of opioid analgesics outweigh
the risks of addiction, abuse, and misuse,
the FDA has required a REMS for these
products. Under the requirements of the
REMS, drug companies with approved opioid analgesic products must make REMS-
compliant education programs available
to health care providers. Further information on the Opioid Analgesic REMS is
available by calling 1-800-503-0784 or at
www.opioidanalgesicrems.com. ∎
• Give drug without regard for meals in a
consistent manner.
• Extended-release capsules and tablets
must be swallowed whole; don't break or
crush tablets.

ACTION
Unknown. Thought to bind to opioid receptors and inhibit reuptake of norepinephrine
and serotonin.

Route	Onset	Peak	Duration
PO	1 hr	2–3 hr	Unknown
PO (extended-release)	Unknown	10–12 hr	Unknown

Half-life: 6 to 7 hours; extended-release, 8 to
10 hours.

ADVERSE REACTIONS
CNS: dizziness, headache, somnolence,
vertigo, *seizures,* anxiety, asthenia, CNS
stimulation, confusion, coordination disturbance, euphoria, malaise, nervousness,
sleep disorder, fever, paresthesia, tremor,
depression, agitation, apathy. **CV:** vasodilation, HTN, peripheral edema. **EENT:** visual
disturbances, nasopharyngitis, pharyngitis,
rhinitis, sinusitis. **GI:** constipation, nausea,
vomiting, abdominal pain, anorexia, diarrhea, dry mouth, dyspepsia, flatulence. **GU:**
menopausal symptoms, proteinuria, urinary
frequency, urine retention, pelvic pain, UTI,
prostate disorder. **Metabolic:** weight loss.
Musculoskeletal: hypertonia, arthralgia,
neck pain, myalgia. **Respiratory:** bronchitis, *respiratory depression.* **Skin:** diaphoresis, pruritus, rash. **Other:** chills, withdrawal
syndrome, accidental injury.

INTERACTIONS
Drug-drug. **Black Box Warning** *Benzodiazepines, CNS depressants:* May cause
slow or difficult breathing, sedation, and
death. Avoid use together. If use together is
necessary, limit dosage and duration of each

Reactions in bold italics are *life-threatening*. Interactions may have a *rapid onset* or a *delayed onset*.

drug to minimum necessary for desired effect. ■

Carbamazepine: May increase tramadol metabolism. Patients receiving long-term carbamazepine therapy up to 800 mg daily may need up to twice the recommended tramadol dose.

CNS depressants, opioids: May cause additive effects. Use together cautiously; tramadol dosage may need to be reduced.

Cyclobenzaprine, MAO inhibitors, neuroleptics, other opioids, SSNRIs, SSRIs, TCAs: May increase risk of seizures. Monitor patient closely.

Black Box Warning *CYP2D6 inhibitors:* May decrease therapeutic effect of tramadol. Monitor therapy closely. ■

Black Box Warning *CYP3A4 inducers:* May decrease tramadol serum concentration. Monitor therapy closely. ■

Black Box Warning *CYP3A4 inhibitors:* May increase tramadol serum concentration. Monitor therapy closely. ■

Quinidine: May increase level of tramadol. Monitor patient closely.

🕒 *Alert:* *Serotonergic drugs (amoxapine, antiemetics [dolasetron, granisetron, ondansetron, palonosetron], antimigraine drugs, buspirone, cyclobenzaprine, dextromethorphan, linezolid, lithium, MAO inhibitors, maprotiline, methylene blue, mirtazapine, nefazodone, SSNRIs, SSRIs, TCAs, trazodone, tryptophan, vilazodone):* May increase risk of serotonin syndrome. Use together cautiously and monitor patient for serotonin syndrome.

Vitamin K antagonists (warfarin): May increase anticoagulant effects. Monitor therapy closely.

Drug-herb. *Kava kava:* May increase CNS depression. Monitor therapy closely.

🕒 *Alert:* *St. John's wort:* May increase risk of serotonin syndrome. Use together cautiously and monitor patient for serotonin syndrome.

Drug-lifestyle. **Black Box Warning** *Alcohol use:* May have additive effects. Don't use together. ■

EFFECTS ON LAB TEST RESULTS
• May increase creatinine, GGT, and liver enzyme levels.
• May decrease Hb level.

CONTRAINDICATIONS & CAUTIONS
• Contraindicated in patients hypersensitive to drug or opioids, in patients with severe renal or hepatic impairment, suicidal patients, and in those with acute intoxication from alcohol, hypnotics, centrally acting analgesics, opioids, or psychotropic drugs.
• Contraindicated in patients with GI obstruction, including paralytic ileus.
• Contraindicated with concomitant use or within 14 days of MAO inhibitor therapy.
• Contraindicated in patients with significant respiratory depression or acute or severe bronchial asthma or hypercapnia in unmonitored settings or where resuscitative equipment isn't available.

Black Box Warning Contraindicated for use to treat pain in children younger than age 12 and to treat pain in children younger than age 18 after surgery to remove tonsils or adenoids. ■

Black Box Warning May cause fatal respiratory depression, especially during initiation or dosage increase. ■

Black Box Warning The effects of concomitant use or discontinuation of CYP3A4 inducers or inhibitors, or CYP2D6 inhibitors with tramadol are complex and require careful consideration of the effects on parent drug, tramadol, and the active metabolite, M1. ■

Black Box Warning Opioids should only be prescribed with benzodiazepines or other CNS depressants to patients for whom alternative treatment options are inadequate. ■

🕒 *Alert:* Serious hypersensitivity reactions can occur, usually after the first dose. Patients with history of anaphylactic reaction to codeine and opioids may be at increased risk.

🕒 *Alert:* Patients are at increased risk for oversedation and respiratory depression if they snore or have a history of sleep apnea, haven't used opioids recently or are first-time opioid users, have increased opioid dosage requirements or opioid habituation, have received general anesthesia for longer lengths of time or received other sedating drugs, have preexisting pulmonary or cardiac disease, or have thoracic or other surgical incisions that may impair breathing. Monitor patients carefully.

• Use cautiously in patients at risk for seizures or respiratory depression; in patients with increased ICP or head injury, acute abdominal conditions, or renal or hepatic impairment; and in patients with physical dependence on opioids. Withdrawal symptoms may occur if drug is abruptly discontinued.

◐ *Alert:* Drug can cause life-threatening serotonin syndrome.

◐ *Alert:* Use cautiously in patients who are experiencing depression or an emotional disturbance because of the increased risk of suicide.

◐ *Alert:* Drug may lead to rare but serious decrease in adrenal gland cortisol production.

◐ *Alert:* Drug may cause decreased sex hormone levels with long-term use.

Black Box Warning Avoid use in adolescents ages 12 to 18 who are obese or have such conditions as obstructive sleep apnea or severe lung disease or other risk factors that may increase their sensitivity to tramadol's respiratory depressant effects. ■

▓ **Black Box Warning** Patients who are CYP2D6 ultrarapid metabolizers shouldn't use tramadol because of the risk of life-threatening or fatal respiratory depression. ■

• Use with extreme caution in elderly patients, especially those older than age 75.

Dialyzable drug: 7%.

⚠ *Overdose S&S:* Lethargy, somnolence, stupor, coma, seizures, skeletal muscle flaccidity, respiratory depression, cool clammy skin, miosis, bradycardia, hypotension, cardiac arrest, death.

PREGNANCY-LACTATION-REPRODUCTION

• Safe use in pregnant women hasn't been established. Use only if potential benefit justifies potential risk to the fetus.

Black Box Warning Prolonged use during pregnancy can result in neonatal opioid withdrawal syndrome, which may be life-threatening if not recognized and treated according to neonatology expert protocols. If opioid use is required for a prolonged period during pregnancy, advise patient of the risk of neonatal opioid withdrawal syndrome; ensure her that appropriate treatment will be available. ■

• Use in breastfeeding women isn't recommended due to the risk of serious adverse reactions in breastfed infants, such as excess sleepiness, difficulty breastfeeding, or serious breathing problems that could result in death.

NURSING CONSIDERATIONS

Black Box Warning Caution patient or caregiver of patient taking an opioid with a benzodiazepine, CNS depressant, or alcohol to seek immediate medical attention for dizziness, light-headedness, extreme sleepiness, slowed or difficult breathing, or unresponsiveness. ■

Black Box Warning Tramadol exposes patients to the risk of addiction, abuse, and misuse, which can lead to overdose and death. Assess each patient's risk before prescribing; monitor patient regularly for development of abnormal behaviors. ■

• Reassess patient's level of pain at least 30 minutes after administration.

• Monitor CV and respiratory status, especially within first 24 to 72 hours of therapy initiation and after dosage increases; adjust dosage accordingly. Withhold dose and notify prescriber if respirations are shallow or rate is below 12 breaths/minute.

◐ *Alert:* Carefully monitor vital signs, pain level, respiratory status, and sedation level in all patients receiving opioids, especially those receiving IV drugs, even those given postoperatively.

• Monitor bowel and bladder function. Anticipate need for stimulant laxative.

• For better analgesic effect, give drug before onset of intense pain.

• Monitor patients at risk for seizures. Drug may reduce seizure threshold.

• In the case of an overdose, naloxone may also increase risk of seizures.

• Monitor patient for drug dependence. Drug can produce dependence similar to that of codeine and thus has potential for abuse.

◐ *Alert:* Don't stop drug abruptly; withdraw slowly and individualize the gradual tapering plan to prevent signs and symptoms of withdrawal, worsening pain, and psychological distress in physically dependent patients. Refer to manufacturer's label for specific tapering instructions.

Alert: When tapering opioids, monitor patient closely for signs and symptoms of opioid withdrawal (restlessness, lacrimation, rhinorrhea, yawning, perspiration, chills, myalgia, mydriasis, irritability, anxiety, insomnia, backache, joint pain, weakness, abdominal cramps, anorexia, nausea, vomiting, diarrhea, increased BP or HR, increased respiratory rate). Such signs and symptoms may indicate a need to taper more slowly. Also monitor patient for suicidal thoughts, use of other substances, and mood changes.

Alert: If patient is taking opioids with serotonergic drugs, watch for signs and symptoms of serotonin syndrome (agitation, hallucinations, rapid HR, fever, excessive sweating, shivering or shaking, muscle twitching or stiffness, trouble with coordination, nausea, vomiting, diarrhea), especially when starting treatment or increasing dosages. Signs and symptoms may occur within several hours of coadministration but may also occur later, especially after dosage increase. Discontinue the opioid, serotonergic drug, or both if serotonin syndrome is suspected.

Alert: Monitor patient for signs and symptoms of adrenal insufficiency (nausea, vomiting, loss of appetite, fatigue, weakness, dizziness, low BP). Perform diagnostic testing if adrenal insufficiency is suspected. If adrenal insufficiency is confirmed, treat with corticosteroids and wean patient off opioids if appropriate. Discontinue corticosteroids when clinically appropriate.

Alert: Monitor patient for signs and symptoms of decreased sex hormone levels (low libido, erectile dysfunction, amenorrhea, infertility). If signs and symptoms occur, evaluate patient and obtain lab testing.

• **Look alike–sound alike:** Don't confuse tramadol with trazodone or trandolapril.

PATIENT TEACHING

Black Box Warning Caution patient or caregiver of patient taking an opioid with a benzodiazepine, CNS depressant, or alcohol to seek immediate medical attention if patient experiences dizziness, lightheadedness, extreme sleepiness, slowed or difficult breathing, or unresponsiveness. ▪

Black Box Warning Advise patient that crushing, chewing, or dissolving extended-release form can cause rapid release of the drug and a potentially fatal dose. ▪

Black Box Warning Tell patient to keep drug away from children. Accidental ingestion of even one dose of tramadol, especially in children, can result in fatal overdose. ▪

Alert: Warn patient and caregivers of patient taking tramadol to watch for slow or shallow breathing, difficulty or noisy breathing, confusion, excessive sleepiness, trouble breastfeeding, or limpness. If any of these signs or symptoms occur, tell them to stop drug and seek immediate emergency medical attention.

• Explain assessment and monitoring process to patient and family. Instruct them to immediately report difficulty breathing or other signs or symptoms of a potential adverse opioid-related reaction.

• Tell patient to take drug as prescribed and not to increase dose or dosage interval unless ordered by prescriber.

• Caution ambulatory patient to be careful when rising and walking. Warn outpatient to avoid driving and other potentially hazardous activities that require mental alertness until drug's CNS effects are known.

• Advise patient to check with prescriber before taking OTC drugs because drug interactions can occur.

Alert: Counsel patient not to discontinue opioids without first discussing the need for a gradual tapering regimen with prescriber.

Alert: Encourage patient to report all medications being taken, including prescription and OTC medications and supplements.

• Advise patient that drug may cause constipation.

Alert: Caution patient to immediately report signs and symptoms of serotonin syndrome, adrenal insufficiency, and decreased sex hormone levels.

trastuzumab ⊠
trass-too-ZOO-mab

Herceptin

trastuzumab-anns
Kanjinti

trastuzumab-dkst
Ogivri

trastuzumab-dttb
Ontruzant

trastuzumab-pkrb
Herzuma

trastuzumab-qyyp
Trazimera

Therapeutic class: Antineoplastics
Pharmacologic class: Monoclonal
antibodies

AVAILABLE FORMS
Lyophilized powder for injection: 150-mg
single-dose vial, 420-mg multiple-dose vial

INDICATIONS & DOSAGES
Adjust-a-dose (for all indications): If patient
misses a dose by 1 week or less, give usual
maintenance dose as soon as possible. Don't
wait until next planned cycle. Give subsequent maintenance doses 7 or 21 days later
according to the weekly or 3-weekly schedules, respectively. If patient misses a dose by
more than 1 week, give a reloading dose as
soon as possible followed by maintenance
doses 7 or 21 days later according to the
weekly or 3-weekly schedules.

    If LVEF decreased 16% or more from
baseline or if LVEF is below normal limits with a 10% or more decrease from baseline, withhold treatment for at least 4 weeks
and repeat LVEF every 4 weeks. May resume treatment if LVEF returns to normal
within 4 to 8 weeks and remains at 15% or
less decrease from baseline. Discontinue
drug permanently for persistent (more than
8 weeks) LVEF decline or for more than

three incidents of treatment interruptions for
cardiomyopathy.

➤ **HER2-overexpressing metastatic gastric or gastroesophageal junction adenocarcinoma in patients not previously
treated for metastatic disease in combination with cisplatin and capecitabine or
5-FU** ⊠
Adults: Initially, 8 mg/kg IV. Then, 6 mg/kg
IV every 3 weeks until disease progression
or intolerable toxicity develops.
➤ **Metastatic breast cancer in patients whose tumors overexpress HER2
protein** ⊠
Adults: Loading dose of 4 mg/kg IV over
90 minutes. If tolerated, continue with
2 mg/kg IV weekly. If patient hasn't previously received one or more chemotherapy
regimens for their metastatic disease, drug is
given with paclitaxel.
➤ **After surgical resection of HER2-
overexpressing node-positive or node-
negative breast cancer** ⊠
Adults: During treatment with paclitaxel,
docetaxel, or docetaxel–carboplatin, give
loading dose of 4 mg/kg IV. Then, 2 mg/kg
IV weekly during chemotherapy for the
first 12 weeks (paclitaxel or docetaxel) or
18 weeks (docetaxel–carboplatin). Continue
trastuzumab 6 mg/kg IV every 3 weeks for a
total of 52 weeks.
➤ **As single agent after surgical resection of HER2-overexpressing breast
cancer within 3 weeks of completion
of multimodality, anthracycline-based
chemotherapy** ⊠
Adults: Initial dose, 8 mg/kg IV. Then,
6 mg/kg IV every 3 weeks for a total of
52 weeks.
➤ **Neoadjuvant treatment of HER2-
positive locally advanced, inflammatory,
or early breast cancer** ⊠ ◆
Adults: Initially, 8 mg/kg IV (cycle 1) followed by 6 mg/kg IV every 3 weeks for a
total of four neoadjuvant cycles; postoperatively, administer three cycles of adjuvant FEC (5-FU, epirubicin, and cyclophosphamide) chemotherapy and continue
trastuzumab to complete 1 year of treatment.
➤ **HER2-positive metastatic breast cancer (in combination with pertuzumab
and docetaxel) in patients without prior**

---

anti-HER2 therapy or chemotherapy to treat metastatic disease ⌧ ♦
Adults: Initially, 8 mg/kg IV followed by a maintenance dose of 6 mg/kg IV every 3 weeks until disease progression or unacceptable toxicity.

➤ **HER2-positive metastatic breast cancer (in combination with either docetaxel or vinorelbine)** ⌧ ♦
Adults: Initially, 8 mg/kg IV followed by a maintenance dose of 6 mg/kg IV every 3 weeks until disease progression or unacceptable toxicity (in combination with docetaxel or vinorelbine), or 4 mg/kg IV loading dose followed by a maintenance dose of 2 mg/kg IV weekly until disease progression (in combination with docetaxel).

➤ **HER2-positive, hormone receptor–positive metastatic breast cancer (in combination with an aromatase inhibitor) when chemotherapy isn't immediately indicated** ⌧ ♦
Adults: Initially, 4 mg/kg IV followed by a maintenance dose of 2 mg/kg IV weekly until disease progression (in combination with anastrozole).

➤ **HER2-overexpressing metastatic breast cancer (in combination with lapatinib) that had progressed on prior trastuzumab-containing therapy** ⌧ ♦
Adults: Initially, 4 mg/kg IV followed by a maintenance dose of 2 mg/kg IV every week.

ADMINISTRATION
IV
▼ Hazardous drug; use safe handling and disposal precautions.
▼ Reconstitute drug in 420-mg vial with 20 mL of bacteriostatic water for injection, 1.1% benzyl alcohol preserved, as supplied, to yield a multidose solution containing 21 mg/mL. Don't shake vial during reconstitution. Make sure reconstituted preparation is colorless to pale yellow and free of particulates. Immediately after reconstitution, label vial with expiration 28 days from date of reconstitution and refrigerate at 36° to 46° F (2° to 8° C).
▼ If patient is hypersensitive to benzyl alcohol, reconstitute drug with sterile water for injection, use immediately, and discard unused portion. Avoid use of other reconstitution diluents.

▼ Determine dose and calculate volume of 21-mg/mL solution needed. Withdraw this amount from vial and add it to an infusion bag containing 250 mL of NSS. Don't use D_5W or dextrose-containing solutions. Gently invert bag to mix solution. Store diluted solution in infusion bag containing NSS at 36° to 46° F (2° to 8° C) for no more than 24 hours before use. Don't freeze.
▼ If using 150-mg vial, reconstitute with 7.4 mL of sterile water for injection to yield a concentration of 21 mg/mL; add to 250-mL NSS infusion bag. Use immediately or refrigerate at 36° to 46° F (2° to 8° C) for no more than 24 hours.
▼ Don't give as IV push or bolus.
▼ Infuse loading dose over 90 minutes. If well tolerated, infuse maintenance doses over 30 to 90 minutes.
▼ Before reconstitution, store vials in refrigerator at 36° to 46° F (2° to 8° C).
▼ **Incompatibilities:** Other IV drugs or dextrose solutions.

ACTION
A recombinant DNA-derived monoclonal antibody that selectively binds to HER2, inhibiting proliferation of tumor cells that overexpress HER2.

Route	Onset	Peak	Duration
IV	Unknown	Unknown	Unknown

Half-life: Unknown.

ADVERSE REACTIONS
CNS: asthenia, dizziness, fever, headache, insomnia, pain, depression, neuropathy, paresthesia, peripheral neuritis, fatigue. **CV:** peripheral edema, edema, *HF*, hypotension, HTN, arrhythmias, tachycardia, decreased LVEF, palpitations. **EENT:** pharyngitis, rhinitis, sinusitis. **GI:** abdominal pain, anorexia, diarrhea, nausea, vomiting, stomatitis, mucosal inflammation, dysgeusia. **GU:** UTI, *renal failure.* **Hematologic:** *leukopenia,* anemia, *neutropenia, thrombocytopenia.* **Metabolic:** weight loss, *hypokalemia.* **Musculoskeletal:** back pain, arthralgia, bone pain, myalgia. **Respiratory:** dyspnea, increased cough, URI. **Skin:**

T

rash, acne. **Other:** *anaphylaxis,* chills, flu-like syndrome, infection, allergic reaction, herpes simplex, infusion-related reaction.

INTERACTIONS
Drug-drug. *Anthracyclines, cyclophosphamide:* May increase cardiotoxicity, even if started after trastuzumab is discontinued. Consider therapy modification.
Immunosuppressants: May increase neutropenic effect of immunosuppressants. Monitor therapy closely.
Paclitaxel: May decrease paclitaxel serum concentration; may increase trastuzumab serum concentration. Monitor therapy closely.

EFFECTS ON LAB TEST RESULTS
• May decrease potassium level.
• May decrease Hb level and platelet and WBC counts.

CONTRAINDICATIONS & CAUTIONS
• Contraindicated in patients hypersensitive to the drug.
• Use cautiously in elderly patients, in patients hypersensitive to drug or its components, and in those with cardiac dysfunction.
• Use with extreme caution in patients with pulmonary compromise, symptomatic intrinsic pulmonary disease (such as asthma, COPD), or extensive tumor involvement of the lungs.
• Patients who receive anthracycline after stopping trastuzumab may be at increased risk for cardiac dysfunction. If possible, avoid anthracycline-based therapy for up to 7 months after stopping trastuzumab. Carefully monitor patient's cardiac function.
• Safety and effectiveness in children haven't been established.
Dialyzable drug: Unknown.

PREGNANCY-LACTATION-REPRODUCTION
Black Box Warning Exposure to drug during pregnancy can result in oligohydramnios, in some cases complicated by pulmonary hypoplasia, skeletal abnormalities, and neonatal death. Patient must use effective contraception. ■
• Verify pregnancy status of females of childbearing potential before start of therapy.

• If drug is used during pregnancy, or if patient becomes pregnant during therapy or within 7 months after last dose, fetal harm can occur. Immediately report exposure to the Genentech Adverse Event Line (1-888-835-2555).
• Encourage women who may be exposed to drug during pregnancy or within 7 months after last dose to enroll in the MotHER Pregnancy Registry (1-800-690-6720).
• It isn't known if drug appears in human milk. Patient should discontinue breastfeeding or discontinue drug.

NURSING CONSIDERATIONS
Black Box Warning Drug can cause HF, especially when used with anthracycline-containing chemotherapy regimens. Evaluate LVEF before and during treatment. Discontinue drug in patients receiving adjuvant therapy and withhold drug in those with metastatic disease for clinically significant decreases in LVEF. ■
• Assess LVEF before therapy, every 3 months during therapy, and when therapy ends. If decreased LVEF occurs, assess LVEF every month; assess LVEF every 6 months for 2 years after therapy ends when drug is used in adjuvant therapy.
• Monitor patient receiving both drug and chemotherapy closely for cardiac dysfunction or failure, anemia, renal toxicity, leukopenia, diarrhea, and infection.
⚕ When used in metastatic breast cancer, drug is only indicated in tumors with HER2 protein overexpression. Assessment of HER2 protein overexpression and *HER2* gene amplification should be performed using FDA-approved tests specific for breast or gastric cancers by labs with demonstrated proficiency to obtain reliable results.
Black Box Warning Drug can cause serious infusion reactions and pulmonary toxicity. Interrupt infusion if patient experiences dyspnea or clinically significant hypotension. Strongly consider discontinuation for patients who develop anaphylaxis, angioedema, pneumonitis, or ARDS. ■
• Check for first-infusion symptom complex, commonly consisting of chills or fever. Give acetaminophen, meperidine, and diphenhydramine (with or without reducing rate of infusion). Other signs or

---

Reactions in bold italics are *life-threatening*. Interactions may have a *rapid onset* or a *delayed onset*.

symptoms include nausea, vomiting, pain, rigors, headache, dizziness, dyspnea, hypotension, rash, and asthenia and occur infrequently with subsequent infusions.

• For mild to moderate infusion reaction, decrease infusion rate. For dyspnea and hypotension, interrupt infusion. For severe infusion reaction, discontinue drug.

• *Look alike–sound alike:* Don't confuse trastuzumab with ado-trastuzumab emtansine.

PATIENT TEACHING
• Tell patient about risk of first-dose infusion-related adverse reactions and to report all adverse reactions to prescriber.

• Urge patient to notify prescriber immediately if signs or symptoms of heart problems occur, such as shortness of breath, increased cough, or swelling in arms or legs. Tell patient that these effects can occur after therapy ends.

• Advise female patient to stop breastfeeding during therapy and for 7 months after last dose.

• Tell patient to avoid pregnancy during therapy and for 7 months after last dose and to notify prescriber immediately if pregnancy occurs during this time.

traZODone hydrochloride
TRAYZ-oh-dohn

Therapeutic class: Antidepressants
Pharmacologic class: Triazolopyridine derivatives

AVAILABLE FORMS
Tablets⊚: 50 mg, 100 mg, 150 mg, 300 mg

INDICATIONS & DOSAGES
➤ **Depression**
Adults: Initially, 150 mg PO daily in divided doses; then increased by 50 mg daily every 3 to 4 days, as needed. Dose ranges from 150 to 400 mg daily. Maximum, 600 mg daily for inpatients and 400 mg daily for outpatients.

ADMINISTRATION
PO
• Give drug after meals or a light snack for optimal absorption and to decrease risk of dizziness.

• If drowsiness occurs, may give a large portion of the dose at bedtime.

• Make sure patient swallows tablets whole or breaks them along the score lines. Tablets shouldn't be chewed or crushed.

ACTION
Unknown. Inhibits CNS neuronal uptake of serotonin; not a tricyclic derivative.

Route	Onset	Peak	Duration
PO	Unknown	1–2 hr	Unknown

Half-life: 5 to 9 hours.

ADVERSE REACTIONS
CNS: drowsiness, dizziness, nervousness, fatigue, confusion, tremor, weakness, hostility, anger, nightmares, vivid dreams, headache, insomnia, syncope, disorientation, incoordination. **CV:** orthostatic hypotension, tachycardia, HTN, shortness of breath, ECG changes, edema, palpitations. **EENT:** blurred vision, red or itchy eyes, tinnitus, nasal congestion. **GI:** dry mouth, dysgeusia, constipation, nausea, vomiting, anorexia, diarrhea. **GU:** urine retention, priapism possibly leading to impotence, hematuria, increased libido. **Hematologic:** anemia. **Metabolic:** weight gain or loss. **Musculoskeletal:** aches, pains. **Skin:** rash, urticaria, diaphoresis.

INTERACTIONS
Drug-drug. *Amphetamines, antipsychotics, buspirone, dextromethorphan, dihydroergotamine, lithium salts, meperidine, opioid analgesics, SSRIs or SSNRIs (duloxetine, venlafaxine), sumatriptan (and other 5-HT$_3$ antagonists), TCAs, tramadol, tryptophan:* May increase the risk of serotonin syndrome. Avoid combining drugs that increase the availability of serotonin in the CNS; monitor patient closely if used together.
Antihypertensives: May increase hypotensive effect of trazodone. Antihypertensive dosage may need to be decreased.

T

Clonidine, CNS depressants: May enhance CNS depression. Avoid using together.

CYP3A4 inducers (carbamazepine): May reduce trazodone level. Monitor patient closely; may need to increase trazodone dose.

CYP3A4 inhibitors (conivaptan, ketoconazole, and others): May slow the clearance of trazodone and increase trazodone level. May cause nausea, hypotension, and fainting. Consider decreasing trazodone dose. Avoid combination with conivaptan.

Digoxin, fosphenytoin, phenytoin: May increase levels of these drugs. Watch for toxicity.

Drugs that prolong QTc interval: May increase QTc-interval prolonging effect and risk of ventricular arrhythmias. Consider therapy modification.

Linezolid, methylene blue: May cause serotonin syndrome. Don't use together.

❸ *Alert:* **MAO inhibitors:** Serious and sometimes fatal reactions have occurred. Allow at least 14 days between discontinuing an MAO inhibitor and starting trazodone and at least 14 days after stopping trazodone before starting an MAO inhibitor.

Protease inhibitors (amprenavir, atazanavir, fosamprenavir, indinavir, lopinavir–ritonavir, nelfinavir, ritonavir, saquinavir): May increase trazodone levels and adverse effects. Monitor patient and adjust trazodone dose, as needed.

Warfarin: May decrease anticoagulant effect of warfarin. Adjust warfarin dosage as needed.

Drug-herb. *Ginkgo biloba:* May cause sedation. Discourage use together.

St. John's wort: May cause serotonin syndrome. Discourage use together.

Drug-lifestyle. *Alcohol use:* May enhance CNS depression. Discourage use together.

EFFECTS ON LAB TEST RESULTS
• May increase ALT and AST levels. May decrease Hb and sodium levels.
• May cause false-positive urine test for amphetamine/methamphetamine.

CONTRAINDICATIONS & CAUTIONS
• Contraindicated in patients hypersensitive to drug.

❸ *Alert:* Concomitant use with linezolid or methylene blue can cause serotonin syndrome. Use drug with linezolid or methylene blue only for life-threatening or urgent conditions when the potential benefits outweigh the risks of toxicity.

• Use cautiously in patients with cardiac disease or in the initial recovery phase of MI, as drug can prolong QTc interval.

• Use cautiously in patients at risk for suicide, in patients with renal or hepatic impairment, in those with a history of seizures, and with medications that may lower seizure threshold.

• May cause mild pupillary dilation, which may trigger an angle-closure attack in patient with anatomically narrow angles who doesn't have a patent iridectomy.

Dialyzable drug: Unlikely.

⚠ Overdose S&S: Priapism, respiratory arrest, seizures, ECG changes, drowsiness, vomiting.

PREGNANCY-LACTATION-REPRODUCTION
• There are no adequate studies in pregnant women. Use only if clearly needed and potential benefit justifies potential risk to the fetus.
• Drug may appear in human milk. Use cautiously in breastfeeding women.

NURSING CONSIDERATIONS
• Monitor patient for signs and symptoms of serotonin syndrome (mental status changes, tachycardia, labile BP, hyperreflexia, incoordination, nausea, vomiting, diarrhea) or NMS (hyperthermia, muscle rigidity, rapidly fluctuating vital signs, mental status change). If these signs and symptoms occur, immediately discontinue trazodone and any other serotonergic, antidopaminergic, or antipsychotic drugs.

• Using trazodone in a bipolar patient for depression can trigger a mixed/manic episode. If patient develops manic symptoms, withhold trazodone and initiate appropriate therapy.

❸ *Alert:* If linezolid or methylene blue must be given, stop trazodone and monitor patient for serotonin toxicity for 2 weeks, or until 24 hours after the last dose of methylene blue or linezolid, whichever comes first. May

---

Reactions in bold italics are *life-threatening*. Interactions may have a *rapid onset* or a ***delayed onset***.

resume trazodone 24 hours after last dose of methylene blue or linezolid.

• Record mood changes. Monitor patient for suicidal tendencies and allow only minimum supply of drug.

Black Box Warning Drug may increase the risk of suicidal thinking and behavior in children, adolescents, and young adults ages 18 to 24, especially during the first few months of treatment, especially those with major depressive disorder or other psychiatric disorder. Drug isn't approved for use in children. ∎

• Consider evaluating patients who haven't had an iridectomy for narrow-angle glaucoma risk factors.

• *Look alike–sound alike:* Don't confuse trazodone hydrochloride with tramadol hydrochloride. Don't confuse trazodone with ziprasidone.

PATIENT TEACHING

• Advise patient to take trazodone after a meal or light snack.

• Advise patient not to crush or chew tablets. Tell patient that if needed, tablets can be broken in half along the score line.

ⓤ *Alert:* Tell patient to report a persistent, painful erection (priapism); immediate intervention may be needed.

ⓤ *Alert:* Tell patient to immediately report signs and symptoms of serotonin toxicity and NMS.

• Warn patient to avoid activities that require alertness and good coordination until effects of drug are known.

Black Box Warning Teach caregivers to recognize and report signs and symptoms of suicidal tendency or suicidal thoughts. ∎

• Tell patient that it might take up to 6 weeks to see therapeutic effect if used for depression.

• Advise patient not to stop drug abruptly in order to avoid withdrawal symptoms.

• Advise patient to avoid alcohol because it will increase sedation.

tretinoin (retinoic acid, vitamin A acid)
TRET-i-noyn

Altreno, Atralin, Avita, ReFissa, Renova, Retin-A, Retin-A Micro, StieVA-A✤, Vitamin A Acid✤

Therapeutic class: Antiacne drugs
Pharmacologic class: Retinoids

AVAILABLE FORMS
Cream: 0.01%✤, 0.02%, 0.025%, 0.05%, 0.1%
Gel: 0.04%, 0.05%, 0.01%, 0.025%
Lotion: 0.05%
Microsphere gel: 0.04%, 0.06%, 0.08%, 0.1%

INDICATIONS & DOSAGES
➤ **Acne vulgaris (except ReFissa and Renova)**
Adults: Clean affected area and lightly apply once daily at bedtime.
Children age 12 and older (Retin-A Micro): Clean affected area and lightly apply once daily at bedtime.
Children age 10 and older (Atralin): Clean affected area and lightly apply once daily at bedtime.
Children age 9 and older (Altreno): Apply a thin layer to the affected areas once daily.
➤ **Adjunctive use in the mitigation of fine facial wrinkles in patients who use comprehensive skin care and sunlight avoidance programs (Renova); adjunctive treatment for mitigation of fine wrinkles, mottled hyperpigmentation, and tactile roughness of facial skin in patients who don't achieve such palliation using comprehensive skin care and sun avoidance programs alone (ReFissa)**
Adults: Apply a small, pea-sized amount (¼ inch or 5 mm in diameter) to cover the entire face lightly, once daily in the evening.

ADMINISTRATION
Topical
• Clean area thoroughly before application, and avoid getting drug in eyes, mouth, paranasal creases, or mucous membranes.

✤Canada ◇OTC ◆Off-label use ✐Photoguide ⬤Do not crush *Liquid contains alcohol ▓Genetic

• Patients using ReFissa or Renova should gently wash their faces with a mild soap, pat the skin dry, and wait 20 to 30 minutes before applying medication.

ACTION
Inhibits comedones by increasing epidermal cell mitosis and turnover.

Route	Onset	Peak	Duration
Topical	Unknown	Unknown	Unknown

Half-life: Unknown.

ADVERSE REACTIONS
Skin: feeling of warmth, slight stinging, local erythema, peeling, chapping, swelling, blistering, crusting, temporary hyperpigmentation or hypopigmentation, burning sensation, skin irritation, dermatitis, photosensitivity.

INTERACTIONS
Drug-drug. *Multivitamins:* May increase adverse effects of retinoic acid. Avoid combination.
Topical drugs containing benzoyl peroxide, resorcinol, salicylic acid, or sulfur: May increase risk of skin irritation. Avoid using together.
Topical minoxidil or photosensitizing drugs (fluoroquinolones, phenothiazines, sulfonamides, tetracyclines, thiazides): May increase risk of skin irritation. Avoid using together.
Drug-food. *Vitamin A:* Vitamin A supplementation can cause toxicity. Avoid excessive intake of vitamin A (cod liver oil, halibut fish oil).
Drug-lifestyle. *Abrasive cleansers, cream depilatories, medicated cosmetics, skin preparations containing alcohol, waxes:* May increase risk of skin irritation. Discourage use together.
Sun exposure, tanning lamps: May increase photosensitivity reaction. Advise patient to avoid excessive exposure.

EFFECTS ON LAB TEST RESULTS
None reported.

CONTRAINDICATIONS & CAUTIONS
• Contraindicated in patients hypersensitive to drug or its components and in those with sunburn.
• Use cautiously in patients with eczema.
• Use Atralin gel and Altreno lotion with caution in patients with known sensitivities or allergies to fish because gel contains soluble fish proteins.
• Don't use ReFissa or Renova if patient is sunburned or has eczema or other chronic skin conditions of the face, is inherently sensitive to sunlight, or is also taking drugs known to be photosensitizers, because of the possibility of augmented phototoxicity.
Dialyzable drug: Unknown.
⚠ *Overdose S&S:* Marked redness, skin peeling, skin discomfort.

PREGNANCY-LACTATION-REPRODUCTION
🚼 **Alert:** Don't use ReFissa or Renova if patient is pregnant, is attempting to become pregnant, or is at high risk for pregnancy.
• There are no adequate studies in pregnant women. Use only if potential benefit justifies potential risk to the fetus.
• It isn't known if drug appears in human milk. Use cautiously in breastfeeding women.

NURSING CONSIDERATIONS
• Initially, drug may be applied every 2 to 3 days using a lower concentration to reduce irritation.
• Relapses typically occur within 3 to 6 weeks after therapy is stopped.
• *Look alike–sound alike:* Don't confuse tretinoin with trientine, Tenormin, triamcinolone, or isotretinoin.

PATIENT TEACHING
• Instruct patient to clean area thoroughly before application and to avoid getting drug in eyes, mouth, paranasal creases, or mucous membranes.
• Tell patient to apply with fingertips, gauze pad, or cotton swab.
• Tell patient to wash hands after application.
• Tell patient to wash face with mild soap no more than b.i.d. or t.i.d. Warn patient against using strong or medicated cosmetics, soaps, or other skin cleansers. Also advise patient

---

to avoid topical products containing alcohol, astringents, spices, and lime because they may interfere with drug's actions.

• Caution patient not to apply to sunburned skin.

• Tell patient using drug for treatment of fine wrinkles to wait 20 to 30 minutes after washing face to apply drug, and to avoid washing face or applying another skin product or cosmetic for 1 hour after application.

• Tell patient that normal use of cosmetics is allowed.

• Advise patient not to stop drug if temporary worsening of inflammatory lesions occurs. If severe local irritation develops, advise patient to stop drug temporarily and notify prescriber. Dosage will be readjusted when application is resumed. Some redness and scaling are normal reactions.

• Warn patient that increased sensitivity to wind or cold temperatures may occur.

• Instruct patient to minimize exposure to sunlight or ultraviolet rays during treatment. If a sunburn develops, advise patient to delay therapy until sunburn subsides. Tell patient who can't avoid exposure to sunlight to use SPF-15 sunblock and to wear protective clothing.

• Warn patient that a temporary increase in lesions may occur, which will improve in 2 to 3 weeks.

• Tell patient not to use ReFissa or Renova if she is pregnant or trying to become pregnant. Advise patient to stop use and notify prescriber if pregnancy is suspected.

triamcinolone acetonide (injection)
trye-am-SIN-oh-lone

Kenalog-10*, Kenalog-40*, Triesence, Zilretta

Therapeutic class: Corticosteroids
Pharmacologic class: Glucocorticoids

AVAILABLE FORMS
Injection (extended-release powder): 32 mg per vial
Injection (suspension): 10 mg/mL, 40 mg/mL
Injection (intravitreal): 40 mg/mL

INDICATIONS & DOSAGES
➤ **Severe inflammation, immunosuppression**
Adults: 60 mg IM, then 20 to 100 mg IM as needed every 6 weeks, if possible. Or, individualize initial intralesional dose depending on the specific disease and lesion. For maintenance, use the lowest dosage and time intervals to maintain an adequate clinical response. Or, initially, 2.5 to 15 mg into joints (depending on joint size) or soft tissue; then may increase to 10 mg for smaller areas and 40 mg for larger areas. Maximum dose (several joints at one time) is 80 mg. A local anesthetic is commonly injected with triamcinolone into the joint.
Children: Dosage may vary depending on the specific disease. Range of initial dose is 0.11 to 1.6 mg/kg/day IM in three or four divided doses (3.2 to 48 mg/m² BSA/day). Or, 2.5 to 5 mg for smaller joints and from 5 to 15 mg for larger joints, depending on the specific disease.

➤ **Management of osteoarthritis pain of the knee (Zilretta extended-release)**
Adults: 32 mg (5 mL) as a single intra-articular injection. Drug isn't intended for repeat administration.

➤ **Ophthalmic diseases (sympathetic ophthalmia, temporal arteritis, uveitis, ocular inflammatory conditions unresponsive to topical corticosteroids)**
Adults and children: 4 mg (100 mcL of 40 mg/mL suspension) injected intravitreally, with subsequent doses as needed during the course of treatment.

➤ **Visualization during vitrectomy**
Adults and children: 1 to 4 mg (25 to 100 mcL of 40 mg/mL suspension) injected intravitreally.

ADMINISTRATION
IM
• Give deep into gluteal muscle. Rotate injection sites to prevent muscle atrophy.
• Don't use 10 mg/mL strength for this route.
• Shake well before use and ensure there's no clumping.
• Administer immediately after withdrawal to prevent settling in the syringe.
• Don't administer IV or via epidural or intrathecal route.

T

Intra-articular

• Prepare extended-release product only using the diluent supplied in the kit. Refer to manufacturer labeling for preparation instructions and administration techniques.

• Promptly inject after preparation.

• If needed, may store in vial for up to 4 hours at ambient conditions. Gently swirl vial to resuspend any settled microspheres before preparing syringe for injection.

• Extended-release form isn't interchangeable with other formulations of injectable triamcinolone acetonide.

• Strict aseptic technique is mandatory.

• Prior use of a local anesthetic may be desirable.

Intralesional

• Strict aseptic technique is mandatory.

• Inject directly into the lesion intradermally or subcutaneously.

• It is preferable to use a tuberculin syringe and small-bore needle (23G to 25G).

Intravitreal

• Before injecting, give adequate anesthesia and a broad-spectrum microbicide.

• Shake vial vigorously for 10 seconds to ensure a uniform suspension. Inspect suspension for clumping or granules. If present, don't use.

• Inject drug without delay under controlled aseptic conditions.

• Each vial is for the treatment of a single eye only.

• Protect from light. Don't freeze. Store between 39° and 77° F (4° and 25° C).

ACTION

Not clearly defined. Decreases inflammation, mainly by stabilizing leukocyte lysosomal membranes; suppresses immune response; stimulates bone marrow; influences protein, fat, and carbohydrate metabolism; and suppresses adrenal function at high doses.

Route	Onset	Peak	Duration
IM, intra-articular, intralesional	12–48 hr	Unknown	30–42 days
Intra-articular (extended-release)	Unknown	7 hr	Unknown
Intravitreal	Unknown	Unknown	Unknown

Half-life: 300 minutes; intravitreal, 13 to 24 days.

ADVERSE REACTIONS

Systemic reactions associated with corticosteroid therapy are possible. Refer to manufacturer's prescribing information for additional adverse reactions not listed here.

CNS: euphoria, insomnia, *pseudotumor cerebri, seizures,* headache, paresthesia, psychotic behavior, vertigo, *stroke.* **CV:** *arrhythmias, HF, thromboembolism,* HTN, edema, thrombophlebitis. **EENT:** cataracts, glaucoma, increased IOP, eye inflammation, conjunctival hemorrhage, reduced visual acuity, sinusitis. **GI:** *pancreatitis,* peptic ulceration, GI irritation, increased appetite, nausea, vomiting. **GU:** menstrual irregularities, increased urine calcium level. **Metabolic:** *hypokalemia,* hyperglycemia and carbohydrate intolerance, hypercholesterolemia, hypocalcemia. **Musculoskeletal:** growth suppression in children, muscle weakness, osteoporosis, acute myopathy, knee joint swelling. **Respiratory:** cough. **Skin:** hirsutism, delayed wound healing, acne, various skin eruptions, contusions. **Other:** *acute adrenal insufficiency,* cushingoid state, susceptibility to infections after increased stress or abrupt withdrawal after long-term therapy.

INTERACTIONS

Drug-drug. *Antidiabetics:* May increase blood glucose level. Adjust dosage of antidiabetics as needed.

Aspirin, indomethacin, other NSAIDs: May increase risk of GI distress and bleeding. Use together cautiously.

Barbiturates, carbamazepine, fosphenytoin, phenytoin, rifampin: May decrease corticosteroid effect. Increase corticosteroid dosage.

Cyclosporine: May increase toxicity and seizures. Monitor patient closely.

Ketoconazole, macrolide antibiotics: May decrease metabolism or clearance of triamcinolone, respectively. Decrease triamcinolone dose or dosage interval if needed.

Oral anticoagulants: May alter dosage requirements. Monitor PT and INR closely.

Potassium-depleting drugs, such as thiazide and loop diuretics and amphotericin B: May enhance potassium-wasting effects of triamcinolone. Monitor potassium level.

Reactions in bold italics are *life-threatening.* Interactions may have a *rapid onset* or a *delayed onset.*

Salicylates: May decrease salicylate level. Monitor patient for lack of salicylate effectiveness.

Skin-test antigens: May decrease response. Postpone skin testing until after therapy.

Toxoids, vaccines: May decrease antibody response and increase risk of neurologic complications. Defer routine administration of vaccines or toxoids until corticosteroid therapy is discontinued, if possible.

Drug-herb. *Echinacea:* May decrease therapeutic effect of immunosuppressants. Avoid combination.

EFFECTS ON LAB TEST RESULTS

• May increase sodium, glucose, and cholesterol levels. May decrease potassium and calcium levels.

• May alter thyroid function tests. May alter reactions to skin tests.

CONTRAINDICATIONS & CAUTIONS

• Contraindicated in patients hypersensitive to drug or its ingredients, in patients with cerebral malaria, in those with systemic fungal infections, and in those receiving immunosuppressive doses together with live-virus vaccines.

• Intravitreal injections are also contraindicated in patients with active ocular HSV.

• Extended-release form is for intra-articular use only for osteoarthritis pain of the knee.

• Safety and effectiveness of extended-release form in children haven't been established.

• Use cautiously in patients with recent MI, GI ulcer, renal disease, HTN, osteoporosis, diabetes mellitus, hypothyroidism, cirrhosis, diverticulitis, nonspecific ulcerative colitis, recent intestinal anastomoses, thromboembolic disorders, seizures, myasthenia gravis, active hepatitis, lactation, HF, TB, ocular herpes simplex, emotional instability, or psychotic tendencies.

⚕ *Alert:* Use of corticosteroids increases risk of cataracts.

Dialyzable drug: Unknown.

PREGNANCY-LACTATION-REPRODUCTION

• Some manufacturers report that human studies show that triamcinolone acetonide can cause fetal harm when administered to a pregnant woman. Use only if potential benefit justifies potential risk to the fetus.

• Carefully observe infants born to mothers who have received corticosteroids during pregnancy for signs and symptoms of hypoadrenalism.

• Drug appears in human milk and could suppress infant growth, interfere with endogenous corticosteroid production, or cause other untoward effects. Use cautiously in breastfeeding women.

NURSING CONSIDERATIONS

• Determine whether patient is sensitive to other corticosteroids.

• Drug isn't used for alternate-day therapy.

• Always adjust to lowest effective dose.

• Most adverse reactions to corticosteroids are dose- or duration-dependent.

• Monitor patient's weight, BP, and glucose and electrolyte levels. If used for more than 6 weeks, monitor IOP.

• Monitor patient for cushingoid effects, such as moon face, buffalo hump, central obesity, thinning hair, HTN, and increased susceptibility to infection.

• Watch for depression or psychotic episodes, especially during high-dose therapy.

• Diabetic patient may need increased insulin dosage; monitor glucose level.

• Drug may mask or worsen infections, including latent amebiasis.

• Elderly patients may be more susceptible to osteoporosis with long-term use.

• Unless contraindicated, give low-sodium diet that's high in potassium and protein. Give potassium supplements as needed.

• Gradually reduce dosage after long-term (more than 10 to 14 days) therapy. Drug may affect patient's sleep.

⚕ *Alert:* Intravitreal injections must be performed under mandatory aseptic technique, which includes the use of sterile gloves, sterile drape, and sterile eyelid speculum.

⚕ *Alert:* Monitor patients receiving intravitreal injections for increased IOP, which can lead to glaucoma and damage to the optic nerve.

• Intra-articular injection may be complicated by joint infection; increased pain accompanied by local swelling, further restriction of joint motion, fever, and malaise

T

suggest septic arthritis. If diagnosis of septic arthritis is confirmed, institute appropriate antimicrobial therapy.

• *Look alike–sound alike:* Don't confuse triamcinolone with Triaminic. Don't confuse Kenalog with Ketalar.

PATIENT TEACHING

• Tell patient not to stop drug abruptly or without prescriber's consent.

• Teach patient signs and symptoms of early adrenal insufficiency: fatigue, muscle weakness, joint pain, fever, anorexia, nausea, shortness of breath, dizziness, and fainting.

• Instruct patient to carry medical identification that includes prescriber's name and drug's name and dosage and indicates patient's need for supplemental systemic glucocorticoids during stress.

• Warn patient on long-term therapy about cushingoid effects (moon face, buffalo hump) and the need to notify prescriber about sudden weight gain and swelling.

• Tell patient to report slow wound healing.

• Advise patient receiving long-term therapy to consider exercise or physical therapy. Also, tell patient to ask prescriber about vitamin D or calcium supplement.

• Instruct patient to avoid exposure to infections and to notify prescriber if exposure occurs.

• Tell patient to report ophthalmic signs and symptoms (eye pain, redness, sensitivity to light, vision loss or disturbance) to prescriber and to seek immediate care from an ophthalmologist if these occur.

triamcinolone acetonide (intranasal)
trye-am-SIN-oh-lone

Children's Nasacort Allergy 24 Hour ◇, Nasacort Allergy 24 Hour ◇, Nasacort AQ � ◇

Therapeutic class: Corticosteroids
Pharmacologic class: Corticosteroids

AVAILABLE FORMS
Nasal spray: 55 mcg/spray

INDICATIONS & DOSAGES
➤ **Treatment of nasal symptoms of seasonal and perennial allergic rhinitis**
Adults and children age 12 and older:
2 sprays in each nostril once daily while sniffing gently; may decrease to 1 spray in each nostril once daily for allergic disorders. Adjust to minimum effective dosage.
Children ages 6 to 11: 1 spray in each nostril once daily while sniffing gently. Maximum dosage is 2 sprays in each nostril once daily. Adjust to minimum effective dosage.
Children ages 2 to 5: 1 spray in each nostril once daily while sniffing gently.
Adjust-a-dose: Start elderly patients at lower end of dosing range.

ADMINISTRATION
Intranasal
• Shake well before each use.
• Release 5 sprays into the air to prime before first use. Reprime with 1 spray if not used for 2 weeks or more.
• Patient should gently blow nose to clear nostrils.
• Insert nozzle into nostril, pointing away from septum. Hold other nostril closed and have patient sniff gently while spraying.

ACTION
Controls the rate of protein synthesis, depresses the migration of polymorphonuclear leukocytes and fibroblasts, reverses capillary permeability, and stabilizes lysosomal membranes at the cellular level.

Route	Onset	Peak	Duration
Intranasal	Unknown	1½–4 hr	Unknown

Half-life: About 3 hours.

ADVERSE REACTIONS
CNS: headache, fever. **EENT:** otitis media, nasal irritation, burning, dry mucous membranes, epistaxis, nasal and sinus congestion, rhinitis, nasopharyngitis, sinusitis, sneezing, stinging, throat pain, rhinorrhea, excoriation. **GI:** dyspepsia, nausea, vomiting, tooth disorder, upper abdominal pain, diarrhea. **Respiratory:** *asthma symptoms,* cough, bronchitis. **Skin:** rash. **Other:** flulike syndrome.

Reactions in bold italics are *life-threatening.* Interactions may have a *rapid onset* or a *delayed onset.*

INTERACTIONS
None significant.

EFFECTS ON LAB TEST RESULTS
None reported.

CONTRAINDICATIONS & CAUTIONS
• Contraindicated in patients hypersensitive to drug or its components and in those with untreated mucosal infection.
• Use with caution, if at all, in patients with active or quiescent tuberculous infection of respiratory tract, glaucoma, cataracts, increased IOP, ocular herpes simplex, eye infection, or untreated fungal, bacterial, or systemic viral infection.
• Use cautiously in patients already receiving systemic corticosteroids because of increased likelihood of HPA axis suppression.
• Use cautiously in patients with recent nasal septal ulcers, nasal surgery, or trauma because drug may inhibit wound healing.
• Use cautiously in patients with severe or recurrent nosebleeds.
Dialyzable drug: Unknown.
⚠ *Overdose S&S:* GI upset, nasal irritation, headache.

PREGNANCY-LACTATION-REPRODUCTION
• There are no adequate studies in pregnant women. Use only if potential benefit justifies potential risk to the fetus.
• It isn't known if drug appears in human milk. Use cautiously in breastfeeding women.

NURSING CONSIDERATIONS
❸ *Alert:* Excessive doses may cause signs and symptoms of hyperadrenocorticism and adrenal axis suppression; stop drug slowly.
• To decrease risk of adverse effects, individualize drug dosage and titrate to minimum effective dosage.
• Monitor growth rate in children, which may be slower while using this product, especially if child needs to use spray for longer than 2 months a year.
• Discontinue drug if symptom relief hasn't occurred after 1 week of treatment.
• *Look alike–sound alike:* Don't confuse triamcinolone with Triaminicin.

PATIENT TEACHING
• Teach patient to prime pump before first use and how to use nasal spray.
• Instruct patient to avoid getting aerosol in eyes or mouth. If this occurs, tell patient to rinse with copious amounts of cool tap water.
• Tell patient not to blow nose for 15 minutes after use.
• Stress importance of using drug on a regular schedule because its effectiveness depends on regular use. Warn patient not to exceed prescribed dosage.
• Tell patient to notify prescriber if signs and symptoms don't diminish or if condition worsens in 1 week.
• Warn patient to avoid exposure to chickenpox or measles and, if exposed, to notify prescriber.
• Instruct patient to watch for and report signs and symptoms of nasal infection. Drug may need to be stopped.

triamcinolone acetonide (topical)
trye-am-SIN-oh-lone

Kenalog, Oracort✺, Trianex, Triderm

Therapeutic class: Corticosteroids
Pharmacologic class: Corticosteroids

AVAILABLE FORMS
Aerosol*: 0.2 mg/2-second spray (0.147 mg/g)
Cream: 0.025%, 0.1%, 0.5%
Dental paste: 0.1%
Lotion: 0.025%, 0.1%
Ointment: 0.025%, 0.05%, 0.1%, 0.5%

INDICATIONS & DOSAGES
➤ **Inflammation and pruritus from corticosteroid-responsive dermatoses**
Adults and children: Clean area; apply aerosol, cream, lotion, or ointment sparingly b.i.d. to q.i.d. Rub in lightly. Or, 3 or 4 applications of spray daily.
➤ **Inflammation from oral lesions**
Adults and children: Apply paste at bedtime and, if needed, b.i.d. or t.i.d., preferably after meals. Apply small amount without rubbing;

T

press to lesion in mouth until thin film develops.

ADMINISTRATION
Topical
• Gently wash skin before applying. To avoid skin damage, rub in gently, leaving a thin coat. When treating hairy sites, part hair and apply directly to lesions.
• Don't apply near eyes or in ear canal.
• When using aerosol near the face, cover patient's eyes and warn against inhaling spray. Aerosol contains alcohol and may cause irritation or burning when used on open lesions. Spray at a distance of 3 to 6 inches (7.6 to 15.25 cm) from affected area.
• Occlusive dressings may be used in severe or resistant dermatoses.

ACTION
Unclear. Diffuses across cell membranes to form complexes with cytoplasmic receptors, showing anti-inflammatory, antipruritic, vasoconstrictive, and antiproliferative activity.

Route	Onset	Peak	Duration
Topical	Several hr	Unknown	1 wk

Half-life: Biologic, 18 to 36 hours.

ADVERSE REACTIONS
GU: glycosuria. **Metabolic:** hyperglycemia. **Skin:** burning, pruritus, irritation, dryness, erythema, folliculitis, hypertrichosis, hypopigmentation, acneiform eruptions, perioral dermatitis, allergic contact dermatitis, maceration, secondary infection, atrophy, striae, miliaria with occlusive dressings. **Other:** *HPA axis suppression,* Cushing syndrome.

INTERACTIONS
Drug-drug. *Aldesleukin:* Corticosteroids may decrease antineoplastic effect. Avoid combination.

EFFECTS ON LAB TEST RESULTS
• May increase glucose level.

CONTRAINDICATIONS & CAUTIONS
• Contraindicated in patients hypersensitive to drug or its components.

• Contraindicated in the presence of fungal, viral, or bacterial infections of the mouth or throat (paste).
• Don't use as monotherapy in primary bacterial infections (impetigo, paronychia, erysipelas, cellulitis, angular cheilitis), treatment of rosacea, perioral dermatitis, or acne.
• Considered a medium-potency (0.025% and 0.1% cream, ointment, lotion) and high-potency (0.5% cream, ointment) drug, according to vasoconstrictive properties.
• Don't use very-high-potency or high-potency agents on the face, groin, or axilla areas.
• Drug isn't for ophthalmic use.
• Prolonged corticosteroid therapy may interfere with growth and development in children.
• Use cautiously in elderly patients because of age-related changes in skin integrity and risks associated with systemic absorption.
Dialyzable drug: Unknown.
⚠ **Overdose S&S:** Systemic effects (including reversible HPA axis suppression, Cushing syndrome, hyperglycemia, glycosuria).

PREGNANCY-LACTATION-REPRODUCTION
• There are no adequate studies in pregnant women. Use only if potential benefit justifies potential risk to the fetus. Don't use extensively in pregnant patients in large amounts or for prolonged periods.
• It isn't known if drug appears in human milk. Use cautiously in breastfeeding women.

NURSING CONSIDERATIONS
• Stop drug and tell prescriber if skin infection, striae, or atrophy occur.
• If antifungal or antibiotic combined with corticosteroid fails to provide prompt improvement, stop corticosteroid until infection is controlled.
• Systemic absorption is more likely with the use of occlusive dressings, prolonged treatment, or extensive body surface treatment.
• Avoid using plastic pants or tight-fitting diapers on treated areas in young children. Children may absorb larger amounts of drug and be more susceptible to systemic toxicity.
• Monitor skin integrity.

Reactions in bold italics are *life-threatening*. Interactions may have a *rapid onset* or a **delayed onset**.

• If used for long time and on large skin areas, monitor patient for HPA axis suppression.
• When used in oral cavity, reevaluate if no improvement in 7 days.
• When using aerosol solution, reevaluate if no improvement in 2 weeks.

PATIENT TEACHING
• Teach patient or family member how to apply drug.
• Advise patient not to use an occlusive dressing unless instructed to. If an occlusive dressing is ordered, advise patient to leave it in place for no longer than 12 hours each day and not to use the dressing on infected or weeping lesions.
• Instruct patient spray is flammable.
• Tell patient to stop drug and report signs of systemic absorption, skin irritation or ulceration, hypersensitivity, infection, or lack of improvement.

triamterene–hydrochlorothiazide
try-AM-tur-een/hye-droe-klor-oh-THYE-a-zide

Dyazide, Maxzide, Maxzide-25

Therapeutic class: Antihypertensives–diuretics
Pharmacologic class: Thiazide diuretics–potassium-sparing diuretics

AVAILABLE FORMS
Capsules: triamterene 37.5 mg/hydrochlorothiazide 25 mg
Tablets: triamterene 37.5 mg/hydrochlorothiazide 25 mg, triamterene 75 mg/hydrochlorothiazide 50 mg

INDICATIONS & DOSAGES
➤ **HTN or edema in patients who develop hypokalemia on hydrochlorothiazide alone, or who require a thiazide diuretic and in whom development of hypokalemia can't be risked**
Adults: Triamterene 37.5 mg/hydrochlorothiazide 25 mg, PO once daily or b.i.d.

ADMINISTRATION
PO
• May give without regard to meals. Give drug with food to minimize GI upset.
• To prevent nocturia, give drug in the morning. If second dose is needed, give in early afternoon.

ACTION
Triamterene works on distal tubule and collecting duct to inhibit reabsorption of sodium in exchange for potassium and hydrogen; hydrochlorothiazide increases excretion of sodium, chloride, potassium, hydrogen, and water by inhibiting reabsorption in distal segment of the nephron.

Route	Onset	Peak	Duration
PO (triamterene)	2–4 hr	3 hr	7–9 hr
PO (hydrochlorothiazide)	2 hr	1–5 hr	6–12 hr

Half-life: Triamterene, 1½ to 2½ hours; hydrochlorothiazide, 6 to 15 hours.

ADVERSE REACTIONS
CNS: weakness, fatigue, dizziness, fever, headache, drowsiness, insomnia, depression, anxiety, vertigo, restlessness, paresthesia. **CV:** arrhythmia, orthostatic hypotension, chest pain, tachycardia. **EENT:** xanthopsia, transient blurred vision, dry mouth, sialadenitis. **GI:** diarrhea, nausea, vomiting, constipation, abdominal pain, pancreatitis, change in appetite, taste alteration, anorexia, gastric irritation, cramping. **GU:** erectile dysfunction, *acute renal failure,* glycosuria, interstitial nephritis, renal calculi, urine discoloration. **Hematologic:** *leukopenia, thrombocytopenia,* purpura, anemia, agranulocytosis. **Hepatic:** jaundice, altered LFT results. **Metabolic:** diabetes mellitus, *hyperkalemia,* hyperglycemia, hyperuricemia, *hypokalemia,* hyponatremia, *metabolic acidosis,* hypochloremic alkalosis, hypercalcemia, *hypomagnesemia.* **Musculoskeletal:** muscle cramps. **Respiratory:** shortness of breath, *pulmonary edema.* **Skin:** rash, urticaria, photosensitivity. **Other:** hypersensitivity reaction, anaphylaxis.

INTERACTIONS
Drug-drug. *ACE inhibitors and ARBs, potassium-containing medications (such as*

T

penicillin G potassium), potassium supplements: May increase risk of hyperkalemia. Avoid concurrent use.

Adrenocorticotropic hormone, amphotericin B, beta$_2$-agonists, corticosteroids: May increase electrolyte depletion, particularly potassium. Use together carefully.

Amiloride, spironolactone, triamterene-containing agents: May increase risk of hyperkalemia. Use together is contraindicated.

Antidiabetics (oral agents and insulin): May increase or decrease blood glucose level. Dosage adjustment of antidiabetic may be required.

Antigout drugs: May increase uric acid level. Increase dosage of antigout medication if indicated.

Barbiturates, opioids: May increase risk of orthostatic hypotension. Use together cautiously.

Bile acid sequestrants: May decrease absorption of thiazide diuretics. Consider therapy modification.

Calcium salts, multivitamins: May decrease calcium excretion. Monitor therapy closely.

Dofetilide: May increase QTc interval–prolonging effect of dofetilide. Avoid combination.

Laxatives: May increase potassium loss. Avoid use together.

Lithium: May increase lithium level, especially in patients with renal insufficiency. Avoid use together.

NSAIDs: May diminish antihypertensive effects and increase risk of acute renal failure. Use together cautiously.

Oral anticoagulants: May decrease anticoagulant effect. Adjust anticoagulant dosage as necessary.

Other antihypertensives: May increase risk of hypotension. Use together carefully and adjust dosage as appropriate.

Polystyrene, other exchange resins: May reduce potassium level, increase sodium retention, and increase edema. Avoid use together unless in setting of hyperkalemia.

Skeletal muscle relaxants, nondepolarizing (tubocurarine): May increase responsiveness to muscle relaxant. Avoid concurrent use.

Vitamin D analogues: May increase hypercalcemic effect of vitamin D. Monitor therapy closely.

Drug-herb. *Yohimbe:* May decrease antihypertensive effect of hydrochlorothiazide. Monitor therapy closely.

Drug-food. *Salt substitutes with potassium:* May increase risk of hyperkalemia. Discourage use together.

Drug-lifestyle. *Alcohol use:* May increase risk of orthostatic hypotension. Discourage use together.

Sun exposure: May increase risk of photosensitivity. Discourage sun exposure.

EFFECTS ON LAB TEST RESULTS

• May increase BUN, creatinine, liver enzyme, calcium, uric acid, cholesterol, and triglyceride levels.
• May decrease sodium, chloride, magnesium, and phosphate levels.
• May increase or decrease potassium or glucose level.
• May increase glucose level in the urine.
• May decrease protein-bound iodine level without signs of thyroid imbalance.
• May decrease leukocyte and platelet counts.
• May interfere with quinidine assays and parathyroid function tests.

CONTRAINDICATIONS & CAUTIONS

Black Box Warning Abnormal elevation of serum potassium levels (5.5 mEq/L or more) can occur and is more likely in patients with renal impairment or diabetes (even without concurrent renal impairment) and in elderly and severely ill patients. ■

• Contraindicated in patients hypersensitive to either drug or to sulfonamides; in those with preexisting hyperkalemia, anuria, acute and chronic renal insufficiency or significant renal impairment, or severe hepatic disease; and in those at risk for metabolic or respiratory acidosis.

• Use cautiously in patients with impaired hepatic function, electrolyte imbalance, or lupus and in those with a history of kidney stones or gout.

Dialyzable drug: Unlikely.

⚠ *Overdose S&S:* Hyperkalemia or hypokalemia, dehydration, nausea, vomiting, weakness, hypotension, lethargy, GI irritation, coma.

Reactions in bold italics are *life-threatening*. Interactions may have a *rapid onset* or a **delayed onset**.

PREGNANCY-LACTATION-REPRODUCTION

• There are no adequate studies in pregnant women. Use only if potential benefit justifies potential risk to the fetus.

• Both drugs may appear in human milk. Patient should discontinue breastfeeding or discontinue drug.

NURSING CONSIDERATIONS

Black Box Warning Monitor potassium level at initiation of therapy, with dosage changes, and with any illness that may influence renal function. ∎

• Warning signs and symptoms of hyperkalemia include paresthesia, muscular weakness, fatigue, flaccid paralysis, bradycardia, and shock.

• Fixed-dose combinations aren't to be used for initial therapy except in patients in whom development of hyperkalemia can't be risked (patients taking cardiac glycosides and those with history of cardiac arrhythmias).

• Monitor potassium level carefully in patients using this combination; if hyperkalemia is suspected, obtain ECG and monitor levels.

• If hyperkalemia is present, stop combination and use thiazide alone.

• If potassium level is greater than 6.5 mEq/L, consider IV calcium chloride, sodium bicarbonate, glucose, or sodium polystyrene sulfonate; consider dialysis if no improvement.

• Monitor patient for infection (sore throat, fever), which could be a sign of leukopenia, or for bruising, which could be a sign of thrombocytopenia.

• Monitor patient for acute myopia and secondary angle-closure glaucoma (acute vision changes, ocular pain usually within hours to weeks of drug ingestion), especially in patient with a history of possible sulfonamide or penicillin allergy. Discontinue drug as soon as possible if symptoms occur.

• Monitor patient for hyperuricemia or acute gout.

• Thiazides may alter calcium and phosphate levels. Discontinue drug before testing parathyroid function.

• Monitor diabetic patients for changes in antidiabetic agent or insulin requirements. Patients with latent diabetes may become fully diabetic during therapy.

• Monitor BP, LFT values, and electrolyte levels.

• *Look alike–sound alike:* Don't confuse Maxzide with Maxidex or Microzide.

PATIENT TEACHING

• Teach patient to report light-headedness, especially during first few days of therapy. Warn patient to discontinue drug and notify prescriber if syncope occurs.

• Caution patient to notify prescriber if fluid loss occurs from excessive perspiration, dehydration, vomiting, or diarrhea.

• Advise patient not to use salt substitutes containing potassium.

• Instruct patient to promptly report signs and symptoms of infection (sore throat, fever) or bruising.

• Inform patient that to be effective, drug must be taken daily as prescribed, and to continue to take drug even if feeling well.

• Advise patient to avoid taking drug at bedtime, to prevent nighttime diuresis.

• Teach patient the warning signs and symptoms of fluid and electrolyte imbalance (decreased urine production, drowsiness, dry mouth, fast HR, fatigue, low BP, muscular fatigue, muscle pain or cramps, restlessness, stomach disturbances, thirst, and weakness).

• Advise patient to keep follow-up appointments to monitor electrolyte levels.

• Warn patient to avoid sun exposure.

• Caution patient to avoid alcohol, to decrease risk of a sudden drop in BP.

• Instruct patient to consult prescriber before taking other prescription or OTC medications, herbal products, or vitamin and mineral supplements.

SAFETY ALERT!

triazolam
trye-AY-zoe-lam

Halcion

Therapeutic class: Hypnotics
Pharmacologic class: Benzodiazepines
Controlled substance schedule: IV

AVAILABLE FORMS
Tablets: 0.125 mg, 0.25 mg

T

INDICATIONS & DOSAGES
➤ **Short-term treatment (7 to 10 days) of insomnia**
Adults: 0.125 to 0.5 mg PO at bedtime.
Elderly or debilitated patients: 0.125 mg PO at bedtime. Maximum dose is 0.25 mg.

ADMINISTRATION
PO
• Don't give drug with or right after a meal.

ACTION
Unknown. Probably acts on the limbic system, thalamus, and hypothalamus of the CNS to produce hypnotic effects by increasing levels of inhibitory neurotransmitter GABA.

Route	Onset	Peak	Duration
PO	15–30 min	<2 hr	6–7 hr

Half-life: 1½ to 5½ hours.

ADVERSE REACTIONS
CNS: drowsiness, ataxia, dizziness, headache, nervousness. **GI:** nausea, vomiting.

INTERACTIONS
Drug-drug. *Anticonvulsants, antihistamines, CNS depressants, dronabinol, magnesium sulfate, psychotropics:* May cause excessive CNS depression. Use together cautiously.
Cimetidine, fluvoxamine, isoniazid, macrolide antibiotics (clarithromycin, erythromycin), oral contraceptives, ranitidine: May increase triazolam level. Monitor patient closely and consider triazolam dosage reduction.
CYP3A4 inducers: May decrease triazolam serum concentration. Consider alternative drug (strong inducers) or monitor therapy closely (moderate inducers).
Diltiazem: May increase CNS depression and prolong effects of triazolam. Reduce triazolam dose.
Black Box Warning *Opioids:* May cause slow or difficult breathing, sedation, and death. Avoid use together. If use together is necessary, limit dosage and duration of each drug to minimum necessary for desired effect. ■

Potent CYP3A inhibitors (azole antifungals [fluconazole, itraconazole, ketoconazole, miconazole], indinavir, lopinavir, nefazodone, nelfinavir, ritonavir, saquinavir): May increase and prolong triazolam level. Use together is contraindicated.
Drug-herb. *Calendula, hops, kava kava, lemon balm, passion flower, skullcap, valerian:* May enhance sedative effect of drug. Discourage use together.
St. John's wort: May decrease triazolam serum concentration. Consider therapy modification.
Yohimbe: May decrease effect of antianxiety agents. Monitor therapy closely.
Drug-food. *Grapefruit:* May delay onset and increase drug effects. Discourage use together.
Drug-lifestyle. ❸ *Alert: Alcohol use:* May cause additive CNS effects. Discourage use together.

EFFECTS ON LAB TEST RESULTS
• May increase LFT values.

CONTRAINDICATIONS & CAUTIONS
• Contraindicated in patients hypersensitive to benzodiazepines.
Black Box Warning Opioids should only be prescribed with benzodiazepines or other CNS depressants to patients for whom alternative treatment options are inadequate. ■
• Use cautiously in patients with impaired hepatic or renal function, chronic pulmonary insufficiency, sleep apnea, mental depression, suicidal tendencies, or history of drug abuse.
Dialyzable drug: Unlikely.
⚠ *Overdose S&S:* Somnolence, impaired coordination, slurred speech, confusion, coma, decreased reflexes, hypotension, seizures, respiratory depression, apnea.

PREGNANCY-LACTATION-REPRODUCTION
• Drug may cause fetal harm and is contraindicated in pregnant women.
• Patient should stop drug before becoming pregnant. If patient becomes pregnant, apprise her of risk to the fetus.
• Drug may appear in human milk. Use in breastfeeding women isn't recommended.

NURSING CONSIDERATIONS

❶ *Alert:* Anaphylaxis and angioedema may occur as early as the first dose; monitor patient closely.

• Assess mental status before starting therapy, and reduce doses in elderly patients.

• Take precautions to prevent hoarding or overdosing by patients who are depressed, suicidal, or drug-dependent or who have history of drug abuse.

• Minor changes in EEG patterns (usually low-voltage fast activity) may occur during and after therapy.

• *Look alike–sound alike:* Don't confuse triazolam with alprazolam. Don't confuse Halcion with Haldol or halcinonide.

PATIENT TEACHING

Black Box Warning Caution patient or caregiver of patient taking an opioid with a benzodiazepine, CNS depressant, or alcohol to seek immediate medical attention if patient experiences dizziness, lightheadedness, extreme sleepiness, slowed or difficult breathing, or unresponsiveness. ∎

❶ *Alert:* Warn patient that drug may cause allergic reactions, facial swelling, and complex sleep-related behaviors (driving, eating, and making phone calls while asleep). Advise patient to report these effects.

• Warn patient not to take more than prescribed amount; overdose can occur at total daily dose of 2 mg (or four times highest recommended amount).

• Tell patient to avoid alcohol use while taking drug.

• Warn patient not to stop drug abruptly after taking for 2 weeks or longer.

• Caution patient to avoid performing activities that require mental alertness or physical coordination.

• Inform patient that drug doesn't tend to cause morning drowsiness.

• Tell patient that rebound insomnia may occur for 1 or 2 nights after stopping therapy.

• Tell patient to avoid pregnancy and breast-feeding while taking drug.

• Advise patient to take drug immediately before bedtime and not with, or immediately after, a meal.

• Instruct patient to consult prescriber before taking other prescription or OTC medications or herbal products.

trospium chloride
TROZ-pee-um

Trosec✦

Therapeutic class: Urinary antispasmodics
Pharmacologic class: Antimuscarinics

AVAILABLE FORMS
Capsules (extended-release): 60 mg
Tablets: 20 mg

INDICATIONS & DOSAGES
➤ **Overactive bladder (urinary urge incontinence, urgency, frequency)**
Adults younger than age 75: 20 mg (immediate-release) PO b.i.d. taken on an empty stomach or at least 1 hour before a meal. Or 60 mg extended-release capsule PO once daily in morning.
Adjust-a-dose: For adults age 75 and older, reduce dosage to 20 mg (immediate-release) PO once daily based on patient tolerance. For CrCl of less than 30 mL/minute, give 20 mg (immediate-release) PO once daily at bedtime. Extended-release form isn't recommended if CrCl is less than 30 mL/minute.

ADMINISTRATION
PO
• Give at least 1 hour before meals or on an empty stomach.
• Give extended-release form with water on an empty stomach at least 1 hour before meal.

ACTION
Relaxes smooth muscle of bladder by antagonizing muscarinic receptors, relieving symptoms of overactive bladder.

Route	Onset	Peak	Duration
PO	Unknown	5–6 hr	Unknown

Half-life: About 20 hours (immediate-release); 35 hours (extended-release).

ADVERSE REACTIONS
CNS: fatigue, headache. **EENT:** dry eyes and nose, nasopharyngitis. **GI:** constipation, dry mouth, abdominal pain and distention, dyspepsia, flatulence, nausea. **GU:** urine retention, UTI. **Other:** flulike symptoms.

INTERACTIONS

Drug-drug. *Anticholinergics:* May increase dry mouth, constipation, or other adverse effects. Monitor patient.

Metformin, morphine, procainamide, pancuronium, tenofovir, vancomycin: May alter elimination of these drugs or trospium, increasing levels. Monitor patient closely.

Opioid analgesics: May increase risk of constipation and urine retention. Monitor therapy closely.

Prokinetic GI agents: May decrease therapeutic effect of GI prokinetic agents. Monitor therapy closely.

Drug-food. *High-fat foods:* May significantly decrease absorption. Give drug at least 1 hour before meals or on an empty stomach.

Drug-lifestyle. *Alcohol use:* May increase drowsiness. Use of alcoholic beverages within 2 hours of taking extended-release capsules isn't recommended. Discourage use together.

EFFECTS ON LAB TEST RESULTS

None reported.

CONTRAINDICATIONS & CAUTIONS

• Contraindicated in patients hypersensitive to the drug or any of its ingredients and in those with or at risk for urine retention, gastric retention, or uncontrolled narrow-angle glaucoma.

• Use cautiously in patients with significant bladder outflow obstruction, obstructive GI disorders, ulcerative colitis, intestinal atony, myasthenia gravis, renal insufficiency, moderate or severe hepatic impairment, or controlled narrow-angle glaucoma.

Dialyzable drug: Unknown.

⚠ **Overdose S&S:** Severe anticholinergic effects, tachycardia, mydriasis.

PREGNANCY-LACTATION-REPRODUCTION

• There are no adequate studies in pregnant women. Use only if potential benefit justifies potential risk to the fetus.

• It isn't known if drug appears in human milk. Use during breastfeeding only if potential benefit justifies potential risk to the infant.

NURSING CONSIDERATIONS

• Assess patient to determine baseline bladder function, and monitor patient for therapeutic effects.

• Angioedema of the face, lips, tongue, or larynx, which may be life-threatening, can occur after first dose. Discontinue drug and promptly provide treatment to ensure a patent airway.

• Various CNS anticholinergic effects have been reported, including dizziness, confusion, hallucinations, and somnolence. Monitor patients for signs and symptoms of anticholinergic CNS effects, particularly after beginning treatment or increasing dosage. Dosage may need to be reduced or drug discontinued.

• If patient has bladder outflow obstruction, watch for evidence of urine retention.

• Monitor patient for decreased gastric motility and constipation.

• Monitor renal and hepatic function periodically during therapy.

PATIENT TEACHING

• Tell patient to take drug on an empty stomach or at least 1 hour before meals.

• Tell patient to take extended-release form with water in the morning on an empty stomach, at least 1 hour before a meal.

• Discourage use of other drugs that may cause dry mouth, constipation, blurred vision, or urine retention.

• Tell patient that alcohol use may increase drowsiness and fatigue. Discourage alcohol consumption. Advise patient not to use alcohol within 2 hours of taking extended-release capsules.

• Explain that drug may decrease sweating and increase the risk of heatstroke when used in hot environments or during strenuous activities.

• Urge patient to avoid activities that are hazardous or require mental alertness until drug's effects are known.

ulipristal acetate ▧
UE-li-PRIS-tal

ella, Fibristal ✤

Therapeutic class: Contraceptives
Pharmacologic class: Progesterone agonists–antagonists

AVAILABLE FORMS

Tablets: 5 mg ✤, 30 mg

Reactions in bold italics are *life-threatening*. Interactions may have a *rapid onset* or a *delayed onset*.

INDICATIONS & DOSAGES
➤ **Prevention of pregnancy following un-protected intercourse or a known or suspected contraceptive failure**
Women and postmenarchal adolescents:
30 mg (1 tablet) PO as soon as possible within 120 hours (5 days) after unprotected intercourse or a known or suspected contraceptive failure.

ADMINISTRATION
PO
• May give without regard for food.
• May give at any time during the menstrual cycle.

ACTION
Inhibits or delays ovulation and alters endometrium to avoid egg implantation; prevents progestin from binding to progesterone receptor.

Route	Onset	Peak	Duration
PO	Unknown	1 hr	Unknown

Half-life: 32 to 38 hours.

ADVERSE REACTIONS
CNS: headache, fatigue, dizziness. **GI:** nausea, abdominal pain. **GU:** dysmenorrhea, intermenstrual bleeding, irregular menses. **Skin:** acne.

INTERACTIONS
Drug-drug. *CYP3A4 inducers (barbiturates, bosentan, carbamazepine, efavirenz, felbamate, griseofulvin, oxcarbazepine, phenytoin, rifampin, topiramate):* May decrease effectiveness of contraceptive. Avoid concurrent use.
CYP3A4 inhibitors (itraconazole, ketoconazole): May increase serum ulipristal levels and risk of adverse reactions. Monitor clinical response and adjust dosage if needed.
Hormonal contraceptives: May impair ability of ulipristal to delay ovulation or decrease effectiveness of regular hormonal contraceptives. Avoid coadministration.
Drug-herb. *St. John's wort:* May decrease effectiveness of contraceptive. Avoid concurrent use.

EFFECTS ON LAB TEST RESULTS
None reported.

CONTRAINDICATIONS & CAUTIONS
• Contraindicated for use as routine contraception.
• Contraindicated in prepubescent and postmenopausal females.
• Drug isn't indicated for termination of an existing pregnancy.
• Safety and effectiveness of repeated use within the same menstrual cycle aren't known; repeat use isn't recommended.
▧ Drug exposure in South Asian patients may exceed that in white and black patients; however, no difference in effectiveness and safety was observed.
Dialyzable drug: Unknown.

PREGNANCY-LACTATION-REPRODUCTION
• There are no adequate studies in pregnant women. Drug is contraindicated in women who are pregnant or may be pregnant.
• Drug appears in human milk. Effect of drug exposure on newborns or infants hasn't been studied; risk to breastfed infants can't be excluded. Use by breastfeeding women isn't recommended.

NURSING CONSIDERATIONS
• If vomiting occurs within 3 hours of taking drug, prescriber should consider repeating dose.
• Rule out pregnancy by obtaining history and physical exam before drug administration. If pregnancy isn't ruled out, perform pregnancy test.
• Perform follow-up physical and pelvic exam if there is concern about patient's health or pregnancy status after drug administration.
• Ulipristal won't terminate existing pregnancy.
• Rule out ectopic pregnancy in those who become pregnant or complain of lower abdominal pain 3 to 5 weeks after ulipristal use.
• Fertility returns rapidly after drug administration; routine contraceptives should be initiated or continued as soon as possible but not sooner than 5 days after emergency contraception.
• Drug may reduce effectiveness of regular hormonal contraceptives; additional use of a barrier method is recommended for subsequent intercourse during the same menstrual cycle.

U

✦Canada   ◇OTC   ◆Off-label use   ℘Photoguide   ⊞Do not crush   *Liquid contains alcohol   ▧Genetic

• After drug administration, menses can occur a few days earlier or later than usual. If menses is late (beyond 1 week), rule out pregnancy.

• Drug doesn't protect against HIV infection (AIDS) or other sexually transmitted infections.

• *Look alike–sound alike:* Don't confuse ulipristal with ursodiol.

PATIENT TEACHING

• Educate patient that drug isn't intended for routine use as a contraceptive, won't terminate an existing pregnancy, and should only be used once per menstrual cycle.

• Warn patient not to use ulipristal if she suspects she is pregnant or is breastfeeding because potential risks to the infant are unknown.

• Tell patient to report lower abdominal pain immediately.

• Instruct patient to resume routine contraceptives no sooner than 5 days after ulipristal and to use a barrier method during the same menstrual cycle.

• Advise patient that after drug administration, menses can occur a few days earlier or later than usual and that she should report if menses is late (beyond 1 week) because pregnancy will have to be ruled out.

• Warn patient that drug doesn't protect against HIV infection (AIDS) or other sexually transmitted infections.

ustekinumab
US-te-KIN-ue-mab

Stelara

Therapeutic class: Immunomodulators
Pharmacologic class: Monoclonal antibodies

AVAILABLE FORMS

Injection: 45 mg/0.5 mL, 90 mg/mL prefilled syringes; 45 mg/0.5 mL in single-use vials
IV infusion: 130 mg/26 mL in single-use vials

INDICATIONS & DOSAGES

➤ **Moderate to severe plaque psoriasis in patients who are candidates for phototherapy or systemic therapy**
Adults and adolescents age 12 and older weighing more than 100 kg: Initially, 90 mg subcut; repeat dose in 4 weeks, followed by maintenance dose of 90 mg subcut every 12 weeks.
Adults weighing 100 kg or less and adolescents age 12 and older weighing 60 to 100 kg: Initially, 45 mg subcut; repeat dose in 4 weeks, followed by maintenance dose of 45 mg subcut every 12 weeks.
Adolescents age 12 and older weighing less than 60 kg: Initially, 0.75 mg/kg subcut; repeat dose in 4 weeks, followed by maintenance dose of 0.75 mg/kg subcut every 12 weeks.

➤ **Psoriatic arthritis as monotherapy or in combination with methotrexate**
Adults: Initially, 45 mg subcut; repeat in 4 weeks. Then maintenance dose of 45 mg subcut every 12 weeks.

➤ **Psoriatic arthritis with coexistent moderate to severe plaque psoriasis as monotherapy or in combination with methotrexate**
Adults weighing more than 100 kg: Initially, 90 mg subcut; repeat dose in 4 weeks. Then maintenance dose of 90 mg subcut every 12 weeks.

➤ **Moderate to severe active Crohn disease in patients who failed or were intolerant to treatment with immunomodulators or corticosteroids, but never failed treatment with a TNF blocker or failed or were intolerant to treatment with one or more TNF blockers**
Adults: For induction as a single dose: If patient weighs more than 85 kg, 520 mg IV; if patient weighs more than 55 to 85 kg, 390 mg IV; if patient weighs 55 kg or less, 260 mg IV. Maintenance dose is 90 mg subcut every 8 weeks. Begin maintenance dose 8 weeks after induction.

ADMINISTRATION

IV
▼ Refrigerate vials upright at 36° to 46° F (2° to 8° C) and protected from light; don't freeze or shake.

▼ After calculating dosage and volume, withdraw an equal amount of fluid from 250-mL bag of NSS and discard. Add drug to the NSS bag and gently mix.

▼ Each vial is for single use only. Discard any remaining solution.

▼ May store diluted solution up to 4 hours at room temperature.

▼ Infuse over 1 hour using an in-line 0.2-micron, low-protein-binding filter.

▼ **Incompatibilities:** Don't infuse in same IV line with other drugs.

Subcutaneous

• Refrigerate vials (upright) and syringes at 36° to 46° F (2° to 8° C) and protected from light; don't freeze or shake.

• Discard any unused portion.

• Before administration, inspect ustekinumab for particulate matter and discoloration. Drug is colorless to light yellow and may contain a few small translucent or white particles. Don't use if discolored or cloudy or if other particulate matter is present.

⚠ *Alert:* The needle cover on the prefilled syringe contains dry natural rubber (a derivative of latex). Persons sensitive to latex shouldn't handle needle cover.

• Give each subcut injection at a different anatomic location (such as upper arms, gluteal regions, top of thighs, or any quadrant of abdomen) than the previous injection; don't administer into areas where psoriasis is present or the skin is tender, bruised, erythematous, or indurated.

• Drug should only be administered under the guidance and supervision of a health care provider and to patients who will be closely monitored and have regular follow-up visits with a health care provider.

ACTION

Antagonizes interleukin 12 and 23 cytokines by binding to an interleukin-specific P40 protein subunit that disrupts interleukin-based inflammatory and immune responses.

Route	Onset	Peak	Duration
Subcut	Unknown	7–13½ days	Unknown
IV	Unknown	Unknown	Unknown

Half-life: 10 to 126 days.

ADVERSE REACTIONS

CNS: depression, dizziness, fatigue, headache, asthenia. **EENT:** nasopharyngitis, pharyngolaryngeal pain, sinusitis. **GI:** diarrhea, nausea, vomiting, dental infections. **GU:** vulvovaginal candidiasis/mycotic infection, UTI. **Musculoskeletal:** back pain, myalgia, arthralgia. **Respiratory:** URI, bronchitis. **Skin:** injection-site erythema, pruritus, acne. **Other:** malignancies, antibody development, *severe infection.*

INTERACTIONS

Drug-drug. *CYP450 substrates (cyclosporine, warfarin):* May alter drug concentrations. Monitor patient for clinical effects and adjust dosage as needed.

Live-virus vaccines: May transmit infection. Use together is contraindicated.

Pimecrolimus, tacrolimus (topical): May enhance adverse/toxic effect of ustekinumab. Avoid combination.

Drug-herb. *Echinacea:* May decrease therapeutic effect of ustekinumab. Consider therapy modification.

EFFECTS ON LAB TEST RESULTS

None reported.

CONTRAINDICATIONS & CAUTIONS

⚠ *Alert:* Don't administer live-virus vaccines during or after treatment.

• Contraindicated in patients with clinically significant hypersensitivity to drug or its components. Hypersensitivity reactions, including anaphylaxis and angioedema, have been reported.

• Drug may increase risk of infections and reactivation of latent infections, including serious bacterial, fungal, and viral infections.

• Drug is contraindicated in patients with a clinically important active infection. Don't administer ustekinumab until the infection resolves or is adequately treated. Instruct patients to seek medical advice if signs or symptoms suggestive of an infection occur. Exercise caution when considering the use of ustekinumab in patients with a chronic infection or a history of recurrent infection.

• Don't administer to patients with active TB. Initiate treatment of latent TB before

U

administering ustekinumab. Consider anti-TB therapy before initiation of ustekinumab in patients with a history of latent or active TB in which an adequate course of treatment can't be confirmed.

• Drug may increase the risk of malignancy. Safety of ustekinumab hasn't been evaluated in patients with a history of malignancy or a known malignancy.

• Safety of use in combination with other immunosuppressants or phototherapy hasn't been evaluated in psoriasis studies.

• Drug may decrease the protective effect of allergen immunotherapy, which may increase the risk of an allergic reaction to a dose of allergen immunotherapy. Use cautiously in patients receiving or who have received allergen immunotherapy, particularly for anaphylaxis.

• The rapid appearance of multiple cutaneous squamous cell carcinomas in patients with preexisting risk factors for developing nonmelanoma skin cancer has been reported.

• Drug may cause reversible posterior leukoencephalopathy syndrome (RPLS). Signs and symptoms include headache, seizures, confusion, and visual disturbances. If RPLS is suspected, discontinue drug and administer appropriate treatment.

• Cases of interstitial pneumonia, eosinophilic pneumonia, and cryptogenic organizing pneumonia have been reported with serious outcomes, including respiratory failure and prolonged hospitalization.
Dialyzable drug: Unknown.

PREGNANCY-LACTATION-REPRODUCTION
• Drug hasn't been studied in pregnant women. Use only if potential benefit outweighs potential risk to the fetus.

• Encourage women exposed to ustekinumab during pregnancy to enroll in the OTIS Autoimmune Diseases in Pregnancy Study (1-877-311-8972).

• It isn't known if drug appears in human milk. Use cautiously in breastfeeding women.

NURSING CONSIDERATIONS
• Evaluate patients for TB before initiating drug. Closely monitor patients receiving drug for signs and symptoms of active TB

(fever, cough, night sweats, fatigue, and unexplained weight loss) during and after treatment.

• Patients should receive all immunizations appropriate for age as recommended by current immunization guidelines before starting treatment. Patients being treated with ustekinumab shouldn't receive live-virus vaccines. Don't give bacillus Calmette-Guérin vaccines for 1 year before initiating treatment, during treatment, or for 1 year after discontinuation of treatment.

• In adolescents, it's recommended that drug be administered by a health care provider.

• Use caution when administering live-virus vaccines to household contacts of patient receiving drug because of the potential risk of shedding from the household contact and transmission to patient.

• Non-live-virus vaccinations received by patient during a course of ustekinumab may not elicit an immune response sufficient to prevent disease.

• Monitor patients for signs and symptoms of infection (fever, fatigue, sore throat, erythema, pain, cough). If infection develops, withhold drug and treat infection.

• Monitor patient for signs and symptoms of RPLS (headache, seizures, confusion, visual disturbances).

• Monitor all patients for the appearance of nonmelanoma skin cancer. Patients older than age 60, those with a medical history of prolonged immunosuppressive therapy, and those with a history of psoralen–ultraviolet A treatment should be followed closely.

• Monitor patient for cough, dyspnea, and interstitial infiltrates after one to three doses. If diagnosis of noninfectious pneumonia is confirmed, discontinue drug and institute appropriate treatment.

• After proper training in subcut injection technique, patient may self-inject.

• *Look alike–sound alike:* Don't confuse ustekinumab with infliximab or rituximab. Don't confuse Stelara with Aldara.

PATIENT TEACHING
• Instruct patient or caregiver to follow directions provided in the Medication Guide.

• Instruct patient to immediately report signs or symptoms of RPLS or pneumonia.

Reactions in bold italics are *life-threatening*. Interactions may have a *rapid onset* or a *delayed onset*.

• Inform patient that drug may lower the ability of the immune system to fight infections. Stress importance of communicating any history of infections to health care provider and reporting signs or symptoms of infection.

• Advise patient to seek immediate medical attention if signs or symptoms of serious allergic reactions occur (wheezing, chest tightness, fever, itching, cough, blue skin color, seizures, facial swelling).

• Instruct patient or caregiver in injection techniques. Assess their ability to inject subcutaneously to ensure proper administration. The first self-injection should be performed under the supervision of a qualified health care professional.

• Advise patient that the needle cover on the prefilled syringe contains dry natural rubber (a derivative of latex), which may cause allergic reactions in latex-sensitive individuals.

• Instruct patient or caregiver in proper technique for syringe and needle disposal. Advise patient not to reuse or share needles or syringes.

• Caution patient to avoid live-virus vaccines during and after therapy.

• Warn patient that drug may increase the risk of malignancy.

---

valACYclovir hydrochloride
val-ah-SYE-kloe-vir

Valtrex⚕

Therapeutic class: Antivirals
Pharmacologic class: Nucleosides–nucleotides

AVAILABLE FORMS
Tablets: 500 mg, 1 g

INDICATIONS & DOSAGES
➤ **Herpes zoster infection (shingles)**
Adults: 1 g PO t.i.d. for 7 days.
Adjust-a-dose: For patients with CrCl of 30 to 49 mL/minute, give 1 g PO every 12 hours; if CrCl is 10 to 29 mL/minute, give 1 g PO every 24 hours; if CrCl is less than 10 mL/minute, give 500 mg PO every 24 hours.

➤ **First episode of genital herpes**
Adults: 1 g PO b.i.d. for 10 days.
Adjust-a-dose: For patients with CrCl of 10 to 29 mL/minute, give 1 g PO every 24 hours; if CrCl is less than 10 mL/minute, give 500 mg PO every 24 hours.

➤ **Recurrent genital herpes in immuno-competent patients**
Adults: 500 mg PO b.i.d. for 3 days, given at the first sign or symptom of an episode.
Adjust-a-dose: For patients with CrCl of 29 mL/minute or less, give 500 mg PO every 24 hours.

➤ **Long-term suppression of recurrent genital herpes**
Adults: 1 g PO once daily. In patients with a history of nine or fewer recurrences per year, use alternative dose of 500 mg once daily.
Adjust-a-dose: For patients with CrCl of 29 mL/minute or less, give 500 mg PO every 24 hours (every 48 hours if patient has nine or fewer occurrences per year).

➤ **Long-term suppression of recurrent genital herpes in patients with HIV and CD4$^+$ cell count of 100/mm^3 or greater**
Adults: 500 mg PO b.i.d.
Adjust-a-dose: For patients with CrCl of 29 mL/minute or less, give 500 mg PO every 24 hours (every 48 hours if patient has nine or fewer occurrences per year).

➤ **Cold sores (herpes labialis)**
Adults and children age 12 and older: 2 g PO b.i.d. for 1 day taken 12 hours apart.
Adjust-a-dose: For patients with CrCl of 30 to 49 mL/minute, give 1 g every 12 hours for two doses; if CrCl is 10 to 29 mL/minute, give 500 mg every 12 hours for two doses; if CrCl is less than 10 mL/minute, give 500 mg as a single dose.

➤ **To reduce transmission of genital herpes in patients with history of nine or fewer occurrences per year**
Adults: 500 mg PO daily for source partner.

➤ **Chickenpox**
Children ages 2 to younger than 18: 20 mg/kg PO t.i.d. for 5 days. Maximum dose is 1 g t.i.d.

ADMINISTRATION
PO
• Give drug without regard for meals.
• An oral suspension may be compounded by a pharmacist if needed.

V

• Suspension must be refrigerated then shaken before each dose. Discard unused portion after 28 days.

ACTION
Rapidly converts to acyclovir, which in turn becomes incorporated into viral DNA, thereby terminating growth of the DNA chain; inhibits viral DNA polymerase, causing inhibition of viral replication.

Route	Onset	Peak	Duration
PO	30 min	1.4–2.6 hr	Unknown

Half-life: 2½ to 3¼ hours.

ADVERSE REACTIONS
CNS: headache, depression, dizziness. **EENT:** nasopharyngitis, rhinorrhea. **GI:** nausea, abdominal pain, diarrhea, vomiting. **GU:** dysmenorrhea. **Hematologic:** *thrombocytopenia.* **Musculoskeletal:** arthralgia. **Respiratory:** URI. **Skin:** rash.

INTERACTIONS
Drug-drug. *Foscarnet:* May increase risk of nephrotoxicity. Avoid use together.
Vaccines (varicella virus, zoster [live/attenuated]): May diminish therapeutic effect of these vaccines. Avoid using drug within 24 hours before vaccination and for 14 days after vaccination.

EFFECTS ON LAB TEST RESULTS
• May increase alkaline phosphatase, ALT, AST, and creatinine levels.
• May decrease Hb level and platelet and WBC counts.

CONTRAINDICATIONS & CAUTIONS
• Contraindicated in patients hypersensitive to or intolerant of valacyclovir, acyclovir, or components of the formulation.
🔇 **Alert:** Thrombotic thrombocytopenic purpura (TTP) and hemolytic-uremic syndrome (HUS) may occur in allogeneic bone marrow or renal transplant recipients and patients with advanced HIV at doses of 8 g/day. Discontinue drug if signs or symptoms or lab findings of TTP or HUS occur.
• Use cautiously in elderly or dehydrated patients, in those with renal impairment, and in those receiving other nephrotoxic drugs.

• Safety and effectiveness in prepubertal children haven't been established except for in chickenpox.
Dialyzable drug: 33%.
⚠ *Overdose S&S:* Precipitation of acyclovir in renal tubules.

PREGNANCY-LACTATION-REPRODUCTION
• There are no adequate studies in pregnant women. Use in pregnant women only if potential benefits outweigh potential risk to the fetus.
• Drug appears in human milk. Use cautiously in breastfeeding women.

NURSING CONSIDERATIONS
• Safety and effectiveness of therapy beyond 12 months (beyond 6 months in HIV-1–infected patients) haven't been established.
• Start treatment for herpes zoster infection at earliest signs or symptoms. It's most effective when started within 48 hours of onset of rash.
• Monitor renal function; give appropriate dose adjusted for renal status.
• If renal failure and anuria occur, hemodialysis may be beneficial until renal function returns.
• Monitor patient for CNS changes (agitation, hallucinations, confusion, delirium, seizures, and encephalopathy). Discontinue drug if changes occur.
• *Look alike–sound alike:* Don't confuse valacyclovir (Valtrex) with valganciclovir (Valcyte) or acyclovir. Don't confuse Valtrex with Keflex or Zovirax.

PATIENT TEACHING
• Inform patient that drug may be taken without regard for meals.
• Teach patient signs and symptoms of herpes infection (rash, tingling, itching, and pain), and to notify prescriber immediately if they occur. Treatment should begin as soon as possible after symptoms appear, preferably within 48 hours of the onset of zoster rash.
• Caution patient to immediately report CNS changes, kidney problems, and any adverse reactions.
• Tell patient that drug isn't a cure for herpes but may decrease length and severity of symptoms.

Reactions in bold italics are *life-threatening*. Interactions may have a *rapid onset* or a *delayed onset*.

• Advise patient with genital herpes to use safe sex practices in combination with suppressive therapy, even if no symptoms are apparent.
• Advise patient to maintain adequate hydration.

---

valproate sodium ⚶
val-PROH-ayt

Depacon

valproic acid
Depakene

divalproex sodium
Depakote✑, Depakote ER, Depakote Sprinkle✑, Epival✤

Therapeutic class: Anticonvulsants
Pharmacologic class: Carboxylic acid derivatives

AVAILABLE FORMS
The strengths of valproate sodium and divalproex sodium are expressed in terms of valproic acid.
valproate sodium
Injection: 100 mg/mL
valproic acid
Capsules ⓞ: 250 mg
Syrup: 250 mg/5 mL
divalproex sodium
Capsules (sprinkle) ⓞ: 125 mg
Tablets (delayed-release) ⓞ: 125 mg, 250 mg, 500 mg
Tablets (extended-release) ⓞ: 250 mg, 500 mg

INDICATIONS & DOSAGES
Adjust-a-dose (for all indications): For elderly patients, start at lower dosage. Increase dosage more slowly and with regular monitoring of fluid and nutritional intake, and watch for dehydration, somnolence, and other adverse reactions.
➤ **Simple and complex absence seizures, mixed seizure types (including absence seizures)**
Adults and children age 2 and older: Initially, 15 mg/kg PO or IV daily; then

increase by 5 to 10 mg/kg daily at weekly intervals up to maximum of 60 mg/kg daily. Don't use Depakote ER in children younger than age 10.
➤ **Complex partial seizures**
Adults and children age 10 and older: 10 to 15 mg/kg Depakene, Depakote, or Depakote ER PO or valproate sodium IV daily; then increase by 5 to 10 mg/kg daily at weekly intervals, up to 60 mg/kg daily.
➤ **Mania**
Adults: Initially, 750 mg Depakote PO daily in divided doses, or 25 mg/kg Depakote ER PO once daily. Adjust dosage based on patient's response; maximum dose for either form is 60 mg/kg daily.
➤ **To prevent migraine headache**
Adults: Initially, 250 mg delayed-release divalproex sodium PO b.i.d. Some patients may need up to 1,000 mg daily. Or, 500 mg Depakote ER PO daily for 1 week; then 1,000 mg PO daily. Maximum recommended dosage is 60 mg/kg/day.

ADMINISTRATION
PO
• Don't crush delayed- or extended-release tablets.
• Give drug with food or milk to reduce adverse GI effects.
• Don't mix syrup with carbonated beverages; mixture may be irritating to oral mucosa.
• Don't give syrup to patients who need sodium restriction. Check with prescriber.
• Sprinkle capsules may be swallowed whole or opened and contents sprinkled on a teaspoonful of soft food. Patient should swallow immediately without chewing.
IV
▼ IV use is indicated only in patients who can't take drug orally. Switch patient to oral form as soon as feasible; effects of IV use for longer than 14 days are unknown.
▼ Dilute valproate sodium injection with at least 50 mL of a compatible diluent. It's physically compatible and chemically stable in D_5W, NSS, and lactated Ringer solution for 24 hours.
▼ Infuse drug over 60 minutes at no more than 20 mg/minute and at the same frequency as oral dosage.

V

▼ Monitor drug level, and adjust dosage as needed.

▼ **Incompatibilities:** None listed by manufacturer. Consult a drug incompatibility reference for more information.

ACTION

Hasn't been established. Activity in epilepsy is thought to be related to increased brain concentrations of GABA.

Route	Onset	Peak	Duration
PO	Unknown	Variable	Unknown
IV	Unknown	1 hr	Unknown

Half-life: Adults, 9 to 16 hours; children, 3½ to 67 hours based on age.

ADVERSE REACTIONS

CNS: asthenia, dizziness, drowsiness, headache, insomnia, nervousness, somnolence, tremor, abnormal thinking, amnesia, ataxia, depression, emotional upset, fever, abnormal dreams. **CV:** chest pain, edema, HTN, hypotension, tachycardia, palpitations. **EENT:** blurred vision, diplopia, nystagmus, pharyngitis, rhinitis, tinnitus. **GI:** abdominal pain, anorexia, diarrhea, dyspepsia, nausea, vomiting, *pancreatitis,* constipation, increased appetite. **GU:** UTI, vaginitis, dysmenorrhea, dysuria, urinary frequency, urinary incontinence. **Hematologic:** *bone marrow suppression, hemorrhage, thrombocytopenia,* bruising, petechiae. **Hepatic:** *hepatotoxicity.* **Metabolic:** hyperammonemia, weight gain or loss. **Musculoskeletal:** back and neck pain, arthralgia. **Respiratory:** bronchitis, dyspnea. **Skin:** alopecia, *erythema multiforme, hypersensitivity reactions, SJS,* rash, photosensitivity reactions, pruritus. **Other:** flulike syndrome, infection, chills.

INTERACTIONS

Drug-drug. *Aspirin, erythromycin, felbamate:* May cause valproic acid toxicity. Use together cautiously and monitor drug level.
Benzodiazepines, other CNS depressants: May cause excessive CNS depression. Avoid using together.
Carbamazepine: May cause carbamazepine CNS toxicity; may decrease valproic acid level and cause loss of seizure control. Use together cautiously, if at all. Monitor patient for seizure activity and toxicity during therapy and for at least 1 month after stopping either drug.
Carbapenem antibiotics (ertapenem, imipenem, meropenem): May decrease valproic acid level and cause loss of seizure control. Consider alternative antimicrobial agent. Monitor levels closely.
Estrogen-containing hormonal contraceptives: May decrease valproate concentration and increase seizure frequency. Monitor valproate level and clinical response.
Fosphenytoin, phenytoin: May increase or decrease phenytoin level; may decrease valproate level. Monitor patient closely.
Lamotrigine: May increase lamotrigine level and decrease valproate level; serious skin reactions may occur. Monitor levels closely.
Phenobarbital: May increase phenobarbital level; may increase clearance of valproate. Monitor patient closely.
Rifampin: May decrease valproate level. Monitor level of valproate.
Rufinamide: May increase rufinamide serum concentration. Begin valproate therapy at a low dosage, and titrate to a clinically effective dosage.
TCAs (amitriptyline, nortriptyline): May increase TCA level. Monitor drug level.
Topiramate: May cause hyperammonemia with and without encephalopathy. Concomitant use has been associated with hypothermia. Check blood ammonia levels in patients reporting hypothermia.
Warfarin: May displace warfarin from binding sites. Monitor PT and INR.
Zidovudine: May decrease zidovudine clearance. Avoid using together.
Drug-lifestyle. *Alcohol use:* May cause excessive CNS depression. Discourage use together.

EFFECTS ON LAB TEST RESULTS

• May increase ammonia, ALT, AST, and bilirubin levels.
• May increase eosinophil count and bleeding time. May decrease platelet, RBC, and WBC counts.
• May cause false-positive results for urine ketone levels.

Reactions in bold italics are *life-threatening*. Interactions may have a *rapid onset* or a *delayed onset*.

CONTRAINDICATIONS & CAUTIONS

• Contraindicated in patients hypersensitive to drug and in those with hepatic disease or significant hepatic dysfunction, and in patients with a urea cycle disorder (UCD).

Black Box Warning Patients with hereditary neurometabolic syndromes caused by DNA mutations of the mitochondrial DNA polymerase gamma (*POLG*) gene such as Alpers-Huttenlocher syndrome are at high risk for acute liver failure and fatalities. Drug is contraindicated in patients known to have mitochondrial disorders caused by *POLG* mutations and in children younger than age 2 who are suspected of having a mitochondrial disorder. In patients older than age 2 who are clinically suspected of having a hereditary mitochondrial disease, use only after other anticonvulsants have failed. ■

Black Box Warning Cases of life-threatening pancreatitis have been reported in children and adults receiving valproate shortly after initial use as well as after several years of use. ■

• Safety and effectiveness of Depakote ER in children younger than age 10 haven't been established.

🛑 *Alert:* Drug is associated with a rare but serious reaction known as DRESS syndrome, which may be fatal. DRESS syndrome is the presence of three or more symptoms, including cutaneous reactions (rash, exfoliative dermatitis), eosinophilia, fever, lymphadenopathy, and one or more systemic complications (hepatitis, nephritis, pneumonitis, myocarditis, pericarditis). Immediately discontinue drug if DRESS syndrome is suspected.

Dialyzable drug: 20%.

⚠ *Overdose S&S:* Somnolence, heart block, deep coma, hypernatremia.

PREGNANCY-LACTATION-REPRODUCTION

Black Box Warning Avoid use in women who may become pregnant. Valproate can cause teratogenic effects, such as neural tube defects and other organ system malformations. Drug is contraindicated for use in pregnancy for the prevention of migraines. ■

Black Box Warning There is an increased risk of lower cognitive test scores in children born to mothers who took drug during pregnancy. Consider alternative medication in

pregnant women unless use of drug is essential. Women of childbearing potential should use effective contraception during therapy. ■

Black Box Warning Use in pregnant women with epilepsy or bipolar disorder only if other drugs have failed to control symptoms. Drug is contraindicated for use in pregnancy for reversible conditions not associated with permanent injury or death. ■

• To prevent major seizures, pregnant women with epilepsy shouldn't discontinue drug abruptly.

• Pregnant women taking valproate may develop hepatic failure or clotting abnormalities, including thrombocytopenia, hypofibrinogenemia, or decrease in other coagulation factors, which may result in hemorrhagic complications in the neonate, including death.

• Offer prenatal diagnostic testing to pregnant women using drug, to detect neural tube and other defects.

• Hypoglycemia in neonates and fatal cases of hepatic failure in infants after maternal use during pregnancy have been reported.

• Pregnant patients should enroll in the North American AED (Antiepileptic Drug) Pregnancy Registry (1-888-233-2334).

• Drug appears in human milk. Use cautiously in breastfeeding women.

NURSING CONSIDERATIONS

Black Box Warning During treatment, closely monitor patients older than age 2 who are suspected of having a mitochondrial disorder for development of acute liver injury; perform regular clinical assessments and serum liver testing. Perform *POLG* mutation screening in accordance with current clinical practice. ■

Black Box Warning Fatal hepatotoxicity may follow nonspecific signs and symptoms, such as malaise, fever, anorexia, facial edema, vomiting, weakness, and lethargy. If these signs and symptoms occur during therapy, notify prescriber at once because patient who might be developing hepatic dysfunction must stop drug. Monitor LFT values before therapy initiation and at frequent intervals, especially during first 6 months. ■

Black Box Warning Patients at high risk for fatal hepatotoxicity include those with congenital metabolic disorders, mental

V

retardation, or organic brain disease; those taking multiple anticonvulsants; and children younger than age 2. In children younger than age 2, use with extreme caution and as a sole agent, weighing benefits of therapy against risks. ■

⊕ Alert: Closely monitor all patients taking or starting antiepileptic drugs for changes in behavior indicating worsening of suicidal thoughts or behavior or depression. Symptoms such as anxiety, agitation, hostility, mania, and hypomania may be precursors to emerging suicidality.

⊕ Alert: Dose-related thrombocytopenia can occur. Monitor CBC, platelet count, PT, and INR before starting therapy and at frequent intervals. Decrease dose or discontinue drug if hemorrhage, bruising, or coagulation disorder occurs.

⊕ Alert: Monitor patients and immediately report symptoms of DRESS syndrome (rash, fever, swollen glands). Discontinue drug if DRESS syndrome is suspected.

• Adverse reactions may not be caused by valproic acid alone because it's usually used with other anticonvulsants.

• When converting adults and children age 10 and older with seizures from Depakote to Depakote ER, make sure the extended-release dose is 8% to 20% higher than the regular dose taken previously. See manufacturer's package insert for more details.

• Never withdraw drug suddenly because sudden withdrawal may worsen seizures. Call prescriber at once if adverse reactions develop.

• Notify prescriber if tremors occur; a dosage reduction may be needed.

• Monitor drug level. Therapeutic level is commonly considered to be 50 to 100 mcg/mL for seizure control and 50 to 125 mcg/mL for mania.

• When converting patients from a brand-name drug to a generic drug, use caution because breakthrough seizures may occur.

⊕ Alert: Sometimes fatal, hyperammonemic encephalopathy may occur when starting valproate therapy in patients with UCD. Evaluate patients with UCD risk factors before starting valproate therapy. Patients who develop symptoms of unexplained hyperammonemic encephalopathy during valproate therapy should stop drug, undergo prompt

appropriate treatment, and be evaluated for underlying UCD.

• **Look alike–sound alike:** Don't confuse Depakote with Depakote ER or Depakene.

PATIENT TEACHING

⊕ Alert: Tell patient and caregivers that drug may increase risk of suicidal thoughts and behavior and to immediately report the emergence or worsening of depression, unusual changes in mood or behavior, or emergence of suicidal thoughts, behavior, or thoughts about self-harm.

• Tell patient to take drug with food or milk to reduce adverse GI effects.

• Advise patient not to chew capsules; irritation of mouth and throat may result.

• Tell patient that sprinkle capsules may be either swallowed whole or carefully opened and contents sprinkled on a teaspoonful of soft food. Tell patient to swallow immediately without chewing.

• Tell patient and parents that syrup shouldn't be mixed with carbonated beverages; mixture may be irritating to mouth and throat.

• Tell patient and parents to keep drug out of children's reach.

• Warn patient and parents not to stop drug therapy abruptly.

⊕ Alert: Tell patient to immediately report rash (with or without blisters), fever, swollen lymph nodes, mouth ulcers, or skin shedding.

Black Box Warning Warn patients and caregivers that abdominal pain, nausea, vomiting, and anorexia can be symptoms of pancreatitis that require prompt medical evaluation. ■

• Advise patient to avoid driving and other potentially hazardous activities that require mental alertness until drug's CNS effects are known.

• Instruct patient or parents to call prescriber if malaise, weakness, lethargy, facial swelling, loss of appetite, or vomiting occurs.

• Tell female patient to call prescriber if she becomes pregnant or plans to become pregnant during therapy.

Reactions in bold italics are *life-threatening*. Interactions may have a *rapid onset* or a *delayed onset*.

valsartan
val-SAR-tan

Diovan✑

Therapeutic class: Antihypertensives
Pharmacologic class: ARBs

AVAILABLE FORMS
Tablets: 40 mg, 80 mg, 160 mg, 320 mg

INDICATIONS & DOSAGES
➤ **HTN (used alone or with other antihypertensives)**
Adults: Initially, 80 or 160 mg PO once daily. Expect to see a reduction in BP in 2 to 4 weeks. If additional antihypertensive effect is needed, dose may be increased to 160 or 320 mg daily, or a diuretic may be added. (Addition of a diuretic has a greater effect than dosage increases beyond 80 mg.) Usual dosage range is 80 to 320 mg daily.
Children ages 6 to 16: Initially, 1.3 mg/kg PO daily (up to 40 mg total). Adjust according to patient response up to 2.7 mg/kg or 160 mg daily.
➤ **NYHA Class II to IV HF**
Adults: Initially, 40 mg PO b.i.d.; increase as tolerated to 80 mg b.i.d., and then to target dose of 160 mg b.i.d.
➤ **To reduce CV death in stable post-MI patients with left ventricular failure or dysfunction**
Adults: 20 mg PO b.i.d. Initial dose may be given as soon as 12 hours after MI. Increase dose to 40 mg b.i.d. within 7 days. Increase subsequent doses, as tolerated, to target dose of 160 mg b.i.d.

ADMINISTRATION
PO
• Give drug without regard for food.
• Pharmacists may prepare suspension for children unable to swallow pills.
• Shake suspension at least 10 seconds before pouring. Store suspension at room temperature for 30 days or in refrigerator for 75 days.

ACTION
Blocks the binding of angiotensin II to receptor sites in vascular smooth muscle and the adrenal gland, which inhibits the pressor effects of the RAAS.

Route	Onset	Peak	Duration
PO	2 hr	2–4 hr	24 hr

Half-life: 6 hours.

ADVERSE REACTIONS
CNS: dizziness, headache, fatigue, vertigo, syncope. **CV:** edema, hypotension, orthostatic hypotension. **EENT:** blurred vision, rhinitis, sinusitis, pharyngitis. **GI:** abdominal pain, diarrhea, nausea. **GU:** renal impairment. **Hematologic:** *neutropenia.* **Metabolic:** hyperkalemia. **Musculoskeletal:** arthralgia, back pain. **Respiratory:** URI, cough. **Other:** viral infection.

INTERACTIONS
Drug-drug. *ACE inhibitors:* May increase risk of renal dysfunction, hypotension, and hyperkalemia. Avoid use together but, if necessary, closely monitor BP, serum potassium level, and renal function.
Aliskiren: May increase risk of renal impairment, hypotension, and hyperkalemia in diabetic patients and those with moderate to severe renal impairment (GFR less than 60 mL/minute). Concomitant use is contraindicated in diabetic patients. Avoid concomitant use in those with moderate to severe renal impairment.
Antihepaciviral combination products: May increase valsartan serum concentration. Consider therapy modification or decrease valsartan dosage and monitor patient for hypotension and worsening renal function.
Canagliflozin: May increase risk of hyperkalemia and hypotension. Monitor therapy.
Lithium: May increase lithium level. Monitor lithium level and patient for toxicity.
NSAIDs: May result in deterioration of renal function in patients who are elderly or volume-depleted or in those with compromised renal function. Monitor renal function. May also decrease antihypertensive effect. Monitor BP.
Potassium supplements, potassium-sparing diuretics, other angiotensin II blockers: May increase potassium level. May also increase creatinine level in HF patients. Avoid using together.

V

Trimethoprim: May increase risk of hyperkalemia, especially in elderly patients. Closely monitor serum potassium level.
Drug-food. *Salt substitutes containing potassium:* May increase potassium level. May also increase creatinine level in HF patients. Discourage use together.

EFFECTS ON LAB TEST RESULTS
• May increase potassium, BUN, and creatinine levels.
• May decrease neutrophil count.

CONTRAINDICATIONS & CAUTIONS
• Contraindicated in patients hypersensitive to drug or its components.
• Angioedema, a rare life-threatening reaction, has been reported. Discontinue drug immediately and treat emergently if angioedema occurs. Don't give drug to patients with history of angioedema.
• Use cautiously in patients with renal or hepatic disease.
• Safety and effectiveness haven't been established in children younger than age 6 and in children of any age with GFR less than 30 mL/minute/1.73 m^2.
Dialyzable drug: No.
⚠ *Overdose S&S:* Hypotension, tachycardia, bradycardia, decreased level of consciousness, circulatory collapse, shock.

PREGNANCY-LACTATION-REPRODUCTION
Black Box Warning Drugs that act directly on the RAAS can cause injury and death to the developing fetus. When pregnancy is detected, stop drug as soon as possible. ∎
• It isn't known if drug appears in human milk. Patient should discontinue breastfeeding or discontinue drug.

NURSING CONSIDERATIONS
• Monitor BP and watch for hypotension. Excessive hypotension can occur when drug is given with high doses of diuretics.
• Correct volume and sodium depletions before starting drug.
• Suspension has 1.6 times greater exposure than tablets. Patients may require a higher dose if switched to tablets.
• Monitor serum BUN, creatinine, and potassium levels.

• **Look alike–sound alike:** Don't confuse Diovan with Zyban.

PATIENT TEACHING
• Advise patient that drug may be taken without regard for food.
• Tell female patient of childbearing potential to notify prescriber if pregnancy occurs. Drug will need to be stopped.
• Advise patient to report all adverse effects, especially dizziness upon standing or other signs and symptoms of hypotension.

vancomycin hydrochloride
van-koh-MYE-sin

Firvanq, Vancocin

Therapeutic class: Antibiotics
Pharmacologic class: Glycopeptides

AVAILABLE FORMS
Capsules: 125 mg, 250 mg
Powder for injection: 500-mg vials, 750-mg vials, 1-g vials
Powder for oral solution: 25 mg/mL, 50 mg/mL
Premixed for injection: 500 mg/100 mL, 750 mg/150 mL, 1 g/200 mL

INDICATIONS & DOSAGES
Adjust-a-dose (for all indications): In renal insufficiency, adjust dosage based on degree of renal impairment, drug level, severity of infection, and susceptibility of causative organism. Initially, give 15 mg/kg, and adjust subsequent doses as needed.
➤ **Serious or severe infections when other antibiotics are ineffective or contraindicated, including those caused by MRSA, *Staphylococcus epidermidis*, or diphtheroid organisms**
Adults: 500 mg IV every 6 hours or 1 g IV every 12 hours.
Children: 10 mg/kg IV every 6 hours.
Neonates and young infants: 15 mg/kg IV loading dose; then 10 mg/kg IV every 12 hours if child is younger than age 1 week or 10 mg/kg IV every 8 hours if older than 1 week but younger than 1 month.

Reactions in bold italics are *life-threatening*. Interactions may have a *rapid onset* or a *delayed onset*.

Elderly patients: 15 mg/kg IV loading dose. Subsequent doses are based on renal function and drug levels.

➤**CDAD**
Adults: 125 mg PO every 6 hours for 10 days.
Children: 40 mg/kg/day PO in three or four divided doses for 7 to 10 days. Maximum daily dose is 2 g.

➤**Staphylococcal enterocolitis**
Adults: 500 mg to 2 g PO in three or four divided doses daily for 7 to 10 days.
Children: 40 mg/kg/day PO in three or four divided doses for 7 to 10 days. Maximum daily dose is 2 g.

ADMINISTRATION
❸ *Alert:* Obtain specimen for culture and sensitivity tests before giving. Because of the emergence of vancomycin-resistant enterococci, reserve use for treatment of serious infections caused by gram-positive bacteria resistant to beta-lactam anti-infectives.
PO
• Powder for oral solution must be reconstituted by the pharmacist before use.
❸ *Alert:* Oral form is ineffective for systemic infections.
IV
▼ This form is ineffective for CDAD and staphylococcal enterocolitis. Reconstitute 500-mg vial with 10 mL, 750-mg vial with 15 mL, or 1-g vial with 20 mL sterile water for injection to provide a solution containing 50 mg/mL.
▼ Refrigerate solution after reconstitution and use within 96 hours.
▼ For infusion, further dilute 500 mg in 100 mL, 750 mg in 150 mL, or 1 g in 200 mL NSS for injection or D₅W, and infuse as soon as possible at no faster than 10 mg/minute or over at least 60 minutes, whichever is longer.
▼ Drug is an irritant; give by secure IV route and ensure proper needle or catheter placement before and during infusion. Pain, tenderness, and necrosis may occur with extravasation. Can minimize frequency and severity of thrombophlebitis by slow infusion of drug and rotation of venous access sites.

▼ Thawed, premixed solution is stable for 72 hours at room temperature or for 30 days in refrigerator. Don't refreeze.
❸ *Alert:* Rapid infusion (over several minutes) has been associated with hypotension, shock and, rarely, cardiac arrest. Check site daily for phlebitis and irritation. Severe irritation and necrosis can result from extravasation.
▼ **Incompatibilities:** Beta-lactam antibiotics, many other drugs (vancomycin has a low pH).

ACTION
Hinders bacterial cell-wall synthesis, damaging the bacterial plasma membrane and making the cell more vulnerable to osmotic pressure. Also interferes with RNA synthesis.

Route	Onset	Peak	Duration
PO	Unknown	Unknown	Unknown
IV	Immediate	Immediate	Unknown

Half-life: 4 to 6 hours (longer in patients with renal impairment).

ADVERSE REACTIONS
CNS: fever, pain, headache, fatigue. **CV:** hypotension, thrombophlebitis at injection site. **EENT:** ototoxicity, tinnitus. **GI:** *pseudomembranous colitis,* nausea, abdominal pain, vomiting, diarrhea, flatulence. **GU:** *nephrotoxicity.* **Hematologic:** *leukopenia, neutropenia,* eosinophilia. **Metabolic:** hypokalemia (PO). **Respiratory:** dyspnea, wheezing. **Skin:** red-man syndrome (with rapid IV infusion). **Other:** *anaphylaxis,* chills, superinfection.

INTERACTIONS
Drug-drug. *Aminoglycosides, amphotericin B, bacitracin, cisplatin, colistin, piperacillin, polymyxin B, viomycin:* May increase risk of nephrotoxicity and ototoxicity. Monitor renal function and hearing function tests.
Nondepolarizing muscle relaxants: May enhance neuromuscular blockade. Monitor patient closely.
NSAIDs: May increase vancomycin serum concentration. Monitor therapy.

V

EFFECTS ON LAB TEST RESULTS
• May increase BUN and creatinine levels. May decrease potassium level.
• May increase eosinophil count. May decrease neutrophil and WBC counts.

CONTRAINDICATIONS & CAUTIONS
• Contraindicated in patients hypersensitive to drug or its components.
• Use cautiously in patients receiving other neurotoxic, nephrotoxic, or ototoxic drugs; in patients older than age 60; and in those with impaired hepatic or renal function, hearing loss, or allergies to other antibiotics.
Dialyzable drug: Poorly dialyzable.

PREGNANCY-LACTATION-REPRODUCTION
• It isn't known if drug causes fetal harm. Use during pregnancy only if clearly needed.
• Drug appears in human milk. Patient should discontinue breastfeeding or discontinue drug.

NURSING CONSIDERATIONS
• Obtain hearing evaluation before and during prolonged therapy.
• Monitor patient's fluid balance and watch for oliguria and cloudy urine.
• Monitor patient carefully for red-man syndrome, which can occur if drug is infused too rapidly. Signs and symptoms include maculopapular rash on face, neck, trunk, and limbs and pruritus and hypotension caused by histamine release. If wheezing, urticaria, or pain and muscle spasm of the chest and back occur, stop infusion and notify prescriber.
• Don't give drug IM.
• Assess renal function (BUN, creatinine level and CrCl, urinalysis, and urine output) before and during therapy.
• Carefully monitor serum concentrations of vancomycin to adjust IV dosage requirements.
• Monitor patient for signs and symptoms of superinfection. CDAD can occur up to 2 months after therapy ends.
• *Look alike–sound alike:* Don't confuse vancomycin with clindamycin, gentamicin, or Vibramycin.

PATIENT TEACHING
• Tell patient to take entire amount of drug exactly as directed, even after feeling better.
• Instruct patient receiving drug IV to report discomfort at IV insertion site.
• Tell patient to report ringing in ears.
• Tell patient to report adverse reactions to prescriber immediately.

vardenafil hydrochloride
var-DEN-ah-fill

Levitra◆, Staxyn

Therapeutic class: Erectile dysfunction drugs
Pharmacologic class: PDE5 inhibitors

AVAILABLE FORMS
Tablets (film-coated): 5 mg, 10 mg, 20 mg
Tablets (ODTs) ⓞⓝⓒ: 10 mg

INDICATIONS & DOSAGES
➤ **Erectile dysfunction**
Adults: 10 mg PO as a single dose, as needed, 1 hour before sexual activity. Dosage range is 5 to 20 mg, based on effectiveness and tolerance. Maximum, 10 mg/day (Staxyn) or 20 mg once daily (Levitra).
Adjust-a-dose: For patients with moderate hepatic impairment (Child-Pugh class B) and patients age 65 and older, first dose of Levitra is 5 mg daily, as needed. Don't exceed 10 mg daily in patients with hepatic impairment. Dosage adjustment may be needed in patients taking potent CYP3A4 inhibitors. Consult manufacturer's instructions for drug-interaction dosage adjustments. Don't use Staxyn in patients with moderate or severe hepatic impairment (Child-Pugh class B or C) or in those taking potent or moderate CYP3A4 inhibitors.

ADMINISTRATION
PO
• Tablets and ODTs aren't interchangeable.
• Give drug without regard for food.
• Don't split or crush ODTs.
• Place ODT on the tongue to disintegrate. Have patient take without water or other liquid.

Reactions in bold italics are *life-threatening*. Interactions may have a *rapid onset* or a *delayed onset*.

• Don't remove ODT from blister pack until ready to use.

ACTION

Increases cyclic guanosine monophosphate levels, prolongs smooth muscle relaxation, and promotes blood flow into the corpus cavernosum by inhibiting PDE5.

Route	Onset	Peak	Duration
PO	60 min	30–120 min	Unknown

Half-life: 4 to 6 hours.

ADVERSE REACTIONS

CNS: headache, dizziness. **CV:** flushing, hypotension, tachycardia. **EENT:** blurred vision, decrease or loss of hearing, tinnitus, rhinitis, sinusitis, nasal congestion. **GI:** dyspepsia, nausea. **Musculoskeletal:** back pain. **Other:** flulike syndrome.

INTERACTIONS

Drug-drug. *Alpha blockers:* May enhance hypotensive effects. Start concomitant treatment at reduced dosage only if patient is stable on alpha-blocker therapy. Don't initiate concomitant treatment with Staxyn.
Antiarrhythmics of Class IA (quinidine, procainamide) and Class III (amiodarone, sotalol): May prolong QTc interval. Avoid using together.
Guanylate cyclase (GC) stimulators (riociguat), nitrates: May enhance hypotensive effects. Use together is contraindicated.
Potent and moderate CYP3A4 inhibitors (erythromycin, indinavir, itraconazole, ketoconazole, ritonavir): May increase vardenafil level. Reduce vardenafil dosage. If taken with ritonavir, reduce dose and extend dosing interval to once every 72 hours. Use with Staxyn is contraindicated.
Drug-food. *Grapefruit, grapefruit juice:* May increase vardenafil level. Avoid use together.
High-fat meals: May reduce peak level of drug. Discourage use with a high-fat meal.
Drug-lifestyle. *Alcohol use:* May increase risk of hypotension and orthostasis. Discourage use together.

EFFECTS ON LAB TEST RESULTS

• May increase CK and liver transaminase levels.

CONTRAINDICATIONS & CAUTIONS

• Contraindicated in patients hypersensitive to drug or its components and in those taking nitrates, nitric oxide donors, or GC stimulators.
• Not recommended in patients with unstable angina, hypotension (systolic less than 90 mm Hg), uncontrolled HTN (over 170/110 mm Hg), stroke, life-threatening arrhythmia, an MI within past 6 months, severe cardiac failure, severe hepatic impairment (Child-Pugh class C), ESRD requiring dialysis, congenital QTc-interval prolongation, or hereditary degenerative retinal disorders.
• Use cautiously in patients with bleeding disorders or significant peptic ulceration.
• Use cautiously in those with anatomic penis abnormalities or conditions that predispose patient to priapism (such as sickle cell anemia, multiple myeloma, or leukemia).
• May cause vision loss and visual disturbances. Use cautiously in patients with or at increased risk for nonarteritic ischemic optic neuropathy, "crowded optic disc."
Dialyzable drug: Unlikely.
⚠ Overdose S&S: Back pain or myalgia, abnormal vision.

PREGNANCY-LACTATION-REPRODUCTION

• Drug isn't indicated for use in women.

NURSING CONSIDERATIONS

⊕ Alert: Sexual activity may increase cardiac risk. Evaluate patient's cardiac risk before start of therapy.
• Before patient starts drug, assess for underlying causes of erectile dysfunction.
• Transient decreases in supine BP may occur.
• Prolonged erections and priapism may occur.

PATIENT TEACHING

• Tell patient that drug doesn't protect against sexually transmitted diseases and to use protective measures.
• Urge patient to seek immediate medical care if erection lasts more than 4 hours.
• Tell patient to take drug 60 minutes before anticipated sexual activity. Explain that drug has no effect without sexual stimulation.

V

- Warn patient not to change dosage unless directed by prescriber.
- Tell patient to stop drug and seek medical attention for sudden vision loss in one or both eyes or sudden decrease in or loss of hearing.
- Tell patient not to split, crush, or chew ODTs and not to take with a liquid.

varenicline tartrate
vah-RENN-ih-kleen

Champix�canada, Chantix✷

Therapeutic class: Smoking cessation aids
Pharmacologic class: Nicotinic acetyl-choline receptor partial agonists

AVAILABLE FORMS
Tablets: 0.5 mg, 1 mg

INDICATIONS & DOSAGES
➤ **Smoking cessation**
Adults: Starting 1 week before patient stops smoking, give 0.5 mg PO once daily on days 1 through 3. Days 4 through 7, give 0.5 mg PO b.i.d. Day 8 through the end of week 12, give 1 mg PO b.i.d. If patient successfully stops smoking, give an additional 12-week course to help with long-term success.
Adjust-a-dose: In patient with severe renal impairment, 0.5 mg PO once daily. Adjust as needed to maximum of 0.5 mg b.i.d. In patient with ESRD who is undergoing dialysis, 0.5 mg once daily.

ADMINISTRATION
PO
- Give drug with full glass of water after a meal.

ACTION
Blocks the effects of nicotine by binding at alpha$_4$ beta$_2$ neuronal nicotinic acetyl-choline receptors. Drug also increases dopamine activity, decreasing craving and withdrawal symptoms.

Route	Onset	Peak	Duration
PO	4 days	3–4 hr	24 hr

Half-life: 24 hours.

ADVERSE REACTIONS
CNS: abnormal dreams, headache, insomnia, altered attention or emotions, asthenia, depression, drowsiness, fatigue, irritability, lethargy, malaise, nightmares, sleep disorder, somnolence. **CV:** chest pain, edema, hot flush, HTN. **EENT:** altered taste. **GI:** nausea, abdominal pain, constipation, diarrhea, dry mouth, dyspepsia, flatulence, vomiting, GERD. **Metabolic:** increased or decreased appetite. **Respiratory:** dyspnea, URI. **Skin:** rash. **Other:** *suicidal ideation.*

INTERACTIONS
Drug-drug. *H$_2$-antagonists (cimetidine), quinolones, trimethoprim:* May increase varenicline serum concentration and decrease its renal clearance. Monitor patient closely.
Nicotine-replacement therapy: May increase nausea, vomiting, dizziness, dyspepsia, and fatigue. Monitor patient closely.
Drug-lifestyle. ⚠ Alert: *Alcohol use:* May decrease alcohol tolerance, with symptoms of increased drunkenness, unusual or aggressive behavior, or amnesia. Caution patient to reduce amount of alcohol consumed until ability to tolerate alcohol is known.

EFFECTS ON LAB TEST RESULTS
- May increase LFT values.

CONTRAINDICATIONS & CAUTIONS
- Contraindicated in patients hypersensitive to drug or its components.
- Consider risks versus benefits before use. Drug increases the likelihood of abstinence from smoking for as long as 1 year. Health benefits of quitting smoking are immediate and substantial.
⚠ Alert: Serious neuropsychiatric events have been reported with use of this drug. Carefully weigh risks versus benefits of smoking cessation.
⚠ Alert: Drug may be associated with increased risk of CV events (stroke, angina, MI, need for coronary revascularization, new diagnosis of PVD, or admission for a procedure to treat PVD) in patients who have CV disease. Consider risks and benefits before prescribing.
⚠ Alert: Drug may increase risk of seizures. Use cautiously in patients with a history

---

of seizures or who are at increased risk for seizures.

• Use cautiously in elderly patients and in patients with severe renal impairment or pre-existing psychiatric illness.

• Not recommended for use in children age 16 or younger.

Dialyzable drug: Yes.

PREGNANCY-LACTATION-REPRODUCTION

• There are no adequate studies in pregnant women. Use during pregnancy only if potential benefit justifies potential risk to the fetus.

• It isn't known if drug appears in human milk. Patient should discontinue breastfeeding or discontinue drug.

NURSING CONSIDERATIONS

• Assess patient's readiness and motivation to stop smoking.

• For patients who are sure they aren't able or willing to quit abruptly, consider a gradual approach by initiating drug and reducing smoking simultaneously until complete abstinence by 12 weeks. Then continue drug for additional 12 weeks.

• Encourage patient who is motivated to quit but didn't succeed during prior therapy or who relapsed after treatment, to make another attempt once factors contributing to the failed attempt have been identified and addressed.

❸ *Alert:* Monitor patient for changes in behavior, agitation, depressed mood, hostility, suicidal ideation, suicidal behavior, and worsening of preexisting psychiatric illness and report immediately.

• Notify prescriber if patient develops intolerable adverse reactions such as nausea; dosage reduction may be needed.

• Life-threatening angioedema and serious skin reactions have been reported. Discontinue drug for such signs and symptoms as swelling of the face, mouth, neck, or extremities or rash with mucosal lesions.

• Temporarily monitor levels of drugs (theophylline, warfarin, and insulin) after patient stops smoking to be sure levels are still within therapeutic range.

PATIENT TEACHING

• Provide patient with educational materials and needed counseling.

• Cases of sleepwalking have been reported in patients taking varenicline. Some patients have described harmful behavior to self, others, or property. Instruct patient to discontinue drug and notify prescriber if such behaviors occur.

• Instruct patient to choose a date to stop smoking and to begin treatment 1 week before this date. Or, patient can begin drug, then quit smoking between days 8 and 35.

• Advise patient to take each dose with a full glass of water after eating.

• Teach patient to gradually increase the dose over the first week to a target of 1 mg in the morning and 1 mg in the evening.

❸ *Alert:* Caution patient that drug can affect reaction to alcohol. Advise patient to reduce amount of alcohol consumed until patient's alcohol tolerance is known.

❸ *Alert:* Warn patient to stop drug and seek medical attention if seizures occur.

• Advise patient to discontinue drug and seek immediate medical care if swelling of the face, mouth, extremities, and neck or a rash with mucosal lesions develops.

• Explain that nausea and insomnia are common and usually temporary. Urge patient to contact prescriber if adverse effects are persistently troubling; a dosage reduction may help.

• Urge patient to continue trying to abstain from smoking if early lapses occur after successfully quitting.

• Tell patient that dosages of other drugs being taken may need adjustment when patient stops smoking.

• Advise patient to use caution when driving or operating machinery until effects of drug are known.

❸ *Alert:* Instruct patient and family to monitor patient for changes in behavior and mood, including agitation, depression, hostility, suicidal ideation or behavior, and worsening of preexisting psychiatric illness; stop drug and report changes to health care provider immediately.

• If female patient plans to become pregnant or to breastfeed, explain the risks of smoking and the risks and benefits of taking drug to aid smoking cessation.

V

vasopressin
vay-soe-PRESS-in

Vasostrict

Therapeutic class: Antidiuretic hormones
Pharmacologic class: Posterior pituitary hormones

AVAILABLE FORMS
Injection: 20 units/mL in 1-mL and 10-mL vials

INDICATIONS & DOSAGES
➤ **Vasodilatory shock in patients who remain hypotensive despite fluids and catecholamines**
Adults: For postcardiotomy shock, begin IV infusion at 0.03 unit/minute; for septic shock begin IV infusion at 0.01 unit/minute. If target BP isn't achieved, titrate dosage up by 0.005 unit/minute at 10- to 15-minute intervals. After target BP has been maintained for 8 hours (without use of catecholamines), taper drug by 0.005 unit/minute every hour as tolerated to maintain BP. Maximum dosage for postcardiotomy shock is 0.1 unit/minute and for septic shock, 0.07 unit/minute.

ADMINISTRATION
IV
▼ For IV infusion, dilute in NSS or D₅W to a concentration of 0.1 to 1 unit/mL. For fluid-restricted patients, mix 5 mL (100 units) in 100 mL; for non-fluid-restricted patients, mix 2.5 mL (50 units) in 500 mL.
▼ Titrate to lowest dosage compatible with a clinically acceptable response. Monitor BP every 10 to 15 minutes.
▼ Administer by CVAD if possible, using an infusion pump.
▼ Intact vials can be stored at 68° to 77° F (20° to 25° C) for up to 12 months.
▼ Discard unused diluted solution after 18 hours at room temperature or 24 hours under refrigeration. Discard vials 48 hours after first entry.
▼ **Incompatibilities:** None listed by manufacturer. Consult a drug incompatibility reference for more information.

ACTION
Causes contraction of smooth muscle in the vascular bed and increases systemic vascular resistance and mean arterial BP and decreases HR and cardiac output.

Route	Onset	Peak	Duration
IV	Rapid	15 min	20 min

Half-life: Less than 10 minutes.

ADVERSE REACTIONS
CNS: headache, vertigo. **CV:** *hemorrhagic shock, HF,* atrial fibrillation, bradycardia, vasoconstriction, *myocardial ischemia, decreased cardiac output, distal limb ischemia.* **Hematologic:** *thrombocytopenia.* **GI:** *mesenteric ischemia.* **GU:** acute renal insufficiency. **Metabolic:** hyponatremia. **Skin:** cutaneous gangrene.

INTERACTIONS
Drug-drug. *Catecholamines:* Causes additive effect on mean arterial pressure and other hemodynamic parameters. Use cautiously.
Drugs suspected of causing diabetes insipidus (clozapine, demeclocycline, foscarnet, lithium): May decrease pressor and antidiuretic effects. Use cautiously.
Drugs suspected of causing SIADH (chlorpropamide, cyclophosphamide, enalapril, felbamate, haloperidol, ifosfamide, methyldopa, pentamidine, SSRIs, TCAs, vincristine): May increase pressor and antidiuretic effects. Use cautiously.
Furosemide: Increases osmolar clearance and urine flow. Monitor urine output and hemodynamic parameters carefully.
Ganglionic blockers: May increase sensitivity to pressor effects. Monitor patient and BP.
Indomethacin: May prolong effect on cardiac index and systemic vascular resistance. Use cautiously.

EFFECTS ON LAB TEST RESULTS
• May increase bilirubin level. May decrease sodium level.
• May decrease platelet count.

CONTRAINDICATIONS & CAUTIONS
• Contraindicated in patients allergic or hypersensitive to 8-arginine vasopressin or

---

Reactions in bold italics are *life-threatening*. Interactions may have a *rapid onset* or a **delayed onset**.

chlorobutanol. Use in patients with impaired cardiac response may worsen cardiac output.
• Use cautiously in elderly patients.
• Safety and effectiveness in children haven't been established.
Dialyzable drug: Unknown.

⚠ *Overdose S&S:* Hyponatremia, ventricular arrhythmias, rhabdomyolysis, nonspecific GI symptoms, peripheral, mesenteric, or coronary ischemia.

PREGNANCY-LACTATION-REPRODUCTION
• There are no adequate studies in pregnant women, and it isn't known whether drug can cause fetal harm. Drug may produce tonic uterine contractions that could threaten continuation of pregnancy. Because of increased clearance during the second and third trimesters, dosage may need to be increased to 0.1 unit/minute when drug is used for postcardiotomy shock and 0.07 unit/minute when used in septic shock.
• It isn't known if drug appears in human milk. Consider advising breastfeeding women to express and discard milk for 1½ hours after receiving vasopressin, to minimize potential exposure to infant.

NURSING CONSIDERATIONS
❸ *Alert:* Extravasation may result in severe tissue damage. Ensure IV catheter is properly placed before and during infusion. If signs or symptoms of extravasation occur, stop infusion immediately and notify prescriber. If possible, withdraw 3 to 5 mL of blood to remove some of the drug and then remove infusion needle. Delineate infiltrated area on patient's skin with felt-tip marker and elevate the arm above the heart. Avoid pressure or friction. The extravasation site may need to be infiltrated with phentolamine or an alternative drug, depending on facility protocol. Signs of necrosis may need surgical treatment.
• Monitor patient for hypersensitivity reactions, including urticaria, angioedema, bronchoconstriction, and anaphylaxis.
• Monitor BP and hemodynamic parameters every 10 to 15 minutes during therapy.
• Monitor urine specific gravity and fluid intake and output to aid evaluation of drug effectiveness.

• Monitor ECG and fluid or electrolyte status periodically.
• Monitor patients for bleeding, palpitations, or signs and symptoms of ischemia (chest pain, limb peripheral pain, paresthesia, coldness, decreased or absent pulses, abdominal pain, nausea, vomiting).
• *Look alike–sound alike:* Don't confuse vasopressin with desmopressin.

PATIENT TEACHING
• Tell patient to immediately report all adverse reactions, especially bleeding, chest pain, palpitations, limb pain, limb coldness and pallor, paresthesia, nausea, vomiting, or abdominal pain.
• Tell patient to immediately report signs or symptoms of hypersensitivity reactions (breathing difficulty, wheezing, hives, nausea, vomiting, or swelling of the face, lips, or tongue).
• Tell patient to immediately report infusion-site symptoms.

SAFETY ALERT!

venetoclax
ven-ET-oh-klax

Venclexta

Therapeutic class: Antineoplastics
Pharmacologic class: BCL-2 inhibitors

AVAILABLE FORMS
Tablets ⓞ: 10 mg, 50 mg, 100 mg

INDICATIONS & DOSAGES
Adjust-a-dose (for all indications): Refer to manufacturer's instructions for TLS, drug interaction, and toxicity-related dosage adjustments and management.
➤ **Chronic lymphocytic leukemia (CLL) or small lymphocytic lymphoma (SLL)**
Adults: Initially, 20 mg PO once daily week 1; increase to 50 mg PO once daily week 2; increase to 100 mg PO once daily week 3; increase to 200 mg PO once daily week 4; then increase to 400 mg PO once daily week 5 and thereafter. Continue until disease progression or unacceptable toxicity occurs.

If drug is used in combination with rituximab, start rituximab after patient has

V

completed the 5-week dose ramp-up schedule with venetoclax and has received the 400-mg dose for 7 days. Give rituximab on day 1 of each 28-day cycle for six cycles, with rituximab dosed at 375 mg/m^2 IV for cycle 1 and 500 mg/m^2 IV for cycles 2 to 6. Continue venetoclax 400 mg once daily for 24 months from cycle 1 day 1 of rituximab.

If drug is used in combination with obinutuzumab, refer to manufacturer's instructions.

➤ **Treatment of newly diagnosed acute myeloid leukemia (AML) in combination with azacitidine or decitabine or low-dose cytarabine in patients age 75 or older, or in patients who have comorbidities that preclude use of intensive induction chemotherapy**

Adults taking venetoclax in combination with azacitidine or decitabine: Initially, on day 1 give 100 mg PO once daily; on day 2 increase to 200 mg PO once daily; on day 3 increase to 400 mg PO once daily and then give 400 mg PO once daily thereafter. Continue until disease progression or unacceptable toxicity occurs.

Adults taking venetoclax in combination with low-dose cytarabine: Initially, on day 1 give 100 mg PO once daily; on day 2 increase to 200 mg PO once daily; on day 3 increase to 400 mg PO once daily; on day 4 increase to 600 mg PO once daily and then give 600 mg PO once daily thereafter. Continue until disease progression or unacceptable toxicity occurs.

ADMINISTRATION
PO
☉ Alert: Hazardous drug; use safe handling and disposal precautions. Wear gloves to handle tablet.
- Give with a meal and water at approximately the same time each day.
- If a dose is missed and it's within 8 hours of the usual dosing time, give missed dose as soon as possible and resume normal daily dosing schedule. If it has been more than 8 hours, don't give missed dose and resume usual dosing schedule the next day.
- If patient vomits after administration of a dose, don't give additional doses that day; give next dose at the usual time.

- Tablets must be swallowed whole; don't crush, break, or allow patient to chew tablets.
- Store at or below 86° F (30° C).

ACTION
An inhibitor of B-cell lymphoma 2 (BCL-2), an antiapoptotic protein. Overexpression of BCL-2 has been demonstrated in CLL cells and has been associated with resistance to chemotherapeutic agents. Venetoclax helps restore apoptosis by binding directly to the BCL-2 protein, displacing proapoptotic proteins and restoring the apoptotic process.

Route	Onset	Peak	Duration
PO	Unknown	5–8 hr	Unknown

Half-life: 26 hours.

ADVERSE REACTIONS
CNS: fatigue, headache, fever. **CV:** peripheral edema. **GI:** diarrhea, nausea, vomiting, constipation. **Hematologic:** *neutropenia,* anemia, *thrombocytopenia, febrile neutropenia, autoimmune hemolytic anemia.* **Metabolic:** *hyperkalemia,* hyperphosphatemia, *hypokalemia, hypocalcemia,* hyperuricemia, *TLS.* **Musculoskeletal:** back pain. **Respiratory:** URI, cough, pneumonia.

INTERACTIONS
Drug-drug. *Live attenuated vaccines:* Safety and effectiveness haven't been studied and vaccines may be less effective. Don't give vaccines before, during, or after treatment until B-cell recovery occurs.
Moderate CYP3A inducers (bosentan, efavirenz, etravirine, modafinil, nafcillin), strong CYP3A inducers (carbamazepine, phenytoin, rifampin): May decrease venetoclax level. Consider alternative treatments.
Moderate CYP3A inhibitors (ciprofloxacin, diltiazem, dronedarone, erythromycin, fluconazole, verapamil), P-gp inhibitors (amiodarone, azithromycin, captopril, carvedilol, cyclosporine, felodipine, quinidine, ranolazine, ticagrelor): May increase venetoclax level and risk of TLS. Consider alternative treatments. If a moderate inhibitor must be used, reduce venetoclax dosage by at least 50%; monitor patient closely. Resume venetoclax dose that was used before initiating

---

Reactions in bold italics are *life-threatening*. Interactions may have a *rapid onset* or a *delayed onset*.

the inhibitor 2 to 3 days after discontinuing inhibitor.

P-gp substrates (digoxin, everolimus, sirolimus): May inhibit absorption of P-gp substrates. Avoid administration of narrow therapeutic index P-gp substrates with venetoclax. If substrate must be used, patient should take it at least 6 hours before venetoclax.

Strong CYP3A inhibitors (clarithromycin, conivaptan, indinavir, itraconazole, ketoconazole, lopinavir, posaconazole, ritonavir, telaprevir, voriconazole): May increase venetoclax level and risk of TLS. Use during initiation and ramp-up phase is contraindicated. For patients who have completed ramp-up phase and are on a steady daily dose of venetoclax, reduce venetoclax dosage by at least 75% when used concomitantly with strong CYP3A inhibitors. Resume venetoclax dose that was used before initiating the CYP3A inhibitor 2 to 3 days after discontinuing inhibitor.

Warfarin: May increase INR. Monitor INR closely.

Drug-herb. *St. John's wort:* May decrease venetoclax level. Don't use together.

Drug-food. *Grapefruit products, Seville oranges, starfruit:* May increase venetoclax level. Avoid use together.

EFFECTS ON LAB TEST RESULTS

• May increase phosphate and uric acid levels. May decrease calcium level. May increase or decrease potassium level.

• May decrease Hb, hematocrit, and neutrophil and platelet counts.

CONTRAINDICATIONS & CAUTIONS

• Contraindicated in patients hypersensitive to drug or its components.

• Contraindicated with strong CYP3A inhibitors at initiation and during ramp-up phase due to the potential for increased risk of TLS.

⊙ **Alert:** Drug may cause a rapid reduction in tumor volume and increases the risk of TLS and renal failure (requiring dialysis); fatalities have been reported. Risk of TLS increases with high tumor burden, concomitant use of CYP3A or P-gp inhibitors, and comorbidities. The 5-week ramp-up dosing

schedule is designed to gradually reduce tumor burden and decrease risk of TLS.

• Use cautiously in patients with hepatic impairment. Adverse events may be increased in patients with moderate impairment; monitor patients closely for toxicity, especially during initiation and ramp-up period. Use hasn't been studied in patients with severe impairment.

• Use cautiously in patients with renal impairment. Patients with decreased renal function (CrCl of less than 80 mL/minute) are at increased risk for TLS and may require more intensive TLS prophylaxis and monitoring during treatment initiation and dosage escalation.

⊙ **Alert:** Drug may cause bone marrow suppression (neutropenia, thrombocytopenia, anemia). Grade 3 and 4 neutropenia occurs in 50% of patients taking drug.

• Fatal and serious infections, such as pneumonia and sepsis, have occurred in patients treated with venetoclax.

• Safety and effectiveness in children haven't been established.

Dialyzable drug: Unlikely.

PREGNANCY-LACTATION-REPRODUCTION

• Drug may cause fetal harm. Women of childbearing potential should have pregnancy testing before therapy and use effective contraception during and for at least 30 days after treatment ends. Women who become pregnant while taking venetoclax should be made aware of risk to the fetus.

• Based on animal data, venetoclax may compromise fertility in males.

• It isn't known if drug appears in human milk. Because of the potential for serious adverse reactions in the breastfed infant, patient should discontinue breastfeeding.

NURSING CONSIDERATIONS

• Patients at high risk for TLS may require hospitalization at treatment initiation.

• Assess patient for risk of TLS before treatment (radiographic evaluation; assessment of potassium, uric acid, phosphorus, calcium, and creatinine levels and renal function). Give prophylactic hydration and antihyperuricemics before first dose of venetoclax as clinically indicated. See prescribing

V

information for recommended TLS prophylaxis and monitoring.
• Monitor serum chemistry values. Changes due to TLS can occur as soon as 6 to 8 hours after first dose and at each dosage increase.
• Monitor CBC with differential throughout treatment; treatment interruption and dosage reduction may be required. Consider WBC growth factor support as clinically indicated.
• Monitor patient for infection, including neutropenic fever. Treat with antimicrobials as appropriate. Withhold drug for grade 3 and higher infection.
• *Look alike–sound alike:* Don't confuse venetoclax with vandetanib, vemurafenib, venlafaxine, or vismodegib. Don't confuse Venclexta with venlafaxine.

PATIENT TEACHING
• Teach patient that treatment may be interrupted, dosage decreased, or treatment stopped due to adverse effects. Tell patient to report all adverse reactions promptly.
• Advise patient of risk of TLS, particularly at treatment initiation and during ramp-up phase, and to immediately report TLS signs and symptoms (fever, chills, nausea, vomiting, confusion, shortness of breath, seizures, irregular heartbeat, dark or cloudy urine, unusual tiredness, muscle pain, joint discomfort).
• Inform patient that it may be necessary to take drug under direct medical supervision to allow for monitoring for TLS.
• Advise patient to maintain adequate hydration to reduce risk of TLS. Recommended intake is 6 to 8 glasses (56 oz) beginning 2 days before treatment, on first day of treatment, and each time dosage is increased.
• Warn patient to immediately report fever or signs and symptoms of infection.
• Remind patient of importance of keeping scheduled appointments for blood work or other lab tests to monitor for adverse effects.
• Caution patient that venetoclax may interact with other drugs. Advise patient to report the use of prescription and OTC medications and supplements and not to start new medications or supplements without first discussing with prescriber.

• Instruct patient to avoid consuming grapefruit products, Seville oranges, or starfruit during treatment.
• Advise patient to avoid vaccination with live-virus vaccines during treatment.
• Teach patient that if a dose is missed by less than 8 hours, to take missed dose right away and take the next dose as usual.
• Advise patient that if vomiting occurs after taking venetoclax, not to take an additional dose that day, but to take the next dose at the usual time the following day.
• Caution female patient of childbearing potential to use effective contraception during and for at least 30 days after therapy ends.
• Instruct female patient to immediately contact prescriber if she becomes pregnant, is planning a pregnancy, or suspects she is pregnant.
• Warn female patient not to breastfeed during treatment.
• Advise male patient of risk of infertility due to treatment and of the option of sperm banking.

venlafaxine hydrochloride
ven-la-FAX-een

Effexor XR⬦

Therapeutic class: Antidepressants
Pharmacologic class: SSNRIs

AVAILABLE FORMS
Capsules (extended-release) ⓄⓃⒸ: 37.5 mg, 75 mg, 150 mg
Tablets: 25 mg, 37.5 mg, 50 mg, 75 mg, 100 mg
Tablets (extended-release) ⓄⓃⒸ: 37.5 mg, 75 mg, 150 mg, 225 mg

INDICATIONS & DOSAGES
Adjust-a-dose (for all indications): For patients with mild to moderate renal impairment (CrCl 30 to 89 mL/minute), reduce daily amount by 25% in patients taking immediate-release tablets. Reduce by 25% to 50% in those taking extended-release form. For those with severe renal impairment (CrCl less than 30 mL/minute) or on hemodialysis, reduce total daily dose by 50% or more and withhold dose until

---

Reactions in bold italics are *life-threatening*. Interactions may have a *rapid onset* or a *delayed onset*.

dialysis is completed. For patients with mild to moderate hepatic impairment (Child-Pugh score 5 to 9), reduce daily amount by 50%. For patients with severe hepatic impairment (Child-Pugh score 10 to 15) or cirrhosis, reduce total daily dose by 50% or more.

> **Depression**

Adults: Initially, 75 mg (immediate-release) PO daily in two or three divided doses with food. Increase as tolerated and needed by 75 mg daily every 4 days. For moderately depressed outpatients, usual maximum is 225 mg daily; in certain severely depressed patients, dose may be as high as 375 mg daily. For extended-release capsules or tablets, 75 mg PO daily in a single dose. For some patients, it may be desirable to start at 37.5 mg PO daily for 4 to 7 days before increasing to 75 mg daily. Dosage may be increased by 75 mg daily every 4 days to maximum of 225 mg daily.

> **Generalized anxiety disorder**

Adults: Initially, 75 mg extended-release capsule PO daily in a single dose. For some patients, it may be desirable to start at 37.5 mg PO daily for 4 to 7 days before increasing to 75 mg daily. Dosage may be increased by 75 mg daily every 4 days to maximum of 225 mg daily.

> **Panic disorder**

Adults: Initially, 37.5 mg extended-release capsule PO daily for 1 week, then increase dose to 75 mg daily. If patient isn't responding, may increase dose by up to 75 mg/day in no less than weekly intervals, as needed, to a maximum dose of 225 mg daily.

> **Social anxiety disorder**

Adults: Initially, 75 mg extended-release capsule or tablet PO daily as a single dose.

> **Hot flashes ◆**

Adults: Initially, 37.5 mg once daily; may increase after 1 week based on response and tolerability to 75 mg once daily for extended-release forms or 75 mg/day in two to three divided doses for immediate-release form.

ADMINISTRATION
PO
• Give drug with food and a full glass of water.

• For extended-release capsules and tablets, don't divide, crush, place in water, or allow patient to chew.
• May give pellet-filled capsules by carefully opening capsule and sprinkling the pellets on a spoonful of applesauce. Patient should swallow applesauce immediately without chewing, then follow with a glass of cool water to ensure that all pellets are swallowed.

ACTION
Potent and selective inhibitor of neuronal serotonin and norepinephrine reuptake and weak inhibitor of dopamine reuptake.

Route	Onset	Peak	Duration
PO (immediate-release)	Unknown	2 hr	Unknown
PO (extended-release)	Unknown	5½ hr	Unknown

Half-life: 3 to 7 hours.

ADVERSE REACTIONS
CNS: asthenia, headache, palpitations, somnolence, dizziness, nervousness, insomnia, anxiety, tremor, abnormal dreams, paresthesia, agitation, weakness. **CV:** HTN, tachycardia, vasodilation, chest pain. **EENT:** blurred vision, mydriasis. **GI:** nausea, constipation, dry mouth, anorexia, vomiting, diarrhea, dyspepsia, flatulence. **GU:** abnormal ejaculation, erectile dysfunction, anorgasmia, urinary frequency, impaired urination, decreased libido. **Metabolic:** weight gain, weight loss, increased appetite, hypercholesterolemia. **Skin:** diaphoresis, ecchymosis, rash. **Other:** yawning, chills, *suicidal behavior.*

INTERACTIONS
Drug-drug. *Anticoagulants, aspirin, NSAIDs:* May increase antiplatelet effect of aspirin and NSAIDs and anticoagulant effect of anticoagulants. Monitor patient for increased risk of bleeding.
Lithium: May increase serotonergic effect of drug. Serotonin syndrome (restlessness, hallucinations, loss of coordination, fast heartbeat, rapid changes in BP, increased body temperature, hyperreflexia, nausea, vomiting, and diarrhea) may occur. Monitor patient closely.

V

♣ Canada   ◇ OTC   ◆ Off-label use   ✐ Photoguide   ⓓ Do not crush   *Liquid contains alcohol   ☒ Genetic

MAO inhibitors (phenelzine, selegiline, tranyl-cypromine): May cause serotonin syndrome and signs and symptoms resembling NMS. Avoid using within 14 days of MAO inhibitor therapy.

Methylene blue (IV), linezolid: May cause serotonin syndrome. Use together is contraindicated.

*Other serotonergic drugs (5-HT$_3$ antagonists, fentanyl, meperidine, **tramadol**, trazodone):* May cause serotonin syndrome. Monitor patient closely.

Triptans: May cause serotonin syndrome or NMS-like reactions. Use cautiously and with increased monitoring at the start of therapy and with dose increase.

Warfarin: May increase PT, PTT, or INR. Monitor these lab values and patient closely.

Drug-herb. *St. John's wort:* May cause serotonin syndrome. Monitor patient closely.

Drug-lifestyle. *Alcohol use:* May increase mental and psychomotor impairment. Avoid alcohol.

EFFECTS ON LAB TEST RESULTS
• May cause false-positive urine immunoassay screening tests for phencyclidine and amphetamine.
• May increase cholesterol and triglyceride levels.

CONTRAINDICATIONS & CAUTIONS
• Contraindicated in patients hypersensitive to drug or within 14 days of stopping MAO inhibitor therapy. Don't start MAO inhibitor less than 7 days after stopping venlafaxine.

Black Box Warning Venlafaxine isn't approved for use in children. ∎

☯ Alert: Concomitant use with serotonergic drugs, linezolid, or methylene blue can cause serotonin syndrome. Concomitant use of these drugs and venlafaxine is recommended only for life-threatening or urgent conditions when the potential benefits outweigh the risks of toxicity.
• Concomitant use with tryptophan supplements isn't recommended.
• Use cautiously in patients with renal impairment, diseases or conditions that could affect hemodynamic responses or metabolism, and in those with history of mania or seizures.

• May trigger an angle-closure attack. Use cautiously in patients at risk for acute narrow-angle glaucoma.
• Hyponatremia can occur, which may be a result of SIADH. Elderly, volume-depleted patients and those taking diuretics are at increased risk. Discontinue drug if patient develops symptomatic hyponatremia.

Dialyzable drug: Unlikely.

⚠ Overdose S&S: Altered level of consciousness, tachycardia, bradycardia, mydriasis, seizures, vomiting, ECG changes, hypotension, liver necrosis, rhabdomyolysis, serotonin syndrome, vertigo, death.

PREGNANCY-LACTATION-REPRODUCTION
• There are no adequate studies in pregnant women. Use during pregnancy only if clearly needed and potential benefit justifies potential risks to the fetus.

☯ Alert: Neonates exposed to drug during the late third trimester have developed complications (sometimes immediately upon delivery) that require respiratory support, tube feedings, and prolonged hospitalization.
• Drug may appear in human milk. Patient should discontinue breastfeeding or discontinue drug.

NURSING CONSIDERATIONS
Black Box Warning Closely monitor patients being treated for depression for signs and symptoms of clinical worsening and suicidal ideation, especially at the beginning of therapy and with dosage adjustments. Symptoms may include agitation, insomnia, anxiety, aggressiveness, or panic attacks. ∎

Black Box Warning Drug may increase the risk of suicidal thinking and behavior in children, adolescents, and young adults ages 18 to 24, especially during the first few months of treatment, especially those with major depressive disorder or other psychiatric disorder. ∎

☯ Alert: Sudden discontinuation or abrupt decrease in venlafaxine dose can lead to serotonin withdrawal (agitation, confusion, flulike symptoms, sensory disturbances, tremor). Reduce dose gradually and watch for symptoms.

☯ Alert: If linezolid or methylene blue must be given, stop venlafaxine and monitor patient for serotonin toxicity for 2 weeks or

---

until 24 hours after last dose of methylene blue or linezolid, whichever comes first. May resume serotonergic psychiatric drugs 24 hours after last dose of methylene blue or linezolid.
• Carefully monitor BP. Drug therapy may cause sustained, dose-dependent increases in BP.
• Monitor patient's weight, particularly in underweight, depressed patients.
🛈 *Alert:* Combining triptans with an SSRI or an SSNRI may cause serotonin syndrome or NMS-like reactions. Signs and symptoms of serotonin syndrome may include restlessness, hallucinations, loss of coordination, fast heartbeat, rapid changes in BP, increased body temperature, overactive reflexes, nausea, vomiting, and diarrhea. Serotonin syndrome may be more likely to occur when starting or increasing the dose of triptan, SSRI, or SSNRI.

PATIENT TEACHING
• If medication is to be stopped, inform patient who has received drug for 6 weeks or longer that drug will be stopped gradually by tapering dosage over a 2-week period, as instructed by prescriber. Patient shouldn't abruptly stop taking the drug.
▐ Black Box Warning ▐ Warn family members to closely monitor patient for signs of worsening condition or suicidal ideation. ▮
• Warn patient to avoid hazardous activities that require alertness and good coordination until effects of drug are known.
• Tell patient to avoid alcohol and to consult prescriber before taking other prescription or OTC drugs or supplements.
• Teach patient to recognize and immediately report signs and symptoms of serotonin toxicity (fever, mental status changes, muscle twitching, excessive sweating, shivering or shaking, diarrhea, loss of coordination).
• Advise female patient of childbearing potential to contact prescriber if she becomes pregnant or intends to become pregnant during therapy or if she's breastfeeding.
• Tell patient to take each dose with food and a full glass of water.
• Tell patient not to crush, chew, or place extended-release capsules or tablets in water. If patient can't swallow capsule whole, advise patient to carefully open capsule and

sprinkle contents on a spoonful of applesauce, mix and take immediately without chewing pellets, then follow with a full glass of water.

verapamil hydrochloride
ver-AP-a-mill

Calan🖉, Calan SR, Isoptin SR✢, Verelan🖉, Verelan PM

Therapeutic class: Antihypertensives
Pharmacologic class: Calcium channel blockers

AVAILABLE FORMS
Capsules (extended-release) 🄓🄝🄒*:* 100 mg, 120 mg, 180 mg, 200 mg, 240 mg, 300 mg, 360 mg
Injection: 2.5 mg/mL
Tablets: 40 mg, 80 mg, 120 mg
Tablets (extended-release) 🄓🄝🄒*:* 120 mg, 180 mg, 240 mg

INDICATIONS & DOSAGES
Adjust-a-dose (for all indications): In patients with severe liver dysfunction, give 30% of dose. For Verelan PM, reduce dosage to 100 mg once daily in patients with renal or hepatic impairment, in elderly patients, and in those with low weight.
➤ **Vasospastic angina (Prinzmetal or variant angina); unstable angina; classic chronic, stable angina pectoris; chronic atrial fibrillation**
Adults: Starting dose is 80 to 120 mg (immediate-release) PO t.i.d. Increase dosage at daily or weekly intervals as needed. Some patients may require up to 480 mg daily. Don't exceed 480 mg/day.
➤ **To prevent paroxysmal supraventricular tachycardia**
Adults: 240 to 480 mg (immediate-release) PO daily, in three or four divided doses. Don't exceed 480 mg/day.
➤ **Atrial flutter/atrial fibrillation; supraventricular arrhythmias**
Adults: 0.075 to 0.15 mg/kg (5 to 10 mg) by IV push over 2 minutes with ECG and BP monitoring. Repeat dose of 0.15 mg/kg (10 mg) in 30 minutes if response is inadequate.

V

Children ages 1 to 15: Give 0.1 to 0.3 mg/kg as IV bolus over 2 minutes; not to exceed 5 mg. Repeat dose in 30 minutes if response is inadequate. Don't exceed 10 mg as a single dose.

Children younger than age 1: Give 0.1 to 0.2 mg/kg as IV bolus over 2 minutes with continuous ECG monitoring. Repeat dose in 30 minutes if response is inadequate.

➤ **Digitalized patients with chronic atrial fibrillation or flutter**
Adults: 240 to 320 mg (immediate-release) PO daily, in three or four divided doses.

➤ **HTN**
Adults: 240 mg extended-release tablet (Verelan) PO once daily in the morning. If response isn't adequate, may increase by 120 mg daily (maximum, 480 mg). If using Verelan PM, 200 mg PO daily at bedtime. May increase to 300 mg at bedtime if response is inadequate. Maximum dose is 400 mg. If using Calan SR, give 180 mg PO in the morning. Evaluate weekly and approximately 24 hours after previous dose. May increase as follows: 240 mg each morning, 180 mg each morning plus 180 mg each evening, or 240 mg each morning plus 120 mg each evening; 240 mg every 12 hours. For immediate-release, 80 mg PO t.i.d.

ADMINISTRATION
PO
• Pellet-filled capsules may be given by carefully opening the capsule and sprinkling the pellets on a spoonful of applesauce. This should be swallowed immediately without chewing, followed by a glass of cool water to ensure that all the pellets are swallowed.
• An oral suspension may be compounded by a pharmacist if needed.
• Give long-acting forms of the drug whole; don't crush or break tablet.

IV
▼ This form is contraindicated in patients receiving IV beta blockers and in those with ventricular tachycardia.
▼ Inject directly into a vein or into the tubing of a free-flowing, compatible solution, such as D₅W, half-NSS, NSS, Ringer solution, or lactated Ringer solution.

▼ Give doses over at least 2 minutes (3 minutes in elderly patients) to minimize the risk of adverse reactions.
▼ Monitor ECG and BP continuously.
▼ **Incompatibilities:** Albumin, amphotericin B, hydralazine, sodium bicarbonate, solutions with a pH greater than 6, sulfamethoxazole–trimethoprim.

ACTION
A calcium channel blocker that inhibits calcium ion influx across cardiac and smooth-muscle cells, thus decreasing myocardial contractility and oxygen demand; it also dilates coronary arteries and arterioles.

Route	Onset	Peak	Duration
PO	1–2 hr	1–2 hr	8–10 hr
PO (extended)	30 min	5–9 hr	24 hr
IV	Immediate	1–5 min	½–6 hr

Half-life: 2.8 to 12 hours (varies by product).

ADVERSE REACTIONS
CNS: dizziness, headache, asthenia, fatigue, sleep disturbances. **CV:** transient hypotension, *HF, bradycardia, AV block, ventricular asystole, ventricular fibrillation,* peripheral edema. **GI:** constipation, nausea, diarrhea, dyspepsia, gingival hyperplasia. **Respiratory:** dyspnea, pharyngitis, *pulmonary edema,* rhinitis, sinusitis, URI. **Skin:** rash.

INTERACTIONS
Drug-drug. *Amiodarone:* May cause bradycardia and decrease cardiac output. Monitor patient closely.
Antihypertensives, quinidine: May cause hypotension. Monitor BP.
Barbiturates (phenobarbital): May increase verapamil clearance. Monitor response and adjust verapamil dose as needed.
Beta blockers (oral), **digoxin:** May increase digoxin level and effects of both drugs. Monitor digoxin level and cardiac function closely and decrease doses as needed.
Betrixaban: May increase betrixaban serum concentration. Consider therapy modification.
Carbamazepine: May increase levels of carbamazepine. Monitor patient for toxicity and adjust dosage as needed.

Reactions in bold italics are *life-threatening*. Interactions may have a *rapid onset* or a *delayed onset*.

Cyclosporine: May increase cyclosporine level. Monitor cyclosporine level.

Disopyramide, flecainide: May cause HF. Avoid using together.

Dofetilide: May increase dofetilide level. Avoid using together.

HMG-CoA reductase inhibitors (atorvastatin, lovastatin, simvastatin): May elevate plasma concentrations of these drugs. If coadministration can't be avoided, administer conservative dose of the HMG-CoA reductase inhibitor.

Inhalation anesthetics (enflurane): May potentiate cardiac effects. Titrate doses carefully to avoid excessive CV depression.

Lithium: May decrease or increase lithium level. Monitor lithium level.

Macrolide antibiotics (clarithromycin, erythromycin): May increase erythromycin and verapamil levels. Monitor cardiac function closely and adjust doses as needed.

Neuromuscular blockers: May potentiate the activity of these drugs. Monitor neuromuscular function, and adjust dosages of either drug as needed.

Phenytoin: May increase phenytoin level and decrease effects of verapamil. Monitor patient closely and adjust dosage as needed.

Rifampin: May decrease oral bioavailability of verapamil. Monitor patient for lack of effect.

Sirolimus, tacrolimus: May increase levels of these drugs. Monitor drug levels closely and adjust dosage as needed.

Theophylline: May decrease clearance of theophylline. Monitor for signs of theophylline toxicity.

Drug-herb. *St. John's wort:* May decrease drug level and effect. Discourage use together.

Drug-food. *Grapefruit juice:* May increase drug level. Discourage use together.

Drug-lifestyle. *Alcohol use:* May increase serum concentration of alcohol. Discourage use together.

EFFECTS ON LAB TEST RESULTS

• May increase ALT, AST, alkaline phosphatase, and bilirubin levels.

• May cause false-positive urine detection of methadone.

CONTRAINDICATIONS & CAUTIONS

• Oral and IV forms are contraindicated in patients hypersensitive to drug and in those with severe left ventricular dysfunction, cardiogenic shock, second- or third-degree AV block, or sick sinus syndrome except in presence of functioning pacemaker, atrial flutter or fibrillation and accessory bypass tract syndrome, severe HF (unless secondary to therapy), and severe hypotension.

• IV form is contraindicated in patients receiving IV beta blockers and in those with ventricular tachycardia.

• Use cautiously in elderly patients, children, and those with increased ICP or hepatic or renal disease.

Dialyzable drug: No.

⚠ **Overdose S&S:** Hypotension, bradycardia, arrhythmias, hyperglycemia, depressed mental status, noncardiogenic pulmonary edema, increasing AV block.

PREGNANCY-LACTATION-REPRODUCTION

• There are no adequate studies in pregnant women. Use during pregnancy only if clearly needed. Fetal monitoring is recommended.

• Drug appears in human milk. Some manufacturers recommend that patients stop breastfeeding.

NURSING CONSIDERATIONS

• Patients receiving beta blockers should receive lower doses of oral drug. Monitor these patients closely.

• Frequently monitor PR interval.

• Monitor BP at the start of therapy and during dosage adjustments. Assist patient with walking because dizziness may occur.

• If signs and symptoms of HF occur, such as swelling of hands and feet and shortness of breath, notify prescriber.

• Monitor renal function test and LFT results during prolonged treatment.

• *Look alike–sound alike:* Don't confuse Verelan with Vivarin or Voltaren.

PATIENT TEACHING

• Tell patient to report all adverse reactions, especially palpitations, slow heartbeat, dizziness, dyspnea, or swelling.

• Instruct patient to take oral form of drug exactly as prescribed.

V

• Tell patient not to crush or chew extended-release forms.

• Caution patient against abruptly stopping drug.

• If patient continues nitrate therapy during oral verapamil dosage adjustment, urge continued compliance. SL nitroglycerin may be taken, as needed, for acute chest pain.

• Drug significantly inhibits alcohol elimination. Advise patient to avoid or severely limit alcohol use.

vigabatrin
veye-gah-BA-trin

Sabril, Vigadrone

Therapeutic class: Anticonvulsants
Pharmacologic class: GABA transaminase inhibitors

AVAILABLE FORMS
Powder for oral solution: 500 mg
Tablets: 500 mg

INDICATIONS & DOSAGES
➤ **Refractory complex partial seizures in patients with inadequate response to several alternative treatments**
Adults and children age 17 and older and children ages 10 to 16 weighing more than 60 kg: Initially, 500 mg PO b.i.d. May increase dosage by 500 mg weekly to maximum of 1,500 mg PO b.i.d.
Children ages 10 to 16 weighing 25 to 60 kg: Initially, 250 mg PO b.i.d. Increase weekly in 500-mg/day (250 mg b.i.d.) increments to a total maintenance dose of 2,000 mg/day (1,000 mg b.i.d.).
Adjust-a-dose: For patients with CrCl of 51 to 80 mL/minute, reduce dosage by 25%; for CrCl of 31 to 50 mL/minute, decrease dosage by 50%; for CrCl of 11 to 30 mL/minute, decrease dosage by 75%.
➤ **Infantile spasms**
Infants and children ages 1 month to 2 years: 50 mg/kg/day PO given in two divided doses. Titrate in 25- to 50-mg/kg/day increments every 3 days as needed. Maximum dose is 150 mg/kg/day.

ADMINISTRATION
PO
• Hazardous drug; use safe handling and disposal precautions.

• Drug may be given with or without food.

• The entire contents of the appropriate number of packets (500 mg/packet) of powder should be emptied into an empty cup, and should be dissolved in 10 mL of cold or room-temperature water per packet using the 10-mL oral syringe supplied with the medication. The concentration of the final solution is 50 mg/mL. Use immediately after reconstitution and discard any unused portion.

• Discard solution if it isn't clear, colorless, and free of particles.

ACTION
Precise mechanism unknown. Thought to control seizures by inhibiting GABA transaminase, the enzyme responsible for metabolizing the inhibitory neurotransmitter GABA, thereby increasing GABA levels in the CNS.

Route	Onset	Peak	Duration
PO	Unknown	1–2½ hr	Unknown

Half-life: 5½ to 10½ hours.

ADVERSE REACTIONS
CNS: abnormal behavior, abnormal coordination, abnormal dreams, abnormal thinking, anxiety, asthenia, attention disturbance, confusion, *seizures,* depression, dizziness, dysarthria, expressive language disorder, fatigue, fever, headache, hyperreflexia, hypoesthesia, hyporeflexia, insomnia, irritability, lethargy, malaise, memory impairment, nervousness, paresthesia, peripheral neuropathy, postictal state, sedation, sensory disturbance, sensory loss, sinus headache, somnolence, ***status epilepticus,*** tremor, vertigo, dystonia, hypotonia, hypertonia. **CV:** chest pain, peripheral edema. **EENT:** asthenopia, blurred vision, diplopia, nystagmus, eye pain, strabismus, conjunctivitis, visual field defect, permanent vision loss, tinnitus, otitis media, nasopharyngitis, pharyngolaryngeal pain, sinusitis, toothache. **GI:** abdominal distention, constipation, diarrhea, dyspepsia, nausea, stomach discomfort, upper abdominal pain, vomiting,

gastroenteritis. **GU:** dysmenorrhea, erectile dysfunction, UTI. **Metabolic:** increased appetite, weight gain. **Musculoskeletal:** arthralgia, back pain, contusion, extremity pain, gait disturbance, joint sprain, myalgia, muscle spasm, muscle twitching. **Respiratory:** bronchitis, cough, pulmonary congestion, URI, pneumonia, infectious croup. **Skin:** rash, wound secretion, acne. **Other:** thirst, flulike syndrome, viral infection.

INTERACTIONS

Drug-drug. *Cannabidiol, cannabis:* May enhance CNS depressant effect of vigabatrin. Monitor therapy.
Clonazepam: May increase clonazepam level. Use together cautiously.
Drugs associated with serious adverse ophthalmic effects, such as retinopathy (hydroxychloroquine) or glaucoma (corticosteroids, TCAs): May increase risk of serious adverse ophthalmic effects. Avoid coadministration unless benefits clearly outweigh risks.
Fosphenytoin, phenytoin: May decrease phenytoin level, especially when drug is started or stopped. Monitor drug levels.
Drug-lifestyle. *Alcohol use:* May increase CNS depression. Patient should avoid alcohol.

EFFECTS ON LAB TEST RESULTS

• May decrease ALT and AST levels.
• May decrease Hb level, hematocrit, and RBC count.
• May increase amino acid levels in urine and lead to false-positive tests for genetic metabolic disorders.

CONTRAINDICATIONS & CAUTIONS

• Contraindicated in patients hypersensitive to drug or its components and as first-line therapy for complex partial seizures.
Black Box Warning Drug may cause progressive and permanent bilateral concentric visual field constriction and may reduce visual acuity. Risk of visual impairment increases with increasing dosage and cumulative exposure, but no dosage or exposure is known to be free of risk of vision loss, which may continue after drug is discontinued. Because of risk of permanent vision loss, drug is available only through the Vigabatrin REMS program. Prescribers,

pharmacists, and patients must enroll by calling 1-866-244-8175. A visual exam should be performed before, every 3 months during, and 3 to 6 months after therapy. ■
Black Box Warning Due to risk of vision loss, withdraw drug in patients who don't show substantial benefit within 3 months of initiation for refractory complex partial seizures and within 2 to 4 weeks of initiation in patients with infantile spasms, or sooner if treatment failure becomes obvious. Periodically reassess patient response to and continued need for drug. Use drug at lowest dosage with shortest exposure time as clinically necessary. ■
Black Box Warning Don't use drug in patients who have or are at high risk for other types of irreversible vision loss unless benefits clearly outweigh risks. Don't use vigabatrin with other drugs associated with serious ophthalmic effects, such as retinopathy or glaucoma, unless benefits clearly outweigh risks. ■
• Use cautiously in patients with a history of abnormalities noted on MRI, neurotoxicity, depression, suicidal behavior or ideation, or anemia.
Dialyzable drug: 40% to 60%.
⚠ *Overdose S&S:* Unconsciousness, coma, drowsiness, vertigo, psychosis, apnea, respiratory depression, bradycardia, agitation, irritability, confusion, headache, hypotension, abnormal behavior, increased seizure activity, status epilepticus, speech disorder.

PREGNANCY-LACTATION-REPRODUCTION

• There are no adequate studies in pregnant women; animal studies suggest drug may cause fetal harm. Use during pregnancy only if potential benefit justifies potential risk to the fetus.
• Pregnant patients taking drug should enroll in the North American AED (Antiepileptic Drug) Pregnancy Registry (1-888-233-2334).
• Drug appears in human milk. Patient should discontinue breastfeeding or discontinue drug.

NURSING CONSIDERATIONS

🕒 *Alert:* Closely monitor all patients taking or starting therapy with antiepileptics for changes in behavior indicating worsening suicidal thoughts or behavior or depression. Symptoms such as anxiety, agitation, hostility, mania, and hypomania may be precursors to emerging suicidality.

• Discontinue drug if patient fails to comply with therapy.

❸ **Alert:** Don't withdraw drug suddenly. For adults, taper by decreasing daily dose by 1,000 mg/day weekly until discontinued. For children with complex partial seizures, taper daily dose by one third every week for 3 weeks. For infantile spasms, decrease daily dose at a rate of 25 to 50 mg/kg every 3 to 4 days.

• Monitor patient closely for such adverse effects as dizziness, which may lead to falls.

• Drug may cause anemia, somnolence, fatigue, peripheral neuropathy, peripheral edema, and weight gain. Monitor patient closely.

• Monitor ALT and AST levels; drug decreases levels, making these measurements unreliable for detecting early hepatic injury.

PATIENT TEACHING

• Advise patient that drug may be taken without regard to food.

• Instruct patient to read the manufacturer's medication guide before starting treatment and before each prescription refill.

• Warn patient that drug may cause dizziness and somnolence and to avoid driving or other hazardous activities until drug's effects are known.

Black Box Warning Inform patient that drug may cause vision loss, and explain the importance of regular eye exams and of the need for immediately reporting vision changes. Counsel patient that signs and symptoms of vision loss may be difficult to recognize before vision loss is severe. ■

• Advise patient to call prescriber and not to stop drug suddenly if adverse reactions occur.

• Tell female patient of childbearing potential to notify prescriber if she becomes pregnant or plans to become pregnant during therapy.

• Inform patient who is breastfeeding that drug appears in human milk and that she shouldn't breastfeed.

vilazodone hydrochloride
vil-AZ-oh-dohne

Viibryd❧

Therapeutic class: Antidepressants
Pharmacologic class: SSRIs–partial 5-HT$_{1A}$ receptor agonists

AVAILABLE FORMS
Tablets: 10 mg, 20 mg, 40 mg

INDICATIONS & DOSAGES
➤ **Major depressive disorder**
Adults: Initially, 10 mg PO daily for 7 days, then 20 mg PO daily for 7 days, then 40 mg PO daily thereafter.
Adjust-a-dose: Don't exceed 20 mg once daily when drug is used with a strong CYP3A4 inhibitor. Based on clinical response, consider increasing dosage twofold, up to a maximum 80 mg once daily, over 1 to 2 weeks in patients taking strong CYP3A4 inducers for more than 14 days.

ADMINISTRATION
PO
• Give drug with food.

ACTION
Binds to serotonin reuptake sites and 5-HT$_{1A}$ receptors; is a partial agonist at serotonergic 5-HT$_{1A}$ receptors.

Route	Onset	Peak	Duration
PO	Unknown	4–5 hr	Unknown

Half-life: 25 hours.

ADVERSE REACTIONS
CNS: dizziness, headache, somnolence, paresthesia, insomnia, abnormal dreams, restlessness, fatigue, sedation, tremor. **CV:** palpitations. **GI:** abdominal pain, diarrhea, nausea, dry mouth, vomiting, dyspepsia, flatulence, gastroenteritis, increased appetite. **GU:** delayed ejaculation, erectile dysfunction, sexual dysfunction, abnormal orgasm, decreased libido. **Musculoskeletal:** arthralgia.

INTERACTIONS

Drug-drug. *Aspirin, NSAIDs, warfarin:* May increase risk of bleeding. Monitor patient closely; adjust dosages of these drugs, or discontinue them.

CNS drugs: May cause additive effects. Use together cautiously.

CYP3A4 inducers: May decrease vilazodone level. Monitor patient for effectiveness.

CYP3A4 inhibitors (moderate to strong, such as erythromycin, ketoconazole): May increase vilazodone level. Reduce vilazodone dosage to 20 mg daily.

Digoxin: May increase digoxin level. Monitor levels before and during use with vilazodone. Reduce digoxin dose as necessary.

Drugs metabolized by CYP2C8 (thiazolidinedione class of antidiabetics, such as pioglitazone, rosiglitazone): May increase levels of these drugs. Monitor patient closely.

Highly protein-bound drugs (aripiprazole, diazepam, fluoxetine): May increase levels of these drugs. Monitor patient closely.

MAO inhibitors, linezolid, methylene blue: May increase risk of serious or fatal adverse effects. Don't use concurrently with MAO inhibitor or within 14 days of starting or discontinuing an MAO inhibitor.

Serotonergics (buspirone, MAO inhibitors, SSNRIs, SSRIs, tramadol, triptans): May cause serotonin syndrome. Use together with extreme caution.

Triptans (almotriptan, sumatriptan): May increase risk of serotonin syndrome or NMS. Use together isn't recommended. If coadministration can't be avoided, closely monitor patient for emergence of serotonin syndrome or NMS-like signs or symptoms. If signs or symptoms occur, discontinue both drugs immediately and initiate supportive symptomatic treatment.

Drug-herb. *Herbs with anticoagulant/antiplatelet properties (alfalfa, anise, bilberry):* May increase bleeding risk. Consider therapy modification.

St. John's wort: May increase risk of serotonin syndrome. Avoid use together.

Drug-lifestyle. *Alcohol use:* May increase bioavailability of vilazodone. Discourage use together.

EFFECTS ON LAB TEST RESULTS

• May decrease sodium level.

CONTRAINDICATIONS & CAUTIONS

۞ Alert: Life-threatening serotonin syndrome (fever, mental status changes, muscle twitching, excessive sweating, shivering or shaking, diarrhea, loss of coordination) and NMS (hyperthermia, muscle rigidity, autonomic instability with possible rapid fluctuation of vital signs, mental status changes) have been reported with antidepressant use. Risk increases when antidepressants are used with other serotonergic drugs and with drugs that impair serotonin metabolism.

۞ Alert: Concomitant use with methylene blue or linezolid can cause serotonin syndrome. Don't initiate drug in patients receiving linezolid or methylene blue.

• Contraindicated in patients hypersensitive to drug or its inactive components and with concurrent use or within 14 days of starting or stopping MAO inhibitor therapy.

• Use cautiously in patients with history or family history of depression, hypomania, severe hepatic dysfunction, seizure disorder, acute angle-closure glaucoma, or hyponatremia and in patients taking NSAIDs, aspirin, or warfarin.

Dialyzable drug: Unlikely.

⚠ Overdose S&S: Serotonin syndrome, lethargy, restlessness, hallucinations, disorientation.

PREGNANCY-LACTATION-REPRODUCTION

• Neonates born to women who used drug in the third trimester can develop complications (including persistent pulmonary HTN of the newborn) upon delivery requiring prolonged hospitalization, respiratory support, and tube feedings. Use drug during pregnancy only if potential benefits outweigh risks to the fetus.

• Drug may appear in human milk. Use only when benefit to mother outweighs risk to infant.

NURSING CONSIDERATIONS

• Evaluate patients for the diagnosis of major depressive disorder according to established guidelines.

Black Box Warning Drug may increase the risk of suicidal thinking and behavior in children, adolescents, and young adults with major depressive disorder or other

V

psychiatric disorders. Drug isn't approved for use in children. ∎

• Screen patients for risk of bipolar disorder. Vilazodone isn't approved for treatment of bipolar depression. Use of an antidepressant in bipolar patients may precipitate mixed or manic episodes.

❸ *Alert:* If linezolid or methylene blue must be given concurrently with vilazodone (or other serotonergic drug), stop serotonergic drug and monitor patient for serotonin toxicity for 2 weeks (5 weeks if fluoxetine was taken) or until 24 hours after the last dose of methylene blue or linezolid, whichever comes first. May resume vilazodone 24 hours after last dose of methylene blue or linezolid.

• Evaluate patient for history of drug abuse, and watch closely for signs and symptoms of misuse or abuse (increased tolerance, drug-seeking behavior, requests for dosage increase).

• Closely monitor patient who had recently been taking MAO inhibitors for tremor, myoclonus, diaphoresis, nausea, vomiting, flushing, dizziness, hyperthermia with features that resemble NMS, seizures, rigidity, autonomic instability with possible rapid fluctuations of vital signs, and mental status changes that include extreme agitation progressing to delirium and coma.

• Monitor patient for signs and symptoms of NMS (hyperthermia, rigidity, autonomic instability with possible rapid fluctuations of vital signs, mental status changes).

• Drug hasn't been studied in patients with severe hepatic dysfunction. Closely monitor patient with hepatic impairment for excessive fatigue or yellowing of the eyes or skin.

• Monitor patients taking aspirin, NSAIDs, or warfarin for signs and symptoms of bleeding.

• When discontinuing vilazodone, avoid abrupt discontinuation. Gradually reduce dosage and monitor patient for adverse events. If withdrawal symptoms are intolerable, consider resuming the previous prescribed dosage and decreasing the dosage at a more gradual rate. Wait at least 14 days before starting an MAO inhibitor.

• Hyponatremia, which may be life-threatening, has occurred as a result of treatment with other SSRIs and SSNRIs, especially in elderly patients and in patients taking diuretics or who are otherwise volume-depleted. Discontinue vilazodone in patients with symptomatic hyponatremia and treat appropriately. Monitor patient for signs and symptoms of hyponatremia, such as headache, difficulty concentrating, memory impairment, confusion, weakness, unsteadiness, hallucinations, syncope, seizures, coma, and respiratory arrest.

• Monitor patients for acute-angle glaucoma. Many antidepressants, including vilazodone, may trigger an angle-closure attack in patients with anatomically narrow angles who don't have a patent iridectomy.

PATIENT TEACHING

Black Box Warning Advise families and caregivers to closely observe patient for increased suicidal thinking and behavior. ∎

❸ *Alert:* Teach patient to recognize and immediately report signs and symptoms of serotonin toxicity (fever, mental status changes, muscle twitching, excessive sweating, shivering or shaking, diarrhea, and loss of coordination) and NMS (hyperthermia, rigidity, autonomic instability with possible rapid fluctuations of vital signs, and mental status changes).

• Teach patient to take drug with food.

• Warn patient not to stop drug abruptly.

• Instruct patient to inform prescriber of all other medicines being taken to avoid dangerous interactions.

• Tell patient to immediately seek medical attention if fever, rigidity, rapid changes in pulse rate or BP, sweating, or confusion occurs.

• Counsel patient to keep all appointments for monitoring blood work and for follow-up care.

• Advise patient to use caution when driving or operating hazardous equipment until effects of drug are known; drug may impair judgment, thinking, and motor skills.

• Advise patient and caregivers to watch for signs and symptoms of the onset of manic or hypomanic episodes.

• Warn patient to avoid alcohol during drug therapy.

• Advise female patient to notify her health care provider if she becomes pregnant or intends to become pregnant during therapy.

Counsel her to consult prescriber before breastfeeding.

SAFETY ALERT!

vinBLAStine sulfate (VLB)
vin-BLAS-teen

Therapeutic class: Antineoplastics
Pharmacologic class: Vinca alkaloids

AVAILABLE FORMS
Injection: 1 mg/mL in 10-mL vials

INDICATIONS & DOSAGES
Adjust-a-dose (for all indications): For patients with serum bilirubin level above 3 mg/dL, give 50% of usual dose. Once a dose is determined to produce a WBC count below 3,000/mm^3, give maintenance doses of one increment less than this amount at weekly intervals.

➤ **Breast or testicular cancer, Hodgkin and malignant lymphoma, choriocarcinoma, lymphosarcoma, mycosis fungoides, Kaposi sarcoma, histiocytosis**
Adults: 3.7 mg/m^2 IV weekly. May increase to maximum dose of 18.5 mg/m^2 IV weekly based on response. Don't repeat dose if WBC count is below 4,000/mm^3. Increase dosage at weekly intervals in increments of 1.8 mg/m^2 until desired therapeutic response is obtained, WBC count decreases to 3,000/mm^3, or maximum weekly dose of 18.5 mg/m^2 is reached.

➤ **Hodgkin disease**
Children: 6 mg/m^2 IV in combination with other chemotherapeutic drugs.

➤ **Letterer-Siwe disease (histiocytosis X)**
Children: 6.5 mg/m^2 IV as a single agent.

➤ **Testicular germ-cell carcinomas**
Children: 3 mg/m^2/day IV on days 1 through 5 of each cycle in combination with other chemotherapeutic drugs.

ADMINISTRATION
IV
▼ Preparing and giving drug may be mutagenic, teratogenic, or carcinogenic. Follow institutional policy to reduce risks.
Black Box Warning Drug is fatal if given intrathecally; it's for IV use only. ∎

☉ *Alert:* When drug is dispensed in other than the original container, it must be packaged in the overwrap provided and labeled, using the auxiliary sticker provided and must state "Do not remove covering until moment of injection. For intravenous use only. Fatal if given by other routes." A syringe containing a specific dose must be labeled, using the auxiliary sticker provided to state: "For intravenous use only. Fatal if given by other routes."
☉ *Alert:* The Institute for Safe Medication Practices strongly recommends dispensing vinblastine in a minibag (NOT in a syringe) to prevent inadvertent intrathecal use.
▼ If a minibag isn't possible, inject drug directly into tubing of running IV line over 1 minute.
Black Box Warning Make sure catheter is properly positioned in vein. Drug is a vesicant; if extravasation occurs, stop infusion immediately and notify prescriber. The manufacturer recommends that moderate heat be applied to area of leakage. Local injection of hyaluronidase may help disperse drug. ∎
▼ Warm compresses may be applied to the area for 15 minutes every 6 hours for 48 hours.
▼ **Incompatibilities:** Cefepime, furosemide, pantoprazole.

ACTION
Arrests mitosis in metaphase, blocking cell division.

Route	Onset	Peak	Duration
IV	Unknown	Unknown	Unknown

Half-life: Initial phase, 3½ minutes; second phase, 1½ hours; terminal phase, 25 hours.

ADVERSE REACTIONS
CNS: numbness, paresthesia, peripheral neuropathy and neuritis, *seizures, stroke,* depression, headache. **CV:** *MI,* HTN. **EENT:** pharyngitis. **GI:** anorexia, constipation, ileus, nausea, stomatitis, vomiting, abdominal pain, bleeding ulcer, diarrhea. **Hematologic:** anemia, *leukopenia, thrombocytopenia.* **Musculoskeletal:** loss of deep tendon reflexes, muscle pain and weakness, jaw pain. **Respiratory:** *acute bronchospasm,* shortness of breath. **Skin:** irritation,

V

phlebitis, cellulitis, reversible alopecia, vesiculation and necrosis with extravasation.

INTERACTIONS

Drug-drug. *Azole antifungals, erythromycin, other drugs that inhibit cytochrome P-450 pathway:* May increase vinblastine toxicity. Avoid combination if possible. Monitor patient closely for toxicity.

Mitomycin: May increase risk of bronchospasm and shortness of breath. Monitor patient's respiratory status.

Ototoxic drugs, such as platinum-containing antineoplastics: May cause temporary or permanent hearing impairment. Monitor hearing function.

Phenytoin: May decrease plasma phenytoin level. Monitor phenytoin level closely.

Vaccines (inactivated): May diminish therapeutic effect of vaccines. Complete all age-appropriate vaccinations at least 2 weeks before starting vinblastine. If patient is vaccinated during therapy, revaccinate at least 3 months after drug is stopped.

Vaccines (live): May enhance adverse/toxic effect of live-virus vaccines and diminish their therapeutic effect. Avoid use with vinblastine; don't vaccinate for at least 3 months after drug is stopped.

Drug-herb. *St. John's wort:* May decrease vinblastine concentration. Avoid use together.

EFFECTS ON LAB TEST RESULTS

• May decrease Hb level and WBC and platelet counts.

CONTRAINDICATIONS & CAUTIONS

• Contraindicated in patients hypersensitive to drug and in those with severe leukopenia or bacterial infection or significant granulocytopenia unless it's a result of the disease being treated.

• Use cautiously in patients with hepatic dysfunction or CV disease.

Dialyzable drug: No.

⚠ *Overdose S&S:* Exaggerated effects, neurotoxicity.

PREGNANCY-LACTATION-REPRODUCTION

• There are no adequate studies in pregnant women, but drug can cause fetal harm.

If drug is used during pregnancy or if patient becomes pregnant during therapy, inform her of potential hazard to the fetus. Women of childbearing potential should avoid becoming pregnant during therapy.

• It isn't known if drug appears in human milk. Patient should discontinue breastfeeding or discontinue drug.

NURSING CONSIDERATIONS

Black Box Warning Drug should be administered by personnel experienced in the administration of vinblastine sulfate. ∎

• To reduce nausea, give antiemetic before drug.

• Don't give drug into a limb with compromised circulation.

❸ Alert: After giving drug, be alert for development of life-threatening acute bronchospasm. If this occurs, notify prescriber immediately. Reaction is most likely to occur in patients who are also receiving mitomycin.

• Monitor patient for stomatitis. If stomatitis occurs, stop drug and notify prescriber.

• Assess bowel activity. Give laxatives as indicated. Stool softeners may be used prophylactically.

• Don't repeat dosage more frequently than every 7 days or severe leukopenia will occur. Nadir occurs on days 5 to 10. Recovery of WBC count is fairly rapid and usually complete within another 7 to 14 days.

• Assess patient for numbness and tingling in hands and feet. Assess gait for early evidence of footdrop.

• Drug is less neurotoxic than related drug vincristine.

• Stop drugs known to cause urine retention for first few days after therapy, particularly in elderly patients.

• **Look alike–sound alike:** Don't confuse vinblastine with vincristine or vinorelbine.

PATIENT TEACHING

• Tell patient to report evidence of infection (fever, sore throat, fatigue) and bleeding (easy bruising, nosebleeds, bleeding gums, tarry stools). Tell patient to take temperature daily.

• Urge patient to report pain, swelling, burning, or any unusual feeling at injection site during infusion.

Reactions in bold italics are *life-threatening*. Interactions may have a *rapid onset* or a *delayed onset*.

• Warn patient that hair loss may occur but that it's usually temporary.
• Caution female patient to avoid pregnancy during therapy.
• Tell patient that pain may occur in jaw and in the organ with the tumor.

SAFETY ALERT!

vinCRIStine sulfate (VCR)
vin-KRIS-teen

Therapeutic class: Antineoplastics
Pharmacologic class: Vinca alkaloids

AVAILABLE FORMS
Injection: 1 mg/mL in 1-mL, 2-mL preservative-free vials

INDICATIONS & DOSAGES
➤ **Acute lymphoblastic and other leukemias, Hodgkin lymphoma, malignant lymphoma, neuroblastoma, rhabdomyosarcoma, Wilms tumor**
Adults: 1.4 mg/m² IV weekly.
Children weighing more than 10 kg: 1.5 to 2 mg/m² IV weekly.
Children weighing 10 kg and less or with BSA less than 1 m²: Initially, 0.05 mg/kg IV weekly. Titrate dosage as tolerated, up to 2 mg/dose.
Adjust-a-dose: For patients with direct bilirubin level above 3 mg/dL, reduce dosage by 50%.

ADMINISTRATION
IV
▼ Preparing and giving drug may be mutagenic, teratogenic, or carcinogenic. Follow institutional policy to reduce risks.
▼ Inject directly into tube of running IV line of NSS or D₅W only, slowly over 1 minute.
۞ Alert: To prevent inadvertent intrathecal administration, WHO and the Institute for Safe Medication Practices strongly recommend dispensing vincristine in a minibag (not in a syringe).
Black Box Warning Make sure catheter is positioned correctly in vein. Drug is a vesicant; if it extravasates, stop infusion immediately and notify prescriber. Apply heat on and off every 2 hours for 24 hours. ∎

Black Box Warning Drug is fatal if given intrathecally; it's for IV use only. ∎
Black Box Warning Syringes containing this product should be labeled, using the auxiliary sticker provided, to state, "For intravenous use only. Fatal if given by other routes." Extemporaneously prepared syringes containing this product must be packaged in an overwrap that's labeled, "Do not remove covering until moment of injection. For intravenous use only. Fatal if given by other routes." ∎
▼ If protocol requires a continuous infusion, use a central line. Give as a short 5- to 10-minute infusion in 25 to 50 mL of NSS or D₅W.
▼ All vials contain 1 mg/mL solution; refrigerate them.
▼ **Incompatibilities:** Cefepime, furosemide, idarubicin, pantoprazole, phenytoin, sodium bicarbonate.

ACTION
Arrests mitosis in metaphase, blocking cell division.

Route	Onset	Peak	Duration
IV	Unknown	Unknown	Unknown

Half-life: Initial phase, 5 minutes; second phase, 2¼ hours; terminal phase, 3½ days.

ADVERSE REACTIONS
CNS: loss of deep tendon reflexes, paresthesia, peripheral neuropathy, *coma, seizures,* ataxia, cranial nerve palsies, fever, headache, sensory loss. **CV:** HTN, hypotension. **EENT:** blindness, diplopia, hoarseness, optic and extraocular neuropathy, photophobia, ptosis, visual disturbances, vocal cord paralysis. **GI:** constipation, cramps, nausea, stomatitis, vomiting, *intestinal necrosis,* anorexia, diarrhea, dysphagia, ileus that mimics surgical paralytic ileus. **GU:** dysuria, polyuria, urine retention. **Hematologic:** *leukopenia, thrombocytopenia,* anemia. **Metabolic:** weight loss. **Musculoskeletal:** cramps, jaw pain, muscle weakness. **Respiratory:** *acute bronchospasm,* dyspnea. **Skin:** phlebitis, cellulitis at injection site, rash, reversible alopecia, severe local reaction following extravasation.

V

INTERACTIONS

Drug-drug. *Digoxin:* May decrease digoxin's effects. Monitor digoxin level.

Fosphenytoin, phenytoin: May reduce phenytoin level. Monitor phenytoin level closely.

HIV protease inhibitors (atazanavir, ritonavir): May increase pharmacologic effects of vincristine. Monitor patient for profound neutropenia and severe neuropathy. Temporarily suspend HIV protease inhibitor or reduce vincristine dosage if significant hematologic or GI toxicity occurs.

Mitomycin: May increase frequency of bronchospasm and acute pulmonary reactions. Monitor patient's respiratory status.

Ototoxic drugs: May potentiate loss of hearing. Use together with caution.

Triazole antifungals (itraconazole, posaconazole, voriconazole): Concomitant use may increase risk of neurotoxicity. Consider therapy modification.

Vaccines (inactivated): May diminish therapeutic effect of vaccines. Complete all age-appropriate vaccinations at least 2 weeks before starting vincristine. If patient is vaccinated during therapy, revaccinate at least 3 months after drug is stopped.

Vaccines (live): May enhance adverse/toxic effect of live-virus vaccines and diminish their therapeutic effect. Avoid use with vincristine; don't vaccinate for at least 3 months after drug is stopped.

Warfarin: May increase anticoagulant effects. Monitor INR and adjust warfarin dose as needed.

Drug-herb. *Echinacea, St. John's wort:* May decrease vincristine concentration. Avoid use together.

EFFECTS ON LAB TEST RESULTS

• May decrease sodium and Hb levels. May increase uric acid level.

• May decrease WBC and platelet counts.

CONTRAINDICATIONS & CAUTIONS

• Contraindicated in patients hypersensitive to drug and in those with demyelinating form of Charcot-Marie-Tooth syndrome.

• Don't give to patients who are receiving radiation therapy through ports that include the liver.

• Use cautiously in patients with hepatic dysfunction, neuromuscular disease, or infection.

Dialyzable drug: No.

⚠ *Overdose S&S:* Exaggerated effects, death.

PREGNANCY-LACTATION-REPRODUCTION

• There are no adequate studies in pregnant women, but drug may cause fetal harm. If drug is used during pregnancy or if patient becomes pregnant during therapy, inform her of potential hazard to the fetus. Women of childbearing potential should use effective contraception during therapy.

• It isn't known if drug appears in human milk. Patient should discontinue breastfeeding or discontinue drug.

NURSING CONSIDERATIONS

Black Box Warning Drug should be administered by personnel experienced in the administration of vincristine sulfate. ▮

🕙 *Alert:* Patient also taking mitomycin has a higher risk of life-threatening bronchospasm. Monitor patient after dose, and notify prescriber immediately if bronchospasm occurs.

🕙 *Alert:* Drug is considered a vesicant. If signs or symptoms of extravasation occur, stop infusion immediately and notify prescriber. Extravasation site may need to be injected with hyaluronidase.

• Watch for hyperuricemia, especially in patients with leukemia or lymphoma. Maintain hydration and give allopurinol to prevent uric acid nephropathy. Watch for toxicity.

• If SIADH (rare) develops, fluid restriction may be needed. Monitor fluid intake and output.

• Because of risk of neurotoxicity, don't give drug more often than once weekly. Children are more resistant to neurotoxicity than adults. Neurotoxicity is dose related and usually reversible.

• Elderly patients and those with underlying neurologic disease may be more susceptible to neurotoxic effects.

• Monitor patient for depression of Achilles tendon reflex, numbness, tingling, footdrop or wristdrop, difficulty walking, ataxia, and slapping gait. Monitor patient's ability to walk on heels. Support patient while walking.

Reactions in bold italics are *life-threatening*. Interactions may have a *rapid onset* or a *delayed onset*.

• Monitor bowel function. Constipation may be an early sign of neurotoxicity.
• Stop drugs known to cause urine retention, particularly in elderly patients, for first few days after therapy.
• **Look alike–sound alike:** Don't confuse vincristine with vinblastine or vinorelbine.

PATIENT TEACHING

• Advise patient to report all adverse reactions, especially pain or burning at injection site during or after administration.
• Tell patient to report increased shortness of breath and evidence of infection (fever, sore throat, fatigue) and bleeding (easy bruising, nosebleeds, bleeding gums, tarry stools). Tell patient to take temperature daily.
• Warn patient that hair loss may occur, but explain that it's usually temporary.
• Caution female patient not to breastfeed and to avoid becoming pregnant during therapy and to consult prescriber before becoming pregnant.

SAFETY ALERT!

vinorelbine tartrate
vin-oh-REL-been

Therapeutic class: Antineoplastics
Pharmacologic class: Semisynthetic vinca alkaloids

AVAILABLE FORMS
Injection: 10 mg/mL, 50 mg/5 mL

INDICATIONS & DOSAGES
Adjust-a-dose (for all indications): Refer to manufacturer's instructions for toxicity-related dosage adjustments.
➤ **In combination with cisplatin for first-line treatment of patients with locally advanced or metastatic NSCLC; as a single agent for the treatment of patients with metastatic NSCLC**
Adults: 30 mg/m^2 IV weekly as monotherapy. In combination treatment, 25 mg/m^2 IV weekly with cisplatin 100 mg/m^2 given every 4 weeks. Or, 30 mg/m^2 IV weekly in combination with cisplatin 120 mg/m^2 given on days 1 and 29, then every 6 weeks.
➤ **HER-2 positive advanced or metastatic breast cancer ◆**

Adults: 25 or 30 mg/m^2 IV every 7 days (as a single agent) until disease progression or unacceptable toxicity.

ADMINISTRATION
IV
▼ Drug may be a contact irritant; handle and give with care. Wear gloves. Avoid inhaling vapors and allowing contact with skin or mucous membranes, especially those of the eyes. In case of contact, wash with generous amounts of water for at least 15 minutes.
▼ Dilute drug before use to 1.5 to 3 mg/mL with D$_5$W or NSS in a syringe. Or, dilute to 0.5 to 2 mg/mL in an IV bag of D$_5$W, NSS, half-NSS, or D$_5$W half-NSS.
▼ Give drug IV over 6 to 10 minutes into side port of a free-flowing IV line that is closest to IV bag; then flush with 75 to 125 mL or more of D$_5$W or NSS.
▼ Monitor site for irritation and infiltration because drug can cause localized tissue damage, necrosis, and thrombophlebitis.
❸ **Alert:** Make sure catheter is properly positioned in vein. If extravasation occurs, stop drug immediately and inject remaining dose into a different vein; notify prescriber.
▼ Diluted drug may be stored for up to 24 hours at room temperature.
▼ **Incompatibilities:** None listed by manufacturer. Consult a drug incompatibility reference for more information.

ACTION
Exerts its primary antineoplastic effect by disrupting microtubule assembly, which in turn disrupts spindle formation and prevents mitosis.

Route	Onset	Peak	Duration
IV	Unknown	Unknown	Unknown

Half-life: About 27½ to 43½ hours.

ADVERSE REACTIONS
CNS: asthenia, fatigue, peripheral neuropathy, fever, paresthesia, hyperesthesia, hyporeflexia. **CV:** chest pain, phlebitis. **GI:** anorexia, constipation, diarrhea, nausea, stomatitis, vomiting. **Hematologic:** anemia, *agranulocytosis, neutropenia, bone marrow suppression, granulocytopenia, thrombocytopenia, leukopenia.* **Hepatic:**

V

hyperbilirubinemia. **Musculoskeletal:** arthralgia, jaw pain, loss of deep tendon reflexes, myalgia. **Respiratory:** dyspnea. **Skin:** alopecia, injection-site pain or reaction, rash. **Other:** sepsis.

INTERACTIONS
Drug-drug. *Cisplatin:* May increase risk of bone marrow suppression when used with cisplatin. Monitor hematologic status closely.
Cyclosporine: May increase therapeutic and toxic effects of vinorelbine. Close clinical and lab monitoring is indicated.
Cytochrome P-450 inhibitors: May decrease metabolism of vinorelbine. Watch for increased adverse effects.
Macrolide antibiotics (clarithromycin, erythromycin): May increase vinorelbine level. Consider therapy modification.
Mitomycin: May cause pulmonary reactions. Monitor respiratory status closely.
Paclitaxel: May increase risk of neuropathy. Monitor patient closely.
Posaconazole: May increase risk of neurotoxicity. Monitor patient closely.
Vaccines (inactivated): May diminish therapeutic effect of vaccines. Complete all age-appropriate vaccinations at least 2 weeks before starting vinorelbine. If patient is vaccinated during therapy, revaccinate at least 3 months after drug is stopped.
Vaccines, live-virus: May increase risk of live-virus vaccine–induced adverse reactions. Concurrent use isn't recommended.
Drug-herb. *Echinacea:* May diminish therapeutic effect of vinorelbine. Consider therapy modification.

EFFECTS ON LAB TEST RESULTS
• May increase bilirubin level and LFT values.
• May decrease Hb level. May decrease granulocyte, WBC, and platelet counts.

CONTRAINDICATIONS & CAUTIONS
• Contraindicated in patients hypersensitive to the drug.
• Monitor CBC before each dose. Don't give drug to patients with neutrophil counts less than 1,000 cells/mm³. Adjust dosage based on neutrophil counts obtained on day of treatment.

• Use with caution in patients whose bone marrow may have been compromised by previous exposure to radiation therapy or chemotherapy or whose bone marrow is still recovering from chemotherapy.
• Use with caution in patients with hepatic impairment.
• Safety and effectiveness in children haven't been established.
Dialyzable drug: 0% to 24%.
⚠ *Overdose S&S:* Paralytic ileus, stomatitis, esophagitis, bone marrow aplasia, sepsis, paresis, death.

PREGNANCY-LACTATION-REPRODUCTION
• Drug can cause fetal harm when used during pregnancy. Advise women of childbearing potential to use highly effective contraception during therapy. If drug is used during pregnancy or patient becomes pregnant during therapy, inform her of potential hazard to the fetus.
• Advise males with female sexual partners of childbearing potential to use highly effective contraception during therapy and for 3 months after final dose.
• It isn't known if drug appears in human milk. Patient should discontinue breastfeeding or discontinue drug.

NURSING CONSIDERATIONS
Black Box Warning Severe myelosuppression resulting in serious infection, septic shock, hospitalization, and death may occur. ∎
Black Box Warning Decrease dosage or withhold drug in accordance with recommended dosage modifications. Neutrophil count should be 1,000/mm³ or more before administration. ∎
🖐 *Alert:* Drug is considered a vesicant. If signs or symptoms of extravasation occur, stop infusion immediately and notify prescriber. Initiate appropriate management measures in accordance with institutional policies.
• If neutrophil count is less than 1,000/mm³, withhold drug and notify prescriber. Neutrophil count nadir occurs between days 7 and 10.
• In patients with hepatic impairment, monitor liver enzyme levels.

Reactions in bold italics are *life-threatening*. Interactions may have a *rapid onset* or a *delayed onset*.

• Patient may receive injections of G-CSF to promote cell growth and decrease risk of infection.

⟲ Alert: Monitor deep tendon reflexes; loss may represent cumulative toxicity.

• Monitor patients closely for hypersensitivity and new or worsening signs and symptoms of neuropathy in those with prior history of or preexisting neuropathy.

• Severe acute bronchospasm, interstitial pneumonitis, and ARDS have been reported. Monitor patient for unexplained dyspnea or other signs and symptoms of pulmonary toxicity.

• As a guide to the effects of therapy, monitor patient's peripheral blood count and bone marrow.

• **Look alike–sound alike:** Don't confuse vinorelbine with vinblastine or vincristine.

PATIENT TEACHING

• Advise patient to report any pain or burning at site of injection.

• Instruct patient not to take other drugs, including OTC preparations, until approved by prescriber.

• Tell patient to report all adverse reactions, especially evidence of infection (fever, sore throat, fatigue) and bleeding (easy bruising, nosebleeds, bleeding gums, tarry stools). Tell patient to take temperature daily.

• Advise patient to report increased shortness of breath, cough, abdominal pain, or constipation.

• Advise female patient of childbearing potential to use highly effective contraception during therapy and male patient with female sexual partner of childbearing potential to use highly effective contraception during therapy and for 3 months after final dose.

• Advise patient not to breastfeed during therapy.

SAFETY ALERT!

vismodegib
VIS-moe-DEG-ib

Erivedge

Therapeutic class: Antineoplastics
Pharmacologic class: Hedgehog pathway inhibitors

AVAILABLE FORMS
Capsules ⊕: 150 mg

INDICATIONS & DOSAGES
➤ **Metastatic basal cell carcinoma; locally advanced basal cell carcinoma that has recurred following surgery or in patients who aren't candidates for surgery or radiation**

Adults: 150 mg PO once daily until disease progression or unacceptable toxicity.

Adjust-a-dose: Withhold drug for up to 8 weeks for intolerable adverse reactions until improvement or resolution. Treatment durations shorter than 8 weeks before interruptions haven't been studied.

ADMINISTRATION
PO
• Hazardous agent; use safe handling precautions.
• May give with or without food.
• Store capsules at room temperature.
• Don't open, crush, or allow patient to chew capsules.

ACTION
Inhibits Hedgehog signaling pathway by binding to and inhibiting Smoothened, a transmembrane protein involved in Hedgehog signal transmission. Inhibition of this protein slows pathway for tumor growth.

Route	Onset	Peak	Duration
PO	Unknown	2.4 days	Unknown

Half-life: 4 days with continued dosing; 12 days after one dose.

ADVERSE REACTIONS
CNS: fatigue. **GI:** nausea, diarrhea, vomiting, constipation, taste perversion, absence of taste, decreased appetite. **GU:** azotemia,

amenorrhea. **Metabolic:** weight loss, hyponatremia, *hypokalemia.* **Musculoskeletal:** muscle spasms, arthralgia. **Skin:** alopecia.

INTERACTIONS

Drug-drug. *Antacids, H_2-receptor antagonists, PPIs:* May decrease vismodegib exposure and its effects. Avoid use together.
P-gp inhibitors (macrolides such as azithromycin, clarithromycin, erythromycin): May increase vismodegib exposure and adverse effects. Avoid use together.

EFFECTS ON LAB TEST RESULTS

• May increase BUN and creatinine levels.
• May decrease sodium and potassium levels.

CONTRAINDICATIONS & CAUTIONS

• Contraindicated in patients hypersensitive to drug.
• Premature fusion of the epiphyses has been reported in children taking drug. In some cases, fusion progressed after drug was discontinued. Drug isn't indicated for children.
Dialyzable drug: Unknown.

PREGNANCY-LACTATION-REPRODUCTION

Black Box Warning Contraindicated in pregnant women. Drug can cause embryofetal death or severe birth defects. ∎
Black Box Warning Verify pregnancy status within 7 days before start of therapy. ∎
Black Box Warning Females of childbearing potential should use effective contraception during therapy and for 24 months after final dose; male patients should use condoms, even after a vasectomy, to avoid drug exposure to pregnant partners and female partners of childbearing potential during therapy and for 3 months after final dose. ∎
• Drug is present in semen but it isn't known if the amount in semen can cause embryofetal harm. Men shouldn't donate semen during therapy and for 3 months after therapy ends.
• Report exposure during pregnancy (directly or from seminal fluid) or within 7 months after treatment ends to Genentech at 1-888-835-2555.

• It isn't known if drug appears in human milk. Breastfeeding isn't recommended during therapy and for 24 months after final dose.
• Drug may cause amenorrhea, which may be irreversible.

NURSING CONSIDERATIONS

• Monitor patient for GI toxicities (decreased appetite, nausea, diarrhea, vomiting, abdominal pain, constipation).
• *Look alike–sound alike:* Don't confuse vismodegib with vemurafenib or vandetanib.

PATIENT TEACHING

Black Box Warning Advise male and female patients of the risks to an embryo or fetus, the need for contraception during and after therapy, and the potential risk of drug exposure through semen. ∎
Black Box Warning Tell female patient to use highly effective contraception during therapy and for 24 months after final dose; advise male patient to use condoms, even after a vasectomy, to avoid drug exposure to pregnant partners and female partners of childbearing potential during therapy and for 3 months after final dose. ∎
• Instruct patient that if a dose is missed, not to make up that dose but to resume dosing with the next scheduled dose.
• Instruct patient to immediately contact health care provider if pregnancy occurs or is suspected after exposure to drug, or if patient has unprotected sex.
• Advise female patient experiencing drug-induced amenorrhea that it's unknown if amenorrhea will be reversed after drug discontinuation.
• Caution patient not to donate blood or blood products while taking drug and for at least 24 months (or semen for 3 months) after last dose.
• Teach patient to swallow capsules whole and not to crush, chew, or open them.

Reactions in bold italics are *life-threatening*. Interactions may have a *rapid onset* or a *delayed onset*.

vorapaxar sulfate
VOR-a-PAX-ar

Zontivity

Therapeutic class: Antiplatelet drugs
Pharmacologic class: Platelet aggregation inhibitors

AVAILABLE FORMS
Tablets: 2.08 mg

INDICATIONS & DOSAGES
➤ **To reduce thrombotic CV events in patients with history of MI or peripheral arterial disease, in combination with aspirin or clopidogrel**
Adults: 1 tablet (2.08 mg) PO once daily.

ADMINISTRATION
PO
• Store tablets in original package at room temperature. Keep the desiccant packet in the bottle to protect from moisture.
• May give with or without food.

ACTION
Inhibits platelet aggregation. Drug is a reversible antagonist of the protease-activated receptor-1 expressed on platelets.

Route	Onset	Peak	Duration
PO	Unknown	1–2 hr	Unknown

Half-life: 5 to 13 days.

ADVERSE REACTIONS
CNS: depression, *intracranial bleeding.*
EENT: retinopathy, retinal disorders. **GI:** *GI bleeding.* **Hematologic:** *hemorrhage,* anemia, iron deficiency. **Skin:** rash, eruption, exanthemas.

INTERACTIONS
Drug-drug. *Drugs known to cause bleeding (anticoagulants, fibrinolytics, NSAIDs [long-term], SSNRIs, SSRIs, warfarin):* Increase risk of bleeding, including intracranial hemorrhage and fatal bleeding. Avoid use together.
Strong CYP3A inducers (carbamazepine, phenytoin, rifampin): May decrease vorapaxar level. Avoid use together.

Strong CYP3A inhibitors (clarithromycin, ketoconazole, nefazodone, ritonavir): May increase vorapaxar level. Avoid use together.
Drug-herb. *Herbs with anticoagulant/antiplatelet properties (alfalfa, anise, bilberry):* May increase bleeding risk. Consider therapy modification.
St. John's wort: May decrease vorapaxar level. Avoid use together.

EFFECTS ON LAB TEST RESULTS
• May decrease RBC count.

CONTRAINDICATIONS & CAUTIONS
Black Box Warning Don't use in patients with history of intracranial hemorrhage, pathological bleeding, stroke, or TIA. Antiplatelet drugs, including vorapaxar, increase risk of bleeding, including intracranial hemorrhage and fatal bleeding. ∎
• Drug has only been studied in combination with aspirin or clopidogrel.
• Use cautiously in elderly patients; in those with low body weight, reduced renal or hepatic function, or history of bleeding disorder; and in patients concomitantly using drugs known to increase bleeding.
• Use isn't recommended in patients with severe hepatic impairment.
• There are no overall differences in safety or effectiveness between younger and older patients. Since elderly patients are at higher risk for bleeding, consider patient's age before administering drug.
• Safety and effectiveness in children haven't been established.
Dialyzable drug: Unlikely.

PREGNANCY-LACTATION-REPRODUCTION
• Use cautiously in pregnant women and only if potential benefits outweigh risk to the fetus.
• It isn't known if drug appears in human milk. Use in breastfeeding women isn't recommended.

NURSING CONSIDERATIONS
⊘ *Alert:* Stopping drug briefly during an episode of acute bleeding won't be useful in managing bleeding, because of drug's long half-life. There's no known treatment to reverse the antiplatelet effect; drug will

V

♣Canada   ◇OTC   ◆Off-label use   ℰPhotoguide   ⓜDo not crush   *Liquid contains alcohol   ☒Genetic significantly inhibit platelet aggregation for 4 weeks after discontinuation.

• Discontinue drug if patient experiences a stroke, TIA, or intracranial hemorrhage.

• Monitor Hb level and hematocrit periodically. Monitor patient for bleeding.

• Evaluate hypotensive patients who have had recent coronary angiography, PCI, CABG, or other surgical procedure for possible bleeding.

PATIENT TEACHING

Black Box Warning Caution patient that drug increases risk of bleeding, including intracranial hemorrhage and fatal bleeding. ∎

• Advise patient to tell other providers about taking drug, especially before any surgery or dental procedure.

• Instruct patient to take drug exactly as prescribed in addition to aspirin or clopidogrel, and not to discontinue drug without first consulting prescriber.

• Instruct patient to report bruising or severe prolonged or excessive unexplained bleeding (blood in stool, vomit, or urine and coughing up blood or blood clots).

• Advise patient to report all prescription and OTC medications, vitamins, herbs, and other dietary supplements being taken to prescriber and pharmacist so that they are aware of other treatment that may affect bleeding risk.

• Warn female patient that drug is used during pregnancy only if potential benefits outweigh risks.

• Tell female patient that breastfeeding isn't recommended during therapy.

---

voriconazole ℞
vor-ah-KON-ah-zole

Vfend

Therapeutic class: Antifungals
Pharmacologic class: Synthetic triazoles

AVAILABLE FORMS
Oral suspension: 200 mg/5 mL (40 mg/mL after reconstitution)
Powder for injection: 200 mg/vial
Tablets: 50 mg, 200 mg

INDICATIONS & DOSAGES
Adjust-a-dose (for all indications): For adults with mild or moderate hepatic impairment (Child-Pugh class A or B), decrease the maintenance dosage by 50%. In adults with a CrCl of less than 50 mL/minute, use PO form instead of IV form to prevent accumulation of a component of the IV mixture. In adults also receiving phenytoin, increase maintenance dose of voriconazole to 5 mg/kg IV every 12 hours, or increase PO dose from 100 mg to 200 mg (in adults weighing 40 kg or less) or from 200 mg to 400 mg (in adults weighing more than 40 kg). In adults also receiving efavirenz, increase voriconazole dosage to 400 mg PO every 12 hours and decrease efavirenz dosage to 300 mg PO every 24 hours. When treatment with voriconazole is stopped, restore initial dosage of efavirenz.

➤ **Esophageal candidiasis**
Adults, children ages 12 to 14 weighing 50 kg or more, and children age 15 and older regardless of body weight: 200 mg PO every 12 hours.
Adults weighing less than 40 kg: 100 mg PO every 12 hours.
Children ages 2 to younger than 12 and children ages 12 to 14 weighing less than 50 kg: Initially, 4 mg/kg IV every 12 hours. If patient can't tolerate 4-mg/kg IV dose, reduce dose by 1-mg/kg steps. If patient response is inadequate and patient is able to tolerate initial IV dose, increase dose by 1-mg/kg steps. After at least 5 days of IV therapy and only after there is significant clinical improvement, consider an oral regimen of 9 mg/kg PO every 12 hours. If patient can't tolerate 9-mg/kg PO dose, reduce dose by 1-mg/kg or 50-mg steps. If patient response is inadequate and patient is able to tolerate initial PO dose, increase dose by 1-mg/kg or 50-mg steps to a maximum of 350 mg PO every 12 hours.

For all patients, treat for a minimum of 14 days and for at least 7 days after symptoms resolve.

➤ **Invasive aspergillosis; serious infections caused by *Fusarium* species and *Scedosporium apiospermum* in patients intolerant of or refractory to other therapy**
Adults, children ages 12 to 14 weighing 50 kg or more, and children age 15 and

---

older regardless of body weight: Initially, 6 mg/kg IV every 12 hours for two doses; then maintenance dose of 4 mg/kg IV every 12 hours. If patient can't tolerate 4-mg/kg dose, decrease to 3 mg/kg. Continue IV therapy for at least 7 days. Switch to PO form as tolerated, using the maintenance dosages shown here.

Adults weighing 40 kg or more, children ages 12 to 14 weighing 50 kg or more, and children age 15 and older regardless of body weight: 200 mg PO every 12 hours. May increase to 300 mg PO every 12 hours, if needed. If unable to tolerate the 300-mg dose, reduce dose in 50-mg decrements to a minimum of 200 mg every 12 hours.

Adults weighing less than 40 kg: 100 mg PO every 12 hours. May increase to 150 mg PO every 12 hours, if needed. If unable to tolerate the 150-mg dose, reduce dose to 100 mg every 12 hours.

Children ages 2 to younger than 12 and children ages 12 to 14 weighing less than 50 kg: Initially, 9 mg/kg IV every 12 hours for two doses; then maintenance dose of 8 mg/kg IV every 12 hours. If patient can't tolerate 8-mg/kg IV dose, reduce dose by 1-mg/kg steps. If patient response is inadequate and patient is able to tolerate initial IV maintenance dose, increase dose by 1-mg/kg steps. Continue IV therapy for at least 7 days; then switch to 9 mg/kg PO every 12 hours. If patient can't tolerate 9-mg/kg PO dose, reduce dose by 1-mg/kg or 50-mg steps. If patient response is inadequate and patient is able to tolerate initial PO maintenance dose, increase dose by 1-mg/kg or 50-mg steps to a maximum of 350 mg PO every 12 hours.

➤ **Candidemia in nonneutropenic patients;** *Candida* **infections of the kidney, abdomen, bladder wall, or wounds and disseminated skin infections**

Adults, children ages 12 to 14 weighing 50 kg or more, and children age 15 and older regardless of body weight: Initially, 6 mg/kg IV every 12 hours for two doses, then 3 to 4 mg/kg IV every 12 hours for maintenance, depending on severity of the infection. If patient can't tolerate 4-mg/kg dose, decrease to 3 mg/kg. Switch to PO form as tolerated, using the maintenance dosages shown here.

Adults weighing 40 kg or more, children ages 12 to 14 weighing 50 kg or more, and children age 15 and older regardless of body weight: 200 mg PO every 12 hours. May increase to 300 mg PO every 12 hours, if needed. If unable to tolerate the 300-mg dose, reduce dose in 50-mg decrements to a minimum of 200 mg every 12 hours.

Adults weighing less than 40 kg: 100 mg PO every 12 hours. May increase to 150 mg PO every 12 hours, if needed. If unable to tolerate the 150-mg dose, reduce dose to 100 mg every 12 hours.

Treat patients with candidemia for at least 14 days after symptoms resolve or after the last positive culture result, whichever is longer.

Children ages 2 to younger than 12 and children ages 12 to 14 weighing less than 50 kg: Initially, 9 mg/kg IV every 12 hours for two doses; then maintenance dose of 8 mg/kg IV every 12 hours. If patient can't tolerate 8-mg/kg IV dose, reduce dose by 1-mg/kg steps. If patient response is inadequate and patient is able to tolerate initial IV maintenance dose, increase dose by 1-mg/kg steps. Continue IV therapy for at least 5 days; then switch to 9 mg/kg PO every 12 hours. If patient can't tolerate 9-mg/kg PO dose, reduce dose by 1-mg/kg or 50-mg steps. If patient response is inadequate and patient is able to tolerate initial PO maintenance dose, increase dose by 1-mg/kg or 50-mg steps to a maximum of 350 mg PO every 12 hours.

ADMINISTRATION
• Obtain specimens for fungal culture and other relevant lab studies (including histopathology) before starting therapy to isolate and identify causative organism(s). May start drug before study results are known. Adjust therapy when results become available if necessary.

PO
• Give tablets or oral suspension at least 1 hour before or 1 hour after a meal or enteral tube feeding.
• For the oral suspension, use only the dispenser provided in the medication package.
• Don't mix oral suspension with other drugs or beverages.
• Shake suspension for 10 seconds before each use. Store at room temperature.

Discard unused portion of suspension after 14 days.

IV

▼ In patients with CrCl less than 50 mL/minute, use IV form cautiously and closely monitor serum creatinine level. Change to PO form is recommended.

▼ Reconstitute the powder with 19 mL of water for injection to obtain a volume of 20 mL of clear concentrate containing 10 mg/mL of drug. Discard the vial if a vacuum doesn't pull the diluent into the vial. Shake the vial until all the powder is dissolved. Use the reconstituted solution immediately.

▼ Further dilute the 10-mg/mL solution to 5 mg/mL or less. Follow manufacturer's instructions for diluting. Stable in NSS, lactated Ringer solution, and D_5W.

▼ Infuse over 1 to 2 hours at 5 mg/mL or less and a maximum hourly rate of 3 mg/kg/hour.

◑ *Alert:* Don't administer as an IV bolus injection.

▼ Don't infuse concomitantly with any blood product or short-term infusion of concentrated electrolytes, even if the two infusions are running in separate IV lines (or cannulas).

▼ **Incompatibilities:** Blood products, electrolyte supplements, 4.2% sodium bicarbonate infusion.

ACTION

Inhibits the cytochrome P-450–dependent synthesis of ergosterol, a vital component of fungal cell membranes.

Route	Onset	Peak	Duration
PO, IV	Immediate	1–2 hr	12 hr

Half-life: Variable depending on dose.

ADVERSE REACTIONS

CNS: fever, headache, hallucinations. **CV:** tachycardia, HTN, peripheral edema. **EENT:** abnormal vision, photophobia, chromatopsia, epistaxis. **GI:** nausea, vomiting, abdominal pain, diarrhea, constipation, mucosal inflammation. **GU:** renal dysfunction. **Hematologic:** *thrombocytopenia.* **Hepatic:** cholestatic jaundice. **Metabolic:** *hypokalemia.* **Respiratory:** cough, dyspnea, URI, hemoptysis. **Skin:** rash. **Other:** chills.

INTERACTIONS

Drug-drug. *Astemizole, pimozide, quinidine, sirolimus, terfenadine:* May increase levels of these drugs, leading to torsades de pointes and prolonged QT interval. Use together is contraindicated.

Benzodiazepines, calcium channel blockers, methadone, NSAIDs, sulfonylureas, vinca alkaloids: May increase levels of these drugs. Adjust dosages of these drugs; monitor patient for adverse reactions.

Carbamazepine, long-acting barbiturates, rifabutin, rifampin, *ritonavir (high-dose therapy):* May decrease voriconazole level. Use together is contraindicated.

Cyclosporine, tacrolimus: May increase levels of these drugs. Adjust dosages; monitor levels.

Efavirenz: May significantly decrease voriconazole level while significantly increasing efavirenz level. Adjust dosage of both drugs. Use of voriconazole when efavirenz dosage is 400 mg or more/day is contraindicated.

Ergot alkaloids (such as ergotamine), sirolimus: May increase levels of these drugs. Use together is contraindicated.

Fluconazole: May increase voriconazole level. Avoid use together. Monitor patient for adverse effects 24 hours after last fluconazole.

HIV protease inhibitors (amprenavir, nelfinavir, saquinavir), NNRTIs (delavirdine): May increase levels of both drugs. Monitor patient for adverse reactions and toxicity.

HMG-CoA reductase inhibitors (atorvastatin, fluvastatin, lovastatin, pravastatin, rosuvastatin, simvastatin): May increase levels and adverse effects, including rhabdomyolysis, of these drugs. Monitor patient closely and reduce dose of HMG-CoA reductase inhibitor as needed.

Omeprazole: May increase omeprazole level. When initiating voriconazole therapy in patients already receiving omeprazole doses of 40 mg or greater, reduce omeprazole dose by half.

Opioids, long-acting (fentanyl, oxycodone): May increase levels of these drugs. Adjust doses of these drugs; monitor patient for adverse reactions.

Oral contraceptives containing ethinyl estradiol and norethindrone: May increase levels

---

Reactions in bold italics are *life-threatening*. Interactions may have a *rapid onset* or a ***delayed onset***.

and adverse effects of these drugs. Monitor patient closely.

Phenytoin: May decrease voriconazole level and increase phenytoin level. Increase voriconazole maintenance dose; monitor phenytoin level.

Ritonavir: May decrease voriconazole level. Use with ritonavir dosages of 400 mg b.i.d. is contraindicated. Avoid using with low-dose ritonavir (100 mg b.i.d.) unless benefits outweigh risks.

Warfarin: May significantly prolong PT and increase INR. Monitor PT, INR, and bleeding.

Drug-herb. *St. John's wort:* May increase drug level. Use together is contraindicated.

Drug-lifestyle. *Sun exposure:* May cause photosensitivity. Advise patient to avoid excessive sunlight exposure.

EFFECTS ON LAB TEST RESULTS

• May increase alkaline phosphatase, AST, ALT, bilirubin, glucose, and creatinine levels.

• May decrease albumin, magnesium, calcium, phosphorus, and potassium levels.

• May decrease Hb level, hematocrit, and platelet, WBC, and RBC counts.

CONTRAINDICATIONS & CAUTIONS

• Contraindicated in patients hypersensitive to drug or its components and in those taking astemizole, carbamazepine, efavirenz (400-mg dose or higher), ergot alkaloid, a long-acting barbiturate, pimozide, quinidine, rifabutin, rifampin, ritonavir (high dose, 400 mg b.i.d.), terfenadine, or sirolimus.

🖾 Contraindicated in patients with rare hereditary galactose intolerance, Lapp lactase deficiency, or glucose-galactose malabsorption.

• May prolong QT interval. Rare cases of torsades de pointes, cardiac arrest, and sudden death have been reported. Use cautiously in patients with proarrhythmic conditions and in those taking concomitant drugs that can prolong QT interval.

• Use cautiously in patients hypersensitive to other azoles.

• Serious reactions, including SJS, toxic epidermal necrolysis, and erythema multiforme, have been reported. Discontinue drug for exfoliative cutaneous reactions.

• IV administration is recommended in children ages 2 to 12 with malabsorption and very low body weight for age, because oral bioavailability may be limited.

Dialyzable drug: Unlikely.

⚠ *Overdose S&S:* Photophobia.

PREGNANCY-LACTATION-REPRODUCTION

• Drug can cause fetal harm when used in pregnant women. Use during pregnancy only if benefit to mother clearly outweighs potential risk to the fetus. If used during pregnancy, inform patient of potential hazard to the fetus.

• It isn't known if drug appears in human milk. Patient should discontinue breastfeeding or discontinue drug.

NURSING CONSIDERATIONS

• Correct electrolyte disturbances before initiation of and during therapy.

• Infusion reactions, including flushing, fever, sweating, tachycardia, chest tightness, dyspnea, faintness, nausea, pruritus, and rash, may occur as soon as infusion starts. If reaction occurs, notify prescriber; infusion may need to be stopped.

• Drug hasn't been studied in children with hepatic or renal impairment. Closely monitor hepatic function and serum creatinine levels in children.

• Monitor LFT results at start of and during therapy. Monitor patients who develop abnormal LFT results for more severe hepatic injury. If patient develops signs and symptoms of liver disease, drug may need to be stopped. A higher frequency of liver enzyme elevations was observed in children.

• Monitor patient for serious exfoliative cutaneous reactions and photosensitivity skin reactions that could lead to melanoma or squamous cell carcinoma of the skin. The frequency of phototoxicity reactions is higher in children. Discontinue drug if patient develops a skin lesion consistent with squamous cell carcinoma or melanoma.

• If treatment lasts longer than 28 days, vision changes may occur.

• *Look alike–sound alike:* Don't confuse voriconazole with fluconazole.

V

PATIENT TEACHING

- Tell patient to take PO form at least 1 hour before or 1 hour after a meal.
- Tell patient taking the oral suspension to only use the dispenser provided with the medication pack.
- Advise patient not to mix oral suspension with other drugs or beverages.
- Tell patient to discard any unused portion of suspension after 14 days.
- Advise patient to avoid driving or operating machinery while taking drug, especially at night, because vision changes, including blurring, photophobia, and changes in color perception, may occur.
- Tell patient to avoid strong, direct sunlight and to use sun-protective measures.
- Advise female patient to avoid becoming pregnant during therapy because of the risk of harm to the fetus.

---

vortioxetine hydrobromide ▨
vor-tie-OX-e-teen

Trintellix

Therapeutic class: Antidepressants
Pharmacologic class: Multimodal antidepressants

AVAILABLE FORMS
Tablets: 5 mg, 10 mg, 20 mg

INDICATIONS & DOSAGES
➤ **Major depressive disorder**
Adults: 10 mg PO once daily. Increase as tolerated to targeted dose of 20 mg once daily.
Adjust-a-dose: If 10 mg once daily isn't tolerated, decrease dosage to 5 mg once daily. If discontinuing drug when patient is taking 15 or 20 mg daily, first decrease dosage to 10 mg daily for 1 week, then stop drug to avoid adverse reactions. For patients who are known CYP2D6 poor metabolizers, maximum recommended dose is 10 mg daily. ▨

ADMINISTRATION
PO
- Give drug without regard to meals.
- Store tablets at room temperature.

ACTION
Antidepressant effect of vortioxetine isn't fully understood, but is thought to be related to its enhancement of serotonergic activity in the CNS through inhibition of the reuptake of serotonin (5-HT), as well as $5\text{-}HT_3$ receptor antagonism and $5\text{-}HT_{1A}$ receptor agonism.

Route	Onset	Peak	Duration
PO	2–4 wk	7–11 hr	Unknown

Half-life: 66 hours.

ADVERSE REACTIONS
CNS: dizziness, abnormal dreams. **GI:** nausea, diarrhea, dry mouth, constipation, vomiting, taste perversion, flatulence. **GU:** sexual dysfunction. **Skin:** pruritus.

INTERACTIONS
Drug-drug. *Aspirin, NSAIDs, warfarin:* May increase risk of upper GI bleeding. Use together cautiously.
Diuretics: May increase risk of hyponatremia. Monitor patient carefully.
Linezolid, methylene blue: May increase risk of serotonin syndrome. Don't use together. Monitor patient for serotonin syndrome for 21 days or until 24 hours after last dose of linezolid or methylene blue, whichever comes first. Resume vortioxetine 24 hours after last dose of linezolid or methylene blue.
MAO inhibitors: May cause severe adverse effects from impaired serotonin metabolism. Concurrent use is contraindicated. Don't restart MAO inhibitor for at least 21 days after vortioxetine has been stopped. Start vortioxetine at least 14 days after MAO inhibitor has been stopped.
Serotonergics (buspirone, fentanyl, lithium, SSNRIs, SSRIs, TCAs, tramadol, triptans, tryptophan products): May increase risk of serotonin syndrome. Monitor patient carefully.
Strong CYP inducers (carbamazepine, phenytoin, rifampin): May decrease vortioxetine level if coadministered for more than 14 days. Consider increasing vortioxetine dosage with concurrent use, to maximum of three times original dose. Decrease vortioxetine dosage to original level within 14 days when strong CYP inducer is discontinued.

Reactions in bold italics are *life-threatening*. Interactions may have a *rapid onset* or a ***delayed onset***.

Strong CYP2D6 inhibitors (bupropion, flu-oxetine, paroxetine, quinidine): May increase vortioxetine level. Decrease vortioxetine dosage by half when given together. Increase vortioxetine dosage to original level when CYP2D6 inhibitor is discontinued.

Drug-herb. *Herbs with anticoagulant/antiplatelet properties (alfalfa, anise, bilberry):* May increase bleeding risk. Consider therapy modification.

St. John's wort: May increase risk of serotonin syndrome. Don't use together.

Drug-lifestyle. *Alcohol use:* May increase psychomotor impairment. Patient should avoid alcohol.

EFFECTS ON LAB TEST RESULTS
• May decrease sodium level.

CONTRAINDICATIONS & CAUTIONS
• Contraindicated in patients hypersensitive to drug or its components.

Black Box Warning Safety and effectiveness haven't been established in children. ■
• Use cautiously in patients with a history or family history of bipolar disorder, mania, or hypomania.
• Use cautiously in patients taking diuretics or who are otherwise volume-depleted because of increased risk of hyponatremia.
• Drug may increase bleeding risk, particularly if used with aspirin, NSAIDs, warfarin, or other drugs or herbs that interfere with hemostasis.
• Drug may cause withdrawal syndrome (dysphoric mood, irritability, agitation, dizziness, sensory disturbances, anxiety, confusion, headache, lethargy, emotional lability, insomnia, hypomania, tinnitus, and seizures). At discontinuation of therapy, it's recommended that dosages of 15 mg once daily or more be decreased to 10 mg once daily for 1 week before full discontinuation to prevent withdrawal signs and symptoms. If intolerable signs and symptoms occur after a dosage decrease or upon discontinuation of therapy, consider resuming previous dosage with a more gradual taper.

Dialyzable drug: Unknown.

⚠ Overdose S&S: Dizziness, diarrhea, abdominal discomfort, generalized pruritus, somnolence, flushing, nausea.

PREGNANCY-LACTATION-REPRODUCTION
• Drug's effects during pregnancy are unknown. Use only if potential benefits outweigh potential risks to the fetus.
• It isn't known if drug appears in human milk. Patient should discontinue breastfeeding or discontinue drug.

NURSING CONSIDERATIONS
• Abrupt discontinuation is possible, but may cause headache, muscle tension, mood swings, and outbursts of anger.

Black Box Warning Drug increases risk of suicidal thoughts and behavior in children, adolescents, and young adults. ■

Black Box Warning Monitor patients for signs and symptoms of worsening depression, emergence of suicidal ideation and behavior (suicidality), or unusual changes in behavior, especially during initial treatment or with dosage changes, either increases or decreases. ■
• Screen patients for bipolar disorder before drug initiation. Drug isn't approved for use in bipolar depression.
• Monitor patients for signs and symptoms of hyponatremia and SIADH (headache, difficulty concentrating, memory impairment, confusion, weakness, unsteadiness, hallucination, syncope, seizure, coma, respiratory arrest, death). Discontinue drug if hyponatremia occurs.
• Monitor patients for signs and symptoms of serotonin syndrome, including mental status changes (agitation, hallucinations, delirium, coma), autonomic instability (tachycardia, labile blood pressure, dizziness, diaphoresis, flushing, hyperthermia), neuromuscular symptoms (tremor, rigidity, myoclonus, hyperreflexia, incoordination), seizures, or severe GI symptoms (nausea, vomiting, diarrhea). Discontinue drug immediately if signs and symptoms occur.

PATIENT TEACHING
Black Box Warning Advise patient and caregivers to watch for signs and symptoms of suicidal ideation and behavior, especially when dosage is being adjusted. ■
• Tell patient to report all adverse reactions to prescriber.
• Warn patient about signs and symptoms of serotonin syndrome or autonomic instability.

V

• Advise patient that nausea, xerostomia, dizziness, constipation, diarrhea, or sexual dysfunction may occur.

• Tell patient to immediately report behavioral changes, insomnia, or signs and symptoms of hyponatremia, hemorrhaging, or serotonin syndrome.

• Warn patient not to stop drug abruptly or without discussing with prescriber.

• Caution patient about operating machinery or doing tasks that require alertness while taking drug.

SAFETY ALERT!

warfarin sodium ☒
WAR-far-in

Coumadin✎, Jantoven

Therapeutic class: Anticoagulants
Pharmacologic class: Coumarin derivatives

AVAILABLE FORMS
Tablets: 1 mg, 2 mg, 2.5 mg, 3 mg, 4 mg, 5 mg, 6 mg, 7.5 mg, 10 mg

INDICATIONS & DOSAGES
➤ **PE, DVT, MI, rheumatic heart disease with heart valve damage, prosthetic heart valves, chronic atrial fibrillation**
Adults: 2 to 5 mg PO daily for 2 to 4 days; then dosage based on daily PT and INR until stable in the therapeutic range. Usual maintenance dosage is 2 to 10 mg PO daily. Base dosages on INR target goals and other clinical factors.
Adjust-a-dose: Consider lower initiation and maintenance doses for Asian and elderly patients and those with CYP2C9 and VKORC1 genotypes. ☒

ADMINISTRATION
PO
• Establish baseline coagulation parameters before therapy. PT and INR determinations are essential for proper control. Recommended INR range is usually 2 to 3 for most patients. Target INR in patients with tilting disk valves and bileaflet mechanical valves in mitral position or caged ball or caged disk valves is 2.5 to 3.5.
• Give drug at same time daily.

ACTION ▮▮▮▮
Inhibits vitamin K-dependent activation of clotting factors II, VII, IX, and X, formed in the liver. Also inhibits anticoagulant proteins C and S.

Route	Onset	Peak	Duration
PO	Within 24 hr	4 hr	2–5 days

Half-life: 20 to 60 hours.

ADVERSE REACTIONS
CV: vasculitis. **GI:** abdominal pain, diarrhea, flatulence, bloating, nausea, taste perversion, vomiting. **Hematologic:** *hemorrhage.* **Hepatic:** hepatitis. **Respiratory:** tracheal or tracheobronchial calcification. **Skin:** alopecia, pruritus, rash, dermatitis, bullous eruptions. **Other:** chills, hypersensitivity or allergic reactions, including *anaphylactic reactions* and urticaria.

INTERACTIONS
Drug-drug. *Acetaminophen:* May increase bleeding with long-term therapy (more than 2 weeks) at high doses (more than 2 g/day) of acetaminophen. Monitor therapy.
Allopurinol, **amiodarone, anabolic steroids,** *anticoagulants (argatroban, bivalirudin),* **azole antifungals,** *aspirin, beta blockers (atenolol, propranolol), cephalosporins, chloramphenicol, cimetidine,* **danazol,** *diazoxide, diflunisal, disulfiram, erythromycin, ethacrynic acid, felbamate,* **fibric acids, fluoxymesterone,** *fluoroquinolones, furosemide, glucagon, HMG-CoA reductase inhibitors (fluvastatin, lovastatin, simvastatin), heparin, influenza virus vaccine, isoniazid,* **lansoprazole,** *macrolide antibiotics (azithromycin, clarithromycin, erythromycin), meclofenamate, methimazole, methyldopa, methylphenidate,* **methyltestosterone, metronidazole, nalidixic acid,** *neomycin (oral),* **NSAIDs,** *omeprazole,* **oxandrolone,** *pentoxifylline, propafenone, propylthiouracil, quinidine, quinolones (ciprofloxacin, levofloxacin, ofloxacin),* **salicylates,** *selective cyclo-oxygenase-2 inhibitors (celecoxib), SSRIs,* **sulfamethoxazole–trimethoprim, sulfonamides,** *tamoxifen, tetracyclines, thiazides, thrombolytics,* **thyroid drugs,** *ticlopidine, tramadol, vitamin E, valproic acid, zafirlukast:* May increase anticoagulant effect.

Reactions in bold italics are *life-threatening*. Interactions may have a *rapid onset* or a **delayed onset**.

Monitor patient carefully for bleeding. Reduce anticoagulant dosage as directed.

Aprepitant, ascorbic acid, **barbiturates,** *bosentan, carbamazepine, clozapine, corticosteroids, corticotropin, cyclosporine, dicloxacillin, griseofulvin, haloperidol, meprobamate, mercaptopurine, nafcillin, oral contraceptives containing estrogen, protease inhibitors (indinavir, ritonavir), raloxifene, ribavirin, rifampin, spironolactone, sucralfate, thiazide diuretics, trazodone, vitamin K:* May reduce the PT and thereby decrease the INR, which reduces the anticoagulant effect. Monitor PT and INR carefully. Increase warfarin dosage, as needed.

Cyclophosphamide, phenytoin, propylthiouracil, ranitidine: May affect PT and INR. Monitor PT and INR carefully.

Sulfonylureas (oral antidiabetics): May increase hypoglycemic response. Monitor glucose levels.

Drug-herb. *Coenzyme Q10, ginseng, St. John's wort:* May reduce action of warfarin. Modify therapy.

Green tea: May decrease anticoagulant effect caused by vitamin K content of green tea. Advise patient to minimize variable consumption of green tea.

Herbs with anticoagulant properties (dong quai, fenugreek, feverfew, garlic, ginger, **ginkgo,** *willow bark):* May increase risk of bleeding. Discourage use together.

Drug-food. **Cranberry juice:** May increase risk of severe bleeding. Discourage use together.

Foods, multivitamins, and other enteral products containing vitamin K: May impair anticoagulation. Tell patient to maintain consistent daily intake of foods containing vitamin K.

Drug-lifestyle. *Alcohol use:* May enhance anticoagulant effects. Tell patient to avoid large amounts of alcohol.

EFFECTS ON LAB TEST RESULTS
- May increase ALT and AST levels.
- May increase INR, and prolong PT and PTT.
- May falsely decrease theophylline level.

CONTRAINDICATIONS & CAUTIONS
Black Box Warning Drugs, dietary changes, and other factors affect INR levels achieved with warfarin therapy. ∎
- Contraindicated in patients hypersensitive to drug and in those with bleeding from the GI, GU, or respiratory tract; aneurysm; cerebrovascular hemorrhage; severe or malignant HTN; severe renal or hepatic disease; subacute bacterial endocarditis, pericarditis, or pericardial effusion; or blood dyscrasias or hemorrhagic tendencies.
- Contraindicated after recent surgery involving large open areas, eye, brain, or spinal cord; recent prostatectomy; or major regional lumbar block anesthesia, spinal puncture, or diagnostic or therapeutic invasive procedures.
- Fatal and serious calciphylaxis (calcium uremic arteriolopathy) has been reported in patients with and without ESRD. If calciphylaxis is diagnosed, stop drug and treat calciphylaxis. Consider alternative anticoagulation.
- Avoid using in patients with a history of warfarin-induced necrosis; in unsupervised patients with senility, alcoholism, or psychosis; or in situations in which there are inadequate lab facilities for coagulation testing.
- Use cautiously in patients with diverticulitis, colitis, mild or moderate HTN, or mild or moderate hepatic or renal disease; with drainage tubes in any orifice; with regional or lumbar block anesthesia; with heparin-induced thrombocytopenia and deep venous thrombosis; and in conditions that increase risk of hemorrhage.
- Acute kidney injury may occur in patients with altered glomerular integrity or with a history of kidney disease, possibly in relation to episodes of excessive anticoagulation and hematuria.
Dialyzable drug: Unknown.
⚠ **Overdose S&S:** Blood in stools or urine, excessive bruising, persistent oozing from superficial injuries, excessive menstrual bleeding, melena, petechiae.

PREGNANCY-LACTATION-REPRODUCTION
- Drug can cause fetal harm. Contraindicated in pregnant women except those with mechanical heart valves, who are at high risk

W

for thromboembolism and for whom benefits of warfarin may outweigh risks.
• Verify pregnancy status of women of childbearing potential before starting drug.
• Women of childbearing potential should use effective contraception during therapy and for 1 month after final dose.
• Drug hasn't been detected in human milk. Use cautiously in breastfeeding women. Monitor breastfed infants for bruising or bleeding.

NURSING CONSIDERATIONS
Black Box Warning Warfarin can cause major or fatal bleeding, which is more likely to occur during the starting period and with a higher dose. Regularly monitor INR in all patients. Consider more frequent INR monitoring in those at high risk for bleeding. ■
• Obtain daily INR determinations upon initiation until stable in the therapeutic range; then, every 1 to 4 weeks.
• Avoid IM injections when possible.
• Regularly inspect patient for bleeding gums, bruises on arms or legs, petechiae, nosebleeds, melena, tarry stools, hematuria, and hematemesis.
• Check for unexpected bleeding in breastfed children of women who take this drug.
• Monitor patient for purple-toes syndrome, characterized by a dark purple or mottled color of the toes; may occur 3 to 10 weeks, or even later, after starting therapy.
○ *Alert:* Withhold drug and call prescriber at once in the event of fever or rash (signs of severe adverse reactions).
• No dosage adjustment is necessary for patients with renal failure. Monitor INR more frequently in patients with compromised renal function to maintain INR within therapeutic range.
• Effect can be neutralized by oral or parenteral vitamin K.
• Elderly patients and patients with renal or hepatic failure are especially sensitive to drug's effect.
• Make sure that patient isn't taking additional anticoagulants unless instructed by prescriber.
• *Look alike–sound alike:* Don't confuse Coumadin with Avandia or Cardura. Don't confuse Jantoven with Janumet or Januvia.

PATIENT TEACHING
• Stress importance of complying with prescribed dosage and follow-up appointments. Tell patient to carry a card that identifies patient's increased risk of bleeding.
Black Box Warning Tell patient and family about measures to prevent bleeding, to watch for signs of bleeding or abnormal bruising, and to call prescriber at once if they occur. ■
• Warn patient to avoid OTC products containing aspirin, other salicylates, or drugs that may interact with warfarin unless ordered by prescriber.
○ *Alert:* Advise patient to consult prescriber before initiating any herbal therapy as many herbs have anticoagulant, antiplatelet, or fibrinolytic properties.
• Tell patient to consult prescriber before using miconazole vaginal cream or suppositories. Abnormal bleeding and bruising have occurred.
• Instruct female patient to notify prescriber if menstruation is heavier than usual; she may need dosage adjustment.
• Tell patient to use electric razor when shaving and to use a soft toothbrush.
• Tell patient to read food labels. Food, nutritional supplements, and multivitamins that contain vitamin K may impair anticoagulation.
• Tell patient that consuming foods high in vitamin K can decrease anticoagulant effects. Tell patient to eat a balanced diet without large amounts of green, leafy vegetables and to notify prescriber before making any dietary changes.
• Tell patient to inform all health care providers about taking warfarin and to inform warfarin prescriber of new medication orders and upcoming surgeries or procedures.

zafirlukast
zah-FUR-luh-kast

Accolate⊘

Therapeutic class: Antiasthmatics
Pharmacologic class: Leukotriene receptor antagonists

AVAILABLE FORMS
Tablets: 10 mg, 20 mg

INDICATIONS & DOSAGES
➤ **Prevention and long-term treatment of asthma**
Adults and children age 12 and older: 20 mg PO b.i.d.
Children ages 5 to 11: 10 mg PO b.i.d.

ADMINISTRATION
PO
• Give drug 1 hour before or 2 hours after meals.

ACTION
Selectively competes for leukotriene receptor sites, blocking inflammatory action.

Route	Onset	Peak	Duration
PO	Rapid	2–3 hr	12 hr

Half-life: 10 hours.

ADVERSE REACTIONS
CNS: headache, asthenia, dizziness, pain, fever. **GI:** abdominal pain, diarrhea, dyspepsia, gastritis, nausea, vomiting. **Musculoskeletal:** back pain, myalgia. **Other:** accidental injury, infection.

INTERACTIONS
Drug-drug. *Aspirin:* May increase zafirlukast level. Monitor patient for adverse effects.
Erythromycin, theophylline: May decrease zafirlukast level. Monitor patient for decreased effectiveness.
Lumacaftor: May increase or decrease serum concentration of CYP2C9 substrates (high risk with inhibitors or inducers). Monitor therapy.
Warfarin: May increase warfarin concentration, prolonging PT. Monitor PT and INR, and adjust anticoagulant dosage.
Drug-food. *Any food:* May reduce rate and extent of drug absorption. Advise patient to take drug 1 hour before or 2 hours after a meal.

EFFECTS ON LAB TEST RESULTS
• May increase liver enzyme levels.

CONTRAINDICATIONS & CAUTIONS
• Contraindicated in patients hypersensitive to drug and in those with hepatic impairment, including hepatic cirrhosis.

• Use cautiously in elderly patients.
Dialyzable drug: Unknown.
⚠ *Overdose S&S:* Rash, upset stomach.

PREGNANCY-LACTATION-REPRODUCTION
• There are no adequate studies in pregnant women. Use during pregnancy only if clearly needed.
• Drug appears in human milk. Don't use in breastfeeding women because of potential for tumorigenicity shown in animal studies.

NURSING CONSIDERATIONS
⚠ *Alert:* Reducing oral corticosteroid dose has been followed in rare cases by eosinophilia, vasculitic rash, worsening pulmonary symptoms, cardiac complications, or neuropathy, sometimes known as Churg-Strauss syndrome.
• Drug isn't indicated to reverse bronchospasm in acute asthma attacks, including status asthmaticus.
⚠ *Alert:* Drug may cause behavior and mood changes, including agitation, depression, insomnia, and suicidal thinking and behavior. Monitor patient and consider discontinuing drug if neuropsychiatric symptoms develop.
⚠ *Alert:* Life-threatening hepatic failure has been noted in postmarketing reports. If liver dysfunction is suspected (right upper quadrant abdominal pain, nausea, fatigue, lethargy, pruritus, jaundice, flulike symptoms, anorexia, enlarged liver), discontinue drug immediately.
• *Look alike–sound alike:* Don't confuse Accolate with Accupril or Accutane.

PATIENT TEACHING
• Tell patient that drug is used for long-term treatment of asthma and to keep taking it even if symptoms resolve.
• Advise patient that drug isn't indicated for use in reversal of bronchospasm in acute asthma attacks, including status asthmaticus.
• Advise patient to continue taking other antiasthmatics, as prescribed.
• Instruct patient to take drug 1 hour before or 2 hours after meals.
• Warn patient that drug may cause behavior and mood changes (agitation, insomnia, depression, suicidal thinking and behavior), and to report development of these symptoms to prescriber.

• Teach patient to report rare but serious signs and symptoms of hepatic dysfunction.

zaleplon
ZAL-ah-plon

Sonata

Therapeutic class: Hypnotics
Pharmacologic class: Pyrazolopyrimidines
Controlled substance schedule: IV

AVAILABLE FORMS
Capsules: 5 mg, 10 mg

INDICATIONS & DOSAGES
➤ **Short-term treatment (7 to 10 days) of insomnia**
Adults: 10 mg PO daily at bedtime; may increase to 20 mg as needed. Low-weight adults may respond to 5-mg dose. Limit use to 7 to 10 days. Reevaluate patient if drug is used for more than 2 to 3 weeks.
Adjust-a-dose: For elderly or debilitated patients, initially, 5 mg PO daily at bedtime; doses of more than 10 mg aren't recommended. For patients with mild to moderate hepatic impairment or those also taking cimetidine, 5 mg PO daily at bedtime.

ADMINISTRATION
PO
• Give drug immediately before bed or after patient has gone to bed and has experienced difficulty falling asleep.
• Don't give drug after a high-fat or heavy meal (may delay onset).

ACTION
A hypnotic with chemical structure unrelated to benzodiazepines that interacts with the GABA–benzodiazepine receptor complex in the CNS. Modulation of this complex is thought to be responsible for sedative, anxiolytic, muscle relaxant, and anticonvulsant effects of benzodiazepines.

Route	Onset	Peak	Duration
PO	Rapid	1 hr	Unknown

Half-life: 1 hour.

ADVERSE REACTIONS
CNS: complex sleep-related behaviors, amnesia, anxiety, asthenia, confusion, depersonalization, depression, difficulty concentrating, dizziness, drowsiness, fever, hallucinations, headache, hypertonia, hypoesthesia, malaise, migraine, nervousness, paresthesia, somnolence, tremor, vertigo. **CV:** chest pain, peripheral edema. **EENT:** abnormal vision, conjunctivitis, eye discomfort, ear discomfort, hyperacusis, epistaxis, smell alteration. **GI:** abdominal pain, anorexia, colitis, constipation, dry mouth, dysgeusia, dyspepsia, nausea, taste perversion. **GU:** dysmenorrhea. **Musculoskeletal:** arthralgia, arthritis, back pain, myalgia. **Respiratory:** bronchitis. **Skin:** photosensitivity reactions, pruritus, rash.

INTERACTIONS
Drug-drug. *Carbamazepine, phenobarbital, phenytoin, rifampin, other CYP3A4 inducers:* May reduce zaleplon bioavailability and peak level by 80%. Consider using a different hypnotic.
Cimetidine: May increase zaleplon bioavailability and peak level by 85%. Use an initial zaleplon dose of 5 mg.
CNS depressants (imipramine, thioridazine): May cause additive CNS effects. Use together cautiously.
Black Box Warning *Opioid class warning:* May cause slow or difficult breathing, sedation, and death. Avoid use together. If use together is necessary, limit dosage and duration of each drug to minimum necessary for desired effect. ∎
Promethazine: May decrease zaleplon plasma level. Use together cautiously.
Drug-food. *Heavy meals, high-fat foods:* May prolong absorption, delaying peak drug level by about 2 hours; may delay sleep onset. Advise patient not to take with meals.
Drug-lifestyle. *Alcohol use:* May increase CNS effects. Discourage use together.

EFFECTS ON LAB TEST RESULTS
• May increase lipid levels.

CONTRAINDICATIONS & CAUTIONS
• Contraindicated in patients hypersensitive to drug or its components and in those with severe hepatic impairment.

Reactions in bold italics are *life-threatening*. Interactions may have a *rapid onset* or a *delayed onset*.

• If hypersensitivity reactions occur, don't rechallenge patient.

Black Box Warning *Opioid class warning:* Opioids should only be prescribed with benzodiazepines or other CNS depressants to patients for whom alternative treatment options are inadequate. ■

Black Box Warning Drug may cause rare but serious injury, including death, due to complex sleep behaviors, such as sleepwalking, sleep driving, and engaging in other activities while not fully awake. These behaviors can occur even at the lowest recommended doses and after just one dose. Drug is contraindicated in patients with a history of complex sleep behavior while taking drug. ■

• Avoid use in patients with sensitivity to tartrazine (FD&C Yellow No. 5), which is contained in capsules. Reactions may occur more frequently in patients with aspirin hypersensitivity.

• Use cautiously in elderly, depressed, or debilitated patients; in patients with history of drug dependence, benzodiazepine abuse, or benzodiazepine-like hypnotic abuse; and in patients with compromised respiratory function or asthma.

• Drug may cause changes in behavior and thinking, including out-of-character extroversion or aggressive behavior, loss of personal identity, confusion, strange behavior, agitation, hallucinations, worsening of depression, or suicidal thoughts.

Dialyzable drug: Unknown.

⚠ Overdose S&S: Drowsiness, confusion, lethargy, ataxia, hypotension, respiratory depression, coma, death.

PREGNANCY-LACTATION-REPRODUCTION

• There are no adequate studies in pregnant women. Use during pregnancy isn't recommended.

• Drug appears in human milk in a small amount, with highest amount occurring during a feeding at about 1 hour after administration. Use in breastfeeding women isn't recommended.

NURSING CONSIDERATIONS

• Closely monitor patients who have compromised respiratory function caused by illness or who are elderly or debilitated

because they are more sensitive to respiratory depression.

• Start treatment only after carefully evaluating patient because sleep disturbances may be a symptom of an underlying physical or psychiatric disorder.

• Adverse reactions are usually dose-related. Consult prescriber about dose reduction if adverse reactions occur.

• *Look alike–sound alike:* Don't confuse zaleplon with Zelapar, Zemplar, or zolpidem.

PATIENT TEACHING

Black Box Warning *Opioid class warning:* Caution patient or caregiver of patient taking an opioid with a benzodiazepine, CNS depressant, or alcohol to seek immediate medical attention for dizziness, lightheadedness, extreme sleepiness, slowed or difficult breathing, or unresponsiveness. ■

Black Box Warning Warn patient of risk of injury or death related to complex sleep behaviors. Direct patient to stop drug and immediately report an episode of complex sleep behavior or if patient doesn't remember activities performed while taking drug. ■

☙ Alert: Warn patient that drug may cause allergic reactions. Advise patient to report these adverse effects.

• Advise patient that drug works rapidly and should only be taken immediately before bedtime or after going to bed when patient has had trouble falling asleep.

• Advise patient to take drug only if patient will be able to sleep for at least 4 undisturbed hours.

• Caution patient that drowsiness, dizziness, light-headedness, and coordination problems occur most often within 1 hour after taking drug.

• Advise patient to avoid alcohol use while taking drug and to notify prescriber before taking other prescription or OTC drugs.

• Tell patient not to take drug after a high-fat or heavy meal.

• Advise patient to report sleep problems that continue despite use of drug.

• Notify patient that dependence can occur and that drug is recommended for short-term use only.

• Warn patient not to abruptly stop drug because of risk of withdrawal symptoms, including unpleasant feelings, stomach and

Z

muscle cramps, vomiting, sweating, shakiness, and seizures.

• Notify patient that insomnia may recur for a few nights after stopping drug but should resolve on its own.

• Warn patient that drug may cause changes in behavior and thinking, including complex behaviors, out-of-character extroversion or aggressive behavior, loss of personal identity, confusion, strange behavior, agitation, hallucinations, worsening of depression, or suicidal thoughts. Tell patient to notify prescriber immediately if these symptoms occur as drug may need to be discontinued.

• Advise female patient to consult prescriber before becoming pregnant or breastfeeding.

zidovudine (azidothymidine, AZT, Compound S)

zid-oh-VEW-den

Retrovir⬦

Therapeutic class: Antiretrovirals
Pharmacologic class: Nucleoside–nucleotide reverse transcriptase inhibitors

AVAILABLE FORMS

Capsules🅾🅽🅲*:* 100 mg
Injection: 10 mg/mL
Syrup: 50 mg/5 mL
Tablets🅾🅽🅲*:* 300 mg

INDICATIONS & DOSAGES

Adjust-a-dose (for all indications): In patients with significant anemia (Hb level less than 7.5 g/dL or more than 25% below baseline) or significant neutropenia (granulocyte count less than 750/mm³ or more than 50% below baseline), interrupt therapy until evidence proves marrow has recovered. In patients receiving hemodialysis or peritoneal dialysis, or with CrCl less than 15 mL/minute, give 100 mg PO or 1 mg/kg IV every 6 to 8 hours. For patients with mild to moderate hepatic dysfunction or liver cirrhosis, daily dose may need to be reduced.

➤ **HIV infection, with other antiretrovirals**

Adults: 300 mg PO b.i.d. with other antiretrovirals. If patient is unable to tolerate oral drug, give 1 mg/kg IV infused over 1 hour every 4 hours until PO form can be given.

Children ages 4 weeks to less than 18 years: Do not exceed the recommended adult dose. For patients weighing 30 kg or more, 300 mg PO b.i.d. or 200 mg PO t.i.d. For patients weighing 9 to less than 30 kg, 9 mg/kg PO b.i.d. or 6 mg/kg PO t.i.d. For patients weighing 4 to less than 9 kg, 12 mg/kg PO b.i.d. or 8 mg/kg PO t.i.d.

➤ **To prevent maternal-fetal transmission of HIV**

Pregnant women at more than 14 weeks' gestation: 100 mg PO five times daily until the start of labor. Then, 2 mg/kg IV over 1 hour followed by a continuous IV infusion of 1 mg/kg/hour until the umbilical cord is clamped.

Neonates: 2 mg/kg PO every 6 hours starting within 12 hours after birth and continuing until 6 weeks old. Or, give 1.5 mg/kg via IV infusion over 30 minutes every 6 hours.

ADMINISTRATION
PO

• Give drug PO without regard to meals.

• Capsules shouldn't be kept in places that may be damp or hot. Heat and moisture may cause the drug to break down.

• Drug is considered hazardous; use safe handling precautions.

IV

▼ Give by this route only until oral drug can be tolerated.

🟢 *Alert:* Vial stoppers contain natural rubber latex, which may cause allergic reactions in latex-sensitive individuals.

▼ Remove the calculated dose from the vial; add to D₅W to achieve a concentration no greater than 4 mg/mL.

▼ Infuse drug over 1 hour (adults) or 30 minutes (neonates) at a constant rate. Avoid rapid infusion or bolus injection.

▼ Don't give by IM injection.

▼ Protect undiluted vials from light.

▼ After dilution, solution is physically and chemically stable for 24 hours at room temperature and for 48 hours if refrigerated at 36° to 46° F (2° to 8° C). Administer diluted solution within 8 hours if stored at 77° F (25° C) or within 24 hours if refrigerated at 36° to 46° F.

▼ **Incompatibilities:** None listed by manufacturer. Consult a drug incompatibility reference for more information.

ACTION
NRTI that inhibits replication of HIV by blocking DNA synthesis.

Route	Onset	Peak	Duration
PO, IV	Unknown	30–90 min	Unknown

Half-life: ½ to 3 hours.

ADVERSE REACTIONS
CNS: asthenia, dizziness, fever, fatigue, headache, malaise, neuropathy, *seizures,* insomnia, paresthesia, somnolence. **GI:** anorexia, nausea, vomiting, *pancreatitis,* abdominal pain, constipation, diarrhea, dyspepsia, taste perversion. **Hematologic:** *agranulocytosis, neutropenia, severe bone marrow suppression, thrombocytopenia,* anemia. **Hepatic:** altered LFT values, hepatomegaly. **Metabolic:** *lactic acidosis.* **Musculoskeletal:** arthralgia, myalgia, myopathy. **Respiratory:** cough, wheezing. **Skin:** rash, diaphoresis.

INTERACTIONS
Drug-drug. *Atovaquone, fluconazole, methadone, probenecid, trimethoprim, valproic acid:* May increase bioavailability of zidovudine. May need to adjust dosage.
Clarithromycin: May enhance myelosuppressive effect of zidovudine and decrease zidovudine serum concentration. Closely monitor response to zidovudine and consider staggering zidovudine and clarithromycin doses when possible to minimize potential for interaction. Consider therapy modification.
Doxorubicin, ribavirin, stavudine: May have antagonistic effects. Avoid using together.
Ganciclovir, interferon alfa, other bone marrow suppressive or cytotoxic drugs: May increase hematologic toxicity of zidovudine. Use together cautiously.
Orlistat: May decrease serum concentration of antiretrovirals. Monitor therapy.
Phenytoin: May alter phenytoin level and decrease zidovudine clearance by 30%. Monitor patient closely.

EFFECTS ON LAB TEST RESULTS
• May increase ALT, AST, alkaline phosphatase, and LDH levels.
• May decrease RBC, WBC, granulocyte, neutrophil, and platelet counts and Hb level.

CONTRAINDICATIONS & CAUTIONS
• Contraindicated in patients who have had a potentially life-threatening hypersensitivity reaction to drug or its components.
• Potentially life-threatening hypersensitivity reactions, such as anaphylaxis and SJS, can occur.
Black Box Warning Use cautiously and with close monitoring in patients with advanced symptomatic HIV infection and in those with severe bone marrow depression. Use of this drug has been associated with hematologic toxicity, including neutropenia and severe anemia. ▮
• Use cautiously in patients with hepatomegaly, hepatitis, or other risk factors for liver disease and in those with renal insufficiency. Monitor renal function tests and LFTs.
• Use cautiously in patients with granulocyte count less than 1,000 cells/mm³ or Hb level less than 9.5 g/dL.
Black Box Warning Prolonged use has been associated with myopathy. ▮
Dialyzable drug: Unlikely.
⚠ *Overdose S&S:* Fatigue, headache, vomiting, hematologic disturbances.

PREGNANCY-LACTATION-REPRODUCTION
• U.S. Department of Health and Human Services Perinatal HIV Guidelines consider zidovudine in combination with lamivudine to be an alternative regimen for use in antiretroviral-naive pregnant women.
• Administer zidovudine IV near delivery regardless of antepartum regimen or mode of delivery in women with HIV RNA greater than 1,000 copies/mL or unknown HIV RNA status.
• Register patients in the Antiretroviral Pregnancy Registry (1-800-258-4263) that monitors pregnant women exposed to zidovudine.
• Drug appears in human milk. Because of potential for postnatal HIV-1 transmission, breastfeeding is contraindicated.

Z

• In couples who want to conceive, the HIV-infected partner should attain maximum viral suppression before conception.

NURSING CONSIDERATIONS

Black Box Warning Although rare, lactic acidosis without hypoxemia and severe hepatomegaly with steatosis may occur. Notify prescriber if patient develops unexplained tachypnea, dyspnea, or a decrease in bicarbonate level. Therapy may need to be suspended until lactic acidosis is ruled out. ■

• Frequently monitor blood studies to detect anemia or agranulocytosis or hepatic decompensation. Patients may need reduced dosage or temporary stop to therapy.

• Monitor patient for signs and symptoms of immune reconstitution syndrome (fever, pain, erythema, wound drainage, swollen lymph nodes, rash) and autoimmune disorders, which have been reported in patients treated with combination antiretroviral therapy.

• Monitor patient for signs of lipoatrophy (localized dents in the skin where fatty tissue is lost) during therapy. If feasible, switch to an alternative regimen if lipoatrophy is suspected.

• Drug may temporarily decrease morbidity and mortality in certain patients with AIDS.

• Health care providers caring for HIV-infected women and their infants may call the National Perinatal HIV Hotline for clinical consultations (888-448-8765).

• *Look alike–sound alike:* Don't confuse Retrovir with ritonavir.

PATIENT TEACHING

• Tell patient to take drug without regard to meals.

• Tell patient to take drug exactly as directed and not to share it with others.

• Remind patient to comply with the dosage schedule. Suggest ways to avoid missing doses, perhaps by using an alarm clock.

• Tell patient that dosages vary among patients and not to change dosing instructions unless directed to do so by prescriber.

• Warn patient not to take other drugs for AIDS unless prescriber has approved them.

• Advise patient that monotherapy isn't recommended and to discuss any questions with prescriber.

• Advise patient that blood transfusions may be needed during therapy because of drug-related anemia and of the importance of complying with frequent lab testing.

• Advise pregnant, HIV-infected patient that drug therapy only reduces the risk of HIV transmission to her newborn. Long-term risks to infants are unknown.

• Inform pregnant patient considering use of zidovudine for prevention of HIV-1 transmission to her infant that transmission may still occur in some cases despite therapy.

• Advise pregnant patient infected with HIV-1 not to breastfeed, to avoid postnatal transmission of HIV.

• Tell patient not to keep capsules in the kitchen, bathroom, or other places that may be damp or hot. Heat and moisture may cause the drug to break down and affect the intended results.

• Advise health care worker considering prophylactic use after occupational exposure (such as needlestick injury) that drug's safety and effectiveness haven't been established.

• Tell patient to report loss of subcutaneous fat, most evident in face, limbs, and buttocks, which may be only partially reversible over months to years if therapy is changed to a non-zidovudine-containing regimen.

• Advise patient to report signs and symptoms of lactic acidosis (nausea, vomiting, shortness of breath, weakness).

• Advise patient that potentially life-threatening hypersensitivity reactions can occur and to immediately report any rash.

ziprasidone hydrochloride
zih-PRAZ-i-done

Geodon◆, Zeldox✤

ziprasidone mesylate
Geodon

Therapeutic class: Antipsychotics
Pharmacologic class: Benzisoxazole derivatives

AVAILABLE FORMS
Capsules ⬤: 20 mg, 40 mg, 60 mg, 80 mg
IM injection: 20 mg/mL single-dose vials (after reconstitution)

Reactions in bold italics are *life-threatening*. Interactions may have a *rapid onset* or a *delayed onset*.

INDICATIONS & DOSAGES
➤ **Symptomatic treatment of schizophrenia**
Adults: Initially, 20 mg PO b.i.d. with food. Dosages are highly individualized. Adjust dosage, if necessary, no more frequently than every 2 days; to allow for lowest possible doses, the interval should be several weeks to assess symptom response.

Effective dosage range is usually 20 to 100 mg b.i.d., but an increase to a dosage greater than 80 mg b.i.d. generally isn't recommended. Safety of dosages exceeding 100 mg b.i.d. hasn't been established.
➤ **Rapid control of acute agitation in schizophrenic patients**
Adults: 10 to 20 mg IM as needed, up to a maximum dose of 40 mg daily. Doses of 10 mg may be given every 2 hours; doses of 20 mg may be given every 4 hours. If long-term therapy is indicated, replace with oral ziprasidone as soon as possible.
➤ **Acute bipolar I mania, including manic and mixed episodes, as monotherapy; maintenance treatment of bipolar I disorder as an adjunct to lithium or valproate**
Adults: 40 mg PO b.i.d. with food on day 1. Increase to 60 to 80 mg PO b.i.d. with food on day 2; then adjust dosage based on patient response from 40 to 80 mg b.i.d. with food.

ADMINISTRATION
PO
• Always give drug with food (at least 500 calories) for optimal effect.
• Capsules must be swallowed whole.
IM
• To prepare IM ziprasidone, add 1.2 mL of sterile water for injection to the vial and shake vigorously until drug is completely dissolved. Each milliliter of reconstituted solution contains 20 mg ziprasidone.
• Don't mix injection with other medicinal products or solvents other than sterile water for injection.
• Inspect parenteral drug products for particulate matter and discoloration before administration. Discard unused portion of reconstituted solution.
• The effects of giving IM for more than 3 consecutive days are unknown. If long-term therapy is necessary, switch to PO as soon as possible.

• Store injection at controlled room temperature of 77° F (25° C), excursions permitted to 59° to 86° F (15° to 30° C) in dry form, and protect from light. After reconstituting, it may be stored away from light for up to 24 hours at 59° to 86° F (15° to 30° C) or up to 7 days refrigerated, 36° to 46° F (2° to 8° C).

ACTION
May inhibit dopamine and serotonin-2 receptors, causing reduction in schizophrenia symptoms.

Route	Onset	Peak	Duration
PO	Unknown	6–8 hr	12 hr
IM	Unknown	1 hr	Unknown

Half-life: PO, about 7 hours; IM, 2 to 5 hours.

ADVERSE REACTIONS
CNS: confusion, headache, somnolence, *suicide attempt,* akathisia, dizziness, extrapyramidal symptoms, hypertonia, asthenia, dystonia (PO); tremor, twitching, fever, hypoesthesia, ataxia, amnesia, delirium, akinesia, dysarthria, choreoathetosis, incoordination, neuropathy, anxiety, insomnia, hypertonia, agitation, cogwheel rigidity, paresthesia, personality disorder, psychosis, speech disorder (IM). **CV:** *bradycardia, QT-interval prolongation,* orthostatic hypotension, tachycardia, chest pain (PO); HTN, vasodilation (IM). **EENT:** rhinitis, abnormal vision (PO). **GI:** nausea, constipation, dyspepsia, diarrhea, dry mouth, anorexia, abdominal pain, *rectal hemorrhage,* vomiting, tooth disorder (IM). **GU:** dysmenorrhea, priapism (IM). **Metabolic:** hyperglycemia. **Musculoskeletal:** myalgia (PO), back pain (IM). **Respiratory:** cough, infection (PO). **Skin:** rash (PO); injection-site pain, furunculosis, sweating (IM). **Other:** flulike syndrome (IM).

INTERACTIONS
Drug-drug. *Antihypertensives:* May enhance hypotensive effects. Monitor BP.
Carbamazepine: May decrease ziprasidone level. May need to increase ziprasidone dose to achieve desired effect.
CYP3A4 inhibitors (itraconazole, ketoconazole): May increase ziprasidone level.

Z

Ziprasidone dosage reduction may be needed to achieve desired effect.

Drugs that decrease potassium or magnesium, such as diuretics: May increase risk of arrhythmias. Monitor potassium and magnesium levels if using these drugs together.

Black Box Warning *Opioid class warning:* May cause slow or difficult breathing, sedation, and death. Avoid use together. If use together is necessary, limit dosage and duration of each drug to minimum necessary for desired effect. ∎

QT interval–prolonging drugs such as antiarrhythmics (amiodarone, bretylium, disopyramide, dofetilide, procainamide, quinidine, sotalol), arsenic trioxide, dolasetron, droperidol, mefloquine, pentamidine, phenothiazines, pimozide, quinolones, tacrolimus: May increase risk of life-threatening arrhythmias. Use together is contraindicated.

Serotonin modulators (nefazodone, trazodone, vilazodone, vortioxetine): May increase risk of serotonin syndrome and NMS. Monitor therapy.

Drug-lifestyle. *Alcohol use:* May increase dizziness, drowsiness, confusion, and difficulty concentrating. Don't use together.

EFFECTS ON LAB TEST RESULTS
• May increase glucose and lipid levels.
• May decrease WBC count.

CONTRAINDICATIONS & CAUTIONS
• Contraindicated in patients hypersensitive to drug and in those with recent MI or uncompensated HF.
• Contraindicated in patients with history of prolonged QT interval or congenital long QT syndrome and in those taking other drugs that prolong QT interval, such as dofetilide, sotalol, quinidine, other Class IA and III antiarrhythmics, thioridazine, chlorpromazine, droperidol, pimozide, gatifloxacin, moxifloxacin, mefloquine, pentamidine, arsenic trioxide, dolasetron mesylate, and tacrolimus.

Black Box Warning Elderly patients with dementia-related psychosis treated with antipsychotics are at increased risk for death. ∎

Black Box Warning *Opioid class warning:* Opioids should only be prescribed with benzodiazepines or other CNS depressants to patients for whom alternative treatment options are inadequate. ∎

⟁ *Alert:* Drug is associated with a rare but serious skin reaction known as DRESS syndrome, which may be fatal. DRESS syndrome is the presence of three or more symptoms, including cutaneous reactions (rash, exfoliative dermatitis), eosinophilia, fever, lymphadenopathy, and one or more systemic complications (hepatitis, nephritis, pneumonitis, myocarditis, pericarditis). Immediately discontinue drug if DRESS syndrome is suspected.

• Use cautiously in patients with history of seizures, bradycardia, hypokalemia, or hypomagnesemia; in those with acute diarrhea; and in those with conditions that may lower the seizure threshold (such as Alzheimer dementia).
• Use cautiously in patients at risk for aspiration pneumonia.
• Use cautiously in patients at risk for falls, including elderly patients and those with diseases or conditions that may cause somnolence, orthostatic hypotension, or motor or sensory instability and those taking medications that may cause the same.
• Don't use IM form in schizophrenic patients already taking oral ziprasidone.
• Use cautiously in elderly patients and in patients with renal or hepatic impairment.
Dialyzable drug: No.

⚠ *Overdose S&S:* Sedation, slurred speech, transitory HTN, anxiety, extrapyramidal symptoms, somnolence, tremor.

PREGNANCY-LACTATION-REPRODUCTION
• There are no adequate studies in pregnant women. Use in pregnancy only if potential benefit justifies potential risk to the fetus.
⟁ *Alert:* Neonates exposed to antipsychotics during the third trimester are at risk for developing extrapyramidal signs and symptoms (repetitive movements of the face and body) and withdrawal symptoms (agitation, abnormally increased or decreased muscle tone, tremors, sleepiness, severe difficulty breathing, difficulty feeding) after delivery.
• Enroll women ages 18 to 45 exposed to drug during pregnancy in the National Pregnancy Registry for Atypical Antipsychotics (1-866-961-2388).

Reactions in bold italics are *life-threatening*. Interactions may have a *rapid onset* or a *delayed onset*.

• It isn't known if drug or its metabolites appear in human milk. Breastfeeding isn't recommended.

NURSING CONSIDERATIONS
Black Box Warning Drug isn't approved for use in elderly patients with dementia-related psychosis because of increased risk of death from CV events or infection. ∎

☯ Alert: Monitor patients and immediately report signs and symptoms of DRESS syndrome (rash, fever, swollen glands), as drug will be discontinued if DRESS syndrome is suspected.

☯ Alert: Severe and sometimes fatal cutaneous adverse reactions such as SJS have been reported in patients taking ziprasidone. Discontinue drug if a severe cutaneous adverse reaction is suspected.

☯ Alert: Hyperglycemia may occur. Monitor patients with diabetes regularly. Patients with risk factors for diabetes should undergo fasting blood glucose testing at baseline and periodically. Monitor all patients for symptoms of hyperglycemia, including excessive hunger or thirst, frequent urination, and weakness. Hyperglycemia may be reversible when drug is stopped.

☯ Alert: Monitor patient for symptoms of metabolic syndrome (significant weight gain and increased BMI, HTN, hyperglycemia, hypercholesterolemia, and hypertriglyceridemia).

• Stop drug in patients with a QTc interval longer than 500 msec.

• Dizziness, palpitations, or syncope may be symptoms of a life-threatening arrhythmia such as torsades de pointes. Provide CV evaluation and monitoring in patients who experience these symptoms.

• Don't give to patients with electrolyte disturbances, such as hypokalemia or hypomagnesemia, because these increase the risk of arrhythmia. Monitor serum electrolyte levels periodically.

☯ Alert: Patient taking an antipsychotic may develop life-threatening NMS (hyperpyrexia, muscle rigidity, altered mental status, and autonomic instability) or tardive dyskinesia. Assess abnormal involuntary movement before starting therapy, at dosage changes, and periodically thereafter, to monitor patient for tardive dyskinesia.

• Monitor patient for abnormal body temperature regulation, especially if patient is exercising strenuously, is exposed to extreme heat, is also receiving anticholinergics, or is subject to dehydration.

• Complete fall risk assessments when initiating treatment and recurrently for patients on long-term therapy, especially for elderly patients and patients with diseases or conditions or who are taking other drugs that could increase fall risk.

• Closely monitor patients at risk for suicide.

• Symptoms may not improve for 4 to 6 weeks.

• **Look alike–sound alike:** Don't confuse ziprasidone with trazodone, zafirlukast, zidovudine, zonisamide, or Zyprexa.

PATIENT TEACHING
Black Box Warning *Opioid class warning:* Caution patient or caregiver of patient taking an opioid with a benzodiazepine, CNS depressant, or alcohol to seek immediate medical attention for dizziness, lightheadedness, extreme sleepiness, slowed or difficult breathing, or unresponsiveness. ∎

• Tell patient to take drug with food and to swallow capsules whole.

• Tell patient to immediately report signs or symptoms of dizziness, fainting, irregular heartbeat, or relevant heart problems.

• Advise patient to report recent episodes of diarrhea, abnormal movements, sudden fever, muscle rigidity, or change in mental status.

☯ Alert: Tell patient to immediately report rash (with or without blisters), fever, swollen lymph nodes, mouth ulcers, skin shedding, or targetlike spots in the skin.

• Advise female patient to consult prescriber if she is pregnant or plans to become pregnant.

• Tell female patient that breastfeeding isn't recommended during therapy.

• Advise patient that drug can cause sleepiness and to use care when operating machinery or driving a motor vehicle.

• Advise patient that drug may cause somnolence, orthostatic hypotension, and motor and sensory instability, which may lead to falls and, consequently, fractures or other injuries.

• Advise patient that symptoms may not improve for 4 to 6 weeks.

ZOLMitriptan
zohl-mah-TRIP-tan

Zomig, Zomig-ZMT

Therapeutic class: Antimigraine drugs
Pharmacologic class: Serotonin 5-HT$_1$ receptor agonists

AVAILABLE FORMS
Nasal spray: 2.5 mg, 5 mg
Tablets (immediate-release): 2.5 mg, 5 mg
Tablets (ODTs) ⬛: 2.5 mg, 5 mg

INDICATIONS & DOSAGES
➤ **Acute migraine headaches**
Adults: Initially, 2.5 mg or less PO. Break a 2.5-mg immediate-release tablet in half if a lower dose is needed. Increase to 5 mg per dose, as needed. If using ODTs, initially, 2.5 mg PO. If headache returns after first dose, give a second dose no sooner than 2 hours after first dose. Maximum dosage is 10 mg in 24 hours.
Adjust-a-dose: In patients with moderate to severe hepatic impairment, give 1.25 mg (half of one 2.5-mg tablet). Don't use ODTs because they shouldn't be broken in half. Limit total daily dose in patients with severe hepatic impairment to no more than 5 mg/day. In patients taking cimetidine, limit maximum single dose to 2.5 mg, not to exceed 5 mg in any 24-hour period.
Adults and children age 12 and older: Initially, 1 spray (2.5 mg) into nostril; may increase to maximum 5-mg single dose if needed. If headache returns after first dose, give a second dose no sooner than 2 hours after first dose. Maximum dose is 10 mg in 24 hours.
Adjust-a-dose: Nasal spray isn't recommended in patients with moderate or severe hepatic impairment. In patients taking cimetidine, limit maximum single dose to 2.5 mg, not to exceed 5 mg in any 24-hour period.
➤ **Short-term prevention of menstrual migraines ◆**
Adults: 2.5-mg tablet (immediate-release) or ODT two to three times daily starting 2 days before expected onset of menses and continued through to 5 days after onset of menses (7 days total).

ADMINISTRATION
PO
• Give ODT immediately after opening.
• Don't break or crush ODT.
• ODT dissolves on tongue and is swallowed with saliva; fluid isn't needed.
Intranasal
• Patient should gently blow nose before use.
• Remove cap and insert device into nostril and block the opposite nostril.
• Press plunger device while patient breathes gently in through the nose. Patient should then breathe gently through the mouth for 5 to 10 seconds.
• Don't test or prime spray before use; nasal sprayer contains only one dose.
• Discard after use.

ACTION
May act as an agonist at serotonin receptors on extracerebral intracranial blood vessels, which constricts the affected vessels, inhibits neuropeptide release, and reduces pain transmission in the trigeminal pathways.

Route	Onset	Peak	Duration
PO	Unknown	1½–3 hr	Unknown
Intranasal	5 min	3 hr	Unknown

Half-life: 3 hours.

ADVERSE REACTIONS
CNS: dizziness, somnolence, vertigo, paresthesia, asthenia, pain, drowsiness, depersonalization, headache, chills, insomnia. **CV:** palpitations; chest pain, pressure, tightness, or heaviness; facial edema. **EENT:** pain, tightness, or pressure in the neck, throat, or jaw; nasal irritation. **GI:** dry mouth, dysgeusia, dyspepsia, dysphagia, nausea, abdominal pain, vomiting. **Musculoskeletal:** myalgia. **Skin:** sweating. **Other:** warm or cold sensations, hypersensitivity reaction.

INTERACTIONS
Drug-drug. *Cimetidine:* May double half-life of zolmitriptan. Limit maximum single dose of zolmitriptan to 2.5 mg, not to exceed 5 mg in any 24-hour period. Monitor patient closely.
Ergot-containing drugs, other triptans: May exacerbate headaches and increase

---

Reactions in bold italics are *life-threatening*. Interactions may have a *rapid onset* or a *delayed onset*.

vasoconstricting effects. Avoid using within 24 hours of zolmitriptan.

Hormonal contraceptives, propranolol: May increase zolmitriptan level. Monitor patient closely.

MAO inhibitors: May increase zolmitriptan level. Avoid using within 2 weeks of MAO inhibitor.

Methylene blue: May enhance serotonergic effect and result in serotonin syndrome. Avoid combination.

SSRIs: May cause additive serotonin effects, resulting in weakness, hyperreflexia, or incoordination. Monitor patient closely.

Tramadol: May enhance adverse/toxic effect of tramadol, increasing risk of seizures; may increase risk of serotonin syndrome. Monitor patient closely.

EFFECTS ON LAB TEST RESULTS
• May increase alkaline phosphatase level.

CONTRAINDICATIONS & CAUTIONS
• Contraindicated in patients hypersensitive to drug or its components, within 24 hours of treatment with another 5-HT$_1$ agonist or ergot-type drug, and in patients with uncontrolled HTN, hemiplegic or basilar migraine, stroke, TIA history, PVD, ischemic bowel disease, Wolff-Parkinson-White syndrome or arrhythmias associated with other cardiac accessory conduction pathway disorders, ischemic heart disease (angina pectoris, history of MI or documented silent ischemia), symptoms of ischemic heart disease (coronary artery vasospasm, including Prinzmetal variant angina), or other significant heart disease.
• Use cautiously in patients with liver disease and in those who may be at risk for CAD (such as postmenopausal women or men older than age 40) or those with risk factors, such as HTN, hypercholesterolemia, obesity, diabetes, smoking, or family history.
Dialyzable drug: Unknown.
⚠ *Overdose S&S:* Sedation.

PREGNANCY-LACTATION-REPRODUCTION
• Drug has caused fetal harm in animal studies, but there are no adequate studies in pregnant women. Use during pregnancy only if clearly needed and potential benefit justifies potential risk to the fetus.

• It isn't known if drug appears in human milk. Patient should discontinue breastfeeding or discontinue drug.

NURSING CONSIDERATIONS
• Drug isn't intended for preventing migraines or treating hemiplegic or basilar migraines.
• Safety of drug hasn't been established for cluster headaches or for treatment of an average of more than three headaches (oral formulation) or four headaches (intranasal formulation) in a 30-day period.
❶ *Alert:* Combining drug with an SSRI or an SSNRI may cause serotonin syndrome. Signs and symptoms may include restlessness, hallucinations, loss of coordination, fast heartbeat, rapid changes in BP, increased body temperature, overactive reflexes, nausea, vomiting, and diarrhea. Serotonin syndrome may be more likely to occur when starting or increasing the dose of drug, SSRI, or SSNRI.
• Watch for serotonin syndrome in patients taking other drugs that increase serotonin level.
• Zomig ODT tablets contain phenylalanine, which can be harmful to patients with phenylketonuria.
• *Look alike–sound alike:* Don't confuse Zomig with Zoloft or Zonegran. Don't confuse zolmitriptan with rizatriptan, sumatriptan, or zolpidem.

PATIENT TEACHING
• Tell patient that drug is intended to relieve, not prevent, signs and symptoms of migraine. It isn't used to treat other types of headaches, and misuse of drug to treat more than 10 headaches per month may lead to worsening of headaches.
• Advise patient to take drug as prescribed and not to take a second dose unless instructed by prescriber. Tell patient that if a second dose is indicated and permitted, to take it 2 hours after first dose.
• Warn patient that maximum total daily dose is 10 mg.
• Instruct patient not to remove grey cap on nasal spray until just before dosing.
• Instruct patient to release the ODTs from the blister pack just before taking; tablet should dissolve on tongue.

Z

• Advise patient not to chew or break ODTs in half.
• Advise patient to immediately report pain or tightness in the chest or throat, heart throbbing, shortness of breath, slurred speech, rash, skin lumps, or swelling of the face, lips, or eyelids.
• Tell female patient not to take drug if she is or may become pregnant or is breastfeeding.
• Warn patient that serotonin syndrome may occur if drug is used in combination with other drugs that increase serotonin level (SSRIs, SSNRIs).

SAFETY ALERT!

zolpidem tartrate
ZOL-pih-dem

Ambien✒, Ambien CR, Edluar, Zolpimist

Therapeutic class: Hypnotics
Pharmacologic class: Imidazopyridines
Controlled substance schedule: IV

AVAILABLE FORMS
Oral spray: 5 mg/actuation
Tablets: 5 mg, 10 mg
Tablets (extended-release): 6.25 mg, 12.5 mg
Tablets (SL) ⓒ: 1.75 mg, 3.5 mg, 5 mg, 10 mg

INDICATIONS & DOSAGES
➤ **Short-term management of insomnia**
Adults: 5 or 10 mg (men) or 5 mg (women) immediate-release or 6.25 or 12.5 mg (men) or 6.25 mg (women) extended-release PO immediately before bedtime. Or, Edluar 5 or 10 mg (men) or 5 mg (women) SL once per night immediately before bedtime with at least 7 to 8 hours remaining before planned time of awakening. Or, Zolpimist 5 or 10 mg (men) or 5 mg (women) once per night immediately before bedtime with at least 7 to 8 hours remaining before planned time of awakening. May increase to 10 mg as needed.
Adjust-a-dose: For elderly or debilitated patients and those with mild to moderate hepatic insufficiency, 5 mg PO or SL

immediately before bedtime. Or, 6.25 mg of extended-release form. Maximum daily dose is 10 mg immediate-release and 12.5 mg extended-release.

ADMINISTRATION
PO
• For rapid sleep onset, drug should not be taken with or immediately after meals.
• Don't crush, break, or divide extended-release tablets.
• Place SL tablet under tongue to disintegrate. Patient shouldn't swallow tablet whole or take with water.
• Prime oral spray pump with 5 sprays before first use or with 1 spray if pump hasn't been used for 14 days.
• Pump spray directly over tongue. Have patient press down fully to make sure full dose is delivered.

ACTION
Although drug interacts with one of three identified GABA–benzodiazepine receptor complexes, it isn't a benzodiazepine. It exhibits hypnotic activity and minimal muscle relaxant and anticonvulsant properties.

Route	Onset	Peak	Duration
PO	30 min	30–120 min	6–8 hr

Half-life: 1½ to 8½ hours.

ADVERSE REACTIONS
CNS: headache, amnesia, abnormal dreams, complex sleep-related behaviors, ataxia, drowsiness, depression, dizziness, drugged feeling, lethargy, light-headedness, nervousness, sleep disorder, euphoria, mood swings, memory disorder. **CV:** palpitations, chest pain. **EENT:** diplopia, abnormal vision, pharyngitis, sinusitis. **GI:** abdominal pain, constipation, diarrhea, dry mouth, dyspepsia, nausea. **GU:** UTI. **Musculoskeletal:** arthralgia, myalgia, back pain. **Respiratory:** respiratory tract infection, bronchitis, cough, dyspnea. **Skin:** rash, urticaria. **Other:** flulike syndrome, hypersensitivity reactions.

INTERACTIONS
Drug-drug. *Chlorpromazine, imipramine:* May cause additive effect of decreased alertness. Monitor patient closely.

CNS depressants: May cause excessive CNS depression. Use together cautiously.

CYP3A4 inducers (rifampin): May decrease effects of zolpidem. Avoid use together.

CYP3A4 inhibitors (itraconazole, ketoconazole, verapamil): May increase zolpidem level. Use a low zolpidem dosage and monitor therapy.

Black Box Warning *Opioid class warning:* May cause slow or difficult breathing, sedation, and death. Avoid use together. If use together is necessary, limit dosage and duration of each drug to minimum necessary for desired effect. ■

Drug-herb. *Calendula, chamomile, gotu kola, kava, valerian:* May increase risk of CNS depression. Avoid concomitant use.

St. John's wort: May decrease zolpidem level and effects. Avoid concomitant use.

Drug-food. *Grapefruit juice:* May decrease zolpidem metabolism. Avoid grapefruit juice.

Drug-lifestyle. *Alcohol use:* May cause excessive CNS depression. Discourage use together.

EFFECTS ON LAB TEST RESULTS

• May increase ALT, AST, and bilirubin levels.

• May decrease radioactive iodine uptake.

CONTRAINDICATIONS & CAUTIONS

• Contraindicated in patients hypersensitive to drug or its components.

Black Box Warning *Opioid class warning:* Opioids should only be prescribed with benzodiazepines or other CNS depressants to patients for whom alternative treatment options are inadequate. ■

Black Box Warning Drug may cause rare but serious injury, including death, due to complex sleep behaviors, such as sleepwalking, sleep driving, and engaging in other activities while not fully awake. These behaviors can occur even at the lowest recommended doses and after just one dose. Drug is contraindicated in patients with a history of complex sleep behavior while taking drug. ■

• Avoid use in patients with severe hepatic impairment as it may contribute to encephalopathy.

• Use cautiously in patients with compromised respiratory status or a history of depression or worsening depression.

🌗 *Alert:* Drug level may remain elevated the day after drug use, impairing mental alertness. Risk increases if patient sleeps for less than 7 hours, takes drug with other CNS depressants including alcohol, or takes higher than recommended dose.

🌗 *Alert:* Patients taking extended-release formulation shouldn't drive or engage in other activities that require complete mental alertness the day after taking drug because drug level can remain high enough to impair these activities.

🌗 *Alert:* Drug can cause drowsiness and decreased level of consciousness, which may lead to falls and severe injuries, such as hip fractures and intracranial hemorrhage.

• Abnormal thinking and behavior changes have been reported in patients treated with zolpidem. Some of these changes included decreased inhibition (e.g., aggressiveness and extroversion that seemed out of character), bizarre behavior, agitation, and depersonalization. Visual and auditory hallucinations have been reported. Immediately evaluate signs or symptoms of new behaviors.

Dialyzable drug: No.

⚠ *Overdose S&S:* Impaired consciousness, somnolence, coma, CV or respiratory compromise, death.

PREGNANCY-LACTATION-REPRODUCTION

• There are no adequate studies in pregnant women, but drug may cause fetal or neonatal harm. Use during pregnancy only if potential benefit outweighs potential risk to the fetus.

• Monitor neonates exposed to zolpidem during pregnancy and labor for excess sedation, hypotonia, and respiratory depression and manage accordingly.

• Drug appears in human milk. Use cautiously in breastfeeding women.

• Monitor infants exposed to zolpidem through human milk for excess sedation, hypotonia, and respiratory depression. Patient may consider expressing and discarding milk during treatment and for 23 hours after zolpidem administration to minimize infant's drug exposure.

Z

NURSING CONSIDERATIONS

◐ *Alert:* Anaphylaxis and angioedema may occur as early as the first dose. Monitor patient closely. Discontinue drug and don't restart if these occur.

• Use drug only for short-term management of insomnia, usually 7 to 10 days. Reevaluate patient if insomnia persists.

• Use the smallest effective dose in all patients.

• Take precautions to prevent hoarding by patients who are depressed, suicidal, or drug-dependent, or who have a history of drug abuse.

• *Look alike–sound alike:* Don't confuse Ambien with Abilify, Ativan, or Coumadin. Don't confuse zolpidem with lorazepam, zaleplon, or zolmitriptan.

PATIENT TEACHING

Black Box Warning *Opioid class warning:* Caution patient or caregiver of patient taking an opioid with a benzodiazepine, CNS depressant, or alcohol to seek immediate medical attention for dizziness, lightheadedness, extreme sleepiness, slowed or difficult breathing, or unresponsiveness. ∎

Black Box Warning Warn patient of risk of injury or death related to complex sleep behaviors. Direct patient to stop drug and immediately report an episode of complex sleep behavior or if patient doesn't remember activities done while taking drug. ∎

◐ *Alert:* Warn patient that drug may cause allergic reactions, facial swelling, and complex sleep-related behaviors, such as driving, eating, and making phone calls while asleep. Advise patient to immediately report these adverse effects.

◐ *Alert:* Tell patient that drug has the potential to cause next-day impairment, and that this risk increases if dosing instructions aren't carefully followed. Tell patient to wait for at least 8 hours after dosing before driving or engaging in other activities requiring full mental alertness. Inform patient that impairment can be present even if patient may feel fully awake.

◐ *Alert:* Tell patient that drug can cause drowsiness and decreased level of consciousness, which may lead to falls and severe injuries.

• For rapid sleep onset, instruct patient not to take drug with or immediately after meals.

• Instruct patient to take drug immediately before going to bed; onset of action is rapid.

• Tell patient to avoid alcohol use while taking drug.

• Tell patient to place the SL tablet under the tongue and allow the tablet to disintegrate. Tell patient not to swallow, chew, break, or split the tablet, or take the tablet with water.

◐ *Alert:* Tell patient not to crush, chew, or divide the extended-release tablets.

• Instruct patient to prime spray pump with 5 sprays before first use or with 1 spray if pump hasn't been used for 14 days.

• Tell patient to aim the spray directly over the tongue and press down fully to make sure the full dose is delivered.

• Caution patient to avoid performing activities that require mental alertness or physical coordination during therapy.

zonisamide
zoh-NISS-a-mide

Zonegran

Therapeutic class: Anticonvulsants
Pharmacologic class: Sulfonamides

AVAILABLE FORMS
Capsules ⒹⓃⒼ: 25 mg, 50 mg, 100 mg

INDICATIONS & DOSAGES
➤ **Adjunctive therapy for partial seizures in adults with epilepsy**
Adults and children older than age 16: Initially, 100 mg PO daily for 2 weeks. Then, may increase dosage to 200 mg daily for at least 2 weeks. May increase dosage to 300 mg and then to 400 mg PO daily, with the dose stable for at least 2 weeks to achieve steady state at each level. May give doses once daily or b.i.d. Maximum recommended dose is 600 mg daily; however, there is no evidence of increased response with doses above 400 mg/day.
Adjust-a-dose: For patients with renal or hepatic impairment, titrate dosages more slowly and monitor patients more frequently. Use isn't recommended in patients with GFR of less than 50 mL/minute.

ADMINISTRATION
PO
- Hazardous drug; use safe handling and disposal precautions.
- Give drug without regard for food.
- Don't crush or open capsule.

ACTION
May stabilize neuronal membranes and suppress neuronal hypersynchronization at sodium and calcium channels, which prevents seizures.

Route	Onset	Peak	Duration
PO	Unknown	2–6 hr	Unknown

Half-life: 63 hours.

ADVERSE REACTIONS
CNS: dizziness, headache, somnolence, *seizures, status epilepticus,* agitation or irritability, anxiety, asthenia, ataxia, confusion, depression, difficulties in concentration or memory, difficulties in verbal expression, fatigue, hyperesthesia, incoordination, insomnia, mental slowing, nervousness, paresthesia, schizophrenic or schizophreniform behavior, speech disorders, tremor. **EENT:** amblyopia, diplopia, pharyngitis, rhinitis, taste perversion, tinnitus, nystagmus. **GI:** anorexia, abdominal pain, constipation, diarrhea, dry mouth, dyspepsia, nausea, vomiting. **GU:** kidney stones. **Hematologic:** ecchymoses. **Metabolic:** weight loss. **Respiratory:** cough. **Skin:** pruritus, rash. **Other:** accidental injury, flulike syndrome.

INTERACTIONS
Drug-drug. *CYP3A4 inducers or inhibitors:* May change zonisamide level; phenytoin, carbamazepine, phenobarbital, and valproate increase zonisamide clearance. Monitor patient closely.
Other carbonic anhydrase inhibitors (acetazolamide, dichlorphenamide, topiramate): May increase severity of metabolic acidosis; may increase risk of kidney stone formation. Monitor patient for development or worsening of metabolic acidosis.
Other CNS depressants: May cause CNS depression and other cognitive or neuropsychiatric adverse events. Use together cautiously.

Drug-herb. *Kava kava:* May enhance adverse/toxic effects of zonisamide. Monitor therapy.
Drug-lifestyle. *Alcohol use:* May cause CNS depression and other cognitive or neuropsychiatric adverse events. Use together cautiously.

EFFECTS ON LAB TEST RESULTS
- May increase chloride, alkaline phosphatase, BUN, and creatinine levels.
- May decrease serum bicarbonate, phosphorus, calcium, and albumin levels.

CONTRAINDICATIONS & CAUTIONS
- Contraindicated in patients hypersensitive to drug or to sulfonamides.
- Use cautiously in patients with renal and hepatic dysfunction or kidney stones.
- Use cautiously in patients with history of psychiatric symptoms.
- Use cautiously with other drugs that predispose patients to heat-related disorders, including but not limited to carbonic anhydrase inhibitors and drugs with anticholinergic activity.
- Safety and effectiveness in children younger than age 16 haven't been established; children are at increased risk for oligohidrosis and hyperthermia.
Dialyzable drug: Yes.
⚠ **Overdose S&S:** CNS symptoms, coma, bradycardia, hypotension, respiratory depression.

PREGNANCY-LACTATION-REPRODUCTION
- Use during pregnancy may present a significant fetal risk; a variety of fetal abnormalities can occur. Use in pregnant women only if potential benefit justifies potential risk to the fetus. Women of childbearing potential should use effective contraception.
- Monitor neonates of mothers treated with zonisamide during pregnancy for metabolic acidosis; transient metabolic acidosis may occur after birth.
- Encourage pregnant patients taking drug to enroll in the North American AED (Antiepileptic Drug) Pregnancy Registry (1-888-233-2334).
- Drug appears in human milk. Patient should discontinue breastfeeding or discontinue drug.

Z

NURSING CONSIDERATIONS

⚠️ **Alert:** Rarely, patients receiving sulfonamides have died because of severe reactions, such as SJS, fulminant hepatic necrosis, aplastic anemia, otherwise unexplained rashes, and agranulocytosis. If signs and symptoms of hypersensitivity or other serious reactions occur, stop drug immediately and notify prescriber.

⚠️ **Alert:** Closely monitor all patients taking or starting AEDs for changes in behavior indicating worsening of suicidal thoughts or behavior or depression. Symptoms such as anxiety, agitation, hostility, mania, and hypomania may be precursors to emerging suicidality.

• If patient develops acute renal failure or a significant sustained increase in creatinine or BUN level, stop drug and notify prescriber. Periodically monitor renal function.

• Drug can cause metabolic acidosis, especially in those with predisposing conditions or therapies. This risk is more frequent and severe in younger patients. Measure serum bicarbonate level before starting treatment and periodically during treatment, even in the absence of symptoms.

• Don't stop drug abruptly because this may cause increased seizures or status epilepticus; reduce dosage or stop drug gradually.

• Achieving steady-state levels may take 2 weeks.

• Monitor patient for signs and symptoms of hypersensitivity.

• Increase fluid intake and urine output to help prevent kidney stones, especially in patients with predisposing factors.

• Monitor patient for cognitive and neuropsychiatric adverse reactions, including psychomotor slowing, difficulty with concentration, speech or language problems (especially word-finding difficulties), somnolence or fatigue, depression, and psychosis.

PATIENT TEACHING

• Tell patient to take drug with or without food and to swallow capsule whole.

• Advise patient to call prescriber immediately if rash develops or seizures worsen.

• Advise patient and family that drug may increase risk of suicidal thoughts and behavior and to be alert for new or worsening symptoms of depression, unusual changes in mood or behavior, or the emergence of suicidal thoughts, behavior, or thoughts about self-harm. Tell them to report these signs or symptoms to prescriber immediately.

• Tell patient to immediately report sudden back or abdominal pain, pain when urinating, bloody or dark urine, fever, sore throat, mouth sores or easy bruising, decreased sweating, fever, depression, or speech or language problems.

• Tell patient to avoid dehydration and to maintain adequate fluid intake.

• Caution patient that drug can cause drowsiness and not to drive or operate dangerous machinery until drug's effects are known.

• Advise patient not to stop taking drug without prescriber's approval because abrupt withdrawal can cause seizures.

• Instruct female patient of childbearing potential to inform prescriber if she is pregnant, plans to become pregnant, or is breastfeeding and to use contraception during therapy.

alpelisib ✂

al-pe-LIS-ib

Piqray

Therapeutic class: Antineoplastics
Pharmacologic class: Kinase inhibitors

AVAILABLE FORMS
Tablets ⓐⓝⓓ: 50 mg, 150 mg, 200 mg

INDICATIONS & DOSAGES
➤ **Hormone receptor (HR)-positive, HER2-negative, *PIK3CA*-mutated, advanced, or metastatic breast cancer as detected by an FDA-approved test following progression on or after an endocrine-based regimen** ✂

Postmenopausal women, and men: 300 mg PO once daily. Continue treatment until disease progression or unacceptable toxicity occurs. When fulvestrant is given with alpelisib, recommended fulvestrant dosage is 500 mg IM on days 1, 15, and 29, and once monthly thereafter.

Adjust-a-dose: Refer to manufacturer's instructions for toxicity-related dosage adjustments of alpelisib and fulvestrant.

ADMINISTRATION
PO
• Drug may be considered hazardous; use safe handling precautions.
• Give at approximately the same time each day with food.
• Patient should swallow tablets whole and not chew, crush, or split them. Don't give tablets that are broken, cracked, or otherwise not intact.
• If a dose is missed, give within 9 hours after the usual time. If it has been more than 9 hours, skip the dose for that day. The next day, give drug at the usual time.
• If patient vomits after taking the dose, don't give an additional dose on that day, and resume the dosing schedule the next day at the usual time.
• Store at 68° to 77° F (20° to 25° C).

ACTION
A phosphatidylinositol-3-kinase inhibitor that induces an increase in estrogen receptor transcription in breast cancer cells. The combination of alpelisib and fulvestrant provided greater antitumor activity compared with either treatment alone.

Route	Onset	Peak	Duration
PO	Unknown	2–4 hr	Unknown

Half-life: 8 to 9 hours.

ADVERSE REACTIONS
CNS: fatigue, pyrexia, dysgeusia, headache. **CV:** peripheral edema. **GI:** diarrhea, stomatitis, vomiting, nausea, abdominal pain, dyspepsia, mucosal inflammation, mucosal dryness, decreased appetite. **GU:** UTI, *acute kidney injury*. **Hematologic:** decreased lymphocyte count, anemia, prolonged aPTT, decreased platelet count. **Metabolic:** weight loss, hyperglycemia. **Musculoskeletal:** osteonecrosis of the jaw. **Skin:** rash, alopecia, pruritus, dry skin.

INTERACTIONS
Drug-drug. *BCRP inhibitors (estrone, omeprazole, saquinavir, verapamil):* May increase alpelisib level and risk of toxicity. Avoid use together. If use together can't be avoided, closely monitor patient for adverse reactions.
CYP2C9 substrates (bosentan, candesartan, celecoxib, diclofenac, glipizide, indomethacin, losartan, phenobarbital, phenytoin, rosuvastatin, warfarin): May decrease substrate plasma concentration and therapeutic effects. Monitor patient closely.
CYP3A4 inducers (carbamazepine, efavirenz, phenytoin, rifampin): May decrease alpelisib level and therapeutic effect. Avoid use together.

EFFECTS ON LAB TEST RESULTS
• May increase creatinine, GGT, ALT, and lipase levels.
• May decrease calcium, potassium, albumin, and magnesium levels.
• May increase or decrease glucose level.
• May prolong aPTT interval.
• May decrease Hb level and lymphocyte and platelet counts.

CONTRAINDICATIONS & CAUTIONS
• Contraindicated in patients with severe hypersensitivity to drug or its components; severe reactions, including anaphylaxis and anaphylactic shock, have been reported.
• Contraindicated in patients with a history of SJS, erythema multiforme (EM), or toxic epidermal necrolysis (TEN). Severe cutaneous reactions have been reported.
• Severe hyperglycemia, including ketoacidosis, has been reported.
• Use cautiously in patients with diabetes. The safety of drug in patients with type 1 and uncontrolled type 2 diabetes hasn't been established. Patients with a history of diabetes may require intensified diabetic treatment.
• Drug may increase risk of severe pneumonitis, including acute interstitial pneumonitis and interstitial lung disease. Consider a diagnosis of noninfectious pneumonitis in patients with nonspecific respiratory signs and symptoms (hypoxia, cough, dyspnea, or interstitial infiltrates on radiologic exams) and in whom infectious, neoplastic, and other causes have been excluded by means of appropriate investigations.
• Safety and effectiveness in children haven't been established.
Dialyzable drug: Unknown.

NEW DRUGS

⚠ Overdose S&S: Hyperglycemia, nausea, asthenia, rash.

PREGNANCY-LACTATION-REPRODUCTION

• Drug can cause fetal harm. Advise pregnant women and women of childbearing potential of the risk to a fetus.
• Verify pregnancy status before starting therapy.
• Advise women of childbearing potential to use effective contraception during therapy and for 1 week after final dose.
• Advise males with female partners of childbearing potential to use condoms and effective contraception during treatment and for 1 week after final dose.
• Drug may impair fertility in males and females of reproductive potential.
• It isn't known if drug appears in human milk. Because of the potential for serious adverse reactions in the breastfed infant, patients shouldn't breastfeed during treatment and for 1 week after final dose.

NURSING CONSIDERATIONS

• Monitor patient for hypersensitivity reactions, such as dyspnea, flushing, rash, fever, or tachycardia. Permanently discontinue drug for severe hypersensitivity reactions.
• Monitor patient for severe cutaneous reactions, including SJS, EM, and TEN. If signs or symptoms of severe cutaneous reactions occur (severe rash, worsening rash, reddened skin, peeling skin; blistering of the lips, eyes, mouth, or skin; flulike symptoms, fever), interrupt therapy and consult a dermatologist. If SJS, TEN, or EM is confirmed, permanently discontinue drug. If SJS, TEN, or EM isn't confirmed, dosage modifications and management of rash may be required per the manufacturer's instructions.
• Monitor patient for hyperglycemia, including ketoacidosis. If hyperglycemia occurs, therapy interruption, dosage reduction, or drug discontinuation may be required per the manufacturer's instructions.
• Before starting drug, obtain fasting plasma glucose (FPG) and HbA_{1c} levels and optimize blood glucose level. After initiating drug, monitor blood glucose level, FPG, or both, at least once every week for the first 2 weeks, then at least once every 4 weeks, and as clinically indicated. Monitor HbA_{1c} every 3 months and as clinically indicated.
• If hyperglycemia occurs during therapy, monitor blood glucose or FPG level as clinically indicated, and at least twice weekly until blood glucose or FPG level decreases to normal. During treatment with antidiabetic medication, continue monitoring blood glucose or FPG level at least once a week for 8 weeks, then once every 2 weeks and as clinically indicated.
• Monitor patient for new or worsening respiratory signs and symptoms or for development of pneumonitis. If signs or symptoms occur, immediately interrupt therapy and evaluate for pneumonitis. Permanently discontinue drug in patients with confirmed pneumonitis.
• Monitor patient for severe diarrhea, including dehydration and acute kidney injury. If diarrhea occurs, therapy interruption, dosage reduction, or drug discontinuation may be required. Treat diarrhea as clinically indicated.

PATIENT TEACHING

• Teach patient to report all adverse reactions.
• Inform patient to immediately report signs and symptoms of hypersensitivity.
• Caution patient that severe skin reactions can occur and to immediately report signs and symptoms of severe cutaneous reactions (flulike symptoms; severe rash or rash that worsens; reddened skin; blistering of the lips, eyes or mouth; blisters on the skin or peeling skin, with or without fever).
• Warn patient that hyperglycemia may develop. Advise patient to closely monitor blood glucose level during therapy and to report signs and symptoms of hyperglycemia (increased thirst, dry mouth, frequent urination, and increased appetite with weight loss).
• Inform patient to immediately report respiratory problems, as drug can increase risk of pneumonitis.
• Advise patient that drug may cause diarrhea, which may be severe. Inform patient to start antidiarrheal treatment, increase fluid intake, and notify prescriber if diarrhea occurs.
• Warn female patient of childbearing potential that drug can cause fetal harm and that pregnancy testing will be performed before therapy begins. Advise her to immediately report a known or suspected pregnancy.
• Advise female patient of childbearing potential to use effective contraception during therapy and for 1 week after final dose.
• Advise male patient with female partners of childbearing potential to use condoms and effective contraception during therapy and for 1 week after final dose.
• Advise patient not to breastfeed during treatment and for 1 week after final dose.
• Advise male patient and female patient of childbearing potential that drug may impair fertility.

amikacin liposome inhalation suspension
am-i-KAY-sin

Arikayce

Therapeutic class: Antibacterials
Pharmacologic class: Aminoglycosides

AVAILABLE FORMS
Inhalation: 590 mg/8.4 mL unit-dose vial

Reactions in bold italics are *life-threatening.* Interactions may have a *rapid onset* or a **delayed onset.**

NEW DRUGS

INDICATIONS & DOSAGES

➤ Treatment of *Mycobacterium avium* complex (MAC) lung disease as part of a combination antibacterial drug regimen in patients who don't achieve negative sputum cultures after a minimum of 6 consecutive months of a multidrug background regimen therapy and who have limited or no alternative treatment options

Adults: 590 mg/8.4 mL oral inhalation once daily using the Lamira Nebulizer System.

ADMINISTRATION
Inhalational
• Patients using a bronchodilator should use the bronchodilator before Arikayce inhalation. Consider pretreatment with short-acting selective beta₂ agonists for patients with COPD, asthma, or bronchospasm.
• If drug has been refrigerated, allow it to come to room temperature before use.
• Before opening, shake vial well for at least 10 to 15 seconds until contents appear uniform and well mixed.
• Flip up the plastic top of vial; then pull downward to loosen the metal ring. Remove the metal ring and the rubber stopper carefully; then pour contents of vial into the medication reservoir of the Lamira Nebulizer System handset.
• Administer with the Lamira Nebulizer System only according to manufacturer's instructions. Inhalation treatment should take between 14 and 20 minutes.
• If a daily dose is missed, give the next dose the next day; don't double doses.
• Store vials refrigerated at 36° to 46° F (2° to 8° C) until expiration date on vial; don't freeze.
• May store at room temperature for up to 4 weeks; once drug is at room temperature, discard any unused drug at the end of 4 weeks.

ACTION
Disrupts and inhibits protein synthesis in the target bacteria by binding to the 30S ribosomal subunit, leading to an antibacterial effect.

Route	Onset	Peak	Duration
Inhalation	Unknown	Unknown	Unknown

Half-life: 5.9 to 19.5 hours.

ADVERSE REACTIONS
CNS: fatigue, asthenia, anxiety, fever, headache, peripheral neuropathy, dizziness, balance disorder. **CV:** chest discomfort. **EENT:** dysphonia, ototoxicity, tinnitus, epistaxis, oral fungal infection, dysgeusia, dry mouth. **GI:** diarrhea, nausea, vomiting. **Metabolic:** weight loss. **Musculoskeletal:** pain, muscular weakness. **Respiratory:** cough, hemoptysis, upper airway irritation, exacerbation of underlying pulmonary disease, pneumonia, change in sputum, bronchitis, *hypersensitivity pneumonitis, respiratory failure, pneumothorax.* **Skin:** rash. **Other:** exercise intolerance.

INTERACTIONS
Drug-drug. *Drugs with neurotoxic, nephrotoxic, or ototoxic potential*: May cause additive effects. Avoid concurrent use.
Ethacrynic acid, furosemide, mannitol, urea: May increase aminoglycoside levels in serum and tissue, and increase risk of toxicity. Avoid concurrent use.

EFFECTS ON LAB TEST RESULTS
None reported.

CONTRAINDICATIONS & CAUTIONS
• Contraindicated in patients hypersensitive to any aminoglycoside.
• Drug isn't approved for use in patients with non-refractory MAC lung disease.
Black Box Warning Drug has been associated with an increased risk of respiratory adverse reactions, including hypersensitivity pneumonitis, hemoptysis, bronchospasm, and exacerbation of underlying pulmonary disease, that have led to hospitalizations in some cases. ■
• Use cautiously in patients with known or suspected renal impairment. Drug may cause nephrotoxicity.
• Use cautiously in patients with known or suspected neuromuscular disorders such as myasthenia gravis. Aminoglycosides may aggravate muscle weakness because of a potential curare-like effect on neuromuscular function. If neuromuscular blockade occurs, it may be reversed by administering calcium salts; however, mechanical ventilation may be necessary.
• Use cautiously in elderly patients. Monitor these patients for decreased renal function.
• Safety and effectiveness in children haven't been established.
Dialyzable drug: Yes.

PREGNANCY-LACTATION-REPRODUCTION
• Drug can cause fetal harm, including total, irreversible bilateral congenital deafness. Before use in pregnant women, consider the risks to the fetus versus benefits to the mother; inform women of childbearing potential of the fetal risks.
• There are no data regarding the presence of drug in human milk or drug's effects on the breast-fed infant or on milk production. Amikacin appears in human milk when administered by other routes. Before using drug in breastfeeding women, consider the risks to the infant versus benefits to the mother.

NURSING CONSIDERATIONS
• Refer to manufacturer's instructions for use of the Lamira Nebulizer System.
Black Box Warning Monitor patient for respiratory adverse reactions, such as hypersensitivity pneumonitis (fever, cough, tachypnea, wheezing, shortness of breath), hemoptysis, bronchospasm (shortness of breath, dyspnea, wheezing, coughing, chest tightness), and exacerbation of

NEW DRUGS

underlying pulmonary disease. Discontinue drug or manage patients as medically appropriate. ∎
• Discontinue drug for hypersensitivity reaction. Manage respiratory reactions as clinically indicated.
• Monitor patient for signs and symptoms of ototoxicity (deafness, dizziness, presyncope, tinnitus, vertigo). Manage as clinically indicated; discontinue drug if necessary.
• Monitor laboratory tests for decline in renal function, which can indicate drug-induced nephrotoxicity.

PATIENT TEACHING
Black Box Warning Warn patient to immediately report serious adverse reactions, including blood in sputum, episodic cough during or after drug administration (particularly in the first month after starting drug), or worsening of lung disease. ∎
• Teach patient to report all adverse reactions and to immediately report signs and symptoms of ototoxicity (ringing or hissing in the ears, problems with balance, dizziness).
• Demonstrate proper drug administration using the Lamira Nebulizer System according to the manufacturer's instructions. Caution patient not to use the nebulizer with any other drug.
• Advise patient to immediately report shortness of breath or wheezing after administration.
• Teach patient with a history of reactive airway disease, asthma, or bronchospasm to administer drug after using a short-acting bronchodilator.
• Advise patient not to operate heavy machinery or engage in dangerous activities while inhaling drug because dizziness or respiratory symptoms can occur.
• Advise patient that blood laboratory studies will be needed during therapy to monitor for nephrotoxicity.
• Advise pregnant patient that drug may cause irreversible congenital deafness if used during pregnancy.
• Before starting drug, advise female patient of childbearing potential who is or plans to become pregnant to discuss pregnancy with prescriber.
• Caution patient not to stop drug or other medicines to treat MAC lung disease unless directed by health care provider.

---

baloxavir marboxil
bal-OX-a-vir mar-BOX-il

Xofluza

Therapeutic class: Antivirals
Pharmacologic class: Endonuclease inhibitors

AVAILABLE FORMS
Tablets: 20 mg, 40 mg

INDICATIONS & DOSAGES
➤ **Treatment of acute, uncomplicated influenza in patients who have been symptomatic for no more than 48 hours**
Adults and children age 12 and older weighing 80 kg or more: 80 mg PO as a single dose.
Adults and children age 12 and older weighing 40 to less than 80 kg: 40 mg PO as a single dose.

ADMINISTRATION
PO
• Give drug with or without food.
• Give drug within 48 hours of symptom onset.
• Store drug in original blister card at 68° to 77° F (20° to 25° C).

ACTION
An antiviral that inhibits the activity of polymerase acidic protein to halt viral gene transcription.

Route	Onset	Peak	Duration
PO	Unknown	4 hr	Unknown

Half-life: 79.1 hours.

ADVERSE REACTIONS
CNS: headache. **EENT:** nasopharyngitis. **GI:** diarrhea, nausea. **Respiratory:** bronchitis.

INTERACTIONS
Drug-drug. *Live attenuated influenza vaccine:* May decrease effectiveness of the vaccine. Avoid concurrent use.
Polyvalent cation–containing antacids, laxatives, or oral supplements (calcium, iron, magnesium, selenium, zinc): May decrease baloxavir level and effectiveness. Avoid concurrent use.
Drug-food. *Calcium-fortified beverages, dairy products, milk:* May decrease baloxavir concentration and effectiveness. Avoid use together.

EFFECTS ON LAB TEST RESULTS
None reported.

CONTRAINDICATIONS & CAUTIONS
• Contraindicated in patients hypersensitive to drug or its components.
• Safety and effectiveness in children younger than age 12 or weighing less than 40 kg haven't been established.
Dialyzable drug: Unlikely.

PREGNANCY-LACTATION-REPRODUCTION
• No data exist on the use of drug in pregnant women or on developmental risk to a fetus.
• Pregnant women may be at higher risk for severe complications from influenza, including maternal death, stillbirth, birth defects, preterm delivery, and low-birthweight and small-for-gestational-age infants.
• It isn't known if drug appears in human milk. Consider the benefits of breastfeeding and the

---

potential adverse effects on the infant before using drug.

NURSING CONSIDERATIONS

• Monitor patient for secondary bacterial infection, which may begin with influenza-like symptoms or coexist with or occur as a complication of influenza. Treat bacterial infections as clinically appropriate.

PATIENT TEACHING

• Tell patient to report all adverse reactions.
• Instruct patient that drug should be given as soon as possible after first appearance of influenza symptoms and within 48 hours of onset of symptoms.
• Counsel patient on drug administration.
• Teach patient to avoid milk, dairy products, and calcium-fortified beverages, and laxatives, antacids, or supplements containing iron, zinc, selenium, calcium, or magnesium while taking drug.
• Advise patient to consider postponing receiving live attenuated influenza vaccine while taking drug.

---

brexanolone
brex-AN-oh-lone

Zulresso

Therapeutic class: Antidepressants
Pharmacologic class: GABA_A receptor modulators
Controlled substance schedule: IV

AVAILABLE FORMS
Injection: 100 mg/20 mL single-dose vial

INDICATIONS & DOSAGES
➤ **Treatment of postpartum depression**
Women: Give as a continuous IV infusion over a total of 60 hours, titrating dosage as follows: 0 to 4 hours, 30 mcg/kg/hour; 4 to 24 hours, increase infusion rate to 60 mcg/kg/hour; 24 to 52 hours, increase infusion rate to 90 mcg/kg/hour or consider a dosage of 60 mcg/kg/hr; 52 to 56 hours, decrease infusion rate to 60 mcg/kg/hour; 56 to 60 hours, decrease infusion rate to 30 mcg/kg/hour.
Adjust-a-dose: For excessive sedation, stop the infusion until symptoms resolve and resume at the same or lower infusion rate.

ADMINISTRATION
IV
▼ Visually inspect vials. Don't use if solution is discolored or particulate matter is present.
▼ The 60-hour infusing will require preparation of five infusion bags; additional bags will be needed for patients weighing 90 kg or more.
▼ Withdraw 20 mL from vial and place in a polyolefin, non-DEHP, nonlatex bag. Dilute with 40 mL of sterile water for injection; then further

dilute with 40 mL of NSS to a concentration of 1 mg/mL. Immediately refrigerate the infusion bag for up to 96 hours.
▼ Each bag of diluted drug may be infused for up to 12 hours at room temperature; discard any unused drug after 12 hours.
▼ Use a polyvinyl chloride, non-DEHP, nonlatex infusion set without in-line filter.
▼ Administer via a dedicated line through a peristaltic infusion pump.
▼ Store undiluted drug at 36° to 46° F (2° to 8° C). Don't freeze. Store protected from light.
▼ **Incompatibilities:** Don't mix with other drugs or place other drugs in infusion bag.

ACTION
Thought to be related to positive modulation of GABA_A receptors.

Route	Onset	Peak	Duration
IV	Unknown	Unknown	Unknown

Half-life: 9 hours.

ADVERSE REACTIONS
CNS: dizziness, presyncope, vertigo, loss of consciousness, sedation, somnolence, fatigue. **CV:** tachycardia, flushing, hot flush, BP changes. **EENT:** oropharyngeal pain. **GI:** diarrhea, dry mouth, dyspepsia. **Other:** infusion-site pain.

INTERACTIONS
Drug-drug. *Antidepressants, CNS depressants (benzodiazepines, opioids):* May increase the likelihood or severity of sedation. Use cautiously together and monitor patient carefully.
Drug-lifestyle. *Alcohol use:* May increase the likelihood or severity of sedation. Discourage use together.

EFFECTS ON LAB TEST RESULTS
None reported.

CONTRAINDICATIONS & CAUTIONS
Black Box Warning There is a risk of excessive sedation or sudden loss of consciousness during administration. Monitor patient closely and include continuous pulse oximetry monitoring. ■
Black Box Warning Patients must be accompanied during interactions with their children, as excessive sedation may occur. ■
Black Box Warning Drug is available only through a Zulresso REMS program. Information can be found at www.zulressorems.com or by calling 1-844-472-4379. ■
• Drug can lead to dependence or abuse.
• Avoid use in patients with ESRD with eGFR of <15 mL/minute/1.73 m².
• Safety and effectiveness in children or elderly patients haven't been established.
Dialyzable drug: Unknown.
⚠ Overdose S&S: Loss of consciousness, excessive sedation.

NEW DRUGS

PREGNANCY-LACTATION-REPRODUCTION

• Based on animal studies, drug may cause fetal harm. Before use in pregnant women, weigh the potential benefits to the mother and risks to the infant.

• Health care providers are encouraged to register patients exposed to drug during pregnancy by calling the National Pregnancy Registry for Antidepressants at 1-844-405-6185 or https://womensmentalhealth.org/clinical-and-research-programs/pregnancyregistry/antidepressants/.

• Drug appears in human milk. However, there are no data on drug's effects on a breastfed infant. Before use in a breastfeeding patient, consider the mother's clinical need for the drug, developmental and health benefits of breastfeeding, and risk to the infant.

NURSING CONSIDERATIONS

• A health care provider must be on site for the duration of the infusion to continuously monitor patients and intervene as necessary.

• Monitor patients for hypoxia using continuous pulse oximetry. Immediately stop the infusion if pulse oximetry reveals hypoxia. Don't resume the infusion.

• Initiate treatment early enough during the day to allow for recognition of excessive sedation.

Black Box Warning Assess for excessive sedation every 2 hours during planned, nonsleep periods. ■

☉ Alert: Monitor patients for worsening of depression or emergence of suicidal thoughts and behaviors. Consider changing to another therapy as clinically indicated.

• Taper drug according to the dosage recommendations, unless signs and symptoms warrant immediate discontinuation.

• After infusion, patients shouldn't engage in potentially hazardous activities requiring mental alertness such as driving until sedative effects have dissipated.

PATIENT TEACHING

Black Box Warning Warn patient of the risk of loss of consciousness or altered states of consciousness during infusion. ■

Black Box Warning Stress that patient will be monitored during administration. Advise patient to immediately report signs and symptoms of excessive sedation. ■

Black Box Warning Emphasize that because of the risk of sedation, patient must not be the primary caregiver of dependents during the infusion and that patient must be accompanied during interactions with children. ■

Black Box Warning Inform patient that drug is available only through the Zulresso REMS program. ■

• Alert patient that drug can be abused or lead to dependence.

• Tell patient to not drive or engage in hazardous activity until drug's effects have dissipated.

☉ Alert: Advise patient and caregivers to look for the emergence of suicidal thoughts and behaviors. Instruct them to report such symptoms to prescriber.

• Advise female patient to report if she is or could be pregnant before starting drug. Also caution her about the possible risk to a fetus.

• Instruct patient who is breastfeeding to discuss risks and benefits of drug with prescriber.

SAFETY ALERT!

calaspargase pegol-mknl
kal-AS-par-jase PEG-ol

Asparlas

Therapeutic class: Antineoplastics
Pharmacologic class: Amino acid enzymes

AVAILABLE FORMS
Injection: 3,750 units/5 mL (750 units/mL) single-dose vial

INDICATIONS & DOSAGES
➤ **Acute lymphoblastic leukemia as part of a multi-agent regimen**
Adults ages 18 to 21 and children age 1 month and older: 2,500 units/m^2 IV infusion no more frequently than once every 21 days.
Adjust-a-dose: Refer to manufacturer's instructions for toxicity-related and infusion reaction adjustments.

ADMINISTRATION
IV
▼ Visually inspect vial for particulate matter, cloudiness, or discoloration before administration. If present, discard.
▼ Dilute in 100 mL NSS or D₅W. Discard any drug remaining in the vial.
▼ After dilution, administer immediately into an infusion of the same type of solution as used for vial dilution.
▼ Infuse over 1 hour.
▼ May store diluted solution for up to 4 hours at room temperature (59° to 77° F [15° to 25° C]) or refrigerated at 36° to 46° F (2° to 8° C) for up to 24 hours.
▼ Refrigerate vials and protect from light. Don't use if vial has been shaken or vigorously agitated, frozen, or stored at room temperature for more than 48 hours.
▼ **Incompatibilities:** Don't infuse other drugs or solutions through the same IV line during administration.

ACTION
An enzyme that converts ʟ-asparagine into aspartic acid and ammonia and depletes plasma

---

Reactions in bold italics are *life-threatening*. Interactions may have a *rapid* onset or a **delayed** onset.

L-asparagine levels. This decreases the amount of L-asparagine available to leukemia cells and leads to cell death.

Route	Onset	Peak	Duration
IV	Unknown	1 hr	Unknown

Half-life: 16 days.

ADVERSE REACTIONS

CV: *cardiac failure,* arrhythmia, *embolic and thrombotic events.* **GI:** *pancreatitis,* diarrhea. **Hematologic:** *hemorrhage,* abnormal clotting studies. **Hepatic:** *hepatotoxicity,* elevated transaminase levels, hyperbilirubinemia. **Respiratory:** dyspnea, pneumonia. **Other:** hypersensitivity, *anaphylaxis, sepsis,* fungal infection.

INTERACTIONS

Drug-drug. *Oral contraceptives:* May decrease efficacy of contraceptive. Patient should use a nonoral contraceptive method.

EFFECTS ON LAB TEST RESULTS

• May increase ALT, AST, bilirubin, amylase, and lipase levels.
• May decrease fibrinogen and albumin levels.
• May prolong PT and aPTT.

CONTRAINDICATIONS & CAUTIONS

• Contraindicated in patients with a history of serious hypersensitivity reactions, including anaphylaxis, to pegylated L-asparaginase therapy.
• Contraindicated in patients with a history of serious pancreatitis, thrombosis, or hemorrhage during previous L-asparaginase therapy.
• Contraindicated in patients with severe hepatic impairment.
• Use isn't indicated in adults older than age 21.
Dialyzable drug: Unknown.

PREGNANCY-LACTATION-REPRODUCTION

• Drug may cause fetal harm. Advise pregnant women of fetal risk before use.
• It isn't known if drug appears in human milk. Women shouldn't breastfeed during therapy and for 3 months after final dose.
• Females of childbearing potential should use effective nonoral contraception, including a barrier method, during treatment and for at least 3 months after final dose.

NURSING CONSIDERATIONS

• Monitor bilirubin and transaminases levels at least weekly during treatment and for at least 6 weeks after final dose. Provide supportive care and discontinue drug for serious liver toxicity.
🔴 **Alert:** Administer drug in a setting with available resuscitation equipment and agents to treat anaphylaxis (epinephrine, oxygen, IV steroids, antihistamines).
• Observe patients for 1 hour after administration. Watch for hypersensitivity reactions (angioedema,

lip or eye swelling, erythema, decreased BP, bronchospasm, dyspnea, pruritus, rash). Discontinue drug in patients with serious hypersensitivity reactions.
• Monitor patients for signs and symptoms of pancreatitis (upper abdominal pain, fever, rapid HR, nausea, vomiting, steatorrhea). Assess amylase or lipase level to confirm signs and symptoms. Withhold drug if pancreatitis is suspected and discontinue if confirmed.
• Monitor patients for hyperglycemia and glucose intolerance related to pancreatitis (excessive thirst, increase in urine volume or frequency of urination).
• Monitor patients for thrombotic events (severe headache, arm or leg swelling, dyspnea, chest pain); discontinue drug if serious event occurs.
• Monitor PT, aPTT, and fibrinogen level and watch for signs and symptoms of hemorrhage (unusual bleeding or bruising). Consider replacement therapy in patients with severe or symptomatic coagulopathy.
• Monitor patients for signs and symptoms of hepatotoxicity (jaundice, severe nausea, vomiting, bruising, bleeding).
• Obtain pregnancy test in women of childbearing potential before starting drug.
• **Look alike-sound alike:** Don't confuse calaspargase with L-asparaginase.

PATIENT TEACHING

• Advise patient to report all adverse reactions.
• Teach patient to recognize and immediately report signs or symptoms of hypersensitivity, pancreatitis, thrombosis, hemorrhage, and hepatotoxicity.
• Advise female patient of childbearing potential to use effective nonoral contraception, including a barrier method, during treatment and for at least 3 months after final dose.
• Caution female patient to immediately contact prescriber if she is pregnant or suspects she is pregnant during therapy.
• Instruct breastfeeding patient not to breastfeed during treatment and for at least 3 months after final dose.

caplacizumab-yhdp
kap-la-SIZ-ue-mab

Cablivi

Therapeutic class: Immunomodulators
Pharmacologic class: Anti–von Willebrand factors

AVAILABLE FORMS
Injection: 11 mg single-dose vial

INDICATIONS & DOSAGES
➤ **Treatment of acquired thrombotic thrombocytopenic purpura (aTTP), in combination with plasma exchange and immunosuppressive therapy**
Adults: On day 1 of plasma exchange therapy, give 11 mg IV bolus at least 15 minutes before plasma exchange, followed by 11 mg subcut after completion of plasma exchange. On subsequent days during daily plasma exchange, give 11 mg subcut once daily following plasma exchange. Continue 11 mg subcut once daily for 30 days following the last daily plasma exchange. After initial treatment course, if signs and symptoms of persistent underlying disease such as suppressed ADAMTS13 activity levels remain, may extend treatment for a maximum of 28 days. Discontinue drug if patient experiences more than two recurrences of aTTP during therapy.

ADMINISTRATION
• Bring vial and provided diluent syringe to room temperature.
• Reconstitute by attaching the adapter to the vial, then attaching the provided prefilled glass syringe of 1 mL sterile water and slowly emptying the syringe into the vial. Leaving the syringe in place, gently swirl the vial until the cake or powder is completely dissolved; don't shake.
• Visually inspect to ensure the solution is clear and colorless.
• Withdraw all of the solution from the vial into the attached syringe and label.
• Use solution immediately or refrigerate for up to 4 hours at 36° to 46° F (2° to 8° C).
• Store vials refrigerated at 36° to 46° F (2° to 8° C) in original carton to protect from light; don't freeze. May store unopened vials in original carton at room temperature up to 86° F (30° C) for a single period up to 2 months. Don't return drug to refrigerator after it has been stored at room temperature.
IV
▼ Give bolus using an IV line by connecting the syringe containing reconstituted solution using a luer-lock (not a needleless connector) and flush with NSS or D_5W.
▼ **Incompatibilities:** Don't mix drug with other drugs or solutions other than NSS or D_5W.
Subcutaneous
• Detach the filled syringe from the adapter, and attach appropriate needle. Discard the vial and attached adapter.
• Give into the abdomen, alternating abdominal quadrants with each injection. Avoid the 2-inch area around the navel.
• If a dose is missed during the plasma exchange period, give it as soon as possible. If a dose is missed after the plasma exchange period, give it within 12 hours of the scheduled time of administration. Beyond 12 hours, skip the missed dose; administer the next daily dose according to the usual dosing schedule.

ACTION
Drug is a von Willebrand factor (vWF)-directed antibody fragment that inhibits interaction between vWF and platelets decreasing platelet adhesion and consumption.

Route	Onset	Peak	Duration
IV	Unknown	Unknown	Unknown
Subcut	Unknown	6–7 hr	Unknown

Half-life: Dependent on drug concentration and target level.

ADVERSE REACTIONS
CNS: headache, *subarachnoid hemorrhage*, fatigue, pyrexia, paresthesia. **EENT:** epistaxis, gingival bleeding. **GI:** *upper GI bleeding*, *rectal hemorrhage*, abdominal wall hematoma. **GU:** UTI, hematuria, *vaginal hemorrhage*, menorrhagia, metrorrhagia. **Musculoskeletal:** back pain, myalgia. **Respiratory:** dyspnea. **Skin:** injection-site hemorrhage, catheter-site hemorrhage, injection-site pruritus, urticaria.

INTERACTIONS
Drug-drug. *Anticoagulants:* May increase risk of bleeding. Monitor patient closely.

EFFECTS ON LAB TEST RESULTS
• May transiently decrease von Willebrand factor antigen and factor VIII:C levels.

CONTRAINDICATIONS & CAUTIONS
• Contraindicated in patients with a previous severe hypersensitivity reaction to drug or its components.
🌢 **Alert:** Use cautiously in patients with underlying coagulopathies or increased risk of bleeding (hemophilia, other coagulation factor deficiencies) or severe hepatic impairment and with use of drugs affecting hemostasis and coagulation.
• Safety and effectiveness in children haven't been established.
Dialyzable drug: Unknown.

PREGNANCY-LACTATION-REPRODUCTION
• There are no available data on use in pregnant women; however, a risk of hemorrhage in the mother and fetus is associated with use of this drug. Mother and fetus or neonate should be monitored for bleeding.
• It isn't known if drug appears in human milk. Before use in breastfeeding women, consider the benefits of therapy and potential adverse effects on the infant.

NURSING CONSIDERATIONS
🌢 **Alert:** Monitor patients and interrupt treatment if clinically significant bleeding occurs. If required, administer von Willebrand factor concentrate to rapidly correct hemostasis. If drug is restarted, monitor patients for bleeding.

Reactions in bold italics are *life-threatening*. Interactions may have a *rapid onset* or a **delayed onset**.

• Withhold drug 7 days before elective surgery, dental procedures, or other invasive interventions. If emergency surgery is required, use von Willebrand factor concentrate to rapidly correct hemostasis.
• Monitor patients for hypersensitivity reactions.

PATIENT TEACHING
• Advise patient to report all adverse reactions.
• Teach patient or caregivers the proper aseptic technique for subcut administration.
• Warn patient that drug will need to be stopped 7 days before elective surgery, dental procedures, or other invasive interventions.
• Advise patient to watch for signs and symptoms of bruising or bleeding (nosebleeds, bleeding of the gums). Inform patient that if bleeding occurs, it may take longer for the bleeding to stop.
• Warn patient to immediately report severe bleeding or bruising.

SAFETY ALERT!

cemiplimab-rwlc
se-MIP-li-mab

Libtayo

Therapeutic class: Antineoplastics
Pharmacologic class: Programmed death receptor-1 blocking antibodies

AVAILABLE FORMS
Injection: 350 mg/7 mL (50 mg/mL) single-dose vial

INDICATIONS & DOSAGES
➤**Metastatic cutaneous squamous cell carcinoma (CSCC) or locally advanced CSCC in patients who aren't candidates for curative surgery or curative radiation**
Adults: 350 mg I.V. infusion every 3 weeks until disease progression or unacceptable toxicity occurs.
Adjust-a-dose: Refer to manufacturer's instructions for toxicity-related dosage adjustments.

ADMINISTRATION
IV
▼ Store unopened vials in refrigerator at 36° to 46° F (2° to 8° C) in original carton and protected from light; don't freeze or shake.
▼ Inspect vial for particulate matter and discoloration. Drug should appear clear to slightly opalescent, colorless to pale yellow, and may contain trace amounts of translucent to white particles. Discard vial if solution is cloudy, discolored, or contains other particulate matter.
▼ Withdraw 7 mL from vial and dilute with NSS or D₅W to a final concentration between 1 mg/mL and 20 mg/mL; mix diluted solution by gentle inversion but don't shake; discard any unused drug.

▼ Infuse over 30 minutes through an I.V. line containing an in-line filter or add-on 0.2- to 5-micron filter.
▼ Store at room temperature up to 77° F (25° C) for no more than 8 hours or refrigerate at 36° to 46° F (2° to 8° C) for no more than 24 hours from the time of preparation to the end of infusion. Diluted solution should come to room temperature before administration; don't freeze.
▼ **Incompatibilities:** Don't give with solutions other than NSS or D₅W.

ACTION
IgG4 monoclonal antibody that binds to programmed death-receptor (PD) antibodies, thereby blocking PD-1 activity and decreasing tumor growth.

Route	Onset	Peak	Duration
IV	Unknown	Unknown	Unknown

Half-life: 19 days.

ADVERSE REACTIONS
CNS: *aseptic meningitis,* complex regional pain syndrome, fatigue. **CV:** HTN. **GI:** diarrhea, nausea, constipation. **GU:** UTI. **Hematologic:** anemia, *lymphocytopenia.* **Hepatic:** *hepatitis.* **Metabolic:** decreased appetite, *endocrinopathies,* hypophosphatemia, hypercalcemia, hypoalbuminemia. **Musculoskeletal:** pain, muscular weakness. **Respiratory:** pneumonia, *pneumonitis,* cough. **Skin:** rash, pruritus, cellulitis, skin infection, *erythema multiforme,* pemphigoid. **Other:** *sepsis,* antibody development.

INTERACTIONS
None reported.

EFFECTS ON LAB TEST RESULTS
• May increase AST and calcium levels.
• May decrease albumin, phosphate, and sodium levels.
• May increase INR.
• May decrease Hb level and hematocrit and lymphocyte and RBC counts.

CONTRAINDICATIONS & CAUTIONS
❸ *Alert:* Immune-mediated adverse reactions, which may be severe or fatal, can occur in any organ system or tissue and include pneumonitis, GI toxicities (colitis, hepatitis, pancreatitis), endocrinopathies (adrenal insufficiency, hypophysitis, hypothyroidism, hyperthyroidism, type 1 diabetes), nephritis with renal dysfunction, dermatologic toxicities (erythema multiforme, Stevens-Johnson syndrome, pemphigoid, toxic epidermal necrolysis), myocarditis, neurologic toxicities (meningitis, encephalitis, myelitis and demyelination, myasthenic syndrome, myasthenia gravis, Guillain-Barré syndrome, nerve paresis, autoimmune neuropathy), ocular inflammatory toxicities (uveitis, iritis, retinal detachment, vision loss), musculoskeletal toxicities

NEW DRUGS

(myositis, rhabdomyolysis, arthritis, polymyalgia rheumatica), and hematologic and immunologic toxicities (hemolytic anemia, aplastic anemia, hemophagocytic lymphohistiocytosis, systemic inflammatory response syndrome, histiocytic necrotizing lymphadenitis, Kikuchi lymphadenitis, sarcoidosis, and immune thrombocytopenic purpura [solid]). Monitor patient closely.
• Drug may cause rejection of a transplanted organ. Monitor patient closely.
• Safety and effectiveness in children haven't been established.
Dialyzable drug: Unknown.

PREGNANCY-LACTATION-REPRODUCTION
• Drug can cause fetal harm based on mechanism of action. Advise females of childbearing potential about fetal risk and the need to use effective contraception during treatment and for at least 4 months after final dose.
• Test for pregnancy before starting drug.
• It isn't known if drug appears in human milk. Women shouldn't breastfeed during treatment and for at least 4 months after final dose.

NURSING CONSIDERATIONS
• Monitor patient for infusion-related reactions (chills, rash, pruritus, flushing, shortness of breath, dizziness, fever, syncope, back or neck pain, facial swelling). Interrupt or slow rate of infusion, or permanently discontinue infusion based on severity of the reaction.
• Monitor patient for development of immune-mediated adverse reactions, such as pneumonitis (new or worsening cough, chest pain, shortness of breath), GI toxicities (diarrhea, blood or mucus in stools, severe abdominal pain), hepatitis (jaundice, severe nausea or vomiting, drowsiness, dark urine, bleeding or easy bruising, anorexia, abdominal pain), endocrinopathies (signs or symptoms of hypothyroidism, hyperthyroidism, adrenal insufficiency, hypophysitis, type 1 diabetes mellitus), nephritis (hematuria, edema, anorexia, decreased urine output), neurologic toxicities (confusion, fever, weakness, balance disorder, nausea, vomiting, stiff neck, seizures), dermatologic toxicities (rash, pruritus, blisters, sores, ulcers), and organ transplant rejection.
• When immune-mediated adverse reactions occur, withhold or discontinue drug as needed and administer corticosteroids until resolved, followed by a corticosteroid taper over 1 month.
• Consider use of other systemic immunosuppressants when immune-mediated adverse reactions aren't controlled with corticosteroids and begin hormone replacement therapy for endocrinopathies as warranted.
• Evaluate LFTs and thyroid function tests at baseline and periodically during treatment.
• Assess pregnancy status before start of treatment.

PATIENT TEACHING
• Teach patient to report all adverse reactions.
• Counsel patient to immediately report immune-mediated adverse reactions or infusion-related reactions.
• Advise female patient of childbearing potential that drug can cause harm to a fetus and to inform prescriber of a known or suspected pregnancy.
• Warn female patient of childbearing potential to use effective contraception during treatment and for at least 4 months after final dose.
• Instruct female patient not to breastfeed while taking drug and for at least 4 months after final dose.

SAFETY ALERT!

dacomitinib ☒
dak-oh-MI-ti-nib

Vizimpro

Therapeutic class: Antineoplastics
Pharmacologic class: Epidermal growth factor receptor inhibitors

AVAILABLE FORMS
Tablets: 15 mg, 30 mg, 45 mg

INDICATIONS & DOSAGES
➤ **First-line treatment of patients with metastatic NSCLC with epidermal growth factor receptor (EGFR) exon 19 deletion or exon 21 L858R substitution mutations as detected by an FDA-approved test**☒
Adults: 45 mg PO once daily until disease progression or unacceptable toxicity.
Adjust-a-dose: Refer to manufacturer's instructions for toxicity-related dosage adjustments.

ADMINISTRATION
PO
• Use appropriate precautions for handling and disposal of a hazardous drug.
• Give at the same time each day with or without food.
• If a dose is missed or is vomited, don't give an additional dose or make up a missed dose; continue with the next scheduled dose.
• Store at 68° to 77° F (20° to 25° C).

ACTION
An irreversible inhibitor of the kinase activity of the human EGFR family (EGFR/HER1, HER2, and HER4) and certain EGFR activating mutations (exon 19 deletion or the exon 21 L858R substitution mutation).

Route	Onset	Peak	Duration
PO	Unknown	6 hr	Unknown

Half-life: 70 hours.

---

*Reactions in bold italics are **life-threatening**. Interactions may have a *rapid onset* or a **delayed onset**.*

ADVERSE REACTIONS
CNS: asthenia, insomnia, fatigue. **CV:** chest pain. **EENT:** ocular keratitis, conjunctivitis, nasal mucosal disorder, mouth ulcer. **GI:** diarrhea, stomatitis, nausea, constipation, vomiting, dysgeusia, decreased appetite. **GU:** increased creatinine level. **Hematologic:** anemia, *lymphopenia*. **Hepatic:** increased ALT, AST, and alkaline phosphatase levels; hyperbilirubinemia. **Metabolic:** weight loss, dehydration, *hypocalcemia, hypokalemia, hypomagnesemia*, hyponatremia, hyperglycemia, hypoalbuminemia. **Musculoskeletal:** extremity pain, musculoskeletal pain. **Respiratory:** cough, dyspnea, URI, ILD. **Skin:** rash, paronychia, dry skin, pruritus, hand-foot syndrome, dermatitis, skin fissures, hypertrichosis, exfoliative skin reactions, alopecia.

INTERACTIONS
Drug-drug. *CYP2D6 substrates (dextromethorphan):* May increase level of CYP2D6 substrates, increasing risk of toxicity. Avoid concomitant use if minimal increase in substrate level could lead to serious or life-threatening toxicity.
PPIs (esomeprazole): May decrease dacomitinib level. Avoid concomitant use. Alternative therapy includes locally acting antacids or an H_2-receptor antagonist. Give dacomitinib at least 6 hours before or 10 hours after the H_2-receptor antagonist.
Drug-lifestyle. *Sun exposure:* May increase incidence and severity of rash and exfoliative skin reactions. Limit sun exposure.

EFFECTS ON LAB TEST RESULTS
• May increase ALT, AST, creatinine, alkaline phosphatase, bilirubin, and glucose levels.
• May decrease albumin, calcium, potassium, sodium, and magnesium levels.
• May decrease RBC and WBC counts.

CONTRAINDICATIONS & CAUTIONS
• Severe and fatal ILD/pneumonitis has occurred in patients treated with drug.
• Severe and fatal diarrhea has occurred in patients treated with dacomitinib. Withhold drug for grade 2 or greater diarrhea until recovery to grade 1 severity or less; then resume at the same or reduced dosage depending on severity.
• Rash and exfoliative skin reactions have occurred in patients treated with dacomitinib. Upon starting treatment, patients should use moisturizers and limit sun exposure. Treat skin reactions with topical antibiotics, topical steroids, or oral antibiotics as clinically indicated.
• Safety and effectiveness in children haven't been established.
• Use cautiously in patients age 65 and older as they may experience a higher incidence of adverse events.
Dialyzable drug: Unknown.

PREGNANCY-LACTATION-REPRODUCTION
• Drug can cause fetal harm.
• Verify pregnancy status of women of childbearing potential before start of therapy.
• Advise women of childbearing potential to use effective contraception during treatment and for at least 17 days after the final dose.
• It isn't known if drug appears in human milk. Women shouldn't breastfeed during treatment and for at least 17 days after the final dose.

NURSING CONSIDERATIONS
• Monitor patients for signs and symptoms of ILD and pneumonitis (dyspnea, cough, fever). If ILD or pneumonitis is suspected, withhold drug and investigate. If confirmed, permanently discontinue drug.
• Monitor patients for diarrhea and promptly initiate treatment with antidiarrheals and fluids as indicated.
• Monitor patients for skin reactions (dry skin, redness, rash, acne, itching, peeling or blistering).
• *Look alike-sound alike:* Don't confuse dacomitinib with dabrafenib or dasatinib.

PATIENT TEACHING
• Advise patient to report all adverse reactions.
• Teach patient safe drug administration.
• Caution patient about the risks of severe or fatal ILD, including pneumonitis. Instruct patient to immediately report new or worsening respiratory signs and symptoms.
• Advise patient to immediately contact prescriber at first sign of diarrhea. Inform patient that increased oral fluid intake, IV hydration, or antidiarrheals (loperamide) may be required.
• Warn patient that dermatologic reactions can occur. Instruct patient to immediately report new or worsening rash and erythematous and exfoliative reactions.
• Advise patient to use moisturizers and to minimize sun exposure by using protective clothing and sunscreen during treatment.
• Inform female patient of childbearing potential that drug can cause fetal harm and to use effective contraception during treatment and for 17 days after the final dose.
• Instruct female patient of childbearing potential to contact prescriber if she is pregnant or plans to become pregnant during therapy.
• Advise patient not to breastfeed during treatment and for 17 days after final dose.

NEW DRUGS

eravacycline
er-a-va-SYE-kleen

Xerava

Therapeutic class: Antibiotics
Pharmacologic class: Tetracyclines

AVAILABLE FORMS
Injection: 50-mg single-dose vial

INDICATIONS & DOSAGES
➤ **Treatment of complicated intra-abdominal infections caused by susceptible microorganisms** (*Escherichia coli, Klebsiella pneumoniae, Citrobacter freundii, Enterobacter cloacae, Klebsiella oxytoca, Enterococcus faecalis, Enterococcus faecium, Staphylococcus aureus, Streptococcus anginosus* group, *Clostridium perfringens, Bacteroides* **species, and** *Parabacteroides distasonis*)
Adults: 1 mg/kg IV over 60 minutes every 12 hours for 4 to 14 days as determined by the severity and location of the infection and clinical response.
Adjust-a-dose: For patients with severe hepatic impairment (Child-Pugh class C), give 1 mg/kg IV every 12 hours on day 1 followed by 1 mg/kg IV every 24 hours starting on day 2 for 4 to 14 days. If drug is used with a strong CYP3A inducer, give 1.5 mg/kg IV every 12 hours for 4 to 14 days.

ADMINISTRATION
IV
▼ Reconstitute each vial with 5 mL of sterile water to yield 50 mg (10 mg/mL) of drug.
▼ Swirl vial gently until contents are entirely dissolved. Don't shake, as rapid movement may cause foaming.
▼ The reconstituted solution should be clear and pale yellow to orange. Don't use if solution is cloudy or contains particles.
▼ Don't administer drug by direct injection. Add the reconstituted solution to an NSS infusion bag to generate an infusion solution with a target concentration of 0.3 mg/mL (within a range of 0.2 to 0.6 mg/mL). Don't shake the bag.
▼ Infuse drug over 60 minutes.
▼ Visually inspect the diluted solution for particulate matter and discoloration before administration. Solution should be clear to light yellow or orange.
▼ Discard unused portion of the reconstituted and diluted solution.
▼ Administer IV through a dedicated line or through a Y-site. If the same IV line is used for sequential infusion of several drugs, flush the line with NSS before and after infusion of eravacycline.
▼ Infuse the diluted solution within 6 hours if stored at room temperature or within 24 hours if refrigerated at 36° to 46° F (2° to 8° C). Don't freeze.

▼ Before reconstitution, store vials at 36° to 46° F (2° to 8° C). Keep vials in carton until ready to use.
▼ **Incompatibilities:** Don't mix eravacycline with other infusion solutions or drugs or add to solutions containing other drugs.

ACTION
A fluorocycline antibiotic within the tetracycline class that inhibits protein synthesis by binding to the 30S and possibly the 50S ribosomal subunit(s) of susceptible bacteria.

Route	Onset	Peak	Duration
IV	Unknown	Unknown	Unknown

Half-life: 20 hours.

ADVERSE REACTIONS
CV: hypotension. **GI:** nausea, vomiting, diarrhea. **Skin:** infusion-site reactions, wound dehiscence.

INTERACTIONS
Drug-drug. *Anticoagulants:* May depress plasma prothrombin activity. Anticoagulant dosage reduction may be needed.
Strong CYP3A inducers (rifampin): May decrease eravacycline concentration and therapeutic effects. Increase eravacycline dosage as needed.
Drug-lifestyle. *Sun exposure:* May cause photosensitivity. Discontinue drug if photosensitivity occurs.

EFFECTS ON LAB TEST RESULTS
• May increase amylase, lipase, ALT, GGT, and creatinine levels. May decrease serum calcium level.
• May prolonged aPTT interval.
• May decrease WBC and neutrophil counts.

CONTRAINDICATIONS & CAUTIONS
• Contraindicated in known hypersensitivity to eravacycline, tetracyclines, or any of the components.
• Life-threatening anaphylactic hypersensitivity reactions have been reported with tetracyclines, including eravacycline. Avoid use in patients with known hypersensitivity to tetracyclines and discontinue therapy if an allergic reaction occurs.
• Drug is similar to tetracycline-class drugs and may have similar adverse reactions, such as pseudotumor cerebri and antianabolic action leading to increased BUN level, azotemia, acidosis, hyperphosphatemia, pancreatitis, and abnormal LFT values. Discontinue drug if these adverse reactions occur.
• Drug isn't indicated for treatment of complicated UTI.
• Use only to treat or prevent infections proven or strongly suspected to be caused by susceptible bacteria.
• Use of eravacycline during tooth development (last half of pregnancy, infancy, and childhood to age 8) may cause permanent teeth discoloration and enamel hypoplasia.

NEW DRUGS

• Use of eravacycline during the second and third trimesters of pregnancy, infancy, and childhood up to age 8 may cause reversible inhibition of bone growth.

• Drug may increase risk of CDAD, ranging in severity from mild diarrhea to fatal colitis. CDAD can occur up to 2 months after therapy ends.

• Safety and effectiveness in children haven't been established.

Dialyzable drug: No.

PREGNANCY-LACTATION-REPRODUCTION

• Tetracyclines may cause discoloration of deciduous teeth and reversible inhibition of bone growth when administered during the second and third trimesters. Avoid use.

• It's isn't known if drug appears in human milk; however, tetracyclines appear in human milk. Breastfeeding isn't recommended during treatment and for 4 days after final dose.

• Drug may impair male fertility. Long-term effects haven't been studied.

NURSING CONSIDERATIONS

• Monitor patient for allergic reactions, including serious allergic reactions that could require immediate emergency treatment.

• Monitor patient for diarrhea, including watery and bloody stools, which may indicate CDAD. Treat CDAD as clinically indicated. If CDAD is suspected or confirmed, discontinue drug.

• Monitor patient for tetracycline-class adverse reactions, including photosensitivity, pseudotumor cerebri, and antianabolic action (increased BUN level, azotemia, acidosis, hyperphosphatemia, pancreatitis, abnormal LFT values). Discontinue drug if these adverse reactions are suspected.

• Monitor patient for microbial overgrowth, including fungal infections. Discontinue drug and treat as clinically indicated if infection occurs.

PATIENT TEACHING

• Teach patient to report all adverse reactions

• Advise patient that allergic reactions, including life-threatening reactions, can occur and that serious reactions require immediate treatment.

• Inform patient that CDAD can occur as late as 2 or more months after therapy ends and to immediately report watery and bloody stools, with or without stomach cramps and fever.

• Warn patient that antibacterial drugs may promote the overgrowth of nonsusceptible microorganisms, including fungi, and to report signs and symptoms of infection.

• Inform patient that antibacterial drugs should only be used to treat bacterial infections and that these drugs aren't used to treat viral infections (for example, the common cold).

• Teach patient to take drug exactly as directed and to complete the full course of treatment, even if feeling better early in the course of therapy.

• Inform patient that skipping doses or not completing the full course of therapy may decrease effectiveness of the immediate treatment and increase the likelihood that bacteria will develop resistance and won't be treatable by antibacterial drugs in the future.

• Inform female patient of childbearing potential that tetracyclines may cause permanent discoloration of deciduous teeth and reversible inhibition of bone growth when administered during the second and third trimesters of pregnancy. Advise her to immediately report suspected pregnancy.

• Caution patient not to breastfeed during treatment and for 4 days after final dose.

esketamine
es-KET-a-meen

Spravato

Therapeutic class: Antidepressants
Pharmacologic class: Noncompetitive N-methyl-D-aspartate receptor antagonists
Controlled substance schedule: III

AVAILABLE FORMS
Nasal spray: 28 mg (2 sprays)/device

INDICATIONS & DOSAGES
➤ **Treatment-resistant depression in conjunction with an oral antidepressant**
Adults: Induction phase (weeks 1 to 4): On day 1, starting dose is 56 mg intranasal with a subsequent dose that week of 56 mg or 84 mg based on efficacy and tolerability. For maintenance phase (weeks 2 to 4), give 56 mg or 84 mg intranasal twice per week. For maintenance phase weeks 5 to 8, give 56 mg or 84 mg intranasal once weekly. For maintenance phase week 9 and after, give 56 mg or 84 mg intranasal once weekly or once every 2 weeks. Individualized to the least frequent dosing to maintain response.

Adjust-a-dose: If patient misses treatment sessions and there is worsening of depression symptoms, consider returning patient to previous dosing schedule.

ADMINISTRATION
Intranasal
• Drug must be administered under the direct supervision of a health care provider.

• A treatment session consists of nasal administration and postadministration observation under supervision.

• Patients should avoid food for at least 2 hours and liquids for at least 30 minutes before administration.

• Patients should blow their nose before the first dose only to clear the nasal passages but not between doses.

NEW DRUGS

• Patients who require a nasal corticosteroid or nasal decongestant on a dosing day should administer these medications at least 1 hour before administration of esketamine.

• Don't prime device before use.

• Use two devices for a 56-mg dose or three devices for an 84-mg dose, with a 5-minute rest period between use of each device.

• Recline head to about 45 degrees during administration.

• Insert the tip straight into the nostril until the nose rest touches the skin between the nostrils; close the opposite nostril. Patient should inhale while pushing the plunger in until it stops. Repeat to deliver dose to the other nostril. Instruct patient to sniff gently to keep drug inside nose.

• Ensure administration by confirming that the indicator shows no green dots when the device is empty. When one dose is delivered, one green dot will indicate that a dose remains in the device.

• Dab nose with a tissue if liquid drops out. Patient shouldn't blow nose.

• Store at room temperature at 68° to 77° F (20° to 25° C).

ACTION
Unknown.

Route	Onset	Peak	Duration
Intranasal	Unknown	20–40 min	Unknown

Half-life: 7 to 12 hours.

ADVERSE REACTIONS
CNS: dissociation, dizziness, sedation, vertigo, hypoesthesia, anxiety, depression, lethargy, feeling drunk, feeling abnormal, dysarthria, headache, tremor, euphoric mood, insomnia, mental impairment. **CV:** increase in BP, tachycardia. **EENT:** nasal discomfort, oropharyngeal pain, throat irritation. **GI:** dysgeusia, dry mouth, nausea, vomiting, constipation, diarrhea. **GU:** urinary frequency. **Skin:** hyperhidrosis.

INTERACTIONS
Drug-drug. *CNS depressants (benzodiazepines, opioids):* May increase sedation. Use cautiously together and monitor patient closely for additive sedative effects.
MAO inhibitors (rasagiline, selegiline), psychostimulants (amphetamines, armodafinil, methylphenidate, modafinil): May increase BP. Use cautiously together and monitor patient closely.
Drug-lifestyle. *Alcohol use:* May increase sedation. Avoid use together.

EFFECTS ON LAB TEST RESULTS
None reported.

CONTRAINDICATIONS & CAUTIONS
• Contraindicated in patients with aneurysmal vascular disease (including thoracic and abdominal aorta and intracranial and peripheral arterial vessels) or arteriovenous malformation, history of intracerebral hemorrhage; and hypersensitivity to esketamine or ketamine, or its components.

• Use cautiously in patients with history of hypertensive encephalopathy.

Black Box Warning Drug can cause delayed or prolonged sedation. Closely monitor patients for sedation with concomitant use of CNS depressants. ■

Black Box Warning Dissociative or perceptual changes (including distortion of time and space and illusions), derealization, and depersonalization may occur. Because of drug's potential to induce dissociative effects, carefully assess patients with psychosis before administering drug. Initiate treatment only if benefit outweighs risk. ■

Black Box Warning Because of risks of sedation and dissociation, patients must be monitored by a health care provider for at least 2 hours at each treatment session, and assessed to determine whether they are clinically stable and ready to leave the health care setting. ■

Black Box Warning Drug is a controlled substance (CIII) with potential for abuse, misuse, and diversion. Assess each patient's risk of abuse or misuse before prescribing and monitor all patients for the development of these behaviors or conditions, including drug-seeking behavior, during therapy. Individuals with a history of drug abuse or dependence are at greater risk. ■

Black Box Warning Drug is only available through a REMS program because of the risks of serious adverse outcomes from sedation, dissociation, and abuse and misuse. ■

Black Box Warning There is increased risk of suicidal thoughts and behaviors in children and young adults taking antidepressants. Closely monitor all patients treated with antidepressants for clinical worsening and emergence of suicidal thoughts and behaviors. Drug isn't approved for use in children. ■

• Drug may increase risk of short- or long-term cognitive or memory impairment.

• Use cautiously in patients with moderate hepatic impairment because of increased risk of adverse reactions.

• Drug hasn't been studied in patients on dialysis or in those with severe (Child-Pugh class C) hepatic impairment.

• Drug hasn't been studied or approved for use as an anesthetic.
Dialyzable drug: Unknown.

PREGNANCY-LACTATION-REPRODUCTION
• May cause fetal harm and isn't recommended for use in pregnant women.

• If pregnancy occurs during treatment, discontinue drug and counsel patient about the risk to the fetus.

• Women of childbearing potential should consider pregnancy planning and prevention during treatment.

Reactions in bold italics are *life-threatening*. Interactions may have a *rapid onset* or a **delayed onset**.

• Health care providers are encouraged to register patients in the antidepressant exposure registry by contacting the National Pregnancy Registry for Antidepressants (1-844-405-6185).

• Drug is present in human milk. Breastfeeding isn't recommended during treatment.

NURSING CONSIDERATIONS

• Assess BP before administration. If baseline BP is elevated (greater than 140 mm Hg systolic or 90 mm Hg diastolic), consider the risks of short-term increases in BP and benefit of treatment.

• Don't administer if an increase in BP or ICP poses a serious risk.

• After administration, reassess BP for at least 2 hours, beginning at approximately 40 minutes. If BP is decreasing and patient appears clinically stable for at least 2 hours, patient may be discharged at the end of the post-dose monitoring period; if not, continue to monitor.

• Assess for hypertensive crisis (chest pain, shortness of breath) or hypertensive encephalopathy (sudden severe headache, visual disturbances, seizures, diminished consciousness or focal neurologic deficits) and provide emergency care as indicated.

 Black Box Warning Monitor patient for sedation and dissociation for at least 2 hours after administration. ▮

 Black Box Warning Monitor all patients for signs and symptoms of abuse, misuse, dependence, and tolerance. ▮

 Black Box Warning Closely monitor all patients for clinical worsening and emergence of suicidal thoughts and behaviors. Consider changing the therapeutic regimen, including possibly discontinuing drug or the concomitant oral antidepressant, in patients whose depression is persistently worse, or who are experiencing emergent suicidal thoughts or behaviors. ▮

• Drug may increase the risk of ulcerative or interstitial cystitis. Monitor patients for urinary tract and bladder signs and symptoms (urinary frequency, dysuria, urinary urgency, nocturia, cystitis) and refer for appropriate follow-up as clinically indicated.

• **Look alike–sound alike:** Don't confuse esketamine with ketamine or escitalopram.

PATIENT TEACHING

• Advise patient to report all adverse reactions.

 Black Box Warning Inform patient that sedation, dissociative symptoms, perception disturbances, dizziness, vertigo, anxiety, and increased BP may occur and that monitoring by a health care provider will be needed until these effects resolve. ▮

 Black Box Warning Advise patient that drug is a federally controlled substance because it can be abused, misused, or lead to dependence. ▮

 Black Box Warning Tell patient that drug is available only through a REMS program. Inform patient that enrollment in the REMS program is necessary before drug administration, that drug must be administered under the direct observation of a health care provider, and that patient will need to be monitored by a health care provider for at least 2 hours after administration. ▮

 Black Box Warning Advise patient and caregivers to look for the emergence of suicidality, especially early during treatment and when the dosage is adjusted, and to immediately contact prescriber if changes occur. ▮

• Because drug may impair the ability to drive or operate machinery, caution patient to avoid potentially hazardous activities requiring complete mental alertness and motor coordination (driving, operating machinery) until the next day after a restful sleep.

• Warn patient that someone must be available to drive patient home after each treatment session.

• Caution female patient of childbearing potential about the risk to a fetus. Advise her to tell prescriber if she is pregnant or plans to become pregnant during treatment.

• Advise patient not to breastfeed during treatment.

SAFETY ALERT!

gilteritinib ℞
GIL-te-ri-ti-nib

Xospata

Therapeutic class: Antineoplastics
Pharmacologic class: Kinase inhibitors

AVAILABLE FORMS
Tablets⬛: 40 mg

INDICATIONS & DOSAGES

➤ **Treatment of relapsed or refractory acute myeloid leukemia (AML) with a *FLT3* mutation as detected by an FDA-approved test**℞

Adults: 120 mg PO once daily for a minimum of 6 months.

Adjust-a-dose: If QTc interval increases to greater than 500 msec, interrupt therapy and resume at 80 mg daily when QTc interval returns to within 30 msec of baseline or 480 msec or less. If QTc interval increased by more than 30 msec on ECG on day 8 of cycle 1, confirm with ECG on day 9; if confirmed, consider dosage reduction to 80 mg daily. If pancreatitis occurs, interrupt therapy until resolved; then resume at 80 mg daily. For other grade 3 or life-threatening toxicities considered related to treatment, interrupt therapy until toxicity resolves or improves to grade 1; then resume at 80 mg daily.

ADMINISTRATION
PO
• May give with or without food at about the same time each day.
• Don't break or crush tablets.

* If a dose is missed or not taken at the usual time, give dose as soon as possible on the same day, and at least 12 hours before next scheduled dose. Return to the normal schedule the following day. Don't administer two doses within 12 hours.
* Store tablets at 68° to 77° F (20° to 25° C) in original container.

ACTION

Inhibits multiple receptor tyrosine kinases, thereby inhibiting receptor signaling and cell proliferation and inducing cellular death in leukemic cells expressing FLT3-ITD.

Route	Onset	Peak	Duration
PO	Within 24 hr	4–6 hr	Unknown

Half-life: 113 hours.

ADVERSE REACTIONS

CNS: fatigue, malaise, fever, headache, dizziness, insomnia, *posterior reversible encephalopathy syndrome (PRES)*. **CV:** hypotension, HTN, *prolonged QT interval*, edema, *HF, pericardial effusion*, pericarditis. **GI:** diarrhea, nausea, stomatitis, vomiting, dysgeusia, abdominal pain, decreased appetite. **GU:** *renal impairment*. **Hepatic:** elevated liver enzyme levels. **Musculoskeletal:** myalgia, arthralgia. **Respiratory:** dyspnea, pneumonia, cough. **Skin:** rash. **Other:** *sepsis, anaphylactic reaction, differentiation syndrome*.

INTERACTIONS

Drug-drug. *Combined P-gp and strong CYP3A inducers (rifampin):* May decrease gilteritinib level and therapeutic effect. Avoid concomitant use with combined P-gp and strong CYP3A inducers. *Drugs that target 5HT$_{2B}$ receptor or sigma nonspecific receptor (escitalopram, fluoxetine, sertraline):* May reduce effects of these drugs. Avoid use together unless their use is essential. *Strong CYP3A inhibitors (itraconazole):* May increase gilteritinib level. Consider alternative therapies other than strong CYP3A inhibitors. If use together is essential, monitor patient more frequently for gilteritinib-related adverse reactions. Interrupt therapy and reduce gilteritinib dosage in patients with serious or life-threatening toxicity.

EFFECTS ON LAB TEST RESULTS

* May increase AST, ALT, alkaline phosphatase, creatinine, glucose, triglyceride, and CK levels.
* May decrease calcium, albumin, phosphate, potassium, and sodium levels.

CONTRAINDICATIONS & CAUTIONS

* Contraindicated in patients hypersensitive to drug or its components. Anaphylactic reactions have been observed in clinical trials.
* PRES can occur.
* QT-interval prolongation can occur. Interrupt therapy and reduce dosage in patients with a QTcF

greater than 500 msec. Correct hypokalemia or hypomagnesemia before and during therapy.
* Safety and effectiveness in children haven't been established.
Dialyzable drug: Unknown.

PREGNANCY-LACTATION-REPRODUCTION

* Drug can cause fetal harm. Women of childbearing potential should use effective contraception during and for at least 6 months after final dose.
* Obtain pregnancy test within 7 days before start of treatment in women of childbearing potential.
* Males with female partners of childbearing potential should use effective contraception during treatment and for at least 4 months after final dose.
* It isn't known if drug appears in human milk. Women shouldn't breastfeed during treatment and for at least 2 months after final dose.

NURSING CONSIDERATIONS

* Patients must be selected for treatment with gilteritinib based on the presence of *FLT3* mutations in their blood or bone marrow. Information on FDA-approved tests for the detection of a *FLT3* mutation in AML is available at www.fda.gov/medical-devices/vitro-diagnostics/companion-diagnostics.
* Response to drug may be delayed. In the absence of disease progression or unacceptable toxicity, treatment for a minimum of 6 months is recommended to allow time for a clinical response.
* Monitor patients for hypersensitivity reactions, including anaphylactic reactions.
* Assess blood counts and blood chemistries, including CK, before start of therapy, at least once weekly for the first month, once every other week for the second month, and once monthly for the duration of therapy.
* Correct hypokalemia or hypomagnesemia before and during treatment to decrease risk of QT-interval prolongation.
* Monitor patients for prolonged QT interval with ECGs before start of treatment, on days 8 and 15 of cycle 1, and before start of the next two cycles.
* Monitor patients for signs and symptoms of PRES (headache, decreased alertness, confusion, seizures, vision problems). Discontinue drug if PRES is confirmed.
* Monitor patients for signs and symptoms of pancreatitis, such as severe and persistent stomach pain with or without nausea and vomiting.

PATIENT TEACHING

* Tell patient to report all adverse reactions.
* Advise patient of the risk of developing PRES and to immediately report signs and symptoms suggestive of PRES.
* Instruct patient to immediately report signs and symptoms of arrhythmia (feeling faint, loss of consciousness, abnormal heartbeat).
* Advise patient that ECGs will be performed periodically.

NEW DRUGS

• Stress importance of electrolyte monitoring, especially for patient with a history of low potassium or low magnesium level.
• Advise patient of risk of pancreatitis and to contact prescriber if signs or symptoms occur.
• Tell female patient of childbearing potential that pregnancy testing will be performed before therapy begins.
• Advise female patient of childbearing potential that drug can cause fetal harm and to use effective contraception during therapy and for 6 months after final dose.
• Advise male patient with female partner of childbearing potential that drug can cause fetal harm and to use effective contraception during treatment and for at least 4 months after final dose.
• Caution female patient to notify prescriber if pregnancy is suspected.
• Warn patient not to breastfeed during treatment and for at least 2 months after final dose.

---

lanadelumab-flyo ⅺ
LAN-a-del-ue-mab

Takhzyro

Therapeutic class: Prophylaxis drugs
Pharmacologic class: Monoclonal antibodies

AVAILABLE FORMS
Injection: 300 mg/2 mL single-dose vial

INDICATIONS & DOSAGES
➤ **Prevention of hereditary angioedema (HAE) attacks** ⅺ
Adults and children age 12 and older: Initially, 300 mg subcut every 2 weeks. If patient is attack free for more than 6 months, may consider decreasing dosing to 300 mg subcut every 4 weeks.

ADMINISTRATION
Subcutaneous
• Remove vial or prepared syringe from refrigerator 15 minutes before injection to allow solution to come to room temperature.
• Don't shake vial.
• Solution should be clear to slightly opalescent, colorless to slightly yellow; don't use if solution is discolored or contains visible particles.
• Withdraw dose from vial using an 18G needle; then, change to a 27G, ½-inch needle or other needle suitable for subcut injection.
• Inject into the abdomen, thigh, or upper arm. Rotate sites.
• Give drug within 2 hours of syringe preparation if kept at room temperature or use within 8 hours if prepared syringe has been refrigerated.
• Discard unused portion of drug remaining in vial and syringe.

• Store in refrigerator in the original carton to protect from light. Don't freeze.

ACTION
A human monoclonal antibody that inhibits plasma kallikrein activity to decrease bradykinin generation. This decreases bradykinin-induced vasodilation and vascular permeability, resulting in decreased HAE-associated swelling and pain.

Route	Onset	Peak	Duration
Subcut.	Unknown	5 days	Unknown

Half-life: About 2 weeks.

ADVERSE REACTIONS
CNS: headache, dizziness. **GI:** diarrhea. **Hepatic:** elevated ALT and AST levels. **Musculoskeletal:** myalgia. **Respiratory:** URI. **Skin:** rash, injection-site reaction. **Other:** hypersensitivity reactions, antibody development.

INTERACTIONS
None reported.

EFFECTS ON LAB TEST RESULTS
• May increase ALT and AST levels.
• May increase aPTT.

CONTRAINDICATIONS & CAUTIONS
• Hypersensitivity reactions can occur.
• Patients may develop antidrug antibodies to lanadelumab.
• Safety and effectiveness in children younger than age 12 are unknown.
Dialyzable drug: Unknown.

PREGNANCY-LACTATION-REPRODUCTION
• There are no available data on use of drug in pregnant women. Monoclonal antibodies are known to cross the placental barrier during the third trimester; therefore, potential effects on a fetus are likely to be greater during the third trimester.
• It isn't known if drug appears in human milk. Before using in breastfeeding women, consider the benefits of the drug and breastfeeding along with the potential adverse effects on the infant.

NURSING CONSIDERATIONS
• Observe patient for hypersensitivity reaction after injection of drug. If severe reactions (dyspnea, wheezing, chest tightness, tachycardia, rash, hives, feeling faint) occur, discontinue drug and start appropriate treatment.
• Patient or caregiver may administer drug after appropriate training.

PATIENT TEACHING
• Teach patient to report all adverse reactions.
• Warn patient to immediately seek medical attention for signs and symptoms of a hypersensitivity reaction.

♣Canada   ◇OTC   ◆Off-label use   ✐Photoguide   ⓓⓝⓒDo not crush   *Liquid contains alcohol   ⅺGenetic

• Teach patient or caregiver proper aseptic, administration, and disposal techniques. Refer patient to manufacturer's Patient Information Instructions for Use.
• Teach patient to rotate injection sites (abdomen, thighs, and upper arms [if drug is administered by a caregiver]). Advise patient to inject at least 2 inches from scars or the navel and not to inject into areas that are bruised, painful, or swollen.

SAFETY ALERT!

larotrectinib ⚇
lar-oh-TREK-ti-nib

Vitrakvi

Therapeutic class: Antineoplastics
Pharmacologic class: Kinase inhibitors

AVAILABLE FORMS
Capsules⚇: 25 mg, 100 mg
Oral solution: 20 mg/mL

INDICATIONS & DOSAGES
➤ Treatment of patients with solid tumors that have a neurotrophic receptor tyrosine kinase (*NTRK*) gene fusion without a known acquired resistance mutation, are metastatic or where surgical resection is likely to result in severe morbidity, or have no satisfactory alternative treatments or have progressed after treatment⚇
Adults and children with a BSA of at least 1 m²:
100 mg PO b.i.d., until disease progression or unacceptable toxicity.
Children with a BSA less than 1 m²: 100 mg/m² PO b.i.d., until disease progression or unacceptable toxicity.
Adjust-a-dose: For moderate (Child-Pugh class B) to severe (Child-Pugh class C) hepatic impairment, reduce the starting dose by 50%. Refer to manufacturer's instructions for toxicity-related dosage adjustment.

ADMINISTRATION
PO
• May use capsule or oral solution interchangeably.
• May give with or without food.
• Don't make up a missed dose if it's within 6 hours of the next scheduled dose.
• If vomiting occurs after a dose, give the next dose at the scheduled time.
• Patients must swallow capsules whole with water and not chew or crush them.
• Use an oral syringe to draw up and administer the oral solution to ensure proper dosing.
• Discard any unused oral solution remaining after 90 days of first opening the bottle.
• Store capsules at room temperature 68° to 77° F (20° to 25° C).
• Refrigerate oral solution at 36° to 46° F (2° to 8° C). Don't freeze.

ACTION
Inhibits the tropomyosin receptor kinases TRKA, TRKB, and TRKC, resulting in antitumor activity.

Route	Onset	Peak	Duration
PO	Unknown	1 hr	Unknown

Half-life: 2.9 hours.

ADVERSE REACTIONS
CNS: fatigue, dizziness, pyrexia, *brain edema*, asthenia, syncope, delirium, dysarthria, gait disturbance, paresthesia, memory impairment, tremor. **CV:** pericardial effusion, HTN, peripheral edema. **EENT:** nasal congestion. **GI:** nausea, vomiting, constipation, diarrhea, abdominal pain, *intestinal perforation*, small intestinal obstruction, enterocutaneous fistula, decreased appetite. **Hematologic:** anemia, *acute myeloid leukemia, neutropenia.* **Hepatic:** *hepatotoxicity*, jaundice. **Metabolic:** weight gain, dehydration, hyponatremia. **Musculoskeletal:** muscular weakness, arthralgia, myalgia, muscular weakness, back pain, extremity pain. **Respiratory:** pleural effusion, dyspnea, cough. **Skin:** cellulitis. **Other:** *sepsis*, falls.

INTERACTIONS
Drug-drug. *Sensitive CYP3A4 substrates (midazolam):* May increase plasma concentrations of these drugs, which may increase the incidence or severity of adverse reactions Avoid use together. If coadministration can't be avoided, monitor patients for increased adverse reactions related to both drugs.
Strong CYP3A4 inducers (rifampin): May decrease larotrectinib plasma concentration and efficacy. Avoid coadministration. If use together can't be avoided, double the larotrectinib dose. After the inducer has been discontinued for three to five elimination half-lives, resume the original dose given before initiation of the CYP3A4 inducer.
Strong CYP3A4 inhibitors (itraconazole): May increase larotrectinib level and risk of larotrectinib-related adverse reactions. Avoid coadministration. If use together can't be avoided, reduce the larotrectinib dose by 50%. After the inhibitor has been discontinued for three to five elimination half-lives, resume the original dose given before initiation of the CYP3A4 inhibitor.
Drug-herb. *St. John's wort:* May decrease drug plasma concentration and therapeutic effects. Discourage use together.
Drug-food. *Grapefruit juice:* May increase drug plasma concentration and risk of adverse reactions. Discourage use together.

EFFECTS ON LAB TEST RESULTS
• May increase AST, ALT, alkaline phosphatase, amylase, and lipase levels.
• May decrease sodium and albumin levels.
• May decrease Hb level and neutrophil cell count.

Reactions in bold italics are *life-threatening*. Interactions may have a *rapid onset* or a **delayed onset**.

CONTRAINDICATIONS & CAUTIONS
• Drug should only be used in patients with *NTRK* gene fusion in the tumor specimens.
• Drug can cause neurotoxicity, hepatotoxicity, GI toxicity, and bone marrow suppression.
• Some dosage forms may contain propylene glycol, which can be toxic in large amounts.
Dialyzable drug: Unknown.

PREGNANCY-LACTATION-REPRODUCTION
• There are no data on the use of drug in pregnant women. Based on mechanism of action and animal studies, drug can cause fetal harm.
• Women of childbearing potential should use effective contraception during treatment and for at least 1 week after final dose.
• Advise males with female partners of childbearing potential to use effective contraception during treatment and for 1 week after final dose.
• It isn't known if drug appears in human milk. Because of potential adverse effects in breastfed infants, women shouldn't breastfeed during therapy and for 1 week after final dose.
• Drug may reduce fertility in women.

NURSING CONSIDERATIONS
• Monitor LFT values, including ALT, AST, amylase, lipase, and albumin levels, every 2 weeks during the first month of treatment, then monthly and as clinically indicated. Withhold drug and modify dosage, or permanently discontinue drug based on severity.
• Monitor patient for signs and symptoms of hepatotoxicity (loss of appetite, nausea, vomiting, abdominal pain, jaundice).
• Monitor sodium level, Hb level, and WBC count routinely during treatment.
• Monitor patient for signs and symptoms of neurotoxicity (limb paralysis or weakness, tingling, numbness, headache, vision changes, confusion, difficulty speaking, dizziness, coordination changes, burning sensation in hands or feet).
• Verify pregnancy status in women of childbearing potential before starting treatment.

PATIENT TEACHING
• Teach patient to report all adverse reactions.
• Demonstrate safe drug administration.
• Inform patient that neurotoxicity can occur and to report new or worsening signs and symptoms of neurotoxicity.
• Advise patient that blood laboratory testing will be needed to monitor therapy.
• Warn patient not to drive or operate hazardous machinery until drug's effects are known or if neurologic adverse reactions occur.
• Caution patient that liver toxicity can occur and to report signs and symptoms of liver toxicity.
• Advise males and females of childbearing potential of the possible risks to a fetus.

• Advise female patient of childbearing potential that pregnancy testing will be needed before start of therapy.
• Caution female patient of childbearing potential to use effective contraception during treatment and for at least 1 week after final dose.
• Advise male patient with female partners of childbearing potential to use effective contraception during treatment and for at least 1 week after final dose.
• Instruct female patient to tell prescriber if she is pregnant or suspects she is pregnant.
• Advise patient not to breastfeed during treatment and for 1 week after final dose.
• Warn female patient of childbearing potential that drug may impair fertility.

migalastat hydrochloride ✂
mi-GAL-a-stat

Galafold

Therapeutic class: Metabolic agents
Pharmacologic class: Pharmacological chaperones

AVAILABLE FORMS
Capsules ⓐ 123 mg

INDICATIONS & DOSAGES
➤ **Treatment of confirmed Fabry disease with an amenable galactosidase alpha gene (*GLA*) variant** ✂
Adults: 123 mg P.O. once every other day, at the same time of day.

ADMINISTRATION
PO
• Give drug on an empty stomach. Patient shouldn't consume food for at least 2 hours before and 2 hours after taking drug. Patient can consume clear liquids during this 4-hour fasting period.
• Give drug every other day; don't give drug on 2 consecutive days.
• If a dose is missed entirely for the day, give the missed dose only if it's within 12 hours of the normal time that the dose should have been taken. If more than 12 hours have passed, give drug at the next normal dosing day and time while maintaining the every-other-day dosing schedule.
• Make sure patient swallows capsules whole and doesn't cut, crush, or chew them.
• Store at room temperature.

ACTION
Reversibly binds to the active site of abnormally folded and unstable forms of alpha-galactosidase A protein (encoded by the *GLA* gene), which is deficient in Fabry disease. Migalastat restores the enzymatic activity of these proteins.

NEW DRUGS

Route	Onset	Peak	Duration
PO	Unknown	3 hr	Unknown

Half-life: 4 hours.

ADVERSE REACTIONS
CNS: headache, fever. **EENT:** nasopharyngitis, epistaxis. **GI:** nausea, vomiting, abdominal pain, diarrhea, vomiting. **GU:** UTI. **Musculoskeletal:** back pain. **Respiratory:** cough.

INTERACTIONS
None reported.

EFFECTS ON LAB TEST RESULTS
None reported.

CONTRAINDICATIONS & CAUTIONS
▨ Drug is only indicated for patients with a confirmed diagnosis of Fabry disease with an amenable *GLA* variant that is causing Fabry disease (pathogenic, likely pathogenic). Consider genetic consultation in cases in which the amenable *GLA* variant is of uncertain clinical significance or may be benign (not causing Fabry disease).
• Drug isn't recommended in patients with severe renal impairment or ESRD requiring dialysis.
• Safety and effectiveness in children haven't been established.
Dialyzable drug: Unknown.

PREGNANCY-LACTATION-REPRODUCTION
• There is insufficient data to assess drug-associated risks during pregnancy.
• Drug is likely to appear in human milk. Before using in breastfeeding women, consider the benefits of breastfeeding and the possible adverse effects to the infant.
• Drug's effects on fertility in humans are unknown. Drug caused reversible infertility in male rats.

NURSING CONSIDERATIONS
• Monitor patient for adverse effects, such as fever, headache, nasopharyngitis, UTI, and GI reactions.

PATIENT TEACHING
• Instruct patient on proper administration of drug and what to do if a dose is missed.
• Teach patient to report all adverse reactions.

SAFETY ALERT!

mogamulizumab-kpkc
moe-GAM-ue-LIZ-ue-mab

Poteligeo

Therapeutic class: Antineoplastics
Pharmacologic class: Monoclonal antibodies

AVAILABLE FORMS
Injection: 4 mg/mL in 5-mL single-use vial

INDICATIONS & DOSAGES
➤ **Treatment of relapsed or refractory mycosis fungoides or Sézary syndrome after at least one prior systemic therapy**
Adults: Initially, 1 mg/kg IV infusion on days 1, 8, 15, and 22 of the first 28-day cycle; then on days 1 and 15 of each subsequent 28-day cycle until disease progression or unacceptable toxicity occurs.
Adjust-a-dose: Refer to manufacturer's instructions for toxicity-related dosage adjustments.

ADMINISTRATION
IV
▼ Premedication with diphenhydramine and acetaminophen is recommended for the first infusion, and subsequent infusions as needed.
▼ Visually inspect vial and discard if cloudiness, discoloration, or particulates are seen.
▼ Withdraw proper dose and transfer into an NSS IV bag. The final concentration of the diluted solution should be between 0.1 mg/mL and 3 mg/mL.
▼ Discard any unused portion left in vial.
▼ Mix diluted solution by gentle inversion. Don't shake.
▼ Don't administer subcut or by rapid IV.
▼ Infuse solution immediately, or store refrigerated at 36° to 46° F (2° to 8° C) for no more than 4 hours from the time of infusion preparation. Don't freeze.
▼ Infuse over 60 minutes through a low-protein-binding, 0.22 micron (or equivalent) in-line filter.
▼ Diluted solution is compatible with polyvinyl chloride or polyolefin infusion bags.
▼ If a dose is missed, give the next dose as soon as possible and resume dosing schedule.
▼ Keep unopened vials under refrigeration at 36° to 46° F (2° to 8° C) in original package to protect from light until time of use. Don't freeze or shake.
▼ **Incompatibilities:** Don't mix with or infuse through same IV line as other drugs.

ACTION
A humanized IgG1 monoclonal antibody that binds to CC chemokine receptor 4 (CCR4). CCR4 is expressed on regulatory T-cells, some Th2 T-cells, and on the surface of some T-cell malignancies. Mogamulizumab-kpkc binding targets a cell for antibody-dependent cellular cytotoxicity, resulting in depletion of the target cells.

Route	Onset	Peak	Duration
IV	Unknown	Unknown	Unknown

Half-life: 17 days.

ADVERSE REACTIONS
CNS: fatigue, headache, dizziness, peripheral neuropathy, fever, insomnia, depression. **CV:** edema, HTN, *arrhythmias*. **EENT:** conjunctivitis, otitis. **GI:** diarrhea, nausea, mucositis, constipation, vomiting, abdominal pain, decreased appetite. **GU:** UTI,

Reactions in bold italics are *life-threatening*. Interactions may have a *rapid onset* or a **delayed onset**.

vaginal candidiasis, renal insufficiency. **Hematologic:** *neutropenia, thrombocytopenia*, anemia. **Metabolic:** hyperglycemia, weight gain or loss, hyperuricemia, hypothyroidism, *hypomagnesemia*. **Musculoskeletal:** pain, muscle spasms, falls. **Respiratory:** URI, lower respiratory tract infection, cough, dyspnea, pneumonia, pneumonitis. **Skin:** rash, skin infection, alopecia, dry skin, folliculitis. **Other:** antibody development, chills, infection, infusion reaction, candidiasis, herpes simplex, *sepsis*.

INTERACTIONS
None reported.

EFFECTS ON LAB TEST RESULTS
• May increase uric acid, AST, ALT, and alkaline phosphatase levels.
• May decrease phosphate, albumin, and magnesium levels.
• May increase or decrease calcium and glucose levels.
• May decrease Hb level and lymphocyte, leukocyte, platelet, and neutrophil counts.

CONTRAINDICATIONS & CAUTIONS
• Life-threatening and fatal infusion reactions have been reported and may occur during or shortly after the first infusion but may also occur with subsequent infusions.
• Fatal and life-threatening immune-mediated complications have been reported. Use cautiously in patients with a history of autoimmune disease.
• Cases of Stevens-Johnson syndrome (SJS), toxic epidermal necrolysis (TEN), TLS, and hepatitis have been reported.
• May increase risk of transplant complications in patients receiving allogeneic hematopoietic stem cell transplant after treatment with drug.
• Safety and effectiveness in children haven't been established.
Dialyzable drug: Unknown.

PREGNANCY-LACTATION-REPRODUCTION
• Drug hasn't been studied in pregnant women. IgG molecules are known to cross the placental barrier; therefore, drug isn't recommended during pregnancy or in women of childbearing potential not using contraception.
• Verify pregnancy status before starting drug. Patients should use effective contraception during treatment and for at least 3 months after final dose.
• It isn't known if drug appears in human milk. Before using in breastfeeding women, consider the benefits of drug and the potential adverse effects on the infant.

NURSING CONSIDERATIONS
• Monitor patient for development of infusion reactions (fever, chills, HTN or hypotension, bradycardia, nausea, tachycardia, headache, vomiting). Interrupt infusion for reaction and treat promptly.

• Monitor patient for rash; manage as clinically indicated. Permanently discontinue treatment for confirmed SJS or TEN.
• Monitor patient for development of infection, including sepsis, pneumonia, and skin infections; treat promptly.
• Monitor patient for immune-mediated complications (myositis, myocarditis, polymyositis, hepatitis, pneumonitis, and Guillain-Barré syndrome).
• Monitor patient for TLS (abdominal or flank pain, distension, hypocalcemia, hyperkalemia, dysuria, oliguria, hematuria); treat as clinically indicated.

PATIENT TEACHING
• Teach patient to report all adverse reactions.
• Teach patient to immediately report signs and symptoms of infusion reaction (chills, shaking, facial flushing, itching, rash, difficulty breathing, coughing, wheezing, dizziness, tiredness, fever), which can occur during or shortly after infusion.
• Advise patient to contact prescriber immediately for new or worsening rash at any time during therapy.
• Caution patient to immediately report fever or evidence of infection (chills, sweats, nausea, sore throat, difficulty swallowing, breathing problems, cough, diarrhea, abdominal pain).
• Alert patient of the potential risk of posttransplant complications if receiving stem cell transplantation after receiving drug.
• Alert female patient of childbearing potential to use effective contraception during treatment and for at least 3 months after final dose.
• Advise patient that laboratory testing will be needed to monitor treatment.

netarsudil–latanoprost
ne-TAR-soo-dil/la-TAN-oh-prost

Rocklatan

Therapeutic class: Antiglaucoma drugs
Pharmacologic class: Rho kinase inhibitors–prostaglandin F2 alpha analogues

AVAILABLE FORMS
Ophthalmic solution: netarsudil 0.2 mg/mL (0.02%)/latanoprost 0.05 mg/mL (0.005%)

INDICATIONS & DOSAGES
➤ **To reduce elevated IOP in patients with open-angle glaucoma or ocular HTN**
Adults: Instill 1 drop into affected eye(s) once daily in the evening.

ADMINISTRATION
Ophthalmic
• If additional topical ophthalmic medications must be administered, allow at least 5 minutes between each product.

• Patient must remove contact lenses before administration. Lenses may be reinserted 15 minutes after dose.
• If a dose is missed, give missed dose the next evening. Don't exceed once-daily dosing.
• Store at 36° to 46° F (2° to 8° C); protect from light.

ACTION
Thought to decrease elevated IOP by increasing the outflow of aqueous humor.

Route	Onset	Peak	Duration
Ophthalmic	Unknown	Unknown	Unknown

Half-life: 17 minutes.

ADVERSE REACTIONS
EENT: conjunctival hyperemia, instillation-site pain, corneal verticillata, conjunctival hemorrhage, instillation-site erythema, blurred vision, decreased visual acuity, corneal staining, increased lacrimation, erythema of eyelid, eye itching, burning and stinging of the eye, foreign body sensation, increased pigmentation of the iris, punctate keratitis, eyelid discomfort, eyelid margin crusting, photophobia, eyelid edema, dry eye, nasopharyngitis. **Musculoskeletal:** myalgia, arthralgia, back pain. **Respiratory:** URI. **Skin:** rash. **Other:** flulike symptoms, allergic reaction.

INTERACTIONS
Drug-drug. *Ophthalmic drops that contain thimerosal:* May cause precipitation of latanoprost. Separate administration by 5 minutes if used together. *Prostaglandin or prostaglandin analogue ophthalmic drugs (bimatoprost, tafluprost, travoprost):* May decrease IOP-lowering effect or cause paradoxical elevations in IOP. Avoid use together.

EFFECTS ON LAB TEST RESULTS
None reported.

CONTRAINDICATIONS & CAUTIONS
• Contraindicated in patients hypersensitive to drug or its components.
• Drug may increase pigmentation of the iris, eyelid, and eyelashes. Iris changes may be permanent; eyelid and eyelash pigmentation changes may reverse after drug is discontinued. Long-term effects of increased pigmentation aren't known.
• Drug may increase length, thickness, pigmentation, and number of lashes and may cause misdirected growth of eyelashes of the treated eye.
• Use cautiously in patients with a history of intraocular inflammation. Avoid use in patients with active intraocular inflammation, as inflammation may worsen.
• Drug may increase risk of macular edema. Use cautiously in aphakic patients, pseudophakic patients with torn posterior lens capsule, and in patients with known risk factors for macular edema.

• Use cautiously in patients with history of herpetic simplex keratitis; reactivation is possible.
• Avoid use in patients with active herpes simplex keratitis, as drug may exacerbate inflammation.
• Safety and effectiveness in children haven't been established.
Dialyzable drug: Unknown.

PREGNANCY-LACTATION-REPRODUCTION
• There are no adequate and well-controlled studies in pregnant women. Use during pregnancy only if potential benefits outweigh potential risk to the fetus.
• It isn't known if drug appears in human milk. Consider benefits of breastfeeding along with potential adverse risks to the breastfed infant.

NURSING CONSIDERATIONS
• Monitor patient for bacterial keratitis due to inadvertent contamination, especially in patients with multidose containers of topical ophthalmic products.
• Monitor IOP.
• Patients with increased iris pigmentation should have regular ophthalmic exams.

PATIENT TEACHING
• Teach patient safe drug administration and to avoid allowing tip of the dispensing container to contact the eye or surrounding structures.
• Teach patient to report all adverse effects.
• Caution patient to report development of other ocular conditions, such as trauma or infection, if ocular surgery is scheduled, or if ocular reactions occur, such as conjunctivitis and eyelid reactions.
• Advise patient of the potential for pigmentation of the iris, which may be permanent, and that long-term effects of pigmentation aren't known.
• Inform patient of the potential for eyelid skin darkening, which may be reversible after drug is discontinued.
• Tell patient of the potential for eyelash and vellus hair changes, including excess length and number of lashes or hairs, misdirected growth, thickening, and pigmentation. Changes are usually reversible if drug is discontinued.

omadacycline
oh-MAD-a-sye-kleen

Nuzyra

Therapeutic class: Antibiotics
Pharmacologic class: Tetracyclines

AVAILABLE FORMS
Injection: 100 mg single-dose vial
Tablets: 150-mg base

Reactions in bold italics are *life-threatening.* Interactions may have a *rapid onset* or a **delayed onset**.

INDICATIONS & DOSAGES

➤ **Treatment of community-acquired bacterial pneumonia (CABP) caused by** *Streptococcus pneumoniae,* *Staphylococcus aureus* **(methicillin-susceptible isolates),** *Haemophilus influenzae,* *Haemophilus parainfluenzae,* *Klebsiella pneumoniae,* *Legionella pneumophila,* *Mycoplasma pneumoniae,* **and** *Chlamydophila pneumoniae*

Adults: Initially, 200 mg IV infusion once or 100 mg IV infusion b.i.d. on day 1; then 100 mg IV infusion once daily or 300 mg PO once daily. Treat for 7 to 14 days.

➤ **Treatment of acute bacterial skin and skin-structure infections caused by** *S. aureus* **(methicillin-susceptible and methicillin-resistant isolates),** *Staphylococcus lugdunensis,* *Streptococcus pyogenes,* *Streptococcus anginosus* **group (includes** *S. anginosus,* *S. intermedius,* *S. constellatus***),** *Enterococcus faecalis,* *Enterobacter cloacae,* **and** *K. pneumoniae*

Adults: Initially, 200 mg IV infusion once or 100 mg IV infusion b.i.d. on day 1; then 100 mg IV infusion once daily or 300 mg PO once daily. Or, initially, 450 mg PO once daily on days 1 and 2; then 300 mg PO once daily beginning on day 3. Treat for 7 to 14 days.

ADMINISTRATION

PO

• Patient should fast for at least 4 hours before dose; then take with water. Patient shouldn't eat or drink (except water) for 2 hours after dose or ingest dairy products, antacids, or multivitamins for 4 hours after dose.

IV

▼ Reconstitute each 100-mg vial with 5 mL sterile water for injection.

▼ Gently swirl contents and let stand until the drug cake has completely dissolved and foam disperses. Don't shake.

▼ Reconstituted solution should be yellow to dark orange; if not, discard it. Visually inspect the vial for particulate matter and discoloration before further dilution and administration. If necessary, invert the vial to dissolve remaining powder and swirl gently to prevent foaming.

▼ Within 1 hour of reconstitution, withdraw 5 mL or 10 mL of the solution and further dilute in a 100-mL bag of NSS or D_5W, for a final concentration of either 1 mg/mL or 2 mg/mL. Discard any unused portion of the solution.

▼ Infuse diluted solution within 24 hours if kept at room temperature or within 48 hours when refrigerated. Don't freeze.

▼ If refrigerated, place diluted solution in a vertical position. Remove from refrigerator and allow solution to warm to room temperature 60 minutes before use.

▼ Administer through a dedicated line or Y-site. If the same IV line is used for infusion of other drugs, flush the line with NSS or D_5W before and after infusion of omadacycline.

▼ Administer infusion over 60 minutes for 200-mg dose or 30 minutes for 100-mg dose.

▼ Store vials at room temperature.

▼ **Incompatibilities:** Don't administer solutions containing multivalent cations (calcium, magnesium) through the same IV line. Infusion with other medications and infusion solutions other than NSS or D_5W hasn't been studied.

ACTION

A tetracycline antibiotic that exerts its bacteriostatic effect by inhibiting bacterial protein synthesis.

Route	Onset	Peak	Duration
PO	Unknown	2½ hr	Unknown
IV	Unknown	30 min	Unknown

Half-life: 15 to 17 hours.

ADVERSE REACTIONS

CNS: insomnia, headache, fatigue, lethargy, vertigo. **CV:** HTN, tachycardia, atrial fibrillation. **EENT:** oral candidiasis, oral pharyngeal pain. **GI:** vomiting, constipation, nausea, diarrhea, abdominal pain, dyspepsia, dysgeusia. **GU:** vulvovaginal mycotic infection. **Hematologic:** anemia, thrombocytosis. **Hepatic:** elevated LFT values. **Skin:** pruritus, erythema, hyperhidrosis, urticaria. **Other:** infusion-site reaction, hypersensitivity.

INTERACTIONS

Drug-drug. *Antacids containing aluminum, calcium, or magnesium; bismuth subsalicylate; iron-containing preparations; iron supplements:* May decrease omadacycline absorption. Separate doses by at least 4 hours before and 4 hours after omadacycline. *Anticoagulants (warfarin):* May increase anticoagulant effects. Monitor patient closely and decrease anticoagulant dosage if needed.

Drug-food. *Dairy products:* May decrease omadacycline absorption. Separate dairy product use by at least 4 hours before and 4 hours after omadacycline.

Food, nondairy drinks (except water): May decrease omadacycline absorption. Avoid for at least 4 hours before and 2 hours after omadacycline.

Drug-lifestyle. *Sun exposure:* May cause photosensitivity. Advise patient to avoid sun exposure and to wear sun-protective clothing and sunscreen.

EFFECTS ON LAB TEST RESULTS

• May increase ALT, AST, GGT, CK, bilirubin, alkaline phosphatase, and lipase levels.

CONTRAINDICATIONS & CAUTIONS

• Contraindicated in patients hypersensitive to drug or its components or tetracycline class drugs.
• Use only to treat or prevent infections proven or strongly suspected to be caused by susceptible bacteria to reduce development of drug-resistance.
• **Alert:** In clinical trials, when drug was used to treat CABP, there was a higher mortality rate than for moxifloxacin-treated patients. All deaths

NEW DRUGS

occurred in patients older than age 65 and most had multiple comorbid conditions. The cause of the mortality imbalance isn't known.

🜂 Alert: CDAD has been reported and may range from mild diarrhea to fatal colitis.

• Use of tetracycline class drugs during the last half (second or third trimester) of pregnancy, during infancy, and in children younger than age 8 may cause permanent yellow-gray-brown discoloration of the teeth or tooth enamel hypoplasia, and may cause reversible inhibition of bone growth.

• Safety and effectiveness in patients younger than age 18 haven't been established. Use in children younger than age 8 isn't recommended.

Dialyzable drug: 8.9%.

PREGNANCY-LACTATION-REPRODUCTION

• Drug may cause fetal harm. Advise women of childbearing potential to use contraception during therapy.

• Tetracyclines appear in human milk. Breastfeeding isn't recommended during treatment and for 4 days after final dose.

• Based on animal studies, drug may affect male and female fertility.

NURSING CONSIDERATIONS

• Confirm that patients don't have an allergy to any tetracycline class drug before starting therapy.

• Monitor patients for hypersensitivity reactions, including anaphylaxis.

🜂 Alert: Use drug cautiously for CABP in patients age 65 and older, especially if they have multiple comorbid conditions.

• Monitor patients for signs and symptoms of CDAD (watery or bloody stools [with or without stomach cramps or fever]) during and for several months after treatment with antibacterial drugs. If CDAD is suspected or confirmed, antibiotic use other than for treatment of *Clostridium difficile* may need to be discontinued. Initiate appropriate treatment.

• Monitor patients for tetracycline class adverse reactions, including photosensitivity, pseudotumor cerebri, and antianabolic activity (increased BUN level, azotemia, acidosis, hyperphosphatemia, pancreatitis, abnormal LFT values). Discontinue drug if any of these are suspected.

• *Look alike-sound alike:* Don't confuse omadacycline with omacetaxine.

PATIENT TEACHING

• Warn patient that antibacterial drugs should only be used to treat bacterial infections and shouldn't be used to treat viral infections such as the common cold.

• Advise patient to report all adverse reactions.

• Caution patient to seek immediate medical attention for serious allergic reactions.

• Teach patient safe drug administration.

• Caution patient to take drug exactly as directed even if feeling better. Stress importance of not skipping doses and completing therapy as prescribed.

• Warn patient that nonadherence may decrease effectiveness of treatment and risk that the bacteria will develop resistance and not be treatable by antibacterial drugs in the future.

🜂 Alert: Instruct patient to immediately report watery or bloody stools (with or without stomach cramps or fever) as these may indicate CDAD.

• Advise patient that drug can cause photosensitivity and to avoid sun exposure and wear sun-protective clothing and sunscreen during treatment.

• Advise female patient of childbearing potential of the risk to the fetus if drug is used during pregnancy. Caution her to use contraceptives during treatment and to immediately contact prescriber if pregnancy is suspected.

• Teach breastfeeding patient that breastfeeding isn't recommended during treatment and for 4 days after final dose.

---

onasemnogene abeparvovec-xioi 🜂
on-a-SEM-noe-jeen a-be-PAR-voe-vek

Zolgensma

Therapeutic class: CNS agents
Pharmacologic class: Gene therapies

AVAILABLE FORMS

Injection: 2.0×10^{13} vector genomes (vg)/mL in vials of 5.5 mL or 8.3 mL in a kit of two to nine vials

INDICATIONS & DOSAGES

➤ **Treatment of patients with spinal muscular atrophy (SMA) with bi-allelic mutations in the survival motor neuron 1 (*SMN1*) gene** 🜂

Children younger than age 2: 1.1×10^{14} vg/kg body weight as a single IV infusion.

ADMINISTRATION

IV

Black Box Warning One day before gene infusion, begin systemic corticosteroids equivalent to 1 mg/kg/day oral prednisolone for a total of 30 days. ■

▼ Thaw before use over approximately 12 hours in refrigerator or 4 hours at room temperature. If thawed in refrigerator, remove from refrigerator on day of dosing. Don't refreeze.

▼ When thawed, liquid is clear to slightly opaque, colorless to faint white, and free of particles. Visually inspect vials before infusion. Don't use if particulates or discoloration is present. Don't shake.

▼ Calculate the appropriate dose according to manufacturer's instructions and draw into a syringe.

▼ Infuse drug through a primary catheter in a peripheral vein in arm or leg. Insertion of a back-up catheter is recommended.

▼ Program syringe pump for saline priming or prime tubing manually with saline. Administer dose as single IV infusion over 60 minutes. Don't give as an IV push or bolus.

▼ Flush line with saline after completion of infusion.

▼ Use drug within 8 hours of drawing into syringe. Discard if not infused within 8 hours.

▼ Drug is shipped and delivered frozen. Upon receipt, store refrigerated at 36° to 46° F (2° to 8° C). Use within 14 days of receipt.

▼ **Incompatibilities:** Don't administer with other drugs or solutions.

ACTION

SMA is caused by a mutation in the *SMN1* gene, which results in insufficient SMN protein expression. Drug is a recombinant gene therapy that delivers copies of the gene encoding the SMN protein and results in *SMN1* gene expression.

Route	Onset	Peak	Duration
IV	N/A	N/A	N/A

Half-life: N/A.

ADVERSE REACTIONS

GI: vomiting. **Hepatic:** increased aminotransferase levels.

INTERACTIONS

Drug-drug. *Vaccines:* Certain vaccines (such as MMR and varicella) are contraindicated in patients receiving immunosuppressive steroid doses. When feasible, adjust patient's vaccination schedule to accommodate corticosteroid administration before and after gene therapy.

EFFECTS ON LAB TEST RESULTS

• May increase AST, ALT, and cardiac troponin-I levels.
• May increase anti-adeno-associated virus type 9 (AAV9) titers.
• May decrease platelet count.

CONTRAINDICATIONS & CAUTIONS

Black Box Warning Acute serious liver injury and elevated aminotransferase levels can occur. Patients with preexisting liver impairment may be at higher risk for liver injury. ▉
• Safety and effectiveness of repeat administration haven't been evaluated.
• Use in patients with advanced SMA (complete paralysis of limbs, permanent ventilator-dependence) hasn't been evaluated.
• Readministration of drug in the presence of a high anti-AAV9 antibody titer hasn't been evaluated.
• Use in premature neonates before they have reached full-term gestational age isn't recommended because corticosteroids may adversely affect neurologic development. Delay treatment until full-term gestational age is attained.
Dialyzable drug: Unknown.

PREGNANCY-LACTATION-REPRODUCTION

• There are no data on the use of this gene therapy in pregnant women.
• It isn't known if drug appears in human milk. Consider the benefits of breastfeeding along with potential adverse effects on the breastfed infant.

NURSING CONSIDERATIONS

• Obtain baseline anti-AAV9 antibody testing before infusion. Retesting may be performed if anti-AAV9 antibody titer is greater than 1:50.
Black Box Warning Assess liver function by clinical exam and blood work (AST, ALT, total bilirubin, PT) before infusion; monitor liver function for at least 3 months after infusion. ▉
• Reassess liver function weekly for the first month, then every other week for the second and third months until the clinical exam is normal and total bilirubin, PT, ALT, and AST levels are less than $2 \times$ ULN.
• Obtain platelet count at baseline and weekly for the first month, then every other week for the second and third months until platelet count returns to baseline.
• Measure troponin-I level at baseline and weekly for the first month, then monthly for the second and third months until troponin-I level returns to baseline.
• After 30 days of corticosteroid treatment, may taper the corticosteroid over 28 days in patients with normal clinical exam and acceptable blood test results. If liver function abnormalities persist, continue the corticosteroid (equivalent to oral prednisolone 1 mg/kg/day) until AST and ALT levels are below $2 \times$ ULN and clinical exam, total bilirubin, and PT return to normal; then taper the corticosteroid over 28 days.
• Consult specialists if patient doesn't adequately respond to the equivalent of oral prednisolone 1 mg/kg/day.
• Follow facility guidelines for handwashing and body waste management for 1 month after drug infusion since vector shedding occurs through body waste.

PATIENT TEACHING

• Inform caregivers to report all adverse reactions.
Black Box Warning Inform caregivers that patient will receive an oral corticosteroid before and after drug infusion. ▉
Black Box Warning Warn caregivers that drug may increase liver enzyme levels and cause serious liver injury. Inform them that regular lab blood tests are needed to monitor liver function. ▉
Black Box Warning Advise caregivers to immediately report signs or symptoms of liver injury (yellowing of the skin or whites of the eyes)

NEW DRUGS

or if patient vomits or misses a corticosteroid dose. ∎

• Inform caregivers to immediately report unexpected bruising or bleeding, as drug can decrease platelet count.

• Advise caregivers to consult prescriber to determine if adjustments to patient's vaccination schedule are necessary during corticosteroid use.

• Counsel caregivers to discuss prophylaxis against RSV with health care provider since RSV infection (cold, flulike symptoms, bronchiolitis) before or after drug infusion could lead to more serious complications.

• Tell caregivers to immediately contact health care provider if signs or symptoms of a viral respiratory infection (coughing, wheezing, sneezing, runny nose, sore throat, fever) occur.

• Teach caregivers and family members the proper handling of patient feces (seal disposable diapers in disposable trash bags and discard into regular trash), because temporary vector shedding of drug occurs primarily through body waste, and to practice proper hand hygiene if they've had direct contact with patient's body waste. Tell them to follow these precautions for 1 month after drug infusion.

patisiran ⚠
PAT-i-sir-an

Onpattro

Therapeutic class: Metabolic agents
Pharmacologic class: Anti-transthyretin small interfering RNA (siRNA) agents

AVAILABLE FORMS
Injection: 2 mg/mL in 5-mL single-dose vials

INDICATIONS & DOSAGES
➤ **Treatment of the polyneuropathy of hereditary transthyretin-mediated amyloidosis** ⚠
Adults weighing 100 kg or more: 30 mg IV infusion once every 3 weeks.
Adults weighing less than 100 kg: 0.3 mg/kg IV infusion once every 3 weeks.

ADMINISTRATION
IV
✪ Alert: To reduce the risk of infusion-related reactions, premedicate all patients at least 60 minutes before the start of each infusion. Treatment should include an IV corticosteroid (dexamethasone 10 mg, or equivalent), 500 mg oral acetaminophen, an IV H₁ blocker (diphenhydramine 50 mg, or equivalent), and an IV H₂ blocker (ranitidine 50 mg, or equivalent).
▼ If premedications aren't available or aren't tolerated by IV route, may administer equivalents orally. For patients with corticosteroid adverse reactions, may decrease the corticosteroid dose

by 2.5-mg increments to a minimum dose of dexamethasone 5 mg IV, or equivalent. Add or increase doses of one or more of the premedications as needed to reduce the risk of infusion-related reactions.
▼ Allow vial to come to room temperature; don't shake or swirl.
▼ Visually inspect vial. Solution should be white to off-white, opalescent, and homogeneous. Discard if particulate matter or discoloration is seen.
▼ Calculate the dose required and withdraw the contents into a single sterile syringe.
▼ Filter drug through a sterile 0.45-micron polyethersulfone (PES) syringe filter into a sterile container.
▼ Dilute in an infusion bag (di(2-ethylhexyl) phthalate [DEHP]-free) containing NSS for a total volume of 200 mL. Gently invert the bag to mix; don't shake.
▼ Discard any unused portion of drug.
▼ Drug is preservative free. Give diluted solution immediately after preparation. If not used immediately, store in the infusion bag at room temperature (up to 86° F [30° C]) for up to 16 hours, including infusion time. Don't freeze.
▼ Infuse through a dedicated line with a DEHP-free infusion set containing a 1.2-micron PES in-line infusion filter through a free-flowing venous access site.
▼ Infuse the diluted solution via an infusion pump over approximately 80 minutes at an initial infusion rate of 1 mL/minute for the first 15 minutes; then increase to approximately 3 mL/minute for the remainder of the infusion. If an infusion-related reaction occurs, may decrease the infusion rate.
▼ After the infusion is completed, flush the IV administration set with NSS to ensure that all of the drug has been administered.
▼ If a dose is missed, give as soon as possible. If drug is given within 3 days of the missed dose, continue dosing according to patient's original schedule; if given more than 3 days after the missed dose, continue dosing every 3 weeks thereafter.
▼ Store vials at 36° to 46° F (2° to 8° C). Discard vial if it has been frozen.
▼ If refrigeration isn't available, store vials at room temperature up to 77° F (25° C) for up to 14 days.
▼ **Incompatibilities:** Don't mix or dilute with other drugs.

ACTION
A double-stranded siRNA that causes degradation of mutant and wild-type *TTR* mRNA through RNA interference, which results in a reduction of serum TTR protein and TTR protein deposits in tissues.

Route	Onset	Peak	Duration
IV	Unknown	Unknown	Unknown

Half-life: 3.2 days.

Reactions in bold italics are *life-threatening*. Interactions may have a *rapid onset* or a **delayed onset**.

ADVERSE REACTIONS
CNS: vertigo. **CV:** *AV heart block.* **EENT:** dry eye, blurred vision, vitreous floaters. **GI:** dyspepsia, abdominal pain, nausea. **Musculoskeletal:** muscle spasms, arthralgia, back pain. **Respiratory:** dyspnea, URI, bronchitis. **Skin:** erythema. **Other:** infusion-related reactions, antibody development.

INTERACTIONS
None reported.

EFFECTS ON LAB TEST RESULTS
• May decrease serum vitamin A and serum retinol-binding protein levels.

CONTRAINDICATIONS & CAUTIONS
• Serious infusion-related reactions can occur, often within the first two infusions; the frequency decreases with additional infusions. Patients should be premedicated before infusions.
• Drug decreases serum vitamin A level. Patients should supplement with the recommended daily allowance of vitamin A.
• Safety and effectiveness in children haven't been established.
Dialyzable drug: Unknown.

PREGNANCY-LACTATION-REPRODUCTION
• Data aren't available on the use of drug in pregnant women, and the risk of adverse developmental outcomes hasn't been determined. However, adverse events were observed in some animal studies.
• Supplementation with vitamin A is recommended during therapy, as it's required for normal embryo-fetal development. Women should avoid excessive vitamin A intake, which can result in adverse developmental effects. There are no data regarding the fetal effects of reduced maternal serum transthyretin (TTR) or vitamin A supplementation.
• It isn't known if drug appears in human milk or how it affects milk production or a breastfed infant. Consider the benefits of breastfeeding along with the mother's clinical need for drug and potential adverse effects on the infant.

NURSING CONSIDERATIONS
• Monitor patient during the infusion for signs and symptoms of infusion-related reaction (flushing, back pain, nausea, abdominal pain, dyspnea, headache, chest pain, rash, increased HR, facial edema). Interrupt the infusion and manage as clinically indicated.
• Monitor infusion site for infiltration. Manage suspected extravasation according to local standard practice for nonvesicants.
• Monitor vitamin A level and observe patient for ocular signs and symptoms suggestive of vitamin A deficiency (night blindness). Refer patient to an ophthalmologist as needed.
• *Look alike–sound alike:* Don't confuse patisiran with patiromer.

PATIENT TEACHING
• Teach patient to report all adverse reactions and to immediately report signs and symptoms of infusion-related reaction.
• Advise patient that drug leads to a decrease in serum vitamin A level. Instruct patient to take the recommended daily allowance of vitamin A.
• Instruct patient to report ocular signs and symptoms suggestive of vitamin A deficiency (such as night blindness), as patient should be referred to an ophthalmologist.
• Instruct female patient to report if she becomes pregnant or plans to become pregnant during treatment.
• Advise female patient of childbearing potential of the potential risk to the fetus.

polatuzumab vedotin-piiq
poe-la-TOOZ-ue-mab ve-DOE-tin

Polivy

Therapeutic class: Antineoplastics
Pharmacologic class: Antibodies–drug conjugates

AVAILABLE FORMS
Injection: 140 mg single-dose vial

INDICATIONS & DOSAGES
➤ **Treatment of patients with relapsed or refractory diffuse large B-cell lymphoma, not otherwise specified, in combination with bendamustine and a rituximab product, after at least two prior therapies**
Adults: 1.8 mg/kg IV infusion every 21 days for six cycles in combination with bendamustine and a rituximab product in any order on day 1 of each cycle. Recommended bendamustine dose is 90 mg/m²/day on days 1 and 2 when administered with polatuzumab vedotin and a rituximab product. Recommended dose of the rituximab product is 375 mg/m² IV on day 1 of each cycle.
Adjust-a-dose: Refer to manufacturer's instructions for toxicity-related dosage adjustments.

ADMINISTRATION
IV
▼ If patient isn't already premedicated, administer an antihistamine and antipyretic at least 30 minutes before infusion.
▼ Drug is cytotoxic; follow special handling and disposal procedures for cytotoxic agents.
▼ Reconstitute each vial immediately before use with 7.2 mL of sterile water for injection, with the stream directed toward the inside wall of the vial.
▼ Gently swirl vial until completely dissolved. Don't shake.
▼ Inspect reconstituted solution for discoloration and particulate matter. Solution should be

NEW DRUGS

colorless to slightly brown, clear to slightly opalescent. Don't use if solution is discolored, cloudy, or contains visible particulates. Don't freeze or expose to direct sunlight.

▼ Store unused reconstituted solution refrigerated at 36° to 46° F (2° to 8° C) for up to 48 hours or at room temperature for up to 8 hours before dilution. Discard vial when cumulative storage time before dilution exceeds 48 hours.

▼ Dilute drug to a final concentration of 0.72 to 2.7 mg/mL in an IV infusion bag with a minimum volume of 50 mL NSS, ½ NSS, or D₅W.

▼ Gently mix IV bag by slowly inverting the bag. Don't shake. Inspect for particulates and discard if present.

▼ Limit agitation of diluted product during preparation and transportation to administration site. Don't transport diluted product through an automated system, such as a pneumatic tube or automated cart.

▼ Administer via a dedicated line with a nonpyrogenic, low-protein-binding in-line or add-on filter (0.2- or 0.22-micron pore size) and catheter.

▼ If patient tolerates initial infusion over 90 minutes, may give subsequent infusions over 30 minutes.

▼ If not used immediately, store the diluted solution as specified in the manufacturer's information. Discard if storage time exceeds these limits. Don't freeze or expose to direct sunlight.

▼ Give missed dose as soon as possible. Adjust the administration schedule to maintain a 21-day interval between doses.

▼ Store vials refrigerated at 36° to 46° F (2° to 8° C) in original carton to protect from light. Don't freeze or shake.

▼ **Incompatibilities:** Don't mix with or administer as an infusion with other drugs.

ACTION

An antibody-drug conjugate that binds to CD79b (a B-cell surface protein), resulting in death of dividing cells through inhibition of cell division and apoptosis.

Route	Onset	Peak	Duration
IV	Unknown	Unknown	Unknown

Half-life: About 12 days.

ADVERSE REACTIONS

CNS: peripheral neuropathy, dizziness, fever, fatigue. **EENT:** blurred vision. **GI:** diarrhea, vomiting, decreased appetite. **Hematologic:** *neutropenia, febrile neutropenia, thrombocytopenia,* anemia, *lymphopenia, pancytopenia.* **Hepatic:** transaminase elevation. **Metabolic:** *hypokalemia,* weight loss. **Musculoskeletal:** arthralgia. **Respiratory:** pneumonia, URI, pneumonitis, lower respiratory tract infection, dyspnea. **Other:** infusion-related reaction, *sepsis,* herpesvirus infection, CMV infection.

INTERACTIONS

Drug-drug. *Strong CYP3A inducers (rifampin):* May decrease effectiveness of polatuzumab vedotin. Monitor patient for therapeutic effectiveness.
Strong CYP3A inhibitors (ketoconazole): May increase toxicity of polatuzumab vedotin. Monitor patient for toxicity.

EFFECTS ON LAB TEST RESULTS

• May increase ALT, AST, lipase, amylase, and creatinine levels.
• May decrease potassium, albumin, calcium, and phosphorus levels.
• May decrease Hb level and neutrophil, platelet, and lymphocyte counts.

CONTRAINDICATIONS & CAUTIONS

• Peripheral neuropathy, including severe cases, may occur as early as the first cycle of treatment and is a cumulative effect. Exacerbation of preexisting peripheral neuropathy may also occur.
• Infusion-related reactions, including severe cases, may occur. Delayed infusion-related reactions have occurred as late as 24 hours after drug administration.
• Treatment can cause serious or severe myelosuppression, including neutropenia, thrombocytopenia, and anemia.
• Fatal or serious infections, including opportunistic infections such as sepsis, pneumonia (including *Pneumocystis jiroveci* and other fungal pneumonia), herpesvirus infection, and CMV infection, have occurred.
• Progressive multifocal leukoencephalopathy (PML) has been reported after treatment.
• Drug may cause TLS. Use cautiously in patients with high tumor burden and rapidly proliferative tumor; these patients are at increased risk.
• Serious cases of hepatotoxicity consistent with hepatocellular injury have occurred. Use cautiously in patients with preexisting liver disease or elevated baseline liver enzyme levels and in those taking concomitant medications.
• Safety and effectiveness in children haven't been established.
Dialyzable drug: Unknown.

PREGNANCY-LACTATION-REPRODUCTION

• Drug may cause fetal harm. Advise pregnant women of the risk to a fetus.
• Test women of childbearing potential for pregnancy before starting treatment.
• Women of childbearing potential should use effective contraception during treatment and for at least 3 months after final dose.
• Male patients with female partners of childbearing potential should use effective contraception during treatment and for at least 5 months after final dose.
• It isn't known if drug appears in human milk. Advise patients not to breastfeed during treatment and for at least 2 months after final dose.

Reactions in bold italics are *life-threatening.* Interactions may have a *rapid onset* or a **delayed onset.**

• Drug may impair male fertility; reversal of this effect is unknown.

NURSING CONSIDERATIONS

• Monitor patients for infusion-related reactions during the infusion and for a minimum of 90 minutes after completion of the initial dose. If the previous infusion was well tolerated, monitor patients during the infusion and for at least 30 minutes after completion of the infusion.

• If an infusion-related reaction occurs, interrupt the infusion and institute appropriate medical management.

• Monitor CBC throughout treatment. Cytopenias may require a therapy interruption, dosage reduction, or drug discontinuation. Consider prophylactic granulocyte colony stimulating factor administration for neutropenia.

• Closely monitor patients during treatment for signs and symptoms of infection. Administer prophylaxis for *P. jiroveci* pneumonia and herpesvirus infection.

• Monitor patients for new or worsening neurologic, cognitive, or behavioral changes. Withhold drug and any concomitant chemotherapy if PML is suspected; permanently discontinue drug if the diagnosis is confirmed.

• Monitor patients for TLS and administer TLS prophylaxis for patients at increased risk for TLS.

• Monitor patients for new or worsening peripheral neuropathy (hypoesthesia, hyperesthesia, paresthesia, dysesthesia, neuropathic pain, burning sensation, weakness, gait disturbance). Interrupt therapy, reduce dosage, or discontinue drug as clinically indicated.

• Monitor liver enzyme and bilirubin levels throughout treatment.

• **Look alike–sound alike:** Don't confuse polatuzumab vedotin-piiq with other monoclonal antibodies.

PATIENT TEACHING

• Advise patient that drug can cause peripheral neuropathy and to report numbness or tingling of the hands or feet or muscle weakness to prescriber.

• Tell patient to report signs and symptoms of infusion reactions (fever, chills, rash, or breathing problems) within 24 hours of infusion.

• Counsel patient to immediately report signs or symptoms of bleeding.

• Instruct patient to contact prescriber for a fever (temperature of 100.4° F [38° C] or greater) or other evidence of infection (chills, cough, pain on urination).

• Inform patient that lab blood work will be needed periodically to monitor for adverse effects.

• Advise patient to seek immediate medical attention for signs and symptoms of PML (new-onset or changes in neurologic signs and symptoms, e.g., confusion, dizziness, loss of balance, difficulty talking or walking, changes in vision).

• Direct patient to seek immediate medical attention for signs and symptoms of TLS (nausea, vomiting, diarrhea, lethargy).

• Tell patient to report signs and symptoms of liver injury (fatigue, anorexia, right upper abdominal discomfort, dark urine, jaundice).

• Warn female patient of childbearing potential of the potential risk to a fetus. Advise her that she will be tested for pregnancy before therapy and to contact prescriber if she becomes pregnant or suspects she is pregnant during therapy.

• Instruct female patient of childbearing potential to use effective contraception during treatment and for at least 3 months after final dose.

• Instruct male patient with female partner of childbearing potential to use effective contraception during treatment and for 5 months after final dose.

• Counsel patient not to breastfeed during therapy and for at least 2 months after final dose.

prucalopride succinate
proo-KAL-oh-pride

Motegrity

Therapeutic class: GI drugs
Pharmacologic class: Selective serotonin type 4 (5-HT$_4$) receptor agonists

AVAILABLE FORMS
Tablets: 1 mg, 2 mg

INDICATIONS & DOSAGES
➤ **Chronic idiopathic constipation**
Adults: 2 mg PO once daily.
Adjust-a-dose: For severe renal impairment (CrCl less than 30 mL/minute), decrease dose to 1 mg PO once daily.

ADMINISTRATION
PO
• Give without regard for food.
• Store in original container to protect from moisture.
• Store at 68° to 77° F (20° to 25° C).

ACTION
A 5-HT$_4$ receptor agonist that stimulates colonic peristalsis, which increases bowel motility.

Route	Onset	Peak	Duration
PO	Unknown	2–3 hr	Unknown

Half-life: About 24 hours.

ADVERSE REACTIONS
CNS: headache, dizziness, fatigue, migraine. **GI:** abdominal pain, nausea, diarrhea, abdominal distension, vomiting, flatulence, abnormal GI sounds, decreased appetite. **GU:** frequent urination.

NEW DRUGS

INTERACTIONS
None reported.

EFFECTS ON LAB TEST RESULTS
None reported.

CONTRAINDICATIONS & CAUTIONS
• Contraindicated in patients hypersensitive to drug or its components.
• Contraindicated in patients with intestinal perforation or obstruction due to structural or functional disorder of the gut wall, obstructive ileus, severe inflammatory conditions of the intestinal tract (Crohn disease, ulcerative colitis, toxic megacolon/megarectum).
◑ **Alert:** Suicides, suicide attempts, and suicidal ideation were reported during clinical trials. A causal association hasn't been established.
• Avoid use in patients with ESRD requiring dialysis.
• Safety and effectiveness in children haven't been evaluated.
• Use cautiously in elderly patients and adjust the dosage based on renal function.
Dialyzable drug: Unknown.
⚠ **Overdose S&S:** Headache, nausea, diarrhea.

PREGNANCY-LACTATION-REPRODUCTION
• It isn't known if drug causes fetal harm. Use in pregnant women only if the benefit to the mother outweighs the potential fetal risk.
• Drug appears in human milk but there are no data on the drug's effects on the breastfed infant or on milk production. Consider the benefits of breastfeeding, the mother's need for the drug, and potential adverse effects on the breastfed infant or from the mother's condition.

NURSING CONSIDERATIONS
• Monitor patients for hypersensitivity reactions (dyspnea, rash, pruritus, urticaria, facial edema).
◑ **Alert:** Monitor patients for worsening depression and suicidal thoughts and behavior.

PATIENT TEACHING
• Advise patient to report all adverse reactions.
• Teach patient safe drug administration.
◑ **Alert:** Inform patient, family members, and caregivers to immediately report unusual changes in mood or behavior, persistent worsening of symptoms of depression, or suicidal thoughts or behavior and to discontinue drug.
• Inform patient that drug may cause diarrhea, which generally occurs during the first week of treatment and then resolves after a few days.
• Advise patient to immediately report signs and symptoms of hypersensitivity reactions.
• Caution female patient that it isn't known if drug can cause fetal harm. Advise her to tell prescriber if she is pregnant or plans to become pregnant before using drug.

• Warn patient who is breastfeeding or plans to breastfeed that drug can appear in human milk and to discuss the best way to feed the infant with prescriber.

rifamycin
rif-a-MYE-sin

Aemcolo

Therapeutic class: Antibiotics
Pharmacologic class: Ansamycins

AVAILABLE FORMS
Tablets (delayed-release) ⒹⓇ: 194 mg

INDICATIONS & DOSAGES
➤ **Travelers' diarrhea caused by noninvasive strains of** *Escherichia coli*
Adults: 388 mg PO b.i.d. for 3 days.

ADMINISTRATION
PO
• Give with 6 to 8 oz of liquid. Patient shouldn't take with alcohol.
• May give with or without food.
• Patient must swallow tablets whole and not crush, break, or chew them.
• Store at 68° to 77° F (20° to 25° C).

ACTION
Ansamycin class of antibacterial drugs act by blocking a step in DNA transcription, inhibiting bacterial synthesis and therefore bacterial growth.

Route	Onset	Peak	Duration
PO	Unknown	Unknown	Unknown

Half-life: Unknown.

ADVERSE REACTIONS
CNS: headache. **GI:** constipation, dyspepsia.

INTERACTIONS
None reported.

EFFECTS ON LAB TEST RESULTS
None reported.

CONTRAINDICATIONS & CAUTIONS
• Contraindicated in patients with known hypersensitivity to drug, its components, or any other rifamycin class antibacterials.
• Drug isn't indicated for diarrhea complicated by fever or bloody stool or from diarrhea due to pathogens other than noninvasive strains of *E. coli.*
• Only use drug to treat or prevent infections proven or strongly suspected to be caused by susceptible bacteria, to decrease the risk of development of drug-resistant bacteria.
◑ **Alert:** CDAD has been associated with almost all antibacterial agents. Diarrhea may range in

NEW DRUGS

severity from mild to fatal colitis. Evaluate patient if diarrhea occurs after therapy, doesn't improve, or worsens during therapy.
• Safety and effectiveness in children younger than age 18 haven't been established.
Dialyzable drug: Unknown.

PREGNANCY-LACTATION-REPRODUCTION
• Drug hasn't been studied in pregnant women. Systemic absorption is negligible and it isn't expected to result in fetal exposure.
• It isn't known if drug appears in human milk. Systemic absorption is negligible, and exposure to the breastfed infant is expected to be negligible. Before use in breastfeeding women, consider the benefits of breastfeeding, the mother's need for the drug, and potential adverse effects on the breastfed infant or from the mother's condition.

NURSING CONSIDERATIONS
• Monitor patient for worsening or persistent diarrhea of more than 48 hours. If diarrhea persists, discontinue drug and consider alternative therapy.
• Monitor patient for diarrhea that persists after therapy and evaluate for possible CDAD. If CDAD is confirmed, treat as clinically indicated.
• Prophylactic use is unlikely to provide a benefit to patient and will increase risk of development of drug-resistant bacteria.
• *Look alike–sound alike:* Don't confuse rifamycin with rifampin, rifaximin, or rifabutin.

PATIENT TEACHING
• Advise patient to report all adverse reactions.
• Teach patient safe drug administration.
• Instruct patient to discontinue drug and report diarrhea persisting for more than 48 hours or diarrhea that worsens (watery or bloody stools with or without stomach cramps and fever) during or even as late as 2 or more months after therapy ends.
• Counsel patient to complete the whole course of therapy as prescribed, as skipping doses or not completing the whole course may decrease effectiveness of treatment and increase the likelihood that bacteria will develop resistance and won't be treatable in the future.

segesterone acetate–ethinyl estradiol
se-JES-ter-one/ETH-i-nill es-tra-DYE-ole

Annovera

Therapeutic class: Contraceptives
Pharmacologic class: Progestin-estrogen combinations

AVAILABLE FORMS
Vaginal ring: 103 mg segesterone acetate and 17.4 mg ethinyl estradiol delivering an average of 0.15 mg segesterone acetate and 0.013 mg ethinyl estradiol daily

INDICATIONS & DOSAGES
➤ Contraception
Women of childbearing potential: 1 vaginal ring inserted into the vagina and left in place continuously for 21 days, followed by a 7-day vaginal ring–free interval. One vaginal ring provides contraception for 13 28-day cycles (1 year).

ADMINISTRATION
Vaginal
• Insert the ring with patient in a comfortable position, such as lying down, squatting, or standing. Press the sides of the vaginal ring together and insert the ring into the vagina. With proper insertion, the ring is entirely inside the vagina and behind the pelvic bone.
• Document the day and time of insertion so the vaginal ring can be removed at the same time 21 days later. Before initial use, label the storage case with the discard date to avoid using the product beyond 13 cycles.
• Remove the ring by hooking an index finger into the ring inside the vagina and gently pulling.
• Wash the ring with mild soap and water, and rinse and pat dry with a clean cloth towel or paper towel before each insertion and at each removal. Place the ring in the provided storage case between uses.
• If the ring is accidentally expelled, wash and dry the device and replace it as soon as possible. If the ring is replaced within 2 hours, no backup contraception is needed.
• Protect from direct sunlight. Store at room temperature; don't refrigerate or freeze.

ACTION
Suppresses gonadotropins, thereby inhibiting ovulation, increasing the viscosity of cervical mucus, and altering the endometrial lining.

Route	Onset	Peak	Duration
Vaginal	Day of insertion	2 hr	Unknown

Half-life: Segesterone acetate, 4.5 hours; ethinyl estradiol, 15.1 hours.

ADVERSE REACTIONS
CNS: headache, migraine, *stroke,* psychiatric disturbance. **CV:** *CV events, venous thromboembolism (DVT, cerebral vein thrombosis, PE).* **GI:** nausea, vomiting, abdominal pain, diarrhea. **GU:** vulvovaginal candidiasis, vaginitis, vaginal discharge, dysmenorrhea, genital pruritus, UTI (cystitis, pyelonephritis), amenorrhea, metrorrhagia, menorrhagia, vaginal and cervical erosion or ulceration, spontaneous abortion. **Other:** breast pain, *hypersensitivity reaction.*

NEW DRUGS

INTERACTIONS

Drug-drug. *Acetaminophen:* May decrease acetaminophen level and increase ethinyl estradiol level. Monitor patient for hormone-related effects.

Aprepitant, barbiturates, bosentan, carbamazepine, efavirenz, felbamate, griseofulvin, oxcarbazepine, phenytoin, rifabutin, rifampin, rufinamide, topiramate: May decrease contraceptive effect and increase risk of pregnancy, breakthrough bleeding, or both. An additional form of contraception should be used if drugs are used together and for 28 days after the inducer drug is discontinued.

Atorvastatin, rosuvastatin: May increase ethinyl estradiol level. Monitor patient for hormone-related adverse effects.

Combined hormonal contraceptives: May increase ethinyl estradiol level. Use together for emergency contraception isn't recommended.

Cyclosporine, prednisolone, theophylline, tizanidine: Combined hormonal contraceptive may increase systemic exposure of these drugs. Refer to prescribing information for dosage adjustments for each drug.

Fluconazole, itraconazole, ketoconazole, voriconazole: May increase ethinyl estradiol or progestin level. Monitor patient for hormone-related adverse effects.

HIV/HCV protease inhibitors: May increase or decrease contraceptive effect. Refer to the specific protease inhibitor prescribing information. Backup methods of contraception may be needed.

Lamotrigine: May decrease lamotrigine level, reducing seizure control. Adjust lamotrigine dosage as needed.

Morphine, salicylic acid, temazepam: Combined hormonal contraceptive may increase levels of these drugs. Use together cautiously.

Oil-based miconazole suppository: May increase segesterone and ethinyl estradiol levels and affect long-term vaginal ring performance. Patient should use water-based cream or oral therapy.

Ombitasvir/paritaprevir/ritonavir with or without dasabuvir: May elevate liver enzyme levels. Don't use together. Discontinue vaginal ring before hepatitis C treatment and restart approximately 2 weeks after completion of hepatitis C treatment.

Thyroid hormone replacement therapy/corticosteroid replacement therapy: May decrease thyroid hormone or corticosteroid level. Increase thyroid hormone dosage or cortisol therapy as clinically indicated.

Drug-herb. *St. John's wort:* May reduce drug effectiveness and increase risk of breakthrough bleeding and pregnancy. Discourage use together.

Drug-food. *Ascorbic acid (vitamin C):* May increase ethinyl estradiol level. Use together cautiously.

Grapefruit juice: May increase ethinyl estradiol or progestin level. Monitor patient for hormone-related adverse effects.

Drug-lifestyle. **Black Box Warning** *Smoking:* May increase risk of serious CV adverse effects, especially in patients older than age 35. Don't use drug in patients older than age 35 who smoke. Urge patient to avoid smoking. ■

EFFECTS ON LAB TEST RESULTS

• May alter the results of certain laboratory tests, such as coagulation factors, lipids, and glucose tolerance.

• May increase thyroxine-binding globulin, sex hormone–binding globulin, and cortisol-binding globulin levels.

CONTRAINDICATIONS & CAUTIONS

Black Box Warning Contraindicated in females older than age 35 who smoke. Smoking increases risk of serious CV events when used in combination with hormonal contraceptives. ■

🜉 **Alert:** Patients taking combination hormonal contraceptives may be at increased risk for thrombophlebitis, DVT, PE, MI, cerebral hemorrhage, cerebral thrombosis, HTN, gallbladder disease, hepatic adenomas, benign liver tumors, mesenteric thrombosis, and retinal thrombosis.

• Contraindicated in patients with high risk of arterial or venous thrombotic diseases, including smokers older than age 35; patients who have a current or history of DVT or PE; cerebrovascular disease; CAD; thrombogenic valvular or thrombogenic rhythm diseases of the heart (subacute bacterial endocarditis with valvular disease or atrial fibrillation); inherited or acquired hypercoagulopathies; uncontrolled HTN or HTN with vascular disease.

• Contraindicated in patients with diabetes mellitus who are older than age 35; in patients with diabetes mellitus with HTN or vascular disease or other end-organ damage; and in those with diabetes mellitus of more than 20 years' duration.

• Contraindicated in patients with headaches with focal neurologic symptoms; in patients with migraine headaches with aura; and in those with migraine headaches who are older than age 35.

• Contraindicated in patients with current or history of breast cancer or other estrogen- or progestin-sensitive cancer; in patients with liver tumors, acute hepatitis, or severe (decompensated) cirrhosis; and in patients with undiagnosed abnormal uterine bleeding.

• Contraindicated in patients hypersensitive to the drugs or other components of the vaginal ring.

• Use cautiously in patients with a history of gallbladder disease, depression, HTN, hyperlipidemias, obesity, or diabetes (age younger than 35).

• Use cautiously in patients with personal or family history of hypertriglyceridemia, because of increased risk of pancreatitis.

• Use cautiously in patients with hereditary angioedema; symptoms may be induced or exacerbated.

• Safety and effectiveness in women with a BMI greater than 29 kg/m² haven't been established; however, higher body weight is associated with lower systemic exposure.

Reactions in bold italics are *life-threatening*. Interactions may have a *rapid onset* or a **delayed onset**.

• Use before menarche and post menopause isn't indicated.
Dialyzable drug: No.
⚠ ***Overdose S&S:*** Vaginal bleeding, nausea.

PREGNANCY-LACTATION-REPRODUCTION
• Not indicated for use in pregnancy; discontinue use if pregnancy is confirmed.
• Rule out pregnancy if patient hasn't adhered to the prescribed regimen and a period is missed, or if prescribed regimen has been adhered to and two periods are missed.
• There is little or no increased risk of birth defects in women who accidently use combined hormonal contraceptives during early pregnancy.
• Drug may appear in breast milk and may decrease milk production. Advise breastfeeding patients to use another method of contraception until breastfeeding is discontinued.
• Resumption of fertility after drug discontinuation is expected by 6 months after discontinuation.

NURSING CONSIDERATIONS
• In patient who didn't use hormonal contraception in the preceding month or after copper IUD removal, initiate therapy between days 2 and 5 of her regular menstrual bleeding; no backup contraception needed. If menstrual cycles are irregular or if initial use is more than 5 days from the last menstrual bleeding, patient should use an additional barrier method for the first 7 days of use.
• A patient who has been using her combined hormonal contraceptive method consistently and correctly and who isn't already pregnant may switch on any day, but no more than 7 hormone-free days should occur before starting drug.
• Switching from a progestin-only method should begin on the next scheduled timing of either oral pill or injection. If switching from a progestin-only implant, begin at the time of implant removal. Patient should use an additional barrier method for 7 days after starting drug.
• After childbirth, don't start drug sooner than 4 weeks postpartum in patients who choose not to breastfeed. If initiated 4 weeks or more postpartum, patient should use an additional method of contraception for the first 7 days of use.
• May start drug within the first 5 days after a complete first trimester abortion or miscarriage without additional backup contraception. If more than 5 days have elapsed, patient should use an additional barrier method for the first 7 days of use.
🚫 ***Alert:*** Don't initiate therapy sooner than 4 weeks postpartum or sooner than 4 weeks after a second trimester abortion or miscarriage, because of the increased risk of thromboembolism.
• Withdrawal bleeding usually occurs during the 1-week dose-free interval. If bleeding doesn't occur between cycles, consider the possibility of pregnancy.
• Assess for breakthrough bleeding and spotting that persist or occur after previously regular cycles

on drug. Assess for pregnancy or malignancy if bleeding irregularities occur. Amenorrhea may occur with vaginal ring use.
• Effectiveness may be reduced if drug isn't used as directed. May adjust change day for vaginal ring if there are deviations from the recommended use.
• If vaginal ring is out of the vagina for more than 2 continuous or cumulative hours during the 21-day insertion period, patient should use backup barrier contraception until the system has been in the vagina for 7 consecutive days.
• If vaginal ring "free-interval" is longer than recommended, patient should use barrier contraception until the system has been in place for 7 consecutive days.
• If vaginal ring has been in place for more than 21 days, the system should be removed for 7 days then reinserted to resume prescribed schedule.
• Assess patient for medical history or family history of thrombotic or thromboembolic disorders that may suggest inherited or acquired hypercoagulopathy.
• Monitor patient for arterial or DVT events. Stop drug and notify prescriber if an event occurs.
• Increased risk of thromboembolism is greatest after initially starting a combined hormonal contraceptive or restarting (after a 4-week or greater dose-free interval) the same or a different combined hormonal contraceptive.
• Monitor BP; stop drug if BP rises significantly.
• Stop drug at least 4 weeks before and for 2 weeks after procedures that may increase risk of thromboembolism, and during and after prolonged immobilization.
• Monitor patient for unexplained changes in the eye or vision (vision loss, proptosis, diplopia, papilledema, retinal vascular lesions). Immediately evaluate patient for retinal vein thrombosis if changes occur.
• Carefully monitor glucose levels in prediabetic and diabetic patients.
• Monitor patient for new-onset headaches that are recurrent, persistent, or severe; evaluate the cause and discontinue use if indicated.
• Observe patients with a history of depression and discontinue drug if depression recurs to a serious degree.
• Monitor thyroid hormone or cortisol therapy; replacement dosages may need to be increased.
• Monitor patient for signs and symptoms of toxic shock syndrome (TSS) (sudden high fever, vomiting, diarrhea, fainting, light-headedness, sunburnlike rash, muscle aches, dizziness). If TSS occurs, remove vaginal ring and initiate appropriate treatment.
• Monitor patient for jaundice and other signs and symptoms of liver disease. Discontinue drug until LFTs return to normal and drug has been excluded as the cause of disease.

NEW DRUGS

PATIENT TEACHING

Black Box Warning Advise patient older than age 35 and who smokes not to use this contraceptive. ■

• Advise all patients taking drug not to smoke.

• Caution patient that vaginal ring doesn't protect against HIV and other sexually transmitted infections.

• Inform patient the ring is compatible with male condoms made with natural rubber latex, polyisoprene, and polyurethane. Use of water-based lubricant is appropriate.

• Teach patient not to use oil-based and silicone-based vaginal lubricants, as they may alter the vaginal ring or increase exposure to ethinyl estradiol. Advise patient to use water-based lubricants instead.

• Advise patient of the increased risk of venous thromboembolism while using vaginal ring. Instruct patient to seek immediate medical attention for persistent leg pain, sudden shortness of breath, vision changes, chest pain or pressure, sudden severe headache, arm or leg weakness or numbness, or trouble speaking.

• Educate patient to remove vaginal ring if pregnancy is confirmed during treatment, as there is no indication for use during pregnancy.

• Caution patient that if scheduled bleeding doesn't occur between cycles, to consider the possibility of pregnancy, especially if patient is experiencing symptoms such as morning sickness or unusual breast tenderness.

• Tell patient to avoid oil-based and silicone-based vaginal products.

• Warn patient to use backup contraception if vaginal ring has been out for more than 2 hours cumulative during 21 days of continuous use or if vaginal ring–free interval exceeds 7 days.

• Instruct patient to replace ring as soon as possible if it's accidentally expelled (such as during sex or when removing a tampon or straining during a bowel movement).

• Inform patient that vaginal ring may be felt during coitus.

• Advise patient that resumption of fertility after drug discontinuation is expected by 6 months after discontinuation.

• Caution patient who tends to develop chloasma to avoid exposure to the sun or UV radiation, and to use sunscreen.

• Instruct patient in proper insertion, removal, and care of vaginal ring.

• Warn patient not to flush ring down the toilet and to discard either at a drug take-back option or in a waste receptacle out of reach of children and pets.

tafamidis ⚕
ta-FAM-id-is

Vyndamax

tafamidis meglumine ⚕
Vyndaqel

Therapeutic class: Endocrine-metabolic agents
Pharmacologic class: Transthyretin stabilizers

AVAILABLE FORMS
tafamidis
Capsules ⒪: 61 mg
tafamidis meglumine
Capsules ⒪: 20 mg

INDICATIONS & DOSAGES
➤ **Treatment of the cardiomyopathy of wild type or hereditary transthyretin-mediated amyloidosis (ATTR-CM) to reduce CV mortality and CV-related hospitalization** ⚕
Adults: 80 mg tafamidis meglumine (four 20-mg capsules) PO once daily, or 61 mg tafamidis PO once daily.

ADMINISTRATION
PO
• May give without regard for food.
• Patient should swallow capsules whole and not crush or cut them.
• Give a missed dose as soon as possible or omit the missed dose and give at the next regularly schedule time. Don't double the dose.
• Store at 68° to 77° F (20° to 25° C).

ACTION
Binds to the *TTR* gene at thyroxine binding sites to stabilize and slow dissociation of tetramers into monomers, the rate-limiting step in the amyloidogenic process.

Route	Onset	Peak	Duration
PO	Unknown	4 hr	Unknown

Half-life: About 49 hours.

ADVERSE REACTIONS
None reported.

INTERACTIONS
Drug-drug. *BCRP substrates (imatinib, methotrexate, rosuvastatin):* May increase levels of BCRP substrates. Dosage adjustment of the substrates may be needed.

EFFECTS ON LAB TEST RESULTS
• May decrease total thyroxine level.

Reactions in bold italics are *life-threatening*. Interactions may have a *rapid onset* or a **delayed onset**.

CONTRAINDICATIONS & CAUTIONS

• Use in patients with severe hepatic impairment hasn't been studied.
• Safety and effectiveness in children haven't been established.
Dialyzable drug: Unknown.
⚠ *Overdose S&S:* Hordeolum.

PREGNANCY-LACTATION-REPRODUCTION

• Drug may cause fetal harm based on adverse events observed in animal reproduction studies.
• It isn't known if drug appears in human milk. Due to the risk of serious adverse reactions in a breastfed infant, patient shouldn't breastfeed during therapy.
• Women of childbearing potential should consider pregnancy planning and prevention.

NURSING CONSIDERATIONS

❸ *Alert:* Vyndamax and Vyndaqel aren't substitutable on a per mg basis.
• *Look alike–sound alike:* Don't confuse Vyndamax with Vyndaqel.

PATIENT TEACHING

• Tell patient about the Transthyretin Amyloidosis Outcome Survey registry, an international disease registry to assess disease progression, genotype/phenotype relationships, and the impact of interventions such as this drug on disease progression. Advise patient that participation is voluntary and that more information is available at www.thaos.net.
• Caution female patient who is pregnant or plans to become pregnant of the potential risk to a fetus. Advise her to consider family planning and contraception during therapy.
• Warn female patient not to breastfeed during treatment.

SAFETY ALERT!

trastuzumab–hyaluronidase-oysk ▧
tras-TOOZ-ue-mab/hye-al-ur-ON-i-dase

Herceptin Hylecta

Therapeutic class: Antineoplastics
Pharmacologic class: Monoclonal antibodies–endoglycosidases

AVAILABLE FORMS

Injection: 600 mg trastuzumab and 10,000 units hyaluronidase/5 mL in single-dose vial

INDICATIONS & DOSAGES

Adjust-a-dose (for all indications): Withhold drug for at least 4 weeks if there is a 16% or more absolute decrease in LVEF from pretreatment values or if LVEF is below institutional limits of normal and there is a 10% or more absolute decrease in LVEF from pretreatment values. May resume therapy within 4 to 8 weeks if LVEF returns to normal limits and the absolute decrease in LVEF from baseline is 15% or less. Permanently discontinue therapy for a persistent (more than 8 weeks) LVEF decline or for suspension of therapy on more than three occasions for cardiomyopathy.

➤ **Adjuvant treatment of HER2 overexpressing node-positive or node-negative (ER/PR-negative or with one high risk feature) breast cancer as part of a treatment regimen consisting of doxorubicin, cyclophosphamide, and either paclitaxel or docetaxel; as part of a treatment regimen with docetaxel and carboplatin; or as a single agent after multimodality anthracycline-based therapy** ▧
Adults: 600 mg trastuzumab/10,000 units hyaluronidase subcut once every 3 weeks for 52 weeks or until disease recurrence. Extending treatment in adjuvant breast cancer beyond 1 year isn't recommended.

➤ **First-line treatment of HER2-overexpressing metastatic breast cancer in combination with paclitaxel or as a single agent for treatment of HER2-overexpressing breast cancer in patients who have received one or more chemotherapy regimens for metastatic disease** ▧
Adults: 600 mg trastuzumab/10,000 units hyaluronidase subcut once every 3 weeks until disease progression.

ADMINISTRATION

Subcutaneous

• Hazardous drug; use safe handling and disposal precautions.
• Don't administer intravenously.
• Drug isn't interchangeable with conventional trastuzumab products or ado-trastuzumab.
• Drug should be administered by a health care professional.
• Inspect visually for particulate matter and discoloration before administration; don't use vial if abnormalities are present.
• Discard any unused portion remaining in the vial; vial is for single use only.
• To avoid needle clogging, attach the hypodermic injection needle to the syringe immediately before administration. Drug is compatible with syringes made with polypropylene and polycarbonate and with stainless steel transfer and injection needles.
• Withdraw solution from the vial and into the syringe, replace the transfer needle with a syringe closing cap. Label the syringe with the peel-off sticker.
• Alternate injection site between left and right thigh.
• Give new injections at least 1 inch (2.5 cm) from the old previous site on healthy skin and never into areas where the skin is red, bruised, tender, or hard, or where there are moles or scars.
• Administer dose subcut over approximately 2 to 5 minutes.

NEW DRUGS

• Can store the prepared syringe in the refrigerator at 36° to 46° F (2° to 8° C) for up to 24 hours and subsequently at 68° to 77° F (20° to 25° C) for up to 4 hours. Protect from light. Don't shake or freeze.
• If one dose is missed, give the next dose as soon as possible. The interval between doses shouldn't be less than 3 weeks.

ACTION
Trastuzumab is a HER2/neu receptor antagonist that inhibits the proliferation of human tumor cells that overexpress HER2. Hyaluronidase is an enzyme shown to increase the absorption rate of a trastuzumab product into the systemic circulation.

Route	Onset	Peak	Duration
Subcut (trastuzumab)	Unknown	3 days	Unknown
Subcut (hyaluronidase)	Unknown	Unknown	24–48 hr

Half-life: trastuzumab, unknown; hyaluronidase, ½ day.

ADVERSE REACTIONS
CNS: asthenia, fatigue, headache, pyrexia, chills, dizziness, insomnia, peripheral sensory neuropathy, paresthesia, pain, depression. **CV:** HTN, left ventricular dysfunction, HF, flushing, arrhythmia, tachycardia, edema. **EENT:** epistaxis, nasal inflammation/discomfort, sinusitis. **GI:** nausea, diarrhea, dysgeusia, vomiting, stomatitis, constipation, mucosal inflammation, abdominal pain, dyspepsia, decreased appetite. **GU:** UTI, irregular menstruation, amenorrhea. **Hematologic:** *neutropenia,* anemia, *leukopenia, granulocytopenia, febrile neutropenia.* **Hepatic:** abnormal LFT values. **Musculoskeletal:** myalgia, arthralgia, back pain, extremity pain, bone pain. **Respiratory:** cough, dyspnea, URI, bronchitis. **Skin:** alopecia, rash, radiation skin injury, incision-site pain and complications, cellulitis, nail disorder, pruritus, skin discoloration, herpes simplex, acne. injection-site reactions, pain, or erythema. **Other:** *hypersensitivity reactions,* viral infection, infection, flulike syndrome.

INTERACTIONS
Drug-drug. ▓Black Box Warning▓ *Anthracyclines (daunorubicin, doxorubicin):* May increase risk of cardiac dysfunction. Avoid anthracycline-based therapy for up to 7 months after stopping trastuzumab–hyaluronidase. If used together, carefully monitor patient's cardiac function. ■

EFFECTS ON LAB TEST RESULTS
• May increase ALT level.
• May decrease WBC and RBC counts.

CONTRAINDICATIONS & CAUTIONS
▓Black Box Warning▓ Drug can cause left ventricular cardiac dysfunction, arrhythmias, HTN, disabling cardiac failure, cardiomyopathy, and death. ■

▓Black Box Warning▓ Can cause serious and fatal pulmonary toxicity, including dyspnea, interstitial pneumonitis, pulmonary infiltrates, pleural effusions, noncardiogenic pulmonary edema, pulmonary insufficiency and hypoxia, ARDS, and pulmonary fibrosis. Patients with symptomatic intrinsic lung disease or with extensive tumor involvement of the lungs, resulting in dyspnea at rest, appear to have more severe toxicity. ■
• May exacerbate chemotherapy-induced neutropenia.
• Severe administration-related reactions, including hypersensitivity and anaphylaxis, have been reported. Patients experiencing dyspnea at rest due to complications of advanced malignancy and comorbidities may be at increased risk for a severe or fatal administration-related reaction.
• Safety and effectiveness in children haven't been studied.
• Patients age 65 and older are at increased risk for cardiac dysfunction.
Dialyzable drug: Unknown.

PREGNANCY-LACTATION-REPRODUCTION
▓Black Box Warning▓ Drug can cause fetal harm (oligohydramnios and pulmonary hypoplasia, skeletal abnormalities) and fetal death. Verify pregnancy status of women of childbearing potential before initiation of therapy. Pregnant women and women of childbearing potential should be made aware that exposure to these drugs during pregnancy or within 7 months before conception can result in fetal harm. ■
▓Black Box Warning▓ Women of childbearing potential should use effective contraception during treatment and for 7 months after the final dose. ■
• There is no information regarding the presence of trastuzumab or hyaluronidase in human milk, the effects on the breastfed infant, or the effects on milk production.
• If drug is administered during pregnancy, or if patient becomes pregnant while receiving therapy or within 7 months after the final dose, health care providers and patients should immediately report exposure to Genentech pregnancy pharmacovigilance program (1-888-835-2555).

NURSING CONSIDERATIONS
▓Black Box Warning▓ Obtain pregnancy test for women of childbearing potential before starting therapy. ■
▓Black Box Warning▓ Monitor patients for systemic hypersensitivity reactions, especially during the first dose. Permanently discontinue drug in patients who experience anaphylaxis or severe hypersensitivity reactions. Medications and emergency equipment should be immediately available. ■
▓Black Box Warning▓ Monitor patients for pulmonary toxicity, which usually occurs during or within 24 hours of administration. Discontinue drug for anaphylaxis, angioedema, interstitial

NEW DRUGS

pneumonitis, or ARDS and monitor patient until symptoms completely resolve. ▮

• Obtain thorough baseline cardiac assessment, including history, physical examination, and determination of LVEF by echocardiogram or MUGA scan. Obtain baseline LVEF measurement immediately before initiation of therapy, then every 3 months during and upon completion of therapy. Repeat LVEF measurement at 4-week intervals if therapy is withheld for significant left ventricular cardiac dysfunction. Obtain LVEF measurements every 6 months for at least 2 years after completion of therapy as a component of adjuvant therapy.

• *Look alike–sound alike:* Don't confuse trastuzumab–hyaluronidase-oysk with ado-trastuzumab emtansine or intravenous trastuzumab.

PATIENT TEACHING

▪Black Box Warning▪ Advise patient to immediately report signs and symptoms of cardiotoxicity, including new-onset or worsening shortness of breath, cough, swelling of the ankles or legs, swelling of the face, palpitations, weight gain of more than 5 pounds in 24 hours, dizziness, or loss of consciousness. ▮

▪Black Box Warning▪ Warn female patient who is pregnant and female patient of childbearing potential of risk to the fetus from exposure to drug during pregnancy or within 7 months before conception. Teach her that pregnancy testing will be needed before therapy begins and to immediately contact prescriber with a known or suspected pregnancy. ▮

▪Black Box Warning▪ Caution female patient of childbearing potential to use effective contraception during treatment and for 7 months after the final dose. ▮

• Advise patient to immediately report signs and symptoms of hypersensitivity and administration-related reactions, including dizziness, nausea, chills, fever, vomiting, diarrhea, urticaria, angioedema, breathing problems, or chest pain.

Appendices

Avoiding common drug errors:
Best practices and prevention

In addition to following your institution's administration policies, you can help prevent errors in drug administration by reviewing these common errors and ways to prevent them. The Joint Commission, the Institute for Safe Medication Practices (ISMP), and the FDA also maintain resources to help improve drug safety.

Topic	Error	Best practices and prevention
Drug orders		
Pharmacy computer system	The system may not detect all unsafe orders.	• Don't rely on the pharmacy computer system to detect all unsafe orders. • Before giving a drug, understand the correct indication, dosage, route, and potential adverse effects. • Consult the pharmacist if there is any question, and verify the information using an approved current drug reference.
Confusing drug names	Many drugs have names that look alike–sound alike and may easily be mistaken one for the other.	• Perform a medication reconciliation upon admission, at each transition of care, and when the practitioner prescribes a new medication. Question any deviations from patient's routine. • Take your time and read the label carefully. • Consult the ISMP "List of Confused Drug Names" (https://www.ismp.org/recommendations/confused-drug-names-list). • Be aware of tall man lettering, which helps differentiate similar drug names.
Abbreviations	Using dangerous abbreviations can result in giving the wrong drug or wrong dose, by the wrong route, or at the wrong time.	• Don't abbreviate drug names. • Be aware of The Joint Commission's official "Do Not Use" list of drug abbreviations to avoid (see *Appendix 4: Abbreviations to avoid [The Joint Commission]*, page 1710). • Consult your facility's list of approved abbreviations and the ISMP's "List of Error-Prone Abbreviations, Symbols, and Dose Designations" (www.ismp.org/recommendations/error-prone-abbreviations-list)
Unclear order	A drug order with incomplete or unclear information can result in giving the wrong drug or wrong dose, by the wrong route, or at the wrong time.	• Ensure that each order specifies the correct drug name, concentration, dosage, route, and frequency of administration. • Clarify all incomplete or unclear orders with the prescriber. Utilize read-back and verify when taking phone and verbal orders.
Inadvertent overdose	A prescriber may write an order for a combination drug such as acetaminophen–opioid analgesic tablets without realizing the total acetaminophen dose could be toxic (don't exceed 4 g daily).	• Note the amount of acetaminophen in each combined formulation. • Warn patients not to take additional drugs that contain acetaminophen. • Verify any "as needed" pain or fever medication orders to check if they contain acetaminophen. Monitor patient's use of "as needed" drugs as prescribed.

Topic	Error	Best practices and prevention
Anticoagulants	Lack of standardization for drug naming, labeling, and packaging can create confusion. Dosing regimens, assay methods, narrow therapeutic ranges, complex drug interactions, and drug monitoring methods create high potential for complications.	• Keep current with your facility's anticoagulant therapy protocol, the different dosing regimens, assay methods and their standardized range of normal values, drug interactions, monitoring methods, and reversal regimens for each anticoagulant given. • Don't confuse direct oral anticoagulants with one another because the drug names are similar, such as confusing rivaroxaban with edoxaban. • Use only unit-dose products if available. • Be especially aware of the correct doses and indications for neonates and children. • Teach patients to manage their therapy appropriately.

Drug preparation

Topic	Error	Best practices and prevention
Crushing drugs for oral or enteral administration	Crushing certain oral or enteral drugs may: • alter the drug's effects, causing overdose or other adverse reactions • result in skin irritation or other adverse reactions for the preparer • produce teratogenic effects in pregnant women (through exposure) • be hazardous if not done in an appropriate environment (e.g., chemotherapy and other hazardous drugs).	• Use a liquid formulation instead of crushing a drug whenever possible. • Before crushing a drug, always check with the pharmacist and established references, such as the ISMP's list of "Oral Dosage Forms That Should Not Be Crushed" (https://www.ismp.org/recommendations/do-not-crush).
Solution color change or particulate matter	Unusual appearance may indicate that: • the drug has been improperly stored or manufactured • the drug has expired • the wrong drug has been provided by the pharmacy • the wrong liquid was chosen out of patient's medication supply.	• Closely examine all solutions before giving them, and know what their appearance should be. • If you note a color change, contact the pharmacist who dispensed the solution and report it. • Don't give a drug until verifying that the drug has been correctly labeled and that it is safe to give. • Verify that you have chosen the correct solution from patient's supply if patient is on more than one liquid drug.
Incorrect drug storage	Incorrect storage may change a drug's physical properties or result in its being inadvertently administered.	• Follow your facility's policy for storing drugs. • Always store drugs in the appropriate container, in the appropriate place, at the appropriate temperature, for the appropriate duration.
Incomplete or incorrect drug labels	Incorrect or incomplete labeling can result in giving the wrong drug, formulation, or dose.	• Never give a drug whose label is incomplete or incorrect. Notify the pharmacy immediately and obtain the correctly labeled drug. • Properly label and verify all medications, medication containers, and other solutions on and off the sterile field.

(continued)

Topic	Error	Best practices and prevention
Drug administration		
Using a parenteral syringe for oral or enteral drugs	Using a parenteral syringe with a luer-lock to prepare small amounts of oral or enteral drugs can result in misadministration because the drug could be accidentally injected into an IV line.	• Always use special oral syringes to give oral or enteral drugs. Their hubs won't support a needle and they don't have a luer-lock, so they can't be attached to IV lines. • Always properly label syringes (if they aren't thrown away immediately).
Infusion pump safety problems	Problems with infusion pumps (used to deliver controlled fluids, drugs, and nutrients) can cause fluid overload or administration of inaccurate doses.	• Make sure you know how to safely operate an infusion pump. Consult your facility's policy on proper usage. • Before beginning an infusion, always verify that the pump is working properly. Make sure all alarms are functional and never bypass them. • Double-check all dosing to include the infusion rate. • Always double-check that the correct medication bag is hanging in the pump.
Calculation errors	Dosage calculation errors can cause significant patient harm, especially with "high alert" medications, and in neonates and children.	• Be aware of medications that are considered high alert. • Write out the mg/kg or mg/m^2 dose and the calculated dose as a safeguard. • Whenever a prescriber provides a calculation, double-check it and document that the dose was verified in the medical record. • Use only approved abbreviations, and be aware of the placement of decimal points.
OTC products/ supplements (herbal supplements and vitamins)	Because OTC products, herbal supplements, and vitamins aren't subject to the same quality assurance standards as drugs, their labels may be misrepresented and their effects and interactions with drugs may not be well studied.	• Always assess and document all OTC drugs, herbal supplements, and vitamins patient is taking in patient's medical record. • Monitor patient carefully, and report unusual adverse reactions. • Consult an evidence-based drug reference for known drug-herb interactions. • Use extra care when combining herbal supplements with anticoagulants because bleeding times may increase.

Pregnancy risk categories: The FDA's Final Rule

In December 2014, the FDA published the *Content and Format of Labeling for Human Prescription Drug and Biological Products; Requirements for Pregnancy and Lactation Labeling*, referred to as the "Pregnancy and Lactation Labeling Rule," a final rule that set new standards for how information about using medications during pregnancy and breastfeeding is presented in the labels of biological products and prescription drugs. These new standards went into effect June 30, 2015, for all newly approved drug and biological products; the new labeling requirements are being phased in gradually for previously approved products.

The final rule recognizes that decisions for medication use during pregnancy and breastfeeding involve complex risk-benefit considerations and must be individualized because many pregnant and breastfeeding patients need medications to manage acute and chronic conditions. According to the final rule, the letter category system was often misinterpreted as a grading system and provided oversimplified information about a drug's risk. Consequently, the current pregnancy risk categories (A, B, C, D, X) were replaced with three labeled subsections titled "Pregnancy," "Lactation," and "Females and Males of Reproductive Potential." These subsections provide more consistent, relevant explanations and information about a drug's risks and benefits in the real-world context of caring for patients. Pregnant and breastfeeding women should always consult their health care professionals before taking any prescription or OTC medication or supplements.

Controlled substance schedules

Drugs regulated under the jurisdiction of the Controlled Substances Act of 1970 are divided into the following groups or schedules:

- Schedule I: High abuse potential, lack of accepted safety, and no accepted medical use. Examples include heroin and LSD.
- Schedule II/IIN: High abuse potential with severe dependence liability. Has an accepted medical use for treatment in the United States. Examples include opioids, amphetamines, and some barbiturates.
- Schedule III/IIIN: Less abuse potential than Schedule I or II drugs; abuse may cause moderate to low physical dependence or high psychological dependence. Has an accepted medical use for treatment in the United States. Examples include nonbarbiturate sedatives, nonamphetamine stimulants, anabolic steroids, and limited amounts of certain opioids.
- Schedule IV: Less abuse potential than Schedule III drugs and limited dependence liability. Has an accepted medical use for treatment in the United States. Examples include some sedatives, anxiolytics, and nonopioid analgesics.
- Schedule V: Less abuse potential with limited physical or psychological dependence compared to Schedule IV drugs. Has an accepted medical use for treatment in the United States. This category mainly includes small amounts of opioids, such as codeine, used in antitussives or antidiarrheals. Under federal law, limited quantities of certain Schedule V drugs may be purchased without a prescription directly from a pharmacist if allowed under specific state statutes. Legal purchasing age is generally age 18 with valid identification. All such transactions and relevant personal information must be recorded by the dispensing pharmacist.

Abbreviations to avoid (The Joint Commission)

The Joint Commission requires every health care facility to develop a list of approved abbreviations for staff use. Certain abbreviations should be avoided because they're easily misunderstood, especially when handwritten. The Joint Commission has identified a minimum list of dangerous abbreviations, acronyms, and symbols. This do-not-use list includes the following items.

Official "Do Not Use" List[1]		
Do not use	**Potential problem**	**Use instead**
U, u (unit)	Mistaken for "0" (zero), the number "4" (four), or "cc"	Write "unit"
IU (International Unit)	Mistaken for "IV" (intravenous) or the number "10" (ten)	Write "International Unit"
Q.D., QD, q.d., qd (daily)	Mistaken for each other	Write "daily"
Q.O.D., QOD, q.o.d, qod (every other day)	Period after the Q mistaken for "I" and the "O" mistaken for "I"	Write "every other day"
Trailing zero (X.0 mg)* Lack of leading zero (.X mg)	Decimal point is missed	Write "X mg" Write "0.X mg"
MS	Can mean morphine sulfate or magnesium sulfate	Write "morphine sulfate"
MSO_4 and $MgSO_4$	Confused for one another	Write "magnesium sulfate"

[1]Applies to all orders and all medication-related documentation that is handwritten (including free-text computer entry) or on preprinted forms.

*Exception: A "trailing zero" may be used only where required to demonstrate the level of precision of the value being reported, such as for laboratory results, imaging studies that report size of lesions, or catheter/tube size. It may not be used in medication orders or other medication-related documentation.

Pediatric drugs commonly involved in drug errors

According to The Joint Commission, the rate of medication errors for pediatric and adult inpatients is similar, but potentially harmful errors occur almost three times as frequently in children. One of the most common errors that occur in hospitalized children is administering the incorrect pediatric dosage. Here are some of the medications most commonly involved in medication errors as reported to the national voluntary medication error reporting system, MEDMARX, with their FDA-approved dosages.

Medication	Indication	Route	Usual dosage
albuterol sulfate	Bronchospasm in children with reversible obstructive airway disease	PO (immediate-release tablets and extended-release tablets)	• *Children older than age 12:* Initially, 2 or 4 mg (immediate-release tablets) PO t.i.d. or q.i.d. If patient fails to respond, may increase dosage to maximum of 8 mg PO q.i.d. Or, 8 mg (extended-release tablets) PO every 12 hours. If patient fails to respond, increase dosage cautiously to maximum of 16 mg PO every 12 hours. • *Children ages 6 to 12:* Initially, 2 mg (immediate-release tablets) PO t.i.d. or q.i.d. May increase dosage cautiously, but total daily dosage shouldn't exceed 24 mg/day (given in divided doses). Or, 4 mg (extended-release tablets) PO every 12 hours. If control of reversible airway spasm isn't achieved with optimized asthma therapy, may cautiously increase dosage to maximum of 12 mg PO every 12 hours.
	Bronchospasm in children with reversible obstructive airway disease	PO (syrup)	• *Children older than age 14:* Initially, 2 mg (1 tsp) or 4 mg (2 tsp) PO t.i.d. or q.i.d. If patient fails to respond, dosage may be cautiously increased to maximum of 8 mg PO q.i.d. • *Children ages 6 to 14:* Initially, 2 mg (1 tsp) PO t.i.d. or q.i.d. If patient fails to respond, dosage may be increased to maximum of 24 mg/day given in divided doses. • *Children ages 2 to younger than 6:* Initially, 0.1 mg/kg PO t.i.d. Initial dose shouldn't exceed 2 mg (1 teaspoonful) PO t.i.d. If patient fails to respond, may increase dosage to 0.2 mg/kg PO t.i.d. Maximum dosage is 4 mg (2 tsp) PO t.i.d.
cefTRIAXone sodium	Acute bacterial otitis media in children younger than age 12	IM	• *Children:* Give single dose of 50 mg/kg IM. Maximum dosage is 1 g.
	Serious infections (including skin and skin-structure infections) other than meningitis	IV infusion over at least 30 minutes or IM	• *Children:* 50 to 75 mg/kg IM or IV once daily or in divided doses every 12 hours. Continue for at least 2 days after signs and symptoms of infection have disappeared. Usual duration of therapy is 4 to 14 days. Maximum dosage is 2 g/day.
	Meningitis	IV infusion over at least 30 minutes or IM	• *Children:* Initially, 100 mg/kg (not to exceed 4 g) IM or IV. Thereafter, give total daily dose of 100 mg/kg/day IM or IV for 7 to 14 days. Maximum dosage is 4 g daily. Daily dose may be administered once a day or in equally divided doses every 12 hours.

(continued)

Medication	Indication	Route	Usual dosage
fentaNYL	To manage persistent, chronic pain only in opioid-tolerant patients (children receiving, for 1 week or longer, at least 60 mg/day of morphine PO or an equianalgesic dose of another opioid)	Transdermal	• *Children age 2 and older:* When converting to transdermal system, base first dose on the daily dose, potency, and characteristics of the current opioid therapy; reliability of the relative potency estimates used to calculate the needed dose; degree of opioid tolerance; and patient's condition. It's preferable to underestimate patient's 24-hour fentanyl requirements and provide rescue medication than to overestimate the 24-hour fentanyl requirements, which could result in adverse reactions. Each patch is worn for 72 hours; dosage may be increased 3 days after first dose and then no sooner than every 6 days thereafter.
gentamicin sulfate	Serious infections caused by sensitive strains of *Pseudomonas aeruginosa, Escherichia coli, Proteus, Klebsiella, Serratia,* or *Staphylococcus*	IV infusion over 30 minutes to 2 hours or IM	• *Children:* 2 to 2.5 mg/kg IV or IM every 8 hours, usually for 7 to 10 days. • *Infants and neonates:* 2.5 mg/kg IV or IM every 8 hours, usually for 7 to 10 days. • *Premature or full-term neonates age 1 week or younger:* 2.5 mg/kg IV or IM every 12 hours, usually for 7 to 10 days.
heparin sodium (unfractionated)	Thrombosis	IV	• According to prescribing information, there are no adequate and well-controlled studies on heparin use in children. In general, the following dosage schedule may be used as a guideline: *Children:* Initially, 75 to 100 units/kg IV bolus over 10 minutes, followed by continuous IV infusion of 25 to 30 units/kg/hour (infants) or 18 to 20 units/kg/hour (children older than age 1). Adjust dosage to maintain aPTT of 60 to 85 seconds, assuming this reflects an anti-factor Xa level of 0.35 to 0.70. Refer to current clinical practice guidelines for additional information.
vancomycin	Treatment of serious or severe infections caused by susceptible strains of methicillin-resistant (beta-lactam-resistant) staphylococci	IV	• *Neonates:* Initially, 15 mg/kg IV, followed by 10 mg/kg IV every 12 hours for neonates in the first week of life and every 8 hours thereafter up to the age of 1 month. Administer over 60 minutes. In premature infants, longer dosing intervals may be necessary. • *Children age 1 month and older:* 10 mg/kg/dose IV every 6 hours. Administer over at least 60 minutes. Individualize dosage and frequency based on serum concentrations.
	Pseudomembranous colitis or staphylococcal enterocolitis	PO	• *Children:* 40 mg/kg/day PO in three or four divided doses for 7 to 10 days. Maximum dosage is 2 g/day.

Elder care medication tips

Age-related changes can alter the way older people absorb, distribute, metabolize, and eliminate medications compared to younger adults or children. Medication dosages and routes may need adjustment to optimize the patient's response to medication and help prevent adverse reactions. Understanding how age-related factors can alter how an older patient's body uses medication will help you plan and implement your patient's medication regimen and monitor the patient's response appropriately. The table below describes how age-related factors can change the pharmacokinetics of medications in older adults.

Pharmacokinetics	Age-related change	Effect on pharmacokinetics
Absorption	Diminished quality and quantity of digestive enzymes	↓
	Increased gastric pH	↑ or ↓
	Decreased GI motility and emptying time	↓
	Decreased GI blood flow	↓
	Diminished number of absorbing cells	↓
Distribution	Diminished cardiac output and reserve	↓
	Diminished blood flow to target organs and tissues	↓
	Decreased lean body mass	↓
	Increased adipose tissue	↑ or ↓
	Decreased circulating plasma proteins	↓
	Decreased total body water	↓
Metabolism	Decreased liver size	↓
	Diminished intestinal and portal vein blood flow	↓
Excretion	Decreased GFR	↓
	Decreased renal tubular secretion	↓
	Decreased renal blood flow from renovascular occlusive disease, microvascular nephropathy, or HF	↓

Prescription drug abuse:
Identifying and treating toxicity

Prescription drugs have CNS effects that can be used or altered in order to achieve stimulant, euphoric, or mind-altering effects. Commonly used preparations (e.g., tablets and capsules) can be crushed, inhaled, or injected to produce quicker results. The table below lists commonly abused prescription drugs with examples of brand names, along with signs and symptoms of toxicity, potential adverse health effects, and treatment/reversal care. Not all drugs have reversal agents that can be used to rapidly counteract adverse effects. General supportive care measures (respiratory and cardiac function support and IV fluids) are needed to improve clinical outcomes when prescription drugs are abused.

Substance	Toxicity signs & symptoms	Possible health effects	Toxicity care and treatment
Anesthetics			
cocaine • Medical uses: topical (ENT) anesthesia • Generic/brand names: cocaine • Routes: inhalation (nasal/oral), injection	↑HR, ↑BP, arrhythmias, chest pain, nosebleeds, vomiting, ↓appetite, dilated pupils, euphoria, insomnia, restlessness, anxiety, erratic behavior, paranoia, seizures	MI, stroke, cardiomyopathy, coma, ↑HIV risk from shared needles, ↓birth weight/premature delivery (if used during pregnancy), psychosis, hyperthermia, rhabdomyolysis	General supportive care; seizure control with IV benzodiazepines (e.g., diazepam, lorazepam). Dialysis and hemoperfusion are ineffective.
propofol • Medical uses: general anesthesia/sedation • Generic/brand names: propofol (Diprivan) • Routes: injection	Hyperthermia, ↓HR, ↓BP, ↑LFTs, nausea, vomiting, itching, wheezing, hypoxia, ↓consciousness, stupor, anxiety, confusion, delirium, seizures	MI, HF, metabolic acidosis, pancreatitis, liver damage, renal failure, respiratory depression, ↑HIV risk from shared needles	General supportive care; seizure control with IV benzodiazepines (e.g., diazepam, lorazepam). May consider hemofiltration for metabolic acidosis. Monitor urine output (urine may be rusty, tea-colored, or green/olive). Mechanical ventilation may be required.
ketamine • Medical uses: anesthesia, analgesia, sedation • Generic/brand names: ketamine (Ketalar) • Routes: injection, inhalation (nasal/oral)	↑HR, ↑BP, ↓respiratory rate, dysuria, diplopia, nystagmus, abnormal dreams, ↓consciousness, hallucinations, dysphoria, sedation, dizziness, palpitations, inability to speak, ↓coordination, seizures	Renal impairment, bladder dysfunction, respiratory depression, loss of memory, ↑HIV risk from shared needles	General supportive care; seizure control with IV benzodiazepines (e.g., diazepam, lorazepam). Treat dystonia with diphenhydramine.

Substance	Toxicity signs & symptoms	Possible health effects	Toxicity care and treatment
Opioid analgesics			
• Medical uses: pain treatment • Generic/brand names: codeine, fentanyl (Duragesic), hydrocodone bitartrate–acetaminophen (Norco), hydromorphone hydrochloride (Dilaudid), meperidine (Demerol), methadone hydrochloride (Methadose), morphine sulfate (MS Contin), oxycodone hydrochloride (OxyContin, Roxicodone), oxycodone hydrochloride–acetaminophen (Percocet), oxycodone–aspirin (Percodan), oxymorphone hydrochloride (Opana), tapentadol (Nucynta), tramadol hydrochloride (Ultram) • Routes: oral, inhalation (nasal), injection, transdermal, buccal, sublingual	↓BP, ↓HR, ↓respiratory rate, nausea, vomiting, constipation, drowsiness, euphoria, ↓GI motility, sedation, seizures	Apnea, hypoxia, coma, CNS depression, respiratory depression, liver function abnormality/liver damage (associated with long-term acetaminophen use), death	General supportive care; seizure control with IV benzodiazepines (e.g., diazepam, lorazepam). Naloxone is the preferred reversal agent for opioids. Activated charcoal isn't recommended due to risk of CNS depression and aspiration. Mechanical ventilation may be required.
Stimulants			
Amphetamines • Medical uses: ADHD, narcolepsy • Generic/brand names: dextroamphetamine (Dexedrine), amphetamine–dextroamphetamine (Adderall XR), lisdexamfetamine (Vyvanse) • Routes: oral, inhalation (nasal/oral), injection	Hyperthermia, ↑HR, ↑BP, arrhythmias, palpitations, chest pain, diaphoresis, flushing, paranoia, agitation, abnormal behavior, dehydration, seizures	HF, MI, psychosis, renal/hepatic failure, serotonin syndrome, coma, ↑HIV risk from shared needles, rhabdomyolysis	General supportive care; seizure control with IV benzodiazepines (e.g., diazepam, lorazepam). Consider activated charcoal (most effective within 1 hour of toxic ingestion); dialysis and hemoperfusion are ineffective.
methylphenidate • Medical uses: ADHD, narcolepsy • Generic/brand names: methylphenidate (Ritalin LA/SR) • Routes: oral, transdermal	Hyperthermia, ↑HR, ↑BP, arrhythmias, palpitations, chest pain, diaphoresis, flushing, nausea, headache, tremor, paranoia, agitation, abnormal behavior, euphoria, seizures, serotonin syndrome	HF, MI, pulmonary HTN, psychosis, renal/hepatic failure, coma, sudden death, rhabdomyolysis	General supportive care; seizure control with IV benzodiazepines (e.g., diazepam, lorazepam). Consider activated charcoal (most effective within 1 hour of toxic ingestion); dialysis and hemoperfusion are ineffective.
Sedatives			
Barbiturates • Medical uses: sedation, seizures, hypnotic • Generic/brand names: pentobarbital (Nembutal), secobarbital (Seconal), amobarbital (Amytal), butabarbital (Butisol), mephobarbital (Mebaral) • Routes: oral, injection	Hypothermia, ↓BP, ↓respiratory rate, ↓reflexes, drowsiness, slurred speech, nystagmus, confusion, ataxia	Respiratory failure, CV collapse, coma	General supportive care. Activated charcoal, urine alkalinization, hemoperfusion/hemofiltration, and dialysis have all been used with some success to increase elimination of barbiturates.

(continued)

Substance	Toxicity signs & symptoms	Possible health effects	Toxicity care and treatment
Sedatives (*continued*)			
Benzodiazepines • Medical uses: alcohol withdrawal, anxiety/panic disorder, insomnia, preoperative/moderate sedation, seizure disorder • Generic/brand names: alprazolam (Xanax), chlordiazepoxide (Librium), clonazepam (Klonopin), diazepam (Valium), lorazepam (Ativan), oxazepam, temazepam (Restoril), midazolam, triazolam (Halcion) • Routes: oral, injection	Hypothermia, ↓BP, ↓respiratory rate, sedation, confusion, slurred speech, ataxia	Metabolic acidosis (from propylene glycol diluent used in Valium and Ativan injection preparations), respiratory failure, coma, rhabdomyolysis	General supportive care. Consider activated charcoal (most effective within 1 hour of toxic oral ingestion); hemodialysis and forced/enhanced diuresis are ineffective. Flumazenil is the reversal agent for benzodiazepines.
Sleep drugs • Medical uses: insomnia • Generic/brand names: zolpidem (Ambien CR), zaleplon (Sonata), eszopiclone (Lunesta) • Routes: oral	↓BP, ↓respiratory rate, nausea, vomiting, abdominal pain, dizziness, confusion, ↓coordination, delusions, headache, sleep-eating/sleep-driving, slurred speech, somnolence	Respiratory depression, CV collapse, coma	General supportive care. Consider activated charcoal (most effective within 1 hour of toxic oral ingestion); hemodialysis is ineffective.
Miscellaneous drugs			
Cannabinoids • Medical uses: treatment of nausea/vomiting, appetite stimulant, epilepsy • Generic/brand names: nabilone (Cesamet), dronabinol (Marinol) • Routes: oral, inhalation (oral), injection (rare)	Lethargy, ↑HR, ataxia, muscle tremors, pulmonary irritation, sore throat, rhinitis, coughing, mydriasis, somnolence, euphoria, depersonalization, alteration of time sense, loss of social inhibition, mood alterations, memory impairment	• Oral: significant altered mental status, hypotonia, coma • Injection (extract or oil): shock, DIC, rhabdomyolysis, acute renal failure, death	General supportive care; seizure control with IV benzodiazepines (e.g., diazepam, lorazepam). Absorption/elimination techniques (e.g., activated charcoal, hemodialysis, hemoperfusion, urine alkalinization) are ineffective.
Anabolic steroids • Medical uses: breast cancer, delayed puberty, hypogonadism • Generic/brand names: testosterone cypionate/enanthate (Aveed), oxandrolone (Oxandrin), oxymetholone (Anadrol-50) • Routes: oral, injection, transdermal	↑BP, acne, fluid retention, ↑lipid levels, jaundice, tendon rupture, breast enlargement (men), male-pattern baldness, changes in sex organs, infertility, libido changes, rage, aggression, mania, delusions, mood swings, insomnia, weight gain	Short stature, MI, hepatitis, hepatic tumors, hepatic failure, thrombosis, stroke, ↑HIV risk from shared needles	General supportive care. Absorption/elimination techniques (e.g., activated charcoal, hemodialysis, hemoperfusion, urine alkalinization) are ineffective. Benzodiazepines and antipsychotics may be considered for extreme aggression.

Understanding biosimilar drugs

What are nonbiologic drug products and how are they approved?

Most drugs on the market are nonbiologic drugs, which are made from chemicals with known structures that can be identically re-created. Brand-name nonbiologic drugs are first approved by the FDA through a New Drug Application approval process that requires evidence of safety and effectiveness of the drug, the quality of the product, and the accuracy of its labeling. Pharmaceutical companies file for patents or exclusive marketing rights with the FDA for each drug.

Once these patents expire, other pharmaceutical companies can manufacture the brand-name nonbiologic drug by making an identical (bioequivalent), less expensive, generic formulation (called an "innovator drug" by the FDA) of the same brand-name drug. Generic formulations are less expensive because the pharmaceutical companies file for an Abbreviated New Drug Application (ANDA) approval process, which doesn't require the pharmaceutical company to perform clinical trials and submit evidence of safety and effectiveness of the generic drug. The FDA's *Approved Drug Products with Therapeutic Equivalence Evaluations* (also known as the Orange Book) contains all of the FDA-approved drugs and identifies which drugs are therapeutically equivalent. If drugs are deemed therapeutically equivalent, a less costly drug may be able to be substituted for a higher-cost drug.

What are biological drug products?

In contrast to conventional drug products, which are pure chemical substances, biological drugs are made from living organisms (human or animal cells or tissues, proteins, microorganisms), and their manufacturing processes are more complex than those for conventional drugs and are also proprietary. Examples of biological products include vaccines, blood and blood products, and recombinant therapeutic proteins. Biological drugs work by targeting a certain biological structure, enzyme, pathway, or other mechanism; for example, they may change the way the immune system reacts to a virus or change cells and proteins involved in inflammation.

What are biosimilar drugs and how are they approved?

Just as nonbiologic drugs have brand-name and generic forms, biological drugs have brand-name and biosimilar forms. Unlike generic drugs, which are chemical replicas of the original brand-name drug, biosimilar drugs are similar to but not exact duplicates of the brand-name drug (biological reference product) because they are made from tissues and other nonchemical components. Each pharmaceutical company must demonstrate that its biosimilar drug is highly similar to a biological reference product that has already been FDA-approved. According to the FDA, biosimilar drugs must demonstrate they have "no clinically meaningful differences in terms of safety and effectiveness from the reference product. Minor differences in clinically inactive components are allowed."

As with nonbiologic drugs, brand-name biological drugs are approved by the FDA through a Biologics License Application, which requires evidence of safety, purity, potency, and effectiveness of the biological drug.

An abbreviated licensure pathway for biological products is described in The Patient Protection and Affordable Care Act (Affordable Care Act) of 2010. Similar to the ANDA approval process, biological drugs have an abbreviated licensure pathway for biological products that are demonstrated to be "biosimilar" to or "interchangeable" with an FDA-licensed biological product. The Biologics Price Competition and Innovation Act (BPCI Act), part of the Affordable Care Act, provides this licensure pathway. According to the BPCI Act, an interchangeable biological drug may be substituted for the reference product by a pharmacist without the consultation or intervention of the prescriber.

Similar to the Orange Book for nonbiologic drugs, the FDA's *Lists of Licensed Biological Products with Reference Product*

Exclusivity and Biosimilarity or Inter-changeability Evaluations (also known as the Purple Book) states whether a biological product has been determined by the FDA to be biosimilar to or interchangeable with a biological reference product.

Why are biosimilar drugs important?

The FDA is expected to approve an increasing number of biosimilar drugs, as these drugs are expected to compete with each other in the medical marketplace and decrease consumer costs. The first approved biosimilar drug, Zarxio, cost 15% less than its biological reference drug, Neupogen. Some pharmaceutical companies have embraced the new technology of biosimilar drugs and have a pipeline of biosimilar drugs in the development or approval stage. Just like generics, biosimilar drugs can be made by more than one pharmaceutical company, thereby increasing competition and hopefully lowering overall health care costs.

What is important to know about biosimilar and biological reference drugs?

Biosimilarity is based on the product being highly similar to the biological reference product as determined by toxicity studies in animals and one or more clinical studies demonstrating the safety, purity, and potency of the product.

Biosimilar drugs:
• may be approved for the same or fewer indications as the biological reference drug. The number of approved indications may not exceed the number of approved indications for the reference drug.
• must have the same mechanism of action, route of administration, dosage forms, and strength as the reference drug.
• are expected to have no differences in safety and effectiveness compared to the reference drug.

How are biosimilar drug names determined?

Biological products and their biosimilar drugs share a nonproprietary name (also referred to as a "proper name"). Biosimilar drugs use the nonproprietary name plus a suffix composed of four lowercase letters,

separated from the core name by a hyphen. These four letters are proposed by the manufacturer at the time of application or submission. Older suffixes may represent the name of the pharmaceutical company that holds the biosimilar drug's licensing agreement. On March 6, 2015, the FDA approved the very first biosimilar drug, which is named filgrastim-sndz (Zarxio); Zarxio is licensed by the Sandoz Company. It's a biosimilar drug to the biological reference product filgrastim (Neupogen).

Additional information may be found at www.biosimilarsresourcecenter.org/fda-releases-final-biologics-naming-guidance/.

Nursing process: Patient safety during drug therapy

Drug therapy is a complex process that can easily lead to adverse patient events. In 2007, the Institute of Medicine (IOM) released its report on the drug safety system, *The Future of Drug Safety: Promoting and Protecting the Health of the Public*. The IOM reported that approximately 400,000 preventable adverse drug events occurred each year in the United States. The IOM also estimated that preventable hospital medication errors occurred at a rate of one/patient/day and contributed to 7,000 patient deaths/year. Although much progress has been made, problems with using medications safely remain. Medication errors are one of the top 10 most frequently reviewed sentinel events by The Joint Commission. Applying the nursing process (assessment, nursing diagnosis, planning, intervention, and evaluation) during drug therapy enables the nurse to systematically identify the drug therapy needs of each patient, thereby reducing the number of adverse events and providing safe patient care.

Nursing process step	Key points

Assessment	• Collect data—subjective and objective
	  ○ Current/previous health status
	  ○ Cultural considerations
	  ○ Lab values
	  ○ Allergies
	  ○ Physical assessment
	  ○ Medication history
	    ■ Prescriptions/OTC drugs
	    ■ Herbal supplements
	    ■ Response to medications
	    ■ Knowledge of medications.

Nursing diagnosis/problem	• Identify all associated nursing diagnoses.
Planning	• Review prescribed medications. • Identify possible adverse effects of medications. • Identify potential interactions with other medications. • Determine route of administration. • Determine time of administration. • Develop patient education regarding medication administration. • Review patient allergies.

Intervention	• Administer medication utilizing the "eight rights"
	  ○ Right patient
	  ○ Right drug
	  ○ Right dose
	  ○ Right time
	  ○ Right route
	  ○ Right reason
	  ○ Right response
	  ○ Right documentation.
	• Use technology such as bar coding to ensure safe and correct administration.
	• Educate patient about each medication at time of administration.

Evaluation	• Monitor patient's response to medication. • Monitor for possible adverse effects of medication. • Monitor for unexpected effects of medication. • Document medication administration.

Serotonin syndrome: What you should know to protect your patient

Serotonin is a neurotransmitter involved in the conduction of nerve impulses. Serotonin syndrome is a drug reaction resulting from an increase in plasma serotonin levels and can range in severity from mild to life-threatening to fatal. It frequently occurs when drugs that affect serotonin levels are given together, causing serotonin levels to rise. Serotonin syndrome can occur within minutes or hours of drug administration and may cause ARDS, DIC, liver and renal failure, rhabdomyolysis, intractable myoclonus, and seizures. Identifying the symptoms and initiating prompt treatment can prevent a potentially fatal outcome. Some drugs commonly associated with serotonin syndrome include SSRIs (fluoxetine), SSNRIs (duloxetine), MAO inhibitors (phenelzine), methylene blue, opiates (methadone), antiemetics (ondansetron), antibiotics (linezolid), antiretrovirals (ritonavir), dextromethorphan, and herbal supplements (St. John's wort).

Key points	What you need to know or do
Risk factors	• Coadministration of medications that affect serotonin levels • Overdose of medications that affect serotonin levels
Signs and symptoms	• Agitation, restlessness, mental status changes, hallucinations • Headache, muscle pain • Loss of muscle coordination, muscle rigidity, seizures, muscle spasms, tremor • Fever, shivering, goose bumps, HTN, tachycardia, arrhythmia • Profound diaphoresis • Nausea, vomiting, diarrhea
Preventive measures	• Review medication history and drug therapy for potential interactions. • Identify patients at risk for serotonin syndrome. • Perform thorough baseline assessment.
Monitoring	• Monitor patient's condition closely. • Monitor temperature, HR (continuous cardiac monitoring), BP, fluid status, and urine output frequently. • Monitor oxygenation, mental status, and pain levels. • Monitor serum serotonin levels. • Monitor electrolyte and CK levels.
Treatment and interventions	• Discontinue drugs associated with serotonin syndrome. • Administer oxygen therapy, ventilation, and paralytics (succinylcholine chloride) as needed to maintain adequate ventilation. • Institute cooling measures (i.e., cooling baths, blankets) for fever. • Administer IV fluids to maintain hydration. • Administer medications to block serotonin production (antihistamines [cyproheptadine hydrochloride]), to control seizures and myoclonus (benzodiazepines [diazepam]), and to control HTN (nitroprusside), tachycardia (beta blockers [esmolol]), and pain (opioids if needed).

Tumor lysis syndrome: A life-threatening emergency

Tumor lysis syndrome (TLS) is a potentially life-threatening oncologic emergency caused by a rapid and massive breakdown of tumor cells, either immediately or within 48 to 72 hours, usually after chemotherapy administration. The release of tumor cell debris into the bloodstream causes an array of metabolic disturbances, such as hyperkalemia, hyperphosphatemia, hyperuricemia, and hypocalcemia, which can lead to seizures, acute kidney injury, fluid overload, cardiac arrhythmias, cardiopulmonary arrest, and death. TLS is associated with treatment for hematologic cancers, including some leukemias and lymphomas, and with the use of such chemotherapeutic drugs as paclitaxel, fludarabine, etoposide, bortezomib, zoledronic acid, and hydroxyurea.

Key considerations	What you need to know or do
Risk factors	• Disease with high tumor-cell proliferation rate • Chemosensitivity of the malignancy, bulky tumor, or extensive metastasis; organ infiltration; bone marrow involvement • Pretreatment hyperuricemia, elevated LDH levels, renal impairment, nephrotoxic drugs
Signs and symptoms	• Lethargy, syncope, seizures, altered mental state • HF, arrhythmias, sudden death • Edema, weight gain, fluid overload • Renal failure, metabolic acidosis, decreased or absent urine output, urine sediment, flank pain, hematuria • Anorexia, nausea, vomiting, constipation, diarrhea • Muscle cramping, tetany • Hyperkalemia, hypocalcemia, hyperphosphatemia, hyperuricemia
Preventive measures	• Identify at-risk patients as soon as possible. • Obtain central venous access. • Obtain baseline ECG, vital signs, and hemodynamic status. • Administer IV hydration to improve renal perfusion and GFR. • Administer sodium bicarbonate for metabolic acidosis and to promote alkaline urine diuresis. • Administer pretreatment hypouricemics (allopurinol or rasburicase). • Avoid potassium-sparing diuretics. • Consider phosphate-binding agents for hyperphosphatemia.
Treatment and monitoring	• Monitor mental status. • Monitor respiratory status and oxygenation. Administer oxygen therapy as prescribed. • Institute continuous cardiac monitoring. • Closely monitor vital signs and fluid volume status (fluid intake, urine output, weight, edema). • Monitor serial electrolytes, acid-base balance, and BUN, creatinine, and uric acid levels every 4 to 6 hours. Monitor calcium, phosphate, and LDH levels. Correct abnormalities. • Monitor fluid volume and administer diuretics. • Possible renal replacement therapy or hemodialysis may be needed.

Antidiarrheals: Indications and dosages

Refer to manufacturer's instructions for complete prescribing and safety information.

bismuth subsalicylate
BIS-mith sub-sal-LIS-a-late

Bismatrol ◇, Kaopectate ◇, Kao-Tin ◇, Peptic Relief ◇, Pepto-Bismol ◇, Pink Bismuth ◇, Stomach Relief ◇

Therapeutic class: Antidiarrheals
Pharmacologic class: Adsorbents

AVAILABLE FORMS
Caplets ⓄⓉⒸ 262 mg ◇
Oral suspension: 262 mg/15 mL (regular strength), 525 mg/15 mL (maximum strength)
Tablets (chewable): 262 mg ◇

INDICATIONS & DOSAGES
➤ **Mild, nonspecific diarrhea; gas, indigestion, heartburn, nausea**
Adults and children age 12 and older: 525 mg PO every 30 to 60 minutes or 1,050 mg PO every 60 minutes as needed for up to 2 days. Maximum, 4,200 mg/24 hours.

crofelemer
kro-FEL-e-mer

Mytesi

Therapeutic class: Antidiarrheals
Pharmacologic class: Antidiarrheals

AVAILABLE FORMS
Tablets (delayed-release) ⓄⓉⒸ 125 mg

INDICATIONS & DOSAGES
➤ **Noninfectious diarrhea in patients with HIV/AIDS on antiretroviral therapy**
Adults: 125 mg PO b.i.d.

diphenoxylate hydrochloride–atropine sulfate
dye-fen-OKS-ul-ate/A-troe-peen

Lomotil*

Therapeutic class: Antidiarrheals
Pharmacologic class: Opioids
Controlled substance schedule: V

AVAILABLE FORMS
Liquid: 2.5 mg diphenoxylate and 0.025 mg atropine/5 mL*
Tablets: 2.5 mg diphenoxylate and 0.025 mg atropine

INDICATIONS & DOSAGES
➤ **Acute, nonspecific diarrhea**
Adults and children age 13 and older: Initially, 5 mg diphenoxylate PO q.i.d.; reduce dosage as soon as initial control of symptoms is achieved. Maximum dosage, 20 mg/day.
Children ages 2 to 12: 0.3 to 0.4 mg/kg diphenoxylate liquid form PO daily in four divided doses. Maintenance, reduce dose when initial control of symptoms is achieved; may reduce dosage by as much as 75%. Maximum, 10 mg/day. Don't use tablets in children younger than age 13.

loperamide hydrochloride
loe-PER-a-mide

Diamode ◇, Imodium A-D ◇

Therapeutic class: Antidiarrheals
Pharmacologic class: Piperidine derivatives

AVAILABLE FORMS
Capsules: 2 mg
Oral liquid: 1 mg/5 mL ◇, 1 mg/7.5 mL ◇
Tablets: 2 mg ◇

INDICATIONS & DOSAGES
Black Box Warning Don't exceed recommended dosages due to risk of torsades de pointes, cardiac arrest, and death. Capsules are contraindicated in children younger than age 2. ■
➤ **Acute, nonspecific diarrhea; reducing volume of discharge from ileostomies**
Adults and children older than age 12: Initially, give 4 mg PO; then 2 mg after each unformed stool. Maximum, 16 mg/day (prescription strength) or 8 mg/day (OTC) unless otherwise directed.
Children ages 8 to 12 weighing more than 30 kg: 2 mg PO t.i.d. on first day. After first treatment day, give 1 mg/10 kg body weight only after a loose stool. Maximum, 6 mg daily.
Children ages 6 to younger than 8 weighing 20 to 30 kg: 2 mg PO b.i.d. on first day. After first treatment day, give 1 mg/10 kg body weight only after a loose stool. Maximum, 4 mg daily.
Children ages 2 to 5 weighing 13 to 20 kg: 1 mg PO t.i.d. for first day. After first treatment day, give 1 mg/10 kg only after a loose stool. Maximum, 3 mg/day.
➤ **Chronic diarrhea associated with inflammatory bowel disease**
Adults: Initially, 4 mg PO; then 2 mg after each unformed stool until diarrhea subsides. Adjust dosage to individual response. Maximum, 16 mg/day (prescription strength).
➤ **Diarrhea, traveler's diarrhea (OTC)**
Adults and children age 12 and older: 4 mg PO followed by 2 mg after each subsequent loose stool for a maximum of 8 mg/24 hours.

Antidotes: Indications and dosages

Refer to manufacturer's instructions for complete prescribing and safety information.

activated charcoal
Charac, Charactol, EZ Char, Insta-Char Aqueous, Insta-Char in Sorbitol

Therapeutic class: Antidotes
Pharmacologic class: Adsorbents

AVAILABLE FORMS
Liquid: 15 g*; 25 g*; 30 g*; 50 g*
Oral suspension: 15 g; 25 g
Pellets for reconstitution: 25 g

INDICATIONS & DOSAGES
➤ **Poisoning**
Adults and children age 12 and older weighing more than 32 kg: 50 to 100 g or 1 to 2 g/kg of body weight PO (in aqueous or sorbitol base).
Adults and children older than age 1: 5 to 60 g PO (aqueous base). Dosage should be 10 times by volume the amount of poison ingested, if known. If amount of poison ingested isn't known, base dosage on weight, size, and age of patient. Initial dosage should be at least 20 to 30 g.
Adults and children (EZ Char): For patients weighing 22 kg or more, give entire amount of reconstituted liquid; for those weighing 11 to less than 22 kg, give 60 to 120 mL (4 to 8 tablespoons) of reconstituted liquid; for those weighing 5.5 to less than 11 kg, give 30 to 60 mL (2 to 4 tablespoons) of reconstituted liquid; for those weighing 2.7 to less than 5.5 kg, give 15 to 30 mL (1 to 2 tablespoons) of reconstituted liquid. Repeat dose immediately, if necessary.

amifostine
am-i-FOS-steen

Ethyol

Therapeutic class: Cytoprotective drugs
Pharmacologic class: Organic thiophosphates

AVAILABLE FORMS
Injection: 500 mg in single-use vials

INDICATIONS & DOSAGES
➤ **Reduction of cumulative renal toxicity associated with repeated administration of cisplatin in patients with advanced ovarian cancer**
Adults: 910 mg/m² once daily as a 15-minute IV infusion, starting 30 minutes before chemotherapy. Antiemetics, including dexamethasone 20 mg IV and a serotonin 5-HT₃ receptor antagonist, are recommended before and in conjunction with drug.

Adjust-a-dose: Refer to manufacturer's instructions for interrupting therapy if hypotension occurs.
➤ **Moderate to severe xerostomia in patients undergoing postoperative radiation treatment for head and neck cancer, when the radiation port includes a substantial portion of the parotid glands**
Adults: 200 mg/m² once daily as a 3-minute IV infusion, starting 15 to 30 minutes before standard fraction radiation therapy. Oral 5-HT₃ receptor antagonists, alone or in combination with other antiemetics, are recommended before and in conjunction with drug.

deferasirox
de-FER-a-sir-ox

Exjade, Jadenu, Jadenu Sprinkle

Therapeutic class: Chelating agents
Pharmacologic class: Heavy metal antagonists

AVAILABLE FORMS
Sprinkles: 90 mg, 180 mg, 360 mg
Tablets: 90 mg, 180 mg, 360 mg
Tablets for oral suspension ⚫: 125 mg, 250 mg, 500 mg

INDICATIONS & DOSAGES
Black Box Warning Drug can cause fatal renal failure, hepatic failure, and GI hemorrhage. Monitor patient carefully. Contraindicated in adults and children with eGFR less than 40 mL/minute/1.73 m². Evaluate baseline renal function before starting drug or increasing dosage in all patients. ■
Adjust-a-dose (for all indications): When converting therapy from Exjade to Jadenu, the dose of Jadenu should be approximately 30% lower (rounded to the nearest whole tablet) than the current dose of Exjade.

Contraindicated in patients with eGFR less than 40 mL/minute/1.73 m² or platelet count less than 50,000/mm³. Discontinue drug if necessary.

Start elderly patients at low end of dosing range.

Avoid use in patients with severe (Child-Pugh class C) hepatic impairment. Reduce starting dose by 50% in patients with moderate (Child-Pugh class B) hepatic impairment. Closely monitor all patients with mild (Child-Pugh class A) or moderate hepatic impairment for effectiveness and adverse reactions. Reduce starting dose by 50% in patients with eGFR of 40 to 60 mL/minute/1.73 m². Use cautiously in children with eGFR between 40 and 60 mL/minute/1.73 m². If treatment is needed, use the minimum effective dose and monitor renal function frequently.
➤ **Chronic iron overload caused by blood transfusions (transfusional hemosiderosis)**
Adults and children age 2 and older with eGFR greater than 60 mL/minute/1.73 m²: Exjade: Initially, 20 mg/kg PO daily on an empty stomach 30 minutes

before eating. Disperse tablets in water, orange juice, or apple juice. Avoid dispersion in milk and carbonated drinks. Monitor serum ferritin level monthly, and adjust dose every 3 to 6 months by 5 or 10 mg/kg based on ferritin trends. Don't exceed 40 mg/kg daily. Interrupt therapy and continue monthly monitoring if serum ferritin level drops below 500 mcg/L.

Jadenu: Initially, 14 mg/kg PO once daily on an empty stomach or with a light meal. Monitor serum ferritin level monthly, and adjust dose every 3 to 6 months by increments of 3.5 or 7 mg/kg, based on serum ferritin trends. Don't exceed 28 mg/kg. If serum ferritin level falls below 1,000 mcg/L at two consecutive visits, consider dosage reduction, especially if dose is greater than 17.5 mg/kg/day. Interrupt therapy if serum ferritin level drops below 500 mcg/L and continue monthly monitoring.

Adjust-a-dose: Interrupt therapy for children who have acute illnesses that can cause volume depletion and monitor more frequently. Resume therapy as appropriate.

For adults: If serum creatinine level increases by 33% or more above the average baseline measurement, repeat serum creatinine within 1 week and, if still elevated by 33% or more, reduce Exjade dose by 10 mg/kg or Jadenu dose by 7 mg/kg.

For children ages 2 to 17: Reduce Exjade dose by 10 mg/kg/day or Jadenu dose by 7 mg/kg if eGFR decreases by greater than 33% below the average baseline measurement and repeat eGFR within 1 week.

For all patients: Discontinue therapy for eGFR less than 40 mL/minute/1.73 m^2.

➤ **Chronic iron overload in patients with non-transfusion-dependent thalassemia syndromes and with a liver iron (Fe) concentration (LIC) of at least 5 mg Fe per gram of dry weight (dw) and a serum ferritin level greater than 300 mcg/L**

Adults and children age 10 and older with eGFR greater than 60 mL/minute/1.73 m^2: Exjade: Initially, 10 mg/kg PO once daily 30 minutes before food and dispersed in water, orange juice, or apple juice. Avoid dispersion in milk and carbonated drinks. Calculate dose to the nearest whole tablet. If baseline LIC is greater than 15 mg Fe/g dw, may increase to 20 mg/kg/day after 4 weeks. Interrupt treatment when serum ferritin level is less than 300 mcg/L, and obtain LIC to determine if LIC is less than 3 mg Fe/g dw. If LIC remains greater than 7 mg Fe/g dw after 6 months of therapy, increase dosage to maximum of 20 mg/kg/day. If LIC is 3 to 7 mg Fe/g dw after 6 months, continue treatment at maximum of 10 mg/kg/day. If LIC is less than 3 mg Fe/g dw, stop treatment. Continue to monitor LIC, and restart treatment when LIC rises again to more than 5 mg Fe/g dw.

Jadenu: Initially, 7 mg/kg PO once daily on an empty stomach or with a light meal. Calculate dose to the nearest whole tablet. If baseline LIC is greater than 15 mg Fe/g dw, may increase to 14 mg/kg/day after 4 weeks. Interrupt treatment when serum ferritin level is less than 300 mcg/L, and obtain LIC to determine if LIC is less than 3 mg Fe/g dw. If LIC remains greater

than 7 mg Fe/g dw after 6 months of therapy, increase dosage to maximum of 14 mg/kg/day. If LIC is 3 to 7 mg Fe/g dw after 6 months, continue treatment at maximum of 7 mg/kg/day. If LIC is less than 3 mg Fe/g dw, stop treatment. Continue to monitor LIC and restart treatment when LIC rises again to more than 5 mg Fe/g dw.

Adjust-a-dose: Increase monitoring frequency and consider dose interruption for children who have acute illness that can cause volume depletion.

For adults: If serum creatinine level increases by 33% or more above the average baseline measurement, repeat serum creatinine within 1 week and, if still elevated by 33% or more, interrupt Exjade therapy if dose is 5 mg/kg, or reduce by 50% if dose is 10 or 20 mg/kg; interrupt Jadenu therapy if dose is 3.5 mg/kg, or reduce by 50% if dose is 7 or 14 mg/kg.

For children ages 10 to 17: Reduce Exjade dose by 5 mg/kg/day or Jadenu dose by 3.5 mg/kg if eGFR decreases by greater than 33% below the average baseline measurement and repeat eGFR within 1 week.

For all patients: Discontinue therapy for eGFR less than 40 mL/minute/1.73 m^2.

deferiprone
de-FER-i-prone

Ferriprox

Therapeutic class: Chelating drugs
Pharmacologic class: Heavy metal antagonists

AVAILABLE FORMS
Solution: 100 mg/mL, 800 mg/mL
Tablets: 500 mg, 1 g

INDICATIONS & DOSAGES
Black Box Warning Drug can cause agranulocytosis that can lead to serious infections and death. Measure ANC before therapy and weekly during therapy. Interrupt therapy for neutropenia or infection. ■

➤ **Treatment of transfusional iron overload due to thalassemia syndromes when current chelation therapy is inadequate**

Adults: Initially, 25 mg/kg PO t.i.d. for a total of 75 mg/kg/day. May titrate to maximum dosage of 33 mg/kg t.i.d. for a total of 99 mg/kg/day based on patient response and therapeutic goals. Round dose to nearest 250 mg (half tablet).

Adjust-a-dose: Withhold drug for ANC less than 1,500/mm^3, if infection develops, or if serum ferritin level is consistently below 500 mcg/L. Allow at least 4 hours between administration of this drug and other medications or supplements containing polyvalent cations, such as iron, aluminum, and zinc.

digoxin immune Fab (ovine)
di-JOX-in

DigiFab

Therapeutic class: Antidotes
Pharmacologic class: Antibody fragments

AVAILABLE FORMS
Injection: 40-mg vial

INDICATIONS & DOSAGES
➤ **Life-threatening digoxin toxicity**
Adults and children: Base dosage on ingested amount or level of digoxin. When calculating amount of antidote, round up to the nearest whole number. For digoxin tablets, calculate number of antidote vials as follows: multiply ingested amount by 0.8; then divide answer by 0.5. For example, if patient takes 25 tablets of 0.25 mg digoxin, the ingested amount is 6.25 mg. Multiply 6.25 mg by 0.8 and divide answer by 0.5 to obtain 10 vials of antidote. If digoxin level is known, determine the number of antidote vials as follows: multiply the digoxin level in nanograms per milliliter by patient's weight in kilograms; then divide by 100.
➤ **Acute toxicity or if estimated ingested amount or digoxin level is unknown**
Adults and children: Consider giving 10 vials of digoxin immune Fab and observing patient's response. Follow with another 10 vials if indicated. Dosage should be effective in most life-threatening cases in adults and children but may cause volume overload in young children.
➤ **Toxicity during prolonged therapy if digoxin level is unknown**
Adults and children: 6 vials of antidote in patients weighing 20 kg or more, or 1 vial of antidote in patients weighing less than 20 kg.

dimercaprol
dye-mer-KAP-role

BAL in Oil

Therapeutic class: Chelating drugs
Pharmacologic class: Heavy metal antagonists

AVAILABLE FORMS
Injection: 100 mg/mL

INDICATIONS & DOSAGES
➤ **Severe arsenic or gold poisoning**
Adults and children: 3 mg/kg deep IM every 4 hours for 2 days; then q.i.d. on third day; then b.i.d. for 10 days.
➤ **Mild arsenic or gold poisoning**
Adults and children: 2.5 mg/kg deep IM q.i.d. for 2 days; then b.i.d. on third day; then once daily for 10 days.
➤ **Mercury poisoning**
Adults and children: Initially, 5 mg/kg deep IM; then 2.5 mg/kg daily or b.i.d. for 10 days.

➤ **Acute lead encephalopathy**
Adults and children: 4 mg/kg given alone by deep IM; then every 4 hours with edetate calcium disodium administered at a separate site for 2 to 7 days. For less severe poisoning, reduce dose to 3 mg/kg after first dose.

doxapram hydrochloride
DOCKS-a-pram

Dopram

Therapeutic class: CNS stimulants
Pharmacologic class: Analeptics

AVAILABLE FORMS
Injection: 20 mg/mL (benzyl alcohol 0.9%)

INDICATIONS & DOSAGES
➤ **Postanesthesia respiratory stimulation**
Adults: 0.5 to 1 mg/kg as a single IV injection (not to exceed 1.5 mg/kg) or as multiple injections every 5 minutes, total not to exceed 2 mg/kg or 3 g daily. Or, 250 mg in 250 mL of NSS, D_5W, or $D_{10}W$ infused at initial rate of 5 mg/minute IV until satisfactory response is achieved. Maintain at 1 to 3 mg/minute. Don't exceed total dose for infusion of 4 mg/kg or 3 g daily.
➤ **Drug-induced CNS depression**
Adults: For injection, priming dose of 1 to 2 mg/kg IV, repeated in 5 minutes and again every 1 to 2 hours until patient awakens (and if relapse occurs). Maximum daily dose is 3 g.
    For infusion, priming dose of 1 to 2 mg/kg IV, repeated in 5 minutes and again in 1 to 2 hours, if needed. If response occurs, give IV infusion (1 mg/mL) at 1 to 3 mg/minute until patient awakens. Don't infuse for longer than 2 hours or give more than 3 g/day. May resume IV infusion after rest period of 30 minutes to 2 hours, if needed.
➤ **COPD related to acute hypercapnia**
Adults: 1 to 2 mg/minute by IV infusion using 2 mg/mL solution. Maximum, 3 mg/minute. Don't infuse for longer than 2 hours. Discontinue infusion if blood gas levels deteriorate.

edetate calcium disodium
ED-e-tate

Calcium Disodium Versenate

Therapeutic class: Chelating drugs
Pharmacologic class: Heavy metal antagonists

AVAILABLE FORMS
Injection: 200 mg/mL

INDICATIONS & DOSAGES
Black Box Warning Toxic effects of drug can be fatal. Use with extreme caution in patients with lead

encephalopathy and cerebral edema. Never exceed the recommended daily dosage. ∎

➤ **Acute lead encephalopathy or lead level greater than 70 mcg/dL**
Adults and children: Use in conjunction with dimercaprol. Consult published protocols and specialized references for dosage recommendations.

➤ **Lead poisoning without encephalopathy or asymptomatic with lead level less than 70 mcg/dL but greater than 20 mcg/dL**
Adults and children: 1 g/m^2/day IV infused over 8 to 12 hours once daily or 1 g/m^2 IM daily in divided doses spaced 8 to 12 hours apart for 5 days. Or, for adults with lead nephropathy, give as follows: If serum creatinine level is 2 to 3 mg/dL, give 500 mg/m^2 every 24 hours for 5 days; if serum creatinine level is 3 to 4 mg/dL, give 500 mg/m^2 every 48 hours for three doses; if serum creatinine level is more than 4 mg/dL, give 500 mg/m^2 once weekly. These regimens may be repeated at 1-month intervals.

glucarpidase
gloo-CAR-pi-daze

Voraxaze

Therapeutic class: Antidotes
Pharmacologic class: Recombinant bacterial enzymes

AVAILABLE FORMS
Powder for injection: 1,000 units/vial

INDICATIONS & DOSAGES
➤ **Methotrexate toxicity (more than 1 micromole/L) in patients with impaired renal function**
Adults and children age 1 month and older: 50 units/kg as a single IV injection over 5 minutes.

lanthanum carbonate
LAN-thah-num

Fosrenol

Therapeutic class: Antihyperphosphatemics
Pharmacologic class: Non-calcium, non-aluminum phosphate binders

AVAILABLE FORMS
Oral powder: 750 mg, 1,000 mg
Tablets (chewable): 500 mg, 750 mg, 1 g

INDICATIONS & DOSAGES
➤ **Reduction of serum phosphate level in patients with ESRD**
Adults: Initially, 500 mg PO t.i.d. with meals. Adjust every 2 to 3 weeks by 750 mg daily until reaching desired phosphate level. Reducing phosphate level to less than 6 mg/dL usually requires 1,500 to 3,000 mg daily. Maximum daily dose is 4,500 mg.

mesna
MES-na

Mesnex

Therapeutic class: Cytoprotective drugs
Pharmacologic class: Antidotes

AVAILABLE FORMS
Injection: 100 mg/mL in 1-g multidose vial*
Tablets: 400 mg

INDICATIONS & DOSAGES
➤ **Prophylaxis of ifosfamide-induced hemorrhagic cystitis**
Adults (IV only regimen): Total daily mesna dose is 60% of ifosfamide dose. Give 20% of ifosfamide dose weight by weight (w/w) IV bolus injection at the time of ifosfamide administration, then at 4 and 8 hours after ifosfamide dose. For example, if ifosfamide dose is 1.2 g/m^2, the mesna dose is 240 mg/m^2 given at the same time as ifosfamide and then 4 hours and 8 hours after ifosfamide. Dosing schedule is repeated each day ifosfamide is given.
Adults (IV and PO dosing regimen): Total daily mesna dose is 100% of ifosfamide dose. Give 20% of ifosfamide dose (w/w) IV bolus injection at the same time ifosfamide is given. Then give 40% of ifosfamide dose (w/w) as PO tablets at 2 hours and 6 hours after ifosfamide dose. Dosing schedule is repeated each day ifosfamide is given. This ratio of IV and oral dosing hasn't been established as effective for daily ifosfamide doses higher than 2 g/m^2.
Adjust-a-dose: If ifosfamide dosage is increased or decreased, the mesna dosage should also be modified to maintain the mesna-to-ifosfamide ratio.
➤ **Prevention of cyclophosphamide-induced hemorrhagic cystitis (with high-dose cyclophosphamide)** ◆
Adults younger than age 40: 2,100 mg/m^2/day continuous IV infusion (mesna dose is equivalent to the cyclophosphamide dose) for 2 days with cyclophosphamide infusion during cycles 1, 2, 3, and 6.

naloxegol oxalate
nal-OX-ee-gol

Movantik

Therapeutic class: Antidotes
Pharmacologic class: Opioid antagonists

AVAILABLE FORMS
Tablets: 12.5 mg, 25 mg

INDICATIONS & DOSAGES
➤ **Opioid-induced constipation in patients with chronic noncancer pain, including patients with chronic pain related to prior cancer or its treatment who don't require frequent opioid dosage escalation**

◆ Off-label use   ⓓⓝⓒ Do not crush   *Liquid contains alcohol

Adults: 25 mg PO once daily in the morning at least 1 hour before or 2 hours after the first meal of the day. If 25 mg isn't tolerated, reduce to 12.5 mg once daily.
Adjust-a-dose: For CrCl less than 60 mL/minute, decrease starting dose to 12.5 mg; if tolerated, may increase to 25 mg if needed. If use with a moderate CYP3A4 inhibitor is necessary, decrease dosage to 12.5 mg daily.

phentolamine mesylate
fen-TOLE-a-meen

OraVerse

Therapeutic class: Antidotes
Pharmacologic class: Alpha blockers

AVAILABLE FORMS
Injection: 0.4 mg/1.7 mL, 5 mg/mL

INDICATIONS & DOSAGES
➤**Prevention of dermal necrosis from norepinephrine extravasation**
Adults: Add 10 mg of phentolamine to each liter of solution containing norepinephrine; the pressor effect of norepinephrine is unaffected.
➤**Dermal necrosis and sloughing after IV extravasation of norepinephrine or dopamine**
Adults: Infiltrate area with 5 to 10 mg phentolamine in 10 mL of NSS within 12 hours of extravasation.
➤**Reversal of soft-tissue anesthesia**
Adults and children age 6 and older weighing more than 30 kg: Dosage depends on amount of anesthetic used. Refer to manufacturer's instructions.
➤**Diagnosis of pheochromocytoma, to control or prevent hypertension before or during pheochromocytomectomy**
Adults: IV or IM diagnostic dose is 5 mg with close monitoring of BP. Give 5 mg IV or IM 1 to 2 hours before surgical removal of tumor. During surgery, patient may need an additional 5 mg IV.
Children: IV diagnostic dose is 1 mg, and IM diagnostic dose is 3 mg with close monitoring of BP. Give 1 mg IV or IM 1 to 2 hours before surgical removal of tumor. During surgery, patient may need an additional 1 mg IV.

pralidoxime chloride (2-PAM chloride, 2-pyridine-aldoxime methochloride)
pra-li-DOX-eem

Protopam Chloride

Therapeutic class: Antidotes
Pharmacologic class: Quaternary ammonium oximes

AVAILABLE FORMS
Injection: 1 g/20 mL in 20-mL vial
Injection (for IM use): 300 mg/mL

INDICATIONS & DOSAGES
➤**Antidote for organophosphate poisoning in combination with atropine**
Adults: 1 to 2 g in 100 mL of NSS by IV infusion over 15 to 30 minutes. If not practical or if pulmonary edema is present, give dose as a 5% solution in sterile water by slow IV push over at least 5 minutes. Repeat in 1 hour if muscle weakness persists. May give additional doses cautiously. May use IM or subcut injection if IV isn't feasible.
For IM dosing: *For mild symptoms,* give 600 mg (2 mL) IM. Wait 15 minutes; if symptoms persist, give a second dose. May give a third dose after an additional 15 minutes. If at any time after the first dose patient develops severe symptoms, give two additional 600-mg doses in rapid succession for a total cumulative dose of 1,800 mg. *For severe symptoms,* give three 600-mg doses (three doses of 2 mL each) in rapid succession. If symptoms persist after the complete 1,800-mg regimen (three injections of 600 mg each), may repeat the series beginning approximately 1 hour after the last injection.
Children age 16 and younger (IV dosing): Give loading dose of 20 to 50 mg/kg (maximum 2 g) IV over 15 to 30 minutes, followed by 10 to 20 mg/kg/hour by continuous IV infusion. Or, give initial dose of 20 to 50 mg/kg IV over 15 to 30 minutes, then give second dose of 20 to 50 mg/kg IV in 1 hour if muscle weakness persists. May repeat dose every 10 to 12 hours p.r.n. Maximum is 2 g/dose. Or, if pulmonary edema is present or it isn't practical to give intermittent or continuous IV infusions, give dose of 20 to 50 mg/kg as 50-mg/mL solution in water by IV push slowly over 5 minutes. If muscle weakness persists, may give additional doses every 10 to 12 hours.
Children age 16 and younger with mild symptoms who weigh 40 kg or more (IM dosing): Give 600 mg IM. If symptoms persist after 15 minutes, give second dose of 600 mg IM. If symptoms persist 15 minutes after second dose, give third dose of 600 mg IM. Maximum combined dose for three injections is 1,800 mg. If patient develops severe symptoms at any time after first dose, administer second and third doses in rapid succession. For severe symptoms, give all three doses of 600 mg IM each in rapid succession for total combined dose of 1,800 mg.
Children age 16 and younger with mild symptoms who weigh less than 40 kg (IM dosing): Give 15 mg/kg IM in anterolateral thigh. If symptoms persist after 15 minutes, give second dose of 15 mg/kg IM. If symptoms persist after second dose, give third dose of 15 mg/kg IM. If patient develops severe symptoms at any time after first dose, give second and third doses in rapid succession. For severe symptoms, give all three doses of 15 mg/kg IM each in rapid succession. Maximum combined dose for three injections is 45 mg/kg.
➤**Control of overdosage by anticholinesterase drugs used in the treatment of myasthenia gravis**
Adults: 1 to 2 g IV; then 250 mg IV every 5 minutes, p.r.n.

protamine sulfate
PROE-ta-meen

Therapeutic class: Antidotes
Pharmacologic class: Heparin antagonists

AVAILABLE FORMS
Injection: 10 mg/mL

INDICATIONS & DOSAGES
Black Box Warning Drug can cause severe hypotension, CV collapse, noncardiogenic pulmonary edema, catastrophic pulmonary vasoconstriction, and pulmonary HTN. Keep vasopressors and resuscitation equipment immediately available. ■
➤ **Heparin overdose**
Adults: Dosage should be guided by blood coagulation studies. 1 mg of protamine sulfate neutralizes not less than 100 USP heparin units. Give by slow IV injection over 10 minutes in doses not to exceed 50 mg.

rasburicase
ras-BUR-ih-kase

Elitek

Therapeutic class: Replacement enzymes
Pharmacologic class: Recombinant urate-oxidases

AVAILABLE FORMS
Injection: 1.5 mg, 7.5 mg in single-dose vials with diluent

INDICATIONS & DOSAGES
Black Box Warning Drug can cause serious and fatal hypersensitivity reactions. Don't give to patients with G6PD deficiency; screen those at higher risk before starting therapy. Immediately and permanently discontinue drug if a serious hypersensitivity reaction, hemolysis, or methemoglobinemia occurs. ■
➤ **Initial management of plasma uric acid levels in patients with leukemia, lymphoma, and solid tumor malignancies who are receiving chemotherapy that's expected to result in tumor lysis and subsequent elevation of plasma uric acid level**
Adults and children: 0.2 mg/kg IV infusion over 30 minutes daily for up to 5 days.

sodium polystyrene sulfonate
pol-ee-STYE-reen

Kionex, SPS

Therapeutic class: Potassium-removing resins
Pharmacologic class: Cation-exchange resins

AVAILABLE FORMS
Powder: 3.5 g/tsp in 1-lb jar
Suspension: 15 g/60 mL*

INDICATIONS & DOSAGES
➤ **Hyperkalemia**
Adults: 15 g PO daily to q.i.d. in water or syrup (3 to 4 mL/g of resin). Or, mix powder with appropriate medium (aqueous suspension or diet appropriate for renal failure) and instill through NG tube. Or, 30 to 50 g as a suspension or in 100 mL of an aqueous vehicle every 6 hours as warm emulsion (at body temperature) deep into sigmoid colon (20 cm).

succimer
SUX-i-mer

Chemet

Therapeutic class: Chelating drugs
Pharmacologic class: Heavy metal chelators

AVAILABLE FORMS
Capsules: 100 mg

INDICATIONS & DOSAGES
➤ **Lead poisoning in children with lead levels greater than 45 mcg/dL**
Children age 12 months and older: Initially, 10 mg/kg or 350 mg/m^2 PO every 8 hours for 5 days. Then reduce to 10 mg/kg or 350 mg/m^2 PO every 12 hours for additional 14 days. Maximum, 500 mg/dose.

sugammadex sodium
su-GAM-ma-dex

Bridion

Therapeutic class: Antidotes
Pharmacologic class: Modified gamma cyclodextrins

AVAILABLE FORMS
Injection: 200 mg/2 mL, 500 mg/5 mL single-dose vials

INDICATIONS & DOSAGES
➤ **Reversal of neuromuscular blockade induced by rocuronium bromide and vecuronium bromide in adults undergoing surgery**
Adults (routine reversal of rocuronium- and vecuronium-induced neuromuscular blockade): Base doses and timing of drug administration on monitoring for twitch responses and extent of spontaneous recovery that has occurred. Give 4 mg/kg IV bolus over 10 seconds if recovery of the twitch response has reached 1 to 2 posttetanic counts (PTC) and there are no twitch responses to train-of-four (TOF) stimulation. Give 2 mg/kg IV over 10 seconds if spontaneous recovery has reached the reappearance of the second twitch (T_2) in response to TOF stimulation.
Adults (immediate reversal of rocuronium-induced neuromuscular blockade): If there is a clinical need to reverse neuromuscular blockade (approximately 3 minutes) after administration of a single 1.2-mg/kg dose of rocuronium, give sugammadex 16 mg/kg IV over 10 seconds.

♦ Off-label use   ⒹⒸDo not crush   *Liquid contains alcohol

Selected biologicals and blood derivatives: Indications and dosages

albumin 5%
al-BYOO-min

Albuked-5, Albuminar-5, Albuminex 5%, AlbuRx 5%, Albutein 5%, Buminate 5%, Flexbumin 5%, Plasbumin-5

albumin 25%
Albuked-25, Albuminar-25, Albuminex 25%, Albutein 25%, Buminate 25%, Flexbumin 25%, Human Albumin Grifols 25%, Kedbumin 25%, Plasbumin-25

Therapeutic class: Plasma volume expanders
Pharmacologic class: Blood derivatives

AVAILABLE FORMS
albumin 5%
Injection: 50 mg/mL in 50-mL, 250-mL, 500-mL vials
albumin 25%
Injection: 250 mg/mL in 20-mL, 50-mL, 100-mL vials

INDICATIONS & DOSAGES
➤ **Hypovolemic shock**
Adults: Initially, 12.5 to 25 g (250 to 500 mL) of 5% solution by IV infusion, repeated every 15 to 30 minutes, as needed. As plasma volume approaches normal, rate of infusion of 5% solution shouldn't exceed 2 to 4 mL/minute. Dosage of 25% solution varies with patient's condition and response. As plasma volume approaches normal, rate of infusion of 25% solution shouldn't exceed 1 mL/minute.
Infants and younger children: Initially, 0.5 to 1 g/kg/dose IV (10 to 20 mL/kg/dose of albumin 5%); repeat in 30-minute intervals as needed.
Older children and adolescents: Initially, 12.5 to 25 g IV (250 to 500 mL of albumin 5%); repeat in 30-minute intervals as needed.
➤ **Burns**
Adults: 25% solution infused no faster than 2 to 3 mL/minute (for Flexbumin, 1 mL/minute) to maintain plasma albumin concentration at approximately 2.5 ± 0.5 g/100 mL with a plasma oncotic pressure of 20 mm Hg (equal to a total plasma protein concentration of 5.2 g/100 mL). The duration of therapy is determined by the loss of protein from burned areas and in the urine.
➤ **Hypoproteinemia**
Adults: 200 to 300 mL of 25% albumin. Dosage varies with patient's condition and response. Usual daily

dose is 50 to 75 g. Rate of infusion shouldn't exceed 2 to 3 mL/minute.
Children: Usual daily dosage is 25 g or 25% albumin. Rate of infusion shouldn't exceed 2 mL/minute.
➤ **Acute nephrosis**
Adults: 100 mL of 25% albumin daily for 7 to 10 days in combination with a loop diuretic.
➤ **Hemolytic disease of the newborn**
Children: 1 g/kg body weight of 25% albumin IV before or during exchange transfusion.

antihemophilic factor (AHF factor VIII)
Advate, Adynovate, Afstyla, Eloctate, Helixate FS, Hemofil M, Koate-DVI, Kogenate FS, Kovaltry, Monoclate-P, Novoeight, Nuwiq, Obizur, Recombinate, ReFacto, Xyntha

Therapeutic class: Clotting factors
Pharmacologic class: Plasma proteins

AVAILABLE FORMS
Injection: Vials, with diluent; units specified on label

INDICATIONS & DOSAGES
Drug provides hemostasis in factor VIII deficiency, hemophilia A. Specific dosage depends on patient's weight, severity of hemorrhage, and presence of inhibitors. Mild bleeding episodes require a circulating factor VIII level 20% to 40% of normal; moderate to major bleeding episodes and minor surgery, a level 30% to 60% of normal; severe bleeding or major surgery, a level 60% to 100% of normal depending on product used. Refer to specific brand for actual dosage.

anti-inhibitor coagulant complex
Feiba, Feiba NF✱

Therapeutic class: Clotting factors
Pharmacologic class: Plasma proteins

AVAILABLE FORMS
Injection: Number of units of factor VIII correctional activity indicated on label of vial
Black Box Warning Thrombotic and thromboembolic events have been reported during postmarketing surveillance. ■

INDICATIONS & DOSAGES

➤ **To prevent or control hemorrhagic episodes in patients with hemophilia A and B with inhibitors**
Adults and children age 31 days and older: For joint hemorrhage, 50 to 100 units/kg IV every 12 hours until pain and acute disabilities improve. For mucous membrane hemorrhage, 50 to 100 units/kg IV every 6 hours for at least 1 day or until bleeding resolves. For soft-tissue hemorrhage, 100 units/kg IV every 12 hours until bleeding resolves. For other severe hemorrhage, 100 units/kg IV every 6 to 12 hours until bleeding resolves. For all indications, don't exceed a single dose of 100 units/kg body weight or a daily dose of 200 units/kg body weight.

➤ **Management of perioperative bleeding in patients with hemophilia A and B with inhibitors**
Adults and children age 31 days and older: 50 to 100 units/kg IV immediately before surgery as a one-time dose; then 50 to 100 units/kg IV every 6 to 12 hours postoperatively until bleeding resolves and healing is achieved. Don't exceed a single dose of 100 units/kg body weight or a daily dose of 200 units/kg body weight.

➤ **Routine prophylaxis to prevent or reduce frequency of bleeding episodes in patients with hemophilia A and B with inhibitors**
Adults and children age 31 days and older: 85 units/kg IV every other day.

beractant (natural lung surfactant)
ber-AKT-ant

Survanta

Therapeutic class: Lung surfactants
Pharmacologic class: Bovine lung extracts

AVAILABLE FORMS
Suspension for intratracheal instillation: 25 mg/mL

INDICATIONS & DOSAGES

➤ **To prevent respiratory distress syndrome (RDS), also known as hyaline membrane disease, in premature neonates weighing 1,250 g (2 lb, 12 oz) or less at birth or having symptoms consistent with surfactant deficiency**
Neonates: 4 mL/kg intratracheally. Divide each dose into four quarter-doses and give each quarter-dose with infant in a different position to ensure even distribution of drug; between quarter-doses, use a hand-held resuscitation bag at 60 breaths/minute and sufficient oxygen to prevent cyanosis. Give drug as soon as possible, preferably within 15 minutes of birth. Repeat in 6 hours if respiratory distress continues. Give no more than four doses in 48 hours.

➤ **Rescue treatment of RDS in premature infants**
Neonates: 4 mL/kg intratracheally; before giving, increase ventilator rate to 60 breaths/minute with an inspiratory time of 0.5 second and a fraction of inspired

oxygen of 1. Divide each dose into four quarter-doses and give each quarter-dose with infant in a different position to ensure even distribution of drug; between quarter doses, continue mechanical ventilation for at least 30 seconds or until stable. Give dose as soon as RDS is confirmed by X-ray, preferably within 8 hours of birth. Repeat in 6 hours if respiratory distress continues. Give no more than four doses in 48 hours.

calfactant
kal-FAK-tant

Infasurf

Therapeutic class: Lung surfactants
Pharmacologic class: Bovine lung extracts

AVAILABLE FORMS
Intratracheal suspension: 35 mg phospholipids and 0.7 mg proteins/mL in 3-mL, 6-mL vials

INDICATIONS & DOSAGES

➤ **To prevent respiratory distress syndrome (RDS) in premature infants younger than 29 weeks' gestational age at high risk for RDS; to treat infants younger than age 72 hours who develop RDS (confirmed by clinical and radiologic findings) and need an endotracheal tube**
Neonates: 3 mL/kg of body weight at birth intratracheally, given in two aliquots of 1.5 mL/kg each, every 12 hours for a total of up to three doses.

SAFETY ALERT!

cobimetinib fumarate
koe-bi-ME-ti-nib

Cotellic

Therapeutic class: Antineoplastics
Pharmacologic class: Kinase inhibitors

AVAILABLE FORMS
Tablets: 20 mg

INDICATIONS & DOSAGES

➤ **Unresectable or metastatic melanoma with a *BRAF* V600E or V600K mutation in combination with vemurafenib**
Adults: 60 mg PO once daily for first 21 days of each 28-day treatment cycle until disease progression or unacceptable toxicity.

Adjust-a-dose: Refer to manufacturer's instructions for toxicity-related dosage adjustments.

crizotinib

kriz-OH-ti-nib

Xalkori

Therapeutic class: Antineoplastics
Pharmacologic class: Tyrosine kinase inhibitors

AVAILABLE FORMS

Capsules: 200 mg, 250 mg

INDICATIONS & DOSAGES

➤ **Metastatic NSCLC that is anaplastic lymphoma kinase (ALK)– or ROS1-positive as detected by an FDA-approved test**
Adults: 250 mg PO b.i.d. until disease progression or intolerance occurs.
Adjust-a-dose: For patients with CrCl less than 30 mL/minute (not requiring dialysis), give 250 mg once daily. For patients with preexisting moderate hepatic impairment, give 200 mg b.i.d. For patients with preexisting severe hepatic impairment, give 250 mg once daily. Refer to manufacturer's instructions for toxicity-related dosage adjustments or discontinuance.

durvalumab

dur-VAL-ue-mab

Imfinzi

Therapeutic class: Antineoplastics
Pharmacologic class: Monoclonal antibodies

AVAILABLE FORMS

Injection: 500 mg/10 mL, 120 mg/2.4 mL single-dose vials

INDICATIONS & DOSAGES

Adjust-a-dose (for all indications): Refer to manufacturer's instructions for toxicity-related withholding or drug discontinuation.
➤ **Locally advanced or metastatic urothelial carcinoma in patients who have disease progression during or after platinum-containing chemotherapy or have disease progression within 12 months of neoadjuvant or adjuvant treatment with platinum-containing chemotherapy**
Adults: 10 mg/kg IV infusion every 2 weeks until disease progression or unacceptable toxicity occurs.
➤ **Unresectable, stage III NSCLC in patients whose disease hasn't progressed after concurrent platinum-based chemotherapy and radiation therapy**

Adults: 10 mg/kg IV infusion every 2 weeks until disease progression, unacceptable toxicity, or a maximum of 12 months.

eltrombopag �േ

ell-trom-BOW-pag

Promacta

Therapeutic class: Hematopoietics
Pharmacologic class: Thrombopoietin receptor agonists

AVAILABLE FORMS

Powder for oral suspension: 25-mg packet
Tablets ⓒⓡⓤ *:* 12.5 mg, 25 mg, 50 mg, 75 mg

INDICATIONS & DOSAGES

Black Box Warning   Drug increases risk of hepatotoxicity and hepatic decompensation when used in patients with HCV infection. Consult prescribing information for specific monitoring guidelines. ∎
➤ **Thrombocytopenia associated with chronic immune thrombocytopenic purpura when response to corticosteroids, immunoglobulins, or splenectomy is inadequate**
Adults and children age 6 and older: Initially, 50 mg PO once daily.
Children ages 1 to 5: Initially, 25 mg PO once daily.
Adjust-a-dose: Adjust dosage as necessary to achieve and maintain platelet count at 50×10^9/L or greater; maximum dosage is 75 mg daily. For patients older than age 6 and of East Asian descent or those with mild, moderate, or severe hepatic impairment, reduce dosage to 25 mg once daily. For patients older than age 6 of East Asian descent and any hepatic impairment, reduce dosage to 12.5 mg once daily. Refer to manufacturer's instructions for dosage adjustments based on hematologic parameters.
➤ **Thrombocytopenia in patients with chronic HCV infection to allow use of interferon-based therapy**
Adults: Initially, 25 mg PO once daily. Increase by 25-mg increments every 2 weeks as necessary to achieve target platelet count required to initiate antiviral therapy. Maximum dose is 100 mg daily.
Adjust-a-dose: During antiviral therapy, adjust dosage to avoid dose reduction of peginterferon. Refer to manufacturer's instruction for dosage adjustments based on hematologic parameters. Discontinue drug when antiviral treatment is stopped.
➤ **Severe aplastic anemia when response to immunosuppressive therapy is insufficient** ✻
Adults: Initially, 50 mg PO once daily. Adjust dosage as necessary in 50-mg increments every 2 weeks to achieve target platelet count of 50×10^9/L or greater. Maximum dosage is 150 mg daily.
Adjust-a-dose: In patients of East Asian descent or those with mild, moderate, or severe hepatic impairment, reduce initial dosage to 25 mg once daily. Refer

to manufacturer's instructions for dosage adjustments based on hematologic parameters.

If no hematologic response has occurred after 16 weeks of therapy, or new cytogenetic abnormalities are observed, discontinue drug.

➤ **First-line treatment of severe aplastic anemia in combination with standard immunosuppressive therapy** 𝕏

Adults and children age 12 and older: 150 mg PO once daily for 6 months.

Children ages 6 to 11: 75 mg PO once daily for 6 months.

Children ages 2 to 5: 2.5 mg/kg PO once daily for 6 months.

Adjust-a-dose: In patients of East Asian descent or those with mild, moderate, or severe hepatic impairment (Child-Pugh class A, B, C), reduce initial dosage by 50%. Don't initiate if baseline ALT or AST level is more than 6 × ULN. Refer to manufacturer's instructions for toxicity-related dosage adjustments.

factor IX complex
Profilnine, Profilnine SD

factor IX (human)
AlphaNine SD, Mononine

factor IX (recombinant)
Alprolix, BeneFIX, Ixinity, Rixubis

Therapeutic class: Clotting factors
Pharmacologic class: Plasma proteins

AVAILABLE FORMS
Injection: Vials, with diluent; international units specified on label

INDICATIONS & DOSAGES
➤ **Factor IX deficiency (also called hemophilia B or Christmas disease)**

Adults and children: Dosage is highly individualized, depending on degree of deficiency, level of factor IX desired, patient's weight and condition, and severity of bleeding. Infusion rates vary with product and patient comfort. Refer to manufacturer's instructions for each product to calculate dosage.

hepatitis B immune globulin (human)
hep-ah-TYE-tis

HepaGam B, HyperHEP B S/D, Nabi-HB

Therapeutic class: Prophylaxis drugs
Pharmacologic class: Immune serums

AVAILABLE FORMS
Injection: 1-mL, 5-mL vials; 0.5-mL neonatal single-dose syringe; 1-mL single-dose syringe

INDICATIONS & DOSAGES
➤ **HBV exposure in high-risk patients**

Adults and children: 0.06 mL/kg (usual dose is 3 to 5 mL) IM as soon as possible (within 24 hours if possible) but within 7 days after exposure (within 14 days if sexual exposure). Repeat dose 28 days after exposure if patient doesn't elect to receive the hepatitis B vaccine.

Neonates born to HBsAg-positive patients: 0.5 mL IM within 12 hours of birth. Active vaccination with hepatitis B vaccine may begin at the same time.

➤ **To prevent recurrence of HBV infection after liver transplantation in HBsAg-positive liver transplant patients (HepaGam B only)**

Adults: 20,000 international units IV at rate of 2 mL/minute. Give first dose simultaneously with the grafting of the transplanted liver (anhepatic phase); then give daily on days 1 through 7, every 2 weeks from day 14 through 12 weeks, and monthly from month 4 onward.

Adjust-a-dose: Adjust dose in patients who don't reach anti-HBs levels of 500 international units/L within the first week after transplantation. Give 10,000 international units IV until target level is reached.

immune globulin intramuscular (gamma globulin, IG, IGIM)
GamaSTAN S/D

immune globulin intravenous (IGIV)
Bivigam, Carimune NF, Flebogamma DIF, Gammagard Liquid, Gammagard S/D, Gammaked, Gammaplex, Gamunex-C, Octagam, Panzyga, Privigen

immune globulin subcutaneous (IGSC, SCIG)
Cuvitru, Gammagard, Gamunex-C, Hizentra, HyQvia

Therapeutic class: Antibodies
Pharmacologic class: Immune serums

AVAILABLE FORMS
immune globulin intramuscular
Injection: 15% to 18% in 2-mL, 10-mL single-dose vials
immune globulin intravenous
Powder for injection (preservative free): 2.5-g, 3-g, 5-g, 6-g, 10-g, 12-g vials
Solution, injection (preservative free): 5% in 10-mL, 25-mL, 50-mL, 100-mL, 200-mL, 400-mL, 500-mL vials; 10% in 10-mL, 20-mL, 50-mL, 100-mL, 200-mL, 300-mL, 400-mL vials

immune globulin subcutaneous
Solution, injection (kit): 10% in 25-mL, 50-mL, 200-mL, 300-mL vials
Solution, injection (preservative free): 20% in 5-mL, 10-mL, 20-mL, 50-mL vials

INDICATIONS & DOSAGES
■ **Black Box Warning** Increases risk of thrombosis; may occur in the absence of known risk factors. Don't exceed recommended dosage. ∎
■ **Black Box Warning** Renal dysfunction and acute renal failure (excluding Cuvitru, Hizentra, HyQvia, Gammastan, and GamaSTAN S/D): Renal dysfunction, acute renal failure, osmotic nephrosis, and death may occur in predisposed patients with IGIV products. ∎
➤ **Primary immunodeficiency**
Bivigam
Adults and children age 6 and older: 300 to 800 mg/kg IV every 3 to 4 weeks. Begin IV infusion at a rate of 0.5 mg/kg/minute for the first 10 minutes. Increase every 20 minutes, if tolerated, by 0.8 mg/kg/minute, up to a maximum rate of 6 mg/kg/minute.
Carimune NF
Adults and children: 400 to 800 mg/kg IV every 3 to 4 weeks. First infusion in previously untreated patients must be given as a 3% Ig solution at initial infusion rate of 0.5 mg/kg/minute. If tolerated, after 30 minutes the rate may be increased to 1 mg/kg/minute for the next 30 minutes, then gradually increased in a stepwise manner up to a maximum of 3 mg/kg/minute as tolerated. See package insert for infusion rates in mL/kg/minute.
Flebogamma DIF
Adults: 300 to 600 mg/kg 10% solution IV every 3 to 4 weeks. Infuse at 1 mg/kg/minute. If tolerated after 30 minutes, may gradually increase rate to 4 mg/kg/minute; then to a maximum of 8 mg/kg/minute.
Adults and children age 2 and older: 300 to 600 mg/kg 5% solution IV every 3 to 4 weeks. Infuse at 0.5 mg/kg/minute; may gradually increase after 30 minutes to 5 mg/kg/minute.
Gammagard Liquid
Adults and children age 2 and older: 300 to 600 mg/kg IV every 3 to 4 weeks. Infuse at 0.8 mg/kg/minute and increase every 30 minutes to 8 mg/kg/minute. Maintenance therapy may be given subcut starting 1 week after last IGIV infusion. Initial subcut dose is 1.37 × current IV dose in mg/kg ÷ number of weeks between IV doses.
Gammagard S/D
Adults and children age 2 and older: 300 to 600 mg/kg IV every 3 to 4 weeks depending on patient response, initially infused in a 5% solution at 0.5 mL/kg/hour that may be increased gradually if patient doesn't experience distress to a maximum rate of 4 mL/kg/hour for patients with no history of adverse reactions to IGIV and no significant risk factors for renal dysfunction or thrombotic complications. See package insert for subsequent solution concentration and infusion-rate increases.

Gammaked
Adults and children age 2 and older: 300 to 600 mg/kg IV every 3 to 4 weeks. Initially (first 30 minutes), 1 mg/kg/minute, increased gradually (if tolerated) up to 8 mg/kg/minute. Maintenance therapy may be given subcut starting 1 week after last IGIV infusion. Initial subcut dose is 1.37 × current IV dose in mg/kg ÷ number of weeks between IV doses.
Gammaplex 5%
Adults and children age 2 and older: 300 to 800 mg/kg IV every 3 to 4 weeks. Initially (first 15 minutes), 0.5 mg/kg/minute, increased every 15 minutes (if tolerated) up to 4 mg/kg/minute.
Gammaplex 10%
Adults: 300 to 800 mg/kg IV every 3 to 4 weeks. Initially (first 15 minutes), 0.5 mg/kg/minute; increase every 15 minutes (if tolerated) up to 8 mg/kg/minute.
Gamunex-C
Adults and children age 2 and older: 300 to 600 mg/kg IV every 3 to 4 weeks. Initially (first 30 minutes), 1 mg/kg/minute; increase (if tolerated) up to 8 mg/kg/minute. May give maintenance therapy subcut starting 1 week after last IGIV infusion. Initial subcut dose is 1.37 × current IV dose in mg/kg ÷ number of weeks between IV doses.
Hizentra
Adults and children age 2 and older: Initial weekly dose is the previous IGIV dose in grams ÷ number of weeks between IGIV doses × 1.37. Multiply dose in grams by 5 to obtain dose in milliliters.

When switching to biweekly dosing, multiply the calculated Hizentra weekly dose by 2. Adjust dose based on clinical response and IgG trough levels. Give by subcut infusion weekly, biweekly, or more frequently. See package insert for full dosage adjustment guidelines, recommended number of subcut sites, and infusion rates.
HyQvia
Adults: See manufacturer's labeling for initial ramp-up schedule.
Patients naive to IgG therapy or switching from IG subcutaneous therapy: 300 to 600 mg/kg subcut infusion every 3 to 4 weeks, after the initial dose ramp-up.
Patients switching from IGIV therapy: Administer the same dose and frequency as the previous IGIV therapy by subcut infusion every 3 to 4 weeks after the initial dose ramp-up. For subsequent dose adjustments, refer to manufacturer's instructions.
Octagam (5%)
Adults and children age 6 and older: 300 to 600 mg/kg IV every 3 to 4 weeks. Start infusion at 30 mg/kg/hour for 30 minutes. May double mg/kg/hour rate every 30 minutes until a maximum rate of 200 mg/kg/hour is reached.
Privigen
Adults: 200 to 800 mg/kg IV every 3 to 4 weeks. Start infusion at 0.5 mg/kg/minute and increase slowly to 8 mg/kg/minute.

➤ **Chronic inflammatory demyelinating polyneuropathy**
Gamunex-C, Gammaked
Adults: 2,000 mg/kg IV in divided doses over 2 to 4 days every 3 weeks. Maintenance dose, 1,000 mg/kg IV over 1 day every 3 weeks or 500 mg/kg IV on 2 consecutive days every 3 weeks.

Hizentra
Adults: For maintenance therapy, begin subcut infusion 1 week after the last IGIV infusion. Give 200 to 400 mg/kg/week subcut using an infusion pump, in one or two sessions over 1 or 2 consecutive days to prevent relapse. Refer to package insert for recommended number of subcut sites, infusion rates, and dosage adjustments if symptoms worsen during treatment.

Privigen
Adults: Initial loading dose is 2,000 mg/kg IV infusion in divided doses over 2 to 5 consecutive days. Maintenance dose, 1,000 mg/kg IV as one to two infusions on consecutive days, every 3 weeks for 6 months.

➤ **ITP (acute)**
Carimune NF
Adults and children: 400 mg/kg/day IV for 2 to 5 consecutive days, depending on platelet count and immune response.

Gammagard S/D
Adults: 1,000 mg/kg IV. May give up to three separate doses on alternate days, if needed, as determined by clinical response and platelet count.

Gamunex-C, Gammaked
Adults: 2,000 mg/kg IV in divided doses over 2 days or 400 mg/kg IV in five doses over 5 days.

➤ **ITP (chronic)**
Gammaplex 5% or 10%, Octagam (10%), Privigen, Panzyga
Adults: 1,000 mg/kg/day IV for 2 consecutive days.

➤ **Chronic primary immune thrombocytopenia**
Flebogamma DIF 10%
Adults and children age 2 and older: 1 g/kg body weight (10 mL/kg) IV infusion daily for 2 consecutive days.

➤ **Multifocal motor neuropathy**
Gammagard Liquid
Adults: 500 to 2,400 mg/kg/month IV based on response.

➤ **Kawasaki syndrome**
Gammagard S/D
Children: 400 mg/kg IV daily over 2 hours for 4 consecutive days, or a single dose of 1,000 mg/kg over 10 hours. Start within 7 days of fever onset. Give with aspirin (80 to 100 mg/kg PO daily in four divided doses).

➤ **Hepatitis A exposure (IGIM)**
Adults and children: 0.1 mL/kg IM as soon as possible after household or institutional exposure. Not indicated in persons with signs and symptoms of hepatitis A or in those exposed more than 2 weeks previously. Refer to product insert for dosages for persons who plan to travel in areas where hepatitis A is common.

➤ **Measles exposure (IGIM)**
Adults and children: 0.25 mL/kg IM within 6 days after exposure.

➤ **Measles postexposure prophylaxis (IGIM)**
Immunocompromised children: 0.5 mL/kg IM (maximum, 15 mL) immediately after exposure (within 6 days).

➤ **Chickenpox exposure (IGIM)**
Adults and children: 0.6 to 1.2 mL/kg IM as soon as possible after exposure (within 3 days).

➤ **Rubella exposure in first trimester of pregnancy (IGIM)**
Women: 0.55 mL/kg IM as soon as possible after exposure (within 72 hours).

➤ **B-cell chronic lymphocytic leukemia**
Adults and children: 400 mg/kg IV Gammagard S/D every 3 to 4 weeks for patients with hypogammaglobulinemia or recurrent bacterial infections.

➤ **Guillain-Barré syndrome (IGIV)** ◆
Adults: 2,000 mg/kg IV over 2 to 5 days within 2 to 4 weeks of onset.

➤ **Acquired hypogammaglobulinemia secondary to malignancy** ◆
Adults: 400 mg/kg/dose IV every 3 weeks. Reevaluate every 4 to 6 months.

---

lymphocyte immune globulin (antithymocyte globulin [equine], ATG, LIG)

LIM-foh-site

Atgam

Therapeutic class: Immunosuppressants
Pharmacologic class: Immunoglobulins

AVAILABLE FORMS
Injection: 50 mg of equine IgG/mL in 5-mL ampules

INDICATIONS & DOSAGES
Black Box Warning Drug can cause anaphylaxis. Only use drug in facilities with adequate laboratory and supportive medical resources. ■

➤ **Acute renal allograft rejection**
Adults and children: 10 to 15 mg/kg IV daily for 14 days. Additional alternate-day therapy to total of 21 doses can be given. Start therapy when rejection is diagnosed.

➤ **Aplastic anemia**
Adults and children: 10 to 20 mg/kg IV daily for 8 to 14 days. Additional alternate-day therapy to total of 21 doses can be given.

plasma protein fraction
Plasmanate

Therapeutic class: Plasma volume expanders
Pharmacologic class: Plasma proteins

AVAILABLE FORMS
Injection: 5% (50 mg/mL) solution in 50-mL, 250-mL vials

INDICATIONS & DOSAGES
➤ **Shock**
Adults: Dosage varies with patient's condition and response.

SAFETY ALERT!

protein C concentrate ▨
Ceprotin

Therapeutic class: Anticoagulants
Pharmacologic class: Protein C replacements

AVAILABLE FORMS
Injection: 500 international units/vial, 1,000 international units/vial

INDICATIONS & DOSAGES
Adjust-a-dose (for all indications): Dose is adjusted based on severity of protein C deficiency, plasma level of protein C, and patient's age and condition.
➤ **Venous thrombosis and purpura fulminans in patients with severe congenital protein C deficiency** ▨
Adults, neonates, and children: Initially for acute episodes and short-term prophylaxis, 100 to 120 international units/kg IV; then, 60 to 80 international units/kg IV every 6 hours for subsequent three doses to maintain peak protein C activity of 100%. Maintenance dose of 45 to 60 international units/kg IV every 6 to 12 hours to maintain trough protein C activity levels above 25%.
➤ **Long-term prevention of venous thrombosis and purpura fulminans** ▨
Adults, neonates, and children: 45 to 60 international units/kg IV every 12 hours to maintain trough protein C activity levels above 25%.

rabies immune globulin (human)
RAY-beez

HyperRAB, Imogam Rabies-HT, Kedrab

Therapeutic class: Antibodies
Pharmacologic class: Immunoglobulins

AVAILABLE FORMS
Injection: 150 international units/mL in 2-mL, 10-mL vials; 300 international units/mL in 1-mL, 5-mL vials

INDICATIONS & DOSAGES
➤ **Rabies exposure**
Adults and children: 20 international units/kg IM at time of first dose of rabies vaccine. If anatomically feasible, up to the full dose is used to infiltrate wound area; remainder is given IM in a different site.

Rh₀(D) immune globulin intramuscular (human) (IGIM)
HyperRHO S/D Full Dose, HyperRHO S/D Mini-Dose, MICRhoGAM, RhoGAM

Rh₀(D) immune globulin intravenous (human) (IGIV)
Rhophylac, WinRho SDF

Therapeutic class: Immune globulins
Pharmacologic class: Immunoglobulins

AVAILABLE FORMS
IGIM
Injection: 300-mcg syringe (1,500 international units, standard dose); 50-mcg syringe (250 international units, microdose)
IGIV
Injection: 120-mcg (600 international units), 300-mcg (1,500 international units), 500-mcg (2,500 international units), 1,000-mcg (5,000 international units), 3,000-mcg (15,000 international units) vials; 300-mcg (1,500 international units) syringe

INDICATIONS & DOSAGES
Black Box Warning Intravascular hemolysis leading to ARDS and death has been reported in patients treated for ITP with IGIV. ■
➤ **Rh exposure after abortion, miscarriage, ectopic pregnancy, or childbirth**
Adults: Transfusion unit or blood bank determines fetal packed RBC volume entering patient's blood; one vial IGIM is given IM if fetal packed RBC volume is less than 15 mL. More than one vial IM may be needed if severe fetomaternal hemorrhage occurs; must be given within 72 hours after delivery or miscarriage.

➤ **To prevent Rh antibody formation after abortion or miscarriage**
Adults: Consult transfusion unit or blood bank. Up to and including 12 weeks' gestation, one IGIM microdose vial IM will suppress immune reaction to 2.5 mL $Rh_0(D)$-positive RBCs. At 13 weeks' gestation and later, use one vial IGIM standard dose. Ideally, give within 3 hours, but may be given up to 72 hours after abortion or miscarriage.

➤ **Rh exposure after abortion, amniocentesis after 34 weeks' gestation, or other manipulations past 34 weeks' gestation with increased risk of Rh isoimmunization**
Adults: 120 mcg IGIV, given IV or IM within 72 hours of delivery, miscarriage, or manipulation.

➤ **To suppress Rh isoimmunization during pregnancy**
Adults: 300 mcg IV or IM at 28 weeks' gestation. If given early in pregnancy, give additional doses at 12-week intervals to maintain adequate levels of passively acquired anti-Rh antibodies. Then, within 72 hours of delivery, give 120 mcg WinRho or 300 mcg HyperRHO, RhoGAM, or Rhophylac IM or IV. If 72 hours have elapsed, give drug as soon as possible, up to 28 days.

➤ **Incompatible blood transfusion**
Adults: 600 mcg IV every 8 hours or 1,200 mcg IM every 12 hours until total dose given. Total dose depends on volume of packed RBCs or whole blood infused. Consult blood bank or transfusion unit at once; must be given within 72 hours.

➤ **$Rh_0(D)$ antigen–positive patients with chronic ITP; ITP secondary to HIV; children with acute ITP**
Adults and children: Initially, 50 mcg/kg IV as single dose or divided into two doses on separate days. If Hb level is less than 10 g/dL, reduce first dose to 25 to 40 mcg/kg. Then, give 25 to 60 mcg/kg IV as needed to elevate platelet count with specific individually determined dosage.

romiPLOStim
roh-mih-PLOH-stim

Nplate

Therapeutic class: Hematopoietics
Pharmacologic class: Thrombopoietin receptor agonists

AVAILABLE FORMS
Injection: 125-mcg, 250-mcg, 500-mcg single-use vials

INDICATIONS & DOSAGES
➤ **Thrombocytopenia in patients with chronic immune ITP who have had an insufficient response to corticosteroids, immunoglobulins, or splenectomy**
Adults: Initially, 1 mcg/kg subcut once weekly. Adjust dosage in increments of 1 mcg/kg/week to maintain platelet count of 50×10^9/L or higher, as needed, to

reduce the risk of bleeding. Maximum dose, 10 mcg/kg weekly. Refer to manufacturer's instructions for dosage adjustments for platelet counts. Discontinue if platelet count doesn't increase after 4 weeks at maximum dose.

tetanus immune globulin (human)
HyperTET S/D

Therapeutic class: Prophylaxis drugs
Pharmacologic class: Immunoglobulins

AVAILABLE FORMS
Injection: 250-unit vial or syringe

INDICATIONS & DOSAGES
➤ **Postexposure prevention of tetanus after injury, in patients whose immunization is incomplete or unknown**
Adults and children: 250 units deep IM injection.

Common combination drugs: Indications and dosages

Refer to manufacturer's instructions for complete prescribing and safety information.

Analgesics

acetaminophen–butalbital–caffeine–codeine phosphate
Fioricet with Codeine ☒
Controlled Substance Schedule: III
AVAILABLE FORMS
Capsules
325 mg acetaminophen, 50 mg butalbital, 40 mg caffeine, and 30 mg codeine phosphate
INDICATIONS & DOSAGES
Black Box Warning Acetaminophen has been associated with cases of acute liver failure and death. Codeine can cause respiratory depression and death in children. Opioids combined with benzodiazepines or CNS depressants can cause death. Use during pregnancy can cause neonatal opioid withdrawal. ■
➤ **Tension headache**
Adults: 1 to 2 capsules PO every 4 hours. Maximum dosage, 6 capsules in 24 hours.

codeine phosphate–aspirin–butalbital–caffeine
Fiorinal with Codeine ☒
Controlled Substance Schedule: III
AVAILABLE FORMS
Capsules
30 mg codeine phosphate, 325 mg aspirin, 50 mg butalbital, and 40 mg caffeine
INDICATIONS & DOSAGES
Black Box Warning Opioids combined with benzodiazepines or CNS depressants can cause death. Accidental ingestion by children can cause death. Use during pregnancy can cause neonatal opioid withdrawal. ■
➤ **Headache, mild to moderate pain**
Adults: 1 to 2 capsules PO every 4 hours. Maximum dosage, 6 capsules in 24 hours.

hydrocodone bitartrate–ibuprofen
Ibudone, Reprexain
Controlled Substance Schedule: II
AVAILABLE FORMS
Tablets
2.5 mg hydrocodone bitartrate and 200 mg ibuprofen
5 mg hydrocodone bitartrate and 200 mg ibuprofen
7.5 mg hydrocodone bitartrate and 200 mg ibuprofen
10 mg hydrocodone bitartrate and 200 mg ibuprofen
INDICATIONS & DOSAGES
Black Box Warning Opioids combined with benzodiazepines or CNS depressants can cause death. Use during pregnancy can cause neonatal opioid withdrawal. Accidental ingestion by children can cause death. Fatal CV and GI events can occur. ■

➤ **Acute pain (short-term)**
Adults and children age 16 and older: 1 tablet PO every 4 to 6 hours p.r.n. Maximum dosage, 5 tablets in 24 hours.

ibuprofen–famotidine
Duexis
AVAILABLE FORMS
Tablets ⓄⓃⒸ
800 mg ibuprofen and 26.6 mg famotidine
INDICATIONS & DOSAGES
Black Box Warning NSAIDs are contraindicated after CABG surgery and may cause an increased risk of serious CV thrombotic events, MI, stroke, and GI adverse reactions (bleeding, ulceration, and perforation), which can be fatal. ■
➤ **RA and osteoarthritis**
Adults: 1 tablet PO t.i.d. Elderly patients may need reduced dosages. Use not recommended in patients with CrCl less than 50 mL/minute.

naproxen–esomeprazole
Vimovo
AVAILABLE FORMS
Tablets ⓄⓃⒸ
375 mg naproxen and 20 mg esomeprazole
500 mg naproxen and 20 mg esomeprazole
INDICATIONS & DOSAGES
Black Box Warning Contraindicated for use in CABG surgery. Drug may cause an increased risk of serious CV thrombotic events, MI, stroke, and GI adverse reactions (bleeding, ulceration, and perforation), which can be fatal. ■
➤ **Osteoarthritis, RA, ankylosing spondylitis; to decrease risk of gastric ulcer development**
Adults: 1 tablet PO b.i.d.
➤ **Juvenile idiopathic arthritis**
Adults and adolescents age 12 and older weighing more than 50 kg: 1 tablet PO b.i.d.
Adolescents age 12 and older weighing 38 to less than 50 kg: 1 tablet (375 naproxen/20 mg esomeprazole) PO b.i.d.

oxyCODONE hydrochloride–aspirin
Controlled Substance Schedule: II
AVAILABLE FORMS
Tablets
4.8355 mg oxycodone hydrochloride and 325 mg aspirin
INDICATIONS & DOSAGES
Black Box Warning Opioids combined with benzodiazepines or CNS depressants can cause death. Use during pregnancy can cause neonatal opioid withdrawal. Accidental ingestion by children can cause death. ■
➤ **Moderate to moderately severe pain**
Adults: 1 tablet PO every 6 hours. Maximum dosage, 12 tablets in 24 hours.

pentazocine–naloxone hydrochloride
Controlled Substance Schedule: IV
AVAILABLE FORMS
Tablets
50 mg pentazocine and 0.5 mg naloxone hydrochloride
INDICATIONS & DOSAGES
Black Box Warning Drug is for oral use only; severe, potentially lethal, reactions may result from misuse by injection. Opioids combined with benzodiazepines or CNS depressants can cause death. Use during pregnancy can cause neonatal opioid withdrawal. Accidental ingestion by children can cause death. ■
➤ **Moderate to severe pain**
Adults and children age 12 and older: 1 tablet PO every 3 to 4 hours. May increase to 2 tablets if necessary. Maximum dosage, 12 tablets in 24 hours.

tramadol hydrochloride–acetaminophen
Ultracet 🖉 🗵
Controlled Substance Schedule: IV
AVAILABLE FORMS
Tablets
37.5 mg tramadol hydrochloride and 325 mg acetaminophen
INDICATIONS & DOSAGES
Black Box Warning Acetaminophen has been associated with acute liver failure and death. Opioids combined with benzodiazepines or CNS depressants can cause death. Use during pregnancy can cause neonatal opioid withdrawal. Accidental ingestion by children can cause death. Drug exposes users to risks of addiction, abuse, and misuse. May cause serious, life-threatening, or fatal respiratory depression. Use with CYP3A4 inducers or inhibitors or CYP2D6 inhibitors requires careful consideration of the effects on the parent drug and active metabolite. ■
➤ **Acute pain**
Adults: 2 tablets PO every 4 to 6 hours as needed for up to 5 days. Maximum dosage, 8 tablets in 24 hours.

Antiacne drugs

benzoyl peroxide–adapalene
Epiduo, Epiduo Forte
AVAILABLE FORMS
Topical gel
2.5% benzoyl peroxide and 0.1% adapalene
2.5% benzoyl peroxide and 0.3% adapalene
INDICATIONS & DOSAGES
➤ **Acne vulgaris**
Adults and children age 9 and older (Epiduo): Apply a thin film to affected areas of face or trunk once daily after washing.
Adults and children age 12 and older (Epiduo Forte): Apply a thin film to affected areas of face or trunk once daily after washing.

clindamycin phosphate–tretinoin
Veltin, Ziana
AVAILABLE FORMS
Topical gel
Clindamycin phosphate 1.2% and tretinoin 0.025%
INDICATIONS & DOSAGES
➤ **Acne vulgaris**
Adults and children age 12 and older: Apply pea-size amount to cover entire affected area once daily in the evening or at bedtime. Avoid eyes, lips, and mucous membranes.

norethindrone–ethinyl estradiol
norethindrone–ethinyl estradiol–ferrous fumarate
Estrostep Fe
AVAILABLE FORMS
Tablets
1 mg norethindrone and 20 mcg ethinyl estradiol
1 mg norethindrone and 30 mcg ethinyl estradiol
1 mg norethindrone, 35 mcg ethinyl estradiol, and 75 mg ferrous fumarate
INDICATIONS & DOSAGES
Black Box Warning Risk of serious CV events; not for use by women older than age 35 who smoke. ■
➤ **Acne vulgaris**
Women older than age 15: 1 tablet PO daily.

norgestimate–ethinyl estradiol
Ortho Tri-Cyclen
AVAILABLE FORMS
Tablets
0.18 mg norgestimate and 35 mcg ethinyl estradiol
0.215 mg norgestimate and 35 mcg ethinyl estradiol
0.25 mg norgestimate and 35 mcg ethinyl estradiol
INDICATIONS & DOSAGES
Black Box Warning Risk of serious CV events; not for use by women older than age 35 who smoke. ■
➤ **Acne vulgaris**
Women older than age 15: 1 tablet PO daily.

Antidiabetics

alogliptin benzoate–metFORMIN hydrochloride
Kazano
AVAILABLE FORMS
Tablets
12.5 mg alogliptin benzoate and 500 mg metformin
12.5 mg alogliptin benzoate and 1,000 mg metformin
INDICATIONS & DOSAGES
Black Box Warning Metformin can cause serious and sometimes fatal lactic acidosis; prompt hemodialysis is recommended. ■
➤ **Adjunct to diet and exercise to improve glycemic control in adults with type 2 diabetes**
Adults: 1 tablet PO b.i.d. with food. Adjust dosage based on effectiveness and tolerability. Maximum daily dose, 25 mg alogliptin and 2,000 mg metformin.
Adjust-a-dose: Discontinue drug if eGFR falls below 30 mL/minute/1.73 m^2.

alogliptin benzoate–pioglitazone hydrochloride

Oseni

AVAILABLE FORMS

Tablets

12.5 mg alogliptin benzoate and 15 mg pioglitazone hydrochloride

12.5 mg alogliptin benzoate and 30 mg pioglitazone hydrochloride

12.5 mg alogliptin benzoate and 45 mg pioglitazone hydrochloride

25 mg alogliptin benzoate and 15 mg pioglitazone hydrochloride

25 mg alogliptin benzoate and 30 mg pioglitazone hydrochloride

25 mg alogliptin benzoate and 45 mg pioglitazone hydrochloride

INDICATIONS & DOSAGES

Black Box Warning Pioglitazone can cause or exacerbate HF. Drug isn't recommended in patients with symptomatic HF and is contraindicated in patients with NYHA Class III or IV HF. ∎

➤ **Adjunct to diet and exercise to improve glycemic control in adults with type 2 diabetes mellitus when treatment with both alogliptin and pioglitazone is appropriate**

Adults inadequately controlled on diet and exercise, inadequately controlled on metformin monotherapy, or who require additional glycemic control on alogliptin: Alogliptin 25 mg/pioglitazone 15 mg or alogliptin 25 mg/pioglitazone 30 mg PO once daily. May titrate to a maximum of alogliptin 25 mg/pioglitazone 45 mg once daily based on glycemic response as determined by HbA$_{1c}$.

Adults who require additional glycemic control on pioglitazone: Alogliptin 25 mg/pioglitazone 15 mg, alogliptin 25 mg/pioglitazone 30 mg, or alogliptin 25 mg/pioglitazone 45 mg PO once daily as appropriate based on current therapy. May titrate to a maximum of alogliptin 25 mg/pioglitazone 45 mg once daily based on glycemic response as determined by HbA$_{1c}$.

Adults switching from alogliptin administered with pioglitazone: Initiate at the dosage of alogliptin and pioglitazone based on current therapy. May titrate to a maximum of alogliptin 25 mg/pioglitazone 45 mg once daily based on glycemic response as determined by HbA$_{1c}$.

Adults with HF (NYHA Class I or II): Alogliptin 25 mg/pioglitazone 15 mg PO once daily. May titrate to a maximum of alogliptin 25 mg/pioglitazone 45 mg once daily based on glycemic response as determined by HbA$_{1c}$.

canagliflozin–metFORMIN hydrochloride

Invokamet, Invokamet XR

AVAILABLE FORMS

Tablets (immediate-release)

50 mg canagliflozin and 500 mg metformin

50 mg canagliflozin and 1,000 mg metformin

150 mg canagliflozin and 500 mg metformin

150 mg canagliflozin and 1,000 mg metformin

Tablets (extended-release) 🞜

50 mg canagliflozin and 500 mg extended-release metformin

50 mg canagliflozin and 1,000 mg extended-release metformin

150 mg canagliflozin and 500 mg extended-release metformin

150 mg canagliflozin and 1,000 mg extended-release metformin

INDICATIONS & DOSAGES

Black Box Warning Canagliflozin is associated with increased risk of lower limb amputations in patients with type 2 diabetes who have, or are at risk for, CV disease. Metformin can cause serious and sometimes fatal lactic acidosis; prompt hemodialysis is recommended. ∎

➤ **Adjunct to diet and exercise to improve glycemic control in adults with type 2 diabetes when treatment with both canagliflozin and metformin is appropriate**

Adults not on canagliflozin or metformin: Initiate therapy with 50 mg canagliflozin and 500 mg metformin PO b.i.d. with meals. Or, 2 extended-release tablets, each containing 50 mg canagliflozin and 500 mg metformin, once daily with morning meal.

Adults already on metformin: 50 mg canagliflozin plus previously prescribed dose of metformin PO b.i.d. with meals. Or, extended-release tablets containing 100 mg canagliflozin plus previously prescribed dose of metformin PO once daily with morning meal.

Adults already on canagliflozin: 500 mg metformin plus previously prescribed dose of canagliflozin PO b.i.d. with meals. Or, extended-release tablets containing 1,000 mg metformin plus previously prescribed dose of canagliflozin PO once daily with morning meal.

Adults already on canagliflozin and metformin: Switch to the same total daily doses of each component PO b.i.d. with meals. Or, use extended-release product once daily with morning meal.

Adjust-a-dose: Increase dosage gradually if needed to reduce metformin's GI adverse effects. Don't exceed maximum daily dose of 2,000 mg of metformin and 300 mg of canagliflozin. Limit dose of the canagliflozin component to 50 mg b.i.d. in patients with moderate renal impairment with an eGFR of 45 to less than 60 mL/minute/1.73 m^2. Discontinue drug if eGFR falls below 45 mL/minute/1.73 m^2.

dapagliflozin–sAXagliptin

Qtern

AVAILABLE FORMS

Tablets 🞜

10 mg dapagliflozin/5 mg saxagliptin

INDICATIONS & DOSAGES

➤ **Adjunct to diet and exercise to improve glycemic control in patients with type 2 diabetes who have inadequate control with dapagliflozin or who are already treated with dapagliflozin and saxagliptin**

Adults: 1 tablet PO once daily in the morning.

glipiZIDE–metFORMIN hydrochloride

AVAILABLE FORMS
Tablets
2.5 mg glipizide and 250 mg metformin hydrochloride
2.5 mg glipizide and 500 mg metformin hydrochloride
5 mg glipizide and 500 mg metformin hydrochloride

INDICATIONS & DOSAGES
Black Box Warning Metformin can cause serious and sometimes fatal lactic acidosis; prompt hemodialysis is recommended. ∎

Adjust-a-dose (for all indications): Discontinue drug if eGFR falls below 30 mL/minute/1.73 m^2.

➤ **As initial adjunctive therapy to diet and exercise to improve glycemic control in adults with type 2 diabetes**

Adults: Initially, glipizide 2.5 mg/metformin 250 mg once a day with a meal. In patients with fasting plasma glucose level of 280 to 320 mg/dL, consider initiating therapy with glipizide 2.5 mg/metformin 500 mg b.i.d. May increase dosage every 2 weeks per glycemic response to maximum daily dose of 10 mg glipizide with 2,000 mg metformin in divided doses.

➤ **Second-line therapy when diet, exercise, and initial treatment with a sulfonylurea or metformin don't achieve glycemic control**

Adults: Initially, 2.5 mg glipizide/500 mg metformin or 5 mg glipizide/500 mg metformin PO b.i.d. Increase dosage in increments of no more than glipizide 5 mg/metformin 500 mg up to a maximum daily dose of glipizide 20 mg/metformin 2,000 mg.

glyBURIDE–metFORMIN hydrochloride

AVAILABLE FORMS
Tablets
1.25 mg glyburide and 250 mg metformin hydrochloride
2.5 mg glyburide and 500 mg metformin hydrochloride
5 mg glyburide and 500 mg metformin hydrochloride

INDICATIONS & DOSAGES
Black Box Warning Metformin can cause serious and sometimes fatal lactic acidosis; prompt hemodialysis is recommended. ∎

➤ **As initial adjunctive therapy to diet and exercise to improve glycemic control in adults with type 2 diabetes; as second-line therapy when diet, exercise, and initial treatment with a sulfonylurea or metformin don't achieve glycemic control**

Adults: 1 or 2 tablets PO daily or b.i.d. with meals. Maximum dosage, glyburide 20 mg and metformin 2,000 mg for treatment of type 2 diabetes, as second-line therapy.

Adjust-a-dose: Discontinue drug if eGFR falls below 30 mL/minute/1.73 m^2.

linagliptin–metFORMIN hydrochloride
Jentadueto, Jentadueto XR

AVAILABLE FORMS
Tablets
2.5 mg linagliptin and 500 mg metformin hydrochloride
2.5 mg linagliptin and 850 mg metformin hydrochloride

2.5 mg linagliptin and 1,000 mg metformin hydrochloride

Tablets (extended-release) **ⓄⓃⒸ**
2.5 mg linagliptin and 1,000 mg extended-release metformin hydrochloride
5 mg linagliptin and 1,000 mg extended-release metformin hydrochloride

INDICATIONS & DOSAGES
Black Box Warning Metformin can cause serious and sometimes fatal lactic acidosis; prompt hemodialysis is recommended. ∎

➤ **Adjunct to diet and exercise to improve glycemic control in adults with type 2 diabetes when treatment with both linagliptin and metformin is appropriate**

Adults already on metformin: 2.5 mg linagliptin PO b.i.d. or 5 mg linagliptin extended-release PO once daily plus current dose of metformin already being taken.

Adults not on metformin: 2.5 mg linagliptin/500 mg metformin PO b.i.d. or 5 mg linagliptin/1,000 mg metformin extended-release PO once daily. Maximum dose, 2.5 mg linagliptin and 1,000 mg metformin b.i.d.

Adjust-a-dose: Discontinue drug if eGFR falls below 30 mL/minute/1.73 m^2.

pioglitazone hydrochloride–metFORMIN hydrochloride
ActoPlus Met, ActoPlus Met XR

AVAILABLE FORMS
Tablets
15 mg pioglitazone and 500 mg metformin hydrochloride
15 mg pioglitazone and 850 mg metformin hydrochloride

Tablets (extended-release) **ⓄⓃⒸ**
15 mg pioglitazone and 1,000 mg extended-release metformin hydrochloride
30 mg pioglitazone and 1,000 mg extended-release metformin hydrochloride

INDICATIONS & DOSAGES
Black Box Warning May cause or exacerbate HF in some patients; drug isn't recommended in patients with symptomatic HF. Metformin can cause serious and sometimes fatal lactic acidosis; prompt hemodialysis is recommended. ∎

➤ **Adjunct to diet and exercise to improve glycemic control in adults with type 2 diabetes**

Adults: 15 mg pioglitazone/500 mg metformin or 15 mg pioglitazone/850 mg metformin PO once daily or b.i.d. with food. Maximum dosage, 45 mg pioglitazone/2,550 mg metformin per day. Or, 15 mg pioglitazone/1,000 mg extended-release metformin or 30 mg pioglitazone/1,000 mg extended-release metformin PO once daily or b.i.d. with meals. Maximum dosage of extended-release formula, 45 mg pioglitazone and 2,000 mg extended-release metformin per day.

Adjust-a-dose: Discontinue drug if eGFR falls below 30 mL/minute/1.73 m^2.

repaglinide–metFORMIN hydrochloride

AVAILABLE FORMS
Tablets

1 mg repaglinide and 500 mg metformin hydrochloride

2 mg repaglinide and 500 mg metformin hydrochloride

INDICATIONS & DOSAGES
Black Box Warning Metformin can cause serious and sometimes fatal lactic acidosis; prompt hemodialysis is recommended. ■

➤ **Adjunct to diet and exercise to improve glycemic control in adults with type 2 diabetes**

Adults: Individualize dosage based on patient's current regimen. Can be administered b.i.d. to t.i.d. within 30 minutes before meals. Maximum daily dose, 10 mg repaglinide and 2,500 mg metformin or 4 mg repaglinide and 1,000 mg metformin per meal.

Adjust-a-dose: Discontinue drug if eGFR falls below 30 mL/minute/1.73 m^2.

sitagliptin phosphate–metFORMIN hydrochloride

Janumet, Janumet XR

AVAILABLE FORMS
Tablets

50 mg sitagliptin phosphate and 500 mg metformin hydrochloride

50 mg sitagliptin phosphate and 1,000 mg metformin hydrochloride

Tablets (extended-release) **ᴰᴺᶜ**

50 mg sitagliptin phosphate and 500 mg extended-release metformin hydrochloride

50 mg sitagliptin phosphate and 1,000 mg extended-release metformin hydrochloride

100 mg sitagliptin phosphate and 1,000 mg extended-release metformin hydrochloride

INDICATIONS & DOSAGES
Black Box Warning Metformin can cause serious and sometimes fatal lactic acidosis; prompt hemodialysis is recommended. ■

➤ **Adjunct to diet and exercise to improve glycemic control in adults with type 2 diabetes when treatment with both sitagliptin and metformin is appropriate**

Adults already on metformin (immediate-release): 50 mg sitagliptin PO b.i.d. plus the dose of metformin already being taken. For patients taking 850 mg metformin PO b.i.d., recommended starting dosage is 50 mg sitagliptin/1,000 mg metformin PO b.i.d.

Adults already on metformin (extended-release): 100 mg/day sitagliptin plus previously prescribed dose of metformin. For patients taking 850 mg immediate-release metformin PO b.i.d. or 1,000 mg metformin PO b.i.d., recommended starting dosage is 100 mg sitagliptin/2,000 mg extended-release metformin PO once daily.

Adults not on metformin: 50 mg sitagliptin/500 mg metformin PO b.i.d. or 100 mg sitagliptin/1,000 mg extended-release metformin PO once daily.

Adjust-a-dose: Discontinue drug if eGFR falls below 30 mL/minute/1.73 m^2.

probenecid–colchicine

AVAILABLE FORMS
Tablets

500 mg probenecid and 0.5 mg colchicine

INDICATIONS & DOSAGES
➤ **Chronic gouty arthritis**

Adults: 1 tablet PO daily for 1 week; then 1 tablet PO b.i.d. If necessary, increase daily dosage by 1 tablet every 4 weeks within tolerance (usually not above 4 tablets daily) if symptoms aren't controlled or 24-hour uric acid excretion isn't above 700 mg.

Adjust-a-dose: Probenecid may not be effective if eGFR falls below 30 mL/minute/1.73 m^2.

aliskiren hemifumarate–hydroCHLOROthiazide

Tekturna HCT

AVAILABLE FORMS
Tablets

150 mg aliskiren hemifumarate and 12.5 mg hydrochlorothiazide

150 mg aliskiren hemifumarate and 25 mg hydrochlorothiazide

300 mg aliskiren hemifumarate and 12.5 mg hydrochlorothiazide

300 mg aliskiren hemifumarate and 25 mg hydrochlorothiazide

INDICATIONS & DOSAGES
Black Box Warning Can cause fetal harm; when pregnancy is detected, discontinue drug as soon as possible. ■

➤ **HTN**

Adults: Initially, 150 mg aliskiren/12.5 mg hydrochlorothiazide PO daily. Titrate up as needed after 2 to 4 weeks to a maximum of 300 mg aliskiren/25 mg hydrochlorothiazide.

amLODIPine besylate–benazepril hydrochloride

Lotrel

AVAILABLE FORMS
Capsules

2.5 mg amlodipine besylate and 10 mg benazepril hydrochloride

5 mg amlodipine besylate and 10 mg benazepril hydrochloride

5 mg amlodipine besylate and 20 mg benazepril hydrochloride

5 mg amlodipine besylate and 40 mg benazepril hydrochloride

10 mg amlodipine besylate and 20 mg benazepril hydrochloride

10 mg amlodipine besylate and 40 mg benazepril hydrochloride

INDICATIONS & DOSAGES
Black Box Warning Can cause fetal harm; when pregnancy is detected, discontinue drug as soon as possible. ■

➤ **HTN**

Adults: Initially, 2.5 mg amlodipine/10 mg benazepril PO daily in morning. Titrate dosage based on BP response. Maximum dosage, 10 mg amlodipine and 40 mg benazepril.

Adjust-a-dose: Consider lower initial doses for elderly patients and patients with hepatic impairment. Drug isn't recommended in patients with CrCl of 30 mL/minute or less.

amLODIPine besylate–hydroCHLOROthiazide–olmesartan medoxomil

Tribenzor

AVAILABLE FORMS

Tablets

5 mg amlodipine besylate, 12.5 mg hydrochlorothiazide, and 20 mg olmesartan medoxomil

5 mg amlodipine besylate, 12.5 mg hydrochlorothiazide, and 40 mg olmesartan medoxomil

5 mg amlodipine besylate, 25 mg hydrochlorothiazide, and 40 mg olmesartan medoxomil

10 mg amlodipine besylate, 12.5 mg hydrochlorothiazide, and 40 mg olmesartan medoxomil

10 mg amlodipine besylate, 25 mg hydrochlorothiazide, and 40 mg olmesartan medoxomil

INDICATIONS & DOSAGES

Black Box Warning Can cause fetal harm; when pregnancy is detected, discontinue drug as soon as possible. ∎

➤ **HTN**

Adults: Adjust dosage of individual products; then switch to appropriate combination product. One tablet PO daily. Or, initiate in patients not adequately controlled on any two of the following antihypertensive classes: calcium channel blockers, ARBs, and diuretic drugs. May increase dosage after 2 weeks. Maximum recommended dose, 10 mg amlodipine/25 mg hydrochlorothiazide/40 mg olmesartan.

Adjust-a-dose: Drug isn't recommended in patients with CrCl of 30 mL/minute or less.

amLODIPine besylate–olmesartan medoxomil

Azor

AVAILABLE FORMS

Tablets

5 mg amlodipine besylate and 20 mg olmesartan medoxomil

5 mg amlodipine besylate and 40 mg olmesartan medoxomil

10 mg amlodipine besylate and 20 mg olmesartan medoxomil

10 mg amlodipine besylate and 40 mg olmesartan medoxomil

INDICATIONS & DOSAGES

Black Box Warning Can cause fetal harm; when pregnancy is detected, discontinue drug as soon as possible. ∎

➤ **HTN**

Adults: Initially, 5 mg amlodipine/20 mg olmesartan PO once daily for 1 to 2 weeks. Titrate as needed up

to maximum of 10 mg amlodipine/40 mg olmesartan once daily.

amLODIPine besylate–telmisartan

Twynsta

AVAILABLE FORMS

Tablets

5 mg amlodipine besylate and 40 mg telmisartan

5 mg amlodipine besylate and 80 mg telmisartan

10 mg amlodipine besylate and 40 mg telmisartan

10 mg amlodipine besylate and 80 mg telmisartan

INDICATIONS & DOSAGES

Black Box Warning Can cause fetal harm; when pregnancy is detected, discontinue drug as soon as possible. ∎

➤ **HTN**

Adults: 1 tablet PO daily. Substitute for its individually titrated components or initiate therapy with 5 mg amlodipine/40 mg telmisartan or 5 mg amlodipine/80 mg telmisartan. May increase dosage after at least 2 weeks to maximum dose of 10 mg amlodipine/80 mg telmisartan.

amLODIPine besylate–valsartan

Exforge

AVAILABLE FORMS

Tablets

5 mg amlodipine besylate and 160 mg valsartan

5 mg amlodipine besylate and 320 mg valsartan

10 mg amlodipine besylate and 160 mg valsartan

10 mg amlodipine besylate and 320 mg valsartan

INDICATIONS & DOSAGES

Black Box Warning Can cause fetal harm; when pregnancy is detected, discontinue drug as soon as possible. ∎

➤ **HTN**

Adults: Initially, 5 mg amlodipine/160 mg valsartan PO once daily if patient isn't volume depleted. Increase after 1 to 2 weeks to desired effect or a maximum of 10 mg amlodipine/320 mg valsartan daily.

amLODIPine besylate–valsartan–hydroCHLOROthiazide

Exforge HCT

AVAILABLE FORMS

Tablets

5 mg amlodipine besylate, 160 mg valsartan, and 12.5 mg hydrochlorothiazide

10 mg amlodipine besylate, 160 mg valsartan, and 12.5 mg hydrochlorothiazide

5 mg amlodipine besylate, 160 mg valsartan, and 25 mg hydrochlorothiazide

10 mg amlodipine besylate, 160 mg valsartan, and 25 mg hydrochlorothiazide

10 mg amlodipine besylate, 320 mg valsartan, and 25 mg hydrochlorothiazide

INDICATIONS & DOSAGES

Black Box Warning Can cause fetal harm; when pregnancy is detected, discontinue drug as soon as possible. ∎

➤ **HTN**
Adults: Give 1 tablet PO once daily. Dosage may be increased after 2 weeks. Maximum recommended dosage, 10 mg amlodipine/320 mg valsartan/25 mg hydrochlorothiazide.
Adjust-a-dose: In elderly patients and patients with hepatic impairment, initiate drug with lower doses and titrate cautiously.

atenolol–chlorthalidone
Tenoretic
AVAILABLE FORMS
Tablets
50 mg atenolol and 25 mg chlorthalidone
100 mg atenolol and 25 mg chlorthalidone
INDICATIONS & DOSAGES
➤ **HTN**
Adults: Initially, 50 mg atenolol/25 mg chlorthalidone PO daily in the morning. May increase to 100 mg atenolol/25 mg chlorthalidone if needed.
Adjust-a-dose: If CrCl is 15 to 35 mL/minute/1.73 m^2, maximum dose is 50 mg atenolol/25 mg chlorthalidone daily. If CrCl is less than 15 mL/minute/1.73 m^2, maximum dose is 50 mg atenolol/25 mg chlorthalidone every other day.

benazepril hydrochloride–hydroCHLOROthiazide
Lotensin HCT
AVAILABLE FORMS
Tablets
10 mg benazepril and 12.5 mg hydrochlorothiazide
20 mg benazepril and 12.5 mg hydrochlorothiazide
20 mg benazepril and 25 mg hydrochlorothiazide
INDICATIONS & DOSAGES
Black Box Warning Can cause fetal harm; when pregnancy is detected, discontinue drug as soon as possible. ▪
➤ **HTN**
Adults: 1 tablet PO daily in the morning. Adjust dosage using individual products; then switch to appropriate combination product. Wait 2 to 3 weeks before increasing hydrochlorothiazide dose. Maximum dose is 20 mg benazepril and 25 mg hydrochlorothiazide daily.
Adjust-a-dose: Drug isn't recommended in patients with CrCl of 30 mL/minute/1.73 m^2 or less.

bisoprolol fumarate–hydroCHLOROthiazide
Ziac
AVAILABLE FORMS
Tablets
2.5 mg bisoprolol fumarate and 6.25 mg hydrochlorothiazide
5 mg bisoprolol fumarate and 6.25 mg hydrochlorothiazide
10 mg bisoprolol fumarate and 6.25 mg hydrochlorothiazide
INDICATIONS & DOSAGES
➤ **HTN**
Adults: Initially, 2.5 mg bisoprolol/6.25 mg hydrochlorothiazide PO daily. Increase dosage in 14-day

intervals; optimal antihypertensive effect may require 2 to 3 weeks. Maximum dosage, 20 mg bisoprolol and 12.5 mg hydrochlorothiazide daily.
Adjust-a-dose: Use caution when titrating drug in patients with renal or hepatic impairment. Drug is contraindicated in patients with anuria.

candesartan cilexetil–hydroCHLOROthiazide
Atacand HCT
AVAILABLE FORMS
Tablets
16 mg candesartan cilexetil and 12.5 mg hydrochlorothiazide
32 mg candesartan cilexetil and 12.5 mg hydrochlorothiazide
32 mg candesartan cilexetil and 25 mg hydrochlorothiazide
INDICATIONS & DOSAGES
Black Box Warning Can cause fetal harm; when pregnancy is detected, discontinue drug as soon as possible. ▪
➤ **HTN**
Adults: Initially, 16 mg candesartan/12.5 mg hydrochlorothiazide PO daily in one or two divided doses in patients who aren't volume-depleted. Adjust dosage using individual products; then switch to appropriate dosage of combination product.

captopril and hydroCHLOROthiazide
AVAILABLE FORMS
Tablets
25 mg captopril and 15 mg hydrochlorothiazide
50 mg captopril and 15 mg hydrochlorothiazide
25 mg captopril and 25 mg hydrochlorothiazide
50 mg captopril and 25 mg hydrochlorothiazide
INDICATIONS & DOSAGES
Black Box Warning Can cause fetal harm; when pregnancy is detected, discontinue drug as soon as possible. ▪
➤ **HTN**
Adults: Initially, 25 mg captopril/15 mg hydrochlorothiazide PO daily; titrate dosage at 6-week intervals based on patient response. Adjust dosage using individual products; then switch to combination product when patient's adjustment schedule is stable. Maximum daily dose, 150 mg captopril or 50 mg hydrochlorothiazide.

enalapril maleate–hydroCHLOROthiazide
Vaseretic
AVAILABLE FORMS
Tablets
5 mg enalapril maleate and 12.5 mg hydrochlorothiazide
10 mg enalapril maleate and 25 mg hydrochlorothiazide
INDICATIONS & DOSAGES
Black Box Warning Can cause fetal harm; when pregnancy is detected, discontinue drug as soon as possible. ▪

➤**HTN**

Adults: Initially, 10 mg enalapril/25 mg hydrochlorothiazide PO daily. Increase dosage based on response after 2 to 3 weeks. Adjust dosage using individual products; then switch to appropriate combination product. Maximum dosage, 20 mg enalapril and 50 mg hydrochlorothiazide daily.

fosinopril and hydroCHLOROthiazide
AVAILABLE FORMS
Tablets
10 mg fosinopril sodium and 12.5 mg hydrochlorothiazide
20 mg fosinopril sodium and 12.5 mg hydrochlorothiazide
INDICATIONS & DOSAGES
Black Box Warning Can cause fetal harm; when pregnancy is detected, discontinue drug as soon as possible. ∎
➤**HTN**
Adults: 1 tablet PO per day in the morning. Adjust dosage using individual products; then switch to appropriate combination product.

irbesartan–hydroCHLOROthiazide
Avalide
AVAILABLE FORMS
Tablets
150 mg irbesartan and 12.5 mg hydrochlorothiazide
300 mg irbesartan and 12.5 mg hydrochlorothiazide
INDICATIONS & DOSAGES
Black Box Warning Can cause fetal harm; when pregnancy is detected, discontinue drug as soon as possible. ∎
➤**HTN**
Adults: Initially, 150 mg irbesartan/12.5 mg hydrochlorothiazide PO daily. Adjust dosage with individual products; then switch to combination product when patient's condition is stabilized. Maximum daily dose, 300 mg irbesartan and 25 mg hydrochlorothiazide.

losartan potassium–hydroCHLOROthiazide
Hyzaar
AVAILABLE FORMS
Tablets
100 mg losartan potassium and 12.5 mg hydrochlorothiazide
INDICATIONS & DOSAGES
Black Box Warning Can cause fetal harm; when pregnancy is detected, discontinue drug as soon as possible. ∎
➤**HTN**
Adults: 1 tablet PO daily as a substitute for individual titrated components in patients not adequately controlled with monotherapy with either of the component products. May use as initial therapy in severe HTN when benefits outweigh risk.

methyldopa and hydroCHLOROthiazide
AVAILABLE FORMS
Tablets
250 mg methyldopa and 15 mg hydrochlorothiazide
250 mg methyldopa and 25 mg hydrochlorothiazide

INDICATIONS & DOSAGES
Black Box Warning Not indicated for initial therapy of HTN. ∎
➤**HTN**
Adults: Initially, 250 mg methyldopa/15 mg hydrochlorothiazide PO b.i.d. or t.i.d. or 250 mg methyldopa/25 mg hydrochlorothiazide PO b.i.d. Adjust dosage using individual products; then switch to appropriate combination product. Maximum dosage, 3,000 mg methyldopa and 50 mg hydrochlorothiazide daily.

metoprolol succinate–hydroCHLOROthiazide
Dutoprol
AVAILABLE FORMS
Tablets (extended-release)
25 mg metoprolol succinate and 12.5 mg hydrochlorothiazide
50 mg metoprolol succinate and 12.5 mg hydrochlorothiazide
100 mg metoprolol succinate and 12.5 mg hydrochlorothiazide
INDICATIONS & DOSAGES
Black Box Warning May exacerbate ischemic heart disease if withdrawn abruptly. ∎
➤**HTN**
Adults: Initially, 25 mg metoprolol/12.5 mg hydrochlorothiazide PO per day. Depending on BP response, may titrate dosage at intervals of 2 weeks to a maximum recommended dose of 200 mg/25 mg (two 100 mg/12.5-mg tablets) once daily.

metoprolol tartrate–hydroCHLOROthiazide
Lopressor HCT
AVAILABLE FORMS
Tablets
50 mg metoprolol tartrate and 25 mg hydrochlorothiazide
100 mg metoprolol tartrate and 25 mg hydrochlorothiazide
INDICATIONS & DOSAGES
Black Box Warning May exacerbate ischemic heart disease if withdrawn abruptly. ∎
➤**HTN**
Adults: 100 to 200 mg metoprolol/25 to 50 mg hydrochlorothiazide PO once daily or 50 to 100 mg metoprolol/12.5 to 50 mg hydrochlorothiazide PO b.i.d. Adjust dosage using individual products; then switch to appropriate combination product.

moexipril hydrochloride–hydroCHLOROthiazide
AVAILABLE FORMS
Tablets
7.5 mg moexipril hydrochloride and 12.5 mg hydrochlorothiazide
15 mg moexipril hydrochloride and 12.5 mg hydrochlorothiazide
15 mg moexipril hydrochloride and 25 mg hydrochlorothiazide

INDICATIONS & DOSAGES
Black Box Warning Can cause fetal harm; when pregnancy is detected, discontinue drug as soon as possible. ∎

➤ **HTN**
Adults: Initially, 7.5 mg moexipril/12.5 mg hydrochlorothiazide, or 15 mg moexipril/12.5 mg hydrochlorothiazide, or 15 mg moexipril/25 mg hydrochlorothiazide PO once daily. Not for initial therapy. Adjust dosage based on clinical response.

nadolol–bendroflumethiazide
Corzide
AVAILABLE FORMS
Tablets
40 mg nadolol and 5 mg bendroflumethiazide
80 mg nadolol and 5 mg bendroflumethiazide
INDICATIONS & DOSAGES
Black Box Warning May exacerbate ischemic heart disease if withdrawn abruptly. ∎

➤ **HTN**
Adults: Individualize dosage. Initially, 40 mg nadolol/5 mg bendroflumethiazide PO daily in the morning. When antihypertensive response isn't satisfactory, may increase to nadolol 80 mg/bendroflumethiazide 5 mg once daily.
Adjust-a-dose: If CrCl (mL/minute/1.73 m^2) is 31 to 50, give dose every 24 to 36 hours; for CrCl of 10 to 30, give dose every 24 to 48 hours; for CrCl less than 10, give dose every 40 to 60 hours.

nebivolol hydrochloride–valsartan
Byvalson
AVAILABLE FORMS
Tablets
5 mg nebivolol and 80 mg valsartan
INDICATIONS & DOSAGES
Black Box Warning Can cause fetal harm; when pregnancy is detected, discontinue drug as soon as possible. ∎

➤ **HTN**
Adults for initial therapy and in patients not controlled on valsartan 80 mg or nebivolol 10 mg: 1 tablet PO once daily.

olmesartan medoxomil–hydroCHLOROthiazide
Benicar HCT 🖉
AVAILABLE FORMS
Tablets
20 mg olmesartan medoxomil and 12.5 mg hydrochlorothiazide
40 mg olmesartan medoxomil and 12.5 mg hydrochlorothiazide
40 mg olmesartan medoxomil and 25 mg hydrochlorothiazide
INDICATIONS & DOSAGES
Black Box Warning Can cause fetal harm; when pregnancy is detected, discontinue drug as soon as possible. ∎

➤ **HTN**
Adults: 1 tablet PO daily in the morning. Adjust dosage using individual products; then switch

to combination product when patient's adjustment schedule is stable. Dosage may be titrated at 2- to 4-week intervals. Maximum dosage, 40 mg olmesartan/25 mg hydrochlorothiazide.

propranolol and hydroCHLOROthiazide
AVAILABLE FORMS
Tablets
40 mg propranolol hydrochloride and 25 mg hydrochlorothiazide
80 mg propranolol hydrochloride and 25 mg hydrochlorothiazide
INDICATIONS & DOSAGES
➤ **HTN**
Adults: 1 tablet PO b.i.d. Adjust dosage using individual products; then switch to appropriate combination product. Maximum daily dose, 160 mg propranolol and 50 mg hydrochlorothiazide.

quinapril hydrochloride–hydroCHLOROthiazide
Accuretic, Quinaretic
AVAILABLE FORMS
Tablets
10 mg quinapril hydrochloride and 12.5 mg hydrochlorothiazide
20 mg quinapril hydrochloride and 12.5 mg hydrochlorothiazide
20 mg quinapril hydrochloride and 25 mg hydrochlorothiazide
INDICATIONS & DOSAGES
Black Box Warning Can cause fetal harm; when pregnancy is detected, discontinue drug as soon as possible. ∎

➤ **HTN**
Adults: 1 tablet PO per day in the morning. Adjust drug using the individual products; then switch to appropriate dosage of the combination product. Correct volume and salt depletion before initiating therapy.
Adjust-a-dose: Discontinue drug if eGFR falls below 30 mL/minute/1.73 m^2 or serum creatinine level is more than 3 mg/dL.

telmisartan–hydroCHLOROthiazide
Micardis HCT
AVAILABLE FORMS
Tablets
40 mg telmisartan and 12.5 mg hydrochlorothiazide
80 mg telmisartan and 12.5 mg hydrochlorothiazide
80 mg telmisartan and 25 mg hydrochlorothiazide
INDICATIONS & DOSAGES
Black Box Warning Can cause fetal harm; when pregnancy is detected, discontinue drug as soon as possible. ∎

➤ **HTN**
Adult without adequate control with monotherapy on either of the component drugs, or as substitute for individual titrated components: Initially, 80 mg telmisartan/12.5 mg hydrochlorothiazide PO per day; may adjust up to 160 mg telmisartan and 25 mg hydrochlorothiazide, based on patient's response after 2 to 4 weeks of therapy. Not for use as initial therapy.

Adjust-a-dose: In patients with mild to moderate hepatic impairment or biliary obstructive disorders, begin therapy with 40 mg telmisartan/12.5 mg hydrochlorothiazide PO once daily. Don't use in patients with severe hepatic impairment. Drug isn't recommended in patients with CrCl of 30 mL/minute/1.73 m² or less.

trandolapril–verapamil hydrochloride
Tarka
AVAILABLE FORMS
Tablets (extended-release)
1 mg trandolapril and 240 mg verapamil hydrochloride
2 mg trandolapril and 180 mg verapamil hydrochloride
2 mg trandolapril and 240 mg verapamil hydrochloride
4 mg trandolapril and 240 mg verapamil hydrochloride
INDICATIONS & DOSAGES
Black Box Warning Can cause fetal harm; when pregnancy is detected, discontinue drug as soon as possible. ∎
➤ HTN
Adults: 1 tablet PO per day with food. Adjust dosage using the individual products; then switch to appropriate combination product.
Adjust-a-dose: In patients with hepatic or renal impairment (CrCl of less than 30 mL/minute), lower doses are recommended.

valsartan–hydroCHLOROthiazide
Diovan HCT 🖉
AVAILABLE FORMS
Tablets
80 mg valsartan and 12.5 mg hydrochlorothiazide
160 mg valsartan and 12.5 mg hydrochlorothiazide
160 mg valsartan and 25 mg hydrochlorothiazide
320 mg valsartan and 12.5 mg hydrochlorothiazide
320 mg valsartan and 25 mg hydrochlorothiazide
INDICATIONS & DOSAGES
Black Box Warning Can cause fetal harm; when pregnancy is detected, discontinue drug as soon as possible. ∎
➤ HTN
Adults: Initially, 160 mg valsartan/12.5 mg hydrochlorothiazide PO daily. Titrate to desired effect after 1 to 2 weeks. Maximum dose, 320 mg valsartan/25 mg hydrochlorothiazide.

Antimigraine drugs

ergotamine tartrate–caffeine
Cafergot, Migergot
AVAILABLE FORMS
Tablets
1 mg ergotamine tartrate and 100 mg caffeine
Suppositories
2 mg ergotamine tartrate and 100 mg caffeine
INDICATIONS & DOSAGES
Black Box Warning Use with potent CYP3A4 inhibitors, including protease inhibitors and macrolide antibiotics, can cause serious vasospasm and is contraindicated. ∎
➤ **Prevention and treatment of vascular headache**
Adults: 2 tablets PO at first sign of attack. Follow with 1 tablet every 30 minutes, if needed. Maximum dose is 6 tablets per attack. Don't exceed 10 tablets per week. Or, 1 suppository PR at first sign of attack; follow with second dose after 1 hour, if needed. Maximum dose is 2 suppositories per attack. Don't exceed 5 suppositories per week.

SUMAtriptan succinate–naproxen sodium
Treximet
AVAILABLE FORMS
Tablets
85 mg sumatriptan succinate and 500 mg naproxen sodium
10 mg sumatriptan succinate and 60 mg naproxen sodium
INDICATIONS & DOSAGES
Black Box Warning NSAIDs may cause an increased risk of serious and sometimes fatal CV thrombotic events, MI, stroke, and GI adverse reactions. Contraindicated after CABG surgery. ∎
➤ **Migraine headache**
Adults: One 85 mg sumatriptan/500 mg naproxen tablet PO at first sign of migraine. May follow with a second dose 2 hours later. Maximum dosage, 2 tablets in 24 hours.
Children age 12 and older: 10 mg sumatriptan/60 mg naproxen PO at first sign of migraine. Maximum dose, 85 mg/500 mg tablet in 24 hours.
Adjust-a-dose: Use isn't recommended in patients with CrCl less than 30 mL/minute.

Antiplatelet drugs

dipyridamole–aspirin
Aggrenox
AVAILABLE FORMS
Capsules (DNC)
200 mg dipyridamole and 25 mg aspirin
INDICATIONS & DOSAGES
➤ **To reduce stroke risk**
Adults: 1 capsule PO b.i.d. in morning and evening. Not interchangeable with the individual components of aspirin and dipyridamole tablets.

Antiretrovirals

abacavir sulfate–lamiVUDine
Epzicom ⚠
AVAILABLE FORMS
Tablets
600 mg abacavir and 300 mg lamivudine
INDICATIONS & DOSAGES
⚠ **Black Box Warning** Contraindicated in patients with prior hypersensitivity reaction to abacavir and in HLA-B*5701-positive patients; screen for the HLA-B*5701 allele before starting drug. Never restart drug in patients who have had a hypersensitivity reaction to abacavir; severe signs and symptoms, including death, can occur

within hours. Severe acute exacerbations of HBV infection have been reported in patients coinfected with HBV and HIV who have discontinued lamivudine. Monitor patients closely for at least several months after stopping drug. ∎

➤ **Treatment of HIV infection**
Adults and children weighing 25 kg or more: 1 tablet PO daily in combination with other antiretrovirals.
Adjust-a-dose: Use isn't recommended in patients with CrCl less than 50 mL/minute or moderate to severe hepatic impairment.

abacavir sulfate–lamiVUDine–zidovudine
Trizivir ▨
AVAILABLE FORMS
Tablets
300 mg abacavir sulfate, 150 mg lamivudine, and 300 mg zidovudine
INDICATIONS & DOSAGES
▨ **Black Box Warning** Contraindicated in patients with prior hypersensitivity reaction to abacavir and in HLA-B*5701-positive patients; screen for the HLA-B*5701 allele before starting drug. Never restart drug in patients who have had a hypersensitivity reaction to abacavir; severe signs and symptoms, including death, can occur within hours. Hematologic toxicity, myopathy, lactic acidosis, and severe hepatomegaly with steatosis, including fatal cases, have been reported. Severe acute exacerbations of HBV infection have been reported in patients coinfected with HBV and HIV who have discontinued lamivudine. Monitor patients closely for at least several months after stopping drug. ∎

➤ **Treatment of HIV infection**
Adults and children weighing 40 kg or more: 1 tablet PO b.i.d., alone or with other antiretrovirals.
Adjust-a-dose: Use isn't recommended in patients with CrCl less than 50 mL/minute or moderate to severe hepatic impairment.

efavirenz–emtricitabine–tenofovir disoproxil fumarate
Atripla
AVAILABLE FORMS
600 mg efavirenz, 200 mg emtricitabine, and 300 mg tenofovir disoproxil fumarate
INDICATIONS & DOSAGES
Black Box Warning Not approved for treatment of chronic HBV infection. ∎

➤ **Treatment of HIV infection**
Adults and children weighing at least 40 kg: 1 tablet PO daily on empty stomach. Dosing at bedtime may improve tolerability of nervous system symptoms.
Adjust-a-dose: Use isn't recommended in patients with CrCl less than 50 mL/minute or moderate to severe hepatic impairment.

emtricitabine–rilpivirine–tenofovir disoproxil fumarate
Complera
AVAILABLE FORMS
Tablets
200 mg emtricitabine, 25 mg rilpivirine, and 300 mg tenofovir disoproxil fumarate
INDICATIONS & DOSAGES
Black Box Warning Not approved for treatment of chronic HBV infection.

➤ **Treatment of HIV infection**
Adults and children age 12 and older weighing 35 kg or more: 1 tablet PO once daily with food.
Adjust-a-dose: Use isn't recommended in patients with CrCl less than 50 mL/minute.

emtricitabine–tenofovir disoproxil fumarate
Truvada
AVAILABLE FORMS
Tablets
100 mg emtricitabine and 150 mg tenofovir disoproxil fumarate
133 mg emtricitabine and 200 mg tenofovir disoproxil fumarate
167 mg emtricitabine and 250 mg tenofovir disoproxil fumarate
200 mg emtricitabine and 300 mg tenofovir disoproxil fumarate
INDICATIONS & DOSAGES
Black Box Warning Not approved for treatment of chronic HBV infection. For preexposure prophylaxis, confirm that patient is HIV-negative immediately before initiating and periodically (at least every 3 months) during use. Severe acute exacerbations of HBV infection have been reported in HBV-infected patients who have discontinued drug. Monitor patients closely for at least several months after stopping drug. ∎

➤ **Preexposure prophylaxis (adults and adolescents) and treatment of HIV infection (adults and children) in combination with other retrovirals**
Adults and adolescents (preexposure prophylaxis and treatment) and children (treatment) weighing 35 kg or more: 200 mg emtricitabine/300 mg tenofovir disoproxil fumarate PO daily.
Children weighing 28 to less than 35 kg: 167 mg emtricitabine/250 mg tenofovir disoproxil fumarate PO daily.
Children weighing 22 to less than 28 kg: 133 mg emtricitabine/200 mg tenofovir disoproxil fumarate PO daily.
Children weighing 17 to less than 22 kg: 100 mg emtricitabine/150 mg tenofovir disoproxil fumarate PO daily.
Adjust-a-dose: For CrCl of 30 to 49 mL/minute, give dose every 48 hours. Withhold drug for CrCl of less than 30 mL/minute. Not recommended for preexposure prophylaxis in individuals with estimated CrCl below 60 mL/minute.

lamiVUDine–zidovudine
Combivir ✑
AVAILABLE FORMS
Tablets
150 mg lamivudine and 300 mg zidovudine
INDICATIONS & DOSAGES
Black Box Warning Hematologic toxicity, myopathy, lactic acidosis, and severe hepatomegaly, including fatal cases, and exacerbations of HBV infection have been reported. ■
➤ **Treatment of HIV infection**
Adults and children weighing 30 kg or more: 1 tablet PO b.i.d.
Adjust-a-dose: Use isn't recommended in patients with CrCl less than 50 mL/minute or hepatic impairment.

Antiulcer drugs

bismuth subcitrate potassium–metroNIDAZOLE–tetracycline hydrochloride
Pylera
AVAILABLE FORMS
Capsules
140 mg bismuth subcitrate potassium, 125 mg metronidazole, and 125 mg tetracycline hydrochloride
INDICATIONS & DOSAGES
Black Box Warning Metronidazole has been shown to be carcinogenic in mice and rats. It's unknown if it's carcinogenic in humans. ■
➤ **Eradication of *Helicobacter pylori* infection; active duodenal ulcers associated with *H. pylori* infection**
Adults: Give each dose (which includes all 3 capsules) PO q.i.d. after meals and at bedtime for 10 days with omeprazole 20 mg PO b.i.d. (after the morning and evening meals) for 10 days.

lansoprazole–amoxicillin–clarithromycin
AVAILABLE FORMS
Daily administration pack
Two 30-mg lansoprazole capsules, four 500-mg amoxicillin capsules, and two 500-mg clarithromycin tablets
INDICATIONS & DOSAGES
➤ **Eradication of *Helicobacter pylori* infection**
Adults: 30 mg lansoprazole, 1 g amoxicillin, 500 mg clarithromycin b.i.d. before eating (morning and evening) for 10 to 14 days
☉ *Alert:* Clarithromycin may increase risk of death, especially in patients with heart disease. Avoid use in patients at high risk, and weigh risks and benefits of therapy in all patients. In patients with heart disease, consider the use of alternative antibiotics.

Benign prostatic hyperplasia drugs

dutasteride–tamsulosin hydrochloride
Jalyn
AVAILABLE FORMS
Capsules 🏵
0.5 mg dutasteride and 0.4 mg tamsulosin hydrochloride

INDICATIONS & DOSAGES
➤ **Treatment of symptomatic BPH**
Adult men: 1 capsule PO daily 30 minutes after same meal each day.

Diuretics

aMILoride and hydroCHLOROthiazide
AVAILABLE FORMS
Tablets
5 mg amiloride hydrochloride and 50 mg hydrochlorothiazide
INDICATIONS & DOSAGES
Black Box Warning May cause potentially fatal hyperkalemia; monitor serum potassium levels carefully. ■
➤ **Edema or HTN**
Adults: 1 to 2 tablets PO per day as a single daily dose or in divided dose with food.

spironolactone–hydrochlorothiazide
Aldactazide
AVAILABLE FORMS
Tablets
25 mg spironolactone and 25 mg hydrochlorothiazide
50 mg spironolactone and 50 mg hydrochlorothiazide
INDICATIONS & DOSAGES
➤ **Edema**
Adults: 25 to 200 mg spironolactone/25 to 200 mg hydrochlorothiazide PO in single or divided doses daily.
➤ **HTN**
Adults: 50 to 100 mg spironolactone/50 to 100 mg hydrochlorothiazide PO daily.
Adjust-a-dose: In elderly patients, initiate with lowest available dose. Avoid spironolactone doses of more than 25 mg/day in elderly patients with HF or renal impairment.

Heart failure drugs

isosorbide dinitrate–hydrALAZINE hydrochloride
BiDil 🎍
AVAILABLE FORMS
Tablets
20 mg isosorbide dinitrate and 37.5 mg hydralazine
INDICATIONS & DOSAGES
➤ **Adjunct to standard HF therapy in self-identified black patients** 🎍
Adults: 1 to 2 tablets PO t.i.d. Maximum, 2 tablets PO t.i.d.

Lipid-lowering drugs

ezetimibe–simvastatin
Vytorin ✑ 🎍
AVAILABLE FORMS
Tablets
10 mg ezetimibe with 10, 20, 40, or 80 mg simvastatin
INDICATIONS & DOSAGES
➤ **Homozygous familial hypercholesterolemia and primary hyperlipidemia** 🎍

Adults: 1 tablet PO daily in the evening in combination with a cholesterol-lowering diet and exercise. May adjust dosage of simvastatin in combination based on patient response.

Only use 10 mg ezetimibe/80 mg simvastatin in patients who have been taking drug long-term without evidence of muscle toxicity. In patients unable to achieve their LDL cholesterol goal using 10 mg ezetimibe/40 mg simvastatin, don't titrate to the 10 mg ezetimibe/80 mg simvastatin dose; use an alternative therapy.

If giving drug with a bile acid sequestrant, give drug at least 2 hours before or 4 hours after the bile acid sequestrant.

Adjust-a-dose: For patients with moderate to severe renal impairment (GFR less than 60 mL/minute), give 10 mg ezetimibe/20 mg simvastatin once daily in the evening. If patient is also taking diltiazem, dronedarone, or verapamil, don't exceed 10 mg ezetimibe/10 mg simvastatin daily. If patient is also taking amiodarone, amlodipine, or ranolazine, don't exceed 10 mg ezetimibe/20 mg simvastatin daily. If patient is also taking lomitapide, reduce simvastatin dosage by 50%.

Use cautiously when treating Chinese patients with doses exceeding 10 mg ezetimibe/20 mg simvastatin when administered with lipid-modifying doses of niacin-containing products because of an increased risk of myopathy; don't use 10 mg ezetimibe/80 mg simvastatin in such patients. ✂

Menopause drugs

conjugated estrogens–bazedoxifene acetate
Duavee
AVAILABLE FORMS
Tablets
0.45 mg conjugated estrogens and 20 mg bazedoxifene acetate
INDICATIONS & DOSAGES
Black Box Warning Risk of endometrial cancer and CV disease; not for preventing dementia; use at lowest effective doses, for the shortest duration, consistent with treatment goals and risks for the individual woman. ∎
➤ **Vasomotor symptoms; postmenopausal osteoporosis prevention**
Adults: 1 tablet PO once daily.

conjugated estrogens/conjugated estrogens–medroxyPROGESTERone
Premphase
AVAILABLE FORMS
Tablets
0.625 mg conjugated estrogens; 0.625 mg conjugated estrogens and 5 mg medroxyprogesterone
INDICATIONS & DOSAGES
Black Box Warning Risk of endometrial and breast cancer and CV disease; not for preventing dementia; use at lowest effective doses, for the shortest duration, consistent with treatment goals and risks for the individual woman. ∎

➤ **Moderate to severe symptoms (vasomotor, vulvar, and vaginal atrophy) of menopause; to prevent osteoporosis**
Women with intact uterus: 1 tablet PO per day. Use estrogen (maroon tablet) alone on days 1 to 14 and estrogen–medroxyprogesterone (light blue tablet) on days 15 to 28.

conjugated estrogens–medroxyPROGESTERone
Prempro
AVAILABLE FORMS
Tablets
0.3 mg conjugated estrogens and 1.5 mg medroxyprogesterone
0.45 mg conjugated estrogens and 1.5 mg medroxyprogesterone
0.625 mg conjugated estrogens and 2.5 mg medroxyprogesterone
0.625 mg conjugated estrogens and 5 mg medroxyprogesterone
INDICATIONS & DOSAGES
Black Box Warning Risk of endometrial and breast cancer and CV disease; not for preventing dementia; use at lowest effective doses, for the shortest duration, consistent with treatment goals and risks for the individual woman. ∎
➤ **Symptoms of menopause (vasomotor, vulvar, and vaginal atrophy); to prevent osteoporosis**
Women with intact uterus: 1 tablet PO per day.

Miscellaneous cardiac drugs

amLODIPine besylate–atorvastatin calcium
Caduet ✂
AVAILABLE FORMS
Tablets
2.5 mg amlodipine besylate with 10 mg, 20 mg, or 40 mg atorvastatin calcium
5 mg amlodipine besylate with 10 mg, 20 mg, 40 mg, or 80 mg atorvastatin calcium
10 mg amlodipine besylate with 10 mg, 20 mg, 40 mg, or 80 mg atorvastatin calcium
INDICATIONS & DOSAGES
Adjust-a-dose (for all indications): For small or fragile patients, initially, 2.5 mg amlodipine once daily. Atorvastatin is contraindicated in patients with active liver disease or unexplained LFT elevations. Refer to manufacturer's instructions for dosage adjustments when used with concomitant drugs.
➤ **Treatment of HTN, chronic stable angina, or suspected vasospastic angina in patients with primary hypercholesterolemia and mixed dyslipidemia or hypertriglyceridemia**
Adults: Determine the most effective dose for each component; then select the most appropriate combination product. Titrate dosage over 7 to 14 days. Maximum dose, amlodipine 10 mg and atorvastatin 80 mg daily.
➤ **Treatment of HTN; adjunct to diet to reduce total cholesterol, LDL cholesterol in children with heterozygous familial hypercholesterolemia** ✂

Boys and postmenarchal girls age 10 and older: Initially 2.5 amlodipine/10 mg atorvastatin PO once daily. Maintenance dosage, 2.5 to 5 mg amlodipine PO once daily. Atorvastatin maximum dose, 20 mg/day. When titrating amlodipine, wait 7 to 14 days between titration steps. When titrating atorvastatin, adjust dosage at intervals of 4 weeks or more.

aspirin–omeprazole
Yosprala
AVAILABLE FORMS
Tablets (delayed-release) 💿
81 mg delayed-release aspirin and 40 mg immediate-release omeprazole
325 mg delayed-release aspirin and 40 mg immediate-release omeprazole
INDICATIONS & DOSAGES
➤ **To reduce risk of aspirin-associated gastric ulcers in patients who require aspirin for the secondary prevention of CV and cerebrovascular events**
Adults: 1 tablet (81 mg delayed-release aspirin/40 mg immediate-release omeprazole or 325 mg delayed-release aspirin/40 mg immediate-release omeprazole) PO once daily.

Opioid agonists

buprenorphine hydrochloride–naloxone hydrochloride
Bunavail, Cassipa, Suboxone, Zubsolv
Controlled Substance Schedule: III
AVAILABLE FORMS
Sublingual tablets
2 mg buprenorphine and 0.5 mg naloxone
8 mg buprenorphine and 2 mg naloxone
Sublingual tablets (Zubsolv)
0.7 mg buprenorphine and 0.18 mg naloxone
1.4 mg buprenorphine and 0.36 mg naloxone
2.9 buprenorphine and 0.71 mg naloxone
5.7 mg buprenorphine and 1.4 mg naloxone
8.6 buprenorphine and 2.1 mg naloxone
11.4 buprenorphine and 2.9 mg naloxone
Sublingual film (Suboxone)
2 mg buprenorphine and 0.5 mg naloxone
4 mg buprenorphine and 1 mg naloxone
8 mg buprenorphine and 2 mg naloxone
12 mg buprenorphine and 3 mg naloxone
Sublingual film (Cassipa)
16 mg buprenorphine and 4 mg naloxone
Buccal film (Bunavail)
2.1 mg buprenorphine and 0.3 mg naloxone
4.2 mg buprenorphine and 0.7 mg naloxone
6.3 mg buprenorphine and 1 mg naloxone
INDICATIONS & DOSAGES
Black Box Warning *Opioid class warning:*
Opioids combined with benzodiazepines or CNS depressants can cause death. Patients physically dependent on opioid pain medications shouldn't suddenly have these medications discontinued or dosage rapidly decreased.
➤ **Induction of opioid dependence treatment**
Adults: On day 1, when objective and clear signs of moderate withdrawal are evident, initial dose is

1.4 mg buprenorphine/0.36 mg naloxone SL. Remainder of day 1 dose of up to 4.2 mg buprenorphine/1.08 mg naloxone should be divided into doses of 1 to 2 tablets of 1.4 mg buprenorphine/0.36 mg naloxone SL at 1.5- to 2-hour intervals up to a total day 1 dosage of 5.7 mg buprenorphine/1.4 mg naloxone. On day 2, give up to 11.4 mg buprenorphine/2.9 mg naloxone SL as a single dose. Maintenance treatment is 11.4 mg buprenorphine/2.9 mg naloxone SL daily. Adjust dosage based on clinical need to control acute withdrawal symptoms.
➤ **Opioid dependence**
Adults: Maintenance dose is based on buprenorphine. Give 12 to 16 mg (buprenorphine) SL tablet once daily, after induction with SL buprenorphine (one Zubsolv 5.7-mg buprenorphine/1.4-mg naloxone SL tablet is equivalent to one 8-mg buprenorphine/2-mg naloxone tablet). Or, buprenorphine 4 to 24 mg with naloxone 1 to 6 mg SL film as a single daily maintenance dose after buprenorphine induction. Or, 2.1 to 12.6 mg buprenorphine/0.3 to 2 mg naloxone buccal film as a single daily maintenance dose after SL buprenorphine induction (4.2-mg buprenorphine/0.7-mg naloxone buccal film is equivalent to one 8-mg buprenorphine/2-mg naloxone tablet).
➤ **Induction treatment of heroin or short-acting opioid dependence (Bunavail)**
Adults: Give initial dose not less than 6 hours after patient's last dose of heroin or short-acting opioid and when objective and clear signs and symptoms of moderate opioid withdrawal appear. Initially, on day 1, give 2.1 mg buprenorphine/0.3 mg naloxone buccally and repeat in 2 hours based on control of acute withdrawal symptoms. On day 2, give a single dose of up to 8.4 mg buprenorphine/1.4 mg naloxone buccally based on withdrawal symptoms. Transition to a clinically effective maintenance dose as soon as possible to decrease patient drop-out rate.

Psychotherapeutics

chlordiazePOXIDE–amitriptyline
Controlled Substance Schedule: IV
AVAILABLE FORMS
Tablets
5 mg chlordiazepoxide and 12.5 mg amitriptyline
10 mg chlordiazepoxide and 25 mg amitriptyline
INDICATIONS & DOSAGES
Black Box Warning Not approved for use in children because of suicide risk. Opioids combined with benzodiazepines or CNS depressants can cause death. ∎
➤ **Severe depression**
Adults: 10 mg chlordiazepoxide/25 mg amitriptyline PO t.i.d. to up to six times daily. For patients who don't tolerate higher doses, 5 mg chlordiazepoxide/12.5 mg amitriptyline PO t.i.d. to q.i.d. Reduce dosage after initial response. Maximum daily dose, amitriptyline 150 mg/chlordiazepoxide 60 mg.
Adjust-a-dose: Elderly patients may need lower dosages.

◇ OTC   ✐ Photoguide   💿 Do not crush   ✄ Genetic

OLANZapine–FLUoxetine hydrochloride
Symbyax
AVAILABLE FORMS
Capsules
3 mg olanzapine and 25 mg fluoxetine
6 mg olanzapine and 25 mg fluoxetine
6 mg olanzapine and 50 mg fluoxetine
12 mg olanzapine and 25 mg fluoxetine
12 mg olanzapine and 50 mg fluoxetine
INDICATIONS & DOSAGES
Black Box Warning Drug increases risk of suicidal thoughts and behavior. Not approved for
use in children younger than age 10 because of
suicide risk or in patients with dementia-related
psychosis because of increased risk of death. ■
➤ **Treatment of bipolar I disorder or depression**
Adults: 1 capsule PO daily in the evening. Begin with
6 mg olanzapine/25 mg fluoxetine capsule and adjust
according to effectiveness and tolerability.
Children age 10 and older with bipolar depression:
Initially, 3 mg olanzapine/25 mg fluoxetine PO daily
in the evening, adjusted according to effectiveness
and tolerability.

perphenazine–amitriptyline hydrochloride
AVAILABLE FORMS
Tablets
2 mg perphenazine and 10 mg amitriptyline hydrochloride
2 mg perphenazine and 25 mg amitriptyline hydrochloride
4 mg perphenazine and 10 mg amitriptyline hydrochloride
4 mg perphenazine and 25 mg amitriptyline hydrochloride
4 mg perphenazine and 50 mg amitriptyline hydrochloride
INDICATIONS & DOSAGES
Black Box Warning Drug increases risk of suicidal thinking and behavior. Not approved for use
in children because of suicide risk or in patients
with dementia-related psychosis because of increased risk of death. ■
➤ **Treatment of anxiety, agitation, or depression**
Adults: 2 to 4 mg perphenazine/10 to 25 mg amitriptyline PO t.i.d. to q.i.d. or 4 mg perphenazine/50 mg
amitriptyline PO b.i.d. Reduce dosage after initial
response. In severely ill patients with schizophrenia,
give initial dose of 2 tablets (4 mg perphenazine/25 mg
amitriptyline) PO t.i.d.; if needed, a fourth dose may
be added at bedtime.

Respiratory tract drugs

budesonide–formoterol fumarate dihydrate
Symbicort
AVAILABLE FORMS
Aerosol inhalation
80 mcg budesonide and 4.5 mcg formoterol fumarate
dihydrate per actuation

160 mcg budesonide and 4.5 mcg formoterol fumarate dihydrate per actuation
INDICATIONS & DOSAGES
➤ **Asthma, COPD**
Adults and children age 12 and older: Initially, 2 inhalations b.i.d. approximately 12 hours apart.
Children ages 6 to younger than age 12: 2 inhalations
of 80 mcg budesonide and 4.5 mcg formoterol fumarate dihydrate b.i.d.

chlorpheniramine polistirex– HYDROcodone polistirex
Tussionex Pennkinetic ER
Controlled Substance Schedule: II
AVAILABLE FORMS
Oral solution (extended-release)
8 mg chlorpheniramine polisterix and 10 mg hydrocodone polistirex (equivalent to 10 mg hydrocodone
bitartrate)/5 mL
INDICATIONS & DOSAGES
Black Box Warning *Opioid class warning:*
Opioids combined with benzodiazepines or CNS
depressants can cause death. Serious, life-
threatening, or fatal respiratory depression may
occur. Drug exposes users to risks of addiction,
abuse, and misuse, which can lead to overdose
and death. Dosing errors can result in accidental
overdose and death. Avoid use in patients taking
CYP3A4 inhibitors or inducers. Accidental ingestion, especially by children, can result in a fatal
overdose. Prolonged use during pregnancy can
result in neonatal opioid withdrawal syndrome. ■
➤ **Cough and URI signs and symptoms**
Adults: 8 mg chlorpheniramine polisterix/10 mg hydrocodone polisterix PO every 12 hours. Maximum
dose, 16 mg chlorpheniramine polisterix and 20 mg
hydrocodone polisterix in 24 hours.

ipratropium bromide–albuterol sulfate
Combivent Respimat
AVAILABLE FORMS
Metered-dose inhaler
20 mcg ipratropium bromide and 100 mcg albuterol
INDICATIONS & DOSAGES
**Bronchospasm with COPD in patients who
require more than a single bronchodilator**
Adults: 1 inhalation q.i.d. May give additional doses
as needed up to maximum of 6 total inhalations in
24 hours.

loratadine–pseudoephedrine sulfate
Claritin-D ◊, Claritin-D 24 Hour ◊
AVAILABLE FORMS
Tablets (extended-release) OTC
5 mg loratadine and 120 mg pseudoephedrine
10 mg loratadine and 240 mg pseudoephedrine
INDICATIONS & DOSAGES
➤ **Seasonal allergic rhinitis**
Adults and children age 12 and older: 5 mg loratadine/
120 mg pseudoephedrine PO b.i.d., or 10 mg loratadine/
240 mg pseudoephedrine PO daily. Maximum dosage,
10 mg loratadine/240 mg pseudoephedrine per day.

mometasone furoate–formoterol fumarate dihydrate

Dulera

AVAILABLE FORMS

Oral inhalation

100 mcg mometasone furoate and 5 mcg formoterol fumarate dihydrate

200 mcg mometasone furoate and 5 mcg formoterol fumarate dihydrate

INDICATIONS & DOSAGES

➤ **Asthma**

Adults and children over age 12: 2 inhalations b.i.d. Base starting dose on prior therapy with inhaled corticosteroids.

Vaccines and toxoids: Indications and dosages

Refer to manufacturer's instructions for complete prescribing and safety information.

anthrax vaccine, adsorbed
BioThrax

Pharmacologic class: Vaccines

AVAILABLE FORMS
Injection: 0.5 mL/dose in 5-mL multidose vial

INDICATIONS & DOSAGES
➤ **Preexposure prophylaxis of disease caused by *Bacillus anthracis* in persons at high risk of exposure**
Adults ages 18 through 65: 0.5 mL IM at day 0, month 1, and then 6, 12, and 18 months. Yearly booster injections of 0.5 mL IM are recommended for those who remain at risk. Or, 0.5 mL subcut at 0, 2, and 4 weeks and 6 months, with booster doses at 12 and 18 months and at 1-year intervals thereafter.
➤ **Postexposure prophylaxis of disease following suspected or confirmed *B. anthracis* exposure, in conjunction with recommended antibacterial drugs**
Adults ages 18 through 65: 0.5 mL subcut 0, 2, and 4 weeks after exposure. Administer with concomitant antibiotic therapy.

cholera vaccine, live
Vaxchora

Pharmacologic class: Vaccines

AVAILABLE FORMS
Suspension: 100-mL package

INDICATIONS & DOSAGES
➤ **Active immunization against disease caused by *Vibrio cholerae***
Adults age 18 through 64: One dose (100 mL) PO 10 days before potential exposure.

diphtheria and tetanus toxoids and acellular pertussis vaccine adsorbed (DTaP)
Daptacel, Infanrix

tetanus toxoid and reduced diphtheria toxoid and acellular pertussis vaccine adsorbed (Tdap)
Adacel, Boostrix

Pharmacologic class: Vaccines/toxoids

AVAILABLE FORMS
DTaP
Daptacel
Injection: 15 limit flocculation (Lf) units diphtheria toxoid, 5 Lf units tetanus toxoid, and 10 mcg pertussis toxoid adsorbed per 0.5 mL
Infanrix
Injection: 25 Lf units diphtheria toxoid, 10 Lf units tetanus toxoid, and 25 mcg inactivated pertussis toxins adsorbed per 0.5 mL
Tdap
Adacel
Injection: 5 Lf units tetanus toxoid, 2 Lf units diphtheria toxoid, and 2.5 mcg detoxified pertussis toxins adsorbed per 0.5 mL
Boostrix
Injection: 5 Lf units tetanus toxoid, 2.5 Lf units diphtheria toxoid, and 8 mcg inactivated pertussis toxins adsorbed per 0.5 mL

INDICATIONS & DOSAGES
➤ **Primary immunization (Daptacel, Infanrix)**
Children ages 6 weeks to 6 years (prior to 7th birthday): 0.5 mL IM 4 to 8 weeks apart for three doses (6 to 8 weeks for Daptacel) and a fourth dose at least 6 months after the third dose.
➤ **Booster immunization**
Children ages 6 weeks to 7 years: Daptacel may be given to complete the immunization series in children who have received at least one dose of whole-cell DTP vaccine.
    Infanrix is indicated as a fifth dose in children ages 4 to 6 before entering school in those who received at least one dose of whole-cell DTP vaccine, unless the fourth dose was given after the fourth birthday.
Adults and children ages 10 to 64 (Adacel): 0.5 mL IM as a single dose at least 5 years after the last DTaP vaccination.
Adults and children age 10 and older (Boostrix): 0.5 mL IM as a single dose at least 5 years after the last DTaP vaccination.

diphtheria and tetanus toxoids, acellular pertussis adsorbed, hepatitis B (recombinant), and inactivated poliovirus vaccine combined
Pediarix

Pharmacologic class: Vaccines/toxoids

AVAILABLE FORMS
Injection: 0.5-mL single-dose vials and disposable, prefilled Tip-Lok syringes

INDICATIONS & DOSAGES
➤ Active immunization

Children ages 6 weeks to 7 years: Primary series is three 0.5-mL doses IM at 6- to 8-week intervals (preferably 8), usually starting at age 2 months; may start at age 6 weeks.

diphtheria and tetanus toxoids, acellular pertussis adsorbed, and inactivated poliovirus combination vaccine (DTaP/IPV)
Kinrix, Quadracel

Pharmacologic class: Vaccines/toxoids

AVAILABLE FORMS
Injection (Kinrix): 25 limit flocculation (Lf) units diphtheria toxoid, 10 Lf units tetanus toxoid, 25 mcg inactivated pertussis toxin (PT), 25 mcg filamentous hemagglutinin, 8 mcg pertactin, 40 D-antigen units type 1 poliovirus (Mahoney), 8 D-antigen units type 2 poliovirus (MEF-1), and 32 D-antigen units/0.5 mL type 3 poliovirus (Saukett)
Injection (Quadracel): 15 Lf units diphtheria toxoid, 5 Lf units tetanus toxoid, acellular pertussis antigens [detoxified 20 mcg pertussis toxin, 20 mcg filamentous hemagglutinin, 3 mcg pertactin, 5 mcg fimbriae (types 2 and 3)], 40 D-antigen units type 1 poliovirus, 8 D-antigen units type 2 poliovirus, and 32 D-antigen units type 3 poliovirus per 0.5 mL

INDICATIONS & DOSAGES
➤ Active immunization against diphtheria, tetanus, pertussis, and poliomyelitis as the fifth dose in the DTaP vaccine series and the fourth dose in the IPV series (Kinrix), or as the fifth dose in the DTaP vaccine series and as a fourth or fifth dose in the IPV series (Quadracel)

Children ages 4 through 6: 0.5 mL IM, preferably in the deltoid muscle of the upper arm as a single dose. Refer to manufacturer's instructions for use with prior specific vaccine products.

diphtheria and tetanus toxoids, acellular pertussis adsorbed, inactivated poliovirus, and *Haemophilus influenzae* type b conjugate vaccine combined
Pentacel

Pharmacologic class: Vaccines/toxoids

AVAILABLE FORMS
Injection: 15 limit flocculation (Lf) units diphtheria toxoid, 5 Lf units tetanus toxoid, 20 mcg pertussis toxin detoxified, 20 mcg filamentous hemagglutinin, 3 mcg pertactin, 5 mcg fimbriae types 2 and 3, 40 D-antigen units type 1 inactivated poliovirus (Mahoney), 8 D-antigen units type 2 inactivated poliovirus (MEF-1), 32 D-antigen units type 3 inactivated poliovirus (Saukett), and 10 mcg lyophilized polyribosylribitol-phosphate of *H. influenzae* type b bound to tetanus toxoid 24 mcg per 0.5 mL

INDICATIONS & DOSAGES
➤ Active immunization against diphtheria, tetanus, pertussis, poliomyelitis, and invasive disease caused by *H. influenzae* type b

Children ages 6 weeks to 4 years (prior to 5th birthday): 0.5 mL IM. Approved for administration as a four-dose series at ages 2, 4, 6, and 15 through 18 months. The first dose may be given as early as age 6 weeks.

Haemophilus b conjugate vaccine, meningococcal protein conjugate (PRP-OMP)
PedvaxHIB

Haemophilus b conjugate, tetanus toxoid conjugate (PRP-T)
ActHIB, Hiberix

Pharmacologic class: Vaccines

AVAILABLE FORMS
Hib conjugate vaccine, meningococcal protein conjugate
Injection: 7.5 mcg of Hib PRP and 125 mcg *N. meningitides* OMPC per 0.5 mL
Hib conjugate vaccine, tetanus toxoid conjugate
Injection: 10 mcg Hib capsular polysaccharide and 24 mcg tetanus toxoid (ActHIB) or 10 mcg Hib capsular polysaccharide and 25 mcg tetanus toxoid (Hiberix)

INDICATIONS & DOSAGES
➤ Active immunization for the prevention of invasive disease caused by Hib (PedvaxHIB)

Infants: 0.5 mL IM at age 2 months; repeat at age 4 months. Give booster dose at age 12 months. May give first dose as early as age 6 weeks.

Previously unvaccinated children ages 15 months to 6 years: 0.5 mL IM. Booster dose isn't needed. Premature infants follow same schedule as full-term infants.

➤ **Active immunization for the prevention of invasive disease caused by Hib (ActHIB, Hiberix)**
Infants: 0.5 mL IM at age 2 months. Repeat at ages 4 and 6 months. Give booster doses at ages 15 to 18 months. May give first dose as early as age 6 weeks.

hepatitis A vaccine, inactivated
Havrix, Vaqta

Pharmacologic class: Vaccines

AVAILABLE FORMS
Havrix
Injection: 720 enzyme-linked immunosorbent assay (ELISA) units (ELU)/0.5 mL, 1,440 ELU/mL
Vaqta
Injection: 25 units/0.5 mL, 50 units/mL

INDICATIONS & DOSAGES
➤ **Active immunization against hepatitis A virus; with immune globulin, to prevent hepatitis A in those exposed to virus or who travel to endemic areas**
Adults: 1,440 ELU Havrix or 50 units Vaqta IM as single dose. For booster dose, give 1,440 ELU Havrix 6 to 12 months after first dose or 50 units Vaqta IM 6 to 18 months after first dose. Booster is recommended for prolonged immunity.
Children ages 12 months to 18 years: 720 ELU Havrix or 25 units Vaqta IM as single dose. Then, give booster dose of 720 ELU Havrix 6 to 12 months after first dose or 25 units Vaqta IM 6 to 18 months after first dose. Booster is recommended for prolonged immunity.

hepatitis B vaccine, recombinant
Engerix-B, Recombivax HB, Recombivax HB Dialysis Formulation

Pharmacologic class: Vaccines

AVAILABLE FORMS
Injection: 5 mcg HBsAg/0.5 mL (Recombivax HB, pediatric and adolescent form with or without preservative); 10 mcg HBsAg/0.5 mL (Engerix-B, pediatric and adolescent form); 10 mcg HBsAg/mL (Recombivax HB, adult form); 20 mcg HBsAg/mL (Engerix-B, adult form); 40 mcg HBsAg/mL (Recombivax HB Dialysis Formulation)

INDICATIONS & DOSAGES
➤ **Immunization against infection from all known subtypes of HBV, primary preexposure prophylaxis against HBV, postexposure prophylaxis when given with hepatitis B immune globulin (HBIG)**
Engerix-B
Adults age 20 and older: Initially, 20 mcg IM; then second dose of 20 mcg IM after 30 days. A third dose of 20 mcg IM is given 6 months after the first dose.
Adjust-a-dose: For adults undergoing dialysis or receiving immunosuppressants, initially, 40 mcg IM (divided into two 20-mcg doses and given at different sites). Then second dose of 40 mcg IM in 30 days, a third dose after 2 months, and final dose of 40 mcg IM 6 months after first dose.
Adolescents ages 11 to 19: Initially, 10 mcg (pediatric and adolescent form) IM; then second dose of 10 mcg IM 30 days later. Give third dose of 10 mcg IM 6 months after first dose. Or, 20 mcg (adult form) IM; then second dose of 20 mcg IM 30 days later. Give third dose of 20 mcg IM 6 months after first dose.
Neonates and children up to age 10: Initially, 10 mcg IM; then second dose of 10 mcg IM 30 days later. Give third dose of 10 mcg IM 6 months after first dose.
➤ **Recombivax HB**
Adults age 20 and older: Initially, 10 mcg IM; then second dose of 10 mcg IM after 30 days. Give third dose of 10 mcg IM 6 months after first dose.
Adjust-a-dose: For adults undergoing dialysis, initially, 40 mcg IM (use dialysis form, which contains 40 mcg/mL); then second dose of 40 mcg IM in 30 days, and final dose of 40 mcg IM 6 months after first dose. A booster or revaccination may be indicated if anti-HBs titer is below 10 mIU/mL 1 to 2 months after third dose.
Infants, children, and adolescents age 19 or younger: Initially, 5 mcg IM; then second dose of 5 mcg IM after 30 days. Give third dose of 5 mcg IM 6 months after first dose. Or, in adolescents ages 11 to 15, give 10 mcg (1 mL adult form) IM; then second dose of 10 mcg IM 4 to 6 months later.
Infants born of HBsAg-positive mothers or mothers of unknown HBsAg status: Initially, 5 mcg IM; then second dose of 5 mcg IM after 30 days. Give third dose of 5 mcg IM 6 months after first dose.
Infants born of HBsAg-negative mothers: Initially, 5 mcg IM; then second dose of 5 mcg IM after 30 days. Give third dose of 5 mcg IM 6 months after first dose.
Note: If the mother is found to be HBsAg-positive within 7 days of delivery, also give the infant a dose of HBIG (0.5 mL) in the opposite anterolateral thigh.

human papillomavirus recombinant vaccine, 9-valent
Gardasil 9

Pharmacologic class: Virus antigens

AVAILABLE FORMS
Injection: 0.5 mL single-dose vial, prefilled syringe

INDICATIONS & DOSAGES
➤ **To prevent cervical, vulvar, vaginal, and anal cancer caused by human papillomavirus (HPV) types 16, 18, 31, 33, 45, 52, and 58; genital warts caused by HPV types 6 and 11; cervical adenocarcinoma in situ, and cervical, vulval, vaginal, and anal intraepithelial neoplasias caused by HPV types 6, 11, 16, 18, 31, 33, 45, 52, and 58**
Women and girls ages 9 to 45: Three separate IM injections of 0.5 mL each. Give second injection 2 months after first; then give third injection 6 months after the first. If second dose is given more than a month after first dose, the minimum interval between second and third dose is 3 months.
➤ **To prevent genital warts caused by HPV types 6 and 11; anal cancer caused by HPV types 6, 18, 31, 33, 45, 52, and 58; anal intraepithelial neoplasia caused by HPV types 6, 11, 16, 18, 31, 33, 45, 52, and 58**
Men and boys ages 9 to 45: Three separate IM injections of 0.5 mL each. Give second injection 2 months after first; then give third injection 6 months after first. If second dose is given more than a month after first dose, the minimum interval between second and third dose is 3 months.

influenza virus vaccine, live
Afluria Quadrivalent, Fluad, Fluarix Quadrivalent, Flublok, Flucelvax Quadrivalent, FluLaval Quadrivalent, Fluvirin, Fluzone High-Dose, Fluzone Intradermal Quadrivalent, Fluzone Quadrivalent

Pharmacologic class: Vaccines

AVAILABLE FORMS
Injection: 0.1-mL pen-injectors, 0.25-mL prefilled syringes, 0.5-mL prefilled syringes, 0.5-mL single-dose vials, 0.5 mL/dose in 5-mL multidose vials

INDICATIONS & DOSAGES
➤ **Active immunization to prevent disease caused by influenza A and B viruses**
Adults ages 18 to 64: 0.5 mL IM as a single dose or 0.1 mL intradermally as a single dose (Fluzone Intradermal Quadrivalent).

Children age 9 and older: 0.5 mL IM as a single dose (Afluria Quadrivalent, Fluarix Quadrivalent, Flucelvax Quadrivalent, FluLaval Quadrivalent, Fluvirin, Fluzone Quadrivalent).
Children ages 3 to 8: 0.5 mL IM as a single dose (Fluarix Quadrivalent, FluLaval Quadrivalent, Fluzone Quadrivalent). Dose may need repeating based on previous vaccination status.
Children ages 4 to 8: 0.5 mL IM as a single dose (Flucelvax Quadrivalent, Fluvirin). Dose may need repeating based on previous vaccination status.
Children ages 5 to 8: 0.5 mL (Afluria Quadrivalent) IM as a single dose.
Children ages 3 to 8: 0.5 mL (Fluzone Quadrivalent) IM as a single dose.
Children ages 6 to 35 months: 0.25 mL IM as a single dose (Fluzone Quadrivalent). Dose may need repeating based on previous vaccination status.
Children age 6 months to less than 9 years: 0.5 mL (FluLaval Quadrivalent) IM as a single dose. Dose may need repeating based on previous vaccination status.
Elderly patients (age 65 and older) (except Fluzone Intradermal Quadrivalent): 0.5 mL IM as a single dose.

Japanese encephalitis virus vaccine
Ixiaro

Pharmacologic class: Vaccines

AVAILABLE FORMS
Injection: 6 mcg/0.5 mL

INDICATIONS & DOSAGES
➤ **To prevent disease caused by Japanese encephalitis virus**
Adults and children age 3 and older: Two doses of 0.5 mL IM 28 days apart. Complete immunization at least 1 week before exposure. If primary series of two doses was completed more than a year previously, may give a booster dose if ongoing exposure or reexposure is expected.
Children ages 2 months to younger than 3 years: Two doses of 0.25 mL IM 28 days apart.

measles, mumps, and rubella virus vaccine, live
M-M-R II, Priorix✤

Pharmacologic class: Vaccines

AVAILABLE FORMS
Injection: Single-dose vial containing at least 1,000 tissue culture infective doses ($TCID_{50}$) of measles, 12,500 $TCID_{50}$ of mumps strain, and 1,000 $TCID_{50}$ rubella virus per 0.5-mL dose

INDICATIONS & DOSAGES

➤ **Routine immunization**

Adults: 0.5 mL subcut.

Children age 12 months and older: 0.5 mL subcut. A two-dose schedule is recommended, with first dose given between ages 12 and 15 months (between ages 6 and 12 months in high-risk areas) and second dose given at ages 4 to 6 before elementary school entry.

measles, mumps, rubella, and varicella (MMRV) virus vaccine, live, attenuated
ProQuad

Pharmacologic class: Vaccines

AVAILABLE FORMS

Injection: Single-dose vial containing at least 3.00 $\log_{10}$ measles tissue culture infective doses (TCID$_{50}$), 4.30 $\log_{10}$ mumps TCID$_{50}$, 3.00 $\log_{10}$ rubella TCID$_{50}$, and at least 3.99 $\log_{10}$ varicella plaque-forming units (PFU) per 0.5-mL dose

INDICATIONS & DOSAGES

➤ **Routine immunization**

Children ages 12 months to 12 years: 0.5 mL subcut. The first dose is usually given between ages 12 and 15 months but may be given any time through age 12. A second dose, if needed, is usually given between ages 4 and 6. At least 1 month should elapse between a dose of a measles-containing vaccine and a dose of MMRV vaccine. If a second dose of a varicella-containing vaccine is required, at least 3 months should elapse between administration of the two doses.

meningococcal (groups A, C, Y, and W-135) polysaccharide diphtheria toxoid conjugate vaccine (MCV4)
Menactra

meningococcal polysaccharide vaccine, groups A, C, Y, and W-135 combined (MPSV4)
Menveo (Men ACWY-CRM)

meningococcal (group B) vaccine
Bexsero, Trumenba

Pharmacologic class: Vaccines

AVAILABLE FORMS

Injection: 0.5 mL single-dose vials and prefilled syringes

INDICATIONS & DOSAGES

➤ **Active immunization for the prevention of invasive meningococcal disease caused by *Neisseria meningitidis* serogroups A, C, Y, and W-135**

Adults and children ages 2 to 55: 0.5 mL MCV4 IM as a single dose, preferably in the deltoid muscle.

Adults and children ages 15 to 55 who are at continued risk for meningococcal disease: 0.5 mL Menactra as a booster at least 4 years after prior dose.

Children ages 9 to 23 months: 0.5 mL Menactra IM given as a two-dose series 3 months apart.

Adults and children older than age 2: 0.5 mL MPSV4 subcut as a single dose, preferably in the upper-outer triceps area.

Adults and children ages 2 to 55: 0.5 mL Menveo IM as single dose, preferably into deltoid muscle. For children ages 2 to 5 at continued high risk for meningococcal disease, a second dose may be given 2 months after the first dose.

Children ages 7 to 23 months: 0.5 mL Menveo IM given as a two-dose series with second dose in the second year of life and at least 3 months after first dose.

Infants: 0.5 mL Menveo IM given as a four-dose series at 2, 4, 6, and 12 months.

➤ **Active immunization for the prevention of invasive meningococcal disease caused by *N. meningitidis* serogroup B**

Adults and children age 10 and older: 0.5 mL/dose (Bexsero) IM as a two-dose series at least 1 month apart. Or, 0.5 mL/dose (Trumenba) IM at 0 and 6 months (two-dose schedule), or at 0 month and then a second dose at either 1 or 2 months and then a third dose at 6 months (three-dose schedule).

palivizumab
Synagis

Pharmacologic class: Monoclonal antibodies

AVAILABLE FORMS

Injection: 50-mg, 100-mg vials

INDICATIONS & DOSAGES

➤ **Prevention of serious lower respiratory tract disease caused by RSV**

High-risk infants age 24 months and younger: 15 mg/kg IM monthly throughout RSV season. Give first dose before commencement of RSV season.

pneumococcal vaccine, polyvalent
Pneumovax 23

13-valent conjugate vaccine
Prevnar 13

Pharmacologic class: Vaccines

AVAILABLE FORMS
Injection: 25 mcg each of 23 polysaccharide isolates/ 0.5 mL (Pneumovax 23); 2.2 mcg each of *Streptococcus pneumoniae* serotypes 1, 3, 4, 5, 6A, 7F, 9V, 14, 18C, 19A, 19F, and 23F saccharides and 4.4 mcg of serotype 6B saccharides (Prevnar 13)

INDICATIONS & DOSAGES
➤ **Pneumococcal immunization**
Adults age 50 and older; children age 2 and older at high risk: 0.5 mL Pneumovax IM or subcut. Adults younger than age 50 who are at high risk may be immunized following Advisory Committee on Immunization Practices guidelines.
➤ **Immunization against *S. pneumoniae* and otitis media (Prevnar 13)**
Infants ages 6 weeks to 15 months: 0.5 mL IM for a total of four doses at ages 2, 4, 6, and 12 to 15 months.
Children ages 7 to 11 months, previously unvaccinated: 0.5 mL IM; three doses with at least 4 weeks between first and second doses, and 8 weeks between second and third doses.
Children ages 12 to 23 months, previously unvaccinated: Two doses of 0.5 mL IM at least 2 months apart.
Children ages 24 months to 5 years, previously unvaccinated: 0.5 mL IM as a single dose.
Children ages 6 to 17 (before the 18th birthday): 0.5 mL IM as a single dose. For children previously vaccinated with PCV7, wait at least 8 weeks.
Children who have received one or more doses of Prevnar (7-valent conjugate vaccine): Complete the four-dose immunization series with 13-valent conjugate vaccine.
Children ages 15 months through 5 years who have previously received four doses of Prevnar: 0.5 mL IM as a single dose.
➤ **Immunization against *S. pneumoniae* (Prevnar 13)**
Adults age 65 and older: 0.5 mL IM as a single dose. Adults ages 19 to 64 who are at high risk may be immunized following Advisory Committee on Immunization Practices guidelines.

poliovirus vaccine, inactivated (IPV)
IPOL

Pharmacologic class: Vaccines

AVAILABLE FORMS
0.5-mL prefilled syringe: Mixture of three types of poliovirus (types 1, 2, and 3) grown in tissue culture

INDICATIONS & DOSAGES
➤ **Poliovirus immunization**
Unvaccinated adults: 0.5 mL subcut or IM; give second dose 4 to 8 weeks later. Give third dose 6 to 12 months later.
Children: 0.5 mL subcut or IM at ages 2 months and 4 months. Give third dose at ages 6 to 18 months. Give a reinforcing dose of 0.5 mL subcut before entry into school at ages 4 to 6.

rabies vaccine
Imovax Rabies, RabAvert

Pharmacologic class: Vaccines

AVAILABLE FORMS
Injection: 2.5 international units rabies antigen/mL, in single-dose vial with diluent

INDICATIONS & DOSAGES
➤ **Postexposure antirabies immunization**
Adults and children: Five 1-mL doses IM. Give first dose as soon as possible after exposure in conjunction with rabies immune globulin; give additional doses on days 3, 7, 14, and 28 after first dose. If no antibody response occurs after this primary series, booster dose is recommended.
➤ **Postexposure antirabies immunization in previously immunized people**
Adults and children: 1 mL IM immediately and 1 mL IM 3 days later.
➤ **Preexposure preventive immunization for persons in high-risk groups**
Adults and children: Three 1-mL injections IM. Give first dose on day 0 (first day of therapy), second dose on day 7, and third dose on day 21 or 28.

rotavirus, live
Rotarix, RotaTeq

Pharmacologic class: Vaccines

AVAILABLE FORMS
Lyophilized powder for oral suspension: Rotavirus human 89-12 strain (G1P[8] type); $\geq 10^6$ cell culture infective dose per 1 mL (after reconstitution)

Oral suspension: Rotavirus outer capsid protein (2.2 ×10^6 infectious units of G1, 2.8 × 10^6 infectious units of G2, 2.2 × 10^6 infectious units of G3, 2 × 10^6 infectious units of G4, and 2.3 × 10^6 infectious units of rotavirus attachment protein P1A[8]) per 2 mL

INDICATIONS & DOSAGES
➤ **Prevention of rotavirus gastroenteritis**
RotaTeq
Children ages 6 to 32 weeks: 2 mL PO. Give second dose 4 weeks later, followed by third dose at 10 weeks. Don't give third dose after the patient reaches age 32 weeks.
Rotarix
Infants ages 6 to 24 weeks: Give first dose of 1 mL PO at age 6 weeks. Give another 1-mL dose PO after at least 4 weeks. The two-dose series should be completed by age 24 weeks.

tetanus toxoid, adsorbed

Pharmacologic class: Vaccines

AVAILABLE FORMS
Injection: 5 limit flocculation (Lf) units inactivated tetanus/0.5 mL, in 0.5-mL syringes and 5-mL vials

INDICATIONS & DOSAGES
➤ **Primary immunization to prevent tetanus**
Adults and children age 7 and older: 0.5 mL IM 4 to 8 weeks apart for two doses; then give third dose 6 to 12 months after second.
➤ **Booster dose to prevent tetanus**
Adults and children age 7 and older: 0.5 mL IM at 10-year intervals.
➤ **Postexposure prevention of tetanus**
Adults and children age 7 and older: For a clean, minor wound, give emergency booster dose if more than 10 years have elapsed since last dose. For all other wounds, give booster dose if more than 5 years have elapsed since last dose.

varicella virus vaccine
Varivax

Pharmacologic class: Vaccines

AVAILABLE FORMS
Injection: 1,350 plaque-forming units of Oka/Merck varicella virus (live) in single-dose vials

INDICATIONS & DOSAGES
➤ **To prevent varicella zoster (chickenpox) infections**
Adults and children age 13 and older: 0.5 mL subcut; then, second 0.5-mL dose 4 to 8 weeks later.
Children ages 1 to 12: 0.5 mL subcut. If a second dose is given, allow a minimum interval of 3 months between doses.

zoster vaccine, live
Zostavax

zoster vaccine recombinant, adjuvanted
Shingrix

Pharmacologic class: Vaccines, live attenuated

AVAILABLE FORMS
Injection (Shingrix): Lyophilized varicella zoster virus glycoprotein E (gE) antigen component; after reconstitution, each 0.5-mL dose contains 50 mcg of the recombinant gE antigen
Injection (Zostavax): Lyophilized vaccine of 19,400 plaque-forming units/0.65 mL

INDICATIONS & DOSAGES
➤ **Prevention of herpes zoster (shingles)**
Adults age 50 and older: 0.65 mL Zostavax subcut as a single dose, preferably in the upper arm. Or, 0.5 mL Shingrix IM as a two-dose series, with first dose given at month 0 and second dose given anytime between 2 and 6 months later.

Vitamins and minerals: Indications and dosages

Refer to manufacturer's instructions for complete prescribing and safety information.

ferrous fumarate
FAIR-us

Ferretts ◇, Ferrocite ◇, Hemocyte ◇, Iron ◇

Therapeutic class: Iron supplements
Pharmacologic class: Hematinics

AVAILABLE FORMS
Each 100 mg of ferrous fumarate provides 33 mg of elemental iron.
Tablets ⓞⓣⓒ: 29 mg ◇, 150 mg ◇, 324 mg ◇, 325 mg ◇

INDICATIONS & DOSAGES
➤ **Iron deficiency**
Adults: 1 or 2 tablets PO daily between meals or as directed by prescriber.
Children: 3 to 6 mg/kg/day of elemental iron PO in three divided doses.

ferrous gluconate
FER-us

Ferate ◇, Fergon ◇

Therapeutic class: Iron supplements
Pharmacologic class: Hematinics

AVAILABLE FORMS
Each 100 mg of ferrous gluconate provides 11.6 mg of elemental iron.
Tablets ⓞⓣⓒ: 240 mg ◇, 324 mg ◇

INDICATIONS & DOSAGES
➤ **Iron deficiency**
Adults: 100 to 200 mg of elemental iron PO daily in two to three divided doses or as directed by prescriber.
Children: 3 to 6 mg/kg/day of elemental iron PO in three divided doses.

ferrous sulfate
FER-us

Ferro-Bob, Ferosol ◇ *, Fer-Iron ◇, Fer-In-Sol ◇, FeroSul ◇

ferrous sulfate (dried)
Feratab ◇, Slow FE ◇, Slow Release Iron ◇

Therapeutic class: Iron supplements
Pharmacologic class: Hematinics

AVAILABLE FORMS
Each 100 mg of ferrous sulfate provides 20 mg of elemental iron or 30 mg of elemental iron in ferrous sulfate dried products.
Elixir: 220 mg/5 mL ◇ *
Liquid: 75 mg/mL ◇, 300 mg/5 mL ◇
Tablets: 325 mg ◇
Tablets (extended-release) ⓞⓣⓒ: 140 mg ◇, 142 mg ◇, 160 mg (dried) ◇

INDICATIONS & DOSAGES
➤ **Iron deficiency**
Adults, infants, and children: Refer to individual manufacturer's instructions for dosages. Immediate-release products are usually given in divided doses daily. Extended-release formulations are given once daily. Lower daily doses may cause less GI adverse events in elderly patients.

vitamin A
A-25 ◇, Vitamin A Fish ◇

vitamin A palmitate
Aquasol A

AVAILABLE FORMS
Capsules: 7,500 international units ◇, 8,000 international units ◇, 10,000 international units ◇, 25,000 international units
Injection: 50,000 international units/mL in 2-mL vials
Tablets: 10,000 international units ◇, 15,000 international units ◇

INDICATIONS & DOSAGES
➤ **RDA**
Men and boys older than age 14: 900 mcg retinol equivalent (RE).
Women and girls older than age 14: 700 mcg RE.
Children ages 9 to 13: 600 mcg RE.
Children ages 4 to 8: 400 mcg RE.
Children ages 1 to 3: 300 mcg RE.
Infants ages 7 to 12 months: 500 mcg RE.

Neonates and infants younger than age 6 months:
400 mcg RE.
Pregnant women ages 14 to 18: 750 mcg RE.
Pregnant women ages 19 to 50: 770 mcg RE.
Breastfeeding women ages 14 to 18: 1,200 mcg RE.
Breastfeeding women ages 19 to 50: 1,300 mcg RE.
➤ **Severe vitamin A deficiency**
Adults and children older than age 8: 100,000 international units IM or 100,000 to 500,000 international units PO for 3 days; then 50,000 international units PO or IM daily for 2 weeks, followed by 10,000 to 20,000 international units PO for 2 months. Follow with adequate dietary nutrition and RE vitamin A supplements.
Children ages 1 to 8: 17,500 to 35,000 international units IM daily for 10 days.
Infants: 7,500 to 15,000 international units IM daily for 10 days.
➤ **Maintenance dose to prevent recurrence of vitamin A deficiency**
Adults and children older than age 8: 10,000 to 20,000 international units PO daily for 2 months.
Children infants to age 8: Give 5,000 to 10,000 international units PO daily for 2 months; then adequate dietary nutrition and RE vitamin A supplements.

vitamin B₁₂ (cyanocobalamin)

B-12 Compliance Injection, Nascobal, Physicians EZ Use B-12, Vitamin Deficiency System-B12, Vibisone

hydroxocobalamin (vitamin B₁₂)

Cyanokit

AVAILABLE FORMS
cyanocobalamin
Injection*: 1,000 mcg/mL
Intranasal spray: 500 mcg/spray
Liquid (S.L.): 3,000 mcg ◇
Lozenges: 50 mcg ◇, 100 mcg ◇, 250 mcg ◇, 500 mcg ◇
Tablets: 100 mcg ◇, 250 mcg ◇, 500 mcg ◇, 1,000 mcg ◇
Tablets (extended-release): 1,000 mcg ◇
Tablets (S.L.): 2,500 mcg ◇
hydroxocobalamin
Injection: 1,000 mcg/mL, 5 g/vial

INDICATIONS & DOSAGES
➤ **RDA for cyanocobalamin**
Adults and children age 14 and older: 2.4 mcg.
Children ages 9 to 13: 1.8 mcg.
Children ages 4 to 8: 1.2 mcg.
Children ages 1 to 3: 0.9 mcg.
Infants ages 7 months to 1 year: 0.5 mcg.

Neonates and infants age 6 months and younger: 0.4 mcg.
Pregnant women: 2.6 mcg.
Breastfeeding women: 2.8 mcg.
➤ **Vitamin B₁₂ deficiency from inadequate diet, subtotal gastrectomy, or other condition, disorder, or disease, except malabsorption, related to pernicious anemia or other GI disease**
Adults: 30 mcg hydroxocobalamin IM daily for 5 to 10 days, depending on severity of deficiency. Maintenance dose is 100 to 200 mcg IM. For subsequent prophylaxis, advise adequate nutrition and daily RDA vitamin B₁₂ supplements.
Children: 1 to 5 mg hydroxocobalamin in single doses of 100 mcg IM over 2 or more weeks, depending on severity of deficiency. Maintenance dose is 30 to 50 mcg IM every 4 weeks. For subsequent prophylaxis, advise adequate nutrition and daily RDA vitamin B₁₂ supplements.
➤ **Pernicious anemia or vitamin B₁₂ malabsorption**
Adults: Initially, 100 mcg cyanocobalamin IM or subcut daily for 6 to 7 days. If response is observed, 100 mcg IM or subcut every other day for 7 doses, then 100 mcg every 3 to 4 days for 2 to 3 weeks; then 100 mcg IM or subcut once monthly.
➤ **Maintenance therapy for remission of pernicious anemia after IM vitamin B₁₂ therapy in patients without nervous system involvement; dietary deficiency, malabsorption disorders, and inadequate secretion of intrinsic factor**
Adults: Initially, 1 spray in one nostril once weekly (Nascobal). Give at least 1 hour before or after hot foods or liquids.
➤ **Schilling test flushing dose**
Adults and children: 1,000 mcg hydroxocobalamin IM as single dose.
➤ **Cyanide poisoning**
Adults: Initially, 5 g hydroxocobalamin IV over 15 minutes. Based on patient's condition, may repeat 5 g dose IV over 15 minutes to 2 hours.

coenzyme Q10

Chew Q ◇, CoQ10 ◇, H₂Q, LiQsorb ◇, Mega CoQ10 ◇, Vitaline CoQ10 ◇

AVAILABLE FORMS
Capsules: 10 mg ◇, 30 mg ◇, 50 mg ◇, 60 mg ◇, 75 mg ◇, 100 mg ◇, 120 mg ◇, 125 mg ◇, 150 mg ◇, 200 mg ◇, 400 mg ◇
Capsules (extended-release): 100 mg ◇
Oral liquid: 6 mg/mL ◇, 20 mg/mL ◇
Tablets: 50 mg ◇, 60 mg ◇, 100 mg ◇
Tablets (chewable): 30 mg ◇, 100 mg ◇
Wafers: 60 mg ◇, 100 mg ◇, 300 mg ◇, 400 mg ◇, 600 mg ◇

INDICATIONS & DOSAGES
➤ **Dietary supplement for conditions associated with coenzyme Q10 deficiency**
Adults: 10 to 300 mg/day PO in one or divided doses. Higher doses (up to 3,000 mg/day) have been used.

folic acid (vitamin B₉)
FA-8 ◇

AVAILABLE FORMS
Injection: 10-mL vials (5 mg/mL with 1.5% benzyl alcohol, and 0.2% ethylenediaminetetraacetic acid)
Capsules: 0.8 mg ◇, 5 mg ◇, 20 mg ◇
Tablets: 0.4 mg ◇, 0.8 mg ◇, 1 mg

INDICATIONS & DOSAGES
➤ **RDA**
Adults and children age 14 and older: 400 mcg.
Children ages 9 to 13: 300 mcg.
Children ages 4 to 8: 200 mcg.
Children ages 1 to 3: 150 mcg.
Infants ages 7 months to 1 year: 80 mcg.
Neonates and infants younger than age 6 months: 65 mcg.
Pregnant women: 600 mcg.
Breastfeeding women: 500 mcg.
➤ **Megaloblastic or macrocytic anemia from folic acid or other nutritional deficiency, hepatic disease, alcoholism, intestinal obstruction, or excessive hemolysis**
Adults and children age 4 and older: 0.4 to 1 mg PO, IM, or subcut daily. After anemia caused by folic acid deficiency is corrected, proper diet and RDA supplements are needed to prevent recurrence.
Children younger than age 4: Up to 0.3 mg PO, IM, or subcut daily.
Pregnant and breastfeeding women: 0.8 mg PO, IM, or subcut daily.
➤ **To prevent fetal neural tube defects during pregnancy ◆**
Adults: 0.4 to 0.8 mg PO daily before conception through at least first 4 to 12 weeks of fetal formation. For women at high risk, recommended dosage is 4 mg daily starting up to 3 months before conception and through first 3 months of pregnancy.

leucovorin calcium (citrovorum factor, folinic acid)

AVAILABLE FORMS
Injection: 50-mg, 100-mg, 200-mg, 350-mg, 500-mg vials for reconstitution (contains no preservatives)
Tablets: 5 mg, 10 mg, 15 mg, 25 mg

INDICATIONS & DOSAGES
➤ **Leucovorin rescue after high-dose methotrexate therapy**
Adults: 15 mg (approximately 10 mg/m²) PO, IM, or IV every 6 hours for 10 doses starting 24 hours after start of methotrexate infusion. Continue treatment until methotrexate level is less than 5×10^{-8} M. See manufacturer's instructions for dosage adjustment guidelines for methotrexate toxicity.
➤ **Impaired methotrexate elimination or inadvertent overdose**
Adults: 10 mg/m² PO, IM, or IV every 6 hours until serum methotrexate level is less than 10^{-8} M. If 24-hour serum creatinine level increases 50% over baseline or if 24-hour methotrexate level is greater than 5×10^{-6} M or 48-hour level is greater than 9×10^{-7} M, increase dosage to 100 mg/m² IV every 3 hours until methotrexate level is less than 10^{-8} M.
➤ **Folate-deficient megaloblastic anemia**
Adults and children: Up to 1 mg IM daily.
➤ **Palliative treatment of advanced colorectal cancer**
Adults: 20 mg/m² IV daily followed by 5-FU 425 mg/m² IV. Or, 200 mg/m² IV daily for 5 days (over 3 minutes or longer) followed by 5-FU 370 mg/m² daily for 5 consecutive days. Repeat at 4-week intervals for two additional courses; then at intervals of 4 to 5 weeks, if tolerated. Give 5-FU and leucovorin separately to avoid precipitate formation.

niacin (nicotinic acid, vitamin B₃)
Endur-Acin ◇, Niacor, Niaspan, Slo-Niacin ◇

niacinamide ◇ (nicotinamide ◇)

AVAILABLE FORMS
niacin
Capsules (extended-release): 250 mg ◇, 500 mg
Tablets: 50 mg ◇, 100 mg ◇, 250 mg ◇, 500 mg
Tablets (extended-release): 250 mg ◇, 500 mg ◇, 750 mg ◇, 1,000 mg ◇
niacinamide
Tablets: 100 mg ◇, 500 mg ◇

INDICATIONS & DOSAGES
➤ **RDA**
Adult men and boys ages 14 to 18: 16 mg.
Adult women and girls ages 14 to 18: 14 mg.
Children ages 9 to 13: 12 mg.
Children ages 4 to 8: 8 mg.
Children ages 1 to 3: 6 mg.
Infants ages 7 months to 1 year: 3 mg.
Neonates and infants younger than age 6 months: 2 mg.
Pregnant women: 18 mg.
Breastfeeding women: 17 mg.

➤ **Niacin deficiency**
Adults: Up to 100 mg PO daily.
➤ **Hyperlipidemias, especially with hypercholesterolemia**
Adults: 250 mg Niacor PO daily after evening meal. Increase at 4- to 7-day intervals up to 1 to 2 g PO daily in two or three divided doses. Maximum 6 g daily. Or, 1 to 2 g extended-release tablets PO daily at bedtime.

paricalcitol
Zemplar

AVAILABLE FORMS
Capsules: 1 mcg, 2 mcg, 4 mcg
Injection: 2 mcg/mL, 5 mcg/mL

INDICATIONS & DOSAGES
➤ **To prevent or treat secondary hyperparathyroidism in patients with stage 3 or 4 chronic kidney disease**
Adults: Initial dose is based on baseline intact parathyroid hormone (iPTH) levels. If iPTH is less than or equal to 500 picograms (pg)/mL, give 1 mcg PO daily or 2 mcg PO three times weekly, no more often than every other day. If iPTH is greater than 500 pg/mL, give 2 mcg PO daily or 4 mcg PO three times weekly, no more often than every other day. Adjust dose at 2- to 4-week intervals, based on iPTH levels.
Children ages 10 to 16: Initially, 1 mcg PO three times weekly, no more frequently than every other day. As indicated, increase each dose every 4 weeks or decrease each dose at any time based on iPTH, serum calcium, and phosphorus levels.
➤ **To prevent or treat secondary hyperparathyroidism in patients with chronic renal failure**
Adults: 0.04 to 0.1 mcg/kg (2.8 to 7 mcg) IV no more often than every other day during dialysis. May safely give doses as high as 0.24 mcg/kg. If satisfactory response isn't observed, increase dosage by 2 to 4 mcg at 2- to 4-week intervals. Or, calculate initial PO dose in mcg, based on baseline iPTH level divided by 80 and administered three times weekly, no more frequently than every other day. Initiate only after baseline serum calcium level has been adjusted to 9.5 mg/dL or less. Titrate as indicated by using most recent iPTH level divided by 80. Decrease dosage by 2 to 4 mcg if serum calcium level is elevated.
Children ages 10 to 16: Calculate initial PO dose in mcg, rounded down to the nearest whole number, based on baseline iPTH level divided by 120 and administered three times weekly, no more frequently than every other day. As indicated, increase each dose every 4 weeks or decrease each dose at any time to maintain iPTH within target range.

pyridoxine hydrochloride (vitamin B₆)
Neuro-K-250 ◊, Neuro-K-250 TD ◊, Pyri 500 ◊

AVAILABLE FORMS
Capsules: 250 mg ◊
Injection: 100 mg/mL
Tablets: 25 mg ◊, 50 mg ◊, 100 mg ◊, 250 mg ◊, 500 mg ◊
Tablets (extended-release): 200 mg ◊

INDICATIONS & DOSAGES
➤ **RDA**
Adults ages 19 to 50: 1.3 mg.
Men age 51 and older: 1.7 mg.
Women age 51 and older: 1.5 mg.
Boys ages 14 to 18: 1.3 mg.
Girls ages 14 to 18: 1.2 mg.
Children ages 9 to 13: 1 mg.
Children ages 4 to 8: 0.6 mg.
Children ages 1 to 3: 0.5 mg.
Infants ages 7 months to 1 year: 0.3 mg (0.03 mg/kg).
Neonates and infants younger than age 6 months: 0.1 mg (0.01 mg/kg).
Pregnant women: 1.9 mg.
Breastfeeding women: 2 mg.
➤ **Dietary vitamin B₆ deficiency**
Adults: 100 to 200 mg PO daily. Or, 10 to 20 mg IM or IV daily for 3 weeks; then maintenance dose is 2 to 5 mg PO daily for several weeks.

sodium fluoride
Fluoritab, Flura, Flura-Loz, Ludent, Luride, Lozi-Flur, Pharmaflur df, Pharmaflur 1.1, Phos-Flur ◊

sodium fluoride, topical
ACT ◊, Denta5000 Plus, EtheDent, Fluoridex, Fluorigard ◊, Fluorinse, Gel-Kam, Gel-Tin ◊, Just For Kids ◊, Karigel, Karigel-N, Listerine Tooth Defense ◊, Luride, MouthKote F/R ◊, NeutraCare, Point-Two, Prevident, SF 5000 Plus, Stop Gel ◊, Thera-Flur, Thera-Flur-N

AVAILABLE FORMS
sodium fluoride
Drops: 0.125 mg/drop, 0.25 mg/drop, 0.2 mg/mL, 0.5 mg/mL
Lozenges: 1 mg
Tablets: 1 mg
Tablets (chewable): 0.25 mg, 0.5 mg, 1 mg

sodium fluoride, topical
Cream: 1.1%
Gel: 0.1%◇, 0.4%, 0.5%, 1.1%, 1.2%, 1.23%
Paste: 0.454%, 1.1%
Rinse: 0.02%◇, 0.04%◇, 0.05%

INDICATIONS & DOSAGES
➤ **To prevent dental caries**
Adults and children older than age 6: 5 to 10 mL of rinse once daily or b.i.d. (see product instructions) for 1 minute, or thin ribbon of gel applied to teeth with toothbrush or mouth trays. Or, 1 lozenge PO once daily (adults only).
If fluoride ion level in drinking water is less than 0.3 parts/million (ppm)
Children ages 6 to 16: 1 mg PO daily.
Children ages 3 to 5: 0.5 mg PO daily.
Infants and children ages 6 months to 2 years: 0.25 mg PO daily.
If fluoride ion level in drinking water is 0.3 to 0.6 ppm
Children ages 6 to 16: 0.5 mg PO daily.
Children ages 3 to 5: 0.25 mg PO daily.

thiamine hydrochloride (vitamin B$_1$)
Thiamiject ✦

AVAILABLE FORMS
Capsules: 50 mg
Injection: 100 mg/mL
Tablets: 50 mg◇, 100 mg◇, 250 mg◇

INDICATIONS & DOSAGES
➤ **RDA**
Adult men: 1.2 mg.
Adult women: 1.1 mg.
Boys ages 14 to 18: 1.2 mg.
Girls ages 14 to 18: 1 mg.
Children ages 9 to 13: 0.9 mg.
Children ages 4 to 8: 0.6 mg.
Children ages 1 to 3: 0.5 mg.
Infants ages 7 months to 1 year: 0.3 mg.
Neonates and infants younger than age 6 months: 0.2 mg.
Pregnant women: 1.4 mg.
Breastfeeding women: 1.4 mg.
➤ **Beriberi**
Adults: Depending on severity, 10 to 20 mg IM t.i.d. for 2 weeks; then dietary correction and multivitamin supplement containing 5 to 10 mg thiamine daily for 1 month.
Children: 25 mg IV daily.
➤ **Wet beriberi with myocardial failure**
Adults and children: 10 to 20 mg IV t.i.d. given slowly.
➤ **Wernicke encephalopathy**
Adults: Initially, 100 mg IV; then 50 to 100 mg IM daily until patient is consuming a regular balanced diet.

➤ **Thiamine deficiency**
Adults: 100 mg/L IV as rapidly as possible. Continue daily parenteral doses at RDA if GI disturbances prevent adequate oral absorption. Or, 1 tablet or capsule PO daily.
➤ **Neuritis of pregnancy in patients unable to take adequate oral therapy due to vomiting**
Adults: 5 to 10 mg IM daily.

vitamin C (ascorbic acid)
Acerola◇, Ascocid◇, Ascor, Asco-Tabs◇, C-Caps◇, Cemill◇, Chew-C◇, Halls Defense Vitamin C Drops◇

AVAILABLE FORMS
Capsules: 500 mg◇
Capsules (timed-release): 500 mg◇
Crystals: 1,000 mg/½ tsp
Injection: 500 mg/mL
Lozenges: 60 mg◇
Oral solution: 100 mg/mL◇, 500 mg/15 mL◇
Powder: 60 mg/¼ tsp◇, 1,060 mg/¼ tsp◇
Tablets: 250 mg◇, 500 mg◇, 1,000 mg◇, 1,500 mg◇
Tablets (chewable): 100 mg◇, 250 mg◇, 500 mg◇
Tablets (timed-release): 500 mg◇
Wafer: 500 mg◇

INDICATIONS & DOSAGES
➤ **RDA**
Men age 19 and older: 90 mg.
Women age 19 and older: 75 mg.
Boys ages 14 to 18: 75 mg.
Girls ages 14 to 18: 65 mg.
Children ages 9 to 13: 45 mg.
Children ages 4 to 8: 25 mg.
Children ages 1 to 3: 15 mg.
Infants ages 7 months to 1 year: 50 mg.
Neonates and infants up to age 6 months: 40 mg.
Pregnant women: 80 to 85 mg.
Breastfeeding women: 115 to 120 mg.
Adult smokers: Add an extra 35 mg daily.
➤ **Frank and subclinical scurvy**
Adults: Depending on severity, 100 to 300 mg PO or 300 to 1,000 mg IV, IM, or subcut daily.
Children: Depending on severity, 100 to 300 mg PO daily.
➤ **Extensive burns**
Adults and children: 200 to 500 mg IV, IM, or subcut daily for 7 to 10 days; 1 to 2 g daily for extensive burns.
➤ **Postoperative wound healing**
Adults and children: 300 to 500 mg IV once daily for 1 week to 10 days.

vitamin D cholecalciferol (vitamin D₃)
Bio-D-Mulsion ◇ , Decara, Delta-D3 ◇ , Dialyvite Vitamin D3 Max ◇ , D-Vita ◇ , VitaMelts ◇

ergocalciferol (vitamin D₂)
Calcidol ◇ , Calciferol, Drisdol

AVAILABLE FORMS
cholecalciferol
Capsules: 10 mcg (400 international units), 25 mcg (1,000 international units), 50 mcg (2,000 international units), 125 mcg (5,000 international units), 250 mcg (10,000 international units), 625 mcg (25,000 international units), 1.25 mg (50,000 international units)
Liquid: 400 international units/mL ◇ , 400 international units/0.03 mL ◇ , 2,000 international units/0.03 mL ◇ , 5,000 international units/mL ◇
Tablets: 10 mcg (400 international units) ◇ , 25 mcg (1,000 international units) ◇ , 50 mcg (2,000 international units) ◇ , 75 mcg (3,000 international units) ◇ , 125 mcg (5,000 international units) ◇
Tablets (chewable): 10 mcg (400 international units) ◇
Tablets (dispersible): 25 mcg (1,000 international units)
ergocalciferol
Capsules: 1.25 mg (50,000 international units)
Oral liquid: 200 mcg (8,000 international units)/mL in 60-mL dropper bottle ◇
Tablets: 10 mcg (400 international units) ◇ , 50 mcg (2,000 international units) ◇

INDICATIONS & DOSAGES
➤ **RDA for cholecalciferol**
Adults older than age 70: 15 mcg (800 international units).
Adults ages 51 to 70: 10 mcg (600 international units).
Infants, children, and adults up to age 50: 5 mcg (200 international units).
Pregnant or breastfeeding women: 15 mcg (600 international units).
➤ **RDA for ergocalciferol**
Adults older than age 70: 20 mcg (800 international units).
Adults up to age 70 and children age 1 and older: 15 mcg (600 international units).
Children from birth to less than 12 months: 10 mcg (400 international units).
Pregnant or breastfeeding women: 15 mcg (600 international units).
➤ **Rickets and other vitamin D deficiency diseases**
Adults and children: For cholecalciferol, give 6,000 units PO daily or 50,000 international units PO once weekly for 8 weeks, followed by maintenance dose of 1,500 to 2,000 units daily. For ergocalciferol, give 12,000 to 500,000 international units PO daily.

After correction of deficiency, maintenance includes adequate diet and RDA supplements.
➤ **Hypoparathyroidism**
Adults and children: 1.25 to 5 mg (50,000 to 200,000 international units) ergocalciferol PO daily with calcium supplement.

vitamin D analogue doxercalciferol
Hectorol

AVAILABLE FORMS
Capsules: 0.5 mcg, 1 mcg, 2.5 mcg
Injection: 2 mcg/mL in 1-mL, 2-mL vials

INDICATIONS & DOSAGES
➤ **Secondary hyperparathyroidism in dialysis patients with chronic kidney disease**
Adults: Initially, 10 mcg PO three times weekly at dialysis. Adjust dosage as needed to lower intact parathyroid hormone (iPTH) levels to 150 to 300 picograms (pg)/mL. Increase dose by 2.5 mcg at 8-week intervals if iPTH level hasn't decreased by 50% and fails to reach target range. Maximum dose is 20 mcg PO three times weekly. If iPTH levels fall below 100 pg/mL, suspend drug for 1 week; then give dose of at least 2.5 mcg less than last dose. Or, 4 mcg IV bolus three times a week at the end of dialysis, about every other day. Adjust dose as needed to lower iPTH levels to 150 to 300 pg/mL. Dosage may be increased by 1 to 2 mcg at 8-week intervals if the iPTH level isn't decreased by 50% and fails to reach target range. Maximum dose is 18 mcg weekly. If iPTH levels go below 100 pg/mL, suspend drug for 1 week, then resume at a dose that's at least 1 mcg PO lower than the last dose.
➤ **Secondary hyperparathyroidism in predialysis patients with stage 3 or 4 chronic kidney disease**
Adults: 1 mcg PO daily. Adjust dosage as needed to lower iPTH levels to 35 to 70 pg/mL for stage 3 or 70 to 110 pg/mL for stage 4. Increase dosage at 2-week intervals by 0.5 mcg if levels are above 70 pg/mL for stage 3 or above 110 pg/mL for stage 4. If level falls below 35 pg/mL for stage 3 or 70 pg/mL for stage 4, suspend treatment for 1 week, then give dose at least 0.5 mcg lower than last dose. Maximum dose, 3.5 mcg daily.

vitamin E (tocopherols)
Alpha-E ◇ , E 1000 ◇ , Formula E, Nutr-E-Sol ◇

AVAILABLE FORMS
Capsules ⓓⓝ: 100 international units ◇ , 200 international units ◇ , 400 international units ◇ , 1,000 international units ◇
Liquid: 15 international units/0.3 mL ◇ , 400 international units/15 mL ◇

Tablets: 100 international units ◇, 200 international units ◇, 400 international units ◇

INDICATIONS & DOSAGES
Note: RDAs for vitamin E have been converted to α-tocopherol equivalents (α-TE). One α-TE equals 1 mg of D-α tocopherol, or 1.49 international units.
➤ **RDA**
Adults and children ages 14 to 18: 15 mg.
Children ages 9 to 13: 11 mg.
Children ages 4 to 8: 7 mg.
Children ages 1 to 3: 6 mg.
Infants ages 7 months to 1 year: 5 mg.
Neonates and infants younger than age 6 months: 4 mg.
Pregnant women: 15 mg.
Breastfeeding women: 19 mg.
➤ **Dietary supplement**
Adults: Dosage of tablets and capsules varies by product and ranges from 100 to 1,000 mg/day. Or, 30 units (0.6 mL of the 15 units/0.3 mL drops) PO daily. Or, 100 units (0.25 mL of the 100 units/0.25 mL) PO daily.
Children (using the 15 units/0.3 mL drops): For children age 4 and older, give 30 units (0.6 mL) PO daily. For those ages 1 to 3, give 10 units (0.2 mL) PO daily. For those younger than age 1, give 5 units (0.1 mL) PO daily.

vitamin K analogue phytonadione (vitamin K₁)
K-100 ◇, Mephyton, Phytonadione, Vitamin K₁

AVAILABLE FORMS
Injection (emulsion): 1 mg/0.5 mL, 10 mg/mL
Tablets: 100 mcg ◇, 5 mg

INDICATIONS & DOSAGES
Black Box Warning Risk of severe and even fatal reactions using IV or IM routes; restrict their use to situations in which the subcut route isn't feasible and the serious risk is justified. ∎
➤ **RDA**
Men age 19 and older: 120 mcg.
Women age 19 and older, including pregnant and breastfeeding women: 90 mcg.
Children ages 14 to 18: 75 mcg.
Children ages 9 to 13: 60 mcg.
Children ages 4 to 8: 55 mcg.
Children ages 1 to 3: 30 mcg.
Infants ages 7 months to 1 year: 2.5 mcg.
Neonates and infants younger than age 6 months: 2 mcg.
➤ **Hypoprothrombinemia caused by vitamin K malabsorption, drug therapy, or excessive vitamin A dosage**
Adults: Depending on severity, 2.5 to 25 mg PO, IM, or subcut; may repeat in 6 to 8 hours.

➤ **Hypoprothrombinemia caused by effect of oral anticoagulants**
Adults: 2.5 to 25 mg PO, IM, or subcut, based on PT and INR.
➤ **To prevent hemorrhagic disease of newborn**
Neonates: 0.5 to 1 mg IM within 1 hour after birth.
➤ **Hemorrhagic disease of newborn**
Neonates: 1 mg subcut or IM. Higher doses may be needed if mother has been receiving oral anticoagulants.

Antacids: Indications and dosages

Refer to manufacturer's instructions for complete prescribing and safety information.

aluminum hydroxide
a-LOO-mi-num

Therapeutic class: Antacids
Pharmacologic class: Aluminum salts

AVAILABLE FORMS
Oral suspension: 320 mg/5 mL

INDICATIONS & DOSAGES
➤ **Acid indigestion**
Adults: 640 mg PO five to six times daily after meals and at bedtime. Maximum dose, 3,840 mg/day.

aluminum hydroxide–magnesium carbonate
a-LOO-mi-num

Acid Gone ◊, Gavis-Care ◊, Gaviscon ◊, Gaviscon Extra Strength ◊

Therapeutic class: Antacids
Pharmacologic class: Aluminum salts

AVAILABLE FORMS
Oral suspension: 31.7 mg aluminum hydroxide/ 119.3 mg magnesium carbonate in 5 mL; 254 mg aluminum hydroxide/237.5 mg magnesium carbonate in 5 mL
Tablets (chewable): 160 mg aluminum hydroxide/ 105 mg magnesium carbonate

INDICATIONS & DOSAGES
➤ **Acid indigestion, heartburn, sour stomach, GI upset**
Adults: 2 to 4 chewable tablets PO q.i.d.; maximum dose, 16 tablets/24 hours.
Adults and children age 12 and older: 15 to 30 mL (31.7 mg aluminum hydroxide/119.3 mg magnesium carbonate/5 mL) PO q.i.d.; maximum dose, 120 mL/ 24 hours. Or, 10 to 20 mL (254 mg aluminum hydroxide/237.5 mg magnesium carbonate/5 mL) PO q.i.d.; maximum dose, 80 mL/24 hours.

calcium carbonate
KAL-see-um

Cal-Carb Forte ◊, Calci-Chew ◊, Cal-Gest ◊, Caltrate ◊, Maalox ◊, Maalox Children's ◊, Mylanta ◊, Oystercal ◊, Rolaids ◊, Titralac ◊, Tums ◊, Tums Smoothies ◊

Therapeutic class: Antacids
Pharmacologic class: Calcium salts

AVAILABLE FORMS
Calcium carbonate contains 40% calcium; 20 mEq calcium per gram.
Oral suspension: 1,250 mg/5 mL ◊
Tablets: 648 mg ◊, 1,250 mg ◊, 1,500 mg ◊
Tablets (chewable): 260 mg ◊, 400 mg ◊, 420 mg ◊, 500 mg ◊, 600 mg ◊, 750 mg ◊, 1,000 mg ◊, 1,177 mg ◊, 1,250 mg

INDICATIONS & DOSAGES
➤ **Acid indigestion, calcium supplement**
Adults and children age 12 and older: 1 to 4 tablets PO when symptomatic. Maximum dose, 8,000 mg daily for up to 2 weeks. Calcium supplement use is 500 mg to 4 g daily in one to three divided doses.
Children ages 6 to 11, weighing at least 21.8 kg: 750 to 800 mg PO when symptomatic. Maximum dose, 3,000 mg daily for up to 2 weeks.
Children ages 4 and older (calcium supplementation): 750 mg PO t.i.d.
Children ages 2 to 5 weighing 10.9 to 21.3 kg: 375 to 400 mg PO when symptomatic. Maximum dose, 1,500 mg daily for up to 2 weeks. Calcium supplement use is 750 mg b.i.d.

magnesium oxide
mag-NEE-see-um

Mag-200 ◊, Mag-Ox 400 ◊, Maox ◊, Uro-Mag ◊

Therapeutic class: Antacids
Pharmacologic class: Magnesium salts

AVAILABLE FORMS
Capsules: 140 mg
Tablets: 200 mg, 400 mg, 420 mg, 500 mg

INDICATIONS & DOSAGES
➤ **Acid indigestion**
Adults: 1 tablet PO once daily or b.i.d. Maximum dosage, 2 tablets/day.
➤ **Dietary supplement**
Adults: 1 to 2 tablets or 1 to 5 capsules PO daily. Maximum dose, 800 mg/24 hours.

Laxatives: Indications and dosages

Refer to manufacturer's instructions for complete prescribing and safety information.

bisacodyl
bye-suh-KOH-dil

Bisacodyl EC ◇, Biscolax ◇, Codulax✦ ◇, Correct ◇, Dulcolax ◇, Ex-Lax Ultra ◇, Feen-a-Mint ◇, Fleet Bisacodyl ◇, Fleet Laxative ◇, Silver Bullet✦ ◇, Soflax EX✦ ◇, The Magic Bullet ◇, Woman's Laxative ◇

Therapeutic class: Laxatives
Pharmacologic class: Diphenylmethane derivatives

AVAILABLE FORMS
Enema: 10 mg/30 mL ◇
Suppositories: 10 mg ◇
Tablets (delayed-release) ⓄⓉⒸ: 5 mg ◇

INDICATIONS & DOSAGES
➤ **Chronic constipation; preparation for childbirth, surgery, or rectal or bowel examination**
Adults and children age 12 and older: 5 to 15 mg PO in evening or before breakfast. Or, 10 mg PR for evacuation before examination or surgery. Enema may be given as a single daily dose.
Children ages 6 to 11: 5 mg PO or PR (suppository) at bedtime or before breakfast. Oral dose isn't recommended if child can't swallow tablet whole. Don't give enema in children younger than age 12.

calcium polycarbophil
KAL-see-um

FiberCon ◇, Fiber-Lax ◇

Therapeutic class: Laxatives
Pharmacologic class: Hydrophilic drugs

AVAILABLE FORMS
Tablets: 625 mg ◇

INDICATIONS & DOSAGES
➤ **Constipation**
Adults and children older than age 12: 2 tablets (1,250 mg) PO once daily to q.i.d., p.r.n.
Children ages 6 to 12: 1 tablet (625 mg) PO once daily to q.i.d., p.r.n.

docusate calcium (dioctyl calcium sulfosuccinate)
DOK-yoo-sayt

Kao-Tin Capsule ◇, Surfak ◇

docusate sodium (dioctyl sodium sulfosuccinate)
Colace ◇, Correctol Extra Gentle ◇, Diocto ◇, Docuprene ◇, Docusoft-S ◇, DocuSol Kids Enema ◇, DOK ◇, D.O.S. ◇, Dulcocomfort✦ ◇, Dulcolax Stool Softener ◇, Enemeez Mini ◇, Pedia-Lax Liquid Stool Softener ◇, Phillips Stool Softener ◇, Promolaxin ◇, Selax✦ ◇, Silace ◇, Sof-Lax ◇

Therapeutic class: Laxatives
Pharmacologic class: Surfactants

AVAILABLE FORMS
docusate calcium
Capsules: 240 mg ◇
docusate sodium
Capsules: 50 mg ◇, 100 mg ◇, 200 mg ◇, 240 mg, 250 mg
Oral liquid: 50 mg/15 mL ◇, 150 mg/15 mL ◇
Rectal suspension: 100 mg/5 mL ◇, 283 mg/4 mL ◇
Syrup: 60 mg/15 mL ◇
Tablets: 100 mg ◇

INDICATIONS & DOSAGES
➤ **Constipation (stool softener)**
Adults and children older than age 12: 50 to 360 mg docusate sodium or 240 mg docusate calcium PO daily until bowel movements are normal. Or, give enema. Administer contents of 1 bottle PR as a single dose.
Children ages 2 to 11: 50 to 150 mg docusate sodium PO daily as a single dose or in divided doses.

glycerin
GLI-ser-in

Fleet ◇, Fleet Babylax ◇, Pedia-Lax ◇, Sani-Supp ◇

Therapeutic class: Laxatives
Pharmacologic class: Trihydric alcohols

AVAILABLE FORMS
Enema: 5.4 g
Enema (pediatric): 4 mL/applicator ◇
Suppositories: Adult, children, and infant sizes (1 and 2 g) ◇

INDICATIONS & DOSAGES
➤ **Constipation**
Adults and children age 6 and older: 1 rectal suppository/day, or 5 to 15 mL PR as enema.
Children ages 2 to 6: 1 rectal suppository/day, or 2 mL PR as enema.

lactulose
LAK-tyoo-lose

Constilac, Constulose, Enulose, Generlac, Kristalose

Therapeutic class: Laxatives
Pharmacologic class: Disaccharides

AVAILABLE FORMS
Oral solution: 10 g/15 mL
Packets: 10 g, 20 g
Rectal solution: 10 g/15 mL, 20 g/30 mL

INDICATIONS & DOSAGES
➤ **Constipation**
Adults: 10 to 20 g or 15 to 30 mL PO daily, increased to 40 g or 60 mL/day, if needed.
➤ **To prevent and treat hepatic encephalopathy, including hepatic precoma and coma in patients with severe hepatic disease**
Adults: Initially, 20 to 30 g or 30 to 45 mL PO t.i.d. or q.i.d., until two or three soft stools are produced daily. Usual dose is 60 to 100 g daily in divided doses. Or, 200 g or 300 mL diluted with 700 mL of water or NSS and given as retention enema PR every 4 to 6 hours, as needed.
Older children and adolescents: 26.7 to 60 g/day (40 to 90 mL/day) PO in divided doses to produce two or three soft stools daily.
Infants: Initially, 1.7 to 6.7 g/day (2.5 to 10 mL/day) PO in divided doses to produce two or three soft stools daily.
➤ **Treatment of subclinical hepatic encephalopathy** ◆
Adults: 20 to 40 g or 30 to 60 mL/day PO in two to three divided doses to maintain two or three daily bowel movements for up to 3 months.

linaclotide
LIN-a-KLOE-tide

Constella ✦, Linzess

Therapeutic class: Laxatives
Pharmacologic class: Guanylate cyclase-C agonists

AVAILABLE FORMS
Capsules ⓞⓝⓒ: 72 mcg, 145 mcg, 290 mcg

INDICATIONS & DOSAGES
Black Box Warning Safety and effectiveness in children younger than age 18 haven't been established. Contraindicated in children younger than age 6 due to dehydration risk. Avoid use in children age 6 to younger than 18. ∎
➤ **IBS with constipation**
Adults: 290 mcg PO once daily on an empty stomach at least 30 minutes before first meal of the day.
➤ **Chronic idiopathic constipation**
Adults: 72 to 145 mcg PO once daily on an empty stomach at least 30 minutes before first meal of the day.

lubiprostone
loo-bee-PRAHS-tohn

Amitiza ✔

Therapeutic class: Laxatives
Pharmacologic class: Chloride channel activators

AVAILABLE FORMS
Capsules ⓞⓝⓒ: 8 mcg, 24 mcg

INDICATIONS & DOSAGES
➤ **Chronic idiopathic constipation**
Adults: 24 mcg PO b.i.d. with food and water.
Adjust-a-dose: For patients with moderately impaired hepatic function (Child-Pugh class B), starting dose is 16 mcg b.i.d.; for those with severely impaired hepatic function (Child-Pugh class C), starting dose is 8 mcg b.i.d. May increase to full dose after appropriate interval if tolerated and an adequate response hasn't been obtained at initial dose. Monitor patient response.
➤ **IBS with constipation**
Women age 18 and older: 8 mcg PO b.i.d. with food and water.
Adjust-a-dose: For patients with severely impaired hepatic function (Child-Pugh class C), starting dose is 8 mcg once daily. May increase to full dose after appropriate interval if tolerated and an adequate response hasn't been obtained at initial dose. Monitor patient response.
➤ **Opioid-induced constipation in patients with chronic, noncancer pain**
Adults: 24 mcg PO b.i.d. with food and water.
Adjust-a-dose: For patients with moderately impaired hepatic function (Child-Pugh class B), starting dose is 16 mcg b.i.d.; for those with severely impaired hepatic function (Child-Pugh class C), starting dose is 8 mcg b.i.d. May increase to full dose after appropriate interval if tolerated and an adequate response hasn't been obtained at initial dose. Monitor patient response.

magnesium citrate (citrate of magnesia)
Citroma◇, GoodSense Magnesium Citrate◇

magnesium hydroxide (milk of magnesia)
Dulcolax Milk of Magnesia◇, Milk of Magnesia◇, Milk of Magnesia-Concentrate◇, Pedia-Lax Chewable Tablets◇, Phillips' Milk of Magnesia◇

magnesium sulfate◇ (Epsom salts◇)

Therapeutic class: Laxatives
Pharmacologic class: Magnesium salts

AVAILABLE FORMS
magnesium citrate
Oral solution: 1.75 g/30 mL◇
Tablets: 100 mg
magnesium hydroxide
Chewable tablets: 400 mg◇
Oral suspension: 400 mg/5 mL◇, 800 mg/5 mL◇, 1,200 mg/15 mL◇, 2,400 mg/10 mL◇
magnesium sulfate
Granules: About 40 mEq magnesium/5 g◇

INDICATIONS & DOSAGES
➤ **Constipation; to evacuate bowel before surgery**
Adults and children age 12 and older: 6.5 to 10 fluid oz magnesium citrate with 8 oz water PO in single or divided doses in 24 hours. Or, 2 to 4 tablets magnesium citrate PO daily at bedtime or in divided doses. Or, 8 chewable magnesium hydroxide tablets PO at bedtime or in divided doses. Or, 30 to 60 mL magnesium hydroxide liquid (400 mg/5 mL) PO as a single daily dose at bedtime or in divided doses. Or, 15 to 30 mL magnesium hydroxide liquid (800 mg/5 mL) PO as a single daily dose at bedtime or in divided doses. Or, 10 to 20 mL magnesium hydroxide (1,200 mg/5 mL) PO as a single daily dose at bedtime or in divided doses. Or, 10 to 30 g magnesium sulfate granules dissolved in 8 fluid oz water PO daily as a single dose or divided doses.
Children ages 6 to 11: 3 to 7 fluid oz magnesium citrate with 8 oz water PO in 24 hours as a single daily dose or in divided doses. Or, 4 chewable tablets magnesium hydroxide PO as a single daily dose at bedtime or in divided doses. Or, 15 to 30 mL magnesium hydroxide liquid (400 mg/5 mL) as a single daily dose at bedtime or in divided doses. Or, 7.5 to 15 mL magnesium hydroxide liquid (800 mg/5 mL) PO as a single daily dose at bedtime or in divided doses. Or, 5 to 10 mL magnesium hydroxide liquid (1,200 mg/5 mL) PO as a single daily dose at bedtime or in divided doses. Or, 5 to 10 g magnesium sulfate dissolved in 8 fluid oz water PO daily as a single dose or in divided doses.

Children ages 3 to 5: 2 magnesium hydroxide chewable tablets PO as a single daily dose or in divided doses. Or, 5 to 15 mL magnesium hydroxide liquid (400 mg/5 mL) PO as a single daily dose or in two to four divided doses. Or, 2.5 to 7.5 mL magnesium hydroxide liquid (800 mg/5 mL) PO as a single daily dose at bedtime or in divided doses.

polyethylene glycol 3350 (PEG)
pol-ee-ETH-ih-leen

Clearlax✦◇, GaviLAX◇, GlycoLax, Lax-A-Day✦◇, MiraLax◇, PEG 3350✦◇, Pegalax✦◇, Relaxa✦◇, Restoralax✦◇

Therapeutic class: Laxatives
Pharmacologic class: Osmotic drugs

AVAILABLE FORMS
Powder: 17 g in single-dose packets

INDICATIONS & DOSAGES
➤ **Short-term (1 to 2 weeks) treatment of occasional constipation**
Adults: 17 g (about 1 heaping tablespoon or one individual dose packet) powder PO dissolved in 120 to 240 mL beverage once daily.

polyethylene glycol-electrolyte solution (PEG-ES)
pol-ee-ETH-ih-leen

Colyte, GaviLyte-C, GaviLyte-G, GaviLyte-N, GoLYTELY, MoviPrep, NuLYTELY, TriLyte

Therapeutic class: Laxatives
Pharmacologic class: Osmotic laxatives

AVAILABLE FORMS
Oral solution: PEG 3350 (refer to individual manufacturer for strength and dosage of electrolytes)
Powder for oral solution: 4-L dose of solution contains PEG 3350 (refer to individual manufacturer for strength and dosage of electrolytes)

INDICATIONS & DOSAGES
➤ **Bowel preparation before GI examination**
Adults: 240 mL PO every 10 minutes until 4 L are consumed or rectal effluent is clear. Typically, give 4 hours before examination, allowing 3 hours for drinking and 1 hour for bowel evacuation. May give via NG tube: 20 to 30 mL/minute (1.2 to 1.8 L/hour) until 4 L is administered or rectal effluent is clear. Or, for MoviPrep and Suclear, refer to package instructions for split-dose or full-dose regimen.

Children age 6 months and older (GaviLyte-N, NuLYTELY, TriLyte): 25 mL/kg/hour PO or via NG tube until rectal effluent is clear and free of solid matter.

sodium phosphate monobasic monohydrate–sodium phosphate dibasic anhydrous
OsmoPrep

Therapeutic class: Laxatives
Pharmacologic class: Osmotic laxatives

AVAILABLE FORMS
Tablets: 1.5 g sodium phosphate (1.102 g sodium phosphate monobasic monohydrate and 0.398 g sodium phosphate dibasic anhydrous)

INDICATIONS & DOSAGES
Black Box Warning Acute phosphate nephropathy has been reported. Use the dose and dosing regimen as recommended (p.m./a.m. split dose). ▌
► **To cleanse bowel before colonoscopy**
Adults age 18 and older: 32 tablets taken in the following manner: The evening before the procedure, 4 tablets PO with 8 oz of clear liquid every 15 minutes for a total of 20 tablets (five doses); 3 to 5 hours before the procedure, 4 tablets PO with at least 8 oz of clear liquid every 15 minutes for a total of 12 tablets (three doses). A minimum of 7 days should elapse before repeating usage.

sodium phosphates
Fleet Enema◇, Fleet Enema Extra◇, Fleet For Children◇, LaCrosse Complete◇, Pedia-Lax◇

Therapeutic class: Laxatives
Pharmacologic class: Acid salts

AVAILABLE FORMS
Enema solution: 19 g monobasic sodium phosphate monohydrate and 7 g dibasic sodium phosphate heptahydrate/118 mL◇, 19 g monobasic sodium phosphate monohydrate and 7 g dibasic sodium phosphate heptahydrate/197 mL◇
Enema solution (pediatric use): 9.5 g monobasic sodium phosphate monohydrate and 3.5 g dibasic sodium phosphate heptahydrate/59 mL◇

INDICATIONS & DOSAGES
► **Constipation**
Adults and children age 12 and older: 1 bottle PR as an enema once in 24 hours.
Children ages 5 to 11: 66 mL (1 bottle enema for pediatric use) PR as an enema once in 24 hours.

Children ages 2 to younger than 5: 33 mL (½ bottle enema for pediatric use) PR as an enema once in 24 hours.

sodium picosulfate–magnesium oxide–anhydrous citric acid
Clenpiq, Prepopik

Therapeutic class: Laxatives
Pharmacologic class: Peristaltic stimulants–osmotic agents

AVAILABLE FORMS
Oral solution: 10 mg sodium picosulfate, 3.5 g magnesium oxide, and 12 g anhydrous citric acid/160-mL bottle
Powder for oral solution (16.1 g/packet, 2 packets/dosing carton): 10 mg sodium picosulfate, 3.5 g magnesium oxide, and 12 g anhydrous citric acid

INDICATIONS & DOSAGES
► **To cleanse colon in preparation for colonoscopy**
Adults (Clenpiq), adults and children age 9 and older (Prepopik): The split-dose method is preferred. Give first dose (1 bottle Clenpiq or 1 packet Prepopik reconstituted with 160 mL cold water) during the evening before colonoscopy (5 p.m. to 9 p.m.) followed by five 8-oz drinks of clear liquids within 5 hours and before bed. Give second dose (1 bottle Clenpiq or 1 packet Prepopik reconstituted with 160 mL cold water) next day, during the morning approximately 5 hours before colonoscopy. Follow dose with at least three 8-oz drinks of clear liquids before colonoscopy; continue with clear liquids within 5 hours and up to 2 hours before colonoscopy. If split-dose method isn't appropriate, use the "day before" method: Give first dose (1 bottle Clenpiq or 1 packet Prepopik reconstituted with 160 mL cold water) in the afternoon or early evening (4 p.m. to 6 p.m.) before colonoscopy followed by five 8-oz drinks of clear liquids within 5 hours and before next dose. Give second dose (1 bottle Clenpiq or 1 packet Prepopik reconstituted with 160 mL cold water) approximately 6 hours later in the late evening (10 p.m. to 12 a.m.) the night before colonoscopy, followed by three 8-oz drinks of clear liquids within 5 hours and before bed.

Additional OTC drugs: Indications and dosages

Refer to manufacturer's instructions for complete prescribing and safety information.

benzocaine
ben-ZOH-cane

Anacaine ◇, Cepacol Extra Strength Sore Throat ◇, Dermoplast ◇, Hurricaine ◇, Ivy-Rid ◇, Trocaine Throat ◇

Therapeutic class: Dermatologic agents
Pharmacologic class: Topical anesthetics

AVAILABLE FORMS
Gel: 7.5%, 10% ◇, 20% ◇
Lozenge: 10 mg ◇, 15 mg ◇
Ointment: 2% ◇, 5% ◇, 10%, 20% ◇
Spray (aerosol): 2% ◇, 5% ◇, 20% ◇
Spray (dental): 5% ◇, 20% ◇

INDICATIONS & DOSAGES
Refer to individual manufacturer's instructions for use.
➤ **Sore throat**
Adults and children age 5 and older: Allow 1 lozenge to dissolve slowly in mouth. May repeat every 2 hours as needed.
➤ **Mouth and gum irritation**
Adults: 1 spray or thin layer of gel or ointment in the mouth up to q.i.d. as needed.
Children age 2 and older: Apply thin layer of gel or ointment to affected area up to q.i.d. as needed.
➤ **Dermal irritation**
Adults and children age 2 and older: Apply ointment to affected area or use 1 spray up to q.i.d.

cetirizine hydrochloride
se-TEER-i-zeen

All Day Allergy ◇, Zyrtec ◇, Zyrtec Children's Allergy ◇

Therapeutic class: Antihistamines
Pharmacologic class: Piperazine derivatives

AVAILABLE FORMS
Capsules: 10 mg ◇
Syrup: 5 mg/5 mL ◇
Tablets: 5 mg ◇, 10 mg ◇
Tablets (chewable): 5 mg ◇, 10 mg ◇
Tablets (ODTs): 10 mg ◇

INDICATIONS & DOSAGES
Adjust-a-dose (for all indications): For adults and children age 6 and older receiving hemodialysis, those with hepatic impairment, those with CrCl less than 31 mL/minute, and patients age 65 and older, give 5 mg PO daily. Don't use in children younger than age 6 with renal or hepatic impairment.
➤ **Seasonal allergic rhinitis**
Adults and children age 6 and older: 5 to 10 mg PO once daily.
Children ages 2 to 5: 2.5 mg PO once daily. Maximum daily dose is 5 mg.
➤ **Perennial allergic rhinitis; chronic urticaria**
Adults and children age 6 and older: 5 to 10 mg PO once daily.
Children ages 1 to 5 years: 2.5 mg PO once daily; increase to maximum of 5 mg daily. Children ages 12 to 23 months should receive the 5-mg dose as two divided doses.
Children ages 6 to 11 months: 2.5 mg PO once daily.

chlorpheniramine maleate
klor-fen-IR-a-meen

Allergy Relief ◇, Allergy Time ◇, ChlorTabs ◇, Chlor-Trimeton ◇, Chlor-Trimeton Allergy 12 Hour ◇, Diabetic Tussin Allergy ◇

Therapeutic class: Antihistamines
Pharmacologic class: Alkylamines

AVAILABLE FORMS
Liquid: 2 mg/mL ◇
Syrup: 2 mg/5 mL ◇ *
Tablets: 4 mg ◇
Tablets (extended-release) ⊚: 12 mg ◇

INDICATIONS & DOSAGES
➤ **Allergic rhinitis**
Adults and children age 12 and older: 4 mg PO every 4 to 6 hours, not to exceed 24 mg daily. Or, 12 mg extended-release PO every 12 hours, not to exceed 24 mg daily.
Children ages 6 to 12: 2 mg PO every 4 to 6 hours, not to exceed 12 mg daily.
Children ages 2 to 6: 1 mg PO every 4 to 6 hours, not to exceed 6 mg daily.

dextromethorphan hydrobromide
dex-troe-meth-OR-fan

Balminil DM✤ ◇, Buckley's Cough Mixture ◇, Children's Robitussin Cough Long-Acting ◇, Creomulsion ◇, Creo-Terpin ◇ *, Delsym ◇, ElixSure Cough ◇, Hold DM ◇, Koffex DM✤ ◇, Little Colds Cough Formula ◇, Robitussin ◇, Scot-Tussin ◇, Triaminic Long Acting Cough ◇ *, Trocal ◇, Vicks Formula 44 ◇

Therapeutic class: Antitussives
Pharmacologic class: Levorphanol derivatives

AVAILABLE FORMS
Gelcaps: 5 mg ◇, 15 mg ◇
Liquid (extended-release): 15 mg/10 mL, 30 mg/5 mL ◇
Lozenges: 5 mg ◇
Solution: 3 mg/mL ◇ ✤, 7.5 mg/5 mL ◇, 10 mg/5 mL ◇ *, 12.5 mg/5 mL ◇, 15 mg/5 mL ◇ *
Strips (orally disintegrating): 7.5 mg ◇ *

INDICATIONS & DOSAGES
➤ **Nonproductive cough**
Adults and children age 12 and older: 10 to 20 mg PO every 4 hours, or 20 to 30 mg every 6 to 8 hours. Or, 60 mg extended-release liquid PO b.i.d. Maximum, 120 mg daily. Or 5 to 15 mg lozenges PO every 4 hours, up to 120 mg/day.
Children ages 6 to 11: 5 to 10 mg PO every 4 hours, or 15 mg every 6 to 8 hours. Or, 30 mg extended-release liquid PO b.i.d. Maximum, 60 mg daily. Or 5 to 10 mg lozenges PO every 4 hours, up to 60 mg/day. Don't exceed four doses in 24 hours.
Children ages 4 to younger than 6: 2.5 to 5 mg PO every 4 hours, or 7.5 mg every 6 to 8 hours. Or, 15 mg extended-release liquid PO b.i.d. Maximum, 30 mg daily.

fexofenadine hydrochloride
fecks-oh-FEN-a-deen

Allegra 12 Hour✤ ◇, Allegra 24 Hour✤ ◇, Allegra Allergy ◇, Allegra Allergy Children's ◇

Therapeutic class: Antihistamines
Pharmacologic class: Piperidines

AVAILABLE FORMS
Oral suspension: 30 mg/5 mL ◇
Tablets: 60 mg ◇, 120 mg✤, 180 mg ◇
Tablets (ODTs): 30 mg ◇

INDICATIONS & DOSAGES
Adjust-a-dose (for all indications): For patients with impaired renal function or need for dialysis, give adults and children age 12 and older 60 mg PO daily, children ages 2 to 11, 30 mg daily.
➤ **Seasonal allergies/hay fever**
Adults and children age 12 and older: 60 mg PO b.i.d. or 180 mg PO once daily.
Children ages 2 to 11: 30 mg PO every 12 hours. Maximum, 60 mg daily.
➤ **Chronic idiopathic urticaria ◆**
Adults and children age 12 and older: 60 mg PO b.i.d., or 180 mg PO once daily.

guaiFENesin (glyceryl guaiacolate)
gwye-FEN-e-sin

Altarussin ◇, Balminil✤ ◇, Children's Mucinex Chest Congestion Mini-Melts ◇, Diabetic Tussin ◇, Fenesin IR ◇, Geri-Tussin ◇, Liquibid ◇, Mucinex ◇, Mucinex Maximum Strength ◇, Mucosa ◇, Mucus Relief ◇, Organ-I NR ◇, Q-Tussin ◇, Refenesen ◇, Robafen ◇, Robitussin Chest Congestion ◇, Tussin ◇

Therapeutic class: Expectorants
Pharmacologic class: Propanediol derivatives

AVAILABLE FORMS
Granules: 100 mg ◇
Liquid: 100 mg/5 mL ◇ *, 200 mg/5 mL ◇, 200 mg/10 mL ◇
Syrup: 100 mg/5 mL ◇
Tablets: 200 mg ◇, 400 mg
Tablets (extended-release) ⓪: 600 mg ◇, 1,200 mg ◇

INDICATIONS & DOSAGES
➤ **Expectorant**
Adults and children age 12 and older: 200 to 400 mg PO every 4 hours, or 600 to 1,200 mg (extended-release tablets) PO every 12 hours. Maximum, 2,400 mg daily.
Children ages 6 to 11: 100 to 200 mg PO every 4 hours. Maximum, 1,200 mg daily.
Children ages 4 to 5: 50 to 100 mg granules, syrup, or liquid every 4 hours as needed. Maximum, 600 mg daily.

ketotifen fumarate
kee-toe-TYE-fen

Alaway ◇ , Zaditor ◇

Therapeutic class: Antihistamines (ophthalmic)
Pharmacologic class: H_1-receptor antagonists–mast cell stabilizers

AVAILABLE FORMS
Ophthalmic solution: 0.025%

INDICATIONS & DOSAGES
➤ **To temporarily prevent eye itching from allergic conjunctivitis or temporarily relieve itchy eyes due to pollen, ragweed, grass, animal hair, and dander**
Adults and children age 3 and older: Instill 1 drop in each affected eye every 8 to 12 hours but not more than b.i.d.

loratadine
lor-AT-a-deen

Alavert Allergy ◇ , Children's Claritin ◇ , Children's Loratadine ◇ , Claritin ◇ , Claritin Liqui-Gels ◇ , Claritin RediTabs ◇ , Claritin 24-Hour Allergy ◇

Therapeutic class: Antihistamines
Pharmacologic class: Piperidines

AVAILABLE FORMS
Capsules: 10 mg ◇
Syrup: 1 mg/mL ◇
Tablets: 10 mg ◇
Tablets (chewable): 5 mg ◇
Tablets (ODTs): 5 mg ◇ , 10 mg ◇

INDICATIONS & DOSAGES
Adjust-a-dose (for all indications): For adults with CrCl of 10 to 50 mL/minute, give 5 to 10 mg every 24 to 48 hours. For adults with CrCl less than 10 mL/minute, give dose every 48 hours.

➤ **Allergic rhinitis**
Adults and children age 6 and older: 10 mg PO daily. Or, 5 mg Claritin RediTabs every 12 hours.
Children ages 2 to 5: 5 mg chewable tablets or syrup PO daily.
➤ **To relieve itching due to hives (urticaria)**
Adults and children age 6 and older: 10 mg PO daily.

meclizine hydrochloride (meclozine hydrochloride)
MEK-li-zeen

Bonine ◇ , Dramamine Less Drowsy Formula ◇ , Motion-Time ◇ , Travel-Ease, Travel Sickness ◇

Therapeutic class: Antivertigo drugs
Pharmacologic class: Anticholinergics

AVAILABLE FORMS
Tablets: 12.5 mg, 25 mg ◇
Tablets (chewable): 25 mg ◇

INDICATIONS & DOSAGES
➤ **Vertigo**
Adults and children age 12 and older: 25 to 100 mg PO daily in divided doses. Dosage varies with response.
➤ **Motion sickness**
Adults and children age 12 and older: 25 to 50 mg PO 1 hour before travel; then daily for duration of trip.

minoxidil (topical)
mi-NOX-i-dill

Men's Rogaine ◇ , Minoxidil Extra Strength for Men ◇ , Theroxidil ◇ , Women's Rogaine ◇

Therapeutic class: Hair-growth stimulants
Pharmacologic class: Direct-acting vasodilators

AVAILABLE FORMS
Topical foam: 5% ◇
Topical solution: 2% ◇ , 5% ◇

INDICATIONS & DOSAGES
➤ **Androgenetic alopecia**
Adults: 1 mL of solution or half a capful of foam applied to affected area b.i.d. Maximum daily dose is 2 mL of solution.

oxymetazoline hydrochloride (intranasal)
ox-i-met-AZ-oh-leen

Afrin Sinus ◊ , Dristan ◊ , Duration Spray ◊ , Nasal Spray ◊ , Neo-Synephrine 12 Hour Spray ◊

Therapeutic class: Decongestants
Pharmacologic class: Sympathomimetics

AVAILABLE FORMS
Nasal solution: 0.05% ◊

INDICATIONS & DOSAGES
➤ **Nasal congestion**
Adults and children age 6 and older: 2 to 3 sprays of 0.05% solution in each nostril b.i.d. Don't use for more than 3 days.

phenylephrine hydrochloride (intranasal)
fen-ill-EF-rin

4-Way Fast Acting ◊ , 4-Way Menthol ◊ , Little Noses Decongestant ◊ , Nasal Four ◊ , Neo-Synephrine Cold and Sinus ◊ , Rhinall ◊

Therapeutic class: Vasoconstrictors
Pharmacologic class: Adrenergics

AVAILABLE FORMS
Nasal solution: 0.25% ◊ , 0.5% ◊ , 1% ◊

INDICATIONS & DOSAGES
➤ **Nasal congestion**
Adults and children age 12 and older: 2 to 3 drops or 2 to 3 sprays of 0.25% to 1% solution in each nostril every 4 hours, p.r.n. Don't use for longer than 3 days.
Children ages 6 to 11: 2 to 3 drops or 2 to 3 sprays of 0.25% solution in each nostril every 4 hours, p.r.n. Don't use for longer than 3 days.
Children ages 2 to 5: 2 to 3 drops of 0.125% solution in each nostril every 4 hours, p.r.n. Don't use for longer than 3 days.

pseudoephedrine hydrochloride
soo-dow-e-FED-rin

Children's Silfedrine ◊ , Children's Sudafed ◊ , Genaphed, Nexafed ◊ , Sudafed ◊ , Sudafed 12 Hour ◊ , Sudafed 24 Hour ◊ , SudoGest ◊ , Zephrex-D ◊

Therapeutic class: Decongestants
Pharmacologic class: Adrenergics

AVAILABLE FORMS
Oral solution: 15 mg/5 mL ◊ , 30 mg/5 mL ◊
Syrup: 15 mg/5 mL ◊ , 30 mg/5 mL ◊
Tablets: 30 mg ◊ , 60 mg ◊
Tablets (abuse-deterrent) ⒹⓃⓒ*:* 30 mg ◊
Tablets (extended-release) ⒹⓃⓒ*:* 120 mg ◊ , 240 mg ◊

INDICATIONS & DOSAGES
⟳ *Alert:* Don't use drug with an MAO inhibitor or within 2 weeks of stopping an MAO inhibitor.
➤ **Nasal decongestant**
Adults and children age 12 and older: 60 mg PO every 4 to 6 hours; or 120 mg extended-release tablet PO every 12 hours; or 240 mg extended-release tablet PO once daily. Maximum dosage, 240 mg daily.
Children ages 6 to 11 (immediate-release products only): 30 mg PO every 4 to 6 hours. Maximum dosage, 120 mg daily.
Children ages 4 to 5 (immediate-release products only): 15 mg PO every 4 to 6 hours or 1 mg/kg/dose every 6 hours. Maximum dosage, 60 mg daily.

pyrethrins–piperonyl butoxide
pi-RETH-rinz/PI-per-oh-nel

Lice Shampoo✦ ◊ , RID ◊

Therapeutic class: Pediculicides
Pharmacologic class: Pyrethrins

AVAILABLE FORMS
Shampoo: pyrethrins 0.33% and piperonyl butoxide 4% ◊

INDICATIONS & DOSAGES
➤ **Treatment of *Pediculus humanus* infestations**
Adults and children age 2 years and older: Apply to hair, scalp, or other infested areas until entirely wet. Allow to remain for 10 minutes but no longer. Wash thoroughly with warm water and soap or shampoo. Remove dead lice and eggs with fine-toothed comb. Repeat treatment in 7 to 10 days to kill newly hatched lice.

simethicone
sye-METH-ih-kone

Gas Relief ◇ , Gas-X ◇ , Gas-X Extra Strength ◇ , Genasyme ◇ , Infacol✤ ◇ , Mylicon ◇ , Ovol✤ ◇ , Ovol Drops✤ ◇ , Pediacol✤ ◇ , Phazyme Maximum Strength ◇

Therapeutic class: Antiflatulents
Pharmacologic class:
Polydimethylsiloxanes

AVAILABLE FORMS
Capsules: 125 mg ◇ , 180 mg ◇ , 250 mg ◇
Drops: 40 mg/mL✤ , 40 mg/0.6 mL ◇
Liquid: 20 mg/0.3 mL ◇
Strips (orally disintegrating): 40 mg ◇ , 62.5 mg ◇
Tablets: 80 mg ◇ , 125 mg ◇
Tablets (chewable): 80 mg ◇ , 125 mg ◇

INDICATIONS & DOSAGES
➤ **Flatulence, functional gastric bloating**
Adults and children older than age 12: 40 to 125 mg PO q.i.d. as needed after each meal and at bedtime; may give single doses of up to 160 to 500 mg after meals or at bedtime, up to 500 mg daily. For drops, 40 to 80 mg PO as needed after each meal and at bedtime, up to 500 mg daily.
Children ages 2 to 12 or weighing more than 11 kg: 40 mg PO q.i.d. as needed after meals and at bedtime, up to 480 mg daily.
Children younger than age 2 or weighing less than 11 kg: 20 mg PO q.i.d. as needed after meals and at bedtime, up to 240 mg daily.

terbinafine hydrochloride (topical)
ter-BIN-ah-fin

Antifungal Foot ◇ , Lamisil ◇ , Lamisil AT ◇

Therapeutic class: Antifungals
Pharmacologic class: Allylamine derivatives

AVAILABLE FORMS
Cream: 1% ◇
Gel: 1% ◇
Solution: 1% ◇
Spray: 1% ◇

INDICATIONS & DOSAGES
➤ **Athlete's foot**
Adults and children age 12 and older: For athlete's foot between the toes, apply b.i.d. (morning and night) for 1 week or as directed by prescriber. For athlete's foot on the bottom or sides of the foot, apply b.i.d. (morning and night) for 2 weeks or as directed by prescriber.
➤ **Jock itch, ringworm**
Adults and children age 12 and older: Apply once daily for 1 week or as directed by prescriber.

tetrahydrozoline hydrochloride (ophthalmic)
tet-rah-hi-DRAZ-oh-leen

Murine Tears Plus ◇ , Opti-Clear ◇ , Visine

Therapeutic class: Vasoconstrictors
Pharmacologic class: Sympathomimetics

AVAILABLE FORMS
Ophthalmic solution: 0.05% ◇

INDICATIONS & DOSAGES
➤ **Conjunctival congestion, irritation, and allergic conditions**
Adults (all products) and children age 6 and older (Visine products): Instill 1 to 2 drops in affected eye up to q.i.d., or as directed by prescriber.

witch hazel
wich HA-zel

A.E.R. Witch Hazel, Medi Pads, Preparation H Wipes ◇ , Preparation H Wipes for Women ◇

Therapeutic class: Dermatologic agents
Pharmacologic class: Astringents

AVAILABLE FORMS
External pads: 20%, 50% ◇ , 86% ◇

INDICATIONS & DOSAGES
➤ **Anal or vaginal irritation**
Adults and children age 12 and older: Apply to affected area up to six times daily or after each bowel movement.

Selected ophthalmic drugs: Indications and dosages

Refer to manufacturer's instructions for complete prescribing and safety information.

alcaftadine
al-CAFF-tuh-deen

Lastacaft

Therapeutic class: Antihistamines
Pharmacologic class: Histamine$_1$-receptor antagonists

AVAILABLE FORMS
Ophthalmic solution: 0.25% (2.5 mg/mL)

INDICATIONS & DOSAGES
➤ **Prevention of itching associated with allergic conjunctivitis**
Adults and children age 2 and older: Instill 1 drop in each eye once daily.

bepotastine besilate
beh-POT-uh-steen

Bepreve

Therapeutic class: Antihistamines (ophthalmic)
Pharmacologic class: Histamine$_1$-receptor antagonists

AVAILABLE FORMS
Ophthalmic solution: 1.5%

INDICATIONS & DOSAGES
➤ **Itching associated with conjunctivitis**
Adults and children age 2 and older: Instill 1 drop into affected eye(s) b.i.d.

besifloxacin hydrochloride
beh-sih-FLOX-ah-sin

Besivance

Therapeutic class: Antibiotics
Pharmacologic class: Fluoroquinolones

AVAILABLE FORMS
Ophthalmic suspension: 0.6%

INDICATIONS & DOSAGES
➤ **Conjunctivitis caused by CDC coryneform group G,** *Aerococcus viridans, Corynebacterium pseudodiphtheriticum, Corynebacterium striatum, Haemophilus influenzae, Moraxella catarrhalis,* *Moraxella lacunata, Pseudomonas aeruginosa, Staphylococcus aureus, Staphylococcus epidermidis, Staphylococcus hominis, Staphylococcus lugdunensis, Staphylococcus warneri, Streptococcus mitis* **group,** *Streptococcus oralis, Streptococcus pneumoniae,* **or** *Streptococcus salivarius*
Adults and children age 1 and older: Instill 1 drop into affected eye t.i.d., 4 to 12 hours apart, for 7 days.

bimatoprost
by-MAT-oh-prost

Latisse, Lumigan

Therapeutic class: Antiglaucoma drugs
Pharmacologic class: Prostaglandin analogues

AVAILABLE FORMS
Ophthalmic solution: 0.01%, 0.03%
Topical ophthalmic solution: 0.03%

INDICATIONS & DOSAGES
➤ **Increased IOP in patients with open-angle glaucoma or ocular HTN**
Adults: Instill 1 drop ophthalmic solution in conjunctival sac of affected eye(s) once daily in the evening.
➤ **Hypotrichosis of the eyelashes**
Adults: Apply 1 drop topical ophthalmic solution nightly directly to skin of upper eyelid margin at base of eyelashes with single-use applicator, using a second applicator for a second eye (if needed).

brinzolamide–brimonidine tartrate
brin-ZOL-ah-mide/brih-MOE-neh-deen

Simbrinza

Therapeutic class: Antiglaucoma drugs
Pharmacologic class: Carbonic anhydrase inhibitors–alpha$_2$ adrenergic receptor agonists

AVAILABLE FORMS
Ophthalmic suspension: brinzolamide 1% and brimonidine 0.2%

INDICATIONS & DOSAGES
➤ **Reduction of IOP in patients with open-angle glaucoma or ocular HTN**
Adults and children age 2 and older: Instill 1 drop into affected eye(s) t.i.d.
Adjust-a-dose: Use not recommended if eGFR falls below 30 mL/minute/1.73 m^2.

bromfenac sodium
BROM-fen-ak

BromSite, Prolensa

Therapeutic class: Anti-inflammatory drugs (ophthalmic)
Pharmacologic class: NSAIDs

AVAILABLE FORMS
Ophthalmic solution: 0.07%, 0.075%, 0.09%

INDICATIONS & DOSAGES
➤ **Inflammation and pain after cataract surgery**
Adults: For 0.07% solution (Prolensa) and 0.09% generic formulation solution, 1 drop in affected eye(s) once daily beginning 1 day before surgery, continued on the day of surgery and for the first 14 days after surgery. For 0.075% solution (BromSite), 1 drop in affected eye(s) b.i.d. (morning and evening) beginning 1 day before surgery, continued on the day of surgery and for the first 14 days after surgery.

carteolol hydrochloride
KAR-tee-oh-lol

Therapeutic class: Antiglaucoma drugs
Pharmacologic class: Nonselective beta blockers

AVAILABLE FORMS
Ophthalmic solution: 1%

INDICATIONS & DOSAGES
➤ **Chronic open-angle glaucoma, intraocular HTN**
Adults: Instill 1 drop into conjunctival sac of each affected eye b.i.d.

ciprofloxacin hydrochloride (ophthalmic)
si-proe-FLOX-a-sin

Ciloxan

Therapeutic class: Antibiotics
Pharmacologic class: Fluoroquinolones

AVAILABLE FORMS
Ophthalmic ointment: 0.3% (base)
Ophthalmic solution: 0.3% (base)

INDICATIONS & DOSAGES
➤ **Corneal ulcers caused by *Pseudomonas aeruginosa*, *Staphylococcus aureus*, *Staphylococcus epidermidis*, *Streptococcus pneumoniae*, or possibly *Serratia marcescens* or *Streptococcus viridans***

Adults and children older than age 1: Give 2 drops in affected eye every 15 minutes for first 6 hours; then 2 drops every 30 minutes for remainder of first day. On the second day, 2 drops hourly. On days 3 to 14, 2 drops every 4 hours. Treatment may be continued after day 14 if reepithelialization hasn't occurred.
➤ **Bacterial conjunctivitis caused by *Haemophilus influenzae*, *S. aureus*, *S. epidermidis*, or possibly *S. pneumoniae***
Adults and children older than age 1: Give 1 or 2 drops into conjunctival sac of affected eye every 2 hours while awake for first 2 days. Then, 1 or 2 drops every 4 hours while awake for next 5 days.
Adults and children older than age 2: ½-inch (1.27-cm) ribbon of ointment into conjunctival sac t.i.d. for the first 2 days, then ½-inch ribbon b.i.d. for next 5 days.

cycloSPORINE (ophthalmic emulsion)
cy-cloh-SPORE-inn

Cequa, Restasis

Therapeutic class: Immunomodulators
Pharmacologic class: Calcineurin inhibitors

AVAILABLE FORMS
Ophthalmic emulsion: 0.5 mg/mL in single-use and multiuse vials
Ophthalmic solution: 0.09%

INDICATIONS & DOSAGES
➤ **To increase tear production in patients whose tear production is presumed to be suppressed due to ocular inflammation associated with keratoconjunctivitis sicca**
Adults: Instill 1 drop in each eye b.i.d. approximately 12 hours apart.

dexamethasone (ophthalmic)
dex-a-METH-a-sone

Dextenza, Dexycu, Maxidex, Ozurdex

dexamethasone sodium phosphate

Therapeutic class: Anti-inflammatory drugs (ophthalmic)
Pharmacologic class: Corticosteroids

AVAILABLE FORMS
dexamethasone
Insert (ophthalmic): 0.4 mg
Intraocular implant: 0.7 mg
Ophthalmic suspension: 0.1%, 0.9%
dexamethasone sodium phosphate
Ophthalmic solution: 0.1%

INDICATIONS & DOSAGES
➤ **Uveitis; iridocyclitis; inflammatory conditions of eyelids, conjunctiva, cornea, and anterior segment of globe; corneal injury from chemical or thermal burns or penetration of foreign bodies; allergic conjunctivitis; suppression of graft rejection after keratoplasty; acne rosacea**
Adults and children: Initially, 1 or 2 drops of solution into conjunctival sac every hour during the day and every 2 hours during the night. Decrease to 1 drop every 4 hours when favorable response is noted. As condition improves, taper to 1 drop t.i.d. or q.i.d. to control symptoms. Treatment may extend from a few days to several weeks. Or, give 1 or 2 drops of suspension in the conjunctival sac up to six times daily. In severe disease, drops may be used hourly, being tapered to discontinuation as inflammation subsides.

Or, apply thin coating of ointment into conjunctival sac b.i.d. to t.i.d., with reduced application frequency to once daily.
➤ **Macular edema; posterior-segment uveitis; diabetic macular edema**
Adults: 1 implant (0.7 mg) injected intravitreally into each affected eye.
➤ **Ocular postoperative inflammation**
Adults: Inject 0.005 mL (517 mcg) of 9% suspension into posterior chamber at the end of ocular surgery.

difluprednate
die-FLU-pred-nate

Durezol

Therapeutic class: Anti-inflammatory drugs (ophthalmic)
Pharmacologic class: Corticosteroids

AVAILABLE FORMS
Ophthalmic emulsion: 0.05%

INDICATIONS & DOSAGES
➤ **Inflammation and pain associated with ocular surgery**
Adults: 1 drop into the conjunctival sac of the affected eye q.i.d. beginning 24 hours after surgery for 2 weeks, then decrease to b.i.d. for 1 week, and then taper according to response.
➤ **Endogenous anterior uveitis**
Adults: 1 drop into the conjunctival sac of the affected eye q.i.d. for 14 days, then taper as clinically indicated.

dorzolamide hydrochloride
dor-ZOLE-ah-mide

Trusopt

Therapeutic class: Antiglaucoma drugs
Pharmacologic class: Carbonic anhydrase inhibitors–sulfonamides

AVAILABLE FORMS
Ophthalmic solution: 2%

INDICATIONS & DOSAGES
➤ **Increased IOP in patients with ocular HTN or open-angle glaucoma**
Adults and children: 1 drop into conjunctival sac of each affected eye t.i.d.

epinastine hydrochloride
ep-ih-NAS-teen

Elestat

Therapeutic class: Antihistamines
Pharmacologic class: H_1-receptor antagonists–mast cell stabilizers

AVAILABLE FORMS
Ophthalmic solution: 0.05%

INDICATIONS & DOSAGES
➤ **To prevent pruritus from allergic conjunctivitis**
Adults and children age 2 and older: Instill 1 drop into each eye b.i.d. Continue treatment as long as allergen is present, even if symptoms resolve.

fluorometholone
flur-oh-METH-oh-lone

FML, FML Forte

fluorometholone acetate
Flarex

Therapeutic class: Anti-inflammatory drugs (ophthalmic)
Pharmacologic class: Corticosteroids

AVAILABLE FORMS
fluorometholone
Ophthalmic ointment: 0.1%
Ophthalmic suspension: 0.1%, 0.25%
fluorometholone acetate
Ophthalmic suspension: 0.1%

INDICATIONS & DOSAGES
➤ **Inflammatory and allergic conditions of cornea, conjunctiva, sclera, or anterior uvea**

Adults and children older than age 2 (acetate form not for use in children of any age): 1 drop b.i.d. to q.i.d. or ½-inch ointment once daily to t.i.d. For first 24 to 48 hours, may increase dosing frequency to every 4 hours. For fluorometholone acetate, 1 to 2 drops q.i.d.; may give 2 drops every 2 hours during initial 24 to 48 hours of treatment.

gatifloxacin
ga-ti-FLOKS-a-sin

Zymar✤, Zymaxid

Therapeutic class: Antibiotics
Pharmacologic class: Fluoroquinolones

AVAILABLE FORMS
Solution: 0.3%✤, 0.5%

INDICATIONS & DOSAGES
➤ **Bacterial conjunctivitis caused by** *Corynebacterium propinquum, Streptococcus mitis, Staphylococcus aureus, Staphylococcus epidermidis, Streptococcus pneumoniae,* **or** *Haemophilus influenzae*
Adults and children age 1 and older: Instill 1 drop of Zymar into affected eye every 2 hours while patient is awake, up to eight times daily for 2 days. Then instill 1 drop up to q.i.d. while patient is awake for 5 more days.
➤ **Bacterial conjunctivitis caused by** *S. mitis, S. aureus, S. epidermidis, S. pneumoniae,* **or** *H. influenzae*
Adults and children age 1 and older: Instill 1 drop Zymaxid into affected eye every 2 hours while patient is awake, up to eight times on day 1. Then instill 1 drop b.i.d. to q.i.d. while patient is awake on days 2 to 7.

gentamicin sulfate (ophthalmic)
jen-ta-MYE-sin

Gentak

Therapeutic class: Antibiotics
Pharmacologic class: Aminoglycosides

AVAILABLE FORMS
Ophthalmic ointment: 0.3% (base)
Ophthalmic solution: 0.3% (base)

INDICATIONS & DOSAGES
➤ **External ocular infections (conjunctivitis, keratoconjunctivitis, corneal ulcers, blepharitis, blepharoconjunctivitis, acute meibomianitis, and dacryocystitis) caused by susceptible organisms (***Staphylococcus aureus, Staphylococcus epidermidis, Streptococcus pyogenes, Streptococcus pneumoniae, Enterobacter aerogenes, Escherichia coli,*

*Haemophilus influenzae, Klebsiella pneumoniae, Neisseria gonorrhoeae, Pseudomonas aeruginosa, Serratia marcescens***)**
Adults and children: 1 to 2 drops in affected eye every 4 hours. In severe infections, up to 2 drops every hour. Or, apply ointment (approximately ½ inch [1.25 cm]) to lower conjunctival sac b.i.d. or t.i.d.

ketorolac tromethamine (ophthalmic)
KEE-toe-role-ak

Acular, Acular LS, Acuvail

Therapeutic class: Anti-inflammatory drugs (ophthalmic)
Pharmacologic class: NSAIDs

AVAILABLE FORMS
Ophthalmic solution: 0.4%, 0.45%, 0.5%

INDICATIONS & DOSAGES
➤ **Relief from ocular itching caused by seasonal allergic conjunctivitis (Acular)**
Adults and children age 2 and older: 1 drop into conjunctival sac in each eye q.i.d.
➤ **Relief of postoperative inflammation in patients who have had cataract extraction (Acular)**
Adults and children age 2 and older: 1 drop to affected eye q.i.d. beginning 24 hours after cataract surgery and continuing through first 2 weeks of postoperative period.
➤ **Reduce ocular pain, burning, and stinging after corneal refractive surgery (Acular LS)**
Adults and children age 3 and older: 1 drop q.i.d. to affected eye, as needed, for up to 4 days after surgery.
➤ **Reduce pain and inflammation after cataract surgery (Acuvail)**
Adults: 1 drop b.i.d. to affected eye beginning 1 day before surgery, continuing on day of surgery, and through first 2 weeks after surgery.

latanoprost
lah-TAN-oh-prost

Xalatan

Therapeutic class: Antiglaucoma drugs
Pharmacologic class: Prostaglandin analogues

AVAILABLE FORMS
Ophthalmic solution: 0.005% (50 mcg/mL)

INDICATIONS & DOSAGES
➤ **Increased IOP in patients with ocular HTN or open-angle glaucoma**
Adults: Instill 1 drop in conjunctival sac of each affected eye once daily in the evening.

levobunolol hydrochloride
LEE-voe-BYOO-no-lahl

Betagan

Therapeutic class: Antiglaucoma drugs
Pharmacologic class: Nonselective beta blockers

AVAILABLE FORMS
Ophthalmic solution: 0.5%

INDICATIONS & DOSAGES
➤ **Chronic open-angle glaucoma, ocular HTN**
Adults: 1 or 2 drops 0.5% solution once daily. May give 1 drop of 0.5% solution b.i.d. in patients with more severe or uncontrolled glaucoma.

lifitegrast
LIF-i-teg-rast

Xiidra

Therapeutic class: Anti-inflammatory drugs (ophthalmic)
Pharmacologic class: Lymphocyte function-associated antigen 1 antagonists

AVAILABLE FORMS
Ophthalmic solution: 5% (50 mg/mL)

INDICATIONS & DOSAGES
➤ **Dry eye disease**
Adults: Instill 1 drop into each eye b.i.d., approximately 12 hours apart.

naphazoline hydrochloride
naf-AZ-oh-leen

Clear Eyes◇, Clear Eyes Redness Relief◇

Therapeutic class: Vasoconstrictors
Pharmacologic class: Alpha-1 agonists

AVAILABLE FORMS
Ophthalmic solution: 0.0125%◇, 0.03%, 0.1%

INDICATIONS & DOSAGES
➤ **Ocular congestion, irritation, itching**
Adults: Instill 1 or 2 drops into the conjunctival sac of affected eye(s) every 3 to 4 hours as needed (0.1% solution), or up to q.i.d. (0.0125% or 0.03%).

ofloxacin (ophthalmic)
oh-FLOX-a-sin

Ocuflox

Therapeutic class: Antibiotics
Pharmacologic class: Fluoroquinolones

AVAILABLE FORMS
Ophthalmic solution: 0.3%

INDICATIONS & DOSAGES
➤ **Conjunctivitis caused by** *Staphylococcus aureus, Staphylococcus epidermidis, Streptococcus pneumoniae, Enterobacter cloacae, Haemophilus influenzae, Proteus mirabilis,* **or** *Pseudomonas aeruginosa*
Adults and children older than age 1: Give 1 or 2 drops in conjunctival sac every 2 to 4 hours daily while patient is awake, for first 2 days; then q.i.d. for up to 5 additional days.
➤ **Bacterial corneal ulcer caused by** *S. aureus, S. epidermidis, S. pneumoniae, P. aeruginosa, Serratia marcescens,* **or** *Propionibacterium acnes*
Adults and children older than age 1: Give 1 or 2 drops every 30 minutes while patient is awake and 1 or 2 drops every 4 to 6 hours after patient goes to bed on days 1 and 2. On day 3, 1 or 2 drops hourly while patient is awake; continue for 4 to 6 days. Then, 1 or 2 drops q.i.d. for an additional 3 days or until cured.

phenylephrine hydrochloride (ophthalmic)
fen-ill-EF-rin

Mydfrin✽

Therapeutic class: Mydriatics
Pharmacologic class: Sympathomimetic amines–adrenergics

AVAILABLE FORMS
Ophthalmic solution: 2.5%, 10%

INDICATIONS & DOSAGES
➤ **Mydriasis**
Adults and children age 1 and older: Instill 1 drop of 2.5% or 10% solution every 3 to 5 minutes, up to 3 drops per eye. May repeat dose.
Children younger than age 1: Instill 1 drop of 2.5% solution every 3 to 5 minutes, up to 3 drops per eye.

pilocarpine hydrochloride (ophthalmic)
pie-low-KAR-peen

Isopto Carpine

Therapeutic class: Miotics
Pharmacologic class: Direct-acting parasympathomimetics

AVAILABLE FORMS
Ophthalmic solution: 1%, 2%, 4%

INDICATIONS & DOSAGES
➤ **Primary open-angle glaucoma or ocular HTN**
Adults and children age 2 and older: Instill 1 drop daily up to q.i.d.; adjust concentration and frequency to control IOP. Start pilocarpine-naive patients on the 1% concentration.
Children younger than age 2: Instill 1 drop of 1% solution in eye t.i.d.
➤ **Management of acute angle-closure glaucoma**
Adults and children age 2 and older: Instill 1 drop of 1% or 2% solution in affected eye up to three times in a 30-minute period.
Children younger than age 2: Instill 1 drop of 1% solution in eye t.i.d.
➤ **Prevention of postoperative elevated IOP associated with laser surgery**
Adults and children age 2 and older: Instill 1 drop of 1%, 2%, or 4% solution in affected eye 15 to 60 minutes before surgery. May give 2 drops, but give them at least 5 minutes apart.
➤ **Induction of miosis**
Adults and children age 2 and older: Instill 1 drop of 1%, 2%, or 4% solution in the eye. May give 2 drops, but give them at least 5 minutes apart.
➤ **Induction of miosis before goniotomy or trabeculotomy**
Children: Instill 1 drop of 1% or 2% solution in eye 15 to 60 minutes before surgery.

sulfacetamide sodium 10%
sul-fah-SEE-tah-mide

Bleph-10

Therapeutic class: Antibiotics
Pharmacologic class: Sulfonamides

AVAILABLE FORMS
Ophthalmic ointment: 10%
Ophthalmic solution: 10%

INDICATIONS & DOSAGES
➤ **Treatment of conjunctivitis and other superficial ocular infections due to susceptible microorganisms**

Adults and children age 2 months and older: 1 or 2 drops into lower conjunctival sac every 2 to 3 hours. Increase interval as condition responds. Or, apply ½ inch of 10% ointment into conjunctival sac every 3 to 4 hours and at bedtime. Ointment may be used at night along with drops during the day. Usual duration of treatment is 7 to 10 days.
➤ **Trachoma**
Adults and children age 2 months and older: 2 drops into lower conjunctival sac every 2 hours with systemic sulfonamide therapy.

tafluprost
TA-floo-prost

Zioptan

Therapeutic class: Antiglaucoma drugs
Pharmacologic class: Prostaglandin analogues

AVAILABLE FORMS
Ophthalmic solution: 0.0015%

INDICATIONS & DOSAGES
➤ **Increased IOP in patients with open-angle glaucoma or ocular HTN**
Adults: 1 drop instilled in conjunctival sac of affected eye once daily in the evening.

timolol maleate
tye-MOE-lol

Betimol, Istalol, Timoptic in Ocudose, Timoptic-XE

Therapeutic class: Antiglaucoma drugs
Pharmacologic class: Nonselective beta blockers

AVAILABLE FORMS
Ophthalmic gel-forming solution: 0.25%, 0.5%
Ophthalmic solution: 0.25%, 0.5%
Ophthalmic solution (preservative-free): 0.25%, 0.5%

INDICATIONS & DOSAGES
➤ **To reduce IOP in ocular HTN or open-angle glaucoma**
Adults: Initially, 1 drop of 0.25% solution in each affected eye b.i.d.; maintenance dosage is 1 drop once daily. If no response, instill 1 drop of 0.5% solution in each affected eye b.i.d. If IOP is controlled, reduce dosage to 1 drop daily. Or, 1 drop of gel-forming solution (0.25% or 0.5%) in each affected eye once daily. Or, for Istalol, initially 1 drop 0.5% solution in each affected eye once daily in the morning. If response is unsatisfactory, concomitant therapy may be considered.

Children age 2 and older: Initially, 1 drop of 0.25%
Timoptic in Ocudose or timolol generic solution in
each affected eye b.i.d. If no response, increase to
1 drop of 0.5% solution in each affected eye b.i.d. If
IOP is controlled, reduce dosage to 1 drop daily.

travoprost
TRA-voe-prost

Travatan Z

Therapeutic class: Antiglaucoma drugs
Pharmacologic class: Prostaglandin
analogues

AVAILABLE FORMS
Ophthalmic solution: 0.004%

INDICATIONS & DOSAGES
➤ **To reduce IOP in patients with open-angle
glaucoma or ocular HTN**
Adults and children age 16 and older: 1 drop in each
affected eye once daily in the evening.

Do not use: Dangerous abbreviations, symbols, and dose designations (ISMP Canada)

The abbreviations, symbols, and dose designations found in this table have been reported as being frequently misinterpreted and involved in harmful medication errors. They should NEVER be used when communicating medication information.

Abbreviation	Intended meaning	Problem	Correction
U	unit	Mistaken for "0" (zero), "4" (four), or "cc"	Use "unit."
IU	international unit	Mistaken for "IV" (intravenous) or "10" (ten)	Use "unit."
Abbreviations for drug names		Misinterpreted because of similar abbreviations for multiple drugs; e.g., MS, MSO$_4$ (morphine sulphate), MgSO$_4$ (magnesium sulphate) may be confused for one another	Do not abbreviate drug names.
QD	every day	Mistaken for QOD, or as "qid."	Use "daily."
QOD	every other day	Q has also been misinterpreted as "2" (two)	Use "every other day."
OD	every day	Mistaken for "right eye" (OD = oculus dexter)	Use "daily."
OS, OD, OU	left eye, right eye, both eyes	May be confused with one another	Use "left eye," "right eye," or "both eyes."
D/C	discharge	Interpreted as "discontinue whatever medications follow" (typically discharge medications)	Use "discharge."
cc	cubic centimetre	Mistaken for "u" (units)	Use "mL" or "millilitre."
μg	microgram	Mistaken for "mg" (milligram) resulting in one thousand-fold overdose	Use "mcg."

Symbol	Intended meaning	Potential problem	Correction
@	at	Mistaken for "2" (two) or "5" (five)	Use "at."
>	greater than	Mistaken for "7" (seven) or confused with < (less than)	Use "greater than/more than."
<	less than	Mistaken for the letter "L" or confused with > (greater than)	Use "less than/lower than."

Dose designation	Intended meaning	Potential problem	Correction
Trailing zero	X.0 mg	Decimal point is overlooked, resulting in 10-fold dose error	Never use a zero by itself after a decimal point. Use "X mg."
Lack of leading zero	.X mg	Decimal point is overlooked, resulting in 10-fold dose error	Always use a zero before a decimal point. Use "0.X mg."

Adapted from ISMP's *List of Error-Prone Abbreviations, Symbols, and Dose Designations 2015.*
Available from: https://www.ismp-canada.org/download/ISMPCanadaListOfDangerousAbbreviations.pdf
Reprinted with permission from ISMP Canada, 2020.

Decision tree: Deciding about medication administration

Use this tool to help you determine whether or not to administer a medication. Be sure to consider all of the phases of medication administration in this document.

Complete order or Directive?

NO

YES

Assessed client factors?

For example, client condition, verified consent

NO

YES

Do not administer medication.

Take appropriate action to safeguard client interest and ensure continued care, for example, follow-up with prescriber.

Assessed your abilities?

For example, your knowledge of medication, skills to reconstitute and administer, judgment to identify and respond to outcomes

NO

YES

Assessed environmental supports?

For example, human and technological resources to monitor and intervene if needed, systems in place to support safe medication administration

NO

YES

Administer medication.

Verifying:
- the right client
- the right drug
- the right dosage
- the right time
- the right route

YES

Evaluate outcomes.

If an adverse reaction occurs, take appropriate action.

Note: Document during and/or after administering medication, according to documentation standards.
© Nurses Association of New Brunswick. Reproduced with permission. Further reproduction prohibited.

Canadian National Drug Schedules

The Canadian National Drug Schedules (NDS), issued by the National Association of Pharmacy Regulatory Authorities (NAPRA), is the regulatory model that defines the conditions of sale for all drug products sold in Canada. NAPRA assigns each drug product to one of four categories (Schedule I, II, III, or Unscheduled) depending on various factors, including the level of professional intervention required, public safety, and the drug's level of toxicity. The NDS is based on a cascading structure that allows regulators to use clinical judgment to determine market placement of the drug product: Schedule I products are considered the most highly regulated, and Unscheduled products have the least restrictions at point of sale.

Schedule	Description of regulatory drug categories
Schedule I drugs	• Drug requires a prescription by a licensed practitioner. • Ongoing drug monitoring and evaluation is required. • Appropriate drug use may cause dependency. • Serious drug reactions may occur at normal therapeutic dosages. • Narrow margin of safety exists between therapeutic and toxic dosages. • Serious drug interactions are known or may occur. • Drug's use may promote development of resistant strains of microorganisms. • Drug is new or the indication isn't appropriate for self-treatment and its safety in widespread use hasn't been established.
Schedule II drugs	• Drug isn't included in Schedule I and the initial need for the drug is identified or confirmed by a regulated health professional (i.e., pharmacist, physician). Prescription not required. • Drug should be administered in a health care setting or under the direction of a regulated health professional. • Drug must be readily available under exceptional circumstances when a prescription isn't practical. • Chronic therapy or subsequent retreatment requires monitoring by a pharmacist. • Drug requires intervention by a pharmacist to confirm that the patient has made an appropriate self-assessment, the condition is new to patient self-assessment, or the condition generally isn't appropriate for patient self-assessment. • Drug has significant potential for abuse or misuse. • Drug may cause serious adverse reactions not completely addressed in product label. • Safe use of drug requires a pharmacist to provide more detailed information and education than appear on the product label. • Drug may mask or delay signs and symptoms of a serious disease. • Drug is new or is in a new drug delivery system, for self-medication.
Schedule III drugs	• Drug isn't in Schedule I or II and is a new ingredient for self-medication, and advice from a pharmacist can support safe use. • Drug is used to treat a chronic or persistent condition, and advice from a pharmacist can support safe use. Prescription not required. • There is potential for abuse or misuse. • Drug may mask or delay signs and symptoms of a serious disease. • Advice from a pharmacist to explain, reinforce, or expand on product labeling information, or when product selection is likely to cause confusion, can promote safe use of drug. • Products may be located in the self-selection area of the pharmacy but must be under direct supervision of the pharmacist and clearly identified as the "professional services area" of the pharmacy.
Unscheduled drugs	• Drug can be sold from any retail outlet without professional supervision. • Acceptable and adequate label information is available for patients to make a safe drug choice. • Drug isn't included in Schedule I, II, or III.

Safe disposal of unused drugs:
What patients need to know

Why is the safe disposal of unused drugs important?

It's reported that Americans fill more than 4 billion prescriptions annually, and many new drugs are approved each year. More drugs available and the saving of unused drugs create an increased potential for drug abuse, misuse, dependence, overdose, and accidental poisoning.

According to data from the 2016 National Survey on Drug Use and Health, almost 6.2 million Americans age 12 and older have misused prescription psychotherapeutic drugs (pain relievers, tranquilizers, stimulants, and sedatives) at least once in the past month; of these, 3.3 million people misused pain relievers. The Substance Abuse and Mental Health Services Administration reports that more than 50% of opioid abusers were first exposed by trying someone else's medication. Presently, steps are being taken to combat the growing epidemic of opioid abuse, dependence, and overdose in the United States: An FDA advisory committee will assess New Drug Applications for opioids that don't have abuse-deterrent formulations; the pharmaceutical industry is developing technologies to develop abuse-deterrent formulations; prescribers will have more training on long-acting and immediate-release opioid use and prescribing; immediate-release opioids will have stronger warnings similar to the warnings enacted for the long-acting formulations; and the FDA will require more postmarketing data to assess misuse and abuse of long-acting opioids. This ongoing assessment has recently resulted in naloxone, a life-saving drug, becoming more readily available to consumers and consumers' families (e.g., OTC programs).

Other important drug safety considerations include unused drugs leading to harmful drug misuse and abuse, as well as accidental drug exposure and poisoning, particularly in children and pets. The U.S. Poison Control Center reported that in 2016, 77.8% of all reported poison exposures were unintentional. The most common substance linked to poison exposure in adults age 20 or older is pain medication, followed by sedatives and sleeping medications, antidepressants, and CV medications. According to Poison Control, analgesic drugs are the most frequent cause of fatal poisonings in children. Since 1997, the FDA has documented more than 32 cases of accidental exposure to transdermal fentanyl pain patches. Most of these cases occurred in children younger than age 2, and 12 of these exposures resulted in death. Child-resistant containers are no guarantee that the container is child-proof; one study reported that 45% of accidental drug exposures in children were to drugs stored in child-resistant containers.

Now, more than ever, it's important for you as a health care provider to discuss the critical issue of safe disposal of prescribed drugs with all patients. Be sure to remind patients about the safe disposal of unused drugs at follow-up visits. Teaching patients to safely dispose of unused drugs is an important strategy to protect household members and pets from accidental drug exposure and poisoning.

Patient-teaching points

Here are some important patient-teaching points about safe disposal of unused drugs:
- Tell patients that the FDA doesn't recommend the reuse or redistribution of an unused drug, because the safety and effectiveness of the drug can't be guaranteed once it's dispensed. Such factors as improper drug storage and possible drug tampering can alter the drug's safety and effectiveness.
- Counsel patients, caregivers, or family members to dispose of all unused drugs as soon as they are no longer needed.
- Advise patients to check for community drug take-back programs. These programs are especially important for the convenient disposal of drugs that can be harmful to others, such as psychotherapeutic drugs. Drug take-back programs have been designed by the U.S. Drug Enforcement Administration and are administered in conjunction with

local law enforcement, usually twice a year. Patients can mail in their unused drugs or drop them off in person to local law enforcement personnel. Or, they can dispose of the drugs in a special receptacle (known as a "drop-box") located in local clinics or retail pharmacies. If drug take-back programs aren't locally available, advise patients to check with community resources or their pharmacist or prescriber to see if they may dispose of drugs themselves.

• Instruct patients that certain drugs considered harmful if ingested by others may be flushed down the sink or toilet; tell them to check the following resources to see if flushing is appropriate:

    ○ Medicines Recommended for Disposal by Flushing: https://www.fda.gov/drugs/safe-disposal-medicines/disposal-unused-medicines-what-you-should-know

    ○ DailyMed (official FDA drug label information and package inserts): https://dailymed.nlm.nih.gov/dailymed/.

Search for the drug's name; then look for the following sections within the label:

    – Information for Patients and Caregivers

    – Patient Information

    – Patient Counseling Information

    – Safety and Handling Instructions

    – Medication Guide.

• Advise patients that nonharmful drugs may be disposed of by placing them intact (don't crush capsules or tablets) in a plastic bag or container filled with an undesirable substance, such as dirt, cat litter, or coffee grounds, and then placing the container in the household trash. Tell patients to make sure that children and pets can't access the trash receptacle.

• Warn patients to remove and destroy all labels from medication containers before recycling or disposing of them, to maintain privacy.

• Instruct patients to safely dispose of transdermal drug patches by folding them in half (sticky sides together) while avoiding contact with the sticky sides. Fentanyl patches should be immediately flushed down the toilet. Patches containing nitroglycerin or testosterone may be placed in the household trash.

Additional resources

Here are additional resources to find out more information about safe drug disposal of unused drugs:

• DEA Diversion Control Division–Drug Disposal Information: www.deadiversion.usdoj.gov/drug_disposal/index.html

• DEA Diversion Control Division–Controlled Substance Public Disposal Locations: https:/apps.deadiversion.usdoj.gov/pubdispsearch/spring/main?execution=e1s1

• DEA Diversion Control Division–Registration call center: 1-800-882-9539

• FDA. Disposal of Unused Medicines: What You Should Know www.fda.gov/drugs/safe-disposal-medicines/disposal-unused-medicines-what-you-should-know

• FDA. Drug Disposal: Questions and Answers www.fda.gov/drugs/disposal-unused-medicines-what-you-should-know/drug-disposal-questions-and-answers

• FDA. Contact number: 1-888-INFO-FDA (1-888-463-6332).

Therapeutic drug monitoring guidelines

Lab value ranges may vary among labs. Be sure to compare test results with the normal values of the lab that did the test.

Drug	Laboratory test monitored	Therapeutic ranges of test
ACE inhibitors (benazepril, captopril, enalapril, enalaprilat, fosinopril, lisinopril, moexipril, quinapril, ramipril, trandolapril)	Creatinine	Men: 0.9–1.3 mg/dL Women: 0.6–1.1 mg/dL
	BUN	6–20 mg/dL
	Potassium	3.5–5.2 mEq/L
	WBC with differential	*****
aminoglycoside antibiotics (amikacin, gentamicin, tobramycin)	Amikacin peak	20–30 mcg/mL
	Amikacin trough	1–8 mcg/mL
	Creatinine	Men: 0.9–1.3 mg/dL Women: 0.6–1.1 mg/dL
	Gentamicin peak	6–10 mcg/mL
	Tobramycin peak	5–10 mcg/mL
	Gentamicin, tobramycin trough	<2 mcg/mL
amphotericin B	BUN	6–20 mg/dL
	CBC with differential and platelets	*****
	Creatinine	Men: 0.9–1.3 mg/dL Women: 0.6–1.1 mg/dL
	Electrolytes (especially potassium and magnesium)	Potassium: 3.5–5.2 mEq/L Magnesium: 1.3–2.2 mEq/L Sodium: 135–147 mEq/L Chloride: 95–110 mEq/L
	Liver function	*
antibiotics	Cultures and sensitivities	
	WBC with differential	*****
biguanides (metformin)	CBC	*****
	Creatinine	Men: 0.9–1.3 mg/dL Women: 0.6–1.1 mg/dL
	Fasting glucose	≤100 mg/dL
	HbA$_{1c}$	5.0%–7.0% of total Hb
	Vitamin B$_{12}$ level	190–900 ng/mL
carbamazepine	BUN	6–20 mg/dL
	Carbamazepine	4–12 mcg/mL
	CBC with differential	*****
	Liver function	*
	Platelet count	140–400 × 10^3/mm^3
corticosteroids (betamethasone, cortisone, dexamethasone, hydrocortisone, methylPREDNISolone, predniSONE, prednisoLONE, triamcinolone)	Electrolytes (especially potassium)	Potassium: 3.5–5.2 mEq/L Magnesium: 1.8–2.6 mEq/L Sodium: 136–145 mEq/L Chloride: 96–106 mEq/L Calcium: 8.8–10.4 mg/dL
	Fasting glucose	≤100/dL

*****For those areas marked with asterisks, the following values can be used:

Hb: Women: 12–16 g/dL	Differential: Neutrophils: 45%–74%
Men: 14–18 g/dL	Bands: 0%–8%
Hematocrit: Women: 37%–48%	Lymphocytes: 16%–45%
Men: 42%–52%	Monocytes: 4%–10%
RBCs: 4–5.5 × 10^3/mm^3	Eosinophils: 0%–7%
WBCs: 5–10 × 10^3/mm^3	Basophils: 0%–2%

Monitoring guidelines

Monitor WBC with differential before therapy, monthly during first 3 months, then periodically for first year. Monitor renal function and potassium level closely at start of therapy, after dosage changes, and periodically during therapy.

Wait until after third dose is given to check drug levels. Obtain blood for peak level 30 minutes after IV infusion ends or 60 minutes after IM administration. For trough levels, draw blood just before next dose. Dosage may need to be adjusted accordingly. Recheck after three doses. For extended-interval (once-daily) amikacin dosing, obtain a random amikacin level between 6 and 14 hours after start of amikacin infusion. Monitor creatinine and BUN levels and urine output for signs of decreasing renal function. Monitor urine for increased proteins, cells, and casts.

Monitor creatinine, BUN, and electrolyte levels at least daily at start of therapy, then as clinically indicated. Regularly monitor blood counts and LFT results during therapy.

Monitor WBC with differential weekly during therapy. Specimen cultures and sensitivities will determine cause of the infection and the best treatment.

Check renal function and hematologic values before starting therapy and at least annually thereafter. If patient has impaired renal function, don't use metformin because it may cause lactic acidosis. Monitor response to therapy by periodically evaluating fasting glucose and HbA_{1c} levels; a patient's home monitoring of glucose level helps monitor compliance and response. Monitor vitamin B_{12} level every 2 to 3 years.

Monitor blood counts and platelets before therapy; monitor closely during therapy. Check LFTs and BUN before and periodically during therapy.

Monitor electrolyte and glucose levels regularly during long-term therapy.

(continued)

*For those areas marked with one asterisk, the following values can be used:
ALT: 7–56 units/L
AST: 5–40 units/L
Alkaline phosphatase: 17–142 units/L
LDH: 140–280 units/L
GGT: <40 units/L
Total bilirubin: 0.2–1 mg/dL

Drug	Laboratory test monitored	Therapeutic ranges of test
digoxin	Creatinine	Men: 0.9–1.3 mg/dL Women: 0.6–1.1 mg/dL
	Digoxin	0.8–2 nanograms/mL
	Digoxin in HF	0.5–0.9 nanograms/mL
	Electrolytes	Potassium: 3.5–5.2 mEq/L Magnesium: 1.8–2.6 mEq/L Sodium: 136–145 mEq/L Chloride: 96–106 mEq/L Calcium: 8.8–10.4 mg/dL
epoetin alfa	CBC with differential	*****
	Hematocrit	Women: 36%–48% Men: 42%–52%
	Platelet count	$140–400 \times 10^3/mm^3$
	Serum ferritin	18–270 nanograms/mL
	Transferrin	250–425 mg/dL
ethosuximide	CBC with differential	******
	Ethosuximide	40–100 mcg/mL
	Liver function	*
gemfibrozil	CBC	*****
	Lipids	Total cholesterol: <200 mg/dL LDL: <130 mg/dL HDL: ≥35 mg/dL Triglycerides: <150 mg/dL
	Liver function	*
	Serum glucose	<100 mg/dL
	CK	26–174 units/L
heparin (unfractionated)	aPTT	1.5–2 × control
	Hematocrit	*****
	Platelet count	$140–400 \times 10^3/mm^3$
HMG-CoA reductase inhibitors (atorvastatin, fluvastatin, lovastatin, pravastatin, rosuvastatin, simvastatin)	Lipids	Total cholesterol: <200 mg/dL LDL: <130 mg/dL HDL: ≥35 mg/dL Triglycerides: <150 mg/dL
	Liver function	*
insulin	Fasting glucose	≤100 mg/dL
	HbA$_{1c}$	<5%–7% of total Hb
isotretinoin	CBC with differential	*****
	Liver function	*
	Lipids	Total cholesterol: <200 mg/dL LDL: <130 mg/dL HDL: ≥35 mg/dL Triglycerides: <150 mg/dL
	Platelet count	$140–400 \times 10^3/mm^3$
	Pregnancy test	Negative

*****For those areas marked with asterisks, the following values can be used:

Hb: Women: 12–16 g/dL
   Men: 14–18 g/dL
Hematocrit: Women: 37%–48%
   Men: 42%–52%
RBCs: $4–5.5 \times 10^3/mm^3$
WBCs: $5–10 \times 10^3/mm^3$

Differential: Neutrophils: 45%–74%
   Bands: 0%–8%
   Lymphocytes: 16%–45%
   Monocytes: 4%–10%
   Eosinophils: 0%–7%
   Basophils: 0%–2%

Monitoring guidelines

Check digoxin level just before next dose or at least 6 to 8 hours after last dose. To monitor maintenance therapy, check drug level at least 1 to 2 weeks after therapy is initiated or changed. Make any adjustments in therapy based on entire clinical picture, not solely on drug level. Also, check electrolyte levels and renal function periodically during therapy.

After therapy is initiated or changed, monitor hematocrit twice weekly for 2 to 6 weeks until stabilized in target range and a maintenance dose has been determined. Monitor hematocrit regularly thereafter.

Check drug level 8 to 10 days after therapy is initiated or changed. Periodically monitor CBC with differential and LFTs.

Therapy is usually withdrawn after 3 months if response is inadequate. Patient must be fasting to measure triglyceride levels. Periodically obtain blood counts and LFT values during first 12 months. Obtain CK for muscle pain or weakness.

When drug is given by continuous IV infusion, check aPTT every 4 hours or according to facility policy in early stages of therapy, and daily thereafter. Check platelet counts and hematocrit, and test for occult blood in stools periodically during therapy.

Perform LFTs at baseline, 2 to 4 weeks after therapy is initiated or changed (depending on drug), and periodically thereafter.

A patient's home monitoring of glucose level helps measure compliance and response. HbA_{1c} level is a good measure of long-term control.

Use a serum or urine pregnancy test with a sensitivity of at least 25 milli-international units/mL. Perform one test before therapy and a second test during first 5 days of the menstrual cycle before therapy begins or at least 11 days after last unprotected act of sexual intercourse, whichever is later. Repeat pregnancy tests monthly. Obtain baseline LFTs and lipid levels; repeat every 1 to 2 weeks until response to treatment is established (usually 4 weeks).

(continued)

*For those areas marked with one asterisk, the following values can be used:
ALT: 7–56 units/L
AST: 5–40 units/L
Alkaline phosphatase: 17–142 units/L
LDH: 140–280 units/L
GGT: <40 units/L
Total bilirubin: 0.2–1 mg/dL

Drug	Laboratory test monitored	Therapeutic ranges of test
linezolid	Amylase	25–125 international units/L
	CBC with differential	******
	Cultures and sensitivities	
	Liver function	*
	Lipase	10–140 units/L
	Platelet count	140–400 × 10³/mm³
lithium	Creatinine	Men: 0.9–1.3 mg/dL
		Women: 0.6–1.1 mg/dL
	CBC	*****
	Electrolytes (especially potassium and sodium)	Potassium: 3.5–5.2 mEq/L
		Magnesium: 1.8–2.6 mEq/L
		Sodium: 136–145 mEq/L
		Chloride: 96–106 mEq/L
	Fasting glucose	≤100 mg/dL
	Lithium	0.6–1.2 mEq/L
	Thyroid function tests	TSH: 0.45–4.5 microunits/mL
		T₃: 80–200 nanograms/dL
		T₄: 5.4–11.5 mcg/dL
methotrexate	CBC with differential	*****
	Creatinine	Men: 0.9–1.3 mg/dL
		Women: 0.6–1.1 mg/dL
	Liver function	*
	Methotrexate	Normal elimination:
		~ 5 micromol/L 24 hours postdose
		~ 0.5 micromol/L 48 hours postdose
		~ <0.2 micromol/L 72 hours postdose
	Platelet count	140–400 × 10³/mm³
NNRTIs (delavirdine, efavirenz, nevirapine)	Amylase	25–125 international units/L
	CBC with differential and platelets	*****
	Liver function	*
	Lipids (efavirenz)	Total cholesterol: <200 mg/dL
		LDL: <130 mg/dL
		HDL: ≥35 mg/dL
		Triglycerides: <150 mg/dL
phenytoin	Albumin	3.5–5.2 g/dL
	CBC	*****
	Phenytoin	10–20 mcg/mL
procainamide	ANA titer	Negative
	CBC	*****
	Liver function	*
	N-acetylprocainamide (NAPA)	15–25 mcg/mL
	Procainamide	3–10 mcg/mL

*****For those areas marked with asterisks, the following values can be used:

Hb: Women: 12–16 g/dL
 Men: 14–18 g/dL
Hematocrit: Women: 37%–48%
 Men: 42%–52%
RBCs: 4–5.5 × 10³/mm³
WBCs: 5–10 × 10³/mm³

Differential: Neutrophils: 45%–74%
 Bands: 0%–8%
 Lymphocytes: 16%–45%
 Monocytes: 4%–10%
 Eosinophils: 0%–7%
 Basophils: 0%–2%

Monitoring guidelines

Obtain baseline CBC with differential and platelet count weekly during therapy. Monitor LFTs and amylase and lipase levels during therapy.

Checking drug levels is crucial to safe use of drug. Consult prescribing information for optimal lithium therapeutic range for acute and maintenance treatment. Obtain level immediately before next dose. Monitor level twice weekly until stable. Once at steady state, check level weekly; when patient is on appropriate maintenance dose, check level every 2 or 3 months. Monitor CBC; creatinine, electrolyte, and fasting glucose levels; and thyroid function test results before therapy starts and periodically thereafter.

Monitor drug level according to dosing protocol. Monitor CBC with differential, platelet count, and LFT and renal function test results more frequently when therapy starts or changes, and when methotrexate levels may be elevated, such as when patient is dehydrated.

Obtain baseline LFTs and monitor closely during first 12 weeks of therapy. Continue to monitor regularly during therapy. Check CBC with differential and platelet count before therapy and periodically during therapy. Monitor lipid levels during efavirenz therapy. Monitor amylase level during efavirenz and delavirdine therapy.

Monitor drug level immediately before next dose and 7 to 10 days after therapy starts or changes. Obtain a CBC at baseline and monthly early in therapy. Watch for toxic effects at therapeutic levels. Adjust the measured level for hypoalbuminemia or renal impairment, which can increase free drug levels.

Measure drug level 6 to 12 hours after a continuous infusion is started or immediately before next oral dose. Combined procainamide and NAPA levels can be used as an index of toxicity when renal impairment exists. Obtain CBC, LFTs, and ANA titer periodically during longer-term therapy.

(continued)

*For those areas marked with one asterisk, the following values can be used:
ALT: 7–56 units/L
AST: 5–40 units/L
Alkaline phosphatase: 17–142 units/L
LDH: 140–280 units/L
GGT: <40 units/L
Total bilirubin: 0.2–1 mg/dL

Drug	Laboratory test monitored	Therapeutic ranges of test
quinidine	CBC	*****
	Creatinine	Men: 0.9–1.3 mg/dL
		Women: 0.6–1.1 mg/dL
	Electrolytes (especially potassium)	Potassium: 3.5–5.2 mEq/L
		Magnesium: 1.8–2.6 mEq/L
		Sodium: 136–145 mEq/L
		Chloride: 96–106 mEq/L
	Liver function	*
	Quinidine	2–6 mg/L
sulfonylureas	Fasting glucose	≤100 mg/dL
	HbA_1c	5%–7% of total Hb
	Creatinine	Men: 0.9–1.3 mg/dL
		Women: 0.6–1.1 mg/dL
theophylline	Theophylline	10–20 mcg/mL
thiazolidinediones (piogli-tazone, rosiglitazone)	Fasting glucose	≤100 mg/dL
	HbA_1c	5%–7% of total Hb
	Liver function	*
thyroid hormones	Thyroid function tests	TSH: 0.45–5.4 microunits/mL
		T_3: 80–200 nanograms/dL
		T_4: 5.4–11.5 mcg/dL
valproate sodium, valproic acid, divalproex sodium	Ammonia	15–45 mcg/dL
	Amylase	25–125 international units/L
	BUN	8–25 mg/dL
	CBC with differential	*****
	Creatinine	Men: 0.9–1.3 mg/dL
		Women: 0.6–1.1 mg/dL
	Liver function	*
	Platelet count	$140–400 \times 10^3/mm^3$
	PT	11–13 seconds
	Valproic acid	50–100 mcg/mL
vancomycin	Creatinine	Men: 0.9–1.3 mg/dL
		Women: 0.6–1.1 mg/dL
	Vancomycin	25–40 mcg/mL (peak)
		10–20 mcg/mL (trough)
warfarin	INR	For an acute MI, atrial fibrillation, treatment of pulmonary embolism, prevention of systemic embolism, tissue heart valves, valvular heart disease, or prophylaxis or treatment of venous thrombosis: 2–3
		For mechanical prosthetic valves or recurrent systemic embolism: 2.5–3.5

*****For those areas marked with asterisks, the following values can be used:

Hb: Women: 12–16 g/dL
    Men: 14–18 g/dL
Hematocrit: Women: 37%–48%
    Men: 42%–52%
RBCs: $4–5.5 \times 10^3/mm^3$
WBCs: $5–10 \times 10^3/mm^3$

Differential: Neutrophils: 45%–74%
    Bands: 0%–8%
    Lymphocytes: 16%–45%
    Monocytes: 4%–10%
    Eosinophils: 0%–7%
    Basophils: 0%–2%

Monitoring guidelines

Obtain level immediately before next oral dose and 30 to 35 hours after therapy starts or changes. Periodically obtain blood counts, LFT and renal function test results, and electrolyte levels.

Monitor response to therapy by periodically evaluating fasting glucose and HbA$_{1c}$ levels. Patient should monitor glucose levels at home to help measure compliance and response.

Obtain drug level right before next dose of sustained-release oral product and at least 2 days after therapy starts or changes.

Monitor response by evaluating fasting glucose and HbA$_{1c}$ levels. Obtain baseline LFT results, and repeat tests periodically during therapy. Don't initiate therapy with pioglitazone or rosiglitazone if ALT level is more than $2.5 \times$ ULN.

Monitor thyroid function test results every 2 to 3 weeks until appropriate maintenance dose is determined and annually thereafter.

Monitor LFT results, ammonia level, coagulation test results, renal function test results, CBC, and platelet count at baseline and periodically during therapy. Closely monitor LFT results during first 6 months.

May check drug level with third dose administered, at the earliest. Draw peak level 1.5 to 2.5 hours after a 1-hour infusion or IV infusion is complete. Draw trough level within 1 hour of next dose administered. Renal function can be used to adjust dosing and intervals.

Check INR daily, beginning 3 days after therapy starts. Continue checking it until therapeutic goal is achieved, and monitor it periodically thereafter. Also check level 7 days after change in dose or start of a potentially interacting therapy.

*For those areas marked with one asterisk, the following values can be used:
ALT: 7–56 units/L
AST: 5–40 units/L
Alkaline phosphatase: 17–142 units/L
LDH: 140–280 units/L
GGT: <40 units/L
Total bilirubin: 0.2–1 mg/dL

Less commonly used drugs: Indications and dosages

Refer to manufacturer's instructions for complete pre-scribing and safety information.

SAFETY ALERT!

abciximab
ab-SIX-ah-mab

ReoPro

Therapeutic class: Antiplatelet drugs
Pharmacologic class: Glycoprotein IIb/IIIa inhibitors

AVAILABLE FORMS
Injection: 2 mg/mL

INDICATIONS & DOSAGES
➤ **Adjunct to PCI to prevent acute cardiac ischemic complications**
Adults: 0.25 mg/kg as IV bolus given 10 to 60 minutes before start of PCI; then, continuous IV infusion of 0.125 mcg/kg/minute to maximum of 10 mcg/minute for 12 hours.
➤ **Unstable angina not responding to conventional medical therapy in patients scheduled for PCI within 24 hours**
Adults: 0.25 mg/kg as IV bolus; then 18- to 24-hour infusion of 10 mcg/minute concluding 1 hour after PCI.

SAFETY ALERT!

acarbose
a-KAR-boz

Glucobay✤, Precose

Therapeutic class: Antidiabetics
Pharmacologic class: Alpha-glucosidase inhibitors

AVAILABLE FORMS
Tablets: 25 mg, 50 mg, 100 mg

INDICATIONS & DOSAGES
➤ **Adjunct to diet and exercise to improve glycemic control in patients with non-insulin-dependent type 2 diabetes**
Adults: Individualized. Initially, 25 mg PO t.i.d. with first bite of each main meal. Adjust dosage every 4 to 8 weeks, based on 1-hour postprandial glucose level or HbA$_{1c}$ levels and tolerance. Maintenance dosage is 50 to 100 mg PO t.i.d. For patients who weigh less than 60 kg, don't exceed 50 mg PO t.i.d. For patients who weigh more than 60 kg, don't exceed 100 mg PO t.i.d.

acetaZOLAMIDE
ah-set-a-ZOLE-ah-mide

acetaZOLAMIDE sodium
Therapeutic class: Diuretics
Pharmacologic class: Carbonic anhydrase inhibitors

AVAILABLE FORMS
acetazolamide
Capsules (extended-release) ⓞⓝⓖ: 500 mg
Tablets: 125 mg, 250 mg
acetazolamide sodium
Powder for injection: 500-mg vial

INDICATIONS & DOSAGES
➤ **Secondary glaucoma; preoperative treatment of acute angle-closure glaucoma**
Adults: 250 mg PO every 4 hours or 250 mg PO b.i.d. for short-term therapy. In acute cases, 500 mg PO; then 125 to 250 mg PO every 4 hours. Or, for extended-release capsules, 500 mg PO b.i.d. To rapidly lower IOP, initially, 250 mg IV every 4 hours. Or, 500 mg IV followed by 125 to 250 mg every 4 hours.
➤ **Chronic open-angle glaucoma**
Adults: 250 mg to 1 g PO daily in divided doses q.i.d., or 250 mg IV every 4 hours, or 500 mg extended-release PO b.i.d.
➤ **To prevent or treat acute mountain sickness (high-altitude sickness)**
Adults and children age 12 and older: 500 mg to 1 g (regular or extended-release) PO daily in divided doses. Start 24 to 48 hours before ascent and continue for 48 hours while at high altitude. When rapid ascent is required, start with 1,000 mg PO daily.
➤ **Adjunct for epilepsy and myoclonic, refractory, generalized tonic-clonic, absence, or mixed seizures**
Adults: 8 to 30 mg/kg PO or IV daily in divided doses; optimum range is 375 mg to 1 g daily. If given with other anticonvulsants, start at 250 mg PO or IV once daily, and increase to 375 mg to 1 g daily.
➤ **Edema caused by HF; drug-induced edema**
Adults: 250 to 375 mg (5 mg/kg) PO daily in the morning. For best results, use every other day or 2 days on followed by 1 to 2 days off. Or, 250 to 375 mg IV once daily for 1 or 2 days, alternating with a day of rest.

aclidinium bromide
a-cli-DIN-ee-um

Tudorza Pressair

Therapeutic class: Miscellaneous respiratory drugs
Pharmacologic class: Anticholinergics

AVAILABLE FORMS
Dry powder inhaler: 400 mcg/actuation

INDICATIONS & DOSAGES
➤ **Long-term maintenance treatment of broncho-spasm associated with COPD, including chronic bronchitis and emphysema**
Adults: 400 mcg (1 inhalation) b.i.d.

SAFETY ALERT!

afatinib dimaleate ☒

a-FA-ti-nib

Gilotrif

Therapeutic class: Antineoplastics
Pharmacologic class: Tyrosine kinase
inhibitors

AVAILABLE FORMS
Tablets: 20 mg, 30 mg, 40 mg

INDICATIONS & DOSAGES
Adjust-a-dose (for all indications): For patients
with preexisting renal impairment and eGFR of 15 to
29 mL/minute/1.73 m^2, give 30 mg PO once daily.
For patients who require long-term therapy with a
P-gp inducer, increase afatinib daily dose by 10 mg as
tolerated. Resume the previous dose 2 to 3 days after
discontinuation of the P-gp inducer.

For patients who require therapy with a P-gp inhibitor, reduce afatinib daily dose by 10 mg if concomitant therapy isn't tolerated. Resume previous dose
after discontinuation of the P-gp inhibitor as tolerated.
Refer to manufacturer's instructions for toxicity-
related dosage adjustments.
➤ **Metastatic, squamous NSCLC that has progressed after platinum-based chemotherapy; first-
line treatment of patients with metastatic NSCLC
whose tumors have epidermal growth factor receptor exon 19 deletions or exon 21 (*L858R*) substitution mutations detected by FDA-approved test** ☒
Adults: 40 mg PO once a day on an empty stomach
until disease progression or intolerability occurs.

aflibercept

a-FLIB-er-sept

Eylea

Therapeutic class: Vascular endothelial
growth factor inhibitors
Pharmacologic class: Antiangiogenetic drugs

AVAILABLE FORMS
Intravitreal injection: 2 mg in 0.05-mL single-use vial

INDICATIONS & DOSAGES
➤ **Neovascular (wet) age-related macular degeneration**
Adults: 2 mg (0.05 mL) intravitreal injection every
4 weeks for first 12 weeks; then 2 mg (0.05 mL) once
every 8 weeks. Some patients may need every-4-week
dosing after first 12 weeks.
➤ **Macular edema (following retinal vein occlusion)**
Adults: 2 mg (0.05 mL) intravitreal injection once
every 4 weeks.
➤ **Diabetic macular edema (DME) and diabetic
retinopathy in patients with DME**
Adults: 2 mg (0.05 mL) intravitreal injection every
4 weeks for first 5 injections; then 2 mg (0.05 mL)
every 8 weeks. Some patients may need every-4-week
dosing after first five injections.

alfuzosin hydrochloride

al-foo-ZOE-sin

Uroxatral, Xatral

Therapeutic class: BPH drugs
Pharmacologic class: Alpha$_1$ blockers

AVAILABLE FORMS
Tablets (extended-release): 10 mg

INDICATIONS & DOSAGES
➤ **BPH**
Men: 10 mg PO once daily.

alirocumab ☒

AL-i-rok-ue-mab

Praluent

Therapeutic class: Antilipemics
Pharmacologic class: Proprotein convertase
subtilisin/kexin type 9 antibody inhibitors

AVAILABLE FORMS
Injection: 75 mg/mL, 150 mg/mL in single-dose prefilled pens or syringes

INDICATIONS & DOSAGES
➤ **Adjunct to diet and maximally tolerated statin
therapy for treatment of heterozygous familial hypercholesterolemia (HeFH) or clinical atherosclerotic CV disease in patients who require additional
lowering of LDL cholesterol (LDL-C) levels** ☒
Adults: 75 mg subcut every 2 weeks or 300 mg every
4 weeks. If LDL-C response is inadequate (within
4 to 8 weeks), may increase dosage to maximum of
150 mg every 2 weeks. Recommended dosage in
patients with HeFH undergoing LDL apheresis is
150 mg subcut every 2 weeks, without regard to the
timing of apheresis.

alosetron hydrochloride

ah-LOSS-e-tron

Lotronex

Therapeutic class: Anti-IBS drugs
Pharmacologic class: Selective 5-HT$_3$
receptor antagonists

AVAILABLE FORMS
Tablets: 0.5 mg, 1 mg

INDICATIONS & DOSAGES
Black Box Warning Drug is only appropriate for
women with severe diarrhea-predominant IBS who
haven't responded to conventional therapy. Infrequent but serious GI adverse reactions have been reported and resulted in hospitalization and, rarely,
blood transfusion, surgery, and death. ■
➤ **Severe diarrhea-predominant IBS**
Women: 0.5 mg PO b.i.d. If, after 4 weeks, drug is
well tolerated but doesn't adequately control IBS
symptoms, increase to 1 mg b.i.d. (maximum dose,
2 mg/day). After 4 weeks at this dosage, if symptoms
aren't controlled, stop drug.

alprostadil (injection)
al-PROSS-ta-dil

Prostin VR Pediatric

Therapeutic class: Prostaglandins
Pharmacologic class: Prostaglandins

AVAILABLE FORMS
Injection: 500 mcg/mL

INDICATIONS & DOSAGES
➤ **Palliative therapy for temporary maintenance of patency of ductus arteriosus until surgery can be performed**
Neonates: 0.05 to 0.1 mcg/kg/minute by IV infusion. When therapeutic response is achieved, reduce infusion rate to lowest dose that will maintain response. Maximum dose is 0.4 mcg/kg/minute. Or, give drug through umbilical artery catheter placed at ductal opening.

alprostadil (intracavernosal injection; urogenital suppository)
al-PROSS-ta-dil

Caverject, Caverject Impulse, Edex, Muse

Therapeutic class: Erectile dysfunction drugs
Pharmacologic class: Prostaglandins

AVAILABLE FORMS
Intracavernosal injection: 10 mcg/vial, 20 mcg/vial, 40 mcg/vial
Urethral suppository: 125 mcg, 250 mcg, 500 mcg, 1,000 mcg

INDICATIONS & DOSAGES
➤ **Erectile dysfunction of vasculogenic, psychogenic, or mixed causes**
Injection
Men: Dosages highly individualized; initially, inject 2.5 mcg intracavernosally. If partial response occurs, give second dose of 2.5 mcg; increase by 5 to 10 mcg until patient achieves erection suitable for intercourse lasting no longer than 1 hour. If no response to first dose, increase second dose to 7.5 mcg within 1 hour; then increase by 5 to 10 mcg until patient achieves suitable erection. After initial doses, patient must remain in prescriber's office until complete detumescence occurs. Don't repeat for at least 24 hours. For Edex, give 1 to 40 mcg by intracavernosal injection over 5 to 10 seconds. Use the lowest effective dose no more than three times per week with at least 24 hours between doses.
Urethral suppository
Men: Initially, 125 to 250 mcg, under supervision of prescriber. Adjust dosage as needed until response is sufficient for sexual intercourse. Maximum of two administrations in 24 hours; maximum dose is 1,000 mcg.
➤ **Erectile dysfunction of neurogenic cause (spinal cord injury)**
Men: Dosages highly individualized; initially, inject 1.25 mcg intracavernosally. If partial response occurs,

give second dose of 1.25 mcg. Increase in increments of 2.5 mcg, to dose of 5 mcg; then increase in increments of 5 mcg until patient achieves erection suitable for intercourse lasting no longer than 1 hour. If no response to first dose, give next higher dose within 1 hour. After initial doses, patient must remain in prescriber's office until complete detumescence occurs. Don't repeat procedure for at least 24 hours. For Edex, give 1 to 40 mcg by intracavernosal injection over 5 to 10 seconds. Use the lowest effective dose no more than three times per week with at least 24 hours between doses.

alvimopan
al-VIM-oh-pan

Entereg

Therapeutic class: Bowel restorative drugs
Pharmacologic class: Peripherally acting mu-opioid receptor antagonists

AVAILABLE FORMS
Capsules: 12 mg

INDICATIONS & DOSAGES
Black Box Warning Drug is for short-term use in hospitalized patients due to MI risk. ■
➤ **Acceleration of recovery after partial large- or small-bowel resection surgery with primary anastomosis**
Adults: 12 mg PO 30 minutes to 5 hours before surgery, followed by 12 mg PO b.i.d. beginning day after surgery for up to 7 days or maximum of 15 in-hospital doses (180 mg).

anakinra
ann-ACK-in-rah

Kineret

Therapeutic class: Immunomodulators
Pharmacologic class: Interleukin-1 receptor antagonists

AVAILABLE FORMS
Injection: 100 mg/0.67 mL in a prefilled glass syringe

INDICATIONS & DOSAGES
Adjust-a-dose (for all indications): In severe renal insufficiency or ESRD (CrCl less than 30 mL/minute), consider every-other-day dosing.
➤ **Neonatal-onset multisystem inflammatory disease**
Adults and children: Initially, 1 to 2 mg/kg subcut once daily. May increase in 0.5- to 1-mg/kg increments to maximum dose of 8 mg/kg daily. Maintenance dose is 3 to 4 mg/kg daily. May divide total daily dose into two equal doses.
➤ **To reduce signs and symptoms and slow progression of structural damage in moderately to severely active RA after one or more failures with DMARDs, alone or combined with DMARDs other than TNF blockers**
Adults: 100 mg subcut daily at the same time each day.

angiotensin II
an-jee-oh-TEN-sin

Giapreza

Therapeutic class: Vasoconstrictors
Pharmacologic class: Angiotensin II
analogues

AVAILABLE FORMS
Injection: 2.5 mg/mL in 1- and 2-mL single-dose vials

INDICATIONS & DOSAGES
➤ **To increase BP in patients with septic or other
distributive shock**
Adults: Initially, 20 nanograms/kg/minute IV infusion. May titrate by up to 15 nanograms/kg/minute
every 5 minutes as needed to achieve or maintain target BP. Don't exceed 80 nanograms/kg/minute during
first 3 hours of treatment. Doses as low as 1.25 nano-
grams/kg/minute may be effective. Maintenance doses shouldn't exceed 40 nanograms/kg/minute. Once
shock has sufficiently improved, wean patient by
down-titrating every 5 to 15 minutes by increments of
up to 15 nanograms/kg/minute.

apomorphine hydrochloride
ah-poe-MORE-feen

Apokyn

Therapeutic class: Antiparkinsonians
Pharmacologic class: Nonergot-derivative
dopamine agonists

AVAILABLE FORMS
Solution for injection: 10 mg/mL (contains benzyl
alcohol)

INDICATIONS & DOSAGES
➤ **Intermittent hypomobility, "off" episodes
caused by advanced Parkinson disease (given with
an antiemetic)**
Adults: Initially, give a 2-mg subcut test dose when
patient is in an "off" episode. Measure supine and
standing BP before first dose and every 20 minutes for
at least the first hour. If patient tolerates and responds
to drug, start with 2 mg subcut as needed as outpatient.
Separate doses by at least 2 hours. Increase by 1 mg
every few days, if needed.

If initial 2-mg dose is ineffective but tolerated, give
4 mg at next "off" period, but no sooner than 2 hours
after the initial test dose of 2 mg. Measure supine and
standing BP every 20 minutes for first hour. If drug
is tolerated, start with 3 mg subcut as outpatient. If
needed, increase by 1 mg every few days.

If patient doesn't tolerate 4-mg dose, give 3 mg as
test dose at next "off" period, measuring supine and
standing BP every 20 minutes for first hour. If drug is
tolerated, give 2 mg as outpatient. Increase by 1 mg
every few days, as needed; doses higher than 4 mg
usually not tolerated if 2 mg is starting dose.

Maximum recommended dose is usually 6 mg
as needed. Most patients use drug t.i.d. If therapy is
interrupted for more than 1 week, restart at 2 mg and
gradually titrate dosage. Experience is limited at more
than five times daily or more than 20 mg daily.
Adjust-a-dose: In patients with mild to moderate
renal impairment, give test and starting doses of 1 mg
subcut.

arformoterol tartrate
arr-fohr-MOH-tur-ahl

Brovana

Therapeutic class: Bronchodilators
Pharmacologic class: Long-acting selective
beta$_2$ agonists

AVAILABLE FORMS
Solution for inhalation: 15 mcg/2-mL vials

INDICATIONS & DOSAGES
➤ **Long-term maintenance treatment of bronchoconstriction in patients with COPD, including
chronic bronchitis and emphysema**
Adults: 15 mcg inhaled via nebulizer b.i.d. (morning
and evening). Maximum dose is 30 mcg daily.

artemether–lumefantrine
art-TEM-mah-ther/loo-meh-FAN-treen

Coartem

Therapeutic class: Antimalarials
Pharmacologic class: Schizontocides

AVAILABLE FORMS
Tablets: artemether 20 mg and lumefantrine 120 mg

INDICATIONS & DOSAGES
➤ **Uncomplicated malaria caused by** *Plasmodium
falciparum*
Adults and children weighing 35 kg or more: Initially,
4 tablets PO, followed by 4 tablets in 8 hours, then
4 tablets b.i.d. for the next 2 days. Total course is
24 tablets.
Children weighing 25 to 34 kg: Initially, 3 tablets PO,
followed by 3 tablets in 8 hours, then 3 tablets b.i.d.
for the next 2 days. Total course is 18 tablets.
Children weighing 15 to 24 kg: Initially, 2 tablets PO,
followed by 2 tablets in 8 hours, then 2 tablets b.i.d.
for the next 2 days. Total course is 12 tablets.
Children weighing 5 to 14 kg: Initially, 1 tablet PO,
followed by 1 tablet in 8 hours, then 1 tablet b.i.d. for
the next 2 days. Total course is 6 tablets.

SAFETY ALERT!

asparaginase *Erwinia
chrysanthemi*
as-PAR-a-jin-ase er-WIN-ee-uh
chris-AN-tha-me

Erwinase✦, Erwinaze

Therapeutic class: Antineoplastics
Pharmacologic class: Enzyme inhibitors

AVAILABLE FORMS
Powder for injection: 10,000 international units/vial

INDICATIONS & DOSAGES

➤ **Acute lymphoblastic leukemia in patients who have developed hypersensitivity to *Escherichia coli*–derived asparaginase as part of a multiagent chemotherapy regimen**

Adults and children age 1 and older: When substituting for pegaspargase, give 25,000 international units/m^2 IM or IV three times a week (Monday/Wednesday/Friday) for six doses. When substituting for native *E. coli* asparaginase, give 25,000 international units/m^2 IM or IV for each scheduled dose of native *E. coli* asparaginase within a treatment. When giving IV, consider monitoring (predose) nadir serum asparaginase activity (NSAA) levels and switching to IM administration if desired NSAA levels aren't achieved.

Adjust-a-dose: Refer to manufacturer's instructions for toxicity-related dosage adjustments.

SAFETY ALERT!

atracurium besylate
at-truh-KYOO-ree-um

Therapeutic class: Skeletal muscle relaxants
Pharmacologic class: Nondepolarizing neuromuscular blockers

AVAILABLE FORMS
Injection: 10 mg/mL

INDICATIONS & DOSAGES

➤ **Adjunct to general anesthesia to facilitate ET intubation and relax skeletal muscles during surgery or mechanical ventilation**

Adults and children age 2 and older: 0.4 to 0.5 mg/kg by IV bolus. Give maintenance dose of 0.08 to 0.1 mg/kg within 20 to 45 minutes during prolonged surgery and every 15 to 25 minutes in patients receiving balanced anesthesia. For prolonged procedures, use a constant infusion at 9 to 10 mcg/kg/minute initially; then reduce to 5 to 9 mcg/kg/minute. For infusion in the ICU, an infusion rate of 11 to 13 mcg/kg/minute should provide adequate neuromuscular blockade.

Children ages 1 month to 2 years: First dose, 0.3 to 0.4 mg/kg IV for children under halothane anesthesia. Frequent maintenance doses may be needed.

Adjust-a-dose: In adults, adolescents, children, or infants with significant CV disease or history suggesting a greater risk of histamine release (anaphylactic reaction, asthma), give initial dose of 0.3 to 0.4 mg/kg slowly or in divided doses over 1 minute. In adults receiving enflurane or isoflurane at the same time, reduce initial atracurium dose by 33% (0.25 to 0.35 mg/kg). In adults receiving atracurium following succinylcholine, initial dose is 0.3 to 0.4 mg/kg.

avanafil
a-VAN-a-fill

Stendra

Therapeutic class: Erectile dysfunction drugs
Pharmacologic class: PDE5 inhibitors

AVAILABLE FORMS
Tablets: 50 mg, 100 mg, 200 mg

INDICATIONS & DOSAGES
➤ **Erectile dysfunction**

Adult men: 100 mg PO daily as needed 15 minutes before sexual activity. May increase to a maximum of 200 mg daily 15 minutes before sexual activity or decrease to 50 mg daily 30 minutes before sexual activity. Use lowest effective dosage.

Adjust-a-dose: In patients taking moderate CYP3A4 inhibitors, maximum dosage is 50 mg PO daily. Don't use in patients taking strong CYP3A4 inhibitors. In patients taking a stable dose of alpha blocker, initially give 50 mg PO daily; adjust as needed and tolerated.

SAFETY ALERT!

avatrombopag maleate
a-va-TROM-boe-PAG

Doptelet

Therapeutic class: Hematopoietics
Pharmacologic class: Thrombopoietin receptor agonists

AVAILABLE FORMS
Tablets: 20 mg

INDICATIONS & DOSAGES
➤ **Thrombocytopenia in patients with chronic liver disease scheduled to undergo a procedure**

Adults: Begin dosing 10 to 13 days before scheduled procedure. For platelet count of 40×10^9/L to less than 50×10^9/L, give 40 mg PO once daily for 5 consecutive days. For platelet count less than 40×10^9/L, give 60 mg PO once daily for 5 consecutive days. Patient should undergo procedure within 5 to 8 days after final dose.

SAFETY ALERT!

axicabtagene ciloleucel
ax-i-KAB-ta-jeen sye-LO-loo-sel

Yescarta

Therapeutic class: Antineoplastics
Pharmacologic class: T-cell immunotherapies

AVAILABLE FORMS
Infusion bag: 2×10^6 chimeric antigen receptor (CAR)-positive T cells/kg body weight (or maximum of 2×10^8 CAR-positive viable T cells for patients 100 kg and above) in suspension (approximately 68 mL)

INDICATIONS & DOSAGES
➤ **Relapsed or refractory large B-cell lymphoma after two or more lines of systemic therapy, including diffuse large B-cell lymphoma (DLBCL) not otherwise specified, primary mediastinal large B-cell lymphoma, high-grade B-cell lymphoma, and DLBCL arising from follicular lymphoma**

Adults: Target dose is 2×10^6 CAR-positive viable T cells/kg body weight (or a maximum of 2×10^8 CAR-positive viable T cells for patients weighing 100 kg or more).

✙Canada ◇ OTC ◆ Off-label use ✐Photoguide 🆖Do not crush *Liquid contains alcohol ▓Genetic

Adjust-a-dose: Refer to manufacturer's instructions for toxicity-related dosage adjustments.

azelaic acid
aze-eh-LAY-ik

Azelex, Finacea

Therapeutic class: Antiacne drugs
Pharmacologic class: Dicarboxylic acids

AVAILABLE FORMS
Cream: 20%
Foam: 15%
Gel: 15%

INDICATIONS & DOSAGES
➤ **Mild to moderate inflammatory acne vulgaris**
Adults and children age 12 and older: Apply thin film of cream (Azelex) and gently but thoroughly massage into affected areas b.i.d., in morning and evening. Can reduce to once daily if persistent skin irritation occurs.
➤ **Mild to moderate rosacea**
Adults: Apply thin film of foam or gel (Finacea) and gently but thoroughly massage into affected areas b.i.d., in morning and evening. Reassess if no improvement in 12 weeks.

azilsartan kamedoxomil
ay-zil-SAR-tan

Edarbi

Therapeutic class: Antihypertensives
Pharmacologic class: ARBs

AVAILABLE FORMS
Tablets: 40 mg, 80 mg

INDICATIONS & DOSAGES
➤ **HTN (alone or in combination with other antihypertensives)**
Adults: 80 mg PO once daily.
Adjust-a-dose: For patients treated with high doses of diuretics, consider initiating therapy at 40 mg PO daily.

basiliximab
ba-sil-IK-si-mab

Simulect

Therapeutic class: Immunosuppressants
Pharmacologic class: Monoclonal antibodies

AVAILABLE FORMS
Injection: 10-mg, 20-mg vials

INDICATIONS & DOSAGES
Black Box Warning Drug should only be prescribed by physicians experienced in management of organ transplant and immunosuppression therapy and only in facilities equipped and staffed with adequate laboratory and supportive medical resources. ∎
➤ **To prevent acute organ rejection in patients receiving renal transplantation when used as part of an immunosuppressive regimen that includes cyclosporine and corticosteroids**

Adults and children weighing 35 kg or more: 20 mg IV given within 2 hours before transplant surgery and 20 mg IV given 4 days after transplantation.
Children weighing less than 35 kg: 10 mg IV given within 2 hours before transplant surgery and 10 mg IV given 4 days after transplantation.
Adjust-a-dose: Withhold second dose if complications, such as a severe hypersensitivity reaction or graft loss, occur.

bedaquiline fumarate
bed-AK-wi-leen

Sirturo

Therapeutic class: Antituberculotics
Pharmacologic class: Diarylquinolines

AVAILABLE FORMS
Tablets: 100 mg

INDICATIONS & DOSAGES
Black Box Warning Due to increased risk of death, drug should be reserved for use when an effective treatment regimen can't otherwise be provided. ∎
➤ **Pulmonary multidrug-resistant TB as part of combination therapy**
Adults: Weeks 1 and 2, 400 mg PO once daily. Weeks 3 to 24, 200 mg PO three times a week (48 hours between doses) for a total of 600 mg/week.
Adjust-a-dose: In first 2 weeks, if a dose is missed, don't make it up but continue the dosing schedule. From 3 weeks on, if a dose is missed, have patient take dose as soon as possible, then resume the three-times-a-week schedule.

SAFETY ALERT!

bendamustine hydrochloride
ben-dah-MOO-steen

Bendeka, Treanda

Therapeutic class: Antineoplastics
Pharmacologic class: Mechlorethamine derivatives

AVAILABLE FORMS
Injection solution: 100 mg/4 mL in vials
Lyophilized powder for injection: 25 mg, 100 mg in single-use vials

INDICATIONS & DOSAGES
Adjust-a-dose (for all indications): Refer to manufacturer's instructions for dosage adjustments for hematologic and nonhematologic toxicities.
☉ Alert: Available formulations have different concentrations; don't mix or combine. See manufacturer's instructions for preparation.
➤ **Chronic lymphocytic leukemia**
Adults: 100 mg/m^2 IV on days 1 and 2 of a 28-day cycle, given for up to six cycles.
➤ **Indolent B-cell non-Hodgkin lymphoma that has progressed during or within 6 months of treatment with rituximab or a rituximab-containing regimen**
Adults: 120 mg/m^2 IV on days 1 and 2 of a 21-day cycle, given in up to eight cycles.

✦Canada ◇OTC ◆Off-label use ✐Photoguide ⊕Do not crush *Liquid contains alcohol ⚥Genetic

benzonatate
ben-ZOE-na-tate

Tessalon

Therapeutic class: Antitussives
Pharmacologic class: Local anesthetics

AVAILABLE FORMS
Capsules ⓒ: 100 mg, 150 mg, 200 mg

INDICATIONS & DOSAGES
➤ **Symptomatic relief of cough**
Adults and children older than age 10: 100 to 200 mg
PO t.i.d.; up to 600 mg daily.

benzyl alcohol
ben-zill AL-ko-hall

Ulesfia

Therapeutic class: Scabicides–pediculicides
Pharmacologic class: Topical alcohols

AVAILABLE FORMS
Lotion: 5%

INDICATIONS & DOSAGES
➤ **Head lice infestation**
*Adults age 60 and younger and children age 6 months
and older:* Apply to hair and scalp until completely
saturated. Allow to remain for 10 minutes; then rinse
thoroughly with warm water. Remove dead lice and
nits with fine-toothed comb. Repeat treatment after
7 days. For each treatment, refer to manufacturer's
instructions for the appropriate volume to use based
on hair length.

betaxolol hydrochloride
beh-TAX-oh-lol

Betoptic, Betoptic S

Therapeutic class: Antiglaucoma drugs–
antihypertensives
Pharmacologic class: Beta blockers

AVAILABLE FORMS
Ophthalmic solution: 0.5%
Ophthalmic suspension: 0.25%
Tablets: 10 mg, 20 mg

INDICATIONS & DOSAGES
➤ **Chronic open-angle glaucoma, ocular HTN
(ophthalmic only)**
Adults: Instill 1 or 2 drops in the affected eye(s) b.i.d.
➤ **HTN with or without diuretic therapy**
Adults: 5 to 10 mg PO once daily. May increase dose
to 20 mg if desired response isn't achieved after 7 to
14 days.
Adjust-a-dose: To prevent bradycardia, reduce
starting dose to 5 mg in elderly patients. In patients
with severe renal impairment and those on dialysis,
reduce initial dose to 5 mg daily. May increase dosage by 5 mg/day every 2 weeks to a maximum dose
of 20 mg/day.

bexarotene
bex-AR-oh-teen

Targretin

Therapeutic class: Antineoplastics
Pharmacologic class: Retinoids

AVAILABLE FORMS
Capsules: 75 mg
Topical gel: 1%

INDICATIONS & DOSAGES
Black Box Warning Drugs in the retinoid class are
associated with birth defects in humans; don't give
during pregnancy. ▪
Adjust-a-dose (for all indications): Refer to manufacturer's instructions for toxicity-related dosage
adjustments.
➤ **Cutaneous manifestations of cutaneous T-cell
lymphoma (CTCL) in patients refractory to at
least one prior systemic therapy**
Adults: Initially, 300 mg/m² PO once daily. If no
tumor response after 8 weeks and if initial dose of
300 mg/m²/day is well tolerated, may increase dosage
to 400 mg/m²/day with careful monitoring. Continue
until disease progression or unacceptable toxicity.
➤ **Cutaneous lesions in patients with CTCL
(Stage IA and IB) with refractory or persistent disease after other therapies or who haven't tolerated
other therapies**
Adults: Apply sufficient gel to cover lesion with a
generous coating. Initially apply once every other day
for first week. Increase application frequency at weekly intervals to once daily, then b.i.d., then t.i.d., and
finally q.i.d. according to individual lesion tolerance;
continue as long as patient derives benefits. Most patients can tolerate a dosing frequency of two to four
times per day.

bezlotoxumab
BEZ-loe-tox-ue-mab

Zinplava

Therapeutic class: Toxin binders
Pharmacologic class: Monoclonal antibodies

AVAILABLE FORMS
Injection: 1,000 mg/40 mL (25 mg/mL) in single-dose
vials

INDICATIONS & DOSAGES
➤ **To reduce recurrence of *Clostridium difficile*
infection (CDI) in patients receiving antibacterial treatment for CDI and who are at high risk for
CDI recurrence**
Adults: 10 mg/kg by IV infusion as a one-time dose
during antibacterial treatment for CDI.

SAFETY ALERT!

bicalutamide
bye-ka-LOO-ta-mide

Casodex

Therapeutic class: Antineoplastics
Pharmacologic class: Androgen receptor inhibitors

AVAILABLE FORMS
Tablets: 50 mg

INDICATIONS & DOSAGES
➤ **Metastatic prostate cancer in combination with a luteinizing hormone-releasing hormone analogue**
Adult males: 50 mg PO once daily.

blinatumomab ⚙
BLIN-a-TOOM-oh-mab

Blincyto

Therapeutic class: Antineoplastics
Pharmacologic class: Monoclonal antibodies

AVAILABLE FORMS
Injection: 35-mcg single-use vial

INDICATIONS & DOSAGES
Black Box Warning Drug can cause fatal cytokine release syndrome and neurologic toxicities. ■
🕭 *Alert:* Strictly follow instructions for preparation (including admixing) and administration to minimize medication errors.
Adjust-a-dose (for all indications): If the interruption after an adverse event is no longer than 7 days, continue the same cycle to a total of 28 days of infusion inclusive of days before and after the interruption in that cycle. If an interruption due to an adverse event is longer than 7 days, start a new cycle. Refer to manufacturer's instructions for toxicity-related dosage adjustments.
➤ **Relapsed or refractory B-cell precursor acute lymphoblastic leukemia (ALL)** ⚙
Adults and children: A treatment course consists of up to two induction cycles followed by three additional consolidation cycles and up to four additional cycles of continued therapy. A single cycle of treatment induction or consolidation consists of 28 days of continuous IV infusion followed by a 14-day treatment-free interval (total 42 days). A single cycle of continued therapy consists of 28 days of continuous IV infusion followed by a 56-day treatment-free interval (total 84 days).
For patients weighing 45 kg or more, for cycle 1, initially give 9 mcg/day by continuous IV infusion on days 1 through 7, then 28 mcg/day by continuous IV infusion on days 8 through 28, followed by a 14-day treatment-free interval (total 42 days). For subsequent induction and consolidation cycles, give 28 mcg/day on days 1 through 28, each cycle followed by a 14-day treatment-free interval (total 42 days). For each cycle of continued therapy, give 28 mcg/day, followed by a 56-day treatment-free interval (total 84 days).
For patients weighing 22 to less than 45 kg, the dose is calculated using patient's BSA. For cycle 1,

initially give 5 mcg/m^2/day (not to exceed 9 mcg/day) by continuous IV infusion on days 1 through 7, then 15 mcg/m^2/day (not to exceed 28 mcg/day) by continuous IV infusion on days 8 through 28, followed by a 14-day treatment-free interval (total 42 days). For subsequent induction and consolidation cycles, give 15 mcg/m^2/day (not to exceed 28 mcg/day) on days 1 through 28, each cycle followed by a 14-day treatment-free interval (total 42 days). For each cycle of continued therapy, give 15 mcg/m^2/day (not to exceed 28 mcg/day), followed by a 56-day treatment-free interval (total 84 days). Drug isn't recommended for use in patients weighing less than 22 kg.
➤ **B-cell precursor ALL in first or second complete remission with minimal residual disease greater than or equal to 0.1%**
Adults and children: A treatment course consists of one induction cycle followed by up to three additional cycles for consolidation.
For patients weighing 45 kg or more, the dose for a single cycle of treatment induction or consolidation is 28 mcg/day continuous IV infusion for 28 days, followed by a 14-day treatment-free interval (total 42 days). For patients weighing 22 to less than 45 kg, the dose for a single cycle of treatment induction or consolidation, calculated using patient's BSA, is 15 mcg/m^2/day (not to exceed 28 mcg/day) continuous IV infusion for 28 days, followed by a 14-day treatment-free interval (total 42 days). Drug isn't recommended for use in patients weighing less than 22 kg.

bosutinib ⚙
boe-SUE-ti-nib

Bosulif

Therapeutic class: Antineoplastics
Pharmacologic class: Kinase inhibitors

AVAILABLE FORMS
Tablets 🕭🕭: 100 mg, 400 mg, 500 mg

INDICATIONS & DOSAGES
Adjust-a-dose (for all indications): If CrCl is 30 to 50 mL/minute at start of therapy, give 400 mg once daily for resistant therapy and 300 mg once daily for newly diagnosed chronic phase; if CrCl is less than 30 mL/minute, give 300 mg once daily for resistant therapy and 200 mg once daily for newly diagnosed chronic phase. For preexisting hepatic impairment (Child-Pugh class A, B, or C) at start of therapy, give 200 mg once daily. Refer to manufacturer's instructions for dosage adjustments based on hematologic and nonhematologic toxicities.
➤ **Chronic, accelerated, or blast-phase Philadelphia chromosome–positive (Ph+) chronic myelogenous leukemia (CML) with resistance or intolerance to prior therapy** ⚙
Adults: 500 mg PO once daily with food. Consider dosage escalation to 600 mg once daily in patients who don't reach complete hematologic response by week 8 or a complete cytogenetic response by week 12, who didn't have grade 3 or higher adverse reactions, and who are currently taking 500 mg daily.

♣ Canada   ◇ OTC   ♦ Off-label use   🖉 Photoguide   🕭 Do not crush   *Liquid contains alcohol   ⚙ Genetic

➤**Newly diagnosed chronic phase Ph+ CML** ✂
Adults: 400 mg PO once daily with food until disease progression or unacceptable toxicity occurs. Consider dosage escalation by 100-mg increments to a maximum of 600 mg once daily in patients who don't achieve or maintain a hematologic, cytogenetic, or molecular response and who don't have grade 3 or higher adverse reactions at the recommended starting dosage.

SAFETY ALERT!

brigatinib
bri-GA-ti-nib

Alunbrig

Therapeutic class: Antineoplastics
Pharmacologic class: Tyrosine kinase inhibitors

AVAILABLE FORMS
Tablets: 30 mg, 90 mg, 180 mg

INDICATIONS & DOSAGES
➤**Treatment of anaplastic lymphoma kinase–positive metastatic NSCLC in patients who have progressed on or are intolerant to crizotinib**
Adults: 90 mg PO once daily for 7 days. If tolerated, increase dosage to 180 mg once daily. Continue until disease progression or unacceptable toxicity occurs. If drug is interrupted for 14 days or more for reasons other than toxicity, resume treatment at 90 mg once daily for 7 days before escalating dosage to the previously tolerated dose.
Adjust-a-dose: If concomitant use of a strong CYP3A inhibitor is unavoidable, reduce brigatinib once-daily dose by approximately 50%. After a strong CYP3A inhibitor is discontinued, resume the brigatinib dose that was tolerated before initiating the strong CYP3A inhibitor.

If CrCl is 15 to 30 mL/minute, reduce dose from 180 to 90 mg daily or from 90 to 60 mg daily. For severe hepatic impairment (Child-Pugh class C), reduce dose from 180 to 120 mg daily, or 120 to 90 mg daily, or 90 to 60 mg daily.

Refer to manufacturer's instructions for toxicity-related dosage adjustments and drug discontinuation.

SAFETY ALERT!

busulfan
byoo-SUL-fan

Busulfex, Myleran

Therapeutic class: Antineoplastics
Pharmacologic class: Alkyl sulfonates

AVAILABLE FORMS
Injection: 6 mg/mL
Tablets: ⓞⓝⓒ 2 mg

INDICATIONS & DOSAGES
Black Box Warning Injection causes severe and prolonged myelosuppression at recommended dosage. Hematopoietic progenitor cell transplantation is required to prevent potentially fatal complications. ∎

➤**Chronic myelocytic (granulocytic) leukemia**
Adults: 4 to 8 mg PO daily until WBC count falls to 15,000/mm^3; stop drug until WBC count rises to approximately 50,000/mm^3; then resume dosage as before. When remission is shorter than 3 months, may give maintenance therapy of 1 to 3 mg PO daily. Or, 0.8 mg/kg IV (ideal or actual body weight, whichever is lower) every 6 hours for 4 days (a total of 16 doses) beginning 7 days before transplant. Give cyclophosphamide 60 mg/kg IV over 1 hour daily for 2 days beginning 6 hours after 16th dose of IV busulfan.

C1 esterase inhibitor subcutaneous (human) ✂
ES-ter-ase in-HIB-a-tor

Berinert, Cinryze, Haegarda

Therapeutic class: Miscellaneous hematologic agents
Pharmacologic class: Serine protease inhibitors

AVAILABLE FORMS
Injection: 500 international units (Berinert, Cinryze), 2,000 international units, 3,000 international units (Haegarda) in single-use vials packaged with sterile water for injection

INDICATIONS & DOSAGES
➤**Routine prophylaxis to prevent hereditary angioedema (HAE) attack (except Berinert)**
Adults and adolescents age 12 and older: 60 international units/kg Haegarda subcut twice weekly (every 3 or 4 days). Or, 1,000 international units Cinryze IV at a rate of 1 mL/minute (10 minutes) every 3 or 4 days. May consider doses up to 2,500 international units (not exceeding 100 units/kg) IV based on individual patient response.
Children ages 6 to 11: 500 international units Cinryze IV at a rate of 1 mL/minute (5 minutes) every 3 or 4 days. May consider doses up to 1,000 international units IV based on individual patient response.
➤**Treatment of HAE attack (Berinert only)** ✂
Adults and children age 5 and older: 20 international units/kg by slow IV injection at a rate of approximately 4 mL/minute.

SAFETY ALERT!

cabazitaxel
ka-baz-ih-TAX-el

Jevtana

Therapeutic class: Antineoplastics
Pharmacologic class: Taxoids

AVAILABLE FORMS
Injection: 60 mg/1.5 mL

INDICATIONS & DOSAGES
Black Box Warning Drug is associated with severe hypersensitivity and neutropenic deaths. Monitor patient and blood cell counts closely and provide appropriate therapy. ∎

➤ **In combination with prednisone for hormone-refractory metastatic prostate cancer previously treated with docetaxel-containing treatment regimen**

Adults: 20 mg/m^2 IV over 1 hour every 3 weeks. A dose of 25 mg/m^2 can be used in select patients at the discretion of the treating health care provider. Give oral prednisone 10 mg daily throughout cabazitaxel therapy. Premedicate at least 30 minutes before each dose of cabazitaxel with the following IV medications to reduce risk or severity of hypersensitivity: antihistamine (5 mg dexchlorpheniramine, or 25 mg diphenhydramine or equivalent antihistamine), corticosteroid (8 mg dexamethasone or equivalent steroid), and H$_2$ antagonist (50 mg ranitidine or equivalent H$_2$ antagonist). Antiemetic prophylaxis is recommended and can be given PO or IV as needed.

Adjust-a-dose: Refer to manufacturer's instructions for dosage adjustments due to hematologic and nonhematologic toxicities, hepatic impairment, and use with strong CYP3A inhibitors.

canakinumab ✂

kan-ah-KIN-yoo-mab

Ilaris

Therapeutic class: Anti-autoimmune agents
Pharmacologic class: Monoclonal antibodies

AVAILABLE FORMS
Injection: 150 mg in single-use vials

INDICATIONS & DOSAGES

➤ **Cryopyrin-associated periodic syndromes (familial cold autoinflammatory syndrome and Muckle-Wells syndrome)** ✂

Adults and children age 4 and older weighing more than 40 kg: 150 mg subcut every 8 weeks.

Adults and children age 4 and older weighing 15 to 40 kg: 2 mg/kg subcut every 8 weeks; may increase dosage to 3 mg/kg in children weighing 15 to 40 kg who have an inadequate response.

➤ **Active systemic juvenile idiopathic arthritis** ✂

Children age 2 and older weighing at least 7.5 kg: 4 mg/kg subcut every 4 weeks. Maximum dose is 300 mg.

➤ **TNF receptor-associated periodic syndrome; hyperimmunoglobulin D syndrome/mevalonate kinase deficiency; familial Mediterranean fever** ✂

Adults and children age 2 and older weighing more than 40 kg: Initially, 150 mg subcut every 4 weeks; may increase to 300 mg every 4 weeks if clinical response is inadequate.

Adults and children age 2 and older weighing 15 to 40 kg: Initially, 2 mg/kg subcut every 4 weeks; may increase dosage to 4 mg/kg every 4 weeks if clinical response isn't adequate.

cannabidiol

kan-a-bi-DYE-ol

Epidiolex

Therapeutic class: Anticonvulsants
Pharmacologic class: Cannabinoids
Controlled substance schedule: V

AVAILABLE FORMS
Oral solution: 100 mg/mL

INDICATIONS & DOSAGES

➤ **Treatment of seizures associated with Lennox-Gastaut syndrome or Dravet syndrome**

Adults and children age 2 and older: Initially, 2.5 mg/kg PO b.i.d. After 1 week, increase to a maintenance dosage of 5 mg/kg PO b.i.d. If necessary, may further increase dose, as tolerated, in weekly increments of 2.5 mg/kg b.i.d. to a maximum maintenance dosage of 10 mg/kg b.i.d. For patients in whom a more rapid titration is warranted from 5 mg/kg b.i.d. to 10 mg/kg b.i.d., may increase dosage no more frequently than every other day.

Adjust-a-dose: For moderate (Child-Pugh class B) hepatic impairment, initiate therapy at 1.25 mg/kg PO b.i.d. Increase to maintenance dose of 2.5 mg/kg PO b.i.d. Maximum dosage is 5 mg/kg PO b.i.d. For severe (Child-Pugh class C) hepatic impairment, initiate therapy at 0.5 mg/kg PO b.i.d. Increase to maintenance dose of 1 mg/kg PO b.i.d. Maximum dosage is 2 mg/kg PO b.i.d. Discontinue drug in patients with transaminase elevations greater than 3 × ULN, bilirubin levels greater than 2 × ULN, and sustained transaminase elevations greater than 5 × ULN.

carboprost tromethamine

KAR-boe-prost

Hemabate

Therapeutic class: Oxytocics
Pharmacologic class: Prostaglandins

AVAILABLE FORMS
Injection: 250 mcg/mL

INDICATIONS & DOSAGES

Black Box Warning Strictly adhere to recommended dosages and only use in a hospital that can provide immediate intensive and acute surgical care. ∎

➤ **To terminate pregnancy between weeks 13 and 20 of gestation**

Adults: Initially, 250 mcg deep IM; optionally, a 100-mcg IM test dose may be given. Give subsequent doses of 250 mcg at intervals of 1½ to 3½ hours, depending on uterine response. Dosage may be increased in increments to 500 mcg if contractility is inadequate after several 250-mcg doses. Total dose shouldn't exceed 12 mg or continuous administration for more than 2 days.

➤ **Refractory postpartum hemorrhage**

Adults: 250 mcg by deep IM injection. Repeat doses every 15 to 90 minutes as needed. Maximum total dose is 2 mg (eight doses).

SAFETY ALERT!

carfilzomib
car-FIL-zoe-mib

Kyprolis

Therapeutic class: Antineoplastics
Pharmacologic class: Proteasome inhibitors

AVAILABLE FORMS
Powder for injection: 10 mg, 30 mg, 60 mg in single-use vials

INDICATIONS & DOSAGES
✪ *Alert:* See manufacturer's instructions for administration precautions.

➤ **Relapsed or refractory multiple myeloma (monotherapy) in patients who have received one or more prior therapies; multiple myeloma in combination with lenalidomide and dexamethasone in patients who have received one to three prior therapies**

Adults: Calculate dosage using patient's actual BSA at baseline. In patients with BSA greater than 2.2 m², calculate dosage based on BSA of 2.2 m². For monotherapy, 20 mg/m² IV over 10 minutes on 2 consecutive days each week for 3 weeks (days 1, 2, 8, 9, 15, and 16), followed by 12-day rest period (days 17 to 28). If tolerated, may increase to 27 mg/m² in cycle 1 days 8, 9, 15, and 16 and to 27 mg/m² for subsequent cycles. From cycle 13 on, omit day 8 and 9 doses.

Or, 20 mg/m² IV over 30 minutes on 2 consecutive days each week for 3 weeks (days 1, 2, 8, 9, 15, and 16), followed by 12-day rest period (days 17 to 28). If tolerated, may increase to 56 mg/m² in cycle 1 days 8, 9, 15, and 16 and to 56 mg/m² for subsequent cycles. From cycle 13 on, omit day 8 and 9 doses. Treatment may continue until disease progression or unacceptable toxicity occurs.

For the combination regimen with lenalidomide and dexamethasone, give 20 mg/m² carfilzomib IV as a 10-minute infusion on 2 consecutive days, each week for 3 weeks, followed by a 12-day rest period. If tolerated, escalate to a target dose of 27 mg/m² on days 8, 9, 15, and 16 in cycle 1 and to 27 mg/m² for subsequent cycles. From cycle 13 on, omit day 8 and 9 doses. Treatment may continue until disease progression or unacceptable toxicity occurs. Discontinue drug after cycle 18.

For the combination regimen with dexamethasone, give 20 mg/m² carfilzomib IV as a 30-minute infusion on 2 consecutive days, each week for 3 weeks, followed by a 12-day rest period. If tolerated, escalate to a target dose of 56 mg/m² on days 8, 9, 15, and 16 in cycle 1 and to 56 mg/m² for subsequent cycles. From cycle 13 on, omit day 8 and 9 doses. Treatment may continue until disease progression or unacceptable toxicity occurs.

See manufacturer's instructions for dosing of other medications.

Adjust-a-dose: For patients with mild or moderate hepatic impairment, reduce dosage by 25%. In patients with ESRD on dialysis, give drug after hemodialysis.

Adjust dosage for weight change of more than 20% from baseline. Refer to manufacturer's instructions for dosage adjustments based on toxicities.

ceftaroline fosamil
sef-TAR-oh-leen

Teflaro

Therapeutic class: Antibiotics
Pharmacologic class: Fifth-generation cephalosporins

AVAILABLE FORMS
Injection: 400 mg, 600 mg in single-use vials

INDICATIONS & DOSAGES
➤ **Acute bacterial skin and skin-structure infections caused by susceptible isolates of *Staphylococcus aureus*, *Streptococcus pyogenes*, *Streptococcus agalactiae*, *Escherichia coli*, *Klebsiella pneumoniae*, or *Klebsiella oxytoca*; community-acquired bacterial pneumonia (CABP) caused by susceptible isolates of *Streptococcus pneumoniae*, *S. aureus*, *Haemophilus influenzae*, *K. pneumoniae*, *K. oxytoca*, or *E. coli***

Adults: 600 mg IV over 5 to 60 minutes every 12 hours. For skin and skin-structure infections, continue treatment for 5 to 14 days; for CABP, continue treatment for 5 to 7 days.

Children older than age 2 and younger than 18 weighing more than 33 kg: 400 mg IV every 8 hours or 600 mg IV every 12 hours for 5 to 14 days.

Children older than age 2 and younger than 18 weighing 33 kg or less: 12 mg/kg IV every 8 hours for 5 to 14 days.

Children age 2 months to younger than 2 years: 8 mg/kg IV every 8 hours for 5 to 14 days.

Adjust-a-dose: For adults with CrCl of 31 to 50 mL/minute, give 400 mg IV every 12 hours. If CrCl is 15 to 30 mL/minute, give 300 mg IV every 12 hours. For patients with ESRD, including those on hemodialysis, give 200 mg IV every 12 hours. Administer after dialysis treatment.

SAFETY ALERT!

ceritinib
se-RI-ti-nib

Zykadia

Therapeutic class: Antineoplastics
Pharmacologic class: Kinase inhibitors

AVAILABLE FORMS
Capsules: 150 mg

INDICATIONS & DOSAGES
➤ **Anaplastic lymphoma kinase-positive metastatic NSCLC**

Adults: 450 mg PO once daily with food until disease progression or unacceptable toxicity occurs.

Adjust-a-dose: Refer to manufacturer's instructions for toxicity-related dosage adjustments and discontinuation.

---

cetrorelix acetate

SE-troe-REL-ix

Cetrotide

Therapeutic class: Infertility drugs
Pharmacologic class: Gonadotropin-releasing hormone antagonists

AVAILABLE FORMS
Powder for injection: 0.25 mg

INDICATIONS & DOSAGES
➤ **To inhibit premature luteinizing hormone surges in women undergoing controlled ovarian stimulation**
Women: Ovarian stimulation therapy with gonadotropins is started on cycle day 2 or 3. Give cetrorelix acetate 0.25 mg subcut on stimulation day 5 (morning or evening) or day 6 (morning), and continue once daily until day of hCG administration.

cevimeline hydrochloride

seh-vih-MEH-leen

Evoxac

Therapeutic class: Cholinergic agonists
Pharmacologic class: Cholinergic agonists

AVAILABLE FORMS
Capsules: 30 mg

INDICATIONS & DOSAGES
➤ **Dry mouth in patients with Sjögren syndrome**
Adults: 30 mg PO t.i.d.

SAFETY ALERT!

chlorambucil

klor-AM-byoo-sill

Leukeran

Therapeutic class: Antineoplastics
Pharmacologic class: Nitrogen mustards

AVAILABLE FORMS
Tablets: 2 mg

INDICATIONS & DOSAGES
Black Box Warning Drug can severely suppress bone marrow function; is a carcinogen, and probably mutagenic and teratogenic; and produces human infertility. ∎
➤ **Chronic lymphocytic leukemia; malignant lymphomas, including lymphosarcoma, giant follicular lymphoma, and Hodgkin lymphoma**
Adults: For initiation of therapy or for short courses of treatment, 0.1 to 0.2 mg/kg PO daily for 3 to 6 weeks (usually 4 to 10 mg daily). Maintenance dosage shouldn't exceed 0.1 mg/kg/day and may be as low as 0.03 mg/kg/day. Adjust dosage according to patient response; reduce when WBC count falls abruptly. For pulse dosage, give initial single dose of 0.4 mg/kg. Then give doses at biweekly or monthly intervals, increasing by 0.1-mg/kg increments until lymphocytosis is controlled or toxicity occurs.

Adjust-a-dose: Reduce first dose if given within 4 weeks after a full course of radiation therapy or myelosuppressive drugs, or if pretreatment WBC or platelet count is depressed from bone marrow disease.

chloramphenicol sodium succinate

klor-am-FEN-i-kole

Therapeutic class: Antibiotics
Pharmacologic class: Dichloroacetic acid derivatives

AVAILABLE FORMS
Injection: 1-g vials

INDICATIONS & DOSAGES
Black Box Warning Drug is associated with serious and fatal blood dyscrasias. Use alternative therapies when possible. Patient should be hospitalized during therapy to closely monitor blood laboratory levels. ∎
➤ ***Haemophilus influenzae* meningitis, acute *Salmonella typhi* infection, and meningitis, bacteremia, or other severe infections caused by sensitive *Salmonella* species, rickettsia, lymphogranuloma, psittacosis, or various sensitive gram-negative organisms**
Adults: 50 to 100 mg/kg IV daily, divided every 6 hours. Increased dosage, up to 100 mg/kg daily, may be needed.
Full-term infants older than age 2 weeks with normal metabolic processes and children: Up to 50 mg/kg IV daily, divided every 6 hours. May use up to 100 mg/kg/day in four divided doses for meningitis.
Preterm infants, neonates age 2 weeks and younger, and children and infants with suspected immature metabolic processes: 25 mg/kg IV once daily.
Adjust-a-dose: For patients with renal or hepatic impairment, excessive blood levels may result from administration of the recommended dosage. Determine drug blood concentration at appropriate intervals and adjust dosage accordingly.

SAFETY ALERT!

chlordiazePOXIDE hydrochloride

klor-dye-az-e-POX-ide

Therapeutic class: Anxiolytics
Pharmacologic class: Benzodiazepines
Controlled substance schedule: IV

AVAILABLE FORMS
Capsules: 5 mg, 10 mg, 25 mg

INDICATIONS & DOSAGES
Black Box Warning Opioids used with benzodiazepines or CNS depressants can cause death. ∎
Adjust-a-dose (for all indications): In elderly or debilitated patients, give 5 mg PO b.i.d. to q.i.d. Use smallest effective dose, to prevent oversedation or ataxia.
➤ **Mild to moderate anxiety**
Adults: 5 to 10 mg PO t.i.d. or q.i.d.
Children older than age 6: 5 mg PO b.i.d. to q.i.d. Maximum, 10 mg PO b.i.d. or t.i.d.

➤ **Severe anxiety**
Adults: 20 to 25 mg PO t.i.d. or q.i.d.
➤ **Withdrawal symptoms of acute alcoholism**
Adults: 50 to 100 mg PO. Repeat as needed, up to 300 mg daily.
➤ **Preoperative apprehension and anxiety**
Adults: 5 to 10 mg PO t.i.d. or q.i.d. on days before surgery.

chlorproMAZINE hydrochloride
klor-PROE-ma-zeen

Therapeutic class: Antipsychotics
Pharmacologic class: Phenothiazines

AVAILABLE FORMS
Injection: 25 mg/mL
Tablets: 10 mg, 25 mg, 50 mg, 100 mg, 200 mg

INDICATIONS & DOSAGES
Black Box Warning Elderly patients with dementia-related psychosis treated with antipsychotics are at an increased risk of death. Drug isn't approved to treat these patients. ∎
➤ **Psychosis, mania**
Adults and children older than age 12: For hospitalized patients with acute disease, 25 mg IM; may give an additional 25 to 50 mg IM in 1 hour if needed. Increase over several days to 400 mg every 4 to 6 hours. Switch to oral therapy as soon as possible. Or, 25 mg PO t.i.d. initially; then gradually increase to 500 mg (400 mg in less acutely disturbed patients) daily in divided doses. For outpatients, 30 to 75 mg daily in two to four divided doses. Increase dosage by 20 to 50 mg twice weekly until symptoms are controlled.
➤ **Nausea and vomiting**
Adults and children older than age 12: 10 to 25 mg PO every 4 to 6 hours, p.r.n. Or, 25 mg IM initially. If no hypotension occurs, 25 to 50 mg IM every 3 to 4 hours may be given, p.r.n., until vomiting stops.
Children ages 6 months to 12 years: 0.55 mg/kg PO every 4 to 6 hours or IM every 6 to 8 hours. Maximum IM dose in children younger than age 5 or weighing less than 23 kg is 40 mg. Maximum IM dose in children ages 5 to 12 or weighing 23 to 45 kg is 75 mg.
➤ **Acute intermittent porphyria, intractable hiccups**
Adults and children older than age 12: 25 to 50 mg PO t.i.d. or q.i.d. If hiccups persist for 2 to 3 days on oral therapy, give 25 to 50 mg IM. If hiccups still persist, give 25 to 50 mg diluted in 500 to 1,000 mL of NSS and infused slowly with patient in supine position. For porphyria, give 25 mg IM t.i.d. or q.i.d. until patient can take oral therapy.
➤ **Tetanus**
Adults and children older than age 12: 25 to 50 mg IV or IM t.i.d. or q.i.d.
Children ages 6 months to 12 years: 0.55 mg/kg IM or IV every 6 to 8 hours. Maximum parenteral dosage in children weighing less than 23 kg is 40 mg daily; for children weighing 23 to 45 kg, 75 mg, except in severe cases. If giving IV, dilute to 1 mg/mL with NSS and give at a rate of 0.5 mg/minute.

➤ **Behavioral disorders, hyperactivity**
Children ages 6 months to 12 years: For outpatients, 0.55 mg/kg PO every 4 to 6 hours or IM every 6 to 8 hours, as needed. For hospitalized patients, start with low oral doses and increase gradually. In severe behavioral disorders, 50 to 100 mg PO daily or, in older children, 200 mg/day or more PO may be necessary. There is little evidence that improvement in severely disturbed mentally retarded patients is enhanced by doses beyond 500 mg/day. In hospitalized patients age 5 or younger or weighing less than 23 kg, don't exceed 40 mg/day IM. In children ages 5 to 12 weighing 23 to 45 kg, don't exceed 75 mg/day IM, except in unmanageable cases.
➤ **Surgery**
Adults and children older than age 12: Preoperatively, 25 to 50 mg PO 2 to 3 hours before surgery or 12.5 to 25 mg IM 1 to 2 hours before surgery; during surgery, 12.5 mg IM, repeated in 30 minutes, if needed, or fractional 2-mg doses IV at 2-minute intervals to maximum dose of 25 mg.
Children ages 6 months to 12 years: Preoperatively, 0.55 mg/kg PO 2 to 3 hours before surgery or IM 1 to 2 hours before surgery. During surgery, 0.25 mg/kg IM, repeated in 30 minutes if needed, or fractional 1-mg doses IV at 2-minute intervals to maximum of 0.25 mg/kg. May repeat fractional IV regimen in 30 minutes if needed.
Elderly patients: Lower dosages are sufficient; dosage increments should be more gradual than in adults.

chlorthalidone
klor-THAL-i-done

Therapeutic class: Antihypertensives
Pharmacologic class: Thiazide diuretics

AVAILABLE FORMS
Tablets: 25 mg, 50 mg

INDICATIONS & DOSAGES
➤ **Edema**
Adults: 50 to 100 mg PO daily, or 100 mg PO on alternating days (maximum, 200 mg/day).
➤ **HTN**
Adults: 12.5 to 25 mg PO daily. May increase to 50 mg, then 100 mg daily as needed.

ciprofloxacin hydrochloride (otic)
si-proe-FLOX-a-sin

Cetraxal

Therapeutic class: Antibiotics
Pharmacologic class: Fluoroquinolones

AVAILABLE FORMS
Otic solution: 0.2% (0.25 mL single-use container)

INDICATIONS & DOSAGES
➤ **Acute otitis externa caused by susceptible isolates of** *P. aeruginosa* **or** *S. aureus*
Adults and children age 1 and older: Instill 0.5 mg (contents of one single-dose container) into affected ear b.i.d. for 7 days.

clomiPHENE citrate
KLOE-mi-feen

Therapeutic class: Ovulation stimulants
Pharmacologic class: Chlorotrianisene derivatives

AVAILABLE FORMS
Tablets: 50 mg

INDICATIONS & DOSAGES
➤ **To induce ovulation**
Women: 50 mg PO daily for 5 days, starting on day 5 of menstrual cycle (first day of menstrual flow is day 1) if bleeding occurs, or at any time if patient hasn't had recent uterine bleeding. If ovulation doesn't occur, may increase dosage to 100 mg PO daily for 5 days as soon as 30 days after first course. Repeat until conception occurs or until three courses of therapy are completed.

clomiPRAMINE hydrochloride
kloe-MI-pra-meen

Anafranil

Therapeutic class: Antidepressants
Pharmacologic class: TCAs

AVAILABLE FORMS
Capsules: 25 mg, 50 mg, 75 mg

INDICATIONS & DOSAGES
Black Box Warning Drug increases risk of suicidal thoughts and behavior in children, adolescents, and young adults. ∎
➤ **OCD**
Adults: Initially, 25 mg PO daily with meals, gradually increased to 100 mg/day in divided doses during first 2 weeks. Thereafter, increase to maximum dose of 250 mg/day in divided doses with meals, as needed. After adjustment, may give total daily dose at bedtime.
Children age 10 and older and adolescents: Initially, 25 mg PO daily with meals, gradually increased over first 2 weeks to maximum of 3 mg/kg daily or 100 mg PO daily in divided doses, whichever is smaller. Maximum daily dose is 3 mg/kg or 200 mg, whichever is smaller; give at bedtime after adjustment. Reassess and adjust dosage periodically. Allow at least 14 days before starting if patient was previously on an MAO inhibitor.

collagenase *Clostridium histolyticum*
kuh-LAJ-eh-nase klos-TRID-ee-um hiss-toe-LIH-teh-kum

Xiaflex

Therapeutic class: Anticollagen drugs
Pharmacologic class: Enzymes

AVAILABLE FORMS
Injection: 0.9 mg single-use vials

INDICATIONS & DOSAGES
Black Box Warning Drug is associated with penile fracture and other related penile injuries, which may require surgery. ∎
➤ **Dupuytren contracture with palpable cord**
Adults: 0.58 mg injected into palpable cord with contracture of metacarpophalangeal joint or proximal interphalangeal joint. May repeat up to three times per cord at 4-week intervals.
➤ **Peyronie disease with palpable plaque and curvature deformity of at least 30 degrees at start of therapy**
Adults: Initially, 0.58 mg injected into the target plaque once; then repeat injection 1 to 3 days later. May repeat up to four treatment cycles of two injections at approximately 6-week intervals. Discontinue treatment if curvature deformity is less than 15 degrees after any cycle.

SAFETY ALERT!

copanlisib dihydrochloride
ko-PAN-li-sib

Aliqopa

Therapeutic class: Antineoplastics
Pharmacologic class: Kinase inhibitors

AVAILABLE FORMS
Injection (lyophilized, preservative-free): 60 mg single-dose vials

INDICATIONS & DOSAGES
➤ **Treatment of relapsed follicular lymphoma in patients who have received at least two prior systemic therapies**
Adults: 60 mg IV infusion over 1 hour on days 1, 8, and 15 of a 28-day treatment cycle on an intermittent schedule (3 weeks on and 1 week off). Continue until disease progression or unacceptable toxicity occurs.
Adjust-a-dose: If concomitant use of a strong CYP3A inhibitor is unavoidable, reduce copanlisib dosage to 45 mg. Refer to manufacturer's instructions for toxicity-related dosage adjustments and drug discontinuation.

crotamiton
kroe-TAM-ih-tuhn

Crotan, Eurax

Therapeutic class: Scabicides–pediculicides
Pharmacologic class: Scabicides

AVAILABLE FORMS
Cream: 10%
Lotion: 10%

INDICATIONS & DOSAGES
➤ **Parasitic infestation (scabies)**
Adults: Scrub entire body with soap and water. Remove scales or crusts. Then apply thin layer of cream over entire body, from chin down (with special attention to skinfolds, creases, interdigital spaces, and genital area). Apply second coat in 24 hours. Change clothing and bed linen the next morning. Wait another

48 hours after last application; then wash off. If retreatment is needed, use an alternative regimen.

➤ **Itching**
Adults: Apply locally, massaging gently into affected area until completely absorbed; repeat p.r.n.

dalfampridine
dal-FAM-prih-deen

Ampyra

Therapeutic class: MS drugs
Pharmacologic class: Potassium channel blockers

AVAILABLE FORMS
Tablets (extended-release) ⓞⓡⓒ: 10 mg

INDICATIONS & DOSAGES
➤ **To improve walking in patients with MS**
Adults: 10 mg PO every 12 hours (maximum, 20 mg daily).

dantrolene sodium
DAN-troe-leen

Dantrium, Dantrium IV, Revonto, Ryanodex

Therapeutic class: Skeletal muscle relaxants
Pharmacologic class: Hydantoin derivatives

AVAILABLE FORMS
Capsules: 25 mg, 50 mg, 100 mg
Injection: 20 mg/vial, 250 mg/vial

INDICATIONS & DOSAGES
Black Box Warning *Opioid class warning:* Opioids combined with benzodiazepines or CNS depressants can cause death. Drug can cause hepatotoxicity; only use for indicated conditions and at recommended dosages. ∎

➤ **Spasticity and sequelae from severe chronic disorders, such as MS, cerebral palsy, spinal cord injury, and stroke**
Adults: Initially, 25 mg PO daily; then 25 mg t.i.d., 50 mg t.i.d., and finally, 100 mg t.i.d. Maintain each dosage level for 7 days to determine response. May increase t.i.d. to q.i.d. if necessary. Maximum, 400 mg daily.
Children age 5 and older: Initially, 0.5 mg/kg PO daily; then 0.5 mg/kg t.i.d., 1 mg/kg t.i.d., and finally, 2 mg/kg t.i.d. Maintain each dosage level for 7 days to determine response. May increase t.i.d. to q.i.d. if necessary. Maximum, 100 mg q.i.d.
Adjust-a-dose: If no further benefit is observed at the next higher dose, decrease dosage to the previous lower dose. Stop drug if benefits aren't evident within 45 days.

➤ **To manage malignant hyperthermic crisis**
Adults and children: Initially, 1 mg/kg IV push. Repeat, as needed, up to cumulative dose of 10 mg/kg.

➤ **To prevent or attenuate malignant hyperthermic crisis in susceptible patients who need surgery**
Adults and children age 5 and older: 4 to 8 mg/kg PO daily in three or four divided doses for 1 or 2 days

before procedure. Give final dose 3 or 4 hours before procedure. Or, 2.5 mg/kg IV about 1.25 hours before anesthesia; infuse Dantrium or Revonto over 1 hour or Ryanodex over at least 1 minute.

➤ **To prevent recurrence of malignant hyperthermic crisis**
Adults and children age 5 and older: 4 to 8 mg/kg PO daily in four divided doses for up to 3 days after hyperthermic crisis.

darunavir ethanolate ☒
duh-ROO-nah-veer

Prezista

Therapeutic class: Antiretrovirals
Pharmacologic class: Protease inhibitors

AVAILABLE FORMS
Oral suspension: 100 mg/mL
Tablets ⓞⓡⓒ: 75 mg, 150 mg, 600 mg, 800 mg

INDICATIONS & DOSAGES
➤ **HIV infection, with ritonavir and other antiretrovirals** ☒
Adults who are treatment-experienced with at least one darunavir resistance–associated substitution or when genotypic testing isn't feasible (testing is recommended): 600 mg PO b.i.d., given with 100 mg ritonavir PO b.i.d.
Adults who are treatment-naive or treatment-experienced with no darunavir resistance–associated substitutions: 800 mg PO once daily, given with ritonavir 100 mg PO once daily.
Pregnant patients: 600 mg PO b.i.d., given with ritonavir 100 mg or cobicistat 150 mg PO b.i.d. May consider 800 mg PO once daily, given with ritonavir 100 mg PO once daily only in certain pregnant patients who are already on a stable 800-mg dose with ritonavir 100 mg once-daily regimen before pregnancy, are virologically suppressed (HIV-1 RNA less than 50 copies/mL), and in whom a change to twice-daily darunavir 600 mg with ritonavir 100 mg may compromise tolerability or compliance.
Children ages 3 to younger than 18 who are treatment-naive or treatment-experienced with no darunavir resistance–associated substitutions: Don't exceed recommended dosage for treatment-experienced adults. For those weighing 40 kg or more, 800 mg PO once daily with ritonavir 100 mg once daily; for those weighing 30 to less than 40 kg, 675 mg (may round dose to 680 mg for oral suspension) PO once daily with ritonavir 100 mg once daily; for those weighing 15 to less than 30 kg, 600 mg PO once daily with ritonavir 100 mg once daily; for those weighing 14 to less than 15 kg, 490 mg (may round dose to 500 mg for oral suspension) PO once daily with ritonavir 96 mg once daily; for those weighing 13 to less than 14 kg, 455 mg (may round dose to 460 mg for oral suspension) PO once daily with ritonavir 80 mg once daily; for those weighing 12 to less than 13 kg, 420 mg PO once daily with ritonavir 80 mg once daily; for those weighing 11 to less than 12 kg, 385 mg (may round dose to 400 mg for oral suspension) PO once

daily with ritonavir 64 mg once daily; for those weighing 10 to less than 11 kg, 350 mg (may round dose to 360 mg for oral suspension) PO once daily with ritonavir 64 mg once daily.

Children ages 3 to younger than 18 who are treatment-experienced with at least one darunavir resistance–associated substitution: Don't exceed recommended dosage for treatment-experienced adults. For those weighing 40 kg or more, 600 mg PO b.i.d. with ritonavir 100 mg b.i.d.; for those weighing 30 to less than 40 kg, 450 mg (may round dose to 460 mg for oral suspension) PO b.i.d. with ritonavir 60 mg b.i.d.; for those weighing 15 to less than 30 kg, 375 mg (may round dose to 380 mg for oral suspension) PO b.i.d. with ritonavir 48 mg b.i.d.; for those weighing 14 to less than 15 kg, 280 mg PO b.i.d. with ritonavir 48 mg b.i.d. and food; for those weighing 13 to less than 14 kg, 260 mg PO b.i.d. with ritonavir 40 mg b.i.d.; for those weighing 12 to less than 13 kg, 240 mg PO b.i.d. with ritonavir 40 mg b.i.d.; for those weighing 11 to less than 12 kg, 220 mg PO b.i.d. with ritonavir 32 mg b.i.d.; for those weighing 10 to less than 11 kg, 200 mg PO b.i.d. with ritonavir 32 mg b.i.d.

SAFETY ALERT!

dasatinib ▨
duh-SAH-tin-nib

Sprycel

Therapeutic class: Antineoplastics
Pharmacologic class: Protein–tyrosine kinase inhibitors

AVAILABLE FORMS
Tablets ⓘ: 20 mg, 50 mg, 70 mg, 80 mg, 100 mg, 140 mg

INDICATIONS & DOSAGES
Adjust-a-dose (for all indications): If patient has hematologic toxicity, such as neutropenia or thrombocytopenia, consider reducing dose or interrupting or stopping therapy. If patient has severe, nonhematologic toxicity, withhold dose until condition resolves; then resume at previous or reduced dose as appropriate. Refer to manufacturer's instructions for toxicity-related dosage adjustments. Continue until disease progresses or intolerable adverse effects occur.
➤ **Chronic, accelerated, or myeloid or lymphoid blast phase Philadelphia chromosome–positive (Ph+) chronic myeloid leukemia (CML) with resistance or intolerance to earlier treatment, including imatinib; Ph+ acute lymphoblastic leukemia with resistance or intolerance to prior therapy** ▨
Adults: 140 mg PO once daily. If patient tolerates this dose but fails to respond to treatment, increase to 180 mg PO once daily.
➤ **Newly diagnosed Ph+ chronic-phase CML; children with Ph+ CML in chronic phase** ▨
Adults: 100 mg PO daily. May increase to 140 mg daily.
Children weighing 45 kg or more: 100 mg PO once daily. May increase to 120 mg daily.
Children weighing 30 to less than 45 kg: 70 mg PO once daily. May increase to 90 mg daily.

Children weighing 20 to less than 30 kg: 60 mg PO once daily. May increase to 70 mg daily.
Children weighing 10 to less than 20 kg: 40 mg PO once daily. May increase to 50 mg daily.
Adjust-a-dose: Recalculate pediatric dose every 3 months, or more often if necessary, based on changes in body weight.

SAFETY ALERT!

DAUNOrubicin hydrochloride
daw-nah-ROO-buh-sin

Therapeutic class: Antineoplastics
Pharmacologic class: Anthracycline glycoside antibiotics

AVAILABLE FORMS
Injection: 5 mg/mL

INDICATIONS & DOSAGES
Black Box Warning Inject into a rapidly flowing IV infusion; never give by IM or subcut route as severe local tissue necrosis may result. Drug may cause severe myelosuppression or myocardial toxicity in the form of potentially fatal HF, during therapy or months to years afterward. Reduce dosage for renal or hepatic impairment. ∎
Adjust-a-dose (for all indications): For patients with impaired hepatic and renal function, reduce dosage as follows: If bilirubin level is 1.2 to 3 mg/dL, give three-fourths normal dose; if bilirubin or creatinine level exceeds 3 mg/dL, give half normal dose. Dosages vary. Check treatment protocol with prescriber.
➤ **To induce remission in acute nonlymphocytic (myelogenous, monocytic, erythroid) leukemia**
Adults age 60 and older: In combination, 30 mg/m^2/day IV on days 1, 2, and 3 of first course and on days 1 and 2 of subsequent courses with cytarabine infusions. Maximum lifetime cumulative dose is 550 mg/m^2; in patients who received mediastinal radiation, maximum lifetime cumulative dose is 400 mg/m^2.
Adults younger than age 60: In combination, 45 mg/m^2/day IV on days 1, 2, and 3 of first course and on days 1 and 2 of subsequent courses with cytarabine infusions. Maximum lifetime cumulative dose is 550 mg/m^2; in patients who received mediastinal radiation, maximum lifetime cumulative dose is 400 mg/m^2.
➤ **To induce remission in acute lymphocytic leukemia (with combination therapy)**
Adults: 45 mg/m^2/day IV on days 1, 2, and 3 of first course. Maximum lifetime cumulative dose is 550 mg/m^2; in patients who received mediastinal radiation, maximum lifetime cumulative dose is 400 mg/m^2.
Children age 2 and older: 25 mg/m^2 IV on day 1 every week for up to 6 weeks, if needed. Maximum lifetime cumulative dose is 300 mg/m^2.
Children younger than age 2 or with BSA less than 0.5 m^2: 1 mg/kg/dose for 1 to 3 days (dose based on body weight, not BSA). Administration frequency is specific to each combination chemotherapy regimen. Maximum lifetime cumulative dose is 10 mg/kg.

✦Canada ◇OTC ◆Off-label use ✐Photoguide ⓘⓘⓒDo not crush *Liquid contains alcohol ▨Genetic

daunorubicin liposome–cytarabine liposome
daw-nah-ROO-buh-sin/sye-TARE-a-been

Vyxeos

Therapeutic class: Antineoplastics
Pharmacologic class: Anthracycline topoisomerase inhibitors–nucleoside metabolic inhibitors

AVAILABLE FORMS
Injection (liposomes as a lyophilized cake): 44 mg daunorubicin/100 mg cytarabine in single-dose vials

INDICATIONS & DOSAGES
Black Box Warning Verify drug name and dosage before preparation and administration to avoid dosing errors. ■

➤ **Newly diagnosed, therapy-related acute myeloid leukemia (t-AML) or AML with myelodysplasia-related changes (AML-MRC)**
Adults: A full course of therapy consists of one to two induction cycles followed by up to two consolidation cycles.

For initial induction cycle, 44 mg/m^2 daunorubicin/100 mg/m^2 cytarabine IV infusion on days 1, 3, and 5. For patients who fail to achieve a response with first induction cycle, give a second induction cycle of 44 mg/m^2 daunorubicin/100 mg/m^2 cytarabine IV infusion on days 1 and 3. May give second induction cycle 2 to 5 weeks after first induction cycle if no unacceptable toxicity occurred with previous cycle.

Give first consolidation cycle 5 to 8 weeks after start of the last induction. Recommended dose for each consolidation cycle is 29 mg/m^2 daunorubicin/65 mg/m^2 cytarabine IV infusion on days 1 and 3. Give second consolidation cycle 5 to 8 weeks after start of first consolidation cycle in patients without disease progression or unacceptable toxicity.

Adjust-a-dose: Refer to manufacturer's instructions for toxicity-related dosage adjustments.

defibrotide sodium
dee-FIB-roe-tide

Defitelio

Therapeutic class: Thrombolytics
Pharmacologic class: Thrombolytics

AVAILABLE FORMS
Injection: 200 mg/2.5 mL (80 mg/mL)

INDICATIONS & DOSAGES
➤ **Hepatic veno-occlusive disease (VOD), also known as sinusoidal obstruction syndrome, with renal or pulmonary dysfunction after hematopoietic stem-cell transplantation**
Adults and children: 6.25 mg/kg IV given as a 2-hour infusion every 6 hours. Administer for a minimum of 21 days; if after 21 days signs and symptoms of hepatic VOD haven't resolved, continue until resolution of VOD or to a maximum of 60 days.

Adjust-a-dose: Refer to manufacturer's instructions for toxicity-related dosage interruption and discontinuation.

deflazacort
de-FLAZE-a-kort

Emflaza

Therapeutic class: Muscular dystrophy drugs
Pharmacologic class: Corticosteroids

AVAILABLE FORMS
Oral suspension*: 22.75 mg/mL
Tablets: 6 mg, 18 mg, 30 mg, 36 mg

INDICATIONS & DOSAGES
➤ **Duchenne muscular dystrophy**
Adults and children age 5 and older: 0.9 mg/kg PO once daily.

Adjust-a-dose: Decrease dosage to one-third of recommended dosage when used with moderate or strong CYP3A4 inhibitors (clarithromycin, diltiazem, fluconazole, verapamil).

deoxycholic acid
dee-OX-i-koe-lik

Kybella

Therapeutic class: Lipolytic agents
Pharmacologic class: Lipolytics

AVAILABLE FORMS
Injection: 10 mg/mL in 2-mL single-use vials*

INDICATIONS & DOSAGES
➤ **Improvement in appearance of moderate to severe convexity or fullness associated with submental fat**
Adults: Inject subcut into the submental region using an area-adjusted dose of 2 mg/cm^2. A single treatment consists of a maximum of 50 injections (up to a total of 10 mL), 0.2 mL each, spaced 1 cm apart. A maximum of six single treatments may be administered at intervals no less than 1 month apart. Tailor the number of injections and the number of treatments to patient's submental fat distribution and treatment goals.

deutetrabenazine
doo-tet-ra-BEN-a-zeen

Austedo

Therapeutic class: Antichorea drugs
Pharmacologic class: Vesicular monoamine transporter 2 inhibitors

AVAILABLE FORMS
Tablets: 6 mg, 9 mg, 12 mg

INDICATIONS & DOSAGES
➤ **Chorea associated with Huntington disease or tardive dyskinesia**
Adults: Initially, 6 mg PO (Huntington disease) once daily or 6 mg PO b.i.d. (tardive dyskinesia). Titrate up at weekly intervals by 6 mg/day to a tolerated dose that reduces chorea, up to a maximum of 48 mg/day.

If total daily dose is 12 mg or more, give in two divided doses. Can discontinue drug without tapering. To resume after treatment interruption of more than 1 week, retitrate dosage. To resume after treatment interruption of less than 1 week, resume at previous dosage without titration.

Adjust-a-dose: In patients currently receiving strong CYP2D6 inhibitors or for those who are known poor CYP2D6 metabolizers, don't exceed 36 mg/day (or 18 mg as a single dose). If switching from tetrabenazine to deutetrabenazine, stop tetrabenazine and initiate deutetrabenazine the next day. Refer to manufacturer's prescribing information for deutetrabenazine dosage based on last tetrabenazine dose.

SAFETY ALERT!

dexmedetomidine hydrochloride
deks-MED-e-toe-mi-deen

Precedex

Therapeutic class: Sedatives
Pharmacologic class: Alpha$_2$-adrenergic agonists

AVAILABLE FORMS
Injection (concentrate): 200 mcg/2 mL (100 mcg/mL) in single-use vials
Injection (ready-to-use): 80 mcg/20 mL (4 mcg/mL single-use vials); 200 mcg/50 mL (4 mcg/mL single-use bottles); 400 mcg/100 mL (4 mcg/mL single-use bottles)

INDICATIONS & DOSAGES
Adjust-a-dose (for all indications): In patients with impaired hepatic function (Child-Pugh class A, B, or C) and in those older than age 65, consider reducing dosage.
➤ **ICU sedation**
Adults: Loading infusion of 1 mcg/kg IV over 10 minutes, then maintenance infusion of 0.2 to 0.7 mcg/kg/hour adjusted to achieve desired level of sedation.
Adjust-a-dose: For conversion from alternative sedative therapy, a loading infusion may not be needed.
➤ **Procedural sedation**
Adults: Loading infusion of 1 mcg/kg IV over 10 minutes. Then give maintenance infusion, generally initiated at 0.6 mcg/kg/hour and adjusted to achieve desired clinical effect; dosages range from 0.2 to 1 mcg/kg/hour.
Adjust-a-dose: For less invasive procedures such as ophthalmic surgery, a loading infusion of 0.5 mcg/kg IV given over 10 minutes may be suitable. In patients older than age 65, give a loading infusion of 0.5 mcg/kg IV over 10 minutes.
➤ **Awake fiber optic intubation**
Adults: Initial loading infusion of 1 mcg/kg IV over 10 minutes, then maintenance infusion of 0.7 mcg/kg/hour until endotracheal tube is secured.

dimenhyDRINATE
dye-men-HYE-dri-nate

Dramamine◇, Driminate◇, Gravol✢◇, Travel Tabs✢◇

Therapeutic class: Antivertigo drugs
Pharmacologic class: Anticholinergics

AVAILABLE FORMS
Capsules: 50 mg ◇ ✢
Injection: 50 mg/mL
Oral solution: 15 mg/5 mL ◇ ✢
Suppositories: 25 mg ◇ ✢, 100 mg ◇ ✢
Tablets: 15 mg ◇ ✢, 50 mg ◇
Tablets (chewable): 15 mg ◇ ✢, 50 mg ◇

INDICATIONS & DOSAGES
➤ **To prevent and treat motion sickness**
Adults and children age 12 and older: 50 to 100 mg PO every 4 to 6 hours; 50 mg IM, as needed; or 50 mg IV diluted in 10 mL NSS for injection, injected over 2 minutes. Maximum, 400 mg daily. For prevention, use drug at least 30 minutes before motion exposure.
Children ages 6 to 11: 25 to 50 mg PO every 6 to 8 hours, not to exceed 150 mg in 24 hours. Or, 1.25 mg/kg or 37.5 mg/m^2 IM q.i.d.
Children ages 2 to 5: 12.5 to 25 mg PO every 6 to 8 hours, not to exceed 75 mg in 24 hours. Or, 1.25 mg/kg or 37.5 mg/m^2 IM q.i.d. Maximum, 300 mg daily.

dimethyl fumarate
dye-METH-il

Tecfidera

Therapeutic class: Immunomodulators
Pharmacologic class: Nuclear factor–like 2 pathway activators

AVAILABLE FORMS
Capsules (delayed-release): 120 mg, 240 mg

INDICATIONS & DOSAGES
➤ **Relapsing MS**
Adults: Initially, 120 mg PO b.i.d. for 7 days; then increase to maintenance dosage of 240 mg b.i.d.
Adjust-a-dose: Consider temporary dosage reduction to 120 mg b.i.d. for patient who can't tolerate maintenance dose. Resume recommended dose of 240 mg b.i.d. within 4 weeks; then consider discontinuing drug if patient is unable to tolerate return to maintenance dose.

Consider interrupting or discontinuing therapy in patients with lymphocyte count of less than 500/mm^3 persisting for more than 6 months. Consider withholding drug in patients with serious infections until resolution. Individualize decisions about restarting therapy based on clinical circumstances.

dinoprostone
dye-noe-PROST-ohn

Cervidil, Prepidil, Prostin E2

Therapeutic class: Oxytocics
Pharmacologic class: Prostaglandins

AVAILABLE FORMS
Endocervical gel: 0.5 mg/application (2.5-mL syringe)
Vaginal insert: 10 mg
Vaginal suppositories: 20 mg

INDICATIONS & DOSAGES
Black Box Warning Strictly adhere to recommended dosages. ∎

➤ **To terminate second-trimester pregnancy; to evacuate uterine contents in missed abortion, intrauterine fetal death up to 28 weeks' gestation, or benign hydatidiform mole (vaginal suppository only)**
Women: Insert 20-mg suppository high into posterior vaginal fornix; repeat every 3 to 5 hours until abortion is complete, for a maximum of 2 days.
➤ **To ripen an unfavorable cervix in pregnant woman at or near term (endocervical gel and vaginal insert only)**
Women: Apply 0.5 mg endocervical gel intravaginally; if cervix remains unfavorable after 6 hours, repeat dose. Don't exceed 1.5 mg (three applications) within 24 hours. After obtaining desired response, wait 6 to 12 hours before giving IV oxytocin. Or, place 10-mg vaginal insert transversely in posterior vaginal fornix immediately after removing insert from foil. Take insert out when active labor begins or after 12 hours have passed, whichever occurs first. After insert removal, wait at least 30 minutes before giving oxytocin.

SAFETY ALERT!

dinutuximab
DIN-ue-TUX-i-mab

Unituxin

Therapeutic class: Antineoplastics
Pharmacologic class: GD2-binding monoclonal antibodies

AVAILABLE FORMS
Injection: 17.5 mg/5 mL (3.5 mg/mL) in single-use vials

INDICATIONS & DOSAGES
Black Box Warning Life-threatening infusion reactions can occur. Give required prehydration and premedication before each infusion and monitor patient for infusion reaction during and for at least 4 hours after infusion. Interrupt drug for infusion reaction and permanently discontinue for anaphylaxis. Drug causes severe neuropathic pain and requires IV opioids before, during, and after infusion. Discontinue drug for severe unresponsive pain and severe sensory or motor neuropathy. ∎

➤ **High-risk neuroblastoma, in combination with granulocyte-macrophage colony-stimulating factor, interleukin-2, and 13-*cis*-retinoic acid, in**

patients who achieved at least a partial response to prior first-line multiagent, multimodality therapy
Children: 17.5 mg/m^2/day IV over 10 to 20 hours for 4 consecutive days for up to five cycles. Cycles 1, 3, and 5 are 24 days in duration, and drug is administered on days 4, 5, 6, and 7. Cycles 2 and 4 are 32 days in duration, and drug is administered on days 8, 9, 10, and 11.
Adjust-a-dose: Refer to manufacturer's instructions for toxicity-related dosage adjustments and drug discontinuation.

disulfiram
dye-SUL-fi-ram

Antabuse

Therapeutic class: Alcohol deterrents
Pharmacologic class: Aldehyde dehydrogenase inhibitors

AVAILABLE FORMS
Tablets: 250 mg, 500 mg

INDICATIONS & DOSAGES
Black Box Warning Never give drug to an intoxicated patient or without patient's full knowledge. ∎
➤ **Adjunct to management of alcohol abstinence**
Adults: 250 to 500 mg PO as single dose in morning for 1 to 2 weeks (or in evening if drowsiness occurs) after patient has abstained from alcohol for at least 12 hours. Maintenance dosage is 125 to 500 mg PO daily (average 250 mg) until permanent self-control is established. Treatment may continue for months or years.

dolutegravir sodium
doe-loo-TEG-ra-vir

Tivicay

Therapeutic class: Antiretrovirals
Pharmacologic class: Integrase strand transfer inhibitors

AVAILABLE FORMS
Tablets: 10 mg, 25 mg, 50 mg

INDICATIONS & DOSAGES
🚫 *Alert:* Embryo-fetal toxicity may occur when drug is used at the time of conception and in early pregnancy. Perform pregnancy testing before starting drug in adolescents and adults of childbearing potential.
➤ **HIV-1 infection in treatment-naive or treatment-experienced integrase strand transfer inhibitor (INSTI)-naive patients, in combination with other antiretrovirals**
Adults and children weighing 40 kg or more: 50 mg PO once daily.
Children weighing 30 to less than 40 kg: 35 mg PO once daily.
Adjust-a-dose: If administered with the potent UGT1A/CYP3A inducers carbamazepine, efavirenz, fosamprenavir/ritonavir, tipranavir/ritonavir, or rifampin, for adults give dolutegravir 50 mg b.i.d. For children, increase the weight-based dose of dolutegravir to b.i.d.

➤ HIV-1 infection in patients who are INSTI-experienced with certain INSTI-associated resistance substitutions or clinically suspected INSTI resistance, or in patients who are treatment-naive or treatment-experienced INSTI-naive when administered with certain UGT1A or CYP3A inducers
Adults: 50 mg PO b.i.d.

➤ HIV-1 infection with rilpivirine as a complete regimen to replace the current antiretroviral regimen in patients who are virologically suppressed (HIV-1 RNA less than 50 copies/mL) on a stable antiretroviral regimen for at least 6 months with no history of treatment failure or known substitutions associated with resistance to either antiretroviral
Adults: 50 mg PO once daily with rilpivirine PO once daily.

dupilumab
doo-PIL-ue-mab

Dupixent

Therapeutic class: Immunomodulators
Pharmacologic class: Monoclonal antibodies

AVAILABLE FORMS
Injection: 300 mg/2 mL in single-dose prefilled syringes

INDICATIONS & DOSAGES
➤ Moderate to severe atopic dermatitis not adequately controlled with topical therapy or when other therapies aren't advisable
Adults: Initially, 600 mg subcut given as two 300-mg injections in different sites followed by 300 mg subcut every other week.
Adolescents older than age 12 but younger than age 17 and weighing less than 60 kg: Initially, 400 mg subcut given as two 200-mg injections in different sites followed by 200 mg subcut every other week.

ecallantide ⚥
ee-KAL-lan-tide

Kalbitor

Therapeutic class: Protein inhibitors
Pharmacologic class: Human plasma kallikrein inhibitors

AVAILABLE FORMS
Injection: 10 mg/mL vials

INDICATIONS & DOSAGES
Black Box Warning Anaphylaxis has been reported after administration. ∎
➤ Acute attacks of hereditary angioedema ⚥
Adults and adolescents age 12 and older: 30 mg subcut given as three 10-mg injections; give additional 30-mg dose within 24 hours if attack persists.

econazole nitrate
ee-KOE-na-zole

Ecoza

Therapeutic class: Antifungals
Pharmacologic class: Imidazole derivatives

AVAILABLE FORMS
Cream: 1%
Foam: 1%

INDICATIONS & DOSAGES
➤ Tinea corporis, tinea cruris, tinea pedis, tinea versicolor
Adults and children: Rub cream into affected areas daily for at least 2 weeks (1 month for tinea pedis).
Adults and children age 12 and older (tinea pedis only): Apply foam to affected areas daily for 4 weeks.
➤ Cutaneous candidiasis
Adults and children: Rub cream into affected areas b.i.d. (morning and evening) for 2 weeks.

SAFETY ALERT!

eculizumab
eck-u-LIZ-uh-mob

Soliris

Therapeutic class: Hemolysis inhibitors
Pharmacologic class: Monoclonal IgG antibodies

AVAILABLE FORMS
Injection: 10 mg/mL in 300-mg single-use vials

INDICATIONS & DOSAGES
Black Box Warning Life-threatening and fatal meningococcal infections have occurred. Meningococcal vaccine is required at least 2 weeks before administration of eculizumab. Access is restricted through a REMS program and prescribers must be enrolled. ∎
➤ Hemolysis in patients with paroxysmal nocturnal hemoglobinuria
Adults: 600 mg IV every 7 days for 4 weeks, 900 mg 7 days later, then 900 mg every 14 days thereafter.
➤ Atypical hemolytic-uremic syndrome
Adults and children weighing 40 kg or more: 900 mg IV weekly for 4 weeks, then 1,200 mg at week 5, then 1,200 mg every 2 weeks.
Children weighing 30 to 39 kg: 600 mg IV weekly for 2 weeks, then 900 mg at week 3, then 900 mg every 2 weeks.
Children weighing 20 to 29 kg: 600 mg IV weekly for 2 weeks, then 600 mg at week 3, then 600 mg every 2 weeks.
Children weighing 10 to 19 kg: 600 mg IV weekly for one dose, then 300 mg at week 2, then 300 mg every 2 weeks.
Children weighing 5 to 9 kg: 300 mg IV weekly for one dose, then 300 mg at week 2, then 300 mg every 3 weeks.
Adjust-a-dose: Supplemental dosing is required in the setting of concomitant plasmapheresis or plasma exchange, or fresh frozen plasma infusion.

✦Canada   ◇OTC   ◆Off-label use   ✐Photoguide   ⊕Do not crush   *Liquid contains alcohol   ⚥Genetic

➤ **Generalized myasthenia gravis in patients who are anti-acetylcholine receptor (AchR) antibody positive**

Adults: 900 mg IV weekly for 4 weeks; then 1,200 mg at week 5; then 1,200 mg every 2 weeks.

Adjust-a-dose: Supplemental dosing is required in the setting of concomitant plasmapheresis or plasma exchange, or fresh frozen plasma infusion.

edaravone
ed-a-RAV-one

Radicava

Therapeutic class: Miscellaneous CNS drugs
Pharmacologic class: Free radical scavengers

AVAILABLE FORMS
Injection: 30 mg/100 mL premixed bags

INDICATIONS & DOSAGES
➤ **Amyotrophic lateral sclerosis**
Adults: For initial treatment cycle, give 60 mg IV infusion daily for 14 days, followed by a 14-day drug-free period. For all subsequent treatment cycles, give 60 mg IV infusion daily for 10 out of 14 days, followed by a 14-day drug-free period.

efinaconazole
EF-in-a-KON-a-zole

Jublia

Therapeutic class: Antifungals
Pharmacologic class: Azole antifungals

AVAILABLE FORMS
Topical solution: 10%

INDICATIONS & DOSAGES
➤ **Toenail onychomycosis due to *Trichophyton rubrum* or *Trichophyton mentagrophytes***
Adults: Apply solution to affected toenails using the brush applicator once daily for 48 weeks.

emicizumab-kxwh
EM-i-SIZ-ue-mab

Hemlibra

Therapeutic class: Antibodies
Pharmacologic class: Monoclonal IgG4 antibodies

AVAILABLE FORMS
Injection: 30 mg/mL, 60 mg/0.4 mL, 105 mg/0.7 mL, 150 mg/mL single-dose vials

INDICATIONS & DOSAGES
➤ **Routine prophylaxis to prevent or reduce frequency of bleeding episodes in patients with hemophilia A (congenital factor VIII deficiency) with or without factor VIII inhibitors**
Adults and children: 3 mg/kg subcut once weekly for 4 weeks; then 1.5 mg/kg once weekly or 3 mg/kg subcut once every 2 weeks or 6 mg subcut once every 4 weeks.

SAFETY ALERT!

enasidenib ☒
en-a-SID-e-nib

Idhifa

Therapeutic class: Antineoplastics
Pharmacologic class: Isocitrate dehydrogenase-2 inhibitors

AVAILABLE FORMS
Tablets: 50 mg, 100 mg

INDICATIONS & DOSAGES
Black Box Warning Patients treated with enasidenib have experienced signs and symptoms of differentiation syndrome, which can be fatal if not treated. ∎
➤ **Relapsed or refractory acute myeloid leukemia in patients with an isocitrate dehydrogenase-2 mutation as detected by an FDA-approved test** ☒
Adults: 100 mg PO once daily until disease progression or unacceptable toxicity. For patients without disease progression or unacceptable toxicity, treat for at least 6 months to allow time for clinical response.
Adjust-a-dose: Refer to manufacturer's instructions for toxicity-related dosage adjustments.

entacapone
en-tah-KAP-own

Comtan

Therapeutic class: Antiparkinsonians
Pharmacologic class: Catechol-O-methyltransferase inhibitors

AVAILABLE FORMS
Tablets ⓒ: 200 mg

INDICATIONS & DOSAGES
➤ **Adjunct to levodopa–carbidopa for treatment of idiopathic Parkinson disease in patients with signs and symptoms of end-of-dose wearing-off**
Adults: 200 mg PO with each dose of levodopa–carbidopa, up to eight times daily. Maximum, 1,600 mg daily. May need to reduce daily levodopa dose or extend the interval between levodopa doses to optimize patient's response.

SAFETY ALERT!

enzalutamide
EN-za-LOO-ta-mide

Xtandi

Therapeutic class: Antineoplastics
Pharmacologic class: Androgen receptor inhibitors

AVAILABLE FORMS
Capsules ⓒ: 40 mg

INDICATIONS & DOSAGES
➤ **Castration-resistant prostate cancer**
Adults: 160 mg PO once daily after a bilateral orchiectomy or with a gonadotropin-releasing hormone analogue.

♣Canada   ◇ OTC   ◆ Off-label use   ✐Photoguide   ⓒDo not crush   *Liquid contains alcohol   ☒Genetic

Adjust-a-dose: For grade 3 or 4 toxicity or an intolerable adverse effect, withhold drug for 1 week or until symptoms improve to grade 2 or less. Resume at same or reduced dosage as appropriate. If use with strong CYP3A4 inducers is unavoidable, increase dose to 240 mg once daily. If use with strong CYP2C8 inhibitors is unavoidable, reduce dosage to 80 mg once daily.

eprosartan mesylate
ep-row-SAR-tan

Therapeutic class: Antihypertensives
Pharmacologic class: Angiotensin II receptor antagonists

AVAILABLE FORMS
Tablets: 400 mg, 600 mg

INDICATIONS & DOSAGES
Black Box Warning Can cause fetal harm; don't use during pregnancy. ∎
➤ **HTN (alone or with other antihypertensives)**
Adults: Initially, 600 mg PO daily. Dosage ranges from 400 to 800 mg daily, given as single daily dose or two divided doses. Maximum dose is 800 mg/day (600 mg in patients with moderate or severe renal impairment).

etelcalcetide
e-tel-KAL-se-tide

Parsabiv

Therapeutic class: Hyperparathyroidism drugs
Pharmacologic class: Calcimimetics

AVAILABLE FORMS
Injection: 2.5 mg/0.5 mL, 5 mg/mL, 10 mg/2 mL in single-dose vials

INDICATIONS & DOSAGES
➤ **Secondary hyperparathyroidism in patients with chronic kidney disease on hemodialysis**
Adults: Initially, 5 mg IV bolus injection three times per week at end of hemodialysis treatment; maintenance dosage is individualized and determined by titration based on parathyroid hormone (PTH) level and corrected serum calcium response. Dosage range is 2.5 to 15 mg three times weekly. Increase dosage in 2.5- or 5-mg increments based on PTH level in patients with corrected serum calcium level within the normal range and PTH level above recommended target range. Increase dosage no more frequently than every 4 weeks.
Adjust-a-dose: If PTH level is below target range, decrease dosage or temporarily discontinue drug. In patients with corrected serum calcium level below lower limit of normal (LLN), but at or above 7.5 mg/dL without symptoms of hypocalcemia, consider decreasing dosage or temporarily discontinuing drug or use concomitant therapies to increase corrected serum calcium level.

If drug is stopped, reinitiate at a lower dose when PTH level is within target range and hypocalcemia has been corrected. If corrected serum calcium level

falls below LLN or signs or symptoms of hypocalcemia develop, start or increase calcium supplementation (calcium, calcium-containing phosphate binders, or vitamin D sterols or increases in dialysate calcium concentration). Etelcalcetide dosage reduction or discontinuation may be necessary.

If corrected serum calcium level falls below 7.5 mg/dL or patient reports signs and symptoms of hypocalcemia, stop drug and treat hypocalcemia; when corrected serum calcium level is within normal limits, signs and symptoms of hypocalcemia have resolved, and predisposing factors for hypocalcemia have been addressed, reinitiate at a dose 5 mg lower than last administered dose. If last administered dose was 2.5 or 5 mg, reinitiate at 2.5-mg dose.

etodolac
ee-toe-DOE-lak

Therapeutic class: NSAIDs
Pharmacologic class: NSAIDs

AVAILABLE FORMS
Capsules: 200 mg, 300 mg
Tablets: 400 mg, 500 mg
Tablets (extended-release): 400 mg, 500 mg, 600 mg

INDICATIONS & DOSAGES
➤ **Acute pain**
Adults: 200 to 400 mg (immediate-release) PO every 6 to 8 hours, not to exceed 1,000 mg daily.
➤ **Short- and long-term management of osteoarthritis and RA**
Adults: 600 to 1,000 mg (immediate-release) PO daily, divided into two or three doses. Maximum daily dose is 1,000 mg. For extended-release tablets, 400 to 1,000 mg PO daily.
➤ **Juvenile RA**
Children ages 6 to 16 weighing 20 to 30 kg: 400 mg (extended-release) PO once daily.
Children ages 6 to 16 weighing 31 to 45 kg: 600 mg (extended-release) PO once daily.
Children ages 6 to 16 weighing 46 to 60 kg: 800 mg (extended-release) PO once daily.
Children ages 6 to 16 weighing more than 60 kg) or more: 1,000 mg (extended-release) PO once daily.

evolocumab
E-voe-lok-ue-mab

Repatha

Therapeutic class: Antilipemics
Pharmacologic class: Proprotein convertase subtilisin kexin type 9 (PCSK9) antibody inhibitors

AVAILABLE FORMS
Injection: 140 mg/mL solution in single-dose prefilled syringe or autoinjector
Injection (Pushtronex system): 420 mg/3.5 mL

INDICATIONS & DOSAGES
➤ **Adjunct to diet and maximally tolerated statin therapy for treatment of heterozygous familial**

hypercholesterolemia or primary hyperlipidemia in patients with established clinical atherosclerotic CV disease who require additional lowering of LDL cholesterol (LDL-C)

Adults: 140 mg subcut every 2 weeks or 420 mg subcut once monthly. When switching dosage regimens, give first dose of new regimen on next scheduled date of prior regimen.

➤ **Adjunct to diet and other LDL-lowering therapies (statins, ezetimibe, LDL apheresis) for treatment of homozygous familial hypercholesterolemia in patients who require additional lowering of LDL-C**

Adults and adolescents age 13 and older: 420 mg subcut once monthly.

➤ **To reduce risk of MI, stroke, and coronary revascularization in patients with established CV disease**

Adults: 140 mg subcut every 2 weeks or 420 mg subcut once monthly. When switching dosage regimens, give first dose of new regimen on next scheduled date of prior regimen.

SAFETY ALERT!

exemestane
ecks-eh-MES-tayn

Aromasin

Therapeutic class: Antineoplastics
Pharmacologic class: Aromatase inhibitors

AVAILABLE FORMS
Tablets: 25 mg

INDICATIONS & DOSAGES
Adjust-a-dose (for all indications): In patients also taking strong CYP3A4 inducers (rifampin, phenytoin), increase daily dose to 50 mg.

➤ **Advanced breast cancer in postmenopausal women whose disease has progressed after treatment with tamoxifen**

Adults: 25 mg PO once daily after a meal.

➤ **Early-stage breast cancer in postmenopausal women who have taken tamoxifen for 2 to 3 years**

Adults: 25 mg PO once daily after a meal to complete a 5-year course, unless cancer recurs or is found in the other breast.

➤ **First-line adjuvant treatment of estrogen receptor–positive early breast cancer in postmenopausal women ♦**

Adults: 25 mg PO once daily after a meal.

➤ **To reduce risk of breast cancer ♦**

Postmenopausal women age 35 and older: 25 mg PO once daily after a meal for 5 years.

ferumoxytol
fer-yoo-MOX-i-tol

Feraheme

Therapeutic class: Iron supplements
Pharmacologic class: Iron salts

AVAILABLE FORMS
Injection: 510 mg elemental iron per 17 mL (30 mg/mL) single-dose vial

INDICATIONS & DOSAGES
➤ **Treatment of iron deficiency anemia (IDA) in patients intolerant of or who have had an unsatisfactory response to oral iron, or who have chronic kidney disease**

Adults: 510 mg IV infusion over at least 15 minutes. Repeat in 3 to 8 days. If IDA persists or recurs 1 month after the second infusion, may repeat the two-dose treatment course.

fish oil triglycerides emulsion
fish oyl try-GLYC-e-rides

Omegaven

Therapeutic class: Nutritional supplements
Pharmacologic class: Essential fatty acid supplements

AVAILABLE FORMS
Injection: 5 g/50 mL, 10 g/100 mL single-dose bottles

INDICATIONS & DOSAGES
➤ **Source of calories and fatty acids in patients with parenteral nutrition–associated cholestasis**

Children: Recommended and maximum dosage is 1 g/kg/day by IV infusion. Initial rate of infusion shouldn't exceed 0.05 mL/minute for first 15 to 30 minutes of infusion; if tolerated, gradually increase until reaching the required rate after 30 minutes. Maximum infusion rate shouldn't exceed 1.5 mL/kg/hour.

Adjust-a-dose: If triglyceride levels are greater than 250 mg/dL in neonates and infants or greater than 400 mg/dL in older children, consider stopping drug for 4 hours and obtain a repeat serum triglyceride level. Resume therapy based on new result as indicated. If triglyceride levels remain elevated, consider a reduced dose of 0.5 to 0.75 g/kg/day with an incremental increase to 1 g/kg/day.

flibanserin ▨
flib-AN-ser-in

Addyi

Therapeutic class: Miscellaneous sexual dysfunction aids
Pharmacologic class: Serotonin agonist/antagonist agents

AVAILABLE FORMS
Tablets: 100 mg

INDICATIONS & DOSAGES
➤ **Acquired, generalized hypoactive sexual desire disorder in premenopausal women, as characterized by low sexual desire that causes marked distress or interpersonal difficulty and isn't due to a coexisting medical or psychiatric condition, problems within the relationship, or effects of a drug or other substance**

Adults: 100 mg PO once daily at bedtime. If no improvement after 8 weeks, discontinue drug. Use cautiously in poor metabolizers of CYP2C19. ▨

fludrocortisone acetate
floo-droe-KOR-ti-sone

Florinef

Therapeutic class: Mineralocorticoids
Pharmacologic class: Mineralocorticoids

AVAILABLE FORMS
Tablets: 0.1 mg

INDICATIONS & DOSAGES
➤ **Salt-losing adrenogenital syndrome**
Adults: 0.1 to 0.2 mg PO daily.
➤ **Addison disease (adrenocortical insufficiency)**
Adults: 0.1 mg PO daily. Usual dosage range is 0.1 mg
three times weekly to 0.2 mg daily. Decrease dosage
to 0.05 mg daily if transient HTN develops.

fosamprenavir calcium
foss-am-PREN-ah-ver

Lexiva, Telzir

Therapeutic class: Antiretrovirals
Pharmacologic class: Protease inhibitors

AVAILABLE FORMS
Oral suspension: 50 mg/mL
Tablets: 700 mg

INDICATIONS & DOSAGES
*Adjust-a-dose (for all indications excluding
adults):* There are no dosing recommendations for
children with hepatic impairment. Dosage for children
shouldn't exceed recommended adult dosage of 700 mg
fosamprenavir with ritonavir 100 mg b.i.d. Drug isn't
approved for once-daily dosing in children.
➤ **HIV infection, with other antiretrovirals**
Adults: In patients not previously treated, 1,400 mg
PO b.i.d. (without ritonavir). Or, 1,400 mg PO once
daily with ritonavir 100 to 200 mg PO once daily. Or,
700 mg PO b.i.d. with ritonavir 100 mg PO b.i.d. In
patients previously treated with a protease inhibitor,
700 mg PO b.i.d. plus ritonavir 100 mg PO b.i.d.
Adjust-a-dose: If patient has mild hepatic impairment
(Child-Pugh score of 5 to 6), reduce dosage to 700 mg
PO b.i.d. without ritonavir (in therapy-naive patients)
or 700 mg b.i.d. plus ritonavir 100 mg once daily (in
therapy-naive or protease inhibitor–experienced patients). If patient has moderate hepatic impairment
(Child-Pugh score of 7 to 9), reduce dosage to 700 mg
b.i.d. (in therapy-naive patients) without ritonavir or
450 mg b.i.d. plus ritonavir 100 mg once daily (in therapy-naive or protease inhibitor–experienced patients).
If patient has severe hepatic impairment (Child-Pugh
score of 10 to 15), reduce dosage to 350 mg b.i.d.
without ritonavir (in therapy-naive patients) or 300 mg
b.i.d. plus ritonavir 100 mg once daily (therapy-naive
or protease inhibitor–experienced patients).
➤ **HIV infection with other antiretrovirals for
protease inhibitor–naive children age 4 weeks and
older**
*Children ages 4 weeks to 18 years weighing 20 kg or
more:* 18 mg/kg PO with ritonavir 3 mg/kg b.i.d.

*Children ages 4 weeks to 18 years weighing 15 to less
than 20 kg:* 23 mg/kg PO with ritonavir 3 mg/kg b.i.d.
*Children ages 4 weeks to 18 years weighing 11 to less
than 15 kg:* 30 mg/kg PO with ritonavir 3 mg/kg b.i.d.
*Children ages 4 weeks to 18 years weighing less than
11 kg:* 45 mg/kg PO with ritonavir 7 mg/kg b.i.d.
➤ **HIV infection with other antiretrovirals for
protease inhibitor–experienced children age
6 months and older**
*Children ages 6 months to 18 years weighing 20 kg or
more:* 18 mg/kg PO with ritonavir 3 mg/kg b.i.d.
*Children ages 6 months to 18 years weighing 15 to
less than 20 kg:* 23 mg/kg PO with ritonavir 3 mg/kg
b.i.d.
*Children ages 6 months to 18 years weighing 11 to
less than 15 kg:* 30 mg/kg PO with ritonavir 3 mg/kg
b.i.d.
*Children ages 6 months to 18 years weighing less than
11 kg:* 45 mg/kg PO with ritonavir 7 mg/kg b.i.d.
➤ **HIV infection without ritonavir in protease
inhibitor–naive children**
Children age 2 years and older: 30 mg/kg PO b.i.d.
For patients weighing at least 47 kg, may use the adult
regimen of fosamprenavir 1,400 mg b.i.d. Maximum
dose is 1,400 mg b.i.d.

fostamatinib disodium hexahydrate
FOS-tam-A-ti-nib

Tavalisse

Therapeutic class: Immunomodulators
Pharmacologic class: Spleen tyrosine kinase
inhibitors

AVAILABLE FORMS
Tablets: 100 mg, 150 mg

INDICATIONS & DOSAGES
➤ **Treatment of thrombocytopenia in patients
with chronic ITP who have had an insufficient
response to previous treatment**
Adults: Initially, 100 mg PO b.i.d. If platelet count
hasn't increased to at least 50×10^9/L after 4 weeks,
increase dosage to 150 mg b.i.d. Use lowest dosage
possible to achieve and maintain platelet count of at
least 50×10^9/L as necessary to reduce the risk of
bleeding. Discontinue fostamatinib after 12 weeks if
platelet count hasn't increased to a level adequate to
avoid clinically important bleeding.
Adjust-a-dose: Refer to manufacturer's instructions
for toxicity-related dosage adjustments.

glucagon
GLOO-ka-gon

GlucaGen Diagnostic Kit, GlucaGen
HypoKit, Glucagon Emergency Kit

Therapeutic class: Diagnostic agents
Pharmacologic class: Antihypoglycemics

AVAILABLE FORMS
Powder for injection: 1-mg (1-unit) vials

INDICATIONS & DOSAGES

➤ **Hypoglycemia**

Glucagon

Adults and children weighing more than 20 kg or older than age 6: 1 mg (1 unit) IV, IM, or subcut. May repeat in 15 minutes, if needed. IV glucose must be given if patient fails to respond.

Children weighing 20 kg or less: 0.5 mg (0.5 unit) or 20 to 30 mcg/kg IV, IM, or subcut; maximum dose, 1 mg. May repeat in 15 minutes, if needed. IV glucose must be given if patient fails to respond.

GlucaGen

Adults and children weighing more than 25 kg and age 6 or older or when weight is unknown: 1 mL IV, IM, or subcut.

Children weighing less than 25 kg or younger than age 6 when weight is unknown: 0.5 mL IV, IM, or subcut.

➤ **Diagnostic aid for radiologic examination of the GI tract**

Adults: 0.2 to 0.75 mg IV or 1 to 2 mg IM before radiologic examination.

SAFETY ALERT!

goserelin acetate
GOE-se-REL-in

Zoladex

Therapeutic class: Antineoplastics
Pharmacologic class: Gonadotropin-releasing hormone analogues

AVAILABLE FORMS
Implants: 3.6 mg, 10.8 mg

INDICATIONS & DOSAGES

➤ **Endometriosis, including pain relief and lesion reduction**

Women: 3.6 mg subcut every 28 days into the anterior abdominal wall below the navel. Maximum length of therapy is 6 months.

➤ **Endometrial thinning before endometrial ablation**

Women: 3.6 mg subcut into the anterior abdominal wall below the navel. Give one or two implants, 4 weeks apart.

➤ **Palliative treatment of advanced breast cancer in premenopausal and postmenopausal women**

Women: 3.6 mg subcut every 28 days into anterior abdominal wall below navel.

➤ **Palliative treatment of advanced prostate cancer**

Men: 3.6 mg subcut every 28 days or 10.8 mg subcut every 12 weeks into anterior abdominal wall below navel.

➤ **Stage B2-C prostate cancer in combination with radiotherapy and flutamide**

Men: Start 8 weeks before initiating radiotherapy and continue during radiation therapy. Give 3.6 mg subcut into anterior abdominal wall below navel 8 weeks before radiotherapy, followed in 28 days by 10.8 mg subcut. Or, give four injections of 3.6 mg at 28-day intervals, two injections preceding and two during radiotherapy.

guanFACINE hydrochloride
GWAHN-fa-seen

Intuniv

Therapeutic class: Antihypertensives
Pharmacologic class: Centrally acting antiadrenergics

AVAILABLE FORMS
Tablets: 1 mg, 2 mg
Tablets (extended-release) 🔵: 1 mg, 2 mg, 3 mg, 4 mg

INDICATIONS & DOSAGES

➤ **HTN**

Adults and children age 12 and older: Initially, 1 mg immediate-release tablet PO once daily at bedtime. If response isn't adequate after 3 to 4 weeks, may increase dosage to 2 mg daily. Higher doses have been used, but adverse effects increase significantly with dosages of more than 3 mg/day.

➤ **ADHD**

Children ages 6 to 17: Extended-release form only. Initially, 1 mg PO once daily in a.m. or p.m. at approximately same time each day. Adjust dosage in increments of 1 mg/week as needed. Doses above 4 mg/day haven't been evaluated in children ages 6 to 12 or above 7 mg/day in adolescents ages 13 to 17. Or, initially, 0.05 to 0.12 mg/kg PO once daily. Adjust dosage up to 0.12 mg/kg once daily if well tolerated and necessary.

Adjust-a-dose: Refer to manufacturer's instructions for dosage adjustment for use with CYP3A4 inhibitors or inducers.

HYDROXYprogesterone caproate
hye-drox-ee-proh-JESS-te-rone

Makena

Therapeutic class: Hormones
Pharmacologic class: Progestins

AVAILABLE FORMS
Injection: 250 mg/mL in single-dose and multidose vials; 275 mg/1.1 mL autoinjector

INDICATIONS & DOSAGES

➤ **To reduce risk of preterm birth in women with singleton pregnancy and history of singleton spontaneous preterm birth**

Pregnant adolescents and women age 16 and older: 250 mg IM (if using vial) or 275 mg IM (if using autoinjector) once weekly starting between 16 weeks, 0 days and 20 weeks, 6 days of gestation and continuing until week 37 (through 36 weeks, 6 days) of gestation or delivery, whichever occurs first.

ibalizumab-uiyk
eye-ba-LIZ-ue-mab

Trogarzo

Therapeutic class: Antiretrovirals
Pharmacologic class: CD4-directed postattachment HIV-1 inhibitors

---

AVAILABLE FORMS
Injection: 200 mg/1.33 mL (150 mg/mL) single-dose vials

INDICATIONS & DOSAGES
➤ **HIV-1 infection in heavily treatment-experienced adults with multidrug-resistant HIV-1 infection failing their current antiretroviral regimen**
Adults: 2,000 mg IV infusion loading dose followed by 800 mg IV infusion maintenance doses every 2 weeks.

icosapent ethyl
eye-KOE-sa-pent

Vascepa

Therapeutic class: Antilipemics
Pharmacologic class: Ethyl esters

AVAILABLE FORMS
Capsules ⓞⓣⓒ: 500 mg, 1 g

INDICATIONS & DOSAGES
➤ **Adjunct to diet to reduce triglyceride levels 500 mg/dL or more**
Adults: 2 g PO b.i.d. with food.

imiquimod
ih-mih-KWI-mahd

Aldara, Vyloma✤, Zyclara

Therapeutic class: Immunosuppressants (topical)
Pharmacologic class: Immune response modifiers

AVAILABLE FORMS
Cream: 2.5%, 3.75%, 5% in single-use packets containing 12.5 mg imiquimod

INDICATIONS & DOSAGES
➤ **External genital and perianal warts**
Adults and adolescents age 12 and older: Apply thin layer of 3.75% cream once daily before sleep; leave on for 8 hours. Continue up to 8 weeks. Or, apply thin layer of 5% cream three times per week before sleep; leave on for 6 to 10 hours. Continue for up to 16 weeks.
➤ **Typical, nonhyperkeratotic, nonhypertrophic actinic keratoses on the face or scalp in immunocompetent adults**
Adults: Wash area with mild soap and water, and allow to dry for at least 10 minutes. Apply Aldara cream to face or scalp, but not both concurrently, twice weekly at bedtime; wash off after about 8 hours. Treat for 16 weeks. Or, apply Zyclara 3.75% cream once daily at bedtime for two 2-week cycles. Separate cycles by a 2-week no-treatment period.
➤ **Superficial basal cell carcinoma**
Adults: Wash area with mild soap and water, and allow to dry thoroughly. Apply a thin layer of 5% cream to the biopsy-confirmed area, including 1 cm of skin surrounding tumor, five times a week at bedtime; wash off after about 8 hours. Treat for 6 weeks.

indacaterol maleate–glycopyrrolate
in-da-KAT-er-ol/glye-koe-PIR-oh-late

Utibron Neohaler

Therapeutic class: Bronchodilators
Pharmacologic class: Beta₂ adrenergic agonists–anticholinergics

AVAILABLE FORMS
Capsules (powder for inhalation): 27.5 mcg indacaterol maleate/15.6 mcg glycopyrrolate

INDICATIONS & DOSAGES
Black Box Warning Long-acting beta₂-adrenergic agonists increase the risk of asthma-related death. Drug isn't indicated for asthma treatment. ■
➤ **Long-term maintenance treatment of airflow obstruction in patients with COPD, including chronic bronchitis and emphysema**
Adults: 1 capsule b.i.d. by oral inhalation.

SAFETY ALERT!

inotuzumab ozogamicin
in-oh-TOOZ-ue-mab

Besponsa

Therapeutic class: Antineoplastics
Pharmacologic class: Antibody–drug conjugates

AVAILABLE FORMS
Injection (lyophilized): 0.9 mg lyophilized powder in single-dose vials

INDICATIONS & DOSAGES
Black Box Warning Hepatotoxicity, including fatal and life-threatening hepatic veno-occlusive disease (VOD), has occurred. Permanently discontinue drug if VOD occurs. A higher posthematopoietic stem cell transplant (HSCT) nonrelapse mortality rate occurred in patients receiving inotuzumab. ■
➤ **Treatment of relapsed or refractory B-cell precursor acute lymphoblastic leukemia**
Adults: Premedicate with a corticosteroid, antipyretic, and antihistamine. For cycle 1, total dose is 1.8 mg/m² given as three divided doses on days 1, 8, and 15 of a 21-day treatment cycle. On day 1, give 0.8 mg/m² IV infusion; on days 8 and 15, give 0.5 mg/m² IV infusion. Cycle 1 is 3 weeks in duration, but may be extended to 4 weeks if patient achieves a complete remission (CR) or CR with incomplete hematologic recovery (Cri), or to allow recovery from toxicity.

For subsequent cycles in patients who achieve a CR or CRi, total dose per cycle is 1.5 mg/m² given as three divided doses on days 1, 8, and 15 of a 28-day treatment cycle. On days 1, 8, and 15, give 0.5 mg/m² IV infusion. Subsequent cycles are 4 weeks in duration.

For subsequent cycles in patients who don't achieve a CR or CRi, total dose per cycle is 1.8 mg/m² given as three divided doses on days, 1, 8, and 15 of a 28-day treatment cycle. On day 1, give 0.8 mg/m² IV infusion; on days 8 and 15, give 0.5 mg/m² IV infusion. Subsequent cycles are 4 weeks in duration, but discontinue drug in patients who don't achieve CR or CRi within three cycles.

For patients proceeding to HSCT, recommended treatment duration is two cycles. May consider a third cycle for those who don't achieve CR or CRi and minimal residual disease negativity after two cycles.

For patients not proceeding to HSCT, may give additional cycles of treatment, up to a maximum of six cycles.

Adjust-a-dose: Refer to manufacturer's instructions for toxicity-related dosage adjustments and drug discontinuation.

SAFETY ALERT!

interferon gamma-1b
in-ter-FEER-on

Actimmune

Therapeutic class: Immune response modifiers
Pharmacologic class: Biological response modifiers

AVAILABLE FORMS
Injection: 100 mcg (2 million international units) in 0.5-mL vials

INDICATIONS & DOSAGES
➤ **Chronic granulomatous disease in adults and children age 1 year and older, severe malignant osteopetrosis in adults and children age 1 month and older**
Adults and children with BSA greater than 0.5 m²: Give 50 mcg/m² (1 million international units/m²) subcut three times weekly, preferably at bedtime.
Adults and children with a BSA of 0.5 m² or less: 1.5 mcg/kg subcut three times weekly.
Adjust-a-dose: If patient has severe reaction, decrease dosage by 50% or stop drug until reaction subsides.

SAFETY ALERT!

irinotecan liposome ☒
eh-rin-OH-te-kan

Onivyde

Therapeutic class: Antineoplastics
Pharmacologic class: DNA topoisomerase inhibitors

AVAILABLE FORMS
Injection: 43 mg/10 mL in single-use vials

INDICATIONS & DOSAGES
Black Box Warning Withhold drug and initiate loperamide for late-onset diarrhea of any severity. Administer IV or subcut atropine 0.25 to 1 mg (unless clinically contraindicated) for early-onset diarrhea of any severity. Drug may cause fatal neutropenic sepsis and severe or life-threatening neutropenic fever. Withhold drug for ANC below 1,500/mm³ or neutropenic fever. Monitor CBC periodically during treatment. ■
➤ **Metastatic adenocarcinoma of the pancreas after disease progression after gemcitabine-based therapy, in combination with 5-FU and leucovorin** ☒

Adults: 70 mg/m² IV infusion over 90 minutes every 2 weeks. Premedicate with a corticosteroid and an antiemetic 30 minutes before infusion.
Adjust-a-dose: Refer to manufacturer's instructions for patients known to be homozygous for the UGT1A1*28 allele and for toxicity-related dosage adjustments and discontinuation.

isoproterenol hydrochloride
eye-soe-proe-TER-e-nole

Isuprel

Therapeutic class: Bronchodilators
Pharmacologic class: Nonselective beta-adrenergic agonists

AVAILABLE FORMS
Injection: 200 mcg/mL in 1-mL, 5-mL ampules

INDICATIONS & DOSAGES
➤ **Bronchospasm during anesthesia**
Adults: Dilute 1 mL (0.2 mg) with 9 mL of NSS or D₅W. Give 0.01 to 0.02 mg IV and repeat as necessary.
➤ **Heart block, ventricular arrhythmias**
Adults: Initially, 0.02 to 0.06 mg IV; then 0.01 to 0.2 mg IV or via infusion at 5 mcg/minute IV. Or, initially, 0.2 mg IM or subcut; then 0.02 to 1 mg IM or 0.15 to 0.3 mg subcut as needed.
➤ **Shock**
Adults: 0.5 to 5 mcg/minute by continuous IV infusion. Usual concentration is 1 mg in 500 mL D₅W. Titrate infusion rate according to HR, central venous pressure, BP, and urine flow.

SAFETY ALERT!

ivosidenib
EYE-voe-SID-e-nib

Tibsovo

Therapeutic class: Antineoplastics
Pharmacologic class: Isocitrate dehydrogenase-1 inhibitors

AVAILABLE FORMS
Tablets: 250 mg

INDICATIONS & DOSAGES
Adjust-a-dose (for all indications): Refer to manufacturer's instructions for toxicity-related dosage adjustments. Treat for a minimum of 6 months to allow time for clinical response.
➤ **Treatment of relapsed or refractory acute myeloid leukemia (AML) with a susceptible *IDH1* mutation as detected by an FDA-approved test**
Adults: 500 mg PO daily until disease progression or unacceptable toxicity.
✳ ***NEW INDICATION:* Treatment of newly diagnosed AML with a susceptible *IDH1* mutation as detected by an FDA-approved test in patients age 75 and older or who have comorbidities that preclude use of intensive induction chemotherapy**
Adults: 500 mg PO daily until disease progression or unacceptable toxicity.

SAFETY ALERT!

ixabepilone
ecks-ah-BEH-pill-own

Ixempra Kit

Therapeutic class: Antineoplastics
Pharmacologic class: Microtubule inhibitors

AVAILABLE FORMS
Injection: 15-mg, 45-mg vials

INDICATIONS & DOSAGES
Black Box Warning Drug is contraindicated in patients with AST or ALT greater than 2.5 × ULN or bilirubin 1 × ULN when used with capecitabine. ■
➤ **With capecitabine for metastatic or locally advanced breast cancer, after failure of anthracycline and a taxane, or in patients whose cancer is taxane-resistant and for whom further anthracycline therapy is contraindicated; or alone for metastatic or locally advanced breast cancer, after failure of anthracycline, taxanes, and capecitabine**
Adults: 40 mg/m² IV over 3 hours every 3 weeks. Doses for patients with BSA greater than 2.2 m² should be calculated based on 2.2 m². Premedicate with an H_1-receptor antagonist, such as diphenhydramine 50 mg PO (or equivalent), and an H_2-receptor antagonist, such as ranitidine 150 to 300 mg PO, 1 hour before ixabepilone infusion. For patients who experienced a prior hypersensitivity reaction, premedicate with corticosteroids (such as dexamethasone 20 mg IV 30 minutes before infusion or PO 60 minutes before infusion) in addition to the H_1- and H_2-receptor antagonists.
Adjust-a-dose: Refer to manufacturer's instructions for monotherapy and combination therapy dosage adjustments for toxicities and hepatic failure.

SAFETY ALERT!

lapatinib ☒
lah-PAH-tih-nihb

Tykerb

Therapeutic class: Antineoplastics
Pharmacologic class: Kinase inhibitors

AVAILABLE FORMS
Tablets: 250 mg

INDICATIONS & DOSAGES
Black Box Warning Severe and fatal hepatotoxicity has been observed in clinical trials and postmarketing experience. ■
Adjust-a-dose (for all indications): Refer to manufacturer's instructions for toxicity-related dosage adjustments and use with strong CYP34A4 inhibitors and CYP3A4 inducers.
➤ **Advanced or metastatic breast cancer with capecitabine when tumors overexpress HER2 and patient has had prior therapy, including an anthracycline, a taxane, and trastuzumab** ☒
Adults: 1,250 mg (5 tablets) PO once daily as a single dose on days 1 through 21, with 2,000 mg/m²/day capecitabine given PO in two doses 12 hours apart on

days 1 to 14. Repeat 21-day cycle. Continue until disease progression or unacceptable toxicity occurs.
➤ **HER2-positive, hormone receptor–positive metastatic breast cancer in postmenopausal women** ☒
Adults: 1,500 mg PO once daily with letrozole 2.5 mg once daily.

lenvatinib mesylate
len-VA-ti-nib

Lenvima

Therapeutic class: Antineoplastics
Pharmacologic class: Kinase inhibitors

AVAILABLE FORMS
Capsules: 4 mg, 10 mg

INDICATIONS & DOSAGES
Adjust-a-dose (for all indications): See manufacturer's instructions for toxicity-related dosage adjustments and management.
➤ **Locally recurrent or metastatic, progressive, radioactive iodine-refractory differentiated thyroid cancer**
Adults: 24 mg PO daily until disease progression or unacceptable toxicity occurs.
Adjust-a-dose: For preexisting severe renal impairment (CrCl less than 30 mL/minute) or severe hepatic impairment (Child-Pugh class C), decrease dosage to 14 mg PO daily.
➤ **Advanced renal cell carcinoma after one prior antiangiogenic therapy, in combination with everolimus**
Adults: 18 mg PO once daily with everolimus 5 mg PO once daily until disease progression or unacceptable toxicity occurs.
Adjust-a-dose: For preexisting severe renal impairment (CrCl less than 30 mL/minute) or severe hepatic impairment (Child-Pugh class C), decrease lenvatinib dosage to 10 mg PO daily.
✳ *NEW INDICATION:* **Unresectable hepatocellular carcinoma, first-line treatment**
Adults weighing 60 kg or more: 12 mg PO once daily.
Adults weighing less than 60 kg: 8 mg PO once daily.
✳ *NEW INDICATION:* **Advanced endometrial carcinoma in patients who have disease progression after prior systemic therapy and aren't candidates for curative surgery or radiation, in combination with pembrolizumab**
Adults: 20 mg PO once daily with pembrolizumab 200 mg IV infusion every 3 weeks until disease progression or unacceptable toxicity. Refer to pembrolizumab prescribing information for recommended dosage information.

letermovir
let-ER-moe-vir

Prevymis

Therapeutic class: Antivirals
Pharmacologic class: CMV DNA terminase complex inhibitors

AVAILABLE FORMS

Injection: 240 mg/12 mL, 480 mg/24 mL single-use vials
Tablets: 240 mg, 480 mg

INDICATIONS & DOSAGES

➤ **Prophylaxis of CMV infection and disease in CMV-seropositive recipients [R+] of an allogeneic hematopoietic stem cell transplant**

Adults: 480 mg PO or 480-mg IV infusion once daily beginning between day 0 and day 28 posttransplant and continuing through day 100 posttransplant.

Adjust-a-dose: If drug is administered with cyclosporine, decrease dose to 240 mg PO or IV once daily. If cyclosporine is initiated after start of letermovir, decrease next dose of letermovir to 240 mg once daily. If cyclosporine is discontinued after start of letermovir, increase next dose of letermovir to 480 mg once daily. If cyclosporine dosing is interrupted due to high cyclosporine level, no letermovir dosage adjustment is needed.

L-glutamine
ell-GLOO-ta-meen

Endari

Therapeutic class: Miscellaneous hematologic drugs
Pharmacologic class: Amino acids

AVAILABLE FORMS

Oral powder: 5 g per packet

INDICATIONS & DOSAGES

➤ **To reduce acute complications of sickle cell disease**

Adults and children age 5 and older weighing more than 65 kg: 15 g (3 packets) PO b.i.d.
Adults and children age 5 and older weighing 30 to 65 kg: 10 g (2 packets) PO b.i.d.
Children age 5 and older weighing less than 30 kg: 5 g (1 packet) PO b.i.d.

---

lidocaine (intradermal, ophthalmic, topical)
LYE-doe-kane

Lidocaine, Lidoderm

lidocaine hydrochloride
Akten, AneCream◇, AneCream 5, Glydo, Larng-O-Jet Kit, LTA Kit II, Lidocaine Viscous, Lidodan♣◇, Maxilene♣◇, Predator◇, RectiCare◇, Regenecare HA◇, Solarcaine Aloe Extra Burn Relief◇, Xolido◇, Xylocaine, Zingo

Therapeutic class: Analgesics
Pharmacologic class: Local anesthetics

AVAILABLE FORMS

Cream: 2%◇, 3%, 3.88%, 4%◇, 5%◇
Gel: 2%◇, 5%◇
Jelly: 2%
Ointment: 5%
Ophthalmic gel: 3.5%
Patch: 5%
Powder for injection: 0.5-mg single-use intradermal injection system
Topical solution: 2%, 4%
Topical spray: 0.5%
Viscous oral solution: 2%, 4%

INDICATIONS & DOSAGES

Black Box Warning Postmarketing cases of seizures, cardiopulmonary arrest, and death in patients younger than age 3 have been reported with use of lidocaine 2% viscous solution when it wasn't administered in strict adherence to the dosing and administration recommendations. Lidocaine 2% viscous solution isn't approved for teething pain. ■

Adjust-a-dose (for all indications): Decrease dosage as needed based on patient's age, weight, and physical condition.

➤ **Urethra anesthesia and treatment of painful urethritis**

Male adults and children: Slowly instill 15 mL (300 mg lidocaine) 2% jelly into urethra using an easy syringelike action, until patient has a feeling of tension or until about 15 mL is instilled. Apply penile clamp for 5 to 10 minutes at the corona then, if needed, an additional 15 mL may be instilled as needed for adequate anesthesia. Before catheterization, 5 to 10 mL (100 to 200 mg) is usually adequate. Maximum dose for adults is 600 g in any 12-hour period. Maximum dose for children is 4.5 mg/kg.

Female adults and children: Slowly instill 3 to 5 mL (60 to 100 mg) of 2% jelly into urethra. A small amount of jelly may be applied to cotton swab and deposited into the urethral opening before instillation. Allow several minutes for anesthetic effect to occur. Maximum dose for adults is 600 g in any 12-hour period. Maximum dose for children is 4.5 mg/kg.

➤ **Anesthetic lubricant for ET intubation**

Adults and children: Apply moderate amount of 2% jelly to external surface of ET tube shortly before use. Maximum adult dose is 30 mL (600 mg) in any 12-hour period. Maximum dose in children is 4.5 mg/kg. Or, apply up to 5 g per single application, approximately 6 inches, of 5% ointment to external surface of ET tube shortly before use. Maximum adult dose of 5% ointment is 20 g (equivalent to lidocaine base 1,000 mg) per day. Maximum dose in children is 4.5 mg/kg.

➤ **Topical anesthesia of accessible mucous membranes of oral and nasal cavities and proximal portions of digestive tract**

Adults and children age 10 and older: Apply 1 to 5 mL (40 to 200 mg) 4% oral topical solution to affected area as a spray, applied with cotton applicators or packs, as when instilled into a cavity. Maximum dose is 4.5 mg/kg, not to exceed 300 mg/dose.

Children younger than age 10 who have a normal lean body mass and normal body development: Apply 4% oral topical solution to affected area as a spray, applied with cotton applicators or packs, as when instilled into a cavity. May determine dose by applying one of the standard pediatric drug formulas. Maximum dose is 4.5 mg/kg.

♣Canada   ◇OTC   ◆Off-label use   ✏Photoguide   ⓓⓝⓒDo not crush   *Liquid contains alcohol   ❄Genetic

➤ **Oropharynx anesthetic**

Adults and children (used in dentistry): Apply 5% ointment to previously dried oral mucosa. For use in adults with the insertion of new dentures, apply to all denture surfaces with mucosal contact. Maximum dose for adults is 5 g/single application (equivalent to lidocaine base 250 mg or 6 inches of ointment) or 20 g of ointment (equivalent to 1,000 g lidocaine base) per day. Patient should consult a dentist at least every 48 hours throughout denture-fitting period. Maximum dose for children is 5 g/single application (equivalent to 250 mg lidocaine base or approximately 6 inches of ointment) or 4.5 mg/kg lidocaine base.

Adults: 15 mL 2% solution swished in the mouth and spit out or gargled and swallowed no more frequently than every 3 hours. Maximum dose for adults is 4.5 mg/kg/dose (or 300 mg/dose); eight doses per 24 hours.

Children age 3 and older: Don't exceed 4.5 mg/kg/dose (or 300 mg/dose) swished in the mouth and spit out no more frequently than every 3 hours (four doses in 12 hours).

Children younger than age 3: 1.2 mL 2% solution applied to immediate area with a cotton-tipped applicator no more frequently than every 3 hours. Maximum is four doses in 12 hours and 1.2 mL/dose.

➤ **Skin discomfort (irritation, itching, pain)**

☝ *Alert:* For children weighing less than 10 kg, a single application should be applied over an area no greater than 100 cm². For children weighing between 10 and 20 kg, a single application should be applied over an area no greater than 600 cm².

Adults and children (5% ointment): Apply ointment topically for adequate control of symptoms. Maximum dose for adults is 5 g/single application (equivalent to lidocaine base 250 mg or approximately 6 inches of ointment) or 20 g of ointment (equivalent to lidocaine base 1,000 mg)/day. Maximum dose for children is 5 g/single application (equivalent to lidocaine base 250 mg or approximately 6 inches of ointment), or 4.5 mg/kg lidocaine base.

Adults and children age 2 and older (cream, gel, spray): Apply 4% cream or 4% gel or spray to affected areas t.i.d. to q.i.d. Or apply 2% gel to affected areas t.i.d. as needed.

➤ **Local analgesia for venipuncture (Zingo)**

Adults and children age 3 and older: Apply one intradermal lidocaine (0.5 mg) device to site planned for venipuncture 1 to 3 minutes before needle insertion.

➤ **Anorectal discomfort**

Adults and children age 12 and older: Apply 5% cream or 5% gel up to six times a day.

➤ **Postherpetic neuralgia**

Adults: Apply 5% patch to most painful area for up to 12 hours in any 24-hour period. Maximum dose is 3 patches in a single application.

➤ **Ocular surface anesthesia (Akten)**

Adults and children: Apply 2 drops to ocular surface in area of planned procedure. Reapply as needed to maintain anesthetic effect.

lindane
LIN-dayn

Therapeutic class: Scabicides–pediculicides
Pharmacologic class: Ectoparasiticides–ovicides

AVAILABLE FORMS
Shampoo: 1%

INDICATIONS & DOSAGES
Black Box Warning Only use drug in patients who can't tolerate or have failed first-line treatment with safer medications. Drug can cause seizures and death. Use with caution in infants, children, elderly patients, individuals with other skin conditions, and those who weigh less than 50 kg; they may be at risked for serious neurotoxicity. ■

➤ **Head lice, crab lice, and their ova in patients who can't tolerate other therapies or have failed treatment with other therapies**

Adults and children age 10 and older: Apply shampoo undiluted to dry hair and work into lather for 4 minutes; small amounts of water may increase lathering. Give special attention to the fine hairs along the neck. Apply 30 mL of shampoo for short hair, 45 mL for medium-length hair, or 60 mL for long hair. Allow shampoo to remain in place for 4 minutes only. Rinse thoroughly and rub dry briskly with towel. Comb with a fine-tooth comb and remove nits with a nit comb or tweezers.

Elderly patients: May need to reduce dosage because of increased skin absorption.

liothyronine sodium (T₃)
lye-oh-THYE-roe-neen

Cytomel, Triostat

Therapeutic class: Thyroid hormone replacements
Pharmacologic class: Thyroid hormones

AVAILABLE FORMS
Injection: 10 mcg/mL in 1-mL vials*
Tablets: 5 mcg, 25 mcg, 50 mcg

INDICATIONS & DOSAGES
Black Box Warning Large doses of drug are toxic, particularly in combination with sympathomimetic amines commonly used in treatment of obesity. Drug is ineffective in weight loss for patients who are euthyroid. ■

➤ **Congenital hypothyroidism**

Children: Initially, 5 mcg PO daily; increase by 5 mcg every 3 to 4 days until desired response is achieved. For maintenance: Infants may require only 20 mcg daily; children ages 1 to 3 may require 50 mcg daily; and children older than age 3 may require full adult dosage.

➤ **Myxedema**

Adults: Initially, 5 mcg PO daily; increase by 5 to 10 mcg every 1 to 2 weeks until daily dose reaches 25 mcg. Then increase by 5 to 25 mcg daily every 1 to 2 weeks. Maintenance dosage, 50 to 100 mcg daily.

➤ **Myxedema coma, premyxedema coma**

Adults: Initially, 10 to 20 mcg IV for patients with CV disease; 25 to 50 mcg IV for patients who don't have CV disease. Adjust dosage based on patient's condition and response. Switch patient to oral therapy as soon as possible.

➤ **Simple (nontoxic) goiter**

Adults: Initially, 5 mcg PO daily; may increase by 5 to 10 mcg daily every 1 to 2 weeks until daily dose reaches 25 mcg. Then increase by 12.5 to 25 mcg daily every 1 to 2 weeks. Usual maintenance dosage, 75 mcg daily.

Patients older than age 65 and children: 5 mcg daily; increase by 5 mcg daily every 1 to 2 weeks.

➤ **Thyroid hormone replacement**

Adults: Initially, 25 mcg PO daily; increase by up to 25 mcg every 1 to 2 weeks until satisfactory response occurs. Usual maintenance dosage, 25 to 75 mcg daily.

Adjust-a-dose: In patients with CV disease, give 5 mcg once daily; may increase by 5 mcg/day every 2 weeks.

➤ **T_3 suppression test to differentiate hyperthyroidism from euthyroidism**

Adults: 75 to 100 mcg PO daily for 7 days; radioactive iodine uptake is determined before and after hormone administration.

SAFETY ALERT!

lomustine (CCNU)
loe-MUS-teen

Gleostine

Therapeutic class: Antineoplastics
Pharmacologic class: Nitrosoureas

AVAILABLE FORMS
Capsules: 10 mg, 40 mg, 100 mg

INDICATIONS & DOSAGES

▪ **Black Box Warning** ▪ Drug can cause severe and fatal myelosuppression. Monitor blood cell counts weekly for at least 6 weeks after a dose. Ensure that patient is prescribed and takes only a single dose every 6 weeks. ▪

➤ **Brain tumor, Hodgkin lymphoma**

Adults and children: 130 mg/m^2 PO as single dose every 6 weeks. Round doses to nearest 5 mg. Don't give repeat doses until WBC exceeds 4,000/mm^3 and platelet count is greater than 100,000/mm^3.

Adjust-a-dose: Reduce dosage to 100 mg/m^2 once every 6 weeks in patients with compromised bone marrow function. Refer to manufacturer's instructions for dosage adjustments for hematologic toxicity or when used with other myelosuppressive drugs.

luliconazole
loo-li-KON-a-zole

Luzu

Therapeutic class: Antifungals
Pharmacologic class: Azole antifungals

AVAILABLE FORMS
Cream: 1%

INDICATIONS & DOSAGES

➤ **Interdigital tinea pedis (athlete's foot) caused by *Trichophyton rubrum* or *Epidermophyton floccosum***

Adults: Apply thin layer to affected area and approximately 1 inch (2.5 cm) of surrounding area once daily for 2 weeks.

➤ **Tinea cruris (jock itch) and tinea corporis (ringworm) caused by *T. rubrum* or *E. floccosum***

Adults: Apply thin layer to affected area and approximately 1 inch (2.5 cm) of surrounding area once daily for 1 week.

lumacaftor–ivacaftor
LOO-ma-kaf-tor/EYE-va-kaf-tor

Orkambi

Therapeutic class: Metabolic agents
Pharmacologic class: Cystic fibrosis transmembrane conductance regulator (CFTR) potentiators

AVAILABLE FORMS
Granules: 100 mg lumacaftor/125 mg ivacaftor, 150 mg lumacaftor/188 mg ivacaftor
Tablets: 100 mg lumacaftor/125 mg ivacaftor, 200 mg lumacaftor/125 mg ivacaftor

INDICATIONS & DOSAGES

➤ **Treatment of cystic fibrosis in patients who are homozygous for the F508del mutation in the *CFTR* gene**

Adults and children age 12 and older: 400 mg lumacaftor/250 mg ivacaftor PO every 12 hours with fat-containing food.

Children ages 6 to 11: 200 mg lumacaftor/250 mg ivacaftor PO every 12 hours with fat-containing food.

Children ages 2 to 5 weighing 14 kg or more: 150 mg lumacaftor/188 mg ivacaftor packet of granules every 12 hours with fat-containing food.

Children ages 2 to 5 weighing less than 14 kg: 100 mg lumacaftor/125 mg ivacaftor PO every 12 hours with fat-containing food.

Adjust-a-dose: Refer to manufacturer's instructions for hepatic impairment, drug-interaction, and toxicity-related dosage adjustments.

mecasermin ▨
meh-KAH-sur-men

Increlex

Therapeutic class: Growth factors
Pharmacologic class: Human insulin growth factors

AVAILABLE FORMS
Injection: 10 mg/mL

INDICATIONS & DOSAGES

➤ **Growth failure in children with severe primary insulin growth factor-1 deficiency or children with**

growth hormone gene deletion who have developed neutralizing antibodies to growth hormone 🧬
Children age 2 and older: Initially, 0.04 to 0.08 mg/kg subcut b.i.d. If well tolerated for at least 1 week, may increase by 0.04 mg/kg per dose, to the maximum dose of 0.12 mg/kg b.i.d.

meloxicam
mel-OX-i-kam

Mobic, Qmiiz ODT, Vivlodex

Therapeutic class: Antirheumatics
Pharmacologic class: NSAIDs

AVAILABLE FORMS
Capsules: 5 mg, 10 mg
Tablets: 7.5 mg, 15 mg
Tablets (ODTs): 7.5 mg, 15 mg

INDICATIONS & DOSAGES
Black Box Warning NSAIDs may increase risk of serious CV thrombotic events, MI, stroke, and GI adverse reactions. Contraindicated for use in CABG surgery. ■
Adjust-a-dose (for all indications): Use isn't recommended in patients with CrCl of less than 20 mL/minute as drug hasn't been studied in this population. If patient is receiving hemodialysis, give no more than 7.5 mg tablet/ODT or 5-mg capsule once daily.
➤ **To relieve signs and symptoms of osteoarthritis or RA**
Adults: 7.5 mg PO once daily. May increase as needed to maximum dosage of 15 mg daily. For osteoarthritis only, give 5 mg Vivlodex PO once daily. May increase to 10 mg in patients who require additional analgesia. Use lowest effective dose for shortest duration consistent with individual patient treatment goals.
➤ **To relieve signs and symptoms of pauciarticular or polyarticular course juvenile RA**
Children weighing 60 kg or more: 7.5 mg PO daily.

menotropins
men-oh-TROE-pins

Menopur

Therapeutic class: Ovulation stimulants
Pharmacologic class: Gonadotropins

AVAILABLE FORMS
Injection: 75 international units of luteinizing hormone and 75 international units of FSH activity per vial

INDICATIONS & DOSAGES
➤ **Assisted reproductive technologies**
Adults: Initially, 225 units subcut into lower abdomen starting on cycle day 2 or 3. Menopur may be used in combination with urofollitropin, but total initial dose of both shouldn't exceed 225 units (150 international units of menotropins and 75 international units of urofollitropin or 75 international units of menotropins and 150 international units of urofollitropin). Adjust dosage after 5 days, based on ovarian response as determined by ultrasound evaluation of follicular growth and serum estradiol levels. Don't make additional

adjustments more frequently than every 2 days and not to exceed 150 units per adjustment. Maximum daily dosage is 450 units. Use for maximum of 20 days.

mepolizumab
meh-po-LIZZ-ue-mabb

Nucala

Therapeutic class: Miscellaneous respiratory drugs
Pharmacologic class: Monoclonal antibodies

AVAILABLE FORMS
Injection: 100-mg single-dose vials

INDICATIONS & DOSAGES
➤ **Add-on maintenance treatment of severe asthma in patients with an eosinophilic phenotype**
Adults and children age 12 and older: 100 mg subcut every 4 weeks into upper arm, thigh, or abdomen.
➤ **Eosinophilic granulomatosis with polyangiitis**
Adults: 300 mg given as three separate 100-mg subcut injections into the upper arm, thigh, or abdomen once every 4 weeks.

methylergonovine maleate
meth-ill-er-goe-NOE-veen

Methergine

Therapeutic class: Oxytocics
Pharmacologic class: Ergot alkaloids

AVAILABLE FORMS
Injection: 0.2 mg/mL in 1-mL vials
Tablets: 0.2 mg

INDICATIONS & DOSAGES
➤ **To prevent and treat postpartum hemorrhage caused by uterine atony or subinvolution**
Adults: 0.2 mg IM or IV after delivery of the anterior shoulder, after delivery of the placenta, or during the puerperium. May repeat every 2 to 4 hours as needed. During life-threatening emergencies, 0.2 mg IV over at least 1 minute while monitoring BP and uterine contractions. After first IM or IV dose, 0.2 mg PO every 6 to 8 hours for up to 7 days. Decrease dosage if severe cramping occurs.

SAFETY ALERT!

midostaurin 🧬
mi-doe-STOR-in

Rydapt

Therapeutic class: Antineoplastics
Pharmacologic class: Tyrosine kinase inhibitors

AVAILABLE FORMS
Capsules: 25 mg

INDICATIONS & DOSAGES
Adjust-a-dose (for all indications): Refer to manufacturer's instructions for toxicity-related adjustments.

♣Canada ◇OTC ◆ Off-label use ✐Photoguide ⊕Do not crush *Liquid contains alcohol 🧬Genetic

➤ **Newly diagnosed acute myeloid leukemia in patients with *FLT3* mutation in combination with daunorubicin and cytarabine** ☒

Adults: 50 mg PO b.i.d. with food on days 8 to 21 of each induction cycle (in combination with dauno-rubicin and cytarabine) and on days 8 to 21 of each consolidation cycle (in combination with high-dose cytarabine).

➤ **Aggressive systemic mastocytosis, systemic mastocytosis with associated hematologic neoplasm, or mast cell leukemia**

Adults: 100 mg PO b.i.d. with food until disease pro-gression or unacceptable toxicity occurs.

misoprostol
mye-soe-PROST-ole

Cytotec

Therapeutic class: Antiulcer drugs
Pharmacologic class: Prostaglandin E₁ analogues

AVAILABLE FORMS
Tablets: 100 mcg, 200 mcg

INDICATIONS & DOSAGES
Black Box Warning Drug can cause abortion, pre-mature birth, birth defects, and uterine rupture and is contraindicated during pregnancy. ■

➤ **To prevent NSAID-induced gastric ulcer in pa-tients at high risk for complications from gastric ulcer and in patients with history of NSAID-induced ulcer**

Adults: 200 mcg PO q.i.d. with food; if not tolerated, decrease to 100 mcg PO q.i.d. Give dosage for dura-tion of NSAID therapy.

moexipril hydrochloride
moe-EX-eh-pril

Therapeutic class: Antihypertensives
Pharmacologic class: ACE inhibitors

AVAILABLE FORMS
Tablets: 7.5 mg, 15 mg

INDICATIONS & DOSAGES
Black Box Warning Drug can cause fetal harm; when pregnancy is detected, discontinue as soon as possible. ■

➤ **HTN, alone or in combination with thiazide diuretics**

Adults: Initially, 7.5 mg PO once daily as monotherapy, given 1 hour before a meal. Or initially, 3.75 mg if di-uretic therapy can't be discontinued. Increase dosage incrementally according to BP response. Maximum dosage is 60 mg/day in one or two divided doses.

Adjust-a-dose: For patients currently being treated with a diuretic, if possible stop diuretic 2 to 3 days before therapy is initiated to reduce likelihood of hypotension. If BP isn't adequately controlled with moexipril alone, may reinstitute diuretic therapy. For patients with CrCl of 40 mL/minute/1.73 m² or less, cautiously give initial dose of 3.75 mg once daily.

May titrate dosage upward to a maximum daily dosage of 15 mg.

nafarelin acetate
nah-FAR-eh-lin

Synarel

Therapeutic class: Endocrine-metabolic agents
Pharmacologic class: Gonadotropin-releasing hormone analogues

AVAILABLE FORMS
Nasal spray: 2 mg/mL (200 mcg/spray)

INDICATIONS & DOSAGES
➤ **Central precocious puberty** ☒

Children age 8 years or younger (female), or age 9 or younger (male): 2 sprays (400 mcg) into each nos-tril in the morning and evening for a total of 8 sprays (1,600 mcg) per day. If necessary, may increase dos-age to a total of 9 sprays (1,800 mcg) per day, admin-istered as 3 sprays (600 mcg) into alternating nostrils t.i.d. Continue treatment until resumption of puberty is desired.

➤ **Endometriosis**

Adults: Begin treatment between days 2 and 4 of menstrual cycle. Administer 1 spray (200 mcg) into one nostril in the morning and 1 spray (200 mcg) into the other nostril in the evening for a total of 2 sprays (400 mcg) per day. If persistent regular menstruation continues after 2 months of treatment, increase dose to 1 spray (200 mcg) into each nostril in the morning and 1 spray (200 mcg) into each nostril in the evening for a total of 4 sprays (800 mcg) per day. Recommended duration of treatment is 6 months.

nefazodone hydrochloride
ne-FAZ-oh-done

Therapeutic class: Antidepressants
Pharmacologic class: Antidepressants

AVAILABLE FORMS
Tablets: 50 mg, 100 mg, 150 mg, 200 mg, 250 mg

INDICATIONS & DOSAGES
Black Box Warning Drug increases risk of suicidal thoughts and behavior in children, adolescents, and young adults. Life-threatening hepatic failure has been reported; discontinue drug if clinical signs or symp-toms suggest liver failure or hepatocellular injury. ■

➤ **Depression**

Adults: Initially, 100 mg/day PO b.i.d. Increase dos-age in increments of 100 to 200 mg/day in two divid-ed doses at intervals of no less than 1 week. Effective dosage range is 300 to 600 mg/day.

Adjust-a-dose: In elderly or debilitated patients, es-pecially women, initially 50 mg PO b.i.d. Don't start drug until 14 days after administration of an MAO inhibitor.

SAFETY ALERT!

nelarabine
neh-LAR-uh-been

Arranon, Atriance ✤

Therapeutic class: Antineoplastics
Pharmacologic class: DNA demethylation agents; prodrugs of cytotoxic deoxyguanosine

AVAILABLE FORMS
Injection: 5 mg/mL in 50-mL vials

INDICATIONS & DOSAGES
Black Box Warning Severe neurologic adverse reactions have been reported, including altered mental states (e.g., severe somnolence), CNS effects (e.g., seizures), and peripheral neuropathy, ranging from numbness and paresthesia to motor weakness and paralysis. ▪

➤ **T-cell acute lymphoblastic leukemia and T-cell lymphoblastic lymphoma in patients whose disease hasn't responded to or has relapsed after treatment with at least two chemotherapy regimens**
Adults: 1,500 mg/m^2 IV over 2 hours on days 1, 3, and 5. Repeat every 21 days.
Children: 650 mg/m^2 IV over 1 hour daily for 5 consecutive days. Repeat every 21 days.
Adjust-a-dose: Discontinue drug for neurologic adverse reactions of NCI CTCAE grade 2 or greater. Dosage may be delayed for other toxicities, including hematologic toxicity. Refer to prescribing information for more information.

netarsudil
ne-TAR-soo-dil

Rhopressa

Therapeutic class: Antiglaucoma drugs
Pharmacologic class: Rho kinase inhibitors

AVAILABLE FORMS
Ophthalmic solution: 0.02%

INDICATIONS & DOSAGES
➤ **To reduce elevated IOP in patients with open-angle glaucoma or ocular HTN**
Adults: Instill 1 drop into affected eye(s) once daily in the evening.

niMODipine
nye-MOE-dih-peen

Nymalize

Therapeutic class: Vasodilators
Pharmacologic class: Calcium channel blockers

AVAILABLE FORMS
Capsules: 30 mg
Oral solution: 30 mg/10 mL, 60 mg/20 mL

INDICATIONS & DOSAGES
Black Box Warning Don't administer parenterally; may cause life-threatening reactions and death. ▪

➤ **To improve neurologic deficits after subarachnoid hemorrhage from ruptured intracranial berry aneurysm**
Adults: 60 mg PO every 4 hours, given 1 hour before or 2 hours after a meal, for 21 days. Begin therapy within 96 hours after subarachnoid hemorrhage.
Adjust-a-dose: For patients with hepatic failure or cirrhosis, 30 mg PO every 4 hours for 21 days.

nintedanib esylate
nin-TED-a-nib

Ofev

Therapeutic class: Miscellaneous respiratory drugs
Pharmacologic class: Tyrosine kinase inhibitors

AVAILABLE FORMS
Capsules ⓞⓝⓒ: 100 mg, 150 mg

INDICATIONS & DOSAGES
ⓘ *Alert:* Obtain LFT and pregnancy test results before treatment starts.
➤ **Idiopathic pulmonary fibrosis**
Adults: 150 mg PO b.i.d. approximately 12 hours apart with food.
Adjust-a-dose: In patients with mild hepatic impairment (Child-Pugh class A), give 100 mg b.i.d. approximately 12 hours apart with food. Refer to manufacturer's instructions for toxicity-related dosage adjustments.

nisoldipine
nye-SOHL-di-peen

Sular

Therapeutic class: Antihypertensives
Pharmacologic class: Calcium channel blockers

AVAILABLE FORMS
Tablets (extended-release) ⓞⓝⓒ: 8.5 mg, 17 mg, 20 mg, 25.5 mg, 30 mg, 34 mg, 40 mg

INDICATIONS & DOSAGES
➤ **HTN**
Adults: Dosage must be adjusted to each patient's needs. Initially, 17 mg PO once daily, 1 hour before or 2 hours after a meal, increased by 8.5 mg/week or at longer intervals, as needed. Usual maintenance dose is 17 to 34 mg daily. Doses of more than 34 mg daily aren't recommended. Or, initially, 20 mg PO once daily, 1 hour before or 2 hours after a meal, increased by 10 mg/week or at longer intervals, as needed. Usual maintenance dose is 20 to 40 mg daily. Doses of more than 60 mg daily aren't recommended.
Patients older than age 65: Initially, 8.5 mg PO once daily; adjust dosage as for other adults.
Adjust-a-dose: For patients with hepatic impairment, initially 8.5 mg PO once daily; dosage is adjusted as for adults.

✤Canada   ◇OTC   ◆Off-label use   ✐Photoguide   ⓞⓝⓒDo not crush   *Liquid contains alcohol   ⚕Genetic

nitazoxanide
nye-te-ZOCKS-a-nide

Alinia

Therapeutic class: Antiprotozoals
Pharmacologic class: Antiprotozoals

AVAILABLE FORMS
Oral suspension: 100 mg/5 mL
Tablets: 500 mg

INDICATIONS & DOSAGES
➤ **Diarrhea caused by** *Cryptosporidium parvum* **or** *Giardia lamblia*
Adults and children age 12 and older: 500 mg PO with food every 12 hours for 3 days.
Children ages 4 to 11: 200 mg (10 mL) PO with food every 12 hours for 3 days.
Children ages 1 to 3: 100 mg (5 mL) PO with food every 12 hours for 3 days.

nusinersen sodium
neu-si-NER-sen

Spinraza

Therapeutic class: Miscellaneous CNS agents
Pharmacologic class: Antisense oligonucleotides

AVAILABLE FORMS
Injection: 12 mg/5 mL single-use vials

INDICATIONS & DOSAGES
➤ **Spinal muscular atrophy**
Adults and children: Initially, 12 mg (5 mL) intrathecally once every 14 days for three doses; then 12 mg intrathecally once 30 days after third dose. Administer a maintenance dose of 12 mg intrathecally once every 4 months thereafter.

obeticholic acid
oh-BET-i-kol-ik

Ocaliva

Therapeutic class: Miscellaneous GI drugs
Pharmacologic class: Farnesoid X receptor agonists

AVAILABLE FORMS
Tablets: 5 mg, 10 mg

INDICATIONS & DOSAGES
Black Box Warning Hepatic decompensation and failure, in some cases fatal, have been reported in patients with primary biliary cholangitis with decompensated cirrhosis or Child-Pugh class B or C hepatic impairment when drug was given more frequently than recommended. ■
➤ **Primary biliary cholangitis in combination with ursodeoxycholic acid (UDCA) in adults with an inadequate response to UDCA, or as monotherapy in adults unable to tolerate UDCA**

Adults: Before starting drug in patients with suspected cirrhosis, refer to manufacturer's instructions to determine their Child-Pugh classification and appropriate starting dosage.

Give 5 mg PO once daily in patients who are noncirrhotic or compensated Child-Pugh class A who haven't achieved an adequate biochemical response to an appropriate dosage of UDCA for at least 1 year or are intolerant to UDCA. If an adequate reduction in alkaline phosphatase or total bilirubin level hasn't been achieved after 3 months and patient is tolerating drug, increase to maximum dosage of 10 mg once daily. Before dosage adjustment, recalculate Child-Pugh classification.
Adjust-a-dose: **Black Box Warning** Recommended starting dosage for patients with Child-Pugh class B or C hepatic impairment or a prior decompensation event is 5 mg once weekly. ■

If an adequate reduction in alkaline phosphatase or total bilirubin level hasn't been achieved after 3 months and patient is tolerating drug, increase to maximum dosage of 5 mg twice weekly, with doses given at least 3 days apart. May titrate to 10 mg twice weekly based on response and tolerability.

Reduce dosing frequency from once daily to once weekly as appropriate for patients who progress to advanced disease. Refer to manufacturer's instructions for toxicity-related dosage adjustments.

obiltoxaximab
oh-bil-tox-AX-i-mab

Anthim

Therapeutic class: Antibodies
Pharmacologic class: Monoclonal antibodies

AVAILABLE FORMS
Injection: 600 mg/6 mL single-dose vials

INDICATIONS & DOSAGES
Black Box Warning Because of risk of hypersensitivity and anaphylaxis, administer drug in a setting monitored by trained personnel and equipped to manage anaphylaxis. ■
➤ **Inhalational anthrax due to** *Bacillus anthracis* **in combination with appropriate antibacterial drugs; prophylaxis of inhalational anthrax due to** *B. anthracis* **when alternative therapies aren't available or aren't appropriate**
Adults weighing more than 40 kg: 16 mg/kg/dose IV over 90 minutes as a single dose.
Adults and children weighing more than 15 to 40 kg: 24 mg/kg/dose IV over 90 minutes as a single dose.
Children weighing 15 kg or less: 32 mg/kg/dose IV over 90 minutes as a single dose.

ofloxacin (otic)
Therapeutic class: Antibiotics
Pharmacologic class: Fluoroquinolones

AVAILABLE FORMS
Otic solution: 0.3%

✚ Canada   ◇ OTC   ◆ Off-label use   ⚕ Photoguide   ⓓ Do not crush   *Liquid contains alcohol   ❀ Genetic

INDICATIONS & DOSAGES
➤ **Chronic suppurative otitis media with perforated tympanic membrane**
Adults and children age 12 and older: 10 drops instilled into the affected ear b.i.d. for 14 days.
➤ **Otitis externa**
Adults and children age 13 and older: 10 drops instilled into the affected ear once daily for 7 days.
Children ages 6 months to younger than 13 years: 5 drops into the affected ear once daily for 7 days.
➤ **Acute otitis media in children with tympanostomy tubes**
Children ages 1 to 12: 5 drops instilled into the affected ear b.i.d. for 10 days.

SAFETY ALERT!

olaparib ☒
oh-LAP-a-rib

Lynparza

Therapeutic class: Antineoplastics
Pharmacologic class: Poly ADP-ribose polymerase inhibitors

AVAILABLE FORMS
Tablets ⓓ*:* 100 mg, 150 mg

INDICATIONS & DOSAGES
Adjust-a-dose (for all indications): For patients with moderate renal impairment (CrCl of 31 to 50 mL/minute), reduce dosage to 200 mg PO b.i.d. Refer to manufacturer's instructions for toxicity-related dosage adjustments and drug's use with CYP3A inhibitors.
➤ **Deleterious or suspected deleterious germline or somatic *BRCA*-mutated advanced ovarian cancer, as detected by FDA-approved test, in women who have been treated with three or more prior lines of chemotherapy** ☒
Adults: 300 mg PO b.i.d. Continue treatment until disease progression or unacceptable toxicity occurs.
➤ **Deleterious or suspected deleterious germline *BRCA*-mutated, HER2-negative metastatic breast cancer in patients who have previously been treated with chemotherapy in the neoadjuvant, adjuvant, or metastatic setting** ☒
Adults: 300 mg PO b.i.d. for a total daily dose of 600 mg until disease progression or unacceptable toxicity occurs.
➤ **Maintenance treatment of recurrent epithelial ovarian, fallopian tube, or primary peritoneal cancer in patients who are in a complete or partial response to platinum-based chemotherapy**
Adults: 300 mg PO b.i.d. Continue treatment until disease progression or unacceptable toxicity occurs.

SAFETY ALERT!

olaratumab
oh-LAR-a-tue-mab

Lartruvo

Therapeutic class: Antineoplastics
Pharmacologic class: Recombinant human IgG1 monoclonal blocking antibodies

AVAILABLE FORMS
Injection: 190 mg/19 mL, 500 mg/50 mL in single-use vials

INDICATIONS & DOSAGES
➤ **Soft-tissue sarcoma with a histologic subtype appropriate for an anthracycline-containing regimen, when radiotherapy or surgery isn't a curative option**
Adults: 15 mg/kg IV over 60 minutes on days 1 and 8 of each 21-day cycle until disease progression or unacceptable toxicity occurs. For first eight cycles, give with doxorubicin.
Adjust-a-dose: Refer to manufacturer's instructions for toxicity-related dosage adjustments.

olopatadine hydrochloride
oh-loh-PAT-ah-dine

Pataday, Patanase, Patanol, Pazeo

Therapeutic class: Antihistamines
Pharmacologic class: H_1-receptor antagonists

AVAILABLE FORMS
Nasal spray: 0.6%
Ophthalmic solution: 0.1%, 0.2%, 0.7%

INDICATIONS & DOSAGES
➤ **Seasonal allergic rhinitis (nasal)**
Adults and children age 12 and older: 2 sprays into each nostril b.i.d.
Children ages 6 to 11: 1 spray into each nostril b.i.d.
➤ **Allergic conjunctivitis**
Adults and children age 3 and older (Patanol): 1 drop (0.1%) in each affected eye b.i.d. at an interval of 6 to 8 hours.
Adults and children age 2 and older (Pataday, Pazeo): 1 drop (0.2%, 0.7%) in each affected eye once a day.

orlistat
ORE-lah-stat

Alli ◇, Xenical

Therapeutic class: Antiobesity drugs
Pharmacologic class: Lipase inhibitors

AVAILABLE FORMS
Capsules: 60 mg ◇, 120 mg

INDICATIONS & DOSAGES
➤ **To manage obesity, including weight loss and weight maintenance with a reduced-calorie diet; to reduce risk of weight gain after previous weight loss**
Adults and children ages 12 and older: 120 mg PO t.i.d. with or up to 1 hour after each main meal containing fat.
➤ **Weight loss (OTC formulation)**
Adults age 18 and older: One 60-mg capsule PO with each meal containing fat. Dosage shouldn't exceed 3 capsules a day.

---

oxacillin sodium
oks-a-SIL-in

Bactocill in Dextrose

Therapeutic class: Antibiotics
Pharmacologic class: Penicillins

AVAILABLE FORMS
Injection: 1-g, 2-g, 10-g vials; 1 g/50 mL, 2 g/50 mL premixed solution

INDICATIONS & DOSAGES
➤ **Infections caused by penicillinase-producing staphylococci that have demonstrated susceptibility to the drug; empirical therapy in suspected cases of resistant staphylococcal infections**
Adults: For mild to moderate infections, 250 to 500 mg IV or IM every 4 to 6 hours. For severe infections, 1 g IV or IM every 4 to 6 hours.
Infants and children weighing less than 40 kg: For mild to moderate infections, 50 mg/kg/day IV or IM in equally divided doses every 6 hours. For severe infections, 100 mg/kg/day IV or IM in equally divided doses every 4 to 6 hours.
Adjust-a-dose: Duration of therapy depends on type and severity of the infection and overall condition of patient. In severe infections, continue drug for at least 14 days. Continue drug for at least 48 hours after patient is afebrile and asymptomatic and cultures are negative. Treatment of endocarditis and osteomyelitis may require a longer duration of therapy. Consider dosage reduction in patients with known or suspected renal impairment.

ozenoxacin
oz-en-OX-a-sin

Xepi

Therapeutic class: Antibiotics
Pharmacologic class: Quinolone antibiotics

AVAILABLE FORMS
Cream: 1%

INDICATIONS & DOSAGES
➤ **Impetigo due to *Staphylococcus aureus* or *Streptococcus pyogenes***
Adults and children age 2 months and older: Apply a thin layer topically to affected areas b.i.d. for 5 days.

SAFETY ALERT!

panitumumab ⚛
pan-eh-TOO-moo-mab

Vectibix

Therapeutic class: Antineoplastics
Pharmacologic class: Monoclonal antibodies

AVAILABLE FORMS
Solution for infusion: 20 mg/mL

INDICATIONS & DOSAGES
Black Box Warning Dermatologic toxicities occur in 90% of patients and are severe in 15%. ■

➤ **Wild-type RAS (defined as wild-type in both KRAS and NRAS as determined by an FDA-approved test) metastatic colorectal cancer as first-line therapy in combination with FOLFOX (5-FU, leucovorin, oxaliplatin); as monotherapy following disease progression during or after fluoropyrimidine-, oxaliplatin-, and irinotecan-containing regimens ⚛**
Adults: 6 mg/kg IV infusion over 60 minutes every 14 days as a single agent or in combination with FOLFOX. For doses greater than 1,000 mg, infuse over 90 minutes.
Adjust-a-dose: For patients with mild or moderate (grade 1 or 2) infusion reactions, reduce infusion rate by 50%. For patients with severe infusion reactions, stop drug permanently. Refer to manufacturer's instructions for toxicity-related dosage adjustments and drug discontinuation.

parathyroid hormone
par-a-THYE-roid

Natpara

Therapeutic class: Hormone replacements
Pharmacologic class: Parathyroid hormone analogues

AVAILABLE FORMS
Injection: 25 mcg, 50 mcg, 75 mcg, 100 mcg multi-dose cartridges

INDICATIONS & DOSAGES
Black Box Warning May increase risk of osteosarcoma. Reserve use for patients for whom the potential benefits outweigh this potential risk. ■
➤ **Adjunct to calcium and vitamin D to control hypocalcemia in patients with hypoparathyroidism who can't be well controlled on calcium supplements and active forms of vitamin D alone**
Adults: Initially, 50 mcg subcut once daily. Titrate maintenance dose to lowest dose that achieves a total albumin-corrected serum calcium level within the lower half of the normal total serum calcium range (between 8 and 9 mg/dL) without the need for active forms of vitamin D and with calcium supplementation sufficient to meet daily requirements. Maximum dose is 100 mcg daily.
Adjust-a-dose: If albumin-corrected serum calcium level can't be maintained above 8 mg/dL without an active form of vitamin D or oral calcium supplementation, may increase Natpara dosage in increments of 25 mcg every 4 weeks to a maximum daily dose of 100 mcg. If total serum calcium level is repeatedly above 9 mg/dL after active form of vitamin D has been discontinued and calcium supplement has been decreased to a dosage sufficient to meet daily requirements, may decrease Natpara dosage to 25 mcg/day.

patiromer sorbitex calcium
pa-TIR-oh-mer

Veltassa

Therapeutic class: Potassium-removing resins
Pharmacologic class: Cation exchange polymers

AVAILABLE FORMS
Oral powder: 8.4-g, 16.8-g, 25.2-g packets

INDICATIONS & DOSAGES
➤ **Nonemergency treatment of hyperkalemia**
Adults: Initially, 8.4 g PO once daily. Monitor serum potassium level and adjust dosage based on potassium level at intervals of 1 week or longer, in increments of 8.4 g, to reach desired potassium concentration. Maximum dosage is 25.2 g once daily.

SAFETY ALERT!

PAZOPanib
paz-OH-pa-nib

Votrient

Therapeutic class: Antineoplastics
Pharmacologic class: Multi-tyrosine kinase inhibitors

AVAILABLE FORMS
Tablets: 200 mg

INDICATIONS & DOSAGES
Black Box Warning Severe and fatal hepatotoxicity has been observed in clinical trials. ■
➤ **Advanced renal cell carcinoma, soft-tissue sarcoma in patients who have received prior chemotherapy**
Adults: 800 mg PO daily at least 1 hour before or 2 hours after a meal.
Adjust-a-dose: For patients with moderate hepatic impairment, 200 mg PO daily. Drug isn't recommended for patients with severe hepatic impairment. When coadministration of strong CYP3A4 inhibitors (clarithromycin, ketoconazole, ritonavir) is necessary, decrease pazopanib dosage to 400 mg PO daily.

peginterferon beta-1a
peg-in-ter-FEER-on

Plegridy, Plegridy Starter

Therapeutic class: Antivirals
Pharmacologic class: Biological response modifiers

AVAILABLE FORMS
Injection: 125 mcg/0.5 mL in single-dose prefilled syringes; 63 mcg/0.5 mL, 94 mcg/0.5 mL pen-injector, prefilled syringes

INDICATIONS & DOSAGES
➤ **Relapsing forms of MS**
Adults: On day 1, 63 mcg subcut. On day 15, 94 mcg subcut. On day 29 and every 14 days thereafter, 125 mcg subcut.

pegloticase
peg-LOE-ti-kase

Krystexxa

Therapeutic class: Antigout agents
Pharmacologic class: Uric acid–specific enzymes

AVAILABLE FORMS
Injection: 8 mg/mL in 2-mL single-use vial

INDICATIONS & DOSAGES
➤ **Treatment of chronic gout in patients refractory to conventional therapy**
Adults: 8 mg by IV infusion every 2 weeks.

pegvaliase-pqpz
peg-VAL-i-ase pqpz

Palynziq

Therapeutic class: Phenylalanine reducers
Pharmacologic class: Phenylalanine-metabolizing enzymes

AVAILABLE FORMS
Injection: 2.5 mg/0.5 mL, 10 mg/0.5 mL, 20 mg/mL in single-dose prefilled syringes

INDICATIONS & DOSAGES
➤ **To reduce blood phenylalanine concentrations in patients with phenylketonuria (PKU) who have uncontrolled blood phenylalanine concentrations greater than 600 micromol/L on existing management**
Adults: Initially, 2.5 mg subcut once weekly for 4 weeks. Then titrate dosage in step-wise fashion over at least 5 weeks to achieve a dosage of 20 mg subcut once daily. After giving 2.5 mg once weekly for 4 weeks, titrate as follows: 2.5 mg subcut twice weekly for 1 week, then 10 mg subcut once weekly for 1 week, then 10 mg subcut twice weekly for 1 week, then 10 mg subcut four times per week for 1 week, then 10 mg subcut once daily for 1 week, then maintenance dose of 20 mg subcut once daily for at least 24 weeks.

Consider a dosage increase to a maximum dose of 40 mg subcut once daily in patients who have been maintained continuously on 20 mg once daily for at least 24 weeks and who haven't achieved a response of at least a 20% reduction in blood phenylalanine concentration from pretreatment baseline or a blood phenylalanine concentration of 600 micromol/L or less. Use lowest effective and tolerated dosage.
Adjust-a-dose: For patients with blood phenylalanine concentrations less than 30 micromol/L, may reduce dosage with or without dietary protein and phenylalanine intake modification to maintain phenylalanine level above 30 micromol/L. Discontinue drug in patients who haven't achieved a response after 16 weeks of continuous treatment with 40 mg subcut once daily.

✦Canada   ◇OTC   ◆Off-label use   ✐Photoguide   ⊕Do not crush   *Liquid contains alcohol   ▓Genetic

pentoxifylline
pen-tox-IH-fi-leen

Therapeutic class: Hemorrheologic drugs
Pharmacologic class: Xanthine derivatives

AVAILABLE FORMS
Tablets (extended-release): 400 mg

INDICATIONS & DOSAGES
➤ **Intermittent claudication from chronic occlusive vascular disease**
Adults: 400 mg PO t.i.d. with meals for at least 8 weeks. May decrease to 400 mg b.i.d. if GI and CNS adverse effects occur. If adverse effects persist, discontinue drug.
Adjust-a-dose: For CrCl less than 30 mL/minute, reduce dosage to 400 mg once daily.

perampanel
per-AMP-an-ell

Fycompa

Therapeutic class: Anticonvulsants
Pharmacologic class: Noncompetitive AMPA receptor antagonists
Controlled substance schedule: III

AVAILABLE FORMS
Oral suspension: 0.5 mg/mL
Tablets: 2 mg, 4 mg, 6 mg, 8 mg, 10 mg, 12 mg

INDICATIONS & DOSAGES
Black Box Warning Serious or life-threatening psychiatric and behavioral adverse reactions have been reported in patients with and without prior psychiatric history. ■
Adjust-a-dose (for all indications): In elderly patients, don't increase dosage more frequently than every 2 weeks. In patients with mild hepatic impairment, increase daily dose by 2 mg no more frequently than every 2 weeks; maximum is 6 mg once daily. In patients with moderate hepatic impairment, increase daily dose by 2 mg no more frequently than every 2 weeks; maximum is 4 mg once daily. Refer to manufacturer's instructions for use with CYP3A4 inducers.
➤ **Monotherapy or adjunctive therapy for partial-onset seizures with or without secondarily generalized seizures in patients with epilepsy**
Adults and children age 12 and older: Initially, 2 mg PO once daily at bedtime. Increase dosage in increments of 2 mg once daily based on clinical response and tolerability and not more frequently than at weekly intervals. Recommended maintenance dose is 8 to 12 mg once daily at bedtime, although some patients may respond to 4 mg once daily.
➤ **Adjunctive therapy in treatment of primary generalized tonic-clonic seizures in patients with epilepsy**
Adults and children age 12 and older: Initially, 2 mg PO once daily at bedtime. Increase dosage in increments of 2 mg once daily based on clinical response

and tolerability and not more frequently than at weekly intervals. Recommended maintenance dose in monotherapy or adjunctive therapy is 8 mg once daily at bedtime, although if needed, may increase dosage to 12 mg once daily.

peramivir
per-AM-i-vir

Rapivab

Therapeutic class: Antivirals
Pharmacologic class: Neuraminidase inhibitors

AVAILABLE FORMS
Injection: 200 mg/20 mL (10 mg/mL) vials

INDICATIONS & DOSAGES
➤ **Acute uncomplicated influenza in patients who have been symptomatic for no more than 2 days**
Adults and adolescents age 13 and older: 600 mg IV infusion over 15 to 30 minutes as a single dose.
Adjust-a-dose: For patients with CrCl of 30 to 49 mL/minute, dose is 200 mg; for patients with CrCl of 10 to 29 mL/minute, dose is 100 mg. For patients with ESRD requiring dialysis, give after dialysis at a dose adjusted for renal function.
Children ages 2 to 12: 12 mg/kg (up to 600 mg) IV infusion over 15 to 30 minutes as a single dose.
Adjust-a-dose: For patients with CrCl of 30 to 49 mL/minute, dose is 4 mg/kg; for patients with CrCl of 10 to 29 mL/minute, dose is 2 mg/kg. For patients with ESRD requiring dialysis, give after dialysis at a dose adjusted for renal function.

perindopril erbumine
pur-IN-doh-pril

Coversyl✦, Coversyl Plus✦

Therapeutic class: Antihypertensives
Pharmacologic class: ACE inhibitors

AVAILABLE FORMS
Tablets: 2 mg, 4 mg, 8 mg

INDICATIONS & DOSAGES
Black Box Warning May cause fetal harm; when pregnancy is detected, discontinue drug as soon as possible. ■
Adjust-a-dose (for all indications): For patients with renal insufficiency and CrCl of 30 mL/minute or greater, initially 2 mg PO daily. Maximum daily maintenance dose is 8 mg. Not recommended for patients with CrCl of less than 30 mL/minute. For patients taking diuretics, consider reducing the diuretic dose before initiating drug. If diuretic therapy can't be altered, monitor patient closely for at least 2 hours after initiating perindopril and until BP has stabilized for another hour. Adjust dosage based on patient's BP response.
➤ **To reduce the risk of CV death or nonfatal MI in patients with stable CAD**
Adults age 70 or younger: 4 mg PO once daily for 2 weeks; then, increase as tolerated to 8 mg once daily.

Adults older than age 70: Initially, 2 mg PO once daily for the first week; then, 4 mg once daily for the second week and 8 mg once daily after that, if tolerated.

➤ **Essential HTN**

Adults: Initially, 4 mg PO once daily. Increase dosage until BP is controlled or to maximum of 16 mg/day; usual maintenance dosage is 4 to 8 mg once daily; may be given in two divided doses.

Adults older than age 65: Initially, 4 mg PO daily as one dose or in two divided doses. May increase dosage by more than 8 mg/day with careful BP monitoring.

---

permethrin
per-METH-rin

Elimite, Kwellada-P✽◇, Nix◇

Therapeutic class: Scabicides–pediculicides
Pharmacologic class: Pyrethroids

AVAILABLE FORMS
Cream: 5%
Lotion: 1%◇✽

INDICATIONS & DOSAGES
➤ **Infestation with *Pediculus humanus capitis* (head louse) and its nits (lotion)**

Adults and children age 2 months and older: Use after hair has been washed with conditioner-free shampoo, rinsed with water, and towel dried. Apply a sufficient amount (25 to 50 mL) of liquid to saturate hair and scalp. Allow drug to remain on hair for 10 minutes before rinsing off with warm water. Remove remaining nits with comb. Usually only one application is needed. May repeat 7 days after first treatment if lice or nits are still present.

➤ **Infestation with *Sarcoptes scabiei* (cream)**

Adults and children age 2 months and older: Thoroughly massage into the skin from the head to the soles of feet. Treat infants on hairline, neck, scalp, temple, and forehead. Wash cream off after 8 to 14 hours. Usually one application is needed. May retreat if living mites are observed 14 days after first treatment.

---

perphenazine
per-FEN-uh-zeen

Therapeutic class: Antipsychotics
Pharmacologic class: Phenothiazines

AVAILABLE FORMS
Tablets: 2 mg, 4 mg, 8 mg, 16 mg

INDICATIONS & DOSAGES
Black Box Warning Not approved to treat patients with dementia-related psychosis. Use with opioids can cause death. ■

➤ **Schizophrenia in nonhospitalized patients**

Adults and children older than age 12: Initially, 4 to 8 mg PO t.i.d.; reduce as soon as possible to minimum effective dose.

➤ **Schizophrenia in hospitalized patients**

Adults and children older than age 12: Initially, 8 to 16 mg PO b.i.d., t.i.d., or q.i.d.; increase to 64 mg daily, as needed.

➤ **Severe nausea and vomiting**

Adults: 8 to 16 mg PO daily in divided doses to maximum of 24 mg.

---

pirfenidone
peer-FEH-nih-dohn

Esbriet

Therapeutic class: Miscellaneous respiratory drugs
Pharmacologic class: Antifibrotics

AVAILABLE FORMS
Capsules 🅓🅒: 267 mg
Tablets: 267 mg, 801 mg

INDICATIONS & DOSAGES
➤ **Idiopathic pulmonary fibrosis**

Adults: Initially, 267 mg PO t.i.d. days 1 to 7 of therapy; then increase to 534 mg PO t.i.d. for 7 more days (days 8 to 14); then increase to 801 mg PO t.i.d. starting on day 15 of therapy. Maintenance dosage is 801 mg PO t.i.d. Maximum dose is 2,403 mg/day.

Adjust-a-dose: Refer to manufacturer's instructions for toxicity-related dosage adjustments and use with CYP1A2 inhibitors.

---

plerixafor
pleh-RIX-uh-for

Mozobil

Therapeutic class: Hematopoietics
Pharmacologic class: CXCR4 chemokine receptor inhibitors

AVAILABLE FORMS
Injection: 24 mg/1.2 mL in single-use vials

INDICATIONS & DOSAGES
➤ **To mobilize hematopoietic stem cells for collection and subsequent autologous transplantation in patients with non-Hodgkin lymphoma and multiple myeloma**

Adults: Initiate plerixafor treatment once daily, 0.24 mg/kg (actual body weight) subcut; or for patients weighing 83 kg or less, give 20 mg fixed dose subcut, in the evening or approximately 11 hours before initiation of each apheresis, after patient has received G-CSF 10 mcg/kg once daily in the morning for 4 days. Repeat plerixafor dose for up to 4 consecutive evenings and administer G-CSF 10 mcg/kg on each day before apheresis. Don't exceed 40 mg/day.

Adjust-a-dose: For patients with CrCl of 50 mL/minute or less, give 0.16 mg/kg once daily (not to exceed 27 mg/day), or for patients weighing 83 kg or less, give fixed dose of 13 mg.

---

potassium iodide
po-TASS-ee-um

Iosat◇, ThyroSafe◇, ThyroShield◇

Therapeutic class: Antihyperthyroid drugs
Pharmacologic class: Salts of stable iodine

AVAILABLE FORMS
Oral solution: 65 mg/mL
Tablets: 65 mg, 130 mg

INDICATIONS & DOSAGES
➤ **Radiation protectant for thyroid gland (Iosat, ThyroSafe, ThyroShield)**
Adults and children ages 12 to 18 weighing at least 68 kg: 130 mg PO every 24 hours for 10 to 14 days as directed by public health authorities. Start no later than 3 to 4 hours after exposure. Avoid repeat dosing in pregnant or breastfeeding women.
Children ages 3 to 12 or children ages 12 to 18 weighing less than 68 kg: 65 mg PO every 24 hours as directed by public health authorities. Start no later than 3 to 4 hours after exposure.
Children older than 1 month to 3 years: 32.5 mg PO every 24 hours as directed by public health authorities. Start no later than 3 to 4 hours after exposure.
Neonates from birth to 1 month: 16.25 mg PO every 24 hours as directed by public health authorities. Start no later than 3 to 4 hours after exposure. Avoid repeat dosing, if possible.

SAFETY ALERT!

PRALAtrexate
PRAL-ah-TREX-ate

Folotyn

Therapeutic class: Antineoplastics
Pharmacologic class: Folate analogue metabolic inhibitors

AVAILABLE FORMS
Injection: 20 mg/mL, 40 mg/2 mL in single-use vials

INDICATIONS & DOSAGES
➤ **Relapsed or refractory peripheral T-cell lymphoma**
Adults: 30 mg/m^2 IV push over 3 to 5 minutes weekly for 6 weeks in 7-week cycles until disease progresses or unacceptable toxicity develops. Initiate supplementation with folic acid and vitamin B_{12} before treatment.
Adjust-a-dose: Refer to manufacturer's instructions for dosage adjustments for hematologic and nonhematologic toxicities.

prasterone
PRAS-ter-one

Intrarosa

Therapeutic class: Hormone replacements
Pharmacologic class: Synthetic steroids

AVAILABLE FORMS
Vaginal insert: 6.5 mg

INDICATIONS & DOSAGES
➤ **Treatment of moderate to severe dyspareunia, a symptom of vulvar and vaginal atrophy, due to menopause**
Adults: 1 vaginal insert intravaginally once daily at bedtime.

primidone
PRI-mi-done

Mysoline

Therapeutic class: Anticonvulsants
Pharmacologic class: Barbiturate analogues

AVAILABLE FORMS
Tablets: 50 mg, 250 mg

INDICATIONS & DOSAGES
➤ **Grand mal, psychomotor, and focal epileptic seizures**
Adults and children age 8 and older: Initially, 100 to 125 mg PO at bedtime on days 1 to 3; then 100 to 125 mg PO b.i.d. on days 4 to 6; then 100 to 125 mg PO t.i.d. on days 7 to 9, followed by maintenance dose of 250 mg PO t.i.d. May increase maintenance dose to 250 mg q.i.d., if needed. May increase dosage to maximum of 2 g daily in divided doses. See manufacturer's instructions for beginning therapy in patients already receiving other anticonvulsants.
Children younger than age 8: Initially, 50 mg PO at bedtime for 3 days; then 50 mg PO b.i.d. for days 4 to 6; then 100 mg PO b.i.d. for days 7 to 9, followed by maintenance dose of 125 to 250 mg PO t.i.d. or 10 to 25 mg/kg daily in divided doses.

probenecid
proe-BEN-e-sid

Therapeutic class: Uricosurics
Pharmacologic class: Sulfonamide derivatives

AVAILABLE FORMS
Tablets: 500 mg

INDICATIONS & DOSAGES
➤ **Adjunct to penicillin therapy**
Adults and children age 15 and older weighing more than 50 kg: 500 mg PO q.i.d.
Children ages 2 to 14 or weighing 50 kg or less: Initially, 25 mg/kg or 0.7 g/m^2 PO; then 40 mg/kg/day or 1.2 g/m^2 in four divided doses daily.
➤ **Hyperuricemia of gout, gouty arthritis**
Adults: 250 mg PO b.i.d. for first week; then 500 mg b.i.d. Review maintenance dose every 6 months and reduce daily dosage by increments of 500 mg, if indicated.

pyrazinamide
peer-a-ZIN-a-mide

Therapeutic class: Antituberculotics
Pharmacologic class: Nicotinamide analogues

AVAILABLE FORMS
Tablets: 500 mg

INDICATIONS & DOSAGES
➤ **Initial treatment of active TB with other antituberculotics or after treatment failure with other primary drugs in any form of active TB**

Adults and children: 15 to 30 mg/kg PO once daily. Don't exceed 3 g/day. Or, 50 to 70 mg/kg lean body weight PO twice weekly. This dosage may exceed the recommended 3-g/day maximum dose, but an increased incidence of adverse reactions hasn't been reported. Administer pyrazinamide for first 2 months of a 6-month or longer treatment regimen for drug-susceptible tuberculosis. Treat known or suspected drug-resistant infections with individualized regimens, which may frequently include pyrazinamide.

HIV-infected patients may need longer courses of therapy. Refer to the CDC (www.CDC.gov) for current treatment recommendations and complete drug regimens.

Adjust-a-dose: For elderly patients, use doses at the low end of the dosing range.

pyrimethamine
pihr-ih-METH-ah-meen

Daraprim

Therapeutic class: Antimalarials
Pharmacologic class: Folate antagonists

AVAILABLE FORMS
Tablets: 25 mg

INDICATIONS & DOSAGES
➤ **Treatment of toxoplasmosis**
Adults: Initially, 50 to 75 mg PO with 1 to 4 g of a sulfonamide (such as sulfadiazine) and leucovorin calcium daily; continue for 1 to 3 weeks. After 3 weeks, reduce dosage of pyrimethamine and the sulfonamide by half and continue for 4 to 5 weeks.
Children: Initially, 1 mg/kg/day PO in two equally divided doses for 2 to 4 days with a sulfonamide and leucovorin calcium at a pediatric dosage; then 0.5 mg/kg daily divided into two equal doses for 4 weeks, along with a sulfonamide and leucovorin.

quinupristin–dalfopristin
QUIN-uh-pris-tin/DALF-oh-pris-tin

Synercid

Therapeutic class: Antibiotics
Pharmacologic class: Streptogramins

AVAILABLE FORMS
Injection: 500-mg vials (150 mg quinupristin and 350 mg dalfopristin)

INDICATIONS & DOSAGES
➤ **Complicated skin and skin-structure infections caused by methicillin-susceptible *Staphylococcus aureus* or *Streptococcus pyogenes***
Adults and adolescents age 12 and older: 7.5 mg/kg IV over 1 hour every 12 hours for at least 7 days.

radioactive iodine
(sodium iodide, 131I)
Hicon, Sodium Iodide 131I Therapeutic

Therapeutic class: Radiopharmaceuticals
Pharmacologic class: Antithyroid drugs

AVAILABLE FORMS
All radioactivity concentrations are determined at time of calibration.
Capsules: Radioactivity range, 0.75 to 100 mCi/capsule
Concentrated oral solution: 1,000 mCi/mL
Oral solution: Radioactivity range, 5 to 150 mCi/vial

INDICATIONS & DOSAGES
➤ **Hyperthyroidism**
Adults: Usual dosage is 4 to 10 mCi PO. Dosage is based on estimated weight of thyroid gland and thyroid uptake. Repeat treatment after 6 weeks, based on T_4 level as needed.
➤ **Thyroid cancer**
Adults: Initially, 30 to 100 mCi PO, with subsequent doses of 100 to 200 mCi for metastases. Dosage is based on estimated malignant thyroid tissue and metastatic tissue as determined by total body scan. Repeat treatment according to clinical status.
➤ **Thyroid function evaluation**
Adults: Dosage ranges from 5 to 100 mCi PO based on patient's weight and type of procedure.

regorafenib 🍽
RE-goe-RAF-e-nib

Stivarga

Therapeutic class: Antineoplastics
Pharmacologic class: Kinase inhibitors

AVAILABLE FORMS
Tablets: 40 mg

INDICATIONS & DOSAGES
Black Box Warning May cause severe or fatal hepatotoxicity. Monitor closely. ∎
Adjust-a-dose (for all indications): Refer to manufacturer's instructions for toxicity-related dosage adjustments and discontinuation.
➤ **Metastatic colorectal cancer previously treated with fluoropyrimidine-, oxaliplatin-, and irinotecan-based chemotherapy, an anti–vascular endothelial growth factor therapy and, if *KRAS* wild type, an anti–epidermal growth factor receptor therapy 🍽**
Adults: 160 mg PO once a day for first 21 days of each 28-day cycle. Continue therapy until disease progression or unacceptable toxicity occurs.
➤ **Locally advanced, unresectable, or metastatic GI stromal tumor previously treated with imatinib mesylate and sunitinib malate**
Adults: 160 mg PO once daily for first 21 days of each 28-day cycle. Continue therapy until disease progression or unacceptable toxicity occurs.

➤ **Hepatocellular carcinoma in patients previously treated with sorafenib**
Adults: 160 mg PO once daily for first 21 days of each 28-day cycle. Continue treatment until progression or unacceptable toxicity occurs.

retapamulin
re-te-PAM-ue-lin

Altabax

Therapeutic class: Antibiotics
Pharmacologic class: Pleuromutilins

AVAILABLE FORMS
Topical ointment: 1%

INDICATIONS & DOSAGES
➤ **Impetigo due to** *Staphylococcus aureus* **(methicillin-susceptible isolates only) or** *Streptococcus pyogenes*
Adults and children age 9 months and older: Apply a thin layer to affected area (up to 100 cm² in total BSA in adults or 2% total BSA in children) b.i.d. for 5 days.

SAFETY ALERT!

reteplase (recombinant)
RET-ah-place

Retavase

Therapeutic class: Thrombolytics
Pharmacologic class: Tissue plasminogen activators

AVAILABLE FORMS
Injection: 10.4 units (18.1 mg)/vial, in a kit with components for reconstitution for two single-use vials

INDICATIONS & DOSAGES
➤ **To manage acute MI**
Adults: Double-bolus injection of 10 + 10 units. Give each bolus IV over 2 minutes. If complications, such as serious bleeding or anaphylactoid reaction, don't occur after first bolus, give second bolus 30 minutes after start of first.

rifabutin
rif-ah-BYOO-tin

Mycobutin

Therapeutic class: Antituberculotics
Pharmacologic class: Semisynthetic ansamycins

AVAILABLE FORMS
Capsules: 150 mg

INDICATIONS & DOSAGES
Adjust-a-dose (for all indications): For patients with CrCl of less than 30 mL/minute, reduce rifabutin dosage by 50%.
➤ **To prevent disseminated** *Mycobacterium avium* **complex in patients with advanced HIV infection**
Adults: 300 mg PO daily as a single dose or in two divided doses. May give with food or give 150 mg b.i.d. to minimize GI distress.

riluzole
RILL-yoo-zole

Rilutek

Therapeutic class: Neuroprotectors
Pharmacologic class: Benzothiazoles

AVAILABLE FORMS
Tablets: 50 mg

INDICATIONS & DOSAGES
➤ **Amyotrophic lateral sclerosis**
Adults: 50 mg PO every 12 hours, taken on empty stomach 1 hour before or 2 hours after a meal.

riociguat
RYE-oh-sig-ue-at

Adempas

Therapeutic class: Vasodilators
Pharmacologic class: Soluble guanylate cyclase stimulators

AVAILABLE FORMS
Tablets: 0.5 mg, 1 mg, 1.5 mg, 2 mg, 2.5 mg

INDICATIONS & DOSAGES
Black Box Warning Drug may cause fetal harm. Exclude pregnancy before treatment; patient should avoid pregnancy for 1 month after treatment. For females, Adempas is available only through a restricted program called the Adempas REMS Program. ∎
➤ **Chronic thromboembolic pulmonary HTN (CTEPH) (WHO Group 4), after surgical treatment, or inoperable CTEPH, to improve exercise capacity and WHO functional class; pulmonary artery HTN (WHO Group 1) to improve exercise capacity and WHO functional class and to delay clinical worsening**
Adults: Initially, 1 mg PO t.i.d. Increase dosage by 0.5 mg t.i.d. if systolic BP remains greater than 95 mm Hg and patient has no signs or symptoms of hypotension. Dosage increases should occur no less than 2 weeks apart. Titrate to highest tolerated dosage; maximum dose is 2.5 mg PO t.i.d.
Adjust-a-dose: Patients unable to tolerate initial 1-mg dosage due to hypotension may start at 0.5 mg PO t.i.d. Decrease dosage by 0.5 mg PO t.i.d. in patients experiencing hypotension. Patients who smoke may need dosages titrated higher than 2.5 mg PO t.i.d. Patients who quit smoking during treatment may need a dosage decrease. Consider a starting dose of 0.5 mg PO t.i.d. for patients taking strong CYP and P-gp/BCRP inhibitors (ketoconazole, itraconazole, ritonavir).

SAFETY ALERT!

romiDEPsin
roh-mih-DEP-sin

Istodax

Therapeutic class: Antineoplastics
Pharmacologic class: Histone deacetylase inhibitors

AVAILABLE FORMS
Injection: 10-mg vials

INDICATIONS & DOSAGES
Adjust-a-dose (for all indications): Refer to manufacturer's instructions for toxicity-related dosage adjustments and discontinuation.
➤ **Cutaneous T-cell lymphoma and peripheral T-cell lymphoma in patients who have received at least one prior systemic therapy**
Adults: 14 mg/m^2 by IV infusion over 4 hours on days 1, 8, and 15 of 28-day cycle. Repeat every 28 days if effective and well tolerated.

rufinamide
roo-FIN-ah-mide

Banzel

Therapeutic class: Anticonvulsants
Pharmacologic class: Triazole derivatives

AVAILABLE FORMS
Suspension: 40 mg/mL
Tablets: 200 mg, 400 mg

INDICATIONS & DOSAGES
➤ **Adjunct treatment of seizures associated with Lennox-Gastaut syndrome**
Adults and children age 17 and older: Initially, 400 to 800 mg PO daily in two equally divided doses. Increase dosage by 400 to 800 mg/day every 2 days to 3,200 mg PO daily in divided doses.
Children ages 1 to less than 17: Initially, 10 mg/kg/day PO in two equally divided doses. Increase dosage by 10 mg/kg every other day to 45 mg/kg/day or 3,200 mg (whichever is less) PO daily in divided doses.
Adjust-a-dose: Dialysis clears drug by 30%; dosage adjustment may be necessary. For patients taking valproate, start rufinamide at dosages less than 400 mg/day (adults) or less than 10 mg/kg/day (children).

saquinavir mesylate
sa-KWEN-ah-veer

Invirase

Therapeutic class: Antiretrovirals
Pharmacologic class: Protease inhibitors

AVAILABLE FORMS
Capsules (hard gelatin): 200 mg
Tablets (film-coated): 500 mg

INDICATIONS & DOSAGES
➤ **Adjunctive treatment of advanced HIV infection in selected patients, in combination with ritonavir and other retrovirals**

Adults and adolescents age 16 and older: Initially, in treatment-naive patients or patients switching from a regimen containing delavirdine or rilpivirine, give 500 mg PO b.i.d. with ritonavir 100 mg b.i.d. within 2 hours after a meal for first 7 days. In patients switching from a regimen that doesn't contain delavirdine or rilpivirine, give 1,000 mg PO b.i.d. with ritonavir 100 mg b.i.d. within 2 hours after a meal. Maintenance dosage after 7 days is 1,000 mg PO b.i.d. given at the same time with 100 mg ritonavir PO b.i.d. within 2 hours after a meal.

SAFETY ALERT!

scopolamine (hyoscine)
skoe-POL-a-meen

Transderm-Scop

Therapeutic class: Antispasmodics
Pharmacologic class: Belladonna alkaloids–antimuscarinics

AVAILABLE FORMS
Transdermal patch: 1.5 mg/2.5 cm^2 (1 mg/72 hours)

INDICATIONS & DOSAGES
➤ **To prevent postoperative nausea and vomiting**
Adults: Apply 1 transdermal patch the evening before scheduled surgery. To minimize exposure to newborns, apply patch 1 hour before cesarean birth. Keep patch in place for 24 hours after surgery, then remove and discard.
➤ **To prevent nausea and vomiting from motion sickness**
Adults: One transdermal patch, formulated to deliver 1 mg scopolamine over 3 days, applied to the skin behind the ear at least 4 hours before antiemetic effect is needed. Replace patch every 3 days if needed.

secnidazole
sek-NID-a-zole

Solosec

Therapeutic class: Antibiotics
Pharmacologic class: Nitroimidazoles

AVAILABLE FORMS
Oral granules: 2 g

INDICATIONS & DOSAGES
➤ **Bacterial vaginosis**
Adult women: One single dose of 2 g PO.

secukinumab
SEK-ue-KIN-ue-mab

Cosentyx, Cosentyx Sensoready Pen

Therapeutic class: Immunomodulators
Pharmacologic class: Human IgG1 monoclonal antibodies

AVAILABLE FORMS
Injection: 150 mg/mL auto-injector or prefilled syringes
Injection (lyophilized powder): 150 mg in single-use vials

✦Canada   ◇ OTC   ◆ Off-label use   ✐Photoguide   ⓝⓓⓒ Do not crush   *Liquid contains alcohol   ▨ Genetic

INDICATIONS & DOSAGES

➤ **Moderate to severe plaque psoriasis in patients who are candidates for systemic therapy or phototherapy; psoriatic arthritis in patients with coexistent moderate to severe plaque psoriasis**

Adults: 300 mg as two subcut injections of 150 mg each on weeks 0, 1, 2, 3, and 4; then 300 mg every 4 weeks thereafter. If clinically indicated, a 150-mg dose may be acceptable for some patients with plaque psoriasis.

➤ **Active psoriatic arthritis; active ankylosing spondylitis**

Adults: To use with a loading dose, give 150 mg subcut once weekly at weeks 0, 1, 2, 3, and 4; then 150 mg subcut every 4 weeks. To use without a loading dose, give 150 mg subcut every 4 weeks. For active psoriatic arthritis, may consider increasing dosage to 300 mg subcut every 4 weeks.

selexipag
se-LEX-i-pag

Uptravi

Therapeutic class: Vasodilators
Pharmacologic class: Prostacyclin receptor agonists

AVAILABLE FORMS

Tablets (extended-release) ⓓⓝⓒ: 200 mcg, 400 mcg, 600 mcg, 800 mcg, 1,000 mcg, 1,200 mcg, 1,400 mcg, 1,600 mcg

INDICATIONS & DOSAGES

➤ **Pulmonary arterial HTN (WHO Group I) to delay disease progression and reduce risk of hospitalization**

Adults: Initially, 200 mcg PO b.i.d. Increase dosage by increments of 200 mcg b.i.d. at weekly intervals to the highest tolerated dose. If dose isn't tolerated, decrease dosage to the previous tolerated dose. Maximum dose is 1,600 mcg b.i.d.

Adjust-a-dose: For patients with moderate hepatic impairment (Child-Pugh class B), initiate therapy at 200 mcg once daily and increase by 200-mcg increments once daily at weekly intervals, as tolerated. Avoid use in patients with severe hepatic impairment (Child-Pugh class C).

sertaconazole nitrate
sir-tah-KAHN-uh-zole

Ertaczo

Therapeutic class: Antifungals
Pharmacologic class: Imidazoles

AVAILABLE FORMS

Topical cream: 2%

INDICATIONS & DOSAGES

➤ **Interdigital tinea pedis caused by *Trichophyton rubrum*, *Trichophyton mentagrophytes*, or *Epidermophyton floccosum* in immunocompetent patients**

Adults and children age 12 and older: Apply cream b.i.d. to affected areas between toes and healthy surrounding areas for 4 weeks.

silver sulfadiazine
sul-fa-DYE-a-zeen

Flamazine ✤, Hydrogel Ag ◊, Silvadene, SSD, Thermazene

Therapeutic class: Antibacterials (topical)
Pharmacologic class: Broad-spectrum sulfonamides

AVAILABLE FORMS

Cream: 1%

INDICATIONS & DOSAGES

➤ **To prevent or treat wound infection in second- and third-degree burns**

Adults: Apply one-sixteenth-inch ribbon of cream to clean, debrided wound daily or b.i.d. Burn areas should be covered with cream at all times. Reapply to areas from which it has been removed by patient activity.

sodium bicarbonate

Therapeutic class: Antacids
Pharmacologic class: Alkalinizers

AVAILABLE FORMS

Injection: 4.2% (0.5 mEq/1 mL), 7.5% (8.92 mEq/10 mL), 44.6 mEq/50 mL), 8.4% (10 mEq/10 mL, 50 mEq/50 mL)
Powder: 30 mg/½ tsp ◊
Tablets: 325 mg ◊, 650 mg ◊

INDICATIONS & DOSAGES

➤ **Metabolic acidosis**

Adults and children: Dosage depends on blood carbon dioxide content, pH, and patient's condition; usually, 2 to 5 mEq/kg IV infused over 4- to 8-hour period.

➤ **Urinary alkalinization**

Adults: Initially, 4,000 mg PO; then 1,000 to 2,000 mg PO every 4 hours; dosage based on urine pH.
Children: 84 to 840 mg/kg PO daily in four divided doses. Titrate based on urine pH.

➤ **Antacid**

Adults: 650 mg to 2,600 mg PO up to every 4 hours taken with glass of water.
Adults and children older than age 12: 30 mg (½ tsp) oral powder in 120 mL water PO every 2 hours up to six doses daily for patients under age 60, or three doses daily for patients over age 60.

➤ **Cardiac arrest**

Adults and children age 2 and older: Administer according to results of arterial blood pH, partial pressure of arterial carbon dioxide, and calculated base deficit. Initially, 200 to 300 mEq of bicarbonate given as 7.5% or 8.4% solution. Then redetermine serum pH and bicarbonate concentration.
Children younger than age 2: 1 mEq/kg (1 mL/kg of 8.4% solution) IV slowly followed by 1 mEq/kg every 10 minutes of arrest. Don't give more than 8 mEq/kg IV total; a 4.2% solution may be preferred.

➤ **Prevention of contrast media nephrotoxicity** ◆
Adults: 154 mEq/L in dextrose 5% infusion as an IV
bolus of 3 mL/kg/hour for 1 hour immediately before
contrast administration, followed by an infusion of
1 mL/kg/hour for 6 hours after the procedure.

SAFETY ALERT!

sonidegib phosphate
SOE-ni-deg-ib

Odomzo

Therapeutic class: Antineoplastics
Pharmacologic class: Hedgehog pathway
inhibitors

AVAILABLE FORMS
Capsules: 200 mg

INDICATIONS & DOSAGES
Black Box Warning Drug can cause birth defects
or embryo-fetal death if used during pregnancy. Female patients must use contraception during therapy
and for 20 months after last dose. Male patients must
use condoms and shouldn't donate sperm during
therapy and for at least 8 months after last dose. ∎
➤ **Locally advanced basal cell carcinoma that has
recurred after surgery or radiation therapy, or in
patients who aren't candidates for surgery or radiation therapy**
Adults: 200 mg PO once daily at least 1 hour before or
2 hours after a meal. Administer until disease progression or unacceptable toxicity occurs.
Adjust-a-dose: Refer to manufacturer's instructions
for toxicity-related dosage adjustments and discontinuation.

SAFETY ALERT!

SORAfenib tosylate
sohr-uh-FEN-ib

NexAVAR

Therapeutic class: Antineoplastics
Pharmacologic class: Multi-kinase inhibitors

AVAILABLE FORMS
Tablets: 200 mg

INDICATIONS & DOSAGES
➤ **Advanced renal cell carcinoma; unresectable
hepatocellular carcinoma; locally advanced or
metastatic, progressive, differentiated thyroid
carcinoma refractory to radioactive iodine
treatment**
Adults: 400 mg PO b.i.d. at least 1 hour before or
2 hours after eating. Continue until disease progresses
or unacceptable toxicity occurs.
Adjust-a-dose: Refer to manufacturer's instructions
for dosage adjustments for dermatologic and other
toxicities.

spinosad
SPIN-oh-sad

Natroba

Therapeutic class: Scabicides–pediculicides
Pharmacologic class: Topical actinomyce
bacterium derivatives

AVAILABLE FORMS
Topical solution: 0.9%*

INDICATIONS & DOSAGES
➤ **Head lice infestation**
Adults and children age 6 months and older: Apply
only amount needed to adequately cover scalp and
hair, up to 120 mL. Leave on for 10 minutes (start
timing after scalp and hair have been completely covered); then thoroughly rinse off with warm water. If
live lice are seen 7 days after first treatment, apply a
second treatment.

tacrolimus ▨
tack-ROW-lim-us

Advagraf❧, Astagraf XL, Envarsus XR,
Prograf

Therapeutic class: Immunosuppressants
Pharmacologic class: Calcineurin inhibitors

AVAILABLE FORMS
Capsules ⊕*:* 0.5 mg, 1 mg, 5 mg
Capsules (extended-release) ⊕*:* 0.5 mg, 1 mg, 3 mg❧,
5 mg
Granules for oral suspension: 0.2 mg, 1 mg unit-dose
packets
Injection: 5 mg/mL*
Tablets (extended-release) ⊕*:* 0.75 mg, 1 mg, 4 mg

INDICATIONS & DOSAGES
Adjust-a-dose (for all indications): Give lowest
recommended oral and IV dosages to elderly patients
and patients with renal or hepatic impairment. Black
patients with renal transplants may need higher dosages than white patients to attain comparable trough
concentrations. ▨
❸ Alert: Individualizing dosing regimen is necessary
for optimal therapy. Frequently monitor trough concentrations in the early transplant period to ensure adequate drug exposure. Extended-release capsules aren't
interchangeable or substitutable with other tacrolimus
extended-release or immediate-release products.
➤ **To prevent organ rejection in allogenic liver,
kidney, or heart transplant (with other immunosuppressants)**
Adults: For patients who can't take drug PO, 0.03 to
0.05 mg/kg/day (liver or kidney) or 0.01 mg/kg/day
(heart) IV as continuous infusion at least 6 hours after
liver or heart transplant or within 24 hours of kidney
transplant if renal function has recovered. Switch to
oral therapy as soon as possible, with first dose 8 to
12 hours after stopping IV infusion. For renal transplant, give oral dose within 24 hours of transplantation

---

❧ Canada   ◇ OTC   ◆ Off-label use   ✐ Photoguide   ⊕ Do not crush   *Liquid contains alcohol   ▨ Genetic after renal function has recovered. Initial immediate-release oral dosages: For liver transplant, 0.1 to 0.15 mg/kg PO daily in two divided doses every 12 hours; for kidney transplant, 0.2 mg/kg PO daily (in combination with azathioprine) or 0.1 mg/kg PO daily (in combination with mycophenolate mofetil and interleukin-2 receptor agonist) in two divided doses every 12 hours; for heart transplant, 0.075 mg/kg PO daily in two divided doses every 12 hours (in combination with azathioprine or mycophenolate mofetil). Adjust dosages based on patient response. Adjunct therapy with adrenal corticosteroids is recommended early posttransplant.

For Astagraf XL extended-release (ER) form (renal transplant only): When using with basiliximab induction, mycophenolate mofetil, and corticosteroids, administer initial dose of 0.15 to 0.2 mg/kg PO once daily before or within 48 hours of completion of transplant procedure, but may delay until renal function has recovered. When using in combination with corticosteroids and mycophenolate without basiliximab induction, give 0.1 mg/kg PO once daily (preoperative within 12 hours before reperfusion); 0.2 mg/kg PO once daily (postoperative at least 4 hours after preoperative dose and within 12 hours of reperfusion).

To convert from immediate-release form to Astagraf XL, initiate ER treatment in a 1:1 ratio (mg:mg) using previously established total daily dose of immediate-release form. Give once daily. To convert from immediate-release form to Envarsus XR, initiate ER treatment with a once-daily dose that's 80% of the total daily dose of the immediate-release product.
Children (liver transplant only): 0.03 to 0.05 mg/kg IV daily as continuous infusion.
Children (liver, kidney, or heart transplant): For kidney transplant, 0.3 mg/kg/day immediate-release capsules or oral suspension, divided in two doses, administered every 12 hours or, within 24 hours of reperfusion, give 0.3 mg/kg Astagraf XL PO once daily in combination with basiliximab induction, mycophenolate mofetil, and corticosteroids; for liver transplant, 0.15 to 0.2 mg/kg/day immediate-release capsules or 0.2 mg/kg/day oral suspension, divided in two doses, administered every 12 hours; for heart transplant, 0.3 mg/kg/day immediate-release capsules or oral suspension or 0.1 mg/kg/day if cell-depleting induction treatment is administered, divided in two doses, administered every 12 hours. Children in general need higher tacrolimus doses compared to adults: The higher dose requirements may decrease as the child grows older.
✳ *NEW INDICATION:* **To prevent organ rejection in de novo kidney transplant patients in combination with other immunosuppressants (Envarsus XR)**
Adults: Initially, 0.14 mg/kg/day PO. Titrate dosage based on clinical assessments of rejection and tolerability and to achieve tacrolimus whole blood trough concentration range of 6 to 11 ng/mL during the first month, then 4 to 11 ng/mL during all subsequent months.
➤ **Immunosuppression (maintenance) after lung transplant** ◆

Adults: 0.05 to 0.3 mg/kg/day (immediate-release) PO or by NG tube in two divided doses every 12 hours (usual dose, 0.05 mg/kg every 12 hours); titrate to target trough concentrations. May also administer sublingually at approximately 50% of the oral/NG dose. Usually used in combination regimen that contains a corticosteroid and either azathioprine or mycophenolate. May convert to once-daily dosing (on a mg-per-mg basis) using extended-release formulation (Astagraf XL) in stable lung transplant recipients. For IV administration, 0.01 to 0.05 mg/kg, usually with a corticosteroid and either azathioprine or mycophenolate, over 24 hours as a continuous infusion; titrate to target trough concentrations. If initial dose is given IV, may begin immediately after transplantation or up to 2 days postoperatively.

AVAILABLE FORMS
Tablets: 100 mg, 150 mg

INDICATIONS & DOSAGES
➤ **Prevention of relapse of *Plasmodium vivax* malaria in patients who have tested negative for G6PD deficiency and who are receiving antimalarial therapy for acute *P. vivax* infection (Krintafel)**
Adults and children age 16 and older: Single dose of 300 mg PO given as two 150-mg tablets taken together. Coadminister on first or second day of appropriate antimalarial therapy for acute *P. vivax* malaria.
➤ **Malaria prophylaxis in patients who have tested negative for G6PD deficiency (Arakoda)**
Adults: 200 mg PO once daily for 3 days before travel to a malarious area; then while patient is in malarious area, 200 mg once weekly beginning 7 days after the last dose of the loading regimen. After patient leaves the malarious area, 200 mg PO as a single dose 7 days after the last dose of maintenance regimen.

SAFETY ALERT!

AVAILABLE FORMS
Tablets: 50 mg, 75 mg, 100 mg
Tablets (extended-release) ⓓⓝⓒ *:* 50 mg, 100 mg, 150 mg, 200 mg, 250 mg

INDICATIONS & DOSAGES
Adjust-a-dose (for all indications): Use lowest effective dosage for shortest duration consistent with individual patient treatment goals.

➤ **Acute pain severe enough to require an opioid analgesic and for which alternative treatments are inadequate (immediate-release only)**

Adults: 50 to 100 mg PO every 4 to 6 hours, as needed, for pain. On day 1, may give second dose in 1 hour if first dose is ineffective. Adjust subsequent dosing to maintain adequate pain control. Maximum daily dose, 700 mg on day 1; 600 mg on subsequent days.

Adjust-a-dose: For patients with moderate hepatic impairment (Child-Pugh class B), initially give 50 mg PO every 8 hours. Maximum, three doses (150 mg) in 24 hours; the interval between doses should be no less than 8 hours.

➤ **Severe chronic pain when continuous, around-the-clock opioid analgesia is needed for an extended period (extended-release); neuropathic pain associated with diabetic peripheral neuropathy (extended-release)**

Adults: Initially, 50 mg PO b.i.d. (approximately every 12 hours). Titrate with dosage increases of 50 mg no more than b.i.d. every 3 days. Therapeutic range is 100 to 250 mg PO b.i.d. Maximum daily dose is 500 mg.

Adjust-a-dose: For patients with moderate hepatic impairment (Child-Pugh class B), initially 50 mg (extended-release) PO once every 24 hours. Maximum dose is 100 mg (extended-release) once daily. Monitor patient closely for respiratory and CNS depression, particularly during initiation and titration.

---

tasimelteon
TAS-i-MEL-tee-on

Hetlioz

Therapeutic class: Hypnotics
Pharmacologic class: Melatonin receptor agonists

AVAILABLE FORMS
Capsules ⓞⓣⓒ: 20 mg

INDICATIONS & DOSAGES
➤ **Non-24-hour sleep-wake disorder**
Adults: 20 mg PO daily at the same time each night at bedtime.

---

tavaborole
tah-vah-BOR-ole

Kerydin

Therapeutic class: Antifungals
Pharmacologic class: Antifungals

AVAILABLE FORMS
Topical solution: 5%

INDICATIONS & DOSAGES
➤ **Onychomycosis of toenails due to *Trichophyton rubrum* or *Trichophyton mentagrophytes***
Adults: Apply once daily for 48 weeks to entire surface of affected toenail and under the tip of affected toenail.

---

tbo-filgrastim
fill-GRASS-tim

Granix

Therapeutic class: Colony stimulating factors
Pharmacologic class: Hematopoietics

AVAILABLE FORMS
Injection: 300 mcg/0.5 mL, 480 mcg/0.8 mL single-use prefilled syringes

INDICATIONS & DOSAGES
➤ **To reduce duration of severe neutropenia in myelosuppressive chemotherapy recipients with nonmyeloid malignancies**
Adults and children age 1 month and older: 5 mcg/kg subcut daily. Give first dose no earlier than 24 hours after myelosuppressive chemotherapy. Don't give drug within 24 hours before chemotherapy. Continue daily dosing until expected neutrophil nadir is passed and neutrophil count has recovered to normal range.

---

tecovirimat
TEK-oh-VIR-i-mat

Tpoxx

Therapeutic class: Antivirals
Pharmacologic class: Antivirals

AVAILABLE FORMS
Capsules: 200 mg

INDICATIONS & DOSAGES
➤ **Treatment of human smallpox disease caused by variola virus**
Adults and children weighing 40 kg or more: 600 mg PO b.i.d. for 14 days.
Children weighing 25 to less than 40 kg: 400 mg PO b.i.d. for 14 days.
Children weighing 13 to less than 25 kg: 200 mg PO b.i.d. for 14 days.

---

tedizolid phosphate
TED-eye-zoe-lid

Sivextro

Therapeutic class: Antibiotics
Pharmacologic class: Oxazolidinones

AVAILABLE FORMS
Injection: 200 mg/vial
Tablets: 200 mg

INDICATIONS & DOSAGES
➤ **Acute bacterial skin and skin-structure infections caused by susceptible gram-positive isolates (*Staphylococcus aureus* [including MRSA and methicillin-susceptible strains], *Streptococcus pyogenes*, *Streptococcus agalactiae*, *Streptococcus anginosus* group [including *S. anginosus*, *Streptococcus intermedius*, and *Streptococcus constellatus*], and *Enterococcus faecalis*)**
Adults: 200 mg PO or IV once daily for 6 days.

---

tegaserod maleate
teg-a-SER-od

Zelnorm

Therapeutic class: Anti-IBS drugs
Pharmacologic class: Serotonin-4 (5-HT₄) receptor agonists

AVAILABLE FORMS
Tablets: 6 mg

INDICATIONS & DOSAGES
➤ IBS with constipation
Women younger than age 65: 6 mg PO b.i.d. 30 minutes before meals. Discontinue in patients with inadequate response after 4 to 6 weeks of treatment.

SAFETY ALERT!

temozolomide
teh-moh-ZOH-loh-mide

Temodal✦, Temodar

Therapeutic class: Antineoplastics
Pharmacologic class: Alkylating drugs

AVAILABLE FORMS
Capsules ⓓ: 5 mg, 20 mg, 100 mg, 140 mg, 180 mg, 250 mg
Injection: 100 mg/vial

INDICATIONS & DOSAGES
Adjust-a-dose (for all indications): Refer to manufacturer's instructions for toxicity-related dosage adjustments.
➤ Newly diagnosed glioblastoma in combination with radiation therapy
Adults: Initially, 75 mg/m² IV infusion or PO once daily for 42 days (up to 49 days if no toxicity). Maintenance dose is 150 mg/m² IV infusion or PO once daily on days 1 to 5 of a 28-day cycle for six cycles; may increase dose to 200 mg/m² for cycles two to six if CTCAE is grade 2 or less, ANC is 1.5×10^9/L or more, and platelet count is 100×10^9/L or more. If dose was increased in cycle two, maintain dose at 200 mg/m² for days 1 to 5 of subsequent cycles, unless toxicity occurs. If dose wasn't increased in cycle two, don't increase in subsequent cycles.
➤ Refractory anaplastic astrocytoma
Adults: Initially, 150 mg/m² IV infusion or PO once daily for 5 days of a 28-day treatment cycle. May increase dose to 200 mg/m² for 5 days of a 28-day treatment cycle, if nadir and day 1 of next cycle ANC is 1.5×10^9/L or more and platelet count is 100×10^9/L or more.

SAFETY ALERT!

temsirolimus
TEM-seer-OLE-ih-muss

Torisel

Therapeutic class: Antineoplastics
Pharmacologic class: Kinase inhibitors

AVAILABLE FORMS
IV solution: 25 mg/mL

INDICATIONS & DOSAGES
➤ Advanced renal cell carcinoma
Adults: 25 mg IV over 30 to 60 minutes once weekly until disease progresses or unacceptable toxicity occurs. Give diphenhydramine 25 to 50 mg IV 30 minutes before each dose.
Adjust-a-dose: Refer to manufacturer's instructions for toxicity-related dosage adjustments.
  If use with a strong CYP3A4 inhibitor is necessary, consider a dosage reduction to 12.5 mg once weekly. If use with a strong CYP3A4 inducer is necessary, increase dosage to 50 mg once weekly.

SAFETY ALERT!

teriflunomide
TER-i-FLOO-noe-mide

Aubagio

Therapeutic class: Immunomodulators
Pharmacologic class: Pyrimidine synthesis inhibitors

AVAILABLE FORMS
Tablets: 7 mg, 14 mg

INDICATIONS & DOSAGES
Black Box Warning Severe and fatal liver injury can occur. May cause major birth defects. Contraindicated during pregnancy. ∎
➤ Relapsing forms of MS
Adults: 7 or 14 mg PO once daily.

tezacaftor–ivacaftor and ivacaftor
tez-a-KAF-tor/eye-va-KAF-tor

Symdeko

Therapeutic class: Metabolic agents
Pharmacologic class: Cystic fibrosis transmembrane conductance regulator (CFTR) facilitators (tezacaftor); CFTR potentiators (ivacaftor)

AVAILABLE FORMS
Tablets: 100 mg tezacaftor/150 mg ivacaftor fixed-dose combination tablet copackaged with ivacaftor 150-mg tablet

INDICATIONS & DOSAGES
➤ Treatment of cystic fibrosis in patients homozygous for the F508del mutation or who have at least one mutation in the *CFTR* gene that's responsive to tezacaftor–ivacaftor based on in vitro data or clinical evidence
Adults and children age 12 and older: 100 mg tezacaftor/150 mg ivacaftor (1 combination tablet) PO in the morning and 150 mg ivacaftor (1 tablet) PO in the evening, approximately 12 hours apart.
Adjust-a-dose: For patients with moderate or severe hepatic impairment (Child-Pugh class B or C), decrease dose to 100 mg tezacaftor/150 mg ivacaftor (1 combination tablet) PO once daily in the morning and omit the 150-mg ivacaftor evening dose. For

patients with Child-Pugh class C hepatic failure, consider giving the morning 100-mg tezacaftor/150-mg ivacaftor dose less frequently. For patients also taking CYP3A inhibitors, refer to manufacturer's instructions for dosage adjustments.

theophylline
thee-OFF-i-lin

Elixophyllin*, Theo-24, Theochron

Therapeutic class: Bronchodilators
Pharmacologic class: Xanthine derivatives

AVAILABLE FORMS
Capsules (extended-release) ⓓ: 100 mg, 200 mg, 300 mg, 400 mg
Syrup: 80 mg/15 mL*
Tablets (extended-release) ⓓ: 100 mg, 200 mg, 300 mg, 400 mg, 450 mg, 600 mg

INDICATIONS & DOSAGES
❸ *Alert:* Don't use extended-release preparations to treat acute bronchospasm.
➤ **Parenteral theophylline (preferred route) for acute bronchospasm in patients not currently receiving theophylline**
Loading dose: 4.6 mg/kg ideal body weight IV over 30 minutes; then maintenance infusion.
Nonsmoking adults younger than age 60 and children older than age 16: 0.4 mg/kg/hour IV (maximum 900 mg daily).
Nonsmoking children ages 12 to 16: 0.5 mg/kg/hour IV (maximum 900 mg daily).
Children ages 12 to 16 who smoke and children ages 9 to 12: 0.7 mg/kg/hour IV.
Children ages 1 to 9: 0.8 mg/kg/hour IV.
Infants ages 6 weeks to 1 year: Calculate mg/kg/hour IV dosage as follows: 0.008 × (age in weeks) + 0.21.
Neonates older than 24 days: 1.5 mg/kg IV every 12 hours to achieve target theophylline concentration of 7.5 mcg/mL.
Neonates 24 days old and younger: 1 mg/kg IV every 12 hours to achieve a target theophylline concentration of 7.5 mcg/mL.
Adjust-a-dose: For adults older than age 60, give 0.3 mg/kg/hour IV, up to a maximum of 17 mg/hour. For adults with HF, cor pulmonale, liver disease, sepsis with multiorgan failure, or shock, give 0.2 mg/kg/hour IV, up to a maximum infusion rate of 17 mg/hour unless serum theophylline concentrations are monitored at 24-hour intervals. Maximum daily dose is 400 mg.
➤ **Oral theophylline for acute bronchospasm in patients not currently receiving theophylline**
Adults age 60 and younger, children ages 16 and older, and children ages 1 to 15 weighing 45 kg or more: 5 mg/kg PO, then 300 mg (immediate-release syrup) PO daily in divided doses every 6 to 8 hours for 3 days. If tolerated, increase to 400 mg PO daily in divided doses every 6 to 8 hours. If necessary, dosage may be increased after 3 days to 600 mg PO daily in divided doses every 6 to 8 hours.

Children ages 1 to 15 weighing less than 45 kg: 5 mg/kg PO, then 12 to 14 mg/kg immediate-release (maximum 300 mg) PO daily in divided doses every 4 to 6 hours for 3 days. If tolerated, increase to 16 mg/kg (maximum 400 mg) PO daily in divided doses every 4 to 6 hours. After 3 days, if necessary, increase to 20 mg/kg (maximum 600 mg) PO daily in divided doses every 4 to 6 hours.
Adjust-a-dose: For children ages 1 to 15 with risk factors for reduced theophylline clearance or for whom serum concentrations can't be monitored, give 5 mg/kg PO, then 12 to 14 mg/kg (maximum 300 mg) PO daily in divided doses every 4 to 6 hours for 3 days. If tolerated, increase to 16 mg/kg (maximum 400 mg) PO daily in divided doses every 4 to 6 hours. For children age 16 and older and adults with risk factors for reduced theophylline clearance or for whom serum concentrations can't be monitored, give 5 mg/kg PO, then 300 mg PO daily in divided doses every 6 to 8 hours for 3 days. If tolerated, increase to 400 mg PO daily in divided doses every 6 to 8 hours.
➤ **Chronic bronchospasm using extended-release preparations**
Adults age 60 or younger, children age 16 and older, and children ages 6 to 15 weighing more than 45 kg: 300 mg PO daily in divided doses every 8 to 12 hours or 300 to 400 mg (24-hour extended-release capsule) PO daily for 3 days. If tolerated, increase to 400 mg PO in divided doses every 8 to 12 hours or 400 to 600 mg (24-hour extended-release capsule) PO daily. After 3 more days, if necessary, increase dose to 600 mg PO daily in divided doses every 8 to 12 hours. Titrate dosages greater than 600 mg according to serum blood levels.
Children ages 6 to 15 weighing less than 45 kg: 12 to 14 mg/kg (maximum 300 mg extended-release tablet) daily in divided doses every 8 to 12 hours for 3 days. If tolerated, increase to 16 mg/kg (maximum 400 mg extended-release tablet) daily in divided doses every 8 to 12 hours. After 3 more days, if necessary, increase to 20 mg/kg (maximum 600 mg extended-release tablet) daily in divided doses every 8 to 12 hours.
Adjust-a-dose: For children ages 6 to 15 with risk factors for reduced theophylline clearance or for whom serum concentrations can't be monitored, give 12 to 14 mg/kg (maximum 300 mg) daily in divided doses for 3 days. If tolerated, increase to a maximum of 16 mg/kg (maximum 400 mg) PO daily in divided doses every 8 to 12 hours. For children age 16 and older and adults age 60 or younger or for whom serum concentrations can't be monitored, give 300 mg PO daily in divided doses every 8 to 12 hours. After 3 days, if necessary, increase to maximum of 400 mg PO daily in divided doses every 8 to 12 hours. For adults older than age 60, the recommended maximum daily dose is 400 mg PO per day in divided doses every 8 to 12 hours unless symptoms continue and peak serum concentration is less than 10 mcg/mL. Administer dosages greater than 400 mg PO daily cautiously.

---

thioridazine hydrochloride
thye-oh-RYE-da-zeen

Therapeutic class: Antipsychotics
Pharmacologic class: Phenothiazines

AVAILABLE FORMS
Tablets: 10 mg, 25 mg, 50 mg, 100 mg

INDICATIONS & DOSAGES
Black Box Warning Prolongs QTc interval and risk for life-threatening ventricular arrhythmias. Drug isn't approved to treat patients with dementia-related psychosis. Opioids combined with benzodiazepines or CNS depressants can cause death. ∎
➤ **Schizophrenia in patients who don't respond to treatment with at least two other antipsychotics**
Adults: Initially, 50 to 100 mg PO t.i.d.; increase gradually to 800 mg daily in divided doses, as needed. Daily maintenance doses range from 200 to 800 mg divided into two to four doses.
Children: Initially, 0.5 mg/kg PO daily in divided doses. Increase gradually to optimal therapeutic effect; maximum dose is 3 mg/kg daily.

ticlopidine hydrochloride
tye-KLOH-pih-deen

Therapeutic class: Antiplatelet drugs
Pharmacologic class: Platelet aggregation inhibitors

AVAILABLE FORMS
Tablets: 250 mg

INDICATIONS & DOSAGES
Black Box Warning Ticlopidine can cause life-threatening hematologic adverse reactions, including neutropenia/agranulocytosis, thrombotic thrombocytopenic purpura, and aplastic anemia. ∎
Adjust-a-dose (for all indications): For patients with renal impairment, it may be necessary to reduce dosage or discontinue drug if hemorrhage or hematopoietic problems occur.
➤ **To reduce risk of thrombotic stroke in patients who have had a stroke or stroke precursors**
Adults: 250 mg PO b.i.d. with meals.
➤ **Adjunct to aspirin to prevent subacute stent thrombosis in patients having coronary stent placement**
Adults: 250 mg PO b.i.d., combined with antiplatelet doses of aspirin. Start therapy after stent placement and continue for up to 30 days. If prescribed longer than 30 days, use is off-label.

tigecycline
tye-gah-SYE-klin

Tygacil

Therapeutic class: Antibiotics
Pharmacologic class: Glycylcycline antibacterials

AVAILABLE FORMS
Lyophilized powder: 50-mg vial

INDICATIONS & DOSAGES
Black Box Warning Compared to other drugs used to treat serious infections, tigecycline has an increased mortality risk. Use only in situations in which alternative treatments aren't suitable. ∎
Adjust-a-dose (for all indications): For adults with severe hepatic impairment (Child-Pugh class C), give initial dose of 100 mg IV; then 25 mg IV every 12 hours.
➤ **Community-acquired bacterial pneumonia**
Adults: Initially, 100 mg IV; then 50 mg IV every 12 hours for 7 to 14 days. Infuse drug over 30 to 60 minutes.
Children ages 12 to 17: 50 mg IV every 12 hours for 7 to 14 days.
Children ages 8 to 11: 1.2 mg/kg IV every 12 hours for 7 to 14 days. Maximum dose, 50 mg every 12 hours.
➤ **Complicated skin or skin-structure infection; complicated intra-abdominal infection**
Adults: Initially 100 mg IV; then 50 mg every 12 hours for 5 to 14 days. Infuse drug over 30 to 60 minutes.
Children ages 12 to 17: 50 mg IV every 12 hours for 5 to 14 days.
Children ages 8 to 11: 1.2 mg/kg IV every 12 hours for 5 to 14 days. Maximum dose, 50 mg every 12 hours.

tildrakizumab-asmn
til-dra-KIZ-ue-mab

Ilumya

Therapeutic class: Antipsoriatics
Pharmacologic class: Interleukin-23 antagonists

AVAILABLE FORMS
Injection: 100 mg/mL single-dose prefilled syringes

INDICATIONS & DOSAGES
➤ **Moderate to severe plaque psoriasis in patients who are candidates for systemic therapy or phototherapy**
Adults: 100 mg subcut at weeks 0, 4, and every 12 weeks thereafter.

SAFETY ALERT!

tisagenlecleucel
tiss-a-GEN-lek-LOO-sel

Kymriah

Therapeutic class: Antineoplastics
Pharmacologic class: CD19-directed genetically modified autologous T-cell immunotherapies

AVAILABLE FORMS
IV infusion: Patient-specific; single-dose 10- to 50-mL infusion bag containing chimeric antigen receptor (CAR)–positive viable T cells

INDICATIONS & DOSAGES
Black Box Warning Don't give drug to patients with active infection or inflammatory disorders. Fatal or life-threatening cytokine release syndrome (CRS)

and neurologic toxicities have occurred. Only available through a restricted program called Kymriah REMS. ■

Adjust-a-dose (for all indications): Refer to manufacturer's instructions for specific lymphodepleting chemotherapy and for management of severe toxicities, including CRS.

➤ **B-cell precursor acute lymphoblastic leukemia that's refractory or in second or later relapse**
Patients younger than age 25 weighing more than 50 kg: 0.1 to 2.5×10^8 total CAR-positive viable T cells IV infusion 2 to 14 days after completion of lymphodepleting chemotherapy. Don't determine dose based on body weight.
Patients younger than age 25 weighing 50 kg or less: 0.2 to 5.0×10^6 CAR-positive viable T cells/kg body weight IV infusion 2 to 14 days after completion of lymphodepleting chemotherapy.

➤ **Relapsed or refractory large B-cell lymphoma after two or more lines of systemic therapy, including diffuse large B-cell lymphoma (DLBCL) not otherwise specified, high-grade B-cell lymphoma, and DLBCL arising from follicular lymphoma**
Adults: 0.6 to 6.0×10^8 CAR-positive viable T cells IV infusion 2 to 11 days after completion of lympho-depleting chemotherapy. May omit lymphodepleting chemotherapy if patient's WBC count is 1×10^9/L or less within 1 week before tisagenlecleucel infusion.

SAFETY ALERT!

toremifene citrate
tore-EM-ah-feen

Fareston

Therapeutic class: Antineoplastics
Pharmacologic class: Nonsteroidal antiestrogens

AVAILABLE FORMS
Tablets: 60 mg

INDICATIONS & DOSAGES
Black Box Warning May prolong QTc interval and risk of fatal ventricular arrhythmias. ■
➤ **Metastatic breast cancer in postmenopausal women with estrogen receptor–positive or estrogen receptor–unknown tumors**
Adults: 60 mg PO once daily. Continue until disease progresses.

trandolapril ▨
tran-DOLE-ah-pril

Therapeutic class: Antihypertensives
Pharmacologic class: ACE inhibitors

AVAILABLE FORMS
Tablets: 1 mg, 2 mg, 4 mg

INDICATIONS & DOSAGES
Black Box Warning May cause fetal harm; when pregnancy is detected, discontinue drug as soon as possible. ■
Adjust-a-dose (for all indications): If CrCl is below 30 mL/minute or patient has hepatic cirrhosis, first dose is 0.5 mg daily.

➤ **HTN**▨
Adults: For patients not taking a diuretic, initially 2 mg PO for a black patient and 1 mg PO for all other patients, once daily. If control isn't adequate, increase dosage at intervals of at least 1 week. Maintenance doses for most patients: 2 to 4 mg daily. Some patients taking once-daily doses of 4 mg may need b.i.d. doses. For patients also taking a diuretic, initially, 0.5 mg PO once daily. Subsequent dosage adjustment is based on BP response.
➤ **HF or left ventricular dysfunction after MI**
Adults: Initially, 1 mg PO daily, adjusted to 4 mg PO daily. If patient can't tolerate 4 mg, continue at highest tolerated dose.

treprostinil
tra-PROS-tin-ill

Remodulin, Tyvaso

treprostinil diolamine
Orenitram

Therapeutic class: Antihypertensives
Pharmacologic class: Vasodilators

AVAILABLE FORMS
Injection: 1 mg/mL, 2.5 mg/mL, 5 mg/mL, 10 mg/mL in 20-mL vials
Solution for inhalation: 1.74 mg/2.9-mL ampule
Tablets (extended-release): 0.125 mg, 0.25 mg, 1 mg, 2.5 mg, 5 mg

INDICATIONS & DOSAGES
➤ **To reduce symptoms caused by exercise in patients with NYHA Class II to IV PAH**
Adults: Initially, 1.25 nanograms/kg/minute by continuous subcut infusion. If patient doesn't tolerate initial dose, reduce infusion rate to 0.625 nanogram/kg/minute. Increase by 1.25 nanograms/kg/minute each week for the first 4 weeks and then by no more than 2.5 nanograms/kg/minute each week for the remaining duration of infusion. Experience with treprostinil dosages exceeding 40 nanograms/kg/minute is limited. May be given IV through a central venous catheter if subcut route isn't tolerated. Or, initially, 3 breaths (18 mcg) per treatment session q.i.d., approximately 4 hours apart. Increase dosage by 3 breaths in 1- to 2-week intervals as tolerated to target maintenance dosage of 9 breaths (54 mcg) q.i.d. If 3 breaths aren't tolerated initially, decrease to 1 or 2 breaths and increase as tolerated.
Adjust-a-dose: For patients with mild or moderate hepatic insufficiency, initially, 0.625 nanogram/kg ideal body weight/minute by continuous IV infusion, and increase cautiously.
➤ **To decrease the rate of clinical deterioration in patients requiring transition from Flolan (epoprostenol sodium)**
Adults: Start treprostinil subcut or IV infusion at 10% of the current IV epoprostenol dose; increase dose as the epoprostenol dose is reduced. Decrease epoprostenol dose in 20% increments and increase treprostinil in 20% increments, always maintaining a total dose of 110% of epoprostenol starting dose. Once epoprostenol is at 20% of starting dose and treprostinil

is at 90%, decrease epoprostenol to 5% and increase treprostinil to 110%. Finally, stop epoprostenol and maintain treprostinil dose at 110% of epoprostenol starting dose plus an additional 5% to 10% as needed. Change rate based on individual patient response. Treat worsening of PAH symptoms with increases in treprostinil dose. Treat adverse effects associated with prostacyclin and prostacyclin analogues with decreases in epoprostenol dose.

➤ **Treatment of PAH in patients with WHO functional class II to III signs and symptoms to improve exercise capacity**
Adults: 0.25 mg PO every 12 hours or 0.125 mg PO every 8 hours. May increase in increments of 0.25 or 0.5 mg every 12 hours or 0.125 mg every 8 hours every 3 to 4 days as tolerated to achieve optimal clinical response. If incremental increases aren't tolerated, consider slower titration. Maximum dose is determined by tolerability. If patient is taking strong CYP2C8 inhibitors (such as gemfibrozil), initiate at 0.125 mg PO every 12 hours; increase in increments of 0.125 mg every 12 hours every 3 to 4 days.

To transition from subcut or IV to PO administration, refer to manufacturer's instructions.
Adjust-a-dose: If intolerable adverse effects occur, decrease dose in 0.25-mg increments. To discontinue therapy, reduce dose in steps of 0.5 to 1 mg/day; avoid discontinuing drug abruptly. If patient is unable to continue oral treatment, consider a temporary infusion of subcut or IV treprostinil. For patients with mild hepatic impairment, initiate drug at 0.125 mg PO every 12 hours and increase in increments of 0.125 mg every 12 hours every 3 to 4 days. Avoid PO use in patients with moderate hepatic impairment; contraindicated in severe hepatic impairment.

SAFETY ALERT!

trifluridine–tipiracil hydrochloride ⚕
trye-FLURE-i-deen/tye-PIR-a-sil

Lonsurf

Therapeutic class: Antineoplastics
Pharmacologic class: Pyrimidine analogues

AVAILABLE FORMS
Tablets: 15 mg trifluridine/6.14 mg tipiracil, 20 mg trifluridine/8.19 mg tipiracil

INDICATIONS & DOSAGES
➤ **Metastatic colorectal cancer in patients previously treated with fluoropyrimidine-, oxaliplatin-, and irinotecan-based chemotherapy, an antivascular endothelial growth factor biological therapy and, if RAS wild-type, an anti-epidermal growth factor receptor therapy** ⚕
Adults: 35 mg/m^2 (based on the trifluridine component) PO b.i.d. with food up to a maximum of 80 mg/dose (based on trifluridine component) on days 1 through 5 and days 8 through 12 of a 28-day cycle. Round doses to nearest 5-mg increment. Continue until disease progression or unacceptable toxicity occurs. Before initiating each drug cycle, ensure that ANC is 1,500/mm^3 or more or febrile neutropenia is resolved,

platelet count is 75,000/mm^3 or greater, and grade 3 or 4 nonhematologic adverse reactions are resolved to grade 0 or 1.
Adjust-a-dose: Refer to manufacturer's instructions for dosage adjustments for hematologic and nonhematologic toxicities.

trimethobenzamide hydrochloride
trye-meth-oh-BEN-za-mide

Tigan

Therapeutic class: Antiemetics
Pharmacologic class: Anticholinergics

AVAILABLE FORMS
Capsules: 300 mg
Injection: 100 mg/mL

INDICATIONS & DOSAGES
➤ **Postoperative nausea and vomiting; nausea associated with gastroenteritis**
Adults: 300 mg PO or 200 mg IM t.i.d. or q.i.d.
Adjust-a-dose: Dosage reduction or increased dosing interval is recommended in elderly patients and patients with renal impairment (CrCl of 70 mL/minute/1.73 m^2).

triptorelin pamoate
trip-toe-REL-in

Trelstar Mixject, Triptodur

Therapeutic class: Hormone analogues
Pharmacologic class: Gonadotropin releasing hormone agonists

AVAILABLE FORMS
Injectable suspension (Trelstar Mixject): 3.75 mg, 11.25 mg, 22.5 mg in Mixjet single-dose delivery systems
Injectable suspension (extended-release) (Triptodur): 22.5 mg single-dose vials packaged with 2 mL of diluent sterile water for injection

INDICATIONS & DOSAGES
➤ **Palliative treatment of advanced prostate cancer (Trelstar Mixject only)**
Adults: 3.75 mg IM once every 4 weeks, or 11.25 mg IM once every 12 weeks, or 22.5 mg IM once every 24 weeks. Because of different release characteristics, dosing schedule depends on the product selected.
➤ **Central precocious puberty (Triptodur only)**
Children age 2 and older: 22.5 mg IM once every 24 weeks. Treatment should be discontinued at the appropriate age of onset of puberty at the discretion of the physician.

uridine triacetate ⚕
URE-i-deen

Xuriden, Vistogard

Therapeutic class: Replacement enzymes
Pharmacologic class: Uridine replacements

AVAILABLE FORMS
Oral granules 🚫: 2-g, 10-g single-use packets

♣Canada   ◇OTC   ◆Off-label use   ✐Photoguide   🚫Do not crush   *Liquid contains alcohol   ⚕Genetic

INDICATIONS & DOSAGES

➤ **Hereditary orotic aciduria (Xuriden)** ▧

Adults and children: 60 mg/kg PO daily; may increase to 120 mg/kg daily for insufficient efficacy. Maximum dose is 8 g/day. See manufacturer's instructions for weight-based dosing tables.

➤ **Fluoropyrimidine overdose (emergency treatment of 5-FU or capecitabine overdose; or early-onset severe or life-threatening cardiac or CNS toxicity; or early-onset, unusually severe adverse reactions [e.g., GI toxicity or neutropenia] within 96 hours after end of 5-FU or capecitabine administration) (Vistogard)**

Adults: 10 g PO every 6 hours for a total of 20 doses beginning as soon as possible after overdose or early-onset toxicity within 96 hours after end of 5-FU or capecitabine administration. Maximum, 10 g/dose.

Children: 6.2 g/m² PO not to exceed 10 g/dose every 6 hours for 20 doses beginning as soon as possible after overdose or early-onset toxicity within 96 hours after end of 5-FU or capecitabine administration. Refer to manufacturer's information for weight-based dosing tables.

---

valbenazine ▧
val-BEN-a-zeen

Ingrezza

Therapeutic class: Neuromuscular transmission blockers
Pharmacologic class: Vesicular monoamine transporter 2 inhibitors

AVAILABLE FORMS
Capsules: 40 mg, 80 mg

INDICATIONS & DOSAGES
➤ **Tardive dyskinesia**

Adults: Initially, 40 mg PO once daily for 1 week, then 80 mg once daily; for some patients, 40 mg once daily may be appropriate.

Adjust-a-dose: For moderate to severe hepatic impairment (Child-Pugh score 7 to 15) or when drug is administered with a strong CYP3A4 inhibitor, give 40 mg once daily. If drug is administered with a strong CYP2D6 inhibitor, or for patients who are known poor metabolizers of CYP2D6, consider a dosage reduction. ▧

---

valGANciclovir hydrochloride
val-gan-SYE-kloe-veer

Valcyte

Therapeutic class: Antivirals
Pharmacologic class: Nucleosides—nucleotides

AVAILABLE FORMS
Oral solution: 50 mg/mL
Tablets ⒹⒸ: 450 mg

INDICATIONS & DOSAGES
Adjust-a-dose (for all indications): For adult patients with CrCl of 40 to 59 mL/minute, induction

dosage is 450 mg b.i.d.; maintenance dosage is 450 mg daily. If CrCl is 25 to 39 mL/minute, induction dosage is 450 mg daily; maintenance dosage is 450 mg every 2 days. If CrCl is 10 to 24 mL/minute, induction dosage is 450 mg every 2 days; maintenance dosage is 450 mg twice weekly. Drug isn't recommended for patients with CrCl of less than 10 mL/minute.

➤ **To prevent CMV disease in heart, kidney, and kidney-pancreas transplantation in patients at high risk (donor CMV-seropositive or recipient CMV-seronegative)**

Adults: For patients with a heart or kidney-pancreas transplant, 900 mg PO once daily starting within 10 days of transplantation until 100 days posttransplantation. For patients with a kidney transplant, 900 mg PO daily starting within 10 days of transplantation until 200 days post-transplantation.

➤ **To prevent CMV disease in pediatric kidney transplant patients at high risk**

Children age 4 months to 16 years: Give dose once daily starting within 10 days of transplantation until 200 days posttransplantation of kidney, based on BSA and CrCl (modified Schwartz formula):

$$\text{Dose (mg)} = 7 \times \text{BSA} \times \text{CrCl}$$

Adjust-a-dose: For pediatric patients, the maximum calculated CrCl (modified Schwartz formula) to be used is 150 mL/minute/1.73 m², even if the calculated value is greater. The maximum pediatric dose is 900 mg, even if the calculated dose is greater.

➤ **To prevent CMV disease in pediatric heart transplant patients at high risk**

Children age 1 month to 16 years: Give dose once daily starting within 10 days of transplantation until 100 days posttransplantation of heart, based on BSA and CrCl (modified Schwartz formula):

$$\text{Dose (mg)} = 7 \times \text{BSA} \times \text{CrCl}$$

Maximum dose is 900 mg once daily.

➤ **CMV retinitis in patients with AIDS**

Adults: For active disease, give 900 mg PO b.i.d. for 21 days; maintenance dose is 900 mg PO daily. For inactive disease, give 900 mg PO once daily.

SAFETY ALERT!

vandetanib
van-DET-a-nib

Caprelsa

Therapeutic class: Antineoplastics
Pharmacologic class: Kinase inhibitors

AVAILABLE FORMS
Tablets: 100 mg, 300 mg

INDICATIONS & DOSAGES
Black Box Warning May prolong QTc interval and increase risk for fatal ventricular arrhythmias. ∎

➤ **Symptomatic or progressive medullary thyroid cancer in patients with unresectable locally advanced or metastatic disease**

Adults: 300 mg PO daily until disease progression or unacceptable toxicity occurs.

Adjust-a-dose: In patients with moderate to severe renal impairment (CrCl of less than 50 mL/minute), initiate therapy at 200 mg PO daily. In the event of corrected QT interval (Fridericia [QTcF]) greater than 500 msec, interrupt therapy until QTcF returns to less than 450 msec; then resume at a reduced dosage. In patients with grade 3 or greater toxicity, stop drug until toxicity resolves or improves to grade 1; resume at reduced dosage of 200 mg, then 100 mg, if necessary.

For recurrent toxicities, reduce dosage to 100 mg once daily after resolution of toxicities or improvement to grade 1, if continued treatment is warranted.

vedolizumab
VE-doe-LIZ-ue-mab

Entyvio

Therapeutic class: Immune response modifiers
Pharmacologic class: Humanized IgG1 monoclonal antibodies

AVAILABLE FORMS
Injection: 300 mg/20 mL single-use vials

INDICATIONS & DOSAGES
➤ **Moderate to severe Crohn disease or ulcerative colitis in patients with inadequate response to, loss of response to, or intolerance to TNF blocker or immunomodulator, or in patients with inadequate response, intolerance to, or demonstrated dependence on corticosteroids**
Adults: 300 mg IV infusion over 30 minutes, administered at weeks 0, 2, and 6, then every 8 weeks thereafter. Discontinue use if no evidence of therapeutic benefit by week 14.

SAFETY ALERT!

vemurafenib ☒
VEM-ue-RAF-e-nib

Zelboraf

Therapeutic class: Antineoplastics
Pharmacologic class: Kinase inhibitors

AVAILABLE FORMS
Tablets ⓪ 240 mg

INDICATIONS & DOSAGES
Adjust-a-dose (for all indications): Avoid concomitant use of strong CYP3A4 inducers during treatment. If use together is unavoidable, increase vemurafenib dosage by 240 mg (1 tablet) as tolerated. After discontinuation of a strong CYP3A4 inducer for 2 weeks, resume prior vemurafenib dosage. Refer to manufacturer's instructions for toxicity-related dosage adjustments. Treat until disease progression or unacceptable toxicity occurs.
➤ **Treatment of unresectable or metastatic melanoma with *BRAF* V600E mutation as detected by an FDA-approved test ☒**
Adults: Usual dosage is 960 mg PO every 12 hours.

➤ **Erdheim-Chester disease with *BRAF* V600 mutation ☒**
Adults: 960 mg PO every 12 hours.

SAFETY ALERT!

vinCRIStine sulfate liposome ☒
vin-KRIS-teen

Marqibo

Therapeutic class: Antineoplastics
Pharmacologic class: Vinca alkaloids

AVAILABLE FORMS
Injection: 5 mg/31 mL in single-dose vials

INDICATIONS & DOSAGES
Black Box Warning Liposomal form has different dosage recommendation than nonliposomal form. To avoid overdose, verify drug name and dose before preparation and administration. For IV use only; fatal if given by other routes. ■
➤ **Patients with Philadelphia chromosome–negative acute lymphoblastic leukemia in second or greater relapse or whose disease has progressed following two or more antileukemia therapies ☒**
Adults: 2.25 mg/m^2 IV over 1 hour every 7 days.
Adjust-a-dose: Refer to manufacturer's instructions for toxicity-related dosage adjustments.

voretigene neparvovec-rzyl
vor-RET-i-jeen ne-PAR-voe-vek

Luxturna

Therapeutic class: Ophthalmic gene therapies
Pharmacologic class: Adeno-associated virus gene therapies

AVAILABLE FORMS
Injection: 0.5 mL single-use vials

INDICATIONS & DOSAGES
➤ **Confirmed biallelic *RPE65* mutation–associated retinal dystrophy**
Adults younger than age 65 and children age 1 and older: Subretinal injection of 0.3 mL (1.5×10^{11} vector genomes [vg]) to each eye on separate days within a close interval, but no fewer than 6 days apart.

zanamivir
zan-AM-ah-veer

Relenza

Therapeutic class: Antiretrovirals
Pharmacologic class: Selective neuraminidase inhibitors

AVAILABLE FORMS
Powder for inhalation: 5 mg/blister

INDICATIONS & DOSAGES
➤ **Uncomplicated acute illness caused by influenza virus A and B in patients who have had symptoms for no longer than 2 days; treatment of H1N1 influenza A**

Adults and children age 7 and older: 2 oral inhalations (one 5-mg blister per inhalation for total dose of 10 mg) b.i.d. using the dry-powder inhalation device for 5 days. Give two doses on first day of treatment, allowing at least 2 hours to elapse between doses. Give subsequent doses about 12 hours apart (in the morning and evening) at about the same time each day. Some guidelines suggest that longer treatment duration may be considered in patients who remain severely ill after 5 days.

➤ **Prevention of influenza in a household setting; prevention of H1N1 influenza A**

Adults and children age 5 and older: 2 oral inhalations (one 5-mg blister per inhalation for total dose of 10 mg) once daily for 10 days.

➤ **Prevention of influenza in a community setting**

Adults and adolescents ages 12 to 16: 2 oral inhalations (one 5-mg blister per inhalation for total dose of 10 mg) once daily for 28 days.

SAFETY ALERT!

ziv-aflibercept
ZIV-a-FLIB-er-sept

Zaltrap

Therapeutic class: Antineoplastics
Pharmacologic class: Vascular endothelial growth factor inhibitors

AVAILABLE FORMS

Injection: 100 mg/4 mL (25 mg/mL), 200 mg/8 mL (25 mg/mL) in single-use vials

INDICATIONS & DOSAGES

`Black Box Warning` May cause severe and fatal GI adverse reactions and compromise wound healing. Don't use for 4 weeks before or after surgery. ∎

`Black Box Warning` Severe and sometimes fatal hemorrhage, especially GI hemorrhage, has occurred with ziv-aflibercept in combination with 5-FU, leucovorin, irinotecan (FOLFIRI) regimen. GI perforation and severely compromised wound healing can occur. ∎

➤ **Metastatic colorectal cancer that is resistant or has progressed after an oxaliplatin-containing regimen in combination with FOLFIRI regimen**

Adults: 4 mg/kg IV infusion over 1 hour every 2 weeks until disease progression or unacceptable toxicity occurs. Give before any component of FOLFIRI regimen on day of treatment. Continue until disease progression or unacceptable toxicity occurs.

Adjust-a-dose: For recurrent or severe HTN, withhold drug until controlled; then permanently reduce dosage to 2 mg/kg every 2 weeks. For proteinuria of 2 g/24 hours or greater, withhold drug until proteinuria is less than 2 g/24 hours; then permanently reduce dosage to 2 mg/kg. For neutropenia, delay treatment until ANC is 1.5×10^9/L or greater.

zoledronic acid
zoh-leh-DROH-nik

Reclast, Zometa

Therapeutic class: Antiosteoporotics
Pharmacologic class: Bisphosphonates

AVAILABLE FORMS

Injection as ready-to-infuse solution: 5 mg/100 mL (Reclast), 4 mg/100 mL (Zometa)
Injection (Zometa): 4 mg/5 mL vial

INDICATIONS & DOSAGES

➤ **Hypercalcemia caused by malignancy**

Adults: 4 mg (Zometa) by IV infusion over at least 15 minutes. If albumin-corrected calcium level doesn't return to normal, may repeat 4 mg. Let at least 7 days pass before retreatment to allow a full response to the first dose.

Adjust-a-dose: Zometa: Assess serum creatinine level before each treatment or retreatment. Dosage adjustments aren't necessary for patients presenting with mild to moderate renal impairment before initiation of therapy (serum creatinine level less than 400 micromol/L or less than 4.5 mg/dL).

➤ **Multiple myeloma and bone metastases of solid tumors in conjunction with standard antineoplastics**

Adults: 4 mg (Zometa) IV infused over at least 15 minutes every 3 to 4 weeks. Treatment duration depends on type of cancer. Use for prostate cancer only after it has progressed after treatment with at least one course of hormonal therapy. Give patients an oral calcium supplement of 500 mg and a multiple vitamin containing 400 international units of vitamin D daily.

Adjust-a-dose: Zometa: For patients with CrCl of 50 to 60 mL/minute, give 3.5 mg. If 40 to 49 mL/minute, give 3.3 mg. If 30 to 39 mL/minute, give 3 mg. For patients with normal baseline creatinine level but an increase of 0.5 mg/dL and in those with abnormal baseline creatinine level who have an increase of 1 mg/dL, withhold drug. Resume treatment at the same dose as that before treatment interruption only when creatinine level has returned to within 10% of baseline value. If CrCl is less than 30 mL/minute, don't give drug.

➤ **Paget disease of bone (osteitis deformans)**

Adults: 5 mg (Reclast) by IV infusion over at least 15 minutes. Give through a vented infusion line. May repeat if relapse occurs. Patient also needs 1,500 mg elemental calcium in divided doses (750 mg b.i.d. or 500 mg t.i.d.) and 800 international units vitamin D daily, especially during the 2 weeks after dosing.

➤ **Treatment of osteoporosis in men; to reduce incidence of fractures in postmenopausal women with osteoporosis, diagnosed by bone mineral density or prevalent vertebral fracture, and in those at high risk for fracture, defined as a recent low-trauma hip fracture; to treat and prevent glucocorticoid-induced osteoporosis in patients taking a daily dosage equivalent to 7.5 mg or greater of prednisone and who are expected to remain on glucocorticoids for at least 12 months**

Adults: 5 mg (Reclast) by IV infusion over no less than 15 minutes once a year.

➤ **Prevention of osteoporosis**

Postmenopausal women: 5 mg (Reclast) by IV infusion over no less than 15 minutes once every 2 years.

➤ **Prevention of osteopenia secondary to androgen-deprivation therapy in prostate cancer ◆**

Adults: 4 mg IV every 3 months for 1 year or 4 mg every 12 months.

➤ **Prevention of osteopenia associated with aromatase inhibitor therapy in women with breast cancer ◆**

Adults: 4 mg IV every 6 months for 5 years.

Additional new drugs: Indications and dosages

amifampridine
AM-i-fam-pri-deen

Ruzurgi

amifampridine phosphate
Firdapse

Therapeutic class: Cholinergic agonists
Pharmacologic class: Potassium channel blockers

AVAILABLE FORMS
Tablets: 10 mg

INDICATIONS & DOSAGES
➤ **Lambert-Eaton myasthenic syndrome**
Adults (Firdapse): 15 to 30 mg/day PO in three to four divided doses. May increase by 5 mg daily every 3 or 4 days. Maximum single dose is 20 mg; maximum daily dose is 80 mg.
Children ages 6 to younger than 17 weighing 45 kg or more (Ruzurgi): Initially, 15 to 30 mg/day PO in two or three divided doses. May increase by 5 to 10 mg daily, with total daily dose divided in up to five doses/day. Maximum single dose is 30 mg; maximum total daily maintenance dose is 100 mg.
Children ages 6 to younger than 17 weighing less than 45 kg (Ruzurgi): Initially, 7.5 to 15 mg/day PO in two or three divided doses. May increase by 2.5 to 5 mg/day, with total daily dose divided in up to five doses/day. Maximum single dose is 15 mg; maximum total daily maintenance dose is 50 mg.
Adjust-a-dose: In adults with renal impairment (CrCl of 15 to 90 mL/minute) or any degree of hepatic impairment, or in known poor metabolizers of N-acetyltransferase, starting dose is 15 mg daily in three divided doses. In children weighing 45 kg or more with renal impairment (CrCl of 15 to 90 mL/minute) or any degree of hepatic impairment, or in known poor metabolizers of N-acetyltransferase, starting dose is 15 mg daily in divided doses. In children weighing less than 45 kg with renal impairment (CrCl of 15 to 90 mL/minute) or any degree of hepatic impairment, or in known poor metabolizers of N-acetyltransferase, starting dose is 7.5 mg daily in divided doses.

bremelanotide
bre-me-LAN-oh-tide

Vyleesi

Therapeutic class: Miscellaneous CNS drugs
Pharmacologic class: Melanocortin receptor agonists

AVAILABLE FORMS
Injection: 1.75 mg/0.3 mL single-dose autoinjector

INDICATIONS & DOSAGES
➤ **Treatment of premenopausal women with acquired, generalized hypoactive sexual desire disorder, as characterized by low sexual desire that causes marked distress or interpersonal difficulty and isn't due to coexisting medical or psychiatric condition, problems with the relationship, or effects of a medication or drug substance**
Women: 1.75 mg subcut in abdomen or thigh as needed, at least 45 minutes before anticipated sexual activity, not to exceed one dose in 24 hours or eight doses in a month. Discontinue if no improvement in symptoms after 8 weeks of treatment.

cenegermin-bkbj
sen-EH-jer-min bkbj

Oxervate

Therapeutic class: Growth factors
Pharmacologic class: Human nerve growth factors

AVAILABLE FORMS
Ophthalmic solution: 0.002% (20 mcg/mL) multidose vial

INDICATIONS & DOSAGES
➤ **Neurotrophic keratitis**
Adults and children age 2 and older: Instill 1 drop into affected eye(s) every 2 hours six times a day for 8 weeks.

SAFETY ALERT!

cladribine
KLA-dri-been

Mavenclad

Therapeutic class: Immunomodulators
Pharmacologic class: Purine antimetabolites

AVAILABLE FORMS
Tablets ⓄⓃⒸ: 10 mg

INDICATIONS & DOSAGES
➤ **Treatment of relapsing forms of MS, including relapsing-remitting disease and active secondary progressive disease in patients who have had inadequate response to, or are unable to tolerate, other MS therapies**
Adults weighing 40 kg or more: 3.5 mg/kg PO over 2 years, given as 1.75 mg/kg each year. Divide the 1.75-mg/kg dose over two cycles, each lasting 4 to 5 consecutive days. Don't give more than 2 tablets (20 mg) daily. For first year of treatment, start first cycle at any time. Give second cycle 23 to 27 days after last dose of first cycle. For second year of treatment, start first cycle at least 43 weeks after last dose of first year's second cycle. Give second cycle 23 to 27 days after last dose of second year's first cycle. After 2 years of treatment, don't give additional doses during the next 2 years.
Adjust-a-dose: Lymphocyte count must be within normal limits before start of treatment. Lymphocyte count must be at least 800 cells/mm³ before start of second treatment course. If needed, delay second

treatment course for up to 6 months to allow lymphocyte recovery to at least 800 cells/mm³. If recovery takes more than 6 months, discontinue treatment.

coagulation factor Xa (recombinant), inactivated-zhzo
Andexxa

Therapeutic class: Antidotes
Pharmacologic class: Factor Xa proteins

AVAILABLE FORMS
Injection: 100-mg, 200-mg vials

INDICATIONS & DOSAGES
➤ **Reversal of anticoagulation in patients treated with rivaroxaban or apixaban in life-threatening or uncontrolled bleeding**
Adults: Base dose on the specific factor Xa inhibitor, dose of factor Xa inhibitor, and time since patient's last dose of factor Xa inhibitor. If last dose of rivaroxaban was 10 mg or less taken less than 8 hours or an unknown time since last dose; apixaban last dose was 5 mg or less and taken less than 8 hours or an unknown time since last dose; or either rivaroxaban or apixaban at any dose was taken 8 hours or more ago, give initial bolus dose of 400 mg IV at a target rate of 30 mg/minute followed 2 minutes later with an IV infusion of 4 mg/minute for up to 120 minutes.

If last dose of rivaroxaban was more than 10 mg or last dose is unknown and taken less than 8 hours or an unknown time since last dose; or apixaban last dose was more than 5 mg or last dose is unknown, give initial bolus dose of 800 mg IV at a target rate of 30 mg/minute followed 2 minutes later with an IV infusion of 8 mg/minute for up to 120 minutes.

dolutegravir–lamivudine
doe-loo-TEG-ra-vir/la-MI-vyoo-deen

Dovato

Therapeutic class: Antiretrovirals
Pharmacologic class: Integrase strand transfer inhibitors–nucleoside analogues–reverse transcriptase inhibitors

AVAILABLE FORMS
Tablets: 50 mg dolutegravir/300 mg lamivudine

INDICATIONS & DOSAGES
➤ **Treatment of HIV-1 infection in patients with no antiretroviral treatment history and with no known substitutions associated with resistance to the individual components**
Adults: One tablet PO once daily.
Adjust-a-dose: If administered with carbamazepine or rifampin, give one tablet PO once daily followed by an additional dolutegravir 50-mg tablet approximately 12 hours from the combination product dose. If lamivudine dosage reduction is needed for patients with CrCl of less than 50 mL/minute, use individual components of this product.

duvelisib
doo-ve-LIS-ib

Copiktra

Therapeutic class: Antineoplastics
Pharmacologic class: Kinase inhibitors

AVAILABLE FORMS
Capsules ⓝ: 15 mg, 25 mg

INDICATIONS & DOSAGES
Adjust-a-dose (for all indications): Refer to manufacturer's instructions for toxicity-related dosage adjustments. If administered with a strong CYP3A4 inhibitor, reduce dosage to 15 mg PO b.i.d.
➤ **Treatment of relapsed or refractory chronic lymphocytic leukemia or small lymphocytic lymphoma after at least two prior therapies**
Adults: 25 mg PO b.i.d. in 28-day treatment cycles.
➤ **Treatment of relapsed or refractory follicular lymphoma after at least two prior systemic therapies**
Adults: 25 mg PO b.i.d. in 28-day treatment cycles.

elapegademase-lvlr ▨
EL-a-peg-ad-e-mase

Revcovi

Therapeutic class: Replacement enzymes
Pharmacologic class: Recombinant adenosine deaminase enzymes

AVAILABLE FORMS
Injection: 2.4 mg/1.5 mL (1.6 mg/mL) single-dose vial

INDICATIONS & DOSAGES
➤ **Adenosine deaminase severe combined immune deficiency** ▨
Adults and children who are pegademase bovine–naive: Initially, 0.2 mg/kg (based on ideal body weight) twice a week for at least 12 to 24 weeks until immune reconstitution is achieved. Then, may gradually decrease dosage to maintain trough adenosine deaminase (ADA) activity greater than 30 mmol/hour/L, trough deoxyadenosine nucleotide (dAXP) levels less than 0.02 mmol/L, or adequate immune reconstitution based on clinical assessment.
Adults and children transitioning from pegademase bovine to elapegademase-lvlr: If weekly pegademase bovine dose is unknown or is 30 units/kg or less, begin elapegademase-lvlr at 0.2 mg/kg IM once weekly. If weekly pegademase bovine dose is more than 30 units/kg, calculate an equivalent weekly elapegademase-lvlr dose (mg/kg) by dividing the elapegademase-lvlr dose (units/kg) by 150. May increase dosage by increments of 0.033 mg/kg weekly if trough ADA activity is less than 30 mmol/hour/L, trough dAXP levels are more than 0.02 mmol/L, or immune reconstitution is inadequate based on clinical assessment. May divide total weekly dose into multiple IM administrations during a week.

ⓝ Do not crush   *Liquid contains alcohol   ▨ Genetic

emapalumab-lzsg
em-a-PAL-ue-mab

Gamifant

Therapeutic class: Immunomodulators
Pharmacologic class: Monoclonal antibodies

AVAILABLE FORMS
Injection: 10 mg/2 mL, 50 mg/10 mL single-dose vials

INDICATIONS & DOSAGES
➤ **Treatment of primary hemophagocytic lymphohistiocytosis (HLH) in patients with refractory, recurrent, or progressive disease or intolerance to conventional HLH therapy**
Adults and children: 1 mg/kg IV infusion twice weekly (every 3 to 4 days) until hematopoietic stem cell transplantation or unacceptable toxicity.
Adjust-a-dose: If unsatisfactory improvement in clinical condition, may increase dose to 3 mg/kg on day 3; to 6 mg/kg from day 6 onwards; to 10 mg/kg on day 9 onwards. See manufacturer's information for specific criteria for dosage increases. After clinical condition is stabilized, decrease dosage to previous level to maintain clinical response.

SAFETY ALERT!

entrectinib ☒
en-TREK-ti-nib

Rozlytrek

Therapeutic class: Antineoplastics
Pharmacologic class: Kinase inhibitors

AVAILABLE FORMS
Capsules ⓓⓃⓒ*:* 100 mg, 200 mg

INDICATIONS & DOSAGES
Adjust-a-dose (for all indications): Refer to manufacturer's instructions for toxicity-related dosage adjustments.
➤ **Treatment of ROS1-positive metastatic NSCLC**☒
Adults: 600 mg PO once daily until disease progression or unacceptable toxicity.
Adjust-a-dose: Decrease entrectinib dose to 200 mg PO once daily if administered with a moderate CYP3A inhibitor or to 100 mg PO once daily if administered with a strong CYP3A inhibitor. After discontinuation of the CYP3A inhibitor for three to five elimination half-lives, resume entrectinib dose given before initiating the CYP3A inhibitor.
➤ **Treatment of solid tumors that have a neurotrophic tyrosine receptor kinase gene fusion without a known acquired resistance mutation, that are metastatic or where surgical resection is likely to result in severe morbidity, and have progressed after treatment or have no satisfactory alternative**☒
Adults and children age 12 and older with BSA greater than 1.50 m²: 600 mg PO once daily until disease progression or unacceptable toxicity.
Adjust-a-dose: Decrease entrectinib dose to 200 mg PO once daily if administered with a moderate CYP3A inhibitor or to 100 mg PO once daily if administered

with a strong CYP3A inhibitor. After discontinuation of the CYP3A inhibitor for three to five elimination half-lives, resume entrectinib dose given before initiating the CYP3A inhibitor.
Children age 12 and older with BSA of 1.11 to 1.50 m²: 500 mg PO once daily until disease progression or unacceptable toxicity.
Children age 12 and older with BSA of 0.91 to 1.10 m²: 400 mg PO once daily until disease progression or unacceptable toxicity.

SAFETY ALERT!

erdafitinib ☒
er-da-FI-ti-nib

Balversa

Therapeutic class: Antineoplastics
Pharmacologic class: Kinase inhibitors

AVAILABLE FORMS
Tablets ⓓⓃⓒ*:* 3 mg, 4 mg, 5 mg

INDICATIONS & DOSAGES
➤ **Treatment of locally advanced or metastatic urothelial carcinoma with susceptible *FGFR3* or *FGFR2* genetic alterations and that has progressed during or after at least one line of prior platinum-containing chemotherapy, including within 12 months of neoadjuvant or adjuvant platinum-containing chemotherapy**☒
Adults: 8 mg PO once daily. May increase to 9 mg once daily if serum phosphate level is less than 5.5 mg/dL and there are no ocular disorders or grade 2 or greater adverse reactions 14 to 21 days after start of treatment. Continue treatment until disease progression or unacceptable toxicity.
Adjust-a-dose: Refer to manufacturer's instructions for toxicity-related dosage adjustments.

SAFETY ALERT!

fedratinib
fed-RA-ti-nib

Inrebic

Therapeutic class: Antineoplastics
Pharmacologic class: Kinase inhibitors

AVAILABLE FORMS
Capsules: 100 mg

INDICATIONS & DOSAGES
➤ **Intermediate-2 or high-risk primary or secondary (post–polycythemia vera or post–essential thrombocythemia) myelofibrosis**
Adults: 400 mg PO once daily if baseline platelet count is 50 × 10⁹/L or greater.
Adjust-a-dose: Reduce fedratinib dose to 200 mg PO once daily when given with strong CYP3A4 inhibitors. When administration with a strong CYP3A4 inhibitor is discontinued, increase dose to 300 mg PO once daily during first 2 weeks after discontinuation of the inhibitor; then increase to 400 mg PO once daily as tolerated. Decrease fedratinib dose to 200 mg PO once daily in patients with severe renal impairment (CrCl of

ⓓⓃⓒ Do not crush　　*Liquid contains alcohol　　☒ Genetic

15 to 29 mL/minute). Refer to manufacturer's instructions for toxicity-related dosage adjustments.

fremanezumab-vfrm
FRE-ma-nez-ue-mab

Ajovy

Therapeutic class: Antimigraine drugs
Pharmacologic class: Calcitonin gene-related peptide antagonists

AVAILABLE FORMS
Injection: 225 mg/1.5 mL single-dose prefilled syringe

INDICATIONS & DOSAGES
➤ **Prevention of migraine headache**
Adults: 225 mg subcut once a month or 675 mg (three consecutive injections of 225 mg each) subcut every 3 months (quarterly).

galcanezumab-gnlm
GAL-ka-nez-ue-mab

Emgality

Therapeutic class: Antimigraine drugs
Pharmacologic class: Monoclonal antibodies

AVAILABLE FORMS
Injection: 120 mg/mL in single-dose pen or syringe

INDICATIONS & DOSAGES
➤ **Prevention of migraine headache**
Adults: Initially, 240 mg subcut (administered as two consecutive injections of 120 mg each) once as a loading dose, followed by 120 mg subcut once monthly.
➤ **Treatment of episodic cluster headache**
Adults: Initially, 300 mg subcut (three consecutive injections of 100 mg) at onset of the cluster period, then monthly until end of the cluster period.

SAFETY ALERT!

glasdegib
glas-DEG-ib

Daurismo

Therapeutic class: Antineoplastics
Pharmacologic class: Hedgehog pathway inhibitors

AVAILABLE FORMS
Tablets ⓓⓝⓒ: 25 mg, 100 mg

INDICATIONS & DOSAGES
➤ **Treatment of newly diagnosed acute myeloid leukemia, in combination with low-dose cytarabine, in patients who are age 75 and older or who have comorbidities that preclude use of intensive induction chemotherapy**
Adults: 100 mg PO once daily on days 1 to 28, in combination with cytarabine 20 mg subcut b.i.d. on days 1 to 10 of each 28-day cycle. Treat for a minimum of six cycles to allow time for clinical response or until unacceptable toxicity or loss of disease control.

Adjust-a-dose: Refer to glasdegib manufacturer's instructions for toxicity-related dosage adjustments. Refer to cytarabine manufacturer's instructions for dosing and toxicity-related information.

imipenem–cilastatin sodium–relebactam
im-ih PEN-em/sye-la-STAT-in/rel-e-BAK-tam

Recarbrio

Therapeutic class: Anti-infectives
Pharmacologic class: Penem antibacterials–renal dehydropeptidase inhibitors–beta-lactamase inhibitors

AVAILABLE FORMS
Injection: 1.25 g (imipenem 500 mg, cilastatin 500 mg, relebactam 250 mg)/vial

INDICATIONS & DOSAGES
➤ **Complicated UTIs, including pyelonephritis, caused by susceptible gram-negative microorganisms (*Enterobacter cloacae, Escherichia coli, Klebsiella aerogenes, Klebsiella pneumoniae,* and *Pseudomonas aeruginosa*); complicated intra-abdominal infections caused by susceptible gram-negative microorganisms (*Bacteroides caccae, Bacteroides fragilis, Bacteroides ovatus, Bacteroides thetaiotaomicron, Bacteroides uniformis, Bacteroides vulgatus, Bifidobacterium stercoris, Citrobacter freundii, E. cloacae, E. coli, Fusobacterium nucleatum, K. aerogenes, Klebsiella oxytoca, K. pneumoniae, Parabacteroides distasonis,* and *P. aeruginosa*) in patients with limited or no alternative treatment options**
Adults: 1.25 g by IV infusion over 30 minutes every 6 hours for 4 to 14 days. Base treatment duration on severity and location of the infection, and clinical response.

Adjust-a-dose: For patients with CrCl of 60 to 89 mL/minute, give 1 g IV every 6 hours (imipenem 400 mg, cilastatin 400 mg, relebactam 200 mg); for CrCl of 30 to 59 mL/minute, give 750 mg IV every 6 hours (imipenem 300 mg, cilastatin 300 mg, relebactam 150 mg); for CrCl of 15 to 29 mL/minute, give 500 mg IV every 6 hours (imipenem 200 mg, cilastatin 200 g, relebactam 100 mg); for CrCl less than 15 mL/minute, don't give unless hemodialysis is instituted within 48 hours. For patients with ESRD on hemodialysis, give 500 mg IV every 6 hours. Give after hemodialysis and at intervals timed from the end of that hemodialysis session.

inotersen
in-oh-TER-sen

Tegsedi

Therapeutic class: Endocrine-metabolic agents
Pharmacologic class: Antisense oligonucleotides

AVAILABLE FORMS
Injection: 284 mg/1.5 mL single-dose prefilled syringe

INDICATIONS & DOSAGES
➤ **Polyneuropathy of hereditary transthyretin–mediated amyloidosis**
Adults: 284 mg subcut once weekly on same day every week.
Adjust-a-dose: Refer to manufacturer's instructions for monitoring and dosage adjustments based on platelet count.
Black Box Warning If urine protein to creatine ratio (UPCR) is 1,000 mg/g or higher, or eGFR is below 45 mL/minute/1.73 m², withhold drug pending further evaluation of the cause. If a dose is withheld, once eGFR is at least 45 mL/minute/1.73 m², UPCR decreases to below 1,000 mg/g, or the underlying cause of the decline in renal function is corrected, may reinitiate weekly dosing. If UPCR is 2,000 mg/g or higher, evaluate for acute glomerulonephritis and if confirmed, permanently discontinue drug. ∎

istradefylline
is-trah-DEF-ah-lin

Nourianz

Therapeutic class: Antiparkinsonians
Pharmacologic class: Adenosine receptor antagonists

AVAILABLE FORMS
Tablets: 20 mg, 40 mg

INDICATIONS & DOSAGES
➤ **Adjunctive treatment to levodopa/carbidopa in adults with Parkinson disease experiencing "off" episodes**
Adults: 20 mg PO once daily; may increase to a maximum of 40 mg PO once daily based on individual need and tolerability.
Adjust-a-dose: For patients with moderate hepatic impairment (Child-Pugh class B) or who are using strong CYP3A4 inhibitors concomitantly, maximum recommended dose is 20 mg once daily. For patients who use tobacco in amounts of 20 or more cigarettes per day (or the equivalent of another tobacco product), dose is 40 mg PO once daily.

lefamulin acetate
lef-a-MOO-lin

Xenleta

Therapeutic class: Antibacterials
Pharmacologic class: Pleuromutilin anti infectives

AVAILABLE FORMS
Injection: 150 mg/15 mL vial
Tablets ⓞⓝⓒ: 600 mg

INDICATIONS & DOSAGES
➤ **Community-acquired bacterial pneumonia caused by** *Streptococcus pneumoniae, Staphylococcus aureus* **(methicillin-susceptible isolates),** *Haemophilus influenzae, Legionella pneumophila,* *Mycoplasma pneumoniae,* **and** *Chlamydophila pneumoniae*
Adults: 150 mg IV infusion over 60 minutes every 12 hours for 5 to 7 days, or 600 mg PO every 12 hours for 5 days. May switch from IV form to oral form to complete treatment course.
Adjust-a-dose: In patients with severe hepatic impairment (Child-Pugh class C), reduce IV dose to 150 mg infused every 24 hours. Use of tablets hasn't been studied in and aren't recommended for patients with moderate (Child-Pugh class B) or severe (Child-Pugh class C) hepatic impairment.

SAFETY ALERT!

lorlatinib ⚥
lor-LA-ti-nib

Lorbrena

Therapeutic class: Antineoplastics
Pharmacologic class: Tyrosine kinase inhibitors

AVAILABLE FORMS
Tablets ⓞⓝⓒ: 25 mg, 100 mg

INDICATIONS & DOSAGES
➤ **Treatment of patients with anaplastic lymphoma kinase (ALK)-positive metastatic NSCLC whose disease has progressed on crizotinib and at least one other ALK inhibitor for metastatic disease, or progressed on alectinib or ceritinib as the first ALK inhibitor for metastatic disease** ⚥
Adults: 100 mg PO once daily until disease progression or unacceptable toxicity.
Adjust-a-dose: Refer to manufacturer's instructions for toxicity-related dosage adjustments. If use with CYP3A inhibitors can't be avoided, reduce lorlatinib starting dose to 75 mg once daily. In patients who have had a lorlatinib dosage reduction to 75 mg once daily due to adverse reactions and who begin a strong CYP3A inhibitor, reduce dose to 50 mg once daily. If the strong CYP3A inhibitor is discontinued, increase the lorlatinib dose (after three plasma half-lives of the strong CYP3A inhibitor) to the dose that was used before initiation of the strong CYP3A inhibitor.

lusutrombopag
loo-soo-TROM-boe-pag

Mulpleta

Therapeutic class: Hematopoietics
Pharmacologic class: Thrombopoietin receptor agonists

AVAILABLE FORMS
Tablets: 3 mg

INDICATIONS & DOSAGES
➤ **Thrombocytopenia in patients with chronic liver disease scheduled to undergo a procedure**
Adults: 3 mg PO once daily for 7 days, beginning 8 to 14 days before procedure.

moxetumomab pasudotox-tdfk
MOX-e-toom-oh-mab pa-SOO-doe-tox

Lumoxiti

Therapeutic class: Antineoplastics
Pharmacologic class: Anti-CD22s

AVAILABLE FORMS
Injection (lyophilized cake or powder): 1 mg/mL
single-dose vial

INDICATIONS & DOSAGES
➤ **Treatment of patients with relapsed or refractory hairy cell leukemia who received at least two prior systemic therapies, including treatment with a purine nucleoside analogue**
Adults: 0.04 mg/kg IV infusion on days 1, 3, and 5 of each 28-day cycle. Continue treatment for a maximum of six cycles, unless disease progression or unacceptable toxicity occurs.
Adjust-a-dose: Refer to manufacturer's information for toxicity-related dosage adjustments.

SAFETY ALERT!

pexidartinib
pex-i-DAR-ti-nib

Turalio

Therapeutic class: Antineoplastics
Pharmacologic class: Kinase inhibitors

AVAILABLE FORMS
Capsules ⓓⓝⓒ: 200 mg

INDICATIONS & DOSAGES
➤ **Symptomatic tenosynovial giant cell tumor associated with severe morbidity or functional limitations and not amenable to improvement with surgery**
Adults: 400 mg PO b.i.d.
Adjust-a-dose: Refer to manufacturer's instructions for toxicity-related dosage adjustments and for dosage adjustments when drug is used with strong CYP3A inhibitors or UGT inhibitors.

pitolisant hydrochloride
pi-TOL-i-sant

Wakix

Therapeutic class: Stimulants
Pharmacologic class: Histamine-3 receptor antagonist/inverse agonists

AVAILABLE FORMS
Tablets: 4.45 mg, 17.8 mg

INDICATIONS & DOSAGES
➤ **Treatment of excessive daytime sleepiness in adults with narcolepsy**
Adults: Dosage range is 17.8 to 35.6 mg PO once daily in the morning upon awakening. Titrate dosage as follows: week 1, 8.9 mg (two 4.45-mg tablets) PO once daily; week 2, increase dosage to 17.8 mg (one 17.8-mg tablet) PO once daily; week 3, may increase

to maximum dosage of 35.6 mg (two 17.8-mg tablets) PO once daily based on tolerability.
Adjust-a-dose: In patients with moderate hepatic impairment, initial dose is 8.9 mg PO once daily; may titrate to maximum dose of 17.8 mg once daily after 14 days. In patients with moderate and severe renal impairment and in patients known to be poor CYP2D6 metabolizers, initial dose is 8.9 mg PO once daily; may titrate to maximum dose of 17.8 mg PO once daily after 7 days.

prabotulinumtoxinA-xvfs
pra-bot-ue-LYE-num-TOX-in-A

Jeuveau

Therapeutic class: Neuromuscular transmission blockers
Pharmacologic class: Acetylcholine release inhibitors

AVAILABLE FORMS
Injection: 100 units/single-dose vial

INDICATIONS & DOSAGES
➤ **Temporary improvement in appearance of moderate to severe glabellar lines associated with corrugator or procerus muscle activity**
Adults: 0.1 mL (4 units) IM into each of the five sites for a total dose of 20 units. See prescribing information for diagram and complete administration instructions. May retreat no less than 3 months from prior dose. Consider cumulative dose if other botulinum toxin agents have been used to treat other conditions.

pretomanid
pre-TOE-ma-nid

Therapeutic class: Antituberculotics
Pharmacologic class: Nitroimidazoles

AVAILABLE FORMS
Tablets ⓓⓝⓒ: 200 mg

INDICATIONS & DOSAGES
➤ **Pulmonary extensively drug-resistant, treatment-intolerant, or nonresponsive multidrug-resistant TB, in combination with bedaquiline and linezolid**
Adults: 200 mg PO once daily for 26 weeks in combination with bedaquiline 400 mg PO once daily for 2 weeks followed by bedaquiline 200 mg three times per week, with at least 48 hours between bedaquiline doses, for 24 weeks for a total of 26 weeks; and linezolid 1,200 mg PO daily for up to 26 weeks. May extend therapy beyond 26 weeks if necessary. Pretomanid must be used only in combination with bedaquiline and linezolid as part of the recommended dosing regimen.
Adjust-a-dose: Refer to manufacturer's instructions for pretomanid, bedaquiline, and linezolid for toxicity-related dosage adjustments and drug discontinuation.

ravulizumab-cwvz
rav-ue-LIZ-ue-mab

Ultomiris

Therapeutic class: Immunomodulators
Pharmacologic class: Complement inhibitors

AVAILABLE FORMS
Injection: 300 mg/30 mL (10 mg/mL) single-dose vial

INDICATIONS & DOSAGES
➤ **Paroxysmal nocturnal hemoglobinuria**
Adults weighing 100 kg or more: 3,000 mg IV infusion loading dose, followed in 2 weeks by maintenance dose of 3,600 mg IV infusion once every 8 weeks.
Adults weighing 60 to less than 100 kg: 2,700 mg IV infusion loading dose, followed in 2 weeks by maintenance dose of 3,300 mg IV infusion once every 8 weeks.
Adults weighing 40 to less than 60 kg: 2,400 mg IV infusion loading dose, followed in 2 weeks by maintenance dose of 3,000 mg IV infusion once every 8 weeks.
Patients switching from eculizumab to ravulizumab: Administer a ravulizumab loading dose 2 weeks after last eculizumab infusion; then follow maintenance dosing according to patient's weight.
➤ **Atypical hemolytic-uremic syndrome to inhibit complement-mediated thrombotic microangiopathy**
Adults: Loading dose: 40 to less than 60 kg, 2,400 mg IV; 60 to less than 100 kg, 2,700 mg IV; 100 kg or more, 3,000 mg IV. Start maintenance doses 2 weeks after loading dose. Refer to manufacturer's instructions for specific maintenance information and dosage adjustments.

revefenacin
REV-e-fen-a-sin

Yupelri

Therapeutic class: Bronchodilators
Pharmacologic class: Anticholinergics

AVAILABLE FORMS
Solution for inhalation: 175 mcg/3 mL unit-dose vial

INDICATIONS & DOSAGES
➤ **Maintenance treatment of COPD**
Adults: 175 mcg oral inhalation via nebulizer once daily.

risankizumab-rzaa
ris-an-KIZ-ue-mab

Skyrizi

Therapeutic class: Immunomodulators
Pharmacologic class: Interleukin-23 receptor antagonists

AVAILABLE FORMS
Injection: 75 mg/0.83 mL prefilled syringe

INDICATIONS & DOSAGES
➤ **Treatment of moderate to severe plaque psoriasis in patients who are candidates for systemic therapy or phototherapy**
Adults: 150 mg (two 75-mg injections) subcut at weeks 0 and 4 and every 12 weeks thereafter.

romosozumab-aqqg
roe-moe-SOZ-ue-mab

Evenity

Therapeutic class: Antiosteoporotics
Pharmacologic class: Sclerostin inhibitors

AVAILABLE FORMS
Injection: 105 mg/1.17 mL single-use prefilled syringe

INDICATIONS & DOSAGES
➤ **Treatment of osteoporosis in postmenopausal women at high risk for fracture (history of osteoporotic fracture or multiple risk factors for fracture); or in patients who have failed or are intolerant of other osteoporosis therapy**
Adult women: 210 mg (two syringes) subcut once every month for 12 months.

sarecycline
sar-e-SYE-kleen

Seysara

Therapeutic class: Antibiotics
Pharmacologic class: Tetracyclines

AVAILABLE FORMS
Tablets: 60 mg, 100 mg, 150 mg

INDICATIONS & DOSAGES
➤ **Inflammatory lesions of nonnodular moderate to severe acne vulgaris**
Adults and children age 9 and older weighing 85 to 136 kg: 150 mg PO once daily.
Adults and children age 9 and older weighing 55 to 84 kg: 100 mg PO once daily.
Adults and children age 9 and older weighing 33 to 54 kg: 60 mg PO once daily.

SAFETY ALERT!

selinexor
sel-i-NEX-or

Xpovio

Therapeutic class: Antineoplastics
Pharmacologic class: Nuclear export inhibitors

AVAILABLE FORMS
Tablets ⓝ: 20 mg

INDICATIONS & DOSAGES
➤ **Relapsed or refractory multiple myeloma in combination with dexamethasone in patients who have had at least four prior therapies and whose disease is refractory to at least two proteasome inhibitors, at least two immunomodulatory agents, and an anti-CD38 monoclonal antibody**

Adults: 80 mg (four 20-mg tablets) PO with dexa-methasone 20 mg PO on days 1 and 3 of each week until disease progression or unacceptable toxicity.
Adjust-a-dose: Refer to manufacturer's instructions for toxicity-related dosage adjustments.

siponimod ☒
si-PON-i-mod

Mayzent

Therapeutic class: MS drugs
Pharmacologic class: Sphingosine 1-phosphate receptor modulators

AVAILABLE FORMS
Tablets: 0.25 mg, 2 mg

INDICATIONS & DOSAGES
➤ **Relapsing forms of MS with CYP2C9 genotype *1/*1, *1/*2, or *2/*2** ☒
Adults: Start drug with a 5-day titration to help reduce cardiac effects. Initially, on days 1 and 2, give 0.25 mg PO once daily; on day 3, give 0.5 mg PO once daily; on day 4, give 0.75 mg PO once daily: on day 5, give 1.25 mg PO once daily, on day 6, begin maintenance dosage of 2 mg PO once daily.
➤ **Relapsing forms of MS with CYP2C9 genotype *1/*3 or *2/*3** ☒
Adults: Start drug with a 4-day titration to help reduce cardiac effects. Initially, on days 1 and 2, give 0.25 mg PO once daily; on day 3, give 0.5 mg PO once daily; on day 4, give 0.75 mg PO once daily; on day 5, begin maintenance dosage of 1 mg PO once daily.

stiripentol
stir-i-PEN-tol

Diacomit

Therapeutic class: Anticonvulsants
Pharmacologic class: Anticonvulsants

AVAILABLE FORMS
Capsules ⓒ: 250 mg, 500 mg
Powder for oral suspension: 250 mg, 500 mg

INDICATIONS & DOSAGES
➤ **Treatment of seizures associated with Dravet syndrome in patients taking clobazam**
Adults and children age 2 and older: 50 mg/kg/day PO in two or three divided doses. If exact dosage isn't available with the available strengths, round to the nearest possible dosage, which is usually within 50 to 150 mg of the recommended 50 mg/kg/day. Maximum daily dose is 3,000 mg/day.
Adjust-a-dose: If somnolence occurs, consider reducing clobazam dosage by 25%. If somnolence persists, consider decreasing clobazam dosage by an additional 25%. Consider adjusting dosage of other concomitant anticonvulsants with sedating properties.

tagraxofusp-erzs
tag-RAX-oh-fusp

Elzonris

Therapeutic class: Antineoplastics
Pharmacologic class: Anti-CD123 agents

AVAILABLE FORMS
Injection: 1,000 mcg/mL single-dose vial

INDICATIONS & DOSAGES
➤ **Blastic plasmacytoid dendritic cell neoplasm**
Adults and children age 2 and older: 12 mcg/kg IV infusion once daily on days 1 to 5 of a 21-day cycle. May extend dosing period for dose delays up to day 10. Continue treatment until disease progression or unacceptable toxicity.
Adjust-a-dose: Refer to manufacturer's instructions for toxicity-related dosage adjustments.

triclabendazole
tri-kla-BEN-da-zole

Egaten

Therapeutic class: Anthelmintics
Pharmacologic class: Anthelmintics

AVAILABLE FORMS
Tablets: 250 mg

INDICATIONS & DOSAGES
➤ **Treatment of fascioliasis**
Adults and children age 6 and older: 10 mg/kg PO every 12 hours for two doses.

upadacitinib
ue-pah-dah-SYE-ti-nib

Rinvoq

Therapeutic class: Antiarthritics
Pharmacologic class: Janus kinase inhibitors

AVAILABLE FORMS
Tablets (extended-release) ⓒ: 15 mg

INDICATIONS & DOSAGES
➤ **Moderately to severely active RA in patients who have had an inadequate response to or are intolerant of methotrexate, as monotherapy or in combination with methotrexate or other nonbiologic DMARDs**
Adults: 15 mg PO once daily.
Adjust-a-dose: If serious infections develop, interrupt therapy until the infection is controlled. If ANC is less than 1,000 cells/mm^3, interrupt therapy and restart once ANC returns above this value. If absolute lymphocyte count (ALC) is less than 500 cells/mm^3, interrupt therapy and restart once ALC returns above this value. If Hb is less than 8 g/dL, interrupt therapy and restart once Hb returns above this value. If hepatic transaminase levels rise and drug-induced liver injury is suspected, interrupt therapy.

Index

Boldface refers to full color photographs.

Boldface refers to full color photographs.